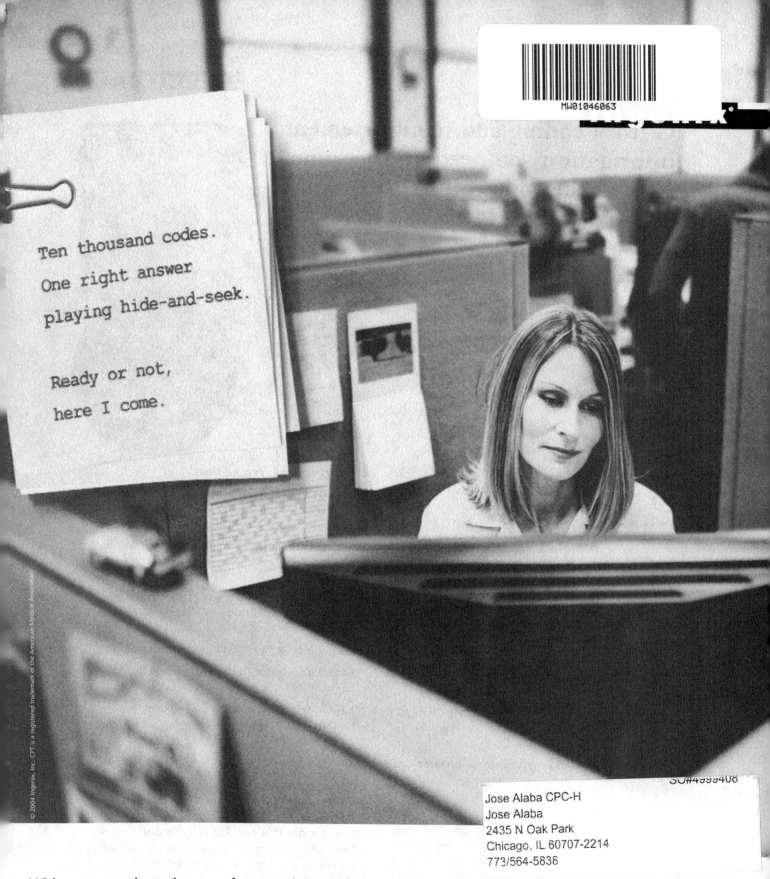
Ten thousand codes.
One right answer
playing hide-and-seek.
Ready or not,
here I come.
MW01046063
© 2004 Ingenix, Inc. CPT is a registered trademark of the American Medical Association
Jose Alaba CPC-H
Jose Alaba
2435 N Oak Park
Chicago, IL 60707-2214
773/564-5836

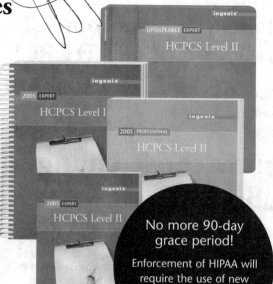

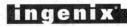

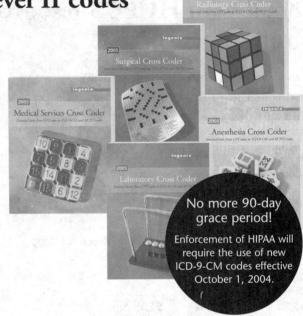

Your Master Code Finder for All Specialties

2005 Code Compass

Item No.: 5759 **$129.95**

Available: December 2004 ISBN: 1-56337-581-8

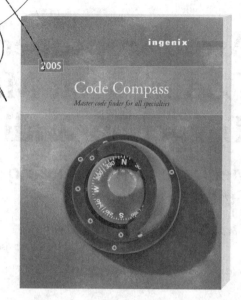

This coding resource presents a unique compendium of code selection grids that allow coders to choose, at a glance, from among several codes available for a single diagnosis or procedure. It's a useful tool for the experienced coder looking for a shortcut, and it is also an ideal tool for the "visual" reader, since the information is organized in easy-lookup grids instead of lists of codes.

- **New—Additional grids have been added to cover more diagnoses and procedures.**
- **Speed up the coding process.** A master alphabetized list of the code selection grids appears at the front of the book, to allow even faster code selection.
- **Quickly find the codes you need with intuitive, easy-to-use CPT®, ICD-9-CM and HCPCS grids.** A series of grids organized by CPT®, ICD-9-CM and HCPCS sections guide the user to possible code selections.
- **Save time with easy organization.** Numerically ordered by code set, similar to CPT® and ICD-9-CM books.
- **Key concepts to use as a refresher or training tool.** A brief introduction with each chapter to remind the coder of specific coding guidelines as well as an anatomical illustration and terminology relating to each specific section of CPT®, ICD-9-CM and HCPCS coding guidelines.

100% Money Back Guarantee:
If our merchandise* ever fails to meet your expectations, please contact our Customer Service Department toll-free at 1.800.INGENIX (464.3649), option 1, for an immediate response.
*Software: Credit will be granted for unopened packages only.

CPT is a registered trademark of the American Medical Association.

SAVE 5% when you order at www.ingenixonline.com (reference source code FOBW5)

or call toll-free 1.800.INGENIX (464.3649), option 1.

Also available from your medical bookstore or distributor.

2005 Publications

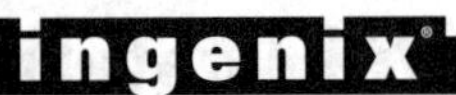

Avoid Improper Coding That May Trigger an Audit

Medicare Correct Coding Guide

Item No.: 3024

$229.95*

*Call for multi-user pricing.

Available: Now

ISBN: 1-56329-864-3

The most comprehensive and current manual of rules, payment restrictions, and claim submission edits, *Medicare Correct Coding Guide* is critical for correctly reporting Part B procedures and services.

- **Exclusive–Stay current as CMS implements changes.** Free updates for one full year.
- **Exclusive–Easily calculate payments, determine CCI edits, and more.** Free *Medicare Reimbursement Pro* CD. Use this CD for both facility and physician office settings based on your geographic area.
- **Know what the OIG is looking for.** Overview of CMS's campaign against fraud and abuse.
- **Better understanding of claim denials.** General correct coding policies help you understand coding methodologies.
- **Become more efficient and effective at coding claims.** Complete list of CPT® and HCPCS Level II codes helps you code correctly for reimbursement of Medicare-covered services and supplies.
- **Help with billing and payment projection.** Medicare physician fee schedule includes status indicators, global periods, supply codes, and more.
- **Complete RVUs and GPCIs.** So you can adjust fees for your geographic area, evaluate managed care contracts, and check code selection and sequencing for each service.
- **Quickly identify edit definitions for each code—eliminating confusion, reducing time and preventing claims denials.** Current CCI edits with policy icons help you understand the policy that determines the edit.
- **Save time.** Transition practice expense RVU adjustments. This information helps you calculate your payments quickly and accurately according to your setting.
- **Gauge pricing.** National average payment allows you to gauge individual pricing standards against national Medicare standards.
- **Continuing Education Units (CEUs).** Earn 5 CEUs from AAPC.

100% Money Back Guarantee:
If our merchandise* ever fails to meet your expectations, please contact our Customer Service Department toll-free at 1.800.INGENIX (464.3649), option 1, for an immediate response.
*Software: Credit will be granted for unopened packages only.

CPT is a registered trademark of the American Medical Association.

SAVE 5% when you order at www.ingenixonline.com (reference source code FOBW5)

or call toll-free 1.800.INGENIX (464.3649), option 1.

Also available from your medical bookstore or distributor.

FOBA5

Specialty-Specific Comprehensive Illustrated Guides to Coding and Reimbursement

2005 Coding Companions

$189.95 each

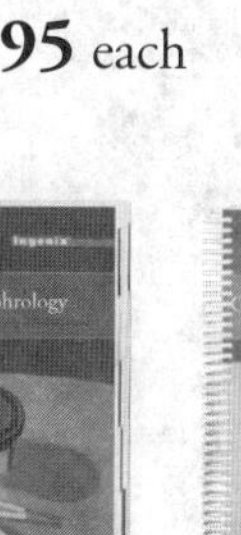

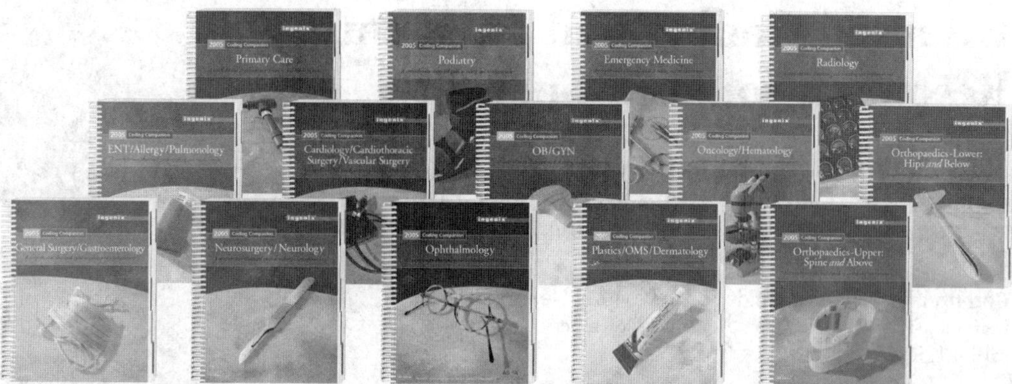

ISBN No.	Item Description	Item No.	Available
1-56337-601-6	Coding Companion for Cardiology/Cardiothoracic Surgery/Vascular Surgery	1528	December 2004
1-56337-602-4	Coding Companion for ENT/Allergy/Pulmonology **Special discount for AAO-HNS members**	1529	December 2004
1-56337-603-2	Coding Companion for General Surgery/ Gastroenterology	1530	December 2004
1-56337-604-0	Coding Companion for Neurosurgery/Neurology	1531	December 2004
1-56337-605-9	Coding Companion for OB/GYN	1532	December 2004
1-56337-606-7	Coding Companion for Ophthalmology **Special discount for ASOA members**	1533	December 2004
1-56337-607-5	Coding Companion for Orthopaedics—Lower: Hips & Below	1534	December 2004
1-56337-608-3	Coding Companion for Orthopaedics—Upper: Spine & Above	1535	December 2004
1-56337-609-1	Coding Companion for Plastics/OMS/Dermatology	1536	December 2004
1-56337-610-5	Coding Companion for Urology/Nephrology	1537	December 2004
1-56337-611-3	Coding Companion for Oncology/Hematology	1538	January 2005
1-56337-612-1	Coding Companion for Primary Care **NEW!**	1539	January 2005
1-56337-615-6	Coding Companion for Podiatry **NEW! Special discount for APMA members**	1542	December 2004
1-56337-613-X	Coding Companion for Emergency Medicine **NEW!**	1540	January 2005
1-56337-614-8	Coding Companion for Radiology **NEW!**	1541	December 2004

Coding Companions provide the comprehensive information a coder/biller needs—CPT codes with ICD-9-CM, HCPCS Level II, and anesthesia crosswalks—along with procedural definitions, coding and reimbursement tips, clinical and procedural information, CCI edits, Pubs 100 issues and illustrations—all in a one-page format for surgical codes, along with most medicine codes, related to each specific specialty.

- **New!—Pubs 100 references (formerly known as MCM/CIM references).** Keep current with Medicare coverage issues with Pubs 100 information specific to your specialty.
- **Submit claims with current, comprehensive code sets.** Updated 2005 surgery, medicine, E/M, radiology and lab/path CPT® codes are included.
- **Facilitate your coding with helpful illustrations.** Medical illustrations help link operative report language to code definitions.
- **Prevent unbundling mistakes by staying current with CCI edits.** Updates sent quarterly via e-mail help identify which code combinations cannot be billed together. A set of CCI edits is published in the guide, followed by three FREE quarterly e-mail updates.

100% Money Back Guarantee:
If our merchandise* ever fails to meet your expectations, please contact our Customer Service Department toll-free at 1.800.INGENIX (464.3649), option 1, for an immediate response.
*Software: Credit will be granted for unopened packages only.

SAVE 5% when you order at www.ingenixonline.com (reference source code FOBW5)

or call toll-free 1.800.INGENIX (464.3649), option 1.

Also available from your medical bookstore or distributor.

FOBA5

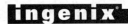

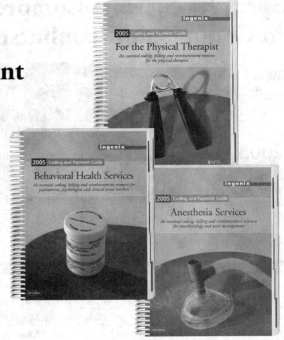

2005 Publications

ingenix

Save Time and Money with These Handy "Cheat Sheets"

2005 Fast Finders

$24.95 Each

order any 4 for only $40

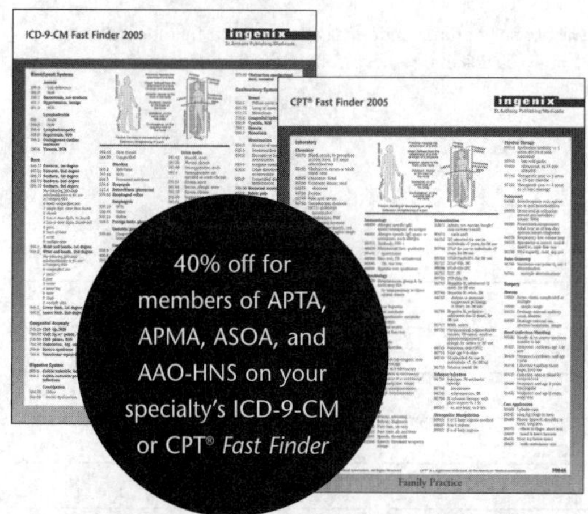

Fast Finders make frequently used codes available on double-sided, laminated "cheat sheets" to speed up your coding. You can now review the abbreviated list before resorting to the larger, more complex code books.

- **New!—Fast Finders for 2005.** Chiropractic Medicine ICD-9-CM and CPT®, Modifiers CPT® and HCPCS, and HIPAA Security Provision.
- **Save coding time with clinically and statistically sound codes.** The comprehensive sets are based on actual specialty billing frequencies.
- **Quickly orient yourself with anatomical illustrations.** Illustrations help you visually orient to your specific specialty.
- **Instant portability.** These two-sided sheets are sized to slip easily into your ICD-9-CM or CPT® book for convenient storage.
- ***HIPAA Privacy and Security Fast Finder.*** Look up essential HIPAA privacy and security terms and definitions in seconds.

Fast Finder Description	ICD-9-CM Item#	CPT® Item#	HCPCS Item#	HIPAA Item#
Allergy/Immunology	10000	10036		
Anesthesiology		10037		
Behavioral Health	10001	10038		
Cardiology	10002	10039		
Cardiovascular/Thoracic Surgery	10003	10040		
Chiropractic Medicine NEW	10004	10041		
Dental/OMS	10005	10042		
Dermatology	10006	10043		
Drug Codes			10027	
Emergency Medicine	10007	10044		
ENT	10008	10045		
External Causes—E Codes	10009			
Family Practice	10010	10046		
Gastroenterology	10011	10047		
General Surgery	10012	10048		
Hematology/Oncology	10013	10049		
HIPAA Privacy				10034
HIPAA Security NEW				10035
Home Health			10028	
Laboratory/Pathology		10050		
Modifiers NEW		10051	10029	
Neurology/Neurosurgery	10014	10052		
Ob/Gyn	10015			
Obstetrics, Gynecology, and Infertility		10053		
Ophthalmology/Optometry	10016	10054		
Orthopaedics	10017	10055		
Orthotics			10030	
Pain Management	10018	10056		
Pediatrics	10019	10057		
Physical Medicine/Rehabilitation	10020	10058		
Physical Therapy	10021	10059		
Physician Office Supplies			10031	
Plastic/Reconstructive Surgery	10022	10060		
Podiatry	10023	10061		
Primary Care/Internal Medicine	10024	10062		
Prosthetics			10032	
Radiology		10063		
Urology/Nephrology	10025	10064		
V Codes	10026			
Vision and Hearing			10033	
Available	Aug. 2004	Dec. 2004	Dec. 2004	Sept. 2004

100% Money Back Guarantee:
If our merchandise* ever fails to meet your expectations, please contact our Customer Service Department toll-free at 1.800.INGENIX (464.3649), option 1, for an immediate response.
*Software: Credit will be granted for unopened packages only.

CPT is a registered trademark of the American Medical Association.

SAVE 5% when you order at www.ingenixonline.com (reference source code FOBW5)

or call toll-free 1.800.INGENIX (464.3649), option 1.

Also available from your medical bookstore or distributor.

FOBA5

Four simple ways to place an order.

Call

1.800.ingenix (464.3649), option 1. Mention source code FOBA5 when ordering.

Mail

PO Box 27116
Salt Lake City, UT 84127-0116
With payment and/or purchase order.

Fax

801.982.4033
With credit card information and/or purchase order.

Click

www.ingenixonline.com
Save 5% when you order online today—use source code FOBW5.

ingenix*e*smart
ingenix online frequent buyer program

GET REWARDS FOR SHOPPING ONLINE!
To find out more, visit IngenixOnline.com

E-Smart program available only to Ingenix customers who are not part of Medallion, Gold Medallion or Partner Accounts programs. You must be registered at Ingenix Online to have your online purchases tracked for rewards purposes. Shipping charges and taxes still apply and cannot be used for rewards. Offer valid online only.

100% Money Back Guarantee

If our merchandise* ever fails to meet your expectations, please contact our Customer Service Department toll-free at 1.800.ingenix (464.3649), option 1 for an immediate response.

*Software: Credit will be granted for unopened packages only.

Customer Service Hours

7:00 am - 5:00 pm Mountain Time
9:00 am - 7:00 pm Eastern Time

Shipping and Handling

no. of items	fee
1	$10.95
2-4	$12.95
5-7	$14.95
8-10	$19.95
11+	Call

ingenix

Order Form

Information

Customer No. ____ Contact No. ____

Source Code ____

Contact Name ____

Title ____ Specialty ____

Company ____

Street Address ____
NO PO BOXES, PLEASE

City ____ State ____ Zip ____

Telephone (   ) ____ Fax (   ) ____
IN CASE WE HAVE QUESTIONS ABOUT YOUR ORDER

E-mail ____ @ ____
REQUIRED FOR ORDER CONFIRMATION AND SELECT PRODUCT DELIVERY.

Ingenix respects your right to privacy. We will not sell or rent your e-mail address or fax number to anyone outside Ingenix and its business partners. If you would like to remove your name from Ingenix promotion, please call 1.800.ingenix (464.3649), option 1.

Product

Item No.	Qty	Description	Price	Total

Subtotal ____

UT, OH, & VA residents, please add applicable Sales tax ____

(See chart on the left) Shipping & handling charges ____
All foreign orders, please call for shipping costs

Total ____

Payment

○Please bill my credit card ○MasterCard ○VISA ○Amex ○Discover

Card No. ____ Expires ____
MONTH YEAR

Signature ____

○Check enclosed, made payable to: Ingenix, Inc. ○Please bill my office

Purchase Order No. ____
ATTACH COPY OF PURCHASE ORDER

FOBA5

ingenix™

Surgical Cross Coder

Essential Links from CPT® codes to ICD-9-CM and HCPCS codes

2005

Publisher's Notice

American Medical Association Notice

Continuing Education Units for AAPC Certified Members

This publication has prior approval by the American Academy of Professional Coders for continuing education units. Granting of prior approval in no way constitutes endorsement by AAPC of the publication content nor the publisher. Instructions to submit CEUs are available at www.aapc.com/education/ceus/ceus.html

Made in the USA

ISBN 1-56337-573-7

Acknowledgments

Bonnie Schreck, CCS, CPC, CPC Product Manager
Lynn Speirs, Senior Director, Publishing Services
Sheri Poe Bernard, CPC, Senior Product Director
Karen Schmidt, BSN, Technical Director
Lori Becks, RHIA, Clinical/Technical Editor
Kristin Hodkinson, RHIT, CPC, CPC-H, CIC, Clinical/Technical Editor
Jean Parkinson, Project Editor
Kerrie Hornsby, Desktop Publishing Manager
Gregory Kemp, Desktop Publishing Specialist

Special thanks to Dana Wagner, CPC

Technical Editors

Lori Becks, RHIA

Ms. Becks has functioned as a coding specialist at the University of Utah and served as Assistant Director of Health Information Management. Her areas of expertise include the ICD-9-CM and CPT coding systems. She also has a background in teaching English to foreign speakers and technical writing.

Kristin Hodkinson, RHIT, CPC, CPC-H, CIC

Ms. Hodkinson has more than 10 years of experience in the health care profession including commercial insurance payers, health information management, and patient accounts. She has extensive background in both the professional and technical components of CPT/HCPCS and ICD-9-CM coding. Her areas of expertise include interventional radiology and cardiology, hospital chargemaster, and the Outpatient Prospective Payment System (OPPS). She recently served as the APC coordinator for a health care system in Florida. She is a member of the American Academy of Professional Coders (AAPC) and the American Health Information Management Association (AHIMA).

Contents

Illustrations

Introduction

Ingenix is proud to present the 2005 *Surgical Cross Coder*. The popularity of *Surgical Cross Coder* in recent years indicates that it has become the quintessential one-stop reference for medical coders. Fully comprehensive and illustrated, *Surgical Cross Coder* links more than 4,000 CPT surgical codes to corresponding diagnosis, procedure, and medical supply codes. This reference is embraced by professional coders working in clinical outpatient, hospital, as well as payer settings.

Surgical Cross Coder has been said to be in pursuit of medical coding's Holy Grail: a single repository where every CPT code instantly reveals the correct diagnosis code, the corresponding inpatient procedure code, as well as appropriate codes for ancillary supplies and pharmaceuticals. *Surgical Cross Coder* is based on the Surgery Section of the *Current Procedural Terminology* (CPT™). Up-to-date CPT surgery codes link to the following related medical coding systems:

- *International Classification of Diseases, 9th Revision, Clinical Modification* (ICD-9-CM)
- *Healthcare Common Procedural Coding System* (HCPCS) Level II

All coding relationships in *Surgical Cross Coder* spring from CPT's surgery codes, and the term "CPT-driven" is sometimes heard; but it is perhaps more appropriate to think of this reference book as "data driven." A team of clinical and coding experts launched *Surgical Cross Coder* by first reviewing surgery data drawn from the Ingenix information base of nationwide medical claims. Pertinent surgery related coding relationships were drawn from the data stream and processed for coding errors and other anomalies. From this early cut of data emerged a general clinical picture of each surgery code; but data analysis for *Surgical Cross Coder* had hardly begun.

All data was carefully screened for appropriate surgery-related information only. For example, it is statistically and clinically unusual for a closed fracture procedure to be performed when an open fracture diagnosis code is reported. This type of unusual association is eliminated from the listing along with other outliers.

Perhaps more significantly, many acute and chronic medical conditions may eventually lead to surgical intervention. Raw data reflects this. Yet, clinical analysts pointed out that chronic and acute conditions are nearly always aggressively approached medically before surgery is even considered. For this reason, the number of cross-coded chronic and acute conditions is selectively culled in this reference book.

In some instances the data is abridged simply due to the enormity of the listings. For example, diagnosis codes for infections call for additional codes to identify specific organisms. The possible associations are simply too numerous and do not appear in *Surgical Cross Coder*. In a similar vein, *Surgical Cross Coder* features codes that require accompanying etiologies or manifestations (examples include "Code first underlying disease..."). However, associated infectious and parasitic diseases are, once again, simply too numerous to list and do not appear in *Surgical Cross Coder*. For further discussion on secondary diagnosis codes, see the ICD-9-CM section later in this introduction.

Some CPT codes are omitted from the listing because consistent and reliable cross links are almost impossible to establish. Unlisted procedure codes are an obvious example. Certain types of add-on codes are also treated somewhat differently in *Surgical Cross Coder*. These codes are discussed in greater detail under the CPT Codes section later in this introduction. Unlisted and add-on codes are listed with full descriptions in the appendix, *Excluded Codes*.

As a data-driven coding reference, *Surgical Cross Coder* presents "most likely" scenarios as derived from clinical statistics. Because the presented scenarios statistically occur so often points to a level of clinical appropriateness and, therefore, of coding accuracy. However, *Surgical Cross Coder* is not a substitute for ICD-9-CM, or any other medical coding reference, and users are urged to regularly consult all available sources. The absence of any specific code does not necessarily indicate that its association to the base procedure code is inappropriate. Assuming all rules of medical coding are followed, excepted diagnosis codes may prove appropriate to a specific code scenario.

Surgical Cross Coder does not include coding rules and guidelines. Once again, the user is urged to consult the original coding reference (i.e., CPT, ICD-9, HCPCS Level II, etc.) or one of several reputable medical coding instruction manuals. This may prove poignant advice when sorting through codes for wounds, burns, fractures, and complications.

Format

An understanding of the *Surgical Cross Coder* format allows users to easily navigate its content. Information within the main section ties to the CPT book and the codes are presented in the numeric order of the Surgery section.

Sections

Surgical Cross Coder provides linked information to the CPT code range 10021 to 69990 — the surgical portion of CPT. The codes are divided into the same sections and subsections of the Surgery part of CPT. For example, the Respiratory System section is divided into anatomical subsections including Nose, Accessory Sinuses, and Larynx. Larynx is further divided into Excision, Introduction, Endoscopy, Repair, and Destruction.

Users will find pertinent procedural and anatomical illustrations within each section. A complete listing is found in the Index of Illustrations on page iii.

Codes and Code Ranges

The data within each CPT code set of *Surgical Cross Coder* is presented as follows:

- CPT code or code range
- CPT code(s) and description(s)

- ICD-9-CM diagnostic code(s)and description(s)
- ICD-9-CM procedural code(s)and description(s)
- HCPCS code(s)and description(s)

For example:

21400–21401

21400	Closed treatment of fracture of orbit, except blowout; without manipulation
21401	with manipulation

ICD-9-CM Diagnostic

801.00	Closed fracture of base of skull without mention of intracranial injury, unspecified state of consciousness
801.01	Closed fracture of base of skull without mention of intracranial injury, no loss of consciousness
801.02	Closed fracture of base of skull without mention of intracranial injury, brief (less than one hour) loss of consciousness
801.03	Closed fracture of base of skull without mention of intracranial injury, moderate (1-24 hours) loss of consciousness
801.04	Closed fracture of base of skull without mention of intracranial injury, prolonged (more than 24 hours) loss of consciousness and return to pre-existing conscious level
801.05	Closed fracture of base of skull without mention of intracranial injury, prolonged (more than 24 hours) loss of consciousness, without return to pre-existing conscious level
801.06	Closed fracture of base of skull without mention of intracranial injury, loss of consciousness of unspecified duration
801.09	Closed fracture of base of skull without mention of intracranial injury, unspecified concussion
801.10	Closed fracture of base of skull with cerebral laceration and contusion, unspecified state of consciousness
801.12	Closed fracture of base of skull with cerebral laceration and contusion, brief (less than one hour) loss of consciousness
801.13	Closed fracture of base of skull with cerebral laceration and contusion, moderate (1-24 hours) loss of consciousness
801.14	Closed fracture of base of skull with cerebral laceration and contusion, prolonged (more than 24 hours) loss of consciousness and return to pre-existing conscious level
801.15	Closed fracture of base of skull with cerebral laceration and contusion, prolonged (more than 24 hours) loss of consciousness, without return to pre-existing conscious level
801.16	Closed fracture of base of skull with cerebral laceration and contusion, loss of consciousness of unspecified duration
801.19	Closed fracture of base of skull with cerebral laceration and contusion, unspecified concussion
801.20	Closed fracture of base of skull with subarachnoid, subdural, and extradural hemorrhage, unspecified state of consciousness
801.30	Closed fracture of base of skull with other and unspecified intracranial hemorrhage, unspecified state of consciousness
801.40	Closed fracture of base of skull with intracranial injury of other and unspecified nature, unspecified state of consciousness
802.4	Malar and maxillary bones, closed fracture
802.8	Other facial bones, closed fracture

ICD-9-CM Procedural

76.78	Other closed reduction of facial fracture

HCPCS

A4305	Disposable drug delivery system, flow rate of 50 ml or greater per hour
A4306	Disposable drug delivery system, flow rate of 5 ml or less per hour
A4550	Surgical trays

Each CPT code or code range is followed by its specific ICD-9-CM, HCPCS. *Surgical Cross Coder* presents full descriptions for all CPT codes and their links.

Keep in mind, though, that ICD-9-CM codes are hierarchical and their "full descriptions" are by nature incomplete. Information on a specific five-digit code is found under its three-digit or four-digit category. Medicode's database and *Surgical Cross Coder* feature complete descriptions for ICD-9-CM codes. For example, the official ICD-9-CM description for 810.03 is a fifth-digit subclassification for use with category 810 and appears as follows:

810 Fracture of clavicle
- **0 unspecified part**
  Clavicle NOS
- **1 sternal end of clavicle**
- **2 shaft of clavicle**
- **3 acromial end of clavicle**

810.0 Closed

Surgical Cross Coder presents a closed clavicle fracture involving the acromial end as the following:

810.03 Closed fracture of the acromial end of clavicle

Complete descriptions are presented throughout this book.

Icon Key

An icon key is provided in the bottom margin on each page. These icons, or symbols, can be found next to particular ICD-9-CM diagnosis codes listed in the crosswalk, as appropriate. These icons warn of coding edits which apply to that particular code and must be followed. For instance, a procedure done on the prostate would list diagnosis codes for prostate conditions supporting medical necessity. These codes would never be assigned to a female patient and these codes appear with the icon denoting a male only diagnosis. The icons appear in the *Surgical Cross Coder*:

♀ **Female Diagnosis.** Codes appearing with this symbol should only be used to report a diagnosis for a female patient.

♂ **Male Diagnosis.** Codes appearing with this symbol should only be used to report a diagnosis for a male patient.

Unspecified Code. Codes denoted as unspecified should only be used when the medical information to substantiate a more specific code is not available. Review the medical record documentation and/or query the physician to determine whether a more specific diagnosis is available for coding to the highest level of specificity.

Manifestation Code. A manifestation code is not allowed to be reported as the primary diagnosis since it describes a manifestation of some other underlying disease, not the disease itself. The underlying disease is coded first and the manifestation code second. This is referred to as mandatory multiple coding of etiology and manifestation.

CPT Codes

CPT is a standardized system of five-digit codes and descriptive terms developed, maintained, and copyrighted by the American Medical Association (AMA). CPT codes are the most widely accepted procedure codes for reporting medical services performed by physicians. Federal law requires Medicare and Medicaid carriers to use CPT codes on health care claims. Commercial insurance payers often recognize only CPT. CPT is a trademark of the American Medical Association.

Although *Surgical Cross Coder* is organized numerically by CPT code, not all codes are presented separately. In many cases, several codes within a CPT code set have similar ICD-9-CM diagnosis or ICD-9-CM procedural codes. In these cases, a range of CPT codes is listed, followed by each individual code and its description.

59840–59841

59840	Induced abortion, by dilation and curettage
59841	Induced abortion, by dilation and evacuation

Indented Procedures

As experienced coders know, each surgical procedure embraces two components in CPT: the five-digit reporting code and its precise, formal description. A simple rule of CPT allows each description to stand alone while also saving space on the printed page. Codes that share a common description are grouped together. The common description is listed in its entirety as the first code. The following codes in the group are indented to indicate that they share the common descriptive portion with the preceding fully described code. For example:

49020–49021

49020	Drainage of peritoneal abscess or localized peritonitis, exclusive of appendiceal abscess; open
49021	percutaneous

The common portion of these two codes precedes the semicolon (;) in the full description of 49020. Terminology following the semicolon is unique to that code. The complete description of 49021 is:

49021 Drainage of peritoneal abscess or localized peritonitis, exclusive of appendiceal abscess; percutaneous

Surgical Cross Coder also employs this methodology with only minor adjustment. When the code links for indented procedures are the same as for the main code, *Surgical Cross Coder* presents the material concurrently. As in the CPT book, the description terminology following the semicolon describes the indented code.

When the cross coding links of an indented procedure vary from those of the main code, the indented code description appears in its entirety. Subsequent indented codes appear indented and are grouped if the links are the same. For example, code range 65270–65286 appears as follows in the CPT book:

65270	Repair of laceration; conjunctiva, with or without nonperforating laceration sclera, direct closure
65272	conjunctiva, by mobilization and rearrangement, without hospitalization
65273	conjunctiva, by mobilization and rearrangement, with hospitalization
65275	cornea, nonperforating, with or without removal foreign body
65280	cornea, and/or sclera, perforating, not involving uveal tissue
65285	cornea and/or sclera, perforating, with reposition or resection of uveal tissue
65286	application of tissue glue, wounds of cornea and/or sclera

Based on diagnostic links, *Surgical Cross Coder* groups these codes as follows:

65270–65273

65270*	Repair of laceration; conjunctiva, with or without nonperforating laceration sclera, direct closure
65272	conjunctiva, by mobilization and rearran
65273	conjunctiva, by mobilization and rearrangement, with hospitalization

65275–65285

65275	Repair of laceration; cornea, nonperforating, with or without removal foreign body
65280	cornea and/or sclera, perforating, not involving uveal tissue
65285	cornea and/or sclera, perforating, with reposition or resection of uveal tissue

65286

65286	Repair of laceration; application of tissue glue, wounds of cornea and/or sclera

Not every code within a CPT surgical code set can be addressed appropriately in a cross-coding publication. Examples are found among add-on and unlisted codes.

Unlisted Procedure Codes

Unlisted codes are reported for procedures not adequately addressed by any other CPT codes. Unlisted codes are classified by general anatomy and no further description is offered. Often classified "by report" payers may require extensive documentation to accompany these manually processed claims. For obvious reasons, unlisted procedure codes cannot be reliably linked to the other medical coding systems. Consequently, *Surgical Cross Coder* does not include unlisted procedure codes from the Surgery portion of the CPT book. A complete listing of these codes and their descriptions may be found in the Appendix, Unlisted Codes.

Add-On Codes

Add-on codes represent procedures performed in addition to the primary procedure and as a rule are never reported separately. Three types exist: 1) those linked exclusively to one primary code; 2) those linked to a variety of primary codes; and 3) those representing procedures unrelated to the primary code, but performed concurrent to the primary procedure.

Add-on Codes Associated with Specific Primary Codes

Many add-on codes report services that are simple extensions of the primary procedure. Consider code 11732 *Avulsion of nail plate, partial or complete, simple; each additional nail plate (List separately in addition to code for primary procedure)*. This code is an "add-on" to the preceding avulsion code and reporting 11732 without 11730 is a fundamental error.

Surgical Cross Coder usually groups this type of add-on code in a range with the primary procedure because the links to diagnosis codes are almost always identical. The preceding example is listed as 11730–11732.

Add-on Codes Appropriate to Various Primary Codes
These codes report "in addition to" procedures. However, each code in this category can apply to multiple primary codes. For example, 67335 *Placement of adjustable suture(s) during strabismus surgery, including postoperative adjustment(s) of suture(s) (List separately in addition to code for specific strabismus surgery)* can be reported with any code in the range 67311–67334.

The primary procedure must be identified before establishing any link between the add-on code and a diagnosis. Coders should consult the instructions and references under the primary code for information also applicable to the add-on code.

Add-on codes as Unrelated Procedures
A set of add-on codes represents procedures that are "in addition to" other surgeries, but performed for unrelated reasons.

Consider 58611 *Ligation or transection of fallopian tube(s) when done at the time of cesarean section or intra-abdominal surgery (not a separate procedure) (List separately in addition to code for primary procedure)*. The tubal ligation is performed for a reason different from that for the primary procedure. The primary procedure (for example, cesarean) is performed for a distinct diagnosis (for example, previous cesarean scar). The cesarean is unrelated to a diagnosis linked to tubal ligation, typically performed for sterilization.

Surgical Cross Coder includes this type of unrelated add-on code as a single entry, since these codes have identifiable code-link relationships independent of the parent procedures.

A complete listing of surgical add-on codes, identified by CPT, is found in the Appendix, Add-on Codes.

Code Links
An extensive review process by Ingenix links each CPT code to corresponding codes in the other major medical coding systems. But not all CPT codes link to every coding system and the listings reflect this fact. For instance, no ADA headings appear in the Urinary System section since no urinary code requires a dental procedure.

ICD-9-CM Diagnostic Codes
ICD-9-CM, Volumes 1 and 2, is a systematic listing of codes that describe the incredible variety of medical conditions known to man. The system used in this country was developed and is maintained by the National Center for Health Statistics. Though designed primarily to track health statistics, ICD-9-CM diagnosis codes serve payers as a check to ensure that medical services provided are warranted.

Selective manipulation of the Ingenix database links each CPT surgical code with the ICD-9-CM diagnoses that would warrant such a procedure. Code associations are edited for most appropriate usage, though Ingenix cannot guarantee that every possible diagnosis for a given procedure is included. This crosswalk is extensive — in some instances more than 400 appropriate diagnosis codes are listed for a single procedure. In some cases the following statement appears:

This code is too broadly diagnostic to adequately present diagnosis codes here. Refer to your ICD-9-CM.

Invalid ICD-9-CM codes identify disease categories, yet do not give the level of detail available and necessary for processing. Valid ICD-9-CM codes can contain three, four, or five digits, which makes for a difficult job to recognize whether a code is at its highest level of specificity. To simplify the coder's job, *Surgical Cross Coder* includes only valid ICD-9-CM codes.

Diagnostic Coding Considerations
Surgical Cross Coder simplifies medical coding for those in physician, hospital, or payer offices. Keep in mind, though, that diagnostic coding practices in clinical settings vary from those in hospitals. The surgical facility influences coding and coders should learn the rules applicable to their medical environment. Consider this example:

A patient presents with a nasal hemorrhage. The physician, using a nasal speculum, identifies a bleeding polyp in the nasopharyngeal cavity. The polyp is removed by snare; the wound is cauterized and packed. The patient is sent home.

This procedure would be reported with CPT code 30110 *Excision, nasal polyp(s), simple*. The procedure is normally performed in an office setting. The place of service, however, could alter the reporting of the diagnostic codes.

An emergency department (ED) coder might order the diagnosis codes as follows:

784.7 Epistaxis
471.0 Polyp of nasal cavity

This coding supports medical necessity for an ED service. A nasal polyp does not justify an ED service; nasal hemorrhage does. Similarly, chest pain is listed before heart disease on an ED claim form, since pain, not the heart condition, prompted the ED visit.

A surgeon excising the polyp in an ambulatory surgical center may report the scenario as follows:

471.0 Polyp of nasal cavity
784.7 Epistaxis

In most sites outside the hospital, the diagnosis applicable to the procedure — the nasal polyp — is generally coded first. Coexisting conditions, like the nosebleed, are considered supplemental information. An unscheduled patient presenting with epistaxis at the physician office may be an exception. If the physician performs a polypectomy on site, the coder may report 99058 *Office services provided on an emergency basis* in addition to 30110. In this case, 784.7 is reported first on the claim form.

Comorbidities
Comorbidities are preexisting conditions or chronic diseases, (e.g., malignant neoplasms, diabetes, or some mental disorders) that occur in background to another, significant diagnostic event. These conditions can affect the care a patient may require.

Comorbidities rarely affect physician reimbursement. The Centers for Medicare and Medicaid Services, or CMS (formerly the Health Care Financing Administration (HCFA)) advises physician coders to submit chronic disease codes only as they apply to a current patient encounter.

Hospitals are reimbursed by Diagnosis Related Groups (DRGs) that are contingent on comorbidity information. For instance, the claims for two patients who undergo similar labor and delivery care are not paid the same when one patient has Type I diabetes. Due to the extreme variability represented by comorbid diagnoses, *Surgical Cross Coder* does not link Type I diabetes to a labor and delivery code.

Coders in physician, hospital, or payer offices should reference ICD-9-CM and their own facility protocols for the role comorbidity codes should play in the patient record.

Secondary Codes

Many ICD-9-CM codes cannot be used as the primary or principal diagnosis. These codes are called secondary diagnosis codes. ICD-9-CM notations specify to "code first" the underlying disease.

443.81 *Peripheral angiopathy in diseases classified elsewhere*
Code first underlying disease, as:
diabetes mellitus (250.7)

The coder turns to 250.7 in ICD-9-CM to find, in addition to fifth-digit subclassification, information required for 250.7 *Diabetes with peripheral circulatory disorders*.

Use additional code to identify manifestations, as:
diabetic:
gangrene (785.4)
peripheral angiopathy (443.81)

When ICD-9-CM provides specific printed code links between primary and secondary codes, those links appear in *Surgical Cross Coder* as a statement (in this case, "Code first 250.7") in parenthesis following the code description. Code 443.81 appears in the crosswalk as follows:

443.81 Peripheral angiopathy in diseases classified elsewhere — (Code first 250.7)

If 443.81 appears in a crosswalk, the primary code 250.7 is listed with its complete description in the numerically ordered crosswalk.

Codes appearing with parenthetical information that begins "Code first..." are secondary codes and, consequently, not listed first on the claim form. Primary or principal diagnosis codes are identified in the parenthetical notation.

Other Related ICD-9-CM Codes

ICD-9-CM notations instruct readers to "Code also" or to "Use additional code" to give more information about the patient's condition. For example:

365.64 Glaucoma associated with tumors or cysts
Use additional code for associated disorder, as:
benign neoplasm (224.0–224.9)
epithelial down-growth (364.61)
malignant neoplasm (190.0–190.9)

The *Surgical Cross Coder* includes specific linking data provided in ICD-9-CM. However, each of these codes may not apply to the CPT code serving as the basis for a crosswalk. In the case of 65900 *Removal of epithelial down-growth, anterior chamber eye*, appropriate ICD-9-CM codes listed include the following:

364.61 Implantation cysts
365.64 Glaucoma associated with tumors or cysts

Note that the two neoplasm codes linked in ICD-9-CM to 365.64 are inappropriate to 65900. A clinical edit has removed these diagnostic links to 365.64 when it is linked with CPT code 65900, so that it reads:

365.64 Glaucoma associated with tumors or cysts

Sometimes, ICD-9-CM makes general references to other codes, such as "use additional E code to identify cause," or "use additional code to identify organism." General notes in *Surgical Cross Coder* address these situations. Consult ICD-9-CM for information about infective agents, toxic drugs or agents, E codes identifying circumstances, hypertension and neoplasm tables, or other codes broadly associated or linked to a diagnosis or procedure.

ICD-9-CM Procedural Codes

ICD-9-CM, Volume 3, is a systematic listing of procedural codes for inpatient hospital coding. CMS developed and maintains these codes. *Surgical Cross Coder* cross-references each CPT procedural code to its corresponding ICD-9-CM Volume 3 code or codes. The Volume 3 codes are somewhat more general than CPT procedural codes, so in some cases numerous CPT codes link to a solitary ICD-9-CM procedural code, each remaining a one-to-one relationship.

Conversely, one CPT code may link to several ICD-9-CM Volume 3, codes. For example, four ICD-9-CM procedure codes are appropriate to 59510 *Routine obstetric care including antepartum care, cesarean delivery, and postpartum care.* The following codes represent the possible choices listed:

74.0 Classical cesarean section
74.1 Low cervical cesarean section
74.2 Extraperitoneal cesarean section
74.4 Cesarean section of other specified type

In other cases, one CPT code may cross to several ICD-9-CM codes, each of which is a component of the CPT code.

42953
42953 Pharyngoesophageal repair

ICD-9-CM Procedural
29.51 Suture of laceration of pharynx
42.82 Suture of laceration of esophagus

The coder is responsible for determining from the patient record which ICD-9-CM procedure code, or codes, apply.

HCPCS Level II Codes

HCPCS is an acronym (pronounced "hick-picks") for the Healthcare Common Procedure Coding System. This field presents national codes to report medical supplies and equipment, as well as select services provided on an outpatient basis. CMS developed and maintains Level II codes for Medicare and Medicaid reporting.

In this field of *Surgical Cross Coder*, Ingenix provides common HCPCS supply codes linked to each CPT code. For example:

65101–65105

65103 Enucleation of eye; with implant, muscles not attached to implant

HCPCS

V2623 Prosthetic eye, plastic, custom
V2628 Fabrication and fitting of ocular conformer
V2629 Prosthetic eye, other type

Site of Service

Someone other than the physician may supply many of the HCPCS supplies and services linked to codes in this crosswalk. For clarity, the crosswalk includes only those HCPCS Level II codes issued during the global period of surgery. Supplies such as mastectomy prosthetics are not included, since postoperative swelling generally pushes the fitting for the prosthesis beyond the surgery's global period.

Sometimes, multi-specialty clinics or other free-standing facilities have in-house equipment suppliers. Always verify the patient's record before billing supplies and report only appropriate supplies issued through that facility.

While supply houses and physicians depend on HCPCS codes to report supplies, the same reporting system is gaining favor for different reasons among hospitals and other inpatient facilities. Although these latter sites report supplies to Medicare with revenue codes instead of HCPCS codes, HCPCS codes are popular for inventory control, patient billing, and related purposes. *Surgical Cross Coder* provides links to appropriate HCPCS Level II codes regardless of place of service.

J Codes

The HCPCS J codes generally report drugs administered other than by an oral method. The clinical editors of *Surgical Cross Coder* have determined that consistent links to pharmaceuticals are extremely difficult to establish and only very specifically linked listings appear in this reference.

Summary

Based on the AMA's CPT code set of 10021 to 69990, *Surgical Cross Coder*, links surgical procedures to appropriate ICD-9-CM diagnostic and procedural codes, HCPCS supply codes, and ADA CDT codes. As a useful adjunct to these coding systems, *Surgical Cross Coder* presents a more accurate and efficient way for professional coders to link CPT surgical codes to other important medical codes. The result is a broader, comprehensive picture of a surgical event.

The Ingenix *Surgical Cross Coder* serves coders' needs by helping providers comply with ever emerging standards for coding, reporting, and reimbursing medical procedures. The Ingenix database and nationally known coding expertise combine to offer a coding book that is as accurate as possible at publication.

Ingenix recognizes the subjective nature of procedural coding and encourages comments or suggestions to improve the product or to illustrate regional idiosyncrasies of the reimbursement process.

As with all medical coding resources, *Surgical Cross Coder* is designed as a post-procedural reference for billing purposes only. The use of any of these listings to select surgical treatment is entirely inappropriate.

General

10021–10022

10021 Fine needle aspiration; without imaging guidance
10022 with imaging guidance

ICD-9-CM Diagnostic

135 Sarcoidosis
155.0 Malignant neoplasm of liver, primary
155.1 Malignant neoplasm of intrahepatic bile ducts
155.2 Malignant neoplasm of liver, not specified as primary or secondary ▽
157.0 Malignant neoplasm of head of pancreas
157.1 Malignant neoplasm of body of pancreas
157.2 Malignant neoplasm of tail of pancreas
157.3 Malignant neoplasm of pancreatic duct
157.4 Malignant neoplasm of islets of Langerhans — (Use additional code to identify any functional activity)
157.8 Malignant neoplasm of other specified sites of pancreas
157.9 Malignant neoplasm of pancreas, part unspecified ▽
158.0 Malignant neoplasm of retroperitoneum
158.8 Malignant neoplasm of specified parts of peritoneum
158.9 Malignant neoplasm of peritoneum, unspecified ▽
159.8 Malignant neoplasm of other sites of digestive system and intra-abdominal organs
162.2 Malignant neoplasm of main bronchus
162.3 Malignant neoplasm of upper lobe, bronchus, or lung
162.4 Malignant neoplasm of middle lobe, bronchus, or lung
162.5 Malignant neoplasm of lower lobe, bronchus, or lung
162.8 Malignant neoplasm of other parts of bronchus or lung
162.9 Malignant neoplasm of bronchus and lung, unspecified site ▽
163.0 Malignant neoplasm of parietal pleura
163.8 Malignant neoplasm of other specified sites of pleura
163.9 Malignant neoplasm of pleura, unspecified site ▽
164.2 Malignant neoplasm of anterior mediastinum
164.3 Malignant neoplasm of posterior mediastinum
164.8 Malignant neoplasm of other parts of mediastinum
164.9 Malignant neoplasm of mediastinum, part unspecified ▽
172.5 Malignant melanoma of skin of trunk, except scrotum
172.6 Malignant melanoma of skin of upper limb, including shoulder
172.7 Malignant melanoma of skin of lower limb, including hip
172.8 Malignant melanoma of other specified sites of skin
173.5 Other malignant neoplasm of skin of trunk, except scrotum
174.0 Malignant neoplasm of nipple and areola of female breast ♀
174.1 Malignant neoplasm of central portion of female breast ♀
174.2 Malignant neoplasm of upper-inner quadrant of female breast ♀
174.3 Malignant neoplasm of lower-inner quadrant of female breast ♀
174.4 Malignant neoplasm of upper-outer quadrant of female breast ♀
174.5 Malignant neoplasm of lower-outer quadrant of female breast ♀
174.6 Malignant neoplasm of axillary tail of female breast ♀
174.8 Malignant neoplasm of other specified sites of female breast ♀
175.0 Malignant neoplasm of nipple and areola of male breast ♂
175.9 Malignant neoplasm of other and unspecified sites of male breast ▽ ♂
176.4 Kaposi's sarcoma of lung
180.9 Malignant neoplasm of cervix uteri, unspecified site ▽ ♀
182.0 Malignant neoplasm of corpus uteri, except isthmus ♀
183.0 Malignant neoplasm of ovary — (Use additional code to identify any functional activity) ♀
183.2 Malignant neoplasm of fallopian tube ♀
183.8 Malignant neoplasm of other specified sites of uterine adnexa ♀
185 Malignant neoplasm of prostate ♂
186.0 Malignant neoplasm of undescended testis — (Use additional code to identify any functional activity) ♂
186.9 Malignant neoplasm of other and unspecified testis — (Use additional code to identify any functional activity) ▽ ♂
187.5 Malignant neoplasm of epididymis ♂
188.9 Malignant neoplasm of bladder, part unspecified ▽
189.0 Malignant neoplasm of kidney, except pelvis
189.1 Malignant neoplasm of renal pelvis
193 Malignant neoplasm of thyroid gland — (Use additional code to identify any functional activity)
195.1 Malignant neoplasm of thorax
195.2 Malignant neoplasm of abdomen
196.0 Secondary and unspecified malignant neoplasm of lymph nodes of head, face, and neck
196.1 Secondary and unspecified malignant neoplasm of intrathoracic lymph nodes
196.2 Secondary and unspecified malignant neoplasm of intra-abdominal lymph nodes
196.3 Secondary and unspecified malignant neoplasm of lymph nodes of axilla and upper limb
196.5 Secondary and unspecified malignant neoplasm of lymph nodes of inguinal region and lower limb
196.6 Secondary and unspecified malignant neoplasm of intrapelvic lymph nodes
196.8 Secondary and unspecified malignant neoplasm of lymph nodes of multiple sites
196.9 Secondary and unspecified malignant neoplasm of lymph nodes, site unspecified ▽
197.0 Secondary malignant neoplasm of lung
197.1 Secondary malignant neoplasm of mediastinum
197.2 Secondary malignant neoplasm of pleura
197.6 Secondary malignant neoplasm of retroperitoneum and peritoneum
197.7 Secondary malignant neoplasm of liver
197.8 Secondary malignant neoplasm of other digestive organs and spleen
198.0 Secondary malignant neoplasm of kidney
198.81 Secondary malignant neoplasm of breast
198.82 Secondary malignant neoplasm of genital organs
198.89 Secondary malignant neoplasm of other specified sites
199.0 Disseminated malignant neoplasm
199.1 Other malignant neoplasm of unspecified site
200.00 Reticulosarcoma, unspecified site, extranodal and solid organ sites ▽
200.01 Reticulosarcoma of lymph nodes of head, face, and neck
200.04 Reticulosarcoma of lymph nodes of axilla and upper limb
200.05 Reticulosarcoma of lymph nodes of inguinal region and lower limb
200.08 Reticulosarcoma of lymph nodes of multiple sites
200.10 Lymphosarcoma, unspecified site, extranodal and solid organ sites ▽
200.14 Lymphosarcoma of lymph nodes of axilla and upper limb
200.15 Lymphosarcoma of lymph nodes of inguinal region and lower limb
200.18 Lymphosarcoma of lymph nodes of multiple sites
200.20 Burkitt's tumor or lymphoma, unspecified site, extranodal and solid organ sites ▽
200.21 Burkitt's tumor or lymphoma of lymph nodes of head, face, and neck
200.24 Burkitt's tumor or lymphoma of lymph nodes of axilla and upper limb
200.25 Burkitt's tumor or lymphoma of lymph nodes of inguinal region and lower limb
200.28 Burkitt's tumor or lymphoma of lymph nodes of multiple sites
201.00 Hodgkin's paragranuloma, unspecified site, extranodal and solid organ sites ▽
201.01 Hodgkin's paragranuloma of lymph nodes of head, face, and neck
201.04 Hodgkin's paragranuloma of lymph nodes of axilla and upper limb
201.05 Hodgkin's paragranuloma of lymph nodes of inguinal region and lower limb
201.08 Hodgkin's paragranuloma of lymph nodes of multiple sites
201.10 Hodgkin's granuloma, unspecified site, extranodal and solid organ sites ▽
201.11 Hodgkin's granuloma of lymph nodes of head, face, and neck
201.14 Hodgkin's granuloma of lymph nodes of axilla and upper limb
201.15 Hodgkin's granuloma of lymph nodes of inguinal region and lower limb
201.18 Hodgkin's granuloma of lymph nodes of multiple sites
201.20 Hodgkin's sarcoma, unspecified site, extranodal and solid organ sites ▽
201.24 Hodgkin's sarcoma of lymph nodes of axilla and upper limb
201.25 Hodgkin's sarcoma of lymph nodes of inguinal region and lower limb
201.28 Hodgkin's sarcoma of lymph nodes of multiple sites
201.40 Hodgkin's disease, lymphocytic-histiocytic predominance, unspecified site, extranodal and solid organ sites ▽
201.44 Hodgkin's disease, lymphocytic-histiocytic predominance of lymph nodes of axilla and upper limb
201.45 Hodgkin's disease, lymphocytic-histiocytic predominance of lymph nodes of inguinal region and lower limb
201.48 Hodgkin's disease, lymphocytic-histiocytic predominance of lymph nodes of multiple sites

▽ Unspecified code
♀ Female diagnosis
☒ Manifestation code
♂ Male diagnosis

201.51 Hodgkin's disease, nodular sclerosis, of lymph nodes of head, face, and neck
201.54 Hodgkin's disease, nodular sclerosis, of lymph nodes of axilla and upper limb
201.55 Hodgkin's disease, nodular sclerosis, of lymph nodes of inguinal region and lower limb
201.58 Hodgkin's disease, nodular sclerosis, of lymph nodes of multiple sites
201.60 Hodgkin's disease, mixed cellularity, unspecified site, extranodal and solid organ sites ▽
201.61 Hodgkin's disease, mixed cellularity, involving lymph nodes of head, face, and neck
201.65 Hodgkin's disease, mixed cellularity, of lymph nodes of inguinal region and lower limb
201.68 Hodgkin's disease, mixed cellularity, of lymph nodes of multiple sites
201.70 Hodgkin's disease, lymphocytic depletion, unspecified site, extranodal and solid organ sites ▽
201.71 Hodgkin's disease, lymphocytic depletion, of lymph nodes of head, face, and neck
201.74 Hodgkin's disease, lymphocytic depletion, of lymph nodes of axilla and upper limb
201.75 Hodgkin's disease, lymphocytic depletion, of lymph nodes of inguinal region and lower limb
201.78 Hodgkin's disease, lymphocytic depletion, of lymph nodes of multiple sites
201.90 Hodgkin's disease, unspecified type, unspecified site, extranodal and solid organ sites ▽
201.91 Hodgkin's disease, unspecified type, of lymph nodes of head, face, and neck ▽
201.94 Hodgkin's disease, unspecified type, of lymph nodes of axilla and upper limb ▽
201.95 Hodgkin's disease, unspecified type, of lymph nodes of inguinal region and lower limb ▽
201.98 Hodgkin's disease, unspecified type, of lymph nodes of multiple sites ▽
202.00 Nodular lymphoma, unspecified site, extranodal and solid organ sites ▽
202.01 Nodular lymphoma of lymph nodes of head, face, and neck
202.04 Nodular lymphoma of lymph nodes of axilla and upper limb
202.05 Nodular lymphoma of lymph nodes of inguinal region and lower limb
202.08 Nodular lymphoma of lymph nodes of multiple sites
202.10 Mycosis fungoides, unspecified site, extranodal and solid organ sites ▽
202.11 Mycosis fungoides of lymph nodes of head, face, and neck
202.14 Mycosis fungoides of lymph nodes of axilla and upper limb
202.15 Mycosis fungoides of lymph nodes of inguinal region and lower limb
202.18 Mycosis fungoides of lymph nodes of multiple sites
202.20 Sezary's disease, unspecified site, extranodal and solid organ sites ▽
202.21 Sezary's disease of lymph nodes of head, face, and neck
202.28 Sezary's disease of lymph nodes of multiple sites
202.30 Malignant histiocytosis, unspecified site, extranodal and solid organ sites ▽
202.31 Malignant histiocytosis of lymph nodes of head, face, and neck
202.34 Malignant histiocytosis of lymph nodes of axilla and upper limb
202.35 Malignant histiocytosis of lymph nodes of inguinal region and lower limb
202.38 Malignant histiocytosis of lymph nodes of multiple sites
202.40 Leukemic reticuloendotheliosis, unspecified site, extranodal and solid organ sites ▽
202.41 Leukemic reticuloendotheliosis of lymph nodes of head, face, and neck
202.44 Leukemic reticuloendotheliosis of lymph nodes of axilla and upper limb
202.45 Leukemic reticuloendotheliosis of lymph nodes of inguinal region and lower limb
202.48 Leukemic reticuloendotheliosis of lymph nodes of multipes sites
202.50 Letterer-Siwe disease, unspecified site, extranodal and solid organ sites ▽
202.51 Letterer-Siwe disease of lymph nodes of head, face, and neck
202.54 Letterer-Siwe disease of lymph nodes of axilla and upper limb
202.55 Letterer-Siwe disease of lymph nodes of inguinal region and lower limb
202.58 Letterer-Siwe disease of lymph nodes of multiple sites
202.60 Malignant mast cell tumors, unspecified site, extranodal and solid organ sites ▽
202.61 Malignant mast cell tumors of lymph nodes of head, face, and neck
202.64 Malignant mast cell tumors of lymph nodes of axilla and upper limb
202.65 Malignant mast cell tumors of lymph nodes of inguinal region and lower limb
202.68 Malignant mast cell tumors of lymph nodes of multiple sites
202.80 Other malignant lymphomas, unspecified site, extranodal and solid organ sites ▽
202.81 Other malignant lymphomas of lymph nodes of head, face, and neck
202.84 Other malignant lymphomas of lymph nodes of axilla and upper limb
202.85 Other malignant lymphomas of lymph nodes of inguinal region and lower limb
202.88 Other malignant lymphomas of lymph nodes of multiple sites
202.91 Other and unspecified malignant neoplasms of lymphoid and histiocytic tissue of lymph nodes of head, face, and neck ▽
202.94 Other and unspecified malignant neoplasms of lymphoid and histiocytic tissue of lymph nodes of axilla and upper limb ▽
202.95 Other and unspecified malignant neoplasms of lymphoid and histiocytic tissue of lymph nodes of inguinal region and lower limb ▽
202.98 Other and unspecified malignant neoplasms of lymphoid and histiocytic tissue of lymph nodes of multiple sites ▽
211.5 Benign neoplasm of liver and biliary passages
211.6 Benign neoplasm of pancreas, except islets of Langerhans
211.7 Benign neoplasm of islets of Langerhans — (Use additional code to identify any functional activity)
211.8 Benign neoplasm of retroperitoneum and peritoneum
211.9 Benign neoplasm of other and unspecified site of the digestive system ▽
212.3 Benign neoplasm of bronchus and lung
212.4 Benign neoplasm of pleura
212.5 Benign neoplasm of mediastinum
212.8 Benign neoplasm of other specified sites of respiratory and intrathoracic organs
214.2 Lipoma of intrathoracic organs
215.0 Other benign neoplasm of connective and other soft tissue of head, face, and neck
215.5 Other benign neoplasm of connective and other soft tissue of abdomen
217 Benign neoplasm of breast
220 Benign neoplasm of ovary — (Use additional code to identify any functional activity: 256.0-256.1) ♀
221.0 Benign neoplasm of fallopian tube and uterine ligaments ♀
222.0 Benign neoplasm of testis — (Use additional code to identify any functional activity) ♂
222.2 Benign neoplasm of prostate ♂
222.3 Benign neoplasm of epididymis ♂
223.0 Benign neoplasm of kidney, except pelvis
223.1 Benign neoplasm of renal pelvis
226 Benign neoplasm of thyroid glands — (Use additional code to identify any functional activity)
227.6 Benign neoplasm of aortic body and other paraganglia — (Use additional code to identify any functional activity)
228.04 Hemangioma of intra-abdominal structures
228.09 Hemangioma of other sites
229.0 Benign neoplasm of lymph nodes
230.1 Carcinoma in situ of esophagus
230.8 Carcinoma in situ of liver and biliary system
231.2 Carcinoma in situ of bronchus and lung
231.8 Carcinoma in situ of other specified parts of respiratory system
231.9 Carcinoma in situ of respiratory system, part unspecified ▽
233.0 Carcinoma in situ of breast
233.1 Carcinoma in situ of cervix uteri ♀
233.3 Carcinoma in situ of other and unspecified female genital organs ▽ ♀
233.4 Carcinoma in situ of prostate ♂
233.6 Carcinoma in situ of other and unspecified male genital organs ▽ ♂
233.9 Carcinoma in situ of other and unspecified urinary organs ▽
234.8 Carcinoma in situ of other specified sites
235.3 Neoplasm of uncertain behavior of liver and biliary passages
235.4 Neoplasm of uncertain behavior of retroperitoneum and peritoneum
235.5 Neoplasm of uncertain behavior of other and unspecified digestive organs ▽
235.7 Neoplasm of uncertain behavior of trachea, bronchus, and lung
235.8 Neoplasm of uncertain behavior of pleura, thymus, and mediastinum
235.9 Neoplasm of uncertain behavior of other and unspecified respiratory organs ▽
236.2 Neoplasm of uncertain behavior of ovary — (Use additional code to identify any functional activity) ♀
236.3 Neoplasm of uncertain behavior of other and unspecified female genital organs ▽ ♀
236.4 Neoplasm of uncertain behavior of testis — (Use additional code to identify any functional activity) ♂
236.5 Neoplasm of uncertain behavior of prostate ♂
236.6 Neoplasm of uncertain behavior of other and unspecified male genital organs ▽ ♂
236.91 Neoplasm of uncertain behavior of kidney and ureter
237.3 Neoplasm of uncertain behavior of paraganglia
237.4 Neoplasm of uncertain behavior of other and unspecified endocrine glands ▽
238.1 Neoplasm of uncertain behavior of connective and other soft tissue ▽
238.3 Neoplasm of uncertain behavior of breast
238.8 Neoplasm of uncertain behavior of other specified sites
238.9 Neoplasm of uncertain behavior, site unspecified ▽
239.0 Neoplasm of unspecified nature of digestive system
239.1 Neoplasm of unspecified nature of respiratory system
239.2 Neoplasms of unspecified nature of bone, soft tissue, and skin
239.3 Neoplasm of unspecified nature of breast
239.5 Neoplasm of unspecified nature of other genitourinary organs
239.7 Neoplasm of unspecified nature of endocrine glands and other parts of nervous system
239.8 Neoplasm of unspecified nature of other specified sites
239.9 Neoplasm of unspecified nature, site unspecified ▽

240.0 Goiter, specified as simple

240.9 Goiter, unspecified ▽

241.0 Nontoxic uninodular goiter

241.1 Nontoxic multinodular goiter

241.9 Unspecified nontoxic nodular goiter ▽

242.00 Toxic diffuse goiter without mention of thyrotoxic crisis or storm

242.01 Toxic diffuse goiter with mention of thyrotoxic crisis or storm

242.10 Toxic uninodular goiter without mention of thyrotoxic crisis or storm

242.11 Toxic uninodular goiter with mention of thyrotoxic crisis or storm

242.20 Toxic multinodular goiter without mention of thyrotoxic crisis or storm

242.21 Toxic multinodular goiter with mention of thyrotoxic crisis or storm

242.30 Toxic nodular goiter, unspecified type, without mention of thyrotoxic crisis or storm ▽

242.31 Toxic nodular goiter, unspecified type, with mention of thyrotoxic crisis or storm ▽

242.40 Thyrotoxicosis from ectopic thyroid nodule without mention of thyrotoxic crisis or storm

242.41 Thyrotoxicosis from ectopic thyroid nodule with mention of thyrotoxic crisis or storm

245.0 Acute thyroiditis — (Use additional code to identify organism)

245.1 Subacute thyroiditis

245.2 Chronic lymphocytic thyroiditis

245.3 Chronic fibrous thyroiditis

245.4 Iatrogenic thyroiditis — (Use additional code to identify cause)

245.8 Other and unspecified chronic thyroiditis ▽

245.9 Unspecified thyroiditis ▽

246.2 Cyst of thyroid

246.8 Other specified disorders of thyroid

250.40 Diabetes with renal manifestations, type II or unspecified type, not stated as uncontrolled — (Use additional code to identify manifestation: 581.81, 583.81)

250.41 Diabetes with renal manifestations, type I [juvenile type], not stated as uncontrolled — (Use additional code to identify manifestation: 581.81, 583.81)

250.42 Diabetes with renal manifestations, type II or unspecified type, uncontrolled — (Use additional code to identify manifestation: 581.81, 583.81)

250.43 Diabetes with renal manifestations, type I [juvenile type], uncontrolled — (Use additional code to identify manifestation: 581.81, 583.81)

257.2 Other testicular hypofunction ♂

277.3 Amyloidosis — (Use additional code to identify any associated mental retardation)

277.4 Disorders of bilirubin excretion — (Use additional code to identify any associated mental retardation)

289.1 Chronic lymphadenitis

289.3 Lymphadenitis, unspecified, except mesenteric ▽

376.00 Unspecified acute inflammation of orbit ▽

376.01 Orbital cellulitis

376.02 Orbital periostitis

376.10 Unspecified chronic inflammation of orbit ▽

376.11 Orbital granuloma

376.12 Orbital myositis

379.92 Swelling or mass of eye

457.8 Other noninfectious disorders of lymphatic channels

482.84 Legionnaires' disease

486 Pneumonia, organism unspecified ▽

511.0 Pleurisy without mention of effusion or current tuberculosis

518.89 Other diseases of lung, not elsewhere classified

570 Acute and subacute necrosis of liver

571.0 Alcoholic fatty liver

571.1 Acute alcoholic hepatitis

571.2 Alcoholic cirrhosis of liver

571.3 Unspecified alcoholic liver damage ▽

571.41 Chronic persistent hepatitis

571.49 Other chronic hepatitis

571.5 Cirrhosis of liver without mention of alcohol

571.6 Biliary cirrhosis

571.8 Other chronic nonalcoholic liver disease

571.9 Unspecified chronic liver disease without mention of alcohol ▽

572.0 Abscess of liver

572.1 Portal pyemia

572.2 Hepatic coma

572.4 Hepatorenal syndrome

572.8 Other sequelae of chronic liver disease

573.0 Chronic passive congestion of liver

573.1 Hepatitis in viral diseases classified elsewhere — (Code first underlying disease: 074.8, 075, 078.5) ☒

573.2 Hepatitis in other infectious diseases classified elsewhere — (Code first underlying disease, 084.9) ☒

573.3 Unspecified hepatitis — (Use additional E code to identify cause) ▽

573.4 Hepatic infarction

573.8 Other specified disorders of liver

576.8 Other specified disorders of biliary tract

577.0 Acute pancreatitis

577.1 Chronic pancreatitis

577.2 Cyst and pseudocyst of pancreas

577.8 Other specified disease of pancreas

579.4 Pancreatic steatorrhea

580.0 Acute glomerulonephritis with lesion of proliferative glomerulonephritis

580.89 Other acute glomerulonephritis with other specified pathological lesion in kidney

580.9 Acute glomerulonephritis with unspecified pathological lesion in kidney ▽

581.0 Nephrotic syndrome with lesion of proliferative glomerulonephritis

581.3 Nephrotic syndrome with lesion of minimal change glomerulonephritis

581.81 Nephrotic syndrome with other specified pathological lesion in kidney in diseases classified elsewhere — (Code first underlying disease: 084.9, 250.4, 277.3, 446.0, 710.0) ☒

581.9 Nephrotic syndrome with unspecified pathological lesion in kidney ▽

582.0 Chronic glomerulonephritis with lesion of proliferative glomerulonephritis

582.2 Chronic glomerulonephritis with lesion of membranoproliferative glomerulonephritis

582.4 Chronic glomerulonephritis with lesion of rapidly progressive glomerulonephritis

582.9 Chronic glomerulonephritis with unspecified pathological lesion in kidney ▽

583.0 Nephritis and nephropathy, not specified as acute or chronic, with lesion of proliferative glomerulonephritis

583.7 Nephritis and nephropathy, not specified as acute or chronic, with lesion of renal medullary necrosis

583.81 Nephritis and nephropathy, not specified as acute or chronic, with other specified pathological lesion in kidney, in diseases classified elsewhere — (Code first underlying disease: 016.0, 098.19, 250.4, 277.3, 446.21, 710.0) ☒

583.9 Nephritis and nephropathy, not specified as acute or chronic, with unspecified pathological lesion in kidney ▽

584.5 Acute renal failure with lesion of tubular necrosis

584.6 Acute renal failure with lesion of renal cortical necrosis

584.8 Acute renal failure with other specified pathological lesion in kidney

585 Chronic renal failure — (Use additional code to identify manifestation: 357.4, 420.0)

586 Unspecified renal failure ▽

588.0 Renal osteodystrophy

593.2 Acquired cyst of kidney

593.70 Vesicoureteral reflux, unspecified or without reflex nephropathy

593.9 Unspecified disorder of kidney and ureter ▽

599.7 Hematuria

600.00 Hypertrophy (benign) of prostate without urinary obstruction — (Use additional code to identify urinary incontinence: 788.30-788.39) ♂

600.01 Hypertrophy (benign) of prostate with urinary obstruction — (Use additional code to identify urinary incontinence: 788.30-788.39) ♂

600.10 Nodular prostate without urinary obstruction — (Use additional code to identify urinary incontinence: 788.30-788.39) ♂

600.11 Nodular prostate with urinary obstruction — (Use additional code to identify urinary incontinence: 788.30-788.39) ♂

600.20 Benign localized hyperplasia of prostate without urinary obstruction — (Use additional code to identify urinary incontinence: 788.30-788.39) ♂

600.21 Benign localized hyperplasia of prostate with urinary obstruction — (Use additional code to identify urinary incontinence: 788.30-788.39) ♂

600.3 Cyst of prostate — (Use additional code to identify urinary incontinence: 788.30-788.39) ♂

600.90 Hyperplasia of prostate, unspecified, without urinary obstruction — (Use additional code to identify urinary incontinence: 788.30-788.39) ▽ ♂

600.91 Hyperplasia of prostate, unspecified, with urinary obstruction — (Use additional code to identify urinary incontinence: 788.30-788.39) ▽ ♂

601.0 Acute prostatitis — (Use additional code to identify organism: 041.0, 041.1) ♂

601.1 Chronic prostatitis — (Use additional code to identify organism: 041.0, 041.1) ♂

601.2 Abscess of prostate — (Use additional code to identify organism: 041.0, 041.1) ♂

601.3 Prostatocystitis — (Use additional code to identify organism: 041.0, 041.1) ♂

601.4 Prostatitis in diseases classified elsewhere — (Code first underlying disease: 016.5, 039.8, 095.8, 116.0. Use additional code to identify organism: 041.0, 041.1) ☒ ♂

601.8 Other specified inflammatory disease of prostate — (Use additional code to identify organism: 041.0, 041.1) ♂

602.0 Calculus of prostate ♂

602.1 Congestion or hemorrhage of prostate ♂

▽ Unspecified code
♀ Female diagnosis
☒ Manifestation code
♂ Male diagnosis

602.2 Atrophy of prostate ♂
602.3 Dysplasia of prostate ♂
602.8 Other specified disorder of prostate ♂
604.90 Unspecified orchitis and epididymitis — (Use additional code to identify organism: 041.0, 041.1, 041.4) ▽ ♂
604.91 Orchitis and epididymitis in disease classified elsewhere — (Code first underlying disease: 032.89, 095.8, 125.0-125.9. Use additional code to identify organism: 041.0, 041.1, 041.4) ☒ ♂
606.0 Azoospermia ♂
606.1 Oligospermia ♂
608.2 Torsion of testis ♂
608.3 Atrophy of testis ♂
608.81 Specified disorder of male genital organs in diseases classified elsewhere — (Code first underlying disease: 016.5, 125.0-125.9) ☒ ♂
608.82 Hematospermia ♂
608.89 Other specified disorder of male genital organs ♂
610.0 Solitary cyst of breast
610.1 Diffuse cystic mastopathy
610.2 Fibroadenosis of breast
610.3 Fibrosclerosis of breast
610.8 Other specified benign mammary dysplasias
611.0 Inflammatory disease of breast
611.72 Lump or mass in breast
614.6 Pelvic peritoneal adhesions, female (postoperative) (postinfection) — (Use additional code to identify any associated infertility, 628.2. Use additional code to identify organism: 041.0, 041.1) ♀
648.10 Maternal thyroid dysfunction complicating pregnancy, childbirth, or the puerperium, unspecified as to episode of care or not applicable — (Use additional code(s) to identify the condition) ▽ ♀
648.11 Maternal thyroid dysfunction with delivery, with or without mention of antepartum condition — (Use additional code(s) to identify the condition) ♀
648.12 Maternal thyroid dysfunction with delivery, with current postpartum complication — (Use additional code(s) to identify the condition) ♀
648.13 Maternal thyroid dysfunction, antepartum condition or complication — (Use additional code(s) to identify the condition) ♀
648.14 Maternal thyroid dysfunction, previous postpartum condition or complication — (Use additional code(s) to identify the condition) ♀
682.2 Cellulitis and abscess of trunk — (Use additional code to identify organism)
683 Acute lymphadenitis — (Use additional code to identify organism)
751.61 Congenital biliary atresia
751.62 Congenital cystic disease of liver
753.0 Congenital renal agenesis and dysgenesis
753.10 Unspecified congenital cystic kidney disease ▽
759.2 Congenital anomalies of other endocrine glands
780.6 Fever
782.2 Localized superficial swelling, mass, or lump
782.4 Jaundice, unspecified, not of newborn ▽
784.2 Swelling, mass, or lump in head and neck
785.6 Enlargement of lymph nodes
786.09 Other dyspnea and respiratory abnormalities
786.2 Cough
786.3 Hemoptysis
786.52 Painful respiration
786.6 Swelling, mass, or lump in chest
786.7 Abnormal chest sounds
786.9 Other symptoms involving respiratory system and chest
788.0 Renal colic
788.29 Other specified retention of urine
788.41 Urinary frequency
788.42 Polyuria
788.43 Nocturia
789.00 Abdominal pain, unspecified site ▽
789.01 Abdominal pain, right upper quadrant
789.02 Abdominal pain, left upper quadrant
789.03 Abdominal pain, right lower quadrant
789.04 Abdominal pain, left lower quadrant
789.05 Abdominal pain, periumbilic
789.06 Abdominal pain, epigastric
789.07 Abdominal pain, generalized
789.09 Abdominal pain, other specified site
789.1 Hepatomegaly
789.30 Abdominal or pelvic swelling, mass or lump, unspecified site ▽
789.31 Abdominal or pelvic swelling, mass, or lump, right upper quadrant
789.32 Abdominal or pelvic swelling, mass, or lump, left upper quadrant
789.33 Abdominal or pelvic swelling, mass, or lump, right lower quadrant
789.34 Abdominal or pelvic swelling, mass, or lump, left lower quadrant
789.35 Abdominal or pelvic swelling, mass or lump, periumbilic
789.36 Abdominal or pelvic swelling, mass, or lump, epigastric
789.37 Abdominal or pelvic swelling, mass, or lump, epigastric, generalized
789.39 Abdominal or pelvic swelling, mass, or lump, other specified site
790.93 Elevated prostate specific antigen (PSA) ♂
791.0 Proteinuria
793.1 Nonspecific abnormal findings on radiological and other examination of lung field
793.5 Nonspecific abnormal findings on radiological and other examination of genitourinary organs
793.6 Nonspecific abnormal findings on radiological and other examination of abdominal area, including retroperitoneum
794.2 Nonspecific abnormal results of pulmonary system function study
794.5 Nonspecific abnormal results of thyroid function study
794.6 Nonspecific abnormal results of other endocrine function study
794.8 Nonspecific abnormal results of liver function study
864.01 Liver hematoma and contusion without mention of open wound into cavity
996.80 Complications of transplanted organ, unspecified site — (Use additional code to identify nature of complication, 078.5) ▽
996.81 Complications of transplanted kidney — (Use additional code to identify nature of complication, 078.5)
996.82 Complications of transplanted liver — (Use additional code to identify nature of complication, 078.5)
V10.29 Personal history of malignant neoplasm of other respiratory and intrathoracic organs
V10.3 Personal history of malignant neoplasm of breast
V10.46 Personal history of malignant neoplasm of prostate ♂
V15.82 Personal history of tobacco use, presenting hazards to health
V16.3 Family history of malignant neoplasm of breast
V42.0 Kidney replaced by transplant — (This code is intended for use when these conditions are recorded as diagnoses or problems)
V42.7 Liver replaced by transplant — (This code is intended for use when these conditions are recorded as diagnoses or problems)
V71.1 Observation for suspected malignant neoplasm

ICD-9-CM Procedural

This code is too broad to adequately present ICD-9-CM procedural code links here. Refer to your ICD-9-CM Volume 3 in the appropriate anatomical site.

HCPCS Level II Supplies & Services

A4550 Surgical trays

▽ Unspecified code
♀ Female diagnosis
☒ Manifestation code
♂ Male diagnosis

Integumentary System

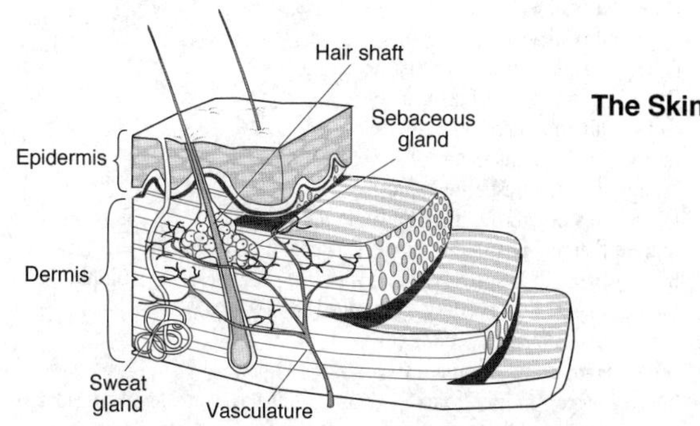

The skin is composed of epidermis and dermis; subcutaneous tissue refers to fatty tissues beneath the skin.

Skin, Subcutaneous and Accessory Structures

10040

10040 Acne surgery (eg, marsupialization, opening or removal of multiple milia, comedones, cysts, pustules)

ICD-9-CM Diagnostic

680.0 Carbuncle and furuncle of face
686.00 Unspecified pyoderma
686.01 Pyoderma gangrenosum
686.09 Other pyoderma
695.3 Rosacea
704.8 Other specified disease of hair and hair follicles
706.0 Acne varioliformis
706.1 Other acne
706.2 Sebaceous cyst
706.8 Other specified disease of sebaceous glands
709.3 Degenerative skin disorder

ICD-9-CM Procedural

86.04 Other incision with drainage of skin and subcutaneous tissue

HCPCS Level II Supplies & Services

A4550 Surgical trays

10060–10061

10060 Incision and drainage of abscess (eg, carbuncle, suppurative hidradenitis, cutaneous or subcutaneous abscess, cyst, furuncle, or paronychia); simple or single
10061 complicated or multiple

ICD-9-CM Diagnostic

110.1 Dermatophytosis of nail — (Use additional code to identify manifestation: 321.0-321.1, 380.15, 711.6)
680.0 Carbuncle and furuncle of face
680.1 Carbuncle and furuncle of neck
680.2 Carbuncle and furuncle of trunk
680.3 Carbuncle and furuncle of upper arm and forearm
680.4 Carbuncle and furuncle of hand
680.5 Carbuncle and furuncle of buttock
680.6 Carbuncle and furuncle of leg, except foot
680.7 Carbuncle and furuncle of foot
680.8 Carbuncle and furuncle of other specified sites
680.9 Carbuncle and furuncle of unspecified site
681.01 Felon — (Use additional code to identify organism)
681.02 Onychia and paronychia of finger — (Use additional code to identify organism)
681.11 Onychia and paronychia of toe — (Use additional code to identify organism)
681.9 Cellulitis and abscess of unspecified digit — (Use additional code to identify organism)
682.0 Cellulitis and abscess of face — (Use additional code to identify organism)
682.1 Cellulitis and abscess of neck — (Use additional code to identify organism)
682.2 Cellulitis and abscess of trunk — (Use additional code to identify organism)
682.3 Cellulitis and abscess of upper arm and forearm — (Use additional code to identify organism)
682.4 Cellulitis and abscess of hand, except fingers and thumb — (Use additional code to identify organism)
682.5 Cellulitis and abscess of buttock — (Use additional code to identify organism)
682.6 Cellulitis and abscess of leg, except foot — (Use additional code to identify organism)
682.7 Cellulitis and abscess of foot, except toes — (Use additional code to identify organism)
682.8 Cellulitis and abscess of other specified site — (Use additional code to identify organism)
682.9 Cellulitis and abscess of unspecified site — (Use additional code to identify organism)
686.00 Unspecified pyoderma
686.01 Pyoderma gangrenosum
686.09 Other pyoderma
686.1 Pyogenic granuloma of skin and subcutaneous tissue
686.8 Other specified local infections of skin and subcutaneous tissue
705.83 Hidradenitis
705.89 Other specified disorder of sweat glands
706.2 Sebaceous cyst
709.8 Other specified disorder of skin
782.2 Localized superficial swelling, mass, or lump
958.3 Posttraumatic wound infection not elsewhere classified
998.51 Infected postoperative seroma — (Use additional code to identify organism)
998.59 Other postoperative infection — (Use additional code to identify infection)

ICD-9-CM Procedural

08.09 Other incision of eyelid
21.1 Incision of nose
27.0 Drainage of face and floor of mouth
86.04 Other incision with drainage of skin and subcutaneous tissue

HCPCS Level II Supplies & Services

A4550 Surgical trays

10080–10081

10080 Incision and drainage of pilonidal cyst; simple
10081 complicated

ICD-9-CM Diagnostic

685.0 Pilonidal cyst with abscess
685.1 Pilonidal cyst without mention of abscess

ICD-9-CM Procedural

86.03 Incision of pilonidal sinus or cyst

HCPCS Level II Supplies & Services

A4550 Surgical trays

10120–10121

10120 Incision and removal of foreign body, subcutaneous tissues; simple
10121 complicated

ICD-9-CM Diagnostic

910.6 Face, neck, and scalp, except eye, superficial foreign body (splinter), without major open wound or mention of infection
910.7 Face, neck, and scalp except eye, superficial foreign body (splinter), without major open wound, infected

911.6 Trunk, superficial foreign body (splinter), without major open wound and without mention of infection
911.7 Trunk, superficial foreign body (splinter), without major open wound, infected
912.6 Shoulder and upper arm, superficial foreign body (splinter), without major open wound and without mention of infection
912.7 Shoulder and upper arm, superficial foreign body (splinter), without major open wound, infected
913.6 Elbow, forearm, and wrist, superficial foreign body (splinter), without major open wound and without mention of infection
913.7 Elbow, forearm, and wrist, superficial foreign body (splinter), without major open wound, infected
914.6 Hand(s) except finger(s) alone, superficial foreign body (splinter), without major open wound and without mention of infection
914.7 Hand(s) except finger(s) alone, superficial foreign body (splinter) without major open wound, infected
915.6 Finger, superficial foreign body (splinter), without major open wound and without mention of infection
915.7 Finger, superficial foreign body (splinter), without major open wound, infected
916.6 Hip, thigh, leg, and ankle, superficial foreign body (splinter), without major open wound and without mention of infection
916.7 Hip, thigh, leg, and ankle, superficial foreign body (splinter), without major open wound, infected
998.4 Foreign body accidentally left during procedure, not elsewhere classified

ICD-9-CM Procedural

86.05 Incision with removal of foreign body or device from skin and subcutaneous tissue

HCPCS Level II Supplies & Services

A4550 Surgical trays

10140

10140 Incision and drainage of hematoma, seroma or fluid collection

ICD-9-CM Diagnostic

674.30 Other complication of obstetrical surgical wounds, unspecified as to episode of care ▽ ♀
674.32 Other complication of obstetrical surgical wounds, with delivery, with mention of postpartum complication ♀
674.34 Other complication of obstetrical surgical wounds, postpartum condition or complication ♀
767.11 Birth trauma, Epicranial subaponeurotic hemorrhage (massive)
767.19 Birth trauma, Other injuries to scalp
767.8 Other specified birth trauma
802.0 Nasal bones, closed fracture
802.1 Nasal bones, open fracture
873.20 Open wound of nose, unspecified site, without mention of complication — (Use additional code to identify infection) ▽
873.30 Open wound of nose, unspecified site, complicated — (Use additional code to identify infection) ▽
873.31 Open wound of nasal septum, complicated — (Use additional code to identify infection)
873.32 Open wound of nasal cavity, complicated — (Use additional code to identify infection)
906.3 Late effect of contusion
920 Contusion of face, scalp, and neck except eye(s)
922.1 Contusion of chest wall
922.2 Contusion of abdominal wall
922.31 Contusion of back
922.32 Contusion of buttock
922.33 Contusion of interscapular region
922.4 Contusion of genital organs
923.00 Contusion of shoulder region
923.01 Contusion of scapular region
923.03 Contusion of upper arm
923.09 Contusion of multiple sites of shoulder and upper arm
923.10 Contusion of forearm
923.11 Contusion of elbow
923.20 Contusion of hand(s)
923.21 Contusion of wrist
923.3 Contusion of finger
923.8 Contusion of multiple sites of upper limb
923.9 Contusion of unspecified part of upper limb
924.00 Contusion of thigh
924.01 Contusion of hip
924.10 Contusion of lower leg
924.11 Contusion of knee
924.20 Contusion of foot
924.3 Contusion of toe
924.4 Contusion of multiple sites of lower limb
924.5 Contusion of unspecified part of lower limb ▽
924.8 Contusion of multiple sites, not elsewhere classified
924.9 Contusion of unspecified site ▽
959.01 Head injury, unspecified ▽
959.09 Injury of face and neck, other and unspecified
959.11 Other injury of chest wall
959.12 Other injury of abdomen
959.13 Other injury, Fracture of corpus cavernosum penis
959.14 Other injury of external genitals
959.19 Other injury of other sites of trunk
959.4 Injury, other and unspecified, hand, except finger
959.5 Injury, other and unspecified, finger
959.6 Injury, other and unspecified, hip and thigh
959.7 Injury, other and unspecified, knee, leg, ankle, and foot
959.8 Injury, other and unspecified, other specified sites, including multiple
959.9 Injury, other and unspecified, unspecified site ▽
998.12 Hematoma complicating a procedure
998.13 Seroma complicating a procedure
998.51 Infected postoperative seroma — (Use additional code to identify organism)

ICD-9-CM Procedural

86.04 Other incision with drainage of skin and subcutaneous tissue

HCPCS Level II Supplies & Services

A4462 Abdominal dressing holder, each
A4550 Surgical trays

10160

10160 Puncture aspiration of abscess, hematoma, bulla, or cyst

ICD-9-CM Diagnostic

528.3 Cellulitis and abscess of oral soft tissues
528.4 Cysts of oral soft tissues
528.5 Diseases of lips
608.89 Other specified disorder of male genital organs ♂
674.30 Other complication of obstetrical surgical wounds, unspecified as to episode of care ▽ ♀
674.32 Other complication of obstetrical surgical wounds, with delivery, with mention of postpartum complication ♀
674.34 Other complication of obstetrical surgical wounds, postpartum condition or complication ♀
680.0 Carbuncle and furuncle of face
681.11 Onychia and paronychia of toe — (Use additional code to identify organism)
682.0 Cellulitis and abscess of face — (Use additional code to identify organism)
682.1 Cellulitis and abscess of neck — (Use additional code to identify organism)
682.2 Cellulitis and abscess of trunk — (Use additional code to identify organism)
682.3 Cellulitis and abscess of upper arm and forearm — (Use additional code to identify organism)
682.4 Cellulitis and abscess of hand, except fingers and thumb — (Use additional code to identify organism)
682.5 Cellulitis and abscess of buttock — (Use additional code to identify organism)
682.6 Cellulitis and abscess of leg, except foot — (Use additional code to identify organism)
682.7 Cellulitis and abscess of foot, except toes — (Use additional code to identify organism)
705.89 Other specified disorder of sweat glands
706.2 Sebaceous cyst
709.8 Other specified disorder of skin
767.11 Birth trauma, Epicranial subaponeurotic hemorrhage (massive)
767.19 Birth trauma, Other injuries to scalp
767.8 Other specified birth trauma
906.3 Late effect of contusion
920 Contusion of face, scalp, and neck except eye(s)
922.1 Contusion of chest wall
922.2 Contusion of abdominal wall
922.31 Contusion of back
922.32 Contusion of buttock
922.33 Contusion of interscapular region
922.4 Contusion of genital organs
923.00 Contusion of shoulder region
923.03 Contusion of upper arm
923.09 Contusion of multiple sites of shoulder and upper arm

923.11 Contusion of elbow
923.20 Contusion of hand(s)
923.21 Contusion of wrist
923.3 Contusion of finger
923.8 Contusion of multiple sites of upper limb
924.00 Contusion of thigh
924.01 Contusion of hip
924.10 Contusion of lower leg
924.20 Contusion of foot
924.3 Contusion of toe
924.4 Contusion of multiple sites of lower limb
959.01 Head injury, unspecified ▽
959.09 Injury of face and neck, other and unspecified
959.11 Other injury of chest wall
959.12 Other injury of abdomen
959.14 Other injury of external genitals
959.19 Other injury of other sites of trunk
959.3 Injury, other and unspecified, elbow, forearm, and wrist
959.6 Injury, other and unspecified, hip and thigh
959.7 Injury, other and unspecified, knee, leg, ankle, and foot
998.12 Hematoma complicating a procedure

ICD-9-CM Procedural

75.91 Evacuation of obstetrical incisional hematoma of perineum
75.92 Evacuation of other hematoma of vulva or vagina
86.01 Aspiration of skin and subcutaneous tissue

HCPCS Level II Supplies & Services

A4550 Surgical trays

10180

10180 Incision and drainage, complex, postoperative wound infection

ICD-9-CM Diagnostic

674.30 Other complication of obstetrical surgical wounds, unspecified as to episode of care ▽ ♀
674.32 Other complication of obstetrical surgical wounds, with delivery, with mention of postpartum complication ♀
674.34 Other complication of obstetrical surgical wounds, postpartum condition or complication ♀
998.51 Infected postoperative seroma — (Use additional code to identify organism)
998.59 Other postoperative infection — (Use additional code to identify infection)

ICD-9-CM Procedural

86.04 Other incision with drainage of skin and subcutaneous tissue

HCPCS Level II Supplies & Services

A4462 Abdominal dressing holder, each

11000–11001

11000 Debridement of extensive eczematous or infected skin; up to 10% of body surface
11001 each additional 10% of the body surface (List separately in addition to code for primary procedure)

ICD-9-CM Diagnostic

681.00 Unspecified cellulitis and abscess of finger — (Use additional code to identify organism) ▽
681.10 Unspecified cellulitis and abscess of toe — (Use additional code to identify organism) ▽
682.0 Cellulitis and abscess of face — (Use additional code to identify organism)
682.1 Cellulitis and abscess of neck — (Use additional code to identify organism)
682.2 Cellulitis and abscess of trunk — (Use additional code to identify organism)
682.3 Cellulitis and abscess of upper arm and forearm — (Use additional code to identify organism)
682.4 Cellulitis and abscess of hand, except fingers and thumb — (Use additional code to identify organism)
682.5 Cellulitis and abscess of buttock — (Use additional code to identify organism)
682.6 Cellulitis and abscess of leg, except foot — (Use additional code to identify organism)
682.7 Cellulitis and abscess of foot, except toes — (Use additional code to identify organism)
682.8 Cellulitis and abscess of other specified site — (Use additional code to identify organism)
684 Impetigo
686.00 Unspecified pyoderma ▽
686.01 Pyoderma gangrenosum
686.09 Other pyoderma
686.1 Pyogenic granuloma of skin and subcutaneous tissue
686.8 Other specified local infections of skin and subcutaneous tissue
686.9 Unspecified local infection of skin and subcutaneous tissue ▽
691.8 Other atopic dermatitis and related conditions
692.9 Contact dermatitis and other eczema, due to unspecified cause ▽
707.00 Decubitus ulcer, unspecified site
707.01 Decubitus ulcer, elbow
707.02 Decubitus ulcer, upper back
707.03 Decubitus ulcer, lower back
707.04 Decubitus ulcer, hip
707.05 Decubitus ulcer, buttock
707.06 Decubitus ulcer, ankle
707.07 Decubitus ulcer, heel
707.09 Decubitus ulcer, other site
707.10 Ulcer of lower limb, unspecified ▽
707.11 Ulcer of thigh
707.12 Ulcer of calf
707.13 Ulcer of ankle
707.14 Ulcer of heel and midfoot
707.15 Ulcer of other part of foot
707.19 Ulcer of other part of lower limb
707.8 Chronic ulcer of other specified site
757.1 Ichthyosis congenita
785.4 Gangrene — (Code first any associated underlying condition:250.7, 443.0)
910.1 Face, neck, and scalp except eye, abrasion or friction burn, infected
911.1 Trunk abrasion or friction burn, infected
912.1 Shoulder and upper arm, abrasion or friction burn, infected
913.1 Elbow, forearm, and wrist, abrasion or friction burn, infected
914.1 Hand(s) except finger(s) alone, abrasion or friction burn, infected
916.1 Hip, thigh, leg, and ankle, abrasion or friction burn, infected
991.0 Frostbite of face
991.1 Frostbite of hand
991.2 Frostbite of foot
991.3 Frostbite of other and unspecified sites
991.5 Effects of chilblains

ICD-9-CM Procedural

86.22 Excisional debridement of wound, infection, or burn

HCPCS Level II Supplies & Services

A4305 Disposable drug delivery system, flow rate of 50 ml or greater per hour
A4306 Disposable drug delivery system, flow rate of 5 ml or less per hour
A4550 Surgical trays

11004–11006

11004 Debridement of skin, subcutaneous tissue, muscle and fascia for necrotizing soft tissue infection; external genitalia and perineum
11005 abdominal wall, with or without fascial closure
11006 external genitalia, perineum and abdominal wall, with or without fascial closure

ICD-9-CM Diagnostic

035 Erysipelas
040.0 Gas gangrene
040.3 Necrobacillosis
041.01 Streptococcus infection in conditions classified elsewhere and of unspecified site, group A — (Note: This code is to be used as an additional code to identify the bacterial agent in diseases classified elsewhere and bacterial infections of unspecified nature or site)
041.04 Streptococcus infection in conditions classified elsewhere and of unspecified site, group D [Enterococcus] — (Note: This code is to be used as an additional code to identify the bacterial agent in diseases classified elsewhere and bacterial infections of unspecified nature or site)
041.09 Other streptococcus infection in conditions classified elsewhere and of unspecified site — (Note: This code is to be used as an additional code to identify the bacterial agent in diseases classified elsewhere and bacterial infections of unspecified nature or site)
041.11 Staphylococcus aureus infection in conditions classified elsewhere and of unspecified site — (Note: This code is to be used as an additional code to identify the bacterial agent in diseases classified elsewhere and bacterial infections of unspecified nature or site)

041.19 Other staphylococcus infection in conditions classified elsewhere and of unspecified site — (Note: This code is to be used as an additional code to identify the bacterial agent in diseases classified elsewhere and bacterial infections of unspecified nature or site)
041.3 Friedländer's bacillus infection in conditions classified elsewhere and of unspecified site — (Note: This code is to be used as an additional code to identify the bacterial agent in diseases classified elsewhere and bacterial infections of unspecified nature or site)
041.4 Escherichia coli (E. coli) infection in conditions classified elsewhere and of unspecified site — (Note: This code is to be used as an additional code to identify the bacterial agent in diseases classified elsewhere and bacterial infections of unspecified nature or site)
041.6 Proteus (mirabilis) (morganii) infection in conditions classified elsewhere and of unspecified site — (Note: This code is to be used as an additional code to identify the bacterial agent in diseases classified elsewhere and bacterial infections of unspecified nature or site)
041.7 Pseudomonas infection in conditions classified elsewhere and of unspecified site — (Note: This code is to be used as an additional code to identify the bacterial agent in diseases classified elsewhere and bacterial infections of unspecified nature or site)
041.82 Bacterial infection in conditions classified elsewhere, Bacteroides fragilis — (Note: This code is to be used as an additional code to identify the bacterial agent in diseases classified elsewhere and bacterial infections of unspecified nature or site)
041.83 Clostridium perfringens infection in conditions classified elsewhere and of unspecified site — (Note: This code is to be used as an additional code to identify the bacterial agent in diseases classified elsewhere and bacterial infections of unspecified nature or site)
041.84 Infection due to other anaerobes in conditions classified elsewhere and of unspecified site — (Note: This code is to be used as an additional code to identify the bacterial agent in diseases classified elsewhere and bacterial infections of unspecified nature or site)
041.85 Infection due to other gram-negative organisms in conditions classified elsewhere and of unspecified site — (Note: This code is to be used as an additional code to identify the bacterial agent in diseases classified elsewhere and bacterial infections of unspecified nature or site)
569.49 Other specified disorder of rectum and anus
604.0 Orchitis, epididymitis, and epididymo-orchitis, with abscess — (Use additional code to identify organism: 041.0, 041.1, 041.4) ♂
604.90 Unspecified orchitis and epididymitis — (Use additional code to identify organism: 041.0, 041.1, 041.4) ▽ ♂
604.99 Other orchitis, epididymitis, and epididymo-orchitis, without mention of abscess — (Use additional code to identify organism: 041.0, 041.1, 041.4) ♂
607.2 Other inflammatory disorders of penis — (Use additional code to identify organism) ♂
608.4 Other inflammatory disorder of male genital organs — (Use additional code to identify organism) ♂
616.10 Unspecified vaginitis and vulvovaginitis — (Use additional code to identify organism: 041.0, 041.1, 041.4) ▽ ♀
616.11 Vaginitis and vulvovaginitis in diseases classified elsewhere — (Code first underlying disease, 127.4.) ☒ ♀
616.4 Other abscess of vulva — (Use additional code to identify organism: 041.0, 041.1) ♀
616.50 Unspecified ulceration of vulva — (Use additional code to identify organism: 041.0, 041.1) ▽ ♀
616.51 Ulceration of vulva in disease classified elsewhere — (Code first underlying disease: 016.7, 136.1.) ☒ ♀
616.8 Other specified inflammatory disease of cervix, vagina, and vulva — (Use additional code to identify organism: 041.0, 041.1) ♀
616.9 Unspecified inflammatory disease of cervix, vagina, and vulva — (Use additional code to identify organism: 041.0, 041.1) ▽ ♀
707.8 Chronic ulcer of other specified site
728.86 Necrotizing fasciitis — (Use additional code to identify infectious organism, 041.00-041.89, 785.4, if applicable)
785.4 Gangrene — (Code first any associated underlying condition:250.7, 443.0)

ICD-9-CM Procedural

54.3 Excision or destruction of lesion or tissue of abdominal wall or umbilicus
83.44 Other fasciectomy
83.45 Other myectomy
86.22 Excisional debridement of wound, infection, or burn

11008

11008 Removal of prosthetic material or mesh, abdominal wall for necrotizing soft tissue infection (List separately in addition to code for primary procedure)

ICD-9-CM Diagnostic

This is an add-on code. Refer to the corresponding primary procedure code for ICD-9 diagnosis code links.

ICD-9-CM Procedural

54.0 Incision of abdominal wall

11010–11012

11010 Debridement including removal of foreign material associated with open fracture(s) and/or dislocation(s); skin and subcutaneous tissues
11011 skin, subcutaneous tissue, muscle fascia, and muscle
11012 skin, subcutaneous tissue, muscle fascia, muscle, and bone

ICD-9-CM Diagnostic

800.50 Open fracture of vault of skull without mention of intracranial injury, unspecified state of consciousness ▽
800.51 Open fracture of vault of skull without mention of intracranial injury, no loss of consciousness
800.52 Open fracture of vault of skull without mention of intracranial injury, brief (less than one hour) loss of consciousness
800.53 Open fracture of vault of skull without mention of intracranial injury, moderate (1-24 hours) loss of consciousness
800.54 Open fracture of vault of skull without mention of intracranial injury, prolonged (more than 24 hours) loss of consciousness and return to pre-existing conscious level
800.55 Open fracture of vault of skull without mention of intracranial injury, prolonged (more than 24 hours) loss of consciousness, without return to pre-existing conscious level
800.56 Open fracture of vault of skull without mention of intracranial injury, loss of consciousness of unspecified duration ▽
800.60 Open fracture of vault of skull with cerebral laceration and contusion, unspecified state of consciousness ▽
800.61 Open fracture of vault of skull with cerebral laceration and contusion, no loss of consciousness
800.62 Open fracture of vault of skull with cerebral laceration and contusion, brief (less than one hour) loss of consciousness
800.63 Open fracture of vault of skull with cerebral laceration and contusion, moderate (1-24 hours) loss of consciousness
800.64 Open fracture of vault of skull with cerebral laceration and contusion, prolonged (more than 24 hours) loss of consciousness and return to pre-existing conscious level
800.65 Open fracture of vault of skull with cerebral laceration and contusion, prolonged (more than 24 hours) loss of consciousness, without return to pre-existing conscious level
800.66 Open fracture of vault of skull with cerebral laceration and contusion, loss of consciousness of unspecified duration ▽
800.70 Open fracture of vault of skull with subarachnoid, subdural, and extradural hemorrhage, unspecified state of consciousness ▽
800.71 Open fracture of vault of skull with subarachnoid, subdural, and extradural hemorrhage, no loss of consciousness
800.72 Open fracture of vault of skull with subarachnoid, subdural, and extradural hemorrhage, brief (less than one hour) loss of consciousness
800.73 Open fracture of vault of skull with subarachnoid, subdural, and extradural hemorrhage, moderate (1-24 hours) loss of consciousness
800.74 Open fracture of vault of skull with subarachnoid, subdural, and extradural hemorrhage, prolonged (more than 24 hours) loss of consciousness and return to pre-existing conscious level
800.75 Open fracture of vault of skull with subarachnoid, subdural, and extradural hemorrhage, prolonged (more than 24 hours) loss of consciousness, without return to pre-existing conscious level
800.76 Open fracture of vault of skull with subarachnoid, subdural, and extradural hemorrhage, loss of consciousness of unspecified duration ▽
800.80 Open fracture of vault of skull with other and unspecified intracranial hemorrhage, unspecified state of consciousness ▽
800.81 Open fracture of vault of skull with other and unspecified intracranial hemorrhage, no loss of consciousness ▽
800.82 Open fracture of vault of skull with other and unspecified intracranial hemorrhage, brief (less than one hour) loss of consciousness ▽
800.83 Open fracture of vault of skull with other and unspecified intracranial hemorrhage, moderate (1-24 hours) loss of consciousness ▽

▽ Unspecified code ☒ Manifestation code
♀ Female diagnosis ♂ Male diagnosis

800.84 Open fracture of vault of skull with other and unspecified intracranial hemorrhage, prolonged (more than 24 hours) loss of consciousness and return to pre-existing conscious level ▽
800.85 Open fracture of vault of skull with other and unspecified intracranial hemorrhage, prolonged (more than 24 hours) loss of consciousness, without return to pre-existing conscious level ▽
800.86 Open fracture of vault of skull with other and unspecified intracranial hemorrhage, loss of consciousness of unspecified duration ▽
801.50 Open fracture of base of skull without mention of intracranial injury, unspecified state of consciousness ▽
801.51 Open fracture of base of skull without mention of intracranial injury, no loss of consciousness
801.52 Open fracture of base of skull without mention of intracranial injury, brief (less than one hour) loss of consciousness
801.53 Open fracture of base of skull without mention of intracranial injury, moderate (1-24 hours) loss of consciousness
801.54 Open fracture of base of skull without mention of intracranial injury, prolonged (more than 24 hours) loss of consciousness and return to pre-existing conscious level
801.55 Open fracture of base of skull without mention of intracranial injury, prolonged (more than 24 hours) loss of consciousness, without return to pre-existing conscious level
801.56 Open fracture of base of skull without mention of intracranial injury, loss of consciousness of unspecified duration ▽
801.60 Open fracture of base of skull with cerebral laceration and contusion, unspecified state of consciousness ▽
801.61 Open fracture of base of skull with cerebral laceration and contusion, no loss of consciousness
801.62 Open fracture of base of skull with cerebral laceration and contusion, brief (less than one hour) loss of consciousness
801.63 Open fracture of base of skull with cerebral laceration and contusion, moderate (1-24 hours) loss of consciousness
801.64 Open fracture of base of skull with cerebral laceration and contusion, prolonged (more than 24 hours) loss of consciousness and return to pre-existing conscious level
801.65 Open fracture of base of skull with cerebral laceration and contusion, prolonged (more than 24 hours) loss of consciousness, without return to pre-existing conscious level
801.66 Open fracture of base of skull with cerebral laceration and contusion, loss of consciousness of unspecified duration ▽
801.70 Open fracture of base of skull with subarachnoid, subdural, and extradural hemorrhage, unspecified state of consciousness ▽
801.71 Open fracture of base of skull with subarachnoid, subdural, and extradural hemorrhage, no loss of consciousness
801.72 Open fracture of base of skull with subarachnoid, subdural, and extradural hemorrhage, brief (less than one hour) loss of consciousness
801.73 Open fracture of base of skull with subarachnoid, subdural, and extradural hemorrhage, moderate (1-24 hours) loss of consciousness
801.74 Open fracture of base of skull with subarachnoid, subdural, and extradural hemorrhage, prolonged (more than 24 hours) loss of consciousness and return to pre-existing conscious level
801.75 Open fracture of base of skull with subarachnoid, subdural, and extradural hemorrhage, prolonged (more than 24 hours) loss of consciousness, without return to pre-existing conscious level
801.76 Open fracture of base of skull with subarachnoid, subdural, and extradural hemorrhage, loss of consciousness of unspecified duration ▽
801.80 Open fracture of base of skull with other and unspecified intracranial hemorrhage, unspecified state of consciousness ▽
801.81 Open fracture of base of skull with other and unspecified intracranial hemorrhage, no loss of consciousness ▽
801.82 Open fracture of base of skull with other and unspecified intracranial hemorrhage, brief (less than one hour) loss of consciousness ▽
801.83 Open fracture of base of skull with other and unspecified intracranial hemorrhage, moderate (1-24 hours) loss of consciousness ▽
801.84 Open fracture of base of skull with other and unspecified intracranial hemorrhage, prolonged (more than 24 hours) loss of consciousness and return to pre-existing conscious level ▽
801.85 Open fracture of base of skull with other and unspecified intracranial hemorrhage, prolonged (more than 24 hours) loss of consciousness, without return to pre-existing conscious level ▽
801.86 Open fracture of base of skull with other and unspecified intracranial hemorrhage, loss of consciousness of unspecified duration ▽
802.1 Nasal bones, open fracture
802.30 Open fracture of unspecified site of mandible ▽
802.31 Open fracture of condylar process of mandible
802.32 Open fracture of subcondylar process of mandible
802.33 Open fracture of coronoid process of mandible
802.34 Open fracture of unspecified part of ramus of mandible ▽
802.35 Open fracture of angle of jaw
802.36 Open fracture of symphysis of body of mandible
802.37 Open fracture of alveolar border of body of mandible
802.38 Open fracture of other and unspecified part of body of mandible
802.39 Open fracture of multiple sites of mandible
802.5 Malar and maxillary bones, open fracture
802.7 Orbital floor (blow-out), open fracture
802.9 Other facial bones, open fracture
803.50 Other open skull fracture without mention of injury, state of consciousness unspecified ▽
803.51 Other open skull fracture without mention of intracranial injury, no loss of consciousness
803.52 Other open skull fracture without mention of intracranial injury, brief (less than one hour) loss of consciousness
803.53 Other open skull fracture without mention of intracranial injury, moderate (1-24 hours) loss of consciousness
803.54 Other open skull fracture without mention of intracranial injury, prolonged (more than 24 hours) loss of consciousness and return to pre-existing conscious level
803.55 Other open skull fracture without mention of intracranial injury, prolonged (more than 24 hours) loss of consciousness, without return to pre-existing conscious level
803.56 Other open skull fracture without mention of intracranial injury, loss of consciousness of unspecified duration ▽
803.60 Other open skull fracture with cerebral laceration and contusion, unspecified state of consciousness ▽
803.61 Other open skull fracture with cerebral laceration and contusion, no loss of consciousness
803.62 Other open skull fracture with cerebral laceration and contusion, brief (less than one hour) loss of consciousness
803.63 Other open skull fracture with cerebral laceration and contusion, moderate (1-24 hours) loss of consciousness
803.64 Other open skull fracture with cerebral laceration and contusion, prolonged (more than 24 hours) loss of consciousness and return to pre-existing conscious level
803.65 Other open skull fracture with cerebral laceration and contusion, prolonged (more than 24 hours) loss of consciousness, without return to pre-existing conscious level
803.66 Other open skull fracture with cerebral laceration and contusion, loss of consciousness of unspecified duration ▽
803.70 Other open skull fracture with subarachnoid, subdural, and extradural hemorrhage, unspecified state of consciousness ▽
803.71 Other open skull fracture with subarachnoid, subdural, and extradural hemorrhage, no loss of consciousness
803.72 Other open skull fracture with subarachnoid, subdural, and extradural hemorrhage, brief (less than one hour) loss of consciousness
803.73 Other open skull fracture with subarachnoid, subdural, and extradural hemorrhage, moderate (1-24 hours) loss of consciousness
803.74 Other open skull fracture with subarachnoid, subdural, and extradural hemorrhage, prolonged (more than 24 hours) loss of consciousness and return to pre-existing conscious level
803.75 Other open skull fracture with subarachnoid, subdural, and extradural hemorrhage, prolonged (more than 24 hours) loss of consciousness, without return to pre-existing conscious level
803.76 Other open skull fracture with subarachnoid, subdural, and extradural hemorrhage, loss of consciousness of unspecified duration ▽
803.79 Other open skull fracture with subarachnoid, subdural, and extradural hemorrhage, unspecified concussion ▽
803.80 Other open skull fracture with other and unspecified intracranial hemorrhage, unspecified state of consciousness ▽
803.81 Other open skull fracture with other and unspecified intracranial hemorrhage, no loss of consciousness ▽
803.82 Other open skull fracture with other and unspecified intracranial hemorrhage, brief (less than one hour) loss of consciousness ▽
803.83 Other open skull fracture with other and unspecified intracranial hemorrhage, moderate (1-24 hours) loss of consciousness ▽
803.84 Other open skull fracture with other and unspecified intracranial hemorrhage, prolonged (more than 24 hours) loss of consciousness and return to pre-existing conscious level ▽
803.85 Other open skull fracture with other and unspecified intracranial hemorrhage, prolonged (more than 24 hours) loss of consciousness, without return to pre-existing conscious level ▽
803.86 Other open skull fracture with other and unspecified intracranial hemorrhage, loss of consciousness of unspecified duration ▽

▽ Unspecified code
♀ Female diagnosis
☒ Manifestation code
♂ Male diagnosis

803.89 Other open skull fracture with other and unspecified intracranial hemorrhage, unspecified concussion ▽

803.90 Other open skull fracture with intracranial injury of other and unspecified nature, unspecified state of consciousness ▽

803.91 Other open skull fracture with intracranial injury of other and unspecified nature, no loss of consciousness ▽

803.92 Other open skull fracture with intracranial injury of other and unspecified nature, brief (less than one hour) loss of consciousness ▽

803.93 Other open skull fracture with intracranial injury of other and unspecified nature, moderate (1-24 hours) loss of consciousness ▽

803.94 Other open skull fracture with intracranial injury of other and unspecified nature, prolonged (more than 24 hours) loss of consciousness and return to pre-existing conscious level ▽

803.95 Other open skull fracture with intracranial injury of other and unspecified nature, prolonged (more than 24 hours) loss of consciousness, without return to pre-existing conscious level ▽

803.96 Other open skull fracture with intracranial injury of other and unspecified nature, loss of consciousness of unspecified duration ▽

803.99 Other open skull fracture with intracranial injury of other and unspecified nature, unspecified concussion ▽

804.51 Open fractures involving skull or face with other bones, without mention of intracranial injury, no loss of consciousness

804.52 Open fractures involving skull or face with other bones, without mention of intracranial injury, brief (less than one hour) loss of consciousness

804.53 Open fractures involving skull or face with other bones, without mention of intracranial injury, moderate (1-24 hours) loss of consciousness

804.54 Open fractures involving skull or face with other bones, without mention of intracranial injury, prolonged (more than 24 hours) loss of consciousness and return to pre-existing conscious level

804.55 Open fractures involving skull or face with other bones, without mention of intracranial injury, prolonged (more than 24 hours) loss of consciousness, without return to pre-existing conscious level

804.56 Open fractures involving skull or face with other bones, without mention of intracranial injury, loss of consciousness of unspecified duration ▽

804.59 Open fractures involving skull or face with other bones, without mention of intracranial injury, unspecified concussion ▽

804.60 Open fractures involving skull or face with other bones, with cerebral laceration and contusion, unspecified state of consciousness ▽

804.61 Open fractures involving skull or face with other bones, with cerebral laceration and contusion, no loss of consciousness

804.62 Open fractures involving skull or face with other bones, with cerebral laceration and contusion, brief (less than one hour) loss of consciousness

804.63 Open fractures involving skull or face with other bones, with cerebral laceration and contusion, moderate (1-24 hours) loss of consciousness

804.64 Open fractures involving skull or face with other bones, with cerebral laceration and contusion, prolonged (more than 24 hours) loss of consciousness and return to pre-existing conscious level

804.65 Open fractures involving skull or face with other bones, with cerebral laceration and contusion, prolonged (more than 24 hours) loss of consciousness, without return to pre-existing conscious level

804.66 Open fractures involving skull or face with other bones, with cerebral laceration and contusion, loss of consciousness of unspecified duration ▽

804.69 Open fractures involving skull or face with other bones, with cerebral laceration and contusion, unspecified concussion ▽

804.70 Open fractures involving skull or face with other bones with subarachnoid, subdural, and extradural hemorrhage, unspecified state of consciousness ▽

804.71 Open fractures involving skull or face with other bones with subarachnoid, subdural, and extradural hemorrhage, no loss of consciousness

804.72 Open fractures involving skull or face with other bones with subarachnoid, subdural, and extradural hemorrhage, brief (less than one hour) loss of consciousness

804.73 Open fractures involving skull or face with other bones with subarachnoid, subdural, and extradural hemorrhage, moderate (1-24 hours) loss of consciousness

804.74 Open fractures involving skull or face with other bones with subarachnoid, subdural, and extradural hemorrhage, prolonged (more than 24 hours) loss of consciousness and return to pre-existing conscious level

804.75 Open fractures involving skull or face with other bones with subarachnoid, subdural, and extradural hemorrhage, prolonged (more than 24 hours) loss of consciousness, without return to pre-existing conscious level

804.76 Open fractures involving skull or face with other bones with subarachnoid, subdural, and extradural hemorrhage, loss of consciousness of unspecified duration ▽

804.79 Open fractures involving skull or face with other bones with subarachnoid, subdural, and extradural hemorrhage, unspecified concussion ▽

804.80 Open fractures involving skull or face with other bones, with other and unspecified intracranial hemorrhage, unspecified state of consciousness ▽

804.81 Open fractures involving skull or face with other bones, with other and unspecified intracranial hemorrhage, no loss of consciousness ▽

804.82 Open fractures involving skull or face with other bones, with other and unspecified intracranial hemorrhage, brief (less than one hour) loss of consciousness ▽

804.83 Open fractures involving skull or face with other bones, with other and unspecified intracranial hemorrhage, moderate (1-24 hours) loss of consciousness ▽

804.84 Open fractures involving skull or face with other bones, with other and unspecified intracranial hemorrhage, prolonged (more than 24 hours) loss of consciousness and return to pre-existing conscious level ▽

804.85 Open fractures involving skull or face with other bones, with other and unspecified intracranial hemorrhage, prolonged (more than 24 hours) loss of consciousness, without return to pre-existing conscious level ▽

804.86 Open fractures involving skull or face with other bones, with other and unspecified intracranial hemorrhage, loss of consciousness of unspecified duration ▽

804.89 Open fractures involving skull or face with other bones, with other and unspecified intracranial hemorrhage, unspecified concussion ▽

804.90 Open fractures involving skull or face with other bones, with intracranial injury of other and unspecified nature, unspecified state of consciousness ▽

804.91 Open fractures involving skull or face with other bones, with intracranial injury of other and unspecified nature, no loss of consciousness ▽

804.92 Open fractures involving skull or face with other bones, with intracranial injury of other and unspecified nature, brief (less than one hour) loss of consciousness ▽

804.93 Open fractures involving skull or face with other bones, with intracranial injury of other and unspecified nature, moderate (1-24 hours) loss of consciousness ▽

804.94 Open fractures involving skull or face with other bones, with intracranial injury of other and unspecified nature, prolonged (more than 24 hours) loss of consciousness and return to pre-existing conscious level ▽

804.95 Open fractures involving skull or face with other bones, with intracranial injury of other and unspecified nature, prolonged (more than 24 hours) loss of consciousness, without return to pre-existing level ▽

804.96 Open fractures involving skull or face with other bones, with intracranial injury of other and unspecified nature, loss of consciousness of unspecified duration ▽

804.99 Open fractures involving skull or face with other bones, with intracranial injury of other and unspecified nature, unspecified concussion ▽

805.10 Open fracture of cervical vertebra, unspecified level without mention of spinal cord injury ▽

805.11 Open fracture of first cervical vertebra without mention of spinal cord injury

805.12 Open fracture of second cervical vertebra without mention of spinal cord injury

805.13 Open fracture of third cervical vertebra without mention of spinal cord injury

805.14 Open fracture of fourth cervical vertebra without mention of spinal cord injury

805.15 Open fracture of fifth cervical vertebra without mention of spinal cord injury

805.16 Open fracture of sixth cervical vertebra without mention of spinal cord injury

805.17 Open fracture of seventh cervical vertebra without mention of spinal cord injury

805.18 Open fracture of multiple cervical vertebrae without mention of spinal cord injury

805.3 Open fracture of dorsal (thoracic) vertebra without mention of spinal cord injury

805.5 Open fracture of lumbar vertebra without mention of spinal cord injury

805.7 Open fracture of sacrum and coccyx without mention of spinal cord injury

805.9 Open fracture of unspecified part of vertebral column without mention of spinal cord injury ▽

806.10 Open fracture of C1-C4 level with unspecified spinal cord injury ▽

806.11 Open fracture of C1-C4 level with complete lesion of cord

806.12 Open fracture of C1-C4 level with anterior cord syndrome

806.13 Open fracture of C1-C4 level with central cord syndrome

806.14 Open fracture of C1-C4 level with other specified spinal cord injury

806.15 Open fracture of C5-C7 level with unspecified spinal cord injury ▽

806.16 Open fracture of C5-C7 level with complete lesion of cord

806.17 Open fracture of C5-C7 level with anterior cord syndrome

806.18 Open fracture of C5-C7 level with central cord syndrome

806.19 Open fracture of C5-C7 level with other specified spinal cord injury

806.30 Open fracture of T1-T6 level with unspecified spinal cord injury ▽

806.31 Open fracture of T1-T6 level with complete lesion of cord

806.32 Open fracture of T1-T6 level with anterior cord syndrome

806.33 Open fracture of T1-T6 level with central cord syndrome

806.34 Open fracture of T1-T6 level with other specified spinal cord injury

806.35 Open fracture of T7-T12 level with unspecified spinal cord injury ▽

▽ Unspecified code
♀ Female diagnosis

☒ Manifestation code
♂ Male diagnosis

806.36 Open fracture of T7-T12 level with complete lesion of cord
806.37 Open fracture of T7-T12 level with anterior cord syndrome
806.38 Open fracture of T7-T12 level with central cord syndrome
806.39 Open fracture of T7-T12 level with other specified spinal cord injury
806.5 Open fracture of lumbar spine with spinal cord injury
806.70 Open fracture of sacrum and coccyx with unspecified spinal cord injury ▽
806.71 Open fracture of sacrum and coccyx with complete cauda equina lesion
806.72 Open fracture of sacrum and coccyx with other cauda equina injury
806.79 Open fracture of sacrum and coccyx with other spinal cord injury
806.9 Open fracture of unspecified vertebra with spinal cord injury ▽
807.11 Open fracture of one rib
807.12 Open fracture of two ribs
807.13 Open fracture of three ribs
807.14 Open fracture of four ribs
807.15 Open fracture of five ribs
807.16 Open fracture of six ribs
807.17 Open fracture of seven ribs
807.18 Open fracture of eight or more ribs
807.6 Open fracture of larynx and trachea
808.1 Open fracture of acetabulum
808.3 Open fracture of pubis
808.51 Open fracture of ilium
808.52 Open fracture of ischium
808.53 Multiple open pelvic fractures with disruption of pelvic circle
808.59 Open fracture of other specified part of pelvis
808.9 Unspecified open fracture of pelvis ▽
809.1 Fracture of bones of trunk, open
810.10 Unspecified part of open fracture of clavicle ▽
810.11 Open fracture of sternal end of clavicle
810.12 Open fracture of shaft of clavicle
810.13 Open fracture of acromial end of clavicle
811.10 Open fracture of unspecified part of scapula ▽
811.11 Open fracture of acromial process of scapula
811.12 Open fracture of coracoid process
811.13 Open fracture of glenoid cavity and neck of scapula
811.19 Open fracture of other part of scapula
812.10 Open fracture of unspecified part of upper end of humerus ▽
812.11 Open fracture of surgical neck of humerus
812.12 Open fracture of anatomical neck of humerus
812.13 Open fracture of greater tuberosity of humerus
812.19 Other open fracture of upper end of humerus
812.30 Open fracture of unspecified part of humerus ▽
812.31 Open fracture of shaft of humerus
812.50 Open fracture of unspecified part of lower end of humerus ▽
812.51 Open fracture of supracondylar humerus
812.52 Open fracture of lateral condyle of humerus
812.53 Open fracture of medial condyle of humerus
812.54 Open fracture of unspecified condyle(s) of humerus ▽
812.59 Other open fracture of lower end of humerus
813.10 Unspecified open fracture of upper end of forearm ▽
813.11 Open fracture of olecranon process of ulna
813.12 Open fracture of coronoid process of ulna
813.13 Open Monteggia's fracture
813.14 Other and unspecified open fractures of proximal end of ulna (alone) ▽
813.15 Open fracture of head of radius
813.17 Other and unspecified open fractures of proximal end of radius (alone) ▽
813.18 Open fracture of radius with ulna, upper end (any part)
813.30 Unspecified open fracture of shaft of radius or ulna ▽
813.31 Open fracture of shaft of radius (alone)
813.32 Open fracture of shaft of ulna (alone)
813.33 Open fracture of shaft of radius with ulna
813.50 Unspecified open fracture of lower end of forearm ▽
813.51 Open Colles' fracture
813.52 Other open fractures of distal end of radius (alone)
813.53 Open fracture of distal end of ulna (alone)
813.54 Open fracture of lower end of radius with ulna
813.90 Open fracture of unspecified part of forearm ▽
813.91 Open fracture of unspecified part of radius (alone) ▽
813.92 Open fracture of unspecified part of ulna (alone) ▽
813.93 Open fracture of unspecified part of radius with ulna ▽
814.10 Unspecified open fracture of carpal bone ▽
814.11 Open fracture of navicular (scaphoid) bone of wrist
814.12 Open fracture of lunate (semilunar) bone of wrist
814.13 Open fracture of triquetral (cuneiform) bone of wrist
814.14 Open fracture of pisiform bone of wrist
814.15 Open fracture of trapezium bone (larger multangular) of wrist
814.16 Open fracture of trapezoid bone (smaller multangular) of wrist
814.17 Open fracture of capitate bone (os magnum) of wrist
814.18 Open fracture of hamate (unciform) bone of wrist
814.19 Open fracture of other bone of wrist
815.10 Open fracture of metacarpal bone(s), site unspecified ▽
815.11 Open fracture of base of thumb (first) metacarpal bone(s)
815.12 Open fracture of base of other metacarpal bone(s)
815.13 Open fracture of shaft of metacarpal bone(s)
815.14 Open fracture of neck of metacarpal bone(s)
815.19 Open fracture of multiple sites of metacarpus
816.10 Open fracture of phalanx or phalanges of hand, unspecified ▽
816.11 Open fracture of middle or proximal phalanx or phalanges of hand
816.12 Open fracture of distal phalanx or phalanges of hand
816.13 Open fractures of multiple sites of phalanx or phalanges of hand
817.1 Multiple open fractures of hand bones
818.1 Ill-defined open fractures of upper limb
819.1 Multiple open fractures involving both upper limbs, and upper limb with rib(s) and sternum
820.10 Open fracture of unspecified intracapsular section of neck of femur ▽
820.11 Open fracture of epiphysis (separation) (upper) of neck of femur
820.12 Open fracture of midcervical section of femur
820.13 Open fracture of base of neck of femur
820.19 Other open transcervical fracture of femur
820.30 Open fracture of unspecified trochanteric section of femur ▽
820.31 Open fracture of intertrochanteric section of femur
820.32 Open fracture of subtrochanteric section of femur
820.9 Open fracture of unspecified part of neck of femur ▽
821.10 Open fracture of unspecified part of femur ▽
821.11 Open fracture of shaft of femur
821.30 Open fracture of unspecified part of lower end of femur ▽
821.31 Open fracture of femoral condyle
821.32 Open fracture of lower epiphysis of femur
821.33 Open supracondylar fracture of femur
821.39 Other open fracture of lower end of femur
822.1 Open fracture of patella
823.10 Open fracture of upper end of tibia
823.11 Open fracture of upper end of fibula
823.12 Open fracture of upper end of fibula with tibia
823.30 Open fracture of shaft of tibia
823.31 Open fracture of shaft of fibula
823.32 Open fracture of shaft of fibula with tibia
823.90 Open fracture of unspecified part of tibia ▽
823.91 Open fracture of unspecified part of fibula ▽
823.92 Open fracture of unspecified part of fibula with tibia ▽
824.1 Open fracture of medial malleolus
824.3 Open fracture of lateral malleolus
824.5 Open bimalleolar fracture
824.7 Open trimalleolar fracture
825.1 Open fracture of calcaneus
825.30 Open fracture of unspecified bone(s) of foot (except toes) ▽
825.31 Open fracture of astragalus
825.32 Open fracture of navicular (scaphoid) bone of foot
825.33 Open fracture of cuboid bone
825.34 Open fracture of cuneiform bone of foot,
825.35 Open fracture of metatarsal bone(s)
825.39 Other open fractures of tarsal and metatarsal bones
826.1 Open fracture of one or more phalanges of foot
827.1 Other, multiple and ill-defined open fractures of lower limb
828.1 Multiple fractures involving both lower limbs, lower with upper limb, and lower limb(s) with rib(s) and sternum, open
829.1 Open fracture of unspecified bone ▽
830.1 Open dislocation of jaw
831.10 Open unspecified dislocation of shoulder ▽
831.11 Open anterior dislocation of humerus
831.12 Open posterior dislocation of humerus
831.13 Open inferior dislocation of humerus
831.14 Open dislocation of acromioclavicular (joint)
831.19 Open dislocation of other site of shoulder
832.10 Open unspecified dislocation of elbow ▽
832.11 Open anterior dislocation of elbow
832.12 Open posterior dislocation of elbow
832.13 Open medial dislocation of elbow
832.14 Open lateral dislocation of elbow
832.19 Open dislocation of other site of elbow
833.10 Open dislocation of wrist, unspecified part ▽
833.11 Open dislocation of distal radioulnar (joint)

▽ Unspecified code
♀ Female diagnosis
Manifestation code
♂ Male diagnosis

833.12 Open dislocation of radiocarpal (joint)
833.13 Open dislocation of midcarpal (joint)
833.14 Open dislocation of carpometacarpal (joint)
833.15 Open dislocation of proximal end of metacarpal (bone)
833.19 Open dislocation of other part of wrist
834.10 Open dislocation of finger, unspecified part ▽
834.11 Open dislocation of metacarpophalangeal (joint)
834.12 Open dislocation interphalangeal (joint), hand
835.10 Open dislocation of hip, unspecified site ▽
835.11 Open posterior dislocation of hip
835.12 Open obturator dislocation of hip
835.13 Other open anterior dislocation of hip
836.4 Open dislocation of patella
836.60 Open dislocation of knee unspecified part ▽
836.61 Open anterior dislocation of tibia, proximal end
836.62 Open posterior dislocation of tibia, proximal end
836.63 Open medial dislocation of tibia, proximal end
836.64 Open lateral dislocation of tibia, proximal end
836.69 Other open dislocation of knee
837.1 Open dislocation of ankle
838.10 Open dislocation of foot, unspecified part ▽
838.11 Open dislocation of tarsal (bone), joint unspecified ▽
838.12 Open dislocation of midtarsal (joint)
838.13 Open dislocation of tarsometatarsal (joint)
838.14 Open dislocation of metatarsal (bone), joint unspecified ▽
838.15 Open dislocation of metatarsophalangeal (joint)
838.16 Open dislocation of interphalangeal (joint), foot
838.19 Open dislocation of other part of foot
839.10 Open dislocation, unspecified cervical vertebra ▽
839.11 Open dislocation, first cervical vertebra
839.12 Open dislocation, second cervical vertebra
839.13 Open dislocation, third cervical vertebra
839.14 Open dislocation, fourth cervical vertebra
839.15 Open dislocation, fifth cervical vertebra
839.16 Open dislocation, sixth cervical vertebra
839.17 Open dislocation, seventh cervical vertebra
839.18 Open dislocation, multiple cervical vertebrae
839.30 Open dislocation, lumbar vertebra
839.31 Open dislocation, thoracic vertebra
839.50 Open dislocation, vertebra, unspecified site ▽
839.51 Open dislocation, coccyx
839.52 Open dislocation, sacrum
839.59 Open dislocation, other vertebra
839.71 Open dislocation, sternum

ICD-9-CM Procedural

76.2 Local excision or destruction of lesion of facial bone
79.60 Debridement of open fracture, unspecified site
79.61 Debridement of open fracture of humerus
79.62 Debridement of open fracture of radius and ulna
79.63 Debridement of open fracture of carpals and metacarpals
79.64 Debridement of open fracture of phalanges of hand
79.65 Debridement of open fracture of femur
79.66 Debridement of open fracture of tibia and fibula
79.67 Debridement of open fracture of tarsals and metatarsals
79.68 Debridement of open fracture of phalanges of foot
79.69 Debridement of open fracture of other specified bone, except facial bones

11040–11044

11040 Debridement; skin, partial thickness
11041 skin, full thickness
11042 skin, and subcutaneous tissue
11043 skin, subcutaneous tissue, and muscle
11044 subcutaneous tissue, muscle, and bone

ICD-9-CM Diagnostic

250.70 Diabetes with peripheral circulatory disorders, type II or unspecified type, not stated as uncontrolled — (Use additional code to identify manifestation: 443.81, 785.4)
250.71 Diabetes with peripheral circulatory disorders, type I [juvenile type], not stated as uncontrolled — (Use additional code to identify manifestation: 443.81, 785.4)
250.72 Diabetes with peripheral circulatory disorders, type II or unspecified type, uncontrolled — (Use additional code to identify manifestation: 443.81, 785.4)
250.73 Diabetes with peripheral circulatory disorders, type I [juvenile type], uncontrolled — (Use additional code to identify manifestation: 443.81, 785.4)
443.81 Peripheral angiopathy in diseases classified elsewhere — (Code first underlying disease, 250.7) ☒
681.00 Unspecified cellulitis and abscess of finger — (Use additional code to identify organism) ▽
681.10 Unspecified cellulitis and abscess of toe — (Use additional code to identify organism) ▽
681.11 Onychia and paronychia of toe — (Use additional code to identify organism)
682.0 Cellulitis and abscess of face — (Use additional code to identify organism)
682.1 Cellulitis and abscess of neck — (Use additional code to identify organism)
682.2 Cellulitis and abscess of trunk — (Use additional code to identify organism)
682.3 Cellulitis and abscess of upper arm and forearm — (Use additional code to identify organism)
682.4 Cellulitis and abscess of hand, except fingers and thumb — (Use additional code to identify organism)
682.5 Cellulitis and abscess of buttock — (Use additional code to identify organism)
682.6 Cellulitis and abscess of leg, except foot — (Use additional code to identify organism)
682.7 Cellulitis and abscess of foot, except toes — (Use additional code to identify organism)
682.8 Cellulitis and abscess of other specified site — (Use additional code to identify organism)
686.1 Pyogenic granuloma of skin and subcutaneous tissue
701.5 Other abnormal granulation tissue
707.00 Decubitus ulcer, unspecified site
707.01 Decubitus ulcer, elbow
707.02 Decubitus ulcer, upper back
707.03 Decubitus ulcer, lower back
707.04 Decubitus ulcer, hip
707.05 Decubitus ulcer, buttock
707.06 Decubitus ulcer, ankle
707.07 Decubitus ulcer, heel
707.09 Decubitus ulcer, other site
707.10 Ulcer of lower limb, unspecified ▽
707.11 Ulcer of thigh
707.12 Ulcer of calf
707.13 Ulcer of ankle
707.14 Ulcer of heel and midfoot
707.15 Ulcer of other part of foot
707.19 Ulcer of other part of lower limb
707.8 Chronic ulcer of other specified site
728.0 Infective myositis
728.86 Necrotizing fasciitis — (Use additional code to identify infectious organism, 041.00-041.89, 785.4, if applicable)
728.88 Rhabdomyolysis
729.4 Unspecified fasciitis ▽
785.4 Gangrene — (Code first any associated underlying condition:250.7, 443.0)
872.10 Open wound of external ear, unspecified site, complicated — (Use additional code to identify infection) ▽
872.11 Open wound of auricle, complicated — (Use additional code to identify infection)
873.1 Open wound of scalp, complicated — (Use additional code to identify infection)
873.30 Open wound of nose, unspecified site, complicated — (Use additional code to identify infection) ▽
873.50 Open wound of face, unspecified site, complicated — (Use additional code to identify infection) ▽
873.51 Open wound of cheek, complicated — (Use additional code to identify infection)
873.52 Open wound of forehead, complicated — (Use additional code to identify infection)
873.54 Open wound of jaw, complicated — (Use additional code to identify infection)
873.59 Open wound of face, other and multiple sites, complicated — (Use additional code to identify infection)
873.9 Other and unspecified open wound of head, complicated — (Use additional code to identify infection) ▽
875.1 Open wound of chest (wall), complicated — (Use additional code to identify infection)
876.1 Open wound of back, complicated — (Use additional code to identify infection)
877.1 Open wound of buttock, complicated — (Use additional code to identify infection)
879.1 Open wound of breast, complicated — (Use additional code to identify infection)
879.3 Open wound of abdominal wall, anterior, complicated — (Use additional code to identify infection)
879.5 Open wound of abdominal wall, lateral, complicated — (Use additional code to identify infection)

879.7 Open wound of other and unspecified parts of trunk, complicated — (Use additional code to identify infection) ▽
879.9 Open wound(s) (multiple) of unspecified site(s), complicated — (Use additional code to identify infection) ▽
880.11 Open wound of scapular region, complicated — (Use additional code to identify infection)
880.12 Open wound of axillary region, complicated — (Use additional code to identify infection)
880.13 Open wound of upper arm, complicated — (Use additional code to identify infection)
880.19 Open wound of multiple sites of shoulder and upper arm, complicated — (Use additional code to identify infection)
881.10 Open wound of forearm, complicated — (Use additional code to identify infection)
881.11 Open wound of elbow, complicated — (Use additional code to identify infection)
881.12 Open wound of wrist, complicated — (Use additional code to identify infection)
881.22 Open wound of wrist, with tendon involvement — (Use additional code to identify infection)
882.1 Open wound of hand except finger(s) alone, complicated — (Use additional code to identify infection)
883.1 Open wound of finger(s), complicated — (Use additional code to identify infection)
884.1 Multiple and unspecified open wound of upper limb, complicated — (Use additional code to identify infection)
885.1 Traumatic amputation of thumb (complete) (partial), complicated — (Use additional code to identify infection)
886.1 Traumatic amputation of other finger(s) (complete) (partial), complicated — (Use additional code to identify infection)
887.1 Traumatic amputation of arm and hand (complete) (partial), unilateral, below elbow, complicated — (Use additional code to identify infection)
887.3 Traumatic amputation of arm and hand (complete) (partial), unilateral, at or above elbow, complicated — (Use additional code to identify infection)
887.5 Traumatic amputation of arm and hand (complete) (partial), unilateral, level not specified, complicated — (Use additional code to identify infection) ▽
887.7 Traumatic amputation of arm and hand (complete) (partial), bilateral (any level), complicated — (Use additional code to identify infection)
890.1 Open wound of hip and thigh, complicated — (Use additional code to identify infection)
891.1 Open wound of knee, leg (except thigh), and ankle, complicated — (Use additional code to identify infection)
892.1 Open wound of foot except toe(s) alone, complicated — (Use additional code to identify infection)
893.1 Open wound of toe(s), complicated — (Use additional code to identify infection)
894.1 Multiple and unspecified open wound of lower limb, complicated — (Use additional code to identify infection)
895.1 Traumatic amputation of toe(s) (complete) (partial), complicated — (Use additional code to identify infection)
896.1 Traumatic amputation of foot (complete) (partial), unilateral, complicated — (Use additional code to identify infection)
896.3 Traumatic amputation of foot (complete) (partial), bilateral, complicated — (Use additional code to identify infection)
897.1 Traumatic amputation of leg(s) (complete) (partial), unilateral, below knee, complicated — (Use additional code to identify infection)
897.3 Traumatic amputation of leg(s) (complete) (partial), unilateral, at or above knee, complicated — (Use additional code to identify infection)
897.5 Traumatic amputation of leg(s) (complete) (partial), unilateral, level not specified, complicated — (Use additional code to identify infection) ▽
897.7 Traumatic amputation of leg(s) (complete) (partial), bilateral (any level), complicated — (Use additional code to identify infection)
925.1 Crushing injury of face and scalp — (Use additional code to identify any associated injuries: 800-829, 850.0-854.1, 860.0-869.1)
925.2 Crushing injury of neck — (Use additional code to identify any associated injuries: 800-829, 850.0-854.1, 860.0-869.1)
926.0 Crushing injury of external genitalia — (Use additional code to identify any associated injuries: 800-829, 850.0-854.1, 860.0-869.1)
926.11 Crushing injury of back — (Use additional code to identify any associated injuries: 800-829, 850.0-854.1, 860.0-869.1)
926.12 Crushing injury of buttock — (Use additional code to identify any associated injuries: 800-829, 850.0-854.1, 860.0-869.1)
926.19 Crushing injury of other specified sites of trunk — (Use additional code to identify any associated injuries: 800-829, 850.0-854.1, 860.0-869.1)
926.8 Crushing injury of multiple sites of trunk — (Use additional code to identify any associated injuries: 800-829, 850.0-854.1, 860.0-869.1)
926.9 Crushing injury of unspecified site of trunk — (Use additional code to identify any associated injuries: 800-829, 850.0-854.1, 860.0-869.1) ▽
927.00 Crushing injury of shoulder region — (Use additional code to identify any associated injuries: 800-829, 850.0-854.1, 860.0-869.1)
927.01 Crushing injury of scapular region — (Use additional code to identify any associated injuries: 800-829, 850.0-854.1, 860.0-869.1)
927.02 Crushing injury of axillary region — (Use additional code to identify any associated injuries: 800-829, 850.0-854.1, 860.0-869.1)
927.03 Crushing injury of upper arm — (Use additional code to identify any associated injuries: 800-829, 850.0-854.1, 860.0-869.1)
927.09 Crushing injury of multiple sites of upper arm — (Use additional code to identify any associated injuries: 800-829, 850.0-854.1, 860.0-869.1)
927.10 Crushing injury of forearm — (Use additional code to identify any associated injuries: 800-829, 850.0-854.1, 860.0-869.1)
927.11 Crushing injury of elbow — (Use additional code to identify any associated injuries: 800-829, 850.0-854.1, 860.0-869.1)
927.20 Crushing injury of hand(s) — (Use additional code to identify any associated injuries: 800-829, 850.0-854.1, 860.0-869.1)
927.21 Crushing injury of wrist — (Use additional code to identify any associated injuries: 800-829, 850.0-854.1, 860.0-869.1)
927.3 Crushing injury of finger(s) — (Use additional code to identify any associated injuries: 800-829, 850.0-854.1, 860.0-869.1)
927.8 Crushing injury of multiple sites of upper limb — (Use additional code to identify any associated injuries: 800-829, 850.0-854.1, 860.0-869.1)
928.00 Crushing injury of thigh — (Use additional code to identify any associated injuries: 800-829, 850.0-854.1, 860.0-869.1)
928.01 Crushing injury of hip — (Use additional code to identify any associated injuries: 800-829, 850.0-854.1, 860.0-869.1)
928.11 Crushing injury of knee — (Use additional code to identify any associated injuries: 800-829, 850.0-854.1, 860.0-869.1)
928.20 Crushing injury of foot — (Use additional code to identify any associated injuries: 800-829, 850.0-854.1, 860.0-869.1)
928.21 Crushing injury of ankle — (Use additional code to identify any associated injuries: 800-829, 850.0-854.1, 860.0-869.1)
928.3 Crushing injury of toe(s) — (Use additional code to identify any associated injuries: 800-829, 850.0-854.1, 860.0-869.1)
928.8 Crushing injury of multiple sites of lower limb — (Use additional code to identify any associated injuries: 800-829, 850.0-854.1, 860.0-869.1)
928.9 Crushing injury of unspecified site of lower limb — (Use additional code to identify any associated injuries: 800-829, 850.0-854.1, 860.0-869.1) ▽
929.0 Crushing injury of multiple sites, not elsewhere classified — (Use additional code to identify any associated injuries: 800-829, 850.0-854.1, 860.0-869.1)
929.9 Crushing injury of unspecified site — (Use additional code to identify any associated injuries: 800-829, 850.0-854.1, 860.0-869.1) ▽
958.3 Posttraumatic wound infection not elsewhere classified
991.0 Frostbite of face
991.1 Frostbite of hand
991.2 Frostbite of foot
991.3 Frostbite of other and unspecified sites
997.62 Infection (chronic) of amputation stump — (Use additional code to identify organism. Use additional code to identify complications)
998.2 Accidental puncture or laceration during procedure
998.59 Other postoperative infection — (Use additional code to identify infection)
998.83 Non-healing surgical wound

ICD-9-CM Procedural

77.60 Local excision of lesion or tissue of bone, unspecified site
77.61 Local excision of lesion or tissue of scapula, clavicle, and thorax (ribs and sternum)
77.62 Local excision of lesion or tissue of humerus
77.63 Local excision of lesion or tissue of radius and ulna
77.64 Local excision of lesion or tissue of carpals and metacarpals
77.65 Local excision of lesion or tissue of femur
77.66 Local excision of lesion or tissue of patella
77.67 Local excision of lesion or tissue of tibia and fibula
77.68 Local excision of lesion or tissue of tarsals and metatarsals
77.69 Local excision of lesion or tissue of other bone, except facial bones
82.36 Other myectomy of hand
83.45 Other myectomy
86.22 Excisional debridement of wound, infection, or burn

HCPCS Level II Supplies & Services

A4305 Disposable drug delivery system, flow rate of 50 ml or greater per hour
A4306 Disposable drug delivery system, flow rate of 5 ml or less per hour
A4550 Surgical trays

11055–11057

11055 Paring or cutting of benign hyperkeratotic lesion (eg, corn or callus); single lesion
11056 two to four lesions
11057 more than four lesions

ICD-9-CM Diagnostic

700 Corns and callosities
702.0 Actinic keratosis
702.11 Inflamed seborrheic keratosis
702.19 Other seborrheic keratosis
702.8 Other specified dermatoses
757.39 Other specified congenital anomaly of skin

ICD-9-CM Procedural

86.3 Other local excision or destruction of lesion or tissue of skin and subcutaneous tissue

HCPCS Level II Supplies & Services

A4550 Surgical trays
S0390 Routine foot care; removal and/or trimming of corns, calluses and/or nails and preventive maintenance in specific medical conditions (e.g., diabetes), per visit

11100–11101

11100 Biopsy of skin, subcutaneous tissue and/or mucous membrane (including simple closure), unless otherwise listed; single lesion
11101 each separate/additional lesion (List separately in addition to code for primary procedure)

ICD-9-CM Diagnostic

145.9 Malignant neoplasm of mouth, unspecified site ▽
171.0 Malignant neoplasm of connective and other soft tissue of head, face, and neck
172.3 Malignant melanoma of skin of other and unspecified parts of face
172.4 Malignant melanoma of skin of scalp and neck
172.5 Malignant melanoma of skin of trunk, except scrotum
172.6 Malignant melanoma of skin of upper limb, including shoulder
172.7 Malignant melanoma of skin of lower limb, including hip
172.8 Malignant melanoma of other specified sites of skin
173.3 Other malignant neoplasm of skin of other and unspecified parts of face ▽
173.4 Other malignant neoplasm of scalp and skin of neck
173.5 Other malignant neoplasm of skin of trunk, except scrotum
173.6 Other malignant neoplasm of skin of upper limb, including shoulder
173.7 Other malignant neoplasm of skin of lower limb, including hip
173.8 Other malignant neoplasm of other specified sites of skin
176.0 Kaposi's sarcoma of skin
195.0 Malignant neoplasm of head, face, and neck
198.2 Secondary malignant neoplasm of skin
215.0 Other benign neoplasm of connective and other soft tissue of head, face, and neck
216.3 Benign neoplasm of skin of other and unspecified parts of face ▽
216.4 Benign neoplasm of scalp and skin of neck
216.5 Benign neoplasm of skin of trunk, except scrotum
216.6 Benign neoplasm of skin of upper limb, including shoulder
216.7 Benign neoplasm of skin of lower limb, including hip
216.8 Benign neoplasm of other specified sites of skin
228.01 Hemangioma of skin and subcutaneous tissue
232.3 Carcinoma in situ of skin of other and unspecified parts of face ▽
232.4 Carcinoma in situ of scalp and skin of neck
232.5 Carcinoma in situ of skin of trunk, except scrotum
232.6 Carcinoma in situ of skin of upper limb, including shoulder
232.7 Carcinoma in situ of skin of lower limb, including hip
232.8 Carcinoma in situ of other specified sites of skin
238.2 Neoplasm of uncertain behavior of skin
239.2 Neoplasms of unspecified nature of bone, soft tissue, and skin
448.1 Nevus, non-neoplastic
694.4 Pemphigus
696.1 Other psoriasis and similar disorders
701.5 Other abnormal granulation tissue
702.8 Other specified dermatoses
709.09 Other dyschromia
709.4 Foreign body granuloma of skin and subcutaneous tissue
709.9 Unspecified disorder of skin and subcutaneous tissue ▽
757.32 Congenital vascular hamartomas
757.33 Congenital pigmentary anomaly of skin

ICD-9-CM Procedural

08.11 Biopsy of eyelid
21.22 Biopsy of nose
27.23 Biopsy of lip
49.22 Biopsy of perianal tissue
61.11 Biopsy of scrotum or tunica vaginalis
86.11 Biopsy of skin and subcutaneous tissue

HCPCS Level II Supplies & Services

The HCPCS Level II code(s) would be the same as the actual procedure performed because these are in-addition-to codes.

11200–11201

11200 Removal of skin tags, multiple fibrocutaneous tags, any area; up to and including 15 lesions
11201 each additional ten lesions (List separately in addition to code for primary procedure)

ICD-9-CM Diagnostic

701.9 Unspecified hypertrophic and atrophic condition of skin ▽
757.39 Other specified congenital anomaly of skin

ICD-9-CM Procedural

86.3 Other local excision or destruction of lesion or tissue of skin and subcutaneous tissue

HCPCS Level II Supplies & Services

A4550 Surgical trays

11300–11303

11300 Shaving of epidermal or dermal lesion, single lesion, trunk, arms or legs; lesion diameter 0.5 cm or less
11301 lesion diameter 0.6 to 1.0 cm
11302 lesion diameter 1.1 to 2.0 cm
11303 lesion diameter over 2.0 cm

ICD-9-CM Diagnostic

173.5 Other malignant neoplasm of skin of trunk, except scrotum
173.6 Other malignant neoplasm of skin of upper limb, including shoulder
173.7 Other malignant neoplasm of skin of lower limb, including hip
216.5 Benign neoplasm of skin of trunk, except scrotum
216.6 Benign neoplasm of skin of upper limb, including shoulder
216.7 Benign neoplasm of skin of lower limb, including hip
228.01 Hemangioma of skin and subcutaneous tissue
232.5 Carcinoma in situ of skin of trunk, except scrotum
232.6 Carcinoma in situ of skin of upper limb, including shoulder
232.7 Carcinoma in situ of skin of lower limb, including hip
238.2 Neoplasm of uncertain behavior of skin
239.2 Neoplasms of unspecified nature of bone, soft tissue, and skin
686.1 Pyogenic granuloma of skin and subcutaneous tissue
701.1 Acquired keratoderma
702.0 Actinic keratosis
702.11 Inflamed seborrheic keratosis
709.00 Dyschromia, unspecified ▽
709.9 Unspecified disorder of skin and subcutaneous tissue ▽
757.39 Other specified congenital anomaly of skin

ICD-9-CM Procedural

86.3 Other local excision or destruction of lesion or tissue of skin and subcutaneous tissue

HCPCS Level II Supplies & Services

A4550 Surgical trays

11305–11308

11305 Shaving of epidermal or dermal lesion, single lesion, scalp, neck, hands, feet, genitalia; lesion diameter 0.5 cm or less
11306 lesion diameter 0.6 to 1.0 cm
11307 lesion diameter 1.1 to 2.0 cm
11308 lesion diameter over 2.0 cm

ICD-9-CM Diagnostic

173.4 Other malignant neoplasm of scalp and skin of neck
173.6 Other malignant neoplasm of skin of upper limb, including shoulder
173.7 Other malignant neoplasm of skin of lower limb, including hip
184.1 Malignant neoplasm of labia majora ♀

184.2 Malignant neoplasm of labia minora ♀
184.4 Malignant neoplasm of vulva, unspecified site ▽ ♀
187.4 Malignant neoplasm of penis, part unspecified ▽ ♂
187.7 Malignant neoplasm of scrotum ♂
216.4 Benign neoplasm of scalp and skin of neck
216.6 Benign neoplasm of skin of upper limb, including shoulder
216.7 Benign neoplasm of skin of lower limb, including hip
221.1 Benign neoplasm of vagina ♀
221.2 Benign neoplasm of vulva ♀
221.8 Benign neoplasm of other specified sites of female genital organs ♀
221.9 Benign neoplasm of female genital organ, site unspecified ▽ ♀
222.4 Benign neoplasm of scrotum ♂
228.01 Hemangioma of skin and subcutaneous tissue
232.4 Carcinoma in situ of scalp and skin of neck
232.6 Carcinoma in situ of skin of upper limb, including shoulder
232.7 Carcinoma in situ of skin of lower limb, including hip
232.8 Carcinoma in situ of other specified sites of skin
233.3 Carcinoma in situ of other and unspecified female genital organs ▽ ♀
233.5 Carcinoma in situ of penis ♂
233.6 Carcinoma in situ of other and unspecified male genital organs ▽ ♂
236.3 Neoplasm of uncertain behavior of other and unspecified female genital organs ▽ ♀
236.6 Neoplasm of uncertain behavior of other and unspecified male genital organs ▽ ♂
238.2 Neoplasm of uncertain behavior of skin
239.2 Neoplasms of unspecified nature of bone, soft tissue, and skin
239.5 Neoplasm of unspecified nature of other genitourinary organs
686.1 Pyogenic granuloma of skin and subcutaneous tissue
701.1 Acquired keratoderma
701.5 Other abnormal granulation tissue
702.0 Actinic keratosis
702.11 Inflamed seborrheic keratosis
702.19 Other seborrheic keratosis
706.2 Sebaceous cyst
709.00 Dyschromia, unspecified ▽
709.9 Unspecified disorder of skin and subcutaneous tissue ▽
757.39 Other specified congenital anomaly of skin

ICD-9-CM Procedural

71.09 Other incision of vulva and perineum
86.3 Other local excision or destruction of lesion or tissue of skin and subcutaneous tissue

HCPCS Level II Supplies & Services

A4550 Surgical trays

11310–11313

11310 Shaving of epidermal or dermal lesion, single lesion, face, ears, eyelids, nose, lips, mucous membrane; lesion diameter 0.5 cm or less
11311 lesion diameter 0.6 to 1.0 cm
11312 lesion diameter 1.1 to 2.0 cm
11313 lesion diameter over 2.0 cm

ICD-9-CM Diagnostic

173.0 Other malignant neoplasm of skin of lip
173.1 Other malignant neoplasm of skin of eyelid, including canthus
173.2 Other malignant neoplasm of skin of ear and external auditory canal
173.3 Other malignant neoplasm of skin of other and unspecified parts of face ▽
198.2 Secondary malignant neoplasm of skin
198.89 Secondary malignant neoplasm of other specified sites
216.0 Benign neoplasm of skin of lip
216.1 Benign neoplasm of eyelid, including canthus
216.2 Benign neoplasm of ear and external auditory canal
216.3 Benign neoplasm of skin of other and unspecified parts of face ▽
228.01 Hemangioma of skin and subcutaneous tissue
232.0 Carcinoma in situ of skin of lip
232.1 Carcinoma in situ of eyelid, including canthus
232.2 Carcinoma in situ of skin of ear and external auditory canal
232.3 Carcinoma in situ of skin of other and unspecified parts of face ▽
238.2 Neoplasm of uncertain behavior of skin
239.2 Neoplasms of unspecified nature of bone, soft tissue, and skin
239.8 Neoplasm of unspecified nature of other specified sites
380.14 Malignant otitis externa
686.1 Pyogenic granuloma of skin and subcutaneous tissue
701.1 Acquired keratoderma
702.0 Actinic keratosis
702.11 Inflamed seborrheic keratosis
702.19 Other seborrheic keratosis
709.9 Unspecified disorder of skin and subcutaneous tissue ▽
757.39 Other specified congenital anomaly of skin

ICD-9-CM Procedural

18.29 Excision or destruction of other lesion of external ear
21.32 Local excision or destruction of other lesion of nose
86.3 Other local excision or destruction of lesion or tissue of skin and subcutaneous tissue

HCPCS Level II Supplies & Services

A4550 Surgical trays

11400–11406

11400 Excision, benign lesion including margins, except skin tag (unless listed elsewhere), trunk, arms or legs; excised diameter 0.5 cm or less
11401 excised diameter 0.6 to 1.0 cm
11402 excised diameter 1.1 to 2.0 cm
11403 excised diameter 2.1 to 3.0 cm
11404 excised diameter 3.1 to 4.0 cm
11406 excised diameter over 4.0 cm

ICD-9-CM Diagnostic

214.1 Lipoma of other skin and subcutaneous tissue
216.5 Benign neoplasm of skin of trunk, except scrotum
216.6 Benign neoplasm of skin of upper limb, including shoulder
216.7 Benign neoplasm of skin of lower limb, including hip
228.01 Hemangioma of skin and subcutaneous tissue
238.2 Neoplasm of uncertain behavior of skin
239.2 Neoplasms of unspecified nature of bone, soft tissue, and skin
448.1 Nevus, non-neoplastic
686.1 Pyogenic granuloma of skin and subcutaneous tissue
701.1 Acquired keratoderma
701.3 Striae atrophicae
701.4 Keloid scar
701.5 Other abnormal granulation tissue
702.11 Inflamed seborrheic keratosis
702.19 Other seborrheic keratosis
706.2 Sebaceous cyst
709.01 Vitiligo
709.09 Other dyschromia
709.1 Vascular disorder of skin
709.2 Scar condition and fibrosis of skin
709.4 Foreign body granuloma of skin and subcutaneous tissue
757.32 Congenital vascular hamartomas

ICD-9-CM Procedural

85.21 Local excision of lesion of breast
86.3 Other local excision or destruction of lesion or tissue of skin and subcutaneous tissue

HCPCS Level II Supplies & Services

A4305 Disposable drug delivery system, flow rate of 50 ml or greater per hour
A4306 Disposable drug delivery system, flow rate of 5 ml or less per hour
A4550 Surgical trays

11420–11426

11420 Excision, benign lesion including margins, except skin tag (unless listed elsewhere), scalp, neck, hands, feet, genitalia; excised diameter 0.5 cm or less
11421 excised diameter 0.6 to 1.0 cm
11422 excised diameter 1.1 to 2.0 cm
11423 excised diameter 2.1 to 3.0 cm
11424 excised diameter 3.1 to 4.0 cm
11426 excised diameter over 4.0 cm

ICD-9-CM Diagnostic

214.1 Lipoma of other skin and subcutaneous tissue
216.4 Benign neoplasm of scalp and skin of neck
216.6 Benign neoplasm of skin of upper limb, including shoulder
216.7 Benign neoplasm of skin of lower limb, including hip
216.8 Benign neoplasm of other specified sites of skin
221.2 Benign neoplasm of vulva ♀
221.8 Benign neoplasm of other specified sites of female genital organs ♀
221.9 Benign neoplasm of female genital organ, site unspecified ▽ ♀
222.1 Benign neoplasm of penis ♂

▽ Unspecified code ♀ Female diagnosis ☒ Manifestation code ♂ Male diagnosis

222.4 Benign neoplasm of scrotum ♂
222.9 Benign neoplasm of male genital organ, site unspecified ▽ ♂
228.01 Hemangioma of skin and subcutaneous tissue
236.3 Neoplasm of uncertain behavior of other and unspecified female genital organs ▽ ♀
236.6 Neoplasm of uncertain behavior of other and unspecified male genital organs ▽ ♂
238.2 Neoplasm of uncertain behavior of skin
239.2 Neoplasms of unspecified nature of bone, soft tissue, and skin
448.1 Nevus, non-neoplastic
614.6 Pelvic peritoneal adhesions, female (postoperative) (postinfection) — (Use additional code to identify any associated infertility, 628.2. Use additional code to identify organism: 041.0, 041.1) ♀
624.4 Old laceration or scarring of vulva ♀
686.1 Pyogenic granuloma of skin and subcutaneous tissue
686.9 Unspecified local infection of skin and subcutaneous tissue ▽
700 Corns and callosities
701.1 Acquired keratoderma
701.4 Keloid scar
701.5 Other abnormal granulation tissue
701.8 Other specified hypertrophic and atrophic condition of skin
702.0 Actinic keratosis
702.11 Inflamed seborrheic keratosis
702.19 Other seborrheic keratosis
702.8 Other specified dermatoses
706.2 Sebaceous cyst
709.00 Dyschromia, unspecified ▽
709.01 Vitiligo
709.09 Other dyschromia
709.1 Vascular disorder of skin
709.2 Scar condition and fibrosis of skin
709.4 Foreign body granuloma of skin and subcutaneous tissue
709.9 Unspecified disorder of skin and subcutaneous tissue ▽
757.32 Congenital vascular hamartomas
757.33 Congenital pigmentary anomaly of skin
757.39 Other specified congenital anomaly of skin
782.2 Localized superficial swelling, mass, or lump

ICD-9-CM Procedural

61.3 Excision or destruction of lesion or tissue of scrotum
64.2 Local excision or destruction of lesion of penis
71.3 Other local excision or destruction of vulva and perineum
86.3 Other local excision or destruction of lesion or tissue of skin and subcutaneous tissue

HCPCS Level II Supplies & Services

A4305 Disposable drug delivery system, flow rate of 50 ml or greater per hour
A4306 Disposable drug delivery system, flow rate of 5 ml or less per hour
A4550 Surgical trays

11440–11446

11440 Excision, other benign lesion including margins (unless listed elsewhere), face, ears, eyelids, nose, lips, mucous membrane; excised diameter 0.5 cm or less
11441 excised diameter 0.6 to 1.0 cm
11442 excised diameter 1.1 to 2.0 cm
11443 excised diameter 2.1 to 3.0 cm
11444 excised diameter 3.1 to 4.0 cm
11446 excised diameter over 4.0 cm

ICD-9-CM Diagnostic

210.0 Benign neoplasm of lip
214.0 Lipoma of skin and subcutaneous tissue of face
214.1 Lipoma of other skin and subcutaneous tissue
215.0 Other benign neoplasm of connective and other soft tissue of head, face, and neck
216.0 Benign neoplasm of skin of lip
216.2 Benign neoplasm of ear and external auditory canal
216.3 Benign neoplasm of skin of other and unspecified parts of face ▽
228.01 Hemangioma of skin and subcutaneous tissue
238.1 Neoplasm of uncertain behavior of connective and other soft tissue ▽
238.2 Neoplasm of uncertain behavior of skin
239.2 Neoplasms of unspecified nature of bone, soft tissue, and skin
448.1 Nevus, non-neoplastic
528.79 Other disturbances of oral epithelium, including tongue
686.1 Pyogenic granuloma of skin and subcutaneous tissue
701.1 Acquired keratoderma
701.4 Keloid scar
701.5 Other abnormal granulation tissue
701.8 Other specified hypertrophic and atrophic condition of skin
702.0 Actinic keratosis
702.11 Inflamed seborrheic keratosis
702.19 Other seborrheic keratosis
706.2 Sebaceous cyst
709.2 Scar condition and fibrosis of skin
709.4 Foreign body granuloma of skin and subcutaneous tissue
757.32 Congenital vascular hamartomas
757.33 Congenital pigmentary anomaly of skin
757.39 Other specified congenital anomaly of skin

ICD-9-CM Procedural

08.20 Removal of lesion of eyelid, not otherwise specified
08.23 Excision of major lesion of eyelid, partial-thickness
18.29 Excision or destruction of other lesion of external ear
21.30 Excision or destruction of lesion of nose, not otherwise specified
21.32 Local excision or destruction of other lesion of nose
27.43 Other excision of lesion or tissue of lip
86.3 Other local excision or destruction of lesion or tissue of skin and subcutaneous tissue

HCPCS Level II Supplies & Services

A4305 Disposable drug delivery system, flow rate of 50 ml or greater per hour
A4306 Disposable drug delivery system, flow rate of 5 ml or less per hour
A4550 Surgical trays

11450–11471

11450 Excision of skin and subcutaneous tissue for hidradenitis, axillary; with simple or intermediate repair
11451 with complex repair
11462 Excision of skin and subcutaneous tissue for hidradenitis, inguinal; with simple or intermediate repair
11463 with complex repair
11470 Excision of skin and subcutaneous tissue for hidradenitis, perianal, perineal, or umbilical; with simple or intermediate repair
11471 with complex repair

ICD-9-CM Diagnostic

705.83 Hidradenitis

ICD-9-CM Procedural

86.3 Other local excision or destruction of lesion or tissue of skin and subcutaneous tissue

HCPCS Level II Supplies & Services

A4305 Disposable drug delivery system, flow rate of 50 ml or greater per hour
A4306 Disposable drug delivery system, flow rate of 5 ml or less per hour
A4550 Surgical trays

11600–11606

11600 Excision, malignant lesion including margins, trunk, arms, or legs; excised diameter 0.5 cm or less
11601 excised diameter 0.6 to 1.0 cm
11602 excised diameter 1.1 to 2.0 cm
11603 excised diameter 2.1 to 3.0 cm
11604 excised diameter 3.1 to 4.0 cm
11606 excised diameter over 4.0 cm

ICD-9-CM Diagnostic

172.5 Malignant melanoma of skin of trunk, except scrotum
172.6 Malignant melanoma of skin of upper limb, including shoulder
172.7 Malignant melanoma of skin of lower limb, including hip
172.8 Malignant melanoma of other specified sites of skin
173.5 Other malignant neoplasm of skin of trunk, except scrotum
173.6 Other malignant neoplasm of skin of upper limb, including shoulder
173.7 Other malignant neoplasm of skin of lower limb, including hip
173.8 Other malignant neoplasm of other specified sites of skin
195.4 Malignant neoplasm of upper limb
198.2 Secondary malignant neoplasm of skin
232.5 Carcinoma in situ of skin of trunk, except scrotum
232.6 Carcinoma in situ of skin of upper limb, including shoulder
232.7 Carcinoma in situ of skin of lower limb, including hip
238.2 Neoplasm of uncertain behavior of skin

▽ Unspecified code
♀ Female diagnosis
☒ Manifestation code
♂ Male diagnosis

ICD-9-CM Procedural
85.21 Local excision of lesion of breast
86.3 Other local excision or destruction of lesion or tissue of skin and subcutaneous tissue

HCPCS Level II Supplies & Services
A4305 Disposable drug delivery system, flow rate of 50 ml or greater per hour
A4306 Disposable drug delivery system, flow rate of 5 ml or less per hour
A4550 Surgical trays

11620–11626
11620 Excision, malignant lesion including margins, scalp, neck, hands, feet, genitalia; excised diameter 0.5 cm or less
11621 excised diameter 0.6 to 1.0 cm
11622 excised diameter 1.1 to 2.0 cm
11623 excised diameter 2.1 to 3.0 cm
11624 excised diameter 3.1 to 4.0 cm
11626 excised diameter over 4.0 cm

ICD-9-CM Diagnostic
171.6 Malignant neoplasm of connective and other soft tissue of pelvis
171.8 Malignant neoplasm of other specified sites of connective and other soft tissue
172.4 Malignant melanoma of skin of scalp and neck
172.6 Malignant melanoma of skin of upper limb, including shoulder
172.7 Malignant melanoma of skin of lower limb, including hip
172.8 Malignant melanoma of other specified sites of skin
173.4 Other malignant neoplasm of scalp and skin of neck
173.5 Other malignant neoplasm of skin of trunk, except scrotum
173.6 Other malignant neoplasm of skin of upper limb, including shoulder
173.7 Other malignant neoplasm of skin of lower limb, including hip
184.0 Malignant neoplasm of vagina ♀
184.1 Malignant neoplasm of labia majora ♀
184.2 Malignant neoplasm of labia minora ♀
184.3 Malignant neoplasm of clitoris ♀
184.4 Malignant neoplasm of vulva, unspecified site ▽ ♀
184.8 Malignant neoplasm of other specified sites of female genital organs ♀
187.1 Malignant neoplasm of prepuce ♂
187.2 Malignant neoplasm of glans penis ♂
187.3 Malignant neoplasm of body of penis ♂
187.4 Malignant neoplasm of penis, part unspecified ▽ ♂
187.7 Malignant neoplasm of scrotum ♂
187.8 Malignant neoplasm of other specified sites of male genital organs ♂
195.4 Malignant neoplasm of upper limb
195.5 Malignant neoplasm of lower limb
198.2 Secondary malignant neoplasm of skin
198.82 Secondary malignant neoplasm of genital organs
232.4 Carcinoma in situ of scalp and skin of neck
232.6 Carcinoma in situ of skin of upper limb, including shoulder
232.7 Carcinoma in situ of skin of lower limb, including hip
232.8 Carcinoma in situ of other specified sites of skin
233.3 Carcinoma in situ of other and unspecified female genital organs ▽ ♀
233.5 Carcinoma in situ of penis ♂
233.6 Carcinoma in situ of other and unspecified male genital organs ▽ ♂
236.3 Neoplasm of uncertain behavior of other and unspecified female genital organs ▽ ♀
236.6 Neoplasm of uncertain behavior of other and unspecified male genital organs ▽ ♂

ICD-9-CM Procedural
61.3 Excision or destruction of lesion or tissue of scrotum
64.2 Local excision or destruction of lesion of penis
71.3 Other local excision or destruction of vulva and perineum
86.3 Other local excision or destruction of lesion or tissue of skin and subcutaneous tissue

HCPCS Level II Supplies & Services
A4305 Disposable drug delivery system, flow rate of 50 ml or greater per hour
A4306 Disposable drug delivery system, flow rate of 5 ml or less per hour
A4550 Surgical trays

11640–11646
11640 Excision, malignant lesion including margins, face, ears, eyelids, nose, lips; excised diameter 0.5 cm or less
11641 excised diameter 0.6 to 1.0 cm
11642 excised diameter 1.1 to 2.0 cm
11643 excised diameter 2.1 to 3.0 cm
11644 excised diameter 3.1 to 4.0 cm
11646 excised diameter over 4.0 cm

ICD-9-CM Diagnostic
140.0 Malignant neoplasm of upper lip, vermilion border
140.1 Malignant neoplasm of lower lip, vermilion border
140.3 Malignant neoplasm of upper lip, inner aspect
140.4 Malignant neoplasm of lower lip, inner aspect
140.8 Malignant neoplasm of other sites of lip
140.9 Malignant neoplasm of lip, vermilion border, unspecified as to upper or lower ▽
171.0 Malignant neoplasm of connective and other soft tissue of head, face, and neck
172.0 Malignant melanoma of skin of lip
172.1 Malignant melanoma of skin of eyelid, including canthus
172.2 Malignant melanoma of skin of ear and external auditory canal
172.3 Malignant melanoma of skin of other and unspecified parts of face
173.0 Other malignant neoplasm of skin of lip
173.1 Other malignant neoplasm of skin of eyelid, including canthus
173.2 Other malignant neoplasm of skin of ear and external auditory canal
173.3 Other malignant neoplasm of skin of other and unspecified parts of face ▽
173.8 Other malignant neoplasm of other specified sites of skin
195.0 Malignant neoplasm of head, face, and neck
198.2 Secondary malignant neoplasm of skin
198.89 Secondary malignant neoplasm of other specified sites
230.0 Carcinoma in situ of lip, oral cavity, and pharynx
232.0 Carcinoma in situ of skin of lip
232.1 Carcinoma in situ of eyelid, including canthus
232.2 Carcinoma in situ of skin of ear and external auditory canal
232.3 Carcinoma in situ of skin of other and unspecified parts of face ▽
235.1 Neoplasm of uncertain behavior of lip, oral cavity, and pharynx
238.2 Neoplasm of uncertain behavior of skin
V84.09 Genetic susceptibility to other malignant neoplasm

ICD-9-CM Procedural
08.20 Removal of lesion of eyelid, not otherwise specified
08.23 Excision of major lesion of eyelid, partial-thickness
08.24 Excision of major lesion of eyelid, full-thickness
18.29 Excision or destruction of other lesion of external ear
21.30 Excision or destruction of lesion of nose, not otherwise specified
21.32 Local excision or destruction of other lesion of nose
27.42 Wide excision of lesion of lip
27.43 Other excision of lesion or tissue of lip
86.3 Other local excision or destruction of lesion or tissue of skin and subcutaneous tissue

HCPCS Level II Supplies & Services
A4305 Disposable drug delivery system, flow rate of 50 ml or greater per hour
A4306 Disposable drug delivery system, flow rate of 5 ml or less per hour
A4550 Surgical trays

Nails

11719
11719 Trimming of nondystrophic nails, any number

ICD-9-CM Diagnostic
250.00 Diabetes mellitus without mention of complication, type II or unspecified type, not stated as uncontrolled
250.01 Diabetes mellitus without mention of complication, type I [juvenile type], not stated as uncontrolled
250.02 Diabetes mellitus without mention of complication, type II or unspecified type, uncontrolled
250.03 Diabetes mellitus without mention of complication, type I [juvenile type], uncontrolled
278.01 Morbid obesity — (Use additional code to identify any associated mental retardation)
342.01 Flacid hemiplegia affecting dominant side
342.11 Spastic hemiplegia affecting dominant side

342.81 Other specified hemiplegia affecting dominant side
342.91 Unspecified hemiplegia affecting dominant side ▽
344.00 Unspecified quadriplegia ▽
344.01 Quadriplegia and quadriparesis, C1-C4, complete
344.02 Quadriplegia and quadriparesis, C1-C4, incomplete
344.03 Quadriplegia and quadriparesis, C5-C7, complete
344.04 C5-C7, incomplete
344.09 Other quadriplegia and quadriparesis
344.1 Paraplegia
344.2 Diplegia of upper limbs
344.41 Monoplegia of upper limb affecting dominant side
438.20 Hemiplegia affecting unspecified side due to cerebrovascular disease — (Use additional code to identify presence of hypertension) ▽
438.31 Monoplegia of upper limb affecting dominant side due to cerebrovascular disease — (Use additional code to identify presence of hypertension)
438.51 Other paralytic syndrome affecting dominant side due to cerebrovascular disease — (Use additional code to identify type of paralytic syndrome: 344.81, 344.00-344.09. Use additional code to identify presence of hypertension)
438.84 Ataxia as late effect of cerebrovascular disease — (Use additional code to identify presence of hypertension)

ICD-9-CM Procedural

89.01 Interview and evaluation, described as brief

HCPCS Level II Supplies & Services

A4649 Surgical supply; miscellaneous
S0390 Routine foot care; removal and/or trimming of corns, calluses and/or nails and preventive maintenance in specific medical conditions (e.g., diabetes), per visit

11720–11721

11720 Debridement of nail(s) by any method(s); one to five
11721 six or more

ICD-9-CM Diagnostic

250.70 Diabetes with peripheral circulatory disorders, type II or unspecified type, not stated as uncontrolled — (Use additional code to identify manifestation: 443.81, 785.4)
250.71 Diabetes with peripheral circulatory disorders, type I [juvenile type], not stated as uncontrolled — (Use additional code to identify manifestation: 443.81, 785.4)
250.72 Diabetes with peripheral circulatory disorders, type II or unspecified type, uncontrolled — (Use additional code to identify manifestation: 443.81, 785.4)
250.73 Diabetes with peripheral circulatory disorders, type I [juvenile type], uncontrolled — (Use additional code to identify manifestation: 443.81, 785.4)
443.81 Peripheral angiopathy in diseases classified elsewhere — (Code first underlying disease, 250.7) ☒
443.89 Other peripheral vascular disease
681.00 Unspecified cellulitis and abscess of finger — (Use additional code to identify organism) ▽
681.02 Onychia and paronychia of finger — (Use additional code to identify organism)
681.10 Unspecified cellulitis and abscess of toe — (Use additional code to identify organism) ▽
681.11 Onychia and paronychia of toe — (Use additional code to identify organism)
681.9 Cellulitis and abscess of unspecified digit — (Use additional code to identify organism) ▽
703.8 Other specified disease of nail
991.1 Frostbite of hand
991.2 Frostbite of foot

ICD-9-CM Procedural

86.27 Debridement of nail, nail bed, or nail fold

HCPCS Level II Supplies & Services

A4649 Surgical supply; miscellaneous

11730–11732

11730 Avulsion of nail plate, partial or complete, simple; single
11732 each additional nail plate (List separately in addition to code for primary procedure)

ICD-9-CM Diagnostic

250.70 Diabetes with peripheral circulatory disorders, type II or unspecified type, not stated as uncontrolled — (Use additional code to identify manifestation: 443.81, 785.4)
250.71 Diabetes with peripheral circulatory disorders, type I [juvenile type], not stated as uncontrolled — (Use additional code to identify manifestation: 443.81, 785.4)
250.72 Diabetes with peripheral circulatory disorders, type II or unspecified type, uncontrolled — (Use additional code to identify manifestation: 443.81, 785.4)
250.73 Diabetes with peripheral circulatory disorders, type I [juvenile type], uncontrolled — (Use additional code to identify manifestation: 443.81, 785.4)
443.81 Peripheral angiopathy in diseases classified elsewhere — (Code first underlying disease, 250.7) ☒
443.89 Other peripheral vascular disease
681.00 Unspecified cellulitis and abscess of finger — (Use additional code to identify organism) ▽
681.02 Onychia and paronychia of finger — (Use additional code to identify organism)
681.10 Unspecified cellulitis and abscess of toe — (Use additional code to identify organism) ▽
681.11 Onychia and paronychia of toe — (Use additional code to identify organism)
681.9 Cellulitis and abscess of unspecified digit — (Use additional code to identify organism) ▽
682.8 Cellulitis and abscess of other specified site — (Use additional code to identify organism)
703.0 Ingrowing nail
703.8 Other specified disease of nail
757.5 Specified congenital anomalies of nails
785.4 Gangrene — (Code first any associated underlying condition:250.7, 443.0)
816.02 Closed fracture of distal phalanx or phalanges of hand
816.03 Closed fracture of multiple sites of phalanx or phalanges of hand
816.12 Open fracture of distal phalanx or phalanges of hand
816.13 Open fractures of multiple sites of phalanx or phalanges of hand
826.0 Closed fracture of one or more phalanges of foot
826.1 Open fracture of one or more phalanges of foot
883.0 Open wound of finger(s), without mention of complication — (Use additional code to identify infection)
883.1 Open wound of finger(s), complicated — (Use additional code to identify infection)
883.2 Open wound of finger(s), with tendon involvement — (Use additional code to identify infection)
893.0 Open wound of toe(s), without mention of complication — (Use additional code to identify infection)
893.1 Open wound of toe(s), complicated — (Use additional code to identify infection)
893.2 Open wound of toe(s), with tendon involvement — (Use additional code to identify infection)
923.3 Contusion of finger
924.3 Contusion of toe
927.3 Crushing injury of finger(s) — (Use additional code to identify any associated injuries: 800-829, 850.0-854.1, 860.0-869.1)
928.3 Crushing injury of toe(s) — (Use additional code to identify any associated injuries: 800-829, 850.0-854.1, 860.0-869.1)
991.1 Frostbite of hand
991.2 Frostbite of foot

ICD-9-CM Procedural

86.23 Removal of nail, nailbed, or nail fold

HCPCS Level II Supplies & Services

A4550 Surgical trays

11740

11740 Evacuation of subungual hematoma

ICD-9-CM Diagnostic

816.02 Closed fracture of distal phalanx or phalanges of hand
816.03 Closed fracture of multiple sites of phalanx or phalanges of hand
816.12 Open fracture of distal phalanx or phalanges of hand
816.13 Open fractures of multiple sites of phalanx or phalanges of hand
826.0 Closed fracture of one or more phalanges of foot
826.1 Open fracture of one or more phalanges of foot
883.0 Open wound of finger(s), without mention of complication — (Use additional code to identify infection)
883.1 Open wound of finger(s), complicated — (Use additional code to identify infection)
893.0 Open wound of toe(s), without mention of complication — (Use additional code to identify infection)
893.1 Open wound of toe(s), complicated — (Use additional code to identify infection)

893.2 Open wound of toe(s), with tendon involvement — (Use additional code to identify infection)
923.20 Contusion of hand(s)
923.3 Contusion of finger
924.3 Contusion of toe
927.3 Crushing injury of finger(s) — (Use additional code to identify any associated injuries: 800-829, 850.0-854.1, 860.0-869.1)
928.3 Crushing injury of toe(s) — (Use additional code to identify any associated injuries: 800-829, 850.0-854.1, 860.0-869.1)
959.5 Injury, other and unspecified, finger
959.7 Injury, other and unspecified, knee, leg, ankle, and foot
998.12 Hematoma complicating a procedure

ICD-9-CM Procedural
86.04 Other incision with drainage of skin and subcutaneous tissue

HCPCS Level II Supplies & Services
A4649 Surgical supply; miscellaneous

11750–11752
11750 Excision of nail and nail matrix, partial or complete, (eg, ingrown or deformed nail) for permanent removal;
11752 with amputation of tuft of distal phalanx

ICD-9-CM Diagnostic
250.00 Diabetes mellitus without mention of complication, type II or unspecified type, not stated as uncontrolled
250.01 Diabetes mellitus without mention of complication, type I [juvenile type], not stated as uncontrolled
250.02 Diabetes mellitus without mention of complication, type II or unspecified type, uncontrolled
250.03 Diabetes mellitus without mention of complication, type I [juvenile type], uncontrolled
250.70 Diabetes with peripheral circulatory disorders, type II or unspecified type, not stated as uncontrolled — (Use additional code to identify manifestation: 443.81, 785.4)
250.71 Diabetes with peripheral circulatory disorders, type I [juvenile type], not stated as uncontrolled — (Use additional code to identify manifestation: 443.81, 785.4)
250.72 Diabetes with peripheral circulatory disorders, type II or unspecified type, uncontrolled — (Use additional code to identify manifestation: 443.81, 785.4)
250.73 Diabetes with peripheral circulatory disorders, type I [juvenile type], uncontrolled — (Use additional code to identify manifestation: 443.81, 785.4)
443.81 Peripheral angiopathy in diseases classified elsewhere — (Code first underlying disease, 250.7) ☒
681.02 Onychia and paronychia of finger — (Use additional code to identify organism)
681.11 Onychia and paronychia of toe — (Use additional code to identify organism)
703.0 Ingrowing nail
703.8 Other specified disease of nail
785.4 Gangrene — (Code first any associated underlying condition:250.7, 443.0)
883.0 Open wound of finger(s), without mention of complication — (Use additional code to identify infection)
883.1 Open wound of finger(s), complicated — (Use additional code to identify infection)
893.0 Open wound of toe(s), without mention of complication — (Use additional code to identify infection)
893.1 Open wound of toe(s), complicated — (Use additional code to identify infection)
927.3 Crushing injury of finger(s) — (Use additional code to identify any associated injuries: 800-829, 850.0-854.1, 860.0-869.1)
928.3 Crushing injury of toe(s) — (Use additional code to identify any associated injuries: 800-829, 850.0-854.1, 860.0-869.1)

ICD-9-CM Procedural
84.00 Upper limb amputation, not otherwise specified
86.23 Removal of nail, nailbed, or nail fold

HCPCS Level II Supplies & Services
A4305 Disposable drug delivery system, flow rate of 50 ml or greater per hour
A4306 Disposable drug delivery system, flow rate of 5 ml or less per hour
A4550 Surgical trays

11755
11755 Biopsy of nail unit (eg, plate, bed, matrix, hyponychium, proximal and lateral nail folds) (separate procedure)

ICD-9-CM Diagnostic
173.6 Other malignant neoplasm of skin of upper limb, including shoulder
173.7 Other malignant neoplasm of skin of lower limb, including hip
198.2 Secondary malignant neoplasm of skin
216.6 Benign neoplasm of skin of upper limb, including shoulder
216.7 Benign neoplasm of skin of lower limb, including hip
216.9 Benign neoplasm of skin, site unspecified ▽
232.6 Carcinoma in situ of skin of upper limb, including shoulder
232.7 Carcinoma in situ of skin of lower limb, including hip
238.2 Neoplasm of uncertain behavior of skin
239.2 Neoplasms of unspecified nature of bone, soft tissue, and skin
703.8 Other specified disease of nail

ICD-9-CM Procedural
86.11 Biopsy of skin and subcutaneous tissue

HCPCS Level II Supplies & Services
A4550 Surgical trays

11760
11760 Repair of nail bed

ICD-9-CM Diagnostic
816.12 Open fracture of distal phalanx or phalanges of hand
816.13 Open fractures of multiple sites of phalanx or phalanges of hand
826.1 Open fracture of one or more phalanges of foot
883.0 Open wound of finger(s), without mention of complication — (Use additional code to identify infection)
883.1 Open wound of finger(s), complicated — (Use additional code to identify infection)
893.0 Open wound of toe(s), without mention of complication — (Use additional code to identify infection)
893.1 Open wound of toe(s), complicated — (Use additional code to identify infection)
893.2 Open wound of toe(s), with tendon involvement — (Use additional code to identify infection)
927.3 Crushing injury of finger(s) — (Use additional code to identify any associated injuries: 800-829, 850.0-854.1, 860.0-869.1)
928.3 Crushing injury of toe(s) — (Use additional code to identify any associated injuries: 800-829, 850.0-854.1, 860.0-869.1)

ICD-9-CM Procedural
86.86 Onychoplasty

HCPCS Level II Supplies & Services
A4550 Surgical trays

11762
11762 Reconstruction of nail bed with graft

ICD-9-CM Diagnostic
171.2 Malignant neoplasm of connective and other soft tissue of upper limb, including shoulder
171.3 Malignant neoplasm of connective and other soft tissue of lower limb, including hip
172.6 Malignant melanoma of skin of upper limb, including shoulder
172.7 Malignant melanoma of skin of lower limb, including hip
173.6 Other malignant neoplasm of skin of upper limb, including shoulder
173.7 Other malignant neoplasm of skin of lower limb, including hip
232.6 Carcinoma in situ of skin of upper limb, including shoulder
232.7 Carcinoma in situ of skin of lower limb, including hip
757.5 Specified congenital anomalies of nails
816.12 Open fracture of distal phalanx or phalanges of hand
816.13 Open fractures of multiple sites of phalanx or phalanges of hand
826.1 Open fracture of one or more phalanges of foot
883.0 Open wound of finger(s), without mention of complication — (Use additional code to identify infection)
883.1 Open wound of finger(s), complicated — (Use additional code to identify infection)
893.0 Open wound of toe(s), without mention of complication — (Use additional code to identify infection)

▽ Unspecified code ☒ Manifestation code
♀ Female diagnosis ♂ Male diagnosis

893.1 Open wound of toe(s), complicated — (Use additional code to identify infection)
893.2 Open wound of toe(s), with tendon involvement — (Use additional code to identify infection)
906.1 Late effect of open wound of extremities without mention of tendon injury
906.7 Late effect of burn of other extremities
927.3 Crushing injury of finger(s) — (Use additional code to identify any associated injuries: 800-829, 850.0-854.1, 860.0-869.1)
928.3 Crushing injury of toe(s) — (Use additional code to identify any associated injuries: 800-829, 850.0-854.1, 860.0-869.1)
944.01 Burn of unspecified degree of single digit [finger (nail)] other than thumb ▽
944.02 Burn of unspecified degree of thumb (nail) ▽
944.03 Burn of unspecified degree of two or more digits of hand, not including thumb ▽
944.04 Burn of unspecified degree of two or more digits of hand, including thumb ▽
944.20 Blisters with epidermal loss due to burn (second degree) of unspecified site of hand ▽
944.21 Blisters with epidermal loss due to burn (second degree) of single digit [finger (nail)] other than thumb
944.23 Blisters with epidermal loss due to burn (second degree) of two or more digits of hand, not including thumb
944.24 Blisters with epidermal loss due to burn (second degree) of two or more digits of hand including thumb
944.28 Blisters with epidermal loss due to burn (second degree) of multiple sites of wrist(s) and hand(s)
944.30 Full-thickness skin loss due to burn (third degree nos) of unspecified site of hand ▽
944.31 Full-thickness skin loss due to burn (third degree nos) of single digit [finger (nail)] other than thumb
944.32 Full-thickness skin loss due to burn (third degree nos) of thumb (nail)
944.33 Full-thickness skin loss due to burn (third degree nos) of two or more digits of hand, not including thumb
944.34 Full-thickness skin loss due to burn (third degree nos) of two or more digits of hand including thumb
944.38 Full-thickness skin loss due to burn (third degree nos) of multiple sites of wrist(s) and hand(s)
944.41 Deep necrosis of underlying tissues due to burn (deep third degree) of single digit [finger (nail)] other than thumb, without mention of a body part
944.42 Deep necrosis of underlying tissues due to burn (deep third degree) of thumb (nail), without mention of loss of a body part
944.43 Deep necrosis of underlying tissues due to burn (deep third degree) of two or more digits of hand, not including thumb, without mention of a body part
944.44 Deep necrosis of underlying tissues due to burn (deep third degree) of two or more digits of hand including thumb, without mention of a body part
944.48 Deep necrosis of underlying tissues due to burn (deep third degree) of multiple sites of wrist(s) and hand(s), without mention of loss of a body part
945.01 Burn of unspecified degree of toe(s) (nail) ▽

ICD-9-CM Procedural
86.86 Onychoplasty

HCPCS Level II Supplies & Services
A4550 Surgical trays

11765
11765 Wedge excision of skin of nail fold (eg, for ingrown toenail)

ICD-9-CM Diagnostic
681.02 Onychia and paronychia of finger — (Use additional code to identify organism)
681.11 Onychia and paronychia of toe — (Use additional code to identify organism)
686.1 Pyogenic granuloma of skin and subcutaneous tissue
703.0 Ingrowing nail
924.3 Contusion of toe
928.3 Crushing injury of toe(s) — (Use additional code to identify any associated injuries: 800-829, 850.0-854.1, 860.0-869.1)

ICD-9-CM Procedural
86.23 Removal of nail, nailbed, or nail fold

HCPCS Level II Supplies & Services
A4550 Surgical trays

Pilonidal Cyst

11770–11772
11770 Excision of pilonidal cyst or sinus; simple
11771 extensive
11772 complicated

ICD-9-CM Diagnostic
685.0 Pilonidal cyst with abscess
685.1 Pilonidal cyst without mention of abscess

ICD-9-CM Procedural
86.21 Excision of pilonidal cyst or sinus

HCPCS Level II Supplies & Services
A4305 Disposable drug delivery system, flow rate of 50 ml or greater per hour
A4306 Disposable drug delivery system, flow rate of 5 ml or less per hour
A4550 Surgical trays

11900–11901
11900 Injection, intralesional; up to and including seven lesions
11901 more than seven lesions

ICD-9-CM Diagnostic
078.10 Unspecified viral warts ▽
373.12 Hordeolum internum
373.2 Chalazion
692.9 Contact dermatitis and other eczema, due to unspecified cause ▽
695.1 Erythema multiforme
695.2 Erythema nodosum
696.1 Other psoriasis and similar disorders
697.0 Lichen planus
698.3 Lichenification and lichen simplex chronicus
701.4 Keloid scar
706.1 Other acne
709.2 Scar condition and fibrosis of skin

ICD-9-CM Procedural
99.29 Injection or infusion of other therapeutic or prophylactic substance
99.77 Application or administration of adhesion barrier substance

HCPCS Level II Supplies & Services
J3302 Injection, triamcinolone diacetate, per 5 mg
J3303 Injection, triamcinolone hexacetonide, per 5 mg

11920–11922
11920 Tattooing, intradermal introduction of insoluble opaque pigments to correct color defects of skin, including micropigmentation; 6.0 sq. cm or less
11921 6.1 to 20.0 sq. cm
11922 each additional 20.0 sq. cm (List separately in addition to code for primary procedure)

ICD-9-CM Diagnostic
374.53 Hypopigmentation of eyelid
709.00 Dyschromia, unspecified ▽
709.01 Vitiligo
709.09 Other dyschromia
757.33 Congenital pigmentary anomaly of skin
757.6 Specified congenital anomalies of breast
906.0 Late effect of open wound of head, neck, and trunk
906.5 Late effect of burn of eye, face, head, and neck
906.8 Late effect of burns of other specified sites
V10.3 Personal history of malignant neoplasm of breast
V50.1 Other plastic surgery for unacceptable cosmetic appearance
V51 Aftercare involving the use of plastic surgery

ICD-9-CM Procedural
86.02 Injection or tattooing of skin lesion or defect

HCPCS Level II Supplies & Services
The HCPCS Level II code(s) would be the same as the actual procedure performed because these are in-addition-to codes.

▽ Unspecified code
♀ Female diagnosis
☒ Manifestation code
♂ Male diagnosis

11950–11954

11950 Subcutaneous injection of filling material (eg, collagen); 1 cc or less
11951 1.1 to 5.0 cc
11952 5.1 to 10.0 cc
11954 over 10.0 cc

ICD-9-CM Diagnostic

374.89 Other disorders of eyelid
380.32 Acquired deformities of auricle or pinna
528.5 Diseases of lips
611.8 Other specified disorder of breast
701.8 Other specified hypertrophic and atrophic condition of skin
706.1 Other acne
709.2 Scar condition and fibrosis of skin
709.3 Degenerative skin disorder
709.8 Other specified disorder of skin
743.62 Congenital deformity of eyelid
744.3 Unspecified congenital anomaly of ear ▽
744.82 Microcheilia
757.8 Other specified congenital anomalies of the integument
757.9 Unspecified congenital anomaly of the integument ▽
906.0 Late effect of open wound of head, neck, and trunk
906.1 Late effect of open wound of extremities without mention of tendon injury
906.5 Late effect of burn of eye, face, head, and neck
906.6 Late effect of burn of wrist and hand
906.7 Late effect of burn of other extremities
906.8 Late effect of burns of other specified sites
906.9 Late effect of burn of unspecified site ▽
V50.1 Other plastic surgery for unacceptable cosmetic appearance
V51 Aftercare involving the use of plastic surgery

ICD-9-CM Procedural

86.02 Injection or tattooing of skin lesion or defect

HCPCS Level II Supplies & Services

A4649 Surgical supply; miscellaneous

11960–11970

11960 Insertion of tissue expander(s) for other than breast, including subsequent expansion
11970 Replacement of tissue expander with permanent prosthesis

ICD-9-CM Diagnostic

709.2 Scar condition and fibrosis of skin
749.11 Unilateral cleft lip, complete
749.12 Unilateral cleft lip, incomplete
752.40 Unspecified congenital anomaly of cervix, vagina, and external female genitalia ▽ ♀
752.49 Other congenital anomaly of cervix, vagina, and external female genitalia ♀
754.0 Congenital musculoskeletal deformities of skull, face, and jaw
872.00 Open wound of external ear, unspecified site, without mention of complication — (Use additional code to identify infection) ▽
872.01 Open wound of auricle, without mention of complication — (Use additional code to identify infection)
872.10 Open wound of external ear, unspecified site, complicated — (Use additional code to identify infection) ▽
872.11 Open wound of auricle, complicated — (Use additional code to identify infection)
873.0 Open wound of scalp, without mention of complication — (Use additional code to identify infection)
873.1 Open wound of scalp, complicated — (Use additional code to identify infection)
873.20 Open wound of nose, unspecified site, without mention of complication — (Use additional code to identify infection) ▽
873.29 Open wound of nose, multiple sites, without mention of complication — (Use additional code to identify infection)
873.30 Open wound of nose, unspecified site, complicated — (Use additional code to identify infection) ▽
873.39 Open wound of nose, multiple sites, complicated — (Use additional code to identify infection)
873.41 Open wound of cheek, without mention of complication — (Use additional code to identify infection)
873.42 Open wound of forehead, without mention of complication — (Use additional code to identify infection)
873.43 Open wound of lip, without mention of complication — (Use additional code to identify infection)
873.44 Open wound of jaw, without mention of complication — (Use additional code to identify infection)
873.49 Open wound of face, other and multiple sites, without mention of complication — (Use additional code to identify infection)
873.51 Open wound of cheek, complicated — (Use additional code to identify infection)
873.52 Open wound of forehead, complicated — (Use additional code to identify infection)
873.53 Open wound of lip, complicated — (Use additional code to identify infection)
873.54 Open wound of jaw, complicated — (Use additional code to identify infection)
873.59 Open wound of face, other and multiple sites, complicated — (Use additional code to identify infection)
874.8 Open wound of other and unspecified parts of neck, without mention of complication — (Use additional code to identify infection) ▽
906.0 Late effect of open wound of head, neck, and trunk
906.5 Late effect of burn of eye, face, head, and neck
906.6 Late effect of burn of wrist and hand
906.7 Late effect of burn of other extremities
906.8 Late effect of burns of other specified sites
909.2 Late effect of radiation
909.3 Late effect of complications of surgical and medical care
941.30 Full-thickness skin loss due to burn (third degree nos) of unspecified site of face and head ▽
941.31 Full-thickness skin loss due to burn (third degree nos) of ear (any part)
941.32 Full-thickness skin loss due to burn (third degree nos) of eye (with other parts of face, head, and neck)
941.33 Full-thickness skin loss due to burn (third degree nos) of lip(s)
941.34 Full-thickness skin loss due to burn (third degree nos) of chin
941.35 Full-thickness skin loss due to burn (third degree nos) of nose (septum)
941.36 Full-thickness skin loss due to burn (third degree nos) of scalp (any part)
941.38 Full-thickness skin loss due to burn (third degree nos) of neck
941.39 Full-thickness skin loss due to burn (third degree nos) of multiple sites (except with eye) of face, head, and neck
941.40 Deep necrosis of underlying tissues due to burn (deep third degree) of unspecified site of face and head, without mention of loss of a body part ▽
941.41 Deep necrosis of underlying tissues due to burn (deep third degree) of ear (any part), without mention of loss of a body part
941.42 Deep necrosis of underlying tissues due to burn (deep third degree) of eye (with other parts of face, head, and neck), without mention of loss of a body part
941.43 Deep necrosis of underlying tissues due to burn (deep third degree) of lip(s), without mention of loss of a body part
941.44 Deep necrosis of underlying tissues due to burn (deep third degree) of chin, without mention of loss of a body part
941.45 Deep necrosis of underlying tissues due to burn (deep third degree) of nose (septum), without mention of loss of a body part
941.46 Deep necrosis of underlying tissues due to burn (deep third degree) of scalp (any part), without mention of loss of a body part
941.47 Deep necrosis of underlying tissues due to burn (deep third degree) of forehead and cheek, without mention of loss of a body part
941.48 Deep necrosis of underlying tissues due to burn (deep third degree) of neck, without mention of loss of a body part
941.49 Deep necrosis of underlying tissues due to burn (deep third degree) of multiple sites (except with eye) of face, head, and neck, without mention of loss of a body part
941.50 Deep necrosis of underlying tissues due to burn (deep third degree) of face and head, unspecified site, with loss of a body part ▽
941.51 Deep necrosis of underlying tissues due to burn (deep third degree) of ear (any part), with loss of a body part
941.52 Deep necrosis of underlying tissues due to burn (deep third degree) of eye (with other parts of face, head, and neck), with loss of a body part
941.53 Deep necrosis of underlying tissues due to burn (deep third degree) of lip(s), with loss of a body part
941.54 Deep necrosis of underlying tissues due to burn (deep third degree) of chin, with loss of a body part
941.55 Deep necrosis of underlying tissues due to burn (deep third degree) of nose (septum), with loss of a body part
941.56 Deep necrosis of underlying tissues due to burn (deep third degree) of scalp (any part), with loss of a body part
941.57 Deep necrosis of underlying tissues due to burn (deep third degree) of forehead and cheek, with loss of a body part
941.58 Deep necrosis of underlying tissues due to burn (deep third degree) of neck, with loss of a body part
941.59 Deep necrosis of underlying tissues due to burn (deep third degree) of multiple sites (except eye) of face, head, and neck, with loss of a body part

943.30 Full-thickness skin loss due to burn (third degree nos) of unspecified site of upper limb
943.31 Full-thickness skin loss due to burn (third degree nos) of forearm
943.32 Full-thickness skin loss due to burn (third degree nos) of elbow
943.39 Full-thickness skin loss due to burn (third degree nos) of multiple sites of upper limb, except wrist and hand
943.50 Deep necrosis of underlying tissues due to burn (deep third degree) of unspecified site of upper limb, with loss of a body part
943.51 Deep necrosis of underlying tissues due to burn (deep third degree) of forearm, with loss of a body part
943.52 Deep necrosis of underlying tissues due to burn (deep third degree) of elbow, with loss of a body part
943.53 Deep necrosis of underlying tissues due to burn (deep third degree) of upper arm, with loss of upper a body part
943.59 Deep necrosis of underlying tissues due to burn (deep third degree) of multiple sites of upper limb, except wrist and hand, with loss of a body part
945.30 Full-thickness skin loss due to burn (third degree nos) of unspecified site of lower limb
945.34 Full-thickness skin loss due to burn (third degree nos) of lower leg
945.35 Full-thickness skin loss due to burn (third degree nos) of knee
945.36 Full-thickness skin loss due to burn (third degree nos) of thigh (any part)
945.39 Full-thickness skin loss due to burn (third degree nos) of multiple sites of lower limb(s)
945.40 Deep necrosis of underlying tissues due to burn (deep third degree) of unspecified site of lower limb (leg), without mention of loss of a body part
945.44 Deep necrosis of underlying tissues due to burn (deep third degree) of lower leg, without mention of loss of a body part
945.45 Deep necrosis of underlying tissues due to burn (deep third degree) of knee, without mention of loss of a body part
945.46 Deep necrosis of underlying tissues due to burn (deep third degree) of thigh (any part), without mention of loss of a body part
945.49 Deep necrosis of underlying tissues due to burn (deep third degree) of multiple sites of lower limb(s), without mention of loss of a body part
945.50 Deep necrosis of underlying tissues due to burn (deep third degree) of unspecified site lower limb (leg), with loss of a body part
945.52 Deep necrosis of underlying tissues due to burn (deep third degree) of foot, with loss of a body part
945.53 Deep necrosis of underlying tissues due to burn (deep third degree) of ankle, with loss of a body part
945.54 Deep necrosis of underlying tissues due to burn (deep third degree) of lower leg, with loss of a body part
945.55 Deep necrosis of underlying tissues due to burn (deep third degree) of knee, with loss of a body part
945.56 Deep necrosis of underlying tissues due to burn (deep third degree) of thigh (any part), with loss of a body part
945.59 Deep necrosis of underlying tissues due to burn (deep third degree) of multiple sites of lower limb(s), with loss of a body part
946.3 Full-thickness skin loss due to burn (third degree nos) of multiple specified sites
946.4 Deep necrosis of underlying tissues due to burn (deep third degree) of multiple specified sites, without mention of loss of a body part
946.5 Deep necrosis of underlying tissues due to burn (deep third degree) of multiple specified sites, with loss of a body part
997.60 Late complications of amputation stump, unspecified — (Use additional code to identify complications)
997.62 Infection (chronic) of amputation stump — (Use additional code to identify organism. Use additional code to identify complications)
997.69 Other late amputation stump complication — (Use additional code to identify complications)
V10.82 Personal history of malignant melanoma of skin
V10.83 Personal history of other malignant neoplasm of skin
V50.1 Other plastic surgery for unacceptable cosmetic appearance
V51 Aftercare involving the use of plastic surgery

ICD-9-CM Procedural

86.93 Insertion of tissue expander

HCPCS Level II Supplies & Services

A4280 Adhesive skin support attachment for use with external breast prosthesis, each
A4305 Disposable drug delivery system, flow rate of 50 ml or greater per hour
A4306 Disposable drug delivery system, flow rate of 5 ml or less per hour
A4550 Surgical trays
A4649 Surgical supply; miscellaneous

11971

11971 Removal of tissue expander(s) without insertion of prosthesis

ICD-9-CM Diagnostic

709.2 Scar condition and fibrosis of skin
872.00 Open wound of external ear, unspecified site, without mention of complication — (Use additional code to identify infection)
872.01 Open wound of auricle, without mention of complication — (Use additional code to identify infection)
872.10 Open wound of external ear, unspecified site, complicated — (Use additional code to identify infection)
872.11 Open wound of auricle, complicated — (Use additional code to identify infection)
873.0 Open wound of scalp, without mention of complication — (Use additional code to identify infection)
873.1 Open wound of scalp, complicated — (Use additional code to identify infection)
873.20 Open wound of nose, unspecified site, without mention of complication — (Use additional code to identify infection)
873.29 Open wound of nose, multiple sites, without mention of complication — (Use additional code to identify infection)
873.30 Open wound of nose, unspecified site, complicated — (Use additional code to identify infection)
873.39 Open wound of nose, multiple sites, complicated — (Use additional code to identify infection)
873.41 Open wound of cheek, without mention of complication — (Use additional code to identify infection)
873.42 Open wound of forehead, without mention of complication — (Use additional code to identify infection)
873.43 Open wound of lip, without mention of complication — (Use additional code to identify infection)
873.44 Open wound of jaw, without mention of complication — (Use additional code to identify infection)
873.49 Open wound of face, other and multiple sites, without mention of complication — (Use additional code to identify infection)
873.51 Open wound of cheek, complicated — (Use additional code to identify infection)
873.52 Open wound of forehead, complicated — (Use additional code to identify infection)
873.53 Open wound of lip, complicated — (Use additional code to identify infection)
873.54 Open wound of jaw, complicated — (Use additional code to identify infection)
873.59 Open wound of face, other and multiple sites, complicated — (Use additional code to identify infection)
874.8 Open wound of other and unspecified parts of neck, without mention of complication — (Use additional code to identify infection)
906.0 Late effect of open wound of head, neck, and trunk
906.5 Late effect of burn of eye, face, head, and neck
906.6 Late effect of burn of wrist and hand
906.7 Late effect of burn of other extremities
941.30 Full-thickness skin loss due to burn (third degree nos) of unspecified site of face and head
941.31 Full-thickness skin loss due to burn (third degree nos) of ear (any part)
941.32 Full-thickness skin loss due to burn (third degree nos) of eye (with other parts of face, head, and neck)
941.33 Full-thickness skin loss due to burn (third degree nos) of lip(s)
941.34 Full-thickness skin loss due to burn (third degree nos) of chin
941.35 Full-thickness skin loss due to burn (third degree nos) of nose (septum)
941.36 Full-thickness skin loss due to burn (third degree nos) of scalp (any part)
941.38 Full-thickness skin loss due to burn (third degree nos) of neck
941.39 Full-thickness skin loss due to burn (third degree nos) of multiple sites (except with eye) of face, head, and neck
941.40 Deep necrosis of underlying tissues due to burn (deep third degree) of unspecified site of face and head, without mention of loss of a body part
941.41 Deep necrosis of underlying tissues due to burn (deep third degree) of ear (any part), without mention of loss of a body part
941.42 Deep necrosis of underlying tissues due to burn (deep third degree) of eye (with other parts of face, head, and neck), without mention of loss of a body part
941.43 Deep necrosis of underlying tissues due to burn (deep third degree) of lip(s), without mention of loss of a body part
941.44 Deep necrosis of underlying tissues due to burn (deep third degree) of chin, without mention of loss of a body part
941.45 Deep necrosis of underlying tissues due to burn (deep third degree) of nose (septum), without mention of loss of a body part
941.46 Deep necrosis of underlying tissues due to burn (deep third degree) of scalp (any part), without mention of loss of a body part

941.47 Deep necrosis of underlying tissues due to burn (deep third degree) of forehead and cheek, without mention of loss of a body part
941.48 Deep necrosis of underlying tissues due to burn (deep third degree) of neck, without mention of loss of a body part
941.49 Deep necrosis of underlying tissues due to burn (deep third degree) of multiple sites (except with eye) of face, head, and neck, without mention of loss of a body part
941.50 Deep necrosis of underlying tissues due to burn (deep third degree) of face and head, unspecified site, with loss of a body part ▽
941.51 Deep necrosis of underlying tissues due to burn (deep third degree) of ear (any part), with loss of a body part
941.52 Deep necrosis of underlying tissues due to burn (deep third degree) of eye (with other parts of face, head, and neck), with loss of a body part
941.53 Deep necrosis of underlying tissues due to burn (deep third degree) of lip(s), with loss of a body part
941.54 Deep necrosis of underlying tissues due to burn (deep third degree) of chin, with loss of a body part
941.55 Deep necrosis of underlying tissues due to burn (deep third degree) of nose (septum), with loss of a body part
941.56 Deep necrosis of underlying tissues due to burn (deep third degree) of scalp (any part), with loss of a body part
941.57 Deep necrosis of underlying tissues due to burn (deep third degree) of forehead and cheek, with loss of a body part
941.58 Deep necrosis of underlying tissues due to burn (deep third degree) of neck, with loss of a body part
941.59 Deep necrosis of underlying tissues due to burn (deep third degree) of multiple sites (except eye) of face, head, and neck, with loss of a body part
942.30 Full-thickness skin loss due to burn (third degree nos) of unspecified site of trunk ▽
942.32 Full-thickness skin loss due to burn (third degree nos) of chest wall, excluding breast and nipple
942.33 Full-thickness skin loss due to burn (third degree nos) of abdominal wall
942.34 Full-thickness skin loss due to burn (third degree nos) of back (any part)
942.35 Full-thickness skin loss due to burn (third degree nos) of genitalia
942.39 Full-thickness skin loss due to burn (third degree nos) of other and multiple sites of trunk
942.40 Deep necrosis of underlying tissues due to burn (deep third degree) of trunk, unspecified site, without mention of loss of a body part ▽
942.42 Deep necrosis of underlying tissues due to burn (deep third degree) of chest wall, excluding breast and nipple, without mention of loss of a body part
942.43 Deep necrosis of underlying tissues due to burn (deep third degree) of abdominal wall, without mention of loss of a body part
942.44 Deep necrosis of underlying tissues due to burn (deep third degree) of back (any part), without mention of loss of a body part
942.45 Deep necrosis of underlying tissues due to burn (deep third degree) of genitalia, without mention of loss of a body part
942.49 Deep necrosis of underlying tissues due to burn (deep third degree) of other and multiple sites of trunk, without mention of loss of a body part
942.50 Deep necrosis of underlying tissues due to burn (deep third degree) of unspecified site of trunk, with loss of a body part ▽
942.52 Deep necrosis of underlying tissues due to burn (deep third degree) of chest wall, excluding breast and nipple, with loss of a body part
942.53 Deep necrosis of underlying tissues due to burn (deep third degree) of abdominal wall with loss of a body part
942.54 Deep necrosis of underlying tissues due to burn (deep third degree) of back (any part), with loss of a body part
942.55 Deep necrosis of underlying tissues due to burn (deep third degree) of genitalia, with loss of a body part
942.59 Deep necrosis of underlying tissues due to burn (deep third degree) of other and multiple sites of trunk, with loss of a body part
943.30 Full-thickness skin loss due to burn (third degree nos) of unspecified site of upper limb ▽
943.31 Full-thickness skin loss due to burn (third degree nos) of forearm
943.32 Full-thickness skin loss due to burn (third degree nos) of elbow
943.39 Full-thickness skin loss due to burn (third degree nos) of multiple sites of upper limb, except wrist and hand
943.50 Deep necrosis of underlying tissues due to burn (deep third degree) of unspecified site of upper limb, with loss of a body part ▽
943.51 Deep necrosis of underlying tissues due to burn (deep third degree) of forearm, with loss of a body part
943.52 Deep necrosis of underlying tissues due to burn (deep third degree) of elbow, with loss of a body part
943.53 Deep necrosis of underlying tissues due to burn (deep third degree) of upper arm, with loss of upper a body part
943.59 Deep necrosis of underlying tissues due to burn (deep third degree) of multiple sites of upper limb, except wrist and hand, with loss of a body part
945.30 Full-thickness skin loss due to burn (third degree nos) of unspecified site of lower limb ▽
945.34 Full-thickness skin loss due to burn (third degree nos) of lower leg
945.35 Full-thickness skin loss due to burn (third degree nos) of knee
945.36 Full-thickness skin loss due to burn (third degree nos) of thigh (any part)
945.39 Full-thickness skin loss due to burn (third degree nos) of multiple sites of lower limb(s)
945.40 Deep necrosis of underlying tissues due to burn (deep third degree) of unspecified site of lower limb (leg), without mention of loss of a body part ▽
945.44 Deep necrosis of underlying tissues due to burn (deep third degree) of lower leg, without mention of loss of a body part
945.45 Deep necrosis of underlying tissues due to burn (deep third degree) of knee, without mention of loss of a body part
945.46 Deep necrosis of underlying tissues due to burn (deep third degree) of thigh (any part), without mention of loss of a body part
945.49 Deep necrosis of underlying tissues due to burn (deep third degree) of multiple sites of lower limb(s), without mention of loss of a body part
945.50 Deep necrosis of underlying tissues due to burn (deep third degree) of unspecified site lower limb (leg), with loss of a body part ▽
945.52 Deep necrosis of underlying tissues due to burn (deep third degree) of foot, with loss of a body part
945.53 Deep necrosis of underlying tissues due to burn (deep third degree) of ankle, with loss of a body part
945.54 Deep necrosis of underlying tissues due to burn (deep third degree) of lower leg, with loss of a body part
945.55 Deep necrosis of underlying tissues due to burn (deep third degree) of knee, with loss of a body part
945.56 Deep necrosis of underlying tissues due to burn (deep third degree) of thigh (any part), with loss of a body part
945.59 Deep necrosis of underlying tissues due to burn (deep third degree) of multiple sites of lower limb(s), with loss of a body part
946.3 Full-thickness skin loss due to burn (third degree nos) of multiple specified sites
946.4 Deep necrosis of underlying tissues due to burn (deep third degree) of multiple specified sites, without mention of loss of a body part
946.5 Deep necrosis of underlying tissues due to burn (deep third degree) of multiple specified sites, with loss of a body part
997.60 Late complications of amputation stump, unspecified — (Use additional code to identify complications) ▽
997.62 Infection (chronic) of amputation stump — (Use additional code to identify organism. Use additional code to identify complications)
997.69 Other late amputation stump complication — (Use additional code to identify complications)
V51 Aftercare involving the use of plastic surgery

ICD-9-CM Procedural

85.96 Removal of breast tissue expander (s)
86.05 Incision with removal of foreign body or device from skin and subcutaneous tissue

HCPCS Level II Supplies & Services

A4305 Disposable drug delivery system, flow rate of 50 ml or greater per hour
A4306 Disposable drug delivery system, flow rate of 5 ml or less per hour
A4550 Surgical trays

11975

11975 Insertion, implantable contraceptive capsules

ICD-9-CM Diagnostic

V25.5 Insertion of implantable subdermal contraceptive ♀

HCPCS Level II Supplies & Services

A4260 Levonorgestrel (contraceptive) implants system, including implants and supplies
A4550 Surgical trays

11976–11977

11976 Removal, implantable contraceptive capsules
11977 Removal with reinsertion, implantable contraceptive capsules

ICD-9-CM Diagnostic

V25.43 Surveillance of previously prescribed implantable subdermal contraceptive ♀

ICD-9-CM Procedural

86.05 Incision with removal of foreign body or device from skin and subcutaneous tissue

▽ Unspecified code ♀ Female diagnosis ☒ Manifestation code ♂ Male diagnosis

HCPCS Level II Supplies & Services

A4260 Levonorgestrel (contraceptive) implants system, including implants and supplies
A4550 Surgical trays

11980

11980 Subcutaneous hormone pellet implantation (implantation of estradiol and/or testosterone pellets beneath the skin)

ICD-9-CM Diagnostic

185 Malignant neoplasm of prostate ♂
253.4 Other anterior pituitary disorders
253.7 Iatrogenic pituitary disorders — (Use additional E code to identify cause)
256.2 Postablative ovarian failure — (Use additional code for states associated with artificial menopause, 627.4) ♀
256.31 Premature menopause ♀
256.39 Other ovarian failure ♀
256.8 Other ovarian dysfunction ♀
256.9 Unspecified ovarian dysfunction ▽ ♀
257.1 Postablative testicular hypofunction ♂
257.2 Other testicular hypofunction ♂
257.8 Other testicular dysfunction ♂
257.9 Unspecified testicular dysfunction ▽ ♂
597.80 Unspecified urethritis ▽
604.90 Unspecified orchitis and epididymitis — (Use additional code to identify organism: 041.0, 041.1, 041.4) ▽ ♂
606.1 Oligospermia ♂
608.2 Torsion of testis ♂
608.3 Atrophy of testis ♂
627.0 Premenopausal menorrhagia ♀
627.1 Postmenopausal bleeding ♀
627.2 Symptomatic menopausal or female climacteric states ♀
627.3 Postmenopausal atrophic vaginitis ♀
627.4 Symptomatic states associated with artificial menopause ♀
627.8 Other specified menopausal and postmenopausal disorder ♀
627.9 Unspecified menopausal and postmenopausal disorder ▽ ♀
733.00 Unspecified osteoporosis ▽
733.01 Senile osteoporosis
752.51 Undescended testis ♂
758.7 Klinefelter's syndrome ♂

ICD-9-CM Procedural

99.23 Injection of steroid

HCPCS Level II Supplies & Services

A4550 Surgical trays
S0189 Testosterone pellet, 75 mg

11981–11983

11981 Insertion, non-biodegradable drug delivery implant
11982 Removal, non-biodegradable drug delivery implant
11983 Removal with reinsertion, non-biodegradable drug delivery implant

ICD-9-CM Diagnostic

The application of this code is too broad to adequately present ICD-9-CM diagnostic code links here. Refer to your ICD-9-CM book.

ICD-9-CM Procedural

86.05 Incision with removal of foreign body or device from skin and subcutaneous tissue
99.23 Injection of steroid

HCPCS Level II Supplies & Services

A4550 Surgical trays

Repair (Closure)

12001–12007

12001 Simple repair of superficial wounds of scalp, neck, axillae, external genitalia, trunk and/or extremities (including hands and feet); 2.5 cm or less
12002 2.6 cm to 7.5 cm
12004 7.6 cm to 12.5 cm
12005 12.6 cm to 20.0 cm
12006 20.1 cm to 30.0 cm
12007 over 30.0 cm

ICD-9-CM Diagnostic

629.20 Female genital mutilation status, unspecified
873.0 Open wound of scalp, without mention of complication — (Use additional code to identify infection)
874.8 Open wound of other and unspecified parts of neck, without mention of complication — (Use additional code to identify infection) ▽
878.0 Open wound of penis, without mention of complication — (Use additional code to identify infection) ♂
878.2 Open wound of scrotum and testes, without mention of complication — (Use additional code to identify infection) ♂
878.4 Open wound of vulva, without mention of complication — (Use additional code to identify infection) ♀
878.6 Open wound of vagina, without mention of complication — (Use additional code to identify infection) ♀
878.8 Open wound of other and unspecified parts of genital organs, without mention of complication — (Use additional code to identify infection) ▽
879.0 Open wound of breast, without mention of complication — (Use additional code to identify infection)
879.2 Open wound of abdominal wall, anterior, without mention of complication — (Use additional code to identify infection)
879.4 Open wound of abdominal wall, lateral, without mention of complication — (Use additional code to identify infection)
879.6 Open wound of other and unspecified parts of trunk, without mention of complication — (Use additional code to identify infection) ▽
879.8 Open wound(s) (multiple) of unspecified site(s), without mention of complication — (Use additional code to identify infection) ▽
880.00 Open wound of shoulder region, without mention of complication — (Use additional code to identify infection)
880.01 Open wound of scapular region, without mention of complication — (Use additional code to identify infection)
880.02 Open wound of axillary region, without mention of complication — (Use additional code to identify infection)
880.03 Open wound of upper arm, without mention of complication — (Use additional code to identify infection)
880.09 Open wound of multiple sites of shoulder and upper arm, without mention of complication — (Use additional code to identify infection)
881.00 Open wound of forearm, without mention of complication — (Use additional code to identify infection)
881.01 Open wound of elbow, without mention of complication — (Use additional code to identify infection)
881.02 Open wound of wrist, without mention of complication — (Use additional code to identify infection)
882.0 Open wound of hand except finger(s) alone, without mention of complication — (Use additional code to identify infection)
883.0 Open wound of finger(s), without mention of complication — (Use additional code to identify infection)

Closures

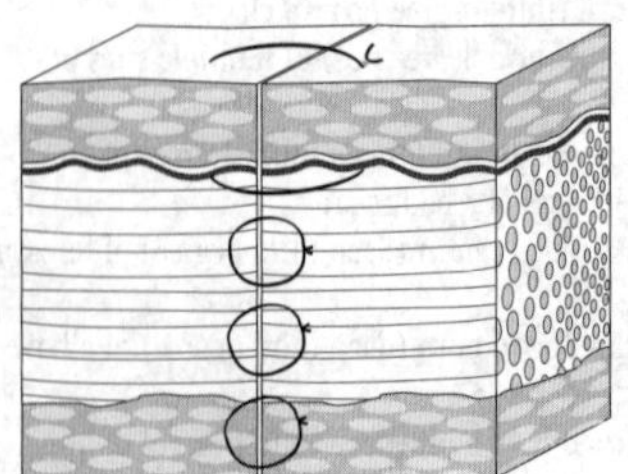
Example of complex layered suturing involving deeper tissues

Simple repair involves superficial repair of the dermis or epidermis without significant involvement of deeper structures

Intermediate repair involves layered suturing of one or more deeper tissue layers or significant debridement before single layer closure

Complex repair generally involves layered suturing of the deeper tissue layers with compounding factors such as scar revision, extensive undermining or retention sutures

884.0 Multiple and unspecified open wound of upper limb, without mention of complication — (Use additional code to identify infection)
890.0 Open wound of hip and thigh, without mention of complication — (Use additional code to identify infection)
891.0 Open wound of knee, leg (except thigh), and ankle, without mention of complication — (Use additional code to identify infection)
892.0 Open wound of foot except toe(s) alone, without mention of complication — (Use additional code to identify infection)
893.0 Open wound of toe(s), without mention of complication — (Use additional code to identify infection)
894.0 Multiple and unspecified open wound of lower limb, without mention of complication — (Use additional code to identify infection)
911.6 Trunk, superficial foreign body (splinter), without major open wound and without mention of infection
911.7 Trunk, superficial foreign body (splinter), without major open wound, infected

ICD-9-CM Procedural

61.41 Suture of laceration of scrotum and tunica vaginalis
64.41 Suture of laceration of penis
71.71 Suture of laceration of vulva or perineum
71.79 Other repair of vulva and perineum
85.81 Suture of laceration of breast
86.59 Closure of skin and subcutaneous tissue of other sites

HCPCS Level II Supplies & Services

A4305 Disposable drug delivery system, flow rate of 50 ml or greater per hour
A4306 Disposable drug delivery system, flow rate of 5 ml or less per hour
A4550 Surgical trays
G0168 Wound closure utilizing tissue adhesive(s) only

12011–12018

12011 Simple repair of superficial wounds of face, ears, eyelids, nose, lips and/or mucous membranes; 2.5 cm or less
12013 2.6 cm to 5.0 cm
12014 5.1 cm to 7.5 cm
12015 7.6 cm to 12.5 cm
12016 12.6 cm to 20.0 cm
12017 20.1 cm to 30.0 cm
12018 over 30.0 cm

ICD-9-CM Diagnostic

870.0 Laceration of skin of eyelid and periocular area — (Use additional code to identify infection)
872.01 Open wound of auricle, without mention of complication — (Use additional code to identify infection)
872.02 Open wound of auditory canal, without mention of complication — (Use additional code to identify infection)
872.8 Open wound of ear, part unspecified, without mention of complication — (Use additional code to identify infection) ▽
873.21 Open wound of nasal septum, without mention of complication — (Use additional code to identify infection)
873.22 Open wound of nasal cavity, without mention of complication — (Use additional code to identify infection)
873.23 Open wound of nasal sinus, without mention of complication — (Use additional code to identify infection)
873.29 Open wound of nose, multiple sites, without mention of complication — (Use additional code to identify infection)
873.40 Open wound of face, unspecified site, without mention of complication — (Use additional code to identify infection) ▽
873.41 Open wound of cheek, without mention of complication — (Use additional code to identify infection)
873.42 Open wound of forehead, without mention of complication — (Use additional code to identify infection)
873.43 Open wound of lip, without mention of complication — (Use additional code to identify infection)
873.44 Open wound of jaw, without mention of complication — (Use additional code to identify infection)
873.49 Open wound of face, other and multiple sites, without mention of complication — (Use additional code to identify infection)
873.60 Open wound of mouth, unspecified site, without mention of complication — (Use additional code to identify infection) ▽

ICD-9-CM Procedural

08.81 Linear repair of laceration of eyelid or eyebrow
18.4 Suture of laceration of external ear
21.81 Suture of laceration of nose
27.51 Suture of laceration of lip
27.52 Suture of laceration of other part of mouth
86.59 Closure of skin and subcutaneous tissue of other sites

HCPCS Level II Supplies & Services

A4305 Disposable drug delivery system, flow rate of 50 ml or greater per hour
A4306 Disposable drug delivery system, flow rate of 5 ml or less per hour
A4550 Surgical trays
G0168 Wound closure utilizing tissue adhesive(s) only

12020–12021

12020 Treatment of superficial wound dehiscence; simple closure
12021 with packing

ICD-9-CM Diagnostic

674.10 Disruption of cesarean wound, unspecified as to episode of care ▽ ♀
674.12 Disruption of cesarean wound, with delivery, with mention of postpartum complication ♀
674.14 Disruption of cesarean wound, postpartum ♀
674.20 Disruption of perineal wound, unspecified as to episode of care in pregnancy ▽ ♀
674.22 Disruption of perineal wound, with delivery, with mention of postpartum complicaton ♀
674.24 Disruption of perineal wound, postpartum ♀
998.32 Disruption of external operation wound
998.59 Other postoperative infection — (Use additional code to identify infection)
998.83 Non-healing surgical wound

ICD-9-CM Procedural

85.81 Suture of laceration of breast
86.59 Closure of skin and subcutaneous tissue of other sites
96.59 Other irrigation of wound

HCPCS Level II Supplies & Services

A4462 Abdominal dressing holder, each
G0168 Wound closure utilizing tissue adhesive(s) only

12031–12037

12031 Layer closure of wounds of scalp, axillae, trunk and/or extremities (excluding hands and feet); 2.5 cm or less
12032 2.6 cm to 7.5 cm
12034 7.6 cm to 12.5 cm
12035 12.6 cm to 20.0 cm
12036 20.1 cm to 30.0 cm
12037 over 30.0 cm

ICD-9-CM Diagnostic

172.4 Malignant melanoma of skin of scalp and neck
172.5 Malignant melanoma of skin of trunk, except scrotum
172.6 Malignant melanoma of skin of upper limb, including shoulder
172.7 Malignant melanoma of skin of lower limb, including hip
172.8 Malignant melanoma of other specified sites of skin
173.4 Other malignant neoplasm of scalp and skin of neck
173.5 Other malignant neoplasm of skin of trunk, except scrotum
173.6 Other malignant neoplasm of skin of upper limb, including shoulder
173.7 Other malignant neoplasm of skin of lower limb, including hip
173.8 Other malignant neoplasm of other specified sites of skin
214.1 Lipoma of other skin and subcutaneous tissue
216.4 Benign neoplasm of scalp and skin of neck
216.5 Benign neoplasm of skin of trunk, except scrotum
216.6 Benign neoplasm of skin of upper limb, including shoulder
216.7 Benign neoplasm of skin of lower limb, including hip
216.8 Benign neoplasm of other specified sites of skin
232.4 Carcinoma in situ of scalp and skin of neck
232.5 Carcinoma in situ of skin of trunk, except scrotum
232.6 Carcinoma in situ of skin of upper limb, including shoulder
232.7 Carcinoma in situ of skin of lower limb, including hip
238.2 Neoplasm of uncertain behavior of skin
448.1 Nevus, non-neoplastic
686.1 Pyogenic granuloma of skin and subcutaneous tissue
701.1 Acquired keratoderma
701.4 Keloid scar
701.5 Other abnormal granulation tissue
701.8 Other specified hypertrophic and atrophic condition of skin
701.9 Unspecified hypertrophic and atrophic condition of skin ▽
702.0 Actinic keratosis
702.11 Inflamed seborrheic keratosis

702.19 Other seborrheic keratosis
702.8 Other specified dermatoses
706.2 Sebaceous cyst
709.1 Vascular disorder of skin
709.2 Scar condition and fibrosis of skin
757.32 Congenital vascular hamartomas
757.33 Congenital pigmentary anomaly of skin
757.39 Other specified congenital anomaly of skin
782.2 Localized superficial swelling, mass, or lump
873.0 Open wound of scalp, without mention of complication — (Use additional code to identify infection)
873.1 Open wound of scalp, complicated — (Use additional code to identify infection)
874.8 Open wound of other and unspecified parts of neck, without mention of complication — (Use additional code to identify infection) ▽
875.0 Open wound of chest (wall), without mention of complication — (Use additional code to identify infection)
876.0 Open wound of back, without mention of complication — (Use additional code to identify infection)
877.0 Open wound of buttock, without mention of complication — (Use additional code to identify infection)
879.0 Open wound of breast, without mention of complication — (Use additional code to identify infection)
879.2 Open wound of abdominal wall, anterior, without mention of complication — (Use additional code to identify infection)
879.4 Open wound of abdominal wall, lateral, without mention of complication — (Use additional code to identify infection)
879.6 Open wound of other and unspecified parts of trunk, without mention of complication — (Use additional code to identify infection) ▽
879.8 Open wound(s) (multiple) of unspecified site(s), without mention of complication — (Use additional code to identify infection) ▽
880.00 Open wound of shoulder region, without mention of complication — (Use additional code to identify infection)
880.03 Open wound of upper arm, without mention of complication — (Use additional code to identify infection)
880.09 Open wound of multiple sites of shoulder and upper arm, without mention of complication — (Use additional code to identify infection)
881.00 Open wound of forearm, without mention of complication — (Use additional code to identify infection)
881.01 Open wound of elbow, without mention of complication — (Use additional code to identify infection)
881.02 Open wound of wrist, without mention of complication — (Use additional code to identify infection)
883.0 Open wound of finger(s), without mention of complication — (Use additional code to identify infection)
884.0 Multiple and unspecified open wound of upper limb, without mention of complication — (Use additional code to identify infection)
890.0 Open wound of hip and thigh, without mention of complication — (Use additional code to identify infection)
891.0 Open wound of knee, leg (except thigh), and ankle, without mention of complication — (Use additional code to identify infection)
894.0 Multiple and unspecified open wound of lower limb, without mention of complication — (Use additional code to identify infection)

ICD-9-CM Procedural

85.81 Suture of laceration of breast
86.59 Closure of skin and subcutaneous tissue of other sites

HCPCS Level II Supplies & Services

A4305 Disposable drug delivery system, flow rate of 50 ml or greater per hour
A4306 Disposable drug delivery system, flow rate of 5 ml or less per hour
A4550 Surgical trays
G0168 Wound closure utilizing tissue adhesive(s) only

12041–12047

12041 Layer closure of wounds of neck, hands, feet and/or external genitalia; 2.5 cm or less
12042 2.6 cm to 7.5 cm
12044 7.6 cm to 12.5 cm
12045 12.6 cm to 20.0 cm
12046 20.1 cm to 30.0 cm
12047 over 30.0 cm

ICD-9-CM Diagnostic

172.4 Malignant melanoma of skin of scalp and neck
172.6 Malignant melanoma of skin of upper limb, including shoulder
172.7 Malignant melanoma of skin of lower limb, including hip
172.8 Malignant melanoma of other specified sites of skin
173.4 Other malignant neoplasm of scalp and skin of neck
173.6 Other malignant neoplasm of skin of upper limb, including shoulder
173.7 Other malignant neoplasm of skin of lower limb, including hip
173.8 Other malignant neoplasm of other specified sites of skin
184.1 Malignant neoplasm of labia majora ♀
184.2 Malignant neoplasm of labia minora ♀
184.4 Malignant neoplasm of vulva, unspecified site ▽ ♀
187.1 Malignant neoplasm of prepuce ♂
187.2 Malignant neoplasm of glans penis ♂
187.3 Malignant neoplasm of body of penis ♂
187.7 Malignant neoplasm of scrotum ♂
187.8 Malignant neoplasm of other specified sites of male genital organs ♂
198.2 Secondary malignant neoplasm of skin
198.82 Secondary malignant neoplasm of genital organs
214.1 Lipoma of other skin and subcutaneous tissue
216.4 Benign neoplasm of scalp and skin of neck
216.6 Benign neoplasm of skin of upper limb, including shoulder
216.7 Benign neoplasm of skin of lower limb, including hip
216.8 Benign neoplasm of other specified sites of skin
221.2 Benign neoplasm of vulva ♀
222.1 Benign neoplasm of penis ♂
222.4 Benign neoplasm of scrotum ♂
228.01 Hemangioma of skin and subcutaneous tissue
232.4 Carcinoma in situ of scalp and skin of neck
232.6 Carcinoma in situ of skin of upper limb, including shoulder
232.7 Carcinoma in situ of skin of lower limb, including hip
232.8 Carcinoma in situ of other specified sites of skin
233.3 Carcinoma in situ of other and unspecified female genital organs ▽ ♀
233.5 Carcinoma in situ of penis ♂
233.6 Carcinoma in situ of other and unspecified male genital organs ▽ ♂
238.2 Neoplasm of uncertain behavior of skin
239.8 Neoplasm of unspecified nature of other specified sites
448.1 Nevus, non-neoplastic
629.20 Female genital mutilation status, unspecified
629.21 Female genital mutilation, Type I status
629.22 Female genital mutilation, Type II status
686.1 Pyogenic granuloma of skin and subcutaneous tissue
701.1 Acquired keratoderma
701.4 Keloid scar
701.5 Other abnormal granulation tissue
701.8 Other specified hypertrophic and atrophic condition of skin
701.9 Unspecified hypertrophic and atrophic condition of skin ▽
702.0 Actinic keratosis
702.11 Inflamed seborrheic keratosis
702.19 Other seborrheic keratosis
702.8 Other specified dermatoses
706.2 Sebaceous cyst
709.1 Vascular disorder of skin
709.2 Scar condition and fibrosis of skin
709.9 Unspecified disorder of skin and subcutaneous tissue ▽
757.32 Congenital vascular hamartomas
757.33 Congenital pigmentary anomaly of skin
757.39 Other specified congenital anomaly of skin
782.2 Localized superficial swelling, mass, or lump
874.8 Open wound of other and unspecified parts of neck, without mention of complication — (Use additional code to identify infection) ▽
878.0 Open wound of penis, without mention of complication — (Use additional code to identify infection) ♂
878.2 Open wound of scrotum and testes, without mention of complication — (Use additional code to identify infection) ♂
878.4 Open wound of vulva, without mention of complication — (Use additional code to identify infection) ♀
878.6 Open wound of vagina, without mention of complication — (Use additional code to identify infection) ♀
878.8 Open wound of other and unspecified parts of genital organs, without mention of complication — (Use additional code to identify infection) ▽
882.0 Open wound of hand except finger(s) alone, without mention of complication — (Use additional code to identify infection)
883.0 Open wound of finger(s), without mention of complication — (Use additional code to identify infection)
892.0 Open wound of foot except toe(s) alone, without mention of complication — (Use additional code to identify infection)
893.0 Open wound of toe(s), without mention of complication — (Use additional code to identify infection)

ICD-9-CM Procedural

61.41 Suture of laceration of scrotum and tunica vaginalis
64.41 Suture of laceration of penis
71.71 Suture of laceration of vulva or perineum
86.59 Closure of skin and subcutaneous tissue of other sites

HCPCS Level II Supplies & Services

A4305 Disposable drug delivery system, flow rate of 50 ml or greater per hour
A4306 Disposable drug delivery system, flow rate of 5 ml or less per hour
A4550 Surgical trays
G0168 Wound closure utilizing tissue adhesive(s) only

12051–12057

12051 Layer closure of wounds of face, ears, eyelids, nose, lips and/or mucous membranes; 2.5 cm or less
12052 2.6 cm to 5.0 cm
12053 5.1 cm to 7.5 cm
12054 7.6 cm to 12.5 cm
12055 12.6 cm to 20.0 cm
12056 20.1 cm to 30.0 cm
12057 over 30.0 cm

ICD-9-CM Diagnostic

172.0 Malignant melanoma of skin of lip
172.1 Malignant melanoma of skin of eyelid, including canthus
172.2 Malignant melanoma of skin of ear and external auditory canal
172.3 Malignant melanoma of skin of other and unspecified parts of face
172.8 Malignant melanoma of other specified sites of skin
173.0 Other malignant neoplasm of skin of lip
173.1 Other malignant neoplasm of skin of eyelid, including canthus
173.2 Other malignant neoplasm of skin of ear and external auditory canal
173.3 Other malignant neoplasm of skin of other and unspecified parts of face ▽
173.8 Other malignant neoplasm of other specified sites of skin
195.0 Malignant neoplasm of head, face, and neck
198.2 Secondary malignant neoplasm of skin
214.0 Lipoma of skin and subcutaneous tissue of face
214.1 Lipoma of other skin and subcutaneous tissue
216.0 Benign neoplasm of skin of lip
216.1 Benign neoplasm of eyelid, including canthus
216.2 Benign neoplasm of ear and external auditory canal
216.3 Benign neoplasm of skin of other and unspecified parts of face ▽
228.01 Hemangioma of skin and subcutaneous tissue
232.0 Carcinoma in situ of skin of lip
232.1 Carcinoma in situ of eyelid, including canthus
232.2 Carcinoma in situ of skin of ear and external auditory canal
232.3 Carcinoma in situ of skin of other and unspecified parts of face ▽
235.1 Neoplasm of uncertain behavior of lip, oral cavity, and pharynx
238.2 Neoplasm of uncertain behavior of skin
239.2 Neoplasms of unspecified nature of bone, soft tissue, and skin
239.8 Neoplasm of unspecified nature of other specified sites
448.1 Nevus, non-neoplastic
686.1 Pyogenic granuloma of skin and subcutaneous tissue
701.1 Acquired keratoderma
701.4 Keloid scar
701.5 Other abnormal granulation tissue
701.8 Other specified hypertrophic and atrophic condition of skin
701.9 Unspecified hypertrophic and atrophic condition of skin ▽
702.0 Actinic keratosis
702.11 Inflamed seborrheic keratosis
702.19 Other seborrheic keratosis
706.2 Sebaceous cyst
709.2 Scar condition and fibrosis of skin
757.32 Congenital vascular hamartomas
757.33 Congenital pigmentary anomaly of skin
757.39 Other specified congenital anomaly of skin
870.0 Laceration of skin of eyelid and periocular area — (Use additional code to identify infection)
870.1 Laceration of eyelid, full-thickness, not involving lacrimal passages — (Use additional code to identify infection)
870.8 Other specified open wound of ocular adnexa — (Use additional code to identify infection)
872.00 Open wound of external ear, unspecified site, without mention of complication — (Use additional code to identify infection) ▽
872.01 Open wound of auricle, without mention of complication — (Use additional code to identify infection)
872.02 Open wound of auditory canal, without mention of complication — (Use additional code to identify infection)
872.69 Open wound of other and multiple sites, without mention of complication — (Use additional code to identify infection)
873.20 Open wound of nose, unspecified site, without mention of complication — (Use additional code to identify infection) ▽
873.21 Open wound of nasal septum, without mention of complication — (Use additional code to identify infection)
873.22 Open wound of nasal cavity, without mention of complication — (Use additional code to identify infection)
873.23 Open wound of nasal sinus, without mention of complication — (Use additional code to identify infection)
873.29 Open wound of nose, multiple sites, without mention of complication — (Use additional code to identify infection)
873.40 Open wound of face, unspecified site, without mention of complication — (Use additional code to identify infection) ▽
873.41 Open wound of cheek, without mention of complication — (Use additional code to identify infection)
873.42 Open wound of forehead, without mention of complication — (Use additional code to identify infection)
873.43 Open wound of lip, without mention of complication — (Use additional code to identify infection)
873.44 Open wound of jaw, without mention of complication — (Use additional code to identify infection)
873.49 Open wound of face, other and multiple sites, without mention of complication — (Use additional code to identify infection)
873.60 Open wound of mouth, unspecified site, without mention of complication — (Use additional code to identify infection) ▽
873.61 Open wound of buccal mucosa, without mention of complication — (Use additional code to identify infection)
873.69 Open wound of mouth, other and multiple sites, without mention of complication — (Use additional code to identify infection)
873.8 Other and unspecified open wound of head without mention of complication — (Use additional code to identify infection) ▽
925.1 Crushing injury of face and scalp — (Use additional code to identify any associated injuries: 800-829, 850.0-854.1, 860.0-869.1)
959.09 Injury of face and neck, other and unspecified

ICD-9-CM Procedural

08.81 Linear repair of laceration of eyelid or eyebrow
18.4 Suture of laceration of external ear
21.81 Suture of laceration of nose
27.51 Suture of laceration of lip
27.52 Suture of laceration of other part of mouth
86.59 Closure of skin and subcutaneous tissue of other sites

HCPCS Level II Supplies & Services

A4305 Disposable drug delivery system, flow rate of 50 ml or greater per hour
A4306 Disposable drug delivery system, flow rate of 5 ml or less per hour
A4550 Surgical trays
G0168 Wound closure utilizing tissue adhesive(s) only

13100–13102

13100 Repair, complex, trunk; 1.1 cm to 2.5 cm
13101 2.6 cm to 7.5 cm
13102 each additional 5 cm or less (List separately in addition to code for primary procedure)

ICD-9-CM Diagnostic

172.5 Malignant melanoma of skin of trunk, except scrotum
173.5 Other malignant neoplasm of skin of trunk, except scrotum
198.2 Secondary malignant neoplasm of skin
214.1 Lipoma of other skin and subcutaneous tissue
216.5 Benign neoplasm of skin of trunk, except scrotum
228.01 Hemangioma of skin and subcutaneous tissue
232.5 Carcinoma in situ of skin of trunk, except scrotum
238.2 Neoplasm of uncertain behavior of skin
448.1 Nevus, non-neoplastic
686.1 Pyogenic granuloma of skin and subcutaneous tissue
701.1 Acquired keratoderma
701.4 Keloid scar
701.5 Other abnormal granulation tissue
702.11 Inflamed seborrheic keratosis
702.19 Other seborrheic keratosis
706.2 Sebaceous cyst
709.1 Vascular disorder of skin

▽ Unspecified code ♀ Female diagnosis ■ Manifestation code ♂ Male diagnosis

709.2 Scar condition and fibrosis of skin
709.4 Foreign body granuloma of skin and subcutaneous tissue
757.32 Congenital vascular hamartomas
875.0 Open wound of chest (wall), without mention of complication — (Use additional code to identify infection)
875.1 Open wound of chest (wall), complicated — (Use additional code to identify infection)
877.0 Open wound of buttock, without mention of complication — (Use additional code to identify infection)
877.1 Open wound of buttock, complicated — (Use additional code to identify infection)
879.0 Open wound of breast, without mention of complication — (Use additional code to identify infection)
879.1 Open wound of breast, complicated — (Use additional code to identify infection)
879.2 Open wound of abdominal wall, anterior, without mention of complication — (Use additional code to identify infection)
879.3 Open wound of abdominal wall, anterior, complicated — (Use additional code to identify infection)
879.4 Open wound of abdominal wall, lateral, without mention of complication — (Use additional code to identify infection)
879.5 Open wound of abdominal wall, lateral, complicated — (Use additional code to identify infection)
879.6 Open wound of other and unspecified parts of trunk, without mention of complication — (Use additional code to identify infection) ▽
879.7 Open wound of other and unspecified parts of trunk, complicated — (Use additional code to identify infection) ▽
879.8 Open wound(s) (multiple) of unspecified site(s), without mention of complication — (Use additional code to identify infection) ▽
879.9 Open wound(s) (multiple) of unspecified site(s), complicated — (Use additional code to identify infection) ▽
880.00 Open wound of shoulder region, without mention of complication — (Use additional code to identify infection)
880.01 Open wound of scapular region, without mention of complication — (Use additional code to identify infection)
880.09 Open wound of multiple sites of shoulder and upper arm, without mention of complication — (Use additional code to identify infection)
880.10 Open wound of shoulder region, complicated — (Use additional code to identify infection)
880.11 Open wound of scapular region, complicated — (Use additional code to identify infection)
880.19 Open wound of multiple sites of shoulder and upper arm, complicated — (Use additional code to identify infection)
906.0 Late effect of open wound of head, neck, and trunk

ICD-9-CM Procedural

85.81 Suture of laceration of breast
86.59 Closure of skin and subcutaneous tissue of other sites

HCPCS Level II Supplies & Services

A4305 Disposable drug delivery system, flow rate of 50 ml or greater per hour
A4306 Disposable drug delivery system, flow rate of 5 ml or less per hour
A4462 Abdominal dressing holder, each
A4550 Surgical trays

13120–13122

13120 Repair, complex, scalp, arms, and/or legs; 1.1 cm to 2.5 cm
13121 2.6 cm to 7.5 cm
13122 each additional 5 cm or less (List separately in addition to code for primary procedure)

ICD-9-CM Diagnostic

172.4 Malignant melanoma of skin of scalp and neck
172.6 Malignant melanoma of skin of upper limb, including shoulder
172.7 Malignant melanoma of skin of lower limb, including hip
172.8 Malignant melanoma of other specified sites of skin
173.4 Other malignant neoplasm of scalp and skin of neck
173.6 Other malignant neoplasm of skin of upper limb, including shoulder
173.7 Other malignant neoplasm of skin of lower limb, including hip
195.4 Malignant neoplasm of upper limb
195.5 Malignant neoplasm of lower limb
198.2 Secondary malignant neoplasm of skin
214.1 Lipoma of other skin and subcutaneous tissue
216.4 Benign neoplasm of scalp and skin of neck
216.6 Benign neoplasm of skin of upper limb, including shoulder
216.7 Benign neoplasm of skin of lower limb, including hip
216.8 Benign neoplasm of other specified sites of skin
228.01 Hemangioma of skin and subcutaneous tissue
232.4 Carcinoma in situ of scalp and skin of neck
232.6 Carcinoma in situ of skin of upper limb, including shoulder
232.7 Carcinoma in situ of skin of lower limb, including hip
232.8 Carcinoma in situ of other specified sites of skin
238.2 Neoplasm of uncertain behavior of skin
448.1 Nevus, non-neoplastic
686.1 Pyogenic granuloma of skin and subcutaneous tissue
701.1 Acquired keratoderma
701.4 Keloid scar
701.5 Other abnormal granulation tissue
701.8 Other specified hypertrophic and atrophic condition of skin
701.9 Unspecified hypertrophic and atrophic condition of skin ▽
702.0 Actinic keratosis
702.11 Inflamed seborrheic keratosis
702.19 Other seborrheic keratosis
702.8 Other specified dermatoses
706.2 Sebaceous cyst
709.1 Vascular disorder of skin
709.2 Scar condition and fibrosis of skin
709.4 Foreign body granuloma of skin and subcutaneous tissue
757.32 Congenital vascular hamartomas
757.33 Congenital pigmentary anomaly of skin
757.39 Other specified congenital anomaly of skin
782.2 Localized superficial swelling, mass, or lump
873.0 Open wound of scalp, without mention of complication — (Use additional code to identify infection)
873.1 Open wound of scalp, complicated — (Use additional code to identify infection)
880.03 Open wound of upper arm, without mention of complication — (Use additional code to identify infection)
880.13 Open wound of upper arm, complicated — (Use additional code to identify infection)
881.00 Open wound of forearm, without mention of complication — (Use additional code to identify infection)
881.01 Open wound of elbow, without mention of complication — (Use additional code to identify infection)
881.02 Open wound of wrist, without mention of complication — (Use additional code to identify infection)
881.10 Open wound of forearm, complicated — (Use additional code to identify infection)
881.11 Open wound of elbow, complicated — (Use additional code to identify infection)
881.12 Open wound of wrist, complicated — (Use additional code to identify infection)
884.0 Multiple and unspecified open wound of upper limb, without mention of complication — (Use additional code to identify infection)
884.1 Multiple and unspecified open wound of upper limb, complicated — (Use additional code to identify infection)
890.0 Open wound of hip and thigh, without mention of complication — (Use additional code to identify infection)
890.1 Open wound of hip and thigh, complicated — (Use additional code to identify infection)
891.0 Open wound of knee, leg (except thigh), and ankle, without mention of complication — (Use additional code to identify infection)
891.1 Open wound of knee, leg (except thigh), and ankle, complicated — (Use additional code to identify infection)
894.0 Multiple and unspecified open wound of lower limb, without mention of complication — (Use additional code to identify infection)
894.1 Multiple and unspecified open wound of lower limb, complicated — (Use additional code to identify infection)
906.0 Late effect of open wound of head, neck, and trunk

ICD-9-CM Procedural

86.51 Replantation of scalp
86.59 Closure of skin and subcutaneous tissue of other sites
86.89 Other repair and reconstruction of skin and subcutaneous tissue

HCPCS Level II Supplies & Services

A4305 Disposable drug delivery system, flow rate of 50 ml or greater per hour
A4306 Disposable drug delivery system, flow rate of 5 ml or less per hour
A4550 Surgical trays
G0168 Wound closure utilizing tissue adhesive(s) only

▽ Unspecified code
♀ Female diagnosis
☒ Manifestation code
♂ Male diagnosis

13131–13133

13131 Repair, complex, forehead, cheeks, chin, mouth, neck, axillae, genitalia, hands and/or feet; 1.1 cm to 2.5 cm
13132 2.6 cm to 7.5 cm
13133 each additional 5 cm or less (List separately in addition to code for primary procedure)

ICD-9-CM Diagnostic

172.3 Malignant melanoma of skin of other and unspecified parts of face
172.4 Malignant melanoma of skin of scalp and neck
172.6 Malignant melanoma of skin of upper limb, including shoulder
172.7 Malignant melanoma of skin of lower limb, including hip
172.8 Malignant melanoma of other specified sites of skin
173.3 Other malignant neoplasm of skin of other and unspecified parts of face ▽
173.4 Other malignant neoplasm of scalp and skin of neck
173.6 Other malignant neoplasm of skin of upper limb, including shoulder
173.7 Other malignant neoplasm of skin of lower limb, including hip
173.8 Other malignant neoplasm of other specified sites of skin
184.4 Malignant neoplasm of vulva, unspecified site ▽ ♀
187.1 Malignant neoplasm of prepuce ♂
187.2 Malignant neoplasm of glans penis ♂
187.3 Malignant neoplasm of body of penis ♂
187.4 Malignant neoplasm of penis, part unspecified ▽ ♂
187.7 Malignant neoplasm of scrotum ♂
187.8 Malignant neoplasm of other specified sites of male genital organs ♂
195.0 Malignant neoplasm of head, face, and neck
195.4 Malignant neoplasm of upper limb
195.5 Malignant neoplasm of lower limb
198.2 Secondary malignant neoplasm of skin
198.82 Secondary malignant neoplasm of genital organs
198.89 Secondary malignant neoplasm of other specified sites
214.0 Lipoma of skin and subcutaneous tissue of face
214.1 Lipoma of other skin and subcutaneous tissue
216.3 Benign neoplasm of skin of other and unspecified parts of face ▽
216.4 Benign neoplasm of scalp and skin of neck
216.6 Benign neoplasm of skin of upper limb, including shoulder
216.7 Benign neoplasm of skin of lower limb, including hip
216.8 Benign neoplasm of other specified sites of skin
221.2 Benign neoplasm of vulva ♀
222.1 Benign neoplasm of penis ♂
222.4 Benign neoplasm of scrotum ♂
228.01 Hemangioma of skin and subcutaneous tissue
230.0 Carcinoma in situ of lip, oral cavity, and pharynx
232.3 Carcinoma in situ of skin of other and unspecified parts of face ▽
232.6 Carcinoma in situ of skin of upper limb, including shoulder
232.7 Carcinoma in situ of skin of lower limb, including hip
232.8 Carcinoma in situ of other specified sites of skin
233.3 Carcinoma in situ of other and unspecified female genital organs ▽ ♀
233.5 Carcinoma in situ of penis ♂
233.6 Carcinoma in situ of other and unspecified male genital organs ▽ ♂
236.3 Neoplasm of uncertain behavior of other and unspecified female genital organs ▽ ♀
236.6 Neoplasm of uncertain behavior of other and unspecified male genital organs ▽ ♂
238.2 Neoplasm of uncertain behavior of skin
239.8 Neoplasm of unspecified nature of other specified sites
448.1 Nevus, non-neoplastic
528.79 Other disturbances of oral epithelium, including tongue
629.20 Female genital mutilation status, unspecified
629.21 Female genital mutilation, Type I status
629.22 Female genital mutilation, Type II status
686.1 Pyogenic granuloma of skin and subcutaneous tissue
701.1 Acquired keratoderma
701.4 Keloid scar
701.5 Other abnormal granulation tissue
701.8 Other specified hypertrophic and atrophic condition of skin
701.9 Unspecified hypertrophic and atrophic condition of skin ▽
702.0 Actinic keratosis
702.11 Inflamed seborrheic keratosis
702.19 Other seborrheic keratosis
702.8 Other specified dermatoses
706.2 Sebaceous cyst
709.1 Vascular disorder of skin
709.2 Scar condition and fibrosis of skin
709.4 Foreign body granuloma of skin and subcutaneous tissue
757.32 Congenital vascular hamartomas
757.33 Congenital pigmentary anomaly of skin
757.39 Other specified congenital anomaly of skin
782.2 Localized superficial swelling, mass, or lump
873.41 Open wound of cheek, without mention of complication — (Use additional code to identify infection)
873.42 Open wound of forehead, without mention of complication — (Use additional code to identify infection)
873.44 Open wound of jaw, without mention of complication — (Use additional code to identify infection)
873.49 Open wound of face, other and multiple sites, without mention of complication — (Use additional code to identify infection)
873.51 Open wound of cheek, complicated — (Use additional code to identify infection)
873.52 Open wound of forehead, complicated — (Use additional code to identify infection)
873.54 Open wound of jaw, complicated — (Use additional code to identify infection)
873.59 Open wound of face, other and multiple sites, complicated — (Use additional code to identify infection)
873.60 Open wound of mouth, unspecified site, without mention of complication — (Use additional code to identify infection) ▽
873.61 Open wound of buccal mucosa, without mention of complication — (Use additional code to identify infection)
873.69 Open wound of mouth, other and multiple sites, without mention of complication — (Use additional code to identify infection)
873.70 Open wound of mouth, unspecified site, complicated — (Use additional code to identify infection) ▽
873.71 Open wound of buccal mucosa, complicated — (Use additional code to identify infection)
873.72 Open wound of gum (alveolar process), complicated — (Use additional code to identify infection)
873.79 Open wound of mouth, other and multiple sites, complicated — (Use additional code to identify infection)
878.0 Open wound of penis, without mention of complication — (Use additional code to identify infection) ♂
878.1 Open wound of penis, complicated — (Use additional code to identify infection) ♂
878.2 Open wound of scrotum and testes, without mention of complication — (Use additional code to identify infection) ♂
878.3 Open wound of scrotum and testes, complicated — (Use additional code to identify infection) ♂
878.4 Open wound of vulva, without mention of complication — (Use additional code to identify infection) ♀
878.5 Open wound of vulva, complicated — (Use additional code to identify infection) ♀
878.8 Open wound of other and unspecified parts of genital organs, without mention of complication — (Use additional code to identify infection) ▽
878.9 Open wound of other and unspecified parts of genital organs, complicated — (Use additional code to identify infection) ▽
880.02 Open wound of axillary region, without mention of complication — (Use additional code to identify infection)
880.12 Open wound of axillary region, complicated — (Use additional code to identify infection)
882.0 Open wound of hand except finger(s) alone, without mention of complication — (Use additional code to identify infection)
882.1 Open wound of hand except finger(s) alone, complicated — (Use additional code to identify infection)
883.0 Open wound of finger(s), without mention of complication — (Use additional code to identify infection)
883.1 Open wound of finger(s), complicated — (Use additional code to identify infection)
892.0 Open wound of foot except toe(s) alone, without mention of complication — (Use additional code to identify infection)
892.1 Open wound of foot except toe(s) alone, complicated — (Use additional code to identify infection)
893.0 Open wound of toe(s), without mention of complication — (Use additional code to identify infection)
893.1 Open wound of toe(s), complicated — (Use additional code to identify infection)

ICD-9-CM Procedural

27.52 Suture of laceration of other part of mouth
61.41 Suture of laceration of scrotum and tunica vaginalis
64.41 Suture of laceration of penis
71.71 Suture of laceration of vulva or perineum
86.59 Closure of skin and subcutaneous tissue of other sites
86.89 Other repair and reconstruction of skin and subcutaneous tissue

▽ Unspecified code
♀ Female diagnosis
☒ Manifestation code
♂ Male diagnosis

HCPCS Level II Supplies & Services

A4305 Disposable drug delivery system, flow rate of 50 ml or greater per hour
A4306 Disposable drug delivery system, flow rate of 5 ml or less per hour
A4550 Surgical trays
G0168 Wound closure utilizing tissue adhesive(s) only

13150–13153

13150 Repair, complex, eyelids, nose, ears and/or lips; 1.0 cm or less
13151 1.1 cm to 2.5 cm
13152 2.6 cm to 7.5 cm
13153 each additional 5 cm or less (List separately in addition to code for primary procedure)

ICD-9-CM Diagnostic

172.0 Malignant melanoma of skin of lip
172.1 Malignant melanoma of skin of eyelid, including canthus
172.2 Malignant melanoma of skin of ear and external auditory canal
172.3 Malignant melanoma of skin of other and unspecified parts of face
172.8 Malignant melanoma of other specified sites of skin
173.0 Other malignant neoplasm of skin of lip
173.1 Other malignant neoplasm of skin of eyelid, including canthus
173.2 Other malignant neoplasm of skin of ear and external auditory canal
173.3 Other malignant neoplasm of skin of other and unspecified parts of face ▽
173.8 Other malignant neoplasm of other specified sites of skin
198.2 Secondary malignant neoplasm of skin
198.89 Secondary malignant neoplasm of other specified sites
214.0 Lipoma of skin and subcutaneous tissue of face
214.1 Lipoma of other skin and subcutaneous tissue
216.0 Benign neoplasm of skin of lip
216.1 Benign neoplasm of eyelid, including canthus
216.2 Benign neoplasm of ear and external auditory canal
216.3 Benign neoplasm of skin of other and unspecified parts of face ▽
228.01 Hemangioma of skin and subcutaneous tissue
232.1 Carcinoma in situ of eyelid, including canthus
232.3 Carcinoma in situ of skin of other and unspecified parts of face ▽
238.2 Neoplasm of uncertain behavior of skin
239.2 Neoplasms of unspecified nature of bone, soft tissue, and skin
239.8 Neoplasm of unspecified nature of other specified sites
448.1 Nevus, non-neoplastic
686.1 Pyogenic granuloma of skin and subcutaneous tissue
701.1 Acquired keratoderma
701.4 Keloid scar
701.5 Other abnormal granulation tissue
701.8 Other specified hypertrophic and atrophic condition of skin
702.0 Actinic keratosis
702.11 Inflamed seborrheic keratosis
702.19 Other seborrheic keratosis
706.2 Sebaceous cyst
709.2 Scar condition and fibrosis of skin
709.4 Foreign body granuloma of skin and subcutaneous tissue
757.32 Congenital vascular hamartomas
757.33 Congenital pigmentary anomaly of skin
757.39 Other specified congenital anomaly of skin
870.0 Laceration of skin of eyelid and periocular area — (Use additional code to identify infection)
870.1 Laceration of eyelid, full-thickness, not involving lacrimal passages — (Use additional code to identify infection)
870.8 Other specified open wound of ocular adnexa — (Use additional code to identify infection)
872.00 Open wound of external ear, unspecified site, without mention of complication — (Use additional code to identify infection) ▽
872.01 Open wound of auricle, without mention of complication — (Use additional code to identify infection)
872.02 Open wound of auditory canal, without mention of complication — (Use additional code to identify infection)
872.10 Open wound of external ear, unspecified site, complicated — (Use additional code to identify infection) ▽
872.11 Open wound of auricle, complicated — (Use additional code to identify infection)
872.12 Open wound of auditory canal, complicated — (Use additional code to identify infection)
873.20 Open wound of nose, unspecified site, without mention of complication — (Use additional code to identify infection) ▽
873.21 Open wound of nasal septum, without mention of complication — (Use additional code to identify infection)
873.22 Open wound of nasal cavity, without mention of complication — (Use additional code to identify infection)
873.29 Open wound of nose, multiple sites, without mention of complication — (Use additional code to identify infection)
873.30 Open wound of nose, unspecified site, complicated — (Use additional code to identify infection) ▽
873.31 Open wound of nasal septum, complicated — (Use additional code to identify infection)
873.32 Open wound of nasal cavity, complicated — (Use additional code to identify infection)
873.39 Open wound of nose, multiple sites, complicated — (Use additional code to identify infection)
873.43 Open wound of lip, without mention of complication — (Use additional code to identify infection)
873.49 Open wound of face, other and multiple sites, without mention of complication — (Use additional code to identify infection)
873.53 Open wound of lip, complicated — (Use additional code to identify infection)
873.59 Open wound of face, other and multiple sites, complicated — (Use additional code to identify infection)
906.0 Late effect of open wound of head, neck, and trunk

ICD-9-CM Procedural

08.72 Other reconstruction of eyelid, partial-thickness
08.81 Linear repair of laceration of eyelid or eyebrow
08.83 Other repair of laceration of eyelid, partial-thickness
18.4 Suture of laceration of external ear
18.72 Reattachment of amputated ear
21.81 Suture of laceration of nose
27.51 Suture of laceration of lip
86.59 Closure of skin and subcutaneous tissue of other sites
86.89 Other repair and reconstruction of skin and subcutaneous tissue

HCPCS Level II Supplies & Services

A4305 Disposable drug delivery system, flow rate of 50 ml or greater per hour
A4306 Disposable drug delivery system, flow rate of 5 ml or less per hour
A4550 Surgical trays
G0168 Wound closure utilizing tissue adhesive(s) only

13160

13160 Secondary closure of surgical wound or dehiscence, extensive or complicated

ICD-9-CM Diagnostic

674.10 Disruption of cesarean wound, unspecified as to episode of care ▽ ♀
674.12 Disruption of cesarean wound, with delivery, with mention of postpartum complication ♀
674.14 Disruption of cesarean wound, postpartum ♀
674.20 Disruption of perineal wound, unspecified as to episode of care in pregnancy ▽ ♀
674.22 Disruption of perineal wound, with delivery, with mention of postpartum complicaton ♀
674.24 Disruption of perineal wound, postpartum ♀
958.3 Posttraumatic wound infection not elsewhere classified
998.31 Disruption of internal operation wound
998.32 Disruption of external operation wound
998.83 Non-healing surgical wound
V58.41 Planned postoperative wound closure — (This code should be used in conjunction with other aftercare codes to fully identify the reason for the aftercare encounter)

ICD-9-CM Procedural

54.62 Delayed closure of granulating abdominal wound
85.81 Suture of laceration of breast

HCPCS Level II Supplies & Services

A4462 Abdominal dressing holder, each

14000–14001

14000 Adjacent tissue transfer or rearrangement, trunk; defect 10 sq. cm or less
14001 defect 10.1 sq. cm to 30.0 sq. cm

ICD-9-CM Diagnostic

172.5 Malignant melanoma of skin of trunk, except scrotum
173.5 Other malignant neoplasm of skin of trunk, except scrotum
216.5 Benign neoplasm of skin of trunk, except scrotum
228.01 Hemangioma of skin and subcutaneous tissue
232.5 Carcinoma in situ of skin of trunk, except scrotum

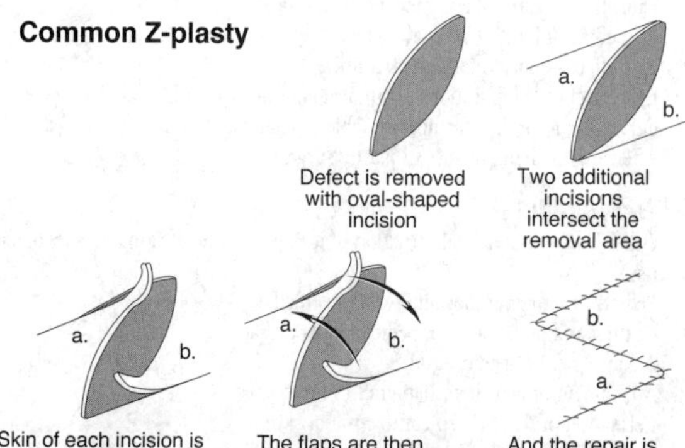
Common Z-plasty
a.
b.
Defect is removed with oval-shaped incision
Two additional incisions intersect the removal area
Skin of each incision is reflected back
The flaps are then transposed
And the repair is closed

238.2 Neoplasm of uncertain behavior of skin
701.4 Keloid scar
701.5 Other abnormal granulation tissue
706.2 Sebaceous cyst
707.00 Decubitus ulcer, unspecified site
707.02 Decubitus ulcer, upper back
707.03 Decubitus ulcer, lower back
707.04 Decubitus ulcer, hip
707.05 Decubitus ulcer, buttock
707.09 Decubitus ulcer, other site
707.8 Chronic ulcer of other specified site
709.2 Scar condition and fibrosis of skin
757.32 Congenital vascular hamartomas
757.6 Specified congenital anomalies of breast
757.8 Other specified congenital anomalies of the integument
757.9 Unspecified congenital anomaly of the integument
875.0 Open wound of chest (wall), without mention of complication — (Use additional code to identify infection)
875.1 Open wound of chest (wall), complicated — (Use additional code to identify infection)
876.0 Open wound of back, without mention of complication — (Use additional code to identify infection)
876.1 Open wound of back, complicated — (Use additional code to identify infection)
877.0 Open wound of buttock, without mention of complication — (Use additional code to identify infection)
877.1 Open wound of buttock, complicated — (Use additional code to identify infection)
879.0 Open wound of breast, without mention of complication — (Use additional code to identify infection)
879.1 Open wound of breast, complicated — (Use additional code to identify infection)
879.2 Open wound of abdominal wall, anterior, without mention of complication — (Use additional code to identify infection)
879.3 Open wound of abdominal wall, anterior, complicated — (Use additional code to identify infection)
879.4 Open wound of abdominal wall, lateral, without mention of complication — (Use additional code to identify infection)
879.5 Open wound of abdominal wall, lateral, complicated — (Use additional code to identify infection)
879.6 Open wound of other and unspecified parts of trunk, without mention of complication — (Use additional code to identify infection)
879.7 Open wound of other and unspecified parts of trunk, complicated — (Use additional code to identify infection)
879.8 Open wound(s) (multiple) of unspecified site(s), without mention of complication — (Use additional code to identify infection)
879.9 Open wound(s) (multiple) of unspecified site(s), complicated — (Use additional code to identify infection)
906.0 Late effect of open wound of head, neck, and trunk
906.8 Late effect of burns of other specified sites
909.3 Late effect of complications of surgical and medical care
942.00 Burn of unspecified degree of trunk, unspecified site
942.01 Burn of trunk, unspecified degree of breast
942.02 Burn of trunk, unspecified degree of chest wall, excluding breast and nipple
942.04 Burn of trunk, unspecified degree of back (any part)
942.09 Burn of trunk, unspecified degree of other and multiple sites
942.23 Blisters with epidermal loss due to burn (second degree) of abdominal wall
942.30 Full-thickness skin loss due to burn (third degree nos) of unspecified site of trunk
942.31 Full-thickness skin loss due to burn (third degree nos) of breast
942.32 Full-thickness skin loss due to burn (third degree nos) of chest wall, excluding breast and nipple
942.34 Full-thickness skin loss due to burn (third degree nos) of back (any part)
942.39 Full-thickness skin loss due to burn (third degree nos) of other and multiple sites of trunk
942.40 Deep necrosis of underlying tissues due to burn (deep third degree) of trunk, unspecified site, without mention of loss of a body part
942.41 Deep necrosis of underlying tissues due to burn (deep third degree) of breast, without mention of loss of a body part
942.42 Deep necrosis of underlying tissues due to burn (deep third degree) of chest wall, excluding breast and nipple, without mention of loss of a body part
942.43 Deep necrosis of underlying tissues due to burn (deep third degree) of abdominal wall, without mention of loss of a body part
942.44 Deep necrosis of underlying tissues due to burn (deep third degree) of back (any part), without mention of loss of a body part
942.49 Deep necrosis of underlying tissues due to burn (deep third degree) of other and multiple sites of trunk, without mention of loss of a body part
998.32 Disruption of external operation wound
V50.1 Other plastic surgery for unacceptable cosmetic appearance
V51 Aftercare involving the use of plastic surgery

ICD-9-CM Procedural

86.3 Other local excision or destruction of lesion or tissue of skin and subcutaneous tissue
86.70 Pedicle or flap graft, not otherwise specified
86.71 Cutting and preparation of pedicle grafts or flaps
86.72 Advancement of pedicle graft
86.74 Attachment of pedicle or flap graft to other sites
86.84 Relaxation of scar or web contracture of skin
86.89 Other repair and reconstruction of skin and subcutaneous tissue

HCPCS Level II Supplies & Services

A4462 Abdominal dressing holder, each

14020–14021

14020 Adjacent tissue transfer or rearrangement, scalp, arms and/or legs; defect 10 sq. cm or less
14021 defect 10.1 sq. cm to 30.0 sq. cm

ICD-9-CM Diagnostic

172.4 Malignant melanoma of skin of scalp and neck
172.6 Malignant melanoma of skin of upper limb, including shoulder
172.7 Malignant melanoma of skin of lower limb, including hip
173.4 Other malignant neoplasm of scalp and skin of neck
173.6 Other malignant neoplasm of skin of upper limb, including shoulder
173.7 Other malignant neoplasm of skin of lower limb, including hip
195.0 Malignant neoplasm of head, face, and neck
214.8 Lipoma of other specified sites
216.4 Benign neoplasm of scalp and skin of neck
216.6 Benign neoplasm of skin of upper limb, including shoulder
216.7 Benign neoplasm of skin of lower limb, including hip
216.8 Benign neoplasm of other specified sites of skin
232.6 Carcinoma in situ of skin of upper limb, including shoulder
238.2 Neoplasm of uncertain behavior of skin
239.2 Neoplasms of unspecified nature of bone, soft tissue, and skin
701.4 Keloid scar
701.9 Unspecified hypertrophic and atrophic condition of skin
706.2 Sebaceous cyst
707.10 Ulcer of lower limb, unspecified
707.11 Ulcer of thigh
707.12 Ulcer of calf
707.13 Ulcer of ankle
707.19 Ulcer of other part of lower limb
709.2 Scar condition and fibrosis of skin
709.4 Foreign body granuloma of skin and subcutaneous tissue
709.9 Unspecified disorder of skin and subcutaneous tissue
757.32 Congenital vascular hamartomas
757.33 Congenital pigmentary anomaly of skin
757.39 Other specified congenital anomaly of skin
757.8 Other specified congenital anomalies of the integument
785.4 Gangrene — (Code first any associated underlying condition:250.7, 443.0)
873.0 Open wound of scalp, without mention of complication — (Use additional code to identify infection)
873.1 Open wound of scalp, complicated — (Use additional code to identify infection)

Unspecified code
♀ Female diagnosis
Manifestation code
♂ Male diagnosis

880.03 Open wound of upper arm, without mention of complication — (Use additional code to identify infection)
880.09 Open wound of multiple sites of shoulder and upper arm, without mention of complication — (Use additional code to identify infection)
880.13 Open wound of upper arm, complicated — (Use additional code to identify infection)
880.19 Open wound of multiple sites of shoulder and upper arm, complicated — (Use additional code to identify infection)
881.00 Open wound of forearm, without mention of complication — (Use additional code to identify infection)
881.01 Open wound of elbow, without mention of complication — (Use additional code to identify infection)
881.02 Open wound of wrist, without mention of complication — (Use additional code to identify infection)
881.10 Open wound of forearm, complicated — (Use additional code to identify infection)
881.11 Open wound of elbow, complicated — (Use additional code to identify infection)
881.12 Open wound of wrist, complicated — (Use additional code to identify infection)
884.0 Multiple and unspecified open wound of upper limb, without mention of complication — (Use additional code to identify infection)
884.1 Multiple and unspecified open wound of upper limb, complicated — (Use additional code to identify infection)
887.0 Traumatic amputation of arm and hand (complete) (partial), unilateral, below elbow, without mention of complication — (Use additional code to identify infection)
887.1 Traumatic amputation of arm and hand (complete) (partial), unilateral, below elbow, complicated — (Use additional code to identify infection)
887.2 Traumatic amputation of arm and hand (complete) (partial), unilateral, at or above elbow, without mention of complication — (Use additional code to identify infection)
887.3 Traumatic amputation of arm and hand (complete) (partial), unilateral, at or above elbow, complicated — (Use additional code to identify infection)
887.4 Traumatic amputation of arm and hand (complete) (partial), unilateral, level not specified, without mention of complication — (Use additional code to identify infection) ▽
887.5 Traumatic amputation of arm and hand (complete) (partial), unilateral, level not specified, complicated — (Use additional code to identify infection) ▽
887.6 Traumatic amputation of arm and hand (complete) (partial), bilateral (any level), without mention of complication — (Use additional code to identify infection)
887.7 Traumatic amputation of arm and hand (complete) (partial), bilateral (any level), complicated — (Use additional code to identify infection)
890.0 Open wound of hip and thigh, without mention of complication — (Use additional code to identify infection)
890.1 Open wound of hip and thigh, complicated — (Use additional code to identify infection)
891.0 Open wound of knee, leg (except thigh), and ankle, without mention of complication — (Use additional code to identify infection)
891.1 Open wound of knee, leg (except thigh), and ankle, complicated — (Use additional code to identify infection)
894.0 Multiple and unspecified open wound of lower limb, without mention of complication — (Use additional code to identify infection)
894.1 Multiple and unspecified open wound of lower limb, complicated — (Use additional code to identify infection)
897.0 Traumatic amputation of leg(s) (complete) (partial), unilateral, below knee, without mention of complication — (Use additional code to identify infection)
897.1 Traumatic amputation of leg(s) (complete) (partial), unilateral, below knee, complicated — (Use additional code to identify infection)
897.2 Traumatic amputation of leg(s) (complete) (partial), unilateral, at or above knee, without mention of complication — (Use additional code to identify infection)
897.3 Traumatic amputation of leg(s) (complete) (partial), unilateral, at or above knee, complicated — (Use additional code to identify infection)
897.4 Traumatic amputation of leg(s) (complete) (partial), unilateral, level not specified, without mention of complication — (Use additional code to identify infection) ▽
897.5 Traumatic amputation of leg(s) (complete) (partial), unilateral, level not specified, complicated — (Use additional code to identify infection) ▽
897.6 Traumatic amputation of leg(s) (complete) (partial), bilateral (any level), without mention of complication — (Use additional code to identify infection)
897.7 Traumatic amputation of leg(s) (complete) (partial), bilateral (any level), complicated — (Use additional code to identify infection)
906.0 Late effect of open wound of head, neck, and trunk
906.1 Late effect of open wound of extremities without mention of tendon injury
906.5 Late effect of burn of eye, face, head, and neck
906.6 Late effect of burn of wrist and hand
906.7 Late effect of burn of other extremities
909.3 Late effect of complications of surgical and medical care
V50.1 Other plastic surgery for unacceptable cosmetic appearance
V51 Aftercare involving the use of plastic surgery

ICD-9-CM Procedural

86.3 Other local excision or destruction of lesion or tissue of skin and subcutaneous tissue
86.70 Pedicle or flap graft, not otherwise specified
86.71 Cutting and preparation of pedicle grafts or flaps
86.72 Advancement of pedicle graft
86.74 Attachment of pedicle or flap graft to other sites
86.84 Relaxation of scar or web contracture of skin
86.89 Other repair and reconstruction of skin and subcutaneous tissue

HCPCS Level II Supplies & Services

A4305 Disposable drug delivery system, flow rate of 50 ml or greater per hour
A4306 Disposable drug delivery system, flow rate of 5 ml or less per hour
A4550 Surgical trays

14040–14041

14040 Adjacent tissue transfer or rearrangement, forehead, cheeks, chin, mouth, neck, axillae, genitalia, hands and/or feet; defect 10 sq. cm or less
14041 defect 10.1 sq. cm to 30.0 sq. cm

ICD-9-CM Diagnostic

171.0 Malignant neoplasm of connective and other soft tissue of head, face, and neck
171.2 Malignant neoplasm of connective and other soft tissue of upper limb, including shoulder
171.3 Malignant neoplasm of connective and other soft tissue of lower limb, including hip
171.8 Malignant neoplasm of other specified sites of connective and other soft tissue
172.0 Malignant melanoma of skin of lip
172.3 Malignant melanoma of skin of other and unspecified parts of face
172.4 Malignant melanoma of skin of scalp and neck
172.5 Malignant melanoma of skin of trunk, except scrotum
172.6 Malignant melanoma of skin of upper limb, including shoulder
172.7 Malignant melanoma of skin of lower limb, including hip
173.3 Other malignant neoplasm of skin of other and unspecified parts of face ▽
173.4 Other malignant neoplasm of scalp and skin of neck
173.5 Other malignant neoplasm of skin of trunk, except scrotum
173.6 Other malignant neoplasm of skin of upper limb, including shoulder
173.7 Other malignant neoplasm of skin of lower limb, including hip
173.8 Other malignant neoplasm of other specified sites of skin
184.0 Malignant neoplasm of vagina ♀
184.1 Malignant neoplasm of labia majora ♀
184.2 Malignant neoplasm of labia minora ♀
184.3 Malignant neoplasm of clitoris ♀
184.4 Malignant neoplasm of vulva, unspecified site ▽ ♀
184.8 Malignant neoplasm of other specified sites of female genital organs ♀
184.9 Malignant neoplasm of female genital organ, site unspecified ▽ ♀
187.1 Malignant neoplasm of prepuce ♂
187.3 Malignant neoplasm of body of penis ♂
187.4 Malignant neoplasm of penis, part unspecified ▽ ♂
187.7 Malignant neoplasm of scrotum ♂
187.8 Malignant neoplasm of other specified sites of male genital organs ♂
195.0 Malignant neoplasm of head, face, and neck
195.1 Malignant neoplasm of thorax
195.3 Malignant neoplasm of pelvis
195.4 Malignant neoplasm of upper limb
195.5 Malignant neoplasm of lower limb
195.8 Malignant neoplasm of other specified sites
198.2 Secondary malignant neoplasm of skin
198.89 Secondary malignant neoplasm of other specified sites
214.0 Lipoma of skin and subcutaneous tissue of face
214.1 Lipoma of other skin and subcutaneous tissue
215.0 Other benign neoplasm of connective and other soft tissue of head, face, and neck
215.2 Other benign neoplasm of connective and other soft tissue of upper limb, including shoulder
215.3 Other benign neoplasm of connective and other soft tissue of lower limb, including hip
215.6 Other benign neoplasm of connective and other soft tissue of pelvis

215.8 Other benign neoplasm of connective and other soft tissue of other specified sites
216.3 Benign neoplasm of skin of other and unspecified parts of face ▽
216.4 Benign neoplasm of scalp and skin of neck
216.5 Benign neoplasm of skin of trunk, except scrotum
216.8 Benign neoplasm of other specified sites of skin
228.01 Hemangioma of skin and subcutaneous tissue
229.8 Benign neoplasm of other specified sites
232.3 Carcinoma in situ of skin of other and unspecified parts of face ▽
232.4 Carcinoma in situ of scalp and skin of neck
232.5 Carcinoma in situ of skin of trunk, except scrotum
232.8 Carcinoma in situ of other specified sites of skin
234.8 Carcinoma in situ of other specified sites
238.2 Neoplasm of uncertain behavior of skin
238.8 Neoplasm of uncertain behavior of other specified sites
239.2 Neoplasms of unspecified nature of bone, soft tissue, and skin
239.8 Neoplasm of unspecified nature of other specified sites
629.20 Female genital mutilation status, unspecified
629.21 Female genital mutilation, Type I status
629.22 Female genital mutilation, Type II status
701.4 Keloid scar
701.5 Other abnormal granulation tissue
707.8 Chronic ulcer of other specified site
709.2 Scar condition and fibrosis of skin
709.4 Foreign body granuloma of skin and subcutaneous tissue
757.32 Congenital vascular hamartomas
757.39 Other specified congenital anomaly of skin
873.40 Open wound of face, unspecified site, without mention of complication — (Use additional code to identify infection) ▽
873.41 Open wound of cheek, without mention of complication — (Use additional code to identify infection)
873.42 Open wound of forehead, without mention of complication — (Use additional code to identify infection)
873.43 Open wound of lip, without mention of complication — (Use additional code to identify infection)
873.44 Open wound of jaw, without mention of complication — (Use additional code to identify infection)
873.49 Open wound of face, other and multiple sites, without mention of complication — (Use additional code to identify infection)
873.50 Open wound of face, unspecified site, complicated — (Use additional code to identify infection) ▽
873.51 Open wound of cheek, complicated — (Use additional code to identify infection)
873.52 Open wound of forehead, complicated — (Use additional code to identify infection)
873.53 Open wound of lip, complicated — (Use additional code to identify infection)
873.54 Open wound of jaw, complicated — (Use additional code to identify infection)
873.59 Open wound of face, other and multiple sites, complicated — (Use additional code to identify infection)
873.70 Open wound of mouth, unspecified site, complicated — (Use additional code to identify infection) ▽
873.71 Open wound of buccal mucosa, complicated — (Use additional code to identify infection)
873.74 Open wound of tongue and floor of mouth, complicated — (Use additional code to identify infection)
873.79 Open wound of mouth, other and multiple sites, complicated — (Use additional code to identify infection)
878.0 Open wound of penis, without mention of complication — (Use additional code to identify infection) ♂
878.1 Open wound of penis, complicated — (Use additional code to identify infection) ♂
878.2 Open wound of scrotum and testes, without mention of complication — (Use additional code to identify infection) ♂
878.3 Open wound of scrotum and testes, complicated — (Use additional code to identify infection) ♂
878.4 Open wound of vulva, without mention of complication — (Use additional code to identify infection) ♀
878.5 Open wound of vulva, complicated — (Use additional code to identify infection) ♀
878.6 Open wound of vagina, without mention of complication — (Use additional code to identify infection) ♀
878.7 Open wound of vagina, complicated — (Use additional code to identify infection) ♀
878.8 Open wound of other and unspecified parts of genital organs, without mention of complication — (Use additional code to identify infection) ▽
878.9 Open wound of other and unspecified parts of genital organs, complicated — (Use additional code to identify infection) ▽
880.02 Open wound of axillary region, without mention of complication — (Use additional code to identify infection)
880.12 Open wound of axillary region, complicated — (Use additional code to identify infection)
882.0 Open wound of hand except finger(s) alone, without mention of complication — (Use additional code to identify infection)
882.1 Open wound of hand except finger(s) alone, complicated — (Use additional code to identify infection)
883.0 Open wound of finger(s), without mention of complication — (Use additional code to identify infection)
883.1 Open wound of finger(s), complicated — (Use additional code to identify infection)
884.0 Multiple and unspecified open wound of upper limb, without mention of complication — (Use additional code to identify infection)
884.1 Multiple and unspecified open wound of upper limb, complicated — (Use additional code to identify infection)
892.0 Open wound of foot except toe(s) alone, without mention of complication — (Use additional code to identify infection)
892.1 Open wound of foot except toe(s) alone, complicated — (Use additional code to identify infection)
893.0 Open wound of toe(s), without mention of complication — (Use additional code to identify infection)
893.1 Open wound of toe(s), complicated — (Use additional code to identify infection)
894.0 Multiple and unspecified open wound of lower limb, without mention of complication — (Use additional code to identify infection)
894.1 Multiple and unspecified open wound of lower limb, complicated — (Use additional code to identify infection)
906.0 Late effect of open wound of head, neck, and trunk
906.1 Late effect of open wound of extremities without mention of tendon injury
906.5 Late effect of burn of eye, face, head, and neck
906.6 Late effect of burn of wrist and hand
906.7 Late effect of burn of other extremities
906.8 Late effect of burns of other specified sites
941.03 Burn of unspecified degree of lip(s) ▽
941.07 Burn of unspecified degree of forehead and cheek ▽
959.09 Injury of face and neck, other and unspecified
959.14 Other injury of external genitals
959.2 Injury, other and unspecified, shoulder and upper arm
959.3 Injury, other and unspecified, elbow, forearm, and wrist
959.4 Injury, other and unspecified, hand, except finger
959.7 Injury, other and unspecified, knee, leg, ankle, and foot
959.8 Injury, other and unspecified, other specified sites, including multiple
996.92 Complications of reattached hand
996.93 Complications of reattached finger(s)
996.95 Complications of reattached foot and toe(s)
997.60 Late complications of amputation stump, unspecified — (Use additional code to identify complications) ▽
997.61 Neuroma of amputation stump — (Use additional code to identify complications)
997.62 Infection (chronic) of amputation stump — (Use additional code to identify organism. Use additional code to identify complications)
997.69 Other late amputation stump complication — (Use additional code to identify complications)
998.32 Disruption of external operation wound
998.59 Other postoperative infection — (Use additional code to identify infection)
998.83 Non-healing surgical wound
V10.44 Personal history of malignant neoplasm of other female genital organs ♀
V10.45 Personal history of malignant neoplasm of unspecified male genital organ ▽ ♂
V10.49 Personal history of malignant neoplasm of other male genital organs ♂
V10.82 Personal history of malignant melanoma of skin
V10.83 Personal history of other malignant neoplasm of skin
V50.1 Other plastic surgery for unacceptable cosmetic appearance
V51 Aftercare involving the use of plastic surgery

ICD-9-CM Procedural

27.57 Attachment of pedicle or flap graft to lip and mouth
86.3 Other local excision or destruction of lesion or tissue of skin and subcutaneous tissue
86.70 Pedicle or flap graft, not otherwise specified
86.71 Cutting and preparation of pedicle grafts or flaps
86.72 Advancement of pedicle graft
86.73 Attachment of pedicle or flap graft to hand
86.74 Attachment of pedicle or flap graft to other sites
86.84 Relaxation of scar or web contracture of skin

▽ Unspecified code
♀ Female diagnosis
☒ Manifestation code
♂ Male diagnosis

86.89 Other repair and reconstruction of skin and subcutaneous tissue

HCPCS Level II Supplies & Services

A4305 Disposable drug delivery system, flow rate of 50 ml or greater per hour
A4306 Disposable drug delivery system, flow rate of 5 ml or less per hour
A4550 Surgical trays

14060–14061

14060 Adjacent tissue transfer or rearrangement, eyelids, nose, ears and/or lips; defect 10 sq. cm or less
14061 defect 10.1 sq. cm to 30.0 sq. cm

ICD-9-CM Diagnostic

171.0 Malignant neoplasm of connective and other soft tissue of head, face, and neck
172.0 Malignant melanoma of skin of lip
172.1 Malignant melanoma of skin of eyelid, including canthus
172.2 Malignant melanoma of skin of ear and external auditory canal
172.3 Malignant melanoma of skin of other and unspecified parts of face
173.0 Other malignant neoplasm of skin of lip
173.1 Other malignant neoplasm of skin of eyelid, including canthus
173.2 Other malignant neoplasm of skin of ear and external auditory canal
173.3 Other malignant neoplasm of skin of other and unspecified parts of face ▽
173.8 Other malignant neoplasm of other specified sites of skin
195.0 Malignant neoplasm of head, face, and neck
198.2 Secondary malignant neoplasm of skin
210.0 Benign neoplasm of lip
214.0 Lipoma of skin and subcutaneous tissue of face
214.1 Lipoma of other skin and subcutaneous tissue
215.0 Other benign neoplasm of connective and other soft tissue of head, face, and neck
216.0 Benign neoplasm of skin of lip
216.1 Benign neoplasm of eyelid, including canthus
216.2 Benign neoplasm of ear and external auditory canal
216.3 Benign neoplasm of skin of other and unspecified parts of face ▽
228.01 Hemangioma of skin and subcutaneous tissue
230.0 Carcinoma in situ of lip, oral cavity, and pharynx
231.8 Carcinoma in situ of other specified parts of respiratory system
232.0 Carcinoma in situ of skin of lip
232.1 Carcinoma in situ of eyelid, including canthus
232.2 Carcinoma in situ of skin of ear and external auditory canal
232.3 Carcinoma in situ of skin of other and unspecified parts of face ▽
235.1 Neoplasm of uncertain behavior of lip, oral cavity, and pharynx
238.2 Neoplasm of uncertain behavior of skin
239.2 Neoplasms of unspecified nature of bone, soft tissue, and skin
373.4 Infective dermatitis of eyelid of types resulting in deformity — (Code first underlying disease: 017.0, 030.0-030.9, 102.0-102.9) ☒
374.50 Unspecified degenerative disorder of eyelid ▽
374.84 Cysts of eyelids
374.86 Retained foreign body of eyelid
374.89 Other disorders of eyelid
701.4 Keloid scar
701.9 Unspecified hypertrophic and atrophic condition of skin ▽
707.8 Chronic ulcer of other specified site
709.2 Scar condition and fibrosis of skin
709.4 Foreign body granuloma of skin and subcutaneous tissue
743.62 Congenital deformity of eyelid
744.21 Congenital absence of ear lobe
744.23 Microtia
749.10 Unspecified cleft lip ▽
749.11 Unilateral cleft lip, complete
749.12 Unilateral cleft lip, incomplete
749.13 Bilateral cleft lip, complete
749.14 Bilateral cleft lip, incomplete
757.32 Congenital vascular hamartomas
757.39 Other specified congenital anomaly of skin
870.0 Laceration of skin of eyelid and periocular area — (Use additional code to identify infection)
870.1 Laceration of eyelid, full-thickness, not involving lacrimal passages — (Use additional code to identify infection)
870.2 Laceration of eyelid involving lacrimal passages — (Use additional code to identify infection)
870.8 Other specified open wound of ocular adnexa — (Use additional code to identify infection)
872.00 Open wound of external ear, unspecified site, without mention of complication — (Use additional code to identify infection) ▽
872.01 Open wound of auricle, without mention of complication — (Use additional code to identify infection)
872.10 Open wound of external ear, unspecified site, complicated — (Use additional code to identify infection) ▽
872.11 Open wound of auricle, complicated — (Use additional code to identify infection)
872.8 Open wound of ear, part unspecified, without mention of complication — (Use additional code to identify infection) ▽
873.20 Open wound of nose, unspecified site, without mention of complication — (Use additional code to identify infection) ▽
873.30 Open wound of nose, unspecified site, complicated — (Use additional code to identify infection) ▽
873.43 Open wound of lip, without mention of complication — (Use additional code to identify infection)
873.53 Open wound of lip, complicated — (Use additional code to identify infection)
906.0 Late effect of open wound of head, neck, and trunk
906.2 Late effect of superficial injury
906.5 Late effect of burn of eye, face, head, and neck
941.09 Burn of unspecified degree of multiple sites (except with eye) of face, head, and neck ▽
959.09 Injury of face and neck, other and unspecified
998.32 Disruption of external operation wound
998.59 Other postoperative infection — (Use additional code to identify infection)
998.83 Non-healing surgical wound
998.89 Other specified complications
V10.02 Personal history of malignant neoplasm of other and unspecified parts of oral cavity and pharynx ▽
V10.82 Personal history of malignant melanoma of skin
V10.83 Personal history of other malignant neoplasm of skin
V50.1 Other plastic surgery for unacceptable cosmetic appearance
V51 Aftercare involving the use of plastic surgery

ICD-9-CM Procedural

08.62 Reconstruction of eyelid with mucous membrane flap or graft
08.63 Reconstruction of eyelid with hair follicle graft
18.72 Reattachment of amputated ear
18.79 Other plastic repair of external ear
27.56 Other skin graft to lip and mouth
27.57 Attachment of pedicle or flap graft to lip and mouth
86.3 Other local excision or destruction of lesion or tissue of skin and subcutaneous tissue
86.70 Pedicle or flap graft, not otherwise specified
86.71 Cutting and preparation of pedicle grafts or flaps
86.72 Advancement of pedicle graft
86.74 Attachment of pedicle or flap graft to other sites
86.84 Relaxation of scar or web contracture of skin
86.89 Other repair and reconstruction of skin and subcutaneous tissue

HCPCS Level II Supplies & Services

A4305 Disposable drug delivery system, flow rate of 50 ml or greater per hour
A4306 Disposable drug delivery system, flow rate of 5 ml or less per hour
A4550 Surgical trays

14300

14300 Adjacent tissue transfer or rearrangement, more than 30 sq. cm, unusual or complicated, any area

ICD-9-CM Diagnostic

140.0 Malignant neoplasm of upper lip, vermilion border
140.1 Malignant neoplasm of lower lip, vermilion border
140.3 Malignant neoplasm of upper lip, inner aspect
140.4 Malignant neoplasm of lower lip, inner aspect
140.5 Malignant neoplasm of lip, inner aspect, unspecified as to upper or lower ▽
140.6 Malignant neoplasm of commissure of lip
140.8 Malignant neoplasm of other sites of lip
140.9 Malignant neoplasm of lip, vermilion border, unspecified as to upper or lower ▽
171.0 Malignant neoplasm of connective and other soft tissue of head, face, and neck
172.0 Malignant melanoma of skin of lip
172.1 Malignant melanoma of skin of eyelid, including canthus
172.2 Malignant melanoma of skin of ear and external auditory canal
172.3 Malignant melanoma of skin of other and unspecified parts of face
172.4 Malignant melanoma of skin of scalp and neck
172.5 Malignant melanoma of skin of trunk, except scrotum
172.6 Malignant melanoma of skin of upper limb, including shoulder
172.7 Malignant melanoma of skin of lower limb, including hip

172.8 Malignant melanoma of other specified sites of skin
173.0 Other malignant neoplasm of skin of lip
173.1 Other malignant neoplasm of skin of eyelid, including canthus
173.2 Other malignant neoplasm of skin of ear and external auditory canal
173.3 Other malignant neoplasm of skin of other and unspecified parts of face ▽
173.4 Other malignant neoplasm of scalp and skin of neck
173.5 Other malignant neoplasm of skin of trunk, except scrotum
173.6 Other malignant neoplasm of skin of upper limb, including shoulder
173.7 Other malignant neoplasm of skin of lower limb, including hip
173.8 Other malignant neoplasm of other specified sites of skin
174.0 Malignant neoplasm of nipple and areola of female breast ♀
174.1 Malignant neoplasm of central portion of female breast ♀
174.2 Malignant neoplasm of upper-inner quadrant of female breast ♀
174.3 Malignant neoplasm of lower-inner quadrant of female breast ♀
174.4 Malignant neoplasm of upper-outer quadrant of female breast ♀
174.5 Malignant neoplasm of lower-outer quadrant of female breast ♀
174.6 Malignant neoplasm of axillary tail of female breast ♀
174.8 Malignant neoplasm of other specified sites of female breast ♀
175.0 Malignant neoplasm of nipple and areola of male breast ♂
175.9 Malignant neoplasm of other and unspecified sites of male breast ▽ ♂
176.0 Kaposi's sarcoma of skin
184.9 Malignant neoplasm of female genital organ, site unspecified ▽ ♀
187.8 Malignant neoplasm of other specified sites of male genital organs ♂
195.0 Malignant neoplasm of head, face, and neck
195.1 Malignant neoplasm of thorax
195.2 Malignant neoplasm of abdomen
195.3 Malignant neoplasm of pelvis
195.4 Malignant neoplasm of upper limb
195.5 Malignant neoplasm of lower limb
195.8 Malignant neoplasm of other specified sites
198.2 Secondary malignant neoplasm of skin
214.0 Lipoma of skin and subcutaneous tissue of face
214.1 Lipoma of other skin and subcutaneous tissue
215.0 Other benign neoplasm of connective and other soft tissue of head, face, and neck
215.2 Other benign neoplasm of connective and other soft tissue of upper limb, including shoulder
215.3 Other benign neoplasm of connective and other soft tissue of lower limb, including hip
215.4 Other benign neoplasm of connective and other soft tissue of thorax
215.5 Other benign neoplasm of connective and other soft tissue of abdomen
215.6 Other benign neoplasm of connective and other soft tissue of pelvis
215.7 Other benign neoplasm of connective and other soft tissue of trunk, unspecified ▽
215.8 Other benign neoplasm of connective and other soft tissue of other specified sites
216.0 Benign neoplasm of skin of lip
216.1 Benign neoplasm of eyelid, including canthus
216.2 Benign neoplasm of ear and external auditory canal
216.3 Benign neoplasm of skin of other and unspecified parts of face ▽
216.4 Benign neoplasm of scalp and skin of neck
216.5 Benign neoplasm of skin of trunk, except scrotum
216.6 Benign neoplasm of skin of upper limb, including shoulder
216.7 Benign neoplasm of skin of lower limb, including hip
216.8 Benign neoplasm of other specified sites of skin
228.01 Hemangioma of skin and subcutaneous tissue
230.0 Carcinoma in situ of lip, oral cavity, and pharynx
232.1 Carcinoma in situ of eyelid, including canthus
232.2 Carcinoma in situ of skin of ear and external auditory canal
232.3 Carcinoma in situ of skin of other and unspecified parts of face ▽
232.4 Carcinoma in situ of scalp and skin of neck
232.5 Carcinoma in situ of skin of trunk, except scrotum
232.6 Carcinoma in situ of skin of upper limb, including shoulder
232.7 Carcinoma in situ of skin of lower limb, including hip
232.8 Carcinoma in situ of other specified sites of skin
235.1 Neoplasm of uncertain behavior of lip, oral cavity, and pharynx
238.2 Neoplasm of uncertain behavior of skin
239.2 Neoplasms of unspecified nature of bone, soft tissue, and skin
701.4 Keloid scar
709.2 Scar condition and fibrosis of skin
709.9 Unspecified disorder of skin and subcutaneous tissue ▽
728.86 Necrotizing fasciitis — (Use additional code to identify infectious organism, 041.00-041.89, 785.4, if applicable)
757.32 Congenital vascular hamartomas
757.39 Other specified congenital anomaly of skin
785.4 Gangrene — (Code first any associated underlying condition:250.7, 443.0)
872.10 Open wound of external ear, unspecified site, complicated — (Use additional code to identify infection) ▽
872.11 Open wound of auricle, complicated — (Use additional code to identify infection)
873.1 Open wound of scalp, complicated — (Use additional code to identify infection)
873.30 Open wound of nose, unspecified site, complicated — (Use additional code to identify infection) ▽
873.49 Open wound of face, other and multiple sites, without mention of complication — (Use additional code to identify infection)
873.50 Open wound of face, unspecified site, complicated — (Use additional code to identify infection) ▽
873.51 Open wound of cheek, complicated — (Use additional code to identify infection)
873.52 Open wound of forehead, complicated — (Use additional code to identify infection)
873.53 Open wound of lip, complicated — (Use additional code to identify infection)
873.54 Open wound of jaw, complicated — (Use additional code to identify infection)
873.59 Open wound of face, other and multiple sites, complicated — (Use additional code to identify infection)
873.9 Other and unspecified open wound of head, complicated — (Use additional code to identify infection) ▽
874.8 Open wound of other and unspecified parts of neck, without mention of complication — (Use additional code to identify infection) ▽
874.9 Open wound of other and unspecified parts of neck, complicated — (Use additional code to identify infection) ▽
875.1 Open wound of chest (wall), complicated — (Use additional code to identify infection)
876.1 Open wound of back, complicated — (Use additional code to identify infection)
877.1 Open wound of buttock, complicated — (Use additional code to identify infection)
878.1 Open wound of penis, complicated — (Use additional code to identify infection) ♂
878.3 Open wound of scrotum and testes, complicated — (Use additional code to identify infection) ♂
878.5 Open wound of vulva, complicated — (Use additional code to identify infection) ♀
878.9 Open wound of other and unspecified parts of genital organs, complicated — (Use additional code to identify infection) ▽
879.1 Open wound of breast, complicated — (Use additional code to identify infection)
879.3 Open wound of abdominal wall, anterior, complicated — (Use additional code to identify infection)
879.5 Open wound of abdominal wall, lateral, complicated — (Use additional code to identify infection)
879.9 Open wound(s) (multiple) of unspecified site(s), complicated — (Use additional code to identify infection) ▽
880.10 Open wound of shoulder region, complicated — (Use additional code to identify infection)
880.11 Open wound of scapular region, complicated — (Use additional code to identify infection)
880.13 Open wound of upper arm, complicated — (Use additional code to identify infection)
880.19 Open wound of multiple sites of shoulder and upper arm, complicated — (Use additional code to identify infection)
882.1 Open wound of hand except finger(s) alone, complicated — (Use additional code to identify infection)
883.1 Open wound of finger(s), complicated — (Use additional code to identify infection)
890.1 Open wound of hip and thigh, complicated — (Use additional code to identify infection)
891.1 Open wound of knee, leg (except thigh), and ankle, complicated — (Use additional code to identify infection)
892.1 Open wound of foot except toe(s) alone, complicated — (Use additional code to identify infection)
893.1 Open wound of toe(s), complicated — (Use additional code to identify infection)
894.1 Multiple and unspecified open wound of lower limb, complicated — (Use additional code to identify infection)
906.0 Late effect of open wound of head, neck, and trunk
906.1 Late effect of open wound of extremities without mention of tendon injury
906.4 Late effect of crushing
906.5 Late effect of burn of eye, face, head, and neck
906.6 Late effect of burn of wrist and hand
906.7 Late effect of burn of other extremities
906.8 Late effect of burns of other specified sites

▽ Unspecified code
♀ Female diagnosis
☒ Manifestation code
♂ Male diagnosis

941.19 Erythema due to burn (first degree) of multiple sites (except with eye) of face, head, and neck
941.20 Blisters, with epidermal loss due to burn (second degree) of face and head, unspecified site ▽
991.0 Frostbite of face
991.1 Frostbite of hand
991.2 Frostbite of foot
991.3 Frostbite of other and unspecified sites
991.6 Effects of hypothermia
991.8 Other specified effects of reduced temperature
997.60 Late complications of amputation stump, unspecified — (Use additional code to identify complications) ▽
997.61 Neuroma of amputation stump — (Use additional code to identify complications)
997.62 Infection (chronic) of amputation stump — (Use additional code to identify organism. Use additional code to identify complications)
997.69 Other late amputation stump complication — (Use additional code to identify complications)
998.32 Disruption of external operation wound
998.59 Other postoperative infection — (Use additional code to identify infection)
998.83 Non-healing surgical wound
V10.02 Personal history of malignant neoplasm of other and unspecified parts of oral cavity and pharynx ▽
V10.82 Personal history of malignant melanoma of skin
V10.83 Personal history of other malignant neoplasm of skin
V51 Aftercare involving the use of plastic surgery
V84.01 Genetic susceptibility to malignant neoplasm of breast
V84.09 Genetic susceptibility to other malignant neoplasm

ICD-9-CM Procedural

21.83 Total nasal reconstruction
27.57 Attachment of pedicle or flap graft to lip and mouth
85.81 Suture of laceration of breast
85.84 Pedicle graft to breast
86.3 Other local excision or destruction of lesion or tissue of skin and subcutaneous tissue
86.70 Pedicle or flap graft, not otherwise specified
86.71 Cutting and preparation of pedicle grafts or flaps
86.72 Advancement of pedicle graft
86.73 Attachment of pedicle or flap graft to hand
86.74 Attachment of pedicle or flap graft to other sites
86.84 Relaxation of scar or web contracture of skin
86.89 Other repair and reconstruction of skin and subcutaneous tissue

14350

14350 Filleted finger or toe flap, including preparation of recipient site

ICD-9-CM Diagnostic

250.70 Diabetes with peripheral circulatory disorders, type II or unspecified type, not stated as uncontrolled — (Use additional code to identify manifestation: 443.81, 785.4)
250.71 Diabetes with peripheral circulatory disorders, type I [juvenile type], not stated as uncontrolled — (Use additional code to identify manifestation: 443.81, 785.4)
250.72 Diabetes with peripheral circulatory disorders, type II or unspecified type, uncontrolled — (Use additional code to identify manifestation: 443.81, 785.4)
250.73 Diabetes with peripheral circulatory disorders, type I [juvenile type], uncontrolled — (Use additional code to identify manifestation: 443.81, 785.4)
443.81 Peripheral angiopathy in diseases classified elsewhere — (Code first underlying disease, 250.7) ☒
707.15 Ulcer of other part of foot
707.8 Chronic ulcer of other specified site
709.2 Scar condition and fibrosis of skin
785.4 Gangrene — (Code first any associated underlying condition:250.7, 443.0)
816.10 Open fracture of phalanx or phalanges of hand, unspecified ▽
816.11 Open fracture of middle or proximal phalanx or phalanges of hand
816.12 Open fracture of distal phalanx or phalanges of hand
816.13 Open fractures of multiple sites of phalanx or phalanges of hand
826.1 Open fracture of one or more phalanges of foot
885.0 Traumatic amputation of thumb (complete) (partial), without mention of complication — (Use additional code to identify infection)
885.1 Traumatic amputation of thumb (complete) (partial), complicated — (Use additional code to identify infection)
886.0 Traumatic amputation of other finger(s) (complete) (partial), without mention of complication — (Use additional code to identify infection)
886.1 Traumatic amputation of other finger(s) (complete) (partial), complicated — (Use additional code to identify infection)
895.0 Traumatic amputation of toe(s) (complete) (partial), without mention of complication — (Use additional code to identify infection)
895.1 Traumatic amputation of toe(s) (complete) (partial), complicated — (Use additional code to identify infection)
928.3 Crushing injury of toe(s) — (Use additional code to identify any associated injuries: 800-829, 850.0-854.1, 860.0-869.1)
944.30 Full-thickness skin loss due to burn (third degree nos) of unspecified site of hand ▽
944.31 Full-thickness skin loss due to burn (third degree nos) of single digit [finger (nail)] other than thumb
944.32 Full-thickness skin loss due to burn (third degree nos) of thumb (nail)
944.33 Full-thickness skin loss due to burn (third degree nos) of two or more digits of hand, not including thumb
944.34 Full-thickness skin loss due to burn (third degree nos) of two or more digits of hand including thumb
944.38 Full-thickness skin loss due to burn (third degree nos) of multiple sites of wrist(s) and hand(s)
944.40 Deep necrosis of underlying tissues due to burn (deep third degree) of unspecified site of hand, without mention of a body part ▽
944.41 Deep necrosis of underlying tissues due to burn (deep third degree) of single digit [finger (nail)] other than thumb, without mention of a body part
944.42 Deep necrosis of underlying tissues due to burn (deep third degree) of thumb (nail), without mention of loss of a body part
944.43 Deep necrosis of underlying tissues due to burn (deep third degree) of two or more digits of hand, not including thumb, without mention of a body part
944.44 Deep necrosis of underlying tissues due to burn (deep third degree) of two or more digits of hand including thumb, without mention of a body part
944.48 Deep necrosis of underlying tissues due to burn (deep third degree) of multiple sites of wrist(s) and hand(s), without mention of loss of a body part
945.10 Erythema due to burn (first degree) of unspecified site of lower limb (leg) ▽
945.41 Deep necrosis of underlying tissues due to burn (deep third degree) of toe(s) (nail), without mention of loss of a body part
945.49 Deep necrosis of underlying tissues due to burn (deep third degree) of multiple sites of lower limb(s), without mention of loss of a body part
V10.82 Personal history of malignant melanoma of skin
V10.83 Personal history of other malignant neoplasm of skin

ICD-9-CM Procedural

86.3 Other local excision or destruction of lesion or tissue of skin and subcutaneous tissue
86.71 Cutting and preparation of pedicle grafts or flaps
86.72 Advancement of pedicle graft
86.73 Attachment of pedicle or flap graft to hand
86.74 Attachment of pedicle or flap graft to other sites

HCPCS Level II Supplies & Services

A4550 Surgical trays

15000–15001

15000 Surgical preparation or creation of recipient site by excision of open wounds, burn eschar, or scar (including subcutaneous tissues); first 100 sq. cm or one percent of body area of infants and children
15001 each additional 100 sq. cm or each additional one percent of body area of infants and children (List separately in addition to code for primary procedure)

ICD-9-CM Diagnostic

140.0 Malignant neoplasm of upper lip, vermilion border
140.1 Malignant neoplasm of lower lip, vermilion border
140.3 Malignant neoplasm of upper lip, inner aspect
140.4 Malignant neoplasm of lower lip, inner aspect
140.5 Malignant neoplasm of lip, inner aspect, unspecified as to upper or lower ▽
140.6 Malignant neoplasm of commissure of lip
140.8 Malignant neoplasm of other sites of lip
140.9 Malignant neoplasm of lip, vermilion border, unspecified as to upper or lower ▽
172.0 Malignant melanoma of skin of lip
172.1 Malignant melanoma of skin of eyelid, including canthus
172.2 Malignant melanoma of skin of ear and external auditory canal
172.3 Malignant melanoma of skin of other and unspecified parts of face
172.4 Malignant melanoma of skin of scalp and neck
172.5 Malignant melanoma of skin of trunk, except scrotum
172.6 Malignant melanoma of skin of upper limb, including shoulder
172.7 Malignant melanoma of skin of lower limb, including hip

172.8 Malignant melanoma of other specified sites of skin
173.0 Other malignant neoplasm of skin of lip
173.1 Other malignant neoplasm of skin of eyelid, including canthus
173.2 Other malignant neoplasm of skin of ear and external auditory canal
173.3 Other malignant neoplasm of skin of other and unspecified parts of face ▽
173.4 Other malignant neoplasm of scalp and skin of neck
173.5 Other malignant neoplasm of skin of trunk, except scrotum
173.6 Other malignant neoplasm of skin of upper limb, including shoulder
173.7 Other malignant neoplasm of skin of lower limb, including hip
173.8 Other malignant neoplasm of other specified sites of skin
174.0 Malignant neoplasm of nipple and areola of female breast ♀
174.1 Malignant neoplasm of central portion of female breast ♀
174.2 Malignant neoplasm of upper-inner quadrant of female breast ♀
174.3 Malignant neoplasm of lower-inner quadrant of female breast ♀
174.4 Malignant neoplasm of upper-outer quadrant of female breast ♀
174.5 Malignant neoplasm of lower-outer quadrant of female breast ♀
174.6 Malignant neoplasm of axillary tail of female breast ♀
174.8 Malignant neoplasm of other specified sites of female breast ♀
175.9 Malignant neoplasm of other and unspecified sites of male breast ▽ ♂
176.0 Kaposi's sarcoma of skin
195.0 Malignant neoplasm of head, face, and neck
195.1 Malignant neoplasm of thorax
195.2 Malignant neoplasm of abdomen
195.3 Malignant neoplasm of pelvis
195.4 Malignant neoplasm of upper limb
195.5 Malignant neoplasm of lower limb
195.8 Malignant neoplasm of other specified sites
198.2 Secondary malignant neoplasm of skin
214.0 Lipoma of skin and subcutaneous tissue of face
214.1 Lipoma of other skin and subcutaneous tissue
215.0 Other benign neoplasm of connective and other soft tissue of head, face, and neck
215.2 Other benign neoplasm of connective and other soft tissue of upper limb, including shoulder
215.3 Other benign neoplasm of connective and other soft tissue of lower limb, including hip
215.4 Other benign neoplasm of connective and other soft tissue of thorax
215.5 Other benign neoplasm of connective and other soft tissue of abdomen
215.6 Other benign neoplasm of connective and other soft tissue of pelvis
215.7 Other benign neoplasm of connective and other soft tissue of trunk, unspecified ▽
215.8 Other benign neoplasm of connective and other soft tissue of other specified sites
216.0 Benign neoplasm of skin of lip
216.1 Benign neoplasm of eyelid, including canthus
216.2 Benign neoplasm of ear and external auditory canal
216.3 Benign neoplasm of skin of other and unspecified parts of face ▽
216.4 Benign neoplasm of scalp and skin of neck
216.5 Benign neoplasm of skin of trunk, except scrotum
216.6 Benign neoplasm of skin of upper limb, including shoulder
216.7 Benign neoplasm of skin of lower limb, including hip
216.8 Benign neoplasm of other specified sites of skin
228.01 Hemangioma of skin and subcutaneous tissue
230.0 Carcinoma in situ of lip, oral cavity, and pharynx
232.0 Carcinoma in situ of skin of lip
232.1 Carcinoma in situ of eyelid, including canthus
232.2 Carcinoma in situ of skin of ear and external auditory canal
232.3 Carcinoma in situ of skin of other and unspecified parts of face ▽
232.4 Carcinoma in situ of scalp and skin of neck
232.5 Carcinoma in situ of skin of trunk, except scrotum
232.6 Carcinoma in situ of skin of upper limb, including shoulder
232.7 Carcinoma in situ of skin of lower limb, including hip
232.8 Carcinoma in situ of other specified sites of skin
235.1 Neoplasm of uncertain behavior of lip, oral cavity, and pharynx
238.2 Neoplasm of uncertain behavior of skin
239.2 Neoplasms of unspecified nature of bone, soft tissue, and skin
701.4 Keloid scar
707.10 Ulcer of lower limb, unspecified ▽
707.11 Ulcer of thigh
707.12 Ulcer of calf
707.13 Ulcer of ankle
707.14 Ulcer of heel and midfoot
707.15 Ulcer of other part of foot
707.19 Ulcer of other part of lower limb
707.8 Chronic ulcer of other specified site
709.2 Scar condition and fibrosis of skin
709.4 Foreign body granuloma of skin and subcutaneous tissue
728.86 Necrotizing fasciitis — (Use additional code to identify infectious organism, 041.00-041.89, 785.4, if applicable)
785.4 Gangrene — (Code first any associated underlying condition:250.7, 443.0)
872.10 Open wound of external ear, unspecified site, complicated — (Use additional code to identify infection) ▽
872.11 Open wound of auricle, complicated — (Use additional code to identify infection)
873.1 Open wound of scalp, complicated — (Use additional code to identify infection)
873.30 Open wound of nose, unspecified site, complicated — (Use additional code to identify infection) ▽
873.49 Open wound of face, other and multiple sites, without mention of complication — (Use additional code to identify infection)
873.50 Open wound of face, unspecified site, complicated — (Use additional code to identify infection) ▽
873.51 Open wound of cheek, complicated — (Use additional code to identify infection)
873.52 Open wound of forehead, complicated — (Use additional code to identify infection)
873.53 Open wound of lip, complicated — (Use additional code to identify infection)
873.54 Open wound of jaw, complicated — (Use additional code to identify infection)
873.59 Open wound of face, other and multiple sites, complicated — (Use additional code to identify infection)
873.9 Other and unspecified open wound of head, complicated — (Use additional code to identify infection) ▽
874.8 Open wound of other and unspecified parts of neck, without mention of complication — (Use additional code to identify infection) ▽
874.9 Open wound of other and unspecified parts of neck, complicated — (Use additional code to identify infection) ▽
875.1 Open wound of chest (wall), complicated — (Use additional code to identify infection)
876.1 Open wound of back, complicated — (Use additional code to identify infection)
877.1 Open wound of buttock, complicated — (Use additional code to identify infection)
878.1 Open wound of penis, complicated — (Use additional code to identify infection) ♂
878.3 Open wound of scrotum and testes, complicated — (Use additional code to identify infection) ♂
878.5 Open wound of vulva, complicated — (Use additional code to identify infection) ♀
878.9 Open wound of other and unspecified parts of genital organs, complicated — (Use additional code to identify infection) ▽
879.1 Open wound of breast, complicated — (Use additional code to identify infection)
879.3 Open wound of abdominal wall, anterior, complicated — (Use additional code to identify infection)
879.5 Open wound of abdominal wall, lateral, complicated — (Use additional code to identify infection)
879.9 Open wound(s) (multiple) of unspecified site(s), complicated — (Use additional code to identify infection) ▽
880.10 Open wound of shoulder region, complicated — (Use additional code to identify infection)
880.11 Open wound of scapular region, complicated — (Use additional code to identify infection)
880.12 Open wound of axillary region, complicated — (Use additional code to identify infection)
880.13 Open wound of upper arm, complicated — (Use additional code to identify infection)
880.19 Open wound of multiple sites of shoulder and upper arm, complicated — (Use additional code to identify infection)
882.1 Open wound of hand except finger(s) alone, complicated — (Use additional code to identify infection)
883.1 Open wound of finger(s), complicated — (Use additional code to identify infection)
890.1 Open wound of hip and thigh, complicated — (Use additional code to identify infection)
891.1 Open wound of knee, leg (except thigh), and ankle, complicated — (Use additional code to identify infection)
892.1 Open wound of foot except toe(s) alone, complicated — (Use additional code to identify infection)
893.1 Open wound of toe(s), complicated — (Use additional code to identify infection)
894.1 Multiple and unspecified open wound of lower limb, complicated — (Use additional code to identify infection)
906.0 Late effect of open wound of head, neck, and trunk

▽ Unspecified code
♀ Female diagnosis
☒ Manifestation code
♂ Male diagnosis

906.1 Late effect of open wound of extremities without mention of tendon injury
906.4 Late effect of crushing
906.5 Late effect of burn of eye, face, head, and neck
909.3 Late effect of complications of surgical and medical care
941.29 Blisters, with epidermal loss due to burn (second degree) of multiple sites (except with eye) of face, head, and neck
941.30 Full-thickness skin loss due to burn (third degree nos) of unspecified site of face and head ▽
941.31 Full-thickness skin loss due to burn (third degree nos) of ear (any part)
941.32 Full-thickness skin loss due to burn (third degree nos) of eye (with other parts of face, head, and neck)
941.33 Full-thickness skin loss due to burn (third degree nos) of lip(s)
941.34 Full-thickness skin loss due to burn (third degree nos) of chin
941.35 Full-thickness skin loss due to burn (third degree nos) of nose (septum)
941.36 Full-thickness skin loss due to burn (third degree nos) of scalp (any part)
941.37 Full-thickness skin loss due to burn (third degree nos) of forehead and cheek
941.38 Full-thickness skin loss due to burn (third degree nos) of neck
941.39 Full-thickness skin loss due to burn (third degree nos) of multiple sites (except with eye) of face, head, and neck
941.40 Deep necrosis of underlying tissues due to burn (deep third degree) of unspecified site of face and head, without mention of loss of a body part ▽
941.41 Deep necrosis of underlying tissues due to burn (deep third degree) of ear (any part), without mention of loss of a body part
941.42 Deep necrosis of underlying tissues due to burn (deep third degree) of eye (with other parts of face, head, and neck), without mention of loss of a body part
941.43 Deep necrosis of underlying tissues due to burn (deep third degree) of lip(s), without mention of loss of a body part
941.44 Deep necrosis of underlying tissues due to burn (deep third degree) of chin, without mention of loss of a body part
941.45 Deep necrosis of underlying tissues due to burn (deep third degree) of nose (septum), without mention of loss of a body part
941.46 Deep necrosis of underlying tissues due to burn (deep third degree) of scalp (any part), without mention of loss of a body part
941.47 Deep necrosis of underlying tissues due to burn (deep third degree) of forehead and cheek, without mention of loss of a body part
941.48 Deep necrosis of underlying tissues due to burn (deep third degree) of neck, without mention of loss of a body part
941.49 Deep necrosis of underlying tissues due to burn (deep third degree) of multiple sites (except with eye) of face, head, and neck, without mention of loss of a body part
942.30 Full-thickness skin loss due to burn (third degree nos) of unspecified site of trunk ▽
942.31 Full-thickness skin loss due to burn (third degree nos) of breast
942.33 Full-thickness skin loss due to burn (third degree nos) of abdominal wall
942.34 Full-thickness skin loss due to burn (third degree nos) of back (any part)
942.35 Full-thickness skin loss due to burn (third degree nos) of genitalia
942.39 Full-thickness skin loss due to burn (third degree nos) of other and multiple sites of trunk
942.40 Deep necrosis of underlying tissues due to burn (deep third degree) of trunk, unspecified site, without mention of loss of a body part ▽
942.41 Deep necrosis of underlying tissues due to burn (deep third degree) of breast, without mention of loss of a body part
942.42 Deep necrosis of underlying tissues due to burn (deep third degree) of chest wall, excluding breast and nipple, without mention of loss of a body part
942.43 Deep necrosis of underlying tissues due to burn (deep third degree) of abdominal wall, without mention of loss of a body part
942.44 Deep necrosis of underlying tissues due to burn (deep third degree) of back (any part), without mention of loss of a body part
942.45 Deep necrosis of underlying tissues due to burn (deep third degree) of genitalia, without mention of loss of a body part
942.49 Deep necrosis of underlying tissues due to burn (deep third degree) of other and multiple sites of trunk, without mention of loss of a body part
943.30 Full-thickness skin loss due to burn (third degree nos) of unspecified site of upper limb ▽
943.31 Full-thickness skin loss due to burn (third degree nos) of forearm
943.32 Full-thickness skin loss due to burn (third degree nos) of elbow
943.33 Full-thickness skin loss due to burn (third degree nos) of upper arm
943.34 Full-thickness skin loss due to burn (third degree nos) of axilla
943.35 Full-thickness skin loss due to burn (third degree nos) of shoulder
943.36 Full-thickness skin loss due to burn (third degree nos) of scapular region
943.39 Full-thickness skin loss due to burn (third degree nos) of multiple sites of upper limb, except wrist and hand
944.30 Full-thickness skin loss due to burn (third degree nos) of unspecified site of hand ▽
944.31 Full-thickness skin loss due to burn (third degree nos) of single digit [finger (nail)] other than thumb
944.32 Full-thickness skin loss due to burn (third degree nos) of thumb (nail)
944.33 Full-thickness skin loss due to burn (third degree nos) of two or more digits of hand, not including thumb
944.34 Full-thickness skin loss due to burn (third degree nos) of two or more digits of hand including thumb
944.37 Full-thickness skin loss due to burn (third degree nos) of wrist
944.38 Full-thickness skin loss due to burn (third degree nos) of multiple sites of wrist(s) and hand(s)
944.40 Deep necrosis of underlying tissues due to burn (deep third degree) of unspecified site of hand, without mention of a body part ▽
944.41 Deep necrosis of underlying tissues due to burn (deep third degree) of single digit [finger (nail)] other than thumb, without mention of a body part
944.42 Deep necrosis of underlying tissues due to burn (deep third degree) of thumb (nail), without mention of loss of a body part
944.43 Deep necrosis of underlying tissues due to burn (deep third degree) of two or more digits of hand, not including thumb, without mention of a body part
944.44 Deep necrosis of underlying tissues due to burn (deep third degree) of two or more digits of hand including thumb, without mention of a body part
944.45 Deep necrosis of underlying tissues due to burn (deep third degree) of palm of hand, without mention of loss of a body part
944.46 Deep necrosis of underlying tissues due to burn (deep third degree) of back of hand, without mention of loss of back of a body part
944.47 Deep necrosis of underlying tissues due to burn (deep third degree) of wrist, without mention of loss of a body part
944.48 Deep necrosis of underlying tissues due to burn (deep third degree) of multiple sites of wrist(s) and hand(s), without mention of loss of a body part
945.30 Full-thickness skin loss due to burn (third degree nos) of unspecified site of lower limb ▽
945.31 Full-thickness skin loss due to burn (third degree nos) of toe(s) (nail)
945.32 Full-thickness skin loss due to burn (third degree nos) of foot
945.33 Full-thickness skin loss due to burn (third degree nos) of ankle
945.34 Full-thickness skin loss due to burn (third degree nos) of lower leg
945.35 Full-thickness skin loss due to burn (third degree nos) of knee
945.36 Full-thickness skin loss due to burn (third degree nos) of thigh (any part)
945.39 Full-thickness skin loss due to burn (third degree nos) of multiple sites of lower limb(s)
945.40 Deep necrosis of underlying tissues due to burn (deep third degree) of unspecified site of lower limb (leg), without mention of loss of a body part ▽
945.41 Deep necrosis of underlying tissues due to burn (deep third degree) of toe(s) (nail), without mention of loss of a body part
945.42 Deep necrosis of underlying tissues due to burn (deep third degree) of foot, without mention of loss of a body part
945.43 Deep necrosis of underlying tissues due to burn (deep third degree) of ankle, without mention of loss of a body part
945.44 Deep necrosis of underlying tissues due to burn (deep third degree) of lower leg, without mention of loss of a body part
945.45 Deep necrosis of underlying tissues due to burn (deep third degree) of knee, without mention of loss of a body part
945.46 Deep necrosis of underlying tissues due to burn (deep third degree) of thigh (any part), without mention of loss of a body part
945.49 Deep necrosis of underlying tissues due to burn (deep third degree) of multiple sites of lower limb(s), without mention of loss of a body part
946.3 Full-thickness skin loss due to burn (third degree nos) of multiple specified sites
946.4 Deep necrosis of underlying tissues due to burn (deep third degree) of multiple specified sites, without mention of loss of a body part
959.01 Head injury, unspecified ▽
959.09 Injury of face and neck, other and unspecified
991.0 Frostbite of face
991.1 Frostbite of hand
991.2 Frostbite of foot
991.3 Frostbite of other and unspecified sites
996.52 Mechanical complication due to other tissue graft, not elsewhere classified
997.60 Late complications of amputation stump, unspecified — (Use additional code to identify complications) ▽
998.32 Disruption of external operation wound
998.59 Other postoperative infection — (Use additional code to identify infection)
V10.82 Personal history of malignant melanoma of skin
V10.83 Personal history of other malignant neoplasm of skin
V84.09 Genetic susceptibility to other malignant neoplasm

ICD-9-CM Procedural

08.20 Removal of lesion of eyelid, not otherwise specified
08.23 Excision of major lesion of eyelid, partial-thickness
08.24 Excision of major lesion of eyelid, full-thickness

▽ Unspecified code ♀ Female diagnosis ☒ Manifestation code ♂ Male diagnosis

18.29 Excision or destruction of other lesion of external ear
21.32 Local excision or destruction of other lesion of nose
27.42 Wide excision of lesion of lip
27.43 Other excision of lesion or tissue of lip
49.39 Other local excision or destruction of lesion or tissue of anus
61.3 Excision or destruction of lesion or tissue of scrotum
64.2 Local excision or destruction of lesion of penis
85.21 Local excision of lesion of breast
86.3 Other local excision or destruction of lesion or tissue of skin and subcutaneous tissue

HCPCS Level II Supplies & Services

A4305 Disposable drug delivery system, flow rate of 50 ml or greater per hour
A4306 Disposable drug delivery system, flow rate of 5 ml or less per hour
A4550 Surgical trays

15050

15050 Pinch graft, single or multiple, to cover small ulcer, tip of digit, or other minimal open area (except on face), up to defect size 2 cm diameter

ICD-9-CM Diagnostic

171.2 Malignant neoplasm of connective and other soft tissue of upper limb, including shoulder
172.6 Malignant melanoma of skin of upper limb, including shoulder
172.7 Malignant melanoma of skin of lower limb, including hip
173.6 Other malignant neoplasm of skin of upper limb, including shoulder
173.7 Other malignant neoplasm of skin of lower limb, including hip
232.8 Carcinoma in situ of other specified sites of skin
238.2 Neoplasm of uncertain behavior of skin
250.70 Diabetes with peripheral circulatory disorders, type II or unspecified type, not stated as uncontrolled — (Use additional code to identify manifestation: 443.81, 785.4)
250.71 Diabetes with peripheral circulatory disorders, type I [juvenile type], not stated as uncontrolled — (Use additional code to identify manifestation: 443.81, 785.4)
250.72 Diabetes with peripheral circulatory disorders, type II or unspecified type, uncontrolled — (Use additional code to identify manifestation: 443.81, 785.4)
250.73 Diabetes with peripheral circulatory disorders, type I [juvenile type], uncontrolled — (Use additional code to identify manifestation: 443.81, 785.4)
443.81 Peripheral angiopathy in diseases classified elsewhere — (Code first underlying disease, 250.7) ☒
681.01 Felon — (Use additional code to identify organism)
707.00 Decubitus ulcer, unspecified site
707.01 Decubitus ulcer, elbow
707.02 Decubitus ulcer, upper back
707.03 Decubitus ulcer, lower back
707.04 Decubitus ulcer, hip
707.05 Decubitus ulcer, buttock
707.06 Decubitus ulcer, ankle
707.07 Decubitus ulcer, heel
707.09 Decubitus ulcer, other site
707.10 Ulcer of lower limb, unspecified ▽
707.11 Ulcer of thigh
707.12 Ulcer of calf
707.13 Ulcer of ankle
707.14 Ulcer of heel and midfoot
707.15 Ulcer of other part of foot
707.19 Ulcer of other part of lower limb
707.8 Chronic ulcer of other specified site
707.9 Chronic ulcer of unspecified site ▽
816.12 Open fracture of distal phalanx or phalanges of hand
882.0 Open wound of hand except finger(s) alone, without mention of complication — (Use additional code to identify infection)
882.1 Open wound of hand except finger(s) alone, complicated — (Use additional code to identify infection)
882.2 Open wound of hand except finger(s) alone, with tendon involvement — (Use additional code to identify infection)
883.0 Open wound of finger(s), without mention of complication — (Use additional code to identify infection)
883.1 Open wound of finger(s), complicated — (Use additional code to identify infection)
883.2 Open wound of finger(s), with tendon involvement — (Use additional code to identify infection)
885.0 Traumatic amputation of thumb (complete) (partial), without mention of complication — (Use additional code to identify infection)
885.1 Traumatic amputation of thumb (complete) (partial), complicated — (Use additional code to identify infection)
886.0 Traumatic amputation of other finger(s) (complete) (partial), without mention of complication — (Use additional code to identify infection)
886.1 Traumatic amputation of other finger(s) (complete) (partial), complicated — (Use additional code to identify infection)
893.0 Open wound of toe(s), without mention of complication — (Use additional code to identify infection)
893.1 Open wound of toe(s), complicated — (Use additional code to identify infection)
893.2 Open wound of toe(s), with tendon involvement — (Use additional code to identify infection)
895.0 Traumatic amputation of toe(s) (complete) (partial), without mention of complication — (Use additional code to identify infection)
895.1 Traumatic amputation of toe(s) (complete) (partial), complicated — (Use additional code to identify infection)
906.4 Late effect of crushing
906.6 Late effect of burn of wrist and hand
906.7 Late effect of burn of other extremities
906.8 Late effect of burns of other specified sites
908.6 Late effect of certain complications of trauma
908.9 Late effect of unspecified injury ▽
909.3 Late effect of complications of surgical and medical care
927.3 Crushing injury of finger(s) — (Use additional code to identify any associated injuries: 800-829, 850.0-854.1, 860.0-869.1)
928.3 Crushing injury of toe(s) — (Use additional code to identify any associated injuries: 800-829, 850.0-854.1, 860.0-869.1)

ICD-9-CM Procedural

86.60 Free skin graft, not otherwise specified
86.62 Other skin graft to hand

HCPCS Level II Supplies & Services

A4550 Surgical trays

15100–15101

15100 Split graft, trunk, arms, legs; first 100 sq. cm or less, or one percent of body area of infants and children (except 15050)
15101 each additional 100 sq. cm, or each additional one percent of body area of infants and children, or part thereof (List separately in addition to code for primary procedure)

ICD-9-CM Diagnostic

172.5 Malignant melanoma of skin of trunk, except scrotum
172.6 Malignant melanoma of skin of upper limb, including shoulder
172.7 Malignant melanoma of skin of lower limb, including hip
172.8 Malignant melanoma of other specified sites of skin
173.5 Other malignant neoplasm of skin of trunk, except scrotum
173.6 Other malignant neoplasm of skin of upper limb, including shoulder
173.7 Other malignant neoplasm of skin of lower limb, including hip
173.8 Other malignant neoplasm of other specified sites of skin
174.0 Malignant neoplasm of nipple and areola of female breast ♀
174.1 Malignant neoplasm of central portion of female breast ♀
174.2 Malignant neoplasm of upper-inner quadrant of female breast ♀
174.3 Malignant neoplasm of lower-inner quadrant of female breast ♀
174.4 Malignant neoplasm of upper-outer quadrant of female breast ♀
174.5 Malignant neoplasm of lower-outer quadrant of female breast ♀
174.6 Malignant neoplasm of axillary tail of female breast ♀
174.8 Malignant neoplasm of other specified sites of female breast ♀
175.0 Malignant neoplasm of nipple and areola of male breast ♂
175.9 Malignant neoplasm of other and unspecified sites of male breast ▽ ♂
195.1 Malignant neoplasm of thorax
195.2 Malignant neoplasm of abdomen
195.3 Malignant neoplasm of pelvis
195.4 Malignant neoplasm of upper limb
195.5 Malignant neoplasm of lower limb
195.8 Malignant neoplasm of other specified sites
198.2 Secondary malignant neoplasm of skin
232.5 Carcinoma in situ of skin of trunk, except scrotum
232.6 Carcinoma in situ of skin of upper limb, including shoulder
232.7 Carcinoma in situ of skin of lower limb, including hip
232.8 Carcinoma in situ of other specified sites of skin
238.2 Neoplasm of uncertain behavior of skin
239.2 Neoplasms of unspecified nature of bone, soft tissue, and skin

250.70 Diabetes with peripheral circulatory disorders, type II or unspecified type, not stated as uncontrolled — (Use additional code to identify manifestation: 443.81, 785.4)
250.71 Diabetes with peripheral circulatory disorders, type I [juvenile type], not stated as uncontrolled — (Use additional code to identify manifestation: 443.81, 785.4)
250.72 Diabetes with peripheral circulatory disorders, type II or unspecified type, uncontrolled — (Use additional code to identify manifestation: 443.81, 785.4)
250.73 Diabetes with peripheral circulatory disorders, type I [juvenile type], uncontrolled — (Use additional code to identify manifestation: 443.81, 785.4)
443.81 Peripheral angiopathy in diseases classified elsewhere — (Code first underlying disease, 250.7) ☒
454.0 Varicose veins of lower extremities with ulcer
454.2 Varicose veins of lower extremities with ulcer and inflammation
454.8 Varicose veins of the lower extremities with other complications
459.11 Postphlebitic syndrome with ulcer
459.13 Postphlebitic syndrome with ulcer and inflammation
459.19 Postphlebitic syndrome with other complication
459.31 Chronic venous hypertension with ulcer
459.33 Chronic venous hypertension with ulcer and inflammation
459.39 Chronic venous hypertension with other complication
682.2 Cellulitis and abscess of trunk — (Use additional code to identify organism)
682.3 Cellulitis and abscess of upper arm and forearm — (Use additional code to identify organism)
682.5 Cellulitis and abscess of buttock — (Use additional code to identify organism)
682.6 Cellulitis and abscess of leg, except foot — (Use additional code to identify organism)
682.8 Cellulitis and abscess of other specified site — (Use additional code to identify organism)
701.4 Keloid scar
701.5 Other abnormal granulation tissue
701.9 Unspecified hypertrophic and atrophic condition of skin ▽
707.00 Decubitus ulcer, unspecified site
707.01 Decubitus ulcer, elbow
707.02 Decubitus ulcer, upper back
707.03 Decubitus ulcer, lower back
707.04 Decubitus ulcer, hip
707.05 Decubitus ulcer, buttock
707.06 Decubitus ulcer, ankle
707.07 Decubitus ulcer, heel
707.09 Decubitus ulcer, other site
707.10 Ulcer of lower limb, unspecified ▽
707.11 Ulcer of thigh
707.12 Ulcer of calf
707.13 Ulcer of ankle
707.8 Chronic ulcer of other specified site
709.2 Scar condition and fibrosis of skin
709.4 Foreign body granuloma of skin and subcutaneous tissue
709.9 Unspecified disorder of skin and subcutaneous tissue ▽
785.4 Gangrene — (Code first any associated underlying condition:250.7, 443.0)
875.0 Open wound of chest (wall), without mention of complication — (Use additional code to identify infection)
875.1 Open wound of chest (wall), complicated — (Use additional code to identify infection)
876.0 Open wound of back, without mention of complication — (Use additional code to identify infection)
876.1 Open wound of back, complicated — (Use additional code to identify infection)
877.0 Open wound of buttock, without mention of complication — (Use additional code to identify infection)
877.1 Open wound of buttock, complicated — (Use additional code to identify infection)
879.0 Open wound of breast, without mention of complication — (Use additional code to identify infection)
879.1 Open wound of breast, complicated — (Use additional code to identify infection)
879.2 Open wound of abdominal wall, anterior, without mention of complication — (Use additional code to identify infection)
879.3 Open wound of abdominal wall, anterior, complicated — (Use additional code to identify infection)
879.4 Open wound of abdominal wall, lateral, without mention of complication — (Use additional code to identify infection)
879.5 Open wound of abdominal wall, lateral, complicated — (Use additional code to identify infection)
879.6 Open wound of other and unspecified parts of trunk, without mention of complication — (Use additional code to identify infection) ▽
879.7 Open wound of other and unspecified parts of trunk, complicated — (Use additional code to identify infection) ▽
879.8 Open wound(s) (multiple) of unspecified site(s), without mention of complication — (Use additional code to identify infection) ▽
879.9 Open wound(s) (multiple) of unspecified site(s), complicated — (Use additional code to identify infection) ▽
880.00 Open wound of shoulder region, without mention of complication — (Use additional code to identify infection)
880.01 Open wound of scapular region, without mention of complication — (Use additional code to identify infection)
880.02 Open wound of axillary region, without mention of complication — (Use additional code to identify infection)
880.03 Open wound of upper arm, without mention of complication — (Use additional code to identify infection)
880.09 Open wound of multiple sites of shoulder and upper arm, without mention of complication — (Use additional code to identify infection)
881.00 Open wound of forearm, without mention of complication — (Use additional code to identify infection)
881.01 Open wound of elbow, without mention of complication — (Use additional code to identify infection)
881.02 Open wound of wrist, without mention of complication — (Use additional code to identify infection)
881.10 Open wound of forearm, complicated — (Use additional code to identify infection)
881.11 Open wound of elbow, complicated — (Use additional code to identify infection)
881.12 Open wound of wrist, complicated — (Use additional code to identify infection)
881.20 Open wound of forearm, with tendon involvement — (Use additional code to identify infection)
881.21 Open wound of elbow, with tendon involvement — (Use additional code to identify infection)
881.22 Open wound of wrist, with tendon involvement — (Use additional code to identify infection)
884.0 Multiple and unspecified open wound of upper limb, without mention of complication — (Use additional code to identify infection)
884.1 Multiple and unspecified open wound of upper limb, complicated — (Use additional code to identify infection)
884.2 Multiple and unspecified open wound of upper limb, with tendon involvement — (Use additional code to identify infection)
887.0 Traumatic amputation of arm and hand (complete) (partial), unilateral, below elbow, without mention of complication — (Use additional code to identify infection)
887.1 Traumatic amputation of arm and hand (complete) (partial), unilateral, below elbow, complicated — (Use additional code to identify infection)
887.2 Traumatic amputation of arm and hand (complete) (partial), unilateral, at or above elbow, without mention of complication — (Use additional code to identify infection)
887.3 Traumatic amputation of arm and hand (complete) (partial), unilateral, at or above elbow, complicated — (Use additional code to identify infection)
887.4 Traumatic amputation of arm and hand (complete) (partial), unilateral, level not specified, without mention of complication — (Use additional code to identify infection) ▽
887.5 Traumatic amputation of arm and hand (complete) (partial), unilateral, level not specified, complicated — (Use additional code to identify infection) ▽
887.6 Traumatic amputation of arm and hand (complete) (partial), bilateral (any level), without mention of complication — (Use additional code to identify infection)
887.7 Traumatic amputation of arm and hand (complete) (partial), bilateral (any level), complicated — (Use additional code to identify infection)
890.0 Open wound of hip and thigh, without mention of complication — (Use additional code to identify infection)
890.1 Open wound of hip and thigh, complicated — (Use additional code to identify infection)
890.2 Open wound of hip and thigh, with tendon involvement — (Use additional code to identify infection)
891.0 Open wound of knee, leg (except thigh), and ankle, without mention of complication — (Use additional code to identify infection)
891.1 Open wound of knee, leg (except thigh), and ankle, complicated — (Use additional code to identify infection)
891.2 Open wound of knee, leg (except thigh), and ankle, with tendon involvement — (Use additional code to identify infection)
894.0 Multiple and unspecified open wound of lower limb, without mention of complication — (Use additional code to identify infection)
894.1 Multiple and unspecified open wound of lower limb, complicated — (Use additional code to identify infection)

▽ Unspecified code ☒ Manifestation code
♀ Female diagnosis ♂ Male diagnosis

894.2 Multiple and unspecified open wound of lower limb, with tendon involvement — (Use additional code to identify infection)
897.0 Traumatic amputation of leg(s) (complete) (partial), unilateral, below knee, without mention of complication — (Use additional code to identify infection)
897.1 Traumatic amputation of leg(s) (complete) (partial), unilateral, below knee, complicated — (Use additional code to identify infection)
897.2 Traumatic amputation of leg(s) (complete) (partial), unilateral, at or above knee, without mention of complication — (Use additional code to identify infection)
897.3 Traumatic amputation of leg(s) (complete) (partial), unilateral, at or above knee, complicated — (Use additional code to identify infection)
897.4 Traumatic amputation of leg(s) (complete) (partial), unilateral, level not specified, without mention of complication — (Use additional code to identify infection)
897.5 Traumatic amputation of leg(s) (complete) (partial), unilateral, level not specified, complicated — (Use additional code to identify infection)
897.6 Traumatic amputation of leg(s) (complete) (partial), bilateral (any level), without mention of complication — (Use additional code to identify infection)
897.7 Traumatic amputation of leg(s) (complete) (partial), bilateral (any level), complicated — (Use additional code to identify infection)
906.0 Late effect of open wound of head, neck, and trunk
906.1 Late effect of open wound of extremities without mention of tendon injury
906.4 Late effect of crushing
906.6 Late effect of burn of wrist and hand
906.7 Late effect of burn of other extremities
906.8 Late effect of burns of other specified sites
908.0 Late effect of internal injury to chest
908.1 Late effect of internal injury to intra-abdominal organs
908.2 Late effect of internal injury to other internal organs
908.3 Late effect of injury to blood vessel of head, neck, and extremities
908.4 Late effect of injury to blood vessel of thorax, abdomen, and pelvis
908.6 Late effect of certain complications of trauma
909.2 Late effect of radiation
948.00 Burn (any degree) involving less than 10% of body surface with third degree burn of less than 10% or unspecified amount
948.10 Burn (any degree) involving 10-19% of body surface with third degree burn of less than 10% or unspecified amount
948.11 Burn (any degree) involving 10-19% of body surface with third degree burn of 10-19%
948.20 Burn (any degree) involving 20-29% of body surface with third degree burn of less than 10% or unspecified amount
948.21 Burn (any degree) involving 20-29% of body surface with third degree burn of 10-19%
948.22 Burn (any degree) involving 20-29% of body surface with third degree burn of 20-29%
948.30 Burn (any degree) involving 30-39% of body surface with third degree burn of less than 10% or unspecified amount
948.31 Burn (any degree) involving 30-39% of body surface with third degree burn of 10-19%
948.32 Burn (any degree) involving 30-39% of body surface with third degree burn of 20-29%
948.33 Burn (any degree) involving 30-39% of body surface with third degree burn of 30-39%
948.40 Burn (any degree) involving 40-49% of body surface with third degree burn of less than 10% or unspecified amount
948.41 Burn (any degree) involving 40-49% of body surface with third degree burn of 10-19%
948.42 Burn (any degree) involving 40-49% of body surface with third degree burn of 20-29%
948.43 Burn (any degree) involving 40-49% of body surface with third degree burn of 30-39%
948.44 Burn (any degree) involving 40-49% of body surface with third degree burn of 40-49%
948.50 Burn (any degree) involving 50-59% of body surface with third degree burn of less than 10% or unspecified amount
948.51 Burn (any degree) involving 50-59% of body surface with third degree burn of 10-19%
948.52 Burn (any degree) involving 50-59% of body surface with third degree burn of 20-29%
948.53 Burn (any degree) involving 50-59% of body surface with third degree burn of 30-39%
948.54 Burn (any degree) involving 50-59% of body surface with third degree burn of 40-49%
948.55 Burn (any degree) involving 50-59% of body surface with third degree burn of 50-59%
948.60 Burn (any degree) involving 60-69% of body surface with third degree burn of less than 10% or unspecified amount
948.61 Burn (any degree) involving 60-69% of body surface with third degree burn of 10-19%
948.62 Burn (any degree) involving 60-69% of body surface with third degree burn of 20-29%
948.63 Burn (any degree) involving 60-69% of body surface with third degree burn of 30-39%
948.64 Burn (any degree) involving 60-69% of body surface with third degree burn of 40-49%
948.65 Burn (any degree) involving 60-69% of body surface with third degree burn of 50-59%
948.66 Burn (any degree) involving 60-69% of body surface with third degree burn of 60-69%
948.70 Burn (any degree) involving 70-79% of body surface with third degree burn of less than 10% or unspecified amount
948.71 Burn (any degree) involving 70-79% of body surface with third degree burn of 10-19%
948.72 Burn (any degree) involving 70-79% of body surface with third degree burn of 20-29%
948.73 Burn (any degree) involving 70-79% of body surface with third degree burn of 30-39%
948.74 Burn (any degree) involving 70-79% of body surface with third degree burn of 40-49%
948.75 Burn (any degree) involving 70-79% of body surface with third degree burn of 50-59%
948.76 Burn (any degree) involving 70-79% of body surface with third degree burn of 60-69%
948.77 Burn (any degree) involving 70-79% of body surface with third degree burn of 70-79%
948.80 Burn (any degree) involving 80-89% of body surface with third degree burn of less than 10% or unspecified amount
948.81 Burn (any degree) involving 80-89% of body surface with third degree burn of 10-19%
948.82 Burn (any degree) involving 80-89% of body surface with third degree burn of 20-29%
948.83 Burn (any degree) involving 80-89% of body surface with third degree burn of 30-39%
948.84 Burn (any degree) involving 80-89% of body surface with third degree burn of 40-49%
948.85 Burn (any degree) involving 80-89% of body surface with third degree burn of 50-59%
948.86 Burn (any degree) involving 80-89% of body surface with third degree burn of 60-69%
948.87 Burn (any degree) involving 80-89% of body surface with third degree burn of 70-79%
948.88 Burn (any degree) involving 80-89% of body surface with third degree burn of 80-89%
958.3 Posttraumatic wound infection not elsewhere classified
991.3 Frostbite of other and unspecified sites
996.52 Mechanical complication due to other tissue graft, not elsewhere classified
996.91 Complications of reattached forearm
996.94 Complications of reattached upper extremity, other and unspecified
996.96 Complications of reattached lower extremity, other and unspecified
997.61 Neuroma of amputation stump — (Use additional code to identify complications)
997.62 Infection (chronic) of amputation stump — (Use additional code to identify organism. Use additional code to identify complications)
997.69 Other late amputation stump complication — (Use additional code to identify complications)
998.32 Disruption of external operation wound
998.59 Other postoperative infection — (Use additional code to identify infection)
998.83 Non-healing surgical wound

ICD-9-CM Procedural

85.82 Split-thickness graft to breast
86.69 Other skin graft to other sites

15120–15121

15120 Split graft, face, scalp, eyelids, mouth, neck, ears, orbits, genitalia, hands, feet and/or multiple digits; first 100 sq. cm or less, or one percent of body area of infants and children (except 15050)

15121 each additional 100 sq. cm, or each additional one percent of body area of infants and children, or part thereof (List separately in addition to code for primary procedure)

ICD-9-CM Diagnostic

145.0 Malignant neoplasm of cheek mucosa
171.0 Malignant neoplasm of connective and other soft tissue of head, face, and neck
171.6 Malignant neoplasm of connective and other soft tissue of pelvis
171.8 Malignant neoplasm of other specified sites of connective and other soft tissue
172.0 Malignant melanoma of skin of lip
172.1 Malignant melanoma of skin of eyelid, including canthus
172.2 Malignant melanoma of skin of ear and external auditory canal
172.4 Malignant melanoma of skin of scalp and neck
172.6 Malignant melanoma of skin of upper limb, including shoulder
172.7 Malignant melanoma of skin of lower limb, including hip
172.8 Malignant melanoma of other specified sites of skin
173.0 Other malignant neoplasm of skin of lip
173.1 Other malignant neoplasm of skin of eyelid, including canthus
173.2 Other malignant neoplasm of skin of ear and external auditory canal
173.3 Other malignant neoplasm of skin of other and unspecified parts of face ▽
173.4 Other malignant neoplasm of scalp and skin of neck
173.6 Other malignant neoplasm of skin of upper limb, including shoulder
173.7 Other malignant neoplasm of skin of lower limb, including hip
173.8 Other malignant neoplasm of other specified sites of skin
184.0 Malignant neoplasm of vagina ♀
184.2 Malignant neoplasm of labia minora ♀
184.3 Malignant neoplasm of clitoris ♀
184.4 Malignant neoplasm of vulva, unspecified site ▽ ♀
184.8 Malignant neoplasm of other specified sites of female genital organs ♀
187.1 Malignant neoplasm of prepuce ♂
187.2 Malignant neoplasm of glans penis ♂
187.3 Malignant neoplasm of body of penis ♂
187.4 Malignant neoplasm of penis, part unspecified ▽ ♂
187.7 Malignant neoplasm of scrotum ♂
187.8 Malignant neoplasm of other specified sites of male genital organs ♂
195.0 Malignant neoplasm of head, face, and neck
195.4 Malignant neoplasm of upper limb
195.5 Malignant neoplasm of lower limb
195.8 Malignant neoplasm of other specified sites
198.2 Secondary malignant neoplasm of skin
198.82 Secondary malignant neoplasm of genital organs
198.89 Secondary malignant neoplasm of other specified sites
210.4 Benign neoplasm of other and unspecified parts of mouth ▽
216.0 Benign neoplasm of skin of lip
216.1 Benign neoplasm of eyelid, including canthus
216.2 Benign neoplasm of ear and external auditory canal
216.3 Benign neoplasm of skin of other and unspecified parts of face ▽
216.4 Benign neoplasm of scalp and skin of neck
216.8 Benign neoplasm of other specified sites of skin
221.2 Benign neoplasm of vulva ♀
221.8 Benign neoplasm of other specified sites of female genital organs ♀
222.1 Benign neoplasm of penis ♂
222.4 Benign neoplasm of scrotum ♂
230.0 Carcinoma in situ of lip, oral cavity, and pharynx
232.0 Carcinoma in situ of skin of lip
232.1 Carcinoma in situ of eyelid, including canthus
232.2 Carcinoma in situ of skin of ear and external auditory canal
232.3 Carcinoma in situ of skin of other and unspecified parts of face ▽
232.4 Carcinoma in situ of scalp and skin of neck
232.8 Carcinoma in situ of other specified sites of skin
233.3 Carcinoma in situ of other and unspecified female genital organs ▽ ♀
233.5 Carcinoma in situ of penis ♂
233.6 Carcinoma in situ of other and unspecified male genital organs ▽ ♂
235.1 Neoplasm of uncertain behavior of lip, oral cavity, and pharynx
236.3 Neoplasm of uncertain behavior of other and unspecified female genital organs ▽ ♀
236.6 Neoplasm of uncertain behavior of other and unspecified male genital organs ▽ ♂
238.2 Neoplasm of uncertain behavior of skin
239.2 Neoplasms of unspecified nature of bone, soft tissue, and skin
239.5 Neoplasm of unspecified nature of other genitourinary organs
250.70 Diabetes with peripheral circulatory disorders, type II or unspecified type, not stated as uncontrolled — (Use additional code to identify manifestation: 443.81, 785.4)
250.71 Diabetes with peripheral circulatory disorders, type I [juvenile type], not stated as uncontrolled — (Use additional code to identify manifestation: 443.81, 785.4)
250.72 Diabetes with peripheral circulatory disorders, type II or unspecified type, uncontrolled — (Use additional code to identify manifestation: 443.81, 785.4)
250.73 Diabetes with peripheral circulatory disorders, type I [juvenile type], uncontrolled — (Use additional code to identify manifestation: 443.81, 785.4)
374.04 Cicatricial entropion
374.50 Unspecified degenerative disorder of eyelid ▽
374.56 Other degenerative disorders of skin affecting eyelid
374.84 Cysts of eyelids
374.85 Vascular anomalies of eyelid
374.86 Retained foreign body of eyelid
380.32 Acquired deformities of auricle or pinna
380.50 Acquired stenosis of external ear canal unspecified as to cause ▽
443.81 Peripheral angiopathy in diseases classified elsewhere — (Code first underlying disease, 250.7) ☒
525.20 Unspecified atrophy of edentulous alveolar ridge
525.21 Minimal atrophy of the mandible
525.22 Moderate atrophy of the mandible
525.23 Severe atrophy of the mandible
525.24 Minimal atrophy of the maxilla
525.25 Moderate atrophy of the maxilla
525.26 Severe atrophy of the maxilla
629.20 Female genital mutilation status, unspecified
629.21 Female genital mutilation, Type I status
629.22 Female genital mutilation, Type II status
629.23 Female genital mutilation, Type III status
682.4 Cellulitis and abscess of hand, except fingers and thumb — (Use additional code to identify organism)
682.7 Cellulitis and abscess of foot, except toes — (Use additional code to identify organism)
701.4 Keloid scar
701.5 Other abnormal granulation tissue
701.9 Unspecified hypertrophic and atrophic condition of skin ▽
707.00 Decubitus ulcer, unspecified site
707.07 Decubitus ulcer, heel
707.09 Decubitus ulcer, other site
707.14 Ulcer of heel and midfoot
707.15 Ulcer of other part of foot
707.8 Chronic ulcer of other specified site
709.2 Scar condition and fibrosis of skin
709.3 Degenerative skin disorder
709.4 Foreign body granuloma of skin and subcutaneous tissue
744.23 Microtia
744.29 Other congenital anomaly of ear
752.40 Unspecified congenital anomaly of cervix, vagina, and external female genitalia ▽ ♀
752.49 Other congenital anomaly of cervix, vagina, and external female genitalia ♀
785.4 Gangrene — (Code first any associated underlying condition:250.7, 443.0)
870.0 Laceration of skin of eyelid and periocular area — (Use additional code to identify infection)
870.1 Laceration of eyelid, full-thickness, not involving lacrimal passages — (Use additional code to identify infection)
870.2 Laceration of eyelid involving lacrimal passages — (Use additional code to identify infection)
872.00 Open wound of external ear, unspecified site, without mention of complication — (Use additional code to identify infection) ▽
872.01 Open wound of auricle, without mention of complication — (Use additional code to identify infection)
872.10 Open wound of external ear, unspecified site, complicated — (Use additional code to identify infection) ▽
872.11 Open wound of auricle, complicated — (Use additional code to identify infection)
872.8 Open wound of ear, part unspecified, without mention of complication — (Use additional code to identify infection) ▽
873.0 Open wound of scalp, without mention of complication — (Use additional code to identify infection)
873.1 Open wound of scalp, complicated — (Use additional code to identify infection)
873.40 Open wound of face, unspecified site, without mention of complication — (Use additional code to identify infection) ▽

873.41 Open wound of cheek, without mention of complication — (Use additional code to identify infection)
873.42 Open wound of forehead, without mention of complication — (Use additional code to identify infection)
873.43 Open wound of lip, without mention of complication — (Use additional code to identify infection)
873.44 Open wound of jaw, without mention of complication — (Use additional code to identify infection)
873.49 Open wound of face, other and multiple sites, without mention of complication — (Use additional code to identify infection)
873.50 Open wound of face, unspecified site, complicated — (Use additional code to identify infection) ▽
873.51 Open wound of cheek, complicated — (Use additional code to identify infection)
873.52 Open wound of forehead, complicated — (Use additional code to identify infection)
873.53 Open wound of lip, complicated — (Use additional code to identify infection)
873.54 Open wound of jaw, complicated — (Use additional code to identify infection)
873.59 Open wound of face, other and multiple sites, complicated — (Use additional code to identify infection)
873.70 Open wound of mouth, unspecified site, complicated — (Use additional code to identify infection) ▽
873.71 Open wound of buccal mucosa, complicated — (Use additional code to identify infection)
873.74 Open wound of tongue and floor of mouth, complicated — (Use additional code to identify infection)
874.8 Open wound of other and unspecified parts of neck, without mention of complication — (Use additional code to identify infection) ▽
878.0 Open wound of penis, without mention of complication — (Use additional code to identify infection) ♂
878.1 Open wound of penis, complicated — (Use additional code to identify infection) ♂
878.2 Open wound of scrotum and testes, without mention of complication — (Use additional code to identify infection) ♂
878.3 Open wound of scrotum and testes, complicated — (Use additional code to identify infection) ♂
878.4 Open wound of vulva, without mention of complication — (Use additional code to identify infection) ♀
878.5 Open wound of vulva, complicated — (Use additional code to identify infection) ♀
878.6 Open wound of vagina, without mention of complication — (Use additional code to identify infection) ♀
878.7 Open wound of vagina, complicated — (Use additional code to identify infection) ♀
878.8 Open wound of other and unspecified parts of genital organs, without mention of complication — (Use additional code to identify infection) ▽
878.9 Open wound of other and unspecified parts of genital organs, complicated — (Use additional code to identify infection) ▽
882.0 Open wound of hand except finger(s) alone, without mention of complication — (Use additional code to identify infection)
882.1 Open wound of hand except finger(s) alone, complicated — (Use additional code to identify infection)
882.2 Open wound of hand except finger(s) alone, with tendon involvement — (Use additional code to identify infection)
883.0 Open wound of finger(s), without mention of complication — (Use additional code to identify infection)
883.1 Open wound of finger(s), complicated — (Use additional code to identify infection)
883.2 Open wound of finger(s), with tendon involvement — (Use additional code to identify infection)
885.0 Traumatic amputation of thumb (complete) (partial), without mention of complication — (Use additional code to identify infection)
885.1 Traumatic amputation of thumb (complete) (partial), complicated — (Use additional code to identify infection)
886.0 Traumatic amputation of other finger(s) (complete) (partial), without mention of complication — (Use additional code to identify infection)
886.1 Traumatic amputation of other finger(s) (complete) (partial), complicated — (Use additional code to identify infection)
892.0 Open wound of foot except toe(s) alone, without mention of complication — (Use additional code to identify infection)
892.1 Open wound of foot except toe(s) alone, complicated — (Use additional code to identify infection)
892.2 Open wound of foot except toe(s) alone, with tendon involvement — (Use additional code to identify infection)
893.0 Open wound of toe(s), without mention of complication — (Use additional code to identify infection)
893.1 Open wound of toe(s), complicated — (Use additional code to identify infection)
893.2 Open wound of toe(s), with tendon involvement — (Use additional code to identify infection)
895.0 Traumatic amputation of toe(s) (complete) (partial), without mention of complication — (Use additional code to identify infection)
895.1 Traumatic amputation of toe(s) (complete) (partial), complicated — (Use additional code to identify infection)
896.0 Traumatic amputation of foot (complete) (partial), unilateral, without mention of complication — (Use additional code to identify infection)
896.1 Traumatic amputation of foot (complete) (partial), unilateral, complicated — (Use additional code to identify infection)
896.2 Traumatic amputation of foot (complete) (partial), bilateral, without mention of complication — (Use additional code to identify infection)
896.3 Traumatic amputation of foot (complete) (partial), bilateral, complicated — (Use additional code to identify infection)
906.0 Late effect of open wound of head, neck, and trunk
906.5 Late effect of burn of eye, face, head, and neck
906.6 Late effect of burn of wrist and hand
906.7 Late effect of burn of other extremities
906.8 Late effect of burns of other specified sites
908.3 Late effect of injury to blood vessel of head, neck, and extremities
926.0 Crushing injury of external genitalia — (Use additional code to identify any associated injuries: 800-829, 850.0-854.1, 860.0-869.1)
940.0 Chemical burn of eyelids and periocular area
940.1 Other burns of eyelids and periocular area
941.01 Burn of unspecified degree of ear (any part) ▽
941.31 Full-thickness skin loss due to burn (third degree nos) of ear (any part)
941.32 Full-thickness skin loss due to burn (third degree nos) of eye (with other parts of face, head, and neck)
941.33 Full-thickness skin loss due to burn (third degree nos) of lip(s)
941.34 Full-thickness skin loss due to burn (third degree nos) of chin
941.35 Full-thickness skin loss due to burn (third degree nos) of nose (septum)
941.36 Full-thickness skin loss due to burn (third degree nos) of scalp (any part)
941.37 Full-thickness skin loss due to burn (third degree nos) of forehead and cheek
941.38 Full-thickness skin loss due to burn (third degree nos) of neck
941.39 Full-thickness skin loss due to burn (third degree nos) of multiple sites (except with eye) of face, head, and neck
941.40 Deep necrosis of underlying tissues due to burn (deep third degree) of unspecified site of face and head, without mention of loss of a body part ▽
941.46 Deep necrosis of underlying tissues due to burn (deep third degree) of scalp (any part), without mention of loss of a body part
941.48 Deep necrosis of underlying tissues due to burn (deep third degree) of neck, without mention of loss of a body part
941.49 Deep necrosis of underlying tissues due to burn (deep third degree) of multiple sites (except with eye) of face, head, and neck, without mention of loss of a body part
947.0 Burn of mouth and pharynx
948.00 Burn (any degree) involving less than 10% of body surface with third degree burn of less than 10% or unspecified amount
948.10 Burn (any degree) involving 10-19% of body surface with third degree burn of less than 10% or unspecified amount
948.11 Burn (any degree) involving 10-19% of body surface with third degree burn of 10-19%
948.20 Burn (any degree) involving 20-29% of body surface with third degree burn of less than 10% or unspecified amount
948.21 Burn (any degree) involving 20-29% of body surface with third degree burn of 10-19%
948.22 Burn (any degree) involving 20-29% of body surface with third degree burn of 20-29%
948.30 Burn (any degree) involving 30-39% of body surface with third degree burn of less than 10% or unspecified amount
948.31 Burn (any degree) involving 30-39% of body surface with third degree burn of 10-19%
948.32 Burn (any degree) involving 30-39% of body surface with third degree burn of 20-29%
948.33 Burn (any degree) involving 30-39% of body surface with third degree burn of 30-39%
948.40 Burn (any degree) involving 40-49% of body surface with third degree burn of less than 10% or unspecified amount
948.41 Burn (any degree) involving 40-49% of body surface with third degree burn of 10-19%
948.42 Burn (any degree) involving 40-49% of body surface with third degree burn of 20-29%
948.43 Burn (any degree) involving 40-49% of body surface with third degree burn of 30-39%

▽ Unspecified code ♀ Female diagnosis ☒ Manifestation code ♂ Male diagnosis

948.44 Burn (any degree) involving 40-49% of body surface with third degree burn of 40-49%
948.50 Burn (any degree) involving 50-59% of body surface with third degree burn of less than 10% or unspecified amount
948.51 Burn (any degree) involving 50-59% of body surface with third degree burn of 10-19%
948.52 Burn (any degree) involving 50-59% of body surface with third degree burn of 20-29%
948.53 Burn (any degree) involving 50-59% of body surface with third degree burn of 30-39%
948.54 Burn (any degree) involving 50-59% of body surface with third degree burn of 40-49%
948.55 Burn (any degree) involving 50-59% of body surface with third degree burn of 50-59%
948.60 Burn (any degree) involving 60-69% of body surface with third degree burn of less than 10% or unspecified amount
948.61 Burn (any degree) involving 60-69% of body surface with third degree burn of 10-19%
948.62 Burn (any degree) involving 60-69% of body surface with third degree burn of 20-29%
948.63 Burn (any degree) involving 60-69% of body surface with third degree burn of 30-39%
948.64 Burn (any degree) involving 60-69% of body surface with third degree burn of 40-49%
948.65 Burn (any degree) involving 60-69% of body surface with third degree burn of 50-59%
948.66 Burn (any degree) involving 60-69% of body surface with third degree burn of 60-69%
948.70 Burn (any degree) involving 70-79% of body surface with third degree burn of less than 10% or unspecified amount
948.71 Burn (any degree) involving 70-79% of body surface with third degree burn of 10-19%
948.72 Burn (any degree) involving 70-79% of body surface with third degree burn of 20-29%
948.73 Burn (any degree) involving 70-79% of body surface with third degree burn of 30-39%
948.74 Burn (any degree) involving 70-79% of body surface with third degree burn of 40-49%
948.75 Burn (any degree) involving 70-79% of body surface with third degree burn of 50-59%
948.76 Burn (any degree) involving 70-79% of body surface with third degree burn of 60-69%
948.77 Burn (any degree) involving 70-79% of body surface with third degree burn of 70-79%
948.80 Burn (any degree) involving 80-89% of body surface with third degree burn of less than 10% or unspecified amount
948.81 Burn (any degree) involving 80-89% of body surface with third degree burn of 10-19%
948.82 Burn (any degree) involving 80-89% of body surface with third degree burn of 20-29%
948.83 Burn (any degree) involving 80-89% of body surface with third degree burn of 30-39%
948.84 Burn (any degree) involving 80-89% of body surface with third degree burn of 40-49%
948.85 Burn (any degree) involving 80-89% of body surface with third degree burn of 50-59%
948.86 Burn (any degree) involving 80-89% of body surface with third degree burn of 60-69%
948.87 Burn (any degree) involving 80-89% of body surface with third degree burn of 70-79%
948.88 Burn (any degree) involving 80-89% of body surface with third degree burn of 80-89%
949.2 Blisters with epidermal loss due to burn (second degree), unspecified site ▽
959.01 Head injury, unspecified ▽
959.09 Injury of face and neck, other and unspecified
959.14 Other injury of external genitals
959.5 Injury, other and unspecified, finger
959.7 Injury, other and unspecified, knee, leg, ankle, and foot
959.8 Injury, other and unspecified, other specified sites, including multiple
991.0 Frostbite of face
991.1 Frostbite of hand
991.2 Frostbite of foot
996.52 Mechanical complication due to other tissue graft, not elsewhere classified
997.62 Infection (chronic) of amputation stump — (Use additional code to identify organism. Use additional code to identify complications)
997.69 Other late amputation stump complication — (Use additional code to identify complications)
998.83 Non-healing surgical wound
V10.02 Personal history of malignant neoplasm of other and unspecified parts of oral cavity and pharynx ▽
V10.21 Personal history of malignant neoplasm of larynx
V51 Aftercare involving the use of plastic surgery

ICD-9-CM Procedural

08.61 Reconstruction of eyelid with skin flap or graft
16.65 Secondary graft to exenteration cavity
18.6 Reconstruction of external auditory canal
18.79 Other plastic repair of external ear
27.56 Other skin graft to lip and mouth
86.62 Other skin graft to hand
86.69 Other skin graft to other sites

15200–15201

15200 Full thickness graft, free, including direct closure of donor site, trunk; 20 sq. cm or less
15201 each additional 20 sq. cm (List separately in addition to code for primary procedure)

ICD-9-CM Diagnostic

171.4 Malignant neoplasm of connective and other soft tissue of thorax
171.5 Malignant neoplasm of connective and other soft tissue of abdomen
171.6 Malignant neoplasm of connective and other soft tissue of pelvis
172.5 Malignant melanoma of skin of trunk, except scrotum
173.5 Other malignant neoplasm of skin of trunk, except scrotum
174.0 Malignant neoplasm of nipple and areola of female breast ♀
174.1 Malignant neoplasm of central portion of female breast ♀
174.2 Malignant neoplasm of upper-inner quadrant of female breast ♀
174.3 Malignant neoplasm of lower-inner quadrant of female breast ♀
174.4 Malignant neoplasm of upper-outer quadrant of female breast ♀
174.5 Malignant neoplasm of lower-outer quadrant of female breast ♀
174.6 Malignant neoplasm of axillary tail of female breast ♀
174.8 Malignant neoplasm of other specified sites of female breast ♀
174.9 Malignant neoplasm of breast (female), unspecified site ▽ ♀
175.0 Malignant neoplasm of nipple and areola of male breast ♂
175.9 Malignant neoplasm of other and unspecified sites of male breast ▽ ♂
215.4 Other benign neoplasm of connective and other soft tissue of thorax
215.5 Other benign neoplasm of connective and other soft tissue of abdomen
215.6 Other benign neoplasm of connective and other soft tissue of pelvis
215.7 Other benign neoplasm of connective and other soft tissue of trunk, unspecified ▽
232.5 Carcinoma in situ of skin of trunk, except scrotum
238.2 Neoplasm of uncertain behavior of skin
239.2 Neoplasms of unspecified nature of bone, soft tissue, and skin
707.00 Decubitus ulcer, unspecified site
707.02 Decubitus ulcer, upper back
707.03 Decubitus ulcer, lower back
707.04 Decubitus ulcer, hip
707.05 Decubitus ulcer, buttock
707.09 Decubitus ulcer, other site
728.86 Necrotizing fasciitis — (Use additional code to identify infectious organism, 041.00-041.89, 785.4, if applicable)
785.4 Gangrene — (Code first any associated underlying condition:250.7, 443.0)
906.8 Late effect of burns of other specified sites
908.0 Late effect of internal injury to chest
908.1 Late effect of internal injury to intra-abdominal organs
908.2 Late effect of internal injury to other internal organs
909.2 Late effect of radiation
909.3 Late effect of complications of surgical and medical care
942.30 Full-thickness skin loss due to burn (third degree nos) of unspecified site of trunk ▽
942.31 Full-thickness skin loss due to burn (third degree nos) of breast
942.32 Full-thickness skin loss due to burn (third degree nos) of chest wall, excluding breast and nipple
942.33 Full-thickness skin loss due to burn (third degree nos) of abdominal wall
942.34 Full-thickness skin loss due to burn (third degree nos) of back (any part)
942.35 Full-thickness skin loss due to burn (third degree nos) of genitalia
942.40 Deep necrosis of underlying tissues due to burn (deep third degree) of trunk, unspecified site, without mention of loss of a body part ▽
942.41 Deep necrosis of underlying tissues due to burn (deep third degree) of breast, without mention of loss of a body part

▽ Unspecified code ♀ Female diagnosis ☒ Manifestation code ♂ Male diagnosis

942.42 Deep necrosis of underlying tissues due to burn (deep third degree) of chest wall, excluding breast and nipple, without mention of loss of a body part
942.43 Deep necrosis of underlying tissues due to burn (deep third degree) of abdominal wall, without mention of loss of a body part
942.44 Deep necrosis of underlying tissues due to burn (deep third degree) of back (any part), without mention of loss of a body part
942.45 Deep necrosis of underlying tissues due to burn (deep third degree) of genitalia, without mention of loss of a body part
943.34 Full-thickness skin loss due to burn (third degree nos) of axilla
943.35 Full-thickness skin loss due to burn (third degree nos) of shoulder
943.36 Full-thickness skin loss due to burn (third degree nos) of scapular region
943.44 Deep necrosis of underlying tissues due to burn (deep third degree) of axilla, without mention of loss of a body part
943.45 Deep necrosis of underlying tissues due to burn (deep third degree) of shoulder, without mention of loss of a body part
943.46 Deep necrosis of underlying tissues due to burn (deep third degree) of scapular region, without mention of loss of a body part
943.54 Deep necrosis of underlying tissues due to burn (deep third degree) of axilla, with loss of a body part
943.56 Deep necrosis of underlying tissues due to burn (deep third degree) of scapular region, with loss of a body part
948.00 Burn (any degree) involving less than 10% of body surface with third degree burn of less than 10% or unspecified amount
948.10 Burn (any degree) involving 10-19% of body surface with third degree burn of less than 10% or unspecified amount
948.11 Burn (any degree) involving 10-19% of body surface with third degree burn of 10-19%
948.20 Burn (any degree) involving 20-29% of body surface with third degree burn of less than 10% or unspecified amount
948.21 Burn (any degree) involving 20-29% of body surface with third degree burn of 10-19%
948.22 Burn (any degree) involving 20-29% of body surface with third degree burn of 20-29%
948.30 Burn (any degree) involving 30-39% of body surface with third degree burn of less than 10% or unspecified amount
948.31 Burn (any degree) involving 30-39% of body surface with third degree burn of 10-19%
948.32 Burn (any degree) involving 30-39% of body surface with third degree burn of 20-29%
948.33 Burn (any degree) involving 30-39% of body surface with third degree burn of 30-39%
948.40 Burn (any degree) involving 40-49% of body surface with third degree burn of less than 10% or unspecified amount
948.41 Burn (any degree) involving 40-49% of body surface with third degree burn of 10-19%
948.42 Burn (any degree) involving 40-49% of body surface with third degree burn of 20-29%
948.43 Burn (any degree) involving 40-49% of body surface with third degree burn of 30-39%
948.44 Burn (any degree) involving 40-49% of body surface with third degree burn of 40-49%
948.50 Burn (any degree) involving 50-59% of body surface with third degree burn of less than 10% or unspecified amount
948.51 Burn (any degree) involving 50-59% of body surface with third degree burn of 10-19%
948.52 Burn (any degree) involving 50-59% of body surface with third degree burn of 20-29%
948.53 Burn (any degree) involving 50-59% of body surface with third degree burn of 30-39%
948.54 Burn (any degree) involving 50-59% of body surface with third degree burn of 40-49%
948.55 Burn (any degree) involving 50-59% of body surface with third degree burn of 50-59%
948.60 Burn (any degree) involving 60-69% of body surface with third degree burn of less than 10% or unspecified amount
948.61 Burn (any degree) involving 60-69% of body surface with third degree burn of 10-19%
948.62 Burn (any degree) involving 60-69% of body surface with third degree burn of 20-29%
948.63 Burn (any degree) involving 60-69% of body surface with third degree burn of 30-39%
948.64 Burn (any degree) involving 60-69% of body surface with third degree burn of 40-49%
948.65 Burn (any degree) involving 60-69% of body surface with third degree burn of 50-59%
948.66 Burn (any degree) involving 60-69% of body surface with third degree burn of 60-69%
948.70 Burn (any degree) involving 70-79% of body surface with third degree burn of less than 10% or unspecified amount
948.71 Burn (any degree) involving 70-79% of body surface with third degree burn of 10-19%
948.72 Burn (any degree) involving 70-79% of body surface with third degree burn of 20-29%
948.73 Burn (any degree) involving 70-79% of body surface with third degree burn of 30-39%
948.74 Burn (any degree) involving 70-79% of body surface with third degree burn of 40-49%
948.75 Burn (any degree) involving 70-79% of body surface with third degree burn of 50-59%
948.76 Burn (any degree) involving 70-79% of body surface with third degree burn of 60-69%
948.77 Burn (any degree) involving 70-79% of body surface with third degree burn of 70-79%
948.80 Burn (any degree) involving 80-89% of body surface with third degree burn of less than 10% or unspecified amount
948.81 Burn (any degree) involving 80-89% of body surface with third degree burn of 10-19%
948.82 Burn (any degree) involving 80-89% of body surface with third degree burn of 20-29%
948.83 Burn (any degree) involving 80-89% of body surface with third degree burn of 30-39%
948.84 Burn (any degree) involving 80-89% of body surface with third degree burn of 40-49%
948.85 Burn (any degree) involving 80-89% of body surface with third degree burn of 50-59%
948.86 Burn (any degree) involving 80-89% of body surface with third degree burn of 60-69%
948.87 Burn (any degree) involving 80-89% of body surface with third degree burn of 70-79%
948.88 Burn (any degree) involving 80-89% of body surface with third degree burn of 80-89%
958.3 Posttraumatic wound infection not elsewhere classified
959.11 Other injury of chest wall
959.12 Other injury of abdomen
959.19 Other injury of other sites of trunk
983.0 Toxic effect of corrosive aromatics — (Use additional code to specify the nature of the toxic effect)
983.1 Toxic effect of acids — (Use additional code to specify the nature of the toxic effect)
983.2 Toxic effect of caustic alkalis — (Use additional code to specify the nature of the toxic effect)
991.3 Frostbite of other and unspecified sites
998.32 Disruption of external operation wound
998.59 Other postoperative infection — (Use additional code to identify infection)
998.83 Non-healing surgical wound
V10.3 Personal history of malignant neoplasm of breast
V10.40 Personal history of malignant neoplasm of unspecified female genital organ ▽ ♀
V10.49 Personal history of malignant neoplasm of other male genital organs ♂
V10.82 Personal history of malignant melanoma of skin
V10.83 Personal history of other malignant neoplasm of skin
V10.84 Personal history of malignant neoplasm of eye
V51 Aftercare involving the use of plastic surgery

ICD-9-CM Procedural

85.83 Full-thickness graft to breast
86.63 Full-thickness skin graft to other sites

15220–15221

15220 Full thickness graft, free, including direct closure of donor site, scalp, arms, and/or legs; 20 sq. cm or less
15221 each additional 20 sq. cm (List separately in addition to code for primary procedure)

ICD-9-CM Diagnostic

172.4 Malignant melanoma of skin of scalp and neck
172.6 Malignant melanoma of skin of upper limb, including shoulder
172.7 Malignant melanoma of skin of lower limb, including hip
172.8 Malignant melanoma of other specified sites of skin
173.4 Other malignant neoplasm of scalp and skin of neck
173.6 Other malignant neoplasm of skin of upper limb, including shoulder

173.7 Other malignant neoplasm of skin of lower limb, including hip
173.8 Other malignant neoplasm of other specified sites of skin
195.0 Malignant neoplasm of head, face, and neck
195.4 Malignant neoplasm of upper limb
195.5 Malignant neoplasm of lower limb
216.4 Benign neoplasm of scalp and skin of neck
216.6 Benign neoplasm of skin of upper limb, including shoulder
216.7 Benign neoplasm of skin of lower limb, including hip
232.4 Carcinoma in situ of scalp and skin of neck
232.6 Carcinoma in situ of skin of upper limb, including shoulder
232.7 Carcinoma in situ of skin of lower limb, including hip
238.2 Neoplasm of uncertain behavior of skin
239.2 Neoplasms of unspecified nature of bone, soft tissue, and skin
454.0 Varicose veins of lower extremities with ulcer
454.2 Varicose veins of lower extremities with ulcer and inflammation
454.8 Varicose veins of the lower extremities with other complications
459.11 Postphlebitic syndrome with ulcer
459.13 Postphlebitic syndrome with ulcer and inflammation
459.19 Postphlebitic syndrome with other complication
459.31 Chronic venous hypertension with ulcer
459.33 Chronic venous hypertension with ulcer and inflammation
459.39 Chronic venous hypertension with other complication
701.4 Keloid scar
707.00 Decubitus ulcer, unspecified site
707.06 Decubitus ulcer, ankle
707.09 Decubitus ulcer, other site
707.10 Ulcer of lower limb, unspecified ▽
707.11 Ulcer of thigh
707.12 Ulcer of calf
707.13 Ulcer of ankle
707.19 Ulcer of other part of lower limb
707.8 Chronic ulcer of other specified site
709.2 Scar condition and fibrosis of skin
728.86 Necrotizing fasciitis — (Use additional code to identify infectious organism, 041.00-041.89, 785.4, if applicable)
785.4 Gangrene — (Code first any associated underlying condition:250.7, 443.0)
873.0 Open wound of scalp, without mention of complication — (Use additional code to identify infection)
873.1 Open wound of scalp, complicated — (Use additional code to identify infection)
880.01 Open wound of scapular region, without mention of complication — (Use additional code to identify infection)
880.02 Open wound of axillary region, without mention of complication — (Use additional code to identify infection)
880.03 Open wound of upper arm, without mention of complication — (Use additional code to identify infection)
880.09 Open wound of multiple sites of shoulder and upper arm, without mention of complication — (Use additional code to identify infection)
880.13 Open wound of upper arm, complicated — (Use additional code to identify infection)
880.19 Open wound of multiple sites of shoulder and upper arm, complicated — (Use additional code to identify infection)
881.00 Open wound of forearm, without mention of complication — (Use additional code to identify infection)
881.01 Open wound of elbow, without mention of complication — (Use additional code to identify infection)
881.02 Open wound of wrist, without mention of complication — (Use additional code to identify infection)
881.10 Open wound of forearm, complicated — (Use additional code to identify infection)
881.11 Open wound of elbow, complicated — (Use additional code to identify infection)
881.12 Open wound of wrist, complicated — (Use additional code to identify infection)
881.21 Open wound of elbow, with tendon involvement — (Use additional code to identify infection)
884.0 Multiple and unspecified open wound of upper limb, without mention of complication — (Use additional code to identify infection)
884.1 Multiple and unspecified open wound of upper limb, complicated — (Use additional code to identify infection)
884.2 Multiple and unspecified open wound of upper limb, with tendon involvement — (Use additional code to identify infection)
887.0 Traumatic amputation of arm and hand (complete) (partial), unilateral, below elbow, without mention of complication — (Use additional code to identify infection)
887.1 Traumatic amputation of arm and hand (complete) (partial), unilateral, below elbow, complicated — (Use additional code to identify infection)
887.2 Traumatic amputation of arm and hand (complete) (partial), unilateral, at or above elbow, without mention of complication — (Use additional code to identify infection)
887.3 Traumatic amputation of arm and hand (complete) (partial), unilateral, at or above elbow, complicated — (Use additional code to identify infection)
887.4 Traumatic amputation of arm and hand (complete) (partial), unilateral, level not specified, without mention of complication — (Use additional code to identify infection) ▽
887.5 Traumatic amputation of arm and hand (complete) (partial), unilateral, level not specified, complicated — (Use additional code to identify infection) ▽
887.6 Traumatic amputation of arm and hand (complete) (partial), bilateral (any level), without mention of complication — (Use additional code to identify infection)
887.7 Traumatic amputation of arm and hand (complete) (partial), bilateral (any level), complicated — (Use additional code to identify infection)
890.0 Open wound of hip and thigh, without mention of complication — (Use additional code to identify infection)
890.1 Open wound of hip and thigh, complicated — (Use additional code to identify infection)
890.2 Open wound of hip and thigh, with tendon involvement — (Use additional code to identify infection)
891.0 Open wound of knee, leg (except thigh), and ankle, without mention of complication — (Use additional code to identify infection)
891.2 Open wound of knee, leg (except thigh), and ankle, with tendon involvement — (Use additional code to identify infection)
892.1 Open wound of foot except toe(s) alone, complicated — (Use additional code to identify infection)
894.0 Multiple and unspecified open wound of lower limb, without mention of complication — (Use additional code to identify infection)
894.1 Multiple and unspecified open wound of lower limb, complicated — (Use additional code to identify infection)
894.2 Multiple and unspecified open wound of lower limb, with tendon involvement — (Use additional code to identify infection)
897.0 Traumatic amputation of leg(s) (complete) (partial), unilateral, below knee, without mention of complication — (Use additional code to identify infection)
897.1 Traumatic amputation of leg(s) (complete) (partial), unilateral, below knee, complicated — (Use additional code to identify infection)
897.3 Traumatic amputation of leg(s) (complete) (partial), unilateral, at or above knee, complicated — (Use additional code to identify infection)
897.4 Traumatic amputation of leg(s) (complete) (partial), unilateral, level not specified, without mention of complication — (Use additional code to identify infection) ▽
897.5 Traumatic amputation of leg(s) (complete) (partial), unilateral, level not specified, complicated — (Use additional code to identify infection) ▽
897.6 Traumatic amputation of leg(s) (complete) (partial), bilateral (any level), without mention of complication — (Use additional code to identify infection)
897.7 Traumatic amputation of leg(s) (complete) (partial), bilateral (any level), complicated — (Use additional code to identify infection)
906.0 Late effect of open wound of head, neck, and trunk
906.1 Late effect of open wound of extremities without mention of tendon injury
906.4 Late effect of crushing
906.5 Late effect of burn of eye, face, head, and neck
906.7 Late effect of burn of other extremities
908.6 Late effect of certain complications of trauma
909.2 Late effect of radiation
941.36 Full-thickness skin loss due to burn (third degree nos) of scalp (any part)
941.46 Deep necrosis of underlying tissues due to burn (deep third degree) of scalp (any part), without mention of loss of a body part
943.30 Full-thickness skin loss due to burn (third degree nos) of unspecified site of upper limb ▽
943.31 Full-thickness skin loss due to burn (third degree nos) of forearm
943.32 Full-thickness skin loss due to burn (third degree nos) of elbow
943.33 Full-thickness skin loss due to burn (third degree nos) of upper arm
943.34 Full-thickness skin loss due to burn (third degree nos) of axilla
943.35 Full-thickness skin loss due to burn (third degree nos) of shoulder
943.36 Full-thickness skin loss due to burn (third degree nos) of scapular region
943.39 Full-thickness skin loss due to burn (third degree nos) of multiple sites of upper limb, except wrist and hand
943.40 Deep necrosis of underlying tissues due to burn (deep third degree) of unspecified site of upper limb, without mention of loss of a body part ▽
943.41 Deep necrosis of underlying tissues due to burn (deep third degree) of forearm, without mention of loss of a body part
943.42 Deep necrosis of underlying tissues due to burn (deep third degree) of elbow, without mention of loss of a body part

▽ Unspecified code
♀ Female diagnosis
☒ Manifestation code
♂ Male diagnosis

943.43 Deep necrosis of underlying tissues due to burn (deep third degree) of upper arm, without mention of loss of a body part
943.49 Deep necrosis of underlying tissues due to burn (deep third degree) of multiple sites of upper limb, except wrist and hand, without mention of loss of a body part
943.50 Deep necrosis of underlying tissues due to burn (deep third degree) of unspecified site of upper limb, with loss of a body part
943.51 Deep necrosis of underlying tissues due to burn (deep third degree) of forearm, with loss of a body part
943.52 Deep necrosis of underlying tissues due to burn (deep third degree) of elbow, with loss of a body part
943.53 Deep necrosis of underlying tissues due to burn (deep third degree) of upper arm, with loss of upper a body part
943.59 Deep necrosis of underlying tissues due to burn (deep third degree) of multiple sites of upper limb, except wrist and hand, with loss of a body part
945.33 Full-thickness skin loss due to burn (third degree nos) of ankle
945.34 Full-thickness skin loss due to burn (third degree nos) of lower leg
945.35 Full-thickness skin loss due to burn (third degree nos) of knee
945.36 Full-thickness skin loss due to burn (third degree nos) of thigh (any part)
945.39 Full-thickness skin loss due to burn (third degree nos) of multiple sites of lower limb(s)
945.40 Deep necrosis of underlying tissues due to burn (deep third degree) of unspecified site of lower limb (leg), without mention of loss of a body part
945.43 Deep necrosis of underlying tissues due to burn (deep third degree) of ankle, without mention of loss of a body part
945.44 Deep necrosis of underlying tissues due to burn (deep third degree) of lower leg, without mention of loss of a body part
945.45 Deep necrosis of underlying tissues due to burn (deep third degree) of knee, without mention of loss of a body part
945.46 Deep necrosis of underlying tissues due to burn (deep third degree) of thigh (any part), without mention of loss of a body part
945.49 Deep necrosis of underlying tissues due to burn (deep third degree) of multiple sites of lower limb(s), without mention of loss of a body part
945.50 Deep necrosis of underlying tissues due to burn (deep third degree) of unspecified site lower limb (leg), with loss of a body part
945.53 Deep necrosis of underlying tissues due to burn (deep third degree) of ankle, with loss of a body part
945.54 Deep necrosis of underlying tissues due to burn (deep third degree) of lower leg, with loss of a body part
945.55 Deep necrosis of underlying tissues due to burn (deep third degree) of knee, with loss of a body part
945.56 Deep necrosis of underlying tissues due to burn (deep third degree) of thigh (any part), with loss of a body part
945.59 Deep necrosis of underlying tissues due to burn (deep third degree) of multiple sites of lower limb(s), with loss of a body part
946.3 Full-thickness skin loss due to burn (third degree nos) of multiple specified sites
946.4 Deep necrosis of underlying tissues due to burn (deep third degree) of multiple specified sites, without mention of loss of a body part
946.5 Deep necrosis of underlying tissues due to burn (deep third degree) of multiple specified sites, with loss of a body part
948.00 Burn (any degree) involving less than 10% of body surface with third degree burn of less than 10% or unspecified amount
948.10 Burn (any degree) involving 10-19% of body surface with third degree burn of less than 10% or unspecified amount
948.11 Burn (any degree) involving 10-19% of body surface with third degree burn of 10-19%
948.20 Burn (any degree) involving 20-29% of body surface with third degree burn of less than 10% or unspecified amount
948.21 Burn (any degree) involving 20-29% of body surface with third degree burn of 10-19%
948.22 Burn (any degree) involving 20-29% of body surface with third degree burn of 20-29%
948.30 Burn (any degree) involving 30-39% of body surface with third degree burn of less than 10% or unspecified amount
948.31 Burn (any degree) involving 30-39% of body surface with third degree burn of 10-19%
948.32 Burn (any degree) involving 30-39% of body surface with third degree burn of 20-29%
948.33 Burn (any degree) involving 30-39% of body surface with third degree burn of 30-39%
948.40 Burn (any degree) involving 40-49% of body surface with third degree burn of less than 10% or unspecified amount
948.41 Burn (any degree) involving 40-49% of body surface with third degree burn of 10-19%
948.42 Burn (any degree) involving 40-49% of body surface with third degree burn of 20-29%
948.43 Burn (any degree) involving 40-49% of body surface with third degree burn of 30-39%
948.44 Burn (any degree) involving 40-49% of body surface with third degree burn of 40-49%
948.50 Burn (any degree) involving 50-59% of body surface with third degree burn of less than 10% or unspecified amount
948.51 Burn (any degree) involving 50-59% of body surface with third degree burn of 10-19%
948.52 Burn (any degree) involving 50-59% of body surface with third degree burn of 20-29%
948.53 Burn (any degree) involving 50-59% of body surface with third degree burn of 30-39%
948.54 Burn (any degree) involving 50-59% of body surface with third degree burn of 40-49%
948.55 Burn (any degree) involving 50-59% of body surface with third degree burn of 50-59%
948.60 Burn (any degree) involving 60-69% of body surface with third degree burn of less than 10% or unspecified amount
948.61 Burn (any degree) involving 60-69% of body surface with third degree burn of 10-19%
948.62 Burn (any degree) involving 60-69% of body surface with third degree burn of 20-29%
948.63 Burn (any degree) involving 60-69% of body surface with third degree burn of 30-39%
948.64 Burn (any degree) involving 60-69% of body surface with third degree burn of 40-49%
948.65 Burn (any degree) involving 60-69% of body surface with third degree burn of 50-59%
948.66 Burn (any degree) involving 60-69% of body surface with third degree burn of 60-69%
948.70 Burn (any degree) involving 70-79% of body surface with third degree burn of less than 10% or unspecified amount
948.71 Burn (any degree) involving 70-79% of body surface with third degree burn of 10-19%
948.72 Burn (any degree) involving 70-79% of body surface with third degree burn of 20-29%
948.73 Burn (any degree) involving 70-79% of body surface with third degree burn of 30-39%
948.74 Burn (any degree) involving 70-79% of body surface with third degree burn of 40-49%
948.75 Burn (any degree) involving 70-79% of body surface with third degree burn of 50-59%
948.76 Burn (any degree) involving 70-79% of body surface with third degree burn of 60-69%
948.77 Burn (any degree) involving 70-79% of body surface with third degree burn of 70-79%
948.80 Burn (any degree) involving 80-89% of body surface with third degree burn of less than 10% or unspecified amount
948.81 Burn (any degree) involving 80-89% of body surface with third degree burn of 10-19%
948.82 Burn (any degree) involving 80-89% of body surface with third degree burn of 20-29%
V51 Aftercare involving the use of plastic surgery

ICD-9-CM Procedural

86.63 Full-thickness skin graft to other sites
86.64 Hair transplant

15240–15241

15240 Full thickness graft, free, including direct closure of donor site, forehead, cheeks, chin, mouth, neck, axillae, genitalia, hands, and/or feet; 20 sq. cm or less

15241 each additional 20 sq. cm (List separately in addition to code for primary procedure)

ICD-9-CM Diagnostic

140.3 Malignant neoplasm of upper lip, inner aspect
140.4 Malignant neoplasm of lower lip, inner aspect
140.5 Malignant neoplasm of lip, inner aspect, unspecified as to upper or lower
145.0 Malignant neoplasm of cheek mucosa
149.8 Malignant neoplasm of other sites within the lip and oral cavity
149.9 Malignant neoplasm of ill-defined sites of lip and oral cavity
171.6 Malignant neoplasm of connective and other soft tissue of pelvis
172.3 Malignant melanoma of skin of other and unspecified parts of face

172.4 Malignant melanoma of skin of scalp and neck
172.5 Malignant melanoma of skin of trunk, except scrotum
172.6 Malignant melanoma of skin of upper limb, including shoulder
172.7 Malignant melanoma of skin of lower limb, including hip
172.8 Malignant melanoma of other specified sites of skin
173.3 Other malignant neoplasm of skin of other and unspecified parts of face ▽
173.4 Other malignant neoplasm of scalp and skin of neck
184.0 Malignant neoplasm of vagina ♀
184.1 Malignant neoplasm of labia majora ♀
184.2 Malignant neoplasm of labia minora ♀
184.3 Malignant neoplasm of clitoris ♀
184.4 Malignant neoplasm of vulva, unspecified site ▽ ♀
184.8 Malignant neoplasm of other specified sites of female genital organs ♀
184.9 Malignant neoplasm of female genital organ, site unspecified ▽ ♀
187.1 Malignant neoplasm of prepuce ♂
187.2 Malignant neoplasm of glans penis ♂
187.3 Malignant neoplasm of body of penis ♂
187.4 Malignant neoplasm of penis, part unspecified ▽ ♂
187.7 Malignant neoplasm of scrotum ♂
187.9 Malignant neoplasm of male genital organ, site unspecified ▽ ♂
198.82 Secondary malignant neoplasm of genital organs
198.89 Secondary malignant neoplasm of other specified sites
210.4 Benign neoplasm of other and unspecified parts of mouth ▽
216.3 Benign neoplasm of skin of other and unspecified parts of face ▽
216.4 Benign neoplasm of scalp and skin of neck
216.6 Benign neoplasm of skin of upper limb, including shoulder
216.7 Benign neoplasm of skin of lower limb, including hip
216.8 Benign neoplasm of other specified sites of skin
222.4 Benign neoplasm of scrotum ♂
230.0 Carcinoma in situ of lip, oral cavity, and pharynx
232.3 Carcinoma in situ of skin of other and unspecified parts of face ▽
232.4 Carcinoma in situ of scalp and skin of neck
232.6 Carcinoma in situ of skin of upper limb, including shoulder
232.7 Carcinoma in situ of skin of lower limb, including hip
232.8 Carcinoma in situ of other specified sites of skin
233.3 Carcinoma in situ of other and unspecified female genital organs ▽ ♀
233.5 Carcinoma in situ of penis ♂
233.6 Carcinoma in situ of other and unspecified male genital organs ▽ ♂
235.1 Neoplasm of uncertain behavior of lip, oral cavity, and pharynx
236.3 Neoplasm of uncertain behavior of other and unspecified female genital organs ▽ ♀
236.6 Neoplasm of uncertain behavior of other and unspecified male genital organs ▽ ♂
238.2 Neoplasm of uncertain behavior of skin
239.5 Neoplasm of unspecified nature of other genitourinary organs
607.2 Other inflammatory disorders of penis — (Use additional code to identify organism) ♂
629.20 Female genital mutilation status, unspecified
629.21 Female genital mutilation, Type I status
629.22 Female genital mutilation, Type II status
629.23 Female genital mutilation, Type III status
707.00 Decubitus ulcer, unspecified site
707.07 Decubitus ulcer, heel
707.09 Decubitus ulcer, other site
707.14 Ulcer of heel and midfoot
707.15 Ulcer of other part of foot
709.2 Scar condition and fibrosis of skin
709.9 Unspecified disorder of skin and subcutaneous tissue ▽
728.86 Necrotizing fasciitis — (Use additional code to identify infectious organism, 041.00-041.89, 785.4, if applicable)
752.40 Unspecified congenital anomaly of cervix, vagina, and external female genitalia ▽ ♀
752.49 Other congenital anomaly of cervix, vagina, and external female genitalia ♀
752.64 Micropenis ♂
752.69 Other penile anomalies ♂
752.7 Indeterminate sex and pseudohermaphroditism
752.81 Scrotal transposition
752.89 Other specified anomalies of genital organs
752.9 Unspecified congenital anomaly of genital organs ▽
757.33 Congenital pigmentary anomaly of skin
873.50 Open wound of face, unspecified site, complicated — (Use additional code to identify infection) ▽
873.51 Open wound of cheek, complicated — (Use additional code to identify infection)
873.52 Open wound of forehead, complicated — (Use additional code to identify infection)
873.54 Open wound of jaw, complicated — (Use additional code to identify infection)
873.59 Open wound of face, other and multiple sites, complicated — (Use additional code to identify infection)
873.70 Open wound of mouth, unspecified site, complicated — (Use additional code to identify infection) ▽
873.71 Open wound of buccal mucosa, complicated — (Use additional code to identify infection)
873.74 Open wound of tongue and floor of mouth, complicated — (Use additional code to identify infection)
878.1 Open wound of penis, complicated — (Use additional code to identify infection) ♂
878.3 Open wound of scrotum and testes, complicated — (Use additional code to identify infection) ♂
878.5 Open wound of vulva, complicated — (Use additional code to identify infection) ♀
878.7 Open wound of vagina, complicated — (Use additional code to identify infection) ♀
878.9 Open wound of other and unspecified parts of genital organs, complicated — (Use additional code to identify infection) ▽
880.12 Open wound of axillary region, complicated — (Use additional code to identify infection)
882.1 Open wound of hand except finger(s) alone, complicated — (Use additional code to identify infection)
882.2 Open wound of hand except finger(s) alone, with tendon involvement — (Use additional code to identify infection)
883.1 Open wound of finger(s), complicated — (Use additional code to identify infection)
883.2 Open wound of finger(s), with tendon involvement — (Use additional code to identify infection)
884.1 Multiple and unspecified open wound of upper limb, complicated — (Use additional code to identify infection)
884.2 Multiple and unspecified open wound of upper limb, with tendon involvement — (Use additional code to identify infection)
885.0 Traumatic amputation of thumb (complete) (partial), without mention of complication — (Use additional code to identify infection)
885.1 Traumatic amputation of thumb (complete) (partial), complicated — (Use additional code to identify infection)
886.0 Traumatic amputation of other finger(s) (complete) (partial), without mention of complication — (Use additional code to identify infection)
886.1 Traumatic amputation of other finger(s) (complete) (partial), complicated — (Use additional code to identify infection)
887.0 Traumatic amputation of arm and hand (complete) (partial), unilateral, below elbow, without mention of complication — (Use additional code to identify infection)
887.1 Traumatic amputation of arm and hand (complete) (partial), unilateral, below elbow, complicated — (Use additional code to identify infection)
887.6 Traumatic amputation of arm and hand (complete) (partial), bilateral (any level), without mention of complication — (Use additional code to identify infection)
887.7 Traumatic amputation of arm and hand (complete) (partial), bilateral (any level), complicated — (Use additional code to identify infection)
892.1 Open wound of foot except toe(s) alone, complicated — (Use additional code to identify infection)
892.2 Open wound of foot except toe(s) alone, with tendon involvement — (Use additional code to identify infection)
893.1 Open wound of toe(s), complicated — (Use additional code to identify infection)
893.2 Open wound of toe(s), with tendon involvement — (Use additional code to identify infection)
894.1 Multiple and unspecified open wound of lower limb, complicated — (Use additional code to identify infection)
894.2 Multiple and unspecified open wound of lower limb, with tendon involvement — (Use additional code to identify infection)
895.0 Traumatic amputation of toe(s) (complete) (partial), without mention of complication — (Use additional code to identify infection)
895.1 Traumatic amputation of toe(s) (complete) (partial), complicated — (Use additional code to identify infection)
896.0 Traumatic amputation of foot (complete) (partial), unilateral, without mention of complication — (Use additional code to identify infection)
896.1 Traumatic amputation of foot (complete) (partial), unilateral, complicated — (Use additional code to identify infection)
896.2 Traumatic amputation of foot (complete) (partial), bilateral, without mention of complication — (Use additional code to identify infection)
896.3 Traumatic amputation of foot (complete) (partial), bilateral, complicated — (Use additional code to identify infection)
906.0 Late effect of open wound of head, neck, and trunk

▽ Unspecified code
♀ Female diagnosis
☒ Manifestation code
♂ Male diagnosis

906.5 Late effect of burn of eye, face, head, and neck
906.6 Late effect of burn of wrist and hand
906.8 Late effect of burns of other specified sites
926.0 Crushing injury of external genitalia — (Use additional code to identify any associated injuries: 800-829, 850.0-854.1, 860.0-869.1)
941.30 Full-thickness skin loss due to burn (third degree nos) of unspecified site of face and head ▽
941.33 Full-thickness skin loss due to burn (third degree nos) of lip(s)
941.34 Full-thickness skin loss due to burn (third degree nos) of chin
941.37 Full-thickness skin loss due to burn (third degree nos) of forehead and cheek
941.38 Full-thickness skin loss due to burn (third degree nos) of neck
941.39 Full-thickness skin loss due to burn (third degree nos) of multiple sites (except with eye) of face, head, and neck
941.40 Deep necrosis of underlying tissues due to burn (deep third degree) of unspecified site of face and head, without mention of loss of a body part ▽
941.44 Deep necrosis of underlying tissues due to burn (deep third degree) of chin, without mention of loss of a body part
941.47 Deep necrosis of underlying tissues due to burn (deep third degree) of forehead and cheek, without mention of loss of a body part
941.48 Deep necrosis of underlying tissues due to burn (deep third degree) of neck, without mention of loss of a body part
941.49 Deep necrosis of underlying tissues due to burn (deep third degree) of multiple sites (except with eye) of face, head, and neck, without mention of loss of a body part
941.50 Deep necrosis of underlying tissues due to burn (deep third degree) of face and head, unspecified site, with loss of a body part ▽
941.57 Deep necrosis of underlying tissues due to burn (deep third degree) of forehead and cheek, with loss of a body part
941.58 Deep necrosis of underlying tissues due to burn (deep third degree) of neck, with loss of a body part
941.59 Deep necrosis of underlying tissues due to burn (deep third degree) of multiple sites (except eye) of face, head, and neck, with loss of a body part
942.05 Burn of trunk, unspecified degree of genitalia ▽
943.34 Full-thickness skin loss due to burn (third degree nos) of axilla
943.44 Deep necrosis of underlying tissues due to burn (deep third degree) of axilla, without mention of loss of a body part
943.54 Deep necrosis of underlying tissues due to burn (deep third degree) of axilla, with loss of a body part
944.30 Full-thickness skin loss due to burn (third degree nos) of unspecified site of hand ▽
944.31 Full-thickness skin loss due to burn (third degree nos) of single digit [finger (nail)] other than thumb
944.32 Full-thickness skin loss due to burn (third degree nos) of thumb (nail)
944.33 Full-thickness skin loss due to burn (third degree nos) of two or more digits of hand, not including thumb
944.34 Full-thickness skin loss due to burn (third degree nos) of two or more digits of hand including thumb
944.35 Full-thickness skin loss due to burn (third degree nos) of palm of hand
944.36 Full-thickness skin loss due to burn (third degree nos) of back of hand
944.37 Full-thickness skin loss due to burn (third degree nos) of wrist
944.38 Full-thickness skin loss due to burn (third degree nos) of multiple sites of wrist(s) and hand(s)
944.40 Deep necrosis of underlying tissues due to burn (deep third degree) of unspecified site of hand, without mention of a body part ▽
944.41 Deep necrosis of underlying tissues due to burn (deep third degree) of single digit [finger (nail)] other than thumb, without mention of a body part
944.42 Deep necrosis of underlying tissues due to burn (deep third degree) of thumb (nail), without mention of loss of a body part
944.43 Deep necrosis of underlying tissues due to burn (deep third degree) of two or more digits of hand, not including thumb, without mention of a body part
944.44 Deep necrosis of underlying tissues due to burn (deep third degree) of two or more digits of hand including thumb, without mention of a body part
944.45 Deep necrosis of underlying tissues due to burn (deep third degree) of palm of hand, without mention of loss of a body part
944.46 Deep necrosis of underlying tissues due to burn (deep third degree) of back of hand, without mention of loss of back of a body part
944.47 Deep necrosis of underlying tissues due to burn (deep third degree) of wrist, without mention of loss of a body part
944.48 Deep necrosis of underlying tissues due to burn (deep third degree) of multiple sites of wrist(s) and hand(s), without mention of loss of a body part
944.50 Deep necrosis of underlying tissues due to burn (deep third degree) of unspecified site of hand, with loss of a body part ▽
944.51 Deep necrosis of underlying tissues due to burn (deep third degree) of single digit (finger (nail)) other than thumb, with loss of a body part
944.52 Deep necrosis of underlying tissues due to burn (deep third degree) of thumb (nail), with loss of a body part
944.53 Deep necrosis of underlying tissues due to burn (deep third degree) of two or more digits of hand, not including thumb, with loss of a body part
944.54 Deep necrosis of underlying tissues due to burn (deep third degree) of two or more digits of hand including thumb, with loss of a body part
944.55 Deep necrosis of underlying tissues due to burn (deep third degree) of palm of hand, with loss of a body part
944.56 Deep necrosis of underlying tissues due to burn (deep third degree) of back of hand, with loss of a body part
944.57 Deep necrosis of underlying tissues due to burn (deep third degree) of wrist, with loss of a body part
944.58 Deep necrosis of underlying tissues due to burn (deep third degree) of multiple sites of wrist(s) and hand(s), with loss of a body part
945.32 Full-thickness skin loss due to burn (third degree nos) of foot
945.42 Deep necrosis of underlying tissues due to burn (deep third degree) of foot, without mention of loss of a body part
945.52 Deep necrosis of underlying tissues due to burn (deep third degree) of foot, with loss of a body part
946.3 Full-thickness skin loss due to burn (third degree nos) of multiple specified sites
946.4 Deep necrosis of underlying tissues due to burn (deep third degree) of multiple specified sites, without mention of loss of a body part
946.5 Deep necrosis of underlying tissues due to burn (deep third degree) of multiple specified sites, with loss of a body part
947.0 Burn of mouth and pharynx
959.09 Injury of face and neck, other and unspecified
959.14 Other injury of external genitals
959.4 Injury, other and unspecified, hand, except finger
959.5 Injury, other and unspecified, finger
959.7 Injury, other and unspecified, knee, leg, ankle, and foot
959.8 Injury, other and unspecified, other specified sites, including multiple
991.0 Frostbite of face
991.1 Frostbite of hand
991.2 Frostbite of foot
996.52 Mechanical complication due to other tissue graft, not elsewhere classified
996.64 Infection and inflammatory reaction due to indwelling urinary catheter — (Use additional code to identify specified infections: 038.0-038.9, 595.0-595.9)
997.60 Late complications of amputation stump, unspecified — (Use additional code to identify complications) ▽
997.62 Infection (chronic) of amputation stump — (Use additional code to identify organism. Use additional code to identify complications)
997.69 Other late amputation stump complication — (Use additional code to identify complications)
998.83 Non-healing surgical wound
V10.02 Personal history of malignant neoplasm of other and unspecified parts of oral cavity and pharynx ▽
V10.21 Personal history of malignant neoplasm of larynx
V51 Aftercare involving the use of plastic surgery

ICD-9-CM Procedural

27.55 Full-thickness skin graft to lip and mouth
86.61 Full-thickness skin graft to hand
86.63 Full-thickness skin graft to other sites

15260–15261

15260 Full thickness graft, free, including direct closure of donor site, nose, ears, eyelids, and/or lips; 20 sq. cm or less

15261 each additional 20 sq. cm (List separately in addition to code for primary procedure)

ICD-9-CM Diagnostic

140.0 Malignant neoplasm of upper lip, vermilion border
140.1 Malignant neoplasm of lower lip, vermilion border
140.3 Malignant neoplasm of upper lip, inner aspect
140.4 Malignant neoplasm of lower lip, inner aspect
140.5 Malignant neoplasm of lip, inner aspect, unspecified as to upper or lower ▽
140.6 Malignant neoplasm of commissure of lip
140.8 Malignant neoplasm of other sites of lip
140.9 Malignant neoplasm of lip, vermilion border, unspecified as to upper or lower ▽
172.0 Malignant melanoma of skin of lip
172.1 Malignant melanoma of skin of eyelid, including canthus
172.2 Malignant melanoma of skin of ear and external auditory canal
172.3 Malignant melanoma of skin of other and unspecified parts of face
172.8 Malignant melanoma of other specified sites of skin
173.0 Other malignant neoplasm of skin of lip
173.1 Other malignant neoplasm of skin of eyelid, including canthus

173.2 Other malignant neoplasm of skin of ear and external auditory canal
173.3 Other malignant neoplasm of skin of other and unspecified parts of face ▽
173.8 Other malignant neoplasm of other specified sites of skin
195.0 Malignant neoplasm of head, face, and neck
198.2 Secondary malignant neoplasm of skin
210.0 Benign neoplasm of lip
210.4 Benign neoplasm of other and unspecified parts of mouth ▽
216.0 Benign neoplasm of skin of lip
216.1 Benign neoplasm of eyelid, including canthus
216.2 Benign neoplasm of ear and external auditory canal
216.3 Benign neoplasm of skin of other and unspecified parts of face ▽
230.0 Carcinoma in situ of lip, oral cavity, and pharynx
232.1 Carcinoma in situ of eyelid, including canthus
232.2 Carcinoma in situ of skin of ear and external auditory canal
232.3 Carcinoma in situ of skin of other and unspecified parts of face ▽
238.2 Neoplasm of uncertain behavior of skin
239.0 Neoplasm of unspecified nature of digestive system
239.2 Neoplasms of unspecified nature of bone, soft tissue, and skin
374.04 Cicatricial entropion
374.14 Cicatricial ectropion
374.41 Eyelid retraction or lag
380.32 Acquired deformities of auricle or pinna
682.0 Cellulitis and abscess of face — (Use additional code to identify organism)
709.2 Scar condition and fibrosis of skin
743.62 Congenital deformity of eyelid
744.01 Congenital absence of external ear causing impairment of hearing
744.09 Other congenital anomalies of ear causing impairment of hearing
744.23 Microtia
744.3 Unspecified congenital anomaly of ear ▽
744.5 Congenital webbing of neck
744.82 Microcheilia
748.1 Other congenital anomaly of nose
749.00 Unspecified cleft palate ▽
749.10 Unspecified cleft lip ▽
749.11 Unilateral cleft lip, complete
749.12 Unilateral cleft lip, incomplete
749.13 Bilateral cleft lip, complete
749.14 Bilateral cleft lip, incomplete
749.20 Unspecified cleft palate with cleft lip ▽
749.21 Unilateral cleft palate with cleft lip, complete
749.22 Unilateral cleft palate with cleft lip, incomplete
749.23 Bilateral cleft palate with cleft lip, complete
749.24 Bilateral cleft palate with cleft lip, incomplete
785.4 Gangrene — (Code first any associated underlying condition:250.7, 443.0)
870.0 Laceration of skin of eyelid and periocular area — (Use additional code to identify infection)
870.1 Laceration of eyelid, full-thickness, not involving lacrimal passages — (Use additional code to identify infection)
870.2 Laceration of eyelid involving lacrimal passages — (Use additional code to identify infection)
872.00 Open wound of external ear, unspecified site, without mention of complication — (Use additional code to identify infection) ▽
872.01 Open wound of auricle, without mention of complication — (Use additional code to identify infection)
872.02 Open wound of auditory canal, without mention of complication — (Use additional code to identify infection)
872.10 Open wound of external ear, unspecified site, complicated — (Use additional code to identify infection) ▽
872.11 Open wound of auricle, complicated — (Use additional code to identify infection)
872.12 Open wound of auditory canal, complicated — (Use additional code to identify infection)
872.8 Open wound of ear, part unspecified, without mention of complication — (Use additional code to identify infection) ▽
872.9 Open wound of ear, part unspecified, complicated — (Use additional code to identify infection) ▽
873.20 Open wound of nose, unspecified site, without mention of complication — (Use additional code to identify infection) ▽
873.23 Open wound of nasal sinus, without mention of complication — (Use additional code to identify infection)
873.30 Open wound of nose, unspecified site, complicated — (Use additional code to identify infection) ▽
873.31 Open wound of nasal septum, complicated — (Use additional code to identify infection)
873.32 Open wound of nasal cavity, complicated — (Use additional code to identify infection)
873.33 Open wound of nasal sinus, complicated — (Use additional code to identify infection)
873.39 Open wound of nose, multiple sites, complicated — (Use additional code to identify infection)
873.43 Open wound of lip, without mention of complication — (Use additional code to identify infection)
873.53 Open wound of lip, complicated — (Use additional code to identify infection)
906.0 Late effect of open wound of head, neck, and trunk
906.5 Late effect of burn of eye, face, head, and neck
941.01 Burn of unspecified degree of ear (any part) ▽
941.02 Burn of unspecified degree of eye (with other parts of face, head, and neck) ▽
941.03 Burn of unspecified degree of lip(s) ▽
941.05 Burn of unspecified degree of nose (septum) ▽
941.09 Burn of unspecified degree of multiple sites (except with eye) of face, head, and neck ▽
941.31 Full-thickness skin loss due to burn (third degree nos) of ear (any part)
941.32 Full-thickness skin loss due to burn (third degree nos) of eye (with other parts of face, head, and neck)
941.33 Full-thickness skin loss due to burn (third degree nos) of lip(s)
941.35 Full-thickness skin loss due to burn (third degree nos) of nose (septum)
941.39 Full-thickness skin loss due to burn (third degree nos) of multiple sites (except with eye) of face, head, and neck
941.49 Deep necrosis of underlying tissues due to burn (deep third degree) of multiple sites (except with eye) of face, head, and neck, without mention of loss of a body part
941.51 Deep necrosis of underlying tissues due to burn (deep third degree) of ear (any part), with loss of a body part
941.52 Deep necrosis of underlying tissues due to burn (deep third degree) of eye (with other parts of face, head, and neck), with loss of a body part
941.53 Deep necrosis of underlying tissues due to burn (deep third degree) of lip(s), with loss of a body part
941.55 Deep necrosis of underlying tissues due to burn (deep third degree) of nose (septum), with loss of a body part
941.59 Deep necrosis of underlying tissues due to burn (deep third degree) of multiple sites (except eye) of face, head, and neck, with loss of a body part
946.3 Full-thickness skin loss due to burn (third degree nos) of multiple specified sites
946.4 Deep necrosis of underlying tissues due to burn (deep third degree) of multiple specified sites, without mention of loss of a body part
946.5 Deep necrosis of underlying tissues due to burn (deep third degree) of multiple specified sites, with loss of a body part
948.00 Burn (any degree) involving less than 10% of body surface with third degree burn of less than 10% or unspecified amount
948.10 Burn (any degree) involving 10-19% of body surface with third degree burn of less than 10% or unspecified amount
948.11 Burn (any degree) involving 10-19% of body surface with third degree burn of 10-19%
948.20 Burn (any degree) involving 20-29% of body surface with third degree burn of less than 10% or unspecified amount
948.21 Burn (any degree) involving 20-29% of body surface with third degree burn of 10-19%
948.22 Burn (any degree) involving 20-29% of body surface with third degree burn of 20-29%
948.30 Burn (any degree) involving 30-39% of body surface with third degree burn of less than 10% or unspecified amount
948.31 Burn (any degree) involving 30-39% of body surface with third degree burn of 10-19%
948.32 Burn (any degree) involving 30-39% of body surface with third degree burn of 20-29%
948.33 Burn (any degree) involving 30-39% of body surface with third degree burn of 30-39%
948.40 Burn (any degree) involving 40-49% of body surface with third degree burn of less than 10% or unspecified amount
948.41 Burn (any degree) involving 40-49% of body surface with third degree burn of 10-19%
948.42 Burn (any degree) involving 40-49% of body surface with third degree burn of 20-29%
948.43 Burn (any degree) involving 40-49% of body surface with third degree burn of 30-39%
948.44 Burn (any degree) involving 40-49% of body surface with third degree burn of 40-49%
948.50 Burn (any degree) involving 50-59% of body surface with third degree burn of less than 10% or unspecified amount
948.51 Burn (any degree) involving 50-59% of body surface with third degree burn of 10-19%

▽ Unspecified code
♀ Female diagnosis
☒ Manifestation code
♂ Male diagnosis

948.52 Burn (any degree) involving 50-59% of body surface with third degree burn of 20-29%
948.53 Burn (any degree) involving 50-59% of body surface with third degree burn of 30-39%
948.54 Burn (any degree) involving 50-59% of body surface with third degree burn of 40-49%
948.55 Burn (any degree) involving 50-59% of body surface with third degree burn of 50-59%
948.60 Burn (any degree) involving 60-69% of body surface with third degree burn of less than 10% or unspecified amount
948.61 Burn (any degree) involving 60-69% of body surface with third degree burn of 10-19%
948.62 Burn (any degree) involving 60-69% of body surface with third degree burn of 20-29%
948.63 Burn (any degree) involving 60-69% of body surface with third degree burn of 30-39%
948.64 Burn (any degree) involving 60-69% of body surface with third degree burn of 40-49%
948.65 Burn (any degree) involving 60-69% of body surface with third degree burn of 50-59%
948.66 Burn (any degree) involving 60-69% of body surface with third degree burn of 60-69%
948.70 Burn (any degree) involving 70-79% of body surface with third degree burn of less than 10% or unspecified amount
948.71 Burn (any degree) involving 70-79% of body surface with third degree burn of 10-19%
948.72 Burn (any degree) involving 70-79% of body surface with third degree burn of 20-29%
948.73 Burn (any degree) involving 70-79% of body surface with third degree burn of 30-39%
948.74 Burn (any degree) involving 70-79% of body surface with third degree burn of 40-49%
948.75 Burn (any degree) involving 70-79% of body surface with third degree burn of 50-59%
948.76 Burn (any degree) involving 70-79% of body surface with third degree burn of 60-69%
948.77 Burn (any degree) involving 70-79% of body surface with third degree burn of 70-79%
948.80 Burn (any degree) involving 80-89% of body surface with third degree burn of less than 10% or unspecified amount
948.81 Burn (any degree) involving 80-89% of body surface with third degree burn of 10-19%
948.82 Burn (any degree) involving 80-89% of body surface with third degree burn of 20-29%
948.83 Burn (any degree) involving 80-89% of body surface with third degree burn of 30-39%
948.84 Burn (any degree) involving 80-89% of body surface with third degree burn of 40-49%
948.85 Burn (any degree) involving 80-89% of body surface with third degree burn of 50-59%
948.86 Burn (any degree) involving 80-89% of body surface with third degree burn of 60-69%
948.87 Burn (any degree) involving 80-89% of body surface with third degree burn of 70-79%
948.88 Burn (any degree) involving 80-89% of body surface with third degree burn of 80-89%
959.01 Head injury, unspecified
959.09 Injury of face and neck, other and unspecified
996.52 Mechanical complication due to other tissue graft, not elsewhere classified
998.59 Other postoperative infection — (Use additional code to identify infection)
998.83 Non-healing surgical wound
V10.02 Personal history of malignant neoplasm of other and unspecified parts of oral cavity and pharynx
V51 Aftercare involving the use of plastic surgery
V84.09 Genetic susceptibility to other malignant neoplasm

ICD-9-CM Procedural

16.63 Revision of enucleation socket with graft
21.89 Other repair and plastic operations on nose
27.55 Full-thickness skin graft to lip and mouth
86.63 Full-thickness skin graft to other sites

15342–15343

15342 Application of bilaminate skin substitute/neodermis; 25 sq. cm
15343 each additional 25 sq. cm (List separately in addition to code for primary procedure)

ICD-9-CM Diagnostic

941.30 Full-thickness skin loss due to burn (third degree nos) of unspecified site of face and head
941.31 Full-thickness skin loss due to burn (third degree nos) of ear (any part)
941.32 Full-thickness skin loss due to burn (third degree nos) of eye (with other parts of face, head, and neck)
941.33 Full-thickness skin loss due to burn (third degree nos) of lip(s)
941.34 Full-thickness skin loss due to burn (third degree nos) of chin
941.35 Full-thickness skin loss due to burn (third degree nos) of nose (septum)
941.36 Full-thickness skin loss due to burn (third degree nos) of scalp (any part)
941.37 Full-thickness skin loss due to burn (third degree nos) of forehead and cheek
941.38 Full-thickness skin loss due to burn (third degree nos) of neck
941.39 Full-thickness skin loss due to burn (third degree nos) of multiple sites (except with eye) of face, head, and neck
941.40 Deep necrosis of underlying tissues due to burn (deep third degree) of unspecified site of face and head, without mention of loss of a body part
941.41 Deep necrosis of underlying tissues due to burn (deep third degree) of ear (any part), without mention of loss of a body part
941.42 Deep necrosis of underlying tissues due to burn (deep third degree) of eye (with other parts of face, head, and neck), without mention of loss of a body part
941.43 Deep necrosis of underlying tissues due to burn (deep third degree) of lip(s), without mention of loss of a body part
941.44 Deep necrosis of underlying tissues due to burn (deep third degree) of chin, without mention of loss of a body part
941.45 Deep necrosis of underlying tissues due to burn (deep third degree) of nose (septum), without mention of loss of a body part
941.46 Deep necrosis of underlying tissues due to burn (deep third degree) of scalp (any part), without mention of loss of a body part
941.47 Deep necrosis of underlying tissues due to burn (deep third degree) of forehead and cheek, without mention of loss of a body part
941.48 Deep necrosis of underlying tissues due to burn (deep third degree) of neck, without mention of loss of a body part
941.49 Deep necrosis of underlying tissues due to burn (deep third degree) of multiple sites (except with eye) of face, head, and neck, without mention of loss of a body part
941.50 Deep necrosis of underlying tissues due to burn (deep third degree) of face and head, unspecified site, with loss of a body part
941.51 Deep necrosis of underlying tissues due to burn (deep third degree) of ear (any part), with loss of a body part
941.52 Deep necrosis of underlying tissues due to burn (deep third degree) of eye (with other parts of face, head, and neck), with loss of a body part
941.53 Deep necrosis of underlying tissues due to burn (deep third degree) of lip(s), with loss of a body part
941.54 Deep necrosis of underlying tissues due to burn (deep third degree) of chin, with loss of a body part
941.55 Deep necrosis of underlying tissues due to burn (deep third degree) of nose (septum), with loss of a body part
941.56 Deep necrosis of underlying tissues due to burn (deep third degree) of scalp (any part), with loss of a body part
941.57 Deep necrosis of underlying tissues due to burn (deep third degree) of forehead and cheek, with loss of a body part
941.58 Deep necrosis of underlying tissues due to burn (deep third degree) of neck, with loss of a body part
941.59 Deep necrosis of underlying tissues due to burn (deep third degree) of multiple sites (except eye) of face, head, and neck, with loss of a body part
942.30 Full-thickness skin loss due to burn (third degree nos) of unspecified site of trunk
942.31 Full-thickness skin loss due to burn (third degree nos) of breast
942.32 Full-thickness skin loss due to burn (third degree nos) of chest wall, excluding breast and nipple
942.33 Full-thickness skin loss due to burn (third degree nos) of abdominal wall
942.34 Full-thickness skin loss due to burn (third degree nos) of back (any part)
942.35 Full-thickness skin loss due to burn (third degree nos) of genitalia
942.39 Full-thickness skin loss due to burn (third degree nos) of other and multiple sites of trunk
942.40 Deep necrosis of underlying tissues due to burn (deep third degree) of trunk, unspecified site, without mention of loss of a body part
942.41 Deep necrosis of underlying tissues due to burn (deep third degree) of breast, without mention of loss of a body part

942.42 Deep necrosis of underlying tissues due to burn (deep third degree) of chest wall, excluding breast and nipple, without mention of loss of a body part
942.43 Deep necrosis of underlying tissues due to burn (deep third degree) of abdominal wall, without mention of loss of a body part
942.44 Deep necrosis of underlying tissues due to burn (deep third degree) of back (any part), without mention of loss of a body part
942.45 Deep necrosis of underlying tissues due to burn (deep third degree) of genitalia, without mention of loss of a body part
942.49 Deep necrosis of underlying tissues due to burn (deep third degree) of other and multiple sites of trunk, without mention of loss of a body part
942.50 Deep necrosis of underlying tissues due to burn (deep third degree) of unspecified site of trunk, with loss of a body part
942.51 Deep necrosis of underlying tissues due to burn (deep third degree) of breast, with loss of a body part
942.52 Deep necrosis of underlying tissues due to burn (deep third degree) of chest wall, excluding breast and nipple, with loss of a body part
942.53 Deep necrosis of underlying tissues due to burn (deep third degree) of abdominal wall with loss of a body part
942.54 Deep necrosis of underlying tissues due to burn (deep third degree) of back (any part), with loss of a body part
942.55 Deep necrosis of underlying tissues due to burn (deep third degree) of genitalia, with loss of a body part
942.59 Deep necrosis of underlying tissues due to burn (deep third degree) of other and multiple sites of trunk, with loss of a body part
943.30 Full-thickness skin loss due to burn (third degree nos) of unspecified site of upper limb
943.31 Full-thickness skin loss due to burn (third degree nos) of forearm
943.32 Full-thickness skin loss due to burn (third degree nos) of elbow
943.33 Full-thickness skin loss due to burn (third degree nos) of upper arm
943.34 Full-thickness skin loss due to burn (third degree nos) of axilla
943.35 Full-thickness skin loss due to burn (third degree nos) of shoulder
943.36 Full-thickness skin loss due to burn (third degree nos) of scapular region
943.39 Full-thickness skin loss due to burn (third degree nos) of multiple sites of upper limb, except wrist and hand
943.40 Deep necrosis of underlying tissues due to burn (deep third degree) of unspecified site of upper limb, without mention of loss of a body part
943.41 Deep necrosis of underlying tissues due to burn (deep third degree) of forearm, without mention of loss of a body part
943.42 Deep necrosis of underlying tissues due to burn (deep third degree) of elbow, without mention of loss of a body part
943.43 Deep necrosis of underlying tissues due to burn (deep third degree) of upper arm, without mention of loss of a body part
943.44 Deep necrosis of underlying tissues due to burn (deep third degree) of axilla, without mention of loss of a body part
943.45 Deep necrosis of underlying tissues due to burn (deep third degree) of shoulder, without mention of loss of a body part
943.46 Deep necrosis of underlying tissues due to burn (deep third degree) of scapular region, without mention of loss of a body part
943.49 Deep necrosis of underlying tissues due to burn (deep third degree) of multiple sites of upper limb, except wrist and hand, without mention of loss of a body part
943.50 Deep necrosis of underlying tissues due to burn (deep third degree) of unspecified site of upper limb, with loss of a body part
943.51 Deep necrosis of underlying tissues due to burn (deep third degree) of forearm, with loss of a body part
943.52 Deep necrosis of underlying tissues due to burn (deep third degree) of elbow, with loss of a body part
943.53 Deep necrosis of underlying tissues due to burn (deep third degree) of upper arm, with loss of upper a body part
943.54 Deep necrosis of underlying tissues due to burn (deep third degree) of axilla, with loss of a body part
943.55 Deep necrosis of underlying tissues due to burn (deep third degree) of shoulder, with loss of a body part
943.56 Deep necrosis of underlying tissues due to burn (deep third degree) of scapular region, with loss of a body part
943.59 Deep necrosis of underlying tissues due to burn (deep third degree) of multiple sites of upper limb, except wrist and hand, with loss of a body part
944.30 Full-thickness skin loss due to burn (third degree nos) of unspecified site of hand
944.31 Full-thickness skin loss due to burn (third degree nos) of single digit [finger (nail)] other than thumb
944.32 Full-thickness skin loss due to burn (third degree nos) of thumb (nail)
944.33 Full-thickness skin loss due to burn (third degree nos) of two or more digits of hand, not including thumb
944.34 Full-thickness skin loss due to burn (third degree nos) of two or more digits of hand including thumb
944.35 Full-thickness skin loss due to burn (third degree nos) of palm of hand
944.36 Full-thickness skin loss due to burn (third degree nos) of back of hand
944.37 Full-thickness skin loss due to burn (third degree nos) of wrist
944.38 Full-thickness skin loss due to burn (third degree nos) of multiple sites of wrist(s) and hand(s)
944.40 Deep necrosis of underlying tissues due to burn (deep third degree) of unspecified site of hand, without mention of a body part
944.41 Deep necrosis of underlying tissues due to burn (deep third degree) of single digit [finger (nail)] other than thumb, without mention of a body part
944.42 Deep necrosis of underlying tissues due to burn (deep third degree) of thumb (nail), without mention of loss of a body part
944.43 Deep necrosis of underlying tissues due to burn (deep third degree) of two or more digits of hand, not including thumb, without mention of a body part
944.44 Deep necrosis of underlying tissues due to burn (deep third degree) of two or more digits of hand including thumb, without mention of a body part
944.45 Deep necrosis of underlying tissues due to burn (deep third degree) of palm of hand, without mention of loss of a body part
944.46 Deep necrosis of underlying tissues due to burn (deep third degree) of back of hand, without mention of loss of back of a body part
944.47 Deep necrosis of underlying tissues due to burn (deep third degree) of wrist, without mention of loss of a body part
944.48 Deep necrosis of underlying tissues due to burn (deep third degree) of multiple sites of wrist(s) and hand(s), without mention of loss of a body part
944.50 Deep necrosis of underlying tissues due to burn (deep third degree) of unspecified site of hand, with loss of a body part
944.51 Deep necrosis of underlying tissues due to burn (deep third degree) of single digit (finger (nail)) other than thumb, with loss of a body part
944.52 Deep necrosis of underlying tissues due to burn (deep third degree) of thumb (nail), with loss of a body part
944.53 Deep necrosis of underlying tissues due to burn (deep third degree) of two or more digits of hand, not including thumb, with loss of a body part
944.54 Deep necrosis of underlying tissues due to burn (deep third degree) of two or more digits of hand including thumb, with loss of a body part
944.55 Deep necrosis of underlying tissues due to burn (deep third degree) of palm of hand, with loss of a body part
944.56 Deep necrosis of underlying tissues due to burn (deep third degree) of back of hand, with loss of a body part
944.57 Deep necrosis of underlying tissues due to burn (deep third degree) of wrist, with loss of a body part
944.58 Deep necrosis of underlying tissues due to burn (deep third degree) of multiple sites of wrist(s) and hand(s), with loss of a body part
945.30 Full-thickness skin loss due to burn (third degree nos) of unspecified site of lower limb
945.31 Full-thickness skin loss due to burn (third degree nos) of toe(s) (nail)
945.32 Full-thickness skin loss due to burn (third degree nos) of foot
945.33 Full-thickness skin loss due to burn (third degree nos) of ankle
945.34 Full-thickness skin loss due to burn (third degree nos) of lower leg
945.35 Full-thickness skin loss due to burn (third degree nos) of knee
945.36 Full-thickness skin loss due to burn (third degree nos) of thigh (any part)
945.39 Full-thickness skin loss due to burn (third degree nos) of multiple sites of lower limb(s)
945.40 Deep necrosis of underlying tissues due to burn (deep third degree) of unspecified site of lower limb (leg), without mention of loss of a body part
945.41 Deep necrosis of underlying tissues due to burn (deep third degree) of toe(s) (nail), without mention of loss of a body part
945.42 Deep necrosis of underlying tissues due to burn (deep third degree) of foot, without mention of loss of a body part
945.43 Deep necrosis of underlying tissues due to burn (deep third degree) of ankle, without mention of loss of a body part
945.44 Deep necrosis of underlying tissues due to burn (deep third degree) of lower leg, without mention of loss of a body part
945.45 Deep necrosis of underlying tissues due to burn (deep third degree) of knee, without mention of loss of a body part
945.46 Deep necrosis of underlying tissues due to burn (deep third degree) of thigh (any part), without mention of loss of a body part
945.49 Deep necrosis of underlying tissues due to burn (deep third degree) of multiple sites of lower limb(s), without mention of loss of a body part
945.50 Deep necrosis of underlying tissues due to burn (deep third degree) of unspecified site lower limb (leg), with loss of a body part
945.51 Deep necrosis of underlying tissues due to burn (deep third degree) of toe(s) (nail), with loss of a body part
945.52 Deep necrosis of underlying tissues due to burn (deep third degree) of foot, with loss of a body part
945.53 Deep necrosis of underlying tissues due to burn (deep third degree) of ankle, with loss of a body part

Unspecified code
♀ Female diagnosis
Manifestation code
♂ Male diagnosis

945.54 Deep necrosis of underlying tissues due to burn (deep third degree) of lower leg, with loss of a body part
945.55 Deep necrosis of underlying tissues due to burn (deep third degree) of knee, with loss of a body part
945.56 Deep necrosis of underlying tissues due to burn (deep third degree) of thigh (any part), with loss of a body part
945.59 Deep necrosis of underlying tissues due to burn (deep third degree) of multiple sites of lower limb(s), with loss of a body part
946.3 Full-thickness skin loss due to burn (third degree nos) of multiple specified sites
946.4 Deep necrosis of underlying tissues due to burn (deep third degree) of multiple specified sites, without mention of loss of a body part
946.5 Deep necrosis of underlying tissues due to burn (deep third degree) of multiple specified sites, with loss of a body part
948.00 Burn (any degree) involving less than 10% of body surface with third degree burn of less than 10% or unspecified amount
948.10 Burn (any degree) involving 10-19% of body surface with third degree burn of less than 10% or unspecified amount
948.11 Burn (any degree) involving 10-19% of body surface with third degree burn of 10-19%
948.20 Burn (any degree) involving 20-29% of body surface with third degree burn of less than 10% or unspecified amount
948.21 Burn (any degree) involving 20-29% of body surface with third degree burn of 10-19%
948.22 Burn (any degree) involving 20-29% of body surface with third degree burn of 20-29%
948.30 Burn (any degree) involving 30-39% of body surface with third degree burn of less than 10% or unspecified amount
948.31 Burn (any degree) involving 30-39% of body surface with third degree burn of 10-19%
948.32 Burn (any degree) involving 30-39% of body surface with third degree burn of 20-29%
948.33 Burn (any degree) involving 30-39% of body surface with third degree burn of 30-39%
948.40 Burn (any degree) involving 40-49% of body surface with third degree burn of less than 10% or unspecified amount
948.41 Burn (any degree) involving 40-49% of body surface with third degree burn of 10-19%
948.42 Burn (any degree) involving 40-49% of body surface with third degree burn of 20-29%
948.43 Burn (any degree) involving 40-49% of body surface with third degree burn of 30-39%
948.44 Burn (any degree) involving 40-49% of body surface with third degree burn of 40-49%
948.50 Burn (any degree) involving 50-59% of body surface with third degree burn of less than 10% or unspecified amount
948.51 Burn (any degree) involving 50-59% of body surface with third degree burn of 10-19%
948.52 Burn (any degree) involving 50-59% of body surface with third degree burn of 20-29%
948.53 Burn (any degree) involving 50-59% of body surface with third degree burn of 30-39%
948.54 Burn (any degree) involving 50-59% of body surface with third degree burn of 40-49%
948.55 Burn (any degree) involving 50-59% of body surface with third degree burn of 50-59%
948.60 Burn (any degree) involving 60-69% of body surface with third degree burn of less than 10% or unspecified amount
948.61 Burn (any degree) involving 60-69% of body surface with third degree burn of 10-19%
948.62 Burn (any degree) involving 60-69% of body surface with third degree burn of 20-29%
948.63 Burn (any degree) involving 60-69% of body surface with third degree burn of 30-39%
948.64 Burn (any degree) involving 60-69% of body surface with third degree burn of 40-49%
948.65 Burn (any degree) involving 60-69% of body surface with third degree burn of 50-59%
948.70 Burn (any degree) involving 70-79% of body surface with third degree burn of less than 10% or unspecified amount
948.71 Burn (any degree) involving 70-79% of body surface with third degree burn of 10-19%
948.72 Burn (any degree) involving 70-79% of body surface with third degree burn of 20-29%
948.73 Burn (any degree) involving 70-79% of body surface with third degree burn of 30-39%
948.74 Burn (any degree) involving 70-79% of body surface with third degree burn of 40-49%
948.75 Burn (any degree) involving 70-79% of body surface with third degree burn of 50-59%
948.76 Burn (any degree) involving 70-79% of body surface with third degree burn of 60-69%
948.77 Burn (any degree) involving 70-79% of body surface with third degree burn of 70-79%
948.80 Burn (any degree) involving 80-89% of body surface with third degree burn of less than 10% or unspecified amount
948.81 Burn (any degree) involving 80-89% of body surface with third degree burn of 10-19%
948.82 Burn (any degree) involving 80-89% of body surface with third degree burn of 20-29%
948.83 Burn (any degree) involving 80-89% of body surface with third degree burn of 30-39%
948.84 Burn (any degree) involving 80-89% of body surface with third degree burn of 40-49%
948.85 Burn (any degree) involving 80-89% of body surface with third degree burn of 50-59%
948.86 Burn (any degree) involving 80-89% of body surface with third degree burn of 60-69%
948.87 Burn (any degree) involving 80-89% of body surface with third degree burn of 70-79%
948.88 Burn (any degree) involving 80-89% of body surface with third degree burn of 80-89%
948.90 Burn (any degree) involving 90% or more of body surface with third degree burn of less than 10% or unspecified amount
948.91 Burn (any degree) involving 90% or more of body surface with third degree burn of 10-19%
948.92 Burn (any degree) involving 90% or more of body surface with third degree burn of 20-29%
948.93 Burn (any degree) involving 90% or more of body surface with third degree burn of 30-39%
948.94 Burn (any degree) involving 90% or more of body surface with third degree burn of 40-49%
948.95 Burn (any degree) involving 90% or more of body surface with third degree burn of 50-59%
948.96 Burn (any degree) involving 90% or more of body surface with third degree burn of 60-69%
948.97 Burn (any degree) involving 90% or more of body surface with third degree burn of 70-79%
948.98 Burn (any degree) involving 90% or more of body surface with third degree burn of 80-89%
948.99 Burn (any degree) involving 90% or more of body surface with third degree burn of 90% or more of body surface
949.3 Full-thickness skin loss due to burn (third degree nos), unspecified site
949.4 Deep necrosis of underlying tissue due to burn (deep third degree), unspecified site without mention of loss of body part
949.5 Deep necrosis of underlying tissues due to burn (deep third degree, unspecified site with loss of body part

ICD-9-CM Procedural

86.67 Dermal regenerative graft

HCPCS Level II Supplies & Services

J7340 Dermal and epidermal tissue of human origin, with or without bioengineered or processed elements, with metabolically active elements, per sq. centimeter
J7342 Dermal tissue, of human origin, with or without other bioengineered or processed elements, with metabolically active elements, per sq. centimeter
J7343 Dermal and epidermal, tissue of non-human origin, with or without other bioengineered or processed elements, without metabolically active elements, per square centimeter
J7344 Dermal tissue, of human origin, with or without other bioengineered or processed elements, without metabolically active elements, per square centimeter
J7350 Dermal tissue of human origin, injectable, with or without other bioengineered or processed elements, but without metabolized active elements, per 10 mg

15350–15351

15350 Application of allograft, skin; 100 sq. cm or less
15351 each additional 100 sq. cm (List separately in addition to code for primary procedure)

ICD-9-CM Diagnostic

172.0 Malignant melanoma of skin of lip

172.1 Malignant melanoma of skin of eyelid, including canthus
172.2 Malignant melanoma of skin of ear and external auditory canal
172.3 Malignant melanoma of skin of other and unspecified parts of face
172.4 Malignant melanoma of skin of scalp and neck
172.5 Malignant melanoma of skin of trunk, except scrotum
172.6 Malignant melanoma of skin of upper limb, including shoulder
172.7 Malignant melanoma of skin of lower limb, including hip
172.8 Malignant melanoma of other specified sites of skin
173.0 Other malignant neoplasm of skin of lip
173.1 Other malignant neoplasm of skin of eyelid, including canthus
173.2 Other malignant neoplasm of skin of ear and external auditory canal
173.3 Other malignant neoplasm of skin of other and unspecified parts of face ▽
173.4 Other malignant neoplasm of scalp and skin of neck
173.5 Other malignant neoplasm of skin of trunk, except scrotum
173.6 Other malignant neoplasm of skin of upper limb, including shoulder
173.7 Other malignant neoplasm of skin of lower limb, including hip
173.8 Other malignant neoplasm of other specified sites of skin
174.0 Malignant neoplasm of nipple and areola of female breast ♀
175.0 Malignant neoplasm of nipple and areola of male breast ♂
198.2 Secondary malignant neoplasm of skin
210.0 Benign neoplasm of lip
232.0 Carcinoma in situ of skin of lip
232.1 Carcinoma in situ of eyelid, including canthus
232.2 Carcinoma in situ of skin of ear and external auditory canal
232.3 Carcinoma in situ of skin of other and unspecified parts of face ▽
232.4 Carcinoma in situ of scalp and skin of neck
232.5 Carcinoma in situ of skin of trunk, except scrotum
232.6 Carcinoma in situ of skin of upper limb, including shoulder
232.7 Carcinoma in situ of skin of lower limb, including hip
232.8 Carcinoma in situ of other specified sites of skin
235.1 Neoplasm of uncertain behavior of lip, oral cavity, and pharynx
238.2 Neoplasm of uncertain behavior of skin
239.0 Neoplasm of unspecified nature of digestive system
239.2 Neoplasms of unspecified nature of bone, soft tissue, and skin
250.70 Diabetes with peripheral circulatory disorders, type II or unspecified type, not stated as uncontrolled — (Use additional code to identify manifestation: 443.81, 785.4)
250.71 Diabetes with peripheral circulatory disorders, type I [juvenile type], not stated as uncontrolled — (Use additional code to identify manifestation: 443.81, 785.4)
250.72 Diabetes with peripheral circulatory disorders, type II or unspecified type, uncontrolled — (Use additional code to identify manifestation: 443.81, 785.4)
250.73 Diabetes with peripheral circulatory disorders, type I [juvenile type], uncontrolled — (Use additional code to identify manifestation: 443.81, 785.4)
443.81 Peripheral angiopathy in diseases classified elsewhere — (Code first underlying disease, 250.7) ☒
454.0 Varicose veins of lower extremities with ulcer
454.2 Varicose veins of lower extremities with ulcer and inflammation
454.8 Varicose veins of the lower extremities with other complications
459.11 Postphlebitic syndrome with ulcer
459.13 Postphlebitic syndrome with ulcer and inflammation
459.19 Postphlebitic syndrome with other complication
459.31 Chronic venous hypertension with ulcer
459.33 Chronic venous hypertension with ulcer and inflammation
459.39 Chronic venous hypertension with other complication
681.00 Unspecified cellulitis and abscess of finger — (Use additional code to identify organism) ▽
681.01 Felon — (Use additional code to identify organism)
681.02 Onychia and paronychia of finger — (Use additional code to identify organism)
681.10 Unspecified cellulitis and abscess of toe — (Use additional code to identify organism) ▽
681.11 Onychia and paronychia of toe — (Use additional code to identify organism)
682.0 Cellulitis and abscess of face — (Use additional code to identify organism)
682.1 Cellulitis and abscess of neck — (Use additional code to identify organism)
682.2 Cellulitis and abscess of trunk — (Use additional code to identify organism)
682.3 Cellulitis and abscess of upper arm and forearm — (Use additional code to identify organism)
682.4 Cellulitis and abscess of hand, except fingers and thumb — (Use additional code to identify organism)
682.5 Cellulitis and abscess of buttock — (Use additional code to identify organism)
682.6 Cellulitis and abscess of leg, except foot — (Use additional code to identify organism)
682.7 Cellulitis and abscess of foot, except toes — (Use additional code to identify organism)
682.8 Cellulitis and abscess of other specified site — (Use additional code to identify organism)
707.00 Decubitus ulcer, unspecified site
707.01 Decubitus ulcer, elbow
707.02 Decubitus ulcer, upper back
707.03 Decubitus ulcer, lower back
707.04 Decubitus ulcer, hip
707.05 Decubitus ulcer, buttock
707.06 Decubitus ulcer, ankle
707.07 Decubitus ulcer, heel
707.09 Decubitus ulcer, other site
707.10 Ulcer of lower limb, unspecified ▽
707.11 Ulcer of thigh
707.12 Ulcer of calf
707.13 Ulcer of ankle
707.14 Ulcer of heel and midfoot
707.15 Ulcer of other part of foot
707.19 Ulcer of other part of lower limb
707.8 Chronic ulcer of other specified site
707.9 Chronic ulcer of unspecified site ▽
709.2 Scar condition and fibrosis of skin
709.9 Unspecified disorder of skin and subcutaneous tissue ▽
728.86 Necrotizing fasciitis — (Use additional code to identify infectious organism, 041.00-041.89, 785.4, if applicable)
754.0 Congenital musculoskeletal deformities of skull, face, and jaw
756.70 Unspecified congenital anomaly of abdominal wall ▽
756.71 Prune belly syndrome
756.79 Other congenital anomalies of abdominal wall
785.4 Gangrene — (Code first any associated underlying condition:250.7, 443.0)
880.00 Open wound of shoulder region, without mention of complication — (Use additional code to identify infection)
880.01 Open wound of scapular region, without mention of complication — (Use additional code to identify infection)
880.02 Open wound of axillary region, without mention of complication — (Use additional code to identify infection)
880.03 Open wound of upper arm, without mention of complication — (Use additional code to identify infection)
880.09 Open wound of multiple sites of shoulder and upper arm, without mention of complication — (Use additional code to identify infection)
880.10 Open wound of shoulder region, complicated — (Use additional code to identify infection)
880.11 Open wound of scapular region, complicated — (Use additional code to identify infection)
880.12 Open wound of axillary region, complicated — (Use additional code to identify infection)
880.13 Open wound of upper arm, complicated — (Use additional code to identify infection)
880.19 Open wound of multiple sites of shoulder and upper arm, complicated — (Use additional code to identify infection)
880.20 Open wound of shoulder region, with tendon involvement — (Use additional code to identify infection)
880.21 Open wound of scapular region, with tendon involvement — (Use additional code to identify infection)
880.22 Open wound of axillary region, with tendon involvement — (Use additional code to identify infection)
880.23 Open wound of upper arm, with tendon involvement — (Use additional code to identify infection)
880.29 Open wound of multiple sites of shoulder and upper arm, with tendon involvement — (Use additional code to identify infection)
881.00 Open wound of forearm, without mention of complication — (Use additional code to identify infection)
881.01 Open wound of elbow, without mention of complication — (Use additional code to identify infection)
881.02 Open wound of wrist, without mention of complication — (Use additional code to identify infection)
881.10 Open wound of forearm, complicated — (Use additional code to identify infection)
881.11 Open wound of elbow, complicated — (Use additional code to identify infection)
881.12 Open wound of wrist, complicated — (Use additional code to identify infection)
881.20 Open wound of forearm, with tendon involvement — (Use additional code to identify infection)
881.21 Open wound of elbow, with tendon involvement — (Use additional code to identify infection)
881.22 Open wound of wrist, with tendon involvement — (Use additional code to identify infection)

▽ Unspecified code ☒ Manifestation code
♀ Female diagnosis ♂ Male diagnosis

882.0 Open wound of hand except finger(s) alone, without mention of complication — (Use additional code to identify infection)
882.1 Open wound of hand except finger(s) alone, complicated — (Use additional code to identify infection)
882.2 Open wound of hand except finger(s) alone, with tendon involvement — (Use additional code to identify infection)
883.0 Open wound of finger(s), without mention of complication — (Use additional code to identify infection)
883.1 Open wound of finger(s), complicated — (Use additional code to identify infection)
883.2 Open wound of finger(s), with tendon involvement — (Use additional code to identify infection)
884.0 Multiple and unspecified open wound of upper limb, without mention of complication — (Use additional code to identify infection)
884.1 Multiple and unspecified open wound of upper limb, complicated — (Use additional code to identify infection)
884.2 Multiple and unspecified open wound of upper limb, with tendon involvement — (Use additional code to identify infection)
885.0 Traumatic amputation of thumb (complete) (partial), without mention of complication — (Use additional code to identify infection)
885.1 Traumatic amputation of thumb (complete) (partial), complicated — (Use additional code to identify infection)
886.0 Traumatic amputation of other finger(s) (complete) (partial), without mention of complication — (Use additional code to identify infection)
886.1 Traumatic amputation of other finger(s) (complete) (partial), complicated — (Use additional code to identify infection)
887.2 Traumatic amputation of arm and hand (complete) (partial), unilateral, at or above elbow, without mention of complication — (Use additional code to identify infection)
887.3 Traumatic amputation of arm and hand (complete) (partial), unilateral, at or above elbow, complicated — (Use additional code to identify infection)
887.4 Traumatic amputation of arm and hand (complete) (partial), unilateral, level not specified, without mention of complication — (Use additional code to identify infection) ▽
887.5 Traumatic amputation of arm and hand (complete) (partial), unilateral, level not specified, complicated — (Use additional code to identify infection) ▽
887.6 Traumatic amputation of arm and hand (complete) (partial), bilateral (any level), without mention of complication — (Use additional code to identify infection)
887.7 Traumatic amputation of arm and hand (complete) (partial), bilateral (any level), complicated — (Use additional code to identify infection)
890.0 Open wound of hip and thigh, without mention of complication — (Use additional code to identify infection)
890.1 Open wound of hip and thigh, complicated — (Use additional code to identify infection)
890.2 Open wound of hip and thigh, with tendon involvement — (Use additional code to identify infection)
891.0 Open wound of knee, leg (except thigh), and ankle, without mention of complication — (Use additional code to identify infection)
891.1 Open wound of knee, leg (except thigh), and ankle, complicated — (Use additional code to identify infection)
891.2 Open wound of knee, leg (except thigh), and ankle, with tendon involvement — (Use additional code to identify infection)
892.0 Open wound of foot except toe(s) alone, without mention of complication — (Use additional code to identify infection)
892.1 Open wound of foot except toe(s) alone, complicated — (Use additional code to identify infection)
892.2 Open wound of foot except toe(s) alone, with tendon involvement — (Use additional code to identify infection)
893.0 Open wound of toe(s), without mention of complication — (Use additional code to identify infection)
893.1 Open wound of toe(s), complicated — (Use additional code to identify infection)
893.2 Open wound of toe(s), with tendon involvement — (Use additional code to identify infection)
894.0 Multiple and unspecified open wound of lower limb, without mention of complication — (Use additional code to identify infection)
894.1 Multiple and unspecified open wound of lower limb, complicated — (Use additional code to identify infection)
894.2 Multiple and unspecified open wound of lower limb, with tendon involvement — (Use additional code to identify infection)
895.0 Traumatic amputation of toe(s) (complete) (partial), without mention of complication — (Use additional code to identify infection)
895.1 Traumatic amputation of toe(s) (complete) (partial), complicated — (Use additional code to identify infection)
896.0 Traumatic amputation of foot (complete) (partial), unilateral, without mention of complication — (Use additional code to identify infection)
896.1 Traumatic amputation of foot (complete) (partial), unilateral, complicated — (Use additional code to identify infection)
896.2 Traumatic amputation of foot (complete) (partial), bilateral, without mention of complication — (Use additional code to identify infection)
896.3 Traumatic amputation of foot (complete) (partial), bilateral, complicated — (Use additional code to identify infection)
897.0 Traumatic amputation of leg(s) (complete) (partial), unilateral, below knee, without mention of complication — (Use additional code to identify infection)
897.1 Traumatic amputation of leg(s) (complete) (partial), unilateral, below knee, complicated — (Use additional code to identify infection)
897.2 Traumatic amputation of leg(s) (complete) (partial), unilateral, at or above knee, without mention of complication — (Use additional code to identify infection)
897.3 Traumatic amputation of leg(s) (complete) (partial), unilateral, at or above knee, complicated — (Use additional code to identify infection)
897.4 Traumatic amputation of leg(s) (complete) (partial), unilateral, level not specified, without mention of complication — (Use additional code to identify infection) ▽
897.5 Traumatic amputation of leg(s) (complete) (partial), unilateral, level not specified, complicated — (Use additional code to identify infection) ▽
897.6 Traumatic amputation of leg(s) (complete) (partial), bilateral (any level), without mention of complication — (Use additional code to identify infection)
897.7 Traumatic amputation of leg(s) (complete) (partial), bilateral (any level), complicated — (Use additional code to identify infection)
906.0 Late effect of open wound of head, neck, and trunk
906.1 Late effect of open wound of extremities without mention of tendon injury
906.5 Late effect of burn of eye, face, head, and neck
906.6 Late effect of burn of wrist and hand
906.7 Late effect of burn of other extremities
906.8 Late effect of burns of other specified sites
906.9 Late effect of burn of unspecified site ▽
941.30 Full-thickness skin loss due to burn (third degree nos) of unspecified site of face and head ▽
941.31 Full-thickness skin loss due to burn (third degree nos) of ear (any part)
941.32 Full-thickness skin loss due to burn (third degree nos) of eye (with other parts of face, head, and neck)
941.33 Full-thickness skin loss due to burn (third degree nos) of lip(s)
941.34 Full-thickness skin loss due to burn (third degree nos) of chin
941.35 Full-thickness skin loss due to burn (third degree nos) of nose (septum)
941.36 Full-thickness skin loss due to burn (third degree nos) of scalp (any part)
941.37 Full-thickness skin loss due to burn (third degree nos) of forehead and cheek
941.38 Full-thickness skin loss due to burn (third degree nos) of neck
941.39 Full-thickness skin loss due to burn (third degree nos) of multiple sites (except with eye) of face, head, and neck
941.40 Deep necrosis of underlying tissues due to burn (deep third degree) of unspecified site of face and head, without mention of loss of a body part ▽
941.41 Deep necrosis of underlying tissues due to burn (deep third degree) of ear (any part), without mention of loss of a body part
941.42 Deep necrosis of underlying tissues due to burn (deep third degree) of eye (with other parts of face, head, and neck), without mention of loss of a body part
941.43 Deep necrosis of underlying tissues due to burn (deep third degree) of lip(s), without mention of loss of a body part
941.44 Deep necrosis of underlying tissues due to burn (deep third degree) of chin, without mention of loss of a body part
941.45 Deep necrosis of underlying tissues due to burn (deep third degree) of nose (septum), without mention of loss of a body part
941.46 Deep necrosis of underlying tissues due to burn (deep third degree) of scalp (any part), without mention of loss of a body part
941.47 Deep necrosis of underlying tissues due to burn (deep third degree) of forehead and cheek, without mention of loss of a body part
941.48 Deep necrosis of underlying tissues due to burn (deep third degree) of neck, without mention of loss of a body part
941.49 Deep necrosis of underlying tissues due to burn (deep third degree) of multiple sites (except with eye) of face, head, and neck, without mention of loss of a body part
941.50 Deep necrosis of underlying tissues due to burn (deep third degree) of face and head, unspecified site, with loss of a body part ▽
941.51 Deep necrosis of underlying tissues due to burn (deep third degree) of ear (any part), with loss of a body part
941.52 Deep necrosis of underlying tissues due to burn (deep third degree) of eye (with other parts of face, head, and neck), with loss of a body part
941.53 Deep necrosis of underlying tissues due to burn (deep third degree) of lip(s), with loss of a body part

▽ Unspecified code ♀ Female diagnosis ☒ Manifestation code ♂ Male diagnosis

941.54 Deep necrosis of underlying tissues due to burn (deep third degree) of chin, with loss of a body part
941.55 Deep necrosis of underlying tissues due to burn (deep third degree) of nose (septum), with loss of a body part
941.56 Deep necrosis of underlying tissues due to burn (deep third degree) of scalp (any part), with loss of a body part
941.57 Deep necrosis of underlying tissues due to burn (deep third degree) of forehead and cheek, with loss of a body part
941.58 Deep necrosis of underlying tissues due to burn (deep third degree) of neck, with loss of a body part
941.59 Deep necrosis of underlying tissues due to burn (deep third degree) of multiple sites (except eye) of face, head, and neck, with loss of a body part
942.30 Full-thickness skin loss due to burn (third degree nos) of unspecified site of trunk
942.31 Full-thickness skin loss due to burn (third degree nos) of breast
942.32 Full-thickness skin loss due to burn (third degree nos) of chest wall, excluding breast and nipple
942.33 Full-thickness skin loss due to burn (third degree nos) of abdominal wall
942.34 Full-thickness skin loss due to burn (third degree nos) of back (any part)
942.35 Full-thickness skin loss due to burn (third degree nos) of genitalia
942.39 Full-thickness skin loss due to burn (third degree nos) of other and multiple sites of trunk
942.40 Deep necrosis of underlying tissues due to burn (deep third degree) of trunk, unspecified site, without mention of loss of a body part
942.41 Deep necrosis of underlying tissues due to burn (deep third degree) of breast, without mention of loss of a body part
942.42 Deep necrosis of underlying tissues due to burn (deep third degree) of chest wall, excluding breast and nipple, without mention of loss of a body part
942.43 Deep necrosis of underlying tissues due to burn (deep third degree) of abdominal wall, without mention of loss of a body part
942.44 Deep necrosis of underlying tissues due to burn (deep third degree) of back (any part), without mention of loss of a body part
942.45 Deep necrosis of underlying tissues due to burn (deep third degree) of genitalia, without mention of loss of a body part
942.49 Deep necrosis of underlying tissues due to burn (deep third degree) of other and multiple sites of trunk, without mention of loss of a body part
942.50 Deep necrosis of underlying tissues due to burn (deep third degree) of unspecified site of trunk, with loss of a body part
942.51 Deep necrosis of underlying tissues due to burn (deep third degree) of breast, with loss of a body part
942.52 Deep necrosis of underlying tissues due to burn (deep third degree) of chest wall, excluding breast and nipple, with loss of a body part
942.53 Deep necrosis of underlying tissues due to burn (deep third degree) of abdominal wall with loss of a body part
942.54 Deep necrosis of underlying tissues due to burn (deep third degree) of back (any part), with loss of a body part
942.55 Deep necrosis of underlying tissues due to burn (deep third degree) of genitalia, with loss of a body part
942.59 Deep necrosis of underlying tissues due to burn (deep third degree) of other and multiple sites of trunk, with loss of a body part
943.30 Full-thickness skin loss due to burn (third degree nos) of unspecified site of upper limb
943.31 Full-thickness skin loss due to burn (third degree nos) of forearm
943.32 Full-thickness skin loss due to burn (third degree nos) of elbow
943.33 Full-thickness skin loss due to burn (third degree nos) of upper arm
943.34 Full-thickness skin loss due to burn (third degree nos) of axilla
943.35 Full-thickness skin loss due to burn (third degree nos) of shoulder
943.36 Full-thickness skin loss due to burn (third degree nos) of scapular region
943.39 Full-thickness skin loss due to burn (third degree nos) of multiple sites of upper limb, except wrist and hand
943.40 Deep necrosis of underlying tissues due to burn (deep third degree) of unspecified site of upper limb, without mention of loss of a body part
943.41 Deep necrosis of underlying tissues due to burn (deep third degree) of forearm, without mention of loss of a body part
943.42 Deep necrosis of underlying tissues due to burn (deep third degree) of elbow, without mention of loss of a body part
943.43 Deep necrosis of underlying tissues due to burn (deep third degree) of upper arm, without mention of loss of a body part
943.44 Deep necrosis of underlying tissues due to burn (deep third degree) of axilla, without mention of loss of a body part
943.45 Deep necrosis of underlying tissues due to burn (deep third degree) of shoulder, without mention of loss of a body part
943.46 Deep necrosis of underlying tissues due to burn (deep third degree) of scapular region, without mention of loss of a body part
943.49 Deep necrosis of underlying tissues due to burn (deep third degree) of multiple sites of upper limb, except wrist and hand, without mention of loss of a body part
943.50 Deep necrosis of underlying tissues due to burn (deep third degree) of unspecified site of upper limb, with loss of a body part
943.51 Deep necrosis of underlying tissues due to burn (deep third degree) of forearm, with loss of a body part
943.52 Deep necrosis of underlying tissues due to burn (deep third degree) of elbow, with loss of a body part
943.53 Deep necrosis of underlying tissues due to burn (deep third degree) of upper arm, with loss of upper a body part
943.54 Deep necrosis of underlying tissues due to burn (deep third degree) of axilla, with loss of a body part
943.55 Deep necrosis of underlying tissues due to burn (deep third degree) of shoulder, with loss of a body part
943.56 Deep necrosis of underlying tissues due to burn (deep third degree) of scapular region, with loss of a body part
943.59 Deep necrosis of underlying tissues due to burn (deep third degree) of multiple sites of upper limb, except wrist and hand, with loss of a body part
944.30 Full-thickness skin loss due to burn (third degree nos) of unspecified site of hand
944.31 Full-thickness skin loss due to burn (third degree nos) of single digit [finger (nail)] other than thumb
944.32 Full-thickness skin loss due to burn (third degree nos) of thumb (nail)
944.33 Full-thickness skin loss due to burn (third degree nos) of two or more digits of hand, not including thumb
944.34 Full-thickness skin loss due to burn (third degree nos) of two or more digits of hand including thumb
944.35 Full-thickness skin loss due to burn (third degree nos) of palm of hand
944.36 Full-thickness skin loss due to burn (third degree nos) of back of hand
944.37 Full-thickness skin loss due to burn (third degree nos) of wrist
944.38 Full-thickness skin loss due to burn (third degree nos) of multiple sites of wrist(s) and hand(s)
944.40 Deep necrosis of underlying tissues due to burn (deep third degree) of unspecified site of hand, without mention of a body part
944.41 Deep necrosis of underlying tissues due to burn (deep third degree) of single digit [finger (nail)] other than thumb, without mention of a body part
944.42 Deep necrosis of underlying tissues due to burn (deep third degree) of thumb (nail), without mention of loss of a body part
944.43 Deep necrosis of underlying tissues due to burn (deep third degree) of two or more digits of hand, not including thumb, without mention of a body part
944.44 Deep necrosis of underlying tissues due to burn (deep third degree) of two or more digits of hand including thumb, without mention of a body part
944.45 Deep necrosis of underlying tissues due to burn (deep third degree) of palm of hand, without mention of loss of a body part
944.46 Deep necrosis of underlying tissues due to burn (deep third degree) of back of hand, without mention of loss of back of a body part
944.47 Deep necrosis of underlying tissues due to burn (deep third degree) of wrist, without mention of loss of a body part
944.48 Deep necrosis of underlying tissues due to burn (deep third degree) of multiple sites of wrist(s) and hand(s), without mention of loss of a body part
944.50 Deep necrosis of underlying tissues due to burn (deep third degree) of unspecified site of hand, with loss of a body part
944.51 Deep necrosis of underlying tissues due to burn (deep third degree) of single digit (finger (nail)) other than thumb, with loss of a body part
944.52 Deep necrosis of underlying tissues due to burn (deep third degree) of thumb (nail), with loss of a body part
944.53 Deep necrosis of underlying tissues due to burn (deep third degree) of two or more digits of hand, not including thumb, with loss of a body part
944.54 Deep necrosis of underlying tissues due to burn (deep third degree) of two or more digits of hand including thumb, with loss of a body part
944.55 Deep necrosis of underlying tissues due to burn (deep third degree) of palm of hand, with loss of a body part
944.56 Deep necrosis of underlying tissues due to burn (deep third degree) of back of hand, with loss of a body part
944.57 Deep necrosis of underlying tissues due to burn (deep third degree) of wrist, with loss of a body part
944.58 Deep necrosis of underlying tissues due to burn (deep third degree) of multiple sites of wrist(s) and hand(s), with loss of a body part
945.30 Full-thickness skin loss due to burn (third degree nos) of unspecified site of lower limb
945.31 Full-thickness skin loss due to burn (third degree nos) of toe(s) (nail)
945.32 Full-thickness skin loss due to burn (third degree nos) of foot
945.33 Full-thickness skin loss due to burn (third degree nos) of ankle
945.34 Full-thickness skin loss due to burn (third degree nos) of lower leg
945.35 Full-thickness skin loss due to burn (third degree nos) of knee

945.36 Full-thickness skin loss due to burn (third degree nos) of thigh (any part)
945.39 Full-thickness skin loss due to burn (third degree nos) of multiple sites of lower limb(s)
945.40 Deep necrosis of underlying tissues due to burn (deep third degree) of unspecified site of lower limb (leg), without mention of loss of a body part
945.41 Deep necrosis of underlying tissues due to burn (deep third degree) of toe(s) (nail), without mention of loss of a body part
945.42 Deep necrosis of underlying tissues due to burn (deep third degree) of foot, without mention of loss of a body part
945.43 Deep necrosis of underlying tissues due to burn (deep third degree) of ankle, without mention of loss of a body part
945.44 Deep necrosis of underlying tissues due to burn (deep third degree) of lower leg, without mention of loss of a body part
945.45 Deep necrosis of underlying tissues due to burn (deep third degree) of knee, without mention of loss of a body part
945.46 Deep necrosis of underlying tissues due to burn (deep third degree) of thigh (any part), without mention of loss of a body part
945.49 Deep necrosis of underlying tissues due to burn (deep third degree) of multiple sites of lower limb(s), without mention of loss of a body part
945.50 Deep necrosis of underlying tissues due to burn (deep third degree) of unspecified site lower limb (leg), with loss of a body part
945.51 Deep necrosis of underlying tissues due to burn (deep third degree) of toe(s) (nail), with loss of a body part
945.52 Deep necrosis of underlying tissues due to burn (deep third degree) of foot, with loss of a body part
945.53 Deep necrosis of underlying tissues due to burn (deep third degree) of ankle, with loss of a body part
945.54 Deep necrosis of underlying tissues due to burn (deep third degree) of lower leg, with loss of a body part
945.55 Deep necrosis of underlying tissues due to burn (deep third degree) of knee, with loss of a body part
945.56 Deep necrosis of underlying tissues due to burn (deep third degree) of thigh (any part), with loss of a body part
945.59 Deep necrosis of underlying tissues due to burn (deep third degree) of multiple sites of lower limb(s), with loss of a body part
946.3 Full-thickness skin loss due to burn (third degree nos) of multiple specified sites
946.4 Deep necrosis of underlying tissues due to burn (deep third degree) of multiple specified sites, without mention of loss of a body part
946.5 Deep necrosis of underlying tissues due to burn (deep third degree) of multiple specified sites, with loss of a body part
948.00 Burn (any degree) involving less than 10% of body surface with third degree burn of less than 10% or unspecified amount
948.10 Burn (any degree) involving 10-19% of body surface with third degree burn of less than 10% or unspecified amount
948.11 Burn (any degree) involving 10-19% of body surface with third degree burn of 10-19%
948.20 Burn (any degree) involving 20-29% of body surface with third degree burn of less than 10% or unspecified amount
948.21 Burn (any degree) involving 20-29% of body surface with third degree burn of 10-19%
948.22 Burn (any degree) involving 20-29% of body surface with third degree burn of 20-29%
948.30 Burn (any degree) involving 30-39% of body surface with third degree burn of less than 10% or unspecified amount
948.31 Burn (any degree) involving 30-39% of body surface with third degree burn of 10-19%
948.32 Burn (any degree) involving 30-39% of body surface with third degree burn of 20-29%
948.33 Burn (any degree) involving 30-39% of body surface with third degree burn of 30-39%
948.40 Burn (any degree) involving 40-49% of body surface with third degree burn of less than 10% or unspecified amount
948.41 Burn (any degree) involving 40-49% of body surface with third degree burn of 10-19%
948.42 Burn (any degree) involving 40-49% of body surface with third degree burn of 20-29%
948.43 Burn (any degree) involving 40-49% of body surface with third degree burn of 30-39%
948.44 Burn (any degree) involving 40-49% of body surface with third degree burn of 40-49%
948.50 Burn (any degree) involving 50-59% of body surface with third degree burn of less than 10% or unspecified amount
948.51 Burn (any degree) involving 50-59% of body surface with third degree burn of 10-19%
948.52 Burn (any degree) involving 50-59% of body surface with third degree burn of 20-29%
948.53 Burn (any degree) involving 50-59% of body surface with third degree burn of 30-39%
948.54 Burn (any degree) involving 50-59% of body surface with third degree burn of 40-49%
948.55 Burn (any degree) involving 50-59% of body surface with third degree burn of 50-59%
948.60 Burn (any degree) involving 60-69% of body surface with third degree burn of less than 10% or unspecified amount
948.61 Burn (any degree) involving 60-69% of body surface with third degree burn of 10-19%
948.62 Burn (any degree) involving 60-69% of body surface with third degree burn of 20-29%
948.63 Burn (any degree) involving 60-69% of body surface with third degree burn of 30-39%
948.64 Burn (any degree) involving 60-69% of body surface with third degree burn of 40-49%
948.65 Burn (any degree) involving 60-69% of body surface with third degree burn of 50-59%
948.66 Burn (any degree) involving 60-69% of body surface with third degree burn of 60-69%
948.70 Burn (any degree) involving 70-79% of body surface with third degree burn of less than 10% or unspecified amount
948.71 Burn (any degree) involving 70-79% of body surface with third degree burn of 10-19%
948.72 Burn (any degree) involving 70-79% of body surface with third degree burn of 20-29%
948.73 Burn (any degree) involving 70-79% of body surface with third degree burn of 30-39%
948.74 Burn (any degree) involving 70-79% of body surface with third degree burn of 40-49%
948.75 Burn (any degree) involving 70-79% of body surface with third degree burn of 50-59%
948.76 Burn (any degree) involving 70-79% of body surface with third degree burn of 60-69%
948.77 Burn (any degree) involving 70-79% of body surface with third degree burn of 70-79%
948.80 Burn (any degree) involving 80-89% of body surface with third degree burn of less than 10% or unspecified amount
948.81 Burn (any degree) involving 80-89% of body surface with third degree burn of 10-19%
948.82 Burn (any degree) involving 80-89% of body surface with third degree burn of 20-29%
948.83 Burn (any degree) involving 80-89% of body surface with third degree burn of 30-39%
948.84 Burn (any degree) involving 80-89% of body surface with third degree burn of 40-49%
948.85 Burn (any degree) involving 80-89% of body surface with third degree burn of 50-59%
948.86 Burn (any degree) involving 80-89% of body surface with third degree burn of 60-69%
948.87 Burn (any degree) involving 80-89% of body surface with third degree burn of 70-79%
948.88 Burn (any degree) involving 80-89% of body surface with third degree burn of 80-89%
948.90 Burn (any degree) involving 90% or more of body surface with third degree burn of less than 10% or unspecified amount
948.91 Burn (any degree) involving 90% or more of body surface with third degree burn of 10-19%
948.92 Burn (any degree) involving 90% or more of body surface with third degree burn of 20-29%
948.93 Burn (any degree) involving 90% or more of body surface with third degree burn of 30-39%
948.94 Burn (any degree) involving 90% or more of body surface with third degree burn of 40-49%
948.95 Burn (any degree) involving 90% or more of body surface with third degree burn of 50-59%
948.96 Burn (any degree) involving 90% or more of body surface with third degree burn of 60-69%
948.97 Burn (any degree) involving 90% or more of body surface with third degree burn of 70-79%
948.98 Burn (any degree) involving 90% or more of body surface with third degree burn of 80-89%
948.99 Burn (any degree) involving 90% or more of body surface with third degree burn of 90% or more of body surface

Unspecified code
♀ Female diagnosis
Manifestation code
♂ Male diagnosis

991.0 Frostbite of face
991.1 Frostbite of hand
991.2 Frostbite of foot
991.3 Frostbite of other and unspecified sites
996.52 Mechanical complication due to other tissue graft, not elsewhere classified
998.59 Other postoperative infection — (Use additional code to identify infection)
998.83 Non-healing surgical wound

ICD-9-CM Procedural

86.66 Homograft to skin

HCPCS Level II Supplies & Services

A4305 Disposable drug delivery system, flow rate of 50 ml or greater per hour
A4306 Disposable drug delivery system, flow rate of 5 ml or less per hour
A4550 Surgical trays
J7340 Dermal and epidermal tissue of human origin, with or without bioengineered or processed elements, with metabolically active elements, per sq. centimeter
J7342 Dermal tissue, of human origin, with or without other bioengineered or processed elements, with metabolically active elements, per sq. centimeter
J7343 Dermal and epidermal, tissue of non-human origin, with or without other bioengineered or processed elements, without metabolically active elements, per square centimeter
J7344 Dermal tissue, of human origin, with or without other bioengineered or processed elements, without metabolically active elements, per square centimeter
J7350 Dermal tissue of human origin, injectable, with or without other bioengineered or processed elements, but without metabolized active elements, per 10 mg

15400–15401

15400 Application of xenograft, skin; 100 sq. cm or less
15401 each additional 100 sq. cm (List separately in addition to code for primary procedure)

ICD-9-CM Diagnostic

172.0 Malignant melanoma of skin of lip
172.1 Malignant melanoma of skin of eyelid, including canthus
172.2 Malignant melanoma of skin of ear and external auditory canal
172.3 Malignant melanoma of skin of other and unspecified parts of face
172.4 Malignant melanoma of skin of scalp and neck
172.5 Malignant melanoma of skin of trunk, except scrotum
172.6 Malignant melanoma of skin of upper limb, including shoulder
172.7 Malignant melanoma of skin of lower limb, including hip
172.8 Malignant melanoma of other specified sites of skin
173.0 Other malignant neoplasm of skin of lip
173.1 Other malignant neoplasm of skin of eyelid, including canthus
173.2 Other malignant neoplasm of skin of ear and external auditory canal
173.3 Other malignant neoplasm of skin of other and unspecified parts of face ▽
173.4 Other malignant neoplasm of scalp and skin of neck
173.5 Other malignant neoplasm of skin of trunk, except scrotum
173.6 Other malignant neoplasm of skin of upper limb, including shoulder
173.7 Other malignant neoplasm of skin of lower limb, including hip
173.8 Other malignant neoplasm of other specified sites of skin
174.0 Malignant neoplasm of nipple and areola of female breast ♀
175.0 Malignant neoplasm of nipple and areola of male breast ♂
198.2 Secondary malignant neoplasm of skin
210.0 Benign neoplasm of lip
232.0 Carcinoma in situ of skin of lip
232.1 Carcinoma in situ of eyelid, including canthus
232.2 Carcinoma in situ of skin of ear and external auditory canal
232.3 Carcinoma in situ of skin of other and unspecified parts of face ▽
232.4 Carcinoma in situ of scalp and skin of neck
232.5 Carcinoma in situ of skin of trunk, except scrotum
232.6 Carcinoma in situ of skin of upper limb, including shoulder
232.7 Carcinoma in situ of skin of lower limb, including hip
232.8 Carcinoma in situ of other specified sites of skin
235.1 Neoplasm of uncertain behavior of lip, oral cavity, and pharynx
238.2 Neoplasm of uncertain behavior of skin
239.2 Neoplasms of unspecified nature of bone, soft tissue, and skin
250.70 Diabetes with peripheral circulatory disorders, type II or unspecified type, not stated as uncontrolled — (Use additional code to identify manifestation: 443.81, 785.4)
250.71 Diabetes with peripheral circulatory disorders, type I [juvenile type], not stated as uncontrolled — (Use additional code to identify manifestation: 443.81, 785.4)
250.72 Diabetes with peripheral circulatory disorders, type II or unspecified type, uncontrolled — (Use additional code to identify manifestation: 443.81, 785.4)
250.73 Diabetes with peripheral circulatory disorders, type I [juvenile type], uncontrolled — (Use additional code to identify manifestation: 443.81, 785.4)
443.81 Peripheral angiopathy in diseases classified elsewhere — (Code first underlying disease, 250.7) ☒
454.0 Varicose veins of lower extremities with ulcer
454.2 Varicose veins of lower extremities with ulcer and inflammation
454.8 Varicose veins of the lower extremities with other complications
459.11 Postphlebitic syndrome with ulcer
459.13 Postphlebitic syndrome with ulcer and inflammation
459.19 Postphlebitic syndrome with other complication
459.31 Chronic venous hypertension with ulcer
459.33 Chronic venous hypertension with ulcer and inflammation
459.39 Chronic venous hypertension with other complication
681.00 Unspecified cellulitis and abscess of finger — (Use additional code to identify organism) ▽
681.01 Felon — (Use additional code to identify organism)
681.02 Onychia and paronychia of finger — (Use additional code to identify organism)
681.10 Unspecified cellulitis and abscess of toe — (Use additional code to identify organism) ▽
681.11 Onychia and paronychia of toe — (Use additional code to identify organism)
682.0 Cellulitis and abscess of face — (Use additional code to identify organism)
682.1 Cellulitis and abscess of neck — (Use additional code to identify organism)
682.2 Cellulitis and abscess of trunk — (Use additional code to identify organism)
682.3 Cellulitis and abscess of upper arm and forearm — (Use additional code to identify organism)
682.4 Cellulitis and abscess of hand, except fingers and thumb — (Use additional code to identify organism)
682.5 Cellulitis and abscess of buttock — (Use additional code to identify organism)
682.6 Cellulitis and abscess of leg, except foot — (Use additional code to identify organism)
682.7 Cellulitis and abscess of foot, except toes — (Use additional code to identify organism)
682.8 Cellulitis and abscess of other specified site — (Use additional code to identify organism)
707.00 Decubitus ulcer, unspecified site
707.01 Decubitus ulcer, elbow
707.02 Decubitus ulcer, upper back
707.03 Decubitus ulcer, lower back
707.04 Decubitus ulcer, hip
707.05 Decubitus ulcer, buttock
707.06 Decubitus ulcer, ankle
707.07 Decubitus ulcer, heel
707.09 Decubitus ulcer, other site
707.10 Ulcer of lower limb, unspecified ▽
707.11 Ulcer of thigh
707.12 Ulcer of calf
707.13 Ulcer of ankle
707.14 Ulcer of heel and midfoot
707.15 Ulcer of other part of foot
707.19 Ulcer of other part of lower limb
707.8 Chronic ulcer of other specified site
707.9 Chronic ulcer of unspecified site ▽
709.2 Scar condition and fibrosis of skin
709.9 Unspecified disorder of skin and subcutaneous tissue ▽
728.86 Necrotizing fasciitis — (Use additional code to identify infectious organism, 041.00-041.89, 785.4, if applicable)
754.0 Congenital musculoskeletal deformities of skull, face, and jaw
756.70 Unspecified congenital anomaly of abdominal wall ▽
756.71 Prune belly syndrome
756.79 Other congenital anomalies of abdominal wall
785.4 Gangrene — (Code first any associated underlying condition:250.7, 443.0)
880.00 Open wound of shoulder region, without mention of complication — (Use additional code to identify infection)
880.01 Open wound of scapular region, without mention of complication — (Use additional code to identify infection)
880.02 Open wound of axillary region, without mention of complication — (Use additional code to identify infection)
880.03 Open wound of upper arm, without mention of complication — (Use additional code to identify infection)
880.09 Open wound of multiple sites of shoulder and upper arm, without mention of complication — (Use additional code to identify infection)
880.10 Open wound of shoulder region, complicated — (Use additional code to identify infection)
880.11 Open wound of scapular region, complicated — (Use additional code to identify infection)

▽ Unspecified code
♀ Female diagnosis
☒ Manifestation code
♂ Male diagnosis

880.12 Open wound of axillary region, complicated — (Use additional code to identify infection)
880.13 Open wound of upper arm, complicated — (Use additional code to identify infection)
880.19 Open wound of multiple sites of shoulder and upper arm, complicated — (Use additional code to identify infection)
880.20 Open wound of shoulder region, with tendon involvement — (Use additional code to identify infection)
880.21 Open wound of scapular region, with tendon involvement — (Use additional code to identify infection)
880.22 Open wound of axillary region, with tendon involvement — (Use additional code to identify infection)
880.23 Open wound of upper arm, with tendon involvement — (Use additional code to identify infection)
880.29 Open wound of multiple sites of shoulder and upper arm, with tendon involvement — (Use additional code to identify infection)
881.00 Open wound of forearm, without mention of complication — (Use additional code to identify infection)
881.01 Open wound of elbow, without mention of complication — (Use additional code to identify infection)
881.02 Open wound of wrist, without mention of complication — (Use additional code to identify infection)
881.10 Open wound of forearm, complicated — (Use additional code to identify infection)
881.11 Open wound of elbow, complicated — (Use additional code to identify infection)
881.12 Open wound of wrist, complicated — (Use additional code to identify infection)
881.20 Open wound of forearm, with tendon involvement — (Use additional code to identify infection)
881.21 Open wound of elbow, with tendon involvement — (Use additional code to identify infection)
881.22 Open wound of wrist, with tendon involvement — (Use additional code to identify infection)
882.0 Open wound of hand except finger(s) alone, without mention of complication — (Use additional code to identify infection)
882.1 Open wound of hand except finger(s) alone, complicated — (Use additional code to identify infection)
882.2 Open wound of hand except finger(s) alone, with tendon involvement — (Use additional code to identify infection)
883.0 Open wound of finger(s), without mention of complication — (Use additional code to identify infection)
883.1 Open wound of finger(s), complicated — (Use additional code to identify infection)
883.2 Open wound of finger(s), with tendon involvement — (Use additional code to identify infection)
884.0 Multiple and unspecified open wound of upper limb, without mention of complication — (Use additional code to identify infection)
884.1 Multiple and unspecified open wound of upper limb, complicated — (Use additional code to identify infection)
884.2 Multiple and unspecified open wound of upper limb, with tendon involvement — (Use additional code to identify infection)
885.0 Traumatic amputation of thumb (complete) (partial), without mention of complication — (Use additional code to identify infection)
885.1 Traumatic amputation of thumb (complete) (partial), complicated — (Use additional code to identify infection)
886.0 Traumatic amputation of other finger(s) (complete) (partial), without mention of complication — (Use additional code to identify infection)
886.1 Traumatic amputation of other finger(s) (complete) (partial), complicated — (Use additional code to identify infection)
887.2 Traumatic amputation of arm and hand (complete) (partial), unilateral, at or above elbow, without mention of complication — (Use additional code to identify infection)
887.3 Traumatic amputation of arm and hand (complete) (partial), unilateral, at or above elbow, complicated — (Use additional code to identify infection)
887.4 Traumatic amputation of arm and hand (complete) (partial), unilateral, level not specified, without mention of complication — (Use additional code to identify infection) ▽
887.5 Traumatic amputation of arm and hand (complete) (partial), unilateral, level not specified, complicated — (Use additional code to identify infection) ▽
887.6 Traumatic amputation of arm and hand (complete) (partial), bilateral (any level), without mention of complication — (Use additional code to identify infection)
887.7 Traumatic amputation of arm and hand (complete) (partial), bilateral (any level), complicated — (Use additional code to identify infection)
890.0 Open wound of hip and thigh, without mention of complication — (Use additional code to identify infection)
890.1 Open wound of hip and thigh, complicated — (Use additional code to identify infection)
890.2 Open wound of hip and thigh, with tendon involvement — (Use additional code to identify infection)
891.0 Open wound of knee, leg (except thigh), and ankle, without mention of complication — (Use additional code to identify infection)
891.1 Open wound of knee, leg (except thigh), and ankle, complicated — (Use additional code to identify infection)
891.2 Open wound of knee, leg (except thigh), and ankle, with tendon involvement — (Use additional code to identify infection)
892.0 Open wound of foot except toe(s) alone, without mention of complication — (Use additional code to identify infection)
892.1 Open wound of foot except toe(s) alone, complicated — (Use additional code to identify infection)
892.2 Open wound of foot except toe(s) alone, with tendon involvement — (Use additional code to identify infection)
893.0 Open wound of toe(s), without mention of complication — (Use additional code to identify infection)
893.1 Open wound of toe(s), complicated — (Use additional code to identify infection)
893.2 Open wound of toe(s), with tendon involvement — (Use additional code to identify infection)
894.0 Multiple and unspecified open wound of lower limb, without mention of complication — (Use additional code to identify infection)
894.1 Multiple and unspecified open wound of lower limb, complicated — (Use additional code to identify infection)
894.2 Multiple and unspecified open wound of lower limb, with tendon involvement — (Use additional code to identify infection)
895.0 Traumatic amputation of toe(s) (complete) (partial), without mention of complication — (Use additional code to identify infection)
895.1 Traumatic amputation of toe(s) (complete) (partial), complicated — (Use additional code to identify infection)
896.0 Traumatic amputation of foot (complete) (partial), unilateral, without mention of complication — (Use additional code to identify infection)
896.1 Traumatic amputation of foot (complete) (partial), unilateral, complicated — (Use additional code to identify infection)
896.2 Traumatic amputation of foot (complete) (partial), bilateral, without mention of complication — (Use additional code to identify infection)
896.3 Traumatic amputation of foot (complete) (partial), bilateral, complicated — (Use additional code to identify infection)
897.0 Traumatic amputation of leg(s) (complete) (partial), unilateral, below knee, without mention of complication — (Use additional code to identify infection)
897.1 Traumatic amputation of leg(s) (complete) (partial), unilateral, below knee, complicated — (Use additional code to identify infection)
897.2 Traumatic amputation of leg(s) (complete) (partial), unilateral, at or above knee, without mention of complication — (Use additional code to identify infection)
897.3 Traumatic amputation of leg(s) (complete) (partial), unilateral, at or above knee, complicated — (Use additional code to identify infection)
897.4 Traumatic amputation of leg(s) (complete) (partial), unilateral, level not specified, without mention of complication — (Use additional code to identify infection) ▽
897.5 Traumatic amputation of leg(s) (complete) (partial), unilateral, level not specified, complicated — (Use additional code to identify infection) ▽
897.6 Traumatic amputation of leg(s) (complete) (partial), bilateral (any level), without mention of complication — (Use additional code to identify infection)
897.7 Traumatic amputation of leg(s) (complete) (partial), bilateral (any level), complicated — (Use additional code to identify infection)
906.0 Late effect of open wound of head, neck, and trunk
906.1 Late effect of open wound of extremities without mention of tendon injury
906.5 Late effect of burn of eye, face, head, and neck
906.6 Late effect of burn of wrist and hand
906.7 Late effect of burn of other extremities
906.8 Late effect of burns of other specified sites
906.9 Late effect of burn of unspecified site ▽
941.30 Full-thickness skin loss due to burn (third degree nos) of unspecified site of face and head ▽
941.31 Full-thickness skin loss due to burn (third degree nos) of ear (any part)
941.32 Full-thickness skin loss due to burn (third degree nos) of eye (with other parts of face, head, and neck)
941.33 Full-thickness skin loss due to burn (third degree nos) of lip(s)
941.34 Full-thickness skin loss due to burn (third degree nos) of chin
941.35 Full-thickness skin loss due to burn (third degree nos) of nose (septum)
941.36 Full-thickness skin loss due to burn (third degree nos) of scalp (any part)

▽ Unspecified code
♀ Female diagnosis
☒ Manifestation code
♂ Male diagnosis

941.37 Full-thickness skin loss due to burn (third degree nos) of forehead and cheek
941.38 Full-thickness skin loss due to burn (third degree nos) of neck
941.39 Full-thickness skin loss due to burn (third degree nos) of multiple sites (except with eye) of face, head, and neck
941.40 Deep necrosis of underlying tissues due to burn (deep third degree) of unspecified site of face and head, without mention of loss of a body part ▽
941.41 Deep necrosis of underlying tissues due to burn (deep third degree) of ear (any part), without mention of loss of a body part
941.42 Deep necrosis of underlying tissues due to burn (deep third degree) of eye (with other parts of face, head, and neck), without mention of loss of a body part
941.43 Deep necrosis of underlying tissues due to burn (deep third degree) of lip(s), without mention of loss of a body part
941.44 Deep necrosis of underlying tissues due to burn (deep third degree) of chin, without mention of loss of a body part
941.45 Deep necrosis of underlying tissues due to burn (deep third degree) of nose (septum), without mention of loss of a body part
941.46 Deep necrosis of underlying tissues due to burn (deep third degree) of scalp (any part), without mention of loss of a body part
941.47 Deep necrosis of underlying tissues due to burn (deep third degree) of forehead and cheek, without mention of loss of a body part
941.48 Deep necrosis of underlying tissues due to burn (deep third degree) of neck, without mention of loss of a body part
941.49 Deep necrosis of underlying tissues due to burn (deep third degree) of multiple sites (except with eye) of face, head, and neck, without mention of loss of a body part
941.50 Deep necrosis of underlying tissues due to burn (deep third degree) of face and head, unspecified site, with loss of a body part ▽
941.51 Deep necrosis of underlying tissues due to burn (deep third degree) of ear (any part), with loss of a body part
941.52 Deep necrosis of underlying tissues due to burn (deep third degree) of eye (with other parts of face, head, and neck), with loss of a body part
941.53 Deep necrosis of underlying tissues due to burn (deep third degree) of lip(s), with loss of a body part
941.54 Deep necrosis of underlying tissues due to burn (deep third degree) of chin, with loss of a body part
941.55 Deep necrosis of underlying tissues due to burn (deep third degree) of nose (septum), with loss of a body part
941.56 Deep necrosis of underlying tissues due to burn (deep third degree) of scalp (any part), with loss of a body part
941.57 Deep necrosis of underlying tissues due to burn (deep third degree) of forehead and cheek, with loss of a body part
941.58 Deep necrosis of underlying tissues due to burn (deep third degree) of neck, with loss of a body part
941.59 Deep necrosis of underlying tissues due to burn (deep third degree) of multiple sites (except eye) of face, head, and neck, with loss of a body part
942.30 Full-thickness skin loss due to burn (third degree nos) of unspecified site of trunk ▽
942.31 Full-thickness skin loss due to burn (third degree nos) of breast
942.32 Full-thickness skin loss due to burn (third degree nos) of chest wall, excluding breast and nipple
942.33 Full-thickness skin loss due to burn (third degree nos) of abdominal wall
942.34 Full-thickness skin loss due to burn (third degree nos) of back (any part)
942.35 Full-thickness skin loss due to burn (third degree nos) of genitalia
942.39 Full-thickness skin loss due to burn (third degree nos) of other and multiple sites of trunk
942.40 Deep necrosis of underlying tissues due to burn (deep third degree) of trunk, unspecified site, without mention of loss of a body part ▽
942.41 Deep necrosis of underlying tissues due to burn (deep third degree) of breast, without mention of loss of a body part
942.42 Deep necrosis of underlying tissues due to burn (deep third degree) of chest wall, excluding breast and nipple, without mention of loss of a body part
942.43 Deep necrosis of underlying tissues due to burn (deep third degree) of abdominal wall, without mention of loss of a body part
942.44 Deep necrosis of underlying tissues due to burn (deep third degree) of back (any part), without mention of loss of a body part
942.45 Deep necrosis of underlying tissues due to burn (deep third degree) of genitalia, without mention of loss of a body part
942.49 Deep necrosis of underlying tissues due to burn (deep third degree) of other and multiple sites of trunk, without mention of loss of a body part
942.50 Deep necrosis of underlying tissues due to burn (deep third degree) of unspecified site of trunk, with loss of a body part ▽
942.51 Deep necrosis of underlying tissues due to burn (deep third degree) of breast, with loss of a body part
942.52 Deep necrosis of underlying tissues due to burn (deep third degree) of chest wall, excluding breast and nipple, with loss of a body part
942.53 Deep necrosis of underlying tissues due to burn (deep third degree) of abdominal wall with loss of a body part
942.54 Deep necrosis of underlying tissues due to burn (deep third degree) of back (any part), with loss of a body part
942.55 Deep necrosis of underlying tissues due to burn (deep third degree) of genitalia, with loss of a body part
942.59 Deep necrosis of underlying tissues due to burn (deep third degree) of other and multiple sites of trunk, with loss of a body part
943.30 Full-thickness skin loss due to burn (third degree nos) of unspecified site of upper limb ▽
943.31 Full-thickness skin loss due to burn (third degree nos) of forearm
943.32 Full-thickness skin loss due to burn (third degree nos) of elbow
943.33 Full-thickness skin loss due to burn (third degree nos) of upper arm
943.34 Full-thickness skin loss due to burn (third degree nos) of axilla
943.35 Full-thickness skin loss due to burn (third degree nos) of shoulder
943.36 Full-thickness skin loss due to burn (third degree nos) of scapular region
943.39 Full-thickness skin loss due to burn (third degree nos) of multiple sites of upper limb, except wrist and hand
943.40 Deep necrosis of underlying tissues due to burn (deep third degree) of unspecified site of upper limb, without mention of loss of a body part ▽
943.41 Deep necrosis of underlying tissues due to burn (deep third degree) of forearm, without mention of loss of a body part
943.42 Deep necrosis of underlying tissues due to burn (deep third degree) of elbow, without mention of loss of a body part
943.43 Deep necrosis of underlying tissues due to burn (deep third degree) of upper arm, without mention of loss of a body part
943.44 Deep necrosis of underlying tissues due to burn (deep third degree) of axilla, without mention of loss of a body part
943.45 Deep necrosis of underlying tissues due to burn (deep third degree) of shoulder, without mention of loss of a body part
943.46 Deep necrosis of underlying tissues due to burn (deep third degree) of scapular region, without mention of loss of a body part
943.49 Deep necrosis of underlying tissues due to burn (deep third degree) of multiple sites of upper limb, except wrist and hand, without mention of loss of a body part
943.50 Deep necrosis of underlying tissues due to burn (deep third degree) of unspecified site of upper limb, with loss of a body part ▽
943.51 Deep necrosis of underlying tissues due to burn (deep third degree) of forearm, with loss of a body part
943.52 Deep necrosis of underlying tissues due to burn (deep third degree) of elbow, with loss of a body part
943.53 Deep necrosis of underlying tissues due to burn (deep third degree) of upper arm, with loss of upper a body part
943.54 Deep necrosis of underlying tissues due to burn (deep third degree) of axilla, with loss of a body part
943.55 Deep necrosis of underlying tissues due to burn (deep third degree) of shoulder, with loss of a body part
943.56 Deep necrosis of underlying tissues due to burn (deep third degree) of scapular region, with loss of a body part
943.59 Deep necrosis of underlying tissues due to burn (deep third degree) of multiple sites of upper limb, except wrist and hand, with loss of a body part
944.30 Full-thickness skin loss due to burn (third degree nos) of unspecified site of hand ▽
944.31 Full-thickness skin loss due to burn (third degree nos) of single digit [finger (nail)] other than thumb
944.32 Full-thickness skin loss due to burn (third degree nos) of thumb (nail)
944.33 Full-thickness skin loss due to burn (third degree nos) of two or more digits of hand, not including thumb
944.34 Full-thickness skin loss due to burn (third degree nos) of two or more digits of hand including thumb
944.35 Full-thickness skin loss due to burn (third degree nos) of palm of hand
944.36 Full-thickness skin loss due to burn (third degree nos) of back of hand
944.37 Full-thickness skin loss due to burn (third degree nos) of wrist
944.38 Full-thickness skin loss due to burn (third degree nos) of multiple sites of wrist(s) and hand(s)
944.40 Deep necrosis of underlying tissues due to burn (deep third degree) of unspecified site of hand, without mention of a body part ▽
944.41 Deep necrosis of underlying tissues due to burn (deep third degree) of single digit [finger (nail)] other than thumb, without mention of a body part
944.42 Deep necrosis of underlying tissues due to burn (deep third degree) of thumb (nail), without mention of loss of a body part
944.43 Deep necrosis of underlying tissues due to burn (deep third degree) of two or more digits of hand, not including thumb, without mention of a body part
944.44 Deep necrosis of underlying tissues due to burn (deep third degree) of two or more digits of hand including thumb, without mention of a body part

▽ Unspecified code
♀ Female diagnosis
☒ Manifestation code
♂ Male diagnosis

944.45 Deep necrosis of underlying tissues due to burn (deep third degree) of palm of hand, without mention of loss of a body part
944.46 Deep necrosis of underlying tissues due to burn (deep third degree) of back of hand, without mention of loss of back of a body part
944.47 Deep necrosis of underlying tissues due to burn (deep third degree) of wrist, without mention of loss of a body part
944.48 Deep necrosis of underlying tissues due to burn (deep third degree) of multiple sites of wrist(s) and hand(s), without mention of loss of a body part
944.50 Deep necrosis of underlying tissues due to burn (deep third degree) of unspecified site of hand, with loss of a body part ▽
944.51 Deep necrosis of underlying tissues due to burn (deep third degree) of single digit (finger (nail)) other than thumb, with loss of a body part
944.52 Deep necrosis of underlying tissues due to burn (deep third degree) of thumb (nail), with loss of a body part
944.53 Deep necrosis of underlying tissues due to burn (deep third degree) of two or more digits of hand, not including thumb, with loss of a body part
944.54 Deep necrosis of underlying tissues due to burn (deep third degree) of two or more digits of hand including thumb, with loss of a body part
944.55 Deep necrosis of underlying tissues due to burn (deep third degree) of palm of hand, with loss of a body part
944.56 Deep necrosis of underlying tissues due to burn (deep third degree) of back of hand, with loss of a body part
944.57 Deep necrosis of underlying tissues due to burn (deep third degree) of wrist, with loss of a body part
944.58 Deep necrosis of underlying tissues due to burn (deep third degree) of multiple sites of wrist(s) and hand(s), with loss of a body part
945.30 Full-thickness skin loss due to burn (third degree nos) of unspecified site of lower limb ▽
945.31 Full-thickness skin loss due to burn (third degree nos) of toe(s) (nail)
945.32 Full-thickness skin loss due to burn (third degree nos) of foot
945.33 Full-thickness skin loss due to burn (third degree nos) of ankle
945.34 Full-thickness skin loss due to burn (third degree nos) of lower leg
945.35 Full-thickness skin loss due to burn (third degree nos) of knee
945.36 Full-thickness skin loss due to burn (third degree nos) of thigh (any part)
945.39 Full-thickness skin loss due to burn (third degree nos) of multiple sites of lower limb(s)
945.40 Deep necrosis of underlying tissues due to burn (deep third degree) of unspecified site of lower limb (leg), without mention of loss of a body part ▽
945.41 Deep necrosis of underlying tissues due to burn (deep third degree) of toe(s) (nail), without mention of loss of a body part
945.42 Deep necrosis of underlying tissues due to burn (deep third degree) of foot, without mention of loss of a body part
945.43 Deep necrosis of underlying tissues due to burn (deep third degree) of ankle, without mention of loss of a body part
945.44 Deep necrosis of underlying tissues due to burn (deep third degree) of lower leg, without mention of loss of a body part
945.45 Deep necrosis of underlying tissues due to burn (deep third degree) of knee, without mention of loss of a body part
945.46 Deep necrosis of underlying tissues due to burn (deep third degree) of thigh (any part), without mention of loss of a body part
945.49 Deep necrosis of underlying tissues due to burn (deep third degree) of multiple sites of lower limb(s), without mention of loss of a body part
945.50 Deep necrosis of underlying tissues due to burn (deep third degree) of unspecified site lower limb (leg), with loss of a body part ▽
945.51 Deep necrosis of underlying tissues due to burn (deep third degree) of toe(s) (nail), with loss of a body part
945.52 Deep necrosis of underlying tissues due to burn (deep third degree) of foot, with loss of a body part
945.53 Deep necrosis of underlying tissues due to burn (deep third degree) of ankle, with loss of a body part
945.54 Deep necrosis of underlying tissues due to burn (deep third degree) of lower leg, with loss of a body part
945.55 Deep necrosis of underlying tissues due to burn (deep third degree) of knee, with loss of a body part
945.56 Deep necrosis of underlying tissues due to burn (deep third degree) of thigh (any part), with loss of a body part
945.59 Deep necrosis of underlying tissues due to burn (deep third degree) of multiple sites of lower limb(s), with loss of a body part
946.3 Full-thickness skin loss due to burn (third degree nos) of multiple specified sites
946.4 Deep necrosis of underlying tissues due to burn (deep third degree) of multiple specified sites, without mention of loss of a body part
946.5 Deep necrosis of underlying tissues due to burn (deep third degree) of multiple specified sites, with loss of a body part
948.00 Burn (any degree) involving less than 10% of body surface with third degree burn of less than 10% or unspecified amount
948.10 Burn (any degree) involving 10-19% of body surface with third degree burn of less than 10% or unspecified amount
948.11 Burn (any degree) involving 10-19% of body surface with third degree burn of 10-19%
948.20 Burn (any degree) involving 20-29% of body surface with third degree burn of less than 10% or unspecified amount
948.21 Burn (any degree) involving 20-29% of body surface with third degree burn of 10-19%
948.22 Burn (any degree) involving 20-29% of body surface with third degree burn of 20-29%
948.30 Burn (any degree) involving 30-39% of body surface with third degree burn of less than 10% or unspecified amount
948.31 Burn (any degree) involving 30-39% of body surface with third degree burn of 10-19%
948.32 Burn (any degree) involving 30-39% of body surface with third degree burn of 20-29%
948.33 Burn (any degree) involving 30-39% of body surface with third degree burn of 30-39%
948.40 Burn (any degree) involving 40-49% of body surface with third degree burn of less than 10% or unspecified amount
948.41 Burn (any degree) involving 40-49% of body surface with third degree burn of 10-19%
948.42 Burn (any degree) involving 40-49% of body surface with third degree burn of 20-29%
948.43 Burn (any degree) involving 40-49% of body surface with third degree burn of 30-39%
948.44 Burn (any degree) involving 40-49% of body surface with third degree burn of 40-49%
948.50 Burn (any degree) involving 50-59% of body surface with third degree burn of less than 10% or unspecified amount
948.51 Burn (any degree) involving 50-59% of body surface with third degree burn of 10-19%
948.52 Burn (any degree) involving 50-59% of body surface with third degree burn of 20-29%
948.53 Burn (any degree) involving 50-59% of body surface with third degree burn of 30-39%
948.54 Burn (any degree) involving 50-59% of body surface with third degree burn of 40-49%
948.55 Burn (any degree) involving 50-59% of body surface with third degree burn of 50-59%
948.60 Burn (any degree) involving 60-69% of body surface with third degree burn of less than 10% or unspecified amount
948.61 Burn (any degree) involving 60-69% of body surface with third degree burn of 10-19%
948.62 Burn (any degree) involving 60-69% of body surface with third degree burn of 20-29%
948.63 Burn (any degree) involving 60-69% of body surface with third degree burn of 30-39%
948.64 Burn (any degree) involving 60-69% of body surface with third degree burn of 40-49%
948.65 Burn (any degree) involving 60-69% of body surface with third degree burn of 50-59%
948.66 Burn (any degree) involving 60-69% of body surface with third degree burn of 60-69%
948.70 Burn (any degree) involving 70-79% of body surface with third degree burn of less than 10% or unspecified amount
948.71 Burn (any degree) involving 70-79% of body surface with third degree burn of 10-19%
948.72 Burn (any degree) involving 70-79% of body surface with third degree burn of 20-29%
948.73 Burn (any degree) involving 70-79% of body surface with third degree burn of 30-39%
948.74 Burn (any degree) involving 70-79% of body surface with third degree burn of 40-49%
948.75 Burn (any degree) involving 70-79% of body surface with third degree burn of 50-59%
948.76 Burn (any degree) involving 70-79% of body surface with third degree burn of 60-69%
948.77 Burn (any degree) involving 70-79% of body surface with third degree burn of 70-79%
948.80 Burn (any degree) involving 80-89% of body surface with third degree burn of less than 10% or unspecified amount
948.81 Burn (any degree) involving 80-89% of body surface with third degree burn of 10-19%
948.82 Burn (any degree) involving 80-89% of body surface with third degree burn of 20-29%

948.83 Burn (any degree) involving 80-89% of body surface with third degree burn of 30-39%
948.84 Burn (any degree) involving 80-89% of body surface with third degree burn of 40-49%
948.85 Burn (any degree) involving 80-89% of body surface with third degree burn of 50-59%
948.86 Burn (any degree) involving 80-89% of body surface with third degree burn of 60-69%
948.87 Burn (any degree) involving 80-89% of body surface with third degree burn of 70-79%
948.88 Burn (any degree) involving 80-89% of body surface with third degree burn of 80-89%
948.90 Burn (any degree) involving 90% or more of body surface with third degree burn of less than 10% or unspecified amount
948.91 Burn (any degree) involving 90% or more of body surface with third degree burn of 10-19%
948.92 Burn (any degree) involving 90% or more of body surface with third degree burn of 20-29%
948.93 Burn (any degree) involving 90% or more of body surface with third degree burn of 30-39%
948.94 Burn (any degree) involving 90% or more of body surface with third degree burn of 40-49%
948.95 Burn (any degree) involving 90% or more of body surface with third degree burn of 50-59%
948.96 Burn (any degree) involving 90% or more of body surface with third degree burn of 60-69%
948.97 Burn (any degree) involving 90% or more of body surface with third degree burn of 70-79%
948.98 Burn (any degree) involving 90% or more of body surface with third degree burn of 80-89%
948.99 Burn (any degree) involving 90% or more of body surface with third degree burn of 90% or more of body surface
991.0 Frostbite of face
991.1 Frostbite of hand
991.2 Frostbite of foot
991.3 Frostbite of other and unspecified sites
996.52 Mechanical complication due to other tissue graft, not elsewhere classified
998.59 Other postoperative infection — (Use additional code to identify infection)
998.83 Non-healing surgical wound

ICD-9-CM Procedural

85.84 Pedicle graft to breast
86.65 Heterograft to skin
86.71 Cutting and preparation of pedicle grafts or flaps
86.74 Attachment of pedicle or flap graft to other sites

HCPCS Level II Supplies & Services

A4305 Disposable drug delivery system, flow rate of 50 ml or greater per hour
A4306 Disposable drug delivery system, flow rate of 5 ml or less per hour
A4550 Surgical trays

15570

15570 Formation of direct or tubed pedicle, with or without transfer; trunk

ICD-9-CM Diagnostic

171.4 Malignant neoplasm of connective and other soft tissue of thorax
171.6 Malignant neoplasm of connective and other soft tissue of pelvis
171.7 Malignant neoplasm of connective and other soft tissue of trunk, unspecified site ▽
171.8 Malignant neoplasm of other specified sites of connective and other soft tissue
172.5 Malignant melanoma of skin of trunk, except scrotum
173.5 Other malignant neoplasm of skin of trunk, except scrotum
174.0 Malignant neoplasm of nipple and areola of female breast ♀
174.1 Malignant neoplasm of central portion of female breast ♀
174.2 Malignant neoplasm of upper-inner quadrant of female breast ♀
174.3 Malignant neoplasm of lower-inner quadrant of female breast ♀
174.4 Malignant neoplasm of upper-outer quadrant of female breast ♀
174.5 Malignant neoplasm of lower-outer quadrant of female breast ♀
174.6 Malignant neoplasm of axillary tail of female breast ♀
174.8 Malignant neoplasm of other specified sites of female breast ♀
175.9 Malignant neoplasm of other and unspecified sites of male breast ▽ ♂
198.81 Secondary malignant neoplasm of breast
233.0 Carcinoma in situ of breast
238.3 Neoplasm of uncertain behavior of breast
239.2 Neoplasms of unspecified nature of bone, soft tissue, and skin
239.3 Neoplasm of unspecified nature of breast

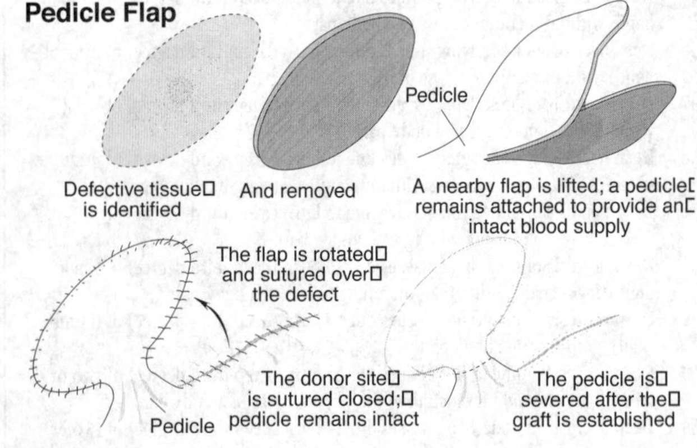
Pedicle Flap
Pedicle
Defective tissue is identified
And removed
A nearby flap is lifted; a pedicle remains attached to provide an intact blood supply
The flap is rotated and sutured over the defect
The donor site is sutured closed; pedicle remains intact
The pedicle is severed after the graft is established
Pedicle

519.2 Mediastinitis
682.2 Cellulitis and abscess of trunk — (Use additional code to identify organism)
682.5 Cellulitis and abscess of buttock — (Use additional code to identify organism)
707.00 Decubitus ulcer, unspecified site
707.02 Decubitus ulcer, upper back
707.03 Decubitus ulcer, lower back
707.04 Decubitus ulcer, hip
707.05 Decubitus ulcer, buttock
707.09 Decubitus ulcer, other site
707.8 Chronic ulcer of other specified site
709.2 Scar condition and fibrosis of skin
738.3 Acquired deformity of chest and rib
741.00 Spina bifida with hydrocephalus, unspecified region ▽
754.81 Pectus excavatum
875.0 Open wound of chest (wall), without mention of complication — (Use additional code to identify infection)
875.1 Open wound of chest (wall), complicated — (Use additional code to identify infection)
876.0 Open wound of back, without mention of complication — (Use additional code to identify infection)
876.1 Open wound of back, complicated — (Use additional code to identify infection)
877.0 Open wound of buttock, without mention of complication — (Use additional code to identify infection)
877.1 Open wound of buttock, complicated — (Use additional code to identify infection)
879.0 Open wound of breast, without mention of complication — (Use additional code to identify infection)
879.1 Open wound of breast, complicated — (Use additional code to identify infection)
879.2 Open wound of abdominal wall, anterior, without mention of complication — (Use additional code to identify infection)
879.3 Open wound of abdominal wall, anterior, complicated — (Use additional code to identify infection)
879.4 Open wound of abdominal wall, lateral, without mention of complication — (Use additional code to identify infection)
879.5 Open wound of abdominal wall, lateral, complicated — (Use additional code to identify infection)
879.6 Open wound of other and unspecified parts of trunk, without mention of complication — (Use additional code to identify infection) ▽
879.7 Open wound of other and unspecified parts of trunk, complicated — (Use additional code to identify infection) ▽
942.30 Full-thickness skin loss due to burn (third degree nos) of unspecified site of trunk ▽
942.31 Full-thickness skin loss due to burn (third degree nos) of breast
942.33 Full-thickness skin loss due to burn (third degree nos) of abdominal wall
942.34 Full-thickness skin loss due to burn (third degree nos) of back (any part)
942.39 Full-thickness skin loss due to burn (third degree nos) of other and multiple sites of trunk
942.40 Deep necrosis of underlying tissues due to burn (deep third degree) of trunk, unspecified site, without mention of loss of a body part ▽
942.41 Deep necrosis of underlying tissues due to burn (deep third degree) of breast, without mention of loss of a body part
942.42 Deep necrosis of underlying tissues due to burn (deep third degree) of chest wall, excluding breast and nipple, without mention of loss of a body part
942.43 Deep necrosis of underlying tissues due to burn (deep third degree) of abdominal wall, without mention of loss of a body part
942.44 Deep necrosis of underlying tissues due to burn (deep third degree) of back (any part), without mention of loss of a body part

▽ Unspecified code
♀ Female diagnosis
☒ Manifestation code
♂ Male diagnosis

942.49 Deep necrosis of underlying tissues due to burn (deep third degree) of other and multiple sites of trunk, without mention of loss of a body part
942.50 Deep necrosis of underlying tissues due to burn (deep third degree) of unspecified site of trunk, with loss of a body part ▽
942.51 Deep necrosis of underlying tissues due to burn (deep third degree) of breast, with loss of a body part
942.52 Deep necrosis of underlying tissues due to burn (deep third degree) of chest wall, excluding breast and nipple, with loss of a body part
942.53 Deep necrosis of underlying tissues due to burn (deep third degree) of abdominal wall with loss of a body part
942.54 Deep necrosis of underlying tissues due to burn (deep third degree) of back (any part), with loss of a body part
942.59 Deep necrosis of underlying tissues due to burn (deep third degree) of other and multiple sites of trunk, with loss of a body part

ICD-9-CM Procedural

85.84 Pedicle graft to breast
86.74 Attachment of pedicle or flap graft to other sites

15572

15572 Formation of direct or tubed pedicle, with or without transfer; scalp, arms, or legs

ICD-9-CM Diagnostic

171.0 Malignant neoplasm of connective and other soft tissue of head, face, and neck
171.2 Malignant neoplasm of connective and other soft tissue of upper limb, including shoulder
171.3 Malignant neoplasm of connective and other soft tissue of lower limb, including hip
172.4 Malignant melanoma of skin of scalp and neck
173.4 Other malignant neoplasm of scalp and skin of neck
216.4 Benign neoplasm of scalp and skin of neck
232.4 Carcinoma in situ of scalp and skin of neck
238.1 Neoplasm of uncertain behavior of connective and other soft tissue ▽
238.2 Neoplasm of uncertain behavior of skin
239.2 Neoplasms of unspecified nature of bone, soft tissue, and skin
682.3 Cellulitis and abscess of upper arm and forearm — (Use additional code to identify organism)
682.6 Cellulitis and abscess of leg, except foot — (Use additional code to identify organism)
682.8 Cellulitis and abscess of other specified site — (Use additional code to identify organism)
701.4 Keloid scar
707.00 Decubitus ulcer, unspecified site
707.01 Decubitus ulcer, elbow
707.06 Decubitus ulcer, ankle
707.07 Decubitus ulcer, heel
707.09 Decubitus ulcer, other site
707.10 Ulcer of lower limb, unspecified ▽
707.11 Ulcer of thigh
707.12 Ulcer of calf
707.13 Ulcer of ankle
707.19 Ulcer of other part of lower limb
707.8 Chronic ulcer of other specified site
709.2 Scar condition and fibrosis of skin
754.0 Congenital musculoskeletal deformities of skull, face, and jaw
873.0 Open wound of scalp, without mention of complication — (Use additional code to identify infection)
873.1 Open wound of scalp, complicated — (Use additional code to identify infection)
880.12 Open wound of axillary region, complicated — (Use additional code to identify infection)
880.13 Open wound of upper arm, complicated — (Use additional code to identify infection)
880.19 Open wound of multiple sites of shoulder and upper arm, complicated — (Use additional code to identify infection)
880.20 Open wound of shoulder region, with tendon involvement — (Use additional code to identify infection)
880.21 Open wound of scapular region, with tendon involvement — (Use additional code to identify infection)
880.22 Open wound of axillary region, with tendon involvement — (Use additional code to identify infection)
880.23 Open wound of upper arm, with tendon involvement — (Use additional code to identify infection)
880.29 Open wound of multiple sites of shoulder and upper arm, with tendon involvement — (Use additional code to identify infection)
881.11 Open wound of elbow, complicated — (Use additional code to identify infection)
881.12 Open wound of wrist, complicated — (Use additional code to identify infection)
881.20 Open wound of forearm, with tendon involvement — (Use additional code to identify infection)
881.21 Open wound of elbow, with tendon involvement — (Use additional code to identify infection)
881.22 Open wound of wrist, with tendon involvement — (Use additional code to identify infection)
884.1 Multiple and unspecified open wound of upper limb, complicated — (Use additional code to identify infection)
884.2 Multiple and unspecified open wound of upper limb, with tendon involvement — (Use additional code to identify infection)
890.1 Open wound of hip and thigh, complicated — (Use additional code to identify infection)
890.2 Open wound of hip and thigh, with tendon involvement — (Use additional code to identify infection)
891.1 Open wound of knee, leg (except thigh), and ankle, complicated — (Use additional code to identify infection)
891.2 Open wound of knee, leg (except thigh), and ankle, with tendon involvement — (Use additional code to identify infection)
894.1 Multiple and unspecified open wound of lower limb, complicated — (Use additional code to identify infection)
894.2 Multiple and unspecified open wound of lower limb, with tendon involvement — (Use additional code to identify infection)
906.0 Late effect of open wound of head, neck, and trunk
906.5 Late effect of burn of eye, face, head, and neck
941.36 Full-thickness skin loss due to burn (third degree nos) of scalp (any part)
941.46 Deep necrosis of underlying tissues due to burn (deep third degree) of scalp (any part), without mention of loss of a body part
941.56 Deep necrosis of underlying tissues due to burn (deep third degree) of scalp (any part), with loss of a body part
943.30 Full-thickness skin loss due to burn (third degree nos) of unspecified site of upper limb ▽
943.31 Full-thickness skin loss due to burn (third degree nos) of forearm
943.32 Full-thickness skin loss due to burn (third degree nos) of elbow
943.33 Full-thickness skin loss due to burn (third degree nos) of upper arm
943.39 Full-thickness skin loss due to burn (third degree nos) of multiple sites of upper limb, except wrist and hand
944.40 Deep necrosis of underlying tissues due to burn (deep third degree) of unspecified site of hand, without mention of a body part ▽
944.41 Deep necrosis of underlying tissues due to burn (deep third degree) of single digit [finger (nail)] other than thumb, without mention of a body part
944.42 Deep necrosis of underlying tissues due to burn (deep third degree) of thumb (nail), without mention of loss of a body part
944.43 Deep necrosis of underlying tissues due to burn (deep third degree) of two or more digits of hand, not including thumb, without mention of a body part
945.30 Full-thickness skin loss due to burn (third degree nos) of unspecified site of lower limb ▽
945.33 Full-thickness skin loss due to burn (third degree nos) of ankle
945.34 Full-thickness skin loss due to burn (third degree nos) of lower leg
945.35 Full-thickness skin loss due to burn (third degree nos) of knee
945.36 Full-thickness skin loss due to burn (third degree nos) of thigh (any part)
945.39 Full-thickness skin loss due to burn (third degree nos) of multiple sites of lower limb(s)
945.40 Deep necrosis of underlying tissues due to burn (deep third degree) of unspecified site of lower limb (leg), without mention of loss of a body part ▽
945.43 Deep necrosis of underlying tissues due to burn (deep third degree) of ankle, without mention of loss of a body part
945.44 Deep necrosis of underlying tissues due to burn (deep third degree) of lower leg, without mention of loss of a body part
945.45 Deep necrosis of underlying tissues due to burn (deep third degree) of knee, without mention of loss of a body part
945.46 Deep necrosis of underlying tissues due to burn (deep third degree) of thigh (any part), without mention of loss of a body part
945.49 Deep necrosis of underlying tissues due to burn (deep third degree) of multiple sites of lower limb(s), without mention of loss of a body part

ICD-9-CM Procedural

86.71 Cutting and preparation of pedicle grafts or flaps
86.74 Attachment of pedicle or flap graft to other sites

15574

15574 Formation of direct or tubed pedicle, with or without transfer; forehead, cheeks, chin, mouth, neck, axillae, genitalia, hands or feet

ICD-9-CM Diagnostic

145.0 Malignant neoplasm of cheek mucosa

171.0 Malignant neoplasm of connective and other soft tissue of head, face, and neck

171.2 Malignant neoplasm of connective and other soft tissue of upper limb, including shoulder

171.3 Malignant neoplasm of connective and other soft tissue of lower limb, including hip

171.4 Malignant neoplasm of connective and other soft tissue of thorax

172.3 Malignant melanoma of skin of other and unspecified parts of face

172.4 Malignant melanoma of skin of scalp and neck

173.0 Other malignant neoplasm of skin of lip

173.3 Other malignant neoplasm of skin of other and unspecified parts of face ▽

173.4 Other malignant neoplasm of scalp and skin of neck

173.5 Other malignant neoplasm of skin of trunk, except scrotum

195.0 Malignant neoplasm of head, face, and neck

195.3 Malignant neoplasm of pelvis

195.4 Malignant neoplasm of upper limb

198.89 Secondary malignant neoplasm of other specified sites

210.0 Benign neoplasm of lip

210.3 Benign neoplasm of floor of mouth

210.4 Benign neoplasm of other and unspecified parts of mouth ▽

216.8 Benign neoplasm of other specified sites of skin

221.2 Benign neoplasm of vulva ♀

222.1 Benign neoplasm of penis ♂

222.4 Benign neoplasm of scrotum ♂

230.0 Carcinoma in situ of lip, oral cavity, and pharynx

233.3 Carcinoma in situ of other and unspecified female genital organs ▽ ♀

233.5 Carcinoma in situ of penis ♂

233.6 Carcinoma in situ of other and unspecified male genital organs ▽ ♂

235.1 Neoplasm of uncertain behavior of lip, oral cavity, and pharynx

236.3 Neoplasm of uncertain behavior of other and unspecified female genital organs ▽ ♀

236.6 Neoplasm of uncertain behavior of other and unspecified male genital organs ▽ ♂

239.0 Neoplasm of unspecified nature of digestive system

239.2 Neoplasms of unspecified nature of bone, soft tissue, and skin

629.20 Female genital mutilation status, unspecified

629.21 Female genital mutilation, Type I status

629.22 Female genital mutilation, Type II status

629.23 Female genital mutilation, Type III status

682.0 Cellulitis and abscess of face — (Use additional code to identify organism)

682.1 Cellulitis and abscess of neck — (Use additional code to identify organism)

682.4 Cellulitis and abscess of hand, except fingers and thumb — (Use additional code to identify organism)

682.7 Cellulitis and abscess of foot, except toes — (Use additional code to identify organism)

707.00 Decubitus ulcer, unspecified site

707.07 Decubitus ulcer, heel

707.09 Decubitus ulcer, other site

707.14 Ulcer of heel and midfoot

707.15 Ulcer of other part of foot

709.2 Scar condition and fibrosis of skin

741.01 Spina bifida with hydrocephalus, cervical region

741.91 Spina bifida without mention of hydrocephalus, cervical region

754.0 Congenital musculoskeletal deformities of skull, face, and jaw

754.1 Congenital musculoskeletal deformity of sternocleidomastoid muscle

873.20 Open wound of nose, unspecified site, without mention of complication — (Use additional code to identify infection) ▽

873.30 Open wound of nose, unspecified site, complicated — (Use additional code to identify infection) ▽

873.41 Open wound of cheek, without mention of complication — (Use additional code to identify infection)

873.42 Open wound of forehead, without mention of complication — (Use additional code to identify infection)

873.43 Open wound of lip, without mention of complication — (Use additional code to identify infection)

873.44 Open wound of jaw, without mention of complication — (Use additional code to identify infection)

873.49 Open wound of face, other and multiple sites, without mention of complication — (Use additional code to identify infection)

873.51 Open wound of cheek, complicated — (Use additional code to identify infection)

873.52 Open wound of forehead, complicated — (Use additional code to identify infection)

873.53 Open wound of lip, complicated — (Use additional code to identify infection)

873.54 Open wound of jaw, complicated — (Use additional code to identify infection)

873.59 Open wound of face, other and multiple sites, complicated — (Use additional code to identify infection)

873.70 Open wound of mouth, unspecified site, complicated — (Use additional code to identify infection) ▽

873.71 Open wound of buccal mucosa, complicated — (Use additional code to identify infection)

873.79 Open wound of mouth, other and multiple sites, complicated — (Use additional code to identify infection)

874.8 Open wound of other and unspecified parts of neck, without mention of complication — (Use additional code to identify infection) ▽

874.9 Open wound of other and unspecified parts of neck, complicated — (Use additional code to identify infection) ▽

878.0 Open wound of penis, without mention of complication — (Use additional code to identify infection) ♂

878.1 Open wound of penis, complicated — (Use additional code to identify infection) ♂

878.2 Open wound of scrotum and testes, without mention of complication — (Use additional code to identify infection) ♂

878.3 Open wound of scrotum and testes, complicated — (Use additional code to identify infection) ♂

878.4 Open wound of vulva, without mention of complication — (Use additional code to identify infection) ♀

878.5 Open wound of vulva, complicated — (Use additional code to identify infection) ♀

878.7 Open wound of vagina, complicated — (Use additional code to identify infection) ♀

878.8 Open wound of other and unspecified parts of genital organs, without mention of complication — (Use additional code to identify infection) ▽

878.9 Open wound of other and unspecified parts of genital organs, complicated — (Use additional code to identify infection) ▽

882.0 Open wound of hand except finger(s) alone, without mention of complication — (Use additional code to identify infection)

882.1 Open wound of hand except finger(s) alone, complicated — (Use additional code to identify infection)

882.2 Open wound of hand except finger(s) alone, with tendon involvement — (Use additional code to identify infection)

883.0 Open wound of finger(s), without mention of complication — (Use additional code to identify infection)

883.1 Open wound of finger(s), complicated — (Use additional code to identify infection)

883.2 Open wound of finger(s), with tendon involvement — (Use additional code to identify infection)

885.0 Traumatic amputation of thumb (complete) (partial), without mention of complication — (Use additional code to identify infection)

885.1 Traumatic amputation of thumb (complete) (partial), complicated — (Use additional code to identify infection)

886.0 Traumatic amputation of other finger(s) (complete) (partial), without mention of complication — (Use additional code to identify infection)

886.1 Traumatic amputation of other finger(s) (complete) (partial), complicated — (Use additional code to identify infection)

887.0 Traumatic amputation of arm and hand (complete) (partial), unilateral, below elbow, without mention of complication — (Use additional code to identify infection)

887.1 Traumatic amputation of arm and hand (complete) (partial), unilateral, below elbow, complicated — (Use additional code to identify infection)

887.4 Traumatic amputation of arm and hand (complete) (partial), unilateral, level not specified, without mention of complication — (Use additional code to identify infection) ▽

887.5 Traumatic amputation of arm and hand (complete) (partial), unilateral, level not specified, complicated — (Use additional code to identify infection) ▽

887.6 Traumatic amputation of arm and hand (complete) (partial), bilateral (any level), without mention of complication — (Use additional code to identify infection)

887.7 Traumatic amputation of arm and hand (complete) (partial), bilateral (any level), complicated — (Use additional code to identify infection)

892.0 Open wound of foot except toe(s) alone, without mention of complication — (Use additional code to identify infection)

892.1 Open wound of foot except toe(s) alone, complicated — (Use additional code to identify infection)

892.2 Open wound of foot except toe(s) alone, with tendon involvement — (Use additional code to identify infection)

893.0 Open wound of toe(s), without mention of complication — (Use additional code to identify infection)
893.1 Open wound of toe(s), complicated — (Use additional code to identify infection)
893.2 Open wound of toe(s), with tendon involvement — (Use additional code to identify infection)
895.0 Traumatic amputation of toe(s) (complete) (partial), without mention of complication — (Use additional code to identify infection)
895.1 Traumatic amputation of toe(s) (complete) (partial), complicated — (Use additional code to identify infection)
896.0 Traumatic amputation of foot (complete) (partial), unilateral, without mention of complication — (Use additional code to identify infection)
896.1 Traumatic amputation of foot (complete) (partial), unilateral, complicated — (Use additional code to identify infection)
896.2 Traumatic amputation of foot (complete) (partial), bilateral, without mention of complication — (Use additional code to identify infection)
906.0 Late effect of open wound of head, neck, and trunk
906.1 Late effect of open wound of extremities without mention of tendon injury
906.4 Late effect of crushing
906.5 Late effect of burn of eye, face, head, and neck
906.6 Late effect of burn of wrist and hand
906.7 Late effect of burn of other extremities
906.8 Late effect of burns of other specified sites
925.1 Crushing injury of face and scalp — (Use additional code to identify any associated injuries: 800-829, 850.0-854.1, 860.0-869.1)
925.2 Crushing injury of neck — (Use additional code to identify any associated injuries: 800-829, 850.0-854.1, 860.0-869.1)
926.0 Crushing injury of external genitalia — (Use additional code to identify any associated injuries: 800-829, 850.0-854.1, 860.0-869.1)
927.20 Crushing injury of hand(s) — (Use additional code to identify any associated injuries: 800-829, 850.0-854.1, 860.0-869.1)
927.21 Crushing injury of wrist — (Use additional code to identify any associated injuries: 800-829, 850.0-854.1, 860.0-869.1)
928.20 Crushing injury of foot — (Use additional code to identify any associated injuries: 800-829, 850.0-854.1, 860.0-869.1)
928.3 Crushing injury of toe(s) — (Use additional code to identify any associated injuries: 800-829, 850.0-854.1, 860.0-869.1)
928.8 Crushing injury of multiple sites of lower limb — (Use additional code to identify any associated injuries: 800-829, 850.0-854.1, 860.0-869.1)
941.30 Full-thickness skin loss due to burn (third degree nos) of unspecified site of face and head ▽
941.33 Full-thickness skin loss due to burn (third degree nos) of lip(s)
941.35 Full-thickness skin loss due to burn (third degree nos) of nose (septum)
941.37 Full-thickness skin loss due to burn (third degree nos) of forehead and cheek
941.38 Full-thickness skin loss due to burn (third degree nos) of neck
941.39 Full-thickness skin loss due to burn (third degree nos) of multiple sites (except with eye) of face, head, and neck
941.40 Deep necrosis of underlying tissues due to burn (deep third degree) of unspecified site of face and head, without mention of loss of a body part ▽
941.43 Deep necrosis of underlying tissues due to burn (deep third degree) of lip(s), without mention of loss of a body part
941.44 Deep necrosis of underlying tissues due to burn (deep third degree) of chin, without mention of loss of a body part
941.45 Deep necrosis of underlying tissues due to burn (deep third degree) of nose (septum), without mention of loss of a body part
941.47 Deep necrosis of underlying tissues due to burn (deep third degree) of forehead and cheek, without mention of loss of a body part
941.48 Deep necrosis of underlying tissues due to burn (deep third degree) of neck, without mention of loss of a body part
941.49 Deep necrosis of underlying tissues due to burn (deep third degree) of multiple sites (except with eye) of face, head, and neck, without mention of loss of a body part
941.50 Deep necrosis of underlying tissues due to burn (deep third degree) of face and head, unspecified site, with loss of a body part ▽
941.53 Deep necrosis of underlying tissues due to burn (deep third degree) of lip(s), with loss of a body part
941.54 Deep necrosis of underlying tissues due to burn (deep third degree) of chin, with loss of a body part
941.55 Deep necrosis of underlying tissues due to burn (deep third degree) of nose (septum), with loss of a body part
941.57 Deep necrosis of underlying tissues due to burn (deep third degree) of forehead and cheek, with loss of a body part
941.58 Deep necrosis of underlying tissues due to burn (deep third degree) of neck, with loss of a body part
941.59 Deep necrosis of underlying tissues due to burn (deep third degree) of multiple sites (except eye) of face, head, and neck, with loss of a body part
942.35 Full-thickness skin loss due to burn (third degree nos) of genitalia
942.45 Deep necrosis of underlying tissues due to burn (deep third degree) of genitalia, without mention of loss of a body part
942.52 Deep necrosis of underlying tissues due to burn (deep third degree) of chest wall, excluding breast and nipple, with loss of a body part
942.55 Deep necrosis of underlying tissues due to burn (deep third degree) of genitalia, with loss of a body part
944.30 Full-thickness skin loss due to burn (third degree nos) of unspecified site of hand ▽
944.31 Full-thickness skin loss due to burn (third degree nos) of single digit [finger (nail)] other than thumb
944.32 Full-thickness skin loss due to burn (third degree nos) of thumb (nail)
944.33 Full-thickness skin loss due to burn (third degree nos) of two or more digits of hand, not including thumb
944.34 Full-thickness skin loss due to burn (third degree nos) of two or more digits of hand including thumb
944.35 Full-thickness skin loss due to burn (third degree nos) of palm of hand
944.36 Full-thickness skin loss due to burn (third degree nos) of back of hand
944.37 Full-thickness skin loss due to burn (third degree nos) of wrist
944.38 Full-thickness skin loss due to burn (third degree nos) of multiple sites of wrist(s) and hand(s)
944.40 Deep necrosis of underlying tissues due to burn (deep third degree) of unspecified site of hand, without mention of a body part ▽
944.41 Deep necrosis of underlying tissues due to burn (deep third degree) of single digit [finger (nail)] other than thumb, without mention of a body part
944.42 Deep necrosis of underlying tissues due to burn (deep third degree) of thumb (nail), without mention of loss of a body part
944.43 Deep necrosis of underlying tissues due to burn (deep third degree) of two or more digits of hand, not including thumb, without mention of a body part
944.44 Deep necrosis of underlying tissues due to burn (deep third degree) of two or more digits of hand including thumb, without mention of a body part
944.45 Deep necrosis of underlying tissues due to burn (deep third degree) of palm of hand, without mention of loss of a body part
944.46 Deep necrosis of underlying tissues due to burn (deep third degree) of back of hand, without mention of loss of back of a body part
944.47 Deep necrosis of underlying tissues due to burn (deep third degree) of wrist, without mention of loss of a body part
944.48 Deep necrosis of underlying tissues due to burn (deep third degree) of multiple sites of wrist(s) and hand(s), without mention of loss of a body part
944.50 Deep necrosis of underlying tissues due to burn (deep third degree) of unspecified site of hand, with loss of a body part ▽
944.51 Deep necrosis of underlying tissues due to burn (deep third degree) of single digit (finger (nail)) other than thumb, with loss of a body part
944.52 Deep necrosis of underlying tissues due to burn (deep third degree) of thumb (nail), with loss of a body part
945.32 Full-thickness skin loss due to burn (third degree nos) of foot
945.42 Deep necrosis of underlying tissues due to burn (deep third degree) of foot, without mention of loss of a body part
947.0 Burn of mouth and pharynx
959.09 Injury of face and neck, other and unspecified
959.14 Other injury of external genitals
997.62 Infection (chronic) of amputation stump — (Use additional code to identify organism. Use additional code to identify complications)
997.69 Other late amputation stump complication — (Use additional code to identify complications)
998.83 Non-healing surgical wound
V10.02 Personal history of malignant neoplasm of other and unspecified parts of oral cavity and pharynx ▽
V10.21 Personal history of malignant neoplasm of larynx
V51 Aftercare involving the use of plastic surgery

ICD-9-CM Procedural

27.57 Attachment of pedicle or flap graft to lip and mouth
71.9 Other operations on female genital organs
86.71 Cutting and preparation of pedicle grafts or flaps
86.73 Attachment of pedicle or flap graft to hand
86.74 Attachment of pedicle or flap graft to other sites

15576

15576 Formation of direct or tubed pedicle, with or without transfer; eyelids, nose, ears, lips, or intraoral

ICD-9-CM Diagnostic

140.0 Malignant neoplasm of upper lip, vermilion border
140.1 Malignant neoplasm of lower lip, vermilion border
140.3 Malignant neoplasm of upper lip, inner aspect

140.4 Malignant neoplasm of lower lip, inner aspect
140.5 Malignant neoplasm of lip, inner aspect, unspecified as to upper or lower ▽
140.6 Malignant neoplasm of commissure of lip
140.8 Malignant neoplasm of other sites of lip
140.9 Malignant neoplasm of lip, vermilion border, unspecified as to upper or lower ▽
144.0 Malignant neoplasm of anterior portion of floor of mouth
144.1 Malignant neoplasm of lateral portion of floor of mouth
144.8 Malignant neoplasm of other sites of floor of mouth
144.9 Malignant neoplasm of floor of mouth, part unspecified ▽
145.0 Malignant neoplasm of cheek mucosa
145.1 Malignant neoplasm of vestibule of mouth
145.2 Malignant neoplasm of hard palate
145.3 Malignant neoplasm of soft palate
145.8 Malignant neoplasm of other specified parts of mouth
145.9 Malignant neoplasm of mouth, unspecified site ▽
172.0 Malignant melanoma of skin of lip
172.1 Malignant melanoma of skin of eyelid, including canthus
172.2 Malignant melanoma of skin of ear and external auditory canal
172.3 Malignant melanoma of skin of other and unspecified parts of face
172.8 Malignant melanoma of other specified sites of skin
173.0 Other malignant neoplasm of skin of lip
173.1 Other malignant neoplasm of skin of eyelid, including canthus
173.2 Other malignant neoplasm of skin of ear and external auditory canal
173.3 Other malignant neoplasm of skin of other and unspecified parts of face ▽
173.8 Other malignant neoplasm of other specified sites of skin
195.0 Malignant neoplasm of head, face, and neck
198.2 Secondary malignant neoplasm of skin
210.0 Benign neoplasm of lip
210.4 Benign neoplasm of other and unspecified parts of mouth ▽
216.0 Benign neoplasm of skin of lip
216.1 Benign neoplasm of eyelid, including canthus
216.2 Benign neoplasm of ear and external auditory canal
216.3 Benign neoplasm of skin of other and unspecified parts of face ▽
230.0 Carcinoma in situ of lip, oral cavity, and pharynx
232.1 Carcinoma in situ of eyelid, including canthus
232.2 Carcinoma in situ of skin of ear and external auditory canal
232.3 Carcinoma in situ of skin of other and unspecified parts of face ▽
235.1 Neoplasm of uncertain behavior of lip, oral cavity, and pharynx
238.1 Neoplasm of uncertain behavior of connective and other soft tissue ▽
238.2 Neoplasm of uncertain behavior of skin
239.0 Neoplasm of unspecified nature of digestive system
239.2 Neoplasms of unspecified nature of bone, soft tissue, and skin
380.32 Acquired deformities of auricle or pinna
682.0 Cellulitis and abscess of face — (Use additional code to identify organism)
709.2 Scar condition and fibrosis of skin
709.9 Unspecified disorder of skin and subcutaneous tissue ▽
743.62 Congenital deformity of eyelid
744.01 Congenital absence of external ear causing impairment of hearing
744.02 Other congenital anomaly of external ear causing impairment of hearing
744.09 Other congenital anomalies of ear causing impairment of hearing
744.23 Microtia
744.3 Unspecified congenital anomaly of ear ▽
744.5 Congenital webbing of neck
744.82 Microcheilia
748.1 Other congenital anomaly of nose
749.01 Unilateral cleft palate, complete
749.02 Unilateral cleft palate, incomplete
749.03 Bilateral cleft palate, complete
749.04 Bilateral cleft palate, incomplete
749.10 Unspecified cleft lip ▽
749.11 Unilateral cleft lip, complete
749.12 Unilateral cleft lip, incomplete
749.13 Bilateral cleft lip, complete
749.14 Bilateral cleft lip, incomplete
749.20 Unspecified cleft palate with cleft lip ▽
749.21 Unilateral cleft palate with cleft lip, complete
749.22 Unilateral cleft palate with cleft lip, incomplete
749.23 Bilateral cleft palate with cleft lip, complete
749.24 Bilateral cleft palate with cleft lip, incomplete
785.4 Gangrene — (Code first any associated underlying condition:250.7, 443.0)
870.0 Laceration of skin of eyelid and periocular area — (Use additional code to identify infection)
870.1 Laceration of eyelid, full-thickness, not involving lacrimal passages — (Use additional code to identify infection)
870.2 Laceration of eyelid involving lacrimal passages — (Use additional code to identify infection)
872.00 Open wound of external ear, unspecified site, without mention of complication — (Use additional code to identify infection) ▽
872.01 Open wound of auricle, without mention of complication — (Use additional code to identify infection)
872.02 Open wound of auditory canal, without mention of complication — (Use additional code to identify infection)
872.10 Open wound of external ear, unspecified site, complicated — (Use additional code to identify infection) ▽
872.11 Open wound of auricle, complicated — (Use additional code to identify infection)
872.12 Open wound of auditory canal, complicated — (Use additional code to identify infection)
872.8 Open wound of ear, part unspecified, without mention of complication — (Use additional code to identify infection) ▽
872.9 Open wound of ear, part unspecified, complicated — (Use additional code to identify infection) ▽
873.20 Open wound of nose, unspecified site, without mention of complication — (Use additional code to identify infection) ▽
873.30 Open wound of nose, unspecified site, complicated — (Use additional code to identify infection) ▽
873.31 Open wound of nasal septum, complicated — (Use additional code to identify infection)
873.32 Open wound of nasal cavity, complicated — (Use additional code to identify infection)
873.33 Open wound of nasal sinus, complicated — (Use additional code to identify infection)
873.39 Open wound of nose, multiple sites, complicated — (Use additional code to identify infection)
873.43 Open wound of lip, without mention of complication — (Use additional code to identify infection)
873.53 Open wound of lip, complicated — (Use additional code to identify infection)
906.0 Late effect of open wound of head, neck, and trunk
906.5 Late effect of burn of eye, face, head, and neck
941.01 Burn of unspecified degree of ear (any part) ▽
941.02 Burn of unspecified degree of eye (with other parts of face, head, and neck) ▽
941.03 Burn of unspecified degree of lip(s) ▽
941.05 Burn of unspecified degree of nose (septum) ▽
941.09 Burn of unspecified degree of multiple sites (except with eye) of face, head, and neck ▽
941.31 Full-thickness skin loss due to burn (third degree nos) of ear (any part)
941.32 Full-thickness skin loss due to burn (third degree nos) of eye (with other parts of face, head, and neck)
941.33 Full-thickness skin loss due to burn (third degree nos) of lip(s)
941.35 Full-thickness skin loss due to burn (third degree nos) of nose (septum)
941.39 Full-thickness skin loss due to burn (third degree nos) of multiple sites (except with eye) of face, head, and neck
941.41 Deep necrosis of underlying tissues due to burn (deep third degree) of ear (any part), without mention of loss of a body part
941.45 Deep necrosis of underlying tissues due to burn (deep third degree) of nose (septum), without mention of loss of a body part
941.49 Deep necrosis of underlying tissues due to burn (deep third degree) of multiple sites (except with eye) of face, head, and neck, without mention of loss of a body part
941.51 Deep necrosis of underlying tissues due to burn (deep third degree) of ear (any part), with loss of a body part
941.52 Deep necrosis of underlying tissues due to burn (deep third degree) of eye (with other parts of face, head, and neck), with loss of a body part
941.53 Deep necrosis of underlying tissues due to burn (deep third degree) of lip(s), with loss of a body part
941.55 Deep necrosis of underlying tissues due to burn (deep third degree) of nose (septum), with loss of a body part
941.59 Deep necrosis of underlying tissues due to burn (deep third degree) of multiple sites (except eye) of face, head, and neck, with loss of a body part
946.3 Full-thickness skin loss due to burn (third degree nos) of multiple specified sites
946.4 Deep necrosis of underlying tissues due to burn (deep third degree) of multiple specified sites, without mention of loss of a body part
946.5 Deep necrosis of underlying tissues due to burn (deep third degree) of multiple specified sites, with loss of a body part
947.0 Burn of mouth and pharynx
948.00 Burn (any degree) involving less than 10% of body surface with third degree burn of less than 10% or unspecified amount
948.10 Burn (any degree) involving 10-19% of body surface with third degree burn of less than 10% or unspecified amount

▽ Unspecified code
♀ Female diagnosis
☒ Manifestation code
♂ Male diagnosis

948.11 Burn (any degree) involving 10-19% of body surface with third degree burn of 10-19%
948.20 Burn (any degree) involving 20-29% of body surface with third degree burn of less than 10% or unspecified amount
948.21 Burn (any degree) involving 20-29% of body surface with third degree burn of 10-19%
948.22 Burn (any degree) involving 20-29% of body surface with third degree burn of 20-29%
948.30 Burn (any degree) involving 30-39% of body surface with third degree burn of less than 10% or unspecified amount
948.31 Burn (any degree) involving 30-39% of body surface with third degree burn of 10-19%
948.32 Burn (any degree) involving 30-39% of body surface with third degree burn of 20-29%
948.33 Burn (any degree) involving 30-39% of body surface with third degree burn of 30-39%
948.40 Burn (any degree) involving 40-49% of body surface with third degree burn of less than 10% or unspecified amount
948.41 Burn (any degree) involving 40-49% of body surface with third degree burn of 10-19%
948.42 Burn (any degree) involving 40-49% of body surface with third degree burn of 20-29%
948.43 Burn (any degree) involving 40-49% of body surface with third degree burn of 30-39%
948.44 Burn (any degree) involving 40-49% of body surface with third degree burn of 40-49%
948.50 Burn (any degree) involving 50-59% of body surface with third degree burn of less than 10% or unspecified amount
948.51 Burn (any degree) involving 50-59% of body surface with third degree burn of 10-19%
948.52 Burn (any degree) involving 50-59% of body surface with third degree burn of 20-29%
948.53 Burn (any degree) involving 50-59% of body surface with third degree burn of 30-39%
948.54 Burn (any degree) involving 50-59% of body surface with third degree burn of 40-49%
948.55 Burn (any degree) involving 50-59% of body surface with third degree burn of 50-59%
948.60 Burn (any degree) involving 60-69% of body surface with third degree burn of less than 10% or unspecified amount
948.61 Burn (any degree) involving 60-69% of body surface with third degree burn of 10-19%
948.62 Burn (any degree) involving 60-69% of body surface with third degree burn of 20-29%
948.63 Burn (any degree) involving 60-69% of body surface with third degree burn of 30-39%
948.64 Burn (any degree) involving 60-69% of body surface with third degree burn of 40-49%
948.65 Burn (any degree) involving 60-69% of body surface with third degree burn of 50-59%
948.66 Burn (any degree) involving 60-69% of body surface with third degree burn of 60-69%
948.70 Burn (any degree) involving 70-79% of body surface with third degree burn of less than 10% or unspecified amount
948.71 Burn (any degree) involving 70-79% of body surface with third degree burn of 10-19%
948.72 Burn (any degree) involving 70-79% of body surface with third degree burn of 20-29%
948.73 Burn (any degree) involving 70-79% of body surface with third degree burn of 30-39%
948.74 Burn (any degree) involving 70-79% of body surface with third degree burn of 40-49%
948.75 Burn (any degree) involving 70-79% of body surface with third degree burn of 50-59%
948.76 Burn (any degree) involving 70-79% of body surface with third degree burn of 60-69%
948.77 Burn (any degree) involving 70-79% of body surface with third degree burn of 70-79%
948.80 Burn (any degree) involving 80-89% of body surface with third degree burn of less than 10% or unspecified amount
948.81 Burn (any degree) involving 80-89% of body surface with third degree burn of 10-19%
948.82 Burn (any degree) involving 80-89% of body surface with third degree burn of 20-29%
948.83 Burn (any degree) involving 80-89% of body surface with third degree burn of 30-39%
948.84 Burn (any degree) involving 80-89% of body surface with third degree burn of 40-49%
948.85 Burn (any degree) involving 80-89% of body surface with third degree burn of 50-59%
948.86 Burn (any degree) involving 80-89% of body surface with third degree burn of 60-69%
948.87 Burn (any degree) involving 80-89% of body surface with third degree burn of 70-79%
948.88 Burn (any degree) involving 80-89% of body surface with third degree burn of 80-89%
959.09 Injury of face and neck, other and unspecified
996.52 Mechanical complication due to other tissue graft, not elsewhere classified
998.59 Other postoperative infection — (Use additional code to identify infection)
998.83 Non-healing surgical wound
V10.02 Personal history of malignant neoplasm of other and unspecified parts of oral cavity and pharynx ▽
V51 Aftercare involving the use of plastic surgery
V84.09 Genetic susceptibility to other malignant neoplasm

ICD-9-CM Procedural

18.71 Construction of auricle of ear
18.79 Other plastic repair of external ear
27.56 Other skin graft to lip and mouth
27.57 Attachment of pedicle or flap graft to lip and mouth
86.71 Cutting and preparation of pedicle grafts or flaps
86.74 Attachment of pedicle or flap graft to other sites

15600

15600 Delay of flap or sectioning of flap (division and inset); at trunk

ICD-9-CM Diagnostic

171.4 Malignant neoplasm of connective and other soft tissue of thorax
171.6 Malignant neoplasm of connective and other soft tissue of pelvis
171.7 Malignant neoplasm of connective and other soft tissue of trunk, unspecified site ▽
171.8 Malignant neoplasm of other specified sites of connective and other soft tissue
172.5 Malignant melanoma of skin of trunk, except scrotum
173.5 Other malignant neoplasm of skin of trunk, except scrotum
174.0 Malignant neoplasm of nipple and areola of female breast ♀
174.1 Malignant neoplasm of central portion of female breast ♀
174.2 Malignant neoplasm of upper-inner quadrant of female breast ♀
174.3 Malignant neoplasm of lower-inner quadrant of female breast ♀
174.4 Malignant neoplasm of upper-outer quadrant of female breast ♀
174.5 Malignant neoplasm of lower-outer quadrant of female breast ♀
174.6 Malignant neoplasm of axillary tail of female breast ♀
174.8 Malignant neoplasm of other specified sites of female breast ♀
175.9 Malignant neoplasm of other and unspecified sites of male breast ▽ ♂
198.81 Secondary malignant neoplasm of breast
233.0 Carcinoma in situ of breast
238.2 Neoplasm of uncertain behavior of skin
238.3 Neoplasm of uncertain behavior of breast
239.2 Neoplasms of unspecified nature of bone, soft tissue, and skin
239.3 Neoplasm of unspecified nature of breast
519.2 Mediastinitis
682.2 Cellulitis and abscess of trunk — (Use additional code to identify organism)
682.5 Cellulitis and abscess of buttock — (Use additional code to identify organism)
707.00 Decubitus ulcer, unspecified site
707.02 Decubitus ulcer, upper back
707.03 Decubitus ulcer, lower back
707.04 Decubitus ulcer, hip
707.05 Decubitus ulcer, buttock
707.09 Decubitus ulcer, other site
707.8 Chronic ulcer of other specified site
709.2 Scar condition and fibrosis of skin
738.3 Acquired deformity of chest and rib
741.00 Spina bifida with hydrocephalus, unspecified region ▽
754.81 Pectus excavatum
875.0 Open wound of chest (wall), without mention of complication — (Use additional code to identify infection)
875.1 Open wound of chest (wall), complicated — (Use additional code to identify infection)
876.0 Open wound of back, without mention of complication — (Use additional code to identify infection)
876.1 Open wound of back, complicated — (Use additional code to identify infection)
877.0 Open wound of buttock, without mention of complication — (Use additional code to identify infection)

877.1 Open wound of buttock, complicated — (Use additional code to identify infection)
879.0 Open wound of breast, without mention of complication — (Use additional code to identify infection)
879.1 Open wound of breast, complicated — (Use additional code to identify infection)
879.2 Open wound of abdominal wall, anterior, without mention of complication — (Use additional code to identify infection)
879.3 Open wound of abdominal wall, anterior, complicated — (Use additional code to identify infection)
879.4 Open wound of abdominal wall, lateral, without mention of complication — (Use additional code to identify infection)
879.5 Open wound of abdominal wall, lateral, complicated — (Use additional code to identify infection)
879.6 Open wound of other and unspecified parts of trunk, without mention of complication — (Use additional code to identify infection)
879.7 Open wound of other and unspecified parts of trunk, complicated — (Use additional code to identify infection)
942.30 Full-thickness skin loss due to burn (third degree nos) of unspecified site of trunk
942.31 Full-thickness skin loss due to burn (third degree nos) of breast
942.33 Full-thickness skin loss due to burn (third degree nos) of abdominal wall
942.34 Full-thickness skin loss due to burn (third degree nos) of back (any part)
942.39 Full-thickness skin loss due to burn (third degree nos) of other and multiple sites of trunk
942.40 Deep necrosis of underlying tissues due to burn (deep third degree) of trunk, unspecified site, without mention of loss of a body part
942.41 Deep necrosis of underlying tissues due to burn (deep third degree) of breast, without mention of loss of a body part
942.42 Deep necrosis of underlying tissues due to burn (deep third degree) of chest wall, excluding breast and nipple, without mention of loss of a body part
942.43 Deep necrosis of underlying tissues due to burn (deep third degree) of abdominal wall, without mention of loss of a body part
942.44 Deep necrosis of underlying tissues due to burn (deep third degree) of back (any part), without mention of loss of a body part
942.49 Deep necrosis of underlying tissues due to burn (deep third degree) of other and multiple sites of trunk, without mention of loss of a body part
942.50 Deep necrosis of underlying tissues due to burn (deep third degree) of unspecified site of trunk, with loss of a body part
942.51 Deep necrosis of underlying tissues due to burn (deep third degree) of breast, with loss of a body part
942.52 Deep necrosis of underlying tissues due to burn (deep third degree) of chest wall, excluding breast and nipple, with loss of a body part
942.53 Deep necrosis of underlying tissues due to burn (deep third degree) of abdominal wall with loss of a body part
942.54 Deep necrosis of underlying tissues due to burn (deep third degree) of back (any part), with loss of a body part
942.59 Deep necrosis of underlying tissues due to burn (deep third degree) of other and multiple sites of trunk, with loss of a body part

ICD-9-CM Procedural

86.71 Cutting and preparation of pedicle grafts or flaps

15610

15610 Delay of flap or sectioning of flap (division and inset); at scalp, arms, or legs

ICD-9-CM Diagnostic

171.0 Malignant neoplasm of connective and other soft tissue of head, face, and neck
171.2 Malignant neoplasm of connective and other soft tissue of upper limb, including shoulder
171.3 Malignant neoplasm of connective and other soft tissue of lower limb, including hip
172.4 Malignant melanoma of skin of scalp and neck
173.4 Other malignant neoplasm of scalp and skin of neck
216.4 Benign neoplasm of scalp and skin of neck
232.4 Carcinoma in situ of scalp and skin of neck
238.1 Neoplasm of uncertain behavior of connective and other soft tissue
238.2 Neoplasm of uncertain behavior of skin
239.2 Neoplasms of unspecified nature of bone, soft tissue, and skin
682.3 Cellulitis and abscess of upper arm and forearm — (Use additional code to identify organism)
682.6 Cellulitis and abscess of leg, except foot — (Use additional code to identify organism)
682.8 Cellulitis and abscess of other specified site — (Use additional code to identify organism)
701.4 Keloid scar
707.00 Decubitus ulcer, unspecified site
707.01 Decubitus ulcer, elbow
707.06 Decubitus ulcer, ankle
707.09 Decubitus ulcer, other site
707.10 Ulcer of lower limb, unspecified
707.11 Ulcer of thigh
707.12 Ulcer of calf
707.13 Ulcer of ankle
707.19 Ulcer of other part of lower limb
707.8 Chronic ulcer of other specified site
709.2 Scar condition and fibrosis of skin
754.0 Congenital musculoskeletal deformities of skull, face, and jaw
873.0 Open wound of scalp, without mention of complication — (Use additional code to identify infection)
873.1 Open wound of scalp, complicated — (Use additional code to identify infection)
880.12 Open wound of axillary region, complicated — (Use additional code to identify infection)
880.13 Open wound of upper arm, complicated — (Use additional code to identify infection)
880.19 Open wound of multiple sites of shoulder and upper arm, complicated — (Use additional code to identify infection)
880.20 Open wound of shoulder region, with tendon involvement — (Use additional code to identify infection)
880.21 Open wound of scapular region, with tendon involvement — (Use additional code to identify infection)
880.22 Open wound of axillary region, with tendon involvement — (Use additional code to identify infection)
880.23 Open wound of upper arm, with tendon involvement — (Use additional code to identify infection)
880.29 Open wound of multiple sites of shoulder and upper arm, with tendon involvement — (Use additional code to identify infection)
881.11 Open wound of elbow, complicated — (Use additional code to identify infection)
881.12 Open wound of wrist, complicated — (Use additional code to identify infection)
881.20 Open wound of forearm, with tendon involvement — (Use additional code to identify infection)
881.21 Open wound of elbow, with tendon involvement — (Use additional code to identify infection)
881.22 Open wound of wrist, with tendon involvement — (Use additional code to identify infection)
884.1 Multiple and unspecified open wound of upper limb, complicated — (Use additional code to identify infection)
884.2 Multiple and unspecified open wound of upper limb, with tendon involvement — (Use additional code to identify infection)
890.1 Open wound of hip and thigh, complicated — (Use additional code to identify infection)
890.2 Open wound of hip and thigh, with tendon involvement — (Use additional code to identify infection)
891.1 Open wound of knee, leg (except thigh), and ankle, complicated — (Use additional code to identify infection)
891.2 Open wound of knee, leg (except thigh), and ankle, with tendon involvement — (Use additional code to identify infection)
894.1 Multiple and unspecified open wound of lower limb, complicated — (Use additional code to identify infection)
894.2 Multiple and unspecified open wound of lower limb, with tendon involvement — (Use additional code to identify infection)
906.0 Late effect of open wound of head, neck, and trunk
906.5 Late effect of burn of eye, face, head, and neck
941.36 Full-thickness skin loss due to burn (third degree nos) of scalp (any part)
941.46 Deep necrosis of underlying tissues due to burn (deep third degree) of scalp (any part), without mention of loss of a body part
941.56 Deep necrosis of underlying tissues due to burn (deep third degree) of scalp (any part), with loss of a body part
943.30 Full-thickness skin loss due to burn (third degree nos) of unspecified site of upper limb
943.31 Full-thickness skin loss due to burn (third degree nos) of forearm
943.32 Full-thickness skin loss due to burn (third degree nos) of elbow
943.33 Full-thickness skin loss due to burn (third degree nos) of upper arm
943.39 Full-thickness skin loss due to burn (third degree nos) of multiple sites of upper limb, except wrist and hand
945.30 Full-thickness skin loss due to burn (third degree nos) of unspecified site of lower limb
945.33 Full-thickness skin loss due to burn (third degree nos) of ankle
945.34 Full-thickness skin loss due to burn (third degree nos) of lower leg

945.35 Full-thickness skin loss due to burn (third degree nos) of knee
945.36 Full-thickness skin loss due to burn (third degree nos) of thigh (any part)
945.39 Full-thickness skin loss due to burn (third degree nos) of multiple sites of lower limb(s)
945.40 Deep necrosis of underlying tissues due to burn (deep third degree) of unspecified site of lower limb (leg), without mention of loss of a body part ▽
945.43 Deep necrosis of underlying tissues due to burn (deep third degree) of ankle, without mention of loss of a body part
945.44 Deep necrosis of underlying tissues due to burn (deep third degree) of lower leg, without mention of loss of a body part
945.45 Deep necrosis of underlying tissues due to burn (deep third degree) of knee, without mention of loss of a body part
945.46 Deep necrosis of underlying tissues due to burn (deep third degree) of thigh (any part), without mention of loss of a body part
945.49 Deep necrosis of underlying tissues due to burn (deep third degree) of multiple sites of lower limb(s), without mention of loss of a body part
948.00 Burn (any degree) involving less than 10% of body surface with third degree burn of less than 10% or unspecified amount
V51 Aftercare involving the use of plastic surgery

ICD-9-CM Procedural

86.71 Cutting and preparation of pedicle grafts or flaps
86.74 Attachment of pedicle or flap graft to other sites

15620

15620 Delay of flap or sectioning of flap (division and inset); at forehead, cheeks, chin, neck, axillae, genitalia, hands, or feet

ICD-9-CM Diagnostic

171.0 Malignant neoplasm of connective and other soft tissue of head, face, and neck
171.2 Malignant neoplasm of connective and other soft tissue of upper limb, including shoulder
171.3 Malignant neoplasm of connective and other soft tissue of lower limb, including hip
171.4 Malignant neoplasm of connective and other soft tissue of thorax
172.0 Malignant melanoma of skin of lip
172.3 Malignant melanoma of skin of other and unspecified parts of face
172.4 Malignant melanoma of skin of scalp and neck
173.0 Other malignant neoplasm of skin of lip
173.3 Other malignant neoplasm of skin of other and unspecified parts of face ▽
173.4 Other malignant neoplasm of scalp and skin of neck
173.5 Other malignant neoplasm of skin of trunk, except scrotum
184.0 Malignant neoplasm of vagina ♀
184.1 Malignant neoplasm of labia majora ♀
184.2 Malignant neoplasm of labia minora ♀
184.3 Malignant neoplasm of clitoris ♀
184.4 Malignant neoplasm of vulva, unspecified site ▽ ♀
184.8 Malignant neoplasm of other specified sites of female genital organs ♀
184.9 Malignant neoplasm of female genital organ, site unspecified ▽ ♀
186.9 Malignant neoplasm of other and unspecified testis — (Use additional code to identify any functional activity) ▽ ♂
187.3 Malignant neoplasm of body of penis ♂
187.4 Malignant neoplasm of penis, part unspecified ▽ ♂
187.7 Malignant neoplasm of scrotum ♂
187.8 Malignant neoplasm of other specified sites of male genital organs ♂
187.9 Malignant neoplasm of male genital organ, site unspecified ▽ ♂
195.0 Malignant neoplasm of head, face, and neck
195.3 Malignant neoplasm of pelvis
195.4 Malignant neoplasm of upper limb
198.2 Secondary malignant neoplasm of skin
210.0 Benign neoplasm of lip
210.3 Benign neoplasm of floor of mouth
210.4 Benign neoplasm of other and unspecified parts of mouth ▽
216.5 Benign neoplasm of skin of trunk, except scrotum
216.8 Benign neoplasm of other specified sites of skin
221.2 Benign neoplasm of vulva ♀
222.1 Benign neoplasm of penis ♂
222.4 Benign neoplasm of scrotum ♂
230.0 Carcinoma in situ of lip, oral cavity, and pharynx
232.0 Carcinoma in situ of skin of lip
232.5 Carcinoma in situ of skin of trunk, except scrotum
233.3 Carcinoma in situ of other and unspecified female genital organs ▽ ♀
233.5 Carcinoma in situ of penis ♂
233.6 Carcinoma in situ of other and unspecified male genital organs ▽ ♂
235.1 Neoplasm of uncertain behavior of lip, oral cavity, and pharynx
236.3 Neoplasm of uncertain behavior of other and unspecified female genital organs ▽ ♀
236.6 Neoplasm of uncertain behavior of other and unspecified male genital organs ▽ ♂
238.1 Neoplasm of uncertain behavior of connective and other soft tissue ▽
239.2 Neoplasms of unspecified nature of bone, soft tissue, and skin
619.2 Genital tract-skin fistula, female ♀
619.8 Other specified fistula involving female genital tract ♀
629.20 Female genital mutilation status, unspecified
629.21 Female genital mutilation, Type I status
629.22 Female genital mutilation, Type II status
629.23 Female genital mutilation, Type III status
681.00 Unspecified cellulitis and abscess of finger — (Use additional code to identify organism) ▽
681.10 Unspecified cellulitis and abscess of toe — (Use additional code to identify organism) ▽
682.0 Cellulitis and abscess of face — (Use additional code to identify organism)
682.1 Cellulitis and abscess of neck — (Use additional code to identify organism)
682.4 Cellulitis and abscess of hand, except fingers and thumb — (Use additional code to identify organism)
682.7 Cellulitis and abscess of foot, except toes — (Use additional code to identify organism)
707.00 Decubitus ulcer, unspecified site
707.07 Decubitus ulcer, heel
707.09 Decubitus ulcer, other site
707.14 Ulcer of heel and midfoot
707.15 Ulcer of other part of foot
709.2 Scar condition and fibrosis of skin
752.40 Unspecified congenital anomaly of cervix, vagina, and external female genitalia ▽ ♀
752.69 Other penile anomalies ♂
752.81 Scrotal transposition
752.89 Other specified anomalies of genital organs
754.0 Congenital musculoskeletal deformities of skull, face, and jaw
754.1 Congenital musculoskeletal deformity of sternocleidomastoid muscle
755.10 Syndactyly of multiple and unspecified sites
755.11 Syndactyly of fingers without fusion of bone
755.12 Syndactyly of fingers with fusion of bone
873.41 Open wound of cheek, without mention of complication — (Use additional code to identify infection)
873.42 Open wound of forehead, without mention of complication — (Use additional code to identify infection)
873.43 Open wound of lip, without mention of complication — (Use additional code to identify infection)
873.44 Open wound of jaw, without mention of complication — (Use additional code to identify infection)
873.49 Open wound of face, other and multiple sites, without mention of complication — (Use additional code to identify infection)
873.51 Open wound of cheek, complicated — (Use additional code to identify infection)
873.52 Open wound of forehead, complicated — (Use additional code to identify infection)
873.53 Open wound of lip, complicated — (Use additional code to identify infection)
873.54 Open wound of jaw, complicated — (Use additional code to identify infection)
873.59 Open wound of face, other and multiple sites, complicated — (Use additional code to identify infection)
874.8 Open wound of other and unspecified parts of neck, without mention of complication — (Use additional code to identify infection) ▽
874.9 Open wound of other and unspecified parts of neck, complicated — (Use additional code to identify infection) ▽
878.0 Open wound of penis, without mention of complication — (Use additional code to identify infection) ♂
878.1 Open wound of penis, complicated — (Use additional code to identify infection) ♂
878.2 Open wound of scrotum and testes, without mention of complication — (Use additional code to identify infection) ♂
878.3 Open wound of scrotum and testes, complicated — (Use additional code to identify infection) ♂
878.4 Open wound of vulva, without mention of complication — (Use additional code to identify infection) ♀
878.5 Open wound of vulva, complicated — (Use additional code to identify infection) ♀
878.7 Open wound of vagina, complicated — (Use additional code to identify infection) ♀
878.8 Open wound of other and unspecified parts of genital organs, without mention of complication — (Use additional code to identify infection) ▽

▽ Unspecified code
♀ Female diagnosis
■ Manifestation code
♂ Male diagnosis

878.9 Open wound of other and unspecified parts of genital organs, complicated — (Use additional code to identify infection) ▽
882.0 Open wound of hand except finger(s) alone, without mention of complication — (Use additional code to identify infection)
882.1 Open wound of hand except finger(s) alone, complicated — (Use additional code to identify infection)
882.2 Open wound of hand except finger(s) alone, with tendon involvement — (Use additional code to identify infection)
883.0 Open wound of finger(s), without mention of complication — (Use additional code to identify infection)
883.1 Open wound of finger(s), complicated — (Use additional code to identify infection)
883.2 Open wound of finger(s), with tendon involvement — (Use additional code to identify infection)
885.0 Traumatic amputation of thumb (complete) (partial), without mention of complication — (Use additional code to identify infection)
885.1 Traumatic amputation of thumb (complete) (partial), complicated — (Use additional code to identify infection)
886.0 Traumatic amputation of other finger(s) (complete) (partial), without mention of complication — (Use additional code to identify infection)
886.1 Traumatic amputation of other finger(s) (complete) (partial), complicated — (Use additional code to identify infection)
887.0 Traumatic amputation of arm and hand (complete) (partial), unilateral, below elbow, without mention of complication — (Use additional code to identify infection)
887.1 Traumatic amputation of arm and hand (complete) (partial), unilateral, below elbow, complicated — (Use additional code to identify infection)
887.4 Traumatic amputation of arm and hand (complete) (partial), unilateral, level not specified, without mention of complication — (Use additional code to identify infection) ▽
887.5 Traumatic amputation of arm and hand (complete) (partial), unilateral, level not specified, complicated — (Use additional code to identify infection) ▽
887.6 Traumatic amputation of arm and hand (complete) (partial), bilateral (any level), without mention of complication — (Use additional code to identify infection)
887.7 Traumatic amputation of arm and hand (complete) (partial), bilateral (any level), complicated — (Use additional code to identify infection)
892.0 Open wound of foot except toe(s) alone, without mention of complication — (Use additional code to identify infection)
892.1 Open wound of foot except toe(s) alone, complicated — (Use additional code to identify infection)
892.2 Open wound of foot except toe(s) alone, with tendon involvement — (Use additional code to identify infection)
893.0 Open wound of toe(s), without mention of complication — (Use additional code to identify infection)
893.1 Open wound of toe(s), complicated — (Use additional code to identify infection)
893.2 Open wound of toe(s), with tendon involvement — (Use additional code to identify infection)
895.0 Traumatic amputation of toe(s) (complete) (partial), without mention of complication — (Use additional code to identify infection)
895.1 Traumatic amputation of toe(s) (complete) (partial), complicated — (Use additional code to identify infection)
896.0 Traumatic amputation of foot (complete) (partial), unilateral, without mention of complication — (Use additional code to identify infection)
896.1 Traumatic amputation of foot (complete) (partial), unilateral, complicated — (Use additional code to identify infection)
896.2 Traumatic amputation of foot (complete) (partial), bilateral, without mention of complication — (Use additional code to identify infection)
906.0 Late effect of open wound of head, neck, and trunk
906.1 Late effect of open wound of extremities without mention of tendon injury
906.4 Late effect of crushing
906.5 Late effect of burn of eye, face, head, and neck
906.6 Late effect of burn of wrist and hand
906.7 Late effect of burn of other extremities
906.8 Late effect of burns of other specified sites
909.3 Late effect of complications of surgical and medical care
925.2 Crushing injury of neck — (Use additional code to identify any associated injuries: 800-829, 850.0-854.1, 860.0-869.1)
926.0 Crushing injury of external genitalia — (Use additional code to identify any associated injuries: 800-829, 850.0-854.1, 860.0-869.1)
927.20 Crushing injury of hand(s) — (Use additional code to identify any associated injuries: 800-829, 850.0-854.1, 860.0-869.1)
927.21 Crushing injury of wrist — (Use additional code to identify any associated injuries: 800-829, 850.0-854.1, 860.0-869.1)
928.20 Crushing injury of foot — (Use additional code to identify any associated injuries: 800-829, 850.0-854.1, 860.0-869.1)
928.3 Crushing injury of toe(s) — (Use additional code to identify any associated injuries: 800-829, 850.0-854.1, 860.0-869.1)
928.8 Crushing injury of multiple sites of lower limb — (Use additional code to identify any associated injuries: 800-829, 850.0-854.1, 860.0-869.1)
941.30 Full-thickness skin loss due to burn (third degree nos) of unspecified site of face and head ▽
941.33 Full-thickness skin loss due to burn (third degree nos) of lip(s)
941.35 Full-thickness skin loss due to burn (third degree nos) of nose (septum)
941.37 Full-thickness skin loss due to burn (third degree nos) of forehead and cheek
941.38 Full-thickness skin loss due to burn (third degree nos) of neck
941.39 Full-thickness skin loss due to burn (third degree nos) of multiple sites (except with eye) of face, head, and neck
941.40 Deep necrosis of underlying tissues due to burn (deep third degree) of unspecified site of face and head, without mention of loss of a body part ▽
941.43 Deep necrosis of underlying tissues due to burn (deep third degree) of lip(s), without mention of loss of a body part
941.44 Deep necrosis of underlying tissues due to burn (deep third degree) of chin, without mention of loss of a body part
941.45 Deep necrosis of underlying tissues due to burn (deep third degree) of nose (septum), without mention of loss of a body part
941.47 Deep necrosis of underlying tissues due to burn (deep third degree) of forehead and cheek, without mention of loss of a body part
941.48 Deep necrosis of underlying tissues due to burn (deep third degree) of neck, without mention of loss of a body part
941.49 Deep necrosis of underlying tissues due to burn (deep third degree) of multiple sites (except with eye) of face, head, and neck, without mention of loss of a body part
941.50 Deep necrosis of underlying tissues due to burn (deep third degree) of face and head, unspecified site, with loss of a body part ▽
941.53 Deep necrosis of underlying tissues due to burn (deep third degree) of lip(s), with loss of a body part
941.54 Deep necrosis of underlying tissues due to burn (deep third degree) of chin, with loss of a body part
941.55 Deep necrosis of underlying tissues due to burn (deep third degree) of nose (septum), with loss of a body part
941.57 Deep necrosis of underlying tissues due to burn (deep third degree) of forehead and cheek, with loss of a body part
941.58 Deep necrosis of underlying tissues due to burn (deep third degree) of neck, with loss of a body part
941.59 Deep necrosis of underlying tissues due to burn (deep third degree) of multiple sites (except eye) of face, head, and neck, with loss of a body part
942.35 Full-thickness skin loss due to burn (third degree nos) of genitalia
942.45 Deep necrosis of underlying tissues due to burn (deep third degree) of genitalia, without mention of loss of a body part
942.52 Deep necrosis of underlying tissues due to burn (deep third degree) of chest wall, excluding breast and nipple, with loss of a body part
942.55 Deep necrosis of underlying tissues due to burn (deep third degree) of genitalia, with loss of a body part
944.30 Full-thickness skin loss due to burn (third degree nos) of unspecified site of hand ▽
944.31 Full-thickness skin loss due to burn (third degree nos) of single digit [finger (nail)] other than thumb
944.32 Full-thickness skin loss due to burn (third degree nos) of thumb (nail)
944.33 Full-thickness skin loss due to burn (third degree nos) of two or more digits of hand, not including thumb
944.34 Full-thickness skin loss due to burn (third degree nos) of two or more digits of hand including thumb
944.35 Full-thickness skin loss due to burn (third degree nos) of palm of hand
944.36 Full-thickness skin loss due to burn (third degree nos) of back of hand
944.37 Full-thickness skin loss due to burn (third degree nos) of wrist
944.38 Full-thickness skin loss due to burn (third degree nos) of multiple sites of wrist(s) and hand(s)
944.40 Deep necrosis of underlying tissues due to burn (deep third degree) of unspecified site of hand, without mention of a body part ▽
944.41 Deep necrosis of underlying tissues due to burn (deep third degree) of single digit [finger (nail)] other than thumb, without mention of a body part
944.42 Deep necrosis of underlying tissues due to burn (deep third degree) of thumb (nail), without mention of loss of a body part
944.43 Deep necrosis of underlying tissues due to burn (deep third degree) of two or more digits of hand, not including thumb, without mention of a body part
944.44 Deep necrosis of underlying tissues due to burn (deep third degree) of two or more digits of hand including thumb, without mention of a body part
944.45 Deep necrosis of underlying tissues due to burn (deep third degree) of palm of hand, without mention of loss of a body part

▽ Unspecified code
♀ Female diagnosis
☒ Manifestation code
♂ Male diagnosis

944.46 Deep necrosis of underlying tissues due to burn (deep third degree) of back of hand, without mention of loss of back of a body part
944.47 Deep necrosis of underlying tissues due to burn (deep third degree) of wrist, without mention of loss of a body part
944.48 Deep necrosis of underlying tissues due to burn (deep third degree) of multiple sites of wrist(s) and hand(s), without mention of loss of a body part
944.50 Deep necrosis of underlying tissues due to burn (deep third degree) of unspecified site of hand, with loss of a body part ▽
944.51 Deep necrosis of underlying tissues due to burn (deep third degree) of single digit (finger (nail)) other than thumb, with loss of a body part
944.52 Deep necrosis of underlying tissues due to burn (deep third degree) of thumb (nail), with loss of a body part
945.32 Full-thickness skin loss due to burn (third degree nos) of foot
945.42 Deep necrosis of underlying tissues due to burn (deep third degree) of foot, without mention of loss of a body part
959.09 Injury of face and neck, other and unspecified
959.14 Other injury of external genitals
991.1 Frostbite of hand
996.52 Mechanical complication due to other tissue graft, not elsewhere classified
997.62 Infection (chronic) of amputation stump — (Use additional code to identify organism. Use additional code to identify complications)
997.69 Other late amputation stump complication — (Use additional code to identify complications)
998.59 Other postoperative infection — (Use additional code to identify infection)
998.83 Non-healing surgical wound
V10.02 Personal history of malignant neoplasm of other and unspecified parts of oral cavity and pharynx ▽
V10.21 Personal history of malignant neoplasm of larynx
V51 Aftercare involving the use of plastic surgery

ICD-9-CM Procedural

86.71 Cutting and preparation of pedicle grafts or flaps
86.74 Attachment of pedicle or flap graft to other sites

15630

15630 Delay of flap or sectioning of flap (division and inset); at eyelids, nose, ears, or lips

ICD-9-CM Diagnostic

140.0 Malignant neoplasm of upper lip, vermilion border
140.1 Malignant neoplasm of lower lip, vermilion border
140.3 Malignant neoplasm of upper lip, inner aspect
140.4 Malignant neoplasm of lower lip, inner aspect
140.5 Malignant neoplasm of lip, inner aspect, unspecified as to upper or lower ▽
140.6 Malignant neoplasm of commissure of lip
140.8 Malignant neoplasm of other sites of lip
140.9 Malignant neoplasm of lip, vermilion border, unspecified as to upper or lower ▽
172.0 Malignant melanoma of skin of lip
172.1 Malignant melanoma of skin of eyelid, including canthus
172.2 Malignant melanoma of skin of ear and external auditory canal
172.8 Malignant melanoma of other specified sites of skin
173.0 Other malignant neoplasm of skin of lip
173.1 Other malignant neoplasm of skin of eyelid, including canthus
173.2 Other malignant neoplasm of skin of ear and external auditory canal
173.3 Other malignant neoplasm of skin of other and unspecified parts of face ▽
173.8 Other malignant neoplasm of other specified sites of skin
195.0 Malignant neoplasm of head, face, and neck
210.0 Benign neoplasm of lip
210.4 Benign neoplasm of other and unspecified parts of mouth ▽
216.0 Benign neoplasm of skin of lip
216.1 Benign neoplasm of eyelid, including canthus
216.2 Benign neoplasm of ear and external auditory canal
216.3 Benign neoplasm of skin of other and unspecified parts of face ▽
230.0 Carcinoma in situ of lip, oral cavity, and pharynx
232.1 Carcinoma in situ of eyelid, including canthus
232.2 Carcinoma in situ of skin of ear and external auditory canal
232.3 Carcinoma in situ of skin of other and unspecified parts of face ▽
238.2 Neoplasm of uncertain behavior of skin
239.0 Neoplasm of unspecified nature of digestive system
239.2 Neoplasms of unspecified nature of bone, soft tissue, and skin
380.32 Acquired deformities of auricle or pinna
682.0 Cellulitis and abscess of face — (Use additional code to identify organism)
709.2 Scar condition and fibrosis of skin
709.9 Unspecified disorder of skin and subcutaneous tissue ▽
744.01 Congenital absence of external ear causing impairment of hearing
744.09 Other congenital anomalies of ear causing impairment of hearing
744.23 Microtia
744.3 Unspecified congenital anomaly of ear ▽
744.5 Congenital webbing of neck
744.82 Microcheilia
748.1 Other congenital anomaly of nose
749.01 Unilateral cleft palate, complete
749.02 Unilateral cleft palate, incomplete
749.03 Bilateral cleft palate, complete
749.04 Bilateral cleft palate, incomplete
749.10 Unspecified cleft lip ▽
749.11 Unilateral cleft lip, complete
749.12 Unilateral cleft lip, incomplete
749.13 Bilateral cleft lip, complete
749.14 Bilateral cleft lip, incomplete
749.20 Unspecified cleft palate with cleft lip ▽
749.21 Unilateral cleft palate with cleft lip, complete
749.22 Unilateral cleft palate with cleft lip, incomplete
749.23 Bilateral cleft palate with cleft lip, complete
749.24 Bilateral cleft palate with cleft lip, incomplete
785.4 Gangrene — (Code first any associated underlying condition:250.7, 443.0)
870.0 Laceration of skin of eyelid and periocular area — (Use additional code to identify infection)
870.1 Laceration of eyelid, full-thickness, not involving lacrimal passages — (Use additional code to identify infection)
870.2 Laceration of eyelid involving lacrimal passages — (Use additional code to identify infection)
872.00 Open wound of external ear, unspecified site, without mention of complication — (Use additional code to identify infection) ▽
872.01 Open wound of auricle, without mention of complication — (Use additional code to identify infection)
872.02 Open wound of auditory canal, without mention of complication — (Use additional code to identify infection)
872.10 Open wound of external ear, unspecified site, complicated — (Use additional code to identify infection) ▽
872.11 Open wound of auricle, complicated — (Use additional code to identify infection)
872.12 Open wound of auditory canal, complicated — (Use additional code to identify infection)
872.8 Open wound of ear, part unspecified, without mention of complication — (Use additional code to identify infection) ▽
872.9 Open wound of ear, part unspecified, complicated — (Use additional code to identify infection) ▽
873.20 Open wound of nose, unspecified site, without mention of complication — (Use additional code to identify infection) ▽
873.30 Open wound of nose, unspecified site, complicated — (Use additional code to identify infection) ▽
873.31 Open wound of nasal septum, complicated — (Use additional code to identify infection)
873.32 Open wound of nasal cavity, complicated — (Use additional code to identify infection)
873.33 Open wound of nasal sinus, complicated — (Use additional code to identify infection)
873.39 Open wound of nose, multiple sites, complicated — (Use additional code to identify infection)
873.41 Open wound of cheek, without mention of complication — (Use additional code to identify infection)
873.42 Open wound of forehead, without mention of complication — (Use additional code to identify infection)
873.43 Open wound of lip, without mention of complication — (Use additional code to identify infection)
873.44 Open wound of jaw, without mention of complication — (Use additional code to identify infection)
873.51 Open wound of cheek, complicated — (Use additional code to identify infection)
873.52 Open wound of forehead, complicated — (Use additional code to identify infection)
873.53 Open wound of lip, complicated — (Use additional code to identify infection)
873.54 Open wound of jaw, complicated — (Use additional code to identify infection)
874.8 Open wound of other and unspecified parts of neck, without mention of complication — (Use additional code to identify infection) ▽
906.0 Late effect of open wound of head, neck, and trunk
906.5 Late effect of burn of eye, face, head, and neck
941.01 Burn of unspecified degree of ear (any part) ▽
941.02 Burn of unspecified degree of eye (with other parts of face, head, and neck) ▽
941.03 Burn of unspecified degree of lip(s) ▽

941.05 Burn of unspecified degree of nose (septum) ▽
941.09 Burn of unspecified degree of multiple sites (except with eye) of face, head, and neck ▽
941.31 Full-thickness skin loss due to burn (third degree nos) of ear (any part)
941.32 Full-thickness skin loss due to burn (third degree nos) of eye (with other parts of face, head, and neck)
941.33 Full-thickness skin loss due to burn (third degree nos) of lip(s)
941.35 Full-thickness skin loss due to burn (third degree nos) of nose (septum)
941.39 Full-thickness skin loss due to burn (third degree nos) of multiple sites (except with eye) of face, head, and neck
941.49 Deep necrosis of underlying tissues due to burn (deep third degree) of multiple sites (except with eye) of face, head, and neck, without mention of loss of a body part
941.51 Deep necrosis of underlying tissues due to burn (deep third degree) of ear (any part), with loss of a body part
941.52 Deep necrosis of underlying tissues due to burn (deep third degree) of eye (with other parts of face, head, and neck), with loss of a body part
941.53 Deep necrosis of underlying tissues due to burn (deep third degree) of lip(s), with loss of a body part
941.55 Deep necrosis of underlying tissues due to burn (deep third degree) of nose (septum), with loss of a body part
941.59 Deep necrosis of underlying tissues due to burn (deep third degree) of multiple sites (except eye) of face, head, and neck, with loss of a body part
946.3 Full-thickness skin loss due to burn (third degree nos) of multiple specified sites
946.4 Deep necrosis of underlying tissues due to burn (deep third degree) of multiple specified sites, without mention of loss of a body part
946.5 Deep necrosis of underlying tissues due to burn (deep third degree) of multiple specified sites, with loss of a body part
948.00 Burn (any degree) involving less than 10% of body surface with third degree burn of less than 10% or unspecified amount
948.10 Burn (any degree) involving 10-19% of body surface with third degree burn of less than 10% or unspecified amount
948.11 Burn (any degree) involving 10-19% of body surface with third degree burn of 10-19%
948.20 Burn (any degree) involving 20-29% of body surface with third degree burn of less than 10% or unspecified amount
948.21 Burn (any degree) involving 20-29% of body surface with third degree burn of 10-19%
948.22 Burn (any degree) involving 20-29% of body surface with third degree burn of 20-29%
948.30 Burn (any degree) involving 30-39% of body surface with third degree burn of less than 10% or unspecified amount
948.31 Burn (any degree) involving 30-39% of body surface with third degree burn of 10-19%
948.32 Burn (any degree) involving 30-39% of body surface with third degree burn of 20-29%
948.33 Burn (any degree) involving 30-39% of body surface with third degree burn of 30-39%
948.40 Burn (any degree) involving 40-49% of body surface with third degree burn of less than 10% or unspecified amount
948.41 Burn (any degree) involving 40-49% of body surface with third degree burn of 10-19%
948.42 Burn (any degree) involving 40-49% of body surface with third degree burn of 20-29%
948.43 Burn (any degree) involving 40-49% of body surface with third degree burn of 30-39%
948.44 Burn (any degree) involving 40-49% of body surface with third degree burn of 40-49%
948.50 Burn (any degree) involving 50-59% of body surface with third degree burn of less than 10% or unspecified amount
948.51 Burn (any degree) involving 50-59% of body surface with third degree burn of 10-19%
948.52 Burn (any degree) involving 50-59% of body surface with third degree burn of 20-29%
948.53 Burn (any degree) involving 50-59% of body surface with third degree burn of 30-39%
948.54 Burn (any degree) involving 50-59% of body surface with third degree burn of 40-49%
948.55 Burn (any degree) involving 50-59% of body surface with third degree burn of 50-59%
948.60 Burn (any degree) involving 60-69% of body surface with third degree burn of less than 10% or unspecified amount
948.61 Burn (any degree) involving 60-69% of body surface with third degree burn of 10-19%
948.62 Burn (any degree) involving 60-69% of body surface with third degree burn of 20-29%
948.63 Burn (any degree) involving 60-69% of body surface with third degree burn of 30-39%
948.64 Burn (any degree) involving 60-69% of body surface with third degree burn of 40-49%
948.65 Burn (any degree) involving 60-69% of body surface with third degree burn of 50-59%
948.66 Burn (any degree) involving 60-69% of body surface with third degree burn of 60-69%
948.70 Burn (any degree) involving 70-79% of body surface with third degree burn of less than 10% or unspecified amount
948.71 Burn (any degree) involving 70-79% of body surface with third degree burn of 10-19%
948.72 Burn (any degree) involving 70-79% of body surface with third degree burn of 20-29%
948.73 Burn (any degree) involving 70-79% of body surface with third degree burn of 30-39%
948.74 Burn (any degree) involving 70-79% of body surface with third degree burn of 40-49%
948.75 Burn (any degree) involving 70-79% of body surface with third degree burn of 50-59%
948.76 Burn (any degree) involving 70-79% of body surface with third degree burn of 60-69%
948.77 Burn (any degree) involving 70-79% of body surface with third degree burn of 70-79%
948.80 Burn (any degree) involving 80-89% of body surface with third degree burn of less than 10% or unspecified amount
948.81 Burn (any degree) involving 80-89% of body surface with third degree burn of 10-19%
948.82 Burn (any degree) involving 80-89% of body surface with third degree burn of 20-29%
948.83 Burn (any degree) involving 80-89% of body surface with third degree burn of 30-39%
948.84 Burn (any degree) involving 80-89% of body surface with third degree burn of 40-49%
948.85 Burn (any degree) involving 80-89% of body surface with third degree burn of 50-59%
948.86 Burn (any degree) involving 80-89% of body surface with third degree burn of 60-69%
948.87 Burn (any degree) involving 80-89% of body surface with third degree burn of 70-79%
948.88 Burn (any degree) involving 80-89% of body surface with third degree burn of 80-89%
959.09 Injury of face and neck, other and unspecified
996.52 Mechanical complication due to other tissue graft, not elsewhere classified
998.59 Other postoperative infection — (Use additional code to identify infection)
998.83 Non-healing surgical wound
V10.02 Personal history of malignant neoplasm of other and unspecified parts of oral cavity and pharynx ▽
V51 Aftercare involving the use of plastic surgery
V84.09 Genetic susceptibility to other malignant neoplasm

ICD-9-CM Procedural

18.79 Other plastic repair of external ear
27.57 Attachment of pedicle or flap graft to lip and mouth
86.71 Cutting and preparation of pedicle grafts or flaps

15650

15650 Transfer, intermediate, of any pedicle flap (eg, abdomen to wrist, Walking tube), any location

ICD-9-CM Diagnostic

172.0 Malignant melanoma of skin of lip
172.1 Malignant melanoma of skin of eyelid, including canthus
172.2 Malignant melanoma of skin of ear and external auditory canal
172.3 Malignant melanoma of skin of other and unspecified parts of face
172.4 Malignant melanoma of skin of scalp and neck
172.5 Malignant melanoma of skin of trunk, except scrotum
172.6 Malignant melanoma of skin of upper limb, including shoulder
172.7 Malignant melanoma of skin of lower limb, including hip
172.8 Malignant melanoma of other specified sites of skin
173.0 Other malignant neoplasm of skin of lip
173.1 Other malignant neoplasm of skin of eyelid, including canthus
173.2 Other malignant neoplasm of skin of ear and external auditory canal
173.3 Other malignant neoplasm of skin of other and unspecified parts of face ▽

▽ Unspecified code
♀ Female diagnosis
⊠ Manifestation code
♂ Male diagnosis

173.4 Other malignant neoplasm of scalp and skin of neck
173.5 Other malignant neoplasm of skin of trunk, except scrotum
173.6 Other malignant neoplasm of skin of upper limb, including shoulder
173.7 Other malignant neoplasm of skin of lower limb, including hip
173.8 Other malignant neoplasm of other specified sites of skin
174.0 Malignant neoplasm of nipple and areola of female breast ♀
175.0 Malignant neoplasm of nipple and areola of male breast ♂
198.2 Secondary malignant neoplasm of skin
210.0 Benign neoplasm of lip
232.0 Carcinoma in situ of skin of lip
232.1 Carcinoma in situ of eyelid, including canthus
232.2 Carcinoma in situ of skin of ear and external auditory canal
232.3 Carcinoma in situ of skin of other and unspecified parts of face ▽
232.4 Carcinoma in situ of scalp and skin of neck
232.5 Carcinoma in situ of skin of trunk, except scrotum
232.6 Carcinoma in situ of skin of upper limb, including shoulder
232.7 Carcinoma in situ of skin of lower limb, including hip
232.8 Carcinoma in situ of other specified sites of skin
235.1 Neoplasm of uncertain behavior of lip, oral cavity, and pharynx
238.2 Neoplasm of uncertain behavior of skin
239.0 Neoplasm of unspecified nature of digestive system
239.2 Neoplasms of unspecified nature of bone, soft tissue, and skin
250.70 Diabetes with peripheral circulatory disorders, type II or unspecified type, not stated as uncontrolled — (Use additional code to identify manifestation: 443.81, 785.4)
250.71 Diabetes with peripheral circulatory disorders, type I [juvenile type], not stated as uncontrolled — (Use additional code to identify manifestation: 443.81, 785.4)
250.72 Diabetes with peripheral circulatory disorders, type II or unspecified type, uncontrolled — (Use additional code to identify manifestation: 443.81, 785.4)
250.73 Diabetes with peripheral circulatory disorders, type I [juvenile type], uncontrolled — (Use additional code to identify manifestation: 443.81, 785.4)
443.81 Peripheral angiopathy in diseases classified elsewhere — (Code first underlying disease, 250.7) ☒
454.0 Varicose veins of lower extremities with ulcer
454.2 Varicose veins of lower extremities with ulcer and inflammation
454.8 Varicose veins of the lower extremities with other complications
459.11 Postphlebitic syndrome with ulcer
459.13 Postphlebitic syndrome with ulcer and inflammation
459.19 Postphlebitic syndrome with other complication
459.31 Chronic venous hypertension with ulcer
459.33 Chronic venous hypertension with ulcer and inflammation
459.39 Chronic venous hypertension with other complication
681.00 Unspecified cellulitis and abscess of finger — (Use additional code to identify organism) ▽
681.01 Felon — (Use additional code to identify organism)
681.02 Onychia and paronychia of finger — (Use additional code to identify organism)
681.10 Unspecified cellulitis and abscess of toe — (Use additional code to identify organism) ▽
681.11 Onychia and paronychia of toe — (Use additional code to identify organism)
682.0 Cellulitis and abscess of face — (Use additional code to identify organism)
682.1 Cellulitis and abscess of neck — (Use additional code to identify organism)
682.2 Cellulitis and abscess of trunk — (Use additional code to identify organism)
682.3 Cellulitis and abscess of upper arm and forearm — (Use additional code to identify organism)
682.4 Cellulitis and abscess of hand, except fingers and thumb — (Use additional code to identify organism)
682.5 Cellulitis and abscess of buttock — (Use additional code to identify organism)
682.6 Cellulitis and abscess of leg, except foot — (Use additional code to identify organism)
682.7 Cellulitis and abscess of foot, except toes — (Use additional code to identify organism)
682.8 Cellulitis and abscess of other specified site — (Use additional code to identify organism)
707.00 Decubitus ulcer, unspecified site
707.01 Decubitus ulcer, elbow
707.02 Decubitus ulcer, upper back
707.03 Decubitus ulcer, lower back
707.04 Decubitus ulcer, hip
707.05 Decubitus ulcer, buttock
707.06 Decubitus ulcer, ankle
707.07 Decubitus ulcer, heel
707.09 Decubitus ulcer, other site
707.10 Ulcer of lower limb, unspecified ▽
707.11 Ulcer of thigh
707.12 Ulcer of calf
707.13 Ulcer of ankle
707.14 Ulcer of heel and midfoot
707.15 Ulcer of other part of foot
707.19 Ulcer of other part of lower limb
707.8 Chronic ulcer of other specified site
707.9 Chronic ulcer of unspecified site ▽
709.2 Scar condition and fibrosis of skin
709.9 Unspecified disorder of skin and subcutaneous tissue ▽
728.86 Necrotizing fasciitis — (Use additional code to identify infectious organism, 041.00-041.89, 785.4, if applicable)
754.0 Congenital musculoskeletal deformities of skull, face, and jaw
756.70 Unspecified congenital anomaly of abdominal wall ▽
756.71 Prune belly syndrome
756.79 Other congenital anomalies of abdominal wall
785.4 Gangrene — (Code first any associated underlying condition:250.7, 443.0)
880.00 Open wound of shoulder region, without mention of complication — (Use additional code to identify infection)
880.01 Open wound of scapular region, without mention of complication — (Use additional code to identify infection)
880.02 Open wound of axillary region, without mention of complication — (Use additional code to identify infection)
880.03 Open wound of upper arm, without mention of complication — (Use additional code to identify infection)
880.09 Open wound of multiple sites of shoulder and upper arm, without mention of complication — (Use additional code to identify infection)
880.10 Open wound of shoulder region, complicated — (Use additional code to identify infection)
880.11 Open wound of scapular region, complicated — (Use additional code to identify infection)
880.12 Open wound of axillary region, complicated — (Use additional code to identify infection)
880.13 Open wound of upper arm, complicated — (Use additional code to identify infection)
880.19 Open wound of multiple sites of shoulder and upper arm, complicated — (Use additional code to identify infection)
880.20 Open wound of shoulder region, with tendon involvement — (Use additional code to identify infection)
880.21 Open wound of scapular region, with tendon involvement — (Use additional code to identify infection)
880.22 Open wound of axillary region, with tendon involvement — (Use additional code to identify infection)
880.23 Open wound of upper arm, with tendon involvement — (Use additional code to identify infection)
880.29 Open wound of multiple sites of shoulder and upper arm, with tendon involvement — (Use additional code to identify infection)
881.00 Open wound of forearm, without mention of complication — (Use additional code to identify infection)
881.01 Open wound of elbow, without mention of complication — (Use additional code to identify infection)
881.02 Open wound of wrist, without mention of complication — (Use additional code to identify infection)
881.10 Open wound of forearm, complicated — (Use additional code to identify infection)
881.11 Open wound of elbow, complicated — (Use additional code to identify infection)
881.12 Open wound of wrist, complicated — (Use additional code to identify infection)
881.20 Open wound of forearm, with tendon involvement — (Use additional code to identify infection)
881.21 Open wound of elbow, with tendon involvement — (Use additional code to identify infection)
881.22 Open wound of wrist, with tendon involvement — (Use additional code to identify infection)
882.0 Open wound of hand except finger(s) alone, without mention of complication — (Use additional code to identify infection)
882.1 Open wound of hand except finger(s) alone, complicated — (Use additional code to identify infection)
882.2 Open wound of hand except finger(s) alone, with tendon involvement — (Use additional code to identify infection)
883.0 Open wound of finger(s), without mention of complication — (Use additional code to identify infection)
883.1 Open wound of finger(s), complicated — (Use additional code to identify infection)
883.2 Open wound of finger(s), with tendon involvement — (Use additional code to identify infection)

▽ Unspecified code
♀ Female diagnosis
☒ Manifestation code
♂ Male diagnosis

884.0 Multiple and unspecified open wound of upper limb, without mention of complication — (Use additional code to identify infection)
884.1 Multiple and unspecified open wound of upper limb, complicated — (Use additional code to identify infection)
884.2 Multiple and unspecified open wound of upper limb, with tendon involvement — (Use additional code to identify infection)
885.0 Traumatic amputation of thumb (complete) (partial), without mention of complication — (Use additional code to identify infection)
885.1 Traumatic amputation of thumb (complete) (partial), complicated — (Use additional code to identify infection)
886.0 Traumatic amputation of other finger(s) (complete) (partial), without mention of complication — (Use additional code to identify infection)
886.1 Traumatic amputation of other finger(s) (complete) (partial), complicated — (Use additional code to identify infection)
887.2 Traumatic amputation of arm and hand (complete) (partial), unilateral, at or above elbow, without mention of complication — (Use additional code to identify infection)
887.3 Traumatic amputation of arm and hand (complete) (partial), unilateral, at or above elbow, complicated — (Use additional code to identify infection)
887.4 Traumatic amputation of arm and hand (complete) (partial), unilateral, level not specified, without mention of complication — (Use additional code to identify infection) ▽
887.5 Traumatic amputation of arm and hand (complete) (partial), unilateral, level not specified, complicated — (Use additional code to identify infection) ▽
887.6 Traumatic amputation of arm and hand (complete) (partial), bilateral (any level), without mention of complication — (Use additional code to identify infection)
887.7 Traumatic amputation of arm and hand (complete) (partial), bilateral (any level), complicated — (Use additional code to identify infection)
890.0 Open wound of hip and thigh, without mention of complication — (Use additional code to identify infection)
890.1 Open wound of hip and thigh, complicated — (Use additional code to identify infection)
890.2 Open wound of hip and thigh, with tendon involvement — (Use additional code to identify infection)
891.0 Open wound of knee, leg (except thigh), and ankle, without mention of complication — (Use additional code to identify infection)
891.1 Open wound of knee, leg (except thigh), and ankle, complicated — (Use additional code to identify infection)
891.2 Open wound of knee, leg (except thigh), and ankle, with tendon involvement — (Use additional code to identify infection)
892.0 Open wound of foot except toe(s) alone, without mention of complication — (Use additional code to identify infection)
892.1 Open wound of foot except toe(s) alone, complicated — (Use additional code to identify infection)
892.2 Open wound of foot except toe(s) alone, with tendon involvement — (Use additional code to identify infection)
893.0 Open wound of toe(s), without mention of complication — (Use additional code to identify infection)
893.1 Open wound of toe(s), complicated — (Use additional code to identify infection)
893.2 Open wound of toe(s), with tendon involvement — (Use additional code to identify infection)
894.0 Multiple and unspecified open wound of lower limb, without mention of complication — (Use additional code to identify infection)
894.1 Multiple and unspecified open wound of lower limb, complicated — (Use additional code to identify infection)
894.2 Multiple and unspecified open wound of lower limb, with tendon involvement — (Use additional code to identify infection)
895.0 Traumatic amputation of toe(s) (complete) (partial), without mention of complication — (Use additional code to identify infection)
895.1 Traumatic amputation of toe(s) (complete) (partial), complicated — (Use additional code to identify infection)
896.0 Traumatic amputation of foot (complete) (partial), unilateral, without mention of complication — (Use additional code to identify infection)
896.1 Traumatic amputation of foot (complete) (partial), unilateral, complicated — (Use additional code to identify infection)
896.2 Traumatic amputation of foot (complete) (partial), bilateral, without mention of complication — (Use additional code to identify infection)
896.3 Traumatic amputation of foot (complete) (partial), bilateral, complicated — (Use additional code to identify infection)
897.0 Traumatic amputation of leg(s) (complete) (partial), unilateral, below knee, without mention of complication — (Use additional code to identify infection)
897.1 Traumatic amputation of leg(s) (complete) (partial), unilateral, below knee, complicated — (Use additional code to identify infection)
897.2 Traumatic amputation of leg(s) (complete) (partial), unilateral, at or above knee, without mention of complication — (Use additional code to identify infection)
897.3 Traumatic amputation of leg(s) (complete) (partial), unilateral, at or above knee, complicated — (Use additional code to identify infection)
897.4 Traumatic amputation of leg(s) (complete) (partial), unilateral, level not specified, without mention of complication — (Use additional code to identify infection) ▽
897.5 Traumatic amputation of leg(s) (complete) (partial), unilateral, level not specified, complicated — (Use additional code to identify infection) ▽
897.6 Traumatic amputation of leg(s) (complete) (partial), bilateral (any level), without mention of complication — (Use additional code to identify infection)
897.7 Traumatic amputation of leg(s) (complete) (partial), bilateral (any level), complicated — (Use additional code to identify infection)
906.0 Late effect of open wound of head, neck, and trunk
906.1 Late effect of open wound of extremities without mention of tendon injury
906.5 Late effect of burn of eye, face, head, and neck
906.6 Late effect of burn of wrist and hand
906.7 Late effect of burn of other extremities
906.8 Late effect of burns of other specified sites
906.9 Late effect of burn of unspecified site ▽
941.30 Full-thickness skin loss due to burn (third degree nos) of unspecified site of face and head ▽
941.31 Full-thickness skin loss due to burn (third degree nos) of ear (any part)
941.32 Full-thickness skin loss due to burn (third degree nos) of eye (with other parts of face, head, and neck)
941.33 Full-thickness skin loss due to burn (third degree nos) of lip(s)
941.34 Full-thickness skin loss due to burn (third degree nos) of chin
941.35 Full-thickness skin loss due to burn (third degree nos) of nose (septum)
941.36 Full-thickness skin loss due to burn (third degree nos) of scalp (any part)
941.37 Full-thickness skin loss due to burn (third degree nos) of forehead and cheek
941.38 Full-thickness skin loss due to burn (third degree nos) of neck
941.39 Full-thickness skin loss due to burn (third degree nos) of multiple sites (except with eye) of face, head, and neck
941.40 Deep necrosis of underlying tissues due to burn (deep third degree) of unspecified site of face and head, without mention of loss of a body part ▽
941.41 Deep necrosis of underlying tissues due to burn (deep third degree) of ear (any part), without mention of loss of a body part
941.42 Deep necrosis of underlying tissues due to burn (deep third degree) of eye (with other parts of face, head, and neck), without mention of loss of a body part
941.43 Deep necrosis of underlying tissues due to burn (deep third degree) of lip(s), without mention of loss of a body part
941.44 Deep necrosis of underlying tissues due to burn (deep third degree) of chin, without mention of loss of a body part
941.45 Deep necrosis of underlying tissues due to burn (deep third degree) of nose (septum), without mention of loss of a body part
941.46 Deep necrosis of underlying tissues due to burn (deep third degree) of scalp (any part), without mention of loss of a body part
941.47 Deep necrosis of underlying tissues due to burn (deep third degree) of forehead and cheek, without mention of loss of a body part
941.48 Deep necrosis of underlying tissues due to burn (deep third degree) of neck, without mention of loss of a body part
941.49 Deep necrosis of underlying tissues due to burn (deep third degree) of multiple sites (except with eye) of face, head, and neck, without mention of loss of a body part
941.50 Deep necrosis of underlying tissues due to burn (deep third degree) of face and head, unspecified site, with loss of a body part ▽
941.51 Deep necrosis of underlying tissues due to burn (deep third degree) of ear (any part), with loss of a body part
941.52 Deep necrosis of underlying tissues due to burn (deep third degree) of eye (with other parts of face, head, and neck), with loss of a body part
941.53 Deep necrosis of underlying tissues due to burn (deep third degree) of lip(s), with loss of a body part
941.54 Deep necrosis of underlying tissues due to burn (deep third degree) of chin, with loss of a body part
941.55 Deep necrosis of underlying tissues due to burn (deep third degree) of nose (septum), with loss of a body part
941.56 Deep necrosis of underlying tissues due to burn (deep third degree) of scalp (any part), with loss of a body part
941.57 Deep necrosis of underlying tissues due to burn (deep third degree) of forehead and cheek, with loss of a body part
941.58 Deep necrosis of underlying tissues due to burn (deep third degree) of neck, with loss of a body part
941.59 Deep necrosis of underlying tissues due to burn (deep third degree) of multiple sites (except eye) of face, head, and neck, with loss of a body part

▽ Unspecified code
♀ Female diagnosis
☒ Manifestation code
♂ Male diagnosis

942.30 Full-thickness skin loss due to burn (third degree nos) of unspecified site of trunk ▽
942.31 Full-thickness skin loss due to burn (third degree nos) of breast
942.32 Full-thickness skin loss due to burn (third degree nos) of chest wall, excluding breast and nipple
942.33 Full-thickness skin loss due to burn (third degree nos) of abdominal wall
942.34 Full-thickness skin loss due to burn (third degree nos) of back (any part)
942.35 Full-thickness skin loss due to burn (third degree nos) of genitalia
942.39 Full-thickness skin loss due to burn (third degree nos) of other and multiple sites of trunk
942.40 Deep necrosis of underlying tissues due to burn (deep third degree) of trunk, unspecified site, without mention of loss of a body part ▽
942.41 Deep necrosis of underlying tissues due to burn (deep third degree) of breast, without mention of loss of a body part
942.42 Deep necrosis of underlying tissues due to burn (deep third degree) of chest wall, excluding breast and nipple, without mention of loss of a body part
942.43 Deep necrosis of underlying tissues due to burn (deep third degree) of abdominal wall, without mention of loss of a body part
942.44 Deep necrosis of underlying tissues due to burn (deep third degree) of back (any part), without mention of loss of a body part
942.45 Deep necrosis of underlying tissues due to burn (deep third degree) of genitalia, without mention of loss of a body part
942.49 Deep necrosis of underlying tissues due to burn (deep third degree) of other and multiple sites of trunk, without mention of loss of a body part
942.50 Deep necrosis of underlying tissues due to burn (deep third degree) of unspecified site of trunk, with loss of a body part ▽
942.51 Deep necrosis of underlying tissues due to burn (deep third degree) of breast, with loss of a body part
942.52 Deep necrosis of underlying tissues due to burn (deep third degree) of chest wall, excluding breast and nipple, with loss of a body part
942.53 Deep necrosis of underlying tissues due to burn (deep third degree) of abdominal wall with loss of a body part
942.54 Deep necrosis of underlying tissues due to burn (deep third degree) of back (any part), with loss of a body part
942.55 Deep necrosis of underlying tissues due to burn (deep third degree) of genitalia, with loss of a body part
942.59 Deep necrosis of underlying tissues due to burn (deep third degree) of other and multiple sites of trunk, with loss of a body part
943.30 Full-thickness skin loss due to burn (third degree nos) of unspecified site of upper limb ▽
943.31 Full-thickness skin loss due to burn (third degree nos) of forearm
943.32 Full-thickness skin loss due to burn (third degree nos) of elbow
943.33 Full-thickness skin loss due to burn (third degree nos) of upper arm
943.34 Full-thickness skin loss due to burn (third degree nos) of axilla
943.35 Full-thickness skin loss due to burn (third degree nos) of shoulder
943.36 Full-thickness skin loss due to burn (third degree nos) of scapular region
943.39 Full-thickness skin loss due to burn (third degree nos) of multiple sites of upper limb, except wrist and hand
943.40 Deep necrosis of underlying tissues due to burn (deep third degree) of unspecified site of upper limb, without mention of loss of a body part ▽
943.41 Deep necrosis of underlying tissues due to burn (deep third degree) of forearm, without mention of loss of a body part
943.42 Deep necrosis of underlying tissues due to burn (deep third degree) of elbow, without mention of loss of a body part
943.43 Deep necrosis of underlying tissues due to burn (deep third degree) of upper arm, without mention of loss of a body part
943.44 Deep necrosis of underlying tissues due to burn (deep third degree) of axilla, without mention of loss of a body part
943.45 Deep necrosis of underlying tissues due to burn (deep third degree) of shoulder, without mention of loss of a body part
943.46 Deep necrosis of underlying tissues due to burn (deep third degree) of scapular region, without mention of loss of a body part
943.49 Deep necrosis of underlying tissues due to burn (deep third degree) of multiple sites of upper limb, except wrist and hand, without mention of loss of a body part
943.50 Deep necrosis of underlying tissues due to burn (deep third degree) of unspecified site of upper limb, with loss of a body part ▽
943.51 Deep necrosis of underlying tissues due to burn (deep third degree) of forearm, with loss of a body part
943.52 Deep necrosis of underlying tissues due to burn (deep third degree) of elbow, with loss of a body part
943.53 Deep necrosis of underlying tissues due to burn (deep third degree) of upper arm, with loss of upper a body part
943.54 Deep necrosis of underlying tissues due to burn (deep third degree) of axilla, with loss of a body part
943.55 Deep necrosis of underlying tissues due to burn (deep third degree) of shoulder, with loss of a body part
943.56 Deep necrosis of underlying tissues due to burn (deep third degree) of scapular region, with loss of a body part
943.59 Deep necrosis of underlying tissues due to burn (deep third degree) of multiple sites of upper limb, except wrist and hand, with loss of a body part
944.30 Full-thickness skin loss due to burn (third degree nos) of unspecified site of hand ▽
944.31 Full-thickness skin loss due to burn (third degree nos) of single digit [finger (nail)] other than thumb
944.32 Full-thickness skin loss due to burn (third degree nos) of thumb (nail)
944.33 Full-thickness skin loss due to burn (third degree nos) of two or more digits of hand, not including thumb
944.34 Full-thickness skin loss due to burn (third degree nos) of two or more digits of hand including thumb
944.35 Full-thickness skin loss due to burn (third degree nos) of palm of hand
944.36 Full-thickness skin loss due to burn (third degree nos) of back of hand
944.37 Full-thickness skin loss due to burn (third degree nos) of wrist
944.38 Full-thickness skin loss due to burn (third degree nos) of multiple sites of wrist(s) and hand(s)
944.40 Deep necrosis of underlying tissues due to burn (deep third degree) of unspecified site of hand, without mention of a body part ▽
944.41 Deep necrosis of underlying tissues due to burn (deep third degree) of single digit [finger (nail)] other than thumb, without mention of a body part
944.42 Deep necrosis of underlying tissues due to burn (deep third degree) of thumb (nail), without mention of loss of a body part
944.43 Deep necrosis of underlying tissues due to burn (deep third degree) of two or more digits of hand, not including thumb, without mention of a body part
944.44 Deep necrosis of underlying tissues due to burn (deep third degree) of two or more digits of hand including thumb, without mention of a body part
944.45 Deep necrosis of underlying tissues due to burn (deep third degree) of palm of hand, without mention of loss of a body part
944.46 Deep necrosis of underlying tissues due to burn (deep third degree) of back of hand, without mention of loss of back of a body part
944.47 Deep necrosis of underlying tissues due to burn (deep third degree) of wrist, without mention of loss of a body part
944.48 Deep necrosis of underlying tissues due to burn (deep third degree) of multiple sites of wrist(s) and hand(s), without mention of loss of a body part
944.50 Deep necrosis of underlying tissues due to burn (deep third degree) of unspecified site of hand, with loss of a body part ▽
944.51 Deep necrosis of underlying tissues due to burn (deep third degree) of single digit (finger (nail)) other than thumb, with loss of a body part
944.52 Deep necrosis of underlying tissues due to burn (deep third degree) of thumb (nail), with loss of a body part
944.53 Deep necrosis of underlying tissues due to burn (deep third degree) of two or more digits of hand, not including thumb, with loss of a body part
944.54 Deep necrosis of underlying tissues due to burn (deep third degree) of two or more digits of hand including thumb, with loss of a body part
944.55 Deep necrosis of underlying tissues due to burn (deep third degree) of palm of hand, with loss of a body part
944.56 Deep necrosis of underlying tissues due to burn (deep third degree) of back of hand, with loss of a body part
944.57 Deep necrosis of underlying tissues due to burn (deep third degree) of wrist, with loss of a body part
944.58 Deep necrosis of underlying tissues due to burn (deep third degree) of multiple sites of wrist(s) and hand(s), with loss of a body part
945.30 Full-thickness skin loss due to burn (third degree nos) of unspecified site of lower limb ▽
945.31 Full-thickness skin loss due to burn (third degree nos) of toe(s) (nail)
945.32 Full-thickness skin loss due to burn (third degree nos) of foot
945.33 Full-thickness skin loss due to burn (third degree nos) of ankle
945.34 Full-thickness skin loss due to burn (third degree nos) of lower leg
945.35 Full-thickness skin loss due to burn (third degree nos) of knee
945.36 Full-thickness skin loss due to burn (third degree nos) of thigh (any part)
945.39 Full-thickness skin loss due to burn (third degree nos) of multiple sites of lower limb(s)
945.40 Deep necrosis of underlying tissues due to burn (deep third degree) of unspecified site of lower limb (leg), without mention of loss of a body part ▽
945.41 Deep necrosis of underlying tissues due to burn (deep third degree) of toe(s) (nail), without mention of loss of a body part
945.42 Deep necrosis of underlying tissues due to burn (deep third degree) of foot, without mention of loss of a body part
945.43 Deep necrosis of underlying tissues due to burn (deep third degree) of ankle, without mention of loss of a body part
945.44 Deep necrosis of underlying tissues due to burn (deep third degree) of lower leg, without mention of loss of a body part

▽ Unspecified code
♀ Female diagnosis
☒ Manifestation code
♂ Male diagnosis

945.45 Deep necrosis of underlying tissues due to burn (deep third degree) of knee, without mention of loss of a body part
945.46 Deep necrosis of underlying tissues due to burn (deep third degree) of thigh (any part), without mention of loss of a body part
945.49 Deep necrosis of underlying tissues due to burn (deep third degree) of multiple sites of lower limb(s), without mention of loss of a body part
945.50 Deep necrosis of underlying tissues due to burn (deep third degree) of unspecified site lower limb (leg), with loss of a body part
945.51 Deep necrosis of underlying tissues due to burn (deep third degree) of toe(s) (nail), with loss of a body part
945.52 Deep necrosis of underlying tissues due to burn (deep third degree) of foot, with loss of a body part
945.53 Deep necrosis of underlying tissues due to burn (deep third degree) of ankle, with loss of a body part
945.54 Deep necrosis of underlying tissues due to burn (deep third degree) of lower leg, with loss of a body part
945.55 Deep necrosis of underlying tissues due to burn (deep third degree) of knee, with loss of a body part
945.56 Deep necrosis of underlying tissues due to burn (deep third degree) of thigh (any part), with loss of a body part
945.59 Deep necrosis of underlying tissues due to burn (deep third degree) of multiple sites of lower limb(s), with loss of a body part
946.3 Full-thickness skin loss due to burn (third degree nos) of multiple specified sites
946.4 Deep necrosis of underlying tissues due to burn (deep third degree) of multiple specified sites, without mention of loss of a body part
946.5 Deep necrosis of underlying tissues due to burn (deep third degree) of multiple specified sites, with loss of a body part
948.00 Burn (any degree) involving less than 10% of body surface with third degree burn of less than 10% or unspecified amount
948.10 Burn (any degree) involving 10-19% of body surface with third degree burn of less than 10% or unspecified amount
948.11 Burn (any degree) involving 10-19% of body surface with third degree burn of 10-19%
948.20 Burn (any degree) involving 20-29% of body surface with third degree burn of less than 10% or unspecified amount
948.21 Burn (any degree) involving 20-29% of body surface with third degree burn of 10-19%
948.22 Burn (any degree) involving 20-29% of body surface with third degree burn of 20-29%
948.30 Burn (any degree) involving 30-39% of body surface with third degree burn of less than 10% or unspecified amount
948.31 Burn (any degree) involving 30-39% of body surface with third degree burn of 10-19%
948.32 Burn (any degree) involving 30-39% of body surface with third degree burn of 20-29%
948.33 Burn (any degree) involving 30-39% of body surface with third degree burn of 30-39%
948.40 Burn (any degree) involving 40-49% of body surface with third degree burn of less than 10% or unspecified amount
948.41 Burn (any degree) involving 40-49% of body surface with third degree burn of 10-19%
948.42 Burn (any degree) involving 40-49% of body surface with third degree burn of 20-29%
948.43 Burn (any degree) involving 40-49% of body surface with third degree burn of 30-39%
948.44 Burn (any degree) involving 40-49% of body surface with third degree burn of 40-49%
948.50 Burn (any degree) involving 50-59% of body surface with third degree burn of less than 10% or unspecified amount
948.51 Burn (any degree) involving 50-59% of body surface with third degree burn of 10-19%
948.52 Burn (any degree) involving 50-59% of body surface with third degree burn of 20-29%
948.53 Burn (any degree) involving 50-59% of body surface with third degree burn of 30-39%
948.54 Burn (any degree) involving 50-59% of body surface with third degree burn of 40-49%
948.55 Burn (any degree) involving 50-59% of body surface with third degree burn of 50-59%
948.60 Burn (any degree) involving 60-69% of body surface with third degree burn of less than 10% or unspecified amount
948.61 Burn (any degree) involving 60-69% of body surface with third degree burn of 10-19%
948.62 Burn (any degree) involving 60-69% of body surface with third degree burn of 20-29%
948.63 Burn (any degree) involving 60-69% of body surface with third degree burn of 30-39%
948.64 Burn (any degree) involving 60-69% of body surface with third degree burn of 40-49%
948.65 Burn (any degree) involving 60-69% of body surface with third degree burn of 50-59%
948.66 Burn (any degree) involving 60-69% of body surface with third degree burn of 60-69%
948.70 Burn (any degree) involving 70-79% of body surface with third degree burn of less than 10% or unspecified amount
948.71 Burn (any degree) involving 70-79% of body surface with third degree burn of 10-19%
948.72 Burn (any degree) involving 70-79% of body surface with third degree burn of 20-29%
948.73 Burn (any degree) involving 70-79% of body surface with third degree burn of 30-39%
948.74 Burn (any degree) involving 70-79% of body surface with third degree burn of 40-49%
948.75 Burn (any degree) involving 70-79% of body surface with third degree burn of 50-59%
948.76 Burn (any degree) involving 70-79% of body surface with third degree burn of 60-69%
948.77 Burn (any degree) involving 70-79% of body surface with third degree burn of 70-79%
948.80 Burn (any degree) involving 80-89% of body surface with third degree burn of less than 10% or unspecified amount
948.81 Burn (any degree) involving 80-89% of body surface with third degree burn of 10-19%
948.82 Burn (any degree) involving 80-89% of body surface with third degree burn of 20-29%
948.83 Burn (any degree) involving 80-89% of body surface with third degree burn of 30-39%
948.84 Burn (any degree) involving 80-89% of body surface with third degree burn of 40-49%
948.85 Burn (any degree) involving 80-89% of body surface with third degree burn of 50-59%
948.86 Burn (any degree) involving 80-89% of body surface with third degree burn of 60-69%
948.87 Burn (any degree) involving 80-89% of body surface with third degree burn of 70-79%
948.88 Burn (any degree) involving 80-89% of body surface with third degree burn of 80-89%
948.90 Burn (any degree) involving 90% or more of body surface with third degree burn of less than 10% or unspecified amount
948.91 Burn (any degree) involving 90% or more of body surface with third degree burn of 10-19%
948.92 Burn (any degree) involving 90% or more of body surface with third degree burn of 20-29%
948.93 Burn (any degree) involving 90% or more of body surface with third degree burn of 30-39%
948.94 Burn (any degree) involving 90% or more of body surface with third degree burn of 40-49%
948.95 Burn (any degree) involving 90% or more of body surface with third degree burn of 50-59%
948.96 Burn (any degree) involving 90% or more of body surface with third degree burn of 60-69%
948.97 Burn (any degree) involving 90% or more of body surface with third degree burn of 70-79%
948.98 Burn (any degree) involving 90% or more of body surface with third degree burn of 80-89%
948.99 Burn (any degree) involving 90% or more of body surface with third degree burn of 90% or more of body surface
991.0 Frostbite of face
991.1 Frostbite of hand
991.2 Frostbite of foot
991.3 Frostbite of other and unspecified sites
996.52 Mechanical complication due to other tissue graft, not elsewhere classified
998.59 Other postoperative infection — (Use additional code to identify infection)
998.83 Non-healing surgical wound

ICD-9-CM Procedural

85.84 Pedicle graft to breast
86.72 Advancement of pedicle graft
86.73 Attachment of pedicle or flap graft to hand
86.74 Attachment of pedicle or flap graft to other sites

15732

15732 Muscle, myocutaneous, or fasciocutaneous flap; head and neck (eg, temporalis, masseter muscle, sternocleidomastoid, levator scapulae)

ICD-9-CM Diagnostic

142.0 Malignant neoplasm of parotid gland
142.1 Malignant neoplasm of submandibular gland
142.2 Malignant neoplasm of sublingual gland
143.0 Malignant neoplasm of upper gum
143.1 Malignant neoplasm of lower gum
143.8 Malignant neoplasm of other sites of gum
144.8 Malignant neoplasm of other sites of floor of mouth
145.0 Malignant neoplasm of cheek mucosa
145.1 Malignant neoplasm of vestibule of mouth
145.5 Malignant neoplasm of palate, unspecified
145.8 Malignant neoplasm of other specified parts of mouth
147.0 Malignant neoplasm of superior wall of nasopharynx
147.1 Malignant neoplasm of posterior wall of nasopharynx
147.2 Malignant neoplasm of lateral wall of nasopharynx
147.3 Malignant neoplasm of anterior wall of nasopharynx
148.0 Malignant neoplasm of postcricoid region of hypopharynx
148.1 Malignant neoplasm of pyriform sinus
148.2 Malignant neoplasm of aryepiglottic fold, hypopharyngeal aspect
148.3 Malignant neoplasm of posterior hypopharyngeal wall
148.8 Malignant neoplasm of other specified sites of hypopharynx
149.0 Malignant neoplasm of pharynx, unspecified
149.8 Malignant neoplasm of other sites within the lip and oral cavity
160.0 Malignant neoplasm of nasal cavities
160.1 Malignant neoplasm of auditory tube, middle ear, and mastoid air cells
160.2 Malignant neoplasm of maxillary sinus
160.3 Malignant neoplasm of ethmoidal sinus
160.4 Malignant neoplasm of frontal sinus
160.5 Malignant neoplasm of sphenoidal sinus
160.8 Malignant neoplasm of other sites of nasal cavities, middle ear, and accessory sinuses
161.8 Malignant neoplasm of other specified sites of larynx
170.0 Malignant neoplasm of bones of skull and face, except mandible
170.1 Malignant neoplasm of mandible
171.0 Malignant neoplasm of connective and other soft tissue of head, face, and neck
172.2 Malignant melanoma of skin of ear and external auditory canal
172.3 Malignant melanoma of skin of other and unspecified parts of face
172.4 Malignant melanoma of skin of scalp and neck
173.4 Other malignant neoplasm of scalp and skin of neck
195.0 Malignant neoplasm of head, face, and neck
196.0 Secondary and unspecified malignant neoplasm of lymph nodes of head, face, and neck
215.0 Other benign neoplasm of connective and other soft tissue of head, face, and neck
230.0 Carcinoma in situ of lip, oral cavity, and pharynx
232.1 Carcinoma in situ of eyelid, including canthus
232.2 Carcinoma in situ of skin of ear and external auditory canal
234.8 Carcinoma in situ of other specified sites
235.0 Neoplasm of uncertain behavior of major salivary glands
235.1 Neoplasm of uncertain behavior of lip, oral cavity, and pharynx
235.9 Neoplasm of uncertain behavior of other and unspecified respiratory organs
238.0 Neoplasm of uncertain behavior of bone and articular cartilage
238.1 Neoplasm of uncertain behavior of connective and other soft tissue
238.2 Neoplasm of uncertain behavior of skin
239.0 Neoplasm of unspecified nature of digestive system
239.1 Neoplasm of unspecified nature of respiratory system
239.2 Neoplasms of unspecified nature of bone, soft tissue, and skin
873.0 Open wound of scalp, without mention of complication — (Use additional code to identify infection)
873.1 Open wound of scalp, complicated — (Use additional code to identify infection)
873.40 Open wound of face, unspecified site, without mention of complication — (Use additional code to identify infection)
873.41 Open wound of cheek, without mention of complication — (Use additional code to identify infection)
873.42 Open wound of forehead, without mention of complication — (Use additional code to identify infection)
873.44 Open wound of jaw, without mention of complication — (Use additional code to identify infection)
873.49 Open wound of face, other and multiple sites, without mention of complication — (Use additional code to identify infection)
873.50 Open wound of face, unspecified site, complicated — (Use additional code to identify infection)
873.51 Open wound of cheek, complicated — (Use additional code to identify infection)
873.52 Open wound of forehead, complicated — (Use additional code to identify infection)
873.54 Open wound of jaw, complicated — (Use additional code to identify infection)
873.59 Open wound of face, other and multiple sites, complicated — (Use additional code to identify infection)
874.8 Open wound of other and unspecified parts of neck, without mention of complication — (Use additional code to identify infection)
874.9 Open wound of other and unspecified parts of neck, complicated — (Use additional code to identify infection)
905.0 Late effect of fracture of skull and face bones
906.5 Late effect of burn of eye, face, head, and neck
909.2 Late effect of radiation
909.3 Late effect of complications of surgical and medical care
925.1 Crushing injury of face and scalp — (Use additional code to identify any associated injuries: 800-829, 850.0-854.1, 860.0-869.1)
925.2 Crushing injury of neck — (Use additional code to identify any associated injuries: 800-829, 850.0-854.1, 860.0-869.1)
941.30 Full-thickness skin loss due to burn (third degree nos) of unspecified site of face and head
941.34 Full-thickness skin loss due to burn (third degree nos) of chin
941.36 Full-thickness skin loss due to burn (third degree nos) of scalp (any part)
941.37 Full-thickness skin loss due to burn (third degree nos) of forehead and cheek
941.38 Full-thickness skin loss due to burn (third degree nos) of neck
941.39 Full-thickness skin loss due to burn (third degree nos) of multiple sites (except with eye) of face, head, and neck
941.40 Deep necrosis of underlying tissues due to burn (deep third degree) of unspecified site of face and head, without mention of loss of a body part
941.44 Deep necrosis of underlying tissues due to burn (deep third degree) of chin, without mention of loss of a body part
941.46 Deep necrosis of underlying tissues due to burn (deep third degree) of scalp (any part), without mention of loss of a body part
941.47 Deep necrosis of underlying tissues due to burn (deep third degree) of forehead and cheek, without mention of loss of a body part
941.48 Deep necrosis of underlying tissues due to burn (deep third degree) of neck, without mention of loss of a body part
941.49 Deep necrosis of underlying tissues due to burn (deep third degree) of multiple sites (except with eye) of face, head, and neck, without mention of loss of a body part
941.50 Deep necrosis of underlying tissues due to burn (deep third degree) of face and head, unspecified site, with loss of a body part
941.54 Deep necrosis of underlying tissues due to burn (deep third degree) of chin, with loss of a body part
941.56 Deep necrosis of underlying tissues due to burn (deep third degree) of scalp (any part), with loss of a body part
941.58 Deep necrosis of underlying tissues due to burn (deep third degree) of neck, with loss of a body part
959.01 Head injury, unspecified
959.09 Injury of face and neck, other and unspecified
V10.02 Personal history of malignant neoplasm of other and unspecified parts of oral cavity and pharynx
V51 Aftercare involving the use of plastic surgery

ICD-9-CM Procedural

18.71 Construction of auricle of ear
18.79 Other plastic repair of external ear
27.57 Attachment of pedicle or flap graft to lip and mouth
83.82 Graft of muscle or fascia
86.71 Cutting and preparation of pedicle grafts or flaps
86.74 Attachment of pedicle or flap graft to other sites

15734

15734 Muscle, myocutaneous, or fasciocutaneous flap; trunk

ICD-9-CM Diagnostic

171.4 Malignant neoplasm of connective and other soft tissue of thorax
171.6 Malignant neoplasm of connective and other soft tissue of pelvis
171.7 Malignant neoplasm of connective and other soft tissue of trunk, unspecified site
171.8 Malignant neoplasm of other specified sites of connective and other soft tissue
172.5 Malignant melanoma of skin of trunk, except scrotum
173.5 Other malignant neoplasm of skin of trunk, except scrotum
174.0 Malignant neoplasm of nipple and areola of female breast ♀

174.1 Malignant neoplasm of central portion of female breast ♀
174.2 Malignant neoplasm of upper-inner quadrant of female breast ♀
174.3 Malignant neoplasm of lower-inner quadrant of female breast ♀
174.4 Malignant neoplasm of upper-outer quadrant of female breast ♀
174.5 Malignant neoplasm of lower-outer quadrant of female breast ♀
174.6 Malignant neoplasm of axillary tail of female breast ♀
174.8 Malignant neoplasm of other specified sites of female breast ♀
175.9 Malignant neoplasm of other and unspecified sites of male breast ▽ ♂
197.0 Secondary malignant neoplasm of lung
197.1 Secondary malignant neoplasm of mediastinum
197.3 Secondary malignant neoplasm of other respiratory organs
197.8 Secondary malignant neoplasm of other digestive organs and spleen
198.2 Secondary malignant neoplasm of skin
198.81 Secondary malignant neoplasm of breast
232.5 Carcinoma in situ of skin of trunk, except scrotum
233.0 Carcinoma in situ of breast
235.7 Neoplasm of uncertain behavior of trachea, bronchus, and lung
235.8 Neoplasm of uncertain behavior of pleura, thymus, and mediastinum
238.2 Neoplasm of uncertain behavior of skin
238.3 Neoplasm of uncertain behavior of breast
239.2 Neoplasms of unspecified nature of bone, soft tissue, and skin
239.3 Neoplasm of unspecified nature of breast
519.2 Mediastinitis
682.2 Cellulitis and abscess of trunk — (Use additional code to identify organism)
682.5 Cellulitis and abscess of buttock — (Use additional code to identify organism)
707.00 Decubitus ulcer, unspecified site
707.02 Decubitus ulcer, upper back
707.03 Decubitus ulcer, lower back
707.04 Decubitus ulcer, hip
707.05 Decubitus ulcer, buttock
707.09 Decubitus ulcer, other site
707.8 Chronic ulcer of other specified site
709.2 Scar condition and fibrosis of skin
728.82 Foreign body granuloma of muscle
728.86 Necrotizing fasciitis — (Use additional code to identify infectious organism, 041.00-041.89, 785.4, if applicable)
728.88 Rhabdomyolysis
729.4 Unspecified fasciitis ▽
730.15 Chronic osteomyelitis, pelvic region and thigh — (Use additional code to identify organism, 041.1)
730.18 Chronic osteomyelitis, other specified sites — (Use additional code to identify organism, 041.1)
738.3 Acquired deformity of chest and rib
741.00 Spina bifida with hydrocephalus, unspecified region ▽
754.81 Pectus excavatum
810.11 Open fracture of sternal end of clavicle
810.12 Open fracture of shaft of clavicle
810.13 Open fracture of acromial end of clavicle
811.10 Open fracture of unspecified part of scapula ▽
811.11 Open fracture of acromial process of scapula
811.12 Open fracture of coracoid process
811.13 Open fracture of glenoid cavity and neck of scapula
811.19 Open fracture of other part of scapula
860.1 Traumatic pneumothorax with open wound into thorax
860.3 Traumatic hemothorax with open wound into thorax
860.5 Traumatic pneumohemothorax with open wound into thorax
861.30 Unspecified lung injury with open wound into thorax ▽
861.31 Lung contusion with open wound into thorax
861.32 Lung laceration with open wound into thorax
862.1 Diaphragm injury with open wound into cavity
862.31 Bronchus injury with open wound into cavity
862.32 Esophagus injury with open wound into cavity
862.39 Injury to other specified intrathoracic organs with open wound into cavity
863.30 Small intestine injury, unspecified site, with open wound into cavity ▽
863.31 Duodenum injury with open wound into cavity
863.39 Other injury to small intestine with open wound into cavity
863.50 Colon injury, unspecified site, with open wound into cavity ▽
863.51 Ascending (right) colon injury with open wound into cavity
863.52 Transverse colon injury with open wound into cavity
863.53 Descending (left) colon injury with open wound into cavity
863.54 Sigmoid colon injury with open wound into cavity
863.55 Rectum injury with open wound into cavity
863.56 Injury to multiple sites in colon and rectum with open wound into cavity
863.59 Other injury to colon and rectum with open wound into cavity
863.90 Gastrointestinal tract injury, unspecified site, with open wound into cavity ▽
863.91 Pancreas head injury with open wound into cavity
863.92 Pancreas body injury with open wound into cavity
863.93 Pancreas tail injury with open wound into cavity
863.94 Pancreas injury, multiple and unspecified sites, with open wound into cavity
863.95 Appendix injury with open wound into cavity
863.99 Injury to other and unspecified gastrointestinal sites with open wound into cavity
864.10 Unspecified liver injury with open wound into cavity ▽
864.11 Liver hematoma and contusion with open wound into cavity
864.12 Liver laceration, minor, with open wound into cavity
864.13 Liver laceration, moderate, with open wound into cavity
864.14 Liver laceration, major, with open wound into cavity
864.15 Liver injury with open wound into cavity, unspecified laceration ▽
864.19 Other liver injury with open wound into cavity
865.10 Unspecified spleen injury with open wound into cavity ▽
865.11 Spleen hematoma, without rupture of capsule, with open wound into cavity
865.12 Capsular tears to spleen, without major disruption of parenchyma, with open wound into cavity
865.13 Spleen laceration extending into parenchyma, with open wound into cavity
865.14 Massive parenchyma disruption of spleen with open wound into cavity
865.19 Other spleen injury with open wound into cavity
866.10 Unspecified ikidney injury with open wound into cavity ▽
866.11 Kidney hematoma, without rupture of capsule, with open wound into cavity
866.12 Kidney laceration with open wound into cavity
866.13 Complete disruption of kidney parenchyma, with open wound into cavity
867.1 Bladder and urethra injury with open wound into cavity
867.3 Ureter injury with open wound into cavity
867.5 Uterus injury with open wound into cavity ♀
867.7 Injury to other specified pelvic organs with open wound into cavity
868.10 Injury to unspecified intra-abdominal organ, with open wound into cavity ▽
868.11 Adrenal gland injury, with open wound into cavity
868.12 Bile duct and gallbladder injury, with open wound into cavity
868.13 Peritoneum injury with open wound into cavity
868.14 Retroperitoneum injury with open wound into cavity
868.19 Injury to other and multiple intra-abdominal organs, with open wound into cavity
869.1 Internal injury to unspecified or ill-defined organs with open wound into cavity
875.1 Open wound of chest (wall), complicated — (Use additional code to identify infection)
876.0 Open wound of back, without mention of complication — (Use additional code to identify infection)
876.1 Open wound of back, complicated — (Use additional code to identify infection)
877.1 Open wound of buttock, complicated — (Use additional code to identify infection)
879.5 Open wound of abdominal wall, lateral, complicated — (Use additional code to identify infection)
879.8 Open wound(s) (multiple) of unspecified site(s), without mention of complication — (Use additional code to identify infection) ▽
879.9 Open wound(s) (multiple) of unspecified site(s), complicated — (Use additional code to identify infection) ▽
906.0 Late effect of open wound of head, neck, and trunk
906.4 Late effect of crushing
906.8 Late effect of burns of other specified sites
908.0 Late effect of internal injury to chest
908.1 Late effect of internal injury to intra-abdominal organs
908.2 Late effect of internal injury to other internal organs
908.4 Late effect of injury to blood vessel of thorax, abdomen, and pelvis
908.6 Late effect of certain complications of trauma
926.0 Crushing injury of external genitalia — (Use additional code to identify any associated injuries: 800-829, 850.0-854.1, 860.0-869.1)
926.11 Crushing injury of back — (Use additional code to identify any associated injuries: 800-829, 850.0-854.1, 860.0-869.1)
926.12 Crushing injury of buttock — (Use additional code to identify any associated injuries: 800-829, 850.0-854.1, 860.0-869.1)
926.19 Crushing injury of other specified sites of trunk — (Use additional code to identify any associated injuries: 800-829, 850.0-854.1, 860.0-869.1)
942.30 Full-thickness skin loss due to burn (third degree nos) of unspecified site of trunk ▽
942.31 Full-thickness skin loss due to burn (third degree nos) of breast
942.33 Full-thickness skin loss due to burn (third degree nos) of abdominal wall
942.34 Full-thickness skin loss due to burn (third degree nos) of back (any part)
942.35 Full-thickness skin loss due to burn (third degree nos) of genitalia
942.39 Full-thickness skin loss due to burn (third degree nos) of other and multiple sites of trunk
942.40 Deep necrosis of underlying tissues due to burn (deep third degree) of trunk, unspecified site, without mention of loss of a body part ▽

▽ Unspecified code
♀ Female diagnosis
☒ Manifestation code
♂ Male diagnosis

942.41 Deep necrosis of underlying tissues due to burn (deep third degree) of breast, without mention of loss of a body part
942.42 Deep necrosis of underlying tissues due to burn (deep third degree) of chest wall, excluding breast and nipple, without mention of loss of a body part
942.43 Deep necrosis of underlying tissues due to burn (deep third degree) of abdominal wall, without mention of loss of a body part
942.44 Deep necrosis of underlying tissues due to burn (deep third degree) of back (any part), without mention of loss of a body part
942.45 Deep necrosis of underlying tissues due to burn (deep third degree) of genitalia, without mention of loss of a body part
942.49 Deep necrosis of underlying tissues due to burn (deep third degree) of other and multiple sites of trunk, without mention of loss of a body part
942.50 Deep necrosis of underlying tissues due to burn (deep third degree) of unspecified site of trunk, with loss of a body part ▽
942.51 Deep necrosis of underlying tissues due to burn (deep third degree) of breast, with loss of a body part
942.52 Deep necrosis of underlying tissues due to burn (deep third degree) of chest wall, excluding breast and nipple, with loss of a body part
942.53 Deep necrosis of underlying tissues due to burn (deep third degree) of abdominal wall with loss of a body part
942.54 Deep necrosis of underlying tissues due to burn (deep third degree) of back (any part), with loss of a body part
942.55 Deep necrosis of underlying tissues due to burn (deep third degree) of genitalia, with loss of a body part
942.59 Deep necrosis of underlying tissues due to burn (deep third degree) of other and multiple sites of trunk, with loss of a body part
996.52 Mechanical complication due to other tissue graft, not elsewhere classified
998.31 Disruption of internal operation wound
998.32 Disruption of external operation wound
998.59 Other postoperative infection — (Use additional code to identify infection)
998.83 Non-healing surgical wound

ICD-9-CM Procedural

83.82 Graft of muscle or fascia
86.71 Cutting and preparation of pedicle grafts or flaps
86.74 Attachment of pedicle or flap graft to other sites

15736

15736 Muscle, myocutaneous, or fasciocutaneous flap; upper extremity

ICD-9-CM Diagnostic

171.2 Malignant neoplasm of connective and other soft tissue of upper limb, including shoulder
172.6 Malignant melanoma of skin of upper limb, including shoulder
173.6 Other malignant neoplasm of skin of upper limb, including shoulder
198.2 Secondary malignant neoplasm of skin
232.6 Carcinoma in situ of skin of upper limb, including shoulder
232.8 Carcinoma in situ of other specified sites of skin
682.3 Cellulitis and abscess of upper arm and forearm — (Use additional code to identify organism)
682.4 Cellulitis and abscess of hand, except fingers and thumb — (Use additional code to identify organism)
701.5 Other abnormal granulation tissue
709.2 Scar condition and fibrosis of skin
728.82 Foreign body granuloma of muscle
728.86 Necrotizing fasciitis — (Use additional code to identify infectious organism, 041.00-041.89, 785.4, if applicable)
728.88 Rhabdomyolysis
812.10 Open fracture of unspecified part of upper end of humerus ▽
812.12 Open fracture of anatomical neck of humerus
812.13 Open fracture of greater tuberosity of humerus
812.19 Other open fracture of upper end of humerus
812.30 Open fracture of unspecified part of humerus ▽
812.31 Open fracture of shaft of humerus
812.50 Open fracture of unspecified part of lower end of humerus ▽
812.51 Open fracture of supracondylar humerus
812.52 Open fracture of lateral condyle of humerus
812.53 Open fracture of medial condyle of humerus
812.54 Open fracture of unspecified condyle(s) of humerus ▽
812.59 Other open fracture of lower end of humerus
813.10 Unspecified open fracture of upper end of forearm ▽
813.11 Open fracture of olecranon process of ulna
813.12 Open fracture of coronoid process of ulna
813.13 Open Monteggia's fracture
813.14 Other and unspecified open fractures of proximal end of ulna (alone) ▽
813.15 Open fracture of head of radius
813.16 Open fracture of neck of radius
813.17 Other and unspecified open fractures of proximal end of radius (alone) ▽
813.18 Open fracture of radius with ulna, upper end (any part)
813.30 Unspecified open fracture of shaft of radius or ulna ▽
813.31 Open fracture of shaft of radius (alone)
813.32 Open fracture of shaft of ulna (alone)
813.33 Open fracture of shaft of radius with ulna
813.50 Unspecified open fracture of lower end of forearm ▽
813.51 Open Colles' fracture
813.52 Other open fractures of distal end of radius (alone)
813.53 Open fracture of distal end of ulna (alone)
813.54 Open fracture of lower end of radius with ulna
813.90 Open fracture of unspecified part of forearm ▽
813.91 Open fracture of unspecified part of radius (alone) ▽
813.92 Open fracture of unspecified part of ulna (alone) ▽
813.93 Open fracture of unspecified part of radius with ulna ▽
819.1 Multiple open fractures involving both upper limbs, and upper limb with rib(s) and sternum
880.03 Open wound of upper arm, without mention of complication — (Use additional code to identify infection)
880.09 Open wound of multiple sites of shoulder and upper arm, without mention of complication — (Use additional code to identify infection)
880.13 Open wound of upper arm, complicated — (Use additional code to identify infection)
880.19 Open wound of multiple sites of shoulder and upper arm, complicated — (Use additional code to identify infection)
880.23 Open wound of upper arm, with tendon involvement — (Use additional code to identify infection)
880.29 Open wound of multiple sites of shoulder and upper arm, with tendon involvement — (Use additional code to identify infection)
881.00 Open wound of forearm, without mention of complication — (Use additional code to identify infection)
881.01 Open wound of elbow, without mention of complication — (Use additional code to identify infection)
881.02 Open wound of wrist, without mention of complication — (Use additional code to identify infection)
881.10 Open wound of forearm, complicated — (Use additional code to identify infection)
881.11 Open wound of elbow, complicated — (Use additional code to identify infection)
881.12 Open wound of wrist, complicated — (Use additional code to identify infection)
881.20 Open wound of forearm, with tendon involvement — (Use additional code to identify infection)
881.21 Open wound of elbow, with tendon involvement — (Use additional code to identify infection)
881.22 Open wound of wrist, with tendon involvement — (Use additional code to identify infection)
882.0 Open wound of hand except finger(s) alone, without mention of complication — (Use additional code to identify infection)
882.1 Open wound of hand except finger(s) alone, complicated — (Use additional code to identify infection)
882.2 Open wound of hand except finger(s) alone, with tendon involvement — (Use additional code to identify infection)
883.0 Open wound of finger(s), without mention of complication — (Use additional code to identify infection)
883.1 Open wound of finger(s), complicated — (Use additional code to identify infection)
883.2 Open wound of finger(s), with tendon involvement — (Use additional code to identify infection)
884.0 Multiple and unspecified open wound of upper limb, without mention of complication — (Use additional code to identify infection)
884.1 Multiple and unspecified open wound of upper limb, complicated — (Use additional code to identify infection)
884.2 Multiple and unspecified open wound of upper limb, with tendon involvement — (Use additional code to identify infection)
885.0 Traumatic amputation of thumb (complete) (partial), without mention of complication — (Use additional code to identify infection)
885.1 Traumatic amputation of thumb (complete) (partial), complicated — (Use additional code to identify infection)
886.0 Traumatic amputation of other finger(s) (complete) (partial), without mention of complication — (Use additional code to identify infection)
886.1 Traumatic amputation of other finger(s) (complete) (partial), complicated — (Use additional code to identify infection)

887.0 Traumatic amputation of arm and hand (complete) (partial), unilateral, below elbow, without mention of complication — (Use additional code to identify infection)
887.1 Traumatic amputation of arm and hand (complete) (partial), unilateral, below elbow, complicated — (Use additional code to identify infection)
887.2 Traumatic amputation of arm and hand (complete) (partial), unilateral, at or above elbow, without mention of complication — (Use additional code to identify infection)
887.3 Traumatic amputation of arm and hand (complete) (partial), unilateral, at or above elbow, complicated — (Use additional code to identify infection)
887.4 Traumatic amputation of arm and hand (complete) (partial), unilateral, level not specified, without mention of complication — (Use additional code to identify infection) ▽
887.5 Traumatic amputation of arm and hand (complete) (partial), unilateral, level not specified, complicated — (Use additional code to identify infection) ▽
887.6 Traumatic amputation of arm and hand (complete) (partial), bilateral (any level), without mention of complication — (Use additional code to identify infection)
887.7 Traumatic amputation of arm and hand (complete) (partial), bilateral (any level), complicated — (Use additional code to identify infection)
906.1 Late effect of open wound of extremities without mention of tendon injury
906.6 Late effect of burn of wrist and hand
906.7 Late effect of burn of other extremities
908.6 Late effect of certain complications of trauma
909.3 Late effect of complications of surgical and medical care
927.03 Crushing injury of upper arm — (Use additional code to identify any associated injuries: 800-829, 850.0-854.1, 860.0-869.1)
927.09 Crushing injury of multiple sites of upper arm — (Use additional code to identify any associated injuries: 800-829, 850.0-854.1, 860.0-869.1)
927.10 Crushing injury of forearm — (Use additional code to identify any associated injuries: 800-829, 850.0-854.1, 860.0-869.1)
927.11 Crushing injury of elbow — (Use additional code to identify any associated injuries: 800-829, 850.0-854.1, 860.0-869.1)
927.20 Crushing injury of hand(s) — (Use additional code to identify any associated injuries: 800-829, 850.0-854.1, 860.0-869.1)
927.21 Crushing injury of wrist — (Use additional code to identify any associated injuries: 800-829, 850.0-854.1, 860.0-869.1)
927.3 Crushing injury of finger(s) — (Use additional code to identify any associated injuries: 800-829, 850.0-854.1, 860.0-869.1)
927.8 Crushing injury of multiple sites of upper limb — (Use additional code to identify any associated injuries: 800-829, 850.0-854.1, 860.0-869.1)
943.30 Full-thickness skin loss due to burn (third degree nos) of unspecified site of upper limb ▽
943.31 Full-thickness skin loss due to burn (third degree nos) of forearm
943.32 Full-thickness skin loss due to burn (third degree nos) of elbow
943.33 Full-thickness skin loss due to burn (third degree nos) of upper arm
943.39 Full-thickness skin loss due to burn (third degree nos) of multiple sites of upper limb, except wrist and hand
943.40 Deep necrosis of underlying tissues due to burn (deep third degree) of unspecified site of upper limb, without mention of loss of a body part ▽
943.41 Deep necrosis of underlying tissues due to burn (deep third degree) of forearm, without mention of loss of a body part
943.42 Deep necrosis of underlying tissues due to burn (deep third degree) of elbow, without mention of loss of a body part
943.44 Deep necrosis of underlying tissues due to burn (deep third degree) of axilla, without mention of loss of a body part
943.49 Deep necrosis of underlying tissues due to burn (deep third degree) of multiple sites of upper limb, except wrist and hand, without mention of loss of a body part
943.50 Deep necrosis of underlying tissues due to burn (deep third degree) of unspecified site of upper limb, with loss of a body part ▽
943.51 Deep necrosis of underlying tissues due to burn (deep third degree) of forearm, with loss of a body part
943.52 Deep necrosis of underlying tissues due to burn (deep third degree) of elbow, with loss of a body part
943.53 Deep necrosis of underlying tissues due to burn (deep third degree) of upper arm, with loss of upper a body part
943.59 Deep necrosis of underlying tissues due to burn (deep third degree) of multiple sites of upper limb, except wrist and hand, with loss of a body part
944.30 Full-thickness skin loss due to burn (third degree nos) of unspecified site of hand ▽
944.31 Full-thickness skin loss due to burn (third degree nos) of single digit [finger (nail)] other than thumb
944.32 Full-thickness skin loss due to burn (third degree nos) of thumb (nail)
944.33 Full-thickness skin loss due to burn (third degree nos) of two or more digits of hand, not including thumb
944.34 Full-thickness skin loss due to burn (third degree nos) of two or more digits of hand including thumb
944.35 Full-thickness skin loss due to burn (third degree nos) of palm of hand
944.36 Full-thickness skin loss due to burn (third degree nos) of back of hand
944.37 Full-thickness skin loss due to burn (third degree nos) of wrist
944.38 Full-thickness skin loss due to burn (third degree nos) of multiple sites of wrist(s) and hand(s)
944.40 Deep necrosis of underlying tissues due to burn (deep third degree) of unspecified site of hand, without mention of a body part ▽
944.41 Deep necrosis of underlying tissues due to burn (deep third degree) of single digit [finger (nail)] other than thumb, without mention of a body part
944.42 Deep necrosis of underlying tissues due to burn (deep third degree) of thumb (nail), without mention of loss of a body part
944.43 Deep necrosis of underlying tissues due to burn (deep third degree) of two or more digits of hand, not including thumb, without mention of a body part
944.44 Deep necrosis of underlying tissues due to burn (deep third degree) of two or more digits of hand including thumb, without mention of a body part
944.46 Deep necrosis of underlying tissues due to burn (deep third degree) of back of hand, without mention of loss of back of a body part
944.47 Deep necrosis of underlying tissues due to burn (deep third degree) of wrist, without mention of loss of a body part
944.48 Deep necrosis of underlying tissues due to burn (deep third degree) of multiple sites of wrist(s) and hand(s), without mention of loss of a body part
944.50 Deep necrosis of underlying tissues due to burn (deep third degree) of unspecified site of hand, with loss of a body part ▽
944.51 Deep necrosis of underlying tissues due to burn (deep third degree) of single digit (finger (nail)) other than thumb, with loss of a body part
944.52 Deep necrosis of underlying tissues due to burn (deep third degree) of thumb (nail), with loss of a body part
944.53 Deep necrosis of underlying tissues due to burn (deep third degree) of two or more digits of hand, not including thumb, with loss of a body part
944.54 Deep necrosis of underlying tissues due to burn (deep third degree) of two or more digits of hand including thumb, with loss of a body part
944.55 Deep necrosis of underlying tissues due to burn (deep third degree) of palm of hand, with loss of a body part
944.56 Deep necrosis of underlying tissues due to burn (deep third degree) of back of hand, with loss of a body part
944.57 Deep necrosis of underlying tissues due to burn (deep third degree) of wrist, with loss of a body part
944.58 Deep necrosis of underlying tissues due to burn (deep third degree) of multiple sites of wrist(s) and hand(s), with loss of a body part
995.4 Shock due to anesthesia not elsewhere classified
997.60 Late complications of amputation stump, unspecified — (Use additional code to identify complications) ▽
997.62 Infection (chronic) of amputation stump — (Use additional code to identify organism. Use additional code to identify complications)
997.69 Other late amputation stump complication — (Use additional code to identify complications)
998.59 Other postoperative infection — (Use additional code to identify infection)
998.83 Non-healing surgical wound
V10.82 Personal history of malignant melanoma of skin
V51 Aftercare involving the use of plastic surgery

ICD-9-CM Procedural

83.82 Graft of muscle or fascia
86.71 Cutting and preparation of pedicle grafts or flaps
86.74 Attachment of pedicle or flap graft to other sites

15738

15738 Muscle, myocutaneous, or fasciocutaneous flap; lower extremity

ICD-9-CM Diagnostic

171.3 Malignant neoplasm of connective and other soft tissue of lower limb, including hip
172.7 Malignant melanoma of skin of lower limb, including hip
173.7 Other malignant neoplasm of skin of lower limb, including hip
195.5 Malignant neoplasm of lower limb
707.00 Decubitus ulcer, unspecified site
707.06 Decubitus ulcer, ankle
707.07 Decubitus ulcer, heel
707.09 Decubitus ulcer, other site
707.10 Ulcer of lower limb, unspecified ▽
707.11 Ulcer of thigh
707.12 Ulcer of calf
707.13 Ulcer of ankle
707.14 Ulcer of heel and midfoot

▽ Unspecified code
♀ Female diagnosis
☒ Manifestation code
♂ Male diagnosis

707.15 Ulcer of other part of foot
707.19 Ulcer of other part of lower limb
730.16 Chronic osteomyelitis, lower leg — (Use additional code to identify organism, 041.1)
730.17 Chronic osteomyelitis, ankle and foot — (Use additional code to identify organism, 041.1)
730.26 Unspecified osteomyelitis, lower leg — (Use additional code to identify organism, 041.1) ▽
821.10 Open fracture of unspecified part of femur ▽
823.92 Open fracture of unspecified part of fibula with tibia ▽
825.1 Open fracture of calcaneus
825.30 Open fracture of unspecified bone(s) of foot (except toes) ▽
826.1 Open fracture of one or more phalanges of foot
827.1 Other, multiple and ill-defined open fractures of lower limb
828.1 Multiple fractures involving both lower limbs, lower with upper limb, and lower limb(s) with rib(s) and sternum, open
829.1 Open fracture of unspecified bone ▽
890.1 Open wound of hip and thigh, complicated — (Use additional code to identify infection)
891.0 Open wound of knee, leg (except thigh), and ankle, without mention of complication — (Use additional code to identify infection)
891.1 Open wound of knee, leg (except thigh), and ankle, complicated — (Use additional code to identify infection)
892.1 Open wound of foot except toe(s) alone, complicated — (Use additional code to identify infection)
896.1 Traumatic amputation of foot (complete) (partial), unilateral, complicated — (Use additional code to identify infection)

ICD-9-CM Procedural

83.82 Graft of muscle or fascia
86.71 Cutting and preparation of pedicle grafts or flaps
86.74 Attachment of pedicle or flap graft to other sites

15740

15740 Flap; island pedicle

ICD-9-CM Diagnostic

140.9 Malignant neoplasm of lip, vermilion border, unspecified as to upper or lower ▽
149.8 Malignant neoplasm of other sites within the lip and oral cavity
149.9 Malignant neoplasm of ill-defined sites of lip and oral cavity
172.1 Malignant melanoma of skin of eyelid, including canthus
172.2 Malignant melanoma of skin of ear and external auditory canal
172.4 Malignant melanoma of skin of scalp and neck
172.6 Malignant melanoma of skin of upper limb, including shoulder
172.7 Malignant melanoma of skin of lower limb, including hip
173.0 Other malignant neoplasm of skin of lip
173.1 Other malignant neoplasm of skin of eyelid, including canthus
173.2 Other malignant neoplasm of skin of ear and external auditory canal
173.4 Other malignant neoplasm of scalp and skin of neck
173.8 Other malignant neoplasm of other specified sites of skin
184.0 Malignant neoplasm of vagina ♀
184.1 Malignant neoplasm of labia majora ♀
184.2 Malignant neoplasm of labia minora ♀
184.3 Malignant neoplasm of clitoris ♀
184.4 Malignant neoplasm of vulva, unspecified site ▽ ♀
184.8 Malignant neoplasm of other specified sites of female genital organs ♀
187.1 Malignant neoplasm of prepuce ♂
187.2 Malignant neoplasm of glans penis ♂
187.3 Malignant neoplasm of body of penis ♂
187.4 Malignant neoplasm of penis, part unspecified ▽ ♂
187.7 Malignant neoplasm of scrotum ♂
187.9 Malignant neoplasm of male genital organ, site unspecified ▽ ♂
195.0 Malignant neoplasm of head, face, and neck
198.2 Secondary malignant neoplasm of skin
210.0 Benign neoplasm of lip
210.4 Benign neoplasm of other and unspecified parts of mouth ▽
216.1 Benign neoplasm of eyelid, including canthus
216.2 Benign neoplasm of ear and external auditory canal
216.4 Benign neoplasm of scalp and skin of neck
216.6 Benign neoplasm of skin of upper limb, including shoulder
216.7 Benign neoplasm of skin of lower limb, including hip
216.8 Benign neoplasm of other specified sites of skin
232.0 Carcinoma in situ of skin of lip
232.1 Carcinoma in situ of eyelid, including canthus
232.2 Carcinoma in situ of skin of ear and external auditory canal
232.4 Carcinoma in situ of scalp and skin of neck
232.6 Carcinoma in situ of skin of upper limb, including shoulder
232.7 Carcinoma in situ of skin of lower limb, including hip
232.8 Carcinoma in situ of other specified sites of skin
238.1 Neoplasm of uncertain behavior of connective and other soft tissue ▽
239.0 Neoplasm of unspecified nature of digestive system
239.2 Neoplasms of unspecified nature of bone, soft tissue, and skin
380.32 Acquired deformities of auricle or pinna
607.2 Other inflammatory disorders of penis — (Use additional code to identify organism) ♂
629.20 Female genital mutilation status, unspecified
629.21 Female genital mutilation, Type I status
629.22 Female genital mutilation, Type II status
629.23 Female genital mutilation, Type III status
682.0 Cellulitis and abscess of face — (Use additional code to identify organism)
707.00 Decubitus ulcer, unspecified site
707.01 Decubitus ulcer, elbow
707.02 Decubitus ulcer, upper back
707.03 Decubitus ulcer, lower back
707.04 Decubitus ulcer, hip
707.05 Decubitus ulcer, buttock
707.06 Decubitus ulcer, ankle
707.07 Decubitus ulcer, heel
707.09 Decubitus ulcer, other site
707.10 Ulcer of lower limb, unspecified ▽
707.11 Ulcer of thigh
707.12 Ulcer of calf
707.13 Ulcer of ankle
707.14 Ulcer of heel and midfoot
707.15 Ulcer of other part of foot
707.19 Ulcer of other part of lower limb
707.8 Chronic ulcer of other specified site
728.86 Necrotizing fasciitis — (Use additional code to identify infectious organism, 041.00-041.89, 785.4, if applicable)
743.62 Congenital deformity of eyelid
744.01 Congenital absence of external ear causing impairment of hearing
744.09 Other congenital anomalies of ear causing impairment of hearing
744.23 Microtia
744.3 Unspecified congenital anomaly of ear ▽
744.5 Congenital webbing of neck
744.82 Microcheilia
748.1 Other congenital anomaly of nose
749.10 Unspecified cleft lip ▽
749.11 Unilateral cleft lip, complete
749.12 Unilateral cleft lip, incomplete
749.13 Bilateral cleft lip, complete
749.14 Bilateral cleft lip, incomplete
749.20 Unspecified cleft palate with cleft lip ▽
749.21 Unilateral cleft palate with cleft lip, complete
749.22 Unilateral cleft palate with cleft lip, incomplete
749.23 Bilateral cleft palate with cleft lip, complete
749.24 Bilateral cleft palate with cleft lip, incomplete
752.40 Unspecified congenital anomaly of cervix, vagina, and external female genitalia ▽ ♀
752.49 Other congenital anomaly of cervix, vagina, and external female genitalia ♀
752.64 Micropenis ♂
752.69 Other penile anomalies ♂
752.7 Indeterminate sex and pseudohermaphroditism
752.81 Scrotal transposition
752.89 Other specified anomalies of genital organs
752.9 Unspecified congenital anomaly of genital organs ▽
757.33 Congenital pigmentary anomaly of skin
785.4 Gangrene — (Code first any associated underlying condition:250.7, 443.0)
870.0 Laceration of skin of eyelid and periocular area — (Use additional code to identify infection)
870.1 Laceration of eyelid, full-thickness, not involving lacrimal passages — (Use additional code to identify infection)
870.2 Laceration of eyelid involving lacrimal passages — (Use additional code to identify infection)
872.00 Open wound of external ear, unspecified site, without mention of complication — (Use additional code to identify infection) ▽
872.01 Open wound of auricle, without mention of complication — (Use additional code to identify infection)
872.02 Open wound of auditory canal, without mention of complication — (Use additional code to identify infection)

▽ Unspecified code ♀ Female diagnosis ☒ Manifestation code ♂ Male diagnosis

872.10 Open wound of external ear, unspecified site, complicated — (Use additional code to identify infection) ▽

872.11 Open wound of auricle, complicated — (Use additional code to identify infection)

872.8 Open wound of ear, part unspecified, without mention of complication — (Use additional code to identify infection) ▽

872.9 Open wound of ear, part unspecified, complicated — (Use additional code to identify infection) ▽

873.30 Open wound of nose, unspecified site, complicated — (Use additional code to identify infection) ▽

873.31 Open wound of nasal septum, complicated — (Use additional code to identify infection)

873.32 Open wound of nasal cavity, complicated — (Use additional code to identify infection)

873.33 Open wound of nasal sinus, complicated — (Use additional code to identify infection)

873.39 Open wound of nose, multiple sites, complicated — (Use additional code to identify infection)

873.43 Open wound of lip, without mention of complication — (Use additional code to identify infection)

873.50 Open wound of face, unspecified site, complicated — (Use additional code to identify infection) ▽

873.52 Open wound of forehead, complicated — (Use additional code to identify infection)

873.54 Open wound of jaw, complicated — (Use additional code to identify infection)

873.59 Open wound of face, other and multiple sites, complicated — (Use additional code to identify infection)

874.8 Open wound of other and unspecified parts of neck, without mention of complication — (Use additional code to identify infection) ▽

874.9 Open wound of other and unspecified parts of neck, complicated — (Use additional code to identify infection) ▽

876.0 Open wound of back, without mention of complication — (Use additional code to identify infection)

876.1 Open wound of back, complicated — (Use additional code to identify infection)

878.1 Open wound of penis, complicated — (Use additional code to identify infection) ♂

878.3 Open wound of scrotum and testes, complicated — (Use additional code to identify infection) ♂

878.5 Open wound of vulva, complicated — (Use additional code to identify infection) ♀

878.7 Open wound of vagina, complicated — (Use additional code to identify infection) ♀

878.9 Open wound of other and unspecified parts of genital organs, complicated — (Use additional code to identify infection) ▽

880.12 Open wound of axillary region, complicated — (Use additional code to identify infection)

882.1 Open wound of hand except finger(s) alone, complicated — (Use additional code to identify infection)

882.2 Open wound of hand except finger(s) alone, with tendon involvement — (Use additional code to identify infection)

883.1 Open wound of finger(s), complicated — (Use additional code to identify infection)

883.2 Open wound of finger(s), with tendon involvement — (Use additional code to identify infection)

884.1 Multiple and unspecified open wound of upper limb, complicated — (Use additional code to identify infection)

884.2 Multiple and unspecified open wound of upper limb, with tendon involvement — (Use additional code to identify infection)

885.0 Traumatic amputation of thumb (complete) (partial), without mention of complication — (Use additional code to identify infection)

885.1 Traumatic amputation of thumb (complete) (partial), complicated — (Use additional code to identify infection)

886.0 Traumatic amputation of other finger(s) (complete) (partial), without mention of complication — (Use additional code to identify infection)

886.1 Traumatic amputation of other finger(s) (complete) (partial), complicated — (Use additional code to identify infection)

887.0 Traumatic amputation of arm and hand (complete) (partial), unilateral, below elbow, without mention of complication — (Use additional code to identify infection)

887.1 Traumatic amputation of arm and hand (complete) (partial), unilateral, below elbow, complicated — (Use additional code to identify infection)

887.6 Traumatic amputation of arm and hand (complete) (partial), bilateral (any level), without mention of complication — (Use additional code to identify infection)

887.7 Traumatic amputation of arm and hand (complete) (partial), bilateral (any level), complicated — (Use additional code to identify infection)

892.1 Open wound of foot except toe(s) alone, complicated — (Use additional code to identify infection)

892.2 Open wound of foot except toe(s) alone, with tendon involvement — (Use additional code to identify infection)

893.1 Open wound of toe(s), complicated — (Use additional code to identify infection)

893.2 Open wound of toe(s), with tendon involvement — (Use additional code to identify infection)

894.1 Multiple and unspecified open wound of lower limb, complicated — (Use additional code to identify infection)

894.2 Multiple and unspecified open wound of lower limb, with tendon involvement — (Use additional code to identify infection)

895.0 Traumatic amputation of toe(s) (complete) (partial), without mention of complication — (Use additional code to identify infection)

895.1 Traumatic amputation of toe(s) (complete) (partial), complicated — (Use additional code to identify infection)

896.0 Traumatic amputation of foot (complete) (partial), unilateral, without mention of complication — (Use additional code to identify infection)

896.1 Traumatic amputation of foot (complete) (partial), unilateral, complicated — (Use additional code to identify infection)

896.2 Traumatic amputation of foot (complete) (partial), bilateral, without mention of complication — (Use additional code to identify infection)

896.3 Traumatic amputation of foot (complete) (partial), bilateral, complicated — (Use additional code to identify infection)

906.0 Late effect of open wound of head, neck, and trunk

906.6 Late effect of burn of wrist and hand

941.01 Burn of unspecified degree of ear (any part) ▽

941.02 Burn of unspecified degree of eye (with other parts of face, head, and neck) ▽

941.03 Burn of unspecified degree of lip(s) ▽

941.05 Burn of unspecified degree of nose (septum) ▽

941.09 Burn of unspecified degree of multiple sites (except with eye) of face, head, and neck ▽

941.30 Full-thickness skin loss due to burn (third degree nos) of unspecified site of face and head ▽

941.31 Full-thickness skin loss due to burn (third degree nos) of ear (any part)

941.32 Full-thickness skin loss due to burn (third degree nos) of eye (with other parts of face, head, and neck)

941.34 Full-thickness skin loss due to burn (third degree nos) of chin

941.35 Full-thickness skin loss due to burn (third degree nos) of nose (septum)

941.37 Full-thickness skin loss due to burn (third degree nos) of forehead and cheek

941.38 Full-thickness skin loss due to burn (third degree nos) of neck

941.40 Deep necrosis of underlying tissues due to burn (deep third degree) of unspecified site of face and head, without mention of loss of a body part ▽

941.43 Deep necrosis of underlying tissues due to burn (deep third degree) of lip(s), without mention of loss of a body part

941.44 Deep necrosis of underlying tissues due to burn (deep third degree) of chin, without mention of loss of a body part

941.47 Deep necrosis of underlying tissues due to burn (deep third degree) of forehead and cheek, without mention of loss of a body part

941.48 Deep necrosis of underlying tissues due to burn (deep third degree) of neck, without mention of loss of a body part

941.49 Deep necrosis of underlying tissues due to burn (deep third degree) of multiple sites (except with eye) of face, head, and neck, without mention of loss of a body part

941.50 Deep necrosis of underlying tissues due to burn (deep third degree) of face and head, unspecified site, with loss of a body part ▽

941.51 Deep necrosis of underlying tissues due to burn (deep third degree) of ear (any part), with loss of a body part

941.52 Deep necrosis of underlying tissues due to burn (deep third degree) of eye (with other parts of face, head, and neck), with loss of a body part

941.55 Deep necrosis of underlying tissues due to burn (deep third degree) of nose (septum), with loss of a body part

941.57 Deep necrosis of underlying tissues due to burn (deep third degree) of forehead and cheek, with loss of a body part

941.58 Deep necrosis of underlying tissues due to burn (deep third degree) of neck, with loss of a body part

943.34 Full-thickness skin loss due to burn (third degree nos) of axilla

943.44 Deep necrosis of underlying tissues due to burn (deep third degree) of axilla, without mention of loss of a body part

943.54 Deep necrosis of underlying tissues due to burn (deep third degree) of axilla, with loss of a body part

944.30 Full-thickness skin loss due to burn (third degree nos) of unspecified site of hand ▽

944.31 Full-thickness skin loss due to burn (third degree nos) of single digit [finger (nail)] other than thumb

944.32 Full-thickness skin loss due to burn (third degree nos) of thumb (nail)

▽ Unspecified code
♀ Female diagnosis
⊠ Manifestation code
♂ Male diagnosis

944.33 Full-thickness skin loss due to burn (third degree nos) of two or more digits of hand, not including thumb
944.34 Full-thickness skin loss due to burn (third degree nos) of two or more digits of hand including thumb
944.35 Full-thickness skin loss due to burn (third degree nos) of palm of hand
944.36 Full-thickness skin loss due to burn (third degree nos) of back of hand
944.37 Full-thickness skin loss due to burn (third degree nos) of wrist
944.38 Full-thickness skin loss due to burn (third degree nos) of multiple sites of wrist(s) and hand(s)
944.40 Deep necrosis of underlying tissues due to burn (deep third degree) of unspecified site of hand, without mention of a body part
944.41 Deep necrosis of underlying tissues due to burn (deep third degree) of single digit [finger (nail)] other than thumb, without mention of a body part
944.42 Deep necrosis of underlying tissues due to burn (deep third degree) of thumb (nail), without mention of loss of a body part
944.43 Deep necrosis of underlying tissues due to burn (deep third degree) of two or more digits of hand, not including thumb, without mention of a body part
944.44 Deep necrosis of underlying tissues due to burn (deep third degree) of two or more digits of hand including thumb, without mention of a body part
944.45 Deep necrosis of underlying tissues due to burn (deep third degree) of palm of hand, without mention of loss of a body part
944.46 Deep necrosis of underlying tissues due to burn (deep third degree) of back of hand, without mention of loss of back of a body part
944.47 Deep necrosis of underlying tissues due to burn (deep third degree) of wrist, without mention of loss of a body part
944.48 Deep necrosis of underlying tissues due to burn (deep third degree) of multiple sites of wrist(s) and hand(s), without mention of loss of a body part
944.50 Deep necrosis of underlying tissues due to burn (deep third degree) of unspecified site of hand, with loss of a body part
944.51 Deep necrosis of underlying tissues due to burn (deep third degree) of single digit (finger (nail)) other than thumb, with loss of a body part
944.52 Deep necrosis of underlying tissues due to burn (deep third degree) of thumb (nail), with loss of a body part
944.53 Deep necrosis of underlying tissues due to burn (deep third degree) of two or more digits of hand, not including thumb, with loss of a body part
944.54 Deep necrosis of underlying tissues due to burn (deep third degree) of two or more digits of hand including thumb, with loss of a body part
944.55 Deep necrosis of underlying tissues due to burn (deep third degree) of palm of hand, with loss of a body part
944.56 Deep necrosis of underlying tissues due to burn (deep third degree) of back of hand, with loss of a body part
944.57 Deep necrosis of underlying tissues due to burn (deep third degree) of wrist, with loss of a body part
944.58 Deep necrosis of underlying tissues due to burn (deep third degree) of multiple sites of wrist(s) and hand(s), with loss of a body part
945.32 Full-thickness skin loss due to burn (third degree nos) of foot
945.42 Deep necrosis of underlying tissues due to burn (deep third degree) of foot, without mention of loss of a body part
945.52 Deep necrosis of underlying tissues due to burn (deep third degree) of foot, with loss of a body part
948.00 Burn (any degree) involving less than 10% of body surface with third degree burn of less than 10% or unspecified amount
948.10 Burn (any degree) involving 10-19% of body surface with third degree burn of less than 10% or unspecified amount
948.11 Burn (any degree) involving 10-19% of body surface with third degree burn of 10-19%
948.20 Burn (any degree) involving 20-29% of body surface with third degree burn of less than 10% or unspecified amount
948.21 Burn (any degree) involving 20-29% of body surface with third degree burn of 10-19%
948.22 Burn (any degree) involving 20-29% of body surface with third degree burn of 20-29%
948.30 Burn (any degree) involving 30-39% of body surface with third degree burn of less than 10% or unspecified amount
948.31 Burn (any degree) involving 30-39% of body surface with third degree burn of 10-19%
948.32 Burn (any degree) involving 30-39% of body surface with third degree burn of 20-29%
948.33 Burn (any degree) involving 30-39% of body surface with third degree burn of 30-39%
948.40 Burn (any degree) involving 40-49% of body surface with third degree burn of less than 10% or unspecified amount
948.41 Burn (any degree) involving 40-49% of body surface with third degree burn of 10-19%
948.42 Burn (any degree) involving 40-49% of body surface with third degree burn of 20-29%
948.43 Burn (any degree) involving 40-49% of body surface with third degree burn of 30-39%
948.44 Burn (any degree) involving 40-49% of body surface with third degree burn of 40-49%
948.50 Burn (any degree) involving 50-59% of body surface with third degree burn of less than 10% or unspecified amount
948.51 Burn (any degree) involving 50-59% of body surface with third degree burn of 10-19%
948.52 Burn (any degree) involving 50-59% of body surface with third degree burn of 20-29%
948.53 Burn (any degree) involving 50-59% of body surface with third degree burn of 30-39%
948.54 Burn (any degree) involving 50-59% of body surface with third degree burn of 40-49%
948.55 Burn (any degree) involving 50-59% of body surface with third degree burn of 50-59%
948.60 Burn (any degree) involving 60-69% of body surface with third degree burn of less than 10% or unspecified amount
948.61 Burn (any degree) involving 60-69% of body surface with third degree burn of 10-19%
948.62 Burn (any degree) involving 60-69% of body surface with third degree burn of 20-29%
948.63 Burn (any degree) involving 60-69% of body surface with third degree burn of 30-39%
948.64 Burn (any degree) involving 60-69% of body surface with third degree burn of 40-49%
948.65 Burn (any degree) involving 60-69% of body surface with third degree burn of 50-59%
948.66 Burn (any degree) involving 60-69% of body surface with third degree burn of 60-69%
948.70 Burn (any degree) involving 70-79% of body surface with third degree burn of less than 10% or unspecified amount
948.71 Burn (any degree) involving 70-79% of body surface with third degree burn of 10-19%
948.72 Burn (any degree) involving 70-79% of body surface with third degree burn of 20-29%
948.73 Burn (any degree) involving 70-79% of body surface with third degree burn of 30-39%
948.74 Burn (any degree) involving 70-79% of body surface with third degree burn of 40-49%
948.75 Burn (any degree) involving 70-79% of body surface with third degree burn of 50-59%
948.76 Burn (any degree) involving 70-79% of body surface with third degree burn of 60-69%
948.77 Burn (any degree) involving 70-79% of body surface with third degree burn of 70-79%
948.80 Burn (any degree) involving 80-89% of body surface with third degree burn of less than 10% or unspecified amount
948.81 Burn (any degree) involving 80-89% of body surface with third degree burn of 10-19%
948.82 Burn (any degree) involving 80-89% of body surface with third degree burn of 20-29%
948.83 Burn (any degree) involving 80-89% of body surface with third degree burn of 30-39%
948.84 Burn (any degree) involving 80-89% of body surface with third degree burn of 40-49%
948.85 Burn (any degree) involving 80-89% of body surface with third degree burn of 50-59%
948.86 Burn (any degree) involving 80-89% of body surface with third degree burn of 60-69%
948.87 Burn (any degree) involving 80-89% of body surface with third degree burn of 70-79%
948.88 Burn (any degree) involving 80-89% of body surface with third degree burn of 80-89%
959.11 Other injury of chest wall
959.12 Other injury of abdomen
959.14 Other injury of external genitals
959.19 Other injury of other sites of trunk
959.4 Injury, other and unspecified, hand, except finger
959.5 Injury, other and unspecified, finger
959.7 Injury, other and unspecified, knee, leg, ankle, and foot
959.8 Injury, other and unspecified, other specified sites, including multiple
991.0 Frostbite of face
991.1 Frostbite of hand
991.2 Frostbite of foot

997.60 Late complications of amputation stump, unspecified — (Use additional code to identify complications) ▽
997.62 Infection (chronic) of amputation stump — (Use additional code to identify organism. Use additional code to identify complications)
997.69 Other late amputation stump complication — (Use additional code to identify complications)
998.59 Other postoperative infection — (Use additional code to identify infection)
V51 Aftercare involving the use of plastic surgery

ICD-9-CM Procedural

85.84 Pedicle graft to breast

15750

15750 Flap; neurovascular pedicle

ICD-9-CM Diagnostic

142.0 Malignant neoplasm of parotid gland
142.1 Malignant neoplasm of submandibular gland
142.2 Malignant neoplasm of sublingual gland
143.0 Malignant neoplasm of upper gum
143.1 Malignant neoplasm of lower gum
143.8 Malignant neoplasm of other sites of gum
144.8 Malignant neoplasm of other sites of floor of mouth
145.0 Malignant neoplasm of cheek mucosa
145.1 Malignant neoplasm of vestibule of mouth
145.8 Malignant neoplasm of other specified parts of mouth
145.9 Malignant neoplasm of mouth, unspecified site ▽
146.9 Malignant neoplasm of oropharynx, unspecified site ▽
147.0 Malignant neoplasm of superior wall of nasopharynx
147.1 Malignant neoplasm of posterior wall of nasopharynx
147.2 Malignant neoplasm of lateral wall of nasopharynx
147.3 Malignant neoplasm of anterior wall of nasopharynx
149.8 Malignant neoplasm of other sites within the lip and oral cavity
160.0 Malignant neoplasm of nasal cavities
160.1 Malignant neoplasm of auditory tube, middle ear, and mastoid air cells
160.2 Malignant neoplasm of maxillary sinus
160.3 Malignant neoplasm of ethmoidal sinus
160.4 Malignant neoplasm of frontal sinus
160.5 Malignant neoplasm of sphenoidal sinus
160.8 Malignant neoplasm of other sites of nasal cavities, middle ear, and accessory sinuses
161.8 Malignant neoplasm of other specified sites of larynx
161.9 Malignant neoplasm of larynx, unspecified site ▽
170.0 Malignant neoplasm of bones of skull and face, except mandible
170.1 Malignant neoplasm of mandible
171.0 Malignant neoplasm of connective and other soft tissue of head, face, and neck
171.2 Malignant neoplasm of connective and other soft tissue of upper limb, including shoulder
171.4 Malignant neoplasm of connective and other soft tissue of thorax
171.6 Malignant neoplasm of connective and other soft tissue of pelvis
171.7 Malignant neoplasm of connective and other soft tissue of trunk, unspecified site ▽
171.8 Malignant neoplasm of other specified sites of connective and other soft tissue
172.2 Malignant melanoma of skin of ear and external auditory canal
172.3 Malignant melanoma of skin of other and unspecified parts of face
172.5 Malignant melanoma of skin of trunk, except scrotum
172.6 Malignant melanoma of skin of upper limb, including shoulder
173.5 Other malignant neoplasm of skin of trunk, except scrotum
173.6 Other malignant neoplasm of skin of upper limb, including shoulder
173.7 Other malignant neoplasm of skin of lower limb, including hip
174.0 Malignant neoplasm of nipple and areola of female breast ♀
174.1 Malignant neoplasm of central portion of female breast ♀
174.2 Malignant neoplasm of upper-inner quadrant of female breast ♀
174.3 Malignant neoplasm of lower-inner quadrant of female breast ♀
174.4 Malignant neoplasm of upper-outer quadrant of female breast ♀
174.5 Malignant neoplasm of lower-outer quadrant of female breast ♀
174.6 Malignant neoplasm of axillary tail of female breast ♀
174.8 Malignant neoplasm of other specified sites of female breast ♀
175.9 Malignant neoplasm of other and unspecified sites of male breast ▽ ♂
195.0 Malignant neoplasm of head, face, and neck
195.5 Malignant neoplasm of lower limb
196.0 Secondary and unspecified malignant neoplasm of lymph nodes of head, face, and neck
197.1 Secondary malignant neoplasm of mediastinum
197.8 Secondary malignant neoplasm of other digestive organs and spleen
198.2 Secondary malignant neoplasm of skin
198.81 Secondary malignant neoplasm of breast
215.0 Other benign neoplasm of connective and other soft tissue of head, face, and neck
230.0 Carcinoma in situ of lip, oral cavity, and pharynx
232.1 Carcinoma in situ of eyelid, including canthus
232.2 Carcinoma in situ of skin of ear and external auditory canal
232.5 Carcinoma in situ of skin of trunk, except scrotum
232.6 Carcinoma in situ of skin of upper limb, including shoulder
232.8 Carcinoma in situ of other specified sites of skin
233.0 Carcinoma in situ of breast
234.8 Carcinoma in situ of other specified sites
235.0 Neoplasm of uncertain behavior of major salivary glands
235.1 Neoplasm of uncertain behavior of lip, oral cavity, and pharynx
235.9 Neoplasm of uncertain behavior of other and unspecified respiratory organs ▽
238.0 Neoplasm of uncertain behavior of bone and articular cartilage
238.1 Neoplasm of uncertain behavior of connective and other soft tissue ▽
238.2 Neoplasm of uncertain behavior of skin
238.3 Neoplasm of uncertain behavior of breast
239.0 Neoplasm of unspecified nature of digestive system
239.1 Neoplasm of unspecified nature of respiratory system
239.2 Neoplasms of unspecified nature of bone, soft tissue, and skin
239.3 Neoplasm of unspecified nature of breast
519.2 Mediastinitis
682.2 Cellulitis and abscess of trunk — (Use additional code to identify organism)
682.3 Cellulitis and abscess of upper arm and forearm — (Use additional code to identify organism)
682.4 Cellulitis and abscess of hand, except fingers and thumb — (Use additional code to identify organism)
682.5 Cellulitis and abscess of buttock — (Use additional code to identify organism)
701.5 Other abnormal granulation tissue
707.00 Decubitus ulcer, unspecified site
707.01 Decubitus ulcer, elbow
707.02 Decubitus ulcer, upper back
707.03 Decubitus ulcer, lower back
707.04 Decubitus ulcer, hip
707.05 Decubitus ulcer, buttock
707.06 Decubitus ulcer, ankle
707.07 Decubitus ulcer, heel
707.09 Decubitus ulcer, other site
707.10 Ulcer of lower limb, unspecified ▽
707.11 Ulcer of thigh
707.12 Ulcer of calf
707.13 Ulcer of ankle
707.14 Ulcer of heel and midfoot
707.15 Ulcer of other part of foot
707.19 Ulcer of other part of lower limb
707.8 Chronic ulcer of other specified site
709.2 Scar condition and fibrosis of skin
728.82 Foreign body granuloma of muscle
728.86 Necrotizing fasciitis — (Use additional code to identify infectious organism, 041.00-041.89, 785.4, if applicable)
729.4 Unspecified fasciitis ▽
730.16 Chronic osteomyelitis, lower leg — (Use additional code to identify organism, 041.1)
730.17 Chronic osteomyelitis, ankle and foot — (Use additional code to identify organism, 041.1)
730.26 Unspecified osteomyelitis, lower leg — (Use additional code to identify organism, 041.1) ▽
738.3 Acquired deformity of chest and rib
741.00 Spina bifida with hydrocephalus, unspecified region ▽
754.81 Pectus excavatum
810.10 Unspecified part of open fracture of clavicle ▽
810.11 Open fracture of sternal end of clavicle
810.12 Open fracture of shaft of clavicle
810.13 Open fracture of acromial end of clavicle
811.10 Open fracture of unspecified part of scapula ▽
811.11 Open fracture of acromial process of scapula
811.12 Open fracture of coracoid process
811.13 Open fracture of glenoid cavity and neck of scapula
811.19 Open fracture of other part of scapula
812.10 Open fracture of unspecified part of upper end of humerus ▽
812.12 Open fracture of anatomical neck of humerus
812.13 Open fracture of greater tuberosity of humerus
812.19 Other open fracture of upper end of humerus
812.30 Open fracture of unspecified part of humerus ▽
812.31 Open fracture of shaft of humerus

▽ Unspecified code
♀ Female diagnosis
☒ Manifestation code
♂ Male diagnosis

812.50	Open fracture of unspecified part of lower end of humerus ▽
812.51	Open fracture of supracondylar humerus
812.52	Open fracture of lateral condyle of humerus
812.53	Open fracture of medial condyle of humerus
812.54	Open fracture of unspecified condyle(s) of humerus ▽
812.59	Other open fracture of lower end of humerus
813.10	Unspecified open fracture of upper end of forearm ▽
813.11	Open fracture of olecranon process of ulna
813.12	Open fracture of coronoid process of ulna
813.13	Open Monteggia's fracture
813.14	Other and unspecified open fractures of proximal end of ulna (alone) ▽
813.15	Open fracture of head of radius
813.16	Open fracture of neck of radius
813.17	Other and unspecified open fractures of proximal end of radius (alone) ▽
813.18	Open fracture of radius with ulna, upper end (any part)
813.30	Unspecified open fracture of shaft of radius or ulna ▽
813.31	Open fracture of shaft of radius (alone)
813.32	Open fracture of shaft of ulna (alone)
813.33	Open fracture of shaft of radius with ulna
813.50	Unspecified open fracture of lower end of forearm ▽
813.51	Open Colles' fracture
813.52	Other open fractures of distal end of radius (alone)
813.53	Open fracture of distal end of ulna (alone)
813.54	Open fracture of lower end of radius with ulna
813.90	Open fracture of unspecified part of forearm ▽
813.91	Open fracture of unspecified part of radius (alone) ▽
813.92	Open fracture of unspecified part of ulna (alone) ▽
813.93	Open fracture of unspecified part of radius with ulna ▽
819.1	Multiple open fractures involving both upper limbs, and upper limb with rib(s) and sternum
823.92	Open fracture of unspecified part of fibula with tibia ▽
860.1	Traumatic pneumothorax with open wound into thorax
860.3	Traumatic hemothorax with open wound into thorax
860.5	Traumatic pneumohemothorax with open wound into thorax
861.30	Unspecified lung injury with open wound into thorax ▽
861.31	Lung contusion with open wound into thorax
861.32	Lung laceration with open wound into thorax
862.1	Diaphragm injury with open wound into cavity
862.31	Bronchus injury with open wound into cavity
862.32	Esophagus injury with open wound into cavity
862.39	Injury to other specified intrathoracic organs with open wound into cavity
863.30	Small intestine injury, unspecified site, with open wound into cavity ▽
863.31	Duodenum injury with open wound into cavity
863.39	Other injury to small intestine with open wound into cavity
863.50	Colon injury, unspecified site, with open wound into cavity ▽
863.51	Ascending (right) colon injury with open wound into cavity
863.52	Transverse colon injury with open wound into cavity
863.53	Descending (left) colon injury with open wound into cavity
863.54	Sigmoid colon injury with open wound into cavity
863.55	Rectum injury with open wound into cavity
863.56	Injury to multiple sites in colon and rectum with open wound into cavity
863.59	Other injury to colon and rectum with open wound into cavity
863.91	Pancreas head injury with open wound into cavity
863.92	Pancreas body injury with open wound into cavity
863.93	Pancreas tail injury with open wound into cavity
863.94	Pancreas injury, multiple and unspecified sites, with open wound into cavity
863.95	Appendix injury with open wound into cavity
863.99	Injury to other and unspecified gastrointestinal sites with open wound into cavity
864.10	Unspecified liver injury with open wound into cavity ▽
864.11	Liver hematoma and contusion with open wound into cavity
864.12	Liver laceration, minor, with open wound into cavity
864.13	Liver laceration, moderate, with open wound into cavity
864.14	Liver laceration, major, with open wound into cavity
864.15	Liver injury with open wound into cavity, unspecified laceration ▽
864.19	Other liver injury with open wound into cavity
865.10	Unspecified spleen injury with open wound into cavity ▽
865.11	Spleen hematoma, without rupture of capsule, with open wound into cavity
865.12	Capsular tears to spleen, without major disruption of parenchyma, with open wound into cavity
865.13	Spleen laceration extending into parenchyma, with open wound into cavity
865.14	Massive parenchyma disruption of spleen with open wound into cavity
865.19	Other spleen injury with open wound into cavity
866.11	Kidney hematoma, without rupture of capsule, with open wound into cavity
866.12	Kidney laceration with open wound into cavity
866.13	Complete disruption of kidney parenchyma, with open wound into cavity
867.1	Bladder and urethra injury with open wound into cavity
867.3	Ureter injury with open wound into cavity
867.5	Uterus injury with open wound into cavity ♀
867.7	Injury to other specified pelvic organs with open wound into cavity
868.10	Injury to unspecified intra-abdominal organ, with open wound into cavity ▽
868.11	Adrenal gland injury, with open wound into cavity
868.12	Bile duct and gallbladder injury, with open wound into cavity
868.13	Peritoneum injury with open wound into cavity
868.14	Retroperitoneum injury with open wound into cavity
868.19	Injury to other and multiple intra-abdominal organs, with open wound into cavity
869.1	Internal injury to unspecified or ill-defined organs with open wound into cavity
873.0	Open wound of scalp, without mention of complication — (Use additional code to identify infection)
873.1	Open wound of scalp, complicated — (Use additional code to identify infection)
873.40	Open wound of face, unspecified site, without mention of complication — (Use additional code to identify infection) ▽
873.41	Open wound of cheek, without mention of complication — (Use additional code to identify infection)
873.42	Open wound of forehead, without mention of complication — (Use additional code to identify infection)
873.49	Open wound of face, other and multiple sites, without mention of complication — (Use additional code to identify infection)
873.50	Open wound of face, unspecified site, complicated — (Use additional code to identify infection) ▽
873.51	Open wound of cheek, complicated — (Use additional code to identify infection)
873.52	Open wound of forehead, complicated — (Use additional code to identify infection)
873.54	Open wound of jaw, complicated — (Use additional code to identify infection)
873.59	Open wound of face, other and multiple sites, complicated — (Use additional code to identify infection)
874.8	Open wound of other and unspecified parts of neck, without mention of complication — (Use additional code to identify infection) ▽
875.1	Open wound of chest (wall), complicated — (Use additional code to identify infection)
876.0	Open wound of back, without mention of complication — (Use additional code to identify infection)
876.1	Open wound of back, complicated — (Use additional code to identify infection)
877.1	Open wound of buttock, complicated — (Use additional code to identify infection)
879.5	Open wound of abdominal wall, lateral, complicated — (Use additional code to identify infection)
879.8	Open wound(s) (multiple) of unspecified site(s), without mention of complication — (Use additional code to identify infection) ▽
879.9	Open wound(s) (multiple) of unspecified site(s), complicated — (Use additional code to identify infection) ▽
880.03	Open wound of upper arm, without mention of complication — (Use additional code to identify infection)
880.09	Open wound of multiple sites of shoulder and upper arm, without mention of complication — (Use additional code to identify infection)
880.13	Open wound of upper arm, complicated — (Use additional code to identify infection)
880.19	Open wound of multiple sites of shoulder and upper arm, complicated — (Use additional code to identify infection)
880.23	Open wound of upper arm, with tendon involvement — (Use additional code to identify infection)
880.29	Open wound of multiple sites of shoulder and upper arm, with tendon involvement — (Use additional code to identify infection)
881.00	Open wound of forearm, without mention of complication — (Use additional code to identify infection)
881.01	Open wound of elbow, without mention of complication — (Use additional code to identify infection)
881.02	Open wound of wrist, without mention of complication — (Use additional code to identify infection)
881.10	Open wound of forearm, complicated — (Use additional code to identify infection)
881.11	Open wound of elbow, complicated — (Use additional code to identify infection)
881.12	Open wound of wrist, complicated — (Use additional code to identify infection)
881.20	Open wound of forearm, with tendon involvement — (Use additional code to identify infection)
881.21	Open wound of elbow, with tendon involvement — (Use additional code to identify infection)

▽ Unspecified code
♀ Female diagnosis
☒ Manifestation code
♂ Male diagnosis

881.22 Open wound of wrist, with tendon involvement — (Use additional code to identify infection)
882.0 Open wound of hand except finger(s) alone, without mention of complication — (Use additional code to identify infection)
882.1 Open wound of hand except finger(s) alone, complicated — (Use additional code to identify infection)
882.2 Open wound of hand except finger(s) alone, with tendon involvement — (Use additional code to identify infection)
883.0 Open wound of finger(s), without mention of complication — (Use additional code to identify infection)
883.1 Open wound of finger(s), complicated — (Use additional code to identify infection)
883.2 Open wound of finger(s), with tendon involvement — (Use additional code to identify infection)
884.0 Multiple and unspecified open wound of upper limb, without mention of complication — (Use additional code to identify infection)
884.1 Multiple and unspecified open wound of upper limb, complicated — (Use additional code to identify infection)
884.2 Multiple and unspecified open wound of upper limb, with tendon involvement — (Use additional code to identify infection)
885.0 Traumatic amputation of thumb (complete) (partial), without mention of complication — (Use additional code to identify infection)
885.1 Traumatic amputation of thumb (complete) (partial), complicated — (Use additional code to identify infection)
886.0 Traumatic amputation of other finger(s) (complete) (partial), without mention of complication — (Use additional code to identify infection)
886.1 Traumatic amputation of other finger(s) (complete) (partial), complicated — (Use additional code to identify infection)
887.0 Traumatic amputation of arm and hand (complete) (partial), unilateral, below elbow, without mention of complication — (Use additional code to identify infection)
887.1 Traumatic amputation of arm and hand (complete) (partial), unilateral, below elbow, complicated — (Use additional code to identify infection)
887.2 Traumatic amputation of arm and hand (complete) (partial), unilateral, at or above elbow, without mention of complication — (Use additional code to identify infection)
887.3 Traumatic amputation of arm and hand (complete) (partial), unilateral, at or above elbow, complicated — (Use additional code to identify infection)
887.4 Traumatic amputation of arm and hand (complete) (partial), unilateral, level not specified, without mention of complication — (Use additional code to identify infection) ▽
887.5 Traumatic amputation of arm and hand (complete) (partial), unilateral, level not specified, complicated — (Use additional code to identify infection) ▽
887.6 Traumatic amputation of arm and hand (complete) (partial), bilateral (any level), without mention of complication — (Use additional code to identify infection)
887.7 Traumatic amputation of arm and hand (complete) (partial), bilateral (any level), complicated — (Use additional code to identify infection)
890.1 Open wound of hip and thigh, complicated — (Use additional code to identify infection)
891.0 Open wound of knee, leg (except thigh), and ankle, without mention of complication — (Use additional code to identify infection)
891.1 Open wound of knee, leg (except thigh), and ankle, complicated — (Use additional code to identify infection)
892.1 Open wound of foot except toe(s) alone, complicated — (Use additional code to identify infection)
896.1 Traumatic amputation of foot (complete) (partial), unilateral, complicated — (Use additional code to identify infection)
905.0 Late effect of fracture of skull and face bones
906.0 Late effect of open wound of head, neck, and trunk
906.1 Late effect of open wound of extremities without mention of tendon injury
906.4 Late effect of crushing
906.6 Late effect of burn of wrist and hand
906.7 Late effect of burn of other extremities
906.8 Late effect of burns of other specified sites
908.0 Late effect of internal injury to chest
908.1 Late effect of internal injury to intra-abdominal organs
908.2 Late effect of internal injury to other internal organs
908.4 Late effect of injury to blood vessel of thorax, abdomen, and pelvis
908.6 Late effect of certain complications of trauma
909.2 Late effect of radiation
909.3 Late effect of complications of surgical and medical care
925.1 Crushing injury of face and scalp — (Use additional code to identify any associated injuries: 800-829, 850.0-854.1, 860.0-869.1)
925.2 Crushing injury of neck — (Use additional code to identify any associated injuries: 800-829, 850.0-854.1, 860.0-869.1)
926.0 Crushing injury of external genitalia — (Use additional code to identify any associated injuries: 800-829, 850.0-854.1, 860.0-869.1)
926.11 Crushing injury of back — (Use additional code to identify any associated injuries: 800-829, 850.0-854.1, 860.0-869.1)
926.12 Crushing injury of buttock — (Use additional code to identify any associated injuries: 800-829, 850.0-854.1, 860.0-869.1)
926.19 Crushing injury of other specified sites of trunk — (Use additional code to identify any associated injuries: 800-829, 850.0-854.1, 860.0-869.1)
927.03 Crushing injury of upper arm — (Use additional code to identify any associated injuries: 800-829, 850.0-854.1, 860.0-869.1)
927.09 Crushing injury of multiple sites of upper arm — (Use additional code to identify any associated injuries: 800-829, 850.0-854.1, 860.0-869.1)
927.10 Crushing injury of forearm — (Use additional code to identify any associated injuries: 800-829, 850.0-854.1, 860.0-869.1)
927.11 Crushing injury of elbow — (Use additional code to identify any associated injuries: 800-829, 850.0-854.1, 860.0-869.1)
927.20 Crushing injury of hand(s) — (Use additional code to identify any associated injuries: 800-829, 850.0-854.1, 860.0-869.1)
927.21 Crushing injury of wrist — (Use additional code to identify any associated injuries: 800-829, 850.0-854.1, 860.0-869.1)
927.3 Crushing injury of finger(s) — (Use additional code to identify any associated injuries: 800-829, 850.0-854.1, 860.0-869.1)
927.8 Crushing injury of multiple sites of upper limb — (Use additional code to identify any associated injuries: 800-829, 850.0-854.1, 860.0-869.1)
941.30 Full-thickness skin loss due to burn (third degree nos) of unspecified site of face and head ▽
941.36 Full-thickness skin loss due to burn (third degree nos) of scalp (any part)
941.37 Full-thickness skin loss due to burn (third degree nos) of forehead and cheek
941.38 Full-thickness skin loss due to burn (third degree nos) of neck
941.39 Full-thickness skin loss due to burn (third degree nos) of multiple sites (except with eye) of face, head, and neck
941.40 Deep necrosis of underlying tissues due to burn (deep third degree) of unspecified site of face and head, without mention of loss of a body part ▽
941.44 Deep necrosis of underlying tissues due to burn (deep third degree) of chin, without mention of loss of a body part
941.46 Deep necrosis of underlying tissues due to burn (deep third degree) of scalp (any part), without mention of loss of a body part
941.47 Deep necrosis of underlying tissues due to burn (deep third degree) of forehead and cheek, without mention of loss of a body part
941.48 Deep necrosis of underlying tissues due to burn (deep third degree) of neck, without mention of loss of a body part
941.49 Deep necrosis of underlying tissues due to burn (deep third degree) of multiple sites (except with eye) of face, head, and neck, without mention of loss of a body part
941.50 Deep necrosis of underlying tissues due to burn (deep third degree) of face and head, unspecified site, with loss of a body part ▽
941.54 Deep necrosis of underlying tissues due to burn (deep third degree) of chin, with loss of a body part
941.56 Deep necrosis of underlying tissues due to burn (deep third degree) of scalp (any part), with loss of a body part
941.58 Deep necrosis of underlying tissues due to burn (deep third degree) of neck, with loss of a body part
942.30 Full-thickness skin loss due to burn (third degree nos) of unspecified site of trunk ▽
942.31 Full-thickness skin loss due to burn (third degree nos) of breast
942.33 Full-thickness skin loss due to burn (third degree nos) of abdominal wall
942.34 Full-thickness skin loss due to burn (third degree nos) of back (any part)
942.35 Full-thickness skin loss due to burn (third degree nos) of genitalia
942.39 Full-thickness skin loss due to burn (third degree nos) of other and multiple sites of trunk
942.40 Deep necrosis of underlying tissues due to burn (deep third degree) of trunk, unspecified site, without mention of loss of a body part ▽
942.41 Deep necrosis of underlying tissues due to burn (deep third degree) of breast, without mention of loss of a body part
942.42 Deep necrosis of underlying tissues due to burn (deep third degree) of chest wall, excluding breast and nipple, without mention of loss of a body part
942.43 Deep necrosis of underlying tissues due to burn (deep third degree) of abdominal wall, without mention of loss of a body part
942.44 Deep necrosis of underlying tissues due to burn (deep third degree) of back (any part), without mention of loss of a body part
942.45 Deep necrosis of underlying tissues due to burn (deep third degree) of genitalia, without mention of loss of a body part
942.49 Deep necrosis of underlying tissues due to burn (deep third degree) of other and multiple sites of trunk, without mention of loss of a body part
942.50 Deep necrosis of underlying tissues due to burn (deep third degree) of unspecified site of trunk, with loss of a body part ▽

▽ Unspecified code
♀ Female diagnosis
☒ Manifestation code
♂ Male diagnosis

942.51 Deep necrosis of underlying tissues due to burn (deep third degree) of breast, with loss of a body part
942.52 Deep necrosis of underlying tissues due to burn (deep third degree) of chest wall, excluding breast and nipple, with loss of a body part
942.53 Deep necrosis of underlying tissues due to burn (deep third degree) of abdominal wall with loss of a body part
942.54 Deep necrosis of underlying tissues due to burn (deep third degree) of back (any part), with loss of a body part
942.55 Deep necrosis of underlying tissues due to burn (deep third degree) of genitalia, with loss of a body part
942.59 Deep necrosis of underlying tissues due to burn (deep third degree) of other and multiple sites of trunk, with loss of a body part
943.30 Full-thickness skin loss due to burn (third degree nos) of unspecified site of upper limb ▽
943.31 Full-thickness skin loss due to burn (third degree nos) of forearm
943.32 Full-thickness skin loss due to burn (third degree nos) of elbow
943.33 Full-thickness skin loss due to burn (third degree nos) of upper arm
943.39 Full-thickness skin loss due to burn (third degree nos) of multiple sites of upper limb, except wrist and hand
943.40 Deep necrosis of underlying tissues due to burn (deep third degree) of unspecified site of upper limb, without mention of loss of a body part ▽
943.41 Deep necrosis of underlying tissues due to burn (deep third degree) of forearm, without mention of loss of a body part
943.42 Deep necrosis of underlying tissues due to burn (deep third degree) of elbow, without mention of loss of a body part
943.44 Deep necrosis of underlying tissues due to burn (deep third degree) of axilla, without mention of loss of a body part
943.49 Deep necrosis of underlying tissues due to burn (deep third degree) of multiple sites of upper limb, except wrist and hand, without mention of loss of a body part
943.50 Deep necrosis of underlying tissues due to burn (deep third degree) of unspecified site of upper limb, with loss of a body part ▽
943.51 Deep necrosis of underlying tissues due to burn (deep third degree) of forearm, with loss of a body part
943.52 Deep necrosis of underlying tissues due to burn (deep third degree) of elbow, with loss of a body part
943.53 Deep necrosis of underlying tissues due to burn (deep third degree) of upper arm, with loss of upper a body part
943.59 Deep necrosis of underlying tissues due to burn (deep third degree) of multiple sites of upper limb, except wrist and hand, with loss of a body part
944.30 Full-thickness skin loss due to burn (third degree nos) of unspecified site of hand ▽
944.31 Full-thickness skin loss due to burn (third degree nos) of single digit [finger (nail)] other than thumb
944.32 Full-thickness skin loss due to burn (third degree nos) of thumb (nail)
944.33 Full-thickness skin loss due to burn (third degree nos) of two or more digits of hand, not including thumb
944.34 Full-thickness skin loss due to burn (third degree nos) of two or more digits of hand including thumb
944.35 Full-thickness skin loss due to burn (third degree nos) of palm of hand
944.36 Full-thickness skin loss due to burn (third degree nos) of back of hand
944.37 Full-thickness skin loss due to burn (third degree nos) of wrist
944.38 Full-thickness skin loss due to burn (third degree nos) of multiple sites of wrist(s) and hand(s)
944.40 Deep necrosis of underlying tissues due to burn (deep third degree) of unspecified site of hand, without mention of a body part ▽
944.41 Deep necrosis of underlying tissues due to burn (deep third degree) of single digit [finger (nail)] other than thumb, without mention of a body part
944.42 Deep necrosis of underlying tissues due to burn (deep third degree) of thumb (nail), without mention of loss of a body part
944.43 Deep necrosis of underlying tissues due to burn (deep third degree) of two or more digits of hand, not including thumb, without mention of a body part
944.44 Deep necrosis of underlying tissues due to burn (deep third degree) of two or more digits of hand including thumb, without mention of a body part
944.46 Deep necrosis of underlying tissues due to burn (deep third degree) of back of hand, without mention of loss of back of a body part
944.47 Deep necrosis of underlying tissues due to burn (deep third degree) of wrist, without mention of loss of a body part
944.48 Deep necrosis of underlying tissues due to burn (deep third degree) of multiple sites of wrist(s) and hand(s), without mention of loss of a body part
944.50 Deep necrosis of underlying tissues due to burn (deep third degree) of unspecified site of hand, with loss of a body part ▽
944.51 Deep necrosis of underlying tissues due to burn (deep third degree) of single digit (finger (nail)) other than thumb, with loss of a body part
944.52 Deep necrosis of underlying tissues due to burn (deep third degree) of thumb (nail), with loss of a body part
944.53 Deep necrosis of underlying tissues due to burn (deep third degree) of two or more digits of hand, not including thumb, with loss of a body part
944.54 Deep necrosis of underlying tissues due to burn (deep third degree) of two or more digits of hand including thumb, with loss of a body part
944.55 Deep necrosis of underlying tissues due to burn (deep third degree) of palm of hand, with loss of a body part
944.56 Deep necrosis of underlying tissues due to burn (deep third degree) of back of hand, with loss of a body part
944.57 Deep necrosis of underlying tissues due to burn (deep third degree) of wrist, with loss of a body part
944.58 Deep necrosis of underlying tissues due to burn (deep third degree) of multiple sites of wrist(s) and hand(s), with loss of a body part
996.52 Mechanical complication due to other tissue graft, not elsewhere classified
997.60 Late complications of amputation stump, unspecified — (Use additional code to identify complications) ▽
997.62 Infection (chronic) of amputation stump — (Use additional code to identify organism. Use additional code to identify complications)
997.69 Other late amputation stump complication — (Use additional code to identify complications)
998.31 Disruption of internal operation wound
998.32 Disruption of external operation wound
998.59 Other postoperative infection — (Use additional code to identify infection)
998.83 Non-healing surgical wound
V10.02 Personal history of malignant neoplasm of other and unspecified parts of oral cavity and pharynx ▽
V10.82 Personal history of malignant melanoma of skin
V51 Aftercare involving the use of plastic surgery

ICD-9-CM Procedural

04.5 Cranial or peripheral nerve graft

15756

15756 Free muscle or myocutaneous flap with microvascular anastomosis

ICD-9-CM Diagnostic

140.3 Malignant neoplasm of upper lip, inner aspect
140.5 Malignant neoplasm of lip, inner aspect, unspecified as to upper or lower ▽
140.8 Malignant neoplasm of other sites of lip
141.0 Malignant neoplasm of base of tongue
142.0 Malignant neoplasm of parotid gland
142.1 Malignant neoplasm of submandibular gland
142.2 Malignant neoplasm of sublingual gland
142.8 Malignant neoplasm of other major salivary glands
143.0 Malignant neoplasm of upper gum
143.1 Malignant neoplasm of lower gum
143.8 Malignant neoplasm of other sites of gum
143.9 Malignant neoplasm of gum, unspecified site ▽
144.0 Malignant neoplasm of anterior portion of floor of mouth
144.1 Malignant neoplasm of lateral portion of floor of mouth
144.8 Malignant neoplasm of other sites of floor of mouth
145.0 Malignant neoplasm of cheek mucosa
145.1 Malignant neoplasm of vestibule of mouth
145.8 Malignant neoplasm of other specified parts of mouth
146.3 Malignant neoplasm of vallecula
146.4 Malignant neoplasm of anterior aspect of epiglottis
146.5 Malignant neoplasm of junctional region of oropharynx
146.6 Malignant neoplasm of lateral wall of oropharynx
146.7 Malignant neoplasm of posterior wall of oropharynx
146.8 Malignant neoplasm of other specified sites of oropharynx
147.0 Malignant neoplasm of superior wall of nasopharynx
147.1 Malignant neoplasm of posterior wall of nasopharynx
147.2 Malignant neoplasm of lateral wall of nasopharynx
147.3 Malignant neoplasm of anterior wall of nasopharynx
149.8 Malignant neoplasm of other sites within the lip and oral cavity
149.9 Malignant neoplasm of ill-defined sites of lip and oral cavity
150.0 Malignant neoplasm of cervical esophagus
150.1 Malignant neoplasm of thoracic esophagus
160.0 Malignant neoplasm of nasal cavities
160.1 Malignant neoplasm of auditory tube, middle ear, and mastoid air cells
160.2 Malignant neoplasm of maxillary sinus
160.3 Malignant neoplasm of ethmoidal sinus
160.4 Malignant neoplasm of frontal sinus
160.5 Malignant neoplasm of sphenoidal sinus
160.8 Malignant neoplasm of other sites of nasal cavities, middle ear, and accessory sinuses
171.0 Malignant neoplasm of connective and other soft tissue of head, face, and neck

171.2 Malignant neoplasm of connective and other soft tissue of upper limb, including shoulder
171.3 Malignant neoplasm of connective and other soft tissue of lower limb, including hip
171.4 Malignant neoplasm of connective and other soft tissue of thorax
171.7 Malignant neoplasm of connective and other soft tissue of trunk, unspecified site
171.8 Malignant neoplasm of other specified sites of connective and other soft tissue
172.0 Malignant melanoma of skin of lip
172.1 Malignant melanoma of skin of eyelid, including canthus
172.2 Malignant melanoma of skin of ear and external auditory canal
172.4 Malignant melanoma of skin of scalp and neck
172.5 Malignant melanoma of skin of trunk, except scrotum
172.6 Malignant melanoma of skin of upper limb, including shoulder
172.7 Malignant melanoma of skin of lower limb, including hip
172.8 Malignant melanoma of other specified sites of skin
193 Malignant neoplasm of thyroid gland — (Use additional code to identify any functional activity)
195.0 Malignant neoplasm of head, face, and neck
195.1 Malignant neoplasm of thorax
196.0 Secondary and unspecified malignant neoplasm of lymph nodes of head, face, and neck
196.1 Secondary and unspecified malignant neoplasm of intrathoracic lymph nodes
235.0 Neoplasm of uncertain behavior of major salivary glands
235.1 Neoplasm of uncertain behavior of lip, oral cavity, and pharynx
238.1 Neoplasm of uncertain behavior of connective and other soft tissue
239.2 Neoplasms of unspecified nature of bone, soft tissue, and skin
682.2 Cellulitis and abscess of trunk — (Use additional code to identify organism)
707.00 Decubitus ulcer, unspecified site
707.01 Decubitus ulcer, elbow
707.02 Decubitus ulcer, upper back
707.03 Decubitus ulcer, lower back
707.04 Decubitus ulcer, hip
707.05 Decubitus ulcer, buttock
707.06 Decubitus ulcer, ankle
707.07 Decubitus ulcer, heel
707.09 Decubitus ulcer, other site
810.10 Unspecified part of open fracture of clavicle
810.11 Open fracture of sternal end of clavicle
810.12 Open fracture of shaft of clavicle
810.13 Open fracture of acromial end of clavicle
813.10 Unspecified open fracture of upper end of forearm
813.11 Open fracture of olecranon process of ulna
813.12 Open fracture of coronoid process of ulna
813.13 Open Monteggia's fracture
813.14 Other and unspecified open fractures of proximal end of ulna (alone)
813.15 Open fracture of head of radius
813.16 Open fracture of neck of radius
813.17 Other and unspecified open fractures of proximal end of radius (alone)
813.18 Open fracture of radius with ulna, upper end (any part)
813.30 Unspecified open fracture of shaft of radius or ulna
813.31 Open fracture of shaft of radius (alone)
813.32 Open fracture of shaft of ulna (alone)
813.33 Open fracture of shaft of radius with ulna
813.50 Unspecified open fracture of lower end of forearm
813.51 Open Colles' fracture
813.52 Other open fractures of distal end of radius (alone)
813.53 Open fracture of distal end of ulna (alone)
813.54 Open fracture of lower end of radius with ulna
813.90 Open fracture of unspecified part of forearm
813.91 Open fracture of unspecified part of radius (alone)
813.92 Open fracture of unspecified part of ulna (alone)
813.93 Open fracture of unspecified part of radius with ulna
823.10 Open fracture of upper end of tibia
823.11 Open fracture of upper end of fibula
823.12 Open fracture of upper end of fibula with tibia
823.30 Open fracture of shaft of tibia
823.31 Open fracture of shaft of fibula
823.32 Open fracture of shaft of fibula with tibia
823.90 Open fracture of unspecified part of tibia
823.91 Open fracture of unspecified part of fibula
823.92 Open fracture of unspecified part of fibula with tibia
873.50 Open wound of face, unspecified site, complicated — (Use additional code to identify infection)
873.51 Open wound of cheek, complicated — (Use additional code to identify infection)
873.52 Open wound of forehead, complicated — (Use additional code to identify infection)
873.53 Open wound of lip, complicated — (Use additional code to identify infection)
873.54 Open wound of jaw, complicated — (Use additional code to identify infection)
873.9 Other and unspecified open wound of head, complicated — (Use additional code to identify infection)
874.10 Open wound of larynx with trachea, complicated — (Use additional code to identify infection)
874.11 Open wound of larynx, complicated — (Use additional code to identify infection)
874.12 Open wound of trachea, complicated — (Use additional code to identify infection)
874.3 Open wound of thyroid gland, complicated — (Use additional code to identify infection)
874.5 Open wound of pharynx, complicated — (Use additional code to identify infection)
874.9 Open wound of other and unspecified parts of neck, complicated — (Use additional code to identify infection)
875.1 Open wound of chest (wall), complicated — (Use additional code to identify infection)
876.1 Open wound of back, complicated — (Use additional code to identify infection)
880.10 Open wound of shoulder region, complicated — (Use additional code to identify infection)
880.11 Open wound of scapular region, complicated — (Use additional code to identify infection)
880.12 Open wound of axillary region, complicated — (Use additional code to identify infection)
880.13 Open wound of upper arm, complicated — (Use additional code to identify infection)
880.19 Open wound of multiple sites of shoulder and upper arm, complicated — (Use additional code to identify infection)
881.10 Open wound of forearm, complicated — (Use additional code to identify infection)
881.11 Open wound of elbow, complicated — (Use additional code to identify infection)
881.12 Open wound of wrist, complicated — (Use additional code to identify infection)
882.1 Open wound of hand except finger(s) alone, complicated — (Use additional code to identify infection)
884.1 Multiple and unspecified open wound of upper limb, complicated — (Use additional code to identify infection)
891.1 Open wound of knee, leg (except thigh), and ankle, complicated — (Use additional code to identify infection)
959.01 Head injury, unspecified
959.09 Injury of face and neck, other and unspecified
959.11 Other injury of chest wall
959.12 Other injury of abdomen
959.19 Other injury of other sites of trunk
998.83 Non-healing surgical wound
V51 Aftercare involving the use of plastic surgery

ICD-9-CM Procedural

39.31 Suture of artery
39.32 Suture of vein
82.72 Plastic operation on hand with graft of muscle or fascia
83.77 Muscle transfer or transplantation
86.61 Full-thickness skin graft to hand
86.63 Full-thickness skin graft to other sites

15757

15757 Free skin flap with microvascular anastomosis

ICD-9-CM Diagnostic

140.9 Malignant neoplasm of lip, vermilion border, unspecified as to upper or lower
149.8 Malignant neoplasm of other sites within the lip and oral cavity
149.9 Malignant neoplasm of ill-defined sites of lip and oral cavity
172.1 Malignant melanoma of skin of eyelid, including canthus
172.2 Malignant melanoma of skin of ear and external auditory canal
172.4 Malignant melanoma of skin of scalp and neck
172.5 Malignant melanoma of skin of trunk, except scrotum
172.6 Malignant melanoma of skin of upper limb, including shoulder
172.7 Malignant melanoma of skin of lower limb, including hip
173.0 Other malignant neoplasm of skin of lip
173.1 Other malignant neoplasm of skin of eyelid, including canthus
173.2 Other malignant neoplasm of skin of ear and external auditory canal

Unspecified code
Female diagnosis
Manifestation code
Male diagnosis

173.4 Other malignant neoplasm of scalp and skin of neck
173.5 Other malignant neoplasm of skin of trunk, except scrotum
173.8 Other malignant neoplasm of other specified sites of skin
184.0 Malignant neoplasm of vagina ♀
184.1 Malignant neoplasm of labia majora ♀
184.2 Malignant neoplasm of labia minora ♀
184.3 Malignant neoplasm of clitoris ♀
184.4 Malignant neoplasm of vulva, unspecified site ▽ ♀
184.8 Malignant neoplasm of other specified sites of female genital organs ♀
187.1 Malignant neoplasm of prepuce ♂
187.2 Malignant neoplasm of glans penis ♂
187.3 Malignant neoplasm of body of penis ♂
187.4 Malignant neoplasm of penis, part unspecified ▽ ♂
187.7 Malignant neoplasm of scrotum ♂
187.9 Malignant neoplasm of male genital organ, site unspecified ▽ ♂
195.0 Malignant neoplasm of head, face, and neck
198.2 Secondary malignant neoplasm of skin
210.0 Benign neoplasm of lip
210.4 Benign neoplasm of other and unspecified parts of mouth ▽
216.1 Benign neoplasm of eyelid, including canthus
216.2 Benign neoplasm of ear and external auditory canal
216.4 Benign neoplasm of scalp and skin of neck
216.6 Benign neoplasm of skin of upper limb, including shoulder
216.7 Benign neoplasm of skin of lower limb, including hip
216.8 Benign neoplasm of other specified sites of skin
232.0 Carcinoma in situ of skin of lip
232.1 Carcinoma in situ of eyelid, including canthus
232.2 Carcinoma in situ of skin of ear and external auditory canal
232.4 Carcinoma in situ of scalp and skin of neck
232.6 Carcinoma in situ of skin of upper limb, including shoulder
232.7 Carcinoma in situ of skin of lower limb, including hip
232.8 Carcinoma in situ of other specified sites of skin
239.0 Neoplasm of unspecified nature of digestive system
239.2 Neoplasms of unspecified nature of bone, soft tissue, and skin
380.32 Acquired deformities of auricle or pinna
607.2 Other inflammatory disorders of penis — (Use additional code to identify organism) ♂
682.0 Cellulitis and abscess of face — (Use additional code to identify organism)
682.2 Cellulitis and abscess of trunk — (Use additional code to identify organism)
707.00 Decubitus ulcer, unspecified site
707.01 Decubitus ulcer, elbow
707.02 Decubitus ulcer, upper back
707.03 Decubitus ulcer, lower back
707.04 Decubitus ulcer, hip
707.05 Decubitus ulcer, buttock
707.06 Decubitus ulcer, ankle
707.07 Decubitus ulcer, heel
707.09 Decubitus ulcer, other site
707.10 Ulcer of lower limb, unspecified ▽
707.11 Ulcer of thigh
707.12 Ulcer of calf
707.13 Ulcer of ankle
707.14 Ulcer of heel and midfoot
707.15 Ulcer of other part of foot
707.19 Ulcer of other part of lower limb
707.8 Chronic ulcer of other specified site
728.86 Necrotizing fasciitis — (Use additional code to identify infectious organism, 041.00-041.89, 785.4, if applicable)
743.62 Congenital deformity of eyelid
744.01 Congenital absence of external ear causing impairment of hearing
744.09 Other congenital anomalies of ear causing impairment of hearing
744.23 Microtia
744.3 Unspecified congenital anomaly of ear ▽
744.5 Congenital webbing of neck
744.82 Microcheilia
748.1 Other congenital anomaly of nose
749.11 Unilateral cleft lip, complete
749.12 Unilateral cleft lip, incomplete
749.13 Bilateral cleft lip, complete
749.14 Bilateral cleft lip, incomplete
749.20 Unspecified cleft palate with cleft lip ▽
749.21 Unilateral cleft palate with cleft lip, complete
749.22 Unilateral cleft palate with cleft lip, incomplete
749.23 Bilateral cleft palate with cleft lip, complete
749.24 Bilateral cleft palate with cleft lip, incomplete
752.40 Unspecified congenital anomaly of cervix, vagina, and external female genitalia ▽ ♀
752.49 Other congenital anomaly of cervix, vagina, and external female genitalia ♀
752.64 Micropenis ♂
752.69 Other penile anomalies ♂
752.7 Indeterminate sex and pseudohermaphroditism
752.81 Scrotal transposition
752.89 Other specified anomalies of genital organs
752.9 Unspecified congenital anomaly of genital organs ▽
757.33 Congenital pigmentary anomaly of skin
785.4 Gangrene — (Code first any associated underlying condition:250.7, 443.0)
870.0 Laceration of skin of eyelid and periocular area — (Use additional code to identify infection)
870.1 Laceration of eyelid, full-thickness, not involving lacrimal passages — (Use additional code to identify infection)
870.2 Laceration of eyelid involving lacrimal passages — (Use additional code to identify infection)
872.00 Open wound of external ear, unspecified site, without mention of complication — (Use additional code to identify infection) ▽
872.01 Open wound of auricle, without mention of complication — (Use additional code to identify infection)
872.02 Open wound of auditory canal, without mention of complication — (Use additional code to identify infection)
872.10 Open wound of external ear, unspecified site, complicated — (Use additional code to identify infection) ▽
872.11 Open wound of auricle, complicated — (Use additional code to identify infection)
872.12 Open wound of auditory canal, complicated — (Use additional code to identify infection)
872.8 Open wound of ear, part unspecified, without mention of complication — (Use additional code to identify infection) ▽
872.9 Open wound of ear, part unspecified, complicated — (Use additional code to identify infection) ▽
873.30 Open wound of nose, unspecified site, complicated — (Use additional code to identify infection) ▽
873.31 Open wound of nasal septum, complicated — (Use additional code to identify infection)
873.32 Open wound of nasal cavity, complicated — (Use additional code to identify infection)
873.33 Open wound of nasal sinus, complicated — (Use additional code to identify infection)
873.39 Open wound of nose, multiple sites, complicated — (Use additional code to identify infection)
873.43 Open wound of lip, without mention of complication — (Use additional code to identify infection)
873.50 Open wound of face, unspecified site, complicated — (Use additional code to identify infection) ▽
873.52 Open wound of forehead, complicated — (Use additional code to identify infection)
873.54 Open wound of jaw, complicated — (Use additional code to identify infection)
873.59 Open wound of face, other and multiple sites, complicated — (Use additional code to identify infection)
874.8 Open wound of other and unspecified parts of neck, without mention of complication — (Use additional code to identify infection) ▽
874.9 Open wound of other and unspecified parts of neck, complicated — (Use additional code to identify infection) ▽
876.0 Open wound of back, without mention of complication — (Use additional code to identify infection)
876.1 Open wound of back, complicated — (Use additional code to identify infection)
878.1 Open wound of penis, complicated — (Use additional code to identify infection) ♂
878.3 Open wound of scrotum and testes, complicated — (Use additional code to identify infection) ♂
878.5 Open wound of vulva, complicated — (Use additional code to identify infection) ♀
878.7 Open wound of vagina, complicated — (Use additional code to identify infection) ♀
878.9 Open wound of other and unspecified parts of genital organs, complicated — (Use additional code to identify infection) ▽
880.12 Open wound of axillary region, complicated — (Use additional code to identify infection)
882.1 Open wound of hand except finger(s) alone, complicated — (Use additional code to identify infection)
882.2 Open wound of hand except finger(s) alone, with tendon involvement — (Use additional code to identify infection)

883.1 Open wound of finger(s), complicated — (Use additional code to identify infection)
883.2 Open wound of finger(s), with tendon involvement — (Use additional code to identify infection)
884.1 Multiple and unspecified open wound of upper limb, complicated — (Use additional code to identify infection)
884.2 Multiple and unspecified open wound of upper limb, with tendon involvement — (Use additional code to identify infection)
885.0 Traumatic amputation of thumb (complete) (partial), without mention of complication — (Use additional code to identify infection)
885.1 Traumatic amputation of thumb (complete) (partial), complicated — (Use additional code to identify infection)
886.0 Traumatic amputation of other finger(s) (complete) (partial), without mention of complication — (Use additional code to identify infection)
886.1 Traumatic amputation of other finger(s) (complete) (partial), complicated — (Use additional code to identify infection)
887.0 Traumatic amputation of arm and hand (complete) (partial), unilateral, below elbow, without mention of complication — (Use additional code to identify infection)
887.1 Traumatic amputation of arm and hand (complete) (partial), unilateral, below elbow, complicated — (Use additional code to identify infection)
887.6 Traumatic amputation of arm and hand (complete) (partial), bilateral (any level), without mention of complication — (Use additional code to identify infection)
887.7 Traumatic amputation of arm and hand (complete) (partial), bilateral (any level), complicated — (Use additional code to identify infection)
892.1 Open wound of foot except toe(s) alone, complicated — (Use additional code to identify infection)
892.2 Open wound of foot except toe(s) alone, with tendon involvement — (Use additional code to identify infection)
893.1 Open wound of toe(s), complicated — (Use additional code to identify infection)
893.2 Open wound of toe(s), with tendon involvement — (Use additional code to identify infection)
894.1 Multiple and unspecified open wound of lower limb, complicated — (Use additional code to identify infection)
894.2 Multiple and unspecified open wound of lower limb, with tendon involvement — (Use additional code to identify infection)
895.0 Traumatic amputation of toe(s) (complete) (partial), without mention of complication — (Use additional code to identify infection)
895.1 Traumatic amputation of toe(s) (complete) (partial), complicated — (Use additional code to identify infection)
896.0 Traumatic amputation of foot (complete) (partial), unilateral, without mention of complication — (Use additional code to identify infection)
896.1 Traumatic amputation of foot (complete) (partial), unilateral, complicated — (Use additional code to identify infection)
896.2 Traumatic amputation of foot (complete) (partial), bilateral, without mention of complication — (Use additional code to identify infection)
896.3 Traumatic amputation of foot (complete) (partial), bilateral, complicated — (Use additional code to identify infection)
906.0 Late effect of open wound of head, neck, and trunk
906.6 Late effect of burn of wrist and hand
941.01 Burn of unspecified degree of ear (any part) ▽
941.02 Burn of unspecified degree of eye (with other parts of face, head, and neck) ▽
941.03 Burn of unspecified degree of lip(s) ▽
941.05 Burn of unspecified degree of nose (septum) ▽
941.09 Burn of unspecified degree of multiple sites (except with eye) of face, head, and neck ▽
941.30 Full-thickness skin loss due to burn (third degree nos) of unspecified site of face and head ▽
941.31 Full-thickness skin loss due to burn (third degree nos) of ear (any part)
941.32 Full-thickness skin loss due to burn (third degree nos) of eye (with other parts of face, head, and neck)
941.34 Full-thickness skin loss due to burn (third degree nos) of chin
941.35 Full-thickness skin loss due to burn (third degree nos) of nose (septum)
941.37 Full-thickness skin loss due to burn (third degree nos) of forehead and cheek
941.38 Full-thickness skin loss due to burn (third degree nos) of neck
941.40 Deep necrosis of underlying tissues due to burn (deep third degree) of unspecified site of face and head, without mention of loss of a body part ▽
941.43 Deep necrosis of underlying tissues due to burn (deep third degree) of lip(s), without mention of loss of a body part
941.44 Deep necrosis of underlying tissues due to burn (deep third degree) of chin, without mention of loss of a body part
941.47 Deep necrosis of underlying tissues due to burn (deep third degree) of forehead and cheek, without mention of loss of a body part
941.48 Deep necrosis of underlying tissues due to burn (deep third degree) of neck, without mention of loss of a body part
941.49 Deep necrosis of underlying tissues due to burn (deep third degree) of multiple sites (except with eye) of face, head, and neck, without mention of loss of a body part
941.50 Deep necrosis of underlying tissues due to burn (deep third degree) of face and head, unspecified site, with loss of a body part ▽
941.51 Deep necrosis of underlying tissues due to burn (deep third degree) of ear (any part), with loss of a body part
941.52 Deep necrosis of underlying tissues due to burn (deep third degree) of eye (with other parts of face, head, and neck), with loss of a body part
941.55 Deep necrosis of underlying tissues due to burn (deep third degree) of nose (septum), with loss of a body part
941.57 Deep necrosis of underlying tissues due to burn (deep third degree) of forehead and cheek, with loss of a body part
941.58 Deep necrosis of underlying tissues due to burn (deep third degree) of neck, with loss of a body part
943.34 Full-thickness skin loss due to burn (third degree nos) of axilla
943.44 Deep necrosis of underlying tissues due to burn (deep third degree) of axilla, without mention of loss of a body part
943.54 Deep necrosis of underlying tissues due to burn (deep third degree) of axilla, with loss of a body part
944.30 Full-thickness skin loss due to burn (third degree nos) of unspecified site of hand ▽
944.31 Full-thickness skin loss due to burn (third degree nos) of single digit [finger (nail)] other than thumb
944.32 Full-thickness skin loss due to burn (third degree nos) of thumb (nail)
944.33 Full-thickness skin loss due to burn (third degree nos) of two or more digits of hand, not including thumb
944.34 Full-thickness skin loss due to burn (third degree nos) of two or more digits of hand including thumb
944.35 Full-thickness skin loss due to burn (third degree nos) of palm of hand
944.36 Full-thickness skin loss due to burn (third degree nos) of back of hand
944.37 Full-thickness skin loss due to burn (third degree nos) of wrist
944.38 Full-thickness skin loss due to burn (third degree nos) of multiple sites of wrist(s) and hand(s)
944.40 Deep necrosis of underlying tissues due to burn (deep third degree) of unspecified site of hand, without mention of loss of a body part ▽
944.41 Deep necrosis of underlying tissues due to burn (deep third degree) of single digit [finger (nail)] other than thumb, without mention of a body part
944.42 Deep necrosis of underlying tissues due to burn (deep third degree) of thumb (nail), without mention of loss of a body part
944.43 Deep necrosis of underlying tissues due to burn (deep third degree) of two or more digits of hand, not including thumb, without mention of a body part
944.44 Deep necrosis of underlying tissues due to burn (deep third degree) of two or more digits of hand including thumb, without mention of a body part
944.45 Deep necrosis of underlying tissues due to burn (deep third degree) of palm of hand, without mention of loss of a body part
944.46 Deep necrosis of underlying tissues due to burn (deep third degree) of back of hand, without mention of loss of back of a body part
944.47 Deep necrosis of underlying tissues due to burn (deep third degree) of wrist, without mention of loss of a body part
944.48 Deep necrosis of underlying tissues due to burn (deep third degree) of multiple sites of wrist(s) and hand(s), without mention of loss of a body part
944.50 Deep necrosis of underlying tissues due to burn (deep third degree) of unspecified site of hand, with loss of a body part ▽
944.51 Deep necrosis of underlying tissues due to burn (deep third degree) of single digit (finger (nail)) other than thumb, with loss of a body part
944.52 Deep necrosis of underlying tissues due to burn (deep third degree) of thumb (nail), with loss of a body part
944.53 Deep necrosis of underlying tissues due to burn (deep third degree) of two or more digits of hand, not including thumb, with loss of a body part
944.54 Deep necrosis of underlying tissues due to burn (deep third degree) of two or more digits of hand including thumb, with loss of a body part
944.55 Deep necrosis of underlying tissues due to burn (deep third degree) of palm of hand, with loss of a body part
944.56 Deep necrosis of underlying tissues due to burn (deep third degree) of back of hand, with loss of a body part
944.57 Deep necrosis of underlying tissues due to burn (deep third degree) of wrist, with loss of a body part
944.58 Deep necrosis of underlying tissues due to burn (deep third degree) of multiple sites of wrist(s) and hand(s), with loss of a body part
945.32 Full-thickness skin loss due to burn (third degree nos) of foot
945.42 Deep necrosis of underlying tissues due to burn (deep third degree) of foot, without mention of loss of a body part

▽ Unspecified code
♀ Female diagnosis
☒ Manifestation code
♂ Male diagnosis

945.52 Deep necrosis of underlying tissues due to burn (deep third degree) of foot, with loss of a body part
948.00 Burn (any degree) involving less than 10% of body surface with third degree burn of less than 10% or unspecified amount
948.10 Burn (any degree) involving 10-19% of body surface with third degree burn of less than 10% or unspecified amount
948.11 Burn (any degree) involving 10-19% of body surface with third degree burn of 10-19%
948.20 Burn (any degree) involving 20-29% of body surface with third degree burn of less than 10% or unspecified amount
948.21 Burn (any degree) involving 20-29% of body surface with third degree burn of 10-19%
948.22 Burn (any degree) involving 20-29% of body surface with third degree burn of 20-29%
948.30 Burn (any degree) involving 30-39% of body surface with third degree burn of less than 10% or unspecified amount
948.31 Burn (any degree) involving 30-39% of body surface with third degree burn of 10-19%
948.32 Burn (any degree) involving 30-39% of body surface with third degree burn of 20-29%
948.33 Burn (any degree) involving 30-39% of body surface with third degree burn of 30-39%
948.40 Burn (any degree) involving 40-49% of body surface with third degree burn of less than 10% or unspecified amount
948.41 Burn (any degree) involving 40-49% of body surface with third degree burn of 10-19%
948.42 Burn (any degree) involving 40-49% of body surface with third degree burn of 20-29%
948.43 Burn (any degree) involving 40-49% of body surface with third degree burn of 30-39%
948.44 Burn (any degree) involving 40-49% of body surface with third degree burn of 40-49%
948.50 Burn (any degree) involving 50-59% of body surface with third degree burn of less than 10% or unspecified amount
948.51 Burn (any degree) involving 50-59% of body surface with third degree burn of 10-19%
948.52 Burn (any degree) involving 50-59% of body surface with third degree burn of 20-29%
948.53 Burn (any degree) involving 50-59% of body surface with third degree burn of 30-39%
948.54 Burn (any degree) involving 50-59% of body surface with third degree burn of 40-49%
948.55 Burn (any degree) involving 50-59% of body surface with third degree burn of 50-59%
948.60 Burn (any degree) involving 60-69% of body surface with third degree burn of less than 10% or unspecified amount
948.61 Burn (any degree) involving 60-69% of body surface with third degree burn of 10-19%
948.62 Burn (any degree) involving 60-69% of body surface with third degree burn of 20-29%
948.63 Burn (any degree) involving 60-69% of body surface with third degree burn of 30-39%
948.64 Burn (any degree) involving 60-69% of body surface with third degree burn of 40-49%
948.65 Burn (any degree) involving 60-69% of body surface with third degree burn of 50-59%
948.66 Burn (any degree) involving 60-69% of body surface with third degree burn of 60-69%
948.70 Burn (any degree) involving 70-79% of body surface with third degree burn of less than 10% or unspecified amount
948.71 Burn (any degree) involving 70-79% of body surface with third degree burn of 10-19%
948.72 Burn (any degree) involving 70-79% of body surface with third degree burn of 20-29%
948.73 Burn (any degree) involving 70-79% of body surface with third degree burn of 30-39%
948.74 Burn (any degree) involving 70-79% of body surface with third degree burn of 40-49%
948.75 Burn (any degree) involving 70-79% of body surface with third degree burn of 50-59%
948.76 Burn (any degree) involving 70-79% of body surface with third degree burn of 60-69%
948.77 Burn (any degree) involving 70-79% of body surface with third degree burn of 70-79%
948.80 Burn (any degree) involving 80-89% of body surface with third degree burn of less than 10% or unspecified amount
948.81 Burn (any degree) involving 80-89% of body surface with third degree burn of 10-19%
948.82 Burn (any degree) involving 80-89% of body surface with third degree burn of 20-29%
948.83 Burn (any degree) involving 80-89% of body surface with third degree burn of 30-39%
948.84 Burn (any degree) involving 80-89% of body surface with third degree burn of 40-49%
948.85 Burn (any degree) involving 80-89% of body surface with third degree burn of 50-59%
948.86 Burn (any degree) involving 80-89% of body surface with third degree burn of 60-69%
948.87 Burn (any degree) involving 80-89% of body surface with third degree burn of 70-79%
948.88 Burn (any degree) involving 80-89% of body surface with third degree burn of 80-89%
959.01 Head injury, unspecified ♥
959.09 Injury of face and neck, other and unspecified
959.11 Other injury of chest wall
959.12 Other injury of abdomen
959.14 Other injury of external genitals
959.19 Other injury of other sites of trunk
959.4 Injury, other and unspecified, hand, except finger
959.5 Injury, other and unspecified, finger
959.7 Injury, other and unspecified, knee, leg, ankle, and foot
959.8 Injury, other and unspecified, other specified sites, including multiple
991.0 Frostbite of face
991.1 Frostbite of hand
991.2 Frostbite of foot
996.64 Infection and inflammatory reaction due to indwelling urinary catheter — (Use additional code to identify specified infections: 038.0-038.9, 595.0-595.9)
997.60 Late complications of amputation stump, unspecified — (Use additional code to identify complications) ♥
997.61 Neuroma of amputation stump — (Use additional code to identify complications)
997.62 Infection (chronic) of amputation stump — (Use additional code to identify organism. Use additional code to identify complications)
997.69 Other late amputation stump complication — (Use additional code to identify complications)
998.59 Other postoperative infection — (Use additional code to identify infection)
998.83 Non-healing surgical wound
V10.21 Personal history of malignant neoplasm of larynx
V51 Aftercare involving the use of plastic surgery

ICD-9-CM Procedural

39.31 Suture of artery
39.32 Suture of vein
86.70 Pedicle or flap graft, not otherwise specified
86.71 Cutting and preparation of pedicle grafts or flaps
86.73 Attachment of pedicle or flap graft to hand
86.74 Attachment of pedicle or flap graft to other sites
86.75 Revision of pedicle or flap graft

15758

15758 Free fascial flap with microvascular anastomosis

ICD-9-CM Diagnostic

881.10 Open wound of forearm, complicated — (Use additional code to identify infection)
881.11 Open wound of elbow, complicated — (Use additional code to identify infection)
881.12 Open wound of wrist, complicated — (Use additional code to identify infection)
881.20 Open wound of forearm, with tendon involvement — (Use additional code to identify infection)
881.21 Open wound of elbow, with tendon involvement — (Use additional code to identify infection)
881.22 Open wound of wrist, with tendon involvement — (Use additional code to identify infection)
882.1 Open wound of hand except finger(s) alone, complicated — (Use additional code to identify infection)
882.2 Open wound of hand except finger(s) alone, with tendon involvement — (Use additional code to identify infection)
883.1 Open wound of finger(s), complicated — (Use additional code to identify infection)

883.2 Open wound of finger(s), with tendon involvement — (Use additional code to identify infection)
892.1 Open wound of foot except toe(s) alone, complicated — (Use additional code to identify infection)
892.2 Open wound of foot except toe(s) alone, with tendon involvement — (Use additional code to identify infection)
893.1 Open wound of toe(s), complicated — (Use additional code to identify infection)
893.2 Open wound of toe(s), with tendon involvement — (Use additional code to identify infection)
906.1 Late effect of open wound of extremities without mention of tendon injury
906.4 Late effect of crushing
906.6 Late effect of burn of wrist and hand
906.7 Late effect of burn of other extremities
927.10 Crushing injury of forearm — (Use additional code to identify any associated injuries: 800-829, 850.0-854.1, 860.0-869.1)
927.11 Crushing injury of elbow — (Use additional code to identify any associated injuries: 800-829, 850.0-854.1, 860.0-869.1)
927.20 Crushing injury of hand(s) — (Use additional code to identify any associated injuries: 800-829, 850.0-854.1, 860.0-869.1)
927.21 Crushing injury of wrist — (Use additional code to identify any associated injuries: 800-829, 850.0-854.1, 860.0-869.1)
927.3 Crushing injury of finger(s) — (Use additional code to identify any associated injuries: 800-829, 850.0-854.1, 860.0-869.1)
927.8 Crushing injury of multiple sites of upper limb — (Use additional code to identify any associated injuries: 800-829, 850.0-854.1, 860.0-869.1)
928.10 Crushing injury of lower leg — (Use additional code to identify any associated injuries: 800-829, 850.0-854.1, 860.0-869.1)
928.11 Crushing injury of knee — (Use additional code to identify any associated injuries: 800-829, 850.0-854.1, 860.0-869.1)
928.20 Crushing injury of foot — (Use additional code to identify any associated injuries: 800-829, 850.0-854.1, 860.0-869.1)
928.21 Crushing injury of ankle — (Use additional code to identify any associated injuries: 800-829, 850.0-854.1, 860.0-869.1)
928.3 Crushing injury of toe(s) — (Use additional code to identify any associated injuries: 800-829, 850.0-854.1, 860.0-869.1)
928.8 Crushing injury of multiple sites of lower limb — (Use additional code to identify any associated injuries: 800-829, 850.0-854.1, 860.0-869.1)
928.9 Crushing injury of unspecified site of lower limb — (Use additional code to identify any associated injuries: 800-829, 850.0-854.1, 860.0-869.1) ▽
943.31 Full-thickness skin loss due to burn (third degree nos) of forearm
943.39 Full-thickness skin loss due to burn (third degree nos) of multiple sites of upper limb, except wrist and hand
943.41 Deep necrosis of underlying tissues due to burn (deep third degree) of forearm, without mention of loss of a body part
943.49 Deep necrosis of underlying tissues due to burn (deep third degree) of multiple sites of upper limb, except wrist and hand, without mention of loss of a body part
944.30 Full-thickness skin loss due to burn (third degree nos) of unspecified site of hand ▽
944.31 Full-thickness skin loss due to burn (third degree nos) of single digit [finger (nail)] other than thumb
944.32 Full-thickness skin loss due to burn (third degree nos) of thumb (nail)
944.33 Full-thickness skin loss due to burn (third degree nos) of two or more digits of hand, not including thumb
944.34 Full-thickness skin loss due to burn (third degree nos) of two or more digits of hand including thumb
944.35 Full-thickness skin loss due to burn (third degree nos) of palm of hand
944.36 Full-thickness skin loss due to burn (third degree nos) of back of hand
944.37 Full-thickness skin loss due to burn (third degree nos) of wrist
944.38 Full-thickness skin loss due to burn (third degree nos) of multiple sites of wrist(s) and hand(s)
944.41 Deep necrosis of underlying tissues due to burn (deep third degree) of single digit [finger (nail)] other than thumb, without mention of a body part
944.42 Deep necrosis of underlying tissues due to burn (deep third degree) of thumb (nail), without mention of loss of a body part
944.43 Deep necrosis of underlying tissues due to burn (deep third degree) of two or more digits of hand, not including thumb, without mention of a body part
944.44 Deep necrosis of underlying tissues due to burn (deep third degree) of two or more digits of hand including thumb, without mention of a body part
944.45 Deep necrosis of underlying tissues due to burn (deep third degree) of palm of hand, without mention of loss of a body part
944.46 Deep necrosis of underlying tissues due to burn (deep third degree) of back of hand, without mention of loss of back of a body part
944.47 Deep necrosis of underlying tissues due to burn (deep third degree) of wrist, without mention of loss of a body part
944.48 Deep necrosis of underlying tissues due to burn (deep third degree) of multiple sites of wrist(s) and hand(s), without mention of loss of a body part
959.3 Injury, other and unspecified, elbow, forearm, and wrist
959.4 Injury, other and unspecified, hand, except finger
959.5 Injury, other and unspecified, finger
959.7 Injury, other and unspecified, knee, leg, ankle, and foot

ICD-9-CM Procedural

08.32 Repair of blepharoptosis by frontalis muscle technique with fascial sling
08.69 Other reconstruction of eyelid with flaps or grafts
39.31 Suture of artery
39.32 Suture of vein
82.72 Plastic operation on hand with graft of muscle or fascia
83.82 Graft of muscle or fascia

15760

15760 Graft; composite (eg, full thickness of external ear or nasal ala), including primary closure, donor area

ICD-9-CM Diagnostic

The application of this code is too broad to adequately present ICD-9-CM diagnostic code links here. Refer to your ICD-9-CM book.

ICD-9-CM Procedural

18.71 Construction of auricle of ear
18.79 Other plastic repair of external ear
21.89 Other repair and plastic operations on nose
86.89 Other repair and reconstruction of skin and subcutaneous tissue

15770

15770 Graft; derma-fat-fascia

ICD-9-CM Diagnostic

The application of this code is too broad to adequately present ICD-9-CM diagnostic code links here. Refer to your ICD-9-CM book.

ICD-9-CM Procedural

83.82 Graft of muscle or fascia
86.69 Other skin graft to other sites
86.71 Cutting and preparation of pedicle grafts or flaps

15775–15776

15775 Punch graft for hair transplant; 1 to 15 punch grafts
15776 more than 15 punch grafts

ICD-9-CM Diagnostic

374.55 Hypotrichosis of eyelid
704.00 Unspecified alopecia ▽
704.01 Alopecia areata
704.02 Telogen effluvium
757.4 Specified congenital anomalies of hair
873.0 Open wound of scalp, without mention of complication — (Use additional code to identify infection)
873.1 Open wound of scalp, complicated — (Use additional code to identify infection)
941.32 Full-thickness skin loss due to burn (third degree nos) of eye (with other parts of face, head, and neck)
941.36 Full-thickness skin loss due to burn (third degree nos) of scalp (any part)
941.42 Deep necrosis of underlying tissues due to burn (deep third degree) of eye (with other parts of face, head, and neck), without mention of loss of a body part
941.46 Deep necrosis of underlying tissues due to burn (deep third degree) of scalp (any part), without mention of loss of a body part
941.49 Deep necrosis of underlying tissues due to burn (deep third degree) of multiple sites (except with eye) of face, head, and neck, without mention of loss of a body part
V50.0 Elective hair transplant for purposes other than remedying health states

ICD-9-CM Procedural

86.64 Hair transplant

HCPCS Level II Supplies & Services

A4550 Surgical trays

▽ Unspecified code
♀ Female diagnosis
☒ Manifestation code
♂ Male diagnosis

15780–15781

15780 Dermabrasion; total face (eg, for acne scarring, fine wrinkling, rhytids, general keratosis)
15781 segmental, face

ICD-9-CM Diagnostic

695.3 Rosacea
701.5 Other abnormal granulation tissue
701.8 Other specified hypertrophic and atrophic condition of skin
701.9 Unspecified hypertrophic and atrophic condition of skin ▽
702.0 Actinic keratosis
702.11 Inflamed seborrheic keratosis
706.0 Acne varioliformis
706.1 Other acne
709.2 Scar condition and fibrosis of skin
906.0 Late effect of open wound of head, neck, and trunk
908.6 Late effect of certain complications of trauma
909.3 Late effect of complications of surgical and medical care
V50.1 Other plastic surgery for unacceptable cosmetic appearance

ICD-9-CM Procedural

86.25 Dermabrasion

HCPCS Level II Supplies & Services

A4305 Disposable drug delivery system, flow rate of 50 ml or greater per hour
A4306 Disposable drug delivery system, flow rate of 5 ml or less per hour
A4550 Surgical trays

15782

15782 Dermabrasion; regional, other than face

ICD-9-CM Diagnostic

701.4 Keloid scar
701.5 Other abnormal granulation tissue
701.8 Other specified hypertrophic and atrophic condition of skin
701.9 Unspecified hypertrophic and atrophic condition of skin ▽
706.0 Acne varioliformis
706.1 Other acne
709.09 Other dyschromia
709.2 Scar condition and fibrosis of skin
906.8 Late effect of burns of other specified sites
909.3 Late effect of complications of surgical and medical care

ICD-9-CM Procedural

86.25 Dermabrasion

HCPCS Level II Supplies & Services

A4305 Disposable drug delivery system, flow rate of 50 ml or greater per hour
A4306 Disposable drug delivery system, flow rate of 5 ml or less per hour
A4550 Surgical trays

15783

15783 Dermabrasion; superficial, any site, (eg, tattoo removal)

ICD-9-CM Diagnostic

701.1 Acquired keratoderma
702.0 Actinic keratosis
702.19 Other seborrheic keratosis
706.0 Acne varioliformis
706.1 Other acne
709.09 Other dyschromia
709.2 Scar condition and fibrosis of skin
906.0 Late effect of open wound of head, neck, and trunk
908.6 Late effect of certain complications of trauma
V50.1 Other plastic surgery for unacceptable cosmetic appearance

ICD-9-CM Procedural

86.25 Dermabrasion

HCPCS Level II Supplies & Services

A4305 Disposable drug delivery system, flow rate of 50 ml or greater per hour
A4306 Disposable drug delivery system, flow rate of 5 ml or less per hour
A4550 Surgical trays

15786–15787

15786 Abrasion; single lesion (eg, keratosis, scar)
15787 each additional four lesions or less (List separately in addition to code for primary procedure)

ICD-9-CM Diagnostic

701.1 Acquired keratoderma
701.4 Keloid scar
702.0 Actinic keratosis
709.09 Other dyschromia
709.2 Scar condition and fibrosis of skin
757.32 Congenital vascular hamartomas
757.39 Other specified congenital anomaly of skin
906.0 Late effect of open wound of head, neck, and trunk
906.8 Late effect of burns of other specified sites

ICD-9-CM Procedural

86.25 Dermabrasion

HCPCS Level II Supplies & Services

The HCPCS Level II code(s) would be the same as the actual procedure performed because these are in-addition-to codes.

15788–15789

15788 Chemical peel, facial; epidermal
15789 dermal

ICD-9-CM Diagnostic

701.4 Keloid scar
701.5 Other abnormal granulation tissue
701.8 Other specified hypertrophic and atrophic condition of skin
701.9 Unspecified hypertrophic and atrophic condition of skin ▽
706.0 Acne varioliformis
706.1 Other acne
709.09 Other dyschromia
709.2 Scar condition and fibrosis of skin
757.32 Congenital vascular hamartomas
757.39 Other specified congenital anomaly of skin
V50.1 Other plastic surgery for unacceptable cosmetic appearance

ICD-9-CM Procedural

86.24 Chemosurgery of skin

HCPCS Level II Supplies & Services

A4305 Disposable drug delivery system, flow rate of 50 ml or greater per hour
A4306 Disposable drug delivery system, flow rate of 5 ml or less per hour
A4550 Surgical trays

15792–15793

15792 Chemical peel, nonfacial; epidermal
15793 dermal

ICD-9-CM Diagnostic

173.4 Other malignant neoplasm of scalp and skin of neck
701.4 Keloid scar
701.5 Other abnormal granulation tissue
701.8 Other specified hypertrophic and atrophic condition of skin
706.0 Acne varioliformis
706.1 Other acne
709.09 Other dyschromia
709.2 Scar condition and fibrosis of skin
757.32 Congenital vascular hamartomas
757.39 Other specified congenital anomaly of skin
V50.1 Other plastic surgery for unacceptable cosmetic appearance

ICD-9-CM Procedural

86.24 Chemosurgery of skin

HCPCS Level II Supplies & Services

A4305 Disposable drug delivery system, flow rate of 50 ml or greater per hour
A4306 Disposable drug delivery system, flow rate of 5 ml or less per hour
A4550 Surgical trays

15810–15811

15810 Salabrasion; 20 sq. cm or less
15811 over 20 sq. cm

ICD-9-CM Diagnostic

701.4 Keloid scar
706.0 Acne varioliformis
706.1 Other acne
709.09 Other dyschromia
709.2 Scar condition and fibrosis of skin
757.32 Congenital vascular hamartomas
757.39 Other specified congenital anomaly of skin
906.0 Late effect of open wound of head, neck, and trunk
906.8 Late effect of burns of other specified sites
V50.1 Other plastic surgery for unacceptable cosmetic appearance

ICD-9-CM Procedural

86.25 Dermabrasion

HCPCS Level II Supplies & Services

A4305 Disposable drug delivery system, flow rate of 50 ml or greater per hour
A4306 Disposable drug delivery system, flow rate of 5 ml or less per hour
A4550 Surgical trays

15819

15819 Cervicoplasty

ICD-9-CM Diagnostic

214.1 Lipoma of other skin and subcutaneous tissue
701.8 Other specified hypertrophic and atrophic condition of skin
709.2 Scar condition and fibrosis of skin
906.0 Late effect of open wound of head, neck, and trunk
V10.83 Personal history of other malignant neoplasm of skin
V10.89 Personal history of malignant neoplasm of other site
V50.1 Other plastic surgery for unacceptable cosmetic appearance

ICD-9-CM Procedural

86.89 Other repair and reconstruction of skin and subcutaneous tissue

15820–15823

15820 Blepharoplasty, lower eyelid;
15821 with extensive herniated fat pad
15822 Blepharoplasty, upper eyelid;
15823 with excessive skin weighting down lid

ICD-9-CM Diagnostic

351.8 Other facial nerve disorders
374.01 Senile entropion
374.03 Spastic entropion
374.11 Senile ectropion
374.30 Unspecified ptosis of eyelid ▽
374.31 Paralytic ptosis
374.32 Myogenic ptosis
374.34 Blepharochalasis
374.87 Dermatochalasis
374.89 Other disorders of eyelid
701.8 Other specified hypertrophic and atrophic condition of skin
701.9 Unspecified hypertrophic and atrophic condition of skin ▽
709.2 Scar condition and fibrosis of skin
743.62 Congenital deformity of eyelid
V50.1 Other plastic surgery for unacceptable cosmetic appearance
V51 Aftercare involving the use of plastic surgery

ICD-9-CM Procedural

08.70 Reconstruction of eyelid, not otherwise specified
08.86 Lower eyelid rhytidectomy

15824

15824 Rhytidectomy; forehead

ICD-9-CM Diagnostic

374.34 Blepharochalasis
692.79 Other dermatitis due to solar radiation
701.8 Other specified hypertrophic and atrophic condition of skin
709.2 Scar condition and fibrosis of skin
709.3 Degenerative skin disorder
906.0 Late effect of open wound of head, neck, and trunk
V50.1 Other plastic surgery for unacceptable cosmetic appearance

ICD-9-CM Procedural

86.82 Facial rhytidectomy

15825

15825 Rhytidectomy; neck with platysmal tightening (platysmal flap, P-flap)

ICD-9-CM Diagnostic

701.8 Other specified hypertrophic and atrophic condition of skin
701.9 Unspecified hypertrophic and atrophic condition of skin ▽
V50.1 Other plastic surgery for unacceptable cosmetic appearance
V51 Aftercare involving the use of plastic surgery

ICD-9-CM Procedural

86.82 Facial rhytidectomy
86.89 Other repair and reconstruction of skin and subcutaneous tissue

15826

15826 Rhytidectomy; glabellar frown lines

ICD-9-CM Diagnostic

692.79 Other dermatitis due to solar radiation
701.8 Other specified hypertrophic and atrophic condition of skin
709.3 Degenerative skin disorder
V50.1 Other plastic surgery for unacceptable cosmetic appearance

ICD-9-CM Procedural

86.82 Facial rhytidectomy
86.89 Other repair and reconstruction of skin and subcutaneous tissue

15828–15829

15828 Rhytidectomy; cheek, chin, and neck
15829 superficial musculoaponeurotic system (SMAS) flap

ICD-9-CM Diagnostic

692.79 Other dermatitis due to solar radiation
701.8 Other specified hypertrophic and atrophic condition of skin
701.9 Unspecified hypertrophic and atrophic condition of skin ▽
V50.1 Other plastic surgery for unacceptable cosmetic appearance

ICD-9-CM Procedural

86.82 Facial rhytidectomy

15831–15839

15831 Excision, excessive skin and subcutaneous tissue (including lipectomy); abdomen (abdominoplasty)
15832 thigh
15833 leg
15834 hip
15835 buttock
15836 arm
15837 forearm or hand
15838 submental fat pad
15839 other area

ICD-9-CM Diagnostic

278.00 Obesity, unspecified — (Use additional code to identify any associated mental retardation) ▽
278.01 Morbid obesity — (Use additional code to identify any associated mental retardation)
278.1 Localized adiposity — (Use additional code to identify any associated mental retardation)
701.9 Unspecified hypertrophic and atrophic condition of skin ▽
729.39 Panniculitis of other sites
V50.1 Other plastic surgery for unacceptable cosmetic appearance
V51 Aftercare involving the use of plastic surgery

ICD-9-CM Procedural

86.83 Size reduction plastic operation

HCPCS Level II Supplies & Services

A4462 Abdominal dressing holder, each

15840–15845

15840 Graft for facial nerve paralysis; free fascia graft (including obtaining fascia)
15841 free muscle graft (including obtaining graft)
15842 free muscle flap by microsurgical technique
15845 regional muscle transfer

ICD-9-CM Diagnostic

350.1 Trigeminal neuralgia
350.8 Other specified trigeminal nerve disorders
351.0 Bell's palsy
351.1 Geniculate ganglionitis
351.8 Other facial nerve disorders
742.8 Other specified congenital anomalies of nervous system
767.5 Facial nerve injury, birth trauma
906.0 Late effect of open wound of head, neck, and trunk
906.5 Late effect of burn of eye, face, head, and neck
909.3 Late effect of complications of surgical and medical care
951.4 Injury to facial nerve

ICD-9-CM Procedural

83.82 Graft of muscle or fascia
86.81 Repair for facial weakness

15850–15851

15850 Removal of sutures under anesthesia (other than local), same surgeon
15851 Removal of sutures under anesthesia (other than local), other surgeon

ICD-9-CM Diagnostic

998.31 Disruption of internal operation wound
998.32 Disruption of external operation wound
998.51 Infected postoperative seroma — (Use additional code to identify organism)
998.59 Other postoperative infection — (Use additional code to identify infection)
V58.3 Attention to surgical dressings and sutures

ICD-9-CM Procedural

97.38 Removal of sutures from head and neck
97.43 Removal of sutures from thorax
97.83 Removal of abdominal wall sutures
97.84 Removal of sutures from trunk, not elsewhere classified
97.89 Removal of other therapeutic device

HCPCS Level II Supplies & Services

A4649 Surgical supply; miscellaneous

15852

15852 Dressing change (for other than burns) under anesthesia (other than local)

ICD-9-CM Diagnostic

440.23 Atherosclerosis of native arteries of the extremities with ulceration — (Use additional code for any associated ulceration: 707.10-707.9)
440.24 Atherosclerosis of native arteries of the extremities with gangrene
707.00 Decubitus ulcer, unspecified site
707.01 Decubitus ulcer, elbow
707.02 Decubitus ulcer, upper back
707.03 Decubitus ulcer, lower back
707.04 Decubitus ulcer, hip
707.05 Decubitus ulcer, buttock
707.06 Decubitus ulcer, ankle
707.07 Decubitus ulcer, heel
707.09 Decubitus ulcer, other site
707.10 Ulcer of lower limb, unspecified ▽
707.11 Ulcer of thigh
707.12 Ulcer of calf
707.13 Ulcer of ankle
707.14 Ulcer of heel and midfoot
707.15 Ulcer of other part of foot
707.19 Ulcer of other part of lower limb
707.9 Chronic ulcer of unspecified site ▽
709.8 Other specified disorder of skin
785.4 Gangrene — (Code first any associated underlying condition:250.7, 443.0)
872.01 Open wound of auricle, without mention of complication — (Use additional code to identify infection)
872.10 Open wound of external ear, unspecified site, complicated — (Use additional code to identify infection) ▽
872.11 Open wound of auricle, complicated — (Use additional code to identify infection)
872.12 Open wound of auditory canal, complicated — (Use additional code to identify infection)
872.9 Open wound of ear, part unspecified, complicated — (Use additional code to identify infection) ▽
873.30 Open wound of nose, unspecified site, complicated — (Use additional code to identify infection) ▽
873.31 Open wound of nasal septum, complicated — (Use additional code to identify infection)
873.32 Open wound of nasal cavity, complicated — (Use additional code to identify infection)
873.33 Open wound of nasal sinus, complicated — (Use additional code to identify infection)
873.39 Open wound of nose, multiple sites, complicated — (Use additional code to identify infection)
873.43 Open wound of lip, without mention of complication — (Use additional code to identify infection)
873.50 Open wound of face, unspecified site, complicated — (Use additional code to identify infection) ▽
873.52 Open wound of forehead, complicated — (Use additional code to identify infection)
873.54 Open wound of jaw, complicated — (Use additional code to identify infection)
873.59 Open wound of face, other and multiple sites, complicated — (Use additional code to identify infection)
878.1 Open wound of penis, complicated — (Use additional code to identify infection) ♂
878.3 Open wound of scrotum and testes, complicated — (Use additional code to identify infection) ♂
878.5 Open wound of vulva, complicated — (Use additional code to identify infection) ♀
878.7 Open wound of vagina, complicated — (Use additional code to identify infection) ♀
878.9 Open wound of other and unspecified parts of genital organs, complicated — (Use additional code to identify infection) ▽
880.12 Open wound of axillary region, complicated — (Use additional code to identify infection)
882.1 Open wound of hand except finger(s) alone, complicated — (Use additional code to identify infection)
882.2 Open wound of hand except finger(s) alone, with tendon involvement — (Use additional code to identify infection)
883.1 Open wound of finger(s), complicated — (Use additional code to identify infection)
883.2 Open wound of finger(s), with tendon involvement — (Use additional code to identify infection)
884.1 Multiple and unspecified open wound of upper limb, complicated — (Use additional code to identify infection)
884.2 Multiple and unspecified open wound of upper limb, with tendon involvement — (Use additional code to identify infection)
892.1 Open wound of foot except toe(s) alone, complicated — (Use additional code to identify infection)
892.2 Open wound of foot except toe(s) alone, with tendon involvement — (Use additional code to identify infection)
893.2 Open wound of toe(s), with tendon involvement — (Use additional code to identify infection)
894.1 Multiple and unspecified open wound of lower limb, complicated — (Use additional code to identify infection)
894.2 Multiple and unspecified open wound of lower limb, with tendon involvement — (Use additional code to identify infection)
925.1 Crushing injury of face and scalp — (Use additional code to identify any associated injuries: 800-829, 850.0-854.1, 860.0-869.1)
925.2 Crushing injury of neck — (Use additional code to identify any associated injuries: 800-829, 850.0-854.1, 860.0-869.1)
926.0 Crushing injury of external genitalia — (Use additional code to identify any associated injuries: 800-829, 850.0-854.1, 860.0-869.1)
926.11 Crushing injury of back — (Use additional code to identify any associated injuries: 800-829, 850.0-854.1, 860.0-869.1)
926.12 Crushing injury of buttock — (Use additional code to identify any associated injuries: 800-829, 850.0-854.1, 860.0-869.1)
926.19 Crushing injury of other specified sites of trunk — (Use additional code to identify any associated injuries: 800-829, 850.0-854.1, 860.0-869.1)
926.8 Crushing injury of multiple sites of trunk — (Use additional code to identify any associated injuries: 800-829, 850.0-854.1, 860.0-869.1)
926.9 Crushing injury of unspecified site of trunk — (Use additional code to identify any associated injuries: 800-829, 850.0-854.1, 860.0-869.1) ▽
927.00 Crushing injury of shoulder region — (Use additional code to identify any associated injuries: 800-829, 850.0-854.1, 860.0-869.1)

▽ Unspecified code
♀ Female diagnosis
☒ Manifestation code
♂ Male diagnosis

927.01 Crushing injury of scapular region — (Use additional code to identify any associated injuries: 800-829, 850.0-854.1, 860.0-869.1)
927.02 Crushing injury of axillary region — (Use additional code to identify any associated injuries: 800-829, 850.0-854.1, 860.0-869.1)
927.03 Crushing injury of upper arm — (Use additional code to identify any associated injuries: 800-829, 850.0-854.1, 860.0-869.1)
927.09 Crushing injury of multiple sites of upper arm — (Use additional code to identify any associated injuries: 800-829, 850.0-854.1, 860.0-869.1)
927.10 Crushing injury of forearm — (Use additional code to identify any associated injuries: 800-829, 850.0-854.1, 860.0-869.1)
927.11 Crushing injury of elbow — (Use additional code to identify any associated injuries: 800-829, 850.0-854.1, 860.0-869.1)
927.20 Crushing injury of hand(s) — (Use additional code to identify any associated injuries: 800-829, 850.0-854.1, 860.0-869.1)
927.21 Crushing injury of wrist — (Use additional code to identify any associated injuries: 800-829, 850.0-854.1, 860.0-869.1)
927.3 Crushing injury of finger(s) — (Use additional code to identify any associated injuries: 800-829, 850.0-854.1, 860.0-869.1)
927.8 Crushing injury of multiple sites of upper limb — (Use additional code to identify any associated injuries: 800-829, 850.0-854.1, 860.0-869.1)
927.9 Crushing injury of unspecified site of upper limb — (Use additional code to identify any associated injuries: 800-829, 850.0-854.1, 860.0-869.1) ▽
928.00 Crushing injury of thigh — (Use additional code to identify any associated injuries: 800-829, 850.0-854.1, 860.0-869.1)
928.01 Crushing injury of hip — (Use additional code to identify any associated injuries: 800-829, 850.0-854.1, 860.0-869.1)
928.11 Crushing injury of knee — (Use additional code to identify any associated injuries: 800-829, 850.0-854.1, 860.0-869.1)
928.20 Crushing injury of foot — (Use additional code to identify any associated injuries: 800-829, 850.0-854.1, 860.0-869.1)
928.21 Crushing injury of ankle — (Use additional code to identify any associated injuries: 800-829, 850.0-854.1, 860.0-869.1)
928.3 Crushing injury of toe(s) — (Use additional code to identify any associated injuries: 800-829, 850.0-854.1, 860.0-869.1)
928.8 Crushing injury of multiple sites of lower limb — (Use additional code to identify any associated injuries: 800-829, 850.0-854.1, 860.0-869.1)
928.9 Crushing injury of unspecified site of lower limb — (Use additional code to identify any associated injuries: 800-829, 850.0-854.1, 860.0-869.1) ▽
929.0 Crushing injury of multiple sites, not elsewhere classified — (Use additional code to identify any associated injuries: 800-829, 850.0-854.1, 860.0-869.1)
983.1 Toxic effect of acids — (Use additional code to specify the nature of the toxic effect)
998.32 Disruption of external operation wound
998.51 Infected postoperative seroma — (Use additional code to identify organism)
998.59 Other postoperative infection — (Use additional code to identify infection)
998.6 Persistent postoperative fistula, not elsewhere classified
V58.3 Attention to surgical dressings and sutures
V58.49 Other specified aftercare following surgery — (This code should be used in conjunction with other aftercare codes to fully identify the reason for the aftercare encounter)

ICD-9-CM Procedural

93.57 Application of other wound dressing

HCPCS Level II Supplies & Services

A4462 Abdominal dressing holder, each

15860

15860 Intravenous injection of agent (eg, fluorescein) to test vascular flow in flap or graft

ICD-9-CM Diagnostic

140.9 Malignant neoplasm of lip, vermilion border, unspecified as to upper or lower ▽
149.8 Malignant neoplasm of other sites within the lip and oral cavity
149.9 Malignant neoplasm of ill-defined sites of lip and oral cavity
172.1 Malignant melanoma of skin of eyelid, including canthus
172.2 Malignant melanoma of skin of ear and external auditory canal
172.6 Malignant melanoma of skin of upper limb, including shoulder
172.7 Malignant melanoma of skin of lower limb, including hip
173.0 Other malignant neoplasm of skin of lip
173.1 Other malignant neoplasm of skin of eyelid, including canthus
173.2 Other malignant neoplasm of skin of ear and external auditory canal
173.4 Other malignant neoplasm of scalp and skin of neck
173.8 Other malignant neoplasm of other specified sites of skin
184.0 Malignant neoplasm of vagina ♀
184.1 Malignant neoplasm of labia majora ♀
184.2 Malignant neoplasm of labia minora ♀
184.3 Malignant neoplasm of clitoris ♀
184.4 Malignant neoplasm of vulva, unspecified site ▽ ♀
184.8 Malignant neoplasm of other specified sites of female genital organs ♀
187.1 Malignant neoplasm of prepuce ♂
187.2 Malignant neoplasm of glans penis ♂
187.3 Malignant neoplasm of body of penis ♂
187.4 Malignant neoplasm of penis, part unspecified ▽ ♂
187.7 Malignant neoplasm of scrotum ♂
195.0 Malignant neoplasm of head, face, and neck
198.2 Secondary malignant neoplasm of skin
210.0 Benign neoplasm of lip
216.1 Benign neoplasm of eyelid, including canthus
216.2 Benign neoplasm of ear and external auditory canal
216.4 Benign neoplasm of scalp and skin of neck
216.6 Benign neoplasm of skin of upper limb, including shoulder
216.7 Benign neoplasm of skin of lower limb, including hip
216.8 Benign neoplasm of other specified sites of skin
232.0 Carcinoma in situ of skin of lip
232.1 Carcinoma in situ of eyelid, including canthus
232.2 Carcinoma in situ of skin of ear and external auditory canal
232.4 Carcinoma in situ of scalp and skin of neck
232.6 Carcinoma in situ of skin of upper limb, including shoulder
232.7 Carcinoma in situ of skin of lower limb, including hip
232.8 Carcinoma in situ of other specified sites of skin
239.0 Neoplasm of unspecified nature of digestive system
239.2 Neoplasms of unspecified nature of bone, soft tissue, and skin
374.04 Cicatricial entropion
374.14 Cicatricial ectropion
374.41 Eyelid retraction or lag
380.32 Acquired deformities of auricle or pinna
607.2 Other inflammatory disorders of penis — (Use additional code to identify organism) ♂
682.0 Cellulitis and abscess of face — (Use additional code to identify organism)
728.86 Necrotizing fasciitis — (Use additional code to identify infectious organism, 041.00-041.89, 785.4, if applicable)
743.62 Congenital deformity of eyelid
744.01 Congenital absence of external ear causing impairment of hearing
744.09 Other congenital anomalies of ear causing impairment of hearing
744.23 Microtia
744.5 Congenital webbing of neck
744.82 Microcheilia
748.1 Other congenital anomaly of nose
749.00 Unspecified cleft palate ▽
749.10 Unspecified cleft lip ▽
749.11 Unilateral cleft lip, complete
749.12 Unilateral cleft lip, incomplete
749.13 Bilateral cleft lip, complete
749.14 Bilateral cleft lip, incomplete
749.21 Unilateral cleft palate with cleft lip, complete
749.22 Unilateral cleft palate with cleft lip, incomplete
749.23 Bilateral cleft palate with cleft lip, complete
749.24 Bilateral cleft palate with cleft lip, incomplete
752.49 Other congenital anomaly of cervix, vagina, and external female genitalia ♀
752.64 Micropenis ♂
752.69 Other penile anomalies ♂
752.7 Indeterminate sex and pseudohermaphroditism
752.89 Other specified anomalies of genital organs
752.9 Unspecified congenital anomaly of genital organs ▽
757.33 Congenital pigmentary anomaly of skin
785.4 Gangrene — (Code first any associated underlying condition:250.7, 443.0)
870.0 Laceration of skin of eyelid and periocular area — (Use additional code to identify infection)
870.1 Laceration of eyelid, full-thickness, not involving lacrimal passages — (Use additional code to identify infection)
870.2 Laceration of eyelid involving lacrimal passages — (Use additional code to identify infection)
872.00 Open wound of external ear, unspecified site, without mention of complication — (Use additional code to identify infection) ▽
872.01 Open wound of auricle, without mention of complication — (Use additional code to identify infection)
872.02 Open wound of auditory canal, without mention of complication — (Use additional code to identify infection)
872.10 Open wound of external ear, unspecified site, complicated — (Use additional code to identify infection) ▽

▽ Unspecified code ♀ Female diagnosis ☒ Manifestation code ♂ Male diagnosis

872.11 Open wound of auricle, complicated — (Use additional code to identify infection)
872.12 Open wound of auditory canal, complicated — (Use additional code to identify infection)
872.8 Open wound of ear, part unspecified, without mention of complication — (Use additional code to identify infection) ▽
872.9 Open wound of ear, part unspecified, complicated — (Use additional code to identify infection) ▽
873.30 Open wound of nose, unspecified site, complicated — (Use additional code to identify infection) ▽
873.31 Open wound of nasal septum, complicated — (Use additional code to identify infection)
873.32 Open wound of nasal cavity, complicated — (Use additional code to identify infection)
873.33 Open wound of nasal sinus, complicated — (Use additional code to identify infection)
873.39 Open wound of nose, multiple sites, complicated — (Use additional code to identify infection)
873.43 Open wound of lip, without mention of complication — (Use additional code to identify infection)
873.50 Open wound of face, unspecified site, complicated — (Use additional code to identify infection) ▽
873.52 Open wound of forehead, complicated — (Use additional code to identify infection)
873.54 Open wound of jaw, complicated — (Use additional code to identify infection)
873.59 Open wound of face, other and multiple sites, complicated — (Use additional code to identify infection)
878.1 Open wound of penis, complicated — (Use additional code to identify infection) ♂
878.3 Open wound of scrotum and testes, complicated — (Use additional code to identify infection) ♂
878.5 Open wound of vulva, complicated — (Use additional code to identify infection) ♀
878.7 Open wound of vagina, complicated — (Use additional code to identify infection) ♀
878.9 Open wound of other and unspecified parts of genital organs, complicated — (Use additional code to identify infection) ▽
880.12 Open wound of axillary region, complicated — (Use additional code to identify infection)
882.1 Open wound of hand except finger(s) alone, complicated — (Use additional code to identify infection)
882.2 Open wound of hand except finger(s) alone, with tendon involvement — (Use additional code to identify infection)
883.1 Open wound of finger(s), complicated — (Use additional code to identify infection)
883.2 Open wound of finger(s), with tendon involvement — (Use additional code to identify infection)
884.1 Multiple and unspecified open wound of upper limb, complicated — (Use additional code to identify infection)
884.2 Multiple and unspecified open wound of upper limb, with tendon involvement — (Use additional code to identify infection)
885.0 Traumatic amputation of thumb (complete) (partial), without mention of complication — (Use additional code to identify infection)
885.1 Traumatic amputation of thumb (complete) (partial), complicated — (Use additional code to identify infection)
886.0 Traumatic amputation of other finger(s) (complete) (partial), without mention of complication — (Use additional code to identify infection)
886.1 Traumatic amputation of other finger(s) (complete) (partial), complicated — (Use additional code to identify infection)
887.0 Traumatic amputation of arm and hand (complete) (partial), unilateral, below elbow, without mention of complication — (Use additional code to identify infection)
887.1 Traumatic amputation of arm and hand (complete) (partial), unilateral, below elbow, complicated — (Use additional code to identify infection)
887.6 Traumatic amputation of arm and hand (complete) (partial), bilateral (any level), without mention of complication — (Use additional code to identify infection)
887.7 Traumatic amputation of arm and hand (complete) (partial), bilateral (any level), complicated — (Use additional code to identify infection)
892.1 Open wound of foot except toe(s) alone, complicated — (Use additional code to identify infection)
892.2 Open wound of foot except toe(s) alone, with tendon involvement — (Use additional code to identify infection)
893.1 Open wound of toe(s), complicated — (Use additional code to identify infection)
893.2 Open wound of toe(s), with tendon involvement — (Use additional code to identify infection)
894.1 Multiple and unspecified open wound of lower limb, complicated — (Use additional code to identify infection)
894.2 Multiple and unspecified open wound of lower limb, with tendon involvement — (Use additional code to identify infection)
895.0 Traumatic amputation of toe(s) (complete) (partial), without mention of complication — (Use additional code to identify infection)
895.1 Traumatic amputation of toe(s) (complete) (partial), complicated — (Use additional code to identify infection)
896.0 Traumatic amputation of foot (complete) (partial), unilateral, without mention of complication — (Use additional code to identify infection)
896.1 Traumatic amputation of foot (complete) (partial), unilateral, complicated — (Use additional code to identify infection)
896.2 Traumatic amputation of foot (complete) (partial), bilateral, without mention of complication — (Use additional code to identify infection)
896.3 Traumatic amputation of foot (complete) (partial), bilateral, complicated — (Use additional code to identify infection)
906.0 Late effect of open wound of head, neck, and trunk
906.6 Late effect of burn of wrist and hand
941.01 Burn of unspecified degree of ear (any part) ▽
941.02 Burn of unspecified degree of eye (with other parts of face, head, and neck) ▽
941.03 Burn of unspecified degree of lip(s) ▽
941.05 Burn of unspecified degree of nose (septum) ▽
941.09 Burn of unspecified degree of multiple sites (except with eye) of face, head, and neck ▽
941.30 Full-thickness skin loss due to burn (third degree nos) of unspecified site of face and head ▽
941.31 Full-thickness skin loss due to burn (third degree nos) of ear (any part)
941.32 Full-thickness skin loss due to burn (third degree nos) of eye (with other parts of face, head, and neck)
941.34 Full-thickness skin loss due to burn (third degree nos) of chin
941.35 Full-thickness skin loss due to burn (third degree nos) of nose (septum)
941.37 Full-thickness skin loss due to burn (third degree nos) of forehead and cheek
941.38 Full-thickness skin loss due to burn (third degree nos) of neck
941.40 Deep necrosis of underlying tissues due to burn (deep third degree) of unspecified site of face and head, without mention of loss of a body part ▽
941.43 Deep necrosis of underlying tissues due to burn (deep third degree) of lip(s), without mention of loss of a body part
941.44 Deep necrosis of underlying tissues due to burn (deep third degree) of chin, without mention of loss of a body part
941.47 Deep necrosis of underlying tissues due to burn (deep third degree) of forehead and cheek, without mention of loss of a body part
941.48 Deep necrosis of underlying tissues due to burn (deep third degree) of neck, without mention of loss of a body part
941.49 Deep necrosis of underlying tissues due to burn (deep third degree) of multiple sites (except with eye) of face, head, and neck, without mention of loss of a body part
941.50 Deep necrosis of underlying tissues due to burn (deep third degree) of face and head, unspecified site, with loss of a body part ▽
941.51 Deep necrosis of underlying tissues due to burn (deep third degree) of ear (any part), with loss of a body part
941.52 Deep necrosis of underlying tissues due to burn (deep third degree) of eye (with other parts of face, head, and neck), with loss of a body part
941.55 Deep necrosis of underlying tissues due to burn (deep third degree) of nose (septum), with loss of a body part
941.57 Deep necrosis of underlying tissues due to burn (deep third degree) of forehead and cheek, with loss of a body part
941.58 Deep necrosis of underlying tissues due to burn (deep third degree) of neck, with loss of a body part
943.34 Full-thickness skin loss due to burn (third degree nos) of axilla
943.44 Deep necrosis of underlying tissues due to burn (deep third degree) of axilla, without mention of loss of a body part
943.54 Deep necrosis of underlying tissues due to burn (deep third degree) of axilla, with loss of a body part
944.30 Full-thickness skin loss due to burn (third degree nos) of unspecified site of hand ▽
944.31 Full-thickness skin loss due to burn (third degree nos) of single digit [finger (nail)] other than thumb
944.32 Full-thickness skin loss due to burn (third degree nos) of thumb (nail)
944.33 Full-thickness skin loss due to burn (third degree nos) of two or more digits of hand, not including thumb
944.34 Full-thickness skin loss due to burn (third degree nos) of two or more digits of hand including thumb
944.35 Full-thickness skin loss due to burn (third degree nos) of palm of hand
944.36 Full-thickness skin loss due to burn (third degree nos) of back of hand

▽ Unspecified code
♀ Female diagnosis
☒ Manifestation code
♂ Male diagnosis

944.37 Full-thickness skin loss due to burn (third degree nos) of wrist
944.38 Full-thickness skin loss due to burn (third degree nos) of multiple sites of wrist(s) and hand(s)
944.40 Deep necrosis of underlying tissues due to burn (deep third degree) of unspecified site of hand, without mention of a body part
944.41 Deep necrosis of underlying tissues due to burn (deep third degree) of single digit [finger (nail)] other than thumb, without mention of a body part
944.42 Deep necrosis of underlying tissues due to burn (deep third degree) of thumb (nail), without mention of loss of a body part
944.43 Deep necrosis of underlying tissues due to burn (deep third degree) of two or more digits of hand, not including thumb, without mention of a body part
944.44 Deep necrosis of underlying tissues due to burn (deep third degree) of two or more digits of hand including thumb, without mention of a body part
944.45 Deep necrosis of underlying tissues due to burn (deep third degree) of palm of hand, without mention of loss of a body part
944.46 Deep necrosis of underlying tissues due to burn (deep third degree) of back of hand, without mention of loss of back of a body part
944.47 Deep necrosis of underlying tissues due to burn (deep third degree) of wrist, without mention of loss of a body part
944.48 Deep necrosis of underlying tissues due to burn (deep third degree) of multiple sites of wrist(s) and hand(s), without mention of loss of a body part
944.50 Deep necrosis of underlying tissues due to burn (deep third degree) of unspecified site of hand, with loss of a body part
944.51 Deep necrosis of underlying tissues due to burn (deep third degree) of single digit (finger (nail)) other than thumb, with loss of a body part
944.52 Deep necrosis of underlying tissues due to burn (deep third degree) of thumb (nail), with loss of a body part
944.53 Deep necrosis of underlying tissues due to burn (deep third degree) of two or more digits of hand, not including thumb, with loss of a body part
944.54 Deep necrosis of underlying tissues due to burn (deep third degree) of two or more digits of hand including thumb, with loss of a body part
944.55 Deep necrosis of underlying tissues due to burn (deep third degree) of palm of hand, with loss of a body part
944.56 Deep necrosis of underlying tissues due to burn (deep third degree) of back of hand, with loss of a body part
944.57 Deep necrosis of underlying tissues due to burn (deep third degree) of wrist, with loss of a body part
944.58 Deep necrosis of underlying tissues due to burn (deep third degree) of multiple sites of wrist(s) and hand(s), with loss of a body part
945.32 Full-thickness skin loss due to burn (third degree nos) of foot
945.42 Deep necrosis of underlying tissues due to burn (deep third degree) of foot, without mention of loss of a body part
945.52 Deep necrosis of underlying tissues due to burn (deep third degree) of foot, with loss of a body part
948.00 Burn (any degree) involving less than 10% of body surface with third degree burn of less than 10% or unspecified amount
948.10 Burn (any degree) involving 10-19% of body surface with third degree burn of less than 10% or unspecified amount
948.11 Burn (any degree) involving 10-19% of body surface with third degree burn of 10-19%
948.20 Burn (any degree) involving 20-29% of body surface with third degree burn of less than 10% or unspecified amount
948.21 Burn (any degree) involving 20-29% of body surface with third degree burn of 10-19%
948.22 Burn (any degree) involving 20-29% of body surface with third degree burn of 20-29%
948.30 Burn (any degree) involving 30-39% of body surface with third degree burn of less than 10% or unspecified amount
948.31 Burn (any degree) involving 30-39% of body surface with third degree burn of 10-19%
948.32 Burn (any degree) involving 30-39% of body surface with third degree burn of 20-29%
948.33 Burn (any degree) involving 30-39% of body surface with third degree burn of 30-39%
948.40 Burn (any degree) involving 40-49% of body surface with third degree burn of less than 10% or unspecified amount
948.41 Burn (any degree) involving 40-49% of body surface with third degree burn of 10-19%
948.42 Burn (any degree) involving 40-49% of body surface with third degree burn of 20-29%
948.43 Burn (any degree) involving 40-49% of body surface with third degree burn of 30-39%
948.44 Burn (any degree) involving 40-49% of body surface with third degree burn of 40-49%
948.50 Burn (any degree) involving 50-59% of body surface with third degree burn of less than 10% or unspecified amount
948.51 Burn (any degree) involving 50-59% of body surface with third degree burn of 10-19%
948.52 Burn (any degree) involving 50-59% of body surface with third degree burn of 20-29%
948.53 Burn (any degree) involving 50-59% of body surface with third degree burn of 30-39%
948.54 Burn (any degree) involving 50-59% of body surface with third degree burn of 40-49%
948.55 Burn (any degree) involving 50-59% of body surface with third degree burn of 50-59%
948.60 Burn (any degree) involving 60-69% of body surface with third degree burn of less than 10% or unspecified amount
948.61 Burn (any degree) involving 60-69% of body surface with third degree burn of 10-19%
948.62 Burn (any degree) involving 60-69% of body surface with third degree burn of 20-29%
948.63 Burn (any degree) involving 60-69% of body surface with third degree burn of 30-39%
948.64 Burn (any degree) involving 60-69% of body surface with third degree burn of 40-49%
948.65 Burn (any degree) involving 60-69% of body surface with third degree burn of 50-59%
948.66 Burn (any degree) involving 60-69% of body surface with third degree burn of 60-69%
948.70 Burn (any degree) involving 70-79% of body surface with third degree burn of less than 10% or unspecified amount
948.71 Burn (any degree) involving 70-79% of body surface with third degree burn of 10-19%
948.72 Burn (any degree) involving 70-79% of body surface with third degree burn of 20-29%
948.73 Burn (any degree) involving 70-79% of body surface with third degree burn of 30-39%
948.74 Burn (any degree) involving 70-79% of body surface with third degree burn of 40-49%
948.75 Burn (any degree) involving 70-79% of body surface with third degree burn of 50-59%
948.76 Burn (any degree) involving 70-79% of body surface with third degree burn of 60-69%
948.77 Burn (any degree) involving 70-79% of body surface with third degree burn of 70-79%
948.80 Burn (any degree) involving 80-89% of body surface with third degree burn of less than 10% or unspecified amount
948.81 Burn (any degree) involving 80-89% of body surface with third degree burn of 10-19%
948.82 Burn (any degree) involving 80-89% of body surface with third degree burn of 20-29%
948.83 Burn (any degree) involving 80-89% of body surface with third degree burn of 30-39%
948.84 Burn (any degree) involving 80-89% of body surface with third degree burn of 40-49%
948.85 Burn (any degree) involving 80-89% of body surface with third degree burn of 50-59%
948.86 Burn (any degree) involving 80-89% of body surface with third degree burn of 60-69%
948.87 Burn (any degree) involving 80-89% of body surface with third degree burn of 70-79%
948.88 Burn (any degree) involving 80-89% of body surface with third degree burn of 80-89%
959.4 Injury, other and unspecified, hand, except finger
959.5 Injury, other and unspecified, finger
959.7 Injury, other and unspecified, knee, leg, ankle, and foot
959.8 Injury, other and unspecified, other specified sites, including multiple
991.0 Frostbite of face
991.1 Frostbite of hand
991.2 Frostbite of foot
997.60 Late complications of amputation stump, unspecified — (Use additional code to identify complications)
997.62 Infection (chronic) of amputation stump — (Use additional code to identify organism. Use additional code to identify complications)
997.69 Other late amputation stump complication — (Use additional code to identify complications)

ICD-9-CM Procedural

86.89 Other repair and reconstruction of skin and subcutaneous tissue

HCPCS Level II Supplies & Services

A4649 Surgical supply; miscellaneous

15876

15876 Suction assisted lipectomy; head and neck

ICD-9-CM Diagnostic

214.0 Lipoma of skin and subcutaneous tissue of face
214.1 Lipoma of other skin and subcutaneous tissue
272.6 Lipodystrophy — (Use additional code to identify any associated mental retardation. Use additional E code to identify cause, if iatrogenic)
272.8 Other disorders of lipoid metabolism — (Use additional code to identify any associated mental retardation)
278.1 Localized adiposity — (Use additional code to identify any associated mental retardation)
V50.1 Other plastic surgery for unacceptable cosmetic appearance

ICD-9-CM Procedural

86.83 Size reduction plastic operation

HCPCS Level II Supplies & Services

A4305 Disposable drug delivery system, flow rate of 50 ml or greater per hour
A4306 Disposable drug delivery system, flow rate of 5 ml or less per hour
A4550 Surgical trays

15877–15879

15877 Suction assisted lipectomy; trunk
15878 upper extremity
15879 lower extremity

ICD-9-CM Diagnostic

214.1 Lipoma of other skin and subcutaneous tissue
272.6 Lipodystrophy — (Use additional code to identify any associated mental retardation. Use additional E code to identify cause, if iatrogenic)
272.8 Other disorders of lipoid metabolism — (Use additional code to identify any associated mental retardation)
278.1 Localized adiposity — (Use additional code to identify any associated mental retardation)
V50.1 Other plastic surgery for unacceptable cosmetic appearance

ICD-9-CM Procedural

86.83 Size reduction plastic operation

HCPCS Level II Supplies & Services

A4305 Disposable drug delivery system, flow rate of 50 ml or greater per hour
A4306 Disposable drug delivery system, flow rate of 5 ml or less per hour
A4462 Abdominal dressing holder, each
A4550 Surgical trays

15920–15922

15920 Excision, coccygeal pressure ulcer, with coccygectomy; with primary suture
15922 with flap closure

ICD-9-CM Diagnostic

707.00 Decubitus ulcer, unspecified site
707.05 Decubitus ulcer, buttock
707.09 Decubitus ulcer, other site
730.18 Chronic osteomyelitis, other specified sites — (Use additional code to identify organism, 041.1)
785.4 Gangrene — (Code first any associated underlying condition:250.7, 443.0)

ICD-9-CM Procedural

77.99 Total ostectomy of other bone, except facial bones
86.3 Other local excision or destruction of lesion or tissue of skin and subcutaneous tissue
86.4 Radical excision of skin lesion
86.74 Attachment of pedicle or flap graft to other sites

15931–15933

15931 Excision, sacral pressure ulcer, with primary suture;
15933 with ostectomy

ICD-9-CM Diagnostic

707.00 Decubitus ulcer, unspecified site
707.05 Decubitus ulcer, buttock
707.09 Decubitus ulcer, other site
730.18 Chronic osteomyelitis, other specified sites — (Use additional code to identify organism, 041.1)
785.4 Gangrene — (Code first any associated underlying condition:250.7, 443.0)

ICD-9-CM Procedural

77.89 Other partial ostectomy of other bone, except facial bones
86.3 Other local excision or destruction of lesion or tissue of skin and subcutaneous tissue
86.4 Radical excision of skin lesion

15934–15935

15934 Excision, sacral pressure ulcer, with skin flap closure;
15935 with ostectomy

ICD-9-CM Diagnostic

707.00 Decubitus ulcer, unspecified site
707.05 Decubitus ulcer, buttock
707.09 Decubitus ulcer, other site
730.18 Chronic osteomyelitis, other specified sites — (Use additional code to identify organism, 041.1)
785.4 Gangrene — (Code first any associated underlying condition:250.7, 443.0)

ICD-9-CM Procedural

77.89 Other partial ostectomy of other bone, except facial bones
86.3 Other local excision or destruction of lesion or tissue of skin and subcutaneous tissue
86.4 Radical excision of skin lesion
86.74 Attachment of pedicle or flap graft to other sites

15936–15937

15936 Excision, sacral pressure ulcer, in preparation for muscle or myocutaneous flap or skin graft closure;
15937 with ostectomy

ICD-9-CM Diagnostic

707.00 Decubitus ulcer, unspecified site
707.05 Decubitus ulcer, buttock
707.09 Decubitus ulcer, other site
730.18 Chronic osteomyelitis, other specified sites — (Use additional code to identify organism, 041.1)
785.4 Gangrene — (Code first any associated underlying condition:250.7, 443.0)

ICD-9-CM Procedural

77.89 Other partial ostectomy of other bone, except facial bones
83.82 Graft of muscle or fascia
86.3 Other local excision or destruction of lesion or tissue of skin and subcutaneous tissue
86.4 Radical excision of skin lesion
86.74 Attachment of pedicle or flap graft to other sites

15940–15941

15940 Excision, ischial pressure ulcer, with primary suture;
15941 with ostectomy (ischiectomy)

ICD-9-CM Diagnostic

707.00 Decubitus ulcer, unspecified site
707.04 Decubitus ulcer, hip
707.09 Decubitus ulcer, other site
730.15 Chronic osteomyelitis, pelvic region and thigh — (Use additional code to identify organism, 041.1)
785.4 Gangrene — (Code first any associated underlying condition:250.7, 443.0)

ICD-9-CM Procedural

77.89 Other partial ostectomy of other bone, except facial bones
77.99 Total ostectomy of other bone, except facial bones
86.3 Other local excision or destruction of lesion or tissue of skin and subcutaneous tissue
86.4 Radical excision of skin lesion

15944–15945

15944 Excision, ischial pressure ulcer, with skin flap closure;
15945 with ostectomy

ICD-9-CM Diagnostic

707.00 Decubitus ulcer, unspecified site
707.04 Decubitus ulcer, hip
707.09 Decubitus ulcer, other site
730.15 Chronic osteomyelitis, pelvic region and thigh — (Use additional code to identify organism, 041.1)

785.4 Gangrene — (Code first any associated underlying condition:250.7, 443.0)

ICD-9-CM Procedural

77.89 Other partial ostectomy of other bone, except facial bones
77.99 Total ostectomy of other bone, except facial bones
86.3 Other local excision or destruction of lesion or tissue of skin and subcutaneous tissue
86.4 Radical excision of skin lesion
86.74 Attachment of pedicle or flap graft to other sites

15946

15946 Excision, ischial pressure ulcer, with ostectomy, in preparation for muscle or myocutaneous flap or skin graft closure

ICD-9-CM Diagnostic

707.00 Decubitus ulcer, unspecified site
707.04 Decubitus ulcer, hip
707.09 Decubitus ulcer, other site
730.15 Chronic osteomyelitis, pelvic region and thigh — (Use additional code to identify organism, 041.1)
785.4 Gangrene — (Code first any associated underlying condition:250.7, 443.0)

ICD-9-CM Procedural

77.89 Other partial ostectomy of other bone, except facial bones
77.99 Total ostectomy of other bone, except facial bones
83.82 Graft of muscle or fascia
86.3 Other local excision or destruction of lesion or tissue of skin and subcutaneous tissue
86.4 Radical excision of skin lesion
86.74 Attachment of pedicle or flap graft to other sites

15950–15951

15950 Excision, trochanteric pressure ulcer, with primary suture;
15951 with ostectomy

ICD-9-CM Diagnostic

707.00 Decubitus ulcer, unspecified site
707.04 Decubitus ulcer, hip
707.09 Decubitus ulcer, other site
730.15 Chronic osteomyelitis, pelvic region and thigh — (Use additional code to identify organism, 041.1)
785.4 Gangrene — (Code first any associated underlying condition:250.7, 443.0)

ICD-9-CM Procedural

77.85 Other partial ostectomy of femur
86.3 Other local excision or destruction of lesion or tissue of skin and subcutaneous tissue
86.4 Radical excision of skin lesion

15952–15953

15952 Excision, trochanteric pressure ulcer, with skin flap closure;
15953 with ostectomy

ICD-9-CM Diagnostic

707.00 Decubitus ulcer, unspecified site
707.04 Decubitus ulcer, hip
707.09 Decubitus ulcer, other site
730.15 Chronic osteomyelitis, pelvic region and thigh — (Use additional code to identify organism, 041.1)
785.4 Gangrene — (Code first any associated underlying condition:250.7, 443.0)

ICD-9-CM Procedural

77.85 Other partial ostectomy of femur
86.3 Other local excision or destruction of lesion or tissue of skin and subcutaneous tissue
86.4 Radical excision of skin lesion
86.74 Attachment of pedicle or flap graft to other sites

15956–15958

15956 Excision, trochanteric pressure ulcer, in preparation for muscle or myocutaneous flap or skin graft closure;
15958 with ostectomy

ICD-9-CM Diagnostic

707.00 Decubitus ulcer, unspecified site
707.04 Decubitus ulcer, hip
707.09 Decubitus ulcer, other site
730.15 Chronic osteomyelitis, pelvic region and thigh — (Use additional code to identify organism, 041.1)
785.4 Gangrene — (Code first any associated underlying condition:250.7, 443.0)

ICD-9-CM Procedural

77.85 Other partial ostectomy of femur
83.82 Graft of muscle or fascia
86.3 Other local excision or destruction of lesion or tissue of skin and subcutaneous tissue
86.4 Radical excision of skin lesion
86.74 Attachment of pedicle or flap graft to other sites

16000

16000 Initial treatment, first degree burn, when no more than local treatment is required

ICD-9-CM Diagnostic

941.10 Erythema due to burn (first degree) of unspecified site of face and head ▽
941.11 Erythema due to burn (first degree) of ear (any part)
941.12 Erythema due to burn (first degree) of eye (with other parts face, head, and neck)
941.13 Erythema due to burn (first degree) of lip(s)
941.14 Erythema due to burn (first degree) of chin
941.15 Erythema due to burn (first degree) of nose (septum)
941.16 Erythema due to burn (first degree) of scalp (any part)
941.17 Erythema due to burn (first degree) of forehead and cheek
941.18 Erythema due to burn (first degree) of neck
941.19 Erythema due to burn (first degree) of multiple sites (except with eye) of face, head, and neck
942.10 Erythema due to burn (first degree) of unspecified site of trunk ▽
942.11 Erythema due to burn (first degree) of breast
942.12 Erythema due to burn (first degree) of chest wall, excluding breast and nipple
942.13 Erythema due to burn (first degree) of abdominal wall
942.14 Erythema due to burn (first degree) of back (any part)

Rule of Nines for Burns

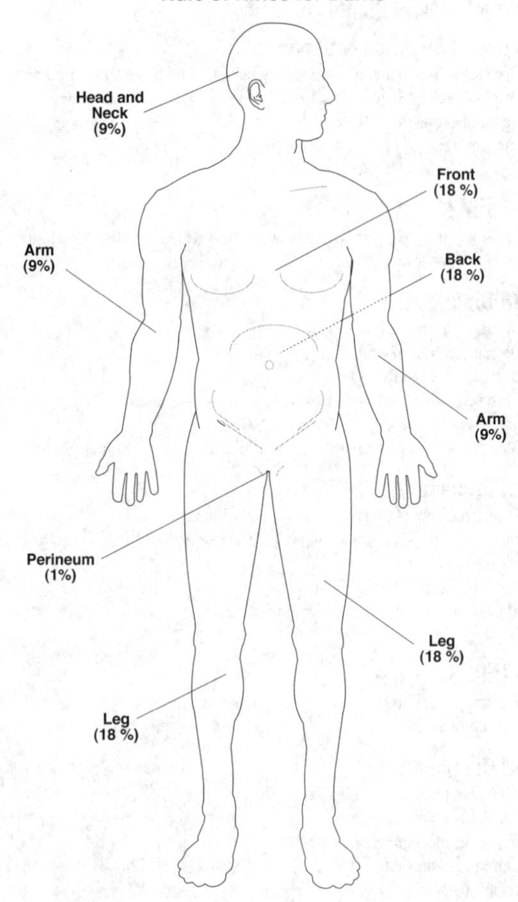

▽ Unspecified code ♀ Female diagnosis ☒ Manifestation code ♂ Male diagnosis

942.15 Erythema due to burn (first degree) of genitalia
942.19 Erythema due to burn (first degree) of other and multiple sites of trunk
943.10 Erythema due to burn (first degree) of unspecified site of upper limb
943.11 Erythema due to burn (first degree) of forearm
943.12 Erythema due to burn (first degree) of elbow
943.13 Erythema due to burn (first degree) of upper arm
943.14 Erythema due to burn (first degree) of axilla
943.15 Erythema due to burn (first degree) of shoulder
943.16 Erythema due to burn (first degree) of scapular region
943.19 Erythema due to burn (first degree) of multiple sites of upper limb, except wrist and hand
944.10 Erythema due to burn (first degree) of unspecified site of hand
944.11 Erythema due to burn (first degree) of single digit [finger (nail)] other than thumb
944.12 Erythema due to burn (first degree) of thumb (nail)
944.13 Erythema due to burn (first degree) of two or more digits of hand, not including thumb
944.14 Erythema due to burn (first degree) of two or more digits of hand including thumb
944.15 Erythema due to burn (first degree) of palm of hand
944.16 Erythema due to burn (first degree) of back of hand
944.17 Erythema due to burn (first degree) of wrist
944.18 Erythema due to burn (first degree) of multiple sites of wrist(s) and hand(s)
945.10 Erythema due to burn (first degree) of unspecified site of lower limb (leg)
945.11 Erythema due to burn (first degree) of toe(s) (nail)
945.12 Erythema due to burn (first degree) of foot
945.13 Erythema due to burn (first degree) of ankle
945.14 Erythema due to burn (first degree) of lower leg
945.15 Erythema due to burn (first degree) of knee
945.16 Erythema due to burn (first degree) of thigh (any part)
945.19 Erythema due to burn (first degree) of multiple sites of lower limb(s)
946.1 Erythema due to burn (first degree) of multiple specified sites
947.0 Burn of mouth and pharynx
948.00 Burn (any degree) involving less than 10% of body surface with third degree burn of less than 10% or unspecified amount

ICD-9-CM Procedural

89.01 Interview and evaluation, described as brief
89.02 Interview and evaluation, described as limited
93.57 Application of other wound dressing

HCPCS Level II Supplies & Services

A4649 Surgical supply; miscellaneous

16010–16030

16010 Dressings and/or debridement, initial or subsequent; under anesthesia, small
16015 under anesthesia, medium or large, or with major debridement
16020 without anesthesia, office or hospital, small
16025 without anesthesia, medium (eg, whole face or whole extremity)
16030 without anesthesia, large (eg, more than one extremity)

ICD-9-CM Diagnostic

941.20 Blisters, with epidermal loss due to burn (second degree) of face and head, unspecified site
941.21 Blisters, with epidermal loss due to burn (second degree) of ear (any part)
941.22 Blisters, with epidermal loss due to burn (second degree) of eye (with other parts of face, head, and neck)
941.23 Blisters, with epidermal loss due to burn (second degree) of lip(s)
941.24 Blisters, with epidermal loss due to burn (second degree) of chin
941.25 Blisters, with epidermal loss due to burn (second degree) of nose (septum)
941.26 Blisters, with epidermal loss due to burn (second degree) of scalp (any part)
941.27 Blisters, with epidermal loss due to burn (second degree) of forehead and cheek
941.28 Blisters, with epidermal loss due to burn (second degree) of neck
941.29 Blisters, with epidermal loss due to burn (second degree) of multiple sites (except with eye) of face, head, and neck
941.30 Full-thickness skin loss due to burn (third degree nos) of unspecified site of face and head
941.31 Full-thickness skin loss due to burn (third degree nos) of ear (any part)
941.32 Full-thickness skin loss due to burn (third degree nos) of eye (with other parts of face, head, and neck)
941.33 Full-thickness skin loss due to burn (third degree nos) of lip(s)
941.34 Full-thickness skin loss due to burn (third degree nos) of chin
941.35 Full-thickness skin loss due to burn (third degree nos) of nose (septum)
941.36 Full-thickness skin loss due to burn (third degree nos) of scalp (any part)
941.37 Full-thickness skin loss due to burn (third degree nos) of forehead and cheek
941.38 Full-thickness skin loss due to burn (third degree nos) of neck
941.39 Full-thickness skin loss due to burn (third degree nos) of multiple sites (except with eye) of face, head, and neck
941.40 Deep necrosis of underlying tissues due to burn (deep third degree) of unspecified site of face and head, without mention of loss of a body part
941.41 Deep necrosis of underlying tissues due to burn (deep third degree) of ear (any part), without mention of loss of a body part
941.42 Deep necrosis of underlying tissues due to burn (deep third degree) of eye (with other parts of face, head, and neck), without mention of loss of a body part
941.43 Deep necrosis of underlying tissues due to burn (deep third degree) of lip(s), without mention of loss of a body part
941.44 Deep necrosis of underlying tissues due to burn (deep third degree) of chin, without mention of loss of a body part
941.45 Deep necrosis of underlying tissues due to burn (deep third degree) of nose (septum), without mention of loss of a body part
941.46 Deep necrosis of underlying tissues due to burn (deep third degree) of scalp (any part), without mention of loss of a body part
941.47 Deep necrosis of underlying tissues due to burn (deep third degree) of forehead and cheek, without mention of loss of a body part
941.48 Deep necrosis of underlying tissues due to burn (deep third degree) of neck, without mention of loss of a body part
941.49 Deep necrosis of underlying tissues due to burn (deep third degree) of multiple sites (except with eye) of face, head, and neck, without mention of loss of a body part
942.20 Blisters with epidermal loss due to burn (second degree) of unspecified site of trunk
942.21 Blisters with epidermal loss due to burn (second degree) of breast
942.22 Blisters with epidermal loss due to burn (second degree) of chest wall, excluding breast and nipple
942.23 Blisters with epidermal loss due to burn (second degree) of abdominal wall
942.24 Blisters with epidermal loss due to burn (second degree) of back (any part)
942.25 Blisters with epidermal loss due to burn (second degree) of genitalia
942.30 Full-thickness skin loss due to burn (third degree nos) of unspecified site of trunk
942.31 Full-thickness skin loss due to burn (third degree nos) of breast
942.32 Full-thickness skin loss due to burn (third degree nos) of chest wall, excluding breast and nipple
942.33 Full-thickness skin loss due to burn (third degree nos) of abdominal wall
942.34 Full-thickness skin loss due to burn (third degree nos) of back (any part)
942.35 Full-thickness skin loss due to burn (third degree nos) of genitalia
942.40 Deep necrosis of underlying tissues due to burn (deep third degree) of trunk, unspecified site, without mention of loss of a body part
942.41 Deep necrosis of underlying tissues due to burn (deep third degree) of breast, without mention of loss of a body part
942.42 Deep necrosis of underlying tissues due to burn (deep third degree) of chest wall, excluding breast and nipple, without mention of loss of a body part
942.43 Deep necrosis of underlying tissues due to burn (deep third degree) of abdominal wall, without mention of loss of a body part
942.44 Deep necrosis of underlying tissues due to burn (deep third degree) of back (any part), without mention of loss of a body part
942.45 Deep necrosis of underlying tissues due to burn (deep third degree) of genitalia, without mention of loss of a body part
942.50 Deep necrosis of underlying tissues due to burn (deep third degree) of unspecified site of trunk, with loss of a body part
942.51 Deep necrosis of underlying tissues due to burn (deep third degree) of breast, with loss of a body part
942.52 Deep necrosis of underlying tissues due to burn (deep third degree) of chest wall, excluding breast and nipple, with loss of a body part
942.53 Deep necrosis of underlying tissues due to burn (deep third degree) of abdominal wall with loss of a body part
942.54 Deep necrosis of underlying tissues due to burn (deep third degree) of back (any part), with loss of a body part
942.55 Deep necrosis of underlying tissues due to burn (deep third degree) of genitalia, with loss of a body part
943.20 Blisters with epidermal loss due to burn (second degree) of unspecified site of upper limb
943.21 Blisters with epidermal loss due to burn (second degree) of forearm
943.22 Blisters with epidermal loss due to burn (second degree) of elbow
943.23 Blisters with epidermal loss due to burn (second degree) of upper arm
943.24 Blisters with epidermal loss due to burn (second degree) of axilla
943.25 Blisters with epidermal loss due to burn (second degree) of shoulder
943.26 Blisters with epidermal loss due to burn (second degree) of scapular region
943.29 Blisters with epidermal loss due to burn (second degree) of multiple sites of upper limb, except wrist and hand
943.30 Full-thickness skin loss due to burn (third degree nos) of unspecified site of upper limb

943.31 Full-thickness skin loss due to burn (third degree nos) of forearm
943.32 Full-thickness skin loss due to burn (third degree nos) of elbow
943.33 Full-thickness skin loss due to burn (third degree nos) of upper arm
943.34 Full-thickness skin loss due to burn (third degree nos) of axilla
943.35 Full-thickness skin loss due to burn (third degree nos) of shoulder
943.36 Full-thickness skin loss due to burn (third degree nos) of scapular region
943.39 Full-thickness skin loss due to burn (third degree nos) of multiple sites of upper limb, except wrist and hand
943.40 Deep necrosis of underlying tissues due to burn (deep third degree) of unspecified site of upper limb, without mention of loss of a body part ▽
943.41 Deep necrosis of underlying tissues due to burn (deep third degree) of forearm, without mention of loss of a body part
943.42 Deep necrosis of underlying tissues due to burn (deep third degree) of elbow, without mention of loss of a body part
943.43 Deep necrosis of underlying tissues due to burn (deep third degree) of upper arm, without mention of loss of a body part
943.44 Deep necrosis of underlying tissues due to burn (deep third degree) of axilla, without mention of loss of a body part
943.45 Deep necrosis of underlying tissues due to burn (deep third degree) of shoulder, without mention of loss of a body part
943.46 Deep necrosis of underlying tissues due to burn (deep third degree) of scapular region, without mention of loss of a body part
943.49 Deep necrosis of underlying tissues due to burn (deep third degree) of multiple sites of upper limb, except wrist and hand, without mention of loss of a body part
943.50 Deep necrosis of underlying tissues due to burn (deep third degree) of unspecified site of upper limb, with loss of a body part ▽
943.51 Deep necrosis of underlying tissues due to burn (deep third degree) of forearm, with loss of a body part
943.52 Deep necrosis of underlying tissues due to burn (deep third degree) of elbow, with loss of a body part
943.53 Deep necrosis of underlying tissues due to burn (deep third degree) of upper arm, with loss of upper a body part
943.54 Deep necrosis of underlying tissues due to burn (deep third degree) of axilla, with loss of a body part
943.55 Deep necrosis of underlying tissues due to burn (deep third degree) of shoulder, with loss of a body part
943.56 Deep necrosis of underlying tissues due to burn (deep third degree) of scapular region, with loss of a body part
943.59 Deep necrosis of underlying tissues due to burn (deep third degree) of multiple sites of upper limb, except wrist and hand, with loss of a body part
944.20 Blisters with epidermal loss due to burn (second degree) of unspecified site of hand ▽
944.21 Blisters with epidermal loss due to burn (second degree) of single digit [finger (nail)] other than thumb
944.22 Blisters with epidermal loss due to burn of (second degree) of thumb (nail)
944.23 Blisters with epidermal loss due to burn (second degree) of two or more digits of hand, not including thumb
944.24 Blisters with epidermal loss due to burn (second degree) of two or more digits of hand including thumb
944.25 Blisters with epidermal loss due to burn (second degree) of palm of hand
944.26 Blisters with epidermal loss due to burn (second degree) of back of hand
944.27 Blisters with epidermal loss due to burn (second degree) of wrist
944.28 Blisters with epidermal loss due to burn (second degree) of multiple sites of wrist(s) and hand(s)
944.30 Full-thickness skin loss due to burn (third degree nos) of unspecified site of hand ▽
944.31 Full-thickness skin loss due to burn (third degree nos) of single digit [finger (nail)] other than thumb
944.32 Full-thickness skin loss due to burn (third degree nos) of thumb (nail)
944.33 Full-thickness skin loss due to burn (third degree nos) of two or more digits of hand, not including thumb
944.34 Full-thickness skin loss due to burn (third degree nos) of two or more digits of hand including thumb
944.35 Full-thickness skin loss due to burn (third degree nos) of palm of hand
944.36 Full-thickness skin loss due to burn (third degree nos) of back of hand
944.37 Full-thickness skin loss due to burn (third degree nos) of wrist
944.38 Full-thickness skin loss due to burn (third degree nos) of multiple sites of wrist(s) and hand(s)
944.40 Deep necrosis of underlying tissues due to burn (deep third degree) of unspecified site of hand, without mention of a body part ▽
944.41 Deep necrosis of underlying tissues due to burn (deep third degree) of single digit [finger (nail)] other than thumb, without mention of a body part
944.42 Deep necrosis of underlying tissues due to burn (deep third degree) of thumb (nail), without mention of loss of a body part
944.43 Deep necrosis of underlying tissues due to burn (deep third degree) of two or more digits of hand, not including thumb, without mention of a body part
944.44 Deep necrosis of underlying tissues due to burn (deep third degree) of two or more digits of hand including thumb, without mention of a body part
944.45 Deep necrosis of underlying tissues due to burn (deep third degree) of palm of hand, without mention of loss of a body part
944.46 Deep necrosis of underlying tissues due to burn (deep third degree) of back of hand, without mention of loss of back of a body part
944.47 Deep necrosis of underlying tissues due to burn (deep third degree) of wrist, without mention of loss of a body part
944.48 Deep necrosis of underlying tissues due to burn (deep third degree) of multiple sites of wrist(s) and hand(s), without mention of loss of a body part
944.50 Deep necrosis of underlying tissues due to burn (deep third degree) of unspecified site of hand, with loss of a body part ▽
944.51 Deep necrosis of underlying tissues due to burn (deep third degree) of single digit (finger (nail)) other than thumb, with loss of a body part
944.52 Deep necrosis of underlying tissues due to burn (deep third degree) of thumb (nail), with loss of a body part
944.53 Deep necrosis of underlying tissues due to burn (deep third degree) of two or more digits of hand, not including thumb, with loss of a body part
944.54 Deep necrosis of underlying tissues due to burn (deep third degree) of two or more digits of hand including thumb, with loss of a body part
944.55 Deep necrosis of underlying tissues due to burn (deep third degree) of palm of hand, with loss of a body part
944.56 Deep necrosis of underlying tissues due to burn (deep third degree) of back of hand, with loss of a body part
944.57 Deep necrosis of underlying tissues due to burn (deep third degree) of wrist, with loss of a body part
944.58 Deep necrosis of underlying tissues due to burn (deep third degree) of multiple sites of wrist(s) and hand(s), with loss of a body part
945.20 Blisters with epidermal loss due to burn (second degree) of unspecified site of lower limb (leg) ▽
945.21 Blisters with epidermal loss due to burn (second degree) of toe(s) (nail)
945.22 Blisters with epidermal loss due to burn (second degree) of foot
945.23 Blisters with epidermal loss due to burn (second degree) of ankle
945.24 Blisters with epidermal loss due to burn (second degree) of lower leg
945.25 Blisters with epidermal loss due to burn (second degree) of knee
945.26 Blisters with epidermal loss due to burn (second degree) of thigh (any part)
945.29 Blisters with epidermal loss due to burn (second degree) of multiple sites of lower limb(s)
945.30 Full-thickness skin loss due to burn (third degree nos) of unspecified site of lower limb ▽
945.31 Full-thickness skin loss due to burn (third degree nos) of toe(s) (nail)
945.32 Full-thickness skin loss due to burn (third degree nos) of foot
945.33 Full-thickness skin loss due to burn (third degree nos) of ankle
945.34 Full-thickness skin loss due to burn (third degree nos) of lower leg
945.35 Full-thickness skin loss due to burn (third degree nos) of knee
945.36 Full-thickness skin loss due to burn (third degree nos) of thigh (any part)
945.39 Full-thickness skin loss due to burn (third degree nos) of multiple sites of lower limb(s)
945.40 Deep necrosis of underlying tissues due to burn (deep third degree) of unspecified site of lower limb (leg), without mention of loss of a body part ▽
945.41 Deep necrosis of underlying tissues due to burn (deep third degree) of toe(s) (nail), without mention of loss of a body part
945.42 Deep necrosis of underlying tissues due to burn (deep third degree) of foot, without mention of loss of a body part
945.49 Deep necrosis of underlying tissues due to burn (deep third degree) of multiple sites of lower limb(s), without mention of loss of a body part
945.50 Deep necrosis of underlying tissues due to burn (deep third degree) of unspecified site lower limb (leg), with loss of a body part ▽
945.51 Deep necrosis of underlying tissues due to burn (deep third degree) of toe(s) (nail), with loss of a body part
945.52 Deep necrosis of underlying tissues due to burn (deep third degree) of foot, with loss of a body part
945.53 Deep necrosis of underlying tissues due to burn (deep third degree) of ankle, with loss of a body part
945.54 Deep necrosis of underlying tissues due to burn (deep third degree) of lower leg, with loss of a body part
945.55 Deep necrosis of underlying tissues due to burn (deep third degree) of knee, with loss of a body part
945.56 Deep necrosis of underlying tissues due to burn (deep third degree) of thigh (any part), with loss of a body part
945.59 Deep necrosis of underlying tissues due to burn (deep third degree) of multiple sites of lower limb(s), with loss of a body part
947.0 Burn of mouth and pharynx

▽ Unspecified code
♀ Female diagnosis
☒ Manifestation code
♂ Male diagnosis

948.00 Burn (any degree) involving less than 10% of body surface with third degree burn of less than 10% or unspecified amount
948.11 Burn (any degree) involving 10-19% of body surface with third degree burn of 10-19%
948.20 Burn (any degree) involving 20-29% of body surface with third degree burn of less than 10% or unspecified amount
948.21 Burn (any degree) involving 20-29% of body surface with third degree burn of 10-19%
948.22 Burn (any degree) involving 20-29% of body surface with third degree burn of 20-29%

ICD-9-CM Procedural

86.22 Excisional debridement of wound, infection, or burn
86.28 Nonexcisional debridement of wound, infection, or burn
93.56 Application of pressure dressing
93.57 Application of other wound dressing

HCPCS Level II Supplies & Services

A4305 Disposable drug delivery system, flow rate of 50 ml or greater per hour
A4306 Disposable drug delivery system, flow rate of 5 ml or less per hour
A4462 Abdominal dressing holder, each
A4550 Surgical trays

16035–16036

16035 Escharotomy; initial incision
16036 each additional incision (List separately in addition to code for primary procedure)

ICD-9-CM Diagnostic

709.2 Scar condition and fibrosis of skin
906.5 Late effect of burn of eye, face, head, and neck
906.6 Late effect of burn of wrist and hand
906.7 Late effect of burn of other extremities
906.8 Late effect of burns of other specified sites
940.0 Chemical burn of eyelids and periocular area
940.1 Other burns of eyelids and periocular area
941.20 Blisters, with epidermal loss due to burn (second degree) of face and head, unspecified site ▽
941.21 Blisters, with epidermal loss due to burn (second degree) of ear (any part)
941.22 Blisters, with epidermal loss due to burn (second degree) of eye (with other parts of face, head, and neck)
941.23 Blisters, with epidermal loss due to burn (second degree) of lip(s)
941.24 Blisters, with epidermal loss due to burn (second degree) of chin
941.25 Blisters, with epidermal loss due to burn (second degree) of nose (septum)
941.26 Blisters, with epidermal loss due to burn (second degree) of scalp (any part)
941.27 Blisters, with epidermal loss due to burn (second degree) of forehead and cheek
941.28 Blisters, with epidermal loss due to burn (second degree) of neck
941.29 Blisters, with epidermal loss due to burn (second degree) of multiple sites (except with eye) of face, head, and neck
941.30 Full-thickness skin loss due to burn (third degree nos) of unspecified site of face and head ▽
941.31 Full-thickness skin loss due to burn (third degree nos) of ear (any part)
941.32 Full-thickness skin loss due to burn (third degree nos) of eye (with other parts of face, head, and neck)
941.33 Full-thickness skin loss due to burn (third degree nos) of lip(s)
941.34 Full-thickness skin loss due to burn (third degree nos) of chin
941.35 Full-thickness skin loss due to burn (third degree nos) of nose (septum)
941.36 Full-thickness skin loss due to burn (third degree nos) of scalp (any part)
941.37 Full-thickness skin loss due to burn (third degree nos) of forehead and cheek
941.38 Full-thickness skin loss due to burn (third degree nos) of neck
941.39 Full-thickness skin loss due to burn (third degree nos) of multiple sites (except with eye) of face, head, and neck
941.40 Deep necrosis of underlying tissues due to burn (deep third degree) of unspecified site of face and head, without mention of loss of a body part ▽
941.41 Deep necrosis of underlying tissues due to burn (deep third degree) of ear (any part), without mention of loss of a body part
941.42 Deep necrosis of underlying tissues due to burn (deep third degree) of eye (with other parts of face, head, and neck), without mention of loss of a body part
941.43 Deep necrosis of underlying tissues due to burn (deep third degree) of lip(s), without mention of loss of a body part
941.44 Deep necrosis of underlying tissues due to burn (deep third degree) of chin, without mention of loss of a body part
941.45 Deep necrosis of underlying tissues due to burn (deep third degree) of nose (septum), without mention of loss of a body part
941.46 Deep necrosis of underlying tissues due to burn (deep third degree) of scalp (any part), without mention of loss of a body part
941.47 Deep necrosis of underlying tissues due to burn (deep third degree) of forehead and cheek, without mention of loss of a body part
941.48 Deep necrosis of underlying tissues due to burn (deep third degree) of neck, without mention of loss of a body part
941.49 Deep necrosis of underlying tissues due to burn (deep third degree) of multiple sites (except with eye) of face, head, and neck, without mention of loss of a body part
941.50 Deep necrosis of underlying tissues due to burn (deep third degree) of face and head, unspecified site, with loss of a body part ▽
941.51 Deep necrosis of underlying tissues due to burn (deep third degree) of ear (any part), with loss of a body part
941.52 Deep necrosis of underlying tissues due to burn (deep third degree) of eye (with other parts of face, head, and neck), with loss of a body part
941.53 Deep necrosis of underlying tissues due to burn (deep third degree) of lip(s), with loss of a body part
941.54 Deep necrosis of underlying tissues due to burn (deep third degree) of chin, with loss of a body part
941.55 Deep necrosis of underlying tissues due to burn (deep third degree) of nose (septum), with loss of a body part
941.56 Deep necrosis of underlying tissues due to burn (deep third degree) of scalp (any part), with loss of a body part
941.57 Deep necrosis of underlying tissues due to burn (deep third degree) of forehead and cheek, with loss of a body part
941.58 Deep necrosis of underlying tissues due to burn (deep third degree) of neck, with loss of a body part
941.59 Deep necrosis of underlying tissues due to burn (deep third degree) of multiple sites (except eye) of face, head, and neck, with loss of a body part
942.20 Blisters with epidermal loss due to burn (second degree) of unspecified site of trunk ▽
942.21 Blisters with epidermal loss due to burn (second degree) of breast
942.22 Blisters with epidermal loss due to burn (second degree) of chest wall, excluding breast and nipple
942.23 Blisters with epidermal loss due to burn (second degree) of abdominal wall
942.24 Blisters with epidermal loss due to burn (second degree) of back (any part)
942.25 Blisters with epidermal loss due to burn (second degree) of genitalia
942.29 Blisters with epidermal loss due to burn (second degree) of other and multiple sites of trunk
942.30 Full-thickness skin loss due to burn (third degree nos) of unspecified site of trunk ▽
942.31 Full-thickness skin loss due to burn (third degree nos) of breast
942.32 Full-thickness skin loss due to burn (third degree nos) of chest wall, excluding breast and nipple
942.33 Full-thickness skin loss due to burn (third degree nos) of abdominal wall
942.34 Full-thickness skin loss due to burn (third degree nos) of back (any part)
942.35 Full-thickness skin loss due to burn (third degree nos) of genitalia
942.39 Full-thickness skin loss due to burn (third degree nos) of other and multiple sites of trunk
942.40 Deep necrosis of underlying tissues due to burn (deep third degree) of trunk, unspecified site, without mention of loss of a body part ▽
942.41 Deep necrosis of underlying tissues due to burn (deep third degree) of breast, without mention of loss of a body part
942.42 Deep necrosis of underlying tissues due to burn (deep third degree) of chest wall, excluding breast and nipple, without mention of loss of a body part
942.43 Deep necrosis of underlying tissues due to burn (deep third degree) of abdominal wall, without mention of loss of a body part
942.44 Deep necrosis of underlying tissues due to burn (deep third degree) of back (any part), without mention of loss of a body part
942.45 Deep necrosis of underlying tissues due to burn (deep third degree) of genitalia, without mention of loss of a body part
942.49 Deep necrosis of underlying tissues due to burn (deep third degree) of other and multiple sites of trunk, without mention of loss of a body part
943.20 Blisters with epidermal loss due to burn (second degree) of unspecified site of upper limb ▽
943.21 Blisters with epidermal loss due to burn (second degree) of forearm
943.22 Blisters with epidermal loss due to burn (second degree) of elbow
943.23 Blisters with epidermal loss due to burn (second degree) of upper arm
943.24 Blisters with epidermal loss due to burn (second degree) of axilla
943.25 Blisters with epidermal loss due to burn (second degree) of shoulder
943.26 Blisters with epidermal loss due to burn (second degree) of scapular region
943.29 Blisters with epidermal loss due to burn (second degree) of multiple sites of upper limb, except wrist and hand
943.30 Full-thickness skin loss due to burn (third degree nos) of unspecified site of upper limb ▽
943.31 Full-thickness skin loss due to burn (third degree nos) of forearm

943.32 Full-thickness skin loss due to burn (third degree nos) of elbow
943.33 Full-thickness skin loss due to burn (third degree nos) of upper arm
943.34 Full-thickness skin loss due to burn (third degree nos) of axilla
943.35 Full-thickness skin loss due to burn (third degree nos) of shoulder
943.36 Full-thickness skin loss due to burn (third degree nos) of scapular region
943.39 Full-thickness skin loss due to burn (third degree nos) of multiple sites of upper limb, except wrist and hand
943.40 Deep necrosis of underlying tissues due to burn (deep third degree) of unspecified site of upper limb, without mention of loss of a body part
943.41 Deep necrosis of underlying tissues due to burn (deep third degree) of forearm, without mention of loss of a body part
943.42 Deep necrosis of underlying tissues due to burn (deep third degree) of elbow, without mention of loss of a body part
943.43 Deep necrosis of underlying tissues due to burn (deep third degree) of upper arm, without mention of loss of a body part
943.44 Deep necrosis of underlying tissues due to burn (deep third degree) of axilla, without mention of loss of a body part
943.45 Deep necrosis of underlying tissues due to burn (deep third degree) of shoulder, without mention of loss of a body part
943.46 Deep necrosis of underlying tissues due to burn (deep third degree) of scapular region, without mention of loss of a body part
943.49 Deep necrosis of underlying tissues due to burn (deep third degree) of multiple sites of upper limb, except wrist and hand, without mention of loss of a body part
943.50 Deep necrosis of underlying tissues due to burn (deep third degree) of unspecified site of upper limb, with loss of a body part
943.51 Deep necrosis of underlying tissues due to burn (deep third degree) of forearm, with loss of a body part
943.52 Deep necrosis of underlying tissues due to burn (deep third degree) of elbow, with loss of a body part
943.53 Deep necrosis of underlying tissues due to burn (deep third degree) of upper arm, with loss of upper a body part
943.54 Deep necrosis of underlying tissues due to burn (deep third degree) of axilla, with loss of a body part
943.55 Deep necrosis of underlying tissues due to burn (deep third degree) of shoulder, with loss of a body part
943.56 Deep necrosis of underlying tissues due to burn (deep third degree) of scapular region, with loss of a body part
943.59 Deep necrosis of underlying tissues due to burn (deep third degree) of multiple sites of upper limb, except wrist and hand, with loss of a body part
944.20 Blisters with epidermal loss due to burn (second degree) of unspecified site of hand
944.21 Blisters with epidermal loss due to burn (second degree) of single digit [finger (nail)] other than thumb
944.22 Blisters with epidermal loss due to burn of (second degree) of thumb (nail)
944.23 Blisters with epidermal loss due to burn (second degree) of two or more digits of hand, not including thumb
944.24 Blisters with epidermal loss due to burn (second degree) of two or more digits of hand including thumb
944.25 Blisters with epidermal loss due to burn (second degree) of palm of hand
944.26 Blisters with epidermal loss due to burn (second degree) of back of hand
944.27 Blisters with epidermal loss due to burn (second degree) of wrist
944.28 Blisters with epidermal loss due to burn (second degree) of multiple sites of wrist(s) and hand(s)
944.30 Full-thickness skin loss due to burn (third degree nos) of unspecified site of hand
944.31 Full-thickness skin loss due to burn (third degree nos) of single digit [finger (nail)] other than thumb
944.32 Full-thickness skin loss due to burn (third degree nos) of thumb (nail)
944.33 Full-thickness skin loss due to burn (third degree nos) of two or more digits of hand, not including thumb
944.34 Full-thickness skin loss due to burn (third degree nos) of two or more digits of hand including thumb
944.35 Full-thickness skin loss due to burn (third degree nos) of palm of hand
944.36 Full-thickness skin loss due to burn (third degree nos) of back of hand
944.37 Full-thickness skin loss due to burn (third degree nos) of wrist
944.38 Full-thickness skin loss due to burn (third degree nos) of multiple sites of wrist(s) and hand(s)
944.40 Deep necrosis of underlying tissues due to burn (deep third degree) of unspecified site of hand, without mention of a body part
944.41 Deep necrosis of underlying tissues due to burn (deep third degree) of single digit [finger (nail)] other than thumb, without mention of a body part
944.42 Deep necrosis of underlying tissues due to burn (deep third degree) of thumb (nail), without mention of loss of a body part
944.43 Deep necrosis of underlying tissues due to burn (deep third degree) of two or more digits of hand, not including thumb, without mention of a body part
944.44 Deep necrosis of underlying tissues due to burn (deep third degree) of two or more digits of hand including thumb, without mention of a body part
944.45 Deep necrosis of underlying tissues due to burn (deep third degree) of palm of hand, without mention of loss of a body part
944.46 Deep necrosis of underlying tissues due to burn (deep third degree) of back of hand, without mention of loss of back of a body part
944.47 Deep necrosis of underlying tissues due to burn (deep third degree) of wrist, without mention of loss of a body part
944.48 Deep necrosis of underlying tissues due to burn (deep third degree) of multiple sites of wrist(s) and hand(s), without mention of loss of a body part
944.50 Deep necrosis of underlying tissues due to burn (deep third degree) of unspecified site of hand, with loss of a body part
944.51 Deep necrosis of underlying tissues due to burn (deep third degree) of single digit (finger (nail)) other than thumb, with loss of a body part
944.52 Deep necrosis of underlying tissues due to burn (deep third degree) of thumb (nail), with loss of a body part
944.53 Deep necrosis of underlying tissues due to burn (deep third degree) of two or more digits of hand, not including thumb, with loss of a body part
944.54 Deep necrosis of underlying tissues due to burn (deep third degree) of two or more digits of hand including thumb, with loss of a body part
944.55 Deep necrosis of underlying tissues due to burn (deep third degree) of palm of hand, with loss of a body part
944.56 Deep necrosis of underlying tissues due to burn (deep third degree) of back of hand, with loss of a body part
944.57 Deep necrosis of underlying tissues due to burn (deep third degree) of wrist, with loss of a body part
944.58 Deep necrosis of underlying tissues due to burn (deep third degree) of multiple sites of wrist(s) and hand(s), with loss of a body part
945.20 Blisters with epidermal loss due to burn (second degree) of unspecified site of lower limb (leg)
945.21 Blisters with epidermal loss due to burn (second degree) of toe(s) (nail)
945.22 Blisters with epidermal loss due to burn (second degree) of foot
945.23 Blisters with epidermal loss due to burn (second degree) of ankle
945.24 Blisters with epidermal loss due to burn (second degree) of lower leg
945.25 Blisters with epidermal loss due to burn (second degree) of knee
945.26 Blisters with epidermal loss due to burn (second degree) of thigh (any part)
945.29 Blisters with epidermal loss due to burn (second degree) of multiple sites of lower limb(s)
945.30 Full-thickness skin loss due to burn (third degree nos) of unspecified site of lower limb
945.31 Full-thickness skin loss due to burn (third degree nos) of toe(s) (nail)
945.32 Full-thickness skin loss due to burn (third degree nos) of foot
945.33 Full-thickness skin loss due to burn (third degree nos) of ankle
945.34 Full-thickness skin loss due to burn (third degree nos) of lower leg
945.35 Full-thickness skin loss due to burn (third degree nos) of knee
945.36 Full-thickness skin loss due to burn (third degree nos) of thigh (any part)
945.39 Full-thickness skin loss due to burn (third degree nos) of multiple sites of lower limb(s)
945.40 Deep necrosis of underlying tissues due to burn (deep third degree) of unspecified site of lower limb (leg), without mention of loss of a body part
945.41 Deep necrosis of underlying tissues due to burn (deep third degree) of toe(s) (nail), without mention of loss of a body part
945.42 Deep necrosis of underlying tissues due to burn (deep third degree) of foot, without mention of loss of a body part
945.43 Deep necrosis of underlying tissues due to burn (deep third degree) of ankle, without mention of loss of a body part
945.44 Deep necrosis of underlying tissues due to burn (deep third degree) of lower leg, without mention of loss of a body part
945.45 Deep necrosis of underlying tissues due to burn (deep third degree) of knee, without mention of loss of a body part
945.46 Deep necrosis of underlying tissues due to burn (deep third degree) of thigh (any part), without mention of loss of a body part
945.49 Deep necrosis of underlying tissues due to burn (deep third degree) of multiple sites of lower limb(s), without mention of loss of a body part
945.50 Deep necrosis of underlying tissues due to burn (deep third degree) of unspecified site lower limb (leg), with loss of a body part
945.51 Deep necrosis of underlying tissues due to burn (deep third degree) of toe(s) (nail), with loss of a body part
945.52 Deep necrosis of underlying tissues due to burn (deep third degree) of foot, with loss of a body part
945.53 Deep necrosis of underlying tissues due to burn (deep third degree) of ankle, with loss of a body part
945.54 Deep necrosis of underlying tissues due to burn (deep third degree) of lower leg, with loss of a body part
945.55 Deep necrosis of underlying tissues due to burn (deep third degree) of knee, with loss of a body part

945.56 Deep necrosis of underlying tissues due to burn (deep third degree) of thigh (any part), with loss of a body part
945.59 Deep necrosis of underlying tissues due to burn (deep third degree) of multiple sites of lower limb(s), with loss of a body part
946.2 Blisters with epidermal loss due to burn (second degree) of multiple specified sites
946.3 Full-thickness skin loss due to burn (third degree nos) of multiple specified sites
946.4 Deep necrosis of underlying tissues due to burn (deep third degree) of multiple specified sites, without mention of loss of a body part
946.5 Deep necrosis of underlying tissues due to burn (deep third degree) of multiple specified sites, with loss of a body part
948.00 Burn (any degree) involving less than 10% of body surface with third degree burn of less than 10% or unspecified amount
948.10 Burn (any degree) involving 10-19% of body surface with third degree burn of less than 10% or unspecified amount
948.11 Burn (any degree) involving 10-19% of body surface with third degree burn of 10-19%
948.20 Burn (any degree) involving 20-29% of body surface with third degree burn of less than 10% or unspecified amount
948.21 Burn (any degree) involving 20-29% of body surface with third degree burn of 10-19%
948.22 Burn (any degree) involving 20-29% of body surface with third degree burn of 20-29%
948.30 Burn (any degree) involving 30-39% of body surface with third degree burn of less than 10% or unspecified amount
948.31 Burn (any degree) involving 30-39% of body surface with third degree burn of 10-19%
948.32 Burn (any degree) involving 30-39% of body surface with third degree burn of 20-29%
948.33 Burn (any degree) involving 30-39% of body surface with third degree burn of 30-39%
948.40 Burn (any degree) involving 40-49% of body surface with third degree burn of less than 10% or unspecified amount
948.41 Burn (any degree) involving 40-49% of body surface with third degree burn of 10-19%
948.42 Burn (any degree) involving 40-49% of body surface with third degree burn of 20-29%
948.43 Burn (any degree) involving 40-49% of body surface with third degree burn of 30-39%
948.44 Burn (any degree) involving 40-49% of body surface with third degree burn of 40-49%
948.50 Burn (any degree) involving 50-59% of body surface with third degree burn of less than 10% or unspecified amount
948.51 Burn (any degree) involving 50-59% of body surface with third degree burn of 10-19%
948.52 Burn (any degree) involving 50-59% of body surface with third degree burn of 20-29%
948.53 Burn (any degree) involving 50-59% of body surface with third degree burn of 30-39%
948.54 Burn (any degree) involving 50-59% of body surface with third degree burn of 40-49%
948.55 Burn (any degree) involving 50-59% of body surface with third degree burn of 50-59%
948.60 Burn (any degree) involving 60-69% of body surface with third degree burn of less than 10% or unspecified amount
948.61 Burn (any degree) involving 60-69% of body surface with third degree burn of 10-19%
948.62 Burn (any degree) involving 60-69% of body surface with third degree burn of 20-29%
948.63 Burn (any degree) involving 60-69% of body surface with third degree burn of 30-39%
948.64 Burn (any degree) involving 60-69% of body surface with third degree burn of 40-49%
948.65 Burn (any degree) involving 60-69% of body surface with third degree burn of 50-59%
948.66 Burn (any degree) involving 60-69% of body surface with third degree burn of 60-69%
948.70 Burn (any degree) involving 70-79% of body surface with third degree burn of less than 10% or unspecified amount
948.71 Burn (any degree) involving 70-79% of body surface with third degree burn of 10-19%
948.72 Burn (any degree) involving 70-79% of body surface with third degree burn of 20-29%
948.73 Burn (any degree) involving 70-79% of body surface with third degree burn of 30-39%
948.74 Burn (any degree) involving 70-79% of body surface with third degree burn of 40-49%
948.75 Burn (any degree) involving 70-79% of body surface with third degree burn of 50-59%
948.76 Burn (any degree) involving 70-79% of body surface with third degree burn of 60-69%
948.77 Burn (any degree) involving 70-79% of body surface with third degree burn of 70-79%
948.80 Burn (any degree) involving 80-89% of body surface with third degree burn of less than 10% or unspecified amount
948.81 Burn (any degree) involving 80-89% of body surface with third degree burn of 10-19%
948.82 Burn (any degree) involving 80-89% of body surface with third degree burn of 20-29%
948.83 Burn (any degree) involving 80-89% of body surface with third degree burn of 30-39%
948.84 Burn (any degree) involving 80-89% of body surface with third degree burn of 40-49%
948.85 Burn (any degree) involving 80-89% of body surface with third degree burn of 50-59%
948.86 Burn (any degree) involving 80-89% of body surface with third degree burn of 60-69%
948.87 Burn (any degree) involving 80-89% of body surface with third degree burn of 70-79%
948.88 Burn (any degree) involving 80-89% of body surface with third degree burn of 80-89%
948.90 Burn (any degree) involving 90% or more of body surface with third degree burn of less than 10% or unspecified amount
948.91 Burn (any degree) involving 90% or more of body surface with third degree burn of 10-19%
948.92 Burn (any degree) involving 90% or more of body surface with third degree burn of 20-29%
948.93 Burn (any degree) involving 90% or more of body surface with third degree burn of 30-39%
948.94 Burn (any degree) involving 90% or more of body surface with third degree burn of 40-49%
948.95 Burn (any degree) involving 90% or more of body surface with third degree burn of 50-59%
948.96 Burn (any degree) involving 90% or more of body surface with third degree burn of 60-69%
948.97 Burn (any degree) involving 90% or more of body surface with third degree burn of 70-79%
948.98 Burn (any degree) involving 90% or more of body surface with third degree burn of 80-89%
948.99 Burn (any degree) involving 90% or more of body surface with third degree burn of 90% or more of body surface

ICD-9-CM Procedural

86.09 Other incision of skin and subcutaneous tissue

Destruction

17000–17004

17000 Destruction (eg, laser surgery, electrosurgery, cryosurgery, chemosurgery, surgical curettement), all benign or premalignant lesions (eg, actinic keratoses) other than skin tags or cutaneous vascular proliferative lesions; first lesion
17003 second through 14 lesions, each (List separately in addition to code for first lesion)
17004 Destruction (eg, laser surgery, electrosurgery, cryosurgery, chemosurgery, surgical curettement), all benign or premalignant lesions (eg, actinic keratoses) other than skin tags or cutaneous vascular proliferative lesions, 15 or more lesions

ICD-9-CM Diagnostic

078.11 Condyloma acuminatum
078.19 Other specified viral warts
216.0 Benign neoplasm of skin of lip
216.1 Benign neoplasm of eyelid, including canthus
216.2 Benign neoplasm of ear and external auditory canal
216.3 Benign neoplasm of skin of other and unspecified parts of face ▽
216.4 Benign neoplasm of scalp and skin of neck
216.5 Benign neoplasm of skin of trunk, except scrotum
216.6 Benign neoplasm of skin of upper limb, including shoulder
216.7 Benign neoplasm of skin of lower limb, including hip

238.2 Neoplasm of uncertain behavior of skin
239.2 Neoplasms of unspecified nature of bone, soft tissue, and skin
239.8 Neoplasm of unspecified nature of other specified sites
608.89 Other specified disorder of male genital organs ♂
629.8 Other specified disorder of female genital organs ♀
695.3 Rosacea
701.1 Acquired keratoderma
701.4 Keloid scar
701.5 Other abnormal granulation tissue
701.8 Other specified hypertrophic and atrophic condition of skin
702.0 Actinic keratosis
702.11 Inflamed seborrheic keratosis
702.19 Other seborrheic keratosis
709.2 Scar condition and fibrosis of skin
709.8 Other specified disorder of skin
757.31 Congenital ectodermal dysplasia
757.33 Congenital pigmentary anomaly of skin
757.39 Other specified congenital anomaly of skin
757.8 Other specified congenital anomalies of the integument

ICD-9-CM Procedural

08.25 Destruction of lesion of eyelid
18.29 Excision or destruction of other lesion of external ear
21.32 Local excision or destruction of other lesion of nose
86.3 Other local excision or destruction of lesion or tissue of skin and subcutaneous tissue

HCPCS Level II Supplies & Services

A4257 Replacement lens shield cartridge for use with laser skin piercing device, each
A4305 Disposable drug delivery system, flow rate of 50 ml or greater per hour
A4306 Disposable drug delivery system, flow rate of 5 ml or less per hour
A4550 Surgical trays

17106–17108

17106 Destruction of cutaneous vascular proliferative lesions (eg, laser technique); less than 10 sq. cm
17107 10.0 - 50.0 sq. cm
17108 over 50.0 sq. cm

ICD-9-CM Diagnostic

216.1 Benign neoplasm of eyelid, including canthus
216.2 Benign neoplasm of ear and external auditory canal
216.3 Benign neoplasm of skin of other and unspecified parts of face ▽
216.4 Benign neoplasm of scalp and skin of neck
216.5 Benign neoplasm of skin of trunk, except scrotum
216.6 Benign neoplasm of skin of upper limb, including shoulder
216.7 Benign neoplasm of skin of lower limb, including hip
216.8 Benign neoplasm of other specified sites of skin
228.01 Hemangioma of skin and subcutaneous tissue
228.09 Hemangioma of other sites
448.1 Nevus, non-neoplastic
448.9 Other and unspecified capillary diseases ▽
709.1 Vascular disorder of skin
757.32 Congenital vascular hamartomas

ICD-9-CM Procedural

08.25 Destruction of lesion of eyelid
18.29 Excision or destruction of other lesion of external ear
21.32 Local excision or destruction of other lesion of nose
86.3 Other local excision or destruction of lesion or tissue of skin and subcutaneous tissue

HCPCS Level II Supplies & Services

A4257 Replacement lens shield cartridge for use with laser skin piercing device, each
A4305 Disposable drug delivery system, flow rate of 50 ml or greater per hour
A4306 Disposable drug delivery system, flow rate of 5 ml or less per hour
A4550 Surgical trays

17110–17111

17110 Destruction (eg, laser surgery, electrosurgery, cryosurgery, chemosurgery, surgical curettement), of flat warts, molluscum contagiosum, or milia; up to 14 lesions
17111 15 or more lesions

ICD-9-CM Diagnostic

078.0 Molluscum contagiosum
078.10 Unspecified viral warts ▽
078.19 Other specified viral warts
706.2 Sebaceous cyst
709.3 Degenerative skin disorder

ICD-9-CM Procedural

08.25 Destruction of lesion of eyelid
18.29 Excision or destruction of other lesion of external ear
21.32 Local excision or destruction of other lesion of nose
86.3 Other local excision or destruction of lesion or tissue of skin and subcutaneous tissue

HCPCS Level II Supplies & Services

A4257 Replacement lens shield cartridge for use with laser skin piercing device, each
A4550 Surgical trays

17250

17250 Chemical cauterization of granulation tissue (proud flesh, sinus or fistula)

ICD-9-CM Diagnostic

701.5 Other abnormal granulation tissue
909.3 Late effect of complications of surgical and medical care
998.59 Other postoperative infection — (Use additional code to identify infection)
998.6 Persistent postoperative fistula, not elsewhere classified
998.83 Non-healing surgical wound

ICD-9-CM Procedural

18.29 Excision or destruction of other lesion of external ear
86.24 Chemosurgery of skin
86.3 Other local excision or destruction of lesion or tissue of skin and subcutaneous tissue

HCPCS Level II Supplies & Services

A4550 Surgical trays

17260–17266

17260 Destruction, malignant lesion (eg, laser surgery, electrosurgery, cryosurgery, chemosurgery, surgical curettement), trunk, arms or legs; lesion diameter 0.5 cm or less
17261 lesion diameter 0.6 to 1.0 cm
17262 lesion diameter 1.1 to 2.0 cm
17263 lesion diameter 2.1 to 3.0 cm
17264 lesion diameter 3.1 to 4.0 cm
17266 lesion diameter over 4.0 cm

ICD-9-CM Diagnostic

173.5 Other malignant neoplasm of skin of trunk, except scrotum
173.6 Other malignant neoplasm of skin of upper limb, including shoulder
173.7 Other malignant neoplasm of skin of lower limb, including hip
232.5 Carcinoma in situ of skin of trunk, except scrotum
232.6 Carcinoma in situ of skin of upper limb, including shoulder
232.7 Carcinoma in situ of skin of lower limb, including hip
238.2 Neoplasm of uncertain behavior of skin

ICD-9-CM Procedural

86.3 Other local excision or destruction of lesion or tissue of skin and subcutaneous tissue

HCPCS Level II Supplies & Services

A4305 Disposable drug delivery system, flow rate of 50 ml or greater per hour
A4306 Disposable drug delivery system, flow rate of 5 ml or less per hour
A4550 Surgical trays

17270–17276

17270 Destruction, malignant lesion (eg, laser surgery, electrosurgery, cryosurgery, chemosurgery, surgical curettement), scalp, neck, hands, feet, genitalia; lesion diameter 0.5 cm or less
17271 lesion diameter 0.6 to 1.0 cm
17272 lesion diameter 1.1 to 2.0 cm
17273 lesion diameter 2.1 to 3.0 cm
17274 lesion diameter 3.1 to 4.0 cm
17276 lesion diameter over 4.0 cm

ICD-9-CM Diagnostic

173.4 Other malignant neoplasm of scalp and skin of neck

▽ Unspecified code ♀ Female diagnosis ☒ Manifestation code ♂ Male diagnosis

173.6 Other malignant neoplasm of skin of upper limb, including shoulder
173.7 Other malignant neoplasm of skin of lower limb, including hip
184.0 Malignant neoplasm of vagina ♀
184.1 Malignant neoplasm of labia majora ♀
184.2 Malignant neoplasm of labia minora ♀
184.3 Malignant neoplasm of clitoris ♀
184.4 Malignant neoplasm of vulva, unspecified site ▽ ♀
184.8 Malignant neoplasm of other specified sites of female genital organs ♀
187.1 Malignant neoplasm of prepuce ♂
187.2 Malignant neoplasm of glans penis ♂
187.3 Malignant neoplasm of body of penis ♂
187.4 Malignant neoplasm of penis, part unspecified ▽ ♂
187.7 Malignant neoplasm of scrotum ♂
187.8 Malignant neoplasm of other specified sites of male genital organs ♂
232.4 Carcinoma in situ of scalp and skin of neck
232.6 Carcinoma in situ of skin of upper limb, including shoulder
232.7 Carcinoma in situ of skin of lower limb, including hip
232.8 Carcinoma in situ of other specified sites of skin
233.3 Carcinoma in situ of other and unspecified female genital organs ▽ ♀
233.5 Carcinoma in situ of penis ♂
233.6 Carcinoma in situ of other and unspecified male genital organs ▽ ♂
236.3 Neoplasm of uncertain behavior of other and unspecified female genital organs ▽ ♀
236.6 Neoplasm of uncertain behavior of other and unspecified male genital organs ▽ ♂
238.2 Neoplasm of uncertain behavior of skin

ICD-9-CM Procedural

61.3 Excision or destruction of lesion or tissue of scrotum
64.2 Local excision or destruction of lesion of penis
71.3 Other local excision or destruction of vulva and perineum
86.3 Other local excision or destruction of lesion or tissue of skin and subcutaneous tissue

HCPCS Level II Supplies & Services

A4305 Disposable drug delivery system, flow rate of 50 ml or greater per hour
A4306 Disposable drug delivery system, flow rate of 5 ml or less per hour
A4550 Surgical trays

17280–17286

17280 Destruction, malignant lesion (eg, laser surgery, electrosurgery, cryosurgery, chemosurgery, surgical curettement), face, ears, eyelids, nose, lips, mucous membrane; lesion diameter 0.5 cm or less
17281 lesion diameter 0.6 to 1.0 cm
17282 lesion diameter 1.1 to 2.0 cm
17283 lesion diameter 2.1 to 3.0 cm
17284 lesion diameter 3.1 to 4.0 cm
17286 lesion diameter over 4.0 cm

ICD-9-CM Diagnostic

140.0 Malignant neoplasm of upper lip, vermilion border
140.1 Malignant neoplasm of lower lip, vermilion border
140.3 Malignant neoplasm of upper lip, inner aspect
140.4 Malignant neoplasm of lower lip, inner aspect
140.5 Malignant neoplasm of lip, inner aspect, unspecified as to upper or lower ▽
140.6 Malignant neoplasm of commissure of lip
140.8 Malignant neoplasm of other sites of lip
143.0 Malignant neoplasm of upper gum
143.1 Malignant neoplasm of lower gum
143.8 Malignant neoplasm of other sites of gum
143.9 Malignant neoplasm of gum, unspecified site ▽
144.0 Malignant neoplasm of anterior portion of floor of mouth
144.1 Malignant neoplasm of lateral portion of floor of mouth
144.8 Malignant neoplasm of other sites of floor of mouth
145.0 Malignant neoplasm of cheek mucosa
145.1 Malignant neoplasm of vestibule of mouth
145.2 Malignant neoplasm of hard palate
145.3 Malignant neoplasm of soft palate
145.4 Malignant neoplasm of uvula
145.5 Malignant neoplasm of palate, unspecified ▽
145.6 Malignant neoplasm of retromolar area
145.8 Malignant neoplasm of other specified parts of mouth
145.9 Malignant neoplasm of mouth, unspecified site ▽
171.0 Malignant neoplasm of connective and other soft tissue of head, face, and neck
172.0 Malignant melanoma of skin of lip
172.1 Malignant melanoma of skin of eyelid, including canthus
172.2 Malignant melanoma of skin of ear and external auditory canal
172.3 Malignant melanoma of skin of other and unspecified parts of face
173.0 Other malignant neoplasm of skin of lip
173.1 Other malignant neoplasm of skin of eyelid, including canthus
173.2 Other malignant neoplasm of skin of ear and external auditory canal
173.3 Other malignant neoplasm of skin of other and unspecified parts of face ▽
198.2 Secondary malignant neoplasm of skin
198.89 Secondary malignant neoplasm of other specified sites
232.0 Carcinoma in situ of skin of lip
232.1 Carcinoma in situ of eyelid, including canthus
232.2 Carcinoma in situ of skin of ear and external auditory canal
232.3 Carcinoma in situ of skin of other and unspecified parts of face ▽
235.1 Neoplasm of uncertain behavior of lip, oral cavity, and pharynx
238.2 Neoplasm of uncertain behavior of skin
V84.09 Genetic susceptibility to other malignant neoplasm

ICD-9-CM Procedural

08.25 Destruction of lesion of eyelid
18.29 Excision or destruction of other lesion of external ear
21.32 Local excision or destruction of other lesion of nose
86.3 Other local excision or destruction of lesion or tissue of skin and subcutaneous tissue

HCPCS Level II Supplies & Services

A4305 Disposable drug delivery system, flow rate of 50 ml or greater per hour
A4306 Disposable drug delivery system, flow rate of 5 ml or less per hour
A4550 Surgical trays

17304–17310

17304 Chemosurgery (Mohs micrographic technique), including removal of all gross tumor, surgical excision of tissue specimens, mapping, color coding of specimens, microscopic examination of specimens by the surgeon, and complete histopathologic preparation including the first routine stain (eg, hematoxylin and eosin, toluidine blue); first stage, fresh tissue technique, up to 5 specimens
17305 second stage, fixed or fresh tissue, up to 5 specimens
17306 third stage, fixed or fresh tissue, up to 5 specimens
17307 additional stage(s), up to 5 specimens, each stage
17310 each additional specimen, after the first 5 specimens, fixed or fresh tissue, any stage (List separately in addition to code for primary procedure)

ICD-9-CM Diagnostic

140.0 Malignant neoplasm of upper lip, vermilion border
140.1 Malignant neoplasm of lower lip, vermilion border
140.3 Malignant neoplasm of upper lip, inner aspect
140.4 Malignant neoplasm of lower lip, inner aspect
140.5 Malignant neoplasm of lip, inner aspect, unspecified as to upper or lower ▽
140.6 Malignant neoplasm of commissure of lip
140.8 Malignant neoplasm of other sites of lip
143.0 Malignant neoplasm of upper gum
143.1 Malignant neoplasm of lower gum
143.8 Malignant neoplasm of other sites of gum
144.0 Malignant neoplasm of anterior portion of floor of mouth
144.1 Malignant neoplasm of lateral portion of floor of mouth
144.8 Malignant neoplasm of other sites of floor of mouth
145.0 Malignant neoplasm of cheek mucosa
145.1 Malignant neoplasm of vestibule of mouth
145.2 Malignant neoplasm of hard palate
145.3 Malignant neoplasm of soft palate
145.4 Malignant neoplasm of uvula
145.5 Malignant neoplasm of palate, unspecified ▽
145.6 Malignant neoplasm of retromolar area
145.8 Malignant neoplasm of other specified parts of mouth
145.9 Malignant neoplasm of mouth, unspecified site ▽
171.0 Malignant neoplasm of connective and other soft tissue of head, face, and neck
172.0 Malignant melanoma of skin of lip
172.1 Malignant melanoma of skin of eyelid, including canthus
172.2 Malignant melanoma of skin of ear and external auditory canal
172.3 Malignant melanoma of skin of other and unspecified parts of face
172.4 Malignant melanoma of skin of scalp and neck
172.5 Malignant melanoma of skin of trunk, except scrotum
172.6 Malignant melanoma of skin of upper limb, including shoulder
172.7 Malignant melanoma of skin of lower limb, including hip
172.8 Malignant melanoma of other specified sites of skin
172.9 Melanoma of skin, site unspecified ▽
173.0 Other malignant neoplasm of skin of lip

173.1 Other malignant neoplasm of skin of eyelid, including canthus
173.2 Other malignant neoplasm of skin of ear and external auditory canal
173.3 Other malignant neoplasm of skin of other and unspecified parts of face ▽
173.4 Other malignant neoplasm of scalp and skin of neck
173.5 Other malignant neoplasm of skin of trunk, except scrotum
173.6 Other malignant neoplasm of skin of upper limb, including shoulder
173.7 Other malignant neoplasm of skin of lower limb, including hip
173.8 Other malignant neoplasm of other specified sites of skin
173.9 Other malignant neoplasm of skin, site unspecified ▽
184.0 Malignant neoplasm of vagina ♀
184.1 Malignant neoplasm of labia majora ♀
184.2 Malignant neoplasm of labia minora ♀
184.3 Malignant neoplasm of clitoris ♀
184.8 Malignant neoplasm of other specified sites of female genital organs ♀
184.9 Malignant neoplasm of female genital organ, site unspecified ▽ ♀
187.1 Malignant neoplasm of prepuce ♂
187.2 Malignant neoplasm of glans penis ♂
187.3 Malignant neoplasm of body of penis ♂
187.7 Malignant neoplasm of scrotum ♂
187.8 Malignant neoplasm of other specified sites of male genital organs ♂
195.0 Malignant neoplasm of head, face, and neck
195.1 Malignant neoplasm of thorax
195.2 Malignant neoplasm of abdomen
195.3 Malignant neoplasm of pelvis
195.4 Malignant neoplasm of upper limb
195.8 Malignant neoplasm of other specified sites
232.0 Carcinoma in situ of skin of lip
232.1 Carcinoma in situ of eyelid, including canthus
232.2 Carcinoma in situ of skin of ear and external auditory canal
232.4 Carcinoma in situ of scalp and skin of neck
232.5 Carcinoma in situ of skin of trunk, except scrotum
232.8 Carcinoma in situ of other specified sites of skin
233.3 Carcinoma in situ of other and unspecified female genital organs ▽ ♀
233.5 Carcinoma in situ of penis ♂
233.6 Carcinoma in situ of other and unspecified male genital organs ▽ ♂
V84.09 Genetic susceptibility to other malignant neoplasm

ICD-9-CM Procedural

86.24 Chemosurgery of skin

HCPCS Level II Supplies & Services

A4305 Disposable drug delivery system, flow rate of 50 ml or greater per hour
A4306 Disposable drug delivery system, flow rate of 5 ml or less per hour
A4550 Surgical trays

17340–17360

17340 Cryotherapy (CO2 slush, liquid N2) for acne
17360 Chemical exfoliation for acne (eg, acne paste, acid)

ICD-9-CM Diagnostic

695.3 Rosacea
706.0 Acne varioliformis
706.1 Other acne

ICD-9-CM Procedural

86.24 Chemosurgery of skin
86.3 Other local excision or destruction of lesion or tissue of skin and subcutaneous tissue

HCPCS Level II Supplies & Services

A4550 Surgical trays

17380

17380 Electrolysis epilation, each 1/2 hour

ICD-9-CM Diagnostic

704.1 Hirsutism
V50.1 Other plastic surgery for unacceptable cosmetic appearance

ICD-9-CM Procedural

86.92 Electrolysis and other epilation of skin

HCPCS Level II Supplies & Services

A4550 Surgical trays

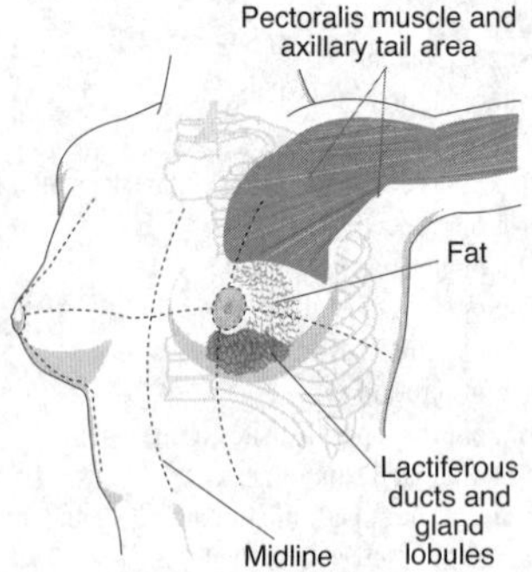

Breast

19000–19001

19000 Puncture aspiration of cyst of breast;
19001 each additional cyst (List separately in addition to code for primary procedure)

ICD-9-CM Diagnostic

610.0 Solitary cyst of breast
610.1 Diffuse cystic mastopathy
610.8 Other specified benign mammary dysplasias
611.5 Galactocele ♀
611.72 Lump or mass in breast
611.8 Other specified disorder of breast
793.80 Unspecified abnormal mammogram ▽
793.89 Other abnormal findings on radiological examination of breast

ICD-9-CM Procedural

85.91 Aspiration of breast

HCPCS Level II Supplies & Services

A4550 Surgical trays

19020

19020 Mastotomy with exploration or drainage of abscess, deep

ICD-9-CM Diagnostic

610.0 Solitary cyst of breast
610.1 Diffuse cystic mastopathy
610.4 Mammary duct ectasia
610.8 Other specified benign mammary dysplasias
611.0 Inflammatory disease of breast
611.71 Mastodynia
611.72 Lump or mass in breast
611.8 Other specified disorder of breast
675.10 Abscess of breast associated with childbirth, unspecified as to episode of care ▽ ♀
675.11 Abscess of breast associated with childbirth, delivered, with or without mention of antepartum condition ♀
675.12 Abscess of breast associated with childbirth, delivered, with mention of postpartum complication ♀
675.13 Abscess of breast, antepartum ♀
675.14 Abscess of breast, postpartum ♀
675.20 Nonpurulent mastitis, unspecified as to episode of prenatal or postnatal care ▽ ♀

ICD-9-CM Procedural

85.0 Mastotomy

HCPCS Level II Supplies & Services

A4550 Surgical trays

▽ Unspecified code ☒ Manifestation code
♀ Female diagnosis ♂ Male diagnosis

19030

19030 Injection procedure only for mammary ductogram or galactogram

ICD-9-CM Diagnostic

610.1 Diffuse cystic mastopathy
610.4 Mammary duct ectasia
611.1 Hypertrophy of breast
611.71 Mastodynia
611.8 Other specified disorder of breast

ICD-9-CM Procedural

85.92 Injection of therapeutic agent into breast
87.35 Contrast radiogram of mammary ducts

HCPCS Level II Supplies & Services

A9525 Supply of low or iso-osmolar contrast material, 10 mg of iodine

19100–19103

19100 Biopsy of breast; percutaneous, needle core, not using imaging guidance (separate procedure)
19101 open, incisional
19102 percutaneous, needle core, using imaging guidance
19103 percutaneous, automated vacuum assisted or rotating biopsy device, using imaging guidance

ICD-9-CM Diagnostic

174.0 Malignant neoplasm of nipple and areola of female breast ♀
174.1 Malignant neoplasm of central portion of female breast ♀
174.2 Malignant neoplasm of upper-inner quadrant of female breast ♀
174.3 Malignant neoplasm of lower-inner quadrant of female breast ♀
174.4 Malignant neoplasm of upper-outer quadrant of female breast ♀
174.5 Malignant neoplasm of lower-outer quadrant of female breast ♀
174.6 Malignant neoplasm of axillary tail of female breast ♀
174.8 Malignant neoplasm of other specified sites of female breast ♀
175.0 Malignant neoplasm of nipple and areola of male breast ♂
175.9 Malignant neoplasm of other and unspecified sites of male breast ▽ ♂
198.81 Secondary malignant neoplasm of breast
217 Benign neoplasm of breast
233.0 Carcinoma in situ of breast
238.3 Neoplasm of uncertain behavior of breast
239.3 Neoplasm of unspecified nature of breast
610.0 Solitary cyst of breast
610.1 Diffuse cystic mastopathy
610.2 Fibroadenosis of breast
610.3 Fibrosclerosis of breast
610.8 Other specified benign mammary dysplasias
611.0 Inflammatory disease of breast
611.72 Lump or mass in breast
793.80 Unspecified abnormal mammogram ▽
793.81 Mammographic microcalcification
793.89 Other abnormal findings on radiological examination of breast
V10.3 Personal history of malignant neoplasm of breast
V16.3 Family history of malignant neoplasm of breast
V84.01 Genetic susceptibility to malignant neoplasm of breast

ICD-9-CM Procedural

85.11 Closed (percutaneous) (needle) biopsy of breast
85.12 Open biopsy of breast
87.37 Other mammography

HCPCS Level II Supplies & Services

A4550 Surgical trays

19110

19110 Nipple exploration, with or without excision of a solitary lactiferous duct or a papilloma lactiferous duct

ICD-9-CM Diagnostic

174.0 Malignant neoplasm of nipple and areola of female breast ♀
174.8 Malignant neoplasm of other specified sites of female breast ♀
217 Benign neoplasm of breast
233.0 Carcinoma in situ of breast
238.3 Neoplasm of uncertain behavior of breast
239.3 Neoplasm of unspecified nature of breast
610.4 Mammary duct ectasia
611.5 Galactocele ♀
611.72 Lump or mass in breast
611.79 Other sign and symptom in breast
611.8 Other specified disorder of breast

ICD-9-CM Procedural

85.0 Mastotomy
85.20 Excision or destruction of breast tissue, not otherwise specified
85.25 Excision of nipple

HCPCS Level II Supplies & Services

A4550 Surgical trays

19112

19112 Excision of lactiferous duct fistula

ICD-9-CM Diagnostic

611.0 Inflammatory disease of breast
611.72 Lump or mass in breast
675.10 Abscess of breast associated with childbirth, unspecified as to episode of care ▽ ♀
675.11 Abscess of breast associated with childbirth, delivered, with or without mention of antepartum condition ♀
675.12 Abscess of breast associated with childbirth, delivered, with mention of postpartum complication ♀
675.13 Abscess of breast, antepartum ♀
675.14 Abscess of breast, postpartum ♀

ICD-9-CM Procedural

85.20 Excision or destruction of breast tissue, not otherwise specified

HCPCS Level II Supplies & Services

A4550 Surgical trays

19120

19120 Excision of cyst, fibroadenoma, or other benign or malignant tumor, aberrant breast tissue, duct lesion, nipple or areolar lesion (except 19140), open, male or female, one or more lesions

ICD-9-CM Diagnostic

174.0 Malignant neoplasm of nipple and areola of female breast ♀
174.1 Malignant neoplasm of central portion of female breast ♀
174.2 Malignant neoplasm of upper-inner quadrant of female breast ♀
174.3 Malignant neoplasm of lower-inner quadrant of female breast ♀
174.4 Malignant neoplasm of upper-outer quadrant of female breast ♀
174.5 Malignant neoplasm of lower-outer quadrant of female breast ♀
174.6 Malignant neoplasm of axillary tail of female breast ♀
174.8 Malignant neoplasm of other specified sites of female breast ♀
175.0 Malignant neoplasm of nipple and areola of male breast ♂
175.9 Malignant neoplasm of other and unspecified sites of male breast ▽ ♂
198.81 Secondary malignant neoplasm of breast
217 Benign neoplasm of breast
233.0 Carcinoma in situ of breast
238.3 Neoplasm of uncertain behavior of breast
239.3 Neoplasm of unspecified nature of breast
610.0 Solitary cyst of breast
610.1 Diffuse cystic mastopathy
610.2 Fibroadenosis of breast
610.3 Fibrosclerosis of breast
610.4 Mammary duct ectasia
610.8 Other specified benign mammary dysplasias
611.0 Inflammatory disease of breast
611.72 Lump or mass in breast
611.79 Other sign and symptom in breast
611.8 Other specified disorder of breast
V10.3 Personal history of malignant neoplasm of breast
V16.3 Family history of malignant neoplasm of breast
V84.01 Genetic susceptibility to malignant neoplasm of breast

ICD-9-CM Procedural

85.20 Excision or destruction of breast tissue, not otherwise specified
85.21 Local excision of lesion of breast
85.24 Excision of ectopic breast tissue
85.25 Excision of nipple

HCPCS Level II Supplies & Services

A4280 Adhesive skin support attachment for use with external breast prosthesis, each
A4305 Disposable drug delivery system, flow rate of 50 ml or greater per hour

▽ Unspecified code
♀ Female diagnosis
☒ Manifestation code
♂ Male diagnosis

A4306 Disposable drug delivery system, flow rate of 5 ml or less per hour
A4550 Surgical trays

19125–19126

19125 Excision of breast lesion identified by preoperative placement of radiological marker, open; single lesion
19126 each additional lesion separately identified by a preoperative radiological marker (List separately in addition to code for primary procedure)

ICD-9-CM Diagnostic

174.0 Malignant neoplasm of nipple and areola of female breast ♀
174.1 Malignant neoplasm of central portion of female breast ♀
174.2 Malignant neoplasm of upper-inner quadrant of female breast ♀
174.3 Malignant neoplasm of lower-inner quadrant of female breast ♀
174.4 Malignant neoplasm of upper-outer quadrant of female breast ♀
174.5 Malignant neoplasm of lower-outer quadrant of female breast ♀
174.6 Malignant neoplasm of axillary tail of female breast ♀
174.8 Malignant neoplasm of other specified sites of female breast ♀
175.0 Malignant neoplasm of nipple and areola of male breast ♂
175.9 Malignant neoplasm of other and unspecified sites of male breast ▽ ♂
198.81 Secondary malignant neoplasm of breast
217 Benign neoplasm of breast
233.0 Carcinoma in situ of breast
238.3 Neoplasm of uncertain behavior of breast
239.3 Neoplasm of unspecified nature of breast
610.0 Solitary cyst of breast
610.1 Diffuse cystic mastopathy
610.3 Fibrosclerosis of breast
611.0 Inflammatory disease of breast
611.72 Lump or mass in breast
611.79 Other sign and symptom in breast
611.8 Other specified disorder of breast
V10.3 Personal history of malignant neoplasm of breast
V16.3 Family history of malignant neoplasm of breast
V84.01 Genetic susceptibility to malignant neoplasm of breast

ICD-9-CM Procedural

85.21 Local excision of lesion of breast

HCPCS Level II Supplies & Services

A4305 Disposable drug delivery system, flow rate of 50 ml or greater per hour
A4306 Disposable drug delivery system, flow rate of 5 ml or less per hour
A4550 Surgical trays

19140

19140 Mastectomy for gynecomastia

ICD-9-CM Diagnostic

611.1 Hypertrophy of breast

ICD-9-CM Procedural

85.31 Unilateral reduction mammoplasty
85.32 Bilateral reduction mammoplasty
85.34 Other unilateral subcutaneous mammectomy
85.36 Other bilateral subcutaneous mammectomy

19160–19162

19160 Mastectomy, partial (eg, lumpectomy, tylectomy, quadrantectomy, segmentectomy);
19162 with axillary lymphadenectomy

ICD-9-CM Diagnostic

174.0 Malignant neoplasm of nipple and areola of female breast ♀
174.1 Malignant neoplasm of central portion of female breast ♀
174.2 Malignant neoplasm of upper-inner quadrant of female breast ♀
174.3 Malignant neoplasm of lower-inner quadrant of female breast ♀
174.4 Malignant neoplasm of upper-outer quadrant of female breast ♀
174.5 Malignant neoplasm of lower-outer quadrant of female breast ♀
174.6 Malignant neoplasm of axillary tail of female breast ♀
174.8 Malignant neoplasm of other specified sites of female breast ♀
175.0 Malignant neoplasm of nipple and areola of male breast ♂
175.9 Malignant neoplasm of other and unspecified sites of male breast ▽ ♂
196.3 Secondary and unspecified malignant neoplasm of lymph nodes of axilla and upper limb
198.81 Secondary malignant neoplasm of breast
238.3 Neoplasm of uncertain behavior of breast
239.3 Neoplasm of unspecified nature of breast
V10.3 Personal history of malignant neoplasm of breast
V16.3 Family history of malignant neoplasm of breast
V45.71 Acquired absence of breast — (This code is intended for use when these conditions are recorded as diagnoses or problems)
V84.01 Genetic susceptibility to malignant neoplasm of breast

ICD-9-CM Procedural

40.23 Excision of axillary lymph node
85.22 Resection of quadrant of breast
85.23 Subtotal mastectomy

19180

19180 Mastectomy, simple, complete

ICD-9-CM Diagnostic

174.0 Malignant neoplasm of nipple and areola of female breast ♀
174.1 Malignant neoplasm of central portion of female breast ♀
174.2 Malignant neoplasm of upper-inner quadrant of female breast ♀
174.3 Malignant neoplasm of lower-inner quadrant of female breast ♀
174.4 Malignant neoplasm of upper-outer quadrant of female breast ♀
174.5 Malignant neoplasm of lower-outer quadrant of female breast ♀
174.6 Malignant neoplasm of axillary tail of female breast ♀
174.8 Malignant neoplasm of other specified sites of female breast ♀
175.0 Malignant neoplasm of nipple and areola of male breast ♂
175.9 Malignant neoplasm of other and unspecified sites of male breast ▽ ♂
198.81 Secondary malignant neoplasm of breast
233.0 Carcinoma in situ of breast
238.3 Neoplasm of uncertain behavior of breast
239.3 Neoplasm of unspecified nature of breast
610.1 Diffuse cystic mastopathy
611.1 Hypertrophy of breast
611.72 Lump or mass in breast
793.89 Other abnormal findings on radiological examination of breast
V10.3 Personal history of malignant neoplasm of breast
V16.3 Family history of malignant neoplasm of breast
V45.71 Acquired absence of breast — (This code is intended for use when these conditions are recorded as diagnoses or problems)
V50.41 Prophylactic breast removal
V84.01 Genetic susceptibility to malignant neoplasm of breast

ICD-9-CM Procedural

85.41 Unilateral simple mastectomy
85.42 Bilateral simple mastectomy

19182

19182 Mastectomy, subcutaneous

ICD-9-CM Diagnostic

173.5 Other malignant neoplasm of skin of trunk, except scrotum
174.0 Malignant neoplasm of nipple and areola of female breast ♀
174.1 Malignant neoplasm of central portion of female breast ♀
174.2 Malignant neoplasm of upper-inner quadrant of female breast ♀
174.3 Malignant neoplasm of lower-inner quadrant of female breast ♀
174.4 Malignant neoplasm of upper-outer quadrant of female breast ♀
174.5 Malignant neoplasm of lower-outer quadrant of female breast ♀
174.6 Malignant neoplasm of axillary tail of female breast ♀
174.8 Malignant neoplasm of other specified sites of female breast ♀
175.0 Malignant neoplasm of nipple and areola of male breast ♂
175.9 Malignant neoplasm of other and unspecified sites of male breast ▽ ♂
198.81 Secondary malignant neoplasm of breast
233.0 Carcinoma in situ of breast
238.3 Neoplasm of uncertain behavior of breast
239.2 Neoplasms of unspecified nature of bone, soft tissue, and skin
239.3 Neoplasm of unspecified nature of breast
757.6 Specified congenital anomalies of breast
V10.3 Personal history of malignant neoplasm of breast
V16.3 Family history of malignant neoplasm of breast
V45.71 Acquired absence of breast — (This code is intended for use when these conditions are recorded as diagnoses or problems)
V50.41 Prophylactic breast removal
V84.01 Genetic susceptibility to malignant neoplasm of breast

ICD-9-CM Procedural

85.33 Unilateral subcutaneous mammectomy with synchronous implant

▽ Unspecified code ♀ Female diagnosis ☒ Manifestation code ♂ Male diagnosis

85.34 Other unilateral subcutaneous mammectomy
85.35 Bilateral subcutaneous mammectomy with synchronous implant
85.36 Other bilateral subcutaneous mammectomy

19200–19220

19200 Mastectomy, radical, including pectoral muscles, axillary lymph nodes
19220 Mastectomy, radical, including pectoral muscles, axillary and internal mammary lymph nodes (Urban type operation)

ICD-9-CM Diagnostic

174.0 Malignant neoplasm of nipple and areola of female breast ♀
174.1 Malignant neoplasm of central portion of female breast ♀
174.2 Malignant neoplasm of upper-inner quadrant of female breast ♀
174.3 Malignant neoplasm of lower-inner quadrant of female breast ♀
174.4 Malignant neoplasm of upper-outer quadrant of female breast ♀
174.5 Malignant neoplasm of lower-outer quadrant of female breast ♀
174.6 Malignant neoplasm of axillary tail of female breast ♀
174.8 Malignant neoplasm of other specified sites of female breast ♀
175.0 Malignant neoplasm of nipple and areola of male breast ♂
175.9 Malignant neoplasm of other and unspecified sites of male breast ▽ ♂
196.3 Secondary and unspecified malignant neoplasm of lymph nodes of axilla and upper limb
198.81 Secondary malignant neoplasm of breast
233.0 Carcinoma in situ of breast
238.3 Neoplasm of uncertain behavior of breast
239.3 Neoplasm of unspecified nature of breast
V10.3 Personal history of malignant neoplasm of breast
V16.3 Family history of malignant neoplasm of breast
V45.71 Acquired absence of breast — (This code is intended for use when these conditions are recorded as diagnoses or problems)
V84.01 Genetic susceptibility to malignant neoplasm of breast

ICD-9-CM Procedural

85.45 Unilateral radical mastectomy
85.46 Bilateral radical mastectomy

19240

19240 Mastectomy, modified radical, including axillary lymph nodes, with or without pectoralis minor muscle, but excluding pectoralis major muscle

ICD-9-CM Diagnostic

174.0 Malignant neoplasm of nipple and areola of female breast ♀
174.1 Malignant neoplasm of central portion of female breast ♀
174.2 Malignant neoplasm of upper-inner quadrant of female breast ♀
174.3 Malignant neoplasm of lower-inner quadrant of female breast ♀
174.4 Malignant neoplasm of upper-outer quadrant of female breast ♀
174.5 Malignant neoplasm of lower-outer quadrant of female breast ♀
174.6 Malignant neoplasm of axillary tail of female breast ♀
174.8 Malignant neoplasm of other specified sites of female breast ♀
175.0 Malignant neoplasm of nipple and areola of male breast ♂
175.9 Malignant neoplasm of other and unspecified sites of male breast ▽ ♂
196.3 Secondary and unspecified malignant neoplasm of lymph nodes of axilla and upper limb
198.81 Secondary malignant neoplasm of breast
233.0 Carcinoma in situ of breast
238.3 Neoplasm of uncertain behavior of breast
239.3 Neoplasm of unspecified nature of breast
V10.3 Personal history of malignant neoplasm of breast
V16.3 Family history of malignant neoplasm of breast
V45.71 Acquired absence of breast — (This code is intended for use when these conditions are recorded as diagnoses or problems)
V84.01 Genetic susceptibility to malignant neoplasm of breast

ICD-9-CM Procedural

85.43 Unilateral extended simple mastectomy
85.44 Bilateral extended simple mastectomy

19260–19272

19260 Excision of chest wall tumor including ribs
19271 Excision of chest wall tumor involving ribs, with plastic reconstruction; without mediastinal lymphadenectomy
19272 with mediastinal lymphadenectomy

ICD-9-CM Diagnostic

170.3 Malignant neoplasm of ribs, sternum, and clavicle
171.4 Malignant neoplasm of connective and other soft tissue of thorax
195.1 Malignant neoplasm of thorax
196.1 Secondary and unspecified malignant neoplasm of intrathoracic lymph nodes
198.5 Secondary malignant neoplasm of bone and bone marrow
198.89 Secondary malignant neoplasm of other specified sites
214.8 Lipoma of other specified sites
229.8 Benign neoplasm of other specified sites
234.8 Carcinoma in situ of other specified sites
238.0 Neoplasm of uncertain behavior of bone and articular cartilage
238.1 Neoplasm of uncertain behavior of connective and other soft tissue ▽
239.2 Neoplasms of unspecified nature of bone, soft tissue, and skin
V10.3 Personal history of malignant neoplasm of breast
V16.3 Family history of malignant neoplasm of breast
V45.71 Acquired absence of breast — (This code is intended for use when these conditions are recorded as diagnoses or problems)
V84.09 Genetic susceptibility to other malignant neoplasm

ICD-9-CM Procedural

34.4 Excision or destruction of lesion of chest wall
40.3 Regional lymph node excision
40.59 Radical excision of other lymph nodes
77.61 Local excision of lesion or tissue of scapula, clavicle, and thorax (ribs and sternum)

19290–19291

19290 Preoperative placement of needle localization wire, breast;
19291 each additional lesion (List separately in addition to code for primary procedure)

ICD-9-CM Diagnostic

174.0 Malignant neoplasm of nipple and areola of female breast ♀
174.1 Malignant neoplasm of central portion of female breast ♀
174.2 Malignant neoplasm of upper-inner quadrant of female breast ♀
174.3 Malignant neoplasm of lower-inner quadrant of female breast ♀
174.4 Malignant neoplasm of upper-outer quadrant of female breast ♀
174.5 Malignant neoplasm of lower-outer quadrant of female breast ♀
174.6 Malignant neoplasm of axillary tail of female breast ♀
174.8 Malignant neoplasm of other specified sites of female breast ♀
175.0 Malignant neoplasm of nipple and areola of male breast ♂
175.9 Malignant neoplasm of other and unspecified sites of male breast ▽ ♂
198.81 Secondary malignant neoplasm of breast
217 Benign neoplasm of breast
233.0 Carcinoma in situ of breast
238.3 Neoplasm of uncertain behavior of breast
239.3 Neoplasm of unspecified nature of breast
610.0 Solitary cyst of breast
610.1 Diffuse cystic mastopathy
610.3 Fibrosclerosis of breast
611.0 Inflammatory disease of breast
611.72 Lump or mass in breast
611.79 Other sign and symptom in breast
611.8 Other specified disorder of breast
V10.3 Personal history of malignant neoplasm of breast
V16.3 Family history of malignant neoplasm of breast
V84.01 Genetic susceptibility to malignant neoplasm of breast

ICD-9-CM Procedural

85.19 Other diagnostic procedures on breast

HCPCS Level II Supplies & Services

A4550 Surgical trays

19295

19295 Image guided placement, metallic localization clip, percutaneous, during breast biopsy (List separately in addition to code for primary procedure)

ICD-9-CM Diagnostic

This is an add-on code. Refer to the corresponding primary procedure code for ICD-9 diagnosis code links.

ICD-9-CM Procedural

85.11 Closed (percutaneous) (needle) biopsy of breast
87.37 Other mammography
88.73 Diagnostic ultrasound of other sites of thorax

▽ Unspecified code
♀ Female diagnosis
☒ Manifestation code
♂ Male diagnosis

HCPCS Level II Supplies & Services

The HCPCS Level II code(s) would be the same as the actual procedure performed because these are in-addition-to codes.

19296–19297

19296 Placement of radiotherapy afterloading balloon catheter into the breast for interstitial radioelement application following partial mastectomy, includes imaging guidance; on date separate from partial mastectomy

19297 concurrent with partial mastectomy (List separately in addition to code for primary procedure)

ICD-9-CM Diagnostic

174.0 Malignant neoplasm of nipple and areola of female breast ♀
174.1 Malignant neoplasm of central portion of female breast ♀
174.2 Malignant neoplasm of upper-inner quadrant of female breast ♀
174.3 Malignant neoplasm of lower-inner quadrant of female breast ♀
174.4 Malignant neoplasm of upper-outer quadrant of female breast ♀
174.5 Malignant neoplasm of lower-outer quadrant of female breast ♀
174.6 Malignant neoplasm of axillary tail of female breast ♀
174.8 Malignant neoplasm of other specified sites of female breast ♀
175.0 Malignant neoplasm of nipple and areola of male breast ♂
175.9 Malignant neoplasm of other and unspecified sites of male breast ▽ ♂
196.3 Secondary and unspecified malignant neoplasm of lymph nodes of axilla and upper limb
198.81 Secondary malignant neoplasm of breast
238.3 Neoplasm of uncertain behavior of breast
239.3 Neoplasm of unspecified nature of breast
V10.3 Personal history of malignant neoplasm of breast
V16.3 Family history of malignant neoplasm of breast
V45.71 Acquired absence of breast — (This code is intended for use when these conditions are recorded as diagnoses or problems)
V84.01 Genetic susceptibility to malignant neoplasm of breast

ICD-9-CM Procedural

85.0 Mastotomy
92.27 Implantation or insertion of radioactive elements

19298

19298 Placement of radiotherapy afterloading brachytherapy catheters (multiple tube and button type) into the breast for interstitial radioelement application following (at the time of or subsequent to) partial mastectomy, includes imaging guidance

ICD-9-CM Diagnostic

174.0 Malignant neoplasm of nipple and areola of female breast ♀
174.1 Malignant neoplasm of central portion of female breast ♀
174.2 Malignant neoplasm of upper-inner quadrant of female breast ♀
174.3 Malignant neoplasm of lower-inner quadrant of female breast ♀
174.4 Malignant neoplasm of upper-outer quadrant of female breast ♀
174.5 Malignant neoplasm of lower-outer quadrant of female breast ♀
174.6 Malignant neoplasm of axillary tail of female breast ♀
174.8 Malignant neoplasm of other specified sites of female breast ♀
175.0 Malignant neoplasm of nipple and areola of male breast ♂
175.9 Malignant neoplasm of other and unspecified sites of male breast ▽ ♂
196.3 Secondary and unspecified malignant neoplasm of lymph nodes of axilla and upper limb
198.81 Secondary malignant neoplasm of breast
238.3 Neoplasm of uncertain behavior of breast
239.3 Neoplasm of unspecified nature of breast
V10.3 Personal history of malignant neoplasm of breast
V16.3 Family history of malignant neoplasm of breast
V45.71 Acquired absence of breast — (This code is intended for use when these conditions are recorded as diagnoses or problems)
V84.01 Genetic susceptibility to malignant neoplasm of breast

ICD-9-CM Procedural

85.0 Mastotomy
92.27 Implantation or insertion of radioactive elements

19316

19316 Mastopexy

ICD-9-CM Diagnostic

611.1 Hypertrophy of breast
611.4 Atrophy of breast

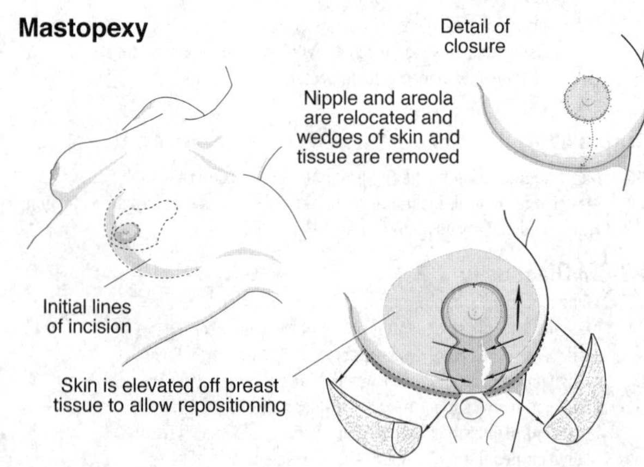
Mastopexy
Detail of closure
Nipple and areola are relocated and wedges of skin and tissue are removed
Initial lines of incision
Skin is elevated off breast tissue to allow repositioning

611.8 Other specified disorder of breast
V50.1 Other plastic surgery for unacceptable cosmetic appearance
V51 Aftercare involving the use of plastic surgery

ICD-9-CM Procedural

85.6 Mastopexy

19318

19318 Reduction mammaplasty

ICD-9-CM Diagnostic

611.1 Hypertrophy of breast
611.4 Atrophy of breast
611.8 Other specified disorder of breast
V50.1 Other plastic surgery for unacceptable cosmetic appearance

ICD-9-CM Procedural

85.31 Unilateral reduction mammoplasty
85.32 Bilateral reduction mammoplasty

19324–19325

19324 Mammaplasty, augmentation; without prosthetic implant
19325 with prosthetic implant

ICD-9-CM Diagnostic

611.4 Atrophy of breast
611.8 Other specified disorder of breast
757.6 Specified congenital anomalies of breast
757.8 Other specified congenital anomalies of the integument
V50.1 Other plastic surgery for unacceptable cosmetic appearance

ICD-9-CM Procedural

85.50 Augmentation mammoplasty, not otherwise specified
85.53 Unilateral breast implant
85.54 Bilateral breast implant

19328–19330

19328 Removal of intact mammary implant
19330 Removal of mammary implant material

ICD-9-CM Diagnostic

611.71 Mastodynia
686.1 Pyogenic granuloma of skin and subcutaneous tissue
909.3 Late effect of complications of surgical and medical care
996.54 Mechanical complication due to breast prosthesis
996.69 Infection and inflammatory reaction due to other internal prosthetic device, implant, and graft — (Use additional code to identify specified infections)
996.79 Other complications due to other internal prosthetic device, implant, and graft
998.51 Infected postoperative seroma — (Use additional code to identify organism)
998.59 Other postoperative infection — (Use additional code to identify infection)
998.83 Non-healing surgical wound
V10.3 Personal history of malignant neoplasm of breast
V45.71 Acquired absence of breast — (This code is intended for use when these conditions are recorded as diagnoses or problems)
V50.1 Other plastic surgery for unacceptable cosmetic appearance

▽ Unspecified code ♀ Female diagnosis ☒ Manifestation code ♂ Male diagnosis

ICD-9-CM Procedural

85.94 Removal of implant of breast

19340

19340 Immediate insertion of breast prosthesis following mastopexy, mastectomy or in reconstruction

ICD-9-CM Diagnostic

174.0 Malignant neoplasm of nipple and areola of female breast ♀
174.1 Malignant neoplasm of central portion of female breast ♀
174.2 Malignant neoplasm of upper-inner quadrant of female breast ♀
174.3 Malignant neoplasm of lower-inner quadrant of female breast ♀
174.4 Malignant neoplasm of upper-outer quadrant of female breast ♀
174.5 Malignant neoplasm of lower-outer quadrant of female breast ♀
174.6 Malignant neoplasm of axillary tail of female breast ♀
174.8 Malignant neoplasm of other specified sites of female breast ♀
174.9 Malignant neoplasm of breast (female), unspecified site ▽ ♀
233.0 Carcinoma in situ of breast
610.1 Diffuse cystic mastopathy
611.1 Hypertrophy of breast
611.4 Atrophy of breast
611.8 Other specified disorder of breast
757.6 Specified congenital anomalies of breast
V10.3 Personal history of malignant neoplasm of breast
V16.3 Family history of malignant neoplasm of breast
V45.71 Acquired absence of breast — (This code is intended for use when these conditions are recorded as diagnoses or problems)
V50.1 Other plastic surgery for unacceptable cosmetic appearance
V50.41 Prophylactic breast removal
V51 Aftercare involving the use of plastic surgery
V84.01 Genetic susceptibility to malignant neoplasm of breast

ICD-9-CM Procedural

85.33 Unilateral subcutaneous mammectomy with synchronous implant
85.35 Bilateral subcutaneous mammectomy with synchronous implant

HCPCS Level II Supplies & Services

A4280 Adhesive skin support attachment for use with external breast prosthesis, each

19342

19342 Delayed insertion of breast prosthesis following mastopexy, mastectomy or in reconstruction

ICD-9-CM Diagnostic

611.8 Other specified disorder of breast
757.6 Specified congenital anomalies of breast
V10.3 Personal history of malignant neoplasm of breast
V16.3 Family history of malignant neoplasm of breast
V45.71 Acquired absence of breast — (This code is intended for use when these conditions are recorded as diagnoses or problems)
V50.1 Other plastic surgery for unacceptable cosmetic appearance
V51 Aftercare involving the use of plastic surgery
V84.01 Genetic susceptibility to malignant neoplasm of breast

ICD-9-CM Procedural

85.53 Unilateral breast implant
85.54 Bilateral breast implant

HCPCS Level II Supplies & Services

A4280 Adhesive skin support attachment for use with external breast prosthesis, each

19350

19350 Nipple/areola reconstruction

ICD-9-CM Diagnostic

611.2 Fissure of nipple
611.8 Other specified disorder of breast
757.6 Specified congenital anomalies of breast
V10.3 Personal history of malignant neoplasm of breast
V16.3 Family history of malignant neoplasm of breast
V45.71 Acquired absence of breast — (This code is intended for use when these conditions are recorded as diagnoses or problems)
V50.1 Other plastic surgery for unacceptable cosmetic appearance
V51 Aftercare involving the use of plastic surgery
V84.01 Genetic susceptibility to malignant neoplasm of breast

ICD-9-CM Procedural

85.87 Other repair or reconstruction of nipple

19355

19355 Correction of inverted nipples

ICD-9-CM Diagnostic

611.79 Other sign and symptom in breast
676.31 Other and unspecified disorder of breast associated with childbirth, delivered, with or without mention of antepartum condition ▽ ♀
676.32 Other and unspecified disorder of breast associated with childbirth, delivered, with mention of postpartum complication ▽ ♀
676.34 Other and unspecified disorder of breast associated with childbirth, postpartum condition or complication ▽ ♀
757.6 Specified congenital anomalies of breast

ICD-9-CM Procedural

85.87 Other repair or reconstruction of nipple

19357

19357 Breast reconstruction, immediate or delayed, with tissue expander, including subsequent expansion

ICD-9-CM Diagnostic

174.0 Malignant neoplasm of nipple and areola of female breast ♀
174.1 Malignant neoplasm of central portion of female breast ♀
174.2 Malignant neoplasm of upper-inner quadrant of female breast ♀
174.3 Malignant neoplasm of lower-inner quadrant of female breast ♀
174.4 Malignant neoplasm of upper-outer quadrant of female breast ♀
174.5 Malignant neoplasm of lower-outer quadrant of female breast ♀
174.6 Malignant neoplasm of axillary tail of female breast ♀
174.8 Malignant neoplasm of other specified sites of female breast ♀
198.81 Secondary malignant neoplasm of breast
233.0 Carcinoma in situ of breast
610.1 Diffuse cystic mastopathy
610.3 Fibrosclerosis of breast
611.0 Inflammatory disease of breast
611.72 Lump or mass in breast
611.8 Other specified disorder of breast
V10.3 Personal history of malignant neoplasm of breast
V16.3 Family history of malignant neoplasm of breast
V45.71 Acquired absence of breast — (This code is intended for use when these conditions are recorded as diagnoses or problems)
V50.1 Other plastic surgery for unacceptable cosmetic appearance
V51 Aftercare involving the use of plastic surgery
V84.01 Genetic susceptibility to malignant neoplasm of breast

ICD-9-CM Procedural

85.51 Unilateral injection into breast for augmentation
85.52 Bilateral injection into breast for augmentation
85.95 Insertion of breast tissue expander

HCPCS Level II Supplies & Services

A4280 Adhesive skin support attachment for use with external breast prosthesis, each

19361

19361 Breast reconstruction with latissimus dorsi flap, with or without prosthetic implant

ICD-9-CM Diagnostic

174.0 Malignant neoplasm of nipple and areola of female breast ♀
174.1 Malignant neoplasm of central portion of female breast ♀
174.2 Malignant neoplasm of upper-inner quadrant of female breast ♀
174.3 Malignant neoplasm of lower-inner quadrant of female breast ♀
174.4 Malignant neoplasm of upper-outer quadrant of female breast ♀
174.5 Malignant neoplasm of lower-outer quadrant of female breast ♀
174.6 Malignant neoplasm of axillary tail of female breast ♀
174.8 Malignant neoplasm of other specified sites of female breast ♀
198.81 Secondary malignant neoplasm of breast
233.0 Carcinoma in situ of breast
610.1 Diffuse cystic mastopathy
610.3 Fibrosclerosis of breast
611.0 Inflammatory disease of breast
611.72 Lump or mass in breast
611.8 Other specified disorder of breast

▽ Unspecified code ♀ Female diagnosis ☒ Manifestation code ♂ Male diagnosis

V10.3 Personal history of malignant neoplasm of breast
V16.3 Family history of malignant neoplasm of breast
V45.71 Acquired absence of breast — (This code is intended for use when these conditions are recorded as diagnoses or problems)
V50.1 Other plastic surgery for unacceptable cosmetic appearance
V51 Aftercare involving the use of plastic surgery
V84.01 Genetic susceptibility to malignant neoplasm of breast

ICD-9-CM Procedural

85.53 Unilateral breast implant
85.54 Bilateral breast implant
85.7 Total reconstruction of breast

HCPCS Level II Supplies & Services

A4280 Adhesive skin support attachment for use with external breast prosthesis, each

19364

19364 Breast reconstruction with free flap

ICD-9-CM Diagnostic

174.0 Malignant neoplasm of nipple and areola of female breast ♀
174.1 Malignant neoplasm of central portion of female breast ♀
174.2 Malignant neoplasm of upper-inner quadrant of female breast ♀
174.3 Malignant neoplasm of lower-inner quadrant of female breast ♀
174.4 Malignant neoplasm of upper-outer quadrant of female breast ♀
174.5 Malignant neoplasm of lower-outer quadrant of female breast ♀
174.6 Malignant neoplasm of axillary tail of female breast ♀
174.8 Malignant neoplasm of other specified sites of female breast ♀
198.81 Secondary malignant neoplasm of breast
233.0 Carcinoma in situ of breast
610.1 Diffuse cystic mastopathy
610.3 Fibrosclerosis of breast
611.0 Inflammatory disease of breast
611.72 Lump or mass in breast
611.8 Other specified disorder of breast
V10.3 Personal history of malignant neoplasm of breast
V16.3 Family history of malignant neoplasm of breast
V45.71 Acquired absence of breast — (This code is intended for use when these conditions are recorded as diagnoses or problems)
V84.01 Genetic susceptibility to malignant neoplasm of breast

ICD-9-CM Procedural

85.7 Total reconstruction of breast

HCPCS Level II Supplies & Services

A4280 Adhesive skin support attachment for use with external breast prosthesis, each

19366

19366 Breast reconstruction with other technique

ICD-9-CM Diagnostic

174.0 Malignant neoplasm of nipple and areola of female breast ♀
174.1 Malignant neoplasm of central portion of female breast ♀
174.2 Malignant neoplasm of upper-inner quadrant of female breast ♀
174.3 Malignant neoplasm of lower-inner quadrant of female breast ♀
174.4 Malignant neoplasm of upper-outer quadrant of female breast ♀
174.5 Malignant neoplasm of lower-outer quadrant of female breast ♀
174.6 Malignant neoplasm of axillary tail of female breast ♀
174.8 Malignant neoplasm of other specified sites of female breast ♀
198.81 Secondary malignant neoplasm of breast
233.0 Carcinoma in situ of breast
610.1 Diffuse cystic mastopathy
610.3 Fibrosclerosis of breast
611.0 Inflammatory disease of breast
611.72 Lump or mass in breast
611.8 Other specified disorder of breast
V10.3 Personal history of malignant neoplasm of breast
V16.3 Family history of malignant neoplasm of breast
V45.71 Acquired absence of breast — (This code is intended for use when these conditions are recorded as diagnoses or problems)
V84.01 Genetic susceptibility to malignant neoplasm of breast

ICD-9-CM Procedural

85.7 Total reconstruction of breast
85.85 Muscle flap graft to breast

HCPCS Level II Supplies & Services

A4280 Adhesive skin support attachment for use with external breast prosthesis, each

19367–19369

19367 Breast reconstruction with transverse rectus abdominis myocutaneous flap (TRAM), single pedicle, including closure of donor site;
19368 with microvascular anastomosis (supercharging)
19369 Breast reconstruction with transverse rectus abdominis myocutaneous flap (TRAM), double pedicle, including closure of donor site

ICD-9-CM Diagnostic

174.0 Malignant neoplasm of nipple and areola of female breast ♀
174.1 Malignant neoplasm of central portion of female breast ♀
174.2 Malignant neoplasm of upper-inner quadrant of female breast ♀
174.3 Malignant neoplasm of lower-inner quadrant of female breast ♀
174.4 Malignant neoplasm of upper-outer quadrant of female breast ♀
174.5 Malignant neoplasm of lower-outer quadrant of female breast ♀
174.6 Malignant neoplasm of axillary tail of female breast ♀
174.8 Malignant neoplasm of other specified sites of female breast ♀
198.81 Secondary malignant neoplasm of breast
233.0 Carcinoma in situ of breast
610.1 Diffuse cystic mastopathy
610.3 Fibrosclerosis of breast
611.0 Inflammatory disease of breast
611.72 Lump or mass in breast
611.8 Other specified disorder of breast
V10.3 Personal history of malignant neoplasm of breast
V16.3 Family history of malignant neoplasm of breast
V45.71 Acquired absence of breast — (This code is intended for use when these conditions are recorded as diagnoses or problems)
V50.1 Other plastic surgery for unacceptable cosmetic appearance
V51 Aftercare involving the use of plastic surgery
V84.01 Genetic susceptibility to malignant neoplasm of breast

ICD-9-CM Procedural

85.7 Total reconstruction of breast

HCPCS Level II Supplies & Services

A4280 Adhesive skin support attachment for use with external breast prosthesis, each

19370–19371

19370 Open periprosthetic capsulotomy, breast
19371 Periprosthetic capsulectomy, breast

ICD-9-CM Diagnostic

611.71 Mastodynia
686.1 Pyogenic granuloma of skin and subcutaneous tissue
909.3 Late effect of complications of surgical and medical care
996.54 Mechanical complication due to breast prosthesis
996.69 Infection and inflammatory reaction due to other internal prosthetic device, implant, and graft — (Use additional code to identify specified infections)
996.79 Other complications due to other internal prosthetic device, implant, and graft
998.51 Infected postoperative seroma — (Use additional code to identify organism)
998.59 Other postoperative infection — (Use additional code to identify infection)
998.83 Non-healing surgical wound
V10.3 Personal history of malignant neoplasm of breast
V45.71 Acquired absence of breast — (This code is intended for use when these conditions are recorded as diagnoses or problems)
V50.1 Other plastic surgery for unacceptable cosmetic appearance
V84.01 Genetic susceptibility to malignant neoplasm of breast

ICD-9-CM Procedural

85.0 Mastotomy
85.20 Excision or destruction of breast tissue, not otherwise specified

HCPCS Level II Supplies & Services

A4280 Adhesive skin support attachment for use with external breast prosthesis, each

19380

19380 Revision of reconstructed breast

ICD-9-CM Diagnostic

611.8 Other specified disorder of breast
709.2 Scar condition and fibrosis of skin
909.3 Late effect of complications of surgical and medical care
996.54 Mechanical complication due to breast prosthesis
996.79 Other complications due to other internal prosthetic device, implant, and graft
998.9 Unspecified complication of procedure, not elsewhere classified
V10.3 Personal history of malignant neoplasm of breast
V16.3 Family history of malignant neoplasm of breast
V45.71 Acquired absence of breast — (This code is intended for use when these conditions are recorded as diagnoses or problems)
V50.1 Other plastic surgery for unacceptable cosmetic appearance
V51 Aftercare involving the use of plastic surgery
V84.01 Genetic susceptibility to malignant neoplasm of breast

ICD-9-CM Procedural

85.93 Revision of implant of breast
85.99 Other operations on the breast

HCPCS Level II Supplies & Services

A4280 Adhesive skin support attachment for use with external breast prosthesis, each

19396

19396 Preparation of moulage for custom breast implant

ICD-9-CM Diagnostic

611.8 Other specified disorder of breast
V10.3 Personal history of malignant neoplasm of breast
V16.3 Family history of malignant neoplasm of breast
V45.71 Acquired absence of breast — (This code is intended for use when these conditions are recorded as diagnoses or problems)
V50.1 Other plastic surgery for unacceptable cosmetic appearance
V51 Aftercare involving the use of plastic surgery
V52.4 Fitting and adjustment of breast prosthesis and implant ♀
V84.01 Genetic susceptibility to malignant neoplasm of breast

ICD-9-CM Procedural

99.99 Other miscellaneous procedures

HCPCS Level II Supplies & Services

A4649 Surgical supply; miscellaneous

Musculoskeletal System

General

20000–20005

20000 Incision of soft tissue abscess (eg, secondary to osteomyelitis); superficial
20005 deep or complicated

ICD-9-CM Diagnostic

383.20 Unspecified petrositis ▽
383.21 Acute petrositis
383.22 Chronic petrositis
526.4 Inflammatory conditions of jaw
682.0 Cellulitis and abscess of face — (Use additional code to identify organism)
682.1 Cellulitis and abscess of neck — (Use additional code to identify organism)
682.2 Cellulitis and abscess of trunk — (Use additional code to identify organism)
682.3 Cellulitis and abscess of upper arm and forearm — (Use additional code to identify organism)
682.4 Cellulitis and abscess of hand, except fingers and thumb — (Use additional code to identify organism)
682.5 Cellulitis and abscess of buttock — (Use additional code to identify organism)
682.6 Cellulitis and abscess of leg, except foot — (Use additional code to identify organism)
682.7 Cellulitis and abscess of foot, except toes — (Use additional code to identify organism)
682.8 Cellulitis and abscess of other specified site — (Use additional code to identify organism)
730.00 Acute osteomyelitis, site unspecified — (Use additional code to identify organism, 041.1) ▽
730.01 Acute osteomyelitis, shoulder region — (Use additional code to identify organism, 041.1)
730.02 Acute osteomyelitis, upper arm — (Use additional code to identify organism, 041.1)
730.03 Acute osteomyelitis, forearm — (Use additional code to identify organism, 041.1)
730.04 Acute osteomyelitis, hand — (Use additional code to identify organism, 041.1)
730.05 Acute osteomyelitis, pelvic region and thigh — (Use additional code to identify organism, 041.1)
730.06 Acute osteomyelitis, lower leg — (Use additional code to identify organism, 041.1)
730.07 Acute osteomyelitis, ankle and foot — (Use additional code to identify organism, 041.1)
730.08 Acute osteomyelitis, other specified site — (Use additional code to identify organism, 041.1)
730.09 Acute osteomyelitis, multiple sites — (Use additional code to identify organism, 041.1)
730.10 Chronic osteomyelitis, site unspecified — (Use additional code to identify organism, 041.1) ▽
730.11 Chronic osteomyelitis, shoulder region — (Use additional code to identify organism, 041.1)
730.12 Chronic osteomyelitis, upper arm — (Use additional code to identify organism, 041.1)
730.13 Chronic osteomyelitis, forearm — (Use additional code to identify organism, 041.1)
730.14 Chronic osteomyelitis, hand — (Use additional code to identify organism, 041.1)
730.15 Chronic osteomyelitis, pelvic region and thigh — (Use additional code to identify organism, 041.1)
730.16 Chronic osteomyelitis, lower leg — (Use additional code to identify organism, 041.1)
730.17 Chronic osteomyelitis, ankle and foot — (Use additional code to identify organism, 041.1)
730.18 Chronic osteomyelitis, other specified sites — (Use additional code to identify organism, 041.1)
730.19 Chronic osteomyelitis, multiple sites — (Use additional code to identify organism, 041.1)
730.21 Unspecified osteomyelitis, shoulder region — (Use additional code to identify organism, 041.1) ▽
730.22 Unspecified osteomyelitis, upper arm — (Use additional code to identify organism, 041.1) ▽
730.23 Unspecified osteomyelitis, forearm — (Use additional code to identify organism, 041.1) ▽
730.24 Unspecified osteomyelitis, hand — (Use additional code to identify organism, 041.1) ▽
730.25 Unspecified osteomyelitis, pelvic region and thigh — (Use additional code to identify organism, 041.1) ▽
730.26 Unspecified osteomyelitis, lower leg — (Use additional code to identify organism, 041.1) ▽
730.27 Unspecified osteomyelitis, ankle and foot — (Use additional code to identify organism, 041.1) ▽
730.28 Unspecified osteomyelitis, other specified sites — (Use additional code to identify organism, 041.1) ▽
730.29 Unspecified osteomyelitis, multiple sites — (Use additional code to identify organism, 041.1) ▽
730.30 Periostitis, without mention of osteomyelitis, unspecified site — (Use additional code to identify organism, 041.1) ▽
730.31 Periostitis, without mention of osteomyelitis, shoulder region — (Use additional code to identify organism, 041.1)
730.32 Periostitis, without mention of osteomyelitis, upper arm — (Use additional code to identify organism, 041.1)
730.33 Periostitis, without mention of osteomyelitis, forearm — (Use additional code to identify organism, 041.1)
730.34 Periostitis, without mention of osteomyelitis, hand — (Use additional code to identify organism, 041.1)
730.35 Periostitis, without mention of osteomyelitis, pelvic region and thigh — (Use additional code to identify organism, 041.1)
730.36 Periostitis, without mention of osteomyelitis, lower leg — (Use additional code to identify organism, 041.1)
730.37 Periostitis, without mention of osteomyelitis, ankle and foot — (Use additional code to identify organism, 041.1)
730.38 Periostitis, without mention of osteomyelitis, other specified sites — (Use additional code to identify organism, 041.1)
730.39 Periostitis, without mention of osteomyelitis, multiple sites — (Use additional code to identify organism, 041.1)
730.80 Other infections involving bone in diseases classified elsewhere, site unspecified — (Code first underlying disease: 002.0, 015.0-015.9. Use additional code to identify organism) ▽ ⊠
730.81 Other infections involving bone diseases classified elsewhere, shoulder region — (Code first underlying disease: 002.0, 015.0-015.9. Use additional code to identify organism) ⊠
730.82 Other infections involving bone diseases classified elsewhere, upper arm — (Code first underlying disease: 002.0, 015.0-015.9. Use additional code to identify organism) ⊠
730.83 Other infections involving bone in diseases classified elsewhere, forearm — (Code first underlying disease: 002.0, 015.0-015.9. Use additional code to identify organism) ⊠
730.84 Other infections involving diseases classified elsewhere, hand bone — (Code first underlying disease: 002.0, 015.0-015.9. Use additional code to identify organism) ⊠
730.85 Other infections involving bone diseases classified elsewhere, pelvic region and thigh — (Code first underlying disease: 002.0, 015.0-015.9. Use additional code to identify organism) ⊠
730.86 Other infections involving bone diseases classified elsewhere, lower leg — (Code first underlying disease: 002.0, 015.0-015.9. Use additional code to identify organism) ⊠
730.87 Other infections involving bone diseases classified elsewhere, ankle and foot — (Code first underlying disease: 002.0, 015.0-015.9. Use additional code to identify organism) ⊠
730.88 Other infections involving bone diseases classified elsewhere, other specified sites — (Code first underlying disease: 002.0, 015.0-015.9. Use additional code to identify organism) ⊠
730.89 Other infections involving bone diseases classified elsewhere, multiple sites — (Code first underlying disease: 002.0, 015.0-015.9. Use additional code to identify organism) ⊠

▽ Unspecified code
♀ Female diagnosis
⊠ Manifestation code
♂ Male diagnosis

996.66 Infection and inflammatory reaction due to internal joint prosthesis — (Use additional code to identify specified infections)

ICD-9-CM Procedural

83.09 Other incision of soft tissue

HCPCS Level II Supplies & Services

A4550 Surgical trays

20100

20100 Exploration of penetrating wound (separate procedure); neck

ICD-9-CM Diagnostic

874.8 Open wound of other and unspecified parts of neck, without mention of complication — (Use additional code to identify infection) ▽

874.9 Open wound of other and unspecified parts of neck, complicated — (Use additional code to identify infection) ▽

959.09 Injury of face and neck, other and unspecified

959.8 Injury, other and unspecified, other specified sites, including multiple

ICD-9-CM Procedural

83.09 Other incision of soft tissue

83.65 Other suture of muscle or fascia

84.99 Other operations on musculoskeletal system

86.09 Other incision of skin and subcutaneous tissue

86.22 Excisional debridement of wound, infection, or burn

86.28 Nonexcisional debridement of wound, infection, or burn

HCPCS Level II Supplies & Services

A4305 Disposable drug delivery system, flow rate of 50 ml or greater per hour

A4306 Disposable drug delivery system, flow rate of 5 ml or less per hour

A4550 Surgical trays

20101

20101 Exploration of penetrating wound (separate procedure); chest

ICD-9-CM Diagnostic

875.0 Open wound of chest (wall), without mention of complication — (Use additional code to identify infection)

875.1 Open wound of chest (wall), complicated — (Use additional code to identify infection)

879.0 Open wound of breast, without mention of complication — (Use additional code to identify infection)

879.1 Open wound of breast, complicated — (Use additional code to identify infection)

879.8 Open wound(s) (multiple) of unspecified site(s), without mention of complication — (Use additional code to identify infection) ▽

879.9 Open wound(s) (multiple) of unspecified site(s), complicated — (Use additional code to identify infection) ▽

959.11 Other injury of chest wall

959.8 Injury, other and unspecified, other specified sites, including multiple

ICD-9-CM Procedural

34.71 Suture of laceration of chest wall

34.79 Other repair of chest wall

83.09 Other incision of soft tissue

83.65 Other suture of muscle or fascia

84.99 Other operations on musculoskeletal system

85.0 Mastotomy

86.09 Other incision of skin and subcutaneous tissue

86.22 Excisional debridement of wound, infection, or burn

86.28 Nonexcisional debridement of wound, infection, or burn

HCPCS Level II Supplies & Services

A4305 Disposable drug delivery system, flow rate of 50 ml or greater per hour

A4306 Disposable drug delivery system, flow rate of 5 ml or less per hour

A4550 Surgical trays

20102

20102 Exploration of penetrating wound (separate procedure); abdomen/flank/back

ICD-9-CM Diagnostic

876.0 Open wound of back, without mention of complication — (Use additional code to identify infection)

876.1 Open wound of back, complicated — (Use additional code to identify infection)

879.2 Open wound of abdominal wall, anterior, without mention of complication — (Use additional code to identify infection)

879.3 Open wound of abdominal wall, anterior, complicated — (Use additional code to identify infection)

879.4 Open wound of abdominal wall, lateral, without mention of complication — (Use additional code to identify infection)

879.5 Open wound of abdominal wall, lateral, complicated — (Use additional code to identify infection)

879.7 Open wound of other and unspecified parts of trunk, complicated — (Use additional code to identify infection) ▽

879.8 Open wound(s) (multiple) of unspecified site(s), without mention of complication — (Use additional code to identify infection) ▽

879.9 Open wound(s) (multiple) of unspecified site(s), complicated — (Use additional code to identify infection) ▽

959.12 Other injury of abdomen

959.19 Other injury of other sites of trunk

959.8 Injury, other and unspecified, other specified sites, including multiple

ICD-9-CM Procedural

54.0 Incision of abdominal wall

54.63 Other suture of abdominal wall

54.72 Other repair of abdominal wall

83.09 Other incision of soft tissue

83.65 Other suture of muscle or fascia

84.99 Other operations on musculoskeletal system

86.09 Other incision of skin and subcutaneous tissue

86.22 Excisional debridement of wound, infection, or burn

86.28 Nonexcisional debridement of wound, infection, or burn

HCPCS Level II Supplies & Services

A4305 Disposable drug delivery system, flow rate of 50 ml or greater per hour

A4306 Disposable drug delivery system, flow rate of 5 ml or less per hour

A4462 Abdominal dressing holder, each

A4550 Surgical trays

20103

20103 Exploration of penetrating wound (separate procedure); extremity

ICD-9-CM Diagnostic

880.00 Open wound of shoulder region, without mention of complication — (Use additional code to identify infection)

880.01 Open wound of scapular region, without mention of complication — (Use additional code to identify infection)

880.02 Open wound of axillary region, without mention of complication — (Use additional code to identify infection)

880.03 Open wound of upper arm, without mention of complication — (Use additional code to identify infection)

880.09 Open wound of multiple sites of shoulder and upper arm, without mention of complication — (Use additional code to identify infection)

880.10 Open wound of shoulder region, complicated — (Use additional code to identify infection)

880.11 Open wound of scapular region, complicated — (Use additional code to identify infection)

880.12 Open wound of axillary region, complicated — (Use additional code to identify infection)

880.13 Open wound of upper arm, complicated — (Use additional code to identify infection)

880.19 Open wound of multiple sites of shoulder and upper arm, complicated — (Use additional code to identify infection)

881.00 Open wound of forearm, without mention of complication — (Use additional code to identify infection)

881.01 Open wound of elbow, without mention of complication — (Use additional code to identify infection)

881.02 Open wound of wrist, without mention of complication — (Use additional code to identify infection)

881.10 Open wound of forearm, complicated — (Use additional code to identify infection)

881.11 Open wound of elbow, complicated — (Use additional code to identify infection)

881.12 Open wound of wrist, complicated — (Use additional code to identify infection)

882.0 Open wound of hand except finger(s) alone, without mention of complication — (Use additional code to identify infection)

882.1 Open wound of hand except finger(s) alone, complicated — (Use additional code to identify infection)

▽ Unspecified code ♀ Female diagnosis ☒ Manifestation code ♂ Male diagnosis

883.0 Open wound of finger(s), without mention of complication — (Use additional code to identify infection)
883.1 Open wound of finger(s), complicated — (Use additional code to identify infection)
884.0 Multiple and unspecified open wound of upper limb, without mention of complication — (Use additional code to identify infection)
884.1 Multiple and unspecified open wound of upper limb, complicated — (Use additional code to identify infection)
890.0 Open wound of hip and thigh, without mention of complication — (Use additional code to identify infection)
890.1 Open wound of hip and thigh, complicated — (Use additional code to identify infection)
891.0 Open wound of knee, leg (except thigh), and ankle, without mention of complication — (Use additional code to identify infection)
891.1 Open wound of knee, leg (except thigh), and ankle, complicated — (Use additional code to identify infection)
892.0 Open wound of foot except toe(s) alone, without mention of complication — (Use additional code to identify infection)
892.1 Open wound of foot except toe(s) alone, complicated — (Use additional code to identify infection)
893.0 Open wound of toe(s), without mention of complication — (Use additional code to identify infection)
893.1 Open wound of toe(s), complicated — (Use additional code to identify infection)
894.0 Multiple and unspecified open wound of lower limb, without mention of complication — (Use additional code to identify infection)
894.1 Multiple and unspecified open wound of lower limb, complicated — (Use additional code to identify infection)
959.2 Injury, other and unspecified, shoulder and upper arm
959.3 Injury, other and unspecified, elbow, forearm, and wrist
959.4 Injury, other and unspecified, hand, except finger
959.5 Injury, other and unspecified, finger
959.6 Injury, other and unspecified, hip and thigh
959.7 Injury, other and unspecified, knee, leg, ankle, and foot
959.8 Injury, other and unspecified, other specified sites, including multiple

ICD-9-CM Procedural

83.09 Other incision of soft tissue
83.65 Other suture of muscle or fascia
84.99 Other operations on musculoskeletal system
86.09 Other incision of skin and subcutaneous tissue
86.22 Excisional debridement of wound, infection, or burn
86.28 Nonexcisional debridement of wound, infection, or burn

HCPCS Level II Supplies & Services

A4305 Disposable drug delivery system, flow rate of 50 ml or greater per hour
A4306 Disposable drug delivery system, flow rate of 5 ml or less per hour
A4550 Surgical trays

20150

20150 Excision of epiphyseal bar, with or without autogenous soft tissue graft obtained through same fascial incision

ICD-9-CM Diagnostic

733.91 Arrest of bone development or growth
736.00 Unspecified deformity of forearm, excluding fingers ▽
736.30 Unspecified acquired deformity of hip ▽
736.39 Other acquired deformities of hip
736.6 Other acquired deformities of knee
736.70 Unspecified deformity of ankle and foot, acquired ▽
736.79 Other acquired deformity of ankle and foot
736.81 Unequal leg length (acquired)
736.89 Other acquired deformity of other parts of limb
905.2 Late effect of fracture of upper extremities
905.3 Late effect of fracture of neck of femur
905.4 Late effect of fracture of lower extremities
906.4 Late effect of crushing

ICD-9-CM Procedural

78.42 Other repair or plastic operation on humerus
78.43 Other repair or plastic operations on radius and ulna
78.45 Other repair or plastic operations on femur
78.47 Other repair or plastic operations on tibia and fibula
78.49 Other repair or plastic operations on other bone, except facial bones

20200–20206

20200 Biopsy, muscle; superficial
20205 deep
20206 Biopsy, muscle, percutaneous needle

ICD-9-CM Diagnostic

171.0 Malignant neoplasm of connective and other soft tissue of head, face, and neck
171.2 Malignant neoplasm of connective and other soft tissue of upper limb, including shoulder
171.3 Malignant neoplasm of connective and other soft tissue of lower limb, including hip
171.4 Malignant neoplasm of connective and other soft tissue of thorax
171.5 Malignant neoplasm of connective and other soft tissue of abdomen
171.6 Malignant neoplasm of connective and other soft tissue of pelvis
171.7 Malignant neoplasm of connective and other soft tissue of trunk, unspecified site ▽
171.8 Malignant neoplasm of other specified sites of connective and other soft tissue
198.89 Secondary malignant neoplasm of other specified sites
215.0 Other benign neoplasm of connective and other soft tissue of head, face, and neck
215.2 Other benign neoplasm of connective and other soft tissue of upper limb, including shoulder
215.3 Other benign neoplasm of connective and other soft tissue of lower limb, including hip
215.4 Other benign neoplasm of connective and other soft tissue of thorax
215.5 Other benign neoplasm of connective and other soft tissue of abdomen
215.6 Other benign neoplasm of connective and other soft tissue of pelvis
215.7 Other benign neoplasm of connective and other soft tissue of trunk, unspecified ▽
215.8 Other benign neoplasm of connective and other soft tissue of other specified sites
229.8 Benign neoplasm of other specified sites
238.1 Neoplasm of uncertain behavior of connective and other soft tissue ▽
239.2 Neoplasms of unspecified nature of bone, soft tissue, and skin
277.3 Amyloidosis — (Use additional code to identify any associated mental retardation)
277.81 Primary carnitine deficiency — (Use additional code to identify any associated mental retardation)
277.82 Carnitine deficiency due to inborn errors of metabolism — (Use additional code to identify any associated mental retardation)
277.83 Iatrogenic carnitine deficiency — (Use additional code to identify any associated mental retardation)
277.84 Other secondary carnitine deficiency — (Use additional code to identify any associated mental retardation)
277.89 Other specified disorders of metabolism — (Use additional code to identify any associated mental retardation)
359.0 Congenital hereditary muscular dystrophy
359.1 Hereditary progressive muscular dystrophy
359.6 Symptomatic inflammatory myopathy in diseases classified elsewhere — (Code first underlying disease: 135, 140.0-208.9, 277.3, 446.0, 710.0, 710.1, 710.2, 714.0) ☒
359.81 Critical illness myopathy
359.89 Other myopathies
446.0 Polyarteritis nodosa
710.0 Systemic lupus erythematosus — (Use additional code to identify manifestation: 424.91, 581.81, 582.81, 583.81)
710.1 Systemic sclerosis — (Use additional code to identify manifestation: 359.6, 517.2)
710.2 Sicca syndrome
714.0 Rheumatoid arthritis — (Use additional code to identify manifestation: 357.1, 359.6)
728.0 Infective myositis
728.19 Other muscular calcification and ossification
728.79 Other fibromatoses of muscle, ligament, and fascia
728.81 Interstitial myositis
728.87 Muscle weakness
728.88 Rhabdomyolysis
729.1 Unspecified myalgia and myositis ▽

ICD-9-CM Procedural

83.21 Biopsy of soft tissue

HCPCS Level II Supplies & Services

A4550 Surgical trays

20220–20225

20220 Biopsy, bone, trocar, or needle; superficial (eg, ilium, sternum, spinous process, ribs)
20225 deep (eg, vertebral body, femur)

ICD-9-CM Diagnostic

170.0 Malignant neoplasm of bones of skull and face, except mandible
170.1 Malignant neoplasm of mandible
170.2 Malignant neoplasm of vertebral column, excluding sacrum and coccyx
170.3 Malignant neoplasm of ribs, sternum, and clavicle
170.4 Malignant neoplasm of scapula and long bones of upper limb
170.5 Malignant neoplasm of short bones of upper limb
170.6 Malignant neoplasm of pelvic bones, sacrum, and coccyx
170.7 Malignant neoplasm of long bones of lower limb
170.8 Malignant neoplasm of short bones of lower limb
174.9 Malignant neoplasm of breast (female), unspecified site ♀
198.5 Secondary malignant neoplasm of bone and bone marrow
202.80 Other malignant lymphomas, unspecified site, extranodal and solid organ sites
203.11 Plasma cell leukemia in remission
204.10 Chronic lymphoid leukemia without mention of remission
205.10 Chronic myeloid leukemia without mention of remission
213.0 Benign neoplasm of bones of skull and face
213.1 Benign neoplasm of lower jaw bone
213.2 Benign neoplasm of vertebral column, excluding sacrum and coccyx
213.3 Benign neoplasm of ribs, sternum, and clavicle
213.4 Benign neoplasm of scapula and long bones of upper limb
213.5 Benign neoplasm of short bones of upper limb
213.6 Benign neoplasm of pelvic bones, sacrum, and coccyx
213.7 Benign neoplasm of long bones of lower limb
213.8 Benign neoplasm of short bones of lower limb
238.0 Neoplasm of uncertain behavior of bone and articular cartilage
239.2 Neoplasms of unspecified nature of bone, soft tissue, and skin
273.1 Monoclonal paraproteinemia — (Use additional code to identify any associated mental retardation)
284.8 Other specified aplastic anemias — (Use additional E code to identify cause)
285.9 Unspecified anemia
730.10 Chronic osteomyelitis, site unspecified — (Use additional code to identify organism, 041.1)
730.11 Chronic osteomyelitis, shoulder region — (Use additional code to identify organism, 041.1)
730.12 Chronic osteomyelitis, upper arm — (Use additional code to identify organism, 041.1)
730.13 Chronic osteomyelitis, forearm — (Use additional code to identify organism, 041.1)
730.14 Chronic osteomyelitis, hand — (Use additional code to identify organism, 041.1)
730.15 Chronic osteomyelitis, pelvic region and thigh — (Use additional code to identify organism, 041.1)
730.16 Chronic osteomyelitis, lower leg — (Use additional code to identify organism, 041.1)
730.17 Chronic osteomyelitis, ankle and foot — (Use additional code to identify organism, 041.1)
730.18 Chronic osteomyelitis, other specified sites — (Use additional code to identify organism, 041.1)
730.19 Chronic osteomyelitis, multiple sites — (Use additional code to identify organism, 041.1)
730.20 Unspecified osteomyelitis, site unspecified — (Use additional code to identify organism, 041.1)
730.21 Unspecified osteomyelitis, shoulder region — (Use additional code to identify organism, 041.1)
730.22 Unspecified osteomyelitis, upper arm — (Use additional code to identify organism, 041.1)
730.23 Unspecified osteomyelitis, forearm — (Use additional code to identify organism, 041.1)
730.24 Unspecified osteomyelitis, hand — (Use additional code to identify organism, 041.1)
730.25 Unspecified osteomyelitis, pelvic region and thigh — (Use additional code to identify organism, 041.1)
730.26 Unspecified osteomyelitis, lower leg — (Use additional code to identify organism, 041.1)
730.27 Unspecified osteomyelitis, ankle and foot — (Use additional code to identify organism, 041.1)
730.28 Unspecified osteomyelitis, other specified sites — (Use additional code to identify organism, 041.1)
730.29 Unspecified osteomyelitis, multiple sites — (Use additional code to identify organism, 041.1)
730.80 Other infections involving bone in diseases classified elsewhere, site unspecified — (Code first underlying disease: 002.0, 015.0-015.9. Use additional code to identify organism) ☒
730.81 Other infections involving bone diseases classified elsewhere, shoulder region — (Code first underlying disease: 002.0, 015.0-015.9. Use additional code to identify organism) ☒
730.82 Other infections involving bone diseases classified elsewhere, upper arm — (Code first underlying disease: 002.0, 015.0-015.9. Use additional code to identify organism) ☒
730.83 Other infections involving bone in diseases classified elsewhere, forearm — (Code first underlying disease: 002.0, 015.0-015.9. Use additional code to identify organism) ☒
730.84 Other infections involving diseases classified elsewhere, hand bone — (Code first underlying disease: 002.0, 015.0-015.9. Use additional code to identify organism) ☒
730.85 Other infections involving bone diseases classified elsewhere, pelvic region and thigh — (Code first underlying disease: 002.0, 015.0-015.9. Use additional code to identify organism) ☒
730.86 Other infections involving bone diseases classified elsewhere, lower leg — (Code first underlying disease: 002.0, 015.0-015.9. Use additional code to identify organism) ☒
730.87 Other infections involving bone diseases classified elsewhere, ankle and foot — (Code first underlying disease: 002.0, 015.0-015.9. Use additional code to identify organism) ☒
730.88 Other infections involving bone diseases classified elsewhere, other specified sites — (Code first underlying disease: 002.0, 015.0-015.9. Use additional code to identify organism) ☒
730.89 Other infections involving bone diseases classified elsewhere, multiple sites — (Code first underlying disease: 002.0, 015.0-015.9. Use additional code to identify organism) ☒
V10.00 Personal history of malignant neoplasm of unspecified site in gastrointestinal tract
V10.01 Personal history of malignant neoplasm of tongue
V10.02 Personal history of malignant neoplasm of other and unspecified parts of oral cavity and pharynx
V10.03 Personal history of malignant neoplasm of esophagus
V10.04 Personal history of malignant neoplasm of stomach
V10.05 Personal history of malignant neoplasm of large intestine
V10.06 Personal history of malignant neoplasm of rectum, rectosigmoid junction, and anus
V10.07 Personal history of malignant neoplasm of liver
V10.09 Personal history of malignant neoplasm of other site in gastrointestinal tract
V10.11 Personal history of malignant neoplasm of bronchus and lung
V10.12 Personal history of malignant neoplasm of trachea
V10.3 Personal history of malignant neoplasm of breast
V10.40 Personal history of malignant neoplasm of unspecified female genital organ ♀
V10.41 Personal history of malignant neoplasm of cervix uteri ♀
V10.42 Personal history of malignant neoplasm of other parts of uterus ♀
V10.43 Personal history of malignant neoplasm of ovary ♀
V10.44 Personal history of malignant neoplasm of other female genital organs ♀
V10.45 Personal history of malignant neoplasm of unspecified male genital organ ♂
V10.46 Personal history of malignant neoplasm of prostate ♂
V10.47 Personal history of malignant neoplasm of testis ♂
V10.49 Personal history of malignant neoplasm of other male genital organs ♂
V10.50 Personal history of malignant neoplasm of unspecified urinary organ
V10.51 Personal history of malignant neoplasm of bladder
V10.52 Personal history of malignant neoplasm of kidney
V10.53 Personal history of malignant neoplasm, renal pelvis
V10.59 Personal history of malignant neoplasm of other urinary organ
V10.81 Personal history of malignant neoplasm of bone
V10.9 Unspecified personal history of malignant neoplasm

ICD-9-CM Procedural

01.15 Biopsy of skull
76.11 Biopsy of facial bone
77.40 Biopsy of bone, unspecified site
77.41 Biopsy of scapula, clavicle, and thorax (ribs and sternum)
77.42 Biopsy of humerus
77.43 Biopsy of radius and ulna
77.44 Biopsy of carpals and metacarpals
77.45 Biopsy of femur
77.46 Biopsy of patella
77.47 Biopsy of tibia and fibula

Unspecified code
♀ Female diagnosis
☒ Manifestation code
♂ Male diagnosis

77.48 Biopsy of tarsals and metatarsals
77.49 Biopsy of other bone, except facial bones

HCPCS Level II Supplies & Services

A4550 Surgical trays

20240–20245

20240 Biopsy, bone, open; superficial (eg, ilium, sternum, spinous process, ribs, trochanter of femur)
20245 deep (eg, humerus, ischium, femur)

ICD-9-CM Diagnostic

170.0 Malignant neoplasm of bones of skull and face, except mandible
170.1 Malignant neoplasm of mandible
170.2 Malignant neoplasm of vertebral column, excluding sacrum and coccyx
170.3 Malignant neoplasm of ribs, sternum, and clavicle
170.4 Malignant neoplasm of scapula and long bones of upper limb
170.5 Malignant neoplasm of short bones of upper limb
170.6 Malignant neoplasm of pelvic bones, sacrum, and coccyx
170.7 Malignant neoplasm of long bones of lower limb
170.8 Malignant neoplasm of short bones of lower limb
170.9 Malignant neoplasm of bone and articular cartilage, site unspecified ▽
174.9 Malignant neoplasm of breast (female), unspecified site ▽ ♀
198.5 Secondary malignant neoplasm of bone and bone marrow
213.0 Benign neoplasm of bones of skull and face
213.1 Benign neoplasm of lower jaw bone
213.2 Benign neoplasm of vertebral column, excluding sacrum and coccyx
213.3 Benign neoplasm of ribs, sternum, and clavicle
213.4 Benign neoplasm of scapula and long bones of upper limb
213.5 Benign neoplasm of short bones of upper limb
213.6 Benign neoplasm of pelvic bones, sacrum, and coccyx
213.7 Benign neoplasm of long bones of lower limb
213.8 Benign neoplasm of short bones of lower limb
238.0 Neoplasm of uncertain behavior of bone and articular cartilage
239.2 Neoplasms of unspecified nature of bone, soft tissue, and skin
730.10 Chronic osteomyelitis, site unspecified — (Use additional code to identify organism, 041.1) ▽
730.11 Chronic osteomyelitis, shoulder region — (Use additional code to identify organism, 041.1)
730.12 Chronic osteomyelitis, upper arm — (Use additional code to identify organism, 041.1)
730.13 Chronic osteomyelitis, forearm — (Use additional code to identify organism, 041.1)
730.14 Chronic osteomyelitis, hand — (Use additional code to identify organism, 041.1)
730.15 Chronic osteomyelitis, pelvic region and thigh — (Use additional code to identify organism, 041.1)
730.16 Chronic osteomyelitis, lower leg — (Use additional code to identify organism, 041.1)
730.17 Chronic osteomyelitis, ankle and foot — (Use additional code to identify organism, 041.1)
730.18 Chronic osteomyelitis, other specified sites — (Use additional code to identify organism, 041.1)
730.19 Chronic osteomyelitis, multiple sites — (Use additional code to identify organism, 041.1)
730.20 Unspecified osteomyelitis, site unspecified — (Use additional code to identify organism, 041.1) ▽
730.21 Unspecified osteomyelitis, shoulder region — (Use additional code to identify organism, 041.1) ▽
730.22 Unspecified osteomyelitis, upper arm — (Use additional code to identify organism, 041.1) ▽
730.23 Unspecified osteomyelitis, forearm — (Use additional code to identify organism, 041.1) ▽
730.24 Unspecified osteomyelitis, hand — (Use additional code to identify organism, 041.1) ▽
730.25 Unspecified osteomyelitis, pelvic region and thigh — (Use additional code to identify organism, 041.1) ▽
730.26 Unspecified osteomyelitis, lower leg — (Use additional code to identify organism, 041.1) ▽
730.27 Unspecified osteomyelitis, ankle and foot — (Use additional code to identify organism, 041.1) ▽
730.28 Unspecified osteomyelitis, other specified sites — (Use additional code to identify organism, 041.1) ▽
730.29 Unspecified osteomyelitis, multiple sites — (Use additional code to identify organism, 041.1) ▽
730.80 Other infections involving bone in diseases classified elsewhere, site unspecified — (Code first underlying disease: 002.0, 015.0-015.9. Use additional code to identify organism) ▽ ☒
730.81 Other infections involving bone diseases classified elsewhere, shoulder region — (Code first underlying disease: 002.0, 015.0-015.9. Use additional code to identify organism) ☒
730.82 Other infections involving bone diseases classified elsewhere, upper arm — (Code first underlying disease: 002.0, 015.0-015.9. Use additional code to identify organism) ☒
730.83 Other infections involving bone in diseases classified elsewhere, forearm — (Code first underlying disease: 002.0, 015.0-015.9. Use additional code to identify organism) ☒
730.84 Other infections involving diseases classified elsewhere, hand bone — (Code first underlying disease: 002.0, 015.0-015.9. Use additional code to identify organism) ☒
730.85 Other infections involving bone diseases classified elsewhere, pelvic region and thigh — (Code first underlying disease: 002.0, 015.0-015.9. Use additional code to identify organism) ☒
730.86 Other infections involving bone diseases classified elsewhere, lower leg — (Code first underlying disease: 002.0, 015.0-015.9. Use additional code to identify organism) ☒
730.87 Other infections involving bone diseases classified elsewhere, ankle and foot — (Code first underlying disease: 002.0, 015.0-015.9. Use additional code to identify organism) ☒
730.88 Other infections involving bone diseases classified elsewhere, other specified sites — (Code first underlying disease: 002.0, 015.0-015.9. Use additional code to identify organism) ☒
730.89 Other infections involving bone diseases classified elsewhere, multiple sites — (Code first underlying disease: 002.0, 015.0-015.9. Use additional code to identify organism) ☒
731.0 Osteitis deformans without mention of bone tumor
731.1 Osteitis deformans in diseases classified elsewhere — (Code first underlying disease: 170.0-170.9) ☒
731.2 Hypertrophic pulmonary osteoarthropathy
731.8 Other bone involvement in diseases classified elsewhere — (Code first underlying disease, 250.8. Use additional code to specify bone condition: 730.00-730.09) ☒
V10.00 Personal history of malignant neoplasm of unspecified site in gastrointestinal tract ▽
V10.03 Personal history of malignant neoplasm of esophagus
V10.04 Personal history of malignant neoplasm of stomach
V10.05 Personal history of malignant neoplasm of large intestine
V10.06 Personal history of malignant neoplasm of rectum, rectosigmoid junction, and anus
V10.07 Personal history of malignant neoplasm of liver
V10.09 Personal history of malignant neoplasm of other site in gastrointestinal tract
V10.11 Personal history of malignant neoplasm of bronchus and lung
V10.12 Personal history of malignant neoplasm of trachea
V10.20 Personal history of malignant neoplasm of unspecified respiratory organ ▽
V10.3 Personal history of malignant neoplasm of breast
V10.40 Personal history of malignant neoplasm of unspecified female genital organ ▽ ♀
V10.41 Personal history of malignant neoplasm of cervix uteri ♀
V10.42 Personal history of malignant neoplasm of other parts of uterus ♀
V10.43 Personal history of malignant neoplasm of ovary ♀
V10.44 Personal history of malignant neoplasm of other female genital organs ♀
V10.45 Personal history of malignant neoplasm of unspecified male genital organ ▽ ♂
V10.46 Personal history of malignant neoplasm of prostate ♂
V10.47 Personal history of malignant neoplasm of testis ♂
V10.49 Personal history of malignant neoplasm of other male genital organs ♂
V10.50 Personal history of malignant neoplasm of unspecified urinary organ ▽
V10.51 Personal history of malignant neoplasm of bladder
V10.52 Personal history of malignant neoplasm of kidney
V10.53 Personal history of malignant neoplasm, renal pelvis
V10.59 Personal history of malignant neoplasm of other urinary organ
V10.81 Personal history of malignant neoplasm of bone

ICD-9-CM Procedural

01.15 Biopsy of skull
76.11 Biopsy of facial bone
77.40 Biopsy of bone, unspecified site
77.41 Biopsy of scapula, clavicle, and thorax (ribs and sternum)
77.42 Biopsy of humerus
77.43 Biopsy of radius and ulna
77.44 Biopsy of carpals and metacarpals
77.45 Biopsy of femur
77.46 Biopsy of patella

▽ Unspecified code ♀ Female diagnosis ☒ Manifestation code ♂ Male diagnosis

77.47 Biopsy of tibia and fibula
77.48 Biopsy of tarsals and metatarsals
77.49 Biopsy of other bone, except facial bones

HCPCS Level II Supplies & Services

A4550 Surgical trays

20250–20251

20250 Biopsy, vertebral body, open; thoracic
20251 lumbar or cervical

ICD-9-CM Diagnostic

170.2 Malignant neoplasm of vertebral column, excluding sacrum and coccyx
198.5 Secondary malignant neoplasm of bone and bone marrow
198.89 Secondary malignant neoplasm of other specified sites
213.2 Benign neoplasm of vertebral column, excluding sacrum and coccyx
237.70 Neurofibromatosis, unspecified ▽
237.71 Neurofibromatosis, Type 1 (von Recklinghausen's disease)
237.72 Neurofibromatosis, Type 2 (acoustic neurofibromatosis)
238.0 Neoplasm of uncertain behavior of bone and articular cartilage
239.2 Neoplasms of unspecified nature of bone, soft tissue, and skin
252.00 Hyperparathyroidism, unspecified
252.01 Primary hyperparathyroidism
252.02 Secondary hyperparathyroidism, non-renal
252.08 Other hyperparathyroidism
277.5 Mucopolysaccharidosis — (Use additional code to identify any associated mental retardation)
336.9 Unspecified disease of spinal cord ▽
356.1 Peroneal muscular atrophy
720.81 Inflammatory spondylopathies in diseases classified elsewhere — (Code first underlying disease, 015.0) ☒
720.89 Other inflammatory spondylopathies
723.4 Brachial neuritis or radiculitis nos
724.4 Thoracic or lumbosacral neuritis or radiculitis, unspecified ▽
724.5 Unspecified backache ▽
724.9 Other unspecified back disorder
729.2 Unspecified neuralgia, neuritis, and radiculitis ▽
730.18 Chronic osteomyelitis, other specified sites — (Use additional code to identify organism, 041.1)
730.28 Unspecified osteomyelitis, other specified sites — (Use additional code to identify organism, 041.1) ▽
730.80 Other infections involving bone in diseases classified elsewhere, site unspecified — (Code first underlying disease: 002.0, 015.0-015.9. Use additional code to identify organism) ▽ ☒
730.88 Other infections involving bone diseases classified elsewhere, other specified sites — (Code first underlying disease: 002.0, 015.0-015.9. Use additional code to identify organism) ☒
730.89 Other infections involving bone diseases classified elsewhere, multiple sites — (Code first underlying disease: 002.0, 015.0-015.9. Use additional code to identify organism) ☒
730.98 Unspecified infection of bone of other specified site — (Use additional code to identify organism, 041.1) ▽
731.0 Osteitis deformans without mention of bone tumor
733.00 Unspecified osteoporosis ▽
733.01 Senile osteoporosis
733.02 Idiopathic osteoporosis
733.03 Disuse osteoporosis
733.09 Other osteoporosis — (Use additional E code to identify drug)
737.40 Unspecified curvature of spine associated with other condition — (Code first associated condition: 015.0, 138, 237.7, 252.0, 277.5, 356.1, 731.0, 733.00-733.09) ▽ ☒
737.41 Kyphosis associated with other condition — (Code first associated condition: 015.0, 138, 237.7, 252.0, 277.5, 356.1, 731.0, 733.00-733.09) ☒
737.42 Lordosis associated with other condition — (Code first associated condition: 015.0, 138, 237.7, 252.0, 277.5, 356.1, 731.0, 733.00-733.09) ☒
737.43 Scoliosis associated with other condition — (Code first associated condition: 015.0, 138, 237.7, 252.0, 277.5, 356.1, 731.0, 733.00-733.09) ☒

ICD-9-CM Procedural

77.49 Biopsy of other bone, except facial bones

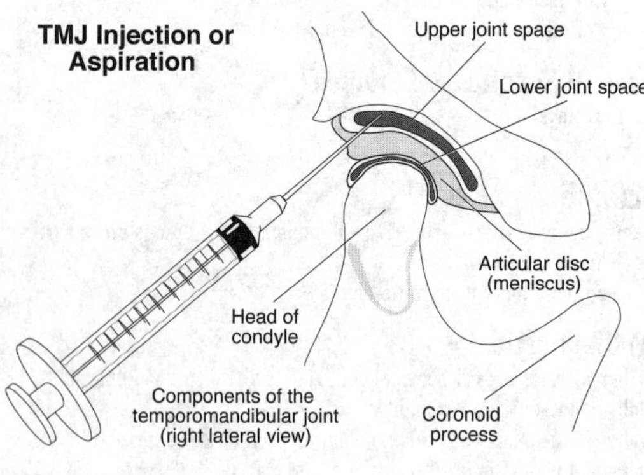

20500

20500 Injection of sinus tract; therapeutic (separate procedure)

ICD-9-CM Diagnostic

510.0 Empyema with fistula — (Use additional code to identify infectious organism: 041.00-041.9)
522.7 Periapical abscess with sinus
527.4 Fistula of salivary gland
528.3 Cellulitis and abscess of oral soft tissues
567.2 Other suppurative peritonitis
685.0 Pilonidal cyst with abscess
685.1 Pilonidal cyst without mention of abscess
686.9 Unspecified local infection of skin and subcutaneous tissue ▽
719.80 Other specified disorders of joint, site unspecified ▽
719.81 Other specified disorders of shoulder joint
719.82 Other specified disorders of upper arm joint
719.83 Other specified disorders of forearm joint
719.84 Other specified disorders of hand joint
719.85 Other specified disorders of pelvic joint
719.86 Other specified disorders of lower leg joint
719.87 Other specified disorders of ankle and foot joint
719.88 Other specified disorders of joint of other specified site
719.89 Other specified disorders of joints of multiple sites
733.99 Other disorders of bone and cartilage
998.6 Persistent postoperative fistula, not elsewhere classified

ICD-9-CM Procedural

83.98 Injection of locally acting therapeutic substance into other soft tissue

HCPCS Level II Supplies & Services

A9525 Supply of low or iso-osmolar contrast material, 10 mg of iodine

20501

20501 Injection of sinus tract; diagnostic (sinogram)

ICD-9-CM Diagnostic

349.81 Cerebrospinal fluid rhinorrhea
360.32 Ocular fistula causing hypotony
375.61 Lacrimal fistula
380.89 Other disorder of external ear
383.81 Postauricular fistula
386.40 Unspecified labyrinthine fistula ▽
386.41 Round window fistula
386.42 Oval window fistula
386.43 Semicircular canal fistula
386.48 Labyrinthine fistula of combined sites
478.79 Other diseases of larynx
510.0 Empyema with fistula — (Use additional code to identify infectious organism: 041.00-041.9)
526.89 Other specified disease of the jaws
528.5 Diseases of lips
530.84 Tracheoesophageal fistula
530.89 Other specified disorder of the esophagus
537.4 Fistula of stomach or duodenum
543.9 Other and unspecified diseases of appendix ▽
569.69 Other complication of colostomy or enterostomy
569.81 Fistula of intestine, excluding rectum and anus
575.5 Fistula of gallbladder

▽ Unspecified code ♀ Female diagnosis ☒ Manifestation code ♂ Male diagnosis

576.4 Fistula of bile duct
577.8 Other specified disease of pancreas
593.81 Vascular disorders of kidney
593.82 Ureteral fistula
596.1 Intestinovesical fistula — (Use additional code to identify urinary incontinence: 625.6, 788.30-788.39)
596.2 Vesical fistula, not elsewhere classified — (Use additional code to identify urinary incontinence: 625.6, 788.30-788.39)
608.89 Other specified disorder of male genital organs ♂
611.0 Inflammatory disease of breast
619.0 Urinary-genital tract fistula, female ♀
619.1 Digestive-genital tract fistula, female ♀
619.2 Genital tract-skin fistula, female ♀
619.8 Other specified fistula involving female genital tract ♀
686.9 Unspecified local infection of skin and subcutaneous tissue
719.80 Other specified disorders of joint, site unspecified
719.81 Other specified disorders of shoulder joint
719.82 Other specified disorders of upper arm joint
719.83 Other specified disorders of forearm joint
719.84 Other specified disorders of hand joint
719.85 Other specified disorders of pelvic joint
719.86 Other specified disorders of lower leg joint
719.87 Other specified disorders of ankle and foot joint
719.88 Other specified disorders of joint of other specified site
719.89 Other specified disorders of joints of multiple sites
733.99 Other disorders of bone and cartilage
744.41 Congenital branchial cleft sinus or fistula
744.46 Congenital preauricular sinus or fistula
744.49 Other congenital branchial cleft cyst or fistula; preauricular sinus
748.3 Other congenital anomaly of larynx, trachea, and bronchus
750.25 Congenital fistula of lip
998.6 Persistent postoperative fistula, not elsewhere classified

ICD-9-CM Procedural
83.98 Injection of locally acting therapeutic substance into other soft tissue
87.38 Sinogram of chest wall
88.03 Sinogram of abdominal wall
88.14 Retroperitoneal fistulogram

HCPCS Level II Supplies & Services
A9525 Supply of low or iso-osmolar contrast material, 10 mg of iodine

20520–20525
20520 Removal of foreign body in muscle or tendon sheath; simple
20525 deep or complicated

ICD-9-CM Diagnostic
709.4 Foreign body granuloma of skin and subcutaneous tissue
728.82 Foreign body granuloma of muscle
729.6 Residual foreign body in soft tissue
870.4 Penetrating wound of orbit with foreign body — (Use additional code to identify infection)
873.50 Open wound of face, unspecified site, complicated — (Use additional code to identify infection)
873.51 Open wound of cheek, complicated — (Use additional code to identify infection)
873.52 Open wound of forehead, complicated — (Use additional code to identify infection)
873.53 Open wound of lip, complicated — (Use additional code to identify infection)
873.54 Open wound of jaw, complicated — (Use additional code to identify infection)
873.59 Open wound of face, other and multiple sites, complicated — (Use additional code to identify infection)
874.9 Open wound of other and unspecified parts of neck, complicated — (Use additional code to identify infection)
875.1 Open wound of chest (wall), complicated — (Use additional code to identify infection)
876.1 Open wound of back, complicated — (Use additional code to identify infection)
879.3 Open wound of abdominal wall, anterior, complicated — (Use additional code to identify infection)
879.5 Open wound of abdominal wall, lateral, complicated — (Use additional code to identify infection)
879.9 Open wound(s) (multiple) of unspecified site(s), complicated — (Use additional code to identify infection)
880.10 Open wound of shoulder region, complicated — (Use additional code to identify infection)
880.11 Open wound of scapular region, complicated — (Use additional code to identify infection)
880.12 Open wound of axillary region, complicated — (Use additional code to identify infection)
880.13 Open wound of upper arm, complicated — (Use additional code to identify infection)
880.19 Open wound of multiple sites of shoulder and upper arm, complicated — (Use additional code to identify infection)
880.20 Open wound of shoulder region, with tendon involvement — (Use additional code to identify infection)
880.21 Open wound of scapular region, with tendon involvement — (Use additional code to identify infection)
880.22 Open wound of axillary region, with tendon involvement — (Use additional code to identify infection)
880.23 Open wound of upper arm, with tendon involvement — (Use additional code to identify infection)
880.29 Open wound of multiple sites of shoulder and upper arm, with tendon involvement — (Use additional code to identify infection)
881.10 Open wound of forearm, complicated — (Use additional code to identify infection)
881.11 Open wound of elbow, complicated — (Use additional code to identify infection)
881.12 Open wound of wrist, complicated — (Use additional code to identify infection)
881.20 Open wound of forearm, with tendon involvement — (Use additional code to identify infection)
881.21 Open wound of elbow, with tendon involvement — (Use additional code to identify infection)
881.22 Open wound of wrist, with tendon involvement — (Use additional code to identify infection)
882.1 Open wound of hand except finger(s) alone, complicated — (Use additional code to identify infection)
882.2 Open wound of hand except finger(s) alone, with tendon involvement — (Use additional code to identify infection)
883.1 Open wound of finger(s), complicated — (Use additional code to identify infection)
883.2 Open wound of finger(s), with tendon involvement — (Use additional code to identify infection)
890.1 Open wound of hip and thigh, complicated — (Use additional code to identify infection)
890.2 Open wound of hip and thigh, with tendon involvement — (Use additional code to identify infection)
891.1 Open wound of knee, leg (except thigh), and ankle, complicated — (Use additional code to identify infection)
891.2 Open wound of knee, leg (except thigh), and ankle, with tendon involvement — (Use additional code to identify infection)
892.1 Open wound of foot except toe(s) alone, complicated — (Use additional code to identify infection)
893.1 Open wound of toe(s), complicated — (Use additional code to identify infection)
893.2 Open wound of toe(s), with tendon involvement — (Use additional code to identify infection)
894.1 Multiple and unspecified open wound of lower limb, complicated — (Use additional code to identify infection)
894.2 Multiple and unspecified open wound of lower limb, with tendon involvement — (Use additional code to identify infection)
930.8 Foreign body in other and combined sites on external eye

ICD-9-CM Procedural
82.01 Exploration of tendon sheath of hand
82.02 Myotomy of hand
83.01 Exploration of tendon sheath
83.02 Myotomy
98.25 Removal of other foreign body without incision from trunk except scrotum, penis, or vulva
98.26 Removal of foreign body from hand without incision
98.27 Removal of foreign body without incision from upper limb, except hand
98.28 Removal of foreign body from foot without incision
98.29 Removal of foreign body without incision from lower limb, except foot

HCPCS Level II Supplies & Services
A4305 Disposable drug delivery system, flow rate of 50 ml or greater per hour
A4306 Disposable drug delivery system, flow rate of 5 ml or less per hour
A4550 Surgical trays

20526

20526 Injection, therapeutic (eg, local anesthetic, corticosteroid), carpal tunnel

ICD-9-CM Diagnostic

354.0 Carpal tunnel syndrome

ICD-9-CM Procedural

99.23 Injection of steroid
99.29 Injection or infusion of other therapeutic or prophylactic substance
99.77 Application or administration of adhesion barrier substance

HCPCS Level II Supplies & Services

J0702 Injection, betamethasone acetate and betamethasone sodium phosphate, per 3 mg
J0704 Injection, betamethasone sodium phosphate, per 4 mg

20550

20550 Injection(s); single tendon sheath, or ligament, aponeurosis (eg, plantar "fascia")

ICD-9-CM Diagnostic

351.1 Geniculate ganglionitis
353.0 Brachial plexus lesions
353.1 Lumbosacral plexus lesions
353.2 Cervical root lesions, not elsewhere classified
353.3 Thoracic root lesions, not elsewhere classified
353.4 Lumbosacral root lesions, not elsewhere classified
353.8 Other nerve root and plexus disorders
354.0 Carpal tunnel syndrome
354.1 Other lesion of median nerve
354.2 Lesion of ulnar nerve
354.3 Lesion of radial nerve
354.5 Mononeuritis multiplex
354.8 Other mononeuritis of upper limb
355.6 Lesion of plantar nerve
357.1 Polyneuropathy in collagen vascular disease — (Code first underlying disease: 446.0, 710.0, 714.0) ☒
359.6 Symptomatic inflammatory myopathy in diseases classified elsewhere — (Code first underlying disease: 135, 140.0-208.9, 277.3, 446.0, 710.0, 710.1, 710.2, 714.0) ☒
714.0 Rheumatoid arthritis — (Use additional code to identify manifestation: 357.1, 359.6)
715.00 Generalized osteoarthrosis, unspecified site ▽
715.04 Generalized osteoarthrosis, involving hand
715.09 Generalized osteoarthrosis, involving multiple sites
716.50 Unspecified polyarthropathy or polyarthritis, site unspecified ▽
716.51 Unspecified polyarthropathy or polyarthritis, shoulder region ▽
716.52 Unspecified polyarthropathy or polyarthritis, upper arm ▽
716.53 Unspecified polyarthropathy or polyarthritis, forearm ▽
716.54 Unspecified polyarthropathy or polyarthritis, hand ▽
716.55 Unspecified polyarthropathy or polyarthritis, pelvic region and thigh ▽
716.56 Unspecified polyarthropathy or polyarthritis, lower leg ▽
716.57 Unspecified polyarthropathy or polyarthritis, ankle and foot ▽
716.58 Unspecified polyarthropathy or polyarthritis, other specified sites ▽
716.59 Unspecified polyarthropathy or polyarthritis, multiple sites ▽
716.60 Unspecified monoarthritis, site unspecified ▽
716.61 Unspecified monoarthritis, shoulder region ▽
716.62 Unspecified monoarthritis, upper arm ▽
716.63 Unspecified monoarthritis, forearm ▽
716.64 Unspecified monoarthritis, hand ▽
716.65 Unspecified monoarthritis, pelvic region and thigh ▽
716.66 Unspecified monoarthritis, lower leg ▽
716.67 Unspecified monoarthritis, ankle and foot ▽
716.68 Unspecified monoarthritis, other specified sites ▽
716.90 Unspecified arthropathy, site unspecified ▽
716.91 Unspecified arthropathy, shoulder region ▽
716.92 Unspecified arthropathy, upper arm ▽
716.93 Unspecified arthropathy, forearm ▽
716.94 Unspecified arthopathy, hand ▽
716.95 Unspecified arthropathy, pelvic region and thigh ▽
716.96 Unspecified arthropathy, lower leg ▽
716.97 Unspecified arthropathy, ankle and foot ▽
716.99 Unspecified arthropathy, multiple sites ▽
719.40 Pain in joint, site unspecified ▽
719.41 Pain in joint, shoulder region
719.42 Pain in joint, upper arm
719.43 Pain in joint, forearm
719.44 Pain in joint, hand
719.45 Pain in joint, pelvic region and thigh
719.46 Pain in joint, lower leg
719.47 Pain in joint, ankle and foot
719.48 Pain in joint, other specified sites
719.49 Pain in joint, multiple sites
720.0 Ankylosing spondylitis
726.10 Unspecified disorders of bursae and tendons in shoulder region ▽
726.32 Lateral epicondylitis of elbow
727.00 Unspecified synovitis and tenosynovitis ▽
727.02 Giant cell tumor of tendon sheath
727.03 Trigger finger (acquired)
727.04 Radial styloid tenosynovitis
727.05 Other tenosynovitis of hand and wrist
727.06 Tenosynovitis of foot and ankle
727.09 Other synovitis and tenosynovitis
727.2 Specific bursitides often of occupational origin
727.3 Other bursitis disorders
728.71 Plantar fascial fibromatosis
729.4 Unspecified fasciitis ▽
729.5 Pain in soft tissues of limb
729.9 Other and unspecified disorders of soft tissue

ICD-9-CM Procedural

81.92 Injection of therapeutic substance into joint or ligament
83.97 Injection of therapeutic substance into tendon

HCPCS Level II Supplies & Services

J0704 Injection, betamethasone sodium phosphate, per 4 mg

20551

20551 Injection(s); single tendon origin/insertion

ICD-9-CM Diagnostic

353.0 Brachial plexus lesions
353.1 Lumbosacral plexus lesions
353.2 Cervical root lesions, not elsewhere classified
353.3 Thoracic root lesions, not elsewhere classified
353.4 Lumbosacral root lesions, not elsewhere classified
353.8 Other nerve root and plexus disorders
354.0 Carpal tunnel syndrome
354.1 Other lesion of median nerve
354.2 Lesion of ulnar nerve
354.3 Lesion of radial nerve
354.5 Mononeuritis multiplex
354.8 Other mononeuritis of upper limb
355.2 Other lesion of femoral nerve
355.3 Lesion of lateral popliteal nerve
355.4 Lesion of medial popliteal nerve
355.5 Tarsal tunnel syndrome
355.6 Lesion of plantar nerve
355.71 Causalgia of lower limb
355.79 Other mononeuritis of lower limb
355.8 Unspecified mononeuritis of lower limb ▽
355.9 Mononeuritis of unspecified site ▽
357.1 Polyneuropathy in collagen vascular disease — (Code first underlying disease: 446.0, 710.0, 714.0) ☒
359.6 Symptomatic inflammatory myopathy in diseases classified elsewhere — (Code first underlying disease: 135, 140.0-208.9, 277.3, 446.0, 710.0, 710.1, 710.2, 714.0) ☒
714.0 Rheumatoid arthritis — (Use additional code to identify manifestation: 357.1, 359.6)
715.00 Generalized osteoarthrosis, unspecified site ▽
715.04 Generalized osteoarthrosis, involving hand
715.09 Generalized osteoarthrosis, involving multiple sites
715.16 Primary localized osteoarthrosis, lower leg
715.17 Primary localized osteoarthrosis, ankle and foot
715.18 Primary localized osteoarthrosis, other specified sites
715.35 Localized osteoarthrosis not specified whether primary or secondary, pelvic region and thigh
715.36 Localized osteoarthrosis not specified whether primary or secondary, lower leg
715.37 Localized osteoarthrosis not specified whether primary or secondary, ankle and foot
715.38 Localized osteoarthrosis not specified whether primary or secondary, other specified sites

716.50 Unspecified polyarthropathy or polyarthritis, site unspecified
716.51 Unspecified polyarthropathy or polyarthritis, shoulder region
716.52 Unspecified polyarthropathy or polyarthritis, upper arm
716.53 Unspecified polyarthropathy or polyarthritis, forearm
716.54 Unspecified polyarthropathy or polyarthritis, hand
716.55 Unspecified polyarthropathy or polyarthritis, pelvic region and thigh
716.56 Unspecified polyarthropathy or polyarthritis, lower leg
716.57 Unspecified polyarthropathy or polyarthritis, ankle and foot
716.58 Unspecified polyarthropathy or polyarthritis, other specified sites
716.59 Unspecified polyarthropathy or polyarthritis, multiple sites
716.60 Unspecified monoarthritis, site unspecified
716.61 Unspecified monoarthritis, shoulder region
716.62 Unspecified monoarthritis, upper arm
716.63 Unspecified monoarthritis, forearm
716.64 Unspecified monoarthritis, hand
716.65 Unspecified monoarthritis, pelvic region and thigh
716.66 Unspecified monoarthritis, lower leg
716.67 Unspecified monoarthritis, ankle and foot
716.68 Unspecified monoarthritis, other specified sites
716.90 Unspecified arthropathy, site unspecified
716.91 Unspecified arthropathy, shoulder region
716.92 Unspecified arthropathy, upper arm
716.93 Unspecified arthropathy, forearm
716.94 Unspecified arthopathy, hand
716.95 Unspecified arthropathy, pelvic region and thigh
716.96 Unspecified arthropathy, lower leg
716.97 Unspecified arthropathy, ankle and foot
716.99 Unspecified arthropathy, multiple sites
719.40 Pain in joint, site unspecified
719.41 Pain in joint, shoulder region
719.42 Pain in joint, upper arm
719.43 Pain in joint, forearm
719.44 Pain in joint, hand
719.45 Pain in joint, pelvic region and thigh
719.46 Pain in joint, lower leg
719.47 Pain in joint, ankle and foot
719.48 Pain in joint, other specified sites
719.49 Pain in joint, multiple sites
720.0 Ankylosing spondylitis
726.10 Unspecified disorders of bursae and tendons in shoulder region
726.32 Lateral epicondylitis of elbow
727.00 Unspecified synovitis and tenosynovitis
727.02 Giant cell tumor of tendon sheath
727.03 Trigger finger (acquired)
727.04 Radial styloid tenosynovitis
727.05 Other tenosynovitis of hand and wrist
727.06 Tenosynovitis of foot and ankle
727.09 Other synovitis and tenosynovitis
727.2 Specific bursitides often of occupational origin
727.3 Other bursitis disorders
728.71 Plantar fascial fibromatosis
729.4 Unspecified fasciitis
729.5 Pain in soft tissues of limb
729.9 Other and unspecified disorders of soft tissue

ICD-9-CM Procedural

82.95 Injection of therapeutic substance into tendon of hand
83.97 Injection of therapeutic substance into tendon

HCPCS Level II Supplies & Services

J0704 Injection, betamethasone sodium phosphate, per 4 mg

20552–20553

20552 Injection(s); single or multiple trigger point(s), one or two muscle(s)
20553 single or multiple trigger point(s), three or more muscle(s)

ICD-9-CM Diagnostic

353.0 Brachial plexus lesions
353.1 Lumbosacral plexus lesions
353.2 Cervical root lesions, not elsewhere classified
353.3 Thoracic root lesions, not elsewhere classified
353.4 Lumbosacral root lesions, not elsewhere classified
353.8 Other nerve root and plexus disorders
354.0 Carpal tunnel syndrome
354.1 Other lesion of median nerve
354.2 Lesion of ulnar nerve
354.3 Lesion of radial nerve
354.5 Mononeuritis multiplex
354.8 Other mononeuritis of upper limb
355.2 Other lesion of femoral nerve
355.3 Lesion of lateral popliteal nerve
355.4 Lesion of medial popliteal nerve
355.5 Tarsal tunnel syndrome
355.6 Lesion of plantar nerve
355.71 Causalgia of lower limb
355.79 Other mononeuritis of lower limb
355.8 Unspecified mononeuritis of lower limb
355.9 Mononeuritis of unspecified site
357.1 Polyneuropathy in collagen vascular disease — (Code first underlying disease: 446.0, 710.0, 714.0)
359.6 Symptomatic inflammatory myopathy in diseases classified elsewhere — (Code first underlying disease: 135, 140.0-208.9, 277.3, 446.0, 710.0, 710.1, 710.2, 714.0)
714.0 Rheumatoid arthritis — (Use additional code to identify manifestation: 357.1, 359.6)
715.00 Generalized osteoarthrosis, unspecified site
715.04 Generalized osteoarthrosis, involving hand
715.09 Generalized osteoarthrosis, involving multiple sites
715.16 Primary localized osteoarthrosis, lower leg
715.17 Primary localized osteoarthrosis, ankle and foot
715.18 Primary localized osteoarthrosis, other specified sites
715.35 Localized osteoarthrosis not specified whether primary or secondary, pelvic region and thigh
715.36 Localized osteoarthrosis not specified whether primary or secondary, lower leg
715.37 Localized osteoarthrosis not specified whether primary or secondary, ankle and foot
715.38 Localized osteoarthrosis not specified whether primary or secondary, other specified sites
716.50 Unspecified polyarthropathy or polyarthritis, site unspecified
716.51 Unspecified polyarthropathy or polyarthritis, shoulder region
716.52 Unspecified polyarthropathy or polyarthritis, upper arm
716.53 Unspecified polyarthropathy or polyarthritis, forearm
716.54 Unspecified polyarthropathy or polyarthritis, hand
716.55 Unspecified polyarthropathy or polyarthritis, pelvic region and thigh
716.56 Unspecified polyarthropathy or polyarthritis, lower leg
716.57 Unspecified polyarthropathy or polyarthritis, ankle and foot
716.58 Unspecified polyarthropathy or polyarthritis, other specified sites
716.59 Unspecified polyarthropathy or polyarthritis, multiple sites
716.60 Unspecified monoarthritis, site unspecified
716.61 Unspecified monoarthritis, shoulder region
716.62 Unspecified monoarthritis, upper arm
716.63 Unspecified monoarthritis, forearm
716.64 Unspecified monoarthritis, hand
716.65 Unspecified monoarthritis, pelvic region and thigh
716.66 Unspecified monoarthritis, lower leg
716.67 Unspecified monoarthritis, ankle and foot
716.68 Unspecified monoarthritis, other specified sites
716.90 Unspecified arthropathy, site unspecified
716.91 Unspecified arthropathy, shoulder region
716.92 Unspecified arthropathy, upper arm
716.93 Unspecified arthropathy, forearm
716.94 Unspecified arthopathy, hand
716.95 Unspecified arthropathy, pelvic region and thigh
716.96 Unspecified arthropathy, lower leg
716.97 Unspecified arthropathy, ankle and foot
716.99 Unspecified arthropathy, multiple sites
719.40 Pain in joint, site unspecified
719.41 Pain in joint, shoulder region
719.42 Pain in joint, upper arm
719.43 Pain in joint, forearm
719.44 Pain in joint, hand
719.45 Pain in joint, pelvic region and thigh
719.46 Pain in joint, lower leg
719.47 Pain in joint, ankle and foot
719.48 Pain in joint, other specified sites
719.49 Pain in joint, multiple sites
720.0 Ankylosing spondylitis
720.2 Sacroiliitis, not elsewhere classified
724.1 Pain in thoracic spine
724.2 Lumbago
724.3 Sciatica
724.4 Thoracic or lumbosacral neuritis or radiculitis, unspecified

724.5 Unspecified backache ▽
724.6 Disorders of sacrum
726.10 Unspecified disorders of bursae and tendons in shoulder region ▽
726.32 Lateral epicondylitis of elbow
727.00 Unspecified synovitis and tenosynovitis ▽
727.02 Giant cell tumor of tendon sheath
727.03 Trigger finger (acquired)
727.04 Radial styloid tenosynovitis
727.05 Other tenosynovitis of hand and wrist
727.06 Tenosynovitis of foot and ankle
727.09 Other synovitis and tenosynovitis
727.2 Specific bursitides often of occupational origin
727.3 Other bursitis disorders
728.71 Plantar fascial fibromatosis
729.2 Unspecified neuralgia, neuritis, and radiculitis ▽
729.4 Unspecified fasciitis ▽
729.5 Pain in soft tissues of limb
729.9 Other and unspecified disorders of soft tissue

ICD-9-CM Procedural

83.98 Injection of locally acting therapeutic substance into other soft tissue

HCPCS Level II Supplies & Services

J0704 Injection, betamethasone sodium phosphate, per 4 mg

20600

20600 Arthrocentesis, aspiration and/or injection; small joint or bursa (eg, fingers, toes)

ICD-9-CM Diagnostic

275.40 Unspecified disorder of calcium metabolism — (Use additional code to identify any associated mental retardation) ▽
275.41 Hypocalcemia — (Use additional code to identify any associated mental retardation)
275.42 Hypercalcemia — (Use additional code to identify any associated mental retardation)
275.49 Other disorders of calcium metabolism — (Use additional code to identify any associated mental retardation)
353.5 Neuralgic amyotrophy
354.0 Carpal tunnel syndrome
354.1 Other lesion of median nerve
354.2 Lesion of ulnar nerve
354.3 Lesion of radial nerve
354.5 Mononeuritis multiplex
354.8 Other mononeuritis of upper limb
354.9 Unspecified mononeuritis of upper limb ▽
355.6 Lesion of plantar nerve
357.1 Polyneuropathy in collagen vascular disease — (Code first underlying disease: 446.0, 710.0, 714.0) ☒
359.6 Symptomatic inflammatory myopathy in diseases classified elsewhere — (Code first underlying disease: 135, 140.0-208.9, 277.3, 446.0, 710.0, 710.1, 710.2, 714.0) ☒
712.17 Chondrocalcinosis due to dicalcium phosphate crystals, ankle and foot — (Code first underlying disease, 275.4) ☒
712.24 Chondrocalcinosis due to pyrophosphate crystals, hand — (Code first underlying disease, 275.4) ☒
712.25 Chondrocalcinosis due to pyrophosphate crystals, pelvic region and thigh — (Code first underlying disease, 275.4) ☒
712.26 Chondrocalcinosis due to pyrophosphate crystals, lower leg — (Code first underlying disease, 275.4) ☒
712.34 Chondrocalcinosis, cause unspecified, involving hand — (Code first underlying disease, 275.4) ▽ ☒
712.35 Chondrocalcinosis, cause unspecified, involving pelvic region and thigh — (Code first underlying disease, 275.4) ▽ ☒
712.36 Chondrocalcinosis, cause unspecified, involving lower leg — (Code first underlying disease, 275.4) ▽ ☒
712.37 Chondrocalcinosis, cause unspecified, involving ankle and foot — (Code first underlying disease, 275.4) ▽ ☒
712.84 Other specified crystal arthropathies, hand
712.85 Other specified crystal arthropathies, pelvic region and thigh
712.86 Other specified crystal arthropathies, lower leg
712.87 Other specified crystal arthropathies, ankle and foot
712.94 Unspecified crystal arthropathy, hand ▽
712.97 Unspecified crystal arthropathy, ankle and foot ▽
714.0 Rheumatoid arthritis — (Use additional code to identify manifestation: 357.1, 359.6)
715.00 Generalized osteoarthrosis, unspecified site ▽
715.04 Generalized osteoarthrosis, involving hand
715.09 Generalized osteoarthrosis, involving multiple sites
716.14 Traumatic arthropathy, hand
716.17 Traumatic arthropathy, ankle and foot
716.18 Traumatic arthropathy, other specified sites
716.19 Traumatic arthropathy, multiple sites
716.27 Allergic arthritis, ankle and foot
716.64 Unspecified monoarthritis, hand ▽
716.68 Unspecified monoarthritis, other specified sites ▽
716.84 Other specified arthropathy, hand
716.85 Other specified arthropathy, pelvic region and thigh
716.86 Other specified arthropathy, lower leg
716.87 Other specified arthropathy, ankle and foot
716.88 Other specified arthropathy, other specified sites
716.89 Other specified arthropathy, multiple sites
716.94 Unspecified arthopathy, hand ▽
716.95 Unspecified arthropathy, pelvic region and thigh ▽
716.96 Unspecified arthropathy, lower leg ▽
716.97 Unspecified arthropathy, ankle and foot ▽
716.98 Unspecified arthropathy, other unspecified sites ▽
716.99 Unspecified arthropathy, multiple sites ▽
719.00 Effusion of joint, site unspecified ▽
719.04 Effusion of hand joint
719.07 Effusion of ankle and foot joint
719.09 Effusion of joint, multiple sites
719.40 Pain in joint, site unspecified ▽
719.41 Pain in joint, shoulder region
719.42 Pain in joint, upper arm
719.43 Pain in joint, forearm
719.44 Pain in joint, hand
719.47 Pain in joint, ankle and foot
719.49 Pain in joint, multiple sites
727.00 Unspecified synovitis and tenosynovitis ▽
727.03 Trigger finger (acquired)
727.05 Other tenosynovitis of hand and wrist
727.06 Tenosynovitis of foot and ankle
727.09 Other synovitis and tenosynovitis
727.2 Specific bursitides often of occupational origin
727.40 Unspecified synovial cyst ▽
727.49 Other ganglion and cyst of synovium, tendon, and bursa

ICD-9-CM Procedural

81.91 Arthrocentesis
81.92 Injection of therapeutic substance into joint or ligament
82.92 Aspiration of bursa of hand
82.94 Injection of therapeutic substance into bursa of hand
82.95 Injection of therapeutic substance into tendon of hand
83.94 Aspiration of bursa
83.96 Injection of therapeutic substance into bursa

HCPCS Level II Supplies & Services

J0704 Injection, betamethasone sodium phosphate, per 4 mg

20605

20605 Arthrocentesis, aspiration and/or injection; intermediate joint or bursa (eg, temporomandibular, acromioclavicular, wrist, elbow or ankle, olecranon bursa)

ICD-9-CM Diagnostic

274.0 Gouty arthropathy — (Use additional code to identify any associated mental retardation)
275.40 Unspecified disorder of calcium metabolism — (Use additional code to identify any associated mental retardation) ▽
275.42 Hypercalcemia — (Use additional code to identify any associated mental retardation)
275.49 Other disorders of calcium metabolism — (Use additional code to identify any associated mental retardation)
277.1 Disorders of porphyrin metabolism — (Use additional code to identify any associated mental retardation)
277.3 Amyloidosis — (Use additional code to identify any associated mental retardation)
357.1 Polyneuropathy in collagen vascular disease — (Code first underlying disease: 446.0, 710.0, 714.0) ☒
359.6 Symptomatic inflammatory myopathy in diseases classified elsewhere — (Code first underlying disease: 135, 140.0-208.9, 277.3, 446.0, 710.0, 710.1, 710.2, 714.0) ☒

524.60 Unspecified temporomandibular joint disorders ▽

524.61 Adhesions and ankylosis (bony or fibrous) of temporomandibular joint

524.62 Arthralgia of temporomandibular joint

524.69 Other specified temporomandibular joint disorders

526.1 Fissural cysts of jaw

526.2 Other cysts of jaws

526.4 Inflammatory conditions of jaw

526.9 Unspecified disease of the jaws ▽

712.12 Chondrocalcinosis due to dicalcium phosphate crystals, upper arm — (Code first underlying disease, 275.4) ☒

712.13 Chondrocalcinosis due to dicalcium phosphate crystals, forearm — (Code first underlying disease, 275.4) ☒

712.17 Chondrocalcinosis due to dicalcium phosphate crystals, ankle and foot — (Code first underlying disease, 275.4) ☒

712.18 Chondrocalcinosis due to dicalcium phosphate crystals, other specified sites — (Code first underlying disease, 275.4) ☒

712.82 Other specified crystal arthropathies, upper arm

712.83 Other specified crystal arthropathies, forearm

712.87 Other specified crystal arthropathies, ankle and foot

712.88 Other specified crystal arthropathies, other specified sites

712.92 Unspecified crystal arthropathy, upper arm ▽

712.93 Unspecified crystal arthropathy, forearm ▽

712.97 Unspecified crystal arthropathy, ankle and foot ▽

712.98 Unspecified crystal arthropathy, other specified sites ▽

714.0 Rheumatoid arthritis — (Use additional code to identify manifestation: 357.1, 359.6)

715.00 Generalized osteoarthrosis, unspecified site ▽

715.04 Generalized osteoarthrosis, involving hand

715.12 Primary localized osteoarthrosis, upper arm

715.13 Primary localized osteoarthrosis, forearm

715.14 Primary localized osteoarthrosis, hand

715.17 Primary localized osteoarthrosis, ankle and foot

715.20 Secondary localized osteoarthrosis, unspecified site ▽

715.22 Secondary localized osteoarthrosis, upper arm

715.23 Secondary localized osteoarthrosis, forearm

715.24 Secondary localized osteoarthrosis, involving hand

715.27 Secondary localized osteoarthrosis, ankle and foot

715.30 Localized osteoarthrosis not specified whether primary or secondary, unspecified site ▽

715.32 Localized osteoarthrosis not specified whether primary or secondary, upper arm

715.33 Localized osteoarthrosis not specified whether primary or secondary, forearm

715.34 Localized osteoarthrosis not specified whether primary or secondary, hand

715.37 Localized osteoarthrosis not specified whether primary or secondary, ankle and foot

715.38 Localized osteoarthrosis not specified whether primary or secondary, other specified sites

715.89 Osteoarthrosis involving multiple sites, but not specified as generalized

715.92 Osteoarthrosis, unspecified whether generalized or localized, upper arm ▽

715.93 Osteoarthrosis, unspecified whether generalized or localized, forearm ▽

715.94 Osteoarthrosis, unspecified whether generalized or localized, hand ▽

715.97 Osteoarthrosis, unspecified whether generalized or localized, ankle and foot ▽

716.10 Traumatic arthropathy, site unspecified ▽

716.12 Traumatic arthropathy, upper arm

716.13 Traumatic arthropathy, forearm

716.14 Traumatic arthropathy, hand

716.17 Traumatic arthropathy, ankle and foot

716.92 Unspecified arthropathy, upper arm ▽

716.93 Unspecified arthropathy, forearm ▽

716.94 Unspecified arthopathy, hand ▽

716.97 Unspecified arthropathy, ankle and foot ▽

719.00 Effusion of joint, site unspecified ▽

719.02 Effusion of upper arm joint

719.03 Effusion of forearm joint

719.04 Effusion of hand joint

719.07 Effusion of ankle and foot joint

719.10 Hemarthrosis, site unspecified ▽

719.12 Hemarthrosis, upper arm

719.13 Hemarthrosis, forearm

719.14 Hemarthrosis, hand

719.17 Hemarthrosis, ankle and foot

719.40 Pain in joint, site unspecified ▽

719.42 Pain in joint, upper arm

719.43 Pain in joint, forearm

719.44 Pain in joint, hand

719.47 Pain in joint, ankle and foot

726.30 Unspecified enthesopathy of elbow ▽

726.31 Medial epicondylitis of elbow

726.32 Lateral epicondylitis of elbow

726.33 Olecranon bursitis

726.39 Other enthesopathy of elbow region

726.4 Enthesopathy of wrist and carpus

726.70 Unspecified enthesopathy of ankle and tarsus ▽

726.71 Achilles bursitis or tendinitis

727.00 Unspecified synovitis and tenosynovitis ▽

727.04 Radial styloid tenosynovitis

727.05 Other tenosynovitis of hand and wrist

727.06 Tenosynovitis of foot and ankle

727.09 Other synovitis and tenosynovitis

830.0 Closed dislocation of jaw

848.1 Sprain and strain of jaw

905.0 Late effect of fracture of skull and face bones

ICD-9-CM Procedural

76.96 Injection of therapeutic substance into temporomandibular joint

81.91 Arthrocentesis

81.92 Injection of therapeutic substance into joint or ligament

83.94 Aspiration of bursa

83.96 Injection of therapeutic substance into bursa

HCPCS Level II Supplies & Services

J0704 Injection, betamethasone sodium phosphate, per 4 mg

20610

20610 Arthrocentesis, aspiration and/or injection; major joint or bursa (eg, shoulder, hip, knee joint, subacromial bursa)

ICD-9-CM Diagnostic

274.0 Gouty arthropathy — (Use additional code to identify any associated mental retardation)

275.40 Unspecified disorder of calcium metabolism — (Use additional code to identify any associated mental retardation) ▽

275.42 Hypercalcemia — (Use additional code to identify any associated mental retardation)

275.49 Other disorders of calcium metabolism — (Use additional code to identify any associated mental retardation)

357.1 Polyneuropathy in collagen vascular disease — (Code first underlying disease: 446.0, 710.0, 714.0) ☒

359.6 Symptomatic inflammatory myopathy in diseases classified elsewhere — (Code first underlying disease: 135, 140.0-208.9, 277.3, 446.0, 710.0, 710.1, 710.2, 714.0) ☒

712.11 Chondrocalcinosis due to dicalcium phosphate crystals, shoulder region — (Code first underlying disease, 275.4) ☒

712.15 Chondrocalcinosis due to dicalcium phosphate crystals, pelvic region and thigh — (Code first underlying disease, 275.4) ☒

712.16 Chondrocalcinosis due to dicalcium phosphate crystals, lower leg — (Code first underlying disease, 275.4) ☒

712.18 Chondrocalcinosis due to dicalcium phosphate crystals, other specified sites — (Code first underlying disease, 275.4) ☒

712.19 Chondrocalcinosis due to dicalcium phosphate crystals, multiple sites — (Code first underlying disease, 275.4) ☒

712.21 Chondrocalcinosis due to pyrophosphate crystals, shoulder region — (Code first underlying disease, 275.4) ☒

712.25 Chondrocalcinosis due to pyrophosphate crystals, pelvic region and thigh — (Code first underlying disease, 275.4) ☒

712.26 Chondrocalcinosis due to pyrophosphate crystals, lower leg — (Code first underlying disease, 275.4) ☒

712.28 Chondrocalcinosis due to pyrophosphate crystals, other specified sites — (Code first underlying disease, 275.4) ☒

712.29 Chondrocalcinosis due to pyrophosphate crystals, multiple sites — (Code first underlying disease, 275.4) ☒

712.31 Chondrocalcinosis, cause unspecified, involving shoulder region — (Code first underlying disease, 275.4) ▽ ☒

712.39 Chondrocalcinosis, cause unspecified, involving multiple sites — (Code first underlying disease, 275.4) ▽ ☒

714.0 Rheumatoid arthritis — (Use additional code to identify manifestation: 357.1, 359.6)

715.00 Generalized osteoarthrosis, unspecified site ▽

715.09 Generalized osteoarthrosis, involving multiple sites

715.11 Primary localized osteoarthrosis, shoulder region

715.15 Primary localized osteoarthrosis, pelvic region and thigh

715.16 Primary localized osteoarthrosis, lower leg

715.18 Primary localized osteoarthrosis, other specified sites

715.91 Osteoarthrosis, unspecified whether generalized or localized, shoulder region
715.95 Osteoarthrosis, unspecified whether generalized or localized, pelvic region and thigh
715.96 Osteoarthrosis, unspecified whether generalized or localized, lower leg
715.98 Osteoarthrosis, unspecified whether generalized or localized, other specified sites
716.90 Unspecified arthropathy, site unspecified
716.91 Unspecified arthropathy, shoulder region
716.95 Unspecified arthropathy, pelvic region and thigh
716.96 Unspecified arthropathy, lower leg
716.98 Unspecified arthropathy, other unspecified sites
716.99 Unspecified arthropathy, multiple sites
717.9 Unspecified internal derangement of knee
719.01 Effusion of shoulder joint
719.05 Effusion of pelvic joint
719.06 Effusion of lower leg joint
719.09 Effusion of joint, multiple sites
719.10 Hemarthrosis, site unspecified
719.11 Herarthrosis, shoulder region
719.15 Hemarthrosis, pelvic region and thigh
719.16 Hemarthrosis, lower leg
719.19 Hemarthrosis, multiple sites
719.20 Villonodular synovitis, site unspecified
719.21 Villonodular synovitis, shoulder region
719.25 Villonodular synovitis, pelvic region and thigh
719.26 Villonodular synovitis, lower leg
719.28 Villonodular synovitis, other specified sites
719.29 Villonodular synovitis, multiple sites
719.41 Pain in joint, shoulder region
719.45 Pain in joint, pelvic region and thigh
719.46 Pain in joint, lower leg
719.49 Pain in joint, multiple sites
726.5 Enthesopathy of hip region
726.60 Unspecified enthesopathy of knee
726.61 Pes anserinus tendinitis or bursitis
726.62 Tibial collateral ligament bursitis
726.63 Fibular collateral ligament bursitis
726.64 Patellar tendinitis
726.65 Prepatellar bursitis
726.69 Other enthesopathy of knee
727.3 Other bursitis disorders

ICD-9-CM Procedural

81.91 Arthrocentesis
81.92 Injection of therapeutic substance into joint or ligament
83.94 Aspiration of bursa
83.96 Injection of therapeutic substance into bursa

HCPCS Level II Supplies & Services

J0704 Injection, betamethasone sodium phosphate, per 4 mg

20612

20612 Aspiration and/or injection of ganglion cyst(s) any location

ICD-9-CM Diagnostic

727.40 Unspecified synovial cyst
727.41 Ganglion of joint
727.42 Ganglion of tendon sheath
727.43 Unspecified ganglion
727.49 Other ganglion and cyst of synovium, tendon, and bursa

ICD-9-CM Procedural

05.39 Other injection into sympathetic nerve or ganglion

HCPCS Level II Supplies & Services

A4550 Surgical trays

20615

20615 Aspiration and injection for treatment of bone cyst

ICD-9-CM Diagnostic

526.0 Developmental odontogenic cysts
526.1 Fissural cysts of jaw
526.2 Other cysts of jaws
526.89 Other specified disease of the jaws
733.20 Unspecified cyst of bone (localized)
733.21 Solitary bone cyst
733.22 Aneurysmal bone cyst
733.29 Other cyst of bone

ICD-9-CM Procedural

78.40 Other repair or plastic operations on bone, unspecified site
78.41 Other repair or plastic operations on scapula, clavicle, and thorax (ribs and sternum)
78.43 Other repair or plastic operations on radius and ulna
78.44 Other repair or plastic operations on carpals and metacarpals
78.45 Other repair or plastic operations on femur
78.46 Other repair or plastic operations on patella
78.47 Other repair or plastic operations on tibia and fibula
78.48 Other repair or plastic operations on tarsals and metatarsals
78.49 Other repair or plastic operations on other bone, except facial bones

HCPCS Level II Supplies & Services

A4550 Surgical trays

20650

20650 Insertion of wire or pin with application of skeletal traction, including removal (separate procedure)

ICD-9-CM Diagnostic

733.93 Stress fracture of tibia or fibula
733.95 Stress fracture of other bone
808.0 Closed fracture of acetabulum
808.1 Open fracture of acetabulum
808.53 Multiple open pelvic fractures with disruption of pelvic circle
812.00 Closed fracture of unspecified part of upper end of humerus
812.01 Closed fracture of surgical neck of humerus
812.02 Closed fracture of anatomical neck of humerus
812.03 Closed fracture of greater tuberosity of humerus
812.09 Other closed fractures of upper end of humerus
812.10 Open fracture of unspecified part of upper end of humerus
812.11 Open fracture of surgical neck of humerus
812.12 Open fracture of anatomical neck of humerus
812.13 Open fracture of greater tuberosity of humerus
812.20 Closed fracture of unspecified part of humerus
812.21 Closed fracture of shaft of humerus
812.30 Open fracture of unspecified part of humerus
812.31 Open fracture of shaft of humerus
812.40 Closed fracture of unspecified part of lower end of humerus
812.41 Closed fracture of supracondylar humerus
812.42 Closed fracture of lateral condyle of humerus
812.43 Closed fracture of medial condyle of humerus
812.44 Closed fracture of unspecified condyle(s) of humerus
812.49 Other closed fracture of lower end of humerus
812.50 Open fracture of unspecified part of lower end of humerus
812.51 Open fracture of supracondylar humerus
812.52 Open fracture of lateral condyle of humerus
812.53 Open fracture of medial condyle of humerus
812.54 Open fracture of unspecified condyle(s) of humerus
812.59 Other open fracture of lower end of humerus
813.07 Other and unspecified closed fractures of proximal end of radius (alone)
813.17 Other and unspecified open fractures of proximal end of radius (alone)
820.00 Closed fracture of unspecified intracapsular section of neck of femur
820.01 Closed fracture of epiphysis (separation) (upper) of neck of femur
820.02 Closed fracture of midcervical section of femur
820.09 Other closed transcervical fracture of femur
820.10 Open fracture of unspecified intracapsular section of neck of femur
820.11 Open fracture of epiphysis (separation) (upper) of neck of femur
820.12 Open fracture of midcervical section of femur
820.13 Open fracture of base of neck of femur
820.19 Other open transcervical fracture of femur
820.20 Closed fracture of unspecified trochanteric section of femur
820.21 Closed fracture of intertrochanteric section of femur
820.22 Closed fracture of subtrochanteric section of femur
820.30 Open fracture of unspecified trochanteric section of femur
820.31 Open fracture of intertrochanteric section of femur
820.8 Closed fracture of unspecified part of neck of femur
820.9 Open fracture of unspecified part of neck of femur
821.00 Closed fracture of unspecified part of femur
821.01 Closed fracture of shaft of femur
821.10 Open fracture of unspecified part of femur

821.11 Open fracture of shaft of femur
821.20 Closed fracture of unspecified part of lower end of femur ▽
821.21 Closed fracture of femoral condyle
821.22 Closed fracture of lower epiphysis of femur
821.23 Closed supracondylar fracture of femur
821.30 Open fracture of unspecified part of lower end of femur ▽
821.31 Open fracture of femoral condyle
821.32 Open fracture of lower epiphysis of femur
821.33 Open supracondylar fracture of femur
821.39 Other open fracture of lower end of femur
823.00 Closed fracture of upper end of tibia
823.01 Closed fracture of upper end of fibula
823.02 Closed fracture of upper end of fibula with tibia
823.10 Open fracture of upper end of tibia
823.11 Open fracture of upper end of fibula
823.12 Open fracture of upper end of fibula with tibia
823.20 Closed fracture of shaft of tibia
823.21 Closed fracture of shaft of fibula
823.22 Closed fracture of shaft of fibula with tibia
823.30 Open fracture of shaft of tibia
823.31 Open fracture of shaft of fibula
823.32 Open fracture of shaft of fibula with tibia
823.80 Closed fracture of unspecified part of tibia ▽
823.81 Closed fracture of unspecified part of fibula ▽
823.82 Closed fracture of unspecified part of fibula with tibia ▽
823.90 Open fracture of unspecified part of tibia ▽
823.91 Open fracture of unspecified part of fibula ▽
823.92 Open fracture of unspecified part of fibula with tibia ▽

ICD-9-CM Procedural
93.44 Other skeletal traction

HCPCS Level II Supplies & Services
A4305 Disposable drug delivery system, flow rate of 50 ml or greater per hour
A4306 Disposable drug delivery system, flow rate of 5 ml or less per hour
A4550 Surgical trays

20660
20660 Application of cranial tongs, caliper, or stereotactic frame, including removal (separate procedure)

ICD-9-CM Diagnostic
805.00 Closed fracture of cervical vertebra, unspecified level without mention of spinal cord injury ▽
805.01 Closed fracture of first cervical vertebra without mention of spinal cord injury
805.02 Closed fracture of second cervical vertebra without mention of spinal cord injury
805.03 Closed fracture of third cervical vertebra without mention of spinal cord injury
805.04 Closed fracture of fourth cervical vertebra without mention of spinal cord injury
805.05 Closed fracture of fifth cervical vertebra without mention of spinal cord injury
805.06 Closed fracture of sixth cervical vertebra without mention of spinal cord injury
805.07 Closed fracture of seventh cervical vertebra without mention of spinal cord injury
805.08 Closed fracture of multiple cervical vertebrae without mention of spinal cord injury
805.10 Open fracture of cervical vertebra, unspecified level without mention of spinal cord injury ▽
805.11 Open fracture of first cervical vertebra without mention of spinal cord injury
805.12 Open fracture of second cervical vertebra without mention of spinal cord injury
805.13 Open fracture of third cervical vertebra without mention of spinal cord injury
805.14 Open fracture of fourth cervical vertebra without mention of spinal cord injury
805.15 Open fracture of fifth cervical vertebra without mention of spinal cord injury
805.16 Open fracture of sixth cervical vertebra without mention of spinal cord injury
805.17 Open fracture of seventh cervical vertebra without mention of spinal cord injury
805.18 Open fracture of multiple cervical vertebrae without mention of spinal cord injury
806.00 Closed fracture of C1-C4 level with unspecified spinal cord injury ▽
806.01 Closed fracture of C1-C4 level with complete lesion of cord
806.02 Closed fracture of C1-C4 level with anterior cord syndrome
806.03 Closed fracture of C1-C4 level with central cord syndrome
806.04 Closed fracture of C1-C4 level with other specified spinal cord injury
806.05 Closed fracture of C5-C7 level with unspecified spinal cord injury ▽
806.06 Closed fracture of C5-C7 level with complete lesion of cord
806.07 Closed fracture of C5-C7 level with anterior cord syndrome
806.08 Closed fracture of C5-C7 level with central cord syndrome
806.09 Closed fracture of C5-C7 level with other specified spinal cord injury
806.10 Open fracture of C1-C4 level with unspecified spinal cord injury ▽
806.11 Open fracture of C1-C4 level with complete lesion of cord
806.12 Open fracture of C1-C4 level with anterior cord syndrome
806.13 Open fracture of C1-C4 level with central cord syndrome
806.14 Open fracture of C1-C4 level with other specified spinal cord injury
806.15 Open fracture of C5-C7 level with unspecified spinal cord injury ▽
806.16 Open fracture of C5-C7 level with complete lesion of cord
806.17 Open fracture of C5-C7 level with anterior cord syndrome
806.18 Open fracture of C5-C7 level with central cord syndrome
806.19 Open fracture of C5-C7 level with other specified spinal cord injury

ICD-9-CM Procedural
02.94 Insertion or replacement of skull tongs or halo traction device
02.95 Removal of skull tongs or halo traction device
93.41 Spinal traction using skull device
93.59 Other immobilization, pressure, and attention to wound

20661
20661 Application of halo, including removal; cranial

ICD-9-CM Diagnostic
805.00 Closed fracture of cervical vertebra, unspecified level without mention of spinal cord injury ▽
805.01 Closed fracture of first cervical vertebra without mention of spinal cord injury
805.02 Closed fracture of second cervical vertebra without mention of spinal cord injury
805.03 Closed fracture of third cervical vertebra without mention of spinal cord injury
805.04 Closed fracture of fourth cervical vertebra without mention of spinal cord injury
805.05 Closed fracture of fifth cervical vertebra without mention of spinal cord injury
805.06 Closed fracture of sixth cervical vertebra without mention of spinal cord injury
805.07 Closed fracture of seventh cervical vertebra without mention of spinal cord injury
805.08 Closed fracture of multiple cervical vertebrae without mention of spinal cord injury
805.10 Open fracture of cervical vertebra, unspecified level without mention of spinal cord injury ▽
805.11 Open fracture of first cervical vertebra without mention of spinal cord injury
805.12 Open fracture of second cervical vertebra without mention of spinal cord injury
805.13 Open fracture of third cervical vertebra without mention of spinal cord injury
805.14 Open fracture of fourth cervical vertebra without mention of spinal cord injury
805.15 Open fracture of fifth cervical vertebra without mention of spinal cord injury
805.16 Open fracture of sixth cervical vertebra without mention of spinal cord injury
805.17 Open fracture of seventh cervical vertebra without mention of spinal cord injury
805.18 Open fracture of multiple cervical vertebrae without mention of spinal cord injury
806.00 Closed fracture of C1-C4 level with unspecified spinal cord injury ▽
806.01 Closed fracture of C1-C4 level with complete lesion of cord
806.02 Closed fracture of C1-C4 level with anterior cord syndrome
806.03 Closed fracture of C1-C4 level with central cord syndrome
806.04 Closed fracture of C1-C4 level with other specified spinal cord injury
806.05 Closed fracture of C5-C7 level with unspecified spinal cord injury ▽
806.06 Closed fracture of C5-C7 level with complete lesion of cord
806.07 Closed fracture of C5-C7 level with anterior cord syndrome
806.08 Closed fracture of C5-C7 level with central cord syndrome
806.09 Closed fracture of C5-C7 level with other specified spinal cord injury
806.10 Open fracture of C1-C4 level with unspecified spinal cord injury ▽
806.11 Open fracture of C1-C4 level with complete lesion of cord
806.12 Open fracture of C1-C4 level with anterior cord syndrome
806.13 Open fracture of C1-C4 level with central cord syndrome
806.14 Open fracture of C1-C4 level with other specified spinal cord injury
806.15 Open fracture of C5-C7 level with unspecified spinal cord injury ▽
806.16 Open fracture of C5-C7 level with complete lesion of cord
806.17 Open fracture of C5-C7 level with anterior cord syndrome
806.18 Open fracture of C5-C7 level with central cord syndrome
806.19 Open fracture of C5-C7 level with other specified spinal cord injury

ICD-9-CM Procedural
02.94 Insertion or replacement of skull tongs or halo traction device
02.95 Removal of skull tongs or halo traction device
93.41 Spinal traction using skull device

HCPCS Level II Supplies & Services
L0810 Halo procedure, cervical halo incorporated into jacket vest

▽ Unspecified code
♀ Female diagnosis
☒ Manifestation code
♂ Male diagnosis

20662

20662 Application of halo, including removal; pelvic

ICD-9-CM Diagnostic

808.0 Closed fracture of acetabulum
808.1 Open fracture of acetabulum
808.2 Closed fracture of pubis
808.3 Open fracture of pubis
808.41 Closed fracture of ilium
808.42 Closed fracture of ischium
808.43 Multiple closed pelvic fractures with disruption of pelvic circle
808.49 Closed fracture of other specified part of pelvis
808.51 Open fracture of ilium
808.52 Open fracture of ischium
808.53 Multiple open pelvic fractures with disruption of pelvic circle
808.59 Open fracture of other specified part of pelvis

ICD-9-CM Procedural

02.94 Insertion or replacement of skull tongs or halo traction device
02.95 Removal of skull tongs or halo traction device
93.41 Spinal traction using skull device

20663

20663 Application of halo, including removal; femoral

ICD-9-CM Diagnostic

820.00 Closed fracture of unspecified intracapsular section of neck of femur ▽
820.01 Closed fracture of epiphysis (separation) (upper) of neck of femur
820.02 Closed fracture of midcervical section of femur
820.03 Closed fracture of base of neck of femur
820.09 Other closed transcervical fracture of femur
820.10 Open fracture of unspecified intracapsular section of neck of femur ▽
820.11 Open fracture of epiphysis (separation) (upper) of neck of femur
820.12 Open fracture of midcervical section of femur
820.13 Open fracture of base of neck of femur
820.19 Other open transcervical fracture of femur
820.20 Closed fracture of unspecified trochanteric section of femur ▽
820.21 Closed fracture of intertrochanteric section of femur
820.22 Closed fracture of subtrochanteric section of femur
820.30 Open fracture of unspecified trochanteric section of femur ▽
820.31 Open fracture of intertrochanteric section of femur
820.32 Open fracture of subtrochanteric section of femur
820.8 Closed fracture of unspecified part of neck of femur ▽
821.01 Closed fracture of shaft of femur
821.11 Open fracture of shaft of femur
821.21 Closed fracture of femoral condyle
821.22 Closed fracture of lower epiphysis of femur
821.23 Closed supracondylar fracture of femur
821.29 Other closed fracture of lower end of femur
821.31 Open fracture of femoral condyle
821.32 Open fracture of lower epiphysis of femur
821.33 Open supracondylar fracture of femur
821.39 Other open fracture of lower end of femur

ICD-9-CM Procedural

02.94 Insertion or replacement of skull tongs or halo traction device
02.95 Removal of skull tongs or halo traction device
93.41 Spinal traction using skull device

20664

20664 Application of halo, including removal, cranial, 6 or more pins placed, for thin skull osteology (eg, pediatric patients, hydrocephalus, osteogenesis imperfecta), requiring general anesthesia

ICD-9-CM Diagnostic

733.90 Disorder of bone and cartilage, unspecified ▽
741.00 Spina bifida with hydrocephalus, unspecified region ▽
741.01 Spina bifida with hydrocephalus, cervical region
741.02 Spina bifida with hydrocephalus, dorsal (thoracic) region
741.03 Spina bifida with hydrocephalus, lumbar region
742.3 Congenital hydrocephalus
756.0 Congenital anomalies of skull and face bones
756.51 Osteogenesis imperfecta
805.01 Closed fracture of first cervical vertebra without mention of spinal cord injury
805.02 Closed fracture of second cervical vertebra without mention of spinal cord injury
805.03 Closed fracture of third cervical vertebra without mention of spinal cord injury
805.04 Closed fracture of fourth cervical vertebra without mention of spinal cord injury
805.05 Closed fracture of fifth cervical vertebra without mention of spinal cord injury
805.06 Closed fracture of sixth cervical vertebra without mention of spinal cord injury
805.07 Closed fracture of seventh cervical vertebra without mention of spinal cord injury
805.08 Closed fracture of multiple cervical vertebrae without mention of spinal cord injury
805.11 Open fracture of first cervical vertebra without mention of spinal cord injury
805.12 Open fracture of second cervical vertebra without mention of spinal cord injury
805.13 Open fracture of third cervical vertebra without mention of spinal cord injury
805.14 Open fracture of fourth cervical vertebra without mention of spinal cord injury
805.15 Open fracture of fifth cervical vertebra without mention of spinal cord injury
805.16 Open fracture of sixth cervical vertebra without mention of spinal cord injury
805.17 Open fracture of seventh cervical vertebra without mention of spinal cord injury
805.18 Open fracture of multiple cervical vertebrae without mention of spinal cord injury
806.00 Closed fracture of C1-C4 level with unspecified spinal cord injury ▽
806.01 Closed fracture of C1-C4 level with complete lesion of cord
806.02 Closed fracture of C1-C4 level with anterior cord syndrome
806.03 Closed fracture of C1-C4 level with central cord syndrome
806.04 Closed fracture of C1-C4 level with other specified spinal cord injury
806.05 Closed fracture of C5-C7 level with unspecified spinal cord injury ▽
806.06 Closed fracture of C5-C7 level with complete lesion of cord
806.07 Closed fracture of C5-C7 level with anterior cord syndrome
806.08 Closed fracture of C5-C7 level with central cord syndrome
806.09 Closed fracture of C5-C7 level with other specified spinal cord injury
806.10 Open fracture of C1-C4 level with unspecified spinal cord injury ▽
806.11 Open fracture of C1-C4 level with complete lesion of cord
806.12 Open fracture of C1-C4 level with anterior cord syndrome
806.13 Open fracture of C1-C4 level with central cord syndrome
806.14 Open fracture of C1-C4 level with other specified spinal cord injury
806.15 Open fracture of C5-C7 level with unspecified spinal cord injury ▽
806.16 Open fracture of C5-C7 level with complete lesion of cord
806.17 Open fracture of C5-C7 level with anterior cord syndrome
806.18 Open fracture of C5-C7 level with central cord syndrome
806.19 Open fracture of C5-C7 level with other specified spinal cord injury

ICD-9-CM Procedural

02.94 Insertion or replacement of skull tongs or halo traction device
02.95 Removal of skull tongs or halo traction device
93.41 Spinal traction using skull device

20665

20665 Removal of tongs or halo applied by another physician

ICD-9-CM Diagnostic

805.01 Closed fracture of first cervical vertebra without mention of spinal cord injury
805.02 Closed fracture of second cervical vertebra without mention of spinal cord injury
805.03 Closed fracture of third cervical vertebra without mention of spinal cord injury
805.04 Closed fracture of fourth cervical vertebra without mention of spinal cord injury
805.05 Closed fracture of fifth cervical vertebra without mention of spinal cord injury
805.06 Closed fracture of sixth cervical vertebra without mention of spinal cord injury
805.07 Closed fracture of seventh cervical vertebra without mention of spinal cord injury
805.08 Closed fracture of multiple cervical vertebrae without mention of spinal cord injury
805.10 Open fracture of cervical vertebra, unspecified level without mention of spinal cord injury ▽
805.11 Open fracture of first cervical vertebra without mention of spinal cord injury
805.12 Open fracture of second cervical vertebra without mention of spinal cord injury
805.13 Open fracture of third cervical vertebra without mention of spinal cord injury
805.14 Open fracture of fourth cervical vertebra without mention of spinal cord injury
805.15 Open fracture of fifth cervical vertebra without mention of spinal cord injury
805.16 Open fracture of sixth cervical vertebra without mention of spinal cord injury
805.17 Open fracture of seventh cervical vertebra without mention of spinal cord injury
805.18 Open fracture of multiple cervical vertebrae without mention of spinal cord injury
806.01 Closed fracture of C1-C4 level with complete lesion of cord
806.02 Closed fracture of C1-C4 level with anterior cord syndrome
806.03 Closed fracture of C1-C4 level with central cord syndrome

806.04 Closed fracture of C1-C4 level with other specified spinal cord injury
806.05 Closed fracture of C5-C7 level with unspecified spinal cord injury
806.06 Closed fracture of C5-C7 level with complete lesion of cord
806.07 Closed fracture of C5-C7 level with anterior cord syndrome
806.08 Closed fracture of C5-C7 level with central cord syndrome
806.09 Closed fracture of C5-C7 level with other specified spinal cord injury
806.10 Open fracture of C1-C4 level with unspecified spinal cord injury
806.11 Open fracture of C1-C4 level with complete lesion of cord
806.12 Open fracture of C1-C4 level with anterior cord syndrome
806.13 Open fracture of C1-C4 level with central cord syndrome
806.14 Open fracture of C1-C4 level with other specified spinal cord injury
806.15 Open fracture of C5-C7 level with unspecified spinal cord injury
806.16 Open fracture of C5-C7 level with complete lesion of cord
806.17 Open fracture of C5-C7 level with anterior cord syndrome
806.18 Open fracture of C5-C7 level with central cord syndrome
806.19 Open fracture of C5-C7 level with other specified spinal cord injury
808.2 Closed fracture of pubis
808.3 Open fracture of pubis
808.41 Closed fracture of ilium
808.42 Closed fracture of ischium
808.43 Multiple closed pelvic fractures with disruption of pelvic circle
808.51 Open fracture of ilium
808.52 Open fracture of ischium
808.53 Multiple open pelvic fractures with disruption of pelvic circle
821.01 Closed fracture of shaft of femur
821.11 Open fracture of shaft of femur
821.20 Closed fracture of unspecified part of lower end of femur
821.29 Other closed fracture of lower end of femur
821.30 Open fracture of unspecified part of lower end of femur
821.39 Other open fracture of lower end of femur
996.4 Mechanical complication of internal orthopedic device, implant, and graft
996.78 Other complications due to other internal orthopedic device, implant, and graft
V54.01 Encounter for removal of internal fixation device
V54.17 Aftercare for healing traumatic fracture of vertebrae
V54.89 Other orthopedic aftercare
V67.4 Treatment of healed fracture follow-up examination

ICD-9-CM Procedural

02.95 Removal of skull tongs or halo traction device

HCPCS Level II Supplies & Services

A4550 Surgical trays

20670–20680

20670 Removal of implant; superficial, (eg, buried wire, pin or rod) (separate procedure)
20680 deep (eg, buried wire, pin, screw, metal band, nail, rod or plate)

ICD-9-CM Diagnostic

996.4 Mechanical complication of internal orthopedic device, implant, and graft
996.59 Mechanical complication due to other implant and internal device, not elsewhere classified
996.66 Infection and inflammatory reaction due to internal joint prosthesis — (Use additional code to identify specified infections)
996.67 Infection and inflammatory reaction due to other internal orthopedic device, implant, and graft — (Use additional code to identify specified infections)
996.77 Other complications due to internal joint prosthesis
996.78 Other complications due to other internal orthopedic device, implant, and graft
V54.01 Encounter for removal of internal fixation device
V54.10 Aftercare for healing traumatic fracture of arm, unspecified
V54.11 Aftercare for healing traumatic fracture of upper arm
V54.12 Aftercare for healing traumatic fracture of lower arm
V54.13 Aftercare for healing traumatic fracture of hip
V54.14 Aftercare for healing traumatic fracture of leg, unspecified
V54.15 Aftercare for healing traumatic fracture of upper leg
V54.16 Aftercare for healing traumatic fracture of lower leg
V54.19 Aftercare for healing traumatic fracture of other bone
V54.20 Aftercare for healing pathologic fracture of arm, unspecified
V54.21 Aftercare for healing pathologic fracture of upper arm
V54.22 Aftercare for healing pathologic fracture of lower arm
V54.23 Aftercare for healing pathologic fracture of hip
V54.24 Aftercare for healing pathologic fracture of leg, unspecified
V54.25 Aftercare for healing pathologic fracture of upper leg
V54.26 Aftercare for healing pathologic fracture of lower leg
V54.29 Aftercare for healing pathologic fracture of other bone
V54.81 Aftercare following joint replacement — (Use additional code to identify joint replacement site: V43.60-V43.69)
V54.89 Other orthopedic aftercare
V67.4 Treatment of healed fracture follow-up examination

ICD-9-CM Procedural

76.97 Removal of internal fixation device from facial bone
78.60 Removal of implanted device, unspecified site
78.61 Removal of implanted device from scapula, clavicle, and thorax (ribs and sternum)
78.62 Removal of implanted device from humerus
78.63 Removal of implanted device from radius and ulna
78.64 Removal of implanted device from carpals and metacarpals
78.65 Removal of implanted device from femur
78.66 Removal of implanted device from patella
78.67 Removal of implanted device from tibia and fibula
78.68 Removal of implanted device from tarsal and metatarsals
78.69 Removal of implanted device from other bone
80.02 Arthrotomy for removal of prosthesis of elbow
97.35 Removal of dental prosthesis
97.36 Removal of other external mandibular fixation device

HCPCS Level II Supplies & Services

A4305 Disposable drug delivery system, flow rate of 50 ml or greater per hour
A4306 Disposable drug delivery system, flow rate of 5 ml or less per hour
A4550 Surgical trays

20690–20692

20690 Application of a uniplane (pins or wires in one plane), unilateral, external fixation system
20692 Application of a multiplane (pins or wires in more than one plane), unilateral, external fixation system (eg, Ilizarov, Monticelli type)

ICD-9-CM Diagnostic

This is designated as an add-on code by Ingenix only. Refer to the corresponding primary procedure code for ICD-9 diagnosis code links.

ICD-9-CM Procedural

78.10 Application of external fixation device, unspecified site
78.11 Application of external fixation device, scapula, clavicle, and thorax (ribs and sternum)
78.12 Application of external fixation device, humerus
78.13 Application of external fixation device, radius and ulna
78.14 Application of external fixation device, carpals and metacarpals
78.15 Application of external fixation device, femur
78.16 Application of external fixation device, patella
78.17 Application of external fixation device, tibia and fibula
78.18 Application of external fixation device, tarsals and metatarsals
78.19 Application of external fixation device, other

HCPCS Level II Supplies & Services

A4305 Disposable drug delivery system, flow rate of 50 ml or greater per hour
A4306 Disposable drug delivery system, flow rate of 5 ml or less per hour
A4550 Surgical trays

20693

20693 Adjustment or revision of external fixation system requiring anesthesia (eg, new pin(s) or wire(s) and/or new ring(s) or bar(s))

ICD-9-CM Diagnostic

733.93 Stress fracture of tibia or fibula
733.95 Stress fracture of other bone
808.0 Closed fracture of acetabulum
808.1 Open fracture of acetabulum
808.2 Closed fracture of pubis
808.3 Open fracture of pubis
808.41 Closed fracture of ilium
808.42 Closed fracture of ischium
808.43 Multiple closed pelvic fractures with disruption of pelvic circle
808.49 Closed fracture of other specified part of pelvis
808.51 Open fracture of ilium
808.52 Open fracture of ischium
808.53 Multiple open pelvic fractures with disruption of pelvic circle
808.59 Open fracture of other specified part of pelvis
812.01 Closed fracture of surgical neck of humerus
812.02 Closed fracture of anatomical neck of humerus

812.09	Other closed fractures of upper end of humerus
812.11	Open fracture of surgical neck of humerus
812.12	Open fracture of anatomical neck of humerus
812.13	Open fracture of greater tuberosity of humerus
812.19	Other open fracture of upper end of humerus
812.21	Closed fracture of shaft of humerus
812.31	Open fracture of shaft of humerus
812.41	Closed fracture of supracondylar humerus
812.42	Closed fracture of lateral condyle of humerus
812.43	Closed fracture of medial condyle of humerus
812.44	Closed fracture of unspecified condyle(s) of humerus
812.49	Other closed fracture of lower end of humerus
812.51	Open fracture of supracondylar humerus
812.52	Open fracture of lateral condyle of humerus
812.53	Open fracture of medial condyle of humerus
812.54	Open fracture of unspecified condyle(s) of humerus
812.59	Other open fracture of lower end of humerus
813.01	Closed fracture of olecranon process of ulna
813.02	Closed fracture of coronoid process of ulna
813.03	Closed Monteggia's fracture
813.04	Other and unspecified closed fractures of proximal end of ulna (alone)
813.05	Closed fracture of head of radius
813.06	Closed fracture of neck of radius
813.07	Other and unspecified closed fractures of proximal end of radius (alone)
813.08	Closed fracture of radius with ulna, upper end (any part)
813.11	Open fracture of olecranon process of ulna
813.12	Open fracture of coronoid process of ulna
813.13	Open Monteggia's fracture
813.14	Other and unspecified open fractures of proximal end of ulna (alone)
813.15	Open fracture of head of radius
813.16	Open fracture of neck of radius
813.17	Other and unspecified open fractures of proximal end of radius (alone)
813.18	Open fracture of radius with ulna, upper end (any part)
813.21	Closed fracture of shaft of radius (alone)
813.22	Closed fracture of shaft of ulna (alone)
813.23	Closed fracture of shaft of radius with ulna
813.31	Open fracture of shaft of radius (alone)
813.32	Open fracture of shaft of ulna (alone)
813.33	Open fracture of shaft of radius with ulna
813.41	Closed Colles' fracture
813.42	Other closed fractures of distal end of radius (alone)
813.43	Closed fracture of distal end of ulna (alone)
813.44	Closed fracture of lower end of radius with ulna
813.51	Open Colles' fracture
813.52	Other open fractures of distal end of radius (alone)
813.53	Open fracture of distal end of ulna (alone)
813.54	Open fracture of lower end of radius with ulna
813.81	Closed fracture of unspecified part of radius (alone)
813.82	Closed fracture of unspecified part of ulna (alone)
813.83	Closed fracture of unspecified part of radius with ulna
813.91	Open fracture of unspecified part of radius (alone)
813.92	Open fracture of unspecified part of ulna (alone)
813.93	Open fracture of unspecified part of radius with ulna
814.00	Unspecified closed fracture of carpal bone
814.10	Unspecified open fracture of carpal bone
815.00	Closed fracture of metacarpal bone(s), site unspecified
815.09	Closed fracture of multiple sites of metacarpus
815.10	Open fracture of metacarpal bone(s), site unspecified
815.19	Open fracture of multiple sites of metacarpus
816.03	Closed fracture of multiple sites of phalanx or phalanges of hand
816.13	Open fractures of multiple sites of phalanx or phalanges of hand
819.0	Multiple closed fractures involving both upper limbs, and upper limb with rib(s) and sternum
819.1	Multiple open fractures involving both upper limbs, and upper limb with rib(s) and sternum
820.00	Closed fracture of unspecified intracapsular section of neck of femur
820.10	Open fracture of unspecified intracapsular section of neck of femur
820.19	Other open transcervical fracture of femur
820.20	Closed fracture of unspecified trochanteric section of femur
820.30	Open fracture of unspecified trochanteric section of femur
821.01	Closed fracture of shaft of femur
821.11	Open fracture of shaft of femur
821.20	Closed fracture of unspecified part of lower end of femur
821.21	Closed fracture of femoral condyle
821.22	Closed fracture of lower epiphysis of femur
821.23	Closed supracondylar fracture of femur
821.29	Other closed fracture of lower end of femur
821.30	Open fracture of unspecified part of lower end of femur
821.31	Open fracture of femoral condyle
821.32	Open fracture of lower epiphysis of femur
821.33	Open supracondylar fracture of femur
821.39	Other open fracture of lower end of femur
823.00	Closed fracture of upper end of tibia
823.01	Closed fracture of upper end of fibula
823.02	Closed fracture of upper end of fibula with tibia
823.10	Open fracture of upper end of tibia
823.11	Open fracture of upper end of fibula
823.12	Open fracture of upper end of fibula with tibia
823.20	Closed fracture of shaft of tibia
823.21	Closed fracture of shaft of fibula
823.22	Closed fracture of shaft of fibula with tibia
823.30	Open fracture of shaft of tibia
823.31	Open fracture of shaft of fibula
823.32	Open fracture of shaft of fibula with tibia
824.0	Closed fracture of medial malleolus
824.1	Open fracture of medial malleolus
824.2	Closed fracture of lateral malleolus
824.3	Open fracture of lateral malleolus
824.4	Closed bimalleolar fracture
824.5	Open bimalleolar fracture
824.6	Closed trimalleolar fracture
824.7	Open trimalleolar fracture
824.8	Unspecified closed fracture of ankle
824.9	Unspecified open fracture of ankle
827.0	Other, multiple and ill-defined closed fractures of lower limb
827.1	Other, multiple and ill-defined open fractures of lower limb
828.0	Multiple closed fractures involving both lower limbs, lower with upper limb, and lower limb(s) with rib(s) and sternum
828.1	Multiple fractures involving both lower limbs, lower with upper limb, and lower limb(s) with rib(s) and sternum, open
996.4	Mechanical complication of internal orthopedic device, implant, and graft
996.67	Infection and inflammatory reaction due to other internal orthopedic device, implant, and graft — (Use additional code to identify specified infections)
996.77	Other complications due to internal joint prosthesis
996.78	Other complications due to other internal orthopedic device, implant, and graft
V53.7	Fitting and adjustment of orthopedic device

ICD-9-CM Procedural

93.44	Other skeletal traction

20694

20694	Removal, under anesthesia, of external fixation system

ICD-9-CM Diagnostic

733.93	Stress fracture of tibia or fibula
733.95	Stress fracture of other bone
808.0	Closed fracture of acetabulum
808.1	Open fracture of acetabulum
808.2	Closed fracture of pubis
808.3	Open fracture of pubis
808.41	Closed fracture of ilium
808.42	Closed fracture of ischium
808.43	Multiple closed pelvic fractures with disruption of pelvic circle
808.49	Closed fracture of other specified part of pelvis
808.51	Open fracture of ilium
808.52	Open fracture of ischium
808.53	Multiple open pelvic fractures with disruption of pelvic circle
808.59	Open fracture of other specified part of pelvis
812.01	Closed fracture of surgical neck of humerus
812.02	Closed fracture of anatomical neck of humerus
812.09	Other closed fractures of upper end of humerus
812.11	Open fracture of surgical neck of humerus
812.12	Open fracture of anatomical neck of humerus
812.13	Open fracture of greater tuberosity of humerus
812.19	Other open fracture of upper end of humerus
812.21	Closed fracture of shaft of humerus
812.31	Open fracture of shaft of humerus
812.41	Closed fracture of supracondylar humerus
812.42	Closed fracture of lateral condyle of humerus
812.43	Closed fracture of medial condyle of humerus
812.44	Closed fracture of unspecified condyle(s) of humerus
812.49	Other closed fracture of lower end of humerus

812.51 Open fracture of supracondylar humerus
812.52 Open fracture of lateral condyle of humerus
812.53 Open fracture of medial condyle of humerus
812.54 Open fracture of unspecified condyle(s) of humerus ▽
812.59 Other open fracture of lower end of humerus
813.01 Closed fracture of olecranon process of ulna
813.02 Closed fracture of coronoid process of ulna
813.03 Closed Monteggia's fracture
813.04 Other and unspecified closed fractures of proximal end of ulna (alone) ▽
813.05 Closed fracture of head of radius
813.06 Closed fracture of neck of radius
813.07 Other and unspecified closed fractures of proximal end of radius (alone) ▽
813.08 Closed fracture of radius with ulna, upper end (any part)
813.11 Open fracture of olecranon process of ulna
813.12 Open fracture of coronoid process of ulna
813.13 Open Monteggia's fracture
813.14 Other and unspecified open fractures of proximal end of ulna (alone) ▽
813.15 Open fracture of head of radius
813.16 Open fracture of neck of radius
813.17 Other and unspecified open fractures of proximal end of radius (alone) ▽
813.18 Open fracture of radius with ulna, upper end (any part)
813.21 Closed fracture of shaft of radius (alone)
813.22 Closed fracture of shaft of ulna (alone)
813.23 Closed fracture of shaft of radius with ulna
813.31 Open fracture of shaft of radius (alone)
813.32 Open fracture of shaft of ulna (alone)
813.33 Open fracture of shaft of radius with ulna
813.41 Closed Colles' fracture
813.42 Other closed fractures of distal end of radius (alone)
813.43 Closed fracture of distal end of ulna (alone)
813.44 Closed fracture of lower end of radius with ulna
813.51 Open Colles' fracture
813.52 Other open fractures of distal end of radius (alone)
813.53 Open fracture of distal end of ulna (alone)
813.54 Open fracture of lower end of radius with ulna
813.81 Closed fracture of unspecified part of radius (alone) ▽
813.82 Closed fracture of unspecified part of ulna (alone) ▽
813.83 Closed fracture of unspecified part of radius with ulna ▽
813.91 Open fracture of unspecified part of radius (alone) ▽
813.92 Open fracture of unspecified part of ulna (alone) ▽
813.93 Open fracture of unspecified part of radius with ulna ▽
814.00 Unspecified closed fracture of carpal bone ▽
814.10 Unspecified open fracture of carpal bone ▽
815.00 Closed fracture of metacarpal bone(s), site unspecified ▽
815.09 Closed fracture of multiple sites of metacarpus
815.10 Open fracture of metacarpal bone(s), site unspecified ▽
815.19 Open fracture of multiple sites of metacarpus
816.03 Closed fracture of multiple sites of phalanx or phalanges of hand
816.13 Open fractures of multiple sites of phalanx or phalanges of hand
819.0 Multiple closed fractures involving both upper limbs, and upper limb with rib(s) and sternum
819.1 Multiple open fractures involving both upper limbs, and upper limb with rib(s) and sternum
820.00 Closed fracture of unspecified intracapsular section of neck of femur ▽
820.10 Open fracture of unspecified intracapsular section of neck of femur ▽
820.19 Other open transcervical fracture of femur
820.20 Closed fracture of unspecified trochanteric section of femur ▽
820.30 Open fracture of unspecified trochanteric section of femur ▽
821.01 Closed fracture of shaft of femur
821.11 Open fracture of shaft of femur
821.20 Closed fracture of unspecified part of lower end of femur ▽
821.21 Closed fracture of femoral condyle
821.22 Closed fracture of lower epiphysis of femur
821.23 Closed supracondylar fracture of femur
821.29 Other closed fracture of lower end of femur
821.30 Open fracture of unspecified part of lower end of femur ▽
821.31 Open fracture of femoral condyle
821.32 Open fracture of lower epiphysis of femur
821.33 Open supracondylar fracture of femur
821.39 Other open fracture of lower end of femur
823.00 Closed fracture of upper end of tibia
823.01 Closed fracture of upper end of fibula
823.02 Closed fracture of upper end of fibula with tibia
823.10 Open fracture of upper end of tibia
823.11 Open fracture of upper end of fibula
823.12 Open fracture of upper end of fibula with tibia
823.20 Closed fracture of shaft of tibia
823.21 Closed fracture of shaft of fibula
823.22 Closed fracture of shaft of fibula with tibia
823.30 Open fracture of shaft of tibia
823.31 Open fracture of shaft of fibula
823.32 Open fracture of shaft of fibula with tibia
824.0 Closed fracture of medial malleolus
824.1 Open fracture of medial malleolus
824.2 Closed fracture of lateral malleolus
824.3 Open fracture of lateral malleolus
824.4 Closed bimalleolar fracture
824.5 Open bimalleolar fracture
824.6 Closed trimalleolar fracture
824.7 Open trimalleolar fracture
824.8 Unspecified closed fracture of ankle ▽
824.9 Unspecified open fracture of ankle ▽
827.0 Other, multiple and ill-defined closed fractures of lower limb
827.1 Other, multiple and ill-defined open fractures of lower limb
828.0 Multiple closed fractures involving both lower limbs, lower with upper limb, and lower limb(s) with rib(s) and sternum
828.1 Multiple fractures involving both lower limbs, lower with upper limb, and lower limb(s) with rib(s) and sternum, open
996.4 Mechanical complication of internal orthopedic device, implant, and graft
996.67 Infection and inflammatory reaction due to other internal orthopedic device, implant, and graft — (Use additional code to identify specified infections)
996.77 Other complications due to internal joint prosthesis
996.78 Other complications due to other internal orthopedic device, implant, and graft
V54.01 Encounter for removal of internal fixation device
V54.10 Aftercare for healing traumatic fracture of arm, unspecified ▽
V54.11 Aftercare for healing traumatic fracture of upper arm
V54.12 Aftercare for healing traumatic fracture of lower arm
V54.14 Aftercare for healing traumatic fracture of leg, unspecified ▽
V54.16 Aftercare for healing traumatic fracture of lower leg
V54.19 Aftercare for healing traumatic fracture of other bone
V54.20 Aftercare for healing pathologic fracture of arm, unspecified ▽
V54.21 Aftercare for healing pathologic fracture of upper arm
V54.22 Aftercare for healing pathologic fracture of lower arm
V54.24 Aftercare for healing pathologic fracture of leg, unspecified ▽
V54.25 Aftercare for healing pathologic fracture of upper leg
V54.26 Aftercare for healing pathologic fracture of lower leg
V54.29 Aftercare for healing pathologic fracture of other bone
V54.89 Other orthopedic aftercare
V67.4 Treatment of healed fracture follow-up examination

ICD-9-CM Procedural

78.60 Removal of implanted device, unspecified site
78.61 Removal of implanted device from scapula, clavicle, and thorax (ribs and sternum)
78.62 Removal of implanted device from humerus
78.63 Removal of implanted device from radius and ulna
78.64 Removal of implanted device from carpals and metacarpals
78.65 Removal of implanted device from femur
78.66 Removal of implanted device from patella
78.67 Removal of implanted device from tibia and fibula
78.68 Removal of implanted device from tarsal and metatarsals
78.69 Removal of implanted device from other bone

20802

20802 Replantation, arm (includes surgical neck of humerus through elbow joint), complete amputation

ICD-9-CM Diagnostic

887.2 Traumatic amputation of arm and hand (complete) (partial), unilateral, at or above elbow, without mention of complication — (Use additional code to identify infection)
887.3 Traumatic amputation of arm and hand (complete) (partial), unilateral, at or above elbow, complicated — (Use additional code to identify infection)
887.6 Traumatic amputation of arm and hand (complete) (partial), bilateral (any level), without mention of complication — (Use additional code to identify infection)
887.7 Traumatic amputation of arm and hand (complete) (partial), bilateral (any level), complicated — (Use additional code to identify infection)

ICD-9-CM Procedural

84.24 Upper arm reattachment

20805

20805 Replantation, forearm (includes radius and ulna to radial carpal joint), complete amputation

ICD-9-CM Diagnostic

887.0 Traumatic amputation of arm and hand (complete) (partial), unilateral, below elbow, without mention of complication — (Use additional code to identify infection)
887.1 Traumatic amputation of arm and hand (complete) (partial), unilateral, below elbow, complicated — (Use additional code to identify infection)
887.6 Traumatic amputation of arm and hand (complete) (partial), bilateral (any level), without mention of complication — (Use additional code to identify infection)
887.7 Traumatic amputation of arm and hand (complete) (partial), bilateral (any level), complicated — (Use additional code to identify infection)

ICD-9-CM Procedural

84.23 Forearm, wrist, or hand reattachment

20808

20808 Replantation, hand (includes hand through metacarpophalangeal joints), complete amputation

ICD-9-CM Diagnostic

887.0 Traumatic amputation of arm and hand (complete) (partial), unilateral, below elbow, without mention of complication — (Use additional code to identify infection)
887.1 Traumatic amputation of arm and hand (complete) (partial), unilateral, below elbow, complicated — (Use additional code to identify infection)
887.4 Traumatic amputation of arm and hand (complete) (partial), unilateral, level not specified, without mention of complication — (Use additional code to identify infection) ▽
887.5 Traumatic amputation of arm and hand (complete) (partial), unilateral, level not specified, complicated — (Use additional code to identify infection) ▽
887.6 Traumatic amputation of arm and hand (complete) (partial), bilateral (any level), without mention of complication — (Use additional code to identify infection)
887.7 Traumatic amputation of arm and hand (complete) (partial), bilateral (any level), complicated — (Use additional code to identify infection)

ICD-9-CM Procedural

84.23 Forearm, wrist, or hand reattachment

20816–20822

20816 Replantation, digit, excluding thumb (includes metacarpophalangeal joint to insertion of flexor sublimis tendon), complete amputation
20822 Replantation, digit, excluding thumb (includes distal tip to sublimis tendon insertion), complete amputation

ICD-9-CM Diagnostic

886.0 Traumatic amputation of other finger(s) (complete) (partial), without mention of complication — (Use additional code to identify infection)
886.1 Traumatic amputation of other finger(s) (complete) (partial), complicated — (Use additional code to identify infection)
895.0 Traumatic amputation of toe(s) (complete) (partial), without mention of complication — (Use additional code to identify infection)
895.1 Traumatic amputation of toe(s) (complete) (partial), complicated — (Use additional code to identify infection)

ICD-9-CM Procedural

84.22 Finger reattachment
84.25 Toe reattachment

20824–20827

20824 Replantation, thumb (includes carpometacarpal joint to MP joint), complete amputation
20827 Replantation, thumb (includes distal tip to MP joint), complete amputation

ICD-9-CM Diagnostic

885.0 Traumatic amputation of thumb (complete) (partial), without mention of complication — (Use additional code to identify infection)
885.1 Traumatic amputation of thumb (complete) (partial), complicated — (Use additional code to identify infection)

ICD-9-CM Procedural

84.21 Thumb reattachment

20838

20838 Replantation, foot, complete amputation

ICD-9-CM Diagnostic

896.0 Traumatic amputation of foot (complete) (partial), unilateral, without mention of complication — (Use additional code to identify infection)
896.1 Traumatic amputation of foot (complete) (partial), unilateral, complicated — (Use additional code to identify infection)
896.2 Traumatic amputation of foot (complete) (partial), bilateral, without mention of complication — (Use additional code to identify infection)
896.3 Traumatic amputation of foot (complete) (partial), bilateral, complicated — (Use additional code to identify infection)

ICD-9-CM Procedural

84.26 Foot reattachment

20900–20902

20900 Bone graft, any donor area; minor or small (eg, dowel or button)
20902 major or large

ICD-9-CM Diagnostic

This is designated as an add-on code by Ingenix only. Refer to the corresponding primary procedure code for ICD-9 diagnosis code links.

ICD-9-CM Procedural

16.81 Repair of wound of orbit
76.91 Bone graft to facial bone
77.70 Excision of bone for graft, unspecified site
77.71 Excision of scapula, clavicle, and thorax (ribs and sternum) for graft
77.72 Excision of humerus for graft
77.73 Excision of radius and ulna for graft
77.74 Excision of carpals and metacarpals for graft
77.76 Excision of patella for graft
78.00 Bone graft, unspecified site
78.01 Bone graft of scapula, clavicle, and thorax (ribs and sternum)
78.02 Bone graft of humerus
78.03 Bone graft of radius and ulna
78.04 Bone graft of carpals and metacarpals
78.05 Bone graft of femur
78.06 Bone graft of patella
78.07 Bone graft of tibia and fibula
78.08 Bone graft of tarsals and metatarsals
78.09 Bone graft of other bone, except facial bones

HCPCS Level II Supplies & Services

A4305 Disposable drug delivery system, flow rate of 50 ml or greater per hour
A4306 Disposable drug delivery system, flow rate of 5 ml or less per hour
A4550 Surgical trays

20910–20912

20910 Cartilage graft; costochondral
20912 nasal septum

ICD-9-CM Diagnostic

This is designated as an add-on code by Ingenix only. Refer to the corresponding primary procedure code for ICD-9 diagnosis code links.

Cartilage for Graft

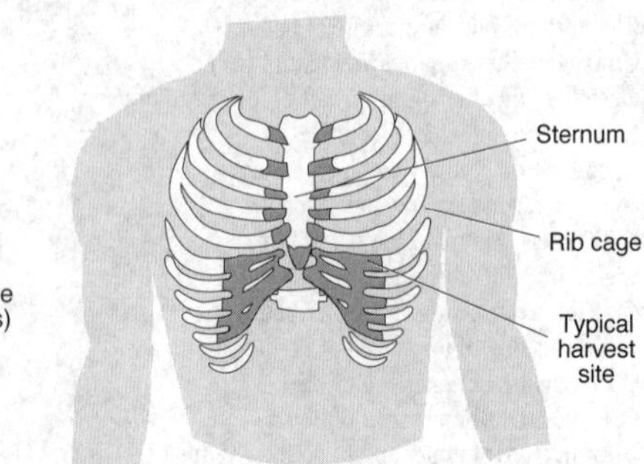

▽ Unspecified code ♀ Female diagnosis ☒ Manifestation code ♂ Male diagnosis

ICD-9-CM Procedural
18.71 Construction of auricle of ear
21.88 Other septoplasty
76.99 Other operations on facial bones and joints

20920–20922
20920 Fascia lata graft; by stripper
20922 by incision and area exposure, complex or sheet

ICD-9-CM Diagnostic
This is designated as an add-on code by Ingenix only. Refer to the corresponding primary procedure code for ICD-9 diagnosis code links.

ICD-9-CM Procedural
83.43 Excision of muscle or fascia for graft

20924
20924 Tendon graft, from a distance (eg, palmaris, toe extensor, plantaris)

ICD-9-CM Diagnostic
This is designated as an add-on code by Ingenix only. Refer to the corresponding primary procedure code for ICD-9 diagnosis code links.

ICD-9-CM Procedural
83.81 Tendon graft

20926
20926 Tissue grafts, other (eg, paratenon, fat, dermis)

ICD-9-CM Diagnostic
This is designated as an add-on code by Ingenix only. Refer to the corresponding primary procedure code for ICD-9 diagnosis code links.

ICD-9-CM Procedural
86.69 Other skin graft to other sites

20930
20930 Allograft for spine surgery only; morselized

ICD-9-CM Diagnostic
This is designated as an add-on code by Ingenix only. Refer to the corresponding primary procedure code for ICD-9 diagnosis code links.

ICD-9-CM Procedural
77.09 Sequestrectomy of other bone, except facial bones
77.70 Excision of bone for graft, unspecified site
77.71 Excision of scapula, clavicle, and thorax (ribs and sternum) for graft
77.79 Excision of other bone for graft, except facial bones

20931
20931 Allograft for spine surgery only; structural

ICD-9-CM Diagnostic
This is designated as an add-on code by Ingenix only. Refer to the corresponding primary procedure code for ICD-9 diagnosis code links.

ICD-9-CM Procedural
77.70 Excision of bone for graft, unspecified site
77.71 Excision of scapula, clavicle, and thorax (ribs and sternum) for graft
77.79 Excision of other bone for graft, except facial bones
78.09 Bone graft of other bone, except facial bones

20936–20938
20936 Autograft for spine surgery only (includes harvesting the graft); local (eg, ribs, spinous process, or laminar fragments) obtained from same incision
20937 morselized (through separate skin or fascial incision)
20938 structural, bicortical or tricortical (through separate skin or fascial incision)

ICD-9-CM Diagnostic
This is designated as an add-on code by Ingenix only. Refer to the corresponding primary procedure code for ICD-9 diagnosis code links.

ICD-9-CM Procedural
77.70 Excision of bone for graft, unspecified site

Autograft of Spine

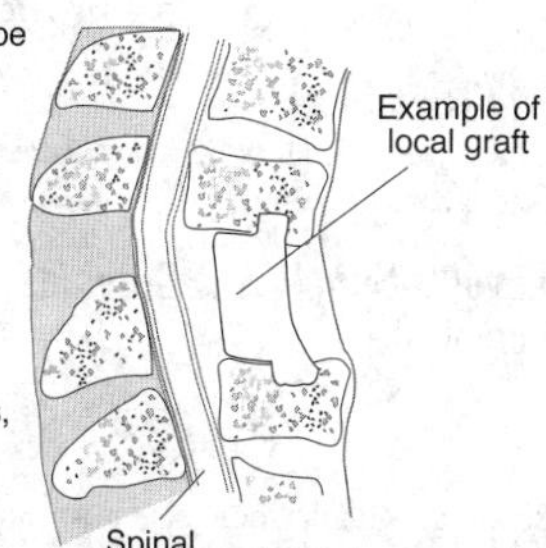
Local autograft is harvested, processed, and placed. Graft may be morselized (chipped), or fashioned into a structural graft.
Example of local graft
Grafts are typically harvested from costal area of ribs, spinous processes, or laminae and are always taken through the main surgical incision
Spinal cord
Lateral cutaway view

77.71 Excision of scapula, clavicle, and thorax (ribs and sternum) for graft
77.79 Excision of other bone for graft, except facial bones
78.09 Bone graft of other bone, except facial bones

20950
20950 Monitoring of interstitial fluid pressure (includes insertion of device, eg, wick catheter technique, needle manometer technique) in detection of muscle compartment syndrome

ICD-9-CM Diagnostic
286.6 Defibrination syndrome
728.86 Necrotizing fasciitis — (Use additional code to identify infectious organism, 041.00-041.89, 785.4, if applicable)
785.4 Gangrene — (Code first any associated underlying condition:250.7, 443.0)
925.1 Crushing injury of face and scalp — (Use additional code to identify any associated injuries: 800-829, 850.0-854.1, 860.0-869.1)
925.2 Crushing injury of neck — (Use additional code to identify any associated injuries: 800-829, 850.0-854.1, 860.0-869.1)
926.0 Crushing injury of external genitalia — (Use additional code to identify any associated injuries: 800-829, 850.0-854.1, 860.0-869.1)
926.11 Crushing injury of back — (Use additional code to identify any associated injuries: 800-829, 850.0-854.1, 860.0-869.1)
926.12 Crushing injury of buttock — (Use additional code to identify any associated injuries: 800-829, 850.0-854.1, 860.0-869.1)
926.19 Crushing injury of other specified sites of trunk — (Use additional code to identify any associated injuries: 800-829, 850.0-854.1, 860.0-869.1)
926.8 Crushing injury of multiple sites of trunk — (Use additional code to identify any associated injuries: 800-829, 850.0-854.1, 860.0-869.1)
927.00 Crushing injury of shoulder region — (Use additional code to identify any associated injuries: 800-829, 850.0-854.1, 860.0-869.1)
927.01 Crushing injury of scapular region — (Use additional code to identify any associated injuries: 800-829, 850.0-854.1, 860.0-869.1)
927.02 Crushing injury of axillary region — (Use additional code to identify any associated injuries: 800-829, 850.0-854.1, 860.0-869.1)
927.03 Crushing injury of upper arm — (Use additional code to identify any associated injuries: 800-829, 850.0-854.1, 860.0-869.1)
927.09 Crushing injury of multiple sites of upper arm — (Use additional code to identify any associated injuries: 800-829, 850.0-854.1, 860.0-869.1)
927.10 Crushing injury of forearm — (Use additional code to identify any associated injuries: 800-829, 850.0-854.1, 860.0-869.1)
927.11 Crushing injury of elbow — (Use additional code to identify any associated injuries: 800-829, 850.0-854.1, 860.0-869.1)
927.3 Crushing injury of finger(s) — (Use additional code to identify any associated injuries: 800-829, 850.0-854.1, 860.0-869.1)
927.8 Crushing injury of multiple sites of upper limb — (Use additional code to identify any associated injuries: 800-829, 850.0-854.1, 860.0-869.1)
928.00 Crushing injury of thigh — (Use additional code to identify any associated injuries: 800-829, 850.0-854.1, 860.0-869.1)
928.01 Crushing injury of hip — (Use additional code to identify any associated injuries: 800-829, 850.0-854.1, 860.0-869.1)
928.10 Crushing injury of lower leg — (Use additional code to identify any associated injuries: 800-829, 850.0-854.1, 860.0-869.1)
928.11 Crushing injury of knee — (Use additional code to identify any associated injuries: 800-829, 850.0-854.1, 860.0-869.1)
928.20 Crushing injury of foot — (Use additional code to identify any associated injuries: 800-829, 850.0-854.1, 860.0-869.1)
928.21 Crushing injury of ankle — (Use additional code to identify any associated injuries: 800-829, 850.0-854.1, 860.0-869.1)

928.3 Crushing injury of toe(s) — (Use additional code to identify any associated injuries: 800-829, 850.0-854.1, 860.0-869.1)
928.8 Crushing injury of multiple sites of lower limb — (Use additional code to identify any associated injuries: 800-829, 850.0-854.1, 860.0-869.1)

ICD-9-CM Procedural
83.29 Other diagnostic procedures on muscle, tendon, fascia, and bursa, including that of hand

HCPCS Level II Supplies & Services
A4550 Surgical trays

20955
20955 Bone graft with microvascular anastomosis; fibula

ICD-9-CM Diagnostic
170.1 Malignant neoplasm of mandible
198.5 Secondary malignant neoplasm of bone and bone marrow
213.0 Benign neoplasm of bones of skull and face
213.1 Benign neoplasm of lower jaw bone
239.2 Neoplasms of unspecified nature of bone, soft tissue, and skin
524.00 Unspecified major anomaly of jaw size
524.03 Maxillary hypoplasia
524.04 Mandibular hypoplasia
524.06 Microgenia
524.07 Excessive tuberosity of jaw
524.09 Other specified major anomaly of jaw size
524.11 Maxillary asymmetry
524.12 Other jaw asymmetry
524.19 Other specified anomaly of relationship of jaw to cranial base
524.69 Other specified temporomandibular joint disorders
524.74 Alveolar mandibular hypoplasia
526.89 Other specified disease of the jaws
730.18 Chronic osteomyelitis, other specified sites — (Use additional code to identify organism, 041.1)
733.49 Aseptic necrosis of other bone site
733.81 Malunion of fracture
733.82 Nonunion of fracture
905.0 Late effect of fracture of skull and face bones
925.1 Crushing injury of face and scalp — (Use additional code to identify any associated injuries: 800-829, 850.0-854.1, 860.0-869.1)
996.4 Mechanical complication of internal orthopedic device, implant, and graft

ICD-9-CM Procedural
76.41 Total mandibulectomy with synchronous reconstruction
76.44 Total ostectomy of other facial bone with synchronous reconstruction
76.91 Bone graft to facial bone
77.77 Excision of tibia and fibula for graft
78.07 Bone graft of tibia and fibula

20956
20956 Bone graft with microvascular anastomosis; iliac crest

ICD-9-CM Diagnostic
170.0 Malignant neoplasm of bones of skull and face, except mandible
170.1 Malignant neoplasm of mandible
170.2 Malignant neoplasm of vertebral column, excluding sacrum and coccyx
170.3 Malignant neoplasm of ribs, sternum, and clavicle
170.4 Malignant neoplasm of scapula and long bones of upper limb
170.5 Malignant neoplasm of short bones of upper limb
170.6 Malignant neoplasm of pelvic bones, sacrum, and coccyx
170.7 Malignant neoplasm of long bones of lower limb
170.8 Malignant neoplasm of short bones of lower limb
198.5 Secondary malignant neoplasm of bone and bone marrow
213.0 Benign neoplasm of bones of skull and face
213.1 Benign neoplasm of lower jaw bone
213.2 Benign neoplasm of vertebral column, excluding sacrum and coccyx
213.3 Benign neoplasm of ribs, sternum, and clavicle
213.4 Benign neoplasm of scapula and long bones of upper limb
213.5 Benign neoplasm of short bones of upper limb
213.6 Benign neoplasm of pelvic bones, sacrum, and coccyx
213.7 Benign neoplasm of long bones of lower limb
213.8 Benign neoplasm of short bones of lower limb
238.0 Neoplasm of uncertain behavior of bone and articular cartilage
239.2 Neoplasms of unspecified nature of bone, soft tissue, and skin
524.00 Unspecified major anomaly of jaw size
524.03 Maxillary hypoplasia
524.04 Mandibular hypoplasia
524.06 Microgenia
524.07 Excessive tuberosity of jaw
524.09 Other specified major anomaly of jaw size
524.11 Maxillary asymmetry
524.12 Other jaw asymmetry
524.19 Other specified anomaly of relationship of jaw to cranial base
524.69 Other specified temporomandibular joint disorders
526.2 Other cysts of jaws
526.4 Inflammatory conditions of jaw
526.89 Other specified disease of the jaws
730.11 Chronic osteomyelitis, shoulder region — (Use additional code to identify organism, 041.1)
730.12 Chronic osteomyelitis, upper arm — (Use additional code to identify organism, 041.1)
730.13 Chronic osteomyelitis, forearm — (Use additional code to identify organism, 041.1)
730.14 Chronic osteomyelitis, hand — (Use additional code to identify organism, 041.1)
730.15 Chronic osteomyelitis, pelvic region and thigh — (Use additional code to identify organism, 041.1)
730.16 Chronic osteomyelitis, lower leg — (Use additional code to identify organism, 041.1)
730.17 Chronic osteomyelitis, ankle and foot — (Use additional code to identify organism, 041.1)
730.18 Chronic osteomyelitis, other specified sites — (Use additional code to identify organism, 041.1)
733.82 Nonunion of fracture
756.9 Other and unspecified congenital anomaly of musculoskeletal system
873.54 Open wound of jaw, complicated — (Use additional code to identify infection)

ICD-9-CM Procedural
76.91 Bone graft to facial bone
77.79 Excision of other bone for graft, except facial bones
78.09 Bone graft of other bone, except facial bones

20957
20957 Bone graft with microvascular anastomosis; metatarsal

ICD-9-CM Diagnostic
170.1 Malignant neoplasm of mandible
170.5 Malignant neoplasm of short bones of upper limb
170.8 Malignant neoplasm of short bones of lower limb
213.0 Benign neoplasm of bones of skull and face
213.1 Benign neoplasm of lower jaw bone
239.2 Neoplasms of unspecified nature of bone, soft tissue, and skin
524.00 Unspecified major anomaly of jaw size
524.03 Maxillary hypoplasia
524.04 Mandibular hypoplasia
524.06 Microgenia
524.07 Excessive tuberosity of jaw
524.09 Other specified major anomaly of jaw size
524.11 Maxillary asymmetry
524.12 Other jaw asymmetry
524.19 Other specified anomaly of relationship of jaw to cranial base
524.69 Other specified temporomandibular joint disorders
730.14 Chronic osteomyelitis, hand — (Use additional code to identify organism, 041.1)
730.17 Chronic osteomyelitis, ankle and foot — (Use additional code to identify organism, 041.1)
730.18 Chronic osteomyelitis, other specified sites — (Use additional code to identify organism, 041.1)
733.19 Pathologic fracture of other specified site
733.81 Malunion of fracture
733.82 Nonunion of fracture
756.9 Other and unspecified congenital anomaly of musculoskeletal system
927.20 Crushing injury of hand(s) — (Use additional code to identify any associated injuries: 800-829, 850.0-854.1, 860.0-869.1)
927.3 Crushing injury of finger(s) — (Use additional code to identify any associated injuries: 800-829, 850.0-854.1, 860.0-869.1)
928.20 Crushing injury of foot — (Use additional code to identify any associated injuries: 800-829, 850.0-854.1, 860.0-869.1)

ICD-9-CM Procedural
76.91 Bone graft to facial bone

77.78 Excision of tarsals and metatarsals for graft
78.08 Bone graft of tarsals and metatarsals

20962

20962 Bone graft with microvascular anastomosis; other than fibula, iliac crest, or metatarsal

ICD-9-CM Diagnostic

170.1 Malignant neoplasm of mandible
170.2 Malignant neoplasm of vertebral column, excluding sacrum and coccyx
170.3 Malignant neoplasm of ribs, sternum, and clavicle
170.4 Malignant neoplasm of scapula and long bones of upper limb
170.5 Malignant neoplasm of short bones of upper limb
170.6 Malignant neoplasm of pelvic bones, sacrum, and coccyx
170.7 Malignant neoplasm of long bones of lower limb
170.8 Malignant neoplasm of short bones of lower limb
213.0 Benign neoplasm of bones of skull and face
213.1 Benign neoplasm of lower jaw bone
213.2 Benign neoplasm of vertebral column, excluding sacrum and coccyx
213.3 Benign neoplasm of ribs, sternum, and clavicle
213.4 Benign neoplasm of scapula and long bones of upper limb
213.5 Benign neoplasm of short bones of upper limb
213.6 Benign neoplasm of pelvic bones, sacrum, and coccyx
213.7 Benign neoplasm of long bones of lower limb
213.8 Benign neoplasm of short bones of lower limb
238.0 Neoplasm of uncertain behavior of bone and articular cartilage
239.2 Neoplasms of unspecified nature of bone, soft tissue, and skin
524.00 Unspecified major anomaly of jaw size ▽
524.03 Maxillary hypoplasia
524.04 Mandibular hypoplasia
524.06 Microgenia
524.07 Excessive tuberosity of jaw
524.09 Other specified major anomaly of jaw size
524.11 Maxillary asymmetry
524.12 Other jaw asymmetry
524.19 Other specified anomaly of relationship of jaw to cranial base
524.69 Other specified temporomandibular joint disorders
730.11 Chronic osteomyelitis, shoulder region — (Use additional code to identify organism, 041.1)
730.12 Chronic osteomyelitis, upper arm — (Use additional code to identify organism, 041.1)
730.13 Chronic osteomyelitis, forearm — (Use additional code to identify organism, 041.1)
730.14 Chronic osteomyelitis, hand — (Use additional code to identify organism, 041.1)
730.15 Chronic osteomyelitis, pelvic region and thigh — (Use additional code to identify organism, 041.1)
730.16 Chronic osteomyelitis, lower leg — (Use additional code to identify organism, 041.1)
730.17 Chronic osteomyelitis, ankle and foot — (Use additional code to identify organism, 041.1)
730.18 Chronic osteomyelitis, other specified sites — (Use additional code to identify organism, 041.1)
733.11 Pathologic fracture of humerus
733.12 Pathologic fracture of distal radius and ulna
733.13 Pathologic fracture of vertebrae
733.14 Pathologic fracture of neck of femur
733.15 Pathologic fracture of other specified part of femur
733.16 Pathologic fracture of tibia or fibula
733.19 Pathologic fracture of other specified site
733.40 Aseptic necrosis of bone, site unspecified ▽
733.42 Aseptic necrosis of head and neck of femur
733.43 Aseptic necrosis of medial femoral condyle
733.44 Aseptic necrosis of talus
733.49 Aseptic necrosis of other bone site
733.81 Malunion of fracture
733.82 Nonunion of fracture
733.93 Stress fracture of tibia or fibula
733.95 Stress fracture of other bone
927.03 Crushing injury of upper arm — (Use additional code to identify any associated injuries: 800-829, 850.0-854.1, 860.0-869.1)
927.10 Crushing injury of forearm — (Use additional code to identify any associated injuries: 800-829, 850.0-854.1, 860.0-869.1)
927.20 Crushing injury of hand(s) — (Use additional code to identify any associated injuries: 800-829, 850.0-854.1, 860.0-869.1)
927.21 Crushing injury of wrist — (Use additional code to identify any associated injuries: 800-829, 850.0-854.1, 860.0-869.1)
928.00 Crushing injury of thigh — (Use additional code to identify any associated injuries: 800-829, 850.0-854.1, 860.0-869.1)
928.10 Crushing injury of lower leg — (Use additional code to identify any associated injuries: 800-829, 850.0-854.1, 860.0-869.1)
928.11 Crushing injury of knee — (Use additional code to identify any associated injuries: 800-829, 850.0-854.1, 860.0-869.1)
928.20 Crushing injury of foot — (Use additional code to identify any associated injuries: 800-829, 850.0-854.1, 860.0-869.1)
928.21 Crushing injury of ankle — (Use additional code to identify any associated injuries: 800-829, 850.0-854.1, 860.0-869.1)

ICD-9-CM Procedural

76.91 Bone graft to facial bone
77.70 Excision of bone for graft, unspecified site
77.71 Excision of scapula, clavicle, and thorax (ribs and sternum) for graft
77.72 Excision of humerus for graft
77.73 Excision of radius and ulna for graft
77.74 Excision of carpals and metacarpals for graft
77.76 Excision of patella for graft
77.78 Excision of tarsals and metatarsals for graft
77.79 Excision of other bone for graft, except facial bones
78.00 Bone graft, unspecified site
78.01 Bone graft of scapula, clavicle, and thorax (ribs and sternum)

20969

20969 Free osteocutaneous flap with microvascular anastomosis; other than iliac crest, metatarsal, or great toe

ICD-9-CM Diagnostic

170.1 Malignant neoplasm of mandible
170.2 Malignant neoplasm of vertebral column, excluding sacrum and coccyx
170.3 Malignant neoplasm of ribs, sternum, and clavicle
170.4 Malignant neoplasm of scapula and long bones of upper limb
170.5 Malignant neoplasm of short bones of upper limb
170.6 Malignant neoplasm of pelvic bones, sacrum, and coccyx
170.7 Malignant neoplasm of long bones of lower limb
170.8 Malignant neoplasm of short bones of lower limb
213.0 Benign neoplasm of bones of skull and face
213.1 Benign neoplasm of lower jaw bone
213.2 Benign neoplasm of vertebral column, excluding sacrum and coccyx
213.3 Benign neoplasm of ribs, sternum, and clavicle
213.4 Benign neoplasm of scapula and long bones of upper limb
213.5 Benign neoplasm of short bones of upper limb
213.6 Benign neoplasm of pelvic bones, sacrum, and coccyx
213.7 Benign neoplasm of long bones of lower limb
213.8 Benign neoplasm of short bones of lower limb
238.0 Neoplasm of uncertain behavior of bone and articular cartilage
239.2 Neoplasms of unspecified nature of bone, soft tissue, and skin
730.11 Chronic osteomyelitis, shoulder region — (Use additional code to identify organism, 041.1)
730.12 Chronic osteomyelitis, upper arm — (Use additional code to identify organism, 041.1)
730.13 Chronic osteomyelitis, forearm — (Use additional code to identify organism, 041.1)
730.14 Chronic osteomyelitis, hand — (Use additional code to identify organism, 041.1)
730.15 Chronic osteomyelitis, pelvic region and thigh — (Use additional code to identify organism, 041.1)
730.16 Chronic osteomyelitis, lower leg — (Use additional code to identify organism, 041.1)
730.17 Chronic osteomyelitis, ankle and foot — (Use additional code to identify organism, 041.1)
730.18 Chronic osteomyelitis, other specified sites — (Use additional code to identify organism, 041.1)
733.11 Pathologic fracture of humerus
733.12 Pathologic fracture of distal radius and ulna
733.13 Pathologic fracture of vertebrae
733.14 Pathologic fracture of neck of femur
733.15 Pathologic fracture of other specified part of femur
733.16 Pathologic fracture of tibia or fibula
733.19 Pathologic fracture of other specified site
733.81 Malunion of fracture
733.82 Nonunion of fracture
733.93 Stress fracture of tibia or fibula

733.95 Stress fracture of other bone
927.03 Crushing injury of upper arm — (Use additional code to identify any associated injuries: 800-829, 850.0-854.1, 860.0-869.1)
927.10 Crushing injury of forearm — (Use additional code to identify any associated injuries: 800-829, 850.0-854.1, 860.0-869.1)
927.20 Crushing injury of hand(s) — (Use additional code to identify any associated injuries: 800-829, 850.0-854.1, 860.0-869.1)
927.21 Crushing injury of wrist — (Use additional code to identify any associated injuries: 800-829, 850.0-854.1, 860.0-869.1)
928.00 Crushing injury of thigh — (Use additional code to identify any associated injuries: 800-829, 850.0-854.1, 860.0-869.1)
928.10 Crushing injury of lower leg — (Use additional code to identify any associated injuries: 800-829, 850.0-854.1, 860.0-869.1)
928.11 Crushing injury of knee — (Use additional code to identify any associated injuries: 800-829, 850.0-854.1, 860.0-869.1)
928.20 Crushing injury of foot — (Use additional code to identify any associated injuries: 800-829, 850.0-854.1, 860.0-869.1)
928.21 Crushing injury of ankle — (Use additional code to identify any associated injuries: 800-829, 850.0-854.1, 860.0-869.1)

ICD-9-CM Procedural

77.70 Excision of bone for graft, unspecified site
77.71 Excision of scapula, clavicle, and thorax (ribs and sternum) for graft
77.72 Excision of humerus for graft
77.73 Excision of radius and ulna for graft
77.74 Excision of carpals and metacarpals for graft
77.75 Excision of femur for graft
77.76 Excision of patella for graft
77.77 Excision of tibia and fibula for graft
77.78 Excision of tarsals and metatarsals for graft
77.79 Excision of other bone for graft, except facial bones
86.09 Other incision of skin and subcutaneous tissue

20970

20970 Free osteocutaneous flap with microvascular anastomosis; iliac crest

ICD-9-CM Diagnostic

170.0 Malignant neoplasm of bones of skull and face, except mandible
170.1 Malignant neoplasm of mandible
170.2 Malignant neoplasm of vertebral column, excluding sacrum and coccyx
170.3 Malignant neoplasm of ribs, sternum, and clavicle
170.4 Malignant neoplasm of scapula and long bones of upper limb
170.5 Malignant neoplasm of short bones of upper limb
170.6 Malignant neoplasm of pelvic bones, sacrum, and coccyx
170.7 Malignant neoplasm of long bones of lower limb
170.8 Malignant neoplasm of short bones of lower limb
198.5 Secondary malignant neoplasm of bone and bone marrow
213.0 Benign neoplasm of bones of skull and face
213.1 Benign neoplasm of lower jaw bone
213.2 Benign neoplasm of vertebral column, excluding sacrum and coccyx
213.3 Benign neoplasm of ribs, sternum, and clavicle
213.4 Benign neoplasm of scapula and long bones of upper limb
213.5 Benign neoplasm of short bones of upper limb
213.6 Benign neoplasm of pelvic bones, sacrum, and coccyx
213.7 Benign neoplasm of long bones of lower limb
213.8 Benign neoplasm of short bones of lower limb
238.0 Neoplasm of uncertain behavior of bone and articular cartilage
239.2 Neoplasms of unspecified nature of bone, soft tissue, and skin
524.03 Maxillary hypoplasia
524.04 Mandibular hypoplasia
524.07 Excessive tuberosity of jaw
524.09 Other specified major anomaly of jaw size
524.11 Maxillary asymmetry
524.12 Other jaw asymmetry
524.69 Other specified temporomandibular joint disorders
526.2 Other cysts of jaws
526.4 Inflammatory conditions of jaw
526.89 Other specified disease of the jaws
730.11 Chronic osteomyelitis, shoulder region — (Use additional code to identify organism, 041.1)
730.12 Chronic osteomyelitis, upper arm — (Use additional code to identify organism, 041.1)
730.13 Chronic osteomyelitis, forearm — (Use additional code to identify organism, 041.1)
730.14 Chronic osteomyelitis, hand — (Use additional code to identify organism, 041.1)
730.15 Chronic osteomyelitis, pelvic region and thigh — (Use additional code to identify organism, 041.1)
730.16 Chronic osteomyelitis, lower leg — (Use additional code to identify organism, 041.1)
730.17 Chronic osteomyelitis, ankle and foot — (Use additional code to identify organism, 041.1)
730.18 Chronic osteomyelitis, other specified sites — (Use additional code to identify organism, 041.1)
733.82 Nonunion of fracture
756.9 Other and unspecified congenital anomaly of musculoskeletal system ▽
873.54 Open wound of jaw, complicated — (Use additional code to identify infection)

ICD-9-CM Procedural

77.79 Excision of other bone for graft, except facial bones
86.09 Other incision of skin and subcutaneous tissue

20972

20972 Free osteocutaneous flap with microvascular anastomosis; metatarsal

ICD-9-CM Diagnostic

170.5 Malignant neoplasm of short bones of upper limb
170.8 Malignant neoplasm of short bones of lower limb
730.14 Chronic osteomyelitis, hand — (Use additional code to identify organism, 041.1)
730.17 Chronic osteomyelitis, ankle and foot — (Use additional code to identify organism, 041.1)
730.18 Chronic osteomyelitis, other specified sites — (Use additional code to identify organism, 041.1)
733.19 Pathologic fracture of other specified site
733.81 Malunion of fracture
733.82 Nonunion of fracture
756.9 Other and unspecified congenital anomaly of musculoskeletal system ▽
927.20 Crushing injury of hand(s) — (Use additional code to identify any associated injuries: 800-829, 850.0-854.1, 860.0-869.1)
927.3 Crushing injury of finger(s) — (Use additional code to identify any associated injuries: 800-829, 850.0-854.1, 860.0-869.1)
928.20 Crushing injury of foot — (Use additional code to identify any associated injuries: 800-829, 850.0-854.1, 860.0-869.1)

ICD-9-CM Procedural

77.78 Excision of tarsals and metatarsals for graft
86.09 Other incision of skin and subcutaneous tissue

20973

20973 Free osteocutaneous flap with microvascular anastomosis; great toe with web space

ICD-9-CM Diagnostic

755.29 Congenital longitudinal deficiency, phalanges, complete or partial
885.0 Traumatic amputation of thumb (complete) (partial), without mention of complication — (Use additional code to identify infection)
885.1 Traumatic amputation of thumb (complete) (partial), complicated — (Use additional code to identify infection)
886.0 Traumatic amputation of other finger(s) (complete) (partial), without mention of complication — (Use additional code to identify infection)
886.1 Traumatic amputation of other finger(s) (complete) (partial), complicated — (Use additional code to identify infection)
927.3 Crushing injury of finger(s) — (Use additional code to identify any associated injuries: 800-829, 850.0-854.1, 860.0-869.1)

ICD-9-CM Procedural

77.79 Excision of other bone for graft, except facial bones
86.09 Other incision of skin and subcutaneous tissue

20974–20975

20974 Electrical stimulation to aid bone healing; noninvasive (nonoperative)
20975 invasive (operative)

ICD-9-CM Diagnostic

733.82 Nonunion of fracture
733.93 Stress fracture of tibia or fibula
733.95 Stress fracture of other bone
805.01 Closed fracture of first cervical vertebra without mention of spinal cord injury
805.02 Closed fracture of second cervical vertebra without mention of spinal cord injury

805.03 Closed fracture of third cervical vertebra without mention of spinal cord injury
805.04 Closed fracture of fourth cervical vertebra without mention of spinal cord injury
805.05 Closed fracture of fifth cervical vertebra without mention of spinal cord injury
805.06 Closed fracture of sixth cervical vertebra without mention of spinal cord injury
805.07 Closed fracture of seventh cervical vertebra without mention of spinal cord injury
805.08 Closed fracture of multiple cervical vertebrae without mention of spinal cord injury
805.11 Open fracture of first cervical vertebra without mention of spinal cord injury
805.12 Open fracture of second cervical vertebra without mention of spinal cord injury
805.13 Open fracture of third cervical vertebra without mention of spinal cord injury
805.14 Open fracture of fourth cervical vertebra without mention of spinal cord injury
805.15 Open fracture of fifth cervical vertebra without mention of spinal cord injury
805.16 Open fracture of sixth cervical vertebra without mention of spinal cord injury
805.17 Open fracture of seventh cervical vertebra without mention of spinal cord injury
805.18 Open fracture of multiple cervical vertebrae without mention of spinal cord injury
805.2 Closed fracture of dorsal (thoracic) vertebra without mention of spinal cord injury
805.3 Open fracture of dorsal (thoracic) vertebra without mention of spinal cord injury
805.4 Closed fracture of lumbar vertebra without mention of spinal cord injury
805.5 Open fracture of lumbar vertebra without mention of spinal cord injury
805.6 Closed fracture of sacrum and coccyx without mention of spinal cord injury
805.7 Open fracture of sacrum and coccyx without mention of spinal cord injury
808.0 Closed fracture of acetabulum
808.1 Open fracture of acetabulum
808.2 Closed fracture of pubis
808.3 Open fracture of pubis
808.41 Closed fracture of ilium
808.42 Closed fracture of ischium
810.01 Closed fracture of sternal end of clavicle
810.02 Closed fracture of shaft of clavicle
810.03 Closed fracture of acromial end of clavicle
810.11 Open fracture of sternal end of clavicle
810.12 Open fracture of shaft of clavicle
810.13 Open fracture of acromial end of clavicle
811.01 Closed fracture of acromial process of scapula
811.02 Closed fracture of coracoid process of scapula
811.03 Closed fracture of glenoid cavity and neck of scapula
811.11 Open fracture of acromial process of scapula
811.12 Open fracture of coracoid process
811.13 Open fracture of glenoid cavity and neck of scapula
812.01 Closed fracture of surgical neck of humerus
812.02 Closed fracture of anatomical neck of humerus
812.03 Closed fracture of greater tuberosity of humerus
812.09 Other closed fractures of upper end of humerus
812.11 Open fracture of surgical neck of humerus
812.12 Open fracture of anatomical neck of humerus
812.13 Open fracture of greater tuberosity of humerus
812.19 Other open fracture of upper end of humerus
812.20 Closed fracture of unspecified part of humerus ▽
812.21 Closed fracture of shaft of humerus
812.30 Open fracture of unspecified part of humerus ▽
812.31 Open fracture of shaft of humerus
812.40 Closed fracture of unspecified part of lower end of humerus ▽
812.41 Closed fracture of supracondylar humerus
812.42 Closed fracture of lateral condyle of humerus
812.43 Closed fracture of medial condyle of humerus
812.44 Closed fracture of unspecified condyle(s) of humerus ▽
812.49 Other closed fracture of lower end of humerus
812.51 Open fracture of supracondylar humerus
812.52 Open fracture of lateral condyle of humerus
812.53 Open fracture of medial condyle of humerus
812.54 Open fracture of unspecified condyle(s) of humerus ▽
812.59 Other open fracture of lower end of humerus
817.0 Multiple closed fractures of hand bones
817.1 Multiple open fractures of hand bones
821.00 Closed fracture of unspecified part of femur ▽
821.01 Closed fracture of shaft of femur
821.20 Closed fracture of unspecified part of lower end of femur ▽
821.21 Closed fracture of femoral condyle
821.22 Closed fracture of lower epiphysis of femur
821.23 Closed supracondylar fracture of femur
821.29 Other closed fracture of lower end of femur
821.30 Open fracture of unspecified part of lower end of femur ▽
821.31 Open fracture of femoral condyle
821.32 Open fracture of lower epiphysis of femur
821.33 Open supracondylar fracture of femur
821.39 Other open fracture of lower end of femur
823.00 Closed fracture of upper end of tibia
823.01 Closed fracture of upper end of fibula
823.02 Closed fracture of upper end of fibula with tibia
823.10 Open fracture of upper end of tibia
823.11 Open fracture of upper end of fibula
823.12 Open fracture of upper end of fibula with tibia
823.20 Closed fracture of shaft of tibia
823.21 Closed fracture of shaft of fibula
823.22 Closed fracture of shaft of fibula with tibia
823.30 Open fracture of shaft of tibia
823.31 Open fracture of shaft of fibula
823.32 Open fracture of shaft of fibula with tibia
823.80 Closed fracture of unspecified part of tibia ▽
823.81 Closed fracture of unspecified part of fibula ▽
823.82 Closed fracture of unspecified part of fibula with tibia ▽
824.0 Closed fracture of medial malleolus
824.1 Open fracture of medial malleolus
824.2 Closed fracture of lateral malleolus
824.3 Open fracture of lateral malleolus
824.4 Closed bimalleolar fracture
824.5 Open bimalleolar fracture
824.6 Closed trimalleolar fracture
824.7 Open trimalleolar fracture
825.0 Closed fracture of calcaneus
825.1 Open fracture of calcaneus

ICD-9-CM Procedural

78.90 Insertion of bone growth stimulator, unspecified site
78.91 Insertion of bone growth stimulator into scapula, clavicle and thorax (ribs and sternum)
78.92 Insertion of bone growth stimulator into humerus
78.93 Insertion of bone growth stimulator into radius and ulna
78.94 Insertion of bone growth stimulator into carpals and metacarpals
78.95 Insertion of bone growth stimulator into femur
78.96 Insertion of bone growth stimulator into patella
78.97 Insertion of bone growth stimulator into tibia and fibula
78.98 Insertion of bone growth stimulator into tarsals and metatarsals
78.99 Insertion of bone growth stimulator into other bone
83.92 Insertion or replacement of skeletal muscle stimulator
99.86 Non-invasive placement of bone growth stimulator

HCPCS Level II Supplies & Services

E0747 Osteogenesis stimulator, electrical, noninvasive, other than spinal applications
E0748 Osteogenesis stimulator, electrical, noninvasive, spinal applications
E0749 Osteogenesis stimulator, electrical, surgically implanted
E0752 Implantable neurostimulator electrode, each
E0754 Patient programmer (external) for use with implantable programmable neurostimulator pulse generator

20979

20979 Low intensity ultrasound stimulation to aid bone healing, noninvasive (nonoperative)

ICD-9-CM Diagnostic

733.82 Nonunion of fracture
733.93 Stress fracture of tibia or fibula
733.95 Stress fracture of other bone
805.01 Closed fracture of first cervical vertebra without mention of spinal cord injury
805.02 Closed fracture of second cervical vertebra without mention of spinal cord injury
805.03 Closed fracture of third cervical vertebra without mention of spinal cord injury
805.04 Closed fracture of fourth cervical vertebra without mention of spinal cord injury
805.05 Closed fracture of fifth cervical vertebra without mention of spinal cord injury
805.06 Closed fracture of sixth cervical vertebra without mention of spinal cord injury
805.07 Closed fracture of seventh cervical vertebra without mention of spinal cord injury
805.08 Closed fracture of multiple cervical vertebrae without mention of spinal cord injury
805.11 Open fracture of first cervical vertebra without mention of spinal cord injury

805.12 Open fracture of second cervical vertebra without mention of spinal cord injury
805.13 Open fracture of third cervical vertebra without mention of spinal cord injury
805.14 Open fracture of fourth cervical vertebra without mention of spinal cord injury
805.15 Open fracture of fifth cervical vertebra without mention of spinal cord injury
805.16 Open fracture of sixth cervical vertebra without mention of spinal cord injury
805.17 Open fracture of seventh cervical vertebra without mention of spinal cord injury
805.18 Open fracture of multiple cervical vertebrae without mention of spinal cord injury
805.2 Closed fracture of dorsal (thoracic) vertebra without mention of spinal cord injury
805.3 Open fracture of dorsal (thoracic) vertebra without mention of spinal cord injury
805.4 Closed fracture of lumbar vertebra without mention of spinal cord injury
805.5 Open fracture of lumbar vertebra without mention of spinal cord injury
805.6 Closed fracture of sacrum and coccyx without mention of spinal cord injury
805.7 Open fracture of sacrum and coccyx without mention of spinal cord injury
808.0 Closed fracture of acetabulum
808.1 Open fracture of acetabulum
808.2 Closed fracture of pubis
808.3 Open fracture of pubis
808.41 Closed fracture of ilium
808.42 Closed fracture of ischium
810.01 Closed fracture of sternal end of clavicle
810.02 Closed fracture of shaft of clavicle
810.03 Closed fracture of acromial end of clavicle
810.11 Open fracture of sternal end of clavicle
810.12 Open fracture of shaft of clavicle
810.13 Open fracture of acromial end of clavicle
811.01 Closed fracture of acromial process of scapula
811.02 Closed fracture of coracoid process of scapula
811.03 Closed fracture of glenoid cavity and neck of scapula
811.11 Open fracture of acromial process of scapula
811.12 Open fracture of coracoid process
811.13 Open fracture of glenoid cavity and neck of scapula
812.01 Closed fracture of surgical neck of humerus
812.02 Closed fracture of anatomical neck of humerus
812.03 Closed fracture of greater tuberosity of humerus
812.09 Other closed fractures of upper end of humerus
812.11 Open fracture of surgical neck of humerus
812.12 Open fracture of anatomical neck of humerus
812.13 Open fracture of greater tuberosity of humerus
812.19 Other open fracture of upper end of humerus
812.20 Closed fracture of unspecified part of humerus ▽
812.21 Closed fracture of shaft of humerus
812.30 Open fracture of unspecified part of humerus ▽
812.31 Open fracture of shaft of humerus
812.40 Closed fracture of unspecified part of lower end of humerus ▽
812.41 Closed fracture of supracondylar humerus
812.42 Closed fracture of lateral condyle of humerus
812.43 Closed fracture of medial condyle of humerus
812.44 Closed fracture of unspecified condyle(s) of humerus ▽
812.49 Other closed fracture of lower end of humerus
812.51 Open fracture of supracondylar humerus
812.52 Open fracture of lateral condyle of humerus
812.53 Open fracture of medial condyle of humerus
812.54 Open fracture of unspecified condyle(s) of humerus ▽
812.59 Other open fracture of lower end of humerus
817.0 Multiple closed fractures of hand bones
817.1 Multiple open fractures of hand bones
821.00 Closed fracture of unspecified part of femur ▽
821.01 Closed fracture of shaft of femur
821.20 Closed fracture of unspecified part of lower end of femur ▽
821.21 Closed fracture of femoral condyle
821.22 Closed fracture of lower epiphysis of femur
821.23 Closed supracondylar fracture of femur
821.29 Other closed fracture of lower end of femur
821.30 Open fracture of unspecified part of lower end of femur ▽
821.31 Open fracture of femoral condyle
821.32 Open fracture of lower epiphysis of femur
821.33 Open supracondylar fracture of femur
821.39 Other open fracture of lower end of femur
823.00 Closed fracture of upper end of tibia
823.01 Closed fracture of upper end of fibula
823.02 Closed fracture of upper end of fibula with tibia
823.10 Open fracture of upper end of tibia
823.11 Open fracture of upper end of fibula
823.12 Open fracture of upper end of fibula with tibia
823.20 Closed fracture of shaft of tibia
823.21 Closed fracture of shaft of fibula
823.22 Closed fracture of shaft of fibula with tibia
823.30 Open fracture of shaft of tibia
823.31 Open fracture of shaft of fibula
823.32 Open fracture of shaft of fibula with tibia
823.80 Closed fracture of unspecified part of tibia ▽
823.81 Closed fracture of unspecified part of fibula ▽
823.82 Closed fracture of unspecified part of fibula with tibia ▽
824.0 Closed fracture of medial malleolus
824.1 Open fracture of medial malleolus
824.2 Closed fracture of lateral malleolus
824.3 Open fracture of lateral malleolus
824.4 Closed bimalleolar fracture
824.5 Open bimalleolar fracture
824.6 Closed trimalleolar fracture
824.7 Open trimalleolar fracture
825.0 Closed fracture of calcaneus
825.1 Open fracture of calcaneus

ICD-9-CM Procedural

93.35 Other heat therapy

HCPCS Level II Supplies & Services

E0760 Osteogenesis stimulator, low intensity ultrasound, non-invasive

20982

20982 Ablation, bone tumor(s) (eg, osteoid osteoma, metastasis) radiofrequency, percutaneous, including computed tomographic guidance

ICD-9-CM Diagnostic

170.0 Malignant neoplasm of bones of skull and face, except mandible
170.1 Malignant neoplasm of mandible
170.2 Malignant neoplasm of vertebral column, excluding sacrum and coccyx
170.3 Malignant neoplasm of ribs, sternum, and clavicle
170.4 Malignant neoplasm of scapula and long bones of upper limb
170.5 Malignant neoplasm of short bones of upper limb
170.6 Malignant neoplasm of pelvic bones, sacrum, and coccyx
170.7 Malignant neoplasm of long bones of lower limb
170.8 Malignant neoplasm of short bones of lower limb
170.9 Malignant neoplasm of bone and articular cartilage, site unspecified ▽
198.5 Secondary malignant neoplasm of bone and bone marrow
213.0 Benign neoplasm of bones of skull and face
213.1 Benign neoplasm of lower jaw bone
213.2 Benign neoplasm of vertebral column, excluding sacrum and coccyx
213.3 Benign neoplasm of ribs, sternum, and clavicle
213.4 Benign neoplasm of scapula and long bones of upper limb
213.5 Benign neoplasm of short bones of upper limb
213.6 Benign neoplasm of pelvic bones, sacrum, and coccyx
213.7 Benign neoplasm of long bones of lower limb
213.8 Benign neoplasm of short bones of lower limb
213.9 Benign neoplasm of bone and articular cartilage, site unspecified ▽
238.0 Neoplasm of uncertain behavior of bone and articular cartilage
239.2 Neoplasms of unspecified nature of bone, soft tissue, and skin

ICD-9-CM Procedural

77.60 Local excision of lesion or tissue of bone, unspecified site
77.61 Local excision of lesion or tissue of scapula, clavicle, and thorax (ribs and sternum)
77.62 Local excision of lesion or tissue of humerus
77.63 Local excision of lesion or tissue of radius and ulna
77.64 Local excision of lesion or tissue of carpals and metacarpals
77.65 Local excision of lesion or tissue of femur
77.66 Local excision of lesion or tissue of patella
77.67 Local excision of lesion or tissue of tibia and fibula
77.68 Local excision of lesion or tissue of tarsals and metatarsals
77.69 Local excision of lesion or tissue of other bone, except facial bones

▽ Unspecified code
♀ Female diagnosis
☒ Manifestation code
♂ Male diagnosis

Head

21010

21010 Arthrotomy, temporomandibular joint

ICD-9-CM Diagnostic

524.60 Unspecified temporomandibular joint disorders ▽
524.61 Adhesions and ankylosis (bony or fibrous) of temporomandibular joint
524.62 Arthralgia of temporomandibular joint
524.69 Other specified temporomandibular joint disorders
526.4 Inflammatory conditions of jaw
715.18 Primary localized osteoarthrosis, other specified sites
715.28 Secondary localized osteoarthrosis, other specified site
718.58 Ankylosis of joint of other specified site
830.0 Closed dislocation of jaw
905.0 Late effect of fracture of skull and face bones
959.09 Injury of face and neck, other and unspecified
V64.43 Arthroscopic surgical procedure converted to open procedure

ICD-9-CM Procedural

80.19 Other arthrotomy of other specified site

21015

21015 Radical resection of tumor (eg, malignant neoplasm), soft tissue of face or scalp

ICD-9-CM Diagnostic

171.0 Malignant neoplasm of connective and other soft tissue of head, face, and neck
171.8 Malignant neoplasm of other specified sites of connective and other soft tissue
172.3 Malignant melanoma of skin of other and unspecified parts of face
172.4 Malignant melanoma of skin of scalp and neck
172.8 Malignant melanoma of other specified sites of skin
173.3 Other malignant neoplasm of skin of other and unspecified parts of face ▽
173.4 Other malignant neoplasm of scalp and skin of neck
173.8 Other malignant neoplasm of other specified sites of skin
238.1 Neoplasm of uncertain behavior of connective and other soft tissue ▽
238.2 Neoplasm of uncertain behavior of skin
239.2 Neoplasms of unspecified nature of bone, soft tissue, and skin

ICD-9-CM Procedural

83.39 Excision of lesion of other soft tissue
83.49 Other excision of soft tissue

21025–21026

21025 Excision of bone (eg, for osteomyelitis or bone abscess); mandible
21026 facial bone(s)

ICD-9-CM Diagnostic

015.60 Tuberculosis of mastoid, confirmation unspecified — (Use additional code to identify manifestation: 711.4, 727.01, 730.8) ▽
015.61 Tuberculosis of mastoid, bacteriological or histological examination not done — (Use additional code to identify manifestation: 711.4, 727.01, 730.8)
015.62 Tuberculosis of mastoid, bacteriological or histological examination unknown (at present) — (Use additional code to identify manifestation: 711.4, 727.01, 730.8)
015.63 Tuberculosis of mastoid, tubercle bacilli found (in sputum) by microscopy — (Use additional code to identify manifestation: 711.4, 727.01, 730.8)
015.65 Tuberculosis of mastoid, tubercle bacilli not found by bacteriological examination, but tuberculosis confirmed histologically — (Use additional code to identify manifestation: 711.4, 727.01, 730.8)
015.66 Tuberculosis of mastoid, tubercle bacilli not found by bacteriological or histological examination but tuberculosis confirmed by other methods [inoculation of animals] — (Use additional code to identify manifestation: 711.4, 727.01, 730.8)
383.01 Subperiosteal abscess of mastoid
383.02 Acute mastoiditis with other complications
383.1 Chronic mastoiditis
383.20 Unspecified petrositis ▽
383.21 Acute petrositis
383.22 Chronic petrositis
383.9 Unspecified mastoiditis ▽
473.0 Chronic maxillary sinusitis
473.1 Chronic frontal sinusitis
473.2 Chronic ethmoidal sinusitis
473.3 Chronic sphenoidal sinusitis
473.9 Unspecified sinusitis (chronic) ▽
526.2 Other cysts of jaws
526.4 Inflammatory conditions of jaw
526.89 Other specified disease of the jaws
730.08 Acute osteomyelitis, other specified site — (Use additional code to identify organism, 041.1)
730.09 Acute osteomyelitis, multiple sites — (Use additional code to identify organism, 041.1)
730.18 Chronic osteomyelitis, other specified sites — (Use additional code to identify organism, 041.1)
730.19 Chronic osteomyelitis, multiple sites — (Use additional code to identify organism, 041.1)
730.28 Unspecified osteomyelitis, other specified sites — (Use additional code to identify organism, 041.1) ▽
730.29 Unspecified osteomyelitis, multiple sites — (Use additional code to identify organism, 041.1) ▽
730.88 Other infections involving bone diseases classified elsewhere, other specified sites — (Code first underlying disease: 002.0, 015.0-015.9. Use additional code to identify organism) ☒
730.89 Other infections involving bone diseases classified elsewhere, multiple sites — (Code first underlying disease: 002.0, 015.0-015.9. Use additional code to identify organism) ☒
906.0 Late effect of open wound of head, neck, and trunk
906.4 Late effect of crushing
906.5 Late effect of burn of eye, face, head, and neck
908.9 Late effect of unspecified injury ▽
909.2 Late effect of radiation
909.3 Late effect of complications of surgical and medical care
996.66 Infection and inflammatory reaction due to internal joint prosthesis — (Use additional code to identify specified infections)
998.59 Other postoperative infection — (Use additional code to identify infection)

ICD-9-CM Procedural

76.31 Partial mandibulectomy
76.39 Partial ostectomy of other facial bone
76.41 Total mandibulectomy with synchronous reconstruction
76.42 Other total mandibulectomy
76.44 Total ostectomy of other facial bone with synchronous reconstruction
76.45 Other total ostectomy of other facial bone

21029

21029 Removal by contouring of benign tumor of facial bone (eg, fibrous dysplasia)

ICD-9-CM Diagnostic

213.0 Benign neoplasm of bones of skull and face
213.1 Benign neoplasm of lower jaw bone
526.0 Developmental odontogenic cysts
526.1 Fissural cysts of jaw
526.2 Other cysts of jaws
526.3 Central giant cell (reparative) granuloma
526.89 Other specified disease of the jaws
733.21 Solitary bone cyst
733.22 Aneurysmal bone cyst
733.29 Other cyst of bone
738.11 Zygomatic hyperplasia
756.54 Polyostotic fibrous dysplasia of bone

ICD-9-CM Procedural

76.2 Local excision or destruction of lesion of facial bone
76.69 Other facial bone repair

21030

21030 Excision of benign tumor or cyst of maxilla or zygoma by enucleation and curettage

ICD-9-CM Diagnostic

213.0 Benign neoplasm of bones of skull and face
521.6 Ankylosis of teeth
526.0 Developmental odontogenic cysts
526.1 Fissural cysts of jaw
526.2 Other cysts of jaws
526.3 Central giant cell (reparative) granuloma
526.81 Exostosis of jaw
526.89 Other specified disease of the jaws
528.1 Cancrum oris

733.20 Unspecified cyst of bone (localized) ▽
733.21 Solitary bone cyst
733.22 Aneurysmal bone cyst
733.29 Other cyst of bone
738.11 Zygomatic hyperplasia

ICD-9-CM Procedural

76.2 Local excision or destruction of lesion of facial bone

HCPCS Level II Supplies & Services

A4305 Disposable drug delivery system, flow rate of 50 ml or greater per hour
A4306 Disposable drug delivery system, flow rate of 5 ml or less per hour
A4550 Surgical trays

21031

21031 Excision of torus mandibularis

ICD-9-CM Diagnostic

526.81 Exostosis of jaw

ICD-9-CM Procedural

76.2 Local excision or destruction of lesion of facial bone

HCPCS Level II Supplies & Services

A4305 Disposable drug delivery system, flow rate of 50 ml or greater per hour
A4306 Disposable drug delivery system, flow rate of 5 ml or less per hour
A4550 Surgical trays

21032

21032 Excision of maxillary torus palatinus

ICD-9-CM Diagnostic

526.81 Exostosis of jaw

ICD-9-CM Procedural

76.2 Local excision or destruction of lesion of facial bone

21034

21034 Excision of malignant tumor of maxilla or zygoma

ICD-9-CM Diagnostic

170.0 Malignant neoplasm of bones of skull and face, except mandible
198.5 Secondary malignant neoplasm of bone and bone marrow

ICD-9-CM Procedural

76.2 Local excision or destruction of lesion of facial bone

21040

21040 Excision of benign tumor or cyst of mandible, by enucleation and/or curettage

ICD-9-CM Diagnostic

213.1 Benign neoplasm of lower jaw bone
521.6 Ankylosis of teeth
526.0 Developmental odontogenic cysts
526.1 Fissural cysts of jaw
526.2 Other cysts of jaws
526.3 Central giant cell (reparative) granuloma
526.81 Exostosis of jaw
526.89 Other specified disease of the jaws
528.1 Cancrum oris
733.20 Unspecified cyst of bone (localized) ▽
733.21 Solitary bone cyst
733.22 Aneurysmal bone cyst
733.29 Other cyst of bone
733.99 Other disorders of bone and cartilage

ICD-9-CM Procedural

24.4 Excision of dental lesion of jaw
76.31 Partial mandibulectomy

HCPCS Level II Supplies & Services

A4305 Disposable drug delivery system, flow rate of 50 ml or greater per hour
A4306 Disposable drug delivery system, flow rate of 5 ml or less per hour
A4550 Surgical trays

21044–21045

21044 Excision of malignant tumor of mandible;
21045 radical resection

ICD-9-CM Diagnostic

170.1 Malignant neoplasm of mandible
195.0 Malignant neoplasm of head, face, and neck
198.5 Secondary malignant neoplasm of bone and bone marrow
199.0 Disseminated malignant neoplasm

ICD-9-CM Procedural

24.4 Excision of dental lesion of jaw
76.31 Partial mandibulectomy
76.41 Total mandibulectomy with synchronous reconstruction
76.42 Other total mandibulectomy

21046–21047

21046 Excision of benign tumor or cyst of mandible; requiring intra-oral osteotomy (eg, locally aggressive or destructive lesion(s))
21047 requiring extra-oral osteotomy and partial mandibulectomy (eg, locally aggressive or destructive lesion(s))

ICD-9-CM Diagnostic

213.1 Benign neoplasm of lower jaw bone
521.6 Ankylosis of teeth
526.0 Developmental odontogenic cysts
526.1 Fissural cysts of jaw
526.2 Other cysts of jaws
526.3 Central giant cell (reparative) granuloma
526.81 Exostosis of jaw
526.89 Other specified disease of the jaws
528.1 Cancrum oris
733.20 Unspecified cyst of bone (localized) ▽
733.21 Solitary bone cyst
733.22 Aneurysmal bone cyst
733.29 Other cyst of bone

ICD-9-CM Procedural

76.2 Local excision or destruction of lesion of facial bone
76.31 Partial mandibulectomy
76.61 Closed osteoplasty (osteotomy) of mandibular ramus
76.62 Open osteoplasty (osteotomy) of mandibular ramus
76.63 Osteoplasty (osteotomy) of body of mandible

HCPCS Level II Supplies & Services

A4550 Surgical trays

21048–21049

21048 Excision of benign tumor or cyst of maxilla; requiring intra-oral osteotomy (eg, locally aggressive or destructive lesion(s))
21049 Excision of benign tumor or cyst of maxilla; requiring extra-oral osteotomy and partial maxillectomy (eg, locally aggressive or destructive lesion(s))

ICD-9-CM Diagnostic

213.0 Benign neoplasm of bones of skull and face
521.6 Ankylosis of teeth
526.0 Developmental odontogenic cysts
526.1 Fissural cysts of jaw
526.2 Other cysts of jaws
526.3 Central giant cell (reparative) granuloma
526.81 Exostosis of jaw
526.89 Other specified disease of the jaws
528.1 Cancrum oris
733.20 Unspecified cyst of bone (localized) ▽
733.21 Solitary bone cyst
733.22 Aneurysmal bone cyst
733.29 Other cyst of bone

ICD-9-CM Procedural

76.2 Local excision or destruction of lesion of facial bone
76.39 Partial ostectomy of other facial bone
76.65 Segmental osteoplasty (osteotomy) of maxilla
76.66 Total osteoplasty (osteotomy) of maxilla

HCPCS Level II Supplies & Services

A4550 Surgical trays

21050
21050 Condylectomy, temporomandibular joint (separate procedure)

ICD-9-CM Diagnostic
170.1 Malignant neoplasm of mandible
357.1 Polyneuropathy in collagen vascular disease — (Code first underlying disease: 446.0, 710.0, 714.0) ☒
359.6 Symptomatic inflammatory myopathy in diseases classified elsewhere — (Code first underlying disease: 135, 140.0-208.9, 277.3, 446.0, 710.0, 710.1, 710.2, 714.0) ☒
524.61 Adhesions and ankylosis (bony or fibrous) of temporomandibular joint
524.62 Arthralgia of temporomandibular joint
524.63 Articular disc disorder (reducing or non-reducing) of temporomandibular joint
524.69 Other specified temporomandibular joint disorders
526.89 Other specified disease of the jaws
714.0 Rheumatoid arthritis — (Use additional code to identify manifestation: 357.1, 359.6)
802.21 Closed fracture of condylar process of mandible
802.31 Open fracture of condylar process of mandible
905.0 Late effect of fracture of skull and face bones

ICD-9-CM Procedural
76.5 Temporomandibular arthroplasty
77.89 Other partial ostectomy of other bone, except facial bones

21060
21060 Meniscectomy, partial or complete, temporomandibular joint (separate procedure)

ICD-9-CM Diagnostic
524.50 Dentofacial functional abnormality, unspecified
524.51 Abnormal jaw closure
524.52 Limited mandibular range of motion
524.53 Deviation in opening and closing of the mandible
524.59 Other dentofacial functional abnormalities
524.60 Unspecified temporomandibular joint disorders ▽
524.61 Adhesions and ankylosis (bony or fibrous) of temporomandibular joint
524.63 Articular disc disorder (reducing or non-reducing) of temporomandibular joint
524.64 Temporomandibular joint sounds on opening and/or closing the jaw
524.69 Other specified temporomandibular joint disorders
715.18 Primary localized osteoarthrosis, other specified sites
715.38 Localized osteoarthrosis not specified whether primary or secondary, other specified sites
830.0 Closed dislocation of jaw
830.1 Open dislocation of jaw
905.0 Late effect of fracture of skull and face bones
906.0 Late effect of open wound of head, neck, and trunk

ICD-9-CM Procedural
76.5 Temporomandibular arthroplasty

21070
21070 Coronoidectomy (separate procedure)

ICD-9-CM Diagnostic
524.02 Mandibular hyperplasia
524.07 Excessive tuberosity of jaw
524.09 Other specified major anomaly of jaw size
524.12 Other jaw asymmetry
524.19 Other specified anomaly of relationship of jaw to cranial base
524.21 Anomaly of dental arch relationship, Angle's class I
524.22 Anomaly of dental arch relationship, Angle's class II
524.23 Anomaly of dental arch relationship, Angle's class III
524.29 Other anomalies of dental arch relationship
524.52 Limited mandibular range of motion
524.53 Deviation in opening and closing of the mandible
524.59 Other dentofacial functional abnormalities
524.89 Other specified dentofacial anomalies
526.89 Other specified disease of the jaws
802.23 Closed fracture of coronoid process of mandible
802.33 Open fracture of coronoid process of mandible
905.0 Late effect of fracture of skull and face bones

ICD-9-CM Procedural
76.31 Partial mandibulectomy

21076
21076 Impression and custom preparation; surgical obturator prosthesis

ICD-9-CM Diagnostic
145.2 Malignant neoplasm of hard palate
145.3 Malignant neoplasm of soft palate
749.01 Unilateral cleft palate, complete
749.02 Unilateral cleft palate, incomplete
749.03 Bilateral cleft palate, complete
749.04 Bilateral cleft palate, incomplete
749.21 Unilateral cleft palate with cleft lip, complete
749.22 Unilateral cleft palate with cleft lip, incomplete
749.23 Bilateral cleft palate with cleft lip, complete
749.24 Bilateral cleft palate with cleft lip, incomplete
749.25 Other combinations of cleft palate with cleft lip
756.0 Congenital anomalies of skull and face bones
873.65 Open wound of palate, without mention of complication — (Use additional code to identify infection)
873.75 Open wound of palate, complicated — (Use additional code to identify infection)
905.0 Late effect of fracture of skull and face bones
V10.02 Personal history of malignant neoplasm of other and unspecified parts of oral cavity and pharynx ▽
V51 Aftercare involving the use of plastic surgery
V52.8 Fitting and adjustment of other specified prosthetic device

ICD-9-CM Procedural
23.6 Prosthetic dental implant
99.99 Other miscellaneous procedures

21077
21077 Impression and custom preparation; orbital prosthesis

ICD-9-CM Diagnostic
170.0 Malignant neoplasm of bones of skull and face, except mandible
730.18 Chronic osteomyelitis, other specified sites — (Use additional code to identify organism, 041.1)
733.49 Aseptic necrosis of other bone site
802.6 Orbital floor (blow-out), closed fracture
802.7 Orbital floor (blow-out), open fracture
802.8 Other facial bones, closed fracture
802.9 Other facial bones, open fracture
870.3 Penetrating wound of orbit, without mention of foreign body — (Use additional code to identify infection)
870.4 Penetrating wound of orbit with foreign body — (Use additional code to identify infection)
905.0 Late effect of fracture of skull and face bones
906.0 Late effect of open wound of head, neck, and trunk
906.4 Late effect of crushing
925.1 Crushing injury of face and scalp — (Use additional code to identify any associated injuries: 800-829, 850.0-854.1, 860.0-869.1)

ICD-9-CM Procedural
95.34 Ocular prosthetics
99.99 Other miscellaneous procedures

HCPCS Level II Supplies & Services
L8042 Orbital prosthesis, provided by a non-physician
L8610 Ocular implant
V2623 Prosthetic eye, plastic, custom

21079–21080
21079 Impression and custom preparation; interim obturator prosthesis
21080 definitive obturator prosthesis

ICD-9-CM Diagnostic
145.2 Malignant neoplasm of hard palate
145.3 Malignant neoplasm of soft palate
170.0 Malignant neoplasm of bones of skull and face, except mandible
749.00 Unspecified cleft palate ▽
749.01 Unilateral cleft palate, complete
749.02 Unilateral cleft palate, incomplete
749.03 Bilateral cleft palate, complete
749.04 Bilateral cleft palate, incomplete
749.21 Unilateral cleft palate with cleft lip, complete
749.22 Unilateral cleft palate with cleft lip, incomplete

749.23	Bilateral cleft palate with cleft lip, complete
749.24	Bilateral cleft palate with cleft lip, incomplete
749.25	Other combinations of cleft palate with cleft lip
756.0	Congenital anomalies of skull and face bones
873.65	Open wound of palate, without mention of complication — (Use additional code to identify infection)
873.75	Open wound of palate, complicated — (Use additional code to identify infection)
905.0	Late effect of fracture of skull and face bones
V10.02	Personal history of malignant neoplasm of other and unspecified parts of oral cavity and pharynx
V52.8	Fitting and adjustment of other specified prosthetic device

ICD-9-CM Procedural

23.6	Prosthetic dental implant
99.99	Other miscellaneous procedures

21081

21081 Impression and custom preparation; mandibular resection prosthesis

ICD-9-CM Diagnostic

170.1	Malignant neoplasm of mandible
213.1	Benign neoplasm of lower jaw bone
524.04	Mandibular hypoplasia
524.12	Other jaw asymmetry
524.74	Alveolar mandibular hypoplasia
526.89	Other specified disease of the jaws
733.91	Arrest of bone development or growth
873.54	Open wound of jaw, complicated — (Use additional code to identify infection)
905.0	Late effect of fracture of skull and face bones
V52.8	Fitting and adjustment of other specified prosthetic device

ICD-9-CM Procedural

23.6	Prosthetic dental implant
99.99	Other miscellaneous procedures

21082–21083

21082 Impression and custom preparation; palatal augmentation prosthesis
21083 palatal lift prosthesis

ICD-9-CM Diagnostic

749.00	Unspecified cleft palate
749.01	Unilateral cleft palate, complete
749.02	Unilateral cleft palate, incomplete
749.03	Bilateral cleft palate, complete
749.04	Bilateral cleft palate, incomplete
749.21	Unilateral cleft palate with cleft lip, complete
749.22	Unilateral cleft palate with cleft lip, incomplete
749.23	Bilateral cleft palate with cleft lip, complete
749.24	Bilateral cleft palate with cleft lip, incomplete
749.25	Other combinations of cleft palate with cleft lip
784.5	Other speech disturbance
787.2	Dysphagia
V52.8	Fitting and adjustment of other specified prosthetic device

ICD-9-CM Procedural

23.6	Prosthetic dental implant
99.99	Other miscellaneous procedures

21084

21084 Impression and custom preparation; speech aid prosthesis

ICD-9-CM Diagnostic

749.00	Unspecified cleft palate
749.01	Unilateral cleft palate, complete
749.02	Unilateral cleft palate, incomplete
749.03	Bilateral cleft palate, complete
749.04	Bilateral cleft palate, incomplete
749.21	Unilateral cleft palate with cleft lip, complete
749.22	Unilateral cleft palate with cleft lip, incomplete
749.23	Bilateral cleft palate with cleft lip, complete
749.24	Bilateral cleft palate with cleft lip, incomplete
749.25	Other combinations of cleft palate with cleft lip
784.5	Other speech disturbance
787.2	Dysphagia
V52.8	Fitting and adjustment of other specified prosthetic device

ICD-9-CM Procedural

23.6	Prosthetic dental implant
99.99	Other miscellaneous procedures

21085

21085 Impression and custom preparation; oral surgical splint

ICD-9-CM Diagnostic

170.0	Malignant neoplasm of bones of skull and face, except mandible
170.1	Malignant neoplasm of mandible
523.4	Chronic periodontitis
524.01	Maxillary hyperplasia
524.02	Mandibular hyperplasia
524.03	Maxillary hypoplasia
524.04	Mandibular hypoplasia
524.12	Other jaw asymmetry
524.28	Anomaly of dental arch relationship, anomalies of interarch distance
524.29	Other anomalies of dental arch relationship
524.51	Abnormal jaw closure
524.59	Other dentofacial functional abnormalities
524.72	Alveolar mandibular hyperplasia
524.74	Alveolar mandibular hypoplasia
526.89	Other specified disease of the jaws
V10.02	Personal history of malignant neoplasm of other and unspecified parts of oral cavity and pharynx
V51	Aftercare involving the use of plastic surgery

ICD-9-CM Procedural

23.6	Prosthetic dental implant
99.99	Other miscellaneous procedures

21086

21086 Impression and custom preparation; auricular prosthesis

ICD-9-CM Diagnostic

171.0	Malignant neoplasm of connective and other soft tissue of head, face, and neck
172.2	Malignant melanoma of skin of ear and external auditory canal
173.2	Other malignant neoplasm of skin of ear and external auditory canal
380.32	Acquired deformities of auricle or pinna
388.8	Other disorders of ear
744.01	Congenital absence of external ear causing impairment of hearing
744.02	Other congenital anomaly of external ear causing impairment of hearing
744.09	Other congenital anomalies of ear causing impairment of hearing
744.23	Microtia
872.11	Open wound of auricle, complicated — (Use additional code to identify infection)
906.5	Late effect of burn of eye, face, head, and neck
925.1	Crushing injury of face and scalp — (Use additional code to identify any associated injuries: 800-829, 850.0-854.1, 860.0-869.1)
941.31	Full-thickness skin loss due to burn (third degree nos) of ear (any part)
941.51	Deep necrosis of underlying tissues due to burn (deep third degree) of ear (any part), with loss of a body part
V10.82	Personal history of malignant melanoma of skin
V10.83	Personal history of other malignant neoplasm of skin
V51	Aftercare involving the use of plastic surgery

ICD-9-CM Procedural

18.71	Construction of auricle of ear
99.99	Other miscellaneous procedures

HCPCS Level II Supplies & Services

L8045	Auricular prosthesis, provided by a non-physician

21087

21087 Impression and custom preparation; nasal prosthesis

ICD-9-CM Diagnostic

738.0	Acquired deformity of nose
748.1	Other congenital anomaly of nose
756.0	Congenital anomalies of skull and face bones
802.0	Nasal bones, closed fracture
802.1	Nasal bones, open fracture
873.30	Open wound of nose, unspecified site, complicated — (Use additional code to identify infection)

873.31 Open wound of nasal septum, complicated — (Use additional code to identify infection)
873.32 Open wound of nasal cavity, complicated — (Use additional code to identify infection)
873.33 Open wound of nasal sinus, complicated — (Use additional code to identify infection)
873.39 Open wound of nose, multiple sites, complicated — (Use additional code to identify infection)
906.5 Late effect of burn of eye, face, head, and neck
V10.22 Personal history of malignant neoplasm of nasal cavities, middle ear, and accessory sinuses
V10.82 Personal history of malignant melanoma of skin
V10.83 Personal history of other malignant neoplasm of skin

ICD-9-CM Procedural

99.99 Other miscellaneous procedures

HCPCS Level II Supplies & Services

L8040 Nasal prosthesis, provided by a non-physician

21088

21088 Impression and custom preparation; facial prosthesis

ICD-9-CM Diagnostic

744.89 Other specified congenital anomaly of face and neck
756.0 Congenital anomalies of skull and face bones
906.5 Late effect of burn of eye, face, head, and neck
V10.81 Personal history of malignant neoplasm of bone
V10.82 Personal history of malignant melanoma of skin
V10.83 Personal history of other malignant neoplasm of skin

ICD-9-CM Procedural

99.99 Other miscellaneous procedures

HCPCS Level II Supplies & Services

L8041 Midfacial prosthesis, provided by a non-physician
L8043 Upper facial prosthesis, provided by a non-physician
L8044 Hemi-facial prosthesis, provided by a non-physician
L8046 Partial facial prosthesis, provided by a non-physician

21100

21100 Application of halo type appliance for maxillofacial fixation, includes removal (separate procedure)

ICD-9-CM Diagnostic

170.0 Malignant neoplasm of bones of skull and face, except mandible
170.1 Malignant neoplasm of mandible
524.01 Maxillary hyperplasia
524.02 Mandibular hyperplasia
524.06 Microgenia
524.07 Excessive tuberosity of jaw
524.09 Other specified major anomaly of jaw size
524.10 Unspecified anomaly of relationship of jaw to cranial base ▽
524.11 Maxillary asymmetry
524.12 Other jaw asymmetry
524.19 Other specified anomaly of relationship of jaw to cranial base
754.0 Congenital musculoskeletal deformities of skull, face, and jaw
756.0 Congenital anomalies of skull and face bones
802.22 Closed fracture of subcondylar process of mandible
802.25 Closed fracture of angle of jaw
802.26 Closed fracture of symphysis of body of mandible
802.28 Closed fracture of other and unspecified part of body of mandible ▽
802.29 Closed fracture of multiple sites of mandible
802.32 Open fracture of subcondylar process of mandible
802.35 Open fracture of angle of jaw
802.36 Open fracture of symphysis of body of mandible
802.38 Open fracture of other and unspecified part of body of mandible
802.39 Open fracture of multiple sites of mandible
802.4 Malar and maxillary bones, closed fracture
802.5 Malar and maxillary bones, open fracture

ICD-9-CM Procedural

78.19 Application of external fixation device, other
97.36 Removal of other external mandibular fixation device

HCPCS Level II Supplies & Services

A4305 Disposable drug delivery system, flow rate of 50 ml or greater per hour
A4306 Disposable drug delivery system, flow rate of 5 ml or less per hour
A4550 Surgical trays

21110

21110 Application of interdental fixation device for conditions other than fracture or dislocation, includes removal

ICD-9-CM Diagnostic

143.0 Malignant neoplasm of upper gum
143.1 Malignant neoplasm of lower gum
143.8 Malignant neoplasm of other sites of gum
143.9 Malignant neoplasm of gum, unspecified site ▽
145.2 Malignant neoplasm of hard palate
145.3 Malignant neoplasm of soft palate
145.5 Malignant neoplasm of palate, unspecified ▽
145.6 Malignant neoplasm of retromolar area
170.0 Malignant neoplasm of bones of skull and face, except mandible
170.1 Malignant neoplasm of mandible
278.00 Obesity, unspecified — (Use additional code to identify any associated mental retardation) ▽
278.01 Morbid obesity — (Use additional code to identify any associated mental retardation)
524.01 Maxillary hyperplasia
524.02 Mandibular hyperplasia
524.06 Microgenia
524.07 Excessive tuberosity of jaw
524.09 Other specified major anomaly of jaw size
524.10 Unspecified anomaly of relationship of jaw to cranial base ▽
524.11 Maxillary asymmetry
524.12 Other jaw asymmetry
524.19 Other specified anomaly of relationship of jaw to cranial base
524.28 Anomaly of dental arch relationship, anomalies of interarch distance
524.29 Other anomalies of dental arch relationship
524.51 Abnormal jaw closure
524.52 Limited mandibular range of motion
524.53 Deviation in opening and closing of the mandible
524.56 Dentofacial functional abnormality, non-working side interference
524.59 Other dentofacial functional abnormalities
524.60 Unspecified temporomandibular joint disorders ▽
524.61 Adhesions and ankylosis (bony or fibrous) of temporomandibular joint
524.62 Arthralgia of temporomandibular joint
524.63 Articular disc disorder (reducing or non-reducing) of temporomandibular joint
524.64 Temporomandibular joint sounds on opening and/or closing the jaw
524.69 Other specified temporomandibular joint disorders
525.0 Exfoliation of teeth due to systemic causes
525.10 Unspecified acquired absence of teeth ▽
525.11 Loss of teeth due to trauma
525.12 Loss of teeth due to periodontal disease
525.13 Loss of teeth due to caries
525.19 Other loss of teeth
525.20 Unspecified atrophy of edentulous alveolar ridge
525.21 Minimal atrophy of the mandible
525.22 Moderate atrophy of the mandible
525.23 Severe atrophy of the mandible
525.24 Minimal atrophy of the maxilla
525.25 Moderate atrophy of the maxilla
525.26 Severe atrophy of the maxilla
525.8 Other specified disorders of the teeth and supporting structures
525.9 Unspecified disorder of the teeth and supporting structures ▽
526.4 Inflammatory conditions of jaw
714.0 Rheumatoid arthritis — (Use additional code to identify manifestation: 357.1, 359.6)
715.80 Osteoarthrosis involving more than one site, but not specified as generalized, unspecified site ▽
715.89 Osteoarthrosis involving multiple sites, but not specified as generalized
715.98 Osteoarthrosis, unspecified whether generalized or localized, other specified sites ▽
716.90 Unspecified arthropathy, site unspecified ▽
716.98 Unspecified arthropathy, other unspecified sites ▽
716.99 Unspecified arthropathy, multiple sites ▽
754.0 Congenital musculoskeletal deformities of skull, face, and jaw
756.0 Congenital anomalies of skull and face bones
905.0 Late effect of fracture of skull and face bones

ICD-9-CM Procedural

24.7 Application of orthodontic appliance

78.59 Internal fixation of other bone, except facial bones, without fracture reduction

HCPCS Level II Supplies & Services

A4305 Disposable drug delivery system, flow rate of 50 ml or greater per hour
A4306 Disposable drug delivery system, flow rate of 5 ml or less per hour
A4550 Surgical trays

21116

21116 Injection procedure for temporomandibular joint arthrography

ICD-9-CM Diagnostic

170.1 Malignant neoplasm of mandible
524.60 Unspecified temporomandibular joint disorders
524.61 Adhesions and ankylosis (bony or fibrous) of temporomandibular joint
524.62 Arthralgia of temporomandibular joint
524.63 Articular disc disorder (reducing or non-reducing) of temporomandibular joint
524.69 Other specified temporomandibular joint disorders
802.21 Closed fracture of condylar process of mandible
802.31 Open fracture of condylar process of mandible
830.0 Closed dislocation of jaw
830.1 Open dislocation of jaw
905.0 Late effect of fracture of skull and face bones

ICD-9-CM Procedural

76.96 Injection of therapeutic substance into temporomandibular joint
87.13 Temporomandibular contrast arthrogram

21120

21120 Genioplasty; augmentation (autograft, allograft, prosthetic material)

ICD-9-CM Diagnostic

170.1 Malignant neoplasm of mandible
524.04 Mandibular hypoplasia
524.06 Microgenia
524.89 Other specified dentofacial anomalies
754.0 Congenital musculoskeletal deformities of skull, face, and jaw
784.5 Other speech disturbance
787.2 Dysphagia
V10.02 Personal history of malignant neoplasm of other and unspecified parts of oral cavity and pharynx
V41.6 Problems with swallowing and mastication — (This code is intended for use when these conditions are recorded as diagnoses or problems)
V50.1 Other plastic surgery for unacceptable cosmetic appearance
V51 Aftercare involving the use of plastic surgery

ICD-9-CM Procedural

76.68 Augmentation genioplasty

21121–21123

21121 Genioplasty; sliding osteotomy, single piece
21122 sliding osteotomies, two or more osteotomies (eg, wedge excision or bone wedge reversal for asymmetrical chin)
21123 sliding, augmentation with interpositional bone grafts (includes obtaining autografts)

ICD-9-CM Diagnostic

524.02 Mandibular hyperplasia
524.04 Mandibular hypoplasia
524.05 Macrogenia
524.06 Microgenia
524.07 Excessive tuberosity of jaw
524.09 Other specified major anomaly of jaw size
524.29 Other anomalies of dental arch relationship
524.30 Anomaly of tooth position, unspecified
524.39 Other anomalies of tooth position
524.89 Other specified dentofacial anomalies
526.89 Other specified disease of the jaws
V50.1 Other plastic surgery for unacceptable cosmetic appearance
V51 Aftercare involving the use of plastic surgery

ICD-9-CM Procedural

76.62 Open osteoplasty (osteotomy) of mandibular ramus
76.68 Augmentation genioplasty
76.91 Bone graft to facial bone

21125–21127

21125 Augmentation, mandibular body or angle; prosthetic material
21127 with bone graft, onlay or interpositional (includes obtaining autograft)

ICD-9-CM Diagnostic

524.04 Mandibular hypoplasia
524.07 Excessive tuberosity of jaw
524.09 Other specified major anomaly of jaw size
524.19 Other specified anomaly of relationship of jaw to cranial base
524.20 Unspecified anomaly of dental arch relationship,
524.21 Anomaly of dental arch relationship, Angle's class I
524.22 Anomaly of dental arch relationship, Angle's class II
524.23 Anomaly of dental arch relationship, Angle's class III
524.28 Anomaly of dental arch relationship, anomalies of interarch distance
524.52 Limited mandibular range of motion
524.53 Deviation in opening and closing of the mandible
524.59 Other dentofacial functional abnormalities
524.89 Other specified dentofacial anomalies
526.89 Other specified disease of the jaws
784.5 Other speech disturbance
787.2 Dysphagia
V50.1 Other plastic surgery for unacceptable cosmetic appearance
V51 Aftercare involving the use of plastic surgery

ICD-9-CM Procedural

76.43 Other reconstruction of mandible
76.68 Augmentation genioplasty
76.91 Bone graft to facial bone
76.92 Insertion of synthetic implant in facial bone

21137

21137 Reduction forehead; contouring only

ICD-9-CM Diagnostic

733.3 Hyperostosis of skull
738.19 Other specified acquired deformity of head
754.0 Congenital musculoskeletal deformities of skull, face, and jaw
756.0 Congenital anomalies of skull and face bones
905.0 Late effect of fracture of skull and face bones
906.3 Late effect of contusion
906.4 Late effect of crushing

ICD-9-CM Procedural

76.99 Other operations on facial bones and joints

21138–21139

21138 Reduction forehead; contouring and application of prosthetic material or bone graft (includes obtaining autograft)
21139 contouring and setback of anterior frontal sinus wall

ICD-9-CM Diagnostic

733.3 Hyperostosis of skull
738.19 Other specified acquired deformity of head
754.0 Congenital musculoskeletal deformities of skull, face, and jaw
756.0 Congenital anomalies of skull and face bones
905.0 Late effect of fracture of skull and face bones
906.4 Late effect of crushing

ICD-9-CM Procedural

76.91 Bone graft to facial bone
76.92 Insertion of synthetic implant in facial bone
76.99 Other operations on facial bones and joints

21141–21143

21141 Reconstruction midface, LeFort 1; single piece, segment movement in any direction (eg, for Long Face Syndrome), without bone graft
21142 two pieces, segment movement in any direction, without bone graft
21143 three or more pieces, segment movement in any direction, without bone graft

ICD-9-CM Diagnostic

524.01 Maxillary hyperplasia
524.03 Maxillary hypoplasia
524.09 Other specified major anomaly of jaw size
524.11 Maxillary asymmetry

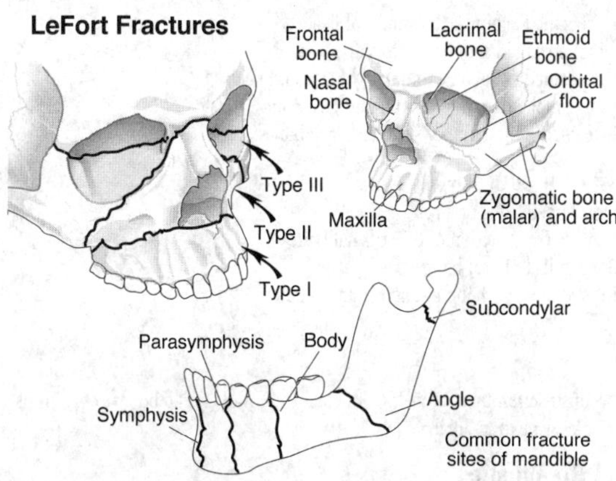

524.12 Other jaw asymmetry
524.19 Other specified anomaly of relationship of jaw to cranial base
524.29 Other anomalies of dental arch relationship
524.9 Unspecified dentofacial anomalies
756.0 Congenital anomalies of skull and face bones

ICD-9-CM Procedural

76.46 Other reconstruction of other facial bone

21145–21147

21145 Reconstruction midface, LeFort I; single piece, segment movement in any direction, requiring bone grafts (includes obtaining autografts)
21146 two pieces, segment movement in any direction, requiring bone grafts (includes obtaining autografts) (eg, ungrafted unilateral alveolar cleft)
21147 three or more pieces, segment movement in any direction, requiring bone grafts (includes obtaining autografts) (eg, ungrafted bilateral alveolar cleft or multiple osteotomies)

ICD-9-CM Diagnostic

524.01 Maxillary hyperplasia
524.03 Maxillary hypoplasia
524.09 Other specified major anomaly of jaw size
524.11 Maxillary asymmetry
524.12 Other jaw asymmetry
524.19 Other specified anomaly of relationship of jaw to cranial base
524.29 Other anomalies of dental arch relationship
524.72 Alveolar mandibular hyperplasia
524.9 Unspecified dentofacial anomalies
756.0 Congenital anomalies of skull and face bones

ICD-9-CM Procedural

76.46 Other reconstruction of other facial bone
76.91 Bone graft to facial bone

21150–21151

21150 Reconstruction midface, LeFort II; anterior intrusion (eg, Treacher-Collins Syndrome)
21151 any direction, requiring bone grafts (includes obtaining autografts)

ICD-9-CM Diagnostic

524.01 Maxillary hyperplasia
524.03 Maxillary hypoplasia
524.09 Other specified major anomaly of jaw size
524.10 Unspecified anomaly of relationship of jaw to cranial base
524.11 Maxillary asymmetry
524.12 Other jaw asymmetry
524.19 Other specified anomaly of relationship of jaw to cranial base
524.29 Other anomalies of dental arch relationship
524.59 Other dentofacial functional abnormalities
524.72 Alveolar mandibular hyperplasia
524.89 Other specified dentofacial anomalies
524.9 Unspecified dentofacial anomalies
733.81 Malunion of fracture
738.10 Unspecified acquired deformity of head
738.11 Zygomatic hyperplasia
738.12 Zygomatic hypoplasia
738.19 Other specified acquired deformity of head
754.0 Congenital musculoskeletal deformities of skull, face, and jaw
756.0 Congenital anomalies of skull and face bones
905.0 Late effect of fracture of skull and face bones

ICD-9-CM Procedural

76.46 Other reconstruction of other facial bone
76.91 Bone graft to facial bone

21154–21155

21154 Reconstruction midface, LeFort III (extracranial), any type, requiring bone grafts (includes obtaining autografts); without LeFort I
21155 with LeFort I

ICD-9-CM Diagnostic

376.40 Unspecified deformity of orbit
376.43 Local deformities of orbit due to bone disease
376.44 Orbital deformities associated with craniofacial deformities
524.01 Maxillary hyperplasia
524.03 Maxillary hypoplasia
524.09 Other specified major anomaly of jaw size
524.11 Maxillary asymmetry
524.12 Other jaw asymmetry
524.19 Other specified anomaly of relationship of jaw to cranial base
524.59 Other dentofacial functional abnormalities
524.72 Alveolar mandibular hyperplasia
524.89 Other specified dentofacial anomalies
524.9 Unspecified dentofacial anomalies
738.19 Other specified acquired deformity of head
743.66 Specified congenital anomaly of orbit
744.9 Unspecified congenital anomaly of face and neck
756.0 Congenital anomalies of skull and face bones

ICD-9-CM Procedural

76.46 Other reconstruction of other facial bone
76.91 Bone graft to facial bone

21159–21160

21159 Reconstruction midface, LeFort III (extra and intracranial) with forehead advancement (eg, mono bloc), requiring bone grafts (includes obtaining autografts); without LeFort I
21160 with LeFort I

ICD-9-CM Diagnostic

376.40 Unspecified deformity of orbit
376.43 Local deformities of orbit due to bone disease
376.44 Orbital deformities associated with craniofacial deformities
376.47 Deformity of orbit due to trauma or surgery
524.01 Maxillary hyperplasia
524.03 Maxillary hypoplasia
524.09 Other specified major anomaly of jaw size
524.11 Maxillary asymmetry
524.12 Other jaw asymmetry
524.19 Other specified anomaly of relationship of jaw to cranial base
524.29 Other anomalies of dental arch relationship
524.70 Unspecified alveolar anomaly
524.71 Alveolar maxillary hyperplasia
524.72 Alveolar mandibular hyperplasia
524.73 Alveolar maxillary hypoplasia

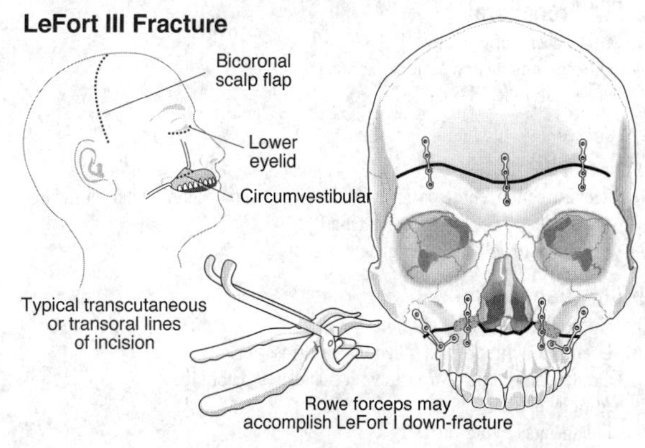

524.79 Other specified alveolar anomaly
524.89 Other specified dentofacial anomalies
524.9 Unspecified dentofacial anomalies
738.10 Unspecified acquired deformity of head
738.11 Zygomatic hyperplasia
738.12 Zygomatic hypoplasia
738.19 Other specified acquired deformity of head
743.66 Specified congenital anomaly of orbit
744.9 Unspecified congenital anomaly of face and neck
756.0 Congenital anomalies of skull and face bones
905.0 Late effect of fracture of skull and face bones

ICD-9-CM Procedural

76.46 Other reconstruction of other facial bone
76.91 Bone graft to facial bone

21172

21172 Reconstruction superior-lateral orbital rim and lower forehead, advancement or alteration, with or without grafts (includes obtaining autografts)

ICD-9-CM Diagnostic

170.0 Malignant neoplasm of bones of skull and face, except mandible
238.0 Neoplasm of uncertain behavior of bone and articular cartilage
239.2 Neoplasms of unspecified nature of bone, soft tissue, and skin
376.40 Unspecified deformity of orbit
376.43 Local deformities of orbit due to bone disease
376.44 Orbital deformities associated with craniofacial deformities
376.45 Atrophy of orbit
376.46 Enlargement of orbit
376.47 Deformity of orbit due to trauma or surgery
738.19 Other specified acquired deformity of head
744.9 Unspecified congenital anomaly of face and neck
756.0 Congenital anomalies of skull and face bones
905.0 Late effect of fracture of skull and face bones

ICD-9-CM Procedural

16.98 Other operations on orbit
76.46 Other reconstruction of other facial bone
76.91 Bone graft to facial bone

21175

21175 Reconstruction, bifrontal, superior-lateral orbital rims and lower forehead, advancement or alteration (eg, plagiocephaly, trigonocephaly, brachycephaly), with or without grafts (includes obtaining autografts)

ICD-9-CM Diagnostic

376.40 Unspecified deformity of orbit
376.43 Local deformities of orbit due to bone disease
376.44 Orbital deformities associated with craniofacial deformities
376.45 Atrophy of orbit
376.46 Enlargement of orbit
376.47 Deformity of orbit due to trauma or surgery
738.10 Unspecified acquired deformity of head
738.19 Other specified acquired deformity of head
744.9 Unspecified congenital anomaly of face and neck
756.0 Congenital anomalies of skull and face bones
905.0 Late effect of fracture of skull and face bones

ICD-9-CM Procedural

16.98 Other operations on orbit
76.46 Other reconstruction of other facial bone
76.91 Bone graft to facial bone

21179–21180

21179 Reconstruction, entire or majority of forehead and/or supraorbital rims; with grafts (allograft or prosthetic material)
21180 with autograft (includes obtaining grafts)

ICD-9-CM Diagnostic

376.40 Unspecified deformity of orbit
376.43 Local deformities of orbit due to bone disease
376.44 Orbital deformities associated with craniofacial deformities
376.45 Atrophy of orbit
376.46 Enlargement of orbit
376.47 Deformity of orbit due to trauma or surgery
738.10 Unspecified acquired deformity of head
738.19 Other specified acquired deformity of head
744.9 Unspecified congenital anomaly of face and neck
756.0 Congenital anomalies of skull and face bones
905.0 Late effect of fracture of skull and face bones

ICD-9-CM Procedural

16.98 Other operations on orbit
76.46 Other reconstruction of other facial bone
76.91 Bone graft to facial bone
76.92 Insertion of synthetic implant in facial bone

21181

21181 Reconstruction by contouring of benign tumor of cranial bones (eg, fibrous dysplasia), extracranial

ICD-9-CM Diagnostic

213.0 Benign neoplasm of bones of skull and face
238.0 Neoplasm of uncertain behavior of bone and articular cartilage
239.2 Neoplasms of unspecified nature of bone, soft tissue, and skin
252.00 Hyperparathyroidism, unspecified
252.01 Primary hyperparathyroidism
252.02 Secondary hyperparathyroidism, non-renal
252.08 Other hyperparathyroidism
733.20 Unspecified cyst of bone (localized)
733.21 Solitary bone cyst
733.22 Aneurysmal bone cyst
733.29 Other cyst of bone
738.11 Zygomatic hyperplasia
756.50 Unspecified congenital osteodystrophy
756.54 Polyostotic fibrous dysplasia of bone
756.59 Other congenital osteodystrophy

ICD-9-CM Procedural

02.99 Other operations on skull, brain, and cerebral meninges
76.91 Bone graft to facial bone

21182–21184

21182 Reconstruction of orbital walls, rims, forehead, nasoethmoid complex following intra- and extracranial excision of benign tumor of cranial bone (eg, fibrous dysplasia), with multiple autografts (includes obtaining grafts); total area of bone grafting less than 40 sq. cm
21183 total area of bone grafting greater than 40 sq. cm but less than 80 sq. cm
21184 total area of bone grafting greater than 80 sq. cm

ICD-9-CM Diagnostic

213.0 Benign neoplasm of bones of skull and face
238.0 Neoplasm of uncertain behavior of bone and articular cartilage
239.2 Neoplasms of unspecified nature of bone, soft tissue, and skin
252.00 Hyperparathyroidism, unspecified
252.01 Primary hyperparathyroidism
252.02 Secondary hyperparathyroidism, non-renal
252.08 Other hyperparathyroidism
376.40 Unspecified deformity of orbit
376.42 Exostosis of orbit
376.43 Local deformities of orbit due to bone disease
376.44 Orbital deformities associated with craniofacial deformities
376.47 Deformity of orbit due to trauma or surgery
733.29 Other cyst of bone
738.11 Zygomatic hyperplasia
738.19 Other specified acquired deformity of head
756.0 Congenital anomalies of skull and face bones
756.54 Polyostotic fibrous dysplasia of bone
756.59 Other congenital osteodystrophy

ICD-9-CM Procedural

16.98 Other operations on orbit
76.46 Other reconstruction of other facial bone
76.91 Bone graft to facial bone

21188

21188 Reconstruction midface, osteotomies (other than LeFort type) and bone grafts (includes obtaining autografts)

ICD-9-CM Diagnostic

143.0 Malignant neoplasm of upper gum
170.0 Malignant neoplasm of bones of skull and face, except mandible
198.5 Secondary malignant neoplasm of bone and bone marrow
238.0 Neoplasm of uncertain behavior of bone and articular cartilage
239.2 Neoplasms of unspecified nature of bone, soft tissue, and skin
524.00 Unspecified major anomaly of jaw size
524.03 Maxillary hypoplasia
524.09 Other specified major anomaly of jaw size
524.11 Maxillary asymmetry
524.12 Other jaw asymmetry
524.19 Other specified anomaly of relationship of jaw to cranial base
738.19 Other specified acquired deformity of head
754.0 Congenital musculoskeletal deformities of skull, face, and jaw
756.0 Congenital anomalies of skull and face bones
802.4 Malar and maxillary bones, closed fracture
802.5 Malar and maxillary bones, open fracture
905.0 Late effect of fracture of skull and face bones
V10.22 Personal history of malignant neoplasm of nasal cavities, middle ear, and accessory sinuses

ICD-9-CM Procedural

76.46 Other reconstruction of other facial bone
76.91 Bone graft to facial bone

21193–21194

21193 Reconstruction of mandibular rami, horizontal, vertical, C, or L osteotomy; without bone graft
21194 with bone graft (includes obtaining graft)

ICD-9-CM Diagnostic

170.1 Malignant neoplasm of mandible
238.0 Neoplasm of uncertain behavior of bone and articular cartilage
239.2 Neoplasms of unspecified nature of bone, soft tissue, and skin
524.02 Mandibular hyperplasia
524.04 Mandibular hypoplasia
524.09 Other specified major anomaly of jaw size
524.19 Other specified anomaly of relationship of jaw to cranial base
524.52 Limited mandibular range of motion
524.53 Deviation in opening and closing of the mandible
524.59 Other dentofacial functional abnormalities
524.69 Other specified temporomandibular joint disorders
524.89 Other specified dentofacial anomalies
526.89 Other specified disease of the jaws
733.81 Malunion of fracture
733.82 Nonunion of fracture
754.0 Congenital musculoskeletal deformities of skull, face, and jaw
784.5 Other speech disturbance
787.2 Dysphagia
905.0 Late effect of fracture of skull and face bones
V50.1 Other plastic surgery for unacceptable cosmetic appearance

ICD-9-CM Procedural

76.43 Other reconstruction of mandible
76.91 Bone graft to facial bone

21195–21196

21195 Reconstruction of mandibular rami and/or body, sagittal split; without internal rigid fixation
21196 with internal rigid fixation

ICD-9-CM Diagnostic

170.1 Malignant neoplasm of mandible
238.0 Neoplasm of uncertain behavior of bone and articular cartilage
239.2 Neoplasms of unspecified nature of bone, soft tissue, and skin
524.00 Unspecified major anomaly of jaw size
524.02 Mandibular hyperplasia
524.04 Mandibular hypoplasia
524.09 Other specified major anomaly of jaw size
524.19 Other specified anomaly of relationship of jaw to cranial base
524.29 Other anomalies of dental arch relationship
524.69 Other specified temporomandibular joint disorders
524.89 Other specified dentofacial anomalies
526.89 Other specified disease of the jaws
754.0 Congenital musculoskeletal deformities of skull, face, and jaw
787.2 Dysphagia
905.0 Late effect of fracture of skull and face bones
V50.1 Other plastic surgery for unacceptable cosmetic appearance

ICD-9-CM Procedural

76.43 Other reconstruction of mandible
76.61 Closed osteoplasty (osteotomy) of mandibular ramus
76.63 Osteoplasty (osteotomy) of body of mandible

21198–21199

21198 Osteotomy, mandible, segmental;
21199 with genioglossus advancement

ICD-9-CM Diagnostic

524.02 Mandibular hyperplasia
524.04 Mandibular hypoplasia
524.12 Other jaw asymmetry
524.72 Alveolar mandibular hyperplasia
524.74 Alveolar mandibular hypoplasia
524.79 Other specified alveolar anomaly
524.89 Other specified dentofacial anomalies
524.9 Unspecified dentofacial anomalies
526.89 Other specified disease of the jaws
754.0 Congenital musculoskeletal deformities of skull, face, and jaw
V50.1 Other plastic surgery for unacceptable cosmetic appearance

ICD-9-CM Procedural

76.63 Osteoplasty (osteotomy) of body of mandible
76.64 Other orthognathic surgery on mandible

21206

21206 Osteotomy, maxilla, segmental (eg, Wassmund or Schuchard)

ICD-9-CM Diagnostic

143.0 Malignant neoplasm of upper gum
170.0 Malignant neoplasm of bones of skull and face, except mandible
198.5 Secondary malignant neoplasm of bone and bone marrow
524.01 Maxillary hyperplasia
524.11 Maxillary asymmetry
524.21 Anomaly of dental arch relationship, Angle's class I
524.22 Anomaly of dental arch relationship, Angle's class II
524.23 Anomaly of dental arch relationship, Angle's class III
524.28 Anomaly of dental arch relationship, anomalies of interarch distance
524.29 Other anomalies of dental arch relationship
524.59 Other dentofacial functional abnormalities
524.9 Unspecified dentofacial anomalies
738.19 Other specified acquired deformity of head
754.0 Congenital musculoskeletal deformities of skull, face, and jaw
756.0 Congenital anomalies of skull and face bones

ICD-9-CM Procedural

76.65 Segmental osteoplasty (osteotomy) of maxilla

21208

21208 Osteoplasty, facial bones; augmentation (autograft, allograft, or prosthetic implant)

ICD-9-CM Diagnostic

524.03 Maxillary hypoplasia
524.04 Mandibular hypoplasia
524.06 Microgenia
524.07 Excessive tuberosity of jaw
524.09 Other specified major anomaly of jaw size
524.11 Maxillary asymmetry
524.12 Other jaw asymmetry
524.19 Other specified anomaly of relationship of jaw to cranial base
524.73 Alveolar maxillary hypoplasia
524.74 Alveolar mandibular hypoplasia
524.79 Other specified alveolar anomaly
524.89 Other specified dentofacial anomalies
526.89 Other specified disease of the jaws
738.12 Zygomatic hypoplasia

Unspecified code
♀ Female diagnosis
Manifestation code
♂ Male diagnosis

738.19 Other specified acquired deformity of head
905.0 Late effect of fracture of skull and face bones
V50.1 Other plastic surgery for unacceptable cosmetic appearance

ICD-9-CM Procedural

76.63 Osteoplasty (osteotomy) of body of mandible
76.66 Total osteoplasty (osteotomy) of maxilla
76.69 Other facial bone repair
76.91 Bone graft to facial bone
76.92 Insertion of synthetic implant in facial bone

21209

21209 Osteoplasty, facial bones; reduction

ICD-9-CM Diagnostic

524.01 Maxillary hyperplasia
524.02 Mandibular hyperplasia
524.05 Macrogenia
524.07 Excessive tuberosity of jaw
524.09 Other specified major anomaly of jaw size
524.10 Unspecified anomaly of relationship of jaw to cranial base ▽
524.11 Maxillary asymmetry
524.12 Other jaw asymmetry
524.19 Other specified anomaly of relationship of jaw to cranial base
524.61 Adhesions and ankylosis (bony or fibrous) of temporomandibular joint
524.69 Other specified temporomandibular joint disorders
524.89 Other specified dentofacial anomalies
526.89 Other specified disease of the jaws
738.11 Zygomatic hyperplasia
738.12 Zygomatic hypoplasia
738.19 Other specified acquired deformity of head
V50.1 Other plastic surgery for unacceptable cosmetic appearance

ICD-9-CM Procedural

76.31 Partial mandibulectomy
76.63 Osteoplasty (osteotomy) of body of mandible
76.66 Total osteoplasty (osteotomy) of maxilla
76.67 Reduction genioplasty
76.69 Other facial bone repair

21210

21210 Graft, bone; nasal, maxillary or malar areas (includes obtaining graft)

ICD-9-CM Diagnostic

160.2 Malignant neoplasm of maxillary sinus
160.8 Malignant neoplasm of other sites of nasal cavities, middle ear, and accessory sinuses
170.0 Malignant neoplasm of bones of skull and face, except mandible
213.0 Benign neoplasm of bones of skull and face
376.50 Enophthalmos, unspecified as to cause ▽
376.51 Enophthalmos due to atrophy of orbital tissue
376.52 Enophthalmos due to trauma or surgery
473.0 Chronic maxillary sinusitis
522.8 Radicular cyst of dental pulp
523.4 Chronic periodontitis
524.03 Maxillary hypoplasia
524.09 Other specified major anomaly of jaw size
524.11 Maxillary asymmetry
524.12 Other jaw asymmetry
524.19 Other specified anomaly of relationship of jaw to cranial base
733.81 Malunion of fracture
738.0 Acquired deformity of nose
748.1 Other congenital anomaly of nose
749.01 Unilateral cleft palate, complete
749.02 Unilateral cleft palate, incomplete
749.03 Bilateral cleft palate, complete
749.04 Bilateral cleft palate, incomplete
749.20 Unspecified cleft palate with cleft lip ▽
749.21 Unilateral cleft palate with cleft lip, complete
749.22 Unilateral cleft palate with cleft lip, incomplete
749.23 Bilateral cleft palate with cleft lip, complete
754.0 Congenital musculoskeletal deformities of skull, face, and jaw
756.0 Congenital anomalies of skull and face bones
802.0 Nasal bones, closed fracture
802.1 Nasal bones, open fracture
802.4 Malar and maxillary bones, closed fracture
802.5 Malar and maxillary bones, open fracture
802.6 Orbital floor (blow-out), closed fracture
802.7 Orbital floor (blow-out), open fracture
802.8 Other facial bones, closed fracture
905.0 Late effect of fracture of skull and face bones
906.5 Late effect of burn of eye, face, head, and neck
996.4 Mechanical complication of internal orthopedic device, implant, and graft
V50.1 Other plastic surgery for unacceptable cosmetic appearance
V51 Aftercare involving the use of plastic surgery

ICD-9-CM Procedural

21.89 Other repair and plastic operations on nose
76.91 Bone graft to facial bone

21215

21215 Graft, bone; mandible (includes obtaining graft)

ICD-9-CM Diagnostic

170.1 Malignant neoplasm of mandible
213.1 Benign neoplasm of lower jaw bone
238.0 Neoplasm of uncertain behavior of bone and articular cartilage
239.2 Neoplasms of unspecified nature of bone, soft tissue, and skin
522.8 Radicular cyst of dental pulp
523.4 Chronic periodontitis
524.04 Mandibular hypoplasia
524.06 Microgenia
524.09 Other specified major anomaly of jaw size
524.10 Unspecified anomaly of relationship of jaw to cranial base ▽
524.12 Other jaw asymmetry
524.19 Other specified anomaly of relationship of jaw to cranial base
524.74 Alveolar mandibular hypoplasia
524.79 Other specified alveolar anomaly
524.89 Other specified dentofacial anomalies
525.20 Unspecified atrophy of edentulous alveolar ridge
525.21 Minimal atrophy of the mandible
525.22 Moderate atrophy of the mandible
525.23 Severe atrophy of the mandible
525.8 Other specified disorders of the teeth and supporting structures
526.89 Other specified disease of the jaws
733.81 Malunion of fracture
733.82 Nonunion of fracture
738.19 Other specified acquired deformity of head
802.20 Closed fracture of unspecified site of mandible ▽
802.22 Closed fracture of subcondylar process of mandible
802.25 Closed fracture of angle of jaw
802.26 Closed fracture of symphysis of body of mandible
802.28 Closed fracture of other and unspecified part of body of mandible ▽
802.30 Open fracture of unspecified site of mandible ▽
802.32 Open fracture of subcondylar process of mandible
802.35 Open fracture of angle of jaw
802.36 Open fracture of symphysis of body of mandible
802.38 Open fracture of other and unspecified part of body of mandible
905.0 Late effect of fracture of skull and face bones
996.4 Mechanical complication of internal orthopedic device, implant, and graft
V50.1 Other plastic surgery for unacceptable cosmetic appearance
V51 Aftercare involving the use of plastic surgery

ICD-9-CM Procedural

76.91 Bone graft to facial bone

21230–21235

21230 Graft; rib cartilage, autogenous, to face, chin, nose or ear (includes obtaining graft)
21235 ear cartilage, autogenous, to nose or ear (includes obtaining graft)

ICD-9-CM Diagnostic

160.0 Malignant neoplasm of nasal cavities
171.0 Malignant neoplasm of connective and other soft tissue of head, face, and neck
172.2 Malignant melanoma of skin of ear and external auditory canal
173.2 Other malignant neoplasm of skin of ear and external auditory canal
198.89 Secondary malignant neoplasm of other specified sites
235.9 Neoplasm of uncertain behavior of other and unspecified respiratory organs ▽
238.1 Neoplasm of uncertain behavior of connective and other soft tissue ▽
239.1 Neoplasm of unspecified nature of respiratory system
239.2 Neoplasms of unspecified nature of bone, soft tissue, and skin
380.32 Acquired deformities of auricle or pinna

524.00 Unspecified major anomaly of jaw size ▽
524.04 Mandibular hypoplasia
524.06 Microgenia
524.09 Other specified major anomaly of jaw size
524.10 Unspecified anomaly of relationship of jaw to cranial base ▽
524.19 Other specified anomaly of relationship of jaw to cranial base
524.89 Other specified dentofacial anomalies
524.9 Unspecified dentofacial anomalies ▽
738.0 Acquired deformity of nose
738.19 Other specified acquired deformity of head
738.7 Cauliflower ear
744.01 Congenital absence of external ear causing impairment of hearing
744.02 Other congenital anomaly of external ear causing impairment of hearing
744.09 Other congenital anomalies of ear causing impairment of hearing
744.23 Microtia
744.3 Unspecified congenital anomaly of ear ▽
748.0 Congenital choanal atresia
748.1 Other congenital anomaly of nose
754.0 Congenital musculoskeletal deformities of skull, face, and jaw
756.0 Congenital anomalies of skull and face bones
872.11 Open wound of auricle, complicated — (Use additional code to identify infection)
905.0 Late effect of fracture of skull and face bones
906.0 Late effect of open wound of head, neck, and trunk
906.5 Late effect of burn of eye, face, head, and neck
925.1 Crushing injury of face and scalp — (Use additional code to identify any associated injuries: 800-829, 850.0-854.1, 860.0-869.1)
996.4 Mechanical complication of internal orthopedic device, implant, and graft
V50.1 Other plastic surgery for unacceptable cosmetic appearance
V51 Aftercare involving the use of plastic surgery

ICD-9-CM Procedural

18.79 Other plastic repair of external ear
76.91 Bone graft to facial bone
76.99 Other operations on facial bones and joints

21240–21242

21240 Arthroplasty, temporomandibular joint, with or without autograft (includes obtaining graft)
21242 Arthroplasty, temporomandibular joint, with allograft

ICD-9-CM Diagnostic

170.1 Malignant neoplasm of mandible
357.1 Polyneuropathy in collagen vascular disease — (Code first underlying disease: 446.0, 710.0, 714.0) ☒
359.6 Symptomatic inflammatory myopathy in diseases classified elsewhere — (Code first underlying disease: 135, 140.0-208.9, 277.3, 446.0, 710.0, 710.1, 710.2, 714.0) ☒
524.60 Unspecified temporomandibular joint disorders ▽
524.61 Adhesions and ankylosis (bony or fibrous) of temporomandibular joint
524.62 Arthralgia of temporomandibular joint
524.63 Articular disc disorder (reducing or non-reducing) of temporomandibular joint
524.64 Temporomandibular joint sounds on opening and/or closing the jaw
524.69 Other specified temporomandibular joint disorders
714.0 Rheumatoid arthritis — (Use additional code to identify manifestation: 357.1, 359.6)
830.0 Closed dislocation of jaw
830.1 Open dislocation of jaw
905.0 Late effect of fracture of skull and face bones
905.6 Late effect of dislocation
996.4 Mechanical complication of internal orthopedic device, implant, and graft
996.66 Infection and inflammatory reaction due to internal joint prosthesis — (Use additional code to identify specified infections)

ICD-9-CM Procedural

76.5 Temporomandibular arthroplasty
76.91 Bone graft to facial bone

21243

21243 Arthroplasty, temporomandibular joint, with prosthetic joint replacement

ICD-9-CM Diagnostic

170.1 Malignant neoplasm of mandible
357.1 Polyneuropathy in collagen vascular disease — (Code first underlying disease: 446.0, 710.0, 714.0) ☒
359.6 Symptomatic inflammatory myopathy in diseases classified elsewhere — (Code first underlying disease: 135, 140.0-208.9, 277.3, 446.0, 710.0, 710.1, 710.2, 714.0) ☒
524.60 Unspecified temporomandibular joint disorders ▽
524.61 Adhesions and ankylosis (bony or fibrous) of temporomandibular joint
524.62 Arthralgia of temporomandibular joint
524.63 Articular disc disorder (reducing or non-reducing) of temporomandibular joint
524.64 Temporomandibular joint sounds on opening and/or closing the jaw
524.69 Other specified temporomandibular joint disorders
714.0 Rheumatoid arthritis — (Use additional code to identify manifestation: 357.1, 359.6)
718.08 Articular cartilage disorder, other specified site
830.0 Closed dislocation of jaw
830.1 Open dislocation of jaw
905.0 Late effect of fracture of skull and face bones
905.6 Late effect of dislocation
996.4 Mechanical complication of internal orthopedic device, implant, and graft
996.66 Infection and inflammatory reaction due to internal joint prosthesis — (Use additional code to identify specified infections)

ICD-9-CM Procedural

76.5 Temporomandibular arthroplasty
76.92 Insertion of synthetic implant in facial bone

21244

21244 Reconstruction of mandible, extraoral, with transosteal bone plate (eg, mandibular staple bone plate)

ICD-9-CM Diagnostic

170.1 Malignant neoplasm of mandible
198.5 Secondary malignant neoplasm of bone and bone marrow
524.04 Mandibular hypoplasia
524.06 Microgenia
524.09 Other specified major anomaly of jaw size
524.12 Other jaw asymmetry
524.19 Other specified anomaly of relationship of jaw to cranial base
524.29 Other anomalies of dental arch relationship
524.52 Limited mandibular range of motion
524.53 Deviation in opening and closing of the mandible
524.59 Other dentofacial functional abnormalities
524.74 Alveolar mandibular hypoplasia
524.79 Other specified alveolar anomaly
525.20 Unspecified atrophy of edentulous alveolar ridge
525.21 Minimal atrophy of the mandible
525.22 Moderate atrophy of the mandible
525.23 Severe atrophy of the mandible
526.4 Inflammatory conditions of jaw
733.81 Malunion of fracture
733.82 Nonunion of fracture
738.19 Other specified acquired deformity of head
905.0 Late effect of fracture of skull and face bones
996.4 Mechanical complication of internal orthopedic device, implant, and graft

ICD-9-CM Procedural

76.43 Other reconstruction of mandible

21245–21246

21245 Reconstruction of mandible or maxilla, subperiosteal implant; partial
21246 complete

ICD-9-CM Diagnostic

170.0 Malignant neoplasm of bones of skull and face, except mandible
170.1 Malignant neoplasm of mandible
198.5 Secondary malignant neoplasm of bone and bone marrow
520.0 Anodontia
520.6 Disturbances in tooth eruption
521.49 Diseases of hard tissues of teeth, other pathological resorption
523.4 Chronic periodontitis
524.12 Other jaw asymmetry
524.39 Other anomalies of tooth position
524.73 Alveolar maxillary hypoplasia
524.74 Alveolar mandibular hypoplasia
524.79 Other specified alveolar anomaly
524.89 Other specified dentofacial anomalies
525.0 Exfoliation of teeth due to systemic causes
525.10 Unspecified acquired absence of teeth ▽

525.11 Loss of teeth due to trauma
525.12 Loss of teeth due to periodontal disease
525.13 Loss of teeth due to caries
525.19 Other loss of teeth
525.20 Unspecified atrophy of edentulous alveolar ridge
525.21 Minimal atrophy of the mandible
525.22 Moderate atrophy of the mandible
525.23 Severe atrophy of the mandible
525.24 Minimal atrophy of the maxilla
525.25 Moderate atrophy of the maxilla
525.26 Severe atrophy of the maxilla
525.8 Other specified disorders of the teeth and supporting structures
526.4 Inflammatory conditions of jaw
738.19 Other specified acquired deformity of head
905.0 Late effect of fracture of skull and face bones
909.3 Late effect of complications of surgical and medical care
996.4 Mechanical complication of internal orthopedic device, implant, and graft
V41.6 Problems with swallowing and mastication — (This code is intended for use when these conditions are recorded as diagnoses or problems)
V51 Aftercare involving the use of plastic surgery

ICD-9-CM Procedural

76.41 Total mandibulectomy with synchronous reconstruction
76.43 Other reconstruction of mandible
76.91 Bone graft to facial bone
76.92 Insertion of synthetic implant in facial bone

21247

21247 Reconstruction of mandibular condyle with bone and cartilage autografts (includes obtaining grafts) (eg, for hemifacial microsomia)

ICD-9-CM Diagnostic

170.1 Malignant neoplasm of mandible
198.5 Secondary malignant neoplasm of bone and bone marrow
524.04 Mandibular hypoplasia
524.09 Other specified major anomaly of jaw size
524.12 Other jaw asymmetry
524.19 Other specified anomaly of relationship of jaw to cranial base
524.52 Limited mandibular range of motion
524.53 Deviation in opening and closing of the mandible
524.59 Other dentofacial functional abnormalities
524.62 Arthralgia of temporomandibular joint
524.63 Articular disc disorder (reducing or non-reducing) of temporomandibular joint
524.89 Other specified dentofacial anomalies
526.89 Other specified disease of the jaws
733.81 Malunion of fracture
733.82 Nonunion of fracture
738.19 Other specified acquired deformity of head
754.0 Congenital musculoskeletal deformities of skull, face, and jaw
905.0 Late effect of fracture of skull and face bones
996.4 Mechanical complication of internal orthopedic device, implant, and graft

ICD-9-CM Procedural

76.46 Other reconstruction of other facial bone
76.91 Bone graft to facial bone

21248–21249

21248 Reconstruction of mandible or maxilla, endosteal implant (eg, blade, cylinder); partial
21249 complete

ICD-9-CM Diagnostic

170.0 Malignant neoplasm of bones of skull and face, except mandible
170.1 Malignant neoplasm of mandible
352.1 Glossopharyngeal neuralgia
520.0 Anodontia
520.6 Disturbances in tooth eruption
521.40 Diseases of hard tissues of teeth, pathological resorption, unspecified
521.41 Diseases of hard tissues of teeth, pathological resorption, internal
521.42 Diseases of hard tissues of teeth, pathological resorption, external
521.49 Diseases of hard tissues of teeth, other pathological resorption
523.4 Chronic periodontitis
524.30 Anomaly of tooth position, unspecified
524.39 Other anomalies of tooth position
524.73 Alveolar maxillary hypoplasia
524.74 Alveolar mandibular hypoplasia
524.79 Other specified alveolar anomaly
524.89 Other specified dentofacial anomalies
525.0 Exfoliation of teeth due to systemic causes
525.10 Unspecified acquired absence of teeth ▽
525.11 Loss of teeth due to trauma
525.12 Loss of teeth due to periodontal disease
525.13 Loss of teeth due to caries
525.19 Other loss of teeth
525.20 Unspecified atrophy of edentulous alveolar ridge
525.21 Minimal atrophy of the mandible
525.22 Moderate atrophy of the mandible
525.23 Severe atrophy of the mandible
525.24 Minimal atrophy of the maxilla
525.25 Moderate atrophy of the maxilla
525.26 Severe atrophy of the maxilla
525.8 Other specified disorders of the teeth and supporting structures
525.9 Unspecified disorder of the teeth and supporting structures ▽
526.4 Inflammatory conditions of jaw
733.99 Other disorders of bone and cartilage
905.0 Late effect of fracture of skull and face bones
996.4 Mechanical complication of internal orthopedic device, implant, and graft
V41.6 Problems with swallowing and mastication — (This code is intended for use when these conditions are recorded as diagnoses or problems)
V51 Aftercare involving the use of plastic surgery

ICD-9-CM Procedural

76.41 Total mandibulectomy with synchronous reconstruction
76.43 Other reconstruction of mandible
76.46 Other reconstruction of other facial bone

21255

21255 Reconstruction of zygomatic arch and glenoid fossa with bone and cartilage (includes obtaining autografts)

ICD-9-CM Diagnostic

170.0 Malignant neoplasm of bones of skull and face, except mandible
198.5 Secondary malignant neoplasm of bone and bone marrow
213.0 Benign neoplasm of bones of skull and face
238.0 Neoplasm of uncertain behavior of bone and articular cartilage
239.2 Neoplasms of unspecified nature of bone, soft tissue, and skin
733.81 Malunion of fracture
733.82 Nonunion of fracture
738.11 Zygomatic hyperplasia
738.12 Zygomatic hypoplasia
738.19 Other specified acquired deformity of head
905.0 Late effect of fracture of skull and face bones
925.1 Crushing injury of face and scalp — (Use additional code to identify any associated injuries: 800-829, 850.0-854.1, 860.0-869.1)
V10.02 Personal history of malignant neoplasm of other and unspecified parts of oral cavity and pharynx ▽
V51 Aftercare involving the use of plastic surgery

ICD-9-CM Procedural

76.46 Other reconstruction of other facial bone
76.91 Bone graft to facial bone

21256

21256 Reconstruction of orbit with osteotomies (extracranial) and with bone grafts (includes obtaining autografts) (eg, micro-ophthalmia)

ICD-9-CM Diagnostic

170.0 Malignant neoplasm of bones of skull and face, except mandible
198.5 Secondary malignant neoplasm of bone and bone marrow
213.0 Benign neoplasm of bones of skull and face
238.0 Neoplasm of uncertain behavior of bone and articular cartilage
239.2 Neoplasms of unspecified nature of bone, soft tissue, and skin
376.40 Unspecified deformity of orbit ▽
376.42 Exostosis of orbit
376.43 Local deformities of orbit due to bone disease
376.44 Orbital deformities associated with craniofacial deformities
376.45 Atrophy of orbit
376.47 Deformity of orbit due to trauma or surgery
376.50 Enophthalmos, unspecified as to cause ▽
376.51 Enophthalmos due to atrophy of orbital tissue
376.52 Enophthalmos due to trauma or surgery
733.21 Solitary bone cyst

733.81 Malunion of fracture
733.82 Nonunion of fracture
738.19 Other specified acquired deformity of head
743.10 Unspecified microphthalmos ▽
743.11 Simple microphthalmos
743.12 Microphthalmos associated with other anomalies of eye and adnexa
756.0 Congenital anomalies of skull and face bones
759.89 Other specified multiple congenital anomalies, so described
905.0 Late effect of fracture of skull and face bones
925.1 Crushing injury of face and scalp — (Use additional code to identify any associated injuries: 800-829, 850.0-854.1, 860.0-869.1)

ICD-9-CM Procedural

76.69 Other facial bone repair
76.91 Bone graft to facial bone

21260–21263

21260 Periorbital osteotomies for orbital hypertelorism, with bone grafts; extracranial approach
21261 combined intra- and extracranial approach
21263 with forehead advancement

ICD-9-CM Diagnostic

376.41 Hypertelorism of orbit
376.44 Orbital deformities associated with craniofacial deformities
754.0 Congenital musculoskeletal deformities of skull, face, and jaw
756.0 Congenital anomalies of skull and face bones

ICD-9-CM Procedural

76.69 Other facial bone repair
76.91 Bone graft to facial bone

21267–21268

21267 Orbital repositioning, periorbital osteotomies, unilateral, with bone grafts; extracranial approach
21268 combined intra- and extracranial approach

ICD-9-CM Diagnostic

376.40 Unspecified deformity of orbit ▽
376.43 Local deformities of orbit due to bone disease
376.44 Orbital deformities associated with craniofacial deformities
376.45 Atrophy of orbit
376.47 Deformity of orbit due to trauma or surgery
376.52 Enophthalmos due to trauma or surgery
733.81 Malunion of fracture
738.10 Unspecified acquired deformity of head ▽
738.11 Zygomatic hyperplasia
738.12 Zygomatic hypoplasia
738.19 Other specified acquired deformity of head
743.10 Unspecified microphthalmos ▽
743.11 Simple microphthalmos
743.12 Microphthalmos associated with other anomalies of eye and adnexa
754.0 Congenital musculoskeletal deformities of skull, face, and jaw
756.0 Congenital anomalies of skull and face bones
756.9 Other and unspecified congenital anomaly of musculoskeletal system ▽
905.0 Late effect of fracture of skull and face bones
925.1 Crushing injury of face and scalp — (Use additional code to identify any associated injuries: 800-829, 850.0-854.1, 860.0-869.1)

ICD-9-CM Procedural

76.69 Other facial bone repair
76.91 Bone graft to facial bone

21270

21270 Malar augmentation, prosthetic material

ICD-9-CM Diagnostic

524.03 Maxillary hypoplasia
524.06 Microgenia
524.07 Excessive tuberosity of jaw
524.09 Other specified major anomaly of jaw size
524.11 Maxillary asymmetry
524.12 Other jaw asymmetry
524.19 Other specified anomaly of relationship of jaw to cranial base
524.73 Alveolar maxillary hypoplasia
524.89 Other specified dentofacial anomalies
526.89 Other specified disease of the jaws
738.12 Zygomatic hypoplasia
754.0 Congenital musculoskeletal deformities of skull, face, and jaw
756.0 Congenital anomalies of skull and face bones
905.0 Late effect of fracture of skull and face bones
925.1 Crushing injury of face and scalp — (Use additional code to identify any associated injuries: 800-829, 850.0-854.1, 860.0-869.1)
V50.1 Other plastic surgery for unacceptable cosmetic appearance

ICD-9-CM Procedural

76.69 Other facial bone repair
76.92 Insertion of synthetic implant in facial bone

21275

21275 Secondary revision of orbitocraniofacial reconstruction

ICD-9-CM Diagnostic

170.0 Malignant neoplasm of bones of skull and face, except mandible
198.5 Secondary malignant neoplasm of bone and bone marrow
376.41 Hypertelorism of orbit
376.42 Exostosis of orbit
376.43 Local deformities of orbit due to bone disease
376.44 Orbital deformities associated with craniofacial deformities
376.45 Atrophy of orbit
376.46 Enlargement of orbit
376.47 Deformity of orbit due to trauma or surgery
376.52 Enophthalmos due to trauma or surgery
738.12 Zygomatic hypoplasia
738.19 Other specified acquired deformity of head
743.10 Unspecified microphthalmos ▽
743.11 Simple microphthalmos
756.0 Congenital anomalies of skull and face bones
756.51 Osteogenesis imperfecta

ICD-9-CM Procedural

76.69 Other facial bone repair

21280

21280 Medial canthopexy (separate procedure)

ICD-9-CM Diagnostic

376.41 Hypertelorism of orbit
376.47 Deformity of orbit due to trauma or surgery
743.11 Simple microphthalmos
743.63 Other specified congenital anomaly of eyelid
756.0 Congenital anomalies of skull and face bones
802.8 Other facial bones, closed fracture
802.9 Other facial bones, open fracture
870.8 Other specified open wound of ocular adnexa — (Use additional code to identify infection)
906.0 Late effect of open wound of head, neck, and trunk
918.0 Superficial injury of eyelids and periocular area
921.1 Contusion of eyelids and periocular area

ICD-9-CM Procedural

08.59 Other adjustment of lid position

21282

21282 Lateral canthopexy

ICD-9-CM Diagnostic

376.47 Deformity of orbit due to trauma or surgery
743.10 Unspecified microphthalmos ▽
743.11 Simple microphthalmos
743.63 Other specified congenital anomaly of eyelid
756.0 Congenital anomalies of skull and face bones
802.4 Malar and maxillary bones, closed fracture
802.5 Malar and maxillary bones, open fracture
802.8 Other facial bones, closed fracture
802.9 Other facial bones, open fracture
870.8 Other specified open wound of ocular adnexa — (Use additional code to identify infection)
906.0 Late effect of open wound of head, neck, and trunk
V50.1 Other plastic surgery for unacceptable cosmetic appearance

ICD-9-CM Procedural
08.59 Other adjustment of lid position

21295–21296
21295 Reduction of masseter muscle and bone (eg, for treatment of benign masseteric hypertrophy); extraoral approach
21296 intraoral approach

ICD-9-CM Diagnostic
728.9 Unspecified disorder of muscle, ligament, and fascia ▽

ICD-9-CM Procedural
76.64 Other orthognathic surgery on mandible
83.49 Other excision of soft tissue

21300
21300 Closed treatment of skull fracture without operation

ICD-9-CM Diagnostic
800.01 Closed fracture of vault of skull without mention of intracranial injury, no loss of consciousness
800.02 Closed fracture of vault of skull without mention of intracranial injury, brief (less than one hour) loss of consciousness
800.03 Closed fracture of vault of skull without mention of intracranial injury, moderate (1-24 hours) loss of consciousness
800.04 Closed fracture of vault of skull without mention of intracranial injury, prolonged (more than 24 hours) loss of consciousness and return to pre-existing conscious level
800.05 Closed fracture of vault of skull without mention of intracranial injury, prolonged (more than 24 hours) loss of consciousness, without return to pre-existing conscious level
800.06 Closed fracture of vault of skull without mention of intracranial injury, loss of consciousness of unspecified duration ▽
801.02 Closed fracture of base of skull without mention of intracranial injury, brief (less than one hour) loss of consciousness
801.03 Closed fracture of base of skull without mention of intracranial injury, moderate (1-24 hours) loss of consciousness
801.04 Closed fracture of base of skull without mention of intracranial injury, prolonged (more than 24 hours) loss of consciousness and return to pre-existing conscious level
801.05 Closed fracture of base of skull without mention of intracranial injury, prolonged (more than 24 hours) loss of consciousness, without return to pre-existing conscious level
801.06 Closed fracture of base of skull without mention of intracranial injury, loss of consciousness of unspecified duration ▽
801.11 Closed fracture of base of skull with cerebral laceration and contusion, no loss of consciousness
803.01 Other closed skull fracture without mention of intracranial injury, no loss of consciousness

ICD-9-CM Procedural
93.59 Other immobilization, pressure, and attention to wound

21310–21320
21310 Closed treatment of nasal bone fracture without manipulation
21315 Closed treatment of nasal bone fracture; without stabilization
21320 with stabilization

ICD-9-CM Diagnostic
802.0 Nasal bones, closed fracture

ICD-9-CM Procedural
21.71 Closed reduction of nasal fracture
21.99 Other operations on nose
93.54 Application of splint

HCPCS Level II Supplies & Services
A4305 Disposable drug delivery system, flow rate of 50 ml or greater per hour
A4306 Disposable drug delivery system, flow rate of 5 ml or less per hour
A4550 Surgical trays
A4570 Splint
A4649 Surgical supply; miscellaneous

21325
21325 Open treatment of nasal fracture; uncomplicated

ICD-9-CM Diagnostic
733.82 Nonunion of fracture
802.0 Nasal bones, closed fracture
802.1 Nasal bones, open fracture

ICD-9-CM Procedural
21.72 Open reduction of nasal fracture

HCPCS Level II Supplies & Services
A4570 Splint

21330
21330 Open treatment of nasal fracture; complicated, with internal and/or external skeletal fixation

ICD-9-CM Diagnostic
733.82 Nonunion of fracture
802.0 Nasal bones, closed fracture
802.1 Nasal bones, open fracture

ICD-9-CM Procedural
21.72 Open reduction of nasal fracture

21335
21335 Open treatment of nasal fracture; with concomitant open treatment of fractured septum

ICD-9-CM Diagnostic
733.82 Nonunion of fracture
802.0 Nasal bones, closed fracture
802.1 Nasal bones, open fracture

ICD-9-CM Procedural
21.5 Submucous resection of nasal septum
21.72 Open reduction of nasal fracture
21.88 Other septoplasty

21336
21336 Open treatment of nasal septal fracture, with or without stabilization

ICD-9-CM Diagnostic
470 Deviated nasal septum
802.0 Nasal bones, closed fracture
802.1 Nasal bones, open fracture

ICD-9-CM Procedural
21.5 Submucous resection of nasal septum
21.72 Open reduction of nasal fracture
21.88 Other septoplasty

21337
21337 Closed treatment of nasal septal fracture, with or without stabilization

ICD-9-CM Diagnostic
470 Deviated nasal septum
802.0 Nasal bones, closed fracture

ICD-9-CM Procedural
21.71 Closed reduction of nasal fracture

21338–21339
21338 Open treatment of nasoethmoid fracture; without external fixation
21339 with external fixation

ICD-9-CM Diagnostic
801.00 Closed fracture of base of skull without mention of intracranial injury, unspecified state of consciousness ▽
801.01 Closed fracture of base of skull without mention of intracranial injury, no loss of consciousness
801.02 Closed fracture of base of skull without mention of intracranial injury, brief (less than one hour) loss of consciousness

801.03 Closed fracture of base of skull without mention of intracranial injury, moderate (1-24 hours) loss of consciousness

801.04 Closed fracture of base of skull without mention of intracranial injury, prolonged (more than 24 hours) loss of consciousness and return to pre-existing conscious level

801.05 Closed fracture of base of skull without mention of intracranial injury, prolonged (more than 24 hours) loss of consciousness, without return to pre-existing conscious level

801.06 Closed fracture of base of skull without mention of intracranial injury, loss of consciousness of unspecified duration ▽

801.09 Closed fracture of base of skull without mention of intracranial injury, unspecified concussion ▽

801.10 Closed fracture of base of skull with cerebral laceration and contusion, unspecified state of consciousness ▽

801.11 Closed fracture of base of skull with cerebral laceration and contusion, no loss of consciousness

801.12 Closed fracture of base of skull with cerebral laceration and contusion, brief (less than one hour) loss of consciousness

801.13 Closed fracture of base of skull with cerebral laceration and contusion, moderate (1-24 hours) loss of consciousness

801.14 Closed fracture of base of skull with cerebral laceration and contusion, prolonged (more than 24 hours) loss of consciousness and return to pre-existing conscious level

801.15 Closed fracture of base of skull with cerebral laceration and contusion, prolonged (more than 24 hours) loss of consciousness, without return to pre-existing conscious level

801.16 Closed fracture of base of skull with cerebral laceration and contusion, loss of consciousness of unspecified duration ▽

801.19 Closed fracture of base of skull with cerebral laceration and contusion, unspecified concussion ▽

801.20 Closed fracture of base of skull with subarachnoid, subdural, and extradural hemorrhage, unspecified state of consciousness ▽

801.21 Closed fracture of base of skull with subarachnoid, subdural, and extradural hemorrhage, no loss of consciousness

801.22 Closed fracture of base of skull with subarachnoid, subdural, and extradural hemorrhage, brief (less than one hour) loss of consciousness

801.23 Closed fracture of base of skull with subarachnoid, subdural, and extradural hemorrhage, moderate (1-24 hours) loss of consciousness

801.24 Closed fracture of base of skull with subarachnoid, subdural, and extradural hemorrhage, prolonged (more than 24 hours) loss of consciousness and return to pre-existing conscious level

801.25 Closed fracture of base of skull with subarachnoid, subdural, and extradural hemorrhage, prolonged (more than 24 hours) loss of consciousness, without return to pre-existing conscious level

801.26 Closed fracture of base of skull with subarachnoid, subdural, and extradural hemorrhage, loss of consciousness of unspecified duration ▽

801.29 Closed fracture of base of skull with subarachnoid, subdural, and extradural hemorrhage, unspecified concussion ▽

801.30 Closed fracture of base of skull with other and unspecified intracranial hemorrhage, unspecified state of consciousness ▽

801.31 Closed fracture of base of skull with other and unspecified intracranial hemorrhage, no loss of consciousness ▽

801.32 Closed fracture of base of skull with other and unspecified intracranial hemorrhage, brief (less than one hour) loss of consciousness ▽

801.33 Closed fracture of base of skull with other and unspecified intracranial hemorrhage, moderate (1-24 hours) loss of consciousness ▽

801.34 Closed fracture of base of skull with other and unspecified intracranial hemorrhage, prolonged (more than 24 hours) loss of consciousness and return to pre-existing conscious level ▽

801.35 Closed fracture of base of skull with other and unspecified intracranial hemorrhage, prolonged (more than 24 hours) loss of consciousness, without return to pre-existing conscious level ▽

801.36 Closed fracture of base of skull with other and unspecified intracranial hemorrhage, loss of consciousness of unspecified duration ▽

801.39 Closed fracture of base of skull with other and unspecified intracranial hemorrhage, unspecified concussion ▽

801.40 Closed fracture of base of skull with intracranial injury of other and unspecified nature, unspecified state of consciousness ▽

801.41 Closed fracture of base of skull with intracranial injury of other and unspecified nature, no loss of consciousness ▽

801.42 Closed fracture of base of skull with intracranial injury of other and unspecified nature, brief (less than one hour) loss of consciousness ▽

801.43 Closed fracture of base of skull with intracranial injury of other and unspecified nature, moderate (1-24 hours) loss of consciousness ▽

801.44 Closed fracture of base of skull with intracranial injury of other and unspecified nature, prolonged (more than 24 hours) loss of consciousness and return to pre-existing conscious level ▽

801.45 Closed fracture of base of skull with intracranial injury of other and unspecified nature, prolonged (more than 24 hours) loss of consciousness, without return to pre-existing conscious level ▽

801.46 Closed fracture of base of skull with intracranial injury of other and unspecified nature, loss of consciousness of unspecified duration ▽

801.49 Closed fracture of base of skull with intracranial injury of other and unspecified nature, unspecified concussion ▽

801.50 Open fracture of base of skull without mention of intracranial injury, unspecified state of consciousness ▽

801.51 Open fracture of base of skull without mention of intracranial injury, no loss of consciousness

801.52 Open fracture of base of skull without mention of intracranial injury, brief (less than one hour) loss of consciousness

801.53 Open fracture of base of skull without mention of intracranial injury, moderate (1-24 hours) loss of consciousness

801.54 Open fracture of base of skull without mention of intracranial injury, prolonged (more than 24 hours) loss of consciousness and return to pre-existing conscious level

801.55 Open fracture of base of skull without mention of intracranial injury, prolonged (more than 24 hours) loss of consciousness, without return to pre-existing conscious level

801.56 Open fracture of base of skull without mention of intracranial injury, loss of consciousness of unspecified duration ▽

801.59 Open fracture of base of skull without mention of intracranial injury, unspecified concussion ▽

801.60 Open fracture of base of skull with cerebral laceration and contusion, unspecified state of consciousness ▽

801.61 Open fracture of base of skull with cerebral laceration and contusion, no loss of consciousness

801.62 Open fracture of base of skull with cerebral laceration and contusion, brief (less than one hour) loss of consciousness

801.63 Open fracture of base of skull with cerebral laceration and contusion, moderate (1-24 hours) loss of consciousness

801.64 Open fracture of base of skull with cerebral laceration and contusion, prolonged (more than 24 hours) loss of consciousness and return to pre-existing conscious level

801.65 Open fracture of base of skull with cerebral laceration and contusion, prolonged (more than 24 hours) loss of consciousness, without return to pre-existing conscious level

801.66 Open fracture of base of skull with cerebral laceration and contusion, loss of consciousness of unspecified duration ▽

801.69 Open fracture of base of skull with cerebral laceration and contusion, unspecified concussion ▽

801.70 Open fracture of base of skull with subarachnoid, subdural, and extradural hemorrhage, unspecified state of consciousness ▽

801.71 Open fracture of base of skull with subarachnoid, subdural, and extradural hemorrhage, no loss of consciousness

801.72 Open fracture of base of skull with subarachnoid, subdural, and extradural hemorrhage, brief (less than one hour) loss of consciousness

801.73 Open fracture of base of skull with subarachnoid, subdural, and extradural hemorrhage, moderate (1-24 hours) loss of consciousness

801.74 Open fracture of base of skull with subarachnoid, subdural, and extradural hemorrhage, prolonged (more than 24 hours) loss of consciousness and return to pre-existing conscious level

801.75 Open fracture of base of skull with subarachnoid, subdural, and extradural hemorrhage, prolonged (more than 24 hours) loss of consciousness, without return to pre-existing conscious level

801.76 Open fracture of base of skull with subarachnoid, subdural, and extradural hemorrhage, loss of consciousness of unspecified duration ▽

801.79 Open fracture of base of skull with subarachnoid, subdural, and extradural hemorrhage, unspecified concussion ▽

801.80 Open fracture of base of skull with other and unspecified intracranial hemorrhage, unspecified state of consciousness ▽

801.81 Open fracture of base of skull with other and unspecified intracranial hemorrhage, no loss of consciousness ▽

801.82 Open fracture of base of skull with other and unspecified intracranial hemorrhage, brief (less than one hour) loss of consciousness ▽

801.83 Open fracture of base of skull with other and unspecified intracranial hemorrhage, moderate (1-24 hours) loss of consciousness ▽

801.84 Open fracture of base of skull with other and unspecified intracranial hemorrhage, prolonged (more than 24 hours) loss of consciousness and return to pre-existing conscious level ▽

▽ Unspecified code
♀ Female diagnosis
☒ Manifestation code
♂ Male diagnosis

801.85 Open fracture of base of skull with other and unspecified intracranial hemorrhage, prolonged (more than 24 hours) loss of consciousness, without return to pre-existing conscious level
801.86 Open fracture of base of skull with other and unspecified intracranial hemorrhage, loss of consciousness of unspecified duration
801.89 Open fracture of base of skull with other and unspecified intracranial hemorrhage, unspecified concussion
801.90 Open fracture of base of skull with intracranial injury of other and unspecified nature, unspecified state of consciousness
801.91 Open fracture of base of skull with intracranial injury of other and unspecified nature, no loss of consciousness
801.92 Open fracture of base of skull with intracranial injury of other and unspecified nature, brief (less than one hour) loss of consciousness
801.93 Open fracture of base of skull with intracranial injury of other and unspecified nature, moderate (1-24 hours) loss of consciousness
801.94 Open fracture of base of skull with intracranial injury of other and unspecified nature, prolonged (more than 24 hours) loss of consciousness and return to pre-existing conscious level
801.95 Open fracture of base of skull with intracranial injury of other and unspecified nature, prolonged (more than 24 hours) loss of consciousness, without return to pre-existing conscious level
801.96 Open fracture of base of skull with intracranial injury of other and unspecified nature, loss of consciousness of unspecified duration
801.99 Open fracture of base of skull with intracranial injury of other and unspecified nature, unspecified concussion
802.0 Nasal bones, closed fracture
802.1 Nasal bones, open fracture

ICD-9-CM Procedural

21.72 Open reduction of nasal fracture
21.99 Other operations on nose
22.79 Other repair of nasal sinus
76.70 Reduction of facial fracture, not otherwise specified

21340

21340 Percutaneous treatment of nasoethmoid complex fracture, with splint, wire or headcap fixation, including repair of canthal ligaments and/or the nasolacrimal apparatus

ICD-9-CM Diagnostic

733.82 Nonunion of fracture
801.00 Closed fracture of base of skull without mention of intracranial injury, unspecified state of consciousness
801.01 Closed fracture of base of skull without mention of intracranial injury, no loss of consciousness
801.02 Closed fracture of base of skull without mention of intracranial injury, brief (less than one hour) loss of consciousness
801.03 Closed fracture of base of skull without mention of intracranial injury, moderate (1-24 hours) loss of consciousness
801.04 Closed fracture of base of skull without mention of intracranial injury, prolonged (more than 24 hours) loss of consciousness and return to pre-existing conscious level
801.05 Closed fracture of base of skull without mention of intracranial injury, prolonged (more than 24 hours) loss of consciousness, without return to pre-existing conscious level
801.06 Closed fracture of base of skull without mention of intracranial injury, loss of consciousness of unspecified duration
801.09 Closed fracture of base of skull without mention of intracranial injury, unspecified concussion
801.10 Closed fracture of base of skull with cerebral laceration and contusion, unspecified state of consciousness
801.11 Closed fracture of base of skull with cerebral laceration and contusion, no loss of consciousness
801.12 Closed fracture of base of skull with cerebral laceration and contusion, brief (less than one hour) loss of consciousness
801.13 Closed fracture of base of skull with cerebral laceration and contusion, moderate (1-24 hours) loss of consciousness
801.14 Closed fracture of base of skull with cerebral laceration and contusion, prolonged (more than 24 hours) loss of consciousness and return to pre-existing conscious level
801.15 Closed fracture of base of skull with cerebral laceration and contusion, prolonged (more than 24 hours) loss of consciousness, without return to pre-existing conscious level
801.16 Closed fracture of base of skull with cerebral laceration and contusion, loss of consciousness of unspecified duration
801.19 Closed fracture of base of skull with cerebral laceration and contusion, unspecified concussion
801.20 Closed fracture of base of skull with subarachnoid, subdural, and extradural hemorrhage, unspecified state of consciousness
801.21 Closed fracture of base of skull with subarachnoid, subdural, and extradural hemorrhage, no loss of consciousness
801.22 Closed fracture of base of skull with subarachnoid, subdural, and extradural hemorrhage, brief (less than one hour) loss of consciousness
801.23 Closed fracture of base of skull with subarachnoid, subdural, and extradural hemorrhage, moderate (1-24 hours) loss of consciousness
801.24 Closed fracture of base of skull with subarachnoid, subdural, and extradural hemorrhage, prolonged (more than 24 hours) loss of consciousness and return to pre-existing conscious level
801.25 Closed fracture of base of skull with subarachnoid, subdural, and extradural hemorrhage, prolonged (more than 24 hours) loss of consciousness, without return to pre-existing conscious level
801.26 Closed fracture of base of skull with subarachnoid, subdural, and extradural hemorrhage, loss of consciousness of unspecified duration
801.29 Closed fracture of base of skull with subarachnoid, subdural, and extradural hemorrhage, unspecified concussion
801.30 Closed fracture of base of skull with other and unspecified intracranial hemorrhage, unspecified state of consciousness
801.31 Closed fracture of base of skull with other and unspecified intracranial hemorrhage, no loss of consciousness
801.32 Closed fracture of base of skull with other and unspecified intracranial hemorrhage, brief (less than one hour) loss of consciousness
801.33 Closed fracture of base of skull with other and unspecified intracranial hemorrhage, moderate (1-24 hours) loss of consciousness
801.34 Closed fracture of base of skull with other and unspecified intracranial hemorrhage, prolonged (more than 24 hours) loss of consciousness and return to pre-existing conscious level
801.35 Closed fracture of base of skull with other and unspecified intracranial hemorrhage, prolonged (more than 24 hours) loss of consciousness, without return to pre-existing conscious level
801.36 Closed fracture of base of skull with other and unspecified intracranial hemorrhage, loss of consciousness of unspecified duration
801.39 Closed fracture of base of skull with other and unspecified intracranial hemorrhage, unspecified concussion
801.40 Closed fracture of base of skull with intracranial injury of other and unspecified nature, unspecified state of consciousness
801.41 Closed fracture of base of skull with intracranial injury of other and unspecified nature, no loss of consciousness
801.42 Closed fracture of base of skull with intracranial injury of other and unspecified nature, brief (less than one hour) loss of consciousness
801.43 Closed fracture of base of skull with intracranial injury of other and unspecified nature, moderate (1-24 hours) loss of consciousness
801.44 Closed fracture of base of skull with intracranial injury of other and unspecified nature, prolonged (more than 24 hours) loss of consciousness and return to pre-existing conscious level
801.45 Closed fracture of base of skull with intracranial injury of other and unspecified nature, prolonged (more than 24 hours) loss of consciousness, without return to pre-existing conscious level
801.46 Closed fracture of base of skull with intracranial injury of other and unspecified nature, loss of consciousness of unspecified duration
801.49 Closed fracture of base of skull with intracranial injury of other and unspecified nature, unspecified concussion
801.50 Open fracture of base of skull without mention of intracranial injury, unspecified state of consciousness
801.51 Open fracture of base of skull without mention of intracranial injury, no loss of consciousness
801.52 Open fracture of base of skull without mention of intracranial injury, brief (less than one hour) loss of consciousness
801.53 Open fracture of base of skull without mention of intracranial injury, moderate (1-24 hours) loss of consciousness
801.54 Open fracture of base of skull without mention of intracranial injury, prolonged (more than 24 hours) loss of consciousness and return to pre-existing conscious level
801.55 Open fracture of base of skull without mention of intracranial injury, prolonged (more than 24 hours) loss of consciousness, without return to pre-existing conscious level
801.56 Open fracture of base of skull without mention of intracranial injury, loss of consciousness of unspecified duration
801.59 Open fracture of base of skull without mention of intracranial injury, unspecified concussion
801.60 Open fracture of base of skull with cerebral laceration and contusion, unspecified state of consciousness

801.61 Open fracture of base of skull with cerebral laceration and contusion, no loss of consciousness
801.62 Open fracture of base of skull with cerebral laceration and contusion, brief (less than one hour) loss of consciousness
801.63 Open fracture of base of skull with cerebral laceration and contusion, moderate (1-24 hours) loss of consciousness
801.64 Open fracture of base of skull with cerebral laceration and contusion, prolonged (more than 24 hours) loss of consciousness and return to pre-existing conscious level
801.65 Open fracture of base of skull with cerebral laceration and contusion, prolonged (more than 24 hours) loss of consciousness, without return to pre-existing conscious level
801.66 Open fracture of base of skull with cerebral laceration and contusion, loss of consciousness of unspecified duration ▽
801.69 Open fracture of base of skull with cerebral laceration and contusion, unspecified concussion ▽
801.70 Open fracture of base of skull with subarachnoid, subdural, and extradural hemorrhage, unspecified state of consciousness ▽
801.71 Open fracture of base of skull with subarachnoid, subdural, and extradural hemorrhage, no loss of consciousness
801.72 Open fracture of base of skull with subarachnoid, subdural, and extradural hemorrhage, brief (less than one hour) loss of consciousness
801.73 Open fracture of base of skull with subarachnoid, subdural, and extradural hemorrhage, moderate (1-24 hours) loss of consciousness
801.74 Open fracture of base of skull with subarachnoid, subdural, and extradural hemorrhage, prolonged (more than 24 hours) loss of consciousness and return to pre-existing conscious level
801.75 Open fracture of base of skull with subarachnoid, subdural, and extradural hemorrhage, prolonged (more than 24 hours) loss of consciousness, without return to pre-existing conscious level
801.76 Open fracture of base of skull with subarachnoid, subdural, and extradural hemorrhage, loss of consciousness of unspecified duration ▽
801.79 Open fracture of base of skull with subarachnoid, subdural, and extradural hemorrhage, unspecified concussion ▽
801.80 Open fracture of base of skull with other and unspecified intracranial hemorrhage, unspecified state of consciousness ▽
801.81 Open fracture of base of skull with other and unspecified intracranial hemorrhage, no loss of consciousness ▽
801.82 Open fracture of base of skull with other and unspecified intracranial hemorrhage, brief (less than one hour) loss of consciousness ▽
801.83 Open fracture of base of skull with other and unspecified intracranial hemorrhage, moderate (1-24 hours) loss of consciousness ▽
801.84 Open fracture of base of skull with other and unspecified intracranial hemorrhage, prolonged (more than 24 hours) loss of consciousness and return to pre-existing conscious level ▽
801.85 Open fracture of base of skull with other and unspecified intracranial hemorrhage, prolonged (more than 24 hours) loss of consciousness, without return to pre-existing conscious level ▽
801.86 Open fracture of base of skull with other and unspecified intracranial hemorrhage, loss of consciousness of unspecified duration ▽
801.89 Open fracture of base of skull with other and unspecified intracranial hemorrhage, unspecified concussion ▽
801.90 Open fracture of base of skull with intracranial injury of other and unspecified nature, unspecified state of consciousness ▽
801.91 Open fracture of base of skull with intracranial injury of other and unspecified nature, no loss of consciousness ▽
801.92 Open fracture of base of skull with intracranial injury of other and unspecified nature, brief (less than one hour) loss of consciousness ▽
801.93 Open fracture of base of skull with intracranial injury of other and unspecified nature, moderate (1-24 hours) loss of consciousness ▽
801.94 Open fracture of base of skull with intracranial injury of other and unspecified nature, prolonged (more than 24 hours) loss of consciousness and return to pre-existing conscious level ▽
801.95 Open fracture of base of skull with intracranial injury of other and unspecified nature, prolonged (more than 24 hours) loss of consciousness, without return to pre-existing conscious level ▽
801.96 Open fracture of base of skull with intracranial injury of other and unspecified nature, loss of consciousness of unspecified duration ▽
801.99 Open fracture of base of skull with intracranial injury of other and unspecified nature, unspecified concussion ▽
802.0 Nasal bones, closed fracture
802.1 Nasal bones, open fracture
802.8 Other facial bones, closed fracture
802.9 Other facial bones, open fracture
870.2 Laceration of eyelid involving lacrimal passages — (Use additional code to identify infection)
870.8 Other specified open wound of ocular adnexa — (Use additional code to identify infection)

ICD-9-CM Procedural

21.71 Closed reduction of nasal fracture
76.78 Other closed reduction of facial fracture

21343

21343 Open treatment of depressed frontal sinus fracture

ICD-9-CM Diagnostic

801.00 Closed fracture of base of skull without mention of intracranial injury, unspecified state of consciousness ▽
801.01 Closed fracture of base of skull without mention of intracranial injury, no loss of consciousness
801.02 Closed fracture of base of skull without mention of intracranial injury, brief (less than one hour) loss of consciousness
801.03 Closed fracture of base of skull without mention of intracranial injury, moderate (1-24 hours) loss of consciousness
801.04 Closed fracture of base of skull without mention of intracranial injury, prolonged (more than 24 hours) loss of consciousness and return to pre-existing conscious level
801.05 Closed fracture of base of skull without mention of intracranial injury, prolonged (more than 24 hours) loss of consciousness, without return to pre-existing conscious level
801.06 Closed fracture of base of skull without mention of intracranial injury, loss of consciousness of unspecified duration ▽
801.09 Closed fracture of base of skull without mention of intracranial injury, unspecified concussion ▽
801.10 Closed fracture of base of skull with cerebral laceration and contusion, unspecified state of consciousness ▽
801.11 Closed fracture of base of skull with cerebral laceration and contusion, no loss of consciousness
801.12 Closed fracture of base of skull with cerebral laceration and contusion, brief (less than one hour) loss of consciousness
801.13 Closed fracture of base of skull with cerebral laceration and contusion, moderate (1-24 hours) loss of consciousness
801.14 Closed fracture of base of skull with cerebral laceration and contusion, prolonged (more than 24 hours) loss of consciousness and return to pre-existing conscious level
801.15 Closed fracture of base of skull with cerebral laceration and contusion, prolonged (more than 24 hours) loss of consciousness, without return to pre-existing conscious level
801.16 Closed fracture of base of skull with cerebral laceration and contusion, loss of consciousness of unspecified duration ▽
801.19 Closed fracture of base of skull with cerebral laceration and contusion, unspecified concussion ▽
801.20 Closed fracture of base of skull with subarachnoid, subdural, and extradural hemorrhage, unspecified state of consciousness ▽
801.21 Closed fracture of base of skull with subarachnoid, subdural, and extradural hemorrhage, no loss of consciousness
801.22 Closed fracture of base of skull with subarachnoid, subdural, and extradural hemorrhage, brief (less than one hour) loss of consciousness
801.23 Closed fracture of base of skull with subarachnoid, subdural, and extradural hemorrhage, moderate (1-24 hours) loss of consciousness
801.24 Closed fracture of base of skull with subarachnoid, subdural, and extradural hemorrhage, prolonged (more than 24 hours) loss of consciousness and return to pre-existing conscious level
801.25 Closed fracture of base of skull with subarachnoid, subdural, and extradural hemorrhage, prolonged (more than 24 hours) loss of consciousness, without return to pre-existing conscious level
801.26 Closed fracture of base of skull with subarachnoid, subdural, and extradural hemorrhage, loss of consciousness of unspecified duration ▽
801.29 Closed fracture of base of skull with subarachnoid, subdural, and extradural hemorrhage, unspecified concussion ▽
801.30 Closed fracture of base of skull with other and unspecified intracranial hemorrhage, unspecified state of consciousness ▽
801.31 Closed fracture of base of skull with other and unspecified intracranial hemorrhage, no loss of consciousness ▽
801.32 Closed fracture of base of skull with other and unspecified intracranial hemorrhage, brief (less than one hour) loss of consciousness ▽
801.33 Closed fracture of base of skull with other and unspecified intracranial hemorrhage, moderate (1-24 hours) loss of consciousness ▽
801.34 Closed fracture of base of skull with other and unspecified intracranial hemorrhage, prolonged (more than 24 hours) loss of consciousness and return to pre-existing conscious level ▽

▽ Unspecified code
♀ Female diagnosis
☒ Manifestation code
♂ Male diagnosis

801.35 Closed fracture of base of skull with other and unspecified intracranial hemorrhage, prolonged (more than 24 hours) loss of consciousness, without return to pre-existing conscious level
801.36 Closed fracture of base of skull with other and unspecified intracranial hemorrhage, loss of consciousness of unspecified duration
801.39 Closed fracture of base of skull with other and unspecified intracranial hemorrhage, unspecified concussion
801.40 Closed fracture of base of skull with intracranial injury of other and unspecified nature, unspecified state of consciousness
801.41 Closed fracture of base of skull with intracranial injury of other and unspecified nature, no loss of consciousness
801.42 Closed fracture of base of skull with intracranial injury of other and unspecified nature, brief (less than one hour) loss of consciousness
801.43 Closed fracture of base of skull with intracranial injury of other and unspecified nature, moderate (1-24 hours) loss of consciousness
801.44 Closed fracture of base of skull with intracranial injury of other and unspecified nature, prolonged (more than 24 hours) loss of consciousness and return to pre-existing conscious level
801.45 Closed fracture of base of skull with intracranial injury of other and unspecified nature, prolonged (more than 24 hours) loss of consciousness, without return to pre-existing conscious level
801.46 Closed fracture of base of skull with intracranial injury of other and unspecified nature, loss of consciousness of unspecified duration
801.49 Closed fracture of base of skull with intracranial injury of other and unspecified nature, unspecified concussion
801.50 Open fracture of base of skull without mention of intracranial injury, unspecified state of consciousness
801.51 Open fracture of base of skull without mention of intracranial injury, no loss of consciousness
801.59 Open fracture of base of skull without mention of intracranial injury, unspecified concussion
801.60 Open fracture of base of skull with cerebral laceration and contusion, unspecified state of consciousness
801.70 Open fracture of base of skull with subarachnoid, subdural, and extradural hemorrhage, unspecified state of consciousness
801.80 Open fracture of base of skull with other and unspecified intracranial hemorrhage, unspecified state of consciousness
801.90 Open fracture of base of skull with intracranial injury of other and unspecified nature, unspecified state of consciousness

ICD-9-CM Procedural

22.41 Frontal sinusotomy
22.79 Other repair of nasal sinus
76.70 Reduction of facial fracture, not otherwise specified

21344

21344 Open treatment of complicated (eg, comminuted or involving posterior wall) frontal sinus fracture, via coronal or multiple approaches

ICD-9-CM Diagnostic

801.00 Closed fracture of base of skull without mention of intracranial injury, unspecified state of consciousness
801.01 Closed fracture of base of skull without mention of intracranial injury, no loss of consciousness
801.02 Closed fracture of base of skull without mention of intracranial injury, brief (less than one hour) loss of consciousness
801.03 Closed fracture of base of skull without mention of intracranial injury, moderate (1-24 hours) loss of consciousness
801.04 Closed fracture of base of skull without mention of intracranial injury, prolonged (more than 24 hours) loss of consciousness and return to pre-existing conscious level
801.05 Closed fracture of base of skull without mention of intracranial injury, prolonged (more than 24 hours) loss of consciousness, without return to pre-existing conscious level
801.06 Closed fracture of base of skull without mention of intracranial injury, loss of consciousness of unspecified duration
801.09 Closed fracture of base of skull without mention of intracranial injury, unspecified concussion
801.10 Closed fracture of base of skull with cerebral laceration and contusion, unspecified state of consciousness
801.11 Closed fracture of base of skull with cerebral laceration and contusion, no loss of consciousness
801.12 Closed fracture of base of skull with cerebral laceration and contusion, brief (less than one hour) loss of consciousness
801.13 Closed fracture of base of skull with cerebral laceration and contusion, moderate (1-24 hours) loss of consciousness
801.14 Closed fracture of base of skull with cerebral laceration and contusion, prolonged (more than 24 hours) loss of consciousness and return to pre-existing conscious level
801.15 Closed fracture of base of skull with cerebral laceration and contusion, prolonged (more than 24 hours) loss of consciousness, without return to pre-existing conscious level
801.16 Closed fracture of base of skull with cerebral laceration and contusion, loss of consciousness of unspecified duration
801.19 Closed fracture of base of skull with cerebral laceration and contusion, unspecified concussion
801.20 Closed fracture of base of skull with subarachnoid, subdural, and extradural hemorrhage, unspecified state of consciousness
801.21 Closed fracture of base of skull with subarachnoid, subdural, and extradural hemorrhage, no loss of consciousness
801.22 Closed fracture of base of skull with subarachnoid, subdural, and extradural hemorrhage, brief (less than one hour) loss of consciousness
801.23 Closed fracture of base of skull with subarachnoid, subdural, and extradural hemorrhage, moderate (1-24 hours) loss of consciousness
801.24 Closed fracture of base of skull with subarachnoid, subdural, and extradural hemorrhage, prolonged (more than 24 hours) loss of consciousness and return to pre-existing conscious level
801.25 Closed fracture of base of skull with subarachnoid, subdural, and extradural hemorrhage, prolonged (more than 24 hours) loss of consciousness, without return to pre-existing conscious level
801.26 Closed fracture of base of skull with subarachnoid, subdural, and extradural hemorrhage, loss of consciousness of unspecified duration
801.29 Closed fracture of base of skull with subarachnoid, subdural, and extradural hemorrhage, unspecified concussion
801.30 Closed fracture of base of skull with other and unspecified intracranial hemorrhage, unspecified state of consciousness
801.31 Closed fracture of base of skull with other and unspecified intracranial hemorrhage, no loss of consciousness
801.32 Closed fracture of base of skull with other and unspecified intracranial hemorrhage, brief (less than one hour) loss of consciousness
801.33 Closed fracture of base of skull with other and unspecified intracranial hemorrhage, moderate (1-24 hours) loss of consciousness
801.34 Closed fracture of base of skull with other and unspecified intracranial hemorrhage, prolonged (more than 24 hours) loss of consciousness and return to pre-existing conscious level
801.35 Closed fracture of base of skull with other and unspecified intracranial hemorrhage, prolonged (more than 24 hours) loss of consciousness, without return to pre-existing conscious level
801.36 Closed fracture of base of skull with other and unspecified intracranial hemorrhage, loss of consciousness of unspecified duration
801.39 Closed fracture of base of skull with other and unspecified intracranial hemorrhage, unspecified concussion
801.40 Closed fracture of base of skull with intracranial injury of other and unspecified nature, unspecified state of consciousness
801.41 Closed fracture of base of skull with intracranial injury of other and unspecified nature, no loss of consciousness
801.42 Closed fracture of base of skull with intracranial injury of other and unspecified nature, brief (less than one hour) loss of consciousness
801.43 Closed fracture of base of skull with intracranial injury of other and unspecified nature, moderate (1-24 hours) loss of consciousness
801.44 Closed fracture of base of skull with intracranial injury of other and unspecified nature, prolonged (more than 24 hours) loss of consciousness and return to pre-existing conscious level
801.45 Closed fracture of base of skull with intracranial injury of other and unspecified nature, prolonged (more than 24 hours) loss of consciousness, without return to pre-existing conscious level
801.46 Closed fracture of base of skull with intracranial injury of other and unspecified nature, loss of consciousness of unspecified duration
801.49 Closed fracture of base of skull with intracranial injury of other and unspecified nature, unspecified concussion
801.50 Open fracture of base of skull without mention of intracranial injury, unspecified state of consciousness
801.51 Open fracture of base of skull without mention of intracranial injury, no loss of consciousness
801.59 Open fracture of base of skull without mention of intracranial injury, unspecified concussion
801.60 Open fracture of base of skull with cerebral laceration and contusion, unspecified state of consciousness
801.70 Open fracture of base of skull with subarachnoid, subdural, and extradural hemorrhage, unspecified state of consciousness
801.80 Open fracture of base of skull with other and unspecified intracranial hemorrhage, unspecified state of consciousness

801.90 Open fracture of base of skull with intracranial injury of other and unspecified nature, unspecified state of consciousness ▽
925.1 Crushing injury of face and scalp — (Use additional code to identify any associated injuries: 800-829, 850.0-854.1, 860.0-869.1)

ICD-9-CM Procedural
22.41 Frontal sinusotomy
22.79 Other repair of nasal sinus
76.70 Reduction of facial fracture, not otherwise specified

21345
21345 Closed treatment of nasomaxillary complex fracture (LeFort II type), with interdental wire fixation or fixation of denture or splint

ICD-9-CM Diagnostic
802.0 Nasal bones, closed fracture
802.4 Malar and maxillary bones, closed fracture

ICD-9-CM Procedural
21.71 Closed reduction of nasal fracture
76.73 Closed reduction of maxillary fracture
76.78 Other closed reduction of facial fracture

21346–21348
21346 Open treatment of nasomaxillary complex fracture (LeFort II type); with wiring and/or local fixation
21347 requiring multiple open approaches
21348 with bone grafting (includes obtaining graft)

ICD-9-CM Diagnostic
733.82 Nonunion of fracture
802.0 Nasal bones, closed fracture
802.1 Nasal bones, open fracture
802.4 Malar and maxillary bones, closed fracture
802.5 Malar and maxillary bones, open fracture

ICD-9-CM Procedural
76.79 Other open reduction of facial fracture
76.91 Bone graft to facial bone

21355
21355 Percutaneous treatment of fracture of malar area, including zygomatic arch and malar tripod, with manipulation

ICD-9-CM Diagnostic
733.82 Nonunion of fracture
802.4 Malar and maxillary bones, closed fracture
802.5 Malar and maxillary bones, open fracture

ICD-9-CM Procedural
76.71 Closed reduction of malar and zygomatic fracture

HCPCS Level II Supplies & Services
A4305 Disposable drug delivery system, flow rate of 50 ml or greater per hour
A4306 Disposable drug delivery system, flow rate of 5 ml or less per hour
A4550 Surgical trays

21356
21356 Open treatment of depressed zygomatic arch fracture (eg, Gillies approach)

ICD-9-CM Diagnostic
733.82 Nonunion of fracture
802.4 Malar and maxillary bones, closed fracture
802.5 Malar and maxillary bones, open fracture

ICD-9-CM Procedural
76.72 Open reduction of malar and zygomatic fracture

21360
21360 Open treatment of depressed malar fracture, including zygomatic arch and malar tripod

ICD-9-CM Diagnostic
733.82 Nonunion of fracture
802.4 Malar and maxillary bones, closed fracture

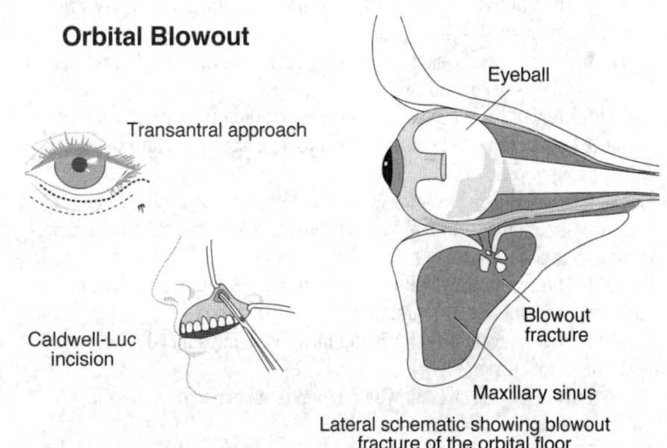

Lateral schematic showing blowout fracture of the orbital floor

802.5 Malar and maxillary bones, open fracture

ICD-9-CM Procedural
76.72 Open reduction of malar and zygomatic fracture

21365–21366
21365 Open treatment of complicated (eg, comminuted or involving cranial nerve foramina) fracture(s) of malar area, including zygomatic arch and malar tripod; with internal fixation and multiple surgical approaches
21366 with bone grafting (includes obtaining graft)

ICD-9-CM Diagnostic
802.4 Malar and maxillary bones, closed fracture
802.5 Malar and maxillary bones, open fracture
951.4 Injury to facial nerve
951.9 Injury to unspecified cranial nerve ▽

ICD-9-CM Procedural
76.71 Closed reduction of malar and zygomatic fracture
76.72 Open reduction of malar and zygomatic fracture
76.91 Bone graft to facial bone

21385–21387
21385 Open treatment of orbital floor blowout fracture; transantral approach (Caldwell-Luc type operation)
21386 periorbital approach
21387 combined approach

ICD-9-CM Diagnostic
802.6 Orbital floor (blow-out), closed fracture
802.7 Orbital floor (blow-out), open fracture

ICD-9-CM Procedural
76.79 Other open reduction of facial fracture

21390–21395
21390 Open treatment of orbital floor blowout fracture; periorbital approach, with alloplastic or other implant
21395 periorbital approach with bone graft (includes obtaining graft)

ICD-9-CM Diagnostic
802.6 Orbital floor (blow-out), closed fracture
802.7 Orbital floor (blow-out), open fracture

ICD-9-CM Procedural
76.79 Other open reduction of facial fracture
76.91 Bone graft to facial bone
76.92 Insertion of synthetic implant in facial bone

21400–21401
21400 Closed treatment of fracture of orbit, except blowout; without manipulation
21401 with manipulation

ICD-9-CM Diagnostic
801.00 Closed fracture of base of skull without mention of intracranial injury, unspecified state of consciousness ▽
801.01 Closed fracture of base of skull without mention of intracranial injury, no loss of consciousness

801.02 Closed fracture of base of skull without mention of intracranial injury, brief (less than one hour) loss of consciousness
801.03 Closed fracture of base of skull without mention of intracranial injury, moderate (1-24 hours) loss of consciousness
801.04 Closed fracture of base of skull without mention of intracranial injury, prolonged (more than 24 hours) loss of consciousness and return to pre-existing conscious level
801.05 Closed fracture of base of skull without mention of intracranial injury, prolonged (more than 24 hours) loss of consciousness, without return to pre-existing conscious level
801.06 Closed fracture of base of skull without mention of intracranial injury, loss of consciousness of unspecified duration ▽
801.09 Closed fracture of base of skull without mention of intracranial injury, unspecified concussion ▽
801.10 Closed fracture of base of skull with cerebral laceration and contusion, unspecified state of consciousness ▽
801.12 Closed fracture of base of skull with cerebral laceration and contusion, brief (less than one hour) loss of consciousness
801.13 Closed fracture of base of skull with cerebral laceration and contusion, moderate (1-24 hours) loss of consciousness
801.14 Closed fracture of base of skull with cerebral laceration and contusion, prolonged (more than 24 hours) loss of consciousness and return to pre-existing conscious level
801.15 Closed fracture of base of skull with cerebral laceration and contusion, prolonged (more than 24 hours) loss of consciousness, without return to pre-existing conscious level
801.16 Closed fracture of base of skull with cerebral laceration and contusion, loss of consciousness of unspecified duration ▽
801.19 Closed fracture of base of skull with cerebral laceration and contusion, unspecified concussion ▽
801.20 Closed fracture of base of skull with subarachnoid, subdural, and extradural hemorrhage, unspecified state of consciousness ▽
801.30 Closed fracture of base of skull with other and unspecified intracranial hemorrhage, unspecified state of consciousness ▽
801.40 Closed fracture of base of skull with intracranial injury of other and unspecified nature, unspecified state of consciousness ▽
802.4 Malar and maxillary bones, closed fracture
802.8 Other facial bones, closed fracture

ICD-9-CM Procedural

76.78 Other closed reduction of facial fracture
93.59 Other immobilization, pressure, and attention to wound

HCPCS Level II Supplies & Services

A4305 Disposable drug delivery system, flow rate of 50 ml or greater per hour
A4306 Disposable drug delivery system, flow rate of 5 ml or less per hour
A4550 Surgical trays

21406–21408

21406 Open treatment of fracture of orbit, except blowout; without implant
21407 with implant
21408 with bone grafting (includes obtaining graft)

ICD-9-CM Diagnostic

801.00 Closed fracture of base of skull without mention of intracranial injury, unspecified state of consciousness ▽
801.01 Closed fracture of base of skull without mention of intracranial injury, no loss of consciousness
801.02 Closed fracture of base of skull without mention of intracranial injury, brief (less than one hour) loss of consciousness
801.03 Closed fracture of base of skull without mention of intracranial injury, moderate (1-24 hours) loss of consciousness
801.04 Closed fracture of base of skull without mention of intracranial injury, prolonged (more than 24 hours) loss of consciousness and return to pre-existing conscious level
801.05 Closed fracture of base of skull without mention of intracranial injury, prolonged (more than 24 hours) loss of consciousness, without return to pre-existing conscious level
801.06 Closed fracture of base of skull without mention of intracranial injury, loss of consciousness of unspecified duration ▽
801.09 Closed fracture of base of skull without mention of intracranial injury, unspecified concussion ▽
801.10 Closed fracture of base of skull with cerebral laceration and contusion, unspecified state of consciousness ▽
801.11 Closed fracture of base of skull with cerebral laceration and contusion, no loss of consciousness
801.12 Closed fracture of base of skull with cerebral laceration and contusion, brief (less than one hour) loss of consciousness
801.13 Closed fracture of base of skull with cerebral laceration and contusion, moderate (1-24 hours) loss of consciousness
801.14 Closed fracture of base of skull with cerebral laceration and contusion, prolonged (more than 24 hours) loss of consciousness and return to pre-existing conscious level
801.15 Closed fracture of base of skull with cerebral laceration and contusion, prolonged (more than 24 hours) loss of consciousness, without return to pre-existing conscious level
801.16 Closed fracture of base of skull with cerebral laceration and contusion, loss of consciousness of unspecified duration ▽
801.19 Closed fracture of base of skull with cerebral laceration and contusion, unspecified concussion ▽
801.50 Open fracture of base of skull without mention of intracranial injury, unspecified state of consciousness ▽
801.51 Open fracture of base of skull without mention of intracranial injury, no loss of consciousness
801.52 Open fracture of base of skull without mention of intracranial injury, brief (less than one hour) loss of consciousness
801.53 Open fracture of base of skull without mention of intracranial injury, moderate (1-24 hours) loss of consciousness
801.54 Open fracture of base of skull without mention of intracranial injury, prolonged (more than 24 hours) loss of consciousness and return to pre-existing conscious level
801.56 Open fracture of base of skull without mention of intracranial injury, loss of consciousness of unspecified duration ▽
801.59 Open fracture of base of skull without mention of intracranial injury, unspecified concussion ▽
802.4 Malar and maxillary bones, closed fracture
802.5 Malar and maxillary bones, open fracture
802.8 Other facial bones, closed fracture
802.9 Other facial bones, open fracture

ICD-9-CM Procedural

76.79 Other open reduction of facial fracture
76.91 Bone graft to facial bone
76.92 Insertion of synthetic implant in facial bone

21421

21421 Closed treatment of palatal or maxillary fracture (LeFort I type), with interdental wire fixation or fixation of denture or splint

ICD-9-CM Diagnostic

802.4 Malar and maxillary bones, closed fracture
802.8 Other facial bones, closed fracture

ICD-9-CM Procedural

76.73 Closed reduction of maxillary fracture
76.78 Other closed reduction of facial fracture

21422

21422 Open treatment of palatal or maxillary fracture (LeFort I type);

ICD-9-CM Diagnostic

802.4 Malar and maxillary bones, closed fracture
802.5 Malar and maxillary bones, open fracture
802.8 Other facial bones, closed fracture
802.9 Other facial bones, open fracture

ICD-9-CM Procedural

76.74 Open reduction of maxillary fracture
76.79 Other open reduction of facial fracture

21423

21423 Open treatment of palatal or maxillary fracture (LeFort I type); complicated (comminuted or involving cranial nerve foramina), multiple approaches

ICD-9-CM Diagnostic

802.4 Malar and maxillary bones, closed fracture
802.5 Malar and maxillary bones, open fracture
802.8 Other facial bones, closed fracture
802.9 Other facial bones, open fracture

ICD-9-CM Procedural

76.74 Open reduction of maxillary fracture

▽ Unspecified code ♀ Female diagnosis ☒ Manifestation code ♂ Male diagnosis

76.78 Other closed reduction of facial fracture

21431

21431 Closed treatment of craniofacial separation (LeFort III type) using interdental wire fixation of denture or splint

ICD-9-CM Diagnostic

800.00 Closed fracture of vault of skull without mention of intracranial injury, unspecified state of consciousness ▽
800.01 Closed fracture of vault of skull without mention of intracranial injury, no loss of consciousness
800.02 Closed fracture of vault of skull without mention of intracranial injury, brief (less than one hour) loss of consciousness
800.03 Closed fracture of vault of skull without mention of intracranial injury, moderate (1-24 hours) loss of consciousness
800.04 Closed fracture of vault of skull without mention of intracranial injury, prolonged (more than 24 hours) loss of consciousness and return to pre-existing conscious level
800.05 Closed fracture of vault of skull without mention of intracranial injury, prolonged (more than 24 hours) loss of consciousness, without return to pre-existing conscious level
800.06 Closed fracture of vault of skull without mention of intracranial injury, loss of consciousness of unspecified duration ▽
800.09 Closed fracture of vault of skull without mention of intracranial injury, unspecified concussion ▽
800.10 Closed fracture of vault of skull with cerebral laceration and contusion, unspecified state of consciousness ▽
800.11 Closed fracture of vault of skull with cerebral laceration and contusion, no loss of consciousness
800.12 Closed fracture of vault of skull with cerebral laceration and contusion, brief (less than one hour) loss of consciousness
800.13 Closed fracture of vault of skull with cerebral laceration and contusion, moderate (1-24 hours) loss of consciousness
800.14 Closed fracture of vault of skull with cerebral laceration and contusion, prolonged (more than 24 hours) loss of consciousness and return to pre-existing conscious level
800.15 Closed fracture of vault of skull with cerebral laceration and contusion, prolonged (more than 24 hours) loss of consciousness, without return to pre-existing conscious level
800.16 Closed fracture of vault of skull with cerebral laceration and contusion, loss of consciousness of unspecified duration ▽
800.19 Closed fracture of vault of skull with cerebral laceration and contusion, unspecified concussion ▽
800.20 Closed fracture of vault of skull with subarachnoid, subdural, and extradural hemorrhage, unspecified state of consciousness ▽
800.21 Closed fracture of vault of skull with subarachnoid, subdural, and extradural hemorrhage, no loss of consciousness
800.22 Closed fracture of vault of skull with subarachnoid, subdural, and extradural hemorrhage, brief (less than one hour) loss of consciousness
800.23 Closed fracture of vault of skull with subarachnoid, subdural, and extradural hemorrhage, moderate (1-24 hours) loss of consciousness
800.24 Closed fracture of vault of skull with subarachnoid, subdural, and extradural hemorrhage, prolonged (more than 24 hours) loss of consciousness and return to pre-existing conscious level
800.25 Closed fracture of vault of skull with subarachnoid, subdural, and extradural hemorrhage, prolonged (more than 24 hours) loss of consciousness, without return to pre-existing conscious level
800.26 Closed fracture of vault of skull with subarachnoid, subdural, and extradural hemorrhage, loss of consciousness of unspecified duration ▽
800.30 Closed fracture of vault of skull with other and unspecified intracranial hemorrhage, unspecified state of consciousness ▽
800.31 Closed fracture of vault of skull with other and unspecified intracranial hemorrhage, no loss of consciousness ▽
800.32 Closed fracture of vault of skull with other and unspecified intracranial hemorrhage, brief (less than one hour) loss of consciousness ▽
800.33 Closed fracture of vault of skull with other and unspecified intracranial hemorrhage, moderate (1-24 hours) loss of consciousness ▽
800.34 Closed fracture of vault of skull with other and unspecified intracranial hemorrhage, prolonged (more than 24 hours) loss of consciousness and return to pre-existing conscious level ▽
800.35 Closed fracture of vault of skull with other and unspecified intracranial hemorrhage, prolonged (more than 24 hours) loss of consciousness, without return to pre-existing conscious level ▽
800.36 Closed fracture of vault of skull with other and unspecified intracranial hemorrhage, loss of consciousness of unspecified duration ▽
800.39 Closed fracture of vault of skull with other and unspecified intracranial hemorrhage, unspecified concussion ▽
800.40 Closed fracture of vault of skull with intracranial injury of other and unspecified nature, unspecified state of consciousness ▽
800.41 Closed fracture of vault of skull with intracranial injury of other and unspecified nature, no loss of consciousness ▽
800.42 Closed fracture of vault of skull with intracranial injury of other and unspecified nature, brief (less than one hour) loss of consciousness ▽
800.43 Closed fracture of vault of skull with intracranial injury of other and unspecified nature, moderate (1-24 hours) loss of consciousness ▽
800.44 Closed fracture of vault of skull with intracranial injury of other and unspecified nature, prolonged (more than 24 hours) loss of consciousness and return to pre-existing conscious level ▽
800.45 Closed fracture of vault of skull with intracranial injury of other and unspecified nature, prolonged (more than 24 hours) loss of consciousness, without return to pre-existing conscious level ▽
800.46 Closed fracture of vault of skull with intracranial injury of other and unspecified nature, loss of consciousness of unspecified duration ▽
800.49 Closed fracture of vault of skull with intracranial injury of other and unspecified nature, unspecified concussion ▽
801.00 Closed fracture of base of skull without mention of intracranial injury, unspecified state of consciousness ▽
801.01 Closed fracture of base of skull without mention of intracranial injury, no loss of consciousness
801.02 Closed fracture of base of skull without mention of intracranial injury, brief (less than one hour) loss of consciousness
801.03 Closed fracture of base of skull without mention of intracranial injury, moderate (1-24 hours) loss of consciousness
801.04 Closed fracture of base of skull without mention of intracranial injury, prolonged (more than 24 hours) loss of consciousness and return to pre-existing conscious level
801.05 Closed fracture of base of skull without mention of intracranial injury, prolonged (more than 24 hours) loss of consciousness, without return to pre-existing conscious level
801.06 Closed fracture of base of skull without mention of intracranial injury, loss of consciousness of unspecified duration ▽
801.09 Closed fracture of base of skull without mention of intracranial injury, unspecified concussion ▽
801.10 Closed fracture of base of skull with cerebral laceration and contusion, unspecified state of consciousness ▽
801.11 Closed fracture of base of skull with cerebral laceration and contusion, no loss of consciousness
801.12 Closed fracture of base of skull with cerebral laceration and contusion, brief (less than one hour) loss of consciousness
801.13 Closed fracture of base of skull with cerebral laceration and contusion, moderate (1-24 hours) loss of consciousness
801.14 Closed fracture of base of skull with cerebral laceration and contusion, prolonged (more than 24 hours) loss of consciousness and return to pre-existing conscious level
801.15 Closed fracture of base of skull with cerebral laceration and contusion, prolonged (more than 24 hours) loss of consciousness, without return to pre-existing conscious level
801.16 Closed fracture of base of skull with cerebral laceration and contusion, loss of consciousness of unspecified duration ▽
801.19 Closed fracture of base of skull with cerebral laceration and contusion, unspecified concussion ▽
801.20 Closed fracture of base of skull with subarachnoid, subdural, and extradural hemorrhage, unspecified state of consciousness ▽
801.21 Closed fracture of base of skull with subarachnoid, subdural, and extradural hemorrhage, no loss of consciousness
801.22 Closed fracture of base of skull with subarachnoid, subdural, and extradural hemorrhage, brief (less than one hour) loss of consciousness
801.23 Closed fracture of base of skull with subarachnoid, subdural, and extradural hemorrhage, moderate (1-24 hours) loss of consciousness
801.24 Closed fracture of base of skull with subarachnoid, subdural, and extradural hemorrhage, prolonged (more than 24 hours) loss of consciousness and return to pre-existing conscious level
801.25 Closed fracture of base of skull with subarachnoid, subdural, and extradural hemorrhage, prolonged (more than 24 hours) loss of consciousness, without return to pre-existing conscious level
801.26 Closed fracture of base of skull with subarachnoid, subdural, and extradural hemorrhage, loss of consciousness of unspecified duration ▽
801.30 Closed fracture of base of skull with other and unspecified intracranial hemorrhage, unspecified state of consciousness ▽
801.31 Closed fracture of base of skull with other and unspecified intracranial hemorrhage, no loss of consciousness ▽

801.32 Closed fracture of base of skull with other and unspecified intracranial hemorrhage, brief (less than one hour) loss of consciousness
801.33 Closed fracture of base of skull with other and unspecified intracranial hemorrhage, moderate (1-24 hours) loss of consciousness
801.34 Closed fracture of base of skull with other and unspecified intracranial hemorrhage, prolonged (more than 24 hours) loss of consciousness and return to pre-existing conscious level
801.35 Closed fracture of base of skull with other and unspecified intracranial hemorrhage, prolonged (more than 24 hours) loss of consciousness, without return to pre-existing conscious level
801.36 Closed fracture of base of skull with other and unspecified intracranial hemorrhage, loss of consciousness of unspecified duration
801.39 Closed fracture of base of skull with other and unspecified intracranial hemorrhage, unspecified concussion
801.40 Closed fracture of base of skull with intracranial injury of other and unspecified nature, unspecified state of consciousness
801.41 Closed fracture of base of skull with intracranial injury of other and unspecified nature, no loss of consciousness
801.42 Closed fracture of base of skull with intracranial injury of other and unspecified nature, brief (less than one hour) loss of consciousness
801.43 Closed fracture of base of skull with intracranial injury of other and unspecified nature, moderate (1-24 hours) loss of consciousness
801.44 Closed fracture of base of skull with intracranial injury of other and unspecified nature, prolonged (more than 24 hours) loss of consciousness and return to pre-existing conscious level
801.45 Closed fracture of base of skull with intracranial injury of other and unspecified nature, prolonged (more than 24 hours) loss of consciousness, without return to pre-existing conscious level
801.46 Closed fracture of base of skull with intracranial injury of other and unspecified nature, loss of consciousness of unspecified duration
801.49 Closed fracture of base of skull with intracranial injury of other and unspecified nature, unspecified concussion
802.4 Malar and maxillary bones, closed fracture
802.5 Malar and maxillary bones, open fracture
802.8 Other facial bones, closed fracture
802.9 Other facial bones, open fracture
804.00 Closed fractures involving skull or face with other bones, without mention of intracranial injury, unspecified state of consciousness
804.01 Closed fractures involving skull or face with other bones, without mention of intracranial injury, no loss of consciousness
804.02 Closed fractures involving skull or face with other bones, without mention of intracranial injury, brief (less than one hour) loss of consciousness
804.03 Closed fractures involving skull or face with other bones, without mention of intracranial injury, moderate (1-24 hours) loss of consciousness
804.04 Closed fractures involving skull or face with other bones, without mention or intracranial injury, prolonged (more than 24 hours) loss of consciousness and return to pre-existing conscious level
804.05 Closed fractures involving skull of face with other bones, without mention of intracranial injury, prolonged (more than 24 hours) loss of consciousness, without return to pre-existing conscious level
804.06 Closed fractures involving skull of face with other bones, without mention of intracranial injury, loss of consciousness of unspecified duration
804.09 Closed fractures involving skull of face with other bones, without mention of intracranial injury, unspecified concussion
804.10 Closed fractures involving skull or face with other bones, with cerebral laceration and contusion, unspecified state of consciousness
804.11 Closed fractures involving skull or face with other bones, with cerebral laceration and contusion, no loss of consciousness
804.12 Closed fractures involving skull or face with other bones, with cerebral laceration and contusion, brief (less than one hour) loss of consciousness
804.13 Closed fractures involving skull or face with other bones, with cerebral laceration and contusion, moderate (1-24 hours) loss of consciousness
804.14 Closed fractures involving skull or face with other bones, with cerebral laceration and contusion, prolonged (more than 24 hours) loss of consciousness and return to pre-existing conscious level
804.15 Closed fractures involving skull or face with other bones, with cerebral laceration and contusion, prolonged (more than 24 hours) loss of consciousness, without return to pre-existing conscious level
804.16 Closed fractures involving skull or face with other bones, with cerebral laceration and contusion, loss of consciousness of unspecified duration
804.19 Closed fractures involving skull or face with other bones, with cerebral laceration and contusion, unspecified concussion
804.20 Closed fractures involving skull or face with other bones with subarachnoid, subdural, and extradural hemorrhage, unspecified state of consciousness
804.21 Closed fractures involving skull or face with other bones with subarachnoid, subdural, and extradural hemorrhage, no loss of consciousness
804.22 Closed fractures involving skull or face with other bones with subarachnoid, subdural, and extradural hemorrhage, brief (less than one hour) loss of consciousness
804.23 Closed fractures involving skull or face with other bones with subarachnoid, subdural, and extradural hemorrhage, moderate (1-24 hours) loss of consciousness
804.24 Closed fractures involving skull or face with other bones with subarachnoid, subdural, and extradural hemorrhage, prolonged (more than 24 hours) loss of consciousness and return to pre-existing conscious level
804.25 Closed fractures involving skull or face with other bones with subarachnoid, subdural, and extradural hemorrhage, prolonged (more than 24 hours) loss of consciousness, without return to pre-existing conscious level
804.26 Closed fractures involving skull or face with other bones with subarachnoid, subdural, and extradural hemorrhage, loss of consciousness of unspecified duration
804.29 Closed fractures involving skull or face with other bones with subarachnoid, subdural, and extradural hemorrhage, unspecified concussion
804.30 Closed fractures involving skull or face with other bones, with other and unspecified intracranial hemorrhage, unspecified state of consciousness
804.31 Closed fractures involving skull or face with other bones, with other and unspecified intracranial hemorrhage, no loss of consciousness
804.32 Closed fractures involving skull or face with other bones, with other and unspecified intracranial hemorrhage, brief (less than one hour) loss of consciousness
804.33 Closed fractures involving skull or face with other bones, with other and unspecified intracranial hemorrrhage, moderate (1-24 hours) loss of consciousness
804.34 Closed fractures involving skull or face with other bones, with other and unspecified intracranial hemorrhage, prolonged (more than 24 hours) loss of consciousness and return to preexisting conscious level
804.35 Closed fractures involving skull or face with other bones, with other and unspecified intracranial hemorrhage, prolonged (more than 24 hours) loss of consciousness, without return to pre-existing conscious level
804.36 Closed fractures involving skull or face with other bones, with other and unspecified intracranial hemorrhage, loss of consciousness of unspecified duration
804.39 Closed fractures involving skull or face with other bones, with other and unspecified intracranial hemorrhage, unspecified concussion
804.40 Closed fractures involving skull or face with other bones, with intracranial injury of other and unspecified nature, unspecified state of consciousness
804.41 Closed fractures involving skull or face with other bones, with intracranial injury of other and unspecified nature, no loss of consciousness
804.42 Closed fractures involving skull or face with other bones, with intracranial injury of other and unspecified nature, brief (less than one hour) loss of consciousness
804.43 Closed fractures involving skull or face with other bones, with intracranial injury of other and unspecified nature, moderate (1-24 hours) loss of consciousness
804.44 Closed fractures involving skull or face with other bones, with intracranial injury of other and unspecified nature, prolonged (more than 24 hours) loss of consciousness and return to pre-existing conscious level
804.45 Closed fractures involving skull or face with other bones, with intracranial injury of other and unspecified nature, prolonged (more than 24 hours) loss of consciousness, without return to pre-existing conscious level
804.46 Closed fractures involving skull or face with other bones, with intracranial injury of other and unspecified nature, loss of consciousness of unspecified duration
804.49 Closed fractures involving skull or face with other bones, with intracranial injury of other and unspecified nature, unspecified concussion

ICD-9-CM Procedural

76.78 Other closed reduction of facial fracture

21432–21436

21432 Open treatment of craniofacial separation (LeFort III type); with wiring and/or internal fixation
21433 complicated (eg, comminuted or involving cranial nerve foramina), multiple surgical approaches
21435 complicated, utilizing internal and/or external fixation techniques (eg, head cap, halo device, and/or intermaxillary fixation)
21436 complicated, multiple surgical approaches, internal fixation, with bone grafting (includes obtaining graft)

ICD-9-CM Diagnostic

733.82 Nonunion of fracture

Unspecified code
♀ Female diagnosis
Manifestation code
♂ Male diagnosis

800.00 Closed fracture of vault of skull without mention of intracranial injury, unspecified state of consciousness ▽

800.01 Closed fracture of vault of skull without mention of intracranial injury, no loss of consciousness

800.02 Closed fracture of vault of skull without mention of intracranial injury, brief (less than one hour) loss of consciousness

800.03 Closed fracture of vault of skull without mention of intracranial injury, moderate (1-24 hours) loss of consciousness

800.04 Closed fracture of vault of skull without mention of intracranial injury, prolonged (more than 24 hours) loss of consciousness and return to pre-existing conscious level

800.05 Closed fracture of vault of skull without mention of intracranial injury, prolonged (more than 24 hours) loss of consciousness, without return to pre-existing conscious level

800.06 Closed fracture of vault of skull without mention of intracranial injury, loss of consciousness of unspecified duration ▽

800.09 Closed fracture of vault of skull without mention of intracranial injury, unspecified concussion ▽

800.10 Closed fracture of vault of skull with cerebral laceration and contusion, unspecified state of consciousness ▽

800.11 Closed fracture of vault of skull with cerebral laceration and contusion, no loss of consciousness

800.12 Closed fracture of vault of skull with cerebral laceration and contusion, brief (less than one hour) loss of consciousness

800.13 Closed fracture of vault of skull with cerebral laceration and contusion, moderate (1-24 hours) loss of consciousness

800.14 Closed fracture of vault of skull with cerebral laceration and contusion, prolonged (more than 24 hours) loss of consciousness and return to pre-existing conscious level

800.15 Closed fracture of vault of skull with cerebral laceration and contusion, prolonged (more than 24 hours) loss of consciousness, without return to pre-existing conscious level

800.16 Closed fracture of vault of skull with cerebral laceration and contusion, loss of consciousness of unspecified duration ▽

800.19 Closed fracture of vault of skull with cerebral laceration and contusion, unspecified concussion ▽

800.20 Closed fracture of vault of skull with subarachnoid, subdural, and extradural hemorrhage, unspecified state of consciousness ▽

800.21 Closed fracture of vault of skull with subarachnoid, subdural, and extradural hemorrhage, no loss of consciousness

800.22 Closed fracture of vault of skull with subarachnoid, subdural, and extradural hemorrhage, brief (less than one hour) loss of consciousness

800.23 Closed fracture of vault of skull with subarachnoid, subdural, and extradural hemorrhage, moderate (1-24 hours) loss of consciousness

800.24 Closed fracture of vault of skull with subarachnoid, subdural, and extradural hemorrhage, prolonged (more than 24 hours) loss of consciousness and return to pre-existing conscious level

800.25 Closed fracture of vault of skull with subarachnoid, subdural, and extradural hemorrhage, prolonged (more than 24 hours) loss of consciousness, without return to pre-existing conscious level

800.26 Closed fracture of vault of skull with subarachnoid, subdural, and extradural hemorrhage, loss of consciousness of unspecified duration ▽

800.30 Closed fracture of vault of skull with other and unspecified intracranial hemorrhage, unspecified state of consciousness ▽

800.31 Closed fracture of vault of skull with other and unspecified intracranial hemorrhage, no loss of consciousness ▽

800.32 Closed fracture of vault of skull with other and unspecified intracranial hemorrhage, brief (less than one hour) loss of consciousness ▽

800.33 Closed fracture of vault of skull with other and unspecified intracranial hemorrhage, moderate (1-24 hours) loss of consciousness ▽

800.34 Closed fracture of vault of skull with other and unspecified intracranial hemorrhage, prolonged (more than 24 hours) loss of consciousness and return to pre-existing conscious level ▽

800.35 Closed fracture of vault of skull with other and unspecified intracranial hemorrhage, prolonged (more than 24 hours) loss of consciousness, without return to pre-existing conscious level ▽

800.36 Closed fracture of vault of skull with other and unspecified intracranial hemorrhage, loss of consciousness of unspecified duration ▽

800.39 Closed fracture of vault of skull with other and unspecified intracranial hemorrhage, unspecified concussion ▽

800.40 Closed fracture of vault of skull with intracranial injury of other and unspecified nature, unspecified state of consciousness ▽

800.41 Closed fracture of vault of skull with intracranial injury of other and unspecified nature, no loss of consciousness ▽

800.42 Closed fracture of vault of skull with intracranial injury of other and unspecified nature, brief (less than one hour) loss of consciousness ▽

800.43 Closed fracture of vault of skull with intracranial injury of other and unspecified nature, moderate (1-24 hours) loss of consciousness ▽

800.44 Closed fracture of vault of skull with intracranial injury of other and unspecified nature, prolonged (more than 24 hours) loss of consciousness and return to pre-existing conscious level ▽

800.45 Closed fracture of vault of skull with intracranial injury of other and unspecified nature, prolonged (more than 24 hours) loss of consciousness, without return to pre-existing conscious level ▽

800.46 Closed fracture of vault of skull with intracranial injury of other and unspecified nature, loss of consciousness of unspecified duration ▽

800.49 Closed fracture of vault of skull with intracranial injury of other and unspecified nature, unspecified concussion ▽

800.50 Open fracture of vault of skull without mention of intracranial injury, unspecified state of consciousness ▽

800.51 Open fracture of vault of skull without mention of intracranial injury, no loss of consciousness

800.52 Open fracture of vault of skull without mention of intracranial injury, brief (less than one hour) loss of consciousness

800.53 Open fracture of vault of skull without mention of intracranial injury, moderate (1-24 hours) loss of consciousness

800.54 Open fracture of vault of skull without mention of intracranial injury, prolonged (more than 24 hours) loss of consciousness and return to pre-existing conscious level

800.55 Open fracture of vault of skull without mention of intracranial injury, prolonged (more than 24 hours) loss of consciousness, without return to pre-existing conscious level

800.56 Open fracture of vault of skull without mention of intracranial injury, loss of consciousness of unspecified duration ▽

800.59 Open fracture of vault of skull without mention of intracranial injury, unspecified concussion ▽

800.60 Open fracture of vault of skull with cerebral laceration and contusion, unspecified state of consciousness ▽

800.61 Open fracture of vault of skull with cerebral laceration and contusion, no loss of consciousness

800.62 Open fracture of vault of skull with cerebral laceration and contusion, brief (less than one hour) loss of consciousness

800.63 Open fracture of vault of skull with cerebral laceration and contusion, moderate (1-24 hours) loss of consciousness

800.64 Open fracture of vault of skull with cerebral laceration and contusion, prolonged (more than 24 hours) loss of consciousness and return to pre-existing conscious level

800.65 Open fracture of vault of skull with cerebral laceration and contusion, prolonged (more than 24 hours) loss of consciousness, without return to pre-existing conscious level

800.66 Open fracture of vault of skull with cerebral laceration and contusion, loss of consciousness of unspecified duration ▽

800.69 Open fracture of vault of skull with cerebral laceration and contusion, unspecified concussion ▽

800.70 Open fracture of vault of skull with subarachnoid, subdural, and extradural hemorrhage, unspecified state of consciousness ▽

800.71 Open fracture of vault of skull with subarachnoid, subdural, and extradural hemorrhage, no loss of consciousness

800.72 Open fracture of vault of skull with subarachnoid, subdural, and extradural hemorrhage, brief (less than one hour) loss of consciousness

800.73 Open fracture of vault of skull with subarachnoid, subdural, and extradural hemorrhage, moderate (1-24 hours) loss of consciousness

800.74 Open fracture of vault of skull with subarachnoid, subdural, and extradural hemorrhage, prolonged (more than 24 hours) loss of consciousness and return to pre-existing conscious level

800.75 Open fracture of vault of skull with subarachnoid, subdural, and extradural hemorrhage, prolonged (more than 24 hours) loss of consciousness, without return to pre-existing conscious level

800.79 Open fracture of vault of skull with subarachnoid, subdural, and extradural hemorrhage, unspecified concussion ▽

800.80 Open fracture of vault of skull with other and unspecified intracranial hemorrhage, unspecified state of consciousness ▽

800.90 Open fracture of vault of skull with intracranial injury of other and unspecified nature, unspecified state of consciousness ▽

800.91 Open fracture of vault of skull with intracranial injury of other and unspecified nature, no loss of consciousness ▽

800.92 Open fracture of vault of skull with intracranial injury of other and unspecified nature, brief (less than one hour) loss of consciousness ▽

800.93 Open fracture of vault of skull with intracranial injury of other and unspecified nature, moderate (1-24 hours) loss of consciousness ▽

800.94 Open fracture of vault of skull with intracranial injury of other and unspecified nature, prolonged (more than 24 hours) loss of consciousness and return to pre-existing conscious level
800.95 Open fracture of vault of skull with intracranial injury of other and unspecified nature, prolonged (more than 24 hours) loss of consciousness, without return to pre-existing conscious level
800.96 Open fracture of vault of skull with intracranial injury of other and unspecified nature, loss of consciousness of unspecified duration
800.99 Open fracture of vault of skull with intracranial injury of other and unspecified nature, unspecified concussion
801.00 Closed fracture of base of skull without mention of intracranial injury, unspecified state of consciousness
801.01 Closed fracture of base of skull without mention of intracranial injury, no loss of consciousness
801.02 Closed fracture of base of skull without mention of intracranial injury, brief (less than one hour) loss of consciousness
801.03 Closed fracture of base of skull without mention of intracranial injury, moderate (1-24 hours) loss of consciousness
801.04 Closed fracture of base of skull without mention of intracranial injury, prolonged (more than 24 hours) loss of consciousness and return to pre-existing conscious level
801.05 Closed fracture of base of skull without mention of intracranial injury, prolonged (more than 24 hours) loss of consciousness, without return to pre-existing conscious level
801.06 Closed fracture of base of skull without mention of intracranial injury, loss of consciousness of unspecified duration
801.09 Closed fracture of base of skull without mention of intracranial injury, unspecified concussion
801.10 Closed fracture of base of skull with cerebral laceration and contusion, unspecified state of consciousness
801.11 Closed fracture of base of skull with cerebral laceration and contusion, no loss of consciousness
801.12 Closed fracture of base of skull with cerebral laceration and contusion, brief (less than one hour) loss of consciousness
801.13 Closed fracture of base of skull with cerebral laceration and contusion, moderate (1-24 hours) loss of consciousness
801.14 Closed fracture of base of skull with cerebral laceration and contusion, prolonged (more than 24 hours) loss of consciousness and return to pre-existing conscious level
801.15 Closed fracture of base of skull with cerebral laceration and contusion, prolonged (more than 24 hours) loss of consciousness, without return to pre-existing conscious level
801.16 Closed fracture of base of skull with cerebral laceration and contusion, loss of consciousness of unspecified duration
801.19 Closed fracture of base of skull with cerebral laceration and contusion, unspecified concussion
801.20 Closed fracture of base of skull with subarachnoid, subdural, and extradural hemorrhage, unspecified state of consciousness
801.21 Closed fracture of base of skull with subarachnoid, subdural, and extradural hemorrhage, no loss of consciousness
801.22 Closed fracture of base of skull with subarachnoid, subdural, and extradural hemorrhage, brief (less than one hour) loss of consciousness
801.23 Closed fracture of base of skull with subarachnoid, subdural, and extradural hemorrhage, moderate (1-24 hours) loss of consciousness
801.24 Closed fracture of base of skull with subarachnoid, subdural, and extradural hemorrhage, prolonged (more than 24 hours) loss of consciousness and return to pre-existing conscious level
801.25 Closed fracture of base of skull with subarachnoid, subdural, and extradural hemorrhage, prolonged (more than 24 hours) loss of consciousness, without return to pre-existing conscious level
801.26 Closed fracture of base of skull with subarachnoid, subdural, and extradural hemorrhage, loss of consciousness of unspecified duration
801.30 Closed fracture of base of skull with other and unspecified intracranial hemorrhage, unspecified state of consciousness
801.31 Closed fracture of base of skull with other and unspecified intracranial hemorrhage, no loss of consciousness
801.32 Closed fracture of base of skull with other and unspecified intracranial hemorrhage, brief (less than one hour) loss of consciousness
801.33 Closed fracture of base of skull with other and unspecified intracranial hemorrhage, moderate (1-24 hours) loss of consciousness
801.34 Closed fracture of base of skull with other and unspecified intracranial hemorrhage, prolonged (more than 24 hours) loss of consciousness and return to pre-existing conscious level
801.35 Closed fracture of base of skull with other and unspecified intracranial hemorrhage, prolonged (more than 24 hours) loss of consciousness, without return to pre-existing conscious level
801.36 Closed fracture of base of skull with other and unspecified intracranial hemorrhage, loss of consciousness of unspecified duration
801.39 Closed fracture of base of skull with other and unspecified intracranial hemorrhage, unspecified concussion
801.41 Closed fracture of base of skull with intracranial injury of other and unspecified nature, no loss of consciousness
801.42 Closed fracture of base of skull with intracranial injury of other and unspecified nature, brief (less than one hour) loss of consciousness
801.43 Closed fracture of base of skull with intracranial injury of other and unspecified nature, moderate (1-24 hours) loss of consciousness
801.44 Closed fracture of base of skull with intracranial injury of other and unspecified nature, prolonged (more than 24 hours) loss of consciousness and return to pre-existing conscious level
801.45 Closed fracture of base of skull with intracranial injury of other and unspecified nature, prolonged (more than 24 hours) loss of consciousness, without return to pre-existing conscious level
801.46 Closed fracture of base of skull with intracranial injury of other and unspecified nature, loss of consciousness of unspecified duration
801.49 Closed fracture of base of skull with intracranial injury of other and unspecified nature, unspecified concussion
802.4 Malar and maxillary bones, closed fracture
802.5 Malar and maxillary bones, open fracture
802.8 Other facial bones, closed fracture
802.9 Other facial bones, open fracture
804.00 Closed fractures involving skull or face with other bones, without mention of intracranial injury, unspecified state of consciousness
804.01 Closed fractures involving skull or face with other bones, without mention of intracranial injury, no loss of consciousness
804.02 Closed fractures involving skull or face with other bones, without mention of intracranial injury, brief (less than one hour) loss of consciousness
804.03 Closed fractures involving skull or face with other bones, without mention of intracranial injury, moderate (1-24 hours) loss of consciousness
804.04 Closed fractures involving skull or face with other bones, without mention or intracranial injury, prolonged (more than 24 hours) loss of consciousness and return to pre-existing conscious level
804.05 Closed fractures involving skull of face with other bones, without mention of intracranial injury, prolonged (more than 24 hours) loss of consciousness, without return to pre-existing conscious level
804.06 Closed fractures involving skull of face with other bones, without mention of intracranial injury, loss of consciousness of unspecified duration
804.09 Closed fractures involving skull of face with other bones, without mention of intracranial injury, unspecified concussion
804.10 Closed fractures involving skull or face with other bones, with cerebral laceration and contusion, unspecified state of consciousness
804.11 Closed fractures involving skull or face with other bones, with cerebral laceration and contusion, no loss of consciousness
804.12 Closed fractures involving skull or face with other bones, with cerebral laceration and contusion, brief (less than one hour) loss of consciousness
804.13 Closed fractures involving skull or face with other bones, with cerebral laceration and contusion, moderate (1-24 hours) loss of consciousness
804.14 Closed fractures involving skull or face with other bones, with cerebral laceration and contusion, prolonged (more than 24 hours) loss of consciousness and return to pre-existing conscious level
804.15 Closed fractures involving skull or face with other bones, with cerebral laceration and contusion, prolonged (more than 24 hours) loss of consciousness, without return to pre-existing conscious level
804.16 Closed fractures involving skull or face with other bones, with cerebral laceration and contusion, loss of consciousness of unspecified duration
804.19 Closed fractures involving skull or face with other bones, with cerebral laceration and contusion, unspecified concussion
804.20 Closed fractures involving skull or face with other bones with subarachnoid, subdural, and extradural hemorrhage, unspecified state of consciousness
804.21 Closed fractures involving skull or face with other bones with subarachnoid, subdural, and extradural hemorrhage, no loss of consciousness
804.22 Closed fractures involving skull or face with other bones with subarachnoid, subdural, and extradural hemorrhage, brief (less than one hour) loss of consciousness
804.23 Closed fractures involving skull or face with other bones with subarachnoid, subdural, and extradural hemorrhage, moderate (1-24 hours) loss of consciousness
804.24 Closed fractures involving skull or face with other bones with subarachnoid, subdural, and extradural hemorrhage, prolonged (more than 24 hours) loss of consciousness and return to pre-existing conscious level
804.25 Closed fractures involving skull or face with other bones with subarachnoid, subdural, and extradural hemorrhage, prolonged (more than 24 hours) loss of consciousness, without return to pre-existing conscious level

Unspecified code
♀ Female diagnosis
Manifestation code
♂ Male diagnosis

804.26 Closed fractures involving skull or face with other bones with subarachnoid, subdural, and extradural hemorrhage, loss of consciousness of unspecified duration ▽
804.29 Closed fractures involving skull or face with other bones with subarachnoid, subdural, and extradural hemorrhage, unspecified concussion ▽
804.30 Closed fractures involving skull or face with other bones, with other and unspecified intracranial hemorrhage, unspecified state of consciousness ▽
804.31 Closed fractures involving skull or face with other bones, with other and unspecified intracranial hemorrhage, no loss of consciousness ▽
804.32 Closed fractures involving skull or face with other bones, with other and unspecified intracranial hemorrhage, brief (less than one hour) loss of consciousness ▽
804.33 Closed fractures involving skull or face with other bones, with other and unspecified intracranial hemorrrhage, moderate (1-24 hours) loss of consciousness ▽
804.34 Closed fractures involving skull or face with other bones, with other and unspecified intracranial hemorrhage, prolonged (more than 24 hours) loss of consciousness and return to preexisting conscious level ▽
804.35 Closed fractures involving skull or face with other bones, with other and unspecified intracranial hemorrhage, prolonged (more than 24 hours) loss of consciousness, without return to pre-existing conscious level ▽
804.36 Closed fractures involving skull or face with other bones, with other and unspecified intracranial hemorrhage, loss of consciousness of unspecified duration ▽
804.39 Closed fractures involving skull or face with other bones, with other and unspecified intracranial hemorrhage, unspecified concussion ▽
804.40 Closed fractures involving skull or face with other bones, with intracranial injury of other and unspecified nature, unspecified state of consciousness ▽
804.41 Closed fractures involving skull or face with other bones, with intracranial injury of other and unspecified nature, no loss of consciousness ▽
804.42 Closed fractures involving skull or face with other bones, with intracranial injury of other and unspecified nature, brief (less than one hour) loss of consciousness ▽
804.43 Closed fractures involving skull or face with other bones, with intracranial injury of other and unspecified nature, moderate (1-24 hours) loss of consciousness ▽
804.44 Closed fractures involving skull or face with other bones, with intracranial injury of other and unspecified nature, prolonged (more than 24 hours) loss of consciousness and return to pre-existing conscious level ▽
804.45 Closed fractures involving skull or face with other bones, with intracranial injury of other and unspecified nature, prolonged (more than 24 hours) loss of consciousness, without return to pre-existing conscious level ▽
804.46 Closed fractures involving skull or face with other bones, with intracranial injury of other and unspecified nature, loss of consciousness of unspecified duration ▽
804.49 Closed fractures involving skull or face with other bones, with intracranial injury of other and unspecified nature, unspecified concussion ▽

ICD-9-CM Procedural

76.79 Other open reduction of facial fracture
76.91 Bone graft to facial bone

21440

21440 Closed treatment of mandibular or maxillary alveolar ridge fracture (separate procedure)

ICD-9-CM Diagnostic

802.27 Closed fracture of alveolar border of body of mandible
802.29 Closed fracture of multiple sites of mandible
802.4 Malar and maxillary bones, closed fracture

ICD-9-CM Procedural

76.73 Closed reduction of maxillary fracture
76.75 Closed reduction of mandibular fracture

HCPCS Level II Supplies & Services

A4570 Splint

21445

21445 Open treatment of mandibular or maxillary alveolar ridge fracture (separate procedure)

ICD-9-CM Diagnostic

802.27 Closed fracture of alveolar border of body of mandible
802.29 Closed fracture of multiple sites of mandible
802.37 Open fracture of alveolar border of body of mandible
802.39 Open fracture of multiple sites of mandible
802.4 Malar and maxillary bones, closed fracture
802.5 Malar and maxillary bones, open fracture

ICD-9-CM Procedural

76.77 Open reduction of alveolar fracture

21450–21451

21450 Closed treatment of mandibular fracture; without manipulation
21451 with manipulation

ICD-9-CM Diagnostic

802.20 Closed fracture of unspecified site of mandible ▽
802.21 Closed fracture of condylar process of mandible
802.22 Closed fracture of subcondylar process of mandible
802.23 Closed fracture of coronoid process of mandible
802.24 Closed fracture of unspecified part of ramus of mandible ▽
802.25 Closed fracture of angle of jaw
802.26 Closed fracture of symphysis of body of mandible
802.29 Closed fracture of multiple sites of mandible

ICD-9-CM Procedural

76.75 Closed reduction of mandibular fracture
93.59 Other immobilization, pressure, and attention to wound

HCPCS Level II Supplies & Services

A4305 Disposable drug delivery system, flow rate of 50 ml or greater per hour
A4306 Disposable drug delivery system, flow rate of 5 ml or less per hour
A4550 Surgical trays

21452

21452 Percutaneous treatment of mandibular fracture, with external fixation

ICD-9-CM Diagnostic

733.82 Nonunion of fracture
802.20 Closed fracture of unspecified site of mandible ▽
802.21 Closed fracture of condylar process of mandible
802.22 Closed fracture of subcondylar process of mandible
802.23 Closed fracture of coronoid process of mandible
802.24 Closed fracture of unspecified part of ramus of mandible ▽
802.25 Closed fracture of angle of jaw
802.26 Closed fracture of symphysis of body of mandible
802.27 Closed fracture of alveolar border of body of mandible
802.28 Closed fracture of other and unspecified part of body of mandible ▽
802.29 Closed fracture of multiple sites of mandible

ICD-9-CM Procedural

76.75 Closed reduction of mandibular fracture
78.19 Application of external fixation device, other

HCPCS Level II Supplies & Services

A4305 Disposable drug delivery system, flow rate of 50 ml or greater per hour
A4306 Disposable drug delivery system, flow rate of 5 ml or less per hour
A4550 Surgical trays

21453

21453 Closed treatment of mandibular fracture with interdental fixation

ICD-9-CM Diagnostic

733.82 Nonunion of fracture
802.20 Closed fracture of unspecified site of mandible ▽
802.21 Closed fracture of condylar process of mandible
802.22 Closed fracture of subcondylar process of mandible
802.23 Closed fracture of coronoid process of mandible
802.24 Closed fracture of unspecified part of ramus of mandible ▽
802.25 Closed fracture of angle of jaw
802.26 Closed fracture of symphysis of body of mandible
802.27 Closed fracture of alveolar border of body of mandible
802.28 Closed fracture of other and unspecified part of body of mandible ▽
802.29 Closed fracture of multiple sites of mandible

ICD-9-CM Procedural

76.75 Closed reduction of mandibular fracture

21454

21454 Open treatment of mandibular fracture with external fixation

ICD-9-CM Diagnostic

733.82 Nonunion of fracture
802.21 Closed fracture of condylar process of mandible
802.22 Closed fracture of subcondylar process of mandible
802.23 Closed fracture of coronoid process of mandible
802.24 Closed fracture of unspecified part of ramus of mandible ▽
802.25 Closed fracture of angle of jaw
802.26 Closed fracture of symphysis of body of mandible
802.27 Closed fracture of alveolar border of body of mandible
802.28 Closed fracture of other and unspecified part of body of mandible ▽
802.29 Closed fracture of multiple sites of mandible
802.31 Open fracture of condylar process of mandible
802.32 Open fracture of subcondylar process of mandible
802.34 Open fracture of unspecified part of ramus of mandible ▽
802.35 Open fracture of angle of jaw
802.36 Open fracture of symphysis of body of mandible
802.37 Open fracture of alveolar border of body of mandible
802.38 Open fracture of other and unspecified part of body of mandible
802.39 Open fracture of multiple sites of mandible

ICD-9-CM Procedural

76.76 Open reduction of mandibular fracture
78.19 Application of external fixation device, other

21461–21462

21461 Open treatment of mandibular fracture; without interdental fixation
21462 with interdental fixation

ICD-9-CM Diagnostic

733.82 Nonunion of fracture
802.21 Closed fracture of condylar process of mandible
802.22 Closed fracture of subcondylar process of mandible
802.23 Closed fracture of coronoid process of mandible
802.24 Closed fracture of unspecified part of ramus of mandible ▽
802.25 Closed fracture of angle of jaw
802.26 Closed fracture of symphysis of body of mandible
802.27 Closed fracture of alveolar border of body of mandible
802.28 Closed fracture of other and unspecified part of body of mandible ▽
802.29 Closed fracture of multiple sites of mandible
802.30 Open fracture of unspecified site of mandible ▽
802.31 Open fracture of condylar process of mandible
802.32 Open fracture of subcondylar process of mandible
802.33 Open fracture of coronoid process of mandible
802.34 Open fracture of unspecified part of ramus of mandible ▽
802.35 Open fracture of angle of jaw
802.36 Open fracture of symphysis of body of mandible
802.37 Open fracture of alveolar border of body of mandible
802.38 Open fracture of other and unspecified part of body of mandible
802.39 Open fracture of multiple sites of mandible

ICD-9-CM Procedural

76.76 Open reduction of mandibular fracture

21465

21465 Open treatment of mandibular condylar fracture

ICD-9-CM Diagnostic

733.82 Nonunion of fracture
802.21 Closed fracture of condylar process of mandible
802.22 Closed fracture of subcondylar process of mandible
802.29 Closed fracture of multiple sites of mandible
802.30 Open fracture of unspecified site of mandible ▽
802.31 Open fracture of condylar process of mandible
802.32 Open fracture of subcondylar process of mandible
802.39 Open fracture of multiple sites of mandible

ICD-9-CM Procedural

76.76 Open reduction of mandibular fracture

21470

21470 Open treatment of complicated mandibular fracture by multiple surgical approaches including internal fixation, interdental fixation, and/or wiring of dentures or splints

ICD-9-CM Diagnostic

733.82 Nonunion of fracture
802.21 Closed fracture of condylar process of mandible
802.22 Closed fracture of subcondylar process of mandible
802.23 Closed fracture of coronoid process of mandible
802.24 Closed fracture of unspecified part of ramus of mandible ▽
802.25 Closed fracture of angle of jaw
802.26 Closed fracture of symphysis of body of mandible
802.27 Closed fracture of alveolar border of body of mandible
802.28 Closed fracture of other and unspecified part of body of mandible ▽
802.29 Closed fracture of multiple sites of mandible
802.30 Open fracture of unspecified site of mandible ▽
802.31 Open fracture of condylar process of mandible
802.32 Open fracture of subcondylar process of mandible
802.33 Open fracture of coronoid process of mandible
802.34 Open fracture of unspecified part of ramus of mandible ▽
802.35 Open fracture of angle of jaw
802.36 Open fracture of symphysis of body of mandible
802.37 Open fracture of alveolar border of body of mandible
802.38 Open fracture of other and unspecified part of body of mandible
802.39 Open fracture of multiple sites of mandible

ICD-9-CM Procedural

76.76 Open reduction of mandibular fracture
78.19 Application of external fixation device, other

21480–21485

21480 Closed treatment of temporomandibular dislocation; initial or subsequent
21485 complicated (eg, recurrent requiring intermaxillary fixation or splinting), initial or subsequent

ICD-9-CM Diagnostic

524.63 Articular disc disorder (reducing or non-reducing) of temporomandibular joint
524.64 Temporomandibular joint sounds on opening and/or closing the jaw
524.69 Other specified temporomandibular joint disorders
830.0 Closed dislocation of jaw
925.1 Crushing injury of face and scalp — (Use additional code to identify any associated injuries: 800-829, 850.0-854.1, 860.0-869.1)

ICD-9-CM Procedural

76.93 Closed reduction of temporomandibular dislocation
76.95 Other manipulation of temporomandibular joint

HCPCS Level II Supplies & Services

A4305 Disposable drug delivery system, flow rate of 50 ml or greater per hour
A4306 Disposable drug delivery system, flow rate of 5 ml or less per hour
A4550 Surgical trays
A4649 Surgical supply; miscellaneous

21490

21490 Open treatment of temporomandibular dislocation

ICD-9-CM Diagnostic

524.63 Articular disc disorder (reducing or non-reducing) of temporomandibular joint
524.64 Temporomandibular joint sounds on opening and/or closing the jaw
524.69 Other specified temporomandibular joint disorders
830.0 Closed dislocation of jaw
830.1 Open dislocation of jaw

ICD-9-CM Procedural

76.94 Open reduction of temporomandibular dislocation

21493–21494

21493 Closed treatment of hyoid fracture; without manipulation
21494 with manipulation

ICD-9-CM Diagnostic

807.5 Closed fracture of larynx and trachea
925.2 Crushing injury of neck — (Use additional code to identify any associated injuries: 800-829, 850.0-854.1, 860.0-869.1)

ICD-9-CM Procedural
79.09 Closed reduction of fracture of other specified bone, except facial bones, without internal fixation
93.52 Application of neck support

21495
21495 Open treatment of hyoid fracture

ICD-9-CM Diagnostic
807.5 Closed fracture of larynx and trachea
807.6 Open fracture of larynx and trachea
925.2 Crushing injury of neck — (Use additional code to identify any associated injuries: 800-829, 850.0-854.1, 860.0-869.1)

ICD-9-CM Procedural
31.64 Repair of laryngeal fracture

21497
21497 Interdental wiring, for condition other than fracture

ICD-9-CM Diagnostic
170.0 Malignant neoplasm of bones of skull and face, except mandible
170.1 Malignant neoplasm of mandible
213.0 Benign neoplasm of bones of skull and face
213.1 Benign neoplasm of lower jaw bone
278.00 Obesity, unspecified — (Use additional code to identify any associated mental retardation) ▽
278.01 Morbid obesity — (Use additional code to identify any associated mental retardation)
524.01 Maxillary hyperplasia
524.02 Mandibular hyperplasia
524.04 Mandibular hypoplasia
524.69 Other specified temporomandibular joint disorders
526.89 Other specified disease of the jaws
830.0 Closed dislocation of jaw
830.1 Open dislocation of jaw
839.8 Closed dislocation, multiple and ill-defined sites
941.09 Burn of unspecified degree of multiple sites (except with eye) of face, head, and neck ▽
V52.3 Fitting and adjustment of dental prosthetic device

ICD-9-CM Procedural
24.7 Application of orthodontic appliance
93.55 Dental wiring

HCPCS Level II Supplies & Services
A4305 Disposable drug delivery system, flow rate of 50 ml or greater per hour
A4306 Disposable drug delivery system, flow rate of 5 ml or less per hour
A4550 Surgical trays

Neck (Soft Tissues) and Thorax

21501–21502
21501 Incision and drainage, deep abscess or hematoma, soft tissues of neck or thorax;
21502 with partial rib ostectomy

ICD-9-CM Diagnostic
682.1 Cellulitis and abscess of neck — (Use additional code to identify organism)
682.2 Cellulitis and abscess of trunk — (Use additional code to identify organism)
784.2 Swelling, mass, or lump in head and neck
920 Contusion of face, scalp, and neck except eye(s)
922.1 Contusion of chest wall
998.51 Infected postoperative seroma — (Use additional code to identify organism)
998.59 Other postoperative infection — (Use additional code to identify infection)

ICD-9-CM Procedural
77.81 Other partial ostectomy of scapula, clavicle, and thorax (ribs and sternum)
83.02 Myotomy
83.09 Other incision of soft tissue

HCPCS Level II Supplies & Services
A4305 Disposable drug delivery system, flow rate of 50 ml or greater per hour
A4306 Disposable drug delivery system, flow rate of 5 ml or less per hour
A4550 Surgical trays

21510
21510 Incision, deep, with opening of bone cortex (eg, for osteomyelitis or bone abscess), thorax

ICD-9-CM Diagnostic
682.2 Cellulitis and abscess of trunk — (Use additional code to identify organism)
730.18 Chronic osteomyelitis, other specified sites — (Use additional code to identify organism, 041.1)
730.19 Chronic osteomyelitis, multiple sites — (Use additional code to identify organism, 041.1)
730.28 Unspecified osteomyelitis, other specified sites — (Use additional code to identify organism, 041.1) ▽
730.29 Unspecified osteomyelitis, multiple sites — (Use additional code to identify organism, 041.1) ▽
786.6 Swelling, mass, or lump in chest
998.51 Infected postoperative seroma — (Use additional code to identify organism)
998.59 Other postoperative infection — (Use additional code to identify infection)

ICD-9-CM Procedural
34.01 Incision of chest wall
77.01 Sequestrectomy of scapula, clavicle, and thorax (ribs and sternum)

21550
21550 Biopsy, soft tissue of neck or thorax

ICD-9-CM Diagnostic
171.0 Malignant neoplasm of connective and other soft tissue of head, face, and neck
171.4 Malignant neoplasm of connective and other soft tissue of thorax
195.0 Malignant neoplasm of head, face, and neck
195.1 Malignant neoplasm of thorax
198.89 Secondary malignant neoplasm of other specified sites
215.0 Other benign neoplasm of connective and other soft tissue of head, face, and neck
215.4 Other benign neoplasm of connective and other soft tissue of thorax
229.8 Benign neoplasm of other specified sites
234.8 Carcinoma in situ of other specified sites
238.1 Neoplasm of uncertain behavior of connective and other soft tissue ▽
239.8 Neoplasm of unspecified nature of other specified sites
709.9 Unspecified disorder of skin and subcutaneous tissue ▽
782.2 Localized superficial swelling, mass, or lump
784.2 Swelling, mass, or lump in head and neck

ICD-9-CM Procedural
34.23 Biopsy of chest wall
83.21 Biopsy of soft tissue

HCPCS Level II Supplies & Services
A4550 Surgical trays

21555–21557
21555 Excision tumor, soft tissue of neck or thorax; subcutaneous
21556 deep, subfascial, intramuscular
21557 Radical resection of tumor (eg, malignant neoplasm), soft tissue of neck or thorax

ICD-9-CM Diagnostic
171.0 Malignant neoplasm of connective and other soft tissue of head, face, and neck
171.4 Malignant neoplasm of connective and other soft tissue of thorax
171.8 Malignant neoplasm of other specified sites of connective and other soft tissue
195.0 Malignant neoplasm of head, face, and neck
195.1 Malignant neoplasm of thorax
198.89 Secondary malignant neoplasm of other specified sites
199.0 Disseminated malignant neoplasm
199.1 Other malignant neoplasm of unspecified site
214.1 Lipoma of other skin and subcutaneous tissue
214.8 Lipoma of other specified sites
215.0 Other benign neoplasm of connective and other soft tissue of head, face, and neck
215.4 Other benign neoplasm of connective and other soft tissue of thorax
229.8 Benign neoplasm of other specified sites
234.8 Carcinoma in situ of other specified sites
238.1 Neoplasm of uncertain behavior of connective and other soft tissue ▽
239.2 Neoplasms of unspecified nature of bone, soft tissue, and skin

782.2 Localized superficial swelling, mass, or lump
784.2 Swelling, mass, or lump in head and neck

ICD-9-CM Procedural
83.32 Excision of lesion of muscle
83.39 Excision of lesion of other soft tissue
83.49 Other excision of soft tissue

HCPCS Level II Supplies & Services
A4550 Surgical trays

21600
21600 Excision of rib, partial

ICD-9-CM Diagnostic
170.3 Malignant neoplasm of ribs, sternum, and clavicle
198.5 Secondary malignant neoplasm of bone and bone marrow
213.3 Benign neoplasm of ribs, sternum, and clavicle
229.8 Benign neoplasm of other specified sites
238.0 Neoplasm of uncertain behavior of bone and articular cartilage
239.2 Neoplasms of unspecified nature of bone, soft tissue, and skin
730.18 Chronic osteomyelitis, other specified sites — (Use additional code to identify organism, 041.1)
730.88 Other infections involving bone diseases classified elsewhere, other specified sites — (Code first underlying disease: 002.0, 015.0-015.9. Use additional code to identify organism) ☒
756.2 Cervical rib
756.3 Other congenital anomaly of ribs and sternum

ICD-9-CM Procedural
77.81 Other partial ostectomy of scapula, clavicle, and thorax (ribs and sternum)

21610
21610 Costotransversectomy (separate procedure)

ICD-9-CM Diagnostic
170.2 Malignant neoplasm of vertebral column, excluding sacrum and coccyx
170.3 Malignant neoplasm of ribs, sternum, and clavicle
198.5 Secondary malignant neoplasm of bone and bone marrow
213.2 Benign neoplasm of vertebral column, excluding sacrum and coccyx
213.3 Benign neoplasm of ribs, sternum, and clavicle
229.8 Benign neoplasm of other specified sites
238.0 Neoplasm of uncertain behavior of bone and articular cartilage
239.2 Neoplasms of unspecified nature of bone, soft tissue, and skin
715.09 Generalized osteoarthrosis, involving multiple sites
715.18 Primary localized osteoarthrosis, other specified sites
715.98 Osteoarthrosis, unspecified whether generalized or localized, other specified sites ▽
730.18 Chronic osteomyelitis, other specified sites — (Use additional code to identify organism, 041.1)
730.88 Other infections involving bone diseases classified elsewhere, other specified sites — (Code first underlying disease: 002.0, 015.0-015.9. Use additional code to identify organism) ☒
756.3 Other congenital anomaly of ribs and sternum

ICD-9-CM Procedural
77.91 Total ostectomy of scapula, clavicle, and thorax (ribs and sternum)

21615–21616
21615 Excision first and/or cervical rib;
21616 with sympathectomy

ICD-9-CM Diagnostic
353.0 Brachial plexus lesions
443.0 Raynaud's syndrome — (Use additional code to identify gangrene, 785.4)
444.21 Embolism and thrombosis of arteries of upper extremity
723.1 Cervicalgia
723.4 Brachial neuritis or radiculitis nos
756.2 Cervical rib
786.52 Painful respiration
786.6 Swelling, mass, or lump in chest

ICD-9-CM Procedural
05.22 Cervical sympathectomy
77.91 Total ostectomy of scapula, clavicle, and thorax (ribs and sternum)

21620
21620 Ostectomy of sternum, partial

ICD-9-CM Diagnostic
170.3 Malignant neoplasm of ribs, sternum, and clavicle
198.5 Secondary malignant neoplasm of bone and bone marrow
213.3 Benign neoplasm of ribs, sternum, and clavicle
238.0 Neoplasm of uncertain behavior of bone and articular cartilage
239.2 Neoplasms of unspecified nature of bone, soft tissue, and skin
519.2 Mediastinitis
730.18 Chronic osteomyelitis, other specified sites — (Use additional code to identify organism, 041.1)
730.28 Unspecified osteomyelitis, other specified sites — (Use additional code to identify organism, 041.1) ▽
730.88 Other infections involving bone diseases classified elsewhere, other specified sites — (Code first underlying disease: 002.0, 015.0-015.9. Use additional code to identify organism) ☒
733.49 Aseptic necrosis of other bone site
733.99 Other disorders of bone and cartilage

ICD-9-CM Procedural
77.81 Other partial ostectomy of scapula, clavicle, and thorax (ribs and sternum)

21627
21627 Sternal debridement

ICD-9-CM Diagnostic
170.3 Malignant neoplasm of ribs, sternum, and clavicle
198.5 Secondary malignant neoplasm of bone and bone marrow
213.3 Benign neoplasm of ribs, sternum, and clavicle
238.0 Neoplasm of uncertain behavior of bone and articular cartilage
239.2 Neoplasms of unspecified nature of bone, soft tissue, and skin
519.2 Mediastinitis
730.18 Chronic osteomyelitis, other specified sites — (Use additional code to identify organism, 041.1)
730.28 Unspecified osteomyelitis, other specified sites — (Use additional code to identify organism, 041.1) ▽
730.88 Other infections involving bone diseases classified elsewhere, other specified sites — (Code first underlying disease: 002.0, 015.0-015.9. Use additional code to identify organism) ☒
733.49 Aseptic necrosis of other bone site
875.1 Open wound of chest (wall), complicated — (Use additional code to identify infection)
998.51 Infected postoperative seroma — (Use additional code to identify organism)
998.59 Other postoperative infection — (Use additional code to identify infection)
998.83 Non-healing surgical wound

ICD-9-CM Procedural
77.61 Local excision of lesion or tissue of scapula, clavicle, and thorax (ribs and sternum)

21630–21632
21630 Radical resection of sternum;
21632 with mediastinal lymphadenectomy

ICD-9-CM Diagnostic
170.3 Malignant neoplasm of ribs, sternum, and clavicle
196.1 Secondary and unspecified malignant neoplasm of intrathoracic lymph nodes
197.1 Secondary malignant neoplasm of mediastinum
198.5 Secondary malignant neoplasm of bone and bone marrow
213.3 Benign neoplasm of ribs, sternum, and clavicle
238.0 Neoplasm of uncertain behavior of bone and articular cartilage
730.18 Chronic osteomyelitis, other specified sites — (Use additional code to identify organism, 041.1)
730.28 Unspecified osteomyelitis, other specified sites — (Use additional code to identify organism, 041.1) ▽
730.88 Other infections involving bone diseases classified elsewhere, other specified sites — (Code first underlying disease: 002.0, 015.0-015.9. Use additional code to identify organism) ☒
733.49 Aseptic necrosis of other bone site
875.1 Open wound of chest (wall), complicated — (Use additional code to identify infection)
998.59 Other postoperative infection — (Use additional code to identify infection)

ICD-9-CM Procedural
40.22 Excision of internal mammary lymph node

▽ Unspecified code
♀ Female diagnosis
☒ Manifestation code
♂ Male diagnosis

40.3 Regional lymph node excision
40.59 Radical excision of other lymph nodes
77.81 Other partial ostectomy of scapula, clavicle, and thorax (ribs and sternum)
77.91 Total ostectomy of scapula, clavicle, and thorax (ribs and sternum)

21685

21685 Hyoid myotomy and suspension

ICD-9-CM Diagnostic

780.50 Unspecified sleep disturbance ▽
780.51 Insomnia with sleep apnea
780.53 Hypersomnia with sleep apnea
780.57 Other and unspecified sleep apnea ▽

ICD-9-CM Procedural

83.02 Myotomy

21700–21705

21700 Division of scalenus anticus; without resection of cervical rib
21705 with resection of cervical rib

ICD-9-CM Diagnostic

353.0 Brachial plexus lesions
728.85 Spasm of muscle
756.2 Cervical rib

ICD-9-CM Procedural

77.81 Other partial ostectomy of scapula, clavicle, and thorax (ribs and sternum)
83.19 Other division of soft tissue

21720–21725

21720 Division of sternocleidomastoid for torticollis, open operation; without cast application
21725 with cast application

ICD-9-CM Diagnostic

333.83 Spasmodic torticollis — (Use additional E code to identify drug, if drug-induced)
723.5 Torticollis, unspecified ▽
754.1 Congenital musculoskeletal deformity of sternocleidomastoid muscle
781.93 Ocular torticollis

ICD-9-CM Procedural

83.19 Other division of soft tissue
93.52 Application of neck support
93.53 Application of other cast

21740–21743

21740 Reconstructive repair of pectus excavatum or carinatum; open
21742 minimally invasive approach (Nuss procedure), without thoracoscopy
21743 minimally invasive approach (Nuss procedure), with thoracoscopy

ICD-9-CM Diagnostic

277.5 Mucopolysaccharidosis — (Use additional code to identify any associated mental retardation)
754.81 Pectus excavatum
754.82 Pectus carinatum
756.51 Osteogenesis imperfecta
758.6 Gonadal dysgenesis
759.82 Marfan's syndrome

ICD-9-CM Procedural

34.21 Transpleural thoracoscopy
34.74 Repair of pectus deformity

HCPCS Level II Supplies & Services

HCPCS Level II codes are used to report the supplies, durable medical equipment, and certain medical services provided on an outpatient basis. Because the procedure(s) represented on this page would be performed in an inpatient facility, no HCPCS Level II codes apply.

21750

21750 Closure of median sternotomy separation with or without debridement (separate procedure)

ICD-9-CM Diagnostic

733.81 Malunion of fracture
733.82 Nonunion of fracture
998.31 Disruption of internal operation wound
998.59 Other postoperative infection — (Use additional code to identify infection)
998.83 Non-healing surgical wound

ICD-9-CM Procedural

77.61 Local excision of lesion or tissue of scapula, clavicle, and thorax (ribs and sternum)
78.49 Other repair or plastic operations on other bone, except facial bones

21800

21800 Closed treatment of rib fracture, uncomplicated, each

ICD-9-CM Diagnostic

786.52 Painful respiration
807.00 Closed fracture of rib(s), unspecified ▽
807.01 Closed fracture of one rib
807.02 Closed fracture of two ribs
807.03 Closed fracture of three ribs
807.04 Closed fracture of four ribs
807.05 Closed fracture of five ribs
807.06 Closed fracture of six ribs
807.07 Closed fracture of seven ribs
807.08 Closed fracture of eight or more ribs
807.09 Closed fracture of multiple ribs, unspecified ▽

ICD-9-CM Procedural

79.09 Closed reduction of fracture of other specified bone, except facial bones, without internal fixation

HCPCS Level II Supplies & Services

L0210 Thoracic, rib belt
L0220 Thoracic, rib belt, custom fabricated

21805

21805 Open treatment of rib fracture without fixation, each

ICD-9-CM Diagnostic

807.01 Closed fracture of one rib
807.02 Closed fracture of two ribs
807.03 Closed fracture of three ribs
807.04 Closed fracture of four ribs
807.05 Closed fracture of five ribs
807.06 Closed fracture of six ribs
807.07 Closed fracture of seven ribs
807.08 Closed fracture of eight or more ribs
807.11 Open fracture of one rib
807.12 Open fracture of two ribs
807.13 Open fracture of three ribs
807.14 Open fracture of four ribs
807.15 Open fracture of five ribs
807.16 Open fracture of six ribs
807.17 Open fracture of seven ribs
807.18 Open fracture of eight or more ribs

ICD-9-CM Procedural

79.29 Open reduction of fracture of other specified bone, except facial bones, without internal fixation

21810

21810 Treatment of rib fracture requiring external fixation (flail chest)

ICD-9-CM Diagnostic

807.4 Flail chest

ICD-9-CM Procedural

78.11 Application of external fixation device, scapula, clavicle, and thorax (ribs and sternum)
79.09 Closed reduction of fracture of other specified bone, except facial bones, without internal fixation

21820

21820 Closed treatment of sternum fracture

ICD-9-CM Diagnostic

807.2 Closed fracture of sternum

ICD-9-CM Procedural

79.09 Closed reduction of fracture of other specified bone, except facial bones, without internal fixation

HCPCS Level II Supplies & Services

A4649 Surgical supply; miscellaneous

21825

21825 Open treatment of sternum fracture with or without skeletal fixation

ICD-9-CM Diagnostic

733.81 Malunion of fracture
733.82 Nonunion of fracture
807.2 Closed fracture of sternum
807.3 Open fracture of sternum

ICD-9-CM Procedural

79.29 Open reduction of fracture of other specified bone, except facial bones, without internal fixation
79.39 Open reduction of fracture of other specified bone, except facial bones, with internal fixation

Back and Flank

21920–21925

21920 Biopsy, soft tissue of back or flank; superficial
21925 deep

ICD-9-CM Diagnostic

171.7 Malignant neoplasm of connective and other soft tissue of trunk, unspecified site ▽
195.8 Malignant neoplasm of other specified sites
198.89 Secondary malignant neoplasm of other specified sites
214.1 Lipoma of other skin and subcutaneous tissue
215.7 Other benign neoplasm of connective and other soft tissue of trunk, unspecified ▽
238.1 Neoplasm of uncertain behavior of connective and other soft tissue ▽
239.2 Neoplasms of unspecified nature of bone, soft tissue, and skin
782.2 Localized superficial swelling, mass, or lump

ICD-9-CM Procedural

83.21 Biopsy of soft tissue

HCPCS Level II Supplies & Services

A4550 Surgical trays

21930

21930 Excision, tumor, soft tissue of back or flank

ICD-9-CM Diagnostic

171.7 Malignant neoplasm of connective and other soft tissue of trunk, unspecified site ▽
172.5 Malignant melanoma of skin of trunk, except scrotum
195.8 Malignant neoplasm of other specified sites
198.89 Secondary malignant neoplasm of other specified sites
214.1 Lipoma of other skin and subcutaneous tissue
215.7 Other benign neoplasm of connective and other soft tissue of trunk, unspecified ▽
228.01 Hemangioma of skin and subcutaneous tissue
238.1 Neoplasm of uncertain behavior of connective and other soft tissue ▽
239.2 Neoplasms of unspecified nature of bone, soft tissue, and skin
782.2 Localized superficial swelling, mass, or lump

ICD-9-CM Procedural

83.32 Excision of lesion of muscle
83.39 Excision of lesion of other soft tissue

HCPCS Level II Supplies & Services

A4305 Disposable drug delivery system, flow rate of 50 ml or greater per hour
A4306 Disposable drug delivery system, flow rate of 5 ml or less per hour
A4550 Surgical trays

21935

21935 Radical resection of tumor (eg, malignant neoplasm), soft tissue of back or flank

ICD-9-CM Diagnostic

171.7 Malignant neoplasm of connective and other soft tissue of trunk, unspecified site ▽
172.5 Malignant melanoma of skin of trunk, except scrotum
195.8 Malignant neoplasm of other specified sites
198.89 Secondary malignant neoplasm of other specified sites

ICD-9-CM Procedural

83.32 Excision of lesion of muscle
83.39 Excision of lesion of other soft tissue
83.49 Other excision of soft tissue

Spine (Vertebral Column)

22100–22103

22100 Partial excision of posterior vertebral component (eg, spinous process, lamina or facet) for intrinsic bony lesion, single vertebral segment; cervical
22101 thoracic
22102 lumbar
22103 each additional segment (List separately in addition to code for primary procedure)

ICD-9-CM Diagnostic

170.2 Malignant neoplasm of vertebral column, excluding sacrum and coccyx
198.5 Secondary malignant neoplasm of bone and bone marrow
213.2 Benign neoplasm of vertebral column, excluding sacrum and coccyx
238.0 Neoplasm of uncertain behavior of bone and articular cartilage
239.2 Neoplasms of unspecified nature of bone, soft tissue, and skin
720.0 Ankylosing spondylitis
720.1 Spinal enthesopathy
720.81 Inflammatory spondylopathies in diseases classified elsewhere — (Code first underlying disease, 015.0) ☒
720.89 Other inflammatory spondylopathies
720.9 Unspecified inflammatory spondylopathy ▽
721.0 Cervical spondylosis without myelopathy
721.1 Cervical spondylosis with myelopathy
721.2 Thoracic spondylosis without myelopathy
721.3 Lumbosacral spondylosis without myelopathy
721.41 Spondylosis with myelopathy, thoracic region
721.42 Spondylosis with myelopathy, lumbar region
721.5 Kissing spine
721.8 Other allied disorders of spine
723.0 Spinal stenosis in cervical region
730.18 Chronic osteomyelitis, other specified sites — (Use additional code to identify organism, 041.1)
730.28 Unspecified osteomyelitis, other specified sites — (Use additional code to identify organism, 041.1) ▽
733.13 Pathologic fracture of vertebrae
733.20 Unspecified cyst of bone (localized) ▽
733.21 Solitary bone cyst
733.22 Aneurysmal bone cyst
733.29 Other cyst of bone
733.95 Stress fracture of other bone
738.5 Other acquired deformity of back or spine
756.15 Congenital fusion of spine (vertebra)

ICD-9-CM Procedural

77.89 Other partial ostectomy of other bone, except facial bones

22110–22116

22110 Partial excision of vertebral body for intrinsic bony lesion, without decompression of spinal cord or nerve root(s), single vertebral segment; cervical
22112 thoracic
22114 lumbar
22116 each additional vertebral segment (List separately in addition to code for primary procedure)

ICD-9-CM Diagnostic

094.0 Tabes dorsalis — (Use additional code to identify any associated mental disorder. Use additional code to identify manifestation, 713.5)
098.53 Gonococcal spondylitis
170.2 Malignant neoplasm of vertebral column, excluding sacrum and coccyx
198.5 Secondary malignant neoplasm of bone and bone marrow
213.2 Benign neoplasm of vertebral column, excluding sacrum and coccyx
238.0 Neoplasm of uncertain behavior of bone and articular cartilage
239.2 Neoplasms of unspecified nature of bone, soft tissue, and skin
721.5 Kissing spine
722.31 Schmorl's nodes, thoracic region
722.32 Schmorl's nodes, lumbar region
722.39 Schmorl's nodes, other spinal region
723.0 Spinal stenosis in cervical region
724.01 Spinal stenosis of thoracic region
724.02 Spinal stenosis of lumbar region
730.18 Chronic osteomyelitis, other specified sites — (Use additional code to identify organism, 041.1)
730.28 Unspecified osteomyelitis, other specified sites — (Use additional code to identify organism, 041.1) ▽
730.88 Other infections involving bone diseases classified elsewhere, other specified sites — (Code first underlying disease: 002.0, 015.0-015.9. Use additional code to identify organism) ⊠
733.21 Solitary bone cyst
733.22 Aneurysmal bone cyst
733.29 Other cyst of bone

ICD-9-CM Procedural

77.89 Other partial ostectomy of other bone, except facial bones

22210–22216

22210 Osteotomy of spine, posterior or posterolateral approach, one vertebral segment; cervical
22212 thoracic
22214 lumbar
22216 each additional vertebral segment (List separately in addition to primary procedure)

ICD-9-CM Diagnostic

138 Late effects of acute poliomyelitis
237.71 Neurofibromatosis, Type 1 (von Recklinghausen's disease)
268.1 Rickets, late effect — (Use additional code to identify the nature of late effect)
720.0 Ankylosing spondylitis
721.7 Traumatic spondylopathy
731.0 Osteitis deformans without mention of bone tumor
732.0 Juvenile osteochondrosis of spine
733.13 Pathologic fracture of vertebrae
733.95 Stress fracture of other bone
737.10 Kyphosis (acquired) (postural)
737.11 Kyphosis due to radiation
737.12 Kyphosis, postlaminectomy

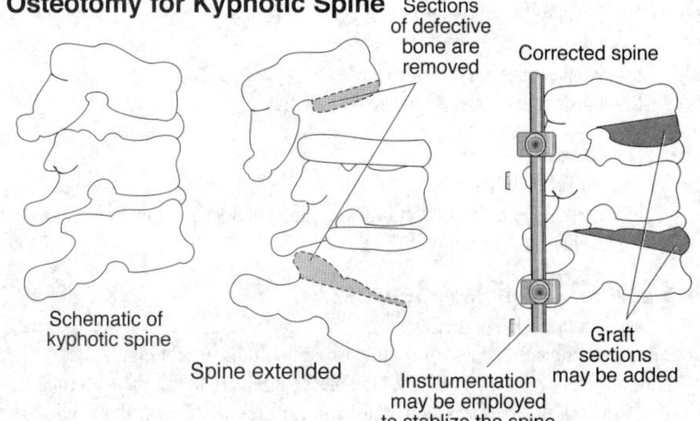
Osteotomy for Kyphotic Spine
Sections of defective bone are removed
Corrected spine
Schematic of kyphotic spine
Spine extended
Instrumentation may be employed to stablize the spine
Graft sections may be added

737.19 Other kyphosis (acquired)
737.20 Lordosis (acquired) (postural)
737.30 Scoliosis (and kyphoscoliosis), idiopathic
737.41 Kyphosis associated with other condition — (Code first associated condition: 015.0, 138, 237.7, 252.0, 277.5, 356.1, 731.0, 733.00-733.09) ⊠
738.5 Other acquired deformity of back or spine
756.12 Congenital spondylolisthesis
756.15 Congenital fusion of spine (vertebra)
756.19 Other congenital anomaly of spine
805.00 Closed fracture of cervical vertebra, unspecified level without mention of spinal cord injury ▽
805.10 Open fracture of cervical vertebra, unspecified level without mention of spinal cord injury ▽
805.2 Closed fracture of dorsal (thoracic) vertebra without mention of spinal cord injury
805.3 Open fracture of dorsal (thoracic) vertebra without mention of spinal cord injury
805.4 Closed fracture of lumbar vertebra without mention of spinal cord injury
805.5 Open fracture of lumbar vertebra without mention of spinal cord injury
905.1 Late effect of fracture of spine and trunk without mention of spinal cord lesion

ICD-9-CM Procedural

77.29 Wedge osteotomy of other bone, except facial bones
77.39 Other division of other bone, except facial bones

22220–22226

22220 Osteotomy of spine, including diskectomy, anterior approach, single vertebral segment; cervical
22222 thoracic
22224 lumbar
22226 each additional vertebral segment (List separately in addition to code for primary procedure)

ICD-9-CM Diagnostic

237.71 Neurofibromatosis, Type 1 (von Recklinghausen's disease)
720.0 Ankylosing spondylitis
721.7 Traumatic spondylopathy
722.0 Displacement of cervical intervertebral disc without myelopathy
722.10 Displacement of lumbar intervertebral disc without myelopathy
722.11 Displacement of thoracic intervertebral disc without myelopathy
722.4 Degeneration of cervical intervertebral disc
722.51 Degeneration of thoracic or thoracolumbar intervertebral disc
722.52 Degeneration of lumbar or lumbosacral intervertebral disc
722.71 Intervertebral cervical disc disorder with myelopathy, cervical region
722.72 Intervertebral thoracic disc disorder with myelopathy, thoracic region
722.73 Intervertebral lumbar disc disorder with myelopathy, lumbar region
731.0 Osteitis deformans without mention of bone tumor
732.0 Juvenile osteochondrosis of spine
733.13 Pathologic fracture of vertebrae
733.95 Stress fracture of other bone
737.10 Kyphosis (acquired) (postural)
737.11 Kyphosis due to radiation
737.12 Kyphosis, postlaminectomy
737.19 Other kyphosis (acquired)
737.20 Lordosis (acquired) (postural)
737.30 Scoliosis (and kyphoscoliosis), idiopathic
737.41 Kyphosis associated with other condition — (Code first associated condition: 015.0, 138, 237.7, 252.0, 277.5, 356.1, 731.0, 733.00-733.09) ⊠
738.5 Other acquired deformity of back or spine
756.12 Congenital spondylolisthesis
756.15 Congenital fusion of spine (vertebra)
756.19 Other congenital anomaly of spine
905.1 Late effect of fracture of spine and trunk without mention of spinal cord lesion
907.2 Late effect of spinal cord injury

ICD-9-CM Procedural

77.29 Wedge osteotomy of other bone, except facial bones
77.39 Other division of other bone, except facial bones
80.51 Excision of intervertebral disc

22305–22310

22305 Closed treatment of vertebral process fracture(s)
22310 Closed treatment of vertebral body fracture(s), without manipulation, requiring and including casting or bracing

ICD-9-CM Diagnostic

336.9 Unspecified disease of spinal cord
733.00 Unspecified osteoporosis
733.01 Senile osteoporosis
733.02 Idiopathic osteoporosis
733.13 Pathologic fracture of vertebrae
733.95 Stress fracture of other bone
805.01 Closed fracture of first cervical vertebra without mention of spinal cord injury
805.02 Closed fracture of second cervical vertebra without mention of spinal cord injury
805.03 Closed fracture of third cervical vertebra without mention of spinal cord injury
805.04 Closed fracture of fourth cervical vertebra without mention of spinal cord injury
805.05 Closed fracture of fifth cervical vertebra without mention of spinal cord injury
805.06 Closed fracture of sixth cervical vertebra without mention of spinal cord injury
805.07 Closed fracture of seventh cervical vertebra without mention of spinal cord injury
805.08 Closed fracture of multiple cervical vertebrae without mention of spinal cord injury
805.2 Closed fracture of dorsal (thoracic) vertebra without mention of spinal cord injury
805.4 Closed fracture of lumbar vertebra without mention of spinal cord injury
805.6 Closed fracture of sacrum and coccyx without mention of spinal cord injury
806.00 Closed fracture of C1-C4 level with unspecified spinal cord injury
806.01 Closed fracture of C1-C4 level with complete lesion of cord
806.02 Closed fracture of C1-C4 level with anterior cord syndrome
806.03 Closed fracture of C1-C4 level with central cord syndrome
806.04 Closed fracture of C1-C4 level with other specified spinal cord injury
806.05 Closed fracture of C5-C7 level with unspecified spinal cord injury
806.06 Closed fracture of C5-C7 level with complete lesion of cord
806.07 Closed fracture of C5-C7 level with anterior cord syndrome
806.08 Closed fracture of C5-C7 level with central cord syndrome
806.09 Closed fracture of C5-C7 level with other specified spinal cord injury
806.20 Closed fracture of T1-T6 level with unspecified spinal cord injury
806.21 Closed fracture of T1-T6 level with complete lesion of cord
806.22 Closed fracture of T1-T6 level with anterior cord syndrome
806.23 Closed fracture of T1-T6 level with central cord syndrome
806.24 Closed fracture of T1-T6 level with other specified spinal cord injury
806.25 Closed fracture of T7-T12 level with unspecified spinal cord injury
806.26 Closed fracture of T7-T12 level with complete lesion of cord
806.27 Closed fracture of T7-T12 level with anterior cord syndrome
806.28 Closed fracture of T7-T12 level with central cord syndrome
806.29 Closed fracture of T7-T12 level with other specified spinal cord injury
806.4 Closed fracture of lumbar spine with spinal cord injury

ICD-9-CM Procedural

03.53 Repair of vertebral fracture
79.09 Closed reduction of fracture of other specified bone, except facial bones, without internal fixation

HCPCS Level II Supplies & Services

A4580 Cast supplies (e.g., plaster)
L0450 TLSO, flexible, provides trunk support, upper thoracic region, produces intracavitary pressure to reduce load on the intervertebral disks with rigid stays or panel(s), includes shoulder straps and closures, prefabricated, includes fitting and adjustment
L0452 TLSO, flexible, provides trunk support, upper thoracic region, produces intracavitary pressure to reduce load on the intervertebral disks with rigid stays or panel(s), includes shoulder straps and closures, custom fabricated
L0454 TLSO flexible, provides trunk support, extends from sacrococcygeal junction to above t-9 vertebra, restricts gross trunk motion in the sagittal plane, produces intracavitary pressure to reduce load on the intervertebral disks with rigid stays or panel(s), includes shoulder straps and closures, prefabricated, includes fitting and adjustment
L0456 TLSO, flexible, provides trunk support, thoracic region, rigid posterior panel and soft anterior apron, extends from the sacrococcygeal junction and terminates just inferior to the scapular spine, restricts gross trunk motion in the sagittal plane, produces intracavitary pressure to reduce load on the intervertebral disks, includes straps and closures, prefabricated, includes fitting and adjustment

22315

22315 Closed treatment of vertebral fracture(s) and/or dislocation(s) requiring casting or bracing, with and including casting and/or bracing, with or without anesthesia, by manipulation or traction

ICD-9-CM Diagnostic

336.9 Unspecified disease of spinal cord
733.00 Unspecified osteoporosis
733.01 Senile osteoporosis
733.02 Idiopathic osteoporosis
733.13 Pathologic fracture of vertebrae
733.95 Stress fracture of other bone
805.00 Closed fracture of cervical vertebra, unspecified level without mention of spinal cord injury
805.01 Closed fracture of first cervical vertebra without mention of spinal cord injury
805.02 Closed fracture of second cervical vertebra without mention of spinal cord injury
805.03 Closed fracture of third cervical vertebra without mention of spinal cord injury
805.04 Closed fracture of fourth cervical vertebra without mention of spinal cord injury
805.05 Closed fracture of fifth cervical vertebra without mention of spinal cord injury
805.06 Closed fracture of sixth cervical vertebra without mention of spinal cord injury
805.07 Closed fracture of seventh cervical vertebra without mention of spinal cord injury
805.08 Closed fracture of multiple cervical vertebrae without mention of spinal cord injury
805.2 Closed fracture of dorsal (thoracic) vertebra without mention of spinal cord injury
805.4 Closed fracture of lumbar vertebra without mention of spinal cord injury
805.6 Closed fracture of sacrum and coccyx without mention of spinal cord injury
806.00 Closed fracture of C1-C4 level with unspecified spinal cord injury
806.01 Closed fracture of C1-C4 level with complete lesion of cord
806.02 Closed fracture of C1-C4 level with anterior cord syndrome
806.03 Closed fracture of C1-C4 level with central cord syndrome
806.04 Closed fracture of C1-C4 level with other specified spinal cord injury
806.05 Closed fracture of C5-C7 level with unspecified spinal cord injury
806.06 Closed fracture of C5-C7 level with complete lesion of cord
806.07 Closed fracture of C5-C7 level with anterior cord syndrome
806.08 Closed fracture of C5-C7 level with central cord syndrome
806.09 Closed fracture of C5-C7 level with other specified spinal cord injury
806.20 Closed fracture of T1-T6 level with unspecified spinal cord injury
806.21 Closed fracture of T1-T6 level with complete lesion of cord
806.22 Closed fracture of T1-T6 level with anterior cord syndrome
806.23 Closed fracture of T1-T6 level with central cord syndrome
806.24 Closed fracture of T1-T6 level with other specified spinal cord injury
806.25 Closed fracture of T7-T12 level with unspecified spinal cord injury
806.26 Closed fracture of T7-T12 level with complete lesion of cord
806.27 Closed fracture of T7-T12 level with anterior cord syndrome
806.28 Closed fracture of T7-T12 level with central cord syndrome
806.29 Closed fracture of T7-T12 level with other specified spinal cord injury
806.4 Closed fracture of lumbar spine with spinal cord injury
806.60 Closed fracture of sacrum and coccyx with unspecified spinal cord injury
839.01 Closed dislocation, first cervical vertebra
839.02 Closed dislocation, second cervical vertebra
839.03 Closed dislocation, third cervical vertebra
839.04 Closed dislocation, fourth cervical vertebra
839.05 Closed dislocation, fifth cervical vertebra
839.06 Closed dislocation, sixth cervical vertebra
839.07 Closed dislocation, seventh cervical vertebra
839.08 Closed dislocation, multiple cervical vertebrae
839.20 Closed dislocation, lumbar vertebra
839.21 Closed dislocation, thoracic vertebra
839.41 Closed dislocation, coccyx
839.42 Closed dislocation, sacrum
839.49 Closed dislocation, other vertebra

ICD-9-CM Procedural

03.53 Repair of vertebral fracture
79.09 Closed reduction of fracture of other specified bone, except facial bones, without internal fixation

HCPCS Level II Supplies & Services

A4580 Cast supplies (e.g., plaster)
L0450 TLSO, flexible, provides trunk support, upper thoracic region, produces intracavitary pressure to reduce load on the intervertebral disks with rigid stays or panel(s), includes shoulder straps and closures, prefabricated, includes fitting and adjustment

Unspecified code
Female diagnosis
Manifestation code
Male diagnosis

L0452 TLSO, flexible, provides trunk support, upper thoracic region, produces intracavitary pressure to reduce load on the intervertebral disks with rigid stays or panel(s), includes shoulder straps and closures, custom fabricated
L0454 TLSO flexible, provides trunk support, extends from sacrococcygeal junction to above t-9 vertebra, restricts gross trunk motion in the sagittal plane, produces intracavitary pressure to reduce load on the intervertebral disks with rigid stays or panel(s), includes shoulder straps and closures, prefabricated, includes fitting and adjustment
L0456 TLSO, flexible, provides trunk support, thoracic region, rigid posterior panel and soft anterior apron, extends from the sacrococcygeal junction and terminates just inferior to the scapular spine, restricts gross trunk motion in the sagittal plane, produces intracavitary pressure to reduce load on the intervertebral disks, includes straps and closures, prefabricated, includes fitting and adjustment

22318–22319

22318 Open treatment and/or reduction of odontoid fracture(s) and or dislocation(s) (including os odontoideum), anterior approach, including placement of internal fixation; without grafting
22319 with grafting

ICD-9-CM Diagnostic

756.10 Congenital anomaly of spine, unspecified ▽
805.02 Closed fracture of second cervical vertebra without mention of spinal cord injury
805.12 Open fracture of second cervical vertebra without mention of spinal cord injury
806.00 Closed fracture of C1-C4 level with unspecified spinal cord injury ▽
806.01 Closed fracture of C1-C4 level with complete lesion of cord
806.02 Closed fracture of C1-C4 level with anterior cord syndrome
806.03 Closed fracture of C1-C4 level with central cord syndrome
806.04 Closed fracture of C1-C4 level with other specified spinal cord injury
806.10 Open fracture of C1-C4 level with unspecified spinal cord injury ▽
806.11 Open fracture of C1-C4 level with complete lesion of cord
806.12 Open fracture of C1-C4 level with anterior cord syndrome
806.13 Open fracture of C1-C4 level with central cord syndrome
806.14 Open fracture of C1-C4 level with other specified spinal cord injury
839.02 Closed dislocation, second cervical vertebra
839.12 Open dislocation, second cervical vertebra

ICD-9-CM Procedural

03.53 Repair of vertebral fracture
78.09 Bone graft of other bone, except facial bones
78.59 Internal fixation of other bone, except facial bones, without fracture reduction
79.39 Open reduction of fracture of other specified bone, except facial bones, with internal fixation
79.89 Open reduction of dislocation of other specified site, except temporomandibular

22325–22328

22325 Open treatment and/or reduction of vertebral fracture(s) and/or dislocation(s); posterior approach, one fractured vertebrae or dislocated segment; lumbar
22326 cervical
22327 thoracic
22328 each additional fractured vertebrae or dislocated segment (List separately in addition to code for primary procedure)

Spinal Fracture with Instrumentation

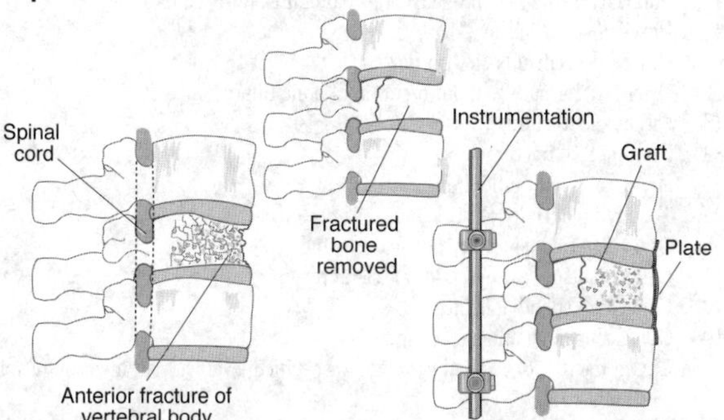

ICD-9-CM Diagnostic

733.13 Pathologic fracture of vertebrae
733.81 Malunion of fracture
733.82 Nonunion of fracture
733.95 Stress fracture of other bone
805.00 Closed fracture of cervical vertebra, unspecified level without mention of spinal cord injury ▽
805.01 Closed fracture of first cervical vertebra without mention of spinal cord injury
805.02 Closed fracture of second cervical vertebra without mention of spinal cord injury
805.03 Closed fracture of third cervical vertebra without mention of spinal cord injury
805.04 Closed fracture of fourth cervical vertebra without mention of spinal cord injury
805.05 Closed fracture of fifth cervical vertebra without mention of spinal cord injury
805.06 Closed fracture of sixth cervical vertebra without mention of spinal cord injury
805.07 Closed fracture of seventh cervical vertebra without mention of spinal cord injury
805.08 Closed fracture of multiple cervical vertebrae without mention of spinal cord injury
805.10 Open fracture of cervical vertebra, unspecified level without mention of spinal cord injury ▽
805.11 Open fracture of first cervical vertebra without mention of spinal cord injury
805.12 Open fracture of second cervical vertebra without mention of spinal cord injury
805.13 Open fracture of third cervical vertebra without mention of spinal cord injury
805.14 Open fracture of fourth cervical vertebra without mention of spinal cord injury
805.15 Open fracture of fifth cervical vertebra without mention of spinal cord injury
805.16 Open fracture of sixth cervical vertebra without mention of spinal cord injury
805.17 Open fracture of seventh cervical vertebra without mention of spinal cord injury
805.18 Open fracture of multiple cervical vertebrae without mention of spinal cord injury
805.2 Closed fracture of dorsal (thoracic) vertebra without mention of spinal cord injury
805.3 Open fracture of dorsal (thoracic) vertebra without mention of spinal cord injury
805.4 Closed fracture of lumbar vertebra without mention of spinal cord injury
805.5 Open fracture of lumbar vertebra without mention of spinal cord injury
806.10 Open fracture of C1-C4 level with unspecified spinal cord injury ▽
806.11 Open fracture of C1-C4 level with complete lesion of cord
806.12 Open fracture of C1-C4 level with anterior cord syndrome
806.13 Open fracture of C1-C4 level with central cord syndrome
806.14 Open fracture of C1-C4 level with other specified spinal cord injury
806.15 Open fracture of C5-C7 level with unspecified spinal cord injury ▽
806.16 Open fracture of C5-C7 level with complete lesion of cord
806.17 Open fracture of C5-C7 level with anterior cord syndrome
806.18 Open fracture of C5-C7 level with central cord syndrome
806.19 Open fracture of C5-C7 level with other specified spinal cord injury
806.20 Closed fracture of T1-T6 level with unspecified spinal cord injury ▽
806.21 Closed fracture of T1-T6 level with complete lesion of cord
806.22 Closed fracture of T1-T6 level with anterior cord syndrome
806.23 Closed fracture of T1-T6 level with central cord syndrome
806.24 Closed fracture of T1-T6 level with other specified spinal cord injury
806.25 Closed fracture of T7-T12 level with unspecified spinal cord injury ▽
806.26 Closed fracture of T7-T12 level with complete lesion of cord
806.27 Closed fracture of T7-T12 level with anterior cord syndrome
806.28 Closed fracture of T7-T12 level with central cord syndrome
806.29 Closed fracture of T7-T12 level with other specified spinal cord injury
806.30 Open fracture of T1-T6 level with unspecified spinal cord injury ▽
806.31 Open fracture of T1-T6 level with complete lesion of cord
806.32 Open fracture of T1-T6 level with anterior cord syndrome
806.33 Open fracture of T1-T6 level with central cord syndrome
806.34 Open fracture of T1-T6 level with other specified spinal cord injury
806.35 Open fracture of T7-T12 level with unspecified spinal cord injury ▽
806.36 Open fracture of T7-T12 level with complete lesion of cord
806.37 Open fracture of T7-T12 level with anterior cord syndrome
806.38 Open fracture of T7-T12 level with central cord syndrome
806.39 Open fracture of T7-T12 level with other specified spinal cord injury
806.4 Closed fracture of lumbar spine with spinal cord injury
806.5 Open fracture of lumbar spine with spinal cord injury
839.00 Closed dislocation, unspecified cervical vertebra ▽
839.01 Closed dislocation, first cervical vertebra
839.02 Closed dislocation, second cervical vertebra
839.03 Closed dislocation, third cervical vertebra
839.04 Closed dislocation, fourth cervical vertebra
839.05 Closed dislocation, fifth cervical vertebra
839.06 Closed dislocation, sixth cervical vertebra

839.07 Closed dislocation, seventh cervical vertebra
839.08 Closed dislocation, multiple cervical vertebrae
839.10 Open dislocation, unspecified cervical vertebra ▽
839.11 Open dislocation, first cervical vertebra
839.12 Open dislocation, second cervical vertebra
839.13 Open dislocation, third cervical vertebra
839.14 Open dislocation, fourth cervical vertebra
839.15 Open dislocation, fifth cervical vertebra
839.16 Open dislocation, sixth cervical vertebra
839.17 Open dislocation, seventh cervical vertebra
839.18 Open dislocation, multiple cervical vertebrae
839.20 Closed dislocation, lumbar vertebra
839.21 Closed dislocation, thoracic vertebra
839.30 Open dislocation, lumbar vertebra
839.31 Open dislocation, thoracic vertebra

ICD-9-CM Procedural

03.53 Repair of vertebral fracture
79.29 Open reduction of fracture of other specified bone, except facial bones, without internal fixation

22505

22505 Manipulation of spine requiring anesthesia, any region

ICD-9-CM Diagnostic

720.2 Sacroiliitis, not elsewhere classified
722.10 Displacement of lumbar intervertebral disc without myelopathy
722.2 Displacement of intervertebral disc, site unspecified, without myelopathy ▽
722.52 Degeneration of lumbar or lumbosacral intervertebral disc
722.93 Other and unspecified disc disorder of lumbar region
723.5 Torticollis, unspecified ▽
724.00 Spinal stenosis, unspecified region other than cervical ▽
724.2 Lumbago
724.3 Sciatica
728.85 Spasm of muscle
729.2 Unspecified neuralgia, neuritis, and radiculitis ▽
739.4 Nonallopathic lesion of sacral region, not elsewhere classified
781.93 Ocular torticollis
839.00 Closed dislocation, unspecified cervical vertebra ▽
839.01 Closed dislocation, first cervical vertebra
839.02 Closed dislocation, second cervical vertebra
839.03 Closed dislocation, third cervical vertebra
839.04 Closed dislocation, fourth cervical vertebra
839.05 Closed dislocation, fifth cervical vertebra
839.06 Closed dislocation, sixth cervical vertebra
839.07 Closed dislocation, seventh cervical vertebra
839.08 Closed dislocation, multiple cervical vertebrae
839.20 Closed dislocation, lumbar vertebra
839.21 Closed dislocation, thoracic vertebra
839.40 Closed dislocation, vertebra, unspecified site ▽
839.41 Closed dislocation, coccyx
839.42 Closed dislocation, sacrum
839.49 Closed dislocation, other vertebra
847.0 Neck sprain and strain
953.0 Injury to cervical nerve root
956.0 Injury to sciatic nerve
996.4 Mechanical complication of internal orthopedic device, implant, and graft

ICD-9-CM Procedural

93.29 Other forcible correction of musculoskeletal deformity

22520–22522

22520 Percutaneous vertebroplasty, one vertebral body, unilateral or bilateral injection; thoracic
22521 lumbar
22522 each additional thoracic or lumbar vertebral body (List separately in addition to code for primary procedure)

ICD-9-CM Diagnostic

170.2 Malignant neoplasm of vertebral column, excluding sacrum and coccyx
198.5 Secondary malignant neoplasm of bone and bone marrow
203.00 Multiple myeloma without mention of remission
203.01 Multiple myeloma in remission
213.2 Benign neoplasm of vertebral column, excluding sacrum and coccyx
238.0 Neoplasm of uncertain behavior of bone and articular cartilage
238.6 Neoplasm of uncertain behavior of plasma cells
239.2 Neoplasms of unspecified nature of bone, soft tissue, and skin
731.0 Osteitis deformans without mention of bone tumor
733.00 Unspecified osteoporosis ▽
733.01 Senile osteoporosis
733.02 Idiopathic osteoporosis
733.03 Disuse osteoporosis
733.09 Other osteoporosis — (Use additional E code to identify drug)
733.13 Pathologic fracture of vertebrae
733.7 Algoneurodystrophy
733.95 Stress fracture of other bone
805.2 Closed fracture of dorsal (thoracic) vertebra without mention of spinal cord injury
805.4 Closed fracture of lumbar vertebra without mention of spinal cord injury

ICD-9-CM Procedural

81.65 Vertebroplasty

22532–22534

22532 Arthrodesis, lateral extracavitary technique, including minimal diskectomy to prepare interspace (other than for decompression); thoracic
22533 lumbar
22534 thoracic or lumbar, each additional vertebral segment (List separately in addition to code for primary procedure)

ICD-9-CM Diagnostic

170.2 Malignant neoplasm of vertebral column, excluding sacrum and coccyx
198.5 Secondary malignant neoplasm of bone and bone marrow
213.2 Benign neoplasm of vertebral column, excluding sacrum and coccyx
238.0 Neoplasm of uncertain behavior of bone and articular cartilage
336.9 Unspecified disease of spinal cord ▽
721.0 Cervical spondylosis without myelopathy
721.1 Cervical spondylosis with myelopathy
721.2 Thoracic spondylosis without myelopathy
721.3 Lumbosacral spondylosis without myelopathy
721.41 Spondylosis with myelopathy, thoracic region
721.42 Spondylosis with myelopathy, lumbar region
721.8 Other allied disorders of spine
722.0 Displacement of cervical intervertebral disc without myelopathy
722.10 Displacement of lumbar intervertebral disc without myelopathy
722.11 Displacement of thoracic intervertebral disc without myelopathy
722.31 Schmorl's nodes, thoracic region
722.4 Degeneration of cervical intervertebral disc
722.51 Degeneration of thoracic or thoracolumbar intervertebral disc
722.52 Degeneration of lumbar or lumbosacral intervertebral disc
722.71 Intervertebral cervical disc disorder with myelopathy, cervical region
722.72 Intervertebral thoracic disc disorder with myelopathy, thoracic region
722.73 Intervertebral lumbar disc disorder with myelopathy, lumbar region
722.81 Postlaminectomy syndrome, cervical region
722.82 Postlaminectomy syndrome, thoracic region
722.83 Postlaminectomy syndrome, lumbar region
722.91 Other and unspecified disc disorder of cervical region
722.92 Other and unspecified disc disorder of thoracic region
722.93 Other and unspecified disc disorder of lumbar region
723.0 Spinal stenosis in cervical region
724.01 Spinal stenosis of thoracic region
724.02 Spinal stenosis of lumbar region
724.2 Lumbago
724.3 Sciatica
724.4 Thoracic or lumbosacral neuritis or radiculitis, unspecified ▽
724.5 Unspecified backache ▽
724.9 Other unspecified back disorder
731.0 Osteitis deformans without mention of bone tumor
733.13 Pathologic fracture of vertebrae
733.82 Nonunion of fracture
733.95 Stress fracture of other bone
738.2 Acquired deformity of neck
738.5 Other acquired deformity of back or spine
756.11 Congenital spondylolysis, lumbosacral region
756.12 Congenital spondylolisthesis
756.19 Other congenital anomaly of spine
805.00 Closed fracture of cervical vertebra, unspecified level without mention of spinal cord injury ▽
805.03 Closed fracture of third cervical vertebra without mention of spinal cord injury
805.04 Closed fracture of fourth cervical vertebra without mention of spinal cord injury
805.05 Closed fracture of fifth cervical vertebra without mention of spinal cord injury

805.06 Closed fracture of sixth cervical vertebra without mention of spinal cord injury
805.07 Closed fracture of seventh cervical vertebra without mention of spinal cord injury
805.08 Closed fracture of multiple cervical vertebrae without mention of spinal cord injury
805.10 Open fracture of cervical vertebra, unspecified level without mention of spinal cord injury ▽
805.13 Open fracture of third cervical vertebra without mention of spinal cord injury
805.14 Open fracture of fourth cervical vertebra without mention of spinal cord injury
805.15 Open fracture of fifth cervical vertebra without mention of spinal cord injury
805.16 Open fracture of sixth cervical vertebra without mention of spinal cord injury
805.17 Open fracture of seventh cervical vertebra without mention of spinal cord injury
805.18 Open fracture of multiple cervical vertebrae without mention of spinal cord injury
805.2 Closed fracture of dorsal (thoracic) vertebra without mention of spinal cord injury
805.3 Open fracture of dorsal (thoracic) vertebra without mention of spinal cord injury
805.4 Closed fracture of lumbar vertebra without mention of spinal cord injury
805.5 Open fracture of lumbar vertebra without mention of spinal cord injury
806.00 Closed fracture of C1-C4 level with unspecified spinal cord injury ▽
806.01 Closed fracture of C1-C4 level with complete lesion of cord
806.02 Closed fracture of C1-C4 level with anterior cord syndrome
806.03 Closed fracture of C1-C4 level with central cord syndrome
806.04 Closed fracture of C1-C4 level with other specified spinal cord injury
806.05 Closed fracture of C5-C7 level with unspecified spinal cord injury ▽
806.06 Closed fracture of C5-C7 level with complete lesion of cord
806.07 Closed fracture of C5-C7 level with anterior cord syndrome
806.08 Closed fracture of C5-C7 level with central cord syndrome
806.09 Closed fracture of C5-C7 level with other specified spinal cord injury
806.10 Open fracture of C1-C4 level with unspecified spinal cord injury ▽
806.11 Open fracture of C1-C4 level with complete lesion of cord
806.12 Open fracture of C1-C4 level with anterior cord syndrome
806.13 Open fracture of C1-C4 level with central cord syndrome
806.14 Open fracture of C1-C4 level with other specified spinal cord injury
806.15 Open fracture of C5-C7 level with unspecified spinal cord injury ▽
806.16 Open fracture of C5-C7 level with complete lesion of cord
806.17 Open fracture of C5-C7 level with anterior cord syndrome
806.18 Open fracture of C5-C7 level with central cord syndrome
806.19 Open fracture of C5-C7 level with other specified spinal cord injury
806.20 Closed fracture of T1-T6 level with unspecified spinal cord injury ▽
806.21 Closed fracture of T1-T6 level with complete lesion of cord
806.22 Closed fracture of T1-T6 level with anterior cord syndrome
806.23 Closed fracture of T1-T6 level with central cord syndrome
806.24 Closed fracture of T1-T6 level with other specified spinal cord injury
806.25 Closed fracture of T7-T12 level with unspecified spinal cord injury ▽
806.26 Closed fracture of T7-T12 level with complete lesion of cord
806.27 Closed fracture of T7-T12 level with anterior cord syndrome
806.28 Closed fracture of T7-T12 level with central cord syndrome
806.29 Closed fracture of T7-T12 level with other specified spinal cord injury
806.30 Open fracture of T1-T6 level with unspecified spinal cord injury ▽
806.31 Open fracture of T1-T6 level with complete lesion of cord
806.32 Open fracture of T1-T6 level with anterior cord syndrome
806.33 Open fracture of T1-T6 level with central cord syndrome
806.34 Open fracture of T1-T6 level with other specified spinal cord injury
806.35 Open fracture of T7-T12 level with unspecified spinal cord injury ▽
806.36 Open fracture of T7-T12 level with complete lesion of cord
806.37 Open fracture of T7-T12 level with anterior cord syndrome
806.38 Open fracture of T7-T12 level with central cord syndrome
806.39 Open fracture of T7-T12 level with other specified spinal cord injury
806.4 Closed fracture of lumbar spine with spinal cord injury
806.5 Open fracture of lumbar spine with spinal cord injury
839.03 Closed dislocation, third cervical vertebra
839.04 Closed dislocation, fourth cervical vertebra
839.05 Closed dislocation, fifth cervical vertebra
839.06 Closed dislocation, sixth cervical vertebra
839.07 Closed dislocation, seventh cervical vertebra
839.08 Closed dislocation, multiple cervical vertebrae
839.13 Open dislocation, third cervical vertebra
839.14 Open dislocation, fourth cervical vertebra
839.15 Open dislocation, fifth cervical vertebra
839.16 Open dislocation, sixth cervical vertebra
839.17 Open dislocation, seventh cervical vertebra
839.18 Open dislocation, multiple cervical vertebrae
839.20 Closed dislocation, lumbar vertebra
839.21 Closed dislocation, thoracic vertebra
839.30 Open dislocation, lumbar vertebra
839.31 Open dislocation, thoracic vertebra
996.4 Mechanical complication of internal orthopedic device, implant, and graft

ICD-9-CM Procedural

81.00 Spinal fusion, not otherwise specified

22548

22548 Arthrodesis, anterior transoral or extraoral technique, clivus-C1-C2 (atlas-axis), with or without excision of odontoid process

ICD-9-CM Diagnostic

170.2 Malignant neoplasm of vertebral column, excluding sacrum and coccyx
198.5 Secondary malignant neoplasm of bone and bone marrow
213.2 Benign neoplasm of vertebral column, excluding sacrum and coccyx
238.0 Neoplasm of uncertain behavior of bone and articular cartilage
721.1 Cervical spondylosis with myelopathy
721.8 Other allied disorders of spine
723.2 Cervicocranial syndrome
723.3 Cervicobrachial syndrome (diffuse)
738.5 Other acquired deformity of back or spine
805.01 Closed fracture of first cervical vertebra without mention of spinal cord injury
805.02 Closed fracture of second cervical vertebra without mention of spinal cord injury
805.08 Closed fracture of multiple cervical vertebrae without mention of spinal cord injury
805.11 Open fracture of first cervical vertebra without mention of spinal cord injury
805.12 Open fracture of second cervical vertebra without mention of spinal cord injury
806.00 Closed fracture of C1-C4 level with unspecified spinal cord injury ▽
806.01 Closed fracture of C1-C4 level with complete lesion of cord
806.02 Closed fracture of C1-C4 level with anterior cord syndrome
806.03 Closed fracture of C1-C4 level with central cord syndrome
806.04 Closed fracture of C1-C4 level with other specified spinal cord injury
806.10 Open fracture of C1-C4 level with unspecified spinal cord injury ▽
806.11 Open fracture of C1-C4 level with complete lesion of cord
806.12 Open fracture of C1-C4 level with anterior cord syndrome
806.13 Open fracture of C1-C4 level with central cord syndrome
806.14 Open fracture of C1-C4 level with other specified spinal cord injury

ICD-9-CM Procedural

81.01 Atlas-axis spinal fusion
81.31 Refusion of Atlas-axis spine
81.62 Fusion or refusion of 2-3 vertebrae

22554–22585

22554 Arthrodesis, anterior interbody technique, including minimal diskectomy to prepare interspace (other than for decompression); cervical below C2
22556 thoracic
22558 lumbar
22585 each additional interspace (List separately in addition to code for primary procedure)

ICD-9-CM Diagnostic

170.2 Malignant neoplasm of vertebral column, excluding sacrum and coccyx
198.5 Secondary malignant neoplasm of bone and bone marrow
213.2 Benign neoplasm of vertebral column, excluding sacrum and coccyx
238.0 Neoplasm of uncertain behavior of bone and articular cartilage
336.9 Unspecified disease of spinal cord ▽
721.0 Cervical spondylosis without myelopathy
721.1 Cervical spondylosis with myelopathy
721.2 Thoracic spondylosis without myelopathy
721.3 Lumbosacral spondylosis without myelopathy
721.41 Spondylosis with myelopathy, thoracic region
721.42 Spondylosis with myelopathy, lumbar region
721.8 Other allied disorders of spine
722.0 Displacement of cervical intervertebral disc without myelopathy
722.10 Displacement of lumbar intervertebral disc without myelopathy
722.11 Displacement of thoracic intervertebral disc without myelopathy
722.31 Schmorl's nodes, thoracic region
722.4 Degeneration of cervical intervertebral disc
722.51 Degeneration of thoracic or thoracolumbar intervertebral disc
722.52 Degeneration of lumbar or lumbosacral intervertebral disc
722.71 Intervertebral cervical disc disorder with myelopathy, cervical region
722.72 Intervertebral thoracic disc disorder with myelopathy, thoracic region
722.73 Intervertebral lumbar disc disorder with myelopathy, lumbar region

722.81 Postlaminectomy syndrome, cervical region

722.82 Postlaminectomy syndrome, thoracic region

722.83 Postlaminectomy syndrome, lumbar region

722.91 Other and unspecified disc disorder of cervical region

722.92 Other and unspecified disc disorder of thoracic region

722.93 Other and unspecified disc disorder of lumbar region

723.0 Spinal stenosis in cervical region

724.01 Spinal stenosis of thoracic region

724.02 Spinal stenosis of lumbar region

724.2 Lumbago

724.3 Sciatica

724.4 Thoracic or lumbosacral neuritis or radiculitis, unspecified ▽

724.5 Unspecified backache ▽

724.9 Other unspecified back disorder

731.0 Osteitis deformans without mention of bone tumor

733.13 Pathologic fracture of vertebrae

733.82 Nonunion of fracture

733.95 Stress fracture of other bone

738.2 Acquired deformity of neck

738.5 Other acquired deformity of back or spine

756.11 Congenital spondylolysis, lumbosacral region

756.12 Congenital spondylolisthesis

756.19 Other congenital anomaly of spine

805.00 Closed fracture of cervical vertebra, unspecified level without mention of spinal cord injury ▽

805.03 Closed fracture of third cervical vertebra without mention of spinal cord injury

805.04 Closed fracture of fourth cervical vertebra without mention of spinal cord injury

805.05 Closed fracture of fifth cervical vertebra without mention of spinal cord injury

805.06 Closed fracture of sixth cervical vertebra without mention of spinal cord injury

805.07 Closed fracture of seventh cervical vertebra without mention of spinal cord injury

805.08 Closed fracture of multiple cervical vertebrae without mention of spinal cord injury

805.10 Open fracture of cervical vertebra, unspecified level without mention of spinal cord injury ▽

805.13 Open fracture of third cervical vertebra without mention of spinal cord injury

805.14 Open fracture of fourth cervical vertebra without mention of spinal cord injury

805.15 Open fracture of fifth cervical vertebra without mention of spinal cord injury

805.16 Open fracture of sixth cervical vertebra without mention of spinal cord injury

805.17 Open fracture of seventh cervical vertebra without mention of spinal cord injury

805.18 Open fracture of multiple cervical vertebrae without mention of spinal cord injury

805.2 Closed fracture of dorsal (thoracic) vertebra without mention of spinal cord injury

805.3 Open fracture of dorsal (thoracic) vertebra without mention of spinal cord injury

805.4 Closed fracture of lumbar vertebra without mention of spinal cord injury

805.5 Open fracture of lumbar vertebra without mention of spinal cord injury

806.00 Closed fracture of C1-C4 level with unspecified spinal cord injury ▽

806.01 Closed fracture of C1-C4 level with complete lesion of cord

806.02 Closed fracture of C1-C4 level with anterior cord syndrome

806.03 Closed fracture of C1-C4 level with central cord syndrome

806.04 Closed fracture of C1-C4 level with other specified spinal cord injury

806.05 Closed fracture of C5-C7 level with unspecified spinal cord injury ▽

806.06 Closed fracture of C5-C7 level with complete lesion of cord

806.07 Closed fracture of C5-C7 level with anterior cord syndrome

806.08 Closed fracture of C5-C7 level with central cord syndrome

806.09 Closed fracture of C5-C7 level with other specified spinal cord injury

806.10 Open fracture of C1-C4 level with unspecified spinal cord injury ▽

806.11 Open fracture of C1-C4 level with complete lesion of cord

806.12 Open fracture of C1-C4 level with anterior cord syndrome

806.13 Open fracture of C1-C4 level with central cord syndrome

806.14 Open fracture of C1-C4 level with other specified spinal cord injury

806.15 Open fracture of C5-C7 level with unspecified spinal cord injury ▽

806.16 Open fracture of C5-C7 level with complete lesion of cord

806.17 Open fracture of C5-C7 level with anterior cord syndrome

806.18 Open fracture of C5-C7 level with central cord syndrome

806.19 Open fracture of C5-C7 level with other specified spinal cord injury

806.20 Closed fracture of T1-T6 level with unspecified spinal cord injury ▽

806.21 Closed fracture of T1-T6 level with complete lesion of cord

806.22 Closed fracture of T1-T6 level with anterior cord syndrome

806.23 Closed fracture of T1-T6 level with central cord syndrome

806.24 Closed fracture of T1-T6 level with other specified spinal cord injury

806.25 Closed fracture of T7-T12 level with unspecified spinal cord injury ▽

806.26 Closed fracture of T7-T12 level with complete lesion of cord

806.27 Closed fracture of T7-T12 level with anterior cord syndrome

806.28 Closed fracture of T7-T12 level with central cord syndrome

806.29 Closed fracture of T7-T12 level with other specified spinal cord injury

806.30 Open fracture of T1-T6 level with unspecified spinal cord injury ▽

806.31 Open fracture of T1-T6 level with complete lesion of cord

806.32 Open fracture of T1-T6 level with anterior cord syndrome

806.33 Open fracture of T1-T6 level with central cord syndrome

806.34 Open fracture of T1-T6 level with other specified spinal cord injury

806.35 Open fracture of T7-T12 level with unspecified spinal cord injury ▽

806.36 Open fracture of T7-T12 level with complete lesion of cord

806.37 Open fracture of T7-T12 level with anterior cord syndrome

806.38 Open fracture of T7-T12 level with central cord syndrome

806.39 Open fracture of T7-T12 level with other specified spinal cord injury

806.4 Closed fracture of lumbar spine with spinal cord injury

806.5 Open fracture of lumbar spine with spinal cord injury

839.03 Closed dislocation, third cervical vertebra

839.04 Closed dislocation, fourth cervical vertebra

839.05 Closed dislocation, fifth cervical vertebra

839.06 Closed dislocation, sixth cervical vertebra

839.07 Closed dislocation, seventh cervical vertebra

839.08 Closed dislocation, multiple cervical vertebrae

839.13 Open dislocation, third cervical vertebra

839.14 Open dislocation, fourth cervical vertebra

839.15 Open dislocation, fifth cervical vertebra

839.16 Open dislocation, sixth cervical vertebra

839.17 Open dislocation, seventh cervical vertebra

839.18 Open dislocation, multiple cervical vertebrae

839.20 Closed dislocation, lumbar vertebra

839.21 Closed dislocation, thoracic vertebra

839.30 Open dislocation, lumbar vertebra

839.31 Open dislocation, thoracic vertebra

996.4 Mechanical complication of internal orthopedic device, implant, and graft

ICD-9-CM Procedural

81.00 Spinal fusion, not otherwise specified

81.02 Other cervical fusion, anterior technique

81.04 Dorsal and dorsolumbar fusion, anterior technique

81.06 Lumbar and lumbosacral fusion, anterior technique

81.32 Refusion of other cervical spine, anterior technique

81.34 Refusion of dorsal and dorsolumbar spine, anterior technique

81.36 Refusion of lumbar and lumbosacral spine, anterior technique

81.62 Fusion or refusion of 2-3 vertebrae

81.63 Fusion or refusion of 4-8 vertebrae

81.64 Fusion or refusion of 9 or more vertebrae

22590

22590 Arthrodesis, posterior technique, craniocervical (occiput-C2)

ICD-9-CM Diagnostic

170.2 Malignant neoplasm of vertebral column, excluding sacrum and coccyx

198.5 Secondary malignant neoplasm of bone and bone marrow

213.2 Benign neoplasm of vertebral column, excluding sacrum and coccyx

238.0 Neoplasm of uncertain behavior of bone and articular cartilage

721.1 Cervical spondylosis with myelopathy

721.8 Other allied disorders of spine

723.2 Cervicocranial syndrome

723.3 Cervicobrachial syndrome (diffuse)

733.81 Malunion of fracture

733.82 Nonunion of fracture

738.5 Other acquired deformity of back or spine

756.12 Congenital spondylolisthesis

805.01 Closed fracture of first cervical vertebra without mention of spinal cord injury

805.02 Closed fracture of second cervical vertebra without mention of spinal cord injury

805.11 Open fracture of first cervical vertebra without mention of spinal cord injury

805.12 Open fracture of second cervical vertebra without mention of spinal cord injury

806.00 Closed fracture of C1-C4 level with unspecified spinal cord injury ▽

806.01 Closed fracture of C1-C4 level with complete lesion of cord

806.02 Closed fracture of C1-C4 level with anterior cord syndrome

806.03 Closed fracture of C1-C4 level with central cord syndrome

806.04 Closed fracture of C1-C4 level with other specified spinal cord injury

806.10 Open fracture of C1-C4 level with unspecified spinal cord injury ▽

806.11 Open fracture of C1-C4 level with complete lesion of cord

806.12 Open fracture of C1-C4 level with anterior cord syndrome

806.13 Open fracture of C1-C4 level with central cord syndrome

▽ Unspecified code ☒ Manifestation code
♀ Female diagnosis ♂ Male diagnosis

806.14 Open fracture of C1-C4 level with other specified spinal cord injury
839.01 Closed dislocation, first cervical vertebra
839.02 Closed dislocation, second cervical vertebra
839.11 Open dislocation, first cervical vertebra
839.12 Open dislocation, second cervical vertebra

ICD-9-CM Procedural

81.01 Atlas-axis spinal fusion
81.03 Other cervical fusion, posterior technique
81.31 Refusion of Atlas-axis spine
81.33 Refusion of other cervical spine, posterior technique
81.62 Fusion or refusion of 2-3 vertebrae

22595

22595 Arthrodesis, posterior technique, atlas-axis (C1-C2)

ICD-9-CM Diagnostic

170.2 Malignant neoplasm of vertebral column, excluding sacrum and coccyx
198.5 Secondary malignant neoplasm of bone and bone marrow
213.2 Benign neoplasm of vertebral column, excluding sacrum and coccyx
238.0 Neoplasm of uncertain behavior of bone and articular cartilage
721.8 Other allied disorders of spine
723.0 Spinal stenosis in cervical region
723.1 Cervicalgia
723.2 Cervicocranial syndrome
723.4 Brachial neuritis or radiculitis nos
733.13 Pathologic fracture of vertebrae
733.81 Malunion of fracture
733.82 Nonunion of fracture
733.95 Stress fracture of other bone
756.12 Congenital spondylolisthesis
756.19 Other congenital anomaly of spine
805.01 Closed fracture of first cervical vertebra without mention of spinal cord injury
805.02 Closed fracture of second cervical vertebra without mention of spinal cord injury
805.11 Open fracture of first cervical vertebra without mention of spinal cord injury
805.12 Open fracture of second cervical vertebra without mention of spinal cord injury
806.00 Closed fracture of C1-C4 level with unspecified spinal cord injury ▽
806.01 Closed fracture of C1-C4 level with complete lesion of cord
806.02 Closed fracture of C1-C4 level with anterior cord syndrome
806.03 Closed fracture of C1-C4 level with central cord syndrome
806.04 Closed fracture of C1-C4 level with other specified spinal cord injury
806.10 Open fracture of C1-C4 level with unspecified spinal cord injury ▽
806.11 Open fracture of C1-C4 level with complete lesion of cord
806.12 Open fracture of C1-C4 level with anterior cord syndrome
806.13 Open fracture of C1-C4 level with central cord syndrome
806.14 Open fracture of C1-C4 level with other specified spinal cord injury
839.01 Closed dislocation, first cervical vertebra
839.02 Closed dislocation, second cervical vertebra
839.11 Open dislocation, first cervical vertebra
839.12 Open dislocation, second cervical vertebra

ICD-9-CM Procedural

81.01 Atlas-axis spinal fusion
81.31 Refusion of Atlas-axis spine
81.62 Fusion or refusion of 2-3 vertebrae

22600–22614

22600 Arthrodesis, posterior or posterolateral technique, single level; cervical below C2 segment
22610 thoracic (with or without lateral transverse technique)
22612 lumbar (with or without lateral transverse technique)
22614 each additional vertebral segment (List separately in addition to code for primary procedure)

ICD-9-CM Diagnostic

170.2 Malignant neoplasm of vertebral column, excluding sacrum and coccyx
198.5 Secondary malignant neoplasm of bone and bone marrow
213.2 Benign neoplasm of vertebral column, excluding sacrum and coccyx
238.0 Neoplasm of uncertain behavior of bone and articular cartilage
336.9 Unspecified disease of spinal cord ▽
721.0 Cervical spondylosis without myelopathy
721.1 Cervical spondylosis with myelopathy
721.2 Thoracic spondylosis without myelopathy
721.3 Lumbosacral spondylosis without myelopathy
721.41 Spondylosis with myelopathy, thoracic region
721.42 Spondylosis with myelopathy, lumbar region
721.8 Other allied disorders of spine
722.0 Displacement of cervical intervertebral disc without myelopathy
722.10 Displacement of lumbar intervertebral disc without myelopathy
722.11 Displacement of thoracic intervertebral disc without myelopathy
722.31 Schmorl's nodes, thoracic region
722.4 Degeneration of cervical intervertebral disc
722.51 Degeneration of thoracic or thoracolumbar intervertebral disc
722.52 Degeneration of lumbar or lumbosacral intervertebral disc
722.71 Intervertebral cervical disc disorder with myelopathy, cervical region
722.72 Intervertebral thoracic disc disorder with myelopathy, thoracic region
722.73 Intervertebral lumbar disc disorder with myelopathy, lumbar region
722.81 Postlaminectomy syndrome, cervical region
722.82 Postlaminectomy syndrome, thoracic region
722.83 Postlaminectomy syndrome, lumbar region
722.91 Other and unspecified disc disorder of cervical region
722.92 Other and unspecified disc disorder of thoracic region
722.93 Other and unspecified disc disorder of lumbar region
723.0 Spinal stenosis in cervical region
724.01 Spinal stenosis of thoracic region
724.02 Spinal stenosis of lumbar region
724.2 Lumbago
724.3 Sciatica
724.4 Thoracic or lumbosacral neuritis or radiculitis, unspecified ▽
724.9 Other unspecified back disorder
731.0 Osteitis deformans without mention of bone tumor
733.13 Pathologic fracture of vertebrae
733.82 Nonunion of fracture
733.95 Stress fracture of other bone
738.2 Acquired deformity of neck
738.5 Other acquired deformity of back or spine
756.11 Congenital spondylolysis, lumbosacral region
756.12 Congenital spondylolisthesis
756.19 Other congenital anomaly of spine
805.00 Closed fracture of cervical vertebra, unspecified level without mention of spinal cord injury ▽
805.03 Closed fracture of third cervical vertebra without mention of spinal cord injury
805.04 Closed fracture of fourth cervical vertebra without mention of spinal cord injury
805.05 Closed fracture of fifth cervical vertebra without mention of spinal cord injury
805.06 Closed fracture of sixth cervical vertebra without mention of spinal cord injury
805.07 Closed fracture of seventh cervical vertebra without mention of spinal cord injury
805.08 Closed fracture of multiple cervical vertebrae without mention of spinal cord injury
805.10 Open fracture of cervical vertebra, unspecified level without mention of spinal cord injury ▽
805.13 Open fracture of third cervical vertebra without mention of spinal cord injury
805.14 Open fracture of fourth cervical vertebra without mention of spinal cord injury
805.15 Open fracture of fifth cervical vertebra without mention of spinal cord injury
805.16 Open fracture of sixth cervical vertebra without mention of spinal cord injury
805.17 Open fracture of seventh cervical vertebra without mention of spinal cord injury
805.18 Open fracture of multiple cervical vertebrae without mention of spinal cord injury
805.2 Closed fracture of dorsal (thoracic) vertebra without mention of spinal cord injury
805.3 Open fracture of dorsal (thoracic) vertebra without mention of spinal cord injury
805.4 Closed fracture of lumbar vertebra without mention of spinal cord injury
805.5 Open fracture of lumbar vertebra without mention of spinal cord injury
806.00 Closed fracture of C1-C4 level with unspecified spinal cord injury ▽
806.01 Closed fracture of C1-C4 level with complete lesion of cord
806.02 Closed fracture of C1-C4 level with anterior cord syndrome
806.03 Closed fracture of C1-C4 level with central cord syndrome
806.04 Closed fracture of C1-C4 level with other specified spinal cord injury
806.05 Closed fracture of C5-C7 level with unspecified spinal cord injury ▽
806.06 Closed fracture of C5-C7 level with complete lesion of cord
806.07 Closed fracture of C5-C7 level with anterior cord syndrome
806.08 Closed fracture of C5-C7 level with central cord syndrome
806.09 Closed fracture of C5-C7 level with other specified spinal cord injury
806.10 Open fracture of C1-C4 level with unspecified spinal cord injury ▽
806.11 Open fracture of C1-C4 level with complete lesion of cord
806.12 Open fracture of C1-C4 level with anterior cord syndrome
806.13 Open fracture of C1-C4 level with central cord syndrome
806.14 Open fracture of C1-C4 level with other specified spinal cord injury

▽ Unspecified code
♀ Female diagnosis
☒ Manifestation code
♂ Male diagnosis

806.15 Open fracture of C5-C7 level with unspecified spinal cord injury ▽
806.16 Open fracture of C5-C7 level with complete lesion of cord
806.17 Open fracture of C5-C7 level with anterior cord syndrome
806.18 Open fracture of C5-C7 level with central cord syndrome
806.19 Open fracture of C5-C7 level with other specified spinal cord injury
806.20 Closed fracture of T1-T6 level with unspecified spinal cord injury ▽
806.21 Closed fracture of T1-T6 level with complete lesion of cord
806.22 Closed fracture of T1-T6 level with anterior cord syndrome
806.23 Closed fracture of T1-T6 level with central cord syndrome
806.24 Closed fracture of T1-T6 level with other specified spinal cord injury
806.25 Closed fracture of T7-T12 level with unspecified spinal cord injury ▽
806.26 Closed fracture of T7-T12 level with complete lesion of cord
806.27 Closed fracture of T7-T12 level with anterior cord syndrome
806.28 Closed fracture of T7-T12 level with central cord syndrome
806.29 Closed fracture of T7-T12 level with other specified spinal cord injury
806.30 Open fracture of T1-T6 level with unspecified spinal cord injury ▽
806.31 Open fracture of T1-T6 level with complete lesion of cord
806.32 Open fracture of T1-T6 level with anterior cord syndrome
806.33 Open fracture of T1-T6 level with central cord syndrome
806.34 Open fracture of T1-T6 level with other specified spinal cord injury
806.35 Open fracture of T7-T12 level with unspecified spinal cord injury ▽
806.36 Open fracture of T7-T12 level with complete lesion of cord
806.37 Open fracture of T7-T12 level with anterior cord syndrome
806.38 Open fracture of T7-T12 level with central cord syndrome
806.39 Open fracture of T7-T12 level with other specified spinal cord injury
806.4 Closed fracture of lumbar spine with spinal cord injury
806.5 Open fracture of lumbar spine with spinal cord injury
839.03 Closed dislocation, third cervical vertebra
839.04 Closed dislocation, fourth cervical vertebra
839.05 Closed dislocation, fifth cervical vertebra
839.06 Closed dislocation, sixth cervical vertebra
839.07 Closed dislocation, seventh cervical vertebra
839.08 Closed dislocation, multiple cervical vertebrae
839.13 Open dislocation, third cervical vertebra
839.14 Open dislocation, fourth cervical vertebra
839.15 Open dislocation, fifth cervical vertebra
839.16 Open dislocation, sixth cervical vertebra
839.17 Open dislocation, seventh cervical vertebra
839.18 Open dislocation, multiple cervical vertebrae
839.20 Closed dislocation, lumbar vertebra
839.21 Closed dislocation, thoracic vertebra
839.30 Open dislocation, lumbar vertebra
839.31 Open dislocation, thoracic vertebra

ICD-9-CM Procedural

81.00 Spinal fusion, not otherwise specified
81.01 Atlas-axis spinal fusion
81.03 Other cervical fusion, posterior technique
81.05 Dorsal and dorsolumbar fusion, posterior technique
81.07 Lumbar and lumbosacral fusion, lateral transverse process technique
81.08 Lumbar and lumbosacral fusion, posterior technique
81.31 Refusion of Atlas-axis spine
81.33 Refusion of other cervical spine, posterior technique
81.35 Refusion of dorsal and dorsolumbar spine, posterior technique
81.37 Refusion of lumbar and lumbosacral spine, lateral transverse process technique
81.38 Refusion of lumbar and lumbosacral spine, posterior technique
81.62 Fusion or refusion of 2-3 vertebrae
81.63 Fusion or refusion of 4-8 vertebrae
81.64 Fusion or refusion of 9 or more vertebrae

22630–22632

22630 Arthrodesis, posterior interbody technique, including laminectomy and/or diskectomy to prepare interspace (other than for decompression), single interspace; lumbar
22632 each additional interspace (List separately in addition to code for primary procedure)

ICD-9-CM Diagnostic

170.2 Malignant neoplasm of vertebral column, excluding sacrum and coccyx
198.5 Secondary malignant neoplasm of bone and bone marrow
213.2 Benign neoplasm of vertebral column, excluding sacrum and coccyx
238.0 Neoplasm of uncertain behavior of bone and articular cartilage
239.2 Neoplasms of unspecified nature of bone, soft tissue, and skin
336.9 Unspecified disease of spinal cord ▽
721.3 Lumbosacral spondylosis without myelopathy
721.42 Spondylosis with myelopathy, lumbar region
722.10 Displacement of lumbar intervertebral disc without myelopathy
722.52 Degeneration of lumbar or lumbosacral intervertebral disc
722.73 Intervertebral lumbar disc disorder with myelopathy, lumbar region
722.83 Postlaminectomy syndrome, lumbar region
722.93 Other and unspecified disc disorder of lumbar region
724.02 Spinal stenosis of lumbar region
724.2 Lumbago
724.3 Sciatica
724.4 Thoracic or lumbosacral neuritis or radiculitis, unspecified ▽
731.0 Osteitis deformans without mention of bone tumor
733.13 Pathologic fracture of vertebrae
733.95 Stress fracture of other bone
756.11 Congenital spondylolysis, lumbosacral region
756.12 Congenital spondylolisthesis
805.4 Closed fracture of lumbar vertebra without mention of spinal cord injury
805.5 Open fracture of lumbar vertebra without mention of spinal cord injury
806.4 Closed fracture of lumbar spine with spinal cord injury
806.5 Open fracture of lumbar spine with spinal cord injury
839.20 Closed dislocation, lumbar vertebra
839.30 Open dislocation, lumbar vertebra

ICD-9-CM Procedural

81.07 Lumbar and lumbosacral fusion, lateral transverse process technique
81.08 Lumbar and lumbosacral fusion, posterior technique
81.37 Refusion of lumbar and lumbosacral spine, lateral transverse process technique
81.38 Refusion of lumbar and lumbosacral spine, posterior technique
81.62 Fusion or refusion of 2-3 vertebrae
81.63 Fusion or refusion of 4-8 vertebrae
81.64 Fusion or refusion of 9 or more vertebrae

22800–22804

22800 Arthrodesis, posterior, for spinal deformity, with or without cast; up to 6 vertebral segments
22802 7 to 12 vertebral segments
22804 13 or more vertebral segments

ICD-9-CM Diagnostic

138 Late effects of acute poliomyelitis
237.70 Neurofibromatosis, unspecified ▽
237.71 Neurofibromatosis, Type 1 (von Recklinghausen's disease)
237.72 Neurofibromatosis, Type 2 (acoustic neurofibromatosis)
252.00 Hyperparathyroidism, unspecified
252.01 Primary hyperparathyroidism
252.02 Secondary hyperparathyroidism, non-renal
252.08 Other hyperparathyroidism
277.5 Mucopolysaccharidosis — (Use additional code to identify any associated mental retardation)
356.1 Peroneal muscular atrophy
731.0 Osteitis deformans without mention of bone tumor
732.0 Juvenile osteochondrosis of spine
732.8 Other specified forms of osteochondropathy
733.00 Unspecified osteoporosis ▽
733.01 Senile osteoporosis
733.02 Idiopathic osteoporosis
733.03 Disuse osteoporosis
733.09 Other osteoporosis — (Use additional E code to identify drug)
737.0 Adolescent postural kyphosis
737.10 Kyphosis (acquired) (postural)
737.20 Lordosis (acquired) (postural)
737.30 Scoliosis (and kyphoscoliosis), idiopathic
737.32 Progressive infantile idiopathic scoliosis
737.33 Scoliosis due to radiation
737.34 Thoracogenic scoliosis
737.40 Unspecified curvature of spine associated with other condition — (Code first associated condition: 015.0, 138, 237.7, 252.0, 277.5, 356.1, 731.0, 733.00-733.09) ▽ ☒
737.41 Kyphosis associated with other condition — (Code first associated condition: 015.0, 138, 237.7, 252.0, 277.5, 356.1, 731.0, 733.00-733.09) ☒
737.42 Lordosis associated with other condition — (Code first associated condition: 015.0, 138, 237.7, 252.0, 277.5, 356.1, 731.0, 733.00-733.09) ☒
737.43 Scoliosis associated with other condition — (Code first associated condition: 015.0, 138, 237.7, 252.0, 277.5, 356.1, 731.0, 733.00-733.09) ☒
737.8 Other curvatures of spine associated with other conditions
737.9 Unspecified curvature of spine associated with other condition ▽
738.5 Other acquired deformity of back or spine
754.2 Congenital musculoskeletal deformity of spine

▽ Unspecified code ☒ Manifestation code
♀ Female diagnosis ♂ Male diagnosis

756.10 Congenital anomaly of spine, unspecified ▽
756.12 Congenital spondylolisthesis

ICD-9-CM Procedural

81.00 Spinal fusion, not otherwise specified
81.01 Atlas-axis spinal fusion
81.03 Other cervical fusion, posterior technique
81.05 Dorsal and dorsolumbar fusion, posterior technique
81.07 Lumbar and lumbosacral fusion, lateral transverse process technique
81.08 Lumbar and lumbosacral fusion, posterior technique
81.31 Refusion of Atlas-axis spine
81.33 Refusion of other cervical spine, posterior technique
81.35 Refusion of dorsal and dorsolumbar spine, posterior technique
81.37 Refusion of lumbar and lumbosacral spine, lateral transverse process technique
81.38 Refusion of lumbar and lumbosacral spine, posterior technique
81.62 Fusion or refusion of 2-3 vertebrae
81.63 Fusion or refusion of 4-8 vertebrae
81.64 Fusion or refusion of 9 or more vertebrae

22808–22812

22808 Arthrodesis, anterior, for spinal deformity, with or without cast; 2 to 3 vertebral segments
22810 4 to 7 vertebral segments
22812 8 or more vertebral segments

ICD-9-CM Diagnostic

138 Late effects of acute poliomyelitis
237.70 Neurofibromatosis, unspecified ▽
237.71 Neurofibromatosis, Type 1 (von Recklinghausen's disease)
237.72 Neurofibromatosis, Type 2 (acoustic neurofibromatosis)
252.00 Hyperparathyroidism, unspecified
252.01 Primary hyperparathyroidism
252.02 Secondary hyperparathyroidism, non-renal
252.08 Other hyperparathyroidism
277.5 Mucopolysaccharidosis — (Use additional code to identify any associated mental retardation)
356.1 Peroneal muscular atrophy
731.0 Osteitis deformans without mention of bone tumor
732.0 Juvenile osteochondrosis of spine
732.8 Other specified forms of osteochondropathy
733.00 Unspecified osteoporosis ▽
733.01 Senile osteoporosis
733.02 Idiopathic osteoporosis
733.03 Disuse osteoporosis
733.09 Other osteoporosis — (Use additional E code to identify drug)
737.0 Adolescent postural kyphosis
737.10 Kyphosis (acquired) (postural)
737.20 Lordosis (acquired) (postural)
737.30 Scoliosis (and kyphoscoliosis), idiopathic
737.32 Progressive infantile idiopathic scoliosis
737.33 Scoliosis due to radiation
737.34 Thoracogenic scoliosis
737.40 Unspecified curvature of spine associated with other condition — (Code first associated condition: 015.0, 138, 237.7, 252.0, 277.5, 356.1, 731.0, 733.00-733.09) ▽ ☒
737.41 Kyphosis associated with other condition — (Code first associated condition: 015.0, 138, 237.7, 252.0, 277.5, 356.1, 731.0, 733.00-733.09) ☒
737.42 Lordosis associated with other condition — (Code first associated condition: 015.0, 138, 237.7, 252.0, 277.5, 356.1, 731.0, 733.00-733.09) ☒
737.43 Scoliosis associated with other condition — (Code first associated condition: 015.0, 138, 237.7, 252.0, 277.5, 356.1, 731.0, 733.00-733.09) ☒
737.8 Other curvatures of spine associated with other conditions
737.9 Unspecified curvature of spine associated with other condition ▽
738.5 Other acquired deformity of back or spine
754.2 Congenital musculoskeletal deformity of spine
756.10 Congenital anomaly of spine, unspecified ▽
756.12 Congenital spondylolisthesis

ICD-9-CM Procedural

81.00 Spinal fusion, not otherwise specified
81.01 Atlas-axis spinal fusion
81.02 Other cervical fusion, anterior technique
81.04 Dorsal and dorsolumbar fusion, anterior technique
81.06 Lumbar and lumbosacral fusion, anterior technique
81.31 Refusion of Atlas-axis spine
81.32 Refusion of other cervical spine, anterior technique
81.34 Refusion of dorsal and dorsolumbar spine, anterior technique
81.36 Refusion of lumbar and lumbosacral spine, anterior technique
81.62 Fusion or refusion of 2-3 vertebrae
81.63 Fusion or refusion of 4-8 vertebrae
81.64 Fusion or refusion of 9 or more vertebrae

22818–22819

22818 Kyphectomy, circumferential exposure of spine and resection of vertebral segment(s) (including body and posterior elements); single or 2 segments
22819 3 or more segments

ICD-9-CM Diagnostic

737.10 Kyphosis (acquired) (postural)
737.30 Scoliosis (and kyphoscoliosis), idiopathic
737.32 Progressive infantile idiopathic scoliosis
737.41 Kyphosis associated with other condition — (Code first associated condition: 015.0, 138, 237.7, 252.0, 277.5, 356.1, 731.0, 733.00-733.09) ☒
737.43 Scoliosis associated with other condition — (Code first associated condition: 015.0, 138, 237.7, 252.0, 277.5, 356.1, 731.0, 733.00-733.09) ☒
738.5 Other acquired deformity of back or spine
741.00 Spina bifida with hydrocephalus, unspecified region ▽
741.02 Spina bifida with hydrocephalus, dorsal (thoracic) region
741.03 Spina bifida with hydrocephalus, lumbar region
741.90 Spina bifida without mention of hydrocephalus, unspecified region ▽
741.92 Spina bifida without mention of hydrocephalus, dorsal (thoracic) region
741.93 Spina bifida without mention of hydrocephalus, lumbar region
742.59 Other specified congenital anomaly of spinal cord
754.2 Congenital musculoskeletal deformity of spine
756.19 Other congenital anomaly of spine

ICD-9-CM Procedural

77.99 Total ostectomy of other bone, except facial bones

22830

22830 Exploration of spinal fusion

ICD-9-CM Diagnostic

324.1 Intraspinal abscess
722.81 Postlaminectomy syndrome, cervical region
722.82 Postlaminectomy syndrome, thoracic region
722.83 Postlaminectomy syndrome, lumbar region
724.4 Thoracic or lumbosacral neuritis or radiculitis, unspecified ▽
733.13 Pathologic fracture of vertebrae
733.81 Malunion of fracture
733.82 Nonunion of fracture
733.95 Stress fracture of other bone
996.4 Mechanical complication of internal orthopedic device, implant, and graft
996.67 Infection and inflammatory reaction due to other internal orthopedic device, implant, and graft — (Use additional code to identify specified infections)
996.78 Other complications due to other internal orthopedic device, implant, and graft
V45.4 Arthrodesis status — (This code is intended for use when these conditions are recorded as diagnoses or problems)

ICD-9-CM Procedural

03.09 Other exploration and decompression of spinal canal

22840

22840 Posterior non-segmental instrumentation (eg, Harrington rod technique, pedicle fixation across one interspace, atlantoaxial transarticular screw fixation, sublaminar wiring at C1, facet screw fixation)

ICD-9-CM Diagnostic

This is designated as an add-on code by Ingenix only. Refer to the corresponding primary procedure code for ICD-9 diagnosis code links.

ICD-9-CM Procedural

81.01 Atlas-axis spinal fusion
81.03 Other cervical fusion, posterior technique
81.31 Refusion of Atlas-axis spine
81.33 Refusion of other cervical spine, posterior technique
81.62 Fusion or refusion of 2-3 vertebrae
81.63 Fusion or refusion of 4-8 vertebrae
81.64 Fusion or refusion of 9 or more vertebrae
84.52 Insertion of recombinant bone morphogenetic protein

▽ Unspecified code ♀ Female diagnosis ☒ Manifestation code ♂ Male diagnosis

22841

22841 Internal spinal fixation by wiring of spinous processes

ICD-9-CM Diagnostic

This is designated as an add-on code by Ingenix only. Refer to the corresponding primary procedure code for ICD-9 diagnosis code links.

ICD-9-CM Procedural

78.59 Internal fixation of other bone, except facial bones, without fracture reduction
84.51 Insertion of interbody spinal fusion device
84.59 Insertion of other spinal devices

22842–22844

22842 Posterior segmental instrumentation (eg, pedicle fixation, dual rods with multiple hooks and sublaminal wires); 3 to 6 vertebral segments
22843 7 to 12 vertebral segments
22844 13 or more vertebral segments

ICD-9-CM Diagnostic

This is designated as an add-on code by Ingenix only. Refer to the corresponding primary procedure code for ICD-9 diagnosis code links.

ICD-9-CM Procedural

78.59 Internal fixation of other bone, except facial bones, without fracture reduction
81.07 Lumbar and lumbosacral fusion, lateral transverse process technique
81.08 Lumbar and lumbosacral fusion, posterior technique
81.37 Refusion of lumbar and lumbosacral spine, lateral transverse process technique
81.38 Refusion of lumbar and lumbosacral spine, posterior technique
81.62 Fusion or refusion of 2-3 vertebrae
81.63 Fusion or refusion of 4-8 vertebrae
81.64 Fusion or refusion of 9 or more vertebrae
84.51 Insertion of interbody spinal fusion device
84.59 Insertion of other spinal devices

22845–22847

22845 Anterior instrumentation; 2 to 3 vertebral segments
22846 4 to 7 vertebral segments
22847 8 or more vertebral segments

ICD-9-CM Diagnostic

This is designated as an add-on code by Ingenix only. Refer to the corresponding primary procedure code for ICD-9 diagnosis code links.

ICD-9-CM Procedural

78.59 Internal fixation of other bone, except facial bones, without fracture reduction
81.62 Fusion or refusion of 2-3 vertebrae
81.63 Fusion or refusion of 4-8 vertebrae
81.64 Fusion or refusion of 9 or more vertebrae
84.51 Insertion of interbody spinal fusion device
84.59 Insertion of other spinal devices

22848

22848 Pelvic fixation (attachment of caudal end of instrumentation to pelvic bony structures) other than sacrum

ICD-9-CM Diagnostic

This is designated as an add-on code by Ingenix only. Refer to the corresponding primary procedure code for ICD-9 diagnosis code links.

ICD-9-CM Procedural

78.59 Internal fixation of other bone, except facial bones, without fracture reduction

22849

22849 Reinsertion of spinal fixation device

ICD-9-CM Diagnostic

996.4 Mechanical complication of internal orthopedic device, implant, and graft
996.67 Infection and inflammatory reaction due to other internal orthopedic device, implant, and graft — (Use additional code to identify specified infections)
996.78 Other complications due to other internal orthopedic device, implant, and graft
V45.4 Arthrodesis status — (This code is intended for use when these conditions are recorded as diagnoses or problems)

ICD-9-CM Procedural

78.59 Internal fixation of other bone, except facial bones, without fracture reduction
84.51 Insertion of interbody spinal fusion device
84.59 Insertion of other spinal devices

22850

22850 Removal of posterior nonsegmental instrumentation (eg, Harrington rod)

ICD-9-CM Diagnostic

996.4 Mechanical complication of internal orthopedic device, implant, and graft
996.67 Infection and inflammatory reaction due to other internal orthopedic device, implant, and graft — (Use additional code to identify specified infections)
996.78 Other complications due to other internal orthopedic device, implant, and graft
V45.4 Arthrodesis status — (This code is intended for use when these conditions are recorded as diagnoses or problems)
V54.01 Encounter for removal of internal fixation device

ICD-9-CM Procedural

78.69 Removal of implanted device from other bone

22851

22851 Application of intervertebral biomechanical device(s) (eg, synthetic cage(s), threaded bone dowel(s), methylmethacrylate) to vertebral defect or interspace

ICD-9-CM Diagnostic

This is designated as an add-on code by Ingenix only. Refer to the corresponding primary procedure code for ICD-9 diagnosis code links.

ICD-9-CM Procedural

81.66 Kyphoplasty
84.51 Insertion of interbody spinal fusion device
84.55 Insertion of bone void filler
84.59 Insertion of other spinal devices

22852

22852 Removal of posterior segmental instrumentation

ICD-9-CM Diagnostic

996.4 Mechanical complication of internal orthopedic device, implant, and graft
996.67 Infection and inflammatory reaction due to other internal orthopedic device, implant, and graft — (Use additional code to identify specified infections)
996.78 Other complications due to other internal orthopedic device, implant, and graft
V45.4 Arthrodesis status — (This code is intended for use when these conditions are recorded as diagnoses or problems)
V54.01 Encounter for removal of internal fixation device

ICD-9-CM Procedural

78.69 Removal of implanted device from other bone

22855

22855 Removal of anterior instrumentation

ICD-9-CM Diagnostic

996.4 Mechanical complication of internal orthopedic device, implant, and graft
996.67 Infection and inflammatory reaction due to other internal orthopedic device, implant, and graft — (Use additional code to identify specified infections)
996.78 Other complications due to other internal orthopedic device, implant, and graft
V45.4 Arthrodesis status — (This code is intended for use when these conditions are recorded as diagnoses or problems)
V54.01 Encounter for removal of internal fixation device

ICD-9-CM Procedural

78.69 Removal of implanted device from other bone

Abdomen

22900

22900 Excision, abdominal wall tumor, subfascial (eg, desmoid)

ICD-9-CM Diagnostic

171.5 Malignant neoplasm of connective and other soft tissue of abdomen
198.89 Secondary malignant neoplasm of other specified sites
214.1 Lipoma of other skin and subcutaneous tissue
215.5 Other benign neoplasm of connective and other soft tissue of abdomen

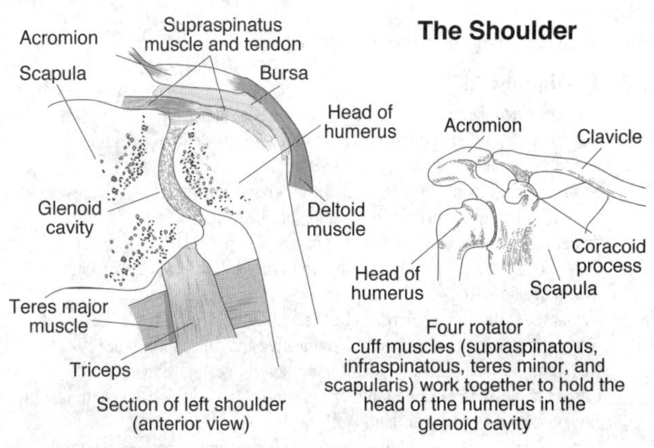

Section of left shoulder (anterior view)

238.1 Neoplasm of uncertain behavior of connective and other soft tissue ▽
239.2 Neoplasms of unspecified nature of bone, soft tissue, and skin

ICD-9-CM Procedural
54.3 Excision or destruction of lesion or tissue of abdominal wall or umbilicus

HCPCS Level II Supplies & Services
A4305 Disposable drug delivery system, flow rate of 50 ml or greater per hour
A4306 Disposable drug delivery system, flow rate of 5 ml or less per hour
A4462 Abdominal dressing holder, each
A4550 Surgical trays

Shoulder

23000
23000 Removal of subdeltoid calcareous deposits, open

ICD-9-CM Diagnostic
726.11 Calcifying tendinitis of shoulder
726.19 Other specified disorders of rotator cuff syndrome of shoulder and allied disorders
726.2 Other affections of shoulder region, not elsewhere classified
727.82 Calcium deposits in tendon and bursa
727.89 Other disorders of synovium, tendon, and bursa
728.11 Progressive myositis ossificans
728.12 Traumatic myositis ossificans
728.13 Postoperative heterotopic calcification
728.19 Other muscular calcification and ossification

ICD-9-CM Procedural
83.39 Excision of lesion of other soft tissue

23020
23020 Capsular contracture release (eg, Sever type procedure)

ICD-9-CM Diagnostic
718.41 Contracture of shoulder joint

ICD-9-CM Procedural
80.41 Division of joint capsule, ligament, or cartilage of shoulder
83.19 Other division of soft tissue

23030
23030 Incision and drainage, shoulder area; deep abscess or hematoma

ICD-9-CM Diagnostic
682.3 Cellulitis and abscess of upper arm and forearm — (Use additional code to identify organism)
711.41 Arthropathy associated with other bacterial diseases, shoulder region — (Code first underlying disease, such as: diseases classifiable to 010-040 (except 036.82), 090-099 (except 098.50)) ☒
719.11 Herarthrosis, shoulder region
727.89 Other disorders of synovium, tendon, and bursa
730.11 Chronic osteomyelitis, shoulder region — (Use additional code to identify organism, 041.1)
730.21 Unspecified osteomyelitis, shoulder region — (Use additional code to identify organism, 041.1) ▽
730.31 Periostitis, without mention of osteomyelitis, shoulder region — (Use additional code to identify organism, 041.1)
923.00 Contusion of shoulder region
998.12 Hematoma complicating a procedure
998.51 Infected postoperative seroma — (Use additional code to identify organism)
998.59 Other postoperative infection — (Use additional code to identify infection)

ICD-9-CM Procedural
83.02 Myotomy

HCPCS Level II Supplies & Services
A4305 Disposable drug delivery system, flow rate of 50 ml or greater per hour
A4306 Disposable drug delivery system, flow rate of 5 ml or less per hour
A4550 Surgical trays

23031
23031 Incision and drainage, shoulder area; infected bursa

ICD-9-CM Diagnostic
726.10 Unspecified disorders of bursae and tendons in shoulder region ▽
727.3 Other bursitis disorders
727.89 Other disorders of synovium, tendon, and bursa
730.01 Acute osteomyelitis, shoulder region — (Use additional code to identify organism, 041.1)
730.11 Chronic osteomyelitis, shoulder region — (Use additional code to identify organism, 041.1)
730.21 Unspecified osteomyelitis, shoulder region — (Use additional code to identify organism, 041.1) ▽
998.51 Infected postoperative seroma — (Use additional code to identify organism)
998.59 Other postoperative infection — (Use additional code to identify infection)

ICD-9-CM Procedural
83.03 Bursotomy

HCPCS Level II Supplies & Services
A4305 Disposable drug delivery system, flow rate of 50 ml or greater per hour
A4306 Disposable drug delivery system, flow rate of 5 ml or less per hour
A4550 Surgical trays

23035
23035 Incision, bone cortex (eg, osteomyelitis or bone abscess), shoulder area

ICD-9-CM Diagnostic
682.3 Cellulitis and abscess of upper arm and forearm — (Use additional code to identify organism)
730.11 Chronic osteomyelitis, shoulder region — (Use additional code to identify organism, 041.1)
730.21 Unspecified osteomyelitis, shoulder region — (Use additional code to identify organism, 041.1) ▽
730.81 Other infections involving bone diseases classified elsewhere, shoulder region — (Code first underlying disease: 002.0, 015.0-015.9. Use additional code to identify organism) ☒
998.51 Infected postoperative seroma — (Use additional code to identify organism)
998.59 Other postoperative infection — (Use additional code to identify infection)

ICD-9-CM Procedural
77.11 Other incision of scapula, clavicle, and thorax (ribs and sternum) without division
77.12 Other incision of humerus without division

23040–23044
23040 Arthrotomy, glenohumeral joint, including exploration, drainage, or removal of foreign body
23044 Arthrotomy, acromioclavicular, sternoclavicular joint, including exploration, drainage, or removal of foreign body

ICD-9-CM Diagnostic
711.01 Pyogenic arthritis, shoulder region — (Use additional code to identify infectious organism: 041.0-041.8)
711.81 Arthropathy associated with other infectious and parasitic diseases, shoulder region — (Code first underlying disease, such as: diseases classifiable to 080-088, 100-104, 130-136) ☒

▽ Unspecified code ♀ Female diagnosis ☒ Manifestation code ♂ Male diagnosis

711.91 Unspecified infective arthritis, shoulder region ▽
715.00 Generalized osteoarthrosis, unspecified site ▽
715.09 Generalized osteoarthrosis, involving multiple sites
715.11 Primary localized osteoarthrosis, shoulder region
716.11 Traumatic arthropathy, shoulder region
718.01 Articular cartilage disorder, shoulder region
718.11 Loose body in shoulder joint
718.21 Pathological dislocation of shoulder joint
718.41 Contracture of shoulder joint
718.51 Ankylosis of joint of shoulder region
718.71 Developmental dislocation of joint, shoulder region
719.01 Effusion of shoulder joint
719.11 Herarthrosis, shoulder region
719.41 Pain in joint, shoulder region
719.81 Other specified disorders of shoulder joint
729.6 Residual foreign body in soft tissue
998.51 Infected postoperative seroma — (Use additional code to identify organism)
998.59 Other postoperative infection — (Use additional code to identify infection)

ICD-9-CM Procedural

80.11 Other arthrotomy of shoulder
80.19 Other arthrotomy of other specified site

23065–23066

23065 Biopsy, soft tissue of shoulder area; superficial
23066 deep

ICD-9-CM Diagnostic

171.2 Malignant neoplasm of connective and other soft tissue of upper limb, including shoulder
198.89 Secondary malignant neoplasm of other specified sites
214.1 Lipoma of other skin and subcutaneous tissue
215.2 Other benign neoplasm of connective and other soft tissue of upper limb, including shoulder
238.1 Neoplasm of uncertain behavior of connective and other soft tissue ▽
239.2 Neoplasms of unspecified nature of bone, soft tissue, and skin
728.82 Foreign body granuloma of muscle
782.2 Localized superficial swelling, mass, or lump

ICD-9-CM Procedural

83.21 Biopsy of soft tissue

HCPCS Level II Supplies & Services

A4550 Surgical trays

23075–23077

23075 Excision, soft tissue tumor, shoulder area; subcutaneous
23076 deep, subfascial or intramuscular
23077 Radical resection of tumor (eg, malignant neoplasm), soft tissue of shoulder area

ICD-9-CM Diagnostic

171.2 Malignant neoplasm of connective and other soft tissue of upper limb, including shoulder
172.6 Malignant melanoma of skin of upper limb, including shoulder
195.4 Malignant neoplasm of upper limb
198.89 Secondary malignant neoplasm of other specified sites
214.1 Lipoma of other skin and subcutaneous tissue
215.2 Other benign neoplasm of connective and other soft tissue of upper limb, including shoulder
228.01 Hemangioma of skin and subcutaneous tissue
238.1 Neoplasm of uncertain behavior of connective and other soft tissue ▽
239.2 Neoplasms of unspecified nature of bone, soft tissue, and skin
728.82 Foreign body granuloma of muscle
782.2 Localized superficial swelling, mass, or lump

ICD-9-CM Procedural

83.32 Excision of lesion of muscle
83.39 Excision of lesion of other soft tissue
86.3 Other local excision or destruction of lesion or tissue of skin and subcutaneous tissue

HCPCS Level II Supplies & Services

A4305 Disposable drug delivery system, flow rate of 50 ml or greater per hour
A4306 Disposable drug delivery system, flow rate of 5 ml or less per hour
A4550 Surgical trays

23100

23100 Arthrotomy, glenohumeral joint, including biopsy

ICD-9-CM Diagnostic

170.4 Malignant neoplasm of scapula and long bones of upper limb
171.2 Malignant neoplasm of connective and other soft tissue of upper limb, including shoulder
198.5 Secondary malignant neoplasm of bone and bone marrow
198.89 Secondary malignant neoplasm of other specified sites
213.4 Benign neoplasm of scapula and long bones of upper limb
215.2 Other benign neoplasm of connective and other soft tissue of upper limb, including shoulder
238.0 Neoplasm of uncertain behavior of bone and articular cartilage
238.1 Neoplasm of uncertain behavior of connective and other soft tissue ▽
239.2 Neoplasms of unspecified nature of bone, soft tissue, and skin
275.40 Unspecified disorder of calcium metabolism — (Use additional code to identify any associated mental retardation) ▽
275.42 Hypercalcemia — (Use additional code to identify any associated mental retardation)
275.49 Other disorders of calcium metabolism — (Use additional code to identify any associated mental retardation)
357.1 Polyneuropathy in collagen vascular disease — (Code first underlying disease: 446.0, 710.0, 714.0) ☒
359.6 Symptomatic inflammatory myopathy in diseases classified elsewhere — (Code first underlying disease: 135, 140.0-208.9, 277.3, 446.0, 710.0, 710.1, 710.2, 714.0) ☒
446.0 Polyarteritis nodosa
710.0 Systemic lupus erythematosus — (Use additional code to identify manifestation: 424.91, 581.81, 582.81, 583.81)
714.0 Rheumatoid arthritis — (Use additional code to identify manifestation: 357.1, 359.6)
998.51 Infected postoperative seroma — (Use additional code to identify organism)
998.59 Other postoperative infection — (Use additional code to identify infection)

ICD-9-CM Procedural

80.11 Other arthrotomy of shoulder
80.31 Biopsy of joint structure of shoulder

23101

23101 Arthrotomy, acromioclavicular joint or sternoclavicular joint, including biopsy and/or excision of torn cartilage

ICD-9-CM Diagnostic

170.4 Malignant neoplasm of scapula and long bones of upper limb
171.2 Malignant neoplasm of connective and other soft tissue of upper limb, including shoulder
195.4 Malignant neoplasm of upper limb
198.89 Secondary malignant neoplasm of other specified sites
213.4 Benign neoplasm of scapula and long bones of upper limb
215.2 Other benign neoplasm of connective and other soft tissue of upper limb, including shoulder
239.2 Neoplasms of unspecified nature of bone, soft tissue, and skin
275.40 Unspecified disorder of calcium metabolism — (Use additional code to identify any associated mental retardation) ▽
275.42 Hypercalcemia — (Use additional code to identify any associated mental retardation)
275.49 Other disorders of calcium metabolism — (Use additional code to identify any associated mental retardation)
357.1 Polyneuropathy in collagen vascular disease — (Code first underlying disease: 446.0, 710.0, 714.0) ☒
359.6 Symptomatic inflammatory myopathy in diseases classified elsewhere — (Code first underlying disease: 135, 140.0-208.9, 277.3, 446.0, 710.0, 710.1, 710.2, 714.0) ☒
446.0 Polyarteritis nodosa
710.0 Systemic lupus erythematosus — (Use additional code to identify manifestation: 424.91, 581.81, 582.81, 583.81)
714.0 Rheumatoid arthritis — (Use additional code to identify manifestation: 357.1, 359.6)
718.01 Articular cartilage disorder, shoulder region
719.41 Pain in joint, shoulder region

ICD-9-CM Procedural

80.31 Biopsy of joint structure of shoulder
80.91 Other excision of shoulder joint

▽ Unspecified code ☒ Manifestation code
♀ Female diagnosis ♂ Male diagnosis

23105–23106

23105 Arthrotomy; glenohumeral joint, with synovectomy, with or without biopsy
23106 sternoclavicular joint, with synovectomy, with or without biopsy

ICD-9-CM Diagnostic

357.1 Polyneuropathy in collagen vascular disease — (Code first underlying disease: 446.0, 710.0, 714.0) ☒
359.6 Symptomatic inflammatory myopathy in diseases classified elsewhere — (Code first underlying disease: 135, 140.0-208.9, 277.3, 446.0, 710.0, 710.1, 710.2, 714.0) ☒
446.0 Polyarteritis nodosa
710.0 Systemic lupus erythematosus — (Use additional code to identify manifestation: 424.91, 581.81, 582.81, 583.81)
714.0 Rheumatoid arthritis — (Use additional code to identify manifestation: 357.1, 359.6)
715.91 Osteoarthrosis, unspecified whether generalized or localized, shoulder region ▽
716.61 Unspecified monoarthritis, shoulder region ▽
719.21 Villonodular synovitis, shoulder region
719.41 Pain in joint, shoulder region
727.00 Unspecified synovitis and tenosynovitis ▽
727.01 Synovitis and tenosynovitis in diseases classified elsewhere — (Code first underlying disease: 015.0-015.9) ☒
727.02 Giant cell tumor of tendon sheath

ICD-9-CM Procedural

80.11 Other arthrotomy of shoulder
80.19 Other arthrotomy of other specified site
80.31 Biopsy of joint structure of shoulder
80.71 Synovectomy of shoulder

23107

23107 Arthrotomy, glenohumeral joint, with joint exploration, with or without removal of loose or foreign body

ICD-9-CM Diagnostic

275.40 Unspecified disorder of calcium metabolism — (Use additional code to identify any associated mental retardation) ▽
275.41 Hypocalcemia — (Use additional code to identify any associated mental retardation)
275.42 Hypercalcemia — (Use additional code to identify any associated mental retardation)
275.49 Other disorders of calcium metabolism — (Use additional code to identify any associated mental retardation)
357.1 Polyneuropathy in collagen vascular disease — (Code first underlying disease: 446.0, 710.0, 714.0) ☒
359.6 Symptomatic inflammatory myopathy in diseases classified elsewhere — (Code first underlying disease: 135, 140.0-208.9, 277.3, 446.0, 710.0, 710.1, 710.2, 714.0) ☒
446.0 Polyarteritis nodosa
710.0 Systemic lupus erythematosus — (Use additional code to identify manifestation: 424.91, 581.81, 582.81, 583.81)
712.11 Chondrocalcinosis due to dicalcium phosphate crystals, shoulder region — (Code first underlying disease, 275.4) ☒
712.21 Chondrocalcinosis due to pyrophosphate crystals, shoulder region — (Code first underlying disease, 275.4) ☒
714.0 Rheumatoid arthritis — (Use additional code to identify manifestation: 357.1, 359.6)
715.91 Osteoarthrosis, unspecified whether generalized or localized, shoulder region ▽
716.61 Unspecified monoarthritis, shoulder region ▽
718.11 Loose body in shoulder joint
719.41 Pain in joint, shoulder region
727.02 Giant cell tumor of tendon sheath
V64.43 Arthroscopic surgical procedure converted to open procedure

ICD-9-CM Procedural

80.11 Other arthrotomy of shoulder

23120–23125

23120 Claviculectomy; partial
23125 total

ICD-9-CM Diagnostic

170.3 Malignant neoplasm of ribs, sternum, and clavicle
196.3 Secondary and unspecified malignant neoplasm of lymph nodes of axilla and upper limb
198.5 Secondary malignant neoplasm of bone and bone marrow
198.89 Secondary malignant neoplasm of other specified sites
213.3 Benign neoplasm of ribs, sternum, and clavicle
238.0 Neoplasm of uncertain behavior of bone and articular cartilage
239.2 Neoplasms of unspecified nature of bone, soft tissue, and skin
715.11 Primary localized osteoarthrosis, shoulder region
715.21 Secondary localized osteoarthrosis, shoulder region
716.11 Traumatic arthropathy, shoulder region
716.61 Unspecified monoarthritis, shoulder region ▽
718.01 Articular cartilage disorder, shoulder region
718.31 Recurrent dislocation of shoulder joint
728.86 Necrotizing fasciitis — (Use additional code to identify infectious organism, 041.00-041.89, 785.4, if applicable)
730.11 Chronic osteomyelitis, shoulder region — (Use additional code to identify organism, 041.1)
733.49 Aseptic necrosis of other bone site
733.90 Disorder of bone and cartilage, unspecified ▽
738.8 Acquired musculoskeletal deformity of other specified site
785.4 Gangrene — (Code first any associated underlying condition:250.7, 443.0)
831.04 Closed dislocation of acromioclavicular (joint)

ICD-9-CM Procedural

77.81 Other partial ostectomy of scapula, clavicle, and thorax (ribs and sternum)
77.91 Total ostectomy of scapula, clavicle, and thorax (ribs and sternum)

23130

23130 Acromioplasty or acromionectomy, partial, with or without coracoacromial ligament release

ICD-9-CM Diagnostic

715.11 Primary localized osteoarthrosis, shoulder region
715.21 Secondary localized osteoarthrosis, shoulder region
716.11 Traumatic arthropathy, shoulder region
716.61 Unspecified monoarthritis, shoulder region ▽
716.91 Unspecified arthropathy, shoulder region ▽
718.01 Articular cartilage disorder, shoulder region
719.41 Pain in joint, shoulder region
726.10 Unspecified disorders of bursae and tendons in shoulder region ▽
726.2 Other affections of shoulder region, not elsewhere classified
727.61 Complete rupture of rotator cuff
811.01 Closed fracture of acromial process of scapula
811.11 Open fracture of acromial process of scapula
831.14 Open dislocation of acromioclavicular (joint)

ICD-9-CM Procedural

77.81 Other partial ostectomy of scapula, clavicle, and thorax (ribs and sternum)
81.81 Partial shoulder replacement
81.82 Repair of recurrent dislocation of shoulder
81.83 Other repair of shoulder

23140–23146

23140 Excision or curettage of bone cyst or benign tumor of clavicle or scapula;
23145 with autograft (includes obtaining graft)
23146 with allograft

ICD-9-CM Diagnostic

213.3 Benign neoplasm of ribs, sternum, and clavicle
213.4 Benign neoplasm of scapula and long bones of upper limb
238.0 Neoplasm of uncertain behavior of bone and articular cartilage
239.2 Neoplasms of unspecified nature of bone, soft tissue, and skin
733.21 Solitary bone cyst
733.22 Aneurysmal bone cyst
733.29 Other cyst of bone

ICD-9-CM Procedural

77.61 Local excision of lesion or tissue of scapula, clavicle, and thorax (ribs and sternum)
77.77 Excision of tibia and fibula for graft
77.79 Excision of other bone for graft, except facial bones
78.01 Bone graft of scapula, clavicle, and thorax (ribs and sternum)

▽ Unspecified code ☒ Manifestation code
♀ Female diagnosis ♂ Male diagnosis

23150–23156

23150 Excision or curettage of bone cyst or benign tumor of proximal humerus;
23155 with autograft (includes obtaining graft)
23156 with allograft

ICD-9-CM Diagnostic

213.4 Benign neoplasm of scapula and long bones of upper limb
238.0 Neoplasm of uncertain behavior of bone and articular cartilage
239.2 Neoplasms of unspecified nature of bone, soft tissue, and skin
733.21 Solitary bone cyst
733.22 Aneurysmal bone cyst
733.29 Other cyst of bone

ICD-9-CM Procedural

77.62 Local excision of lesion or tissue of humerus
77.77 Excision of tibia and fibula for graft
77.79 Excision of other bone for graft, except facial bones
78.02 Bone graft of humerus

23170–23172

23170 Sequestrectomy (eg, for osteomyelitis or bone abscess), clavicle
23172 Sequestrectomy (eg, for osteomyelitis or bone abscess), scapula

ICD-9-CM Diagnostic

730.01 Acute osteomyelitis, shoulder region — (Use additional code to identify organism, 041.1)
730.11 Chronic osteomyelitis, shoulder region — (Use additional code to identify organism, 041.1)
730.21 Unspecified osteomyelitis, shoulder region — (Use additional code to identify organism, 041.1) ▽
730.31 Periostitis, without mention of osteomyelitis, shoulder region — (Use additional code to identify organism, 041.1)
730.88 Other infections involving bone diseases classified elsewhere, other specified sites — (Code first underlying disease: 002.0, 015.0-015.9. Use additional code to identify organism) ☒
733.49 Aseptic necrosis of other bone site

ICD-9-CM Procedural

77.01 Sequestrectomy of scapula, clavicle, and thorax (ribs and sternum)

23174

23174 Sequestrectomy (eg, for osteomyelitis or bone abscess), humeral head to surgical neck

ICD-9-CM Diagnostic

730.02 Acute osteomyelitis, upper arm — (Use additional code to identify organism, 041.1)
730.12 Chronic osteomyelitis, upper arm — (Use additional code to identify organism, 041.1)
730.22 Unspecified osteomyelitis, upper arm — (Use additional code to identify organism, 041.1) ▽
730.32 Periostitis, without mention of osteomyelitis, upper arm — (Use additional code to identify organism, 041.1)
730.82 Other infections involving bone diseases classified elsewhere, upper arm — (Code first underlying disease: 002.0, 015.0-015.9. Use additional code to identify organism) ☒
733.41 Aseptic necrosis of head of humerus

ICD-9-CM Procedural

77.02 Sequestrectomy of humerus

23180–23182

23180 Partial excision (craterization, saucerization, or diaphysectomy) bone (eg, osteomyelitis), clavicle
23182 Partial excision (craterization, saucerization, or diaphysectomy) bone (eg, osteomyelitis), scapula

ICD-9-CM Diagnostic

730.11 Chronic osteomyelitis, shoulder region — (Use additional code to identify organism, 041.1)
730.21 Unspecified osteomyelitis, shoulder region — (Use additional code to identify organism, 041.1) ▽
730.31 Periostitis, without mention of osteomyelitis, shoulder region — (Use additional code to identify organism, 041.1)
730.81 Other infections involving bone diseases classified elsewhere, shoulder region — (Code first underlying disease: 002.0, 015.0-015.9. Use additional code to identify organism) ☒
733.49 Aseptic necrosis of other bone site

ICD-9-CM Procedural

77.81 Other partial ostectomy of scapula, clavicle, and thorax (ribs and sternum)

23184

23184 Partial excision (craterization, saucerization, or diaphysectomy) bone (eg, osteomyelitis), proximal humerus

ICD-9-CM Diagnostic

730.12 Chronic osteomyelitis, upper arm — (Use additional code to identify organism, 041.1)
730.22 Unspecified osteomyelitis, upper arm — (Use additional code to identify organism, 041.1) ▽
730.32 Periostitis, without mention of osteomyelitis, upper arm — (Use additional code to identify organism, 041.1)
730.82 Other infections involving bone diseases classified elsewhere, upper arm — (Code first underlying disease: 002.0, 015.0-015.9. Use additional code to identify organism) ☒
733.41 Aseptic necrosis of head of humerus

ICD-9-CM Procedural

77.82 Other partial ostectomy of humerus

23190

23190 Ostectomy of scapula, partial (eg, superior medial angle)

ICD-9-CM Diagnostic

170.4 Malignant neoplasm of scapula and long bones of upper limb
171.4 Malignant neoplasm of connective and other soft tissue of thorax
195.1 Malignant neoplasm of thorax
198.5 Secondary malignant neoplasm of bone and bone marrow
213.4 Benign neoplasm of scapula and long bones of upper limb
238.0 Neoplasm of uncertain behavior of bone and articular cartilage
239.2 Neoplasms of unspecified nature of bone, soft tissue, and skin
733.90 Disorder of bone and cartilage, unspecified ▽

ICD-9-CM Procedural

77.81 Other partial ostectomy of scapula, clavicle, and thorax (ribs and sternum)

23195

23195 Resection, humeral head

ICD-9-CM Diagnostic

170.4 Malignant neoplasm of scapula and long bones of upper limb
195.4 Malignant neoplasm of upper limb
213.4 Benign neoplasm of scapula and long bones of upper limb
357.1 Polyneuropathy in collagen vascular disease — (Code first underlying disease: 446.0, 710.0, 714.0) ☒
359.6 Symptomatic inflammatory myopathy in diseases classified elsewhere — (Code first underlying disease: 135, 140.0-208.9, 277.3, 446.0, 710.0, 710.1, 710.2, 714.0) ☒
446.0 Polyarteritis nodosa
710.0 Systemic lupus erythematosus — (Use additional code to identify manifestation: 424.91, 581.81, 582.81, 583.81)
714.0 Rheumatoid arthritis — (Use additional code to identify manifestation: 357.1, 359.6)
715.11 Primary localized osteoarthrosis, shoulder region
715.12 Primary localized osteoarthrosis, upper arm
715.31 Localized osteoarthrosis not specified whether primary or secondary, shoulder region
715.32 Localized osteoarthrosis not specified whether primary or secondary, upper arm
716.11 Traumatic arthropathy, shoulder region
716.12 Traumatic arthropathy, upper arm
716.61 Unspecified monoarthritis, shoulder region ▽
716.62 Unspecified monoarthritis, upper arm ▽
718.81 Other joint derangement, not elsewhere classified, shoulder region
718.82 Other joint derangement, not elsewhere classified, upper arm
733.41 Aseptic necrosis of head of humerus
733.82 Nonunion of fracture
812.03 Closed fracture of greater tuberosity of humerus
812.09 Other closed fractures of upper end of humerus

▽ Unspecified code ♀ Female diagnosis ☒ Manifestation code ♂ Male diagnosis

ICD-9-CM Procedural
77.82 Other partial ostectomy of humerus

23200–23210
23200 Radical resection for tumor; clavicle
23210 scapula

ICD-9-CM Diagnostic
170.3 Malignant neoplasm of ribs, sternum, and clavicle
170.4 Malignant neoplasm of scapula and long bones of upper limb
171.4 Malignant neoplasm of connective and other soft tissue of thorax
171.7 Malignant neoplasm of connective and other soft tissue of trunk, unspecified site
198.5 Secondary malignant neoplasm of bone and bone marrow
199.0 Disseminated malignant neoplasm
213.3 Benign neoplasm of ribs, sternum, and clavicle
213.4 Benign neoplasm of scapula and long bones of upper limb
238.0 Neoplasm of uncertain behavior of bone and articular cartilage
239.2 Neoplasms of unspecified nature of bone, soft tissue, and skin

ICD-9-CM Procedural
77.81 Other partial ostectomy of scapula, clavicle, and thorax (ribs and sternum)

23220–23222
23220 Radical resection of bone tumor, proximal humerus;
23221 with autograft (includes obtaining graft)
23222 with prosthetic replacement

ICD-9-CM Diagnostic
170.4 Malignant neoplasm of scapula and long bones of upper limb
171.2 Malignant neoplasm of connective and other soft tissue of upper limb, including shoulder
198.5 Secondary malignant neoplasm of bone and bone marrow
199.0 Disseminated malignant neoplasm
213.4 Benign neoplasm of scapula and long bones of upper limb
238.0 Neoplasm of uncertain behavior of bone and articular cartilage
239.2 Neoplasms of unspecified nature of bone, soft tissue, and skin

ICD-9-CM Procedural
77.82 Other partial ostectomy of humerus
78.02 Bone graft of humerus
84.44 Implantation of prosthetic device of arm

23330
23330 Removal of foreign body, shoulder; subcutaneous

ICD-9-CM Diagnostic
709.4 Foreign body granuloma of skin and subcutaneous tissue
729.6 Residual foreign body in soft tissue
880.10 Open wound of shoulder region, complicated — (Use additional code to identify infection)
912.6 Shoulder and upper arm, superficial foreign body (splinter), without major open wound and without mention of infection
912.7 Shoulder and upper arm, superficial foreign body (splinter), without major open wound, infected

ICD-9-CM Procedural
86.05 Incision with removal of foreign body or device from skin and subcutaneous tissue
98.27 Removal of foreign body without incision from upper limb, except hand

HCPCS Level II Supplies & Services
A4305 Disposable drug delivery system, flow rate of 50 ml or greater per hour

23331–23332
23331 Removal of foreign body, shoulder; deep (eg, Neer hemiarthroplasty removal)
23332 complicated (eg, total shoulder)

ICD-9-CM Diagnostic
719.41 Pain in joint, shoulder region
728.82 Foreign body granuloma of muscle
729.6 Residual foreign body in soft tissue
880.10 Open wound of shoulder region, complicated — (Use additional code to identify infection)
996.4 Mechanical complication of internal orthopedic device, implant, and graft
996.66 Infection and inflammatory reaction due to internal joint prosthesis — (Use additional code to identify specified infections)
996.67 Infection and inflammatory reaction due to other internal orthopedic device, implant, and graft — (Use additional code to identify specified infections)
998.59 Other postoperative infection — (Use additional code to identify infection)

ICD-9-CM Procedural
80.01 Arthrotomy for removal of prosthesis of shoulder

23350
23350 Injection procedure for shoulder arthrography or enhanced CT/MRI shoulder arthrography

ICD-9-CM Diagnostic
275.40 Unspecified disorder of calcium metabolism — (Use additional code to identify any associated mental retardation)
275.42 Hypercalcemia — (Use additional code to identify any associated mental retardation)
275.49 Other disorders of calcium metabolism — (Use additional code to identify any associated mental retardation)
715.11 Primary localized osteoarthrosis, shoulder region
715.21 Secondary localized osteoarthrosis, shoulder region
715.31 Localized osteoarthrosis not specified whether primary or secondary, shoulder region
715.91 Osteoarthrosis, unspecified whether generalized or localized, shoulder region
716.61 Unspecified monoarthritis, shoulder region
716.91 Unspecified arthropathy, shoulder region
718.01 Articular cartilage disorder, shoulder region
718.11 Loose body in shoulder joint
718.21 Pathological dislocation of shoulder joint
718.31 Recurrent dislocation of shoulder joint
718.71 Developmental dislocation of joint, shoulder region
719.01 Effusion of shoulder joint
719.41 Pain in joint, shoulder region
719.42 Pain in joint, upper arm
726.90 Enthesopathy of unspecified site
727.61 Complete rupture of rotator cuff
831.00 Closed dislocation of shoulder, unspecified site
831.01 Closed anterior dislocation of humerus
831.02 Closed posterior dislocation of humerus
831.03 Closed inferior dislocation of humerus
831.04 Closed dislocation of acromioclavicular (joint)
831.09 Closed dislocation of other site of shoulder
831.10 Open unspecified dislocation of shoulder
831.11 Open anterior dislocation of humerus
831.12 Open posterior dislocation of humerus
831.13 Open inferior dislocation of humerus
831.14 Open dislocation of acromioclavicular (joint)
831.19 Open dislocation of other site of shoulder
840.0 Acromioclavicular (joint) (ligament) sprain and strain
840.1 Coracoclavicular (ligament) sprain and strain
840.2 Coracohumeral (ligament) sprain and strain
840.3 Infraspinatus (muscle) (tendon) sprain and strain
840.4 Rotator cuff (capsule) sprain and strain
923.00 Contusion of shoulder region

ICD-9-CM Procedural
81.92 Injection of therapeutic substance into joint or ligament
88.32 Contrast arthrogram

HCPCS Level II Supplies & Services
A9525 Supply of low or iso-osmolar contrast material, 10 mg of iodine

23395–23397
23395 Muscle transfer, any type, shoulder or upper arm; single
23397 multiple

ICD-9-CM Diagnostic
880.10 Open wound of shoulder region, complicated — (Use additional code to identify infection)
880.11 Open wound of scapular region, complicated — (Use additional code to identify infection)
880.12 Open wound of axillary region, complicated — (Use additional code to identify infection)

880.13 Open wound of upper arm, complicated — (Use additional code to identify infection)
880.19 Open wound of multiple sites of shoulder and upper arm, complicated — (Use additional code to identify infection)
880.20 Open wound of shoulder region, with tendon involvement — (Use additional code to identify infection)
880.21 Open wound of scapular region, with tendon involvement — (Use additional code to identify infection)
880.22 Open wound of axillary region, with tendon involvement — (Use additional code to identify infection)
880.23 Open wound of upper arm, with tendon involvement — (Use additional code to identify infection)
880.29 Open wound of multiple sites of shoulder and upper arm, with tendon involvement — (Use additional code to identify infection)
906.1 Late effect of open wound of extremities without mention of tendon injury
906.7 Late effect of burn of other extremities
927.00 Crushing injury of shoulder region — (Use additional code to identify any associated injuries: 800-829, 850.0-854.1, 860.0-869.1)
927.01 Crushing injury of scapular region — (Use additional code to identify any associated injuries: 800-829, 850.0-854.1, 860.0-869.1)
927.02 Crushing injury of axillary region — (Use additional code to identify any associated injuries: 800-829, 850.0-854.1, 860.0-869.1)
927.03 Crushing injury of upper arm — (Use additional code to identify any associated injuries: 800-829, 850.0-854.1, 860.0-869.1)
927.09 Crushing injury of multiple sites of upper arm — (Use additional code to identify any associated injuries: 800-829, 850.0-854.1, 860.0-869.1)
V10.89 Personal history of malignant neoplasm of other site

ICD-9-CM Procedural

83.77 Muscle transfer or transplantation

23400

23400 Scapulopexy (eg, Sprengels deformity or for paralysis)

ICD-9-CM Diagnostic

342.10 Spastic hemiplegia affecting unspecified side ▽
342.11 Spastic hemiplegia affecting dominant side
342.12 Spastic hemiplegia affecting nondominant side
353.0 Brachial plexus lesions
718.41 Contracture of shoulder joint
755.52 Congenital elevation of scapula

ICD-9-CM Procedural

78.41 Other repair or plastic operations on scapula, clavicle, and thorax (ribs and sternum)

23405–23406

23405 Tenotomy, shoulder area; single tendon
23406 multiple tendons through same incision

ICD-9-CM Diagnostic

342.10 Spastic hemiplegia affecting unspecified side ▽
342.11 Spastic hemiplegia affecting dominant side
342.12 Spastic hemiplegia affecting nondominant side
718.41 Contracture of shoulder joint
727.02 Giant cell tumor of tendon sheath
755.52 Congenital elevation of scapula
756.89 Other specified congenital anomaly of muscle, tendon, fascia, and connective tissue

ICD-9-CM Procedural

83.13 Other tenotomy

23410–23412

23410 Repair of ruptured musculotendinous cuff (eg, rotator cuff) open; acute
23412 chronic

ICD-9-CM Diagnostic

715.10 Primary localized osteoarthrosis, specified site ▽
715.11 Primary localized osteoarthrosis, shoulder region
715.21 Secondary localized osteoarthrosis, shoulder region
715.31 Localized osteoarthrosis not specified whether primary or secondary, shoulder region
716.11 Traumatic arthropathy, shoulder region
716.61 Unspecified monoarthritis, shoulder region ▽
719.41 Pain in joint, shoulder region
726.10 Unspecified disorders of bursae and tendons in shoulder region ▽
727.61 Complete rupture of rotator cuff
831.00 Closed dislocation of shoulder, unspecified site ▽
831.01 Closed anterior dislocation of humerus
831.02 Closed posterior dislocation of humerus
831.03 Closed inferior dislocation of humerus
831.10 Open unspecified dislocation of shoulder ▽
831.11 Open anterior dislocation of humerus
831.12 Open posterior dislocation of humerus
831.13 Open inferior dislocation of humerus
840.4 Rotator cuff (capsule) sprain and strain
880.20 Open wound of shoulder region, with tendon involvement — (Use additional code to identify infection)
927.00 Crushing injury of shoulder region — (Use additional code to identify any associated injuries: 800-829, 850.0-854.1, 860.0-869.1)
959.2 Injury, other and unspecified, shoulder and upper arm

ICD-9-CM Procedural

83.63 Rotator cuff repair

23415

23415 Coracoacromial ligament release, with or without acromioplasty

ICD-9-CM Diagnostic

715.11 Primary localized osteoarthrosis, shoulder region
715.31 Localized osteoarthrosis not specified whether primary or secondary, shoulder region
716.11 Traumatic arthropathy, shoulder region
716.91 Unspecified arthropathy, shoulder region ▽
719.41 Pain in joint, shoulder region
726.10 Unspecified disorders of bursae and tendons in shoulder region ▽
726.11 Calcifying tendinitis of shoulder
726.2 Other affections of shoulder region, not elsewhere classified
727.61 Complete rupture of rotator cuff
840.4 Rotator cuff (capsule) sprain and strain

ICD-9-CM Procedural

80.41 Division of joint capsule, ligament, or cartilage of shoulder
81.83 Other repair of shoulder

23420

23420 Reconstruction of complete shoulder (rotator) cuff avulsion, chronic (includes acromioplasty)

ICD-9-CM Diagnostic

719.41 Pain in joint, shoulder region
726.10 Unspecified disorders of bursae and tendons in shoulder region ▽
727.61 Complete rupture of rotator cuff
840.4 Rotator cuff (capsule) sprain and strain
V64.43 Arthroscopic surgical procedure converted to open procedure

ICD-9-CM Procedural

81.82 Repair of recurrent dislocation of shoulder
83.63 Rotator cuff repair

23430

23430 Tenodesis of long tendon of biceps

ICD-9-CM Diagnostic

718.91 Unspecified derangement, shoulder region ▽
719.61 Other symptoms referable to shoulder joint
726.12 Bicipital tenosynovitis
727.62 Nontraumatic rupture of tendons of biceps (long head)
840.8 Sprain and strain of other specified sites of shoulder and upper arm
880.20 Open wound of shoulder region, with tendon involvement — (Use additional code to identify infection)
927.03 Crushing injury of upper arm — (Use additional code to identify any associated injuries: 800-829, 850.0-854.1, 860.0-869.1)

ICD-9-CM Procedural

83.88 Other plastic operations on tendon

23440

23440 Resection or transplantation of long tendon of biceps

ICD-9-CM Diagnostic

726.12 Bicipital tenosynovitis
727.62 Nontraumatic rupture of tendons of biceps (long head)
880.20 Open wound of shoulder region, with tendon involvement — (Use additional code to identify infection)
927.03 Crushing injury of upper arm — (Use additional code to identify any associated injuries: 800-829, 850.0-854.1, 860.0-869.1)

ICD-9-CM Procedural

83.42 Other tenonectomy
83.75 Tendon transfer or transplantation

23450–23455

23450 Capsulorrhaphy, anterior; Putti-Platt procedure or Magnuson type operation
23455 with labral repair (eg, Bankart procedure)

ICD-9-CM Diagnostic

718.21 Pathological dislocation of shoulder joint
718.31 Recurrent dislocation of shoulder joint
831.01 Closed anterior dislocation of humerus
831.11 Open anterior dislocation of humerus
840.5 Subscapularis (muscle) sprain and strain
840.7 Superior glenoid labrum lesions (SLAP)
V64.43 Arthroscopic surgical procedure converted to open procedure

ICD-9-CM Procedural

81.82 Repair of recurrent dislocation of shoulder
81.83 Other repair of shoulder
81.93 Suture of capsule or ligament of upper extremity

23460–23462

23460 Capsulorrhaphy, anterior, any type; with bone block
23462 with coracoid process transfer

ICD-9-CM Diagnostic

718.21 Pathological dislocation of shoulder joint
718.31 Recurrent dislocation of shoulder joint
831.01 Closed anterior dislocation of humerus
831.11 Open anterior dislocation of humerus
840.2 Coracohumeral (ligament) sprain and strain
V64.43 Arthroscopic surgical procedure converted to open procedure

ICD-9-CM Procedural

81.82 Repair of recurrent dislocation of shoulder
81.83 Other repair of shoulder
81.93 Suture of capsule or ligament of upper extremity

23465

23465 Capsulorrhaphy, glenohumeral joint, posterior, with or without bone block

ICD-9-CM Diagnostic

718.21 Pathological dislocation of shoulder joint
718.31 Recurrent dislocation of shoulder joint
831.02 Closed posterior dislocation of humerus
831.12 Open posterior dislocation of humerus
840.4 Rotator cuff (capsule) sprain and strain
V64.43 Arthroscopic surgical procedure converted to open procedure

ICD-9-CM Procedural

81.82 Repair of recurrent dislocation of shoulder
81.83 Other repair of shoulder
81.93 Suture of capsule or ligament of upper extremity

23466

23466 Capsulorrhaphy, glenohumeral joint, any type multi-directional instability

ICD-9-CM Diagnostic

718.21 Pathological dislocation of shoulder joint
718.31 Recurrent dislocation of shoulder joint
831.00 Closed dislocation of shoulder, unspecified site ▽
831.01 Closed anterior dislocation of humerus
831.02 Closed posterior dislocation of humerus
831.03 Closed inferior dislocation of humerus
831.10 Open unspecified dislocation of shoulder ▽
831.11 Open anterior dislocation of humerus
831.12 Open posterior dislocation of humerus
831.13 Open inferior dislocation of humerus
840.4 Rotator cuff (capsule) sprain and strain
V64.43 Arthroscopic surgical procedure converted to open procedure

ICD-9-CM Procedural

81.82 Repair of recurrent dislocation of shoulder
81.83 Other repair of shoulder
81.93 Suture of capsule or ligament of upper extremity

23470

23470 Arthroplasty, glenohumeral joint; hemiarthroplasty

ICD-9-CM Diagnostic

170.4 Malignant neoplasm of scapula and long bones of upper limb
171.2 Malignant neoplasm of connective and other soft tissue of upper limb, including shoulder
198.5 Secondary malignant neoplasm of bone and bone marrow
238.0 Neoplasm of uncertain behavior of bone and articular cartilage
239.2 Neoplasms of unspecified nature of bone, soft tissue, and skin
357.1 Polyneuropathy in collagen vascular disease — (Code first underlying disease: 446.0, 710.0, 714.0) ☒
359.6 Symptomatic inflammatory myopathy in diseases classified elsewhere — (Code first underlying disease: 135, 140.0-208.9, 277.3, 446.0, 710.0, 710.1, 710.2, 714.0) ☒
446.0 Polyarteritis nodosa
710.0 Systemic lupus erythematosus — (Use additional code to identify manifestation: 424.91, 581.81, 582.81, 583.81)
714.0 Rheumatoid arthritis — (Use additional code to identify manifestation: 357.1, 359.6)
715.11 Primary localized osteoarthrosis, shoulder region
715.21 Secondary localized osteoarthrosis, shoulder region
715.31 Localized osteoarthrosis not specified whether primary or secondary, shoulder region
715.91 Osteoarthrosis, unspecified whether generalized or localized, shoulder region ▽
716.11 Traumatic arthropathy, shoulder region
716.61 Unspecified monoarthritis, shoulder region ▽
716.81 Other specified arthropathy, shoulder region
718.01 Articular cartilage disorder, shoulder region
726.10 Unspecified disorders of bursae and tendons in shoulder region ▽
726.19 Other specified disorders of rotator cuff syndrome of shoulder and allied disorders
727.61 Complete rupture of rotator cuff
730.11 Chronic osteomyelitis, shoulder region — (Use additional code to identify organism, 041.1)
730.12 Chronic osteomyelitis, upper arm — (Use additional code to identify organism, 041.1)
730.81 Other infections involving bone diseases classified elsewhere, shoulder region — (Code first underlying disease: 002.0, 015.0-015.9. Use additional code to identify organism) ☒
733.41 Aseptic necrosis of head of humerus
812.00 Closed fracture of unspecified part of upper end of humerus ▽
812.10 Open fracture of unspecified part of upper end of humerus ▽
996.4 Mechanical complication of internal orthopedic device, implant, and graft
998.59 Other postoperative infection — (Use additional code to identify infection)

ICD-9-CM Procedural

81.81 Partial shoulder replacement
81.97 Revision of joint replacement of upper extremity

23472

23472 Arthroplasty, glenohumeral joint; total shoulder (glenoid and proximal humeral replacement (eg, total shoulder))

ICD-9-CM Diagnostic

170.4 Malignant neoplasm of scapula and long bones of upper limb
171.2 Malignant neoplasm of connective and other soft tissue of upper limb, including shoulder
198.5 Secondary malignant neoplasm of bone and bone marrow
238.0 Neoplasm of uncertain behavior of bone and articular cartilage
239.2 Neoplasms of unspecified nature of bone, soft tissue, and skin

357.1 Polyneuropathy in collagen vascular disease — (Code first underlying disease: 446.0, 710.0, 714.0) ☒
359.6 Symptomatic inflammatory myopathy in diseases classified elsewhere — (Code first underlying disease: 135, 140.0-208.9, 277.3, 446.0, 710.0, 710.1, 710.2, 714.0) ☒
446.0 Polyarteritis nodosa
710.0 Systemic lupus erythematosus — (Use additional code to identify manifestation: 424.91, 581.81, 582.81, 583.81)
710.1 Systemic sclerosis — (Use additional code to identify manifestation: 359.6, 517.2)
710.2 Sicca syndrome
714.0 Rheumatoid arthritis — (Use additional code to identify manifestation: 357.1, 359.6)
715.11 Primary localized osteoarthrosis, shoulder region
715.21 Secondary localized osteoarthrosis, shoulder region
715.31 Localized osteoarthrosis not specified whether primary or secondary, shoulder region
715.91 Osteoarthrosis, unspecified whether generalized or localized, shoulder region ▽
716.11 Traumatic arthropathy, shoulder region
718.01 Articular cartilage disorder, shoulder region
730.11 Chronic osteomyelitis, shoulder region — (Use additional code to identify organism, 041.1)
733.41 Aseptic necrosis of head of humerus
733.81 Malunion of fracture
733.82 Nonunion of fracture
927.00 Crushing injury of shoulder region — (Use additional code to identify any associated injuries: 800-829, 850.0-854.1, 860.0-869.1)

ICD-9-CM Procedural
81.80 Total shoulder replacement
81.97 Revision of joint replacement of upper extremity

23480–23485
23480 Osteotomy, clavicle, with or without internal fixation;
23485 with bone graft for nonunion or malunion (includes obtaining graft and/or necessary fixation)

ICD-9-CM Diagnostic
170.3 Malignant neoplasm of ribs, sternum, and clavicle
213.3 Benign neoplasm of ribs, sternum, and clavicle
730.11 Chronic osteomyelitis, shoulder region — (Use additional code to identify organism, 041.1)
733.81 Malunion of fracture
733.82 Nonunion of fracture
738.8 Acquired musculoskeletal deformity of other specified site
755.51 Congenital deformity of clavicle
905.1 Late effect of fracture of spine and trunk without mention of spinal cord lesion

ICD-9-CM Procedural
77.21 Wedge osteotomy of scapula, clavicle, and thorax (ribs and sternum)
77.31 Other division of scapula, clavicle, and thorax (ribs and sternum)
77.71 Excision of scapula, clavicle, and thorax (ribs and sternum) for graft
77.77 Excision of tibia and fibula for graft
77.79 Excision of other bone for graft, except facial bones
78.01 Bone graft of scapula, clavicle, and thorax (ribs and sternum)
78.41 Other repair or plastic operations on scapula, clavicle, and thorax (ribs and sternum)

23490–23491
23490 Prophylactic treatment (nailing, pinning, plating or wiring) with or without methylmethacrylate; clavicle
23491 proximal humerus

ICD-9-CM Diagnostic
170.4 Malignant neoplasm of scapula and long bones of upper limb
198.5 Secondary malignant neoplasm of bone and bone marrow
238.0 Neoplasm of uncertain behavior of bone and articular cartilage
239.2 Neoplasms of unspecified nature of bone, soft tissue, and skin
733.00 Unspecified osteoporosis ▽
733.01 Senile osteoporosis
733.02 Idiopathic osteoporosis
733.7 Algoneurodystrophy

ICD-9-CM Procedural
78.51 Internal fixation of scapula, clavicle, and thorax (ribs and sternum) without fracture reduction
78.52 Internal fixation of humerus without fracture reduction
84.55 Insertion of bone void filler

23500–23505
23500 Closed treatment of clavicular fracture; without manipulation
23505 with manipulation

ICD-9-CM Diagnostic
733.19 Pathologic fracture of other specified site
810.00 Unspecified part of closed fracture of clavicle ▽
810.01 Closed fracture of sternal end of clavicle
810.02 Closed fracture of shaft of clavicle
810.03 Closed fracture of acromial end of clavicle

ICD-9-CM Procedural
79.09 Closed reduction of fracture of other specified bone, except facial bones, without internal fixation
93.54 Application of splint

HCPCS Level II Supplies & Services
A4565 Slings
L3650 SO, figure of eight design abduction re- strainer, prefabricated, includes fitting and adjustment
L3651 Shoulder orthosis, single shoulder, elastic, prefabricated, includes fitting and adjustment (e.g., neoprene, Lycra)
L3652 Shoulder orthosis, double shoulder, elastic, prefabricated, includes fitting and adjustment (e.g., neoprene, Lycra)
L3660 SO, figure of eight design abduction restrainer, canvas and webbing, prefabricated, includes fitting and adjustment

23515
23515 Open treatment of clavicular fracture, with or without internal or external fixation

ICD-9-CM Diagnostic
733.19 Pathologic fracture of other specified site
733.81 Malunion of fracture
733.82 Nonunion of fracture
810.00 Unspecified part of closed fracture of clavicle ▽
810.02 Closed fracture of shaft of clavicle
810.03 Closed fracture of acromial end of clavicle
810.10 Unspecified part of open fracture of clavicle ▽
810.11 Open fracture of sternal end of clavicle
810.12 Open fracture of shaft of clavicle
810.13 Open fracture of acromial end of clavicle

ICD-9-CM Procedural
79.29 Open reduction of fracture of other specified bone, except facial bones, without internal fixation
79.39 Open reduction of fracture of other specified bone, except facial bones, with internal fixation

23520–23525
23520 Closed treatment of sternoclavicular dislocation; without manipulation
23525 with manipulation

ICD-9-CM Diagnostic
718.21 Pathological dislocation of shoulder joint
718.71 Developmental dislocation of joint, shoulder region
839.61 Closed dislocation, sternum

ICD-9-CM Procedural
79.79 Closed reduction of dislocation of other specified site, except temporomandibular
93.54 Application of splint
93.59 Other immobilization, pressure, and attention to wound

HCPCS Level II Supplies & Services
A4565 Slings
A4570 Splint

23530–23532

23530 Open treatment of sternoclavicular dislocation, acute or chronic;
23532 with fascial graft (includes obtaining graft)

ICD-9-CM Diagnostic

718.21 Pathological dislocation of shoulder joint
718.31 Recurrent dislocation of shoulder joint
718.71 Developmental dislocation of joint, shoulder region
718.78 Developmental dislocation of joint, other specified sites
839.61 Closed dislocation, sternum
839.71 Open dislocation, sternum

ICD-9-CM Procedural

79.89 Open reduction of dislocation of other specified site, except temporomandibular
83.82 Graft of muscle or fascia

23540–23545

23540 Closed treatment of acromioclavicular dislocation; without manipulation
23545 with manipulation

ICD-9-CM Diagnostic

718.21 Pathological dislocation of shoulder joint
718.31 Recurrent dislocation of shoulder joint
718.71 Developmental dislocation of joint, shoulder region
831.04 Closed dislocation of acromioclavicular (joint)
840.0 Acromioclavicular (joint) (ligament) sprain and strain

ICD-9-CM Procedural

79.79 Closed reduction of dislocation of other specified site, except temporomandibular
93.59 Other immobilization, pressure, and attention to wound

HCPCS Level II Supplies & Services

A4565 Slings

23550–23552

23550 Open treatment of acromioclavicular dislocation, acute or chronic;
23552 with fascial graft (includes obtaining graft)

ICD-9-CM Diagnostic

718.21 Pathological dislocation of shoulder joint
718.31 Recurrent dislocation of shoulder joint
718.71 Developmental dislocation of joint, shoulder region
831.04 Closed dislocation of acromioclavicular (joint)
831.14 Open dislocation of acromioclavicular (joint)
840.0 Acromioclavicular (joint) (ligament) sprain and strain

ICD-9-CM Procedural

79.89 Open reduction of dislocation of other specified site, except temporomandibular
83.82 Graft of muscle or fascia

HCPCS Level II Supplies & Services

A4565 Slings

23570–23575

23570 Closed treatment of scapular fracture; without manipulation
23575 with manipulation, with or without skeletal traction (with or without shoulder joint involvement)

ICD-9-CM Diagnostic

733.19 Pathologic fracture of other specified site
811.01 Closed fracture of acromial process of scapula
811.02 Closed fracture of coracoid process of scapula
811.03 Closed fracture of glenoid cavity and neck of scapula
811.09 Closed fracture of other part of scapula

ICD-9-CM Procedural

79.09 Closed reduction of fracture of other specified bone, except facial bones, without internal fixation
79.19 Closed reduction of fracture of other specified bone, except facial bones, with internal fixation
93.44 Other skeletal traction
93.54 Application of splint
93.59 Other immobilization, pressure, and attention to wound

HCPCS Level II Supplies & Services

A4565 Slings
A4570 Splint
A4580 Cast supplies (e.g., plaster)
A4590 Special casting material (e.g., fiberglass)
L3650 SO, figure of eight design abduction re- strainer, prefabricated, includes fitting and adjustment

23585

23585 Open treatment of scapular fracture (body, glenoid or acromion) with or without internal fixation

ICD-9-CM Diagnostic

733.19 Pathologic fracture of other specified site
733.81 Malunion of fracture
733.82 Nonunion of fracture
811.01 Closed fracture of acromial process of scapula
811.03 Closed fracture of glenoid cavity and neck of scapula
811.09 Closed fracture of other part of scapula
811.11 Open fracture of acromial process of scapula
811.13 Open fracture of glenoid cavity and neck of scapula
811.19 Open fracture of other part of scapula

ICD-9-CM Procedural

79.29 Open reduction of fracture of other specified bone, except facial bones, without internal fixation
79.39 Open reduction of fracture of other specified bone, except facial bones, with internal fixation

23600–23605

23600 Closed treatment of proximal humeral (surgical or anatomical neck) fracture; without manipulation
23605 with manipulation, with or without skeletal traction

ICD-9-CM Diagnostic

733.11 Pathologic fracture of humerus
812.01 Closed fracture of surgical neck of humerus
812.02 Closed fracture of anatomical neck of humerus

ICD-9-CM Procedural

79.01 Closed reduction of fracture of humerus without internal fixation
79.11 Closed reduction of fracture of humerus with internal fixation
93.54 Application of splint

HCPCS Level II Supplies & Services

A4565 Slings
A4580 Cast supplies (e.g., plaster)

23615–23616

23615 Open treatment of proximal humeral (surgical or anatomical neck) fracture, with or without internal or external fixation, with or without repair of tuberosity(s);
23616 with proximal humeral prosthetic replacement

ICD-9-CM Diagnostic

733.11 Pathologic fracture of humerus
733.81 Malunion of fracture
733.82 Nonunion of fracture
812.01 Closed fracture of surgical neck of humerus
812.02 Closed fracture of anatomical neck of humerus
812.03 Closed fracture of greater tuberosity of humerus
812.09 Other closed fractures of upper end of humerus
812.11 Open fracture of surgical neck of humerus
812.12 Open fracture of anatomical neck of humerus
812.13 Open fracture of greater tuberosity of humerus
812.19 Other open fracture of upper end of humerus

ICD-9-CM Procedural

79.21 Open reduction of fracture of humerus without internal fixation
79.31 Open reduction of fracture of humerus with internal fixation
81.81 Partial shoulder replacement

23620–23625

23620 Closed treatment of greater humeral tuberosity fracture; without manipulation
23625 with manipulation

ICD-9-CM Diagnostic

733.11 Pathologic fracture of humerus
812.03 Closed fracture of greater tuberosity of humerus

ICD-9-CM Procedural

79.01 Closed reduction of fracture of humerus without internal fixation
93.54 Application of splint

HCPCS Level II Supplies & Services

A4565 Slings

23630

23630 Open treatment of greater humeral tuberosity fracture, with or without internal or external fixation

ICD-9-CM Diagnostic

733.19 Pathologic fracture of other specified site
733.81 Malunion of fracture
733.82 Nonunion of fracture
812.03 Closed fracture of greater tuberosity of humerus
812.13 Open fracture of greater tuberosity of humerus

ICD-9-CM Procedural

78.12 Application of external fixation device, humerus
79.21 Open reduction of fracture of humerus without internal fixation
79.31 Open reduction of fracture of humerus with internal fixation

23650–23655

23650 Closed treatment of shoulder dislocation, with manipulation; without anesthesia
23655 requiring anesthesia

ICD-9-CM Diagnostic

718.21 Pathological dislocation of shoulder joint
718.31 Recurrent dislocation of shoulder joint
718.71 Developmental dislocation of joint, shoulder region
831.00 Closed dislocation of shoulder, unspecified site ▽
831.01 Closed anterior dislocation of humerus
831.02 Closed posterior dislocation of humerus
831.03 Closed inferior dislocation of humerus
831.09 Closed dislocation of other site of shoulder

ICD-9-CM Procedural

79.71 Closed reduction of dislocation of shoulder

HCPCS Level II Supplies & Services

A4565 Slings

23660

23660 Open treatment of acute shoulder dislocation

ICD-9-CM Diagnostic

718.21 Pathological dislocation of shoulder joint
718.71 Developmental dislocation of joint, shoulder region
831.00 Closed dislocation of shoulder, unspecified site ▽
831.01 Closed anterior dislocation of humerus
831.02 Closed posterior dislocation of humerus
831.03 Closed inferior dislocation of humerus
831.04 Closed dislocation of acromioclavicular (joint)
831.09 Closed dislocation of other site of shoulder
831.10 Open unspecified dislocation of shoulder ▽
831.11 Open anterior dislocation of humerus
831.12 Open posterior dislocation of humerus
831.13 Open inferior dislocation of humerus
831.14 Open dislocation of acromioclavicular (joint)
831.19 Open dislocation of other site of shoulder

ICD-9-CM Procedural

79.81 Open reduction of dislocation of shoulder

23665

23665 Closed treatment of shoulder dislocation, with fracture of greater humeral tuberosity, with manipulation

ICD-9-CM Diagnostic

733.11 Pathologic fracture of humerus
812.03 Closed fracture of greater tuberosity of humerus
831.00 Closed dislocation of shoulder, unspecified site ▽

ICD-9-CM Procedural

79.01 Closed reduction of fracture of humerus without internal fixation
79.71 Closed reduction of dislocation of shoulder

23670

23670 Open treatment of shoulder dislocation, with fracture of greater humeral tuberosity, with or without internal or external fixation

ICD-9-CM Diagnostic

733.11 Pathologic fracture of humerus
812.03 Closed fracture of greater tuberosity of humerus
812.13 Open fracture of greater tuberosity of humerus
831.00 Closed dislocation of shoulder, unspecified site ▽
831.10 Open unspecified dislocation of shoulder ▽

ICD-9-CM Procedural

78.12 Application of external fixation device, humerus
79.21 Open reduction of fracture of humerus without internal fixation
79.31 Open reduction of fracture of humerus with internal fixation
79.81 Open reduction of dislocation of shoulder

23675

23675 Closed treatment of shoulder dislocation, with surgical or anatomical neck fracture, with manipulation

ICD-9-CM Diagnostic

733.11 Pathologic fracture of humerus
812.01 Closed fracture of surgical neck of humerus
812.02 Closed fracture of anatomical neck of humerus
831.00 Closed dislocation of shoulder, unspecified site ▽

ICD-9-CM Procedural

79.01 Closed reduction of fracture of humerus without internal fixation
79.71 Closed reduction of dislocation of shoulder

23680

23680 Open treatment of shoulder dislocation, with surgical or anatomical neck fracture, with or without internal or external fixation

ICD-9-CM Diagnostic

733.11 Pathologic fracture of humerus
812.01 Closed fracture of surgical neck of humerus
812.02 Closed fracture of anatomical neck of humerus
812.11 Open fracture of surgical neck of humerus
812.12 Open fracture of anatomical neck of humerus
831.00 Closed dislocation of shoulder, unspecified site ▽
831.10 Open unspecified dislocation of shoulder ▽

ICD-9-CM Procedural

79.21 Open reduction of fracture of humerus without internal fixation
79.31 Open reduction of fracture of humerus with internal fixation
79.81 Open reduction of dislocation of shoulder

23700

23700 Manipulation under anesthesia, shoulder joint, including application of fixation apparatus (dislocation excluded)

ICD-9-CM Diagnostic

354.4 Causalgia of upper limb
719.41 Pain in joint, shoulder region
723.4 Brachial neuritis or radiculitis nos
726.0 Adhesive capsulitis of shoulder
726.10 Unspecified disorders of bursae and tendons in shoulder region ▽
726.11 Calcifying tendinitis of shoulder
726.2 Other affections of shoulder region, not elsewhere classified
727.82 Calcium deposits in tendon and bursa

728.85 Spasm of muscle
729.1 Unspecified myalgia and myositis ▽
729.2 Unspecified neuralgia, neuritis, and radiculitis ▽
739.7 Nonallopathic lesion of upper extremities, not elsewhere classified

ICD-9-CM Procedural

78.19 Application of external fixation device, other
93.25 Forced extension of limb
93.26 Manual rupture of joint adhesions

HCPCS Level II Supplies & Services

A4550 Surgical trays

23800–23802

23800 Arthrodesis, glenohumeral joint;
23802 with autogenous graft (includes obtaining graft)

ICD-9-CM Diagnostic

171.2 Malignant neoplasm of connective and other soft tissue of upper limb, including shoulder
198.5 Secondary malignant neoplasm of bone and bone marrow
238.0 Neoplasm of uncertain behavior of bone and articular cartilage
239.2 Neoplasms of unspecified nature of bone, soft tissue, and skin
357.1 Polyneuropathy in collagen vascular disease — (Code first underlying disease: 446.0, 710.0, 714.0) ☒
359.6 Symptomatic inflammatory myopathy in diseases classified elsewhere — (Code first underlying disease: 135, 140.0-208.9, 277.3, 446.0, 710.0, 710.1, 710.2, 714.0) ☒
711.01 Pyogenic arthritis, shoulder region — (Use additional code to identify infectious organism: 041.0-041.8)
714.0 Rheumatoid arthritis — (Use additional code to identify manifestation: 357.1, 359.6)
715.11 Primary localized osteoarthrosis, shoulder region
715.21 Secondary localized osteoarthrosis, shoulder region
715.31 Localized osteoarthrosis not specified whether primary or secondary, shoulder region
715.91 Osteoarthrosis, unspecified whether generalized or localized, shoulder region ▽
716.11 Traumatic arthropathy, shoulder region
718.01 Articular cartilage disorder, shoulder region
718.31 Recurrent dislocation of shoulder joint
730.11 Chronic osteomyelitis, shoulder region — (Use additional code to identify organism, 041.1)

ICD-9-CM Procedural

77.71 Excision of scapula, clavicle, and thorax (ribs and sternum) for graft
77.77 Excision of tibia and fibula for graft
77.79 Excision of other bone for graft, except facial bones
78.02 Bone graft of humerus
81.23 Arthrodesis of shoulder

23900

23900 Interthoracoscapular amputation (forequarter)

ICD-9-CM Diagnostic

170.4 Malignant neoplasm of scapula and long bones of upper limb
171.2 Malignant neoplasm of connective and other soft tissue of upper limb, including shoulder
199.0 Disseminated malignant neoplasm
238.0 Neoplasm of uncertain behavior of bone and articular cartilage
728.86 Necrotizing fasciitis — (Use additional code to identify infectious organism, 041.00-041.89, 785.4, if applicable)
785.4 Gangrene — (Code first any associated underlying condition:250.7, 443.0)
880.10 Open wound of shoulder region, complicated — (Use additional code to identify infection)
880.11 Open wound of scapular region, complicated — (Use additional code to identify infection)
880.12 Open wound of axillary region, complicated — (Use additional code to identify infection)
880.13 Open wound of upper arm, complicated — (Use additional code to identify infection)
880.20 Open wound of shoulder region, with tendon involvement — (Use additional code to identify infection)
880.21 Open wound of scapular region, with tendon involvement — (Use additional code to identify infection)
880.22 Open wound of axillary region, with tendon involvement — (Use additional code to identify infection)
880.23 Open wound of upper arm, with tendon involvement — (Use additional code to identify infection)
887.2 Traumatic amputation of arm and hand (complete) (partial), unilateral, at or above elbow, without mention of complication — (Use additional code to identify infection)
887.3 Traumatic amputation of arm and hand (complete) (partial), unilateral, at or above elbow, complicated — (Use additional code to identify infection)
906.7 Late effect of burn of other extremities
927.00 Crushing injury of shoulder region — (Use additional code to identify any associated injuries: 800-829, 850.0-854.1, 860.0-869.1)
927.01 Crushing injury of scapular region — (Use additional code to identify any associated injuries: 800-829, 850.0-854.1, 860.0-869.1)
927.02 Crushing injury of axillary region — (Use additional code to identify any associated injuries: 800-829, 850.0-854.1, 860.0-869.1)

ICD-9-CM Procedural

84.09 Interthoracoscapular amputation

23920

23920 Disarticulation of shoulder;

ICD-9-CM Diagnostic

170.4 Malignant neoplasm of scapula and long bones of upper limb
171.2 Malignant neoplasm of connective and other soft tissue of upper limb, including shoulder
199.0 Disseminated malignant neoplasm
238.0 Neoplasm of uncertain behavior of bone and articular cartilage
728.86 Necrotizing fasciitis — (Use additional code to identify infectious organism, 041.00-041.89, 785.4, if applicable)
785.4 Gangrene — (Code first any associated underlying condition:250.7, 443.0)
880.10 Open wound of shoulder region, complicated — (Use additional code to identify infection)
880.12 Open wound of axillary region, complicated — (Use additional code to identify infection)
880.13 Open wound of upper arm, complicated — (Use additional code to identify infection)
880.19 Open wound of multiple sites of shoulder and upper arm, complicated — (Use additional code to identify infection)
880.20 Open wound of shoulder region, with tendon involvement — (Use additional code to identify infection)
880.22 Open wound of axillary region, with tendon involvement — (Use additional code to identify infection)
880.23 Open wound of upper arm, with tendon involvement — (Use additional code to identify infection)
880.29 Open wound of multiple sites of shoulder and upper arm, with tendon involvement — (Use additional code to identify infection)
887.2 Traumatic amputation of arm and hand (complete) (partial), unilateral, at or above elbow, without mention of complication — (Use additional code to identify infection)
887.3 Traumatic amputation of arm and hand (complete) (partial), unilateral, at or above elbow, complicated — (Use additional code to identify infection)
906.7 Late effect of burn of other extremities
908.6 Late effect of certain complications of trauma
927.00 Crushing injury of shoulder region — (Use additional code to identify any associated injuries: 800-829, 850.0-854.1, 860.0-869.1)
927.01 Crushing injury of scapular region — (Use additional code to identify any associated injuries: 800-829, 850.0-854.1, 860.0-869.1)
927.02 Crushing injury of axillary region — (Use additional code to identify any associated injuries: 800-829, 850.0-854.1, 860.0-869.1)
927.03 Crushing injury of upper arm — (Use additional code to identify any associated injuries: 800-829, 850.0-854.1, 860.0-869.1)
927.09 Crushing injury of multiple sites of upper arm — (Use additional code to identify any associated injuries: 800-829, 850.0-854.1, 860.0-869.1)

ICD-9-CM Procedural

84.08 Disarticulation of shoulder

23921

23921 Disarticulation of shoulder; secondary closure or scar revision

ICD-9-CM Diagnostic

997.61 Neuroma of amputation stump — (Use additional code to identify complications)

997.62 Infection (chronic) of amputation stump — (Use additional code to identify organism. Use additional code to identify complications)
997.69 Other late amputation stump complication — (Use additional code to identify complications)
V49.67 Upper limb amputation, shoulder — (This code is intended for use when these conditions are recorded as diagnoses or problems)
V51 Aftercare involving the use of plastic surgery

ICD-9-CM Procedural
84.3 Revision of amputation stump

Humerus (Upper Arm) and Elbow

23930
23930 Incision and drainage, upper arm or elbow area; deep abscess or hematoma

ICD-9-CM Diagnostic
682.3 Cellulitis and abscess of upper arm and forearm — (Use additional code to identify organism)
719.12 Hemarthrosis, upper arm
719.82 Other specified disorders of upper arm joint
727.89 Other disorders of synovium, tendon, and bursa
729.4 Unspecified fasciitis ▽
730.12 Chronic osteomyelitis, upper arm — (Use additional code to identify organism, 041.1)
903.1 Brachial blood vessels injury
923.03 Contusion of upper arm
923.11 Contusion of elbow
958.8 Other early complications of trauma
996.1 Mechanical complication of other vascular device, implant, and graft
998.59 Other postoperative infection — (Use additional code to identify infection)

ICD-9-CM Procedural
83.09 Other incision of soft tissue

HCPCS Level II Supplies & Services
A4550 Surgical trays
A4570 Splint

23931
23931 Incision and drainage, upper arm or elbow area; bursa

ICD-9-CM Diagnostic
711.02 Pyogenic arthritis, upper arm — (Use additional code to identify infectious organism: 041.0-041.8)
719.02 Effusion of upper arm joint
726.33 Olecranon bursitis
728.0 Infective myositis
729.5 Pain in soft tissues of limb
730.02 Acute osteomyelitis, upper arm — (Use additional code to identify organism, 041.1)
730.12 Chronic osteomyelitis, upper arm — (Use additional code to identify organism, 041.1)

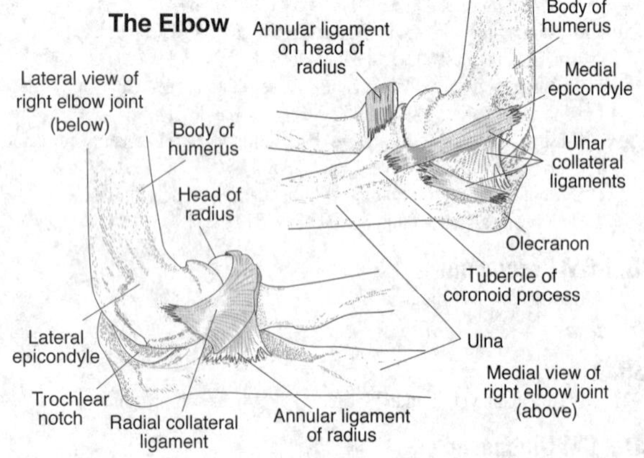

ICD-9-CM Procedural
83.03 Bursotomy

HCPCS Level II Supplies & Services
A4550 Surgical trays
A4570 Splint

23935
23935 Incision, deep, with opening of bone cortex (eg, for osteomyelitis or bone abscess), humerus or elbow

ICD-9-CM Diagnostic
682.3 Cellulitis and abscess of upper arm and forearm — (Use additional code to identify organism)
730.12 Chronic osteomyelitis, upper arm — (Use additional code to identify organism, 041.1)
730.22 Unspecified osteomyelitis, upper arm — (Use additional code to identify organism, 041.1) ▽
730.28 Unspecified osteomyelitis, other specified sites — (Use additional code to identify organism, 041.1) ▽
730.29 Unspecified osteomyelitis, multiple sites — (Use additional code to identify organism, 041.1) ▽
730.30 Periostitis, without mention of osteomyelitis, unspecified site — (Use additional code to identify organism, 041.1) ▽
730.32 Periostitis, without mention of osteomyelitis, upper arm — (Use additional code to identify organism, 041.1)
730.80 Other infections involving bone in diseases classified elsewhere, site unspecified — (Code first underlying disease: 002.0, 015.0-015.9. Use additional code to identify organism) ▽ ☒
730.82 Other infections involving bone diseases classified elsewhere, upper arm — (Code first underlying disease: 002.0, 015.0-015.9. Use additional code to identify organism) ☒
730.88 Other infections involving bone diseases classified elsewhere, other specified sites — (Code first underlying disease: 002.0, 015.0-015.9. Use additional code to identify organism) ☒
730.92 Unspecified infection of bone, upper arm — (Use additional code to identify organism, 041.1) ▽

ICD-9-CM Procedural
77.12 Other incision of humerus without division
77.19 Other incision of other bone, except facial bones, without division

24000
24000 Arthrotomy, elbow, including exploration, drainage, or removal of foreign body

ICD-9-CM Diagnostic
711.02 Pyogenic arthritis, upper arm — (Use additional code to identify infectious organism: 041.0-041.8)
711.92 Unspecified infective arthritis, upper arm ▽
711.98 Unspecified infective arthritis, other specified sites ▽
715.92 Osteoarthrosis, unspecified whether generalized or localized, upper arm ▽
718.12 Loose body in upper arm joint
719.02 Effusion of upper arm joint
719.12 Hemarthrosis, upper arm
726.33 Olecranon bursitis
729.6 Residual foreign body in soft tissue
881.01 Open wound of elbow, without mention of complication — (Use additional code to identify infection)
881.11 Open wound of elbow, complicated — (Use additional code to identify infection)
998.51 Infected postoperative seroma — (Use additional code to identify organism)
998.59 Other postoperative infection — (Use additional code to identify infection)
V64.43 Arthroscopic surgical procedure converted to open procedure

ICD-9-CM Procedural
80.12 Other arthrotomy of elbow

24006
24006 Arthrotomy of the elbow, with capsular excision for capsular release (separate procedure)

ICD-9-CM Diagnostic
718.42 Contracture of upper arm joint
718.52 Ankylosis of upper arm joint
726.30 Unspecified enthesopathy of elbow ▽

▽ Unspecified code ☒ Manifestation code
♀ Female diagnosis ♂ Male diagnosis

726.31 Medial epicondylitis of elbow
726.32 Lateral epicondylitis of elbow
726.33 Olecranon bursitis
726.39 Other enthesopathy of elbow region
V64.43 Arthroscopic surgical procedure converted to open procedure

ICD-9-CM Procedural

80.92 Other excision of elbow joint

24065–24066

24065 Biopsy, soft tissue of upper arm or elbow area; superficial
24066 deep (subfascial or intramuscular)

ICD-9-CM Diagnostic

171.2 Malignant neoplasm of connective and other soft tissue of upper limb, including shoulder
195.4 Malignant neoplasm of upper limb
198.89 Secondary malignant neoplasm of other specified sites
214.1 Lipoma of other skin and subcutaneous tissue
215.2 Other benign neoplasm of connective and other soft tissue of upper limb, including shoulder
238.1 Neoplasm of uncertain behavior of connective and other soft tissue ▽
239.2 Neoplasms of unspecified nature of bone, soft tissue, and skin
682.3 Cellulitis and abscess of upper arm and forearm — (Use additional code to identify organism)
686.8 Other specified local infections of skin and subcutaneous tissue
709.9 Unspecified disorder of skin and subcutaneous tissue ▽
728.82 Foreign body granuloma of muscle

ICD-9-CM Procedural

83.21 Biopsy of soft tissue

HCPCS Level II Supplies & Services

A4570 Splint

24075–24077

24075 Excision, tumor, soft tissue of upper arm or elbow area; subcutaneous
24076 deep, subfascial or intramuscular
24077 Radical resection of tumor (eg, malignant neoplasm), soft tissue of upper arm or elbow area

ICD-9-CM Diagnostic

171.2 Malignant neoplasm of connective and other soft tissue of upper limb, including shoulder
195.4 Malignant neoplasm of upper limb
214.1 Lipoma of other skin and subcutaneous tissue
214.8 Lipoma of other specified sites
215.2 Other benign neoplasm of connective and other soft tissue of upper limb, including shoulder
238.1 Neoplasm of uncertain behavior of connective and other soft tissue ▽
239.2 Neoplasms of unspecified nature of bone, soft tissue, and skin
782.2 Localized superficial swelling, mass, or lump

ICD-9-CM Procedural

80.81 Other local excision or destruction of lesion of shoulder joint
80.82 Other local excision or destruction of lesion of elbow joint
83.31 Excision of lesion of tendon sheath
83.32 Excision of lesion of muscle
83.39 Excision of lesion of other soft tissue

HCPCS Level II Supplies & Services

A4570 Splint

24100–24102

24100 Arthrotomy, elbow; with synovial biopsy only
24101 with joint exploration, with or without biopsy, with or without removal of loose or foreign body
24102 with synovectomy

ICD-9-CM Diagnostic

171.2 Malignant neoplasm of connective and other soft tissue of upper limb, including shoulder
198.89 Secondary malignant neoplasm of other specified sites
215.2 Other benign neoplasm of connective and other soft tissue of upper limb, including shoulder
238.1 Neoplasm of uncertain behavior of connective and other soft tissue ▽
239.2 Neoplasms of unspecified nature of bone, soft tissue, and skin
357.1 Polyneuropathy in collagen vascular disease — (Code first underlying disease: 446.0, 710.0, 714.0) ⊠
359.6 Symptomatic inflammatory myopathy in diseases classified elsewhere — (Code first underlying disease: 135, 140.0-208.9, 277.3, 446.0, 710.0, 710.1, 710.2, 714.0) ⊠
446.0 Polyarteritis nodosa
710.0 Systemic lupus erythematosus — (Use additional code to identify manifestation: 424.91, 581.81, 582.81, 583.81)
710.1 Systemic sclerosis — (Use additional code to identify manifestation: 359.6, 517.2)
710.2 Sicca syndrome
711.02 Pyogenic arthritis, upper arm — (Use additional code to identify infectious organism: 041.0-041.8)
711.32 Postdysenteric arthropathy, upper arm — (Code first underlying disease: 002.0-002.9, 008.0-009.3) ⊠
711.42 Arthropathy associated with other bacterial diseases, upper arm — (Code first underlying disease, such as: diseases classifiable to 010-040 (except 036.82), 090-099 (except 098.50)) ⊠
711.52 Arthropathy associated with other viral diseases, upper arm — (Code first underlying disease, such as: diseases classifiable to 045-049, 050-079 (except 056.71), 480, 487) ⊠
711.62 Arthropathy associated with mycoses, upper arm — (Code first underlying disease: 110.0-118) ⊠
711.82 Arthropathy associated with other infectious and parasitic diseases, upper arm — (Code first underlying disease, such as: diseases classifiable to 080-088, 100-104, 130-136) ⊠
711.92 Unspecified infective arthritis, upper arm ▽
714.0 Rheumatoid arthritis — (Use additional code to identify manifestation: 357.1, 359.6)
714.1 Felty's syndrome
714.30 Polyarticular juvenile rheumatoid arthritis, chronic or unspecified
714.31 Polyarticular juvenile rheumatoid arthritis, acute
714.32 Pauciarticular juvenile rheumatoid arthritis
714.33 Monoarticular juvenile rheumatoid arthritis
714.4 Chronic postrheumatic arthropathy
714.89 Other specified inflammatory polyarthropathies
715.12 Primary localized osteoarthrosis, upper arm
715.22 Secondary localized osteoarthrosis, upper arm
715.32 Localized osteoarthrosis not specified whether primary or secondary, upper arm
716.62 Unspecified monoarthritis, upper arm ▽
716.92 Unspecified arthropathy, upper arm ▽
718.12 Loose body in upper arm joint
719.02 Effusion of upper arm joint
719.22 Villonodular synovitis, upper arm
719.42 Pain in joint, upper arm
719.62 Other symptoms referable to upper arm joint
727.00 Unspecified synovitis and tenosynovitis ▽
727.09 Other synovitis and tenosynovitis
727.9 Unspecified disorder of synovium, tendon, and bursa ▽
732.7 Osteochondritis dissecans
V64.43 Arthroscopic surgical procedure converted to open procedure

ICD-9-CM Procedural

80.32 Biopsy of joint structure of elbow
80.72 Synovectomy of elbow
80.92 Other excision of elbow joint

24105

24105 Excision, olecranon bursa

ICD-9-CM Diagnostic

357.1 Polyneuropathy in collagen vascular disease — (Code first underlying disease: 446.0, 710.0, 714.0) ⊠
359.6 Symptomatic inflammatory myopathy in diseases classified elsewhere — (Code first underlying disease: 135, 140.0-208.9, 277.3, 446.0, 710.0, 710.1, 710.2, 714.0) ⊠
446.0 Polyarteritis nodosa
710.0 Systemic lupus erythematosus — (Use additional code to identify manifestation: 424.91, 581.81, 582.81, 583.81)
710.1 Systemic sclerosis — (Use additional code to identify manifestation: 359.6, 517.2)
710.2 Sicca syndrome
714.0 Rheumatoid arthritis — (Use additional code to identify manifestation: 357.1, 359.6)
719.42 Pain in joint, upper arm

▽ Unspecified code
♀ Female diagnosis
⊠ Manifestation code
♂ Male diagnosis

719.43 Pain in joint, forearm
719.62 Other symptoms referable to upper arm joint
726.33 Olecranon bursitis
727.2 Specific bursitides often of occupational origin
727.3 Other bursitis disorders
727.49 Other ganglion and cyst of synovium, tendon, and bursa

ICD-9-CM Procedural
83.5 Bursectomy

24110–24116
24110 Excision or curettage of bone cyst or benign tumor, humerus;
24115 with autograft (includes obtaining graft)
24116 with allograft

ICD-9-CM Diagnostic
213.4 Benign neoplasm of scapula and long bones of upper limb
238.0 Neoplasm of uncertain behavior of bone and articular cartilage
239.2 Neoplasms of unspecified nature of bone, soft tissue, and skin
726.91 Exostosis of unspecified site ▽
733.21 Solitary bone cyst
733.22 Aneurysmal bone cyst
733.29 Other cyst of bone

ICD-9-CM Procedural
77.62 Local excision of lesion or tissue of humerus
77.77 Excision of tibia and fibula for graft
77.79 Excision of other bone for graft, except facial bones
78.02 Bone graft of humerus

24120–24126
24120 Excision or curettage of bone cyst or benign tumor of head or neck of radius or olecranon process;
24125 with autograft (includes obtaining graft)
24126 with allograft

ICD-9-CM Diagnostic
213.4 Benign neoplasm of scapula and long bones of upper limb
238.0 Neoplasm of uncertain behavior of bone and articular cartilage
239.2 Neoplasms of unspecified nature of bone, soft tissue, and skin
726.91 Exostosis of unspecified site ▽
733.21 Solitary bone cyst
733.22 Aneurysmal bone cyst
733.29 Other cyst of bone

ICD-9-CM Procedural
77.63 Local excision of lesion or tissue of radius and ulna
77.77 Excision of tibia and fibula for graft
77.79 Excision of other bone for graft, except facial bones
78.03 Bone graft of radius and ulna

24130
24130 Excision, radial head

ICD-9-CM Diagnostic
171.2 Malignant neoplasm of connective and other soft tissue of upper limb, including shoulder
195.4 Malignant neoplasm of upper limb
213.4 Benign neoplasm of scapula and long bones of upper limb
238.0 Neoplasm of uncertain behavior of bone and articular cartilage
239.2 Neoplasms of unspecified nature of bone, soft tissue, and skin
277.3 Amyloidosis — (Use additional code to identify any associated mental retardation)
357.1 Polyneuropathy in collagen vascular disease — (Code first underlying disease: 446.0, 710.0, 714.0) ☒
359.6 Symptomatic inflammatory myopathy in diseases classified elsewhere — (Code first underlying disease: 135, 140.0-208.9, 277.3, 446.0, 710.0, 710.1, 710.2, 714.0) ☒
446.0 Polyarteritis nodosa
710.0 Systemic lupus erythematosus — (Use additional code to identify manifestation: 424.91, 581.81, 582.81, 583.81)
710.1 Systemic sclerosis — (Use additional code to identify manifestation: 359.6, 517.2)
710.2 Sicca syndrome
714.0 Rheumatoid arthritis — (Use additional code to identify manifestation: 357.1, 359.6)
715.13 Primary localized osteoarthrosis, forearm
718.93 Unspecified derangement, forearm joint ▽
719.43 Pain in joint, forearm
733.81 Malunion of fracture
754.89 Other specified nonteratogenic anomalies

ICD-9-CM Procedural
77.83 Other partial ostectomy of radius and ulna

24134
24134 Sequestrectomy (eg, for osteomyelitis or bone abscess), shaft or distal humerus

ICD-9-CM Diagnostic
715.12 Primary localized osteoarthrosis, upper arm
715.32 Localized osteoarthrosis not specified whether primary or secondary, upper arm
715.92 Osteoarthrosis, unspecified whether generalized or localized, upper arm ▽
716.62 Unspecified monoarthritis, upper arm ▽
730.12 Chronic osteomyelitis, upper arm — (Use additional code to identify organism, 041.1)
730.22 Unspecified osteomyelitis, upper arm — (Use additional code to identify organism, 041.1) ▽
730.32 Periostitis, without mention of osteomyelitis, upper arm — (Use additional code to identify organism, 041.1)
730.72 Osteopathy resulting from poliomyelitis, upper arm — (Code first underlying disease: 045.0-045.9. Use additional code to identify organism) ☒
730.82 Other infections involving bone diseases classified elsewhere, upper arm — (Code first underlying disease: 002.0, 015.0-015.9. Use additional code to identify organism) ☒
733.49 Aseptic necrosis of other bone site
905.2 Late effect of fracture of upper extremities

ICD-9-CM Procedural
77.02 Sequestrectomy of humerus

24136–24138
24136 Sequestrectomy (eg, for osteomyelitis or bone abscess), radial head or neck
24138 Sequestrectomy (eg, for osteomyelitis or bone abscess), olecranon process

ICD-9-CM Diagnostic
715.12 Primary localized osteoarthrosis, upper arm
715.32 Localized osteoarthrosis not specified whether primary or secondary, upper arm
715.92 Osteoarthrosis, unspecified whether generalized or localized, upper arm ▽
716.62 Unspecified monoarthritis, upper arm ▽
730.12 Chronic osteomyelitis, upper arm — (Use additional code to identify organism, 041.1)
730.22 Unspecified osteomyelitis, upper arm — (Use additional code to identify organism, 041.1) ▽
730.32 Periostitis, without mention of osteomyelitis, upper arm — (Use additional code to identify organism, 041.1)
730.72 Osteopathy resulting from poliomyelitis, upper arm — (Code first underlying disease: 045.0-045.9. Use additional code to identify organism) ☒
730.82 Other infections involving bone diseases classified elsewhere, upper arm — (Code first underlying disease: 002.0, 015.0-015.9. Use additional code to identify organism) ☒
730.92 Unspecified infection of bone, upper arm — (Use additional code to identify organism, 041.1) ▽
733.49 Aseptic necrosis of other bone site
905.2 Late effect of fracture of upper extremities

ICD-9-CM Procedural
77.03 Sequestrectomy of radius and ulna
77.09 Sequestrectomy of other bone, except facial bones

24140
24140 Partial excision (craterization, saucerization, or diaphysectomy) bone (eg, osteomyelitis), humerus

ICD-9-CM Diagnostic
729.5 Pain in soft tissues of limb
730.12 Chronic osteomyelitis, upper arm — (Use additional code to identify organism, 041.1)
730.22 Unspecified osteomyelitis, upper arm — (Use additional code to identify organism, 041.1) ▽

730.32 Periostitis, without mention of osteomyelitis, upper arm — (Use additional code to identify organism, 041.1)
730.72 Osteopathy resulting from poliomyelitis, upper arm — (Code first underlying disease: 045.0-045.9. Use additional code to identify organism) ☒
730.82 Other infections involving bone diseases classified elsewhere, upper arm — (Code first underlying disease: 002.0, 015.0-015.9. Use additional code to identify organism) ☒
730.92 Unspecified infection of bone, upper arm — (Use additional code to identify organism, 041.1) ▽
733.49 Aseptic necrosis of other bone site

ICD-9-CM Procedural

77.82 Other partial ostectomy of humerus

24145–24147

24145 Partial excision (craterization, saucerization, or diaphysectomy) bone (eg, osteomyelitis), radial head or neck
24147 Partial excision (craterization, saucerization, or diaphysectomy) bone (eg, osteomyelitis), olecranon process

ICD-9-CM Diagnostic

729.5 Pain in soft tissues of limb
730.12 Chronic osteomyelitis, upper arm — (Use additional code to identify organism, 041.1)
730.13 Chronic osteomyelitis, forearm — (Use additional code to identify organism, 041.1)
730.22 Unspecified osteomyelitis, upper arm — (Use additional code to identify organism, 041.1) ▽
730.23 Unspecified osteomyelitis, forearm — (Use additional code to identify organism, 041.1) ▽
730.32 Periostitis, without mention of osteomyelitis, upper arm — (Use additional code to identify organism, 041.1)
730.33 Periostitis, without mention of osteomyelitis, forearm — (Use additional code to identify organism, 041.1)
730.73 Osteopathy resulting from poliomyelitis, forearm — (Code first underlying disease: 045.0-045.9. Use additional code to identify organism) ☒
730.82 Other infections involving bone diseases classified elsewhere, upper arm — (Code first underlying disease: 002.0, 015.0-015.9. Use additional code to identify organism) ☒
730.83 Other infections involving bone in diseases classified elsewhere, forearm — (Code first underlying disease: 002.0, 015.0-015.9. Use additional code to identify organism) ☒
730.92 Unspecified infection of bone, upper arm — (Use additional code to identify organism, 041.1) ▽
730.93 Unspecified infection of bone, forearm — (Use additional code to identify organism, 041.1) ▽
733.49 Aseptic necrosis of other bone site

ICD-9-CM Procedural

77.83 Other partial ostectomy of radius and ulna
77.89 Other partial ostectomy of other bone, except facial bones

24149

24149 Radical resection of capsule, soft tissue, and heterotopic bone, elbow, with contracture release (separate procedure)

ICD-9-CM Diagnostic

357.1 Polyneuropathy in collagen vascular disease — (Code first underlying disease: 446.0, 710.0, 714.0) ☒
359.6 Symptomatic inflammatory myopathy in diseases classified elsewhere — (Code first underlying disease: 135, 140.0-208.9, 277.3, 446.0, 710.0, 710.1, 710.2, 714.0) ☒
446.0 Polyarteritis nodosa
710.0 Systemic lupus erythematosus — (Use additional code to identify manifestation: 424.91, 581.81, 582.81, 583.81)
710.1 Systemic sclerosis — (Use additional code to identify manifestation: 359.6, 517.2)
710.2 Sicca syndrome
711.02 Pyogenic arthritis, upper arm — (Use additional code to identify infectious organism: 041.0-041.8)
711.92 Unspecified infective arthritis, upper arm ▽
714.0 Rheumatoid arthritis — (Use additional code to identify manifestation: 357.1, 359.6)
718.52 Ankylosis of upper arm joint
719.22 Villonodular synovitis, upper arm
719.42 Pain in joint, upper arm
730.12 Chronic osteomyelitis, upper arm — (Use additional code to identify organism, 041.1)
730.22 Unspecified osteomyelitis, upper arm — (Use additional code to identify organism, 041.1) ▽
730.92 Unspecified infection of bone, upper arm — (Use additional code to identify organism, 041.1) ▽
733.49 Aseptic necrosis of other bone site
905.2 Late effect of fracture of upper extremities
905.6 Late effect of dislocation
906.4 Late effect of crushing
927.11 Crushing injury of elbow — (Use additional code to identify any associated injuries: 800-829, 850.0-854.1, 860.0-869.1)

ICD-9-CM Procedural

77.62 Local excision of lesion or tissue of humerus
80.42 Division of joint capsule, ligament, or cartilage of elbow
83.49 Other excision of soft tissue

24150–24151

24150 Radical resection for tumor, shaft or distal humerus;
24151 with autograft (includes obtaining graft)

ICD-9-CM Diagnostic

170.4 Malignant neoplasm of scapula and long bones of upper limb
198.5 Secondary malignant neoplasm of bone and bone marrow
238.0 Neoplasm of uncertain behavior of bone and articular cartilage
239.2 Neoplasms of unspecified nature of bone, soft tissue, and skin

ICD-9-CM Procedural

77.77 Excision of tibia and fibula for graft
77.79 Excision of other bone for graft, except facial bones
77.82 Other partial ostectomy of humerus
78.02 Bone graft of humerus

24152–24153

24152 Radical resection for tumor, radial head or neck;
24153 with autograft (includes obtaining graft)

ICD-9-CM Diagnostic

170.4 Malignant neoplasm of scapula and long bones of upper limb
198.5 Secondary malignant neoplasm of bone and bone marrow
238.0 Neoplasm of uncertain behavior of bone and articular cartilage
239.2 Neoplasms of unspecified nature of bone, soft tissue, and skin

ICD-9-CM Procedural

77.77 Excision of tibia and fibula for graft
77.79 Excision of other bone for graft, except facial bones
77.83 Other partial ostectomy of radius and ulna
78.03 Bone graft of radius and ulna

24155

24155 Resection of elbow joint (arthrectomy)

ICD-9-CM Diagnostic

170.4 Malignant neoplasm of scapula and long bones of upper limb
195.4 Malignant neoplasm of upper limb
238.0 Neoplasm of uncertain behavior of bone and articular cartilage
239.2 Neoplasms of unspecified nature of bone, soft tissue, and skin
239.8 Neoplasm of unspecified nature of other specified sites
357.1 Polyneuropathy in collagen vascular disease — (Code first underlying disease: 446.0, 710.0, 714.0) ☒
359.6 Symptomatic inflammatory myopathy in diseases classified elsewhere — (Code first underlying disease: 135, 140.0-208.9, 277.3, 446.0, 710.0, 710.1, 710.2, 714.0) ☒
446.0 Polyarteritis nodosa
710.0 Systemic lupus erythematosus — (Use additional code to identify manifestation: 424.91, 581.81, 582.81, 583.81)
710.1 Systemic sclerosis — (Use additional code to identify manifestation: 359.6, 517.2)
710.2 Sicca syndrome
711.02 Pyogenic arthritis, upper arm — (Use additional code to identify infectious organism: 041.0-041.8)
711.92 Unspecified infective arthritis, upper arm ▽
714.0 Rheumatoid arthritis — (Use additional code to identify manifestation: 357.1, 359.6)

▽ Unspecified code
♀ Female diagnosis
☒ Manifestation code
♂ Male diagnosis

718.52 Ankylosis of upper arm joint
718.72 Developmental dislocation of joint, upper arm
719.22 Villonodular synovitis, upper arm
719.42 Pain in joint, upper arm
730.12 Chronic osteomyelitis, upper arm — (Use additional code to identify organism, 041.1)
730.22 Unspecified osteomyelitis, upper arm — (Use additional code to identify organism, 041.1) ▽
730.92 Unspecified infection of bone, upper arm — (Use additional code to identify organism, 041.1) ▽
733.49 Aseptic necrosis of other bone site
812.41 Closed fracture of supracondylar humerus
812.42 Closed fracture of lateral condyle of humerus
812.43 Closed fracture of medial condyle of humerus
812.44 Closed fracture of unspecified condyle(s) of humerus ▽
812.49 Other closed fracture of lower end of humerus
812.51 Open fracture of supracondylar humerus
812.52 Open fracture of lateral condyle of humerus
812.53 Open fracture of medial condyle of humerus
812.54 Open fracture of unspecified condyle(s) of humerus ▽
812.59 Other open fracture of lower end of humerus
813.01 Closed fracture of olecranon process of ulna
813.02 Closed fracture of coronoid process of ulna
813.04 Other and unspecified closed fractures of proximal end of ulna (alone) ▽
813.05 Closed fracture of head of radius
813.06 Closed fracture of neck of radius
813.07 Other and unspecified closed fractures of proximal end of radius (alone) ▽
813.08 Closed fracture of radius with ulna, upper end (any part)
813.11 Open fracture of olecranon process of ulna
813.12 Open fracture of coronoid process of ulna
813.15 Open fracture of head of radius
813.16 Open fracture of neck of radius
813.17 Other and unspecified open fractures of proximal end of radius (alone) ▽
813.18 Open fracture of radius with ulna, upper end (any part)
832.00 Closed unspecified dislocation of elbow ▽
832.01 Closed anterior dislocation of elbow
832.02 Closed posterior dislocation of elbow
832.10 Open unspecified dislocation of elbow ▽
832.11 Open anterior dislocation of elbow
832.12 Open posterior dislocation of elbow
832.13 Open medial dislocation of elbow
832.14 Open lateral dislocation of elbow
832.19 Open dislocation of other site of elbow
927.11 Crushing injury of elbow — (Use additional code to identify any associated injuries: 800-829, 850.0-854.1, 860.0-869.1)

ICD-9-CM Procedural

80.92 Other excision of elbow joint

24160–24164

24160 Implant removal; elbow joint
24164 radial head

ICD-9-CM Diagnostic

996.4 Mechanical complication of internal orthopedic device, implant, and graft
996.67 Infection and inflammatory reaction due to other internal orthopedic device, implant, and graft — (Use additional code to identify specified infections)
996.77 Other complications due to internal joint prosthesis
998.59 Other postoperative infection — (Use additional code to identify infection)

ICD-9-CM Procedural

78.63 Removal of implanted device from radius and ulna
78.69 Removal of implanted device from other bone

24200–24201

24200 Removal of foreign body, upper arm or elbow area; subcutaneous
24201 deep (subfascial or intramuscular)

ICD-9-CM Diagnostic

709.4 Foreign body granuloma of skin and subcutaneous tissue
728.82 Foreign body granuloma of muscle
729.6 Residual foreign body in soft tissue
733.99 Other disorders of bone and cartilage
880.13 Open wound of upper arm, complicated — (Use additional code to identify infection)
881.11 Open wound of elbow, complicated — (Use additional code to identify infection)
906.1 Late effect of open wound of extremities without mention of tendon injury
913.6 Elbow, forearm, and wrist, superficial foreign body (splinter), without major open wound and without mention of infection
913.7 Elbow, forearm, and wrist, superficial foreign body (splinter), without major open wound, infected
996.4 Mechanical complication of internal orthopedic device, implant, and graft
996.60 Infection and inflammatory reaction due to unspecified device, implant, and graft — (Use additional code to identify specified infections) ▽
996.67 Infection and inflammatory reaction due to other internal orthopedic device, implant, and graft — (Use additional code to identify specified infections)
996.78 Other complications due to other internal orthopedic device, implant, and graft
998.4 Foreign body accidentally left during procedure, not elsewhere classified

ICD-9-CM Procedural

83.02 Myotomy
83.09 Other incision of soft tissue
86.05 Incision with removal of foreign body or device from skin and subcutaneous tissue
98.27 Removal of foreign body without incision from upper limb, except hand

HCPCS Level II Supplies & Services

A4570 Splint
A4580 Cast supplies (e.g., plaster)

24220

24220 Injection procedure for elbow arthrography

ICD-9-CM Diagnostic

275.40 Unspecified disorder of calcium metabolism — (Use additional code to identify any associated mental retardation) ▽
275.42 Hypercalcemia — (Use additional code to identify any associated mental retardation)
275.49 Other disorders of calcium metabolism — (Use additional code to identify any associated mental retardation)
357.1 Polyneuropathy in collagen vascular disease — (Code first underlying disease: 446.0, 710.0, 714.0) ☒
359.6 Symptomatic inflammatory myopathy in diseases classified elsewhere — (Code first underlying disease: 135, 140.0-208.9, 277.3, 446.0, 710.0, 710.1, 710.2, 714.0) ☒
446.0 Polyarteritis nodosa
710.0 Systemic lupus erythematosus — (Use additional code to identify manifestation: 424.91, 581.81, 582.81, 583.81)
710.1 Systemic sclerosis — (Use additional code to identify manifestation: 359.6, 517.2)
710.2 Sicca syndrome
714.0 Rheumatoid arthritis — (Use additional code to identify manifestation: 357.1, 359.6)
715.12 Primary localized osteoarthrosis, upper arm
715.92 Osteoarthrosis, unspecified whether generalized or localized, upper arm ▽
716.12 Traumatic arthropathy, upper arm
718.12 Loose body in upper arm joint
718.72 Developmental dislocation of joint, upper arm
718.82 Other joint derangement, not elsewhere classified, upper arm
719.42 Pain in joint, upper arm
719.52 Stiffness of joint, not elsewhere classified, upper arm
719.82 Other specified disorders of upper arm joint
812.40 Closed fracture of unspecified part of lower end of humerus ▽
812.41 Closed fracture of supracondylar humerus
812.42 Closed fracture of lateral condyle of humerus
812.43 Closed fracture of medial condyle of humerus
812.44 Closed fracture of unspecified condyle(s) of humerus ▽
812.49 Other closed fracture of lower end of humerus
813.01 Closed fracture of olecranon process of ulna
813.02 Closed fracture of coronoid process of ulna
813.04 Other and unspecified closed fractures of proximal end of ulna (alone) ▽
813.05 Closed fracture of head of radius
813.07 Other and unspecified closed fractures of proximal end of radius (alone) ▽
832.00 Closed unspecified dislocation of elbow ▽
832.01 Closed anterior dislocation of elbow
832.02 Closed posterior dislocation of elbow
832.03 Closed medial dislocation of elbow
832.04 Closed lateral dislocation of elbow
832.09 Closed dislocation of other site of elbow

▽ Unspecified code ☒ Manifestation code
♀ Female diagnosis ♂ Male diagnosis

ICD-9-CM Procedural

81.92 Injection of therapeutic substance into joint or ligament
88.32 Contrast arthrogram

HCPCS Level II Supplies & Services

A9525 Supply of low or iso-osmolar contrast material, 10 mg of iodine

24300

24300 Manipulation, elbow, under anesthesia

ICD-9-CM Diagnostic

357.1 Polyneuropathy in collagen vascular disease — (Code first underlying disease: 446.0, 710.0, 714.0) ☒
359.6 Symptomatic inflammatory myopathy in diseases classified elsewhere — (Code first underlying disease: 135, 140.0-208.9, 277.3, 446.0, 710.0, 710.1, 710.2, 714.0) ☒
446.0 Polyarteritis nodosa
710.0 Systemic lupus erythematosus — (Use additional code to identify manifestation: 424.91, 581.81, 582.81, 583.81)
710.1 Systemic sclerosis — (Use additional code to identify manifestation: 359.6, 517.2)
710.2 Sicca syndrome
714.0 Rheumatoid arthritis — (Use additional code to identify manifestation: 357.1, 359.6)
715.12 Primary localized osteoarthrosis, upper arm
715.92 Osteoarthrosis, unspecified whether generalized or localized, upper arm ▽
718.42 Contracture of upper arm joint
718.52 Ankylosis of upper arm joint
719.22 Villonodular synovitis, upper arm
719.52 Stiffness of joint, not elsewhere classified, upper arm
726.30 Unspecified enthesopathy of elbow ▽
726.31 Medial epicondylitis of elbow
726.32 Lateral epicondylitis of elbow
726.33 Olecranon bursitis
726.39 Other enthesopathy of elbow region

ICD-9-CM Procedural

93.25 Forced extension of limb
93.26 Manual rupture of joint adhesions
93.29 Other forcible correction of musculoskeletal deformity

24301

24301 Muscle or tendon transfer, any type, upper arm or elbow, single (excluding 24320-24331)

ICD-9-CM Diagnostic

342.10 Spastic hemiplegia affecting unspecified side ▽
342.11 Spastic hemiplegia affecting dominant side
342.12 Spastic hemiplegia affecting nondominant side
343.0 Diplegic infantile cerebral palsy
343.1 Hemiplegic infantile cerebral palsy
343.2 Quadriplegic infantile cerebral palsy
343.3 Monoplegic infantile cerebral palsy
718.32 Recurrent dislocation of upper arm joint
726.30 Unspecified enthesopathy of elbow ▽
726.39 Other enthesopathy of elbow region
728.4 Laxity of ligament
728.5 Hypermobility syndrome
841.0 Radial collateral ligament sprain and strain
841.1 Ulnar collateral ligament sprain and strain
841.2 Radiohumeral (joint) sprain and strain
841.3 Ulnohumeral (joint) sprain and strain
841.8 Sprain and strain of other specified sites of elbow and forearm
841.9 Sprain and strain of unspecified site of elbow and forearm ▽
881.11 Open wound of elbow, complicated — (Use additional code to identify infection)

ICD-9-CM Procedural

83.75 Tendon transfer or transplantation
83.77 Muscle transfer or transplantation

24305

24305 Tendon lengthening, upper arm or elbow, each tendon

ICD-9-CM Diagnostic

343.0 Diplegic infantile cerebral palsy
715.31 Localized osteoarthrosis not specified whether primary or secondary, shoulder region
718.41 Contracture of shoulder joint
718.42 Contracture of upper arm joint
728.3 Other specific muscle disorders
840.8 Sprain and strain of other specified sites of shoulder and upper arm
840.9 Sprain and strain of unspecified site of shoulder and upper arm ▽
841.0 Radial collateral ligament sprain and strain
841.1 Ulnar collateral ligament sprain and strain
841.2 Radiohumeral (joint) sprain and strain
841.3 Ulnohumeral (joint) sprain and strain
841.8 Sprain and strain of other specified sites of elbow and forearm
841.9 Sprain and strain of unspecified site of elbow and forearm ▽

ICD-9-CM Procedural

83.85 Other change in muscle or tendon length

24310

24310 Tenotomy, open, elbow to shoulder, each tendon

ICD-9-CM Diagnostic

716.51 Unspecified polyarthropathy or polyarthritis, shoulder region ▽
716.52 Unspecified polyarthropathy or polyarthritis, upper arm ▽
718.41 Contracture of shoulder joint
718.42 Contracture of upper arm joint
718.51 Ankylosis of joint of shoulder region
718.52 Ankylosis of upper arm joint
718.81 Other joint derangement, not elsewhere classified, shoulder region
718.82 Other joint derangement, not elsewhere classified, upper arm
718.91 Unspecified derangement, shoulder region ▽
718.92 Unspecified derangement, upper arm joint ▽
728.3 Other specific muscle disorders
840.8 Sprain and strain of other specified sites of shoulder and upper arm

ICD-9-CM Procedural

83.13 Other tenotomy

24320

24320 Tenoplasty, with muscle transfer, with or without free graft, elbow to shoulder, single (Seddon-Brookes type procedure)

ICD-9-CM Diagnostic

343.0 Diplegic infantile cerebral palsy
718.41 Contracture of shoulder joint
718.42 Contracture of upper arm joint
718.81 Other joint derangement, not elsewhere classified, shoulder region
718.82 Other joint derangement, not elsewhere classified, upper arm
718.91 Unspecified derangement, shoulder region ▽
718.92 Unspecified derangement, upper arm joint ▽
718.98 Unspecified derangement of joint, other specified sites ▽
727.62 Nontraumatic rupture of tendons of biceps (long head)
881.21 Open wound of elbow, with tendon involvement — (Use additional code to identify infection)

ICD-9-CM Procedural

83.77 Muscle transfer or transplantation
83.81 Tendon graft
83.88 Other plastic operations on tendon

24330–24331

24330 Flexor-plasty, elbow (eg, Steindler type advancement);
24331 with extensor advancement

ICD-9-CM Diagnostic

343.0 Diplegic infantile cerebral palsy
718.32 Recurrent dislocation of upper arm joint
718.42 Contracture of upper arm joint
718.82 Other joint derangement, not elsewhere classified, upper arm
718.92 Unspecified derangement, upper arm joint ▽
719.42 Pain in joint, upper arm

▽ Unspecified code
♀ Female diagnosis
☒ Manifestation code
♂ Male diagnosis

767.6 Injury to brachial plexus, birth trauma

ICD-9-CM Procedural

83.71 Advancement of tendon
83.77 Muscle transfer or transplantation
83.81 Tendon graft

24332

24332 Tenolysis, triceps

ICD-9-CM Diagnostic

357.1 Polyneuropathy in collagen vascular disease — (Code first underlying disease: 446.0, 710.0, 714.0) ☒
359.6 Symptomatic inflammatory myopathy in diseases classified elsewhere — (Code first underlying disease: 135, 140.0-208.9, 277.3, 446.0, 710.0, 710.1, 710.2, 714.0) ☒
446.0 Polyarteritis nodosa
710.0 Systemic lupus erythematosus — (Use additional code to identify manifestation: 424.91, 581.81, 582.81, 583.81)
710.1 Systemic sclerosis — (Use additional code to identify manifestation: 359.6, 517.2)
710.2 Sicca syndrome
714.0 Rheumatoid arthritis — (Use additional code to identify manifestation: 357.1, 359.6)
718.52 Ankylosis of upper arm joint
719.52 Stiffness of joint, not elsewhere classified, upper arm
727.00 Unspecified synovitis and tenosynovitis ▽
727.01 Synovitis and tenosynovitis in diseases classified elsewhere — (Code first underlying disease: 015.0-015.9) ☒
727.09 Other synovitis and tenosynovitis
727.81 Contracture of tendon (sheath)
727.82 Calcium deposits in tendon and bursa
727.89 Other disorders of synovium, tendon, and bursa
727.9 Unspecified disorder of synovium, tendon, and bursa ▽

ICD-9-CM Procedural

83.91 Lysis of adhesions of muscle, tendon, fascia, and bursa

HCPCS Level II Supplies & Services

HCPCS Level II codes are used to report the supplies, durable medical equipment, and certain medical services provided on an outpatient basis. Because the procedure(s) represented on this page would be performed in an inpatient or outpatient facility, no HCPCS Level II codes apply.

24340

24340 Tenodesis of biceps tendon at elbow (separate procedure)

ICD-9-CM Diagnostic

727.62 Nontraumatic rupture of tendons of biceps (long head)
728.83 Rupture of muscle, nontraumatic
841.8 Sprain and strain of other specified sites of elbow and forearm

ICD-9-CM Procedural

83.88 Other plastic operations on tendon

24341

24341 Repair, tendon or muscle, upper arm or elbow, each tendon or muscle, primary or secondary (excludes rotator cuff)

ICD-9-CM Diagnostic

727.62 Nontraumatic rupture of tendons of biceps (long head)
727.69 Nontraumatic rupture of other tendon
831.00 Closed dislocation of shoulder, unspecified site ▽
831.02 Closed posterior dislocation of humerus
831.03 Closed inferior dislocation of humerus
831.04 Closed dislocation of acromioclavicular (joint)
831.09 Closed dislocation of other site of shoulder
831.10 Open unspecified dislocation of shoulder ▽
831.11 Open anterior dislocation of humerus
831.12 Open posterior dislocation of humerus
831.13 Open inferior dislocation of humerus
831.14 Open dislocation of acromioclavicular (joint)
831.19 Open dislocation of other site of shoulder
832.00 Closed unspecified dislocation of elbow ▽
832.01 Closed anterior dislocation of elbow
832.02 Closed posterior dislocation of elbow
832.03 Closed medial dislocation of elbow
832.04 Closed lateral dislocation of elbow
832.09 Closed dislocation of other site of elbow
832.10 Open unspecified dislocation of elbow ▽
832.11 Open anterior dislocation of elbow
832.12 Open posterior dislocation of elbow
832.13 Open medial dislocation of elbow
832.14 Open lateral dislocation of elbow
832.19 Open dislocation of other site of elbow
840.8 Sprain and strain of other specified sites of shoulder and upper arm
840.9 Sprain and strain of unspecified site of shoulder and upper arm ▽
841.8 Sprain and strain of other specified sites of elbow and forearm
841.9 Sprain and strain of unspecified site of elbow and forearm ▽
880.03 Open wound of upper arm, without mention of complication — (Use additional code to identify infection)
880.09 Open wound of multiple sites of shoulder and upper arm, without mention of complication — (Use additional code to identify infection)
880.19 Open wound of multiple sites of shoulder and upper arm, complicated — (Use additional code to identify infection)
880.23 Open wound of upper arm, with tendon involvement — (Use additional code to identify infection)
880.29 Open wound of multiple sites of shoulder and upper arm, with tendon involvement — (Use additional code to identify infection)
884.1 Multiple and unspecified open wound of upper limb, complicated — (Use additional code to identify infection)
884.2 Multiple and unspecified open wound of upper limb, with tendon involvement — (Use additional code to identify infection)
927.00 Crushing injury of shoulder region — (Use additional code to identify any associated injuries: 800-829, 850.0-854.1, 860.0-869.1)
927.01 Crushing injury of scapular region — (Use additional code to identify any associated injuries: 800-829, 850.0-854.1, 860.0-869.1)
927.02 Crushing injury of axillary region — (Use additional code to identify any associated injuries: 800-829, 850.0-854.1, 860.0-869.1)
927.03 Crushing injury of upper arm — (Use additional code to identify any associated injuries: 800-829, 850.0-854.1, 860.0-869.1)
927.09 Crushing injury of multiple sites of upper arm — (Use additional code to identify any associated injuries: 800-829, 850.0-854.1, 860.0-869.1)
927.11 Crushing injury of elbow — (Use additional code to identify any associated injuries: 800-829, 850.0-854.1, 860.0-869.1)
998.2 Accidental puncture or laceration during procedure

ICD-9-CM Procedural

83.64 Other suture of tendon
83.65 Other suture of muscle or fascia
83.87 Other plastic operations on muscle
83.88 Other plastic operations on tendon

24342

24342 Reinsertion of ruptured biceps or triceps tendon, distal, with or without tendon graft

ICD-9-CM Diagnostic

727.62 Nontraumatic rupture of tendons of biceps (long head)
841.8 Sprain and strain of other specified sites of elbow and forearm

ICD-9-CM Procedural

83.75 Tendon transfer or transplantation
83.82 Graft of muscle or fascia

24343–24346

24343 Repair lateral collateral ligament, elbow, with local tissue
24344 Reconstruction lateral collateral ligament, elbow, with tendon graft (includes harvesting of graft)
24345 Repair medial collateral ligament, elbow, with local tissue
24346 Reconstruction medial collateral ligament, elbow, with tendon graft (includes harvesting of graft)

ICD-9-CM Diagnostic

716.12 Traumatic arthropathy, upper arm
718.02 Articular cartilage disorder, upper arm
718.32 Recurrent dislocation of upper arm joint
718.82 Other joint derangement, not elsewhere classified, upper arm
728.89 Other disorder of muscle, ligament, and fascia — (Use additional E code to identify drug, if drug-induced)
728.9 Unspecified disorder of muscle, ligament, and fascia ▽
812.40 Closed fracture of unspecified part of lower end of humerus ▽

▽ Unspecified code ☒ Manifestation code
♀ Female diagnosis ♂ Male diagnosis

812.41 Closed fracture of supracondylar humerus
812.42 Closed fracture of lateral condyle of humerus
812.43 Closed fracture of medial condyle of humerus
812.44 Closed fracture of unspecified condyle(s) of humerus ▽
812.49 Other closed fracture of lower end of humerus
812.50 Open fracture of unspecified part of lower end of humerus ▽
812.51 Open fracture of supracondylar humerus
812.52 Open fracture of lateral condyle of humerus
812.53 Open fracture of medial condyle of humerus
812.54 Open fracture of unspecified condyle(s) of humerus ▽
812.59 Other open fracture of lower end of humerus
813.00 Unspecified fracture of radius and ulna, upper end of forearm, closed ▽
813.01 Closed fracture of olecranon process of ulna
813.02 Closed fracture of coronoid process of ulna
813.03 Closed Monteggia's fracture
813.04 Other and unspecified closed fractures of proximal end of ulna (alone) ▽
813.05 Closed fracture of head of radius
813.06 Closed fracture of neck of radius
813.07 Other and unspecified closed fractures of proximal end of radius (alone) ▽
813.08 Closed fracture of radius with ulna, upper end (any part)
813.10 Unspecified open fracture of upper end of forearm ▽
813.11 Open fracture of olecranon process of ulna
813.12 Open fracture of coronoid process of ulna
813.13 Open Monteggia's fracture
813.14 Other and unspecified open fractures of proximal end of ulna (alone) ▽
813.15 Open fracture of head of radius
813.16 Open fracture of neck of radius
813.17 Other and unspecified open fractures of proximal end of radius (alone) ▽
813.18 Open fracture of radius with ulna, upper end (any part)
832.00 Closed unspecified dislocation of elbow ▽
832.01 Closed anterior dislocation of elbow
832.02 Closed posterior dislocation of elbow
832.03 Closed medial dislocation of elbow
832.04 Closed lateral dislocation of elbow
832.09 Closed dislocation of other site of elbow
832.10 Open unspecified dislocation of elbow ▽
832.11 Open anterior dislocation of elbow
832.12 Open posterior dislocation of elbow
832.13 Open medial dislocation of elbow
832.14 Open lateral dislocation of elbow
832.19 Open dislocation of other site of elbow
841.0 Radial collateral ligament sprain and strain
841.1 Ulnar collateral ligament sprain and strain
841.2 Radiohumeral (joint) sprain and strain
841.3 Ulnohumeral (joint) sprain and strain
841.8 Sprain and strain of other specified sites of elbow and forearm
841.9 Sprain and strain of unspecified site of elbow and forearm ▽
880.23 Open wound of upper arm, with tendon involvement — (Use additional code to identify infection)
881.21 Open wound of elbow, with tendon involvement — (Use additional code to identify infection)
884.2 Multiple and unspecified open wound of upper limb, with tendon involvement — (Use additional code to identify infection)
927.11 Crushing injury of elbow — (Use additional code to identify any associated injuries: 800-829, 850.0-854.1, 860.0-869.1)

ICD-9-CM Procedural

81.96 Other repair of joint
83.81 Tendon graft

24350–24356

24350 Fasciotomy, lateral or medial (eg, tennis elbow or epicondylitis);
24351 with extensor origin detachment
24352 with annular ligament resection
24354 with stripping
24356 with partial ostectomy

ICD-9-CM Diagnostic

719.42 Pain in joint, upper arm
726.31 Medial epicondylitis of elbow
726.32 Lateral epicondylitis of elbow
726.39 Other enthesopathy of elbow region
726.90 Enthesopathy of unspecified site ▽
727.09 Other synovitis and tenosynovitis

ICD-9-CM Procedural

77.89 Other partial ostectomy of other bone, except facial bones
80.99 Other excision of joint of other specified site
83.14 Fasciotomy
83.82 Graft of muscle or fascia

24360

24360 Arthroplasty, elbow; with membrane (eg, fascial)

ICD-9-CM Diagnostic

357.1 Polyneuropathy in collagen vascular disease — (Code first underlying disease: 446.0, 710.0, 714.0) ☒
359.6 Symptomatic inflammatory myopathy in diseases classified elsewhere — (Code first underlying disease: 135, 140.0-208.9, 277.3, 446.0, 710.0, 710.1, 710.2, 714.0) ☒
446.0 Polyarteritis nodosa
710.0 Systemic lupus erythematosus — (Use additional code to identify manifestation: 424.91, 581.81, 582.81, 583.81)
710.1 Systemic sclerosis — (Use additional code to identify manifestation: 359.6, 517.2)
710.2 Sicca syndrome
711.02 Pyogenic arthritis, upper arm — (Use additional code to identify infectious organism: 041.0-041.8)
711.92 Unspecified infective arthritis, upper arm ▽
714.0 Rheumatoid arthritis — (Use additional code to identify manifestation: 357.1, 359.6)
715.12 Primary localized osteoarthrosis, upper arm
715.32 Localized osteoarthrosis not specified whether primary or secondary, upper arm
716.12 Traumatic arthropathy, upper arm
716.22 Allergic arthritis, upper arm
716.62 Unspecified monoarthritis, upper arm ▽
719.42 Pain in joint, upper arm
730.12 Chronic osteomyelitis, upper arm — (Use additional code to identify organism, 041.1)
730.22 Unspecified osteomyelitis, upper arm — (Use additional code to identify organism, 041.1) ▽
730.32 Periostitis, without mention of osteomyelitis, upper arm — (Use additional code to identify organism, 041.1)
730.82 Other infections involving bone diseases classified elsewhere, upper arm — (Code first underlying disease: 002.0, 015.0-015.9. Use additional code to identify organism) ☒
731.0 Osteitis deformans without mention of bone tumor
733.49 Aseptic necrosis of other bone site
733.82 Nonunion of fracture
736.00 Unspecified deformity of forearm, excluding fingers ▽
754.89 Other specified nonteratogenic anomalies
756.51 Osteogenesis imperfecta
812.40 Closed fracture of unspecified part of lower end of humerus ▽
812.41 Closed fracture of supracondylar humerus
812.42 Closed fracture of lateral condyle of humerus
812.43 Closed fracture of medial condyle of humerus
812.44 Closed fracture of unspecified condyle(s) of humerus ▽
812.49 Other closed fracture of lower end of humerus
812.50 Open fracture of unspecified part of lower end of humerus ▽
812.51 Open fracture of supracondylar humerus
812.52 Open fracture of lateral condyle of humerus
812.53 Open fracture of medial condyle of humerus
812.54 Open fracture of unspecified condyle(s) of humerus ▽
812.59 Other open fracture of lower end of humerus
813.00 Unspecified fracture of radius and ulna, upper end of forearm, closed ▽
813.02 Closed fracture of coronoid process of ulna
813.03 Closed Monteggia's fracture
813.04 Other and unspecified closed fractures of proximal end of ulna (alone) ▽
813.05 Closed fracture of head of radius
813.06 Closed fracture of neck of radius
813.07 Other and unspecified closed fractures of proximal end of radius (alone) ▽
813.08 Closed fracture of radius with ulna, upper end (any part)
813.10 Unspecified open fracture of upper end of forearm ▽
813.11 Open fracture of olecranon process of ulna
813.12 Open fracture of coronoid process of ulna
813.13 Open Monteggia's fracture
813.14 Other and unspecified open fractures of proximal end of ulna (alone) ▽
813.15 Open fracture of head of radius
813.16 Open fracture of neck of radius
813.17 Other and unspecified open fractures of proximal end of radius (alone) ▽
813.18 Open fracture of radius with ulna, upper end (any part)

▽ Unspecified code ☒ Manifestation code
♀ Female diagnosis ♂ Male diagnosis

ICD-9-CM Procedural
81.85 Other repair of elbow

24361–24362
24361 Arthroplasty, elbow; with distal humeral prosthetic replacement
24362 with implant and fascia lata ligament reconstruction

ICD-9-CM Diagnostic
357.1 Polyneuropathy in collagen vascular disease — (Code first underlying disease: 446.0, 710.0, 714.0) ☒
359.6 Symptomatic inflammatory myopathy in diseases classified elsewhere — (Code first underlying disease: 135, 140.0-208.9, 277.3, 446.0, 710.0, 710.1, 710.2, 714.0) ☒
446.0 Polyarteritis nodosa
710.0 Systemic lupus erythematosus — (Use additional code to identify manifestation: 424.91, 581.81, 582.81, 583.81)
710.1 Systemic sclerosis — (Use additional code to identify manifestation: 359.6, 517.2)
710.2 Sicca syndrome
711.02 Pyogenic arthritis, upper arm — (Use additional code to identify infectious organism: 041.0-041.8)
711.92 Unspecified infective arthritis, upper arm ▽
714.0 Rheumatoid arthritis — (Use additional code to identify manifestation: 357.1, 359.6)
715.12 Primary localized osteoarthrosis, upper arm
715.32 Localized osteoarthrosis not specified whether primary or secondary, upper arm
716.12 Traumatic arthropathy, upper arm
716.22 Allergic arthritis, upper arm
716.62 Unspecified monoarthritis, upper arm ▽
719.22 Villonodular synovitis, upper arm
719.42 Pain in joint, upper arm
730.12 Chronic osteomyelitis, upper arm — (Use additional code to identify organism, 041.1)
730.22 Unspecified osteomyelitis, upper arm — (Use additional code to identify organism, 041.1) ▽
730.32 Periostitis, without mention of osteomyelitis, upper arm — (Use additional code to identify organism, 041.1)
730.82 Other infections involving bone diseases classified elsewhere, upper arm — (Code first underlying disease: 002.0, 015.0-015.9. Use additional code to identify organism) ☒
731.0 Osteitis deformans without mention of bone tumor
733.49 Aseptic necrosis of other bone site
733.82 Nonunion of fracture
736.00 Unspecified deformity of forearm, excluding fingers ▽
754.89 Other specified nonteratogenic anomalies
756.51 Osteogenesis imperfecta

ICD-9-CM Procedural
81.85 Other repair of elbow

24363
24363 Arthroplasty, elbow; with distal humerus and proximal ulnar prosthetic replacement (eg, total elbow)

ICD-9-CM Diagnostic
357.1 Polyneuropathy in collagen vascular disease — (Code first underlying disease: 446.0, 710.0, 714.0) ☒
359.6 Symptomatic inflammatory myopathy in diseases classified elsewhere — (Code first underlying disease: 135, 140.0-208.9, 277.3, 446.0, 710.0, 710.1, 710.2, 714.0) ☒
446.0 Polyarteritis nodosa
710.0 Systemic lupus erythematosus — (Use additional code to identify manifestation: 424.91, 581.81, 582.81, 583.81)
710.1 Systemic sclerosis — (Use additional code to identify manifestation: 359.6, 517.2)
710.2 Sicca syndrome
711.02 Pyogenic arthritis, upper arm — (Use additional code to identify infectious organism: 041.0-041.8)
711.92 Unspecified infective arthritis, upper arm ▽
714.0 Rheumatoid arthritis — (Use additional code to identify manifestation: 357.1, 359.6)
715.12 Primary localized osteoarthrosis, upper arm
715.32 Localized osteoarthrosis not specified whether primary or secondary, upper arm
716.12 Traumatic arthropathy, upper arm
716.22 Allergic arthritis, upper arm
716.62 Unspecified monoarthritis, upper arm ▽
719.22 Villonodular synovitis, upper arm
719.42 Pain in joint, upper arm
730.12 Chronic osteomyelitis, upper arm — (Use additional code to identify organism, 041.1)
730.22 Unspecified osteomyelitis, upper arm — (Use additional code to identify organism, 041.1) ▽
730.32 Periostitis, without mention of osteomyelitis, upper arm — (Use additional code to identify organism, 041.1)
730.82 Other infections involving bone diseases classified elsewhere, upper arm — (Code first underlying disease: 002.0, 015.0-015.9. Use additional code to identify organism) ☒
731.0 Osteitis deformans without mention of bone tumor
733.49 Aseptic necrosis of other bone site
733.82 Nonunion of fracture
736.00 Unspecified deformity of forearm, excluding fingers ▽
754.89 Other specified nonteratogenic anomalies
756.51 Osteogenesis imperfecta

ICD-9-CM Procedural
81.84 Total elbow replacement

24365–24366
24365 Arthroplasty, radial head;
24366 with implant

ICD-9-CM Diagnostic
357.1 Polyneuropathy in collagen vascular disease — (Code first underlying disease: 446.0, 710.0, 714.0) ☒
359.6 Symptomatic inflammatory myopathy in diseases classified elsewhere — (Code first underlying disease: 135, 140.0-208.9, 277.3, 446.0, 710.0, 710.1, 710.2, 714.0) ☒
446.0 Polyarteritis nodosa
710.0 Systemic lupus erythematosus — (Use additional code to identify manifestation: 424.91, 581.81, 582.81, 583.81)
710.1 Systemic sclerosis — (Use additional code to identify manifestation: 359.6, 517.2)
710.2 Sicca syndrome
711.02 Pyogenic arthritis, upper arm — (Use additional code to identify infectious organism: 041.0-041.8)
711.92 Unspecified infective arthritis, upper arm ▽
714.0 Rheumatoid arthritis — (Use additional code to identify manifestation: 357.1, 359.6)
715.00 Generalized osteoarthrosis, unspecified site ▽
715.12 Primary localized osteoarthrosis, upper arm
715.32 Localized osteoarthrosis not specified whether primary or secondary, upper arm
716.12 Traumatic arthropathy, upper arm
716.22 Allergic arthritis, upper arm
716.62 Unspecified monoarthritis, upper arm ▽
718.82 Other joint derangement, not elsewhere classified, upper arm
719.22 Villonodular synovitis, upper arm
719.42 Pain in joint, upper arm
719.52 Stiffness of joint, not elsewhere classified, upper arm
730.12 Chronic osteomyelitis, upper arm — (Use additional code to identify organism, 041.1)
730.22 Unspecified osteomyelitis, upper arm — (Use additional code to identify organism, 041.1) ▽
730.32 Periostitis, without mention of osteomyelitis, upper arm — (Use additional code to identify organism, 041.1)
730.82 Other infections involving bone diseases classified elsewhere, upper arm — (Code first underlying disease: 002.0, 015.0-015.9. Use additional code to identify organism) ☒
731.0 Osteitis deformans without mention of bone tumor
733.49 Aseptic necrosis of other bone site
733.82 Nonunion of fracture
736.00 Unspecified deformity of forearm, excluding fingers ▽
756.51 Osteogenesis imperfecta

ICD-9-CM Procedural
81.85 Other repair of elbow

▽ Unspecified code ♀ Female diagnosis ☒ Manifestation code ♂ Male diagnosis

24400

24400 Osteotomy, humerus, with or without internal fixation

ICD-9-CM Diagnostic

170.4 Malignant neoplasm of scapula and long bones of upper limb
213.4 Benign neoplasm of scapula and long bones of upper limb
715.10 Primary localized osteoarthrosis, specified site
715.22 Secondary localized osteoarthrosis, upper arm
715.32 Localized osteoarthrosis not specified whether primary or secondary, upper arm
730.12 Chronic osteomyelitis, upper arm — (Use additional code to identify organism, 041.1)
733.11 Pathologic fracture of humerus
733.41 Aseptic necrosis of head of humerus
733.81 Malunion of fracture
733.82 Nonunion of fracture
736.89 Other acquired deformity of other parts of limb
756.4 Chondrodystrophy
756.51 Osteogenesis imperfecta
812.21 Closed fracture of shaft of humerus
812.31 Open fracture of shaft of humerus
812.49 Other closed fracture of lower end of humerus

ICD-9-CM Procedural

77.22 Wedge osteotomy of humerus
77.32 Other division of humerus

24410

24410 Multiple osteotomies with realignment on intramedullary rod, humeral shaft (Sofield type procedure)

ICD-9-CM Diagnostic

170.4 Malignant neoplasm of scapula and long bones of upper limb
213.4 Benign neoplasm of scapula and long bones of upper limb
715.12 Primary localized osteoarthrosis, upper arm
715.22 Secondary localized osteoarthrosis, upper arm
715.32 Localized osteoarthrosis not specified whether primary or secondary, upper arm
730.12 Chronic osteomyelitis, upper arm — (Use additional code to identify organism, 041.1)
733.11 Pathologic fracture of humerus
733.41 Aseptic necrosis of head of humerus
733.81 Malunion of fracture
733.82 Nonunion of fracture
736.89 Other acquired deformity of other parts of limb
756.4 Chondrodystrophy
756.51 Osteogenesis imperfecta
V54.02 Encounter for lengthening/adjustment of growth rod

ICD-9-CM Procedural

77.32 Other division of humerus

24420

24420 Osteoplasty, humerus (eg, shortening or lengthening) (excluding 64876)

ICD-9-CM Diagnostic

170.4 Malignant neoplasm of scapula and long bones of upper limb
198.5 Secondary malignant neoplasm of bone and bone marrow
213.4 Benign neoplasm of scapula and long bones of upper limb
715.10 Primary localized osteoarthrosis, specified site
715.22 Secondary localized osteoarthrosis, upper arm
715.31 Localized osteoarthrosis not specified whether primary or secondary, shoulder region
715.32 Localized osteoarthrosis not specified whether primary or secondary, upper arm
730.12 Chronic osteomyelitis, upper arm — (Use additional code to identify organism, 041.1)
733.41 Aseptic necrosis of head of humerus
733.81 Malunion of fracture
733.82 Nonunion of fracture
736.89 Other acquired deformity of other parts of limb
756.4 Chondrodystrophy
756.51 Osteogenesis imperfecta

ICD-9-CM Procedural

77.32 Other division of humerus
78.12 Application of external fixation device, humerus
78.22 Limb shortening procedures, humerus
78.32 Limb lengthening procedures, humerus
84.53 Implantation of internal limb lengthening device with kinetic distraction
84.54 Implantation of other internal limb lengthening device

24430–24435

24430 Repair of nonunion or malunion, humerus; without graft (eg, compression technique)
24435 with iliac or other autograft (includes obtaining graft)

ICD-9-CM Diagnostic

733.81 Malunion of fracture
733.82 Nonunion of fracture

ICD-9-CM Procedural

77.79 Excision of other bone for graft, except facial bones
78.02 Bone graft of humerus
78.42 Other repair or plastic operation on humerus

24470

24470 Hemiepiphyseal arrest (eg, cubitus varus or valgus, distal humerus)

ICD-9-CM Diagnostic

268.1 Rickets, late effect — (Use additional code to identify the nature of late effect)
736.01 Cubitus valgus (acquired)
736.02 Cubitus varus (acquired)
755.59 Other congenital anomaly of upper limb, including shoulder girdle

ICD-9-CM Procedural

78.42 Other repair or plastic operation on humerus

24495

24495 Decompression fasciotomy, forearm, with brachial artery exploration

ICD-9-CM Diagnostic

682.3 Cellulitis and abscess of upper arm and forearm — (Use additional code to identify organism)
728.88 Rhabdomyolysis
813.21 Closed fracture of shaft of radius (alone)
813.22 Closed fracture of shaft of ulna (alone)
813.23 Closed fracture of shaft of radius with ulna
813.31 Open fracture of shaft of radius (alone)
813.32 Open fracture of shaft of ulna (alone)
813.33 Open fracture of shaft of radius with ulna
813.80 Closed fracture of unspecified part of forearm
813.90 Open fracture of unspecified part of forearm
832.00 Closed unspecified dislocation of elbow
832.10 Open unspecified dislocation of elbow
881.01 Open wound of elbow, without mention of complication — (Use additional code to identify infection)
881.10 Open wound of forearm, complicated — (Use additional code to identify infection)
881.11 Open wound of elbow, complicated — (Use additional code to identify infection)
881.20 Open wound of forearm, with tendon involvement — (Use additional code to identify infection)
903.1 Brachial blood vessels injury
923.10 Contusion of forearm
923.11 Contusion of elbow
927.10 Crushing injury of forearm — (Use additional code to identify any associated injuries: 800-829, 850.0-854.1, 860.0-869.1)
927.11 Crushing injury of elbow — (Use additional code to identify any associated injuries: 800-829, 850.0-854.1, 860.0-869.1)
958.8 Other early complications of trauma

ICD-9-CM Procedural

83.14 Fasciotomy

24498

24498 Prophylactic treatment (nailing, pinning, plating or wiring), with or without methylmethacrylate, humeral shaft

ICD-9-CM Diagnostic

170.4 Malignant neoplasm of scapula and long bones of upper limb
198.5 Secondary malignant neoplasm of bone and bone marrow
213.4 Benign neoplasm of scapula and long bones of upper limb
238.0 Neoplasm of uncertain behavior of bone and articular cartilage

239.2 Neoplasms of unspecified nature of bone, soft tissue, and skin
732.3 Juvenile osteochondrosis of upper extremity
733.11 Pathologic fracture of humerus
756.4 Chondrodystrophy
756.51 Osteogenesis imperfecta

ICD-9-CM Procedural

78.52 Internal fixation of humerus without fracture reduction
84.55 Insertion of bone void filler

24500–24505

24500 Closed treatment of humeral shaft fracture; without manipulation
24505 with manipulation, with or without skeletal traction

ICD-9-CM Diagnostic

733.11 Pathologic fracture of humerus
812.21 Closed fracture of shaft of humerus

ICD-9-CM Procedural

79.01 Closed reduction of fracture of humerus without internal fixation
93.43 Intermittent skeletal traction
93.44 Other skeletal traction
93.53 Application of other cast
93.54 Application of splint

HCPCS Level II Supplies & Services

A4565 Slings
A4570 Splint
A4580 Cast supplies (e.g., plaster)
A4590 Special casting material (e.g., fiberglass)

24515–24516

24515 Open treatment of humeral shaft fracture with plate/screws, with or without cerclage
24516 Treatment of humeral shaft fracture, with insertion of intramedullary implant, with or without cerclage and/or locking screws

ICD-9-CM Diagnostic

733.11 Pathologic fracture of humerus
812.21 Closed fracture of shaft of humerus
812.31 Open fracture of shaft of humerus

ICD-9-CM Procedural

79.21 Open reduction of fracture of humerus without internal fixation
79.31 Open reduction of fracture of humerus with internal fixation

24530–24535

24530 Closed treatment of supracondylar or transcondylar humeral fracture, with or without intercondylar extension; without manipulation
24535 with manipulation, with or without skin or skeletal traction

ICD-9-CM Diagnostic

733.11 Pathologic fracture of humerus
812.40 Closed fracture of unspecified part of lower end of humerus ▽
812.41 Closed fracture of supracondylar humerus
812.42 Closed fracture of lateral condyle of humerus
812.43 Closed fracture of medial condyle of humerus
812.44 Closed fracture of unspecified condyle(s) of humerus ▽
812.49 Other closed fracture of lower end of humerus

ICD-9-CM Procedural

79.01 Closed reduction of fracture of humerus without internal fixation
79.11 Closed reduction of fracture of humerus with internal fixation
93.43 Intermittent skeletal traction
93.44 Other skeletal traction
93.46 Other skin traction of limbs
93.53 Application of other cast
93.54 Application of splint

HCPCS Level II Supplies & Services

A4570 Splint
A4580 Cast supplies (e.g., plaster)
L3700 EO, elastic with stays, prefabricated, includes fitting and adjustment
L3710 EO, elastic with metal joints, prefabricated, includes fitting and adjustment
L3720 EO, double upright with forearm/arm cuffs, free motion, custom fabricated

24538

24538 Percutaneous skeletal fixation of supracondylar or transcondylar humeral fracture, with or without intercondylar extension

ICD-9-CM Diagnostic

733.11 Pathologic fracture of humerus
812.20 Closed fracture of unspecified part of humerus ▽
812.40 Closed fracture of unspecified part of lower end of humerus ▽
812.41 Closed fracture of supracondylar humerus
812.42 Closed fracture of lateral condyle of humerus
812.43 Closed fracture of medial condyle of humerus
812.49 Other closed fracture of lower end of humerus
812.50 Open fracture of unspecified part of lower end of humerus ▽
812.51 Open fracture of supracondylar humerus
812.52 Open fracture of lateral condyle of humerus
812.53 Open fracture of medial condyle of humerus
812.54 Open fracture of unspecified condyle(s) of humerus ▽
812.59 Other open fracture of lower end of humerus

ICD-9-CM Procedural

79.31 Open reduction of fracture of humerus with internal fixation

HCPCS Level II Supplies & Services

A4565 Slings
A4580 Cast supplies (e.g., plaster)
A4590 Special casting material (e.g., fiberglass)
L3700 EO, elastic with stays, prefabricated, includes fitting and adjustment
L3710 EO, elastic with metal joints, prefabricated, includes fitting and adjustment

24545–24546

24545 Open treatment of humeral supracondylar or transcondylar fracture, with or without internal or external fixation; without intercondylar extension
24546 with intercondylar extension

ICD-9-CM Diagnostic

733.11 Pathologic fracture of humerus
812.40 Closed fracture of unspecified part of lower end of humerus ▽
812.41 Closed fracture of supracondylar humerus
812.42 Closed fracture of lateral condyle of humerus
812.43 Closed fracture of medial condyle of humerus
812.49 Other closed fracture of lower end of humerus
812.50 Open fracture of unspecified part of lower end of humerus ▽
812.51 Open fracture of supracondylar humerus
812.52 Open fracture of lateral condyle of humerus
812.53 Open fracture of medial condyle of humerus
812.54 Open fracture of unspecified condyle(s) of humerus ▽
812.59 Other open fracture of lower end of humerus

ICD-9-CM Procedural

78.12 Application of external fixation device, humerus
79.21 Open reduction of fracture of humerus without internal fixation
79.31 Open reduction of fracture of humerus with internal fixation

24560–24565

24560 Closed treatment of humeral epicondylar fracture, medial or lateral; without manipulation
24565 with manipulation

ICD-9-CM Diagnostic

812.40 Closed fracture of unspecified part of lower end of humerus ▽
812.42 Closed fracture of lateral condyle of humerus
812.43 Closed fracture of medial condyle of humerus
812.44 Closed fracture of unspecified condyle(s) of humerus ▽
812.49 Other closed fracture of lower end of humerus

ICD-9-CM Procedural

79.01 Closed reduction of fracture of humerus without internal fixation
93.54 Application of splint

HCPCS Level II Supplies & Services

A4570 Splint
A4580 Cast supplies (e.g., plaster)

▽ Unspecified code ♀ Female diagnosis ☒ Manifestation code ♂ Male diagnosis

24566

24566 Percutaneous skeletal fixation of humeral epicondylar fracture, medial or lateral, with manipulation

ICD-9-CM Diagnostic

812.40 Closed fracture of unspecified part of lower end of humerus
812.42 Closed fracture of lateral condyle of humerus
812.43 Closed fracture of medial condyle of humerus
812.44 Closed fracture of unspecified condyle(s) of humerus
812.49 Other closed fracture of lower end of humerus
812.50 Open fracture of unspecified part of lower end of humerus
812.52 Open fracture of lateral condyle of humerus
812.53 Open fracture of medial condyle of humerus
812.54 Open fracture of unspecified condyle(s) of humerus
812.59 Other open fracture of lower end of humerus

ICD-9-CM Procedural

79.11 Closed reduction of fracture of humerus with internal fixation

HCPCS Level II Supplies & Services

A4305 Disposable drug delivery system, flow rate of 50 ml or greater per hour
A4306 Disposable drug delivery system, flow rate of 5 ml or less per hour
A4550 Surgical trays

24575

24575 Open treatment of humeral epicondylar fracture, medial or lateral, with or without internal or external fixation

ICD-9-CM Diagnostic

812.40 Closed fracture of unspecified part of lower end of humerus
812.42 Closed fracture of lateral condyle of humerus
812.43 Closed fracture of medial condyle of humerus
812.49 Other closed fracture of lower end of humerus
812.50 Open fracture of unspecified part of lower end of humerus
812.52 Open fracture of lateral condyle of humerus
812.53 Open fracture of medial condyle of humerus
812.54 Open fracture of unspecified condyle(s) of humerus
812.59 Other open fracture of lower end of humerus

ICD-9-CM Procedural

78.12 Application of external fixation device, humerus
79.21 Open reduction of fracture of humerus without internal fixation
79.31 Open reduction of fracture of humerus with internal fixation

24576–24577

24576 Closed treatment of humeral condylar fracture, medial or lateral; without manipulation
24577 with manipulation

ICD-9-CM Diagnostic

812.40 Closed fracture of unspecified part of lower end of humerus
812.41 Closed fracture of supracondylar humerus
812.42 Closed fracture of lateral condyle of humerus
812.43 Closed fracture of medial condyle of humerus
812.44 Closed fracture of unspecified condyle(s) of humerus
812.49 Other closed fracture of lower end of humerus

ICD-9-CM Procedural

79.01 Closed reduction of fracture of humerus without internal fixation
93.54 Application of splint

HCPCS Level II Supplies & Services

A4570 Splint
A4580 Cast supplies (e.g., plaster)

24579

24579 Open treatment of humeral condylar fracture, medial or lateral, with or without internal or external fixation

ICD-9-CM Diagnostic

812.40 Closed fracture of unspecified part of lower end of humerus
812.42 Closed fracture of lateral condyle of humerus
812.43 Closed fracture of medial condyle of humerus
812.44 Closed fracture of unspecified condyle(s) of humerus
812.49 Other closed fracture of lower end of humerus
812.50 Open fracture of unspecified part of lower end of humerus
812.52 Open fracture of lateral condyle of humerus
812.53 Open fracture of medial condyle of humerus
812.54 Open fracture of unspecified condyle(s) of humerus
812.59 Other open fracture of lower end of humerus

ICD-9-CM Procedural

78.12 Application of external fixation device, humerus
79.21 Open reduction of fracture of humerus without internal fixation
79.31 Open reduction of fracture of humerus with internal fixation

24582

24582 Percutaneous skeletal fixation of humeral condylar fracture, medial or lateral, with manipulation

ICD-9-CM Diagnostic

812.40 Closed fracture of unspecified part of lower end of humerus
812.42 Closed fracture of lateral condyle of humerus
812.43 Closed fracture of medial condyle of humerus
812.44 Closed fracture of unspecified condyle(s) of humerus
812.49 Other closed fracture of lower end of humerus
812.50 Open fracture of unspecified part of lower end of humerus
812.52 Open fracture of lateral condyle of humerus
812.53 Open fracture of medial condyle of humerus
812.54 Open fracture of unspecified condyle(s) of humerus
812.59 Other open fracture of lower end of humerus

ICD-9-CM Procedural

79.11 Closed reduction of fracture of humerus with internal fixation

HCPCS Level II Supplies & Services

A4570 Splint
A4580 Cast supplies (e.g., plaster)

24586–24587

24586 Open treatment of periarticular fracture and/or dislocation of the elbow (fracture distal humerus and proximal ulna and/or proximal radius);
24587 with implant arthroplasty

ICD-9-CM Diagnostic

718.72 Developmental dislocation of joint, upper arm
812.40 Closed fracture of unspecified part of lower end of humerus
812.41 Closed fracture of supracondylar humerus
812.42 Closed fracture of lateral condyle of humerus
812.43 Closed fracture of medial condyle of humerus
812.44 Closed fracture of unspecified condyle(s) of humerus
812.49 Other closed fracture of lower end of humerus
812.50 Open fracture of unspecified part of lower end of humerus
812.51 Open fracture of supracondylar humerus
812.52 Open fracture of lateral condyle of humerus
812.53 Open fracture of medial condyle of humerus
812.54 Open fracture of unspecified condyle(s) of humerus
812.59 Other open fracture of lower end of humerus
813.00 Unspecified fracture of radius and ulna, upper end of forearm, closed
813.01 Closed fracture of olecranon process of ulna
813.02 Closed fracture of coronoid process of ulna
813.04 Other and unspecified closed fractures of proximal end of ulna (alone)
813.05 Closed fracture of head of radius
813.06 Closed fracture of neck of radius
813.07 Other and unspecified closed fractures of proximal end of radius (alone)
813.08 Closed fracture of radius with ulna, upper end (any part)
813.10 Unspecified open fracture of upper end of forearm
813.11 Open fracture of olecranon process of ulna
813.12 Open fracture of coronoid process of ulna
813.14 Other and unspecified open fractures of proximal end of ulna (alone)
813.15 Open fracture of head of radius
813.17 Other and unspecified open fractures of proximal end of radius (alone)
813.18 Open fracture of radius with ulna, upper end (any part)
832.01 Closed anterior dislocation of elbow
832.02 Closed posterior dislocation of elbow
832.03 Closed medial dislocation of elbow
832.04 Closed lateral dislocation of elbow
832.09 Closed dislocation of other site of elbow
832.10 Open unspecified dislocation of elbow
832.11 Open anterior dislocation of elbow
832.12 Open posterior dislocation of elbow
832.13 Open medial dislocation of elbow

832.14 Open lateral dislocation of elbow
832.19 Open dislocation of other site of elbow

ICD-9-CM Procedural

79.21 Open reduction of fracture of humerus without internal fixation
79.32 Open reduction of fracture of radius and ulna with internal fixation
79.82 Open reduction of dislocation of elbow
81.84 Total elbow replacement

24600–24605

24600 Treatment of closed elbow dislocation; without anesthesia
24605 requiring anesthesia

ICD-9-CM Diagnostic

718.72 Developmental dislocation of joint, upper arm
832.00 Closed unspecified dislocation of elbow ▽
832.01 Closed anterior dislocation of elbow
832.02 Closed posterior dislocation of elbow
832.03 Closed medial dislocation of elbow
832.04 Closed lateral dislocation of elbow
832.09 Closed dislocation of other site of elbow

ICD-9-CM Procedural

79.72 Closed reduction of dislocation of elbow

HCPCS Level II Supplies & Services

A4570 Splint
A4580 Cast supplies (e.g., plaster)
A4590 Special casting material (e.g., fiberglass)
L3700 EO, elastic with stays, prefabricated, includes fitting and adjustment
L3710 EO, elastic with metal joints, prefabricated, includes fitting and adjustment

24615

24615 Open treatment of acute or chronic elbow dislocation

ICD-9-CM Diagnostic

718.32 Recurrent dislocation of upper arm joint
718.72 Developmental dislocation of joint, upper arm
754.89 Other specified nonteratogenic anomalies
832.01 Closed anterior dislocation of elbow
832.02 Closed posterior dislocation of elbow
832.03 Closed medial dislocation of elbow
832.04 Closed lateral dislocation of elbow
832.09 Closed dislocation of other site of elbow
832.10 Open unspecified dislocation of elbow ▽
832.11 Open anterior dislocation of elbow
832.12 Open posterior dislocation of elbow
832.13 Open medial dislocation of elbow
832.14 Open lateral dislocation of elbow
832.19 Open dislocation of other site of elbow

ICD-9-CM Procedural

79.82 Open reduction of dislocation of elbow

24620

24620 Closed treatment of Monteggia type of fracture dislocation at elbow (fracture proximal end of ulna with dislocation of radial head), with manipulation

ICD-9-CM Diagnostic

813.03 Closed Monteggia's fracture

ICD-9-CM Procedural

79.02 Closed reduction of fracture of radius and ulna without internal fixation
79.72 Closed reduction of dislocation of elbow

HCPCS Level II Supplies & Services

A4570 Splint
A4580 Cast supplies (e.g., plaster)
A4590 Special casting material (e.g., fiberglass)
L3700 EO, elastic with stays, prefabricated, includes fitting and adjustment
L3710 EO, elastic with metal joints, prefabricated, includes fitting and adjustment

24635

24635 Open treatment of Monteggia type of fracture dislocation at elbow (fracture proximal end of ulna with dislocation of radial head), with or without internal or external fixation

ICD-9-CM Diagnostic

813.03 Closed Monteggia's fracture
813.13 Open Monteggia's fracture

ICD-9-CM Procedural

78.13 Application of external fixation device, radius and ulna
79.22 Open reduction of fracture of radius and ulna without internal fixation
79.32 Open reduction of fracture of radius and ulna with internal fixation
79.82 Open reduction of dislocation of elbow
81.85 Other repair of elbow

24640

24640 Closed treatment of radial head subluxation in child, nursemaid elbow, with manipulation

ICD-9-CM Diagnostic

832.01 Closed anterior dislocation of elbow
832.02 Closed posterior dislocation of elbow
832.03 Closed medial dislocation of elbow
832.04 Closed lateral dislocation of elbow
832.09 Closed dislocation of other site of elbow

ICD-9-CM Procedural

79.72 Closed reduction of dislocation of elbow

HCPCS Level II Supplies & Services

A4570 Splint
A4580 Cast supplies (e.g., plaster)
A4590 Special casting material (e.g., fiberglass)

24650–24655

24650 Closed treatment of radial head or neck fracture; without manipulation
24655 with manipulation

ICD-9-CM Diagnostic

813.05 Closed fracture of head of radius
813.06 Closed fracture of neck of radius
813.07 Other and unspecified closed fractures of proximal end of radius (alone) ▽

ICD-9-CM Procedural

79.02 Closed reduction of fracture of radius and ulna without internal fixation
93.54 Application of splint

HCPCS Level II Supplies & Services

A4570 Splint
A4580 Cast supplies (e.g., plaster)
L3700 EO, elastic with stays, prefabricated, includes fitting and adjustment
L3710 EO, elastic with metal joints, prefabricated, includes fitting and adjustment
L3720 EO, double upright with forearm/arm cuffs, free motion, custom fabricated

24665–24666

24665 Open treatment of radial head or neck fracture, with or without internal fixation or radial head excision;
24666 with radial head prosthetic replacement

ICD-9-CM Diagnostic

813.05 Closed fracture of head of radius
813.06 Closed fracture of neck of radius
813.07 Other and unspecified closed fractures of proximal end of radius (alone) ▽
813.15 Open fracture of head of radius
813.16 Open fracture of neck of radius
813.17 Other and unspecified open fractures of proximal end of radius (alone) ▽

ICD-9-CM Procedural

77.83 Other partial ostectomy of radius and ulna
79.22 Open reduction of fracture of radius and ulna without internal fixation
79.32 Open reduction of fracture of radius and ulna with internal fixation
81.85 Other repair of elbow

▽ Unspecified code ♀ Female diagnosis ☒ Manifestation code ♂ Male diagnosis

24670–24675

24670 Closed treatment of ulnar fracture, proximal end (olecranon process); without manipulation
24675 with manipulation

ICD-9-CM Diagnostic

813.01 Closed fracture of olecranon process of ulna
813.02 Closed fracture of coronoid process of ulna
813.04 Other and unspecified closed fractures of proximal end of ulna (alone) ▽

ICD-9-CM Procedural

79.02 Closed reduction of fracture of radius and ulna without internal fixation
93.54 Application of splint

HCPCS Level II Supplies & Services

A4570 Splint
A4580 Cast supplies (e.g., plaster)

24685

24685 Open treatment of ulnar fracture proximal end (olecranon process), with or without internal or external fixation

ICD-9-CM Diagnostic

813.01 Closed fracture of olecranon process of ulna
813.02 Closed fracture of coronoid process of ulna
813.04 Other and unspecified closed fractures of proximal end of ulna (alone) ▽
813.11 Open fracture of olecranon process of ulna
813.12 Open fracture of coronoid process of ulna
813.14 Other and unspecified open fractures of proximal end of ulna (alone) ▽

ICD-9-CM Procedural

78.13 Application of external fixation device, radius and ulna
79.22 Open reduction of fracture of radius and ulna without internal fixation
79.32 Open reduction of fracture of radius and ulna with internal fixation

24800–24802

24800 Arthrodesis, elbow joint; local
24802 with autogenous graft (includes obtaining graft)

ICD-9-CM Diagnostic

171.2 Malignant neoplasm of connective and other soft tissue of upper limb, including shoulder
198.5 Secondary malignant neoplasm of bone and bone marrow
238.0 Neoplasm of uncertain behavior of bone and articular cartilage
239.2 Neoplasms of unspecified nature of bone, soft tissue, and skin
357.1 Polyneuropathy in collagen vascular disease — (Code first underlying disease: 446.0, 710.0, 714.0) ☒
359.6 Symptomatic inflammatory myopathy in diseases classified elsewhere — (Code first underlying disease: 135, 140.0-208.9, 277.3, 446.0, 710.0, 710.1, 710.2, 714.0) ☒
446.0 Polyarteritis nodosa
710.0 Systemic lupus erythematosus — (Use additional code to identify manifestation: 424.91, 581.81, 582.81, 583.81)
710.1 Systemic sclerosis — (Use additional code to identify manifestation: 359.6, 517.2)
710.2 Sicca syndrome
711.02 Pyogenic arthritis, upper arm — (Use additional code to identify infectious organism: 041.0-041.8)
714.0 Rheumatoid arthritis — (Use additional code to identify manifestation: 357.1, 359.6)
714.1 Felty's syndrome
714.2 Other rheumatoid arthritis with visceral or systemic involvement
714.4 Chronic postrheumatic arthropathy
714.9 Unspecified inflammatory polyarthropathy ▽
715.12 Primary localized osteoarthrosis, upper arm
715.32 Localized osteoarthrosis not specified whether primary or secondary, upper arm
716.12 Traumatic arthropathy, upper arm
716.82 Other specified arthropathy, upper arm
716.92 Unspecified arthropathy, upper arm ▽
719.42 Pain in joint, upper arm
728.0 Infective myositis
728.10 Unspecified calcification and ossification ▽
728.11 Progressive myositis ossificans
728.12 Traumatic myositis ossificans
728.13 Postoperative heterotopic calcification
728.19 Other muscular calcification and ossification
728.3 Other specific muscle disorders
728.81 Interstitial myositis
730.12 Chronic osteomyelitis, upper arm — (Use additional code to identify organism, 041.1)

ICD-9-CM Procedural

81.24 Arthrodesis of elbow

24900–24920

24900 Amputation, arm through humerus; with primary closure
24920 open, circular (guillotine)

ICD-9-CM Diagnostic

170.4 Malignant neoplasm of scapula and long bones of upper limb
171.2 Malignant neoplasm of connective and other soft tissue of upper limb, including shoulder
198.5 Secondary malignant neoplasm of bone and bone marrow
250.70 Diabetes with peripheral circulatory disorders, type II or unspecified type, not stated as uncontrolled — (Use additional code to identify manifestation: 443.81, 785.4)
250.71 Diabetes with peripheral circulatory disorders, type I [juvenile type], not stated as uncontrolled — (Use additional code to identify manifestation: 443.81, 785.4)
440.24 Atherosclerosis of native arteries of the extremities with gangrene
443.81 Peripheral angiopathy in diseases classified elsewhere — (Code first underlying disease, 250.7) ☒
443.9 Unspecified peripheral vascular disease ▽
444.21 Embolism and thrombosis of arteries of upper extremity
445.01 Atheroembolism of upper extremity
446.0 Polyarteritis nodosa
728.86 Necrotizing fasciitis — (Use additional code to identify infectious organism, 041.00-041.89, 785.4, if applicable)
730.12 Chronic osteomyelitis, upper arm — (Use additional code to identify organism, 041.1)
731.1 Osteitis deformans in diseases classified elsewhere — (Code first underlying disease: 170.0-170.9) ☒
785.4 Gangrene — (Code first any associated underlying condition:250.7, 443.0)
812.49 Other closed fracture of lower end of humerus
812.59 Other open fracture of lower end of humerus
880.13 Open wound of upper arm, complicated — (Use additional code to identify infection)
880.23 Open wound of upper arm, with tendon involvement — (Use additional code to identify infection)
887.2 Traumatic amputation of arm and hand (complete) (partial), unilateral, at or above elbow, without mention of complication — (Use additional code to identify infection)
887.3 Traumatic amputation of arm and hand (complete) (partial), unilateral, at or above elbow, complicated — (Use additional code to identify infection)
887.6 Traumatic amputation of arm and hand (complete) (partial), bilateral (any level), without mention of complication — (Use additional code to identify infection)
887.7 Traumatic amputation of arm and hand (complete) (partial), bilateral (any level), complicated — (Use additional code to identify infection)
927.03 Crushing injury of upper arm — (Use additional code to identify any associated injuries: 800-829, 850.0-854.1, 860.0-869.1)
943.52 Deep necrosis of underlying tissues due to burn (deep third degree) of elbow, with loss of a body part
943.53 Deep necrosis of underlying tissues due to burn (deep third degree) of upper arm, with loss of upper a body part
996.94 Complications of reattached upper extremity, other and unspecified

ICD-9-CM Procedural

84.07 Amputation through humerus

24925

24925 Amputation, arm through humerus; secondary closure or scar revision

ICD-9-CM Diagnostic

250.70 Diabetes with peripheral circulatory disorders, type II or unspecified type, not stated as uncontrolled — (Use additional code to identify manifestation: 443.81, 785.4)
250.71 Diabetes with peripheral circulatory disorders, type I [juvenile type], not stated as uncontrolled — (Use additional code to identify manifestation: 443.81, 785.4)
440.24 Atherosclerosis of native arteries of the extremities with gangrene

443.81 Peripheral angiopathy in diseases classified elsewhere — (Code first underlying disease, 250.7) ☒
443.9 Unspecified peripheral vascular disease ▽
446.0 Polyarteritis nodosa
682.3 Cellulitis and abscess of upper arm and forearm — (Use additional code to identify organism)
707.00 Decubitus ulcer, unspecified site
707.01 Decubitus ulcer, elbow
707.09 Decubitus ulcer, other site
707.8 Chronic ulcer of other specified site
709.2 Scar condition and fibrosis of skin
728.86 Necrotizing fasciitis — (Use additional code to identify infectious organism, 041.00-041.89, 785.4, if applicable)
730.12 Chronic osteomyelitis, upper arm — (Use additional code to identify organism, 041.1)
785.4 Gangrene — (Code first any associated underlying condition:250.7, 443.0)
880.23 Open wound of upper arm, with tendon involvement — (Use additional code to identify infection)
997.60 Late complications of amputation stump, unspecified — (Use additional code to identify complications) ▽
997.61 Neuroma of amputation stump — (Use additional code to identify complications)
997.62 Infection (chronic) of amputation stump — (Use additional code to identify organism. Use additional code to identify complications)
997.69 Other late amputation stump complication — (Use additional code to identify complications)
998.83 Non-healing surgical wound
V51 Aftercare involving the use of plastic surgery
V58.41 Planned postoperative wound closure — (This code should be used in conjunction with other aftercare codes to fully identify the reason for the aftercare encounter)

ICD-9-CM Procedural

84.3 Revision of amputation stump

24930

24930 Amputation, arm through humerus; re-amputation

ICD-9-CM Diagnostic

785.4 Gangrene — (Code first any associated underlying condition:250.7, 443.0)
997.60 Late complications of amputation stump, unspecified — (Use additional code to identify complications) ▽
997.61 Neuroma of amputation stump — (Use additional code to identify complications)
997.62 Infection (chronic) of amputation stump — (Use additional code to identify organism. Use additional code to identify complications)
997.69 Other late amputation stump complication — (Use additional code to identify complications)
998.59 Other postoperative infection — (Use additional code to identify infection)
998.6 Persistent postoperative fistula, not elsewhere classified
998.83 Non-healing surgical wound
V49.66 Upper limb amputation, above elbow — (This code is intended for use when these conditions are recorded as diagnoses or problems)

ICD-9-CM Procedural

84.07 Amputation through humerus
84.3 Revision of amputation stump

24931

24931 Amputation, arm through humerus; with implant

ICD-9-CM Diagnostic

170.4 Malignant neoplasm of scapula and long bones of upper limb
171.2 Malignant neoplasm of connective and other soft tissue of upper limb, including shoulder
198.5 Secondary malignant neoplasm of bone and bone marrow
440.24 Atherosclerosis of native arteries of the extremities with gangrene
443.9 Unspecified peripheral vascular disease ▽
444.21 Embolism and thrombosis of arteries of upper extremity
445.01 Atheroembolism of upper extremity
728.86 Necrotizing fasciitis — (Use additional code to identify infectious organism, 041.00-041.89, 785.4, if applicable)
785.4 Gangrene — (Code first any associated underlying condition:250.7, 443.0)
812.49 Other closed fracture of lower end of humerus
812.59 Other open fracture of lower end of humerus
880.13 Open wound of upper arm, complicated — (Use additional code to identify infection)
880.23 Open wound of upper arm, with tendon involvement — (Use additional code to identify infection)
887.2 Traumatic amputation of arm and hand (complete) (partial), unilateral, at or above elbow, without mention of complication — (Use additional code to identify infection)
887.3 Traumatic amputation of arm and hand (complete) (partial), unilateral, at or above elbow, complicated — (Use additional code to identify infection)
887.6 Traumatic amputation of arm and hand (complete) (partial), bilateral (any level), without mention of complication — (Use additional code to identify infection)
887.7 Traumatic amputation of arm and hand (complete) (partial), bilateral (any level), complicated — (Use additional code to identify infection)
927.03 Crushing injury of upper arm — (Use additional code to identify any associated injuries: 800-829, 850.0-854.1, 860.0-869.1)
943.52 Deep necrosis of underlying tissues due to burn (deep third degree) of elbow, with loss of a body part
943.53 Deep necrosis of underlying tissues due to burn (deep third degree) of upper arm, with loss of upper a body part
996.94 Complications of reattached upper extremity, other and unspecified

ICD-9-CM Procedural

81.96 Other repair of joint
84.07 Amputation through humerus
84.44 Implantation of prosthetic device of arm

24935

24935 Stump elongation, upper extremity

ICD-9-CM Diagnostic

V51 Aftercare involving the use of plastic surgery
V58.49 Other specified aftercare following surgery — (This code should be used in conjunction with other aftercare codes to fully identify the reason for the aftercare encounter)

ICD-9-CM Procedural

77.77 Excision of tibia and fibula for graft
77.79 Excision of other bone for graft, except facial bones
78.02 Bone graft of humerus
78.03 Bone graft of radius and ulna
78.32 Limb lengthening procedures, humerus
78.33 Limb lengthening procedures, radius and ulna

24940

24940 Cineplasty, upper extremity, complete procedure

ICD-9-CM Diagnostic

170.4 Malignant neoplasm of scapula and long bones of upper limb
170.5 Malignant neoplasm of short bones of upper limb
171.2 Malignant neoplasm of connective and other soft tissue of upper limb, including shoulder
198.5 Secondary malignant neoplasm of bone and bone marrow
250.70 Diabetes with peripheral circulatory disorders, type II or unspecified type, not stated as uncontrolled — (Use additional code to identify manifestation: 443.81, 785.4)
250.71 Diabetes with peripheral circulatory disorders, type I [juvenile type], not stated as uncontrolled — (Use additional code to identify manifestation: 443.81, 785.4)
440.24 Atherosclerosis of native arteries of the extremities with gangrene
443.81 Peripheral angiopathy in diseases classified elsewhere — (Code first underlying disease, 250.7) ☒
443.9 Unspecified peripheral vascular disease ▽
444.21 Embolism and thrombosis of arteries of upper extremity
445.01 Atheroembolism of upper extremity
446.0 Polyarteritis nodosa
728.86 Necrotizing fasciitis — (Use additional code to identify infectious organism, 041.00-041.89, 785.4, if applicable)
730.12 Chronic osteomyelitis, upper arm — (Use additional code to identify organism, 041.1)
731.1 Osteitis deformans in diseases classified elsewhere — (Code first underlying disease: 170.0-170.9) ☒
785.4 Gangrene — (Code first any associated underlying condition:250.7, 443.0)
812.49 Other closed fracture of lower end of humerus
812.59 Other open fracture of lower end of humerus

▽ Unspecified code
♀ Female diagnosis
☒ Manifestation code
♂ Male diagnosis

880.13 Open wound of upper arm, complicated — (Use additional code to identify infection)
880.23 Open wound of upper arm, with tendon involvement — (Use additional code to identify infection)
887.2 Traumatic amputation of arm and hand (complete) (partial), unilateral, at or above elbow, without mention of complication — (Use additional code to identify infection)
887.3 Traumatic amputation of arm and hand (complete) (partial), unilateral, at or above elbow, complicated — (Use additional code to identify infection)
887.6 Traumatic amputation of arm and hand (complete) (partial), bilateral (any level), without mention of complication — (Use additional code to identify infection)
887.7 Traumatic amputation of arm and hand (complete) (partial), bilateral (any level), complicated — (Use additional code to identify infection)
927.03 Crushing injury of upper arm — (Use additional code to identify any associated injuries: 800-829, 850.0-854.1, 860.0-869.1)
943.52 Deep necrosis of underlying tissues due to burn (deep third degree) of elbow, with loss of a body part
943.53 Deep necrosis of underlying tissues due to burn (deep third degree) of upper arm, with loss of upper a body part
996.94 Complications of reattached upper extremity, other and unspecified
V49.66 Upper limb amputation, above elbow — (This code is intended for use when these conditions are recorded as diagnoses or problems)
V51 Aftercare involving the use of plastic surgery
V58.41 Planned postoperative wound closure — (This code should be used in conjunction with other aftercare codes to fully identify the reason for the aftercare encounter)
V58.49 Other specified aftercare following surgery — (This code should be used in conjunction with other aftercare codes to fully identify the reason for the aftercare encounter)

ICD-9-CM Procedural

84.07 Amputation through humerus
84.44 Implantation of prosthetic device of arm

Forearm and Wrist

25000–25001

25000 Incision, extensor tendon sheath, wrist (eg, deQuervain's disease)
25001 Incision, flexor tendon sheath, wrist (eg, flexor carpi radialis)

ICD-9-CM Diagnostic

719.23 Villonodular synovitis, forearm
726.4 Enthesopathy of wrist and carpus
727.00 Unspecified synovitis and tenosynovitis ▽
727.04 Radial styloid tenosynovitis
727.05 Other tenosynovitis of hand and wrist
727.2 Specific bursitides often of occupational origin

ICD-9-CM Procedural

83.01 Exploration of tendon sheath

25020–25023

25020 Decompression fasciotomy, forearm and/or wrist, flexor OR extensor compartment; without debridement of nonviable muscle and/or nerve
25023 with debridement of nonviable muscle and/or nerve

ICD-9-CM Diagnostic

682.3 Cellulitis and abscess of upper arm and forearm — (Use additional code to identify organism)
682.4 Cellulitis and abscess of hand, except fingers and thumb — (Use additional code to identify organism)
728.86 Necrotizing fasciitis — (Use additional code to identify infectious organism, 041.00-041.89, 785.4, if applicable)
728.88 Rhabdomyolysis
729.4 Unspecified fasciitis ▽
785.4 Gangrene — (Code first any associated underlying condition:250.7, 443.0)
813.21 Closed fracture of shaft of radius (alone)
813.22 Closed fracture of shaft of ulna (alone)
813.23 Closed fracture of shaft of radius with ulna
813.31 Open fracture of shaft of radius (alone)
813.32 Open fracture of shaft of ulna (alone)
813.33 Open fracture of shaft of radius with ulna

813.80 Closed fracture of unspecified part of forearm ▽
813.90 Open fracture of unspecified part of forearm ▽
832.00 Closed unspecified dislocation of elbow ▽
832.10 Open unspecified dislocation of elbow ▽
881.01 Open wound of elbow, without mention of complication — (Use additional code to identify infection)
881.10 Open wound of forearm, complicated — (Use additional code to identify infection)
881.11 Open wound of elbow, complicated — (Use additional code to identify infection)
881.12 Open wound of wrist, complicated — (Use additional code to identify infection)
881.20 Open wound of forearm, with tendon involvement — (Use additional code to identify infection)
881.22 Open wound of wrist, with tendon involvement — (Use additional code to identify infection)
923.10 Contusion of forearm
923.11 Contusion of elbow
927.10 Crushing injury of forearm — (Use additional code to identify any associated injuries: 800-829, 850.0-854.1, 860.0-869.1)
927.11 Crushing injury of elbow — (Use additional code to identify any associated injuries: 800-829, 850.0-854.1, 860.0-869.1)
927.21 Crushing injury of wrist — (Use additional code to identify any associated injuries: 800-829, 850.0-854.1, 860.0-869.1)
943.01 Burn of unspecified degree of forearm ▽
943.21 Blisters with epidermal loss due to burn (second degree) of forearm
943.31 Full-thickness skin loss due to burn (third degree nos) of forearm
943.41 Deep necrosis of underlying tissues due to burn (deep third degree) of forearm, without mention of loss of a body part
948.00 Burn (any degree) involving less than 10% of body surface with third degree burn of less than 10% or unspecified amount
958.8 Other early complications of trauma

ICD-9-CM Procedural

04.07 Other excision or avulsion of cranial and peripheral nerves
83.14 Fasciotomy
83.45 Other myectomy

HCPCS Level II Supplies & Services

A4305 Disposable drug delivery system, flow rate of 50 ml or greater per hour
A4306 Disposable drug delivery system, flow rate of 5 ml or less per hour
A4550 Surgical trays

25024–25025

25024 Decompression fasciotomy, forearm and/or wrist, flexor AND extensor compartment; without debridement of nonviable muscle and/or nerve
25025 with debridement of nonviable muscle and/or nerve

ICD-9-CM Diagnostic

682.3 Cellulitis and abscess of upper arm and forearm — (Use additional code to identify organism)
682.4 Cellulitis and abscess of hand, except fingers and thumb — (Use additional code to identify organism)
728.86 Necrotizing fasciitis — (Use additional code to identify infectious organism, 041.00-041.89, 785.4, if applicable)
728.88 Rhabdomyolysis
729.4 Unspecified fasciitis ▽
785.4 Gangrene — (Code first any associated underlying condition:250.7, 443.0)

813.21 Closed fracture of shaft of radius (alone)
813.22 Closed fracture of shaft of ulna (alone)
813.23 Closed fracture of shaft of radius with ulna
813.31 Open fracture of shaft of radius (alone)
813.32 Open fracture of shaft of ulna (alone)
813.33 Open fracture of shaft of radius with ulna
813.80 Closed fracture of unspecified part of forearm ▽
813.90 Open fracture of unspecified part of forearm ▽
832.00 Closed unspecified dislocation of elbow ▽
832.10 Open unspecified dislocation of elbow ▽
881.01 Open wound of elbow, without mention of complication — (Use additional code to identify infection)
881.10 Open wound of forearm, complicated — (Use additional code to identify infection)
881.11 Open wound of elbow, complicated — (Use additional code to identify infection)
881.12 Open wound of wrist, complicated — (Use additional code to identify infection)
881.20 Open wound of forearm, with tendon involvement — (Use additional code to identify infection)
881.22 Open wound of wrist, with tendon involvement — (Use additional code to identify infection)
923.10 Contusion of forearm
923.11 Contusion of elbow
927.10 Crushing injury of forearm — (Use additional code to identify any associated injuries: 800-829, 850.0-854.1, 860.0-869.1)
927.11 Crushing injury of elbow — (Use additional code to identify any associated injuries: 800-829, 850.0-854.1, 860.0-869.1)
927.21 Crushing injury of wrist — (Use additional code to identify any associated injuries: 800-829, 850.0-854.1, 860.0-869.1)
943.01 Burn of unspecified degree of forearm ▽
943.21 Blisters with epidermal loss due to burn (second degree) of forearm
943.31 Full-thickness skin loss due to burn (third degree nos) of forearm
943.41 Deep necrosis of underlying tissues due to burn (deep third degree) of forearm, without mention of loss of a body part
948.00 Burn (any degree) involving less than 10% of body surface with third degree burn of less than 10% or unspecified amount
958.8 Other early complications of trauma

ICD-9-CM Procedural
04.07 Other excision or avulsion of cranial and peripheral nerves
83.14 Fasciotomy
83.45 Other myectomy

HCPCS Level II Supplies & Services
HCPCS Level II codes are used to report the supplies, durable medical equipment, and certain medical services provided on an outpatient basis. Because the procedure(s) represented on this page would be performed in an inpatient or outpatient facility, no HCPCS Level II codes apply.

25028
25028 Incision and drainage, forearm and/or wrist; deep abscess or hematoma

ICD-9-CM Diagnostic
682.3 Cellulitis and abscess of upper arm and forearm — (Use additional code to identify organism)
682.4 Cellulitis and abscess of hand, except fingers and thumb — (Use additional code to identify organism)
727.89 Other disorders of synovium, tendon, and bursa
730.33 Periostitis, without mention of osteomyelitis, forearm — (Use additional code to identify organism, 041.1)
881.10 Open wound of forearm, complicated — (Use additional code to identify infection)
881.12 Open wound of wrist, complicated — (Use additional code to identify infection)
923.10 Contusion of forearm
923.21 Contusion of wrist
927.10 Crushing injury of forearm — (Use additional code to identify any associated injuries: 800-829, 850.0-854.1, 860.0-869.1)
927.21 Crushing injury of wrist — (Use additional code to identify any associated injuries: 800-829, 850.0-854.1, 860.0-869.1)
927.8 Crushing injury of multiple sites of upper limb — (Use additional code to identify any associated injuries: 800-829, 850.0-854.1, 860.0-869.1)
998.59 Other postoperative infection — (Use additional code to identify infection)

ICD-9-CM Procedural
83.02 Myotomy
83.09 Other incision of soft tissue

HCPCS Level II Supplies & Services
A4305 Disposable drug delivery system, flow rate of 50 ml or greater per hour
A4306 Disposable drug delivery system, flow rate of 5 ml or less per hour
A4550 Surgical trays

25031
25031 Incision and drainage, forearm and/or wrist; bursa

ICD-9-CM Diagnostic
711.03 Pyogenic arthritis, forearm — (Use additional code to identify infectious organism: 041.0-041.8)
711.93 Unspecified infective arthritis, forearm ▽
716.93 Unspecified arthropathy, forearm ▽
726.4 Enthesopathy of wrist and carpus
727.2 Specific bursitides often of occupational origin
727.3 Other bursitis disorders
727.89 Other disorders of synovium, tendon, and bursa
906.3 Late effect of contusion
906.4 Late effect of crushing
998.51 Infected postoperative seroma — (Use additional code to identify organism)
998.59 Other postoperative infection — (Use additional code to identify infection)

ICD-9-CM Procedural
83.03 Bursotomy

HCPCS Level II Supplies & Services
A4305 Disposable drug delivery system, flow rate of 50 ml or greater per hour
A4306 Disposable drug delivery system, flow rate of 5 ml or less per hour
A4550 Surgical trays

25035
25035 Incision, deep, bone cortex, forearm and/or wrist (eg, osteomyelitis or bone abscess)

ICD-9-CM Diagnostic
730.13 Chronic osteomyelitis, forearm — (Use additional code to identify organism, 041.1)
730.23 Unspecified osteomyelitis, forearm — (Use additional code to identify organism, 041.1) ▽
730.83 Other infections involving bone in diseases classified elsewhere, forearm — (Code first underlying disease: 002.0, 015.0-015.9. Use additional code to identify organism) ☒
730.88 Other infections involving bone diseases classified elsewhere, other specified sites — (Code first underlying disease: 002.0, 015.0-015.9. Use additional code to identify organism) ☒
998.59 Other postoperative infection — (Use additional code to identify infection)

ICD-9-CM Procedural
77.13 Other incision of radius and ulna without division
77.14 Other incision of carpals and metacarpals without division

25040
25040 Arthrotomy, radiocarpal or midcarpal joint, with exploration, drainage, or removal of foreign body

ICD-9-CM Diagnostic
357.1 Polyneuropathy in collagen vascular disease — (Code first underlying disease: 446.0, 710.0, 714.0) ☒
359.6 Symptomatic inflammatory myopathy in diseases classified elsewhere — (Code first underlying disease: 135, 140.0-208.9, 277.3, 446.0, 710.0, 710.1, 710.2, 714.0) ☒
446.0 Polyarteritis nodosa
710.0 Systemic lupus erythematosus — (Use additional code to identify manifestation: 424.91, 581.81, 582.81, 583.81)
710.1 Systemic sclerosis — (Use additional code to identify manifestation: 359.6, 517.2)
710.2 Sicca syndrome
711.03 Pyogenic arthritis, forearm — (Use additional code to identify infectious organism: 041.0-041.8)
714.0 Rheumatoid arthritis — (Use additional code to identify manifestation: 357.1, 359.6)
715.13 Primary localized osteoarthrosis, forearm
715.33 Localized osteoarthrosis not specified whether primary or secondary, forearm
716.13 Traumatic arthropathy, forearm

▽ Unspecified code ☒ Manifestation code
♀ Female diagnosis ♂ Male diagnosis

716.63 Unspecified monoarthritis, forearm ▽
718.13 Loose body in forearm joint
719.03 Effusion of forearm joint
719.23 Villonodular synovitis, forearm
719.83 Other specified disorders of forearm joint
730.03 Acute osteomyelitis, forearm — (Use additional code to identify organism, 041.1)
730.13 Chronic osteomyelitis, forearm — (Use additional code to identify organism, 041.1)
881.12 Open wound of wrist, complicated — (Use additional code to identify infection)

ICD-9-CM Procedural

80.13 Other arthrotomy of wrist

25065–25066

25065 Biopsy, soft tissue of forearm and/or wrist; superficial
25066 deep (subfascial or intramuscular)

ICD-9-CM Diagnostic

171.2 Malignant neoplasm of connective and other soft tissue of upper limb, including shoulder
195.4 Malignant neoplasm of upper limb
198.89 Secondary malignant neoplasm of other specified sites
215.2 Other benign neoplasm of connective and other soft tissue of upper limb, including shoulder
238.1 Neoplasm of uncertain behavior of connective and other soft tissue ▽
239.2 Neoplasms of unspecified nature of bone, soft tissue, and skin

ICD-9-CM Procedural

83.21 Biopsy of soft tissue

HCPCS Level II Supplies & Services

A4550 Surgical trays

25075–25077

25075 Excision, tumor, soft tissue of forearm and/or wrist area; subcutaneous
25076 deep, subfascial or intramuscular
25077 Radical resection of tumor (eg, malignant neoplasm), soft tissue of forearm and/or wrist area

ICD-9-CM Diagnostic

171.2 Malignant neoplasm of connective and other soft tissue of upper limb, including shoulder
195.4 Malignant neoplasm of upper limb
198.89 Secondary malignant neoplasm of other specified sites
214.1 Lipoma of other skin and subcutaneous tissue
215.2 Other benign neoplasm of connective and other soft tissue of upper limb, including shoulder
238.1 Neoplasm of uncertain behavior of connective and other soft tissue ▽
239.2 Neoplasms of unspecified nature of bone, soft tissue, and skin
782.2 Localized superficial swelling, mass, or lump

ICD-9-CM Procedural

80.83 Other local excision or destruction of lesion of wrist joint
83.31 Excision of lesion of tendon sheath
83.32 Excision of lesion of muscle
83.39 Excision of lesion of other soft tissue

HCPCS Level II Supplies & Services

A4305 Disposable drug delivery system, flow rate of 50 ml or greater per hour
A4306 Disposable drug delivery system, flow rate of 5 ml or less per hour
A4550 Surgical trays

25085

25085 Capsulotomy, wrist (eg, contracture)

ICD-9-CM Diagnostic

718.43 Contracture of forearm joint
728.10 Unspecified calcification and ossification ▽

ICD-9-CM Procedural

80.43 Division of joint capsule, ligament, or cartilage of wrist

25100

25100 Arthrotomy, wrist joint; with biopsy

ICD-9-CM Diagnostic

170.5 Malignant neoplasm of short bones of upper limb
171.2 Malignant neoplasm of connective and other soft tissue of upper limb, including shoulder
195.4 Malignant neoplasm of upper limb
198.5 Secondary malignant neoplasm of bone and bone marrow
213.5 Benign neoplasm of short bones of upper limb
238.0 Neoplasm of uncertain behavior of bone and articular cartilage
239.2 Neoplasms of unspecified nature of bone, soft tissue, and skin
275.40 Unspecified disorder of calcium metabolism — (Use additional code to identify any associated mental retardation) ▽
275.42 Hypercalcemia — (Use additional code to identify any associated mental retardation)
275.49 Other disorders of calcium metabolism — (Use additional code to identify any associated mental retardation)
357.1 Polyneuropathy in collagen vascular disease — (Code first underlying disease: 446.0, 710.0, 714.0) ☒
359.6 Symptomatic inflammatory myopathy in diseases classified elsewhere — (Code first underlying disease: 135, 140.0-208.9, 277.3, 446.0, 710.0, 710.1, 710.2, 714.0) ☒
446.0 Polyarteritis nodosa
710.0 Systemic lupus erythematosus — (Use additional code to identify manifestation: 424.91, 581.81, 582.81, 583.81)
710.1 Systemic sclerosis — (Use additional code to identify manifestation: 359.6, 517.2)
710.2 Sicca syndrome
714.0 Rheumatoid arthritis — (Use additional code to identify manifestation: 357.1, 359.6)
719.23 Villonodular synovitis, forearm
V64.43 Arthroscopic surgical procedure converted to open procedure

ICD-9-CM Procedural

80.13 Other arthrotomy of wrist
80.33 Biopsy of joint structure of wrist

HCPCS Level II Supplies & Services

A4305 Disposable drug delivery system, flow rate of 50 ml or greater per hour
A4306 Disposable drug delivery system, flow rate of 5 ml or less per hour
A4550 Surgical trays

25101–25105

25101 Arthrotomy, wrist joint; with joint exploration, with or without biopsy, with or without removal of loose or foreign body
25105 with synovectomy

ICD-9-CM Diagnostic

170.5 Malignant neoplasm of short bones of upper limb
198.5 Secondary malignant neoplasm of bone and bone marrow
198.89 Secondary malignant neoplasm of other specified sites
213.5 Benign neoplasm of short bones of upper limb
215.2 Other benign neoplasm of connective and other soft tissue of upper limb, including shoulder
238.0 Neoplasm of uncertain behavior of bone and articular cartilage
239.2 Neoplasms of unspecified nature of bone, soft tissue, and skin
357.1 Polyneuropathy in collagen vascular disease — (Code first underlying disease: 446.0, 710.0, 714.0) ☒
359.6 Symptomatic inflammatory myopathy in diseases classified elsewhere — (Code first underlying disease: 135, 140.0-208.9, 277.3, 446.0, 710.0, 710.1, 710.2, 714.0) ☒
446.0 Polyarteritis nodosa
710.0 Systemic lupus erythematosus — (Use additional code to identify manifestation: 424.91, 581.81, 582.81, 583.81)
710.1 Systemic sclerosis — (Use additional code to identify manifestation: 359.6, 517.2)
710.2 Sicca syndrome
711.03 Pyogenic arthritis, forearm — (Use additional code to identify infectious organism: 041.0-041.8)
711.93 Unspecified infective arthritis, forearm ▽
714.0 Rheumatoid arthritis — (Use additional code to identify manifestation: 357.1, 359.6)
715.13 Primary localized osteoarthrosis, forearm
715.33 Localized osteoarthrosis not specified whether primary or secondary, forearm
716.63 Unspecified monoarthritis, forearm ▽

718.13 Loose body in forearm joint
718.93 Unspecified derangement, forearm joint ▽
719.23 Villonodular synovitis, forearm
727.05 Other tenosynovitis of hand and wrist
729.6 Residual foreign body in soft tissue
906.3 Late effect of contusion
906.4 Late effect of crushing
V64.43 Arthroscopic surgical procedure converted to open procedure

ICD-9-CM Procedural

80.13 Other arthrotomy of wrist
80.33 Biopsy of joint structure of wrist
80.73 Synovectomy of wrist

HCPCS Level II Supplies & Services

A4305 Disposable drug delivery system, flow rate of 50 ml or greater per hour
A4306 Disposable drug delivery system, flow rate of 5 ml or less per hour
A4550 Surgical trays

25107

25107 Arthrotomy, distal radioulnar joint including repair of triangular cartilage, complex

ICD-9-CM Diagnostic

718.03 Articular cartilage disorder, forearm
718.73 Developmental dislocation of joint, forearm
718.83 Other joint derangement, not elsewhere classified, forearm
718.93 Unspecified derangement, forearm joint ▽
813.42 Other closed fractures of distal end of radius (alone)
813.52 Other open fractures of distal end of radius (alone)
813.54 Open fracture of lower end of radius with ulna
833.01 Closed dislocation of distal radioulnar (joint)
833.11 Open dislocation of distal radioulnar (joint)
842.09 Other wrist sprain and strain
881.12 Open wound of wrist, complicated — (Use additional code to identify infection)
881.22 Open wound of wrist, with tendon involvement — (Use additional code to identify infection)

ICD-9-CM Procedural

81.96 Other repair of joint

25110

25110 Excision, lesion of tendon sheath, forearm and/or wrist

ICD-9-CM Diagnostic

171.2 Malignant neoplasm of connective and other soft tissue of upper limb, including shoulder
215.2 Other benign neoplasm of connective and other soft tissue of upper limb, including shoulder
216.6 Benign neoplasm of skin of upper limb, including shoulder
238.1 Neoplasm of uncertain behavior of connective and other soft tissue ▽
239.2 Neoplasms of unspecified nature of bone, soft tissue, and skin
719.93 Unspecified disorder of forearm joint ▽
727.02 Giant cell tumor of tendon sheath
727.05 Other tenosynovitis of hand and wrist
782.2 Localized superficial swelling, mass, or lump

ICD-9-CM Procedural

83.31 Excision of lesion of tendon sheath

HCPCS Level II Supplies & Services

A4305 Disposable drug delivery system, flow rate of 50 ml or greater per hour
A4306 Disposable drug delivery system, flow rate of 5 ml or less per hour
A4550 Surgical trays

25111–25112

25111 Excision of ganglion, wrist (dorsal or volar); primary
25112 recurrent

ICD-9-CM Diagnostic

727.41 Ganglion of joint
727.42 Ganglion of tendon sheath

ICD-9-CM Procedural

82.21 Excision of lesion of tendon sheath of hand

HCPCS Level II Supplies & Services

A4305 Disposable drug delivery system, flow rate of 50 ml or greater per hour
A4306 Disposable drug delivery system, flow rate of 5 ml or less per hour
A4550 Surgical trays

25115–25116

25115 Radical excision of bursa, synovia of wrist, or forearm tendon sheaths (eg, tenosynovitis, fungus, Tbc, or other granulomas, rheumatoid arthritis); flexors
25116 extensors, with or without transposition of dorsal retinaculum

ICD-9-CM Diagnostic

357.1 Polyneuropathy in collagen vascular disease — (Code first underlying disease: 446.0, 710.0, 714.0) ☒
359.6 Symptomatic inflammatory myopathy in diseases classified elsewhere — (Code first underlying disease: 135, 140.0-208.9, 277.3, 446.0, 710.0, 710.1, 710.2, 714.0) ☒
446.0 Polyarteritis nodosa
517.8 Lung involvement in other diseases classified elsewhere — (Code first underlying disease: 135, 277.3, 710.0, 710.2, 710.4) ☒
710.0 Systemic lupus erythematosus — (Use additional code to identify manifestation: 424.91, 581.81, 582.81, 583.81)
710.1 Systemic sclerosis — (Use additional code to identify manifestation: 359.6, 517.2)
710.2 Sicca syndrome
710.9 Unspecified diffuse connective tissue disease ▽
711.03 Pyogenic arthritis, forearm — (Use additional code to identify infectious organism: 041.0-041.8)
711.13 Arthropathy associated with Reiter's disease and nonspecific urethritis, forearm — (Code first underlying disease: 099.3, 099.4) ☒
711.93 Unspecified infective arthritis, forearm ▽
714.0 Rheumatoid arthritis — (Use additional code to identify manifestation: 357.1, 359.6)
719.23 Villonodular synovitis, forearm
727.00 Unspecified synovitis and tenosynovitis ▽
727.01 Synovitis and tenosynovitis in diseases classified elsewhere — (Code first underlying disease: 015.0-015.9) ☒
727.02 Giant cell tumor of tendon sheath
727.05 Other tenosynovitis of hand and wrist
727.42 Ganglion of tendon sheath
727.49 Other ganglion and cyst of synovium, tendon, and bursa

ICD-9-CM Procedural

83.31 Excision of lesion of tendon sheath
83.39 Excision of lesion of other soft tissue
83.5 Bursectomy

25118–25119

25118 Synovectomy, extensor tendon sheath, wrist, single compartment;
25119 with resection of distal ulna

ICD-9-CM Diagnostic

171.2 Malignant neoplasm of connective and other soft tissue of upper limb, including shoulder
198.89 Secondary malignant neoplasm of other specified sites
215.2 Other benign neoplasm of connective and other soft tissue of upper limb, including shoulder
238.1 Neoplasm of uncertain behavior of connective and other soft tissue ▽
239.2 Neoplasms of unspecified nature of bone, soft tissue, and skin
354.5 Mononeuritis multiplex
357.1 Polyneuropathy in collagen vascular disease — (Code first underlying disease: 446.0, 710.0, 714.0) ☒
359.6 Symptomatic inflammatory myopathy in diseases classified elsewhere — (Code first underlying disease: 135, 140.0-208.9, 277.3, 446.0, 710.0, 710.1, 710.2, 714.0) ☒
446.0 Polyarteritis nodosa
710.0 Systemic lupus erythematosus — (Use additional code to identify manifestation: 424.91, 581.81, 582.81, 583.81)
710.1 Systemic sclerosis — (Use additional code to identify manifestation: 359.6, 517.2)
710.2 Sicca syndrome
714.0 Rheumatoid arthritis — (Use additional code to identify manifestation: 357.1, 359.6)
715.13 Primary localized osteoarthrosis, forearm
716.13 Traumatic arthropathy, forearm
719.23 Villonodular synovitis, forearm

▽ Unspecified code ♀ Female diagnosis ☒ Manifestation code ♂ Male diagnosis

727.00 Unspecified synovitis and tenosynovitis ▽
727.01 Synovitis and tenosynovitis in diseases classified elsewhere — (Code first underlying disease: 015.0-015.9) ☒
727.04 Radial styloid tenosynovitis
727.05 Other tenosynovitis of hand and wrist
727.40 Unspecified synovial cyst ▽
727.49 Other ganglion and cyst of synovium, tendon, and bursa
881.22 Open wound of wrist, with tendon involvement — (Use additional code to identify infection)
V64.43 Arthroscopic surgical procedure converted to open procedure

ICD-9-CM Procedural
77.83 Other partial ostectomy of radius and ulna
80.73 Synovectomy of wrist
83.42 Other tenonectomy

HCPCS Level II Supplies & Services
A4305 Disposable drug delivery system, flow rate of 50 ml or greater per hour
A4306 Disposable drug delivery system, flow rate of 5 ml or less per hour
A4550 Surgical trays

25120–25126
25120 Excision or curettage of bone cyst or benign tumor of radius or ulna (excluding head or neck of radius and olecranon process);
25125 with autograft (includes obtaining graft)
25126 with allograft

ICD-9-CM Diagnostic
213.4 Benign neoplasm of scapula and long bones of upper limb
238.0 Neoplasm of uncertain behavior of bone and articular cartilage
239.2 Neoplasms of unspecified nature of bone, soft tissue, and skin
726.91 Exostosis of unspecified site ▽
733.21 Solitary bone cyst
733.22 Aneurysmal bone cyst
733.29 Other cyst of bone

ICD-9-CM Procedural
77.79 Excision of other bone for graft, except facial bones
78.03 Bone graft of radius and ulna
80.83 Other local excision or destruction of lesion of wrist joint

25130–25136
25130 Excision or curettage of bone cyst or benign tumor of carpal bones;
25135 with autograft (includes obtaining graft)
25136 with allograft

ICD-9-CM Diagnostic
213.5 Benign neoplasm of short bones of upper limb
238.0 Neoplasm of uncertain behavior of bone and articular cartilage
239.2 Neoplasms of unspecified nature of bone, soft tissue, and skin
726.91 Exostosis of unspecified site ▽
733.21 Solitary bone cyst
733.22 Aneurysmal bone cyst
733.29 Other cyst of bone

ICD-9-CM Procedural
77.77 Excision of tibia and fibula for graft
77.79 Excision of other bone for graft, except facial bones
78.04 Bone graft of carpals and metacarpals
80.83 Other local excision or destruction of lesion of wrist joint

25145
25145 Sequestrectomy (eg, for osteomyelitis or bone abscess), forearm and/or wrist

ICD-9-CM Diagnostic
715.13 Primary localized osteoarthrosis, forearm
715.33 Localized osteoarthrosis not specified whether primary or secondary, forearm
716.63 Unspecified monoarthritis, forearm ▽
730.13 Chronic osteomyelitis, forearm — (Use additional code to identify organism, 041.1)
730.23 Unspecified osteomyelitis, forearm — (Use additional code to identify organism, 041.1) ▽
730.33 Periostitis, without mention of osteomyelitis, forearm — (Use additional code to identify organism, 041.1)
730.83 Other infections involving bone in diseases classified elsewhere, forearm — (Code first underlying disease: 002.0, 015.0-015.9. Use additional code to identify organism) ☒
905.2 Late effect of fracture of upper extremities

ICD-9-CM Procedural
77.03 Sequestrectomy of radius and ulna
77.04 Sequestrectomy of carpals and metacarpals
77.09 Sequestrectomy of other bone, except facial bones

25150–25151
25150 Partial excision (craterization, saucerization or diaphysectomy) of bone (eg, for osteomyelitis); ulna
25151 radius

ICD-9-CM Diagnostic
715.13 Primary localized osteoarthrosis, forearm
715.33 Localized osteoarthrosis not specified whether primary or secondary, forearm
716.63 Unspecified monoarthritis, forearm ▽
730.13 Chronic osteomyelitis, forearm — (Use additional code to identify organism, 041.1)
730.23 Unspecified osteomyelitis, forearm — (Use additional code to identify organism, 041.1) ▽
730.33 Periostitis, without mention of osteomyelitis, forearm — (Use additional code to identify organism, 041.1)
730.83 Other infections involving bone in diseases classified elsewhere, forearm — (Code first underlying disease: 002.0, 015.0-015.9. Use additional code to identify organism) ☒
905.2 Late effect of fracture of upper extremities

ICD-9-CM Procedural
77.83 Other partial ostectomy of radius and ulna

25170
25170 Radical resection for tumor, radius or ulna

ICD-9-CM Diagnostic
170.4 Malignant neoplasm of scapula and long bones of upper limb
198.5 Secondary malignant neoplasm of bone and bone marrow
238.0 Neoplasm of uncertain behavior of bone and articular cartilage
239.2 Neoplasms of unspecified nature of bone, soft tissue, and skin

ICD-9-CM Procedural
77.63 Local excision of lesion or tissue of radius and ulna

25210–25215
25210 Carpectomy; one bone
25215 all bones of proximal row

ICD-9-CM Diagnostic
357.1 Polyneuropathy in collagen vascular disease — (Code first underlying disease: 446.0, 710.0, 714.0) ☒
359.6 Symptomatic inflammatory myopathy in diseases classified elsewhere — (Code first underlying disease: 135, 140.0-208.9, 277.3, 446.0, 710.0, 710.1, 710.2, 714.0) ☒
446.0 Polyarteritis nodosa
710.0 Systemic lupus erythematosus — (Use additional code to identify manifestation: 424.91, 581.81, 582.81, 583.81)
710.1 Systemic sclerosis — (Use additional code to identify manifestation: 359.6, 517.2)
710.2 Sicca syndrome
714.0 Rheumatoid arthritis — (Use additional code to identify manifestation: 357.1, 359.6)
715.04 Generalized osteoarthrosis, involving hand
715.14 Primary localized osteoarthrosis, hand
715.34 Localized osteoarthrosis not specified whether primary or secondary, hand
715.94 Osteoarthrosis, unspecified whether generalized or localized, hand ▽
716.14 Traumatic arthropathy, hand
716.64 Unspecified monoarthritis, hand ▽
716.94 Unspecified arthopathy, hand ▽
718.83 Other joint derangement, not elsewhere classified, forearm
726.91 Exostosis of unspecified site ▽
727.05 Other tenosynovitis of hand and wrist
730.14 Chronic osteomyelitis, hand — (Use additional code to identify organism, 041.1)

730.24 Unspecified osteomyelitis, hand — (Use additional code to identify organism, 041.1)
730.84 Other infections involving diseases classified elsewhere, hand bone — (Code first underlying disease: 002.0, 015.0-015.9. Use additional code to identify organism)
730.94 Unspecified infection of bone, hand — (Use additional code to identify organism, 041.1)
733.49 Aseptic necrosis of other bone site
733.82 Nonunion of fracture
814.00 Unspecified closed fracture of carpal bone
814.01 Closed fracture of navicular (scaphoid) bone of wrist
814.02 Closed fracture of lunate (semilunar) bone of wrist
814.03 Closed fracture of triquetral (cuneiform) bone of wrist
814.04 Closed fracture of pisiform bone of wrist
814.05 Closed fracture of trapezium bone (larger multangular) of wrist
814.06 Closed fracture of trapezoid bone (smaller multangular) of wrist
814.07 Closed fracture of capitate bone (os magnum) of wrist
814.08 Closed fracture of hamate (unciform) bone of wrist
814.09 Closed fracture of other bone of wrist
814.10 Unspecified open fracture of carpal bone
814.11 Open fracture of navicular (scaphoid) bone of wrist
814.12 Open fracture of lunate (semilunar) bone of wrist
814.13 Open fracture of triquetral (cuneiform) bone of wrist
814.14 Open fracture of pisiform bone of wrist
814.15 Open fracture of trapezium bone (larger multangular) of wrist
814.16 Open fracture of trapezoid bone (smaller multangular) of wrist
814.17 Open fracture of capitate bone (os magnum) of wrist
814.18 Open fracture of hamate (unciform) bone of wrist
814.19 Open fracture of other bone of wrist
906.4 Late effect of crushing
927.21 Crushing injury of wrist — (Use additional code to identify any associated injuries: 800-829, 850.0-854.1, 860.0-869.1)

ICD-9-CM Procedural

77.84 Other partial ostectomy of carpals and metacarpals
77.94 Total ostectomy of carpals and metacarpals

25230

25230 Radial styloidectomy (separate procedure)

ICD-9-CM Diagnostic

170.5 Malignant neoplasm of short bones of upper limb
198.5 Secondary malignant neoplasm of bone and bone marrow
213.5 Benign neoplasm of short bones of upper limb
238.0 Neoplasm of uncertain behavior of bone and articular cartilage
239.2 Neoplasms of unspecified nature of bone, soft tissue, and skin
357.1 Polyneuropathy in collagen vascular disease — (Code first underlying disease: 446.0, 710.0, 714.0)
359.6 Symptomatic inflammatory myopathy in diseases classified elsewhere — (Code first underlying disease: 135, 140.0-208.9, 277.3, 446.0, 710.0, 710.1, 710.2, 714.0)
446.0 Polyarteritis nodosa
710.0 Systemic lupus erythematosus — (Use additional code to identify manifestation: 424.91, 581.81, 582.81, 583.81)
710.1 Systemic sclerosis — (Use additional code to identify manifestation: 359.6, 517.2)
710.2 Sicca syndrome
714.0 Rheumatoid arthritis — (Use additional code to identify manifestation: 357.1, 359.6)
715.13 Primary localized osteoarthrosis, forearm
715.93 Osteoarthrosis, unspecified whether generalized or localized, forearm
716.13 Traumatic arthropathy, forearm
716.93 Unspecified arthropathy, forearm
718.83 Other joint derangement, not elsewhere classified, forearm
727.00 Unspecified synovitis and tenosynovitis
727.04 Radial styloid tenosynovitis
727.05 Other tenosynovitis of hand and wrist
729.5 Pain in soft tissues of limb
730.13 Chronic osteomyelitis, forearm — (Use additional code to identify organism, 041.1)
730.23 Unspecified osteomyelitis, forearm — (Use additional code to identify organism, 041.1)
730.83 Other infections involving bone in diseases classified elsewhere, forearm — (Code first underlying disease: 002.0, 015.0-015.9. Use additional code to identify organism)
732.3 Juvenile osteochondrosis of upper extremity
733.81 Malunion of fracture
733.82 Nonunion of fracture

ICD-9-CM Procedural

77.83 Other partial ostectomy of radius and ulna

25240

25240 Excision distal ulna partial or complete (eg, Darrach type or matched resection)

ICD-9-CM Diagnostic

238.0 Neoplasm of uncertain behavior of bone and articular cartilage
239.2 Neoplasms of unspecified nature of bone, soft tissue, and skin
357.1 Polyneuropathy in collagen vascular disease — (Code first underlying disease: 446.0, 710.0, 714.0)
359.6 Symptomatic inflammatory myopathy in diseases classified elsewhere — (Code first underlying disease: 135, 140.0-208.9, 277.3, 446.0, 710.0, 710.1, 710.2, 714.0)
446.0 Polyarteritis nodosa
710.0 Systemic lupus erythematosus — (Use additional code to identify manifestation: 424.91, 581.81, 582.81, 583.81)
710.1 Systemic sclerosis — (Use additional code to identify manifestation: 359.6, 517.2)
710.2 Sicca syndrome
714.0 Rheumatoid arthritis — (Use additional code to identify manifestation: 357.1, 359.6)
715.13 Primary localized osteoarthrosis, forearm
715.93 Osteoarthrosis, unspecified whether generalized or localized, forearm
716.13 Traumatic arthropathy, forearm
716.93 Unspecified arthropathy, forearm
718.83 Other joint derangement, not elsewhere classified, forearm
727.00 Unspecified synovitis and tenosynovitis
727.05 Other tenosynovitis of hand and wrist
730.13 Chronic osteomyelitis, forearm — (Use additional code to identify organism, 041.1)
730.23 Unspecified osteomyelitis, forearm — (Use additional code to identify organism, 041.1)
730.83 Other infections involving bone in diseases classified elsewhere, forearm — (Code first underlying disease: 002.0, 015.0-015.9. Use additional code to identify organism)
732.3 Juvenile osteochondrosis of upper extremity
733.81 Malunion of fracture
733.82 Nonunion of fracture
736.09 Other acquired deformities of forearm, excluding fingers

ICD-9-CM Procedural

77.83 Other partial ostectomy of radius and ulna

25246

25246 Injection procedure for wrist arthrography

ICD-9-CM Diagnostic

275.40 Unspecified disorder of calcium metabolism — (Use additional code to identify any associated mental retardation)
275.42 Hypercalcemia — (Use additional code to identify any associated mental retardation)
275.49 Other disorders of calcium metabolism — (Use additional code to identify any associated mental retardation)
718.03 Articular cartilage disorder, forearm
718.13 Loose body in forearm joint
718.73 Developmental dislocation of joint, forearm
718.93 Unspecified derangement, forearm joint
814.00 Unspecified closed fracture of carpal bone
814.01 Closed fracture of navicular (scaphoid) bone of wrist
814.02 Closed fracture of lunate (semilunar) bone of wrist
814.03 Closed fracture of triquetral (cuneiform) bone of wrist
814.04 Closed fracture of pisiform bone of wrist
814.05 Closed fracture of trapezium bone (larger multangular) of wrist
814.06 Closed fracture of trapezoid bone (smaller multangular) of wrist
814.07 Closed fracture of capitate bone (os magnum) of wrist
814.08 Closed fracture of hamate (unciform) bone of wrist
814.09 Closed fracture of other bone of wrist
814.10 Unspecified open fracture of carpal bone
814.11 Open fracture of navicular (scaphoid) bone of wrist
814.12 Open fracture of lunate (semilunar) bone of wrist
814.13 Open fracture of triquetral (cuneiform) bone of wrist
814.14 Open fracture of pisiform bone of wrist

Unspecified code
Female diagnosis
Manifestation code
Male diagnosis

814.15 Open fracture of trapezium bone (larger multangular) of wrist
814.16 Open fracture of trapezoid bone (smaller multangular) of wrist
814.17 Open fracture of capitate bone (os magnum) of wrist
814.18 Open fracture of hamate (unciform) bone of wrist
814.19 Open fracture of other bone of wrist
833.00 Closed dislocation of wrist, unspecified part ▽
833.01 Closed dislocation of distal radioulnar (joint)
833.02 Closed dislocation of radiocarpal (joint)
833.03 Closed dislocation of midcarpal (joint)
833.04 Closed dislocation of carpometacarpal (joint)
833.05 Closed dislocation of proximal end of metacarpal (bone)
833.09 Closed dislocation of other part of wrist
833.10 Open dislocation of wrist, unspecified part ▽
833.11 Open dislocation of distal radioulnar (joint)
833.12 Open dislocation of radiocarpal (joint)
833.13 Open dislocation of midcarpal (joint)
833.14 Open dislocation of carpometacarpal (joint)
833.15 Open dislocation of proximal end of metacarpal (bone)
833.19 Open dislocation of other part of wrist
842.00 Sprain and strain of unspecified site of wrist ▽
842.01 Sprain and strain of carpal (joint) of wrist
842.02 Sprain and strain of radiocarpal (joint) (ligament) of wrist
842.09 Other wrist sprain and strain
881.12 Open wound of wrist, complicated — (Use additional code to identify infection)
881.22 Open wound of wrist, with tendon involvement — (Use additional code to identify infection)
927.21 Crushing injury of wrist — (Use additional code to identify any associated injuries: 800-829, 850.0-854.1, 860.0-869.1)
959.3 Injury, other and unspecified, elbow, forearm, and wrist

ICD-9-CM Procedural

81.92 Injection of therapeutic substance into joint or ligament
88.32 Contrast arthrogram

HCPCS Level II Supplies & Services

A9525 Supply of low or iso-osmolar contrast material, 10 mg of iodine

25248

25248 Exploration with removal of deep foreign body, forearm or wrist

ICD-9-CM Diagnostic

728.82 Foreign body granuloma of muscle
729.6 Residual foreign body in soft tissue
881.10 Open wound of forearm, complicated — (Use additional code to identify infection)
881.12 Open wound of wrist, complicated — (Use additional code to identify infection)
959.3 Injury, other and unspecified, elbow, forearm, and wrist

ICD-9-CM Procedural

81.91 Arthrocentesis
83.02 Myotomy
83.09 Other incision of soft tissue
98.27 Removal of foreign body without incision from upper limb, except hand

HCPCS Level II Supplies & Services

A4550 Surgical trays

25250–25251

25250 Removal of wrist prosthesis; (separate procedure)
25251 complicated, including total wrist

ICD-9-CM Diagnostic

996.4 Mechanical complication of internal orthopedic device, implant, and graft
996.66 Infection and inflammatory reaction due to internal joint prosthesis — (Use additional code to identify specified infections)
998.6 Persistent postoperative fistula, not elsewhere classified
998.83 Non-healing surgical wound

ICD-9-CM Procedural

80.03 Arthrotomy for removal of prosthesis of wrist

25259

25259 Manipulation, wrist, under anesthesia

ICD-9-CM Diagnostic

357.1 Polyneuropathy in collagen vascular disease — (Code first underlying disease: 446.0, 710.0, 714.0) ☒
359.6 Symptomatic inflammatory myopathy in diseases classified elsewhere — (Code first underlying disease: 135, 140.0-208.9, 277.3, 446.0, 710.0, 710.1, 710.2, 714.0) ☒
446.0 Polyarteritis nodosa
710.0 Systemic lupus erythematosus — (Use additional code to identify manifestation: 424.91, 581.81, 582.81, 583.81)
710.1 Systemic sclerosis — (Use additional code to identify manifestation: 359.6, 517.2)
710.2 Sicca syndrome
714.0 Rheumatoid arthritis — (Use additional code to identify manifestation: 357.1, 359.6)
715.13 Primary localized osteoarthrosis, forearm
715.93 Osteoarthrosis, unspecified whether generalized or localized, forearm ▽
718.43 Contracture of forearm joint
718.53 Ankylosis of forearm joint
719.23 Villonodular synovitis, forearm
719.53 Stiffness of joint, not elsewhere classified, forearm
726.4 Enthesopathy of wrist and carpus

ICD-9-CM Procedural

93.25 Forced extension of limb
93.26 Manual rupture of joint adhesions
93.29 Other forcible correction of musculoskeletal deformity

25260–25265

25260 Repair, tendon or muscle, flexor, forearm and/or wrist; primary, single, each tendon or muscle
25263 secondary, single, each tendon or muscle
25265 secondary, with free graft (includes obtaining graft), each tendon or muscle

ICD-9-CM Diagnostic

727.64 Nontraumatic rupture of flexor tendons of hand and wrist
727.69 Nontraumatic rupture of other tendon
727.9 Unspecified disorder of synovium, tendon, and bursa ▽
841.8 Sprain and strain of other specified sites of elbow and forearm
842.00 Sprain and strain of unspecified site of wrist ▽
842.01 Sprain and strain of carpal (joint) of wrist
842.02 Sprain and strain of radiocarpal (joint) (ligament) of wrist
842.09 Other wrist sprain and strain
881.20 Open wound of forearm, with tendon involvement — (Use additional code to identify infection)
881.22 Open wound of wrist, with tendon involvement — (Use additional code to identify infection)
884.2 Multiple and unspecified open wound of upper limb, with tendon involvement — (Use additional code to identify infection)
905.8 Late effect of tendon injury
959.3 Injury, other and unspecified, elbow, forearm, and wrist

ICD-9-CM Procedural

83.64 Other suture of tendon
83.65 Other suture of muscle or fascia
83.81 Tendon graft
83.82 Graft of muscle or fascia
83.88 Other plastic operations on tendon
83.99 Other operations on muscle, tendon, fascia, and bursa

HCPCS Level II Supplies & Services

A4550 Surgical trays
A4570 Splint
E1805 Dynamic adjustable wrist extension/flexion device, includes soft interface material

25270–25274

25270 Repair, tendon or muscle, extensor, forearm and/or wrist; primary, single, each tendon or muscle
25272 secondary, single, each tendon or muscle
25274 secondary, with free graft (includes obtaining graft), each tendon or muscle

ICD-9-CM Diagnostic

727.63 Nontraumatic rupture of extensor tendons of hand and wrist

▽ Unspecified code ♀ Female diagnosis ☒ Manifestation code ♂ Male diagnosis

727.69 Nontraumatic rupture of other tendon
727.9 Unspecified disorder of synovium, tendon, and bursa ▽
841.8 Sprain and strain of other specified sites of elbow and forearm
842.00 Sprain and strain of unspecified site of wrist ▽
842.01 Sprain and strain of carpal (joint) of wrist
842.02 Sprain and strain of radiocarpal (joint) (ligament) of wrist
842.09 Other wrist sprain and strain
881.20 Open wound of forearm, with tendon involvement — (Use additional code to identify infection)
881.22 Open wound of wrist, with tendon involvement — (Use additional code to identify infection)
884.2 Multiple and unspecified open wound of upper limb, with tendon involvement — (Use additional code to identify infection)
905.7 Late effect of sprain and strain without mention of tendon injury
905.8 Late effect of tendon injury
959.3 Injury, other and unspecified, elbow, forearm, and wrist

ICD-9-CM Procedural

83.64 Other suture of tendon
83.65 Other suture of muscle or fascia
83.81 Tendon graft
83.88 Other plastic operations on tendon
83.99 Other operations on muscle, tendon, fascia, and bursa

HCPCS Level II Supplies & Services

A4570 Splint
E1805 Dynamic adjustable wrist extension/flexion device, includes soft interface material

25275

25275 Repair, tendon sheath, extensor, forearm and/or wrist, with free graft (includes obtaining graft) (eg, for extensor carpi ulnaris subluxation)

ICD-9-CM Diagnostic

727.63 Nontraumatic rupture of extensor tendons of hand and wrist
727.69 Nontraumatic rupture of other tendon
727.9 Unspecified disorder of synovium, tendon, and bursa ▽
841.8 Sprain and strain of other specified sites of elbow and forearm
842.00 Sprain and strain of unspecified site of wrist ▽
842.01 Sprain and strain of carpal (joint) of wrist
842.02 Sprain and strain of radiocarpal (joint) (ligament) of wrist
842.09 Other wrist sprain and strain
881.20 Open wound of forearm, with tendon involvement — (Use additional code to identify infection)
881.22 Open wound of wrist, with tendon involvement — (Use additional code to identify infection)
884.2 Multiple and unspecified open wound of upper limb, with tendon involvement — (Use additional code to identify infection)
905.7 Late effect of sprain and strain without mention of tendon injury
905.8 Late effect of tendon injury
959.3 Injury, other and unspecified, elbow, forearm, and wrist

ICD-9-CM Procedural

83.61 Suture of tendon sheath
83.81 Tendon graft

25280

25280 Lengthening or shortening of flexor or extensor tendon, forearm and/or wrist, single, each tendon

ICD-9-CM Diagnostic

342.10 Spastic hemiplegia affecting unspecified side ▽
342.11 Spastic hemiplegia affecting dominant side
342.12 Spastic hemiplegia affecting nondominant side
342.80 Other specified hemiplegia affecting unspecified side ▽
342.81 Other specified hemiplegia affecting dominant side
342.82 Other specified hemiplegia affecting nondominant side
343.9 Unspecified infantile cerebral palsy ▽
344.89 Other specified paralytic syndrome
718.33 Recurrent dislocation of forearm joint
718.43 Contracture of forearm joint
727.81 Contracture of tendon (sheath)

ICD-9-CM Procedural

83.85 Other change in muscle or tendon length

25290

25290 Tenotomy, open, flexor or extensor tendon, forearm and/or wrist, single, each tendon

ICD-9-CM Diagnostic

718.43 Contracture of forearm joint
726.4 Enthesopathy of wrist and carpus
727.00 Unspecified synovitis and tenosynovitis ▽
727.01 Synovitis and tenosynovitis in diseases classified elsewhere — (Code first underlying disease: 015.0-015.9) ☒
727.02 Giant cell tumor of tendon sheath
727.03 Trigger finger (acquired)
727.04 Radial styloid tenosynovitis
727.05 Other tenosynovitis of hand and wrist
727.81 Contracture of tendon (sheath)

ICD-9-CM Procedural

83.13 Other tenotomy

25295

25295 Tenolysis, flexor or extensor tendon, forearm and/or wrist, single, each tendon

ICD-9-CM Diagnostic

342.10 Spastic hemiplegia affecting unspecified side ▽
342.11 Spastic hemiplegia affecting dominant side
342.12 Spastic hemiplegia affecting nondominant side
343.9 Unspecified infantile cerebral palsy ▽
344.81 Locked-in state
357.1 Polyneuropathy in collagen vascular disease — (Code first underlying disease: 446.0, 710.0, 714.0) ☒
359.6 Symptomatic inflammatory myopathy in diseases classified elsewhere — (Code first underlying disease: 135, 140.0-208.9, 277.3, 446.0, 710.0, 710.1, 710.2, 714.0) ☒
446.0 Polyarteritis nodosa
710.0 Systemic lupus erythematosus — (Use additional code to identify manifestation: 424.91, 581.81, 582.81, 583.81)
710.1 Systemic sclerosis — (Use additional code to identify manifestation: 359.6, 517.2)
710.2 Sicca syndrome
714.0 Rheumatoid arthritis — (Use additional code to identify manifestation: 357.1, 359.6)
727.05 Other tenosynovitis of hand and wrist
727.42 Ganglion of tendon sheath
727.81 Contracture of tendon (sheath)
727.82 Calcium deposits in tendon and bursa
727.89 Other disorders of synovium, tendon, and bursa
727.9 Unspecified disorder of synovium, tendon, and bursa ▽
905.8 Late effect of tendon injury

ICD-9-CM Procedural

83.91 Lysis of adhesions of muscle, tendon, fascia, and bursa

25300–25301

25300 Tenodesis at wrist; flexors of fingers
25301 extensors of fingers

ICD-9-CM Diagnostic

138 Late effects of acute poliomyelitis
343.8 Other specified infantile cerebral palsy
718.73 Developmental dislocation of joint, forearm
718.74 Developmental dislocation of joint, hand
726.4 Enthesopathy of wrist and carpus
727.63 Nontraumatic rupture of extensor tendons of hand and wrist
727.64 Nontraumatic rupture of flexor tendons of hand and wrist
727.9 Unspecified disorder of synovium, tendon, and bursa ▽
833.00 Closed dislocation of wrist, unspecified part ▽
833.01 Closed dislocation of distal radioulnar (joint)
833.02 Closed dislocation of radiocarpal (joint)
833.03 Closed dislocation of midcarpal (joint)
833.04 Closed dislocation of carpometacarpal (joint)
833.05 Closed dislocation of proximal end of metacarpal (bone)
833.09 Closed dislocation of other part of wrist
834.00 Closed dislocation of finger, unspecified part ▽
834.01 Closed dislocation of metacarpophalangeal (joint)
834.02 Closed dislocation of interphalangeal (joint), hand
834.10 Open dislocation of finger, unspecified part ▽

▽ Unspecified code ♀ Female diagnosis ☒ Manifestation code ♂ Male diagnosis

834.11 Open dislocation of metacarpophalangeal (joint)
834.12 Open dislocation interphalangeal (joint), hand
881.22 Open wound of wrist, with tendon involvement — (Use additional code to identify infection)
883.2 Open wound of finger(s), with tendon involvement — (Use additional code to identify infection)
884.2 Multiple and unspecified open wound of upper limb, with tendon involvement — (Use additional code to identify infection)
905.8 Late effect of tendon injury

ICD-9-CM Procedural

82.85 Other tenodesis of hand
83.88 Other plastic operations on tendon

25310–25312

25310 Tendon transplantation or transfer, flexor or extensor, forearm and/or wrist, single; each tendon
25312 with tendon graft(s) (includes obtaining graft), each tendon

ICD-9-CM Diagnostic

138 Late effects of acute poliomyelitis
343.8 Other specified infantile cerebral palsy
357.1 Polyneuropathy in collagen vascular disease — (Code first underlying disease: 446.0, 710.0, 714.0) ☒
359.6 Symptomatic inflammatory myopathy in diseases classified elsewhere — (Code first underlying disease: 135, 140.0-208.9, 277.3, 446.0, 710.0, 710.1, 710.2, 714.0) ☒
446.0 Polyarteritis nodosa
710.0 Systemic lupus erythematosus — (Use additional code to identify manifestation: 424.91, 581.81, 582.81, 583.81)
710.1 Systemic sclerosis — (Use additional code to identify manifestation: 359.6, 517.2)
710.2 Sicca syndrome
714.0 Rheumatoid arthritis — (Use additional code to identify manifestation: 357.1, 359.6)
715.13 Primary localized osteoarthrosis, forearm
715.33 Localized osteoarthrosis not specified whether primary or secondary, forearm
715.93 Osteoarthrosis, unspecified whether generalized or localized, forearm ▽
726.4 Enthesopathy of wrist and carpus
727.63 Nontraumatic rupture of extensor tendons of hand and wrist
727.64 Nontraumatic rupture of flexor tendons of hand and wrist
881.20 Open wound of forearm, with tendon involvement — (Use additional code to identify infection)
881.22 Open wound of wrist, with tendon involvement — (Use additional code to identify infection)
905.8 Late effect of tendon injury

ICD-9-CM Procedural

83.75 Tendon transfer or transplantation
83.81 Tendon graft

25315–25316

25315 Flexor origin slide (eg, for cerebral palsy, Volkmann contracture), forearm and/or wrist;
25316 with tendon(s) transfer

ICD-9-CM Diagnostic

138 Late effects of acute poliomyelitis
343.0 Diplegic infantile cerebral palsy
343.1 Hemiplegic infantile cerebral palsy
343.2 Quadriplegic infantile cerebral palsy
343.3 Monoplegic infantile cerebral palsy
343.4 Infantile hemiplegia
343.8 Other specified infantile cerebral palsy
343.9 Unspecified infantile cerebral palsy ▽
726.4 Enthesopathy of wrist and carpus
728.88 Rhabdomyolysis
755.26 Congenital longitudinal deficiency, radial, complete or partial (with or without distal deficiencies, incomplete)
881.20 Open wound of forearm, with tendon involvement — (Use additional code to identify infection)
881.22 Open wound of wrist, with tendon involvement — (Use additional code to identify infection)
905.8 Late effect of tendon injury
958.6 Volkmann's ischemic contracture

ICD-9-CM Procedural

82.85 Other tenodesis of hand
83.75 Tendon transfer or transplantation
83.88 Other plastic operations on tendon

25320

25320 Capsulorrhaphy or reconstruction, wrist, open (eg, capsulodesis, ligament repair, tendon transfer or graft) (includes synovectomy, capsulotomy and open reduction) for carpal instability

ICD-9-CM Diagnostic

170.5 Malignant neoplasm of short bones of upper limb
357.1 Polyneuropathy in collagen vascular disease — (Code first underlying disease: 446.0, 710.0, 714.0) ☒
359.6 Symptomatic inflammatory myopathy in diseases classified elsewhere — (Code first underlying disease: 135, 140.0-208.9, 277.3, 446.0, 710.0, 710.1, 710.2, 714.0) ☒
446.0 Polyarteritis nodosa
710.0 Systemic lupus erythematosus — (Use additional code to identify manifestation: 424.91, 581.81, 582.81, 583.81)
710.1 Systemic sclerosis — (Use additional code to identify manifestation: 359.6, 517.2)
710.2 Sicca syndrome
710.3 Dermatomyositis
710.4 Polymyositis
710.5 Eosinophilia myalgia syndrome — (Use additional E code to identify drug, if drug-induced)
710.8 Other specified diffuse disease of connective tissue
710.9 Unspecified diffuse connective tissue disease ▽
714.0 Rheumatoid arthritis — (Use additional code to identify manifestation: 357.1, 359.6)
714.9 Unspecified inflammatory polyarthropathy ▽
715.13 Primary localized osteoarthrosis, forearm
715.93 Osteoarthrosis, unspecified whether generalized or localized, forearm ▽
718.03 Articular cartilage disorder, forearm
718.73 Developmental dislocation of joint, forearm
718.83 Other joint derangement, not elsewhere classified, forearm
727.63 Nontraumatic rupture of extensor tendons of hand and wrist
727.64 Nontraumatic rupture of flexor tendons of hand and wrist
727.9 Unspecified disorder of synovium, tendon, and bursa ▽
731.1 Osteitis deformans in diseases classified elsewhere — (Code first underlying disease: 170.0-170.9) ☒
833.00 Closed dislocation of wrist, unspecified part ▽
833.10 Open dislocation of wrist, unspecified part ▽
881.12 Open wound of wrist, complicated — (Use additional code to identify infection)
881.22 Open wound of wrist, with tendon involvement — (Use additional code to identify infection)
884.1 Multiple and unspecified open wound of upper limb, complicated — (Use additional code to identify infection)

ICD-9-CM Procedural

81.75 Arthroplasty of carpocarpal or carpometacarpal joint without implant
81.93 Suture of capsule or ligament of upper extremity
83.73 Reattachment of tendon
83.75 Tendon transfer or transplantation

25332

25332 Arthroplasty, wrist, with or without interposition, with or without external or internal fixation

ICD-9-CM Diagnostic

357.1 Polyneuropathy in collagen vascular disease — (Code first underlying disease: 446.0, 710.0, 714.0) ☒
359.6 Symptomatic inflammatory myopathy in diseases classified elsewhere — (Code first underlying disease: 135, 140.0-208.9, 277.3, 446.0, 710.0, 710.1, 710.2, 714.0) ☒
446.0 Polyarteritis nodosa
710.0 Systemic lupus erythematosus — (Use additional code to identify manifestation: 424.91, 581.81, 582.81, 583.81)
710.1 Systemic sclerosis — (Use additional code to identify manifestation: 359.6, 517.2)
710.2 Sicca syndrome
714.0 Rheumatoid arthritis — (Use additional code to identify manifestation: 357.1, 359.6)

▽ Unspecified code
♀ Female diagnosis
☒ Manifestation code
♂ Male diagnosis

714.9 Unspecified inflammatory polyarthropathy ▽
715.13 Primary localized osteoarthrosis, forearm
715.93 Osteoarthrosis, unspecified whether generalized or localized, forearm ▽
716.93 Unspecified arthropathy, forearm ▽
719.13 Hemarthrosis, forearm
733.81 Malunion of fracture
733.82 Nonunion of fracture
905.2 Late effect of fracture of upper extremities

ICD-9-CM Procedural

81.74 Arthroplasty of carpocarpal or carpometacarpal joint with implant

25335

25335 Centralization of wrist on ulna (eg, radial club hand)

ICD-9-CM Diagnostic

357.1 Polyneuropathy in collagen vascular disease — (Code first underlying disease: 446.0, 710.0, 714.0) ☒
359.6 Symptomatic inflammatory myopathy in diseases classified elsewhere — (Code first underlying disease: 135, 140.0-208.9, 277.3, 446.0, 710.0, 710.1, 710.2, 714.0) ☒
446.0 Polyarteritis nodosa
710.0 Systemic lupus erythematosus — (Use additional code to identify manifestation: 424.91, 581.81, 582.81, 583.81)
710.1 Systemic sclerosis — (Use additional code to identify manifestation: 359.6, 517.2)
710.2 Sicca syndrome
714.0 Rheumatoid arthritis — (Use additional code to identify manifestation: 357.1, 359.6)
736.00 Unspecified deformity of forearm, excluding fingers ▽
736.07 Club hand, acquired
736.09 Other acquired deformities of forearm, excluding fingers
754.89 Other specified nonteratogenic anomalies
755.50 Unspecified congenital anomaly of upper limb ▽

ICD-9-CM Procedural

78.54 Internal fixation of carpals and metacarpals without fracture reduction
80.43 Division of joint capsule, ligament, or cartilage of wrist
81.75 Arthroplasty of carpocarpal or carpometacarpal joint without implant

25337

25337 Reconstruction for stabilization of unstable distal ulna or distal radioulnar joint, secondary by soft tissue stabilization (eg, tendon transfer, tendon graft or weave, or tenodesis) with or without open reduction of distal radioulnar joint

ICD-9-CM Diagnostic

716.13 Traumatic arthropathy, forearm
718.73 Developmental dislocation of joint, forearm
718.83 Other joint derangement, not elsewhere classified, forearm
726.90 Enthesopathy of unspecified site ▽
727.05 Other tenosynovitis of hand and wrist
727.63 Nontraumatic rupture of extensor tendons of hand and wrist
727.64 Nontraumatic rupture of flexor tendons of hand and wrist
728.4 Laxity of ligament
728.5 Hypermobility syndrome
813.43 Closed fracture of distal end of ulna (alone)
813.53 Open fracture of distal end of ulna (alone)
813.92 Open fracture of unspecified part of ulna (alone) ▽
833.01 Closed dislocation of distal radioulnar (joint)
833.09 Closed dislocation of other part of wrist
833.11 Open dislocation of distal radioulnar (joint)
833.19 Open dislocation of other part of wrist
881.20 Open wound of forearm, with tendon involvement — (Use additional code to identify infection)
927.10 Crushing injury of forearm — (Use additional code to identify any associated injuries: 800-829, 850.0-854.1, 860.0-869.1)

ICD-9-CM Procedural

78.43 Other repair or plastic operations on radius and ulna
79.22 Open reduction of fracture of radius and ulna without internal fixation
83.75 Tendon transfer or transplantation
83.81 Tendon graft

25350–25355

25350 Osteotomy, radius; distal third
25355 middle or proximal third

ICD-9-CM Diagnostic

170.4 Malignant neoplasm of scapula and long bones of upper limb
198.5 Secondary malignant neoplasm of bone and bone marrow
213.4 Benign neoplasm of scapula and long bones of upper limb
715.13 Primary localized osteoarthrosis, forearm
715.23 Secondary localized osteoarthrosis, forearm
718.83 Other joint derangement, not elsewhere classified, forearm
731.1 Osteitis deformans in diseases classified elsewhere — (Code first underlying disease: 170.0-170.9) ☒
733.12 Pathologic fracture of distal radius and ulna
733.49 Aseptic necrosis of other bone site
733.81 Malunion of fracture
733.82 Nonunion of fracture
736.89 Other acquired deformity of other parts of limb
755.53 Radioulnar synostosis
756.51 Osteogenesis imperfecta
813.42 Other closed fractures of distal end of radius (alone)
813.43 Closed fracture of distal end of ulna (alone)
813.52 Other open fractures of distal end of radius (alone)
905.2 Late effect of fracture of upper extremities

ICD-9-CM Procedural

77.23 Wedge osteotomy of radius and ulna
77.33 Other division of radius and ulna

25360–25365

25360 Osteotomy; ulna
25365 radius AND ulna

ICD-9-CM Diagnostic

170.4 Malignant neoplasm of scapula and long bones of upper limb
198.5 Secondary malignant neoplasm of bone and bone marrow
213.4 Benign neoplasm of scapula and long bones of upper limb
715.13 Primary localized osteoarthrosis, forearm
715.23 Secondary localized osteoarthrosis, forearm
731.1 Osteitis deformans in diseases classified elsewhere — (Code first underlying disease: 170.0-170.9) ☒
733.49 Aseptic necrosis of other bone site
733.81 Malunion of fracture
733.82 Nonunion of fracture
736.89 Other acquired deformity of other parts of limb
755.53 Radioulnar synostosis
756.51 Osteogenesis imperfecta
905.2 Late effect of fracture of upper extremities

ICD-9-CM Procedural

77.23 Wedge osteotomy of radius and ulna
77.33 Other division of radius and ulna

25370–25375

25370 Multiple osteotomies, with realignment on intramedullary rod (Sofield type procedure); radius OR ulna
25375 radius AND ulna

ICD-9-CM Diagnostic

170.4 Malignant neoplasm of scapula and long bones of upper limb
198.5 Secondary malignant neoplasm of bone and bone marrow
213.4 Benign neoplasm of scapula and long bones of upper limb
715.13 Primary localized osteoarthrosis, forearm
716.13 Traumatic arthropathy, forearm
716.53 Unspecified polyarthropathy or polyarthritis, forearm ▽
716.93 Unspecified arthropathy, forearm ▽
731.1 Osteitis deformans in diseases classified elsewhere — (Code first underlying disease: 170.0-170.9) ☒
736.89 Other acquired deformity of other parts of limb
755.50 Unspecified congenital anomaly of upper limb ▽
755.59 Other congenital anomaly of upper limb, including shoulder girdle
756.51 Osteogenesis imperfecta
756.53 Osteopoikilosis
V54.02 Encounter for lengthening/adjustment of growth rod

▽ Unspecified code ☒ Manifestation code
♀ Female diagnosis ♂ Male diagnosis

ICD-9-CM Procedural
77.23 Wedge osteotomy of radius and ulna
77.33 Other division of radius and ulna
78.43 Other repair or plastic operations on radius and ulna

25390
25390 Osteoplasty, radius OR ulna; shortening

ICD-9-CM Diagnostic
718.83 Other joint derangement, not elsewhere classified, forearm
732.3 Juvenile osteochondrosis of upper extremity
733.99 Other disorders of bone and cartilage
736.00 Unspecified deformity of forearm, excluding fingers ▽
736.09 Other acquired deformities of forearm, excluding fingers
755.50 Unspecified congenital anomaly of upper limb ▽
755.54 Madelung's deformity
755.59 Other congenital anomaly of upper limb, including shoulder girdle

ICD-9-CM Procedural
78.23 Limb shortening procedures, radius and ulna

25391
25391 Osteoplasty, radius OR ulna; lengthening with autograft

ICD-9-CM Diagnostic
718.83 Other joint derangement, not elsewhere classified, forearm
733.81 Malunion of fracture
733.82 Nonunion of fracture
733.99 Other disorders of bone and cartilage
736.00 Unspecified deformity of forearm, excluding fingers ▽
736.09 Other acquired deformities of forearm, excluding fingers
755.20 Congenital unspecified reduction deformity of upper limb ▽
755.26 Congenital longitudinal deficiency, radial, complete or partial (with or without distal deficiencies, incomplete)
755.27 Congenital longitudinal deficiency, ulnar, complete or partial (with or without distal deficiencies, incomplete)
755.50 Unspecified congenital anomaly of upper limb ▽

ICD-9-CM Procedural
77.79 Excision of other bone for graft, except facial bones
78.03 Bone graft of radius and ulna
78.13 Application of external fixation device, radius and ulna
78.33 Limb lengthening procedures, radius and ulna
84.53 Implantation of internal limb lengthening device with kinetic distraction
84.54 Implantation of other internal limb lengthening device

25392
25392 Osteoplasty, radius AND ulna; shortening (excluding 64876)

ICD-9-CM Diagnostic
718.83 Other joint derangement, not elsewhere classified, forearm
732.3 Juvenile osteochondrosis of upper extremity
733.99 Other disorders of bone and cartilage
736.00 Unspecified deformity of forearm, excluding fingers ▽
736.09 Other acquired deformities of forearm, excluding fingers
755.50 Unspecified congenital anomaly of upper limb ▽
755.59 Other congenital anomaly of upper limb, including shoulder girdle

ICD-9-CM Procedural
78.23 Limb shortening procedures, radius and ulna

25393
25393 Osteoplasty, radius AND ulna; lengthening with autograft

ICD-9-CM Diagnostic
718.83 Other joint derangement, not elsewhere classified, forearm
733.81 Malunion of fracture
733.82 Nonunion of fracture
733.99 Other disorders of bone and cartilage
736.00 Unspecified deformity of forearm, excluding fingers ▽
736.09 Other acquired deformities of forearm, excluding fingers
755.20 Congenital unspecified reduction deformity of upper limb ▽
755.26 Congenital longitudinal deficiency, radial, complete or partial (with or without distal deficiencies, incomplete)
755.27 Congenital longitudinal deficiency, ulnar, complete or partial (with or without distal deficiencies, incomplete)
755.50 Unspecified congenital anomaly of upper limb ▽

ICD-9-CM Procedural
77.79 Excision of other bone for graft, except facial bones
78.03 Bone graft of radius and ulna
78.13 Application of external fixation device, radius and ulna
78.33 Limb lengthening procedures, radius and ulna
84.53 Implantation of internal limb lengthening device with kinetic distraction
84.54 Implantation of other internal limb lengthening device

25394
25394 Osteoplasty, carpal bone, shortening

ICD-9-CM Diagnostic
718.83 Other joint derangement, not elsewhere classified, forearm
732.3 Juvenile osteochondrosis of upper extremity
733.99 Other disorders of bone and cartilage
736.00 Unspecified deformity of forearm, excluding fingers ▽
736.09 Other acquired deformities of forearm, excluding fingers
755.50 Unspecified congenital anomaly of upper limb ▽
755.59 Other congenital anomaly of upper limb, including shoulder girdle

ICD-9-CM Procedural
78.24 Limb shortening procedures, carpals and metacarpals

25400–25405
25400 Repair of nonunion or malunion, radius OR ulna; without graft (eg, compression technique)
25405 with autograft (includes obtaining graft)v

ICD-9-CM Diagnostic
733.81 Malunion of fracture
733.82 Nonunion of fracture
905.2 Late effect of fracture of upper extremities

ICD-9-CM Procedural
77.77 Excision of tibia and fibula for graft
77.79 Excision of other bone for graft, except facial bones
78.03 Bone graft of radius and ulna
78.43 Other repair or plastic operations on radius and ulna

25415–25420
25415 Repair of nonunion or malunion, radius AND ulna; without graft (eg, compression technique)
25420 with autograft (includes obtaining graft)

ICD-9-CM Diagnostic
733.81 Malunion of fracture
733.82 Nonunion of fracture
905.2 Late effect of fracture of upper extremities

ICD-9-CM Procedural
77.77 Excision of tibia and fibula for graft
77.79 Excision of other bone for graft, except facial bones
78.03 Bone graft of radius and ulna
78.43 Other repair or plastic operations on radius and ulna

25425–25426
25425 Repair of defect with autograft; radius OR ulna
25426 radius AND ulna

ICD-9-CM Diagnostic
730.13 Chronic osteomyelitis, forearm — (Use additional code to identify organism, 041.1)
730.83 Other infections involving bone in diseases classified elsewhere, forearm — (Code first underlying disease: 002.0, 015.0-015.9. Use additional code to identify organism) ☒
732.3 Juvenile osteochondrosis of upper extremity
733.12 Pathologic fracture of distal radius and ulna
733.49 Aseptic necrosis of other bone site
733.81 Malunion of fracture
733.82 Nonunion of fracture
736.00 Unspecified deformity of forearm, excluding fingers ▽

736.05 Wrist drop (acquired)
736.09 Other acquired deformities of forearm, excluding fingers
755.26 Congenital longitudinal deficiency, radial, complete or partial (with or without distal deficiencies, incomplete)
755.27 Congenital longitudinal deficiency, ulnar, complete or partial (with or without distal deficiencies, incomplete)
905.2 Late effect of fracture of upper extremities
996.4 Mechanical complication of internal orthopedic device, implant, and graft

ICD-9-CM Procedural

77.77 Excision of tibia and fibula for graft
77.79 Excision of other bone for graft, except facial bones
78.03 Bone graft of radius and ulna
78.43 Other repair or plastic operations on radius and ulna

25430

25430 Insertion of vascular pedicle into carpal bone (eg, Hori procedure)

ICD-9-CM Diagnostic

170.5 Malignant neoplasm of short bones of upper limb
198.5 Secondary malignant neoplasm of bone and bone marrow
213.5 Benign neoplasm of short bones of upper limb
238.0 Neoplasm of uncertain behavior of bone and articular cartilage
239.2 Neoplasms of unspecified nature of bone, soft tissue, and skin
730.13 Chronic osteomyelitis, forearm — (Use additional code to identify organism, 041.1)
730.14 Chronic osteomyelitis, hand — (Use additional code to identify organism, 041.1)
730.23 Unspecified osteomyelitis, forearm — (Use additional code to identify organism, 041.1) ▽
730.24 Unspecified osteomyelitis, hand — (Use additional code to identify organism, 041.1) ▽
733.19 Pathologic fracture of other specified site
733.49 Aseptic necrosis of other bone site
733.82 Nonunion of fracture
733.90 Disorder of bone and cartilage, unspecified ▽
733.99 Other disorders of bone and cartilage
814.00 Unspecified closed fracture of carpal bone ▽
814.01 Closed fracture of navicular (scaphoid) bone of wrist
814.02 Closed fracture of lunate (semilunar) bone of wrist
814.03 Closed fracture of triquetral (cuneiform) bone of wrist
814.04 Closed fracture of pisiform bone of wrist
814.05 Closed fracture of trapezium bone (larger multangular) of wrist
814.06 Closed fracture of trapezoid bone (smaller multangular) of wrist
814.07 Closed fracture of capitate bone (os magnum) of wrist
814.08 Closed fracture of hamate (unciform) bone of wrist
814.09 Closed fracture of other bone of wrist
814.10 Unspecified open fracture of carpal bone ▽
814.12 Open fracture of lunate (semilunar) bone of wrist
814.13 Open fracture of triquetral (cuneiform) bone of wrist
814.14 Open fracture of pisiform bone of wrist
814.15 Open fracture of trapezium bone (larger multangular) of wrist
814.16 Open fracture of trapezoid bone (smaller multangular) of wrist
814.17 Open fracture of capitate bone (os magnum) of wrist
814.18 Open fracture of hamate (unciform) bone of wrist
814.19 Open fracture of other bone of wrist
905.2 Late effect of fracture of upper extremities
927.20 Crushing injury of hand(s) — (Use additional code to identify any associated injuries: 800-829, 850.0-854.1, 860.0-869.1)
927.21 Crushing injury of wrist — (Use additional code to identify any associated injuries: 800-829, 850.0-854.1, 860.0-869.1)

ICD-9-CM Procedural

86.73 Attachment of pedicle or flap graft to hand
86.74 Attachment of pedicle or flap graft to other sites

HCPCS Level II Supplies & Services

HCPCS Level II codes are used to report the supplies, durable medical equipment, and certain medical services provided on an outpatient basis. Because the procedure(s) represented on this page would be performed in an inpatient or outpatient facility, no HCPCS Level II codes apply.

25431

25431 Repair of nonunion of carpal bone (excluding carpal scaphoid (navicular)) (includes obtaining graft and necessary fixation), each bone

ICD-9-CM Diagnostic

733.82 Nonunion of fracture
905.2 Late effect of fracture of upper extremities

ICD-9-CM Procedural

77.77 Excision of tibia and fibula for graft
78.04 Bone graft of carpals and metacarpals
78.79 Osteoclasis of other bone, except facial bones

HCPCS Level II Supplies & Services

HCPCS Level II codes are used to report the supplies, durable medical equipment, and certain medical services provided on an outpatient basis. Because the procedure(s) represented on this page would be performed in an inpatient or outpatient facility, no HCPCS Level II codes apply.

25440

25440 Repair of nonunion, scaphoid carpal (navicular) bone, with or without radial styloidectomy (includes obtaining graft and necessary fixation)

ICD-9-CM Diagnostic

733.82 Nonunion of fracture
905.2 Late effect of fracture of upper extremities

ICD-9-CM Procedural

77.77 Excision of tibia and fibula for graft
77.79 Excision of other bone for graft, except facial bones
78.04 Bone graft of carpals and metacarpals

25441

25441 Arthroplasty with prosthetic replacement; distal radius

ICD-9-CM Diagnostic

357.1 Polyneuropathy in collagen vascular disease — (Code first underlying disease: 446.0, 710.0, 714.0) ☒
359.6 Symptomatic inflammatory myopathy in diseases classified elsewhere — (Code first underlying disease: 135, 140.0-208.9, 277.3, 446.0, 710.0, 710.1, 710.2, 714.0) ☒
446.0 Polyarteritis nodosa
710.0 Systemic lupus erythematosus — (Use additional code to identify manifestation: 424.91, 581.81, 582.81, 583.81)
710.1 Systemic sclerosis — (Use additional code to identify manifestation: 359.6, 517.2)
710.2 Sicca syndrome
711.03 Pyogenic arthritis, forearm — (Use additional code to identify infectious organism: 041.0-041.8)
711.93 Unspecified infective arthritis, forearm ▽
714.0 Rheumatoid arthritis — (Use additional code to identify manifestation: 357.1, 359.6)
715.13 Primary localized osteoarthrosis, forearm
715.23 Secondary localized osteoarthrosis, forearm
715.33 Localized osteoarthrosis not specified whether primary or secondary, forearm
716.13 Traumatic arthropathy, forearm
716.23 Allergic arthritis, forearm
716.63 Unspecified monoarthritis, forearm ▽
716.93 Unspecified arthropathy, forearm ▽
730.13 Chronic osteomyelitis, forearm — (Use additional code to identify organism, 041.1)
730.23 Unspecified osteomyelitis, forearm — (Use additional code to identify organism, 041.1) ▽
905.2 Late effect of fracture of upper extremities

ICD-9-CM Procedural

81.74 Arthroplasty of carpocarpal or carpometacarpal joint with implant

25442

25442 Arthroplasty with prosthetic replacement; distal ulna

ICD-9-CM Diagnostic

357.1 Polyneuropathy in collagen vascular disease — (Code first underlying disease: 446.0, 710.0, 714.0) ☒

▽ Unspecified code
♀ Female diagnosis
☒ Manifestation code
♂ Male diagnosis

359.6 Symptomatic inflammatory myopathy in diseases classified elsewhere — (Code first underlying disease: 135, 140.0-208.9, 277.3, 446.0, 710.0, 710.1, 710.2, 714.0) ☒
446.0 Polyarteritis nodosa
710.0 Systemic lupus erythematosus — (Use additional code to identify manifestation: 424.91, 581.81, 582.81, 583.81)
710.1 Systemic sclerosis — (Use additional code to identify manifestation: 359.6, 517.2)
710.2 Sicca syndrome
711.03 Pyogenic arthritis, forearm — (Use additional code to identify infectious organism: 041.0-041.8)
711.04 Pyogenic arthritis, hand — (Use additional code to identify infectious organism: 041.0-041.8)
711.93 Unspecified infective arthritis, forearm ▽
711.94 Unspecified infective arthritis, hand ▽
714.0 Rheumatoid arthritis — (Use additional code to identify manifestation: 357.1, 359.6)
715.13 Primary localized osteoarthrosis, forearm
715.14 Primary localized osteoarthrosis, hand
715.23 Secondary localized osteoarthrosis, forearm
715.24 Secondary localized osteoarthrosis, involving hand
715.33 Localized osteoarthrosis not specified whether primary or secondary, forearm
715.34 Localized osteoarthrosis not specified whether primary or secondary, hand
716.13 Traumatic arthropathy, forearm
716.14 Traumatic arthropathy, hand
716.63 Unspecified monoarthritis, forearm ▽
716.64 Unspecified monoarthritis, hand ▽
716.93 Unspecified arthropathy, forearm ▽
716.94 Unspecified arthopathy, hand ▽
718.83 Other joint derangement, not elsewhere classified, forearm
718.84 Other joint derangement, not elsewhere classified, hand
719.23 Villonodular synovitis, forearm
719.24 Villonodular synovitis, hand
719.63 Other symptoms referable to forearm joint
719.64 Other symptoms referable to hand joint
730.13 Chronic osteomyelitis, forearm — (Use additional code to identify organism, 041.1)
730.14 Chronic osteomyelitis, hand — (Use additional code to identify organism, 041.1)
730.23 Unspecified osteomyelitis, forearm — (Use additional code to identify organism, 041.1) ▽
730.24 Unspecified osteomyelitis, hand — (Use additional code to identify organism, 041.1) ▽
730.33 Periostitis, without mention of osteomyelitis, forearm — (Use additional code to identify organism, 041.1)
730.34 Periostitis, without mention of osteomyelitis, hand — (Use additional code to identify organism, 041.1)
731.0 Osteitis deformans without mention of bone tumor
733.49 Aseptic necrosis of other bone site
733.82 Nonunion of fracture
736.00 Unspecified deformity of forearm, excluding fingers ▽
756.51 Osteogenesis imperfecta
905.2 Late effect of fracture of upper extremities

ICD-9-CM Procedural

81.74 Arthroplasty of carpocarpal or carpometacarpal joint with implant

25443

25443 Arthroplasty with prosthetic replacement; scaphoid carpal (navicular)

ICD-9-CM Diagnostic

357.1 Polyneuropathy in collagen vascular disease — (Code first underlying disease: 446.0, 710.0, 714.0) ☒
359.6 Symptomatic inflammatory myopathy in diseases classified elsewhere — (Code first underlying disease: 135, 140.0-208.9, 277.3, 446.0, 710.0, 710.1, 710.2, 714.0) ☒
446.0 Polyarteritis nodosa
710.0 Systemic lupus erythematosus — (Use additional code to identify manifestation: 424.91, 581.81, 582.81, 583.81)
710.1 Systemic sclerosis — (Use additional code to identify manifestation: 359.6, 517.2)
710.2 Sicca syndrome
711.03 Pyogenic arthritis, forearm — (Use additional code to identify infectious organism: 041.0-041.8)
711.04 Pyogenic arthritis, hand — (Use additional code to identify infectious organism: 041.0-041.8)
711.93 Unspecified infective arthritis, forearm ▽
711.94 Unspecified infective arthritis, hand ▽
714.0 Rheumatoid arthritis — (Use additional code to identify manifestation: 357.1, 359.6)
715.13 Primary localized osteoarthrosis, forearm
715.14 Primary localized osteoarthrosis, hand
715.23 Secondary localized osteoarthrosis, forearm
715.24 Secondary localized osteoarthrosis, involving hand
715.33 Localized osteoarthrosis not specified whether primary or secondary, forearm
715.34 Localized osteoarthrosis not specified whether primary or secondary, hand
716.13 Traumatic arthropathy, forearm
716.14 Traumatic arthropathy, hand
716.63 Unspecified monoarthritis, forearm ▽
716.64 Unspecified monoarthritis, hand ▽
716.93 Unspecified arthropathy, forearm ▽
716.94 Unspecified arthopathy, hand ▽
718.83 Other joint derangement, not elsewhere classified, forearm
718.84 Other joint derangement, not elsewhere classified, hand
719.23 Villonodular synovitis, forearm
719.24 Villonodular synovitis, hand
719.63 Other symptoms referable to forearm joint
719.64 Other symptoms referable to hand joint
730.13 Chronic osteomyelitis, forearm — (Use additional code to identify organism, 041.1)
730.14 Chronic osteomyelitis, hand — (Use additional code to identify organism, 041.1)
730.23 Unspecified osteomyelitis, forearm — (Use additional code to identify organism, 041.1) ▽
730.24 Unspecified osteomyelitis, hand — (Use additional code to identify organism, 041.1) ▽
730.33 Periostitis, without mention of osteomyelitis, forearm — (Use additional code to identify organism, 041.1)
730.34 Periostitis, without mention of osteomyelitis, hand — (Use additional code to identify organism, 041.1)
731.0 Osteitis deformans without mention of bone tumor
733.49 Aseptic necrosis of other bone site
733.82 Nonunion of fracture
736.00 Unspecified deformity of forearm, excluding fingers ▽
756.51 Osteogenesis imperfecta
905.2 Late effect of fracture of upper extremities

ICD-9-CM Procedural

81.74 Arthroplasty of carpocarpal or carpometacarpal joint with implant

25444

25444 Arthroplasty with prosthetic replacement; lunate

ICD-9-CM Diagnostic

357.1 Polyneuropathy in collagen vascular disease — (Code first underlying disease: 446.0, 710.0, 714.0) ☒
359.6 Symptomatic inflammatory myopathy in diseases classified elsewhere — (Code first underlying disease: 135, 140.0-208.9, 277.3, 446.0, 710.0, 710.1, 710.2, 714.0) ☒
446.0 Polyarteritis nodosa
710.0 Systemic lupus erythematosus — (Use additional code to identify manifestation: 424.91, 581.81, 582.81, 583.81)
710.1 Systemic sclerosis — (Use additional code to identify manifestation: 359.6, 517.2)
710.2 Sicca syndrome
711.03 Pyogenic arthritis, forearm — (Use additional code to identify infectious organism: 041.0-041.8)
711.04 Pyogenic arthritis, hand — (Use additional code to identify infectious organism: 041.0-041.8)
711.93 Unspecified infective arthritis, forearm ▽
711.94 Unspecified infective arthritis, hand ▽
714.0 Rheumatoid arthritis — (Use additional code to identify manifestation: 357.1, 359.6)
715.13 Primary localized osteoarthrosis, forearm
715.14 Primary localized osteoarthrosis, hand
715.23 Secondary localized osteoarthrosis, forearm
715.24 Secondary localized osteoarthrosis, involving hand
715.33 Localized osteoarthrosis not specified whether primary or secondary, forearm
715.34 Localized osteoarthrosis not specified whether primary or secondary, hand
716.13 Traumatic arthropathy, forearm
716.14 Traumatic arthropathy, hand
716.63 Unspecified monoarthritis, forearm ▽

716.64 Unspecified monoarthritis, hand ▽
716.93 Unspecified arthropathy, forearm ▽
716.94 Unspecified arthopathy, hand ▽
718.83 Other joint derangement, not elsewhere classified, forearm
718.84 Other joint derangement, not elsewhere classified, hand
719.23 Villonodular synovitis, forearm
719.24 Villonodular synovitis, hand
719.63 Other symptoms referable to forearm joint
719.64 Other symptoms referable to hand joint
730.13 Chronic osteomyelitis, forearm — (Use additional code to identify organism, 041.1)
730.14 Chronic osteomyelitis, hand — (Use additional code to identify organism, 041.1)
730.23 Unspecified osteomyelitis, forearm — (Use additional code to identify organism, 041.1) ▽
730.24 Unspecified osteomyelitis, hand — (Use additional code to identify organism, 041.1) ▽
730.33 Periostitis, without mention of osteomyelitis, forearm — (Use additional code to identify organism, 041.1)
730.34 Periostitis, without mention of osteomyelitis, hand — (Use additional code to identify organism, 041.1)
731.0 Osteitis deformans without mention of bone tumor
733.49 Aseptic necrosis of other bone site
733.82 Nonunion of fracture
736.00 Unspecified deformity of forearm, excluding fingers ▽
756.51 Osteogenesis imperfecta
905.2 Late effect of fracture of upper extremities

ICD-9-CM Procedural

81.74 Arthroplasty of carpocarpal or carpometacarpal joint with implant

25445

25445 Arthroplasty with prosthetic replacement; trapezium

ICD-9-CM Diagnostic

357.1 Polyneuropathy in collagen vascular disease — (Code first underlying disease: 446.0, 710.0, 714.0) ☒
359.6 Symptomatic inflammatory myopathy in diseases classified elsewhere — (Code first underlying disease: 135, 140.0-208.9, 277.3, 446.0, 710.0, 710.1, 710.2, 714.0) ☒
446.0 Polyarteritis nodosa
710.0 Systemic lupus erythematosus — (Use additional code to identify manifestation: 424.91, 581.81, 582.81, 583.81)
710.1 Systemic sclerosis — (Use additional code to identify manifestation: 359.6, 517.2)
710.2 Sicca syndrome
711.03 Pyogenic arthritis, forearm — (Use additional code to identify infectious organism: 041.0-041.8)
711.04 Pyogenic arthritis, hand — (Use additional code to identify infectious organism: 041.0-041.8)
711.93 Unspecified infective arthritis, forearm ▽
711.94 Unspecified infective arthritis, hand ▽
714.0 Rheumatoid arthritis — (Use additional code to identify manifestation: 357.1, 359.6)
715.13 Primary localized osteoarthrosis, forearm
715.14 Primary localized osteoarthrosis, hand
715.23 Secondary localized osteoarthrosis, forearm
715.24 Secondary localized osteoarthrosis, involving hand
715.33 Localized osteoarthrosis not specified whether primary or secondary, forearm
715.34 Localized osteoarthrosis not specified whether primary or secondary, hand
716.13 Traumatic arthropathy, forearm
716.14 Traumatic arthropathy, hand
716.63 Unspecified monoarthritis, forearm ▽
716.64 Unspecified monoarthritis, hand ▽
716.93 Unspecified arthropathy, forearm ▽
716.94 Unspecified arthopathy, hand ▽
718.83 Other joint derangement, not elsewhere classified, forearm
718.84 Other joint derangement, not elsewhere classified, hand
719.23 Villonodular synovitis, forearm
719.24 Villonodular synovitis, hand
719.63 Other symptoms referable to forearm joint
719.64 Other symptoms referable to hand joint
730.13 Chronic osteomyelitis, forearm — (Use additional code to identify organism, 041.1)
730.14 Chronic osteomyelitis, hand — (Use additional code to identify organism, 041.1)
730.23 Unspecified osteomyelitis, forearm — (Use additional code to identify organism, 041.1) ▽
730.24 Unspecified osteomyelitis, hand — (Use additional code to identify organism, 041.1) ▽
730.33 Periostitis, without mention of osteomyelitis, forearm — (Use additional code to identify organism, 041.1)
730.34 Periostitis, without mention of osteomyelitis, hand — (Use additional code to identify organism, 041.1)
731.0 Osteitis deformans without mention of bone tumor
733.49 Aseptic necrosis of other bone site
733.82 Nonunion of fracture
736.00 Unspecified deformity of forearm, excluding fingers ▽
756.51 Osteogenesis imperfecta
905.2 Late effect of fracture of upper extremities

ICD-9-CM Procedural

81.79 Other repair of hand, fingers, and wrist

25446

25446 Arthroplasty with prosthetic replacement; distal radius and partial or entire carpus (total wrist)

ICD-9-CM Diagnostic

357.1 Polyneuropathy in collagen vascular disease — (Code first underlying disease: 446.0, 710.0, 714.0) ☒
359.6 Symptomatic inflammatory myopathy in diseases classified elsewhere — (Code first underlying disease: 135, 140.0-208.9, 277.3, 446.0, 710.0, 710.1, 710.2, 714.0) ☒
446.0 Polyarteritis nodosa
710.0 Systemic lupus erythematosus — (Use additional code to identify manifestation: 424.91, 581.81, 582.81, 583.81)
710.1 Systemic sclerosis — (Use additional code to identify manifestation: 359.6, 517.2)
710.2 Sicca syndrome
711.03 Pyogenic arthritis, forearm — (Use additional code to identify infectious organism: 041.0-041.8)
711.04 Pyogenic arthritis, hand — (Use additional code to identify infectious organism: 041.0-041.8)
711.93 Unspecified infective arthritis, forearm ▽
711.94 Unspecified infective arthritis, hand ▽
714.0 Rheumatoid arthritis — (Use additional code to identify manifestation: 357.1, 359.6)
715.13 Primary localized osteoarthrosis, forearm
715.14 Primary localized osteoarthrosis, hand
715.23 Secondary localized osteoarthrosis, forearm
715.24 Secondary localized osteoarthrosis, involving hand
715.33 Localized osteoarthrosis not specified whether primary or secondary, forearm
715.34 Localized osteoarthrosis not specified whether primary or secondary, hand
716.13 Traumatic arthropathy, forearm
716.14 Traumatic arthropathy, hand
716.63 Unspecified monoarthritis, forearm ▽
716.64 Unspecified monoarthritis, hand ▽
716.93 Unspecified arthropathy, forearm ▽
716.94 Unspecified arthopathy, hand ▽
718.83 Other joint derangement, not elsewhere classified, forearm
718.84 Other joint derangement, not elsewhere classified, hand
719.23 Villonodular synovitis, forearm
719.24 Villonodular synovitis, hand
719.63 Other symptoms referable to forearm joint
719.64 Other symptoms referable to hand joint
730.13 Chronic osteomyelitis, forearm — (Use additional code to identify organism, 041.1)
730.14 Chronic osteomyelitis, hand — (Use additional code to identify organism, 041.1)
730.23 Unspecified osteomyelitis, forearm — (Use additional code to identify organism, 041.1) ▽
730.24 Unspecified osteomyelitis, hand — (Use additional code to identify organism, 041.1) ▽
730.33 Periostitis, without mention of osteomyelitis, forearm — (Use additional code to identify organism, 041.1)
730.34 Periostitis, without mention of osteomyelitis, hand — (Use additional code to identify organism, 041.1)
731.0 Osteitis deformans without mention of bone tumor
733.49 Aseptic necrosis of other bone site
733.82 Nonunion of fracture
736.00 Unspecified deformity of forearm, excluding fingers ▽

▽ Unspecified code
♀ Female diagnosis
☒ Manifestation code
♂ Male diagnosis

756.51 Osteogenesis imperfecta
905.2 Late effect of fracture of upper extremities

ICD-9-CM Procedural
81.73 Total wrist replacement

25447
25447 Arthroplasty, interposition, intercarpal or carpometacarpal joints

ICD-9-CM Diagnostic
357.1 Polyneuropathy in collagen vascular disease — (Code first underlying disease: 446.0, 710.0, 714.0) ☒
359.6 Symptomatic inflammatory myopathy in diseases classified elsewhere — (Code first underlying disease: 135, 140.0-208.9, 277.3, 446.0, 710.0, 710.1, 710.2, 714.0) ☒
446.0 Polyarteritis nodosa
710.0 Systemic lupus erythematosus — (Use additional code to identify manifestation: 424.91, 581.81, 582.81, 583.81)
710.1 Systemic sclerosis — (Use additional code to identify manifestation: 359.6, 517.2)
710.2 Sicca syndrome
714.0 Rheumatoid arthritis — (Use additional code to identify manifestation: 357.1, 359.6)
715.04 Generalized osteoarthrosis, involving hand
715.14 Primary localized osteoarthrosis, hand
715.94 Osteoarthrosis, unspecified whether generalized or localized, hand ▽
716.14 Traumatic arthropathy, hand
716.94 Unspecified arthopathy, hand ▽
814.00 Unspecified closed fracture of carpal bone ▽
905.2 Late effect of fracture of upper extremities

ICD-9-CM Procedural
81.74 Arthroplasty of carpocarpal or carpometacarpal joint with implant

25449
25449 Revision of arthroplasty, including removal of implant, wrist joint

ICD-9-CM Diagnostic
711.03 Pyogenic arthritis, forearm — (Use additional code to identify infectious organism: 041.0-041.8)
711.04 Pyogenic arthritis, hand — (Use additional code to identify infectious organism: 041.0-041.8)
711.83 Arthropathy associated with other infectious and parasitic diseases, forearm — (Code first underlying disease, such as: diseases classifiable to 080-088, 100-104, 130-136) ☒
711.84 Arthropathy associated with other infectious and parasitic diseases, hand — (Code first underlying disease, such as: diseases classifiable to 080-088, 100-104, 130-136) ☒
711.93 Unspecified infective arthritis, forearm ▽
711.94 Unspecified infective arthritis, hand ▽
730.13 Chronic osteomyelitis, forearm — (Use additional code to identify organism, 041.1)
730.14 Chronic osteomyelitis, hand — (Use additional code to identify organism, 041.1)
996.4 Mechanical complication of internal orthopedic device, implant, and graft
996.66 Infection and inflammatory reaction due to internal joint prosthesis — (Use additional code to identify specified infections)
996.67 Infection and inflammatory reaction due to other internal orthopedic device, implant, and graft — (Use additional code to identify specified infections)
998.59 Other postoperative infection — (Use additional code to identify infection)
998.6 Persistent postoperative fistula, not elsewhere classified

ICD-9-CM Procedural
78.64 Removal of implanted device from carpals and metacarpals
81.75 Arthroplasty of carpocarpal or carpometacarpal joint without implant

25450–25455
25450 Epiphyseal arrest by epiphysiodesis or stapling; distal radius OR ulna
25455 distal radius AND ulna

ICD-9-CM Diagnostic
732.3 Juvenile osteochondrosis of upper extremity

ICD-9-CM Procedural
78.23 Limb shortening procedures, radius and ulna

25490–25492
25490 Prophylactic treatment (nailing, pinning, plating or wiring) with or without methylmethacrylate; radius
25491 ulna
25492 radius AND ulna

ICD-9-CM Diagnostic
170.4 Malignant neoplasm of scapula and long bones of upper limb
198.5 Secondary malignant neoplasm of bone and bone marrow
213.4 Benign neoplasm of scapula and long bones of upper limb
238.0 Neoplasm of uncertain behavior of bone and articular cartilage
239.2 Neoplasms of unspecified nature of bone, soft tissue, and skin
733.49 Aseptic necrosis of other bone site

ICD-9-CM Procedural
78.13 Application of external fixation device, radius and ulna
78.53 Internal fixation of radius and ulna without fracture reduction
84.55 Insertion of bone void filler

25500–25505
25500 Closed treatment of radial shaft fracture; without manipulation
25505 with manipulation

ICD-9-CM Diagnostic
733.19 Pathologic fracture of other specified site
813.21 Closed fracture of shaft of radius (alone)

ICD-9-CM Procedural
79.02 Closed reduction of fracture of radius and ulna without internal fixation
93.53 Application of other cast

HCPCS Level II Supplies & Services
A4580 Cast supplies (e.g., plaster)
A4590 Special casting material (e.g., fiberglass)

25515
25515 Open treatment of radial shaft fracture, with or without internal or external fixation

ICD-9-CM Diagnostic
733.10 Pathologic fracture, unspecified site ▽
733.82 Nonunion of fracture
813.21 Closed fracture of shaft of radius (alone)
813.31 Open fracture of shaft of radius (alone)

ICD-9-CM Procedural
78.13 Application of external fixation device, radius and ulna
79.22 Open reduction of fracture of radius and ulna without internal fixation
79.32 Open reduction of fracture of radius and ulna with internal fixation

25520
25520 Closed treatment of radial shaft fracture and closed treatment of dislocation of distal radioulnar joint (Galeazzi fracture/dislocation)

ICD-9-CM Diagnostic
813.00 Unspecified fracture of radius and ulna, upper end of forearm, closed ▽
813.20 Unspecified closed fracture of shaft of radius or ulna ▽
813.21 Closed fracture of shaft of radius (alone)
813.42 Other closed fractures of distal end of radius (alone)
833.01 Closed dislocation of distal radioulnar (joint)

ICD-9-CM Procedural
79.02 Closed reduction of fracture of radius and ulna without internal fixation
79.79 Closed reduction of dislocation of other specified site, except temporomandibular

HCPCS Level II Supplies & Services
A4580 Cast supplies (e.g., plaster)
A4590 Special casting material (e.g., fiberglass)

25525

25525 Open treatment of radial shaft fracture, with internal and/ or external fixation and closed treatment of dislocation of distal radioulnar joint (Galeazzi fracture/dislocation), with or without percutaneous skeletal fixation

ICD-9-CM Diagnostic

733.19 Pathologic fracture of other specified site
813.21 Closed fracture of shaft of radius (alone)
813.31 Open fracture of shaft of radius (alone)
813.42 Other closed fractures of distal end of radius (alone)
833.01 Closed dislocation of distal radioulnar (joint)
833.11 Open dislocation of distal radioulnar (joint)

ICD-9-CM Procedural

78.13 Application of external fixation device, radius and ulna
79.32 Open reduction of fracture of radius and ulna with internal fixation

25526

25526 Open treatment of radial shaft fracture, with internal and/or external fixation and open treatment, with or without internal or external fixation of distal radioulnar joint (Galeazzi fracture/dislocation), includes repair of triangular fibrocartilage complex

ICD-9-CM Diagnostic

733.19 Pathologic fracture of other specified site
813.21 Closed fracture of shaft of radius (alone)
813.31 Open fracture of shaft of radius (alone)
813.42 Other closed fractures of distal end of radius (alone)
833.01 Closed dislocation of distal radioulnar (joint)
833.11 Open dislocation of distal radioulnar (joint)

ICD-9-CM Procedural

79.22 Open reduction of fracture of radius and ulna without internal fixation
79.32 Open reduction of fracture of radius and ulna with internal fixation
79.83 Open reduction of dislocation of wrist

25530–25535

25530 Closed treatment of ulnar shaft fracture; without manipulation
25535 with manipulation

ICD-9-CM Diagnostic

733.19 Pathologic fracture of other specified site
813.22 Closed fracture of shaft of ulna (alone)

ICD-9-CM Procedural

79.02 Closed reduction of fracture of radius and ulna without internal fixation
93.53 Application of other cast

HCPCS Level II Supplies & Services

A4580 Cast supplies (e.g., plaster)
A4590 Special casting material (e.g., fiberglass)

25545

25545 Open treatment of ulnar shaft fracture, with or without internal or external fixation

ICD-9-CM Diagnostic

733.19 Pathologic fracture of other specified site
733.81 Malunion of fracture
733.82 Nonunion of fracture
813.22 Closed fracture of shaft of ulna (alone)
813.32 Open fracture of shaft of ulna (alone)

ICD-9-CM Procedural

78.13 Application of external fixation device, radius and ulna
79.22 Open reduction of fracture of radius and ulna without internal fixation
79.32 Open reduction of fracture of radius and ulna with internal fixation

25560–25565

25560 Closed treatment of radial and ulnar shaft fractures; without manipulation
25565 with manipulation

ICD-9-CM Diagnostic

733.19 Pathologic fracture of other specified site
813.23 Closed fracture of shaft of radius with ulna

ICD-9-CM Procedural

79.02 Closed reduction of fracture of radius and ulna without internal fixation
93.53 Application of other cast

HCPCS Level II Supplies & Services

A4580 Cast supplies (e.g., plaster)
A4590 Special casting material (e.g., fiberglass)

25574–25575

25574 Open treatment of radial AND ulnar shaft fractures, with internal or external fixation; of radius OR ulna
25575 of radius AND ulna

ICD-9-CM Diagnostic

733.19 Pathologic fracture of other specified site
813.23 Closed fracture of shaft of radius with ulna
813.33 Open fracture of shaft of radius with ulna
927.10 Crushing injury of forearm — (Use additional code to identify any associated injuries: 800-829, 850.0-854.1, 860.0-869.1)

ICD-9-CM Procedural

78.13 Application of external fixation device, radius and ulna
79.32 Open reduction of fracture of radius and ulna with internal fixation

25600–25605

25600 Closed treatment of distal radial fracture (eg, Colles or Smith type) or epiphyseal separation, with or without fracture of ulnar styloid; without manipulation
25605 with manipulation

ICD-9-CM Diagnostic

732.9 Unspecified osteochondropathy
733.12 Pathologic fracture of distal radius and ulna
813.41 Closed Colles' fracture
813.42 Other closed fractures of distal end of radius (alone)
813.44 Closed fracture of lower end of radius with ulna
813.45 Torus fracture of lower end of radius

ICD-9-CM Procedural

79.02 Closed reduction of fracture of radius and ulna without internal fixation
79.42 Closed reduction of separated epiphysis of radius and ulna
93.53 Application of other cast
93.54 Application of splint

HCPCS Level II Supplies & Services

A4580 Cast supplies (e.g., plaster)
A4590 Special casting material (e.g., fiberglass)

25611

25611 Percutaneous skeletal fixation of distal radial fracture (eg, Colles or Smith type) or epiphyseal separation, with or without fracture of ulnar styloid, requiring manipulation, with or without external fixation

ICD-9-CM Diagnostic

732.9 Unspecified osteochondropathy
733.12 Pathologic fracture of distal radius and ulna
813.41 Closed Colles' fracture
813.42 Other closed fractures of distal end of radius (alone)
813.44 Closed fracture of lower end of radius with ulna

ICD-9-CM Procedural

78.13 Application of external fixation device, radius and ulna
79.12 Closed reduction of fracture of radius and ulna with internal fixation
79.42 Closed reduction of separated epiphysis of radius and ulna

25620

25620 Open treatment of distal radial fracture (eg, Colles or Smith type) or epiphyseal separation, with or without fracture of ulnar styloid, with or without internal or external fixation

ICD-9-CM Diagnostic

732.9 Unspecified osteochondropathy
733.12 Pathologic fracture of distal radius and ulna
733.82 Nonunion of fracture
813.41 Closed Colles' fracture

Unspecified code
♀ Female diagnosis

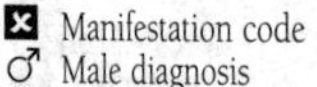
Manifestation code
♂ Male diagnosis

813.42 Other closed fractures of distal end of radius (alone)
813.44 Closed fracture of lower end of radius with ulna
813.51 Open Colles' fracture
813.52 Other open fractures of distal end of radius (alone)
813.54 Open fracture of lower end of radius with ulna

ICD-9-CM Procedural
78.13 Application of external fixation device, radius and ulna
79.22 Open reduction of fracture of radius and ulna without internal fixation
79.32 Open reduction of fracture of radius and ulna with internal fixation
79.52 Open reduction of separated epiphysis of radius and ulna

25622–25624
25622 Closed treatment of carpal scaphoid (navicular) fracture; without manipulation
25624 with manipulation

ICD-9-CM Diagnostic
733.19 Pathologic fracture of other specified site
814.01 Closed fracture of navicular (scaphoid) bone of wrist

ICD-9-CM Procedural
79.03 Closed reduction of fracture of carpals and metacarpals without internal fixation
93.53 Application of other cast

HCPCS Level II Supplies & Services
A4580 Cast supplies (e.g., plaster)
A4590 Special casting material (e.g., fiberglass)

25628
25628 Open treatment of carpal scaphoid (navicular) fracture, with or without internal or external fixation

ICD-9-CM Diagnostic
733.19 Pathologic fracture of other specified site
814.01 Closed fracture of navicular (scaphoid) bone of wrist
814.11 Open fracture of navicular (scaphoid) bone of wrist

ICD-9-CM Procedural
78.14 Application of external fixation device, carpals and metacarpals
79.23 Open reduction of fracture of carpals and metacarpals without internal fixation
79.33 Open reduction of fracture of carpals and metacarpals with internal fixation

HCPCS Level II Supplies & Services
A4305 Disposable drug delivery system, flow rate of 50 ml or greater per hour
A4306 Disposable drug delivery system, flow rate of 5 ml or less per hour
A4550 Surgical trays
A4580 Cast supplies (e.g., plaster)
A4590 Special casting material (e.g., fiberglass)

25630–25635
25630 Closed treatment of carpal bone fracture (excluding carpal scaphoid (navicular)); without manipulation, each bone
25635 with manipulation, each bone

ICD-9-CM Diagnostic
733.19 Pathologic fracture of other specified site
814.02 Closed fracture of lunate (semilunar) bone of wrist
814.03 Closed fracture of triquetral (cuneiform) bone of wrist
814.04 Closed fracture of pisiform bone of wrist
814.05 Closed fracture of trapezium bone (larger multangular) of wrist
814.06 Closed fracture of trapezoid bone (smaller multangular) of wrist
814.07 Closed fracture of capitate bone (os magnum) of wrist
814.08 Closed fracture of hamate (unciform) bone of wrist
814.09 Closed fracture of other bone of wrist

ICD-9-CM Procedural
79.03 Closed reduction of fracture of carpals and metacarpals without internal fixation
93.53 Application of other cast
93.54 Application of splint

HCPCS Level II Supplies & Services
A4580 Cast supplies (e.g., plaster)
A4590 Special casting material (e.g., fiberglass)

25645
25645 Open treatment of carpal bone fracture (other than carpal scaphoid (navicular)), each bone

ICD-9-CM Diagnostic
733.19 Pathologic fracture of other specified site
814.02 Closed fracture of lunate (semilunar) bone of wrist
814.03 Closed fracture of triquetral (cuneiform) bone of wrist
814.04 Closed fracture of pisiform bone of wrist
814.05 Closed fracture of trapezium bone (larger multangular) of wrist
814.06 Closed fracture of trapezoid bone (smaller multangular) of wrist
814.07 Closed fracture of capitate bone (os magnum) of wrist
814.08 Closed fracture of hamate (unciform) bone of wrist
814.09 Closed fracture of other bone of wrist
814.12 Open fracture of lunate (semilunar) bone of wrist
814.13 Open fracture of triquetral (cuneiform) bone of wrist
814.14 Open fracture of pisiform bone of wrist
814.15 Open fracture of trapezium bone (larger multangular) of wrist
814.16 Open fracture of trapezoid bone (smaller multangular) of wrist
814.17 Open fracture of capitate bone (os magnum) of wrist
814.18 Open fracture of hamate (unciform) bone of wrist
814.19 Open fracture of other bone of wrist

ICD-9-CM Procedural
79.23 Open reduction of fracture of carpals and metacarpals without internal fixation
79.33 Open reduction of fracture of carpals and metacarpals with internal fixation

HCPCS Level II Supplies & Services
A4550 Surgical trays
A4580 Cast supplies (e.g., plaster)
A4590 Special casting material (e.g., fiberglass)

25650
25650 Closed treatment of ulnar styloid fracture

ICD-9-CM Diagnostic
733.19 Pathologic fracture of other specified site
813.43 Closed fracture of distal end of ulna (alone)

ICD-9-CM Procedural
93.53 Application of other cast
93.54 Application of splint

HCPCS Level II Supplies & Services
A4580 Cast supplies (e.g., plaster)
A4590 Special casting material (e.g., fiberglass)

25651
25651 Percutaneous skeletal fixation of ulnar styloid fracture

ICD-9-CM Diagnostic
733.19 Pathologic fracture of other specified site
813.43 Closed fracture of distal end of ulna (alone)

ICD-9-CM Procedural
78.13 Application of external fixation device, radius and ulna
79.12 Closed reduction of fracture of radius and ulna with internal fixation

25652
25652 Open treatment of ulnar styloid fracture

ICD-9-CM Diagnostic
733.19 Pathologic fracture of other specified site
733.81 Malunion of fracture
733.82 Nonunion of fracture
813.43 Closed fracture of distal end of ulna (alone)
813.53 Open fracture of distal end of ulna (alone)

ICD-9-CM Procedural
78.13 Application of external fixation device, radius and ulna
79.22 Open reduction of fracture of radius and ulna without internal fixation

25660

25660 Closed treatment of radiocarpal or intercarpal dislocation, one or more bones, with manipulation

ICD-9-CM Diagnostic

718.23 Pathological dislocation of forearm joint
718.24 Pathological dislocation of hand joint
718.33 Recurrent dislocation of forearm joint
718.34 Recurrent dislocation of hand joint
718.73 Developmental dislocation of joint, forearm
833.02 Closed dislocation of radiocarpal (joint)
833.03 Closed dislocation of midcarpal (joint)

ICD-9-CM Procedural

79.73 Closed reduction of dislocation of wrist

HCPCS Level II Supplies & Services

A4580 Cast supplies (e.g., plaster)
A4590 Special casting material (e.g., fiberglass)

25670

25670 Open treatment of radiocarpal or intercarpal dislocation, one or more bones

ICD-9-CM Diagnostic

718.23 Pathological dislocation of forearm joint
718.24 Pathological dislocation of hand joint
718.33 Recurrent dislocation of forearm joint
718.34 Recurrent dislocation of hand joint
718.73 Developmental dislocation of joint, forearm
833.02 Closed dislocation of radiocarpal (joint)
833.03 Closed dislocation of midcarpal (joint)
833.12 Open dislocation of radiocarpal (joint)
833.13 Open dislocation of midcarpal (joint)

ICD-9-CM Procedural

79.83 Open reduction of dislocation of wrist

HCPCS Level II Supplies & Services

A4550 Surgical trays
A4580 Cast supplies (e.g., plaster)
A4590 Special casting material (e.g., fiberglass)

25671

25671 Percutaneous skeletal fixation of distal radioulnar dislocation

ICD-9-CM Diagnostic

718.23 Pathological dislocation of forearm joint
718.33 Recurrent dislocation of forearm joint
718.73 Developmental dislocation of joint, forearm
833.01 Closed dislocation of distal radioulnar (joint)

ICD-9-CM Procedural

79.73 Closed reduction of dislocation of wrist

25675

25675 Closed treatment of distal radioulnar dislocation with manipulation

ICD-9-CM Diagnostic

718.23 Pathological dislocation of forearm joint
718.33 Recurrent dislocation of forearm joint
718.73 Developmental dislocation of joint, forearm
833.01 Closed dislocation of distal radioulnar (joint)

ICD-9-CM Procedural

79.73 Closed reduction of dislocation of wrist

HCPCS Level II Supplies & Services

A4580 Cast supplies (e.g., plaster)
A4590 Special casting material (e.g., fiberglass)

25676

25676 Open treatment of distal radioulnar dislocation, acute or chronic

ICD-9-CM Diagnostic

718.23 Pathological dislocation of forearm joint
718.33 Recurrent dislocation of forearm joint
718.73 Developmental dislocation of joint, forearm
833.01 Closed dislocation of distal radioulnar (joint)
833.11 Open dislocation of distal radioulnar (joint)

ICD-9-CM Procedural

79.83 Open reduction of dislocation of wrist

HCPCS Level II Supplies & Services

A4550 Surgical trays
A4580 Cast supplies (e.g., plaster)
A4590 Special casting material (e.g., fiberglass)

25680

25680 Closed treatment of trans-scaphoperilunar type of fracture dislocation, with manipulation

ICD-9-CM Diagnostic

814.01 Closed fracture of navicular (scaphoid) bone of wrist
833.03 Closed dislocation of midcarpal (joint)

ICD-9-CM Procedural

79.03 Closed reduction of fracture of carpals and metacarpals without internal fixation
79.73 Closed reduction of dislocation of wrist

HCPCS Level II Supplies & Services

A4570 Splint
A4580 Cast supplies (e.g., plaster)

25685

25685 Open treatment of trans-scaphoperilunar type of fracture dislocation

ICD-9-CM Diagnostic

814.01 Closed fracture of navicular (scaphoid) bone of wrist
814.11 Open fracture of navicular (scaphoid) bone of wrist
833.03 Closed dislocation of midcarpal (joint)
833.13 Open dislocation of midcarpal (joint)

ICD-9-CM Procedural

79.83 Open reduction of dislocation of wrist

HCPCS Level II Supplies & Services

A4550 Surgical trays
A4580 Cast supplies (e.g., plaster)
A4590 Special casting material (e.g., fiberglass)

25690

25690 Closed treatment of lunate dislocation, with manipulation

ICD-9-CM Diagnostic

718.24 Pathological dislocation of hand joint
718.34 Recurrent dislocation of hand joint
718.73 Developmental dislocation of joint, forearm
833.03 Closed dislocation of midcarpal (joint)

ICD-9-CM Procedural

79.73 Closed reduction of dislocation of wrist

HCPCS Level II Supplies & Services

A4580 Cast supplies (e.g., plaster)
A4590 Special casting material (e.g., fiberglass)

25695

25695 Open treatment of lunate dislocation

ICD-9-CM Diagnostic

718.24 Pathological dislocation of hand joint
718.34 Recurrent dislocation of hand joint
718.73 Developmental dislocation of joint, forearm
833.03 Closed dislocation of midcarpal (joint)
833.13 Open dislocation of midcarpal (joint)

ICD-9-CM Procedural

79.83 Open reduction of dislocation of wrist

Unspecified code
♀ Female diagnosis
Manifestation code
♂ Male diagnosis

25800–25810

25800 Arthrodesis, wrist; complete, without bone graft (includes radiocarpal and/or intercarpal and/or carpometacarpal joints)
25805 with sliding graft
25810 with iliac or other autograft (includes obtaining graft)

ICD-9-CM Diagnostic

170.4 Malignant neoplasm of scapula and long bones of upper limb
170.5 Malignant neoplasm of short bones of upper limb
171.2 Malignant neoplasm of connective and other soft tissue of upper limb, including shoulder
198.5 Secondary malignant neoplasm of bone and bone marrow
238.0 Neoplasm of uncertain behavior of bone and articular cartilage
239.2 Neoplasms of unspecified nature of bone, soft tissue, and skin
357.1 Polyneuropathy in collagen vascular disease — (Code first underlying disease: 446.0, 710.0, 714.0) ☒
359.6 Symptomatic inflammatory myopathy in diseases classified elsewhere — (Code first underlying disease: 135, 140.0-208.9, 277.3, 446.0, 710.0, 710.1, 710.2, 714.0) ☒
446.0 Polyarteritis nodosa
710.0 Systemic lupus erythematosus — (Use additional code to identify manifestation: 424.91, 581.81, 582.81, 583.81)
710.1 Systemic sclerosis — (Use additional code to identify manifestation: 359.6, 517.2)
710.2 Sicca syndrome
711.03 Pyogenic arthritis, forearm — (Use additional code to identify infectious organism: 041.0-041.8)
711.04 Pyogenic arthritis, hand — (Use additional code to identify infectious organism: 041.0-041.8)
714.0 Rheumatoid arthritis — (Use additional code to identify manifestation: 357.1, 359.6)
714.30 Polyarticular juvenile rheumatoid arthritis, chronic or unspecified
715.13 Primary localized osteoarthrosis, forearm
715.14 Primary localized osteoarthrosis, hand
715.23 Secondary localized osteoarthrosis, forearm
715.24 Secondary localized osteoarthrosis, involving hand
716.04 Kaschin-Beck disease, hand
716.13 Traumatic arthropathy, forearm
716.14 Traumatic arthropathy, hand
716.93 Unspecified arthropathy, forearm ▽
716.94 Unspecified arthopathy, hand ▽
718.03 Articular cartilage disorder, forearm
718.04 Articular cartilage disorder, hand
718.33 Recurrent dislocation of forearm joint
718.34 Recurrent dislocation of hand joint
718.83 Other joint derangement, not elsewhere classified, forearm
718.84 Other joint derangement, not elsewhere classified, hand
719.03 Effusion of forearm joint
719.04 Effusion of hand joint
719.23 Villonodular synovitis, forearm
719.24 Villonodular synovitis, hand
733.81 Malunion of fracture
959.3 Injury, other and unspecified, elbow, forearm, and wrist
996.4 Mechanical complication of internal orthopedic device, implant, and graft

ICD-9-CM Procedural

81.25 Carporadial fusion
81.26 Metacarpocarpal fusion
81.29 Arthrodesis of other specified joint

25820–25825

25820 Arthrodesis, wrist; limited, without bone graft (eg, intercarpal or radiocarpal)
25825 with autograft (includes obtaining graft)

ICD-9-CM Diagnostic

357.1 Polyneuropathy in collagen vascular disease — (Code first underlying disease: 446.0, 710.0, 714.0) ☒
359.6 Symptomatic inflammatory myopathy in diseases classified elsewhere — (Code first underlying disease: 135, 140.0-208.9, 277.3, 446.0, 710.0, 710.1, 710.2, 714.0) ☒
446.0 Polyarteritis nodosa
710.0 Systemic lupus erythematosus — (Use additional code to identify manifestation: 424.91, 581.81, 582.81, 583.81)
710.1 Systemic sclerosis — (Use additional code to identify manifestation: 359.6, 517.2)
710.2 Sicca syndrome
714.0 Rheumatoid arthritis — (Use additional code to identify manifestation: 357.1, 359.6)
714.31 Polyarticular juvenile rheumatoid arthritis, acute
715.04 Generalized osteoarthrosis, involving hand
715.14 Primary localized osteoarthrosis, hand
715.24 Secondary localized osteoarthrosis, involving hand
715.34 Localized osteoarthrosis not specified whether primary or secondary, hand
715.94 Osteoarthrosis, unspecified whether generalized or localized, hand ▽
716.04 Kaschin-Beck disease, hand
716.14 Traumatic arthropathy, hand
718.04 Articular cartilage disorder, hand
718.84 Other joint derangement, not elsewhere classified, hand
733.49 Aseptic necrosis of other bone site
733.81 Malunion of fracture

ICD-9-CM Procedural

81.25 Carporadial fusion
81.29 Arthrodesis of other specified joint

25830

25830 Arthrodesis, distal radioulnar joint with segmental resection of ulna, with or without bone graft (eg, Sauve-Kapandji procedure)

ICD-9-CM Diagnostic

170.5 Malignant neoplasm of short bones of upper limb
198.5 Secondary malignant neoplasm of bone and bone marrow
238.0 Neoplasm of uncertain behavior of bone and articular cartilage
239.2 Neoplasms of unspecified nature of bone, soft tissue, and skin
715.33 Localized osteoarthrosis not specified whether primary or secondary, forearm
715.93 Osteoarthrosis, unspecified whether generalized or localized, forearm ▽
716.13 Traumatic arthropathy, forearm
718.33 Recurrent dislocation of forearm joint
733.49 Aseptic necrosis of other bone site
733.81 Malunion of fracture

ICD-9-CM Procedural

81.29 Arthrodesis of other specified joint

25900–25905

25900 Amputation, forearm, through radius and ulna;
25905 open, circular (guillotine)

ICD-9-CM Diagnostic

170.5 Malignant neoplasm of short bones of upper limb
170.9 Malignant neoplasm of bone and articular cartilage, site unspecified ▽
198.5 Secondary malignant neoplasm of bone and bone marrow
250.70 Diabetes with peripheral circulatory disorders, type II or unspecified type, not stated as uncontrolled — (Use additional code to identify manifestation: 443.81, 785.4)
250.71 Diabetes with peripheral circulatory disorders, type I [juvenile type], not stated as uncontrolled — (Use additional code to identify manifestation: 443.81, 785.4)
440.24 Atherosclerosis of native arteries of the extremities with gangrene
443.81 Peripheral angiopathy in diseases classified elsewhere — (Code first underlying disease, 250.7) ☒
446.0 Polyarteritis nodosa
682.3 Cellulitis and abscess of upper arm and forearm — (Use additional code to identify organism)
728.86 Necrotizing fasciitis — (Use additional code to identify infectious organism, 041.00-041.89, 785.4, if applicable)
730.13 Chronic osteomyelitis, forearm — (Use additional code to identify organism, 041.1)
731.1 Osteitis deformans in diseases classified elsewhere — (Code first underlying disease: 170.0-170.9) ☒
785.4 Gangrene — (Code first any associated underlying condition:250.7, 443.0)
887.0 Traumatic amputation of arm and hand (complete) (partial), unilateral, below elbow, without mention of complication — (Use additional code to identify infection)
887.1 Traumatic amputation of arm and hand (complete) (partial), unilateral, below elbow, complicated — (Use additional code to identify infection)
887.6 Traumatic amputation of arm and hand (complete) (partial), bilateral (any level), without mention of complication — (Use additional code to identify infection)
887.7 Traumatic amputation of arm and hand (complete) (partial), bilateral (any level), complicated — (Use additional code to identify infection)

▽ Unspecified code ♀ Female diagnosis ☒ Manifestation code ♂ Male diagnosis

927.10 Crushing injury of forearm — (Use additional code to identify any associated injuries: 800-829, 850.0-854.1, 860.0-869.1)
927.21 Crushing injury of wrist — (Use additional code to identify any associated injuries: 800-829, 850.0-854.1, 860.0-869.1)
943.51 Deep necrosis of underlying tissues due to burn (deep third degree) of forearm, with loss of a body part
958.3 Posttraumatic wound infection not elsewhere classified

ICD-9-CM Procedural

84.05 Amputation through forearm

25907

25907 Amputation, forearm, through radius and ulna; secondary closure or scar revision

ICD-9-CM Diagnostic

170.5 Malignant neoplasm of short bones of upper limb
170.9 Malignant neoplasm of bone and articular cartilage, site unspecified ▽
198.5 Secondary malignant neoplasm of bone and bone marrow
250.70 Diabetes with peripheral circulatory disorders, type II or unspecified type, not stated as uncontrolled — (Use additional code to identify manifestation: 443.81, 785.4)
250.71 Diabetes with peripheral circulatory disorders, type I [juvenile type], not stated as uncontrolled — (Use additional code to identify manifestation: 443.81, 785.4)
440.24 Atherosclerosis of native arteries of the extremities with gangrene
443.81 Peripheral angiopathy in diseases classified elsewhere — (Code first underlying disease, 250.7) ☒
443.9 Unspecified peripheral vascular disease ▽
446.0 Polyarteritis nodosa
682.3 Cellulitis and abscess of upper arm and forearm — (Use additional code to identify organism)
707.00 Decubitus ulcer, unspecified site
707.01 Decubitus ulcer, elbow
707.09 Decubitus ulcer, other site
707.8 Chronic ulcer of other specified site
709.2 Scar condition and fibrosis of skin
728.86 Necrotizing fasciitis — (Use additional code to identify infectious organism, 041.00-041.89, 785.4, if applicable)
730.12 Chronic osteomyelitis, upper arm — (Use additional code to identify organism, 041.1)
785.4 Gangrene — (Code first any associated underlying condition:250.7, 443.0)
944.58 Deep necrosis of underlying tissues due to burn (deep third degree) of multiple sites of wrist(s) and hand(s), with loss of a body part
997.60 Late complications of amputation stump, unspecified — (Use additional code to identify complications) ▽
997.61 Neuroma of amputation stump — (Use additional code to identify complications)
997.62 Infection (chronic) of amputation stump — (Use additional code to identify organism. Use additional code to identify complications)
997.69 Other late amputation stump complication — (Use additional code to identify complications)
998.83 Non-healing surgical wound
V51 Aftercare involving the use of plastic surgery
V58.41 Planned postoperative wound closure — (This code should be used in conjunction with other aftercare codes to fully identify the reason for the aftercare encounter)

ICD-9-CM Procedural

84.3 Revision of amputation stump

HCPCS Level II Supplies & Services

A4305 Disposable drug delivery system, flow rate of 50 ml or greater per hour
A4306 Disposable drug delivery system, flow rate of 5 ml or less per hour
A4550 Surgical trays
L6382 Immediate postsurgical or early fitting, application of initial rigid dressing including fitting alignment and suspension of components, and one cast change, elbow disarticulation or above elbow
L8415 Prosthetic sheath, upper limb, each

25909

25909 Amputation, forearm, through radius and ulna; re-amputation

ICD-9-CM Diagnostic

250.70 Diabetes with peripheral circulatory disorders, type II or unspecified type, not stated as uncontrolled — (Use additional code to identify manifestation: 443.81, 785.4)
250.71 Diabetes with peripheral circulatory disorders, type I [juvenile type], not stated as uncontrolled — (Use additional code to identify manifestation: 443.81, 785.4)
785.4 Gangrene — (Code first any associated underlying condition:250.7, 443.0)
997.60 Late complications of amputation stump, unspecified — (Use additional code to identify complications) ▽
997.61 Neuroma of amputation stump — (Use additional code to identify complications)
997.62 Infection (chronic) of amputation stump — (Use additional code to identify organism. Use additional code to identify complications)
997.69 Other late amputation stump complication — (Use additional code to identify complications)
998.59 Other postoperative infection — (Use additional code to identify infection)
998.6 Persistent postoperative fistula, not elsewhere classified
998.83 Non-healing surgical wound
V49.66 Upper limb amputation, above elbow — (This code is intended for use when these conditions are recorded as diagnoses or problems)
V51 Aftercare involving the use of plastic surgery

ICD-9-CM Procedural

84.05 Amputation through forearm
84.3 Revision of amputation stump

25915

25915 Krukenberg procedure

ICD-9-CM Diagnostic

170.5 Malignant neoplasm of short bones of upper limb
198.5 Secondary malignant neoplasm of bone and bone marrow
250.70 Diabetes with peripheral circulatory disorders, type II or unspecified type, not stated as uncontrolled — (Use additional code to identify manifestation: 443.81, 785.4)
250.71 Diabetes with peripheral circulatory disorders, type I [juvenile type], not stated as uncontrolled — (Use additional code to identify manifestation: 443.81, 785.4)
440.24 Atherosclerosis of native arteries of the extremities with gangrene
443.81 Peripheral angiopathy in diseases classified elsewhere — (Code first underlying disease, 250.7) ☒
682.3 Cellulitis and abscess of upper arm and forearm — (Use additional code to identify organism)
728.86 Necrotizing fasciitis — (Use additional code to identify infectious organism, 041.00-041.89, 785.4, if applicable)
736.00 Unspecified deformity of forearm, excluding fingers ▽
755.50 Unspecified congenital anomaly of upper limb ▽
785.4 Gangrene — (Code first any associated underlying condition:250.7, 443.0)
997.60 Late complications of amputation stump, unspecified — (Use additional code to identify complications) ▽
997.61 Neuroma of amputation stump — (Use additional code to identify complications)

ICD-9-CM Procedural

82.89 Other plastic operations on hand

25920–25924

25920 Disarticulation through wrist;
25922 secondary closure or scar revision
25924 re-amputation

ICD-9-CM Diagnostic

170.5 Malignant neoplasm of short bones of upper limb
171.2 Malignant neoplasm of connective and other soft tissue of upper limb, including shoulder
195.5 Malignant neoplasm of lower limb
250.70 Diabetes with peripheral circulatory disorders, type II or unspecified type, not stated as uncontrolled — (Use additional code to identify manifestation: 443.81, 785.4)
250.71 Diabetes with peripheral circulatory disorders, type I [juvenile type], not stated as uncontrolled — (Use additional code to identify manifestation: 443.81, 785.4)

▽ Unspecified code ♀ Female diagnosis ☒ Manifestation code ♂ Male diagnosis

440.24 Atherosclerosis of native arteries of the extremities with gangrene
443.81 Peripheral angiopathy in diseases classified elsewhere — (Code first underlying disease, 250.7) ☒
446.0 Polyarteritis nodosa
682.3 Cellulitis and abscess of upper arm and forearm — (Use additional code to identify organism)
707.09 Decubitus ulcer, other site
707.8 Chronic ulcer of other specified site
709.2 Scar condition and fibrosis of skin
728.86 Necrotizing fasciitis — (Use additional code to identify infectious organism, 041.00-041.89, 785.4, if applicable)
785.4 Gangrene — (Code first any associated underlying condition:250.7, 443.0)
817.1 Multiple open fractures of hand bones
887.0 Traumatic amputation of arm and hand (complete) (partial), unilateral, below elbow, without mention of complication — (Use additional code to identify infection)
887.1 Traumatic amputation of arm and hand (complete) (partial), unilateral, below elbow, complicated — (Use additional code to identify infection)
887.6 Traumatic amputation of arm and hand (complete) (partial), bilateral (any level), without mention of complication — (Use additional code to identify infection)
887.7 Traumatic amputation of arm and hand (complete) (partial), bilateral (any level), complicated — (Use additional code to identify infection)
927.21 Crushing injury of wrist — (Use additional code to identify any associated injuries: 800-829, 850.0-854.1, 860.0-869.1)
997.60 Late complications of amputation stump, unspecified — (Use additional code to identify complications) ▽
997.61 Neuroma of amputation stump — (Use additional code to identify complications)
997.62 Infection (chronic) of amputation stump — (Use additional code to identify organism. Use additional code to identify complications)
997.69 Other late amputation stump complication — (Use additional code to identify complications)
998.59 Other postoperative infection — (Use additional code to identify infection)
998.6 Persistent postoperative fistula, not elsewhere classified
998.83 Non-healing surgical wound
V51 Aftercare involving the use of plastic surgery
V58.41 Planned postoperative wound closure — (This code should be used in conjunction with other aftercare codes to fully identify the reason for the aftercare encounter)

ICD-9-CM Procedural

84.04 Disarticulation of wrist
84.3 Revision of amputation stump

HCPCS Level II Supplies & Services

A4305 Disposable drug delivery system, flow rate of 50 ml or greater per hour
A4306 Disposable drug delivery system, flow rate of 5 ml or less per hour
A4550 Surgical trays
L6380 Immediate postsurgical or early fitting, application of initial rigid dressing, including fitting alignment and suspension of components, and one cast change, wrist disarticulation or below elbow
L8415 Prosthetic sheath, upper limb, each

25927–25931

25927 Transmetacarpal amputation;
25929 secondary closure or scar revision
25931 re-amputation

ICD-9-CM Diagnostic

170.5 Malignant neoplasm of short bones of upper limb
171.2 Malignant neoplasm of connective and other soft tissue of upper limb, including shoulder
198.5 Secondary malignant neoplasm of bone and bone marrow
250.70 Diabetes with peripheral circulatory disorders, type II or unspecified type, not stated as uncontrolled — (Use additional code to identify manifestation: 443.81, 785.4)
250.71 Diabetes with peripheral circulatory disorders, type I [juvenile type], not stated as uncontrolled — (Use additional code to identify manifestation: 443.81, 785.4)
440.24 Atherosclerosis of native arteries of the extremities with gangrene
443.81 Peripheral angiopathy in diseases classified elsewhere — (Code first underlying disease, 250.7) ☒
682.3 Cellulitis and abscess of upper arm and forearm — (Use additional code to identify organism)
707.00 Decubitus ulcer, unspecified site
707.09 Decubitus ulcer, other site
707.8 Chronic ulcer of other specified site
709.2 Scar condition and fibrosis of skin
728.86 Necrotizing fasciitis — (Use additional code to identify infectious organism, 041.00-041.89, 785.4, if applicable)
785.4 Gangrene — (Code first any associated underlying condition:250.7, 443.0)
886.0 Traumatic amputation of other finger(s) (complete) (partial), without mention of complication — (Use additional code to identify infection)
886.1 Traumatic amputation of other finger(s) (complete) (partial), complicated — (Use additional code to identify infection)
887.0 Traumatic amputation of arm and hand (complete) (partial), unilateral, below elbow, without mention of complication — (Use additional code to identify infection)
887.1 Traumatic amputation of arm and hand (complete) (partial), unilateral, below elbow, complicated — (Use additional code to identify infection)
927.20 Crushing injury of hand(s) — (Use additional code to identify any associated injuries: 800-829, 850.0-854.1, 860.0-869.1)
944.58 Deep necrosis of underlying tissues due to burn (deep third degree) of multiple sites of wrist(s) and hand(s), with loss of a body part
959.4 Injury, other and unspecified, hand, except finger
997.60 Late complications of amputation stump, unspecified — (Use additional code to identify complications) ▽
997.61 Neuroma of amputation stump — (Use additional code to identify complications)
997.62 Infection (chronic) of amputation stump — (Use additional code to identify organism. Use additional code to identify complications)
997.69 Other late amputation stump complication — (Use additional code to identify complications)
998.59 Other postoperative infection — (Use additional code to identify infection)
998.6 Persistent postoperative fistula, not elsewhere classified
998.83 Non-healing surgical wound
V51 Aftercare involving the use of plastic surgery
V58.41 Planned postoperative wound closure — (This code should be used in conjunction with other aftercare codes to fully identify the reason for the aftercare encounter)

ICD-9-CM Procedural

84.03 Amputation through hand
84.3 Revision of amputation stump

HCPCS Level II Supplies & Services

A4305 Disposable drug delivery system, flow rate of 50 ml or greater per hour
A4306 Disposable drug delivery system, flow rate of 5 ml or less per hour
A4550 Surgical trays

Hand and Fingers

26010–26011

26010 Drainage of finger abscess; simple
26011 complicated (eg, felon)

ICD-9-CM Diagnostic

681.00 Unspecified cellulitis and abscess of finger — (Use additional code to identify organism) ▽
681.01 Felon — (Use additional code to identify organism)
681.02 Onychia and paronychia of finger — (Use additional code to identify organism)

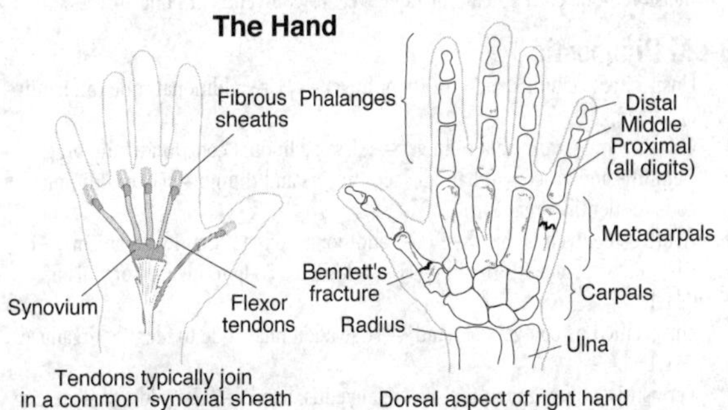

The major muscles of the hand are on the palmar side and their flexor tendons arise in the forearm and extend to the fingertips. Numerous fascial compartments exist in the palm

883.1 Open wound of finger(s), complicated — (Use additional code to identify infection)

ICD-9-CM Procedural
86.04 Other incision with drainage of skin and subcutaneous tissue

HCPCS Level II Supplies & Services
A4550 Surgical trays

26020
26020 Drainage of tendon sheath, digit and/or palm, each

ICD-9-CM Diagnostic
727.05 Other tenosynovitis of hand and wrist
727.89 Other disorders of synovium, tendon, and bursa
882.1 Open wound of hand except finger(s) alone, complicated — (Use additional code to identify infection)
882.2 Open wound of hand except finger(s) alone, with tendon involvement — (Use additional code to identify infection)
883.1 Open wound of finger(s), complicated — (Use additional code to identify infection)
883.2 Open wound of finger(s), with tendon involvement — (Use additional code to identify infection)

ICD-9-CM Procedural
82.01 Exploration of tendon sheath of hand
83.01 Exploration of tendon sheath

HCPCS Level II Supplies & Services
A4305 Disposable drug delivery system, flow rate of 50 ml or greater per hour
A4306 Disposable drug delivery system, flow rate of 5 ml or less per hour
A4550 Surgical trays

26025–26030
26025 Drainage of palmar bursa; single, bursa
26030 multiple bursa

ICD-9-CM Diagnostic
682.4 Cellulitis and abscess of hand, except fingers and thumb — (Use additional code to identify organism)
727.05 Other tenosynovitis of hand and wrist
727.3 Other bursitis disorders
727.89 Other disorders of synovium, tendon, and bursa
882.1 Open wound of hand except finger(s) alone, complicated — (Use additional code to identify infection)
882.2 Open wound of hand except finger(s) alone, with tendon involvement — (Use additional code to identify infection)
958.8 Other early complications of trauma

ICD-9-CM Procedural
82.03 Bursotomy of hand

HCPCS Level II Supplies & Services
A4305 Disposable drug delivery system, flow rate of 50 ml or greater per hour
A4306 Disposable drug delivery system, flow rate of 5 ml or less per hour
A4550 Surgical trays

26034
26034 Incision, bone cortex, hand or finger (eg, osteomyelitis or bone abscess)

ICD-9-CM Diagnostic
681.00 Unspecified cellulitis and abscess of finger — (Use additional code to identify organism) ▽
681.02 Onychia and paronychia of finger — (Use additional code to identify organism)
682.4 Cellulitis and abscess of hand, except fingers and thumb — (Use additional code to identify organism)
730.04 Acute osteomyelitis, hand — (Use additional code to identify organism, 041.1)
730.14 Chronic osteomyelitis, hand — (Use additional code to identify organism, 041.1)
730.24 Unspecified osteomyelitis, hand — (Use additional code to identify organism, 041.1) ▽
730.34 Periostitis, without mention of osteomyelitis, hand — (Use additional code to identify organism, 041.1)
730.84 Other infections involving diseases classified elsewhere, hand bone — (Code first underlying disease: 002.0, 015.0-015.9. Use additional code to identify organism) ☒
730.94 Unspecified infection of bone, hand — (Use additional code to identify organism, 041.1) ▽
883.1 Open wound of finger(s), complicated — (Use additional code to identify infection)

ICD-9-CM Procedural
77.14 Other incision of carpals and metacarpals without division
77.19 Other incision of other bone, except facial bones, without division

HCPCS Level II Supplies & Services
A4305 Disposable drug delivery system, flow rate of 50 ml or greater per hour
A4306 Disposable drug delivery system, flow rate of 5 ml or less per hour
A4550 Surgical trays

26035
26035 Decompression fingers and/or hand, injection injury (eg, grease gun)

ICD-9-CM Diagnostic
882.1 Open wound of hand except finger(s) alone, complicated — (Use additional code to identify infection)
882.2 Open wound of hand except finger(s) alone, with tendon involvement — (Use additional code to identify infection)
883.1 Open wound of finger(s), complicated — (Use additional code to identify infection)
883.2 Open wound of finger(s), with tendon involvement — (Use additional code to identify infection)

ICD-9-CM Procedural
77.14 Other incision of carpals and metacarpals without division
82.96 Other injection of locally-acting therapeutic substance into soft tissue of hand

HCPCS Level II Supplies & Services
A4305 Disposable drug delivery system, flow rate of 50 ml or greater per hour
A4306 Disposable drug delivery system, flow rate of 5 ml or less per hour
A4550 Surgical trays

26037
26037 Decompressive fasciotomy, hand (excludes 26035)

ICD-9-CM Diagnostic
682.4 Cellulitis and abscess of hand, except fingers and thumb — (Use additional code to identify organism)
728.0 Infective myositis
728.86 Necrotizing fasciitis — (Use additional code to identify infectious organism, 041.00-041.89, 785.4, if applicable)
728.88 Rhabdomyolysis
728.89 Other disorder of muscle, ligament, and fascia — (Use additional E code to identify drug, if drug-induced)
729.4 Unspecified fasciitis ▽
882.1 Open wound of hand except finger(s) alone, complicated — (Use additional code to identify infection)
927.20 Crushing injury of hand(s) — (Use additional code to identify any associated injuries: 800-829, 850.0-854.1, 860.0-869.1)
958.8 Other early complications of trauma

ICD-9-CM Procedural
82.12 Fasciotomy of hand

HCPCS Level II Supplies & Services
A4305 Disposable drug delivery system, flow rate of 50 ml or greater per hour
A4306 Disposable drug delivery system, flow rate of 5 ml or less per hour
A4550 Surgical trays

26040–26045
26040 Fasciotomy, palmar (eg, Dupuytrens contracture); percutaneous
26045 open, partial

ICD-9-CM Diagnostic
728.6 Contracture of palmar fascia

ICD-9-CM Procedural
82.12 Fasciotomy of hand

HCPCS Level II Supplies & Services
A4305 Disposable drug delivery system, flow rate of 50 ml or greater per hour
A4306 Disposable drug delivery system, flow rate of 5 ml or less per hour

▽ Unspecified code ☒ Manifestation code
♀ Female diagnosis ♂ Male diagnosis

A4550 Surgical trays

26055

26055 Tendon sheath incision (eg, for trigger finger)

ICD-9-CM Diagnostic

357.1 Polyneuropathy in collagen vascular disease — (Code first underlying disease: 446.0, 710.0, 714.0) ☒
359.6 Symptomatic inflammatory myopathy in diseases classified elsewhere — (Code first underlying disease: 135, 140.0-208.9, 277.3, 446.0, 710.0, 710.1, 710.2, 714.0) ☒
446.0 Polyarteritis nodosa
710.0 Systemic lupus erythematosus — (Use additional code to identify manifestation: 424.91, 581.81, 582.81, 583.81)
710.1 Systemic sclerosis — (Use additional code to identify manifestation: 359.6, 517.2)
710.2 Sicca syndrome
711.04 Pyogenic arthritis, hand — (Use additional code to identify infectious organism: 041.0-041.8)
711.84 Arthropathy associated with other infectious and parasitic diseases, hand — (Code first underlying disease, such as: diseases classifiable to 080-088, 100-104, 130-136) ☒
711.94 Unspecified infective arthritis, hand ▽
714.0 Rheumatoid arthritis — (Use additional code to identify manifestation: 357.1, 359.6)
716.04 Kaschin-Beck disease, hand
716.14 Traumatic arthropathy, hand
716.54 Unspecified polyarthropathy or polyarthritis, hand ▽
716.64 Unspecified monoarthritis, hand ▽
716.84 Other specified arthropathy, hand
716.94 Unspecified arthopathy, hand ▽
718.44 Contracture of hand joint
718.94 Unspecified derangement of hand joint ▽
727.00 Unspecified synovitis and tenosynovitis ▽
727.01 Synovitis and tenosynovitis in diseases classified elsewhere — (Code first underlying disease: 015.0-015.9) ☒
727.03 Trigger finger (acquired)
727.04 Radial styloid tenosynovitis
727.05 Other tenosynovitis of hand and wrist
727.89 Other disorders of synovium, tendon, and bursa
736.20 Unspecified deformity of finger ▽
736.29 Other acquired deformity of finger
756.89 Other specified congenital anomaly of muscle, tendon, fascia, and connective tissue
905.8 Late effect of tendon injury

ICD-9-CM Procedural

83.01 Exploration of tendon sheath

HCPCS Level II Supplies & Services

A4550 Surgical trays

26060

26060 Tenotomy, percutaneous, single, each digit

ICD-9-CM Diagnostic

727.00 Unspecified synovitis and tenosynovitis ▽
727.01 Synovitis and tenosynovitis in diseases classified elsewhere — (Code first underlying disease: 015.0-015.9) ☒
727.02 Giant cell tumor of tendon sheath
727.03 Trigger finger (acquired)
727.04 Radial styloid tenosynovitis
727.05 Other tenosynovitis of hand and wrist
727.09 Other synovitis and tenosynovitis
727.81 Contracture of tendon (sheath)
727.82 Calcium deposits in tendon and bursa
727.89 Other disorders of synovium, tendon, and bursa

ICD-9-CM Procedural

82.11 Tenotomy of hand

HCPCS Level II Supplies & Services

A4550 Surgical trays

26070–26080

26070 Arthrotomy, with exploration, drainage, or removal of loose or foreign body; carpometacarpal joint
26075 metacarpophalangeal joint, each
26080 interphalangeal joint, each

ICD-9-CM Diagnostic

682.4 Cellulitis and abscess of hand, except fingers and thumb — (Use additional code to identify organism)
709.4 Foreign body granuloma of skin and subcutaneous tissue
711.04 Pyogenic arthritis, hand — (Use additional code to identify infectious organism: 041.0-041.8)
716.14 Traumatic arthropathy, hand
728.0 Infective myositis
728.82 Foreign body granuloma of muscle
728.89 Other disorder of muscle, ligament, and fascia — (Use additional E code to identify drug, if drug-induced)
729.4 Unspecified fasciitis ▽
729.6 Residual foreign body in soft tissue
730.04 Acute osteomyelitis, hand — (Use additional code to identify organism, 041.1)
730.14 Chronic osteomyelitis, hand — (Use additional code to identify organism, 041.1)
730.24 Unspecified osteomyelitis, hand — (Use additional code to identify organism, 041.1) ▽
730.34 Periostitis, without mention of osteomyelitis, hand — (Use additional code to identify organism, 041.1)
730.84 Other infections involving diseases classified elsewhere, hand bone — (Code first underlying disease: 002.0, 015.0-015.9. Use additional code to identify organism) ☒
882.1 Open wound of hand except finger(s) alone, complicated — (Use additional code to identify infection)
883.1 Open wound of finger(s), complicated — (Use additional code to identify infection)
V64.43 Arthroscopic surgical procedure converted to open procedure

ICD-9-CM Procedural

80.14 Other arthrotomy of hand and finger

HCPCS Level II Supplies & Services

A4305 Disposable drug delivery system, flow rate of 50 ml or greater per hour
A4306 Disposable drug delivery system, flow rate of 5 ml or less per hour
A4550 Surgical trays

26100–26110

26100 Arthrotomy with biopsy; carpometacarpal joint, each
26105 metacarpophalangeal joint, each
26110 interphalangeal joint, each

ICD-9-CM Diagnostic

357.1 Polyneuropathy in collagen vascular disease — (Code first underlying disease: 446.0, 710.0, 714.0) ☒
359.6 Symptomatic inflammatory myopathy in diseases classified elsewhere — (Code first underlying disease: 135, 140.0-208.9, 277.3, 446.0, 710.0, 710.1, 710.2, 714.0) ☒
446.0 Polyarteritis nodosa
710.0 Systemic lupus erythematosus — (Use additional code to identify manifestation: 424.91, 581.81, 582.81, 583.81)
710.1 Systemic sclerosis — (Use additional code to identify manifestation: 359.6, 517.2)
710.2 Sicca syndrome
711.04 Pyogenic arthritis, hand — (Use additional code to identify infectious organism: 041.0-041.8)
711.44 Arthropathy, associated with other bacterial diseases, hand — (Code first underlying disease, such as: diseases classifiable to 010-040 (except 036.82), 090-099 (except 098.50)) ☒
711.54 Arthropathy associated with other viral diseases, hand — (Code first underlying disease, such as: diseases classifiable to 045-049, 050-079 (except 056.71), 480, 487) ☒
711.64 Arthropathy associated with mycoses, hand — (Code first underlying disease: 110.0-118) ☒
713.8 Arthropathy associated with other conditions classifiable elsewhere — (Code first underlying disease) ☒
714.0 Rheumatoid arthritis — (Use additional code to identify manifestation: 357.1, 359.6)
714.30 Polyarticular juvenile rheumatoid arthritis, chronic or unspecified
714.9 Unspecified inflammatory polyarthropathy ▽

▽ Unspecified code ♀ Female diagnosis ☒ Manifestation code ♂ Male diagnosis

716.04 Kaschin-Beck disease, hand
716.64 Unspecified monoarthritis, hand
719.24 Villonodular synovitis, hand
726.4 Enthesopathy of wrist and carpus
727.00 Unspecified synovitis and tenosynovitis
727.01 Synovitis and tenosynovitis in diseases classified elsewhere — (Code first underlying disease: 015.0-015.9)
727.05 Other tenosynovitis of hand and wrist
V64.43 Arthroscopic surgical procedure converted to open procedure

ICD-9-CM Procedural

80.34 Biopsy of joint structure of hand and finger

HCPCS Level II Supplies & Services

A4305 Disposable drug delivery system, flow rate of 50 ml or greater per hour
A4306 Disposable drug delivery system, flow rate of 5 ml or less per hour
A4550 Surgical trays

26115–26117

26115 Excision, tumor or vascular malformation, soft tissue of hand or finger; subcutaneous
26116 deep (subfascial or intramuscular)
26117 Radical resection of tumor (eg, malignant neoplasm), soft tissue of hand or finger

ICD-9-CM Diagnostic

171.2 Malignant neoplasm of connective and other soft tissue of upper limb, including shoulder
173.6 Other malignant neoplasm of skin of upper limb, including shoulder
195.4 Malignant neoplasm of upper limb
198.89 Secondary malignant neoplasm of other specified sites
214.1 Lipoma of other skin and subcutaneous tissue
215.2 Other benign neoplasm of connective and other soft tissue of upper limb, including shoulder
228.01 Hemangioma of skin and subcutaneous tissue
238.1 Neoplasm of uncertain behavior of connective and other soft tissue
239.2 Neoplasms of unspecified nature of bone, soft tissue, and skin
686.1 Pyogenic granuloma of skin and subcutaneous tissue
727.02 Giant cell tumor of tendon sheath
728.79 Other fibromatoses of muscle, ligament, and fascia
747.63 Congenital upper limb vessel anomaly
747.69 Congenital anomaly of other specified site of peripheral vascular system
782.2 Localized superficial swelling, mass, or lump

ICD-9-CM Procedural

80.84 Other local excision or destruction of lesion of joint of hand and finger
82.21 Excision of lesion of tendon sheath of hand
82.22 Excision of lesion of muscle of hand
82.29 Excision of other lesion of soft tissue of hand

HCPCS Level II Supplies & Services

A4305 Disposable drug delivery system, flow rate of 50 ml or greater per hour
A4306 Disposable drug delivery system, flow rate of 5 ml or less per hour
A4550 Surgical trays

26121–26125

26121 Fasciectomy, palm only, with or without Z-plasty, other local tissue rearrangement, or skin grafting (includes obtaining graft)
26123 Fasciectomy, partial palmar with release of single digit including proximal interphalangeal joint, with or without Z-plasty, other local tissue rearrangement, or skin grafting (includes obtaining graft);
26125 each additional digit (List separately in addition to code for primary procedure)

ICD-9-CM Diagnostic

239.2 Neoplasms of unspecified nature of bone, soft tissue, and skin
682.4 Cellulitis and abscess of hand, except fingers and thumb — (Use additional code to identify organism)
718.44 Contracture of hand joint
727.03 Trigger finger (acquired)
727.81 Contracture of tendon (sheath)
728.0 Infective myositis
728.6 Contracture of palmar fascia
729.4 Unspecified fasciitis
736.29 Other acquired deformity of finger
882.1 Open wound of hand except finger(s) alone, complicated — (Use additional code to identify infection)

ICD-9-CM Procedural

82.35 Other fasciectomy of hand
86.61 Full-thickness skin graft to hand
86.84 Relaxation of scar or web contracture of skin

26130

26130 Synovectomy, carpometacarpal joint

ICD-9-CM Diagnostic

275.40 Unspecified disorder of calcium metabolism — (Use additional code to identify any associated mental retardation)
275.42 Hypercalcemia — (Use additional code to identify any associated mental retardation)
275.49 Other disorders of calcium metabolism — (Use additional code to identify any associated mental retardation)
357.1 Polyneuropathy in collagen vascular disease — (Code first underlying disease: 446.0, 710.0, 714.0)
359.6 Symptomatic inflammatory myopathy in diseases classified elsewhere — (Code first underlying disease: 135, 140.0-208.9, 277.3, 446.0, 710.0, 710.1, 710.2, 714.0)
446.0 Polyarteritis nodosa
710.0 Systemic lupus erythematosus — (Use additional code to identify manifestation: 424.91, 581.81, 582.81, 583.81)
710.1 Systemic sclerosis — (Use additional code to identify manifestation: 359.6, 517.2)
710.2 Sicca syndrome
711.04 Pyogenic arthritis, hand — (Use additional code to identify infectious organism: 041.0-041.8)
711.44 Arthropathy, associated with other bacterial diseases, hand — (Code first underlying disease, such as: diseases classifiable to 010-040 (except 036.82), 090-099 (except 098.50))
711.54 Arthropathy associated with other viral diseases, hand — (Code first underlying disease, such as: diseases classifiable to 045-049, 050-079 (except 056.71), 480, 487)
711.64 Arthropathy associated with mycoses, hand — (Code first underlying disease: 110.0-118)
711.94 Unspecified infective arthritis, hand
712.84 Other specified crystal arthropathies, hand
713.8 Arthropathy associated with other conditions classifiable elsewhere — (Code first underlying disease)
714.0 Rheumatoid arthritis — (Use additional code to identify manifestation: 357.1, 359.6)
714.30 Polyarticular juvenile rheumatoid arthritis, chronic or unspecified
714.31 Polyarticular juvenile rheumatoid arthritis, acute
714.32 Pauciarticular juvenile rheumatoid arthritis
714.33 Monoarticular juvenile rheumatoid arthritis
714.9 Unspecified inflammatory polyarthropathy
716.04 Kaschin-Beck disease, hand
716.14 Traumatic arthropathy, hand
716.64 Unspecified monoarthritis, hand
719.24 Villonodular synovitis, hand
726.4 Enthesopathy of wrist and carpus
727.00 Unspecified synovitis and tenosynovitis
727.50 Unspecified rupture of synovium

ICD-9-CM Procedural

80.79 Synovectomy of other specified site

HCPCS Level II Supplies & Services

A4305 Disposable drug delivery system, flow rate of 50 ml or greater per hour
A4306 Disposable drug delivery system, flow rate of 5 ml or less per hour
A4550 Surgical trays

26135

26135 Synovectomy, metacarpophalangeal joint including intrinsic release and extensor hood reconstruction, each digit

ICD-9-CM Diagnostic

275.40 Unspecified disorder of calcium metabolism — (Use additional code to identify any associated mental retardation)
275.42 Hypercalcemia — (Use additional code to identify any associated mental retardation)

Unspecified code
♀ Female diagnosis
Manifestation code
♂ Male diagnosis

275.49 Other disorders of calcium metabolism — (Use additional code to identify any associated mental retardation)
357.1 Polyneuropathy in collagen vascular disease — (Code first underlying disease: 446.0, 710.0, 714.0) ☒
359.6 Symptomatic inflammatory myopathy in diseases classified elsewhere — (Code first underlying disease: 135, 140.0-208.9, 277.3, 446.0, 710.0, 710.1, 710.2, 714.0) ☒
446.0 Polyarteritis nodosa
710.0 Systemic lupus erythematosus — (Use additional code to identify manifestation: 424.91, 581.81, 582.81, 583.81)
710.1 Systemic sclerosis — (Use additional code to identify manifestation: 359.6, 517.2)
710.2 Sicca syndrome
714.0 Rheumatoid arthritis — (Use additional code to identify manifestation: 357.1, 359.6)
714.31 Polyarticular juvenile rheumatoid arthritis, acute
716.14 Traumatic arthropathy, hand
718.44 Contracture of hand joint
719.24 Villonodular synovitis, hand
727.00 Unspecified synovitis and tenosynovitis ▽
727.01 Synovitis and tenosynovitis in diseases classified elsewhere — (Code first underlying disease: 015.0-015.9) ☒
727.05 Other tenosynovitis of hand and wrist

ICD-9-CM Procedural
80.74 Synovectomy of hand and finger

HCPCS Level II Supplies & Services
A4305 Disposable drug delivery system, flow rate of 50 ml or greater per hour
A4306 Disposable drug delivery system, flow rate of 5 ml or less per hour
A4550 Surgical trays

26140
26140 Synovectomy, proximal interphalangeal joint, including extensor reconstruction, each interphalangeal joint

ICD-9-CM Diagnostic
275.40 Unspecified disorder of calcium metabolism — (Use additional code to identify any associated mental retardation) ▽
275.42 Hypercalcemia — (Use additional code to identify any associated mental retardation)
275.49 Other disorders of calcium metabolism — (Use additional code to identify any associated mental retardation)
277.3 Amyloidosis — (Use additional code to identify any associated mental retardation)
357.1 Polyneuropathy in collagen vascular disease — (Code first underlying disease: 446.0, 710.0, 714.0) ☒
359.6 Symptomatic inflammatory myopathy in diseases classified elsewhere — (Code first underlying disease: 135, 140.0-208.9, 277.3, 446.0, 710.0, 710.1, 710.2, 714.0) ☒
446.0 Polyarteritis nodosa
710.0 Systemic lupus erythematosus — (Use additional code to identify manifestation: 424.91, 581.81, 582.81, 583.81)
710.1 Systemic sclerosis — (Use additional code to identify manifestation: 359.6, 517.2)
710.2 Sicca syndrome
714.0 Rheumatoid arthritis — (Use additional code to identify manifestation: 357.1, 359.6)
714.1 Felty's syndrome
718.44 Contracture of hand joint
727.00 Unspecified synovitis and tenosynovitis ▽
736.21 Boutonniere deformity

ICD-9-CM Procedural
80.74 Synovectomy of hand and finger

HCPCS Level II Supplies & Services
A4305 Disposable drug delivery system, flow rate of 50 ml or greater per hour
A4306 Disposable drug delivery system, flow rate of 5 ml or less per hour
A4550 Surgical trays

26145
26145 Synovectomy, tendon sheath, radical (tenosynovectomy), flexor tendon, palm and/or finger, each tendon

ICD-9-CM Diagnostic
171.2 Malignant neoplasm of connective and other soft tissue of upper limb, including shoulder
238.1 Neoplasm of uncertain behavior of connective and other soft tissue ▽
239.2 Neoplasms of unspecified nature of bone, soft tissue, and skin
357.1 Polyneuropathy in collagen vascular disease — (Code first underlying disease: 446.0, 710.0, 714.0) ☒
359.6 Symptomatic inflammatory myopathy in diseases classified elsewhere — (Code first underlying disease: 135, 140.0-208.9, 277.3, 446.0, 710.0, 710.1, 710.2, 714.0) ☒
446.0 Polyarteritis nodosa
710.0 Systemic lupus erythematosus — (Use additional code to identify manifestation: 424.91, 581.81, 582.81, 583.81)
710.1 Systemic sclerosis — (Use additional code to identify manifestation: 359.6, 517.2)
710.2 Sicca syndrome
714.0 Rheumatoid arthritis — (Use additional code to identify manifestation: 357.1, 359.6)
714.1 Felty's syndrome

ICD-9-CM Procedural
80.74 Synovectomy of hand and finger

26160
26160 Excision of lesion of tendon sheath or joint capsule (eg, cyst, mucous cyst, or ganglion), hand or finger

ICD-9-CM Diagnostic
215.2 Other benign neoplasm of connective and other soft tissue of upper limb, including shoulder
229.8 Benign neoplasm of other specified sites
238.8 Neoplasm of uncertain behavior of other specified sites
239.2 Neoplasms of unspecified nature of bone, soft tissue, and skin
727.00 Unspecified synovitis and tenosynovitis ▽
727.02 Giant cell tumor of tendon sheath
727.04 Radial styloid tenosynovitis
727.41 Ganglion of joint
727.42 Ganglion of tendon sheath
727.9 Unspecified disorder of synovium, tendon, and bursa ▽
782.2 Localized superficial swelling, mass, or lump

ICD-9-CM Procedural
82.21 Excision of lesion of tendon sheath of hand

HCPCS Level II Supplies & Services
A4305 Disposable drug delivery system, flow rate of 50 ml or greater per hour
A4306 Disposable drug delivery system, flow rate of 5 ml or less per hour
A4550 Surgical trays

26170–26180
26170 Excision of tendon, palm, flexor, single (separate procedure), each
26180 Excision of tendon, finger, flexor (separate procedure), each tendon

ICD-9-CM Diagnostic
357.1 Polyneuropathy in collagen vascular disease — (Code first underlying disease: 446.0, 710.0, 714.0) ☒
359.6 Symptomatic inflammatory myopathy in diseases classified elsewhere — (Code first underlying disease: 135, 140.0-208.9, 277.3, 446.0, 710.0, 710.1, 710.2, 714.0) ☒
446.0 Polyarteritis nodosa
682.4 Cellulitis and abscess of hand, except fingers and thumb — (Use additional code to identify organism)
710.0 Systemic lupus erythematosus — (Use additional code to identify manifestation: 424.91, 581.81, 582.81, 583.81)
710.1 Systemic sclerosis — (Use additional code to identify manifestation: 359.6, 517.2)
710.2 Sicca syndrome
714.0 Rheumatoid arthritis — (Use additional code to identify manifestation: 357.1, 359.6)
716.14 Traumatic arthropathy, hand
727.81 Contracture of tendon (sheath)
727.89 Other disorders of synovium, tendon, and bursa

728.6 Contracture of palmar fascia
882.2 Open wound of hand except finger(s) alone, with tendon involvement — (Use additional code to identify infection)
905.8 Late effect of tendon injury

ICD-9-CM Procedural
82.33 Other tenonectomy of hand

HCPCS Level II Supplies & Services
A4305 Disposable drug delivery system, flow rate of 50 ml or greater per hour
A4306 Disposable drug delivery system, flow rate of 5 ml or less per hour
A4550 Surgical trays

26185
26185 Sesamoidectomy, thumb or finger (separate procedure)

ICD-9-CM Diagnostic
170.5 Malignant neoplasm of short bones of upper limb
213.5 Benign neoplasm of short bones of upper limb
357.1 Polyneuropathy in collagen vascular disease — (Code first underlying disease: 446.0, 710.0, 714.0) ☒
359.6 Symptomatic inflammatory myopathy in diseases classified elsewhere — (Code first underlying disease: 135, 140.0-208.9, 277.3, 446.0, 710.0, 710.1, 710.2, 714.0) ☒
446.0 Polyarteritis nodosa
710.0 Systemic lupus erythematosus — (Use additional code to identify manifestation: 424.91, 581.81, 582.81, 583.81)
710.1 Systemic sclerosis — (Use additional code to identify manifestation: 359.6, 517.2)
710.2 Sicca syndrome
714.0 Rheumatoid arthritis — (Use additional code to identify manifestation: 357.1, 359.6)
715.09 Generalized osteoarthrosis, involving multiple sites
715.14 Primary localized osteoarthrosis, hand
726.4 Enthesopathy of wrist and carpus
726.90 Enthesopathy of unspecified site ▽
732.9 Unspecified osteochondropathy ▽
733.99 Other disorders of bone and cartilage

ICD-9-CM Procedural
77.99 Total ostectomy of other bone, except facial bones

HCPCS Level II Supplies & Services
A4305 Disposable drug delivery system, flow rate of 50 ml or greater per hour
A4306 Disposable drug delivery system, flow rate of 5 ml or less per hour
A4550 Surgical trays

26200–26205
26200 Excision or curettage of bone cyst or benign tumor of metacarpal;
26205 with autograft (includes obtaining graft)

ICD-9-CM Diagnostic
213.5 Benign neoplasm of short bones of upper limb
238.0 Neoplasm of uncertain behavior of bone and articular cartilage
239.2 Neoplasms of unspecified nature of bone, soft tissue, and skin
726.91 Exostosis of unspecified site ▽
733.21 Solitary bone cyst
733.22 Aneurysmal bone cyst
733.29 Other cyst of bone

ICD-9-CM Procedural
77.64 Local excision of lesion or tissue of carpals and metacarpals

HCPCS Level II Supplies & Services
A4305 Disposable drug delivery system, flow rate of 50 ml or greater per hour
A4306 Disposable drug delivery system, flow rate of 5 ml or less per hour
A4550 Surgical trays

26210–26215
26210 Excision or curettage of bone cyst or benign tumor of proximal, middle or distal phalanx of finger;
26215 with autograft (includes obtaining graft)

ICD-9-CM Diagnostic
213.5 Benign neoplasm of short bones of upper limb
238.0 Neoplasm of uncertain behavior of bone and articular cartilage
239.2 Neoplasms of unspecified nature of bone, soft tissue, and skin
726.91 Exostosis of unspecified site ▽
733.21 Solitary bone cyst
733.22 Aneurysmal bone cyst
733.29 Other cyst of bone

ICD-9-CM Procedural
77.64 Local excision of lesion or tissue of carpals and metacarpals

HCPCS Level II Supplies & Services
A4305 Disposable drug delivery system, flow rate of 50 ml or greater per hour
A4306 Disposable drug delivery system, flow rate of 5 ml or less per hour
A4550 Surgical trays

26230–26236
26230 Partial excision (craterization, saucerization, or diaphysectomy) bone (eg, osteomyelitis); metacarpal
26235 proximal or middle phalanx of finger
26236 distal phalanx of finger

ICD-9-CM Diagnostic
730.14 Chronic osteomyelitis, hand — (Use additional code to identify organism, 041.1)
730.18 Chronic osteomyelitis, other specified sites — (Use additional code to identify organism, 041.1)
730.24 Unspecified osteomyelitis, hand — (Use additional code to identify organism, 041.1) ▽
730.84 Other infections involving diseases classified elsewhere, hand bone — (Code first underlying disease: 002.0, 015.0-015.9. Use additional code to identify organism) ☒
733.49 Aseptic necrosis of other bone site

ICD-9-CM Procedural
77.89 Other partial ostectomy of other bone, except facial bones

HCPCS Level II Supplies & Services
A4305 Disposable drug delivery system, flow rate of 50 ml or greater per hour
A4306 Disposable drug delivery system, flow rate of 5 ml or less per hour
A4550 Surgical trays

26250–26255
26250 Radical resection, metacarpal (eg, tumor);
26255 with autograft (includes obtaining graft)

ICD-9-CM Diagnostic
170.5 Malignant neoplasm of short bones of upper limb
195.4 Malignant neoplasm of upper limb
198.5 Secondary malignant neoplasm of bone and bone marrow
198.89 Secondary malignant neoplasm of other specified sites
238.0 Neoplasm of uncertain behavior of bone and articular cartilage
238.1 Neoplasm of uncertain behavior of connective and other soft tissue ▽
239.2 Neoplasms of unspecified nature of bone, soft tissue, and skin

ICD-9-CM Procedural
77.64 Local excision of lesion or tissue of carpals and metacarpals

26260–26262
26260 Radical resection, proximal or middle phalanx of finger (eg, tumor);
26261 with autograft (includes obtaining graft)
26262 Radical resection, distal phalanx of finger (eg, tumor)

ICD-9-CM Diagnostic
170.5 Malignant neoplasm of short bones of upper limb
195.4 Malignant neoplasm of upper limb
198.5 Secondary malignant neoplasm of bone and bone marrow
198.89 Secondary malignant neoplasm of other specified sites
238.0 Neoplasm of uncertain behavior of bone and articular cartilage
238.1 Neoplasm of uncertain behavior of connective and other soft tissue ▽
239.2 Neoplasms of unspecified nature of bone, soft tissue, and skin

ICD-9-CM Procedural
77.64 Local excision of lesion or tissue of carpals and metacarpals

HCPCS Level II Supplies & Services
A4305 Disposable drug delivery system, flow rate of 50 ml or greater per hour
A4306 Disposable drug delivery system, flow rate of 5 ml or less per hour

▽ Unspecified code ♀ Female diagnosis ☒ Manifestation code ♂ Male diagnosis

A4550 Surgical trays

26320

26320 Removal of implant from finger or hand

ICD-9-CM Diagnostic

357.1 Polyneuropathy in collagen vascular disease — (Code first underlying disease: 446.0, 710.0, 714.0) ☒
359.6 Symptomatic inflammatory myopathy in diseases classified elsewhere — (Code first underlying disease: 135, 140.0-208.9, 277.3, 446.0, 710.0, 710.1, 710.2, 714.0) ☒
446.0 Polyarteritis nodosa
710.0 Systemic lupus erythematosus — (Use additional code to identify manifestation: 424.91, 581.81, 582.81, 583.81)
710.1 Systemic sclerosis — (Use additional code to identify manifestation: 359.6, 517.2)
710.2 Sicca syndrome
714.0 Rheumatoid arthritis — (Use additional code to identify manifestation: 357.1, 359.6)
905.2 Late effect of fracture of upper extremities
996.4 Mechanical complication of internal orthopedic device, implant, and graft
996.66 Infection and inflammatory reaction due to internal joint prosthesis — (Use additional code to identify specified infections)
996.67 Infection and inflammatory reaction due to other internal orthopedic device, implant, and graft — (Use additional code to identify specified infections)
998.51 Infected postoperative seroma — (Use additional code to identify organism)
998.59 Other postoperative infection — (Use additional code to identify infection)

ICD-9-CM Procedural

78.64 Removal of implanted device from carpals and metacarpals
80.04 Arthrotomy for removal of prosthesis of hand and finger

HCPCS Level II Supplies & Services

A4305 Disposable drug delivery system, flow rate of 50 ml or greater per hour
A4306 Disposable drug delivery system, flow rate of 5 ml or less per hour
A4550 Surgical trays

26340

26340 Manipulation, finger joint, under anesthesia, each joint

ICD-9-CM Diagnostic

357.1 Polyneuropathy in collagen vascular disease — (Code first underlying disease: 446.0, 710.0, 714.0) ☒
359.6 Symptomatic inflammatory myopathy in diseases classified elsewhere — (Code first underlying disease: 135, 140.0-208.9, 277.3, 446.0, 710.0, 710.1, 710.2, 714.0) ☒
446.0 Polyarteritis nodosa
710.0 Systemic lupus erythematosus — (Use additional code to identify manifestation: 424.91, 581.81, 582.81, 583.81)
710.1 Systemic sclerosis — (Use additional code to identify manifestation: 359.6, 517.2)
710.2 Sicca syndrome
714.0 Rheumatoid arthritis — (Use additional code to identify manifestation: 357.1, 359.6)
715.14 Primary localized osteoarthrosis, hand
715.94 Osteoarthrosis, unspecified whether generalized or localized, hand ▽
718.44 Contracture of hand joint
718.54 Ankylosis of hand joint
719.24 Villonodular synovitis, hand
719.54 Stiffness of joint, not elsewhere classified, hand
726.8 Other peripheral enthesopathies

ICD-9-CM Procedural

93.25 Forced extension of limb
93.26 Manual rupture of joint adhesions
93.29 Other forcible correction of musculoskeletal deformity

26350–26352

26350 Repair or advancement, flexor tendon, not in zone 2 digital flexor tendon sheath (eg, no man's land); primary or secondary without free graft, each tendon
26352 secondary with free graft (includes obtaining graft), each tendon

ICD-9-CM Diagnostic

357.1 Polyneuropathy in collagen vascular disease — (Code first underlying disease: 446.0, 710.0, 714.0) ☒
359.6 Symptomatic inflammatory myopathy in diseases classified elsewhere — (Code first underlying disease: 135, 140.0-208.9, 277.3, 446.0, 710.0, 710.1, 710.2, 714.0) ☒
446.0 Polyarteritis nodosa
710.0 Systemic lupus erythematosus — (Use additional code to identify manifestation: 424.91, 581.81, 582.81, 583.81)
710.1 Systemic sclerosis — (Use additional code to identify manifestation: 359.6, 517.2)
710.2 Sicca syndrome
714.0 Rheumatoid arthritis — (Use additional code to identify manifestation: 357.1, 359.6)
727.64 Nontraumatic rupture of flexor tendons of hand and wrist
881.22 Open wound of wrist, with tendon involvement — (Use additional code to identify infection)
882.2 Open wound of hand except finger(s) alone, with tendon involvement — (Use additional code to identify infection)
883.2 Open wound of finger(s), with tendon involvement — (Use additional code to identify infection)
884.2 Multiple and unspecified open wound of upper limb, with tendon involvement — (Use additional code to identify infection)
886.1 Traumatic amputation of other finger(s) (complete) (partial), complicated — (Use additional code to identify infection)
959.4 Injury, other and unspecified, hand, except finger
998.2 Accidental puncture or laceration during procedure

ICD-9-CM Procedural

82.42 Delayed suture of flexor tendon of hand
82.44 Other suture of flexor tendon of hand
82.51 Advancement of tendon of hand
83.71 Advancement of tendon
83.88 Other plastic operations on tendon

26356–26358

26356 Repair or advancement, flexor tendon, in zone 2 digital flexor tendon sheath (eg, no man's land); primary, without free graft, each tendon
26357 secondary, without free graft, each tendon
26358 secondary, with free graft (includes obtaining graft), each tendon

ICD-9-CM Diagnostic

357.1 Polyneuropathy in collagen vascular disease — (Code first underlying disease: 446.0, 710.0, 714.0) ☒
359.6 Symptomatic inflammatory myopathy in diseases classified elsewhere — (Code first underlying disease: 135, 140.0-208.9, 277.3, 446.0, 710.0, 710.1, 710.2, 714.0) ☒
446.0 Polyarteritis nodosa
710.0 Systemic lupus erythematosus — (Use additional code to identify manifestation: 424.91, 581.81, 582.81, 583.81)
710.1 Systemic sclerosis — (Use additional code to identify manifestation: 359.6, 517.2)
710.2 Sicca syndrome
714.0 Rheumatoid arthritis — (Use additional code to identify manifestation: 357.1, 359.6)
727.64 Nontraumatic rupture of flexor tendons of hand and wrist
881.22 Open wound of wrist, with tendon involvement — (Use additional code to identify infection)
882.2 Open wound of hand except finger(s) alone, with tendon involvement — (Use additional code to identify infection)
883.2 Open wound of finger(s), with tendon involvement — (Use additional code to identify infection)
884.2 Multiple and unspecified open wound of upper limb, with tendon involvement — (Use additional code to identify infection)
886.1 Traumatic amputation of other finger(s) (complete) (partial), complicated — (Use additional code to identify infection)
959.4 Injury, other and unspecified, hand, except finger
998.2 Accidental puncture or laceration during procedure

ICD-9-CM Procedural

82.42 Delayed suture of flexor tendon of hand
82.44 Other suture of flexor tendon of hand
82.51 Advancement of tendon of hand
83.71 Advancement of tendon
83.88 Other plastic operations on tendon

26370–26373

26370 Repair or advancement of profundus tendon, with intact superficialis tendon; primary, each tendon
26372 secondary with free graft (includes obtaining graft), each tendon
26373 secondary without free graft, each tendon

ICD-9-CM Diagnostic

357.1 Polyneuropathy in collagen vascular disease — (Code first underlying disease: 446.0, 710.0, 714.0) ☒
359.6 Symptomatic inflammatory myopathy in diseases classified elsewhere — (Code first underlying disease: 135, 140.0-208.9, 277.3, 446.0, 710.0, 710.1, 710.2, 714.0) ☒
446.0 Polyarteritis nodosa
710.0 Systemic lupus erythematosus — (Use additional code to identify manifestation: 424.91, 581.81, 582.81, 583.81)
710.1 Systemic sclerosis — (Use additional code to identify manifestation: 359.6, 517.2)
710.2 Sicca syndrome
714.0 Rheumatoid arthritis — (Use additional code to identify manifestation: 357.1, 359.6)
727.64 Nontraumatic rupture of flexor tendons of hand and wrist
881.22 Open wound of wrist, with tendon involvement — (Use additional code to identify infection)
882.2 Open wound of hand except finger(s) alone, with tendon involvement — (Use additional code to identify infection)
883.2 Open wound of finger(s), with tendon involvement — (Use additional code to identify infection)
884.2 Multiple and unspecified open wound of upper limb, with tendon involvement — (Use additional code to identify infection)
886.1 Traumatic amputation of other finger(s) (complete) (partial), complicated — (Use additional code to identify infection)
959.4 Injury, other and unspecified, hand, except finger
998.2 Accidental puncture or laceration during procedure

ICD-9-CM Procedural

82.42 Delayed suture of flexor tendon of hand
82.44 Other suture of flexor tendon of hand
82.51 Advancement of tendon of hand
83.71 Advancement of tendon
83.88 Other plastic operations on tendon

26390–26392

26390 Excision flexor tendon, with implantation of synthetic rod for delayed tendon graft, hand or finger, each rod
26392 Removal of synthetic rod and insertion of flexor tendon graft, hand or finger (includes obtaining graft), each rod

ICD-9-CM Diagnostic

727.64 Nontraumatic rupture of flexor tendons of hand and wrist
727.69 Nontraumatic rupture of other tendon
881.22 Open wound of wrist, with tendon involvement — (Use additional code to identify infection)
882.2 Open wound of hand except finger(s) alone, with tendon involvement — (Use additional code to identify infection)
883.2 Open wound of finger(s), with tendon involvement — (Use additional code to identify infection)
884.2 Multiple and unspecified open wound of upper limb, with tendon involvement — (Use additional code to identify infection)
906.1 Late effect of open wound of extremities without mention of tendon injury
998.2 Accidental puncture or laceration during procedure
V51 Aftercare involving the use of plastic surgery
V54.01 Encounter for removal of internal fixation device
V54.02 Encounter for lengthening/adjustment of growth rod
V54.09 Other aftercare involving internal fixation device

ICD-9-CM Procedural

78.64 Removal of implanted device from carpals and metacarpals
82.33 Other tenonectomy of hand
82.79 Plastic operation on hand with other graft or implant
83.81 Tendon graft

26410–26412

26410 Repair, extensor tendon, hand, primary or secondary; without free graft, each tendon
26412 with free graft (includes obtaining graft), each tendon

ICD-9-CM Diagnostic

727.63 Nontraumatic rupture of extensor tendons of hand and wrist
881.22 Open wound of wrist, with tendon involvement — (Use additional code to identify infection)
882.2 Open wound of hand except finger(s) alone, with tendon involvement — (Use additional code to identify infection)
884.2 Multiple and unspecified open wound of upper limb, with tendon involvement — (Use additional code to identify infection)
927.20 Crushing injury of hand(s) — (Use additional code to identify any associated injuries: 800-829, 850.0-854.1, 860.0-869.1)
959.4 Injury, other and unspecified, hand, except finger
998.2 Accidental puncture or laceration during procedure

ICD-9-CM Procedural

82.43 Delayed suture of other tendon of hand
82.45 Other suture of other tendon of hand
83.81 Tendon graft
83.88 Other plastic operations on tendon

26415–26416

26415 Excision of extensor tendon, with implantation of synthetic rod for delayed tendon graft, hand or finger, each rod
26416 Removal of synthetic rod and insertion of extensor tendon graft (includes obtaining graft), hand or finger, each rod

ICD-9-CM Diagnostic

727.63 Nontraumatic rupture of extensor tendons of hand and wrist
881.22 Open wound of wrist, with tendon involvement — (Use additional code to identify infection)
882.2 Open wound of hand except finger(s) alone, with tendon involvement — (Use additional code to identify infection)
883.2 Open wound of finger(s), with tendon involvement — (Use additional code to identify infection)
884.2 Multiple and unspecified open wound of upper limb, with tendon involvement — (Use additional code to identify infection)
887.1 Traumatic amputation of arm and hand (complete) (partial), unilateral, below elbow, complicated — (Use additional code to identify infection)
998.2 Accidental puncture or laceration during procedure
V51 Aftercare involving the use of plastic surgery
V54.01 Encounter for removal of internal fixation device
V54.02 Encounter for lengthening/adjustment of growth rod
V54.09 Other aftercare involving internal fixation device

ICD-9-CM Procedural

78.64 Removal of implanted device from carpals and metacarpals
82.33 Other tenonectomy of hand
82.79 Plastic operation on hand with other graft or implant

26418–26420

26418 Repair, extensor tendon, finger, primary or secondary; without free graft, each tendon
26420 with free graft (includes obtaining graft) each tendon

ICD-9-CM Diagnostic

357.1 Polyneuropathy in collagen vascular disease — (Code first underlying disease: 446.0, 710.0, 714.0) ☒
359.6 Symptomatic inflammatory myopathy in diseases classified elsewhere — (Code first underlying disease: 135, 140.0-208.9, 277.3, 446.0, 710.0, 710.1, 710.2, 714.0) ☒
446.0 Polyarteritis nodosa
710.0 Systemic lupus erythematosus — (Use additional code to identify manifestation: 424.91, 581.81, 582.81, 583.81)
710.1 Systemic sclerosis — (Use additional code to identify manifestation: 359.6, 517.2)
710.2 Sicca syndrome
714.0 Rheumatoid arthritis — (Use additional code to identify manifestation: 357.1, 359.6)
727.63 Nontraumatic rupture of extensor tendons of hand and wrist

Unspecified code
♀ Female diagnosis
☒ Manifestation code
♂ Male diagnosis

727.9 Unspecified disorder of synovium, tendon, and bursa ▽
883.2 Open wound of finger(s), with tendon involvement — (Use additional code to identify infection)

ICD-9-CM Procedural

82.43 Delayed suture of other tendon of hand
82.45 Other suture of other tendon of hand
82.51 Advancement of tendon of hand

26426–26428

26426 Repair of extensor tendon, central slip, secondary (eg, boutonniere deformity); using local tissue(s), including lateral band(s), each finger
26428 with free graft (includes obtaining graft), each finger

ICD-9-CM Diagnostic

357.1 Polyneuropathy in collagen vascular disease — (Code first underlying disease: 446.0, 710.0, 714.0) ☒
359.6 Symptomatic inflammatory myopathy in diseases classified elsewhere — (Code first underlying disease: 135, 140.0-208.9, 277.3, 446.0, 710.0, 710.1, 710.2, 714.0) ☒
446.0 Polyarteritis nodosa
710.0 Systemic lupus erythematosus — (Use additional code to identify manifestation: 424.91, 581.81, 582.81, 583.81)
710.1 Systemic sclerosis — (Use additional code to identify manifestation: 359.6, 517.2)
710.2 Sicca syndrome
714.0 Rheumatoid arthritis — (Use additional code to identify manifestation: 357.1, 359.6)
714.1 Felty's syndrome
736.21 Boutonniere deformity
883.2 Open wound of finger(s), with tendon involvement — (Use additional code to identify infection)
905.2 Late effect of fracture of upper extremities

ICD-9-CM Procedural

83.88 Other plastic operations on tendon

26432

26432 Closed treatment of distal extensor tendon insertion, with or without percutaneous pinning (eg, mallet finger)

ICD-9-CM Diagnostic

736.1 Mallet finger

ICD-9-CM Procedural

82.84 Repair of mallet finger
83.88 Other plastic operations on tendon

26433–26434

26433 Repair of extensor tendon, distal insertion, primary or secondary; without graft (eg, mallet finger)
26434 with free graft (includes obtaining graft)

ICD-9-CM Diagnostic

736.1 Mallet finger

ICD-9-CM Procedural

82.84 Repair of mallet finger
83.88 Other plastic operations on tendon

26437

26437 Realignment of extensor tendon, hand, each tendon

ICD-9-CM Diagnostic

357.1 Polyneuropathy in collagen vascular disease — (Code first underlying disease: 446.0, 710.0, 714.0) ☒
359.6 Symptomatic inflammatory myopathy in diseases classified elsewhere — (Code first underlying disease: 135, 140.0-208.9, 277.3, 446.0, 710.0, 710.1, 710.2, 714.0) ☒
446.0 Polyarteritis nodosa
710.0 Systemic lupus erythematosus — (Use additional code to identify manifestation: 424.91, 581.81, 582.81, 583.81)
710.1 Systemic sclerosis — (Use additional code to identify manifestation: 359.6, 517.2)
710.2 Sicca syndrome
714.0 Rheumatoid arthritis — (Use additional code to identify manifestation: 357.1, 359.6)
882.2 Open wound of hand except finger(s) alone, with tendon involvement — (Use additional code to identify infection)

ICD-9-CM Procedural

83.88 Other plastic operations on tendon

26440–26442

26440 Tenolysis, flexor tendon; palm OR finger, each tendon
26442 palm AND finger, each tendon

ICD-9-CM Diagnostic

357.1 Polyneuropathy in collagen vascular disease — (Code first underlying disease: 446.0, 710.0, 714.0) ☒
359.6 Symptomatic inflammatory myopathy in diseases classified elsewhere — (Code first underlying disease: 135, 140.0-208.9, 277.3, 446.0, 710.0, 710.1, 710.2, 714.0) ☒
446.0 Polyarteritis nodosa
710.0 Systemic lupus erythematosus — (Use additional code to identify manifestation: 424.91, 581.81, 582.81, 583.81)
710.1 Systemic sclerosis — (Use additional code to identify manifestation: 359.6, 517.2)
710.2 Sicca syndrome
714.0 Rheumatoid arthritis — (Use additional code to identify manifestation: 357.1, 359.6)
727.00 Unspecified synovitis and tenosynovitis ▽
727.05 Other tenosynovitis of hand and wrist
727.81 Contracture of tendon (sheath)
727.89 Other disorders of synovium, tendon, and bursa
736.29 Other acquired deformity of finger
883.2 Open wound of finger(s), with tendon involvement — (Use additional code to identify infection)
905.8 Late effect of tendon injury

ICD-9-CM Procedural

82.91 Lysis of adhesions of hand
83.91 Lysis of adhesions of muscle, tendon, fascia, and bursa

26445–26449

26445 Tenolysis, extensor tendon, hand OR finger, each tendon
26449 Tenolysis, complex, extensor tendon, finger, including forearm, each tendon

ICD-9-CM Diagnostic

357.1 Polyneuropathy in collagen vascular disease — (Code first underlying disease: 446.0, 710.0, 714.0) ☒
359.6 Symptomatic inflammatory myopathy in diseases classified elsewhere — (Code first underlying disease: 135, 140.0-208.9, 277.3, 446.0, 710.0, 710.1, 710.2, 714.0) ☒
446.0 Polyarteritis nodosa
710.0 Systemic lupus erythematosus — (Use additional code to identify manifestation: 424.91, 581.81, 582.81, 583.81)
710.1 Systemic sclerosis — (Use additional code to identify manifestation: 359.6, 517.2)
710.2 Sicca syndrome
714.0 Rheumatoid arthritis — (Use additional code to identify manifestation: 357.1, 359.6)
727.00 Unspecified synovitis and tenosynovitis ▽
727.04 Radial styloid tenosynovitis
727.05 Other tenosynovitis of hand and wrist
727.89 Other disorders of synovium, tendon, and bursa
736.29 Other acquired deformity of finger
882.2 Open wound of hand except finger(s) alone, with tendon involvement — (Use additional code to identify infection)
883.2 Open wound of finger(s), with tendon involvement — (Use additional code to identify infection)
905.8 Late effect of tendon injury

ICD-9-CM Procedural

82.91 Lysis of adhesions of hand
83.91 Lysis of adhesions of muscle, tendon, fascia, and bursa

▽ Unspecified code ☒ Manifestation code
♀ Female diagnosis ♂ Male diagnosis

26450–26460

26450 Tenotomy, flexor, palm, open, each tendon
26455 Tenotomy, flexor, finger, open, each tendon
26460 Tenotomy, extensor, hand or finger, open, each tendon

ICD-9-CM Diagnostic

718.44 Contracture of hand joint
727.00 Unspecified synovitis and tenosynovitis ▽
727.05 Other tenosynovitis of hand and wrist
727.81 Contracture of tendon (sheath)
728.6 Contracture of palmar fascia
736.29 Other acquired deformity of finger
755.50 Unspecified congenital anomaly of upper limb ▽
905.8 Late effect of tendon injury

ICD-9-CM Procedural

82.11 Tenotomy of hand

HCPCS Level II Supplies & Services

A4305 Disposable drug delivery system, flow rate of 50 ml or greater per hour
A4306 Disposable drug delivery system, flow rate of 5 ml or less per hour
A4550 Surgical trays

26471–26474

26471 Tenodesis; of proximal interphalangeal joint, each joint
26474 of distal joint, each joint

ICD-9-CM Diagnostic

714.1 Felty's syndrome
715.14 Primary localized osteoarthrosis, hand
718.44 Contracture of hand joint
718.84 Other joint derangement, not elsewhere classified, hand
727.64 Nontraumatic rupture of flexor tendons of hand and wrist
816.11 Open fracture of middle or proximal phalanx or phalanges of hand
816.12 Open fracture of distal phalanx or phalanges of hand
833.15 Open dislocation of proximal end of metacarpal (bone)
834.11 Open dislocation of metacarpophalangeal (joint)
883.2 Open wound of finger(s), with tendon involvement — (Use additional code to identify infection)
886.1 Traumatic amputation of other finger(s) (complete) (partial), complicated — (Use additional code to identify infection)
927.3 Crushing injury of finger(s) — (Use additional code to identify any associated injuries: 800-829, 850.0-854.1, 860.0-869.1)

ICD-9-CM Procedural

82.85 Other tenodesis of hand

26476

26476 Lengthening of tendon, extensor, hand or finger, each tendon

ICD-9-CM Diagnostic

715.14 Primary localized osteoarthrosis, hand
718.44 Contracture of hand joint
755.50 Unspecified congenital anomaly of upper limb ▽
816.01 Closed fracture of middle or proximal phalanx or phalanges of hand
816.10 Open fracture of phalanx or phalanges of hand, unspecified ▽
834.01 Closed dislocation of metacarpophalangeal (joint)
883.2 Open wound of finger(s), with tendon involvement — (Use additional code to identify infection)
886.1 Traumatic amputation of other finger(s) (complete) (partial), complicated — (Use additional code to identify infection)
905.2 Late effect of fracture of upper extremities
906.4 Late effect of crushing
927.3 Crushing injury of finger(s) — (Use additional code to identify any associated injuries: 800-829, 850.0-854.1, 860.0-869.1)

ICD-9-CM Procedural

82.55 Other change in muscle or tendon length of hand

26477

26477 Shortening of tendon, extensor, hand or finger, each tendon

ICD-9-CM Diagnostic

715.14 Primary localized osteoarthrosis, hand
755.50 Unspecified congenital anomaly of upper limb ▽
816.11 Open fracture of middle or proximal phalanx or phalanges of hand
833.15 Open dislocation of proximal end of metacarpal (bone)
834.11 Open dislocation of metacarpophalangeal (joint)
842.12 Sprain and strain of metacarpophalangeal (joint) of hand
883.2 Open wound of finger(s), with tendon involvement — (Use additional code to identify infection)
886.1 Traumatic amputation of other finger(s) (complete) (partial), complicated — (Use additional code to identify infection)
905.2 Late effect of fracture of upper extremities
906.4 Late effect of crushing
927.3 Crushing injury of finger(s) — (Use additional code to identify any associated injuries: 800-829, 850.0-854.1, 860.0-869.1)

ICD-9-CM Procedural

82.55 Other change in muscle or tendon length of hand

26478

26478 Lengthening of tendon, flexor, hand or finger, each tendon

ICD-9-CM Diagnostic

718.44 Contracture of hand joint
727.64 Nontraumatic rupture of flexor tendons of hand and wrist
728.6 Contracture of palmar fascia
755.50 Unspecified congenital anomaly of upper limb ▽
816.11 Open fracture of middle or proximal phalanx or phalanges of hand
833.15 Open dislocation of proximal end of metacarpal (bone)
834.11 Open dislocation of metacarpophalangeal (joint)
842.12 Sprain and strain of metacarpophalangeal (joint) of hand
882.2 Open wound of hand except finger(s) alone, with tendon involvement — (Use additional code to identify infection)
883.2 Open wound of finger(s), with tendon involvement — (Use additional code to identify infection)
886.1 Traumatic amputation of other finger(s) (complete) (partial), complicated — (Use additional code to identify infection)
905.2 Late effect of fracture of upper extremities
906.4 Late effect of crushing

ICD-9-CM Procedural

82.55 Other change in muscle or tendon length of hand

26479

26479 Shortening of tendon, flexor, hand or finger, each tendon

ICD-9-CM Diagnostic

727.64 Nontraumatic rupture of flexor tendons of hand and wrist
728.6 Contracture of palmar fascia
755.50 Unspecified congenital anomaly of upper limb ▽
816.11 Open fracture of middle or proximal phalanx or phalanges of hand
833.15 Open dislocation of proximal end of metacarpal (bone)
834.11 Open dislocation of metacarpophalangeal (joint)
842.12 Sprain and strain of metacarpophalangeal (joint) of hand
882.2 Open wound of hand except finger(s) alone, with tendon involvement — (Use additional code to identify infection)
883.2 Open wound of finger(s), with tendon involvement — (Use additional code to identify infection)
886.1 Traumatic amputation of other finger(s) (complete) (partial), complicated — (Use additional code to identify infection)
905.2 Late effect of fracture of upper extremities
906.4 Late effect of crushing

ICD-9-CM Procedural

82.55 Other change in muscle or tendon length of hand

26480–26483

26480 Transfer or transplant of tendon, carpometacarpal area or dorsum of hand; without free graft, each tendon
26483 with free tendon graft (includes obtaining graft), each tendon

ICD-9-CM Diagnostic

138 Late effects of acute poliomyelitis
343.0 Diplegic infantile cerebral palsy
714.4 Chronic postrheumatic arthropathy
716.14 Traumatic arthropathy, hand
718.54 Ankylosis of hand joint
718.84 Other joint derangement, not elsewhere classified, hand

▽ Unspecified code ♀ Female diagnosis ☒ Manifestation code ♂ Male diagnosis

719.14 Hemarthrosis, hand
727.63 Nontraumatic rupture of extensor tendons of hand and wrist
755.50 Unspecified congenital anomaly of upper limb ▽
842.12 Sprain and strain of metacarpophalangeal (joint) of hand
882.2 Open wound of hand except finger(s) alone, with tendon involvement — (Use additional code to identify infection)
883.2 Open wound of finger(s), with tendon involvement — (Use additional code to identify infection)
886.1 Traumatic amputation of other finger(s) (complete) (partial), complicated — (Use additional code to identify infection)
905.2 Late effect of fracture of upper extremities
906.4 Late effect of crushing

ICD-9-CM Procedural

82.56 Other hand tendon transfer or transplantation

26485–26489

26485 Transfer or transplant of tendon, palmar; without free tendon graft, each tendon
26489 with free tendon graft (includes obtaining graft), each tendon

ICD-9-CM Diagnostic

138 Late effects of acute poliomyelitis
343.0 Diplegic infantile cerebral palsy
714.4 Chronic postrheumatic arthropathy
716.14 Traumatic arthropathy, hand
718.54 Ankylosis of hand joint
718.84 Other joint derangement, not elsewhere classified, hand
719.14 Hemarthrosis, hand
727.63 Nontraumatic rupture of extensor tendons of hand and wrist
755.50 Unspecified congenital anomaly of upper limb ▽
842.12 Sprain and strain of metacarpophalangeal (joint) of hand
882.2 Open wound of hand except finger(s) alone, with tendon involvement — (Use additional code to identify infection)
883.2 Open wound of finger(s), with tendon involvement — (Use additional code to identify infection)
886.1 Traumatic amputation of other finger(s) (complete) (partial), complicated — (Use additional code to identify infection)
905.2 Late effect of fracture of upper extremities
906.4 Late effect of crushing

ICD-9-CM Procedural

82.56 Other hand tendon transfer or transplantation
82.79 Plastic operation on hand with other graft or implant

26490–26496

26490 Opponensplasty; superficialis tendon transfer type, each tendon
26492 tendon transfer with graft (includes obtaining graft), each tendon
26494 hypothenar muscle transfer
26496 other methods

ICD-9-CM Diagnostic

138 Late effects of acute poliomyelitis
718.44 Contracture of hand joint
718.84 Other joint derangement, not elsewhere classified, hand
727.63 Nontraumatic rupture of extensor tendons of hand and wrist
728.6 Contracture of palmar fascia
736.29 Other acquired deformity of finger
755.21 Congenital transverse deficiency of upper limb
755.50 Unspecified congenital anomaly of upper limb ▽
883.2 Open wound of finger(s), with tendon involvement — (Use additional code to identify infection)
886.1 Traumatic amputation of other finger(s) (complete) (partial), complicated — (Use additional code to identify infection)
905.2 Late effect of fracture of upper extremities
905.9 Late effect of traumatic amputation
906.4 Late effect of crushing
927.3 Crushing injury of finger(s) — (Use additional code to identify any associated injuries: 800-829, 850.0-854.1, 860.0-869.1)

ICD-9-CM Procedural

82.56 Other hand tendon transfer or transplantation

26497–26498

26497 Transfer of tendon to restore intrinsic function; ring and small finger
26498 all four fingers

ICD-9-CM Diagnostic

138 Late effects of acute poliomyelitis
343.0 Diplegic infantile cerebral palsy
718.44 Contracture of hand joint
718.84 Other joint derangement, not elsewhere classified, hand
727.63 Nontraumatic rupture of extensor tendons of hand and wrist
736.29 Other acquired deformity of finger
755.21 Congenital transverse deficiency of upper limb
816.11 Open fracture of middle or proximal phalanx or phalanges of hand
883.2 Open wound of finger(s), with tendon involvement — (Use additional code to identify infection)
886.1 Traumatic amputation of other finger(s) (complete) (partial), complicated — (Use additional code to identify infection)
905.2 Late effect of fracture of upper extremities
905.9 Late effect of traumatic amputation
906.4 Late effect of crushing
927.3 Crushing injury of finger(s) — (Use additional code to identify any associated injuries: 800-829, 850.0-854.1, 860.0-869.1)

ICD-9-CM Procedural

82.56 Other hand tendon transfer or transplantation

26499

26499 Correction claw finger, other methods

ICD-9-CM Diagnostic

736.06 Claw hand (acquired)

ICD-9-CM Procedural

80.44 Division of joint capsule, ligament, or cartilage of hand and finger
81.28 Interphalangeal fusion
82.55 Other change in muscle or tendon length of hand

26500–26504

26500 Reconstruction of tendon pulley, each tendon; with local tissues (separate procedure)
26502 with tendon or fascial graft (includes obtaining graft) (separate procedure)
26504 with tendon prosthesis (separate procedure)

ICD-9-CM Diagnostic

138 Late effects of acute poliomyelitis
344.89 Other specified paralytic syndrome
715.14 Primary localized osteoarthrosis, hand
718.44 Contracture of hand joint
718.84 Other joint derangement, not elsewhere classified, hand
727.64 Nontraumatic rupture of flexor tendons of hand and wrist
727.89 Other disorders of synovium, tendon, and bursa
816.00 Closed fracture of unspecified phalanx or phalanges of hand ▽
816.01 Closed fracture of middle or proximal phalanx or phalanges of hand
816.02 Closed fracture of distal phalanx or phalanges of hand
816.03 Closed fracture of multiple sites of phalanx or phalanges of hand
816.10 Open fracture of phalanx or phalanges of hand, unspecified ▽
816.11 Open fracture of middle or proximal phalanx or phalanges of hand
816.12 Open fracture of distal phalanx or phalanges of hand
816.13 Open fractures of multiple sites of phalanx or phalanges of hand
842.13 Sprain and strain of interphalangeal (joint) of hand
883.2 Open wound of finger(s), with tendon involvement — (Use additional code to identify infection)
886.1 Traumatic amputation of other finger(s) (complete) (partial), complicated — (Use additional code to identify infection)
905.2 Late effect of fracture of upper extremities
905.8 Late effect of tendon injury
905.9 Late effect of traumatic amputation
927.3 Crushing injury of finger(s) — (Use additional code to identify any associated injuries: 800-829, 850.0-854.1, 860.0-869.1)

ICD-9-CM Procedural

82.71 Tendon pulley reconstruction on hand
82.79 Plastic operation on hand with other graft or implant
83.83 Tendon pulley reconstruction on muscle, tendon, and fascia

26508

26508 Release of thenar muscle(s) (eg, thumb contracture)

ICD-9-CM Diagnostic

344.89 Other specified paralytic syndrome
357.1 Polyneuropathy in collagen vascular disease — (Code first underlying disease: 446.0, 710.0, 714.0) ☒
359.6 Symptomatic inflammatory myopathy in diseases classified elsewhere — (Code first underlying disease: 135, 140.0-208.9, 277.3, 446.0, 710.0, 710.1, 710.2, 714.0) ☒
446.0 Polyarteritis nodosa
710.0 Systemic lupus erythematosus — (Use additional code to identify manifestation: 424.91, 581.81, 582.81, 583.81)
710.1 Systemic sclerosis — (Use additional code to identify manifestation: 359.6, 517.2)
710.2 Sicca syndrome
714.0 Rheumatoid arthritis — (Use additional code to identify manifestation: 357.1, 359.6)
715.14 Primary localized osteoarthrosis, hand
718.44 Contracture of hand joint
728.2 Muscular wasting and disuse atrophy, not elsewhere classified
728.88 Rhabdomyolysis
728.89 Other disorder of muscle, ligament, and fascia — (Use additional E code to identify drug, if drug-induced)
736.29 Other acquired deformity of finger
905.8 Late effect of tendon injury
906.4 Late effect of crushing
906.6 Late effect of burn of wrist and hand
909.3 Late effect of complications of surgical and medical care
958.6 Volkmann's ischemic contracture

ICD-9-CM Procedural

82.19 Other division of soft tissue of hand

26510

26510 Cross intrinsic transfer, each tendon

ICD-9-CM Diagnostic

344.89 Other specified paralytic syndrome
357.1 Polyneuropathy in collagen vascular disease — (Code first underlying disease: 446.0, 710.0, 714.0) ☒
359.6 Symptomatic inflammatory myopathy in diseases classified elsewhere — (Code first underlying disease: 135, 140.0-208.9, 277.3, 446.0, 710.0, 710.1, 710.2, 714.0) ☒
446.0 Polyarteritis nodosa
710.0 Systemic lupus erythematosus — (Use additional code to identify manifestation: 424.91, 581.81, 582.81, 583.81)
710.1 Systemic sclerosis — (Use additional code to identify manifestation: 359.6, 517.2)
710.2 Sicca syndrome
714.0 Rheumatoid arthritis — (Use additional code to identify manifestation: 357.1, 359.6)
715.14 Primary localized osteoarthrosis, hand
718.44 Contracture of hand joint
727.63 Nontraumatic rupture of extensor tendons of hand and wrist
727.64 Nontraumatic rupture of flexor tendons of hand and wrist
728.2 Muscular wasting and disuse atrophy, not elsewhere classified
728.88 Rhabdomyolysis
728.89 Other disorder of muscle, ligament, and fascia — (Use additional E code to identify drug, if drug-induced)
842.12 Sprain and strain of metacarpophalangeal (joint) of hand
883.2 Open wound of finger(s), with tendon involvement — (Use additional code to identify infection)
886.1 Traumatic amputation of other finger(s) (complete) (partial), complicated — (Use additional code to identify infection)
905.8 Late effect of tendon injury
905.9 Late effect of traumatic amputation
906.4 Late effect of crushing
906.6 Late effect of burn of wrist and hand
927.3 Crushing injury of finger(s) — (Use additional code to identify any associated injuries: 800-829, 850.0-854.1, 860.0-869.1)
958.6 Volkmann's ischemic contracture

ICD-9-CM Procedural

83.75 Tendon transfer or transplantation

26516–26518

26516 Capsulodesis, metacarpophalangeal joint; single digit
26517 two digits
26518 three or four digits

ICD-9-CM Diagnostic

343.0 Diplegic infantile cerebral palsy
343.1 Hemiplegic infantile cerebral palsy
343.2 Quadriplegic infantile cerebral palsy
343.3 Monoplegic infantile cerebral palsy
343.4 Infantile hemiplegia
343.8 Other specified infantile cerebral palsy
343.9 Unspecified infantile cerebral palsy ▽
344.81 Locked-in state
344.89 Other specified paralytic syndrome
357.1 Polyneuropathy in collagen vascular disease — (Code first underlying disease: 446.0, 710.0, 714.0) ☒
359.6 Symptomatic inflammatory myopathy in diseases classified elsewhere — (Code first underlying disease: 135, 140.0-208.9, 277.3, 446.0, 710.0, 710.1, 710.2, 714.0) ☒
446.0 Polyarteritis nodosa
710.0 Systemic lupus erythematosus — (Use additional code to identify manifestation: 424.91, 581.81, 582.81, 583.81)
710.1 Systemic sclerosis — (Use additional code to identify manifestation: 359.6, 517.2)
710.2 Sicca syndrome
714.0 Rheumatoid arthritis — (Use additional code to identify manifestation: 357.1, 359.6)
715.14 Primary localized osteoarthrosis, hand
718.44 Contracture of hand joint
718.74 Developmental dislocation of joint, hand
718.84 Other joint derangement, not elsewhere classified, hand
728.2 Muscular wasting and disuse atrophy, not elsewhere classified
728.88 Rhabdomyolysis
728.89 Other disorder of muscle, ligament, and fascia — (Use additional E code to identify drug, if drug-induced)
736.06 Claw hand (acquired)
834.11 Open dislocation of metacarpophalangeal (joint)
882.1 Open wound of hand except finger(s) alone, complicated — (Use additional code to identify infection)
882.2 Open wound of hand except finger(s) alone, with tendon involvement — (Use additional code to identify infection)
883.1 Open wound of finger(s), complicated — (Use additional code to identify infection)
883.2 Open wound of finger(s), with tendon involvement — (Use additional code to identify infection)
886.1 Traumatic amputation of other finger(s) (complete) (partial), complicated — (Use additional code to identify infection)
906.1 Late effect of open wound of extremities without mention of tendon injury
906.4 Late effect of crushing
906.6 Late effect of burn of wrist and hand
927.20 Crushing injury of hand(s) — (Use additional code to identify any associated injuries: 800-829, 850.0-854.1, 860.0-869.1)
927.3 Crushing injury of finger(s) — (Use additional code to identify any associated injuries: 800-829, 850.0-854.1, 860.0-869.1)
944.04 Burn of unspecified degree of two or more digits of hand, including thumb ▽
944.08 Burn of unspecified degree of multiple sites of wrist(s) and hand(s) ▽
944.42 Deep necrosis of underlying tissues due to burn (deep third degree) of thumb (nail), without mention of loss of a body part
955.4 Injury to musculocutaneous nerve
958.6 Volkmann's ischemic contracture

ICD-9-CM Procedural

81.29 Arthrodesis of other specified joint

26520–26525

26520 Capsulectomy or capsulotomy; metacarpophalangeal joint, each joint
26525 interphalangeal joint, each joint

ICD-9-CM Diagnostic

357.1 Polyneuropathy in collagen vascular disease — (Code first underlying disease: 446.0, 710.0, 714.0) ☒
359.6 Symptomatic inflammatory myopathy in diseases classified elsewhere — (Code first underlying disease: 135, 140.0-208.9, 277.3, 446.0, 710.0, 710.1, 710.2, 714.0) ☒
446.0 Polyarteritis nodosa

▽ Unspecified code ☒ Manifestation code
♀ Female diagnosis ♂ Male diagnosis

710.0 Systemic lupus erythematosus — (Use additional code to identify manifestation: 424.91, 581.81, 582.81, 583.81)
710.1 Systemic sclerosis — (Use additional code to identify manifestation: 359.6, 517.2)
710.2 Sicca syndrome
714.0 Rheumatoid arthritis — (Use additional code to identify manifestation: 357.1, 359.6)
714.4 Chronic postrheumatic arthropathy
715.14 Primary localized osteoarthrosis, hand
716.14 Traumatic arthropathy, hand
718.44 Contracture of hand joint
719.54 Stiffness of joint, not elsewhere classified, hand
728.89 Other disorder of muscle, ligament, and fascia — (Use additional E code to identify drug, if drug-induced)
736.20 Unspecified deformity of finger ▽
736.29 Other acquired deformity of finger
756.89 Other specified congenital anomaly of muscle, tendon, fascia, and connective tissue
906.4 Late effect of crushing
959.5 Injury, other and unspecified, finger
996.92 Complications of reattached hand
996.93 Complications of reattached finger(s)
998.59 Other postoperative infection — (Use additional code to identify infection)

ICD-9-CM Procedural

80.44 Division of joint capsule, ligament, or cartilage of hand and finger
80.94 Other excision of joint of hand and finger

26530–26531

26530 Arthroplasty, metacarpophalangeal joint; each joint
26531 with prosthetic implant, each joint

ICD-9-CM Diagnostic

357.1 Polyneuropathy in collagen vascular disease — (Code first underlying disease: 446.0, 710.0, 714.0) ☒
359.6 Symptomatic inflammatory myopathy in diseases classified elsewhere — (Code first underlying disease: 135, 140.0-208.9, 277.3, 446.0, 710.0, 710.1, 710.2, 714.0) ☒
446.0 Polyarteritis nodosa
710.0 Systemic lupus erythematosus — (Use additional code to identify manifestation: 424.91, 581.81, 582.81, 583.81)
710.1 Systemic sclerosis — (Use additional code to identify manifestation: 359.6, 517.2)
710.2 Sicca syndrome
714.0 Rheumatoid arthritis — (Use additional code to identify manifestation: 357.1, 359.6)
714.4 Chronic postrheumatic arthropathy
715.14 Primary localized osteoarthrosis, hand
715.94 Osteoarthrosis, unspecified whether generalized or localized, hand ▽
716.14 Traumatic arthropathy, hand
718.04 Articular cartilage disorder, hand
718.74 Developmental dislocation of joint, hand
730.14 Chronic osteomyelitis, hand — (Use additional code to identify organism, 041.1)
733.82 Nonunion of fracture
815.12 Open fracture of base of other metacarpal bone(s)
834.01 Closed dislocation of metacarpophalangeal (joint)
834.11 Open dislocation of metacarpophalangeal (joint)
882.1 Open wound of hand except finger(s) alone, complicated — (Use additional code to identify infection)
882.2 Open wound of hand except finger(s) alone, with tendon involvement — (Use additional code to identify infection)
905.2 Late effect of fracture of upper extremities
927.20 Crushing injury of hand(s) — (Use additional code to identify any associated injuries: 800-829, 850.0-854.1, 860.0-869.1)
927.3 Crushing injury of finger(s) — (Use additional code to identify any associated injuries: 800-829, 850.0-854.1, 860.0-869.1)

ICD-9-CM Procedural

81.71 Arthroplasty of metacarpophalangeal and interphalangeal joint with implant
81.72 Arthroplasty of metacarpophalangeal and interphalangeal joint without implant

26535–26536

26535 Arthroplasty, interphalangeal joint; each joint
26536 with prosthetic implant, each joint

ICD-9-CM Diagnostic

357.1 Polyneuropathy in collagen vascular disease — (Code first underlying disease: 446.0, 710.0, 714.0) ☒
359.6 Symptomatic inflammatory myopathy in diseases classified elsewhere — (Code first underlying disease: 135, 140.0-208.9, 277.3, 446.0, 710.0, 710.1, 710.2, 714.0) ☒
446.0 Polyarteritis nodosa
710.0 Systemic lupus erythematosus — (Use additional code to identify manifestation: 424.91, 581.81, 582.81, 583.81)
710.1 Systemic sclerosis — (Use additional code to identify manifestation: 359.6, 517.2)
710.2 Sicca syndrome
714.0 Rheumatoid arthritis — (Use additional code to identify manifestation: 357.1, 359.6)
714.4 Chronic postrheumatic arthropathy
715.14 Primary localized osteoarthrosis, hand
715.94 Osteoarthrosis, unspecified whether generalized or localized, hand ▽
716.14 Traumatic arthropathy, hand
718.44 Contracture of hand joint
718.74 Developmental dislocation of joint, hand
730.14 Chronic osteomyelitis, hand — (Use additional code to identify organism, 041.1)
736.29 Other acquired deformity of finger
816.11 Open fracture of middle or proximal phalanx or phalanges of hand
816.12 Open fracture of distal phalanx or phalanges of hand
816.13 Open fractures of multiple sites of phalanx or phalanges of hand
817.1 Multiple open fractures of hand bones
834.02 Closed dislocation of interphalangeal (joint), hand
834.12 Open dislocation interphalangeal (joint), hand
883.1 Open wound of finger(s), complicated — (Use additional code to identify infection)
883.2 Open wound of finger(s), with tendon involvement — (Use additional code to identify infection)
905.2 Late effect of fracture of upper extremities
905.9 Late effect of traumatic amputation
906.4 Late effect of crushing
927.3 Crushing injury of finger(s) — (Use additional code to identify any associated injuries: 800-829, 850.0-854.1, 860.0-869.1)

ICD-9-CM Procedural

81.71 Arthroplasty of metacarpophalangeal and interphalangeal joint with implant
81.72 Arthroplasty of metacarpophalangeal and interphalangeal joint without implant

26540

26540 Repair of collateral ligament, metacarpophalangeal or interphalangeal joint

ICD-9-CM Diagnostic

716.14 Traumatic arthropathy, hand
718.34 Recurrent dislocation of hand joint
718.74 Developmental dislocation of joint, hand
718.84 Other joint derangement, not elsewhere classified, hand
728.89 Other disorder of muscle, ligament, and fascia — (Use additional E code to identify drug, if drug-induced)
816.01 Closed fracture of middle or proximal phalanx or phalanges of hand
816.02 Closed fracture of distal phalanx or phalanges of hand
816.03 Closed fracture of multiple sites of phalanx or phalanges of hand
816.11 Open fracture of middle or proximal phalanx or phalanges of hand
816.12 Open fracture of distal phalanx or phalanges of hand
816.13 Open fractures of multiple sites of phalanx or phalanges of hand
834.01 Closed dislocation of metacarpophalangeal (joint)
834.02 Closed dislocation of interphalangeal (joint), hand
834.11 Open dislocation of metacarpophalangeal (joint)
834.12 Open dislocation interphalangeal (joint), hand
842.12 Sprain and strain of metacarpophalangeal (joint) of hand
842.13 Sprain and strain of interphalangeal (joint) of hand
882.1 Open wound of hand except finger(s) alone, complicated — (Use additional code to identify infection)
882.2 Open wound of hand except finger(s) alone, with tendon involvement — (Use additional code to identify infection)
883.1 Open wound of finger(s), complicated — (Use additional code to identify infection)

▽ Unspecified code ♀ Female diagnosis ☒ Manifestation code ♂ Male diagnosis

883.2 Open wound of finger(s), with tendon involvement — (Use additional code to identify infection)
927.3 Crushing injury of finger(s) — (Use additional code to identify any associated injuries: 800-829, 850.0-854.1, 860.0-869.1)

ICD-9-CM Procedural

81.93 Suture of capsule or ligament of upper extremity

26541–26545

26541 Reconstruction, collateral ligament, metacarpophalangeal joint, single, with tendon or fascial graft (includes obtaining graft)
26542 with local tissue (eg, adductor advancement)
26545 Reconstruction, collateral ligament, interphalangeal joint, single, including graft, each joint

ICD-9-CM Diagnostic

716.14 Traumatic arthropathy, hand
718.34 Recurrent dislocation of hand joint
718.74 Developmental dislocation of joint, hand
718.84 Other joint derangement, not elsewhere classified, hand
728.89 Other disorder of muscle, ligament, and fascia — (Use additional E code to identify drug, if drug-induced)
816.01 Closed fracture of middle or proximal phalanx or phalanges of hand
816.02 Closed fracture of distal phalanx or phalanges of hand
816.03 Closed fracture of multiple sites of phalanx or phalanges of hand
816.11 Open fracture of middle or proximal phalanx or phalanges of hand
816.12 Open fracture of distal phalanx or phalanges of hand
816.13 Open fractures of multiple sites of phalanx or phalanges of hand
834.01 Closed dislocation of metacarpophalangeal (joint)
834.02 Closed dislocation of interphalangeal (joint), hand
834.11 Open dislocation of metacarpophalangeal (joint)
834.12 Open dislocation interphalangeal (joint), hand
842.12 Sprain and strain of metacarpophalangeal (joint) of hand
842.13 Sprain and strain of interphalangeal (joint) of hand
882.1 Open wound of hand except finger(s) alone, complicated — (Use additional code to identify infection)
882.2 Open wound of hand except finger(s) alone, with tendon involvement — (Use additional code to identify infection)
883.1 Open wound of finger(s), complicated — (Use additional code to identify infection)
883.2 Open wound of finger(s), with tendon involvement — (Use additional code to identify infection)
927.3 Crushing injury of finger(s) — (Use additional code to identify any associated injuries: 800-829, 850.0-854.1, 860.0-869.1)

ICD-9-CM Procedural

81.93 Suture of capsule or ligament of upper extremity
82.72 Plastic operation on hand with graft of muscle or fascia
83.41 Excision of tendon for graft
83.81 Tendon graft

26546

26546 Repair non-union, metacarpal or phalanx, (includes obtaining bone graft with or without external or internal fixation)

ICD-9-CM Diagnostic

733.82 Nonunion of fracture
905.2 Late effect of fracture of upper extremities

ICD-9-CM Procedural

77.77 Excision of tibia and fibula for graft
77.78 Excision of tarsals and metatarsals for graft
77.99 Total ostectomy of other bone, except facial bones
78.09 Bone graft of other bone, except facial bones
78.44 Other repair or plastic operations on carpals and metacarpals
78.49 Other repair or plastic operations on other bone, except facial bones

26548

26548 Repair and reconstruction, finger, volar plate, interphalangeal joint

ICD-9-CM Diagnostic

716.14 Traumatic arthropathy, hand
718.04 Articular cartilage disorder, hand
718.24 Pathological dislocation of hand joint
718.34 Recurrent dislocation of hand joint
718.74 Developmental dislocation of joint, hand
718.84 Other joint derangement, not elsewhere classified, hand
816.01 Closed fracture of middle or proximal phalanx or phalanges of hand
816.02 Closed fracture of distal phalanx or phalanges of hand
816.03 Closed fracture of multiple sites of phalanx or phalanges of hand
816.11 Open fracture of middle or proximal phalanx or phalanges of hand
816.12 Open fracture of distal phalanx or phalanges of hand
816.13 Open fractures of multiple sites of phalanx or phalanges of hand
834.02 Closed dislocation of interphalangeal (joint), hand
834.12 Open dislocation interphalangeal (joint), hand
842.13 Sprain and strain of interphalangeal (joint) of hand
883.2 Open wound of finger(s), with tendon involvement — (Use additional code to identify infection)
905.9 Late effect of traumatic amputation
927.3 Crushing injury of finger(s) — (Use additional code to identify any associated injuries: 800-829, 850.0-854.1, 860.0-869.1)

ICD-9-CM Procedural

81.96 Other repair of joint

26550

26550 Pollicization of a digit

ICD-9-CM Diagnostic

755.29 Congenital longitudinal deficiency, phalanges, complete or partial
906.4 Late effect of crushing
906.6 Late effect of burn of wrist and hand
V10.81 Personal history of malignant neoplasm of bone
V49.61 Upper limb amputation, thumb — (This code is intended for use when these conditions are recorded as diagnoses or problems)
V49.62 Upper limb amputation, other finger(s) — (This code is intended for use when these conditions are recorded as diagnoses or problems)
V51 Aftercare involving the use of plastic surgery

ICD-9-CM Procedural

82.61 Pollicization operation carrying over nerves and blood supply

26551

26551 Transfer, toe-to-hand with microvascular anastomosis; great toe wrap-around with bone graft

ICD-9-CM Diagnostic

755.29 Congenital longitudinal deficiency, phalanges, complete or partial
906.4 Late effect of crushing
906.6 Late effect of burn of wrist and hand
V10.81 Personal history of malignant neoplasm of bone
V49.61 Upper limb amputation, thumb — (This code is intended for use when these conditions are recorded as diagnoses or problems)
V51 Aftercare involving the use of plastic surgery

ICD-9-CM Procedural

82.69 Other reconstruction of thumb
84.11 Amputation of toe

26553–26554

26553 Transfer, toe-to-hand with microvascular anastomosis; other than great toe, single
26554 other than great toe, double

ICD-9-CM Diagnostic

755.29 Congenital longitudinal deficiency, phalanges, complete or partial
906.1 Late effect of open wound of extremities without mention of tendon injury
906.4 Late effect of crushing
906.6 Late effect of burn of wrist and hand
V10.81 Personal history of malignant neoplasm of bone
V49.62 Upper limb amputation, other finger(s) — (This code is intended for use when these conditions are recorded as diagnoses or problems)
V51 Aftercare involving the use of plastic surgery

ICD-9-CM Procedural

82.81 Transfer of finger, except thumb
82.89 Other plastic operations on hand

26555

26555 Transfer, finger to another position without microvascular anastomosis

ICD-9-CM Diagnostic

755.29 Congenital longitudinal deficiency, phalanges, complete or partial
906.1 Late effect of open wound of extremities without mention of tendon injury
906.4 Late effect of crushing
906.6 Late effect of burn of wrist and hand
V10.81 Personal history of malignant neoplasm of bone
V49.62 Upper limb amputation, other finger(s) — (This code is intended for use when these conditions are recorded as diagnoses or problems)
V51 Aftercare involving the use of plastic surgery

ICD-9-CM Procedural

82.81 Transfer of finger, except thumb
82.89 Other plastic operations on hand

26556

26556 Transfer, free toe joint, with microvascular anastomosis

ICD-9-CM Diagnostic

755.29 Congenital longitudinal deficiency, phalanges, complete or partial
906.4 Late effect of crushing
906.6 Late effect of burn of wrist and hand
V10.81 Personal history of malignant neoplasm of bone
V49.61 Upper limb amputation, thumb — (This code is intended for use when these conditions are recorded as diagnoses or problems)
V49.62 Upper limb amputation, other finger(s) — (This code is intended for use when these conditions are recorded as diagnoses or problems)
V51 Aftercare involving the use of plastic surgery

ICD-9-CM Procedural

80.98 Other excision of joint of foot and toe
81.72 Arthroplasty of metacarpophalangeal and interphalangeal joint without implant

26560–26562

26560 Repair of syndactyly (web finger) each web space; with skin flaps
26561 with skin flaps and grafts
26562 complex (eg, involving bone, nails)

ICD-9-CM Diagnostic

755.10 Syndactyly of multiple and unspecified sites
755.11 Syndactyly of fingers without fusion of bone
755.12 Syndactyly of fingers with fusion of bone

ICD-9-CM Procedural

86.85 Correction of syndactyly

26565–26567

26565 Osteotomy; metacarpal, each
26567 phalanx of finger, each

ICD-9-CM Diagnostic

357.1 Polyneuropathy in collagen vascular disease — (Code first underlying disease: 446.0, 710.0, 714.0) ☒
359.6 Symptomatic inflammatory myopathy in diseases classified elsewhere — (Code first underlying disease: 135, 140.0-208.9, 277.3, 446.0, 710.0, 710.1, 710.2, 714.0) ☒
446.0 Polyarteritis nodosa
710.0 Systemic lupus erythematosus — (Use additional code to identify manifestation: 424.91, 581.81, 582.81, 583.81)
710.1 Systemic sclerosis — (Use additional code to identify manifestation: 359.6, 517.2)
710.2 Sicca syndrome
714.0 Rheumatoid arthritis — (Use additional code to identify manifestation: 357.1, 359.6)
714.4 Chronic postrheumatic arthropathy
715.14 Primary localized osteoarthrosis, hand
716.14 Traumatic arthropathy, hand
736.00 Unspecified deformity of forearm, excluding fingers ▽
736.07 Club hand, acquired
736.09 Other acquired deformities of forearm, excluding fingers
736.20 Unspecified deformity of finger ▽
736.29 Other acquired deformity of finger
738.9 Acquired musculoskeletal deformity of unspecified site ▽
754.89 Other specified nonteratogenic anomalies
755.28 Congenital longitudinal deficiency, carpals or metacarpals, complete or partial (with or without incomplete phalangeal deficiency)
756.9 Other and unspecified congenital anomaly of musculoskeletal system ▽
905.2 Late effect of fracture of upper extremities
909.3 Late effect of complications of surgical and medical care
998.59 Other postoperative infection — (Use additional code to identify infection)

ICD-9-CM Procedural

77.24 Wedge osteotomy of carpals and metacarpals
77.34 Other division of carpals and metacarpals
77.39 Other division of other bone, except facial bones

26568

26568 Osteoplasty, lengthening, metacarpal or phalanx

ICD-9-CM Diagnostic

714.4 Chronic postrheumatic arthropathy
715.14 Primary localized osteoarthrosis, hand
716.14 Traumatic arthropathy, hand
733.81 Malunion of fracture
736.06 Claw hand (acquired)
736.20 Unspecified deformity of finger ▽
736.29 Other acquired deformity of finger
738.9 Acquired musculoskeletal deformity of unspecified site ▽
755.28 Congenital longitudinal deficiency, carpals or metacarpals, complete or partial (with or without incomplete phalangeal deficiency)
756.9 Other and unspecified congenital anomaly of musculoskeletal system ▽
905.2 Late effect of fracture of upper extremities

ICD-9-CM Procedural

78.14 Application of external fixation device, carpals and metacarpals
78.19 Application of external fixation device, other
78.34 Limb lengthening procedures, carpals and metacarpals
78.39 Other limb lengthening procedures
84.53 Implantation of internal limb lengthening device with kinetic distraction
84.54 Implantation of other internal limb lengthening device

26580

26580 Repair cleft hand

ICD-9-CM Diagnostic

755.58 Congenital cleft hand

ICD-9-CM Procedural

82.82 Repair of cleft hand

26587

26587 Reconstruction of polydactylous digit, soft tissue and bone

ICD-9-CM Diagnostic

755.01 Polydactyly of fingers

ICD-9-CM Procedural

82.89 Other plastic operations on hand

26590

26590 Repair macrodactylia, each digit

ICD-9-CM Diagnostic

755.57 Macrodactylia (fingers)

ICD-9-CM Procedural

82.83 Repair of macrodactyly

26591

26591 Repair, intrinsic muscles of hand, each muscle

ICD-9-CM Diagnostic

727.64 Nontraumatic rupture of flexor tendons of hand and wrist
728.2 Muscular wasting and disuse atrophy, not elsewhere classified
728.83 Rupture of muscle, nontraumatic
842.12 Sprain and strain of metacarpophalangeal (joint) of hand
882.1 Open wound of hand except finger(s) alone, complicated — (Use additional code to identify infection)

▽ Unspecified code ☒ Manifestation code
♀ Female diagnosis ♂ Male diagnosis

882.2 Open wound of hand except finger(s) alone, with tendon involvement — (Use additional code to identify infection)
927.20 Crushing injury of hand(s) — (Use additional code to identify any associated injuries: 800-829, 850.0-854.1, 860.0-869.1)

ICD-9-CM Procedural

82.46 Suture of muscle or fascia of hand
82.72 Plastic operation on hand with graft of muscle or fascia
82.89 Other plastic operations on hand

26593

26593 Release, intrinsic muscles of hand, each muscle

ICD-9-CM Diagnostic

343.0 Diplegic infantile cerebral palsy
343.3 Monoplegic infantile cerebral palsy
344.89 Other specified paralytic syndrome
714.4 Chronic postrheumatic arthropathy
728.6 Contracture of palmar fascia
728.88 Rhabdomyolysis
728.89 Other disorder of muscle, ligament, and fascia — (Use additional E code to identify drug, if drug-induced)
736.06 Claw hand (acquired)
756.89 Other specified congenital anomaly of muscle, tendon, fascia, and connective tissue
905.2 Late effect of fracture of upper extremities
905.7 Late effect of sprain and strain without mention of tendon injury
905.8 Late effect of tendon injury
905.9 Late effect of traumatic amputation
906.1 Late effect of open wound of extremities without mention of tendon injury
906.6 Late effect of burn of wrist and hand
907.4 Late effect of injury to peripheral nerve of shoulder girdle and upper limb
927.20 Crushing injury of hand(s) — (Use additional code to identify any associated injuries: 800-829, 850.0-854.1, 860.0-869.1)
958.6 Volkmann's ischemic contracture

ICD-9-CM Procedural

82.19 Other division of soft tissue of hand

26596

26596 Excision of constricting ring of finger, with multiple Z-plasties

ICD-9-CM Diagnostic

709.2 Scar condition and fibrosis of skin
718.44 Contracture of hand joint
727.81 Contracture of tendon (sheath)
728.6 Contracture of palmar fascia
905.8 Late effect of tendon injury
905.9 Late effect of traumatic amputation
906.1 Late effect of open wound of extremities without mention of tendon injury
906.4 Late effect of crushing
906.6 Late effect of burn of wrist and hand

ICD-9-CM Procedural

86.84 Relaxation of scar or web contracture of skin

26600–26607

26600 Closed treatment of metacarpal fracture, single; without manipulation, each bone
26605 with manipulation, each bone
26607 Closed treatment of metacarpal fracture, with manipulation, with external fixation, each bone

ICD-9-CM Diagnostic

815.00 Closed fracture of metacarpal bone(s), site unspecified ▽
815.02 Closed fracture of base of other metacarpal bone(s)
815.03 Closed fracture of shaft of metacarpal bone(s)
815.04 Closed fracture of neck of metacarpal bone(s)
815.09 Closed fracture of multiple sites of metacarpus
817.0 Multiple closed fractures of hand bones

ICD-9-CM Procedural

79.03 Closed reduction of fracture of carpals and metacarpals without internal fixation
79.13 Closed reduction of fracture of carpals and metacarpals with internal fixation
79.14 Closed reduction of fracture of phalanges of hand with internal fixation
93.54 Application of splint

HCPCS Level II Supplies & Services

A4580 Cast supplies (e.g., plaster)
A4590 Special casting material (e.g., fiberglass)

26608

26608 Percutaneous skeletal fixation of metacarpal fracture, each bone

ICD-9-CM Diagnostic

815.00 Closed fracture of metacarpal bone(s), site unspecified ▽
815.02 Closed fracture of base of other metacarpal bone(s)
815.03 Closed fracture of shaft of metacarpal bone(s)
815.04 Closed fracture of neck of metacarpal bone(s)
815.09 Closed fracture of multiple sites of metacarpus
817.0 Multiple closed fractures of hand bones

ICD-9-CM Procedural

78.54 Internal fixation of carpals and metacarpals without fracture reduction

HCPCS Level II Supplies & Services

A4570 Splint
A4580 Cast supplies (e.g., plaster)

26615

26615 Open treatment of metacarpal fracture, single, with or without internal or external fixation, each bone

ICD-9-CM Diagnostic

815.00 Closed fracture of metacarpal bone(s), site unspecified ▽
815.02 Closed fracture of base of other metacarpal bone(s)
815.03 Closed fracture of shaft of metacarpal bone(s)
815.04 Closed fracture of neck of metacarpal bone(s)
815.09 Closed fracture of multiple sites of metacarpus
815.10 Open fracture of metacarpal bone(s), site unspecified ▽
815.12 Open fracture of base of other metacarpal bone(s)
815.13 Open fracture of shaft of metacarpal bone(s)
815.14 Open fracture of neck of metacarpal bone(s)
815.19 Open fracture of multiple sites of metacarpus
817.0 Multiple closed fractures of hand bones
817.1 Multiple open fractures of hand bones

ICD-9-CM Procedural

78.14 Application of external fixation device, carpals and metacarpals
79.23 Open reduction of fracture of carpals and metacarpals without internal fixation
79.33 Open reduction of fracture of carpals and metacarpals with internal fixation

HCPCS Level II Supplies & Services

A4570 Splint
A4580 Cast supplies (e.g., plaster)

26641–26645

26641 Closed treatment of carpometacarpal dislocation, thumb, with manipulation
26645 Closed treatment of carpometacarpal fracture dislocation, thumb (Bennett fracture), with manipulation

ICD-9-CM Diagnostic

718.24 Pathological dislocation of hand joint
718.30 Recurrent dislocation of joint, site unspecified ▽
718.34 Recurrent dislocation of hand joint
718.74 Developmental dislocation of joint, hand
815.01 Closed fracture of base of thumb (first) metacarpal bone(s)
833.04 Closed dislocation of carpometacarpal (joint)

ICD-9-CM Procedural

79.03 Closed reduction of fracture of carpals and metacarpals without internal fixation
79.13 Closed reduction of fracture of carpals and metacarpals with internal fixation
79.74 Closed reduction of dislocation of hand and finger

HCPCS Level II Supplies & Services

A4570 Splint
A4580 Cast supplies (e.g., plaster)

▽ Unspecified code ♀ Female diagnosis ☒ Manifestation code ♂ Male diagnosis

26650

26650 Percutaneous skeletal fixation of carpometacarpal fracture dislocation, thumb (Bennett fracture), with manipulation, with or without external fixation

ICD-9-CM Diagnostic

815.01 Closed fracture of base of thumb (first) metacarpal bone(s)
815.11 Open fracture of base of thumb (first) metacarpal bone(s)

ICD-9-CM Procedural

78.14 Application of external fixation device, carpals and metacarpals
78.54 Internal fixation of carpals and metacarpals without fracture reduction
79.13 Closed reduction of fracture of carpals and metacarpals with internal fixation
79.73 Closed reduction of dislocation of wrist

HCPCS Level II Supplies & Services

A4570 Splint
A4580 Cast supplies (e.g., plaster)

26665

26665 Open treatment of carpometacarpal fracture dislocation, thumb (Bennett fracture), with or without internal or external fixation

ICD-9-CM Diagnostic

815.01 Closed fracture of base of thumb (first) metacarpal bone(s)
815.11 Open fracture of base of thumb (first) metacarpal bone(s)

ICD-9-CM Procedural

78.14 Application of external fixation device, carpals and metacarpals
79.23 Open reduction of fracture of carpals and metacarpals without internal fixation
79.33 Open reduction of fracture of carpals and metacarpals with internal fixation
79.84 Open reduction of dislocation of hand and finger

HCPCS Level II Supplies & Services

A4570 Splint
A4580 Cast supplies (e.g., plaster)

26670–26675

26670 Closed treatment of carpometacarpal dislocation, other than thumb, with manipulation, each joint; without anesthesia
26675 requiring anesthesia

ICD-9-CM Diagnostic

718.24 Pathological dislocation of hand joint
718.30 Recurrent dislocation of joint, site unspecified ▼
718.34 Recurrent dislocation of hand joint
718.74 Developmental dislocation of joint, hand
833.04 Closed dislocation of carpometacarpal (joint)

ICD-9-CM Procedural

79.74 Closed reduction of dislocation of hand and finger

HCPCS Level II Supplies & Services

A4570 Splint
A4580 Cast supplies (e.g., plaster)

26676

26676 Percutaneous skeletal fixation of carpometacarpal dislocation, other than thumb, with manipulation, each joint

ICD-9-CM Diagnostic

718.24 Pathological dislocation of hand joint
718.34 Recurrent dislocation of hand joint
718.74 Developmental dislocation of joint, hand
833.04 Closed dislocation of carpometacarpal (joint)
833.14 Open dislocation of carpometacarpal (joint)

ICD-9-CM Procedural

78.54 Internal fixation of carpals and metacarpals without fracture reduction
79.74 Closed reduction of dislocation of hand and finger

HCPCS Level II Supplies & Services

A4570 Splint
A4580 Cast supplies (e.g., plaster)

26685–26686

26685 Open treatment of carpometacarpal dislocation, other than thumb; with or without internal or external fixation, each joint
26686 complex, multiple or delayed reduction

ICD-9-CM Diagnostic

718.24 Pathological dislocation of hand joint
718.34 Recurrent dislocation of hand joint
718.74 Developmental dislocation of joint, hand
833.04 Closed dislocation of carpometacarpal (joint)
833.14 Open dislocation of carpometacarpal (joint)

ICD-9-CM Procedural

78.14 Application of external fixation device, carpals and metacarpals
79.84 Open reduction of dislocation of hand and finger

HCPCS Level II Supplies & Services

A4570 Splint
A4580 Cast supplies (e.g., plaster)

26700–26705

26700 Closed treatment of metacarpophalangeal dislocation, single, with manipulation; without anesthesia
26705 requiring anesthesia

ICD-9-CM Diagnostic

718.24 Pathological dislocation of hand joint
718.34 Recurrent dislocation of hand joint
718.74 Developmental dislocation of joint, hand
834.01 Closed dislocation of metacarpophalangeal (joint)

ICD-9-CM Procedural

79.74 Closed reduction of dislocation of hand and finger

HCPCS Level II Supplies & Services

A4570 Splint
A4580 Cast supplies (e.g., plaster)

26706

26706 Percutaneous skeletal fixation of metacarpophalangeal dislocation, single, with manipulation

ICD-9-CM Diagnostic

718.24 Pathological dislocation of hand joint
718.34 Recurrent dislocation of hand joint
718.74 Developmental dislocation of joint, hand
834.01 Closed dislocation of metacarpophalangeal (joint)

ICD-9-CM Procedural

78.54 Internal fixation of carpals and metacarpals without fracture reduction
79.74 Closed reduction of dislocation of hand and finger

HCPCS Level II Supplies & Services

A4570 Splint
A4580 Cast supplies (e.g., plaster)

26715

26715 Open treatment of metacarpophalangeal dislocation, single, with or without internal or external fixation

ICD-9-CM Diagnostic

718.24 Pathological dislocation of hand joint
718.74 Developmental dislocation of joint, hand
834.01 Closed dislocation of metacarpophalangeal (joint)
834.11 Open dislocation of metacarpophalangeal (joint)

ICD-9-CM Procedural

79.84 Open reduction of dislocation of hand and finger

HCPCS Level II Supplies & Services

A4570 Splint
A4580 Cast supplies (e.g., plaster)

26720–26725

26720 Closed treatment of phalangeal shaft fracture, proximal or middle phalanx, finger or thumb; without manipulation, each
26725 with manipulation, with or without skin or skeletal traction, each

ICD-9-CM Diagnostic

816.01 Closed fracture of middle or proximal phalanx or phalanges of hand
816.03 Closed fracture of multiple sites of phalanx or phalanges of hand
817.0 Multiple closed fractures of hand bones
927.3 Crushing injury of finger(s) — (Use additional code to identify any associated injuries: 800-829, 850.0-854.1, 860.0-869.1)

ICD-9-CM Procedural

79.04 Closed reduction of fracture of phalanges of hand without internal fixation
93.54 Application of splint

HCPCS Level II Supplies & Services

A4570 Splint

26727

26727 Percutaneous skeletal fixation of unstable phalangeal shaft fracture, proximal or middle phalanx, finger or thumb, with manipulation, each

ICD-9-CM Diagnostic

816.01 Closed fracture of middle or proximal phalanx or phalanges of hand
816.03 Closed fracture of multiple sites of phalanx or phalanges of hand
817.0 Multiple closed fractures of hand bones
927.3 Crushing injury of finger(s) — (Use additional code to identify any associated injuries: 800-829, 850.0-854.1, 860.0-869.1)

ICD-9-CM Procedural

79.14 Closed reduction of fracture of phalanges of hand with internal fixation

HCPCS Level II Supplies & Services

A4570 Splint

26735

26735 Open treatment of phalangeal shaft fracture, proximal or middle phalanx, finger or thumb, with or without internal or external fixation, each

ICD-9-CM Diagnostic

816.01 Closed fracture of middle or proximal phalanx or phalanges of hand
816.03 Closed fracture of multiple sites of phalanx or phalanges of hand
816.11 Open fracture of middle or proximal phalanx or phalanges of hand
816.13 Open fractures of multiple sites of phalanx or phalanges of hand
817.0 Multiple closed fractures of hand bones
817.1 Multiple open fractures of hand bones
927.3 Crushing injury of finger(s) — (Use additional code to identify any associated injuries: 800-829, 850.0-854.1, 860.0-869.1)

ICD-9-CM Procedural

79.24 Open reduction of fracture of phalanges of hand without internal fixation
79.34 Open reduction of fracture of phalanges of hand with internal fixation
79.80 Open reduction of dislocation of unspecified site

HCPCS Level II Supplies & Services

A4570 Splint

26740–26742

26740 Closed treatment of articular fracture, involving metacarpophalangeal or interphalangeal joint; without manipulation, each
26742 with manipulation, each

ICD-9-CM Diagnostic

815.02 Closed fracture of base of other metacarpal bone(s)
815.04 Closed fracture of neck of metacarpal bone(s)
815.09 Closed fracture of multiple sites of metacarpus
816.01 Closed fracture of middle or proximal phalanx or phalanges of hand
816.03 Closed fracture of multiple sites of phalanx or phalanges of hand
817.0 Multiple closed fractures of hand bones
927.20 Crushing injury of hand(s) — (Use additional code to identify any associated injuries: 800-829, 850.0-854.1, 860.0-869.1)
927.3 Crushing injury of finger(s) — (Use additional code to identify any associated injuries: 800-829, 850.0-854.1, 860.0-869.1)

ICD-9-CM Procedural

79.04 Closed reduction of fracture of phalanges of hand without internal fixation
93.54 Application of splint

HCPCS Level II Supplies & Services

A4570 Splint

26746

26746 Open treatment of articular fracture, involving metacarpophalangeal or interphalangeal joint, with or without internal or external fixation, each

ICD-9-CM Diagnostic

815.02 Closed fracture of base of other metacarpal bone(s)
815.04 Closed fracture of neck of metacarpal bone(s)
815.09 Closed fracture of multiple sites of metacarpus
815.11 Open fracture of base of thumb (first) metacarpal bone(s)
815.14 Open fracture of neck of metacarpal bone(s)
815.19 Open fracture of multiple sites of metacarpus
816.01 Closed fracture of middle or proximal phalanx or phalanges of hand
816.03 Closed fracture of multiple sites of phalanx or phalanges of hand
817.0 Multiple closed fractures of hand bones
817.1 Multiple open fractures of hand bones

ICD-9-CM Procedural

79.24 Open reduction of fracture of phalanges of hand without internal fixation
79.34 Open reduction of fracture of phalanges of hand with internal fixation

HCPCS Level II Supplies & Services

A4570 Splint

26750–26755

26750 Closed treatment of distal phalangeal fracture, finger or thumb; without manipulation, each
26755 with manipulation, each

ICD-9-CM Diagnostic

816.02 Closed fracture of distal phalanx or phalanges of hand
816.03 Closed fracture of multiple sites of phalanx or phalanges of hand
817.0 Multiple closed fractures of hand bones

ICD-9-CM Procedural

79.04 Closed reduction of fracture of phalanges of hand without internal fixation
93.54 Application of splint

HCPCS Level II Supplies & Services

A4570 Splint

26756

26756 Percutaneous skeletal fixation of distal phalangeal fracture, finger or thumb, each

ICD-9-CM Diagnostic

816.02 Closed fracture of distal phalanx or phalanges of hand
816.03 Closed fracture of multiple sites of phalanx or phalanges of hand
816.12 Open fracture of distal phalanx or phalanges of hand
816.13 Open fractures of multiple sites of phalanx or phalanges of hand
817.0 Multiple closed fractures of hand bones

ICD-9-CM Procedural

78.59 Internal fixation of other bone, except facial bones, without fracture reduction

HCPCS Level II Supplies & Services

A4570 Splint

26765

26765 Open treatment of distal phalangeal fracture, finger or thumb, with or without internal or external fixation, each

ICD-9-CM Diagnostic

816.02 Closed fracture of distal phalanx or phalanges of hand
816.03 Closed fracture of multiple sites of phalanx or phalanges of hand
816.12 Open fracture of distal phalanx or phalanges of hand
816.13 Open fractures of multiple sites of phalanx or phalanges of hand
817.0 Multiple closed fractures of hand bones
817.1 Multiple open fractures of hand bones

ICD-9-CM Procedural
78.19 Application of external fixation device, other
79.24 Open reduction of fracture of phalanges of hand without internal fixation
79.34 Open reduction of fracture of phalanges of hand with internal fixation

HCPCS Level II Supplies & Services
A4570 Splint

26770–26775
26770 Closed treatment of interphalangeal joint dislocation, single, with manipulation; without anesthesia
26775 requiring anesthesia

ICD-9-CM Diagnostic
718.24 Pathological dislocation of hand joint
718.34 Recurrent dislocation of hand joint
718.74 Developmental dislocation of joint, hand
834.02 Closed dislocation of interphalangeal (joint), hand

ICD-9-CM Procedural
79.70 Closed reduction of dislocation of unspecified site

HCPCS Level II Supplies & Services
A4570 Splint

26776
26776 Percutaneous skeletal fixation of interphalangeal joint dislocation, single, with manipulation

ICD-9-CM Diagnostic
718.24 Pathological dislocation of hand joint
718.34 Recurrent dislocation of hand joint
718.74 Developmental dislocation of joint, hand
834.02 Closed dislocation of interphalangeal (joint), hand

ICD-9-CM Procedural
78.59 Internal fixation of other bone, except facial bones, without fracture reduction
79.74 Closed reduction of dislocation of hand and finger

HCPCS Level II Supplies & Services
A4570 Splint

26785
26785 Open treatment of interphalangeal joint dislocation, with or without internal or external fixation, single

ICD-9-CM Diagnostic
718.24 Pathological dislocation of hand joint
718.34 Recurrent dislocation of hand joint
718.74 Developmental dislocation of joint, hand
834.02 Closed dislocation of interphalangeal (joint), hand
834.12 Open dislocation interphalangeal (joint), hand

ICD-9-CM Procedural
79.80 Open reduction of dislocation of unspecified site

HCPCS Level II Supplies & Services
A4570 Splint

26820
26820 Fusion in opposition, thumb, with autogenous graft (includes obtaining graft)

ICD-9-CM Diagnostic
357.1 Polyneuropathy in collagen vascular disease — (Code first underlying disease: 446.0, 710.0, 714.0) ☒
359.6 Symptomatic inflammatory myopathy in diseases classified elsewhere — (Code first underlying disease: 135, 140.0-208.9, 277.3, 446.0, 710.0, 710.1, 710.2, 714.0) ☒
446.0 Polyarteritis nodosa
710.0 Systemic lupus erythematosus — (Use additional code to identify manifestation: 424.91, 581.81, 582.81, 583.81)
710.1 Systemic sclerosis — (Use additional code to identify manifestation: 359.6, 517.2)
710.2 Sicca syndrome
714.0 Rheumatoid arthritis — (Use additional code to identify manifestation: 357.1, 359.6)
715.34 Localized osteoarthrosis not specified whether primary or secondary, hand
716.14 Traumatic arthropathy, hand
718.24 Pathological dislocation of hand joint
718.34 Recurrent dislocation of hand joint
726.4 Enthesopathy of wrist and carpus
733.81 Malunion of fracture
905.2 Late effect of fracture of upper extremities
905.6 Late effect of dislocation
906.4 Late effect of crushing

ICD-9-CM Procedural
81.29 Arthrodesis of other specified joint

26841–26842
26841 Arthrodesis, carpometacarpal joint, thumb, with or without internal fixation;
26842 with autograft (includes obtaining graft)

ICD-9-CM Diagnostic
357.1 Polyneuropathy in collagen vascular disease — (Code first underlying disease: 446.0, 710.0, 714.0) ☒
359.6 Symptomatic inflammatory myopathy in diseases classified elsewhere — (Code first underlying disease: 135, 140.0-208.9, 277.3, 446.0, 710.0, 710.1, 710.2, 714.0) ☒
446.0 Polyarteritis nodosa
710.0 Systemic lupus erythematosus — (Use additional code to identify manifestation: 424.91, 581.81, 582.81, 583.81)
710.1 Systemic sclerosis — (Use additional code to identify manifestation: 359.6, 517.2)
710.2 Sicca syndrome
714.0 Rheumatoid arthritis — (Use additional code to identify manifestation: 357.1, 359.6)
715.34 Localized osteoarthrosis not specified whether primary or secondary, hand
716.14 Traumatic arthropathy, hand
718.24 Pathological dislocation of hand joint
718.34 Recurrent dislocation of hand joint
726.4 Enthesopathy of wrist and carpus
727.00 Unspecified synovitis and tenosynovitis ▽
733.81 Malunion of fracture
755.56 Accessory carpal bones
905.2 Late effect of fracture of upper extremities
905.6 Late effect of dislocation
906.4 Late effect of crushing

ICD-9-CM Procedural
81.29 Arthrodesis of other specified joint

26843–26844
26843 Arthrodesis, carpometacarpal joint, digit, other than thumb, each;
26844 with autograft (includes obtaining graft)

ICD-9-CM Diagnostic
357.1 Polyneuropathy in collagen vascular disease — (Code first underlying disease: 446.0, 710.0, 714.0) ☒
359.6 Symptomatic inflammatory myopathy in diseases classified elsewhere — (Code first underlying disease: 135, 140.0-208.9, 277.3, 446.0, 710.0, 710.1, 710.2, 714.0) ☒
446.0 Polyarteritis nodosa
710.0 Systemic lupus erythematosus — (Use additional code to identify manifestation: 424.91, 581.81, 582.81, 583.81)
710.1 Systemic sclerosis — (Use additional code to identify manifestation: 359.6, 517.2)
710.2 Sicca syndrome
714.0 Rheumatoid arthritis — (Use additional code to identify manifestation: 357.1, 359.6)
715.34 Localized osteoarthrosis not specified whether primary or secondary, hand
716.14 Traumatic arthropathy, hand
718.24 Pathological dislocation of hand joint
718.34 Recurrent dislocation of hand joint
726.4 Enthesopathy of wrist and carpus
727.00 Unspecified synovitis and tenosynovitis ▽
733.81 Malunion of fracture
755.56 Accessory carpal bones
905.2 Late effect of fracture of upper extremities
905.6 Late effect of dislocation

906.4 Late effect of crushing

ICD-9-CM Procedural

81.29 Arthrodesis of other specified joint

26850–26852

26850 Arthrodesis, metacarpophalangeal joint, with or without internal fixation;
26852 with autograft (includes obtaining graft)

ICD-9-CM Diagnostic

357.1 Polyneuropathy in collagen vascular disease — (Code first underlying disease: 446.0, 710.0, 714.0) ☒
359.6 Symptomatic inflammatory myopathy in diseases classified elsewhere — (Code first underlying disease: 135, 140.0-208.9, 277.3, 446.0, 710.0, 710.1, 710.2, 714.0) ☒
446.0 Polyarteritis nodosa
710.0 Systemic lupus erythematosus — (Use additional code to identify manifestation: 424.91, 581.81, 582.81, 583.81)
710.1 Systemic sclerosis — (Use additional code to identify manifestation: 359.6, 517.2)
710.2 Sicca syndrome
714.0 Rheumatoid arthritis — (Use additional code to identify manifestation: 357.1, 359.6)
715.34 Localized osteoarthrosis not specified whether primary or secondary, hand
716.14 Traumatic arthropathy, hand
718.24 Pathological dislocation of hand joint
718.34 Recurrent dislocation of hand joint
726.91 Exostosis of unspecified site ▽
727.00 Unspecified synovitis and tenosynovitis ▽
733.81 Malunion of fracture
905.2 Late effect of fracture of upper extremities
905.6 Late effect of dislocation
906.4 Late effect of crushing

ICD-9-CM Procedural

81.27 Metacarpophalangeal fusion

26860–26863

26860 Arthrodesis, interphalangeal joint, with or without internal fixation;
26861 each additional interphalangeal joint (List separately in addition to code for primary procedure)
26862 with autograft (includes obtaining graft)
26863 with autograft (includes obtaining graft), each additional joint (List separately in addition to code for primary procedure)

ICD-9-CM Diagnostic

357.1 Polyneuropathy in collagen vascular disease — (Code first underlying disease: 446.0, 710.0, 714.0) ☒
359.6 Symptomatic inflammatory myopathy in diseases classified elsewhere — (Code first underlying disease: 135, 140.0-208.9, 277.3, 446.0, 710.0, 710.1, 710.2, 714.0) ☒
446.0 Polyarteritis nodosa
710.0 Systemic lupus erythematosus — (Use additional code to identify manifestation: 424.91, 581.81, 582.81, 583.81)
710.1 Systemic sclerosis — (Use additional code to identify manifestation: 359.6, 517.2)
710.2 Sicca syndrome
714.0 Rheumatoid arthritis — (Use additional code to identify manifestation: 357.1, 359.6)
715.14 Primary localized osteoarthrosis, hand
715.34 Localized osteoarthrosis not specified whether primary or secondary, hand
716.14 Traumatic arthropathy, hand
718.24 Pathological dislocation of hand joint
718.34 Recurrent dislocation of hand joint
718.94 Unspecified derangement of hand joint ▽
733.81 Malunion of fracture
736.1 Mallet finger
736.20 Unspecified deformity of finger ▽
736.29 Other acquired deformity of finger
905.2 Late effect of fracture of upper extremities
905.6 Late effect of dislocation
906.4 Late effect of crushing
927.3 Crushing injury of finger(s) — (Use additional code to identify any associated injuries: 800-829, 850.0-854.1, 860.0-869.1)
959.5 Injury, other and unspecified, finger

ICD-9-CM Procedural

81.28 Interphalangeal fusion

26910

26910 Amputation, metacarpal, with finger or thumb (ray amputation), single, with or without interosseous transfer

ICD-9-CM Diagnostic

170.5 Malignant neoplasm of short bones of upper limb
198.5 Secondary malignant neoplasm of bone and bone marrow
238.0 Neoplasm of uncertain behavior of bone and articular cartilage
239.2 Neoplasms of unspecified nature of bone, soft tissue, and skin
250.70 Diabetes with peripheral circulatory disorders, type II or unspecified type, not stated as uncontrolled — (Use additional code to identify manifestation: 443.81, 785.4)
250.71 Diabetes with peripheral circulatory disorders, type I [juvenile type], not stated as uncontrolled — (Use additional code to identify manifestation: 443.81, 785.4)
250.72 Diabetes with peripheral circulatory disorders, type II or unspecified type, uncontrolled — (Use additional code to identify manifestation: 443.81, 785.4)
250.73 Diabetes with peripheral circulatory disorders, type I [juvenile type], uncontrolled — (Use additional code to identify manifestation: 443.81, 785.4)
443.81 Peripheral angiopathy in diseases classified elsewhere — (Code first underlying disease, 250.7) ☒
443.9 Unspecified peripheral vascular disease ▽
730.14 Chronic osteomyelitis, hand — (Use additional code to identify organism, 041.1)
755.01 Polydactyly of fingers
785.4 Gangrene — (Code first any associated underlying condition:250.7, 443.0)
882.1 Open wound of hand except finger(s) alone, complicated — (Use additional code to identify infection)
883.1 Open wound of finger(s), complicated — (Use additional code to identify infection)
885.0 Traumatic amputation of thumb (complete) (partial), without mention of complication — (Use additional code to identify infection)
886.0 Traumatic amputation of other finger(s) (complete) (partial), without mention of complication — (Use additional code to identify infection)
906.4 Late effect of crushing
906.6 Late effect of burn of wrist and hand
927.20 Crushing injury of hand(s) — (Use additional code to identify any associated injuries: 800-829, 850.0-854.1, 860.0-869.1)
927.3 Crushing injury of finger(s) — (Use additional code to identify any associated injuries: 800-829, 850.0-854.1, 860.0-869.1)
944.40 Deep necrosis of underlying tissues due to burn (deep third degree) of unspecified site of hand, without mention of a body part ▽
944.41 Deep necrosis of underlying tissues due to burn (deep third degree) of single digit [finger (nail)] other than thumb, without mention of a body part
944.42 Deep necrosis of underlying tissues due to burn (deep third degree) of thumb (nail), without mention of loss of a body part
944.43 Deep necrosis of underlying tissues due to burn (deep third degree) of two or more digits of hand, not including thumb, without mention of a body part
944.44 Deep necrosis of underlying tissues due to burn (deep third degree) of two or more digits of hand including thumb, without mention of a body part
944.45 Deep necrosis of underlying tissues due to burn (deep third degree) of palm of hand, without mention of loss of a body part
944.46 Deep necrosis of underlying tissues due to burn (deep third degree) of back of hand, without mention of loss of back of a body part
948.00 Burn (any degree) involving less than 10% of body surface with third degree burn of less than 10% or unspecified amount
948.10 Burn (any degree) involving 10-19% of body surface with third degree burn of less than 10% or unspecified amount
948.11 Burn (any degree) involving 10-19% of body surface with third degree burn of 10-19%
991.1 Frostbite of hand
998.59 Other postoperative infection — (Use additional code to identify infection)

ICD-9-CM Procedural

84.01 Amputation and disarticulation of finger
84.03 Amputation through hand
84.91 Amputation, not otherwise specified

26951–26952

26951 Amputation, finger or thumb, primary or secondary, any joint or phalanx, single, including neurectomies; with direct closure
26952 with local advancement flaps (V-Y, hood)

ICD-9-CM Diagnostic

170.5 Malignant neoplasm of short bones of upper limb
198.5 Secondary malignant neoplasm of bone and bone marrow
238.0 Neoplasm of uncertain behavior of bone and articular cartilage
239.2 Neoplasms of unspecified nature of bone, soft tissue, and skin
250.70 Diabetes with peripheral circulatory disorders, type II or unspecified type, not stated as uncontrolled — (Use additional code to identify manifestation: 443.81, 785.4)
250.71 Diabetes with peripheral circulatory disorders, type I [juvenile type], not stated as uncontrolled — (Use additional code to identify manifestation: 443.81, 785.4)
250.72 Diabetes with peripheral circulatory disorders, type II or unspecified type, uncontrolled — (Use additional code to identify manifestation: 443.81, 785.4)
250.73 Diabetes with peripheral circulatory disorders, type I [juvenile type], uncontrolled — (Use additional code to identify manifestation: 443.81, 785.4)
443.81 Peripheral angiopathy in diseases classified elsewhere — (Code first underlying disease, 250.7) ☒
443.9 Unspecified peripheral vascular disease ▽
730.14 Chronic osteomyelitis, hand — (Use additional code to identify organism, 041.1)
730.24 Unspecified osteomyelitis, hand — (Use additional code to identify organism, 041.1) ▽
733.49 Aseptic necrosis of other bone site
736.20 Unspecified deformity of finger ▽
755.01 Polydactyly of fingers
785.4 Gangrene — (Code first any associated underlying condition:250.7, 443.0)
883.0 Open wound of finger(s), without mention of complication — (Use additional code to identify infection)
883.1 Open wound of finger(s), complicated — (Use additional code to identify infection)
883.2 Open wound of finger(s), with tendon involvement — (Use additional code to identify infection)
885.0 Traumatic amputation of thumb (complete) (partial), without mention of complication — (Use additional code to identify infection)
886.0 Traumatic amputation of other finger(s) (complete) (partial), without mention of complication — (Use additional code to identify infection)
906.1 Late effect of open wound of extremities without mention of tendon injury
906.4 Late effect of crushing
906.6 Late effect of burn of wrist and hand
927.3 Crushing injury of finger(s) — (Use additional code to identify any associated injuries: 800-829, 850.0-854.1, 860.0-869.1)
944.40 Deep necrosis of underlying tissues due to burn (deep third degree) of unspecified site of hand, without mention of a body part ▽
944.41 Deep necrosis of underlying tissues due to burn (deep third degree) of single digit [finger (nail)] other than thumb, without mention of a body part
944.42 Deep necrosis of underlying tissues due to burn (deep third degree) of thumb (nail), without mention of loss of a body part
944.43 Deep necrosis of underlying tissues due to burn (deep third degree) of two or more digits of hand, not including thumb, without mention of a body part
944.44 Deep necrosis of underlying tissues due to burn (deep third degree) of two or more digits of hand including thumb, without mention of a body part
944.54 Deep necrosis of underlying tissues due to burn (deep third degree) of two or more digits of hand including thumb, with loss of a body part
948.00 Burn (any degree) involving less than 10% of body surface with third degree burn of less than 10% or unspecified amount
948.10 Burn (any degree) involving 10-19% of body surface with third degree burn of less than 10% or unspecified amount
948.11 Burn (any degree) involving 10-19% of body surface with third degree burn of 10-19%
991.1 Frostbite of hand
998.59 Other postoperative infection — (Use additional code to identify infection)

ICD-9-CM Procedural

84.01 Amputation and disarticulation of finger
84.02 Amputation and disarticulation of thumb
84.91 Amputation, not otherwise specified

26989

26989 Unlisted procedure, hands or fingers

ICD-9-CM Diagnostic

The application of this code is too broad to adequately present ICD-9-CM diagnostic code links here. Refer to your ICD-9-CM book.

Pelvis and Hip Joint

26990

26990 Incision and drainage, pelvis or hip joint area; deep abscess or hematoma

ICD-9-CM Diagnostic

682.6 Cellulitis and abscess of leg, except foot — (Use additional code to identify organism)
711.05 Pyogenic arthritis, pelvic region and thigh — (Use additional code to identify infectious organism: 041.0-041.8)
728.89 Other disorder of muscle, ligament, and fascia — (Use additional E code to identify drug, if drug-induced)
730.15 Chronic osteomyelitis, pelvic region and thigh — (Use additional code to identify organism, 041.1)
782.2 Localized superficial swelling, mass, or lump
924.01 Contusion of hip
998.59 Other postoperative infection — (Use additional code to identify infection)

ICD-9-CM Procedural

77.19 Other incision of other bone, except facial bones, without division
83.01 Exploration of tendon sheath
83.02 Myotomy
83.09 Other incision of soft tissue

HCPCS Level II Supplies & Services

A4305 Disposable drug delivery system, flow rate of 50 ml or greater per hour
A4306 Disposable drug delivery system, flow rate of 5 ml or less per hour
A4550 Surgical trays

26991

26991 Incision and drainage, pelvis or hip joint area; infected bursa

ICD-9-CM Diagnostic

726.5 Enthesopathy of hip region

ICD-9-CM Procedural

83.03 Bursotomy

HCPCS Level II Supplies & Services

A4305 Disposable drug delivery system, flow rate of 50 ml or greater per hour
A4306 Disposable drug delivery system, flow rate of 5 ml or less per hour

26992

26992 Incision, bone cortex, pelvis and/or hip joint (eg, osteomyelitis or bone abscess)

ICD-9-CM Diagnostic

730.05 Acute osteomyelitis, pelvic region and thigh — (Use additional code to identify organism, 041.1)
730.15 Chronic osteomyelitis, pelvic region and thigh — (Use additional code to identify organism, 041.1)
730.35 Periostitis, without mention of osteomyelitis, pelvic region and thigh — (Use additional code to identify organism, 041.1)
730.85 Other infections involving bone diseases classified elsewhere, pelvic region and thigh — (Code first underlying disease: 002.0, 015.0-015.9. Use additional code to identify organism) ☒

ICD-9-CM Procedural

77.19 Other incision of other bone, except facial bones, without division

27000

27000 Tenotomy, adductor of hip, percutaneous (separate procedure)

ICD-9-CM Diagnostic

343.9 Unspecified infantile cerebral palsy ▽

357.1 Polyneuropathy in collagen vascular disease — (Code first underlying disease: 446.0, 710.0, 714.0) ☒
359.6 Symptomatic inflammatory myopathy in diseases classified elsewhere — (Code first underlying disease: 135, 140.0-208.9, 277.3, 446.0, 710.0, 710.1, 710.2, 714.0) ☒
714.0 Rheumatoid arthritis — (Use additional code to identify manifestation: 357.1, 359.6)
715.95 Osteoarthrosis, unspecified whether generalized or localized, pelvic region and thigh ▽
718.45 Contracture of pelvic joint
726.5 Enthesopathy of hip region
732.1 Juvenile osteochondrosis of hip and pelvis
754.30 Congenital dislocation of hip, unilateral
996.4 Mechanical complication of internal orthopedic device, implant, and graft

ICD-9-CM Procedural

83.12 Adductor tenotomy of hip

27001–27003

27001 Tenotomy, adductor of hip, open
27003 Tenotomy, adductor, subcutaneous, open, with obturator neurectomy

ICD-9-CM Diagnostic

343.9 Unspecified infantile cerebral palsy ▽
718.45 Contracture of pelvic joint
727.09 Other synovitis and tenosynovitis
727.81 Contracture of tendon (sheath)
732.1 Juvenile osteochondrosis of hip and pelvis
737.32 Progressive infantile idiopathic scoliosis
754.30 Congenital dislocation of hip, unilateral
754.32 Congenital subluxation of hip, unilateral

ICD-9-CM Procedural

04.07 Other excision or avulsion of cranial and peripheral nerves
83.12 Adductor tenotomy of hip

27005

27005 Tenotomy, hip flexor(s), open (separate procedure)

ICD-9-CM Diagnostic

343.9 Unspecified infantile cerebral palsy ▽
718.35 Recurrent dislocation of pelvic region and thigh joint
718.45 Contracture of pelvic joint
726.5 Enthesopathy of hip region
727.81 Contracture of tendon (sheath)
754.30 Congenital dislocation of hip, unilateral
754.32 Congenital subluxation of hip, unilateral

ICD-9-CM Procedural

83.12 Adductor tenotomy of hip
83.13 Other tenotomy

27006

27006 Tenotomy, abductors and/or extensor(s) of hip, open (separate procedure)

ICD-9-CM Diagnostic

343.9 Unspecified infantile cerebral palsy ▽
718.45 Contracture of pelvic joint
727.81 Contracture of tendon (sheath)
737.32 Progressive infantile idiopathic scoliosis

ICD-9-CM Procedural

83.13 Other tenotomy

27025

27025 Fasciotomy, hip or thigh, any type

ICD-9-CM Diagnostic

343.9 Unspecified infantile cerebral palsy ▽
718.35 Recurrent dislocation of pelvic region and thigh joint
718.45 Contracture of pelvic joint
726.5 Enthesopathy of hip region
727.81 Contracture of tendon (sheath)
728.89 Other disorder of muscle, ligament, and fascia — (Use additional E code to identify drug, if drug-induced)
737.32 Progressive infantile idiopathic scoliosis
754.30 Congenital dislocation of hip, unilateral
754.32 Congenital subluxation of hip, unilateral

ICD-9-CM Procedural

83.14 Fasciotomy

27030

27030 Arthrotomy, hip, with drainage (eg, infection)

ICD-9-CM Diagnostic

711.05 Pyogenic arthritis, pelvic region and thigh — (Use additional code to identify infectious organism: 041.0-041.8)
719.85 Other specified disorders of pelvic joint
996.66 Infection and inflammatory reaction due to internal joint prosthesis — (Use additional code to identify specified infections)
996.67 Infection and inflammatory reaction due to other internal orthopedic device, implant, and graft — (Use additional code to identify specified infections)
998.51 Infected postoperative seroma — (Use additional code to identify organism)
998.59 Other postoperative infection — (Use additional code to identify infection)

ICD-9-CM Procedural

80.15 Other arthrotomy of hip

27033

27033 Arthrotomy, hip, including exploration or removal of loose or foreign body

ICD-9-CM Diagnostic

718.15 Loose body in pelvic joint
719.85 Other specified disorders of pelvic joint
728.12 Traumatic myositis ossificans
754.32 Congenital subluxation of hip, unilateral
890.1 Open wound of hip and thigh, complicated — (Use additional code to identify infection)
996.4 Mechanical complication of internal orthopedic device, implant, and graft
996.78 Other complications due to other internal orthopedic device, implant, and graft
V64.43 Arthroscopic surgical procedure converted to open procedure

ICD-9-CM Procedural

80.15 Other arthrotomy of hip

27035

27035 Denervation, hip joint, intrapelvic or extrapelvic intra-articular branches of sciatic, femoral, or obturator nerves

ICD-9-CM Diagnostic

343.9 Unspecified infantile cerebral palsy ▽
355.0 Lesion of sciatic nerve
355.79 Other mononeuritis of lower limb
718.45 Contracture of pelvic joint
737.32 Progressive infantile idiopathic scoliosis

ICD-9-CM Procedural

04.03 Division or crushing of other cranial and peripheral nerves
04.04 Other incision of cranial and peripheral nerves

27036

27036 Capsulectomy or capsulotomy, hip, with or without excision of heterotopic bone, with release of hip flexor muscles (ie, gluteus medius, gluteus minimus, tensor fascia latae, rectus femoris, sartorius, iliopsoas)

ICD-9-CM Diagnostic

719.85 Other specified disorders of pelvic joint
733.90 Disorder of bone and cartilage, unspecified ▽
733.99 Other disorders of bone and cartilage
754.30 Congenital dislocation of hip, unilateral
755.69 Other congenital anomaly of lower limb, including pelvic girdle

ICD-9-CM Procedural

80.45 Division of joint capsule, ligament, or cartilage of hip
80.85 Other local excision or destruction of lesion of hip joint
80.95 Other excision of hip joint
83.19 Other division of soft tissue

▽ Unspecified code
♀ Female diagnosis
☒ Manifestation code
♂ Male diagnosis

27040–27041

27040 Biopsy, soft tissue of pelvis and hip area; superficial
27041 deep, subfascial or intramuscular

ICD-9-CM Diagnostic

171.3 Malignant neoplasm of connective and other soft tissue of lower limb, including hip
171.6 Malignant neoplasm of connective and other soft tissue of pelvis
172.7 Malignant melanoma of skin of lower limb, including hip
198.89 Secondary malignant neoplasm of other specified sites
214.1 Lipoma of other skin and subcutaneous tissue
215.3 Other benign neoplasm of connective and other soft tissue of lower limb, including hip
215.6 Other benign neoplasm of connective and other soft tissue of pelvis
238.1 Neoplasm of uncertain behavior of connective and other soft tissue ▽
239.2 Neoplasms of unspecified nature of bone, soft tissue, and skin
728.82 Foreign body granuloma of muscle
728.89 Other disorder of muscle, ligament, and fascia — (Use additional E code to identify drug, if drug-induced)
729.89 Other musculoskeletal symptoms referable to limbs

ICD-9-CM Procedural

83.21 Biopsy of soft tissue

HCPCS Level II Supplies & Services

A4305 Disposable drug delivery system, flow rate of 50 ml or greater per hour
A4306 Disposable drug delivery system, flow rate of 5 ml or less per hour
A4550 Surgical trays

27047–27049

27047 Excision, tumor, pelvis and hip area; subcutaneous tissue
27048 deep, subfascial, intramuscular
27049 Radical resection of tumor, soft tissue of pelvis and hip area (eg, malignant neoplasm)

ICD-9-CM Diagnostic

171.3 Malignant neoplasm of connective and other soft tissue of lower limb, including hip
171.6 Malignant neoplasm of connective and other soft tissue of pelvis
172.7 Malignant melanoma of skin of lower limb, including hip
195.3 Malignant neoplasm of pelvis
198.89 Secondary malignant neoplasm of other specified sites
214.1 Lipoma of other skin and subcutaneous tissue
215.3 Other benign neoplasm of connective and other soft tissue of lower limb, including hip
215.6 Other benign neoplasm of connective and other soft tissue of pelvis
238.1 Neoplasm of uncertain behavior of connective and other soft tissue ▽
239.2 Neoplasms of unspecified nature of bone, soft tissue, and skin
709.4 Foreign body granuloma of skin and subcutaneous tissue

ICD-9-CM Procedural

80.85 Other local excision or destruction of lesion of hip joint
83.31 Excision of lesion of tendon sheath
83.32 Excision of lesion of muscle
83.39 Excision of lesion of other soft tissue
83.49 Other excision of soft tissue

HCPCS Level II Supplies & Services

A4305 Disposable drug delivery system, flow rate of 50 ml or greater per hour
A4306 Disposable drug delivery system, flow rate of 5 ml or less per hour
A4550 Surgical trays

27050

27050 Arthrotomy, with biopsy; sacroiliac joint

ICD-9-CM Diagnostic

170.6 Malignant neoplasm of pelvic bones, sacrum, and coccyx
198.5 Secondary malignant neoplasm of bone and bone marrow
215.6 Other benign neoplasm of connective and other soft tissue of pelvis
238.0 Neoplasm of uncertain behavior of bone and articular cartilage
239.2 Neoplasms of unspecified nature of bone, soft tissue, and skin
275.40 Unspecified disorder of calcium metabolism — (Use additional code to identify any associated mental retardation) ▽
275.42 Hypercalcemia — (Use additional code to identify any associated mental retardation)
275.49 Other disorders of calcium metabolism — (Use additional code to identify any associated mental retardation)

ICD-9-CM Procedural

80.39 Biopsy of joint structure of other specified site

27052

27052 Arthrotomy, with biopsy; hip joint

ICD-9-CM Diagnostic

170.3 Malignant neoplasm of ribs, sternum, and clavicle
170.6 Malignant neoplasm of pelvic bones, sacrum, and coccyx
170.7 Malignant neoplasm of long bones of lower limb
198.5 Secondary malignant neoplasm of bone and bone marrow
213.6 Benign neoplasm of pelvic bones, sacrum, and coccyx
213.7 Benign neoplasm of long bones of lower limb
215.3 Other benign neoplasm of connective and other soft tissue of lower limb, including hip
238.0 Neoplasm of uncertain behavior of bone and articular cartilage
239.2 Neoplasms of unspecified nature of bone, soft tissue, and skin
275.40 Unspecified disorder of calcium metabolism — (Use additional code to identify any associated mental retardation) ▽
275.42 Hypercalcemia — (Use additional code to identify any associated mental retardation)
275.49 Other disorders of calcium metabolism — (Use additional code to identify any associated mental retardation)
711.05 Pyogenic arthritis, pelvic region and thigh — (Use additional code to identify infectious organism: 041.0-041.8)
727.02 Giant cell tumor of tendon sheath
727.41 Ganglion of joint
727.82 Calcium deposits in tendon and bursa
730.15 Chronic osteomyelitis, pelvic region and thigh — (Use additional code to identify organism, 041.1)
733.20 Unspecified cyst of bone (localized) ▽
733.42 Aseptic necrosis of head and neck of femur

ICD-9-CM Procedural

80.35 Biopsy of joint structure of hip

27054

27054 Arthrotomy with synovectomy, hip joint

ICD-9-CM Diagnostic

274.0 Gouty arthropathy — (Use additional code to identify any associated mental retardation)
275.40 Unspecified disorder of calcium metabolism — (Use additional code to identify any associated mental retardation) ▽
275.42 Hypercalcemia — (Use additional code to identify any associated mental retardation)
275.49 Other disorders of calcium metabolism — (Use additional code to identify any associated mental retardation)
719.25 Villonodular synovitis, pelvic region and thigh
726.5 Enthesopathy of hip region
727.09 Other synovitis and tenosynovitis
727.40 Unspecified synovial cyst ▽
V64.43 Arthroscopic surgical procedure converted to open procedure

ICD-9-CM Procedural

80.75 Synovectomy of hip

27060–27062

27060 Excision; ischial bursa
27062 trochanteric bursa or calcification

ICD-9-CM Diagnostic

215.6 Other benign neoplasm of connective and other soft tissue of pelvis
726.5 Enthesopathy of hip region
727.3 Other bursitis disorders
727.49 Other ganglion and cyst of synovium, tendon, and bursa
727.9 Unspecified disorder of synovium, tendon, and bursa ▽

ICD-9-CM Procedural

83.5 Bursectomy

27065–27067

27065 Excision of bone cyst or benign tumor; superficial (wing of ilium, symphysis pubis, or greater trochanter of femur) with or without autograft
27066 deep, with or without autograft
27067 with autograft requiring separate incision

ICD-9-CM Diagnostic

213.6 Benign neoplasm of pelvic bones, sacrum, and coccyx
213.7 Benign neoplasm of long bones of lower limb
238.0 Neoplasm of uncertain behavior of bone and articular cartilage
239.2 Neoplasms of unspecified nature of bone, soft tissue, and skin
732.1 Juvenile osteochondrosis of hip and pelvis
732.4 Juvenile osteochondrosis of lower extremity, excluding foot
732.9 Unspecified osteochondropathy ▽
733.21 Solitary bone cyst
733.22 Aneurysmal bone cyst
733.29 Other cyst of bone

ICD-9-CM Procedural

77.65 Local excision of lesion or tissue of femur
77.69 Local excision of lesion or tissue of other bone, except facial bones
77.75 Excision of femur for graft
77.79 Excision of other bone for graft, except facial bones
78.05 Bone graft of femur
78.09 Bone graft of other bone, except facial bones

27070–27071

27070 Partial excision (craterization, saucerization) (eg, osteomyelitis or bone abscess); superficial (eg, wing of ilium, symphysis pubis, or greater trochanter of femur)
27071 deep (subfascial or intramuscular)

ICD-9-CM Diagnostic

715.15 Primary localized osteoarthrosis, pelvic region and thigh
728.13 Postoperative heterotopic calcification
730.05 Acute osteomyelitis, pelvic region and thigh — (Use additional code to identify organism, 041.1)
730.15 Chronic osteomyelitis, pelvic region and thigh — (Use additional code to identify organism, 041.1)
730.25 Unspecified osteomyelitis, pelvic region and thigh — (Use additional code to identify organism, 041.1) ▽
730.85 Other infections involving bone diseases classified elsewhere, pelvic region and thigh — (Code first underlying disease: 002.0, 015.0-015.9. Use additional code to identify organism) ☒
733.99 Other disorders of bone and cartilage
996.4 Mechanical complication of internal orthopedic device, implant, and graft

ICD-9-CM Procedural

77.65 Local excision of lesion or tissue of femur
77.69 Local excision of lesion or tissue of other bone, except facial bones
77.85 Other partial ostectomy of femur
77.89 Other partial ostectomy of other bone, except facial bones

27075

27075 Radical resection of tumor or infection; wing of ilium, one pubic or ischial ramus or symphysis pubis

ICD-9-CM Diagnostic

170.6 Malignant neoplasm of pelvic bones, sacrum, and coccyx
170.7 Malignant neoplasm of long bones of lower limb
198.5 Secondary malignant neoplasm of bone and bone marrow
213.7 Benign neoplasm of long bones of lower limb
238.0 Neoplasm of uncertain behavior of bone and articular cartilage
239.2 Neoplasms of unspecified nature of bone, soft tissue, and skin
707.00 Decubitus ulcer, unspecified site
707.04 Decubitus ulcer, hip
707.09 Decubitus ulcer, other site
715.15 Primary localized osteoarthrosis, pelvic region and thigh
716.15 Traumatic arthropathy, pelvic region and thigh
730.15 Chronic osteomyelitis, pelvic region and thigh — (Use additional code to identify organism, 041.1)
730.35 Periostitis, without mention of osteomyelitis, pelvic region and thigh — (Use additional code to identify organism, 041.1)
730.85 Other infections involving bone diseases classified elsewhere, pelvic region and thigh — (Code first underlying disease: 002.0, 015.0-015.9. Use additional code to identify organism) ☒
996.66 Infection and inflammatory reaction due to internal joint prosthesis — (Use additional code to identify specified infections)
996.67 Infection and inflammatory reaction due to other internal orthopedic device, implant, and graft — (Use additional code to identify specified infections)
996.77 Other complications due to internal joint prosthesis

ICD-9-CM Procedural

77.89 Other partial ostectomy of other bone, except facial bones

27076

27076 Radical resection of tumor or infection; ilium, including acetabulum, both pubic rami, or ischium and acetabulum

ICD-9-CM Diagnostic

170.6 Malignant neoplasm of pelvic bones, sacrum, and coccyx
170.7 Malignant neoplasm of long bones of lower limb
198.5 Secondary malignant neoplasm of bone and bone marrow
213.7 Benign neoplasm of long bones of lower limb
238.0 Neoplasm of uncertain behavior of bone and articular cartilage
239.2 Neoplasms of unspecified nature of bone, soft tissue, and skin
707.00 Decubitus ulcer, unspecified site
707.04 Decubitus ulcer, hip
707.09 Decubitus ulcer, other site
715.15 Primary localized osteoarthrosis, pelvic region and thigh
716.15 Traumatic arthropathy, pelvic region and thigh
730.15 Chronic osteomyelitis, pelvic region and thigh — (Use additional code to identify organism, 041.1)
730.35 Periostitis, without mention of osteomyelitis, pelvic region and thigh — (Use additional code to identify organism, 041.1)
730.85 Other infections involving bone diseases classified elsewhere, pelvic region and thigh — (Code first underlying disease: 002.0, 015.0-015.9. Use additional code to identify organism) ☒
996.66 Infection and inflammatory reaction due to internal joint prosthesis — (Use additional code to identify specified infections)
996.67 Infection and inflammatory reaction due to other internal orthopedic device, implant, and graft — (Use additional code to identify specified infections)
996.77 Other complications due to internal joint prosthesis

ICD-9-CM Procedural

77.89 Other partial ostectomy of other bone, except facial bones
80.95 Other excision of hip joint

27077

27077 Radical resection of tumor or infection; innominate bone, total

ICD-9-CM Diagnostic

170.6 Malignant neoplasm of pelvic bones, sacrum, and coccyx
170.7 Malignant neoplasm of long bones of lower limb
198.5 Secondary malignant neoplasm of bone and bone marrow
213.7 Benign neoplasm of long bones of lower limb
238.0 Neoplasm of uncertain behavior of bone and articular cartilage
239.2 Neoplasms of unspecified nature of bone, soft tissue, and skin
707.00 Decubitus ulcer, unspecified site
707.03 Decubitus ulcer, lower back
707.04 Decubitus ulcer, hip
707.09 Decubitus ulcer, other site
715.15 Primary localized osteoarthrosis, pelvic region and thigh
716.15 Traumatic arthropathy, pelvic region and thigh
730.15 Chronic osteomyelitis, pelvic region and thigh — (Use additional code to identify organism, 041.1)
730.35 Periostitis, without mention of osteomyelitis, pelvic region and thigh — (Use additional code to identify organism, 041.1)
730.85 Other infections involving bone diseases classified elsewhere, pelvic region and thigh — (Code first underlying disease: 002.0, 015.0-015.9. Use additional code to identify organism) ☒
996.66 Infection and inflammatory reaction due to internal joint prosthesis — (Use additional code to identify specified infections)
996.67 Infection and inflammatory reaction due to other internal orthopedic device, implant, and graft — (Use additional code to identify specified infections)
996.77 Other complications due to internal joint prosthesis

ICD-9-CM Procedural

77.89 Other partial ostectomy of other bone, except facial bones
77.99 Total ostectomy of other bone, except facial bones

▽ Unspecified code ☒ Manifestation code
♀ Female diagnosis ♂ Male diagnosis

27078–27079

27078 Radical resection of tumor or infection; ischial tuberosity and greater trochanter of femur
27079 ischial tuberosity and greater trochanter of femur, with skin flaps

ICD-9-CM Diagnostic

170.6 Malignant neoplasm of pelvic bones, sacrum, and coccyx
170.7 Malignant neoplasm of long bones of lower limb
198.5 Secondary malignant neoplasm of bone and bone marrow
213.7 Benign neoplasm of long bones of lower limb
238.0 Neoplasm of uncertain behavior of bone and articular cartilage
239.2 Neoplasms of unspecified nature of bone, soft tissue, and skin
707.00 Decubitus ulcer, unspecified site
707.04 Decubitus ulcer, hip
707.09 Decubitus ulcer, other site
715.15 Primary localized osteoarthrosis, pelvic region and thigh
716.15 Traumatic arthropathy, pelvic region and thigh
730.15 Chronic osteomyelitis, pelvic region and thigh — (Use additional code to identify organism, 041.1)
730.35 Periostitis, without mention of osteomyelitis, pelvic region and thigh — (Use additional code to identify organism, 041.1)
730.85 Other infections involving bone diseases classified elsewhere, pelvic region and thigh — (Code first underlying disease: 002.0, 015.0-015.9. Use additional code to identify organism) ☒
996.66 Infection and inflammatory reaction due to internal joint prosthesis — (Use additional code to identify specified infections)
996.67 Infection and inflammatory reaction due to other internal orthopedic device, implant, and graft — (Use additional code to identify specified infections)
996.77 Other complications due to internal joint prosthesis

ICD-9-CM Procedural

77.85 Other partial ostectomy of femur
77.89 Other partial ostectomy of other bone, except facial bones
77.95 Total ostectomy of femur
77.99 Total ostectomy of other bone, except facial bones
86.74 Attachment of pedicle or flap graft to other sites

27080

27080 Coccygectomy, primary

ICD-9-CM Diagnostic

170.6 Malignant neoplasm of pelvic bones, sacrum, and coccyx
198.5 Secondary malignant neoplasm of bone and bone marrow
213.6 Benign neoplasm of pelvic bones, sacrum, and coccyx
238.0 Neoplasm of uncertain behavior of bone and articular cartilage
239.2 Neoplasms of unspecified nature of bone, soft tissue, and skin
707.05 Decubitus ulcer, buttock
707.09 Decubitus ulcer, other site
724.70 Unspecified disorder of coccyx ▽
730.15 Chronic osteomyelitis, pelvic region and thigh — (Use additional code to identify organism, 041.1)
730.35 Periostitis, without mention of osteomyelitis, pelvic region and thigh — (Use additional code to identify organism, 041.1)

ICD-9-CM Procedural

77.99 Total ostectomy of other bone, except facial bones

27086–27087

27086 Removal of foreign body, pelvis or hip; subcutaneous tissue
27087 deep (subfascial or intramuscular)

ICD-9-CM Diagnostic

686.1 Pyogenic granuloma of skin and subcutaneous tissue
709.4 Foreign body granuloma of skin and subcutaneous tissue
718.15 Loose body in pelvic joint
728.82 Foreign body granuloma of muscle
729.6 Residual foreign body in soft tissue
879.7 Open wound of other and unspecified parts of trunk, complicated — (Use additional code to identify infection) ▽
890.1 Open wound of hip and thigh, complicated — (Use additional code to identify infection)
890.2 Open wound of hip and thigh, with tendon involvement — (Use additional code to identify infection)
919.6 Other, multiple, and unspecified sites, superficial foreign body (splinter), without major open wound and without mention of infection
919.7 Other, multiple, and unspecified sites, superficial foreign body (splinter), without major open wound, infected

ICD-9-CM Procedural

83.02 Myotomy
83.09 Other incision of soft tissue
86.05 Incision with removal of foreign body or device from skin and subcutaneous tissue
98.20 Removal of foreign body, not otherwise specified
98.29 Removal of foreign body without incision from lower limb, except foot

HCPCS Level II Supplies & Services

A4305 Disposable drug delivery system, flow rate of 50 ml or greater per hour
A4306 Disposable drug delivery system, flow rate of 5 ml or less per hour
A4550 Surgical trays

27090–27091

27090 Removal of hip prosthesis; (separate procedure)
27091 complicated, including total hip prosthesis, methylmethacrylate with or without insertion of spacer

ICD-9-CM Diagnostic

996.4 Mechanical complication of internal orthopedic device, implant, and graft
996.66 Infection and inflammatory reaction due to internal joint prosthesis — (Use additional code to identify specified infections)
996.67 Infection and inflammatory reaction due to other internal orthopedic device, implant, and graft — (Use additional code to identify specified infections)
996.69 Infection and inflammatory reaction due to other internal prosthetic device, implant, and graft — (Use additional code to identify specified infections)
996.77 Other complications due to internal joint prosthesis
996.78 Other complications due to other internal orthopedic device, implant, and graft
998.51 Infected postoperative seroma — (Use additional code to identify organism)
998.59 Other postoperative infection — (Use additional code to identify infection)
998.7 Acute reaction to foreign substance accidentally left during procedure, not elsewhere classified

ICD-9-CM Procedural

80.05 Arthrotomy for removal of prosthesis of hip

27093–27095

27093 Injection procedure for hip arthrography; without anesthesia
27095 with anesthesia

ICD-9-CM Diagnostic

213.6 Benign neoplasm of pelvic bones, sacrum, and coccyx
357.1 Polyneuropathy in collagen vascular disease — (Code first underlying disease: 446.0, 710.0, 714.0) ☒
359.6 Symptomatic inflammatory myopathy in diseases classified elsewhere — (Code first underlying disease: 135, 140.0-208.9, 277.3, 446.0, 710.0, 710.1, 710.2, 714.0) ☒
446.0 Polyarteritis nodosa
696.0 Psoriatic arthropathy
710.0 Systemic lupus erythematosus — (Use additional code to identify manifestation: 424.91, 581.81, 582.81, 583.81)
710.1 Systemic sclerosis — (Use additional code to identify manifestation: 359.6, 517.2)
710.2 Sicca syndrome
711.05 Pyogenic arthritis, pelvic region and thigh — (Use additional code to identify infectious organism: 041.0-041.8)
711.95 Unspecified infective arthritis, pelvic region and thigh ▽
714.0 Rheumatoid arthritis — (Use additional code to identify manifestation: 357.1, 359.6)
714.9 Unspecified inflammatory polyarthropathy ▽
715.09 Generalized osteoarthrosis, involving multiple sites
715.15 Primary localized osteoarthrosis, pelvic region and thigh
715.35 Localized osteoarthrosis not specified whether primary or secondary, pelvic region and thigh
715.90 Osteoarthrosis, unspecified whether generalized or localized, unspecified site ▽
715.95 Osteoarthrosis, unspecified whether generalized or localized, pelvic region and thigh ▽
716.15 Traumatic arthropathy, pelvic region and thigh
716.95 Unspecified arthropathy, pelvic region and thigh ▽
716.99 Unspecified arthropathy, multiple sites ▽
718.15 Loose body in pelvic joint
718.35 Recurrent dislocation of pelvic region and thigh joint
718.65 Unspecified intrapelvic protrusion acetabulum, pelvic region and thigh ▽

718.75 Developmental dislocation of joint, pelvic region and thigh
718.85 Other joint derangement, not elsewhere classified, pelvic region and thigh
719.05 Effusion of pelvic joint
719.45 Pain in joint, pelvic region and thigh
726.5 Enthesopathy of hip region
727.00 Unspecified synovitis and tenosynovitis ▽
727.09 Other synovitis and tenosynovitis
732.1 Juvenile osteochondrosis of hip and pelvis
733.40 Aseptic necrosis of bone, site unspecified ▽
733.42 Aseptic necrosis of head and neck of femur
733.90 Disorder of bone and cartilage, unspecified ▽
754.30 Congenital dislocation of hip, unilateral
754.31 Congenital dislocation of hip, bilateral
754.32 Congenital subluxation of hip, unilateral
755.62 Congenital coxa vara
755.63 Other congenital deformity of hip (joint)
820.8 Closed fracture of unspecified part of neck of femur ▽
835.00 Closed dislocation of hip, unspecified site ▽
959.6 Injury, other and unspecified, hip and thigh
996.4 Mechanical complication of internal orthopedic device, implant, and graft
996.59 Mechanical complication due to other implant and internal device, not elsewhere classified
996.60 Infection and inflammatory reaction due to unspecified device, implant, and graft — (Use additional code to identify specified infections) ▽
996.66 Infection and inflammatory reaction due to internal joint prosthesis — (Use additional code to identify specified infections)
996.67 Infection and inflammatory reaction due to other internal orthopedic device, implant, and graft — (Use additional code to identify specified infections)
996.77 Other complications due to internal joint prosthesis
996.78 Other complications due to other internal orthopedic device, implant, and graft
V43.64 Hip joint replacement by other means — (This code is intended for use when these conditions are recorded as diagnoses or problems)
V72.5 Radiological examination, not elsewhere classified — (Use additional code(s) to identify any special screening examination(s) performed: V73.0-V82.9)

ICD-9-CM Procedural

81.92 Injection of therapeutic substance into joint or ligament
88.32 Contrast arthrogram

HCPCS Level II Supplies & Services

A9525 Supply of low or iso-osmolar contrast material, 10 mg of iodine

27096

27096 Injection procedure for sacroiliac joint, arthrography and/or anesthetic/steroid

ICD-9-CM Diagnostic

359.6 Symptomatic inflammatory myopathy in diseases classified elsewhere — (Code first underlying disease: 135, 140.0-208.9, 277.3, 446.0, 710.0, 710.1, 710.2, 714.0) ☒
710.0 Systemic lupus erythematosus — (Use additional code to identify manifestation: 424.91, 581.81, 582.81, 583.81)
710.1 Systemic sclerosis — (Use additional code to identify manifestation: 359.6, 517.2)
710.2 Sicca syndrome
711.05 Pyogenic arthritis, pelvic region and thigh — (Use additional code to identify infectious organism: 041.0-041.8)
711.95 Unspecified infective arthritis, pelvic region and thigh ▽
714.0 Rheumatoid arthritis — (Use additional code to identify manifestation: 357.1, 359.6)
714.9 Unspecified inflammatory polyarthropathy ▽
715.09 Generalized osteoarthrosis, involving multiple sites
715.15 Primary localized osteoarthrosis, pelvic region and thigh
715.25 Secondary localized osteoarthrosis, pelvic region and thigh
715.35 Localized osteoarthrosis not specified whether primary or secondary, pelvic region and thigh
715.89 Osteoarthrosis involving multiple sites, but not specified as generalized
715.95 Osteoarthrosis, unspecified whether generalized or localized, pelvic region and thigh ▽
716.15 Traumatic arthropathy, pelvic region and thigh
716.95 Unspecified arthropathy, pelvic region and thigh ▽
718.25 Pathological dislocation of pelvic region and thigh joint
718.35 Recurrent dislocation of pelvic region and thigh joint
718.55 Ankylosis of pelvic region and thigh joint
719.45 Pain in joint, pelvic region and thigh
719.85 Other specified disorders of pelvic joint
719.95 Unspecified disorder of joint of pelvic region and thigh ▽
724.6 Disorders of sacrum
755.69 Other congenital anomaly of lower limb, including pelvic girdle
805.6 Closed fracture of sacrum and coccyx without mention of spinal cord injury
805.7 Open fracture of sacrum and coccyx without mention of spinal cord injury
808.41 Closed fracture of ilium
808.43 Multiple closed pelvic fractures with disruption of pelvic circle
808.51 Open fracture of ilium
808.53 Multiple open pelvic fractures with disruption of pelvic circle
839.42 Closed dislocation, sacrum
839.52 Open dislocation, sacrum

ICD-9-CM Procedural

81.92 Injection of therapeutic substance into joint or ligament
88.32 Contrast arthrogram
99.23 Injection of steroid
99.29 Injection or infusion of other therapeutic or prophylactic substance
99.77 Application or administration of adhesion barrier substance

27097

27097 Release or recession, hamstring, proximal

ICD-9-CM Diagnostic

343.9 Unspecified infantile cerebral palsy ▽
716.15 Traumatic arthropathy, pelvic region and thigh
718.25 Pathological dislocation of pelvic region and thigh joint
718.45 Contracture of pelvic joint
726.5 Enthesopathy of hip region
741.93 Spina bifida without mention of hydrocephalus, lumbar region
890.1 Open wound of hip and thigh, complicated — (Use additional code to identify infection)
890.2 Open wound of hip and thigh, with tendon involvement — (Use additional code to identify infection)
996.4 Mechanical complication of internal orthopedic device, implant, and graft
996.67 Infection and inflammatory reaction due to other internal orthopedic device, implant, and graft — (Use additional code to identify specified infections)

ICD-9-CM Procedural

83.14 Fasciotomy
83.72 Recession of tendon

27098

27098 Transfer, adductor to ischium

ICD-9-CM Diagnostic

343.9 Unspecified infantile cerebral palsy ▽
718.25 Pathological dislocation of pelvic region and thigh joint
718.45 Contracture of pelvic joint
741.93 Spina bifida without mention of hydrocephalus, lumbar region
890.2 Open wound of hip and thigh, with tendon involvement — (Use additional code to identify infection)
996.4 Mechanical complication of internal orthopedic device, implant, and graft

ICD-9-CM Procedural

83.75 Tendon transfer or transplantation

27100

27100 Transfer external oblique muscle to greater trochanter including fascial or tendon extension (graft)

ICD-9-CM Diagnostic

343.9 Unspecified infantile cerebral palsy ▽
718.45 Contracture of pelvic joint
741.93 Spina bifida without mention of hydrocephalus, lumbar region
996.4 Mechanical complication of internal orthopedic device, implant, and graft

ICD-9-CM Procedural

83.77 Muscle transfer or transplantation
83.82 Graft of muscle or fascia

27105

27105 Transfer paraspinal muscle to hip (includes fascial or tendon extension graft)

ICD-9-CM Diagnostic

343.9 Unspecified infantile cerebral palsy ▽
718.25 Pathological dislocation of pelvic region and thigh joint

▽ Unspecified code
♀ Female diagnosis
☒ Manifestation code
♂ Male diagnosis

718.45 Contracture of pelvic joint
741.93 Spina bifida without mention of hydrocephalus, lumbar region
996.4 Mechanical complication of internal orthopedic device, implant, and graft

ICD-9-CM Procedural
83.77 Muscle transfer or transplantation
83.82 Graft of muscle or fascia
83.83 Tendon pulley reconstruction on muscle, tendon, and fascia

27110
27110 Transfer iliopsoas; to greater trochanter of femur

ICD-9-CM Diagnostic
343.9 Unspecified infantile cerebral palsy ▽
718.25 Pathological dislocation of pelvic region and thigh joint
718.45 Contracture of pelvic joint
741.93 Spina bifida without mention of hydrocephalus, lumbar region
996.4 Mechanical complication of internal orthopedic device, implant, and graft

ICD-9-CM Procedural
83.77 Muscle transfer or transplantation

27111
27111 Transfer iliopsoas; to femoral neck

ICD-9-CM Diagnostic
343.9 Unspecified infantile cerebral palsy ▽
718.25 Pathological dislocation of pelvic region and thigh joint
718.45 Contracture of pelvic joint
718.75 Developmental dislocation of joint, pelvic region and thigh
741.93 Spina bifida without mention of hydrocephalus, lumbar region
835.01 Closed posterior dislocation of hip
996.4 Mechanical complication of internal orthopedic device, implant, and graft

ICD-9-CM Procedural
83.77 Muscle transfer or transplantation

27120
27120 Acetabuloplasty; (eg, Whitman, Colonna, Haygroves, or cup type)

ICD-9-CM Diagnostic
715.15 Primary localized osteoarthrosis, pelvic region and thigh
732.1 Juvenile osteochondrosis of hip and pelvis
733.21 Solitary bone cyst
808.0 Closed fracture of acetabulum
808.1 Open fracture of acetabulum

ICD-9-CM Procedural
81.40 Repair of hip, not elsewhere classified

27122
27122 Acetabuloplasty; resection, femoral head (eg, Girdlestone procedure)

ICD-9-CM Diagnostic
718.45 Contracture of pelvic joint
730.15 Chronic osteomyelitis, pelvic region and thigh — (Use additional code to identify organism, 041.1)
733.42 Aseptic necrosis of head and neck of femur
835.12 Open obturator dislocation of hip
996.4 Mechanical complication of internal orthopedic device, implant, and graft
996.77 Other complications due to internal joint prosthesis

ICD-9-CM Procedural
77.85 Other partial ostectomy of femur

27125
27125 Hemiarthroplasty, hip, partial (eg, femoral stem prosthesis, bipolar arthroplasty)

ICD-9-CM Diagnostic
170.1 Malignant neoplasm of mandible
170.7 Malignant neoplasm of long bones of lower limb
198.5 Secondary malignant neoplasm of bone and bone marrow
213.7 Benign neoplasm of long bones of lower limb
238.0 Neoplasm of uncertain behavior of bone and articular cartilage
239.2 Neoplasms of unspecified nature of bone, soft tissue, and skin
357.1 Polyneuropathy in collagen vascular disease — (Code first underlying disease: 446.0, 710.0, 714.0) ☒
359.6 Symptomatic inflammatory myopathy in diseases classified elsewhere — (Code first underlying disease: 135, 140.0-208.9, 277.3, 446.0, 710.0, 710.1, 710.2, 714.0) ☒
446.0 Polyarteritis nodosa
710.0 Systemic lupus erythematosus — (Use additional code to identify manifestation: 424.91, 581.81, 582.81, 583.81)
710.1 Systemic sclerosis — (Use additional code to identify manifestation: 359.6, 517.2)
710.2 Sicca syndrome
714.0 Rheumatoid arthritis — (Use additional code to identify manifestation: 357.1, 359.6)
715.15 Primary localized osteoarthrosis, pelvic region and thigh
715.35 Localized osteoarthrosis not specified whether primary or secondary, pelvic region and thigh
715.95 Osteoarthrosis, unspecified whether generalized or localized, pelvic region and thigh ▽
716.15 Traumatic arthropathy, pelvic region and thigh
716.95 Unspecified arthropathy, pelvic region and thigh ▽
718.05 Articular cartilage disorder, pelvic region and thigh
718.15 Loose body in pelvic joint
718.95 Unspecified pelvic joint derangement ▽
732.1 Juvenile osteochondrosis of hip and pelvis
733.42 Aseptic necrosis of head and neck of femur
733.81 Malunion of fracture
733.82 Nonunion of fracture
733.99 Other disorders of bone and cartilage
905.3 Late effect of fracture of neck of femur
905.4 Late effect of fracture of lower extremities

ICD-9-CM Procedural
81.52 Partial hip replacement

27130
27130 Arthroplasty, acetabular and proximal femoral prosthetic replacement (total hip arthroplasty), with or without autograft or allograft

ICD-9-CM Diagnostic
357.1 Polyneuropathy in collagen vascular disease — (Code first underlying disease: 446.0, 710.0, 714.0) ☒
359.6 Symptomatic inflammatory myopathy in diseases classified elsewhere — (Code first underlying disease: 135, 140.0-208.9, 277.3, 446.0, 710.0, 710.1, 710.2, 714.0) ☒
446.0 Polyarteritis nodosa
710.0 Systemic lupus erythematosus — (Use additional code to identify manifestation: 424.91, 581.81, 582.81, 583.81)
710.1 Systemic sclerosis — (Use additional code to identify manifestation: 359.6, 517.2)
710.2 Sicca syndrome
714.0 Rheumatoid arthritis — (Use additional code to identify manifestation: 357.1, 359.6)
715.09 Generalized osteoarthrosis, involving multiple sites
715.15 Primary localized osteoarthrosis, pelvic region and thigh
715.25 Secondary localized osteoarthrosis, pelvic region and thigh
715.35 Localized osteoarthrosis not specified whether primary or secondary, pelvic region and thigh
715.95 Osteoarthrosis, unspecified whether generalized or localized, pelvic region and thigh ▽

Hip Replacement

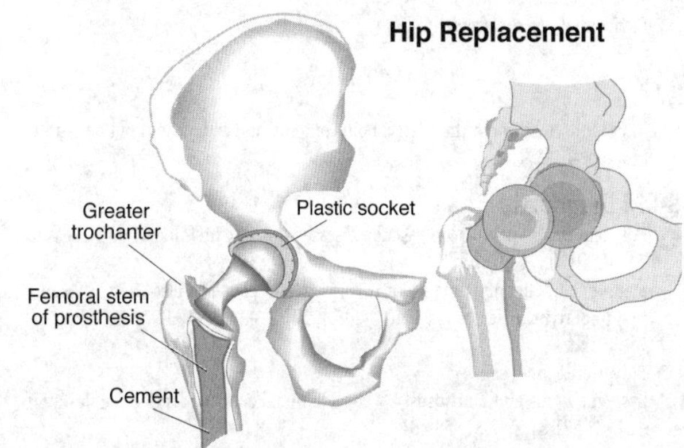

▽ Unspecified code ♀ Female diagnosis ☒ Manifestation code ♂ Male diagnosis

716.05 Kaschin-Beck disease pelvic, region and thigh
716.15 Traumatic arthropathy, pelvic region and thigh
716.95 Unspecified arthropathy, pelvic region and thigh ▽
718.65 Unspecified intrapelvic protrusion acetabulum, pelvic region and thigh ▽
719.35 Palindromic rheumatism, pelvic region and thigh
733.14 Pathologic fracture of neck of femur
733.42 Aseptic necrosis of head and neck of femur
733.82 Nonunion of fracture
754.30 Congenital dislocation of hip, unilateral
755.63 Other congenital deformity of hip (joint)
905.4 Late effect of fracture of lower extremities
996.4 Mechanical complication of internal orthopedic device, implant, and graft

ICD-9-CM Procedural

81.51 Total hip replacement

27132

27132 Conversion of previous hip surgery to total hip arthroplasty, with or without autograft or allograft

ICD-9-CM Diagnostic

357.1 Polyneuropathy in collagen vascular disease — (Code first underlying disease: 446.0, 710.0, 714.0) ☒
359.6 Symptomatic inflammatory myopathy in diseases classified elsewhere — (Code first underlying disease: 135, 140.0-208.9, 277.3, 446.0, 710.0, 710.1, 710.2, 714.0) ☒
446.0 Polyarteritis nodosa
710.0 Systemic lupus erythematosus — (Use additional code to identify manifestation: 424.91, 581.81, 582.81, 583.81)
710.1 Systemic sclerosis — (Use additional code to identify manifestation: 359.6, 517.2)
710.2 Sicca syndrome
714.0 Rheumatoid arthritis — (Use additional code to identify manifestation: 357.1, 359.6)
715.09 Generalized osteoarthrosis, involving multiple sites
715.15 Primary localized osteoarthrosis, pelvic region and thigh
715.25 Secondary localized osteoarthrosis, pelvic region and thigh
715.35 Localized osteoarthrosis not specified whether primary or secondary, pelvic region and thigh
715.95 Osteoarthrosis, unspecified whether generalized or localized, pelvic region and thigh ▽
716.05 Kaschin-Beck disease pelvic, region and thigh
716.15 Traumatic arthropathy, pelvic region and thigh
716.95 Unspecified arthropathy, pelvic region and thigh ▽
718.05 Articular cartilage disorder, pelvic region and thigh
718.25 Pathological dislocation of pelvic region and thigh joint
718.35 Recurrent dislocation of pelvic region and thigh joint
718.85 Other joint derangement, not elsewhere classified, pelvic region and thigh
719.35 Palindromic rheumatism, pelvic region and thigh
719.95 Unspecified disorder of joint of pelvic region and thigh ▽
733.14 Pathologic fracture of neck of femur
733.42 Aseptic necrosis of head and neck of femur
733.82 Nonunion of fracture
754.30 Congenital dislocation of hip, unilateral
755.63 Other congenital deformity of hip (joint)
905.4 Late effect of fracture of lower extremities
996.4 Mechanical complication of internal orthopedic device, implant, and graft

ICD-9-CM Procedural

81.51 Total hip replacement
81.53 Revision of hip replacement

27134

27134 Revision of total hip arthroplasty; both components, with or without autograft or allograft

ICD-9-CM Diagnostic

357.1 Polyneuropathy in collagen vascular disease — (Code first underlying disease: 446.0, 710.0, 714.0) ☒
359.6 Symptomatic inflammatory myopathy in diseases classified elsewhere — (Code first underlying disease: 135, 140.0-208.9, 277.3, 446.0, 710.0, 710.1, 710.2, 714.0) ☒
446.0 Polyarteritis nodosa
710.0 Systemic lupus erythematosus — (Use additional code to identify manifestation: 424.91, 581.81, 582.81, 583.81)
710.1 Systemic sclerosis — (Use additional code to identify manifestation: 359.6, 517.2)
710.2 Sicca syndrome
714.0 Rheumatoid arthritis — (Use additional code to identify manifestation: 357.1, 359.6)
715.09 Generalized osteoarthrosis, involving multiple sites
715.15 Primary localized osteoarthrosis, pelvic region and thigh
715.25 Secondary localized osteoarthrosis, pelvic region and thigh
715.35 Localized osteoarthrosis not specified whether primary or secondary, pelvic region and thigh
715.95 Osteoarthrosis, unspecified whether generalized or localized, pelvic region and thigh ▽
716.05 Kaschin-Beck disease pelvic, region and thigh
716.15 Traumatic arthropathy, pelvic region and thigh
718.05 Articular cartilage disorder, pelvic region and thigh
718.25 Pathological dislocation of pelvic region and thigh joint
718.35 Recurrent dislocation of pelvic region and thigh joint
718.85 Other joint derangement, not elsewhere classified, pelvic region and thigh
719.95 Unspecified disorder of joint of pelvic region and thigh ▽
733.14 Pathologic fracture of neck of femur
996.4 Mechanical complication of internal orthopedic device, implant, and graft
996.66 Infection and inflammatory reaction due to internal joint prosthesis — (Use additional code to identify specified infections)
996.67 Infection and inflammatory reaction due to other internal orthopedic device, implant, and graft — (Use additional code to identify specified infections)
996.77 Other complications due to internal joint prosthesis
998.59 Other postoperative infection — (Use additional code to identify infection)

ICD-9-CM Procedural

81.53 Revision of hip replacement

27137

27137 Revision of total hip arthroplasty; acetabular component only, with or without autograft or allograft

ICD-9-CM Diagnostic

357.1 Polyneuropathy in collagen vascular disease — (Code first underlying disease: 446.0, 710.0, 714.0) ☒
359.6 Symptomatic inflammatory myopathy in diseases classified elsewhere — (Code first underlying disease: 135, 140.0-208.9, 277.3, 446.0, 710.0, 710.1, 710.2, 714.0) ☒
446.0 Polyarteritis nodosa
710.0 Systemic lupus erythematosus — (Use additional code to identify manifestation: 424.91, 581.81, 582.81, 583.81)
710.1 Systemic sclerosis — (Use additional code to identify manifestation: 359.6, 517.2)
710.2 Sicca syndrome
714.0 Rheumatoid arthritis — (Use additional code to identify manifestation: 357.1, 359.6)
714.33 Monoarticular juvenile rheumatoid arthritis
715.09 Generalized osteoarthrosis, involving multiple sites
715.15 Primary localized osteoarthrosis, pelvic region and thigh
715.25 Secondary localized osteoarthrosis, pelvic region and thigh
715.35 Localized osteoarthrosis not specified whether primary or secondary, pelvic region and thigh
715.95 Osteoarthrosis, unspecified whether generalized or localized, pelvic region and thigh ▽
716.05 Kaschin-Beck disease pelvic, region and thigh
716.15 Traumatic arthropathy, pelvic region and thigh
718.05 Articular cartilage disorder, pelvic region and thigh
718.15 Loose body in pelvic joint
718.25 Pathological dislocation of pelvic region and thigh joint
718.35 Recurrent dislocation of pelvic region and thigh joint
718.85 Other joint derangement, not elsewhere classified, pelvic region and thigh
719.95 Unspecified disorder of joint of pelvic region and thigh ▽
733.14 Pathologic fracture of neck of femur
996.4 Mechanical complication of internal orthopedic device, implant, and graft
996.66 Infection and inflammatory reaction due to internal joint prosthesis — (Use additional code to identify specified infections)
996.67 Infection and inflammatory reaction due to other internal orthopedic device, implant, and graft — (Use additional code to identify specified infections)
996.77 Other complications due to internal joint prosthesis
998.59 Other postoperative infection — (Use additional code to identify infection)

ICD-9-CM Procedural

81.53 Revision of hip replacement

▽ Unspecified code
♀ Female diagnosis
☒ Manifestation code
♂ Male diagnosis

27138

27138 Revision of total hip arthroplasty; femoral component only, with or without allograft

ICD-9-CM Diagnostic

357.1 Polyneuropathy in collagen vascular disease — (Code first underlying disease: 446.0, 710.0, 714.0) ☒
359.6 Symptomatic inflammatory myopathy in diseases classified elsewhere — (Code first underlying disease: 135, 140.0-208.9, 277.3, 446.0, 710.0, 710.1, 710.2, 714.0) ☒
446.0 Polyarteritis nodosa
710.0 Systemic lupus erythematosus — (Use additional code to identify manifestation: 424.91, 581.81, 582.81, 583.81)
710.1 Systemic sclerosis — (Use additional code to identify manifestation: 359.6, 517.2)
710.2 Sicca syndrome
714.0 Rheumatoid arthritis — (Use additional code to identify manifestation: 357.1, 359.6)
715.09 Generalized osteoarthrosis, involving multiple sites
715.15 Primary localized osteoarthrosis, pelvic region and thigh
715.25 Secondary localized osteoarthrosis, pelvic region and thigh
715.35 Localized osteoarthrosis not specified whether primary or secondary, pelvic region and thigh
715.95 Osteoarthrosis, unspecified whether generalized or localized, pelvic region and thigh ▽
716.05 Kaschin-Beck disease pelvic, region and thigh
718.25 Pathological dislocation of pelvic region and thigh joint
718.35 Recurrent dislocation of pelvic region and thigh joint
718.85 Other joint derangement, not elsewhere classified, pelvic region and thigh
733.14 Pathologic fracture of neck of femur
996.4 Mechanical complication of internal orthopedic device, implant, and graft
996.66 Infection and inflammatory reaction due to internal joint prosthesis — (Use additional code to identify specified infections)
996.77 Other complications due to internal joint prosthesis
998.59 Other postoperative infection — (Use additional code to identify infection)

ICD-9-CM Procedural

81.53 Revision of hip replacement

27140

27140 Osteotomy and transfer of greater trochanter of femur (separate procedure)

ICD-9-CM Diagnostic

718.25 Pathological dislocation of pelvic region and thigh joint
718.35 Recurrent dislocation of pelvic region and thigh joint
733.15 Pathologic fracture of other specified part of femur
733.81 Malunion of fracture
736.39 Other acquired deformities of hip
996.4 Mechanical complication of internal orthopedic device, implant, and graft
996.77 Other complications due to internal joint prosthesis

ICD-9-CM Procedural

77.35 Other division of femur

27146–27147

27146 Osteotomy, iliac, acetabular or innominate bone;
27147 with open reduction of hip

ICD-9-CM Diagnostic

343.9 Unspecified infantile cerebral palsy ▽
718.35 Recurrent dislocation of pelvic region and thigh joint
718.85 Other joint derangement, not elsewhere classified, pelvic region and thigh
754.30 Congenital dislocation of hip, unilateral
754.31 Congenital dislocation of hip, bilateral
754.32 Congenital subluxation of hip, unilateral
754.33 Congenital subluxation of hip, bilateral
755.61 Congenital coxa valga
755.63 Other congenital deformity of hip (joint)

ICD-9-CM Procedural

77.39 Other division of other bone, except facial bones
77.85 Other partial ostectomy of femur
79.85 Open reduction of dislocation of hip

27151–27156

27151 Osteotomy, iliac, acetabular or innominate bone; with femoral osteotomy
27156 with femoral osteotomy and with open reduction of hip

ICD-9-CM Diagnostic

343.9 Unspecified infantile cerebral palsy ▽
718.35 Recurrent dislocation of pelvic region and thigh joint
718.85 Other joint derangement, not elsewhere classified, pelvic region and thigh
754.30 Congenital dislocation of hip, unilateral
754.31 Congenital dislocation of hip, bilateral
754.32 Congenital subluxation of hip, unilateral
754.33 Congenital subluxation of hip, bilateral
755.61 Congenital coxa valga
755.63 Other congenital deformity of hip (joint)

ICD-9-CM Procedural

77.35 Other division of femur
77.39 Other division of other bone, except facial bones
79.85 Open reduction of dislocation of hip

27158

27158 Osteotomy, pelvis, bilateral (eg, congenital malformation)

ICD-9-CM Diagnostic

755.63 Other congenital deformity of hip (joint)

ICD-9-CM Procedural

77.39 Other division of other bone, except facial bones

27161

27161 Osteotomy, femoral neck (separate procedure)

ICD-9-CM Diagnostic

343.9 Unspecified infantile cerebral palsy ▽
733.14 Pathologic fracture of neck of femur
733.81 Malunion of fracture
736.30 Unspecified acquired deformity of hip ▽
754.32 Congenital subluxation of hip, unilateral

ICD-9-CM Procedural

77.35 Other division of femur

27165

27165 Osteotomy, intertrochanteric or subtrochanteric including internal or external fixation and/or cast

ICD-9-CM Diagnostic

343.9 Unspecified infantile cerebral palsy ▽
715.15 Primary localized osteoarthrosis, pelvic region and thigh
718.25 Pathological dislocation of pelvic region and thigh joint
733.14 Pathologic fracture of neck of femur
733.42 Aseptic necrosis of head and neck of femur
733.82 Nonunion of fracture
754.30 Congenital dislocation of hip, unilateral
754.31 Congenital dislocation of hip, bilateral
754.32 Congenital subluxation of hip, unilateral
754.33 Congenital subluxation of hip, bilateral
755.61 Congenital coxa valga
755.62 Congenital coxa vara

ICD-9-CM Procedural

77.35 Other division of femur
78.15 Application of external fixation device, femur

27170

27170 Bone graft, femoral head, neck, intertrochanteric or subtrochanteric area (includes obtaining bone graft)

ICD-9-CM Diagnostic

239.2 Neoplasms of unspecified nature of bone, soft tissue, and skin
733.14 Pathologic fracture of neck of femur
733.20 Unspecified cyst of bone (localized) ▽
733.21 Solitary bone cyst
733.42 Aseptic necrosis of head and neck of femur
733.82 Nonunion of fracture

▽ Unspecified code
♀ Female diagnosis
☒ Manifestation code
♂ Male diagnosis

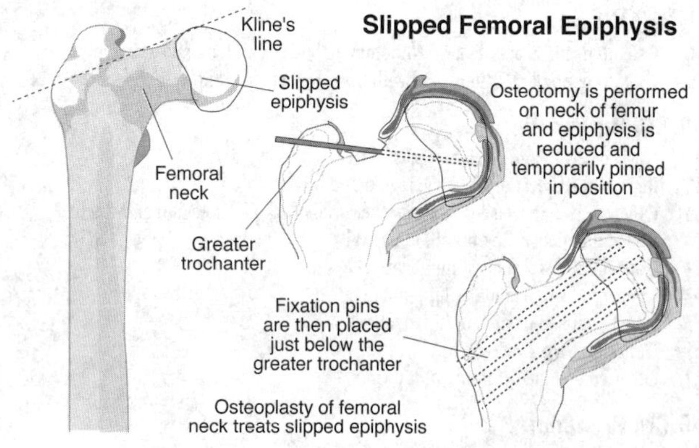
Slipped Femoral Epiphysis
Kline's line
Slipped epiphysis
Femoral neck
Greater trochanter
Osteotomy is performed on neck of femur and epiphysis is reduced and temporarily pinned in position
Fixation pins are then placed just below the greater trochanter
Osteoplasty of femoral neck treats slipped epiphysis

820.01 Closed fracture of epiphysis (separation) (upper) of neck of femur
820.11 Open fracture of epiphysis (separation) (upper) of neck of femur
820.13 Open fracture of base of neck of femur
820.20 Closed fracture of unspecified trochanteric section of femur ▽
820.21 Closed fracture of intertrochanteric section of femur
820.22 Closed fracture of subtrochanteric section of femur

ICD-9-CM Procedural
77.77 Excision of tibia and fibula for graft
77.79 Excision of other bone for graft, except facial bones
78.05 Bone graft of femur

27175–27176
27175 Treatment of slipped femoral epiphysis; by traction, without reduction
27176 by single or multiple pinning, in situ

ICD-9-CM Diagnostic
732.2 Nontraumatic slipped upper femoral epiphysis
732.9 Unspecified osteochondropathy ▽
820.01 Closed fracture of epiphysis (separation) (upper) of neck of femur

ICD-9-CM Procedural
78.55 Internal fixation of femur without fracture reduction
93.44 Other skeletal traction
93.45 Thomas' splint traction

27177
27177 Open treatment of slipped femoral epiphysis; single or multiple pinning or bone graft (includes obtaining graft)

ICD-9-CM Diagnostic
732.2 Nontraumatic slipped upper femoral epiphysis
732.9 Unspecified osteochondropathy ▽
820.01 Closed fracture of epiphysis (separation) (upper) of neck of femur

ICD-9-CM Procedural
77.79 Excision of other bone for graft, except facial bones
78.05 Bone graft of femur
78.55 Internal fixation of femur without fracture reduction
79.55 Open reduction of separated epiphysis of femur

27178
27178 Open treatment of slipped femoral epiphysis; closed manipulation with single or multiple pinning

ICD-9-CM Diagnostic
732.2 Nontraumatic slipped upper femoral epiphysis
732.9 Unspecified osteochondropathy ▽
820.01 Closed fracture of epiphysis (separation) (upper) of neck of femur

ICD-9-CM Procedural
78.55 Internal fixation of femur without fracture reduction
79.55 Open reduction of separated epiphysis of femur

27179
27179 Open treatment of slipped femoral epiphysis; osteoplasty of femoral neck (Heyman type procedure)

ICD-9-CM Diagnostic
732.2 Nontraumatic slipped upper femoral epiphysis
732.9 Unspecified osteochondropathy ▽
820.01 Closed fracture of epiphysis (separation) (upper) of neck of femur

ICD-9-CM Procedural
78.45 Other repair or plastic operations on femur
79.55 Open reduction of separated epiphysis of femur

27181
27181 Open treatment of slipped femoral epiphysis; osteotomy and internal fixation

ICD-9-CM Diagnostic
732.2 Nontraumatic slipped upper femoral epiphysis
732.9 Unspecified osteochondropathy ▽
820.01 Closed fracture of epiphysis (separation) (upper) of neck of femur

ICD-9-CM Procedural
77.25 Wedge osteotomy of femur
78.55 Internal fixation of femur without fracture reduction
79.55 Open reduction of separated epiphysis of femur

27185
27185 Epiphyseal arrest by epiphysiodesis or stapling, greater trochanter of femur

ICD-9-CM Diagnostic
733.91 Arrest of bone development or growth
736.32 Coxa vara (acquired)
755.30 Congenital unspecified reduction deformity of lower limb ▽
755.31 Congenital transverse deficiency of lower limb

ICD-9-CM Procedural
78.25 Limb shortening procedures, femur

27187
27187 Prophylactic treatment (nailing, pinning, plating or wiring) with or without methylmethacrylate, femoral neck and proximal femur

ICD-9-CM Diagnostic
170.7 Malignant neoplasm of long bones of lower limb
198.5 Secondary malignant neoplasm of bone and bone marrow
213.7 Benign neoplasm of long bones of lower limb
238.0 Neoplasm of uncertain behavior of bone and articular cartilage
239.2 Neoplasms of unspecified nature of bone, soft tissue, and skin
733.00 Unspecified osteoporosis ▽
733.09 Other osteoporosis — (Use additional E code to identify drug)

ICD-9-CM Procedural
78.55 Internal fixation of femur without fracture reduction
84.55 Insertion of bone void filler

27193–27194
27193 Closed treatment of pelvic ring fracture, dislocation, diastasis or subluxation; without manipulation
27194 with manipulation, requiring more than local anesthesia

ICD-9-CM Diagnostic
724.6 Disorders of sacrum
805.6 Closed fracture of sacrum and coccyx without mention of spinal cord injury
806.61 Closed fracture of sacrum and coccyx with complete cauda equina lesion
806.62 Closed fracture of sacrum and coccyx with other cauda equina injury
806.79 Open fracture of sacrum and coccyx with other spinal cord injury
808.0 Closed fracture of acetabulum
808.2 Closed fracture of pubis
808.41 Closed fracture of ilium
808.42 Closed fracture of ischium
808.43 Multiple closed pelvic fractures with disruption of pelvic circle
808.49 Closed fracture of other specified part of pelvis
839.41 Closed dislocation, coccyx
839.42 Closed dislocation, sacrum
839.69 Closed dislocation, other location

▽ Unspecified code ♀ Female diagnosis ☒ Manifestation code ♂ Male diagnosis

ICD-9-CM Procedural

79.09 Closed reduction of fracture of other specified bone, except facial bones, without internal fixation
79.79 Closed reduction of dislocation of other specified site, except temporomandibular
93.59 Other immobilization, pressure, and attention to wound

27200

27200 Closed treatment of coccygeal fracture

ICD-9-CM Diagnostic

733.19 Pathologic fracture of other specified site
805.6 Closed fracture of sacrum and coccyx without mention of spinal cord injury
806.60 Closed fracture of sacrum and coccyx with unspecified spinal cord injury
806.61 Closed fracture of sacrum and coccyx with complete cauda equina lesion
806.62 Closed fracture of sacrum and coccyx with other cauda equina injury
806.69 Closed fracture of sacrum and coccyx with other spinal cord injury
839.41 Closed dislocation, coccyx

ICD-9-CM Procedural

79.09 Closed reduction of fracture of other specified bone, except facial bones, without internal fixation
93.59 Other immobilization, pressure, and attention to wound

27202

27202 Open treatment of coccygeal fracture

ICD-9-CM Diagnostic

733.19 Pathologic fracture of other specified site
805.6 Closed fracture of sacrum and coccyx without mention of spinal cord injury
805.7 Open fracture of sacrum and coccyx without mention of spinal cord injury
805.8 Closed fracture of unspecified part of vertebral column without mention of spinal cord injury
806.60 Closed fracture of sacrum and coccyx with unspecified spinal cord injury
806.61 Closed fracture of sacrum and coccyx with complete cauda equina lesion
806.69 Closed fracture of sacrum and coccyx with other spinal cord injury
839.41 Closed dislocation, coccyx
839.51 Open dislocation, coccyx

ICD-9-CM Procedural

77.89 Other partial ostectomy of other bone, except facial bones
79.29 Open reduction of fracture of other specified bone, except facial bones, without internal fixation

27215

27215 Open treatment of iliac spine(s), tuberosity avulsion, or iliac wing fracture(s) (eg, pelvic fracture(s) which do not disrupt the pelvic ring), with internal fixation

ICD-9-CM Diagnostic

733.19 Pathologic fracture of other specified site
808.41 Closed fracture of ilium
808.51 Open fracture of ilium

ICD-9-CM Procedural

79.39 Open reduction of fracture of other specified bone, except facial bones, with internal fixation

27216

27216 Percutaneous skeletal fixation of posterior pelvic ring fracture and/or dislocation (includes ilium, sacroiliac joint and/or sacrum)

ICD-9-CM Diagnostic

724.6 Disorders of sacrum
805.6 Closed fracture of sacrum and coccyx without mention of spinal cord injury
808.41 Closed fracture of ilium
808.49 Closed fracture of other specified part of pelvis
808.51 Open fracture of ilium
839.42 Closed dislocation, sacrum
839.52 Open dislocation, sacrum

ICD-9-CM Procedural

78.59 Internal fixation of other bone, except facial bones, without fracture reduction
79.79 Closed reduction of dislocation of other specified site, except temporomandibular

27217

27217 Open treatment of anterior ring fracture and/or dislocation with internal fixation (includes pubic symphysis and/or rami)

ICD-9-CM Diagnostic

808.2 Closed fracture of pubis
808.3 Open fracture of pubis
808.43 Multiple closed pelvic fractures with disruption of pelvic circle
808.53 Multiple open pelvic fractures with disruption of pelvic circle
839.69 Closed dislocation, other location
839.79 Open dislocation, other location

ICD-9-CM Procedural

79.39 Open reduction of fracture of other specified bone, except facial bones, with internal fixation
79.89 Open reduction of dislocation of other specified site, except temporomandibular

27218

27218 Open treatment of posterior ring fracture and/or dislocation with internal fixation (includes ilium, sacroiliac joint and/or sacrum)

ICD-9-CM Diagnostic

805.6 Closed fracture of sacrum and coccyx without mention of spinal cord injury
806.61 Closed fracture of sacrum and coccyx with complete cauda equina lesion
806.62 Closed fracture of sacrum and coccyx with other cauda equina injury
806.79 Open fracture of sacrum and coccyx with other spinal cord injury
808.41 Closed fracture of ilium
808.43 Multiple closed pelvic fractures with disruption of pelvic circle
808.51 Open fracture of ilium
808.53 Multiple open pelvic fractures with disruption of pelvic circle
839.42 Closed dislocation, sacrum
839.52 Open dislocation, sacrum

ICD-9-CM Procedural

79.39 Open reduction of fracture of other specified bone, except facial bones, with internal fixation
79.89 Open reduction of dislocation of other specified site, except temporomandibular

27220–27222

27220 Closed treatment of acetabulum (hip socket) fracture(s); without manipulation
27222 with manipulation, with or without skeletal traction

ICD-9-CM Diagnostic

808.0 Closed fracture of acetabulum

ICD-9-CM Procedural

79.09 Closed reduction of fracture of other specified bone, except facial bones, without internal fixation
93.44 Other skeletal traction
93.46 Other skin traction of limbs
93.59 Other immobilization, pressure, and attention to wound

27226

27226 Open treatment of posterior or anterior acetabular wall fracture, with internal fixation

ICD-9-CM Diagnostic

808.0 Closed fracture of acetabulum
808.1 Open fracture of acetabulum
808.43 Multiple closed pelvic fractures with disruption of pelvic circle
808.53 Multiple open pelvic fractures with disruption of pelvic circle

ICD-9-CM Procedural

79.39 Open reduction of fracture of other specified bone, except facial bones, with internal fixation

27227

27227 Open treatment of acetabular fracture(s) involving anterior or posterior (one) column, or a fracture running transversely across the acetabulum, with internal fixation

ICD-9-CM Diagnostic

808.0 Closed fracture of acetabulum
808.1 Open fracture of acetabulum
808.43 Multiple closed pelvic fractures with disruption of pelvic circle

808.53 Multiple open pelvic fractures with disruption of pelvic circle

ICD-9-CM Procedural

79.39 Open reduction of fracture of other specified bone, except facial bones, with internal fixation

27228

27228 Open treatment of acetabular fracture(s) involving anterior and posterior (two) columns, includes T-fracture and both column fracture with complete articular detachment, or single column or transverse fracture with associated acetabular wall fracture, with internal fixation

ICD-9-CM Diagnostic

808.0 Closed fracture of acetabulum
808.1 Open fracture of acetabulum
808.43 Multiple closed pelvic fractures with disruption of pelvic circle
808.53 Multiple open pelvic fractures with disruption of pelvic circle

ICD-9-CM Procedural

79.39 Open reduction of fracture of other specified bone, except facial bones, with internal fixation

27230–27232

27230 Closed treatment of femoral fracture, proximal end, neck; without manipulation
27232 with manipulation, with or without skeletal traction

ICD-9-CM Diagnostic

733.14 Pathologic fracture of neck of femur
733.81 Malunion of fracture
820.00 Closed fracture of unspecified intracapsular section of neck of femur ▽
820.01 Closed fracture of epiphysis (separation) (upper) of neck of femur
820.02 Closed fracture of midcervical section of femur
820.03 Closed fracture of base of neck of femur
820.09 Other closed transcervical fracture of femur
820.8 Closed fracture of unspecified part of neck of femur ▽

ICD-9-CM Procedural

79.05 Closed reduction of fracture of femur without internal fixation
93.44 Other skeletal traction
93.46 Other skin traction of limbs
93.53 Application of other cast

27235

27235 Percutaneous skeletal fixation of femoral fracture, proximal end, neck

ICD-9-CM Diagnostic

733.14 Pathologic fracture of neck of femur
820.00 Closed fracture of unspecified intracapsular section of neck of femur ▽
820.01 Closed fracture of epiphysis (separation) (upper) of neck of femur
820.02 Closed fracture of midcervical section of femur
820.03 Closed fracture of base of neck of femur
820.09 Other closed transcervical fracture of femur
820.8 Closed fracture of unspecified part of neck of femur ▽

ICD-9-CM Procedural

78.55 Internal fixation of femur without fracture reduction
79.15 Closed reduction of fracture of femur with internal fixation

27236

27236 Open treatment of femoral fracture, proximal end, neck, internal fixation or prosthetic replacement

ICD-9-CM Diagnostic

733.14 Pathologic fracture of neck of femur
820.01 Closed fracture of epiphysis (separation) (upper) of neck of femur
820.02 Closed fracture of midcervical section of femur
820.03 Closed fracture of base of neck of femur
820.09 Other closed transcervical fracture of femur
820.10 Open fracture of unspecified intracapsular section of neck of femur ▽
820.11 Open fracture of epiphysis (separation) (upper) of neck of femur
820.12 Open fracture of midcervical section of femur
820.13 Open fracture of base of neck of femur
820.19 Other open transcervical fracture of femur
820.8 Closed fracture of unspecified part of neck of femur ▽
820.9 Open fracture of unspecified part of neck of femur ▽
827.0 Other, multiple and ill-defined closed fractures of lower limb
827.1 Other, multiple and ill-defined open fractures of lower limb
828.0 Multiple closed fractures involving both lower limbs, lower with upper limb, and lower limb(s) with rib(s) and sternum
828.1 Multiple fractures involving both lower limbs, lower with upper limb, and lower limb(s) with rib(s) and sternum, open

ICD-9-CM Procedural

79.35 Open reduction of fracture of femur with internal fixation
81.52 Partial hip replacement

27238–27240

27238 Closed treatment of intertrochanteric, pertrochanteric, or subtrochanteric femoral fracture; without manipulation
27240 with manipulation, with or without skin or skeletal traction

ICD-9-CM Diagnostic

733.14 Pathologic fracture of neck of femur
733.15 Pathologic fracture of other specified part of femur
820.20 Closed fracture of unspecified trochanteric section of femur ▽
820.21 Closed fracture of intertrochanteric section of femur
820.22 Closed fracture of subtrochanteric section of femur
820.8 Closed fracture of unspecified part of neck of femur ▽

ICD-9-CM Procedural

79.05 Closed reduction of fracture of femur without internal fixation
93.44 Other skeletal traction
93.46 Other skin traction of limbs
93.53 Application of other cast

27244–27245

27244 Treatment of intertrochanteric, pertrochanteric, or subtrochanteric femoral fracture; with plate/screw type implant, with or without cerclage
27245 with intramedullary implant, with or without interlocking screws and/or cerclage

ICD-9-CM Diagnostic

733.14 Pathologic fracture of neck of femur
733.15 Pathologic fracture of other specified part of femur
733.81 Malunion of fracture
820.20 Closed fracture of unspecified trochanteric section of femur ▽
820.21 Closed fracture of intertrochanteric section of femur
820.22 Closed fracture of subtrochanteric section of femur
820.30 Open fracture of unspecified trochanteric section of femur ▽
820.31 Open fracture of intertrochanteric section of femur
820.32 Open fracture of subtrochanteric section of femur
820.8 Closed fracture of unspecified part of neck of femur ▽
820.9 Open fracture of unspecified part of neck of femur ▽
827.0 Other, multiple and ill-defined closed fractures of lower limb
827.1 Other, multiple and ill-defined open fractures of lower limb
828.0 Multiple closed fractures involving both lower limbs, lower with upper limb, and lower limb(s) with rib(s) and sternum
828.1 Multiple fractures involving both lower limbs, lower with upper limb, and lower limb(s) with rib(s) and sternum, open
829.0 Closed fracture of unspecified bone ▽
996.4 Mechanical complication of internal orthopedic device, implant, and graft
996.78 Other complications due to other internal orthopedic device, implant, and graft

ICD-9-CM Procedural

79.35 Open reduction of fracture of femur with internal fixation

27246–27248

27246 Closed treatment of greater trochanteric fracture, without manipulation
27248 Open treatment of greater trochanteric fracture, with or without internal or external fixation

ICD-9-CM Diagnostic

820.20 Closed fracture of unspecified trochanteric section of femur ▽
820.21 Closed fracture of intertrochanteric section of femur
820.22 Closed fracture of subtrochanteric section of femur
820.30 Open fracture of unspecified trochanteric section of femur ▽
820.31 Open fracture of intertrochanteric section of femur
820.32 Open fracture of subtrochanteric section of femur

ICD-9-CM Procedural

78.15 Application of external fixation device, femur

79.35 Open reduction of fracture of femur with internal fixation
93.46 Other skin traction of limbs
93.53 Application of other cast

27250–27252

27250 Closed treatment of hip dislocation, traumatic; without anesthesia
27252 requiring anesthesia

ICD-9-CM Diagnostic

835.00 Closed dislocation of hip, unspecified site ▽
835.01 Closed posterior dislocation of hip
835.02 Closed obturator dislocation of hip
835.03 Other closed anterior dislocation of hip

ICD-9-CM Procedural

79.75 Closed reduction of dislocation of hip

HCPCS Level II Supplies & Services

A4570 Splint
A4580 Cast supplies (e.g., plaster)
E0112 Crutches, underarm, wood, adjustable or fixed, pair, with pads, tips and handgrips
E0113 Crutch, underarm, wood, adjustable or fixed, each, with pad, tip and handgrip
E0114 Crutches, underarm, other than wood, adjustable or fixed, pair, with pads, tips and handgrips

27253

27253 Open treatment of hip dislocation, traumatic, without internal fixation

ICD-9-CM Diagnostic

835.01 Closed posterior dislocation of hip
835.02 Closed obturator dislocation of hip
835.03 Other closed anterior dislocation of hip
835.11 Open posterior dislocation of hip
835.12 Open obturator dislocation of hip
835.13 Other open anterior dislocation of hip

ICD-9-CM Procedural

79.85 Open reduction of dislocation of hip

27254

27254 Open treatment of hip dislocation, traumatic, with acetabular wall and femoral head fracture, with or without internal or external fixation

ICD-9-CM Diagnostic

808.0 Closed fracture of acetabulum
808.1 Open fracture of acetabulum
820.01 Closed fracture of epiphysis (separation) (upper) of neck of femur
820.02 Closed fracture of midcervical section of femur
820.09 Other closed transcervical fracture of femur
820.11 Open fracture of epiphysis (separation) (upper) of neck of femur
820.12 Open fracture of midcervical section of femur
820.19 Other open transcervical fracture of femur
820.8 Closed fracture of unspecified part of neck of femur ▽
820.9 Open fracture of unspecified part of neck of femur ▽
835.01 Closed posterior dislocation of hip
835.02 Closed obturator dislocation of hip
835.03 Other closed anterior dislocation of hip
835.11 Open posterior dislocation of hip
835.12 Open obturator dislocation of hip
835.13 Other open anterior dislocation of hip

ICD-9-CM Procedural

78.15 Application of external fixation device, femur
79.25 Open reduction of fracture of femur without internal fixation
79.35 Open reduction of fracture of femur with internal fixation
79.85 Open reduction of dislocation of hip

27256–27257

27256 Treatment of spontaneous hip dislocation (developmental, including congenital or pathological), by abduction, splint or traction; without anesthesia, without manipulation
27257 with manipulation, requiring anesthesia

ICD-9-CM Diagnostic

718.25 Pathological dislocation of pelvic region and thigh joint
718.35 Recurrent dislocation of pelvic region and thigh joint
736.31 Coxa valga (acquired)
754.30 Congenital dislocation of hip, unilateral
754.31 Congenital dislocation of hip, bilateral

ICD-9-CM Procedural

79.70 Closed reduction of dislocation of unspecified site
79.75 Closed reduction of dislocation of hip
79.79 Closed reduction of dislocation of other specified site, except temporomandibular
93.44 Other skeletal traction
93.46 Other skin traction of limbs
93.53 Application of other cast

HCPCS Level II Supplies & Services

A4305 Disposable drug delivery system, flow rate of 50 ml or greater per hour
A4306 Disposable drug delivery system, flow rate of 5 ml or less per hour
A4550 Surgical trays
A4570 Splint
A4580 Cast supplies (e.g., plaster)

27258–27259

27258 Open treatment of spontaneous hip dislocation (developmental, including congenital or pathological), replacement of femoral head in acetabulum (including tenotomy, etc.);
27259 with femoral shaft shortening

ICD-9-CM Diagnostic

718.25 Pathological dislocation of pelvic region and thigh joint
718.35 Recurrent dislocation of pelvic region and thigh joint
736.31 Coxa valga (acquired)
754.30 Congenital dislocation of hip, unilateral
754.31 Congenital dislocation of hip, bilateral

ICD-9-CM Procedural

78.25 Limb shortening procedures, femur
79.85 Open reduction of dislocation of hip

27265–27266

27265 Closed treatment of post hip arthroplasty dislocation; without anesthesia
27266 requiring regional or general anesthesia

ICD-9-CM Diagnostic

718.35 Recurrent dislocation of pelvic region and thigh joint
835.00 Closed dislocation of hip, unspecified site ▽
835.01 Closed posterior dislocation of hip
835.02 Closed obturator dislocation of hip
835.03 Other closed anterior dislocation of hip
996.4 Mechanical complication of internal orthopedic device, implant, and graft
996.66 Infection and inflammatory reaction due to internal joint prosthesis — (Use additional code to identify specified infections)
996.77 Other complications due to internal joint prosthesis

ICD-9-CM Procedural

79.75 Closed reduction of dislocation of hip

HCPCS Level II Supplies & Services

A4305 Disposable drug delivery system, flow rate of 50 ml or greater per hour
A4306 Disposable drug delivery system, flow rate of 5 ml or less per hour
A4550 Surgical trays
A4570 Splint
A4580 Cast supplies (e.g., plaster)

27275

27275 Manipulation, hip joint, requiring general anesthesia

ICD-9-CM Diagnostic

718.55 Ankylosis of pelvic region and thigh joint

718.56 Ankylosis of lower leg joint
996.4 Mechanical complication of internal orthopedic device, implant, and graft

ICD-9-CM Procedural

93.26 Manual rupture of joint adhesions
93.29 Other forcible correction of musculoskeletal deformity

27280

27280 Arthrodesis, sacroiliac joint (including obtaining graft)

ICD-9-CM Diagnostic

808.43 Multiple closed pelvic fractures with disruption of pelvic circle
808.53 Multiple open pelvic fractures with disruption of pelvic circle
839.42 Closed dislocation, sacrum
839.52 Open dislocation, sacrum

ICD-9-CM Procedural

81.29 Arthrodesis of other specified joint

27282

27282 Arthrodesis, symphysis pubis (including obtaining graft)

ICD-9-CM Diagnostic

357.1 Polyneuropathy in collagen vascular disease — (Code first underlying disease: 446.0, 710.0, 714.0) ☒
359.6 Symptomatic inflammatory myopathy in diseases classified elsewhere — (Code first underlying disease: 135, 140.0-208.9, 277.3, 446.0, 710.0, 710.1, 710.2, 714.0) ☒
446.0 Polyarteritis nodosa
710.0 Systemic lupus erythematosus — (Use additional code to identify manifestation: 424.91, 581.81, 582.81, 583.81)
710.1 Systemic sclerosis — (Use additional code to identify manifestation: 359.6, 517.2)
710.2 Sicca syndrome
714.0 Rheumatoid arthritis — (Use additional code to identify manifestation: 357.1, 359.6)
730.15 Chronic osteomyelitis, pelvic region and thigh — (Use additional code to identify organism, 041.1)
808.2 Closed fracture of pubis
808.3 Open fracture of pubis
808.43 Multiple closed pelvic fractures with disruption of pelvic circle
808.53 Multiple open pelvic fractures with disruption of pelvic circle
839.69 Closed dislocation, other location
839.79 Open dislocation, other location

ICD-9-CM Procedural

81.29 Arthrodesis of other specified joint

27284–27286

27284 Arthrodesis, hip joint (including obtaining graft);
27286 with subtrochanteric osteotomy

ICD-9-CM Diagnostic

715.35 Localized osteoarthrosis not specified whether primary or secondary, pelvic region and thigh
726.5 Enthesopathy of hip region
730.15 Chronic osteomyelitis, pelvic region and thigh — (Use additional code to identify organism, 041.1)
733.42 Aseptic necrosis of head and neck of femur
733.81 Malunion of fracture
733.82 Nonunion of fracture
808.0 Closed fracture of acetabulum
808.1 Open fracture of acetabulum

ICD-9-CM Procedural

77.39 Other division of other bone, except facial bones
81.21 Arthrodesis of hip

27290

27290 Interpelviabdominal amputation (hindquarter amputation)

ICD-9-CM Diagnostic

170.6 Malignant neoplasm of pelvic bones, sacrum, and coccyx
171.6 Malignant neoplasm of connective and other soft tissue of pelvis
198.5 Secondary malignant neoplasm of bone and bone marrow
200.06 Reticulosarcoma of intrapelvic lymph nodes
200.16 Lymphosarcoma of intrapelvic lymph nodes
730.15 Chronic osteomyelitis, pelvic region and thigh — (Use additional code to identify organism, 041.1)
926.12 Crushing injury of buttock — (Use additional code to identify any associated injuries: 800-829, 850.0-854.1, 860.0-869.1)

ICD-9-CM Procedural

84.19 Abdominopelvic amputation

27295

27295 Disarticulation of hip

ICD-9-CM Diagnostic

170.7 Malignant neoplasm of long bones of lower limb
198.5 Secondary malignant neoplasm of bone and bone marrow
730.15 Chronic osteomyelitis, pelvic region and thigh — (Use additional code to identify organism, 041.1)
890.1 Open wound of hip and thigh, complicated — (Use additional code to identify infection)
897.3 Traumatic amputation of leg(s) (complete) (partial), unilateral, at or above knee, complicated — (Use additional code to identify infection)
897.5 Traumatic amputation of leg(s) (complete) (partial), unilateral, level not specified, complicated — (Use additional code to identify infection) ▽
905.4 Late effect of fracture of lower extremities
928.01 Crushing injury of hip — (Use additional code to identify any associated injuries: 800-829, 850.0-854.1, 860.0-869.1)

ICD-9-CM Procedural

84.18 Disarticulation of hip

Femur (Thigh Region) and Knee Joint

27301

27301 Incision and drainage, deep abscess, bursa, or hematoma, thigh or knee region

ICD-9-CM Diagnostic

680.6 Carbuncle and furuncle of leg, except foot
682.6 Cellulitis and abscess of leg, except foot — (Use additional code to identify organism)
686.9 Unspecified local infection of skin and subcutaneous tissue ▽
696.0 Psoriatic arthropathy
711.06 Pyogenic arthritis, lower leg — (Use additional code to identify infectious organism: 041.0-041.8)
726.60 Unspecified enthesopathy of knee ▽
726.65 Prepatellar bursitis
890.0 Open wound of hip and thigh, without mention of complication — (Use additional code to identify infection)
890.1 Open wound of hip and thigh, complicated — (Use additional code to identify infection)
891.0 Open wound of knee, leg (except thigh), and ankle, without mention of complication — (Use additional code to identify infection)
891.1 Open wound of knee, leg (except thigh), and ankle, complicated — (Use additional code to identify infection)
904.8 Injury to unspecified blood vessel of lower extremity ▽
924.00 Contusion of thigh
924.11 Contusion of knee
928.11 Crushing injury of knee — (Use additional code to identify any associated injuries: 800-829, 850.0-854.1, 860.0-869.1)
958.3 Posttraumatic wound infection not elsewhere classified
996.66 Infection and inflammatory reaction due to internal joint prosthesis — (Use additional code to identify specified infections)
998.11 Hemorrhage complicating a procedure
998.31 Disruption of internal operation wound
998.32 Disruption of external operation wound
998.59 Other postoperative infection — (Use additional code to identify infection)

ICD-9-CM Procedural

83.02 Myotomy
83.03 Bursotomy
83.09 Other incision of soft tissue

HCPCS Level II Supplies & Services

A4305 Disposable drug delivery system, flow rate of 50 ml or greater per hour

▽ Unspecified code
♀ Female diagnosis
☒ Manifestation code
♂ Male diagnosis

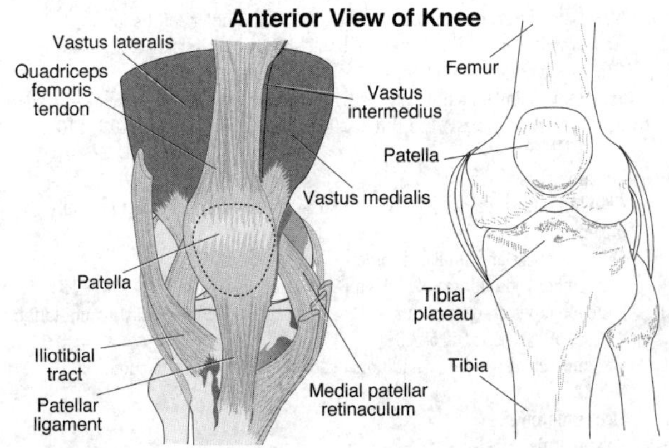

A4306 Disposable drug delivery system, flow rate of 5 ml or less per hour
A4550 Surgical trays
E0112 Crutches, underarm, wood, adjustable or fixed, pair, with pads, tips and handgrips
E0114 Crutches, underarm, other than wood, adjustable or fixed, pair, with pads, tips and handgrips

27303

27303 Incision, deep, with opening of bone cortex, femur or knee (eg, osteomyelitis or bone abscess)

ICD-9-CM Diagnostic

198.5 Secondary malignant neoplasm of bone and bone marrow
213.7 Benign neoplasm of long bones of lower limb
711.05 Pyogenic arthritis, pelvic region and thigh — (Use additional code to identify infectious organism: 041.0-041.8)
711.06 Pyogenic arthritis, lower leg — (Use additional code to identify infectious organism: 041.0-041.8)
730.05 Acute osteomyelitis, pelvic region and thigh — (Use additional code to identify organism, 041.1)
730.06 Acute osteomyelitis, lower leg — (Use additional code to identify organism, 041.1)
730.15 Chronic osteomyelitis, pelvic region and thigh — (Use additional code to identify organism, 041.1)
730.16 Chronic osteomyelitis, lower leg — (Use additional code to identify organism, 041.1)
730.25 Unspecified osteomyelitis, pelvic region and thigh — (Use additional code to identify organism, 041.1) ▽
730.26 Unspecified osteomyelitis, lower leg — (Use additional code to identify organism, 041.1) ▽
730.95 Unspecified infection of bone, pelvic region and thigh — (Use additional code to identify organism, 041.1) ▽
730.96 Unspecified infection of bone, lower leg — (Use additional code to identify organism, 041.1) ▽
733.20 Unspecified cyst of bone (localized) ▽
733.22 Aneurysmal bone cyst
733.49 Aseptic necrosis of other bone site
996.66 Infection and inflammatory reaction due to internal joint prosthesis — (Use additional code to identify specified infections)
996.67 Infection and inflammatory reaction due to other internal orthopedic device, implant, and graft — (Use additional code to identify specified infections)
998.59 Other postoperative infection — (Use additional code to identify infection)

ICD-9-CM Procedural

77.15 Other incision of femur without division
77.16 Other incision of patella without division
77.17 Other incision of tibia and fibula without division

27305

27305 Fasciotomy, iliotibial (tenotomy), open

ICD-9-CM Diagnostic

716.16 Traumatic arthropathy, lower leg
726.69 Other enthesopathy of knee
726.72 Tibialis tendinitis
727.09 Other synovitis and tenosynovitis
727.81 Contracture of tendon (sheath)
728.88 Rhabdomyolysis
736.41 Genu valgum (acquired)
836.51 Closed anterior dislocation of tibia, proximal end
836.52 Closed posterior dislocation of tibia, proximal end
836.61 Open anterior dislocation of tibia, proximal end
836.62 Open posterior dislocation of tibia, proximal end
844.8 Sprain and strain of other specified sites of knee and leg
844.9 Sprain and strain of unspecified site of knee and leg ▽
891.2 Open wound of knee, leg (except thigh), and ankle, with tendon involvement — (Use additional code to identify infection)
958.8 Other early complications of trauma

ICD-9-CM Procedural

83.14 Fasciotomy

27306–27307

27306 Tenotomy, percutaneous, adductor or hamstring; single tendon (separate procedure)
27307 multiple tendons

ICD-9-CM Diagnostic

359.6 Symptomatic inflammatory myopathy in diseases classified elsewhere — (Code first underlying disease: 135, 140.0-208.9, 277.3, 446.0, 710.0, 710.1, 710.2, 714.0) ☒
446.0 Polyarteritis nodosa
710.0 Systemic lupus erythematosus — (Use additional code to identify manifestation: 424.91, 581.81, 582.81, 583.81)
710.1 Systemic sclerosis — (Use additional code to identify manifestation: 359.6, 517.2)
711.05 Pyogenic arthritis, pelvic region and thigh — (Use additional code to identify infectious organism: 041.0-041.8)
714.0 Rheumatoid arthritis — (Use additional code to identify manifestation: 357.1, 359.6)
726.69 Other enthesopathy of knee
727.89 Other disorders of synovium, tendon, and bursa
755.60 Unspecified congenital anomaly of lower limb ▽
755.61 Congenital coxa valga
755.62 Congenital coxa vara
890.2 Open wound of hip and thigh, with tendon involvement — (Use additional code to identify infection)
905.8 Late effect of tendon injury
928.01 Crushing injury of hip — (Use additional code to identify any associated injuries: 800-829, 850.0-854.1, 860.0-869.1)
928.11 Crushing injury of knee — (Use additional code to identify any associated injuries: 800-829, 850.0-854.1, 860.0-869.1)
996.4 Mechanical complication of internal orthopedic device, implant, and graft
996.67 Infection and inflammatory reaction due to other internal orthopedic device, implant, and graft — (Use additional code to identify specified infections)

ICD-9-CM Procedural

83.12 Adductor tenotomy of hip
83.13 Other tenotomy

27310

27310 Arthrotomy, knee, with exploration, drainage, or removal of foreign body (eg, infection)

ICD-9-CM Diagnostic

711.06 Pyogenic arthritis, lower leg — (Use additional code to identify infectious organism: 041.0-041.8)
719.46 Pain in joint, lower leg
726.60 Unspecified enthesopathy of knee ▽
891.0 Open wound of knee, leg (except thigh), and ankle, without mention of complication — (Use additional code to identify infection)
891.1 Open wound of knee, leg (except thigh), and ankle, complicated — (Use additional code to identify infection)
996.66 Infection and inflammatory reaction due to internal joint prosthesis — (Use additional code to identify specified infections)
996.67 Infection and inflammatory reaction due to other internal orthopedic device, implant, and graft — (Use additional code to identify specified infections)
998.4 Foreign body accidentally left during procedure, not elsewhere classified
998.59 Other postoperative infection — (Use additional code to identify infection)

ICD-9-CM Procedural

80.16 Other arthrotomy of knee

▽ Unspecified code
♀ Female diagnosis
☒ Manifestation code
♂ Male diagnosis

27315

27315 Neurectomy, hamstring muscle

ICD-9-CM Diagnostic

250.60 Diabetes with neurological manifestations, type II or unspecified type, not stated as uncontrolled — (Use additional code to identify manifestation: 337.1, 354.0-355.9, 357.2, 358.1, 713.5)
250.61 Diabetes with neurological manifestations, type I [juvenile type], not stated as uncontrolled — (Use additional code to identify manifestation: 337.1, 354.0-355.9, 357.2, 358.1, 713.5)
250.62 Diabetes with neurological manifestations, type II or unspecified type, uncontrolled — (Use additional code to identify manifestation: 337.1, 354.0-355.9, 357.2, 358.1, 713.5)
250.63 Diabetes with neurological manifestations, type I [juvenile type], uncontrolled — (Use additional code to identify manifestation: 337.1, 354.0-355.9, 357.2, 358.1, 713.5)
336.0 Syringomyelia and syringobulbia
337.1 Peripheral autonomic neuropathy in disorders classified elsewhere — (Code first underlying disease: 250.6, 277.3) ☒
355.1 Meralgia paresthetica
355.2 Other lesion of femoral nerve
355.71 Causalgia of lower limb
355.79 Other mononeuritis of lower limb
357.2 Polyneuropathy in diabetes — (Code first underlying disease: 250.6) ☒
713.5 Arthropathy associated with neurological disorders — (Code first underlying disease: 094.0, 250.6, 336.0) ☒
727.42 Ganglion of tendon sheath
729.2 Unspecified neuralgia, neuritis, and radiculitis ▽

ICD-9-CM Procedural

04.07 Other excision or avulsion of cranial and peripheral nerves

27320

27320 Neurectomy, popliteal (gastrocnemius)

ICD-9-CM Diagnostic

250.60 Diabetes with neurological manifestations, type II or unspecified type, not stated as uncontrolled — (Use additional code to identify manifestation: 337.1, 354.0-355.9, 357.2, 358.1, 713.5)
250.61 Diabetes with neurological manifestations, type I [juvenile type], not stated as uncontrolled — (Use additional code to identify manifestation: 337.1, 354.0-355.9, 357.2, 358.1, 713.5)
250.62 Diabetes with neurological manifestations, type II or unspecified type, uncontrolled — (Use additional code to identify manifestation: 337.1, 354.0-355.9, 357.2, 358.1, 713.5)
250.63 Diabetes with neurological manifestations, type I [juvenile type], uncontrolled — (Use additional code to identify manifestation: 337.1, 354.0-355.9, 357.2, 358.1, 713.5)
336.0 Syringomyelia and syringobulbia
355.1 Meralgia paresthetica
355.2 Other lesion of femoral nerve
355.3 Lesion of lateral popliteal nerve
355.4 Lesion of medial popliteal nerve
355.71 Causalgia of lower limb
355.79 Other mononeuritis of lower limb
713.5 Arthropathy associated with neurological disorders — (Code first underlying disease: 094.0, 250.6, 336.0) ☒
727.42 Ganglion of tendon sheath
729.2 Unspecified neuralgia, neuritis, and radiculitis ▽

ICD-9-CM Procedural

04.07 Other excision or avulsion of cranial and peripheral nerves

27323–27324

27323 Biopsy, soft tissue of thigh or knee area; superficial
27324 deep (subfascial or intramuscular)

ICD-9-CM Diagnostic

171.3 Malignant neoplasm of connective and other soft tissue of lower limb, including hip
172.7 Malignant melanoma of skin of lower limb, including hip
195.5 Malignant neoplasm of lower limb
198.89 Secondary malignant neoplasm of other specified sites
214.1 Lipoma of other skin and subcutaneous tissue
215.3 Other benign neoplasm of connective and other soft tissue of lower limb, including hip
238.1 Neoplasm of uncertain behavior of connective and other soft tissue ▽
239.2 Neoplasms of unspecified nature of bone, soft tissue, and skin
355.2 Other lesion of femoral nerve
359.6 Symptomatic inflammatory myopathy in diseases classified elsewhere — (Code first underlying disease: 135, 140.0-208.9, 277.3, 446.0, 710.0, 710.1, 710.2, 714.0) ☒
446.0 Polyarteritis nodosa
682.6 Cellulitis and abscess of leg, except foot — (Use additional code to identify organism)
696.1 Other psoriasis and similar disorders
709.4 Foreign body granuloma of skin and subcutaneous tissue
710.0 Systemic lupus erythematosus — (Use additional code to identify manifestation: 424.91, 581.81, 582.81, 583.81)
710.1 Systemic sclerosis — (Use additional code to identify manifestation: 359.6, 517.2)
710.2 Sicca syndrome
710.4 Polymyositis
710.9 Unspecified diffuse connective tissue disease ▽
714.0 Rheumatoid arthritis — (Use additional code to identify manifestation: 357.1, 359.6)
727.51 Synovial cyst of popliteal space
728.82 Foreign body granuloma of muscle
728.89 Other disorder of muscle, ligament, and fascia — (Use additional E code to identify drug, if drug-induced)
730.26 Unspecified osteomyelitis, lower leg — (Use additional code to identify organism, 041.1) ▽
733.90 Disorder of bone and cartilage, unspecified ▽
782.2 Localized superficial swelling, mass, or lump

ICD-9-CM Procedural

83.21 Biopsy of soft tissue

HCPCS Level II Supplies & Services

A4550 Surgical trays
A4580 Cast supplies (e.g., plaster)

27327–27329

27327 Excision, tumor, thigh or knee area; subcutaneous
27328 deep, subfascial, or intramuscular
27329 Radical resection of tumor (eg, malignant neoplasm), soft tissue of thigh or knee area

ICD-9-CM Diagnostic

171.3 Malignant neoplasm of connective and other soft tissue of lower limb, including hip
172.7 Malignant melanoma of skin of lower limb, including hip
173.7 Other malignant neoplasm of skin of lower limb, including hip
195.5 Malignant neoplasm of lower limb
198.89 Secondary malignant neoplasm of other specified sites
214.1 Lipoma of other skin and subcutaneous tissue
214.8 Lipoma of other specified sites
215.3 Other benign neoplasm of connective and other soft tissue of lower limb, including hip
228.1 Lymphangioma, any site
238.1 Neoplasm of uncertain behavior of connective and other soft tissue ▽
239.2 Neoplasms of unspecified nature of bone, soft tissue, and skin
782.2 Localized superficial swelling, mass, or lump

ICD-9-CM Procedural

83.31 Excision of lesion of tendon sheath
83.32 Excision of lesion of muscle
83.39 Excision of lesion of other soft tissue
83.49 Other excision of soft tissue

HCPCS Level II Supplies & Services

A4305 Disposable drug delivery system, flow rate of 50 ml or greater per hour
A4306 Disposable drug delivery system, flow rate of 5 ml or less per hour
A4550 Surgical trays
A4580 Cast supplies (e.g., plaster)
E0114 Crutches, underarm, other than wood, adjustable or fixed, pair, with pads, tips and handgrips

27330–27331

27330 Arthrotomy, knee; with synovial biopsy only
27331 including joint exploration, biopsy, or removal of loose or foreign bodies

ICD-9-CM Diagnostic

171.3 Malignant neoplasm of connective and other soft tissue of lower limb, including hip
198.89 Secondary malignant neoplasm of other specified sites
215.3 Other benign neoplasm of connective and other soft tissue of lower limb, including hip
238.1 Neoplasm of uncertain behavior of connective and other soft tissue
239.2 Neoplasms of unspecified nature of bone, soft tissue, and skin
275.40 Unspecified disorder of calcium metabolism — (Use additional code to identify any associated mental retardation)
275.42 Hypercalcemia — (Use additional code to identify any associated mental retardation)
275.49 Other disorders of calcium metabolism — (Use additional code to identify any associated mental retardation)
711.06 Pyogenic arthritis, lower leg — (Use additional code to identify infectious organism: 041.0-041.8)
712.96 Unspecified crystal arthropathy, lower leg
714.9 Unspecified inflammatory polyarthropathy
715.96 Osteoarthrosis, unspecified whether generalized or localized, lower leg
717.5 Derangement of meniscus, not elsewhere classified
717.6 Loose body in knee
717.9 Unspecified internal derangement of knee
718.46 Contracture of lower leg joint
718.76 Developmental dislocation of joint, lower leg
719.26 Villonodular synovitis, lower leg
719.46 Pain in joint, lower leg
719.66 Other symptoms referable to lower leg joint
727.50 Unspecified rupture of synovium
727.51 Synovial cyst of popliteal space
727.83 Plica syndrome
727.89 Other disorders of synovium, tendon, and bursa
732.7 Osteochondritis dissecans
836.2 Other tear of cartilage or meniscus of knee, current
891.1 Open wound of knee, leg (except thigh), and ankle, complicated — (Use additional code to identify infection)
996.4 Mechanical complication of internal orthopedic device, implant, and graft
V64.43 Arthroscopic surgical procedure converted to open procedure

ICD-9-CM Procedural

80.16 Other arthrotomy of knee
80.36 Biopsy of joint structure of knee

27332–27333

27332 Arthrotomy, with excision of semilunar cartilage (meniscectomy) knee; medial OR lateral
27333 medial AND lateral

ICD-9-CM Diagnostic

717.0 Old bucket handle tear of medial meniscus
717.1 Derangement of anterior horn of medial meniscus
717.2 Derangement of posterior horn of medial meniscus
717.3 Other and unspecified derangement of medial meniscus
717.40 Unspecified derangement of lateral meniscus
717.41 Bucket handle tear of lateral meniscus
717.42 Derangement of anterior horn of lateral meniscus
717.43 Derangement of posterior horn of lateral meniscus
717.49 Other derangement of lateral meniscus
717.5 Derangement of meniscus, not elsewhere classified
717.9 Unspecified internal derangement of knee
718.76 Developmental dislocation of joint, lower leg
719.66 Other symptoms referable to lower leg joint
719.86 Other specified disorders of lower leg joint
719.96 Unspecified disorder of lower leg joint
836.0 Tear of medial cartilage or meniscus of knee, current
836.1 Tear of lateral cartilage or meniscus of knee, current
836.2 Other tear of cartilage or meniscus of knee, current
836.50 Closed dislocation of knee, unspecified part
836.51 Closed anterior dislocation of tibia, proximal end
836.52 Closed posterior dislocation of tibia, proximal end
836.53 Closed medial dislocation of tibia, proximal end
836.54 Closed lateral dislocation of tibia, proximal end
836.59 Other closed dislocation of knee
959.7 Injury, other and unspecified, knee, leg, ankle, and foot
V64.43 Arthroscopic surgical procedure converted to open procedure

ICD-9-CM Procedural

80.6 Excision of semilunar cartilage of knee
81.42 Five-in-one repair of knee
81.43 Triad knee repair

27334–27335

27334 Arthrotomy, with synovectomy, knee; anterior OR posterior
27335 anterior AND posterior including popliteal area

ICD-9-CM Diagnostic

711.06 Pyogenic arthritis, lower leg — (Use additional code to identify infectious organism: 041.0-041.8)
714.9 Unspecified inflammatory polyarthropathy
715.96 Osteoarthrosis, unspecified whether generalized or localized, lower leg
719.26 Villonodular synovitis, lower leg
719.46 Pain in joint, lower leg
726.60 Unspecified enthesopathy of knee
726.65 Prepatellar bursitis
727.41 Ganglion of joint
727.42 Ganglion of tendon sheath
727.83 Plica syndrome
727.89 Other disorders of synovium, tendon, and bursa
727.9 Unspecified disorder of synovium, tendon, and bursa
996.4 Mechanical complication of internal orthopedic device, implant, and graft
996.77 Other complications due to internal joint prosthesis
V64.43 Arthroscopic surgical procedure converted to open procedure

ICD-9-CM Procedural

80.76 Synovectomy of knee

27340

27340 Excision, prepatellar bursa

ICD-9-CM Diagnostic

726.60 Unspecified enthesopathy of knee
726.65 Prepatellar bursitis
727.3 Other bursitis disorders
727.83 Plica syndrome
727.89 Other disorders of synovium, tendon, and bursa
782.2 Localized superficial swelling, mass, or lump

ICD-9-CM Procedural

83.5 Bursectomy

HCPCS Level II Supplies & Services

A4550 Surgical trays
A4580 Cast supplies (e.g., plaster)
A4590 Special casting material (e.g., fiberglass)
L1800 KO, elastic with stays, prefabricated, includes fitting and adjustment
L1825 KO, elastic knee cap, prefabricated, includes fitting and adjustment

27345

27345 Excision of synovial cyst of popliteal space (eg, Baker's cyst)

ICD-9-CM Diagnostic

727.51 Synovial cyst of popliteal space

ICD-9-CM Procedural

83.39 Excision of lesion of other soft tissue

27347

27347 Excision of lesion of meniscus or capsule (eg, cyst, ganglion), knee

ICD-9-CM Diagnostic

717.0 Old bucket handle tear of medial meniscus
717.1 Derangement of anterior horn of medial meniscus
717.2 Derangement of posterior horn of medial meniscus
717.3 Other and unspecified derangement of medial meniscus
717.40 Unspecified derangement of lateral meniscus
717.41 Bucket handle tear of lateral meniscus
717.42 Derangement of anterior horn of lateral meniscus
717.43 Derangement of posterior horn of lateral meniscus

Unspecified code
♀ Female diagnosis
Manifestation code
♂ Male diagnosis

717.49 Other derangement of lateral meniscus
717.5 Derangement of meniscus, not elsewhere classified
727.40 Unspecified synovial cyst ▽
727.41 Ganglion of joint

ICD-9-CM Procedural

80.6 Excision of semilunar cartilage of knee
80.96 Other excision of knee joint

27350

27350 Patellectomy or hemipatellectomy

ICD-9-CM Diagnostic

713.8 Arthropathy associated with other conditions classifiable elsewhere — (Code first underlying disease) ☒
715.16 Primary localized osteoarthrosis, lower leg
715.36 Localized osteoarthrosis not specified whether primary or secondary, lower leg
715.96 Osteoarthrosis, unspecified whether generalized or localized, lower leg ▽
717.7 Chondromalacia of patella
717.81 Old disruption of lateral collateral ligament
718.76 Developmental dislocation of joint, lower leg
727.65 Nontraumatic rupture of quadriceps tendon
730.16 Chronic osteomyelitis, lower leg — (Use additional code to identify organism, 041.1)
755.64 Congenital deformity of knee (joint)
822.0 Closed fracture of patella
822.1 Open fracture of patella
836.3 Closed dislocation of patella
836.4 Open dislocation of patella
996.4 Mechanical complication of internal orthopedic device, implant, and graft
996.77 Other complications due to internal joint prosthesis

ICD-9-CM Procedural

77.86 Other partial ostectomy of patella
77.96 Total ostectomy of patella

27355–27358

27355 Excision or curettage of bone cyst or benign tumor of femur;
27356 with allograft
27357 with autograft (includes obtaining graft)
27358 Excision or curettage of bone cyst or benign tumor of femur; with internal fixation (List in addition to code for primary procedure)

ICD-9-CM Diagnostic

213.7 Benign neoplasm of long bones of lower limb
238.0 Neoplasm of uncertain behavior of bone and articular cartilage
239.2 Neoplasms of unspecified nature of bone, soft tissue, and skin
733.21 Solitary bone cyst
733.29 Other cyst of bone
733.90 Disorder of bone and cartilage, unspecified ▽
756.4 Chondrodystrophy

ICD-9-CM Procedural

77.65 Local excision of lesion or tissue of femur
77.79 Excision of other bone for graft, except facial bones
78.05 Bone graft of femur
78.55 Internal fixation of femur without fracture reduction

27360

27360 Partial excision (craterization, saucerization, or diaphysectomy) bone, femur, proximal tibia and/or fibula (eg, osteomyelitis or bone abscess)

ICD-9-CM Diagnostic

730.06 Acute osteomyelitis, lower leg — (Use additional code to identify organism, 041.1)
730.16 Chronic osteomyelitis, lower leg — (Use additional code to identify organism, 041.1)
730.26 Unspecified osteomyelitis, lower leg — (Use additional code to identify organism, 041.1) ▽
730.36 Periostitis, without mention of osteomyelitis, lower leg — (Use additional code to identify organism, 041.1)
730.96 Unspecified infection of bone, lower leg — (Use additional code to identify organism, 041.1) ▽
732.4 Juvenile osteochondrosis of lower extremity, excluding foot
732.6 Other juvenile osteochondrosis
732.9 Unspecified osteochondropathy ▽
733.40 Aseptic necrosis of bone, site unspecified ▽
733.92 Chondromalacia

ICD-9-CM Procedural

77.85 Other partial ostectomy of femur
77.87 Other partial ostectomy of tibia and fibula

27365

27365 Radical resection of tumor, bone, femur or knee

ICD-9-CM Diagnostic

170.7 Malignant neoplasm of long bones of lower limb
213.7 Benign neoplasm of long bones of lower limb
238.0 Neoplasm of uncertain behavior of bone and articular cartilage
239.2 Neoplasms of unspecified nature of bone, soft tissue, and skin

ICD-9-CM Procedural

77.65 Local excision of lesion or tissue of femur
77.67 Local excision of lesion or tissue of tibia and fibula
77.85 Other partial ostectomy of femur
77.86 Other partial ostectomy of patella

27370

27370 Injection procedure for knee arthrography

ICD-9-CM Diagnostic

275.40 Unspecified disorder of calcium metabolism — (Use additional code to identify any associated mental retardation) ▽
275.42 Hypercalcemia — (Use additional code to identify any associated mental retardation)
275.49 Other disorders of calcium metabolism — (Use additional code to identify any associated mental retardation)
357.1 Polyneuropathy in collagen vascular disease — (Code first underlying disease: 446.0, 710.0, 714.0) ☒
359.6 Symptomatic inflammatory myopathy in diseases classified elsewhere — (Code first underlying disease: 135, 140.0-208.9, 277.3, 446.0, 710.0, 710.1, 710.2, 714.0) ☒
446.0 Polyarteritis nodosa
710.0 Systemic lupus erythematosus — (Use additional code to identify manifestation: 424.91, 581.81, 582.81, 583.81)
710.1 Systemic sclerosis — (Use additional code to identify manifestation: 359.6, 517.2)
710.2 Sicca syndrome
714.0 Rheumatoid arthritis — (Use additional code to identify manifestation: 357.1, 359.6)
715.16 Primary localized osteoarthrosis, lower leg
715.96 Osteoarthrosis, unspecified whether generalized or localized, lower leg ▽
716.96 Unspecified arthropathy, lower leg ▽
717.1 Derangement of anterior horn of medial meniscus
717.42 Derangement of anterior horn of lateral meniscus
717.6 Loose body in knee
718.76 Developmental dislocation of joint, lower leg
719.06 Effusion of lower leg joint
719.16 Hemarthrosis, lower leg
719.26 Villonodular synovitis, lower leg
719.36 Palindromic rheumatism, lower leg
719.46 Pain in joint, lower leg
719.56 Stiffness of joint, not elsewhere classified, lower leg
719.86 Other specified disorders of lower leg joint
719.96 Unspecified disorder of lower leg joint ▽
725 Polymyalgia rheumatica
836.2 Other tear of cartilage or meniscus of knee, current
836.50 Closed dislocation of knee, unspecified part ▽
836.60 Open dislocation of knee unspecified part ▽

ICD-9-CM Procedural

81.92 Injection of therapeutic substance into joint or ligament
88.32 Contrast arthrogram

HCPCS Level II Supplies & Services

A4550 Surgical trays
A9525 Supply of low or iso-osmolar contrast material, 10 mg of iodine

27372

27372 Removal of foreign body, deep, thigh region or knee area

ICD-9-CM Diagnostic

709.4 Foreign body granuloma of skin and subcutaneous tissue
717.6 Loose body in knee
728.82 Foreign body granuloma of muscle
729.6 Residual foreign body in soft tissue
890.1 Open wound of hip and thigh, complicated — (Use additional code to identify infection)
891.1 Open wound of knee, leg (except thigh), and ankle, complicated — (Use additional code to identify infection)
916.6 Hip, thigh, leg, and ankle, superficial foreign body (splinter), without major open wound and without mention of infection
996.4 Mechanical complication of internal orthopedic device, implant, and graft
996.78 Other complications due to other internal orthopedic device, implant, and graft
998.4 Foreign body accidentally left during procedure, not elsewhere classified

ICD-9-CM Procedural

83.02 Myotomy
83.09 Other incision of soft tissue
98.29 Removal of foreign body without incision from lower limb, except foot

HCPCS Level II Supplies & Services

A4550 Surgical trays
A4580 Cast supplies (e.g., plaster)
A4590 Special casting material (e.g., fiberglass)
E0112 Crutches, underarm, wood, adjustable or fixed, pair, with pads, tips and handgrips
L1800 KO, elastic with stays, prefabricated, includes fitting and adjustment

27380–27381

27380 Suture of infrapatellar tendon; primary
27381 secondary reconstruction, including fascial or tendon graft

ICD-9-CM Diagnostic

717.89 Other internal derangement of knee
718.36 Recurrent dislocation of lower leg joint
727.66 Nontraumatic rupture of patellar tendon
822.0 Closed fracture of patella
822.1 Open fracture of patella
844.8 Sprain and strain of other specified sites of knee and leg
891.2 Open wound of knee, leg (except thigh), and ankle, with tendon involvement — (Use additional code to identify infection)

ICD-9-CM Procedural

83.62 Delayed suture of tendon
83.64 Other suture of tendon
83.81 Tendon graft
83.82 Graft of muscle or fascia

27385–27386

27385 Suture of quadriceps or hamstring muscle rupture; primary
27386 secondary reconstruction, including fascial or tendon graft

ICD-9-CM Diagnostic

727.65 Nontraumatic rupture of quadriceps tendon
821.01 Closed fracture of shaft of femur
822.0 Closed fracture of patella
843.8 Sprain and strain of other specified sites of hip and thigh
844.8 Sprain and strain of other specified sites of knee and leg
890.1 Open wound of hip and thigh, complicated — (Use additional code to identify infection)
890.2 Open wound of hip and thigh, with tendon involvement — (Use additional code to identify infection)
905.7 Late effect of sprain and strain without mention of tendon injury
905.8 Late effect of tendon injury
906.1 Late effect of open wound of extremities without mention of tendon injury
906.3 Late effect of contusion
906.4 Late effect of crushing

ICD-9-CM Procedural

83.65 Other suture of muscle or fascia
83.81 Tendon graft
83.82 Graft of muscle or fascia
83.87 Other plastic operations on muscle

27390–27392

27390 Tenotomy, open, hamstring, knee to hip; single tendon
27391 multiple tendons, one leg
27392 multiple tendons, bilateral

ICD-9-CM Diagnostic

718.45 Contracture of pelvic joint
727.81 Contracture of tendon (sheath)
727.82 Calcium deposits in tendon and bursa
727.89 Other disorders of synovium, tendon, and bursa
727.9 Unspecified disorder of synovium, tendon, and bursa ▽
728.0 Infective myositis
728.13 Postoperative heterotopic calcification
728.85 Spasm of muscle
728.9 Unspecified disorder of muscle, ligament, and fascia ▽
736.89 Other acquired deformity of other parts of limb
785.4 Gangrene — (Code first any associated underlying condition:250.7, 443.0)
924.00 Contusion of thigh

ICD-9-CM Procedural

83.13 Other tenotomy

27393–27395

27393 Lengthening of hamstring tendon; single tendon
27394 multiple tendons, one leg
27395 multiple tendons, bilateral

ICD-9-CM Diagnostic

343.9 Unspecified infantile cerebral palsy ▽
718.45 Contracture of pelvic joint
727.81 Contracture of tendon (sheath)
728.85 Spasm of muscle
728.89 Other disorder of muscle, ligament, and fascia — (Use additional E code to identify drug, if drug-induced)
754.30 Congenital dislocation of hip, unilateral

ICD-9-CM Procedural

83.85 Other change in muscle or tendon length

27396–27397

27396 Transplant, hamstring tendon to patella; single tendon
27397 multiple tendons

ICD-9-CM Diagnostic

333.7 Symptomatic torsion dystonia — (Use additional E code to identify drug, if drug-induced)
343.2 Quadriplegic infantile cerebral palsy
343.9 Unspecified infantile cerebral palsy ▽
355.8 Unspecified mononeuritis of lower limb ▽
718.46 Contracture of lower leg joint
729.9 Other and unspecified disorders of soft tissue
754.89 Other specified nonteratogenic anomalies
785.4 Gangrene — (Code first any associated underlying condition:250.7, 443.0)
843.8 Sprain and strain of other specified sites of hip and thigh
843.9 Sprain and strain of unspecified site of hip and thigh ▽
890.1 Open wound of hip and thigh, complicated — (Use additional code to identify infection)
890.2 Open wound of hip and thigh, with tendon involvement — (Use additional code to identify infection)
928.00 Crushing injury of thigh — (Use additional code to identify any associated injuries: 800-829, 850.0-854.1, 860.0-869.1)
928.10 Crushing injury of lower leg — (Use additional code to identify any associated injuries: 800-829, 850.0-854.1, 860.0-869.1)
928.11 Crushing injury of knee — (Use additional code to identify any associated injuries: 800-829, 850.0-854.1, 860.0-869.1)

ICD-9-CM Procedural

83.75 Tendon transfer or transplantation

27400

27400 Transfer, tendon or muscle, hamstrings to femur (eg, Egger's type procedure)

ICD-9-CM Diagnostic

718.46 Contracture of lower leg joint
726.5 Enthesopathy of hip region

736.41 Genu valgum (acquired)
754.41 Congenital dislocation of knee (with genu recurvatum)
754.42 Congenital bowing of femur
755.35 Congenital longitudinal deficiency, tibiofibular, complete or partial (with or without distal deficiencies, incomplete)
755.61 Congenital coxa valga
781.2 Abnormality of gait
996.4 Mechanical complication of internal orthopedic device, implant, and graft
996.77 Other complications due to internal joint prosthesis

ICD-9-CM Procedural

83.75 Tendon transfer or transplantation
83.79 Other muscle transposition

27403

27403 Arthrotomy with meniscus repair, knee

ICD-9-CM Diagnostic

717.0 Old bucket handle tear of medial meniscus
717.1 Derangement of anterior horn of medial meniscus
717.2 Derangement of posterior horn of medial meniscus
717.3 Other and unspecified derangement of medial meniscus ▽
717.40 Unspecified derangement of lateral meniscus ▽
717.41 Bucket handle tear of lateral meniscus
717.42 Derangement of anterior horn of lateral meniscus
717.43 Derangement of posterior horn of lateral meniscus
717.5 Derangement of meniscus, not elsewhere classified
717.6 Loose body in knee
836.0 Tear of medial cartilage or meniscus of knee, current
836.1 Tear of lateral cartilage or meniscus of knee, current
836.2 Other tear of cartilage or meniscus of knee, current
V64.43 Arthroscopic surgical procedure converted to open procedure

ICD-9-CM Procedural

81.47 Other repair of knee

27405–27409

27405 Repair, primary, torn ligament and/or capsule, knee; collateral
27407 cruciate
27409 collateral and cruciate ligaments

ICD-9-CM Diagnostic

716.16 Traumatic arthropathy, lower leg
717.81 Old disruption of lateral collateral ligament
717.82 Old disruption of medial collateral ligament
717.83 Old disruption of anterior cruciate ligament
717.84 Old disruption of posterior cruciate ligament
717.85 Old disruption of other ligament of knee
717.89 Other internal derangement of knee
836.0 Tear of medial cartilage or meniscus of knee, current
836.1 Tear of lateral cartilage or meniscus of knee, current
844.0 Sprain and strain of lateral collateral ligament of knee
844.1 Sprain and strain of medial collateral ligament of knee
844.2 Sprain and strain of cruciate ligament of knee
844.8 Sprain and strain of other specified sites of knee and leg
844.9 Sprain and strain of unspecified site of knee and leg ▽
891.1 Open wound of knee, leg (except thigh), and ankle, complicated — (Use additional code to identify infection)

ICD-9-CM Procedural

81.42 Five-in-one repair of knee
81.43 Triad knee repair
81.45 Other repair of the cruciate ligaments
81.46 Other repair of the collateral ligaments
81.95 Suture of capsule or ligament of other lower extremity

27412

27412 Autologous chondrocyte implantation, knee

ICD-9-CM Diagnostic

714.30 Polyarticular juvenile rheumatoid arthritis, chronic or unspecified
715.16 Primary localized osteoarthrosis, lower leg
715.26 Secondary localized osteoarthrosis, lower leg
715.36 Localized osteoarthrosis not specified whether primary or secondary, lower leg
715.96 Osteoarthrosis, unspecified whether generalized or localized, lower leg ▽
717.7 Chondromalacia of patella
717.83 Old disruption of anterior cruciate ligament
719.96 Unspecified disorder of lower leg joint ▽
732.4 Juvenile osteochondrosis of lower extremity, excluding foot
732.7 Osteochondritis dissecans
732.9 Unspecified osteochondropathy ▽
844.2 Sprain and strain of cruciate ligament of knee

ICD-9-CM Procedural

81.47 Other repair of knee

27415

27415 Osteochondral allograft, knee, open

ICD-9-CM Diagnostic

714.30 Polyarticular juvenile rheumatoid arthritis, chronic or unspecified
715.16 Primary localized osteoarthrosis, lower leg
715.26 Secondary localized osteoarthrosis, lower leg
715.36 Localized osteoarthrosis not specified whether primary or secondary, lower leg
715.96 Osteoarthrosis, unspecified whether generalized or localized, lower leg ▽
717.7 Chondromalacia of patella
717.83 Old disruption of anterior cruciate ligament
719.96 Unspecified disorder of lower leg joint ▽
732.4 Juvenile osteochondrosis of lower extremity, excluding foot
732.7 Osteochondritis dissecans
732.9 Unspecified osteochondropathy ▽
844.2 Sprain and strain of cruciate ligament of knee

ICD-9-CM Procedural

81.47 Other repair of knee

27418

27418 Anterior tibial tubercleplasty (eg, Maquet type procedure)

ICD-9-CM Diagnostic

713.8 Arthropathy associated with other conditions classifiable elsewhere — (Code first underlying disease) ☒
717.7 Chondromalacia of patella
717.81 Old disruption of lateral collateral ligament
717.82 Old disruption of medial collateral ligament
717.83 Old disruption of anterior cruciate ligament
717.84 Old disruption of posterior cruciate ligament
717.85 Old disruption of other ligament of knee
717.89 Other internal derangement of knee
755.30 Congenital unspecified reduction deformity of lower limb ▽
755.64 Congenital deformity of knee (joint)
755.69 Other congenital anomaly of lower limb, including pelvic girdle
836.3 Closed dislocation of patella
836.4 Open dislocation of patella

ICD-9-CM Procedural

77.87 Other partial ostectomy of tibia and fibula

27420

27420 Reconstruction of dislocating patella; (eg, Hauser type procedure)

ICD-9-CM Diagnostic

713.8 Arthropathy associated with other conditions classifiable elsewhere — (Code first underlying disease) ☒
717.7 Chondromalacia of patella
718.36 Recurrent dislocation of lower leg joint
718.86 Other joint derangement, not elsewhere classified, lower leg
719.46 Pain in joint, lower leg
736.41 Genu valgum (acquired)
736.5 Genu recurvatum (acquired)
754.40 Congenital genu recurvatum
754.41 Congenital dislocation of knee (with genu recurvatum)
755.35 Congenital longitudinal deficiency, tibiofibular, complete or partial (with or without distal deficiencies, incomplete)
755.61 Congenital coxa valga
755.64 Congenital deformity of knee (joint)
755.69 Other congenital anomaly of lower limb, including pelvic girdle
836.3 Closed dislocation of patella
836.4 Open dislocation of patella

▽ Unspecified code ☒ Manifestation code
♀ Female diagnosis ♂ Male diagnosis

ICD-9-CM Procedural
81.44 Patellar stabilization

27422
27422 Reconstruction of dislocating patella; with extensor realignment and/or muscle advancement or release (eg, Campbell, Goldwaite type procedure)

ICD-9-CM Diagnostic
713.8 Arthropathy associated with other conditions classifiable elsewhere — (Code first underlying disease) ☒
717.7 Chondromalacia of patella
718.36 Recurrent dislocation of lower leg joint
718.86 Other joint derangement, not elsewhere classified, lower leg
719.46 Pain in joint, lower leg
736.41 Genu valgum (acquired)
736.5 Genu recurvatum (acquired)
754.40 Congenital genu recurvatum
754.41 Congenital dislocation of knee (with genu recurvatum)
755.35 Congenital longitudinal deficiency, tibiofibular, complete or partial (with or without distal deficiencies, incomplete)
755.61 Congenital coxa valga
755.64 Congenital deformity of knee (joint)
755.69 Other congenital anomaly of lower limb, including pelvic girdle
836.3 Closed dislocation of patella
836.4 Open dislocation of patella

ICD-9-CM Procedural
81.44 Patellar stabilization

27424
27424 Reconstruction of dislocating patella; with patellectomy

ICD-9-CM Diagnostic
713.8 Arthropathy associated with other conditions classifiable elsewhere — (Code first underlying disease) ☒
717.7 Chondromalacia of patella
718.36 Recurrent dislocation of lower leg joint
718.86 Other joint derangement, not elsewhere classified, lower leg
719.46 Pain in joint, lower leg
736.41 Genu valgum (acquired)
736.5 Genu recurvatum (acquired)
754.40 Congenital genu recurvatum
754.41 Congenital dislocation of knee (with genu recurvatum)
755.35 Congenital longitudinal deficiency, tibiofibular, complete or partial (with or without distal deficiencies, incomplete)
755.61 Congenital coxa valga
755.64 Congenital deformity of knee (joint)
755.69 Other congenital anomaly of lower limb, including pelvic girdle
836.3 Closed dislocation of patella
836.4 Open dislocation of patella

ICD-9-CM Procedural
77.96 Total ostectomy of patella
81.44 Patellar stabilization

27425
27425 Lateral retinacular release, open

ICD-9-CM Diagnostic
715.16 Primary localized osteoarthrosis, lower leg
715.96 Osteoarthrosis, unspecified whether generalized or localized, lower leg ▽
717.6 Loose body in knee
717.7 Chondromalacia of patella
717.9 Unspecified internal derangement of knee ▽
718.36 Recurrent dislocation of lower leg joint
718.46 Contracture of lower leg joint
718.56 Ankylosis of lower leg joint
718.86 Other joint derangement, not elsewhere classified, lower leg
719.26 Villonodular synovitis, lower leg
719.86 Other specified disorders of lower leg joint
733.92 Chondromalacia
755.64 Congenital deformity of knee (joint)
822.1 Open fracture of patella
836.3 Closed dislocation of patella
836.50 Closed dislocation of knee, unspecified part ▽
836.54 Closed lateral dislocation of tibia, proximal end
844.2 Sprain and strain of cruciate ligament of knee
996.4 Mechanical complication of internal orthopedic device, implant, and graft
V64.43 Arthroscopic surgical procedure converted to open procedure

ICD-9-CM Procedural
80.46 Division of joint capsule, ligament, or cartilage of knee

27427–27429
27427 Ligamentous reconstruction (augmentation), knee; extra-articular
27428 intra-articular (open)
27429 intra-articular (open) and extra-articular

ICD-9-CM Diagnostic
717.81 Old disruption of lateral collateral ligament
717.82 Old disruption of medial collateral ligament
717.83 Old disruption of anterior cruciate ligament
717.84 Old disruption of posterior cruciate ligament
717.89 Other internal derangement of knee
717.9 Unspecified internal derangement of knee ▽
718.56 Ankylosis of lower leg joint
718.86 Other joint derangement, not elsewhere classified, lower leg
728.89 Other disorder of muscle, ligament, and fascia — (Use additional E code to identify drug, if drug-induced)
728.9 Unspecified disorder of muscle, ligament, and fascia ▽
836.2 Other tear of cartilage or meniscus of knee, current
844.0 Sprain and strain of lateral collateral ligament of knee
844.1 Sprain and strain of medial collateral ligament of knee
844.2 Sprain and strain of cruciate ligament of knee
844.8 Sprain and strain of other specified sites of knee and leg
844.9 Sprain and strain of unspecified site of knee and leg ▽
891.2 Open wound of knee, leg (except thigh), and ankle, with tendon involvement — (Use additional code to identify infection)

ICD-9-CM Procedural
81.45 Other repair of the cruciate ligaments
81.46 Other repair of the collateral ligaments
81.47 Other repair of knee

27430
27430 Quadricepsplasty (eg, Bennett or Thompson type)

ICD-9-CM Diagnostic
713.8 Arthropathy associated with other conditions classifiable elsewhere — (Code first underlying disease) ☒
718.46 Contracture of lower leg joint
890.1 Open wound of hip and thigh, complicated — (Use additional code to identify infection)
996.4 Mechanical complication of internal orthopedic device, implant, and graft
996.66 Infection and inflammatory reaction due to internal joint prosthesis — (Use additional code to identify specified infections)

ICD-9-CM Procedural
83.86 Quadricepsplasty

27435
27435 Capsulotomy, posterior capsular release, knee

ICD-9-CM Diagnostic
715.96 Osteoarthrosis, unspecified whether generalized or localized, lower leg ▽
716.16 Traumatic arthropathy, lower leg
717.41 Bucket handle tear of lateral meniscus
717.7 Chondromalacia of patella
717.81 Old disruption of lateral collateral ligament
719.26 Villonodular synovitis, lower leg
726.60 Unspecified enthesopathy of knee ▽
726.61 Pes anserinus tendinitis or bursitis
727.00 Unspecified synovitis and tenosynovitis ▽
727.60 Nontraumatic rupture of unspecified tendon ▽
727.65 Nontraumatic rupture of quadriceps tendon
727.66 Nontraumatic rupture of patellar tendon
727.9 Unspecified disorder of synovium, tendon, and bursa ▽
844.0 Sprain and strain of lateral collateral ligament of knee
844.1 Sprain and strain of medial collateral ligament of knee
844.2 Sprain and strain of cruciate ligament of knee

844.8 Sprain and strain of other specified sites of knee and leg

ICD-9-CM Procedural
80.46 Division of joint capsule, ligament, or cartilage of knee

27437–27438
27437 Arthroplasty, patella; without prosthesis
27438 with prosthesis

ICD-9-CM Diagnostic
715.09 Generalized osteoarthrosis, involving multiple sites
715.16 Primary localized osteoarthrosis, lower leg
715.89 Osteoarthrosis involving multiple sites, but not specified as generalized
715.96 Osteoarthrosis, unspecified whether generalized or localized, lower leg ▽
717.7 Chondromalacia of patella
718.26 Pathological dislocation of lower leg joint
718.36 Recurrent dislocation of lower leg joint
718.86 Other joint derangement, not elsewhere classified, lower leg
726.64 Patellar tendinitis
730.16 Chronic osteomyelitis, lower leg — (Use additional code to identify organism, 041.1)
732.4 Juvenile osteochondrosis of lower extremity, excluding foot
822.0 Closed fracture of patella
822.1 Open fracture of patella
836.3 Closed dislocation of patella
836.4 Open dislocation of patella
996.4 Mechanical complication of internal orthopedic device, implant, and graft
996.59 Mechanical complication due to other implant and internal device, not elsewhere classified

ICD-9-CM Procedural
81.47 Other repair of knee
81.54 Total knee replacement

27440–27441
27440 Arthroplasty, knee, tibial plateau;
27441 with debridement and partial synovectomy

ICD-9-CM Diagnostic
715.16 Primary localized osteoarthrosis, lower leg
715.96 Osteoarthrosis, unspecified whether generalized or localized, lower leg ▽
716.96 Unspecified arthropathy, lower leg ▽
718.56 Ankylosis of lower leg joint
719.26 Villonodular synovitis, lower leg
719.66 Other symptoms referable to lower leg joint
726.60 Unspecified enthesopathy of knee ▽
726.91 Exostosis of unspecified site ▽
727.00 Unspecified synovitis and tenosynovitis ▽
727.09 Other synovitis and tenosynovitis
730.16 Chronic osteomyelitis, lower leg — (Use additional code to identify organism, 041.1)
730.36 Periostitis, without mention of osteomyelitis, lower leg — (Use additional code to identify organism, 041.1)
733.81 Malunion of fracture
733.82 Nonunion of fracture
733.92 Chondromalacia
823.00 Closed fracture of upper end of tibia

ICD-9-CM Procedural
80.76 Synovectomy of knee
81.47 Other repair of knee

27442–27443
27442 Arthroplasty, femoral condyles or tibial plateau(s), knee;
27443 with debridement and partial synovectomy

ICD-9-CM Diagnostic
357.1 Polyneuropathy in collagen vascular disease — (Code first underlying disease: 446.0, 710.0, 714.0) ☒
359.6 Symptomatic inflammatory myopathy in diseases classified elsewhere — (Code first underlying disease: 135, 140.0-208.9, 277.3, 446.0, 710.0, 710.1, 710.2, 714.0) ☒
446.0 Polyarteritis nodosa
710.0 Systemic lupus erythematosus — (Use additional code to identify manifestation: 424.91, 581.81, 582.81, 583.81)
710.1 Systemic sclerosis — (Use additional code to identify manifestation: 359.6, 517.2)
710.2 Sicca syndrome
714.0 Rheumatoid arthritis — (Use additional code to identify manifestation: 357.1, 359.6)
715.16 Primary localized osteoarthrosis, lower leg
715.96 Osteoarthrosis, unspecified whether generalized or localized, lower leg ▽
716.16 Traumatic arthropathy, lower leg
716.96 Unspecified arthropathy, lower leg ▽
717.41 Bucket handle tear of lateral meniscus
717.42 Derangement of anterior horn of lateral meniscus
717.5 Derangement of meniscus, not elsewhere classified
717.83 Old disruption of anterior cruciate ligament
717.84 Old disruption of posterior cruciate ligament
719.26 Villonodular synovitis, lower leg
726.60 Unspecified enthesopathy of knee ▽
726.91 Exostosis of unspecified site ▽
727.00 Unspecified synovitis and tenosynovitis ▽
727.09 Other synovitis and tenosynovitis

ICD-9-CM Procedural
80.76 Synovectomy of knee
81.47 Other repair of knee

27445
27445 Arthroplasty, knee, hinge prosthesis (eg, Walldius type)

ICD-9-CM Diagnostic
714.4 Chronic postrheumatic arthropathy
715.16 Primary localized osteoarthrosis, lower leg
715.36 Localized osteoarthrosis not specified whether primary or secondary, lower leg
715.96 Osteoarthrosis, unspecified whether generalized or localized, lower leg ▽
716.16 Traumatic arthropathy, lower leg
716.96 Unspecified arthropathy, lower leg ▽
719.46 Pain in joint, lower leg

ICD-9-CM Procedural
81.54 Total knee replacement

27446–27447
27446 Arthroplasty, knee, condyle and plateau; medial OR lateral compartment
27447 medial AND lateral compartments with or without patella resurfacing (total knee arthroplasty)

ICD-9-CM Diagnostic
357.1 Polyneuropathy in collagen vascular disease — (Code first underlying disease: 446.0, 710.0, 714.0) ☒
359.6 Symptomatic inflammatory myopathy in diseases classified elsewhere — (Code first underlying disease: 135, 140.0-208.9, 277.3, 446.0, 710.0, 710.1, 710.2, 714.0) ☒
446.0 Polyarteritis nodosa
710.0 Systemic lupus erythematosus — (Use additional code to identify manifestation: 424.91, 581.81, 582.81, 583.81)
710.1 Systemic sclerosis — (Use additional code to identify manifestation: 359.6, 517.2)
710.2 Sicca syndrome
714.0 Rheumatoid arthritis — (Use additional code to identify manifestation: 357.1, 359.6)
714.30 Polyarticular juvenile rheumatoid arthritis, chronic or unspecified
714.31 Polyarticular juvenile rheumatoid arthritis, acute
714.4 Chronic postrheumatic arthropathy
715.09 Generalized osteoarthrosis, involving multiple sites
715.16 Primary localized osteoarthrosis, lower leg
715.26 Secondary localized osteoarthrosis, lower leg
715.36 Localized osteoarthrosis not specified whether primary or secondary, lower leg
715.96 Osteoarthrosis, unspecified whether generalized or localized, lower leg ▽
716.06 Kaschin-Beck disease, lower leg
716.16 Traumatic arthropathy, lower leg
716.96 Unspecified arthropathy, lower leg ▽
719.46 Pain in joint, lower leg
733.49 Aseptic necrosis of other bone site
755.64 Congenital deformity of knee (joint)
V43.65 Knee joint replacement by other means — (This code is intended for use when these conditions are recorded as diagnoses or problems)

▽ Unspecified code
♀ Female diagnosis
☒ Manifestation code
♂ Male diagnosis

ICD-9-CM Procedural

81.47 Other repair of knee
81.54 Total knee replacement

27448–27450

27448 Osteotomy, femur, shaft or supracondylar; without fixation
27450 with fixation

ICD-9-CM Diagnostic

715.96 Osteoarthrosis, unspecified whether generalized or localized, lower leg ▽
733.81 Malunion of fracture
733.82 Nonunion of fracture
733.91 Arrest of bone development or growth
736.81 Unequal leg length (acquired)
736.89 Other acquired deformity of other parts of limb
755.60 Unspecified congenital anomaly of lower limb ▽
755.61 Congenital coxa valga
755.62 Congenital coxa vara
755.63 Other congenital deformity of hip (joint)

ICD-9-CM Procedural

77.25 Wedge osteotomy of femur
77.35 Other division of femur
78.55 Internal fixation of femur without fracture reduction

27454

27454 Osteotomy, multiple, with realignment on intramedullary rod, femoral shaft (eg, Sofield type procedure)

ICD-9-CM Diagnostic

170.7 Malignant neoplasm of long bones of lower limb
730.05 Acute osteomyelitis, pelvic region and thigh — (Use additional code to identify organism, 041.1)
732.9 Unspecified osteochondropathy ▽
733.81 Malunion of fracture
733.82 Nonunion of fracture
733.91 Arrest of bone development or growth
736.81 Unequal leg length (acquired)
736.89 Other acquired deformity of other parts of limb
755.60 Unspecified congenital anomaly of lower limb ▽
755.61 Congenital coxa valga
755.62 Congenital coxa vara
755.63 Other congenital deformity of hip (joint)
V54.02 Encounter for lengthening/adjustment of growth rod

ICD-9-CM Procedural

77.35 Other division of femur
78.55 Internal fixation of femur without fracture reduction

27455–27457

27455 Osteotomy, proximal tibia, including fibular excision or osteotomy (includes correction of genu varus (bowleg) or genu valgus (knock-knee)); before epiphyseal closure
27457 after epiphyseal closure

ICD-9-CM Diagnostic

268.1 Rickets, late effect — (Use additional code to identify the nature of late effect)
343.9 Unspecified infantile cerebral palsy ▽
715.16 Primary localized osteoarthrosis, lower leg
715.96 Osteoarthrosis, unspecified whether generalized or localized, lower leg ▽
716.96 Unspecified arthropathy, lower leg ▽
718.36 Recurrent dislocation of lower leg joint
719.66 Other symptoms referable to lower leg joint
732.4 Juvenile osteochondrosis of lower extremity, excluding foot
732.7 Osteochondritis dissecans
733.81 Malunion of fracture
733.82 Nonunion of fracture
736.41 Genu valgum (acquired)
736.42 Genu varum (acquired)
736.81 Unequal leg length (acquired)
736.89 Other acquired deformity of other parts of limb
754.43 Congenital bowing of tibia and fibula
755.64 Congenital deformity of knee (joint)

ICD-9-CM Procedural

77.37 Other division of tibia and fibula
77.87 Other partial ostectomy of tibia and fibula

27465–27468

27465 Osteoplasty, femur; shortening (excluding 64876)
27466 lengthening
27468 combined, lengthening and shortening with femoral segment transfer

ICD-9-CM Diagnostic

732.2 Nontraumatic slipped upper femoral epiphysis
732.4 Juvenile osteochondrosis of lower extremity, excluding foot
733.15 Pathologic fracture of other specified part of femur
733.81 Malunion of fracture
733.82 Nonunion of fracture
733.99 Other disorders of bone and cartilage
736.81 Unequal leg length (acquired)
754.89 Other specified nonteratogenic anomalies
755.30 Congenital unspecified reduction deformity of lower limb ▽
755.33 Congenital longitudinal deficiency, combined, involving femur, tibia, and fibula (complete or incomplete)

ICD-9-CM Procedural

78.15 Application of external fixation device, femur
78.25 Limb shortening procedures, femur
78.35 Limb lengthening procedures, femur
84.53 Implantation of internal limb lengthening device with kinetic distraction
84.54 Implantation of other internal limb lengthening device

27470–27472

27470 Repair, nonunion or malunion, femur, distal to head and neck; without graft (eg, compression technique)
27472 with iliac or other autogenous bone graft (includes obtaining graft)

ICD-9-CM Diagnostic

733.81 Malunion of fracture
733.82 Nonunion of fracture
996.4 Mechanical complication of internal orthopedic device, implant, and graft
996.67 Infection and inflammatory reaction due to other internal orthopedic device, implant, and graft — (Use additional code to identify specified infections)
996.77 Other complications due to internal joint prosthesis
996.78 Other complications due to other internal orthopedic device, implant, and graft

ICD-9-CM Procedural

77.79 Excision of other bone for graft, except facial bones
78.05 Bone graft of femur
78.45 Other repair or plastic operations on femur
78.75 Osteoclasis of femur

27475–27479

27475 Arrest, epiphyseal, any method (eg, epiphysiodesis); distal femur
27477 tibia and fibula, proximal
27479 combined distal femur, proximal tibia and fibula

ICD-9-CM Diagnostic

715.96 Osteoarthrosis, unspecified whether generalized or localized, lower leg ▽
716.16 Traumatic arthropathy, lower leg
716.96 Unspecified arthropathy, lower leg ▽
718.56 Ankylosis of lower leg joint
730.16 Chronic osteomyelitis, lower leg — (Use additional code to identify organism, 041.1)
736.41 Genu valgum (acquired)
736.42 Genu varum (acquired)
736.81 Unequal leg length (acquired)
755.30 Congenital unspecified reduction deformity of lower limb ▽

ICD-9-CM Procedural

78.25 Limb shortening procedures, femur
78.27 Limb shortening procedures, tibia and fibula

▽ Unspecified code ♀ Female diagnosis ☒ Manifestation code ♂ Male diagnosis

27485

27485 Arrest, hemiepiphyseal, distal femur or proximal tibia or fibula (eg, genu varus or valgus)

ICD-9-CM Diagnostic

718.56 Ankylosis of lower leg joint
736.41 Genu valgum (acquired)
736.42 Genu varum (acquired)
736.81 Unequal leg length (acquired)
755.30 Congenital unspecified reduction deformity of lower limb ▽
755.64 Congenital deformity of knee (joint)

ICD-9-CM Procedural

78.25 Limb shortening procedures, femur
78.27 Limb shortening procedures, tibia and fibula
78.45 Other repair or plastic operations on femur

27486–27487

27486 Revision of total knee arthroplasty, with or without allograft; one component
27487 femoral and entire tibial component

ICD-9-CM Diagnostic

357.1 Polyneuropathy in collagen vascular disease — (Code first underlying disease: 446.0, 710.0, 714.0) ☒
359.6 Symptomatic inflammatory myopathy in diseases classified elsewhere — (Code first underlying disease: 135, 140.0-208.9, 277.3, 446.0, 710.0, 710.1, 710.2, 714.0) ☒
446.0 Polyarteritis nodosa
710.0 Systemic lupus erythematosus — (Use additional code to identify manifestation: 424.91, 581.81, 582.81, 583.81)
710.1 Systemic sclerosis — (Use additional code to identify manifestation: 359.6, 517.2)
710.2 Sicca syndrome
714.0 Rheumatoid arthritis — (Use additional code to identify manifestation: 357.1, 359.6)
715.16 Primary localized osteoarthrosis, lower leg
715.96 Osteoarthrosis, unspecified whether generalized or localized, lower leg ▽
716.16 Traumatic arthropathy, lower leg
716.96 Unspecified arthropathy, lower leg ▽
717.6 Loose body in knee
718.36 Recurrent dislocation of lower leg joint
718.46 Contracture of lower leg joint
718.56 Ankylosis of lower leg joint
718.86 Other joint derangement, not elsewhere classified, lower leg
736.41 Genu valgum (acquired)
996.4 Mechanical complication of internal orthopedic device, implant, and graft
996.66 Infection and inflammatory reaction due to internal joint prosthesis — (Use additional code to identify specified infections)
996.70 Other complications due to unspecified device, implant, and graft ▽
996.77 Other complications due to internal joint prosthesis
V43.65 Knee joint replacement by other means — (This code is intended for use when these conditions are recorded as diagnoses or problems)

ICD-9-CM Procedural

81.55 Revision of knee replacement

27488

27488 Removal of prosthesis, including total knee prosthesis, methylmethacrylate with or without insertion of spacer, knee

ICD-9-CM Diagnostic

711.06 Pyogenic arthritis, lower leg — (Use additional code to identify infectious organism: 041.0-041.8)
711.96 Unspecified infective arthritis, lower leg ▽
715.16 Primary localized osteoarthrosis, lower leg
715.96 Osteoarthrosis, unspecified whether generalized or localized, lower leg ▽
716.86 Other specified arthropathy, lower leg
717.6 Loose body in knee
719.26 Villonodular synovitis, lower leg
730.06 Acute osteomyelitis, lower leg — (Use additional code to identify organism, 041.1)
730.16 Chronic osteomyelitis, lower leg — (Use additional code to identify organism, 041.1)
736.6 Other acquired deformities of knee
996.4 Mechanical complication of internal orthopedic device, implant, and graft
996.66 Infection and inflammatory reaction due to internal joint prosthesis — (Use additional code to identify specified infections)
996.67 Infection and inflammatory reaction due to other internal orthopedic device, implant, and graft — (Use additional code to identify specified infections)
996.77 Other complications due to internal joint prosthesis
996.78 Other complications due to other internal orthopedic device, implant, and graft

ICD-9-CM Procedural

80.06 Arthrotomy for removal of prosthesis of knee

27495

27495 Prophylactic treatment (nailing, pinning, plating or wiring) with or without methylmethacrylate, femur

ICD-9-CM Diagnostic

170.7 Malignant neoplasm of long bones of lower limb
198.5 Secondary malignant neoplasm of bone and bone marrow
213.7 Benign neoplasm of long bones of lower limb
238.0 Neoplasm of uncertain behavior of bone and articular cartilage
239.2 Neoplasms of unspecified nature of bone, soft tissue, and skin
268.1 Rickets, late effect — (Use additional code to identify the nature of late effect)
275.40 Unspecified disorder of calcium metabolism — (Use additional code to identify any associated mental retardation) ▽
275.41 Hypocalcemia — (Use additional code to identify any associated mental retardation)
275.42 Hypercalcemia — (Use additional code to identify any associated mental retardation)
275.49 Other disorders of calcium metabolism — (Use additional code to identify any associated mental retardation)
733.00 Unspecified osteoporosis ▽
733.02 Idiopathic osteoporosis
733.09 Other osteoporosis — (Use additional E code to identify drug)
756.51 Osteogenesis imperfecta
756.52 Osteopetrosis
821.01 Closed fracture of shaft of femur

ICD-9-CM Procedural

78.55 Internal fixation of femur without fracture reduction
84.55 Insertion of bone void filler

27496–27497

27496 Decompression fasciotomy, thigh and/or knee, one compartment (flexor or extensor or adductor);
27497 with debridement of nonviable muscle and/or nerve

ICD-9-CM Diagnostic

287.8 Other specified hemorrhagic conditions
682.6 Cellulitis and abscess of leg, except foot — (Use additional code to identify organism)
728.0 Infective myositis
728.81 Interstitial myositis
728.88 Rhabdomyolysis
906.4 Late effect of crushing
906.7 Late effect of burn of other extremities
928.00 Crushing injury of thigh — (Use additional code to identify any associated injuries: 800-829, 850.0-854.1, 860.0-869.1)
928.01 Crushing injury of hip — (Use additional code to identify any associated injuries: 800-829, 850.0-854.1, 860.0-869.1)
928.10 Crushing injury of lower leg — (Use additional code to identify any associated injuries: 800-829, 850.0-854.1, 860.0-869.1)
928.11 Crushing injury of knee — (Use additional code to identify any associated injuries: 800-829, 850.0-854.1, 860.0-869.1)
945.44 Deep necrosis of underlying tissues due to burn (deep third degree) of lower leg, without mention of loss of a body part
945.45 Deep necrosis of underlying tissues due to burn (deep third degree) of knee, without mention of loss of a body part
945.46 Deep necrosis of underlying tissues due to burn (deep third degree) of thigh (any part), without mention of loss of a body part
958.8 Other early complications of trauma
959.6 Injury, other and unspecified, hip and thigh
998.59 Other postoperative infection — (Use additional code to identify infection)

ICD-9-CM Procedural

83.14 Fasciotomy
83.45 Other myectomy

▽ Unspecified code
♀ Female diagnosis
☒ Manifestation code
♂ Male diagnosis

27498–27499

27498 Decompression fasciotomy, thigh and/or knee, multiple compartments;
27499 with debridement of nonviable muscle and/or nerve

ICD-9-CM Diagnostic

287.8 Other specified hemorrhagic conditions
682.6 Cellulitis and abscess of leg, except foot — (Use additional code to identify organism)
728.0 Infective myositis
728.81 Interstitial myositis
728.88 Rhabdomyolysis
906.4 Late effect of crushing
906.7 Late effect of burn of other extremities
928.00 Crushing injury of thigh — (Use additional code to identify any associated injuries: 800-829, 850.0-854.1, 860.0-869.1)
928.01 Crushing injury of hip — (Use additional code to identify any associated injuries: 800-829, 850.0-854.1, 860.0-869.1)
928.10 Crushing injury of lower leg — (Use additional code to identify any associated injuries: 800-829, 850.0-854.1, 860.0-869.1)
928.11 Crushing injury of knee — (Use additional code to identify any associated injuries: 800-829, 850.0-854.1, 860.0-869.1)
945.44 Deep necrosis of underlying tissues due to burn (deep third degree) of lower leg, without mention of loss of a body part
945.45 Deep necrosis of underlying tissues due to burn (deep third degree) of knee, without mention of loss of a body part
945.46 Deep necrosis of underlying tissues due to burn (deep third degree) of thigh (any part), without mention of loss of a body part
945.49 Deep necrosis of underlying tissues due to burn (deep third degree) of multiple sites of lower limb(s), without mention of loss of a body part
958.8 Other early complications of trauma
959.6 Injury, other and unspecified, hip and thigh

ICD-9-CM Procedural

83.14 Fasciotomy
83.45 Other myectomy

27500

27500 Closed treatment of femoral shaft fracture, without manipulation

ICD-9-CM Diagnostic

733.15 Pathologic fracture of other specified part of femur
756.51 Osteogenesis imperfecta
821.01 Closed fracture of shaft of femur
827.0 Other, multiple and ill-defined closed fractures of lower limb
828.0 Multiple closed fractures involving both lower limbs, lower with upper limb, and lower limb(s) with rib(s) and sternum
928.00 Crushing injury of thigh — (Use additional code to identify any associated injuries: 800-829, 850.0-854.1, 860.0-869.1)

ICD-9-CM Procedural

93.53 Application of other cast

27501

27501 Closed treatment of supracondylar or transcondylar femoral fracture with or without intercondylar extension, without manipulation

ICD-9-CM Diagnostic

733.15 Pathologic fracture of other specified part of femur
733.43 Aseptic necrosis of medial femoral condyle
756.51 Osteogenesis imperfecta
821.20 Closed fracture of unspecified part of lower end of femur ▽
821.21 Closed fracture of femoral condyle
821.22 Closed fracture of lower epiphysis of femur
821.23 Closed supracondylar fracture of femur
821.29 Other closed fracture of lower end of femur
828.0 Multiple closed fractures involving both lower limbs, lower with upper limb, and lower limb(s) with rib(s) and sternum

ICD-9-CM Procedural

93.53 Application of other cast

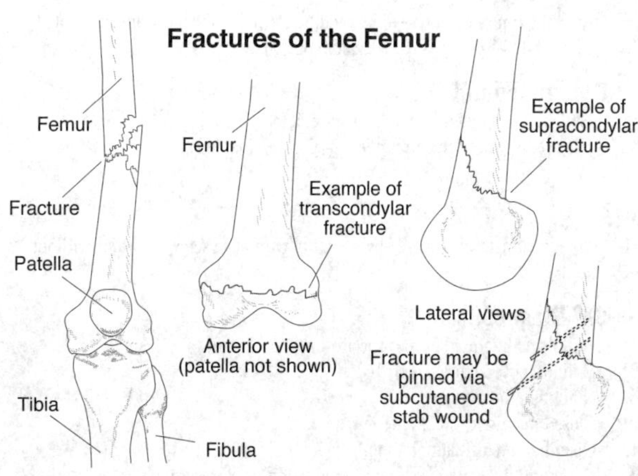

27502

27502 Closed treatment of femoral shaft fracture, with manipulation, with or without skin or skeletal traction

ICD-9-CM Diagnostic

733.15 Pathologic fracture of other specified part of femur
756.51 Osteogenesis imperfecta
821.01 Closed fracture of shaft of femur
827.0 Other, multiple and ill-defined closed fractures of lower limb
828.0 Multiple closed fractures involving both lower limbs, lower with upper limb, and lower limb(s) with rib(s) and sternum

ICD-9-CM Procedural

79.05 Closed reduction of fracture of femur without internal fixation
93.44 Other skeletal traction
93.46 Other skin traction of limbs

27503

27503 Closed treatment of supracondylar or transcondylar femoral fracture with or without intercondylar extension, with manipulation, with or without skin or skeletal traction

ICD-9-CM Diagnostic

733.15 Pathologic fracture of other specified part of femur
733.43 Aseptic necrosis of medial femoral condyle
756.51 Osteogenesis imperfecta
821.20 Closed fracture of unspecified part of lower end of femur ▽
821.21 Closed fracture of femoral condyle
821.22 Closed fracture of lower epiphysis of femur
821.23 Closed supracondylar fracture of femur
821.29 Other closed fracture of lower end of femur
828.0 Multiple closed fractures involving both lower limbs, lower with upper limb, and lower limb(s) with rib(s) and sternum

ICD-9-CM Procedural

79.05 Closed reduction of fracture of femur without internal fixation
93.44 Other skeletal traction
93.46 Other skin traction of limbs

27506

27506 Open treatment of femoral shaft fracture, with or without external fixation, with insertion of intramedullary implant, with or without cerclage and/or locking screws

ICD-9-CM Diagnostic

733.15 Pathologic fracture of other specified part of femur
733.81 Malunion of fracture
733.82 Nonunion of fracture
756.51 Osteogenesis imperfecta
821.01 Closed fracture of shaft of femur
821.10 Open fracture of unspecified part of femur ▽
821.11 Open fracture of shaft of femur
827.0 Other, multiple and ill-defined closed fractures of lower limb
827.1 Other, multiple and ill-defined open fractures of lower limb
828.0 Multiple closed fractures involving both lower limbs, lower with upper limb, and lower limb(s) with rib(s) and sternum

928.00 Crushing injury of thigh — (Use additional code to identify any associated injuries: 800-829, 850.0-854.1, 860.0-869.1)

ICD-9-CM Procedural

78.15 Application of external fixation device, femur
79.35 Open reduction of fracture of femur with internal fixation

27507

27507 Open treatment of femoral shaft fracture with plate/screws, with or without cerclage

ICD-9-CM Diagnostic

733.15 Pathologic fracture of other specified part of femur
733.81 Malunion of fracture
733.82 Nonunion of fracture
821.01 Closed fracture of shaft of femur
821.11 Open fracture of shaft of femur
827.0 Other, multiple and ill-defined closed fractures of lower limb
827.1 Other, multiple and ill-defined open fractures of lower limb
828.0 Multiple closed fractures involving both lower limbs, lower with upper limb, and lower limb(s) with rib(s) and sternum
928.00 Crushing injury of thigh — (Use additional code to identify any associated injuries: 800-829, 850.0-854.1, 860.0-869.1)
996.4 Mechanical complication of internal orthopedic device, implant, and graft

ICD-9-CM Procedural

79.35 Open reduction of fracture of femur with internal fixation

27508

27508 Closed treatment of femoral fracture, distal end, medial or lateral condyle, without manipulation

ICD-9-CM Diagnostic

733.01 Senile osteoporosis
733.15 Pathologic fracture of other specified part of femur
733.43 Aseptic necrosis of medial femoral condyle
756.51 Osteogenesis imperfecta
821.20 Closed fracture of unspecified part of lower end of femur ▽
821.21 Closed fracture of femoral condyle
821.22 Closed fracture of lower epiphysis of femur
821.23 Closed supracondylar fracture of femur
821.29 Other closed fracture of lower end of femur
827.0 Other, multiple and ill-defined closed fractures of lower limb
828.0 Multiple closed fractures involving both lower limbs, lower with upper limb, and lower limb(s) with rib(s) and sternum

ICD-9-CM Procedural

93.53 Application of other cast

HCPCS Level II Supplies & Services

A4550 Surgical trays
A4580 Cast supplies (e.g., plaster)
A4590 Special casting material (e.g., fiberglass)
A6441 Padding bandage, non-elastic, non-woven/non-knitted, width greater than or equal to three inches and less than five inches, per yard

27509

27509 Percutaneous skeletal fixation of femoral fracture, distal end, medial or lateral condyle, or supracondylar or transcondylar, with or without intercondylar extension, or distal femoral epiphyseal separation

ICD-9-CM Diagnostic

733.15 Pathologic fracture of other specified part of femur
733.43 Aseptic necrosis of medial femoral condyle
756.51 Osteogenesis imperfecta
821.20 Closed fracture of unspecified part of lower end of femur ▽
821.21 Closed fracture of femoral condyle
821.22 Closed fracture of lower epiphysis of femur
821.23 Closed supracondylar fracture of femur
821.29 Other closed fracture of lower end of femur
821.30 Open fracture of unspecified part of lower end of femur ▽
821.31 Open fracture of femoral condyle
821.32 Open fracture of lower epiphysis of femur
821.33 Open supracondylar fracture of femur
821.39 Other open fracture of lower end of femur
827.0 Other, multiple and ill-defined closed fractures of lower limb
827.1 Other, multiple and ill-defined open fractures of lower limb
828.0 Multiple closed fractures involving both lower limbs, lower with upper limb, and lower limb(s) with rib(s) and sternum
828.1 Multiple fractures involving both lower limbs, lower with upper limb, and lower limb(s) with rib(s) and sternum, open

ICD-9-CM Procedural

78.55 Internal fixation of femur without fracture reduction

27510

27510 Closed treatment of femoral fracture, distal end, medial or lateral condyle, with manipulation

ICD-9-CM Diagnostic

733.15 Pathologic fracture of other specified part of femur
733.43 Aseptic necrosis of medial femoral condyle
756.51 Osteogenesis imperfecta
821.20 Closed fracture of unspecified part of lower end of femur ▽
821.21 Closed fracture of femoral condyle
821.22 Closed fracture of lower epiphysis of femur
821.23 Closed supracondylar fracture of femur
821.29 Other closed fracture of lower end of femur
821.30 Open fracture of unspecified part of lower end of femur ▽
821.31 Open fracture of femoral condyle
821.32 Open fracture of lower epiphysis of femur
821.33 Open supracondylar fracture of femur
821.39 Other open fracture of lower end of femur
827.0 Other, multiple and ill-defined closed fractures of lower limb
827.1 Other, multiple and ill-defined open fractures of lower limb
828.0 Multiple closed fractures involving both lower limbs, lower with upper limb, and lower limb(s) with rib(s) and sternum
828.1 Multiple fractures involving both lower limbs, lower with upper limb, and lower limb(s) with rib(s) and sternum, open

ICD-9-CM Procedural

79.05 Closed reduction of fracture of femur without internal fixation

HCPCS Level II Supplies & Services

A4550 Surgical trays
A4580 Cast supplies (e.g., plaster)
A4590 Special casting material (e.g., fiberglass)
A6441 Padding bandage, non-elastic, non-woven/non-knitted, width greater than or equal to three inches and less than five inches, per yard

27511–27513

27511 Open treatment of femoral supracondylar or transcondylar fracture without intercondylar extension, with or without internal or external fixation
27513 Open treatment of femoral supracondylar or transcondylar fracture with intercondylar extension, with or without internal or external fixation

ICD-9-CM Diagnostic

732.7 Osteochondritis dissecans
733.15 Pathologic fracture of other specified part of femur
733.43 Aseptic necrosis of medial femoral condyle
733.81 Malunion of fracture
733.82 Nonunion of fracture
756.51 Osteogenesis imperfecta
821.20 Closed fracture of unspecified part of lower end of femur ▽
821.21 Closed fracture of femoral condyle
821.22 Closed fracture of lower epiphysis of femur
821.23 Closed supracondylar fracture of femur
821.29 Other closed fracture of lower end of femur
821.30 Open fracture of unspecified part of lower end of femur ▽
821.31 Open fracture of femoral condyle
821.32 Open fracture of lower epiphysis of femur
821.33 Open supracondylar fracture of femur
821.39 Other open fracture of lower end of femur
827.0 Other, multiple and ill-defined closed fractures of lower limb
827.1 Other, multiple and ill-defined open fractures of lower limb
828.0 Multiple closed fractures involving both lower limbs, lower with upper limb, and lower limb(s) with rib(s) and sternum
828.1 Multiple fractures involving both lower limbs, lower with upper limb, and lower limb(s) with rib(s) and sternum, open

ICD-9-CM Procedural

78.15 Application of external fixation device, femur

▽ Unspecified code ♀ Female diagnosis ⊠ Manifestation code ♂ Male diagnosis

79.25 Open reduction of fracture of femur without internal fixation
79.35 Open reduction of fracture of femur with internal fixation

27514

27514 Open treatment of femoral fracture, distal end, medial or lateral condyle, with or without internal or external fixation

ICD-9-CM Diagnostic

732.7 Osteochondritis dissecans
733.15 Pathologic fracture of other specified part of femur
733.81 Malunion of fracture
733.82 Nonunion of fracture
756.51 Osteogenesis imperfecta
821.20 Closed fracture of unspecified part of lower end of femur ▽
821.21 Closed fracture of femoral condyle
821.22 Closed fracture of lower epiphysis of femur
821.23 Closed supracondylar fracture of femur
821.29 Other closed fracture of lower end of femur
821.30 Open fracture of unspecified part of lower end of femur ▽
821.31 Open fracture of femoral condyle
821.32 Open fracture of lower epiphysis of femur
821.33 Open supracondylar fracture of femur
821.39 Other open fracture of lower end of femur
827.0 Other, multiple and ill-defined closed fractures of lower limb
827.1 Other, multiple and ill-defined open fractures of lower limb
828.0 Multiple closed fractures involving both lower limbs, lower with upper limb, and lower limb(s) with rib(s) and sternum
828.1 Multiple fractures involving both lower limbs, lower with upper limb, and lower limb(s) with rib(s) and sternum, open

ICD-9-CM Procedural

78.15 Application of external fixation device, femur
79.25 Open reduction of fracture of femur without internal fixation
79.35 Open reduction of fracture of femur with internal fixation

27516–27517

27516 Closed treatment of distal femoral epiphyseal separation; without manipulation
27517 with manipulation, with or without skin or skeletal traction

ICD-9-CM Diagnostic

732.2 Nontraumatic slipped upper femoral epiphysis
732.6 Other juvenile osteochondrosis
732.9 Unspecified osteochondropathy ▽
733.15 Pathologic fracture of other specified part of femur
821.22 Closed fracture of lower epiphysis of femur

ICD-9-CM Procedural

79.45 Closed reduction of separated epiphysis of femur
93.44 Other skeletal traction
93.46 Other skin traction of limbs
93.53 Application of other cast

HCPCS Level II Supplies & Services

A4550 Surgical trays
A4580 Cast supplies (e.g., plaster)
A4590 Special casting material (e.g., fiberglass)
E0112 Crutches, underarm, wood, adjustable or fixed, pair, with pads, tips and handgrips
E0113 Crutch, underarm, wood, adjustable or fixed, each, with pad, tip and handgrip

27519

27519 Open treatment of distal femoral epiphyseal separation, with or without internal or external fixation

ICD-9-CM Diagnostic

732.2 Nontraumatic slipped upper femoral epiphysis
732.6 Other juvenile osteochondrosis
732.7 Osteochondritis dissecans
732.9 Unspecified osteochondropathy ▽
733.15 Pathologic fracture of other specified part of femur
821.22 Closed fracture of lower epiphysis of femur
821.32 Open fracture of lower epiphysis of femur

ICD-9-CM Procedural

78.15 Application of external fixation device, femur
79.55 Open reduction of separated epiphysis of femur

27520

27520 Closed treatment of patellar fracture, without manipulation

ICD-9-CM Diagnostic

715.96 Osteoarthrosis, unspecified whether generalized or localized, lower leg ▽
719.46 Pain in joint, lower leg
732.7 Osteochondritis dissecans
733.19 Pathologic fracture of other specified site
756.51 Osteogenesis imperfecta
822.0 Closed fracture of patella

ICD-9-CM Procedural

93.53 Application of other cast
93.54 Application of splint

HCPCS Level II Supplies & Services

A4550 Surgical trays
A4570 Splint
A4580 Cast supplies (e.g., plaster)
A4590 Special casting material (e.g., fiberglass)
E0112 Crutches, underarm, wood, adjustable or fixed, pair, with pads, tips and handgrips

27524

27524 Open treatment of patellar fracture, with internal fixation and/or partial or complete patellectomy and soft tissue repair

ICD-9-CM Diagnostic

732.7 Osteochondritis dissecans
733.19 Pathologic fracture of other specified site
756.51 Osteogenesis imperfecta
822.0 Closed fracture of patella
822.1 Open fracture of patella

ICD-9-CM Procedural

77.86 Other partial ostectomy of patella
77.96 Total ostectomy of patella
79.36 Open reduction of fracture of tibia and fibula with internal fixation
79.39 Open reduction of fracture of other specified bone, except facial bones, with internal fixation
83.09 Other incision of soft tissue

27530–27532

27530 Closed treatment of tibial fracture, proximal (plateau); without manipulation
27532 with or without manipulation, with skeletal traction

ICD-9-CM Diagnostic

733.16 Pathologic fracture of tibia or fibula
733.93 Stress fracture of tibia or fibula
756.51 Osteogenesis imperfecta
823.00 Closed fracture of upper end of tibia
823.02 Closed fracture of upper end of fibula with tibia
823.40 Torus fracture of tibia alone
827.0 Other, multiple and ill-defined closed fractures of lower limb
828.0 Multiple closed fractures involving both lower limbs, lower with upper limb, and lower limb(s) with rib(s) and sternum

ICD-9-CM Procedural

79.06 Closed reduction of fracture of tibia and fibula without internal fixation
93.44 Other skeletal traction
93.53 Application of other cast

HCPCS Level II Supplies & Services

A4550 Surgical trays
A4570 Splint
A4580 Cast supplies (e.g., plaster)
A4590 Special casting material (e.g., fiberglass)
A6441 Padding bandage, non-elastic, non-woven/non-knitted, width greater than or equal to three inches and less than five inches, per yard

27535–27536

27535 Open treatment of tibial fracture, proximal (plateau); unicondylar, with or without internal or external fixation
27536 bicondylar, with or without internal fixation

ICD-9-CM Diagnostic

733.16 Pathologic fracture of tibia or fibula
733.93 Stress fracture of tibia or fibula
756.51 Osteogenesis imperfecta
823.00 Closed fracture of upper end of tibia
823.02 Closed fracture of upper end of fibula with tibia
823.10 Open fracture of upper end of tibia
823.12 Open fracture of upper end of fibula with tibia
827.0 Other, multiple and ill-defined closed fractures of lower limb
827.1 Other, multiple and ill-defined open fractures of lower limb
828.0 Multiple closed fractures involving both lower limbs, lower with upper limb, and lower limb(s) with rib(s) and sternum
828.1 Multiple fractures involving both lower limbs, lower with upper limb, and lower limb(s) with rib(s) and sternum, open

ICD-9-CM Procedural

78.17 Application of external fixation device, tibia and fibula
79.26 Open reduction of fracture of tibia and fibula without internal fixation
79.36 Open reduction of fracture of tibia and fibula with internal fixation
79.89 Open reduction of dislocation of other specified site, except temporomandibular

27538

27538 Closed treatment of intercondylar spine(s) and/or tuberosity fracture(s) of knee, with or without manipulation

ICD-9-CM Diagnostic

733.16 Pathologic fracture of tibia or fibula
733.93 Stress fracture of tibia or fibula
756.51 Osteogenesis imperfecta
823.00 Closed fracture of upper end of tibia
823.02 Closed fracture of upper end of fibula with tibia
827.0 Other, multiple and ill-defined closed fractures of lower limb

ICD-9-CM Procedural

79.06 Closed reduction of fracture of tibia and fibula without internal fixation
93.53 Application of other cast
93.54 Application of splint

HCPCS Level II Supplies & Services

A4550 Surgical trays
A4570 Splint
A4580 Cast supplies (e.g., plaster)
A4590 Special casting material (e.g., fiberglass)
E0112 Crutches, underarm, wood, adjustable or fixed, pair, with pads, tips and handgrips

27540

27540 Open treatment of intercondylar spine(s) and/or tuberosity fracture(s) of the knee, with or without internal or external fixation

ICD-9-CM Diagnostic

733.16 Pathologic fracture of tibia or fibula
733.93 Stress fracture of tibia or fibula
756.51 Osteogenesis imperfecta
823.00 Closed fracture of upper end of tibia
823.10 Open fracture of upper end of tibia
827.0 Other, multiple and ill-defined closed fractures of lower limb
827.1 Other, multiple and ill-defined open fractures of lower limb

ICD-9-CM Procedural

78.17 Application of external fixation device, tibia and fibula
79.26 Open reduction of fracture of tibia and fibula without internal fixation
79.36 Open reduction of fracture of tibia and fibula with internal fixation

27550–27552

27550 Closed treatment of knee dislocation; without anesthesia
27552 requiring anesthesia

ICD-9-CM Diagnostic

717.85 Old disruption of other ligament of knee
718.26 Pathological dislocation of lower leg joint
718.36 Recurrent dislocation of lower leg joint
718.76 Developmental dislocation of joint, lower leg
754.41 Congenital dislocation of knee (with genu recurvatum)
836.0 Tear of medial cartilage or meniscus of knee, current
836.1 Tear of lateral cartilage or meniscus of knee, current
836.2 Other tear of cartilage or meniscus of knee, current
836.3 Closed dislocation of patella
836.50 Closed dislocation of knee, unspecified part ♡
836.51 Closed anterior dislocation of tibia, proximal end
836.52 Closed posterior dislocation of tibia, proximal end
836.53 Closed medial dislocation of tibia, proximal end
836.54 Closed lateral dislocation of tibia, proximal end

ICD-9-CM Procedural

79.76 Closed reduction of dislocation of knee

HCPCS Level II Supplies & Services

A4550 Surgical trays
A4570 Splint
A4580 Cast supplies (e.g., plaster)
A4590 Special casting material (e.g., fiberglass)
E0112 Crutches, underarm, wood, adjustable or fixed, pair, with pads, tips and handgrips

27556–27557

27556 Open treatment of knee dislocation, with or without internal or external fixation; without primary ligamentous repair or augmentation/reconstruction
27557 with primary ligamentous repair

ICD-9-CM Diagnostic

717.81 Old disruption of lateral collateral ligament
717.82 Old disruption of medial collateral ligament
717.83 Old disruption of anterior cruciate ligament
717.84 Old disruption of posterior cruciate ligament
718.26 Pathological dislocation of lower leg joint
718.36 Recurrent dislocation of lower leg joint
718.76 Developmental dislocation of joint, lower leg
754.41 Congenital dislocation of knee (with genu recurvatum)
836.3 Closed dislocation of patella
836.4 Open dislocation of patella
836.50 Closed dislocation of knee, unspecified part ♡
836.51 Closed anterior dislocation of tibia, proximal end
836.52 Closed posterior dislocation of tibia, proximal end
836.53 Closed medial dislocation of tibia, proximal end
836.54 Closed lateral dislocation of tibia, proximal end
836.60 Open dislocation of knee unspecified part ♡
836.61 Open anterior dislocation of tibia, proximal end
836.62 Open posterior dislocation of tibia, proximal end
836.63 Open medial dislocation of tibia, proximal end
836.64 Open lateral dislocation of tibia, proximal end

ICD-9-CM Procedural

79.86 Open reduction of dislocation of knee
81.47 Other repair of knee
81.96 Other repair of joint

27558

27558 Open treatment of knee dislocation, with or without internal or external fixation; with primary ligamentous repair, with augmentation/reconstruction

ICD-9-CM Diagnostic

717.81 Old disruption of lateral collateral ligament
717.82 Old disruption of medial collateral ligament
717.83 Old disruption of anterior cruciate ligament
717.84 Old disruption of posterior cruciate ligament
718.26 Pathological dislocation of lower leg joint
718.36 Recurrent dislocation of lower leg joint
718.76 Developmental dislocation of joint, lower leg
754.41 Congenital dislocation of knee (with genu recurvatum)
836.3 Closed dislocation of patella
836.4 Open dislocation of patella
836.50 Closed dislocation of knee, unspecified part ♡
836.51 Closed anterior dislocation of tibia, proximal end
836.52 Closed posterior dislocation of tibia, proximal end
836.53 Closed medial dislocation of tibia, proximal end

836.54 Closed lateral dislocation of tibia, proximal end
836.60 Open dislocation of knee unspecified part
836.61 Open anterior dislocation of tibia, proximal end
836.62 Open posterior dislocation of tibia, proximal end
836.63 Open medial dislocation of tibia, proximal end
836.64 Open lateral dislocation of tibia, proximal end

ICD-9-CM Procedural
79.86 Open reduction of dislocation of knee
81.47 Other repair of knee
81.96 Other repair of joint

27560–27562
27560 Closed treatment of patellar dislocation; without anesthesia
27562 requiring anesthesia

ICD-9-CM Diagnostic
718.36 Recurrent dislocation of lower leg joint
718.76 Developmental dislocation of joint, lower leg
836.3 Closed dislocation of patella
905.7 Late effect of sprain and strain without mention of tendon injury
905.8 Late effect of tendon injury

ICD-9-CM Procedural
79.79 Closed reduction of dislocation of other specified site, except temporomandibular

HCPCS Level II Supplies & Services
A4550 Surgical trays
A4570 Splint
A4580 Cast supplies (e.g., plaster)
A4590 Special casting material (e.g., fiberglass)
E0112 Crutches, underarm, wood, adjustable or fixed, pair, with pads, tips and handgrips

27566
27566 Open treatment of patellar dislocation, with or without partial or total patellectomy

ICD-9-CM Diagnostic
718.36 Recurrent dislocation of lower leg joint
718.76 Developmental dislocation of joint, lower leg
836.3 Closed dislocation of patella
836.4 Open dislocation of patella

ICD-9-CM Procedural
77.86 Other partial ostectomy of patella
77.96 Total ostectomy of patella
79.89 Open reduction of dislocation of other specified site, except temporomandibular

27570
27570 Manipulation of knee joint under general anesthesia (includes application of traction or other fixation devices)

ICD-9-CM Diagnostic
357.1 Polyneuropathy in collagen vascular disease — (Code first underlying disease: 446.0, 710.0, 714.0) ☒
359.6 Symptomatic inflammatory myopathy in diseases classified elsewhere — (Code first underlying disease: 135, 140.0-208.9, 277.3, 446.0, 710.0, 710.1, 710.2, 714.0) ☒
446.0 Polyarteritis nodosa
710.0 Systemic lupus erythematosus — (Use additional code to identify manifestation: 424.91, 581.81, 582.81, 583.81)
710.1 Systemic sclerosis — (Use additional code to identify manifestation: 359.6, 517.2)
710.2 Sicca syndrome
714.0 Rheumatoid arthritis — (Use additional code to identify manifestation: 357.1, 359.6)
715.16 Primary localized osteoarthrosis, lower leg
715.96 Osteoarthrosis, unspecified whether generalized or localized, lower leg
717.7 Chondromalacia of patella
717.83 Old disruption of anterior cruciate ligament
717.84 Old disruption of posterior cruciate ligament
718.26 Pathological dislocation of lower leg joint
718.46 Contracture of lower leg joint
718.56 Ankylosis of lower leg joint
718.76 Developmental dislocation of joint, lower leg
719.26 Villonodular synovitis, lower leg
719.56 Stiffness of joint, not elsewhere classified, lower leg
726.60 Unspecified enthesopathy of knee
V43.65 Knee joint replacement by other means — (This code is intended for use when these conditions are recorded as diagnoses or problems)

ICD-9-CM Procedural
78.15 Application of external fixation device, femur
78.17 Application of external fixation device, tibia and fibula
93.25 Forced extension of limb
93.26 Manual rupture of joint adhesions
93.44 Other skeletal traction

27580
27580 Arthrodesis, knee, any technique

ICD-9-CM Diagnostic
711.16 Arthropathy associated with Reiter's disease and nonspecific urethritis, lower leg — (Code first underlying disease: 099.3, 099.4) ☒
711.26 Arthropathy in Behcet's syndrome, lower leg — (Code first underlying disease, 136.1) ☒
718.26 Pathological dislocation of lower leg joint
718.36 Recurrent dislocation of lower leg joint
718.46 Contracture of lower leg joint
718.56 Ankylosis of lower leg joint
718.86 Other joint derangement, not elsewhere classified, lower leg
726.60 Unspecified enthesopathy of knee
733.15 Pathologic fracture of other specified part of femur
733.81 Malunion of fracture
733.82 Nonunion of fracture
733.92 Chondromalacia
756.51 Osteogenesis imperfecta
996.4 Mechanical complication of internal orthopedic device, implant, and graft

ICD-9-CM Procedural
81.22 Arthrodesis of knee

27590–27592
27590 Amputation, thigh, through femur, any level;
27591 immediate fitting technique including first cast
27592 open, circular (guillotine)

ICD-9-CM Diagnostic
170.7 Malignant neoplasm of long bones of lower limb
195.5 Malignant neoplasm of lower limb
198.5 Secondary malignant neoplasm of bone and bone marrow
250.70 Diabetes with peripheral circulatory disorders, type II or unspecified type, not stated as uncontrolled — (Use additional code to identify manifestation: 443.81, 785.4)
250.71 Diabetes with peripheral circulatory disorders, type I [juvenile type], not stated as uncontrolled — (Use additional code to identify manifestation: 443.81, 785.4)
250.80 Diabetes with other specified manifestations, type II or unspecified type, not stated as uncontrolled — (Use additional code to identify manifestation: 707.10-707.9, 731.8. Use additional E code to identify cause, if drug-induced)
250.81 Diabetes with other specified manifestations, type I [juvenile type], not stated as uncontrolled — (Use additional code to identify manifestation: 707.10-707.9, 731.8. Use additional E code to identify cause, if drug-induced)
250.82 Diabetes with other specified manifestations, type II or unspecified type, uncontrolled — (Use additional code to identify manifestation: 707.10-707.9, 731.8. Use additional E code to identify cause, if drug-induced)
250.83 Diabetes with other specified manifestations, type I [juvenile type], uncontrolled — (Use additional code to identify manifestation: 707.10-707.9, 731.8. Use additional E code to identify cause, if drug-induced)
440.20 Atherosclerosis of native arteries of the extremities, unspecified
440.21 Atherosclerosis of native arteries of the extremities with intermittent claudication
440.22 Atherosclerosis of native arteries of the extremities with rest pain
440.23 Atherosclerosis of native arteries of the extremities with ulceration — (Use additional code for any associated ulceration: 707.10-707.9)
440.24 Atherosclerosis of native arteries of the extremities with gangrene
443.1 Thromboangiitis obliterans (Buerger's disease)
443.81 Peripheral angiopathy in diseases classified elsewhere — (Code first underlying disease, 250.7) ☒
443.9 Unspecified peripheral vascular disease

444.22 Embolism and thrombosis of arteries of lower extremity
445.02 Atheroembolism of lower extremity
446.0 Polyarteritis nodosa
446.6 Thrombotic microangiopathy
447.5 Necrosis of artery
682.6 Cellulitis and abscess of leg, except foot — (Use additional code to identify organism)
707.10 Ulcer of lower limb, unspecified ▽
707.11 Ulcer of thigh
728.89 Other disorder of muscle, ligament, and fascia — (Use additional E code to identify drug, if drug-induced)
730.16 Chronic osteomyelitis, lower leg — (Use additional code to identify organism, 041.1)
731.1 Osteitis deformans in diseases classified elsewhere — (Code first underlying disease: 170.0-170.9) ☒
731.8 Other bone involvement in diseases classified elsewhere — (Code first underlying disease, 250.8. Use additional code to specify bone condition: 730.00-730.09) ☒
733.43 Aseptic necrosis of medial femoral condyle
785.4 Gangrene — (Code first any associated underlying condition:250.7, 443.0)
890.1 Open wound of hip and thigh, complicated — (Use additional code to identify infection)
897.7 Traumatic amputation of leg(s) (complete) (partial), bilateral (any level), complicated — (Use additional code to identify infection)
928.00 Crushing injury of thigh — (Use additional code to identify any associated injuries: 800-829, 850.0-854.1, 860.0-869.1)

ICD-9-CM Procedural

84.17 Amputation above knee
84.45 Fitting of prosthesis above knee

27594

27594 Amputation, thigh, through femur, any level; secondary closure or scar revision

ICD-9-CM Diagnostic

170.7 Malignant neoplasm of long bones of lower limb
195.5 Malignant neoplasm of lower limb
198.5 Secondary malignant neoplasm of bone and bone marrow
250.70 Diabetes with peripheral circulatory disorders, type II or unspecified type, not stated as uncontrolled — (Use additional code to identify manifestation: 443.81, 785.4)
250.71 Diabetes with peripheral circulatory disorders, type I [juvenile type], not stated as uncontrolled — (Use additional code to identify manifestation: 443.81, 785.4)
440.24 Atherosclerosis of native arteries of the extremities with gangrene
682.6 Cellulitis and abscess of leg, except foot — (Use additional code to identify organism)
707.10 Ulcer of lower limb, unspecified ▽
707.11 Ulcer of thigh
730.16 Chronic osteomyelitis, lower leg — (Use additional code to identify organism, 041.1)
785.4 Gangrene — (Code first any associated underlying condition:250.7, 443.0)
897.3 Traumatic amputation of leg(s) (complete) (partial), unilateral, at or above knee, complicated — (Use additional code to identify infection)
897.7 Traumatic amputation of leg(s) (complete) (partial), bilateral (any level), complicated — (Use additional code to identify infection)
928.00 Crushing injury of thigh — (Use additional code to identify any associated injuries: 800-829, 850.0-854.1, 860.0-869.1)
996.74 Other complications due to other vascular device, implant, and graft
997.60 Late complications of amputation stump, unspecified — (Use additional code to identify complications) ▽
997.61 Neuroma of amputation stump — (Use additional code to identify complications)
997.62 Infection (chronic) of amputation stump — (Use additional code to identify organism. Use additional code to identify complications)
997.69 Other late amputation stump complication — (Use additional code to identify complications)

ICD-9-CM Procedural

84.3 Revision of amputation stump

27596

27596 Amputation, thigh, through femur, any level; re-amputation

ICD-9-CM Diagnostic

440.24 Atherosclerosis of native arteries of the extremities with gangrene
707.10 Ulcer of lower limb, unspecified ▽
707.11 Ulcer of thigh
733.15 Pathologic fracture of other specified part of femur
785.4 Gangrene — (Code first any associated underlying condition:250.7, 443.0)
897.2 Traumatic amputation of leg(s) (complete) (partial), unilateral, at or above knee, without mention of complication — (Use additional code to identify infection)
928.00 Crushing injury of thigh — (Use additional code to identify any associated injuries: 800-829, 850.0-854.1, 860.0-869.1)
997.60 Late complications of amputation stump, unspecified — (Use additional code to identify complications) ▽
997.61 Neuroma of amputation stump — (Use additional code to identify complications)
997.62 Infection (chronic) of amputation stump — (Use additional code to identify organism. Use additional code to identify complications)
997.69 Other late amputation stump complication — (Use additional code to identify complications)

ICD-9-CM Procedural

84.3 Revision of amputation stump

27598

27598 Disarticulation at knee

ICD-9-CM Diagnostic

170.7 Malignant neoplasm of long bones of lower limb
195.5 Malignant neoplasm of lower limb
198.5 Secondary malignant neoplasm of bone and bone marrow
250.70 Diabetes with peripheral circulatory disorders, type II or unspecified type, not stated as uncontrolled — (Use additional code to identify manifestation: 443.81, 785.4)
250.71 Diabetes with peripheral circulatory disorders, type I [juvenile type], not stated as uncontrolled — (Use additional code to identify manifestation: 443.81, 785.4)
250.80 Diabetes with other specified manifestations, type II or unspecified type, not stated as uncontrolled — (Use additional code to identify manifestation: 707.10-707.9, 731.8. Use additional E code to identify cause, if drug-induced)
250.81 Diabetes with other specified manifestations, type I [juvenile type], not stated as uncontrolled — (Use additional code to identify manifestation: 707.10-707.9, 731.8. Use additional E code to identify cause, if drug-induced)
250.82 Diabetes with other specified manifestations, type II or unspecified type, uncontrolled — (Use additional code to identify manifestation: 707.10-707.9, 731.8. Use additional E code to identify cause, if drug-induced)
250.83 Diabetes with other specified manifestations, type I [juvenile type], uncontrolled — (Use additional code to identify manifestation: 707.10-707.9, 731.8. Use additional E code to identify cause, if drug-induced)
440.20 Atherosclerosis of native arteries of the extremities, unspecified ▽
440.21 Atherosclerosis of native arteries of the extremities with intermittent claudication
440.22 Atherosclerosis of native arteries of the extremities with rest pain
440.23 Atherosclerosis of native arteries of the extremities with ulceration — (Use additional code for any associated ulceration: 707.10-707.9)
440.24 Atherosclerosis of native arteries of the extremities with gangrene
443.1 Thromboangiitis obliterans (Buerger's disease)
443.81 Peripheral angiopathy in diseases classified elsewhere — (Code first underlying disease, 250.7) ☒
682.6 Cellulitis and abscess of leg, except foot — (Use additional code to identify organism)
730.16 Chronic osteomyelitis, lower leg — (Use additional code to identify organism, 041.1)
731.1 Osteitis deformans in diseases classified elsewhere — (Code first underlying disease: 170.0-170.9) ☒
731.8 Other bone involvement in diseases classified elsewhere — (Code first underlying disease, 250.8. Use additional code to specify bone condition: 730.00-730.09) ☒
733.43 Aseptic necrosis of medial femoral condyle
785.4 Gangrene — (Code first any associated underlying condition:250.7, 443.0)
891.1 Open wound of knee, leg (except thigh), and ankle, complicated — (Use additional code to identify infection)
897.3 Traumatic amputation of leg(s) (complete) (partial), unilateral, at or above knee, complicated — (Use additional code to identify infection)
928.10 Crushing injury of lower leg — (Use additional code to identify any associated injuries: 800-829, 850.0-854.1, 860.0-869.1)
928.11 Crushing injury of knee — (Use additional code to identify any associated injuries: 800-829, 850.0-854.1, 860.0-869.1)

▽ Unspecified code
♀ Female diagnosis
☒ Manifestation code
♂ Male diagnosis

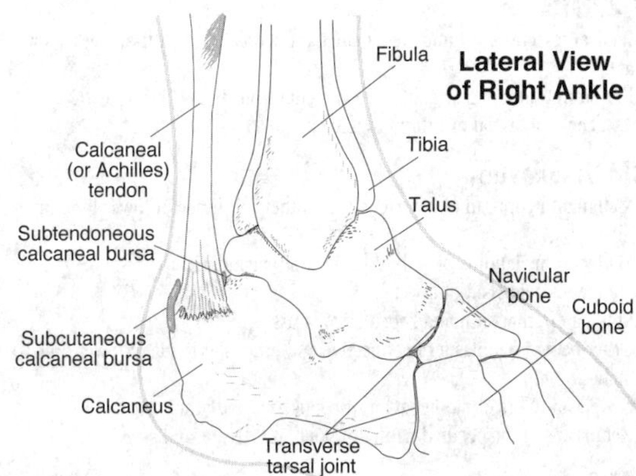

ICD-9-CM Procedural
84.16 Disarticulation of knee

27599
27599 Unlisted procedure, femur or knee

ICD-9-CM Diagnostic
The application of this code is too broad to adequately present ICD-9-CM diagnostic code links here. Refer to your ICD-9-CM book.

Leg (Tibia and Fibula) and Ankle Joint

27600–27602
27600 Decompression fasciotomy, leg; anterior and/or lateral compartments only
27601 posterior compartment(s) only
27602 anterior and/or lateral, and posterior compartment(s)

ICD-9-CM Diagnostic
728.0 Infective myositis
728.81 Interstitial myositis
728.88 Rhabdomyolysis
906.4 Late effect of crushing
906.7 Late effect of burn of other extremities
928.10 Crushing injury of lower leg — (Use additional code to identify any associated injuries: 800-829, 850.0-854.1, 860.0-869.1)
928.11 Crushing injury of knee — (Use additional code to identify any associated injuries: 800-829, 850.0-854.1, 860.0-869.1)
945.44 Deep necrosis of underlying tissues due to burn (deep third degree) of lower leg, without mention of loss of a body part
945.45 Deep necrosis of underlying tissues due to burn (deep third degree) of knee, without mention of loss of a body part
945.49 Deep necrosis of underlying tissues due to burn (deep third degree) of multiple sites of lower limb(s), without mention of loss of a body part
958.8 Other early complications of trauma

ICD-9-CM Procedural
83.14 Fasciotomy

27603
27603 Incision and drainage, leg or ankle; deep abscess or hematoma

ICD-9-CM Diagnostic
682.6 Cellulitis and abscess of leg, except foot — (Use additional code to identify organism)
707.10 Ulcer of lower limb, unspecified ▽
707.11 Ulcer of thigh
707.12 Ulcer of calf
707.13 Ulcer of ankle
719.17 Hemarthrosis, ankle and foot
719.47 Pain in joint, ankle and foot
730.26 Unspecified osteomyelitis, lower leg — (Use additional code to identify organism, 041.1) ▽
891.1 Open wound of knee, leg (except thigh), and ankle, complicated — (Use additional code to identify infection)
924.10 Contusion of lower leg
924.21 Contusion of ankle
998.11 Hemorrhage complicating a procedure
998.12 Hematoma complicating a procedure
998.13 Seroma complicating a procedure

ICD-9-CM Procedural
83.02 Myotomy
83.09 Other incision of soft tissue

HCPCS Level II Supplies & Services
A4305 Disposable drug delivery system, flow rate of 50 ml or greater per hour
A4306 Disposable drug delivery system, flow rate of 5 ml or less per hour
A4550 Surgical trays

27604
27604 Incision and drainage, leg or ankle; infected bursa

ICD-9-CM Diagnostic
726.70 Unspecified enthesopathy of ankle and tarsus ▽
726.71 Achilles bursitis or tendinitis
726.79 Other enthesopathy of ankle and tarsus

ICD-9-CM Procedural
83.03 Bursotomy

HCPCS Level II Supplies & Services
A4305 Disposable drug delivery system, flow rate of 50 ml or greater per hour
A4306 Disposable drug delivery system, flow rate of 5 ml or less per hour
A4550 Surgical trays

27605–27606
27605 Tenotomy, percutaneous, Achilles tendon (separate procedure); local anesthesia
27606 general anesthesia

ICD-9-CM Diagnostic
726.71 Achilles bursitis or tendinitis
727.06 Tenosynovitis of foot and ankle
727.81 Contracture of tendon (sheath)

ICD-9-CM Procedural
83.11 Achillotenotomy

HCPCS Level II Supplies & Services
A4580 Cast supplies (e.g., plaster)
E0112 Crutches, underarm, wood, adjustable or fixed, pair, with pads, tips and handgrips
E0113 Crutch, underarm, wood, adjustable or fixed, each, with pad, tip and handgrip
E0114 Crutches, underarm, other than wood, adjustable or fixed, pair, with pads, tips and handgrips
E0116 Crutch, underarm, other than wood, adjustable or fixed, each, with pad, tip and handgrip

27607
27607 Incision (eg, osteomyelitis or bone abscess), leg or ankle

ICD-9-CM Diagnostic
682.6 Cellulitis and abscess of leg, except foot — (Use additional code to identify organism)
711.06 Pyogenic arthritis, lower leg — (Use additional code to identify infectious organism: 041.0-041.8)
711.07 Pyogenic arthritis, ankle and foot — (Use additional code to identify infectious organism: 041.0-041.8)
730.16 Chronic osteomyelitis, lower leg — (Use additional code to identify organism, 041.1)
730.17 Chronic osteomyelitis, ankle and foot — (Use additional code to identify organism, 041.1)
730.26 Unspecified osteomyelitis, lower leg — (Use additional code to identify organism, 041.1) ▽
730.27 Unspecified osteomyelitis, ankle and foot — (Use additional code to identify organism, 041.1) ▽
730.97 Unspecified infection of bone, ankle and foot — (Use additional code to identify organism, 041.1) ▽
891.1 Open wound of knee, leg (except thigh), and ankle, complicated — (Use additional code to identify infection)

996.66 Infection and inflammatory reaction due to internal joint prosthesis — (Use additional code to identify specified infections)
996.67 Infection and inflammatory reaction due to other internal orthopedic device, implant, and graft — (Use additional code to identify specified infections)
998.59 Other postoperative infection — (Use additional code to identify infection)

ICD-9-CM Procedural
77.17 Other incision of tibia and fibula without division
77.18 Other incision of tarsals and metatarsals without division

27610
27610 Arthrotomy, ankle, including exploration, drainage, or removal of foreign body

ICD-9-CM Diagnostic
711.07 Pyogenic arthritis, ankle and foot — (Use additional code to identify infectious organism: 041.0-041.8)
715.37 Localized osteoarthrosis not specified whether primary or secondary, ankle and foot
718.17 Loose body in ankle and foot joint
719.07 Effusion of ankle and foot joint
730.17 Chronic osteomyelitis, ankle and foot — (Use additional code to identify organism, 041.1)
730.27 Unspecified osteomyelitis, ankle and foot — (Use additional code to identify organism, 041.1) ▽
730.97 Unspecified infection of bone, ankle and foot — (Use additional code to identify organism, 041.1) ▽
996.66 Infection and inflammatory reaction due to internal joint prosthesis — (Use additional code to identify specified infections)
996.67 Infection and inflammatory reaction due to other internal orthopedic device, implant, and graft — (Use additional code to identify specified infections)
V64.43 Arthroscopic surgical procedure converted to open procedure

ICD-9-CM Procedural
80.17 Other arthrotomy of ankle

27612
27612 Arthrotomy, posterior capsular release, ankle, with or without Achilles tendon lengthening

ICD-9-CM Diagnostic
718.47 Contracture of ankle and foot joint
727.81 Contracture of tendon (sheath)
736.71 Acquired equinovarus deformity
736.72 Equinus deformity of foot, acquired
754.50 Congenital talipes varus
754.51 Congenital talipes equinovarus
754.69 Other congenital valgus deformity of feet

ICD-9-CM Procedural
80.47 Division of joint capsule, ligament, or cartilage of ankle
83.85 Other change in muscle or tendon length

27613–27614
27613 Biopsy, soft tissue of leg or ankle area; superficial
27614 deep (subfascial or intramuscular)

ICD-9-CM Diagnostic
171.3 Malignant neoplasm of connective and other soft tissue of lower limb, including hip
172.7 Malignant melanoma of skin of lower limb, including hip
215.3 Other benign neoplasm of connective and other soft tissue of lower limb, including hip
238.1 Neoplasm of uncertain behavior of connective and other soft tissue ▽
239.2 Neoplasms of unspecified nature of bone, soft tissue, and skin
682.6 Cellulitis and abscess of leg, except foot — (Use additional code to identify organism)
782.2 Localized superficial swelling, mass, or lump

ICD-9-CM Procedural
83.21 Biopsy of soft tissue

HCPCS Level II Supplies & Services
A4305 Disposable drug delivery system, flow rate of 50 ml or greater per hour
A4306 Disposable drug delivery system, flow rate of 5 ml or less per hour
A4550 Surgical trays

27615–27619
27615 Radical resection of tumor (eg, malignant neoplasm), soft tissue of leg or ankle area
27618 Excision, tumor, leg or ankle area; subcutaneous tissue
27619 deep (subfascial or intramuscular)

ICD-9-CM Diagnostic
171.3 Malignant neoplasm of connective and other soft tissue of lower limb, including hip
172.7 Malignant melanoma of skin of lower limb, including hip
195.5 Malignant neoplasm of lower limb
214.1 Lipoma of other skin and subcutaneous tissue
215.3 Other benign neoplasm of connective and other soft tissue of lower limb, including hip
238.1 Neoplasm of uncertain behavior of connective and other soft tissue ▽
239.2 Neoplasms of unspecified nature of bone, soft tissue, and skin

ICD-9-CM Procedural
80.87 Other local excision or destruction of lesion of ankle joint
83.31 Excision of lesion of tendon sheath
83.32 Excision of lesion of muscle
83.39 Excision of lesion of other soft tissue
83.49 Other excision of soft tissue

HCPCS Level II Supplies & Services
A4305 Disposable drug delivery system, flow rate of 50 ml or greater per hour
A4306 Disposable drug delivery system, flow rate of 5 ml or less per hour
A4550 Surgical trays

27620
27620 Arthrotomy, ankle, with joint exploration, with or without biopsy, with or without removal of loose or foreign body

ICD-9-CM Diagnostic
275.40 Unspecified disorder of calcium metabolism — (Use additional code to identify any associated mental retardation) ▽
275.42 Hypercalcemia — (Use additional code to identify any associated mental retardation)
275.49 Other disorders of calcium metabolism — (Use additional code to identify any associated mental retardation)
715.17 Primary localized osteoarthrosis, ankle and foot
715.27 Secondary localized osteoarthrosis, ankle and foot
715.97 Osteoarthrosis, unspecified whether generalized or localized, ankle and foot ▽
716.17 Traumatic arthropathy, ankle and foot
716.97 Unspecified arthropathy, ankle and foot ▽
718.17 Loose body in ankle and foot joint
718.87 Other joint derangement, not elsewhere classified, ankle and foot
719.47 Pain in joint, ankle and foot
726.91 Exostosis of unspecified site ▽
732.7 Osteochondritis dissecans
733.82 Nonunion of fracture
733.90 Disorder of bone and cartilage, unspecified ▽
996.4 Mechanical complication of internal orthopedic device, implant, and graft
V64.43 Arthroscopic surgical procedure converted to open procedure

ICD-9-CM Procedural
80.17 Other arthrotomy of ankle
80.37 Biopsy of joint structure of ankle

27625–27626
27625 Arthrotomy, with synovectomy, ankle;
27626 including tenosynovectomy

ICD-9-CM Diagnostic
357.1 Polyneuropathy in collagen vascular disease — (Code first underlying disease: 446.0, 710.0, 714.0) ☒
359.6 Symptomatic inflammatory myopathy in diseases classified elsewhere — (Code first underlying disease: 135, 140.0-208.9, 277.3, 446.0, 710.0, 710.1, 710.2, 714.0) ☒
446.0 Polyarteritis nodosa
710.0 Systemic lupus erythematosus — (Use additional code to identify manifestation: 424.91, 581.81, 582.81, 583.81)
710.1 Systemic sclerosis — (Use additional code to identify manifestation: 359.6, 517.2)
710.2 Sicca syndrome

714.0 Rheumatoid arthritis — (Use additional code to identify manifestation: 357.1, 359.6)
719.27 Villonodular synovitis, ankle and foot
V64.43 Arthroscopic surgical procedure converted to open procedure

ICD-9-CM Procedural

80.77 Synovectomy of ankle
83.42 Other tenonectomy

27630

27630 Excision of lesion of tendon sheath or capsule (eg, cyst or ganglion), leg and/or ankle

ICD-9-CM Diagnostic

215.3 Other benign neoplasm of connective and other soft tissue of lower limb, including hip
719.27 Villonodular synovitis, ankle and foot
727.42 Ganglion of tendon sheath

ICD-9-CM Procedural

83.31 Excision of lesion of tendon sheath

HCPCS Level II Supplies & Services

A4305 Disposable drug delivery system, flow rate of 50 ml or greater per hour
A4306 Disposable drug delivery system, flow rate of 5 ml or less per hour
A4550 Surgical trays

27635–27638

27635 Excision or curettage of bone cyst or benign tumor, tibia or fibula;
27637 with autograft (includes obtaining graft)
27638 with allograft

ICD-9-CM Diagnostic

213.7 Benign neoplasm of long bones of lower limb
238.0 Neoplasm of uncertain behavior of bone and articular cartilage
239.2 Neoplasms of unspecified nature of bone, soft tissue, and skin
730.26 Unspecified osteomyelitis, lower leg — (Use additional code to identify organism, 041.1) ▽
733.21 Solitary bone cyst
733.99 Other disorders of bone and cartilage

ICD-9-CM Procedural

77.67 Local excision of lesion or tissue of tibia and fibula
77.77 Excision of tibia and fibula for graft
78.07 Bone graft of tibia and fibula

HCPCS Level II Supplies & Services

A4305 Disposable drug delivery system, flow rate of 50 ml or greater per hour
A4306 Disposable drug delivery system, flow rate of 5 ml or less per hour
A4550 Surgical trays

27640–27641

27640 Partial excision (craterization, saucerization, or diaphysectomy) bone (eg, osteomyelitis or exostosis); tibia
27641 fibula

ICD-9-CM Diagnostic

726.91 Exostosis of unspecified site ▽
730.16 Chronic osteomyelitis, lower leg — (Use additional code to identify organism, 041.1)

ICD-9-CM Procedural

77.87 Other partial ostectomy of tibia and fibula

27645–27646

27645 Radical resection of tumor, bone; tibia
27646 fibula

ICD-9-CM Diagnostic

170.7 Malignant neoplasm of long bones of lower limb
198.5 Secondary malignant neoplasm of bone and bone marrow
238.0 Neoplasm of uncertain behavior of bone and articular cartilage

ICD-9-CM Procedural

77.97 Total ostectomy of tibia and fibula

27647

27647 Radical resection of tumor, bone; talus or calcaneus

ICD-9-CM Diagnostic

170.8 Malignant neoplasm of short bones of lower limb
198.5 Secondary malignant neoplasm of bone and bone marrow
238.0 Neoplasm of uncertain behavior of bone and articular cartilage

ICD-9-CM Procedural

77.99 Total ostectomy of other bone, except facial bones

27648

27648 Injection procedure for ankle arthrography

ICD-9-CM Diagnostic

275.40 Unspecified disorder of calcium metabolism — (Use additional code to identify any associated mental retardation) ▽
275.42 Hypercalcemia — (Use additional code to identify any associated mental retardation)
275.49 Other disorders of calcium metabolism — (Use additional code to identify any associated mental retardation)
357.1 Polyneuropathy in collagen vascular disease — (Code first underlying disease: 446.0, 710.0, 714.0) ☒
359.6 Symptomatic inflammatory myopathy in diseases classified elsewhere — (Code first underlying disease: 135, 140.0-208.9, 277.3, 446.0, 710.0, 710.1, 710.2, 714.0) ☒
446.0 Polyarteritis nodosa
710.0 Systemic lupus erythematosus — (Use additional code to identify manifestation: 424.91, 581.81, 582.81, 583.81)
710.1 Systemic sclerosis — (Use additional code to identify manifestation: 359.6, 517.2)
710.2 Sicca syndrome
714.0 Rheumatoid arthritis — (Use additional code to identify manifestation: 357.1, 359.6)
715.97 Osteoarthrosis, unspecified whether generalized or localized, ankle and foot ▽
718.17 Loose body in ankle and foot joint
719.07 Effusion of ankle and foot joint
732.7 Osteochondritis dissecans
905.4 Late effect of fracture of lower extremities

ICD-9-CM Procedural

81.92 Injection of therapeutic substance into joint or ligament
88.32 Contrast arthrogram

HCPCS Level II Supplies & Services

A9525 Supply of low or iso-osmolar contrast material, 10 mg of iodine

27650–27652

27650 Repair, primary, open or percutaneous, ruptured Achilles tendon;
27652 with graft (includes obtaining graft)

ICD-9-CM Diagnostic

727.67 Nontraumatic rupture of Achilles tendon
845.09 Other ankle sprain and strain
891.2 Open wound of knee, leg (except thigh), and ankle, with tendon involvement — (Use additional code to identify infection)
928.20 Crushing injury of foot — (Use additional code to identify any associated injuries: 800-829, 850.0-854.1, 860.0-869.1)

ICD-9-CM Procedural

83.64 Other suture of tendon

27654

27654 Repair, secondary, Achilles tendon, with or without graft

ICD-9-CM Diagnostic

727.67 Nontraumatic rupture of Achilles tendon
845.09 Other ankle sprain and strain
892.1 Open wound of foot except toe(s) alone, complicated — (Use additional code to identify infection)
928.20 Crushing injury of foot — (Use additional code to identify any associated injuries: 800-829, 850.0-854.1, 860.0-869.1)

ICD-9-CM Procedural

83.41 Excision of tendon for graft
83.62 Delayed suture of tendon
83.81 Tendon graft

27656

27656 Repair, fascial defect of leg

ICD-9-CM Diagnostic

728.89 Other disorder of muscle, ligament, and fascia — (Use additional E code to identify drug, if drug-induced)
729.4 Unspecified fasciitis ▽

ICD-9-CM Procedural

83.89 Other plastic operations on fascia

27658–27659

27658 Repair, flexor tendon, leg; primary, without graft, each tendon
27659 secondary, with or without graft, each tendon

ICD-9-CM Diagnostic

727.68 Nontraumatic rupture of other tendons of foot and ankle
727.69 Nontraumatic rupture of other tendon
891.2 Open wound of knee, leg (except thigh), and ankle, with tendon involvement — (Use additional code to identify infection)
894.1 Multiple and unspecified open wound of lower limb, complicated — (Use additional code to identify infection)
894.2 Multiple and unspecified open wound of lower limb, with tendon involvement — (Use additional code to identify infection)
905.8 Late effect of tendon injury
906.4 Late effect of crushing

ICD-9-CM Procedural

83.41 Excision of tendon for graft
83.62 Delayed suture of tendon
83.64 Other suture of tendon
83.81 Tendon graft

27664–27665

27664 Repair, extensor tendon, leg; primary, without graft, each tendon
27665 secondary, with or without graft, each tendon

ICD-9-CM Diagnostic

727.68 Nontraumatic rupture of other tendons of foot and ankle
727.69 Nontraumatic rupture of other tendon
891.2 Open wound of knee, leg (except thigh), and ankle, with tendon involvement — (Use additional code to identify infection)
894.2 Multiple and unspecified open wound of lower limb, with tendon involvement — (Use additional code to identify infection)
905.8 Late effect of tendon injury
906.4 Late effect of crushing
959.7 Injury, other and unspecified, knee, leg, ankle, and foot

ICD-9-CM Procedural

83.41 Excision of tendon for graft
83.62 Delayed suture of tendon
83.64 Other suture of tendon
83.81 Tendon graft

27675–27676

27675 Repair, dislocating peroneal tendons; without fibular osteotomy
27676 with fibular osteotomy

ICD-9-CM Diagnostic

718.37 Recurrent dislocation of ankle and foot joint
718.77 Developmental dislocation of joint, ankle and foot
718.87 Other joint derangement, not elsewhere classified, ankle and foot
726.79 Other enthesopathy of ankle and tarsus
727.00 Unspecified synovitis and tenosynovitis ▽
837.0 Closed dislocation of ankle
845.00 Unspecified site of ankle sprain and strain ▽
891.2 Open wound of knee, leg (except thigh), and ankle, with tendon involvement — (Use additional code to identify infection)

ICD-9-CM Procedural

77.17 Other incision of tibia and fibula without division
83.64 Other suture of tendon
83.76 Other tendon transposition
83.88 Other plastic operations on tendon

27680–27681

27680 Tenolysis, flexor or extensor tendon, leg and/or ankle; single, each tendon
27681 multiple tendons (through separate incision(s))

ICD-9-CM Diagnostic

718.57 Ankylosis of ankle and foot joint
719.57 Stiffness of joint, not elsewhere classified, ankle and foot
727.81 Contracture of tendon (sheath)
959.7 Injury, other and unspecified, knee, leg, ankle, and foot

ICD-9-CM Procedural

83.91 Lysis of adhesions of muscle, tendon, fascia, and bursa

27685–27686

27685 Lengthening or shortening of tendon, leg or ankle; single tendon (separate procedure)
27686 multiple tendons (through same incision), each

ICD-9-CM Diagnostic

718.46 Contracture of lower leg joint
718.47 Contracture of ankle and foot joint
727.81 Contracture of tendon (sheath)
736.70 Unspecified deformity of ankle and foot, acquired ▽
736.72 Equinus deformity of foot, acquired
736.79 Other acquired deformity of ankle and foot
754.51 Congenital talipes equinovarus
754.69 Other congenital valgus deformity of feet
754.79 Other congenital deformity of feet

ICD-9-CM Procedural

83.85 Other change in muscle or tendon length

27687

27687 Gastrocnemius recession (eg, Strayer procedure)

ICD-9-CM Diagnostic

343.9 Unspecified infantile cerebral palsy ▽
727.81 Contracture of tendon (sheath)
736.75 Cavovarus deformity of foot, acquired

ICD-9-CM Procedural

83.72 Recession of tendon

27690–27692

27690 Transfer or transplant of single tendon (with muscle redirection or rerouting); superficial (eg, anterior tibial extensors into midfoot)
27691 deep (eg, anterior tibial or posterior tibial through interosseous space, flexor digitorum longus, flexor hallicus longus, or peroneal tendon to midfoot or hindfoot)
27692 each additional tendon (List in addition to code for primary procedure)

ICD-9-CM Diagnostic

718.47 Contracture of ankle and foot joint
726.72 Tibialis tendinitis
726.90 Enthesopathy of unspecified site ▽
727.06 Tenosynovitis of foot and ankle
727.68 Nontraumatic rupture of other tendons of foot and ankle
727.81 Contracture of tendon (sheath)
736.72 Equinus deformity of foot, acquired
754.51 Congenital talipes equinovarus

ICD-9-CM Procedural

83.75 Tendon transfer or transplantation
83.79 Other muscle transposition

27695–27696

27695 Repair, primary, disrupted ligament, ankle; collateral
27696 both collateral ligaments

ICD-9-CM Diagnostic

837.1 Open dislocation of ankle
845.00 Unspecified site of ankle sprain and strain ▽
845.01 Sprain and strain of deltoid (ligament) of ankle
845.02 Sprain and strain of calcaneofibular (ligament)
845.03 Sprain and strain of tibiofibular (ligament)
845.09 Other ankle sprain and strain
891.1 Open wound of knee, leg (except thigh), and ankle, complicated — (Use additional code to identify infection)
959.7 Injury, other and unspecified, knee, leg, ankle, and foot

ICD-9-CM Procedural

81.94 Suture of capsule or ligament of ankle and foot

27698

27698 Repair, secondary, disrupted ligament, ankle, collateral (eg, Watson-Jones procedure)

ICD-9-CM Diagnostic

718.37 Recurrent dislocation of ankle and foot joint
726.79 Other enthesopathy of ankle and tarsus
845.01 Sprain and strain of deltoid (ligament) of ankle
845.02 Sprain and strain of calcaneofibular (ligament)
845.03 Sprain and strain of tibiofibular (ligament)
845.09 Other ankle sprain and strain
959.7 Injury, other and unspecified, knee, leg, ankle, and foot

ICD-9-CM Procedural

81.49 Other repair of ankle
81.94 Suture of capsule or ligament of ankle and foot

27700

27700 Arthroplasty, ankle;

ICD-9-CM Diagnostic

357.1 Polyneuropathy in collagen vascular disease — (Code first underlying disease: 446.0, 710.0, 714.0) ☒
359.6 Symptomatic inflammatory myopathy in diseases classified elsewhere — (Code first underlying disease: 135, 140.0-208.9, 277.3, 446.0, 710.0, 710.1, 710.2, 714.0) ☒
446.0 Polyarteritis nodosa
710.0 Systemic lupus erythematosus — (Use additional code to identify manifestation: 424.91, 581.81, 582.81, 583.81)
710.1 Systemic sclerosis — (Use additional code to identify manifestation: 359.6, 517.2)
710.2 Sicca syndrome
714.0 Rheumatoid arthritis — (Use additional code to identify manifestation: 357.1, 359.6)
715.17 Primary localized osteoarthrosis, ankle and foot
715.97 Osteoarthrosis, unspecified whether generalized or localized, ankle and foot ▽
718.57 Ankylosis of ankle and foot joint
718.87 Other joint derangement, not elsewhere classified, ankle and foot

ICD-9-CM Procedural

81.49 Other repair of ankle

27702

27702 Arthroplasty, ankle; with implant (total ankle)

ICD-9-CM Diagnostic

357.1 Polyneuropathy in collagen vascular disease — (Code first underlying disease: 446.0, 710.0, 714.0) ☒
359.6 Symptomatic inflammatory myopathy in diseases classified elsewhere — (Code first underlying disease: 135, 140.0-208.9, 277.3, 446.0, 710.0, 710.1, 710.2, 714.0) ☒
446.0 Polyarteritis nodosa
710.0 Systemic lupus erythematosus — (Use additional code to identify manifestation: 424.91, 581.81, 582.81, 583.81)
710.1 Systemic sclerosis — (Use additional code to identify manifestation: 359.6, 517.2)
710.2 Sicca syndrome
714.0 Rheumatoid arthritis — (Use additional code to identify manifestation: 357.1, 359.6)
715.17 Primary localized osteoarthrosis, ankle and foot
715.97 Osteoarthrosis, unspecified whether generalized or localized, ankle and foot ▽
718.57 Ankylosis of ankle and foot joint
730.27 Unspecified osteomyelitis, ankle and foot — (Use additional code to identify organism, 041.1) ▽
824.9 Unspecified open fracture of ankle ▽

ICD-9-CM Procedural

81.56 Total ankle replacement

27703

27703 Arthroplasty, ankle; revision, total ankle

ICD-9-CM Diagnostic

357.1 Polyneuropathy in collagen vascular disease — (Code first underlying disease: 446.0, 710.0, 714.0) ☒
359.6 Symptomatic inflammatory myopathy in diseases classified elsewhere — (Code first underlying disease: 135, 140.0-208.9, 277.3, 446.0, 710.0, 710.1, 710.2, 714.0) ☒
446.0 Polyarteritis nodosa
710.0 Systemic lupus erythematosus — (Use additional code to identify manifestation: 424.91, 581.81, 582.81, 583.81)
710.1 Systemic sclerosis — (Use additional code to identify manifestation: 359.6, 517.2)
710.2 Sicca syndrome
714.0 Rheumatoid arthritis — (Use additional code to identify manifestation: 357.1, 359.6)
715.17 Primary localized osteoarthrosis, ankle and foot
715.27 Secondary localized osteoarthrosis, ankle and foot
715.97 Osteoarthrosis, unspecified whether generalized or localized, ankle and foot ▽
718.57 Ankylosis of ankle and foot joint
718.87 Other joint derangement, not elsewhere classified, ankle and foot
733.16 Pathologic fracture of tibia or fibula
996.4 Mechanical complication of internal orthopedic device, implant, and graft

ICD-9-CM Procedural

81.59 Revision of joint replacement of lower extremity, not elsewhere classified

27704

27704 Removal of ankle implant

ICD-9-CM Diagnostic

996.4 Mechanical complication of internal orthopedic device, implant, and graft
996.60 Infection and inflammatory reaction due to unspecified device, implant, and graft — (Use additional code to identify specified infections) ▽
998.59 Other postoperative infection — (Use additional code to identify infection)
V54.01 Encounter for removal of internal fixation device

ICD-9-CM Procedural

80.07 Arthrotomy for removal of prosthesis of ankle

27705–27709

27705 Osteotomy; tibia
27707 fibula
27709 tibia and fibula

ICD-9-CM Diagnostic

733.5 Osteitis condensans
733.81 Malunion of fracture
736.41 Genu valgum (acquired)
736.42 Genu varum (acquired)
736.81 Unequal leg length (acquired)
756.51 Osteogenesis imperfecta

ICD-9-CM Procedural

77.27 Wedge osteotomy of tibia and fibula
77.37 Other division of tibia and fibula

27712

27712 Osteotomy; multiple, with realignment on intramedullary rod (eg, Sofield type procedure)

ICD-9-CM Diagnostic

733.81 Malunion of fracture
736.41 Genu valgum (acquired)
736.42 Genu varum (acquired)
756.51 Osteogenesis imperfecta
V54.02 Encounter for lengthening/adjustment of growth rod

ICD-9-CM Procedural

77.39 Other division of other bone, except facial bones

27715

27715 Osteoplasty, tibia and fibula, lengthening or shortening

ICD-9-CM Diagnostic

733.81 Malunion of fracture
736.81 Unequal leg length (acquired)
755.30 Congenital unspecified reduction deformity of lower limb ▽
755.32 Congenital longitudinal deficiency of lower limb, not elsewhere classified

ICD-9-CM Procedural

78.17 Application of external fixation device, tibia and fibula
78.27 Limb shortening procedures, tibia and fibula
78.37 Limb lengthening procedures, tibia and fibula
84.53 Implantation of internal limb lengthening device with kinetic distraction
84.54 Implantation of other internal limb lengthening device

27720–27725

27720 Repair of nonunion or malunion, tibia; without graft, (eg, compression technique)
27722 with sliding graft
27724 with iliac or other autograft (includes obtaining graft)
27725 by synostosis, with fibula, any method

ICD-9-CM Diagnostic

733.81 Malunion of fracture
733.82 Nonunion of fracture

ICD-9-CM Procedural

77.77 Excision of tibia and fibula for graft
78.07 Bone graft of tibia and fibula
78.47 Other repair or plastic operations on tibia and fibula

27727

27727 Repair of congenital pseudarthrosis, tibia

ICD-9-CM Diagnostic

755.69 Other congenital anomaly of lower limb, including pelvic girdle

ICD-9-CM Procedural

78.47 Other repair or plastic operations on tibia and fibula

27730–27734

27730 Arrest, epiphyseal (epiphysiodesis), open; distal tibia
27732 distal fibula
27734 distal tibia and fibula

ICD-9-CM Diagnostic

733.91 Arrest of bone development or growth
736.81 Unequal leg length (acquired)
755.30 Congenital unspecified reduction deformity of lower limb ▽
755.32 Congenital longitudinal deficiency of lower limb, not elsewhere classified

ICD-9-CM Procedural

78.27 Limb shortening procedures, tibia and fibula

27740–27742

27740 Arrest, epiphyseal (epiphysiodesis), any method, combined, proximal and distal tibia and fibula;
27742 and distal femur

ICD-9-CM Diagnostic

733.91 Arrest of bone development or growth
736.81 Unequal leg length (acquired)
755.30 Congenital unspecified reduction deformity of lower limb ▽
755.32 Congenital longitudinal deficiency of lower limb, not elsewhere classified

ICD-9-CM Procedural

78.25 Limb shortening procedures, femur
78.27 Limb shortening procedures, tibia and fibula

27745

27745 Prophylactic treatment (nailing, pinning, plating or wiring) with or without methylmethacrylate, tibia

ICD-9-CM Diagnostic

170.7 Malignant neoplasm of long bones of lower limb
198.5 Secondary malignant neoplasm of bone and bone marrow
213.7 Benign neoplasm of long bones of lower limb
238.0 Neoplasm of uncertain behavior of bone and articular cartilage
239.2 Neoplasms of unspecified nature of bone, soft tissue, and skin
733.00 Unspecified osteoporosis ▽
733.02 Idiopathic osteoporosis
733.09 Other osteoporosis — (Use additional E code to identify drug)
733.90 Disorder of bone and cartilage, unspecified ▽

ICD-9-CM Procedural

78.47 Other repair or plastic operations on tibia and fibula
84.55 Insertion of bone void filler

27750–27752

27750 Closed treatment of tibial shaft fracture (with or without fibular fracture); without manipulation
27752 with manipulation, with or without skeletal traction

ICD-9-CM Diagnostic

733.16 Pathologic fracture of tibia or fibula
733.93 Stress fracture of tibia or fibula
823.20 Closed fracture of shaft of tibia
823.22 Closed fracture of shaft of fibula with tibia
823.40 Torus fracture of tibia alone
823.42 Torus fracture of fibula with tibia

ICD-9-CM Procedural

79.06 Closed reduction of fracture of tibia and fibula without internal fixation
93.44 Other skeletal traction
93.53 Application of other cast
93.54 Application of splint

HCPCS Level II Supplies & Services

A4570 Splint
A4580 Cast supplies (e.g., plaster)
A4590 Special casting material (e.g., fiberglass)
E0112 Crutches, underarm, wood, adjustable or fixed, pair, with pads, tips and handgrips
E0113 Crutch, underarm, wood, adjustable or fixed, each, with pad, tip and handgrip

27756

27756 Percutaneous skeletal fixation of tibial shaft fracture (with or without fibular fracture) (eg, pins or screws)

ICD-9-CM Diagnostic

733.16 Pathologic fracture of tibia or fibula
733.93 Stress fracture of tibia or fibula
823.21 Closed fracture of shaft of fibula
823.22 Closed fracture of shaft of fibula with tibia

ICD-9-CM Procedural

78.57 Internal fixation of tibia and fibula without fracture reduction

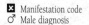

▽ Unspecified code
♀ Female diagnosis
☒ Manifestation code
♂ Male diagnosis

27758–27759

27758 Open treatment of tibial shaft fracture, (with or without fibular fracture) with plate/screws, with or without cerclage
27759 Treatment of tibial shaft fracture (with or without fibular fracture) by intramedullary implant, with or without interlocking screws and/or cerclage

ICD-9-CM Diagnostic

733.16 Pathologic fracture of tibia or fibula
733.93 Stress fracture of tibia or fibula
823.20 Closed fracture of shaft of tibia
823.22 Closed fracture of shaft of fibula with tibia
823.30 Open fracture of shaft of tibia
823.32 Open fracture of shaft of fibula with tibia

ICD-9-CM Procedural

79.36 Open reduction of fracture of tibia and fibula with internal fixation

27760–27762

27760 Closed treatment of medial malleolus fracture; without manipulation
27762 with manipulation, with or without skin or skeletal traction

ICD-9-CM Diagnostic

733.16 Pathologic fracture of tibia or fibula
733.93 Stress fracture of tibia or fibula
824.0 Closed fracture of medial malleolus

ICD-9-CM Procedural

79.09 Closed reduction of fracture of other specified bone, except facial bones, without internal fixation
93.44 Other skeletal traction
93.46 Other skin traction of limbs
93.53 Application of other cast

HCPCS Level II Supplies & Services

A4580 Cast supplies (e.g., plaster)
A4590 Special casting material (e.g., fiberglass)
E0112 Crutches, underarm, wood, adjustable or fixed, pair, with pads, tips and handgrips
E0113 Crutch, underarm, wood, adjustable or fixed, each, with pad, tip and handgrip
E0114 Crutches, underarm, other than wood, adjustable or fixed, pair, with pads, tips and handgrips

27766

27766 Open treatment of medial malleolus fracture, with or without internal or external fixation

ICD-9-CM Diagnostic

733.16 Pathologic fracture of tibia or fibula
733.93 Stress fracture of tibia or fibula
824.0 Closed fracture of medial malleolus
824.1 Open fracture of medial malleolus

ICD-9-CM Procedural

79.29 Open reduction of fracture of other specified bone, except facial bones, without internal fixation
79.39 Open reduction of fracture of other specified bone, except facial bones, with internal fixation

27780–27781

27780 Closed treatment of proximal fibula or shaft fracture; without manipulation
27781 with manipulation

ICD-9-CM Diagnostic

733.16 Pathologic fracture of tibia or fibula
733.93 Stress fracture of tibia or fibula
823.01 Closed fracture of upper end of fibula
823.21 Closed fracture of shaft of fibula
823.41 Torus fracture of fibula alone

ICD-9-CM Procedural

79.06 Closed reduction of fracture of tibia and fibula without internal fixation
93.53 Application of other cast

HCPCS Level II Supplies & Services

A4580 Cast supplies (e.g., plaster)
A4590 Special casting material (e.g., fiberglass)
E0112 Crutches, underarm, wood, adjustable or fixed, pair, with pads, tips and handgrips
E0113 Crutch, underarm, wood, adjustable or fixed, each, with pad, tip and handgrip
E0114 Crutches, underarm, other than wood, adjustable or fixed, pair, with pads, tips and handgrips

27784

27784 Open treatment of proximal fibula or shaft fracture, with or without internal or external fixation

ICD-9-CM Diagnostic

733.16 Pathologic fracture of tibia or fibula
733.93 Stress fracture of tibia or fibula
823.01 Closed fracture of upper end of fibula
823.11 Open fracture of upper end of fibula
823.21 Closed fracture of shaft of fibula
823.31 Open fracture of shaft of fibula

ICD-9-CM Procedural

79.26 Open reduction of fracture of tibia and fibula without internal fixation
79.36 Open reduction of fracture of tibia and fibula with internal fixation

27786–27788

27786 Closed treatment of distal fibular fracture (lateral malleolus); without manipulation
27788 with manipulation

ICD-9-CM Diagnostic

733.16 Pathologic fracture of tibia or fibula
733.93 Stress fracture of tibia or fibula
824.2 Closed fracture of lateral malleolus

ICD-9-CM Procedural

79.06 Closed reduction of fracture of tibia and fibula without internal fixation
93.53 Application of other cast

HCPCS Level II Supplies & Services

A4570 Splint
A4580 Cast supplies (e.g., plaster)
A4590 Special casting material (e.g., fiberglass)
E0112 Crutches, underarm, wood, adjustable or fixed, pair, with pads, tips and handgrips
E0113 Crutch, underarm, wood, adjustable or fixed, each, with pad, tip and handgrip

27792

27792 Open treatment of distal fibular fracture (lateral malleolus), with or without internal or external fixation

ICD-9-CM Diagnostic

733.16 Pathologic fracture of tibia or fibula
733.93 Stress fracture of tibia or fibula
824.2 Closed fracture of lateral malleolus
824.3 Open fracture of lateral malleolus

ICD-9-CM Procedural

79.26 Open reduction of fracture of tibia and fibula without internal fixation
79.36 Open reduction of fracture of tibia and fibula with internal fixation

27808–27810

27808 Closed treatment of bimalleolar ankle fracture, (including Potts); without manipulation
27810 with manipulation

ICD-9-CM Diagnostic

733.16 Pathologic fracture of tibia or fibula
733.93 Stress fracture of tibia or fibula
824.4 Closed bimalleolar fracture

ICD-9-CM Procedural

79.09 Closed reduction of fracture of other specified bone, except facial bones, without internal fixation
93.53 Application of other cast

HCPCS Level II Supplies & Services

A4570 Splint

A4580 Cast supplies (e.g., plaster)
A4590 Special casting material (e.g., fiberglass)
E0112 Crutches, underarm, wood, adjustable or fixed, pair, with pads, tips and handgrips
E0113 Crutch, underarm, wood, adjustable or fixed, each, with pad, tip and handgrip

27814

27814 Open treatment of bimalleolar ankle fracture, with or without internal or external fixation

ICD-9-CM Diagnostic

733.16 Pathologic fracture of tibia or fibula
733.93 Stress fracture of tibia or fibula
824.4 Closed bimalleolar fracture
824.5 Open bimalleolar fracture

ICD-9-CM Procedural

79.29 Open reduction of fracture of other specified bone, except facial bones, without internal fixation
79.39 Open reduction of fracture of other specified bone, except facial bones, with internal fixation

27816–27818

27816 Closed treatment of trimalleolar ankle fracture; without manipulation
27818 with manipulation

ICD-9-CM Diagnostic

733.16 Pathologic fracture of tibia or fibula
733.93 Stress fracture of tibia or fibula
824.6 Closed trimalleolar fracture

ICD-9-CM Procedural

79.09 Closed reduction of fracture of other specified bone, except facial bones, without internal fixation
93.53 Application of other cast

HCPCS Level II Supplies & Services

A4570 Splint
A4580 Cast supplies (e.g., plaster)
A4590 Special casting material (e.g., fiberglass)
E0112 Crutches, underarm, wood, adjustable or fixed, pair, with pads, tips and handgrips
E0113 Crutch, underarm, wood, adjustable or fixed, each, with pad, tip and handgrip

27822–27823

27822 Open treatment of trimalleolar ankle fracture, with or without internal or external fixation, medial and/or lateral malleolus; without fixation of posterior lip
27823 with fixation of posterior lip

ICD-9-CM Diagnostic

733.16 Pathologic fracture of tibia or fibula
733.93 Stress fracture of tibia or fibula
824.6 Closed trimalleolar fracture
824.7 Open trimalleolar fracture

ICD-9-CM Procedural

79.29 Open reduction of fracture of other specified bone, except facial bones, without internal fixation
79.39 Open reduction of fracture of other specified bone, except facial bones, with internal fixation

27824–27825

27824 Closed treatment of fracture of weight bearing articular portion of distal tibia (eg, pilon or tibial plafond), with or without anesthesia; without manipulation
27825 with skeletal traction and/or requiring manipulation

ICD-9-CM Diagnostic

733.93 Stress fracture of tibia or fibula
733.95 Stress fracture of other bone
824.8 Unspecified closed fracture of ankle ▽

ICD-9-CM Procedural

79.06 Closed reduction of fracture of tibia and fibula without internal fixation
93.44 Other skeletal traction
93.53 Application of other cast

27826–27828

27826 Open treatment of fracture of weight bearing articular surface/portion of distal tibia (eg, pilon or tibial plafond), with internal or external fixation; of fibula only
27827 of tibia only
27828 of both tibia and fibula

ICD-9-CM Diagnostic

733.93 Stress fracture of tibia or fibula
733.95 Stress fracture of other bone
823.92 Open fracture of unspecified part of fibula with tibia ▽
824.8 Unspecified closed fracture of ankle ▽
824.9 Unspecified open fracture of ankle ▽

ICD-9-CM Procedural

78.17 Application of external fixation device, tibia and fibula
79.36 Open reduction of fracture of tibia and fibula with internal fixation

27829

27829 Open treatment of distal tibiofibular joint (syndesmosis) disruption, with or without internal or external fixation

ICD-9-CM Diagnostic

718.77 Developmental dislocation of joint, ankle and foot
837.0 Closed dislocation of ankle
837.1 Open dislocation of ankle

ICD-9-CM Procedural

79.26 Open reduction of fracture of tibia and fibula without internal fixation
79.36 Open reduction of fracture of tibia and fibula with internal fixation

27830–27831

27830 Closed treatment of proximal tibiofibular joint dislocation; without anesthesia
27831 requiring anesthesia

ICD-9-CM Diagnostic

718.76 Developmental dislocation of joint, lower leg
836.59 Other closed dislocation of knee

ICD-9-CM Procedural

79.79 Closed reduction of dislocation of other specified site, except temporomandibular

HCPCS Level II Supplies & Services

A4570 Splint
A4580 Cast supplies (e.g., plaster)
A4590 Special casting material (e.g., fiberglass)
E0112 Crutches, underarm, wood, adjustable or fixed, pair, with pads, tips and handgrips
E0113 Crutch, underarm, wood, adjustable or fixed, each, with pad, tip and handgrip

27832

27832 Open treatment of proximal tibiofibular joint dislocation, with or without internal or external fixation, or with excision of proximal fibula

ICD-9-CM Diagnostic

718.76 Developmental dislocation of joint, lower leg
836.59 Other closed dislocation of knee
836.69 Other open dislocation of knee

ICD-9-CM Procedural

79.89 Open reduction of dislocation of other specified site, except temporomandibular

27840–27842

27840 Closed treatment of ankle dislocation; without anesthesia
27842 requiring anesthesia, with or without percutaneous skeletal fixation

ICD-9-CM Diagnostic

718.77 Developmental dislocation of joint, ankle and foot
837.0 Closed dislocation of ankle

▽ Unspecified code ♀ Female diagnosis ☒ Manifestation code ♂ Male diagnosis

ICD-9-CM Procedural

79.09 Closed reduction of fracture of other specified bone, except facial bones, without internal fixation
79.77 Closed reduction of dislocation of ankle

HCPCS Level II Supplies & Services

A4570 Splint
A4580 Cast supplies (e.g., plaster)
A4590 Special casting material (e.g., fiberglass)
E0112 Crutches, underarm, wood, adjustable or fixed, pair, with pads, tips and handgrips
E0113 Crutch, underarm, wood, adjustable or fixed, each, with pad, tip and handgrip

27846–27848

27846 Open treatment of ankle dislocation, with or without percutaneous skeletal fixation; without repair or internal fixation
27848 with repair or internal or external fixation

ICD-9-CM Diagnostic

718.77 Developmental dislocation of joint, ankle and foot
837.0 Closed dislocation of ankle
837.1 Open dislocation of ankle

ICD-9-CM Procedural

79.87 Open reduction of dislocation of ankle
81.49 Other repair of ankle

27860

27860 Manipulation of ankle under general anesthesia (includes application of traction or other fixation apparatus)

ICD-9-CM Diagnostic

718.57 Ankylosis of ankle and foot joint
996.4 Mechanical complication of internal orthopedic device, implant, and graft

ICD-9-CM Procedural

79.79 Closed reduction of dislocation of other specified site, except temporomandibular

HCPCS Level II Supplies & Services

A4305 Disposable drug delivery system, flow rate of 50 ml or greater per hour
A4306 Disposable drug delivery system, flow rate of 5 ml or less per hour
A4550 Surgical trays

27870

27870 Arthrodesis, ankle, open

ICD-9-CM Diagnostic

711.07 Pyogenic arthritis, ankle and foot — (Use additional code to identify infectious organism: 041.0-041.8)
711.67 Arthropathy associated with mycoses, ankle and foot — (Code first underlying disease: 110.0-118) ☒
712.17 Chondrocalcinosis due to dicalcium phosphate crystals, ankle and foot — (Code first underlying disease, 275.4) ☒
712.27 Chondrocalcinosis due to pyrophosphate crystals, ankle and foot — (Code first underlying disease, 275.4) ☒
713.5 Arthropathy associated with neurological disorders — (Code first underlying disease: 094.0, 250.6, 336.0) ☒
714.0 Rheumatoid arthritis — (Use additional code to identify manifestation: 357.1, 359.6)
714.4 Chronic postrheumatic arthropathy
715.17 Primary localized osteoarthrosis, ankle and foot
715.27 Secondary localized osteoarthrosis, ankle and foot
715.97 Osteoarthrosis, unspecified whether generalized or localized, ankle and foot ▽
716.17 Traumatic arthropathy, ankle and foot
718.87 Other joint derangement, not elsewhere classified, ankle and foot
730.17 Chronic osteomyelitis, ankle and foot — (Use additional code to identify organism, 041.1)
733.81 Malunion of fracture
736.70 Unspecified deformity of ankle and foot, acquired ▽
754.51 Congenital talipes equinovarus
905.4 Late effect of fracture of lower extremities
906.4 Late effect of crushing
996.77 Other complications due to internal joint prosthesis
V64.43 Arthroscopic surgical procedure converted to open procedure

ICD-9-CM Procedural

81.29 Arthrodesis of other specified joint

27871

27871 Arthrodesis, tibiofibular joint, proximal or distal

ICD-9-CM Diagnostic

718.36 Recurrent dislocation of lower leg joint
718.87 Other joint derangement, not elsewhere classified, ankle and foot
718.97 Unspecified ankle and foot joint derangement ▽

ICD-9-CM Procedural

81.29 Arthrodesis of other specified joint

27880–27882

27880 Amputation, leg, through tibia and fibula;
27881 with immediate fitting technique including application of first cast
27882 open, circular (guillotine)

ICD-9-CM Diagnostic

170.7 Malignant neoplasm of long bones of lower limb
170.8 Malignant neoplasm of short bones of lower limb
171.3 Malignant neoplasm of connective and other soft tissue of lower limb, including hip
195.5 Malignant neoplasm of lower limb
198.5 Secondary malignant neoplasm of bone and bone marrow
238.0 Neoplasm of uncertain behavior of bone and articular cartilage
250.70 Diabetes with peripheral circulatory disorders, type II or unspecified type, not stated as uncontrolled — (Use additional code to identify manifestation: 443.81, 785.4)
250.71 Diabetes with peripheral circulatory disorders, type I [juvenile type], not stated as uncontrolled — (Use additional code to identify manifestation: 443.81, 785.4)
250.72 Diabetes with peripheral circulatory disorders, type II or unspecified type, uncontrolled — (Use additional code to identify manifestation: 443.81, 785.4)
250.73 Diabetes with peripheral circulatory disorders, type I [juvenile type], uncontrolled — (Use additional code to identify manifestation: 443.81, 785.4)
440.20 Atherosclerosis of native arteries of the extremities, unspecified ▽
440.21 Atherosclerosis of native arteries of the extremities with intermittent claudication
440.22 Atherosclerosis of native arteries of the extremities with rest pain
440.23 Atherosclerosis of native arteries of the extremities with ulceration — (Use additional code for any associated ulceration: 707.10-707.9)
440.24 Atherosclerosis of native arteries of the extremities with gangrene
443.81 Peripheral angiopathy in diseases classified elsewhere — (Code first underlying disease, 250.7) ☒
682.7 Cellulitis and abscess of foot, except toes — (Use additional code to identify organism)
707.10 Ulcer of lower limb, unspecified ▽
707.12 Ulcer of calf
707.13 Ulcer of ankle
730.16 Chronic osteomyelitis, lower leg — (Use additional code to identify organism, 041.1)
730.17 Chronic osteomyelitis, ankle and foot — (Use additional code to identify organism, 041.1)
733.49 Aseptic necrosis of other bone site
785.4 Gangrene — (Code first any associated underlying condition:250.7, 443.0)
897.0 Traumatic amputation of leg(s) (complete) (partial), unilateral, below knee, without mention of complication — (Use additional code to identify infection)
897.1 Traumatic amputation of leg(s) (complete) (partial), unilateral, below knee, complicated — (Use additional code to identify infection)

ICD-9-CM Procedural

84.15 Other amputation below knee
84.46 Fitting of prosthesis below knee

27884

27884 Amputation, leg, through tibia and fibula; secondary closure or scar revision

ICD-9-CM Diagnostic

250.70 Diabetes with peripheral circulatory disorders, type II or unspecified type, not stated as uncontrolled — (Use additional code to identify manifestation: 443.81, 785.4)

250.71 Diabetes with peripheral circulatory disorders, type I [juvenile type], not stated as uncontrolled — (Use additional code to identify manifestation: 443.81, 785.4)
250.72 Diabetes with peripheral circulatory disorders, type II or unspecified type, uncontrolled — (Use additional code to identify manifestation: 443.81, 785.4)
250.73 Diabetes with peripheral circulatory disorders, type I [juvenile type], uncontrolled — (Use additional code to identify manifestation: 443.81, 785.4)
443.81 Peripheral angiopathy in diseases classified elsewhere — (Code first underlying disease, 250.7) ☒
459.89 Other specified circulatory system disorders
682.6 Cellulitis and abscess of leg, except foot — (Use additional code to identify organism)
707.10 Ulcer of lower limb, unspecified ▽
707.12 Ulcer of calf
709.2 Scar condition and fibrosis of skin
785.4 Gangrene — (Code first any associated underlying condition:250.7, 443.0)
997.62 Infection (chronic) of amputation stump — (Use additional code to identify organism. Use additional code to identify complications)
998.51 Infected postoperative seroma — (Use additional code to identify organism)
998.59 Other postoperative infection — (Use additional code to identify infection)

ICD-9-CM Procedural

84.15 Other amputation below knee
84.3 Revision of amputation stump

HCPCS Level II Supplies & Services

A4580 Cast supplies (e.g., plaster)
L5450 Immediate postsurgical or early fitting, application of nonweight bearing rigid dressing, below knee
L5510 Preparatory, below knee "PTB" type socket, non-alignable system, pylon, no cover, SACH foot, plaster socket, molded to model
L5520 Preparatory, below knee "PTB" type socket, non-alignable system, pylon, no cover, SACH foot, thermoplastic or equal, direct formed
L5530 Preparatory, below knee "PTB" type socket, non-alignable system, pylon, no cover, SACH foot, thermoplastic or equal, molded to model

27886

27886 Amputation, leg, through tibia and fibula; re-amputation

ICD-9-CM Diagnostic

250.70 Diabetes with peripheral circulatory disorders, type II or unspecified type, not stated as uncontrolled — (Use additional code to identify manifestation: 443.81, 785.4)
250.71 Diabetes with peripheral circulatory disorders, type I [juvenile type], not stated as uncontrolled — (Use additional code to identify manifestation: 443.81, 785.4)
250.72 Diabetes with peripheral circulatory disorders, type II or unspecified type, uncontrolled — (Use additional code to identify manifestation: 443.81, 785.4)
250.73 Diabetes with peripheral circulatory disorders, type I [juvenile type], uncontrolled — (Use additional code to identify manifestation: 443.81, 785.4)
443.81 Peripheral angiopathy in diseases classified elsewhere — (Code first underlying disease, 250.7) ☒
443.9 Unspecified peripheral vascular disease ▽
682.6 Cellulitis and abscess of leg, except foot — (Use additional code to identify organism)
707.10 Ulcer of lower limb, unspecified ▽
707.12 Ulcer of calf
709.2 Scar condition and fibrosis of skin
785.4 Gangrene — (Code first any associated underlying condition:250.7, 443.0)
997.62 Infection (chronic) of amputation stump — (Use additional code to identify organism. Use additional code to identify complications)
998.51 Infected postoperative seroma — (Use additional code to identify organism)
998.59 Other postoperative infection — (Use additional code to identify infection)

ICD-9-CM Procedural

84.15 Other amputation below knee
84.3 Revision of amputation stump

27888

27888 Amputation, ankle, through malleoli of tibia and fibula (eg, Syme, Pirogoff type procedures), with plastic closure and resection of nerves

ICD-9-CM Diagnostic

170.8 Malignant neoplasm of short bones of lower limb
195.5 Malignant neoplasm of lower limb
198.5 Secondary malignant neoplasm of bone and bone marrow
238.0 Neoplasm of uncertain behavior of bone and articular cartilage
250.70 Diabetes with peripheral circulatory disorders, type II or unspecified type, not stated as uncontrolled — (Use additional code to identify manifestation: 443.81, 785.4)
250.71 Diabetes with peripheral circulatory disorders, type I [juvenile type], not stated as uncontrolled — (Use additional code to identify manifestation: 443.81, 785.4)
250.80 Diabetes with other specified manifestations, type II or unspecified type, not stated as uncontrolled — (Use additional code to identify manifestation: 707.10-707.9, 731.8. Use additional E code to identify cause, if drug-induced)
250.81 Diabetes with other specified manifestations, type I [juvenile type], not stated as uncontrolled — (Use additional code to identify manifestation: 707.10-707.9, 731.8. Use additional E code to identify cause, if drug-induced)
355.79 Other mononeuritis of lower limb
355.8 Unspecified mononeuritis of lower limb ▽
440.20 Atherosclerosis of native arteries of the extremities, unspecified ▽
440.21 Atherosclerosis of native arteries of the extremities with intermittent claudication
440.22 Atherosclerosis of native arteries of the extremities with rest pain
440.23 Atherosclerosis of native arteries of the extremities with ulceration — (Use additional code for any associated ulceration: 707.10-707.9)
440.24 Atherosclerosis of native arteries of the extremities with gangrene
443.81 Peripheral angiopathy in diseases classified elsewhere — (Code first underlying disease, 250.7) ☒
446.0 Polyarteritis nodosa
707.10 Ulcer of lower limb, unspecified ▽
707.13 Ulcer of ankle
707.14 Ulcer of heel and midfoot
707.15 Ulcer of other part of foot
728.86 Necrotizing fasciitis — (Use additional code to identify infectious organism, 041.00-041.89, 785.4, if applicable)
730.17 Chronic osteomyelitis, ankle and foot — (Use additional code to identify organism, 041.1)
731.1 Osteitis deformans in diseases classified elsewhere — (Code first underlying disease: 170.0-170.9) ☒
731.8 Other bone involvement in diseases classified elsewhere — (Code first underlying disease, 250.8. Use additional code to specify bone condition: 730.00-730.09) ☒
785.4 Gangrene — (Code first any associated underlying condition:250.7, 443.0)
896.0 Traumatic amputation of foot (complete) (partial), unilateral, without mention of complication — (Use additional code to identify infection)
896.1 Traumatic amputation of foot (complete) (partial), unilateral, complicated — (Use additional code to identify infection)
928.20 Crushing injury of foot — (Use additional code to identify any associated injuries: 800-829, 850.0-854.1, 860.0-869.1)
945.34 Full-thickness skin loss due to burn (third degree nos) of lower leg
945.44 Deep necrosis of underlying tissues due to burn (deep third degree) of lower leg, without mention of loss of a body part

ICD-9-CM Procedural

84.14 Amputation of ankle through malleoli of tibia and fibula

27889

27889 Ankle disarticulation

ICD-9-CM Diagnostic

170.8 Malignant neoplasm of short bones of lower limb
195.5 Malignant neoplasm of lower limb
198.5 Secondary malignant neoplasm of bone and bone marrow
238.0 Neoplasm of uncertain behavior of bone and articular cartilage
250.70 Diabetes with peripheral circulatory disorders, type II or unspecified type, not stated as uncontrolled — (Use additional code to identify manifestation: 443.81, 785.4)
250.71 Diabetes with peripheral circulatory disorders, type I [juvenile type], not stated as uncontrolled — (Use additional code to identify manifestation: 443.81, 785.4)
250.80 Diabetes with other specified manifestations, type II or unspecified type, not stated as uncontrolled — (Use additional code to identify manifestation: 707.10-707.9, 731.8. Use additional E code to identify cause, if drug-induced)
250.81 Diabetes with other specified manifestations, type I [juvenile type], not stated as uncontrolled — (Use additional code to identify manifestation: 707.10-707.9, 731.8. Use additional E code to identify cause, if drug-induced)
355.79 Other mononeuritis of lower limb
355.8 Unspecified mononeuritis of lower limb ▽
440.20 Atherosclerosis of native arteries of the extremities, unspecified ▽

440.21 Atherosclerosis of native arteries of the extremities with intermittent claudication
440.22 Atherosclerosis of native arteries of the extremities with rest pain
440.23 Atherosclerosis of native arteries of the extremities with ulceration — (Use additional code for any associated ulceration: 707.10-707.9)
440.24 Atherosclerosis of native arteries of the extremities with gangrene
443.81 Peripheral angiopathy in diseases classified elsewhere — (Code first underlying disease, 250.7) ☒
446.0 Polyarteritis nodosa
707.10 Ulcer of lower limb, unspecified ▽
707.13 Ulcer of ankle
707.14 Ulcer of heel and midfoot
707.15 Ulcer of other part of foot
728.86 Necrotizing fasciitis — (Use additional code to identify infectious organism, 041.00-041.89, 785.4, if applicable)
730.17 Chronic osteomyelitis, ankle and foot — (Use additional code to identify organism, 041.1)
731.1 Osteitis deformans in diseases classified elsewhere — (Code first underlying disease: 170.0-170.9) ☒
731.8 Other bone involvement in diseases classified elsewhere — (Code first underlying disease, 250.8. Use additional code to specify bone condition: 730.00-730.09) ☒
785.4 Gangrene — (Code first any associated underlying condition:250.7, 443.0)
896.0 Traumatic amputation of foot (complete) (partial), unilateral, without mention of complication — (Use additional code to identify infection)
896.1 Traumatic amputation of foot (complete) (partial), unilateral, complicated — (Use additional code to identify infection)
928.20 Crushing injury of foot — (Use additional code to identify any associated injuries: 800-829, 850.0-854.1, 860.0-869.1)
945.34 Full-thickness skin loss due to burn (third degree nos) of lower leg
945.44 Deep necrosis of underlying tissues due to burn (deep third degree) of lower leg, without mention of loss of a body part

ICD-9-CM Procedural

84.13 Disarticulation of ankle

27892–27894

27892 Decompression fasciotomy, leg; anterior and/or lateral compartments only, with debridement of nonviable muscle and/or nerve
27893 posterior compartment(s) only, with debridement of nonviable muscle and/or nerve
27894 anterior and/or lateral, and posterior compartment(s), with debridement of nonviable muscle and/or nerve

ICD-9-CM Diagnostic

444.22 Embolism and thrombosis of arteries of lower extremity
445.02 Atheroembolism of lower extremity
682.6 Cellulitis and abscess of leg, except foot — (Use additional code to identify organism)
728.86 Necrotizing fasciitis — (Use additional code to identify infectious organism, 041.00-041.89, 785.4, if applicable)
728.88 Rhabdomyolysis
729.4 Unspecified fasciitis ▽
785.4 Gangrene — (Code first any associated underlying condition:250.7, 443.0)
823.22 Closed fracture of shaft of fibula with tibia
823.30 Open fracture of shaft of tibia
823.32 Open fracture of shaft of fibula with tibia
928.10 Crushing injury of lower leg — (Use additional code to identify any associated injuries: 800-829, 850.0-854.1, 860.0-869.1)
945.34 Full-thickness skin loss due to burn (third degree nos) of lower leg
945.44 Deep necrosis of underlying tissues due to burn (deep third degree) of lower leg, without mention of loss of a body part
958.6 Volkmann's ischemic contracture
958.8 Other early complications of trauma
996.74 Other complications due to other vascular device, implant, and graft

ICD-9-CM Procedural

83.14 Fasciotomy

28001

28001 Incision and drainage, bursa, foot

ICD-9-CM Diagnostic

250.71 Diabetes with peripheral circulatory disorders, type I [juvenile type], not stated as uncontrolled — (Use additional code to identify manifestation: 443.81, 785.4)
250.72 Diabetes with peripheral circulatory disorders, type II or unspecified type, uncontrolled — (Use additional code to identify manifestation: 443.81, 785.4)
443.81 Peripheral angiopathy in diseases classified elsewhere — (Code first underlying disease, 250.7) ☒
681.9 Cellulitis and abscess of unspecified digit — (Use additional code to identify organism) ▽
682.7 Cellulitis and abscess of foot, except toes — (Use additional code to identify organism)
686.1 Pyogenic granuloma of skin and subcutaneous tissue
726.70 Unspecified enthesopathy of ankle and tarsus ▽
726.79 Other enthesopathy of ankle and tarsus
727.3 Other bursitis disorders
727.89 Other disorders of synovium, tendon, and bursa

ICD-9-CM Procedural

83.03 Bursotomy

HCPCS Level II Supplies & Services

A4305 Disposable drug delivery system, flow rate of 50 ml or greater per hour
A4306 Disposable drug delivery system, flow rate of 5 ml or less per hour
A4550 Surgical trays

28002–28003

28002 Incision and drainage below fascia, with or without tendon sheath involvement, foot; single bursal space
28003 multiple areas

ICD-9-CM Diagnostic

250.70 Diabetes with peripheral circulatory disorders, type II or unspecified type, not stated as uncontrolled — (Use additional code to identify manifestation: 443.81, 785.4)
250.71 Diabetes with peripheral circulatory disorders, type I [juvenile type], not stated as uncontrolled — (Use additional code to identify manifestation: 443.81, 785.4)
250.80 Diabetes with other specified manifestations, type II or unspecified type, not stated as uncontrolled — (Use additional code to identify manifestation: 707.10-707.9, 731.8. Use additional E code to identify cause, if drug-induced)
250.81 Diabetes with other specified manifestations, type I [juvenile type], not stated as uncontrolled — (Use additional code to identify manifestation: 707.10-707.9, 731.8. Use additional E code to identify cause, if drug-induced)
443.81 Peripheral angiopathy in diseases classified elsewhere — (Code first underlying disease, 250.7) ☒
682.7 Cellulitis and abscess of foot, except toes — (Use additional code to identify organism)
707.10 Ulcer of lower limb, unspecified ▽
707.14 Ulcer of heel and midfoot
707.15 Ulcer of other part of foot
711.07 Pyogenic arthritis, ankle and foot — (Use additional code to identify infectious organism: 041.0-041.8)
726.70 Unspecified enthesopathy of ankle and tarsus ▽
785.4 Gangrene — (Code first any associated underlying condition:250.7, 443.0)
892.1 Open wound of foot except toe(s) alone, complicated — (Use additional code to identify infection)
998.51 Infected postoperative seroma — (Use additional code to identify organism)
998.59 Other postoperative infection — (Use additional code to identify infection)

ICD-9-CM Procedural

83.01 Exploration of tendon sheath
83.03 Bursotomy

HCPCS Level II Supplies & Services

A4305 Disposable drug delivery system, flow rate of 50 ml or greater per hour
A4306 Disposable drug delivery system, flow rate of 5 ml or less per hour
A4550 Surgical trays

28005

28005 Incision, bone cortex (eg, osteomyelitis or bone abscess), foot

ICD-9-CM Diagnostic

250.70 Diabetes with peripheral circulatory disorders, type II or unspecified type, not stated as uncontrolled — (Use additional code to identify manifestation: 443.81, 785.4)
250.71 Diabetes with peripheral circulatory disorders, type I [juvenile type], not stated as uncontrolled — (Use additional code to identify manifestation: 443.81, 785.4)

250.80 Diabetes with other specified manifestations, type II or unspecified type, not stated as uncontrolled — (Use additional code to identify manifestation: 707.10-707.9, 731.8. Use additional E code to identify cause, if drug-induced)
250.81 Diabetes with other specified manifestations, type I [juvenile type], not stated as uncontrolled — (Use additional code to identify manifestation: 707.10-707.9, 731.8. Use additional E code to identify cause, if drug-induced)
355.79 Other mononeuritis of lower limb
355.8 Unspecified mononeuritis of lower limb ▽
440.20 Atherosclerosis of native arteries of the extremities, unspecified ▽
440.24 Atherosclerosis of native arteries of the extremities with gangrene
443.81 Peripheral angiopathy in diseases classified elsewhere — (Code first underlying disease, 250.7) ☒
446.0 Polyarteritis nodosa
707.10 Ulcer of lower limb, unspecified ▽
707.14 Ulcer of heel and midfoot
707.15 Ulcer of other part of foot
728.86 Necrotizing fasciitis — (Use additional code to identify infectious organism, 041.00-041.89, 785.4, if applicable)
730.17 Chronic osteomyelitis, ankle and foot — (Use additional code to identify organism, 041.1)
731.1 Osteitis deformans in diseases classified elsewhere — (Code first underlying disease: 170.0-170.9) ☒
731.8 Other bone involvement in diseases classified elsewhere — (Code first underlying disease, 250.8. Use additional code to specify bone condition: 730.00-730.09) ☒
785.4 Gangrene — (Code first any associated underlying condition:250.7, 443.0)
896.0 Traumatic amputation of foot (complete) (partial), unilateral, without mention of complication — (Use additional code to identify infection)
896.1 Traumatic amputation of foot (complete) (partial), unilateral, complicated — (Use additional code to identify infection)
928.20 Crushing injury of foot — (Use additional code to identify any associated injuries: 800-829, 850.0-854.1, 860.0-869.1)
945.34 Full-thickness skin loss due to burn (third degree nos) of lower leg
945.44 Deep necrosis of underlying tissues due to burn (deep third degree) of lower leg, without mention of loss of a body part

ICD-9-CM Procedural

77.18 Other incision of tarsals and metatarsals without division

28008

28008 Fasciotomy, foot and/or toe

ICD-9-CM Diagnostic

250.70 Diabetes with peripheral circulatory disorders, type II or unspecified type, not stated as uncontrolled — (Use additional code to identify manifestation: 443.81, 785.4)
250.71 Diabetes with peripheral circulatory disorders, type I [juvenile type], not stated as uncontrolled — (Use additional code to identify manifestation: 443.81, 785.4)
443.81 Peripheral angiopathy in diseases classified elsewhere — (Code first underlying disease, 250.7) ☒
682.6 Cellulitis and abscess of leg, except foot — (Use additional code to identify organism)
726.73 Calcaneal spur
726.91 Exostosis of unspecified site ▽
728.71 Plantar fascial fibromatosis
728.86 Necrotizing fasciitis — (Use additional code to identify infectious organism, 041.00-041.89, 785.4, if applicable)
728.88 Rhabdomyolysis
729.4 Unspecified fasciitis ▽
785.4 Gangrene — (Code first any associated underlying condition:250.7, 443.0)
945.34 Full-thickness skin loss due to burn (third degree nos) of lower leg
945.44 Deep necrosis of underlying tissues due to burn (deep third degree) of lower leg, without mention of loss of a body part
958.6 Volkmann's ischemic contracture
958.8 Other early complications of trauma

ICD-9-CM Procedural

83.14 Fasciotomy

HCPCS Level II Supplies & Services

A4580 Cast supplies (e.g., plaster)
A4590 Special casting material (e.g., fiberglass)
E0112 Crutches, underarm, wood, adjustable or fixed, pair, with pads, tips and handgrips
E0113 Crutch, underarm, wood, adjustable or fixed, each, with pad, tip and handgrip
E0114 Crutches, underarm, other than wood, adjustable or fixed, pair, with pads, tips and handgrips

28010–28011

28010 Tenotomy, percutaneous, toe; single tendon
28011 multiple tendons

ICD-9-CM Diagnostic

735.0 Hallux valgus (acquired)
735.1 Hallux varus (acquired)
735.2 Hallux rigidus
735.3 Hallux malleus
735.4 Other hammer toe (acquired)
735.5 Claw toe (acquired)
735.8 Other acquired deformity of toe
755.66 Other congenital anomaly of toes

ICD-9-CM Procedural

83.13 Other tenotomy

HCPCS Level II Supplies & Services

A4305 Disposable drug delivery system, flow rate of 50 ml or greater per hour
A4306 Disposable drug delivery system, flow rate of 5 ml or less per hour
A4550 Surgical trays

28020–28024

28020 Arthrotomy, including exploration, drainage, or removal of loose or foreign body; intertarsal or tarsometatarsal joint
28022 metatarsophalangeal joint
28024 interphalangeal joint

ICD-9-CM Diagnostic

355.5 Tarsal tunnel syndrome
682.7 Cellulitis and abscess of foot, except toes — (Use additional code to identify organism)
711.07 Pyogenic arthritis, ankle and foot — (Use additional code to identify infectious organism: 041.0-041.8)
718.17 Loose body in ankle and foot joint
726.70 Unspecified enthesopathy of ankle and tarsus ▽
729.6 Residual foreign body in soft tissue
730.17 Chronic osteomyelitis, ankle and foot — (Use additional code to identify organism, 041.1)
892.1 Open wound of foot except toe(s) alone, complicated — (Use additional code to identify infection)
893.0 Open wound of toe(s), without mention of complication — (Use additional code to identify infection)
893.1 Open wound of toe(s), complicated — (Use additional code to identify infection)
996.4 Mechanical complication of internal orthopedic device, implant, and graft

ICD-9-CM Procedural

80.18 Other arthrotomy of foot and toe

HCPCS Level II Supplies & Services

A4305 Disposable drug delivery system, flow rate of 50 ml or greater per hour
A4306 Disposable drug delivery system, flow rate of 5 ml or less per hour
A4550 Surgical trays

28030

28030 Neurectomy, intrinsic musculature of foot

ICD-9-CM Diagnostic

215.3 Other benign neoplasm of connective and other soft tissue of lower limb, including hip
355.6 Lesion of plantar nerve
355.8 Unspecified mononeuritis of lower limb ▽
729.2 Unspecified neuralgia, neuritis, and radiculitis ▽

ICD-9-CM Procedural

04.07 Other excision or avulsion of cranial and peripheral nerves

28035

28035 Release, tarsal tunnel (posterior tibial nerve decompression)

ICD-9-CM Diagnostic

355.5 Tarsal tunnel syndrome

ICD-9-CM Procedural

04.44 Release of tarsal tunnel

28043–28046

28043 Excision, tumor, foot; subcutaneous tissue
28045 deep, subfascial, intramuscular
28046 Radical resection of tumor (eg, malignant neoplasm), soft tissue of foot

ICD-9-CM Diagnostic

171.3 Malignant neoplasm of connective and other soft tissue of lower limb, including hip
172.7 Malignant melanoma of skin of lower limb, including hip
195.5 Malignant neoplasm of lower limb
198.89 Secondary malignant neoplasm of other specified sites
214.1 Lipoma of other skin and subcutaneous tissue
215.3 Other benign neoplasm of connective and other soft tissue of lower limb, including hip
238.1 Neoplasm of uncertain behavior of connective and other soft tissue ▽
239.2 Neoplasms of unspecified nature of bone, soft tissue, and skin
706.2 Sebaceous cyst

ICD-9-CM Procedural

83.31 Excision of lesion of tendon sheath
83.32 Excision of lesion of muscle
83.49 Other excision of soft tissue

HCPCS Level II Supplies & Services

A4305 Disposable drug delivery system, flow rate of 50 ml or greater per hour
A4306 Disposable drug delivery system, flow rate of 5 ml or less per hour
A4550 Surgical trays

28050–28054

28050 Arthrotomy with biopsy; intertarsal or tarsometatarsal joint
28052 metatarsophalangeal joint
28054 interphalangeal joint

ICD-9-CM Diagnostic

170.8 Malignant neoplasm of short bones of lower limb
171.3 Malignant neoplasm of connective and other soft tissue of lower limb, including hip
213.8 Benign neoplasm of short bones of lower limb
215.3 Other benign neoplasm of connective and other soft tissue of lower limb, including hip
238.0 Neoplasm of uncertain behavior of bone and articular cartilage
238.1 Neoplasm of uncertain behavior of connective and other soft tissue ▽
239.2 Neoplasms of unspecified nature of bone, soft tissue, and skin
357.1 Polyneuropathy in collagen vascular disease — (Code first underlying disease: 446.0, 710.0, 714.0) ☒
359.6 Symptomatic inflammatory myopathy in diseases classified elsewhere — (Code first underlying disease: 135, 140.0-208.9, 277.3, 446.0, 710.0, 710.1, 710.2, 714.0) ☒
446.0 Polyarteritis nodosa
710.0 Systemic lupus erythematosus — (Use additional code to identify manifestation: 424.91, 581.81, 582.81, 583.81)
710.1 Systemic sclerosis — (Use additional code to identify manifestation: 359.6, 517.2)
710.2 Sicca syndrome
714.0 Rheumatoid arthritis — (Use additional code to identify manifestation: 357.1, 359.6)
714.1 Felty's syndrome
714.2 Other rheumatoid arthritis with visceral or systemic involvement
714.30 Polyarticular juvenile rheumatoid arthritis, chronic or unspecified
714.31 Polyarticular juvenile rheumatoid arthritis, acute
714.32 Pauciarticular juvenile rheumatoid arthritis
714.33 Monoarticular juvenile rheumatoid arthritis
714.4 Chronic postrheumatic arthropathy
714.89 Other specified inflammatory polyarthropathies
716.07 Kaschin-Beck disease, ankle and foot
719.17 Hemarthrosis, ankle and foot
719.27 Villonodular synovitis, ankle and foot
727.00 Unspecified synovitis and tenosynovitis ▽
732.5 Juvenile osteochondrosis of foot

ICD-9-CM Procedural

80.38 Biopsy of joint structure of foot and toe

HCPCS Level II Supplies & Services

A4305 Disposable drug delivery system, flow rate of 50 ml or greater per hour
A4306 Disposable drug delivery system, flow rate of 5 ml or less per hour
A4550 Surgical trays

28060–28062

28060 Fasciectomy, plantar fascia; partial (separate procedure)
28062 radical (separate procedure)

ICD-9-CM Diagnostic

237.71 Neurofibromatosis, Type 1 (von Recklinghausen's disease)
355.6 Lesion of plantar nerve
728.6 Contracture of palmar fascia
728.71 Plantar fascial fibromatosis

ICD-9-CM Procedural

83.44 Other fasciectomy

HCPCS Level II Supplies & Services

A4305 Disposable drug delivery system, flow rate of 50 ml or greater per hour
A4306 Disposable drug delivery system, flow rate of 5 ml or less per hour
A4550 Surgical trays

28070–28072

28070 Synovectomy; intertarsal or tarsometatarsal joint, each
28072 metatarsophalangeal joint, each

ICD-9-CM Diagnostic

357.1 Polyneuropathy in collagen vascular disease — (Code first underlying disease: 446.0, 710.0, 714.0) ☒
359.6 Symptomatic inflammatory myopathy in diseases classified elsewhere — (Code first underlying disease: 135, 140.0-208.9, 277.3, 446.0, 710.0, 710.1, 710.2, 714.0) ☒
446.0 Polyarteritis nodosa
710.0 Systemic lupus erythematosus — (Use additional code to identify manifestation: 424.91, 581.81, 582.81, 583.81)
710.1 Systemic sclerosis — (Use additional code to identify manifestation: 359.6, 517.2)
710.2 Sicca syndrome
714.0 Rheumatoid arthritis — (Use additional code to identify manifestation: 357.1, 359.6)
719.27 Villonodular synovitis, ankle and foot
727.00 Unspecified synovitis and tenosynovitis ▽

ICD-9-CM Procedural

80.78 Synovectomy of foot and toe

28080

28080 Excision, interdigital (Morton) neuroma, single, each

ICD-9-CM Diagnostic

355.6 Lesion of plantar nerve

ICD-9-CM Procedural

04.07 Other excision or avulsion of cranial and peripheral nerves

HCPCS Level II Supplies & Services

A4305 Disposable drug delivery system, flow rate of 50 ml or greater per hour
A4306 Disposable drug delivery system, flow rate of 5 ml or less per hour
A4550 Surgical trays

28086–28088

28086 Synovectomy, tendon sheath, foot; flexor
28088 extensor

ICD-9-CM Diagnostic

357.1 Polyneuropathy in collagen vascular disease — (Code first underlying disease: 446.0, 710.0, 714.0) ☒

359.6 Symptomatic inflammatory myopathy in diseases classified elsewhere — (Code first underlying disease: 135, 140.0-208.9, 277.3, 446.0, 710.0, 710.1, 710.2, 714.0) ☒
446.0 Polyarteritis nodosa
710.0 Systemic lupus erythematosus — (Use additional code to identify manifestation: 424.91, 581.81, 582.81, 583.81)
710.1 Systemic sclerosis — (Use additional code to identify manifestation: 359.6, 517.2)
710.2 Sicca syndrome
714.0 Rheumatoid arthritis — (Use additional code to identify manifestation: 357.1, 359.6)
726.70 Unspecified enthesopathy of ankle and tarsus ▽
726.71 Achilles bursitis or tendinitis
726.72 Tibialis tendinitis
726.73 Calcaneal spur
726.79 Other enthesopathy of ankle and tarsus
727.42 Ganglion of tendon sheath
727.49 Other ganglion and cyst of synovium, tendon, and bursa

ICD-9-CM Procedural

80.78 Synovectomy of foot and toe
83.42 Other tenonectomy

28090–28092

28090 Excision of lesion, tendon, tendon sheath, or capsule (including synovectomy) (eg, cyst or ganglion); foot
28092 toe(s), each

ICD-9-CM Diagnostic

357.1 Polyneuropathy in collagen vascular disease — (Code first underlying disease: 446.0, 710.0, 714.0) ☒
359.6 Symptomatic inflammatory myopathy in diseases classified elsewhere — (Code first underlying disease: 135, 140.0-208.9, 277.3, 446.0, 710.0, 710.1, 710.2, 714.0) ☒
446.0 Polyarteritis nodosa
701.5 Other abnormal granulation tissue
710.0 Systemic lupus erythematosus — (Use additional code to identify manifestation: 424.91, 581.81, 582.81, 583.81)
710.1 Systemic sclerosis — (Use additional code to identify manifestation: 359.6, 517.2)
710.2 Sicca syndrome
714.0 Rheumatoid arthritis — (Use additional code to identify manifestation: 357.1, 359.6)
716.67 Unspecified monoarthritis, ankle and foot ▽
726.71 Achilles bursitis or tendinitis
727.41 Ganglion of joint
727.42 Ganglion of tendon sheath
727.49 Other ganglion and cyst of synovium, tendon, and bursa
727.82 Calcium deposits in tendon and bursa
728.71 Plantar fascial fibromatosis

ICD-9-CM Procedural

80.78 Synovectomy of foot and toe
80.88 Other local excision or destruction of lesion of joint of foot and toe
83.31 Excision of lesion of tendon sheath
83.39 Excision of lesion of other soft tissue

HCPCS Level II Supplies & Services

A4305 Disposable drug delivery system, flow rate of 50 ml or greater per hour
A4306 Disposable drug delivery system, flow rate of 5 ml or less per hour
A4550 Surgical trays

28100–28103

28100 Excision or curettage of bone cyst or benign tumor, talus or calcaneus;
28102 with iliac or other autograft (includes obtaining graft)
28103 with allograft

ICD-9-CM Diagnostic

213.8 Benign neoplasm of short bones of lower limb
732.5 Juvenile osteochondrosis of foot
733.21 Solitary bone cyst
733.22 Aneurysmal bone cyst
733.29 Other cyst of bone
733.5 Osteitis condensans

ICD-9-CM Procedural

77.68 Local excision of lesion or tissue of tarsals and metatarsals
77.78 Excision of tarsals and metatarsals for graft
78.08 Bone graft of tarsals and metatarsals

HCPCS Level II Supplies & Services

E0112 Crutches, underarm, wood, adjustable or fixed, pair, with pads, tips and handgrips
E0113 Crutch, underarm, wood, adjustable or fixed, each, with pad, tip and handgrip
E0114 Crutches, underarm, other than wood, adjustable or fixed, pair, with pads, tips and handgrips
E0116 Crutch, underarm, other than wood, adjustable or fixed, each, with pad, tip and handgrip
E0117 Crutch, underarm, articulating, spring assisted, each

28104–28108

28104 Excision or curettage of bone cyst or benign tumor, tarsal or metatarsal, except talus or calcaneus;
28106 with iliac or other autograft (includes obtaining graft)
28107 with allograft
28108 Excision or curettage of bone cyst or benign tumor, phalanges of foot

ICD-9-CM Diagnostic

213.8 Benign neoplasm of short bones of lower limb
733.21 Solitary bone cyst
733.22 Aneurysmal bone cyst
733.29 Other cyst of bone
733.5 Osteitis condensans

ICD-9-CM Procedural

77.68 Local excision of lesion or tissue of tarsals and metatarsals
77.69 Local excision of lesion or tissue of other bone, except facial bones
77.78 Excision of tarsals and metatarsals for graft
78.08 Bone graft of tarsals and metatarsals

HCPCS Level II Supplies & Services

E0112 Crutches, underarm, wood, adjustable or fixed, pair, with pads, tips and handgrips
E0113 Crutch, underarm, wood, adjustable or fixed, each, with pad, tip and handgrip
E0114 Crutches, underarm, other than wood, adjustable or fixed, pair, with pads, tips and handgrips
E0116 Crutch, underarm, other than wood, adjustable or fixed, each, with pad, tip and handgrip
E0117 Crutch, underarm, articulating, spring assisted, each

28110

28110 Ostectomy, partial excision, fifth metatarsal head (bunionette) (separate procedure)

ICD-9-CM Diagnostic

726.91 Exostosis of unspecified site ▽
727.1 Bunion
733.99 Other disorders of bone and cartilage
735.4 Other hammer toe (acquired)
736.74 Claw foot, acquired
736.79 Other acquired deformity of ankle and foot
754.52 Congenital metatarsus primus varus

ICD-9-CM Procedural

77.54 Excision or correction of bunionette
77.88 Other partial ostectomy of tarsals and metatarsals

28111–28114

28111 Ostectomy, complete excision; first metatarsal head
28112 other metatarsal head (second, third or fourth)
28113 fifth metatarsal head
28114 all metatarsal heads, with partial proximal phalangectomy, excluding first metatarsal (eg, Clayton type procedure)

ICD-9-CM Diagnostic

213.8 Benign neoplasm of short bones of lower limb
357.1 Polyneuropathy in collagen vascular disease — (Code first underlying disease: 446.0, 710.0, 714.0) ☒

359.6 Symptomatic inflammatory myopathy in diseases classified elsewhere — (Code first underlying disease: 135, 140.0-208.9, 277.3, 446.0, 710.0, 710.1, 710.2, 714.0) ☒
446.0 Polyarteritis nodosa
710.0 Systemic lupus erythematosus — (Use additional code to identify manifestation: 424.91, 581.81, 582.81, 583.81)
710.1 Systemic sclerosis — (Use additional code to identify manifestation: 359.6, 517.2)
710.2 Sicca syndrome
714.0 Rheumatoid arthritis — (Use additional code to identify manifestation: 357.1, 359.6)
714.1 Felty's syndrome
714.2 Other rheumatoid arthritis with visceral or systemic involvement
714.30 Polyarticular juvenile rheumatoid arthritis, chronic or unspecified
714.31 Polyarticular juvenile rheumatoid arthritis, acute
714.32 Pauciarticular juvenile rheumatoid arthritis
714.33 Monoarticular juvenile rheumatoid arthritis
714.4 Chronic postrheumatic arthropathy
715.17 Primary localized osteoarthrosis, ankle and foot
715.27 Secondary localized osteoarthrosis, ankle and foot
727.1 Bunion
730.17 Chronic osteomyelitis, ankle and foot — (Use additional code to identify organism, 041.1)
733.49 Aseptic necrosis of other bone site
733.81 Malunion of fracture
733.82 Nonunion of fracture
733.94 Stress fracture of the metatarsals
733.99 Other disorders of bone and cartilage
735.0 Hallux valgus (acquired)
735.4 Other hammer toe (acquired)
735.8 Other acquired deformity of toe
785.4 Gangrene — (Code first any associated underlying condition:250.7, 443.0)
825.25 Closed fracture of metatarsal bone(s)
825.35 Open fracture of metatarsal bone(s)
905.4 Late effect of fracture of lower extremities
928.20 Crushing injury of foot — (Use additional code to identify any associated injuries: 800-829, 850.0-854.1, 860.0-869.1)

ICD-9-CM Procedural

77.88 Other partial ostectomy of tarsals and metatarsals

28116

28116 Ostectomy, excision of tarsal coalition

ICD-9-CM Diagnostic

755.56 Accessory carpal bones
755.67 Congenital anomalies of foot, not elsewhere classified

ICD-9-CM Procedural

77.98 Total ostectomy of tarsals and metatarsals

28118

28118 Ostectomy, calcaneus;

ICD-9-CM Diagnostic

213.8 Benign neoplasm of short bones of lower limb
726.73 Calcaneal spur
726.91 Exostosis of unspecified site ▽
732.5 Juvenile osteochondrosis of foot
733.90 Disorder of bone and cartilage, unspecified ▽
736.76 Other acquired calcaneus deformity
755.67 Congenital anomalies of foot, not elsewhere classified

ICD-9-CM Procedural

77.88 Other partial ostectomy of tarsals and metatarsals
77.98 Total ostectomy of tarsals and metatarsals

28119

28119 Ostectomy, calcaneus; for spur, with or without plantar fascial release

ICD-9-CM Diagnostic

355.6 Lesion of plantar nerve
726.73 Calcaneal spur
726.79 Other enthesopathy of ankle and tarsus
726.91 Exostosis of unspecified site ▽
729.4 Unspecified fasciitis ▽
729.5 Pain in soft tissues of limb
732.5 Juvenile osteochondrosis of foot
732.6 Other juvenile osteochondrosis
733.99 Other disorders of bone and cartilage
736.76 Other acquired calcaneus deformity

ICD-9-CM Procedural

77.88 Other partial ostectomy of tarsals and metatarsals
83.09 Other incision of soft tissue

28120–28124

28120 Partial excision (craterization, saucerization, sequestrectomy, or diaphysectomy) bone (eg, osteomyelitis or bossing); talus or calcaneus
28122 tarsal or metatarsal bone, except talus or calcaneus
28124 phalanx of toe

ICD-9-CM Diagnostic

213.8 Benign neoplasm of short bones of lower limb
239.2 Neoplasms of unspecified nature of bone, soft tissue, and skin
357.1 Polyneuropathy in collagen vascular disease — (Code first underlying disease: 446.0, 710.0, 714.0) ☒
359.6 Symptomatic inflammatory myopathy in diseases classified elsewhere — (Code first underlying disease: 135, 140.0-208.9, 277.3, 446.0, 710.0, 710.1, 710.2, 714.0) ☒
446.0 Polyarteritis nodosa
681.11 Onychia and paronychia of toe — (Use additional code to identify organism)
703.8 Other specified disease of nail
707.10 Ulcer of lower limb, unspecified ▽
707.13 Ulcer of ankle
707.14 Ulcer of heel and midfoot
707.15 Ulcer of other part of foot
710.0 Systemic lupus erythematosus — (Use additional code to identify manifestation: 424.91, 581.81, 582.81, 583.81)
710.1 Systemic sclerosis — (Use additional code to identify manifestation: 359.6, 517.2)
710.2 Sicca syndrome
714.0 Rheumatoid arthritis — (Use additional code to identify manifestation: 357.1, 359.6)
715.17 Primary localized osteoarthrosis, ankle and foot
719.40 Pain in joint, site unspecified ▽
719.47 Pain in joint, ankle and foot
726.73 Calcaneal spur
726.79 Other enthesopathy of ankle and tarsus
726.8 Other peripheral enthesopathies
726.90 Enthesopathy of unspecified site ▽
726.91 Exostosis of unspecified site ▽
727.1 Bunion
730.17 Chronic osteomyelitis, ankle and foot — (Use additional code to identify organism, 041.1)
730.87 Other infections involving bone diseases classified elsewhere, ankle and foot — (Code first underlying disease: 002.0, 015.0-015.9. Use additional code to identify organism) ☒
732.5 Juvenile osteochondrosis of foot
733.49 Aseptic necrosis of other bone site
733.99 Other disorders of bone and cartilage
735.0 Hallux valgus (acquired)
735.1 Hallux varus (acquired)
735.2 Hallux rigidus
735.3 Hallux malleus
735.4 Other hammer toe (acquired)
735.5 Claw toe (acquired)
735.8 Other acquired deformity of toe
735.9 Unspecified acquired deformity of toe ▽
736.76 Other acquired calcaneus deformity
755.67 Congenital anomalies of foot, not elsewhere classified
785.4 Gangrene — (Code first any associated underlying condition:250.7, 443.0)
826.1 Open fracture of one or more phalanges of foot
905.4 Late effect of fracture of lower extremities
996.66 Infection and inflammatory reaction due to internal joint prosthesis — (Use additional code to identify specified infections)
996.67 Infection and inflammatory reaction due to other internal orthopedic device, implant, and graft — (Use additional code to identify specified infections)

ICD-9-CM Procedural

77.88 Other partial ostectomy of tarsals and metatarsals

77.89 Other partial ostectomy of other bone, except facial bones

HCPCS Level II Supplies & Services

A4580 Cast supplies (e.g., plaster)
A4590 Special casting material (e.g., fiberglass)
E0112 Crutches, underarm, wood, adjustable or fixed, pair, with pads, tips and handgrips
E0113 Crutch, underarm, wood, adjustable or fixed, each, with pad, tip and handgrip
E0114 Crutches, underarm, other than wood, adjustable or fixed, pair, with pads, tips and handgrips

28126

28126 Resection, partial or complete, phalangeal base, each toe

ICD-9-CM Diagnostic

213.8 Benign neoplasm of short bones of lower limb
726.91 Exostosis of unspecified site ▽
727.1 Bunion
733.99 Other disorders of bone and cartilage
735.0 Hallux valgus (acquired)
735.4 Other hammer toe (acquired)
735.8 Other acquired deformity of toe
755.66 Other congenital anomaly of toes

ICD-9-CM Procedural

77.89 Other partial ostectomy of other bone, except facial bones

28130

28130 Talectomy (astragalectomy)

ICD-9-CM Diagnostic

726.70 Unspecified enthesopathy of ankle and tarsus ▽
728.0 Infective myositis
730.17 Chronic osteomyelitis, ankle and foot — (Use additional code to identify organism, 041.1)
730.87 Other infections involving bone diseases classified elsewhere, ankle and foot — (Code first underlying disease: 002.0, 015.0-015.9. Use additional code to identify organism) ☒
733.44 Aseptic necrosis of talus
733.81 Malunion of fracture

ICD-9-CM Procedural

77.98 Total ostectomy of tarsals and metatarsals

28140

28140 Metatarsectomy

ICD-9-CM Diagnostic

170.8 Malignant neoplasm of short bones of lower limb
198.5 Secondary malignant neoplasm of bone and bone marrow
238.0 Neoplasm of uncertain behavior of bone and articular cartilage
707.14 Ulcer of heel and midfoot
726.91 Exostosis of unspecified site ▽
728.0 Infective myositis
730.17 Chronic osteomyelitis, ankle and foot — (Use additional code to identify organism, 041.1)
730.87 Other infections involving bone diseases classified elsewhere, ankle and foot — (Code first underlying disease: 002.0, 015.0-015.9. Use additional code to identify organism) ☒
732.5 Juvenile osteochondrosis of foot
733.49 Aseptic necrosis of other bone site
733.81 Malunion of fracture
733.82 Nonunion of fracture
733.99 Other disorders of bone and cartilage
735.9 Unspecified acquired deformity of toe ▽
755.67 Congenital anomalies of foot, not elsewhere classified
785.4 Gangrene — (Code first any associated underlying condition:250.7, 443.0)
825.35 Open fracture of metatarsal bone(s)
905.4 Late effect of fracture of lower extremities
928.20 Crushing injury of foot — (Use additional code to identify any associated injuries: 800-829, 850.0-854.1, 860.0-869.1)
996.66 Infection and inflammatory reaction due to internal joint prosthesis — (Use additional code to identify specified infections)
996.67 Infection and inflammatory reaction due to other internal orthopedic device, implant, and graft — (Use additional code to identify specified infections)

ICD-9-CM Procedural

77.98 Total ostectomy of tarsals and metatarsals

28150

28150 Phalangectomy, toe, each toe

ICD-9-CM Diagnostic

357.1 Polyneuropathy in collagen vascular disease — (Code first underlying disease: 446.0, 710.0, 714.0) ☒
359.6 Symptomatic inflammatory myopathy in diseases classified elsewhere — (Code first underlying disease: 135, 140.0-208.9, 277.3, 446.0, 710.0, 710.1, 710.2, 714.0) ☒
446.0 Polyarteritis nodosa
707.10 Ulcer of lower limb, unspecified ▽
707.15 Ulcer of other part of foot
710.0 Systemic lupus erythematosus — (Use additional code to identify manifestation: 424.91, 581.81, 582.81, 583.81)
710.1 Systemic sclerosis — (Use additional code to identify manifestation: 359.6, 517.2)
710.2 Sicca syndrome
714.0 Rheumatoid arthritis — (Use additional code to identify manifestation: 357.1, 359.6)
726.91 Exostosis of unspecified site ▽
728.0 Infective myositis
728.12 Traumatic myositis ossificans
730.17 Chronic osteomyelitis, ankle and foot — (Use additional code to identify organism, 041.1)
735.0 Hallux valgus (acquired)
735.1 Hallux varus (acquired)
735.2 Hallux rigidus
735.3 Hallux malleus
735.4 Other hammer toe (acquired)
735.5 Claw toe (acquired)
735.8 Other acquired deformity of toe
755.66 Other congenital anomaly of toes
785.4 Gangrene — (Code first any associated underlying condition:250.7, 443.0)
879.8 Open wound(s) (multiple) of unspecified site(s), without mention of complication — (Use additional code to identify infection) ▽

ICD-9-CM Procedural

77.89 Other partial ostectomy of other bone, except facial bones
77.99 Total ostectomy of other bone, except facial bones

28153

28153 Resection, condyle(s), distal end of phalanx, each toe

ICD-9-CM Diagnostic

213.8 Benign neoplasm of short bones of lower limb
700 Corns and callosities
726.90 Enthesopathy of unspecified site ▽
726.91 Exostosis of unspecified site ▽
727.1 Bunion
728.0 Infective myositis
730.17 Chronic osteomyelitis, ankle and foot — (Use additional code to identify organism, 041.1)
732.5 Juvenile osteochondrosis of foot
733.90 Disorder of bone and cartilage, unspecified ▽
733.99 Other disorders of bone and cartilage
735.0 Hallux valgus (acquired)
735.1 Hallux varus (acquired)
735.2 Hallux rigidus
735.3 Hallux malleus
735.4 Other hammer toe (acquired)
735.5 Claw toe (acquired)
735.8 Other acquired deformity of toe
755.66 Other congenital anomaly of toes
785.4 Gangrene — (Code first any associated underlying condition:250.7, 443.0)

ICD-9-CM Procedural

77.89 Other partial ostectomy of other bone, except facial bones

28160

28160 Hemiphalangectomy or interphalangeal joint excision, toe, proximal end of phalanx, each

ICD-9-CM Diagnostic

357.1 Polyneuropathy in collagen vascular disease — (Code first underlying disease: 446.0, 710.0, 714.0) ☒
359.6 Symptomatic inflammatory myopathy in diseases classified elsewhere — (Code first underlying disease: 135, 140.0-208.9, 277.3, 446.0, 710.0, 710.1, 710.2, 714.0) ☒
446.0 Polyarteritis nodosa
710.0 Systemic lupus erythematosus — (Use additional code to identify manifestation: 424.91, 581.81, 582.81, 583.81)
710.1 Systemic sclerosis — (Use additional code to identify manifestation: 359.6, 517.2)
710.2 Sicca syndrome
714.0 Rheumatoid arthritis — (Use additional code to identify manifestation: 357.1, 359.6)
726.91 Exostosis of unspecified site ▽
733.99 Other disorders of bone and cartilage
735.0 Hallux valgus (acquired)
735.1 Hallux varus (acquired)
735.2 Hallux rigidus
735.3 Hallux malleus
735.4 Other hammer toe (acquired)
735.5 Claw toe (acquired)
735.8 Other acquired deformity of toe
755.66 Other congenital anomaly of toes

ICD-9-CM Procedural

77.89 Other partial ostectomy of other bone, except facial bones

28171–28175

28171 Radical resection of tumor, bone; tarsal (except talus or calcaneus)
28173 metatarsal
28175 phalanx of toe

ICD-9-CM Diagnostic

170.8 Malignant neoplasm of short bones of lower limb
171.3 Malignant neoplasm of connective and other soft tissue of lower limb, including hip
172.7 Malignant melanoma of skin of lower limb, including hip
198.5 Secondary malignant neoplasm of bone and bone marrow
213.8 Benign neoplasm of short bones of lower limb
238.0 Neoplasm of uncertain behavior of bone and articular cartilage
239.2 Neoplasms of unspecified nature of bone, soft tissue, and skin

ICD-9-CM Procedural

77.88 Other partial ostectomy of tarsals and metatarsals
77.98 Total ostectomy of tarsals and metatarsals
77.99 Total ostectomy of other bone, except facial bones

28190–28193

28190 Removal of foreign body, foot; subcutaneous
28192 deep
28193 complicated

ICD-9-CM Diagnostic

709.4 Foreign body granuloma of skin and subcutaneous tissue
728.82 Foreign body granuloma of muscle
729.6 Residual foreign body in soft tissue
892.1 Open wound of foot except toe(s) alone, complicated — (Use additional code to identify infection)
893.1 Open wound of toe(s), complicated — (Use additional code to identify infection)
917.6 Foot and toe(s), superficial foreign body (splinter), without major open wound and without mention of infection
917.7 Foot and toe(s), superficial foreign body (splinter), without major open wound, infected
917.9 Other and unspecified superficial injury of foot and toes, infected ▽

ICD-9-CM Procedural

83.02 Myotomy
83.09 Other incision of soft tissue
86.05 Incision with removal of foreign body or device from skin and subcutaneous tissue
98.28 Removal of foreign body from foot without incision

HCPCS Level II Supplies & Services

A4305 Disposable drug delivery system, flow rate of 50 ml or greater per hour
A4306 Disposable drug delivery system, flow rate of 5 ml or less per hour
A4550 Surgical trays

28200–28202

28200 Repair, tendon, flexor, foot; primary or secondary, without free graft, each tendon
28202 secondary with free graft, each tendon (includes obtaining graft)

ICD-9-CM Diagnostic

727.68 Nontraumatic rupture of other tendons of foot and ankle
845.10 Sprain and strain of unspecified site of foot ▽
845.11 Sprain and strain of tarsometatarsal (joint) (ligament)
845.12 Sprain and strain of metatarsaophalangeal (joint)
845.13 Sprain and strain of interphalangeal (joint), of toe
845.19 Other foot sprain and strain
892.2 Open wound of foot except toe(s) alone, with tendon involvement — (Use additional code to identify infection)
893.2 Open wound of toe(s), with tendon involvement — (Use additional code to identify infection)
905.8 Late effect of tendon injury
928.3 Crushing injury of toe(s) — (Use additional code to identify any associated injuries: 800-829, 850.0-854.1, 860.0-869.1)
998.31 Disruption of internal operation wound

ICD-9-CM Procedural

83.61 Suture of tendon sheath
83.62 Delayed suture of tendon

HCPCS Level II Supplies & Services

A4305 Disposable drug delivery system, flow rate of 50 ml or greater per hour
A4306 Disposable drug delivery system, flow rate of 5 ml or less per hour
A4550 Surgical trays

28208–28210

28208 Repair, tendon, extensor, foot; primary or secondary, each tendon
28210 secondary with free graft, each tendon (includes obtaining graft)

ICD-9-CM Diagnostic

727.68 Nontraumatic rupture of other tendons of foot and ankle
727.69 Nontraumatic rupture of other tendon
845.10 Sprain and strain of unspecified site of foot ▽
845.11 Sprain and strain of tarsometatarsal (joint) (ligament)
845.12 Sprain and strain of metatarsaophalangeal (joint)
845.13 Sprain and strain of interphalangeal (joint), of toe
845.19 Other foot sprain and strain
892.2 Open wound of foot except toe(s) alone, with tendon involvement — (Use additional code to identify infection)
893.2 Open wound of toe(s), with tendon involvement — (Use additional code to identify infection)
905.8 Late effect of tendon injury
928.3 Crushing injury of toe(s) — (Use additional code to identify any associated injuries: 800-829, 850.0-854.1, 860.0-869.1)

ICD-9-CM Procedural

83.61 Suture of tendon sheath
83.62 Delayed suture of tendon

HCPCS Level II Supplies & Services

A4580 Cast supplies (e.g., plaster)
A4590 Special casting material (e.g., fiberglass)
E0112 Crutches, underarm, wood, adjustable or fixed, pair, with pads, tips and handgrips
E0113 Crutch, underarm, wood, adjustable or fixed, each, with pad, tip and handgrip
E0114 Crutches, underarm, other than wood, adjustable or fixed, pair, with pads, tips and handgrips

28220–28222

28220 Tenolysis, flexor, foot; single tendon
28222 multiple tendons

ICD-9-CM Diagnostic

727.01 Synovitis and tenosynovitis in diseases classified elsewhere — (Code first underlying disease: 015.0-015.9) ☒
727.06 Tenosynovitis of foot and ankle
727.82 Calcium deposits in tendon and bursa
727.89 Other disorders of synovium, tendon, and bursa
735.8 Other acquired deformity of toe

ICD-9-CM Procedural

83.91 Lysis of adhesions of muscle, tendon, fascia, and bursa

HCPCS Level II Supplies & Services

A4305 Disposable drug delivery system, flow rate of 50 ml or greater per hour
A4306 Disposable drug delivery system, flow rate of 5 ml or less per hour
A4550 Surgical trays

28225–28226

28225 Tenolysis, extensor, foot; single tendon
28226 multiple tendons

ICD-9-CM Diagnostic

727.01 Synovitis and tenosynovitis in diseases classified elsewhere — (Code first underlying disease: 015.0-015.9) ☒
727.06 Tenosynovitis of foot and ankle
727.82 Calcium deposits in tendon and bursa
727.89 Other disorders of synovium, tendon, and bursa
735.8 Other acquired deformity of toe

ICD-9-CM Procedural

83.91 Lysis of adhesions of muscle, tendon, fascia, and bursa

HCPCS Level II Supplies & Services

A4305 Disposable drug delivery system, flow rate of 50 ml or greater per hour
A4306 Disposable drug delivery system, flow rate of 5 ml or less per hour
A4550 Surgical trays

28230–28232

28230 Tenotomy, open, tendon flexor; foot, single or multiple tendon(s) (separate procedure)
28232 toe, single tendon (separate procedure)

ICD-9-CM Diagnostic

357.1 Polyneuropathy in collagen vascular disease — (Code first underlying disease: 446.0, 710.0, 714.0) ☒
359.6 Symptomatic inflammatory myopathy in diseases classified elsewhere — (Code first underlying disease: 135, 140.0-208.9, 277.3, 446.0, 710.0, 710.1, 710.2, 714.0) ☒
446.0 Polyarteritis nodosa
710.0 Systemic lupus erythematosus — (Use additional code to identify manifestation: 424.91, 581.81, 582.81, 583.81)
710.1 Systemic sclerosis — (Use additional code to identify manifestation: 359.6, 517.2)
710.2 Sicca syndrome
714.0 Rheumatoid arthritis — (Use additional code to identify manifestation: 357.1, 359.6)
718.47 Contracture of ankle and foot joint
727.81 Contracture of tendon (sheath)
735.0 Hallux valgus (acquired)
735.1 Hallux varus (acquired)
735.2 Hallux rigidus
735.3 Hallux malleus
735.4 Other hammer toe (acquired)
735.5 Claw toe (acquired)
735.8 Other acquired deformity of toe
736.71 Acquired equinovarus deformity
736.72 Equinus deformity of foot, acquired
736.73 Cavus deformity of foot, acquired
736.74 Claw foot, acquired
736.75 Cavovarus deformity of foot, acquired
736.79 Other acquired deformity of ankle and foot

ICD-9-CM Procedural

83.13 Other tenotomy

HCPCS Level II Supplies & Services

A4305 Disposable drug delivery system, flow rate of 50 ml or greater per hour
A4306 Disposable drug delivery system, flow rate of 5 ml or less per hour
A4550 Surgical trays

28234

28234 Tenotomy, open, extensor, foot or toe, each tendon

ICD-9-CM Diagnostic

357.1 Polyneuropathy in collagen vascular disease — (Code first underlying disease: 446.0, 710.0, 714.0) ☒
359.6 Symptomatic inflammatory myopathy in diseases classified elsewhere — (Code first underlying disease: 135, 140.0-208.9, 277.3, 446.0, 710.0, 710.1, 710.2, 714.0) ☒
446.0 Polyarteritis nodosa
710.0 Systemic lupus erythematosus — (Use additional code to identify manifestation: 424.91, 581.81, 582.81, 583.81)
710.1 Systemic sclerosis — (Use additional code to identify manifestation: 359.6, 517.2)
710.2 Sicca syndrome
714.0 Rheumatoid arthritis — (Use additional code to identify manifestation: 357.1, 359.6)
718.47 Contracture of ankle and foot joint
727.81 Contracture of tendon (sheath)
735.0 Hallux valgus (acquired)
735.1 Hallux varus (acquired)
735.2 Hallux rigidus
735.3 Hallux malleus
735.4 Other hammer toe (acquired)
735.5 Claw toe (acquired)
735.8 Other acquired deformity of toe
736.71 Acquired equinovarus deformity
736.72 Equinus deformity of foot, acquired
736.73 Cavus deformity of foot, acquired
736.74 Claw foot, acquired
736.75 Cavovarus deformity of foot, acquired
736.79 Other acquired deformity of ankle and foot

ICD-9-CM Procedural

83.13 Other tenotomy

HCPCS Level II Supplies & Services

A4305 Disposable drug delivery system, flow rate of 50 ml or greater per hour
A4306 Disposable drug delivery system, flow rate of 5 ml or less per hour
A4550 Surgical trays

28238

28238 Reconstruction (advancement), posterior tibial tendon with excision of accessory tarsal navicular bone (eg, Kidner type procedure)

ICD-9-CM Diagnostic

138 Late effects of acute poliomyelitis
726.72 Tibialis tendinitis
727.68 Nontraumatic rupture of other tendons of foot and ankle
727.81 Contracture of tendon (sheath)
727.89 Other disorders of synovium, tendon, and bursa
754.50 Congenital talipes varus
754.51 Congenital talipes equinovarus
754.52 Congenital metatarsus primus varus
754.53 Congenital metatarsus varus
754.59 Other congenital varus deformity of feet

ICD-9-CM Procedural

77.68 Local excision of lesion or tissue of tarsals and metatarsals
83.71 Advancement of tendon

28240

28240 Tenotomy, lengthening, or release, abductor hallucis muscle

ICD-9-CM Diagnostic

727.1 Bunion
727.81 Contracture of tendon (sheath)

Unspecified code ☒ Manifestation code
♀ Female diagnosis ♂ Male diagnosis

735.1 Hallux varus (acquired)
735.2 Hallux rigidus
736.71 Acquired equinovarus deformity
736.72 Equinus deformity of foot, acquired
736.73 Cavus deformity of foot, acquired
736.74 Claw foot, acquired
736.75 Cavovarus deformity of foot, acquired
736.76 Other acquired calcaneus deformity
736.79 Other acquired deformity of ankle and foot

ICD-9-CM Procedural
83.19 Other division of soft tissue
83.85 Other change in muscle or tendon length

28250
28250 Division of plantar fascia and muscle (eg, Steindler stripping) (separate procedure)

ICD-9-CM Diagnostic
726.73 Calcaneal spur
728.71 Plantar fascial fibromatosis
736.73 Cavus deformity of foot, acquired
736.75 Cavovarus deformity of foot, acquired
754.50 Congenital talipes varus
754.51 Congenital talipes equinovarus
754.52 Congenital metatarsus primus varus
754.53 Congenital metatarsus varus
754.59 Other congenital varus deformity of feet
754.60 Congenital talipes valgus
754.61 Congenital pes planus
754.62 Talipes calcaneovalgus
754.69 Other congenital valgus deformity of feet
754.71 Talipes cavus
754.79 Other congenital deformity of feet

ICD-9-CM Procedural
83.14 Fasciotomy

28260–28262
28260 Capsulotomy, midfoot; medial release only (separate procedure)
28261 with tendon lengthening
28262 extensive, including posterior talotibial capsulotomy and tendon(s) lengthening (eg, resistant clubfoot deformity)

ICD-9-CM Diagnostic
357.1 Polyneuropathy in collagen vascular disease — (Code first underlying disease: 446.0, 710.0, 714.0) ☒
359.6 Symptomatic inflammatory myopathy in diseases classified elsewhere — (Code first underlying disease: 135, 140.0-208.9, 277.3, 446.0, 710.0, 710.1, 710.2, 714.0) ☒
446.0 Polyarteritis nodosa
710.0 Systemic lupus erythematosus — (Use additional code to identify manifestation: 424.91, 581.81, 582.81, 583.81)
710.1 Systemic sclerosis — (Use additional code to identify manifestation: 359.6, 517.2)
710.2 Sicca syndrome
714.0 Rheumatoid arthritis — (Use additional code to identify manifestation: 357.1, 359.6)
727.1 Bunion
727.81 Contracture of tendon (sheath)
735.4 Other hammer toe (acquired)
754.50 Congenital talipes varus
754.60 Congenital talipes valgus
754.71 Talipes cavus
754.79 Other congenital deformity of feet
755.66 Other congenital anomaly of toes
893.2 Open wound of toe(s), with tendon involvement — (Use additional code to identify infection)

ICD-9-CM Procedural
80.48 Division of joint capsule, ligament, or cartilage of foot and toe
83.84 Release of clubfoot, not elsewhere classified

HCPCS Level II Supplies & Services
A4580 Cast supplies (e.g., plaster)
A4590 Special casting material (e.g., fiberglass)
E0112 Crutches, underarm, wood, adjustable or fixed, pair, with pads, tips and handgrips
E0113 Crutch, underarm, wood, adjustable or fixed, each, with pad, tip and handgrip
E0114 Crutches, underarm, other than wood, adjustable or fixed, pair, with pads, tips and handgrips

28264
28264 Capsulotomy, midtarsal (eg, Heyman type procedure)

ICD-9-CM Diagnostic
727.1 Bunion
735.4 Other hammer toe (acquired)
736.73 Cavus deformity of foot, acquired
754.50 Congenital talipes varus
754.60 Congenital talipes valgus

ICD-9-CM Procedural
80.48 Division of joint capsule, ligament, or cartilage of foot and toe

HCPCS Level II Supplies & Services
A4580 Cast supplies (e.g., plaster)
A4590 Special casting material (e.g., fiberglass)
E0112 Crutches, underarm, wood, adjustable or fixed, pair, with pads, tips and handgrips
E0113 Crutch, underarm, wood, adjustable or fixed, each, with pad, tip and handgrip
E0114 Crutches, underarm, other than wood, adjustable or fixed, pair, with pads, tips and handgrips

28270–28272
28270 Capsulotomy; metatarsophalangeal joint, with or without tenorrhaphy, each joint (separate procedure)
28272 interphalangeal joint, each joint (separate procedure)

ICD-9-CM Diagnostic
357.1 Polyneuropathy in collagen vascular disease — (Code first underlying disease: 446.0, 710.0, 714.0) ☒
359.6 Symptomatic inflammatory myopathy in diseases classified elsewhere — (Code first underlying disease: 135, 140.0-208.9, 277.3, 446.0, 710.0, 710.1, 710.2, 714.0) ☒
446.0 Polyarteritis nodosa
710.0 Systemic lupus erythematosus — (Use additional code to identify manifestation: 424.91, 581.81, 582.81, 583.81)
710.1 Systemic sclerosis — (Use additional code to identify manifestation: 359.6, 517.2)
710.2 Sicca syndrome
714.0 Rheumatoid arthritis — (Use additional code to identify manifestation: 357.1, 359.6)
718.40 Contracture of joint, site unspecified ▽
718.47 Contracture of ankle and foot joint
727.81 Contracture of tendon (sheath)
733.99 Other disorders of bone and cartilage
735.4 Other hammer toe (acquired)
735.5 Claw toe (acquired)
735.8 Other acquired deformity of toe
755.66 Other congenital anomaly of toes
893.2 Open wound of toe(s), with tendon involvement — (Use additional code to identify infection)

ICD-9-CM Procedural
80.48 Division of joint capsule, ligament, or cartilage of foot and toe
83.64 Other suture of tendon

28280
28280 Syndactylization, toes (eg, webbing or Kelikian type procedure)

ICD-9-CM Diagnostic
735.8 Other acquired deformity of toe

ICD-9-CM Procedural
86.89 Other repair and reconstruction of skin and subcutaneous tissue

28285

28285 Correction, hammertoe (eg, interphalangeal fusion, partial or total phalangectomy)

ICD-9-CM Diagnostic

735.3 Hallux malleus
735.4 Other hammer toe (acquired)
735.8 Other acquired deformity of toe
755.66 Other congenital anomaly of toes

ICD-9-CM Procedural

77.56 Repair of hammer toe

28286

28286 Correction, cock-up fifth toe, with plastic skin closure (eg, Ruiz-Mora type procedure)

ICD-9-CM Diagnostic

735.4 Other hammer toe (acquired)
735.8 Other acquired deformity of toe
755.66 Other congenital anomaly of toes

ICD-9-CM Procedural

77.58 Other excision, fusion, and repair of toes

28288

28288 Ostectomy, partial, exostectomy or condylectomy, metatarsal head, each metatarsal head

ICD-9-CM Diagnostic

213.8 Benign neoplasm of short bones of lower limb
357.1 Polyneuropathy in collagen vascular disease — (Code first underlying disease: 446.0, 710.0, 714.0) ☒
359.6 Symptomatic inflammatory myopathy in diseases classified elsewhere — (Code first underlying disease: 135, 140.0-208.9, 277.3, 446.0, 710.0, 710.1, 710.2, 714.0) ☒
446.0 Polyarteritis nodosa
700 Corns and callosities
710.0 Systemic lupus erythematosus — (Use additional code to identify manifestation: 424.91, 581.81, 582.81, 583.81)
710.1 Systemic sclerosis — (Use additional code to identify manifestation: 359.6, 517.2)
710.2 Sicca syndrome
714.0 Rheumatoid arthritis — (Use additional code to identify manifestation: 357.1, 359.6)
727.1 Bunion
733.99 Other disorders of bone and cartilage
735.0 Hallux valgus (acquired)
735.1 Hallux varus (acquired)
735.2 Hallux rigidus
735.3 Hallux malleus
735.4 Other hammer toe (acquired)
735.5 Claw toe (acquired)
735.8 Other acquired deformity of toe
755.66 Other congenital anomaly of toes
755.67 Congenital anomalies of foot, not elsewhere classified
825.35 Open fracture of metatarsal bone(s)

ICD-9-CM Procedural

77.51 Bunionectomy with soft tissue correction and osteotomy of the first metatarsal
77.88 Other partial ostectomy of tarsals and metatarsals

28289

28289 Hallux rigidus correction with cheilectomy, debridement and capsular release of the first metatarsophalangeal joint

ICD-9-CM Diagnostic

The application of this code is too broad to adequately present ICD-9-CM diagnostic code links here. Refer to your ICD-9-CM book.

ICD-9-CM Procedural

77.89 Other partial ostectomy of other bone, except facial bones

28290

28290 Correction, hallux valgus (bunion), with or without sesamoidectomy; simple exostectomy (eg, Silver type procedure)

ICD-9-CM Diagnostic

727.1 Bunion
735.0 Hallux valgus (acquired)
735.2 Hallux rigidus
735.8 Other acquired deformity of toe
755.66 Other congenital anomaly of toes

ICD-9-CM Procedural

77.59 Other bunionectomy

HCPCS Level II Supplies & Services

A4550 Surgical trays

28292

28292 Correction, hallux valgus (bunion), with or without sesamoidectomy; Keller, McBride, or Mayo type procedure

ICD-9-CM Diagnostic

727.1 Bunion
728.13 Postoperative heterotopic calcification
733.99 Other disorders of bone and cartilage
735.0 Hallux valgus (acquired)
735.1 Hallux varus (acquired)
735.2 Hallux rigidus
735.3 Hallux malleus
754.52 Congenital metatarsus primus varus

ICD-9-CM Procedural

77.53 Other bunionectomy with soft tissue correction
77.59 Other bunionectomy

HCPCS Level II Supplies & Services

A4550 Surgical trays

28293

28293 Correction, hallux valgus (bunion), with or without sesamoidectomy; resection of joint with implant

ICD-9-CM Diagnostic

357.1 Polyneuropathy in collagen vascular disease — (Code first underlying disease: 446.0, 710.0, 714.0) ☒
359.6 Symptomatic inflammatory myopathy in diseases classified elsewhere — (Code first underlying disease: 135, 140.0-208.9, 277.3, 446.0, 710.0, 710.1, 710.2, 714.0) ☒
446.0 Polyarteritis nodosa
710.0 Systemic lupus erythematosus — (Use additional code to identify manifestation: 424.91, 581.81, 582.81, 583.81)
710.1 Systemic sclerosis — (Use additional code to identify manifestation: 359.6, 517.2)
710.2 Sicca syndrome
714.0 Rheumatoid arthritis — (Use additional code to identify manifestation: 357.1, 359.6)
714.89 Other specified inflammatory polyarthropathies
715.09 Generalized osteoarthrosis, involving multiple sites
715.17 Primary localized osteoarthrosis, ankle and foot
715.37 Localized osteoarthrosis not specified whether primary or secondary, ankle and foot
715.97 Osteoarthrosis, unspecified whether generalized or localized, ankle and foot ▽
718.47 Contracture of ankle and foot joint
719.57 Stiffness of joint, not elsewhere classified, ankle and foot
726.73 Calcaneal spur
726.91 Exostosis of unspecified site ▽
727.1 Bunion
735.0 Hallux valgus (acquired)
735.1 Hallux varus (acquired)
735.2 Hallux rigidus
735.3 Hallux malleus
735.8 Other acquired deformity of toe
996.4 Mechanical complication of internal orthopedic device, implant, and graft

ICD-9-CM Procedural

77.59 Other bunionectomy

▽ Unspecified code
♀ Female diagnosis
☒ Manifestation code
♂ Male diagnosis

HCPCS Level II Supplies & Services

A4550 Surgical trays

28294

28294 Correction, hallux valgus (bunion), with or without sesamoidectomy; with tendon transplants (eg, Joplin type procedure)

ICD-9-CM Diagnostic

727.06 Tenosynovitis of foot and ankle
727.1 Bunion
733.99 Other disorders of bone and cartilage
735.0 Hallux valgus (acquired)
735.1 Hallux varus (acquired)
735.2 Hallux rigidus
735.3 Hallux malleus
735.4 Other hammer toe (acquired)

ICD-9-CM Procedural

77.53 Other bunionectomy with soft tissue correction

HCPCS Level II Supplies & Services

A4550 Surgical trays

28296

28296 Correction, hallux valgus (bunion), with or without sesamoidectomy; with metatarsal osteotomy (eg, Mitchell, Chevron, or concentric type procedures)

ICD-9-CM Diagnostic

727.1 Bunion
733.99 Other disorders of bone and cartilage
735.0 Hallux valgus (acquired)
735.1 Hallux varus (acquired)
735.2 Hallux rigidus
735.3 Hallux malleus
735.8 Other acquired deformity of toe
754.52 Congenital metatarsus primus varus
755.66 Other congenital anomaly of toes

ICD-9-CM Procedural

77.51 Bunionectomy with soft tissue correction and osteotomy of the first metatarsal
77.59 Other bunionectomy

HCPCS Level II Supplies & Services

A4550 Surgical trays

28297

28297 Correction, hallux valgus (bunion), with or without sesamoidectomy; Lapidus type procedure

ICD-9-CM Diagnostic

727.1 Bunion
733.99 Other disorders of bone and cartilage
735.0 Hallux valgus (acquired)
735.1 Hallux varus (acquired)
735.2 Hallux rigidus
735.3 Hallux malleus
755.66 Other congenital anomaly of toes

ICD-9-CM Procedural

77.51 Bunionectomy with soft tissue correction and osteotomy of the first metatarsal

HCPCS Level II Supplies & Services

A4550 Surgical trays

28298

28298 Correction, hallux valgus (bunion), with or without sesamoidectomy; by phalanx osteotomy

ICD-9-CM Diagnostic

727.1 Bunion
733.99 Other disorders of bone and cartilage
735.0 Hallux valgus (acquired)
735.1 Hallux varus (acquired)
735.2 Hallux rigidus
735.3 Hallux malleus
735.8 Other acquired deformity of toe
755.66 Other congenital anomaly of toes

ICD-9-CM Procedural

77.59 Other bunionectomy

HCPCS Level II Supplies & Services

A4550 Surgical trays

28299

28299 Correction, hallux valgus (bunion), with or without sesamoidectomy; by double osteotomy

ICD-9-CM Diagnostic

727.1 Bunion
733.99 Other disorders of bone and cartilage
735.0 Hallux valgus (acquired)
735.1 Hallux varus (acquired)
735.2 Hallux rigidus
735.3 Hallux malleus
754.52 Congenital metatarsus primus varus
755.66 Other congenital anomaly of toes

ICD-9-CM Procedural

77.59 Other bunionectomy

HCPCS Level II Supplies & Services

A4550 Surgical trays

28300–28302

28300 Osteotomy; calcaneus (eg, Dwyer or Chambers type procedure), with or without internal fixation
28302 talus

ICD-9-CM Diagnostic

239.2 Neoplasms of unspecified nature of bone, soft tissue, and skin
732.5 Juvenile osteochondrosis of foot
736.70 Unspecified deformity of ankle and foot, acquired ▽
736.72 Equinus deformity of foot, acquired
736.73 Cavus deformity of foot, acquired
736.76 Other acquired calcaneus deformity
736.79 Other acquired deformity of ankle and foot
738.9 Acquired musculoskeletal deformity of unspecified site ▽
754.50 Congenital talipes varus
754.59 Other congenital varus deformity of feet
754.60 Congenital talipes valgus
754.62 Talipes calcaneovalgus
754.69 Other congenital valgus deformity of feet

ICD-9-CM Procedural

77.28 Wedge osteotomy of tarsals and metatarsals
77.38 Other division of tarsals and metatarsals
78.58 Internal fixation of tarsals and metatarsals without fracture reduction

28304–28305

28304 Osteotomy, tarsal bones, other than calcaneus or talus;
28305 with autograft (includes obtaining graft) (eg, Fowler type)

ICD-9-CM Diagnostic

732.5 Juvenile osteochondrosis of foot
736.70 Unspecified deformity of ankle and foot, acquired ▽
736.71 Acquired equinovarus deformity
736.73 Cavus deformity of foot, acquired
754.51 Congenital talipes equinovarus
754.53 Congenital metatarsus varus
754.70 Unspecified talipes ▽
754.71 Talipes cavus
754.79 Other congenital deformity of feet
756.89 Other specified congenital anomaly of muscle, tendon, fascia, and connective tissue

ICD-9-CM Procedural

77.28 Wedge osteotomy of tarsals and metatarsals
77.38 Other division of tarsals and metatarsals
77.77 Excision of tibia and fibula for graft
77.79 Excision of other bone for graft, except facial bones

78.08 Bone graft of tarsals and metatarsals

28306–28308

28306 Osteotomy, with or without lengthening, shortening or angular correction, metatarsal; first metatarsal
28307 first metatarsal with autograft (other than first toe)
28308 other than first metatarsal, each

ICD-9-CM Diagnostic

357.1 Polyneuropathy in collagen vascular disease — (Code first underlying disease: 446.0, 710.0, 714.0) ☒
359.6 Symptomatic inflammatory myopathy in diseases classified elsewhere — (Code first underlying disease: 135, 140.0-208.9, 277.3, 446.0, 710.0, 710.1, 710.2, 714.0) ☒
446.0 Polyarteritis nodosa
710.0 Systemic lupus erythematosus — (Use additional code to identify manifestation: 424.91, 581.81, 582.81, 583.81)
710.1 Systemic sclerosis — (Use additional code to identify manifestation: 359.6, 517.2)
710.2 Sicca syndrome
714.0 Rheumatoid arthritis — (Use additional code to identify manifestation: 357.1, 359.6)
715.17 Primary localized osteoarthrosis, ankle and foot
715.97 Osteoarthrosis, unspecified whether generalized or localized, ankle and foot ▽
718.47 Contracture of ankle and foot joint
719.47 Pain in joint, ankle and foot
726.91 Exostosis of unspecified site ▽
727.1 Bunion
733.91 Arrest of bone development or growth
733.99 Other disorders of bone and cartilage
735.0 Hallux valgus (acquired)
735.1 Hallux varus (acquired)
735.2 Hallux rigidus
735.3 Hallux malleus
735.4 Other hammer toe (acquired)
735.5 Claw toe (acquired)
735.8 Other acquired deformity of toe
736.79 Other acquired deformity of ankle and foot
754.50 Congenital talipes varus
754.52 Congenital metatarsus primus varus
754.53 Congenital metatarsus varus
754.59 Other congenital varus deformity of feet
754.60 Congenital talipes valgus
754.71 Talipes cavus
755.38 Congenital longitudinal deficiency, tarsals or metatarsals, complete or partial (with or without incomplete phalangeal deficiency)
755.67 Congenital anomalies of foot, not elsewhere classified

ICD-9-CM Procedural

77.28 Wedge osteotomy of tarsals and metatarsals
77.38 Other division of tarsals and metatarsals
77.79 Excision of other bone for graft, except facial bones
78.08 Bone graft of tarsals and metatarsals
78.18 Application of external fixation device, tarsals and metatarsals
78.28 Limb shortening procedures, tarsals and metatarsals
78.38 Limb lengthening procedures, tarsals and metatarsals
84.53 Implantation of internal limb lengthening device with kinetic distraction
84.54 Implantation of other internal limb lengthening device

28309

28309 Osteotomy, with or without lengthening, shortening or angular correction, metatarsal; multiple (eg, Swanson type cavus foot procedure)

ICD-9-CM Diagnostic

735.8 Other acquired deformity of toe
736.73 Cavus deformity of foot, acquired
736.75 Cavovarus deformity of foot, acquired
754.71 Talipes cavus
755.67 Congenital anomalies of foot, not elsewhere classified

ICD-9-CM Procedural

77.29 Wedge osteotomy of other bone, except facial bones
77.38 Other division of tarsals and metatarsals
78.18 Application of external fixation device, tarsals and metatarsals
78.28 Limb shortening procedures, tarsals and metatarsals
78.38 Limb lengthening procedures, tarsals and metatarsals
84.53 Implantation of internal limb lengthening device with kinetic distraction
84.54 Implantation of other internal limb lengthening device

28310–28312

28310 Osteotomy, shortening, angular or rotational correction; proximal phalanx, first toe (separate procedure)
28312 other phalanges, any toe

ICD-9-CM Diagnostic

357.1 Polyneuropathy in collagen vascular disease — (Code first underlying disease: 446.0, 710.0, 714.0) ☒
359.6 Symptomatic inflammatory myopathy in diseases classified elsewhere — (Code first underlying disease: 135, 140.0-208.9, 277.3, 446.0, 710.0, 710.1, 710.2, 714.0) ☒
446.0 Polyarteritis nodosa
700 Corns and callosities
710.0 Systemic lupus erythematosus — (Use additional code to identify manifestation: 424.91, 581.81, 582.81, 583.81)
710.1 Systemic sclerosis — (Use additional code to identify manifestation: 359.6, 517.2)
710.2 Sicca syndrome
714.0 Rheumatoid arthritis — (Use additional code to identify manifestation: 357.1, 359.6)
727.1 Bunion
733.91 Arrest of bone development or growth
733.99 Other disorders of bone and cartilage
735.0 Hallux valgus (acquired)
735.1 Hallux varus (acquired)
735.2 Hallux rigidus
735.3 Hallux malleus
735.4 Other hammer toe (acquired)
735.5 Claw toe (acquired)
735.8 Other acquired deformity of toe
736.74 Claw foot, acquired
736.79 Other acquired deformity of ankle and foot
754.52 Congenital metatarsus primus varus
754.53 Congenital metatarsus varus
754.69 Other congenital valgus deformity of feet
755.66 Other congenital anomaly of toes
755.67 Congenital anomalies of foot, not elsewhere classified

ICD-9-CM Procedural

77.29 Wedge osteotomy of other bone, except facial bones
78.29 Limb shortening procedures, other

28313

28313 Reconstruction, angular deformity of toe, soft tissue procedures only (eg, overlapping second toe, fifth toe, curly toes)

ICD-9-CM Diagnostic

718.47 Contracture of ankle and foot joint
733.90 Disorder of bone and cartilage, unspecified ▽
735.4 Other hammer toe (acquired)
735.5 Claw toe (acquired)
735.8 Other acquired deformity of toe
755.66 Other congenital anomaly of toes

ICD-9-CM Procedural

83.09 Other incision of soft tissue
83.75 Tendon transfer or transplantation

28315

28315 Sesamoidectomy, first toe (separate procedure)

ICD-9-CM Diagnostic

357.1 Polyneuropathy in collagen vascular disease — (Code first underlying disease: 446.0, 710.0, 714.0) ☒
359.6 Symptomatic inflammatory myopathy in diseases classified elsewhere — (Code first underlying disease: 135, 140.0-208.9, 277.3, 446.0, 710.0, 710.1, 710.2, 714.0) ☒
446.0 Polyarteritis nodosa
710.0 Systemic lupus erythematosus — (Use additional code to identify manifestation: 424.91, 581.81, 582.81, 583.81)
710.1 Systemic sclerosis — (Use additional code to identify manifestation: 359.6, 517.2)

▽ Unspecified code ☒ Manifestation code
♀ Female diagnosis ♂ Male diagnosis

710.2 Sicca syndrome
714.0 Rheumatoid arthritis — (Use additional code to identify manifestation: 357.1, 359.6)
733.99 Other disorders of bone and cartilage
735.0 Hallux valgus (acquired)
735.1 Hallux varus (acquired)
754.52 Congenital metatarsus primus varus
755.67 Congenital anomalies of foot, not elsewhere classified

ICD-9-CM Procedural
77.98 Total ostectomy of tarsals and metatarsals

28320–28322
28320 Repair, nonunion or malunion; tarsal bones
28322 metatarsal, with or without bone graft (includes obtaining graft)

ICD-9-CM Diagnostic
733.81 Malunion of fracture
733.82 Nonunion of fracture
905.4 Late effect of fracture of lower extremities

ICD-9-CM Procedural
77.78 Excision of tarsals and metatarsals for graft
78.08 Bone graft of tarsals and metatarsals
78.48 Other repair or plastic operations on tarsals and metatarsals

28340–28341
28340 Reconstruction, toe, macrodactyly; soft tissue resection
28341 requiring bone resection

ICD-9-CM Diagnostic
755.65 Macrodactylia of toes

ICD-9-CM Procedural
77.39 Other division of other bone, except facial bones
78.48 Other repair or plastic operations on tarsals and metatarsals
83.49 Other excision of soft tissue

28344
28344 Reconstruction, toe(s); polydactyly

ICD-9-CM Diagnostic
755.02 Polydactyly of toes

ICD-9-CM Procedural
77.69 Local excision of lesion or tissue of other bone, except facial bones
78.49 Other repair or plastic operations on other bone, except facial bones

28345
28345 Reconstruction, toe(s); syndactyly, with or without skin graft(s), each web

ICD-9-CM Diagnostic
755.13 Syndactyly of toes without fusion of bone
755.14 Syndactyly of toes with fusion of bone

ICD-9-CM Procedural
77.69 Local excision of lesion or tissue of other bone, except facial bones
78.49 Other repair or plastic operations on other bone, except facial bones

28360
28360 Reconstruction, cleft foot

ICD-9-CM Diagnostic
755.66 Other congenital anomaly of toes
755.67 Congenital anomalies of foot, not elsewhere classified

ICD-9-CM Procedural
83.85 Other change in muscle or tendon length

28400–28405
28400 Closed treatment of calcaneal fracture; without manipulation
28405 with manipulation

ICD-9-CM Diagnostic
733.95 Stress fracture of other bone
825.0 Closed fracture of calcaneus
928.20 Crushing injury of foot — (Use additional code to identify any associated injuries: 800-829, 850.0-854.1, 860.0-869.1)

ICD-9-CM Procedural
79.07 Closed reduction of fracture of tarsals and metatarsals without internal fixation
93.53 Application of other cast
93.54 Application of splint

HCPCS Level II Supplies & Services
A4570 Splint
A4580 Cast supplies (e.g., plaster)
E0112 Crutches, underarm, wood, adjustable or fixed, pair, with pads, tips and handgrips
E0113 Crutch, underarm, wood, adjustable or fixed, each, with pad, tip and handgrip
E0114 Crutches, underarm, other than wood, adjustable or fixed, pair, with pads, tips and handgrips

28406
28406 Percutaneous skeletal fixation of calcaneal fracture, with manipulation

ICD-9-CM Diagnostic
733.95 Stress fracture of other bone
825.0 Closed fracture of calcaneus
928.20 Crushing injury of foot — (Use additional code to identify any associated injuries: 800-829, 850.0-854.1, 860.0-869.1)

ICD-9-CM Procedural
79.17 Closed reduction of fracture of tarsals and metatarsals with internal fixation

HCPCS Level II Supplies & Services
A4550 Surgical trays

28415
28415 Open treatment of calcaneal fracture, with or without internal or external fixation;

ICD-9-CM Diagnostic
733.19 Pathologic fracture of other specified site
733.81 Malunion of fracture
733.82 Nonunion of fracture
733.95 Stress fracture of other bone
825.0 Closed fracture of calcaneus
825.1 Open fracture of calcaneus
825.29 Other closed fracture of tarsal and metatarsal bones
928.20 Crushing injury of foot — (Use additional code to identify any associated injuries: 800-829, 850.0-854.1, 860.0-869.1)

ICD-9-CM Procedural
78.18 Application of external fixation device, tarsals and metatarsals
79.27 Open reduction of fracture of tarsals and metatarsals without internal fixation
79.37 Open reduction of fracture of tarsals and metatarsals with internal fixation

HCPCS Level II Supplies & Services
A4305 Disposable drug delivery system, flow rate of 50 ml or greater per hour
A4306 Disposable drug delivery system, flow rate of 5 ml or less per hour
A4550 Surgical trays

28420
28420 Open treatment of calcaneal fracture, with or without internal or external fixation; with primary iliac or other autogenous bone graft (includes obtaining graft)

ICD-9-CM Diagnostic
733.19 Pathologic fracture of other specified site
733.81 Malunion of fracture
733.82 Nonunion of fracture
733.95 Stress fracture of other bone
825.0 Closed fracture of calcaneus
825.1 Open fracture of calcaneus

825.29 Other closed fracture of tarsal and metatarsal bones
825.39 Other open fractures of tarsal and metatarsal bones
928.20 Crushing injury of foot — (Use additional code to identify any associated injuries: 800-829, 850.0-854.1, 860.0-869.1)

ICD-9-CM Procedural
77.77 Excision of tibia and fibula for graft
77.79 Excision of other bone for graft, except facial bones
78.08 Bone graft of tarsals and metatarsals
78.18 Application of external fixation device, tarsals and metatarsals
79.27 Open reduction of fracture of tarsals and metatarsals without internal fixation
79.37 Open reduction of fracture of tarsals and metatarsals with internal fixation

28430–28435
28430 Closed treatment of talus fracture; without manipulation
28435 with manipulation

ICD-9-CM Diagnostic
733.19 Pathologic fracture of other specified site
733.95 Stress fracture of other bone
825.21 Closed fracture of astragalus
825.29 Other closed fracture of tarsal and metatarsal bones
928.20 Crushing injury of foot — (Use additional code to identify any associated injuries: 800-829, 850.0-854.1, 860.0-869.1)
928.21 Crushing injury of ankle — (Use additional code to identify any associated injuries: 800-829, 850.0-854.1, 860.0-869.1)

ICD-9-CM Procedural
79.07 Closed reduction of fracture of tarsals and metatarsals without internal fixation
93.53 Application of other cast
93.54 Application of splint

HCPCS Level II Supplies & Services
A4570 Splint
A4580 Cast supplies (e.g., plaster)
A4590 Special casting material (e.g., fiberglass)
E0112 Crutches, underarm, wood, adjustable or fixed, pair, with pads, tips and handgrips
E0113 Crutch, underarm, wood, adjustable or fixed, each, with pad, tip and handgrip

28436
28436 Percutaneous skeletal fixation of talus fracture, with manipulation

ICD-9-CM Diagnostic
733.19 Pathologic fracture of other specified site
733.95 Stress fracture of other bone
825.21 Closed fracture of astragalus
825.29 Other closed fracture of tarsal and metatarsal bones
928.20 Crushing injury of foot — (Use additional code to identify any associated injuries: 800-829, 850.0-854.1, 860.0-869.1)
928.21 Crushing injury of ankle — (Use additional code to identify any associated injuries: 800-829, 850.0-854.1, 860.0-869.1)

ICD-9-CM Procedural
79.17 Closed reduction of fracture of tarsals and metatarsals with internal fixation

HCPCS Level II Supplies & Services
A4570 Splint
A4580 Cast supplies (e.g., plaster)
A4590 Special casting material (e.g., fiberglass)
E0112 Crutches, underarm, wood, adjustable or fixed, pair, with pads, tips and handgrips
E0113 Crutch, underarm, wood, adjustable or fixed, each, with pad, tip and handgrip

28445
28445 Open treatment of talus fracture, with or without internal or external fixation

ICD-9-CM Diagnostic
733.19 Pathologic fracture of other specified site
733.81 Malunion of fracture
733.82 Nonunion of fracture
733.95 Stress fracture of other bone
825.21 Closed fracture of astragalus
825.29 Other closed fracture of tarsal and metatarsal bones
825.31 Open fracture of astragalus
825.39 Other open fractures of tarsal and metatarsal bones
905.4 Late effect of fracture of lower extremities
928.20 Crushing injury of foot — (Use additional code to identify any associated injuries: 800-829, 850.0-854.1, 860.0-869.1)
928.21 Crushing injury of ankle — (Use additional code to identify any associated injuries: 800-829, 850.0-854.1, 860.0-869.1)

ICD-9-CM Procedural
78.18 Application of external fixation device, tarsals and metatarsals
79.27 Open reduction of fracture of tarsals and metatarsals without internal fixation
79.37 Open reduction of fracture of tarsals and metatarsals with internal fixation

HCPCS Level II Supplies & Services
A4570 Splint
A4580 Cast supplies (e.g., plaster)
A4590 Special casting material (e.g., fiberglass)
E0112 Crutches, underarm, wood, adjustable or fixed, pair, with pads, tips and handgrips
E0113 Crutch, underarm, wood, adjustable or fixed, each, with pad, tip and handgrip

28450–28455
28450 Treatment of tarsal bone fracture (except talus and calcaneus); without manipulation, each
28455 with manipulation, each

ICD-9-CM Diagnostic
733.19 Pathologic fracture of other specified site
733.95 Stress fracture of other bone
825.22 Closed fracture of navicular (scaphoid) bone of foot
825.23 Closed fracture of cuboid bone
825.24 Closed fracture of cuneiform bone of foot
825.29 Other closed fracture of tarsal and metatarsal bones

ICD-9-CM Procedural
79.07 Closed reduction of fracture of tarsals and metatarsals without internal fixation
79.97 Unspecified operation on bone injury of tarsals and metatarsals
93.53 Application of other cast
93.54 Application of splint

HCPCS Level II Supplies & Services
A4570 Splint
A4580 Cast supplies (e.g., plaster)
A4590 Special casting material (e.g., fiberglass)
E0112 Crutches, underarm, wood, adjustable or fixed, pair, with pads, tips and handgrips
E0113 Crutch, underarm, wood, adjustable or fixed, each, with pad, tip and handgrip

28456
28456 Percutaneous skeletal fixation of tarsal bone fracture (except talus and calcaneus), with manipulation, each

ICD-9-CM Diagnostic
733.19 Pathologic fracture of other specified site
733.95 Stress fracture of other bone
825.22 Closed fracture of navicular (scaphoid) bone of foot
825.23 Closed fracture of cuboid bone
825.24 Closed fracture of cuneiform bone of foot
825.29 Other closed fracture of tarsal and metatarsal bones

ICD-9-CM Procedural
79.17 Closed reduction of fracture of tarsals and metatarsals with internal fixation

HCPCS Level II Supplies & Services
A4570 Splint
A4580 Cast supplies (e.g., plaster)
A4590 Special casting material (e.g., fiberglass)
E0112 Crutches, underarm, wood, adjustable or fixed, pair, with pads, tips and handgrips
E0113 Crutch, underarm, wood, adjustable or fixed, each, with pad, tip and handgrip

28465
28465 Open treatment of tarsal bone fracture (except talus and calcaneus), with or without internal or external fixation, each

ICD-9-CM Diagnostic
733.19 Pathologic fracture of other specified site
733.81 Malunion of fracture

733.82 Nonunion of fracture
733.95 Stress fracture of other bone
825.22 Closed fracture of navicular (scaphoid) bone of foot
825.23 Closed fracture of cuboid bone
825.24 Closed fracture of cuneiform bone of foot
825.29 Other closed fracture of tarsal and metatarsal bones
825.32 Open fracture of navicular (scaphoid) bone of foot
825.33 Open fracture of cuboid bone
825.34 Open fracture of cuneiform bone of foot,
825.39 Other open fractures of tarsal and metatarsal bones
905.4 Late effect of fracture of lower extremities

ICD-9-CM Procedural
78.18 Application of external fixation device, tarsals and metatarsals
79.27 Open reduction of fracture of tarsals and metatarsals without internal fixation
79.37 Open reduction of fracture of tarsals and metatarsals with internal fixation

28470–28475
28470 Closed treatment of metatarsal fracture; without manipulation, each
28475 with manipulation, each

ICD-9-CM Diagnostic
733.94 Stress fracture of the metatarsals
825.25 Closed fracture of metatarsal bone(s)
825.29 Other closed fracture of tarsal and metatarsal bones
928.20 Crushing injury of foot — (Use additional code to identify any associated injuries: 800-829, 850.0-854.1, 860.0-869.1)

ICD-9-CM Procedural
79.07 Closed reduction of fracture of tarsals and metatarsals without internal fixation
93.53 Application of other cast
93.54 Application of splint

HCPCS Level II Supplies & Services
A4570 Splint
A4580 Cast supplies (e.g., plaster)
A4590 Special casting material (e.g., fiberglass)
E0112 Crutches, underarm, wood, adjustable or fixed, pair, with pads, tips and handgrips
E0113 Crutch, underarm, wood, adjustable or fixed, each, with pad, tip and handgrip

28476
28476 Percutaneous skeletal fixation of metatarsal fracture, with manipulation, each

ICD-9-CM Diagnostic
733.94 Stress fracture of the metatarsals
825.25 Closed fracture of metatarsal bone(s)
825.29 Other closed fracture of tarsal and metatarsal bones
928.20 Crushing injury of foot — (Use additional code to identify any associated injuries: 800-829, 850.0-854.1, 860.0-869.1)

ICD-9-CM Procedural
79.17 Closed reduction of fracture of tarsals and metatarsals with internal fixation

HCPCS Level II Supplies & Services
A4570 Splint
A4580 Cast supplies (e.g., plaster)
A4590 Special casting material (e.g., fiberglass)
E0112 Crutches, underarm, wood, adjustable or fixed, pair, with pads, tips and handgrips
E0113 Crutch, underarm, wood, adjustable or fixed, each, with pad, tip and handgrip

28485
28485 Open treatment of metatarsal fracture, with or without internal or external fixation, each

ICD-9-CM Diagnostic
733.19 Pathologic fracture of other specified site
733.81 Malunion of fracture
733.82 Nonunion of fracture
733.94 Stress fracture of the metatarsals
825.25 Closed fracture of metatarsal bone(s)
825.29 Other closed fracture of tarsal and metatarsal bones
825.35 Open fracture of metatarsal bone(s)
825.39 Other open fractures of tarsal and metatarsal bones

ICD-9-CM Procedural
78.18 Application of external fixation device, tarsals and metatarsals
79.27 Open reduction of fracture of tarsals and metatarsals without internal fixation
79.37 Open reduction of fracture of tarsals and metatarsals with internal fixation

HCPCS Level II Supplies & Services
A4570 Splint
A4580 Cast supplies (e.g., plaster)
A4590 Special casting material (e.g., fiberglass)
E0112 Crutches, underarm, wood, adjustable or fixed, pair, with pads, tips and handgrips
E0113 Crutch, underarm, wood, adjustable or fixed, each, with pad, tip and handgrip

28490–28495
28490 Closed treatment of fracture great toe, phalanx or phalanges; without manipulation
28495 with manipulation

ICD-9-CM Diagnostic
733.19 Pathologic fracture of other specified site
733.95 Stress fracture of other bone
826.0 Closed fracture of one or more phalanges of foot

ICD-9-CM Procedural
79.08 Closed reduction of fracture of phalanges of foot without internal fixation
93.53 Application of other cast
93.54 Application of splint

HCPCS Level II Supplies & Services
A4570 Splint
A4580 Cast supplies (e.g., plaster)
A4590 Special casting material (e.g., fiberglass)
E0112 Crutches, underarm, wood, adjustable or fixed, pair, with pads, tips and handgrips
E0113 Crutch, underarm, wood, adjustable or fixed, each, with pad, tip and handgrip

28496
28496 Percutaneous skeletal fixation of fracture great toe, phalanx or phalanges, with manipulation

ICD-9-CM Diagnostic
733.19 Pathologic fracture of other specified site
733.95 Stress fracture of other bone
826.0 Closed fracture of one or more phalanges of foot

ICD-9-CM Procedural
79.18 Closed reduction of fracture of phalanges of foot with internal fixation

HCPCS Level II Supplies & Services
A4570 Splint
A4580 Cast supplies (e.g., plaster)
A4590 Special casting material (e.g., fiberglass)
E0112 Crutches, underarm, wood, adjustable or fixed, pair, with pads, tips and handgrips
E0113 Crutch, underarm, wood, adjustable or fixed, each, with pad, tip and handgrip

28505
28505 Open treatment of fracture great toe, phalanx or phalanges, with or without internal or external fixation

ICD-9-CM Diagnostic
733.81 Malunion of fracture
733.82 Nonunion of fracture
733.95 Stress fracture of other bone
826.0 Closed fracture of one or more phalanges of foot
826.1 Open fracture of one or more phalanges of foot
905.4 Late effect of fracture of lower extremities

ICD-9-CM Procedural
78.18 Application of external fixation device, tarsals and metatarsals
79.28 Open reduction of fracture of phalanges of foot without internal fixation
79.38 Open reduction of fracture of phalanges of foot with internal fixation

HCPCS Level II Supplies & Services

A4570 Splint
A4580 Cast supplies (e.g., plaster)
A4590 Special casting material (e.g., fiberglass)
E0112 Crutches, underarm, wood, adjustable or fixed, pair, with pads, tips and handgrips
E0113 Crutch, underarm, wood, adjustable or fixed, each, with pad, tip and handgrip

28510–28515

28510 Closed treatment of fracture, phalanx or phalanges, other than great toe; without manipulation, each
28515 with manipulation, each

ICD-9-CM Diagnostic

733.19 Pathologic fracture of other specified site
733.95 Stress fracture of other bone
826.0 Closed fracture of one or more phalanges of foot

ICD-9-CM Procedural

79.08 Closed reduction of fracture of phalanges of foot without internal fixation
93.53 Application of other cast
93.54 Application of splint

HCPCS Level II Supplies & Services

A4570 Splint
A4580 Cast supplies (e.g., plaster)
A4590 Special casting material (e.g., fiberglass)
E0112 Crutches, underarm, wood, adjustable or fixed, pair, with pads, tips and handgrips
E0113 Crutch, underarm, wood, adjustable or fixed, each, with pad, tip and handgrip

28525

28525 Open treatment of fracture, phalanx or phalanges, other than great toe, with or without internal or external fixation, each

ICD-9-CM Diagnostic

733.19 Pathologic fracture of other specified site
733.81 Malunion of fracture
733.95 Stress fracture of other bone
826.0 Closed fracture of one or more phalanges of foot
826.1 Open fracture of one or more phalanges of foot
905.4 Late effect of fracture of lower extremities

ICD-9-CM Procedural

78.18 Application of external fixation device, tarsals and metatarsals
79.28 Open reduction of fracture of phalanges of foot without internal fixation
79.38 Open reduction of fracture of phalanges of foot with internal fixation

HCPCS Level II Supplies & Services

A4305 Disposable drug delivery system, flow rate of 50 ml or greater per hour
A4306 Disposable drug delivery system, flow rate of 5 ml or less per hour
A4550 Surgical trays

28530

28530 Closed treatment of sesamoid fracture

ICD-9-CM Diagnostic

733.19 Pathologic fracture of other specified site
733.95 Stress fracture of other bone
825.20 Closed fracture of unspecified bone(s) of foot (except toes) ▽

ICD-9-CM Procedural

79.08 Closed reduction of fracture of phalanges of foot without internal fixation
79.18 Closed reduction of fracture of phalanges of foot with internal fixation

HCPCS Level II Supplies & Services

A4570 Splint
A4580 Cast supplies (e.g., plaster)
A4590 Special casting material (e.g., fiberglass)
E0112 Crutches, underarm, wood, adjustable or fixed, pair, with pads, tips and handgrips
E0113 Crutch, underarm, wood, adjustable or fixed, each, with pad, tip and handgrip

28531

28531 Open treatment of sesamoid fracture, with or without internal fixation

ICD-9-CM Diagnostic

733.19 Pathologic fracture of other specified site
733.81 Malunion of fracture
733.82 Nonunion of fracture
733.95 Stress fracture of other bone
825.20 Closed fracture of unspecified bone(s) of foot (except toes) ▽
825.30 Open fracture of unspecified bone(s) of foot (except toes) ▽
893.1 Open wound of toe(s), complicated — (Use additional code to identify infection)

ICD-9-CM Procedural

79.28 Open reduction of fracture of phalanges of foot without internal fixation
79.38 Open reduction of fracture of phalanges of foot with internal fixation

HCPCS Level II Supplies & Services

A4305 Disposable drug delivery system, flow rate of 50 ml or greater per hour
A4306 Disposable drug delivery system, flow rate of 5 ml or less per hour
A4550 Surgical trays

28540–28545

28540 Closed treatment of tarsal bone dislocation, other than talotarsal; without anesthesia
28545 requiring anesthesia

ICD-9-CM Diagnostic

718.77 Developmental dislocation of joint, ankle and foot
837.0 Closed dislocation of ankle
838.01 Closed dislocation of tarsal (bone), joint unspecified ▽
838.02 Closed dislocation of midtarsal (joint)

ICD-9-CM Procedural

79.78 Closed reduction of dislocation of foot and toe

HCPCS Level II Supplies & Services

A4570 Splint
A4580 Cast supplies (e.g., plaster)
A4590 Special casting material (e.g., fiberglass)
E0112 Crutches, underarm, wood, adjustable or fixed, pair, with pads, tips and handgrips
E0113 Crutch, underarm, wood, adjustable or fixed, each, with pad, tip and handgrip

28546

28546 Percutaneous skeletal fixation of tarsal bone dislocation, other than talotarsal, with manipulation

ICD-9-CM Diagnostic

718.77 Developmental dislocation of joint, ankle and foot
838.02 Closed dislocation of midtarsal (joint)
838.03 Closed dislocation of tarsometatarsal (joint)

ICD-9-CM Procedural

78.58 Internal fixation of tarsals and metatarsals without fracture reduction
79.78 Closed reduction of dislocation of foot and toe

HCPCS Level II Supplies & Services

A4570 Splint
A4580 Cast supplies (e.g., plaster)
A4590 Special casting material (e.g., fiberglass)
E0112 Crutches, underarm, wood, adjustable or fixed, pair, with pads, tips and handgrips
E0113 Crutch, underarm, wood, adjustable or fixed, each, with pad, tip and handgrip

28555

28555 Open treatment of tarsal bone dislocation, with or without internal or external fixation

ICD-9-CM Diagnostic

718.77 Developmental dislocation of joint, ankle and foot
837.0 Closed dislocation of ankle
837.1 Open dislocation of ankle
838.01 Closed dislocation of tarsal (bone), joint unspecified ▽
838.02 Closed dislocation of midtarsal (joint)
838.03 Closed dislocation of tarsometatarsal (joint)

▽ Unspecified code
♀ Female diagnosis
☒ Manifestation code
♂ Male diagnosis

838.11 Open dislocation of tarsal (bone), joint unspecified ▽
838.12 Open dislocation of midtarsal (joint)
838.13 Open dislocation of tarsometatarsal (joint)

ICD-9-CM Procedural
79.88 Open reduction of dislocation of foot and toe

HCPCS Level II Supplies & Services
A4580 Cast supplies (e.g., plaster)
A4590 Special casting material (e.g., fiberglass)
E0112 Crutches, underarm, wood, adjustable or fixed, pair, with pads, tips and handgrips
E0113 Crutch, underarm, wood, adjustable or fixed, each, with pad, tip and handgrip
E0114 Crutches, underarm, other than wood, adjustable or fixed, pair, with pads, tips and handgrips

28570–28575
28570 Closed treatment of talotarsal joint dislocation; without anesthesia
28575 requiring anesthesia

ICD-9-CM Diagnostic
718.77 Developmental dislocation of joint, ankle and foot
837.0 Closed dislocation of ankle
838.02 Closed dislocation of midtarsal (joint)

ICD-9-CM Procedural
79.78 Closed reduction of dislocation of foot and toe

HCPCS Level II Supplies & Services
A4580 Cast supplies (e.g., plaster)
A4590 Special casting material (e.g., fiberglass)
E0112 Crutches, underarm, wood, adjustable or fixed, pair, with pads, tips and handgrips
E0113 Crutch, underarm, wood, adjustable or fixed, each, with pad, tip and handgrip
E0114 Crutches, underarm, other than wood, adjustable or fixed, pair, with pads, tips and handgrips

28576
28576 Percutaneous skeletal fixation of talotarsal joint dislocation, with manipulation

ICD-9-CM Diagnostic
718.77 Developmental dislocation of joint, ankle and foot
837.0 Closed dislocation of ankle
838.02 Closed dislocation of midtarsal (joint)

ICD-9-CM Procedural
78.58 Internal fixation of tarsals and metatarsals without fracture reduction
79.77 Closed reduction of dislocation of ankle

HCPCS Level II Supplies & Services
A4580 Cast supplies (e.g., plaster)
A4590 Special casting material (e.g., fiberglass)
E0112 Crutches, underarm, wood, adjustable or fixed, pair, with pads, tips and handgrips
E0113 Crutch, underarm, wood, adjustable or fixed, each, with pad, tip and handgrip
E0114 Crutches, underarm, other than wood, adjustable or fixed, pair, with pads, tips and handgrips

28585
28585 Open treatment of talotarsal joint dislocation, with or without internal or external fixation

ICD-9-CM Diagnostic
718.77 Developmental dislocation of joint, ankle and foot
837.0 Closed dislocation of ankle
837.1 Open dislocation of ankle
838.02 Closed dislocation of midtarsal (joint)
838.12 Open dislocation of midtarsal (joint)

ICD-9-CM Procedural
78.18 Application of external fixation device, tarsals and metatarsals
79.88 Open reduction of dislocation of foot and toe

HCPCS Level II Supplies & Services
A4580 Cast supplies (e.g., plaster)
A4590 Special casting material (e.g., fiberglass)
E0112 Crutches, underarm, wood, adjustable or fixed, pair, with pads, tips and handgrips
E0113 Crutch, underarm, wood, adjustable or fixed, each, with pad, tip and handgrip
E0114 Crutches, underarm, other than wood, adjustable or fixed, pair, with pads, tips and handgrips

28600–28605
28600 Closed treatment of tarsometatarsal joint dislocation; without anesthesia
28605 requiring anesthesia

ICD-9-CM Diagnostic
718.77 Developmental dislocation of joint, ankle and foot
838.02 Closed dislocation of midtarsal (joint)
838.03 Closed dislocation of tarsometatarsal (joint)

ICD-9-CM Procedural
79.78 Closed reduction of dislocation of foot and toe

HCPCS Level II Supplies & Services
A4580 Cast supplies (e.g., plaster)
A4590 Special casting material (e.g., fiberglass)
E0112 Crutches, underarm, wood, adjustable or fixed, pair, with pads, tips and handgrips
E0113 Crutch, underarm, wood, adjustable or fixed, each, with pad, tip and handgrip
E0114 Crutches, underarm, other than wood, adjustable or fixed, pair, with pads, tips and handgrips

28606
28606 Percutaneous skeletal fixation of tarsometatarsal joint dislocation, with manipulation

ICD-9-CM Diagnostic
718.77 Developmental dislocation of joint, ankle and foot
838.02 Closed dislocation of midtarsal (joint)
838.03 Closed dislocation of tarsometatarsal (joint)

ICD-9-CM Procedural
78.58 Internal fixation of tarsals and metatarsals without fracture reduction
79.78 Closed reduction of dislocation of foot and toe

HCPCS Level II Supplies & Services
A4580 Cast supplies (e.g., plaster)
A4590 Special casting material (e.g., fiberglass)
E0112 Crutches, underarm, wood, adjustable or fixed, pair, with pads, tips and handgrips
E0113 Crutch, underarm, wood, adjustable or fixed, each, with pad, tip and handgrip
E0114 Crutches, underarm, other than wood, adjustable or fixed, pair, with pads, tips and handgrips

28615
28615 Open treatment of tarsometatarsal joint dislocation, with or without internal or external fixation

ICD-9-CM Diagnostic
718.77 Developmental dislocation of joint, ankle and foot
838.02 Closed dislocation of midtarsal (joint)
838.03 Closed dislocation of tarsometatarsal (joint)
838.11 Open dislocation of tarsal (bone), joint unspecified ▽
838.12 Open dislocation of midtarsal (joint)

ICD-9-CM Procedural
79.88 Open reduction of dislocation of foot and toe

HCPCS Level II Supplies & Services
A4580 Cast supplies (e.g., plaster)
A4590 Special casting material (e.g., fiberglass)
E0112 Crutches, underarm, wood, adjustable or fixed, pair, with pads, tips and handgrips
E0113 Crutch, underarm, wood, adjustable or fixed, each, with pad, tip and handgrip
E0114 Crutches, underarm, other than wood, adjustable or fixed, pair, with pads, tips and handgrips

28630–28635

28630 Closed treatment of metatarsophalangeal joint dislocation; without anesthesia
28635 requiring anesthesia

ICD-9-CM Diagnostic

718.77 Developmental dislocation of joint, ankle and foot
838.05 Closed dislocation of metatarsophalangeal (joint)

ICD-9-CM Procedural

79.78 Closed reduction of dislocation of foot and toe

HCPCS Level II Supplies & Services

A4580 Cast supplies (e.g., plaster)
A4590 Special casting material (e.g., fiberglass)
E0112 Crutches, underarm, wood, adjustable or fixed, pair, with pads, tips and handgrips
E0113 Crutch, underarm, wood, adjustable or fixed, each, with pad, tip and handgrip
E0114 Crutches, underarm, other than wood, adjustable or fixed, pair, with pads, tips and handgrips

28636

28636 Percutaneous skeletal fixation of metatarsophalangeal joint dislocation, with manipulation

ICD-9-CM Diagnostic

718.77 Developmental dislocation of joint, ankle and foot
838.05 Closed dislocation of metatarsophalangeal (joint)

ICD-9-CM Procedural

78.58 Internal fixation of tarsals and metatarsals without fracture reduction
79.78 Closed reduction of dislocation of foot and toe

HCPCS Level II Supplies & Services

A4580 Cast supplies (e.g., plaster)
A4590 Special casting material (e.g., fiberglass)
E0112 Crutches, underarm, wood, adjustable or fixed, pair, with pads, tips and handgrips
E0113 Crutch, underarm, wood, adjustable or fixed, each, with pad, tip and handgrip
E0114 Crutches, underarm, other than wood, adjustable or fixed, pair, with pads, tips and handgrips

28645

28645 Open treatment of metatarsophalangeal joint dislocation, with or without internal or external fixation

ICD-9-CM Diagnostic

718.77 Developmental dislocation of joint, ankle and foot
838.05 Closed dislocation of metatarsophalangeal (joint)
838.15 Open dislocation of metatarsophalangeal (joint)

ICD-9-CM Procedural

79.88 Open reduction of dislocation of foot and toe

HCPCS Level II Supplies & Services

A4580 Cast supplies (e.g., plaster)
A4590 Special casting material (e.g., fiberglass)
E0112 Crutches, underarm, wood, adjustable or fixed, pair, with pads, tips and handgrips
E0113 Crutch, underarm, wood, adjustable or fixed, each, with pad, tip and handgrip
E0114 Crutches, underarm, other than wood, adjustable or fixed, pair, with pads, tips and handgrips

28660–28665

28660 Closed treatment of interphalangeal joint dislocation; without anesthesia
28665 requiring anesthesia

ICD-9-CM Diagnostic

718.77 Developmental dislocation of joint, ankle and foot
838.06 Closed dislocation of interphalangeal (joint), foot

ICD-9-CM Procedural

79.78 Closed reduction of dislocation of foot and toe

HCPCS Level II Supplies & Services

A4570 Splint
A4580 Cast supplies (e.g., plaster)

28666

28666 Percutaneous skeletal fixation of interphalangeal joint dislocation, with manipulation

ICD-9-CM Diagnostic

718.77 Developmental dislocation of joint, ankle and foot
838.06 Closed dislocation of interphalangeal (joint), foot

ICD-9-CM Procedural

78.59 Internal fixation of other bone, except facial bones, without fracture reduction
79.78 Closed reduction of dislocation of foot and toe

HCPCS Level II Supplies & Services

A4570 Splint
A4580 Cast supplies (e.g., plaster)

28675

28675 Open treatment of interphalangeal joint dislocation, with or without internal or external fixation

ICD-9-CM Diagnostic

718.77 Developmental dislocation of joint, ankle and foot
838.06 Closed dislocation of interphalangeal (joint), foot
838.16 Open dislocation of interphalangeal (joint), foot

ICD-9-CM Procedural

79.88 Open reduction of dislocation of foot and toe

HCPCS Level II Supplies & Services

A4570 Splint
A4580 Cast supplies (e.g., plaster)

28705

28705 Arthrodesis; pantalar

ICD-9-CM Diagnostic

357.1 Polyneuropathy in collagen vascular disease — (Code first underlying disease: 446.0, 710.0, 714.0) ☒
359.6 Symptomatic inflammatory myopathy in diseases classified elsewhere — (Code first underlying disease: 135, 140.0-208.9, 277.3, 446.0, 710.0, 710.1, 710.2, 714.0) ☒
446.0 Polyarteritis nodosa
710.0 Systemic lupus erythematosus — (Use additional code to identify manifestation: 424.91, 581.81, 582.81, 583.81)
710.1 Systemic sclerosis — (Use additional code to identify manifestation: 359.6, 517.2)
710.2 Sicca syndrome
714.0 Rheumatoid arthritis — (Use additional code to identify manifestation: 357.1, 359.6)
715.17 Primary localized osteoarthrosis, ankle and foot
715.27 Secondary localized osteoarthrosis, ankle and foot
715.37 Localized osteoarthrosis not specified whether primary or secondary, ankle and foot
715.89 Osteoarthrosis involving multiple sites, but not specified as generalized
715.97 Osteoarthrosis, unspecified whether generalized or localized, ankle and foot ▽
716.17 Traumatic arthropathy, ankle and foot
718.87 Other joint derangement, not elsewhere classified, ankle and foot
733.44 Aseptic necrosis of talus
733.81 Malunion of fracture
733.82 Nonunion of fracture

ICD-9-CM Procedural

81.11 Ankle fusion

28715

28715 Arthrodesis; triple

ICD-9-CM Diagnostic

138 Late effects of acute poliomyelitis
356.1 Peroneal muscular atrophy
357.1 Polyneuropathy in collagen vascular disease — (Code first underlying disease: 446.0, 710.0, 714.0) ☒
359.6 Symptomatic inflammatory myopathy in diseases classified elsewhere — (Code first underlying disease: 135, 140.0-208.9, 277.3, 446.0, 710.0, 710.1, 710.2, 714.0) ☒
446.0 Polyarteritis nodosa

▽ Unspecified code
♀ Female diagnosis
☒ Manifestation code
♂ Male diagnosis

710.0 Systemic lupus erythematosus — (Use additional code to identify manifestation: 424.91, 581.81, 582.81, 583.81)
710.1 Systemic sclerosis — (Use additional code to identify manifestation: 359.6, 517.2)
710.2 Sicca syndrome
714.0 Rheumatoid arthritis — (Use additional code to identify manifestation: 357.1, 359.6)
714.1 Felty's syndrome
715.17 Primary localized osteoarthrosis, ankle and foot
715.27 Secondary localized osteoarthrosis, ankle and foot
715.37 Localized osteoarthrosis not specified whether primary or secondary, ankle and foot
715.97 Osteoarthrosis, unspecified whether generalized or localized, ankle and foot
716.17 Traumatic arthropathy, ankle and foot
718.87 Other joint derangement, not elsewhere classified, ankle and foot
719.47 Pain in joint, ankle and foot
733.81 Malunion of fracture
736.71 Acquired equinovarus deformity
736.72 Equinus deformity of foot, acquired
736.73 Cavus deformity of foot, acquired
736.74 Claw foot, acquired
736.75 Cavovarus deformity of foot, acquired
736.76 Other acquired calcaneus deformity
736.79 Other acquired deformity of ankle and foot
754.61 Congenital pes planus
754.62 Talipes calcaneovalgus
754.69 Other congenital valgus deformity of feet
755.67 Congenital anomalies of foot, not elsewhere classified
825.22 Closed fracture of navicular (scaphoid) bone of foot
928.20 Crushing injury of foot — (Use additional code to identify any associated injuries: 800-829, 850.0-854.1, 860.0-869.1)

ICD-9-CM Procedural

81.12 Triple arthrodesis

28725

28725 Arthrodesis; subtalar

ICD-9-CM Diagnostic

357.1 Polyneuropathy in collagen vascular disease — (Code first underlying disease: 446.0, 710.0, 714.0)
359.6 Symptomatic inflammatory myopathy in diseases classified elsewhere — (Code first underlying disease: 135, 140.0-208.9, 277.3, 446.0, 710.0, 710.1, 710.2, 714.0)
446.0 Polyarteritis nodosa
710.0 Systemic lupus erythematosus — (Use additional code to identify manifestation: 424.91, 581.81, 582.81, 583.81)
710.1 Systemic sclerosis — (Use additional code to identify manifestation: 359.6, 517.2)
710.2 Sicca syndrome
714.0 Rheumatoid arthritis — (Use additional code to identify manifestation: 357.1, 359.6)
716.17 Traumatic arthropathy, ankle and foot
733.44 Aseptic necrosis of talus
733.81 Malunion of fracture
736.76 Other acquired calcaneus deformity
736.79 Other acquired deformity of ankle and foot
754.61 Congenital pes planus
754.62 Talipes calcaneovalgus
754.69 Other congenital valgus deformity of feet
755.67 Congenital anomalies of foot, not elsewhere classified
825.0 Closed fracture of calcaneus
825.1 Open fracture of calcaneus
825.20 Closed fracture of unspecified bone(s) of foot (except toes)
928.20 Crushing injury of foot — (Use additional code to identify any associated injuries: 800-829, 850.0-854.1, 860.0-869.1)
928.21 Crushing injury of ankle — (Use additional code to identify any associated injuries: 800-829, 850.0-854.1, 860.0-869.1)

ICD-9-CM Procedural

81.13 Subtalar fusion

28730–28735

28730 Arthrodesis, midtarsal or tarsometatarsal, multiple or transverse;
28735 with osteotomy (eg, flatfoot correction)

ICD-9-CM Diagnostic

357.1 Polyneuropathy in collagen vascular disease — (Code first underlying disease: 446.0, 710.0, 714.0)
359.6 Symptomatic inflammatory myopathy in diseases classified elsewhere — (Code first underlying disease: 135, 140.0-208.9, 277.3, 446.0, 710.0, 710.1, 710.2, 714.0)
446.0 Polyarteritis nodosa
710.0 Systemic lupus erythematosus — (Use additional code to identify manifestation: 424.91, 581.81, 582.81, 583.81)
710.1 Systemic sclerosis — (Use additional code to identify manifestation: 359.6, 517.2)
710.2 Sicca syndrome
714.0 Rheumatoid arthritis — (Use additional code to identify manifestation: 357.1, 359.6)
715.17 Primary localized osteoarthrosis, ankle and foot
715.37 Localized osteoarthrosis not specified whether primary or secondary, ankle and foot
715.97 Osteoarthrosis, unspecified whether generalized or localized, ankle and foot
716.17 Traumatic arthropathy, ankle and foot
718.87 Other joint derangement, not elsewhere classified, ankle and foot
733.49 Aseptic necrosis of other bone site
733.81 Malunion of fracture
733.82 Nonunion of fracture
734 Flat foot
736.71 Acquired equinovarus deformity
736.72 Equinus deformity of foot, acquired
736.73 Cavus deformity of foot, acquired
754.70 Unspecified talipes
825.20 Closed fracture of unspecified bone(s) of foot (except toes)
825.22 Closed fracture of navicular (scaphoid) bone of foot
825.29 Other closed fracture of tarsal and metatarsal bones

ICD-9-CM Procedural

77.38 Other division of tarsals and metatarsals
81.15 Tarsometatarsal fusion

28737

28737 Arthrodesis, with tendon lengthening and advancement, midtarsal, tarsal navicular-cuneiform (eg, Miller type procedure)

ICD-9-CM Diagnostic

715.17 Primary localized osteoarthrosis, ankle and foot
715.97 Osteoarthrosis, unspecified whether generalized or localized, ankle and foot
716.17 Traumatic arthropathy, ankle and foot
754.50 Congenital talipes varus
754.51 Congenital talipes equinovarus
754.52 Congenital metatarsus primus varus
754.53 Congenital metatarsus varus
754.59 Other congenital varus deformity of feet
754.60 Congenital talipes valgus
754.61 Congenital pes planus
754.62 Talipes calcaneovalgus
754.69 Other congenital valgus deformity of feet
754.70 Unspecified talipes
754.71 Talipes cavus

ICD-9-CM Procedural

81.14 Midtarsal fusion
83.71 Advancement of tendon
83.75 Tendon transfer or transplantation

28740

28740 Arthrodesis, midtarsal or tarsometatarsal, single joint

ICD-9-CM Diagnostic

355.5 Tarsal tunnel syndrome
357.1 Polyneuropathy in collagen vascular disease — (Code first underlying disease: 446.0, 710.0, 714.0)
359.6 Symptomatic inflammatory myopathy in diseases classified elsewhere — (Code first underlying disease: 135, 140.0-208.9, 277.3, 446.0, 710.0, 710.1, 710.2, 714.0)
446.0 Polyarteritis nodosa

710.0	Systemic lupus erythematosus — (Use additional code to identify manifestation: 424.91, 581.81, 582.81, 583.81)
710.1	Systemic sclerosis — (Use additional code to identify manifestation: 359.6, 517.2)
710.2	Sicca syndrome
714.0	Rheumatoid arthritis — (Use additional code to identify manifestation: 357.1, 359.6)
715.17	Primary localized osteoarthrosis, ankle and foot
715.37	Localized osteoarthrosis not specified whether primary or secondary, ankle and foot
715.97	Osteoarthrosis, unspecified whether generalized or localized, ankle and foot
716.17	Traumatic arthropathy, ankle and foot
718.47	Contracture of ankle and foot joint
718.77	Developmental dislocation of joint, ankle and foot
719.67	Other symptoms referable to ankle and foot joint
719.87	Other specified disorders of ankle and foot joint
733.81	Malunion of fracture
733.82	Nonunion of fracture
736.74	Claw foot, acquired
754.50	Congenital talipes varus
754.51	Congenital talipes equinovarus
754.59	Other congenital varus deformity of feet
754.60	Congenital talipes valgus
754.70	Unspecified talipes
754.89	Other specified nonteratogenic anomalies
825.25	Closed fracture of metatarsal bone(s)
838.02	Closed dislocation of midtarsal (joint)
905.4	Late effect of fracture of lower extremities

ICD-9-CM Procedural

81.14	Midtarsal fusion

28750

28750 Arthrodesis, great toe; metatarsophalangeal joint

ICD-9-CM Diagnostic

356.1	Peroneal muscular atrophy
357.1	Polyneuropathy in collagen vascular disease — (Code first underlying disease: 446.0, 710.0, 714.0)
359.6	Symptomatic inflammatory myopathy in diseases classified elsewhere — (Code first underlying disease: 135, 140.0-208.9, 277.3, 446.0, 710.0, 710.1, 710.2, 714.0)
446.0	Polyarteritis nodosa
710.0	Systemic lupus erythematosus — (Use additional code to identify manifestation: 424.91, 581.81, 582.81, 583.81)
710.1	Systemic sclerosis — (Use additional code to identify manifestation: 359.6, 517.2)
710.2	Sicca syndrome
714.0	Rheumatoid arthritis — (Use additional code to identify manifestation: 357.1, 359.6)
714.30	Polyarticular juvenile rheumatoid arthritis, chronic or unspecified
714.32	Pauciarticular juvenile rheumatoid arthritis
715.17	Primary localized osteoarthrosis, ankle and foot
715.27	Secondary localized osteoarthrosis, ankle and foot
715.37	Localized osteoarthrosis not specified whether primary or secondary, ankle and foot
715.97	Osteoarthrosis, unspecified whether generalized or localized, ankle and foot
716.17	Traumatic arthropathy, ankle and foot
718.47	Contracture of ankle and foot joint
727.1	Bunion
733.81	Malunion of fracture
733.82	Nonunion of fracture
735.0	Hallux valgus (acquired)
735.1	Hallux varus (acquired)
735.2	Hallux rigidus
735.3	Hallux malleus
735.4	Other hammer toe (acquired)
735.5	Claw toe (acquired)
735.8	Other acquired deformity of toe
735.9	Unspecified acquired deformity of toe
736.70	Unspecified deformity of ankle and foot, acquired
736.71	Acquired equinovarus deformity
736.72	Equinus deformity of foot, acquired
736.73	Cavus deformity of foot, acquired
755.39	Congenital longitudinal deficiency, phalanges, complete or partial
755.67	Congenital anomalies of foot, not elsewhere classified
838.05	Closed dislocation of metatarsophalangeal (joint)
928.3	Crushing injury of toe(s) — (Use additional code to identify any associated injuries: 800-829, 850.0-854.1, 860.0-869.1)

ICD-9-CM Procedural

81.16	Metatarsophalangeal fusion

HCPCS Level II Supplies & Services

A4305	Disposable drug delivery system, flow rate of 50 ml or greater per hour
A4306	Disposable drug delivery system, flow rate of 5 ml or less per hour
A4550	Surgical trays

28755

28755 Arthrodesis, great toe; interphalangeal joint

ICD-9-CM Diagnostic

357.1	Polyneuropathy in collagen vascular disease — (Code first underlying disease: 446.0, 710.0, 714.0)
359.6	Symptomatic inflammatory myopathy in diseases classified elsewhere — (Code first underlying disease: 135, 140.0-208.9, 277.3, 446.0, 710.0, 710.1, 710.2, 714.0)
446.0	Polyarteritis nodosa
710.0	Systemic lupus erythematosus — (Use additional code to identify manifestation: 424.91, 581.81, 582.81, 583.81)
710.1	Systemic sclerosis — (Use additional code to identify manifestation: 359.6, 517.2)
710.2	Sicca syndrome
714.0	Rheumatoid arthritis — (Use additional code to identify manifestation: 357.1, 359.6)
715.97	Osteoarthrosis, unspecified whether generalized or localized, ankle and foot
716.17	Traumatic arthropathy, ankle and foot
718.87	Other joint derangement, not elsewhere classified, ankle and foot
719.57	Stiffness of joint, not elsewhere classified, ankle and foot
735.1	Hallux varus (acquired)
735.2	Hallux rigidus
735.8	Other acquired deformity of toe
755.66	Other congenital anomaly of toes
928.3	Crushing injury of toe(s) — (Use additional code to identify any associated injuries: 800-829, 850.0-854.1, 860.0-869.1)

ICD-9-CM Procedural

77.58	Other excision, fusion, and repair of toes

HCPCS Level II Supplies & Services

A4305	Disposable drug delivery system, flow rate of 50 ml or greater per hour
A4306	Disposable drug delivery system, flow rate of 5 ml or less per hour
A4550	Surgical trays

28760

28760 Arthrodesis, with extensor hallucis longus transfer to first metatarsal neck, great toe, interphalangeal joint (eg, Jones type procedure)

ICD-9-CM Diagnostic

138	Late effects of acute poliomyelitis
715.27	Secondary localized osteoarthrosis, ankle and foot
715.37	Localized osteoarthrosis not specified whether primary or secondary, ankle and foot
715.97	Osteoarthrosis, unspecified whether generalized or localized, ankle and foot
716.17	Traumatic arthropathy, ankle and foot
719.57	Stiffness of joint, not elsewhere classified, ankle and foot
735.1	Hallux varus (acquired)
735.3	Hallux malleus
735.4	Other hammer toe (acquired)
735.5	Claw toe (acquired)
755.66	Other congenital anomaly of toes
826.0	Closed fracture of one or more phalanges of foot
826.1	Open fracture of one or more phalanges of foot
928.3	Crushing injury of toe(s) — (Use additional code to identify any associated injuries: 800-829, 850.0-854.1, 860.0-869.1)

ICD-9-CM Procedural

77.57	Repair of claw toe

HCPCS Level II Supplies & Services

A4305	Disposable drug delivery system, flow rate of 50 ml or greater per hour
A4306	Disposable drug delivery system, flow rate of 5 ml or less per hour
A4550	Surgical trays

Unspecified code
♀ Female diagnosis

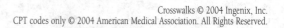

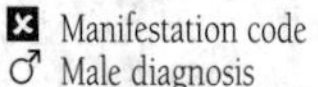
Manifestation code
♂ Male diagnosis

28800

28800 Amputation, foot; midtarsal (eg, Chopart type procedure)

ICD-9-CM Diagnostic

250.70 Diabetes with peripheral circulatory disorders, type II or unspecified type, not stated as uncontrolled — (Use additional code to identify manifestation: 443.81, 785.4)
250.71 Diabetes with peripheral circulatory disorders, type I [juvenile type], not stated as uncontrolled — (Use additional code to identify manifestation: 443.81, 785.4)
440.23 Atherosclerosis of native arteries of the extremities with ulceration — (Use additional code for any associated ulceration: 707.10-707.9)
443.81 Peripheral angiopathy in diseases classified elsewhere — (Code first underlying disease, 250.7) ☒
444.22 Embolism and thrombosis of arteries of lower extremity
445.02 Atheroembolism of lower extremity
447.1 Stricture of artery
707.10 Ulcer of lower limb, unspecified ▽
707.14 Ulcer of heel and midfoot
707.15 Ulcer of other part of foot
730.17 Chronic osteomyelitis, ankle and foot — (Use additional code to identify organism, 041.1)
730.37 Periostitis, without mention of osteomyelitis, ankle and foot — (Use additional code to identify organism, 041.1)
733.49 Aseptic necrosis of other bone site
785.4 Gangrene — (Code first any associated underlying condition:250.7, 443.0)
892.1 Open wound of foot except toe(s) alone, complicated — (Use additional code to identify infection)
895.0 Traumatic amputation of toe(s) (complete) (partial), without mention of complication — (Use additional code to identify infection)
896.0 Traumatic amputation of foot (complete) (partial), unilateral, without mention of complication — (Use additional code to identify infection)
928.20 Crushing injury of foot — (Use additional code to identify any associated injuries: 800-829, 850.0-854.1, 860.0-869.1)

ICD-9-CM Procedural

84.12 Amputation through foot

28805

28805 Amputation, foot; transmetatarsal

ICD-9-CM Diagnostic

250.70 Diabetes with peripheral circulatory disorders, type II or unspecified type, not stated as uncontrolled — (Use additional code to identify manifestation: 443.81, 785.4)
250.71 Diabetes with peripheral circulatory disorders, type I [juvenile type], not stated as uncontrolled — (Use additional code to identify manifestation: 443.81, 785.4)
440.23 Atherosclerosis of native arteries of the extremities with ulceration — (Use additional code for any associated ulceration: 707.10-707.9)
443.81 Peripheral angiopathy in diseases classified elsewhere — (Code first underlying disease, 250.7) ☒
444.22 Embolism and thrombosis of arteries of lower extremity
445.02 Atheroembolism of lower extremity
447.1 Stricture of artery
707.10 Ulcer of lower limb, unspecified ▽
707.14 Ulcer of heel and midfoot
707.15 Ulcer of other part of foot
730.17 Chronic osteomyelitis, ankle and foot — (Use additional code to identify organism, 041.1)
730.37 Periostitis, without mention of osteomyelitis, ankle and foot — (Use additional code to identify organism, 041.1)
733.49 Aseptic necrosis of other bone site
785.4 Gangrene — (Code first any associated underlying condition:250.7, 443.0)
892.1 Open wound of foot except toe(s) alone, complicated — (Use additional code to identify infection)
895.0 Traumatic amputation of toe(s) (complete) (partial), without mention of complication — (Use additional code to identify infection)
896.0 Traumatic amputation of foot (complete) (partial), unilateral, without mention of complication — (Use additional code to identify infection)
928.20 Crushing injury of foot — (Use additional code to identify any associated injuries: 800-829, 850.0-854.1, 860.0-869.1)

ICD-9-CM Procedural

84.12 Amputation through foot

28810

28810 Amputation, metatarsal, with toe, single

ICD-9-CM Diagnostic

250.70 Diabetes with peripheral circulatory disorders, type II or unspecified type, not stated as uncontrolled — (Use additional code to identify manifestation: 443.81, 785.4)
250.71 Diabetes with peripheral circulatory disorders, type I [juvenile type], not stated as uncontrolled — (Use additional code to identify manifestation: 443.81, 785.4)
250.72 Diabetes with peripheral circulatory disorders, type II or unspecified type, uncontrolled — (Use additional code to identify manifestation: 443.81, 785.4)
250.73 Diabetes with peripheral circulatory disorders, type I [juvenile type], uncontrolled — (Use additional code to identify manifestation: 443.81, 785.4)
250.80 Diabetes with other specified manifestations, type II or unspecified type, not stated as uncontrolled — (Use additional code to identify manifestation: 707.10-707.9, 731.8. Use additional E code to identify cause, if drug-induced)
250.81 Diabetes with other specified manifestations, type I [juvenile type], not stated as uncontrolled — (Use additional code to identify manifestation: 707.10-707.9, 731.8. Use additional E code to identify cause, if drug-induced)
250.82 Diabetes with other specified manifestations, type II or unspecified type, uncontrolled — (Use additional code to identify manifestation: 707.10-707.9, 731.8. Use additional E code to identify cause, if drug-induced)
250.83 Diabetes with other specified manifestations, type I [juvenile type], uncontrolled — (Use additional code to identify manifestation: 707.10-707.9, 731.8. Use additional E code to identify cause, if drug-induced)
250.90 Diabetes with unspecified complication, type II or unspecified type, not stated as uncontrolled ▽
250.91 Diabetes with unspecified complication, type I [juvenile type], not stated as uncontrolled ▽
250.92 Diabetes with unspecified complication, type II or unspecified type, uncontrolled ▽
250.93 Diabetes with unspecified complication, type I [juvenile type], uncontrolled ▽
440.24 Atherosclerosis of native arteries of the extremities with gangrene
443.81 Peripheral angiopathy in diseases classified elsewhere — (Code first underlying disease, 250.7) ☒
444.22 Embolism and thrombosis of arteries of lower extremity
445.02 Atheroembolism of lower extremity
682.7 Cellulitis and abscess of foot, except toes — (Use additional code to identify organism)
707.10 Ulcer of lower limb, unspecified ▽
707.14 Ulcer of heel and midfoot
707.15 Ulcer of other part of foot
730.07 Acute osteomyelitis, ankle and foot — (Use additional code to identify organism, 041.1)
730.17 Chronic osteomyelitis, ankle and foot — (Use additional code to identify organism, 041.1)
730.37 Periostitis, without mention of osteomyelitis, ankle and foot — (Use additional code to identify organism, 041.1)
730.87 Other infections involving bone diseases classified elsewhere, ankle and foot — (Code first underlying disease: 002.0, 015.0-015.9. Use additional code to identify organism) ☒
731.8 Other bone involvement in diseases classified elsewhere — (Code first underlying disease, 250.8. Use additional code to specify bone condition: 730.00-730.09) ☒
785.4 Gangrene — (Code first any associated underlying condition:250.7, 443.0)
892.1 Open wound of foot except toe(s) alone, complicated — (Use additional code to identify infection)
895.0 Traumatic amputation of toe(s) (complete) (partial), without mention of complication — (Use additional code to identify infection)
896.0 Traumatic amputation of foot (complete) (partial), unilateral, without mention of complication — (Use additional code to identify infection)
928.3 Crushing injury of toe(s) — (Use additional code to identify any associated injuries: 800-829, 850.0-854.1, 860.0-869.1)

ICD-9-CM Procedural

84.12 Amputation through foot

28820

28820 Amputation, toe; metatarsophalangeal joint

ICD-9-CM Diagnostic

213.8 Benign neoplasm of short bones of lower limb
250.70 Diabetes with peripheral circulatory disorders, type II or unspecified type, not stated as uncontrolled — (Use additional code to identify manifestation: 443.81, 785.4)

▽ Unspecified code ☒ Manifestation code
♀ Female diagnosis ♂ Male diagnosis

250.71 Diabetes with peripheral circulatory disorders, type I [juvenile type], not stated as uncontrolled — (Use additional code to identify manifestation: 443.81, 785.4)
250.72 Diabetes with peripheral circulatory disorders, type II or unspecified type, uncontrolled — (Use additional code to identify manifestation: 443.81, 785.4)
250.73 Diabetes with peripheral circulatory disorders, type I [juvenile type], uncontrolled — (Use additional code to identify manifestation: 443.81, 785.4)
250.80 Diabetes with other specified manifestations, type II or unspecified type, not stated as uncontrolled — (Use additional code to identify manifestation: 707.10-707.9, 731.8. Use additional E code to identify cause, if drug-induced)
250.81 Diabetes with other specified manifestations, type I [juvenile type], not stated as uncontrolled — (Use additional code to identify manifestation: 707.10-707.9, 731.8. Use additional E code to identify cause, if drug-induced)
250.90 Diabetes with unspecified complication, type II or unspecified type, not stated as uncontrolled
250.91 Diabetes with unspecified complication, type I [juvenile type], not stated as uncontrolled
357.1 Polyneuropathy in collagen vascular disease — (Code first underlying disease: 446.0, 710.0, 714.0)
359.6 Symptomatic inflammatory myopathy in diseases classified elsewhere — (Code first underlying disease: 135, 140.0-208.9, 277.3, 446.0, 710.0, 710.1, 710.2, 714.0)
440.21 Atherosclerosis of native arteries of the extremities with intermittent claudication
443.81 Peripheral angiopathy in diseases classified elsewhere — (Code first underlying disease, 250.7)
443.9 Unspecified peripheral vascular disease
444.22 Embolism and thrombosis of arteries of lower extremity
445.02 Atheroembolism of lower extremity
459.9 Unspecified circulatory system disorder
707.10 Ulcer of lower limb, unspecified
707.14 Ulcer of heel and midfoot
707.15 Ulcer of other part of foot
714.0 Rheumatoid arthritis — (Use additional code to identify manifestation: 357.1, 359.6)
730.07 Acute osteomyelitis, ankle and foot — (Use additional code to identify organism, 041.1)
730.17 Chronic osteomyelitis, ankle and foot — (Use additional code to identify organism, 041.1)
731.8 Other bone involvement in diseases classified elsewhere — (Code first underlying disease, 250.8. Use additional code to specify bone condition: 730.00-730.09)
733.40 Aseptic necrosis of bone, site unspecified
735.0 Hallux valgus (acquired)
735.1 Hallux varus (acquired)
735.2 Hallux rigidus
735.3 Hallux malleus
735.4 Other hammer toe (acquired)
735.5 Claw toe (acquired)
735.8 Other acquired deformity of toe
785.4 Gangrene — (Code first any associated underlying condition:250.7, 443.0)
893.0 Open wound of toe(s), without mention of complication — (Use additional code to identify infection)
895.0 Traumatic amputation of toe(s) (complete) (partial), without mention of complication — (Use additional code to identify infection)
895.1 Traumatic amputation of toe(s) (complete) (partial), complicated — (Use additional code to identify infection)
896.0 Traumatic amputation of foot (complete) (partial), unilateral, without mention of complication — (Use additional code to identify infection)
928.3 Crushing injury of toe(s) — (Use additional code to identify any associated injuries: 800-829, 850.0-854.1, 860.0-869.1)

ICD-9-CM Procedural

84.11 Amputation of toe

28825

28825 Amputation, toe; interphalangeal joint

ICD-9-CM Diagnostic

239.2 Neoplasms of unspecified nature of bone, soft tissue, and skin
250.60 Diabetes with neurological manifestations, type II or unspecified type, not stated as uncontrolled — (Use additional code to identify manifestation: 337.1, 354.0-355.9, 357.2, 358.1, 713.5)
250.61 Diabetes with neurological manifestations, type I [juvenile type], not stated as uncontrolled — (Use additional code to identify manifestation: 337.1, 354.0-355.9, 357.2, 358.1, 713.5)
250.70 Diabetes with peripheral circulatory disorders, type II or unspecified type, not stated as uncontrolled — (Use additional code to identify manifestation: 443.81, 785.4)
250.71 Diabetes with peripheral circulatory disorders, type I [juvenile type], not stated as uncontrolled — (Use additional code to identify manifestation: 443.81, 785.4)
250.72 Diabetes with peripheral circulatory disorders, type II or unspecified type, uncontrolled — (Use additional code to identify manifestation: 443.81, 785.4)
250.73 Diabetes with peripheral circulatory disorders, type I [juvenile type], uncontrolled — (Use additional code to identify manifestation: 443.81, 785.4)
250.80 Diabetes with other specified manifestations, type II or unspecified type, not stated as uncontrolled — (Use additional code to identify manifestation: 707.10-707.9, 731.8. Use additional E code to identify cause, if drug-induced)
250.81 Diabetes with other specified manifestations, type I [juvenile type], not stated as uncontrolled — (Use additional code to identify manifestation: 707.10-707.9, 731.8. Use additional E code to identify cause, if drug-induced)
337.1 Peripheral autonomic neuropathy in disorders classified elsewhere — (Code first underlying disease: 250.6, 277.3)
355.0 Lesion of sciatic nerve
355.1 Meralgia paresthetica
355.2 Other lesion of femoral nerve
355.3 Lesion of lateral popliteal nerve
355.4 Lesion of medial popliteal nerve
355.5 Tarsal tunnel syndrome
355.6 Lesion of plantar nerve
355.71 Causalgia of lower limb
355.79 Other mononeuritis of lower limb
355.8 Unspecified mononeuritis of lower limb
355.9 Mononeuritis of unspecified site
357.2 Polyneuropathy in diabetes — (Code first underlying disease: 250.6)
359.6 Symptomatic inflammatory myopathy in diseases classified elsewhere — (Code first underlying disease: 135, 140.0-208.9, 277.3, 446.0, 710.0, 710.1, 710.2, 714.0)
440.21 Atherosclerosis of native arteries of the extremities with intermittent claudication
443.81 Peripheral angiopathy in diseases classified elsewhere — (Code first underlying disease, 250.7)
444.22 Embolism and thrombosis of arteries of lower extremity
445.02 Atheroembolism of lower extremity
703.8 Other specified disease of nail
707.10 Ulcer of lower limb, unspecified
707.14 Ulcer of heel and midfoot
707.15 Ulcer of other part of foot
713.5 Arthropathy associated with neurological disorders — (Code first underlying disease: 094.0, 250.6, 336.0)
714.0 Rheumatoid arthritis — (Use additional code to identify manifestation: 357.1, 359.6)
730.17 Chronic osteomyelitis, ankle and foot — (Use additional code to identify organism, 041.1)
730.37 Periostitis, without mention of osteomyelitis, ankle and foot — (Use additional code to identify organism, 041.1)
730.77 Osteopathy resulting from poliomyelitis, ankle and foot — (Code first underlying disease: 045.0-045.9. Use additional code to identify organism)
731.8 Other bone involvement in diseases classified elsewhere — (Code first underlying disease, 250.8. Use additional code to specify bone condition: 730.00-730.09)
735.8 Other acquired deformity of toe
785.4 Gangrene — (Code first any associated underlying condition:250.7, 443.0)
893.1 Open wound of toe(s), complicated — (Use additional code to identify infection)
895.0 Traumatic amputation of toe(s) (complete) (partial), without mention of complication — (Use additional code to identify infection)
928.3 Crushing injury of toe(s) — (Use additional code to identify any associated injuries: 800-829, 850.0-854.1, 860.0-869.1)

ICD-9-CM Procedural

84.11 Amputation of toe

HCPCS Level II Supplies & Services

A4305 Disposable drug delivery system, flow rate of 50 ml or greater per hour
A4306 Disposable drug delivery system, flow rate of 5 ml or less per hour
A4550 Surgical trays

Application of Casts and Strapping

29000

29000 Application of halo type body cast (see 20661-20663 for insertion)

ICD-9-CM Diagnostic

805.00 Closed fracture of cervical vertebra, unspecified level without mention of spinal cord injury ▽
805.01 Closed fracture of first cervical vertebra without mention of spinal cord injury
805.02 Closed fracture of second cervical vertebra without mention of spinal cord injury
805.03 Closed fracture of third cervical vertebra without mention of spinal cord injury
805.04 Closed fracture of fourth cervical vertebra without mention of spinal cord injury
805.05 Closed fracture of fifth cervical vertebra without mention of spinal cord injury
805.06 Closed fracture of sixth cervical vertebra without mention of spinal cord injury
805.07 Closed fracture of seventh cervical vertebra without mention of spinal cord injury
805.08 Closed fracture of multiple cervical vertebrae without mention of spinal cord injury
805.10 Open fracture of cervical vertebra, unspecified level without mention of spinal cord injury ▽
805.11 Open fracture of first cervical vertebra without mention of spinal cord injury
805.12 Open fracture of second cervical vertebra without mention of spinal cord injury
805.13 Open fracture of third cervical vertebra without mention of spinal cord injury
805.14 Open fracture of fourth cervical vertebra without mention of spinal cord injury
805.15 Open fracture of fifth cervical vertebra without mention of spinal cord injury
805.16 Open fracture of sixth cervical vertebra without mention of spinal cord injury
805.17 Open fracture of seventh cervical vertebra without mention of spinal cord injury
805.18 Open fracture of multiple cervical vertebrae without mention of spinal cord injury
806.00 Closed fracture of C1-C4 level with unspecified spinal cord injury ▽
806.01 Closed fracture of C1-C4 level with complete lesion of cord
806.02 Closed fracture of C1-C4 level with anterior cord syndrome
806.03 Closed fracture of C1-C4 level with central cord syndrome
806.04 Closed fracture of C1-C4 level with other specified spinal cord injury
806.05 Closed fracture of C5-C7 level with unspecified spinal cord injury ▽
806.06 Closed fracture of C5-C7 level with complete lesion of cord
806.07 Closed fracture of C5-C7 level with anterior cord syndrome
806.08 Closed fracture of C5-C7 level with central cord syndrome
806.09 Closed fracture of C5-C7 level with other specified spinal cord injury
806.10 Open fracture of C1-C4 level with unspecified spinal cord injury ▽
806.11 Open fracture of C1-C4 level with complete lesion of cord
806.12 Open fracture of C1-C4 level with anterior cord syndrome
806.13 Open fracture of C1-C4 level with central cord syndrome
806.14 Open fracture of C1-C4 level with other specified spinal cord injury
806.15 Open fracture of C5-C7 level with unspecified spinal cord injury ▽
806.16 Open fracture of C5-C7 level with complete lesion of cord
806.17 Open fracture of C5-C7 level with anterior cord syndrome
806.18 Open fracture of C5-C7 level with central cord syndrome
806.19 Open fracture of C5-C7 level with other specified spinal cord injury

ICD-9-CM Procedural

93.51 Application of plaster jacket
93.52 Application of neck support
97.13 Replacement of other cast

HCPCS Level II Supplies & Services

A6441 Padding bandage, non-elastic, non-woven/non-knitted, width greater than or equal to three inches and less than five inches, per yard
Q4001 Casting supplies, body cast adult, with or without head, plaster
Q4002 Cast supplies, body cast adult, with or without head, fiberglass
Q4050 Cast supplies, for unlisted types and materials of casts
Q4051 Splint supplies, miscellaneous (includes thermoplastics, strapping, fasteners, padding and other supplies)

29010–29015

29010 Application of Risser jacket, localizer, body; only
29015 including head

ICD-9-CM Diagnostic

268.1 Rickets, late effect — (Use additional code to identify the nature of late effect)
737.0 Adolescent postural kyphosis
737.10 Kyphosis (acquired) (postural)
737.11 Kyphosis due to radiation
737.12 Kyphosis, postlaminectomy
737.19 Other kyphosis (acquired)
737.20 Lordosis (acquired) (postural)
737.21 Lordosis, postlaminectomy
737.22 Other postsurgical lordosis
737.29 Other lordosis (acquired)
737.30 Scoliosis (and kyphoscoliosis), idiopathic
737.34 Thoracogenic scoliosis
737.39 Other kyphoscoliosis and scoliosis
738.5 Other acquired deformity of back or spine
756.19 Other congenital anomaly of spine

ICD-9-CM Procedural

93.51 Application of plaster jacket
93.52 Application of neck support
97.13 Replacement of other cast

HCPCS Level II Supplies & Services

A6441 Padding bandage, non-elastic, non-woven/non-knitted, width greater than or equal to three inches and less than five inches, per yard
Q4001 Casting supplies, body cast adult, with or without head, plaster
Q4002 Cast supplies, body cast adult, with or without head, fiberglass
Q4050 Cast supplies, for unlisted types and materials of casts
Q4051 Splint supplies, miscellaneous (includes thermoplastics, strapping, fasteners, padding and other supplies)

29020–29025

29020 Application of turnbuckle jacket, body; only
29025 including head

ICD-9-CM Diagnostic

268.1 Rickets, late effect — (Use additional code to identify the nature of late effect)
737.0 Adolescent postural kyphosis
737.11 Kyphosis due to radiation
737.12 Kyphosis, postlaminectomy
737.19 Other kyphosis (acquired)
737.21 Lordosis, postlaminectomy
737.22 Other postsurgical lordosis
737.29 Other lordosis (acquired)
737.30 Scoliosis (and kyphoscoliosis), idiopathic
737.34 Thoracogenic scoliosis
737.39 Other kyphoscoliosis and scoliosis
738.5 Other acquired deformity of back or spine
756.19 Other congenital anomaly of spine

ICD-9-CM Procedural

93.51 Application of plaster jacket
93.52 Application of neck support
97.13 Replacement of other cast

HCPCS Level II Supplies & Services

A4580 Cast supplies (e.g., plaster)
A4590 Special casting material (e.g., fiberglass)
A6441 Padding bandage, non-elastic, non-woven/non-knitted, width greater than or equal to three inches and less than five inches, per yard
Q4001 Casting supplies, body cast adult, with or without head, plaster
Q4002 Cast supplies, body cast adult, with or without head, fiberglass

29035–29046

29035 Application of body cast, shoulder to hips;
29040 including head, Minerva type
29044 including one thigh
29046 including both thighs

ICD-9-CM Diagnostic

805.00 Closed fracture of cervical vertebra, unspecified level without mention of spinal cord injury ▽
805.01 Closed fracture of first cervical vertebra without mention of spinal cord injury
805.02 Closed fracture of second cervical vertebra without mention of spinal cord injury
805.03 Closed fracture of third cervical vertebra without mention of spinal cord injury
805.04 Closed fracture of fourth cervical vertebra without mention of spinal cord injury
805.05 Closed fracture of fifth cervical vertebra without mention of spinal cord injury

805.06 Closed fracture of sixth cervical vertebra without mention of spinal cord injury
805.07 Closed fracture of seventh cervical vertebra without mention of spinal cord injury
805.08 Closed fracture of multiple cervical vertebrae without mention of spinal cord injury
805.10 Open fracture of cervical vertebra, unspecified level without mention of spinal cord injury ▽
805.11 Open fracture of first cervical vertebra without mention of spinal cord injury
805.12 Open fracture of second cervical vertebra without mention of spinal cord injury
805.13 Open fracture of third cervical vertebra without mention of spinal cord injury
805.14 Open fracture of fourth cervical vertebra without mention of spinal cord injury
805.16 Open fracture of sixth cervical vertebra without mention of spinal cord injury
805.17 Open fracture of seventh cervical vertebra without mention of spinal cord injury
805.18 Open fracture of multiple cervical vertebrae without mention of spinal cord injury
805.2 Closed fracture of dorsal (thoracic) vertebra without mention of spinal cord injury
805.3 Open fracture of dorsal (thoracic) vertebra without mention of spinal cord injury
805.4 Closed fracture of lumbar vertebra without mention of spinal cord injury
805.5 Open fracture of lumbar vertebra without mention of spinal cord injury
805.6 Closed fracture of sacrum and coccyx without mention of spinal cord injury
805.7 Open fracture of sacrum and coccyx without mention of spinal cord injury
805.8 Closed fracture of unspecified part of vertebral column without mention of spinal cord injury ▽
805.9 Open fracture of unspecified part of vertebral column without mention of spinal cord injury ▽
806.00 Closed fracture of C1-C4 level with unspecified spinal cord injury ▽
806.01 Closed fracture of C1-C4 level with complete lesion of cord
806.02 Closed fracture of C1-C4 level with anterior cord syndrome
806.03 Closed fracture of C1-C4 level with central cord syndrome
806.04 Closed fracture of C1-C4 level with other specified spinal cord injury
806.05 Closed fracture of C5-C7 level with unspecified spinal cord injury ▽
806.06 Closed fracture of C5-C7 level with complete lesion of cord
806.07 Closed fracture of C5-C7 level with anterior cord syndrome
806.08 Closed fracture of C5-C7 level with central cord syndrome
806.09 Closed fracture of C5-C7 level with other specified spinal cord injury
806.10 Open fracture of C1-C4 level with unspecified spinal cord injury ▽
806.11 Open fracture of C1-C4 level with complete lesion of cord
806.12 Open fracture of C1-C4 level with anterior cord syndrome
806.13 Open fracture of C1-C4 level with central cord syndrome
806.14 Open fracture of C1-C4 level with other specified spinal cord injury
806.15 Open fracture of C5-C7 level with unspecified spinal cord injury ▽
806.16 Open fracture of C5-C7 level with complete lesion of cord
806.17 Open fracture of C5-C7 level with anterior cord syndrome
806.18 Open fracture of C5-C7 level with central cord syndrome
806.19 Open fracture of C5-C7 level with other specified spinal cord injury
806.20 Closed fracture of T1-T6 level with unspecified spinal cord injury ▽
806.21 Closed fracture of T1-T6 level with complete lesion of cord
806.22 Closed fracture of T1-T6 level with anterior cord syndrome
806.23 Closed fracture of T1-T6 level with central cord syndrome
806.24 Closed fracture of T1-T6 level with other specified spinal cord injury
806.25 Closed fracture of T7-T12 level with unspecified spinal cord injury ▽
806.26 Closed fracture of T7-T12 level with complete lesion of cord
806.27 Closed fracture of T7-T12 level with anterior cord syndrome
806.28 Closed fracture of T7-T12 level with central cord syndrome
806.29 Closed fracture of T7-T12 level with other specified spinal cord injury
806.30 Open fracture of T1-T6 level with unspecified spinal cord injury ▽
806.31 Open fracture of T1-T6 level with complete lesion of cord
806.32 Open fracture of T1-T6 level with anterior cord syndrome
806.33 Open fracture of T1-T6 level with central cord syndrome
806.34 Open fracture of T1-T6 level with other specified spinal cord injury
806.35 Open fracture of T7-T12 level with unspecified spinal cord injury ▽
806.36 Open fracture of T7-T12 level with complete lesion of cord
806.37 Open fracture of T7-T12 level with anterior cord syndrome
806.38 Open fracture of T7-T12 level with central cord syndrome
806.39 Open fracture of T7-T12 level with other specified spinal cord injury
806.4 Closed fracture of lumbar spine with spinal cord injury
806.5 Open fracture of lumbar spine with spinal cord injury
806.60 Closed fracture of sacrum and coccyx with unspecified spinal cord injury ▽
806.61 Closed fracture of sacrum and coccyx with complete cauda equina lesion
806.62 Closed fracture of sacrum and coccyx with other cauda equina injury
806.69 Closed fracture of sacrum and coccyx with other spinal cord injury
806.70 Open fracture of sacrum and coccyx with unspecified spinal cord injury ▽
806.71 Open fracture of sacrum and coccyx with complete cauda equina lesion
806.72 Open fracture of sacrum and coccyx with other cauda equina injury
806.79 Open fracture of sacrum and coccyx with other spinal cord injury
808.0 Closed fracture of acetabulum
808.1 Open fracture of acetabulum
808.2 Closed fracture of pubis
808.3 Open fracture of pubis
808.41 Closed fracture of ilium
808.42 Closed fracture of ischium
808.43 Multiple closed pelvic fractures with disruption of pelvic circle
808.49 Closed fracture of other specified part of pelvis
808.51 Open fracture of ilium
808.52 Open fracture of ischium
808.53 Multiple open pelvic fractures with disruption of pelvic circle
808.59 Open fracture of other specified part of pelvis

ICD-9-CM Procedural

93.52 Application of neck support
93.53 Application of other cast
97.13 Replacement of other cast

HCPCS Level II Supplies & Services

A6441 Padding bandage, non-elastic, non-woven/non-knitted, width greater than or equal to three inches and less than five inches, per yard
Q4001 Casting supplies, body cast adult, with or without head, plaster
Q4002 Cast supplies, body cast adult, with or without head, fiberglass
Q4050 Cast supplies, for unlisted types and materials of casts
Q4051 Splint supplies, miscellaneous (includes thermoplastics, strapping, fasteners, padding and other supplies)

29049–29058

29049 Application, cast; figure-of-eight
29055 shoulder spica
29058 plaster Velpeau

ICD-9-CM Diagnostic

718.71 Developmental dislocation of joint, shoulder region
810.01 Closed fracture of sternal end of clavicle
810.02 Closed fracture of shaft of clavicle
810.03 Closed fracture of acromial end of clavicle
811.00 Closed fracture of unspecified part of scapula ▽
811.01 Closed fracture of acromial process of scapula
811.02 Closed fracture of coracoid process of scapula
811.03 Closed fracture of glenoid cavity and neck of scapula
811.09 Closed fracture of other part of scapula
811.10 Open fracture of unspecified part of scapula ▽
811.11 Open fracture of acromial process of scapula
811.12 Open fracture of coracoid process
811.13 Open fracture of glenoid cavity and neck of scapula
811.19 Open fracture of other part of scapula
812.00 Closed fracture of unspecified part of upper end of humerus ▽
812.01 Closed fracture of surgical neck of humerus
812.02 Closed fracture of anatomical neck of humerus
812.03 Closed fracture of greater tuberosity of humerus
812.09 Other closed fractures of upper end of humerus
831.01 Closed anterior dislocation of humerus
831.02 Closed posterior dislocation of humerus
831.03 Closed inferior dislocation of humerus
831.04 Closed dislocation of acromioclavicular (joint)
831.09 Closed dislocation of other site of shoulder
840.0 Acromioclavicular (joint) (ligament) sprain and strain
840.1 Coracoclavicular (ligament) sprain and strain
840.2 Coracohumeral (ligament) sprain and strain
840.3 Infraspinatus (muscle) (tendon) sprain and strain
840.4 Rotator cuff (capsule) sprain and strain
840.5 Subscapularis (muscle) sprain and strain
840.6 Supraspinatus (muscle) (tendon) sprain and strain
840.8 Sprain and strain of other specified sites of shoulder and upper arm

ICD-9-CM Procedural

93.53 Application of other cast
97.11 Replacement of cast on upper limb

HCPCS Level II Supplies & Services

A4580 Cast supplies (e.g., plaster)
A4590 Special casting material (e.g., fiberglass)
Q4003 Cast supplies, shoulder cast, adult (11 years +), plaster
Q4004 Cast supplies, shoulder cast, adult (11 years +), fiberglass

Q4050 Cast supplies, for unlisted types and materials of casts

29065

29065 Application, cast; shoulder to hand (long arm)

ICD-9-CM Diagnostic

733.81 Malunion of fracture
733.82 Nonunion of fracture
812.00 Closed fracture of unspecified part of upper end of humerus ▽
812.01 Closed fracture of surgical neck of humerus
812.03 Closed fracture of greater tuberosity of humerus
812.09 Other closed fractures of upper end of humerus
812.20 Closed fracture of unspecified part of humerus ▽
812.21 Closed fracture of shaft of humerus
812.40 Closed fracture of unspecified part of lower end of humerus ▽
812.41 Closed fracture of supracondylar humerus
812.42 Closed fracture of lateral condyle of humerus
812.43 Closed fracture of medial condyle of humerus
812.44 Closed fracture of unspecified condyle(s) of humerus ▽
812.49 Other closed fracture of lower end of humerus
813.00 Unspecified fracture of radius and ulna, upper end of forearm, closed ▽
813.01 Closed fracture of olecranon process of ulna
813.02 Closed fracture of coronoid process of ulna
813.03 Closed Monteggia's fracture
813.04 Other and unspecified closed fractures of proximal end of ulna (alone) ▽
813.05 Closed fracture of head of radius
813.06 Closed fracture of neck of radius
813.07 Other and unspecified closed fractures of proximal end of radius (alone) ▽
813.08 Closed fracture of radius with ulna, upper end (any part)

ICD-9-CM Procedural

93.53 Application of other cast
97.11 Replacement of cast on upper limb

HCPCS Level II Supplies & Services

A4580 Cast supplies (e.g., plaster)
A4590 Special casting material (e.g., fiberglass)
A6441 Padding bandage, non-elastic, non-woven/non-knitted, width greater than or equal to three inches and less than five inches, per yard
Q4005 Cast supplies, long arm cast, adult (11 years +), plaster
Q4006 Cast supplies, long arm cast, adult (11 years +), fiberglass

29075

29075 Application, cast; elbow to finger (short arm)

ICD-9-CM Diagnostic

718.23 Pathological dislocation of forearm joint
718.24 Pathological dislocation of hand joint
718.33 Recurrent dislocation of forearm joint
718.34 Recurrent dislocation of hand joint
718.73 Developmental dislocation of joint, forearm
718.74 Developmental dislocation of joint, hand
727.02 Giant cell tumor of tendon sheath
727.03 Trigger finger (acquired)
727.04 Radial styloid tenosynovitis
727.05 Other tenosynovitis of hand and wrist
727.09 Other synovitis and tenosynovitis
727.2 Specific bursitides often of occupational origin
727.59 Other rupture of synovium
727.63 Nontraumatic rupture of extensor tendons of hand and wrist
727.64 Nontraumatic rupture of flexor tendons of hand and wrist
727.69 Nontraumatic rupture of other tendon
727.81 Contracture of tendon (sheath)
727.82 Calcium deposits in tendon and bursa
727.89 Other disorders of synovium, tendon, and bursa
728.4 Laxity of ligament
728.5 Hypermobility syndrome
728.6 Contracture of palmar fascia
733.12 Pathologic fracture of distal radius and ulna
733.19 Pathologic fracture of other specified site
733.21 Solitary bone cyst
733.22 Aneurysmal bone cyst
733.29 Other cyst of bone
733.40 Aseptic necrosis of bone, site unspecified ▽
733.81 Malunion of fracture
733.82 Nonunion of fracture
736.00 Unspecified deformity of forearm, excluding fingers ▽
736.01 Cubitus valgus (acquired)
736.02 Cubitus varus (acquired)
736.03 Valgus deformity of wrist (acquired)
736.04 Varus deformity of wrist (acquired)
736.05 Wrist drop (acquired)
736.06 Claw hand (acquired)
736.07 Club hand, acquired
736.09 Other acquired deformities of forearm, excluding fingers
736.21 Boutonniere deformity
736.22 Swan-neck deformity
736.29 Other acquired deformity of finger
755.53 Radioulnar synostosis
755.56 Accessory carpal bones
755.57 Macrodactylia (fingers)
755.58 Congenital cleft hand
755.59 Other congenital anomaly of upper limb, including shoulder girdle
813.01 Closed fracture of olecranon process of ulna
813.02 Closed fracture of coronoid process of ulna
813.03 Closed Monteggia's fracture
813.05 Closed fracture of head of radius
813.06 Closed fracture of neck of radius
813.08 Closed fracture of radius with ulna, upper end (any part)
813.10 Unspecified open fracture of upper end of forearm ▽
813.11 Open fracture of olecranon process of ulna
813.12 Open fracture of coronoid process of ulna
813.15 Open fracture of head of radius
813.16 Open fracture of neck of radius
813.18 Open fracture of radius with ulna, upper end (any part)
813.21 Closed fracture of shaft of radius (alone)
813.22 Closed fracture of shaft of ulna (alone)
813.23 Closed fracture of shaft of radius with ulna
813.31 Open fracture of shaft of radius (alone)
813.32 Open fracture of shaft of ulna (alone)
813.33 Open fracture of shaft of radius with ulna
813.41 Closed Colles' fracture
813.42 Other closed fractures of distal end of radius (alone)
813.43 Closed fracture of distal end of ulna (alone)
813.44 Closed fracture of lower end of radius with ulna
813.45 Torus fracture of lower end of radius
813.51 Open Colles' fracture
813.52 Other open fractures of distal end of radius (alone)
813.53 Open fracture of distal end of ulna (alone)
813.54 Open fracture of lower end of radius with ulna
813.80 Closed fracture of unspecified part of forearm ▽
813.81 Closed fracture of unspecified part of radius (alone) ▽
813.82 Closed fracture of unspecified part of ulna (alone) ▽
813.83 Closed fracture of unspecified part of radius with ulna ▽
813.91 Open fracture of unspecified part of radius (alone) ▽
813.92 Open fracture of unspecified part of ulna (alone) ▽
814.01 Closed fracture of navicular (scaphoid) bone of wrist
814.02 Closed fracture of lunate (semilunar) bone of wrist
814.03 Closed fracture of triquetral (cuneiform) bone of wrist
814.04 Closed fracture of pisiform bone of wrist
814.05 Closed fracture of trapezium bone (larger multangular) of wrist
814.06 Closed fracture of trapezoid bone (smaller multangular) of wrist
814.07 Closed fracture of capitate bone (os magnum) of wrist
814.08 Closed fracture of hamate (unciform) bone of wrist
814.09 Closed fracture of other bone of wrist
814.11 Open fracture of navicular (scaphoid) bone of wrist
814.12 Open fracture of lunate (semilunar) bone of wrist
814.13 Open fracture of triquetral (cuneiform) bone of wrist
814.14 Open fracture of pisiform bone of wrist
814.15 Open fracture of trapezium bone (larger multangular) of wrist
814.16 Open fracture of trapezoid bone (smaller multangular) of wrist
814.17 Open fracture of capitate bone (os magnum) of wrist
814.18 Open fracture of hamate (unciform) bone of wrist
814.19 Open fracture of other bone of wrist
815.01 Closed fracture of base of thumb (first) metacarpal bone(s)
815.02 Closed fracture of base of other metacarpal bone(s)
815.03 Closed fracture of shaft of metacarpal bone(s)
815.04 Closed fracture of neck of metacarpal bone(s)
815.09 Closed fracture of multiple sites of metacarpus
815.10 Open fracture of metacarpal bone(s), site unspecified ▽
815.11 Open fracture of base of thumb (first) metacarpal bone(s)
815.12 Open fracture of base of other metacarpal bone(s)

815.13 Open fracture of shaft of metacarpal bone(s)
815.14 Open fracture of neck of metacarpal bone(s)
815.19 Open fracture of multiple sites of metacarpus
816.00 Closed fracture of unspecified phalanx or phalanges of hand ▽
816.01 Closed fracture of middle or proximal phalanx or phalanges of hand
816.02 Closed fracture of distal phalanx or phalanges of hand
816.03 Closed fracture of multiple sites of phalanx or phalanges of hand
816.10 Open fracture of phalanx or phalanges of hand, unspecified ▽
816.11 Open fracture of middle or proximal phalanx or phalanges of hand
816.12 Open fracture of distal phalanx or phalanges of hand
816.13 Open fractures of multiple sites of phalanx or phalanges of hand
817.0 Multiple closed fractures of hand bones
817.1 Multiple open fractures of hand bones
818.0 Ill-defined closed fractures of upper limb
818.1 Ill-defined open fractures of upper limb
833.01 Closed dislocation of distal radioulnar (joint)
833.02 Closed dislocation of radiocarpal (joint)
833.03 Closed dislocation of midcarpal (joint)
833.04 Closed dislocation of carpometacarpal (joint)
833.05 Closed dislocation of proximal end of metacarpal (bone)
833.09 Closed dislocation of other part of wrist
833.10 Open dislocation of wrist, unspecified part ▽
833.11 Open dislocation of distal radioulnar (joint)
833.12 Open dislocation of radiocarpal (joint)
833.13 Open dislocation of midcarpal (joint)
833.14 Open dislocation of carpometacarpal (joint)
833.15 Open dislocation of proximal end of metacarpal (bone)
833.19 Open dislocation of other part of wrist
834.00 Closed dislocation of finger, unspecified part ▽
834.01 Closed dislocation of metacarpophalangeal (joint)
834.02 Closed dislocation of interphalangeal (joint), hand
834.11 Open dislocation of metacarpophalangeal (joint)
834.12 Open dislocation interphalangeal (joint), hand
842.01 Sprain and strain of carpal (joint) of wrist
842.02 Sprain and strain of radiocarpal (joint) (ligament) of wrist
842.09 Other wrist sprain and strain
842.11 Sprain and strain of carpometacarpal (joint) of hand
842.12 Sprain and strain of metacarpophalangeal (joint) of hand
842.13 Sprain and strain of interphalangeal (joint) of hand
842.19 Other hand sprain and strain
881.00 Open wound of forearm, without mention of complication — (Use additional code to identify infection)
881.02 Open wound of wrist, without mention of complication — (Use additional code to identify infection)
881.10 Open wound of forearm, complicated — (Use additional code to identify infection)
881.12 Open wound of wrist, complicated — (Use additional code to identify infection)
881.20 Open wound of forearm, with tendon involvement — (Use additional code to identify infection)
881.22 Open wound of wrist, with tendon involvement — (Use additional code to identify infection)
883.0 Open wound of finger(s), without mention of complication — (Use additional code to identify infection)
883.1 Open wound of finger(s), complicated — (Use additional code to identify infection)
883.2 Open wound of finger(s), with tendon involvement — (Use additional code to identify infection)
884.0 Multiple and unspecified open wound of upper limb, without mention of complication — (Use additional code to identify infection)
884.1 Multiple and unspecified open wound of upper limb, complicated — (Use additional code to identify infection)
884.2 Multiple and unspecified open wound of upper limb, with tendon involvement — (Use additional code to identify infection)
905.2 Late effect of fracture of upper extremities
959.3 Injury, other and unspecified, elbow, forearm, and wrist
V54.12 Aftercare for healing traumatic fracture of lower arm
V54.19 Aftercare for healing traumatic fracture of other bone
V54.22 Aftercare for healing pathologic fracture of lower arm
V54.29 Aftercare for healing pathologic fracture of other bone
V54.89 Other orthopedic aftercare
V67.00 Follow-up examination, following unspecified surgery ▽
V67.09 Follow-up examination, following other surgery

ICD-9-CM Procedural

93.53 Application of other cast
97.11 Replacement of cast on upper limb

HCPCS Level II Supplies & Services

A4580 Cast supplies (e.g., plaster)
A4590 Special casting material (e.g., fiberglass)
A6441 Padding bandage, non-elastic, non-woven/non-knitted, width greater than or equal to three inches and less than five inches, per yard
Q4009 Cast supplies, short arm cast, adult (11 years +), plaster
Q4010 Cast supplies, short arm cast, adult (11 years +), fiberglass

29085

29085 Application, cast; hand and lower forearm (gauntlet)

ICD-9-CM Diagnostic

716.13 Traumatic arthropathy, forearm
718.83 Other joint derangement, not elsewhere classified, forearm
718.84 Other joint derangement, not elsewhere classified, hand
733.82 Nonunion of fracture
813.05 Closed fracture of head of radius
813.06 Closed fracture of neck of radius
813.21 Closed fracture of shaft of radius (alone)
813.22 Closed fracture of shaft of ulna (alone)
813.41 Closed Colles' fracture
813.42 Other closed fractures of distal end of radius (alone)
813.43 Closed fracture of distal end of ulna (alone)
813.44 Closed fracture of lower end of radius with ulna
813.45 Torus fracture of lower end of radius
813.51 Open Colles' fracture
813.52 Other open fractures of distal end of radius (alone)
813.53 Open fracture of distal end of ulna (alone)
813.54 Open fracture of lower end of radius with ulna
813.91 Open fracture of unspecified part of radius (alone) ▽
813.92 Open fracture of unspecified part of ulna (alone) ▽
814.01 Closed fracture of navicular (scaphoid) bone of wrist
814.02 Closed fracture of lunate (semilunar) bone of wrist
814.03 Closed fracture of triquetral (cuneiform) bone of wrist
814.04 Closed fracture of pisiform bone of wrist
814.05 Closed fracture of trapezium bone (larger multangular) of wrist
814.06 Closed fracture of trapezoid bone (smaller multangular) of wrist
814.07 Closed fracture of capitate bone (os magnum) of wrist
814.08 Closed fracture of hamate (unciform) bone of wrist
814.09 Closed fracture of other bone of wrist
814.11 Open fracture of navicular (scaphoid) bone of wrist
814.12 Open fracture of lunate (semilunar) bone of wrist
814.13 Open fracture of triquetral (cuneiform) bone of wrist
814.14 Open fracture of pisiform bone of wrist
814.15 Open fracture of trapezium bone (larger multangular) of wrist
814.16 Open fracture of trapezoid bone (smaller multangular) of wrist
814.17 Open fracture of capitate bone (os magnum) of wrist
814.18 Open fracture of hamate (unciform) bone of wrist
814.19 Open fracture of other bone of wrist
815.00 Closed fracture of metacarpal bone(s), site unspecified ▽
815.01 Closed fracture of base of thumb (first) metacarpal bone(s)
815.02 Closed fracture of base of other metacarpal bone(s)
815.03 Closed fracture of shaft of metacarpal bone(s)
815.04 Closed fracture of neck of metacarpal bone(s)
815.09 Closed fracture of multiple sites of metacarpus
815.10 Open fracture of metacarpal bone(s), site unspecified ▽
815.11 Open fracture of base of thumb (first) metacarpal bone(s)
815.12 Open fracture of base of other metacarpal bone(s)
815.13 Open fracture of shaft of metacarpal bone(s)
815.14 Open fracture of neck of metacarpal bone(s)
815.19 Open fracture of multiple sites of metacarpus
816.00 Closed fracture of unspecified phalanx or phalanges of hand ▽
816.01 Closed fracture of middle or proximal phalanx or phalanges of hand
816.02 Closed fracture of distal phalanx or phalanges of hand
816.03 Closed fracture of multiple sites of phalanx or phalanges of hand
816.10 Open fracture of phalanx or phalanges of hand, unspecified ▽
816.11 Open fracture of middle or proximal phalanx or phalanges of hand
816.12 Open fracture of distal phalanx or phalanges of hand
816.13 Open fractures of multiple sites of phalanx or phalanges of hand
817.0 Multiple closed fractures of hand bones
817.1 Multiple open fractures of hand bones
959.4 Injury, other and unspecified, hand, except finger
959.5 Injury, other and unspecified, finger

ICD-9-CM Procedural

93.53 Application of other cast

▽ Unspecified code
♀ Female diagnosis
☒ Manifestation code
♂ Male diagnosis

97.11 Replacement of cast on upper limb

HCPCS Level II Supplies & Services

A4580 Cast supplies (e.g., plaster)
A4590 Special casting material (e.g., fiberglass)
A6441 Padding bandage, non-elastic, non-woven/non-knitted, width greater than or equal to three inches and less than five inches, per yard
Q4013 Cast supplies, gauntlet cast (includes lower forearm and hand), adult (11 years +), plaster
Q4014 Cast supplies, gauntlet cast (includes lower forearm and hand), adult (11 years +), fiberglass

29086

29086 Application, cast; finger (eg, contracture)

ICD-9-CM Diagnostic

718.74 Developmental dislocation of joint, hand
727.03 Trigger finger (acquired)
727.05 Other tenosynovitis of hand and wrist
728.6 Contracture of palmar fascia
736.1 Mallet finger
736.20 Unspecified deformity of finger ▽
736.21 Boutonniere deformity
736.22 Swan-neck deformity
736.29 Other acquired deformity of finger
816.00 Closed fracture of unspecified phalanx or phalanges of hand ▽
816.01 Closed fracture of middle or proximal phalanx or phalanges of hand
816.02 Closed fracture of distal phalanx or phalanges of hand
816.03 Closed fracture of multiple sites of phalanx or phalanges of hand
834.00 Closed dislocation of finger, unspecified part ▽
834.01 Closed dislocation of metacarpophalangeal (joint)
834.02 Closed dislocation of interphalangeal (joint), hand
842.12 Sprain and strain of metacarpophalangeal (joint) of hand
842.13 Sprain and strain of interphalangeal (joint) of hand
883.0 Open wound of finger(s), without mention of complication — (Use additional code to identify infection)
883.1 Open wound of finger(s), complicated — (Use additional code to identify infection)
883.2 Open wound of finger(s), with tendon involvement — (Use additional code to identify infection)
927.3 Crushing injury of finger(s) — (Use additional code to identify any associated injuries: 800-829, 850.0-854.1, 860.0-869.1)
959.5 Injury, other and unspecified, finger

ICD-9-CM Procedural

93.53 Application of other cast

HCPCS Level II Supplies & Services

A4580 Cast supplies (e.g., plaster)
A4590 Special casting material (e.g., fiberglass)

29105

29105 Application of long arm splint (shoulder to hand)

ICD-9-CM Diagnostic

357.1 Polyneuropathy in collagen vascular disease — (Code first underlying disease: 446.0, 710.0, 714.0) ☒
359.6 Symptomatic inflammatory myopathy in diseases classified elsewhere — (Code first underlying disease: 135, 140.0-208.9, 277.3, 446.0, 710.0, 710.1, 710.2, 714.0) ☒
446.0 Polyarteritis nodosa
710.0 Systemic lupus erythematosus — (Use additional code to identify manifestation: 424.91, 581.81, 582.81, 583.81)
710.1 Systemic sclerosis — (Use additional code to identify manifestation: 359.6, 517.2)
710.2 Sicca syndrome
714.0 Rheumatoid arthritis — (Use additional code to identify manifestation: 357.1, 359.6)
718.82 Other joint derangement, not elsewhere classified, upper arm
718.83 Other joint derangement, not elsewhere classified, forearm
726.30 Unspecified enthesopathy of elbow ▽
726.31 Medial epicondylitis of elbow
726.32 Lateral epicondylitis of elbow
726.33 Olecranon bursitis
726.39 Other enthesopathy of elbow region
726.90 Enthesopathy of unspecified site ▽
727.00 Unspecified synovitis and tenosynovitis ▽
727.05 Other tenosynovitis of hand and wrist
810.00 Unspecified part of closed fracture of clavicle ▽
812.00 Closed fracture of unspecified part of upper end of humerus ▽
812.01 Closed fracture of surgical neck of humerus
812.03 Closed fracture of greater tuberosity of humerus
812.09 Other closed fractures of upper end of humerus
812.20 Closed fracture of unspecified part of humerus ▽
812.21 Closed fracture of shaft of humerus
812.40 Closed fracture of unspecified part of lower end of humerus ▽
812.41 Closed fracture of supracondylar humerus
812.42 Closed fracture of lateral condyle of humerus
812.43 Closed fracture of medial condyle of humerus
812.44 Closed fracture of unspecified condyle(s) of humerus ▽
812.49 Other closed fracture of lower end of humerus
813.00 Unspecified fracture of radius and ulna, upper end of forearm, closed ▽
813.01 Closed fracture of olecranon process of ulna
813.02 Closed fracture of coronoid process of ulna
813.03 Closed Monteggia's fracture
813.04 Other and unspecified closed fractures of proximal end of ulna (alone) ▽
813.05 Closed fracture of head of radius
813.06 Closed fracture of neck of radius
813.07 Other and unspecified closed fractures of proximal end of radius (alone) ▽
813.08 Closed fracture of radius with ulna, upper end (any part)
813.21 Closed fracture of shaft of radius (alone)
813.22 Closed fracture of shaft of ulna (alone)
813.40 Unspecified closed fracture of lower end of forearm ▽
813.41 Closed Colles' fracture
813.42 Other closed fractures of distal end of radius (alone)
813.43 Closed fracture of distal end of ulna (alone)
813.44 Closed fracture of lower end of radius with ulna
813.45 Torus fracture of lower end of radius
813.80 Closed fracture of unspecified part of forearm ▽
813.81 Closed fracture of unspecified part of radius (alone) ▽
813.82 Closed fracture of unspecified part of ulna (alone) ▽
813.83 Closed fracture of unspecified part of radius with ulna ▽
814.01 Closed fracture of navicular (scaphoid) bone of wrist
814.08 Closed fracture of hamate (unciform) bone of wrist
815.00 Closed fracture of metacarpal bone(s), site unspecified ▽
815.01 Closed fracture of base of thumb (first) metacarpal bone(s)
815.02 Closed fracture of base of other metacarpal bone(s)
815.03 Closed fracture of shaft of metacarpal bone(s)
815.04 Closed fracture of neck of metacarpal bone(s)
816.00 Closed fracture of unspecified phalanx or phalanges of hand ▽
816.01 Closed fracture of middle or proximal phalanx or phalanges of hand
816.02 Closed fracture of distal phalanx or phalanges of hand

ICD-9-CM Procedural

93.54 Application of splint
97.14 Replacement of other device for musculoskeletal immobilization

HCPCS Level II Supplies & Services

A4570 Splint
A4580 Cast supplies (e.g., plaster)
A4590 Special casting material (e.g., fiberglass)
A6441 Padding bandage, non-elastic, non-woven/non-knitted, width greater than or equal to three inches and less than five inches, per yard
Q4017 Cast supplies, long arm splint, adult (11 years +), plaster

29125–29126

29125 Application of short arm splint (forearm to hand); static
29126 dynamic

ICD-9-CM Diagnostic

354.0 Carpal tunnel syndrome
357.1 Polyneuropathy in collagen vascular disease — (Code first underlying disease: 446.0, 710.0, 714.0) ☒
359.6 Symptomatic inflammatory myopathy in diseases classified elsewhere — (Code first underlying disease: 135, 140.0-208.9, 277.3, 446.0, 710.0, 710.1, 710.2, 714.0) ☒
446.0 Polyarteritis nodosa
710.0 Systemic lupus erythematosus — (Use additional code to identify manifestation: 424.91, 581.81, 582.81, 583.81)
710.1 Systemic sclerosis — (Use additional code to identify manifestation: 359.6, 517.2)
710.2 Sicca syndrome

▽ Unspecified code
♀ Female diagnosis
☒ Manifestation code
♂ Male diagnosis

714.0 Rheumatoid arthritis — (Use additional code to identify manifestation: 357.1, 359.6)
715.14 Primary localized osteoarthrosis, hand
715.93 Osteoarthrosis, unspecified whether generalized or localized, forearm
715.94 Osteoarthrosis, unspecified whether generalized or localized, hand
718.83 Other joint derangement, not elsewhere classified, forearm
718.84 Other joint derangement, not elsewhere classified, hand
726.90 Enthesopathy of unspecified site
727.05 Other tenosynovitis of hand and wrist
729.81 Swelling of limb
813.21 Closed fracture of shaft of radius (alone)
813.22 Closed fracture of shaft of ulna (alone)
813.23 Closed fracture of shaft of radius with ulna
813.41 Closed Colles' fracture
813.42 Other closed fractures of distal end of radius (alone)
813.43 Closed fracture of distal end of ulna (alone)
813.44 Closed fracture of lower end of radius with ulna
813.45 Torus fracture of lower end of radius
813.80 Closed fracture of unspecified part of forearm
813.81 Closed fracture of unspecified part of radius (alone)
813.82 Closed fracture of unspecified part of ulna (alone)
813.83 Closed fracture of unspecified part of radius with ulna
814.01 Closed fracture of navicular (scaphoid) bone of wrist
814.02 Closed fracture of lunate (semilunar) bone of wrist
814.03 Closed fracture of triquetral (cuneiform) bone of wrist
814.04 Closed fracture of pisiform bone of wrist
814.05 Closed fracture of trapezium bone (larger multangular) of wrist
814.06 Closed fracture of trapezoid bone (smaller multangular) of wrist
814.07 Closed fracture of capitate bone (os magnum) of wrist
814.08 Closed fracture of hamate (unciform) bone of wrist
815.00 Closed fracture of metacarpal bone(s), site unspecified
815.01 Closed fracture of base of thumb (first) metacarpal bone(s)
815.02 Closed fracture of base of other metacarpal bone(s)
815.03 Closed fracture of shaft of metacarpal bone(s)
815.04 Closed fracture of neck of metacarpal bone(s)
815.09 Closed fracture of multiple sites of metacarpus
816.00 Closed fracture of unspecified phalanx or phalanges of hand
816.01 Closed fracture of middle or proximal phalanx or phalanges of hand
816.02 Closed fracture of distal phalanx or phalanges of hand
816.03 Closed fracture of multiple sites of phalanx or phalanges of hand
817.0 Multiple closed fractures of hand bones
818.0 Ill-defined closed fractures of upper limb
841.9 Sprain and strain of unspecified site of elbow and forearm
842.00 Sprain and strain of unspecified site of wrist
842.10 Sprain and strain of unspecified site of hand
842.11 Sprain and strain of carpometacarpal (joint) of hand
842.12 Sprain and strain of metacarpophalangeal (joint) of hand
842.13 Sprain and strain of interphalangeal (joint) of hand
842.19 Other hand sprain and strain
923.10 Contusion of forearm
923.20 Contusion of hand(s)
923.21 Contusion of wrist
959.3 Injury, other and unspecified, elbow, forearm, and wrist
959.4 Injury, other and unspecified, hand, except finger
959.5 Injury, other and unspecified, finger
V67.4 Treatment of healed fracture follow-up examination

ICD-9-CM Procedural

93.54 Application of splint
97.14 Replacement of other device for musculoskeletal immobilization

HCPCS Level II Supplies & Services

A4570 Splint
A4580 Cast supplies (e.g., plaster)
A6441 Padding bandage, non-elastic, non-woven/non-knitted, width greater than or equal to three inches and less than five inches, per yard
Q4021 Cast supplies, short arm splint, adult (11 years +), plaster
Q4022 Cast supplies, short arm splint, adult (11 years +), fiberglass

29130–29131

29130 Application of finger splint; static
29131 dynamic

ICD-9-CM Diagnostic

718.74 Developmental dislocation of joint, hand
727.03 Trigger finger (acquired)
727.05 Other tenosynovitis of hand and wrist
728.6 Contracture of palmar fascia
736.1 Mallet finger
736.20 Unspecified deformity of finger
736.21 Boutonniere deformity
736.22 Swan-neck deformity
736.29 Other acquired deformity of finger
816.00 Closed fracture of unspecified phalanx or phalanges of hand
816.01 Closed fracture of middle or proximal phalanx or phalanges of hand
816.02 Closed fracture of distal phalanx or phalanges of hand
816.03 Closed fracture of multiple sites of phalanx or phalanges of hand
834.00 Closed dislocation of finger, unspecified part
834.01 Closed dislocation of metacarpophalangeal (joint)
834.02 Closed dislocation of interphalangeal (joint), hand
842.12 Sprain and strain of metacarpophalangeal (joint) of hand
842.13 Sprain and strain of interphalangeal (joint) of hand
883.0 Open wound of finger(s), without mention of complication — (Use additional code to identify infection)
883.1 Open wound of finger(s), complicated — (Use additional code to identify infection)
883.2 Open wound of finger(s), with tendon involvement — (Use additional code to identify infection)
927.3 Crushing injury of finger(s) — (Use additional code to identify any associated injuries: 800-829, 850.0-854.1, 860.0-869.1)
959.5 Injury, other and unspecified, finger

ICD-9-CM Procedural

93.54 Application of splint
97.14 Replacement of other device for musculoskeletal immobilization

HCPCS Level II Supplies & Services

A4570 Splint
A6441 Padding bandage, non-elastic, non-woven/non-knitted, width greater than or equal to three inches and less than five inches, per yard
Q4049 Finger splint, static
Q4051 Splint supplies, miscellaneous (includes thermoplastics, strapping, fasteners, padding and other supplies)
S8430 Padding for compression bandage, roll

29200

29200 Strapping; thorax

ICD-9-CM Diagnostic

807.01 Closed fracture of one rib
807.02 Closed fracture of two ribs
807.03 Closed fracture of three ribs
807.04 Closed fracture of four ribs
807.05 Closed fracture of five ribs
807.06 Closed fracture of six ribs
807.07 Closed fracture of seven ribs
807.08 Closed fracture of eight or more ribs
807.09 Closed fracture of multiple ribs, unspecified
807.2 Closed fracture of sternum

ICD-9-CM Procedural

93.59 Other immobilization, pressure, and attention to wound
97.14 Replacement of other device for musculoskeletal immobilization

HCPCS Level II Supplies & Services

A4450 Tape, non-waterproof, per 18 sq. inches
A4452 Tape, waterproof, per 18 sq. inches
A4649 Surgical supply; miscellaneous

29220

29220 Strapping; low back

ICD-9-CM Diagnostic

722.10 Displacement of lumbar intervertebral disc without myelopathy
722.2 Displacement of intervertebral disc, site unspecified, without myelopathy
722.52 Degeneration of lumbar or lumbosacral intervertebral disc
724.2 Lumbago
724.3 Sciatica
724.4 Thoracic or lumbosacral neuritis or radiculitis, unspecified
724.6 Disorders of sacrum
724.70 Unspecified disorder of coccyx
724.71 Hypermobility of coccyx

724.79 Other disorder of coccyx
724.8 Other symptoms referable to back
728.85 Spasm of muscle
739.3 Nonallopathic lesion of lumbar region, not elsewhere classified
839.20 Closed dislocation, lumbar vertebra
846.0 Sprain and strain of lumbosacral (joint) (ligament)
847.2 Lumbar sprain and strain

ICD-9-CM Procedural

93.59 Other immobilization, pressure, and attention to wound
97.14 Replacement of other device for musculoskeletal immobilization

HCPCS Level II Supplies & Services

A4450 Tape, non-waterproof, per 18 sq. inches
A4452 Tape, waterproof, per 18 sq. inches
A4649 Surgical supply; miscellaneous

29240

29240 Strapping; shoulder (eg, Velpeau)

ICD-9-CM Diagnostic

718.31 Recurrent dislocation of shoulder joint
719.41 Pain in joint, shoulder region
719.81 Other specified disorders of shoulder joint
726.10 Unspecified disorders of bursae and tendons in shoulder region ▽
726.11 Calcifying tendinitis of shoulder
726.12 Bicipital tenosynovitis
726.19 Other specified disorders of rotator cuff syndrome of shoulder and allied disorders
726.2 Other affections of shoulder region, not elsewhere classified
810.03 Closed fracture of acromial end of clavicle
811.01 Closed fracture of acromial process of scapula
811.03 Closed fracture of glenoid cavity and neck of scapula
812.00 Closed fracture of unspecified part of upper end of humerus ▽
812.01 Closed fracture of surgical neck of humerus
812.02 Closed fracture of anatomical neck of humerus
812.03 Closed fracture of greater tuberosity of humerus
812.09 Other closed fractures of upper end of humerus
812.20 Closed fracture of unspecified part of humerus ▽
812.21 Closed fracture of shaft of humerus
812.40 Closed fracture of unspecified part of lower end of humerus ▽
812.41 Closed fracture of supracondylar humerus

ICD-9-CM Procedural

93.59 Other immobilization, pressure, and attention to wound
97.14 Replacement of other device for musculoskeletal immobilization

HCPCS Level II Supplies & Services

A4450 Tape, non-waterproof, per 18 sq. inches
A4452 Tape, waterproof, per 18 sq. inches
A4649 Surgical supply; miscellaneous

29260–29280

29260 Strapping; elbow or wrist
29280 hand or finger

ICD-9-CM Diagnostic

354.0 Carpal tunnel syndrome
715.94 Osteoarthrosis, unspecified whether generalized or localized, hand ▽
718.72 Developmental dislocation of joint, upper arm
718.73 Developmental dislocation of joint, forearm
718.74 Developmental dislocation of joint, hand
727.05 Other tenosynovitis of hand and wrist
814.01 Closed fracture of navicular (scaphoid) bone of wrist
815.00 Closed fracture of metacarpal bone(s), site unspecified ▽
815.01 Closed fracture of base of thumb (first) metacarpal bone(s)
815.02 Closed fracture of base of other metacarpal bone(s)
815.03 Closed fracture of shaft of metacarpal bone(s)
815.04 Closed fracture of neck of metacarpal bone(s)
815.09 Closed fracture of multiple sites of metacarpus
816.00 Closed fracture of unspecified phalanx or phalanges of hand ▽
816.01 Closed fracture of middle or proximal phalanx or phalanges of hand
816.02 Closed fracture of distal phalanx or phalanges of hand
816.03 Closed fracture of multiple sites of phalanx or phalanges of hand
817.0 Multiple closed fractures of hand bones
833.05 Closed dislocation of proximal end of metacarpal (bone)
834.00 Closed dislocation of finger, unspecified part ▽
834.01 Closed dislocation of metacarpophalangeal (joint)
834.02 Closed dislocation of interphalangeal (joint), hand
834.11 Open dislocation of metacarpophalangeal (joint)
842.10 Sprain and strain of unspecified site of hand ▽
842.11 Sprain and strain of carpometacarpal (joint) of hand
842.12 Sprain and strain of metacarpophalangeal (joint) of hand
842.13 Sprain and strain of interphalangeal (joint) of hand
842.19 Other hand sprain and strain
927.20 Crushing injury of hand(s) — (Use additional code to identify any associated injuries: 800-829, 850.0-854.1, 860.0-869.1)
927.3 Crushing injury of finger(s) — (Use additional code to identify any associated injuries: 800-829, 850.0-854.1, 860.0-869.1)
959.4 Injury, other and unspecified, hand, except finger
959.5 Injury, other and unspecified, finger

ICD-9-CM Procedural

93.59 Other immobilization, pressure, and attention to wound
97.14 Replacement of other device for musculoskeletal immobilization

HCPCS Level II Supplies & Services

A4450 Tape, non-waterproof, per 18 sq. inches
A4452 Tape, waterproof, per 18 sq. inches
A4649 Surgical supply; miscellaneous

29305–29325

29305 Application of hip spica cast; one leg
29325 one and one-half spica or both legs

ICD-9-CM Diagnostic

718.45 Contracture of pelvic joint
718.46 Contracture of lower leg joint
736.89 Other acquired deformity of other parts of limb
754.30 Congenital dislocation of hip, unilateral
754.31 Congenital dislocation of hip, bilateral
754.32 Congenital subluxation of hip, unilateral
756.11 Congenital spondylolysis, lumbosacral region
820.8 Closed fracture of unspecified part of neck of femur ▽
821.00 Closed fracture of unspecified part of femur ▽
821.01 Closed fracture of shaft of femur
821.20 Closed fracture of unspecified part of lower end of femur ▽
827.0 Other, multiple and ill-defined closed fractures of lower limb

ICD-9-CM Procedural

93.53 Application of other cast
97.12 Replacement of cast on lower limb

HCPCS Level II Supplies & Services

A4580 Cast supplies (e.g., plaster)
A4590 Special casting material (e.g., fiberglass)
A6441 Padding bandage, non-elastic, non-woven/non-knitted, width greater than or equal to three inches and less than five inches, per yard
Q4025 Cast supplies, hip spica (one or both legs), adult (11 years +), plaster
Q4026 Cast supplies, hip spica (one or both legs), adult (11 years +), fiberglass

29345–29355

29345 Application of long leg cast (thigh to toes);
29355 walker or ambulatory type

ICD-9-CM Diagnostic

718.46 Contracture of lower leg joint
718.76 Developmental dislocation of joint, lower leg
718.86 Other joint derangement, not elsewhere classified, lower leg
732.4 Juvenile osteochondrosis of lower extremity, excluding foot
733.81 Malunion of fracture
733.82 Nonunion of fracture
733.93 Stress fracture of tibia or fibula
733.95 Stress fracture of other bone
821.01 Closed fracture of shaft of femur
821.20 Closed fracture of unspecified part of lower end of femur ▽
821.21 Closed fracture of femoral condyle
821.22 Closed fracture of lower epiphysis of femur
821.23 Closed supracondylar fracture of femur
821.32 Open fracture of lower epiphysis of femur
821.33 Open supracondylar fracture of femur
822.0 Closed fracture of patella

823.00 Closed fracture of upper end of tibia
823.01 Closed fracture of upper end of fibula
823.02 Closed fracture of upper end of fibula with tibia
823.10 Open fracture of upper end of tibia
823.20 Closed fracture of shaft of tibia
823.21 Closed fracture of shaft of fibula
823.22 Closed fracture of shaft of fibula with tibia
823.30 Open fracture of shaft of tibia
823.32 Open fracture of shaft of fibula with tibia
823.40 Torus fracture of tibia alone
823.41 Torus fracture of fibula alone
823.42 Torus fracture of fibula with tibia
823.80 Closed fracture of unspecified part of tibia ▽
823.81 Closed fracture of unspecified part of fibula ▽
823.82 Closed fracture of unspecified part of fibula with tibia ▽
823.90 Open fracture of unspecified part of tibia ▽
823.91 Open fracture of unspecified part of fibula ▽
823.92 Open fracture of unspecified part of fibula with tibia ▽
836.0 Tear of medial cartilage or meniscus of knee, current
836.1 Tear of lateral cartilage or meniscus of knee, current
836.2 Other tear of cartilage or meniscus of knee, current
836.3 Closed dislocation of patella
836.50 Closed dislocation of knee, unspecified part ▽
V67.00 Follow-up examination, following unspecified surgery ▽
V67.09 Follow-up examination, following other surgery

ICD-9-CM Procedural

93.53 Application of other cast
97.12 Replacement of cast on lower limb

HCPCS Level II Supplies & Services

A4580 Cast supplies (e.g., plaster)
A4590 Special casting material (e.g., fiberglass)
A6441 Padding bandage, non-elastic, non-woven/non-knitted, width greater than or equal to three inches and less than five inches, per yard
Q4029 Cast supplies, long leg cast, adult (11 years +), plaster
Q4030 Cast supplies, long leg cast, adult (11 years +), fiberglass

29358

29358 Application of long leg cast brace

ICD-9-CM Diagnostic

718.76 Developmental dislocation of joint, lower leg
733.93 Stress fracture of tibia or fibula
733.95 Stress fracture of other bone
821.01 Closed fracture of shaft of femur
821.20 Closed fracture of unspecified part of lower end of femur ▽
821.21 Closed fracture of femoral condyle
821.22 Closed fracture of lower epiphysis of femur
821.23 Closed supracondylar fracture of femur
822.0 Closed fracture of patella
823.00 Closed fracture of upper end of tibia
823.01 Closed fracture of upper end of fibula
823.02 Closed fracture of upper end of fibula with tibia
823.20 Closed fracture of shaft of tibia
823.21 Closed fracture of shaft of fibula
823.22 Closed fracture of shaft of fibula with tibia
823.30 Open fracture of shaft of tibia
823.40 Torus fracture of tibia alone
823.41 Torus fracture of fibula alone
823.42 Torus fracture of fibula with tibia
823.80 Closed fracture of unspecified part of tibia ▽
823.81 Closed fracture of unspecified part of fibula ▽
823.82 Closed fracture of unspecified part of fibula with tibia ▽
823.90 Open fracture of unspecified part of tibia ▽
823.91 Open fracture of unspecified part of fibula ▽
823.92 Open fracture of unspecified part of fibula with tibia ▽
836.0 Tear of medial cartilage or meniscus of knee, current
836.1 Tear of lateral cartilage or meniscus of knee, current
836.2 Other tear of cartilage or meniscus of knee, current
836.3 Closed dislocation of patella
836.50 Closed dislocation of knee, unspecified part ▽
V67.00 Follow-up examination, following unspecified surgery ▽
V67.09 Follow-up examination, following other surgery

ICD-9-CM Procedural

93.53 Application of other cast
97.12 Replacement of cast on lower limb

HCPCS Level II Supplies & Services

A4580 Cast supplies (e.g., plaster)
A4590 Special casting material (e.g., fiberglass)

29365

29365 Application of cylinder cast (thigh to ankle)

ICD-9-CM Diagnostic

715.16 Primary localized osteoarthrosis, lower leg
717.3 Other and unspecified derangement of medial meniscus ▽
717.7 Chondromalacia of patella
717.82 Old disruption of medial collateral ligament
717.83 Old disruption of anterior cruciate ligament
718.36 Recurrent dislocation of lower leg joint
718.76 Developmental dislocation of joint, lower leg
727.65 Nontraumatic rupture of quadriceps tendon
727.66 Nontraumatic rupture of patellar tendon
732.4 Juvenile osteochondrosis of lower extremity, excluding foot
733.93 Stress fracture of tibia or fibula
733.95 Stress fracture of other bone
821.01 Closed fracture of shaft of femur
821.20 Closed fracture of unspecified part of lower end of femur ▽
821.21 Closed fracture of femoral condyle
821.22 Closed fracture of lower epiphysis of femur
821.23 Closed supracondylar fracture of femur
821.29 Other closed fracture of lower end of femur
821.30 Open fracture of unspecified part of lower end of femur ▽
821.31 Open fracture of femoral condyle
821.32 Open fracture of lower epiphysis of femur
821.33 Open supracondylar fracture of femur
821.39 Other open fracture of lower end of femur
822.0 Closed fracture of patella
823.00 Closed fracture of upper end of tibia
823.01 Closed fracture of upper end of fibula
823.02 Closed fracture of upper end of fibula with tibia
823.10 Open fracture of upper end of tibia
823.11 Open fracture of upper end of fibula
823.12 Open fracture of upper end of fibula with tibia
823.20 Closed fracture of shaft of tibia
823.21 Closed fracture of shaft of fibula
823.40 Torus fracture of tibia alone
823.41 Torus fracture of fibula alone
823.42 Torus fracture of fibula with tibia
823.80 Closed fracture of unspecified part of tibia ▽
823.81 Closed fracture of unspecified part of fibula ▽
823.82 Closed fracture of unspecified part of fibula with tibia ▽
823.90 Open fracture of unspecified part of tibia ▽
823.91 Open fracture of unspecified part of fibula ▽
823.92 Open fracture of unspecified part of fibula with tibia ▽
836.0 Tear of medial cartilage or meniscus of knee, current
836.2 Other tear of cartilage or meniscus of knee, current
836.3 Closed dislocation of patella
844.1 Sprain and strain of medial collateral ligament of knee
844.2 Sprain and strain of cruciate ligament of knee
V67.00 Follow-up examination, following unspecified surgery ▽
V67.09 Follow-up examination, following other surgery
V67.4 Treatment of healed fracture follow-up examination

ICD-9-CM Procedural

93.53 Application of other cast
97.12 Replacement of cast on lower limb

HCPCS Level II Supplies & Services

A4580 Cast supplies (e.g., plaster)
A4590 Special casting material (e.g., fiberglass)
A6441 Padding bandage, non-elastic, non-woven/non-knitted, width greater than or equal to three inches and less than five inches, per yard
Q4033 Cast supplies, long leg cylinder cast, adult (11 years +), plaster
Q4034 Cast supplies, long leg cylinder cast, adult (11 years +), fiberglass

▽ Unspecified code
♀ Female diagnosis
☒ Manifestation code
♂ Male diagnosis

29405–29425

29405 Application of short leg cast (below knee to toes);
29425 walking or ambulatory type

ICD-9-CM Diagnostic

355.3 Lesion of lateral popliteal nerve
355.4 Lesion of medial popliteal nerve
355.5 Tarsal tunnel syndrome
355.6 Lesion of plantar nerve
718.07 Articular cartilage disorder, ankle and foot
718.17 Loose body in ankle and foot joint
718.27 Pathological dislocation of ankle and foot joint
718.37 Recurrent dislocation of ankle and foot joint
718.40 Contracture of joint, site unspecified ▽
718.47 Contracture of ankle and foot joint
718.57 Ankylosis of ankle and foot joint
718.77 Developmental dislocation of joint, ankle and foot
718.87 Other joint derangement, not elsewhere classified, ankle and foot
719.87 Other specified disorders of ankle and foot joint
726.71 Achilles bursitis or tendinitis
726.72 Tibialis tendinitis
726.73 Calcaneal spur
726.79 Other enthesopathy of ankle and tarsus
726.8 Other peripheral enthesopathies
726.90 Enthesopathy of unspecified site ▽
726.91 Exostosis of unspecified site ▽
727.00 Unspecified synovitis and tenosynovitis ▽
727.01 Synovitis and tenosynovitis in diseases classified elsewhere — (Code first underlying disease: 015.0-015.9) ☒
727.02 Giant cell tumor of tendon sheath
727.06 Tenosynovitis of foot and ankle
727.09 Other synovitis and tenosynovitis
727.1 Bunion
727.3 Other bursitis disorders
727.67 Nontraumatic rupture of Achilles tendon
727.68 Nontraumatic rupture of other tendons of foot and ankle
727.81 Contracture of tendon (sheath)
728.71 Plantar fascial fibromatosis
732.5 Juvenile osteochondrosis of foot
733.16 Pathologic fracture of tibia or fibula
733.19 Pathologic fracture of other specified site
733.21 Solitary bone cyst
733.22 Aneurysmal bone cyst
733.29 Other cyst of bone
733.44 Aseptic necrosis of talus
733.49 Aseptic necrosis of other bone site
733.81 Malunion of fracture
733.82 Nonunion of fracture
733.93 Stress fracture of tibia or fibula
733.94 Stress fracture of the metatarsals
733.95 Stress fracture of other bone
733.99 Other disorders of bone and cartilage
735.0 Hallux valgus (acquired)
735.1 Hallux varus (acquired)
735.2 Hallux rigidus
735.3 Hallux malleus
735.4 Other hammer toe (acquired)
735.5 Claw toe (acquired)
735.8 Other acquired deformity of toe
736.71 Acquired equinovarus deformity
736.72 Equinus deformity of foot, acquired
736.73 Cavus deformity of foot, acquired
736.74 Claw foot, acquired
736.75 Cavovarus deformity of foot, acquired
736.76 Other acquired calcaneus deformity
736.79 Other acquired deformity of ankle and foot
736.81 Unequal leg length (acquired)
736.89 Other acquired deformity of other parts of limb
736.9 Acquired deformity of limb, site unspecified ▽
754.50 Congenital talipes varus
754.51 Congenital talipes equinovarus
754.52 Congenital metatarsus primus varus
754.53 Congenital metatarsus varus
754.59 Other congenital varus deformity of feet
754.60 Congenital talipes valgus
754.61 Congenital pes planus
754.62 Talipes calcaneovalgus
754.69 Other congenital valgus deformity of feet
754.70 Unspecified talipes ▽
754.71 Talipes cavus
754.79 Other congenital deformity of feet
755.66 Other congenital anomaly of toes
755.67 Congenital anomalies of foot, not elsewhere classified
755.69 Other congenital anomaly of lower limb, including pelvic girdle
755.8 Other specified congenital anomalies of unspecified limb
823.20 Closed fracture of shaft of tibia
823.21 Closed fracture of shaft of fibula
823.22 Closed fracture of shaft of fibula with tibia
823.30 Open fracture of shaft of tibia
823.31 Open fracture of shaft of fibula
823.32 Open fracture of shaft of fibula with tibia
823.40 Torus fracture of tibia alone
823.41 Torus fracture of fibula alone
823.42 Torus fracture of fibula with tibia
824.0 Closed fracture of medial malleolus
824.1 Open fracture of medial malleolus
824.2 Closed fracture of lateral malleolus
824.3 Open fracture of lateral malleolus
824.4 Closed bimalleolar fracture
824.5 Open bimalleolar fracture
824.6 Closed trimalleolar fracture
824.7 Open trimalleolar fracture
825.0 Closed fracture of calcaneus
825.1 Open fracture of calcaneus
825.21 Closed fracture of astragalus
825.22 Closed fracture of navicular (scaphoid) bone of foot
825.23 Closed fracture of cuboid bone
825.24 Closed fracture of cuneiform bone of foot
825.25 Closed fracture of metatarsal bone(s)
825.29 Other closed fracture of tarsal and metatarsal bones
825.31 Open fracture of astragalus
825.33 Open fracture of cuboid bone
825.34 Open fracture of cuneiform bone of foot,
825.35 Open fracture of metatarsal bone(s)
825.39 Other open fractures of tarsal and metatarsal bones
826.0 Closed fracture of one or more phalanges of foot
826.1 Open fracture of one or more phalanges of foot
827.0 Other, multiple and ill-defined closed fractures of lower limb
827.1 Other, multiple and ill-defined open fractures of lower limb
837.0 Closed dislocation of ankle
837.1 Open dislocation of ankle
838.01 Closed dislocation of tarsal (bone), joint unspecified ▽
838.02 Closed dislocation of midtarsal (joint)
838.03 Closed dislocation of tarsometatarsal (joint)
838.04 Closed dislocation of metatarsal (bone), joint unspecified ▽
838.05 Closed dislocation of metatarsophalangeal (joint)
838.06 Closed dislocation of interphalangeal (joint), foot
838.09 Closed dislocation of other part of foot
838.10 Open dislocation of foot, unspecified part ▽
838.11 Open dislocation of tarsal (bone), joint unspecified ▽
838.12 Open dislocation of midtarsal (joint)
838.13 Open dislocation of tarsometatarsal (joint)
838.14 Open dislocation of metatarsal (bone), joint unspecified ▽
838.15 Open dislocation of metatarsophalangeal (joint)
838.16 Open dislocation of interphalangeal (joint), foot
838.19 Open dislocation of other part of foot
845.01 Sprain and strain of deltoid (ligament) of ankle
845.02 Sprain and strain of calcaneofibular (ligament)
845.03 Sprain and strain of tibiofibular (ligament)
845.09 Other ankle sprain and strain
845.10 Sprain and strain of unspecified site of foot ▽
845.11 Sprain and strain of tarsometatarsal (joint) (ligament)
845.12 Sprain and strain of metatarsaophalangeal (joint)
845.13 Sprain and strain of interphalangeal (joint), of toe
845.19 Other foot sprain and strain
891.0 Open wound of knee, leg (except thigh), and ankle, without mention of complication — (Use additional code to identify infection)
891.1 Open wound of knee, leg (except thigh), and ankle, complicated — (Use additional code to identify infection)
891.2 Open wound of knee, leg (except thigh), and ankle, with tendon involvement — (Use additional code to identify infection)

892.0 Open wound of foot except toe(s) alone, without mention of complication — (Use additional code to identify infection)
892.1 Open wound of foot except toe(s) alone, complicated — (Use additional code to identify infection)
892.2 Open wound of foot except toe(s) alone, with tendon involvement — (Use additional code to identify infection)
893.0 Open wound of toe(s), without mention of complication — (Use additional code to identify infection)
893.1 Open wound of toe(s), complicated — (Use additional code to identify infection)
893.2 Open wound of toe(s), with tendon involvement — (Use additional code to identify infection)
894.0 Multiple and unspecified open wound of lower limb, without mention of complication — (Use additional code to identify infection)
894.1 Multiple and unspecified open wound of lower limb, complicated — (Use additional code to identify infection)
894.2 Multiple and unspecified open wound of lower limb, with tendon involvement — (Use additional code to identify infection)
905.4 Late effect of fracture of lower extremities
959.7 Injury, other and unspecified, knee, leg, ankle, and foot
V54.16 Aftercare for healing traumatic fracture of lower leg
V54.19 Aftercare for healing traumatic fracture of other bone
V54.26 Aftercare for healing pathologic fracture of lower leg
V54.29 Aftercare for healing pathologic fracture of other bone
V54.89 Other orthopedic aftercare
V67.00 Follow-up examination, following unspecified surgery ▽
V67.09 Follow-up examination, following other surgery

ICD-9-CM Procedural

93.53 Application of other cast
97.12 Replacement of cast on lower limb

HCPCS Level II Supplies & Services

A4580 Cast supplies (e.g., plaster)
A4590 Special casting material (e.g., fiberglass)
Q4037 Cast supplies, short leg cast, adult (11 years +), plaster
Q4038 Cast supplies, short leg cast, adult (11 years +), fiberglass
Q4039 Cast supplies, short leg cast, pediatric (0-10 years), plaster

29435

29435 Application of patellar tendon bearing (PTB) cast

ICD-9-CM Diagnostic

717.83 Old disruption of anterior cruciate ligament
732.4 Juvenile osteochondrosis of lower extremity, excluding foot
733.93 Stress fracture of tibia or fibula
823.20 Closed fracture of shaft of tibia
823.21 Closed fracture of shaft of fibula
823.22 Closed fracture of shaft of fibula with tibia
823.40 Torus fracture of tibia alone
823.41 Torus fracture of fibula alone
823.42 Torus fracture of fibula with tibia
823.80 Closed fracture of unspecified part of tibia ▽
823.81 Closed fracture of unspecified part of fibula ▽
823.82 Closed fracture of unspecified part of fibula with tibia ▽
836.0 Tear of medial cartilage or meniscus of knee, current
V54.16 Aftercare for healing traumatic fracture of lower leg
V54.26 Aftercare for healing pathologic fracture of lower leg
V54.89 Other orthopedic aftercare

ICD-9-CM Procedural

93.53 Application of other cast
97.12 Replacement of cast on lower limb

HCPCS Level II Supplies & Services

A4580 Cast supplies (e.g., plaster)
A4590 Special casting material (e.g., fiberglass)
A6441 Padding bandage, non-elastic, non-woven/non-knitted, width greater than or equal to three inches and less than five inches, per yard
Q4037 Cast supplies, short leg cast, adult (11 years +), plaster
Q4038 Cast supplies, short leg cast, adult (11 years +), fiberglass

29440

29440 Adding walker to previously applied cast

ICD-9-CM Diagnostic

733.93 Stress fracture of tibia or fibula
733.94 Stress fracture of the metatarsals
733.95 Stress fracture of other bone
733.99 Other disorders of bone and cartilage
822.0 Closed fracture of patella
823.01 Closed fracture of upper end of fibula
823.02 Closed fracture of upper end of fibula with tibia
823.20 Closed fracture of shaft of tibia
823.22 Closed fracture of shaft of fibula with tibia
823.32 Open fracture of shaft of fibula with tibia
823.40 Torus fracture of tibia alone
823.41 Torus fracture of fibula alone
823.42 Torus fracture of fibula with tibia
823.80 Closed fracture of unspecified part of tibia ▽
823.81 Closed fracture of unspecified part of fibula ▽
823.82 Closed fracture of unspecified part of fibula with tibia ▽
824.0 Closed fracture of medial malleolus
824.1 Open fracture of medial malleolus
824.2 Closed fracture of lateral malleolus
824.3 Open fracture of lateral malleolus
824.4 Closed bimalleolar fracture
824.5 Open bimalleolar fracture
824.6 Closed trimalleolar fracture
824.7 Open trimalleolar fracture
V54.16 Aftercare for healing traumatic fracture of lower leg
V54.19 Aftercare for healing traumatic fracture of other bone
V54.26 Aftercare for healing pathologic fracture of lower leg
V54.29 Aftercare for healing pathologic fracture of other bone
V54.89 Other orthopedic aftercare

ICD-9-CM Procedural

93.59 Other immobilization, pressure, and attention to wound

HCPCS Level II Supplies & Services

A4580 Cast supplies (e.g., plaster)
A4590 Special casting material (e.g., fiberglass)
A6441 Padding bandage, non-elastic, non-woven/non-knitted, width greater than or equal to three inches and less than five inches, per yard
Q4050 Cast supplies, for unlisted types and materials of casts
S8430 Padding for compression bandage, roll

29445

29445 Application of rigid total contact leg cast

ICD-9-CM Diagnostic

454.0 Varicose veins of lower extremities with ulcer
454.1 Varicose veins of lower extremities with inflammation
454.2 Varicose veins of lower extremities with ulcer and inflammation
454.8 Varicose veins of the lower extremities with other complications
454.9 Asymptomatic varicose veins
459.10 Postphlebitic syndrome without complications
459.11 Postphlebitic syndrome with ulcer
459.12 Postphlebitic syndrome with inflammation
459.13 Postphlebitic syndrome with ulcer and inflammation
459.19 Postphlebitic syndrome with other complication
459.30 Chronic venous hypertension without complications
459.31 Chronic venous hypertension with ulcer
459.32 Chronic venous hypertension with inflammation
459.33 Chronic venous hypertension with ulcer and inflammation
459.39 Chronic venous hypertension with other complication
459.81 Unspecified venous (peripheral) insufficiency — (Use additional code for any associated ulceration: 707.10-707.9) ▽

ICD-9-CM Procedural

93.53 Application of other cast
97.12 Replacement of cast on lower limb

HCPCS Level II Supplies & Services

A4580 Cast supplies (e.g., plaster)
A4590 Special casting material (e.g., fiberglass)
A6441 Padding bandage, non-elastic, non-woven/non-knitted, width greater than or equal to three inches and less than five inches, per yard
Q4037 Cast supplies, short leg cast, adult (11 years +), plaster

Q4038 Cast supplies, short leg cast, adult (11 years +), fiberglass

29450

29450 Application of clubfoot cast with molding or manipulation, long or short leg

ICD-9-CM Diagnostic

736.71 Acquired equinovarus deformity
736.76 Other acquired calcaneus deformity
736.89 Other acquired deformity of other parts of limb
754.50 Congenital talipes varus
754.51 Congenital talipes equinovarus
754.52 Congenital metatarsus primus varus
754.53 Congenital metatarsus varus
754.59 Other congenital varus deformity of feet
754.60 Congenital talipes valgus
754.61 Congenital pes planus
754.62 Talipes calcaneovalgus
754.70 Unspecified talipes ▽
754.79 Other congenital deformity of feet
755.67 Congenital anomalies of foot, not elsewhere classified
V54.89 Other orthopedic aftercare

ICD-9-CM Procedural

93.53 Application of other cast
97.12 Replacement of cast on lower limb

HCPCS Level II Supplies & Services

A4580 Cast supplies (e.g., plaster)
A4590 Special casting material (e.g., fiberglass)
A6441 Padding bandage, non-elastic, non-woven/non-knitted, width greater than or equal to three inches and less than five inches, per yard
Q4035 Cast supplies, long leg cylinder cast, pediatric (0-10 years), plaster
Q4036 Cast supplies, long leg cylinder cast, pediatric (0-10 years), fiberglass

29505

29505 Application of long leg splint (thigh to ankle or toes)

ICD-9-CM Diagnostic

717.7 Chondromalacia of patella
717.83 Old disruption of anterior cruciate ligament
718.36 Recurrent dislocation of lower leg joint
719.06 Effusion of lower leg joint
726.60 Unspecified enthesopathy of knee ▽
726.64 Patellar tendinitis
727.65 Nontraumatic rupture of quadriceps tendon
727.67 Nontraumatic rupture of Achilles tendon
732.4 Juvenile osteochondrosis of lower extremity, excluding foot
733.93 Stress fracture of tibia or fibula
733.95 Stress fracture of other bone
754.42 Congenital bowing of femur
821.01 Closed fracture of shaft of femur
821.22 Closed fracture of lower epiphysis of femur
821.23 Closed supracondylar fracture of femur
822.0 Closed fracture of patella
822.1 Open fracture of patella
823.02 Closed fracture of upper end of fibula with tibia
823.10 Open fracture of upper end of tibia
823.32 Open fracture of shaft of fibula with tibia
836.0 Tear of medial cartilage or meniscus of knee, current
836.2 Other tear of cartilage or meniscus of knee, current
836.3 Closed dislocation of patella
844.0 Sprain and strain of lateral collateral ligament of knee
844.1 Sprain and strain of medial collateral ligament of knee
844.2 Sprain and strain of cruciate ligament of knee
844.3 Sprain and strain of tibiofibular (joint) (ligament) superior, of knee
844.8 Sprain and strain of other specified sites of knee and leg
844.9 Sprain and strain of unspecified site of knee and leg ▽
924.11 Contusion of knee

ICD-9-CM Procedural

93.45 Thomas' splint traction
93.54 Application of splint
97.14 Replacement of other device for musculoskeletal immobilization

HCPCS Level II Supplies & Services

A4570 Splint
A4580 Cast supplies (e.g., plaster)
Q4041 Cast supplies, long leg splint, adult (11 years +), plaster
Q4042 Cast supplies, long leg splint, adult (11 years +), fiberglass
Q4043 Cast supplies, long leg splint, pediatric (0-10 years), plaster

29515

29515 Application of short leg splint (calf to foot)

ICD-9-CM Diagnostic

718.87 Other joint derangement, not elsewhere classified, ankle and foot
845.00 Unspecified site of ankle sprain and strain ▽
845.01 Sprain and strain of deltoid (ligament) of ankle
845.02 Sprain and strain of calcaneofibular (ligament)
845.03 Sprain and strain of tibiofibular (ligament)
845.09 Other ankle sprain and strain

ICD-9-CM Procedural

93.54 Application of splint
97.14 Replacement of other device for musculoskeletal immobilization

HCPCS Level II Supplies & Services

A4570 Splint
A4580 Cast supplies (e.g., plaster)
A6441 Padding bandage, non-elastic, non-woven/non-knitted, width greater than or equal to three inches and less than five inches, per yard
Q4045 Cast supplies, short leg splint, adult (11 years +), plaster
Q4046 Cast supplies, short leg splint, adult (11 years +), fiberglass

29520

29520 Strapping; hip

ICD-9-CM Diagnostic

718.75 Developmental dislocation of joint, pelvic region and thigh
835.00 Closed dislocation of hip, unspecified site ▽
835.01 Closed posterior dislocation of hip
835.02 Closed obturator dislocation of hip
835.03 Other closed anterior dislocation of hip
843.0 Iliofemoral (ligament) sprain and strain
843.1 Ischiocapsular (ligament) sprain and strain
843.8 Sprain and strain of other specified sites of hip and thigh
843.9 Sprain and strain of unspecified site of hip and thigh ▽

ICD-9-CM Procedural

93.59 Other immobilization, pressure, and attention to wound
97.14 Replacement of other device for musculoskeletal immobilization

HCPCS Level II Supplies & Services

A4450 Tape, non-waterproof, per 18 sq. inches
A4452 Tape, waterproof, per 18 sq. inches
A4649 Surgical supply; miscellaneous

29530

29530 Strapping; knee

ICD-9-CM Diagnostic

717.7 Chondromalacia of patella
717.81 Old disruption of lateral collateral ligament
717.82 Old disruption of medial collateral ligament
717.83 Old disruption of anterior cruciate ligament
718.36 Recurrent dislocation of lower leg joint
719.06 Effusion of lower leg joint
726.60 Unspecified enthesopathy of knee ▽
726.64 Patellar tendinitis
726.65 Prepatellar bursitis
729.4 Unspecified fasciitis ▽
729.81 Swelling of limb
836.0 Tear of medial cartilage or meniscus of knee, current
836.1 Tear of lateral cartilage or meniscus of knee, current
836.2 Other tear of cartilage or meniscus of knee, current
836.3 Closed dislocation of patella
844.0 Sprain and strain of lateral collateral ligament of knee
844.1 Sprain and strain of medial collateral ligament of knee
844.2 Sprain and strain of cruciate ligament of knee
844.3 Sprain and strain of tibiofibular (joint) (ligament) superior, of knee
844.8 Sprain and strain of other specified sites of knee and leg
844.9 Sprain and strain of unspecified site of knee and leg ▽

891.0 Open wound of knee, leg (except thigh), and ankle, without mention of complication — (Use additional code to identify infection)
924.11 Contusion of knee

ICD-9-CM Procedural
93.59 Other immobilization, pressure, and attention to wound
97.14 Replacement of other device for musculoskeletal immobilization

HCPCS Level II Supplies & Services
A4450 Tape, non-waterproof, per 18 sq. inches
A4452 Tape, waterproof, per 18 sq. inches
A4649 Surgical supply; miscellaneous

29540
29540 Strapping; ankle and/or foot

ICD-9-CM Diagnostic
718.37 Recurrent dislocation of ankle and foot joint
718.87 Other joint derangement, not elsewhere classified, ankle and foot
719.27 Villonodular synovitis, ankle and foot
726.70 Unspecified enthesopathy of ankle and tarsus ▽
726.73 Calcaneal spur
726.79 Other enthesopathy of ankle and tarsus
727.06 Tenosynovitis of foot and ankle
728.71 Plantar fascial fibromatosis
736.79 Other acquired deformity of ankle and foot
845.01 Sprain and strain of deltoid (ligament) of ankle
924.21 Contusion of ankle
959.7 Injury, other and unspecified, knee, leg, ankle, and foot

ICD-9-CM Procedural
93.59 Other immobilization, pressure, and attention to wound
97.14 Replacement of other device for musculoskeletal immobilization

HCPCS Level II Supplies & Services
A4450 Tape, non-waterproof, per 18 sq. inches
A4452 Tape, waterproof, per 18 sq. inches
A4649 Surgical supply; miscellaneous

29550
29550 Strapping; toes

ICD-9-CM Diagnostic
681.11 Onychia and paronychia of toe — (Use additional code to identify organism)
735.0 Hallux valgus (acquired)
735.1 Hallux varus (acquired)
735.2 Hallux rigidus
735.3 Hallux malleus
735.4 Other hammer toe (acquired)
735.5 Claw toe (acquired)
735.8 Other acquired deformity of toe
826.0 Closed fracture of one or more phalanges of foot
826.1 Open fracture of one or more phalanges of foot
845.10 Sprain and strain of unspecified site of foot ▽
924.3 Contusion of toe

ICD-9-CM Procedural
93.59 Other immobilization, pressure, and attention to wound
97.14 Replacement of other device for musculoskeletal immobilization

HCPCS Level II Supplies & Services
A4450 Tape, non-waterproof, per 18 sq. inches
A4452 Tape, waterproof, per 18 sq. inches
A4649 Surgical supply; miscellaneous

29580
29580 Strapping; Unna boot

ICD-9-CM Diagnostic
250.70 Diabetes with peripheral circulatory disorders, type II or unspecified type, not stated as uncontrolled — (Use additional code to identify manifestation: 443.81, 785.4)
250.71 Diabetes with peripheral circulatory disorders, type I [juvenile type], not stated as uncontrolled — (Use additional code to identify manifestation: 443.81, 785.4)
250.72 Diabetes with peripheral circulatory disorders, type II or unspecified type, uncontrolled — (Use additional code to identify manifestation: 443.81, 785.4)
250.73 Diabetes with peripheral circulatory disorders, type I [juvenile type], uncontrolled — (Use additional code to identify manifestation: 443.81, 785.4)
250.80 Diabetes with other specified manifestations, type II or unspecified type, not stated as uncontrolled — (Use additional code to identify manifestation: 707.10-707.9, 731.8. Use additional E code to identify cause, if drug-induced)
250.82 Diabetes with other specified manifestations, type II or unspecified type, uncontrolled — (Use additional code to identify manifestation: 707.10-707.9, 731.8. Use additional E code to identify cause, if drug-induced)
250.83 Diabetes with other specified manifestations, type I [juvenile type], uncontrolled — (Use additional code to identify manifestation: 707.10-707.9, 731.8. Use additional E code to identify cause, if drug-induced)
443.81 Peripheral angiopathy in diseases classified elsewhere — (Code first underlying disease, 250.7) ☒
443.9 Unspecified peripheral vascular disease ▽
451.9 Phlebitis and thrombophlebitis of unspecified site — (Use additional E code to identify drug, if drug-induced) ▽
454.0 Varicose veins of lower extremities with ulcer
454.1 Varicose veins of lower extremities with inflammation
454.2 Varicose veins of lower extremities with ulcer and inflammation
454.8 Varicose veins of the lower extremities with other complications
457.1 Other noninfectious lymphedema
459.10 Postphlebitic syndrome without complications
459.11 Postphlebitic syndrome with ulcer
459.12 Postphlebitic syndrome with inflammation
459.13 Postphlebitic syndrome with ulcer and inflammation
459.19 Postphlebitic syndrome with other complication
459.30 Chronic venous hypertension without complications
459.31 Chronic venous hypertension with ulcer
459.32 Chronic venous hypertension with inflammation
459.33 Chronic venous hypertension with ulcer and inflammation
459.39 Chronic venous hypertension with other complication
459.81 Unspecified venous (peripheral) insufficiency — (Use additional code for any associated ulceration: 707.10-707.9) ▽
682.7 Cellulitis and abscess of foot, except toes — (Use additional code to identify organism)
707.10 Ulcer of lower limb, unspecified ▽
707.13 Ulcer of ankle
707.14 Ulcer of heel and midfoot
707.15 Ulcer of other part of foot
707.8 Chronic ulcer of other specified site
707.9 Chronic ulcer of unspecified site ▽
728.71 Plantar fascial fibromatosis
731.8 Other bone involvement in diseases classified elsewhere — (Code first underlying disease, 250.8. Use additional code to specify bone condition: 730.00-730.09) ☒
782.3 Edema
785.4 Gangrene — (Code first any associated underlying condition:250.7, 443.0)
891.0 Open wound of knee, leg (except thigh), and ankle, without mention of complication — (Use additional code to identify infection)
891.1 Open wound of knee, leg (except thigh), and ankle, complicated — (Use additional code to identify infection)
892.1 Open wound of foot except toe(s) alone, complicated — (Use additional code to identify infection)

ICD-9-CM Procedural
93.59 Other immobilization, pressure, and attention to wound
97.14 Replacement of other device for musculoskeletal immobilization

HCPCS Level II Supplies & Services
L3260 Surgical boot/shoe, each

29590
29590 Denis-Browne splint strapping

ICD-9-CM Diagnostic
735.0 Hallux valgus (acquired)
735.1 Hallux varus (acquired)
735.2 Hallux rigidus
735.3 Hallux malleus

ICD-9-CM Procedural
93.59 Other immobilization, pressure, and attention to wound
97.14 Replacement of other device for musculoskeletal immobilization

▽ Unspecified code ☒ Manifestation code
♀ Female diagnosis ♂ Male diagnosis

HCPCS Level II Supplies & Services

A4450 Tape, non-waterproof, per 18 sq. inches
A4452 Tape, waterproof, per 18 sq. inches
A4570 Splint

29700–29715

29700 Removal or bivalving; gauntlet, boot or body cast
29705 full arm or full leg cast
29710 shoulder or hip spica, Minerva, or Risser jacket, etc.
29715 turnbuckle jacket

ICD-9-CM Diagnostic

V54.10 Aftercare for healing traumatic fracture of arm, unspecified ▽
V54.11 Aftercare for healing traumatic fracture of upper arm
V54.12 Aftercare for healing traumatic fracture of lower arm
V54.13 Aftercare for healing traumatic fracture of hip
V54.14 Aftercare for healing traumatic fracture of leg, unspecified ▽
V54.15 Aftercare for healing traumatic fracture of upper leg
V54.16 Aftercare for healing traumatic fracture of lower leg
V54.19 Aftercare for healing traumatic fracture of other bone
V54.20 Aftercare for healing pathologic fracture of arm, unspecified ▽
V54.21 Aftercare for healing pathologic fracture of upper arm
V54.22 Aftercare for healing pathologic fracture of lower arm
V54.23 Aftercare for healing pathologic fracture of hip
V54.24 Aftercare for healing pathologic fracture of leg, unspecified ▽
V54.25 Aftercare for healing pathologic fracture of upper leg
V54.26 Aftercare for healing pathologic fracture of lower leg
V54.29 Aftercare for healing pathologic fracture of other bone
V54.89 Other orthopedic aftercare
V67.4 Treatment of healed fracture follow-up examination

ICD-9-CM Procedural

97.88 Removal of external immobilization device

HCPCS Level II Supplies & Services

A4649 Surgical supply; miscellaneous

29720

29720 Repair of spica, body cast or jacket

ICD-9-CM Diagnostic

V54.13 Aftercare for healing traumatic fracture of hip
V54.14 Aftercare for healing traumatic fracture of leg, unspecified ▽
V54.15 Aftercare for healing traumatic fracture of upper leg
V54.16 Aftercare for healing traumatic fracture of lower leg
V54.19 Aftercare for healing traumatic fracture of other bone
V54.23 Aftercare for healing pathologic fracture of hip
V54.24 Aftercare for healing pathologic fracture of leg, unspecified ▽
V54.25 Aftercare for healing pathologic fracture of upper leg
V54.26 Aftercare for healing pathologic fracture of lower leg
V54.29 Aftercare for healing pathologic fracture of other bone
V54.89 Other orthopedic aftercare
V67.4 Treatment of healed fracture follow-up examination

ICD-9-CM Procedural

93.59 Other immobilization, pressure, and attention to wound

HCPCS Level II Supplies & Services

A4580 Cast supplies (e.g., plaster)
A4590 Special casting material (e.g., fiberglass)

29730–29750

29730 Windowing of cast
29740 Wedging of cast (except clubfoot casts)
29750 Wedging of clubfoot cast

ICD-9-CM Diagnostic

V54.10 Aftercare for healing traumatic fracture of arm, unspecified ▽
V54.11 Aftercare for healing traumatic fracture of upper arm
V54.12 Aftercare for healing traumatic fracture of lower arm
V54.13 Aftercare for healing traumatic fracture of hip
V54.14 Aftercare for healing traumatic fracture of leg, unspecified ▽
V54.15 Aftercare for healing traumatic fracture of upper leg
V54.16 Aftercare for healing traumatic fracture of lower leg
V54.19 Aftercare for healing traumatic fracture of other bone
V54.20 Aftercare for healing pathologic fracture of arm, unspecified ▽
V54.21 Aftercare for healing pathologic fracture of upper arm
V54.22 Aftercare for healing pathologic fracture of lower arm
V54.23 Aftercare for healing pathologic fracture of hip
V54.24 Aftercare for healing pathologic fracture of leg, unspecified ▽
V54.25 Aftercare for healing pathologic fracture of upper leg
V54.26 Aftercare for healing pathologic fracture of lower leg
V54.29 Aftercare for healing pathologic fracture of other bone
V54.89 Other orthopedic aftercare

ICD-9-CM Procedural

93.59 Other immobilization, pressure, and attention to wound

HCPCS Level II Supplies & Services

A4580 Cast supplies (e.g., plaster)
A4590 Special casting material (e.g., fiberglass)

Endoscopy/Arthroscopy

29800

29800 Arthroscopy, temporomandibular joint, diagnostic, with or without synovial biopsy (separate procedure)

ICD-9-CM Diagnostic

170.0 Malignant neoplasm of bones of skull and face, except mandible
524.29 Other anomalies of dental arch relationship
524.60 Unspecified temporomandibular joint disorders ▽
524.61 Adhesions and ankylosis (bony or fibrous) of temporomandibular joint
524.62 Arthralgia of temporomandibular joint
524.63 Articular disc disorder (reducing or non-reducing) of temporomandibular joint
524.64 Temporomandibular joint sounds on opening and/or closing the jaw
524.69 Other specified temporomandibular joint disorders
525.8 Other specified disorders of the teeth and supporting structures
526.1 Fissural cysts of jaw
714.0 Rheumatoid arthritis — (Use additional code to identify manifestation: 357.1, 359.6)
830.0 Closed dislocation of jaw

ICD-9-CM Procedural

76.19 Other diagnostic procedures on facial bones and joints
80.29 Arthroscopy of other specified site
80.39 Biopsy of joint structure of other specified site

HCPCS Level II Supplies & Services

A4305 Disposable drug delivery system, flow rate of 50 ml or greater per hour
A4306 Disposable drug delivery system, flow rate of 5 ml or less per hour
A4550 Surgical trays

29804

29804 Arthroscopy, temporomandibular joint, surgical

ICD-9-CM Diagnostic

524.02 Mandibular hyperplasia
524.04 Mandibular hypoplasia
524.11 Maxillary asymmetry
524.59 Other dentofacial functional abnormalities
524.61 Adhesions and ankylosis (bony or fibrous) of temporomandibular joint
524.62 Arthralgia of temporomandibular joint
524.63 Articular disc disorder (reducing or non-reducing) of temporomandibular joint
524.64 Temporomandibular joint sounds on opening and/or closing the jaw
524.69 Other specified temporomandibular joint disorders
714.0 Rheumatoid arthritis — (Use additional code to identify manifestation: 357.1, 359.6)
830.0 Closed dislocation of jaw
830.1 Open dislocation of jaw

ICD-9-CM Procedural

76.2 Local excision or destruction of lesion of facial bone
76.99 Other operations on facial bones and joints

HCPCS Level II Supplies & Services

A4305 Disposable drug delivery system, flow rate of 50 ml or greater per hour
A4306 Disposable drug delivery system, flow rate of 5 ml or less per hour

A4550 Surgical trays

29805

29805 Arthroscopy, shoulder, diagnostic, with or without synovial biopsy (separate procedure)

ICD-9-CM Diagnostic

170.4 Malignant neoplasm of scapula and long bones of upper limb
195.4 Malignant neoplasm of upper limb
213.4 Benign neoplasm of scapula and long bones of upper limb
215.2 Other benign neoplasm of connective and other soft tissue of upper limb, including shoulder
238.0 Neoplasm of uncertain behavior of bone and articular cartilage
239.2 Neoplasms of unspecified nature of bone, soft tissue, and skin
275.40 Unspecified disorder of calcium metabolism — (Use additional code to identify any associated mental retardation) ▽
275.41 Hypocalcemia — (Use additional code to identify any associated mental retardation)
275.42 Hypercalcemia — (Use additional code to identify any associated mental retardation)
275.49 Other disorders of calcium metabolism — (Use additional code to identify any associated mental retardation)
357.1 Polyneuropathy in collagen vascular disease — (Code first underlying disease: 446.0, 710.0, 714.0) ☒
359.6 Symptomatic inflammatory myopathy in diseases classified elsewhere — (Code first underlying disease: 135, 140.0-208.9, 277.3, 446.0, 710.0, 710.1, 710.2, 714.0) ☒
446.0 Polyarteritis nodosa
710.0 Systemic lupus erythematosus — (Use additional code to identify manifestation: 424.91, 581.81, 582.81, 583.81)
710.1 Systemic sclerosis — (Use additional code to identify manifestation: 359.6, 517.2)
710.2 Sicca syndrome
711.01 Pyogenic arthritis, shoulder region — (Use additional code to identify infectious organism: 041.0-041.8)
712.11 Chondrocalcinosis due to dicalcium phosphate crystals, shoulder region — (Code first underlying disease, 275.4) ☒
712.21 Chondrocalcinosis due to pyrophosphate crystals, shoulder region — (Code first underlying disease, 275.4) ☒
714.0 Rheumatoid arthritis — (Use additional code to identify manifestation: 357.1, 359.6)
715.11 Primary localized osteoarthrosis, shoulder region
715.21 Secondary localized osteoarthrosis, shoulder region
715.91 Osteoarthrosis, unspecified whether generalized or localized, shoulder region ▽
716.11 Traumatic arthropathy, shoulder region
716.91 Unspecified arthropathy, shoulder region ▽
718.01 Articular cartilage disorder, shoulder region
718.21 Pathological dislocation of shoulder joint
718.31 Recurrent dislocation of shoulder joint
718.41 Contracture of shoulder joint
718.71 Developmental dislocation of joint, shoulder region
718.81 Other joint derangement, not elsewhere classified, shoulder region
719.01 Effusion of shoulder joint
719.11 Herarthrosis, shoulder region
719.21 Villonodular synovitis, shoulder region
719.31 Palindromic rheumatism, shoulder region
719.41 Pain in joint, shoulder region
719.51 Stiffness of joint, not elsewhere classified, shoulder region
719.81 Other specified disorders of shoulder joint
726.0 Adhesive capsulitis of shoulder
726.11 Calcifying tendinitis of shoulder
726.12 Bicipital tenosynovitis
726.19 Other specified disorders of rotator cuff syndrome of shoulder and allied disorders
726.2 Other affections of shoulder region, not elsewhere classified
727.61 Complete rupture of rotator cuff
755.59 Other congenital anomaly of upper limb, including shoulder girdle
831.00 Closed dislocation of shoulder, unspecified site ▽
831.01 Closed anterior dislocation of humerus
831.03 Closed inferior dislocation of humerus
840.0 Acromioclavicular (joint) (ligament) sprain and strain
840.1 Coracoclavicular (ligament) sprain and strain
840.2 Coracohumeral (ligament) sprain and strain
840.3 Infraspinatus (muscle) (tendon) sprain and strain
840.4 Rotator cuff (capsule) sprain and strain
840.5 Subscapularis (muscle) sprain and strain
840.6 Supraspinatus (muscle) (tendon) sprain and strain
840.9 Sprain and strain of unspecified site of shoulder and upper arm ▽
905.2 Late effect of fracture of upper extremities
905.6 Late effect of dislocation

ICD-9-CM Procedural

80.21 Arthroscopy of shoulder
80.31 Biopsy of joint structure of shoulder

HCPCS Level II Supplies & Services

HCPCS Level II codes are used to report the supplies, durable medical equipment, and certain medical services provided on an outpatient basis. Because the procedure(s) represented on this page would be performed in an inpatient or outpatient facility, no HCPCS Level II codes apply.

29806

29806 Arthroscopy, shoulder, surgical; capsulorrhaphy

ICD-9-CM Diagnostic

718.21 Pathological dislocation of shoulder joint
718.31 Recurrent dislocation of shoulder joint
831.00 Closed dislocation of shoulder, unspecified site ▽
831.01 Closed anterior dislocation of humerus
831.02 Closed posterior dislocation of humerus
831.03 Closed inferior dislocation of humerus
831.10 Open unspecified dislocation of shoulder ▽
831.11 Open anterior dislocation of humerus
831.12 Open posterior dislocation of humerus
831.13 Open inferior dislocation of humerus
840.2 Coracohumeral (ligament) sprain and strain
840.4 Rotator cuff (capsule) sprain and strain
840.5 Subscapularis (muscle) sprain and strain

ICD-9-CM Procedural

81.93 Suture of capsule or ligament of upper extremity

HCPCS Level II Supplies & Services

HCPCS Level II codes are used to report the supplies, durable medical equipment, and certain medical services provided on an outpatient basis. Because the procedure(s) represented on this page would be performed in an inpatient or outpatient facility, no HCPCS Level II codes apply.

29807

29807 Arthroscopy, shoulder, surgical; repair of SLAP lesion

ICD-9-CM Diagnostic

718.31 Recurrent dislocation of shoulder joint
840.7 Superior glenoid labrum lesions (SLAP)

ICD-9-CM Procedural

81.96 Other repair of joint

29819

29819 Arthroscopy, shoulder, surgical; with removal of loose body or foreign body

ICD-9-CM Diagnostic

275.40 Unspecified disorder of calcium metabolism — (Use additional code to identify any associated mental retardation) ▽
275.42 Hypercalcemia — (Use additional code to identify any associated mental retardation)
275.49 Other disorders of calcium metabolism — (Use additional code to identify any associated mental retardation)
718.01 Articular cartilage disorder, shoulder region
718.11 Loose body in shoulder joint
729.6 Residual foreign body in soft tissue

ICD-9-CM Procedural

80.21 Arthroscopy of shoulder

▽ Unspecified code ☒ Manifestation code
♀ Female diagnosis ♂ Male diagnosis

29820–29821

29820 Arthroscopy, shoulder, surgical; synovectomy, partial
29821 synovectomy, complete

ICD-9-CM Diagnostic

170.4 Malignant neoplasm of scapula and long bones of upper limb
195.4 Malignant neoplasm of upper limb
213.4 Benign neoplasm of scapula and long bones of upper limb
215.2 Other benign neoplasm of connective and other soft tissue of upper limb, including shoulder
238.0 Neoplasm of uncertain behavior of bone and articular cartilage
239.2 Neoplasms of unspecified nature of bone, soft tissue, and skin
275.41 Hypocalcemia — (Use additional code to identify any associated mental retardation)
275.42 Hypercalcemia — (Use additional code to identify any associated mental retardation)
357.1 Polyneuropathy in collagen vascular disease — (Code first underlying disease: 446.0, 710.0, 714.0) ☒
359.6 Symptomatic inflammatory myopathy in diseases classified elsewhere — (Code first underlying disease: 135, 140.0-208.9, 277.3, 446.0, 710.0, 710.1, 710.2, 714.0) ☒
446.0 Polyarteritis nodosa
710.0 Systemic lupus erythematosus — (Use additional code to identify manifestation: 424.91, 581.81, 582.81, 583.81)
710.1 Systemic sclerosis — (Use additional code to identify manifestation: 359.6, 517.2)
710.2 Sicca syndrome
712.11 Chondrocalcinosis due to dicalcium phosphate crystals, shoulder region — (Code first underlying disease, 275.4) ☒
712.12 Chondrocalcinosis due to dicalcium phosphate crystals, upper arm — (Code first underlying disease, 275.4) ☒
714.0 Rheumatoid arthritis — (Use additional code to identify manifestation: 357.1, 359.6)
715.11 Primary localized osteoarthrosis, shoulder region
719.21 Villonodular synovitis, shoulder region
726.0 Adhesive capsulitis of shoulder
726.11 Calcifying tendinitis of shoulder
726.12 Bicipital tenosynovitis
727.00 Unspecified synovitis and tenosynovitis ▽

ICD-9-CM Procedural

80.71 Synovectomy of shoulder

29822–29823

29822 Arthroscopy, shoulder, surgical; debridement, limited
29823 debridement, extensive

ICD-9-CM Diagnostic

357.1 Polyneuropathy in collagen vascular disease — (Code first underlying disease: 446.0, 710.0, 714.0) ☒
359.6 Symptomatic inflammatory myopathy in diseases classified elsewhere — (Code first underlying disease: 135, 140.0-208.9, 277.3, 446.0, 710.0, 710.1, 710.2, 714.0) ☒
446.0 Polyarteritis nodosa
710.0 Systemic lupus erythematosus — (Use additional code to identify manifestation: 424.91, 581.81, 582.81, 583.81)
710.1 Systemic sclerosis — (Use additional code to identify manifestation: 359.6, 517.2)
710.2 Sicca syndrome
714.0 Rheumatoid arthritis — (Use additional code to identify manifestation: 357.1, 359.6)
715.11 Primary localized osteoarthrosis, shoulder region
715.31 Localized osteoarthrosis not specified whether primary or secondary, shoulder region
715.91 Osteoarthrosis, unspecified whether generalized or localized, shoulder region ▽
716.01 Kaschin-Beck disease, shoulder region
716.11 Traumatic arthropathy, shoulder region
718.01 Articular cartilage disorder, shoulder region
718.31 Recurrent dislocation of shoulder joint
718.81 Other joint derangement, not elsewhere classified, shoulder region
719.01 Effusion of shoulder joint
719.21 Villonodular synovitis, shoulder region
719.41 Pain in joint, shoulder region
726.0 Adhesive capsulitis of shoulder
726.10 Unspecified disorders of bursae and tendons in shoulder region ▽
726.11 Calcifying tendinitis of shoulder
726.12 Bicipital tenosynovitis
726.19 Other specified disorders of rotator cuff syndrome of shoulder and allied disorders
726.2 Other affections of shoulder region, not elsewhere classified
727.00 Unspecified synovitis and tenosynovitis ▽
733.90 Disorder of bone and cartilage, unspecified ▽
840.0 Acromioclavicular (joint) (ligament) sprain and strain
840.4 Rotator cuff (capsule) sprain and strain
840.6 Supraspinatus (muscle) (tendon) sprain and strain
840.8 Sprain and strain of other specified sites of shoulder and upper arm

ICD-9-CM Procedural

80.81 Other local excision or destruction of lesion of shoulder joint

29824

29824 Arthroscopy, shoulder, surgical; distal claviculectomy including distal articular surface (Mumford procedure)

ICD-9-CM Diagnostic

170.3 Malignant neoplasm of ribs, sternum, and clavicle
196.3 Secondary and unspecified malignant neoplasm of lymph nodes of axilla and upper limb
198.5 Secondary malignant neoplasm of bone and bone marrow
198.89 Secondary malignant neoplasm of other specified sites
213.3 Benign neoplasm of ribs, sternum, and clavicle
238.0 Neoplasm of uncertain behavior of bone and articular cartilage
239.2 Neoplasms of unspecified nature of bone, soft tissue, and skin
715.11 Primary localized osteoarthrosis, shoulder region
715.21 Secondary localized osteoarthrosis, shoulder region
716.11 Traumatic arthropathy, shoulder region
716.61 Unspecified monoarthritis, shoulder region ▽
718.01 Articular cartilage disorder, shoulder region
718.31 Recurrent dislocation of shoulder joint
728.86 Necrotizing fasciitis — (Use additional code to identify infectious organism, 041.00-041.89, 785.4, if applicable)
730.11 Chronic osteomyelitis, shoulder region — (Use additional code to identify organism, 041.1)
733.49 Aseptic necrosis of other bone site
733.90 Disorder of bone and cartilage, unspecified ▽
738.8 Acquired musculoskeletal deformity of other specified site
785.4 Gangrene — (Code first any associated underlying condition:250.7, 443.0)
831.04 Closed dislocation of acromioclavicular (joint)

ICD-9-CM Procedural

77.81 Other partial ostectomy of scapula, clavicle, and thorax (ribs and sternum)

29825

29825 Arthroscopy, shoulder, surgical; with lysis and resection of adhesions, with or without manipulation

ICD-9-CM Diagnostic

357.1 Polyneuropathy in collagen vascular disease — (Code first underlying disease: 446.0, 710.0, 714.0) ☒
359.6 Symptomatic inflammatory myopathy in diseases classified elsewhere — (Code first underlying disease: 135, 140.0-208.9, 277.3, 446.0, 710.0, 710.1, 710.2, 714.0) ☒
446.0 Polyarteritis nodosa
710.0 Systemic lupus erythematosus — (Use additional code to identify manifestation: 424.91, 581.81, 582.81, 583.81)
710.1 Systemic sclerosis — (Use additional code to identify manifestation: 359.6, 517.2)
710.2 Sicca syndrome
714.0 Rheumatoid arthritis — (Use additional code to identify manifestation: 357.1, 359.6)
715.11 Primary localized osteoarthrosis, shoulder region
715.31 Localized osteoarthrosis not specified whether primary or secondary, shoulder region
715.91 Osteoarthrosis, unspecified whether generalized or localized, shoulder region ▽
716.11 Traumatic arthropathy, shoulder region
718.31 Recurrent dislocation of shoulder joint
718.41 Contracture of shoulder joint
718.51 Ankylosis of joint of shoulder region
726.0 Adhesive capsulitis of shoulder
726.10 Unspecified disorders of bursae and tendons in shoulder region ▽

▽ Unspecified code
♀ Female diagnosis
☒ Manifestation code
♂ Male diagnosis

726.11 Calcifying tendinitis of shoulder
726.12 Bicipital tenosynovitis
726.19 Other specified disorders of rotator cuff syndrome of shoulder and allied disorders
726.2 Other affections of shoulder region, not elsewhere classified
840.0 Acromioclavicular (joint) (ligament) sprain and strain
840.4 Rotator cuff (capsule) sprain and strain
840.6 Supraspinatus (muscle) (tendon) sprain and strain
840.9 Sprain and strain of unspecified site of shoulder and upper arm ▽

ICD-9-CM Procedural

80.41 Division of joint capsule, ligament, or cartilage of shoulder

29826

29826 Arthroscopy, shoulder, surgical; decompression of subacromial space with partial acromioplasty, with or without coracoacromial release

ICD-9-CM Diagnostic

353.0 Brachial plexus lesions
715.11 Primary localized osteoarthrosis, shoulder region
715.21 Secondary localized osteoarthrosis, shoulder region
715.31 Localized osteoarthrosis not specified whether primary or secondary, shoulder region
715.91 Osteoarthrosis, unspecified whether generalized or localized, shoulder region ▽
716.11 Traumatic arthropathy, shoulder region
718.01 Articular cartilage disorder, shoulder region
718.31 Recurrent dislocation of shoulder joint
718.51 Ankylosis of joint of shoulder region
718.81 Other joint derangement, not elsewhere classified, shoulder region
726.0 Adhesive capsulitis of shoulder
726.10 Unspecified disorders of bursae and tendons in shoulder region ▽
726.11 Calcifying tendinitis of shoulder
726.12 Bicipital tenosynovitis
726.19 Other specified disorders of rotator cuff syndrome of shoulder and allied disorders
726.2 Other affections of shoulder region, not elsewhere classified
727.61 Complete rupture of rotator cuff
840.0 Acromioclavicular (joint) (ligament) sprain and strain
840.4 Rotator cuff (capsule) sprain and strain
840.8 Sprain and strain of other specified sites of shoulder and upper arm

ICD-9-CM Procedural

81.82 Repair of recurrent dislocation of shoulder
81.83 Other repair of shoulder

29827

29827 Arthroscopy, shoulder, surgical; with rotator cuff repair

ICD-9-CM Diagnostic

715.10 Primary localized osteoarthrosis, specified site ▽
715.11 Primary localized osteoarthrosis, shoulder region
715.21 Secondary localized osteoarthrosis, shoulder region
715.31 Localized osteoarthrosis not specified whether primary or secondary, shoulder region
716.11 Traumatic arthropathy, shoulder region
716.61 Unspecified monoarthritis, shoulder region ▽
719.41 Pain in joint, shoulder region
726.10 Unspecified disorders of bursae and tendons in shoulder region ▽
727.61 Complete rupture of rotator cuff
831.00 Closed dislocation of shoulder, unspecified site ▽
831.01 Closed anterior dislocation of humerus
831.02 Closed posterior dislocation of humerus
831.03 Closed inferior dislocation of humerus
840.4 Rotator cuff (capsule) sprain and strain
927.00 Crushing injury of shoulder region — (Use additional code to identify any associated injuries: 800-829, 850.0-854.1, 860.0-869.1)
959.2 Injury, other and unspecified, shoulder and upper arm

ICD-9-CM Procedural

83.63 Rotator cuff repair

29830

29830 Arthroscopy, elbow, diagnostic, with or without synovial biopsy (separate procedure)

ICD-9-CM Diagnostic

170.4 Malignant neoplasm of scapula and long bones of upper limb
195.4 Malignant neoplasm of upper limb
213.4 Benign neoplasm of scapula and long bones of upper limb
215.2 Other benign neoplasm of connective and other soft tissue of upper limb, including shoulder
238.0 Neoplasm of uncertain behavior of bone and articular cartilage
239.2 Neoplasms of unspecified nature of bone, soft tissue, and skin
275.40 Unspecified disorder of calcium metabolism — (Use additional code to identify any associated mental retardation) ▽
275.41 Hypocalcemia — (Use additional code to identify any associated mental retardation)
275.42 Hypercalcemia — (Use additional code to identify any associated mental retardation)
275.49 Other disorders of calcium metabolism — (Use additional code to identify any associated mental retardation)
357.1 Polyneuropathy in collagen vascular disease — (Code first underlying disease: 446.0, 710.0, 714.0) ☒
359.6 Symptomatic inflammatory myopathy in diseases classified elsewhere — (Code first underlying disease: 135, 140.0-208.9, 277.3, 446.0, 710.0, 710.1, 710.2, 714.0) ☒
446.0 Polyarteritis nodosa
710.0 Systemic lupus erythematosus — (Use additional code to identify manifestation: 424.91, 581.81, 582.81, 583.81)
710.1 Systemic sclerosis — (Use additional code to identify manifestation: 359.6, 517.2)
710.2 Sicca syndrome
714.0 Rheumatoid arthritis — (Use additional code to identify manifestation: 357.1, 359.6)
715.12 Primary localized osteoarthrosis, upper arm
715.22 Secondary localized osteoarthrosis, upper arm
716.12 Traumatic arthropathy, upper arm
718.02 Articular cartilage disorder, upper arm
718.22 Pathological dislocation of upper arm joint
718.32 Recurrent dislocation of upper arm joint
718.42 Contracture of upper arm joint
719.22 Villonodular synovitis, upper arm
727.00 Unspecified synovitis and tenosynovitis ▽

ICD-9-CM Procedural

80.22 Arthroscopy of elbow
80.32 Biopsy of joint structure of elbow

HCPCS Level II Supplies & Services

A4305 Disposable drug delivery system, flow rate of 50 ml or greater per hour
A4306 Disposable drug delivery system, flow rate of 5 ml or less per hour
A4550 Surgical trays

29834

29834 Arthroscopy, elbow, surgical; with removal of loose body or foreign body

ICD-9-CM Diagnostic

718.02 Articular cartilage disorder, upper arm
718.12 Loose body in upper arm joint
729.6 Residual foreign body in soft tissue

ICD-9-CM Procedural

80.22 Arthroscopy of elbow

HCPCS Level II Supplies & Services

A4305 Disposable drug delivery system, flow rate of 50 ml or greater per hour
A4306 Disposable drug delivery system, flow rate of 5 ml or less per hour
A4550 Surgical trays

29835–29836

29835 Arthroscopy, elbow, surgical; synovectomy, partial
29836 synovectomy, complete

ICD-9-CM Diagnostic

275.40 Unspecified disorder of calcium metabolism — (Use additional code to identify any associated mental retardation) ▽

275.41 Hypocalcemia — (Use additional code to identify any associated mental retardation)
275.49 Other disorders of calcium metabolism — (Use additional code to identify any associated mental retardation)
357.1 Polyneuropathy in collagen vascular disease — (Code first underlying disease: 446.0, 710.0, 714.0) ☒
359.6 Symptomatic inflammatory myopathy in diseases classified elsewhere — (Code first underlying disease: 135, 140.0-208.9, 277.3, 446.0, 710.0, 710.1, 710.2, 714.0) ☒
446.0 Polyarteritis nodosa
710.0 Systemic lupus erythematosus — (Use additional code to identify manifestation: 424.91, 581.81, 582.81, 583.81)
710.1 Systemic sclerosis — (Use additional code to identify manifestation: 359.6, 517.2)
710.2 Sicca syndrome
712.12 Chondrocalcinosis due to dicalcium phosphate crystals, upper arm — (Code first underlying disease, 275.4) ☒
712.22 Chondrocalcinosis due to pyrophosphate crystals, upper arm — (Code first underlying disease, 275.4) ☒
714.0 Rheumatoid arthritis — (Use additional code to identify manifestation: 357.1, 359.6)
715.12 Primary localized osteoarthrosis, upper arm
718.32 Recurrent dislocation of upper arm joint
718.82 Other joint derangement, not elsewhere classified, upper arm
719.22 Villonodular synovitis, upper arm
727.00 Unspecified synovitis and tenosynovitis ▽

ICD-9-CM Procedural
80.72 Synovectomy of elbow

HCPCS Level II Supplies & Services
A4305 Disposable drug delivery system, flow rate of 50 ml or greater per hour
A4306 Disposable drug delivery system, flow rate of 5 ml or less per hour
A4550 Surgical trays

29837–29838
29837 Arthroscopy, elbow, surgical; debridement, limited
29838 debridement, extensive

ICD-9-CM Diagnostic
275.41 Hypocalcemia — (Use additional code to identify any associated mental retardation)
275.42 Hypercalcemia — (Use additional code to identify any associated mental retardation)
357.1 Polyneuropathy in collagen vascular disease — (Code first underlying disease: 446.0, 710.0, 714.0) ☒
359.6 Symptomatic inflammatory myopathy in diseases classified elsewhere — (Code first underlying disease: 135, 140.0-208.9, 277.3, 446.0, 710.0, 710.1, 710.2, 714.0) ☒
446.0 Polyarteritis nodosa
710.0 Systemic lupus erythematosus — (Use additional code to identify manifestation: 424.91, 581.81, 582.81, 583.81)
710.1 Systemic sclerosis — (Use additional code to identify manifestation: 359.6, 517.2)
710.2 Sicca syndrome
712.12 Chondrocalcinosis due to dicalcium phosphate crystals, upper arm — (Code first underlying disease, 275.4) ☒
712.22 Chondrocalcinosis due to pyrophosphate crystals, upper arm — (Code first underlying disease, 275.4) ☒
714.0 Rheumatoid arthritis — (Use additional code to identify manifestation: 357.1, 359.6)
715.12 Primary localized osteoarthrosis, upper arm
718.32 Recurrent dislocation of upper arm joint
718.82 Other joint derangement, not elsewhere classified, upper arm
719.22 Villonodular synovitis, upper arm
727.00 Unspecified synovitis and tenosynovitis ▽

ICD-9-CM Procedural
80.82 Other local excision or destruction of lesion of elbow joint

HCPCS Level II Supplies & Services
A4305 Disposable drug delivery system, flow rate of 50 ml or greater per hour
A4306 Disposable drug delivery system, flow rate of 5 ml or less per hour
A4550 Surgical trays

29840
29840 Arthroscopy, wrist, diagnostic, with or without synovial biopsy (separate procedure)

ICD-9-CM Diagnostic
171.2 Malignant neoplasm of connective and other soft tissue of upper limb, including shoulder
198.89 Secondary malignant neoplasm of other specified sites
215.2 Other benign neoplasm of connective and other soft tissue of upper limb, including shoulder
238.1 Neoplasm of uncertain behavior of connective and other soft tissue ▽
239.2 Neoplasms of unspecified nature of bone, soft tissue, and skin
275.40 Unspecified disorder of calcium metabolism — (Use additional code to identify any associated mental retardation) ▽
275.42 Hypercalcemia — (Use additional code to identify any associated mental retardation)
275.49 Other disorders of calcium metabolism — (Use additional code to identify any associated mental retardation)
357.1 Polyneuropathy in collagen vascular disease — (Code first underlying disease: 446.0, 710.0, 714.0) ☒
359.6 Symptomatic inflammatory myopathy in diseases classified elsewhere — (Code first underlying disease: 135, 140.0-208.9, 277.3, 446.0, 710.0, 710.1, 710.2, 714.0) ☒
446.0 Polyarteritis nodosa
710.0 Systemic lupus erythematosus — (Use additional code to identify manifestation: 424.91, 581.81, 582.81, 583.81)
710.1 Systemic sclerosis — (Use additional code to identify manifestation: 359.6, 517.2)
710.2 Sicca syndrome
714.0 Rheumatoid arthritis — (Use additional code to identify manifestation: 357.1, 359.6)
715.23 Secondary localized osteoarthrosis, forearm
716.13 Traumatic arthropathy, forearm
718.03 Articular cartilage disorder, forearm
718.23 Pathological dislocation of forearm joint
718.33 Recurrent dislocation of forearm joint
718.43 Contracture of forearm joint
719.23 Villonodular synovitis, forearm
727.09 Other synovitis and tenosynovitis

ICD-9-CM Procedural
80.23 Arthroscopy of wrist
80.33 Biopsy of joint structure of wrist

HCPCS Level II Supplies & Services
A4305 Disposable drug delivery system, flow rate of 50 ml or greater per hour
A4306 Disposable drug delivery system, flow rate of 5 ml or less per hour
A4550 Surgical trays

29843
29843 Arthroscopy, wrist, surgical; for infection, lavage and drainage

ICD-9-CM Diagnostic
711.03 Pyogenic arthritis, forearm — (Use additional code to identify infectious organism: 041.0-041.8)
711.43 Arthropathy associated with other bacterial diseases, forearm — (Code first underlying disease, such as: diseases classifiable to 010-040 (except 036.82), 090-099 (except 098.50)) ☒
711.53 Arthropathy associated with other viral diseases, forearm — (Code first underlying disease, such as: diseases classifiable to 045-049, 050-079 (except 056.71), 480, 487) ☒
711.63 Arthropathy associated with mycoses, forearm — (Code first underlying disease: 110.0-118) ☒
711.83 Arthropathy associated with other infectious and parasitic diseases, forearm — (Code first underlying disease, such as: diseases classifiable to 080-088, 100-104, 130-136) ☒
996.67 Infection and inflammatory reaction due to other internal orthopedic device, implant, and graft — (Use additional code to identify specified infections)
996.69 Infection and inflammatory reaction due to other internal prosthetic device, implant, and graft — (Use additional code to identify specified infections)
998.51 Infected postoperative seroma — (Use additional code to identify organism)
998.59 Other postoperative infection — (Use additional code to identify infection)

ICD-9-CM Procedural
80.23 Arthroscopy of wrist

▽ Unspecified code ♀ Female diagnosis ☒ Manifestation code ♂ Male diagnosis

HCPCS Level II Supplies & Services

A4305 Disposable drug delivery system, flow rate of 50 ml or greater per hour
A4306 Disposable drug delivery system, flow rate of 5 ml or less per hour
A4550 Surgical trays

29844–29845

29844 Arthroscopy, wrist, surgical; synovectomy, partial
29845 synovectomy, complete

ICD-9-CM Diagnostic

171.2 Malignant neoplasm of connective and other soft tissue of upper limb, including shoulder
198.89 Secondary malignant neoplasm of other specified sites
215.2 Other benign neoplasm of connective and other soft tissue of upper limb, including shoulder
238.1 Neoplasm of uncertain behavior of connective and other soft tissue ▽
239.2 Neoplasms of unspecified nature of bone, soft tissue, and skin
275.40 Unspecified disorder of calcium metabolism — (Use additional code to identify any associated mental retardation) ▽
275.41 Hypocalcemia — (Use additional code to identify any associated mental retardation)
275.49 Other disorders of calcium metabolism — (Use additional code to identify any associated mental retardation)
357.1 Polyneuropathy in collagen vascular disease — (Code first underlying disease: 446.0, 710.0, 714.0) ☒
359.6 Symptomatic inflammatory myopathy in diseases classified elsewhere — (Code first underlying disease: 135, 140.0-208.9, 277.3, 446.0, 710.0, 710.1, 710.2, 714.0) ☒
446.0 Polyarteritis nodosa
710.0 Systemic lupus erythematosus — (Use additional code to identify manifestation: 424.91, 581.81, 582.81, 583.81)
710.1 Systemic sclerosis — (Use additional code to identify manifestation: 359.6, 517.2)
710.2 Sicca syndrome
712.12 Chondrocalcinosis due to dicalcium phosphate crystals, upper arm — (Code first underlying disease, 275.4) ☒
712.23 Chondrocalcinosis due to pyrophosphate crystals, forearm — (Code first underlying disease, 275.4) ☒
714.0 Rheumatoid arthritis — (Use additional code to identify manifestation: 357.1, 359.6)
715.13 Primary localized osteoarthrosis, forearm
719.23 Villonodular synovitis, forearm
727.00 Unspecified synovitis and tenosynovitis ▽

ICD-9-CM Procedural

80.73 Synovectomy of wrist

HCPCS Level II Supplies & Services

A4305 Disposable drug delivery system, flow rate of 50 ml or greater per hour
A4306 Disposable drug delivery system, flow rate of 5 ml or less per hour
A4550 Surgical trays

29846

29846 Arthroscopy, wrist, surgical; excision and/or repair of triangular fibrocartilage and/or joint debridement

ICD-9-CM Diagnostic

718.03 Articular cartilage disorder, forearm
718.83 Other joint derangement, not elsewhere classified, forearm

ICD-9-CM Procedural

80.83 Other local excision or destruction of lesion of wrist joint
81.96 Other repair of joint

HCPCS Level II Supplies & Services

A4305 Disposable drug delivery system, flow rate of 50 ml or greater per hour
A4306 Disposable drug delivery system, flow rate of 5 ml or less per hour
A4550 Surgical trays

29847

29847 Arthroscopy, wrist, surgical; internal fixation for fracture or instability

ICD-9-CM Diagnostic

718.83 Other joint derangement, not elsewhere classified, forearm
733.82 Nonunion of fracture
813.42 Other closed fractures of distal end of radius (alone)
813.82 Closed fracture of unspecified part of ulna (alone) ▽
813.83 Closed fracture of unspecified part of radius with ulna ▽

ICD-9-CM Procedural

78.59 Internal fixation of other bone, except facial bones, without fracture reduction

HCPCS Level II Supplies & Services

A4305 Disposable drug delivery system, flow rate of 50 ml or greater per hour
A4306 Disposable drug delivery system, flow rate of 5 ml or less per hour
A4550 Surgical trays

29848

29848 Endoscopy, wrist, surgical, with release of transverse carpal ligament

ICD-9-CM Diagnostic

354.0 Carpal tunnel syndrome

ICD-9-CM Procedural

04.43 Release of carpal tunnel

HCPCS Level II Supplies & Services

A4305 Disposable drug delivery system, flow rate of 50 ml or greater per hour
A4306 Disposable drug delivery system, flow rate of 5 ml or less per hour
A4550 Surgical trays

29850–29851

29850 Arthroscopically aided treatment of intercondylar spine(s) and/or tuberosity fracture(s) of the knee, with or without manipulation; without internal or external fixation (includes arthroscopy)
29851 with internal or external fixation (includes arthroscopy)

ICD-9-CM Diagnostic

717.81 Old disruption of lateral collateral ligament
717.82 Old disruption of medial collateral ligament
717.83 Old disruption of anterior cruciate ligament
717.84 Old disruption of posterior cruciate ligament
733.93 Stress fracture of tibia or fibula
823.00 Closed fracture of upper end of tibia
823.02 Closed fracture of upper end of fibula with tibia
823.10 Open fracture of upper end of tibia
823.12 Open fracture of upper end of fibula with tibia
836.2 Other tear of cartilage or meniscus of knee, current
844.9 Sprain and strain of unspecified site of knee and leg ▽

ICD-9-CM Procedural

78.17 Application of external fixation device, tibia and fibula
79.26 Open reduction of fracture of tibia and fibula without internal fixation
79.36 Open reduction of fracture of tibia and fibula with internal fixation

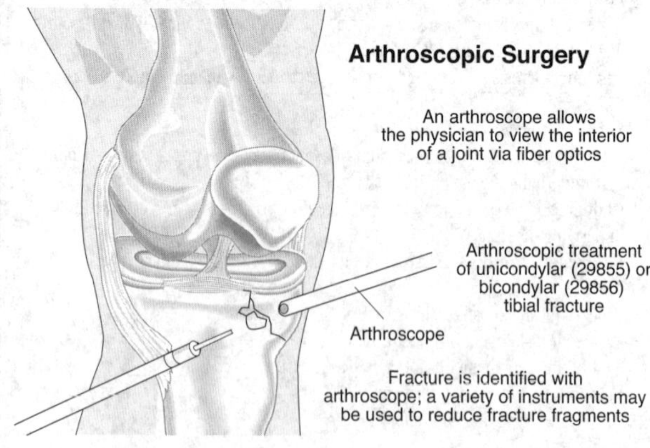

Arthroscopic Surgery
An arthroscope allows the physician to view the interior of a joint via fiber optics
Arthroscopic treatment of unicondylar (29855) or bicondylar (29856) tibial fracture
Arthroscope
Fracture is identified with arthroscope; a variety of instruments may be used to reduce fracture fragments

▽ Unspecified code ♀ Female diagnosis ☒ Manifestation code ♂ Male diagnosis

29855–29856

29855 Arthroscopically aided treatment of tibial fracture, proximal (plateau); unicondylar, with or without internal or external fixation (includes arthroscopy)
29856 bicondylar, with or without internal or external fixation (includes arthroscopy)

ICD-9-CM Diagnostic

733.93 Stress fracture of tibia or fibula
823.00 Closed fracture of upper end of tibia
823.02 Closed fracture of upper end of fibula with tibia
823.10 Open fracture of upper end of tibia
823.12 Open fracture of upper end of fibula with tibia

ICD-9-CM Procedural

78.17 Application of external fixation device, tibia and fibula
79.26 Open reduction of fracture of tibia and fibula without internal fixation
79.36 Open reduction of fracture of tibia and fibula with internal fixation

29860

29860 Arthroscopy, hip, diagnostic with or without synovial biopsy (separate procedure)

ICD-9-CM Diagnostic

171.3 Malignant neoplasm of connective and other soft tissue of lower limb, including hip
198.89 Secondary malignant neoplasm of other specified sites
215.3 Other benign neoplasm of connective and other soft tissue of lower limb, including hip
238.1 Neoplasm of uncertain behavior of connective and other soft tissue ▽
239.2 Neoplasms of unspecified nature of bone, soft tissue, and skin
275.40 Unspecified disorder of calcium metabolism — (Use additional code to identify any associated mental retardation) ▽
275.42 Hypercalcemia — (Use additional code to identify any associated mental retardation)
275.49 Other disorders of calcium metabolism — (Use additional code to identify any associated mental retardation)
711.05 Pyogenic arthritis, pelvic region and thigh — (Use additional code to identify infectious organism: 041.0-041.8)
714.0 Rheumatoid arthritis — (Use additional code to identify manifestation: 357.1, 359.6)
715.15 Primary localized osteoarthrosis, pelvic region and thigh
716.95 Unspecified arthropathy, pelvic region and thigh ▽
718.05 Articular cartilage disorder, pelvic region and thigh
718.15 Loose body in pelvic joint
718.35 Recurrent dislocation of pelvic region and thigh joint
718.75 Developmental dislocation of joint, pelvic region and thigh
719.25 Villonodular synovitis, pelvic region and thigh
719.45 Pain in joint, pelvic region and thigh
719.95 Unspecified disorder of joint of pelvic region and thigh ▽
726.5 Enthesopathy of hip region
727.00 Unspecified synovitis and tenosynovitis ▽
732.1 Juvenile osteochondrosis of hip and pelvis
732.9 Unspecified osteochondropathy ▽
733.90 Disorder of bone and cartilage, unspecified ▽
733.92 Chondromalacia
733.99 Other disorders of bone and cartilage
820.01 Closed fracture of epiphysis (separation) (upper) of neck of femur
835.00 Closed dislocation of hip, unspecified site ▽
835.03 Other closed anterior dislocation of hip
843.8 Sprain and strain of other specified sites of hip and thigh
843.9 Sprain and strain of unspecified site of hip and thigh ▽
905.6 Late effect of dislocation
908.9 Late effect of unspecified injury ▽
959.6 Injury, other and unspecified, hip and thigh

ICD-9-CM Procedural

80.25 Arthroscopy of hip
80.35 Biopsy of joint structure of hip

29861–29862

29861 Arthroscopy, hip, surgical; with removal of loose body or foreign body
29862 Arthroscopy, hip, surgical; with debridement/shaving of articular cartilage (chondroplasty), abrasion arthroplasty, and/or resection of labrum

ICD-9-CM Diagnostic

213.6 Benign neoplasm of pelvic bones, sacrum, and coccyx
213.7 Benign neoplasm of long bones of lower limb
238.0 Neoplasm of uncertain behavior of bone and articular cartilage
275.40 Unspecified disorder of calcium metabolism — (Use additional code to identify any associated mental retardation) ▽
275.42 Hypercalcemia — (Use additional code to identify any associated mental retardation)
275.49 Other disorders of calcium metabolism — (Use additional code to identify any associated mental retardation)
714.0 Rheumatoid arthritis — (Use additional code to identify manifestation: 357.1, 359.6)
715.15 Primary localized osteoarthrosis, pelvic region and thigh
716.95 Unspecified arthropathy, pelvic region and thigh ▽
718.05 Articular cartilage disorder, pelvic region and thigh
718.15 Loose body in pelvic joint
718.35 Recurrent dislocation of pelvic region and thigh joint
719.45 Pain in joint, pelvic region and thigh
719.95 Unspecified disorder of joint of pelvic region and thigh ▽
726.5 Enthesopathy of hip region
732.1 Juvenile osteochondrosis of hip and pelvis
732.9 Unspecified osteochondropathy ▽
733.90 Disorder of bone and cartilage, unspecified ▽
733.92 Chondromalacia
733.99 Other disorders of bone and cartilage
835.00 Closed dislocation of hip, unspecified site ▽
835.03 Other closed anterior dislocation of hip
843.8 Sprain and strain of other specified sites of hip and thigh
843.9 Sprain and strain of unspecified site of hip and thigh ▽
905.6 Late effect of dislocation
908.9 Late effect of unspecified injury ▽
959.6 Injury, other and unspecified, hip and thigh

ICD-9-CM Procedural

80.25 Arthroscopy of hip
80.85 Other local excision or destruction of lesion of hip joint

29863

29863 Arthroscopy, hip, surgical; with synovectomy

ICD-9-CM Diagnostic

171.3 Malignant neoplasm of connective and other soft tissue of lower limb, including hip
198.89 Secondary malignant neoplasm of other specified sites
215.3 Other benign neoplasm of connective and other soft tissue of lower limb, including hip
238.1 Neoplasm of uncertain behavior of connective and other soft tissue ▽
239.2 Neoplasms of unspecified nature of bone, soft tissue, and skin
275.40 Unspecified disorder of calcium metabolism — (Use additional code to identify any associated mental retardation) ▽
275.42 Hypercalcemia — (Use additional code to identify any associated mental retardation)
275.49 Other disorders of calcium metabolism — (Use additional code to identify any associated mental retardation)
711.05 Pyogenic arthritis, pelvic region and thigh — (Use additional code to identify infectious organism: 041.0-041.8)
714.0 Rheumatoid arthritis — (Use additional code to identify manifestation: 357.1, 359.6)
715.15 Primary localized osteoarthrosis, pelvic region and thigh
716.95 Unspecified arthropathy, pelvic region and thigh ▽
719.25 Villonodular synovitis, pelvic region and thigh
719.45 Pain in joint, pelvic region and thigh
726.5 Enthesopathy of hip region
727.00 Unspecified synovitis and tenosynovitis ▽

ICD-9-CM Procedural

80.75 Synovectomy of hip
80.85 Other local excision or destruction of lesion of hip joint

▽ Unspecified code ♀ Female diagnosis
☒ Manifestation code ♂ Male diagnosis

29866–29867

29866 Arthroscopy, knee, surgical; osteochondral autograft(s) (eg, mosaicplasty) (includes harvesting of the autograft)
29867 osteochondral allograft (eg, mosaicplasty)

ICD-9-CM Diagnostic

714.30 Polyarticular juvenile rheumatoid arthritis, chronic or unspecified
715.16 Primary localized osteoarthrosis, lower leg
715.26 Secondary localized osteoarthrosis, lower leg
715.36 Localized osteoarthrosis not specified whether primary or secondary, lower leg
715.96 Osteoarthrosis, unspecified whether generalized or localized, lower leg ▽
717.7 Chondromalacia of patella
717.83 Old disruption of anterior cruciate ligament
719.96 Unspecified disorder of lower leg joint ▽
732.4 Juvenile osteochondrosis of lower extremity, excluding foot
732.7 Osteochondritis dissecans
732.9 Unspecified osteochondropathy ▽
844.2 Sprain and strain of cruciate ligament of knee

ICD-9-CM Procedural

81.47 Other repair of knee

29868

29868 Arthroscopy, knee, surgical; meniscal transplantation (includes arthrotomy for meniscal insertion), medial or lateral

ICD-9-CM Diagnostic

717.0 Old bucket handle tear of medial meniscus
717.1 Derangement of anterior horn of medial meniscus
717.2 Derangement of posterior horn of medial meniscus
717.3 Other and unspecified derangement of medial meniscus ▽
717.40 Unspecified derangement of lateral meniscus ▽
717.41 Bucket handle tear of lateral meniscus
717.42 Derangement of anterior horn of lateral meniscus
717.43 Derangement of posterior horn of lateral meniscus
717.49 Other derangement of lateral meniscus
717.5 Derangement of meniscus, not elsewhere classified
718.36 Recurrent dislocation of lower leg joint
836.0 Tear of medial cartilage or meniscus of knee, current
836.1 Tear of lateral cartilage or meniscus of knee, current
836.2 Other tear of cartilage or meniscus of knee, current

ICD-9-CM Procedural

80.6 Excision of semilunar cartilage of knee
81.47 Other repair of knee

29870

29870 Arthroscopy, knee, diagnostic, with or without synovial biopsy (separate procedure)

ICD-9-CM Diagnostic

171.3 Malignant neoplasm of connective and other soft tissue of lower limb, including hip
198.89 Secondary malignant neoplasm of other specified sites
215.3 Other benign neoplasm of connective and other soft tissue of lower limb, including hip
238.1 Neoplasm of uncertain behavior of connective and other soft tissue ▽
239.2 Neoplasms of unspecified nature of bone, soft tissue, and skin
275.40 Unspecified disorder of calcium metabolism — (Use additional code to identify any associated mental retardation) ▽
275.41 Hypocalcemia — (Use additional code to identify any associated mental retardation)
275.42 Hypercalcemia — (Use additional code to identify any associated mental retardation)
275.49 Other disorders of calcium metabolism — (Use additional code to identify any associated mental retardation)
711.56 Arthropathy associated with other viral diseases, lower leg — (Code first underlying disease, such as: diseases classifiable to 045-049, 050-079 (except 056.71), 480, 487) ☒
712.16 Chondrocalcinosis due to dicalcium phosphate crystals, lower leg — (Code first underlying disease, 275.4) ☒
712.26 Chondrocalcinosis due to pyrophosphate crystals, lower leg — (Code first underlying disease, 275.4) ☒
713.1 Arthropathy associated with gastrointestinal conditions other than infections — (Code first underlying disease: 555.0-555.9, 556.0-556.9) ☒
713.2 Arthropathy associated with hematological disorders — (Code first underlying disease: 202.3, 203.0, 204.0-208.9, 282.4-282.7, 286.0-286.2) ☒
713.3 Arthropathy associated with dermatological disorders — (Code first underlying disease: 695.1, 695.2) ☒
715.09 Generalized osteoarthrosis, involving multiple sites
715.16 Primary localized osteoarthrosis, lower leg
715.96 Osteoarthrosis, unspecified whether generalized or localized, lower leg ▽
716.16 Traumatic arthropathy, lower leg
716.46 Transient arthropathy, lower leg
717.0 Old bucket handle tear of medial meniscus
717.1 Derangement of anterior horn of medial meniscus
717.2 Derangement of posterior horn of medial meniscus
717.3 Other and unspecified derangement of medial meniscus ▽
717.40 Unspecified derangement of lateral meniscus ▽
717.41 Bucket handle tear of lateral meniscus
717.42 Derangement of anterior horn of lateral meniscus
717.43 Derangement of posterior horn of lateral meniscus
717.49 Other derangement of lateral meniscus
717.5 Derangement of meniscus, not elsewhere classified
717.7 Chondromalacia of patella
717.81 Old disruption of lateral collateral ligament
717.82 Old disruption of medial collateral ligament
717.83 Old disruption of anterior cruciate ligament
717.84 Old disruption of posterior cruciate ligament
717.85 Old disruption of other ligament of knee
717.89 Other internal derangement of knee
718.36 Recurrent dislocation of lower leg joint
718.46 Contracture of lower leg joint
718.76 Developmental dislocation of joint, lower leg
718.86 Other joint derangement, not elsewhere classified, lower leg
719.06 Effusion of lower leg joint
719.16 Hemarthrosis, lower leg
719.26 Villonodular synovitis, lower leg
719.86 Other specified disorders of lower leg joint
727.00 Unspecified synovitis and tenosynovitis ▽
727.51 Synovial cyst of popliteal space
733.90 Disorder of bone and cartilage, unspecified ▽
733.92 Chondromalacia
736.6 Other acquired deformities of knee
755.64 Congenital deformity of knee (joint)
755.69 Other congenital anomaly of lower limb, including pelvic girdle
836.0 Tear of medial cartilage or meniscus of knee, current
836.1 Tear of lateral cartilage or meniscus of knee, current
836.2 Other tear of cartilage or meniscus of knee, current
836.3 Closed dislocation of patella
836.4 Open dislocation of patella
836.50 Closed dislocation of knee, unspecified part ▽
844.0 Sprain and strain of lateral collateral ligament of knee
844.1 Sprain and strain of medial collateral ligament of knee
844.2 Sprain and strain of cruciate ligament of knee

ICD-9-CM Procedural

80.26 Arthroscopy of knee
80.36 Biopsy of joint structure of knee

29871

29871 Arthroscopy, knee, surgical; for infection, lavage and drainage

ICD-9-CM Diagnostic

357.1 Polyneuropathy in collagen vascular disease — (Code first underlying disease: 446.0, 710.0, 714.0) ☒
359.6 Symptomatic inflammatory myopathy in diseases classified elsewhere — (Code first underlying disease: 135, 140.0-208.9, 277.3, 446.0, 710.0, 710.1, 710.2, 714.0) ☒
446.0 Polyarteritis nodosa
710.0 Systemic lupus erythematosus — (Use additional code to identify manifestation: 424.91, 581.81, 582.81, 583.81)
710.1 Systemic sclerosis — (Use additional code to identify manifestation: 359.6, 517.2)
710.2 Sicca syndrome
711.06 Pyogenic arthritis, lower leg — (Use additional code to identify infectious organism: 041.0-041.8)
711.46 Arthropathy associated with other bacterial diseases, lower leg — (Code first underlying disease, such as: diseases classifiable to 010-040 (except 036.82), 090-099 (except 098.50)) ☒

▽ Unspecified code
♀ Female diagnosis
☒ Manifestation code
♂ Male diagnosis

711.56 Arthropathy associated with other viral diseases, lower leg — (Code first underlying disease, such as: diseases classifiable to 045-049, 050-079 (except 056.71), 480, 487) ☒
711.66 Arthropathy associated with mycoses, lower leg — (Code first underlying disease: 110.0-118) ☒
711.86 Arthropathy associated with other infectious and parasitic diseases, lower leg — (Code first underlying disease, such as: diseases classifiable to 080-088, 100-104, 130-136) ☒
719.86 Other specified disorders of lower leg joint
727.51 Synovial cyst of popliteal space
730.06 Acute osteomyelitis, lower leg — (Use additional code to identify organism, 041.1)
730.16 Chronic osteomyelitis, lower leg — (Use additional code to identify organism, 041.1)
730.26 Unspecified osteomyelitis, lower leg — (Use additional code to identify organism, 041.1) ▽
730.36 Periostitis, without mention of osteomyelitis, lower leg — (Use additional code to identify organism, 041.1)
996.66 Infection and inflammatory reaction due to internal joint prosthesis — (Use additional code to identify specified infections)
996.67 Infection and inflammatory reaction due to other internal orthopedic device, implant, and graft — (Use additional code to identify specified infections)
998.51 Infected postoperative seroma — (Use additional code to identify organism)
998.59 Other postoperative infection — (Use additional code to identify infection)

ICD-9-CM Procedural
80.26 Arthroscopy of knee

29873
29873 Arthroscopy, knee, surgical; with lateral release

ICD-9-CM Diagnostic
715.16 Primary localized osteoarthrosis, lower leg
715.96 Osteoarthrosis, unspecified whether generalized or localized, lower leg ▽
717.6 Loose body in knee
717.7 Chondromalacia of patella
717.9 Unspecified internal derangement of knee ▽
718.36 Recurrent dislocation of lower leg joint
718.46 Contracture of lower leg joint
718.56 Ankylosis of lower leg joint
718.86 Other joint derangement, not elsewhere classified, lower leg
719.26 Villonodular synovitis, lower leg
719.86 Other specified disorders of lower leg joint
733.92 Chondromalacia
755.64 Congenital deformity of knee (joint)
836.3 Closed dislocation of patella
836.50 Closed dislocation of knee, unspecified part ▽
836.54 Closed lateral dislocation of tibia, proximal end
844.2 Sprain and strain of cruciate ligament of knee
996.4 Mechanical complication of internal orthopedic device, implant, and graft

ICD-9-CM Procedural
80.46 Division of joint capsule, ligament, or cartilage of knee

HCPCS Level II Supplies & Services
HCPCS Level II codes are used to report the supplies, durable medical equipment, and certain medical services provided on an outpatient basis. Because the procedure(s) represented on this page would be performed in an inpatient or outpatient facility, no HCPCS Level II codes apply.

29874
29874 Arthroscopy, knee, surgical; for removal of loose body or foreign body (eg, osteochondritis dissecans fragmentation, chondral fragmentation)

ICD-9-CM Diagnostic
275.40 Unspecified disorder of calcium metabolism — (Use additional code to identify any associated mental retardation) ▽
275.42 Hypercalcemia — (Use additional code to identify any associated mental retardation)
275.49 Other disorders of calcium metabolism — (Use additional code to identify any associated mental retardation)
716.16 Traumatic arthropathy, lower leg
717.6 Loose body in knee
717.7 Chondromalacia of patella
718.18 Loose body in joint of other specified site
718.86 Other joint derangement, not elsewhere classified, lower leg
732.4 Juvenile osteochondrosis of lower extremity, excluding foot
732.6 Other juvenile osteochondrosis
732.7 Osteochondritis dissecans
732.9 Unspecified osteochondropathy ▽
928.11 Crushing injury of knee — (Use additional code to identify any associated injuries: 800-829, 850.0-854.1, 860.0-869.1)

ICD-9-CM Procedural
80.96 Other excision of knee joint

29875–29876
29875 Arthroscopy, knee, surgical; synovectomy, limited (eg, plica or shelf resection) (separate procedure)
29876 synovectomy, major, two or more compartments (eg, medial or lateral)

ICD-9-CM Diagnostic
171.3 Malignant neoplasm of connective and other soft tissue of lower limb, including hip
198.89 Secondary malignant neoplasm of other specified sites
215.3 Other benign neoplasm of connective and other soft tissue of lower limb, including hip
238.1 Neoplasm of uncertain behavior of connective and other soft tissue ▽
239.2 Neoplasms of unspecified nature of bone, soft tissue, and skin
275.41 Hypocalcemia — (Use additional code to identify any associated mental retardation)
275.42 Hypercalcemia — (Use additional code to identify any associated mental retardation)
357.1 Polyneuropathy in collagen vascular disease — (Code first underlying disease: 446.0, 710.0, 714.0) ☒
359.6 Symptomatic inflammatory myopathy in diseases classified elsewhere — (Code first underlying disease: 135, 140.0-208.9, 277.3, 446.0, 710.0, 710.1, 710.2, 714.0) ☒
446.0 Polyarteritis nodosa
710.0 Systemic lupus erythematosus — (Use additional code to identify manifestation: 424.91, 581.81, 582.81, 583.81)
710.1 Systemic sclerosis — (Use additional code to identify manifestation: 359.6, 517.2)
710.2 Sicca syndrome
712.16 Chondrocalcinosis due to dicalcium phosphate crystals, lower leg — (Code first underlying disease, 275.4) ☒
712.26 Chondrocalcinosis due to pyrophosphate crystals, lower leg — (Code first underlying disease, 275.4) ☒
714.0 Rheumatoid arthritis — (Use additional code to identify manifestation: 357.1, 359.6)
714.2 Other rheumatoid arthritis with visceral or systemic involvement
714.31 Polyarticular juvenile rheumatoid arthritis, acute
714.32 Pauciarticular juvenile rheumatoid arthritis
714.33 Monoarticular juvenile rheumatoid arthritis
715.16 Primary localized osteoarthrosis, lower leg
717.7 Chondromalacia of patella
718.36 Recurrent dislocation of lower leg joint
719.26 Villonodular synovitis, lower leg
727.00 Unspecified synovitis and tenosynovitis ▽
727.01 Synovitis and tenosynovitis in diseases classified elsewhere — (Code first underlying disease: 015.0-015.9) ☒
727.09 Other synovitis and tenosynovitis
727.51 Synovial cyst of popliteal space
727.83 Plica syndrome
727.89 Other disorders of synovium, tendon, and bursa
755.64 Congenital deformity of knee (joint)
755.69 Other congenital anomaly of lower limb, including pelvic girdle
836.0 Tear of medial cartilage or meniscus of knee, current

ICD-9-CM Procedural
80.76 Synovectomy of knee

29877
29877 Arthroscopy, knee, surgical; debridement/shaving of articular cartilage (chondroplasty)

ICD-9-CM Diagnostic
275.40 Unspecified disorder of calcium metabolism — (Use additional code to identify any associated mental retardation) ▽
275.41 Hypocalcemia — (Use additional code to identify any associated mental retardation)

▽ Unspecified code ☒ Manifestation code
♀ Female diagnosis ♂ Male diagnosis

275.42 Hypercalcemia — (Use additional code to identify any associated mental retardation)
275.49 Other disorders of calcium metabolism — (Use additional code to identify any associated mental retardation)
357.1 Polyneuropathy in collagen vascular disease — (Code first underlying disease: 446.0, 710.0, 714.0) ☒
359.6 Symptomatic inflammatory myopathy in diseases classified elsewhere — (Code first underlying disease: 135, 140.0-208.9, 277.3, 446.0, 710.0, 710.1, 710.2, 714.0) ☒
446.0 Polyarteritis nodosa
710.0 Systemic lupus erythematosus — (Use additional code to identify manifestation: 424.91, 581.81, 582.81, 583.81)
710.1 Systemic sclerosis — (Use additional code to identify manifestation: 359.6, 517.2)
710.2 Sicca syndrome
712.16 Chondrocalcinosis due to dicalcium phosphate crystals, lower leg — (Code first underlying disease, 275.4) ☒
712.26 Chondrocalcinosis due to pyrophosphate crystals, lower leg — (Code first underlying disease, 275.4) ☒
714.0 Rheumatoid arthritis — (Use additional code to identify manifestation: 357.1, 359.6)
714.1 Felty's syndrome
714.2 Other rheumatoid arthritis with visceral or systemic involvement
714.30 Polyarticular juvenile rheumatoid arthritis, chronic or unspecified
714.31 Polyarticular juvenile rheumatoid arthritis, acute
714.32 Pauciarticular juvenile rheumatoid arthritis
714.33 Monoarticular juvenile rheumatoid arthritis
715.10 Primary localized osteoarthrosis, specified site ▽
715.16 Primary localized osteoarthrosis, lower leg
715.26 Secondary localized osteoarthrosis, lower leg
715.36 Localized osteoarthrosis not specified whether primary or secondary, lower leg
715.96 Osteoarthrosis, unspecified whether generalized or localized, lower leg ▽
716.16 Traumatic arthropathy, lower leg
716.86 Other specified arthropathy, lower leg
717.0 Old bucket handle tear of medial meniscus
717.1 Derangement of anterior horn of medial meniscus
717.2 Derangement of posterior horn of medial meniscus
717.3 Other and unspecified derangement of medial meniscus ▽
717.40 Unspecified derangement of lateral meniscus ▽
717.7 Chondromalacia of patella
718.46 Contracture of lower leg joint
718.56 Ankylosis of lower leg joint
718.86 Other joint derangement, not elsewhere classified, lower leg
719.16 Hemarthrosis, lower leg
719.26 Villonodular synovitis, lower leg
719.86 Other specified disorders of lower leg joint
719.96 Unspecified disorder of lower leg joint ▽
732.7 Osteochondritis dissecans
732.9 Unspecified osteochondropathy ▽
733.92 Chondromalacia
733.99 Other disorders of bone and cartilage
755.64 Congenital deformity of knee (joint)
755.69 Other congenital anomaly of lower limb, including pelvic girdle
836.0 Tear of medial cartilage or meniscus of knee, current
836.1 Tear of lateral cartilage or meniscus of knee, current
836.2 Other tear of cartilage or meniscus of knee, current
844.2 Sprain and strain of cruciate ligament of knee
844.9 Sprain and strain of unspecified site of knee and leg ▽

ICD-9-CM Procedural

80.86 Other local excision or destruction of lesion of knee joint
81.47 Other repair of knee

29879

29879 Arthroscopy, knee, surgical; abrasion arthroplasty (includes chondroplasty where necessary) or multiple drilling or microfracture

ICD-9-CM Diagnostic

275.40 Unspecified disorder of calcium metabolism — (Use additional code to identify any associated mental retardation) ▽
275.41 Hypocalcemia — (Use additional code to identify any associated mental retardation)
275.42 Hypercalcemia — (Use additional code to identify any associated mental retardation)
275.49 Other disorders of calcium metabolism — (Use additional code to identify any associated mental retardation)
357.1 Polyneuropathy in collagen vascular disease — (Code first underlying disease: 446.0, 710.0, 714.0) ☒
359.6 Symptomatic inflammatory myopathy in diseases classified elsewhere — (Code first underlying disease: 135, 140.0-208.9, 277.3, 446.0, 710.0, 710.1, 710.2, 714.0) ☒
712.16 Chondrocalcinosis due to dicalcium phosphate crystals, lower leg — (Code first underlying disease, 275.4) ☒
712.26 Chondrocalcinosis due to pyrophosphate crystals, lower leg — (Code first underlying disease, 275.4) ☒
714.0 Rheumatoid arthritis — (Use additional code to identify manifestation: 357.1, 359.6)
714.1 Felty's syndrome
714.2 Other rheumatoid arthritis with visceral or systemic involvement
714.30 Polyarticular juvenile rheumatoid arthritis, chronic or unspecified
714.31 Polyarticular juvenile rheumatoid arthritis, acute
714.32 Pauciarticular juvenile rheumatoid arthritis
714.33 Monoarticular juvenile rheumatoid arthritis
715.16 Primary localized osteoarthrosis, lower leg
715.26 Secondary localized osteoarthrosis, lower leg
715.36 Localized osteoarthrosis not specified whether primary or secondary, lower leg
715.96 Osteoarthrosis, unspecified whether generalized or localized, lower leg ▽
716.16 Traumatic arthropathy, lower leg
716.66 Unspecified monoarthritis, lower leg ▽
717.0 Old bucket handle tear of medial meniscus
717.1 Derangement of anterior horn of medial meniscus
717.2 Derangement of posterior horn of medial meniscus
717.3 Other and unspecified derangement of medial meniscus ▽
717.40 Unspecified derangement of lateral meniscus ▽
717.7 Chondromalacia of patella
717.9 Unspecified internal derangement of knee ▽
718.46 Contracture of lower leg joint
718.56 Ankylosis of lower leg joint
732.7 Osteochondritis dissecans
733.92 Chondromalacia
836.0 Tear of medial cartilage or meniscus of knee, current

ICD-9-CM Procedural

81.47 Other repair of knee

29880–29881

29880 Arthroscopy, knee, surgical; with meniscectomy (medial AND lateral, including any meniscal shaving)
29881 with meniscectomy (medial OR lateral, including any meniscal shaving)

ICD-9-CM Diagnostic

715.16 Primary localized osteoarthrosis, lower leg
715.26 Secondary localized osteoarthrosis, lower leg
715.36 Localized osteoarthrosis not specified whether primary or secondary, lower leg
715.96 Osteoarthrosis, unspecified whether generalized or localized, lower leg ▽
717.0 Old bucket handle tear of medial meniscus
717.1 Derangement of anterior horn of medial meniscus
717.2 Derangement of posterior horn of medial meniscus
717.3 Other and unspecified derangement of medial meniscus ▽
717.41 Bucket handle tear of lateral meniscus
717.42 Derangement of anterior horn of lateral meniscus
717.43 Derangement of posterior horn of lateral meniscus
717.49 Other derangement of lateral meniscus
717.5 Derangement of meniscus, not elsewhere classified
718.86 Other joint derangement, not elsewhere classified, lower leg
727.83 Plica syndrome
727.89 Other disorders of synovium, tendon, and bursa
836.0 Tear of medial cartilage or meniscus of knee, current
836.1 Tear of lateral cartilage or meniscus of knee, current
836.2 Other tear of cartilage or meniscus of knee, current

ICD-9-CM Procedural

80.6 Excision of semilunar cartilage of knee
81.42 Five-in-one repair of knee
81.43 Triad knee repair

29882–29883

29882 Arthroscopy, knee, surgical; with meniscus repair (medial OR lateral)
29883 with meniscus repair (medial AND lateral)

ICD-9-CM Diagnostic

717.0 Old bucket handle tear of medial meniscus

717.1 Derangement of anterior horn of medial meniscus
717.2 Derangement of posterior horn of medial meniscus
717.3 Other and unspecified derangement of medial meniscus ▽
717.40 Unspecified derangement of lateral meniscus ▽
717.41 Bucket handle tear of lateral meniscus
717.42 Derangement of anterior horn of lateral meniscus
717.43 Derangement of posterior horn of lateral meniscus
717.49 Other derangement of lateral meniscus
717.5 Derangement of meniscus, not elsewhere classified
836.0 Tear of medial cartilage or meniscus of knee, current
836.1 Tear of lateral cartilage or meniscus of knee, current
836.2 Other tear of cartilage or meniscus of knee, current

ICD-9-CM Procedural

81.47 Other repair of knee

29884

29884 Arthroscopy, knee, surgical; with lysis of adhesions, with or without manipulation (separate procedure)

ICD-9-CM Diagnostic

715.96 Osteoarthrosis, unspecified whether generalized or localized, lower leg ▽
717.7 Chondromalacia of patella
717.9 Unspecified internal derangement of knee ▽
718.46 Contracture of lower leg joint
718.56 Ankylosis of lower leg joint
719.56 Stiffness of joint, not elsewhere classified, lower leg
719.86 Other specified disorders of lower leg joint
726.61 Pes anserinus tendinitis or bursitis
726.62 Tibial collateral ligament bursitis
726.63 Fibular collateral ligament bursitis
726.64 Patellar tendinitis
726.65 Prepatellar bursitis
727.81 Contracture of tendon (sheath)
727.83 Plica syndrome
836.0 Tear of medial cartilage or meniscus of knee, current

ICD-9-CM Procedural

80.46 Division of joint capsule, ligament, or cartilage of knee

29885–29887

29885 Arthroscopy, knee, surgical; drilling for osteochondritis dissecans with bone grafting, with or without internal fixation (including debridement of base of lesion)
29886 drilling for intact osteochondritis dissecans lesion
29887 drilling for intact osteochondritis dissecans lesion with internal fixation

ICD-9-CM Diagnostic

717.6 Loose body in knee
732.4 Juvenile osteochondrosis of lower extremity, excluding foot
732.6 Other juvenile osteochondrosis
732.7 Osteochondritis dissecans
732.9 Unspecified osteochondropathy ▽

ICD-9-CM Procedural

78.57 Internal fixation of tibia and fibula without fracture reduction
81.47 Other repair of knee

29888–29889

29888 Arthroscopically aided anterior cruciate ligament repair/augmentation or reconstruction
29889 Arthroscopically aided posterior cruciate ligament repair/augmentation or reconstruction

ICD-9-CM Diagnostic

717.83 Old disruption of anterior cruciate ligament
717.84 Old disruption of posterior cruciate ligament
717.9 Unspecified internal derangement of knee ▽
718.76 Developmental dislocation of joint, lower leg
718.86 Other joint derangement, not elsewhere classified, lower leg
728.4 Laxity of ligament
754.41 Congenital dislocation of knee (with genu recurvatum)
836.0 Tear of medial cartilage or meniscus of knee, current
836.50 Closed dislocation of knee, unspecified part ▽
836.51 Closed anterior dislocation of tibia, proximal end
836.63 Open medial dislocation of tibia, proximal end
844.0 Sprain and strain of lateral collateral ligament of knee
844.1 Sprain and strain of medial collateral ligament of knee
844.2 Sprain and strain of cruciate ligament of knee

ICD-9-CM Procedural

81.45 Other repair of the cruciate ligaments
81.47 Other repair of knee

29891

29891 Arthroscopy, ankle, surgical, excision of osteochondral defect of talus and/or tibia, including drilling of the defect

ICD-9-CM Diagnostic

732.4 Juvenile osteochondrosis of lower extremity, excluding foot
732.5 Juvenile osteochondrosis of foot
732.7 Osteochondritis dissecans
732.9 Unspecified osteochondropathy ▽

ICD-9-CM Procedural

80.87 Other local excision or destruction of lesion of ankle joint

29892

29892 Arthroscopically aided repair of large osteochondritis dissecans lesion, talar dome fracture, or tibial plafond fracture, with or without internal fixation (includes arthroscopy)

ICD-9-CM Diagnostic

732.7 Osteochondritis dissecans
823.80 Closed fracture of unspecified part of tibia ▽
824.0 Closed fracture of medial malleolus
825.21 Closed fracture of astragalus

ICD-9-CM Procedural

78.57 Internal fixation of tibia and fibula without fracture reduction
78.58 Internal fixation of tarsals and metatarsals without fracture reduction
79.26 Open reduction of fracture of tibia and fibula without internal fixation
79.27 Open reduction of fracture of tarsals and metatarsals without internal fixation
79.36 Open reduction of fracture of tibia and fibula with internal fixation
79.37 Open reduction of fracture of tarsals and metatarsals with internal fixation
80.87 Other local excision or destruction of lesion of ankle joint
80.90 Other excision of joint, unspecified site

29893

29893 Endoscopic plantar fasciotomy

ICD-9-CM Diagnostic

728.71 Plantar fascial fibromatosis
728.79 Other fibromatoses of muscle, ligament, and fascia
733.94 Stress fracture of the metatarsals
825.25 Closed fracture of metatarsal bone(s)
825.29 Other closed fracture of tarsal and metatarsal bones
825.39 Other open fractures of tarsal and metatarsal bones
845.19 Other foot sprain and strain
892.0 Open wound of foot except toe(s) alone, without mention of complication — (Use additional code to identify infection)
892.1 Open wound of foot except toe(s) alone, complicated — (Use additional code to identify infection)
892.2 Open wound of foot except toe(s) alone, with tendon involvement — (Use additional code to identify infection)
905.4 Late effect of fracture of lower extremities
905.8 Late effect of tendon injury
906.1 Late effect of open wound of extremities without mention of tendon injury
906.4 Late effect of crushing
928.20 Crushing injury of foot — (Use additional code to identify any associated injuries: 800-829, 850.0-854.1, 860.0-869.1)
997.99 Other complications affecting other specified body systems, NEC — (Use additional code to identify complications)

ICD-9-CM Procedural

83.14 Fasciotomy

29894

29894 Arthroscopy, ankle (tibiotalar and fibulotalar joints), surgical; with removal of loose body or foreign body

ICD-9-CM Diagnostic

275.40 Unspecified disorder of calcium metabolism — (Use additional code to identify any associated mental retardation) ▽
275.42 Hypercalcemia — (Use additional code to identify any associated mental retardation)
275.49 Other disorders of calcium metabolism — (Use additional code to identify any associated mental retardation)
715.17 Primary localized osteoarthrosis, ankle and foot
715.97 Osteoarthrosis, unspecified whether generalized or localized, ankle and foot ▽
716.17 Traumatic arthropathy, ankle and foot
718.17 Loose body in ankle and foot joint
718.87 Other joint derangement, not elsewhere classified, ankle and foot
718.97 Unspecified ankle and foot joint derangement ▽
719.27 Villonodular synovitis, ankle and foot

ICD-9-CM Procedural

80.97 Other excision of ankle joint

HCPCS Level II Supplies & Services

A4305 Disposable drug delivery system, flow rate of 50 ml or greater per hour
A4306 Disposable drug delivery system, flow rate of 5 ml or less per hour
A4550 Surgical trays

29895

29895 Arthroscopy, ankle (tibiotalar and fibulotalar joints), surgical; synovectomy, partial

ICD-9-CM Diagnostic

171.3 Malignant neoplasm of connective and other soft tissue of lower limb, including hip
198.89 Secondary malignant neoplasm of other specified sites
215.3 Other benign neoplasm of connective and other soft tissue of lower limb, including hip
238.1 Neoplasm of uncertain behavior of connective and other soft tissue ▽
239.2 Neoplasms of unspecified nature of bone, soft tissue, and skin
275.40 Unspecified disorder of calcium metabolism — (Use additional code to identify any associated mental retardation) ▽
275.42 Hypercalcemia — (Use additional code to identify any associated mental retardation)
275.49 Other disorders of calcium metabolism — (Use additional code to identify any associated mental retardation)
357.1 Polyneuropathy in collagen vascular disease — (Code first underlying disease: 446.0, 710.0, 714.0) ☒
359.6 Symptomatic inflammatory myopathy in diseases classified elsewhere — (Code first underlying disease: 135, 140.0-208.9, 277.3, 446.0, 710.0, 710.1, 710.2, 714.0) ☒
446.0 Polyarteritis nodosa
710.0 Systemic lupus erythematosus — (Use additional code to identify manifestation: 424.91, 581.81, 582.81, 583.81)
710.1 Systemic sclerosis — (Use additional code to identify manifestation: 359.6, 517.2)
710.2 Sicca syndrome
714.0 Rheumatoid arthritis — (Use additional code to identify manifestation: 357.1, 359.6)
715.17 Primary localized osteoarthrosis, ankle and foot
715.97 Osteoarthrosis, unspecified whether generalized or localized, ankle and foot ▽
716.17 Traumatic arthropathy, ankle and foot
718.07 Articular cartilage disorder, ankle and foot
718.87 Other joint derangement, not elsewhere classified, ankle and foot
718.97 Unspecified ankle and foot joint derangement ▽
719.27 Villonodular synovitis, ankle and foot
719.57 Stiffness of joint, not elsewhere classified, ankle and foot
727.00 Unspecified synovitis and tenosynovitis ▽
727.01 Synovitis and tenosynovitis in diseases classified elsewhere — (Code first underlying disease: 015.0-015.9) ☒
727.06 Tenosynovitis of foot and ankle
959.7 Injury, other and unspecified, knee, leg, ankle, and foot

ICD-9-CM Procedural

80.77 Synovectomy of ankle

HCPCS Level II Supplies & Services

A4305 Disposable drug delivery system, flow rate of 50 ml or greater per hour
A4306 Disposable drug delivery system, flow rate of 5 ml or less per hour
A4550 Surgical trays

29897–29898

29897 Arthroscopy, ankle (tibiotalar and fibulotalar joints), surgical; debridement, limited
29898 debridement, extensive

ICD-9-CM Diagnostic

357.1 Polyneuropathy in collagen vascular disease — (Code first underlying disease: 446.0, 710.0, 714.0) ☒
359.6 Symptomatic inflammatory myopathy in diseases classified elsewhere — (Code first underlying disease: 135, 140.0-208.9, 277.3, 446.0, 710.0, 710.1, 710.2, 714.0) ☒
446.0 Polyarteritis nodosa
710.0 Systemic lupus erythematosus — (Use additional code to identify manifestation: 424.91, 581.81, 582.81, 583.81)
710.1 Systemic sclerosis — (Use additional code to identify manifestation: 359.6, 517.2)
710.2 Sicca syndrome
714.0 Rheumatoid arthritis — (Use additional code to identify manifestation: 357.1, 359.6)
715.17 Primary localized osteoarthrosis, ankle and foot
716.17 Traumatic arthropathy, ankle and foot
718.07 Articular cartilage disorder, ankle and foot
718.87 Other joint derangement, not elsewhere classified, ankle and foot
719.27 Villonodular synovitis, ankle and foot
726.79 Other enthesopathy of ankle and tarsus
727.06 Tenosynovitis of foot and ankle
732.7 Osteochondritis dissecans
732.9 Unspecified osteochondropathy ▽
733.92 Chondromalacia

ICD-9-CM Procedural

80.87 Other local excision or destruction of lesion of ankle joint

HCPCS Level II Supplies & Services

A4305 Disposable drug delivery system, flow rate of 50 ml or greater per hour
A4306 Disposable drug delivery system, flow rate of 5 ml or less per hour
A4550 Surgical trays

29899

29899 Arthroscopy, ankle (tibiotalar and fibulotalar joints), surgical; with ankle arthrodesis

ICD-9-CM Diagnostic

711.07 Pyogenic arthritis, ankle and foot — (Use additional code to identify infectious organism: 041.0-041.8)
711.67 Arthropathy associated with mycoses, ankle and foot — (Code first underlying disease: 110.0-118) ☒
712.17 Chondrocalcinosis due to dicalcium phosphate crystals, ankle and foot — (Code first underlying disease, 275.4) ☒
712.27 Chondrocalcinosis due to pyrophosphate crystals, ankle and foot — (Code first underlying disease, 275.4) ☒
713.5 Arthropathy associated with neurological disorders — (Code first underlying disease: 094.0, 250.6, 336.0) ☒
714.0 Rheumatoid arthritis — (Use additional code to identify manifestation: 357.1, 359.6)
714.4 Chronic postrheumatic arthropathy
715.17 Primary localized osteoarthrosis, ankle and foot
715.27 Secondary localized osteoarthrosis, ankle and foot
715.97 Osteoarthrosis, unspecified whether generalized or localized, ankle and foot ▽
716.17 Traumatic arthropathy, ankle and foot
718.87 Other joint derangement, not elsewhere classified, ankle and foot
730.17 Chronic osteomyelitis, ankle and foot — (Use additional code to identify organism, 041.1)
733.81 Malunion of fracture
736.70 Unspecified deformity of ankle and foot, acquired ▽
754.51 Congenital talipes equinovarus
905.4 Late effect of fracture of lower extremities
906.4 Late effect of crushing
996.77 Other complications due to internal joint prosthesis

ICD-9-CM Procedural

81.29 Arthrodesis of other specified joint

▽ Unspecified code
♀ Female diagnosis
☒ Manifestation code
♂ Male diagnosis

29900

29900 Arthroscopy, metacarpophalangeal joint, diagnostic, includes synovial biopsy

ICD-9-CM Diagnostic

357.1 Polyneuropathy in collagen vascular disease — (Code first underlying disease: 446.0, 710.0, 714.0) ☒
359.6 Symptomatic inflammatory myopathy in diseases classified elsewhere — (Code first underlying disease: 135, 140.0-208.9, 277.3, 446.0, 710.0, 710.1, 710.2, 714.0) ☒
446.0 Polyarteritis nodosa
682.4 Cellulitis and abscess of hand, except fingers and thumb — (Use additional code to identify organism)
709.4 Foreign body granuloma of skin and subcutaneous tissue
710.0 Systemic lupus erythematosus — (Use additional code to identify manifestation: 424.91, 581.81, 582.81, 583.81)
710.1 Systemic sclerosis — (Use additional code to identify manifestation: 359.6, 517.2)
710.2 Sicca syndrome
711.04 Pyogenic arthritis, hand — (Use additional code to identify infectious organism: 041.0-041.8)
714.0 Rheumatoid arthritis — (Use additional code to identify manifestation: 357.1, 359.6)
714.30 Polyarticular juvenile rheumatoid arthritis, chronic or unspecified
714.31 Polyarticular juvenile rheumatoid arthritis, acute
714.9 Unspecified inflammatory polyarthropathy ▽
716.04 Kaschin-Beck disease, hand
716.14 Traumatic arthropathy, hand
716.64 Unspecified monoarthritis, hand ▽
718.74 Developmental dislocation of joint, hand
719.24 Villonodular synovitis, hand
727.00 Unspecified synovitis and tenosynovitis ▽
727.01 Synovitis and tenosynovitis in diseases classified elsewhere — (Code first underlying disease: 015.0-015.9) ☒
727.05 Other tenosynovitis of hand and wrist
728.0 Infective myositis
728.82 Foreign body granuloma of muscle
728.89 Other disorder of muscle, ligament, and fascia — (Use additional E code to identify drug, if drug-induced)
729.4 Unspecified fasciitis ▽
729.6 Residual foreign body in soft tissue
730.04 Acute osteomyelitis, hand — (Use additional code to identify organism, 041.1)
730.14 Chronic osteomyelitis, hand — (Use additional code to identify organism, 041.1)
730.24 Unspecified osteomyelitis, hand — (Use additional code to identify organism, 041.1) ▽
730.34 Periostitis, without mention of osteomyelitis, hand — (Use additional code to identify organism, 041.1)
730.84 Other infections involving diseases classified elsewhere, hand bone — (Code first underlying disease: 002.0, 015.0-015.9. Use additional code to identify organism) ☒
882.1 Open wound of hand except finger(s) alone, complicated — (Use additional code to identify infection)
883.1 Open wound of finger(s), complicated — (Use additional code to identify infection)

ICD-9-CM Procedural

80.24 Arthroscopy of hand and finger
80.34 Biopsy of joint structure of hand and finger

29901

29901 Arthroscopy, metacarpophalangeal joint, surgical; with debridement

ICD-9-CM Diagnostic

682.4 Cellulitis and abscess of hand, except fingers and thumb — (Use additional code to identify organism)
709.4 Foreign body granuloma of skin and subcutaneous tissue
711.04 Pyogenic arthritis, hand — (Use additional code to identify infectious organism: 041.0-041.8)
728.0 Infective myositis
728.82 Foreign body granuloma of muscle
729.4 Unspecified fasciitis ▽
729.6 Residual foreign body in soft tissue
730.04 Acute osteomyelitis, hand — (Use additional code to identify organism, 041.1)
730.14 Chronic osteomyelitis, hand — (Use additional code to identify organism, 041.1)
730.24 Unspecified osteomyelitis, hand — (Use additional code to identify organism, 041.1) ▽
730.34 Periostitis, without mention of osteomyelitis, hand — (Use additional code to identify organism, 041.1)
730.84 Other infections involving diseases classified elsewhere, hand bone — (Code first underlying disease: 002.0, 015.0-015.9. Use additional code to identify organism) ☒
882.1 Open wound of hand except finger(s) alone, complicated — (Use additional code to identify infection)
883.1 Open wound of finger(s), complicated — (Use additional code to identify infection)

ICD-9-CM Procedural

80.84 Other local excision or destruction of lesion of joint of hand and finger

HCPCS Level II Supplies & Services

HCPCS Level II codes are used to report the supplies, durable medical equipment, and certain medical services provided on an outpatient basis. Because the procedure(s) represented on this page would be performed in an inpatient or outpatient facility, no HCPCS Level II codes apply.

29902

29902 Arthroscopy, metacarpophalangeal joint, surgical; with reduction of displaced ulnar collateral ligament (eg, Stenar lesion)

ICD-9-CM Diagnostic

815.01 Closed fracture of base of thumb (first) metacarpal bone(s)
815.11 Open fracture of base of thumb (first) metacarpal bone(s)
834.01 Closed dislocation of metacarpophalangeal (joint)
834.11 Open dislocation of metacarpophalangeal (joint)
841.1 Ulnar collateral ligament sprain and strain
842.12 Sprain and strain of metacarpophalangeal (joint) of hand
883.2 Open wound of finger(s), with tendon involvement — (Use additional code to identify infection)
927.20 Crushing injury of hand(s) — (Use additional code to identify any associated injuries: 800-829, 850.0-854.1, 860.0-869.1)
927.3 Crushing injury of finger(s) — (Use additional code to identify any associated injuries: 800-829, 850.0-854.1, 860.0-869.1)

ICD-9-CM Procedural

81.96 Other repair of joint

Respiratory System

Nose

30000–30020

30000 Drainage abscess or hematoma, nasal, internal approach
30020 Drainage abscess or hematoma, nasal septum

ICD-9-CM Diagnostic

478.1 Other diseases of nasal cavity and sinuses
784.0 Headache
802.0 Nasal bones, closed fracture
802.1 Nasal bones, open fracture
873.20 Open wound of nose, unspecified site, without mention of complication — (Use additional code to identify infection) ▽
873.21 Open wound of nasal septum, without mention of complication — (Use additional code to identify infection)
873.30 Open wound of nose, unspecified site, complicated — (Use additional code to identify infection) ▽
873.31 Open wound of nasal septum, complicated — (Use additional code to identify infection)
873.32 Open wound of nasal cavity, complicated — (Use additional code to identify infection)
906.0 Late effect of open wound of head, neck, and trunk
920 Contusion of face, scalp, and neck except eye(s)
959.01 Head injury, unspecified ▽
959.09 Injury of face and neck, other and unspecified
996.69 Infection and inflammatory reaction due to other internal prosthetic device, implant, and graft — (Use additional code to identify specified infections)
998.12 Hematoma complicating a procedure
998.51 Infected postoperative seroma — (Use additional code to identify organism)
998.59 Other postoperative infection — (Use additional code to identify infection)

ICD-9-CM Procedural

21.1 Incision of nose

HCPCS Level II Supplies & Services

A4550 Surgical trays
A4628 Oropharyngeal suction catheter, each

30100

30100 Biopsy, intranasal

ICD-9-CM Diagnostic

160.0 Malignant neoplasm of nasal cavities
195.0 Malignant neoplasm of head, face, and neck
197.3 Secondary malignant neoplasm of other respiratory organs
212.0 Benign neoplasm of nasal cavities, middle ear, and accessory sinuses
231.8 Carcinoma in situ of other specified parts of respiratory system
235.9 Neoplasm of uncertain behavior of other and unspecified respiratory organs ▽
239.1 Neoplasm of unspecified nature of respiratory system
446.4 Wegener's granulomatosis
471.0 Polyp of nasal cavity
471.9 Unspecified nasal polyp ▽
472.0 Chronic rhinitis
473.9 Unspecified sinusitis (chronic) ▽
478.1 Other diseases of nasal cavity and sinuses
686.1 Pyogenic granuloma of skin and subcutaneous tissue
784.2 Swelling, mass, or lump in head and neck

ICD-9-CM Procedural

21.22 Biopsy of nose
22.12 Open biopsy of nasal sinus

HCPCS Level II Supplies & Services

A4305 Disposable drug delivery system, flow rate of 50 ml or greater per hour
A4306 Disposable drug delivery system, flow rate of 5 ml or less per hour
A4550 Surgical trays
A4628 Oropharyngeal suction catheter, each

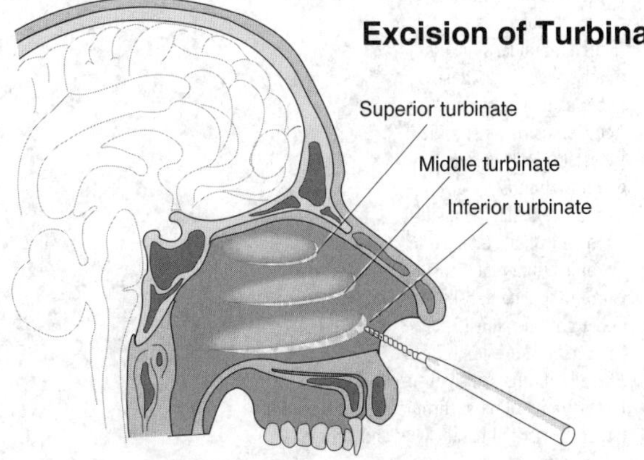

30110–30115

30110 Excision, nasal polyp(s), simple
30115 Excision, nasal polyp(s), extensive

ICD-9-CM Diagnostic

212.0 Benign neoplasm of nasal cavities, middle ear, and accessory sinuses
471.0 Polyp of nasal cavity
471.9 Unspecified nasal polyp ▽
478.1 Other diseases of nasal cavity and sinuses
784.7 Epistaxis

ICD-9-CM Procedural

21.31 Local excision or destruction of intranasal lesion

HCPCS Level II Supplies & Services

A4305 Disposable drug delivery system, flow rate of 50 ml or greater per hour
A4306 Disposable drug delivery system, flow rate of 5 ml or less per hour
A4550 Surgical trays
A4628 Oropharyngeal suction catheter, each

30117–30118

30117 Excision or destruction (eg, laser), intranasal lesion; internal approach
30118 external approach (lateral rhinotomy)

ICD-9-CM Diagnostic

147.9 Malignant neoplasm of nasopharynx, unspecified site ▽
160.0 Malignant neoplasm of nasal cavities
171.0 Malignant neoplasm of connective and other soft tissue of head, face, and neck
195.0 Malignant neoplasm of head, face, and neck
197.3 Secondary malignant neoplasm of other respiratory organs
212.0 Benign neoplasm of nasal cavities, middle ear, and accessory sinuses
228.00 Hemangioma of unspecified site ▽
231.8 Carcinoma in situ of other specified parts of respiratory system
235.9 Neoplasm of uncertain behavior of other and unspecified respiratory organs ▽
239.1 Neoplasm of unspecified nature of respiratory system
471.0 Polyp of nasal cavity
471.9 Unspecified nasal polyp ▽
478.0 Hypertrophy of nasal turbinates
478.1 Other diseases of nasal cavity and sinuses
478.26 Cyst of pharynx or nasopharynx
738.0 Acquired deformity of nose
781.1 Disturbances of sensation of smell and taste

ICD-9-CM Procedural

21.30 Excision or destruction of lesion of nose, not otherwise specified
21.31 Local excision or destruction of intranasal lesion

HCPCS Level II Supplies & Services

A4305 Disposable drug delivery system, flow rate of 50 ml or greater per hour
A4306 Disposable drug delivery system, flow rate of 5 ml or less per hour
A4550 Surgical trays
A4628 Oropharyngeal suction catheter, each

30120

30120 Excision or surgical planing of skin of nose for rhinophyma

ICD-9-CM Diagnostic

695.3 Rosacea

ICD-9-CM Procedural

21.32 Local excision or destruction of other lesion of nose
86.25 Dermabrasion

HCPCS Level II Supplies & Services

A4305 Disposable drug delivery system, flow rate of 50 ml or greater per hour
A4306 Disposable drug delivery system, flow rate of 5 ml or less per hour
A4550 Surgical trays
A4628 Oropharyngeal suction catheter, each

30124–30125

30124 Excision dermoid cyst, nose; simple, skin, subcutaneous
30125 complex, under bone or cartilage

ICD-9-CM Diagnostic

212.0 Benign neoplasm of nasal cavities, middle ear, and accessory sinuses
216.3 Benign neoplasm of skin of other and unspecified parts of face ▽
229.8 Benign neoplasm of other specified sites
709.8 Other specified disorder of skin

ICD-9-CM Procedural

21.32 Local excision or destruction of other lesion of nose

HCPCS Level II Supplies & Services

A4305 Disposable drug delivery system, flow rate of 50 ml or greater per hour
A4306 Disposable drug delivery system, flow rate of 5 ml or less per hour
A4550 Surgical trays

30130–30140

30130 Excision turbinate, partial or complete, any method
30140 Submucous resection turbinate, partial or complete, any method

ICD-9-CM Diagnostic

160.0 Malignant neoplasm of nasal cavities
170.0 Malignant neoplasm of bones of skull and face, except mandible
197.3 Secondary malignant neoplasm of other respiratory organs
198.5 Secondary malignant neoplasm of bone and bone marrow
212.0 Benign neoplasm of nasal cavities, middle ear, and accessory sinuses
213.0 Benign neoplasm of bones of skull and face
231.8 Carcinoma in situ of other specified parts of respiratory system
235.9 Neoplasm of uncertain behavior of other and unspecified respiratory organs ▽
238.0 Neoplasm of uncertain behavior of bone and articular cartilage
239.1 Neoplasm of unspecified nature of respiratory system
239.2 Neoplasms of unspecified nature of bone, soft tissue, and skin
375.22 Epiphora due to insufficient drainage
461.3 Acute sphenoidal sinusitis
461.8 Other acute sinusitis
470 Deviated nasal septum
472.0 Chronic rhinitis
472.2 Chronic nasopharyngitis
473.0 Chronic maxillary sinusitis
473.1 Chronic frontal sinusitis
473.2 Chronic ethmoidal sinusitis
473.3 Chronic sphenoidal sinusitis
473.8 Other chronic sinusitis
473.9 Unspecified sinusitis (chronic) ▽
477.9 Allergic rhinitis, cause unspecified ▽
478.0 Hypertrophy of nasal turbinates
478.1 Other diseases of nasal cavity and sinuses
780.51 Insomnia with sleep apnea
780.57 Other and unspecified sleep apnea ▽
786.09 Other dyspnea and respiratory abnormalities
802.0 Nasal bones, closed fracture
802.1 Nasal bones, open fracture
905.0 Late effect of fracture of skull and face bones

ICD-9-CM Procedural

21.61 Turbinectomy by diathermy or cryosurgery
21.69 Other turbinectomy

30150–30160

30150 Rhinectomy; partial
30160 total

ICD-9-CM Diagnostic

160.0 Malignant neoplasm of nasal cavities
170.0 Malignant neoplasm of bones of skull and face, except mandible
172.3 Malignant melanoma of skin of other and unspecified parts of face
173.3 Other malignant neoplasm of skin of other and unspecified parts of face ▽
195.0 Malignant neoplasm of head, face, and neck
197.3 Secondary malignant neoplasm of other respiratory organs
198.2 Secondary malignant neoplasm of skin
198.89 Secondary malignant neoplasm of other specified sites
212.0 Benign neoplasm of nasal cavities, middle ear, and accessory sinuses
228.01 Hemangioma of skin and subcutaneous tissue
231.8 Carcinoma in situ of other specified parts of respiratory system
232.3 Carcinoma in situ of skin of other and unspecified parts of face ▽
238.0 Neoplasm of uncertain behavior of bone and articular cartilage
238.2 Neoplasm of uncertain behavior of skin
478.1 Other diseases of nasal cavity and sinuses
738.0 Acquired deformity of nose
785.4 Gangrene — (Code first any associated underlying condition:250.7, 443.0)
873.30 Open wound of nose, unspecified site, complicated — (Use additional code to identify infection) ▽
873.31 Open wound of nasal septum, complicated — (Use additional code to identify infection)
873.32 Open wound of nasal cavity, complicated — (Use additional code to identify infection)
873.33 Open wound of nasal sinus, complicated — (Use additional code to identify infection)
873.39 Open wound of nose, multiple sites, complicated — (Use additional code to identify infection)
925.1 Crushing injury of face and scalp — (Use additional code to identify any associated injuries: 800-829, 850.0-854.1, 860.0-869.1)
941.55 Deep necrosis of underlying tissues due to burn (deep third degree) of nose (septum), with loss of a body part
948.00 Burn (any degree) involving less than 10% of body surface with third degree burn of less than 10% or unspecified amount
991.0 Frostbite of face
998.59 Other postoperative infection — (Use additional code to identify infection)
V10.22 Personal history of malignant neoplasm of nasal cavities, middle ear, and accessory sinuses
V10.81 Personal history of malignant neoplasm of bone
V10.82 Personal history of malignant melanoma of skin

ICD-9-CM Procedural

21.4 Resection of nose

30200

30200 Injection into turbinate(s), therapeutic

ICD-9-CM Diagnostic

461.0 Acute maxillary sinusitis
461.1 Acute frontal sinusitis
461.2 Acute ethmoidal sinusitis
461.3 Acute sphenoidal sinusitis
461.8 Other acute sinusitis
461.9 Acute sinusitis, unspecified ▽
470 Deviated nasal septum
472.0 Chronic rhinitis
473.0 Chronic maxillary sinusitis
473.1 Chronic frontal sinusitis
473.2 Chronic ethmoidal sinusitis
473.3 Chronic sphenoidal sinusitis
473.8 Other chronic sinusitis
473.9 Unspecified sinusitis (chronic) ▽
477.9 Allergic rhinitis, cause unspecified ▽
478.0 Hypertrophy of nasal turbinates
478.1 Other diseases of nasal cavity and sinuses

▽ Unspecified code ♀ Female diagnosis ☒ Manifestation code ♂ Male diagnosis

ICD-9-CM Procedural
99.29 Injection or infusion of other therapeutic or prophylactic substance
99.77 Application or administration of adhesion barrier substance

HCPCS Level II Supplies & Services
A4305 Disposable drug delivery system, flow rate of 50 ml or greater per hour
A4306 Disposable drug delivery system, flow rate of 5 ml or less per hour
A4550 Surgical trays
A4628 Oropharyngeal suction catheter, each

30210
30210 Displacement therapy (Proetz type)

ICD-9-CM Diagnostic
461.2 Acute ethmoidal sinusitis
461.3 Acute sphenoidal sinusitis
461.8 Other acute sinusitis
461.9 Acute sinusitis, unspecified ▽
472.0 Chronic rhinitis
473.2 Chronic ethmoidal sinusitis
473.3 Chronic sphenoidal sinusitis
473.8 Other chronic sinusitis
473.9 Unspecified sinusitis (chronic) ▽
477.9 Allergic rhinitis, cause unspecified ▽
478.0 Hypertrophy of nasal turbinates

ICD-9-CM Procedural
22.00 Aspiration and lavage of nasal sinus, not otherwise specified

HCPCS Level II Supplies & Services
A4305 Disposable drug delivery system, flow rate of 50 ml or greater per hour
A4306 Disposable drug delivery system, flow rate of 5 ml or less per hour
A4550 Surgical trays
A4628 Oropharyngeal suction catheter, each

30220
30220 Insertion, nasal septal prosthesis (button)

ICD-9-CM Diagnostic
160.0 Malignant neoplasm of nasal cavities
234.8 Carcinoma in situ of other specified sites
305.60 Nondependent cocaine abuse, unspecified ▽
305.61 Nondependent cocaine abuse, continuous
305.62 Nondependent cocaine abuse, episodic
305.63 Nondependent cocaine abuse, in remission
461.3 Acute sphenoidal sinusitis
470 Deviated nasal septum
473.9 Unspecified sinusitis (chronic) ▽
478.0 Hypertrophy of nasal turbinates
478.1 Other diseases of nasal cavity and sinuses
748.1 Other congenital anomaly of nose
802.0 Nasal bones, closed fracture
802.1 Nasal bones, open fracture
905.0 Late effect of fracture of skull and face bones
906.4 Late effect of crushing
906.5 Late effect of burn of eye, face, head, and neck
959.01 Head injury, unspecified ▽
959.09 Injury of face and neck, other and unspecified
998.12 Hematoma complicating a procedure
998.59 Other postoperative infection — (Use additional code to identify infection)
V10.22 Personal history of malignant neoplasm of nasal cavities, middle ear, and accessory sinuses

ICD-9-CM Procedural
21.89 Other repair and plastic operations on nose

30300–30320
30300 Removal foreign body, intranasal; office type procedure
30310 requiring general anesthesia
30320 by lateral rhinotomy

ICD-9-CM Diagnostic
932 Foreign body in nose

ICD-9-CM Procedural
21.1 Incision of nose
96.53 Irrigation of nasal passages
98.12 Removal of intraluminal foreign body from nose without incision

HCPCS Level II Supplies & Services
A4305 Disposable drug delivery system, flow rate of 50 ml or greater per hour
A4306 Disposable drug delivery system, flow rate of 5 ml or less per hour
A4550 Surgical trays
A4628 Oropharyngeal suction catheter, each

30400–30410
30400 Rhinoplasty, primary; lateral and alar cartilages and/or elevation of nasal tip
30410 complete, external parts including bony pyramid, lateral and alar cartilages, and/or elevation of nasal tip

ICD-9-CM Diagnostic
160.0 Malignant neoplasm of nasal cavities
170.0 Malignant neoplasm of bones of skull and face, except mandible
173.3 Other malignant neoplasm of skin of other and unspecified parts of face ▽
198.2 Secondary malignant neoplasm of skin
212.0 Benign neoplasm of nasal cavities, middle ear, and accessory sinuses
213.0 Benign neoplasm of bones of skull and face
216.3 Benign neoplasm of skin of other and unspecified parts of face ▽
232.3 Carcinoma in situ of skin of other and unspecified parts of face ▽
238.2 Neoplasm of uncertain behavior of skin
239.2 Neoplasms of unspecified nature of bone, soft tissue, and skin
478.1 Other diseases of nasal cavity and sinuses
738.0 Acquired deformity of nose
748.1 Other congenital anomaly of nose
754.0 Congenital musculoskeletal deformities of skull, face, and jaw
785.4 Gangrene — (Code first any associated underlying condition:250.7, 443.0)
802.0 Nasal bones, closed fracture
802.1 Nasal bones, open fracture
873.32 Open wound of nasal cavity, complicated — (Use additional code to identify infection)
905.0 Late effect of fracture of skull and face bones
906.0 Late effect of open wound of head, neck, and trunk
906.5 Late effect of burn of eye, face, head, and neck
925.1 Crushing injury of face and scalp — (Use additional code to identify any associated injuries: 800-829, 850.0-854.1, 860.0-869.1)
991.0 Frostbite of face
V50.1 Other plastic surgery for unacceptable cosmetic appearance
V51 Aftercare involving the use of plastic surgery

ICD-9-CM Procedural
21.83 Total nasal reconstruction
21.86 Limited rhinoplasty
21.87 Other rhinoplasty

30420
30420 Rhinoplasty, primary; including major septal repair

ICD-9-CM Diagnostic
160.0 Malignant neoplasm of nasal cavities
173.3 Other malignant neoplasm of skin of other and unspecified parts of face ▽
197.3 Secondary malignant neoplasm of other respiratory organs
198.2 Secondary malignant neoplasm of skin
198.89 Secondary malignant neoplasm of other specified sites
212.0 Benign neoplasm of nasal cavities, middle ear, and accessory sinuses
216.3 Benign neoplasm of skin of other and unspecified parts of face ▽
231.8 Carcinoma in situ of other specified parts of respiratory system
232.3 Carcinoma in situ of skin of other and unspecified parts of face ▽
235.9 Neoplasm of uncertain behavior of other and unspecified respiratory organs ▽
238.1 Neoplasm of uncertain behavior of connective and other soft tissue ▽
238.2 Neoplasm of uncertain behavior of skin
239.1 Neoplasm of unspecified nature of respiratory system
239.2 Neoplasms of unspecified nature of bone, soft tissue, and skin
470 Deviated nasal septum
478.1 Other diseases of nasal cavity and sinuses
519.8 Other diseases of respiratory system, not elsewhere classified
738.0 Acquired deformity of nose
748.1 Other congenital anomaly of nose
754.0 Congenital musculoskeletal deformities of skull, face, and jaw
786.09 Other dyspnea and respiratory abnormalities
802.0 Nasal bones, closed fracture
802.1 Nasal bones, open fracture
802.5 Malar and maxillary bones, open fracture

873.31 Open wound of nasal septum, complicated — (Use additional code to identify infection)
873.32 Open wound of nasal cavity, complicated — (Use additional code to identify infection)
873.39 Open wound of nose, multiple sites, complicated — (Use additional code to identify infection)
905.0 Late effect of fracture of skull and face bones
906.0 Late effect of open wound of head, neck, and trunk
906.5 Late effect of burn of eye, face, head, and neck
991.0 Frostbite of face
V50.1 Other plastic surgery for unacceptable cosmetic appearance
V51 Aftercare involving the use of plastic surgery

ICD-9-CM Procedural

21.5 Submucous resection of nasal septum
21.87 Other rhinoplasty
21.88 Other septoplasty

30430–30450

30430 Rhinoplasty, secondary; minor revision (small amount of nasal tip work)
30435 intermediate revision (bony work with osteotomies)
30450 major revision (nasal tip work and osteotomies)

ICD-9-CM Diagnostic

738.0 Acquired deformity of nose
748.1 Other congenital anomaly of nose
754.0 Congenital musculoskeletal deformities of skull, face, and jaw
786.09 Other dyspnea and respiratory abnormalities
905.0 Late effect of fracture of skull and face bones
906.0 Late effect of open wound of head, neck, and trunk
906.4 Late effect of crushing
906.5 Late effect of burn of eye, face, head, and neck
996.4 Mechanical complication of internal orthopedic device, implant, and graft
996.52 Mechanical complication due to other tissue graft, not elsewhere classified
996.79 Other complications due to other internal prosthetic device, implant, and graft
V10.22 Personal history of malignant neoplasm of nasal cavities, middle ear, and accessory sinuses
V50.1 Other plastic surgery for unacceptable cosmetic appearance
V51 Aftercare involving the use of plastic surgery

ICD-9-CM Procedural

21.84 Revision rhinoplasty
21.89 Other repair and plastic operations on nose

30460–30462

30460 Rhinoplasty for nasal deformity secondary to congenital cleft lip and/or palate, including columellar lengthening; tip only
30462 tip, septum, osteotomies

ICD-9-CM Diagnostic

470 Deviated nasal septum
748.1 Other congenital anomaly of nose
749.01 Unilateral cleft palate, complete
749.03 Bilateral cleft palate, complete
749.11 Unilateral cleft lip, complete
749.13 Bilateral cleft lip, complete
749.21 Unilateral cleft palate with cleft lip, complete
749.23 Bilateral cleft palate with cleft lip, complete
756.0 Congenital anomalies of skull and face bones
V50.1 Other plastic surgery for unacceptable cosmetic appearance
V51 Aftercare involving the use of plastic surgery

ICD-9-CM Procedural

21.86 Limited rhinoplasty
21.87 Other rhinoplasty
21.88 Other septoplasty

30465

30465 Repair of nasal vestibular stenosis (eg, spreader grafting, lateral nasal wall reconstruction)

ICD-9-CM Diagnostic

478.1 Other diseases of nasal cavity and sinuses
748.0 Congenital choanal atresia

ICD-9-CM Procedural

21.89 Other repair and plastic operations on nose

30520

30520 Septoplasty or submucous resection, with or without cartilage scoring, contouring or replacement with graft

ICD-9-CM Diagnostic

160.0 Malignant neoplasm of nasal cavities
197.3 Secondary malignant neoplasm of other respiratory organs
198.89 Secondary malignant neoplasm of other specified sites
212.0 Benign neoplasm of nasal cavities, middle ear, and accessory sinuses
231.8 Carcinoma in situ of other specified parts of respiratory system
235.9 Neoplasm of uncertain behavior of other and unspecified respiratory organs ▽
239.1 Neoplasm of unspecified nature of respiratory system
305.60 Nondependent cocaine abuse, unspecified ▽
305.61 Nondependent cocaine abuse, continuous
305.62 Nondependent cocaine abuse, episodic
305.63 Nondependent cocaine abuse, in remission
461.2 Acute ethmoidal sinusitis
461.8 Other acute sinusitis
470 Deviated nasal septum
471.0 Polyp of nasal cavity
471.9 Unspecified nasal polyp ▽
472.0 Chronic rhinitis
473.0 Chronic maxillary sinusitis
473.2 Chronic ethmoidal sinusitis
473.9 Unspecified sinusitis (chronic) ▽
478.1 Other diseases of nasal cavity and sinuses
738.0 Acquired deformity of nose
748.1 Other congenital anomaly of nose
754.0 Congenital musculoskeletal deformities of skull, face, and jaw
784.7 Epistaxis
786.02 Orthopnea
786.09 Other dyspnea and respiratory abnormalities
802.0 Nasal bones, closed fracture
802.1 Nasal bones, open fracture
873.31 Open wound of nasal septum, complicated — (Use additional code to identify infection)
905.0 Late effect of fracture of skull and face bones
V10.22 Personal history of malignant neoplasm of nasal cavities, middle ear, and accessory sinuses

ICD-9-CM Procedural

21.5 Submucous resection of nasal septum
21.88 Other septoplasty

30540–30545

30540 Repair choanal atresia; intranasal
30545 transpalatine

ICD-9-CM Diagnostic

738.0 Acquired deformity of nose
748.0 Congenital choanal atresia

ICD-9-CM Procedural

21.89 Other repair and plastic operations on nose

30560

30560 Lysis intranasal synechia

ICD-9-CM Diagnostic

470 Deviated nasal septum
471.1 Polypoid sinus degeneration
471.9 Unspecified nasal polyp ▽
473.0 Chronic maxillary sinusitis
473.1 Chronic frontal sinusitis
473.2 Chronic ethmoidal sinusitis
473.3 Chronic sphenoidal sinusitis
473.8 Other chronic sinusitis
473.9 Unspecified sinusitis (chronic) ▽
478.0 Hypertrophy of nasal turbinates
478.1 Other diseases of nasal cavity and sinuses
738.0 Acquired deformity of nose
748.0 Congenital choanal atresia

▽ Unspecified code
♀ Female diagnosis
☒ Manifestation code
♂ Male diagnosis

905.0 Late effect of fracture of skull and face bones
906.5 Late effect of burn of eye, face, head, and neck

ICD-9-CM Procedural
21.91 Lysis of adhesions of nose

30580–30600
30580 Repair fistula; oromaxillary (combine with 31030 if antrotomy is included)
30600 oronasal

ICD-9-CM Diagnostic
473.0 Chronic maxillary sinusitis
478.1 Other diseases of nasal cavity and sinuses
526.89 Other specified disease of the jaws
528.3 Cellulitis and abscess of oral soft tissues
528.9 Other and unspecified diseases of the oral soft tissues ▽
738.19 Other specified acquired deformity of head
748.1 Other congenital anomaly of nose
749.00 Unspecified cleft palate ▽
749.01 Unilateral cleft palate, complete
749.02 Unilateral cleft palate, incomplete
749.03 Bilateral cleft palate, complete
749.04 Bilateral cleft palate, incomplete
749.20 Unspecified cleft palate with cleft lip ▽
749.21 Unilateral cleft palate with cleft lip, complete
749.22 Unilateral cleft palate with cleft lip, incomplete
749.23 Bilateral cleft palate with cleft lip, complete
749.24 Bilateral cleft palate with cleft lip, incomplete
749.25 Other combinations of cleft palate with cleft lip
905.0 Late effect of fracture of skull and face bones
996.4 Mechanical complication of internal orthopedic device, implant, and graft

ICD-9-CM Procedural
21.82 Closure of nasal fistula
22.71 Closure of nasal sinus fistula

30620
30620 Septal or other intranasal dermatoplasty (does not include obtaining graft)

ICD-9-CM Diagnostic
448.0 Hereditary hemorrhagic telangiectasia
470 Deviated nasal septum
471.0 Polyp of nasal cavity
473.0 Chronic maxillary sinusitis
473.2 Chronic ethmoidal sinusitis
473.3 Chronic sphenoidal sinusitis
473.8 Other chronic sinusitis
473.9 Unspecified sinusitis (chronic) ▽
478.0 Hypertrophy of nasal turbinates
478.1 Other diseases of nasal cavity and sinuses
519.8 Other diseases of respiratory system, not elsewhere classified
738.0 Acquired deformity of nose
748.1 Other congenital anomaly of nose
754.0 Congenital musculoskeletal deformities of skull, face, and jaw
784.7 Epistaxis
802.0 Nasal bones, closed fracture
802.1 Nasal bones, open fracture

ICD-9-CM Procedural
21.07 Control of epistaxis by excision of nasal mucosa and skin grafting of septum and lateral nasal wall
21.89 Other repair and plastic operations on nose

30630
30630 Repair nasal septal perforations

ICD-9-CM Diagnostic
305.60 Nondependent cocaine abuse, unspecified ▽
305.61 Nondependent cocaine abuse, continuous
305.62 Nondependent cocaine abuse, episodic
305.63 Nondependent cocaine abuse, in remission
478.1 Other diseases of nasal cavity and sinuses
748.1 Other congenital anomaly of nose
784.7 Epistaxis
802.0 Nasal bones, closed fracture
802.1 Nasal bones, open fracture
905.0 Late effect of fracture of skull and face bones
906.4 Late effect of crushing
906.5 Late effect of burn of eye, face, head, and neck

ICD-9-CM Procedural
21.88 Other septoplasty

30801–30802
30801 Cautery and/or ablation, mucosa of turbinates, unilateral or bilateral, any method, (separate procedure); superficial
30802 intramural

ICD-9-CM Diagnostic
470 Deviated nasal septum
471.8 Other polyp of sinus
471.9 Unspecified nasal polyp ▽
472.0 Chronic rhinitis
473.0 Chronic maxillary sinusitis
473.2 Chronic ethmoidal sinusitis
473.3 Chronic sphenoidal sinusitis
473.8 Other chronic sinusitis
473.9 Unspecified sinusitis (chronic) ▽
478.0 Hypertrophy of nasal turbinates
478.1 Other diseases of nasal cavity and sinuses
519.8 Other diseases of respiratory system, not elsewhere classified
738.0 Acquired deformity of nose
780.51 Insomnia with sleep apnea
780.57 Other and unspecified sleep apnea ▽
784.7 Epistaxis
786.09 Other dyspnea and respiratory abnormalities

ICD-9-CM Procedural
21.61 Turbinectomy by diathermy or cryosurgery
21.69 Other turbinectomy

HCPCS Level II Supplies & Services
A4305 Disposable drug delivery system, flow rate of 50 ml or greater per hour
A4306 Disposable drug delivery system, flow rate of 5 ml or less per hour
A4550 Surgical trays
A4628 Oropharyngeal suction catheter, each

30901–30903
30901 Control nasal hemorrhage, anterior, simple (limited cautery and/or packing) any method
30903 Control nasal hemorrhage, anterior, complex (extensive cautery and/or packing) any method

ICD-9-CM Diagnostic
448.9 Other and unspecified capillary diseases ▽
478.29 Other disease of pharynx or nasopharynx
772.8 Other specified hemorrhage of fetus or newborn
784.7 Epistaxis
958.2 Secondary and recurrent hemorrhage as an early complication of trauma
998.11 Hemorrhage complicating a procedure
998.2 Accidental puncture or laceration during procedure

ICD-9-CM Procedural
21.00 Control of epistaxis, not otherwise specified
21.01 Control of epistaxis by anterior nasal packing
21.02 Control of epistaxis by posterior (and anterior) packing
21.03 Control of epistaxis by cauterization (and packing)

HCPCS Level II Supplies & Services
A4550 Surgical trays
A4628 Oropharyngeal suction catheter, each

30905–30906
30905 Control nasal hemorrhage, posterior, with posterior nasal packs and/or cautery, any method; initial
30906 subsequent

ICD-9-CM Diagnostic
448.9 Other and unspecified capillary diseases ▽
478.29 Other disease of pharynx or nasopharynx
772.8 Other specified hemorrhage of fetus or newborn

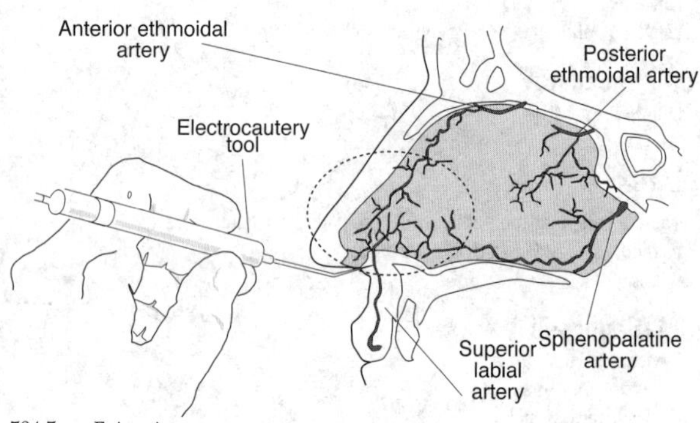

784.7	Epistaxis
958.2	Secondary and recurrent hemorrhage as an early complication of trauma
998.11	Hemorrhage complicating a procedure
998.2	Accidental puncture or laceration during procedure

ICD-9-CM Procedural

21.02	Control of epistaxis by posterior (and anterior) packing
21.03	Control of epistaxis by cauterization (and packing)

HCPCS Level II Supplies & Services

A4550	Surgical trays

30915–30920

30915	Ligation arteries; ethmoidal
30920	internal maxillary artery, transantral

ICD-9-CM Diagnostic

784.7	Epistaxis
802.0	Nasal bones, closed fracture
802.1	Nasal bones, open fracture
802.8	Other facial bones, closed fracture
900.82	Injury to multiple blood vessels of head and neck
958.2	Secondary and recurrent hemorrhage as an early complication of trauma
959.01	Head injury, unspecified ▽
959.09	Injury of face and neck, other and unspecified
998.2	Accidental puncture or laceration during procedure

ICD-9-CM Procedural

21.04	Control of epistaxis by ligation of ethmoidal arteries
21.05	Control of epistaxis by (transantral) ligation of the maxillary artery

30930

30930	Fracture nasal turbinate(s), therapeutic

ICD-9-CM Diagnostic

461.9	Acute sinusitis, unspecified ▽
470	Deviated nasal septum
472.0	Chronic rhinitis
473.0	Chronic maxillary sinusitis
473.1	Chronic frontal sinusitis
473.2	Chronic ethmoidal sinusitis
473.3	Chronic sphenoidal sinusitis
473.8	Other chronic sinusitis
473.9	Unspecified sinusitis (chronic) ▽
477.9	Allergic rhinitis, cause unspecified ▽
478.0	Hypertrophy of nasal turbinates
478.1	Other diseases of nasal cavity and sinuses
519.8	Other diseases of respiratory system, not elsewhere classified
738.0	Acquired deformity of nose
748.1	Other congenital anomaly of nose
780.51	Insomnia with sleep apnea
780.57	Other and unspecified sleep apnea ▽
786.09	Other dyspnea and respiratory abnormalities

ICD-9-CM Procedural

21.62	Fracture of the turbinates

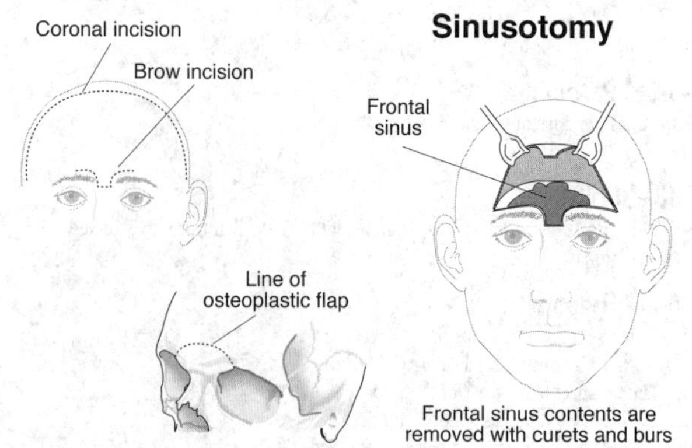

Frontal sinus contents are removed with curets and burs

Accessory Sinuses

31000–31002

31000	Lavage by cannulation; maxillary sinus (antrum puncture or natural ostium)
31002	sphenoid sinus

ICD-9-CM Diagnostic

461.0	Acute maxillary sinusitis
461.3	Acute sphenoidal sinusitis
461.9	Acute sinusitis, unspecified ▽
472.0	Chronic rhinitis
473.0	Chronic maxillary sinusitis
473.3	Chronic sphenoidal sinusitis
473.8	Other chronic sinusitis
473.9	Unspecified sinusitis (chronic) ▽
478.1	Other diseases of nasal cavity and sinuses
784.0	Headache

ICD-9-CM Procedural

22.00	Aspiration and lavage of nasal sinus, not otherwise specified
22.01	Puncture of nasal sinus for aspiration or lavage
22.02	Aspiration or lavage of nasal sinus through natural ostium

HCPCS Level II Supplies & Services

A4550	Surgical trays
A4628	Oropharyngeal suction catheter, each

31020–31032

31020	Sinusotomy, maxillary (antrotomy); intranasal
31030	radical (Caldwell-Luc) without removal of antrochoanal polyps
31032	radical (Caldwell-Luc) with removal of antrochoanal polyps

ICD-9-CM Diagnostic

160.2	Malignant neoplasm of maxillary sinus
197.3	Secondary malignant neoplasm of other respiratory organs
212.0	Benign neoplasm of nasal cavities, middle ear, and accessory sinuses
231.8	Carcinoma in situ of other specified parts of respiratory system
235.9	Neoplasm of uncertain behavior of other and unspecified respiratory organs ▽
238.0	Neoplasm of uncertain behavior of bone and articular cartilage
239.1	Neoplasm of unspecified nature of respiratory system
289.1	Chronic lymphadenitis
446.4	Wegener's granulomatosis
461.0	Acute maxillary sinusitis
461.8	Other acute sinusitis
461.9	Acute sinusitis, unspecified ▽
470	Deviated nasal septum
471.0	Polyp of nasal cavity
471.8	Other polyp of sinus
471.9	Unspecified nasal polyp ▽
473.0	Chronic maxillary sinusitis
473.8	Other chronic sinusitis
473.9	Unspecified sinusitis (chronic) ▽
478.0	Hypertrophy of nasal turbinates
478.1	Other diseases of nasal cavity and sinuses
730.18	Chronic osteomyelitis, other specified sites — (Use additional code to identify organism, 041.1)

▽ Unspecified code ♀ Female diagnosis ☒ Manifestation code ♂ Male diagnosis

730.28 Unspecified osteomyelitis, other specified sites — (Use additional code to identify organism, 041.1)
748.8 Other specified congenital anomaly of respiratory system
784.0 Headache
784.2 Swelling, mass, or lump in head and neck
784.7 Epistaxis
786.09 Other dyspnea and respiratory abnormalities
905.0 Late effect of fracture of skull and face bones
996.60 Infection and inflammatory reaction due to unspecified device, implant, and graft — (Use additional code to identify specified infections)
996.69 Infection and inflammatory reaction due to other internal prosthetic device, implant, and graft — (Use additional code to identify specified infections)

ICD-9-CM Procedural

22.2 Intranasal antrotomy
22.31 Radical maxillary antrotomy
22.39 Other external maxillary antrotomy
22.61 Excision of lesion of maxillary sinus with Caldwell-Luc approach

HCPCS Level II Supplies & Services

A4305 Disposable drug delivery system, flow rate of 50 ml or greater per hour
A4306 Disposable drug delivery system, flow rate of 5 ml or less per hour
A4550 Surgical trays

31040

31040 Pterygomaxillary fossa surgery, any approach

ICD-9-CM Diagnostic

239.1 Neoplasm of unspecified nature of respiratory system
350.1 Trigeminal neuralgia
350.2 Atypical face pain

ICD-9-CM Procedural

22.50 Sinusotomy, not otherwise specified

31050–31051

31050 Sinusotomy, sphenoid, with or without biopsy;
31051 with mucosal stripping or removal of polyp(s)

ICD-9-CM Diagnostic

160.0 Malignant neoplasm of nasal cavities
160.5 Malignant neoplasm of sphenoidal sinus
197.3 Secondary malignant neoplasm of other respiratory organs
212.0 Benign neoplasm of nasal cavities, middle ear, and accessory sinuses
231.8 Carcinoma in situ of other specified parts of respiratory system
235.9 Neoplasm of uncertain behavior of other and unspecified respiratory organs
239.1 Neoplasm of unspecified nature of respiratory system
461.3 Acute sphenoidal sinusitis
461.8 Other acute sinusitis
461.9 Acute sinusitis, unspecified
471.1 Polypoid sinus degeneration
471.8 Other polyp of sinus
471.9 Unspecified nasal polyp
472.0 Chronic rhinitis
473.3 Chronic sphenoidal sinusitis
473.8 Other chronic sinusitis
473.9 Unspecified sinusitis (chronic)
478.0 Hypertrophy of nasal turbinates
478.1 Other diseases of nasal cavity and sinuses
730.18 Chronic osteomyelitis, other specified sites — (Use additional code to identify organism, 041.1)
748.8 Other specified congenital anomaly of respiratory system
784.0 Headache
784.2 Swelling, mass, or lump in head and neck
905.0 Late effect of fracture of skull and face bones

ICD-9-CM Procedural

21.31 Local excision or destruction of intranasal lesion
22.12 Open biopsy of nasal sinus
22.52 Sphenoidotomy

31070

31070 Sinusotomy frontal; external, simple (trephine operation)

ICD-9-CM Diagnostic

160.0 Malignant neoplasm of nasal cavities
160.4 Malignant neoplasm of frontal sinus
160.8 Malignant neoplasm of other sites of nasal cavities, middle ear, and accessory sinuses
197.3 Secondary malignant neoplasm of other respiratory organs
212.0 Benign neoplasm of nasal cavities, middle ear, and accessory sinuses
231.8 Carcinoma in situ of other specified parts of respiratory system
235.9 Neoplasm of uncertain behavior of other and unspecified respiratory organs
239.1 Neoplasm of unspecified nature of respiratory system
376.01 Orbital cellulitis
461.1 Acute frontal sinusitis
461.8 Other acute sinusitis
461.9 Acute sinusitis, unspecified
471.1 Polypoid sinus degeneration
471.8 Other polyp of sinus
472.0 Chronic rhinitis
473.1 Chronic frontal sinusitis
473.8 Other chronic sinusitis
473.9 Unspecified sinusitis (chronic)
478.0 Hypertrophy of nasal turbinates
478.1 Other diseases of nasal cavity and sinuses
905.0 Late effect of fracture of skull and face bones

ICD-9-CM Procedural

22.41 Frontal sinusotomy

31075

31075 Sinusotomy frontal; transorbital, unilateral (for mucocele or osteoma, Lynch type)

ICD-9-CM Diagnostic

212.0 Benign neoplasm of nasal cavities, middle ear, and accessory sinuses
213.0 Benign neoplasm of bones of skull and face
231.8 Carcinoma in situ of other specified parts of respiratory system
235.9 Neoplasm of uncertain behavior of other and unspecified respiratory organs
239.1 Neoplasm of unspecified nature of respiratory system
461.1 Acute frontal sinusitis
461.8 Other acute sinusitis
461.9 Acute sinusitis, unspecified
471.1 Polypoid sinus degeneration
471.8 Other polyp of sinus
472.0 Chronic rhinitis
473.1 Chronic frontal sinusitis
473.8 Other chronic sinusitis
473.9 Unspecified sinusitis (chronic)
478.0 Hypertrophy of nasal turbinates
478.1 Other diseases of nasal cavity and sinuses
905.0 Late effect of fracture of skull and face bones

ICD-9-CM Procedural

22.41 Frontal sinusotomy

31080–31085

31080 Sinusotomy frontal; obliterative without osteoplastic flap, brow incision (includes ablation)
31081 obliterative, without osteoplastic flap, coronal incision (includes ablation)
31084 obliterative, with osteoplastic flap, brow incision
31085 obliterative, with osteoplastic flap, coronal incision

ICD-9-CM Diagnostic

160.0 Malignant neoplasm of nasal cavities
160.4 Malignant neoplasm of frontal sinus
160.8 Malignant neoplasm of other sites of nasal cavities, middle ear, and accessory sinuses
195.0 Malignant neoplasm of head, face, and neck
197.3 Secondary malignant neoplasm of other respiratory organs
198.89 Secondary malignant neoplasm of other specified sites
212.0 Benign neoplasm of nasal cavities, middle ear, and accessory sinuses
213.0 Benign neoplasm of bones of skull and face
231.8 Carcinoma in situ of other specified parts of respiratory system
235.9 Neoplasm of uncertain behavior of other and unspecified respiratory organs
239.1 Neoplasm of unspecified nature of respiratory system
376.01 Orbital cellulitis
461.1 Acute frontal sinusitis
461.8 Other acute sinusitis
461.9 Acute sinusitis, unspecified
471.1 Polypoid sinus degeneration

471.8 Other polyp of sinus
471.9 Unspecified nasal polyp ▽
472.0 Chronic rhinitis
473.1 Chronic frontal sinusitis
473.8 Other chronic sinusitis
473.9 Unspecified sinusitis (chronic) ▽
478.0 Hypertrophy of nasal turbinates
478.1 Other diseases of nasal cavity and sinuses
905.0 Late effect of fracture of skull and face bones

ICD-9-CM Procedural

22.42 Frontal sinusectomy

31086–31087

31086 Sinusotomy frontal; nonobliterative, with osteoplastic flap, brow incision
31087 nonobliterative, with osteoplastic flap, coronal incision

ICD-9-CM Diagnostic

160.0 Malignant neoplasm of nasal cavities
160.4 Malignant neoplasm of frontal sinus
160.8 Malignant neoplasm of other sites of nasal cavities, middle ear, and accessory sinuses
195.0 Malignant neoplasm of head, face, and neck
197.3 Secondary malignant neoplasm of other respiratory organs
198.89 Secondary malignant neoplasm of other specified sites
212.0 Benign neoplasm of nasal cavities, middle ear, and accessory sinuses
213.0 Benign neoplasm of bones of skull and face
231.8 Carcinoma in situ of other specified parts of respiratory system
235.9 Neoplasm of uncertain behavior of other and unspecified respiratory organs ▽
239.1 Neoplasm of unspecified nature of respiratory system
376.01 Orbital cellulitis
461.1 Acute frontal sinusitis
461.8 Other acute sinusitis
461.9 Acute sinusitis, unspecified ▽
471.1 Polypoid sinus degeneration
471.8 Other polyp of sinus
472.0 Chronic rhinitis
473.1 Chronic frontal sinusitis
473.2 Chronic ethmoidal sinusitis
473.8 Other chronic sinusitis
473.9 Unspecified sinusitis (chronic) ▽
478.0 Hypertrophy of nasal turbinates
478.1 Other diseases of nasal cavity and sinuses
905.0 Late effect of fracture of skull and face bones

ICD-9-CM Procedural

22.41 Frontal sinusotomy
22.42 Frontal sinusectomy

31090

31090 Sinusotomy, unilateral, three or more paranasal sinuses (frontal, maxillary, ethmoid, sphenoid)

ICD-9-CM Diagnostic

160.2 Malignant neoplasm of maxillary sinus
160.3 Malignant neoplasm of ethmoidal sinus
160.4 Malignant neoplasm of frontal sinus
160.5 Malignant neoplasm of sphenoidal sinus
160.8 Malignant neoplasm of other sites of nasal cavities, middle ear, and accessory sinuses
160.9 Malignant neoplasm of site of nasal cavities, middle ear, and accessory sinus, unspecified site ▽
195.0 Malignant neoplasm of head, face, and neck
197.3 Secondary malignant neoplasm of other respiratory organs
212.0 Benign neoplasm of nasal cavities, middle ear, and accessory sinuses
213.0 Benign neoplasm of bones of skull and face
231.8 Carcinoma in situ of other specified parts of respiratory system
235.9 Neoplasm of uncertain behavior of other and unspecified respiratory organs ▽
239.1 Neoplasm of unspecified nature of respiratory system
350.2 Atypical face pain
376.01 Orbital cellulitis
461.1 Acute frontal sinusitis
461.8 Other acute sinusitis
461.9 Acute sinusitis, unspecified ▽
470 Deviated nasal septum
471.1 Polypoid sinus degeneration
471.8 Other polyp of sinus
473.0 Chronic maxillary sinusitis
473.1 Chronic frontal sinusitis
473.2 Chronic ethmoidal sinusitis
473.3 Chronic sphenoidal sinusitis
473.8 Other chronic sinusitis
473.9 Unspecified sinusitis (chronic) ▽
477.9 Allergic rhinitis, cause unspecified ▽
478.0 Hypertrophy of nasal turbinates
478.1 Other diseases of nasal cavity and sinuses
786.09 Other dyspnea and respiratory abnormalities

ICD-9-CM Procedural

22.53 Incision of multiple nasal sinuses

31200–31201

31200 Ethmoidectomy; intranasal, anterior
31201 intranasal, total

ICD-9-CM Diagnostic

160.0 Malignant neoplasm of nasal cavities
160.3 Malignant neoplasm of ethmoidal sinus
160.8 Malignant neoplasm of other sites of nasal cavities, middle ear, and accessory sinuses
197.3 Secondary malignant neoplasm of other respiratory organs
212.0 Benign neoplasm of nasal cavities, middle ear, and accessory sinuses
231.8 Carcinoma in situ of other specified parts of respiratory system
235.9 Neoplasm of uncertain behavior of other and unspecified respiratory organs ▽
239.1 Neoplasm of unspecified nature of respiratory system
376.01 Orbital cellulitis
461.2 Acute ethmoidal sinusitis
461.8 Other acute sinusitis
461.9 Acute sinusitis, unspecified ▽
471.1 Polypoid sinus degeneration
471.8 Other polyp of sinus
473.2 Chronic ethmoidal sinusitis
473.8 Other chronic sinusitis
473.9 Unspecified sinusitis (chronic) ▽
478.1 Other diseases of nasal cavity and sinuses
519.8 Other diseases of respiratory system, not elsewhere classified
730.18 Chronic osteomyelitis, other specified sites — (Use additional code to identify organism, 041.1)
784.0 Headache
802.8 Other facial bones, closed fracture
905.0 Late effect of fracture of skull and face bones

ICD-9-CM Procedural

22.63 Ethmoidectomy

31205

31205 Ethmoidectomy; extranasal, total

ICD-9-CM Diagnostic

160.0 Malignant neoplasm of nasal cavities
160.3 Malignant neoplasm of ethmoidal sinus
160.8 Malignant neoplasm of other sites of nasal cavities, middle ear, and accessory sinuses
197.3 Secondary malignant neoplasm of other respiratory organs
212.0 Benign neoplasm of nasal cavities, middle ear, and accessory sinuses
231.8 Carcinoma in situ of other specified parts of respiratory system
235.9 Neoplasm of uncertain behavior of other and unspecified respiratory organs ▽
239.1 Neoplasm of unspecified nature of respiratory system
376.01 Orbital cellulitis
461.2 Acute ethmoidal sinusitis
461.8 Other acute sinusitis
461.9 Acute sinusitis, unspecified ▽
471.1 Polypoid sinus degeneration
471.8 Other polyp of sinus
473.2 Chronic ethmoidal sinusitis
473.8 Other chronic sinusitis
473.9 Unspecified sinusitis (chronic) ▽
478.1 Other diseases of nasal cavity and sinuses
519.8 Other diseases of respiratory system, not elsewhere classified
730.18 Chronic osteomyelitis, other specified sites — (Use additional code to identify organism, 041.1)
784.0 Headache

▽ Unspecified code ♀ Female diagnosis ☒ Manifestation code ♂ Male diagnosis

802.8 Other facial bones, closed fracture
905.0 Late effect of fracture of skull and face bones

ICD-9-CM Procedural

22.63 Ethmoidectomy

31225–31230

31225 Maxillectomy; without orbital exenteration
31230 with orbital exenteration (en bloc)

ICD-9-CM Diagnostic

160.0 Malignant neoplasm of nasal cavities
160.2 Malignant neoplasm of maxillary sinus
160.8 Malignant neoplasm of other sites of nasal cavities, middle ear, and accessory sinuses
170.0 Malignant neoplasm of bones of skull and face, except mandible
173.3 Other malignant neoplasm of skin of other and unspecified parts of face ▽
190.1 Malignant neoplasm of orbit
197.3 Secondary malignant neoplasm of other respiratory organs
198.5 Secondary malignant neoplasm of bone and bone marrow
212.0 Benign neoplasm of nasal cavities, middle ear, and accessory sinuses
213.0 Benign neoplasm of bones of skull and face
231.8 Carcinoma in situ of other specified parts of respiratory system
235.9 Neoplasm of uncertain behavior of other and unspecified respiratory organs ▽
239.1 Neoplasm of unspecified nature of respiratory system
376.01 Orbital cellulitis
471.1 Polypoid sinus degeneration
471.8 Other polyp of sinus
473.0 Chronic maxillary sinusitis
478.1 Other diseases of nasal cavity and sinuses
730.18 Chronic osteomyelitis, other specified sites — (Use additional code to identify organism, 041.1)
802.6 Orbital floor (blow-out), closed fracture
802.7 Orbital floor (blow-out), open fracture

ICD-9-CM Procedural

16.51 Exenteration of orbit with removal of adjacent structures
22.62 Excision of lesion of maxillary sinus with other approach
76.39 Partial ostectomy of other facial bone
76.45 Other total ostectomy of other facial bone

31231–31233

31231 Nasal endoscopy, diagnostic, unilateral or bilateral (separate procedure)
31233 Nasal/sinus endoscopy, diagnostic with maxillary sinusoscopy (via inferior meatus or canine fossa puncture)

ICD-9-CM Diagnostic

147.0 Malignant neoplasm of superior wall of nasopharynx
147.1 Malignant neoplasm of posterior wall of nasopharynx
147.2 Malignant neoplasm of lateral wall of nasopharynx
147.3 Malignant neoplasm of anterior wall of nasopharynx
147.8 Malignant neoplasm of other specified sites of nasopharynx
147.9 Malignant neoplasm of nasopharynx, unspecified site ▽
160.0 Malignant neoplasm of nasal cavities
160.2 Malignant neoplasm of maxillary sinus
160.3 Malignant neoplasm of ethmoidal sinus
160.5 Malignant neoplasm of sphenoidal sinus
160.8 Malignant neoplasm of other sites of nasal cavities, middle ear, and accessory sinuses
170.0 Malignant neoplasm of bones of skull and face, except mandible
210.7 Benign neoplasm of nasopharynx
212.0 Benign neoplasm of nasal cavities, middle ear, and accessory sinuses
228.09 Hemangioma of other sites
230.0 Carcinoma in situ of lip, oral cavity, and pharynx
231.8 Carcinoma in situ of other specified parts of respiratory system
235.1 Neoplasm of uncertain behavior of lip, oral cavity, and pharynx
235.9 Neoplasm of uncertain behavior of other and unspecified respiratory organs ▽
239.1 Neoplasm of unspecified nature of respiratory system
381.81 Dysfunction of Eustachian tube
446.4 Wegener's granulomatosis
461.0 Acute maxillary sinusitis
461.2 Acute ethmoidal sinusitis
461.3 Acute sphenoidal sinusitis
461.8 Other acute sinusitis
461.9 Acute sinusitis, unspecified ▽
470 Deviated nasal septum
471.0 Polyp of nasal cavity
471.1 Polypoid sinus degeneration
471.8 Other polyp of sinus
471.9 Unspecified nasal polyp ▽
472.0 Chronic rhinitis
472.2 Chronic nasopharyngitis
473.0 Chronic maxillary sinusitis
473.1 Chronic frontal sinusitis
473.2 Chronic ethmoidal sinusitis
473.3 Chronic sphenoidal sinusitis
473.8 Other chronic sinusitis
473.9 Unspecified sinusitis (chronic) ▽
477.8 Allergic rhinitis due to other allergen
477.9 Allergic rhinitis, cause unspecified ▽
478.0 Hypertrophy of nasal turbinates
478.1 Other diseases of nasal cavity and sinuses
478.21 Cellulitis of pharynx or nasopharynx
478.25 Edema of pharynx or nasopharynx
478.26 Cyst of pharynx or nasopharynx
478.29 Other disease of pharynx or nasopharynx
478.9 Other and unspecified diseases of upper respiratory tract
738.0 Acquired deformity of nose
748.0 Congenital choanal atresia
748.1 Other congenital anomaly of nose
748.8 Other specified congenital anomaly of respiratory system
748.9 Unspecified congenital anomaly of respiratory system ▽
780.51 Insomnia with sleep apnea
780.57 Other and unspecified sleep apnea ▽
784.0 Headache
784.2 Swelling, mass, or lump in head and neck
784.7 Epistaxis
786.00 Unspecified respiratory abnormality ▽
786.09 Other dyspnea and respiratory abnormalities
793.0 Nonspecific abnormal findings on radiological and other examination of skull and head
802.0 Nasal bones, closed fracture
802.1 Nasal bones, open fracture
905.0 Late effect of fracture of skull and face bones
925.1 Crushing injury of face and scalp — (Use additional code to identify any associated injuries: 800-829, 850.0-854.1, 860.0-869.1)
932 Foreign body in nose
V10.22 Personal history of malignant neoplasm of nasal cavities, middle ear, and accessory sinuses
V10.81 Personal history of malignant neoplasm of bone
V10.82 Personal history of malignant melanoma of skin
V67.00 Follow-up examination, following unspecified surgery ▽
V67.09 Follow-up examination, following other surgery

ICD-9-CM Procedural

21.21 Rhinoscopy
22.19 Other diagnostic procedures on nasal sinuses

HCPCS Level II Supplies & Services

A4305 Disposable drug delivery system, flow rate of 50 ml or greater per hour
A4306 Disposable drug delivery system, flow rate of 5 ml or less per hour
A4550 Surgical trays

31235

31235 Nasal/sinus endoscopy, diagnostic with sphenoid sinusoscopy (via puncture of sphenoidal face or cannulation of ostium)

ICD-9-CM Diagnostic

147.0 Malignant neoplasm of superior wall of nasopharynx
147.1 Malignant neoplasm of posterior wall of nasopharynx
147.2 Malignant neoplasm of lateral wall of nasopharynx
147.3 Malignant neoplasm of anterior wall of nasopharynx
147.8 Malignant neoplasm of other specified sites of nasopharynx
147.9 Malignant neoplasm of nasopharynx, unspecified site ▽
160.0 Malignant neoplasm of nasal cavities
160.5 Malignant neoplasm of sphenoidal sinus
160.8 Malignant neoplasm of other sites of nasal cavities, middle ear, and accessory sinuses
160.9 Malignant neoplasm of site of nasal cavities, middle ear, and accessory sinus, unspecified site ▽
197.3 Secondary malignant neoplasm of other respiratory organs
212.0 Benign neoplasm of nasal cavities, middle ear, and accessory sinuses

212.9 Benign neoplasm of respiratory and intrathoracic organs, site unspecified
231.8 Carcinoma in situ of other specified parts of respiratory system
235.9 Neoplasm of uncertain behavior of other and unspecified respiratory organs
239.1 Neoplasm of unspecified nature of respiratory system
446.4 Wegener's granulomatosis
461.3 Acute sphenoidal sinusitis
461.8 Other acute sinusitis
461.9 Acute sinusitis, unspecified
470 Deviated nasal septum
471.0 Polyp of nasal cavity
471.1 Polypoid sinus degeneration
471.8 Other polyp of sinus
471.9 Unspecified nasal polyp
472.0 Chronic rhinitis
472.2 Chronic nasopharyngitis
473.3 Chronic sphenoidal sinusitis
473.8 Other chronic sinusitis
473.9 Unspecified sinusitis (chronic)
478.0 Hypertrophy of nasal turbinates
478.1 Other diseases of nasal cavity and sinuses
478.21 Cellulitis of pharynx or nasopharynx
478.25 Edema of pharynx or nasopharynx
478.26 Cyst of pharynx or nasopharynx
478.29 Other disease of pharynx or nasopharynx
478.9 Other and unspecified diseases of upper respiratory tract
738.0 Acquired deformity of nose
748.0 Congenital choanal atresia
748.1 Other congenital anomaly of nose
748.8 Other specified congenital anomaly of respiratory system
748.9 Unspecified congenital anomaly of respiratory system
780.51 Insomnia with sleep apnea
780.57 Other and unspecified sleep apnea
784.0 Headache
784.2 Swelling, mass, or lump in head and neck
784.7 Epistaxis
786.00 Unspecified respiratory abnormality
786.09 Other dyspnea and respiratory abnormalities
793.0 Nonspecific abnormal findings on radiological and other examination of skull and head
802.0 Nasal bones, closed fracture
802.1 Nasal bones, open fracture
905.0 Late effect of fracture of skull and face bones
925.1 Crushing injury of face and scalp — (Use additional code to identify any associated injuries: 800-829, 850.0-854.1, 860.0-869.1)
V10.22 Personal history of malignant neoplasm of nasal cavities, middle ear, and accessory sinuses
V10.81 Personal history of malignant neoplasm of bone
V10.82 Personal history of malignant melanoma of skin

ICD-9-CM Procedural

22.19 Other diagnostic procedures on nasal sinuses

31237

31237 Nasal/sinus endoscopy, surgical; with biopsy, polypectomy or debridement (separate procedure)

ICD-9-CM Diagnostic

147.0 Malignant neoplasm of superior wall of nasopharynx
147.1 Malignant neoplasm of posterior wall of nasopharynx
147.2 Malignant neoplasm of lateral wall of nasopharynx
147.3 Malignant neoplasm of anterior wall of nasopharynx
147.8 Malignant neoplasm of other specified sites of nasopharynx
160.0 Malignant neoplasm of nasal cavities
160.2 Malignant neoplasm of maxillary sinus
160.3 Malignant neoplasm of ethmoidal sinus
160.4 Malignant neoplasm of frontal sinus
160.5 Malignant neoplasm of sphenoidal sinus
160.8 Malignant neoplasm of other sites of nasal cavities, middle ear, and accessory sinuses
160.9 Malignant neoplasm of site of nasal cavities, middle ear, and accessory sinus, unspecified site
170.0 Malignant neoplasm of bones of skull and face, except mandible
210.7 Benign neoplasm of nasopharynx
212.0 Benign neoplasm of nasal cavities, middle ear, and accessory sinuses
228.00 Hemangioma of unspecified site
228.09 Hemangioma of other sites
230.0 Carcinoma in situ of lip, oral cavity, and pharynx
231.8 Carcinoma in situ of other specified parts of respiratory system
235.9 Neoplasm of uncertain behavior of other and unspecified respiratory organs
239.1 Neoplasm of unspecified nature of respiratory system
446.4 Wegener's granulomatosis
461.0 Acute maxillary sinusitis
461.1 Acute frontal sinusitis
461.2 Acute ethmoidal sinusitis
461.3 Acute sphenoidal sinusitis
461.8 Other acute sinusitis
461.9 Acute sinusitis, unspecified
470 Deviated nasal septum
471.0 Polyp of nasal cavity
471.1 Polypoid sinus degeneration
471.8 Other polyp of sinus
471.9 Unspecified nasal polyp
472.0 Chronic rhinitis
473.0 Chronic maxillary sinusitis
473.1 Chronic frontal sinusitis
473.2 Chronic ethmoidal sinusitis
473.3 Chronic sphenoidal sinusitis
473.8 Other chronic sinusitis
473.9 Unspecified sinusitis (chronic)
478.0 Hypertrophy of nasal turbinates
478.1 Other diseases of nasal cavity and sinuses
478.20 Unspecified disease of pharynx
478.21 Cellulitis of pharynx or nasopharynx
478.25 Edema of pharynx or nasopharynx
478.26 Cyst of pharynx or nasopharynx
478.29 Other disease of pharynx or nasopharynx
478.9 Other and unspecified diseases of upper respiratory tract
784.0 Headache
784.2 Swelling, mass, or lump in head and neck
784.7 Epistaxis
786.00 Unspecified respiratory abnormality
786.09 Other dyspnea and respiratory abnormalities
786.9 Other symptoms involving respiratory system and chest
793.0 Nonspecific abnormal findings on radiological and other examination of skull and head
802.0 Nasal bones, closed fracture
802.1 Nasal bones, open fracture
905.0 Late effect of fracture of skull and face bones

ICD-9-CM Procedural

21.30 Excision or destruction of lesion of nose, not otherwise specified
21.31 Local excision or destruction of intranasal lesion
21.32 Local excision or destruction of other lesion of nose
22.11 Closed (endoscopic) (needle) biopsy of nasal sinus

HCPCS Level II Supplies & Services

A4305 Disposable drug delivery system, flow rate of 50 ml or greater per hour
A4306 Disposable drug delivery system, flow rate of 5 ml or less per hour
A4550 Surgical trays

31238

31238 Nasal/sinus endoscopy, surgical; with control of nasal hemorrhage

ICD-9-CM Diagnostic

448.0 Hereditary hemorrhagic telangiectasia
456.8 Varices of other sites
784.7 Epistaxis
958.2 Secondary and recurrent hemorrhage as an early complication of trauma
998.11 Hemorrhage complicating a procedure

ICD-9-CM Procedural

21.00 Control of epistaxis, not otherwise specified
21.03 Control of epistaxis by cauterization (and packing)
21.07 Control of epistaxis by excision of nasal mucosa and skin grafting of septum and lateral nasal wall
21.09 Control of epistaxis by other means

HCPCS Level II Supplies & Services

A4305 Disposable drug delivery system, flow rate of 50 ml or greater per hour
A4306 Disposable drug delivery system, flow rate of 5 ml or less per hour
A4550 Surgical trays

Unspecified code
♀ Female diagnosis
Manifestation code
♂ Male diagnosis

31239

31239 Nasal/sinus endoscopy, surgical; with dacryocystorhinostomy

ICD-9-CM Diagnostic

375.11 Dacryops
375.21 Epiphora due to excess lacrimation
375.22 Epiphora due to insufficient drainage
375.30 Unspecified dacryocystitis ▽
375.55 Obstruction of nasolacrimal duct, neonatal
375.56 Stenosis of nasolacrimal duct, acquired
375.81 Granuloma of lacrimal passages
375.9 Unspecified disorder of lacrimal system ▽
743.65 Specified congenital anomaly of lacrimal passages
905.0 Late effect of fracture of skull and face bones

ICD-9-CM Procedural

09.81 Dacryocystorhinostomy (DCR)

31240

31240 Nasal/sinus endoscopy, surgical; with concha bullosa resection

ICD-9-CM Diagnostic

472.0 Chronic rhinitis
472.2 Chronic nasopharyngitis
473.0 Chronic maxillary sinusitis
473.8 Other chronic sinusitis
478.0 Hypertrophy of nasal turbinates
478.1 Other diseases of nasal cavity and sinuses
730.18 Chronic osteomyelitis, other specified sites — (Use additional code to identify organism, 041.1)

ICD-9-CM Procedural

21.30 Excision or destruction of lesion of nose, not otherwise specified
21.32 Local excision or destruction of other lesion of nose
21.61 Turbinectomy by diathermy or cryosurgery
21.69 Other turbinectomy

31254–31255

31254 Nasal/sinus endoscopy, surgical; with ethmoidectomy, partial (anterior)
31255 with ethmoidectomy, total (anterior and posterior)

ICD-9-CM Diagnostic

160.0 Malignant neoplasm of nasal cavities
160.3 Malignant neoplasm of ethmoidal sinus
197.3 Secondary malignant neoplasm of other respiratory organs
212.0 Benign neoplasm of nasal cavities, middle ear, and accessory sinuses
231.8 Carcinoma in situ of other specified parts of respiratory system
235.9 Neoplasm of uncertain behavior of other and unspecified respiratory organs ▽
376.01 Orbital cellulitis
461.2 Acute ethmoidal sinusitis
461.8 Other acute sinusitis
461.9 Acute sinusitis, unspecified ▽
470 Deviated nasal septum
471.1 Polypoid sinus degeneration
471.8 Other polyp of sinus
473.2 Chronic ethmoidal sinusitis
473.8 Other chronic sinusitis
473.9 Unspecified sinusitis (chronic) ▽
478.0 Hypertrophy of nasal turbinates
478.1 Other diseases of nasal cavity and sinuses
519.8 Other diseases of respiratory system, not elsewhere classified
519.9 Unspecified disease of respiratory system ▽
730.18 Chronic osteomyelitis, other specified sites — (Use additional code to identify organism, 041.1)
784.0 Headache
802.8 Other facial bones, closed fracture
905.0 Late effect of fracture of skull and face bones

ICD-9-CM Procedural

22.63 Ethmoidectomy

31256–31267

31256 Nasal/sinus endoscopy, surgical, with maxillary antrostomy;
31267 with removal of tissue from maxillary sinus

ICD-9-CM Diagnostic

160.2 Malignant neoplasm of maxillary sinus
197.3 Secondary malignant neoplasm of other respiratory organs
212.0 Benign neoplasm of nasal cavities, middle ear, and accessory sinuses
231.8 Carcinoma in situ of other specified parts of respiratory system
235.9 Neoplasm of uncertain behavior of other and unspecified respiratory organs ▽
238.0 Neoplasm of uncertain behavior of bone and articular cartilage
239.1 Neoplasm of unspecified nature of respiratory system
461.0 Acute maxillary sinusitis
461.8 Other acute sinusitis
461.9 Acute sinusitis, unspecified ▽
470 Deviated nasal septum
471.1 Polypoid sinus degeneration
471.8 Other polyp of sinus
473.0 Chronic maxillary sinusitis
473.8 Other chronic sinusitis
473.9 Unspecified sinusitis (chronic) ▽
478.0 Hypertrophy of nasal turbinates
478.1 Other diseases of nasal cavity and sinuses
730.18 Chronic osteomyelitis, other specified sites — (Use additional code to identify organism, 041.1)
730.28 Unspecified osteomyelitis, other specified sites — (Use additional code to identify organism, 041.1) ▽
748.8 Other specified congenital anomaly of respiratory system
784.0 Headache
784.2 Swelling, mass, or lump in head and neck
784.7 Epistaxis
786.09 Other dyspnea and respiratory abnormalities
802.4 Malar and maxillary bones, closed fracture
802.5 Malar and maxillary bones, open fracture
802.6 Orbital floor (blow-out), closed fracture
802.7 Orbital floor (blow-out), open fracture
905.0 Late effect of fracture of skull and face bones
996.60 Infection and inflammatory reaction due to unspecified device, implant, and graft — (Use additional code to identify specified infections) ▽
996.69 Infection and inflammatory reaction due to other internal prosthetic device, implant, and graft — (Use additional code to identify specified infections)

ICD-9-CM Procedural

22.2 Intranasal antrotomy
22.62 Excision of lesion of maxillary sinus with other approach

31276

31276 Nasal/sinus endoscopy, surgical with frontal sinus exploration, with or without removal of tissue from frontal sinus

ICD-9-CM Diagnostic

160.4 Malignant neoplasm of frontal sinus
160.8 Malignant neoplasm of other sites of nasal cavities, middle ear, and accessory sinuses
212.0 Benign neoplasm of nasal cavities, middle ear, and accessory sinuses
212.8 Benign neoplasm of other specified sites of respiratory and intrathoracic organs
212.9 Benign neoplasm of respiratory and intrathoracic organs, site unspecified ▽
231.8 Carcinoma in situ of other specified parts of respiratory system
235.9 Neoplasm of uncertain behavior of other and unspecified respiratory organs ▽
239.1 Neoplasm of unspecified nature of respiratory system
461.1 Acute frontal sinusitis
461.9 Acute sinusitis, unspecified ▽
471.1 Polypoid sinus degeneration
471.8 Other polyp of sinus
473.0 Chronic maxillary sinusitis
473.1 Chronic frontal sinusitis
473.2 Chronic ethmoidal sinusitis
473.8 Other chronic sinusitis
473.9 Unspecified sinusitis (chronic) ▽
478.0 Hypertrophy of nasal turbinates
478.1 Other diseases of nasal cavity and sinuses
730.18 Chronic osteomyelitis, other specified sites — (Use additional code to identify organism, 041.1)
748.1 Other congenital anomaly of nose
784.0 Headache
784.2 Swelling, mass, or lump in head and neck

784.7 Epistaxis
802.8 Other facial bones, closed fracture

ICD-9-CM Procedural

22.41 Frontal sinusotomy
22.42 Frontal sinusectomy

31287–31288

31287 Nasal/sinus endoscopy, surgical, with sphenoidotomy;
31288 with removal of tissue from the sphenoid sinus

ICD-9-CM Diagnostic

160.5 Malignant neoplasm of sphenoidal sinus
160.8 Malignant neoplasm of other sites of nasal cavities, middle ear, and accessory sinuses
197.3 Secondary malignant neoplasm of other respiratory organs
212.0 Benign neoplasm of nasal cavities, middle ear, and accessory sinuses
231.8 Carcinoma in situ of other specified parts of respiratory system
235.9 Neoplasm of uncertain behavior of other and unspecified respiratory organs ▽
239.1 Neoplasm of unspecified nature of respiratory system
461.3 Acute sphenoidal sinusitis
461.8 Other acute sinusitis
461.9 Acute sinusitis, unspecified ▽
471.1 Polypoid sinus degeneration
471.8 Other polyp of sinus
473.3 Chronic sphenoidal sinusitis
473.8 Other chronic sinusitis
473.9 Unspecified sinusitis (chronic) ▽
478.0 Hypertrophy of nasal turbinates
478.1 Other diseases of nasal cavity and sinuses
730.18 Chronic osteomyelitis, other specified sites — (Use additional code to identify organism, 041.1)
748.8 Other specified congenital anomaly of respiratory system
784.0 Headache
784.2 Swelling, mass, or lump in head and neck
784.7 Epistaxis
905.0 Late effect of fracture of skull and face bones

ICD-9-CM Procedural

21.31 Local excision or destruction of intranasal lesion
22.52 Sphenoidotomy

31290–31291

31290 Nasal/sinus endoscopy, surgical, with repair of cerebrospinal fluid leak; ethmoid region
31291 sphenoid region

ICD-9-CM Diagnostic

349.81 Cerebrospinal fluid rhinorrhea
473.2 Chronic ethmoidal sinusitis
473.3 Chronic sphenoidal sinusitis
748.1 Other congenital anomaly of nose
801.10 Closed fracture of base of skull with cerebral laceration and contusion, unspecified state of consciousness ▽
801.11 Closed fracture of base of skull with cerebral laceration and contusion, no loss of consciousness
801.12 Closed fracture of base of skull with cerebral laceration and contusion, brief (less than one hour) loss of consciousness
801.13 Closed fracture of base of skull with cerebral laceration and contusion, moderate (1-24 hours) loss of consciousness
801.14 Closed fracture of base of skull with cerebral laceration and contusion, prolonged (more than 24 hours) loss of consciousness and return to pre-existing conscious level
801.15 Closed fracture of base of skull with cerebral laceration and contusion, prolonged (more than 24 hours) loss of consciousness, without return to pre-existing conscious level
801.16 Closed fracture of base of skull with cerebral laceration and contusion, loss of consciousness of unspecified duration ▽
801.19 Closed fracture of base of skull with cerebral laceration and contusion, unspecified concussion ▽
802.0 Nasal bones, closed fracture
802.1 Nasal bones, open fracture
802.6 Orbital floor (blow-out), closed fracture
802.7 Orbital floor (blow-out), open fracture
802.8 Other facial bones, closed fracture
802.9 Other facial bones, open fracture
873.30 Open wound of nose, unspecified site, complicated — (Use additional code to identify infection) ▽
873.31 Open wound of nasal septum, complicated — (Use additional code to identify infection)
873.32 Open wound of nasal cavity, complicated — (Use additional code to identify infection)
873.33 Open wound of nasal sinus, complicated — (Use additional code to identify infection)
998.2 Accidental puncture or laceration during procedure

ICD-9-CM Procedural

22.51 Ethmoidotomy
22.52 Sphenoidotomy

31292–31294

31292 Nasal/sinus endoscopy, surgical; with medial or inferior orbital wall decompression
31293 with medial orbital wall and inferior orbital wall decompression
31294 with optic nerve decompression

ICD-9-CM Diagnostic

376.01 Orbital cellulitis
376.11 Orbital granuloma
376.21 Thyrotoxic exophthalmos ☒
376.30 Unspecified exophthalmos ▽
376.32 Orbital hemorrhage
376.47 Deformity of orbit due to trauma or surgery
377.49 Other disorder of optic nerve
802.6 Orbital floor (blow-out), closed fracture
802.7 Orbital floor (blow-out), open fracture
802.8 Other facial bones, closed fracture
802.9 Other facial bones, open fracture
905.0 Late effect of fracture of skull and face bones
950.0 Optic nerve injury
959.01 Head injury, unspecified ▽
959.09 Injury of face and neck, other and unspecified

ICD-9-CM Procedural

04.42 Other cranial nerve decompression
16.09 Other orbitotomy

31300–31320

31300 Laryngotomy (thyrotomy, laryngofissure); with removal of tumor or laryngocele, cordectomy
31320 diagnostic

ICD-9-CM Diagnostic

148.2 Malignant neoplasm of aryepiglottic fold, hypopharyngeal aspect
161.0 Malignant neoplasm of glottis
161.1 Malignant neoplasm of supraglottis
161.2 Malignant neoplasm of subglottis
161.3 Malignant neoplasm of laryngeal cartilages
161.8 Malignant neoplasm of other specified sites of larynx
197.3 Secondary malignant neoplasm of other respiratory organs
199.1 Other malignant neoplasm of unspecified site
212.1 Benign neoplasm of larynx
231.0 Carcinoma in situ of larynx
235.6 Neoplasm of uncertain behavior of larynx
239.1 Neoplasm of unspecified nature of respiratory system
476.0 Chronic laryngitis
476.1 Chronic laryngotracheitis
478.30 Unspecified paralysis of vocal cords or larynx ▽
478.31 Unilateral partial paralysis of vocal cords or larynx
478.32 Unilateral complete paralysis of vocal cords or larynx
478.33 Bilateral partial paralysis of vocal cords or larynx
478.34 Bilateral complete paralysis of vocal cords or larynx
478.4 Polyp of vocal cord or larynx
478.5 Other diseases of vocal cords
478.6 Edema of larynx
478.71 Cellulitis and perichondritis of larynx
478.74 Stenosis of larynx
478.75 Laryngeal spasm
478.79 Other diseases of larynx
519.8 Other diseases of respiratory system, not elsewhere classified
519.9 Unspecified disease of respiratory system ▽
748.3 Other congenital anomaly of larynx, trachea, and bronchus

▽ Unspecified code ☒ Manifestation code
♀ Female diagnosis ♂ Male diagnosis

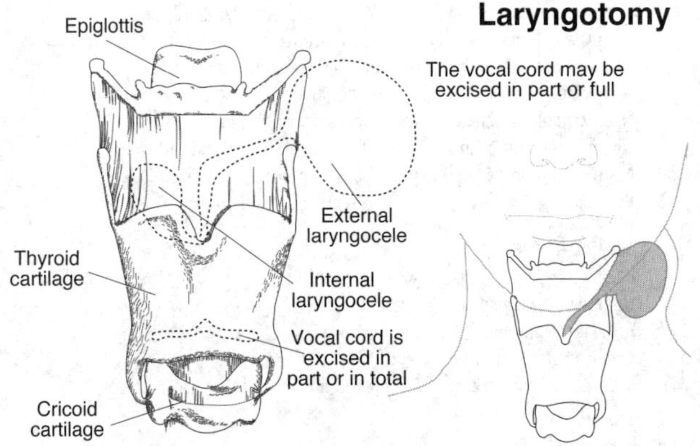
Laryngotomy
The vocal cord may be excised in part or full
Epiglottis
External laryngocele
Thyroid cartilage
Internal laryngocele
Vocal cord is excised in part or in total
Cricoid cartilage

748.8	Other specified congenital anomaly of respiratory system
784.1	Throat pain
784.2	Swelling, mass, or lump in head and neck
784.40	Unspecified voice disturbance
784.41	Aphonia
784.49	Other voice disturbance
784.8	Hemorrhage from throat
785.6	Enlargement of lymph nodes
786.09	Other dyspnea and respiratory abnormalities
786.2	Cough
786.3	Hemoptysis
787.2	Dysphagia
933.0	Foreign body in pharynx
933.1	Foreign body in larynx
947.1	Burn of larynx, trachea, and lung
948.00	Burn (any degree) involving less than 10% of body surface with third degree burn of less than 10% or unspecified amount
V15.82	Personal history of tobacco use, presenting hazards to health

ICD-9-CM Procedural

30.09	Other excision or destruction of lesion or tissue of larynx
30.22	Vocal cordectomy
31.48	Other diagnostic procedures on larynx

31360–31365

31360 Laryngectomy; total, without radical neck dissection
31365 total, with radical neck dissection

ICD-9-CM Diagnostic

141.0	Malignant neoplasm of base of tongue
142.1	Malignant neoplasm of submandibular gland
148.2	Malignant neoplasm of aryepiglottic fold, hypopharyngeal aspect
148.9	Malignant neoplasm of hypopharynx, unspecified site
150.0	Malignant neoplasm of cervical esophagus
150.3	Malignant neoplasm of upper third of esophagus
150.8	Malignant neoplasm of other specified part of esophagus
161.0	Malignant neoplasm of glottis
161.1	Malignant neoplasm of supraglottis
161.2	Malignant neoplasm of subglottis
161.3	Malignant neoplasm of laryngeal cartilages
161.8	Malignant neoplasm of other specified sites of larynx
161.9	Malignant neoplasm of larynx, unspecified site
170.0	Malignant neoplasm of bones of skull and face, except mandible
171.0	Malignant neoplasm of connective and other soft tissue of head, face, and neck
196.0	Secondary and unspecified malignant neoplasm of lymph nodes of head, face, and neck
197.3	Secondary malignant neoplasm of other respiratory organs
197.8	Secondary malignant neoplasm of other digestive organs and spleen
198.5	Secondary malignant neoplasm of bone and bone marrow
198.89	Secondary malignant neoplasm of other specified sites
199.1	Other malignant neoplasm of unspecified site
230.0	Carcinoma in situ of lip, oral cavity, and pharynx
230.1	Carcinoma in situ of esophagus
231.0	Carcinoma in situ of larynx
235.0	Neoplasm of uncertain behavior of major salivary glands
235.1	Neoplasm of uncertain behavior of lip, oral cavity, and pharynx
235.6	Neoplasm of uncertain behavior of larynx
238.0	Neoplasm of uncertain behavior of bone and articular cartilage
238.1	Neoplasm of uncertain behavior of connective and other soft tissue
239.0	Neoplasm of unspecified nature of digestive system
239.1	Neoplasm of unspecified nature of respiratory system
239.2	Neoplasms of unspecified nature of bone, soft tissue, and skin
239.8	Neoplasm of unspecified nature of other specified sites
V15.82	Personal history of tobacco use, presenting hazards to health

ICD-9-CM Procedural

30.3	Complete laryngectomy
30.4	Radical laryngectomy

31367–31368

31367 Laryngectomy; subtotal supraglottic, without radical neck dissection
31368 subtotal supraglottic, with radical neck dissection

ICD-9-CM Diagnostic

141.0	Malignant neoplasm of base of tongue
142.1	Malignant neoplasm of submandibular gland
148.2	Malignant neoplasm of aryepiglottic fold, hypopharyngeal aspect
148.9	Malignant neoplasm of hypopharynx, unspecified site
150.0	Malignant neoplasm of cervical esophagus
150.3	Malignant neoplasm of upper third of esophagus
150.8	Malignant neoplasm of other specified part of esophagus
161.0	Malignant neoplasm of glottis
161.1	Malignant neoplasm of supraglottis
161.2	Malignant neoplasm of subglottis
161.3	Malignant neoplasm of laryngeal cartilages
161.8	Malignant neoplasm of other specified sites of larynx
161.9	Malignant neoplasm of larynx, unspecified site
170.0	Malignant neoplasm of bones of skull and face, except mandible
171.0	Malignant neoplasm of connective and other soft tissue of head, face, and neck
196.0	Secondary and unspecified malignant neoplasm of lymph nodes of head, face, and neck
197.3	Secondary malignant neoplasm of other respiratory organs
197.8	Secondary malignant neoplasm of other digestive organs and spleen
198.5	Secondary malignant neoplasm of bone and bone marrow
198.89	Secondary malignant neoplasm of other specified sites
199.1	Other malignant neoplasm of unspecified site
230.0	Carcinoma in situ of lip, oral cavity, and pharynx
230.1	Carcinoma in situ of esophagus
231.0	Carcinoma in situ of larynx
235.0	Neoplasm of uncertain behavior of major salivary glands
235.1	Neoplasm of uncertain behavior of lip, oral cavity, and pharynx
235.6	Neoplasm of uncertain behavior of larynx
238.0	Neoplasm of uncertain behavior of bone and articular cartilage
238.1	Neoplasm of uncertain behavior of connective and other soft tissue
239.0	Neoplasm of unspecified nature of digestive system
239.1	Neoplasm of unspecified nature of respiratory system
239.2	Neoplasms of unspecified nature of bone, soft tissue, and skin
239.8	Neoplasm of unspecified nature of other specified sites
V15.82	Personal history of tobacco use, presenting hazards to health

ICD-9-CM Procedural

30.3	Complete laryngectomy
30.4	Radical laryngectomy

31370–31382

31370 Partial laryngectomy (hemilaryngectomy); horizontal
31375 laterovertical
31380 anterovertical
31382 antero-latero-vertical

ICD-9-CM Diagnostic

148.2	Malignant neoplasm of aryepiglottic fold, hypopharyngeal aspect
161.0	Malignant neoplasm of glottis
161.1	Malignant neoplasm of supraglottis
161.2	Malignant neoplasm of subglottis
161.3	Malignant neoplasm of laryngeal cartilages
161.8	Malignant neoplasm of other specified sites of larynx
161.9	Malignant neoplasm of larynx, unspecified site
197.3	Secondary malignant neoplasm of other respiratory organs
198.89	Secondary malignant neoplasm of other specified sites
199.1	Other malignant neoplasm of unspecified site
212.1	Benign neoplasm of larynx
230.0	Carcinoma in situ of lip, oral cavity, and pharynx
231.0	Carcinoma in situ of larynx
235.1	Neoplasm of uncertain behavior of lip, oral cavity, and pharynx

Unspecified code
♀ Female diagnosis
Manifestation code
♂ Male diagnosis

235.6 Neoplasm of uncertain behavior of larynx
239.1 Neoplasm of unspecified nature of respiratory system
478.4 Polyp of vocal cord or larynx
478.5 Other diseases of vocal cords
478.71 Cellulitis and perichondritis of larynx
478.74 Stenosis of larynx
478.79 Other diseases of larynx
748.2 Congenital web of larynx
925.2 Crushing injury of neck — (Use additional code to identify any associated injuries: 800-829, 850.0-854.1, 860.0-869.1)
947.1 Burn of larynx, trachea, and lung
948.00 Burn (any degree) involving less than 10% of body surface with third degree burn of less than 10% or unspecified amount
948.10 Burn (any degree) involving 10-19% of body surface with third degree burn of less than 10% or unspecified amount
948.11 Burn (any degree) involving 10-19% of body surface with third degree burn of 10-19%
949.4 Deep necrosis of underlying tissue due to burn (deep third degree), unspecified site without mention of loss of body part ▽
949.5 Deep necrosis of underlying tissues due to burn (deep third degree, unspecified site with loss of body part ▽
V15.82 Personal history of tobacco use, presenting hazards to health

ICD-9-CM Procedural

30.1 Hemilaryngectomy
30.29 Other partial laryngectomy

31390–31395

31390 Pharyngolaryngectomy, with radical neck dissection; without reconstruction
31395 with reconstruction

ICD-9-CM Diagnostic

141.0 Malignant neoplasm of base of tongue
142.1 Malignant neoplasm of submandibular gland
146.5 Malignant neoplasm of junctional region of oropharynx
146.6 Malignant neoplasm of lateral wall of oropharynx
146.7 Malignant neoplasm of posterior wall of oropharynx
146.8 Malignant neoplasm of other specified sites of oropharynx
146.9 Malignant neoplasm of oropharynx, unspecified site ▽
147.0 Malignant neoplasm of superior wall of nasopharynx
147.1 Malignant neoplasm of posterior wall of nasopharynx
147.2 Malignant neoplasm of lateral wall of nasopharynx
147.3 Malignant neoplasm of anterior wall of nasopharynx
147.8 Malignant neoplasm of other specified sites of nasopharynx
147.9 Malignant neoplasm of nasopharynx, unspecified site ▽
148.0 Malignant neoplasm of postcricoid region of hypopharynx
148.1 Malignant neoplasm of pyriform sinus
148.2 Malignant neoplasm of aryepiglottic fold, hypopharyngeal aspect
148.3 Malignant neoplasm of posterior hypopharyngeal wall
148.8 Malignant neoplasm of other specified sites of hypopharynx
148.9 Malignant neoplasm of hypopharynx, unspecified site ▽
149.0 Malignant neoplasm of pharynx, unspecified ▽
149.1 Malignant neoplasm of Waldeyer's ring
149.8 Malignant neoplasm of other sites within the lip and oral cavity
150.0 Malignant neoplasm of cervical esophagus
150.3 Malignant neoplasm of upper third of esophagus
150.8 Malignant neoplasm of other specified part of esophagus
161.0 Malignant neoplasm of glottis
161.1 Malignant neoplasm of supraglottis
161.2 Malignant neoplasm of subglottis
161.3 Malignant neoplasm of laryngeal cartilages
161.8 Malignant neoplasm of other specified sites of larynx
161.9 Malignant neoplasm of larynx, unspecified site ▽
171.0 Malignant neoplasm of connective and other soft tissue of head, face, and neck
196.0 Secondary and unspecified malignant neoplasm of lymph nodes of head, face, and neck
197.3 Secondary malignant neoplasm of other respiratory organs
198.5 Secondary malignant neoplasm of bone and bone marrow
198.89 Secondary malignant neoplasm of other specified sites
199.1 Other malignant neoplasm of unspecified site
230.0 Carcinoma in situ of lip, oral cavity, and pharynx
231.0 Carcinoma in situ of larynx
235.0 Neoplasm of uncertain behavior of major salivary glands
235.1 Neoplasm of uncertain behavior of lip, oral cavity, and pharynx
235.5 Neoplasm of uncertain behavior of other and unspecified digestive organs ▽
235.6 Neoplasm of uncertain behavior of larynx
238.0 Neoplasm of uncertain behavior of bone and articular cartilage
238.1 Neoplasm of uncertain behavior of connective and other soft tissue ▽
238.8 Neoplasm of uncertain behavior of other specified sites
239.0 Neoplasm of unspecified nature of digestive system
239.1 Neoplasm of unspecified nature of respiratory system
239.2 Neoplasms of unspecified nature of bone, soft tissue, and skin
239.8 Neoplasm of unspecified nature of other specified sites
V15.82 Personal history of tobacco use, presenting hazards to health

ICD-9-CM Procedural

29.4 Plastic operation on pharynx
30.3 Complete laryngectomy
30.4 Radical laryngectomy
31.69 Other repair of larynx
31.75 Reconstruction of trachea and construction of artificial larynx

31400

31400 Arytenoidectomy or arytenoidopexy, external approach

ICD-9-CM Diagnostic

148.2 Malignant neoplasm of aryepiglottic fold, hypopharyngeal aspect
150.0 Malignant neoplasm of cervical esophagus
161.1 Malignant neoplasm of supraglottis
161.3 Malignant neoplasm of laryngeal cartilages
161.8 Malignant neoplasm of other specified sites of larynx
197.3 Secondary malignant neoplasm of other respiratory organs
198.89 Secondary malignant neoplasm of other specified sites
212.1 Benign neoplasm of larynx
231.0 Carcinoma in situ of larynx
235.6 Neoplasm of uncertain behavior of larynx
238.0 Neoplasm of uncertain behavior of bone and articular cartilage
478.79 Other diseases of larynx
748.3 Other congenital anomaly of larynx, trachea, and bronchus
784.2 Swelling, mass, or lump in head and neck

ICD-9-CM Procedural

30.29 Other partial laryngectomy
31.69 Other repair of larynx

31420

31420 Epiglottidectomy

ICD-9-CM Diagnostic

146.4 Malignant neoplasm of anterior aspect of epiglottis
146.5 Malignant neoplasm of junctional region of oropharynx
148.2 Malignant neoplasm of aryepiglottic fold, hypopharyngeal aspect
161.0 Malignant neoplasm of glottis
161.1 Malignant neoplasm of supraglottis
161.2 Malignant neoplasm of subglottis
161.3 Malignant neoplasm of laryngeal cartilages
197.3 Secondary malignant neoplasm of other respiratory organs
198.89 Secondary malignant neoplasm of other specified sites
210.6 Benign neoplasm of other parts of oropharynx
212.1 Benign neoplasm of larynx
230.0 Carcinoma in situ of lip, oral cavity, and pharynx
231.0 Carcinoma in situ of larynx
235.1 Neoplasm of uncertain behavior of lip, oral cavity, and pharynx
235.6 Neoplasm of uncertain behavior of larynx
239.0 Neoplasm of unspecified nature of digestive system
239.1 Neoplasm of unspecified nature of respiratory system
748.3 Other congenital anomaly of larynx, trachea, and bronchus

ICD-9-CM Procedural

30.21 Epiglottidectomy

31500

31500 Intubation, endotracheal, emergency procedure

ICD-9-CM Diagnostic

The application of this code is too broad to adequately present ICD-9-CM diagnostic code links here. Refer to your ICD-9-CM book.

ICD-9-CM Procedural

96.04 Insertion of endotracheal tube

▽ Unspecified code ♀ Female diagnosis ☒ Manifestation code ♂ Male diagnosis

31502

31502 Tracheotomy tube change prior to establishment of fistula tract

ICD-9-CM Diagnostic

The application of this code is too broad to adequately present ICD-9-CM diagnostic code links here. Refer to your ICD-9-CM book.

ICD-9-CM Procedural

97.23 Replacement of tracheostomy tube

HCPCS Level II Supplies & Services

A7520 Tracheostomy/laryngectomy tube, non-cuffed, polyvinylchloride (PVC), silicone or equal, each
A7521 Tracheostomy/laryngectomy tube, cuffed, polyvinylchloride (PVC), silicone or equal, each
A7522 Tracheostomy/laryngectomy tube, stainless steel or equal (sterilizable and reusable), each
A7523 Tracheostomy shower protector, each
A7524 Tracheostoma stent/stud/button, each
A7525 Tracheostomy mask, each
A7526 Tracheostomy tube collar/holder, each

31505–31510

31505 Laryngoscopy, indirect; diagnostic (separate procedure)
31510 with biopsy

ICD-9-CM Diagnostic

148.2 Malignant neoplasm of aryepiglottic fold, hypopharyngeal aspect
161.0 Malignant neoplasm of glottis
161.1 Malignant neoplasm of supraglottis
161.2 Malignant neoplasm of subglottis
161.3 Malignant neoplasm of laryngeal cartilages
161.8 Malignant neoplasm of other specified sites of larynx
197.3 Secondary malignant neoplasm of other respiratory organs
198.89 Secondary malignant neoplasm of other specified sites
199.1 Other malignant neoplasm of unspecified site
212.0 Benign neoplasm of nasal cavities, middle ear, and accessory sinuses
212.1 Benign neoplasm of larynx
231.0 Carcinoma in situ of larynx
235.6 Neoplasm of uncertain behavior of larynx
239.1 Neoplasm of unspecified nature of respiratory system
446.4 Wegener's granulomatosis
464.21 Acute laryngotracheitis with obstruction
464.31 Acute epiglottitis with obstruction
465.0 Acute laryngopharyngitis
476.0 Chronic laryngitis
476.1 Chronic laryngotracheitis
478.30 Unspecified paralysis of vocal cords or larynx ▽
478.31 Unilateral partial paralysis of vocal cords or larynx
478.32 Unilateral complete paralysis of vocal cords or larynx
478.33 Bilateral partial paralysis of vocal cords or larynx
478.34 Bilateral complete paralysis of vocal cords or larynx
478.4 Polyp of vocal cord or larynx
478.5 Other diseases of vocal cords
478.6 Edema of larynx
478.71 Cellulitis and perichondritis of larynx
478.74 Stenosis of larynx
478.75 Laryngeal spasm
478.79 Other diseases of larynx
519.8 Other diseases of respiratory system, not elsewhere classified
519.9 Unspecified disease of respiratory system ▽
748.2 Congenital web of larynx
748.3 Other congenital anomaly of larynx, trachea, and bronchus
748.8 Other specified congenital anomaly of respiratory system
784.1 Throat pain
784.2 Swelling, mass, or lump in head and neck
784.3 Aphasia
784.40 Unspecified voice disturbance ▽
784.41 Aphonia
784.49 Other voice disturbance
784.8 Hemorrhage from throat
786.09 Other dyspnea and respiratory abnormalities
786.1 Stridor
786.2 Cough
786.3 Hemoptysis
787.2 Dysphagia

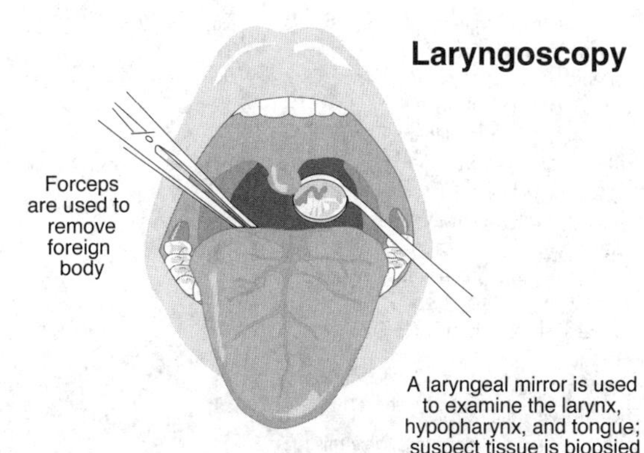
Laryngoscopy
Forceps are used to remove foreign body
A laryngeal mirror is used to examine the larynx, hypopharynx, and tongue; suspect tissue is biopsied

807.5 Closed fracture of larynx and trachea
925.2 Crushing injury of neck — (Use additional code to identify any associated injuries: 800-829, 850.0-854.1, 860.0-869.1)
933.0 Foreign body in pharynx
933.1 Foreign body in larynx
947.1 Burn of larynx, trachea, and lung
948.00 Burn (any degree) involving less than 10% of body surface with third degree burn of less than 10% or unspecified amount
V10.02 Personal history of malignant neoplasm of other and unspecified parts of oral cavity and pharynx ▽
V10.21 Personal history of malignant neoplasm of larynx
V15.82 Personal history of tobacco use, presenting hazards to health
V67.00 Follow-up examination, following unspecified surgery ▽
V67.09 Follow-up examination, following other surgery
V71.1 Observation for suspected malignant neoplasm

ICD-9-CM Procedural

31.42 Laryngoscopy and other tracheoscopy
31.43 Closed (endoscopic) biopsy of larynx
31.48 Other diagnostic procedures on larynx

HCPCS Level II Supplies & Services

A4305 Disposable drug delivery system, flow rate of 50 ml or greater per hour
A4306 Disposable drug delivery system, flow rate of 5 ml or less per hour
A4550 Surgical trays

31511

31511 Laryngoscopy, indirect; with removal of foreign body

ICD-9-CM Diagnostic

787.2 Dysphagia
933.0 Foreign body in pharynx
933.1 Foreign body in larynx

ICD-9-CM Procedural

98.14 Removal of intraluminal foreign body from larynx without incision

HCPCS Level II Supplies & Services

A4305 Disposable drug delivery system, flow rate of 50 ml or greater per hour
A4306 Disposable drug delivery system, flow rate of 5 ml or less per hour
A4550 Surgical trays

31512

31512 Laryngoscopy, indirect; with removal of lesion

ICD-9-CM Diagnostic

148.2 Malignant neoplasm of aryepiglottic fold, hypopharyngeal aspect
161.0 Malignant neoplasm of glottis
161.1 Malignant neoplasm of supraglottis
161.2 Malignant neoplasm of subglottis
161.3 Malignant neoplasm of laryngeal cartilages
161.8 Malignant neoplasm of other specified sites of larynx
197.3 Secondary malignant neoplasm of other respiratory organs
198.89 Secondary malignant neoplasm of other specified sites
199.1 Other malignant neoplasm of unspecified site
212.0 Benign neoplasm of nasal cavities, middle ear, and accessory sinuses
212.1 Benign neoplasm of larynx
231.0 Carcinoma in situ of larynx
235.6 Neoplasm of uncertain behavior of larynx

239.1 Neoplasm of unspecified nature of respiratory system
446.4 Wegener's granulomatosis
476.0 Chronic laryngitis
476.1 Chronic laryngotracheitis
478.4 Polyp of vocal cord or larynx
478.5 Other diseases of vocal cords
748.2 Congenital web of larynx
748.3 Other congenital anomaly of larynx, trachea, and bronchus
784.1 Throat pain
784.2 Swelling, mass, or lump in head and neck
784.3 Aphasia
784.40 Unspecified voice disturbance ▽
784.41 Aphonia
784.49 Other voice disturbance
784.8 Hemorrhage from throat
786.09 Other dyspnea and respiratory abnormalities
786.1 Stridor
786.2 Cough
786.3 Hemoptysis
787.2 Dysphagia
V10.02 Personal history of malignant neoplasm of other and unspecified parts of oral cavity and pharynx ▽
V10.21 Personal history of malignant neoplasm of larynx
V15.82 Personal history of tobacco use, presenting hazards to health
V67.00 Follow-up examination, following unspecified surgery ▽
V67.09 Follow-up examination, following other surgery

ICD-9-CM Procedural

30.09 Other excision or destruction of lesion or tissue of larynx

31513

31513 Laryngoscopy, indirect; with vocal cord injection

ICD-9-CM Diagnostic

476.0 Chronic laryngitis
476.1 Chronic laryngotracheitis
478.31 Unilateral partial paralysis of vocal cords or larynx
478.32 Unilateral complete paralysis of vocal cords or larynx
478.33 Bilateral partial paralysis of vocal cords or larynx
478.34 Bilateral complete paralysis of vocal cords or larynx
478.5 Other diseases of vocal cords
478.75 Laryngeal spasm
784.41 Aphonia
784.49 Other voice disturbance
786.1 Stridor

ICD-9-CM Procedural

31.0 Injection of larynx

HCPCS Level II Supplies & Services

A4305 Disposable drug delivery system, flow rate of 50 ml or greater per hour
A4306 Disposable drug delivery system, flow rate of 5 ml or less per hour
A4550 Surgical trays

31515

31515 Laryngoscopy direct, with or without tracheoscopy; for aspiration

ICD-9-CM Diagnostic

464.00 Acute laryngitis, without mention of obstruction
464.01 Acute laryngitis, with obstruction
478.24 Retropharyngeal abscess
478.5 Other diseases of vocal cords
478.79 Other diseases of larynx
507.0 Pneumonitis due to inhalation of food or vomitus
507.1 Pneumonitis due to inhalation of oils and essences
507.8 Pneumonitis due to other solids and liquids
519.01 Infection of tracheostomy — (Use additional code to identify type of infection: 038.0-038.9, 682.1. Use additional code to identify organism: 041.00-041.9)
519.09 Other tracheostomy complications
519.1 Other diseases of trachea and bronchus, not elsewhere classified
519.8 Other diseases of respiratory system, not elsewhere classified
668.04 Pulmonary complications of the administration of anesthesia or other sedation in labor and delivery, postpartum — (Use additional code(s) to further specify complication) ♀
761.3 Fetus or newborn affected by polyhydramnios
770.1 Meconium aspiration syndrome
770.3 Pulmonary hemorrhage of fetus or newborn
784.2 Swelling, mass, or lump in head and neck
784.49 Other voice disturbance
784.8 Hemorrhage from throat
786.09 Other dyspnea and respiratory abnormalities
786.1 Stridor
786.3 Hemoptysis
786.4 Abnormal sputum
787.2 Dysphagia
933.1 Foreign body in larynx
934.0 Foreign body in trachea
998.51 Infected postoperative seroma — (Use additional code to identify organism)
998.59 Other postoperative infection — (Use additional code to identify infection)

ICD-9-CM Procedural

31.42 Laryngoscopy and other tracheoscopy
31.48 Other diagnostic procedures on larynx

HCPCS Level II Supplies & Services

A4305 Disposable drug delivery system, flow rate of 50 ml or greater per hour
A4306 Disposable drug delivery system, flow rate of 5 ml or less per hour
A4550 Surgical trays

31520–31526

31520 Laryngoscopy direct, with or without tracheoscopy; diagnostic, newborn
31525 diagnostic, except newborn
31526 diagnostic, with operating microscope

ICD-9-CM Diagnostic

148.2 Malignant neoplasm of aryepiglottic fold, hypopharyngeal aspect
161.0 Malignant neoplasm of glottis
161.1 Malignant neoplasm of supraglottis
161.2 Malignant neoplasm of subglottis
161.3 Malignant neoplasm of laryngeal cartilages
161.8 Malignant neoplasm of other specified sites of larynx
161.9 Malignant neoplasm of larynx, unspecified site ▽
197.3 Secondary malignant neoplasm of other respiratory organs
198.89 Secondary malignant neoplasm of other specified sites
199.1 Other malignant neoplasm of unspecified site
212.1 Benign neoplasm of larynx
212.2 Benign neoplasm of trachea
215.0 Other benign neoplasm of connective and other soft tissue of head, face, and neck
231.0 Carcinoma in situ of larynx
231.1 Carcinoma in situ of trachea
234.8 Carcinoma in situ of other specified sites
235.6 Neoplasm of uncertain behavior of larynx
235.7 Neoplasm of uncertain behavior of trachea, bronchus, and lung
239.1 Neoplasm of unspecified nature of respiratory system
464.11 Acute tracheitis with obstruction
464.21 Acute laryngotracheitis with obstruction
464.31 Acute epiglottitis with obstruction
476.0 Chronic laryngitis
476.1 Chronic laryngotracheitis
478.31 Unilateral partial paralysis of vocal cords or larynx
478.32 Unilateral complete paralysis of vocal cords or larynx
478.33 Bilateral partial paralysis of vocal cords or larynx
478.34 Bilateral complete paralysis of vocal cords or larynx
478.4 Polyp of vocal cord or larynx
478.5 Other diseases of vocal cords
478.6 Edema of larynx
478.71 Cellulitis and perichondritis of larynx
478.74 Stenosis of larynx
478.75 Laryngeal spasm
478.79 Other diseases of larynx
518.81 Acute respiratory failure
519.1 Other diseases of trachea and bronchus, not elsewhere classified
519.8 Other diseases of respiratory system, not elsewhere classified
748.2 Congenital web of larynx
748.3 Other congenital anomaly of larynx, trachea, and bronchus
748.8 Other specified congenital anomaly of respiratory system
750.3 Congenital tracheoesophageal fistula, esophageal atresia and stenosis
768.2 Fetal distress before onset of labor, in liveborn infant — (Use only when associated with newborn morbidity classifiable elsewhere)
768.3 Fetal distress first noted during labor, in liveborn infant — (Use only when associated with newborn morbidity classifiable elsewhere)

768.4 Fetal distress, unspecified as to time of onset, in liveborn infant — (Use only when associated with newborn morbidity classifiable elsewhere) ▽
768.5 Severe birth asphyxia — (Use only when associated with newborn morbidity classifiable elsewhere)
768.6 Mild or moderate birth asphyxia — (Use only when associated with newborn morbidity classifiable elsewhere)
769 Respiratory distress syndrome in newborn
770.1 Meconium aspiration syndrome
770.3 Pulmonary hemorrhage of fetus or newborn
770.81 Primary apnea of newborn
770.82 Other apnea of newborn
770.83 Cyanotic attacks of newborn
770.84 Respiratory failure of newborn
770.89 Other respiratory problems of newborn after birth
779.3 Feeding problems in newborn
784.1 Throat pain
784.41 Aphonia
784.49 Other voice disturbance
784.8 Hemorrhage from throat
786.09 Other dyspnea and respiratory abnormalities
786.1 Stridor
786.2 Cough
787.2 Dysphagia
807.5 Closed fracture of larynx and trachea
807.6 Open fracture of larynx and trachea
933.1 Foreign body in larynx
997.3 Respiratory complications — (Use additional code to identify complications)
V10.20 Personal history of malignant neoplasm of unspecified respiratory organ ▽
V10.21 Personal history of malignant neoplasm of larynx
V12.6 Personal history of diseases of respiratory system

ICD-9-CM Procedural

31.42 Laryngoscopy and other tracheoscopy
31.48 Other diagnostic procedures on larynx

HCPCS Level II Supplies & Services

A4305 Disposable drug delivery system, flow rate of 50 ml or greater per hour
A4306 Disposable drug delivery system, flow rate of 5 ml or less per hour
A4550 Surgical trays

31527–31529

31527 Laryngoscopy direct, with or without tracheoscopy; with insertion of obturator
31528 with dilation, initial
31529 with dilation, subsequent

ICD-9-CM Diagnostic

148.2 Malignant neoplasm of aryepiglottic fold, hypopharyngeal aspect
161.0 Malignant neoplasm of glottis
161.1 Malignant neoplasm of supraglottis
161.2 Malignant neoplasm of subglottis
161.3 Malignant neoplasm of laryngeal cartilages
161.8 Malignant neoplasm of other specified sites of larynx
161.9 Malignant neoplasm of larynx, unspecified site ▽
197.3 Secondary malignant neoplasm of other respiratory organs
198.89 Secondary malignant neoplasm of other specified sites
199.1 Other malignant neoplasm of unspecified site
212.1 Benign neoplasm of larynx
212.2 Benign neoplasm of trachea
215.0 Other benign neoplasm of connective and other soft tissue of head, face, and neck
231.0 Carcinoma in situ of larynx
231.1 Carcinoma in situ of trachea
234.8 Carcinoma in situ of other specified sites
235.6 Neoplasm of uncertain behavior of larynx
235.7 Neoplasm of uncertain behavior of trachea, bronchus, and lung
239.1 Neoplasm of unspecified nature of respiratory system
464.11 Acute tracheitis with obstruction
464.21 Acute laryngotracheitis with obstruction
464.31 Acute epiglottitis with obstruction
476.0 Chronic laryngitis
476.1 Chronic laryngotracheitis
478.31 Unilateral partial paralysis of vocal cords or larynx
478.32 Unilateral complete paralysis of vocal cords or larynx
478.33 Bilateral partial paralysis of vocal cords or larynx
478.34 Bilateral complete paralysis of vocal cords or larynx
478.4 Polyp of vocal cord or larynx
478.5 Other diseases of vocal cords
478.6 Edema of larynx
478.71 Cellulitis and perichondritis of larynx
478.74 Stenosis of larynx
478.75 Laryngeal spasm
478.79 Other diseases of larynx
518.81 Acute respiratory failure
519.1 Other diseases of trachea and bronchus, not elsewhere classified
519.8 Other diseases of respiratory system, not elsewhere classified
748.2 Congenital web of larynx
748.3 Other congenital anomaly of larynx, trachea, and bronchus
748.8 Other specified congenital anomaly of respiratory system
784.1 Throat pain
784.41 Aphonia
784.49 Other voice disturbance
784.8 Hemorrhage from throat
786.09 Other dyspnea and respiratory abnormalities
786.1 Stridor
786.2 Cough
787.2 Dysphagia
807.5 Closed fracture of larynx and trachea
807.6 Open fracture of larynx and trachea
933.1 Foreign body in larynx
997.3 Respiratory complications — (Use additional code to identify complications)
V10.20 Personal history of malignant neoplasm of unspecified respiratory organ ▽
V10.21 Personal history of malignant neoplasm of larynx
V12.6 Personal history of diseases of respiratory system

ICD-9-CM Procedural

31.98 Other operations on larynx

HCPCS Level II Supplies & Services

A4305 Disposable drug delivery system, flow rate of 50 ml or greater per hour
A4306 Disposable drug delivery system, flow rate of 5 ml or less per hour
A4550 Surgical trays

31530–31531

31530 Laryngoscopy, direct, operative, with foreign body removal;
31531 with operating microscope

ICD-9-CM Diagnostic

784.41 Aphonia
786.1 Stridor
786.2 Cough
933.1 Foreign body in larynx

ICD-9-CM Procedural

98.14 Removal of intraluminal foreign body from larynx without incision

HCPCS Level II Supplies & Services

A4305 Disposable drug delivery system, flow rate of 50 ml or greater per hour
A4306 Disposable drug delivery system, flow rate of 5 ml or less per hour
A4550 Surgical trays

31535–31536

31535 Laryngoscopy, direct, operative, with biopsy;
31536 with operating microscope

ICD-9-CM Diagnostic

150.0 Malignant neoplasm of cervical esophagus
161.0 Malignant neoplasm of glottis
161.1 Malignant neoplasm of supraglottis
161.2 Malignant neoplasm of subglottis
161.3 Malignant neoplasm of laryngeal cartilages
161.8 Malignant neoplasm of other specified sites of larynx
161.9 Malignant neoplasm of larynx, unspecified site ▽
195.0 Malignant neoplasm of head, face, and neck
196.0 Secondary and unspecified malignant neoplasm of lymph nodes of head, face, and neck
197.3 Secondary malignant neoplasm of other respiratory organs
198.89 Secondary malignant neoplasm of other specified sites
199.1 Other malignant neoplasm of unspecified site
212.1 Benign neoplasm of larynx
212.2 Benign neoplasm of trachea
212.9 Benign neoplasm of respiratory and intrathoracic organs, site unspecified ▽

215.0 Other benign neoplasm of connective and other soft tissue of head, face, and neck
230.0 Carcinoma in situ of lip, oral cavity, and pharynx
231.0 Carcinoma in situ of larynx
231.1 Carcinoma in situ of trachea
234.8 Carcinoma in situ of other specified sites
235.6 Neoplasm of uncertain behavior of larynx
235.7 Neoplasm of uncertain behavior of trachea, bronchus, and lung
239.1 Neoplasm of unspecified nature of respiratory system
464.00 Acute laryngitis, without mention of obstruction
464.01 Acute laryngitis, with obstruction
464.10 Acute tracheitis without mention of obstruction
464.11 Acute tracheitis with obstruction
464.20 Acute laryngotracheitis without mention of obstruction
464.21 Acute laryngotracheitis with obstruction
464.30 Acute epiglottitis without mention of obstruction
464.31 Acute epiglottitis with obstruction
465.0 Acute laryngopharyngitis
465.8 Acute upper respiratory infections of other multiple sites
465.9 Acute upper respiratory infections of unspecified site ▽
476.0 Chronic laryngitis
476.1 Chronic laryngotracheitis
478.30 Unspecified paralysis of vocal cords or larynx ▽
478.31 Unilateral partial paralysis of vocal cords or larynx
478.32 Unilateral complete paralysis of vocal cords or larynx
478.33 Bilateral partial paralysis of vocal cords or larynx
478.4 Polyp of vocal cord or larynx
478.5 Other diseases of vocal cords
478.6 Edema of larynx
478.70 Unspecified disease of larynx ▽
478.71 Cellulitis and perichondritis of larynx
478.74 Stenosis of larynx
478.79 Other diseases of larynx
496 Chronic airway obstruction, not elsewhere classified — (Note: This code is not to be used with any code from 491-493) ▽
519.1 Other diseases of trachea and bronchus, not elsewhere classified
748.2 Congenital web of larynx
748.3 Other congenital anomaly of larynx, trachea, and bronchus
748.8 Other specified congenital anomaly of respiratory system
748.9 Unspecified congenital anomaly of respiratory system ▽
784.1 Throat pain
784.2 Swelling, mass, or lump in head and neck
784.41 Aphonia
784.49 Other voice disturbance
784.8 Hemorrhage from throat
785.6 Enlargement of lymph nodes
786.09 Other dyspnea and respiratory abnormalities
786.1 Stridor
786.2 Cough
786.3 Hemoptysis
786.6 Swelling, mass, or lump in chest
787.2 Dysphagia
V10.20 Personal history of malignant neoplasm of unspecified respiratory organ ▽
V10.21 Personal history of malignant neoplasm of larynx
V12.6 Personal history of diseases of respiratory system
V15.82 Personal history of tobacco use, presenting hazards to health

ICD-9-CM Procedural

31.43 Closed (endoscopic) biopsy of larynx
31.44 Closed (endoscopic) biopsy of trachea

HCPCS Level II Supplies & Services

A4305 Disposable drug delivery system, flow rate of 50 ml or greater per hour
A4306 Disposable drug delivery system, flow rate of 5 ml or less per hour
A4550 Surgical trays

31540–31541

31540 Laryngoscopy, direct, operative, with excision of tumor and/or stripping of vocal cords or epiglottis;
31541 with operating microscope

ICD-9-CM Diagnostic

148.2 Malignant neoplasm of aryepiglottic fold, hypopharyngeal aspect
161.0 Malignant neoplasm of glottis
161.1 Malignant neoplasm of supraglottis
161.2 Malignant neoplasm of subglottis
161.3 Malignant neoplasm of laryngeal cartilages
161.8 Malignant neoplasm of other specified sites of larynx
197.3 Secondary malignant neoplasm of other respiratory organs
198.89 Secondary malignant neoplasm of other specified sites
199.1 Other malignant neoplasm of unspecified site
212.1 Benign neoplasm of larynx
228.09 Hemangioma of other sites
231.0 Carcinoma in situ of larynx
235.6 Neoplasm of uncertain behavior of larynx
239.1 Neoplasm of unspecified nature of respiratory system
352.3 Disorders of pneumogastric (10th) nerve
476.0 Chronic laryngitis
478.31 Unilateral partial paralysis of vocal cords or larynx
478.32 Unilateral complete paralysis of vocal cords or larynx
478.33 Bilateral partial paralysis of vocal cords or larynx
478.34 Bilateral complete paralysis of vocal cords or larynx
478.4 Polyp of vocal cord or larynx
478.5 Other diseases of vocal cords
478.79 Other diseases of larynx
519.8 Other diseases of respiratory system, not elsewhere classified
784.2 Swelling, mass, or lump in head and neck
784.49 Other voice disturbance
787.2 Dysphagia
V15.82 Personal history of tobacco use, presenting hazards to health

ICD-9-CM Procedural

30.09 Other excision or destruction of lesion or tissue of larynx

31545–31546

31545 Laryngoscopy, direct, operative, with operating microscope or telescope, with submucosal removal of non-neoplastic lesion(s) of vocal cord; reconstruction with local tissue flap(s)
31546 reconstruction with graft(s) (includes obtaining autograft)

ICD-9-CM Diagnostic

212.1 Benign neoplasm of larynx
478.4 Polyp of vocal cord or larynx
478.5 Other diseases of vocal cords
478.6 Edema of larynx
478.70 Unspecified disease of larynx ▽
478.71 Cellulitis and perichondritis of larynx
478.79 Other diseases of larynx
748.2 Congenital web of larynx
748.3 Other congenital anomaly of larynx, trachea, and bronchus
784.1 Throat pain
784.2 Swelling, mass, or lump in head and neck
784.40 Unspecified voice disturbance ▽
784.49 Other voice disturbance

ICD-9-CM Procedural

30.09 Other excision or destruction of lesion or tissue of larynx
31.69 Other repair of larynx

31560–31561

31560 Laryngoscopy, direct, operative, with arytenoidectomy;
31561 with operating microscope

ICD-9-CM Diagnostic

148.2 Malignant neoplasm of aryepiglottic fold, hypopharyngeal aspect
150.0 Malignant neoplasm of cervical esophagus
161.1 Malignant neoplasm of supraglottis
161.3 Malignant neoplasm of laryngeal cartilages
161.8 Malignant neoplasm of other specified sites of larynx
197.3 Secondary malignant neoplasm of other respiratory organs
198.89 Secondary malignant neoplasm of other specified sites
212.1 Benign neoplasm of larynx
231.0 Carcinoma in situ of larynx
235.6 Neoplasm of uncertain behavior of larynx
238.0 Neoplasm of uncertain behavior of bone and articular cartilage
478.79 Other diseases of larynx
748.3 Other congenital anomaly of larynx, trachea, and bronchus
784.2 Swelling, mass, or lump in head and neck

ICD-9-CM Procedural

30.29 Other partial laryngectomy

31570–31571

31570 Laryngoscopy, direct, with injection into vocal cord(s), therapeutic;
31571 with operating microscope

ICD-9-CM Diagnostic

476.0 Chronic laryngitis
476.1 Chronic laryngotracheitis
478.31 Unilateral partial paralysis of vocal cords or larynx
478.32 Unilateral complete paralysis of vocal cords or larynx
478.33 Bilateral partial paralysis of vocal cords or larynx
478.34 Bilateral complete paralysis of vocal cords or larynx
478.4 Polyp of vocal cord or larynx
478.6 Edema of larynx
478.75 Laryngeal spasm
784.41 Aphonia
784.49 Other voice disturbance
906.0 Late effect of open wound of head, neck, and trunk
908.6 Late effect of certain complications of trauma

ICD-9-CM Procedural

31.0 Injection of larynx

HCPCS Level II Supplies & Services

A4305 Disposable drug delivery system, flow rate of 50 ml or greater per hour
A4306 Disposable drug delivery system, flow rate of 5 ml or less per hour
A4550 Surgical trays

31575–31576

31575 Laryngoscopy, flexible fiberoptic; diagnostic
31576 with biopsy

ICD-9-CM Diagnostic

148.2 Malignant neoplasm of aryepiglottic fold, hypopharyngeal aspect
161.0 Malignant neoplasm of glottis
161.1 Malignant neoplasm of supraglottis
161.2 Malignant neoplasm of subglottis
161.3 Malignant neoplasm of laryngeal cartilages
161.8 Malignant neoplasm of other specified sites of larynx
197.3 Secondary malignant neoplasm of other respiratory organs
198.89 Secondary malignant neoplasm of other specified sites
199.1 Other malignant neoplasm of unspecified site
212.1 Benign neoplasm of larynx
231.0 Carcinoma in situ of larynx
235.6 Neoplasm of uncertain behavior of larynx
239.1 Neoplasm of unspecified nature of respiratory system
446.4 Wegener's granulomatosis
464.21 Acute laryngotracheitis with obstruction
464.31 Acute epiglottitis with obstruction
465.0 Acute laryngopharyngitis
476.0 Chronic laryngitis
476.1 Chronic laryngotracheitis
478.30 Unspecified paralysis of vocal cords or larynx ▽
478.31 Unilateral partial paralysis of vocal cords or larynx
478.32 Unilateral complete paralysis of vocal cords or larynx
478.33 Bilateral partial paralysis of vocal cords or larynx
478.34 Bilateral complete paralysis of vocal cords or larynx
478.4 Polyp of vocal cord or larynx
478.5 Other diseases of vocal cords
478.6 Edema of larynx
478.75 Laryngeal spasm
478.79 Other diseases of larynx
519.00 Unspecified tracheostomy complication ▽
519.01 Infection of tracheostomy — (Use additional code to identify type of infection: 038.0-038.9, 682.1. Use additional code to identify organism: 041.00-041.9)
519.02 Mechanical complication of tracheostomy
519.09 Other tracheostomy complications
519.8 Other diseases of respiratory system, not elsewhere classified
519.9 Unspecified disease of respiratory system ▽
748.2 Congenital web of larynx
748.3 Other congenital anomaly of larynx, trachea, and bronchus
748.8 Other specified congenital anomaly of respiratory system
749.00 Unspecified cleft palate ▽
780.51 Insomnia with sleep apnea
780.53 Hypersomnia with sleep apnea
780.57 Other and unspecified sleep apnea ▽
784.1 Throat pain
784.2 Swelling, mass, or lump in head and neck
784.41 Aphonia
784.49 Other voice disturbance
784.8 Hemorrhage from throat
786.09 Other dyspnea and respiratory abnormalities
786.1 Stridor
786.2 Cough
786.3 Hemoptysis
787.2 Dysphagia
807.5 Closed fracture of larynx and trachea
925.2 Crushing injury of neck — (Use additional code to identify any associated injuries: 800-829, 850.0-854.1, 860.0-869.1)
933.0 Foreign body in pharynx
933.1 Foreign body in larynx
947.1 Burn of larynx, trachea, and lung
V10.02 Personal history of malignant neoplasm of other and unspecified parts of oral cavity and pharynx ▽
V10.21 Personal history of malignant neoplasm of larynx
V67.00 Follow-up examination, following unspecified surgery ▽
V67.09 Follow-up examination, following other surgery
V71.1 Observation for suspected malignant neoplasm

ICD-9-CM Procedural

31.42 Laryngoscopy and other tracheoscopy
31.43 Closed (endoscopic) biopsy of larynx
31.48 Other diagnostic procedures on larynx

HCPCS Level II Supplies & Services

A4305 Disposable drug delivery system, flow rate of 50 ml or greater per hour
A4306 Disposable drug delivery system, flow rate of 5 ml or less per hour
A4550 Surgical trays

31577

31577 Laryngoscopy, flexible fiberoptic; with removal of foreign body

ICD-9-CM Diagnostic

784.1 Throat pain
786.09 Other dyspnea and respiratory abnormalities
786.1 Stridor
786.2 Cough
787.2 Dysphagia
933.0 Foreign body in pharynx
933.1 Foreign body in larynx

ICD-9-CM Procedural

98.14 Removal of intraluminal foreign body from larynx without incision

HCPCS Level II Supplies & Services

A4305 Disposable drug delivery system, flow rate of 50 ml or greater per hour
A4306 Disposable drug delivery system, flow rate of 5 ml or less per hour
A4550 Surgical trays

31578

31578 Laryngoscopy, flexible fiberoptic; with removal of lesion

ICD-9-CM Diagnostic

148.2 Malignant neoplasm of aryepiglottic fold, hypopharyngeal aspect
161.0 Malignant neoplasm of glottis
161.1 Malignant neoplasm of supraglottis
161.2 Malignant neoplasm of subglottis
161.3 Malignant neoplasm of laryngeal cartilages
161.8 Malignant neoplasm of other specified sites of larynx
197.3 Secondary malignant neoplasm of other respiratory organs
198.89 Secondary malignant neoplasm of other specified sites
199.1 Other malignant neoplasm of unspecified site
212.1 Benign neoplasm of larynx
231.0 Carcinoma in situ of larynx
235.6 Neoplasm of uncertain behavior of larynx
239.1 Neoplasm of unspecified nature of respiratory system
446.4 Wegener's granulomatosis
464.21 Acute laryngotracheitis with obstruction
464.31 Acute epiglottitis with obstruction
465.0 Acute laryngopharyngitis
476.0 Chronic laryngitis
476.1 Chronic laryngotracheitis
478.30 Unspecified paralysis of vocal cords or larynx ▽

478.31 Unilateral partial paralysis of vocal cords or larynx
478.32 Unilateral complete paralysis of vocal cords or larynx
478.33 Bilateral partial paralysis of vocal cords or larynx
478.34 Bilateral complete paralysis of vocal cords or larynx
478.4 Polyp of vocal cord or larynx
478.5 Other diseases of vocal cords
478.6 Edema of larynx
478.75 Laryngeal spasm
478.79 Other diseases of larynx
519.8 Other diseases of respiratory system, not elsewhere classified
519.9 Unspecified disease of respiratory system
748.2 Congenital web of larynx
748.3 Other congenital anomaly of larynx, trachea, and bronchus
748.8 Other specified congenital anomaly of respiratory system
784.1 Throat pain
784.2 Swelling, mass, or lump in head and neck
784.41 Aphonia
784.49 Other voice disturbance
784.8 Hemorrhage from throat
786.09 Other dyspnea and respiratory abnormalities
786.1 Stridor
786.2 Cough
786.3 Hemoptysis
787.2 Dysphagia
947.1 Burn of larynx, trachea, and lung
V10.02 Personal history of malignant neoplasm of other and unspecified parts of oral cavity and pharynx
V10.21 Personal history of malignant neoplasm of larynx
V67.00 Follow-up examination, following unspecified surgery
V67.09 Follow-up examination, following other surgery
V71.1 Observation for suspected malignant neoplasm

ICD-9-CM Procedural
30.09 Other excision or destruction of lesion or tissue of larynx

HCPCS Level II Supplies & Services
A4305 Disposable drug delivery system, flow rate of 50 ml or greater per hour
A4306 Disposable drug delivery system, flow rate of 5 ml or less per hour
A4550 Surgical trays

31579
31579 Laryngoscopy, flexible or rigid fiberoptic, with stroboscopy

ICD-9-CM Diagnostic
148.2 Malignant neoplasm of aryepiglottic fold, hypopharyngeal aspect
161.0 Malignant neoplasm of glottis
161.1 Malignant neoplasm of supraglottis
161.2 Malignant neoplasm of subglottis
161.3 Malignant neoplasm of laryngeal cartilages
161.8 Malignant neoplasm of other specified sites of larynx
197.3 Secondary malignant neoplasm of other respiratory organs
198.89 Secondary malignant neoplasm of other specified sites
199.1 Other malignant neoplasm of unspecified site
212.1 Benign neoplasm of larynx
231.0 Carcinoma in situ of larynx
235.6 Neoplasm of uncertain behavior of larynx
239.1 Neoplasm of unspecified nature of respiratory system
446.4 Wegener's granulomatosis
476.0 Chronic laryngitis
476.1 Chronic laryngotracheitis
478.30 Unspecified paralysis of vocal cords or larynx
478.31 Unilateral partial paralysis of vocal cords or larynx
478.32 Unilateral complete paralysis of vocal cords or larynx
478.33 Bilateral partial paralysis of vocal cords or larynx
478.34 Bilateral complete paralysis of vocal cords or larynx
478.4 Polyp of vocal cord or larynx
478.5 Other diseases of vocal cords
478.6 Edema of larynx
478.75 Laryngeal spasm
478.79 Other diseases of larynx
519.8 Other diseases of respiratory system, not elsewhere classified
519.9 Unspecified disease of respiratory system
748.2 Congenital web of larynx
748.3 Other congenital anomaly of larynx, trachea, and bronchus
748.8 Other specified congenital anomaly of respiratory system
784.1 Throat pain
784.2 Swelling, mass, or lump in head and neck
784.41 Aphonia
784.49 Other voice disturbance
784.8 Hemorrhage from throat
786.09 Other dyspnea and respiratory abnormalities
786.1 Stridor
786.2 Cough
786.3 Hemoptysis
787.2 Dysphagia
947.1 Burn of larynx, trachea, and lung
V10.02 Personal history of malignant neoplasm of other and unspecified parts of oral cavity and pharynx
V10.21 Personal history of malignant neoplasm of larynx
V67.00 Follow-up examination, following unspecified surgery
V67.09 Follow-up examination, following other surgery
V71.1 Observation for suspected malignant neoplasm

ICD-9-CM Procedural
31.42 Laryngoscopy and other tracheoscopy
31.48 Other diagnostic procedures on larynx

HCPCS Level II Supplies & Services
A4305 Disposable drug delivery system, flow rate of 50 ml or greater per hour
A4306 Disposable drug delivery system, flow rate of 5 ml or less per hour
A4550 Surgical trays

31580–31582
31580 Laryngoplasty; for laryngeal web, two stage, with keel insertion and removal
31582 for laryngeal stenosis, with graft or core mold, including tracheotomy

ICD-9-CM Diagnostic
478.74 Stenosis of larynx
748.2 Congenital web of larynx
748.3 Other congenital anomaly of larynx, trachea, and bronchus

ICD-9-CM Procedural
31.69 Other repair of larynx
31.98 Other operations on larynx

31584
31584 Laryngoplasty; with open reduction of fracture

ICD-9-CM Diagnostic
807.5 Closed fracture of larynx and trachea
807.6 Open fracture of larynx and trachea

ICD-9-CM Procedural
31.64 Repair of laryngeal fracture
31.69 Other repair of larynx

31585–31586
31585 Treatment of closed laryngeal fracture; without manipulation
31586 with closed manipulative reduction

ICD-9-CM Diagnostic
807.5 Closed fracture of larynx and trachea

ICD-9-CM Procedural
31.64 Repair of laryngeal fracture
93.52 Application of neck support
93.53 Application of other cast

HCPCS Level II Supplies & Services
A4580 Cast supplies (e.g., plaster)

31587
31587 Laryngoplasty, cricoid split

ICD-9-CM Diagnostic
478.74 Stenosis of larynx
748.3 Other congenital anomaly of larynx, trachea, and bronchus
807.5 Closed fracture of larynx and trachea
807.6 Open fracture of larynx and trachea
874.01 Open wound of larynx, without mention of complication — (Use additional code to identify infection)

Unspecified code
♀ Female diagnosis
Manifestation code
♂ Male diagnosis

874.11 Open wound of larynx, complicated — (Use additional code to identify infection)
925.2 Crushing injury of neck — (Use additional code to identify any associated injuries: 800-829, 850.0-854.1, 860.0-869.1)
959.01 Head injury, unspecified ▽
959.09 Injury of face and neck, other and unspecified

ICD-9-CM Procedural

31.69 Other repair of larynx

31588

31588 Laryngoplasty, not otherwise specified (eg, for burns, reconstruction after partial laryngectomy)

ICD-9-CM Diagnostic

161.0 Malignant neoplasm of glottis
161.1 Malignant neoplasm of supraglottis
161.2 Malignant neoplasm of subglottis
161.3 Malignant neoplasm of laryngeal cartilages
161.8 Malignant neoplasm of other specified sites of larynx
212.1 Benign neoplasm of larynx
231.0 Carcinoma in situ of larynx
235.6 Neoplasm of uncertain behavior of larynx
478.79 Other diseases of larynx
748.3 Other congenital anomaly of larynx, trachea, and bronchus
874.01 Open wound of larynx, without mention of complication — (Use additional code to identify infection)
874.11 Open wound of larynx, complicated — (Use additional code to identify infection)
906.8 Late effect of burns of other specified sites
947.1 Burn of larynx, trachea, and lung
948.00 Burn (any degree) involving less than 10% of body surface with third degree burn of less than 10% or unspecified amount
948.10 Burn (any degree) involving 10-19% of body surface with third degree burn of less than 10% or unspecified amount
948.11 Burn (any degree) involving 10-19% of body surface with third degree burn of 10-19%
949.4 Deep necrosis of underlying tissue due to burn (deep third degree), unspecified site without mention of loss of body part ▽
949.5 Deep necrosis of underlying tissues due to burn (deep third degree, unspecified site with loss of body part ▽
V10.21 Personal history of malignant neoplasm of larynx
V45.89 Other postsurgical status — (This code is intended for use when these conditions are recorded as diagnoses or problems)

ICD-9-CM Procedural

31.61 Suture of laceration of larynx
31.62 Closure of fistula of larynx
31.69 Other repair of larynx
31.92 Lysis of adhesions of trachea or larynx

31590

31590 Laryngeal reinnervation by neuromuscular pedicle

ICD-9-CM Diagnostic

478.30 Unspecified paralysis of vocal cords or larynx ▽
478.31 Unilateral partial paralysis of vocal cords or larynx
478.32 Unilateral complete paralysis of vocal cords or larynx
478.33 Bilateral partial paralysis of vocal cords or larynx
478.34 Bilateral complete paralysis of vocal cords or larynx
478.5 Other diseases of vocal cords
V10.02 Personal history of malignant neoplasm of other and unspecified parts of oral cavity and pharynx ▽
V10.21 Personal history of malignant neoplasm of larynx

ICD-9-CM Procedural

31.69 Other repair of larynx

31595

31595 Section recurrent laryngeal nerve, therapeutic (separate procedure), unilateral

ICD-9-CM Diagnostic

352.3 Disorders of pneumogastric (10th) nerve
478.30 Unspecified paralysis of vocal cords or larynx ▽
478.31 Unilateral partial paralysis of vocal cords or larynx
478.32 Unilateral complete paralysis of vocal cords or larynx
478.33 Bilateral partial paralysis of vocal cords or larynx
478.34 Bilateral complete paralysis of vocal cords or larynx
478.74 Stenosis of larynx
478.75 Laryngeal spasm
748.3 Other congenital anomaly of larynx, trachea, and bronchus
784.41 Aphonia
786.1 Stridor

ICD-9-CM Procedural

05.0 Division of sympathetic nerve or ganglion
31.69 Other repair of larynx
31.91 Division of laryngeal nerve

Trachea and Bronchi

31600–31601

31600 Tracheostomy, planned (separate procedure);
31601 under two years

ICD-9-CM Diagnostic

141.0 Malignant neoplasm of base of tongue
141.5 Malignant neoplasm of junctional zone of tongue
141.6 Malignant neoplasm of lingual tonsil
141.8 Malignant neoplasm of other sites of tongue
146.0 Malignant neoplasm of tonsil
146.1 Malignant neoplasm of tonsillar fossa
146.2 Malignant neoplasm of tonsillar pillars (anterior) (posterior)
146.3 Malignant neoplasm of vallecula
146.4 Malignant neoplasm of anterior aspect of epiglottis
146.5 Malignant neoplasm of junctional region of oropharynx
146.6 Malignant neoplasm of lateral wall of oropharynx
146.7 Malignant neoplasm of posterior wall of oropharynx
146.8 Malignant neoplasm of other specified sites of oropharynx
148.0 Malignant neoplasm of postcricoid region of hypopharynx
148.1 Malignant neoplasm of pyriform sinus
148.2 Malignant neoplasm of aryepiglottic fold, hypopharyngeal aspect
148.3 Malignant neoplasm of posterior hypopharyngeal wall
148.8 Malignant neoplasm of other specified sites of hypopharynx
148.9 Malignant neoplasm of hypopharynx, unspecified site ▽
161.0 Malignant neoplasm of glottis
161.1 Malignant neoplasm of supraglottis
161.2 Malignant neoplasm of subglottis
161.3 Malignant neoplasm of laryngeal cartilages
161.8 Malignant neoplasm of other specified sites of larynx
197.3 Secondary malignant neoplasm of other respiratory organs
197.8 Secondary malignant neoplasm of other digestive organs and spleen
231.0 Carcinoma in situ of larynx
231.1 Carcinoma in situ of trachea
235.6 Neoplasm of uncertain behavior of larynx
348.1 Anoxic brain damage — (Use additional E code to identify cause)
478.74 Stenosis of larynx
518.5 Pulmonary insufficiency following trauma and surgery
518.81 Acute respiratory failure
518.82 Other pulmonary insufficiency, not elsewhere classified
519.00 Unspecified tracheostomy complication ▽
519.1 Other diseases of trachea and bronchus, not elsewhere classified
748.3 Other congenital anomaly of larynx, trachea, and bronchus
765.00 Extreme fetal immaturity, unspecified (weight) — (Use additional code for weeks of gestation: 765.20-765.29) ▽
765.01 Extreme fetal immaturity, less than 500 grams — (Use additional code for weeks of gestation: 765.20-765.29)
765.02 Extreme fetal immaturity, 500-749 grams — (Use additional code for weeks of gestation: 765.20-765.29)
765.03 Extreme fetal immaturity, 750-999 grams — (Use additional code for weeks of gestation: 765.20-765.29)
765.04 Extreme fetal immaturity, 1,000-1,249 grams — (Use additional code for weeks of gestation: 765.20-765.29)
765.05 Extreme fetal immaturity, 1,250-1,499 grams — (Use additional code for weeks of gestation: 765.20-765.29)
765.06 Extreme fetal immaturity, 1,500-1,749 grams — (Use additional code for weeks of gestation: 765.20-765.29)
765.10 Other preterm infants, unspecified (weight) — (Use additional code for weeks of gestation: 765.20-765.29) ▽

▽ Unspecified code ♀ Female diagnosis ☒ Manifestation code ♂ Male diagnosis

765.11 Other preterm infants, less than 500 grams — (Use additional code for weeks of gestation: 765.20-765.29)
765.12 Other preterm infants, 500-749 grams — (Use additional code for weeks of gestation: 765.20-765.29)
765.13 Other preterm infants, 750-999 grams — (Use additional code for weeks of gestation: 765.20-765.29)
765.14 Other preterm infants, 1,000-1,249 grams — (Use additional code for weeks of gestation: 765.20-765.29)
765.15 Other preterm infants, 1,250-1,499 grams — (Use additional code for weeks of gestation: 765.20-765.29)
765.16 Other preterm infants, 1,500-1,749 grams — (Use additional code for weeks of gestation: 765.20-765.29)
765.20 Unspecified weeks of gestation
765.21 Less than 24 completed weeks of gestation
765.22 24 completed weeks of gestation
765.23 25-26 completed weeks of gestation
765.24 27-28 completed weeks of gestation
765.25 29-30 completed weeks of gestation
765.26 31-32 completed weeks of gestation
765.27 33-34 completed weeks of gestation
765.28 35-36 completed weeks of gestation
765.29 37 or more completed weeks of gestation
769 Respiratory distress syndrome in newborn
770.7 Chronic respiratory disease arising in the perinatal period
770.81 Primary apnea of newborn
770.82 Other apnea of newborn
770.83 Cyanotic attacks of newborn
770.84 Respiratory failure of newborn
770.89 Other respiratory problems of newborn after birth
786.09 Other dyspnea and respiratory abnormalities
V10.02 Personal history of malignant neoplasm of other and unspecified parts of oral cavity and pharynx
V10.21 Personal history of malignant neoplasm of larynx

ICD-9-CM Procedural

31.1 Temporary tracheostomy
31.21 Mediastinal tracheostomy
31.29 Other permanent tracheostomy

HCPCS Level II Supplies & Services

A7527 Tracheostomy/laryngectomy tube plug/stop, each

31603–31605

31603 Tracheostomy, emergency procedure; transtracheal
31605 cricothyroid membrane

ICD-9-CM Diagnostic

344.00 Unspecified quadriplegia
344.01 Quadriplegia and quadriparesis, C1-C4, complete
348.1 Anoxic brain damage — (Use additional E code to identify cause)
464.31 Acute epiglottitis with obstruction
478.6 Edema of larynx
478.75 Laryngeal spasm
518.5 Pulmonary insufficiency following trauma and surgery
518.81 Acute respiratory failure
518.82 Other pulmonary insufficiency, not elsewhere classified
519.00 Unspecified tracheostomy complication
519.1 Other diseases of trachea and bronchus, not elsewhere classified
748.3 Other congenital anomaly of larynx, trachea, and bronchus
765.00 Extreme fetal immaturity, unspecified (weight) — (Use additional code for weeks of gestation: 765.20-765.29)
765.01 Extreme fetal immaturity, less than 500 grams — (Use additional code for weeks of gestation: 765.20-765.29)
765.02 Extreme fetal immaturity, 500-749 grams — (Use additional code for weeks of gestation: 765.20-765.29)
765.03 Extreme fetal immaturity, 750-999 grams — (Use additional code for weeks of gestation: 765.20-765.29)
765.04 Extreme fetal immaturity, 1,000-1,249 grams — (Use additional code for weeks of gestation: 765.20-765.29)
765.05 Extreme fetal immaturity, 1,250-1,499 grams — (Use additional code for weeks of gestation: 765.20-765.29)
765.06 Extreme fetal immaturity, 1,500-1,749 grams — (Use additional code for weeks of gestation: 765.20-765.29)
765.10 Other preterm infants, unspecified (weight) — (Use additional code for weeks of gestation: 765.20-765.29)
765.11 Other preterm infants, less than 500 grams — (Use additional code for weeks of gestation: 765.20-765.29)
765.12 Other preterm infants, 500-749 grams — (Use additional code for weeks of gestation: 765.20-765.29)
765.13 Other preterm infants, 750-999 grams — (Use additional code for weeks of gestation: 765.20-765.29)
765.14 Other preterm infants, 1,000-1,249 grams — (Use additional code for weeks of gestation: 765.20-765.29)
765.15 Other preterm infants, 1,250-1,499 grams — (Use additional code for weeks of gestation: 765.20-765.29)
765.16 Other preterm infants, 1,500-1,749 grams — (Use additional code for weeks of gestation: 765.20-765.29)
765.20 Unspecified weeks of gestation
765.21 Less than 24 completed weeks of gestation
765.22 24 completed weeks of gestation
765.23 25-26 completed weeks of gestation
765.24 27-28 completed weeks of gestation
765.25 29-30 completed weeks of gestation
765.26 31-32 completed weeks of gestation
765.27 33-34 completed weeks of gestation
765.28 35-36 completed weeks of gestation
765.29 37 or more completed weeks of gestation
767.0 Subdural and cerebral hemorrhage, birth trauma — (Use additional code to identify cause)
768.5 Severe birth asphyxia — (Use only when associated with newborn morbidity classifiable elsewhere)
769 Respiratory distress syndrome in newborn
770.83 Cyanotic attacks of newborn
770.84 Respiratory failure of newborn
770.89 Other respiratory problems of newborn after birth
772.10 Intraventricular hemorrhage, unspecified grade
772.11 Intraventricular hemorrhage, Grade I
772.12 Intraventricular hemorrhage, Grade II
772.13 Intraventricular hemorrhage, Grade III
772.14 Intraventricular hemorrhage, Grade IV
772.2 Fetal and neonatal subarachnoid hemorrhage of newborn
786.09 Other dyspnea and respiratory abnormalities
799.1 Respiratory arrest
805.00 Closed fracture of cervical vertebra, unspecified level without mention of spinal cord injury
805.01 Closed fracture of first cervical vertebra without mention of spinal cord injury
805.02 Closed fracture of second cervical vertebra without mention of spinal cord injury
805.03 Closed fracture of third cervical vertebra without mention of spinal cord injury
805.04 Closed fracture of fourth cervical vertebra without mention of spinal cord injury
805.10 Open fracture of cervical vertebra, unspecified level without mention of spinal cord injury
805.11 Open fracture of first cervical vertebra without mention of spinal cord injury
805.12 Open fracture of second cervical vertebra without mention of spinal cord injury
805.13 Open fracture of third cervical vertebra without mention of spinal cord injury
805.14 Open fracture of fourth cervical vertebra without mention of spinal cord injury
806.00 Closed fracture of C1-C4 level with unspecified spinal cord injury
806.01 Closed fracture of C1-C4 level with complete lesion of cord
806.02 Closed fracture of C1-C4 level with anterior cord syndrome
806.03 Closed fracture of C1-C4 level with central cord syndrome
806.04 Closed fracture of C1-C4 level with other specified spinal cord injury
806.05 Closed fracture of C5-C7 level with unspecified spinal cord injury
806.06 Closed fracture of C5-C7 level with complete lesion of cord
806.07 Closed fracture of C5-C7 level with anterior cord syndrome
806.08 Closed fracture of C5-C7 level with central cord syndrome
806.09 Closed fracture of C5-C7 level with other specified spinal cord injury
806.10 Open fracture of C1-C4 level with unspecified spinal cord injury
806.11 Open fracture of C1-C4 level with complete lesion of cord
806.12 Open fracture of C1-C4 level with anterior cord syndrome
806.13 Open fracture of C1-C4 level with central cord syndrome
806.14 Open fracture of C1-C4 level with other specified spinal cord injury
806.15 Open fracture of C5-C7 level with unspecified spinal cord injury
806.16 Open fracture of C5-C7 level with complete lesion of cord
806.17 Open fracture of C5-C7 level with anterior cord syndrome
806.18 Open fracture of C5-C7 level with central cord syndrome
806.19 Open fracture of C5-C7 level with other specified spinal cord injury
807.5 Closed fracture of larynx and trachea
807.6 Open fracture of larynx and trachea
873.59 Open wound of face, other and multiple sites, complicated — (Use additional code to identify infection)

873.9 Other and unspecified open wound of head, complicated — (Use additional code to identify infection) ▽
874.10 Open wound of larynx with trachea, complicated — (Use additional code to identify infection)
874.11 Open wound of larynx, complicated — (Use additional code to identify infection)
874.12 Open wound of trachea, complicated — (Use additional code to identify infection)
925.1 Crushing injury of face and scalp — (Use additional code to identify any associated injuries: 800-829, 850.0-854.1, 860.0-869.1)
925.2 Crushing injury of neck — (Use additional code to identify any associated injuries: 800-829, 850.0-854.1, 860.0-869.1)
933.1 Foreign body in larynx
934.0 Foreign body in trachea
934.8 Foreign body in other specified parts of trachea, bronchus, and lung
947.0 Burn of mouth and pharynx
947.1 Burn of larynx, trachea, and lung
995.0 Other anaphylactic shock not else where classifed — (Use additional E code to identify external cause: E930-E949)
995.1 Angioneurotic edema not elsewhere classified
997.3 Respiratory complications — (Use additional code to identify complications)

ICD-9-CM Procedural
31.1 Temporary tracheostomy

HCPCS Level II Supplies & Services
A4624 Tracheal suction catheter, any type other than closed system, each
A7520 Tracheostomy/laryngectomy tube, non-cuffed, polyvinylchloride (PVC), silicone or equal, each
A7521 Tracheostomy/laryngectomy tube, cuffed, polyvinylchloride (PVC), silicone or equal, each
A7522 Tracheostomy/laryngectomy tube, stainless steel or equal (sterilizable and reusable), each
A7523 Tracheostomy shower protector, each
A7524 Tracheostoma stent/stud/button, each
A7525 Tracheostomy mask, each
A7526 Tracheostomy tube collar/holder, each
A7527 Tracheostomy/laryngectomy tube plug/stop, each

31610
31610 Tracheostomy, fenestration procedure with skin flaps

ICD-9-CM Diagnostic
141.0 Malignant neoplasm of base of tongue
141.5 Malignant neoplasm of junctional zone of tongue
141.6 Malignant neoplasm of lingual tonsil
141.8 Malignant neoplasm of other sites of tongue
146.0 Malignant neoplasm of tonsil
146.1 Malignant neoplasm of tonsillar fossa
146.2 Malignant neoplasm of tonsillar pillars (anterior) (posterior)
146.3 Malignant neoplasm of vallecula
146.4 Malignant neoplasm of anterior aspect of epiglottis
146.5 Malignant neoplasm of junctional region of oropharynx
146.6 Malignant neoplasm of lateral wall of oropharynx
146.7 Malignant neoplasm of posterior wall of oropharynx
146.8 Malignant neoplasm of other specified sites of oropharynx
148.0 Malignant neoplasm of postcricoid region of hypopharynx
148.1 Malignant neoplasm of pyriform sinus
148.2 Malignant neoplasm of aryepiglottic fold, hypopharyngeal aspect
148.3 Malignant neoplasm of posterior hypopharyngeal wall
148.8 Malignant neoplasm of other specified sites of hypopharynx
148.9 Malignant neoplasm of hypopharynx, unspecified site ▽
161.0 Malignant neoplasm of glottis
161.1 Malignant neoplasm of supraglottis
161.2 Malignant neoplasm of subglottis
161.3 Malignant neoplasm of laryngeal cartilages
161.8 Malignant neoplasm of other specified sites of larynx
197.3 Secondary malignant neoplasm of other respiratory organs
197.8 Secondary malignant neoplasm of other digestive organs and spleen
231.0 Carcinoma in situ of larynx
231.1 Carcinoma in situ of trachea
235.6 Neoplasm of uncertain behavior of larynx
344.00 Unspecified quadriplegia ▽
344.01 Quadriplegia and quadriparesis, C1-C4, complete
348.1 Anoxic brain damage — (Use additional E code to identify cause)
478.74 Stenosis of larynx
518.5 Pulmonary insufficiency following trauma and surgery
518.81 Acute respiratory failure
518.82 Other pulmonary insufficiency, not elsewhere classified
519.00 Unspecified tracheostomy complication ▽
519.1 Other diseases of trachea and bronchus, not elsewhere classified
748.3 Other congenital anomaly of larynx, trachea, and bronchus
786.09 Other dyspnea and respiratory abnormalities
806.00 Closed fracture of C1-C4 level with unspecified spinal cord injury ▽
806.05 Closed fracture of C5-C7 level with unspecified spinal cord injury ▽
806.10 Open fracture of C1-C4 level with unspecified spinal cord injury ▽
806.15 Open fracture of C5-C7 level with unspecified spinal cord injury ▽
V10.02 Personal history of malignant neoplasm of other and unspecified parts of oral cavity and pharynx ▽
V10.21 Personal history of malignant neoplasm of larynx

ICD-9-CM Procedural
31.29 Other permanent tracheostomy

HCPCS Level II Supplies & Services
A7527 Tracheostomy/laryngectomy tube plug/stop, each

31611
31611 Construction of tracheoesophageal fistula and subsequent insertion of an alaryngeal speech prosthesis (eg, voice button, Blom-Singer prosthesis)

ICD-9-CM Diagnostic
748.3 Other congenital anomaly of larynx, trachea, and bronchus
V10.21 Personal history of malignant neoplasm of larynx

ICD-9-CM Procedural
31.75 Reconstruction of trachea and construction of artificial larynx
31.95 Tracheoesophageal fistulization

31612
31612 Tracheal puncture, percutaneous with transtracheal aspiration and/or injection

ICD-9-CM Diagnostic
162.0 Malignant neoplasm of trachea
197.3 Secondary malignant neoplasm of other respiratory organs
478.32 Unilateral complete paralysis of vocal cords or larynx
478.9 Other and unspecified diseases of upper respiratory tract
482.84 Legionnaires' disease
506.0 Bronchitis and pneumonitis due to fumes and vapors — (Use additional E code to identify cause)
507.0 Pneumonitis due to inhalation of food or vomitus
507.8 Pneumonitis due to other solids and liquids
668.01 Pulmonary complications of the administration of anesthesia or other sedation in labor and delivery, delivered — (Use additional code(s) to further specify complication) ♀
668.02 Pulmonary complications of the administration of anesthesia or other sedation in labor and delivery, delivered, with mention of postpartum complication — (Use additional code(s) to further specify complication) ♀
668.03 Pulmonary complications of the administration of anesthesia or other sedation in labor and delivery, antepartum — (Use additional code(s) to further specify complication) ♀
668.04 Pulmonary complications of the administration of anesthesia or other sedation in labor and delivery, postpartum — (Use additional code(s) to further specify complication) ♀
748.3 Other congenital anomaly of larynx, trachea, and bronchus
770.1 Meconium aspiration syndrome
784.49 Other voice disturbance
958.3 Posttraumatic wound infection not elsewhere classified

ICD-9-CM Procedural
31.94 Injection of locally-acting therapeutic substance into trachea
31.99 Other operations on trachea

HCPCS Level II Supplies & Services
A4305 Disposable drug delivery system, flow rate of 50 ml or greater per hour
A4306 Disposable drug delivery system, flow rate of 5 ml or less per hour
A4550 Surgical trays

31613–31614

31613 Tracheostoma revision; simple, without flap rotation
31614 complex, with flap rotation

ICD-9-CM Diagnostic

348.1 Anoxic brain damage — (Use additional E code to identify cause)
478.74 Stenosis of larynx
478.79 Other diseases of larynx
478.9 Other and unspecified diseases of upper respiratory tract
519.00 Unspecified tracheostomy complication ▽
519.01 Infection of tracheostomy — (Use additional code to identify type of infection: 038.0-038.9, 682.1. Use additional code to identify organism: 041.00-041.9)
519.02 Mechanical complication of tracheostomy
519.09 Other tracheostomy complications
519.1 Other diseases of trachea and bronchus, not elsewhere classified
750.3 Congenital tracheoesophageal fistula, esophageal atresia and stenosis
806.00 Closed fracture of C1-C4 level with unspecified spinal cord injury ▽
806.05 Closed fracture of C5-C7 level with unspecified spinal cord injury ▽
806.10 Open fracture of C1-C4 level with unspecified spinal cord injury ▽
806.15 Open fracture of C5-C7 level with unspecified spinal cord injury ▽
V10.02 Personal history of malignant neoplasm of other and unspecified parts of oral cavity and pharynx ▽
V10.21 Personal history of malignant neoplasm of larynx

ICD-9-CM Procedural

31.74 Revision of tracheostomy

31615

31615 Tracheobronchoscopy through established tracheostomy incision

ICD-9-CM Diagnostic

162.0 Malignant neoplasm of trachea
162.2 Malignant neoplasm of main bronchus
162.3 Malignant neoplasm of upper lobe, bronchus, or lung
162.4 Malignant neoplasm of middle lobe, bronchus, or lung
162.8 Malignant neoplasm of other parts of bronchus or lung
197.0 Secondary malignant neoplasm of lung
197.3 Secondary malignant neoplasm of other respiratory organs
212.2 Benign neoplasm of trachea
212.3 Benign neoplasm of bronchus and lung
231.1 Carcinoma in situ of trachea
231.2 Carcinoma in situ of bronchus and lung
231.9 Carcinoma in situ of respiratory system, part unspecified ▽
235.7 Neoplasm of uncertain behavior of trachea, bronchus, and lung
239.1 Neoplasm of unspecified nature of respiratory system
486 Pneumonia, organism unspecified ▽
510.0 Empyema with fistula — (Use additional code to identify infectious organism: 041.00-041.9)
518.89 Other diseases of lung, not elsewhere classified
519.00 Unspecified tracheostomy complication ▽
519.01 Infection of tracheostomy — (Use additional code to identify type of infection: 038.0-038.9, 682.1. Use additional code to identify organism: 041.00-041.9)
519.02 Mechanical complication of tracheostomy
519.09 Other tracheostomy complications
519.1 Other diseases of trachea and bronchus, not elsewhere classified
519.8 Other diseases of respiratory system, not elsewhere classified
V10.02 Personal history of malignant neoplasm of other and unspecified parts of oral cavity and pharynx ▽
V10.21 Personal history of malignant neoplasm of larynx

ICD-9-CM Procedural

31.41 Tracheoscopy through artificial stoma
33.21 Bronchoscopy through artificial stoma

HCPCS Level II Supplies & Services

A4550 Surgical trays
A4624 Tracheal suction catheter, any type other than closed system, each
A4625 Tracheostomy care kit for new tracheostomy
A7520 Tracheostomy/laryngectomy tube, non-cuffed, polyvinylchloride (PVC), silicone or equal, each
A7521 Tracheostomy/laryngectomy tube, cuffed, polyvinylchloride (PVC), silicone or equal, each
A7522 Tracheostomy/laryngectomy tube, stainless steel or equal (sterilizable and reusable), each
A7523 Tracheostomy shower protector, each
A7524 Tracheostoma stent/stud/button, each
A7525 Tracheostomy mask, each
A7526 Tracheostomy tube collar/holder, each

31620

31620 Endobronchial ultrasound (EBUS) during bronchoscopic diagnostic or therapeutic intervention(s) (List separately in addition to code for primary procedure(s))

ICD-9-CM Diagnostic

This is an add-on code. Refer to the corresponding primary procedure code for ICD-9 diagnosis code links.

ICD-9-CM Procedural

88.73 Diagnostic ultrasound of other sites of thorax

31622–31624

31622 Bronchoscopy, rigid or flexible, with or without fluoroscopic guidance; diagnostic, with or without cell washing (separate procedure)
31623 with brushing or protected brushings
31624 with bronchial alveolar lavage

ICD-9-CM Diagnostic

135 Sarcoidosis
162.2 Malignant neoplasm of main bronchus
162.3 Malignant neoplasm of upper lobe, bronchus, or lung
162.4 Malignant neoplasm of middle lobe, bronchus, or lung
162.5 Malignant neoplasm of lower lobe, bronchus, or lung
162.8 Malignant neoplasm of other parts of bronchus or lung
162.9 Malignant neoplasm of bronchus and lung, unspecified site ▽
197.0 Secondary malignant neoplasm of lung
197.2 Secondary malignant neoplasm of pleura
198.89 Secondary malignant neoplasm of other specified sites
199.1 Other malignant neoplasm of unspecified site
212.2 Benign neoplasm of trachea
212.3 Benign neoplasm of bronchus and lung
212.4 Benign neoplasm of pleura
231.1 Carcinoma in situ of trachea
231.2 Carcinoma in situ of bronchus and lung
235.7 Neoplasm of uncertain behavior of trachea, bronchus, and lung
239.1 Neoplasm of unspecified nature of respiratory system
478.9 Other and unspecified diseases of upper respiratory tract
485 Bronchopneumonia, organism unspecified ▽
486 Pneumonia, organism unspecified ▽
500 Coal workers' pneumoconiosis
501 Asbestosis
502 Pneumoconiosis due to other silica or silicates
503 Pneumoconiosis due to other inorganic dust
504 Pneumonopathy due to inhalation of other dust
505 Unspecified pneumoconiosis ▽
506.4 Chronic respiratory conditions due to fumes and vapors — (Use additional E code to identify cause)
507.0 Pneumonitis due to inhalation of food or vomitus
508.1 Chronic and other pulmonary manifestations due to radiation — (Use additional E code to identify cause)
510.0 Empyema with fistula — (Use additional code to identify infectious organism: 041.00-041.9)
510.9 Empyema without mention of fistula — (Use additional code to identify infectious organism: 041.00-041.9)
512.0 Spontaneous tension pneumothorax
512.1 Iatrogenic pneumothroax
512.8 Other spontaneous pneumothorax
513.0 Abscess of lung
514 Pulmonary congestion and hypostasis
515 Postinflammatory pulmonary fibrosis
516.0 Pulmonary alveolar proteinosis
516.1 Idiopathic pulmonary hemosiderosis — (Code first underlying disease, 275.0) ☒
516.2 Pulmonary alveolar microlithiasis
516.3 Idiopathic fibrosing alveolitis
516.8 Other specified alveolar and parietoalveolar pneumonopathies
517.3 Acute chest syndrome — (Code first sickle-cell disease in crisis: 282.42, 282.62, 282.64, 282.69)
517.8 Lung involvement in other diseases classified elsewhere — (Code first underlying disease: 135, 277.3, 710.0, 710.2, 710.4) ☒
518.0 Pulmonary collapse
518.3 Pulmonary eosinophilia

518.5 Pulmonary insufficiency following trauma and surgery
518.83 Chronic respiratory failure
518.84 Acute and chronic respiratory failure
518.89 Other diseases of lung, not elsewhere classified
770.7 Chronic respiratory disease arising in the perinatal period
786.05 Shortness of breath
786.06 Tachypnea
786.07 Wheezing
786.2 Cough
786.3 Hemoptysis
V10.11 Personal history of malignant neoplasm of bronchus and lung
V10.12 Personal history of malignant neoplasm of trachea
V15.82 Personal history of tobacco use, presenting hazards to health
V15.84 Personal history of exposure to asbestos, presenting hazards to health
V16.2 Family history of malignant neoplasm of other respiratory and intrathoracic organs
V43.89 Other organ or tissue replaced by other means — (This code is intended for use when these conditions are recorded as diagnoses or problems)

ICD-9-CM Procedural

33.24 Closed (endoscopic) biopsy of bronchus
96.56 Other lavage of bronchus and trachea

31625–31629

31625 Bronchoscopy, rigid or flexible, with or without fluoroscopic guidance; with bronchial or endobronchial biopsy(s), single or multiple sites
31628 with transbronchial lung biopsy(s), single lobe
31629 with transbronchial needle aspiration biopsy(s), trachea, main stem and/or lobar bronchus(i)

ICD-9-CM Diagnostic

135 Sarcoidosis
162.0 Malignant neoplasm of trachea
162.2 Malignant neoplasm of main bronchus
162.3 Malignant neoplasm of upper lobe, bronchus, or lung
162.4 Malignant neoplasm of middle lobe, bronchus, or lung
162.5 Malignant neoplasm of lower lobe, bronchus, or lung
162.8 Malignant neoplasm of other parts of bronchus or lung
162.9 Malignant neoplasm of bronchus and lung, unspecified site ▽
197.0 Secondary malignant neoplasm of lung
197.2 Secondary malignant neoplasm of pleura
197.3 Secondary malignant neoplasm of other respiratory organs
198.89 Secondary malignant neoplasm of other specified sites
199.1 Other malignant neoplasm of unspecified site
212.2 Benign neoplasm of trachea
212.3 Benign neoplasm of bronchus and lung
212.4 Benign neoplasm of pleura
231.1 Carcinoma in situ of trachea
231.2 Carcinoma in situ of bronchus and lung
235.7 Neoplasm of uncertain behavior of trachea, bronchus, and lung
239.1 Neoplasm of unspecified nature of respiratory system
478.9 Other and unspecified diseases of upper respiratory tract
485 Bronchopneumonia, organism unspecified ▽
486 Pneumonia, organism unspecified ▽
500 Coal workers' pneumoconiosis
501 Asbestosis
502 Pneumoconiosis due to other silica or silicates
503 Pneumoconiosis due to other inorganic dust
504 Pneumonopathy due to inhalation of other dust
505 Unspecified pneumoconiosis ▽
506.4 Chronic respiratory conditions due to fumes and vapors — (Use additional E code to identify cause)
507.0 Pneumonitis due to inhalation of food or vomitus
508.1 Chronic and other pulmonary manifestations due to radiation — (Use additional E code to identify cause)
510.0 Empyema with fistula — (Use additional code to identify infectious organism: 041.00-041.9)
510.9 Empyema without mention of fistula — (Use additional code to identify infectious organism: 041.00-041.9)
512.0 Spontaneous tension pneumothorax
512.1 Iatrogenic pneumothroax
512.8 Other spontaneous pneumothorax
513.0 Abscess of lung
514 Pulmonary congestion and hypostasis
515 Postinflammatory pulmonary fibrosis
516.0 Pulmonary alveolar proteinosis
516.1 Idiopathic pulmonary hemosiderosis — (Code first underlying disease, 275.0) ☒
516.2 Pulmonary alveolar microlithiasis
516.3 Idiopathic fibrosing alveolitis
516.8 Other specified alveolar and parietoalveolar pneumonopathies
517.8 Lung involvement in other diseases classified elsewhere — (Code first underlying disease: 135, 277.3, 710.0, 710.2, 710.4) ☒
518.0 Pulmonary collapse
518.3 Pulmonary eosinophilia
518.5 Pulmonary insufficiency following trauma and surgery
518.83 Chronic respiratory failure
518.84 Acute and chronic respiratory failure
518.89 Other diseases of lung, not elsewhere classified
519.1 Other diseases of trachea and bronchus, not elsewhere classified
770.7 Chronic respiratory disease arising in the perinatal period
786.05 Shortness of breath
786.06 Tachypnea
786.07 Wheezing
786.2 Cough
786.3 Hemoptysis
V10.11 Personal history of malignant neoplasm of bronchus and lung
V10.12 Personal history of malignant neoplasm of trachea
V15.82 Personal history of tobacco use, presenting hazards to health
V15.84 Personal history of exposure to asbestos, presenting hazards to health
V16.2 Family history of malignant neoplasm of other respiratory and intrathoracic organs
V43.89 Other organ or tissue replaced by other means — (This code is intended for use when these conditions are recorded as diagnoses or problems)

ICD-9-CM Procedural

33.24 Closed (endoscopic) biopsy of bronchus
33.27 Closed endoscopic biopsy of lung

31630–31631

31630 Bronchoscopy, rigid or flexible, with or without fluoroscopic guidance; with tracheal/bronchial dilation or closed reduction of fracture
31631 with placement of tracheal stent(s) (includes tracheal/bronchial dilation as required)

ICD-9-CM Diagnostic

162.0 Malignant neoplasm of trachea
162.2 Malignant neoplasm of main bronchus
162.3 Malignant neoplasm of upper lobe, bronchus, or lung
162.4 Malignant neoplasm of middle lobe, bronchus, or lung
162.5 Malignant neoplasm of lower lobe, bronchus, or lung
162.8 Malignant neoplasm of other parts of bronchus or lung
162.9 Malignant neoplasm of bronchus and lung, unspecified site ▽
197.0 Secondary malignant neoplasm of lung
197.3 Secondary malignant neoplasm of other respiratory organs
212.2 Benign neoplasm of trachea
212.3 Benign neoplasm of bronchus and lung
231.1 Carcinoma in situ of trachea
231.2 Carcinoma in situ of bronchus and lung
235.7 Neoplasm of uncertain behavior of trachea, bronchus, and lung
239.1 Neoplasm of unspecified nature of respiratory system
476.1 Chronic laryngotracheitis
478.74 Stenosis of larynx
515 Postinflammatory pulmonary fibrosis
519.1 Other diseases of trachea and bronchus, not elsewhere classified
519.3 Other diseases of mediastinum, not elsewhere classified
748.3 Other congenital anomaly of larynx, trachea, and bronchus
807.5 Closed fracture of larynx and trachea
V10.11 Personal history of malignant neoplasm of bronchus and lung
V10.12 Personal history of malignant neoplasm of trachea

ICD-9-CM Procedural

31.64 Repair of laryngeal fracture
31.93 Replacement of laryngeal or tracheal stent
31.99 Other operations on trachea
33.91 Bronchial dilation

▽ Unspecified code
♀ Female diagnosis
☒ Manifestation code
♂ Male diagnosis

31632

31632 Bronchoscopy, rigid or flexible, with or without fluoroscopic guidance; with transbronchial lung biopsy(s), each additional lobe (List separately in addition to code for primary procedure)

ICD-9-CM Diagnostic

This is an add-on code. Refer to the corresponding primary procedure code for ICD-9 diagnosis code links.

ICD-9-CM Procedural

33.24 Closed (endoscopic) biopsy of bronchus
33.27 Closed endoscopic biopsy of lung

31633

31633 Bronchoscopy, rigid or flexible, with or without fluoroscopic guidance; with transbronchial needle aspiration biopsy(s), each additional lobe (List separately in addition to code for primary procedure)

ICD-9-CM Diagnostic

This is an add-on code. Refer to the corresponding primary procedure code for ICD-9 diagnosis code links.

ICD-9-CM Procedural

33.24 Closed (endoscopic) biopsy of bronchus
33.27 Closed endoscopic biopsy of lung

31635

31635 Bronchoscopy, rigid or flexible, with or without fluoroscopic guidance; with removal of foreign body

ICD-9-CM Diagnostic

934.1 Foreign body in main bronchus
934.8 Foreign body in other specified parts of trachea, bronchus, and lung
934.9 Foreign body in respiratory tree, unspecified ♥

ICD-9-CM Procedural

98.15 Removal of intraluminal foreign body from trachea and bronchus without incision

31636–31638

31636 Bronchoscopy, rigid or flexible, with or without fluoroscopic guidance; with placement of bronchial stent(s) (includes tracheal/bronchial dilation as required), initial bronchus
31637 each additional major bronchus stented (List separately in addition to code for primary procedure)
31638 with revision of tracheal or bronchial stent inserted at previous session (includes tracheal/bronchial dilation as required)

ICD-9-CM Diagnostic

162.0 Malignant neoplasm of trachea
162.2 Malignant neoplasm of main bronchus
162.3 Malignant neoplasm of upper lobe, bronchus, or lung
162.4 Malignant neoplasm of middle lobe, bronchus, or lung
162.5 Malignant neoplasm of lower lobe, bronchus, or lung
162.8 Malignant neoplasm of other parts of bronchus or lung
162.9 Malignant neoplasm of bronchus and lung, unspecified site ♥
197.0 Secondary malignant neoplasm of lung
197.3 Secondary malignant neoplasm of other respiratory organs
212.2 Benign neoplasm of trachea
212.3 Benign neoplasm of bronchus and lung
231.1 Carcinoma in situ of trachea
231.2 Carcinoma in situ of bronchus and lung
235.7 Neoplasm of uncertain behavior of trachea, bronchus, and lung
239.1 Neoplasm of unspecified nature of respiratory system
476.1 Chronic laryngotracheitis
478.74 Stenosis of larynx
515 Postinflammatory pulmonary fibrosis
519.1 Other diseases of trachea and bronchus, not elsewhere classified
519.3 Other diseases of mediastinum, not elsewhere classified
748.3 Other congenital anomaly of larynx, trachea, and bronchus
807.5 Closed fracture of larynx and trachea
996.59 Mechanical complication due to other implant and internal device, not elsewhere classified
996.69 Infection and inflammatory reaction due to other internal prosthetic device, implant, and graft — (Use additional code to identify specified infections)
996.79 Other complications due to other internal prosthetic device, implant, and graft
V10.11 Personal history of malignant neoplasm of bronchus and lung
V10.12 Personal history of malignant neoplasm of trachea

ICD-9-CM Procedural

31.93 Replacement of laryngeal or tracheal stent
31.99 Other operations on trachea
33.91 Bronchial dilation
96.05 Other intubation of respiratory tract

31640–31641

31640 Bronchoscopy, rigid or flexible, with or without fluoroscopic guidance; with excision of tumor
31641 Bronchoscopy, (rigid or flexible); with destruction of tumor or relief of stenosis by any method other than excision (eg, laser therapy, cryotherapy)

ICD-9-CM Diagnostic

162.2 Malignant neoplasm of main bronchus
162.3 Malignant neoplasm of upper lobe, bronchus, or lung
162.4 Malignant neoplasm of middle lobe, bronchus, or lung
162.5 Malignant neoplasm of lower lobe, bronchus, or lung
162.8 Malignant neoplasm of other parts of bronchus or lung
162.9 Malignant neoplasm of bronchus and lung, unspecified site ♥
197.0 Secondary malignant neoplasm of lung
197.3 Secondary malignant neoplasm of other respiratory organs
212.3 Benign neoplasm of bronchus and lung
212.9 Benign neoplasm of respiratory and intrathoracic organs, site unspecified ♥
231.2 Carcinoma in situ of bronchus and lung
235.7 Neoplasm of uncertain behavior of trachea, bronchus, and lung
239.1 Neoplasm of unspecified nature of respiratory system
519.1 Other diseases of trachea and bronchus, not elsewhere classified
519.8 Other diseases of respiratory system, not elsewhere classified
748.3 Other congenital anomaly of larynx, trachea, and bronchus
786.05 Shortness of breath
786.06 Tachypnea
786.07 Wheezing
786.09 Other dyspnea and respiratory abnormalities
786.6 Swelling, mass, or lump in chest
793.1 Nonspecific abnormal findings on radiological and other examination of lung field
V10.11 Personal history of malignant neoplasm of bronchus and lung
V10.12 Personal history of malignant neoplasm of trachea
V15.82 Personal history of tobacco use, presenting hazards to health
V15.84 Personal history of exposure to asbestos, presenting hazards to health
V16.2 Family history of malignant neoplasm of other respiratory and intrathoracic organs

ICD-9-CM Procedural

32.01 Endoscopic excision or destruction of lesion or tissue of bronchus

31643

31643 Bronchoscopy, (rigid or flexible); with placement of catheter(s) for intracavitary radioelement application

ICD-9-CM Diagnostic

162.2 Malignant neoplasm of main bronchus
162.3 Malignant neoplasm of upper lobe, bronchus, or lung
162.4 Malignant neoplasm of middle lobe, bronchus, or lung
162.5 Malignant neoplasm of lower lobe, bronchus, or lung
162.8 Malignant neoplasm of other parts of bronchus or lung
162.9 Malignant neoplasm of bronchus and lung, unspecified site ♥
197.0 Secondary malignant neoplasm of lung
197.3 Secondary malignant neoplasm of other respiratory organs
231.2 Carcinoma in situ of bronchus and lung
235.7 Neoplasm of uncertain behavior of trachea, bronchus, and lung
239.1 Neoplasm of unspecified nature of respiratory system

ICD-9-CM Procedural

96.05 Other intubation of respiratory tract

31645–31646

31645 Bronchoscopy, (rigid or flexible); with therapeutic aspiration of tracheobronchial tree, initial (eg, drainage of lung abscess)
31646 with therapeutic aspiration of tracheobronchial tree, subsequent

ICD-9-CM Diagnostic

006.4 Amebic lung abscess
480.0 Pneumonia due to adenovirus
480.1 Pneumonia due to respiratory syncytial virus
480.2 Pneumonia due to parainfluenza virus
480.3 Pneumonia due to SARS-associated coronavirus
480.8 Pneumonia due to other virus not elsewhere classified
482.0 Pneumonia due to Klebsiella pneumoniae
482.1 Pneumonia due to Pseudomonas
482.2 Pneumonia due to Hemophilus influenzae (H. influenzae)
482.30 Pneumonia due to unspecified Streptococcus ▽
482.31 Pneumonia due to Streptococcus, group A
482.32 Pneumonia due to Streptococcus, group B
482.39 Pneumonia due to other Streptococcus
482.40 Pneumonia due to Staphylococcus, unspecified ▽
482.49 Other Staphylococcus pneumonia
482.81 Pneumonia due to anaerobes
482.82 Pneumonia due to escherichia coli (E. coli)
482.83 Pneumonia due to other gram-negative bacteria
482.89 Pneumonia due to other specified bacteria
483.0 Pneumonia due to Mycoplasma pneumoniae
483.1 Pneumonia due to Chlamydia
483.8 Pneumonia due to other specified organism
484.1 Pneumonia in cytomegalic inclusion disease — (Code first underlying disease, 078.5) ☒
484.3 Pneumonia in whooping cough — (Code first underlying disease: 033.0-033.9) ☒
484.5 Pneumonia in anthrax — (Code first underlying disease, 022.1) ☒
484.6 Pneumonia in aspergillosis — (Code first underlying disease, 117.3) ☒
484.7 Pneumonia in other systemic mycoses — (Code first underlying disease) ☒
484.8 Pneumonia in other infectious diseases classified elsewhere — (Code first underlying disease: 002.0, 083.0) ☒
485 Bronchopneumonia, organism unspecified ▽
486 Pneumonia, organism unspecified ▽
487.0 Influenza with pneumonia
490 Bronchitis, not specified as acute or chronic ▽
491.0 Simple chronic bronchitis
491.1 Mucopurulent chronic bronchitis
491.20 Obstructive chronic bronchitis, without exacerbation
491.21 Obstructive chronic bronchitis, with (acute) exacerbation
491.8 Other chronic bronchitis
492.0 Emphysematous bleb
492.8 Other emphysema
494.0 Bronchiectasis without acute exacerbation
494.1 Bronchiectasis with acute exacerbation
495.0 Farmers' lung
495.1 Bagassosis
495.2 Bird-fanciers' lung
495.3 Suberosis
495.4 Malt workers' lung
495.5 Mushroom workers' lung
495.6 Maple bark-strippers' lung
495.7 "Ventilation" pneumonitis
495.8 Other specified allergic alveolitis and pneumonitis
495.9 Unspecified allergic alveolitis and pneumonitis ▽
496 Chronic airway obstruction, not elsewhere classified — (Note: This code is not to be used with any code from 491-493) ▽
506.1 Acute pulmonary edema due to fumes and vapors — (Use additional E code to identify cause)
507.0 Pneumonitis due to inhalation of food or vomitus
507.1 Pneumonitis due to inhalation of oils and essences
507.8 Pneumonitis due to other solids and liquids
510.0 Empyema with fistula — (Use additional code to identify infectious organism: 041.00-041.9)
510.9 Empyema without mention of fistula — (Use additional code to identify infectious organism: 041.00-041.9)
513.0 Abscess of lung
513.1 Abscess of mediastinum
514 Pulmonary congestion and hypostasis
515 Postinflammatory pulmonary fibrosis
516.0 Pulmonary alveolar proteinosis
516.1 Idiopathic pulmonary hemosiderosis — (Code first underlying disease, 275.0) ☒
516.2 Pulmonary alveolar microlithiasis
516.3 Idiopathic fibrosing alveolitis
516.8 Other specified alveolar and parietoalveolar pneumonopathies
517.1 Rheumatic pneumonia — (Code first underlying disease, 390) ☒
517.2 Lung involvement in systemic sclerosis — (Code first underlying disease, 710.1) ☒
517.8 Lung involvement in other diseases classified elsewhere — (Code first underlying disease: 135, 277.3, 710.0, 710.2, 710.4) ☒
518.0 Pulmonary collapse
518.3 Pulmonary eosinophilia
518.4 Unspecified acute edema of lung ▽
518.5 Pulmonary insufficiency following trauma and surgery
518.81 Acute respiratory failure
518.82 Other pulmonary insufficiency, not elsewhere classified
518.89 Other diseases of lung, not elsewhere classified
519.1 Other diseases of trachea and bronchus, not elsewhere classified
958.3 Posttraumatic wound infection not elsewhere classified
V15.82 Personal history of tobacco use, presenting hazards to health

ICD-9-CM Procedural

33.93 Puncture of lung
96.05 Other intubation of respiratory tract

31656

31656 Bronchoscopy, (rigid or flexible); with injection of contrast material for segmental bronchography (fiberscope only)

ICD-9-CM Diagnostic

162.2 Malignant neoplasm of main bronchus
162.3 Malignant neoplasm of upper lobe, bronchus, or lung
162.4 Malignant neoplasm of middle lobe, bronchus, or lung
162.5 Malignant neoplasm of lower lobe, bronchus, or lung
162.8 Malignant neoplasm of other parts of bronchus or lung
162.9 Malignant neoplasm of bronchus and lung, unspecified site ▽
197.0 Secondary malignant neoplasm of lung
212.2 Benign neoplasm of trachea
212.3 Benign neoplasm of bronchus and lung
231.2 Carcinoma in situ of bronchus and lung
239.1 Neoplasm of unspecified nature of respiratory system
510.0 Empyema with fistula — (Use additional code to identify infectious organism: 041.00-041.9)
519.1 Other diseases of trachea and bronchus, not elsewhere classified
V10.11 Personal history of malignant neoplasm of bronchus and lung
V10.12 Personal history of malignant neoplasm of trachea
V15.82 Personal history of tobacco use, presenting hazards to health
V16.2 Family history of malignant neoplasm of other respiratory and intrathoracic organs
V43.89 Other organ or tissue replaced by other means — (This code is intended for use when these conditions are recorded as diagnoses or problems)

ICD-9-CM Procedural

87.31 Endotracheal bronchogram

31700

31700 Catheterization, transglottic (separate procedure)

ICD-9-CM Diagnostic

162.2 Malignant neoplasm of main bronchus
162.3 Malignant neoplasm of upper lobe, bronchus, or lung
162.4 Malignant neoplasm of middle lobe, bronchus, or lung
162.5 Malignant neoplasm of lower lobe, bronchus, or lung
212.3 Benign neoplasm of bronchus and lung
231.0 Carcinoma in situ of larynx
231.2 Carcinoma in situ of bronchus and lung
235.7 Neoplasm of uncertain behavior of trachea, bronchus, and lung
478.4 Polyp of vocal cord or larynx
V10.12 Personal history of malignant neoplasm of trachea
V15.82 Personal history of tobacco use, presenting hazards to health
V15.84 Personal history of exposure to asbestos, presenting hazards to health
V16.2 Family history of malignant neoplasm of other respiratory and intrathoracic organs

ICD-9-CM Procedural

96.05 Other intubation of respiratory tract

▽ Unspecified code ☒ Manifestation code
♀ Female diagnosis ♂ Male diagnosis

HCPCS Level II Supplies & Services

A4305 Disposable drug delivery system, flow rate of 50 ml or greater per hour

A4306 Disposable drug delivery system, flow rate of 5 ml or less per hour

A4550 Surgical trays

31708

31708 Instillation of contrast material for laryngography or bronchography, without catheterization

ICD-9-CM Diagnostic

161.0 Malignant neoplasm of glottis

161.1 Malignant neoplasm of supraglottis

161.3 Malignant neoplasm of laryngeal cartilages

161.8 Malignant neoplasm of other specified sites of larynx

161.9 Malignant neoplasm of larynx, unspecified site ▽

162.2 Malignant neoplasm of main bronchus

162.3 Malignant neoplasm of upper lobe, bronchus, or lung

162.4 Malignant neoplasm of middle lobe, bronchus, or lung

162.5 Malignant neoplasm of lower lobe, bronchus, or lung

162.8 Malignant neoplasm of other parts of bronchus or lung

162.9 Malignant neoplasm of bronchus and lung, unspecified site ▽

197.0 Secondary malignant neoplasm of lung

197.3 Secondary malignant neoplasm of other respiratory organs

212.1 Benign neoplasm of larynx

212.3 Benign neoplasm of bronchus and lung

231.0 Carcinoma in situ of larynx

231.2 Carcinoma in situ of bronchus and lung

235.6 Neoplasm of uncertain behavior of larynx

235.7 Neoplasm of uncertain behavior of trachea, bronchus, and lung

239.1 Neoplasm of unspecified nature of respiratory system

510.0 Empyema with fistula — (Use additional code to identify infectious organism: 041.00-041.9)

518.0 Pulmonary collapse

933.1 Foreign body in larynx

V10.11 Personal history of malignant neoplasm of bronchus and lung

V10.12 Personal history of malignant neoplasm of trachea

V15.84 Personal history of exposure to asbestos, presenting hazards to health

V16.2 Family history of malignant neoplasm of other respiratory and intrathoracic organs

V43.89 Other organ or tissue replaced by other means — (This code is intended for use when these conditions are recorded as diagnoses or problems)

ICD-9-CM Procedural

31.48 Other diagnostic procedures on larynx

33.29 Other diagnostic procedures on lung or bronchus

87.07 Contrast laryngogram

87.31 Endotracheal bronchogram

87.32 Other contrast bronchogram

31710–31715

31710 Catheterization for bronchography, with or without instillation of contrast material

31715 Transtracheal injection for bronchography

ICD-9-CM Diagnostic

161.0 Malignant neoplasm of glottis

161.1 Malignant neoplasm of supraglottis

161.3 Malignant neoplasm of laryngeal cartilages

161.8 Malignant neoplasm of other specified sites of larynx

161.9 Malignant neoplasm of larynx, unspecified site ▽

162.2 Malignant neoplasm of main bronchus

162.3 Malignant neoplasm of upper lobe, bronchus, or lung

162.4 Malignant neoplasm of middle lobe, bronchus, or lung

162.5 Malignant neoplasm of lower lobe, bronchus, or lung

162.8 Malignant neoplasm of other parts of bronchus or lung

162.9 Malignant neoplasm of bronchus and lung, unspecified site ▽

197.0 Secondary malignant neoplasm of lung

197.3 Secondary malignant neoplasm of other respiratory organs

212.1 Benign neoplasm of larynx

212.3 Benign neoplasm of bronchus and lung

231.0 Carcinoma in situ of larynx

231.2 Carcinoma in situ of bronchus and lung

235.6 Neoplasm of uncertain behavior of larynx

235.7 Neoplasm of uncertain behavior of trachea, bronchus, and lung

239.1 Neoplasm of unspecified nature of respiratory system

510.0 Empyema with fistula — (Use additional code to identify infectious organism: 041.00-041.9)

518.0 Pulmonary collapse

933.1 Foreign body in larynx

V10.11 Personal history of malignant neoplasm of bronchus and lung

V10.12 Personal history of malignant neoplasm of trachea

V15.84 Personal history of exposure to asbestos, presenting hazards to health

V16.2 Family history of malignant neoplasm of other respiratory and intrathoracic organs

V43.89 Other organ or tissue replaced by other means — (This code is intended for use when these conditions are recorded as diagnoses or problems)

ICD-9-CM Procedural

33.29 Other diagnostic procedures on lung or bronchus

87.31 Endotracheal bronchogram

31717

31717 Catheterization with bronchial brush biopsy

ICD-9-CM Diagnostic

135 Sarcoidosis

162.2 Malignant neoplasm of main bronchus

162.3 Malignant neoplasm of upper lobe, bronchus, or lung

162.4 Malignant neoplasm of middle lobe, bronchus, or lung

162.5 Malignant neoplasm of lower lobe, bronchus, or lung

162.8 Malignant neoplasm of other parts of bronchus or lung

162.9 Malignant neoplasm of bronchus and lung, unspecified site ▽

197.0 Secondary malignant neoplasm of lung

197.2 Secondary malignant neoplasm of pleura

198.89 Secondary malignant neoplasm of other specified sites

199.1 Other malignant neoplasm of unspecified site

212.2 Benign neoplasm of trachea

212.3 Benign neoplasm of bronchus and lung

212.4 Benign neoplasm of pleura

231.1 Carcinoma in situ of trachea

231.2 Carcinoma in situ of bronchus and lung

235.7 Neoplasm of uncertain behavior of trachea, bronchus, and lung

239.1 Neoplasm of unspecified nature of respiratory system

482.84 Legionnaires' disease

485 Bronchopneumonia, organism unspecified ▽

486 Pneumonia, organism unspecified ▽

495.9 Unspecified allergic alveolitis and pneumonitis ▽

500 Coal workers' pneumoconiosis

501 Asbestosis

502 Pneumoconiosis due to other silica or silicates

503 Pneumoconiosis due to other inorganic dust

504 Pneumonopathy due to inhalation of other dust

505 Unspecified pneumoconiosis ▽

506.4 Chronic respiratory conditions due to fumes and vapors — (Use additional E code to identify cause)

507.0 Pneumonitis due to inhalation of food or vomitus

508.1 Chronic and other pulmonary manifestations due to radiation — (Use additional E code to identify cause)

510.0 Empyema with fistula — (Use additional code to identify infectious organism: 041.00-041.9)

510.9 Empyema without mention of fistula — (Use additional code to identify infectious organism: 041.00-041.9)

512.0 Spontaneous tension pneumothorax

512.1 Iatrogenic pneumothroax

512.8 Other spontaneous pneumothorax

513.0 Abscess of lung

514 Pulmonary congestion and hypostasis

515 Postinflammatory pulmonary fibrosis

516.0 Pulmonary alveolar proteinosis

516.1 Idiopathic pulmonary hemosiderosis — (Code first underlying disease, 275.0) ☒

516.2 Pulmonary alveolar microlithiasis

516.3 Idiopathic fibrosing alveolitis

516.8 Other specified alveolar and parietoalveolar pneumonopathies

517.8 Lung involvement in other diseases classified elsewhere — (Code first underlying disease: 135, 277.3, 710.0, 710.2, 710.4) ☒

518.0 Pulmonary collapse

518.3 Pulmonary eosinophilia

518.5 Pulmonary insufficiency following trauma and surgery

518.89 Other diseases of lung, not elsewhere classified

770.7 Chronic respiratory disease arising in the perinatal period

▽ Unspecified code
♀ Female diagnosis
☒ Manifestation code
♂ Male diagnosis

786.2 Cough
786.3 Hemoptysis
V10.11 Personal history of malignant neoplasm of bronchus and lung
V10.12 Personal history of malignant neoplasm of trachea
V15.82 Personal history of tobacco use, presenting hazards to health
V15.84 Personal history of exposure to asbestos, presenting hazards to health
V16.2 Family history of malignant neoplasm of other respiratory and intrathoracic organs
V43.89 Other organ or tissue replaced by other means — (This code is intended for use when these conditions are recorded as diagnoses or problems)

ICD-9-CM Procedural

33.24 Closed (endoscopic) biopsy of bronchus

31720–31725

31720 Catheter aspiration (separate procedure); nasotracheal
31725 tracheobronchial with fiberscope, bedside

ICD-9-CM Diagnostic

277.00 Cystic fibrosis without mention of meconium ileus — (Use additional code to identify any associated mental retardation)
277.02 Cystic fibrosis with pulmonary manifestations — (Use additional code to identify any associated mental retardation. Use additional code to identify any infectious organism present)
277.03 Cystic fibrosis with gastrointestinal manifestations — (Use additional code to identify any associated mental retardation)
277.09 Cystic fibrosis with other manifestations — (Use additional code to identify any associated mental retardation)
480.0 Pneumonia due to adenovirus
480.1 Pneumonia due to respiratory syncytial virus
480.2 Pneumonia due to parainfluenza virus
480.3 Pneumonia due to SARS-associated coronavirus
480.8 Pneumonia due to other virus not elsewhere classified
482.0 Pneumonia due to Klebsiella pneumoniae
482.1 Pneumonia due to Pseudomonas
482.2 Pneumonia due to Hemophilus influenzae (H. influenzae)
482.30 Pneumonia due to unspecified Streptococcus ▽
482.31 Pneumonia due to Streptococcus, group A
482.32 Pneumonia due to Streptococcus, group B
482.39 Pneumonia due to other Streptococcus
482.41 Pneumonia due to Staphylococcus aureus
482.81 Pneumonia due to anaerobes
482.82 Pneumonia due to escherichia coli (E. coli)
482.83 Pneumonia due to other gram-negative bacteria
482.89 Pneumonia due to other specified bacteria
483.0 Pneumonia due to Mycoplasma pneumoniae
483.1 Pneumonia due to Chlamydia
483.8 Pneumonia due to other specified organism
484.1 Pneumonia in cytomegalic inclusion disease — (Code first underlying disease, 078.5) ☒
484.3 Pneumonia in whooping cough — (Code first underlying disease: 033.0-033.9) ☒
484.5 Pneumonia in anthrax — (Code first underlying disease, 022.1) ☒
484.6 Pneumonia in aspergillosis — (Code first underlying disease, 117.3) ☒
484.7 Pneumonia in other systemic mycoses — (Code first underlying disease) ☒
484.8 Pneumonia in other infectious diseases classified elsewhere — (Code first underlying disease: 002.0, 083.0) ☒
485 Bronchopneumonia, organism unspecified ▽
487.0 Influenza with pneumonia
490 Bronchitis, not specified as acute or chronic ▽
491.0 Simple chronic bronchitis
491.1 Mucopurulent chronic bronchitis
491.20 Obstructive chronic bronchitis, without exacerbation
491.21 Obstructive chronic bronchitis, with (acute) exacerbation
491.8 Other chronic bronchitis
492.0 Emphysematous bleb
492.8 Other emphysema
494.0 Bronchiectasis without acute exacerbation
494.1 Bronchiectasis with acute exacerbation
495.0 Farmers' lung
495.1 Bagassosis
495.2 Bird-fanciers' lung
495.3 Suberosis
495.4 Malt workers' lung
495.5 Mushroom workers' lung
495.6 Maple bark-strippers' lung
495.7 "Ventilation" pneumonitis
495.8 Other specified allergic alveolitis and pneumonitis
495.9 Unspecified allergic alveolitis and pneumonitis ▽
496 Chronic airway obstruction, not elsewhere classified — (Note: This code is not to be used with any code from 491-493) ▽
506.1 Acute pulmonary edema due to fumes and vapors — (Use additional E code to identify cause)
507.0 Pneumonitis due to inhalation of food or vomitus
507.1 Pneumonitis due to inhalation of oils and essences
507.8 Pneumonitis due to other solids and liquids
510.0 Empyema with fistula — (Use additional code to identify infectious organism: 041.00-041.9)
513.0 Abscess of lung
513.1 Abscess of mediastinum
514 Pulmonary congestion and hypostasis
515 Postinflammatory pulmonary fibrosis
516.0 Pulmonary alveolar proteinosis
516.1 Idiopathic pulmonary hemosiderosis — (Code first underlying disease, 275.0) ☒
516.2 Pulmonary alveolar microlithiasis
516.3 Idiopathic fibrosing alveolitis
516.8 Other specified alveolar and parietoalveolar pneumonopathies
517.1 Rheumatic pneumonia — (Code first underlying disease, 390) ☒
517.2 Lung involvement in systemic sclerosis — (Code first underlying disease, 710.1) ☒
517.8 Lung involvement in other diseases classified elsewhere — (Code first underlying disease: 135, 277.3, 710.0, 710.2, 710.4) ☒
518.0 Pulmonary collapse
518.3 Pulmonary eosinophilia
518.4 Unspecified acute edema of lung ▽
518.5 Pulmonary insufficiency following trauma and surgery
518.81 Acute respiratory failure
518.82 Other pulmonary insufficiency, not elsewhere classified
518.83 Chronic respiratory failure
518.84 Acute and chronic respiratory failure
518.89 Other diseases of lung, not elsewhere classified
519.1 Other diseases of trachea and bronchus, not elsewhere classified
958.3 Posttraumatic wound infection not elsewhere classified
V15.82 Personal history of tobacco use, presenting hazards to health

ICD-9-CM Procedural

96.05 Other intubation of respiratory tract

HCPCS Level II Supplies & Services

A4305 Disposable drug delivery system, flow rate of 50 ml or greater per hour
A4306 Disposable drug delivery system, flow rate of 5 ml or less per hour
A4550 Surgical trays

31730

31730 Transtracheal (percutaneous) introduction of needle wire dilator/stent or indwelling tube for oxygen therapy

ICD-9-CM Diagnostic

478.6 Edema of larynx
478.71 Cellulitis and perichondritis of larynx
478.74 Stenosis of larynx
478.79 Other diseases of larynx
478.9 Other and unspecified diseases of upper respiratory tract
483.0 Pneumonia due to Mycoplasma pneumoniae
483.8 Pneumonia due to other specified organism
496 Chronic airway obstruction, not elsewhere classified — (Note: This code is not to be used with any code from 491-493) ▽
518.81 Acute respiratory failure
518.82 Other pulmonary insufficiency, not elsewhere classified
518.89 Other diseases of lung, not elsewhere classified
770.7 Chronic respiratory disease arising in the perinatal period

ICD-9-CM Procedural

31.99 Other operations on trachea

HCPCS Level II Supplies & Services

A4305 Disposable drug delivery system, flow rate of 50 ml or greater per hour
A4306 Disposable drug delivery system, flow rate of 5 ml or less per hour
A4550 Surgical trays

▽ Unspecified code ♀ Female diagnosis ☒ Manifestation code ♂ Male diagnosis

31750

31750 Tracheoplasty; cervical

ICD-9-CM Diagnostic

161.0 Malignant neoplasm of glottis
161.1 Malignant neoplasm of supraglottis
161.2 Malignant neoplasm of subglottis
161.3 Malignant neoplasm of laryngeal cartilages
161.8 Malignant neoplasm of other specified sites of larynx
161.9 Malignant neoplasm of larynx, unspecified site ▽
162.0 Malignant neoplasm of trachea
197.3 Secondary malignant neoplasm of other respiratory organs
198.89 Secondary malignant neoplasm of other specified sites
212.2 Benign neoplasm of trachea
231.1 Carcinoma in situ of trachea
235.7 Neoplasm of uncertain behavior of trachea, bronchus, and lung
239.1 Neoplasm of unspecified nature of respiratory system
519.00 Unspecified tracheostomy complication ▽
519.01 Infection of tracheostomy — (Use additional code to identify type of infection: 038.0-038.9, 682.1. Use additional code to identify organism: 041.00-041.9)
519.02 Mechanical complication of tracheostomy
519.09 Other tracheostomy complications
519.1 Other diseases of trachea and bronchus, not elsewhere classified
530.84 Tracheoesophageal fistula
748.3 Other congenital anomaly of larynx, trachea, and bronchus
750.3 Congenital tracheoesophageal fistula, esophageal atresia and stenosis
874.12 Open wound of trachea, complicated — (Use additional code to identify infection)
906.4 Late effect of crushing
906.8 Late effect of burns of other specified sites
925.2 Crushing injury of neck — (Use additional code to identify any associated injuries: 800-829, 850.0-854.1, 860.0-869.1)
947.1 Burn of larynx, trachea, and lung
960.0 Poisoning by penicillins — (Use additional code to specify the effects of the poisoning)
V10.12 Personal history of malignant neoplasm of trachea
V10.21 Personal history of malignant neoplasm of larynx
V15.82 Personal history of tobacco use, presenting hazards to health

ICD-9-CM Procedural

31.73 Closure of other fistula of trachea
31.79 Other repair and plastic operations on trachea

31755

31755 Tracheoplasty; tracheopharyngeal fistulization, each stage

ICD-9-CM Diagnostic

161.0 Malignant neoplasm of glottis
161.1 Malignant neoplasm of supraglottis
161.2 Malignant neoplasm of subglottis
161.3 Malignant neoplasm of laryngeal cartilages
161.8 Malignant neoplasm of other specified sites of larynx
161.9 Malignant neoplasm of larynx, unspecified site ▽
162.0 Malignant neoplasm of trachea
197.3 Secondary malignant neoplasm of other respiratory organs
198.89 Secondary malignant neoplasm of other specified sites
212.2 Benign neoplasm of trachea
231.1 Carcinoma in situ of trachea
235.7 Neoplasm of uncertain behavior of trachea, bronchus, and lung
239.1 Neoplasm of unspecified nature of respiratory system
519.00 Unspecified tracheostomy complication ▽
519.01 Infection of tracheostomy — (Use additional code to identify type of infection: 038.0-038.9, 682.1. Use additional code to identify organism: 041.00-041.9)
519.02 Mechanical complication of tracheostomy
519.09 Other tracheostomy complications
519.1 Other diseases of trachea and bronchus, not elsewhere classified
530.84 Tracheoesophageal fistula
748.3 Other congenital anomaly of larynx, trachea, and bronchus
750.3 Congenital tracheoesophageal fistula, esophageal atresia and stenosis
874.12 Open wound of trachea, complicated — (Use additional code to identify infection)
906.4 Late effect of crushing
906.8 Late effect of burns of other specified sites
925.2 Crushing injury of neck — (Use additional code to identify any associated injuries: 800-829, 850.0-854.1, 860.0-869.1)
947.1 Burn of larynx, trachea, and lung
960.0 Poisoning by penicillins — (Use additional code to specify the effects of the poisoning)
V10.12 Personal history of malignant neoplasm of trachea
V10.21 Personal history of malignant neoplasm of larynx
V15.82 Personal history of tobacco use, presenting hazards to health

ICD-9-CM Procedural

31.5 Local excision or destruction of lesion or tissue of trachea
31.79 Other repair and plastic operations on trachea

31760

31760 Tracheoplasty; intrathoracic

ICD-9-CM Diagnostic

161.0 Malignant neoplasm of glottis
161.1 Malignant neoplasm of supraglottis
161.2 Malignant neoplasm of subglottis
161.3 Malignant neoplasm of laryngeal cartilages
161.8 Malignant neoplasm of other specified sites of larynx
161.9 Malignant neoplasm of larynx, unspecified site ▽
162.0 Malignant neoplasm of trachea
197.3 Secondary malignant neoplasm of other respiratory organs
198.89 Secondary malignant neoplasm of other specified sites
212.2 Benign neoplasm of trachea
231.1 Carcinoma in situ of trachea
235.7 Neoplasm of uncertain behavior of trachea, bronchus, and lung
239.1 Neoplasm of unspecified nature of respiratory system
519.00 Unspecified tracheostomy complication ▽
519.01 Infection of tracheostomy — (Use additional code to identify type of infection: 038.0-038.9, 682.1. Use additional code to identify organism: 041.00-041.9)
519.02 Mechanical complication of tracheostomy
519.09 Other tracheostomy complications
519.1 Other diseases of trachea and bronchus, not elsewhere classified
530.84 Tracheoesophageal fistula
748.3 Other congenital anomaly of larynx, trachea, and bronchus
750.3 Congenital tracheoesophageal fistula, esophageal atresia and stenosis
874.12 Open wound of trachea, complicated — (Use additional code to identify infection)
906.4 Late effect of crushing
906.8 Late effect of burns of other specified sites
925.2 Crushing injury of neck — (Use additional code to identify any associated injuries: 800-829, 850.0-854.1, 860.0-869.1)
947.1 Burn of larynx, trachea, and lung
960.0 Poisoning by penicillins — (Use additional code to specify the effects of the poisoning)
V10.12 Personal history of malignant neoplasm of trachea
V10.21 Personal history of malignant neoplasm of larynx
V15.82 Personal history of tobacco use, presenting hazards to health

ICD-9-CM Procedural

31.79 Other repair and plastic operations on trachea

31766

31766 Carinal reconstruction

ICD-9-CM Diagnostic

162.0 Malignant neoplasm of trachea
162.2 Malignant neoplasm of main bronchus
197.0 Secondary malignant neoplasm of lung
197.3 Secondary malignant neoplasm of other respiratory organs
212.3 Benign neoplasm of bronchus and lung
231.1 Carcinoma in situ of trachea
231.2 Carcinoma in situ of bronchus and lung
235.7 Neoplasm of uncertain behavior of trachea, bronchus, and lung
239.1 Neoplasm of unspecified nature of respiratory system
515 Postinflammatory pulmonary fibrosis
519.00 Unspecified tracheostomy complication ▽
519.01 Infection of tracheostomy — (Use additional code to identify type of infection: 038.0-038.9, 682.1. Use additional code to identify organism: 041.00-041.9)
519.02 Mechanical complication of tracheostomy
519.09 Other tracheostomy complications
519.1 Other diseases of trachea and bronchus, not elsewhere classified
530.84 Tracheoesophageal fistula
748.3 Other congenital anomaly of larynx, trachea, and bronchus
750.3 Congenital tracheoesophageal fistula, esophageal atresia and stenosis
862.21 Bronchus injury without mention of open wound into cavity

▽ Unspecified code
♀ Female diagnosis
☒ Manifestation code
♂ Male diagnosis

862.31 Bronchus injury with open wound into cavity
874.12 Open wound of trachea, complicated — (Use additional code to identify infection)
906.0 Late effect of open wound of head, neck, and trunk
906.4 Late effect of crushing
906.8 Late effect of burns of other specified sites
947.1 Burn of larynx, trachea, and lung
V10.11 Personal history of malignant neoplasm of bronchus and lung
V10.12 Personal history of malignant neoplasm of trachea
V10.21 Personal history of malignant neoplasm of larynx
V15.82 Personal history of tobacco use, presenting hazards to health

ICD-9-CM Procedural
31.79 Other repair and plastic operations on trachea

31770–31775
31770 Bronchoplasty; graft repair
31775 excision stenosis and anastomosis

ICD-9-CM Diagnostic
162.2 Malignant neoplasm of main bronchus
162.3 Malignant neoplasm of upper lobe, bronchus, or lung
162.4 Malignant neoplasm of middle lobe, bronchus, or lung
162.5 Malignant neoplasm of lower lobe, bronchus, or lung
162.8 Malignant neoplasm of other parts of bronchus or lung
165.9 Malignant neoplasm of ill-defined sites within the respiratory system
171.4 Malignant neoplasm of connective and other soft tissue of thorax
197.0 Secondary malignant neoplasm of lung
197.1 Secondary malignant neoplasm of mediastinum
198.89 Secondary malignant neoplasm of other specified sites
212.3 Benign neoplasm of bronchus and lung
231.2 Carcinoma in situ of bronchus and lung
235.7 Neoplasm of uncertain behavior of trachea, bronchus, and lung
519.1 Other diseases of trachea and bronchus, not elsewhere classified
862.21 Bronchus injury without mention of open wound into cavity
862.31 Bronchus injury with open wound into cavity
906.0 Late effect of open wound of head, neck, and trunk
906.4 Late effect of crushing
906.5 Late effect of burn of eye, face, head, and neck
908.0 Late effect of internal injury to chest
934.1 Foreign body in main bronchus
947.1 Burn of larynx, trachea, and lung
V10.11 Personal history of malignant neoplasm of bronchus and lung
V10.12 Personal history of malignant neoplasm of trachea
V15.82 Personal history of tobacco use, presenting hazards to health

ICD-9-CM Procedural
32.1 Other excision of bronchus
33.48 Other repair and plastic operations on bronchus

31780
31780 Excision tracheal stenosis and anastomosis; cervical

ICD-9-CM Diagnostic
519.02 Mechanical complication of tracheostomy
519.1 Other diseases of trachea and bronchus, not elsewhere classified
748.3 Other congenital anomaly of larynx, trachea, and bronchus
906.0 Late effect of open wound of head, neck, and trunk
906.4 Late effect of crushing
906.5 Late effect of burn of eye, face, head, and neck
V16.1 Family history of malignant neoplasm of trachea, bronchus, and lung

ICD-9-CM Procedural
31.5 Local excision or destruction of lesion or tissue of trachea
31.79 Other repair and plastic operations on trachea

31781
31781 Excision tracheal stenosis and anastomosis; cervicothoracic

ICD-9-CM Diagnostic
519.02 Mechanical complication of tracheostomy
519.1 Other diseases of trachea and bronchus, not elsewhere classified
748.3 Other congenital anomaly of larynx, trachea, and bronchus
906.0 Late effect of open wound of head, neck, and trunk
906.4 Late effect of crushing
906.5 Late effect of burn of eye, face, head, and neck
V10.12 Personal history of malignant neoplasm of trachea
V16.1 Family history of malignant neoplasm of trachea, bronchus, and lung

ICD-9-CM Procedural
31.5 Local excision or destruction of lesion or tissue of trachea
31.79 Other repair and plastic operations on trachea

31785
31785 Excision of tracheal tumor or carcinoma; cervical

ICD-9-CM Diagnostic
162.0 Malignant neoplasm of trachea
162.2 Malignant neoplasm of main bronchus
197.0 Secondary malignant neoplasm of lung
197.3 Secondary malignant neoplasm of other respiratory organs
212.2 Benign neoplasm of trachea
212.3 Benign neoplasm of bronchus and lung
231.1 Carcinoma in situ of trachea
231.2 Carcinoma in situ of bronchus and lung
235.7 Neoplasm of uncertain behavior of trachea, bronchus, and lung
239.1 Neoplasm of unspecified nature of respiratory system
V15.82 Personal history of tobacco use, presenting hazards to health

ICD-9-CM Procedural
31.5 Local excision or destruction of lesion or tissue of trachea

31786
31786 Excision of tracheal tumor or carcinoma; thoracic

ICD-9-CM Diagnostic
162.0 Malignant neoplasm of trachea
162.2 Malignant neoplasm of main bronchus
197.0 Secondary malignant neoplasm of lung
197.3 Secondary malignant neoplasm of other respiratory organs
212.2 Benign neoplasm of trachea
212.3 Benign neoplasm of bronchus and lung
231.1 Carcinoma in situ of trachea
231.2 Carcinoma in situ of bronchus and lung
235.7 Neoplasm of uncertain behavior of trachea, bronchus, and lung
239.1 Neoplasm of unspecified nature of respiratory system
V15.82 Personal history of tobacco use, presenting hazards to health

ICD-9-CM Procedural
31.5 Local excision or destruction of lesion or tissue of trachea

31800
31800 Suture of tracheal wound or injury; cervical

ICD-9-CM Diagnostic
862.29 Injury to other specified intrathoracic organs without mention of open wound into cavity
862.39 Injury to other specified intrathoracic organs with open wound into cavity
874.02 Open wound of trachea, without mention of complication — (Use additional code to identify infection)
874.12 Open wound of trachea, complicated — (Use additional code to identify infection)

ICD-9-CM Procedural
31.71 Suture of laceration of trachea

HCPCS Level II Supplies & Services
A4305 Disposable drug delivery system, flow rate of 50 ml or greater per hour
A4306 Disposable drug delivery system, flow rate of 5 ml or less per hour
A4550 Surgical trays

31805
31805 Suture of tracheal wound or injury; intrathoracic

ICD-9-CM Diagnostic
862.29 Injury to other specified intrathoracic organs without mention of open wound into cavity
862.39 Injury to other specified intrathoracic organs with open wound into cavity
874.02 Open wound of trachea, without mention of complication — (Use additional code to identify infection)

874.12 Open wound of trachea, complicated — (Use additional code to identify infection)

ICD-9-CM Procedural

31.71 Suture of laceration of trachea

31820–31825

31820 Surgical closure tracheostomy or fistula; without plastic repair
31825 with plastic repair

ICD-9-CM Diagnostic

V44.0 Tracheostomy status — (This code is intended for use when these conditions are recorded as diagnoses or problems)
V51 Aftercare involving the use of plastic surgery
V55.0 Attention to tracheostomy

ICD-9-CM Procedural

31.72 Closure of external fistula of trachea
31.79 Other repair and plastic operations on trachea

31830

31830 Revision of tracheostomy scar

ICD-9-CM Diagnostic

701.4 Keloid scar
701.5 Other abnormal granulation tissue
709.2 Scar condition and fibrosis of skin
V10.12 Personal history of malignant neoplasm of trachea
V10.21 Personal history of malignant neoplasm of larynx
V51 Aftercare involving the use of plastic surgery
V58.49 Other specified aftercare following surgery — (This code should be used in conjunction with other aftercare codes to fully identify the reason for the aftercare encounter)

ICD-9-CM Procedural

86.3 Other local excision or destruction of lesion or tissue of skin and subcutaneous tissue

Lungs and Pleura

32000

32000 Thoracentesis, puncture of pleural cavity for aspiration, initial or subsequent

ICD-9-CM Diagnostic

162.0 Malignant neoplasm of trachea
162.2 Malignant neoplasm of main bronchus
162.3 Malignant neoplasm of upper lobe, bronchus, or lung
162.4 Malignant neoplasm of middle lobe, bronchus, or lung
162.5 Malignant neoplasm of lower lobe, bronchus, or lung
162.8 Malignant neoplasm of other parts of bronchus or lung
162.9 Malignant neoplasm of bronchus and lung, unspecified site ▽
163.0 Malignant neoplasm of parietal pleura
163.1 Malignant neoplasm of visceral pleura
163.8 Malignant neoplasm of other specified sites of pleura
163.9 Malignant neoplasm of pleura, unspecified site ▽

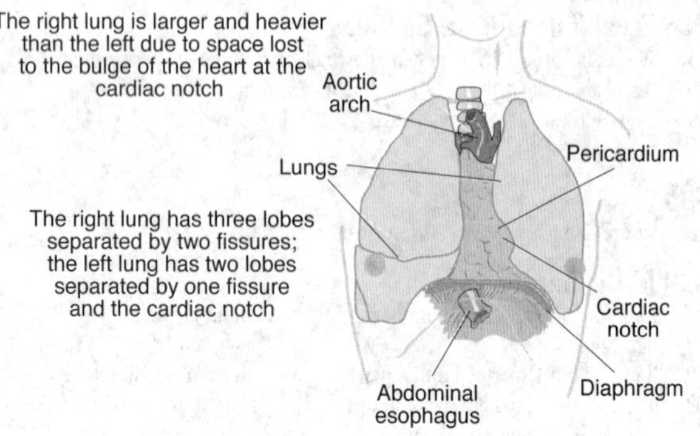
Respiratory System
The right lung is larger and heavier than the left due to space lost to the bulge of the heart at the cardiac notch
Aortic arch
Lungs
Pericardium
The right lung has three lobes separated by two fissures; the left lung has two lobes separated by one fissure and the cardiac notch
Cardiac notch
Abdominal esophagus
Diaphragm

197.0 Secondary malignant neoplasm of lung
197.2 Secondary malignant neoplasm of pleura
212.3 Benign neoplasm of bronchus and lung
212.4 Benign neoplasm of pleura
231.2 Carcinoma in situ of bronchus and lung
231.9 Carcinoma in situ of respiratory system, part unspecified ▽
235.7 Neoplasm of uncertain behavior of trachea, bronchus, and lung
235.8 Neoplasm of uncertain behavior of pleura, thymus, and mediastinum
239.1 Neoplasm of unspecified nature of respiratory system
239.8 Neoplasm of unspecified nature of other specified sites
506.1 Acute pulmonary edema due to fumes and vapors — (Use additional E code to identify cause)
508.1 Chronic and other pulmonary manifestations due to radiation — (Use additional E code to identify cause)
508.8 Respiratory conditions due to other specified external agents — (Use additional E code to identify cause)
511.1 Pleurisy with effusion, with mention of bacterial cause other than tuberculosis
511.8 Pleurisy with other specified forms of effusion, except tuberculous
511.9 Unspecified pleural effusion ▽
514 Pulmonary congestion and hypostasis
518.4 Unspecified acute edema of lung ▽
518.89 Other diseases of lung, not elsewhere classified
519.8 Other diseases of respiratory system, not elsewhere classified
519.9 Unspecified disease of respiratory system ▽
780.6 Fever
786.00 Unspecified respiratory abnormality ▽
786.09 Other dyspnea and respiratory abnormalities
861.22 Lung laceration without mention of open wound into thorax
861.32 Lung laceration with open wound into thorax
862.29 Injury to other specified intrathoracic organs without mention of open wound into cavity
862.39 Injury to other specified intrathoracic organs with open wound into cavity
997.3 Respiratory complications — (Use additional code to identify complications)
998.2 Accidental puncture or laceration during procedure

ICD-9-CM Procedural

34.91 Thoracentesis

HCPCS Level II Supplies & Services

A4550 Surgical trays
A7042 Implanted pleural catheter, each

32002

32002 Thoracentesis with insertion of tube with or without water seal (eg, for pneumothorax) (separate procedure)

ICD-9-CM Diagnostic

511.1 Pleurisy with effusion, with mention of bacterial cause other than tuberculosis
511.8 Pleurisy with other specified forms of effusion, except tuberculous
511.9 Unspecified pleural effusion ▽
512.0 Spontaneous tension pneumothorax
512.1 Iatrogenic pneumothroax
512.8 Other spontaneous pneumothorax
518.0 Pulmonary collapse
518.89 Other diseases of lung, not elsewhere classified
519.8 Other diseases of respiratory system, not elsewhere classified
770.2 Interstitial emphysema and related conditions of newborn
770.5 Other and unspecified atelectasis of newborn ▽
860.0 Traumatic pneumothorax without mention of open wound into thorax
860.1 Traumatic pneumothorax with open wound into thorax
860.2 Traumatic hemothorax without mention of open wound into thorax
860.3 Traumatic hemothorax with open wound into thorax
860.4 Traumatic pneumohemothorax without mention of open wound into thorax
860.5 Traumatic pneumohemothorax with open wound into thorax
862.8 Injury to multiple and unspecified intrathoracic organs without mention of open wound into cavity
862.9 Injury to multiple and unspecified intrathoracic organs with open wound into cavity
997.3 Respiratory complications — (Use additional code to identify complications)
998.2 Accidental puncture or laceration during procedure

ICD-9-CM Procedural

34.04 Insertion of intercostal catheter for drainage
34.91 Thoracentesis

▽ Unspecified code ☒ Manifestation code
♀ Female diagnosis ♂ Male diagnosis

32005

32005 Chemical pleurodesis (eg, for recurrent or persistent pneumothorax)

ICD-9-CM Diagnostic

277.00 Cystic fibrosis without mention of meconium ileus — (Use additional code to identify any associated mental retardation)
277.02 Cystic fibrosis with pulmonary manifestations — (Use additional code to identify any associated mental retardation. Use additional code to identify any infectious organism present)
277.03 Cystic fibrosis with gastrointestinal manifestations — (Use additional code to identify any associated mental retardation)
277.09 Cystic fibrosis with other manifestations — (Use additional code to identify any associated mental retardation)
492.0 Emphysematous bleb
510.0 Empyema with fistula — (Use additional code to identify infectious organism: 041.00-041.9)
511.0 Pleurisy without mention of effusion or current tuberculosis
512.0 Spontaneous tension pneumothorax
512.1 Iatrogenic pneumothroax
512.8 Other spontaneous pneumothorax
518.89 Other diseases of lung, not elsewhere classified
786.09 Other dyspnea and respiratory abnormalities
786.50 Unspecified chest pain ▽
786.52 Painful respiration
786.7 Abnormal chest sounds
V64.42 Thorascopic surgical procedure converted to open procedure

ICD-9-CM Procedural

34.92 Injection into thoracic cavity

32019

32019 Insertion of indwelling tunneled pleural catheter with cuff

ICD-9-CM Diagnostic

162.2 Malignant neoplasm of main bronchus
162.3 Malignant neoplasm of upper lobe, bronchus, or lung
162.4 Malignant neoplasm of middle lobe, bronchus, or lung
162.5 Malignant neoplasm of lower lobe, bronchus, or lung
162.8 Malignant neoplasm of other parts of bronchus or lung
162.9 Malignant neoplasm of bronchus and lung, unspecified site ▽
163.0 Malignant neoplasm of parietal pleura
163.1 Malignant neoplasm of visceral pleura
163.8 Malignant neoplasm of other specified sites of pleura
163.9 Malignant neoplasm of pleura, unspecified site ▽
164.8 Malignant neoplasm of other parts of mediastinum
165.8 Malignant neoplasm of other sites within the respiratory system and intrathoracic organs
165.9 Malignant neoplasm of ill-defined sites within the respiratory system
197.0 Secondary malignant neoplasm of lung
197.1 Secondary malignant neoplasm of mediastinum
197.2 Secondary malignant neoplasm of pleura
197.3 Secondary malignant neoplasm of other respiratory organs
231.2 Carcinoma in situ of bronchus and lung
231.8 Carcinoma in situ of other specified parts of respiratory system
231.9 Carcinoma in situ of respiratory system, part unspecified ▽
235.7 Neoplasm of uncertain behavior of trachea, bronchus, and lung
235.8 Neoplasm of uncertain behavior of pleura, thymus, and mediastinum
235.9 Neoplasm of uncertain behavior of other and unspecified respiratory organs ▽
239.1 Neoplasm of unspecified nature of respiratory system

ICD-9-CM Procedural

34.04 Insertion of intercostal catheter for drainage
34.09 Other incision of pleura

HCPCS Level II Supplies & Services

A7042 Implanted pleural catheter, each

32020

32020 Tube thoracostomy with or without water seal (eg, for abscess, hemothorax, empyema) (separate procedure)

ICD-9-CM Diagnostic

482.84 Legionnaires' disease
486 Pneumonia, organism unspecified ▽
510.0 Empyema with fistula — (Use additional code to identify infectious organism: 041.00-041.9)
510.9 Empyema without mention of fistula — (Use additional code to identify infectious organism: 041.00-041.9)
512.0 Spontaneous tension pneumothorax
512.1 Iatrogenic pneumothroax
512.8 Other spontaneous pneumothorax
513.0 Abscess of lung
513.1 Abscess of mediastinum
518.0 Pulmonary collapse
518.5 Pulmonary insufficiency following trauma and surgery
770.3 Pulmonary hemorrhage of fetus or newborn
770.5 Other and unspecified atelectasis of newborn ▽
786.09 Other dyspnea and respiratory abnormalities
860.0 Traumatic pneumothorax without mention of open wound into thorax
860.1 Traumatic pneumothorax with open wound into thorax
860.2 Traumatic hemothorax without mention of open wound into thorax
860.3 Traumatic hemothorax with open wound into thorax
860.4 Traumatic pneumohemothorax without mention of open wound into thorax
862.29 Injury to other specified intrathoracic organs without mention of open wound into cavity
862.39 Injury to other specified intrathoracic organs with open wound into cavity
862.8 Injury to multiple and unspecified intrathoracic organs without mention of open wound into cavity
862.9 Injury to multiple and unspecified intrathoracic organs with open wound into cavity
958.3 Posttraumatic wound infection not elsewhere classified

ICD-9-CM Procedural

34.04 Insertion of intercostal catheter for drainage

32035–32036

32035 Thoracostomy; with rib resection for empyema
32036 with open flap drainage for empyema

ICD-9-CM Diagnostic

510.0 Empyema with fistula — (Use additional code to identify infectious organism: 041.00-041.9)
510.9 Empyema without mention of fistula — (Use additional code to identify infectious organism: 041.00-041.9)

ICD-9-CM Procedural

34.09 Other incision of pleura

32095

32095 Thoracotomy, limited, for biopsy of lung or pleura

ICD-9-CM Diagnostic

162.0 Malignant neoplasm of trachea
162.2 Malignant neoplasm of main bronchus
162.3 Malignant neoplasm of upper lobe, bronchus, or lung
162.4 Malignant neoplasm of middle lobe, bronchus, or lung
162.5 Malignant neoplasm of lower lobe, bronchus, or lung
162.8 Malignant neoplasm of other parts of bronchus or lung
162.9 Malignant neoplasm of bronchus and lung, unspecified site ▽
163.0 Malignant neoplasm of parietal pleura
163.1 Malignant neoplasm of visceral pleura
163.8 Malignant neoplasm of other specified sites of pleura
163.9 Malignant neoplasm of pleura, unspecified site ▽
164.2 Malignant neoplasm of anterior mediastinum
164.3 Malignant neoplasm of posterior mediastinum
164.8 Malignant neoplasm of other parts of mediastinum
165.8 Malignant neoplasm of other sites within the respiratory system and intrathoracic organs
165.9 Malignant neoplasm of ill-defined sites within the respiratory system
176.4 Kaposi's sarcoma of lung
195.1 Malignant neoplasm of thorax
197.0 Secondary malignant neoplasm of lung
197.1 Secondary malignant neoplasm of mediastinum
197.2 Secondary malignant neoplasm of pleura
198.89 Secondary malignant neoplasm of other specified sites
212.3 Benign neoplasm of bronchus and lung
212.4 Benign neoplasm of pleura
212.5 Benign neoplasm of mediastinum
212.8 Benign neoplasm of other specified sites of respiratory and intrathoracic organs
231.2 Carcinoma in situ of bronchus and lung
231.9 Carcinoma in situ of respiratory system, part unspecified ▽
235.7 Neoplasm of uncertain behavior of trachea, bronchus, and lung

235.8 Neoplasm of uncertain behavior of pleura, thymus, and mediastinum
239.1 Neoplasm of unspecified nature of respiratory system
275.0 Disorders of iron metabolism — (Use additional code to identify any associated mental retardation)
492.0 Emphysematous bleb
510.9 Empyema without mention of fistula — (Use additional code to identify infectious organism: 041.00-041.9)
511.0 Pleurisy without mention of effusion or current tuberculosis
511.1 Pleurisy with effusion, with mention of bacterial cause other than tuberculosis
511.8 Pleurisy with other specified forms of effusion, except tuberculous
511.9 Unspecified pleural effusion ▽
512.8 Other spontaneous pneumothorax
513.0 Abscess of lung
515 Postinflammatory pulmonary fibrosis
516.0 Pulmonary alveolar proteinosis
516.1 Idiopathic pulmonary hemosiderosis — (Code first underlying disease, 275.0) ☒
516.2 Pulmonary alveolar microlithiasis
516.3 Idiopathic fibrosing alveolitis
516.8 Other specified alveolar and parietoalveolar pneumonopathies
516.9 Unspecified alveolar and parietoalveolar pneumonopathy ▽
518.89 Other diseases of lung, not elsewhere classified
519.2 Mediastinitis
519.3 Other diseases of mediastinum, not elsewhere classified
519.8 Other diseases of respiratory system, not elsewhere classified
780.6 Fever
786.09 Other dyspnea and respiratory abnormalities
786.3 Hemoptysis
786.6 Swelling, mass, or lump in chest
786.9 Other symptoms involving respiratory system and chest
793.1 Nonspecific abnormal findings on radiological and other examination of lung field
908.0 Late effect of internal injury to chest
V64.42 Thoracoscopic surgical procedure converted to open procedure

ICD-9-CM Procedural

33.28 Open biopsy of lung
34.24 Pleural biopsy

32100

32100 Thoracotomy, major; with exploration and biopsy

ICD-9-CM Diagnostic

162.0 Malignant neoplasm of trachea
162.2 Malignant neoplasm of main bronchus
162.3 Malignant neoplasm of upper lobe, bronchus, or lung
162.4 Malignant neoplasm of middle lobe, bronchus, or lung
162.5 Malignant neoplasm of lower lobe, bronchus, or lung
162.8 Malignant neoplasm of other parts of bronchus or lung
162.9 Malignant neoplasm of bronchus and lung, unspecified site ▽
163.0 Malignant neoplasm of parietal pleura
163.1 Malignant neoplasm of visceral pleura
163.8 Malignant neoplasm of other specified sites of pleura
163.9 Malignant neoplasm of pleura, unspecified site ▽
164.2 Malignant neoplasm of anterior mediastinum
164.3 Malignant neoplasm of posterior mediastinum
164.8 Malignant neoplasm of other parts of mediastinum
165.8 Malignant neoplasm of other sites within the respiratory system and intrathoracic organs
165.9 Malignant neoplasm of ill-defined sites within the respiratory system
176.4 Kaposi's sarcoma of lung
195.1 Malignant neoplasm of thorax
197.0 Secondary malignant neoplasm of lung
197.1 Secondary malignant neoplasm of mediastinum
197.2 Secondary malignant neoplasm of pleura
198.89 Secondary malignant neoplasm of other specified sites
212.3 Benign neoplasm of bronchus and lung
212.4 Benign neoplasm of pleura
212.5 Benign neoplasm of mediastinum
212.8 Benign neoplasm of other specified sites of respiratory and intrathoracic organs
231.2 Carcinoma in situ of bronchus and lung
231.9 Carcinoma in situ of respiratory system, part unspecified ▽
235.7 Neoplasm of uncertain behavior of trachea, bronchus, and lung
235.8 Neoplasm of uncertain behavior of pleura, thymus, and mediastinum
239.1 Neoplasm of unspecified nature of respiratory system
275.0 Disorders of iron metabolism — (Use additional code to identify any associated mental retardation)
492.0 Emphysematous bleb
510.9 Empyema without mention of fistula — (Use additional code to identify infectious organism: 041.00-041.9)
511.0 Pleurisy without mention of effusion or current tuberculosis
511.1 Pleurisy with effusion, with mention of bacterial cause other than tuberculosis
511.8 Pleurisy with other specified forms of effusion, except tuberculous
511.9 Unspecified pleural effusion ▽
512.8 Other spontaneous pneumothorax
513.0 Abscess of lung
515 Postinflammatory pulmonary fibrosis
516.0 Pulmonary alveolar proteinosis
516.1 Idiopathic pulmonary hemosiderosis — (Code first underlying disease, 275.0) ☒
516.2 Pulmonary alveolar microlithiasis
516.3 Idiopathic fibrosing alveolitis
516.8 Other specified alveolar and parietoalveolar pneumonopathies
516.9 Unspecified alveolar and parietoalveolar pneumonopathy ▽
518.89 Other diseases of lung, not elsewhere classified
519.2 Mediastinitis
519.3 Other diseases of mediastinum, not elsewhere classified
519.8 Other diseases of respiratory system, not elsewhere classified
780.6 Fever
786.09 Other dyspnea and respiratory abnormalities
786.3 Hemoptysis
786.6 Swelling, mass, or lump in chest
786.9 Other symptoms involving respiratory system and chest
793.1 Nonspecific abnormal findings on radiological and other examination of lung field
908.0 Late effect of internal injury to chest

ICD-9-CM Procedural

33.28 Open biopsy of lung
34.02 Exploratory thoracotomy
34.24 Pleural biopsy

32110

32110 Thoracotomy, major; with control of traumatic hemorrhage and/or repair of lung tear

ICD-9-CM Diagnostic

786.3 Hemoptysis
807.10 Open fracture of rib(s), unspecified ▽
860.1 Traumatic pneumothorax with open wound into thorax
860.3 Traumatic hemothorax with open wound into thorax
860.5 Traumatic pneumohemothorax with open wound into thorax
861.22 Lung laceration without mention of open wound into thorax
861.32 Lung laceration with open wound into thorax
862.1 Diaphragm injury with open wound into cavity
901.40 Injury to unspecified pulmonary vessel(s) ▽
901.41 Pulmonary artery injury
901.42 Pulmonary vein injury
901.83 Injury to multiple blood vessels of thorax
901.89 Injury to specified blood vessels of thorax, other
926.11 Crushing injury of back — (Use additional code to identify any associated injuries: 800-829, 850.0-854.1, 860.0-869.1)
926.9 Crushing injury of unspecified site of trunk — (Use additional code to identify any associated injuries: 800-829, 850.0-854.1, 860.0-869.1) ▽
V64.42 Thoracoscopic surgical procedure converted to open procedure

ICD-9-CM Procedural

33.43 Closure of laceration of lung
33.49 Other repair and plastic operations on lung
33.99 Other operations on lung
34.02 Exploratory thoracotomy

32120

32120 Thoracotomy, major; for postoperative complications

ICD-9-CM Diagnostic

510.0 Empyema with fistula — (Use additional code to identify infectious organism: 041.00-041.9)
510.9 Empyema without mention of fistula — (Use additional code to identify infectious organism: 041.00-041.9)
513.0 Abscess of lung

▽ Unspecified code ☒ Manifestation code
♀ Female diagnosis ♂ Male diagnosis

513.1 Abscess of mediastinum
996.59 Mechanical complication due to other implant and internal device, not elsewhere classified
996.60 Infection and inflammatory reaction due to unspecified device, implant, and graft — (Use additional code to identify specified infections)
996.84 Complications of transplanted lung — (Use additional code to identify nature of complication, 078.5)
998.0 Postoperative shock, not elsewhere classified
998.11 Hemorrhage complicating a procedure
998.2 Accidental puncture or laceration during procedure
998.4 Foreign body accidentally left during procedure, not elsewhere classified
998.51 Infected postoperative seroma — (Use additional code to identify organism)
998.59 Other postoperative infection — (Use additional code to identify infection)
998.6 Persistent postoperative fistula, not elsewhere classified
998.7 Acute reaction to foreign substance accidentally left during procedure, not elsewhere classified
998.9 Unspecified complication of procedure, not elsewhere classified
999.2 Other vascular complications of medical care, not elsewhere classified

ICD-9-CM Procedural

34.03 Reopening of recent thoracotomy site

32124

32124 Thoracotomy, major; with open intrapleural pneumonolysis

ICD-9-CM Diagnostic

137.0 Late effects of respiratory or unspecified tuberculosis
492.8 Other emphysema
510.9 Empyema without mention of fistula — (Use additional code to identify infectious organism: 041.00-041.9)
511.0 Pleurisy without mention of effusion or current tuberculosis
512.1 Iatrogenic pneumothroax
515 Postinflammatory pulmonary fibrosis
997.3 Respiratory complications — (Use additional code to identify complications)
V12.09 Personal history of other infectious and parasitic disease

ICD-9-CM Procedural

33.39 Other surgical collapse of lung

32140

32140 Thoracotomy, major; with cyst(s) removal, with or without a pleural procedure

ICD-9-CM Diagnostic

492.0 Emphysematous bleb
515 Postinflammatory pulmonary fibrosis
518.89 Other diseases of lung, not elsewhere classified
748.4 Congenital cystic lung
793.1 Nonspecific abnormal findings on radiological and other examination of lung field

ICD-9-CM Procedural

32.29 Other local excision or destruction of lesion or tissue of lung
33.99 Other operations on lung
34.59 Other excision of pleura

HCPCS Level II Supplies & Services

A7042 Implanted pleural catheter, each

32141

32141 Thoracotomy, major; with excision-plication of bullae, with or without any pleural procedure

ICD-9-CM Diagnostic

492.0 Emphysematous bleb
V64.42 Thoracoscopic surgical procedure converted to open procedure

ICD-9-CM Procedural

32.21 Plication of emphysematous bleb
32.29 Other local excision or destruction of lesion or tissue of lung
34.59 Other excision of pleura

HCPCS Level II Supplies & Services

A7042 Implanted pleural catheter, each

32150–32151

32150 Thoracotomy, major; with removal of intrapleural foreign body or fibrin deposit
32151 with removal of intrapulmonary foreign body

ICD-9-CM Diagnostic

511.0 Pleurisy without mention of effusion or current tuberculosis
513.0 Abscess of lung
515 Postinflammatory pulmonary fibrosis
793.1 Nonspecific abnormal findings on radiological and other examination of lung field
861.30 Unspecified lung injury with open wound into thorax
861.31 Lung contusion with open wound into thorax
861.32 Lung laceration with open wound into thorax
862.31 Bronchus injury with open wound into cavity
862.39 Injury to other specified intrathoracic organs with open wound into cavity
934.1 Foreign body in main bronchus
934.8 Foreign body in other specified parts of trachea, bronchus, and lung
934.9 Foreign body in respiratory tree, unspecified
998.4 Foreign body accidentally left during procedure, not elsewhere classified
V64.42 Thorascopic surgical procedure converted to open procedure

ICD-9-CM Procedural

33.1 Incision of lung
34.09 Other incision of pleura

32160

32160 Thoracotomy, major; with cardiac massage

ICD-9-CM Diagnostic

427.5 Cardiac arrest

ICD-9-CM Procedural

37.91 Open chest cardiac massage

32200–32201

32200 Pneumonostomy; with open drainage of abscess or cyst
32201 with percutaneous drainage of abscess or cyst

ICD-9-CM Diagnostic

492.0 Emphysematous bleb
510.9 Empyema without mention of fistula — (Use additional code to identify infectious organism: 041.00-041.9)
513.0 Abscess of lung
518.89 Other diseases of lung, not elsewhere classified
748.4 Congenital cystic lung
958.3 Posttraumatic wound infection not elsewhere classified
998.59 Other postoperative infection — (Use additional code to identify infection)

ICD-9-CM Procedural

33.1 Incision of lung
33.93 Puncture of lung

32215

32215 Pleural scarification for repeat pneumothorax

ICD-9-CM Diagnostic

512.0 Spontaneous tension pneumothorax
512.1 Iatrogenic pneumothroax
512.8 Other spontaneous pneumothorax

ICD-9-CM Procedural

34.6 Scarification of pleura

HCPCS Level II Supplies & Services

A7042 Implanted pleural catheter, each

32220–32225

32220 Decortication, pulmonary, (separate procedure); total
32225 Decortication, pulmonary (separate procedure); partial

ICD-9-CM Diagnostic

163.0 Malignant neoplasm of parietal pleura
163.8 Malignant neoplasm of other specified sites of pleura
163.9 Malignant neoplasm of pleura, unspecified site
197.2 Secondary malignant neoplasm of pleura

239.1 Neoplasm of unspecified nature of respiratory system
513.0 Abscess of lung
515 Postinflammatory pulmonary fibrosis
516.3 Idiopathic fibrosing alveolitis
V64.42 Thoracoscopic surgical procedure converted to open procedure

ICD-9-CM Procedural

34.51 Decortication of lung

32310–32320

32310 Pleurectomy, parietal (separate procedure)
32320 Decortication and parietal pleurectomy

ICD-9-CM Diagnostic

163.0 Malignant neoplasm of parietal pleura
163.8 Malignant neoplasm of other specified sites of pleura
163.9 Malignant neoplasm of pleura, unspecified site ▽
197.2 Secondary malignant neoplasm of pleura
239.1 Neoplasm of unspecified nature of respiratory system
492.0 Emphysematous bleb
510.0 Empyema with fistula — (Use additional code to identify infectious organism: 041.00-041.9)
511.0 Pleurisy without mention of effusion or current tuberculosis
512.0 Spontaneous tension pneumothorax
513.0 Abscess of lung
515 Postinflammatory pulmonary fibrosis
516.3 Idiopathic fibrosing alveolitis
518.89 Other diseases of lung, not elsewhere classified
V64.42 Thoracoscopic surgical procedure converted to open procedure

ICD-9-CM Procedural

34.51 Decortication of lung
34.59 Other excision of pleura

32400–32402

32400 Biopsy, pleura; percutaneous needle
32402 open

ICD-9-CM Diagnostic

163.0 Malignant neoplasm of parietal pleura
163.8 Malignant neoplasm of other specified sites of pleura
163.9 Malignant neoplasm of pleura, unspecified site ▽
197.2 Secondary malignant neoplasm of pleura
199.0 Disseminated malignant neoplasm
199.1 Other malignant neoplasm of unspecified site
212.4 Benign neoplasm of pleura
231.8 Carcinoma in situ of other specified parts of respiratory system
231.9 Carcinoma in situ of respiratory system, part unspecified ▽
235.8 Neoplasm of uncertain behavior of pleura, thymus, and mediastinum
239.1 Neoplasm of unspecified nature of respiratory system
486 Pneumonia, organism unspecified ▽
518.89 Other diseases of lung, not elsewhere classified
786.09 Other dyspnea and respiratory abnormalities
786.52 Painful respiration
786.7 Abnormal chest sounds
786.9 Other symptoms involving respiratory system and chest
793.1 Nonspecific abnormal findings on radiological and other examination of lung field

ICD-9-CM Procedural

34.24 Pleural biopsy

32405

32405 Biopsy, lung or mediastinum, percutaneous needle

ICD-9-CM Diagnostic

162.2 Malignant neoplasm of main bronchus
162.3 Malignant neoplasm of upper lobe, bronchus, or lung
162.4 Malignant neoplasm of middle lobe, bronchus, or lung
162.5 Malignant neoplasm of lower lobe, bronchus, or lung
162.8 Malignant neoplasm of other parts of bronchus or lung
162.9 Malignant neoplasm of bronchus and lung, unspecified site ▽
164.2 Malignant neoplasm of anterior mediastinum
164.3 Malignant neoplasm of posterior mediastinum
164.8 Malignant neoplasm of other parts of mediastinum
164.9 Malignant neoplasm of mediastinum, part unspecified ▽
176.4 Kaposi's sarcoma of lung
195.1 Malignant neoplasm of thorax
196.1 Secondary and unspecified malignant neoplasm of intrathoracic lymph nodes
197.0 Secondary malignant neoplasm of lung
197.1 Secondary malignant neoplasm of mediastinum
212.3 Benign neoplasm of bronchus and lung
212.5 Benign neoplasm of mediastinum
212.8 Benign neoplasm of other specified sites of respiratory and intrathoracic organs
214.2 Lipoma of intrathoracic organs
215.5 Other benign neoplasm of connective and other soft tissue of abdomen
230.1 Carcinoma in situ of esophagus
231.2 Carcinoma in situ of bronchus and lung
235.7 Neoplasm of uncertain behavior of trachea, bronchus, and lung
235.8 Neoplasm of uncertain behavior of pleura, thymus, and mediastinum
235.9 Neoplasm of uncertain behavior of other and unspecified respiratory organs ▽
239.1 Neoplasm of unspecified nature of respiratory system
239.8 Neoplasm of unspecified nature of other specified sites
482.84 Legionnaires' disease
511.0 Pleurisy without mention of effusion or current tuberculosis
518.89 Other diseases of lung, not elsewhere classified
786.09 Other dyspnea and respiratory abnormalities
786.2 Cough
786.3 Hemoptysis
786.6 Swelling, mass, or lump in chest
786.7 Abnormal chest sounds
786.9 Other symptoms involving respiratory system and chest
793.1 Nonspecific abnormal findings on radiological and other examination of lung field
794.2 Nonspecific abnormal results of pulmonary system function study
V15.82 Personal history of tobacco use, presenting hazards to health

ICD-9-CM Procedural

33.26 Closed (percutaneous)(needle) biopsy of lung
34.25 Closed (percutaneous) (needle) biopsy of mediastinum

32420

32420 Pneumocentesis, puncture of lung for aspiration

ICD-9-CM Diagnostic

482.84 Legionnaires' disease
486 Pneumonia, organism unspecified ▽
507.0 Pneumonitis due to inhalation of food or vomitus
507.1 Pneumonitis due to inhalation of oils and essences
507.8 Pneumonitis due to other solids and liquids
511.1 Pleurisy with effusion, with mention of bacterial cause other than tuberculosis
511.8 Pleurisy with other specified forms of effusion, except tuberculous
511.9 Unspecified pleural effusion ▽
513.0 Abscess of lung
514 Pulmonary congestion and hypostasis

ICD-9-CM Procedural

33.93 Puncture of lung

HCPCS Level II Supplies & Services

A4550 Surgical trays

32440

32440 Removal of lung, total pneumonectomy;

ICD-9-CM Diagnostic

162.2 Malignant neoplasm of main bronchus
162.3 Malignant neoplasm of upper lobe, bronchus, or lung
162.4 Malignant neoplasm of middle lobe, bronchus, or lung
162.5 Malignant neoplasm of lower lobe, bronchus, or lung
165.8 Malignant neoplasm of other sites within the respiratory system and intrathoracic organs
165.9 Malignant neoplasm of ill-defined sites within the respiratory system
197.0 Secondary malignant neoplasm of lung
231.2 Carcinoma in situ of bronchus and lung
235.7 Neoplasm of uncertain behavior of trachea, bronchus, and lung
239.1 Neoplasm of unspecified nature of respiratory system
492.0 Emphysematous bleb
502 Pneumoconiosis due to other silica or silicates
513.0 Abscess of lung

▽ Unspecified code
♀ Female diagnosis
☒ Manifestation code
♂ Male diagnosis

514 Pulmonary congestion and hypostasis
515 Postinflammatory pulmonary fibrosis
518.89 Other diseases of lung, not elsewhere classified
786.3 Hemoptysis
V15.82 Personal history of tobacco use, presenting hazards to health

ICD-9-CM Procedural

32.5 Complete pneumonectomy

32442

32442 Removal of lung, total pneumonectomy; with resection of segment of trachea followed by broncho-tracheal anastomosis (sleeve pneumonectomy)

ICD-9-CM Diagnostic

162.2 Malignant neoplasm of main bronchus
162.3 Malignant neoplasm of upper lobe, bronchus, or lung
162.4 Malignant neoplasm of middle lobe, bronchus, or lung
162.5 Malignant neoplasm of lower lobe, bronchus, or lung
162.8 Malignant neoplasm of other parts of bronchus or lung
165.8 Malignant neoplasm of other sites within the respiratory system and intrathoracic organs
165.9 Malignant neoplasm of ill-defined sites within the respiratory system
176.4 Kaposi's sarcoma of lung
197.0 Secondary malignant neoplasm of lung
198.89 Secondary malignant neoplasm of other specified sites
231.2 Carcinoma in situ of bronchus and lung
235.7 Neoplasm of uncertain behavior of trachea, bronchus, and lung
239.1 Neoplasm of unspecified nature of respiratory system
514 Pulmonary congestion and hypostasis
515 Postinflammatory pulmonary fibrosis
V15.82 Personal history of tobacco use, presenting hazards to health

ICD-9-CM Procedural

32.5 Complete pneumonectomy

32445

32445 Removal of lung, total pneumonectomy; extrapleural

ICD-9-CM Diagnostic

162.2 Malignant neoplasm of main bronchus
162.3 Malignant neoplasm of upper lobe, bronchus, or lung
162.4 Malignant neoplasm of middle lobe, bronchus, or lung
162.5 Malignant neoplasm of lower lobe, bronchus, or lung
162.8 Malignant neoplasm of other parts of bronchus or lung
165.8 Malignant neoplasm of other sites within the respiratory system and intrathoracic organs
165.9 Malignant neoplasm of ill-defined sites within the respiratory system
176.4 Kaposi's sarcoma of lung
197.0 Secondary malignant neoplasm of lung
198.89 Secondary malignant neoplasm of other specified sites
231.2 Carcinoma in situ of bronchus and lung
235.7 Neoplasm of uncertain behavior of trachea, bronchus, and lung
239.1 Neoplasm of unspecified nature of respiratory system
514 Pulmonary congestion and hypostasis
515 Postinflammatory pulmonary fibrosis
V15.82 Personal history of tobacco use, presenting hazards to health

ICD-9-CM Procedural

32.5 Complete pneumonectomy

32480–32488

32480 Removal of lung, other than total pneumonectomy; single lobe (lobectomy)
32482 two lobes (bilobectomy)
32484 single segment (segmentectomy)
32486 with circumferential resection of segment of bronchus followed by broncho-bronchial anastomosis (sleeve lobectomy)
32488 all remaining lung following previous removal of a portion of lung (completion pneumonectomy)

ICD-9-CM Diagnostic

162.2 Malignant neoplasm of main bronchus
162.3 Malignant neoplasm of upper lobe, bronchus, or lung
162.4 Malignant neoplasm of middle lobe, bronchus, or lung
162.5 Malignant neoplasm of lower lobe, bronchus, or lung
162.8 Malignant neoplasm of other parts of bronchus or lung
162.9 Malignant neoplasm of bronchus and lung, unspecified site ▽
176.4 Kaposi's sarcoma of lung
197.0 Secondary malignant neoplasm of lung
198.89 Secondary malignant neoplasm of other specified sites
231.2 Carcinoma in situ of bronchus and lung
235.7 Neoplasm of uncertain behavior of trachea, bronchus, and lung
239.1 Neoplasm of unspecified nature of respiratory system
492.0 Emphysematous bleb
513.0 Abscess of lung
514 Pulmonary congestion and hypostasis
515 Postinflammatory pulmonary fibrosis
518.89 Other diseases of lung, not elsewhere classified
748.5 Congenital agenesis, hypoplasia, and dysplasia of lung
786.3 Hemoptysis
793.1 Nonspecific abnormal findings on radiological and other examination of lung field
861.22 Lung laceration without mention of open wound into thorax
861.32 Lung laceration with open wound into thorax
862.8 Injury to multiple and unspecified intrathoracic organs without mention of open wound into cavity
862.9 Injury to multiple and unspecified intrathoracic organs with open wound into cavity
V15.82 Personal history of tobacco use, presenting hazards to health
V64.42 Thoracoscopic surgical procedure converted to open procedure

ICD-9-CM Procedural

32.1 Other excision of bronchus
32.3 Segmental resection of lung
32.4 Lobectomy of lung

32491

32491 Removal of lung, other than total pneumonectomy; excision-plication of emphysematous lung(s) (bullous or non-bullous) for lung volume reduction, sternal split or transthoracic approach, with or without any pleural procedure

ICD-9-CM Diagnostic

492.0 Emphysematous bleb
492.8 Other emphysema

ICD-9-CM Procedural

32.22 Lung volume reduction surgery

HCPCS Level II Supplies & Services

A7042 Implanted pleural catheter, each

32500

32500 Removal of lung, other than total pneumonectomy; wedge resection, single or multiple

ICD-9-CM Diagnostic

162.2 Malignant neoplasm of main bronchus
162.3 Malignant neoplasm of upper lobe, bronchus, or lung
162.4 Malignant neoplasm of middle lobe, bronchus, or lung
162.5 Malignant neoplasm of lower lobe, bronchus, or lung
162.9 Malignant neoplasm of bronchus and lung, unspecified site ▽
164.8 Malignant neoplasm of other parts of mediastinum
176.4 Kaposi's sarcoma of lung
197.0 Secondary malignant neoplasm of lung
198.89 Secondary malignant neoplasm of other specified sites
212.3 Benign neoplasm of bronchus and lung
231.2 Carcinoma in situ of bronchus and lung
235.7 Neoplasm of uncertain behavior of trachea, bronchus, and lung
239.1 Neoplasm of unspecified nature of respiratory system
492.0 Emphysematous bleb
492.8 Other emphysema
513.0 Abscess of lung
515 Postinflammatory pulmonary fibrosis
518.89 Other diseases of lung, not elsewhere classified
748.5 Congenital agenesis, hypoplasia, and dysplasia of lung
786.3 Hemoptysis
786.6 Swelling, mass, or lump in chest
861.22 Lung laceration without mention of open wound into thorax
861.32 Lung laceration with open wound into thorax
862.8 Injury to multiple and unspecified intrathoracic organs without mention of open wound into cavity

▽ Unspecified code ♀ Female diagnosis ☒ Manifestation code ♂ Male diagnosis

862.9 Injury to multiple and unspecified intrathoracic organs with open wound into cavity
934.8 Foreign body in other specified parts of trachea, bronchus, and lung
947.1 Burn of larynx, trachea, and lung
V15.82 Personal history of tobacco use, presenting hazards to health

ICD-9-CM Procedural

32.29 Other local excision or destruction of lesion or tissue of lung

32501

32501 Resection and repair of portion of bronchus (bronchoplasty) when performed at time of lobectomy or segmentectomy (List separately in addition to code for primary procedure)

ICD-9-CM Diagnostic

This is an add-on code. Refer to the corresponding primary procedure code for ICD-9 diagnosis code links.

ICD-9-CM Procedural

32.1 Other excision of bronchus
33.48 Other repair and plastic operations on bronchus

HCPCS Level II Supplies & Services

The HCPCS Level II code(s) would be the same as the actual procedure performed because these are in-addition-to codes.

32520–32525

32520 Resection of lung; with resection of chest wall
32522 with reconstruction of chest wall, without prosthesis
32525 with major reconstruction of chest wall, with prosthesis

ICD-9-CM Diagnostic

162.2 Malignant neoplasm of main bronchus
162.3 Malignant neoplasm of upper lobe, bronchus, or lung
162.4 Malignant neoplasm of middle lobe, bronchus, or lung
162.5 Malignant neoplasm of lower lobe, bronchus, or lung
162.8 Malignant neoplasm of other parts of bronchus or lung
162.9 Malignant neoplasm of bronchus and lung, unspecified site ▽
170.3 Malignant neoplasm of ribs, sternum, and clavicle
171.4 Malignant neoplasm of connective and other soft tissue of thorax
197.0 Secondary malignant neoplasm of lung
198.5 Secondary malignant neoplasm of bone and bone marrow
198.89 Secondary malignant neoplasm of other specified sites
235.7 Neoplasm of uncertain behavior of trachea, bronchus, and lung
239.1 Neoplasm of unspecified nature of respiratory system
786.6 Swelling, mass, or lump in chest
861.20 Unspecified lung injury without mention of open wound into thorax ▽
861.22 Lung laceration without mention of open wound into thorax
861.30 Unspecified lung injury with open wound into thorax ▽
861.31 Lung contusion with open wound into thorax
861.32 Lung laceration with open wound into thorax
862.39 Injury to other specified intrathoracic organs with open wound into cavity
862.8 Injury to multiple and unspecified intrathoracic organs without mention of open wound into cavity
862.9 Injury to multiple and unspecified intrathoracic organs with open wound into cavity
V15.82 Personal history of tobacco use, presenting hazards to health

ICD-9-CM Procedural

32.29 Other local excision or destruction of lesion or tissue of lung
32.3 Segmental resection of lung
34.79 Other repair of chest wall

32540

32540 Extrapleural enucleation of empyema (empyemectomy)

ICD-9-CM Diagnostic

510.0 Empyema with fistula — (Use additional code to identify infectious organism: 041.00-041.9)
510.9 Empyema without mention of fistula — (Use additional code to identify infectious organism: 041.00-041.9)

ICD-9-CM Procedural

34.3 Excision or destruction of lesion or tissue of mediastinum

32601–32602

32601 Thoracoscopy, diagnostic (separate procedure); lungs and pleural space, without biopsy
32602 lungs and pleural space, with biopsy

ICD-9-CM Diagnostic

162.0 Malignant neoplasm of trachea
162.2 Malignant neoplasm of main bronchus
162.3 Malignant neoplasm of upper lobe, bronchus, or lung
162.4 Malignant neoplasm of middle lobe, bronchus, or lung
162.5 Malignant neoplasm of lower lobe, bronchus, or lung
162.8 Malignant neoplasm of other parts of bronchus or lung
162.9 Malignant neoplasm of bronchus and lung, unspecified site ▽
163.0 Malignant neoplasm of parietal pleura
163.1 Malignant neoplasm of visceral pleura
163.8 Malignant neoplasm of other specified sites of pleura
163.9 Malignant neoplasm of pleura, unspecified site ▽
165.0 Malignant neoplasm of upper respiratory tract, part unspecified ▽
165.8 Malignant neoplasm of other sites within the respiratory system and intrathoracic organs
165.9 Malignant neoplasm of ill-defined sites within the respiratory system
176.4 Kaposi's sarcoma of lung
195.1 Malignant neoplasm of thorax
197.0 Secondary malignant neoplasm of lung
197.2 Secondary malignant neoplasm of pleura
198.89 Secondary malignant neoplasm of other specified sites
212.3 Benign neoplasm of bronchus and lung
212.4 Benign neoplasm of pleura
229.8 Benign neoplasm of other specified sites
231.2 Carcinoma in situ of bronchus and lung
234.8 Carcinoma in situ of other specified sites
235.7 Neoplasm of uncertain behavior of trachea, bronchus, and lung
235.8 Neoplasm of uncertain behavior of pleura, thymus, and mediastinum
238.8 Neoplasm of uncertain behavior of other specified sites
239.1 Neoplasm of unspecified nature of respiratory system
239.8 Neoplasm of unspecified nature of other specified sites
492.0 Emphysematous bleb
510.9 Empyema without mention of fistula — (Use additional code to identify infectious organism: 041.00-041.9)
511.0 Pleurisy without mention of effusion or current tuberculosis
511.1 Pleurisy with effusion, with mention of bacterial cause other than tuberculosis
511.8 Pleurisy with other specified forms of effusion, except tuberculous
511.9 Unspecified pleural effusion ▽
512.8 Other spontaneous pneumothorax
513.0 Abscess of lung
515 Postinflammatory pulmonary fibrosis
516.0 Pulmonary alveolar proteinosis
516.1 Idiopathic pulmonary hemosiderosis — (Code first underlying disease, 275.0) ☒
516.2 Pulmonary alveolar microlithiasis
516.3 Idiopathic fibrosing alveolitis
516.8 Other specified alveolar and parietoalveolar pneumonopathies
516.9 Unspecified alveolar and parietoalveolar pneumonopathy ▽
518.83 Chronic respiratory failure
518.89 Other diseases of lung, not elsewhere classified
519.8 Other diseases of respiratory system, not elsewhere classified
780.6 Fever
786.09 Other dyspnea and respiratory abnormalities
786.3 Hemoptysis
786.59 Other chest pain
786.6 Swelling, mass, or lump in chest
786.9 Other symptoms involving respiratory system and chest
793.1 Nonspecific abnormal findings on radiological and other examination of lung field
908.0 Late effect of internal injury to chest
V15.82 Personal history of tobacco use, presenting hazards to health

ICD-9-CM Procedural

33.27 Closed endoscopic biopsy of lung
34.21 Transpleural thoracoscopy
34.24 Pleural biopsy

HCPCS Level II Supplies & Services

A7042 Implanted pleural catheter, each

▽ Unspecified code ☒ Manifestation code
♀ Female diagnosis ♂ Male diagnosis

32603–32604

32603 Thoracoscopy, diagnostic (separate procedure); pericardial sac, without biopsy
32604 pericardial sac, with biopsy

ICD-9-CM Diagnostic

164.1 Malignant neoplasm of heart
164.8 Malignant neoplasm of other parts of mediastinum
198.89 Secondary malignant neoplasm of other specified sites
212.7 Benign neoplasm of heart
238.8 Neoplasm of uncertain behavior of other specified sites
239.8 Neoplasm of unspecified nature of other specified sites
391.0 Acute rheumatic pericarditis
392.0 Rheumatic chorea with heart involvement
393 Chronic rheumatic pericarditis
411.0 Postmyocardial infarction syndrome — (Use additional code to identify presence of hypertension: 401.0-405.9)
420.0 Acute pericarditis in diseases classified elsewhere — (Code first underlying disease: 017.9, 039.8, 066.8, 585) ☒
420.90 Unspecified acute pericarditis ▽
420.91 Acute idiopathic pericarditis
420.99 Other acute pericarditis
423.0 Hemopericardium
423.1 Adhesive pericarditis
423.2 Constrictive pericarditis
423.8 Other specified diseases of pericardium
423.9 Unspecified disease of pericardium ▽
429.3 Cardiomegaly
585 Chronic renal failure — (Use additional code to identify manifestation: 357.4, 420.0)
786.59 Other chest pain
861.01 Heart contusion without mention of open wound into thorax

ICD-9-CM Procedural

34.21 Transpleural thoracoscopy
37.24 Biopsy of pericardium

32605–32606

32605 Thoracoscopy, diagnostic (separate procedure); mediastinal space, without biopsy
32606 mediastinal space, with biopsy

ICD-9-CM Diagnostic

164.2 Malignant neoplasm of anterior mediastinum
164.3 Malignant neoplasm of posterior mediastinum
164.8 Malignant neoplasm of other parts of mediastinum
164.9 Malignant neoplasm of mediastinum, part unspecified ▽
195.1 Malignant neoplasm of thorax
197.1 Secondary malignant neoplasm of mediastinum
212.5 Benign neoplasm of mediastinum
235.8 Neoplasm of uncertain behavior of pleura, thymus, and mediastinum
239.8 Neoplasm of unspecified nature of other specified sites
786.59 Other chest pain
996.00 Mechanical complication of unspecified cardiac device, implant, and graft ▽

ICD-9-CM Procedural

34.22 Mediastinoscopy
34.25 Closed (percutaneous) (needle) biopsy of mediastinum

32650

32650 Thoracoscopy, surgical; with pleurodesis (eg, mechanical or chemical)

ICD-9-CM Diagnostic

163.0 Malignant neoplasm of parietal pleura
235.8 Neoplasm of uncertain behavior of pleura, thymus, and mediastinum
277.00 Cystic fibrosis without mention of meconium ileus — (Use additional code to identify any associated mental retardation)
277.02 Cystic fibrosis with pulmonary manifestations — (Use additional code to identify any associated mental retardation. Use additional code to identify any infectious organism present)
277.03 Cystic fibrosis with gastrointestinal manifestations — (Use additional code to identify any associated mental retardation)
277.09 Cystic fibrosis with other manifestations — (Use additional code to identify any associated mental retardation)
492.0 Emphysematous bleb
510.0 Empyema with fistula — (Use additional code to identify infectious organism: 041.00-041.9)
511.0 Pleurisy without mention of effusion or current tuberculosis
512.0 Spontaneous tension pneumothorax
512.1 Iatrogenic pneumothroax
512.8 Other spontaneous pneumothorax
518.89 Other diseases of lung, not elsewhere classified
786.09 Other dyspnea and respiratory abnormalities
786.50 Unspecified chest pain ▽
786.52 Painful respiration
786.7 Abnormal chest sounds

ICD-9-CM Procedural

34.6 Scarification of pleura
34.92 Injection into thoracic cavity

32651–32652

32651 Thoracoscopy, surgical; with partial pulmonary decortication
32652 with total pulmonary decortication, including intrapleural pneumonolysis

ICD-9-CM Diagnostic

163.0 Malignant neoplasm of parietal pleura
163.8 Malignant neoplasm of other specified sites of pleura
163.9 Malignant neoplasm of pleura, unspecified site ▽
197.2 Secondary malignant neoplasm of pleura
239.1 Neoplasm of unspecified nature of respiratory system
492.0 Emphysematous bleb
510.0 Empyema with fistula — (Use additional code to identify infectious organism: 041.00-041.9)
511.0 Pleurisy without mention of effusion or current tuberculosis
512.0 Spontaneous tension pneumothorax
513.0 Abscess of lung
515 Postinflammatory pulmonary fibrosis
516.3 Idiopathic fibrosing alveolitis
518.89 Other diseases of lung, not elsewhere classified

ICD-9-CM Procedural

33.39 Other surgical collapse of lung
34.51 Decortication of lung

32653

32653 Thoracoscopy, surgical; with removal of intrapleural foreign body or fibrin deposit

ICD-9-CM Diagnostic

511.0 Pleurisy without mention of effusion or current tuberculosis
513.0 Abscess of lung
515 Postinflammatory pulmonary fibrosis
516.3 Idiopathic fibrosing alveolitis
793.1 Nonspecific abnormal findings on radiological and other examination of lung field
861.30 Unspecified lung injury with open wound into thorax ▽
861.31 Lung contusion with open wound into thorax
861.32 Lung laceration with open wound into thorax
934.8 Foreign body in other specified parts of trachea, bronchus, and lung
998.4 Foreign body accidentally left during procedure, not elsewhere classified

ICD-9-CM Procedural

34.09 Other incision of pleura

32654

32654 Thoracoscopy, surgical; with control of traumatic hemorrhage

ICD-9-CM Diagnostic

786.3 Hemoptysis
807.10 Open fracture of rib(s), unspecified ▽
860.1 Traumatic pneumothorax with open wound into thorax
860.3 Traumatic hemothorax with open wound into thorax
860.5 Traumatic pneumohemothorax with open wound into thorax
861.22 Lung laceration without mention of open wound into thorax
861.32 Lung laceration with open wound into thorax
862.1 Diaphragm injury with open wound into cavity
901.40 Injury to unspecified pulmonary vessel(s) ▽
901.41 Pulmonary artery injury
901.42 Pulmonary vein injury
901.83 Injury to multiple blood vessels of thorax
901.89 Injury to specified blood vessels of thorax, other

926.11 Crushing injury of back — (Use additional code to identify any associated injuries: 800-829, 850.0-854.1, 860.0-869.1)

926.9 Crushing injury of unspecified site of trunk — (Use additional code to identify any associated injuries: 800-829, 850.0-854.1, 860.0-869.1) ▽

ICD-9-CM Procedural

34.03 Reopening of recent thoracotomy site

34.09 Other incision of pleura

32655–32656

32655 Thoracoscopy, surgical; with excision-plication of bullae, including any pleural procedure

32656 with parietal pleurectomy

ICD-9-CM Diagnostic

163.0 Malignant neoplasm of parietal pleura

163.8 Malignant neoplasm of other specified sites of pleura

163.9 Malignant neoplasm of pleura, unspecified site ▽

492.0 Emphysematous bleb

515 Postinflammatory pulmonary fibrosis

518.89 Other diseases of lung, not elsewhere classified

ICD-9-CM Procedural

32.21 Plication of emphysematous bleb

34.59 Other excision of pleura

HCPCS Level II Supplies & Services

A7042 Implanted pleural catheter, each

32657

32657 Thoracoscopy, surgical; with wedge resection of lung, single or multiple

ICD-9-CM Diagnostic

162.2 Malignant neoplasm of main bronchus

162.3 Malignant neoplasm of upper lobe, bronchus, or lung

162.4 Malignant neoplasm of middle lobe, bronchus, or lung

162.5 Malignant neoplasm of lower lobe, bronchus, or lung

162.9 Malignant neoplasm of bronchus and lung, unspecified site ▽

164.8 Malignant neoplasm of other parts of mediastinum

176.4 Kaposi's sarcoma of lung

197.0 Secondary malignant neoplasm of lung

198.89 Secondary malignant neoplasm of other specified sites

212.3 Benign neoplasm of bronchus and lung

235.7 Neoplasm of uncertain behavior of trachea, bronchus, and lung

239.1 Neoplasm of unspecified nature of respiratory system

492.0 Emphysematous bleb

492.8 Other emphysema

513.0 Abscess of lung

515 Postinflammatory pulmonary fibrosis

518.89 Other diseases of lung, not elsewhere classified

748.5 Congenital agenesis, hypoplasia, and dysplasia of lung

786.3 Hemoptysis

786.6 Swelling, mass, or lump in chest

861.22 Lung laceration without mention of open wound into thorax

861.32 Lung laceration with open wound into thorax

862.8 Injury to multiple and unspecified intrathoracic organs without mention of open wound into cavity

862.9 Injury to multiple and unspecified intrathoracic organs with open wound into cavity

934.8 Foreign body in other specified parts of trachea, bronchus, and lung

947.1 Burn of larynx, trachea, and lung

V15.82 Personal history of tobacco use, presenting hazards to health

ICD-9-CM Procedural

32.29 Other local excision or destruction of lesion or tissue of lung

32658

32658 Thoracoscopy, surgical; with removal of clot or foreign body from pericardial sac

ICD-9-CM Diagnostic

420.91 Acute idiopathic pericarditis

420.99 Other acute pericarditis

423.0 Hemopericardium

861.01 Heart contusion without mention of open wound into thorax

861.02 Heart laceration without penetration of heart chambers or mention of open wound into thorax

861.11 Heart contusion with open wound into thorax

861.12 Heart laceration without penetration of heart chambers, with open wound into thorax

862.8 Injury to multiple and unspecified intrathoracic organs without mention of open wound into cavity

908.0 Late effect of internal injury to chest

926.11 Crushing injury of back — (Use additional code to identify any associated injuries: 800-829, 850.0-854.1, 860.0-869.1)

926.8 Crushing injury of multiple sites of trunk — (Use additional code to identify any associated injuries: 800-829, 850.0-854.1, 860.0-869.1)

996.59 Mechanical complication due to other implant and internal device, not elsewhere classified

996.61 Infection and inflammatory reaction due to cardiac device, implant, and graft — (Use additional code to identify specified infections)

ICD-9-CM Procedural

37.12 Pericardiotomy

32659

32659 Thoracoscopy, surgical; with creation of pericardial window or partial resection of pericardial sac for drainage

ICD-9-CM Diagnostic

164.1 Malignant neoplasm of heart

198.89 Secondary malignant neoplasm of other specified sites

212.7 Benign neoplasm of heart

234.8 Carcinoma in situ of other specified sites

238.8 Neoplasm of uncertain behavior of other specified sites

239.8 Neoplasm of unspecified nature of other specified sites

411.0 Postmyocardial infarction syndrome — (Use additional code to identify presence of hypertension: 401.0-405.9)

420.0 Acute pericarditis in diseases classified elsewhere — (Code first underlying disease: 017.9, 039.8, 066.8, 585) ☒

420.90 Unspecified acute pericarditis ▽

420.91 Acute idiopathic pericarditis

420.99 Other acute pericarditis

423.0 Hemopericardium

423.1 Adhesive pericarditis

423.2 Constrictive pericarditis

423.8 Other specified diseases of pericardium

585 Chronic renal failure — (Use additional code to identify manifestation: 357.4, 420.0)

746.89 Other specified congenital anomaly of heart

786.6 Swelling, mass, or lump in chest

908.0 Late effect of internal injury to chest

909.2 Late effect of radiation

996.00 Mechanical complication of unspecified cardiac device, implant, and graft ▽

996.61 Infection and inflammatory reaction due to cardiac device, implant, and graft — (Use additional code to identify specified infections)

998.59 Other postoperative infection — (Use additional code to identify infection)

ICD-9-CM Procedural

37.12 Pericardiotomy

32660

32660 Thoracoscopy, surgical; with total pericardiectomy

ICD-9-CM Diagnostic

164.1 Malignant neoplasm of heart

198.89 Secondary malignant neoplasm of other specified sites

212.7 Benign neoplasm of heart

234.8 Carcinoma in situ of other specified sites

238.8 Neoplasm of uncertain behavior of other specified sites

239.8 Neoplasm of unspecified nature of other specified sites

411.0 Postmyocardial infarction syndrome — (Use additional code to identify presence of hypertension: 401.0-405.9)

420.0 Acute pericarditis in diseases classified elsewhere — (Code first underlying disease: 017.9, 039.8, 066.8, 585) ☒

420.90 Unspecified acute pericarditis ▽

420.91 Acute idiopathic pericarditis

420.99 Other acute pericarditis

423.0 Hemopericardium

423.1 Adhesive pericarditis

423.2 Constrictive pericarditis

▽ Unspecified code ☒ Manifestation code
♀ Female diagnosis ♂ Male diagnosis

423.8 Other specified diseases of pericardium
585 Chronic renal failure — (Use additional code to identify manifestation: 357.4, 420.0)
746.89 Other specified congenital anomaly of heart
786.6 Swelling, mass, or lump in chest
908.0 Late effect of internal injury to chest
909.2 Late effect of radiation
996.00 Mechanical complication of unspecified cardiac device, implant, and graft
996.61 Infection and inflammatory reaction due to cardiac device, implant, and graft — (Use additional code to identify specified infections)
998.59 Other postoperative infection — (Use additional code to identify infection)

ICD-9-CM Procedural
37.31 Pericardiectomy

32661
32661 Thoracoscopy, surgical; with excision of pericardial cyst, tumor, or mass

ICD-9-CM Diagnostic
164.1 Malignant neoplasm of heart
198.89 Secondary malignant neoplasm of other specified sites
212.7 Benign neoplasm of heart
234.8 Carcinoma in situ of other specified sites
238.8 Neoplasm of uncertain behavior of other specified sites
239.8 Neoplasm of unspecified nature of other specified sites
423.8 Other specified diseases of pericardium
746.89 Other specified congenital anomaly of heart
786.6 Swelling, mass, or lump in chest

ICD-9-CM Procedural
37.33 Excision or destruction of other lesion or tissue of heart, open approach

32662
32662 Thoracoscopy, surgical; with excision of mediastinal cyst, tumor, or mass

ICD-9-CM Diagnostic
164.2 Malignant neoplasm of anterior mediastinum
164.3 Malignant neoplasm of posterior mediastinum
164.8 Malignant neoplasm of other parts of mediastinum
164.9 Malignant neoplasm of mediastinum, part unspecified
176.8 Kaposi's sarcoma of other specified sites
195.1 Malignant neoplasm of thorax
197.1 Secondary malignant neoplasm of mediastinum
199.0 Disseminated malignant neoplasm
212.5 Benign neoplasm of mediastinum
238.8 Neoplasm of uncertain behavior of other specified sites
239.8 Neoplasm of unspecified nature of other specified sites
279.8 Other specified disorders involving the immune mechanism — (Use additional code to identify any associated mental retardation)
748.8 Other specified congenital anomaly of respiratory system
786.6 Swelling, mass, or lump in chest

ICD-9-CM Procedural
34.3 Excision or destruction of lesion or tissue of mediastinum

32663
32663 Thoracoscopy, surgical; with lobectomy, total or segmental

ICD-9-CM Diagnostic
162.2 Malignant neoplasm of main bronchus
162.3 Malignant neoplasm of upper lobe, bronchus, or lung
162.4 Malignant neoplasm of middle lobe, bronchus, or lung
162.5 Malignant neoplasm of lower lobe, bronchus, or lung
162.8 Malignant neoplasm of other parts of bronchus or lung
176.4 Kaposi's sarcoma of lung
197.0 Secondary malignant neoplasm of lung
198.89 Secondary malignant neoplasm of other specified sites
231.2 Carcinoma in situ of bronchus and lung
235.7 Neoplasm of uncertain behavior of trachea, bronchus, and lung
239.1 Neoplasm of unspecified nature of respiratory system
492.0 Emphysematous bleb
513.0 Abscess of lung
514 Pulmonary congestion and hypostasis
515 Postinflammatory pulmonary fibrosis
518.89 Other diseases of lung, not elsewhere classified
748.5 Congenital agenesis, hypoplasia, and dysplasia of lung
786.3 Hemoptysis
793.1 Nonspecific abnormal findings on radiological and other examination of lung field
861.22 Lung laceration without mention of open wound into thorax
861.32 Lung laceration with open wound into thorax
862.8 Injury to multiple and unspecified intrathoracic organs without mention of open wound into cavity
862.9 Injury to multiple and unspecified intrathoracic organs with open wound into cavity
V15.82 Personal history of tobacco use, presenting hazards to health

ICD-9-CM Procedural
32.3 Segmental resection of lung
32.4 Lobectomy of lung

32664
32664 Thoracoscopy, surgical; with thoracic sympathectomy

ICD-9-CM Diagnostic
780.8 Generalized hyperhidrosis

ICD-9-CM Procedural
05.29 Other sympathectomy and ganglionectomy

32665
32665 Thoracoscopy, surgical; with esophagomyotomy (Heller type)

ICD-9-CM Diagnostic
530.0 Achalasia and cardiospasm
530.3 Stricture and stenosis of esophagus
530.5 Dyskinesia of esophagus
750.3 Congenital tracheoesophageal fistula, esophageal atresia and stenosis

ICD-9-CM Procedural
42.7 Esophagomyotomy

32800
32800 Repair lung hernia through chest wall

ICD-9-CM Diagnostic
518.89 Other diseases of lung, not elsewhere classified
748.69 Other congenital anomaly of lung

ICD-9-CM Procedural
34.79 Other repair of chest wall

32810
32810 Closure of chest wall following open flap drainage for empyema (Clagett type procedure)

ICD-9-CM Diagnostic
510.0 Empyema with fistula — (Use additional code to identify infectious organism: 041.00-041.9)
510.9 Empyema without mention of fistula — (Use additional code to identify infectious organism: 041.00-041.9)

ICD-9-CM Procedural
34.72 Closure of thoracostomy

32815
32815 Open closure of major bronchial fistula

ICD-9-CM Diagnostic
510.0 Empyema with fistula — (Use additional code to identify infectious organism: 041.00-041.9)
530.89 Other specified disorder of the esophagus
750.3 Congenital tracheoesophageal fistula, esophageal atresia and stenosis
908.0 Late effect of internal injury to chest
998.6 Persistent postoperative fistula, not elsewhere classified

ICD-9-CM Procedural
33.42 Closure of bronchial fistula

32820

32820 Major reconstruction, chest wall (posttraumatic)

ICD-9-CM Diagnostic

807.10 Open fracture of rib(s), unspecified ▽
807.19 Open fracture of multiple ribs, unspecified ▽
807.3 Open fracture of sternum
807.4 Flail chest
809.1 Fracture of bones of trunk, open
860.0 Traumatic pneumothorax without mention of open wound into thorax
860.1 Traumatic pneumothorax with open wound into thorax
860.2 Traumatic hemothorax without mention of open wound into thorax
860.3 Traumatic hemothorax with open wound into thorax
860.4 Traumatic pneumohemothorax without mention of open wound into thorax
860.5 Traumatic pneumohemothorax with open wound into thorax
861.30 Unspecified lung injury with open wound into thorax ▽
861.32 Lung laceration with open wound into thorax
862.39 Injury to other specified intrathoracic organs with open wound into cavity
862.8 Injury to multiple and unspecified intrathoracic organs without mention of open wound into cavity
862.9 Injury to multiple and unspecified intrathoracic organs with open wound into cavity
875.1 Open wound of chest (wall), complicated — (Use additional code to identify infection)
926.8 Crushing injury of multiple sites of trunk — (Use additional code to identify any associated injuries: 800-829, 850.0-854.1, 860.0-869.1)
926.9 Crushing injury of unspecified site of trunk — (Use additional code to identify any associated injuries: 800-829, 850.0-854.1, 860.0-869.1) ▽
942.22 Blisters with epidermal loss due to burn (second degree) of chest wall, excluding breast and nipple
942.32 Full-thickness skin loss due to burn (third degree nos) of chest wall, excluding breast and nipple
942.40 Deep necrosis of underlying tissues due to burn (deep third degree) of trunk, unspecified site, without mention of loss of a body part ▽
942.42 Deep necrosis of underlying tissues due to burn (deep third degree) of chest wall, excluding breast and nipple, without mention of loss of a body part
959.11 Other injury of chest wall
998.31 Disruption of internal operation wound
998.32 Disruption of external operation wound

ICD-9-CM Procedural

34.79 Other repair of chest wall

32850

32850 Donor pneumonectomy (including cold preservation), from cadaver donor

ICD-9-CM Diagnostic

V59.8 Donor of other specified organ or tissue

ICD-9-CM Procedural

32.5 Complete pneumonectomy

32851–32854

32851 Lung transplant, single; without cardiopulmonary bypass
32852 with cardiopulmonary bypass
32853 Lung transplant, double (bilateral sequential or en bloc); without cardiopulmonary bypass
32854 with cardiopulmonary bypass

ICD-9-CM Diagnostic

162.2 Malignant neoplasm of main bronchus
162.3 Malignant neoplasm of upper lobe, bronchus, or lung
162.4 Malignant neoplasm of middle lobe, bronchus, or lung
162.5 Malignant neoplasm of lower lobe, bronchus, or lung
162.8 Malignant neoplasm of other parts of bronchus or lung
162.9 Malignant neoplasm of bronchus and lung, unspecified site ▽
163.0 Malignant neoplasm of parietal pleura
163.1 Malignant neoplasm of visceral pleura
163.8 Malignant neoplasm of other specified sites of pleura
197.0 Secondary malignant neoplasm of lung
231.2 Carcinoma in situ of bronchus and lung
235.7 Neoplasm of uncertain behavior of trachea, bronchus, and lung
239.1 Neoplasm of unspecified nature of respiratory system
273.4 Alpha-1-antitrypsin deficiency
277.00 Cystic fibrosis without mention of meconium ileus — (Use additional code to identify any associated mental retardation)
277.02 Cystic fibrosis with pulmonary manifestations — (Use additional code to identify any associated mental retardation. Use additional code to identify any infectious organism present)
277.03 Cystic fibrosis with gastrointestinal manifestations — (Use additional code to identify any associated mental retardation)
277.09 Cystic fibrosis with other manifestations — (Use additional code to identify any associated mental retardation)
500 Coal workers' pneumoconiosis
501 Asbestosis
502 Pneumoconiosis due to other silica or silicates
503 Pneumoconiosis due to other inorganic dust
506.4 Chronic respiratory conditions due to fumes and vapors — (Use additional E code to identify cause)
506.9 Unspecified respiratory conditions due to fumes and vapors — (Use additional E code to identify cause) ▽
508.1 Chronic and other pulmonary manifestations due to radiation — (Use additional E code to identify cause)
510.9 Empyema without mention of fistula — (Use additional code to identify infectious organism: 041.00-041.9)
513.0 Abscess of lung
515 Postinflammatory pulmonary fibrosis
516.0 Pulmonary alveolar proteinosis
516.3 Idiopathic fibrosing alveolitis
518.5 Pulmonary insufficiency following trauma and surgery
518.81 Acute respiratory failure
518.83 Chronic respiratory failure
518.89 Other diseases of lung, not elsewhere classified
519.1 Other diseases of trachea and bronchus, not elsewhere classified
748.4 Congenital cystic lung
748.5 Congenital agenesis, hypoplasia, and dysplasia of lung
770.3 Pulmonary hemorrhage of fetus or newborn
786.09 Other dyspnea and respiratory abnormalities
909.1 Late effect of toxic effects of nonmedical substances
947.1 Burn of larynx, trachea, and lung
V15.82 Personal history of tobacco use, presenting hazards to health

ICD-9-CM Procedural

00.91 Transplant from live related donor
00.92 Transplant from live non-related donor
00.93 Transplant from cadaver
33.50 Lung transplantation, NOS
33.51 Unilateral lung transplantation
33.52 Bilateral lung transplantation
39.61 Extracorporeal circulation auxiliary to open heart surgery

32855–32856

32855 Backbench standard preparation of cadaver donor lung allograft prior to transplantation, including dissection of allograft from surrounding soft tissues to prepare pulmonary venous/atrial cuff, pulmonary artery, and bronchus; unilateral
32856 bilateral

ICD-9-CM Diagnostic

162.2 Malignant neoplasm of main bronchus
162.3 Malignant neoplasm of upper lobe, bronchus, or lung
162.4 Malignant neoplasm of middle lobe, bronchus, or lung
162.5 Malignant neoplasm of lower lobe, bronchus, or lung
162.8 Malignant neoplasm of other parts of bronchus or lung
162.9 Malignant neoplasm of bronchus and lung, unspecified site ▽
163.0 Malignant neoplasm of parietal pleura
163.1 Malignant neoplasm of visceral pleura
163.8 Malignant neoplasm of other specified sites of pleura
197.0 Secondary malignant neoplasm of lung
231.2 Carcinoma in situ of bronchus and lung
235.7 Neoplasm of uncertain behavior of trachea, bronchus, and lung
239.1 Neoplasm of unspecified nature of respiratory system
273.4 Alpha-1-antitrypsin deficiency
277.00 Cystic fibrosis without mention of meconium ileus — (Use additional code to identify any associated mental retardation)
277.02 Cystic fibrosis with pulmonary manifestations — (Use additional code to identify any associated mental retardation. Use additional code to identify any infectious organism present)
277.03 Cystic fibrosis with gastrointestinal manifestations — (Use additional code to identify any associated mental retardation)
277.09 Cystic fibrosis with other manifestations — (Use additional code to identify any associated mental retardation)

▽ Unspecified code
♀ Female diagnosis
☒ Manifestation code
♂ Male diagnosis

500	Coal workers' pneumoconiosis
501	Asbestosis
502	Pneumoconiosis due to other silica or silicates
503	Pneumoconiosis due to other inorganic dust
506.4	Chronic respiratory conditions due to fumes and vapors — (Use additional E code to identify cause)
506.9	Unspecified respiratory conditions due to fumes and vapors — (Use additional E code to identify cause) ▽
508.1	Chronic and other pulmonary manifestations due to radiation — (Use additional E code to identify cause)
510.9	Empyema without mention of fistula — (Use additional code to identify infectious organism: 041.00-041.9)
513.0	Abscess of lung
515	Postinflammatory pulmonary fibrosis
516.0	Pulmonary alveolar proteinosis
516.3	Idiopathic fibrosing alveolitis
518.5	Pulmonary insufficiency following trauma and surgery
518.81	Acute respiratory failure
518.83	Chronic respiratory failure
518.89	Other diseases of lung, not elsewhere classified
519.1	Other diseases of trachea and bronchus, not elsewhere classified
748.4	Congenital cystic lung
748.5	Congenital agenesis, hypoplasia, and dysplasia of lung
770.3	Pulmonary hemorrhage of fetus or newborn
786.09	Other dyspnea and respiratory abnormalities
909.1	Late effect of toxic effects of nonmedical substances
947.1	Burn of larynx, trachea, and lung
V15.82	Personal history of tobacco use, presenting hazards to health

ICD-9-CM Procedural

00.93	Transplant from cadaver
33.51	Unilateral lung transplantation
33.52	Bilateral lung transplantation
33.99	Other operations on lung

32900

32900 Resection of ribs, extrapleural, all stages

ICD-9-CM Diagnostic

170.3	Malignant neoplasm of ribs, sternum, and clavicle
203.00	Multiple myeloma without mention of remission
213.3	Benign neoplasm of ribs, sternum, and clavicle
238.0	Neoplasm of uncertain behavior of bone and articular cartilage
730.18	Chronic osteomyelitis, other specified sites — (Use additional code to identify organism, 041.1)
733.20	Unspecified cyst of bone (localized) ▽
737.34	Thoracogenic scoliosis
738.3	Acquired deformity of chest and rib
754.81	Pectus excavatum

ICD-9-CM Procedural

77.91	Total ostectomy of scapula, clavicle, and thorax (ribs and sternum)

32905–32906

32905 Thoracoplasty, Schede type or extrapleural (all stages);
32906 with closure of bronchopleural fistula

ICD-9-CM Diagnostic

510.0	Empyema with fistula — (Use additional code to identify infectious organism: 041.00-041.9)
510.9	Empyema without mention of fistula — (Use additional code to identify infectious organism: 041.00-041.9)
512.8	Other spontaneous pneumothorax
738.3	Acquired deformity of chest and rib
807.3	Open fracture of sternum
875.1	Open wound of chest (wall), complicated — (Use additional code to identify infection)

ICD-9-CM Procedural

33.34	Thoracoplasty
34.73	Closure of other fistula of thorax

32940

32940 Pneumonolysis, extraperiosteal, including filling or packing procedures

ICD-9-CM Diagnostic

137.0	Late effects of respiratory or unspecified tuberculosis
492.8	Other emphysema
510.9	Empyema without mention of fistula — (Use additional code to identify infectious organism: 041.00-041.9)
511.0	Pleurisy without mention of effusion or current tuberculosis
515	Postinflammatory pulmonary fibrosis
997.3	Respiratory complications — (Use additional code to identify complications)
V12.09	Personal history of other infectious and parasitic disease

ICD-9-CM Procedural

33.39	Other surgical collapse of lung

32960

32960 Pneumothorax, therapeutic, intrapleural injection of air

ICD-9-CM Diagnostic

511.1	Pleurisy with effusion, with mention of bacterial cause other than tuberculosis
512.1	Iatrogenic pneumothroax
513.0	Abscess of lung
786.3	Hemoptysis
997.3	Respiratory complications — (Use additional code to identify complications)

ICD-9-CM Procedural

33.32	Artificial pneumothorax for collapse of lung

32997

32997 Total lung lavage (unilateral)

ICD-9-CM Diagnostic

482.84	Legionnaires' disease
482.9	Unspecified bacterial pneumonia ▽
486	Pneumonia, organism unspecified ▽
506.0	Bronchitis and pneumonitis due to fumes and vapors — (Use additional E code to identify cause)
507.0	Pneumonitis due to inhalation of food or vomitus
507.1	Pneumonitis due to inhalation of oils and essences
507.8	Pneumonitis due to other solids and liquids
510.0	Empyema with fistula — (Use additional code to identify infectious organism: 041.00-041.9)
510.9	Empyema without mention of fistula — (Use additional code to identify infectious organism: 041.00-041.9)
513.0	Abscess of lung
860.1	Traumatic pneumothorax with open wound into thorax
860.3	Traumatic hemothorax with open wound into thorax
860.5	Traumatic pneumohemothorax with open wound into thorax
861.22	Lung laceration without mention of open wound into thorax
861.32	Lung laceration with open wound into thorax
862.8	Injury to multiple and unspecified intrathoracic organs without mention of open wound into cavity
862.9	Injury to multiple and unspecified intrathoracic organs with open wound into cavity
958.3	Posttraumatic wound infection not elsewhere classified

ICD-9-CM Procedural

96.05	Other intubation of respiratory tract

Cardiovascular System

Heart and Pericardium

33010–33015

33010	Pericardiocentesis; initial
33011	subsequent
33015	Tube pericardiostomy

ICD-9-CM Diagnostic

017.90	Tuberculosis of other specified organs, confirmation unspecified — (Use additional code to identify manifestation: 420.0, 422.0, 424.91)
039.8	Actinomycotic infection of other specified sites
066.8	Other specified arthropod-borne viral diseases — (Use additional code to identify any associated meningitis, 321.2)
164.1	Malignant neoplasm of heart
198.89	Secondary malignant neoplasm of other specified sites
212.7	Benign neoplasm of heart
238.8	Neoplasm of uncertain behavior of other specified sites
391.0	Acute rheumatic pericarditis
393	Chronic rheumatic pericarditis
411.0	Postmyocardial infarction syndrome — (Use additional code to identify presence of hypertension: 401.0-405.9)
420.0	Acute pericarditis in diseases classified elsewhere — (Code first underlying disease: 017.9, 039.8, 066.8, 585)
420.90	Unspecified acute pericarditis
420.91	Acute idiopathic pericarditis
420.99	Other acute pericarditis
423.0	Hemopericardium
423.1	Adhesive pericarditis
423.2	Constrictive pericarditis
423.8	Other specified diseases of pericardium
429.3	Cardiomegaly
585	Chronic renal failure — (Use additional code to identify manifestation: 357.4, 420.0)
786.59	Other chest pain
861.01	Heart contusion without mention of open wound into thorax

ICD-9-CM Procedural

37.0	Pericardiocentesis
37.12	Pericardiotomy

33020

33020	Pericardiotomy for removal of clot or foreign body (primary procedure)

ICD-9-CM Diagnostic

420.91	Acute idiopathic pericarditis
420.99	Other acute pericarditis
423.0	Hemopericardium
861.01	Heart contusion without mention of open wound into thorax
861.02	Heart laceration without penetration of heart chambers or mention of open wound into thorax
861.11	Heart contusion with open wound into thorax
861.12	Heart laceration without penetration of heart chambers, with open wound into thorax
862.8	Injury to multiple and unspecified intrathoracic organs without mention of open wound into cavity
862.9	Injury to multiple and unspecified intrathoracic organs with open wound into cavity
908.0	Late effect of internal injury to chest
926.11	Crushing injury of back — (Use additional code to identify any associated injuries: 800-829, 850.0-854.1, 860.0-869.1)
926.8	Crushing injury of multiple sites of trunk — (Use additional code to identify any associated injuries: 800-829, 850.0-854.1, 860.0-869.1)
996.00	Mechanical complication of unspecified cardiac device, implant, and graft
996.61	Infection and inflammatory reaction due to cardiac device, implant, and graft — (Use additional code to identify specified infections)

ICD-9-CM Procedural

37.12	Pericardiotomy

33025

33025	Creation of pericardial window or partial resection for drainage

ICD-9-CM Diagnostic

164.1	Malignant neoplasm of heart
198.89	Secondary malignant neoplasm of other specified sites
212.7	Benign neoplasm of heart
238.8	Neoplasm of uncertain behavior of other specified sites
239.8	Neoplasm of unspecified nature of other specified sites
391.0	Acute rheumatic pericarditis
411.0	Postmyocardial infarction syndrome — (Use additional code to identify presence of hypertension: 401.0-405.9)
420.0	Acute pericarditis in diseases classified elsewhere — (Code first underlying disease: 017.9, 039.8, 066.8, 585)
420.90	Unspecified acute pericarditis
420.91	Acute idiopathic pericarditis
420.99	Other acute pericarditis
423.0	Hemopericardium
423.1	Adhesive pericarditis
423.2	Constrictive pericarditis
423.8	Other specified diseases of pericardium
585	Chronic renal failure — (Use additional code to identify manifestation: 357.4, 420.0)
908.0	Late effect of internal injury to chest
909.2	Late effect of radiation
996.00	Mechanical complication of unspecified cardiac device, implant, and graft
996.61	Infection and inflammatory reaction due to cardiac device, implant, and graft — (Use additional code to identify specified infections)
998.59	Other postoperative infection — (Use additional code to identify infection)
V64.42	Thorascopic surgical procedure converted to open procedure

ICD-9-CM Procedural

37.12	Pericardiotomy

33030–33031

33030	Pericardiectomy, subtotal or complete; without cardiopulmonary bypass
33031	with cardiopulmonary bypass

ICD-9-CM Diagnostic

164.1	Malignant neoplasm of heart
198.89	Secondary malignant neoplasm of other specified sites
212.7	Benign neoplasm of heart
238.8	Neoplasm of uncertain behavior of other specified sites
239.8	Neoplasm of unspecified nature of other specified sites
391.0	Acute rheumatic pericarditis
411.0	Postmyocardial infarction syndrome — (Use additional code to identify presence of hypertension: 401.0-405.9)
420.0	Acute pericarditis in diseases classified elsewhere — (Code first underlying disease: 017.9, 039.8, 066.8, 585)
420.90	Unspecified acute pericarditis
420.91	Acute idiopathic pericarditis
420.99	Other acute pericarditis
423.0	Hemopericardium
423.1	Adhesive pericarditis
423.2	Constrictive pericarditis
423.8	Other specified diseases of pericardium
585	Chronic renal failure — (Use additional code to identify manifestation: 357.4, 420.0)
908.0	Late effect of internal injury to chest
909.2	Late effect of radiation
996.00	Mechanical complication of unspecified cardiac device, implant, and graft
996.61	Infection and inflammatory reaction due to cardiac device, implant, and graft — (Use additional code to identify specified infections)

998.59 Other postoperative infection — (Use additional code to identify infection)
V64.42 Thoracoscopic surgical procedure converted to open procedure

ICD-9-CM Procedural

37.31 Pericardiectomy
39.61 Extracorporeal circulation auxiliary to open heart surgery

33050

33050 Excision of pericardial cyst or tumor

ICD-9-CM Diagnostic

164.1 Malignant neoplasm of heart
198.89 Secondary malignant neoplasm of other specified sites
212.7 Benign neoplasm of heart
234.8 Carcinoma in situ of other specified sites
238.8 Neoplasm of uncertain behavior of other specified sites
239.8 Neoplasm of unspecified nature of other specified sites
423.8 Other specified diseases of pericardium
746.89 Other specified congenital anomaly of heart
V64.42 Thoracoscopic surgical procedure converted to open procedure

ICD-9-CM Procedural

37.33 Excision or destruction of other lesion or tissue of heart, open approach
39.61 Extracorporeal circulation auxiliary to open heart surgery

33120–33130

33120 Excision of intracardiac tumor, resection with cardiopulmonary bypass
33130 Resection of external cardiac tumor

ICD-9-CM Diagnostic

164.1 Malignant neoplasm of heart
198.89 Secondary malignant neoplasm of other specified sites
212.7 Benign neoplasm of heart
234.8 Carcinoma in situ of other specified sites
238.8 Neoplasm of uncertain behavior of other specified sites
239.8 Neoplasm of unspecified nature of other specified sites

ICD-9-CM Procedural

37.33 Excision or destruction of other lesion or tissue of heart, open approach
39.61 Extracorporeal circulation auxiliary to open heart surgery

33140–33141

33140 Transmyocardial laser revascularization, by thoracotomy (separate procedure)
33141 performed at the time of other open cardiac procedure(s) (List separately in addition to code for primary procedure)

ICD-9-CM Diagnostic

410.01 Acute myocardial infarction of anterolateral wall, initial episode of care — (Use additional code to identify presence of hypertension: 401.0-405.9)
410.02 Acute myocardial infarction of anterolateral wall, subsequent episode of care — (Use additional code to identify presence of hypertension: 401.0-405.9)
410.11 Acute myocardial infarction of other anterior wall, initial episode of care — (Use additional code to identify presence of hypertension: 401.0-405.9)
410.12 Acute myocardial infarction of other anterior wall, subsequent episode of care — (Use additional code to identify presence of hypertension: 401.0-405.9)
410.21 Acute myocardial infarction of inferolateral wall, initial episode of care — (Use additional code to identify presence of hypertension: 401.0-405.9)
410.22 Acute myocardial infarction of inferolateral wall, subsequent episode of care — (Use additional code to identify presence of hypertension: 401.0-405.9)
410.31 Acute myocardial infarction of inferoposterior wall, initial episode of care — (Use additional code to identify presence of hypertension: 401.0-405.9)
410.32 Acute myocardial infarction of inferoposterior wall, subsequent episode of care — (Use additional code to identify presence of hypertension: 401.0-405.9)
410.41 Acute myocardial infarction of other inferior wall, initial episode of care — (Use additional code to identify presence of hypertension: 401.0-405.9)
410.42 Acute myocardial infarction of other inferior wall, subsequent episode of care — (Use additional code to identify presence of hypertension: 401.0-405.9)
410.51 Acute myocardial infarction of other lateral wall, initial episode of care — (Use additional code to identify presence of hypertension: 401.0-405.9)
410.52 Acute myocardial infarction of other lateral wall, subsequent episode of care — (Use additional code to identify presence of hypertension: 401.0-405.9)
410.61 Acute myocardial infarction, true posterior wall infarction, initial episode of care — (Use additional code to identify presence of hypertension: 401.0-405.9)
410.62 Acute myocardial infarction, true posterior wall infarction, subsequent episode of care — (Use additional code to identify presence of hypertension: 401.0-405.9)
410.71 Acute myocardial infarction, subendocardial infarction, initial episode of care — (Use additional code to identify presence of hypertension: 401.0-405.9)
410.72 Acute myocardial infarction, subendocardial infarction, subsequent episode of care — (Use additional code to identify presence of hypertension: 401.0-405.9)
410.81 Acute myocardial infarction of other specified sites, initial episode of care — (Use additional code to identify presence of hypertension: 401.0-405.9)
410.82 Acute myocardial infarction of other specified sites, subsequent episode of care — (Use additional code to identify presence of hypertension: 401.0-405.9)
410.91 Acute myocardial infarction, unspecified site, initial episode of care — (Use additional code to identify presence of hypertension: 401.0-405.9) ▽
410.92 Acute myocardial infarction, unspecified site, subsequent episode of care — (Use additional code to identify presence of hypertension: 401.0-405.9) ▽
411.1 Intermediate coronary syndrome — (Use additional code to identify presence of hypertension: 401.0-405.9)
411.81 Acute coronary occlusion without myocardial infarction — (Use additional code to identify presence of hypertension: 401.0-405.9)
411.89 Other acute and subacute form of ischemic heart disease — (Use additional code to identify presence of hypertension: 401.0-405.9)
413.9 Other and unspecified angina pectoris — (Use additional code to identify presence of hypertension: 401.0-405.9) ▽
414.00 Coronary atherosclerosis of unspecified type of vessel, native or graft — (Use additional code to identify presence of hypertension: 401.0-405.9) ▽
414.01 Coronary atherosclerosis of native coronary artery — (Use additional code to identify presence of hypertension: 401.0-405.9)
414.02 Coronary atherosclerosis of autologous vein bypass graft — (Use additional code to identify presence of hypertension: 401.0-405.9)
414.03 Coronary atherosclerosis of nonautologous biological bypass graft — (Use additional code to identify presence of hypertension: 401.0-405.9)
414.04 Coronary atherosclerosis of artery bypass graft — (Use additional code to identify presence of hypertension: 401.0-405.9)
414.05 Coronary atherosclerosis of unspecified type of bypass graft — (Use additional code to identify presence of hypertension: 401.0-405.9) ▽
414.06 Coronary atherosclerosis, of native coronary artery of transplanted heart — (Use additional code to identify presence of hypertension: 401.0-405.9)
414.07 Coronary atherosclerosis, of bypass graft (artery) (vein) of transplanted heart — (Use additional code to identify presence of hypertension: 401.0-405.9)
414.10 Aneurysm of heart — (Use additional code to identify presence of hypertension: 401.0-405.9)
414.11 Aneurysm of coronary vessels — (Use additional code to identify presence of hypertension: 401.0-405.9)
414.12 Dissection of coronary artery — (Use additional code to identify presence of hypertension: 401.0-405.9)
414.19 Other aneurysm of heart — (Use additional code to identify presence of hypertension: 401.0-405.9)
414.8 Other specified forms of chronic ischemic heart disease — (Use additional code to identify presence of hypertension: 401.0-405.9)
414.9 Unspecified chronic ischemic heart disease — (Use additional code to identify presence of hypertension: 401.0-405.9) ▽
746.85 Congenital coronary artery anomaly

ICD-9-CM Procedural

36.31 Open chest transmyocardial revascularization

33200–33201

33200 Insertion of permanent pacemaker with epicardial electrode(s); by thoracotomy
33201 by xiphoid approach

ICD-9-CM Diagnostic

337.0 Idiopathic peripheral autonomic neuropathy
426.0 Atrioventricular block, complete
426.10 Unspecified atrioventricular block ▽
426.11 First degree atrioventricular block
426.12 Mobitz (type) II atrioventricular block
426.13 Other second degree atrioventricular block
426.6 Other heart block
426.7 Anomalous atrioventricular excitation
426.9 Unspecified conduction disorder ▽
427.0 Paroxysmal supraventricular tachycardia
427.31 Atrial fibrillation
427.81 Sinoatrial node dysfunction
427.89 Other specified cardiac dysrhythmias
746.86 Congenital heart block
996.01 Mechanical complication due to cardiac pacemaker (electrode)

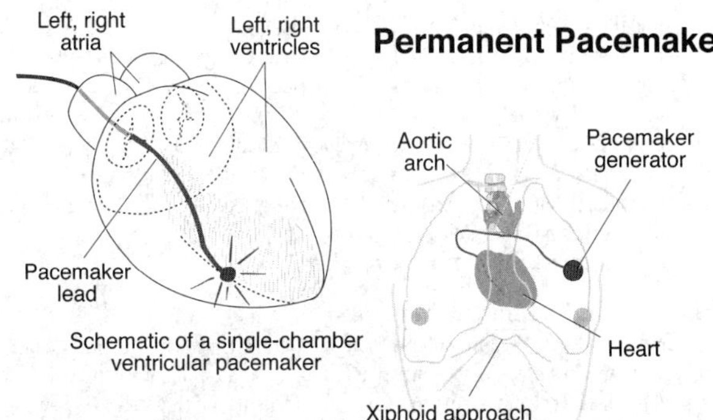

Permanent pacemakers are commonly delivered intravenously via the cephalic or subclavian veins; leads may be placed in an atrium or a ventricle, or both

996.61 Infection and inflammatory reaction due to cardiac device, implant, and graft — (Use additional code to identify specified infections)
V53.31 Fitting and adjustment of cardiac pacemaker

ICD-9-CM Procedural

00.50 Implantation of cardiac resynchronization pacemaker without mention of defibrillation, total system (CRT-P)
00.51 Implantation of cardiac resynchronization defibrillator, total system (CRT-D)
37.74 Insertion or replacement of epicardial lead (electrode) into epicardium
37.80 Insertion of permanent pacemaker, initial or replacement, type of device not specified
37.81 Initial insertion of single-chamber device, not specified as rate responsive
37.82 Initial insertion of single-chamber device, rate responsive

33206–33208

33206 Insertion or replacement of permanent pacemaker with transvenous electrode(s); atrial
33207 ventricular
33208 atrial and ventricular

ICD-9-CM Diagnostic

337.0 Idiopathic peripheral autonomic neuropathy
426.0 Atrioventricular block, complete
426.10 Unspecified atrioventricular block
426.11 First degree atrioventricular block
426.12 Mobitz (type) II atrioventricular block
426.13 Other second degree atrioventricular block
426.6 Other heart block
426.7 Anomalous atrioventricular excitation
426.9 Unspecified conduction disorder
427.0 Paroxysmal supraventricular tachycardia
427.31 Atrial fibrillation
427.81 Sinoatrial node dysfunction
427.89 Other specified cardiac dysrhythmias
427.9 Unspecified cardiac dysrhythmia
746.86 Congenital heart block
996.01 Mechanical complication due to cardiac pacemaker (electrode)
996.72 Other complications due to other cardiac device, implant, and graft
997.1 Cardiac complications — (Use additional code to identify complications)
V45.01 Cardiac pacemaker in situ — (This code is intended for use when these conditions are recorded as diagnoses or problems)
V45.09 Other specified cardiac device in situ — (This code is intended for use when these conditions are recorded as diagnoses or problems)
V53.31 Fitting and adjustment of cardiac pacemaker

ICD-9-CM Procedural

00.50 Implantation of cardiac resynchronization pacemaker without mention of defibrillation, total system (CRT-P)
00.51 Implantation of cardiac resynchronization defibrillator, total system (CRT-D)
37.71 Initial insertion of transvenous lead (electrode) into ventricle
37.72 Initial insertion of transvenous leads (electrodes) into atrium and ventricle
37.73 Initial insertion of transvenous lead (electrode) into atrium
37.76 Replacement of transvenous atrial and/or ventricular lead(s) (electrode(s))
37.80 Insertion of permanent pacemaker, initial or replacement, type of device not specified
37.83 Initial insertion of dual-chamber device

33210–33211

33210 Insertion or replacement of temporary transvenous single chamber cardiac electrode transvenous single chamber cardiac electrode or pacemaker catheter (separate procedure)
33211 Insertion or replacement of temporary transvenous dual chamber pacing electrodes (separate procedure)

ICD-9-CM Diagnostic

337.0 Idiopathic peripheral autonomic neuropathy
410.00 Acute myocardial infarction of anterolateral wall, episode of care unspecified — (Use additional code to identify presence of hypertension: 401.0-405.9)
410.01 Acute myocardial infarction of anterolateral wall, initial episode of care — (Use additional code to identify presence of hypertension: 401.0-405.9)
410.02 Acute myocardial infarction of anterolateral wall, subsequent episode of care — (Use additional code to identify presence of hypertension: 401.0-405.9)
410.10 Acute myocardial infarction of other anterior wall, episode of care unspecified — (Use additional code to identify presence of hypertension: 401.0-405.9)
410.11 Acute myocardial infarction of other anterior wall, initial episode of care — (Use additional code to identify presence of hypertension: 401.0-405.9)
410.12 Acute myocardial infarction of other anterior wall, subsequent episode of care — (Use additional code to identify presence of hypertension: 401.0-405.9)
410.20 Acute myocardial infarction of inferolateral wall, episode of care unspecified — (Use additional code to identify presence of hypertension: 401.0-405.9)
410.21 Acute myocardial infarction of inferolateral wall, initial episode of care — (Use additional code to identify presence of hypertension: 401.0-405.9)
410.22 Acute myocardial infarction of inferolateral wall, subsequent episode of care — (Use additional code to identify presence of hypertension: 401.0-405.9)
410.30 Acute myocardial infarction of inferoposterior wall, episode of care unspecified — (Use additional code to identify presence of hypertension: 401.0-405.9)
410.31 Acute myocardial infarction of inferoposterior wall, initial episode of care — (Use additional code to identify presence of hypertension: 401.0-405.9)
410.32 Acute myocardial infarction of inferoposterior wall, subsequent episode of care — (Use additional code to identify presence of hypertension: 401.0-405.9)
410.40 Acute myocardial infarction of other inferior wall, episode of care unspecified — (Use additional code to identify presence of hypertension: 401.0-405.9)
410.41 Acute myocardial infarction of other inferior wall, initial episode of care — (Use additional code to identify presence of hypertension: 401.0-405.9)
410.42 Acute myocardial infarction of other inferior wall, subsequent episode of care — (Use additional code to identify presence of hypertension: 401.0-405.9)
410.90 Acute myocardial infarction, unspecified site, episode of care unspecified — (Use additional code to identify presence of hypertension: 401.0-405.9)
426.0 Atrioventricular block, complete
426.10 Unspecified atrioventricular block
426.11 First degree atrioventricular block
426.12 Mobitz (type) II atrioventricular block
426.13 Other second degree atrioventricular block
426.51 Right bundle branch block and left posterior fascicular block
426.52 Right bundle branch block and left anterior fascicular block
426.53 Other bilateral bundle branch block
426.54 Trifascicular block
426.6 Other heart block
426.7 Anomalous atrioventricular excitation
426.9 Unspecified conduction disorder
427.0 Paroxysmal supraventricular tachycardia
427.31 Atrial fibrillation
427.32 Atrial flutter
427.5 Cardiac arrest
427.81 Sinoatrial node dysfunction
427.89 Other specified cardiac dysrhythmias
746.86 Congenital heart block
780.2 Syncope and collapse
785.1 Palpitations
785.51 Cardiogenic shock
785.9 Other symptoms involving cardiovascular system
972.1 Poisoning by cardiotonic glycosides and drugs of similar action — (Use additional code to specify the effects of the poisoning)
996.01 Mechanical complication due to cardiac pacemaker (electrode)
996.02 Mechanical complication due to heart valve prosthesis
996.03 Mechanical complication due to coronary bypass graft
996.04 Mechanical complication due to automatic implantable cardiac defibrillator
996.09 Mechanical complication of cardiac device, implant, and graft, other
996.72 Other complications due to other cardiac device, implant, and graft
997.1 Cardiac complications — (Use additional code to identify complications)
V45.01 Cardiac pacemaker in situ — (This code is intended for use when these conditions are recorded as diagnoses or problems)

V45.09 Other specified cardiac device in situ — (This code is intended for use when these conditions are recorded as diagnoses or problems)
V53.31 Fitting and adjustment of cardiac pacemaker

ICD-9-CM Procedural

00.50 Implantation of cardiac resynchronization pacemaker without mention of defibrillation, total system (CRT-P)
00.52 Implantation or replacement of transvenous lead (electrode) into left ventricular coronary venous system
37.72 Initial insertion of transvenous leads (electrodes) into atrium and ventricle
37.76 Replacement of transvenous atrial and/or ventricular lead(s) (electrode(s))
37.78 Insertion of temporary transvenous pacemaker system
39.64 Intraoperative cardiac pacemaker

33212–33213

33212 Insertion or replacement of pacemaker pulse generator only; single chamber, atrial or ventricular
33213 dual chamber

ICD-9-CM Diagnostic

996.01 Mechanical complication due to cardiac pacemaker (electrode)
996.09 Mechanical complication of cardiac device, implant, and graft, other
V45.01 Cardiac pacemaker in situ — (This code is intended for use when these conditions are recorded as diagnoses or problems)
V53.31 Fitting and adjustment of cardiac pacemaker

ICD-9-CM Procedural

00.50 Implantation of cardiac resynchronization pacemaker without mention of defibrillation, total system (CRT-P)
00.51 Implantation of cardiac resynchronization defibrillator, total system (CRT-D)
00.53 Implantation or replacement of cardiac resynchronization pacemaker pulse generator only (CRT-P)
37.75 Revision of lead (electrode)
37.76 Replacement of transvenous atrial and/or ventricular lead(s) (electrode(s))
37.81 Initial insertion of single-chamber device, not specified as rate responsive
37.82 Initial insertion of single-chamber device, rate responsive
37.83 Initial insertion of dual-chamber device
37.86 Replacement of any type of pacemaker device with single-chamber device, rate responsive

33214

33214 Upgrade of implanted pacemaker system, conversion of single chamber system to dual chamber system (includes removal of previously placed pulse generator, testing of existing lead, insertion of new lead, insertion of new pulse generator)

ICD-9-CM Diagnostic

996.01 Mechanical complication due to cardiac pacemaker (electrode)
996.09 Mechanical complication of cardiac device, implant, and graft, other
V45.01 Cardiac pacemaker in situ — (This code is intended for use when these conditions are recorded as diagnoses or problems)
V53.31 Fitting and adjustment of cardiac pacemaker

ICD-9-CM Procedural

00.50 Implantation of cardiac resynchronization pacemaker without mention of defibrillation, total system (CRT-P)
00.51 Implantation of cardiac resynchronization defibrillator, total system (CRT-D)
37.87 Replacement of any type of pacemaker device with dual-chamber device

33215–33217

33216 Insertion of a transvenous electrode; single chamber (one electrode) permanent pacemaker or single chamber pacing cardioverter-defibrillator
33217 dual chamber (two electrodes) permanent pacemaker or dual chamber pacing cardioverter-defibrillator
33215 Repositioning of previously implanted transvenous pacemaker or pacing cardioverter-defibrillator (right atrial or right ventricular) electrode

ICD-9-CM Diagnostic

996.01 Mechanical complication due to cardiac pacemaker (electrode)
996.09 Mechanical complication of cardiac device, implant, and graft, other
V45.01 Cardiac pacemaker in situ — (This code is intended for use when these conditions are recorded as diagnoses or problems)
V53.31 Fitting and adjustment of cardiac pacemaker

ICD-9-CM Procedural

00.52 Implantation or replacement of transvenous lead (electrode) into left ventricular coronary venous system
37.71 Initial insertion of transvenous lead (electrode) into ventricle
37.72 Initial insertion of transvenous leads (electrodes) into atrium and ventricle
37.73 Initial insertion of transvenous lead (electrode) into atrium
37.75 Revision of lead (electrode)
37.76 Replacement of transvenous atrial and/or ventricular lead(s) (electrode(s))
37.81 Initial insertion of single-chamber device, not specified as rate responsive
37.82 Initial insertion of single-chamber device, rate responsive
37.83 Initial insertion of dual-chamber device
37.99 Other operations on heart and pericardium

HCPCS Level II Supplies & Services

HCPCS Level II codes are used to report the supplies, durable medical equipment, and certain medical services provided on an outpatient basis. Because the procedure(s) represented on this page would be performed in an inpatient facility, no HCPCS Level II codes apply.

33218–33220

33218 Repair of single transvenous electrode for a single chamber, permanent pacemaker or single chamber pacing cardioverter-defibrillator
33220 Repair of two transvenous electrodes for a dual chamber permanent pacemaker or dual chamber pacing cardioverter-defibrillator

ICD-9-CM Diagnostic

996.01 Mechanical complication due to cardiac pacemaker (electrode)
996.04 Mechanical complication due to automatic implantable cardiac defibrillator
996.09 Mechanical complication of cardiac device, implant, and graft, other
V45.01 Cardiac pacemaker in situ — (This code is intended for use when these conditions are recorded as diagnoses or problems)
V53.31 Fitting and adjustment of cardiac pacemaker
V53.32 Fitting and adjustment of automatic implantable cardiac defibrillator

ICD-9-CM Procedural

37.75 Revision of lead (electrode)
37.76 Replacement of transvenous atrial and/or ventricular lead(s) (electrode(s))
37.89 Revision or removal of pacemaker device
37.99 Other operations on heart and pericardium

33222–33223

33222 Revision or relocation of skin pocket for pacemaker
33223 Revision of skin pocket for single or dual chamber pacing cardioverter-defibrillator

ICD-9-CM Diagnostic

996.61 Infection and inflammatory reaction due to cardiac device, implant, and graft — (Use additional code to identify specified infections)
996.72 Other complications due to other cardiac device, implant, and graft
998.51 Infected postoperative seroma — (Use additional code to identify organism)
998.59 Other postoperative infection — (Use additional code to identify infection)
998.6 Persistent postoperative fistula, not elsewhere classified
998.83 Non-healing surgical wound
998.89 Other specified complications

ICD-9-CM Procedural

37.79 Revision or relocation of pacemaker pocket
37.99 Other operations on heart and pericardium

33224

33224 Insertion of pacing electrode, cardiac venous system, for left ventricular pacing, with attachment to previously placed pacemaker or pacing cardioverter-defibrillator pulse generator (including revision of pocket, removal, insertion and/or replacement of generator)

ICD-9-CM Diagnostic

996.01 Mechanical complication due to cardiac pacemaker (electrode)
996.04 Mechanical complication due to automatic implantable cardiac defibrillator
996.09 Mechanical complication of cardiac device, implant, and graft, other
996.61 Infection and inflammatory reaction due to cardiac device, implant, and graft — (Use additional code to identify specified infections)
996.72 Other complications due to other cardiac device, implant, and graft
998.51 Infected postoperative seroma — (Use additional code to identify organism)
998.59 Other postoperative infection — (Use additional code to identify infection)
998.6 Persistent postoperative fistula, not elsewhere classified
998.83 Non-healing surgical wound
998.89 Other specified complications

Unspecified code
♀ Female diagnosis
Manifestation code
♂ Male diagnosis

V45.01 Cardiac pacemaker in situ — (This code is intended for use when these conditions are recorded as diagnoses or problems)
V53.32 Fitting and adjustment of automatic implantable cardiac defibrillator

ICD-9-CM Procedural

00.52 Implantation or replacement of transvenous lead (electrode) into left ventricular coronary venous system

HCPCS Level II Supplies & Services

HCPCS Level II codes are used to report the supplies, durable medical equipment, and certain medical services provided on an outpatient basis. Because the procedure(s) represented on this page would be performed in an inpatient facility, no HCPCS Level II codes apply.

33225

33225 Insertion of pacing electrode, cardiac venous system, for left ventricular pacing, at time of insertion of pacing cardioverter-defibrillator or pacemaker pulse generator (including upgrade to dual chamber system) (List separately in addition to code for primary procedure)

ICD-9-CM Diagnostic

This is an add-on code. Refer to the corresponding primary procedure code for ICD-9 diagnosis code links.

ICD-9-CM Procedural

00.52 Implantation or replacement of transvenous lead (electrode) into left ventricular coronary venous system

HCPCS Level II Supplies & Services

The HCPCS Level II code(s) would be the same as the actual procedure performed because these are in-addition-to codes.

33226

33226 Repositioning of previously implanted cardiac venous system (left ventricular) electrode (including removal, insertion and/or replacement of generator)

ICD-9-CM Diagnostic

996.01 Mechanical complication due to cardiac pacemaker (electrode)
996.04 Mechanical complication due to automatic implantable cardiac defibrillator
996.09 Mechanical complication of cardiac device, implant, and graft, other
V45.01 Cardiac pacemaker in situ — (This code is intended for use when these conditions are recorded as diagnoses or problems)
V53.32 Fitting and adjustment of automatic implantable cardiac defibrillator

ICD-9-CM Procedural

37.99 Other operations on heart and pericardium

HCPCS Level II Supplies & Services

HCPCS Level II codes are used to report the supplies, durable medical equipment, and certain medical services provided on an outpatient basis. Because the procedure(s) represented on this page would be performed in an inpatient facility, no HCPCS Level II codes apply.

33233

33233 Removal of permanent pacemaker pulse generator

ICD-9-CM Diagnostic

996.01 Mechanical complication due to cardiac pacemaker (electrode)
996.61 Infection and inflammatory reaction due to cardiac device, implant, and graft — (Use additional code to identify specified infections)

ICD-9-CM Procedural

37.89 Revision or removal of pacemaker device

33234–33235

33234 Removal of transvenous pacemaker electrode(s); single lead system, atrial or ventricular
33235 dual lead system

ICD-9-CM Diagnostic

996.01 Mechanical complication due to cardiac pacemaker (electrode)
996.61 Infection and inflammatory reaction due to cardiac device, implant, and graft — (Use additional code to identify specified infections)

ICD-9-CM Procedural

37.77 Removal of lead(s) (electrodes) without replacement
37.89 Revision or removal of pacemaker device

33236–33238

33236 Removal of permanent epicardial pacemaker and electrodes by thoracotomy; single lead system, atrial or ventricular
33237 dual lead system
33238 Removal of permanent transvenous electrode(s) by thoracotomy

ICD-9-CM Diagnostic

996.01 Mechanical complication due to cardiac pacemaker (electrode)
996.61 Infection and inflammatory reaction due to cardiac device, implant, and graft — (Use additional code to identify specified infections)

ICD-9-CM Procedural

37.77 Removal of lead(s) (electrodes) without replacement
37.89 Revision or removal of pacemaker device

33240–33241

33240 Insertion of single or dual chamber pacing cardioverter-defibrillator pulse generator
33241 Subcutaneous removal of single or dual chamber pacing cardioverter-defibrillator pulse generator

ICD-9-CM Diagnostic

996.04 Mechanical complication due to automatic implantable cardiac defibrillator
996.61 Infection and inflammatory reaction due to cardiac device, implant, and graft — (Use additional code to identify specified infections)
V53.32 Fitting and adjustment of automatic implantable cardiac defibrillator

ICD-9-CM Procedural

00.51 Implantation of cardiac resynchronization defibrillator, total system (CRT-D)
00.54 Implantation or replacement of cardiac resynchronization defibrillator pulse generator device only (CRT-D)
37.95 Implantation of automatic cardioverter/defibrillator leads(s) only
37.96 Implantation of automatic cardioverter/defibrillator pulse generator only
37.98 Replacement of automatic cardioverter/defibrillator pulse generator only
37.99 Other operations on heart and pericardium

33243–33244

33243 Removal of single or dual chamber pacing cardioverter-defibrillator electrode(s); by thoracotomy
33244 by transvenous extraction

ICD-9-CM Diagnostic

996.04 Mechanical complication due to automatic implantable cardiac defibrillator
996.61 Infection and inflammatory reaction due to cardiac device, implant, and graft — (Use additional code to identify specified infections)
V53.32 Fitting and adjustment of automatic implantable cardiac defibrillator

ICD-9-CM Procedural

37.99 Other operations on heart and pericardium

33245–33246

33245 Insertion of epicardial single or dual chamber pacing cardioverter-defibrillator electrodes by thoracotomy;
33246 with insertion of pulse generator

ICD-9-CM Diagnostic

427.0 Paroxysmal supraventricular tachycardia
427.1 Paroxysmal ventricular tachycardia
427.41 Ventricular fibrillation
427.42 Ventricular flutter
427.5 Cardiac arrest
427.89 Other specified cardiac dysrhythmias
996.04 Mechanical complication due to automatic implantable cardiac defibrillator
996.61 Infection and inflammatory reaction due to cardiac device, implant, and graft — (Use additional code to identify specified infections)
V45.02 Automatic implantable cardiac defibrillator in situ — (This code is intended for use when these conditions are recorded as diagnoses or problems)
V53.32 Fitting and adjustment of automatic implantable cardiac defibrillator
V53.39 Fitting and adjustment of other cardiac device

ICD-9-CM Procedural

00.54 Implantation or replacement of cardiac resynchronization defibrillator pulse generator device only (CRT-D)

37.94 Implantation or replacement of automatic cardioverter/ defibrillator, total system (AICD)
37.95 Implantation of automatic cardioverter/defibrillator leads(s) only
37.97 Replacement of automatic cardioverter/defibrillator leads(s) only
37.99 Other operations on heart and pericardium

33249

33249 Insertion or repositioning of electrode lead(s) for single or dual chamber pacing cardioverter-defibrillator and insertion of pulse generator

ICD-9-CM Diagnostic

427.0 Paroxysmal supraventricular tachycardia
427.1 Paroxysmal ventricular tachycardia
427.41 Ventricular fibrillation
427.42 Ventricular flutter
427.5 Cardiac arrest
427.89 Other specified cardiac dysrhythmias
996.04 Mechanical complication due to automatic implantable cardiac defibrillator
996.61 Infection and inflammatory reaction due to cardiac device, implant, and graft — (Use additional code to identify specified infections)
V45.02 Automatic implantable cardiac defibrillator in situ — (This code is intended for use when these conditions are recorded as diagnoses or problems)
V53.32 Fitting and adjustment of automatic implantable cardiac defibrillator
V53.39 Fitting and adjustment of other cardiac device

ICD-9-CM Procedural

00.54 Implantation or replacement of cardiac resynchronization defibrillator pulse generator device only (CRT-D)
37.94 Implantation or replacement of automatic cardioverter/ defibrillator, total system (AICD)
37.96 Implantation of automatic cardioverter/defibrillator pulse generator only
37.98 Replacement of automatic cardioverter/defibrillator pulse generator only
37.99 Other operations on heart and pericardium

33250–33251

33250 Operative ablation of supraventricular arrhythmogenic focus or pathway (eg, Wolff-Parkinson-White, atrioventricular node re-entry), tract(s) and/or focus (foci); without cardiopulmonary bypass
33251 with cardiopulmonary bypass

ICD-9-CM Diagnostic

426.7 Anomalous atrioventricular excitation
427.41 Ventricular fibrillation
427.89 Other specified cardiac dysrhythmias

ICD-9-CM Procedural

37.33 Excision or destruction of other lesion or tissue of heart, open approach
39.61 Extracorporeal circulation auxiliary to open heart surgery

33253

33253 Operative incisions and reconstruction of atria for treatment of atrial fibrillation or atrial flutter (eg, maze procedure)

ICD-9-CM Diagnostic

427.0 Paroxysmal supraventricular tachycardia
427.31 Atrial fibrillation
427.32 Atrial flutter
427.89 Other specified cardiac dysrhythmias

ICD-9-CM Procedural

37.99 Other operations on heart and pericardium
39.61 Extracorporeal circulation auxiliary to open heart surgery

33261

33261 Operative ablation of ventricular arrhythmogenic focus with cardiopulmonary bypass

ICD-9-CM Diagnostic

426.81 Lown-Ganong-Levine syndrome
426.89 Other specified conduction disorder
427.0 Paroxysmal supraventricular tachycardia
427.1 Paroxysmal ventricular tachycardia
427.41 Ventricular fibrillation
427.42 Ventricular flutter
427.89 Other specified cardiac dysrhythmias

ICD-9-CM Procedural

37.33 Excision or destruction of other lesion or tissue of heart, open approach
39.61 Extracorporeal circulation auxiliary to open heart surgery

33282–33284

33282 Implantation of patient-activated cardiac event recorder
33284 Removal of an implantable, patient-activated cardiac event recorder

ICD-9-CM Diagnostic

337.0 Idiopathic peripheral autonomic neuropathy
426.0 Atrioventricular block, complete
426.10 Unspecified atrioventricular block
426.11 First degree atrioventricular block
426.12 Mobitz (type) II atrioventricular block
426.13 Other second degree atrioventricular block
426.6 Other heart block
426.7 Anomalous atrioventricular excitation
426.9 Unspecified conduction disorder
427.0 Paroxysmal supraventricular tachycardia
427.1 Paroxysmal ventricular tachycardia
427.31 Atrial fibrillation
427.32 Atrial flutter
427.41 Ventricular fibrillation
427.42 Ventricular flutter
427.5 Cardiac arrest
427.60 Unspecified premature beats
427.61 Supraventricular premature beats
427.69 Other premature beats
427.81 Sinoatrial node dysfunction
427.89 Other specified cardiac dysrhythmias
427.9 Unspecified cardiac dysrhythmia
746.86 Congenital heart block
780.2 Syncope and collapse
780.4 Dizziness and giddiness
785.0 Unspecified tachycardia
785.1 Palpitations
794.31 Nonspecific abnormal electrocardiogram (ecg) (ekg)
996.09 Mechanical complication of cardiac device, implant, and graft, other
996.61 Infection and inflammatory reaction due to cardiac device, implant, and graft — (Use additional code to identify specified infections)
996.72 Other complications due to other cardiac device, implant, and graft
997.1 Cardiac complications — (Use additional code to identify complications)
998.51 Infected postoperative seroma — (Use additional code to identify organism)
998.59 Other postoperative infection — (Use additional code to identify infection)
998.89 Other specified complications
V45.09 Other specified cardiac device in situ — (This code is intended for use when these conditions are recorded as diagnoses or problems)
V53.39 Fitting and adjustment of other cardiac device

ICD-9-CM Procedural

86.09 Other incision of skin and subcutaneous tissue

33300–33305

33300 Repair of cardiac wound; without bypass
33305 with cardiopulmonary bypass

ICD-9-CM Diagnostic

861.00 Unspecified injury to heart without mention of open wound into thorax
861.01 Heart contusion without mention of open wound into thorax
861.02 Heart laceration without penetration of heart chambers or mention of open wound into thorax
861.03 Heart laceration with penetration of heart chambers, without mention of open wound into thorax
861.10 Unspecified injury to heart with open wound into thorax
861.11 Heart contusion with open wound into thorax
861.12 Heart laceration without penetration of heart chambers, with open wound into thorax
861.13 Heart laceration with penetration of heart chambers and open wound into thorax
862.8 Injury to multiple and unspecified intrathoracic organs without mention of open wound into cavity
862.9 Injury to multiple and unspecified intrathoracic organs with open wound into cavity
998.2 Accidental puncture or laceration during procedure

Unspecified code
♀ Female diagnosis
Manifestation code
♂ Male diagnosis

ICD-9-CM Procedural

35.31 Operations on papillary muscle
35.32 Operations on chordae tendineae
37.4 Repair of heart and pericardium
39.61 Extracorporeal circulation auxiliary to open heart surgery

33310–33315

33310 Cardiotomy, exploratory (includes removal of foreign body, atrial or ventricular thrombus); without bypass
33315 with cardiopulmonary bypass

ICD-9-CM Diagnostic

410.00 Acute myocardial infarction of anterolateral wall, episode of care unspecified — (Use additional code to identify presence of hypertension: 401.0-405.9) ▽
410.01 Acute myocardial infarction of anterolateral wall, initial episode of care — (Use additional code to identify presence of hypertension: 401.0-405.9)
410.02 Acute myocardial infarction of anterolateral wall, subsequent episode of care — (Use additional code to identify presence of hypertension: 401.0-405.9)
410.10 Acute myocardial infarction of other anterior wall, episode of care unspecified — (Use additional code to identify presence of hypertension: 401.0-405.9) ▽
410.11 Acute myocardial infarction of other anterior wall, initial episode of care — (Use additional code to identify presence of hypertension: 401.0-405.9)
410.12 Acute myocardial infarction of other anterior wall, subsequent episode of care — (Use additional code to identify presence of hypertension: 401.0-405.9)
410.20 Acute myocardial infarction of inferolateral wall, episode of care unspecified — (Use additional code to identify presence of hypertension: 401.0-405.9) ▽
410.21 Acute myocardial infarction of inferolateral wall, initial episode of care — (Use additional code to identify presence of hypertension: 401.0-405.9)
410.22 Acute myocardial infarction of inferolateral wall, subsequent episode of care — (Use additional code to identify presence of hypertension: 401.0-405.9)
410.30 Acute myocardial infarction of inferoposterior wall, episode of care unspecified — (Use additional code to identify presence of hypertension: 401.0-405.9) ▽
410.31 Acute myocardial infarction of inferoposterior wall, initial episode of care — (Use additional code to identify presence of hypertension: 401.0-405.9)
410.32 Acute myocardial infarction of inferoposterior wall, subsequent episode of care — (Use additional code to identify presence of hypertension: 401.0-405.9)
410.40 Acute myocardial infarction of other inferior wall, episode of care unspecified — (Use additional code to identify presence of hypertension: 401.0-405.9) ▽
410.41 Acute myocardial infarction of other inferior wall, initial episode of care — (Use additional code to identify presence of hypertension: 401.0-405.9)
410.42 Acute myocardial infarction of other inferior wall, subsequent episode of care — (Use additional code to identify presence of hypertension: 401.0-405.9)
410.50 Acute myocardial infarction of other lateral wall, episode of care unspecified — (Use additional code to identify presence of hypertension: 401.0-405.9) ▽
410.51 Acute myocardial infarction of other lateral wall, initial episode of care — (Use additional code to identify presence of hypertension: 401.0-405.9)
410.52 Acute myocardial infarction of other lateral wall, subsequent episode of care — (Use additional code to identify presence of hypertension: 401.0-405.9)
410.60 Acute myocardial infarction, true posterior wall infarction, episode of care unspecified — (Use additional code to identify presence of hypertension: 401.0-405.9) ▽
410.61 Acute myocardial infarction, true posterior wall infarction, initial episode of care — (Use additional code to identify presence of hypertension: 401.0-405.9)
410.62 Acute myocardial infarction, true posterior wall infarction, subsequent episode of care — (Use additional code to identify presence of hypertension: 401.0-405.9)
410.70 Acute myocardial infarction, subendocardial infarction, episode of care unspecified — (Use additional code to identify presence of hypertension: 401.0-405.9) ▽
410.71 Acute myocardial infarction, subendocardial infarction, initial episode of care — (Use additional code to identify presence of hypertension: 401.0-405.9)
410.72 Acute myocardial infarction, subendocardial infarction, subsequent episode of care — (Use additional code to identify presence of hypertension: 401.0-405.9)
410.80 Acute myocardial infarction of other specified sites, episode of care unspecified — (Use additional code to identify presence of hypertension: 401.0-405.9) ▽
410.81 Acute myocardial infarction of other specified sites, initial episode of care — (Use additional code to identify presence of hypertension: 401.0-405.9)
410.82 Acute myocardial infarction of other specified sites, subsequent episode of care — (Use additional code to identify presence of hypertension: 401.0-405.9)
410.90 Acute myocardial infarction, unspecified site, episode of care unspecified — (Use additional code to identify presence of hypertension: 401.0-405.9) ▽
410.91 Acute myocardial infarction, unspecified site, initial episode of care — (Use additional code to identify presence of hypertension: 401.0-405.9) ▽
410.92 Acute myocardial infarction, unspecified site, subsequent episode of care — (Use additional code to identify presence of hypertension: 401.0-405.9) ▽
424.90 Endocarditis, valve unspecified, unspecified cause ▽
861.00 Unspecified injury to heart without mention of open wound into thorax ▽
861.01 Heart contusion without mention of open wound into thorax
861.02 Heart laceration without penetration of heart chambers or mention of open wound into thorax
861.03 Heart laceration with penetration of heart chambers, without mention of open wound into thorax
861.10 Unspecified injury to heart with open wound into thorax ▽
861.11 Heart contusion with open wound into thorax
861.12 Heart laceration without penetration of heart chambers, with open wound into thorax
861.13 Heart laceration with penetration of heart chambers and open wound into thorax
862.8 Injury to multiple and unspecified intrathoracic organs without mention of open wound into cavity
862.9 Injury to multiple and unspecified intrathoracic organs with open wound into cavity
998.2 Accidental puncture or laceration during procedure

ICD-9-CM Procedural

37.11 Cardiotomy
39.61 Extracorporeal circulation auxiliary to open heart surgery

33320–33322

33320 Suture repair of aorta or great vessels; without shunt or cardiopulmonary bypass
33321 with shunt bypass
33322 with cardiopulmonary bypass

ICD-9-CM Diagnostic

901.0 Thoracic aorta injury
901.2 Superior vena cava injury
901.40 Injury to unspecified pulmonary vessel(s) ▽
901.41 Pulmonary artery injury
901.42 Pulmonary vein injury
902.0 Abdominal aorta injury
902.10 Unspecified inferior vena cava injury ▽
998.2 Accidental puncture or laceration during procedure

ICD-9-CM Procedural

39.0 Systemic to pulmonary artery shunt
39.21 Caval-pulmonary artery anastomosis
39.23 Other intrathoracic vascular shunt or bypass
39.31 Suture of artery
39.32 Suture of vein
39.61 Extracorporeal circulation auxiliary to open heart surgery

33330–33335

33330 Insertion of graft, aorta or great vessels; without shunt, or cardiopulmonary bypass
33332 with shunt bypass
33335 with cardiopulmonary bypass

ICD-9-CM Diagnostic

901.0 Thoracic aorta injury
901.2 Superior vena cava injury
901.40 Injury to unspecified pulmonary vessel(s) ▽
901.41 Pulmonary artery injury
901.42 Pulmonary vein injury
902.0 Abdominal aorta injury
902.10 Unspecified inferior vena cava injury ▽
998.2 Accidental puncture or laceration during procedure

ICD-9-CM Procedural

39.0 Systemic to pulmonary artery shunt
39.21 Caval-pulmonary artery anastomosis
39.23 Other intrathoracic vascular shunt or bypass
39.56 Repair of blood vessel with tissue patch graft
39.57 Repair of blood vessel with synthetic patch graft
39.58 Repair of blood vessel with unspecified type of patch graft
39.61 Extracorporeal circulation auxiliary to open heart surgery

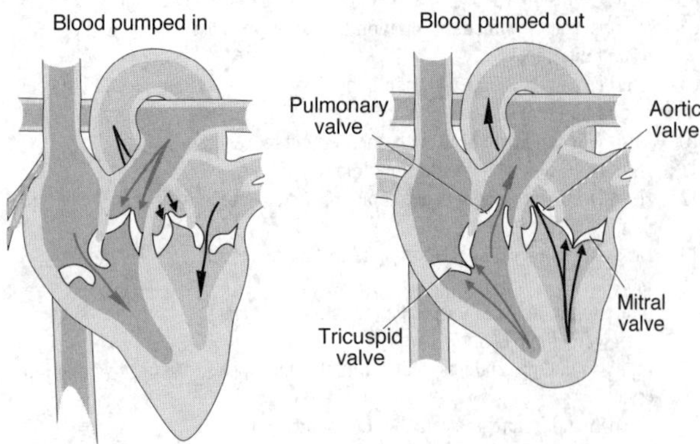

33400–33401

33400 Valvuloplasty, aortic valve; open, with cardiopulmonary bypass
33401 open, with inflow occlusion

ICD-9-CM Diagnostic

395.0 Rheumatic aortic stenosis
395.1 Rheumatic aortic insufficiency
395.2 Rheumatic aortic stenosis with insufficiency
424.1 Aortic valve disorders
446.7 Takayasu's disease
746.3 Congenital stenosis of aortic valve
747.22 Congenital atresia and stenosis of aorta

ICD-9-CM Procedural

35.11 Open heart valvuloplasty of aortic valve without replacement
39.61 Extracorporeal circulation auxiliary to open heart surgery

33403

33403 Valvuloplasty, aortic valve; using transventricular dilation, with cardiopulmonary bypass

ICD-9-CM Diagnostic

395.0 Rheumatic aortic stenosis
395.1 Rheumatic aortic insufficiency
395.2 Rheumatic aortic stenosis with insufficiency
424.1 Aortic valve disorders
446.7 Takayasu's disease
746.3 Congenital stenosis of aortic valve
747.22 Congenital atresia and stenosis of aorta

ICD-9-CM Procedural

35.11 Open heart valvuloplasty of aortic valve without replacement
39.61 Extracorporeal circulation auxiliary to open heart surgery

33404

33404 Construction of apical-aortic conduit

ICD-9-CM Diagnostic

395.0 Rheumatic aortic stenosis
395.1 Rheumatic aortic insufficiency
395.2 Rheumatic aortic stenosis with insufficiency
395.9 Other and unspecified rheumatic aortic diseases ▽
424.1 Aortic valve disorders
446.7 Takayasu's disease
746.3 Congenital stenosis of aortic valve
747.22 Congenital atresia and stenosis of aorta

ICD-9-CM Procedural

35.93 Creation of conduit between left ventricle and aorta
39.61 Extracorporeal circulation auxiliary to open heart surgery

33405–33410

33405 Replacement, aortic valve, with cardiopulmonary bypass; with prosthetic valve other than homograft or stentless valve
33406 with allograft valve (freehand)
33410 with stentless tissue valve

ICD-9-CM Diagnostic

395.0 Rheumatic aortic stenosis
395.1 Rheumatic aortic insufficiency
395.2 Rheumatic aortic stenosis with insufficiency
395.9 Other and unspecified rheumatic aortic diseases ▽
396.1 Mitral valve stenosis and aortic valve insufficiency
396.2 Mitral valve insufficiency and aortic valve stenosis
396.3 Mitral valve insufficiency and aortic valve insufficiency
396.8 Multiple involvement of mitral and aortic valves
424.1 Aortic valve disorders
424.90 Endocarditis, valve unspecified, unspecified cause ▽
746.3 Congenital stenosis of aortic valve
747.22 Congenital atresia and stenosis of aorta
862.9 Injury to multiple and unspecified intrathoracic organs with open wound into cavity
996.02 Mechanical complication due to heart valve prosthesis
996.61 Infection and inflammatory reaction due to cardiac device, implant, and graft — (Use additional code to identify specified infections)
996.71 Other complications due to heart valve prosthesis

ICD-9-CM Procedural

35.21 Replacement of aortic valve with tissue graft
35.22 Other replacement of aortic valve
39.61 Extracorporeal circulation auxiliary to open heart surgery

33411–33412

33411 Replacement, aortic valve; with aortic annulus enlargement, noncoronary cusp
33412 with transventricular aortic annulus enlargement (Konno procedure)

ICD-9-CM Diagnostic

395.0 Rheumatic aortic stenosis
395.1 Rheumatic aortic insufficiency
395.2 Rheumatic aortic stenosis with insufficiency
395.9 Other and unspecified rheumatic aortic diseases ▽
396.1 Mitral valve stenosis and aortic valve insufficiency
396.2 Mitral valve insufficiency and aortic valve stenosis
396.3 Mitral valve insufficiency and aortic valve insufficiency
396.8 Multiple involvement of mitral and aortic valves
424.1 Aortic valve disorders
424.90 Endocarditis, valve unspecified, unspecified cause ▽
746.3 Congenital stenosis of aortic valve
747.22 Congenital atresia and stenosis of aorta
862.9 Injury to multiple and unspecified intrathoracic organs with open wound into cavity
996.02 Mechanical complication due to heart valve prosthesis
996.61 Infection and inflammatory reaction due to cardiac device, implant, and graft — (Use additional code to identify specified infections)
996.71 Other complications due to heart valve prosthesis

ICD-9-CM Procedural

35.21 Replacement of aortic valve with tissue graft
35.22 Other replacement of aortic valve
35.33 Annuloplasty
39.61 Extracorporeal circulation auxiliary to open heart surgery

33413

33413 Replacement, aortic valve; by translocation of autologous pulmonary valve with allograft replacement of pulmonary valve (Ross procedure)

ICD-9-CM Diagnostic

395.0 Rheumatic aortic stenosis
395.1 Rheumatic aortic insufficiency
395.2 Rheumatic aortic stenosis with insufficiency
395.9 Other and unspecified rheumatic aortic diseases ▽
396.1 Mitral valve stenosis and aortic valve insufficiency
396.2 Mitral valve insufficiency and aortic valve stenosis
396.3 Mitral valve insufficiency and aortic valve insufficiency
396.8 Multiple involvement of mitral and aortic valves
424.1 Aortic valve disorders
424.90 Endocarditis, valve unspecified, unspecified cause ▽

▽ Unspecified code
♀ Female diagnosis
☒ Manifestation code
♂ Male diagnosis

746.3 Congenital stenosis of aortic valve
747.22 Congenital atresia and stenosis of aorta
862.9 Injury to multiple and unspecified intrathoracic organs with open wound into cavity
996.02 Mechanical complication due to heart valve prosthesis
996.61 Infection and inflammatory reaction due to cardiac device, implant, and graft — (Use additional code to identify specified infections)
996.71 Other complications due to heart valve prosthesis

ICD-9-CM Procedural
35.21 Replacement of aortic valve with tissue graft
35.25 Replacement of pulmonary valve with tissue graft
35.33 Annuloplasty
39.61 Extracorporeal circulation auxiliary to open heart surgery

33414
33414 Repair of left ventricular outflow tract obstruction by patch enlargement of the outflow tract

ICD-9-CM Diagnostic
395.0 Rheumatic aortic stenosis
395.1 Rheumatic aortic insufficiency
395.2 Rheumatic aortic stenosis with insufficiency
395.9 Other and unspecified rheumatic aortic diseases ▽
424.1 Aortic valve disorders
746.3 Congenital stenosis of aortic valve
747.22 Congenital atresia and stenosis of aorta

ICD-9-CM Procedural
35.35 Operations on trabeculae carneae cordis
35.98 Other operations on septa of heart
39.61 Extracorporeal circulation auxiliary to open heart surgery

33415–33416
33415 Resection or incision of subvalvular tissue for discrete subvalvular aortic stenosis
33416 Ventriculomyotomy (-myectomy) for idiopathic hypertrophic subaortic stenosis (eg, asymmetric septal hypertrophy)

ICD-9-CM Diagnostic
395.0 Rheumatic aortic stenosis
395.1 Rheumatic aortic insufficiency
395.2 Rheumatic aortic stenosis with insufficiency
395.9 Other and unspecified rheumatic aortic diseases ▽
424.1 Aortic valve disorders
746.3 Congenital stenosis of aortic valve
747.22 Congenital atresia and stenosis of aorta

ICD-9-CM Procedural
35.35 Operations on trabeculae carneae cordis
37.11 Cardiotomy
39.61 Extracorporeal circulation auxiliary to open heart surgery

33417
33417 Aortoplasty (gusset) for supravalvular stenosis

ICD-9-CM Diagnostic
395.0 Rheumatic aortic stenosis
395.1 Rheumatic aortic insufficiency
395.2 Rheumatic aortic stenosis with insufficiency
395.9 Other and unspecified rheumatic aortic diseases ▽
424.1 Aortic valve disorders
746.3 Congenital stenosis of aortic valve
747.22 Congenital atresia and stenosis of aorta

ICD-9-CM Procedural
35.11 Open heart valvuloplasty of aortic valve without replacement
39.61 Extracorporeal circulation auxiliary to open heart surgery

33420–33422
33420 Valvotomy, mitral valve; closed heart
33422 open heart, with cardiopulmonary bypass

ICD-9-CM Diagnostic
394.0 Mitral stenosis
394.1 Rheumatic mitral insufficiency
394.2 Mitral stenosis with insufficiency
394.9 Other and unspecified mitral valve diseases ▽
396.1 Mitral valve stenosis and aortic valve insufficiency
396.2 Mitral valve insufficiency and aortic valve stenosis
396.3 Mitral valve insufficiency and aortic valve insufficiency
396.8 Multiple involvement of mitral and aortic valves
424.0 Mitral valve disorders
746.5 Congenital mitral stenosis
746.6 Congenital mitral insufficiency

ICD-9-CM Procedural
35.02 Closed heart valvotomy, mitral valve
35.12 Open heart valvuloplasty of mitral valve without replacement
39.61 Extracorporeal circulation auxiliary to open heart surgery

33425–33427
33425 Valvuloplasty, mitral valve, with cardiopulmonary bypass;
33426 with prosthetic ring
33427 radical reconstruction, with or without ring

ICD-9-CM Diagnostic
394.0 Mitral stenosis
394.1 Rheumatic mitral insufficiency
394.2 Mitral stenosis with insufficiency
394.9 Other and unspecified mitral valve diseases ▽
396.1 Mitral valve stenosis and aortic valve insufficiency
396.2 Mitral valve insufficiency and aortic valve stenosis
396.3 Mitral valve insufficiency and aortic valve insufficiency
396.8 Multiple involvement of mitral and aortic valves
424.0 Mitral valve disorders
746.5 Congenital mitral stenosis
746.6 Congenital mitral insufficiency

ICD-9-CM Procedural
35.12 Open heart valvuloplasty of mitral valve without replacement
35.23 Replacement of mitral valve with tissue graft
35.24 Other replacement of mitral valve
39.61 Extracorporeal circulation auxiliary to open heart surgery

33430
33430 Replacement, mitral valve, with cardiopulmonary bypass

ICD-9-CM Diagnostic
394.0 Mitral stenosis
394.1 Rheumatic mitral insufficiency
394.2 Mitral stenosis with insufficiency
394.9 Other and unspecified mitral valve diseases ▽
396.0 Mitral valve stenosis and aortic valve stenosis
396.1 Mitral valve stenosis and aortic valve insufficiency
396.2 Mitral valve insufficiency and aortic valve stenosis
396.3 Mitral valve insufficiency and aortic valve insufficiency
396.8 Multiple involvement of mitral and aortic valves
424.0 Mitral valve disorders
424.90 Endocarditis, valve unspecified, unspecified cause ▽
710.0 Systemic lupus erythematosus — (Use additional code to identify manifestation: 424.91, 581.81, 582.81, 583.81)
746.5 Congenital mitral stenosis
746.6 Congenital mitral insufficiency
996.02 Mechanical complication due to heart valve prosthesis
996.61 Infection and inflammatory reaction due to cardiac device, implant, and graft — (Use additional code to identify specified infections)
996.71 Other complications due to heart valve prosthesis

ICD-9-CM Procedural
35.23 Replacement of mitral valve with tissue graft
35.24 Other replacement of mitral valve
39.61 Extracorporeal circulation auxiliary to open heart surgery

33460–33464

33460 Valvectomy, tricuspid valve, with cardiopulmonary bypass
33463 Valvuloplasty, tricuspid valve; without ring insertion
33464 with ring insertion

ICD-9-CM Diagnostic

397.0 Diseases of tricuspid valve
424.2 Tricuspid valve disorders, specified as nonrheumatic
424.90 Endocarditis, valve unspecified, unspecified cause ▽
746.1 Congenital tricuspid atresia and stenosis
996.02 Mechanical complication due to heart valve prosthesis
996.61 Infection and inflammatory reaction due to cardiac device, implant, and graft — (Use additional code to identify specified infections)
996.71 Other complications due to heart valve prosthesis

ICD-9-CM Procedural

35.14 Open heart valvuloplasty of tricuspid valve without replacement
35.28 Other replacement of tricuspid valve
39.61 Extracorporeal circulation auxiliary to open heart surgery

33465

33465 Replacement, tricuspid valve, with cardiopulmonary bypass

ICD-9-CM Diagnostic

397.0 Diseases of tricuspid valve
424.2 Tricuspid valve disorders, specified as nonrheumatic
424.90 Endocarditis, valve unspecified, unspecified cause ▽
746.1 Congenital tricuspid atresia and stenosis
996.02 Mechanical complication due to heart valve prosthesis
996.61 Infection and inflammatory reaction due to cardiac device, implant, and graft — (Use additional code to identify specified infections)
996.71 Other complications due to heart valve prosthesis

ICD-9-CM Procedural

35.27 Replacement of tricuspid valve with tissue graft
35.28 Other replacement of tricuspid valve
39.61 Extracorporeal circulation auxiliary to open heart surgery

33468

33468 Tricuspid valve repositioning and plication for Ebstein anomaly

ICD-9-CM Diagnostic

746.2 Ebstein's anomaly

ICD-9-CM Procedural

35.14 Open heart valvuloplasty of tricuspid valve without replacement
39.61 Extracorporeal circulation auxiliary to open heart surgery

33470–33471

33470 Valvotomy, pulmonary valve, closed heart; transventricular
33471 via pulmonary artery

ICD-9-CM Diagnostic

424.3 Pulmonary valve disorders
424.90 Endocarditis, valve unspecified, unspecified cause ▽
746.02 Congenital stenosis of pulmonary valve
996.02 Mechanical complication due to heart valve prosthesis
996.61 Infection and inflammatory reaction due to cardiac device, implant, and graft — (Use additional code to identify specified infections)
996.71 Other complications due to heart valve prosthesis

ICD-9-CM Procedural

35.03 Closed heart valvotomy, pulmonary valve

33472–33474

33472 Valvotomy, pulmonary valve, open heart; with inflow occlusion
33474 with cardiopulmonary bypass

ICD-9-CM Diagnostic

424.3 Pulmonary valve disorders
424.90 Endocarditis, valve unspecified, unspecified cause ▽
746.02 Congenital stenosis of pulmonary valve
996.02 Mechanical complication due to heart valve prosthesis
996.61 Infection and inflammatory reaction due to cardiac device, implant, and graft — (Use additional code to identify specified infections)
996.71 Other complications due to heart valve prosthesis

ICD-9-CM Procedural

35.13 Open heart valvuloplasty of pulmonary valve without replacement
39.61 Extracorporeal circulation auxiliary to open heart surgery

33475

33475 Replacement, pulmonary valve

ICD-9-CM Diagnostic

424.3 Pulmonary valve disorders
424.90 Endocarditis, valve unspecified, unspecified cause ▽
746.02 Congenital stenosis of pulmonary valve
996.02 Mechanical complication due to heart valve prosthesis
996.61 Infection and inflammatory reaction due to cardiac device, implant, and graft — (Use additional code to identify specified infections)
996.71 Other complications due to heart valve prosthesis

ICD-9-CM Procedural

35.25 Replacement of pulmonary valve with tissue graft
35.26 Other replacement of pulmonary valve
39.61 Extracorporeal circulation auxiliary to open heart surgery

33476–33478

33476 Right ventricular resection for infundibular stenosis, with or without commissurotomy
33478 Outflow tract augmentation (gusset), with or without commissurotomy or infundibular resection

ICD-9-CM Diagnostic

746.02 Congenital stenosis of pulmonary valve
746.83 Congenital infundibular pulmonic stenosis
747.3 Congenital anomalies of pulmonary artery

ICD-9-CM Procedural

35.13 Open heart valvuloplasty of pulmonary valve without replacement
35.34 Infundibulectomy
39.61 Extracorporeal circulation auxiliary to open heart surgery

33496

33496 Repair of non-structural prosthetic valve dysfunction with cardiopulmonary bypass (separate procedure)

ICD-9-CM Diagnostic

996.02 Mechanical complication due to heart valve prosthesis
996.74 Other complications due to other vascular device, implant, and graft
V43.3 Heart valve replaced by other means — (This code is intended for use when these conditions are recorded as diagnoses or problems)

ICD-9-CM Procedural

35.95 Revision of corrective procedure on heart
39.61 Extracorporeal circulation auxiliary to open heart surgery

33500–33501

33500 Repair of coronary arteriovenous or arteriocardiac chamber fistula; with cardiopulmonary bypass
33501 without cardiopulmonary bypass

ICD-9-CM Diagnostic

414.19 Other aneurysm of heart — (Use additional code to identify presence of hypertension: 401.0-405.9)
746.85 Congenital coronary artery anomaly

ICD-9-CM Procedural

36.99 Other operations on vessels of heart
39.53 Repair of arteriovenous fistula
39.61 Extracorporeal circulation auxiliary to open heart surgery

33502–33504

33502 Repair of anomalous coronary artery; by ligation
33503 by graft, without cardiopulmonary bypass
33504 by graft, with cardiopulmonary bypass

ICD-9-CM Diagnostic

746.85 Congenital coronary artery anomaly

▽ Unspecified code ♀ Female diagnosis ☒ Manifestation code ♂ Male diagnosis

ICD-9-CM Procedural

36.99 Other operations on vessels of heart
39.61 Extracorporeal circulation auxiliary to open heart surgery

33505–33506

33505 Repair of anomalous coronary artery; with construction of intrapulmonary artery tunnel (Takeuchi procedure)
33506 by translocation from pulmonary artery to aorta

ICD-9-CM Diagnostic

746.85 Congenital coronary artery anomaly

ICD-9-CM Procedural

36.99 Other operations on vessels of heart
39.61 Extracorporeal circulation auxiliary to open heart surgery

33508

33508 Endoscopy, surgical, including video-assisted harvest of vein(s) for coronary artery bypass procedure (List separately in addition to code for primary procedure)

ICD-9-CM Diagnostic

410.00 Acute myocardial infarction of anterolateral wall, episode of care unspecified — (Use additional code to identify presence of hypertension: 401.0-405.9) ▽
410.01 Acute myocardial infarction of anterolateral wall, initial episode of care — (Use additional code to identify presence of hypertension: 401.0-405.9)
410.02 Acute myocardial infarction of anterolateral wall, subsequent episode of care — (Use additional code to identify presence of hypertension: 401.0-405.9)
410.10 Acute myocardial infarction of other anterior wall, episode of care unspecified — (Use additional code to identify presence of hypertension: 401.0-405.9) ▽
410.11 Acute myocardial infarction of other anterior wall, initial episode of care — (Use additional code to identify presence of hypertension: 401.0-405.9)
410.12 Acute myocardial infarction of other anterior wall, subsequent episode of care — (Use additional code to identify presence of hypertension: 401.0-405.9)
410.20 Acute myocardial infarction of inferolateral wall, episode of care unspecified — (Use additional code to identify presence of hypertension: 401.0-405.9) ▽
410.21 Acute myocardial infarction of inferolateral wall, initial episode of care — (Use additional code to identify presence of hypertension: 401.0-405.9)
410.22 Acute myocardial infarction of inferolateral wall, subsequent episode of care — (Use additional code to identify presence of hypertension: 401.0-405.9)
410.30 Acute myocardial infarction of inferoposterior wall, episode of care unspecified — (Use additional code to identify presence of hypertension: 401.0-405.9) ▽
410.31 Acute myocardial infarction of inferoposterior wall, initial episode of care — (Use additional code to identify presence of hypertension: 401.0-405.9)
410.32 Acute myocardial infarction of inferoposterior wall, subsequent episode of care — (Use additional code to identify presence of hypertension: 401.0-405.9)
410.40 Acute myocardial infarction of other inferior wall, episode of care unspecified — (Use additional code to identify presence of hypertension: 401.0-405.9) ▽
410.41 Acute myocardial infarction of other inferior wall, initial episode of care — (Use additional code to identify presence of hypertension: 401.0-405.9)
410.42 Acute myocardial infarction of other inferior wall, subsequent episode of care — (Use additional code to identify presence of hypertension: 401.0-405.9)
410.50 Acute myocardial infarction of other lateral wall, episode of care unspecified — (Use additional code to identify presence of hypertension: 401.0-405.9) ▽
410.51 Acute myocardial infarction of other lateral wall, initial episode of care — (Use additional code to identify presence of hypertension: 401.0-405.9)
410.52 Acute myocardial infarction of other lateral wall, subsequent episode of care — (Use additional code to identify presence of hypertension: 401.0-405.9)
410.60 Acute myocardial infarction, true posterior wall infarction, episode of care unspecified — (Use additional code to identify presence of hypertension: 401.0-405.9) ▽
410.61 Acute myocardial infarction, true posterior wall infarction, initial episode of care — (Use additional code to identify presence of hypertension: 401.0-405.9)
410.62 Acute myocardial infarction, true posterior wall infarction, subsequent episode of care — (Use additional code to identify presence of hypertension: 401.0-405.9)
410.70 Acute myocardial infarction, subendocardial infarction, episode of care unspecified — (Use additional code to identify presence of hypertension: 401.0-405.9) ▽
410.71 Acute myocardial infarction, subendocardial infarction, initial episode of care — (Use additional code to identify presence of hypertension: 401.0-405.9)
410.72 Acute myocardial infarction, subendocardial infarction, subsequent episode of care — (Use additional code to identify presence of hypertension: 401.0-405.9)
410.80 Acute myocardial infarction of other specified sites, episode of care unspecified — (Use additional code to identify presence of hypertension: 401.0-405.9) ▽
410.81 Acute myocardial infarction of other specified sites, initial episode of care — (Use additional code to identify presence of hypertension: 401.0-405.9)
410.82 Acute myocardial infarction of other specified sites, subsequent episode of care — (Use additional code to identify presence of hypertension: 401.0-405.9)
410.90 Acute myocardial infarction, unspecified site, episode of care unspecified — (Use additional code to identify presence of hypertension: 401.0-405.9) ▽
410.91 Acute myocardial infarction, unspecified site, initial episode of care — (Use additional code to identify presence of hypertension: 401.0-405.9) ▽
410.92 Acute myocardial infarction, unspecified site, subsequent episode of care — (Use additional code to identify presence of hypertension: 401.0-405.9) ▽
411.1 Intermediate coronary syndrome — (Use additional code to identify presence of hypertension: 401.0-405.9)
411.81 Acute coronary occlusion without myocardial infarction — (Use additional code to identify presence of hypertension: 401.0-405.9)
411.89 Other acute and subacute form of ischemic heart disease — (Use additional code to identify presence of hypertension: 401.0-405.9)
413.0 Angina decubitus — (Use additional code to identify presence of hypertension: 401.0-405.9)
413.1 Prinzmetal angina — (Use additional code to identify presence of hypertension: 401.0-405.9)
413.9 Other and unspecified angina pectoris — (Use additional code to identify presence of hypertension: 401.0-405.9) ▽
414.00 Coronary atherosclerosis of unspecified type of vessel, native or graft — (Use additional code to identify presence of hypertension: 401.0-405.9) ▽
414.01 Coronary atherosclerosis of native coronary artery — (Use additional code to identify presence of hypertension: 401.0-405.9)
414.02 Coronary atherosclerosis of autologous vein bypass graft — (Use additional code to identify presence of hypertension: 401.0-405.9)
414.03 Coronary atherosclerosis of nonautologous biological bypass graft — (Use additional code to identify presence of hypertension: 401.0-405.9)
414.04 Coronary atherosclerosis of artery bypass graft — (Use additional code to identify presence of hypertension: 401.0-405.9)
414.05 Coronary atherosclerosis of unspecified type of bypass graft — (Use additional code to identify presence of hypertension: 401.0-405.9) ▽
414.06 Coronary atherosclerosis, of native coronary artery of transplanted heart — (Use additional code to identify presence of hypertension: 401.0-405.9)
414.07 Coronary atherosclerosis, of bypass graft (artery) (vein) of transplanted heart — (Use additional code to identify presence of hypertension: 401.0-405.9)
414.10 Aneurysm of heart — (Use additional code to identify presence of hypertension: 401.0-405.9)
414.11 Aneurysm of coronary vessels — (Use additional code to identify presence of hypertension: 401.0-405.9)
414.12 Dissection of coronary artery — (Use additional code to identify presence of hypertension: 401.0-405.9)
414.19 Other aneurysm of heart — (Use additional code to identify presence of hypertension: 401.0-405.9)
414.8 Other specified forms of chronic ischemic heart disease — (Use additional code to identify presence of hypertension: 401.0-405.9)
414.9 Unspecified chronic ischemic heart disease — (Use additional code to identify presence of hypertension: 401.0-405.9) ▽
426.7 Anomalous atrioventricular excitation
428.0 Congestive heart failure, unspecified ▽
428.1 Left heart failure
428.20 Unspecified systolic heart failure ▽
428.21 Acute systolic heart failure
428.22 Chronic systolic heart failure
428.23 Acute on chronic systolic heart failure
428.30 Unspecified diastolic heart failure ▽
428.31 Acute diastolic heart failure
428.32 Chronic diastolic heart failure
428.33 Acute on chronic diastolic heart failure
428.40 Unspecified combined systolic and diastolic heart failure ▽
428.41 Acute combined systolic and diastolic heart failure
428.42 Chronic combined systolic and diastolic heart failure
428.43 Acute on chronic combined systolic and diastolic heart failure
428.9 Unspecified heart failure ▽
746.85 Congenital coronary artery anomaly
747.41 Total congenital anomalous pulmonary venous connection
996.03 Mechanical complication due to coronary bypass graft

ICD-9-CM Procedural

38.63 Other excision of upper limb vessels

HCPCS Level II Supplies & Services

The HCPCS Level II code(s) would be the same as the actual procedure performed because these are in-addition-to codes.

33510–33516

33510 Coronary artery bypass, vein only; single coronary venous graft
33511 two coronary venous grafts
33512 three coronary venous grafts
33513 four coronary venous grafts
33514 five coronary venous grafts
33516 six or more coronary venous grafts

ICD-9-CM Diagnostic

410.00 Acute myocardial infarction of anterolateral wall, episode of care unspecified — (Use additional code to identify presence of hypertension: 401.0-405.9) ▽
410.01 Acute myocardial infarction of anterolateral wall, initial episode of care — (Use additional code to identify presence of hypertension: 401.0-405.9)
410.02 Acute myocardial infarction of anterolateral wall, subsequent episode of care — (Use additional code to identify presence of hypertension: 401.0-405.9)
410.10 Acute myocardial infarction of other anterior wall, episode of care unspecified — (Use additional code to identify presence of hypertension: 401.0-405.9) ▽
410.11 Acute myocardial infarction of other anterior wall, initial episode of care — (Use additional code to identify presence of hypertension: 401.0-405.9)
410.12 Acute myocardial infarction of other anterior wall, subsequent episode of care — (Use additional code to identify presence of hypertension: 401.0-405.9)
410.20 Acute myocardial infarction of inferolateral wall, episode of care unspecified — (Use additional code to identify presence of hypertension: 401.0-405.9) ▽
410.21 Acute myocardial infarction of inferolateral wall, initial episode of care — (Use additional code to identify presence of hypertension: 401.0-405.9)
410.22 Acute myocardial infarction of inferolateral wall, subsequent episode of care — (Use additional code to identify presence of hypertension: 401.0-405.9)
410.30 Acute myocardial infarction of inferoposterior wall, episode of care unspecified — (Use additional code to identify presence of hypertension: 401.0-405.9) ▽
410.31 Acute myocardial infarction of inferoposterior wall, initial episode of care — (Use additional code to identify presence of hypertension: 401.0-405.9)
410.32 Acute myocardial infarction of inferoposterior wall, subsequent episode of care — (Use additional code to identify presence of hypertension: 401.0-405.9)
410.40 Acute myocardial infarction of other inferior wall, episode of care unspecified — (Use additional code to identify presence of hypertension: 401.0-405.9) ▽
410.41 Acute myocardial infarction of other inferior wall, initial episode of care — (Use additional code to identify presence of hypertension: 401.0-405.9)
410.42 Acute myocardial infarction of other inferior wall, subsequent episode of care — (Use additional code to identify presence of hypertension: 401.0-405.9)
410.50 Acute myocardial infarction of other lateral wall, episode of care unspecified — (Use additional code to identify presence of hypertension: 401.0-405.9) ▽
410.51 Acute myocardial infarction of other lateral wall, initial episode of care — (Use additional code to identify presence of hypertension: 401.0-405.9)
410.52 Acute myocardial infarction of other lateral wall, subsequent episode of care — (Use additional code to identify presence of hypertension: 401.0-405.9)
410.60 Acute myocardial infarction, true posterior wall infarction, episode of care unspecified — (Use additional code to identify presence of hypertension: 401.0-405.9) ▽
410.61 Acute myocardial infarction, true posterior wall infarction, initial episode of care — (Use additional code to identify presence of hypertension: 401.0-405.9)
410.62 Acute myocardial infarction, true posterior wall infarction, subsequent episode of care — (Use additional code to identify presence of hypertension: 401.0-405.9)
410.70 Acute myocardial infarction, subendocardial infarction, episode of care unspecified — (Use additional code to identify presence of hypertension: 401.0-405.9) ▽
410.71 Acute myocardial infarction, subendocardial infarction, initial episode of care — (Use additional code to identify presence of hypertension: 401.0-405.9)
410.72 Acute myocardial infarction, subendocardial infarction, subsequent episode of care — (Use additional code to identify presence of hypertension: 401.0-405.9)
410.80 Acute myocardial infarction of other specified sites, episode of care unspecified — (Use additional code to identify presence of hypertension: 401.0-405.9) ▽
410.81 Acute myocardial infarction of other specified sites, initial episode of care — (Use additional code to identify presence of hypertension: 401.0-405.9)
410.82 Acute myocardial infarction of other specified sites, subsequent episode of care — (Use additional code to identify presence of hypertension: 401.0-405.9)
410.90 Acute myocardial infarction, unspecified site, episode of care unspecified — (Use additional code to identify presence of hypertension: 401.0-405.9) ▽
410.91 Acute myocardial infarction, unspecified site, initial episode of care — (Use additional code to identify presence of hypertension: 401.0-405.9) ▽
410.92 Acute myocardial infarction, unspecified site, subsequent episode of care — (Use additional code to identify presence of hypertension: 401.0-405.9) ▽
411.1 Intermediate coronary syndrome — (Use additional code to identify presence of hypertension: 401.0-405.9)
411.81 Acute coronary occlusion without myocardial infarction — (Use additional code to identify presence of hypertension: 401.0-405.9)
411.89 Other acute and subacute form of ischemic heart disease — (Use additional code to identify presence of hypertension: 401.0-405.9)
413.0 Angina decubitus — (Use additional code to identify presence of hypertension: 401.0-405.9)
413.1 Prinzmetal angina — (Use additional code to identify presence of hypertension: 401.0-405.9)
413.9 Other and unspecified angina pectoris — (Use additional code to identify presence of hypertension: 401.0-405.9) ▽
414.00 Coronary atherosclerosis of unspecified type of vessel, native or graft — (Use additional code to identify presence of hypertension: 401.0-405.9) ▽
414.01 Coronary atherosclerosis of native coronary artery — (Use additional code to identify presence of hypertension: 401.0-405.9)
414.03 Coronary atherosclerosis of nonautologous biological bypass graft — (Use additional code to identify presence of hypertension: 401.0-405.9)
414.04 Coronary atherosclerosis of artery bypass graft — (Use additional code to identify presence of hypertension: 401.0-405.9)
414.05 Coronary atherosclerosis of unspecified type of bypass graft — (Use additional code to identify presence of hypertension: 401.0-405.9) ▽
414.06 Coronary atherosclerosis, of native coronary artery of transplanted heart — (Use additional code to identify presence of hypertension: 401.0-405.9)
414.07 Coronary atherosclerosis, of bypass graft (artery) (vein) of transplanted heart — (Use additional code to identify presence of hypertension: 401.0-405.9)
414.10 Aneurysm of heart — (Use additional code to identify presence of hypertension: 401.0-405.9)
414.11 Aneurysm of coronary vessels — (Use additional code to identify presence of hypertension: 401.0-405.9)
414.12 Dissection of coronary artery — (Use additional code to identify presence of hypertension: 401.0-405.9)
414.8 Other specified forms of chronic ischemic heart disease — (Use additional code to identify presence of hypertension: 401.0-405.9)
414.9 Unspecified chronic ischemic heart disease — (Use additional code to identify presence of hypertension: 401.0-405.9) ▽
426.7 Anomalous atrioventricular excitation
428.0 Congestive heart failure, unspecified ▽
428.1 Left heart failure
428.20 Unspecified systolic heart failure ▽
428.21 Acute systolic heart failure
428.22 Chronic systolic heart failure
428.23 Acute on chronic systolic heart failure
428.30 Unspecified diastolic heart failure ▽
428.31 Acute diastolic heart failure
428.32 Chronic diastolic heart failure
428.33 Acute on chronic diastolic heart failure
428.40 Unspecified combined systolic and diastolic heart failure ▽
428.41 Acute combined systolic and diastolic heart failure
428.42 Chronic combined systolic and diastolic heart failure
428.43 Acute on chronic combined systolic and diastolic heart failure
428.9 Unspecified heart failure ▽
746.85 Congenital coronary artery anomaly
747.41 Total congenital anomalous pulmonary venous connection
996.03 Mechanical complication due to coronary bypass graft

ICD-9-CM Procedural

36.11 (Aorto)coronary bypass of one coronary artery
36.12 (Aorto)coronary bypass of two coronary arteries
36.13 (Aorto)coronary bypass of three coronary arteries
36.14 (Aorto)coronary bypass of four or more coronary arteries
39.61 Extracorporeal circulation auxiliary to open heart surgery

33517–33523

33517 Coronary artery bypass, using venous graft(s) and arterial graft(s); single vein graft (list separately in addition to code for arterial graft)
33518 two venous grafts (list separately in addition to code for arterial graft)
33519 three venous grafts (list separately in addition to code for arterial graft)
33521 four venous grafts (list separately in addition to code for arterial graft)
33522 five venous grafts (list separately in addition to code for arterial graft)
33523 six or more venous grafts (list separately in addition to code for arterial graft)

ICD-9-CM Diagnostic

SUB2 This is designated as an add-on code by Ingenix only. Refer to the corresponding primary procedure code for ICD-9 diagnosis code links.

ICD-9-CM Procedural

36.11 (Aorto)coronary bypass of one coronary artery
36.12 (Aorto)coronary bypass of two coronary arteries

▽ Unspecified code ♀ Female diagnosis ☒ Manifestation code ♂ Male diagnosis

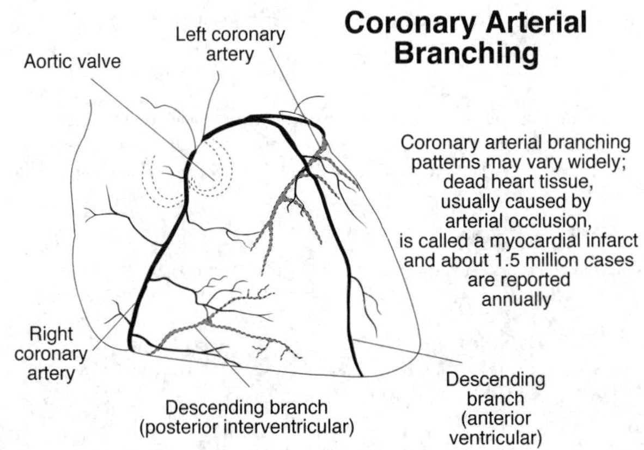
Coronary Arterial Branching
Left coronary artery
Aortic valve
Coronary arterial branching patterns may vary widely; dead heart tissue, usually caused by arterial occlusion, is called a myocardial infarct and about 1.5 million cases are reported annually
Right coronary artery
Descending branch (posterior interventricular)
Descending branch (anterior ventricular)

36.13 (Aorto)coronary bypass of three coronary arteries
36.14 (Aorto)coronary bypass of four or more coronary arteries
39.61 Extracorporeal circulation auxiliary to open heart surgery

33530

33530 Reoperation, coronary artery bypass procedure or valve procedure, more than one month after original operation (List separately in addition to code for primary procedure)

ICD-9-CM Diagnostic

This is an add-on code. Refer to the corresponding primary procedure code for ICD-9 diagnosis code links.

ICD-9-CM Procedural

35.99 Other operations on valves of heart
36.11 (Aorto)coronary bypass of one coronary artery
36.12 (Aorto)coronary bypass of two coronary arteries
36.13 (Aorto)coronary bypass of three coronary arteries
36.14 (Aorto)coronary bypass of four or more coronary arteries
39.61 Extracorporeal circulation auxiliary to open heart surgery

33533–33536

33533 Coronary artery bypass, using arterial graft(s); single arterial graft
33534 two coronary arterial grafts
33535 three coronary arterial grafts
33536 four or more coronary arterial grafts

ICD-9-CM Diagnostic

410.00 Acute myocardial infarction of anterolateral wall, episode of care unspecified — (Use additional code to identify presence of hypertension: 401.0-405.9)
410.01 Acute myocardial infarction of anterolateral wall, initial episode of care — (Use additional code to identify presence of hypertension: 401.0-405.9)
410.02 Acute myocardial infarction of anterolateral wall, subsequent episode of care — (Use additional code to identify presence of hypertension: 401.0-405.9)
410.10 Acute myocardial infarction of other anterior wall, episode of care unspecified — (Use additional code to identify presence of hypertension: 401.0-405.9)
410.11 Acute myocardial infarction of other anterior wall, initial episode of care — (Use additional code to identify presence of hypertension: 401.0-405.9)
410.12 Acute myocardial infarction of other anterior wall, subsequent episode of care — (Use additional code to identify presence of hypertension: 401.0-405.9)
410.20 Acute myocardial infarction of inferolateral wall, episode of care unspecified — (Use additional code to identify presence of hypertension: 401.0-405.9)
410.21 Acute myocardial infarction of inferolateral wall, initial episode of care — (Use additional code to identify presence of hypertension: 401.0-405.9)
410.22 Acute myocardial infarction of inferolateral wall, subsequent episode of care — (Use additional code to identify presence of hypertension: 401.0-405.9)
410.30 Acute myocardial infarction of inferoposterior wall, episode of care unspecified — (Use additional code to identify presence of hypertension: 401.0-405.9)
410.31 Acute myocardial infarction of inferoposterior wall, initial episode of care — (Use additional code to identify presence of hypertension: 401.0-405.9)
410.32 Acute myocardial infarction of inferoposterior wall, subsequent episode of care — (Use additional code to identify presence of hypertension: 401.0-405.9)
410.40 Acute myocardial infarction of other inferior wall, episode of care unspecified — (Use additional code to identify presence of hypertension: 401.0-405.9)
410.41 Acute myocardial infarction of other inferior wall, initial episode of care — (Use additional code to identify presence of hypertension: 401.0-405.9)
410.42 Acute myocardial infarction of other inferior wall, subsequent episode of care — (Use additional code to identify presence of hypertension: 401.0-405.9)
410.50 Acute myocardial infarction of other lateral wall, episode of care unspecified — (Use additional code to identify presence of hypertension: 401.0-405.9)
410.51 Acute myocardial infarction of other lateral wall, initial episode of care — (Use additional code to identify presence of hypertension: 401.0-405.9)
410.52 Acute myocardial infarction of other lateral wall, subsequent episode of care — (Use additional code to identify presence of hypertension: 401.0-405.9)
410.60 Acute myocardial infarction, true posterior wall infarction, episode of care unspecified — (Use additional code to identify presence of hypertension: 401.0-405.9)
410.61 Acute myocardial infarction, true posterior wall infarction, initial episode of care — (Use additional code to identify presence of hypertension: 401.0-405.9)
410.62 Acute myocardial infarction, true posterior wall infarction, subsequent episode of care — (Use additional code to identify presence of hypertension: 401.0-405.9)
410.70 Acute myocardial infarction, subendocardial infarction, episode of care unspecified — (Use additional code to identify presence of hypertension: 401.0-405.9)
410.71 Acute myocardial infarction, subendocardial infarction, initial episode of care — (Use additional code to identify presence of hypertension: 401.0-405.9)
410.72 Acute myocardial infarction, subendocardial infarction, subsequent episode of care — (Use additional code to identify presence of hypertension: 401.0-405.9)
410.80 Acute myocardial infarction of other specified sites, episode of care unspecified — (Use additional code to identify presence of hypertension: 401.0-405.9)
410.81 Acute myocardial infarction of other specified sites, initial episode of care — (Use additional code to identify presence of hypertension: 401.0-405.9)
410.82 Acute myocardial infarction of other specified sites, subsequent episode of care — (Use additional code to identify presence of hypertension: 401.0-405.9)
410.90 Acute myocardial infarction, unspecified site, episode of care unspecified — (Use additional code to identify presence of hypertension: 401.0-405.9)
410.91 Acute myocardial infarction, unspecified site, initial episode of care — (Use additional code to identify presence of hypertension: 401.0-405.9)
410.92 Acute myocardial infarction, unspecified site, subsequent episode of care — (Use additional code to identify presence of hypertension: 401.0-405.9)
411.1 Intermediate coronary syndrome — (Use additional code to identify presence of hypertension: 401.0-405.9)
411.81 Acute coronary occlusion without myocardial infarction — (Use additional code to identify presence of hypertension: 401.0-405.9)
411.89 Other acute and subacute form of ischemic heart disease — (Use additional code to identify presence of hypertension: 401.0-405.9)
413.0 Angina decubitus — (Use additional code to identify presence of hypertension: 401.0-405.9)
413.1 Prinzmetal angina — (Use additional code to identify presence of hypertension: 401.0-405.9)
413.9 Other and unspecified angina pectoris — (Use additional code to identify presence of hypertension: 401.0-405.9)
414.00 Coronary atherosclerosis of unspecified type of vessel, native or graft — (Use additional code to identify presence of hypertension: 401.0-405.9)
414.01 Coronary atherosclerosis of native coronary artery — (Use additional code to identify presence of hypertension: 401.0-405.9)
414.03 Coronary atherosclerosis of nonautologous biological bypass graft — (Use additional code to identify presence of hypertension: 401.0-405.9)
414.04 Coronary atherosclerosis of artery bypass graft — (Use additional code to identify presence of hypertension: 401.0-405.9)
414.05 Coronary atherosclerosis of unspecified type of bypass graft — (Use additional code to identify presence of hypertension: 401.0-405.9)
414.06 Coronary atherosclerosis, of native coronary artery of transplanted heart — (Use additional code to identify presence of hypertension: 401.0-405.9)
414.07 Coronary atherosclerosis, of bypass graft (artery) (vein) of transplanted heart — (Use additional code to identify presence of hypertension: 401.0-405.9)
414.10 Aneurysm of heart — (Use additional code to identify presence of hypertension: 401.0-405.9)
414.11 Aneurysm of coronary vessels — (Use additional code to identify presence of hypertension: 401.0-405.9)
414.12 Dissection of coronary artery — (Use additional code to identify presence of hypertension: 401.0-405.9)
414.8 Other specified forms of chronic ischemic heart disease — (Use additional code to identify presence of hypertension: 401.0-405.9)
414.9 Unspecified chronic ischemic heart disease — (Use additional code to identify presence of hypertension: 401.0-405.9)
426.7 Anomalous atrioventricular excitation
428.0 Congestive heart failure, unspecified
428.1 Left heart failure
428.20 Unspecified systolic heart failure
428.21 Acute systolic heart failure
428.22 Chronic systolic heart failure
428.23 Acute on chronic systolic heart failure

428.30 Unspecified diastolic heart failure ▽
428.31 Acute diastolic heart failure
428.32 Chronic diastolic heart failure
428.33 Acute on chronic diastolic heart failure
428.40 Unspecified combined systolic and diastolic heart failure ▽
428.41 Acute combined systolic and diastolic heart failure
428.42 Chronic combined systolic and diastolic heart failure
428.43 Acute on chronic combined systolic and diastolic heart failure
428.9 Unspecified heart failure ▽
746.85 Congenital coronary artery anomaly
747.41 Total congenital anomalous pulmonary venous connection
996.03 Mechanical complication due to coronary bypass graft

ICD-9-CM Procedural

36.15 Single internal mammary-coronary artery bypass
36.16 Double internal mammary-coronary artery bypass
36.17 Abdominal-coronary artery bypass
36.19 Other bypass anastomosis for heart revascularization
39.61 Extracorporeal circulation auxiliary to open heart surgery

33542

33542 Myocardial resection (eg, ventricular aneurysmectomy)

ICD-9-CM Diagnostic

414.10 Aneurysm of heart — (Use additional code to identify presence of hypertension: 401.0-405.9)
429.3 Cardiomegaly

ICD-9-CM Procedural

37.32 Excision of aneurysm of heart
37.33 Excision or destruction of other lesion or tissue of heart, open approach
39.61 Extracorporeal circulation auxiliary to open heart surgery

33545

33545 Repair of postinfarction ventricular septal defect, with or without myocardial resection

ICD-9-CM Diagnostic

410.10 Acute myocardial infarction of other anterior wall, episode of care unspecified — (Use additional code to identify presence of hypertension: 401.0-405.9) ▽
410.11 Acute myocardial infarction of other anterior wall, initial episode of care — (Use additional code to identify presence of hypertension: 401.0-405.9)
410.12 Acute myocardial infarction of other anterior wall, subsequent episode of care — (Use additional code to identify presence of hypertension: 401.0-405.9)
410.40 Acute myocardial infarction of other inferior wall, episode of care unspecified — (Use additional code to identify presence of hypertension: 401.0-405.9) ▽
410.41 Acute myocardial infarction of other inferior wall, initial episode of care — (Use additional code to identify presence of hypertension: 401.0-405.9)
410.42 Acute myocardial infarction of other inferior wall, subsequent episode of care — (Use additional code to identify presence of hypertension: 401.0-405.9)
410.90 Acute myocardial infarction, unspecified site, episode of care unspecified — (Use additional code to identify presence of hypertension: 401.0-405.9) ▽
410.92 Acute myocardial infarction, unspecified site, subsequent episode of care — (Use additional code to identify presence of hypertension: 401.0-405.9) ▽
414.00 Coronary atherosclerosis of unspecified type of vessel, native or graft — (Use additional code to identify presence of hypertension: 401.0-405.9) ▽
414.01 Coronary atherosclerosis of native coronary artery — (Use additional code to identify presence of hypertension: 401.0-405.9)
414.02 Coronary atherosclerosis of autologous vein bypass graft — (Use additional code to identify presence of hypertension: 401.0-405.9)
414.03 Coronary atherosclerosis of nonautologous biological bypass graft — (Use additional code to identify presence of hypertension: 401.0-405.9)
414.04 Coronary atherosclerosis of artery bypass graft — (Use additional code to identify presence of hypertension: 401.0-405.9)
414.05 Coronary atherosclerosis of unspecified type of bypass graft — (Use additional code to identify presence of hypertension: 401.0-405.9) ▽
414.06 Coronary atherosclerosis, of native coronary artery of transplanted heart — (Use additional code to identify presence of hypertension: 401.0-405.9)
414.07 Coronary atherosclerosis, of bypass graft (artery) (vein) of transplanted heart — (Use additional code to identify presence of hypertension: 401.0-405.9)
429.1 Myocardial degeneration — (Use additional code to identify presence of arteriosclerosis)

ICD-9-CM Procedural

35.72 Other and unspecified repair of ventricular septal defect
39.61 Extracorporeal circulation auxiliary to open heart surgery

33572

33572 Coronary endarterectomy, open, any method, of left anterior descending, circumflex, or right coronary artery performed in conjunction with coronary artery bypass graft procedure, each vessel (List separately in addition to primary procedure)

ICD-9-CM Diagnostic

This is an add-on code. Refer to the corresponding primary procedure code for ICD-9 diagnosis code links.

ICD-9-CM Procedural

36.03 Open chest coronary artery angioplasty
36.09 Other removal of coronary artery obstruction

33600–33602

33600 Closure of atrioventricular valve (mitral or tricuspid) by suture or patch
33602 Closure of semilunar valve (aortic or pulmonary) by suture or patch

ICD-9-CM Diagnostic

424.0 Mitral valve disorders
424.1 Aortic valve disorders
424.2 Tricuspid valve disorders, specified as nonrheumatic
424.3 Pulmonary valve disorders
745.60 Unspecified type congenital endocardial cushion defect ▽
745.61 Ostium primum defect
745.69 Other congenital endocardial cushion defect
745.7 Cor biloculare
746.00 Unspecified congenital pulmonary valve anomaly ▽
746.01 Congenital atresia of pulmonary valve
746.09 Other congenital anomalies of pulmonary valve
746.1 Congenital tricuspid atresia and stenosis
746.2 Ebstein's anomaly
746.4 Congenital insufficiency of aortic valve
746.6 Congenital mitral insufficiency
746.85 Congenital coronary artery anomaly

ICD-9-CM Procedural

35.11 Open heart valvuloplasty of aortic valve without replacement
35.12 Open heart valvuloplasty of mitral valve without replacement
35.13 Open heart valvuloplasty of pulmonary valve without replacement
35.14 Open heart valvuloplasty of tricuspid valve without replacement
39.59 Other repair of vessel
39.61 Extracorporeal circulation auxiliary to open heart surgery

33606

33606 Anastomosis of pulmonary artery to aorta (Damus-Kaye-Stansel procedure)

ICD-9-CM Diagnostic

745.10 Complete transposition of great vessels
745.11 Transposition of great vessels, double outlet right ventricle
745.2 Tetralogy of Fallot
746.01 Congenital atresia of pulmonary valve
746.7 Hypoplastic left heart syndrome

ICD-9-CM Procedural

39.0 Systemic to pulmonary artery shunt
39.61 Extracorporeal circulation auxiliary to open heart surgery

33608

33608 Repair of complex cardiac anomaly other than pulmonary atresia with ventricular septal defect by construction or replacement of conduit from right or left ventricle to pulmonary artery

ICD-9-CM Diagnostic

745.10 Complete transposition of great vessels
745.11 Transposition of great vessels, double outlet right ventricle
745.2 Tetralogy of Fallot

ICD-9-CM Procedural

35.72 Other and unspecified repair of ventricular septal defect
35.82 Total repair of total anomalous pulmonary venous connection
39.61 Extracorporeal circulation auxiliary to open heart surgery

▽ Unspecified code
♀ Female diagnosis

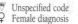

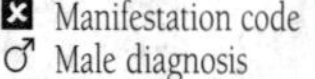
☒ Manifestation code
♂ Male diagnosis

33610

33610 Repair of complex cardiac anomalies (eg, single ventricle with subaortic obstruction) by surgical enlargement of ventricular septal defect

ICD-9-CM Diagnostic

745.3 Bulbus cordis anomalies and anomalies of cardiac septal closure, common ventricle

ICD-9-CM Procedural

35.42 Creation of septal defect in heart
39.61 Extracorporeal circulation auxiliary to open heart surgery

33611–33612

33611 Repair of double outlet right ventricle with intraventricular tunnel repair;
33612 with repair of right ventricular outflow tract obstruction

ICD-9-CM Diagnostic

745.11 Transposition of great vessels, double outlet right ventricle
745.3 Bulbus cordis anomalies and anomalies of cardiac septal closure, common ventricle
746.84 Congenital obstructive anomalies of heart, not elsewhere classified

ICD-9-CM Procedural

35.72 Other and unspecified repair of ventricular septal defect
39.61 Extracorporeal circulation auxiliary to open heart surgery

33615

33615 Repair of complex cardiac anomalies (eg, tricuspid atresia) by closure of atrial septal defect and anastomosis of atria or vena cava to pulmonary artery (simple Fontan procedure)

ICD-9-CM Diagnostic

745.5 Ostium secundum type atrial septal defect
745.61 Ostium primum defect
745.69 Other congenital endocardial cushion defect
746.01 Congenital atresia of pulmonary valve
746.1 Congenital tricuspid atresia and stenosis
746.2 Ebstein's anomaly
747.41 Total congenital anomalous pulmonary venous connection
747.42 Partial congenital anomalous pulmonary venous connection

ICD-9-CM Procedural

35.94 Creation of conduit between atrium and pulmonary artery
39.61 Extracorporeal circulation auxiliary to open heart surgery

33617

33617 Repair of complex cardiac anomalies (eg, single ventricle) by modified Fontan procedure

ICD-9-CM Diagnostic

745.3 Bulbus cordis anomalies and anomalies of cardiac septal closure, common ventricle
745.8 Other bulbus cordis anomalies and anomalies of cardiac septal closure
746.7 Hypoplastic left heart syndrome

ICD-9-CM Procedural

35.94 Creation of conduit between atrium and pulmonary artery
39.61 Extracorporeal circulation auxiliary to open heart surgery

33619

33619 Repair of single ventricle with aortic outflow obstruction and aortic arch hypoplasia (hypoplastic left heart syndrome) (eg, Norwood procedure)

ICD-9-CM Diagnostic

745.3 Bulbus cordis anomalies and anomalies of cardiac septal closure, common ventricle
745.8 Other bulbus cordis anomalies and anomalies of cardiac septal closure
746.7 Hypoplastic left heart syndrome

ICD-9-CM Procedural

39.29 Other (peripheral) vascular shunt or bypass
39.61 Extracorporeal circulation auxiliary to open heart surgery

33641

33641 Repair atrial septal defect, secundum, with cardiopulmonary bypass, with or without patch

ICD-9-CM Diagnostic

410.00 Acute myocardial infarction of anterolateral wall, episode of care unspecified — (Use additional code to identify presence of hypertension: 401.0-405.9) ▽
410.01 Acute myocardial infarction of anterolateral wall, initial episode of care — (Use additional code to identify presence of hypertension: 401.0-405.9)
410.02 Acute myocardial infarction of anterolateral wall, subsequent episode of care — (Use additional code to identify presence of hypertension: 401.0-405.9)
410.10 Acute myocardial infarction of other anterior wall, episode of care unspecified — (Use additional code to identify presence of hypertension: 401.0-405.9) ▽
410.11 Acute myocardial infarction of other anterior wall, initial episode of care — (Use additional code to identify presence of hypertension: 401.0-405.9)
410.12 Acute myocardial infarction of other anterior wall, subsequent episode of care — (Use additional code to identify presence of hypertension: 401.0-405.9)
410.20 Acute myocardial infarction of inferolateral wall, episode of care unspecified — (Use additional code to identify presence of hypertension: 401.0-405.9) ▽
410.21 Acute myocardial infarction of inferolateral wall, initial episode of care — (Use additional code to identify presence of hypertension: 401.0-405.9)
410.22 Acute myocardial infarction of inferolateral wall, subsequent episode of care — (Use additional code to identify presence of hypertension: 401.0-405.9)
410.30 Acute myocardial infarction of inferoposterior wall, episode of care unspecified — (Use additional code to identify presence of hypertension: 401.0-405.9) ▽
410.31 Acute myocardial infarction of inferoposterior wall, initial episode of care — (Use additional code to identify presence of hypertension: 401.0-405.9)
410.32 Acute myocardial infarction of inferoposterior wall, subsequent episode of care — (Use additional code to identify presence of hypertension: 401.0-405.9)
410.40 Acute myocardial infarction of other inferior wall, episode of care unspecified — (Use additional code to identify presence of hypertension: 401.0-405.9) ▽
410.41 Acute myocardial infarction of other inferior wall, initial episode of care — (Use additional code to identify presence of hypertension: 401.0-405.9)
410.42 Acute myocardial infarction of other inferior wall, subsequent episode of care — (Use additional code to identify presence of hypertension: 401.0-405.9)
410.50 Acute myocardial infarction of other lateral wall, episode of care unspecified — (Use additional code to identify presence of hypertension: 401.0-405.9) ▽
410.51 Acute myocardial infarction of other lateral wall, initial episode of care — (Use additional code to identify presence of hypertension: 401.0-405.9)
410.52 Acute myocardial infarction of other lateral wall, subsequent episode of care — (Use additional code to identify presence of hypertension: 401.0-405.9)
410.60 Acute myocardial infarction, true posterior wall infarction, episode of care unspecified — (Use additional code to identify presence of hypertension: 401.0-405.9) ▽
410.61 Acute myocardial infarction, true posterior wall infarction, initial episode of care — (Use additional code to identify presence of hypertension: 401.0-405.9)
410.62 Acute myocardial infarction, true posterior wall infarction, subsequent episode of care — (Use additional code to identify presence of hypertension: 401.0-405.9)
410.70 Acute myocardial infarction, subendocardial infarction, episode of care unspecified — (Use additional code to identify presence of hypertension: 401.0-405.9) ▽
410.71 Acute myocardial infarction, subendocardial infarction, initial episode of care — (Use additional code to identify presence of hypertension: 401.0-405.9)
410.72 Acute myocardial infarction, subendocardial infarction, subsequent episode of care — (Use additional code to identify presence of hypertension: 401.0-405.9)
410.80 Acute myocardial infarction of other specified sites, episode of care unspecified — (Use additional code to identify presence of hypertension: 401.0-405.9) ▽
410.81 Acute myocardial infarction of other specified sites, initial episode of care — (Use additional code to identify presence of hypertension: 401.0-405.9)
410.82 Acute myocardial infarction of other specified sites, subsequent episode of care — (Use additional code to identify presence of hypertension: 401.0-405.9)
410.90 Acute myocardial infarction, unspecified site, episode of care unspecified — (Use additional code to identify presence of hypertension: 401.0-405.9) ▽
410.91 Acute myocardial infarction, unspecified site, initial episode of care — (Use additional code to identify presence of hypertension: 401.0-405.9) ▽
410.92 Acute myocardial infarction, unspecified site, subsequent episode of care — (Use additional code to identify presence of hypertension: 401.0-405.9) ▽
414.8 Other specified forms of chronic ischemic heart disease — (Use additional code to identify presence of hypertension: 401.0-405.9)
429.71 Acquired cardiac septal defect — (Use additional code to identify the associated myocardial infarction: with onset of 8 weeks of less, 410.00-410.92; with onset of more than 8 weeks, 414.8)
745.5 Ostium secundum type atrial septal defect
745.61 Ostium primum defect

ICD-9-CM Procedural

35.51 Repair of atrial septal defect with prosthesis, open technique
35.61 Repair of atrial septal defect with tissue graft
35.71 Other and unspecified repair of atrial septal defect
39.61 Extracorporeal circulation auxiliary to open heart surgery

33645

33645 Direct or patch closure, sinus venosus, with or without anomalous pulmonary venous drainage

ICD-9-CM Diagnostic

410.00 Acute myocardial infarction of anterolateral wall, episode of care unspecified — (Use additional code to identify presence of hypertension: 401.0-405.9) ▽
410.01 Acute myocardial infarction of anterolateral wall, initial episode of care — (Use additional code to identify presence of hypertension: 401.0-405.9)
410.02 Acute myocardial infarction of anterolateral wall, subsequent episode of care — (Use additional code to identify presence of hypertension: 401.0-405.9)
410.10 Acute myocardial infarction of other anterior wall, episode of care unspecified — (Use additional code to identify presence of hypertension: 401.0-405.9) ▽
410.11 Acute myocardial infarction of other anterior wall, initial episode of care — (Use additional code to identify presence of hypertension: 401.0-405.9)
410.12 Acute myocardial infarction of other anterior wall, subsequent episode of care — (Use additional code to identify presence of hypertension: 401.0-405.9)
410.20 Acute myocardial infarction of inferolateral wall, episode of care unspecified — (Use additional code to identify presence of hypertension: 401.0-405.9) ▽
410.21 Acute myocardial infarction of inferolateral wall, initial episode of care — (Use additional code to identify presence of hypertension: 401.0-405.9)
410.22 Acute myocardial infarction of inferolateral wall, subsequent episode of care — (Use additional code to identify presence of hypertension: 401.0-405.9)
410.30 Acute myocardial infarction of inferoposterior wall, episode of care unspecified — (Use additional code to identify presence of hypertension: 401.0-405.9) ▽
410.31 Acute myocardial infarction of inferoposterior wall, initial episode of care — (Use additional code to identify presence of hypertension: 401.0-405.9)
410.32 Acute myocardial infarction of inferoposterior wall, subsequent episode of care — (Use additional code to identify presence of hypertension: 401.0-405.9)
410.40 Acute myocardial infarction of other inferior wall, episode of care unspecified — (Use additional code to identify presence of hypertension: 401.0-405.9) ▽
410.41 Acute myocardial infarction of other inferior wall, initial episode of care — (Use additional code to identify presence of hypertension: 401.0-405.9)
410.42 Acute myocardial infarction of other inferior wall, subsequent episode of care — (Use additional code to identify presence of hypertension: 401.0-405.9)
410.50 Acute myocardial infarction of other lateral wall, episode of care unspecified — (Use additional code to identify presence of hypertension: 401.0-405.9) ▽
410.51 Acute myocardial infarction of other lateral wall, initial episode of care — (Use additional code to identify presence of hypertension: 401.0-405.9)
410.52 Acute myocardial infarction of other lateral wall, subsequent episode of care — (Use additional code to identify presence of hypertension: 401.0-405.9)
410.60 Acute myocardial infarction, true posterior wall infarction, episode of care unspecified — (Use additional code to identify presence of hypertension: 401.0-405.9) ▽
410.61 Acute myocardial infarction, true posterior wall infarction, initial episode of care — (Use additional code to identify presence of hypertension: 401.0-405.9)
410.62 Acute myocardial infarction, true posterior wall infarction, subsequent episode of care — (Use additional code to identify presence of hypertension: 401.0-405.9)
410.70 Acute myocardial infarction, subendocardial infarction, episode of care unspecified — (Use additional code to identify presence of hypertension: 401.0-405.9) ▽
410.71 Acute myocardial infarction, subendocardial infarction, initial episode of care — (Use additional code to identify presence of hypertension: 401.0-405.9)
410.72 Acute myocardial infarction, subendocardial infarction, subsequent episode of care — (Use additional code to identify presence of hypertension: 401.0-405.9)
410.80 Acute myocardial infarction of other specified sites, episode of care unspecified — (Use additional code to identify presence of hypertension: 401.0-405.9) ▽
410.81 Acute myocardial infarction of other specified sites, initial episode of care — (Use additional code to identify presence of hypertension: 401.0-405.9)
410.82 Acute myocardial infarction of other specified sites, subsequent episode of care — (Use additional code to identify presence of hypertension: 401.0-405.9)
410.90 Acute myocardial infarction, unspecified site, episode of care unspecified — (Use additional code to identify presence of hypertension: 401.0-405.9) ▽
410.91 Acute myocardial infarction, unspecified site, initial episode of care — (Use additional code to identify presence of hypertension: 401.0-405.9) ▽
410.92 Acute myocardial infarction, unspecified site, subsequent episode of care — (Use additional code to identify presence of hypertension: 401.0-405.9) ▽
414.8 Other specified forms of chronic ischemic heart disease — (Use additional code to identify presence of hypertension: 401.0-405.9)
429.71 Acquired cardiac septal defect — (Use additional code to identify the associated myocardial infarction: with onset of 8 weeks of less, 410.00-410.92; with onset of more than 8 weeks, 414.8)
745.4 Ventricular septal defect
745.5 Ostium secundum type atrial septal defect
745.61 Ostium primum defect
745.8 Other bulbus cordis anomalies and anomalies of cardiac septal closure
745.9 Unspecified congenital defect of septal closure ▽
747.40 Congenital anomaly of great veins unspecified ▽
747.41 Total congenital anomalous pulmonary venous connection
747.42 Partial congenital anomalous pulmonary venous connection

ICD-9-CM Procedural

35.51 Repair of atrial septal defect with prosthesis, open technique
35.61 Repair of atrial septal defect with tissue graft
35.71 Other and unspecified repair of atrial septal defect
39.61 Extracorporeal circulation auxiliary to open heart surgery

33647

33647 Repair of atrial septal defect and ventricular septal defect, with direct or patch closure

ICD-9-CM Diagnostic

410.00 Acute myocardial infarction of anterolateral wall, episode of care unspecified — (Use additional code to identify presence of hypertension: 401.0-405.9) ▽
410.01 Acute myocardial infarction of anterolateral wall, initial episode of care — (Use additional code to identify presence of hypertension: 401.0-405.9)
410.02 Acute myocardial infarction of anterolateral wall, subsequent episode of care — (Use additional code to identify presence of hypertension: 401.0-405.9)
410.10 Acute myocardial infarction of other anterior wall, episode of care unspecified — (Use additional code to identify presence of hypertension: 401.0-405.9) ▽
410.11 Acute myocardial infarction of other anterior wall, initial episode of care — (Use additional code to identify presence of hypertension: 401.0-405.9)
410.12 Acute myocardial infarction of other anterior wall, subsequent episode of care — (Use additional code to identify presence of hypertension: 401.0-405.9)
410.20 Acute myocardial infarction of inferolateral wall, episode of care unspecified — (Use additional code to identify presence of hypertension: 401.0-405.9) ▽
410.21 Acute myocardial infarction of inferolateral wall, initial episode of care — (Use additional code to identify presence of hypertension: 401.0-405.9)
410.22 Acute myocardial infarction of inferolateral wall, subsequent episode of care — (Use additional code to identify presence of hypertension: 401.0-405.9)
410.30 Acute myocardial infarction of inferoposterior wall, episode of care unspecified — (Use additional code to identify presence of hypertension: 401.0-405.9) ▽
410.31 Acute myocardial infarction of inferoposterior wall, initial episode of care — (Use additional code to identify presence of hypertension: 401.0-405.9)
410.32 Acute myocardial infarction of inferoposterior wall, subsequent episode of care — (Use additional code to identify presence of hypertension: 401.0-405.9)
410.40 Acute myocardial infarction of other inferior wall, episode of care unspecified — (Use additional code to identify presence of hypertension: 401.0-405.9) ▽
410.41 Acute myocardial infarction of other inferior wall, initial episode of care — (Use additional code to identify presence of hypertension: 401.0-405.9)
410.42 Acute myocardial infarction of other inferior wall, subsequent episode of care — (Use additional code to identify presence of hypertension: 401.0-405.9)
410.50 Acute myocardial infarction of other lateral wall, episode of care unspecified — (Use additional code to identify presence of hypertension: 401.0-405.9) ▽
410.51 Acute myocardial infarction of other lateral wall, initial episode of care — (Use additional code to identify presence of hypertension: 401.0-405.9)
410.52 Acute myocardial infarction of other lateral wall, subsequent episode of care — (Use additional code to identify presence of hypertension: 401.0-405.9)
410.60 Acute myocardial infarction, true posterior wall infarction, episode of care unspecified — (Use additional code to identify presence of hypertension: 401.0-405.9) ▽
410.61 Acute myocardial infarction, true posterior wall infarction, initial episode of care — (Use additional code to identify presence of hypertension: 401.0-405.9)
410.62 Acute myocardial infarction, true posterior wall infarction, subsequent episode of care — (Use additional code to identify presence of hypertension: 401.0-405.9)
410.70 Acute myocardial infarction, subendocardial infarction, episode of care unspecified — (Use additional code to identify presence of hypertension: 401.0-405.9) ▽
410.71 Acute myocardial infarction, subendocardial infarction, initial episode of care — (Use additional code to identify presence of hypertension: 401.0-405.9)
410.72 Acute myocardial infarction, subendocardial infarction, subsequent episode of care — (Use additional code to identify presence of hypertension: 401.0-405.9)
410.80 Acute myocardial infarction of other specified sites, episode of care unspecified — (Use additional code to identify presence of hypertension: 401.0-405.9) ▽

▽ Unspecified code
♀ Female diagnosis
☒ Manifestation code
♂ Male diagnosis

410.81 Acute myocardial infarction of other specified sites, initial episode of care — (Use additional code to identify presence of hypertension: 401.0-405.9)
410.82 Acute myocardial infarction of other specified sites, subsequent episode of care — (Use additional code to identify presence of hypertension: 401.0-405.9)
410.90 Acute myocardial infarction, unspecified site, episode of care unspecified — (Use additional code to identify presence of hypertension: 401.0-405.9) ▽
410.91 Acute myocardial infarction, unspecified site, initial episode of care — (Use additional code to identify presence of hypertension: 401.0-405.9) ▽
410.92 Acute myocardial infarction, unspecified site, subsequent episode of care — (Use additional code to identify presence of hypertension: 401.0-405.9) ▽
414.8 Other specified forms of chronic ischemic heart disease — (Use additional code to identify presence of hypertension: 401.0-405.9)
429.71 Acquired cardiac septal defect — (Use additional code to identify the associated myocardial infarction: with onset of 8 weeks of less, 410.00-410.92; with onset of more than 8 weeks, 414.8)
745.5 Ostium secundum type atrial septal defect
745.61 Ostium primum defect
745.69 Other congenital endocardial cushion defect
745.9 Unspecified congenital defect of septal closure ▽
746.9 Unspecified congenital anomaly of heart ▽
786.59 Other chest pain

ICD-9-CM Procedural

35.61 Repair of atrial septal defect with tissue graft
35.62 Repair of ventricular septal defect with tissue graft
35.71 Other and unspecified repair of atrial septal defect
35.72 Other and unspecified repair of ventricular septal defect
39.61 Extracorporeal circulation auxiliary to open heart surgery

33660

33660 Repair of incomplete or partial atrioventricular canal (ostium primum atrial septal defect), with or without atrioventricular valve repair

ICD-9-CM Diagnostic

745.61 Ostium primum defect
745.69 Other congenital endocardial cushion defect
745.9 Unspecified congenital defect of septal closure ▽
746.9 Unspecified congenital anomaly of heart ▽

ICD-9-CM Procedural

35.54 Repair of endocardial cushion defect with prosthesis
35.63 Repair of endocardial cushion defect with tissue graft
35.73 Other and unspecified repair of endocardial cushion defect
39.61 Extracorporeal circulation auxiliary to open heart surgery

33665

33665 Repair of intermediate or transitional atrioventricular canal, with or without atrioventricular valve repair

ICD-9-CM Diagnostic

745.61 Ostium primum defect
745.69 Other congenital endocardial cushion defect
745.9 Unspecified congenital defect of septal closure ▽
746.9 Unspecified congenital anomaly of heart ▽

ICD-9-CM Procedural

35.54 Repair of endocardial cushion defect with prosthesis
35.63 Repair of endocardial cushion defect with tissue graft
35.73 Other and unspecified repair of endocardial cushion defect
39.61 Extracorporeal circulation auxiliary to open heart surgery

33670

33670 Repair of complete atrioventricular canal, with or without prosthetic valve

ICD-9-CM Diagnostic

745.61 Ostium primum defect
745.69 Other congenital endocardial cushion defect
745.9 Unspecified congenital defect of septal closure ▽
746.9 Unspecified congenital anomaly of heart ▽

ICD-9-CM Procedural

35.54 Repair of endocardial cushion defect with prosthesis
35.63 Repair of endocardial cushion defect with tissue graft
35.73 Other and unspecified repair of endocardial cushion defect
39.61 Extracorporeal circulation auxiliary to open heart surgery

33681

33681 Closure of ventricular septal defect, with or without patch;

ICD-9-CM Diagnostic

410.00 Acute myocardial infarction of anterolateral wall, episode of care unspecified — (Use additional code to identify presence of hypertension: 401.0-405.9) ▽
410.01 Acute myocardial infarction of anterolateral wall, initial episode of care — (Use additional code to identify presence of hypertension: 401.0-405.9)
410.02 Acute myocardial infarction of anterolateral wall, subsequent episode of care — (Use additional code to identify presence of hypertension: 401.0-405.9)
410.10 Acute myocardial infarction of other anterior wall, episode of care unspecified — (Use additional code to identify presence of hypertension: 401.0-405.9) ▽
410.11 Acute myocardial infarction of other anterior wall, initial episode of care — (Use additional code to identify presence of hypertension: 401.0-405.9)
410.12 Acute myocardial infarction of other anterior wall, subsequent episode of care — (Use additional code to identify presence of hypertension: 401.0-405.9)
410.20 Acute myocardial infarction of inferolateral wall, episode of care unspecified — (Use additional code to identify presence of hypertension: 401.0-405.9) ▽
410.21 Acute myocardial infarction of inferolateral wall, initial episode of care — (Use additional code to identify presence of hypertension: 401.0-405.9)
410.22 Acute myocardial infarction of inferolateral wall, subsequent episode of care — (Use additional code to identify presence of hypertension: 401.0-405.9)
410.30 Acute myocardial infarction of inferoposterior wall, episode of care unspecified — (Use additional code to identify presence of hypertension: 401.0-405.9) ▽
410.31 Acute myocardial infarction of inferoposterior wall, initial episode of care — (Use additional code to identify presence of hypertension: 401.0-405.9)
410.32 Acute myocardial infarction of inferoposterior wall, subsequent episode of care — (Use additional code to identify presence of hypertension: 401.0-405.9)
410.40 Acute myocardial infarction of other inferior wall, episode of care unspecified — (Use additional code to identify presence of hypertension: 401.0-405.9) ▽
410.41 Acute myocardial infarction of other inferior wall, initial episode of care — (Use additional code to identify presence of hypertension: 401.0-405.9)
410.42 Acute myocardial infarction of other inferior wall, subsequent episode of care — (Use additional code to identify presence of hypertension: 401.0-405.9)
410.50 Acute myocardial infarction of other lateral wall, episode of care unspecified — (Use additional code to identify presence of hypertension: 401.0-405.9) ▽
410.51 Acute myocardial infarction of other lateral wall, initial episode of care — (Use additional code to identify presence of hypertension: 401.0-405.9)
410.52 Acute myocardial infarction of other lateral wall, subsequent episode of care — (Use additional code to identify presence of hypertension: 401.0-405.9)
410.60 Acute myocardial infarction, true posterior wall infarction, episode of care unspecified — (Use additional code to identify presence of hypertension: 401.0-405.9) ▽
410.61 Acute myocardial infarction, true posterior wall infarction, initial episode of care — (Use additional code to identify presence of hypertension: 401.0-405.9)
410.62 Acute myocardial infarction, true posterior wall infarction, subsequent episode of care — (Use additional code to identify presence of hypertension: 401.0-405.9)
410.70 Acute myocardial infarction, subendocardial infarction, episode of care unspecified — (Use additional code to identify presence of hypertension: 401.0-405.9) ▽
410.71 Acute myocardial infarction, subendocardial infarction, initial episode of care — (Use additional code to identify presence of hypertension: 401.0-405.9)
410.72 Acute myocardial infarction, subendocardial infarction, subsequent episode of care — (Use additional code to identify presence of hypertension: 401.0-405.9)
410.80 Acute myocardial infarction of other specified sites, episode of care unspecified — (Use additional code to identify presence of hypertension: 401.0-405.9) ▽
410.81 Acute myocardial infarction of other specified sites, initial episode of care — (Use additional code to identify presence of hypertension: 401.0-405.9)
410.82 Acute myocardial infarction of other specified sites, subsequent episode of care — (Use additional code to identify presence of hypertension: 401.0-405.9)
410.90 Acute myocardial infarction, unspecified site, episode of care unspecified — (Use additional code to identify presence of hypertension: 401.0-405.9) ▽
410.91 Acute myocardial infarction, unspecified site, initial episode of care — (Use additional code to identify presence of hypertension: 401.0-405.9) ▽
410.92 Acute myocardial infarction, unspecified site, subsequent episode of care — (Use additional code to identify presence of hypertension: 401.0-405.9) ▽
414.8 Other specified forms of chronic ischemic heart disease — (Use additional code to identify presence of hypertension: 401.0-405.9)
429.71 Acquired cardiac septal defect — (Use additional code to identify the associated myocardial infarction: with onset of 8 weeks of less, 410.00-410.92; with onset of more than 8 weeks, 414.8)
745.4 Ventricular septal defect
745.7 Cor biloculare
745.8 Other bulbus cordis anomalies and anomalies of cardiac septal closure
745.9 Unspecified congenital defect of septal closure ▽

746.00 Unspecified congenital pulmonary valve anomaly
746.01 Congenital atresia of pulmonary valve
746.02 Congenital stenosis of pulmonary valve
746.09 Other congenital anomalies of pulmonary valve
746.9 Unspecified congenital anomaly of heart

ICD-9-CM Procedural

35.52 Repair of atrial septal defect with prosthesis, closed technique
35.62 Repair of ventricular septal defect with tissue graft
35.72 Other and unspecified repair of ventricular septal defect
39.61 Extracorporeal circulation auxiliary to open heart surgery

33684

33684 Closure of ventricular septal defect, with or without patch; with pulmonary valvotomy or infundibular resection (acyanotic)

ICD-9-CM Diagnostic

410.00 Acute myocardial infarction of anterolateral wall, episode of care unspecified — (Use additional code to identify presence of hypertension: 401.0-405.9)
410.01 Acute myocardial infarction of anterolateral wall, initial episode of care — (Use additional code to identify presence of hypertension: 401.0-405.9)
410.02 Acute myocardial infarction of anterolateral wall, subsequent episode of care — (Use additional code to identify presence of hypertension: 401.0-405.9)
410.10 Acute myocardial infarction of other anterior wall, episode of care unspecified — (Use additional code to identify presence of hypertension: 401.0-405.9)
410.11 Acute myocardial infarction of other anterior wall, initial episode of care — (Use additional code to identify presence of hypertension: 401.0-405.9)
410.12 Acute myocardial infarction of other anterior wall, subsequent episode of care — (Use additional code to identify presence of hypertension: 401.0-405.9)
410.20 Acute myocardial infarction of inferolateral wall, episode of care unspecified — (Use additional code to identify presence of hypertension: 401.0-405.9)
410.21 Acute myocardial infarction of inferolateral wall, initial episode of care — (Use additional code to identify presence of hypertension: 401.0-405.9)
410.22 Acute myocardial infarction of inferolateral wall, subsequent episode of care — (Use additional code to identify presence of hypertension: 401.0-405.9)
410.30 Acute myocardial infarction of inferoposterior wall, episode of care unspecified — (Use additional code to identify presence of hypertension: 401.0-405.9)
410.31 Acute myocardial infarction of inferoposterior wall, initial episode of care — (Use additional code to identify presence of hypertension: 401.0-405.9)
410.32 Acute myocardial infarction of inferoposterior wall, subsequent episode of care — (Use additional code to identify presence of hypertension: 401.0-405.9)
410.40 Acute myocardial infarction of other inferior wall, episode of care unspecified — (Use additional code to identify presence of hypertension: 401.0-405.9)
410.41 Acute myocardial infarction of other inferior wall, initial episode of care — (Use additional code to identify presence of hypertension: 401.0-405.9)
410.42 Acute myocardial infarction of other inferior wall, subsequent episode of care — (Use additional code to identify presence of hypertension: 401.0-405.9)
410.50 Acute myocardial infarction of other lateral wall, episode of care unspecified — (Use additional code to identify presence of hypertension: 401.0-405.9)
410.51 Acute myocardial infarction of other lateral wall, initial episode of care — (Use additional code to identify presence of hypertension: 401.0-405.9)
410.52 Acute myocardial infarction of other lateral wall, subsequent episode of care — (Use additional code to identify presence of hypertension: 401.0-405.9)
410.60 Acute myocardial infarction, true posterior wall infarction, episode of care unspecified — (Use additional code to identify presence of hypertension: 401.0-405.9)
410.61 Acute myocardial infarction, true posterior wall infarction, initial episode of care — (Use additional code to identify presence of hypertension: 401.0-405.9)
410.62 Acute myocardial infarction, true posterior wall infarction, subsequent episode of care — (Use additional code to identify presence of hypertension: 401.0-405.9)
410.70 Acute myocardial infarction, subendocardial infarction, episode of care unspecified — (Use additional code to identify presence of hypertension: 401.0-405.9)
410.71 Acute myocardial infarction, subendocardial infarction, initial episode of care — (Use additional code to identify presence of hypertension: 401.0-405.9)
410.72 Acute myocardial infarction, subendocardial infarction, subsequent episode of care — (Use additional code to identify presence of hypertension: 401.0-405.9)
410.80 Acute myocardial infarction of other specified sites, episode of care unspecified — (Use additional code to identify presence of hypertension: 401.0-405.9)
410.81 Acute myocardial infarction of other specified sites, initial episode of care — (Use additional code to identify presence of hypertension: 401.0-405.9)
410.82 Acute myocardial infarction of other specified sites, subsequent episode of care — (Use additional code to identify presence of hypertension: 401.0-405.9)
410.90 Acute myocardial infarction, unspecified site, episode of care unspecified — (Use additional code to identify presence of hypertension: 401.0-405.9)
410.91 Acute myocardial infarction, unspecified site, initial episode of care — (Use additional code to identify presence of hypertension: 401.0-405.9)
410.92 Acute myocardial infarction, unspecified site, subsequent episode of care — (Use additional code to identify presence of hypertension: 401.0-405.9)
414.8 Other specified forms of chronic ischemic heart disease — (Use additional code to identify presence of hypertension: 401.0-405.9)
429.71 Acquired cardiac septal defect — (Use additional code to identify the associated myocardial infarction: with onset of 8 weeks of less, 410.00-410.92; with onset of more than 8 weeks, 414.8)
745.4 Ventricular septal defect
745.7 Cor biloculare
745.8 Other bulbus cordis anomalies and anomalies of cardiac septal closure
745.9 Unspecified congenital defect of septal closure
746.00 Unspecified congenital pulmonary valve anomaly
746.01 Congenital atresia of pulmonary valve
746.02 Congenital stenosis of pulmonary valve
746.09 Other congenital anomalies of pulmonary valve
746.9 Unspecified congenital anomaly of heart

ICD-9-CM Procedural

35.03 Closed heart valvotomy, pulmonary valve
35.34 Infundibulectomy
35.62 Repair of ventricular septal defect with tissue graft
39.61 Extracorporeal circulation auxiliary to open heart surgery

33688

33688 Closure of ventricular septal defect, with or without patch; with removal of pulmonary artery band, with or without gusset

ICD-9-CM Diagnostic

410.00 Acute myocardial infarction of anterolateral wall, episode of care unspecified — (Use additional code to identify presence of hypertension: 401.0-405.9)
410.01 Acute myocardial infarction of anterolateral wall, initial episode of care — (Use additional code to identify presence of hypertension: 401.0-405.9)
410.02 Acute myocardial infarction of anterolateral wall, subsequent episode of care — (Use additional code to identify presence of hypertension: 401.0-405.9)
410.10 Acute myocardial infarction of other anterior wall, episode of care unspecified — (Use additional code to identify presence of hypertension: 401.0-405.9)
410.11 Acute myocardial infarction of other anterior wall, initial episode of care — (Use additional code to identify presence of hypertension: 401.0-405.9)
410.12 Acute myocardial infarction of other anterior wall, subsequent episode of care — (Use additional code to identify presence of hypertension: 401.0-405.9)
410.20 Acute myocardial infarction of inferolateral wall, episode of care unspecified — (Use additional code to identify presence of hypertension: 401.0-405.9)
410.21 Acute myocardial infarction of inferolateral wall, initial episode of care — (Use additional code to identify presence of hypertension: 401.0-405.9)
410.22 Acute myocardial infarction of inferolateral wall, subsequent episode of care — (Use additional code to identify presence of hypertension: 401.0-405.9)
410.30 Acute myocardial infarction of inferoposterior wall, episode of care unspecified — (Use additional code to identify presence of hypertension: 401.0-405.9)
410.31 Acute myocardial infarction of inferoposterior wall, initial episode of care — (Use additional code to identify presence of hypertension: 401.0-405.9)
410.32 Acute myocardial infarction of inferoposterior wall, subsequent episode of care — (Use additional code to identify presence of hypertension: 401.0-405.9)
410.40 Acute myocardial infarction of other inferior wall, episode of care unspecified — (Use additional code to identify presence of hypertension: 401.0-405.9)
410.41 Acute myocardial infarction of other inferior wall, initial episode of care — (Use additional code to identify presence of hypertension: 401.0-405.9)
410.42 Acute myocardial infarction of other inferior wall, subsequent episode of care — (Use additional code to identify presence of hypertension: 401.0-405.9)
410.50 Acute myocardial infarction of other lateral wall, episode of care unspecified — (Use additional code to identify presence of hypertension: 401.0-405.9)
410.51 Acute myocardial infarction of other lateral wall, initial episode of care — (Use additional code to identify presence of hypertension: 401.0-405.9)
410.52 Acute myocardial infarction of other lateral wall, subsequent episode of care — (Use additional code to identify presence of hypertension: 401.0-405.9)
410.60 Acute myocardial infarction, true posterior wall infarction, episode of care unspecified — (Use additional code to identify presence of hypertension: 401.0-405.9)
410.61 Acute myocardial infarction, true posterior wall infarction, initial episode of care — (Use additional code to identify presence of hypertension: 401.0-405.9)
410.62 Acute myocardial infarction, true posterior wall infarction, subsequent episode of care — (Use additional code to identify presence of hypertension: 401.0-405.9)

Unspecified code
♀ Female diagnosis
Manifestation code
♂ Male diagnosis

410.70 Acute myocardial infarction, subendocardial infarction, episode of care unspecified — (Use additional code to identify presence of hypertension: 401.0-405.9) ▽
410.71 Acute myocardial infarction, subendocardial infarction, initial episode of care — (Use additional code to identify presence of hypertension: 401.0-405.9)
410.72 Acute myocardial infarction, subendocardial infarction, subsequent episode of care — (Use additional code to identify presence of hypertension: 401.0-405.9)
410.80 Acute myocardial infarction of other specified sites, episode of care unspecified — (Use additional code to identify presence of hypertension: 401.0-405.9) ▽
410.81 Acute myocardial infarction of other specified sites, initial episode of care — (Use additional code to identify presence of hypertension: 401.0-405.9)
410.82 Acute myocardial infarction of other specified sites, subsequent episode of care — (Use additional code to identify presence of hypertension: 401.0-405.9)
410.90 Acute myocardial infarction, unspecified site, episode of care unspecified — (Use additional code to identify presence of hypertension: 401.0-405.9) ▽
410.91 Acute myocardial infarction, unspecified site, initial episode of care — (Use additional code to identify presence of hypertension: 401.0-405.9) ▽
410.92 Acute myocardial infarction, unspecified site, subsequent episode of care — (Use additional code to identify presence of hypertension: 401.0-405.9) ▽
414.8 Other specified forms of chronic ischemic heart disease — (Use additional code to identify presence of hypertension: 401.0-405.9)
429.71 Acquired cardiac septal defect — (Use additional code to identify the associated myocardial infarction: with onset of 8 weeks of less, 410.00-410.92; with onset of more than 8 weeks, 414.8)
745.4 Ventricular septal defect
745.7 Cor biloculare
745.8 Other bulbus cordis anomalies and anomalies of cardiac septal closure
745.9 Unspecified congenital defect of septal closure ▽
746.00 Unspecified congenital pulmonary valve anomaly ▽
746.01 Congenital atresia of pulmonary valve
746.02 Congenital stenosis of pulmonary valve
746.09 Other congenital anomalies of pulmonary valve
746.9 Unspecified congenital anomaly of heart ▽

ICD-9-CM Procedural
35.52 Repair of atrial septal defect with prosthesis, closed technique
35.62 Repair of ventricular septal defect with tissue graft
35.72 Other and unspecified repair of ventricular septal defect
39.61 Extracorporeal circulation auxiliary to open heart surgery

33690
33690 Banding of pulmonary artery

ICD-9-CM Diagnostic
745.10 Complete transposition of great vessels
745.11 Transposition of great vessels, double outlet right ventricle
745.69 Other congenital endocardial cushion defect
746.1 Congenital tricuspid atresia and stenosis

ICD-9-CM Procedural
38.85 Other surgical occlusion of other thoracic vessel

33692–33694
33692 Complete repair tetralogy of Fallot without pulmonary atresia;
33694 with transannular patch

ICD-9-CM Diagnostic
745.2 Tetralogy of Fallot
747.3 Congenital anomalies of pulmonary artery

ICD-9-CM Procedural
35.81 Total repair of tetralogy of Fallot
39.61 Extracorporeal circulation auxiliary to open heart surgery

33697
33697 Complete repair tetralogy of Fallot with pulmonary atresia including construction of conduit from right ventricle to pulmonary artery and closure of ventricular septal defect

ICD-9-CM Diagnostic
745.2 Tetralogy of Fallot
747.3 Congenital anomalies of pulmonary artery

ICD-9-CM Procedural
35.81 Total repair of tetralogy of Fallot
39.61 Extracorporeal circulation auxiliary to open heart surgery

33702–33710
33702 Repair sinus of Valsalva fistula, with cardiopulmonary bypass;
33710 with repair of ventricular septal defect

ICD-9-CM Diagnostic
745.4 Ventricular septal defect
745.69 Other congenital endocardial cushion defect
747.29 Other congenital anomaly of aorta

ICD-9-CM Procedural
35.39 Operations on other structures adjacent to valves of heart
35.53 Repair of ventricular septal defect with prosthesis
35.62 Repair of ventricular septal defect with tissue graft
35.72 Other and unspecified repair of ventricular septal defect
39.61 Extracorporeal circulation auxiliary to open heart surgery

33720
33720 Repair sinus of Valsalva aneurysm, with cardiopulmonary bypass

ICD-9-CM Diagnostic
747.29 Other congenital anomaly of aorta

ICD-9-CM Procedural
35.39 Operations on other structures adjacent to valves of heart
39.61 Extracorporeal circulation auxiliary to open heart surgery

33722
33722 Closure of aortico-left ventricular tunnel

ICD-9-CM Diagnostic
745.8 Other bulbus cordis anomalies and anomalies of cardiac septal closure

ICD-9-CM Procedural
35.39 Operations on other structures adjacent to valves of heart
39.61 Extracorporeal circulation auxiliary to open heart surgery

33730
33730 Complete repair of anomalous venous return (supracardiac, intracardiac, or infracardiac types)

ICD-9-CM Diagnostic
747.40 Congenital anomaly of great veins unspecified ▽
747.41 Total congenital anomalous pulmonary venous connection
747.42 Partial congenital anomalous pulmonary venous connection
747.49 Other congenital anomalies of great veins

ICD-9-CM Procedural
35.82 Total repair of total anomalous pulmonary venous connection
39.61 Extracorporeal circulation auxiliary to open heart surgery

33732
33732 Repair of cor triatriatum or supravalvular mitral ring by resection of left atrial membrane

ICD-9-CM Diagnostic
746.5 Congenital mitral stenosis
746.82 Cor triatriatum

ICD-9-CM Procedural
35.12 Open heart valvuloplasty of mitral valve without replacement
39.61 Extracorporeal circulation auxiliary to open heart surgery

33735–33737
33735 Atrial septectomy or septostomy; closed heart (Blalock-Hanlon type operation)
33736 open heart with cardiopulmonary bypass
33737 open heart, with inflow occlusion

ICD-9-CM Diagnostic
745.10 Complete transposition of great vessels
746.1 Congenital tricuspid atresia and stenosis
746.89 Other specified congenital anomaly of heart
747.41 Total congenital anomalous pulmonary venous connection

ICD-9-CM Procedural
35.42 Creation of septal defect in heart

▽ Unspecified code ♀ Female diagnosis ☒ Manifestation code ♂ Male diagnosis

39.61 Extracorporeal circulation auxiliary to open heart surgery

33750

33750 Shunt; subclavian to pulmonary artery (Blalock-Taussig type operation)

ICD-9-CM Diagnostic

424.3 Pulmonary valve disorders
745.2 Tetralogy of Fallot
746.01 Congenital atresia of pulmonary valve
746.02 Congenital stenosis of pulmonary valve
746.09 Other congenital anomalies of pulmonary valve
746.1 Congenital tricuspid atresia and stenosis
746.2 Ebstein's anomaly
746.9 Unspecified congenital anomaly of heart

ICD-9-CM Procedural

39.0 Systemic to pulmonary artery shunt
39.61 Extracorporeal circulation auxiliary to open heart surgery

33755

33755 Shunt; ascending aorta to pulmonary artery (Waterston type operation)

ICD-9-CM Diagnostic

424.3 Pulmonary valve disorders
745.2 Tetralogy of Fallot
746.01 Congenital atresia of pulmonary valve
746.02 Congenital stenosis of pulmonary valve
746.09 Other congenital anomalies of pulmonary valve
746.1 Congenital tricuspid atresia and stenosis
746.2 Ebstein's anomaly
746.9 Unspecified congenital anomaly of heart

ICD-9-CM Procedural

39.0 Systemic to pulmonary artery shunt
39.61 Extracorporeal circulation auxiliary to open heart surgery

33762

33762 Shunt; descending aorta to pulmonary artery (Potts-Smith type operation)

ICD-9-CM Diagnostic

424.3 Pulmonary valve disorders
745.2 Tetralogy of Fallot
746.01 Congenital atresia of pulmonary valve
746.02 Congenital stenosis of pulmonary valve
746.09 Other congenital anomalies of pulmonary valve
746.1 Congenital tricuspid atresia and stenosis
746.2 Ebstein's anomaly
746.9 Unspecified congenital anomaly of heart

ICD-9-CM Procedural

39.0 Systemic to pulmonary artery shunt
39.61 Extracorporeal circulation auxiliary to open heart surgery

33764

33764 Shunt; central, with prosthetic graft

ICD-9-CM Diagnostic

745.2 Tetralogy of Fallot
745.69 Other congenital endocardial cushion defect
746.1 Congenital tricuspid atresia and stenosis
746.9 Unspecified congenital anomaly of heart
747.3 Congenital anomalies of pulmonary artery

ICD-9-CM Procedural

39.0 Systemic to pulmonary artery shunt
39.61 Extracorporeal circulation auxiliary to open heart surgery

33766–33767

33766 Shunt; superior vena cava to pulmonary artery for flow to one lung (classical Glenn procedure)
33767 superior vena cava to pulmonary artery for flow to both lungs (bidirectional Glenn procedure)

ICD-9-CM Diagnostic

745.2 Tetralogy of Fallot
746.02 Congenital stenosis of pulmonary valve
746.1 Congenital tricuspid atresia and stenosis
746.2 Ebstein's anomaly
746.83 Congenital infundibular pulmonic stenosis
746.9 Unspecified congenital anomaly of heart
782.5 Cyanosis

ICD-9-CM Procedural

39.21 Caval-pulmonary artery anastomosis
39.61 Extracorporeal circulation auxiliary to open heart surgery

33770–33771

33770 Repair of transposition of the great arteries with ventricular septal defect and subpulmonary stenosis; without surgical enlargement of ventricular septal defect
33771 with surgical enlargement of ventricular septal defect

ICD-9-CM Diagnostic

745.10 Complete transposition of great vessels
745.11 Transposition of great vessels, double outlet right ventricle
745.19 Other transposition of great vessels

ICD-9-CM Procedural

35.41 Enlargement of existing atrial septal defect
35.84 Total correction of transposition of great vessels, not elsewhere classified
39.61 Extracorporeal circulation auxiliary to open heart surgery

33774–33775

33774 Repair of transposition of the great arteries, atrial baffle procedure (eg, Mustard or Senning type) with cardiopulmonary bypass;
33775 with removal of pulmonary band

ICD-9-CM Diagnostic

745.10 Complete transposition of great vessels
745.11 Transposition of great vessels, double outlet right ventricle
745.19 Other transposition of great vessels

ICD-9-CM Procedural

35.91 Interatrial transposition of venous return
39.61 Extracorporeal circulation auxiliary to open heart surgery

33776

33776 Repair of transposition of the great arteries, atrial baffle procedure (eg, Mustard or Senning type) with cardiopulmonary bypass; with closure of ventricular septal defect

ICD-9-CM Diagnostic

745.10 Complete transposition of great vessels
745.11 Transposition of great vessels, double outlet right ventricle
745.19 Other transposition of great vessels

ICD-9-CM Procedural

35.53 Repair of ventricular septal defect with prosthesis
35.62 Repair of ventricular septal defect with tissue graft
35.72 Other and unspecified repair of ventricular septal defect
35.91 Interatrial transposition of venous return
39.61 Extracorporeal circulation auxiliary to open heart surgery

33777

33777 Repair of transposition of the great arteries, atrial baffle procedure (eg, Mustard or Senning type) with cardiopulmonary bypass; with repair of subpulmonic obstruction

ICD-9-CM Diagnostic

745.10 Complete transposition of great vessels
745.11 Transposition of great vessels, double outlet right ventricle
745.19 Other transposition of great vessels

Unspecified code
♀ Female diagnosis
Manifestation code
♂ Male diagnosis

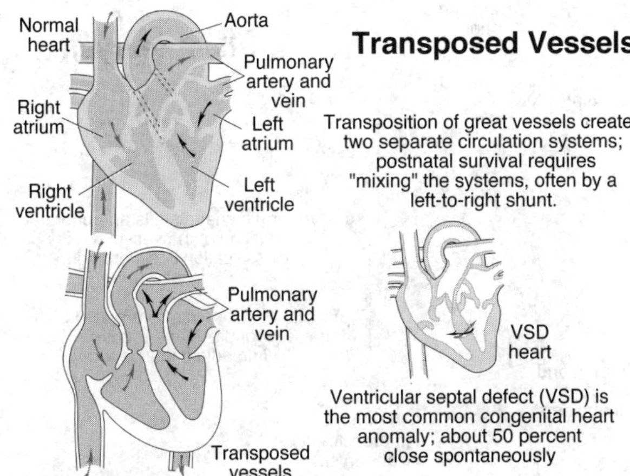

Normal heart
Aorta
Pulmonary artery and vein
Right atrium
Left atrium
Right ventricle
Left ventricle
Transposed Vessels
Transposition of great vessels creates two separate circulation systems; postnatal survival requires "mixing" the systems, often by a left-to-right shunt.
Pulmonary artery and vein
VSD heart
Transposed vessels
Ventricular septal defect (VSD) is the most common congenital heart anomaly; about 50 percent close spontaneously

ICD-9-CM Procedural

35.91 Interatrial transposition of venous return
39.61 Extracorporeal circulation auxiliary to open heart surgery

33778–33779

33778 Repair of transposition of the great arteries, aortic pulmonary artery reconstruction (eg, Jatene type);
33779 with removal of pulmonary band

ICD-9-CM Diagnostic

745.10 Complete transposition of great vessels
745.11 Transposition of great vessels, double outlet right ventricle
745.19 Other transposition of great vessels

ICD-9-CM Procedural

35.84 Total correction of transposition of great vessels, not elsewhere classified
39.61 Extracorporeal circulation auxiliary to open heart surgery

33780

33780 Repair of transposition of the great arteries, aortic pulmonary artery reconstruction (eg, Jatene type); with closure of ventricular septal defect

ICD-9-CM Diagnostic

745.10 Complete transposition of great vessels
745.11 Transposition of great vessels, double outlet right ventricle
745.19 Other transposition of great vessels

ICD-9-CM Procedural

35.53 Repair of ventricular septal defect with prosthesis
35.62 Repair of ventricular septal defect with tissue graft
35.72 Other and unspecified repair of ventricular septal defect
35.84 Total correction of transposition of great vessels, not elsewhere classified
39.61 Extracorporeal circulation auxiliary to open heart surgery

33781

33781 Repair of transposition of the great arteries, aortic pulmonary artery reconstruction (eg, Jatene type); with repair of subpulmonic obstruction

ICD-9-CM Diagnostic

745.10 Complete transposition of great vessels
745.11 Transposition of great vessels, double outlet right ventricle
745.19 Other transposition of great vessels

ICD-9-CM Procedural

35.84 Total correction of transposition of great vessels, not elsewhere classified
39.61 Extracorporeal circulation auxiliary to open heart surgery

33786

33786 Total repair, truncus arteriosus (Rastelli type operation)

ICD-9-CM Diagnostic

745.0 Bulbus cordis anomalies and anomalies of cardiac septal closure, common truncus
747.3 Congenital anomalies of pulmonary artery

ICD-9-CM Procedural

35.83 Total repair of truncus arteriosus
39.61 Extracorporeal circulation auxiliary to open heart surgery

33788

33788 Reimplantation of an anomalous pulmonary artery

ICD-9-CM Diagnostic

747.3 Congenital anomalies of pulmonary artery

ICD-9-CM Procedural

39.59 Other repair of vessel
39.61 Extracorporeal circulation auxiliary to open heart surgery

33800

33800 Aortic suspension (aortopexy) for tracheal decompression (eg, for tracheomalacia) (separate procedure)

ICD-9-CM Diagnostic

519.1 Other diseases of trachea and bronchus, not elsewhere classified
747.29 Other congenital anomaly of aorta
748.3 Other congenital anomaly of larynx, trachea, and bronchus

ICD-9-CM Procedural

39.99 Other operations on vessels

33802–33803

33802 Division of aberrant vessel (vascular ring);
33803 with reanastomosis

ICD-9-CM Diagnostic

747.21 Congenital anomaly of aortic arch
747.3 Congenital anomalies of pulmonary artery

ICD-9-CM Procedural

38.35 Resection of other thoracic vessels with anastomosis
38.85 Other surgical occlusion of other thoracic vessel
39.61 Extracorporeal circulation auxiliary to open heart surgery
99.77 Application or administration of adhesion barrier substance

33813–33814

33813 Obliteration of aortopulmonary septal defect; without cardiopulmonary bypass
33814 with cardiopulmonary bypass

ICD-9-CM Diagnostic

745.0 Bulbus cordis anomalies and anomalies of cardiac septal closure, common truncus

ICD-9-CM Procedural

35.98 Other operations on septa of heart
39.61 Extracorporeal circulation auxiliary to open heart surgery

33820–33824

33820 Repair of patent ductus arteriosus; by ligation
33822 by division, under 18 years
33824 by division, 18 years and older

ICD-9-CM Diagnostic

747.0 Patent ductus arteriosus

ICD-9-CM Procedural

38.85 Other surgical occlusion of other thoracic vessel
39.61 Extracorporeal circulation auxiliary to open heart surgery
99.77 Application or administration of adhesion barrier substance

33840–33851

33840 Excision of coarctation of aorta, with or without associated patent ductus arteriosus; with direct anastomosis
33845 with graft
33851 repair using either left subclavian artery or prosthetic material as gusset for enlargement

ICD-9-CM Diagnostic

747.0 Patent ductus arteriosus

747.10 Coarctation of aorta (preductal) (postductal)

ICD-9-CM Procedural

38.35 Resection of other thoracic vessels with anastomosis
38.45 Resection of other thoracic vessels with replacement
38.85 Other surgical occlusion of other thoracic vessel
39.61 Extracorporeal circulation auxiliary to open heart surgery
99.77 Application or administration of adhesion barrier substance

33852–33853

33852 Repair of hypoplastic or interrupted aortic arch using autogenous or prosthetic material; without cardiopulmonary bypass
33853 with cardiopulmonary bypass

ICD-9-CM Diagnostic

747.10 Coarctation of aorta (preductal) (postductal)
747.11 Congenital interruption of aortic arch
747.22 Congenital atresia and stenosis of aorta

ICD-9-CM Procedural

39.56 Repair of blood vessel with tissue patch graft
39.57 Repair of blood vessel with synthetic patch graft
39.61 Extracorporeal circulation auxiliary to open heart surgery

33860–33863

33860 Ascending aorta graft, with cardiopulmonary bypass, with or without valve suspension;
33861 with coronary reconstruction
33863 with aortic root replacement using composite prosthesis and coronary reconstruction

ICD-9-CM Diagnostic

395.0 Rheumatic aortic stenosis
395.1 Rheumatic aortic insufficiency
395.2 Rheumatic aortic stenosis with insufficiency
441.00 Dissecting aortic aneurysm (any part), unspecified site ▽
441.01 Dissecting aortic aneurysm (any part), thoracic
441.1 Thoracic aneurysm, ruptured
441.2 Thoracic aneurysm without mention of rupture
441.9 Aortic aneurysm of unspecified site without mention of rupture ▽
861.02 Heart laceration without penetration of heart chambers or mention of open wound into thorax
861.12 Heart laceration without penetration of heart chambers, with open wound into thorax
901.0 Thoracic aorta injury

ICD-9-CM Procedural

38.45 Resection of other thoracic vessels with replacement
39.61 Extracorporeal circulation auxiliary to open heart surgery
99.77 Application or administration of adhesion barrier substance

33870

33870 Transverse arch graft, with cardiopulmonary bypass

ICD-9-CM Diagnostic

395.0 Rheumatic aortic stenosis
395.1 Rheumatic aortic insufficiency
395.2 Rheumatic aortic stenosis with insufficiency
441.00 Dissecting aortic aneurysm (any part), unspecified site ▽
441.01 Dissecting aortic aneurysm (any part), thoracic
441.1 Thoracic aneurysm, ruptured
441.2 Thoracic aneurysm without mention of rupture
441.9 Aortic aneurysm of unspecified site without mention of rupture ▽
861.02 Heart laceration without penetration of heart chambers or mention of open wound into thorax
861.12 Heart laceration without penetration of heart chambers, with open wound into thorax
901.0 Thoracic aorta injury

ICD-9-CM Procedural

38.45 Resection of other thoracic vessels with replacement
39.61 Extracorporeal circulation auxiliary to open heart surgery
99.77 Application or administration of adhesion barrier substance

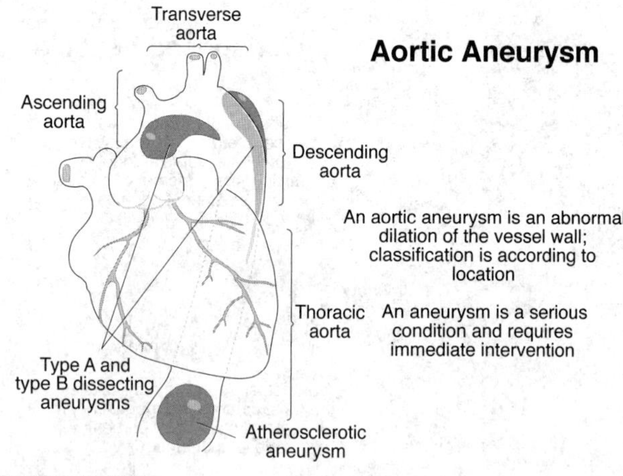
Transverse aorta
Aortic Aneurysm
Ascending aorta
Descending aorta
An aortic aneurysm is an abnormal dilation of the vessel wall; classification is according to location
Thoracic aorta
An aneurysm is a serious condition and requires immediate intervention
Type A and type B dissecting aneurysms
Atherosclerotic aneurysm

33875–33877

33875 Descending thoracic aorta graft, with or without bypass
33877 Repair of thoracoabdominal aortic aneurysm with graft, with or without cardiopulmonary bypass

ICD-9-CM Diagnostic

395.0 Rheumatic aortic stenosis
395.1 Rheumatic aortic insufficiency
395.2 Rheumatic aortic stenosis with insufficiency
441.00 Dissecting aortic aneurysm (any part), unspecified site ▽
441.01 Dissecting aortic aneurysm (any part), thoracic
441.03 Dissecting aortic aneurysm (any part), thoracoabdominal
441.1 Thoracic aneurysm, ruptured
441.2 Thoracic aneurysm without mention of rupture
441.4 Abdominal aneurysm without mention of rupture
441.5 Aortic aneurysm of unspecified site, ruptured ▽
441.6 Thoracoabdominal aneurysm, ruptured
441.7 Thoracoabdominal aneurysm without mention of rupture
441.9 Aortic aneurysm of unspecified site without mention of rupture ▽
861.02 Heart laceration without penetration of heart chambers or mention of open wound into thorax
861.12 Heart laceration without penetration of heart chambers, with open wound into thorax
901.0 Thoracic aorta injury

ICD-9-CM Procedural

38.44 Resection of abdominal aorta with replacement
38.45 Resection of other thoracic vessels with replacement
39.61 Extracorporeal circulation auxiliary to open heart surgery
99.77 Application or administration of adhesion barrier substance

33910–33915

33910 Pulmonary artery embolectomy; with cardiopulmonary bypass
33915 without cardiopulmonary bypass

ICD-9-CM Diagnostic

415.11 Iatrogenic pulmonary embolism and infarction
415.19 Other pulmonary embolism and infarction
901.41 Pulmonary artery injury

ICD-9-CM Procedural

38.05 Incision of other thoracic vessels
39.61 Extracorporeal circulation auxiliary to open heart surgery
99.77 Application or administration of adhesion barrier substance

33916–33917

33916 Pulmonary endarterectomy, with or without embolectomy, with cardiopulmonary bypass
33917 Repair of pulmonary artery stenosis by reconstruction with patch or graft

ICD-9-CM Diagnostic

415.11 Iatrogenic pulmonary embolism and infarction
415.19 Other pulmonary embolism and infarction
746.83 Congenital infundibular pulmonic stenosis
747.3 Congenital anomalies of pulmonary artery
901.41 Pulmonary artery injury

▽ Unspecified code
♀ Female diagnosis
☒ Manifestation code
♂ Male diagnosis

ICD-9-CM Procedural

38.15 Endarterectomy of other thoracic vessels
39.58 Repair of blood vessel with unspecified type of patch graft
39.61 Extracorporeal circulation auxiliary to open heart surgery
99.77 Application or administration of adhesion barrier substance

33918–33919

33918 Repair of pulmonary atresia with ventricular septal defect, by unifocalization of pulmonary arteries; without cardiopulmonary bypass
33919 with cardiopulmonary bypass

ICD-9-CM Diagnostic

745.4 Ventricular septal defect
746.01 Congenital atresia of pulmonary valve
746.83 Congenital infundibular pulmonic stenosis
747.3 Congenital anomalies of pulmonary artery

ICD-9-CM Procedural

35.73 Other and unspecified repair of endocardial cushion defect
39.61 Extracorporeal circulation auxiliary to open heart surgery

33920

33920 Repair of pulmonary atresia with ventricular septal defect, by construction or replacement of conduit from right or left ventricle to pulmonary artery

ICD-9-CM Diagnostic

745.4 Ventricular septal defect
746.01 Congenital atresia of pulmonary valve
746.83 Congenital infundibular pulmonic stenosis
747.3 Congenital anomalies of pulmonary artery

ICD-9-CM Procedural

35.13 Open heart valvuloplasty of pulmonary valve without replacement
39.61 Extracorporeal circulation auxiliary to open heart surgery

33922

33922 Transection of pulmonary artery with cardiopulmonary bypass

ICD-9-CM Diagnostic

417.8 Other specified disease of pulmonary circulation
747.3 Congenital anomalies of pulmonary artery
901.41 Pulmonary artery injury

ICD-9-CM Procedural

38.35 Resection of other thoracic vessels with anastomosis
39.56 Repair of blood vessel with tissue patch graft
39.61 Extracorporeal circulation auxiliary to open heart surgery
99.77 Application or administration of adhesion barrier substance

33924

33924 Ligation and takedown of a systemic-to-pulmonary artery shunt, performed in conjunction with a congenital heart procedure (List separately in addition to code for primary procedure)

ICD-9-CM Diagnostic

This is an add-on code. Refer to the corresponding primary procedure code for ICD-9 diagnosis code links.

ICD-9-CM Procedural

35.81 Total repair of tetralogy of Fallot
39.49 Other revision of vascular procedure

33930

33930 Donor cardiectomy-pneumonectomy (including cold preservation)

ICD-9-CM Diagnostic

V59.8 Donor of other specified organ or tissue

ICD-9-CM Procedural

32.5 Complete pneumonectomy
37.99 Other operations on heart and pericardium

33933

33933 Backbench standard preparation of cadaver donor heart/lung allograft prior to transplantation, including dissection of allograft from surrounding soft tissues to prepare aorta, superior vena cava, inferior vena cava, and trachea for implantation

ICD-9-CM Diagnostic

148.8 Malignant neoplasm of other specified sites of hypopharynx
162.2 Malignant neoplasm of main bronchus
162.3 Malignant neoplasm of upper lobe, bronchus, or lung
162.4 Malignant neoplasm of middle lobe, bronchus, or lung
162.5 Malignant neoplasm of lower lobe, bronchus, or lung
162.8 Malignant neoplasm of other parts of bronchus or lung
163.0 Malignant neoplasm of parietal pleura
163.1 Malignant neoplasm of visceral pleura
163.8 Malignant neoplasm of other specified sites of pleura
164.1 Malignant neoplasm of heart
164.8 Malignant neoplasm of other parts of mediastinum
197.0 Secondary malignant neoplasm of lung
197.1 Secondary malignant neoplasm of mediastinum
198.89 Secondary malignant neoplasm of other specified sites
231.2 Carcinoma in situ of bronchus and lung
398.0 Rheumatic myocarditis
412 Old myocardial infarction — (Use additional code to identify presence of hypertension: 401.0-405.9)
414.00 Coronary atherosclerosis of unspecified type of vessel, native or graft — (Use additional code to identify presence of hypertension: 401.0-405.9) ▽
414.01 Coronary atherosclerosis of native coronary artery — (Use additional code to identify presence of hypertension: 401.0-405.9)
414.02 Coronary atherosclerosis of autologous vein bypass graft — (Use additional code to identify presence of hypertension: 401.0-405.9)
414.03 Coronary atherosclerosis of nonautologous biological bypass graft — (Use additional code to identify presence of hypertension: 401.0-405.9)
414.04 Coronary atherosclerosis of artery bypass graft — (Use additional code to identify presence of hypertension: 401.0-405.9)
414.05 Coronary atherosclerosis of unspecified type of bypass graft — (Use additional code to identify presence of hypertension: 401.0-405.9) ▽
414.8 Other specified forms of chronic ischemic heart disease — (Use additional code to identify presence of hypertension: 401.0-405.9)
416.8 Other chronic pulmonary heart diseases
422.91 Idiopathic myocarditis
422.92 Septic myocarditis — (Use additional code to identify infectious organism)
422.93 Toxic myocarditis
425.0 Endomyocardial fibrosis
425.3 Endocardial fibroelastosis
425.4 Other primary cardiomyopathies
428.0 Congestive heart failure, unspecified ▽
428.1 Left heart failure
428.22 Chronic systolic heart failure
428.23 Acute on chronic systolic heart failure
428.32 Chronic diastolic heart failure
428.33 Acute on chronic diastolic heart failure
428.42 Chronic combined systolic and diastolic heart failure
428.43 Acute on chronic combined systolic and diastolic heart failure
429.0 Unspecified myocarditis — (Use additional code to identify presence of arteriosclerosis) ▽
429.1 Myocardial degeneration — (Use additional code to identify presence of arteriosclerosis)
429.2 Unspecified cardiovascular disease — (Use additional code to identify presence of arteriosclerosis) ▽
496 Chronic airway obstruction, not elsewhere classified — (Note: This code is not to be used with any code from 491-493) ▽
508.1 Chronic and other pulmonary manifestations due to radiation — (Use additional E code to identify cause)
514 Pulmonary congestion and hypostasis
515 Postinflammatory pulmonary fibrosis
516.3 Idiopathic fibrosing alveolitis
518.83 Chronic respiratory failure
518.89 Other diseases of lung, not elsewhere classified
746.9 Unspecified congenital anomaly of heart ▽
748.4 Congenital cystic lung
V15.82 Personal history of tobacco use, presenting hazards to health

ICD-9-CM Procedural

00.93 Transplant from cadaver
33.6 Combined heart-lung transplantation
33.99 Other operations on lung

▽ Unspecified code
♀ Female diagnosis
☒ Manifestation code
♂ Male diagnosis

33935

33935 Heart-lung transplant with recipient cardiectomy-pneumonectomy

ICD-9-CM Diagnostic

148.8 Malignant neoplasm of other specified sites of hypopharynx
162.2 Malignant neoplasm of main bronchus
162.3 Malignant neoplasm of upper lobe, bronchus, or lung
162.4 Malignant neoplasm of middle lobe, bronchus, or lung
162.5 Malignant neoplasm of lower lobe, bronchus, or lung
162.8 Malignant neoplasm of other parts of bronchus or lung
163.0 Malignant neoplasm of parietal pleura
163.1 Malignant neoplasm of visceral pleura
163.8 Malignant neoplasm of other specified sites of pleura
164.1 Malignant neoplasm of heart
164.8 Malignant neoplasm of other parts of mediastinum
197.0 Secondary malignant neoplasm of lung
197.1 Secondary malignant neoplasm of mediastinum
198.89 Secondary malignant neoplasm of other specified sites
231.2 Carcinoma in situ of bronchus and lung
398.0 Rheumatic myocarditis
412 Old myocardial infarction — (Use additional code to identify presence of hypertension: 401.0-405.9)
414.00 Coronary atherosclerosis of unspecified type of vessel, native or graft — (Use additional code to identify presence of hypertension: 401.0-405.9) ▽
414.01 Coronary atherosclerosis of native coronary artery — (Use additional code to identify presence of hypertension: 401.0-405.9)
414.02 Coronary atherosclerosis of autologous vein bypass graft — (Use additional code to identify presence of hypertension: 401.0-405.9)
414.03 Coronary atherosclerosis of nonautologous biological bypass graft — (Use additional code to identify presence of hypertension: 401.0-405.9)
414.04 Coronary atherosclerosis of artery bypass graft — (Use additional code to identify presence of hypertension: 401.0-405.9)
414.05 Coronary atherosclerosis of unspecified type of bypass graft — (Use additional code to identify presence of hypertension: 401.0-405.9) ▽
414.8 Other specified forms of chronic ischemic heart disease — (Use additional code to identify presence of hypertension: 401.0-405.9)
416.8 Other chronic pulmonary heart diseases
422.91 Idiopathic myocarditis
422.92 Septic myocarditis — (Use additional code to identify infectious organism)
422.93 Toxic myocarditis
425.0 Endomyocardial fibrosis
425.3 Endocardial fibroelastosis
425.4 Other primary cardiomyopathies
428.0 Congestive heart failure, unspecified ▽
428.1 Left heart failure
428.22 Chronic systolic heart failure
428.23 Acute on chronic systolic heart failure
428.32 Chronic diastolic heart failure
428.33 Acute on chronic diastolic heart failure
428.42 Chronic combined systolic and diastolic heart failure
428.43 Acute on chronic combined systolic and diastolic heart failure
429.0 Unspecified myocarditis — (Use additional code to identify presence of arteriosclerosis) ▽
429.1 Myocardial degeneration — (Use additional code to identify presence of arteriosclerosis)
429.2 Unspecified cardiovascular disease — (Use additional code to identify presence of arteriosclerosis) ▽
496 Chronic airway obstruction, not elsewhere classified — (Note: This code is not to be used with any code from 491-493) ▽
508.1 Chronic and other pulmonary manifestations due to radiation — (Use additional E code to identify cause)
514 Pulmonary congestion and hypostasis
515 Postinflammatory pulmonary fibrosis
516.3 Idiopathic fibrosing alveolitis
518.83 Chronic respiratory failure
518.89 Other diseases of lung, not elsewhere classified
746.9 Unspecified congenital anomaly of heart ▽
748.4 Congenital cystic lung
V15.82 Personal history of tobacco use, presenting hazards to health

ICD-9-CM Procedural

00.93 Transplant from cadaver
33.6 Combined heart-lung transplantation
39.61 Extracorporeal circulation auxiliary to open heart surgery

33940

33940 Donor cardiectomy (including cold preservation)

ICD-9-CM Diagnostic

V59.8 Donor of other specified organ or tissue

ICD-9-CM Procedural

37.99 Other operations on heart and pericardium

33944

33944 Backbench standard preparation of cadaver donor heart allograft prior to transplantation, including dissection of allograft from surrounding soft tissues to prepare aorta, superior vena cava, inferior vena cava, pulmonary artery, and left atrium for implantation

ICD-9-CM Diagnostic

164.1 Malignant neoplasm of heart
164.8 Malignant neoplasm of other parts of mediastinum
198.89 Secondary malignant neoplasm of other specified sites
398.0 Rheumatic myocarditis
412 Old myocardial infarction — (Use additional code to identify presence of hypertension: 401.0-405.9)
414.00 Coronary atherosclerosis of unspecified type of vessel, native or graft — (Use additional code to identify presence of hypertension: 401.0-405.9) ▽
414.01 Coronary atherosclerosis of native coronary artery — (Use additional code to identify presence of hypertension: 401.0-405.9)
414.02 Coronary atherosclerosis of autologous vein bypass graft — (Use additional code to identify presence of hypertension: 401.0-405.9)
414.03 Coronary atherosclerosis of nonautologous biological bypass graft — (Use additional code to identify presence of hypertension: 401.0-405.9)
414.04 Coronary atherosclerosis of artery bypass graft — (Use additional code to identify presence of hypertension: 401.0-405.9)
414.05 Coronary atherosclerosis of unspecified type of bypass graft — (Use additional code to identify presence of hypertension: 401.0-405.9) ▽
414.8 Other specified forms of chronic ischemic heart disease — (Use additional code to identify presence of hypertension: 401.0-405.9)
422.91 Idiopathic myocarditis
422.92 Septic myocarditis — (Use additional code to identify infectious organism)
422.93 Toxic myocarditis
425.0 Endomyocardial fibrosis
425.3 Endocardial fibroelastosis
425.4 Other primary cardiomyopathies
428.0 Congestive heart failure, unspecified ▽
428.1 Left heart failure
428.22 Chronic systolic heart failure
428.23 Acute on chronic systolic heart failure
428.32 Chronic diastolic heart failure
428.33 Acute on chronic diastolic heart failure
428.42 Chronic combined systolic and diastolic heart failure
428.43 Acute on chronic combined systolic and diastolic heart failure
428.9 Unspecified heart failure ▽
429.0 Unspecified myocarditis — (Use additional code to identify presence of arteriosclerosis) ▽
429.1 Myocardial degeneration — (Use additional code to identify presence of arteriosclerosis)
429.2 Unspecified cardiovascular disease — (Use additional code to identify presence of arteriosclerosis) ▽
429.3 Cardiomegaly
746.9 Unspecified congenital anomaly of heart ▽

ICD-9-CM Procedural

00.93 Transplant from cadaver
37.51 Heart transplantation

33945

33945 Heart transplant, with or without recipient cardiectomy

ICD-9-CM Diagnostic

164.1 Malignant neoplasm of heart
164.8 Malignant neoplasm of other parts of mediastinum
198.89 Secondary malignant neoplasm of other specified sites
398.0 Rheumatic myocarditis
412 Old myocardial infarction — (Use additional code to identify presence of hypertension: 401.0-405.9)
414.00 Coronary atherosclerosis of unspecified type of vessel, native or graft — (Use additional code to identify presence of hypertension: 401.0-405.9) ▽

▽ Unspecified code ♀ Female diagnosis ☒ Manifestation code ♂ Male diagnosis

414.01 Coronary atherosclerosis of native coronary artery — (Use additional code to identify presence of hypertension: 401.0-405.9)
414.02 Coronary atherosclerosis of autologous vein bypass graft — (Use additional code to identify presence of hypertension: 401.0-405.9)
414.03 Coronary atherosclerosis of nonautologous biological bypass graft — (Use additional code to identify presence of hypertension: 401.0-405.9)
414.04 Coronary atherosclerosis of artery bypass graft — (Use additional code to identify presence of hypertension: 401.0-405.9)
414.05 Coronary atherosclerosis of unspecified type of bypass graft — (Use additional code to identify presence of hypertension: 401.0-405.9) ▽
414.8 Other specified forms of chronic ischemic heart disease — (Use additional code to identify presence of hypertension: 401.0-405.9)
422.91 Idiopathic myocarditis
422.92 Septic myocarditis — (Use additional code to identify infectious organism)
422.93 Toxic myocarditis
425.0 Endomyocardial fibrosis
425.3 Endocardial fibroelastosis
425.4 Other primary cardiomyopathies
428.0 Congestive heart failure, unspecified ▽
428.1 Left heart failure
428.22 Chronic systolic heart failure
428.23 Acute on chronic systolic heart failure
428.32 Chronic diastolic heart failure
428.33 Acute on chronic diastolic heart failure
428.42 Chronic combined systolic and diastolic heart failure
428.43 Acute on chronic combined systolic and diastolic heart failure
428.9 Unspecified heart failure ▽
429.0 Unspecified myocarditis — (Use additional code to identify presence of arteriosclerosis) ▽
429.1 Myocardial degeneration — (Use additional code to identify presence of arteriosclerosis)
429.2 Unspecified cardiovascular disease — (Use additional code to identify presence of arteriosclerosis) ▽
429.3 Cardiomegaly
746.9 Unspecified congenital anomaly of heart ▽

ICD-9-CM Procedural

00.93 Transplant from cadaver
37.51 Heart transplantation
39.61 Extracorporeal circulation auxiliary to open heart surgery

33960–33961

33960 Prolonged extracorporeal circulation for cardiopulmonary insufficiency; initial 24 hours
33961 each additional 24 hours (List separately in addition to code for primary procedure)

ICD-9-CM Diagnostic

The application of this code is too broad to adequately present ICD-9-CM diagnostic code links here. Refer to your ICD-9-CM book.

ICD-9-CM Procedural

39.61 Extracorporeal circulation auxiliary to open heart surgery
39.65 Extracorporeal membrane oxygenation (ECMO)
39.66 Percutaneous cardiopulmonary bypass

33967

33967 Insertion of intra-aortic balloon assist device, percutaneous

ICD-9-CM Diagnostic

402.01 Malignant hypertensive heart disease with heart failure
402.11 Benign hypertensive heart disease with heart failure
402.91 Unspecified hypertensive heart disease with heart failure ▽
404.01 Malignant hypertensive heart and renal disease with heart failure
404.03 Malignant hypertensive heart and renal disease with heart failure and renal failure
404.11 Benign hypertensive heart and renal disease with heart failure
404.13 Benign hypertensive heart and renal disease with heart failure and renal failure
404.91 Unspecified hypertensive heart and renal disease with heart failure ▽
404.93 Unspecified hypertensive hear and renal disease with heart failure and renal failure ▽
410.00 Acute myocardial infarction of anterolateral wall, episode of care unspecified — (Use additional code to identify presence of hypertension: 401.0-405.9) ▽
410.01 Acute myocardial infarction of anterolateral wall, initial episode of care — (Use additional code to identify presence of hypertension: 401.0-405.9)
410.02 Acute myocardial infarction of anterolateral wall, subsequent episode of care — (Use additional code to identify presence of hypertension: 401.0-405.9)
410.10 Acute myocardial infarction of other anterior wall, episode of care unspecified — (Use additional code to identify presence of hypertension: 401.0-405.9) ▽
410.11 Acute myocardial infarction of other anterior wall, initial episode of care — (Use additional code to identify presence of hypertension: 401.0-405.9)
410.12 Acute myocardial infarction of other anterior wall, subsequent episode of care — (Use additional code to identify presence of hypertension: 401.0-405.9)
410.20 Acute myocardial infarction of inferolateral wall, episode of care unspecified — (Use additional code to identify presence of hypertension: 401.0-405.9) ▽
410.21 Acute myocardial infarction of inferolateral wall, initial episode of care — (Use additional code to identify presence of hypertension: 401.0-405.9)
410.22 Acute myocardial infarction of inferolateral wall, subsequent episode of care — (Use additional code to identify presence of hypertension: 401.0-405.9)
410.30 Acute myocardial infarction of inferoposterior wall, episode of care unspecified — (Use additional code to identify presence of hypertension: 401.0-405.9) ▽
410.31 Acute myocardial infarction of inferoposterior wall, initial episode of care — (Use additional code to identify presence of hypertension: 401.0-405.9)
410.32 Acute myocardial infarction of inferoposterior wall, subsequent episode of care — (Use additional code to identify presence of hypertension: 401.0-405.9)
410.40 Acute myocardial infarction of other inferior wall, episode of care unspecified — (Use additional code to identify presence of hypertension: 401.0-405.9) ▽
410.41 Acute myocardial infarction of other inferior wall, initial episode of care — (Use additional code to identify presence of hypertension: 401.0-405.9)
410.42 Acute myocardial infarction of other inferior wall, subsequent episode of care — (Use additional code to identify presence of hypertension: 401.0-405.9)
410.50 Acute myocardial infarction of other lateral wall, episode of care unspecified — (Use additional code to identify presence of hypertension: 401.0-405.9) ▽
410.51 Acute myocardial infarction of other lateral wall, initial episode of care — (Use additional code to identify presence of hypertension: 401.0-405.9)
410.52 Acute myocardial infarction of other lateral wall, subsequent episode of care — (Use additional code to identify presence of hypertension: 401.0-405.9)
410.60 Acute myocardial infarction, true posterior wall infarction, episode of care unspecified — (Use additional code to identify presence of hypertension: 401.0-405.9) ▽
410.61 Acute myocardial infarction, true posterior wall infarction, initial episode of care — (Use additional code to identify presence of hypertension: 401.0-405.9)
410.62 Acute myocardial infarction, true posterior wall infarction, subsequent episode of care — (Use additional code to identify presence of hypertension: 401.0-405.9)
410.70 Acute myocardial infarction, subendocardial infarction, episode of care unspecified — (Use additional code to identify presence of hypertension: 401.0-405.9) ▽
410.71 Acute myocardial infarction, subendocardial infarction, initial episode of care — (Use additional code to identify presence of hypertension: 401.0-405.9)
410.72 Acute myocardial infarction, subendocardial infarction, subsequent episode of care — (Use additional code to identify presence of hypertension: 401.0-405.9)
410.80 Acute myocardial infarction of other specified sites, episode of care unspecified — (Use additional code to identify presence of hypertension: 401.0-405.9) ▽
410.81 Acute myocardial infarction of other specified sites, initial episode of care — (Use additional code to identify presence of hypertension: 401.0-405.9)
410.82 Acute myocardial infarction of other specified sites, subsequent episode of care — (Use additional code to identify presence of hypertension: 401.0-405.9)
410.90 Acute myocardial infarction, unspecified site, episode of care unspecified — (Use additional code to identify presence of hypertension: 401.0-405.9) ▽
410.91 Acute myocardial infarction, unspecified site, initial episode of care — (Use additional code to identify presence of hypertension: 401.0-405.9) ▽
410.92 Acute myocardial infarction, unspecified site, subsequent episode of care — (Use additional code to identify presence of hypertension: 401.0-405.9) ▽
411.89 Other acute and subacute form of ischemic heart disease — (Use additional code to identify presence of hypertension: 401.0-405.9)
414.9 Unspecified chronic ischemic heart disease — (Use additional code to identify presence of hypertension: 401.0-405.9) ▽
424.1 Aortic valve disorders
425.4 Other primary cardiomyopathies
427.5 Cardiac arrest
428.0 Congestive heart failure, unspecified ▽
428.1 Left heart failure
428.20 Unspecified systolic heart failure ▽
428.21 Acute systolic heart failure
428.22 Chronic systolic heart failure
428.23 Acute on chronic systolic heart failure
428.30 Unspecified diastolic heart failure ▽
428.31 Acute diastolic heart failure
428.32 Chronic diastolic heart failure
428.33 Acute on chronic diastolic heart failure

428.40 Unspecified combined systolic and diastolic heart failure ▽
428.41 Acute combined systolic and diastolic heart failure
428.42 Chronic combined systolic and diastolic heart failure
428.43 Acute on chronic combined systolic and diastolic heart failure
429.1 Myocardial degeneration — (Use additional code to identify presence of arteriosclerosis)
429.2 Unspecified cardiovascular disease — (Use additional code to identify presence of arteriosclerosis) ▽
429.4 Functional disturbances following cardiac surgery
785.51 Cardiogenic shock
997.1 Cardiac complications — (Use additional code to identify complications)
V45.81 Postsurgical aortocoronary bypass status — (This code is intended for use when these conditions are recorded as diagnoses or problems)

ICD-9-CM Procedural

37.61 Implant of pulsation balloon

33968

33968 Removal of intra-aortic balloon assist device, percutaneous

ICD-9-CM Diagnostic

996.00 Mechanical complication of unspecified cardiac device, implant, and graft ▽
996.1 Mechanical complication of other vascular device, implant, and graft
996.62 Infection and inflammatory reaction due to other vascular device, implant, and graft — (Use additional code to identify specified infections)
997.1 Cardiac complications — (Use additional code to identify complications)
V45.81 Postsurgical aortocoronary bypass status — (This code is intended for use when these conditions are recorded as diagnoses or problems)
V58.81 Fitting and adjustment of vascular catheter

ICD-9-CM Procedural

37.64 Removal of heart assist system
97.44 Nonoperative removal of heart assist system

33970–33971

33970 Insertion of intra-aortic balloon assist device through the femoral artery, open approach
33971 Removal of intra-aortic balloon assist device including repair of femoral artery, with or without graft

ICD-9-CM Diagnostic

402.01 Malignant hypertensive heart disease with heart failure
402.11 Benign hypertensive heart disease with heart failure
402.91 Unspecified hypertensive heart disease with heart failure ▽
404.01 Malignant hypertensive heart and renal disease with heart failure
404.11 Benign hypertensive heart and renal disease with heart failure
404.13 Benign hypertensive heart and renal disease with heart failure and renal failure
404.91 Unspecified hypertensive heart and renal disease with heart failure ▽
404.93 Unspecified hypertensive hear and renal disease with heart failure and renal failure ▽
410.00 Acute myocardial infarction of anterolateral wall, episode of care unspecified — (Use additional code to identify presence of hypertension: 401.0-405.9) ▽
410.01 Acute myocardial infarction of anterolateral wall, initial episode of care — (Use additional code to identify presence of hypertension: 401.0-405.9)
410.02 Acute myocardial infarction of anterolateral wall, subsequent episode of care — (Use additional code to identify presence of hypertension: 401.0-405.9)
410.10 Acute myocardial infarction of other anterior wall, episode of care unspecified — (Use additional code to identify presence of hypertension: 401.0-405.9) ▽
410.11 Acute myocardial infarction of other anterior wall, initial episode of care — (Use additional code to identify presence of hypertension: 401.0-405.9)
410.12 Acute myocardial infarction of other anterior wall, subsequent episode of care — (Use additional code to identify presence of hypertension: 401.0-405.9)
410.20 Acute myocardial infarction of inferolateral wall, episode of care unspecified — (Use additional code to identify presence of hypertension: 401.0-405.9) ▽
410.21 Acute myocardial infarction of inferolateral wall, initial episode of care — (Use additional code to identify presence of hypertension: 401.0-405.9)
410.22 Acute myocardial infarction of inferolateral wall, subsequent episode of care — (Use additional code to identify presence of hypertension: 401.0-405.9)
410.30 Acute myocardial infarction of inferoposterior wall, episode of care unspecified — (Use additional code to identify presence of hypertension: 401.0-405.9) ▽
410.31 Acute myocardial infarction of inferoposterior wall, initial episode of care — (Use additional code to identify presence of hypertension: 401.0-405.9)
410.32 Acute myocardial infarction of inferoposterior wall, subsequent episode of care — (Use additional code to identify presence of hypertension: 401.0-405.9)
410.40 Acute myocardial infarction of other inferior wall, episode of care unspecified — (Use additional code to identify presence of hypertension: 401.0-405.9) ▽
410.41 Acute myocardial infarction of other inferior wall, initial episode of care — (Use additional code to identify presence of hypertension: 401.0-405.9)
410.42 Acute myocardial infarction of other inferior wall, subsequent episode of care — (Use additional code to identify presence of hypertension: 401.0-405.9)
410.50 Acute myocardial infarction of other lateral wall, episode of care unspecified — (Use additional code to identify presence of hypertension: 401.0-405.9) ▽
410.51 Acute myocardial infarction of other lateral wall, initial episode of care — (Use additional code to identify presence of hypertension: 401.0-405.9)
410.52 Acute myocardial infarction of other lateral wall, subsequent episode of care — (Use additional code to identify presence of hypertension: 401.0-405.9)
410.60 Acute myocardial infarction, true posterior wall infarction, episode of care unspecified — (Use additional code to identify presence of hypertension: 401.0-405.9) ▽
410.61 Acute myocardial infarction, true posterior wall infarction, initial episode of care — (Use additional code to identify presence of hypertension: 401.0-405.9)
410.62 Acute myocardial infarction, true posterior wall infarction, subsequent episode of care — (Use additional code to identify presence of hypertension: 401.0-405.9)
410.70 Acute myocardial infarction, subendocardial infarction, episode of care unspecified — (Use additional code to identify presence of hypertension: 401.0-405.9) ▽
410.71 Acute myocardial infarction, subendocardial infarction, initial episode of care — (Use additional code to identify presence of hypertension: 401.0-405.9)
410.72 Acute myocardial infarction, subendocardial infarction, subsequent episode of care — (Use additional code to identify presence of hypertension: 401.0-405.9)
410.80 Acute myocardial infarction of other specified sites, episode of care unspecified — (Use additional code to identify presence of hypertension: 401.0-405.9) ▽
410.81 Acute myocardial infarction of other specified sites, initial episode of care — (Use additional code to identify presence of hypertension: 401.0-405.9)
410.82 Acute myocardial infarction of other specified sites, subsequent episode of care — (Use additional code to identify presence of hypertension: 401.0-405.9)
410.90 Acute myocardial infarction, unspecified site, episode of care unspecified — (Use additional code to identify presence of hypertension: 401.0-405.9) ▽
410.91 Acute myocardial infarction, unspecified site, initial episode of care — (Use additional code to identify presence of hypertension: 401.0-405.9) ▽
410.92 Acute myocardial infarction, unspecified site, subsequent episode of care — (Use additional code to identify presence of hypertension: 401.0-405.9) ▽
411.89 Other acute and subacute form of ischemic heart disease — (Use additional code to identify presence of hypertension: 401.0-405.9)
414.9 Unspecified chronic ischemic heart disease — (Use additional code to identify presence of hypertension: 401.0-405.9) ▽
424.1 Aortic valve disorders
425.4 Other primary cardiomyopathies
427.5 Cardiac arrest
428.0 Congestive heart failure, unspecified ▽
428.1 Left heart failure
428.20 Unspecified systolic heart failure ▽
428.21 Acute systolic heart failure
428.22 Chronic systolic heart failure
428.23 Acute on chronic systolic heart failure
428.30 Unspecified diastolic heart failure ▽
428.31 Acute diastolic heart failure
428.32 Chronic diastolic heart failure
428.33 Acute on chronic diastolic heart failure
428.40 Unspecified combined systolic and diastolic heart failure ▽
428.41 Acute combined systolic and diastolic heart failure
428.42 Chronic combined systolic and diastolic heart failure
428.43 Acute on chronic combined systolic and diastolic heart failure
429.1 Myocardial degeneration — (Use additional code to identify presence of arteriosclerosis)
429.2 Unspecified cardiovascular disease — (Use additional code to identify presence of arteriosclerosis) ▽
429.4 Functional disturbances following cardiac surgery
785.51 Cardiogenic shock
996.00 Mechanical complication of unspecified cardiac device, implant, and graft ▽
996.02 Mechanical complication due to heart valve prosthesis
996.1 Mechanical complication of other vascular device, implant, and graft
996.62 Infection and inflammatory reaction due to other vascular device, implant, and graft — (Use additional code to identify specified infections)
997.1 Cardiac complications — (Use additional code to identify complications)
V45.81 Postsurgical aortocoronary bypass status — (This code is intended for use when these conditions are recorded as diagnoses or problems)
V58.81 Fitting and adjustment of vascular catheter

▽ Unspecified code ♀ Female diagnosis ☒ Manifestation code ♂ Male diagnosis

ICD-9-CM Procedural

37.61 Implant of pulsation balloon
37.64 Removal of heart assist system

33973–33974

33973 Insertion of intra-aortic balloon assist device through the ascending aorta
33974 Removal of intra-aortic balloon assist device from the ascending aorta, including repair of the ascending aorta, with or without graft

ICD-9-CM Diagnostic

402.01 Malignant hypertensive heart disease with heart failure
402.11 Benign hypertensive heart disease with heart failure
402.91 Unspecified hypertensive heart disease with heart failure ▽
404.01 Malignant hypertensive heart and renal disease with heart failure
404.11 Benign hypertensive heart and renal disease with heart failure
404.13 Benign hypertensive heart and renal disease with heart failure and renal failure
404.91 Unspecified hypertensive heart and renal disease with heart failure ▽
404.93 Unspecified hypertensive hear and renal disease with heart failure and renal failure ▽
410.00 Acute myocardial infarction of anterolateral wall, episode of care unspecified — (Use additional code to identify presence of hypertension: 401.0-405.9) ▽
410.01 Acute myocardial infarction of anterolateral wall, initial episode of care — (Use additional code to identify presence of hypertension: 401.0-405.9)
410.02 Acute myocardial infarction of anterolateral wall, subsequent episode of care — (Use additional code to identify presence of hypertension: 401.0-405.9)
410.10 Acute myocardial infarction of other anterior wall, episode of care unspecified — (Use additional code to identify presence of hypertension: 401.0-405.9) ▽
410.11 Acute myocardial infarction of other anterior wall, initial episode of care — (Use additional code to identify presence of hypertension: 401.0-405.9)
410.12 Acute myocardial infarction of other anterior wall, subsequent episode of care — (Use additional code to identify presence of hypertension: 401.0-405.9)
410.20 Acute myocardial infarction of inferolateral wall, episode of care unspecified — (Use additional code to identify presence of hypertension: 401.0-405.9) ▽
410.21 Acute myocardial infarction of inferolateral wall, initial episode of care — (Use additional code to identify presence of hypertension: 401.0-405.9)
410.22 Acute myocardial infarction of inferolateral wall, subsequent episode of care — (Use additional code to identify presence of hypertension: 401.0-405.9)
410.30 Acute myocardial infarction of inferoposterior wall, episode of care unspecified — (Use additional code to identify presence of hypertension: 401.0-405.9) ▽
410.31 Acute myocardial infarction of inferoposterior wall, initial episode of care — (Use additional code to identify presence of hypertension: 401.0-405.9)
410.32 Acute myocardial infarction of inferoposterior wall, subsequent episode of care — (Use additional code to identify presence of hypertension: 401.0-405.9)
410.40 Acute myocardial infarction of other inferior wall, episode of care unspecified — (Use additional code to identify presence of hypertension: 401.0-405.9) ▽
410.41 Acute myocardial infarction of other inferior wall, initial episode of care — (Use additional code to identify presence of hypertension: 401.0-405.9)
410.42 Acute myocardial infarction of other inferior wall, subsequent episode of care — (Use additional code to identify presence of hypertension: 401.0-405.9)
410.50 Acute myocardial infarction of other lateral wall, episode of care unspecified — (Use additional code to identify presence of hypertension: 401.0-405.9) ▽
410.51 Acute myocardial infarction of other lateral wall, initial episode of care — (Use additional code to identify presence of hypertension: 401.0-405.9)
410.52 Acute myocardial infarction of other lateral wall, subsequent episode of care — (Use additional code to identify presence of hypertension: 401.0-405.9)
410.60 Acute myocardial infarction, true posterior wall infarction, episode of care unspecified — (Use additional code to identify presence of hypertension: 401.0-405.9) ▽
410.61 Acute myocardial infarction, true posterior wall infarction, initial episode of care — (Use additional code to identify presence of hypertension: 401.0-405.9)
410.62 Acute myocardial infarction, true posterior wall infarction, subsequent episode of care — (Use additional code to identify presence of hypertension: 401.0-405.9)
410.70 Acute myocardial infarction, subendocardial infarction, episode of care unspecified — (Use additional code to identify presence of hypertension: 401.0-405.9) ▽
410.71 Acute myocardial infarction, subendocardial infarction, initial episode of care — (Use additional code to identify presence of hypertension: 401.0-405.9)
410.72 Acute myocardial infarction, subendocardial infarction, subsequent episode of care — (Use additional code to identify presence of hypertension: 401.0-405.9)
410.80 Acute myocardial infarction of other specified sites, episode of care unspecified — (Use additional code to identify presence of hypertension: 401.0-405.9) ▽
410.81 Acute myocardial infarction of other specified sites, initial episode of care — (Use additional code to identify presence of hypertension: 401.0-405.9)
410.82 Acute myocardial infarction of other specified sites, subsequent episode of care — (Use additional code to identify presence of hypertension: 401.0-405.9)
410.90 Acute myocardial infarction, unspecified site, episode of care unspecified — (Use additional code to identify presence of hypertension: 401.0-405.9) ▽
410.91 Acute myocardial infarction, unspecified site, initial episode of care — (Use additional code to identify presence of hypertension: 401.0-405.9) ▽
410.92 Acute myocardial infarction, unspecified site, subsequent episode of care — (Use additional code to identify presence of hypertension: 401.0-405.9) ▽
411.89 Other acute and subacute form of ischemic heart disease — (Use additional code to identify presence of hypertension: 401.0-405.9)
414.9 Unspecified chronic ischemic heart disease — (Use additional code to identify presence of hypertension: 401.0-405.9) ▽
424.1 Aortic valve disorders
425.4 Other primary cardiomyopathies
427.5 Cardiac arrest
428.0 Congestive heart failure, unspecified ▽
428.1 Left heart failure
428.20 Unspecified systolic heart failure ▽
428.21 Acute systolic heart failure
428.22 Chronic systolic heart failure
428.23 Acute on chronic systolic heart failure
428.30 Unspecified diastolic heart failure ▽
428.31 Acute diastolic heart failure
428.32 Chronic diastolic heart failure
428.33 Acute on chronic diastolic heart failure
428.40 Unspecified combined systolic and diastolic heart failure ▽
428.41 Acute combined systolic and diastolic heart failure
428.42 Chronic combined systolic and diastolic heart failure
428.43 Acute on chronic combined systolic and diastolic heart failure
429.1 Myocardial degeneration — (Use additional code to identify presence of arteriosclerosis)
429.2 Unspecified cardiovascular disease — (Use additional code to identify presence of arteriosclerosis) ▽
429.4 Functional disturbances following cardiac surgery
785.51 Cardiogenic shock
996.00 Mechanical complication of unspecified cardiac device, implant, and graft ▽
996.02 Mechanical complication due to heart valve prosthesis
996.1 Mechanical complication of other vascular device, implant, and graft
996.62 Infection and inflammatory reaction due to other vascular device, implant, and graft — (Use additional code to identify specified infections)
997.1 Cardiac complications — (Use additional code to identify complications)
V45.81 Postsurgical aortocoronary bypass status — (This code is intended for use when these conditions are recorded as diagnoses or problems)
V58.81 Fitting and adjustment of vascular catheter

ICD-9-CM Procedural

37.61 Implant of pulsation balloon
37.64 Removal of heart assist system

33975–33976

33975 Insertion of ventricular assist device; extracorporeal, single ventricle
33976 extracorporeal, biventricular

ICD-9-CM Diagnostic

402.01 Malignant hypertensive heart disease with heart failure
402.11 Benign hypertensive heart disease with heart failure
402.91 Unspecified hypertensive heart disease with heart failure ▽
404.01 Malignant hypertensive heart and renal disease with heart failure
404.03 Malignant hypertensive heart and renal disease with heart failure and renal failure
404.11 Benign hypertensive heart and renal disease with heart failure
404.13 Benign hypertensive heart and renal disease with heart failure and renal failure
404.91 Unspecified hypertensive heart and renal disease with heart failure ▽
404.93 Unspecified hypertensive hear and renal disease with heart failure and renal failure ▽
410.00 Acute myocardial infarction of anterolateral wall, episode of care unspecified — (Use additional code to identify presence of hypertension: 401.0-405.9) ▽
410.01 Acute myocardial infarction of anterolateral wall, initial episode of care — (Use additional code to identify presence of hypertension: 401.0-405.9)
410.02 Acute myocardial infarction of anterolateral wall, subsequent episode of care — (Use additional code to identify presence of hypertension: 401.0-405.9)
410.10 Acute myocardial infarction of other anterior wall, episode of care unspecified — (Use additional code to identify presence of hypertension: 401.0-405.9) ▽
410.11 Acute myocardial infarction of other anterior wall, initial episode of care — (Use additional code to identify presence of hypertension: 401.0-405.9)
410.12 Acute myocardial infarction of other anterior wall, subsequent episode of care — (Use additional code to identify presence of hypertension: 401.0-405.9)

410.20 Acute myocardial infarction of inferolateral wall, episode of care unspecified — (Use additional code to identify presence of hypertension: 401.0-405.9)
410.21 Acute myocardial infarction of inferolateral wall, initial episode of care — (Use additional code to identify presence of hypertension: 401.0-405.9)
410.22 Acute myocardial infarction of inferolateral wall, subsequent episode of care — (Use additional code to identify presence of hypertension: 401.0-405.9)
410.30 Acute myocardial infarction of inferoposterior wall, episode of care unspecified — (Use additional code to identify presence of hypertension: 401.0-405.9)
410.31 Acute myocardial infarction of inferoposterior wall, initial episode of care — (Use additional code to identify presence of hypertension: 401.0-405.9)
410.32 Acute myocardial infarction of inferoposterior wall, subsequent episode of care — (Use additional code to identify presence of hypertension: 401.0-405.9)
410.40 Acute myocardial infarction of other inferior wall, episode of care unspecified — (Use additional code to identify presence of hypertension: 401.0-405.9)
410.41 Acute myocardial infarction of other inferior wall, initial episode of care — (Use additional code to identify presence of hypertension: 401.0-405.9)
410.42 Acute myocardial infarction of other inferior wall, subsequent episode of care — (Use additional code to identify presence of hypertension: 401.0-405.9)
410.50 Acute myocardial infarction of other lateral wall, episode of care unspecified — (Use additional code to identify presence of hypertension: 401.0-405.9)
410.51 Acute myocardial infarction of other lateral wall, initial episode of care — (Use additional code to identify presence of hypertension: 401.0-405.9)
410.52 Acute myocardial infarction of other lateral wall, subsequent episode of care — (Use additional code to identify presence of hypertension: 401.0-405.9)
410.60 Acute myocardial infarction, true posterior wall infarction, episode of care unspecified — (Use additional code to identify presence of hypertension: 401.0-405.9)
410.61 Acute myocardial infarction, true posterior wall infarction, initial episode of care — (Use additional code to identify presence of hypertension: 401.0-405.9)
410.62 Acute myocardial infarction, true posterior wall infarction, subsequent episode of care — (Use additional code to identify presence of hypertension: 401.0-405.9)
410.70 Acute myocardial infarction, subendocardial infarction, episode of care unspecified — (Use additional code to identify presence of hypertension: 401.0-405.9)
410.71 Acute myocardial infarction, subendocardial infarction, initial episode of care — (Use additional code to identify presence of hypertension: 401.0-405.9)
410.72 Acute myocardial infarction, subendocardial infarction, subsequent episode of care — (Use additional code to identify presence of hypertension: 401.0-405.9)
410.80 Acute myocardial infarction of other specified sites, episode of care unspecified — (Use additional code to identify presence of hypertension: 401.0-405.9)
410.81 Acute myocardial infarction of other specified sites, initial episode of care — (Use additional code to identify presence of hypertension: 401.0-405.9)
410.82 Acute myocardial infarction of other specified sites, subsequent episode of care — (Use additional code to identify presence of hypertension: 401.0-405.9)
410.90 Acute myocardial infarction, unspecified site, episode of care unspecified — (Use additional code to identify presence of hypertension: 401.0-405.9)
410.91 Acute myocardial infarction, unspecified site, initial episode of care — (Use additional code to identify presence of hypertension: 401.0-405.9)
410.92 Acute myocardial infarction, unspecified site, subsequent episode of care — (Use additional code to identify presence of hypertension: 401.0-405.9)
411.89 Other acute and subacute form of ischemic heart disease — (Use additional code to identify presence of hypertension: 401.0-405.9)
425.4 Other primary cardiomyopathies
427.5 Cardiac arrest
428.0 Congestive heart failure, unspecified
428.1 Left heart failure
428.20 Unspecified systolic heart failure
428.21 Acute systolic heart failure
428.22 Chronic systolic heart failure
428.23 Acute on chronic systolic heart failure
428.30 Unspecified diastolic heart failure
428.31 Acute diastolic heart failure
428.32 Chronic diastolic heart failure
428.33 Acute on chronic diastolic heart failure
428.40 Unspecified combined systolic and diastolic heart failure
428.41 Acute combined systolic and diastolic heart failure
428.42 Chronic combined systolic and diastolic heart failure
428.43 Acute on chronic combined systolic and diastolic heart failure
428.9 Unspecified heart failure
429.1 Myocardial degeneration — (Use additional code to identify presence of arteriosclerosis)
429.2 Unspecified cardiovascular disease — (Use additional code to identify presence of arteriosclerosis)
429.4 Functional disturbances following cardiac surgery
785.51 Cardiogenic shock
997.1 Cardiac complications — (Use additional code to identify complications)
V45.81 Postsurgical aortocoronary bypass status — (This code is intended for use when these conditions are recorded as diagnoses or problems)

ICD-9-CM Procedural

37.65 Implant of external heart assist system

33977–33978

33977 Removal of ventricular assist device; extracorporeal, single ventricle
33978 extracorporeal, biventricular

ICD-9-CM Diagnostic

996.00 Mechanical complication of unspecified cardiac device, implant, and graft
996.61 Infection and inflammatory reaction due to cardiac device, implant, and graft — (Use additional code to identify specified infections)
V58.81 Fitting and adjustment of vascular catheter
V58.89 Encounter for other specified aftercare

ICD-9-CM Procedural

37.64 Removal of heart assist system

33979

33979 Insertion of ventricular assist device, implantable intracorporeal, single ventricle

ICD-9-CM Diagnostic

402.01 Malignant hypertensive heart disease with heart failure
402.11 Benign hypertensive heart disease with heart failure
402.91 Unspecified hypertensive heart disease with heart failure
404.01 Malignant hypertensive heart and renal disease with heart failure
404.03 Malignant hypertensive heart and renal disease with heart failure and renal failure
404.11 Benign hypertensive heart and renal disease with heart failure
404.13 Benign hypertensive heart and renal disease with heart failure and renal failure
404.91 Unspecified hypertensive heart and renal disease with heart failure
404.93 Unspecified hypertensive hear and renal disease with heart failure and renal failure
410.00 Acute myocardial infarction of anterolateral wall, episode of care unspecified — (Use additional code to identify presence of hypertension: 401.0-405.9)
410.01 Acute myocardial infarction of anterolateral wall, initial episode of care — (Use additional code to identify presence of hypertension: 401.0-405.9)
410.02 Acute myocardial infarction of anterolateral wall, subsequent episode of care — (Use additional code to identify presence of hypertension: 401.0-405.9)
410.10 Acute myocardial infarction of other anterior wall, episode of care unspecified — (Use additional code to identify presence of hypertension: 401.0-405.9)
410.11 Acute myocardial infarction of other anterior wall, initial episode of care — (Use additional code to identify presence of hypertension: 401.0-405.9)
410.12 Acute myocardial infarction of other anterior wall, subsequent episode of care — (Use additional code to identify presence of hypertension: 401.0-405.9)
410.20 Acute myocardial infarction of inferolateral wall, episode of care unspecified — (Use additional code to identify presence of hypertension: 401.0-405.9)
410.21 Acute myocardial infarction of inferolateral wall, initial episode of care — (Use additional code to identify presence of hypertension: 401.0-405.9)
410.22 Acute myocardial infarction of inferolateral wall, subsequent episode of care — (Use additional code to identify presence of hypertension: 401.0-405.9)
410.30 Acute myocardial infarction of inferoposterior wall, episode of care unspecified — (Use additional code to identify presence of hypertension: 401.0-405.9)
410.31 Acute myocardial infarction of inferoposterior wall, initial episode of care — (Use additional code to identify presence of hypertension: 401.0-405.9)
410.32 Acute myocardial infarction of inferoposterior wall, subsequent episode of care — (Use additional code to identify presence of hypertension: 401.0-405.9)
410.40 Acute myocardial infarction of other inferior wall, episode of care unspecified — (Use additional code to identify presence of hypertension: 401.0-405.9)
410.41 Acute myocardial infarction of other inferior wall, initial episode of care — (Use additional code to identify presence of hypertension: 401.0-405.9)
410.42 Acute myocardial infarction of other inferior wall, subsequent episode of care — (Use additional code to identify presence of hypertension: 401.0-405.9)
410.50 Acute myocardial infarction of other lateral wall, episode of care unspecified — (Use additional code to identify presence of hypertension: 401.0-405.9)
410.51 Acute myocardial infarction of other lateral wall, initial episode of care — (Use additional code to identify presence of hypertension: 401.0-405.9)
410.52 Acute myocardial infarction of other lateral wall, subsequent episode of care — (Use additional code to identify presence of hypertension: 401.0-405.9)
410.60 Acute myocardial infarction, true posterior wall infarction, episode of care unspecified — (Use additional code to identify presence of hypertension: 401.0-405.9)

410.61 Acute myocardial infarction, true posterior wall infarction, initial episode of care — (Use additional code to identify presence of hypertension: 401.0-405.9)
410.62 Acute myocardial infarction, true posterior wall infarction, subsequent episode of care — (Use additional code to identify presence of hypertension: 401.0-405.9)
410.70 Acute myocardial infarction, subendocardial infarction, episode of care unspecified — (Use additional code to identify presence of hypertension: 401.0-405.9) ▽
410.71 Acute myocardial infarction, subendocardial infarction, initial episode of care — (Use additional code to identify presence of hypertension: 401.0-405.9)
410.72 Acute myocardial infarction, subendocardial infarction, subsequent episode of care — (Use additional code to identify presence of hypertension: 401.0-405.9)
410.80 Acute myocardial infarction of other specified sites, episode of care unspecified — (Use additional code to identify presence of hypertension: 401.0-405.9) ▽
410.81 Acute myocardial infarction of other specified sites, initial episode of care — (Use additional code to identify presence of hypertension: 401.0-405.9)
410.82 Acute myocardial infarction of other specified sites, subsequent episode of care — (Use additional code to identify presence of hypertension: 401.0-405.9)
410.90 Acute myocardial infarction, unspecified site, episode of care unspecified — (Use additional code to identify presence of hypertension: 401.0-405.9) ▽
410.91 Acute myocardial infarction, unspecified site, initial episode of care — (Use additional code to identify presence of hypertension: 401.0-405.9) ▽
410.92 Acute myocardial infarction, unspecified site, subsequent episode of care — (Use additional code to identify presence of hypertension: 401.0-405.9) ▽
411.89 Other acute and subacute form of ischemic heart disease — (Use additional code to identify presence of hypertension: 401.0-405.9)
425.4 Other primary cardiomyopathies
427.5 Cardiac arrest
428.0 Congestive heart failure, unspecified ▽
428.1 Left heart failure
428.20 Unspecified systolic heart failure ▽
428.21 Acute systolic heart failure
428.22 Chronic systolic heart failure
428.23 Acute on chronic systolic heart failure
428.30 Unspecified diastolic heart failure ▽
428.31 Acute diastolic heart failure
428.32 Chronic diastolic heart failure
428.33 Acute on chronic diastolic heart failure
428.40 Unspecified combined systolic and diastolic heart failure ▽
428.41 Acute combined systolic and diastolic heart failure
428.42 Chronic combined systolic and diastolic heart failure
428.43 Acute on chronic combined systolic and diastolic heart failure
428.9 Unspecified heart failure ▽
429.1 Myocardial degeneration — (Use additional code to identify presence of arteriosclerosis)
429.2 Unspecified cardiovascular disease — (Use additional code to identify presence of arteriosclerosis) ▽
429.4 Functional disturbances following cardiac surgery
785.51 Cardiogenic shock
997.1 Cardiac complications — (Use additional code to identify complications)
V45.81 Postsurgical aortocoronary bypass status — (This code is intended for use when these conditions are recorded as diagnoses or problems)

ICD-9-CM Procedural

37.66 Insertion of implantable heart assist system

HCPCS Level II Supplies & Services

HCPCS Level II codes are used to report the supplies, durable medical equipment, and certain medical services provided on an outpatient basis. Because the procedure(s) represented on this page would be performed in an inpatient facility, no HCPCS Level II codes apply.

33980

33980 Removal of ventricular assist device, implantable intracorporeal, single ventricle

ICD-9-CM Diagnostic

996.00 Mechanical complication of unspecified cardiac device, implant, and graft ▽
996.09 Mechanical complication of cardiac device, implant, and graft, other
996.61 Infection and inflammatory reaction due to cardiac device, implant, and graft — (Use additional code to identify specified infections)
996.62 Infection and inflammatory reaction due to other vascular device, implant, and graft — (Use additional code to identify specified infections)
V58.81 Fitting and adjustment of vascular catheter
V58.89 Encounter for other specified aftercare

ICD-9-CM Procedural

37.64 Removal of heart assist system

Arteries and Veins

34001

34001 Embolectomy or thrombectomy, with or without catheter; carotid, subclavian or innominate artery, by neck incision

ICD-9-CM Diagnostic

433.10 Occlusion and stenosis of carotid artery without mention of cerebral infarction — (Use additional code to identify presence of hypertension)
433.11 Occlusion and stenosis of carotid artery with cerebral infarction — (Use additional code to identify presence of hypertension)
433.30 Occlusion and stenosis of multiple and bilateral precerebral arteries without mention of cerebral infarction — (Use additional code to identify presence of hypertension)
433.31 Occlusion and stenosis of multiple and bilateral precerebral arteries with cerebral infarction — (Use additional code to identify presence of hypertension)
433.80 Occlusion and stenosis of other specified precerebral artery without mention of cerebral infarction — (Use additional code to identify presence of hypertension)
433.81 Occlusion and stenosis of other specified precerebral artery with cerebral infarction — (Use additional code to identify presence of hypertension)
435.0 Basilar artery syndrome — (Use additional code to identify presence of hypertension)
435.1 Vertebral artery syndrome — (Use additional code to identify presence of hypertension)
435.2 Subclavian steal syndrome — (Use additional code to identify presence of hypertension)
435.3 Vertebrobasilar artery syndrome — (Use additional code to identify presence of hypertension)
435.8 Other specified transient cerebral ischemias — (Use additional code to identify presence of hypertension)
435.9 Unspecified transient cerebral ischemia — (Use additional code to identify presence of hypertension) ▽
438.10 Unspecified speech and language deficit due to cerebrovascular disease — (Use additional code to identify presence of hypertension) ▽
438.12 Dysphasia due to cerebrovascular disease — (Use additional code to identify presence of hypertension)
438.20 Hemiplegia affecting unspecified side due to cerebrovascular disease — (Use additional code to identify presence of hypertension) ▽
438.22 Hemiplegia affecting nondominant side due to cerebrovascular disease — (Use additional code to identify presence of hypertension)
438.31 Monoplegia of upper limb affecting dominant side due to cerebrovascular disease — (Use additional code to identify presence of hypertension)
438.40 Monoplegia of lower limb affecting unspecified side due to cerebrovascular disease — (Use additional code to identify presence of hypertension) ▽
438.42 Monoplegia of lower limb affecting nondominant side due to cerebrovascular disease — (Use additional code to identify presence of hypertension)
438.51 Other paralytic syndrome affecting dominant side due to cerebrovascular disease — (Use additional code to identify type of paralytic syndrome: 344.81, 344.00-344.09. Use additional code to identify presence of hypertension)
438.81 Apraxia due to cerebrovascular disease — (Use additional code to identify presence of hypertension)
438.9 Unspecified late effects of cerebrovascular disease due to cerebrovascular disease — (Use additional code to identify presence of hypertension) ▽
441.1 Thoracic aneurysm, ruptured
443.21 Dissection of carotid artery
443.29 Dissection of other artery
900.01 Common carotid artery injury
900.02 External carotid artery injury
900.03 Internal carotid artery injury
901.1 Innominate and subclavian artery injury
996.71 Other complications due to heart valve prosthesis
996.72 Other complications due to other cardiac device, implant, and graft
996.74 Other complications due to other vascular device, implant, and graft
997.79 Vascular complications of other vessels — (Use additional code to identify complications)

ICD-9-CM Procedural

38.02 Incision of other vessels of head and neck
38.05 Incision of other thoracic vessels

▽ Unspecified code ♀ Female diagnosis ☒ Manifestation code ♂ Male diagnosis

34051

34051 Embolectomy or thrombectomy, with or without catheter; innominate, subclavian artery, by thoracic incision

ICD-9-CM Diagnostic

433.30 Occlusion and stenosis of multiple and bilateral precerebral arteries without mention of cerebral infarction — (Use additional code to identify presence of hypertension)
433.31 Occlusion and stenosis of multiple and bilateral precerebral arteries with cerebral infarction — (Use additional code to identify presence of hypertension)
433.80 Occlusion and stenosis of other specified precerebral artery without mention of cerebral infarction — (Use additional code to identify presence of hypertension)
433.81 Occlusion and stenosis of other specified precerebral artery with cerebral infarction — (Use additional code to identify presence of hypertension)
435.0 Basilar artery syndrome — (Use additional code to identify presence of hypertension)
435.1 Vertebral artery syndrome — (Use additional code to identify presence of hypertension)
435.2 Subclavian steal syndrome — (Use additional code to identify presence of hypertension)
435.3 Vertebrobasilar artery syndrome — (Use additional code to identify presence of hypertension)
435.8 Other specified transient cerebral ischemias — (Use additional code to identify presence of hypertension)
435.9 Unspecified transient cerebral ischemia — (Use additional code to identify presence of hypertension) ▽
438.10 Unspecified speech and language deficit due to cerebrovascular disease — (Use additional code to identify presence of hypertension) ▽
438.12 Dysphasia due to cerebrovascular disease — (Use additional code to identify presence of hypertension)
438.20 Hemiplegia affecting unspecified side due to cerebrovascular disease — (Use additional code to identify presence of hypertension) ▽
438.22 Hemiplegia affecting nondominant side due to cerebrovascular disease — (Use additional code to identify presence of hypertension)
438.31 Monoplegia of upper limb affecting dominant side due to cerebrovascular disease — (Use additional code to identify presence of hypertension)
438.40 Monoplegia of lower limb affecting unspecified side due to cerebrovascular disease — (Use additional code to identify presence of hypertension) ▽
438.42 Monoplegia of lower limb affecting nondominant side due to cerebrovascular disease — (Use additional code to identify presence of hypertension)
438.51 Other paralytic syndrome affecting dominant side due to cerebrovascular disease — (Use additional code to identify type of paralytic syndrome: 344.81, 344.00-344.09. Use additional code to identify presence of hypertension)
438.81 Apraxia due to cerebrovascular disease — (Use additional code to identify presence of hypertension)
438.9 Unspecified late effects of cerebrovascular disease due to cerebrovascular disease — (Use additional code to identify presence of hypertension) ▽
443.29 Dissection of other artery
901.1 Innominate and subclavian artery injury
996.71 Other complications due to heart valve prosthesis
996.72 Other complications due to other cardiac device, implant, and graft
996.74 Other complications due to other vascular device, implant, and graft
997.79 Vascular complications of other vessels — (Use additional code to identify complications)

ICD-9-CM Procedural

38.05 Incision of other thoracic vessels

34101–34111

34101 Embolectomy or thrombectomy, with or without catheter; axillary, brachial, innominate, subclavian artery, by arm incision
34111 radial or ulnar artery, by arm incision

ICD-9-CM Diagnostic

444.21 Embolism and thrombosis of arteries of upper extremity
444.9 Embolism and thrombosis of unspecified artery ▽
445.01 Atheroembolism of upper extremity
901.1 Innominate and subclavian artery injury
903.01 Axillary artery injury
903.1 Brachial blood vessels injury
903.2 Radial blood vessels injury
903.3 Ulnar blood vessels injury
903.8 Injury to specified blood vessels of upper extremity, other
996.62 Infection and inflammatory reaction due to other vascular device, implant, and graft — (Use additional code to identify specified infections)
996.74 Other complications due to other vascular device, implant, and graft
999.2 Other vascular complications of medical care, not elsewhere classified

ICD-9-CM Procedural

38.03 Incision of upper limb vessels
38.05 Incision of other thoracic vessels

34151

34151 Embolectomy or thrombectomy, with or without catheter; renal, celiac, mesentery, aortoiliac artery, by abdominal incision

ICD-9-CM Diagnostic

440.0 Atherosclerosis of aorta
440.1 Atherosclerosis of renal artery
444.0 Embolism and thrombosis of abdominal aorta
444.81 Embolism and thrombosis of iliac artery
444.89 Embolism and thrombosis of other specified artery
445.81 Atheroembolism of kidney — (Use additional code for any associated kidney failure: 584, 585)
445.89 Atheroembolism of other site
557.0 Acute vascular insufficiency of intestine
557.9 Unspecified vascular insufficiency of intestine ▽
593.81 Vascular disorders of kidney
673.24 Obstetrical blood-clot embolism, postpartum ♀
902.24 Injury to specified branches of celiac axis, other
902.25 Superior mesenteric artery (trunk) injury
902.26 Injury to primary branches of superior mesenteric artery
902.27 Inferior mesenteric artery injury
902.41 Renal artery injury
902.49 Renal blood vessel injury, other
902.59 Injury to iliac blood vessels, other
908.4 Late effect of injury to blood vessel of thorax, abdomen, and pelvis
996.62 Infection and inflammatory reaction due to other vascular device, implant, and graft — (Use additional code to identify specified infections)
996.74 Other complications due to other vascular device, implant, and graft
997.71 Vascular complications of mesenteric artery — (Use additional code to identify complications)
997.72 Vascular complications of renal artery — (Use additional code to identify complications)
997.79 Vascular complications of other vessels — (Use additional code to identify complications)
999.2 Other vascular complications of medical care, not elsewhere classified

ICD-9-CM Procedural

38.04 Incision of aorta
38.06 Incision of abdominal arteries

34201

34201 Embolectomy or thrombectomy, with or without catheter; femoropopliteal, aortoiliac artery, by leg incision

ICD-9-CM Diagnostic

444.0 Embolism and thrombosis of abdominal aorta
444.22 Embolism and thrombosis of arteries of lower extremity
445.02 Atheroembolism of lower extremity
733.93 Stress fracture of tibia or fibula
733.95 Stress fracture of other bone
821.00 Closed fracture of unspecified part of femur ▽
823.80 Closed fracture of unspecified part of tibia ▽
823.81 Closed fracture of unspecified part of fibula ▽
823.82 Closed fracture of unspecified part of fibula with tibia ▽
824.8 Unspecified closed fracture of ankle ▽
902.59 Injury to iliac blood vessels, other
904.0 Common femoral artery injury
904.41 Popliteal artery injury
996.74 Other complications due to other vascular device, implant, and graft
996.77 Other complications due to internal joint prosthesis
996.79 Other complications due to other internal prosthetic device, implant, and graft
997.79 Vascular complications of other vessels — (Use additional code to identify complications)
999.2 Other vascular complications of medical care, not elsewhere classified

ICD-9-CM Procedural

38.04 Incision of aorta
38.06 Incision of abdominal arteries
38.08 Incision of lower limb arteries

▽ Unspecified code ♀ Female diagnosis ☒ Manifestation code ♂ Male diagnosis

34203

34203 Embolectomy or thrombectomy, with or without catheter; popliteal-tibio-peroneal artery, by leg incision

ICD-9-CM Diagnostic

444.22 Embolism and thrombosis of arteries of lower extremity
445.02 Atheroembolism of lower extremity
733.93 Stress fracture of tibia or fibula
733.95 Stress fracture of other bone
823.80 Closed fracture of unspecified part of tibia
823.81 Closed fracture of unspecified part of fibula
823.82 Closed fracture of unspecified part of fibula with tibia
824.8 Unspecified closed fracture of ankle
904.41 Popliteal artery injury
904.51 Anterior tibial artery injury
904.53 Posterior tibial artery injury
904.7 Injury to specified blood vessels of lower extremity, other
996.74 Other complications due to other vascular device, implant, and graft
996.77 Other complications due to internal joint prosthesis
996.79 Other complications due to other internal prosthetic device, implant, and graft
999.2 Other vascular complications of medical care, not elsewhere classified

ICD-9-CM Procedural

38.08 Incision of lower limb arteries

34401

34401 Thrombectomy, direct or with catheter; vena cava, iliac vein, by abdominal incision

ICD-9-CM Diagnostic

451.81 Phlebitis and thrombophlebitis of iliac vein — (Use additional E code to identify drug, if drug-induced)
453.2 Embolism and thrombosis of vena cava
671.44 Deep phlebothrombosis, postpartum ♀
785.9 Other symptoms involving cardiovascular system
789.00 Abdominal pain, unspecified site
793.6 Nonspecific abnormal findings on radiological and other examination of abdominal area, including retroperitoneum
902.54 Iliac vein injury
908.4 Late effect of injury to blood vessel of thorax, abdomen, and pelvis
908.6 Late effect of certain complications of trauma
996.70 Other complications due to unspecified device, implant, and graft
996.74 Other complications due to other vascular device, implant, and graft
996.79 Other complications due to other internal prosthetic device, implant, and graft
997.2 Peripheral vascular complications — (Use additional code to identify complications)
997.79 Vascular complications of other vessels — (Use additional code to identify complications)
999.2 Other vascular complications of medical care, not elsewhere classified

ICD-9-CM Procedural

38.07 Incision of abdominal veins

34421–34451

34421 Thrombectomy, direct or with catheter; vena cava, iliac, femoropopliteal vein, by leg incision
34451 vena cava, iliac, femoropopliteal vein, by abdominal and leg incision

ICD-9-CM Diagnostic

451.0 Phlebitis and thrombophlebitis of superficial vessels of lower extremities — (Use additional E code to identify drug, if drug-induced)
451.11 Phlebitis and thrombophlebitis of femoral vein (deep) (superficial) — (Use additional E code to identify drug, if drug-induced)
451.19 Phlebitis and thrombophlebitis of other deep vessels of lower extremities — (Use additional E code to identify drug, if drug-induced)
451.81 Phlebitis and thrombophlebitis of iliac vein — (Use additional E code to identify drug, if drug-induced)
453.2 Embolism and thrombosis of vena cava
453.40 Venous embolism and thrombosis of unspecified deep vessels of lower extremity
453.41 Venous embolism and thrombosis of deep vessels of proximal lower extremity
453.42 Venous embolism and thrombosis of deep vessels of distal lower extremity
453.8 Embolism and thrombosis of other specified veins
733.93 Stress fracture of tibia or fibula
733.95 Stress fracture of other bone
821.00 Closed fracture of unspecified part of femur
823.80 Closed fracture of unspecified part of tibia

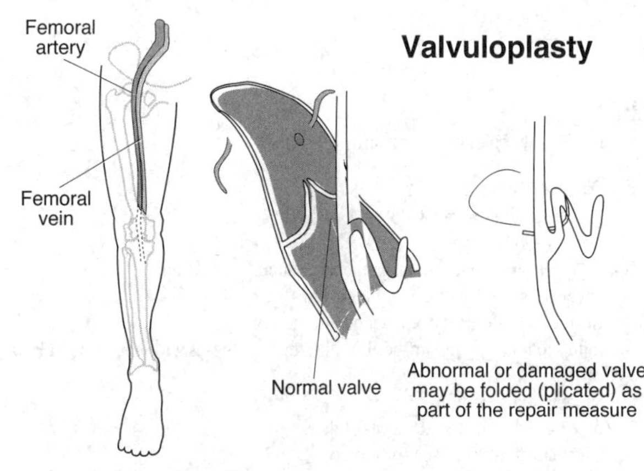
Femoral artery
Valvuloplasty
Femoral vein
Normal valve
Abnormal or damaged valve may be folded (plicated) as part of the repair measure

823.81 Closed fracture of unspecified part of fibula
823.82 Closed fracture of unspecified part of fibula with tibia
824.8 Unspecified closed fracture of ankle
902.54 Iliac vein injury
904.2 Femoral vein injury
996.70 Other complications due to unspecified device, implant, and graft
996.74 Other complications due to other vascular device, implant, and graft
997.79 Vascular complications of other vessels — (Use additional code to identify complications)
999.2 Other vascular complications of medical care, not elsewhere classified

ICD-9-CM Procedural

38.07 Incision of abdominal veins
38.09 Incision of lower limb veins

34471–34490

34471 Thrombectomy, direct or with catheter; subclavian vein, by neck incision
34490 axillary and subclavian vein, by arm incision

ICD-9-CM Diagnostic

451.89 Phlebitis and thrombophlebitis of other site — (Use additional E code to identify drug, if drug-induced)
453.40 Venous embolism and thrombosis of unspecified deep vessels of lower extremity
453.41 Venous embolism and thrombosis of deep vessels of proximal lower extremity
453.42 Venous embolism and thrombosis of deep vessels of distal lower extremity
453.8 Embolism and thrombosis of other specified veins
453.9 Embolism and thrombosis of unspecified site
901.3 Innominate and subclavian vein injury
903.02 Axillary vein injury
996.74 Other complications due to other vascular device, implant, and graft
997.79 Vascular complications of other vessels — (Use additional code to identify complications)

ICD-9-CM Procedural

38.02 Incision of other vessels of head and neck
38.03 Incision of upper limb vessels
38.05 Incision of other thoracic vessels

34501

34501 Valvuloplasty, femoral vein

ICD-9-CM Diagnostic

454.0 Varicose veins of lower extremities with ulcer
454.1 Varicose veins of lower extremities with inflammation
454.2 Varicose veins of lower extremities with ulcer and inflammation
454.8 Varicose veins of the lower extremities with other complications
454.9 Asymptomatic varicose veins
459.10 Postphlebitic syndrome without complications
459.11 Postphlebitic syndrome with ulcer
459.12 Postphlebitic syndrome with inflammation
459.13 Postphlebitic syndrome with ulcer and inflammation
459.19 Postphlebitic syndrome with other complication
459.81 Unspecified venous (peripheral) insufficiency — (Use additional code for any associated ulceration: 707.10-707.9)
747.60 Congenital anomaly of the peripheral vascular system, unspecified site
747.64 Congenital lower limb vessel anomaly
904.2 Femoral vein injury

ICD-9-CM Procedural
39.59 Other repair of vessel

34502
34502 Reconstruction of vena cava, any method

ICD-9-CM Diagnostic
453.2 Embolism and thrombosis of vena cava
459.2 Compression of vein
747.41 Total congenital anomalous pulmonary venous connection
747.49 Other congenital anomalies of great veins
861.11 Heart contusion with open wound into thorax
862.9 Injury to multiple and unspecified intrathoracic organs with open wound into cavity
901.2 Superior vena cava injury
901.83 Injury to multiple blood vessels of thorax
902.10 Unspecified inferior vena cava injury ▽
902.19 Injury to specified branches of inferior vena cava, other
908.4 Late effect of injury to blood vessel of thorax, abdomen, and pelvis
997.79 Vascular complications of other vessels — (Use additional code to identify complications)

ICD-9-CM Procedural
38.47 Resection of abdominal veins with replacement
39.57 Repair of blood vessel with synthetic patch graft
39.59 Other repair of vessel

34510
34510 Venous valve transposition, any vein donor

ICD-9-CM Diagnostic
454.0 Varicose veins of lower extremities with ulcer
454.1 Varicose veins of lower extremities with inflammation
454.2 Varicose veins of lower extremities with ulcer and inflammation
454.8 Varicose veins of the lower extremities with other complications
454.9 Asymptomatic varicose veins
459.10 Postphlebitic syndrome without complications
459.11 Postphlebitic syndrome with ulcer
459.12 Postphlebitic syndrome with inflammation
459.13 Postphlebitic syndrome with ulcer and inflammation
459.19 Postphlebitic syndrome with other complication
459.81 Unspecified venous (peripheral) insufficiency — (Use additional code for any associated ulceration: 707.10-707.9) ▽
747.60 Congenital anomaly of the peripheral vascular system, unspecified site ▽
747.64 Congenital lower limb vessel anomaly
904.2 Femoral vein injury

ICD-9-CM Procedural
38.40 Resection of vessel with replacement, unspecified site
38.42 Resection of other vessels of head and neck with replacement
38.43 Resection of upper limb vessels with replacement
38.45 Resection of other thoracic vessels with replacement

34520
34520 Cross-over vein graft to venous system

ICD-9-CM Diagnostic
454.0 Varicose veins of lower extremities with ulcer
454.1 Varicose veins of lower extremities with inflammation
454.2 Varicose veins of lower extremities with ulcer and inflammation
454.8 Varicose veins of the lower extremities with other complications
454.9 Asymptomatic varicose veins
459.10 Postphlebitic syndrome without complications
459.11 Postphlebitic syndrome with ulcer
459.12 Postphlebitic syndrome with inflammation
459.13 Postphlebitic syndrome with ulcer and inflammation
459.19 Postphlebitic syndrome with other complication
459.2 Compression of vein
459.81 Unspecified venous (peripheral) insufficiency — (Use additional code for any associated ulceration: 707.10-707.9) ▽
747.49 Other congenital anomalies of great veins
747.60 Congenital anomaly of the peripheral vascular system, unspecified site ▽
747.64 Congenital lower limb vessel anomaly
904.2 Femoral vein injury

ICD-9-CM Procedural
39.23 Other intrathoracic vascular shunt or bypass
39.29 Other (peripheral) vascular shunt or bypass

34530
34530 Saphenopopliteal vein anastomosis

ICD-9-CM Diagnostic
454.0 Varicose veins of lower extremities with ulcer
454.1 Varicose veins of lower extremities with inflammation
454.2 Varicose veins of lower extremities with ulcer and inflammation
454.8 Varicose veins of the lower extremities with other complications
454.9 Asymptomatic varicose veins
459.10 Postphlebitic syndrome without complications
459.11 Postphlebitic syndrome with ulcer
459.12 Postphlebitic syndrome with inflammation
459.13 Postphlebitic syndrome with ulcer and inflammation
459.19 Postphlebitic syndrome with other complication
459.2 Compression of vein
459.81 Unspecified venous (peripheral) insufficiency — (Use additional code for any associated ulceration: 707.10-707.9) ▽
891.1 Open wound of knee, leg (except thigh), and ankle, complicated — (Use additional code to identify infection)
904.3 Saphenous vein injury
904.42 Popliteal vein injury
904.7 Injury to specified blood vessels of lower extremity, other
998.2 Accidental puncture or laceration during procedure

ICD-9-CM Procedural
38.39 Resection of lower limb veins with anastomosis

34800–34805
34800 Endovascular repair of infrarenal abdominal aortic aneurysm or dissection; using aorto-aortic tube prosthesis
34802 using modular bifurcated prosthesis (one docking limb)
34803 using modular bifurcated prosthesis (two docking limbs)
34804 using unibody bifurcated prosthesis
34805 using aorto-uniiliac or aorto-unifemoral prosthesis

ICD-9-CM Diagnostic
440.0 Atherosclerosis of aorta
440.1 Atherosclerosis of renal artery
440.8 Atherosclerosis of other specified arteries
441.02 Dissecting aortic aneurysm (any part), abdominal
441.4 Abdominal aneurysm without mention of rupture
442.1 Aneurysm of renal artery
442.2 Aneurysm of iliac artery
444.0 Embolism and thrombosis of abdominal aorta
557.0 Acute vascular insufficiency of intestine
557.1 Chronic vascular insufficiency of intestine
593.81 Vascular disorders of kidney
747.89 Other specified congenital anomaly of circulatory system
902.50 Unspecified iliac vessel(s) injury ▽
902.51 Hypogastric artery injury
902.53 Iliac artery injury
908.4 Late effect of injury to blood vessel of thorax, abdomen, and pelvis
997.4 Digestive system complication — (Use additional code to identify complications)
997.79 Vascular complications of other vessels — (Use additional code to identify complications)

ICD-9-CM Procedural
39.71 Endovascular implantation of graft in abdominal aorta

34808
34808 Endovascular placement of iliac artery occlusion device (List separately in addition to code for primary procedure)

ICD-9-CM Diagnostic
This is an add-on code. Refer to the corresponding primary procedure code for ICD-9 diagnosis code links.

ICD-9-CM Procedural
39.79 Other endovascular repair (of aneurysm) of other vessels

▽ Unspecified code
♀ Female diagnosis
☒ Manifestation code
♂ Male diagnosis

34812

34812 Open femoral artery exposure for delivery of endovascular prosthesis, by groin incision, unilateral

ICD-9-CM Diagnostic

440.0 Atherosclerosis of aorta
440.1 Atherosclerosis of renal artery
440.8 Atherosclerosis of other specified arteries
441.02 Dissecting aortic aneurysm (any part), abdominal
441.4 Abdominal aneurysm without mention of rupture
442.1 Aneurysm of renal artery
442.2 Aneurysm of iliac artery
444.0 Embolism and thrombosis of abdominal aorta
557.0 Acute vascular insufficiency of intestine
557.1 Chronic vascular insufficiency of intestine
593.81 Vascular disorders of kidney
747.89 Other specified congenital anomaly of circulatory system
902.50 Unspecified iliac vessel(s) injury ▽
902.51 Hypogastric artery injury
902.53 Iliac artery injury
908.4 Late effect of injury to blood vessel of thorax, abdomen, and pelvis
997.4 Digestive system complication — (Use additional code to identify complications)
997.79 Vascular complications of other vessels — (Use additional code to identify complications)

ICD-9-CM Procedural

39.71 Endovascular implantation of graft in abdominal aorta

34813

34813 Placement of femoral-femoral prosthetic graft during endovascular aortic aneurysm repair (List separately in addition to code for primary procedure)

ICD-9-CM Diagnostic

440.20 Atherosclerosis of native arteries of the extremities, unspecified ▽
440.21 Atherosclerosis of native arteries of the extremities with intermittent claudication
440.24 Atherosclerosis of native arteries of the extremities with gangrene
442.3 Aneurysm of artery of lower extremity
443.29 Dissection of other artery
443.9 Unspecified peripheral vascular disease ▽
447.1 Stricture of artery
459.9 Unspecified circulatory system disorder ▽
747.69 Congenital anomaly of other specified site of peripheral vascular system
904.0 Common femoral artery injury
904.1 Superficial femoral artery injury
908.3 Late effect of injury to blood vessel of head, neck, and extremities
996.1 Mechanical complication of other vascular device, implant, and graft
996.74 Other complications due to other vascular device, implant, and graft
997.79 Vascular complications of other vessels — (Use additional code to identify complications)

ICD-9-CM Procedural

39.79 Other endovascular repair (of aneurysm) of other vessels

34820

34820 Open iliac artery exposure for delivery of endovascular prosthesis or iliac occlusion during endovascular therapy, by abdominal or retroperitoneal incision, unilateral

ICD-9-CM Diagnostic

440.0 Atherosclerosis of aorta
440.1 Atherosclerosis of renal artery
440.8 Atherosclerosis of other specified arteries
441.02 Dissecting aortic aneurysm (any part), abdominal
441.4 Abdominal aneurysm without mention of rupture
442.1 Aneurysm of renal artery
442.2 Aneurysm of iliac artery
443.22 Dissection of iliac artery
444.0 Embolism and thrombosis of abdominal aorta
557.0 Acute vascular insufficiency of intestine
557.1 Chronic vascular insufficiency of intestine
593.81 Vascular disorders of kidney
747.89 Other specified congenital anomaly of circulatory system
902.50 Unspecified iliac vessel(s) injury ▽
902.51 Hypogastric artery injury
902.53 Iliac artery injury
908.4 Late effect of injury to blood vessel of thorax, abdomen, and pelvis
997.4 Digestive system complication — (Use additional code to identify complications)
997.79 Vascular complications of other vessels — (Use additional code to identify complications)

ICD-9-CM Procedural

38.87 Other surgical occlusion of abdominal veins
39.79 Other endovascular repair (of aneurysm) of other vessels

34825–34826

34825 Placement of proximal or distal extension prosthesis for endovascular repair of infrarenal abdominal aortic or iliac aneurysm, false aneurysm, or dissection; initial vessel
34826 each additional vessel (List separately in addition to code for primary procedure)

ICD-9-CM Diagnostic

440.0 Atherosclerosis of aorta
440.8 Atherosclerosis of other specified arteries
441.02 Dissecting aortic aneurysm (any part), abdominal
441.3 Abdominal aneurysm, ruptured
441.4 Abdominal aneurysm without mention of rupture
442.2 Aneurysm of iliac artery
443.22 Dissection of iliac artery
444.0 Embolism and thrombosis of abdominal aorta
444.81 Embolism and thrombosis of iliac artery
902.50 Unspecified iliac vessel(s) injury ▽
902.53 Iliac artery injury
908.4 Late effect of injury to blood vessel of thorax, abdomen, and pelvis
997.79 Vascular complications of other vessels — (Use additional code to identify complications)

ICD-9-CM Procedural

39.71 Endovascular implantation of graft in abdominal aorta

34830–34832

34830 Open repair of infrarenal aortic aneurysm or dissection, plus repair of associated arterial trauma, following unsuccessful endovascular repair; tube prosthesis
34831 aorto-bi-iliac prosthesis
34832 aorto-bifemoral prosthesis

ICD-9-CM Diagnostic

440.0 Atherosclerosis of aorta
440.1 Atherosclerosis of renal artery
440.8 Atherosclerosis of other specified arteries
441.02 Dissecting aortic aneurysm (any part), abdominal
441.4 Abdominal aneurysm without mention of rupture
442.1 Aneurysm of renal artery
442.2 Aneurysm of iliac artery
443.22 Dissection of iliac artery
444.0 Embolism and thrombosis of abdominal aorta
557.0 Acute vascular insufficiency of intestine
557.1 Chronic vascular insufficiency of intestine
593.81 Vascular disorders of kidney
747.89 Other specified congenital anomaly of circulatory system
902.50 Unspecified iliac vessel(s) injury ▽
902.51 Hypogastric artery injury
902.53 Iliac artery injury
908.4 Late effect of injury to blood vessel of thorax, abdomen, and pelvis
997.4 Digestive system complication — (Use additional code to identify complications)
997.79 Vascular complications of other vessels — (Use additional code to identify complications)
998.11 Hemorrhage complicating a procedure
998.12 Hematoma complicating a procedure
998.2 Accidental puncture or laceration during procedure

ICD-9-CM Procedural

38.44 Resection of abdominal aorta with replacement

34833–34834

34833 Open iliac artery exposure with creation of conduit for delivery of infrarenal aortic or iliac endovascular prosthesis, by abdominal or retroperitoneal incision, unilateral

34834 Open brachial artery exposure to assist in the deployment of infrarenal aortic or iliac endovascular prosthesis by arm incision, unilateral

ICD-9-CM Diagnostic

440.0 Atherosclerosis of aorta
440.8 Atherosclerosis of other specified arteries
441.02 Dissecting aortic aneurysm (any part), abdominal
441.3 Abdominal aneurysm, ruptured
441.4 Abdominal aneurysm without mention of rupture
442.2 Aneurysm of iliac artery
444.0 Embolism and thrombosis of abdominal aorta
444.81 Embolism and thrombosis of iliac artery
444.89 Embolism and thrombosis of other specified artery
557.0 Acute vascular insufficiency of intestine
557.1 Chronic vascular insufficiency of intestine
747.89 Other specified congenital anomaly of circulatory system
902.50 Unspecified iliac vessel(s) injury ▽
902.51 Hypogastric artery injury
902.53 Iliac artery injury
908.4 Late effect of injury to blood vessel of thorax, abdomen, and pelvis
997.71 Vascular complications of mesenteric artery — (Use additional code to identify complications)
997.79 Vascular complications of other vessels — (Use additional code to identify complications)
998.11 Hemorrhage complicating a procedure
998.2 Accidental puncture or laceration during procedure

ICD-9-CM Procedural

39.79 Other endovascular repair (of aneurysm) of other vessels

HCPCS Level II Supplies & Services

HCPCS Level II codes are used to report the supplies, durable medical equipment, and certain medical services provided on an outpatient basis. Because the procedure(s) represented on this page would be performed in an inpatient facility, no HCPCS Level II codes apply.

34900

34900 Endovascular graft placement for repair of iliac artery (eg, aneurysm, pseudoaneurysm, arteriovenous malformation, trauma)

ICD-9-CM Diagnostic

442.2 Aneurysm of iliac artery
443.22 Dissection of iliac artery
444.81 Embolism and thrombosis of iliac artery
747.64 Congenital lower limb vessel anomaly
747.89 Other specified congenital anomaly of circulatory system
902.50 Unspecified iliac vessel(s) injury ▽
902.51 Hypogastric artery injury
902.53 Iliac artery injury
908.4 Late effect of injury to blood vessel of thorax, abdomen, and pelvis
997.79 Vascular complications of other vessels — (Use additional code to identify complications)
998.11 Hemorrhage complicating a procedure
998.12 Hematoma complicating a procedure
998.2 Accidental puncture or laceration during procedure

ICD-9-CM Procedural

39.79 Other endovascular repair (of aneurysm) of other vessels

HCPCS Level II Supplies & Services

HCPCS Level II codes are used to report the supplies, durable medical equipment, and certain medical services provided on an outpatient basis. Because the procedure(s) represented on this page would be performed in an inpatient facility, no HCPCS Level II codes apply.

35001–35002

35001 Direct repair of aneurysm, pseudoaneurysm, or excision (partial or total) and graft insertion, with or without patch graft; for aneurysm and associated occlusive disease, carotid, subclavian artery, by neck incision

35002 for ruptured aneurysm, carotid, subclavian artery, by neck incision

ICD-9-CM Diagnostic

433.10 Occlusion and stenosis of carotid artery without mention of cerebral infarction — (Use additional code to identify presence of hypertension)
433.11 Occlusion and stenosis of carotid artery with cerebral infarction — (Use additional code to identify presence of hypertension)
433.30 Occlusion and stenosis of multiple and bilateral precerebral arteries without mention of cerebral infarction — (Use additional code to identify presence of hypertension)
435.2 Subclavian steal syndrome — (Use additional code to identify presence of hypertension)
442.81 Aneurysm of artery of neck
442.82 Aneurysm of subclavian artery
443.21 Dissection of carotid artery
443.29 Dissection of other artery
447.1 Stricture of artery
747.89 Other specified congenital anomaly of circulatory system
900.00 Injury to carotid artery, unspecified ▽
900.01 Common carotid artery injury
900.02 External carotid artery injury
900.03 Internal carotid artery injury
900.82 Injury to multiple blood vessels of head and neck
901.1 Innominate and subclavian artery injury
908.3 Late effect of injury to blood vessel of head, neck, and extremities

ICD-9-CM Procedural

38.42 Resection of other vessels of head and neck with replacement
38.45 Resection of other thoracic vessels with replacement
39.51 Clipping of aneurysm
39.52 Other repair of aneurysm

35005

35005 Direct repair of aneurysm, pseudoaneurysm, or excision (partial or total) and graft insertion, with or without patch graft; for aneurysm, pseudoaneurysm, and associated occlusive disease, vertebral artery

ICD-9-CM Diagnostic

433.20 Occlusion and stenosis of vertebral artery without mention of cerebral infarction — (Use additional code to identify presence of hypertension)
433.30 Occlusion and stenosis of multiple and bilateral precerebral arteries without mention of cerebral infarction — (Use additional code to identify presence of hypertension)
435.2 Subclavian steal syndrome — (Use additional code to identify presence of hypertension)
442.81 Aneurysm of artery of neck
442.89 Aneurysm of other specified artery
443.24 Dissection of vertebral artery
447.1 Stricture of artery
908.3 Late effect of injury to blood vessel of head, neck, and extremities

ICD-9-CM Procedural

38.32 Resection of other vessels of head and neck with anastomosis
38.42 Resection of other vessels of head and neck with replacement
39.51 Clipping of aneurysm
39.52 Other repair of aneurysm

35011–35013

35011 Direct repair of aneurysm, pseudoaneurysm, or excision (partial or total) and graft insertion, with or without patch graft; for aneurysm and associated occlusive disease, axillary-brachial artery, by arm incision

35013 for ruptured aneurysm, axillary-brachial artery, by arm incision

ICD-9-CM Diagnostic

440.20 Atherosclerosis of native arteries of the extremities, unspecified ▽
440.21 Atherosclerosis of native arteries of the extremities with intermittent claudication
440.22 Atherosclerosis of native arteries of the extremities with rest pain
442.0 Aneurysm of artery of upper extremity
443.29 Dissection of other artery
444.21 Embolism and thrombosis of arteries of upper extremity
445.01 Atheroembolism of upper extremity

447.1 Stricture of artery
747.63 Congenital upper limb vessel anomaly
903.01 Axillary artery injury
903.1 Brachial blood vessels injury
908.3 Late effect of injury to blood vessel of head, neck, and extremities

ICD-9-CM Procedural

38.33 Resection of upper limb vessels with anastomosis
38.43 Resection of upper limb vessels with replacement
39.51 Clipping of aneurysm
39.52 Other repair of aneurysm

35021–35022

35021 Direct repair of aneurysm, pseudoaneurysm, or excision (partial or total) and graft insertion, with or without patch graft; for aneurysm, pseudoaneurysm, and associated occlusive disease, innominate, subclavian artery, by thoracic incision
35022 for ruptured aneurysm, innominate, subclavian artery, by thoracic incision

ICD-9-CM Diagnostic

435.2 Subclavian steal syndrome — (Use additional code to identify presence of hypertension)
440.8 Atherosclerosis of other specified arteries
442.82 Aneurysm of subclavian artery
442.89 Aneurysm of other specified artery
443.29 Dissection of other artery
447.2 Rupture of artery
447.8 Other specified disorders of arteries and arterioles
747.89 Other specified congenital anomaly of circulatory system
901.1 Innominate and subclavian artery injury
908.3 Late effect of injury to blood vessel of head, neck, and extremities

ICD-9-CM Procedural

38.35 Resection of other thoracic vessels with anastomosis
38.45 Resection of other thoracic vessels with replacement
39.51 Clipping of aneurysm
39.52 Other repair of aneurysm

35045

35045 Direct repair of aneurysm, pseudoaneurysm, or excision (partial or total) and graft insertion, with or without patch graft; for aneurysm, pseudoaneurysm, and associated occlusive disease, radial or ulnar artery

ICD-9-CM Diagnostic

440.20 Atherosclerosis of native arteries of the extremities, unspecified ▽
440.21 Atherosclerosis of native arteries of the extremities with intermittent claudication
440.22 Atherosclerosis of native arteries of the extremities with rest pain
442.0 Aneurysm of artery of upper extremity
443.29 Dissection of other artery
444.21 Embolism and thrombosis of arteries of upper extremity
445.01 Atheroembolism of upper extremity
447.1 Stricture of artery
729.5 Pain in soft tissues of limb
747.63 Congenital upper limb vessel anomaly
785.9 Other symptoms involving cardiovascular system
903.2 Radial blood vessels injury
903.3 Ulnar blood vessels injury
903.8 Injury to specified blood vessels of upper extremity, other
908.3 Late effect of injury to blood vessel of head, neck, and extremities

ICD-9-CM Procedural

38.33 Resection of upper limb vessels with anastomosis
38.43 Resection of upper limb vessels with replacement
39.51 Clipping of aneurysm
39.52 Other repair of aneurysm

35081

35081 Direct repair of aneurysm, pseudoaneurysm, or excision (partial or total) and graft insertion, with or without patch graft; for aneurysm, pseudoaneurysm, and associated occlusive disease, abdominal aorta

ICD-9-CM Diagnostic

440.0 Atherosclerosis of aorta
441.4 Abdominal aneurysm without mention of rupture
441.7 Thoracoabdominal aneurysm without mention of rupture
444.0 Embolism and thrombosis of abdominal aorta
458.8 Other specified hypotension
458.9 Unspecified hypotension ▽
557.1 Chronic vascular insufficiency of intestine
789.07 Abdominal pain, generalized
789.09 Abdominal pain, other specified site
902.0 Abdominal aorta injury
908.4 Late effect of injury to blood vessel of thorax, abdomen, and pelvis
996.70 Other complications due to unspecified device, implant, and graft ▽
997.2 Peripheral vascular complications — (Use additional code to identify complications)
V45.89 Other postsurgical status — (This code is intended for use when these conditions are recorded as diagnoses or problems)

ICD-9-CM Procedural

38.34 Resection of aorta with anastomosis
38.44 Resection of abdominal aorta with replacement
38.64 Other excision of abdominal aorta
39.51 Clipping of aneurysm
39.52 Other repair of aneurysm

35082

35082 Direct repair of aneurysm, pseudoaneurysm, or excision (partial or total) and graft insertion, with or without patch graft; for ruptured aneurysm, abdominal aorta

ICD-9-CM Diagnostic

440.0 Atherosclerosis of aorta
441.00 Dissecting aortic aneurysm (any part), unspecified site ▽
441.3 Abdominal aneurysm, ruptured
441.5 Aortic aneurysm of unspecified site, ruptured ▽
557.0 Acute vascular insufficiency of intestine
785.59 Other shock without mention of trauma
788.5 Oliguria and anuria
789.00 Abdominal pain, unspecified site ▽
789.40 Abdominal rigidity, unspecified site ▽
793.6 Nonspecific abnormal findings on radiological and other examination of abdominal area, including retroperitoneum
902.0 Abdominal aorta injury
908.4 Late effect of injury to blood vessel of thorax, abdomen, and pelvis

ICD-9-CM Procedural

38.34 Resection of aorta with anastomosis
38.37 Resection of abdominal veins with anastomosis
38.44 Resection of abdominal aorta with replacement
38.64 Other excision of abdominal aorta
39.51 Clipping of aneurysm
39.52 Other repair of aneurysm

35091

35091 Direct repair of aneurysm, pseudoaneurysm, or excision (partial or total) and graft insertion, with or without patch graft; for aneurysm, pseudoaneurysm, and associated occlusive disease, abdominal aorta involving visceral vessels (mesenteric, celiac, renal)

ICD-9-CM Diagnostic

440.0 Atherosclerosis of aorta
440.1 Atherosclerosis of renal artery
440.8 Atherosclerosis of other specified arteries
441.4 Abdominal aneurysm without mention of rupture
442.1 Aneurysm of renal artery
442.83 Aneurysm of splenic artery
442.84 Aneurysm of other visceral artery
443.23 Dissection of renal artery
443.29 Dissection of other artery
444.0 Embolism and thrombosis of abdominal aorta
445.81 Atheroembolism of kidney — (Use additional code for any associated kidney failure: 584, 585)
445.89 Atheroembolism of other site
557.0 Acute vascular insufficiency of intestine
557.1 Chronic vascular insufficiency of intestine
593.81 Vascular disorders of kidney
747.62 Congenital renal vessel anomaly
747.89 Other specified congenital anomaly of circulatory system
908.4 Late effect of injury to blood vessel of thorax, abdomen, and pelvis

997.4 Digestive system complication — (Use additional code to identify complications)

ICD-9-CM Procedural

38.34 Resection of aorta with anastomosis
38.37 Resection of abdominal veins with anastomosis
38.44 Resection of abdominal aorta with replacement
38.64 Other excision of abdominal aorta
39.51 Clipping of aneurysm
39.52 Other repair of aneurysm

35092

35092 Direct repair of aneurysm, pseudoaneurysm, or excision (partial or total) and graft insertion, with or without patch graft; for ruptured aneurysm, abdominal aorta involving visceral vessels (mesenteric, celiac, renal)

ICD-9-CM Diagnostic

440.0 Atherosclerosis of aorta
440.1 Atherosclerosis of renal artery
440.8 Atherosclerosis of other specified arteries
441.00 Dissecting aortic aneurysm (any part), unspecified site ▽
441.3 Abdominal aneurysm, ruptured
441.5 Aortic aneurysm of unspecified site, ruptured ▽
441.6 Thoracoabdominal aneurysm, ruptured
442.1 Aneurysm of renal artery
442.83 Aneurysm of splenic artery
442.84 Aneurysm of other visceral artery
443.23 Dissection of renal artery
443.29 Dissection of other artery
747.89 Other specified congenital anomaly of circulatory system
902.20 Unspecified celiac and mesenteric artery injury ▽
902.25 Superior mesenteric artery (trunk) injury
902.27 Inferior mesenteric artery injury
908.4 Late effect of injury to blood vessel of thorax, abdomen, and pelvis

ICD-9-CM Procedural

38.34 Resection of aorta with anastomosis
38.37 Resection of abdominal veins with anastomosis
38.44 Resection of abdominal aorta with replacement
38.64 Other excision of abdominal aorta
39.51 Clipping of aneurysm
39.52 Other repair of aneurysm

35102

35102 Direct repair of aneurysm, pseudoaneurysm, or excision (partial or total) and graft insertion, with or without patch graft; for aneurysm, pseudoaneurysm, and associated occlusive disease, abdominal aorta involving iliac vessels (common, hypogastric, external)

ICD-9-CM Diagnostic

440.0 Atherosclerosis of aorta
440.8 Atherosclerosis of other specified arteries
441.02 Dissecting aortic aneurysm (any part), abdominal
441.4 Abdominal aneurysm without mention of rupture
441.9 Aortic aneurysm of unspecified site without mention of rupture ▽
442.2 Aneurysm of iliac artery
443.22 Dissection of iliac artery
747.89 Other specified congenital anomaly of circulatory system
902.50 Unspecified iliac vessel(s) injury ▽
902.51 Hypogastric artery injury
902.53 Iliac artery injury
908.4 Late effect of injury to blood vessel of thorax, abdomen, and pelvis

ICD-9-CM Procedural

38.34 Resection of aorta with anastomosis
38.37 Resection of abdominal veins with anastomosis
38.44 Resection of abdominal aorta with replacement
38.64 Other excision of abdominal aorta
39.51 Clipping of aneurysm
39.52 Other repair of aneurysm

35103

35103 Direct repair of aneurysm, pseudoaneurysm, or excision (partial or total) and graft insertion, with or without patch graft; for ruptured aneurysm, abdominal aorta involving iliac vessels (common, hypogastric, external)

ICD-9-CM Diagnostic

440.0 Atherosclerosis of aorta
440.8 Atherosclerosis of other specified arteries
441.02 Dissecting aortic aneurysm (any part), abdominal
441.3 Abdominal aneurysm, ruptured
442.2 Aneurysm of iliac artery
443.22 Dissection of iliac artery
747.89 Other specified congenital anomaly of circulatory system
902.0 Abdominal aorta injury
902.51 Hypogastric artery injury
902.53 Iliac artery injury
908.3 Late effect of injury to blood vessel of head, neck, and extremities
908.4 Late effect of injury to blood vessel of thorax, abdomen, and pelvis
996.74 Other complications due to other vascular device, implant, and graft

ICD-9-CM Procedural

38.34 Resection of aorta with anastomosis
38.36 Resection of abdominal arteries with anastomosis
38.37 Resection of abdominal veins with anastomosis
38.44 Resection of abdominal aorta with replacement
38.64 Other excision of abdominal aorta
39.51 Clipping of aneurysm
39.52 Other repair of aneurysm

35111–35112

35111 Direct repair of aneurysm, pseudoaneurysm, or excision (partial or total) and graft insertion, with or without patch graft; for aneurysm, pseudoaneurysm, and associated occlusive disease, splenic artery
35112 for ruptured aneurysm, splenic artery

ICD-9-CM Diagnostic

440.8 Atherosclerosis of other specified arteries
442.83 Aneurysm of splenic artery
443.29 Dissection of other artery
747.89 Other specified congenital anomaly of circulatory system
902.23 Splenic artery injury
908.4 Late effect of injury to blood vessel of thorax, abdomen, and pelvis
996.74 Other complications due to other vascular device, implant, and graft

ICD-9-CM Procedural

38.36 Resection of abdominal arteries with anastomosis
38.46 Resection of abdominal arteries with replacement
38.66 Other excision of abdominal arteries
39.51 Clipping of aneurysm
39.52 Other repair of aneurysm

35121–35122

35121 Direct repair of aneurysm, pseudoaneurysm, or excision (partial or total) and graft insertion, with or without patch graft; for aneurysm, pseudoaneurysm, and associated occlusive disease, hepatic, celiac, renal, or mesenteric artery
35122 for ruptured aneurysm, hepatic, celiac, renal, or mesenteric artery

ICD-9-CM Diagnostic

440.1 Atherosclerosis of renal artery
440.8 Atherosclerosis of other specified arteries
442.1 Aneurysm of renal artery
442.84 Aneurysm of other visceral artery
443.23 Dissection of renal artery
443.29 Dissection of other artery
447.3 Hyperplasia of renal artery
747.62 Congenital renal vessel anomaly
747.89 Other specified congenital anomaly of circulatory system
902.22 Hepatic artery injury
902.24 Injury to specified branches of celiac axis, other
902.25 Superior mesenteric artery (trunk) injury
902.26 Injury to primary branches of superior mesenteric artery
902.27 Inferior mesenteric artery injury
902.41 Renal artery injury
908.4 Late effect of injury to blood vessel of thorax, abdomen, and pelvis

ICD-9-CM Procedural
38.36 Resection of abdominal arteries with anastomosis
38.37 Resection of abdominal veins with anastomosis
38.46 Resection of abdominal arteries with replacement
39.51 Clipping of aneurysm
39.52 Other repair of aneurysm

35131–35132
35131 Direct repair of aneurysm, pseudoaneurysm, or excision (partial or total) and graft insertion, with or without patch graft; for aneurysm, pseudoaneurysm, and associated occlusive disease, iliac artery (common, hypogastric, external)
35132 for ruptured aneurysm, iliac artery (common, hypogastric, external)

ICD-9-CM Diagnostic
440.8 Atherosclerosis of other specified arteries
442.2 Aneurysm of iliac artery
443.22 Dissection of iliac artery
747.89 Other specified congenital anomaly of circulatory system
902.51 Hypogastric artery injury
902.53 Iliac artery injury
908.4 Late effect of injury to blood vessel of thorax, abdomen, and pelvis

ICD-9-CM Procedural
38.36 Resection of abdominal arteries with anastomosis
38.37 Resection of abdominal veins with anastomosis
39.51 Clipping of aneurysm
39.52 Other repair of aneurysm

35141–35142
35141 Direct repair of aneurysm, pseudoaneurysm, or excision (partial or total) and graft insertion, with or without patch graft; for aneurysm, pseudoaneurysm, and associated occlusive disease, common femoral artery (profunda femoris, superficial femoral)
35142 for ruptured aneurysm, common femoral artery (profunda femoris, superficial femoral)

ICD-9-CM Diagnostic
440.20 Atherosclerosis of native arteries of the extremities, unspecified ▽
440.21 Atherosclerosis of native arteries of the extremities with intermittent claudication
440.22 Atherosclerosis of native arteries of the extremities with rest pain
442.3 Aneurysm of artery of lower extremity
442.9 Other aneurysm of unspecified site ▽
443.29 Dissection of other artery
747.64 Congenital lower limb vessel anomaly
904.2 Femoral vein injury
908.3 Late effect of injury to blood vessel of head, neck, and extremities

ICD-9-CM Procedural
38.38 Resection of lower limb arteries with anastomosis
38.48 Resection of lower limb arteries with replacement
38.49 Resection of lower limb veins with replacement
39.51 Clipping of aneurysm
39.52 Other repair of aneurysm

35151–35152
35151 Direct repair of aneurysm, pseudoaneurysm, or excision (partial or total) and graft insertion, with or without patch graft; for aneurysm, pseudoaneurysm, and associated occlusive disease, popliteal artery
35152 for ruptured aneurysm, popliteal artery

ICD-9-CM Diagnostic
440.20 Atherosclerosis of native arteries of the extremities, unspecified ▽
440.21 Atherosclerosis of native arteries of the extremities with intermittent claudication
440.22 Atherosclerosis of native arteries of the extremities with rest pain
442.3 Aneurysm of artery of lower extremity
443.29 Dissection of other artery
443.9 Unspecified peripheral vascular disease ▽
444.22 Embolism and thrombosis of arteries of lower extremity
445.02 Atheroembolism of lower extremity
447.1 Stricture of artery
747.64 Congenital lower limb vessel anomaly
785.9 Other symptoms involving cardiovascular system
904.41 Popliteal artery injury

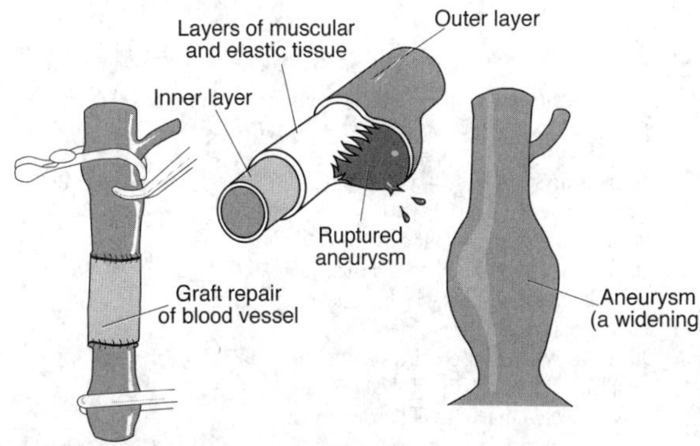

908.3 Late effect of injury to blood vessel of head, neck, and extremities

ICD-9-CM Procedural
38.38 Resection of lower limb arteries with anastomosis
38.48 Resection of lower limb arteries with replacement
38.49 Resection of lower limb veins with replacement
39.51 Clipping of aneurysm
39.52 Other repair of aneurysm

35180
35180 Repair, congenital arteriovenous fistula; head and neck

ICD-9-CM Diagnostic
430 Subarachnoid hemorrhage — (Use additional code to identify presence of hypertension)
437.3 Cerebral aneurysm, nonruptured — (Use additional code to identify presence of hypertension)
747.69 Congenital anomaly of other specified site of peripheral vascular system
747.81 Congenital anomaly of cerebrovascular system

ICD-9-CM Procedural
39.53 Repair of arteriovenous fistula

35182
35182 Repair, congenital arteriovenous fistula; thorax and abdomen

ICD-9-CM Diagnostic
746.85 Congenital coronary artery anomaly
747.3 Congenital anomalies of pulmonary artery
747.49 Other congenital anomalies of great veins
747.61 Congenital gastrointestinal vessel anomaly
747.62 Congenital renal vessel anomaly

ICD-9-CM Procedural
39.53 Repair of arteriovenous fistula

35184
35184 Repair, congenital arteriovenous fistula; extremities

ICD-9-CM Diagnostic
747.63 Congenital upper limb vessel anomaly
747.64 Congenital lower limb vessel anomaly

ICD-9-CM Procedural
39.53 Repair of arteriovenous fistula

35188
35188 Repair, acquired or traumatic arteriovenous fistula; head and neck

ICD-9-CM Diagnostic
430 Subarachnoid hemorrhage — (Use additional code to identify presence of hypertension)
437.3 Cerebral aneurysm, nonruptured — (Use additional code to identify presence of hypertension)
447.0 Arteriovenous fistula, acquired
900.02 External carotid artery injury
908.3 Late effect of injury to blood vessel of head, neck, and extremities

▽ Unspecified code
♀ Female diagnosis
Manifestation code
♂ Male diagnosis

ICD-9-CM Procedural
39.53 Repair of arteriovenous fistula

35189
35189 Repair, acquired or traumatic arteriovenous fistula; thorax and abdomen

ICD-9-CM Diagnostic
414.19 Other aneurysm of heart — (Use additional code to identify presence of hypertension: 401.0-405.9)
417.0 Arteriovenous fistula of pulmonary vessels
417.9 Unspecified disease of pulmonary circulation ▽
440.9 Generalized and unspecified atherosclerosis ▽
442.84 Aneurysm of other visceral artery
442.9 Other aneurysm of unspecified site ▽
444.0 Embolism and thrombosis of abdominal aorta
444.1 Embolism and thrombosis of thoracic aorta
447.0 Arteriovenous fistula, acquired
447.1 Stricture of artery
901.1 Innominate and subclavian artery injury
902.22 Hepatic artery injury
908.4 Late effect of injury to blood vessel of thorax, abdomen, and pelvis

ICD-9-CM Procedural
39.53 Repair of arteriovenous fistula

35190
35190 Repair, acquired or traumatic arteriovenous fistula; extremities

ICD-9-CM Diagnostic
444.21 Embolism and thrombosis of arteries of upper extremity
444.22 Embolism and thrombosis of arteries of lower extremity
447.0 Arteriovenous fistula, acquired
903.1 Brachial blood vessels injury
904.2 Femoral vein injury
908.3 Late effect of injury to blood vessel of head, neck, and extremities

ICD-9-CM Procedural
39.53 Repair of arteriovenous fistula

35201
35201 Repair blood vessel, direct; neck

ICD-9-CM Diagnostic
433.00 Occlusion and stenosis of basilar artery without mention of cerebral infarction — (Use additional code to identify presence of hypertension)
433.10 Occlusion and stenosis of carotid artery without mention of cerebral infarction — (Use additional code to identify presence of hypertension)
433.20 Occlusion and stenosis of vertebral artery without mention of cerebral infarction — (Use additional code to identify presence of hypertension)
433.30 Occlusion and stenosis of multiple and bilateral precerebral arteries without mention of cerebral infarction — (Use additional code to identify presence of hypertension)
433.80 Occlusion and stenosis of other specified precerebral artery without mention of cerebral infarction — (Use additional code to identify presence of hypertension)
433.90 Occlusion and stenosis of unspecified precerebral artery without mention of cerebral infarction — (Use additional code to identify presence of hypertension) ▽
443.21 Dissection of carotid artery
443.29 Dissection of other artery
447.2 Rupture of artery
900.00 Injury to carotid artery, unspecified ▽
900.01 Common carotid artery injury
900.02 External carotid artery injury
900.03 Internal carotid artery injury
900.1 Internal jugular vein injury
900.81 External jugular vein injury
900.82 Injury to multiple blood vessels of head and neck
900.89 Injury to other specified blood vessels of head and neck
998.2 Accidental puncture or laceration during procedure

ICD-9-CM Procedural
39.30 Suture of unspecified blood vessel
39.31 Suture of artery
39.32 Suture of vein
39.59 Other repair of vessel

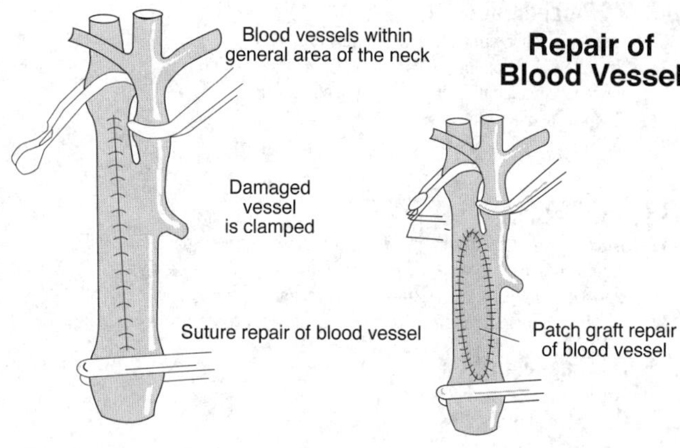

35206
35206 Repair blood vessel, direct; upper extremity

ICD-9-CM Diagnostic
440.20 Atherosclerosis of native arteries of the extremities, unspecified ▽
440.21 Atherosclerosis of native arteries of the extremities with intermittent claudication
440.22 Atherosclerosis of native arteries of the extremities with rest pain
440.23 Atherosclerosis of native arteries of the extremities with ulceration — (Use additional code for any associated ulceration: 707.10-707.9)
440.24 Atherosclerosis of native arteries of the extremities with gangrene
440.30 Atheroslerosis of unspecified bypass graft of extremities ▽
440.31 Atheroslerosis of autologous vein bypass graft of extremities
440.32 Atheroslerosis of nonautologous biological bypass graft of extremities
447.2 Rupture of artery
903.01 Axillary artery injury
903.02 Axillary vein injury
903.1 Brachial blood vessels injury
903.2 Radial blood vessels injury
903.3 Ulnar blood vessels injury
903.8 Injury to specified blood vessels of upper extremity, other
998.2 Accidental puncture or laceration during procedure

ICD-9-CM Procedural
39.30 Suture of unspecified blood vessel
39.31 Suture of artery
39.32 Suture of vein
39.59 Other repair of vessel

35207
35207 Repair blood vessel, direct; hand, finger

ICD-9-CM Diagnostic
447.2 Rupture of artery
883.1 Open wound of finger(s), complicated — (Use additional code to identify infection)
883.2 Open wound of finger(s), with tendon involvement — (Use additional code to identify infection)
903.4 Palmar artery injury
903.5 Digital blood vessels injury
903.8 Injury to specified blood vessels of upper extremity, other
959.5 Injury, other and unspecified, finger
998.2 Accidental puncture or laceration during procedure

ICD-9-CM Procedural
39.30 Suture of unspecified blood vessel
39.31 Suture of artery
39.32 Suture of vein
39.59 Other repair of vessel

35211–35216
35211 Repair blood vessel, direct; intrathoracic, with bypass
35216 intrathoracic, without bypass

ICD-9-CM Diagnostic
440.0 Atherosclerosis of aorta

▽ Unspecified code ♀ Female diagnosis ☒ Manifestation code ♂ Male diagnosis

447.1 Stricture of artery
447.5 Necrosis of artery
451.89 Phlebitis and thrombophlebitis of other site — (Use additional E code to identify drug, if drug-induced)
875.1 Open wound of chest (wall), complicated — (Use additional code to identify infection)
901.0 Thoracic aorta injury
901.1 Innominate and subclavian artery injury
901.2 Superior vena cava injury
901.3 Innominate and subclavian vein injury
901.40 Injury to unspecified pulmonary vessel(s)
901.41 Pulmonary artery injury
901.42 Pulmonary vein injury
901.81 Intercostal artery or vein injury
901.82 Internal mammary artery or vein injury
901.83 Injury to multiple blood vessels of thorax
901.89 Injury to specified blood vessels of thorax, other
901.9 Injury to unspecified blood vessel of thorax
998.2 Accidental puncture or laceration during procedure

ICD-9-CM Procedural
39.30 Suture of unspecified blood vessel
39.31 Suture of artery
39.32 Suture of vein
39.59 Other repair of vessel
39.61 Extracorporeal circulation auxiliary to open heart surgery

35221
35221 Repair blood vessel, direct; intra-abdominal

ICD-9-CM Diagnostic
440.0 Atherosclerosis of aorta
440.1 Atherosclerosis of renal artery
447.1 Stricture of artery
447.6 Unspecified arteritis
453.0 Budd-Chiari syndrome
459.9 Unspecified circulatory system disorder
557.0 Acute vascular insufficiency of intestine
902.0 Abdominal aorta injury
902.10 Unspecified inferior vena cava injury
902.11 Hepatic vein injury
902.20 Unspecified celiac and mesenteric artery injury
902.21 Gastric artery injury
902.22 Hepatic artery injury
902.23 Splenic artery injury
902.33 Portal vein injury
902.34 Splenic vein injury
902.39 Injury to portal and splenic veins, other
902.40 Renal vessel(s) injury, unspecified
902.41 Renal artery injury
902.42 Renal vein injury
902.50 Unspecified iliac vessel(s) injury
902.53 Iliac artery injury
902.55 Uterine artery injury ♀
902.56 Uterine vein injury ♀
902.59 Injury to iliac blood vessels, other
902.81 Ovarian artery injury ♀
902.82 Ovarian vein injury ♀
902.89 Injury to specified blood vessels of abdomen and pelvis, other
902.9 Injury to blood vessel of abdomen and pelvis, unspecified
998.2 Accidental puncture or laceration during procedure

ICD-9-CM Procedural
39.30 Suture of unspecified blood vessel
39.31 Suture of artery
39.32 Suture of vein
39.59 Other repair of vessel

35226
35226 Repair blood vessel, direct; lower extremity

ICD-9-CM Diagnostic
440.20 Atherosclerosis of native arteries of the extremities, unspecified
440.21 Atherosclerosis of native arteries of the extremities with intermittent claudication
440.22 Atherosclerosis of native arteries of the extremities with rest pain
440.23 Atherosclerosis of native arteries of the extremities with ulceration — (Use additional code for any associated ulceration: 707.10-707.9)
440.24 Atherosclerosis of native arteries of the extremities with gangrene
440.30 Atheroslerosis of unspecified bypass graft of extremities
440.31 Atheroslerosis of autologous vein bypass graft of extremities
440.32 Atheroslerosis of nonautologous biological bypass graft of extremities
447.2 Rupture of artery
904.0 Common femoral artery injury
904.1 Superficial femoral artery injury
904.3 Saphenous vein injury
904.41 Popliteal artery injury
904.42 Popliteal vein injury
904.51 Anterior tibial artery injury
904.52 Anterior tibial vein injury
904.53 Posterior tibial artery injury
904.54 Posterior tibial vein injury
904.7 Injury to specified blood vessels of lower extremity, other
904.8 Injury to unspecified blood vessel of lower extremity
998.2 Accidental puncture or laceration during procedure

ICD-9-CM Procedural
39.30 Suture of unspecified blood vessel
39.31 Suture of artery
39.32 Suture of vein
39.59 Other repair of vessel

35231
35231 Repair blood vessel with vein graft; neck

ICD-9-CM Diagnostic
433.00 Occlusion and stenosis of basilar artery without mention of cerebral infarction — (Use additional code to identify presence of hypertension)
433.10 Occlusion and stenosis of carotid artery without mention of cerebral infarction — (Use additional code to identify presence of hypertension)
433.20 Occlusion and stenosis of vertebral artery without mention of cerebral infarction — (Use additional code to identify presence of hypertension)
433.30 Occlusion and stenosis of multiple and bilateral precerebral arteries without mention of cerebral infarction — (Use additional code to identify presence of hypertension)
433.80 Occlusion and stenosis of other specified precerebral artery without mention of cerebral infarction — (Use additional code to identify presence of hypertension)
433.90 Occlusion and stenosis of unspecified precerebral artery without mention of cerebral infarction — (Use additional code to identify presence of hypertension)
443.21 Dissection of carotid artery
443.29 Dissection of other artery
447.2 Rupture of artery
900.00 Injury to carotid artery, unspecified
900.01 Common carotid artery injury
900.02 External carotid artery injury
900.03 Internal carotid artery injury
900.1 Internal jugular vein injury
900.81 External jugular vein injury
900.82 Injury to multiple blood vessels of head and neck
900.89 Injury to other specified blood vessels of head and neck
998.2 Accidental puncture or laceration during procedure

ICD-9-CM Procedural
38.42 Resection of other vessels of head and neck with replacement
39.56 Repair of blood vessel with tissue patch graft

35236
35236 Repair blood vessel with vein graft; upper extremity

ICD-9-CM Diagnostic
440.20 Atherosclerosis of native arteries of the extremities, unspecified
440.21 Atherosclerosis of native arteries of the extremities with intermittent claudication
440.22 Atherosclerosis of native arteries of the extremities with rest pain
440.23 Atherosclerosis of native arteries of the extremities with ulceration — (Use additional code for any associated ulceration: 707.10-707.9)
440.24 Atherosclerosis of native arteries of the extremities with gangrene
440.30 Atheroslerosis of unspecified bypass graft of extremities
440.31 Atheroslerosis of autologous vein bypass graft of extremities
440.32 Atheroslerosis of nonautologous biological bypass graft of extremities
447.2 Rupture of artery

903.01 Axillary artery injury
903.02 Axillary vein injury
903.1 Brachial blood vessels injury
903.2 Radial blood vessels injury
903.3 Ulnar blood vessels injury
903.8 Injury to specified blood vessels of upper extremity, other
998.2 Accidental puncture or laceration during procedure

ICD-9-CM Procedural

38.43 Resection of upper limb vessels with replacement
39.56 Repair of blood vessel with tissue patch graft

35241–35246

35241 Repair blood vessel with vein graft; intrathoracic, with bypass
35246 intrathoracic, without bypass

ICD-9-CM Diagnostic

171.4 Malignant neoplasm of connective and other soft tissue of thorax
215.4 Other benign neoplasm of connective and other soft tissue of thorax
239.2 Neoplasms of unspecified nature of bone, soft tissue, and skin
440.0 Atherosclerosis of aorta
441.1 Thoracic aneurysm, ruptured
447.1 Stricture of artery
447.5 Necrosis of artery
451.89 Phlebitis and thrombophlebitis of other site — (Use additional E code to identify drug, if drug-induced)
459.2 Compression of vein
875.1 Open wound of chest (wall), complicated — (Use additional code to identify infection)
901.0 Thoracic aorta injury
901.1 Innominate and subclavian artery injury
901.2 Superior vena cava injury
901.3 Innominate and subclavian vein injury
901.40 Injury to unspecified pulmonary vessel(s) ▽
901.41 Pulmonary artery injury
901.42 Pulmonary vein injury
901.81 Intercostal artery or vein injury
901.82 Internal mammary artery or vein injury
901.83 Injury to multiple blood vessels of thorax
998.2 Accidental puncture or laceration during procedure

ICD-9-CM Procedural

38.45 Resection of other thoracic vessels with replacement
39.30 Suture of unspecified blood vessel
39.56 Repair of blood vessel with tissue patch graft
39.61 Extracorporeal circulation auxiliary to open heart surgery

35251

35251 Repair blood vessel with vein graft; intra-abdominal

ICD-9-CM Diagnostic

440.0 Atherosclerosis of aorta
440.1 Atherosclerosis of renal artery
447.1 Stricture of artery
453.0 Budd-Chiari syndrome
557.0 Acute vascular insufficiency of intestine
902.0 Abdominal aorta injury
902.10 Unspecified inferior vena cava injury ▽
902.11 Hepatic vein injury
902.20 Unspecified celiac and mesenteric artery injury ▽
902.21 Gastric artery injury
902.22 Hepatic artery injury
902.23 Splenic artery injury
902.33 Portal vein injury
902.34 Splenic vein injury
902.39 Injury to portal and splenic veins, other
902.40 Renal vessel(s) injury, unspecified ▽
902.41 Renal artery injury
902.42 Renal vein injury
902.50 Unspecified iliac vessel(s) injury ▽
902.53 Iliac artery injury
902.55 Uterine artery injury ♀
902.56 Uterine vein injury ♀
902.59 Injury to iliac blood vessels, other
902.81 Ovarian artery injury ♀
902.82 Ovarian vein injury ♀
902.89 Injury to specified blood vessels of abdomen and pelvis, other
902.9 Injury to blood vessel of abdomen and pelvis, unspecified ▽
998.2 Accidental puncture or laceration during procedure

ICD-9-CM Procedural

38.46 Resection of abdominal arteries with replacement
38.47 Resection of abdominal veins with replacement
39.56 Repair of blood vessel with tissue patch graft

35256

35256 Repair blood vessel with vein graft; lower extremity

ICD-9-CM Diagnostic

440.20 Atherosclerosis of native arteries of the extremities, unspecified ▽
440.21 Atherosclerosis of native arteries of the extremities with intermittent claudication
440.22 Atherosclerosis of native arteries of the extremities with rest pain
440.23 Atherosclerosis of native arteries of the extremities with ulceration — (Use additional code for any associated ulceration: 707.10-707.9)
440.24 Atherosclerosis of native arteries of the extremities with gangrene
440.30 Atheroslerosis of unspecified bypass graft of extremities ▽
440.31 Atheroslerosis of autologous vein bypass graft of extremities
440.32 Atheroslerosis of nonautologous biological bypass graft of extremities
447.2 Rupture of artery
904.0 Common femoral artery injury
904.1 Superficial femoral artery injury
904.3 Saphenous vein injury
904.41 Popliteal artery injury
904.42 Popliteal vein injury
904.51 Anterior tibial artery injury
904.52 Anterior tibial vein injury
904.53 Posterior tibial artery injury
904.54 Posterior tibial vein injury
904.7 Injury to specified blood vessels of lower extremity, other
904.8 Injury to unspecified blood vessel of lower extremity ▽
998.2 Accidental puncture or laceration during procedure

ICD-9-CM Procedural

38.48 Resection of lower limb arteries with replacement
38.49 Resection of lower limb veins with replacement
39.56 Repair of blood vessel with tissue patch graft

35261

35261 Repair blood vessel with graft other than vein; neck

ICD-9-CM Diagnostic

433.00 Occlusion and stenosis of basilar artery without mention of cerebral infarction — (Use additional code to identify presence of hypertension)
433.10 Occlusion and stenosis of carotid artery without mention of cerebral infarction — (Use additional code to identify presence of hypertension)
433.20 Occlusion and stenosis of vertebral artery without mention of cerebral infarction — (Use additional code to identify presence of hypertension)
433.30 Occlusion and stenosis of multiple and bilateral precerebral arteries without mention of cerebral infarction — (Use additional code to identify presence of hypertension)
433.80 Occlusion and stenosis of other specified precerebral artery without mention of cerebral infarction — (Use additional code to identify presence of hypertension)
433.90 Occlusion and stenosis of unspecified precerebral artery without mention of cerebral infarction — (Use additional code to identify presence of hypertension) ▽
443.21 Dissection of carotid artery
443.29 Dissection of other artery
447.2 Rupture of artery
900.00 Injury to carotid artery, unspecified ▽
900.01 Common carotid artery injury
900.02 External carotid artery injury
900.03 Internal carotid artery injury
900.1 Internal jugular vein injury
900.81 External jugular vein injury
900.82 Injury to multiple blood vessels of head and neck
900.89 Injury to other specified blood vessels of head and neck
998.2 Accidental puncture or laceration during procedure

ICD-9-CM Procedural

38.42 Resection of other vessels of head and neck with replacement
39.57 Repair of blood vessel with synthetic patch graft

39.58 Repair of blood vessel with unspecified type of patch graft
39.72 Endovascular repair or occlusion of head and neck vessels

35266

35266 Repair blood vessel with graft other than vein; upper extremity

ICD-9-CM Diagnostic

440.20 Atherosclerosis of native arteries of the extremities, unspecified
440.21 Atherosclerosis of native arteries of the extremities with intermittent claudication
440.22 Atherosclerosis of native arteries of the extremities with rest pain
440.23 Atherosclerosis of native arteries of the extremities with ulceration — (Use additional code for any associated ulceration: 707.10-707.9)
440.24 Atherosclerosis of native arteries of the extremities with gangrene
440.30 Atheroslerosis of unspecified bypass graft of extremities
440.31 Atheroslerosis of autologous vein bypass graft of extremities
440.32 Atheroslerosis of nonautologous biological bypass graft of extremities
447.2 Rupture of artery
903.01 Axillary artery injury
903.02 Axillary vein injury
903.1 Brachial blood vessels injury
903.2 Radial blood vessels injury
903.3 Ulnar blood vessels injury
903.8 Injury to specified blood vessels of upper extremity, other
998.2 Accidental puncture or laceration during procedure

ICD-9-CM Procedural

38.43 Resection of upper limb vessels with replacement
39.57 Repair of blood vessel with synthetic patch graft
39.58 Repair of blood vessel with unspecified type of patch graft

35271–35276

35271 Repair blood vessel with graft other than vein; intrathoracic, with bypass
35276 intrathoracic, without bypass

ICD-9-CM Diagnostic

440.0 Atherosclerosis of aorta
447.1 Stricture of artery
447.5 Necrosis of artery
451.89 Phlebitis and thrombophlebitis of other site — (Use additional E code to identify drug, if drug-induced)
459.2 Compression of vein
875.1 Open wound of chest (wall), complicated — (Use additional code to identify infection)
901.0 Thoracic aorta injury
901.2 Superior vena cava injury
901.3 Innominate and subclavian vein injury
901.40 Injury to unspecified pulmonary vessel(s)
901.41 Pulmonary artery injury
901.42 Pulmonary vein injury
901.81 Intercostal artery or vein injury
901.82 Internal mammary artery or vein injury
901.83 Injury to multiple blood vessels of thorax
901.89 Injury to specified blood vessels of thorax, other
901.9 Injury to unspecified blood vessel of thorax
998.2 Accidental puncture or laceration during procedure

ICD-9-CM Procedural

38.45 Resection of other thoracic vessels with replacement
39.56 Repair of blood vessel with tissue patch graft
39.57 Repair of blood vessel with synthetic patch graft
39.58 Repair of blood vessel with unspecified type of patch graft
39.61 Extracorporeal circulation auxiliary to open heart surgery

35281

35281 Repair blood vessel with graft other than vein; intra-abdominal

ICD-9-CM Diagnostic

440.0 Atherosclerosis of aorta
440.1 Atherosclerosis of renal artery
447.2 Rupture of artery
451.81 Phlebitis and thrombophlebitis of iliac vein — (Use additional E code to identify drug, if drug-induced)
452 Portal vein thrombosis
453.0 Budd-Chiari syndrome
557.0 Acute vascular insufficiency of intestine
902.0 Abdominal aorta injury
902.11 Hepatic vein injury
902.20 Unspecified celiac and mesenteric artery injury
902.21 Gastric artery injury
902.22 Hepatic artery injury
902.23 Splenic artery injury
902.33 Portal vein injury
902.34 Splenic vein injury
902.39 Injury to portal and splenic veins, other
902.40 Renal vessel(s) injury, unspecified
902.41 Renal artery injury
902.42 Renal vein injury
902.50 Unspecified iliac vessel(s) injury
902.53 Iliac artery injury
902.55 Uterine artery injury ♀
902.56 Uterine vein injury ♀
902.59 Injury to iliac blood vessels, other
902.81 Ovarian artery injury ♀
902.82 Ovarian vein injury ♀
902.89 Injury to specified blood vessels of abdomen and pelvis, other
902.9 Injury to blood vessel of abdomen and pelvis, unspecified

ICD-9-CM Procedural

38.46 Resection of abdominal arteries with replacement
38.47 Resection of abdominal veins with replacement
39.30 Suture of unspecified blood vessel
39.56 Repair of blood vessel with tissue patch graft
39.57 Repair of blood vessel with synthetic patch graft
39.58 Repair of blood vessel with unspecified type of patch graft

35286

35286 Repair blood vessel with graft other than vein; lower extremity

ICD-9-CM Diagnostic

440.20 Atherosclerosis of native arteries of the extremities, unspecified
440.21 Atherosclerosis of native arteries of the extremities with intermittent claudication
440.22 Atherosclerosis of native arteries of the extremities with rest pain
440.23 Atherosclerosis of native arteries of the extremities with ulceration — (Use additional code for any associated ulceration: 707.10-707.9)
440.24 Atherosclerosis of native arteries of the extremities with gangrene
440.30 Atheroslerosis of unspecified bypass graft of extremities
440.31 Atheroslerosis of autologous vein bypass graft of extremities
440.32 Atheroslerosis of nonautologous biological bypass graft of extremities
447.2 Rupture of artery
904.0 Common femoral artery injury
904.1 Superficial femoral artery injury
904.3 Saphenous vein injury
904.41 Popliteal artery injury
904.42 Popliteal vein injury
904.51 Anterior tibial artery injury
904.52 Anterior tibial vein injury
904.53 Posterior tibial artery injury
904.54 Posterior tibial vein injury
904.7 Injury to specified blood vessels of lower extremity, other
904.8 Injury to unspecified blood vessel of lower extremity
998.2 Accidental puncture or laceration during procedure

ICD-9-CM Procedural

38.48 Resection of lower limb arteries with replacement
38.49 Resection of lower limb veins with replacement
39.30 Suture of unspecified blood vessel
39.57 Repair of blood vessel with synthetic patch graft
39.58 Repair of blood vessel with unspecified type of patch graft

35301

35301 Thromboendarterectomy, with or without patch graft; carotid, vertebral, subclavian, by neck incision

ICD-9-CM Diagnostic

433.00 Occlusion and stenosis of basilar artery without mention of cerebral infarction — (Use additional code to identify presence of hypertension)
433.01 Occlusion and stenosis of basilar artery with cerebral infarction — (Use additional code to identify presence of hypertension)

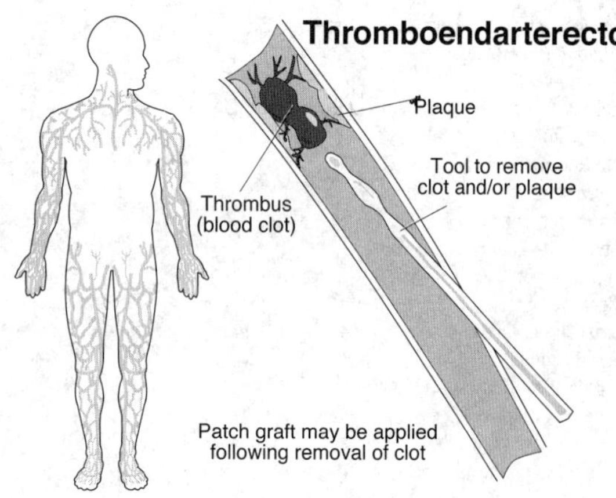

433.10 Occlusion and stenosis of carotid artery without mention of cerebral infarction — (Use additional code to identify presence of hypertension)
433.11 Occlusion and stenosis of carotid artery with cerebral infarction — (Use additional code to identify presence of hypertension)
433.20 Occlusion and stenosis of vertebral artery without mention of cerebral infarction — (Use additional code to identify presence of hypertension)
433.21 Occlusion and stenosis of vertebral artery with cerebral infarction — (Use additional code to identify presence of hypertension)
433.30 Occlusion and stenosis of multiple and bilateral precerebral arteries without mention of cerebral infarction — (Use additional code to identify presence of hypertension)
433.31 Occlusion and stenosis of multiple and bilateral precerebral arteries with cerebral infarction — (Use additional code to identify presence of hypertension)
433.80 Occlusion and stenosis of other specified precerebral artery without mention of cerebral infarction — (Use additional code to identify presence of hypertension)
433.81 Occlusion and stenosis of other specified precerebral artery with cerebral infarction — (Use additional code to identify presence of hypertension)
433.90 Occlusion and stenosis of unspecified precerebral artery without mention of cerebral infarction — (Use additional code to identify presence of hypertension) ▽
433.91 Occlusion and stenosis of unspecified precerebral artery with cerebral infarction — (Use additional code to identify presence of hypertension) ▽
435.0 Basilar artery syndrome — (Use additional code to identify presence of hypertension)
435.1 Vertebral artery syndrome — (Use additional code to identify presence of hypertension)
435.2 Subclavian steal syndrome — (Use additional code to identify presence of hypertension)
435.8 Other specified transient cerebral ischemias — (Use additional code to identify presence of hypertension)
435.9 Unspecified transient cerebral ischemia — (Use additional code to identify presence of hypertension) ▽
437.9 Unspecified cerebrovascular disease — (Use additional code to identify presence of hypertension) ▽
440.8 Atherosclerosis of other specified arteries
443.21 Dissection of carotid artery
443.24 Dissection of vertebral artery
443.29 Dissection of other artery
780.02 Transient alteration of awareness
780.09 Other alteration of consciousness
780.2 Syncope and collapse
780.31 Febrile convulsions
780.39 Other convulsions
780.4 Dizziness and giddiness
784.0 Headache
785.9 Other symptoms involving cardiovascular system

ICD-9-CM Procedural
38.12 Endarterectomy of other vessels of head and neck

35311
35311 Thromboendarterectomy, with or without patch graft; subclavian, innominate, by thoracic incision

ICD-9-CM Diagnostic
435.1 Vertebral artery syndrome — (Use additional code to identify presence of hypertension)
435.2 Subclavian steal syndrome — (Use additional code to identify presence of hypertension)
440.8 Atherosclerosis of other specified arteries
444.89 Embolism and thrombosis of other specified artery
445.89 Atheroembolism of other site

ICD-9-CM Procedural
38.15 Endarterectomy of other thoracic vessels

35321
35321 Thromboendarterectomy, with or without patch graft; axillary-brachial

ICD-9-CM Diagnostic
440.20 Atherosclerosis of native arteries of the extremities, unspecified ▽
440.21 Atherosclerosis of native arteries of the extremities with intermittent claudication
440.22 Atherosclerosis of native arteries of the extremities with rest pain
440.23 Atherosclerosis of native arteries of the extremities with ulceration — (Use additional code for any associated ulceration: 707.10-707.9)
440.24 Atherosclerosis of native arteries of the extremities with gangrene
440.29 Other atherosclerosis of native arteries of the extremities
440.30 Atheroslerosis of unspecified bypass graft of extremities ▽
440.31 Atheroslerosis of autologous vein bypass graft of extremities
440.32 Atheroslerosis of nonautologous biological bypass graft of extremities
444.21 Embolism and thrombosis of arteries of upper extremity
444.9 Embolism and thrombosis of unspecified artery ▽
445.01 Atheroembolism of upper extremity

ICD-9-CM Procedural
38.13 Endarterectomy of upper limb vessels

35331
35331 Thromboendarterectomy, with or without patch graft; abdominal aorta

ICD-9-CM Diagnostic
440.0 Atherosclerosis of aorta
444.0 Embolism and thrombosis of abdominal aorta
444.9 Embolism and thrombosis of unspecified artery ▽

ICD-9-CM Procedural
38.14 Endarterectomy of aorta

35341
35341 Thromboendarterectomy, with or without patch graft; mesenteric, celiac, or renal

ICD-9-CM Diagnostic
440.1 Atherosclerosis of renal artery
440.8 Atherosclerosis of other specified arteries
453.3 Embolism and thrombosis of renal vein
453.8 Embolism and thrombosis of other specified veins
557.0 Acute vascular insufficiency of intestine
557.1 Chronic vascular insufficiency of intestine
997.71 Vascular complications of mesenteric artery — (Use additional code to identify complications)
997.72 Vascular complications of renal artery — (Use additional code to identify complications)
997.79 Vascular complications of other vessels — (Use additional code to identify complications)

ICD-9-CM Procedural
38.16 Endarterectomy of abdominal arteries

35351
35351 Thromboendarterectomy, with or without patch graft; iliac

ICD-9-CM Diagnostic
440.8 Atherosclerosis of other specified arteries
444.81 Embolism and thrombosis of iliac artery
444.89 Embolism and thrombosis of other specified artery
445.89 Atheroembolism of other site
997.79 Vascular complications of other vessels — (Use additional code to identify complications)

▽ Unspecified code ♀ Female diagnosis ☒ Manifestation code ♂ Male diagnosis

ICD-9-CM Procedural

38.16 Endarterectomy of abdominal arteries

35355

35355 Thromboendarterectomy, with or without patch graft; iliofemoral

ICD-9-CM Diagnostic

440.20 Atherosclerosis of native arteries of the extremities, unspecified ▽
440.21 Atherosclerosis of native arteries of the extremities with intermittent claudication
440.22 Atherosclerosis of native arteries of the extremities with rest pain
440.23 Atherosclerosis of native arteries of the extremities with ulceration — (Use additional code for any associated ulceration: 707.10-707.9)
440.24 Atherosclerosis of native arteries of the extremities with gangrene
440.29 Other atherosclerosis of native arteries of the extremities
444.22 Embolism and thrombosis of arteries of lower extremity
444.81 Embolism and thrombosis of iliac artery
445.02 Atheroembolism of lower extremity
445.89 Atheroembolism of other site
997.79 Vascular complications of other vessels — (Use additional code to identify complications)

ICD-9-CM Procedural

38.16 Endarterectomy of abdominal arteries
38.18 Endarterectomy of lower limb arteries

35361

35361 Thromboendarterectomy, with or without patch graft; combined aortoiliac

ICD-9-CM Diagnostic

440.8 Atherosclerosis of other specified arteries
444.0 Embolism and thrombosis of abdominal aorta
444.81 Embolism and thrombosis of iliac artery
445.89 Atheroembolism of other site
997.79 Vascular complications of other vessels — (Use additional code to identify complications)

ICD-9-CM Procedural

38.14 Endarterectomy of aorta
38.16 Endarterectomy of abdominal arteries
38.18 Endarterectomy of lower limb arteries

35363

35363 Thromboendarterectomy, with or without patch graft; combined aortoiliofemoral

ICD-9-CM Diagnostic

440.0 Atherosclerosis of aorta
440.1 Atherosclerosis of renal artery
440.21 Atherosclerosis of native arteries of the extremities with intermittent claudication
440.8 Atherosclerosis of other specified arteries
444.0 Embolism and thrombosis of abdominal aorta
444.22 Embolism and thrombosis of arteries of lower extremity
444.81 Embolism and thrombosis of iliac artery
445.02 Atheroembolism of lower extremity
445.89 Atheroembolism of other site
997.79 Vascular complications of other vessels — (Use additional code to identify complications)

ICD-9-CM Procedural

38.14 Endarterectomy of aorta
38.16 Endarterectomy of abdominal arteries
38.18 Endarterectomy of lower limb arteries

35371–35372

35371 Thromboendarterectomy, with or without patch graft; common femoral
35372 deep (profunda) femoral

ICD-9-CM Diagnostic

250.70 Diabetes with peripheral circulatory disorders, type II or unspecified type, not stated as uncontrolled — (Use additional code to identify manifestation: 443.81, 785.4)
250.71 Diabetes with peripheral circulatory disorders, type I [juvenile type], not stated as uncontrolled — (Use additional code to identify manifestation: 443.81, 785.4)
250.72 Diabetes with peripheral circulatory disorders, type II or unspecified type, uncontrolled — (Use additional code to identify manifestation: 443.81, 785.4)
250.73 Diabetes with peripheral circulatory disorders, type I [juvenile type], uncontrolled — (Use additional code to identify manifestation: 443.81, 785.4)
440.20 Atherosclerosis of native arteries of the extremities, unspecified ▽
440.21 Atherosclerosis of native arteries of the extremities with intermittent claudication
440.22 Atherosclerosis of native arteries of the extremities with rest pain
440.23 Atherosclerosis of native arteries of the extremities with ulceration — (Use additional code for any associated ulceration: 707.10-707.9)
440.24 Atherosclerosis of native arteries of the extremities with gangrene
440.29 Other atherosclerosis of native arteries of the extremities
443.29 Dissection of other artery
443.81 Peripheral angiopathy in diseases classified elsewhere — (Code first underlying disease, 250.7) ☒
443.9 Unspecified peripheral vascular disease ▽
444.22 Embolism and thrombosis of arteries of lower extremity
444.9 Embolism and thrombosis of unspecified artery ▽
445.02 Atheroembolism of lower extremity
447.1 Stricture of artery
447.2 Rupture of artery
785.9 Other symptoms involving cardiovascular system
902.53 Iliac artery injury
904.2 Femoral vein injury

ICD-9-CM Procedural

38.18 Endarterectomy of lower limb arteries

35381

35381 Thromboendarterectomy, with or without patch graft; femoral and/or popliteal, and/or tibioperoneal

ICD-9-CM Diagnostic

250.70 Diabetes with peripheral circulatory disorders, type II or unspecified type, not stated as uncontrolled — (Use additional code to identify manifestation: 443.81, 785.4)
250.71 Diabetes with peripheral circulatory disorders, type I [juvenile type], not stated as uncontrolled — (Use additional code to identify manifestation: 443.81, 785.4)
250.72 Diabetes with peripheral circulatory disorders, type II or unspecified type, uncontrolled — (Use additional code to identify manifestation: 443.81, 785.4)
250.73 Diabetes with peripheral circulatory disorders, type I [juvenile type], uncontrolled — (Use additional code to identify manifestation: 443.81, 785.4)
440.20 Atherosclerosis of native arteries of the extremities, unspecified ▽
440.21 Atherosclerosis of native arteries of the extremities with intermittent claudication
440.22 Atherosclerosis of native arteries of the extremities with rest pain
440.23 Atherosclerosis of native arteries of the extremities with ulceration — (Use additional code for any associated ulceration: 707.10-707.9)
440.24 Atherosclerosis of native arteries of the extremities with gangrene
440.29 Other atherosclerosis of native arteries of the extremities
443.29 Dissection of other artery
443.81 Peripheral angiopathy in diseases classified elsewhere — (Code first underlying disease, 250.7) ☒
443.9 Unspecified peripheral vascular disease ▽
444.22 Embolism and thrombosis of arteries of lower extremity
444.9 Embolism and thrombosis of unspecified artery ▽
445.02 Atheroembolism of lower extremity
447.1 Stricture of artery
447.2 Rupture of artery
785.4 Gangrene — (Code first any associated underlying condition:250.7, 443.0)
785.9 Other symptoms involving cardiovascular system
904.2 Femoral vein injury

ICD-9-CM Procedural

38.18 Endarterectomy of lower limb arteries

▽ Unspecified code ♀ Female diagnosis ☒ Manifestation code ♂ Male diagnosis

Balloon Angioplasty

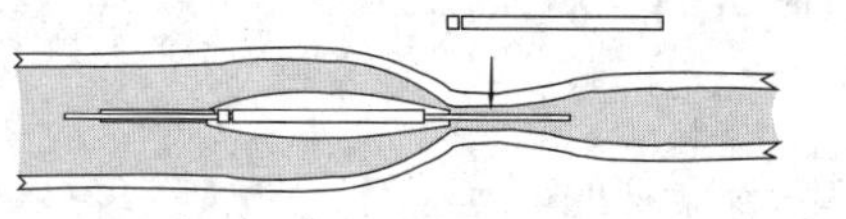
Balloon is delivered by catheter into narrowed section of artery
Access is through brachial artery (occasionally carotid artery)
Balloon is inflated in narrowed section of artery and patency is restored

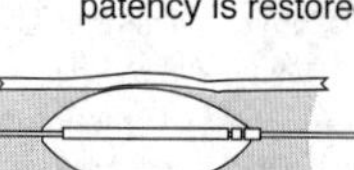

35390

35390 Reoperation, carotid, thromboendarterectomy, more than one month after original operation (List separately in addition to code for primary procedure)

ICD-9-CM Diagnostic

This is an add-on code. Refer to the corresponding primary procedure code for ICD-9 diagnosis code links.

ICD-9-CM Procedural

38.12 Endarterectomy of other vessels of head and neck

35400

35400 Angioscopy (non-coronary vessels or grafts) during therapeutic intervention (List separately in addition to code for primary procedure)

ICD-9-CM Diagnostic

This is an add-on code. Refer to the corresponding primary procedure code for ICD-9 diagnosis code links.

ICD-9-CM Procedural

38.22 Percutaneous angioscopy

35450

35450 Transluminal balloon angioplasty, open; renal or other visceral artery

ICD-9-CM Diagnostic

405.01 Secondary renovascular hypertension, malignant
405.11 Secondary renovascular hypertension, benign
405.91 Secondary renovascular hypertension, unspecified ▽
440.1 Atherosclerosis of renal artery
440.8 Atherosclerosis of other specified arteries
447.1 Stricture of artery
447.4 Celiac artery compression syndrome
557.0 Acute vascular insufficiency of intestine
557.1 Chronic vascular insufficiency of intestine

ICD-9-CM Procedural

39.50 Angioplasty or atherectomy of other non-coronary vessel(s)

35452

35452 Transluminal balloon angioplasty, open; aortic

ICD-9-CM Diagnostic

440.0 Atherosclerosis of aorta
444.89 Embolism and thrombosis of other specified artery
747.22 Congenital atresia and stenosis of aorta

ICD-9-CM Procedural

39.50 Angioplasty or atherectomy of other non-coronary vessel(s)

35454

35454 Transluminal balloon angioplasty, open; iliac

ICD-9-CM Diagnostic

440.8 Atherosclerosis of other specified arteries
443.9 Unspecified peripheral vascular disease ▽
444.81 Embolism and thrombosis of iliac artery
445.89 Atheroembolism of other site
447.1 Stricture of artery
453.41 Venous embolism and thrombosis of deep vessels of proximal lower extremity
453.8 Embolism and thrombosis of other specified veins
747.60 Congenital anomaly of the peripheral vascular system, unspecified site ▽
747.69 Congenital anomaly of other specified site of peripheral vascular system

ICD-9-CM Procedural

39.50 Angioplasty or atherectomy of other non-coronary vessel(s)

35456–35459

35456 Transluminal balloon angioplasty, open; femoral-popliteal
35458 brachiocephalic trunk or branches, each vessel
35459 tibioperoneal trunk and branches

ICD-9-CM Diagnostic

250.70 Diabetes with peripheral circulatory disorders, type II or unspecified type, not stated as uncontrolled — (Use additional code to identify manifestation: 443.81, 785.4)
250.71 Diabetes with peripheral circulatory disorders, type I [juvenile type], not stated as uncontrolled — (Use additional code to identify manifestation: 443.81, 785.4)
250.72 Diabetes with peripheral circulatory disorders, type II or unspecified type, uncontrolled — (Use additional code to identify manifestation: 443.81, 785.4)
250.73 Diabetes with peripheral circulatory disorders, type I [juvenile type], uncontrolled — (Use additional code to identify manifestation: 443.81, 785.4)
433.80 Occlusion and stenosis of other specified precerebral artery without mention of cerebral infarction — (Use additional code to identify presence of hypertension)
433.81 Occlusion and stenosis of other specified precerebral artery with cerebral infarction — (Use additional code to identify presence of hypertension)
440.20 Atherosclerosis of native arteries of the extremities, unspecified ▽
440.21 Atherosclerosis of native arteries of the extremities with intermittent claudication
440.22 Atherosclerosis of native arteries of the extremities with rest pain
440.23 Atherosclerosis of native arteries of the extremities with ulceration — (Use additional code for any associated ulceration: 707.10-707.9)
440.24 Atherosclerosis of native arteries of the extremities with gangrene
440.8 Atherosclerosis of other specified arteries
443.81 Peripheral angiopathy in diseases classified elsewhere — (Code first underlying disease, 250.7) ☒
443.9 Unspecified peripheral vascular disease ▽
444.21 Embolism and thrombosis of arteries of upper extremity
444.22 Embolism and thrombosis of arteries of lower extremity
445.01 Atheroembolism of upper extremity
445.02 Atheroembolism of lower extremity
447.1 Stricture of artery
447.8 Other specified disorders of arteries and arterioles
459.2 Compression of vein
747.63 Congenital upper limb vessel anomaly
747.64 Congenital lower limb vessel anomaly
785.4 Gangrene — (Code first any associated underlying condition:250.7, 443.0)
785.9 Other symptoms involving cardiovascular system
996.74 Other complications due to other vascular device, implant, and graft
999.2 Other vascular complications of medical care, not elsewhere classified

ICD-9-CM Procedural

39.50 Angioplasty or atherectomy of other non-coronary vessel(s)

HCPCS Level II Supplies & Services

C1884 Embolization protective system

35460

35460 Transluminal balloon angioplasty, open; venous

ICD-9-CM Diagnostic

443.89 Other peripheral vascular disease
453.40 Venous embolism and thrombosis of unspecified deep vessels of lower extremity
453.41 Venous embolism and thrombosis of deep vessels of proximal lower extremity
453.42 Venous embolism and thrombosis of deep vessels of distal lower extremity
453.8 Embolism and thrombosis of other specified veins
453.9 Embolism and thrombosis of unspecified site ▽
459.2 Compression of vein
459.81 Unspecified venous (peripheral) insufficiency — (Use additional code for any associated ulceration: 707.10-707.9) ▽

▽ Unspecified code ♀ Female diagnosis ☒ Manifestation code ♂ Male diagnosis

459.89 Other specified circulatory system disorders
747.63 Congenital upper limb vessel anomaly
747.64 Congenital lower limb vessel anomaly
747.69 Congenital anomaly of other specified site of peripheral vascular system

ICD-9-CM Procedural
39.50 Angioplasty or atherectomy of other non-coronary vessel(s)

HCPCS Level II Supplies & Services
C1884 Embolization protective system

35470
35470 Transluminal balloon angioplasty, percutaneous; tibioperoneal trunk or branches, each vessel

ICD-9-CM Diagnostic
250.70 Diabetes with peripheral circulatory disorders, type II or unspecified type, not stated as uncontrolled — (Use additional code to identify manifestation: 443.81, 785.4)
250.71 Diabetes with peripheral circulatory disorders, type I [juvenile type], not stated as uncontrolled — (Use additional code to identify manifestation: 443.81, 785.4)
440.20 Atherosclerosis of native arteries of the extremities, unspecified ▽
440.21 Atherosclerosis of native arteries of the extremities with intermittent claudication
440.22 Atherosclerosis of native arteries of the extremities with rest pain
440.23 Atherosclerosis of native arteries of the extremities with ulceration — (Use additional code for any associated ulceration: 707.10-707.9)
440.24 Atherosclerosis of native arteries of the extremities with gangrene
440.30 Atheroslerosis of unspecified bypass graft of extremities ▽
440.31 Atheroslerosis of autologous vein bypass graft of extremities
440.32 Atheroslerosis of nonautologous biological bypass graft of extremities
440.9 Generalized and unspecified atherosclerosis ▽
442.3 Aneurysm of artery of lower extremity
443.81 Peripheral angiopathy in diseases classified elsewhere — (Code first underlying disease, 250.7) ☒
443.9 Unspecified peripheral vascular disease ▽
444.22 Embolism and thrombosis of arteries of lower extremity
444.89 Embolism and thrombosis of other specified artery
444.9 Embolism and thrombosis of unspecified artery ▽
445.02 Atheroembolism of lower extremity
447.1 Stricture of artery
447.8 Other specified disorders of arteries and arterioles
447.9 Unspecified disorders of arteries and arterioles ▽
459.2 Compression of vein
747.64 Congenital lower limb vessel anomaly
785.4 Gangrene — (Code first any associated underlying condition:250.7, 443.0)
996.62 Infection and inflammatory reaction due to other vascular device, implant, and graft — (Use additional code to identify specified infections)

ICD-9-CM Procedural
39.50 Angioplasty or atherectomy of other non-coronary vessel(s)

HCPCS Level II Supplies & Services
C1884 Embolization protective system

35471
35471 Transluminal balloon angioplasty, percutaneous; renal or visceral artery

ICD-9-CM Diagnostic
277.1 Disorders of porphyrin metabolism — (Use additional code to identify any associated mental retardation)
277.3 Amyloidosis — (Use additional code to identify any associated mental retardation)
357.4 Polyneuropathy in other diseases classified elsewhere — (Code first underlying disease: 032.0-032.9, 135, 251.2, 265.0, 265.2, 266.0-266.9, 277.1, 277.3, 585) ☒
403.00 Malignant hypertensive renal disease without mention of renal failure
403.90 Unspecified hypertensive renal disease without mention of renal failure ▽
405.01 Secondary renovascular hypertension, malignant
405.11 Secondary renovascular hypertension, benign
405.91 Secondary renovascular hypertension, unspecified ▽
440.1 Atherosclerosis of renal artery
440.8 Atherosclerosis of other specified arteries
440.9 Generalized and unspecified atherosclerosis ▽
443.9 Unspecified peripheral vascular disease ▽
444.0 Embolism and thrombosis of abdominal aorta
445.81 Atheroembolism of kidney — (Use additional code for any associated kidney failure: 584, 585)
445.89 Atheroembolism of other site
447.1 Stricture of artery
447.4 Celiac artery compression syndrome
447.9 Unspecified disorders of arteries and arterioles ▽
557.0 Acute vascular insufficiency of intestine
557.1 Chronic vascular insufficiency of intestine
557.9 Unspecified vascular insufficiency of intestine ▽
585 Chronic renal failure — (Use additional code to identify manifestation: 357.4, 420.0)
593.81 Vascular disorders of kidney
747.62 Congenital renal vessel anomaly
996.1 Mechanical complication of other vascular device, implant, and graft

ICD-9-CM Procedural
39.50 Angioplasty or atherectomy of other non-coronary vessel(s)

HCPCS Level II Supplies & Services
C1884 Embolization protective system

35472
35472 Transluminal balloon angioplasty, percutaneous; aortic

ICD-9-CM Diagnostic
440.0 Atherosclerosis of aorta
444.89 Embolism and thrombosis of other specified artery
747.22 Congenital atresia and stenosis of aorta

ICD-9-CM Procedural
39.50 Angioplasty or atherectomy of other non-coronary vessel(s)

HCPCS Level II Supplies & Services
C1884 Embolization protective system

35473
35473 Transluminal balloon angioplasty, percutaneous; iliac

ICD-9-CM Diagnostic
440.8 Atherosclerosis of other specified arteries
443.9 Unspecified peripheral vascular disease ▽
444.81 Embolism and thrombosis of iliac artery
445.89 Atheroembolism of other site
447.1 Stricture of artery
453.41 Venous embolism and thrombosis of deep vessels of proximal lower extremity
453.8 Embolism and thrombosis of other specified veins
747.60 Congenital anomaly of the peripheral vascular system, unspecified site ▽
747.69 Congenital anomaly of other specified site of peripheral vascular system

ICD-9-CM Procedural
39.50 Angioplasty or atherectomy of other non-coronary vessel(s)

HCPCS Level II Supplies & Services
C1884 Embolization protective system

35474–35475
35474 Transluminal balloon angioplasty, percutaneous; femoral-popliteal
35475 brachiocephalic trunk or branches, each vessel

ICD-9-CM Diagnostic
250.70 Diabetes with peripheral circulatory disorders, type II or unspecified type, not stated as uncontrolled — (Use additional code to identify manifestation: 443.81, 785.4)
250.71 Diabetes with peripheral circulatory disorders, type I [juvenile type], not stated as uncontrolled — (Use additional code to identify manifestation: 443.81, 785.4)
250.72 Diabetes with peripheral circulatory disorders, type II or unspecified type, uncontrolled — (Use additional code to identify manifestation: 443.81, 785.4)
250.73 Diabetes with peripheral circulatory disorders, type I [juvenile type], uncontrolled — (Use additional code to identify manifestation: 443.81, 785.4)
433.80 Occlusion and stenosis of other specified precerebral artery without mention of cerebral infarction — (Use additional code to identify presence of hypertension)
433.81 Occlusion and stenosis of other specified precerebral artery with cerebral infarction — (Use additional code to identify presence of hypertension)
440.20 Atherosclerosis of native arteries of the extremities, unspecified ▽

440.21 Atherosclerosis of native arteries of the extremities with intermittent claudication
440.22 Atherosclerosis of native arteries of the extremities with rest pain
440.23 Atherosclerosis of native arteries of the extremities with ulceration — (Use additional code for any associated ulceration: 707.10-707.9)
440.24 Atherosclerosis of native arteries of the extremities with gangrene
440.29 Other atherosclerosis of native arteries of the extremities
440.30 Atheroslerosis of unspecified bypass graft of extremities ▽
440.31 Atheroslerosis of autologous vein bypass graft of extremities
440.32 Atheroslerosis of nonautologous biological bypass graft of extremities
440.8 Atherosclerosis of other specified arteries
440.9 Generalized and unspecified atherosclerosis ▽
442.3 Aneurysm of artery of lower extremity
443.81 Peripheral angiopathy in diseases classified elsewhere — (Code first underlying disease, 250.7) ☒
443.9 Unspecified peripheral vascular disease ▽
444.21 Embolism and thrombosis of arteries of upper extremity
444.22 Embolism and thrombosis of arteries of lower extremity
444.89 Embolism and thrombosis of other specified artery
444.9 Embolism and thrombosis of unspecified artery ▽
445.01 Atheroembolism of upper extremity
445.02 Atheroembolism of lower extremity
447.1 Stricture of artery
447.8 Other specified disorders of arteries and arterioles
447.9 Unspecified disorders of arteries and arterioles ▽
747.63 Congenital upper limb vessel anomaly
747.64 Congenital lower limb vessel anomaly
785.4 Gangrene — (Code first any associated underlying condition:250.7, 443.0)
785.59 Other shock without mention of trauma
785.9 Other symptoms involving cardiovascular system
996.62 Infection and inflammatory reaction due to other vascular device, implant, and graft — (Use additional code to identify specified infections)
996.73 Other complications due to renal dialysis device, implant, and graft
996.74 Other complications due to other vascular device, implant, and graft

ICD-9-CM Procedural

00.61 Percutaneous angioplasty or atherectomy of precerebral (extracranial) vessel(s)
00.62 Percutaneous angioplasty or atherectomy of intracranial vessel(s)
39.50 Angioplasty or atherectomy of other non-coronary vessel(s)

HCPCS Level II Supplies & Services

C1884 Embolization protective system

35476

35476 Transluminal balloon angioplasty, percutaneous; venous

ICD-9-CM Diagnostic

440.30 Atheroslerosis of unspecified bypass graft of extremities ▽
440.31 Atheroslerosis of autologous vein bypass graft of extremities
440.32 Atheroslerosis of nonautologous biological bypass graft of extremities
440.9 Generalized and unspecified atherosclerosis ▽
443.89 Other peripheral vascular disease
443.9 Unspecified peripheral vascular disease ▽
453.40 Venous embolism and thrombosis of unspecified deep vessels of lower extremity
453.41 Venous embolism and thrombosis of deep vessels of proximal lower extremity
453.42 Venous embolism and thrombosis of deep vessels of distal lower extremity
453.8 Embolism and thrombosis of other specified veins
453.9 Embolism and thrombosis of unspecified site ▽
459.2 Compression of vein
459.81 Unspecified venous (peripheral) insufficiency — (Use additional code for any associated ulceration: 707.10-707.9) ▽
459.89 Other specified circulatory system disorders
593.81 Vascular disorders of kidney
729.81 Swelling of limb
747.63 Congenital upper limb vessel anomaly
747.64 Congenital lower limb vessel anomaly
747.69 Congenital anomaly of other specified site of peripheral vascular system
996.1 Mechanical complication of other vascular device, implant, and graft
996.62 Infection and inflammatory reaction due to other vascular device, implant, and graft — (Use additional code to identify specified infections)
996.73 Other complications due to renal dialysis device, implant, and graft
996.74 Other complications due to other vascular device, implant, and graft

ICD-9-CM Procedural

39.50 Angioplasty or atherectomy of other non-coronary vessel(s)

Atherectomy

High blood pressure, cigarette smoking, and high cholestrol levels contribute to the progressive disease of atherosclerosis.

Atherosclerostic plaque is removed by a rotary cutter introduced into the artery through a catheter.

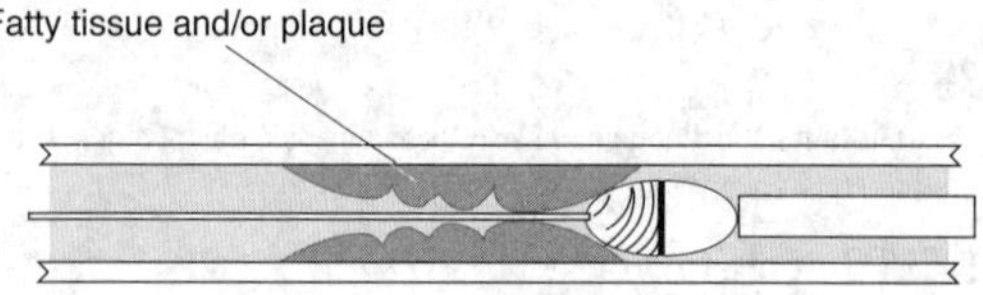

Fatty tissue and/or plaque

HCPCS Level II Supplies & Services

C1884 Embolization protective system

35480

35480 Transluminal peripheral atherectomy, open; renal or other visceral artery

ICD-9-CM Diagnostic

277.1 Disorders of porphyrin metabolism — (Use additional code to identify any associated mental retardation)
277.3 Amyloidosis — (Use additional code to identify any associated mental retardation)
403.00 Malignant hypertensive renal disease without mention of renal failure
403.90 Unspecified hypertensive renal disease without mention of renal failure ▽
405.01 Secondary renovascular hypertension, malignant
405.11 Secondary renovascular hypertension, benign
405.91 Secondary renovascular hypertension, unspecified ▽
440.1 Atherosclerosis of renal artery
440.8 Atherosclerosis of other specified arteries
440.9 Generalized and unspecified atherosclerosis ▽
447.1 Stricture of artery
447.4 Celiac artery compression syndrome
447.9 Unspecified disorders of arteries and arterioles ▽
557.0 Acute vascular insufficiency of intestine
557.1 Chronic vascular insufficiency of intestine
557.9 Unspecified vascular insufficiency of intestine ▽
585 Chronic renal failure — (Use additional code to identify manifestation: 357.4, 420.0)
593.81 Vascular disorders of kidney
996.1 Mechanical complication of other vascular device, implant, and graft

ICD-9-CM Procedural

39.50 Angioplasty or atherectomy of other non-coronary vessel(s)

35481

35481 Transluminal peripheral atherectomy, open; aortic

ICD-9-CM Diagnostic

440.0 Atherosclerosis of aorta

ICD-9-CM Procedural

39.50 Angioplasty or atherectomy of other non-coronary vessel(s)

35482

35482 Transluminal peripheral atherectomy, open; iliac

ICD-9-CM Diagnostic

440.20 Atherosclerosis of native arteries of the extremities, unspecified ▽
440.21 Atherosclerosis of native arteries of the extremities with intermittent claudication
440.22 Atherosclerosis of native arteries of the extremities with rest pain
440.23 Atherosclerosis of native arteries of the extremities with ulceration — (Use additional code for any associated ulceration: 707.10-707.9)
440.24 Atherosclerosis of native arteries of the extremities with gangrene
440.8 Atherosclerosis of other specified arteries
440.9 Generalized and unspecified atherosclerosis ▽
442.2 Aneurysm of iliac artery
443.9 Unspecified peripheral vascular disease ▽

447.1 Stricture of artery
447.9 Unspecified disorders of arteries and arterioles ▽

ICD-9-CM Procedural
39.50 Angioplasty or atherectomy of other non-coronary vessel(s)

35483–35485
35482 Transluminal peripheral atherectomy, open; iliac
35484 brachiocephalic trunk or branches, each vessel
35485 tibioperoneal trunk and branches

ICD-9-CM Diagnostic
250.70 Diabetes with peripheral circulatory disorders, type II or unspecified type, not stated as uncontrolled — (Use additional code to identify manifestation: 443.81, 785.4)
250.71 Diabetes with peripheral circulatory disorders, type I [juvenile type], not stated as uncontrolled — (Use additional code to identify manifestation: 443.81, 785.4)
250.72 Diabetes with peripheral circulatory disorders, type II or unspecified type, uncontrolled — (Use additional code to identify manifestation: 443.81, 785.4)
250.73 Diabetes with peripheral circulatory disorders, type I [juvenile type], uncontrolled — (Use additional code to identify manifestation: 443.81, 785.4)
440.20 Atherosclerosis of native arteries of the extremities, unspecified ▽
440.21 Atherosclerosis of native arteries of the extremities with intermittent claudication
440.22 Atherosclerosis of native arteries of the extremities with rest pain
440.23 Atherosclerosis of native arteries of the extremities with ulceration — (Use additional code for any associated ulceration: 707.10-707.9)
440.24 Atherosclerosis of native arteries of the extremities with gangrene
440.29 Other atherosclerosis of native arteries of the extremities
440.8 Atherosclerosis of other specified arteries
442.0 Aneurysm of artery of upper extremity
442.3 Aneurysm of artery of lower extremity
443.81 Peripheral angiopathy in diseases classified elsewhere — (Code first underlying disease, 250.7) ☒
443.9 Unspecified peripheral vascular disease ▽
447.1 Stricture of artery
747.63 Congenital upper limb vessel anomaly
747.64 Congenital lower limb vessel anomaly

ICD-9-CM Procedural
39.50 Angioplasty or atherectomy of other non-coronary vessel(s)

HCPCS Level II Supplies & Services
C1884 Embolization protective system

35490
35490 Transluminal peripheral atherectomy, percutaneous; renal or other visceral artery

ICD-9-CM Diagnostic
277.1 Disorders of porphyrin metabolism — (Use additional code to identify any associated mental retardation)
277.3 Amyloidosis — (Use additional code to identify any associated mental retardation)
403.00 Malignant hypertensive renal disease without mention of renal failure
405.01 Secondary renovascular hypertension, malignant
405.11 Secondary renovascular hypertension, benign
405.91 Secondary renovascular hypertension, unspecified ▽
440.1 Atherosclerosis of renal artery
442.1 Aneurysm of renal artery
442.84 Aneurysm of other visceral artery
443.9 Unspecified peripheral vascular disease ▽
447.1 Stricture of artery
447.4 Celiac artery compression syndrome
447.9 Unspecified disorders of arteries and arterioles ▽
557.0 Acute vascular insufficiency of intestine
557.1 Chronic vascular insufficiency of intestine
557.9 Unspecified vascular insufficiency of intestine ▽
593.81 Vascular disorders of kidney

ICD-9-CM Procedural
39.50 Angioplasty or atherectomy of other non-coronary vessel(s)

HCPCS Level II Supplies & Services
C1884 Embolization protective system

35491
35491 Transluminal peripheral atherectomy, percutaneous; aortic

ICD-9-CM Diagnostic
440.0 Atherosclerosis of aorta
440.9 Generalized and unspecified atherosclerosis ▽
441.00 Dissecting aortic aneurysm (any part), unspecified site ▽
441.2 Thoracic aneurysm without mention of rupture
441.4 Abdominal aneurysm without mention of rupture
441.7 Thoracoabdominal aneurysm without mention of rupture
441.9 Aortic aneurysm of unspecified site without mention of rupture ▽
443.9 Unspecified peripheral vascular disease ▽

ICD-9-CM Procedural
39.50 Angioplasty or atherectomy of other non-coronary vessel(s)

HCPCS Level II Supplies & Services
C1884 Embolization protective system

35492
35492 Transluminal peripheral atherectomy, percutaneous; iliac

ICD-9-CM Diagnostic
440.20 Atherosclerosis of native arteries of the extremities, unspecified ▽
440.21 Atherosclerosis of native arteries of the extremities with intermittent claudication
440.22 Atherosclerosis of native arteries of the extremities with rest pain
440.23 Atherosclerosis of native arteries of the extremities with ulceration — (Use additional code for any associated ulceration: 707.10-707.9)
440.24 Atherosclerosis of native arteries of the extremities with gangrene
440.8 Atherosclerosis of other specified arteries
440.9 Generalized and unspecified atherosclerosis ▽
442.2 Aneurysm of iliac artery
443.9 Unspecified peripheral vascular disease ▽
447.1 Stricture of artery
447.9 Unspecified disorders of arteries and arterioles ▽

ICD-9-CM Procedural
39.50 Angioplasty or atherectomy of other non-coronary vessel(s)

HCPCS Level II Supplies & Services
C1884 Embolization protective system

35493–35495
35493 Transluminal peripheral atherectomy, percutaneous; femoral-popliteal
35494 brachiocephalic trunk or branches, each vessel
35495 tibioperoneal trunk and branches

ICD-9-CM Diagnostic
250.70 Diabetes with peripheral circulatory disorders, type II or unspecified type, not stated as uncontrolled — (Use additional code to identify manifestation: 443.81, 785.4)
250.71 Diabetes with peripheral circulatory disorders, type I [juvenile type], not stated as uncontrolled — (Use additional code to identify manifestation: 443.81, 785.4)
250.72 Diabetes with peripheral circulatory disorders, type II or unspecified type, uncontrolled — (Use additional code to identify manifestation: 443.81, 785.4)
250.73 Diabetes with peripheral circulatory disorders, type I [juvenile type], uncontrolled — (Use additional code to identify manifestation: 443.81, 785.4)
440.20 Atherosclerosis of native arteries of the extremities, unspecified ▽
440.21 Atherosclerosis of native arteries of the extremities with intermittent claudication
440.22 Atherosclerosis of native arteries of the extremities with rest pain
440.23 Atherosclerosis of native arteries of the extremities with ulceration — (Use additional code for any associated ulceration: 707.10-707.9)
440.24 Atherosclerosis of native arteries of the extremities with gangrene
440.29 Other atherosclerosis of native arteries of the extremities
440.8 Atherosclerosis of other specified arteries
442.0 Aneurysm of artery of upper extremity
442.3 Aneurysm of artery of lower extremity
443.81 Peripheral angiopathy in diseases classified elsewhere — (Code first underlying disease, 250.7) ☒
443.9 Unspecified peripheral vascular disease ▽
447.1 Stricture of artery
447.9 Unspecified disorders of arteries and arterioles ▽
747.63 Congenital upper limb vessel anomaly

▽ Unspecified code ♀ Female diagnosis ☒ Manifestation code ♂ Male diagnosis

747.64 Congenital lower limb vessel anomaly

ICD-9-CM Procedural

00.61 Percutaneous angioplasty or atherectomy of precerebral (extracranial) vessel(s)
00.62 Percutaneous angioplasty or atherectomy of intracranial vessel(s)
39.50 Angioplasty or atherectomy of other non-coronary vessel(s)

HCPCS Level II Supplies & Services

C1884 Embolization protective system

35500

35500 Harvest of upper extremity vein, one segment, for lower extremity or coronary artery bypass procedure (List separately in addition to code for primary procedure)

ICD-9-CM Diagnostic

This is an add-on code. Refer to the corresponding primary procedure code for ICD-9 diagnosis code links.

ICD-9-CM Procedural

38.63 Other excision of upper limb vessels

35501

35501 Bypass graft, with vein; carotid

ICD-9-CM Diagnostic

433.10 Occlusion and stenosis of carotid artery without mention of cerebral infarction — (Use additional code to identify presence of hypertension)
433.11 Occlusion and stenosis of carotid artery with cerebral infarction — (Use additional code to identify presence of hypertension)
433.30 Occlusion and stenosis of multiple and bilateral precerebral arteries without mention of cerebral infarction — (Use additional code to identify presence of hypertension)
433.31 Occlusion and stenosis of multiple and bilateral precerebral arteries with cerebral infarction — (Use additional code to identify presence of hypertension)
433.80 Occlusion and stenosis of other specified precerebral artery without mention of cerebral infarction — (Use additional code to identify presence of hypertension)
433.81 Occlusion and stenosis of other specified precerebral artery with cerebral infarction — (Use additional code to identify presence of hypertension)
435.8 Other specified transient cerebral ischemias — (Use additional code to identify presence of hypertension)
437.1 Other generalized ischemic cerebrovascular disease — (Use additional code to identify presence of hypertension)
437.3 Cerebral aneurysm, nonruptured — (Use additional code to identify presence of hypertension)
440.8 Atherosclerosis of other specified arteries
442.81 Aneurysm of artery of neck
443.21 Dissection of carotid artery
447.1 Stricture of artery
747.81 Congenital anomaly of cerebrovascular system
780.2 Syncope and collapse
785.9 Other symptoms involving cardiovascular system
900.00 Injury to carotid artery, unspecified ▽
900.01 Common carotid artery injury
900.02 External carotid artery injury
900.03 Internal carotid artery injury
906.0 Late effect of open wound of head, neck, and trunk
908.3 Late effect of injury to blood vessel of head, neck, and extremities
925.2 Crushing injury of neck — (Use additional code to identify any associated injuries: 800-829, 850.0-854.1, 860.0-869.1)
996.1 Mechanical complication of other vascular device, implant, and graft
996.74 Other complications due to other vascular device, implant, and graft

ICD-9-CM Procedural

39.22 Aorta-subclavian-carotid bypass

35506

35506 Bypass graft, with vein; carotid-subclavian

ICD-9-CM Diagnostic

433.10 Occlusion and stenosis of carotid artery without mention of cerebral infarction — (Use additional code to identify presence of hypertension)
433.11 Occlusion and stenosis of carotid artery with cerebral infarction — (Use additional code to identify presence of hypertension)
433.30 Occlusion and stenosis of multiple and bilateral precerebral arteries without mention of cerebral infarction — (Use additional code to identify presence of hypertension)
433.31 Occlusion and stenosis of multiple and bilateral precerebral arteries with cerebral infarction — (Use additional code to identify presence of hypertension)
435.2 Subclavian steal syndrome — (Use additional code to identify presence of hypertension)
435.8 Other specified transient cerebral ischemias — (Use additional code to identify presence of hypertension)
440.8 Atherosclerosis of other specified arteries
442.81 Aneurysm of artery of neck
442.82 Aneurysm of subclavian artery
443.21 Dissection of carotid artery
443.29 Dissection of other artery
447.1 Stricture of artery
447.6 Unspecified arteritis ▽
747.69 Congenital anomaly of other specified site of peripheral vascular system
785.9 Other symptoms involving cardiovascular system
874.9 Open wound of other and unspecified parts of neck, complicated — (Use additional code to identify infection) ▽
900.01 Common carotid artery injury
900.02 External carotid artery injury
900.03 Internal carotid artery injury
900.82 Injury to multiple blood vessels of head and neck
901.1 Innominate and subclavian artery injury
906.0 Late effect of open wound of head, neck, and trunk
908.3 Late effect of injury to blood vessel of head, neck, and extremities
925.2 Crushing injury of neck — (Use additional code to identify any associated injuries: 800-829, 850.0-854.1, 860.0-869.1)
996.1 Mechanical complication of other vascular device, implant, and graft
996.74 Other complications due to other vascular device, implant, and graft

ICD-9-CM Procedural

39.22 Aorta-subclavian-carotid bypass

35507

35507 Bypass graft, with vein; subclavian-carotid

ICD-9-CM Diagnostic

433.10 Occlusion and stenosis of carotid artery without mention of cerebral infarction — (Use additional code to identify presence of hypertension)
433.11 Occlusion and stenosis of carotid artery with cerebral infarction — (Use additional code to identify presence of hypertension)
433.30 Occlusion and stenosis of multiple and bilateral precerebral arteries without mention of cerebral infarction — (Use additional code to identify presence of hypertension)
433.31 Occlusion and stenosis of multiple and bilateral precerebral arteries with cerebral infarction — (Use additional code to identify presence of hypertension)
435.2 Subclavian steal syndrome — (Use additional code to identify presence of hypertension)
435.8 Other specified transient cerebral ischemias — (Use additional code to identify presence of hypertension)
440.8 Atherosclerosis of other specified arteries
442.81 Aneurysm of artery of neck
442.82 Aneurysm of subclavian artery
443.21 Dissection of carotid artery
443.29 Dissection of other artery
447.1 Stricture of artery
447.6 Unspecified arteritis ▽
747.69 Congenital anomaly of other specified site of peripheral vascular system
874.9 Open wound of other and unspecified parts of neck, complicated — (Use additional code to identify infection) ▽
900.01 Common carotid artery injury
900.02 External carotid artery injury
900.03 Internal carotid artery injury
900.82 Injury to multiple blood vessels of head and neck
901.1 Innominate and subclavian artery injury
906.0 Late effect of open wound of head, neck, and trunk
908.3 Late effect of injury to blood vessel of head, neck, and extremities
925.2 Crushing injury of neck — (Use additional code to identify any associated injuries: 800-829, 850.0-854.1, 860.0-869.1)
996.1 Mechanical complication of other vascular device, implant, and graft
996.74 Other complications due to other vascular device, implant, and graft

ICD-9-CM Procedural

39.22 Aorta-subclavian-carotid bypass

35508

35508 Bypass graft, with vein; carotid-vertebral

ICD-9-CM Diagnostic

433.20 Occlusion and stenosis of vertebral artery without mention of cerebral infarction — (Use additional code to identify presence of hypertension)
433.21 Occlusion and stenosis of vertebral artery with cerebral infarction — (Use additional code to identify presence of hypertension)
435.1 Vertebral artery syndrome — (Use additional code to identify presence of hypertension)
435.8 Other specified transient cerebral ischemias — (Use additional code to identify presence of hypertension)
440.8 Atherosclerosis of other specified arteries
442.81 Aneurysm of artery of neck
443.21 Dissection of carotid artery
443.24 Dissection of vertebral artery
447.1 Stricture of artery
747.69 Congenital anomaly of other specified site of peripheral vascular system
874.9 Open wound of other and unspecified parts of neck, complicated — (Use additional code to identify infection) ▽
900.82 Injury to multiple blood vessels of head and neck
906.0 Late effect of open wound of head, neck, and trunk

ICD-9-CM Procedural

39.28 Extracranial-intracranial (EC-IC) vascular bypass

35509

35509 Bypass graft, with vein; carotid-carotid

ICD-9-CM Diagnostic

433.10 Occlusion and stenosis of carotid artery without mention of cerebral infarction — (Use additional code to identify presence of hypertension)
433.11 Occlusion and stenosis of carotid artery with cerebral infarction — (Use additional code to identify presence of hypertension)
433.30 Occlusion and stenosis of multiple and bilateral precerebral arteries without mention of cerebral infarction — (Use additional code to identify presence of hypertension)
433.31 Occlusion and stenosis of multiple and bilateral precerebral arteries with cerebral infarction — (Use additional code to identify presence of hypertension)
435.8 Other specified transient cerebral ischemias — (Use additional code to identify presence of hypertension)
442.81 Aneurysm of artery of neck
443.21 Dissection of carotid artery
447.1 Stricture of artery
747.69 Congenital anomaly of other specified site of peripheral vascular system
900.01 Common carotid artery injury
900.02 External carotid artery injury
900.03 Internal carotid artery injury
906.0 Late effect of open wound of head, neck, and trunk
906.4 Late effect of crushing
908.3 Late effect of injury to blood vessel of head, neck, and extremities
925.2 Crushing injury of neck — (Use additional code to identify any associated injuries: 800-829, 850.0-854.1, 860.0-869.1)
996.1 Mechanical complication of other vascular device, implant, and graft
996.74 Other complications due to other vascular device, implant, and graft

ICD-9-CM Procedural

39.22 Aorta-subclavian-carotid bypass

35510

35510 Bypass graft, with vein; carotid-brachial

ICD-9-CM Diagnostic

433.10 Occlusion and stenosis of carotid artery without mention of cerebral infarction — (Use additional code to identify presence of hypertension)
433.11 Occlusion and stenosis of carotid artery with cerebral infarction — (Use additional code to identify presence of hypertension)
433.30 Occlusion and stenosis of multiple and bilateral precerebral arteries without mention of cerebral infarction — (Use additional code to identify presence of hypertension)
433.31 Occlusion and stenosis of multiple and bilateral precerebral arteries with cerebral infarction — (Use additional code to identify presence of hypertension)
433.80 Occlusion and stenosis of other specified precerebral artery without mention of cerebral infarction — (Use additional code to identify presence of hypertension)
433.81 Occlusion and stenosis of other specified precerebral artery with cerebral infarction — (Use additional code to identify presence of hypertension)
435.8 Other specified transient cerebral ischemias — (Use additional code to identify presence of hypertension)
437.1 Other generalized ischemic cerebrovascular disease — (Use additional code to identify presence of hypertension)
440.20 Atherosclerosis of native arteries of the extremities, unspecified ▽
440.8 Atherosclerosis of other specified arteries
442.0 Aneurysm of artery of upper extremity
442.81 Aneurysm of artery of neck
443.21 Dissection of carotid artery
443.29 Dissection of other artery
443.9 Unspecified peripheral vascular disease ▽
444.21 Embolism and thrombosis of arteries of upper extremity
445.01 Atheroembolism of upper extremity
447.1 Stricture of artery
747.81 Congenital anomaly of cerebrovascular system
780.2 Syncope and collapse
785.9 Other symptoms involving cardiovascular system
900.00 Injury to carotid artery, unspecified ▽
900.01 Common carotid artery injury
900.02 External carotid artery injury
900.03 Internal carotid artery injury
903.1 Brachial blood vessels injury
906.0 Late effect of open wound of head, neck, and trunk
908.3 Late effect of injury to blood vessel of head, neck, and extremities
925.2 Crushing injury of neck — (Use additional code to identify any associated injuries: 800-829, 850.0-854.1, 860.0-869.1)
996.1 Mechanical complication of other vascular device, implant, and graft
996.74 Other complications due to other vascular device, implant, and graft

ICD-9-CM Procedural

39.22 Aorta-subclavian-carotid bypass

35511

35511 Bypass graft, with vein; subclavian-subclavian

ICD-9-CM Diagnostic

435.2 Subclavian steal syndrome — (Use additional code to identify presence of hypertension)
435.8 Other specified transient cerebral ischemias — (Use additional code to identify presence of hypertension)
440.8 Atherosclerosis of other specified arteries
442.82 Aneurysm of subclavian artery
443.29 Dissection of other artery
444.89 Embolism and thrombosis of other specified artery
447.1 Stricture of artery
447.6 Unspecified arteritis ▽
747.69 Congenital anomaly of other specified site of peripheral vascular system
785.9 Other symptoms involving cardiovascular system
874.9 Open wound of other and unspecified parts of neck, complicated — (Use additional code to identify infection) ▽
900.82 Injury to multiple blood vessels of head and neck
900.89 Injury to other specified blood vessels of head and neck
901.1 Innominate and subclavian artery injury
901.89 Injury to specified blood vessels of thorax, other
906.0 Late effect of open wound of head, neck, and trunk
906.4 Late effect of crushing
908.3 Late effect of injury to blood vessel of head, neck, and extremities
996.1 Mechanical complication of other vascular device, implant, and graft
996.74 Other complications due to other vascular device, implant, and graft
998.2 Accidental puncture or laceration during procedure

ICD-9-CM Procedural

39.22 Aorta-subclavian-carotid bypass

35512

35512 Bypass graft, with vein; subclavian-brachial

ICD-9-CM Diagnostic

435.2 Subclavian steal syndrome — (Use additional code to identify presence of hypertension)
435.8 Other specified transient cerebral ischemias — (Use additional code to identify presence of hypertension)
440.20 Atherosclerosis of native arteries of the extremities, unspecified ▽
440.8 Atherosclerosis of other specified arteries
442.0 Aneurysm of artery of upper extremity
442.82 Aneurysm of subclavian artery

▽ Unspecified code ♀ Female diagnosis ☒ Manifestation code ♂ Male diagnosis

443.29 Dissection of other artery
443.9 Unspecified peripheral vascular disease ▽
444.21 Embolism and thrombosis of arteries of upper extremity
444.89 Embolism and thrombosis of other specified artery
447.1 Stricture of artery
447.6 Unspecified arteritis ▽
747.69 Congenital anomaly of other specified site of peripheral vascular system
785.9 Other symptoms involving cardiovascular system
874.9 Open wound of other and unspecified parts of neck, complicated — (Use additional code to identify infection) ▽
900.82 Injury to multiple blood vessels of head and neck
900.89 Injury to other specified blood vessels of head and neck
901.1 Innominate and subclavian artery injury
901.89 Injury to specified blood vessels of thorax, other
903.1 Brachial blood vessels injury
906.0 Late effect of open wound of head, neck, and trunk
906.4 Late effect of crushing
908.3 Late effect of injury to blood vessel of head, neck, and extremities
996.1 Mechanical complication of other vascular device, implant, and graft
996.74 Other complications due to other vascular device, implant, and graft

ICD-9-CM Procedural

39.22 Aorta-subclavian-carotid bypass

35515

35515 Bypass graft, with vein; subclavian-vertebral

ICD-9-CM Diagnostic

433.20 Occlusion and stenosis of vertebral artery without mention of cerebral infarction — (Use additional code to identify presence of hypertension)
433.21 Occlusion and stenosis of vertebral artery with cerebral infarction — (Use additional code to identify presence of hypertension)
435.1 Vertebral artery syndrome — (Use additional code to identify presence of hypertension)
435.8 Other specified transient cerebral ischemias — (Use additional code to identify presence of hypertension)
443.24 Dissection of vertebral artery
443.29 Dissection of other artery
447.1 Stricture of artery
447.6 Unspecified arteritis ▽
747.69 Congenital anomaly of other specified site of peripheral vascular system
874.9 Open wound of other and unspecified parts of neck, complicated — (Use additional code to identify infection) ▽
900.82 Injury to multiple blood vessels of head and neck
906.0 Late effect of open wound of head, neck, and trunk
908.3 Late effect of injury to blood vessel of head, neck, and extremities
996.1 Mechanical complication of other vascular device, implant, and graft
996.74 Other complications due to other vascular device, implant, and graft
998.2 Accidental puncture or laceration during procedure

ICD-9-CM Procedural

39.22 Aorta-subclavian-carotid bypass

35516

35516 Bypass graft, with vein; subclavian-axillary

ICD-9-CM Diagnostic

435.2 Subclavian steal syndrome — (Use additional code to identify presence of hypertension)
435.8 Other specified transient cerebral ischemias — (Use additional code to identify presence of hypertension)
440.8 Atherosclerosis of other specified arteries
447.1 Stricture of artery
447.6 Unspecified arteritis ▽
747.69 Congenital anomaly of other specified site of peripheral vascular system
785.9 Other symptoms involving cardiovascular system
874.9 Open wound of other and unspecified parts of neck, complicated — (Use additional code to identify infection) ▽
900.82 Injury to multiple blood vessels of head and neck
901.1 Innominate and subclavian artery injury
906.0 Late effect of open wound of head, neck, and trunk
925.2 Crushing injury of neck — (Use additional code to identify any associated injuries: 800-829, 850.0-854.1, 860.0-869.1)
996.1 Mechanical complication of other vascular device, implant, and graft
996.74 Other complications due to other vascular device, implant, and graft
998.2 Accidental puncture or laceration during procedure

ICD-9-CM Procedural

39.29 Other (peripheral) vascular shunt or bypass

35518

35518 Bypass graft, with vein; axillary-axillary

ICD-9-CM Diagnostic

435.2 Subclavian steal syndrome — (Use additional code to identify presence of hypertension)
440.20 Atherosclerosis of native arteries of the extremities, unspecified ▽
440.8 Atherosclerosis of other specified arteries
442.0 Aneurysm of artery of upper extremity
442.89 Aneurysm of other specified artery
443.29 Dissection of other artery
443.9 Unspecified peripheral vascular disease ▽
444.21 Embolism and thrombosis of arteries of upper extremity
444.89 Embolism and thrombosis of other specified artery
445.01 Atheroembolism of upper extremity
447.1 Stricture of artery
447.5 Necrosis of artery
447.9 Unspecified disorders of arteries and arterioles ▽
459.9 Unspecified circulatory system disorder ▽
747.63 Congenital upper limb vessel anomaly
785.9 Other symptoms involving cardiovascular system
880.02 Open wound of axillary region, without mention of complication — (Use additional code to identify infection)
880.12 Open wound of axillary region, complicated — (Use additional code to identify infection)
901.1 Innominate and subclavian artery injury
903.01 Axillary artery injury
906.1 Late effect of open wound of extremities without mention of tendon injury
906.4 Late effect of crushing
908.3 Late effect of injury to blood vessel of head, neck, and extremities
927.02 Crushing injury of axillary region — (Use additional code to identify any associated injuries: 800-829, 850.0-854.1, 860.0-869.1)
996.1 Mechanical complication of other vascular device, implant, and graft
996.74 Other complications due to other vascular device, implant, and graft

ICD-9-CM Procedural

39.29 Other (peripheral) vascular shunt or bypass

35521

35521 Bypass graft, with vein; axillary-femoral

ICD-9-CM Diagnostic

440.0 Atherosclerosis of aorta
440.8 Atherosclerosis of other specified arteries
440.9 Generalized and unspecified atherosclerosis ▽
441.02 Dissecting aortic aneurysm (any part), abdominal
441.03 Dissecting aortic aneurysm (any part), thoracoabdominal
441.3 Abdominal aneurysm, ruptured
441.4 Abdominal aneurysm without mention of rupture
441.5 Aortic aneurysm of unspecified site, ruptured ▽
441.6 Thoracoabdominal aneurysm, ruptured
441.7 Thoracoabdominal aneurysm without mention of rupture
441.9 Aortic aneurysm of unspecified site without mention of rupture ▽
442.2 Aneurysm of iliac artery
442.3 Aneurysm of artery of lower extremity
443.22 Dissection of iliac artery
443.29 Dissection of other artery
443.9 Unspecified peripheral vascular disease ▽
444.0 Embolism and thrombosis of abdominal aorta
444.81 Embolism and thrombosis of iliac artery
445.02 Atheroembolism of lower extremity
447.1 Stricture of artery
447.5 Necrosis of artery
447.9 Unspecified disorders of arteries and arterioles ▽
747.22 Congenital atresia and stenosis of aorta
747.69 Congenital anomaly of other specified site of peripheral vascular system
785.4 Gangrene — (Code first any associated underlying condition:250.7, 443.0)
785.9 Other symptoms involving cardiovascular system
879.5 Open wound of abdominal wall, lateral, complicated — (Use additional code to identify infection)
902.0 Abdominal aorta injury
902.53 Iliac artery injury

▽ Unspecified code
♀ Female diagnosis
☒ Manifestation code
♂ Male diagnosis

904.7 Injury to specified blood vessels of lower extremity, other
908.3 Late effect of injury to blood vessel of head, neck, and extremities
908.4 Late effect of injury to blood vessel of thorax, abdomen, and pelvis
996.1 Mechanical complication of other vascular device, implant, and graft
996.74 Other complications due to other vascular device, implant, and graft
998.2 Accidental puncture or laceration during procedure

ICD-9-CM Procedural
39.29 Other (peripheral) vascular shunt or bypass

35522
35522 Bypass graft, with vein; axillary-brachial

ICD-9-CM Diagnostic
435.2 Subclavian steal syndrome — (Use additional code to identify presence of hypertension)
440.20 Atherosclerosis of native arteries of the extremities, unspecified ▽
440.8 Atherosclerosis of other specified arteries
442.0 Aneurysm of artery of upper extremity
442.89 Aneurysm of other specified artery
443.29 Dissection of other artery
443.9 Unspecified peripheral vascular disease ▽
444.21 Embolism and thrombosis of arteries of upper extremity
444.89 Embolism and thrombosis of other specified artery
445.01 Atheroembolism of upper extremity
447.1 Stricture of artery
447.5 Necrosis of artery
447.9 Unspecified disorders of arteries and arterioles ▽
459.9 Unspecified circulatory system disorder ▽
747.63 Congenital upper limb vessel anomaly
785.9 Other symptoms involving cardiovascular system
880.02 Open wound of axillary region, without mention of complication — (Use additional code to identify infection)
880.12 Open wound of axillary region, complicated — (Use additional code to identify infection)
901.1 Innominate and subclavian artery injury
903.01 Axillary artery injury
903.1 Brachial blood vessels injury
906.1 Late effect of open wound of extremities without mention of tendon injury
906.4 Late effect of crushing
908.3 Late effect of injury to blood vessel of head, neck, and extremities
927.02 Crushing injury of axillary region — (Use additional code to identify any associated injuries: 800-829, 850.0-854.1, 860.0-869.1)
996.1 Mechanical complication of other vascular device, implant, and graft
996.74 Other complications due to other vascular device, implant, and graft

ICD-9-CM Procedural
39.29 Other (peripheral) vascular shunt or bypass

35525
35525 Bypass graft, with vein; brachial-brachial

ICD-9-CM Diagnostic
435.2 Subclavian steal syndrome — (Use additional code to identify presence of hypertension)
440.20 Atherosclerosis of native arteries of the extremities, unspecified ▽
440.8 Atherosclerosis of other specified arteries
442.0 Aneurysm of artery of upper extremity
442.89 Aneurysm of other specified artery
443.29 Dissection of other artery
443.9 Unspecified peripheral vascular disease ▽
444.21 Embolism and thrombosis of arteries of upper extremity
444.89 Embolism and thrombosis of other specified artery
445.01 Atheroembolism of upper extremity
447.1 Stricture of artery
447.5 Necrosis of artery
447.9 Unspecified disorders of arteries and arterioles ▽
459.9 Unspecified circulatory system disorder ▽
747.63 Congenital upper limb vessel anomaly
785.9 Other symptoms involving cardiovascular system
880.03 Open wound of upper arm, without mention of complication — (Use additional code to identify infection)
880.13 Open wound of upper arm, complicated — (Use additional code to identify infection)
903.1 Brachial blood vessels injury
906.1 Late effect of open wound of extremities without mention of tendon injury
906.4 Late effect of crushing
908.3 Late effect of injury to blood vessel of head, neck, and extremities
927.03 Crushing injury of upper arm — (Use additional code to identify any associated injuries: 800-829, 850.0-854.1, 860.0-869.1)
996.1 Mechanical complication of other vascular device, implant, and graft
996.74 Other complications due to other vascular device, implant, and graft

ICD-9-CM Procedural
39.29 Other (peripheral) vascular shunt or bypass

35526
35526 Bypass graft, with vein; aortosubclavian or carotid

ICD-9-CM Diagnostic
433.10 Occlusion and stenosis of carotid artery without mention of cerebral infarction — (Use additional code to identify presence of hypertension)
433.11 Occlusion and stenosis of carotid artery with cerebral infarction — (Use additional code to identify presence of hypertension)
435.0 Basilar artery syndrome — (Use additional code to identify presence of hypertension)
435.2 Subclavian steal syndrome — (Use additional code to identify presence of hypertension)
437.1 Other generalized ischemic cerebrovascular disease — (Use additional code to identify presence of hypertension)
440.8 Atherosclerosis of other specified arteries
442.81 Aneurysm of artery of neck
442.82 Aneurysm of subclavian artery
443.21 Dissection of carotid artery
443.29 Dissection of other artery
901.0 Thoracic aorta injury
901.1 Innominate and subclavian artery injury
996.1 Mechanical complication of other vascular device, implant, and graft
996.74 Other complications due to other vascular device, implant, and graft
997.79 Vascular complications of other vessels — (Use additional code to identify complications)
998.2 Accidental puncture or laceration during procedure

ICD-9-CM Procedural
39.22 Aorta-subclavian-carotid bypass

35531
35531 Bypass graft, with vein; aortoceliac or aortomesenteric

ICD-9-CM Diagnostic
440.0 Atherosclerosis of aorta
440.8 Atherosclerosis of other specified arteries
441.3 Abdominal aneurysm, ruptured
441.4 Abdominal aneurysm without mention of rupture
441.9 Aortic aneurysm of unspecified site without mention of rupture ▽
442.84 Aneurysm of other visceral artery
443.29 Dissection of other artery
444.89 Embolism and thrombosis of other specified artery
445.89 Atheroembolism of other site
446.0 Polyarteritis nodosa
447.1 Stricture of artery
447.4 Celiac artery compression syndrome
447.5 Necrosis of artery
447.6 Unspecified arteritis ▽
447.9 Unspecified disorders of arteries and arterioles ▽
459.9 Unspecified circulatory system disorder ▽
557.0 Acute vascular insufficiency of intestine
557.1 Chronic vascular insufficiency of intestine
593.81 Vascular disorders of kidney
902.0 Abdominal aorta injury
902.20 Unspecified celiac and mesenteric artery injury ▽
908.4 Late effect of injury to blood vessel of thorax, abdomen, and pelvis
996.1 Mechanical complication of other vascular device, implant, and graft
996.74 Other complications due to other vascular device, implant, and graft
997.71 Vascular complications of mesenteric artery — (Use additional code to identify complications)
997.79 Vascular complications of other vessels — (Use additional code to identify complications)
998.2 Accidental puncture or laceration during procedure

ICD-9-CM Procedural
39.24 Aorta-renal bypass

39.26 Other intra-abdominal vascular shunt or bypass

35533

35533 Bypass graft, with vein; axillary-femoral-femoral

ICD-9-CM Diagnostic

250.70 Diabetes with peripheral circulatory disorders, type II or unspecified type, not stated as uncontrolled — (Use additional code to identify manifestation: 443.81, 785.4)
250.71 Diabetes with peripheral circulatory disorders, type I [juvenile type], not stated as uncontrolled — (Use additional code to identify manifestation: 443.81, 785.4)
440.0 Atherosclerosis of aorta
440.20 Atherosclerosis of native arteries of the extremities, unspecified ▽
440.21 Atherosclerosis of native arteries of the extremities with intermittent claudication
440.22 Atherosclerosis of native arteries of the extremities with rest pain
440.23 Atherosclerosis of native arteries of the extremities with ulceration — (Use additional code for any associated ulceration: 707.10-707.9)
440.8 Atherosclerosis of other specified arteries
441.00 Dissecting aortic aneurysm (any part), unspecified site ▽
441.02 Dissecting aortic aneurysm (any part), abdominal
441.03 Dissecting aortic aneurysm (any part), thoracoabdominal
441.3 Abdominal aneurysm, ruptured
441.4 Abdominal aneurysm without mention of rupture
441.5 Aortic aneurysm of unspecified site, ruptured ▽
441.6 Thoracoabdominal aneurysm, ruptured
441.7 Thoracoabdominal aneurysm without mention of rupture
441.9 Aortic aneurysm of unspecified site without mention of rupture ▽
442.2 Aneurysm of iliac artery
442.3 Aneurysm of artery of lower extremity
443.22 Dissection of iliac artery
443.29 Dissection of other artery
443.81 Peripheral angiopathy in diseases classified elsewhere — (Code first underlying disease, 250.7) ☒
443.9 Unspecified peripheral vascular disease ▽
444.0 Embolism and thrombosis of abdominal aorta
444.22 Embolism and thrombosis of arteries of lower extremity
444.81 Embolism and thrombosis of iliac artery
445.02 Atheroembolism of lower extremity
447.1 Stricture of artery
447.5 Necrosis of artery
447.9 Unspecified disorders of arteries and arterioles ▽
747.22 Congenital atresia and stenosis of aorta
747.64 Congenital lower limb vessel anomaly
747.69 Congenital anomaly of other specified site of peripheral vascular system
785.4 Gangrene — (Code first any associated underlying condition:250.7, 443.0)
785.9 Other symptoms involving cardiovascular system
902.0 Abdominal aorta injury
902.53 Iliac artery injury
904.0 Common femoral artery injury
904.1 Superficial femoral artery injury
906.0 Late effect of open wound of head, neck, and trunk
908.4 Late effect of injury to blood vessel of thorax, abdomen, and pelvis
996.1 Mechanical complication of other vascular device, implant, and graft
996.74 Other complications due to other vascular device, implant, and graft
998.2 Accidental puncture or laceration during procedure

ICD-9-CM Procedural

39.29 Other (peripheral) vascular shunt or bypass

35536

35536 Bypass graft, with vein; splenorenal

ICD-9-CM Diagnostic

405.11 Secondary renovascular hypertension, benign
405.91 Secondary renovascular hypertension, unspecified ▽
440.1 Atherosclerosis of renal artery
440.8 Atherosclerosis of other specified arteries
441.4 Abdominal aneurysm without mention of rupture
442.1 Aneurysm of renal artery
442.83 Aneurysm of splenic artery
443.23 Dissection of renal artery
443.29 Dissection of other artery
443.9 Unspecified peripheral vascular disease ▽
445.81 Atheroembolism of kidney — (Use additional code for any associated kidney failure: 584, 585)
447.1 Stricture of artery
447.3 Hyperplasia of renal artery
447.5 Necrosis of artery
447.9 Unspecified disorders of arteries and arterioles ▽
584.9 Unspecified acute renal failure ▽
593.81 Vascular disorders of kidney
747.62 Congenital renal vessel anomaly
747.69 Congenital anomaly of other specified site of peripheral vascular system
902.23 Splenic artery injury
902.40 Renal vessel(s) injury, unspecified ▽
902.41 Renal artery injury
996.1 Mechanical complication of other vascular device, implant, and graft
996.74 Other complications due to other vascular device, implant, and graft
997.72 Vascular complications of renal artery — (Use additional code to identify complications)

ICD-9-CM Procedural

39.26 Other intra-abdominal vascular shunt or bypass

35541

35541 Bypass graft, with vein; aortoiliac or bi-iliac

ICD-9-CM Diagnostic

440.0 Atherosclerosis of aorta
440.8 Atherosclerosis of other specified arteries
441.00 Dissecting aortic aneurysm (any part), unspecified site ▽
441.02 Dissecting aortic aneurysm (any part), abdominal
441.3 Abdominal aneurysm, ruptured
441.4 Abdominal aneurysm without mention of rupture
441.5 Aortic aneurysm of unspecified site, ruptured ▽
441.9 Aortic aneurysm of unspecified site without mention of rupture ▽
442.2 Aneurysm of iliac artery
443.22 Dissection of iliac artery
443.9 Unspecified peripheral vascular disease ▽
444.0 Embolism and thrombosis of abdominal aorta
444.81 Embolism and thrombosis of iliac artery
445.89 Atheroembolism of other site
447.1 Stricture of artery
447.5 Necrosis of artery
447.9 Unspecified disorders of arteries and arterioles ▽
747.22 Congenital atresia and stenosis of aorta
785.9 Other symptoms involving cardiovascular system
902.0 Abdominal aorta injury
902.53 Iliac artery injury
908.4 Late effect of injury to blood vessel of thorax, abdomen, and pelvis
996.1 Mechanical complication of other vascular device, implant, and graft
996.74 Other complications due to other vascular device, implant, and graft
997.79 Vascular complications of other vessels — (Use additional code to identify complications)
998.2 Accidental puncture or laceration during procedure

ICD-9-CM Procedural

39.25 Aorta-iliac-femoral bypass

35546

35546 Bypass graft, with vein; aortofemoral or bifemoral

ICD-9-CM Diagnostic

250.70 Diabetes with peripheral circulatory disorders, type II or unspecified type, not stated as uncontrolled — (Use additional code to identify manifestation: 443.81, 785.4)
250.71 Diabetes with peripheral circulatory disorders, type I [juvenile type], not stated as uncontrolled — (Use additional code to identify manifestation: 443.81, 785.4)
250.72 Diabetes with peripheral circulatory disorders, type II or unspecified type, uncontrolled — (Use additional code to identify manifestation: 443.81, 785.4)
250.73 Diabetes with peripheral circulatory disorders, type I [juvenile type], uncontrolled — (Use additional code to identify manifestation: 443.81, 785.4)
440.0 Atherosclerosis of aorta
440.20 Atherosclerosis of native arteries of the extremities, unspecified ▽
440.21 Atherosclerosis of native arteries of the extremities with intermittent claudication
440.22 Atherosclerosis of native arteries of the extremities with rest pain

440.23 Atherosclerosis of native arteries of the extremities with ulceration — (Use additional code for any associated ulceration: 707.10-707.9)
440.8 Atherosclerosis of other specified arteries
440.9 Generalized and unspecified atherosclerosis ▽
441.00 Dissecting aortic aneurysm (any part), unspecified site ▽
441.02 Dissecting aortic aneurysm (any part), abdominal
441.3 Abdominal aneurysm, ruptured
441.4 Abdominal aneurysm without mention of rupture
441.5 Aortic aneurysm of unspecified site, ruptured ▽
441.6 Thoracoabdominal aneurysm, ruptured
441.9 Aortic aneurysm of unspecified site without mention of rupture ▽
442.2 Aneurysm of iliac artery
443.22 Dissection of iliac artery
443.29 Dissection of other artery
443.81 Peripheral angiopathy in diseases classified elsewhere — (Code first underlying disease, 250.7) ☒
443.9 Unspecified peripheral vascular disease ▽
444.0 Embolism and thrombosis of abdominal aorta
444.22 Embolism and thrombosis of arteries of lower extremity
444.81 Embolism and thrombosis of iliac artery
445.02 Atheroembolism of lower extremity
447.1 Stricture of artery
447.5 Necrosis of artery
447.9 Unspecified disorders of arteries and arterioles ▽
707.10 Ulcer of lower limb, unspecified ▽
707.11 Ulcer of thigh
707.12 Ulcer of calf
707.13 Ulcer of ankle
707.14 Ulcer of heel and midfoot
707.15 Ulcer of other part of foot
707.19 Ulcer of other part of lower limb
747.22 Congenital atresia and stenosis of aorta
747.64 Congenital lower limb vessel anomaly
747.69 Congenital anomaly of other specified site of peripheral vascular system
785.4 Gangrene — (Code first any associated underlying condition:250.7, 443.0)
785.9 Other symptoms involving cardiovascular system
902.0 Abdominal aorta injury
904.0 Common femoral artery injury
904.1 Superficial femoral artery injury
908.3 Late effect of injury to blood vessel of head, neck, and extremities
908.4 Late effect of injury to blood vessel of thorax, abdomen, and pelvis
928.10 Crushing injury of lower leg — (Use additional code to identify any associated injuries: 800-829, 850.0-854.1, 860.0-869.1)
928.8 Crushing injury of multiple sites of lower limb — (Use additional code to identify any associated injuries: 800-829, 850.0-854.1, 860.0-869.1)
996.1 Mechanical complication of other vascular device, implant, and graft
996.74 Other complications due to other vascular device, implant, and graft
997.79 Vascular complications of other vessels — (Use additional code to identify complications)
998.2 Accidental puncture or laceration during procedure

ICD-9-CM Procedural

39.25 Aorta-iliac-femoral bypass

35548–35549

35548 Bypass graft, with vein; aortoiliofemoral, unilateral
35549 aortoiliofemoral, bilateral

ICD-9-CM Diagnostic

250.70 Diabetes with peripheral circulatory disorders, type II or unspecified type, not stated as uncontrolled — (Use additional code to identify manifestation: 443.81, 785.4)
250.71 Diabetes with peripheral circulatory disorders, type I [juvenile type], not stated as uncontrolled — (Use additional code to identify manifestation: 443.81, 785.4)
250.72 Diabetes with peripheral circulatory disorders, type II or unspecified type, uncontrolled — (Use additional code to identify manifestation: 443.81, 785.4)
250.73 Diabetes with peripheral circulatory disorders, type I [juvenile type], uncontrolled — (Use additional code to identify manifestation: 443.81, 785.4)
440.0 Atherosclerosis of aorta
440.20 Atherosclerosis of native arteries of the extremities, unspecified ▽
440.21 Atherosclerosis of native arteries of the extremities with intermittent claudication
440.22 Atherosclerosis of native arteries of the extremities with rest pain
440.23 Atherosclerosis of native arteries of the extremities with ulceration — (Use additional code for any associated ulceration: 707.10-707.9)
440.9 Generalized and unspecified atherosclerosis ▽
441.00 Dissecting aortic aneurysm (any part), unspecified site ▽
441.02 Dissecting aortic aneurysm (any part), abdominal
441.3 Abdominal aneurysm, ruptured
441.4 Abdominal aneurysm without mention of rupture
441.5 Aortic aneurysm of unspecified site, ruptured ▽
441.6 Thoracoabdominal aneurysm, ruptured
441.9 Aortic aneurysm of unspecified site without mention of rupture ▽
442.2 Aneurysm of iliac artery
443.22 Dissection of iliac artery
443.29 Dissection of other artery
443.81 Peripheral angiopathy in diseases classified elsewhere — (Code first underlying disease, 250.7) ☒
443.9 Unspecified peripheral vascular disease ▽
444.0 Embolism and thrombosis of abdominal aorta
444.22 Embolism and thrombosis of arteries of lower extremity
444.81 Embolism and thrombosis of iliac artery
445.02 Atheroembolism of lower extremity
447.1 Stricture of artery
447.5 Necrosis of artery
447.9 Unspecified disorders of arteries and arterioles ▽
707.10 Ulcer of lower limb, unspecified ▽
707.11 Ulcer of thigh
707.12 Ulcer of calf
707.13 Ulcer of ankle
707.14 Ulcer of heel and midfoot
707.15 Ulcer of other part of foot
707.19 Ulcer of other part of lower limb
747.22 Congenital atresia and stenosis of aorta
747.64 Congenital lower limb vessel anomaly
747.69 Congenital anomaly of other specified site of peripheral vascular system
785.4 Gangrene — (Code first any associated underlying condition:250.7, 443.0)
785.9 Other symptoms involving cardiovascular system
902.0 Abdominal aorta injury
904.0 Common femoral artery injury
904.1 Superficial femoral artery injury
908.3 Late effect of injury to blood vessel of head, neck, and extremities
908.4 Late effect of injury to blood vessel of thorax, abdomen, and pelvis
928.10 Crushing injury of lower leg — (Use additional code to identify any associated injuries: 800-829, 850.0-854.1, 860.0-869.1)
928.8 Crushing injury of multiple sites of lower limb — (Use additional code to identify any associated injuries: 800-829, 850.0-854.1, 860.0-869.1)
996.1 Mechanical complication of other vascular device, implant, and graft
997.79 Vascular complications of other vessels — (Use additional code to identify complications)
998.2 Accidental puncture or laceration during procedure

ICD-9-CM Procedural

39.25 Aorta-iliac-femoral bypass

35551

35551 Bypass graft, with vein; aortofemoral-popliteal

ICD-9-CM Diagnostic

250.70 Diabetes with peripheral circulatory disorders, type II or unspecified type, not stated as uncontrolled — (Use additional code to identify manifestation: 443.81, 785.4)
250.71 Diabetes with peripheral circulatory disorders, type I [juvenile type], not stated as uncontrolled — (Use additional code to identify manifestation: 443.81, 785.4)
250.72 Diabetes with peripheral circulatory disorders, type II or unspecified type, uncontrolled — (Use additional code to identify manifestation: 443.81, 785.4)
250.73 Diabetes with peripheral circulatory disorders, type I [juvenile type], uncontrolled — (Use additional code to identify manifestation: 443.81, 785.4)
440.0 Atherosclerosis of aorta
440.20 Atherosclerosis of native arteries of the extremities, unspecified ▽
440.21 Atherosclerosis of native arteries of the extremities with intermittent claudication
440.22 Atherosclerosis of native arteries of the extremities with rest pain
440.23 Atherosclerosis of native arteries of the extremities with ulceration — (Use additional code for any associated ulceration: 707.10-707.9)
440.24 Atherosclerosis of native arteries of the extremities with gangrene
440.8 Atherosclerosis of other specified arteries
440.9 Generalized and unspecified atherosclerosis ▽
441.00 Dissecting aortic aneurysm (any part), unspecified site ▽
441.02 Dissecting aortic aneurysm (any part), abdominal

441.3 Abdominal aneurysm, ruptured
441.4 Abdominal aneurysm without mention of rupture
441.5 Aortic aneurysm of unspecified site, ruptured ▽
441.6 Thoracoabdominal aneurysm, ruptured
441.9 Aortic aneurysm of unspecified site without mention of rupture ▽
442.2 Aneurysm of iliac artery
442.3 Aneurysm of artery of lower extremity
443.22 Dissection of iliac artery
443.29 Dissection of other artery
443.81 Peripheral angiopathy in diseases classified elsewhere — (Code first underlying disease, 250.7) ☒
443.9 Unspecified peripheral vascular disease ▽
444.0 Embolism and thrombosis of abdominal aorta
444.22 Embolism and thrombosis of arteries of lower extremity
444.81 Embolism and thrombosis of iliac artery
445.02 Atheroembolism of lower extremity
447.1 Stricture of artery
447.5 Necrosis of artery
447.9 Unspecified disorders of arteries and arterioles ▽
707.10 Ulcer of lower limb, unspecified ▽
707.11 Ulcer of thigh
707.12 Ulcer of calf
707.13 Ulcer of ankle
707.14 Ulcer of heel and midfoot
707.15 Ulcer of other part of foot
707.19 Ulcer of other part of lower limb
747.22 Congenital atresia and stenosis of aorta
747.64 Congenital lower limb vessel anomaly
747.69 Congenital anomaly of other specified site of peripheral vascular system
785.4 Gangrene — (Code first any associated underlying condition:250.7, 443.0)
785.9 Other symptoms involving cardiovascular system
902.0 Abdominal aorta injury
904.0 Common femoral artery injury
904.1 Superficial femoral artery injury
908.3 Late effect of injury to blood vessel of head, neck, and extremities
908.4 Late effect of injury to blood vessel of thorax, abdomen, and pelvis
928.10 Crushing injury of lower leg — (Use additional code to identify any associated injuries: 800-829, 850.0-854.1, 860.0-869.1)
928.8 Crushing injury of multiple sites of lower limb — (Use additional code to identify any associated injuries: 800-829, 850.0-854.1, 860.0-869.1)
996.1 Mechanical complication of other vascular device, implant, and graft
996.74 Other complications due to other vascular device, implant, and graft
997.79 Vascular complications of other vessels — (Use additional code to identify complications)

ICD-9-CM Procedural

39.25 Aorta-iliac-femoral bypass
39.29 Other (peripheral) vascular shunt or bypass

35556

35556 Bypass graft, with vein; femoral-popliteal

ICD-9-CM Diagnostic

250.70 Diabetes with peripheral circulatory disorders, type II or unspecified type, not stated as uncontrolled — (Use additional code to identify manifestation: 443.81, 785.4)
250.71 Diabetes with peripheral circulatory disorders, type I [juvenile type], not stated as uncontrolled — (Use additional code to identify manifestation: 443.81, 785.4)
250.72 Diabetes with peripheral circulatory disorders, type II or unspecified type, uncontrolled — (Use additional code to identify manifestation: 443.81, 785.4)
250.73 Diabetes with peripheral circulatory disorders, type I [juvenile type], uncontrolled — (Use additional code to identify manifestation: 443.81, 785.4)
440.20 Atherosclerosis of native arteries of the extremities, unspecified ▽
440.21 Atherosclerosis of native arteries of the extremities with intermittent claudication
440.22 Atherosclerosis of native arteries of the extremities with rest pain
440.23 Atherosclerosis of native arteries of the extremities with ulceration — (Use additional code for any associated ulceration: 707.10-707.9)
440.24 Atherosclerosis of native arteries of the extremities with gangrene
440.29 Other atherosclerosis of native arteries of the extremities
440.30 Atheroslerosis of unspecified bypass graft of extremities ▽
440.31 Atheroslerosis of autologous vein bypass graft of extremities
440.32 Atheroslerosis of nonautologous biological bypass graft of extremities
440.8 Atherosclerosis of other specified arteries
440.9 Generalized and unspecified atherosclerosis ▽
442.3 Aneurysm of artery of lower extremity
442.9 Other aneurysm of unspecified site ▽
443.0 Raynaud's syndrome — (Use additional code to identify gangrene, 785.4)
443.29 Dissection of other artery
443.81 Peripheral angiopathy in diseases classified elsewhere — (Code first underlying disease, 250.7) ☒
443.89 Other peripheral vascular disease
443.9 Unspecified peripheral vascular disease ▽
444.22 Embolism and thrombosis of arteries of lower extremity
445.02 Atheroembolism of lower extremity
447.1 Stricture of artery
447.5 Necrosis of artery
459.9 Unspecified circulatory system disorder ▽
707.10 Ulcer of lower limb, unspecified ▽
707.11 Ulcer of thigh
707.12 Ulcer of calf
707.13 Ulcer of ankle
707.14 Ulcer of heel and midfoot
707.15 Ulcer of other part of foot
707.19 Ulcer of other part of lower limb
747.64 Congenital lower limb vessel anomaly
747.69 Congenital anomaly of other specified site of peripheral vascular system
785.4 Gangrene — (Code first any associated underlying condition:250.7, 443.0)
785.9 Other symptoms involving cardiovascular system
904.1 Superficial femoral artery injury
908.3 Late effect of injury to blood vessel of head, neck, and extremities
928.10 Crushing injury of lower leg — (Use additional code to identify any associated injuries: 800-829, 850.0-854.1, 860.0-869.1)
928.8 Crushing injury of multiple sites of lower limb — (Use additional code to identify any associated injuries: 800-829, 850.0-854.1, 860.0-869.1)
996.1 Mechanical complication of other vascular device, implant, and graft
996.74 Other complications due to other vascular device, implant, and graft

ICD-9-CM Procedural

39.29 Other (peripheral) vascular shunt or bypass

35558

35558 Bypass graft, with vein; femoral-femoral

ICD-9-CM Diagnostic

250.70 Diabetes with peripheral circulatory disorders, type II or unspecified type, not stated as uncontrolled — (Use additional code to identify manifestation: 443.81, 785.4)
250.71 Diabetes with peripheral circulatory disorders, type I [juvenile type], not stated as uncontrolled — (Use additional code to identify manifestation: 443.81, 785.4)
250.72 Diabetes with peripheral circulatory disorders, type II or unspecified type, uncontrolled — (Use additional code to identify manifestation: 443.81, 785.4)
250.73 Diabetes with peripheral circulatory disorders, type I [juvenile type], uncontrolled — (Use additional code to identify manifestation: 443.81, 785.4)
440.20 Atherosclerosis of native arteries of the extremities, unspecified ▽
440.21 Atherosclerosis of native arteries of the extremities with intermittent claudication
440.22 Atherosclerosis of native arteries of the extremities with rest pain
440.23 Atherosclerosis of native arteries of the extremities with ulceration — (Use additional code for any associated ulceration: 707.10-707.9)
440.24 Atherosclerosis of native arteries of the extremities with gangrene
442.3 Aneurysm of artery of lower extremity
443.29 Dissection of other artery
443.81 Peripheral angiopathy in diseases classified elsewhere — (Code first underlying disease, 250.7) ☒
443.9 Unspecified peripheral vascular disease ▽
447.1 Stricture of artery
447.5 Necrosis of artery
459.9 Unspecified circulatory system disorder ▽
707.10 Ulcer of lower limb, unspecified ▽
707.11 Ulcer of thigh
707.12 Ulcer of calf
707.13 Ulcer of ankle
707.14 Ulcer of heel and midfoot
707.15 Ulcer of other part of foot
707.19 Ulcer of other part of lower limb
747.64 Congenital lower limb vessel anomaly
747.69 Congenital anomaly of other specified site of peripheral vascular system
785.4 Gangrene — (Code first any associated underlying condition:250.7, 443.0)
904.0 Common femoral artery injury

904.1 Superficial femoral artery injury
908.3 Late effect of injury to blood vessel of head, neck, and extremities
996.1 Mechanical complication of other vascular device, implant, and graft
996.74 Other complications due to other vascular device, implant, and graft

ICD-9-CM Procedural

39.29 Other (peripheral) vascular shunt or bypass

35560

35560 Bypass graft, with vein; aortorenal

ICD-9-CM Diagnostic

405.11 Secondary renovascular hypertension, benign
405.91 Secondary renovascular hypertension, unspecified ▽
440.0 Atherosclerosis of aorta
440.1 Atherosclerosis of renal artery
441.00 Dissecting aortic aneurysm (any part), unspecified site ▽
441.02 Dissecting aortic aneurysm (any part), abdominal
441.3 Abdominal aneurysm, ruptured
441.4 Abdominal aneurysm without mention of rupture
441.9 Aortic aneurysm of unspecified site without mention of rupture ▽
442.1 Aneurysm of renal artery
443.23 Dissection of renal artery
444.0 Embolism and thrombosis of abdominal aorta
445.81 Atheroembolism of kidney — (Use additional code for any associated kidney failure: 584, 585)
447.1 Stricture of artery
447.3 Hyperplasia of renal artery
447.5 Necrosis of artery
447.9 Unspecified disorders of arteries and arterioles ▽
584.9 Unspecified acute renal failure ▽
593.81 Vascular disorders of kidney
902.0 Abdominal aorta injury
902.40 Renal vessel(s) injury, unspecified ▽
902.41 Renal artery injury
996.1 Mechanical complication of other vascular device, implant, and graft
996.74 Other complications due to other vascular device, implant, and graft
997.72 Vascular complications of renal artery — (Use additional code to identify complications)
998.2 Accidental puncture or laceration during procedure

ICD-9-CM Procedural

39.24 Aorta-renal bypass

35563

35563 Bypass graft, with vein; ilioiliac

ICD-9-CM Diagnostic

440.8 Atherosclerosis of other specified arteries
442.2 Aneurysm of iliac artery
443.22 Dissection of iliac artery
443.9 Unspecified peripheral vascular disease ▽
444.81 Embolism and thrombosis of iliac artery
445.89 Atheroembolism of other site
447.1 Stricture of artery
447.5 Necrosis of artery
902.53 Iliac artery injury
996.1 Mechanical complication of other vascular device, implant, and graft
996.74 Other complications due to other vascular device, implant, and graft
997.79 Vascular complications of other vessels — (Use additional code to identify complications)

ICD-9-CM Procedural

39.26 Other intra-abdominal vascular shunt or bypass

35565

35565 Bypass graft, with vein; iliofemoral

ICD-9-CM Diagnostic

250.70 Diabetes with peripheral circulatory disorders, type II or unspecified type, not stated as uncontrolled — (Use additional code to identify manifestation: 443.81, 785.4)
250.71 Diabetes with peripheral circulatory disorders, type I [juvenile type], not stated as uncontrolled — (Use additional code to identify manifestation: 443.81, 785.4)
250.72 Diabetes with peripheral circulatory disorders, type II or unspecified type, uncontrolled — (Use additional code to identify manifestation: 443.81, 785.4)
250.73 Diabetes with peripheral circulatory disorders, type I [juvenile type], uncontrolled — (Use additional code to identify manifestation: 443.81, 785.4)
440.21 Atherosclerosis of native arteries of the extremities with intermittent claudication
440.22 Atherosclerosis of native arteries of the extremities with rest pain
440.23 Atherosclerosis of native arteries of the extremities with ulceration — (Use additional code for any associated ulceration: 707.10-707.9)
440.24 Atherosclerosis of native arteries of the extremities with gangrene
440.8 Atherosclerosis of other specified arteries
440.9 Generalized and unspecified atherosclerosis ▽
442.2 Aneurysm of iliac artery
442.3 Aneurysm of artery of lower extremity
443.22 Dissection of iliac artery
443.81 Peripheral angiopathy in diseases classified elsewhere — (Code first underlying disease, 250.7) ☒
443.89 Other peripheral vascular disease
443.9 Unspecified peripheral vascular disease ▽
444.22 Embolism and thrombosis of arteries of lower extremity
444.81 Embolism and thrombosis of iliac artery
445.02 Atheroembolism of lower extremity
447.1 Stricture of artery
447.5 Necrosis of artery
459.9 Unspecified circulatory system disorder ▽
707.10 Ulcer of lower limb, unspecified ▽
707.11 Ulcer of thigh
707.12 Ulcer of calf
707.13 Ulcer of ankle
707.14 Ulcer of heel and midfoot
707.15 Ulcer of other part of foot
707.19 Ulcer of other part of lower limb
747.64 Congenital lower limb vessel anomaly
747.69 Congenital anomaly of other specified site of peripheral vascular system
785.4 Gangrene — (Code first any associated underlying condition:250.7, 443.0)
785.9 Other symptoms involving cardiovascular system
894.1 Multiple and unspecified open wound of lower limb, complicated — (Use additional code to identify infection)
902.53 Iliac artery injury
904.7 Injury to specified blood vessels of lower extremity, other
908.3 Late effect of injury to blood vessel of head, neck, and extremities
928.00 Crushing injury of thigh — (Use additional code to identify any associated injuries: 800-829, 850.0-854.1, 860.0-869.1)
996.74 Other complications due to other vascular device, implant, and graft
997.79 Vascular complications of other vessels — (Use additional code to identify complications)

ICD-9-CM Procedural

39.25 Aorta-iliac-femoral bypass

35566

35566 Bypass graft, with vein; femoral-anterior tibial, posterior tibial, peroneal artery or other distal vessels

ICD-9-CM Diagnostic

250.70 Diabetes with peripheral circulatory disorders, type II or unspecified type, not stated as uncontrolled — (Use additional code to identify manifestation: 443.81, 785.4)
250.71 Diabetes with peripheral circulatory disorders, type I [juvenile type], not stated as uncontrolled — (Use additional code to identify manifestation: 443.81, 785.4)
250.72 Diabetes with peripheral circulatory disorders, type II or unspecified type, uncontrolled — (Use additional code to identify manifestation: 443.81, 785.4)
250.73 Diabetes with peripheral circulatory disorders, type I [juvenile type], uncontrolled — (Use additional code to identify manifestation: 443.81, 785.4)
440.21 Atherosclerosis of native arteries of the extremities with intermittent claudication
440.22 Atherosclerosis of native arteries of the extremities with rest pain
440.23 Atherosclerosis of native arteries of the extremities with ulceration — (Use additional code for any associated ulceration: 707.10-707.9)
440.24 Atherosclerosis of native arteries of the extremities with gangrene
440.29 Other atherosclerosis of native arteries of the extremities
440.8 Atherosclerosis of other specified arteries
440.9 Generalized and unspecified atherosclerosis ▽
442.3 Aneurysm of artery of lower extremity
443.29 Dissection of other artery

443.9 Unspecified peripheral vascular disease ▽
447.1 Stricture of artery
459.89 Other specified circulatory system disorders
459.9 Unspecified circulatory system disorder ▽
707.10 Ulcer of lower limb, unspecified ▽
707.11 Ulcer of thigh
707.12 Ulcer of calf
707.13 Ulcer of ankle
707.14 Ulcer of heel and midfoot
707.15 Ulcer of other part of foot
707.19 Ulcer of other part of lower limb
747.64 Congenital lower limb vessel anomaly
785.4 Gangrene — (Code first any associated underlying condition:250.7, 443.0)
785.9 Other symptoms involving cardiovascular system
894.1 Multiple and unspecified open wound of lower limb, complicated — (Use additional code to identify infection)
904.0 Common femoral artery injury
904.1 Superficial femoral artery injury
904.41 Popliteal artery injury
904.42 Popliteal vein injury
904.51 Anterior tibial artery injury
904.52 Anterior tibial vein injury
904.53 Posterior tibial artery injury
904.54 Posterior tibial vein injury
904.7 Injury to specified blood vessels of lower extremity, other
908.3 Late effect of injury to blood vessel of head, neck, and extremities
928.10 Crushing injury of lower leg — (Use additional code to identify any associated injuries: 800-829, 850.0-854.1, 860.0-869.1)
928.8 Crushing injury of multiple sites of lower limb — (Use additional code to identify any associated injuries: 800-829, 850.0-854.1, 860.0-869.1)
996.1 Mechanical complication of other vascular device, implant, and graft
996.74 Other complications due to other vascular device, implant, and graft

ICD-9-CM Procedural

39.29 Other (peripheral) vascular shunt or bypass

35571

35571 Bypass graft, with vein; popliteal-tibial, -peroneal artery or other distal vessels

ICD-9-CM Diagnostic

250.70 Diabetes with peripheral circulatory disorders, type II or unspecified type, not stated as uncontrolled — (Use additional code to identify manifestation: 443.81, 785.4)
250.71 Diabetes with peripheral circulatory disorders, type I [juvenile type], not stated as uncontrolled — (Use additional code to identify manifestation: 443.81, 785.4)
250.72 Diabetes with peripheral circulatory disorders, type II or unspecified type, uncontrolled — (Use additional code to identify manifestation: 443.81, 785.4)
250.73 Diabetes with peripheral circulatory disorders, type I [juvenile type], uncontrolled — (Use additional code to identify manifestation: 443.81, 785.4)
440.20 Atherosclerosis of native arteries of the extremities, unspecified ▽
440.21 Atherosclerosis of native arteries of the extremities with intermittent claudication
440.22 Atherosclerosis of native arteries of the extremities with rest pain
440.23 Atherosclerosis of native arteries of the extremities with ulceration — (Use additional code for any associated ulceration: 707.10-707.9)
440.24 Atherosclerosis of native arteries of the extremities with gangrene
440.8 Atherosclerosis of other specified arteries
442.3 Aneurysm of artery of lower extremity
443.81 Peripheral angiopathy in diseases classified elsewhere — (Code first underlying disease, 250.7) ☒
443.9 Unspecified peripheral vascular disease ▽
444.22 Embolism and thrombosis of arteries of lower extremity
445.02 Atheroembolism of lower extremity
447.1 Stricture of artery
459.9 Unspecified circulatory system disorder ▽
707.10 Ulcer of lower limb, unspecified ▽
707.11 Ulcer of thigh
707.12 Ulcer of calf
707.13 Ulcer of ankle
707.14 Ulcer of heel and midfoot
707.15 Ulcer of other part of foot
707.19 Ulcer of other part of lower limb
747.64 Congenital lower limb vessel anomaly
785.4 Gangrene — (Code first any associated underlying condition:250.7, 443.0)
785.9 Other symptoms involving cardiovascular system
894.1 Multiple and unspecified open wound of lower limb, complicated — (Use additional code to identify infection)
904.41 Popliteal artery injury
904.51 Anterior tibial artery injury
904.53 Posterior tibial artery injury
904.7 Injury to specified blood vessels of lower extremity, other
908.3 Late effect of injury to blood vessel of head, neck, and extremities
928.10 Crushing injury of lower leg — (Use additional code to identify any associated injuries: 800-829, 850.0-854.1, 860.0-869.1)
928.8 Crushing injury of multiple sites of lower limb — (Use additional code to identify any associated injuries: 800-829, 850.0-854.1, 860.0-869.1)
996.1 Mechanical complication of other vascular device, implant, and graft
996.74 Other complications due to other vascular device, implant, and graft

ICD-9-CM Procedural

39.29 Other (peripheral) vascular shunt or bypass

35572

35572 Harvest of femoropopliteal vein, one segment, for vascular reconstruction procedure (eg, aortic, vena caval, coronary, peripheral artery) (List separately in addition to code for primary procedure)

ICD-9-CM Diagnostic

This is an add-on code. Refer to the corresponding primary procedure code for ICD-9 diagnosis code links.

ICD-9-CM Procedural

38.69 Other excision of lower limb veins

HCPCS Level II Supplies & Services

The HCPCS Level II code(s) would be the same as the actual procedure performed because these are in-addition-to codes.

35583

35583 In-situ vein bypass; femoral-popliteal

ICD-9-CM Diagnostic

250.70 Diabetes with peripheral circulatory disorders, type II or unspecified type, not stated as uncontrolled — (Use additional code to identify manifestation: 443.81, 785.4)
250.71 Diabetes with peripheral circulatory disorders, type I [juvenile type], not stated as uncontrolled — (Use additional code to identify manifestation: 443.81, 785.4)
250.72 Diabetes with peripheral circulatory disorders, type II or unspecified type, uncontrolled — (Use additional code to identify manifestation: 443.81, 785.4)
250.73 Diabetes with peripheral circulatory disorders, type I [juvenile type], uncontrolled — (Use additional code to identify manifestation: 443.81, 785.4)
440.21 Atherosclerosis of native arteries of the extremities with intermittent claudication
440.22 Atherosclerosis of native arteries of the extremities with rest pain
440.23 Atherosclerosis of native arteries of the extremities with ulceration — (Use additional code for any associated ulceration: 707.10-707.9)
442.3 Aneurysm of artery of lower extremity
443.0 Raynaud's syndrome — (Use additional code to identify gangrene, 785.4)
443.29 Dissection of other artery
443.81 Peripheral angiopathy in diseases classified elsewhere — (Code first underlying disease, 250.7) ☒
443.89 Other peripheral vascular disease
443.9 Unspecified peripheral vascular disease ▽
444.22 Embolism and thrombosis of arteries of lower extremity
445.02 Atheroembolism of lower extremity
447.1 Stricture of artery
447.5 Necrosis of artery
453.9 Embolism and thrombosis of unspecified site ▽
459.81 Unspecified venous (peripheral) insufficiency — (Use additional code for any associated ulceration: 707.10-707.9) ▽
459.9 Unspecified circulatory system disorder ▽
707.10 Ulcer of lower limb, unspecified ▽
707.11 Ulcer of thigh
707.12 Ulcer of calf
707.13 Ulcer of ankle
707.14 Ulcer of heel and midfoot
707.15 Ulcer of other part of foot
707.19 Ulcer of other part of lower limb
747.64 Congenital lower limb vessel anomaly
747.69 Congenital anomaly of other specified site of peripheral vascular system

785.4 Gangrene — (Code first any associated underlying condition:250.7, 443.0)
785.9 Other symptoms involving cardiovascular system
908.3 Late effect of injury to blood vessel of head, neck, and extremities
996.1 Mechanical complication of other vascular device, implant, and graft
996.74 Other complications due to other vascular device, implant, and graft

ICD-9-CM Procedural

39.29 Other (peripheral) vascular shunt or bypass

35585

35585 In-situ vein bypass; femoral-anterior tibial, posterior tibial, or peroneal artery

ICD-9-CM Diagnostic

250.70 Diabetes with peripheral circulatory disorders, type II or unspecified type, not stated as uncontrolled — (Use additional code to identify manifestation: 443.81, 785.4)
250.71 Diabetes with peripheral circulatory disorders, type I [juvenile type], not stated as uncontrolled — (Use additional code to identify manifestation: 443.81, 785.4)
250.72 Diabetes with peripheral circulatory disorders, type II or unspecified type, uncontrolled — (Use additional code to identify manifestation: 443.81, 785.4)
250.73 Diabetes with peripheral circulatory disorders, type I [juvenile type], uncontrolled — (Use additional code to identify manifestation: 443.81, 785.4)
440.21 Atherosclerosis of native arteries of the extremities with intermittent claudication
440.22 Atherosclerosis of native arteries of the extremities with rest pain
440.23 Atherosclerosis of native arteries of the extremities with ulceration — (Use additional code for any associated ulceration: 707.10-707.9)
440.24 Atherosclerosis of native arteries of the extremities with gangrene
442.3 Aneurysm of artery of lower extremity
443.81 Peripheral angiopathy in diseases classified elsewhere — (Code first underlying disease, 250.7) ☒
443.9 Unspecified peripheral vascular disease ▽
444.22 Embolism and thrombosis of arteries of lower extremity
445.02 Atheroembolism of lower extremity
447.1 Stricture of artery
447.2 Rupture of artery
447.5 Necrosis of artery
447.6 Unspecified arteritis ▽
459.81 Unspecified venous (peripheral) insufficiency — (Use additional code for any associated ulceration: 707.10-707.9) ▽
459.9 Unspecified circulatory system disorder ▽
707.10 Ulcer of lower limb, unspecified ▽
707.11 Ulcer of thigh
707.12 Ulcer of calf
707.13 Ulcer of ankle
707.14 Ulcer of heel and midfoot
707.15 Ulcer of other part of foot
707.19 Ulcer of other part of lower limb
747.64 Congenital lower limb vessel anomaly
785.4 Gangrene — (Code first any associated underlying condition:250.7, 443.0)
785.9 Other symptoms involving cardiovascular system
904.41 Popliteal artery injury
904.51 Anterior tibial artery injury
904.53 Posterior tibial artery injury
908.3 Late effect of injury to blood vessel of head, neck, and extremities
996.1 Mechanical complication of other vascular device, implant, and graft
996.74 Other complications due to other vascular device, implant, and graft

ICD-9-CM Procedural

39.29 Other (peripheral) vascular shunt or bypass

35587

35587 In-situ vein bypass; popliteal-tibial, peroneal

ICD-9-CM Diagnostic

250.70 Diabetes with peripheral circulatory disorders, type II or unspecified type, not stated as uncontrolled — (Use additional code to identify manifestation: 443.81, 785.4)
250.71 Diabetes with peripheral circulatory disorders, type I [juvenile type], not stated as uncontrolled — (Use additional code to identify manifestation: 443.81, 785.4)
250.72 Diabetes with peripheral circulatory disorders, type II or unspecified type, uncontrolled — (Use additional code to identify manifestation: 443.81, 785.4)
250.73 Diabetes with peripheral circulatory disorders, type I [juvenile type], uncontrolled — (Use additional code to identify manifestation: 443.81, 785.4)
440.21 Atherosclerosis of native arteries of the extremities with intermittent claudication
440.22 Atherosclerosis of native arteries of the extremities with rest pain
443.81 Peripheral angiopathy in diseases classified elsewhere — (Code first underlying disease, 250.7) ☒
444.22 Embolism and thrombosis of arteries of lower extremity
445.02 Atheroembolism of lower extremity
447.1 Stricture of artery
459.9 Unspecified circulatory system disorder ▽
707.10 Ulcer of lower limb, unspecified ▽
707.11 Ulcer of thigh
707.12 Ulcer of calf
707.13 Ulcer of ankle
707.14 Ulcer of heel and midfoot
707.15 Ulcer of other part of foot
707.19 Ulcer of other part of lower limb
747.64 Congenital lower limb vessel anomaly
785.4 Gangrene — (Code first any associated underlying condition:250.7, 443.0)
785.9 Other symptoms involving cardiovascular system
996.1 Mechanical complication of other vascular device, implant, and graft
996.74 Other complications due to other vascular device, implant, and graft

ICD-9-CM Procedural

39.29 Other (peripheral) vascular shunt or bypass

35600

35600 Harvest of upper extremity artery, one segment, for coronary artery bypass procedure

ICD-9-CM Diagnostic

410.00 Acute myocardial infarction of anterolateral wall, episode of care unspecified — (Use additional code to identify presence of hypertension: 401.0-405.9) ▽
410.01 Acute myocardial infarction of anterolateral wall, initial episode of care — (Use additional code to identify presence of hypertension: 401.0-405.9)
410.02 Acute myocardial infarction of anterolateral wall, subsequent episode of care — (Use additional code to identify presence of hypertension: 401.0-405.9)
410.10 Acute myocardial infarction of other anterior wall, episode of care unspecified — (Use additional code to identify presence of hypertension: 401.0-405.9) ▽
410.11 Acute myocardial infarction of other anterior wall, initial episode of care — (Use additional code to identify presence of hypertension: 401.0-405.9)
410.12 Acute myocardial infarction of other anterior wall, subsequent episode of care — (Use additional code to identify presence of hypertension: 401.0-405.9)
410.20 Acute myocardial infarction of inferolateral wall, episode of care unspecified — (Use additional code to identify presence of hypertension: 401.0-405.9) ▽
410.21 Acute myocardial infarction of inferolateral wall, initial episode of care — (Use additional code to identify presence of hypertension: 401.0-405.9)
410.22 Acute myocardial infarction of inferolateral wall, subsequent episode of care — (Use additional code to identify presence of hypertension: 401.0-405.9)
410.30 Acute myocardial infarction of inferoposterior wall, episode of care unspecified — (Use additional code to identify presence of hypertension: 401.0-405.9) ▽
410.31 Acute myocardial infarction of inferoposterior wall, initial episode of care — (Use additional code to identify presence of hypertension: 401.0-405.9)
410.32 Acute myocardial infarction of inferoposterior wall, subsequent episode of care — (Use additional code to identify presence of hypertension: 401.0-405.9)
410.40 Acute myocardial infarction of other inferior wall, episode of care unspecified — (Use additional code to identify presence of hypertension: 401.0-405.9) ▽
410.41 Acute myocardial infarction of other inferior wall, initial episode of care — (Use additional code to identify presence of hypertension: 401.0-405.9)
410.42 Acute myocardial infarction of other inferior wall, subsequent episode of care — (Use additional code to identify presence of hypertension: 401.0-405.9)
410.50 Acute myocardial infarction of other lateral wall, episode of care unspecified — (Use additional code to identify presence of hypertension: 401.0-405.9) ▽
410.51 Acute myocardial infarction of other lateral wall, initial episode of care — (Use additional code to identify presence of hypertension: 401.0-405.9)
410.52 Acute myocardial infarction of other lateral wall, subsequent episode of care — (Use additional code to identify presence of hypertension: 401.0-405.9)
410.60 Acute myocardial infarction, true posterior wall infarction, episode of care unspecified — (Use additional code to identify presence of hypertension: 401.0-405.9) ▽
410.61 Acute myocardial infarction, true posterior wall infarction, initial episode of care — (Use additional code to identify presence of hypertension: 401.0-405.9)
410.62 Acute myocardial infarction, true posterior wall infarction, subsequent episode of care — (Use additional code to identify presence of hypertension: 401.0-405.9)

410.70 Acute myocardial infarction, subendocardial infarction, episode of care unspecified — (Use additional code to identify presence of hypertension: 401.0-405.9) ▽
410.71 Acute myocardial infarction, subendocardial infarction, initial episode of care — (Use additional code to identify presence of hypertension: 401.0-405.9)
410.72 Acute myocardial infarction, subendocardial infarction, subsequent episode of care — (Use additional code to identify presence of hypertension: 401.0-405.9)
410.80 Acute myocardial infarction of other specified sites, episode of care unspecified — (Use additional code to identify presence of hypertension: 401.0-405.9) ▽
410.81 Acute myocardial infarction of other specified sites, initial episode of care — (Use additional code to identify presence of hypertension: 401.0-405.9)
410.82 Acute myocardial infarction of other specified sites, subsequent episode of care — (Use additional code to identify presence of hypertension: 401.0-405.9)
410.90 Acute myocardial infarction, unspecified site, episode of care unspecified — (Use additional code to identify presence of hypertension: 401.0-405.9) ▽
410.91 Acute myocardial infarction, unspecified site, initial episode of care — (Use additional code to identify presence of hypertension: 401.0-405.9) ▽
410.92 Acute myocardial infarction, unspecified site, subsequent episode of care — (Use additional code to identify presence of hypertension: 401.0-405.9) ▽
411.1 Intermediate coronary syndrome — (Use additional code to identify presence of hypertension: 401.0-405.9)
411.81 Acute coronary occlusion without myocardial infarction — (Use additional code to identify presence of hypertension: 401.0-405.9)
411.89 Other acute and subacute form of ischemic heart disease — (Use additional code to identify presence of hypertension: 401.0-405.9)
413.0 Angina decubitus — (Use additional code to identify presence of hypertension: 401.0-405.9)
413.1 Prinzmetal angina — (Use additional code to identify presence of hypertension: 401.0-405.9)
413.9 Other and unspecified angina pectoris — (Use additional code to identify presence of hypertension: 401.0-405.9) ▽
414.00 Coronary atherosclerosis of unspecified type of vessel, native or graft — (Use additional code to identify presence of hypertension: 401.0-405.9) ▽
414.01 Coronary atherosclerosis of native coronary artery — (Use additional code to identify presence of hypertension: 401.0-405.9)
414.03 Coronary atherosclerosis of nonautologous biological bypass graft — (Use additional code to identify presence of hypertension: 401.0-405.9)
414.04 Coronary atherosclerosis of artery bypass graft — (Use additional code to identify presence of hypertension: 401.0-405.9)
414.05 Coronary atherosclerosis of unspecified type of bypass graft — (Use additional code to identify presence of hypertension: 401.0-405.9) ▽
414.06 Coronary atherosclerosis, of native coronary artery of transplanted heart — (Use additional code to identify presence of hypertension: 401.0-405.9)
414.07 Coronary atherosclerosis, of bypass graft (artery) (vein) of transplanted heart — (Use additional code to identify presence of hypertension: 401.0-405.9)
414.10 Aneurysm of heart — (Use additional code to identify presence of hypertension: 401.0-405.9)
414.11 Aneurysm of coronary vessels — (Use additional code to identify presence of hypertension: 401.0-405.9)
414.12 Dissection of coronary artery — (Use additional code to identify presence of hypertension: 401.0-405.9)
414.8 Other specified forms of chronic ischemic heart disease — (Use additional code to identify presence of hypertension: 401.0-405.9)
414.9 Unspecified chronic ischemic heart disease — (Use additional code to identify presence of hypertension: 401.0-405.9) ▽
426.7 Anomalous atrioventricular excitation
428.0 Congestive heart failure, unspecified ▽
428.1 Left heart failure
428.20 Unspecified systolic heart failure ▽
428.21 Acute systolic heart failure
428.22 Chronic systolic heart failure
428.23 Acute on chronic systolic heart failure
428.30 Unspecified diastolic heart failure ▽
428.31 Acute diastolic heart failure
428.32 Chronic diastolic heart failure
428.33 Acute on chronic diastolic heart failure
428.40 Unspecified combined systolic and diastolic heart failure ▽
428.41 Acute combined systolic and diastolic heart failure
428.42 Chronic combined systolic and diastolic heart failure
428.43 Acute on chronic combined systolic and diastolic heart failure
428.9 Unspecified heart failure ▽
746.85 Congenital coronary artery anomaly
747.41 Total congenital anomalous pulmonary venous connection
996.03 Mechanical complication due to coronary bypass graft

ICD-9-CM Procedural

36.10 Aortocoronary bypass for heart revascularization, not otherwise specified
36.11 (Aorto)coronary bypass of one coronary artery
36.12 (Aorto)coronary bypass of two coronary arteries
36.13 (Aorto)coronary bypass of three coronary arteries
36.14 (Aorto)coronary bypass of four or more coronary arteries

35601

35601 Bypass graft, with other than vein; carotid

ICD-9-CM Diagnostic

433.10 Occlusion and stenosis of carotid artery without mention of cerebral infarction — (Use additional code to identify presence of hypertension)
433.11 Occlusion and stenosis of carotid artery with cerebral infarction — (Use additional code to identify presence of hypertension)
433.30 Occlusion and stenosis of multiple and bilateral precerebral arteries without mention of cerebral infarction — (Use additional code to identify presence of hypertension)
433.31 Occlusion and stenosis of multiple and bilateral precerebral arteries with cerebral infarction — (Use additional code to identify presence of hypertension)
433.80 Occlusion and stenosis of other specified precerebral artery without mention of cerebral infarction — (Use additional code to identify presence of hypertension)
433.81 Occlusion and stenosis of other specified precerebral artery with cerebral infarction — (Use additional code to identify presence of hypertension)
435.8 Other specified transient cerebral ischemias — (Use additional code to identify presence of hypertension)
440.8 Atherosclerosis of other specified arteries
442.81 Aneurysm of artery of neck
443.21 Dissection of carotid artery
447.1 Stricture of artery
747.81 Congenital anomaly of cerebrovascular system
780.2 Syncope and collapse
785.9 Other symptoms involving cardiovascular system
900.01 Common carotid artery injury
900.03 Internal carotid artery injury
906.0 Late effect of open wound of head, neck, and trunk
908.3 Late effect of injury to blood vessel of head, neck, and extremities
925.2 Crushing injury of neck — (Use additional code to identify any associated injuries: 800-829, 850.0-854.1, 860.0-869.1)
996.1 Mechanical complication of other vascular device, implant, and graft
996.74 Other complications due to other vascular device, implant, and graft

ICD-9-CM Procedural

39.22 Aorta-subclavian-carotid bypass

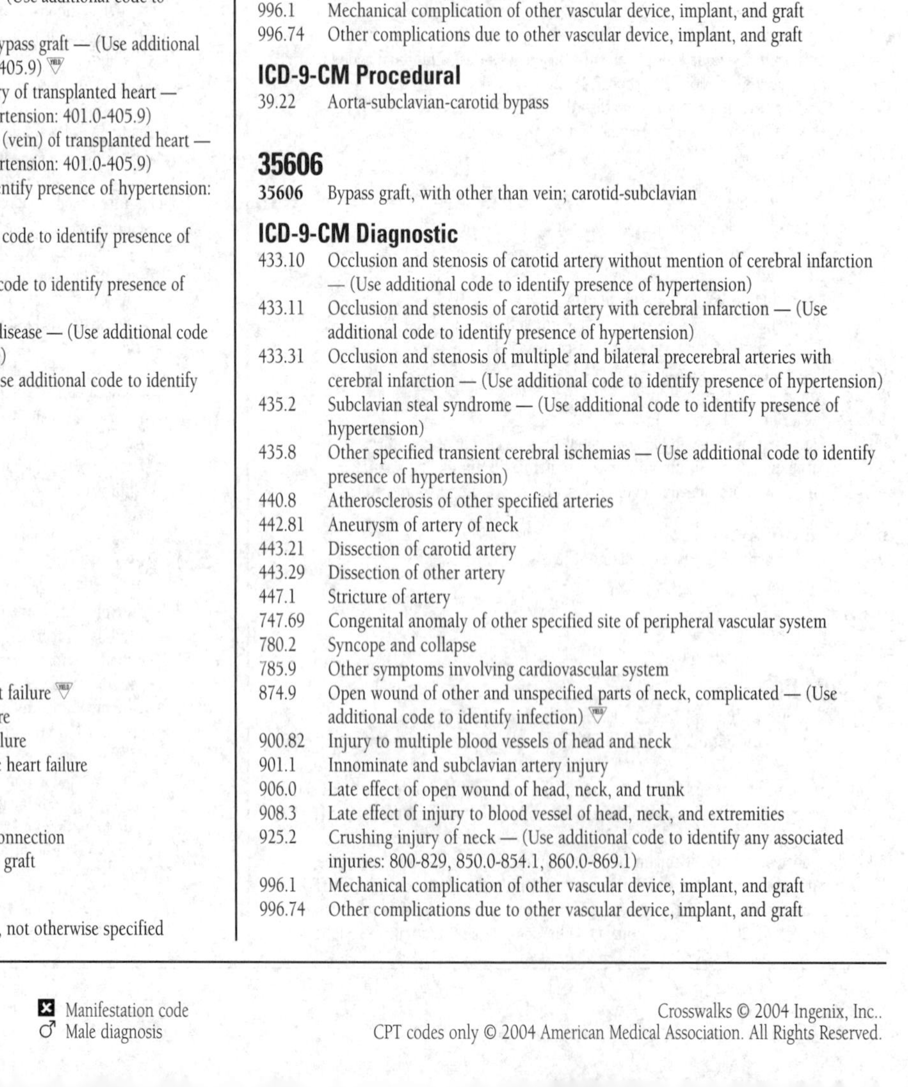

35606

35606 Bypass graft, with other than vein; carotid-subclavian

ICD-9-CM Diagnostic

433.10 Occlusion and stenosis of carotid artery without mention of cerebral infarction — (Use additional code to identify presence of hypertension)
433.11 Occlusion and stenosis of carotid artery with cerebral infarction — (Use additional code to identify presence of hypertension)
433.31 Occlusion and stenosis of multiple and bilateral precerebral arteries with cerebral infarction — (Use additional code to identify presence of hypertension)
435.2 Subclavian steal syndrome — (Use additional code to identify presence of hypertension)
435.8 Other specified transient cerebral ischemias — (Use additional code to identify presence of hypertension)
440.8 Atherosclerosis of other specified arteries
442.81 Aneurysm of artery of neck
443.21 Dissection of carotid artery
443.29 Dissection of other artery
447.1 Stricture of artery
747.69 Congenital anomaly of other specified site of peripheral vascular system
780.2 Syncope and collapse
785.9 Other symptoms involving cardiovascular system
874.9 Open wound of other and unspecified parts of neck, complicated — (Use additional code to identify infection) ▽
900.82 Injury to multiple blood vessels of head and neck
901.1 Innominate and subclavian artery injury
906.0 Late effect of open wound of head, neck, and trunk
908.3 Late effect of injury to blood vessel of head, neck, and extremities
925.2 Crushing injury of neck — (Use additional code to identify any associated injuries: 800-829, 850.0-854.1, 860.0-869.1)
996.1 Mechanical complication of other vascular device, implant, and graft
996.74 Other complications due to other vascular device, implant, and graft

▽ Unspecified code
♀ Female diagnosis
☒ Manifestation code
♂ Male diagnosis

ICD-9-CM Procedural

39.22 Aorta-subclavian-carotid bypass

35612

35612 Bypass graft, with other than vein; subclavian-subclavian

ICD-9-CM Diagnostic

435.2 Subclavian steal syndrome — (Use additional code to identify presence of hypertension)
435.8 Other specified transient cerebral ischemias — (Use additional code to identify presence of hypertension)
440.8 Atherosclerosis of other specified arteries
443.29 Dissection of other artery
447.1 Stricture of artery
447.6 Unspecified arteritis ▽
747.69 Congenital anomaly of other specified site of peripheral vascular system
785.9 Other symptoms involving cardiovascular system
874.9 Open wound of other and unspecified parts of neck, complicated — (Use additional code to identify infection) ▽
900.82 Injury to multiple blood vessels of head and neck
900.89 Injury to other specified blood vessels of head and neck
901.1 Innominate and subclavian artery injury
901.89 Injury to specified blood vessels of thorax, other
906.0 Late effect of open wound of head, neck, and trunk
906.4 Late effect of crushing
908.3 Late effect of injury to blood vessel of head, neck, and extremities
996.1 Mechanical complication of other vascular device, implant, and graft
996.74 Other complications due to other vascular device, implant, and graft

ICD-9-CM Procedural

39.22 Aorta-subclavian-carotid bypass

35616

35616 Bypass graft, with other than vein; subclavian-axillary

ICD-9-CM Diagnostic

435.2 Subclavian steal syndrome — (Use additional code to identify presence of hypertension)
435.8 Other specified transient cerebral ischemias — (Use additional code to identify presence of hypertension)
440.8 Atherosclerosis of other specified arteries
447.1 Stricture of artery
447.6 Unspecified arteritis ▽
747.69 Congenital anomaly of other specified site of peripheral vascular system
785.9 Other symptoms involving cardiovascular system
874.9 Open wound of other and unspecified parts of neck, complicated — (Use additional code to identify infection) ▽
900.82 Injury to multiple blood vessels of head and neck
901.1 Innominate and subclavian artery injury
906.0 Late effect of open wound of head, neck, and trunk
925.2 Crushing injury of neck — (Use additional code to identify any associated injuries: 800-829, 850.0-854.1, 860.0-869.1)
996.1 Mechanical complication of other vascular device, implant, and graft
996.74 Other complications due to other vascular device, implant, and graft
998.2 Accidental puncture or laceration during procedure

ICD-9-CM Procedural

38.53 Ligation and stripping of varicose veins of upper limb vessels
39.29 Other (peripheral) vascular shunt or bypass

35621

35621 Bypass graft, with other than vein; axillary-femoral

ICD-9-CM Diagnostic

440.0 Atherosclerosis of aorta
440.8 Atherosclerosis of other specified arteries
440.9 Generalized and unspecified atherosclerosis ▽
441.02 Dissecting aortic aneurysm (any part), abdominal
441.3 Abdominal aneurysm, ruptured
441.4 Abdominal aneurysm without mention of rupture
441.5 Aortic aneurysm of unspecified site, ruptured ▽
441.9 Aortic aneurysm of unspecified site without mention of rupture ▽
442.2 Aneurysm of iliac artery
442.3 Aneurysm of artery of lower extremity
443.22 Dissection of iliac artery
443.29 Dissection of other artery
443.9 Unspecified peripheral vascular disease ▽
444.0 Embolism and thrombosis of abdominal aorta
444.81 Embolism and thrombosis of iliac artery
445.02 Atheroembolism of lower extremity
447.1 Stricture of artery
447.5 Necrosis of artery
447.9 Unspecified disorders of arteries and arterioles ▽
747.22 Congenital atresia and stenosis of aorta
747.69 Congenital anomaly of other specified site of peripheral vascular system
785.4 Gangrene — (Code first any associated underlying condition:250.7, 443.0)
785.9 Other symptoms involving cardiovascular system
879.5 Open wound of abdominal wall, lateral, complicated — (Use additional code to identify infection)
902.0 Abdominal aorta injury
902.53 Iliac artery injury
904.7 Injury to specified blood vessels of lower extremity, other
908.3 Late effect of injury to blood vessel of head, neck, and extremities
908.4 Late effect of injury to blood vessel of thorax, abdomen, and pelvis
996.1 Mechanical complication of other vascular device, implant, and graft
996.74 Other complications due to other vascular device, implant, and graft
998.2 Accidental puncture or laceration during procedure

ICD-9-CM Procedural

39.29 Other (peripheral) vascular shunt or bypass

35623

35623 Bypass graft, with other than vein; axillary-popliteal or -tibial

ICD-9-CM Diagnostic

250.70 Diabetes with peripheral circulatory disorders, type II or unspecified type, not stated as uncontrolled — (Use additional code to identify manifestation: 443.81, 785.4)
250.71 Diabetes with peripheral circulatory disorders, type I [juvenile type], not stated as uncontrolled — (Use additional code to identify manifestation: 443.81, 785.4)
250.72 Diabetes with peripheral circulatory disorders, type II or unspecified type, uncontrolled — (Use additional code to identify manifestation: 443.81, 785.4)
250.73 Diabetes with peripheral circulatory disorders, type I [juvenile type], uncontrolled — (Use additional code to identify manifestation: 443.81, 785.4)
440.0 Atherosclerosis of aorta
440.20 Atherosclerosis of native arteries of the extremities, unspecified ▽
440.21 Atherosclerosis of native arteries of the extremities with intermittent claudication
440.22 Atherosclerosis of native arteries of the extremities with rest pain
440.23 Atherosclerosis of native arteries of the extremities with ulceration — (Use additional code for any associated ulceration: 707.10-707.9)
440.8 Atherosclerosis of other specified arteries
440.9 Generalized and unspecified atherosclerosis ▽
441.02 Dissecting aortic aneurysm (any part), abdominal
441.03 Dissecting aortic aneurysm (any part), thoracoabdominal
441.3 Abdominal aneurysm, ruptured
441.4 Abdominal aneurysm without mention of rupture
441.5 Aortic aneurysm of unspecified site, ruptured ▽
441.6 Thoracoabdominal aneurysm, ruptured
441.7 Thoracoabdominal aneurysm without mention of rupture
441.9 Aortic aneurysm of unspecified site without mention of rupture ▽
442.2 Aneurysm of iliac artery
442.3 Aneurysm of artery of lower extremity
443.29 Dissection of other artery
443.81 Peripheral angiopathy in diseases classified elsewhere — (Code first underlying disease, 250.7) ☒
443.9 Unspecified peripheral vascular disease ▽
444.0 Embolism and thrombosis of abdominal aorta
444.81 Embolism and thrombosis of iliac artery
445.02 Atheroembolism of lower extremity
447.1 Stricture of artery
447.5 Necrosis of artery
447.9 Unspecified disorders of arteries and arterioles ▽
707.10 Ulcer of lower limb, unspecified ▽
707.11 Ulcer of thigh
707.12 Ulcer of calf
707.13 Ulcer of ankle
707.14 Ulcer of heel and midfoot
707.15 Ulcer of other part of foot
707.19 Ulcer of other part of lower limb

747.22 Congenital atresia and stenosis of aorta
747.69 Congenital anomaly of other specified site of peripheral vascular system
785.4 Gangrene — (Code first any associated underlying condition:250.7, 443.0)
785.9 Other symptoms involving cardiovascular system
879.5 Open wound of abdominal wall, lateral, complicated — (Use additional code to identify infection)
902.0 Abdominal aorta injury
902.53 Iliac artery injury
904.7 Injury to specified blood vessels of lower extremity, other
908.3 Late effect of injury to blood vessel of head, neck, and extremities
908.4 Late effect of injury to blood vessel of thorax, abdomen, and pelvis
996.1 Mechanical complication of other vascular device, implant, and graft
996.74 Other complications due to other vascular device, implant, and graft

ICD-9-CM Procedural

39.29 Other (peripheral) vascular shunt or bypass

35626

35626 Bypass graft, with other than vein; aortosubclavian or carotid

ICD-9-CM Diagnostic

433.10 Occlusion and stenosis of carotid artery without mention of cerebral infarction — (Use additional code to identify presence of hypertension)
433.11 Occlusion and stenosis of carotid artery with cerebral infarction — (Use additional code to identify presence of hypertension)
433.21 Occlusion and stenosis of vertebral artery with cerebral infarction — (Use additional code to identify presence of hypertension)
435.0 Basilar artery syndrome — (Use additional code to identify presence of hypertension)
435.2 Subclavian steal syndrome — (Use additional code to identify presence of hypertension)
437.1 Other generalized ischemic cerebrovascular disease — (Use additional code to identify presence of hypertension)
440.8 Atherosclerosis of other specified arteries
442.81 Aneurysm of artery of neck
442.82 Aneurysm of subclavian artery
443.21 Dissection of carotid artery
443.29 Dissection of other artery
901.0 Thoracic aorta injury
901.1 Innominate and subclavian artery injury
996.1 Mechanical complication of other vascular device, implant, and graft
996.74 Other complications due to other vascular device, implant, and graft
997.79 Vascular complications of other vessels — (Use additional code to identify complications)
998.2 Accidental puncture or laceration during procedure

ICD-9-CM Procedural

39.22 Aorta-subclavian-carotid bypass

35631

35631 Bypass graft, with other than vein; aortoceliac, aortomesenteric, aortorenal

ICD-9-CM Diagnostic

440.0 Atherosclerosis of aorta
440.1 Atherosclerosis of renal artery
440.8 Atherosclerosis of other specified arteries
441.3 Abdominal aneurysm, ruptured
441.4 Abdominal aneurysm without mention of rupture
441.9 Aortic aneurysm of unspecified site without mention of rupture ▽
442.1 Aneurysm of renal artery
442.84 Aneurysm of other visceral artery
443.29 Dissection of other artery
444.89 Embolism and thrombosis of other specified artery
445.81 Atheroembolism of kidney — (Use additional code for any associated kidney failure: 584, 585)
445.89 Atheroembolism of other site
446.0 Polyarteritis nodosa
447.1 Stricture of artery
447.4 Celiac artery compression syndrome
447.6 Unspecified arteritis ▽
447.9 Unspecified disorders of arteries and arterioles ▽
557.0 Acute vascular insufficiency of intestine
557.1 Chronic vascular insufficiency of intestine
593.81 Vascular disorders of kidney
902.0 Abdominal aorta injury
902.20 Unspecified celiac and mesenteric artery injury ▽
908.4 Late effect of injury to blood vessel of thorax, abdomen, and pelvis
996.1 Mechanical complication of other vascular device, implant, and graft
996.74 Other complications due to other vascular device, implant, and graft
997.71 Vascular complications of mesenteric artery — (Use additional code to identify complications)
997.72 Vascular complications of renal artery — (Use additional code to identify complications)
997.79 Vascular complications of other vessels — (Use additional code to identify complications)
998.2 Accidental puncture or laceration during procedure

ICD-9-CM Procedural

39.24 Aorta-renal bypass
39.26 Other intra-abdominal vascular shunt or bypass

35636

35636 Bypass graft, with other than vein; splenorenal (splenic to renal arterial anastomosis)

ICD-9-CM Diagnostic

405.11 Secondary renovascular hypertension, benign
405.91 Secondary renovascular hypertension, unspecified ▽
440.1 Atherosclerosis of renal artery
440.8 Atherosclerosis of other specified arteries
441.4 Abdominal aneurysm without mention of rupture
442.1 Aneurysm of renal artery
442.83 Aneurysm of splenic artery
443.23 Dissection of renal artery
443.29 Dissection of other artery
443.9 Unspecified peripheral vascular disease ▽
445.81 Atheroembolism of kidney — (Use additional code for any associated kidney failure: 584, 585)
447.1 Stricture of artery
447.3 Hyperplasia of renal artery
447.5 Necrosis of artery
447.9 Unspecified disorders of arteries and arterioles ▽
584.9 Unspecified acute renal failure ▽
593.81 Vascular disorders of kidney
747.62 Congenital renal vessel anomaly
747.69 Congenital anomaly of other specified site of peripheral vascular system
902.23 Splenic artery injury
902.41 Renal artery injury
902.42 Renal vein injury
996.1 Mechanical complication of other vascular device, implant, and graft
996.74 Other complications due to other vascular device, implant, and graft
997.72 Vascular complications of renal artery — (Use additional code to identify complications)

ICD-9-CM Procedural

39.26 Other intra-abdominal vascular shunt or bypass

35641

35641 Bypass graft, with other than vein; aortoiliac or bi-iliac

ICD-9-CM Diagnostic

440.0 Atherosclerosis of aorta
440.8 Atherosclerosis of other specified arteries
441.00 Dissecting aortic aneurysm (any part), unspecified site ▽
441.02 Dissecting aortic aneurysm (any part), abdominal
441.3 Abdominal aneurysm, ruptured
441.4 Abdominal aneurysm without mention of rupture
441.5 Aortic aneurysm of unspecified site, ruptured ▽
441.9 Aortic aneurysm of unspecified site without mention of rupture ▽
442.2 Aneurysm of iliac artery
443.22 Dissection of iliac artery
443.9 Unspecified peripheral vascular disease ▽
444.0 Embolism and thrombosis of abdominal aorta
444.81 Embolism and thrombosis of iliac artery
445.89 Atheroembolism of other site
447.1 Stricture of artery
447.5 Necrosis of artery
447.9 Unspecified disorders of arteries and arterioles ▽
747.22 Congenital atresia and stenosis of aorta
785.9 Other symptoms involving cardiovascular system
902.0 Abdominal aorta injury
902.53 Iliac artery injury

▽ Unspecified code
♀ Female diagnosis
☒ Manifestation code
♂ Male diagnosis

908.4 Late effect of injury to blood vessel of thorax, abdomen, and pelvis
996.1 Mechanical complication of other vascular device, implant, and graft
996.74 Other complications due to other vascular device, implant, and graft
997.79 Vascular complications of other vessels — (Use additional code to identify complications)
998.2 Accidental puncture or laceration during procedure

ICD-9-CM Procedural

39.25 Aorta-iliac-femoral bypass

35642–35645

35642 carotid-vertebral
35645 subclavian-vertebral

ICD-9-CM Diagnostic

433.20 Occlusion and stenosis of vertebral artery without mention of cerebral infarction — (Use additional code to identify presence of hypertension)
433.21 Occlusion and stenosis of vertebral artery with cerebral infarction — (Use additional code to identify presence of hypertension)
435.1 Vertebral artery syndrome — (Use additional code to identify presence of hypertension)
435.2 Subclavian steal syndrome — (Use additional code to identify presence of hypertension)
435.8 Other specified transient cerebral ischemias — (Use additional code to identify presence of hypertension)
440.8 Atherosclerosis of other specified arteries
442.81 Aneurysm of artery of neck
442.82 Aneurysm of subclavian artery
443.21 Dissection of carotid artery
443.24 Dissection of vertebral artery
443.29 Dissection of other artery
447.1 Stricture of artery
747.69 Congenital anomaly of other specified site of peripheral vascular system
874.9 Open wound of other and unspecified parts of neck, complicated — (Use additional code to identify infection) ▽
900.82 Injury to multiple blood vessels of head and neck
901.1 Innominate and subclavian artery injury
906.0 Late effect of open wound of head, neck, and trunk
996.1 Mechanical complication of other vascular device, implant, and graft
996.74 Other complications due to other vascular device, implant, and graft

ICD-9-CM Procedural

39.22 Aorta-subclavian-carotid bypass
39.28 Extracranial-intracranial (EC-IC) vascular bypass

35646

35646 Bypass graft, with other than vein; aortobifemoral

ICD-9-CM Diagnostic

250.70 Diabetes with peripheral circulatory disorders, type II or unspecified type, not stated as uncontrolled — (Use additional code to identify manifestation: 443.81, 785.4)
250.71 Diabetes with peripheral circulatory disorders, type I [juvenile type], not stated as uncontrolled — (Use additional code to identify manifestation: 443.81, 785.4)
250.72 Diabetes with peripheral circulatory disorders, type II or unspecified type, uncontrolled — (Use additional code to identify manifestation: 443.81, 785.4)
250.73 Diabetes with peripheral circulatory disorders, type I [juvenile type], uncontrolled — (Use additional code to identify manifestation: 443.81, 785.4)
440.0 Atherosclerosis of aorta
440.20 Atherosclerosis of native arteries of the extremities, unspecified ▽
440.21 Atherosclerosis of native arteries of the extremities with intermittent claudication
440.22 Atherosclerosis of native arteries of the extremities with rest pain
440.23 Atherosclerosis of native arteries of the extremities with ulceration — (Use additional code for any associated ulceration: 707.10-707.9)
440.8 Atherosclerosis of other specified arteries
440.9 Generalized and unspecified atherosclerosis ▽
441.00 Dissecting aortic aneurysm (any part), unspecified site ▽
441.02 Dissecting aortic aneurysm (any part), abdominal
441.3 Abdominal aneurysm, ruptured
441.4 Abdominal aneurysm without mention of rupture
441.5 Aortic aneurysm of unspecified site, ruptured ▽
441.6 Thoracoabdominal aneurysm, ruptured
441.9 Aortic aneurysm of unspecified site without mention of rupture ▽
442.2 Aneurysm of iliac artery
443.22 Dissection of iliac artery
443.29 Dissection of other artery
443.81 Peripheral angiopathy in diseases classified elsewhere — (Code first underlying disease, 250.7) ☒
443.9 Unspecified peripheral vascular disease ▽
444.0 Embolism and thrombosis of abdominal aorta
444.22 Embolism and thrombosis of arteries of lower extremity
444.81 Embolism and thrombosis of iliac artery
445.02 Atheroembolism of lower extremity
447.1 Stricture of artery
447.5 Necrosis of artery
447.9 Unspecified disorders of arteries and arterioles ▽
459.9 Unspecified circulatory system disorder ▽
707.10 Ulcer of lower limb, unspecified ▽
707.11 Ulcer of thigh
707.12 Ulcer of calf
707.13 Ulcer of ankle
707.14 Ulcer of heel and midfoot
707.15 Ulcer of other part of foot
707.19 Ulcer of other part of lower limb
747.22 Congenital atresia and stenosis of aorta
747.64 Congenital lower limb vessel anomaly
747.69 Congenital anomaly of other specified site of peripheral vascular system
785.4 Gangrene — (Code first any associated underlying condition:250.7, 443.0)
785.9 Other symptoms involving cardiovascular system
902.0 Abdominal aorta injury
904.0 Common femoral artery injury
904.1 Superficial femoral artery injury
908.3 Late effect of injury to blood vessel of head, neck, and extremities
908.4 Late effect of injury to blood vessel of thorax, abdomen, and pelvis
928.10 Crushing injury of lower leg — (Use additional code to identify any associated injuries: 800-829, 850.0-854.1, 860.0-869.1)
928.8 Crushing injury of multiple sites of lower limb — (Use additional code to identify any associated injuries: 800-829, 850.0-854.1, 860.0-869.1)
996.1 Mechanical complication of other vascular device, implant, and graft
996.74 Other complications due to other vascular device, implant, and graft
997.79 Vascular complications of other vessels — (Use additional code to identify complications)
998.2 Accidental puncture or laceration during procedure

ICD-9-CM Procedural

39.25 Aorta-iliac-femoral bypass

35647

35647 Bypass graft, with other than vein; aortofemoral

ICD-9-CM Diagnostic

250.70 Diabetes with peripheral circulatory disorders, type II or unspecified type, not stated as uncontrolled — (Use additional code to identify manifestation: 443.81, 785.4)
250.71 Diabetes with peripheral circulatory disorders, type I [juvenile type], not stated as uncontrolled — (Use additional code to identify manifestation: 443.81, 785.4)
250.72 Diabetes with peripheral circulatory disorders, type II or unspecified type, uncontrolled — (Use additional code to identify manifestation: 443.81, 785.4)
250.73 Diabetes with peripheral circulatory disorders, type I [juvenile type], uncontrolled — (Use additional code to identify manifestation: 443.81, 785.4)
440.0 Atherosclerosis of aorta
440.20 Atherosclerosis of native arteries of the extremities, unspecified ▽
440.21 Atherosclerosis of native arteries of the extremities with intermittent claudication
440.22 Atherosclerosis of native arteries of the extremities with rest pain
440.23 Atherosclerosis of native arteries of the extremities with ulceration — (Use additional code for any associated ulceration: 707.10-707.9)
440.8 Atherosclerosis of other specified arteries
440.9 Generalized and unspecified atherosclerosis ▽
441.00 Dissecting aortic aneurysm (any part), unspecified site ▽
441.02 Dissecting aortic aneurysm (any part), abdominal
441.3 Abdominal aneurysm, ruptured
441.4 Abdominal aneurysm without mention of rupture
441.5 Aortic aneurysm of unspecified site, ruptured ▽
441.6 Thoracoabdominal aneurysm, ruptured
441.9 Aortic aneurysm of unspecified site without mention of rupture ▽
442.2 Aneurysm of iliac artery
443.22 Dissection of iliac artery
443.29 Dissection of other artery

443.81 Peripheral angiopathy in diseases classified elsewhere — (Code first underlying disease, 250.7) ☒
443.9 Unspecified peripheral vascular disease ▽
444.0 Embolism and thrombosis of abdominal aorta
444.22 Embolism and thrombosis of arteries of lower extremity
444.81 Embolism and thrombosis of iliac artery
445.02 Atheroembolism of lower extremity
447.1 Stricture of artery
447.5 Necrosis of artery
447.9 Unspecified disorders of arteries and arterioles ▽
459.9 Unspecified circulatory system disorder ▽
707.10 Ulcer of lower limb, unspecified ▽
707.11 Ulcer of thigh
707.12 Ulcer of calf
707.13 Ulcer of ankle
707.14 Ulcer of heel and midfoot
707.15 Ulcer of other part of foot
707.19 Ulcer of other part of lower limb
747.22 Congenital atresia and stenosis of aorta
747.64 Congenital lower limb vessel anomaly
747.69 Congenital anomaly of other specified site of peripheral vascular system
785.4 Gangrene — (Code first any associated underlying condition:250.7, 443.0)
785.9 Other symptoms involving cardiovascular system
902.0 Abdominal aorta injury
904.0 Common femoral artery injury
904.1 Superficial femoral artery injury
908.3 Late effect of injury to blood vessel of head, neck, and extremities
908.4 Late effect of injury to blood vessel of thorax, abdomen, and pelvis
928.10 Crushing injury of lower leg — (Use additional code to identify any associated injuries: 800-829, 850.0-854.1, 860.0-869.1)
928.8 Crushing injury of multiple sites of lower limb — (Use additional code to identify any associated injuries: 800-829, 850.0-854.1, 860.0-869.1)
996.1 Mechanical complication of other vascular device, implant, and graft
996.74 Other complications due to other vascular device, implant, and graft
997.79 Vascular complications of other vessels — (Use additional code to identify complications)
998.2 Accidental puncture or laceration during procedure

ICD-9-CM Procedural

39.25 Aorta-iliac-femoral bypass

HCPCS Level II Supplies & Services

HCPCS Level II codes are used to report the supplies, durable medical equipment, and certain medical services provided on an outpatient basis. Because the procedure(s) represented on this page would be performed in an inpatient facility, no HCPCS Level II codes apply.

35650

35650 Bypass graft, with other than vein; axillary-axillary

ICD-9-CM Diagnostic

435.2 Subclavian steal syndrome — (Use additional code to identify presence of hypertension)
440.20 Atherosclerosis of native arteries of the extremities, unspecified ▽
440.8 Atherosclerosis of other specified arteries
442.0 Aneurysm of artery of upper extremity
442.89 Aneurysm of other specified artery
443.29 Dissection of other artery
443.9 Unspecified peripheral vascular disease ▽
444.21 Embolism and thrombosis of arteries of upper extremity
444.89 Embolism and thrombosis of other specified artery
445.01 Atheroembolism of upper extremity
447.1 Stricture of artery
447.5 Necrosis of artery
447.9 Unspecified disorders of arteries and arterioles ▽
459.9 Unspecified circulatory system disorder ▽
747.63 Congenital upper limb vessel anomaly
747.69 Congenital anomaly of other specified site of peripheral vascular system
785.9 Other symptoms involving cardiovascular system
880.02 Open wound of axillary region, without mention of complication — (Use additional code to identify infection)
880.12 Open wound of axillary region, complicated — (Use additional code to identify infection)
901.1 Innominate and subclavian artery injury
903.01 Axillary artery injury
906.1 Late effect of open wound of extremities without mention of tendon injury
906.4 Late effect of crushing
908.3 Late effect of injury to blood vessel of head, neck, and extremities
927.02 Crushing injury of axillary region — (Use additional code to identify any associated injuries: 800-829, 850.0-854.1, 860.0-869.1)
996.1 Mechanical complication of other vascular device, implant, and graft
996.74 Other complications due to other vascular device, implant, and graft

ICD-9-CM Procedural

39.29 Other (peripheral) vascular shunt or bypass

35651

35651 Bypass graft, with other than vein; aortofemoral-popliteal

ICD-9-CM Diagnostic

250.70 Diabetes with peripheral circulatory disorders, type II or unspecified type, not stated as uncontrolled — (Use additional code to identify manifestation: 443.81, 785.4)
250.71 Diabetes with peripheral circulatory disorders, type I [juvenile type], not stated as uncontrolled — (Use additional code to identify manifestation: 443.81, 785.4)
250.72 Diabetes with peripheral circulatory disorders, type II or unspecified type, uncontrolled — (Use additional code to identify manifestation: 443.81, 785.4)
250.73 Diabetes with peripheral circulatory disorders, type I [juvenile type], uncontrolled — (Use additional code to identify manifestation: 443.81, 785.4)
440.0 Atherosclerosis of aorta
440.20 Atherosclerosis of native arteries of the extremities, unspecified ▽
440.21 Atherosclerosis of native arteries of the extremities with intermittent claudication
440.22 Atherosclerosis of native arteries of the extremities with rest pain
440.23 Atherosclerosis of native arteries of the extremities with ulceration — (Use additional code for any associated ulceration: 707.10-707.9)
440.24 Atherosclerosis of native arteries of the extremities with gangrene
440.8 Atherosclerosis of other specified arteries
440.9 Generalized and unspecified atherosclerosis ▽
441.00 Dissecting aortic aneurysm (any part), unspecified site ▽
441.02 Dissecting aortic aneurysm (any part), abdominal
441.3 Abdominal aneurysm, ruptured
441.4 Abdominal aneurysm without mention of rupture
441.5 Aortic aneurysm of unspecified site, ruptured ▽
441.6 Thoracoabdominal aneurysm, ruptured
441.9 Aortic aneurysm of unspecified site without mention of rupture ▽
442.2 Aneurysm of iliac artery
442.3 Aneurysm of artery of lower extremity
443.22 Dissection of iliac artery
443.29 Dissection of other artery
443.81 Peripheral angiopathy in diseases classified elsewhere — (Code first underlying disease, 250.7) ☒
443.9 Unspecified peripheral vascular disease ▽
444.0 Embolism and thrombosis of abdominal aorta
444.22 Embolism and thrombosis of arteries of lower extremity
444.81 Embolism and thrombosis of iliac artery
445.02 Atheroembolism of lower extremity
447.1 Stricture of artery
447.5 Necrosis of artery
447.9 Unspecified disorders of arteries and arterioles ▽
707.10 Ulcer of lower limb, unspecified ▽
707.11 Ulcer of thigh
707.12 Ulcer of calf
707.13 Ulcer of ankle
707.14 Ulcer of heel and midfoot
707.15 Ulcer of other part of foot
707.19 Ulcer of other part of lower limb
747.22 Congenital atresia and stenosis of aorta
747.64 Congenital lower limb vessel anomaly
747.69 Congenital anomaly of other specified site of peripheral vascular system
785.4 Gangrene — (Code first any associated underlying condition:250.7, 443.0)
785.9 Other symptoms involving cardiovascular system
902.0 Abdominal aorta injury
904.0 Common femoral artery injury
904.1 Superficial femoral artery injury
908.3 Late effect of injury to blood vessel of head, neck, and extremities
908.4 Late effect of injury to blood vessel of thorax, abdomen, and pelvis
928.10 Crushing injury of lower leg — (Use additional code to identify any associated injuries: 800-829, 850.0-854.1, 860.0-869.1)
928.8 Crushing injury of multiple sites of lower limb — (Use additional code to identify any associated injuries: 800-829, 850.0-854.1, 860.0-869.1)

996.1 Mechanical complication of other vascular device, implant, and graft
996.74 Other complications due to other vascular device, implant, and graft
997.79 Vascular complications of other vessels — (Use additional code to identify complications)

ICD-9-CM Procedural

39.25 Aorta-iliac-femoral bypass

35654

35654 Bypass graft, with other than vein; axillary-femoral-femoral

ICD-9-CM Diagnostic

250.70 Diabetes with peripheral circulatory disorders, type II or unspecified type, not stated as uncontrolled — (Use additional code to identify manifestation: 443.81, 785.4)
250.71 Diabetes with peripheral circulatory disorders, type I [juvenile type], not stated as uncontrolled — (Use additional code to identify manifestation: 443.81, 785.4)
250.72 Diabetes with peripheral circulatory disorders, type II or unspecified type, uncontrolled — (Use additional code to identify manifestation: 443.81, 785.4)
250.73 Diabetes with peripheral circulatory disorders, type I [juvenile type], uncontrolled — (Use additional code to identify manifestation: 443.81, 785.4)
440.0 Atherosclerosis of aorta
440.20 Atherosclerosis of native arteries of the extremities, unspecified ▽
440.21 Atherosclerosis of native arteries of the extremities with intermittent claudication
440.22 Atherosclerosis of native arteries of the extremities with rest pain
440.23 Atherosclerosis of native arteries of the extremities with ulceration — (Use additional code for any associated ulceration: 707.10-707.9)
440.8 Atherosclerosis of other specified arteries
441.00 Dissecting aortic aneurysm (any part), unspecified site ▽
441.02 Dissecting aortic aneurysm (any part), abdominal
441.03 Dissecting aortic aneurysm (any part), thoracoabdominal
441.3 Abdominal aneurysm, ruptured
441.4 Abdominal aneurysm without mention of rupture
441.5 Aortic aneurysm of unspecified site, ruptured ▽
441.6 Thoracoabdominal aneurysm, ruptured
441.7 Thoracoabdominal aneurysm without mention of rupture
441.9 Aortic aneurysm of unspecified site without mention of rupture ▽
442.2 Aneurysm of iliac artery
442.3 Aneurysm of artery of lower extremity
443.22 Dissection of iliac artery
443.29 Dissection of other artery
443.81 Peripheral angiopathy in diseases classified elsewhere — (Code first underlying disease, 250.7) ☒
443.9 Unspecified peripheral vascular disease ▽
444.0 Embolism and thrombosis of abdominal aorta
444.22 Embolism and thrombosis of arteries of lower extremity
444.81 Embolism and thrombosis of iliac artery
445.02 Atheroembolism of lower extremity
447.1 Stricture of artery
447.5 Necrosis of artery
447.9 Unspecified disorders of arteries and arterioles ▽
747.22 Congenital atresia and stenosis of aorta
747.64 Congenital lower limb vessel anomaly
747.69 Congenital anomaly of other specified site of peripheral vascular system
785.4 Gangrene — (Code first any associated underlying condition:250.7, 443.0)
785.9 Other symptoms involving cardiovascular system
902.0 Abdominal aorta injury
902.53 Iliac artery injury
904.0 Common femoral artery injury
904.1 Superficial femoral artery injury
906.0 Late effect of open wound of head, neck, and trunk
908.4 Late effect of injury to blood vessel of thorax, abdomen, and pelvis
996.1 Mechanical complication of other vascular device, implant, and graft
996.74 Other complications due to other vascular device, implant, and graft
998.2 Accidental puncture or laceration during procedure

ICD-9-CM Procedural

39.29 Other (peripheral) vascular shunt or bypass

35656

35656 Bypass graft, with other than vein; femoral-popliteal

ICD-9-CM Diagnostic

250.70 Diabetes with peripheral circulatory disorders, type II or unspecified type, not stated as uncontrolled — (Use additional code to identify manifestation: 443.81, 785.4)
250.71 Diabetes with peripheral circulatory disorders, type I [juvenile type], not stated as uncontrolled — (Use additional code to identify manifestation: 443.81, 785.4)
250.72 Diabetes with peripheral circulatory disorders, type II or unspecified type, uncontrolled — (Use additional code to identify manifestation: 443.81, 785.4)
250.73 Diabetes with peripheral circulatory disorders, type I [juvenile type], uncontrolled — (Use additional code to identify manifestation: 443.81, 785.4)
440.20 Atherosclerosis of native arteries of the extremities, unspecified ▽
440.21 Atherosclerosis of native arteries of the extremities with intermittent claudication
440.22 Atherosclerosis of native arteries of the extremities with rest pain
440.23 Atherosclerosis of native arteries of the extremities with ulceration — (Use additional code for any associated ulceration: 707.10-707.9)
440.24 Atherosclerosis of native arteries of the extremities with gangrene
440.29 Other atherosclerosis of native arteries of the extremities
440.30 Atheroslerosis of unspecified bypass graft of extremities ▽
440.31 Atheroslerosis of autologous vein bypass graft of extremities
440.32 Atheroslerosis of nonautologous biological bypass graft of extremities
440.8 Atherosclerosis of other specified arteries
440.9 Generalized and unspecified atherosclerosis ▽
442.3 Aneurysm of artery of lower extremity
443.29 Dissection of other artery
443.81 Peripheral angiopathy in diseases classified elsewhere — (Code first underlying disease, 250.7) ☒
443.89 Other peripheral vascular disease
443.9 Unspecified peripheral vascular disease ▽
444.22 Embolism and thrombosis of arteries of lower extremity
445.02 Atheroembolism of lower extremity
447.1 Stricture of artery
447.5 Necrosis of artery
459.89 Other specified circulatory system disorders
459.9 Unspecified circulatory system disorder ▽
707.10 Ulcer of lower limb, unspecified ▽
707.11 Ulcer of thigh
707.12 Ulcer of calf
707.13 Ulcer of ankle
707.14 Ulcer of heel and midfoot
707.15 Ulcer of other part of foot
707.19 Ulcer of other part of lower limb
747.64 Congenital lower limb vessel anomaly
747.69 Congenital anomaly of other specified site of peripheral vascular system
785.4 Gangrene — (Code first any associated underlying condition:250.7, 443.0)
785.9 Other symptoms involving cardiovascular system
894.1 Multiple and unspecified open wound of lower limb, complicated — (Use additional code to identify infection)
904.1 Superficial femoral artery injury
908.3 Late effect of injury to blood vessel of head, neck, and extremities
928.10 Crushing injury of lower leg — (Use additional code to identify any associated injuries: 800-829, 850.0-854.1, 860.0-869.1)
928.8 Crushing injury of multiple sites of lower limb — (Use additional code to identify any associated injuries: 800-829, 850.0-854.1, 860.0-869.1)
996.1 Mechanical complication of other vascular device, implant, and graft
996.74 Other complications due to other vascular device, implant, and graft

ICD-9-CM Procedural

39.29 Other (peripheral) vascular shunt or bypass

35661

35661 Bypass graft, with other than vein; femoral-femoral

ICD-9-CM Diagnostic

250.70 Diabetes with peripheral circulatory disorders, type II or unspecified type, not stated as uncontrolled — (Use additional code to identify manifestation: 443.81, 785.4)
250.71 Diabetes with peripheral circulatory disorders, type I [juvenile type], not stated as uncontrolled — (Use additional code to identify manifestation: 443.81, 785.4)
250.72 Diabetes with peripheral circulatory disorders, type II or unspecified type, uncontrolled — (Use additional code to identify manifestation: 443.81, 785.4)

250.73 Diabetes with peripheral circulatory disorders, type I [juvenile type], uncontrolled — (Use additional code to identify manifestation: 443.81, 785.4)
440.20 Atherosclerosis of native arteries of the extremities, unspecified
440.21 Atherosclerosis of native arteries of the extremities with intermittent claudication
440.22 Atherosclerosis of native arteries of the extremities with rest pain
440.23 Atherosclerosis of native arteries of the extremities with ulceration — (Use additional code for any associated ulceration: 707.10-707.9)
440.24 Atherosclerosis of native arteries of the extremities with gangrene
440.8 Atherosclerosis of other specified arteries
442.3 Aneurysm of artery of lower extremity
442.9 Other aneurysm of unspecified site
443.29 Dissection of other artery
443.81 Peripheral angiopathy in diseases classified elsewhere — (Code first underlying disease, 250.7)
443.9 Unspecified peripheral vascular disease
447.1 Stricture of artery
447.5 Necrosis of artery
459.9 Unspecified circulatory system disorder
707.10 Ulcer of lower limb, unspecified
707.11 Ulcer of thigh
707.12 Ulcer of calf
707.13 Ulcer of ankle
707.14 Ulcer of heel and midfoot
707.15 Ulcer of other part of foot
707.19 Ulcer of other part of lower limb
747.64 Congenital lower limb vessel anomaly
747.69 Congenital anomaly of other specified site of peripheral vascular system
904.0 Common femoral artery injury
904.1 Superficial femoral artery injury
908.3 Late effect of injury to blood vessel of head, neck, and extremities
996.1 Mechanical complication of other vascular device, implant, and graft
996.74 Other complications due to other vascular device, implant, and graft

ICD-9-CM Procedural

39.29 Other (peripheral) vascular shunt or bypass

35663

35663 Bypass graft, with other than vein; ilioiliac

ICD-9-CM Diagnostic

440.8 Atherosclerosis of other specified arteries
443.22 Dissection of iliac artery
443.9 Unspecified peripheral vascular disease
444.81 Embolism and thrombosis of iliac artery
445.89 Atheroembolism of other site
447.1 Stricture of artery
447.5 Necrosis of artery
902.50 Unspecified iliac vessel(s) injury
902.53 Iliac artery injury
996.1 Mechanical complication of other vascular device, implant, and graft
996.74 Other complications due to other vascular device, implant, and graft
997.79 Vascular complications of other vessels — (Use additional code to identify complications)

ICD-9-CM Procedural

39.26 Other intra-abdominal vascular shunt or bypass

35665

35665 Bypass graft, with other than vein; iliofemoral

ICD-9-CM Diagnostic

250.70 Diabetes with peripheral circulatory disorders, type II or unspecified type, not stated as uncontrolled — (Use additional code to identify manifestation: 443.81, 785.4)
250.71 Diabetes with peripheral circulatory disorders, type I [juvenile type], not stated as uncontrolled — (Use additional code to identify manifestation: 443.81, 785.4)
250.72 Diabetes with peripheral circulatory disorders, type II or unspecified type, uncontrolled — (Use additional code to identify manifestation: 443.81, 785.4)
250.73 Diabetes with peripheral circulatory disorders, type I [juvenile type], uncontrolled — (Use additional code to identify manifestation: 443.81, 785.4)
440.20 Atherosclerosis of native arteries of the extremities, unspecified
440.21 Atherosclerosis of native arteries of the extremities with intermittent claudication
440.22 Atherosclerosis of native arteries of the extremities with rest pain
440.23 Atherosclerosis of native arteries of the extremities with ulceration — (Use additional code for any associated ulceration: 707.10-707.9)
440.24 Atherosclerosis of native arteries of the extremities with gangrene
440.8 Atherosclerosis of other specified arteries
440.9 Generalized and unspecified atherosclerosis
442.2 Aneurysm of iliac artery
442.3 Aneurysm of artery of lower extremity
443.22 Dissection of iliac artery
443.81 Peripheral angiopathy in diseases classified elsewhere — (Code first underlying disease, 250.7)
443.89 Other peripheral vascular disease
443.9 Unspecified peripheral vascular disease
444.22 Embolism and thrombosis of arteries of lower extremity
444.81 Embolism and thrombosis of iliac artery
445.02 Atheroembolism of lower extremity
447.1 Stricture of artery
447.5 Necrosis of artery
459.9 Unspecified circulatory system disorder
707.10 Ulcer of lower limb, unspecified
707.11 Ulcer of thigh
707.12 Ulcer of calf
707.13 Ulcer of ankle
707.14 Ulcer of heel and midfoot
707.15 Ulcer of other part of foot
707.19 Ulcer of other part of lower limb
747.64 Congenital lower limb vessel anomaly
747.69 Congenital anomaly of other specified site of peripheral vascular system
785.4 Gangrene — (Code first any associated underlying condition:250.7, 443.0)
785.9 Other symptoms involving cardiovascular system
894.1 Multiple and unspecified open wound of lower limb, complicated — (Use additional code to identify infection)
902.53 Iliac artery injury
904.7 Injury to specified blood vessels of lower extremity, other
908.3 Late effect of injury to blood vessel of head, neck, and extremities
928.00 Crushing injury of thigh — (Use additional code to identify any associated injuries: 800-829, 850.0-854.1, 860.0-869.1)
996.74 Other complications due to other vascular device, implant, and graft
997.79 Vascular complications of other vessels — (Use additional code to identify complications)

ICD-9-CM Procedural

39.25 Aorta-iliac-femoral bypass

35666

35666 Bypass graft, with other than vein; femoral-anterior tibial, posterior tibial, or peroneal artery

ICD-9-CM Diagnostic

250.70 Diabetes with peripheral circulatory disorders, type II or unspecified type, not stated as uncontrolled — (Use additional code to identify manifestation: 443.81, 785.4)
250.71 Diabetes with peripheral circulatory disorders, type I [juvenile type], not stated as uncontrolled — (Use additional code to identify manifestation: 443.81, 785.4)
250.72 Diabetes with peripheral circulatory disorders, type II or unspecified type, uncontrolled — (Use additional code to identify manifestation: 443.81, 785.4)
250.73 Diabetes with peripheral circulatory disorders, type I [juvenile type], uncontrolled — (Use additional code to identify manifestation: 443.81, 785.4)
440.20 Atherosclerosis of native arteries of the extremities, unspecified
440.21 Atherosclerosis of native arteries of the extremities with intermittent claudication
440.22 Atherosclerosis of native arteries of the extremities with rest pain
440.23 Atherosclerosis of native arteries of the extremities with ulceration — (Use additional code for any associated ulceration: 707.10-707.9)
440.24 Atherosclerosis of native arteries of the extremities with gangrene
440.29 Other atherosclerosis of native arteries of the extremities
440.8 Atherosclerosis of other specified arteries
440.9 Generalized and unspecified atherosclerosis
442.3 Aneurysm of artery of lower extremity
443.29 Dissection of other artery
443.81 Peripheral angiopathy in diseases classified elsewhere — (Code first underlying disease, 250.7)
443.9 Unspecified peripheral vascular disease
447.1 Stricture of artery
459.89 Other specified circulatory system disorders
459.9 Unspecified circulatory system disorder

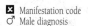

Unspecified code — Female diagnosis — Manifestation code — Male diagnosis

707.10 Ulcer of lower limb, unspecified ▽
707.11 Ulcer of thigh
707.12 Ulcer of calf
707.13 Ulcer of ankle
707.14 Ulcer of heel and midfoot
707.15 Ulcer of other part of foot
707.19 Ulcer of other part of lower limb
747.64 Congenital lower limb vessel anomaly
785.4 Gangrene — (Code first any associated underlying condition:250.7, 443.0)
785.9 Other symptoms involving cardiovascular system
894.1 Multiple and unspecified open wound of lower limb, complicated — (Use additional code to identify infection)
904.0 Common femoral artery injury
904.1 Superficial femoral artery injury
904.41 Popliteal artery injury
904.42 Popliteal vein injury
904.51 Anterior tibial artery injury
904.52 Anterior tibial vein injury
904.53 Posterior tibial artery injury
904.54 Posterior tibial vein injury
904.7 Injury to specified blood vessels of lower extremity, other
908.3 Late effect of injury to blood vessel of head, neck, and extremities
928.10 Crushing injury of lower leg — (Use additional code to identify any associated injuries: 800-829, 850.0-854.1, 860.0-869.1)
928.8 Crushing injury of multiple sites of lower limb — (Use additional code to identify any associated injuries: 800-829, 850.0-854.1, 860.0-869.1)
996.1 Mechanical complication of other vascular device, implant, and graft
996.74 Other complications due to other vascular device, implant, and graft

ICD-9-CM Procedural
39.29 Other (peripheral) vascular shunt or bypass

35671
35671 Bypass graft, with other than vein; popliteal-tibial or -peroneal artery

ICD-9-CM Diagnostic
250.70 Diabetes with peripheral circulatory disorders, type II or unspecified type, not stated as uncontrolled — (Use additional code to identify manifestation: 443.81, 785.4)
250.71 Diabetes with peripheral circulatory disorders, type I [juvenile type], not stated as uncontrolled — (Use additional code to identify manifestation: 443.81, 785.4)
250.72 Diabetes with peripheral circulatory disorders, type II or unspecified type, uncontrolled — (Use additional code to identify manifestation: 443.81, 785.4)
250.73 Diabetes with peripheral circulatory disorders, type I [juvenile type], uncontrolled — (Use additional code to identify manifestation: 443.81, 785.4)
440.20 Atherosclerosis of native arteries of the extremities, unspecified ▽
440.21 Atherosclerosis of native arteries of the extremities with intermittent claudication
440.22 Atherosclerosis of native arteries of the extremities with rest pain
440.23 Atherosclerosis of native arteries of the extremities with ulceration — (Use additional code for any associated ulceration: 707.10-707.9)
440.24 Atherosclerosis of native arteries of the extremities with gangrene
440.8 Atherosclerosis of other specified arteries
442.3 Aneurysm of artery of lower extremity
443.81 Peripheral angiopathy in diseases classified elsewhere — (Code first underlying disease, 250.7) ☒
443.9 Unspecified peripheral vascular disease ▽
444.22 Embolism and thrombosis of arteries of lower extremity
445.02 Atheroembolism of lower extremity
447.1 Stricture of artery
459.9 Unspecified circulatory system disorder ▽
707.10 Ulcer of lower limb, unspecified ▽
707.11 Ulcer of thigh
707.12 Ulcer of calf
707.13 Ulcer of ankle
707.14 Ulcer of heel and midfoot
707.15 Ulcer of other part of foot
707.19 Ulcer of other part of lower limb
747.64 Congenital lower limb vessel anomaly
785.4 Gangrene — (Code first any associated underlying condition:250.7, 443.0)
785.9 Other symptoms involving cardiovascular system
894.1 Multiple and unspecified open wound of lower limb, complicated — (Use additional code to identify infection)
904.41 Popliteal artery injury
904.42 Popliteal vein injury
904.51 Anterior tibial artery injury
904.53 Posterior tibial artery injury
904.7 Injury to specified blood vessels of lower extremity, other
908.3 Late effect of injury to blood vessel of head, neck, and extremities
928.10 Crushing injury of lower leg — (Use additional code to identify any associated injuries: 800-829, 850.0-854.1, 860.0-869.1)
928.8 Crushing injury of multiple sites of lower limb — (Use additional code to identify any associated injuries: 800-829, 850.0-854.1, 860.0-869.1)
996.1 Mechanical complication of other vascular device, implant, and graft
996.74 Other complications due to other vascular device, implant, and graft

ICD-9-CM Procedural
39.29 Other (peripheral) vascular shunt or bypass

35681–35683
35681 Bypass graft; composite, prosthetic and vein (List separately in addition to code for primary procedure)
35682 autogenous composite, two segments of veins from two locations (List separately in addition to code for primary procedure)
35683 autogenous composite, three or more segments of vein from two or more locations (List separately in addition to code for primary procedure)

ICD-9-CM Diagnostic
This is an add-on code. Refer to the corresponding primary procedure code for ICD-9 diagnosis code links.

ICD-9-CM Procedural
38.33 Resection of upper limb vessels with anastomosis
38.39 Resection of lower limb veins with anastomosis
39.56 Repair of blood vessel with tissue patch graft
39.57 Repair of blood vessel with synthetic patch graft

35685
35685 Placement of vein patch or cuff at distal anastomosis of bypass graft, synthetic conduit (List separately in addition to code for primary procedure)

ICD-9-CM Diagnostic
This is an add-on code. Refer to the corresponding primary procedure code for ICD-9 diagnosis code links.

ICD-9-CM Procedural
39.56 Repair of blood vessel with tissue patch graft

HCPCS Level II Supplies & Services
The HCPCS Level II code(s) would be the same as the actual procedure performed because these are in-addition-to codes.

35686
35686 Creation of distal arteriovenous fistula during lower extremity bypass surgery (non-hemodialysis) (List separately in addition to code for primary procedure)

ICD-9-CM Diagnostic
This is an add-on code. Refer to the corresponding primary procedure code for ICD-9 diagnosis code links.

ICD-9-CM Procedural
39.29 Other (peripheral) vascular shunt or bypass

HCPCS Level II Supplies & Services
The HCPCS Level II code(s) would be the same as the actual procedure performed because these are in-addition-to codes.

35691
35691 Transposition and/or reimplantation; vertebral to carotid artery

ICD-9-CM Diagnostic
433.20 Occlusion and stenosis of vertebral artery without mention of cerebral infarction — (Use additional code to identify presence of hypertension)
433.21 Occlusion and stenosis of vertebral artery with cerebral infarction — (Use additional code to identify presence of hypertension)
435.1 Vertebral artery syndrome — (Use additional code to identify presence of hypertension)
440.8 Atherosclerosis of other specified arteries
442.81 Aneurysm of artery of neck
443.24 Dissection of vertebral artery

▽ Unspecified code ☒ Manifestation code
♀ Female diagnosis ♂ Male diagnosis

447.1 Stricture of artery
747.81 Congenital anomaly of cerebrovascular system
747.82 Congenital spinal vessel anomaly
900.00 Injury to carotid artery, unspecified

ICD-9-CM Procedural
39.59 Other repair of vessel

35693
35693 Transposition and/or reimplantation; vertebral to subclavian artery

ICD-9-CM Diagnostic
433.20 Occlusion and stenosis of vertebral artery without mention of cerebral infarction — (Use additional code to identify presence of hypertension)
433.21 Occlusion and stenosis of vertebral artery with cerebral infarction — (Use additional code to identify presence of hypertension)
435.1 Vertebral artery syndrome — (Use additional code to identify presence of hypertension)
435.2 Subclavian steal syndrome — (Use additional code to identify presence of hypertension)
440.8 Atherosclerosis of other specified arteries
442.82 Aneurysm of subclavian artery
443.24 Dissection of vertebral artery
447.1 Stricture of artery
747.81 Congenital anomaly of cerebrovascular system
747.82 Congenital spinal vessel anomaly
901.1 Innominate and subclavian artery injury

ICD-9-CM Procedural
39.59 Other repair of vessel

35694
35694 Transposition and/or reimplantation; subclavian to carotid artery

ICD-9-CM Diagnostic
433.10 Occlusion and stenosis of carotid artery without mention of cerebral infarction — (Use additional code to identify presence of hypertension)
433.11 Occlusion and stenosis of carotid artery with cerebral infarction — (Use additional code to identify presence of hypertension)
433.30 Occlusion and stenosis of multiple and bilateral precerebral arteries without mention of cerebral infarction — (Use additional code to identify presence of hypertension)
433.31 Occlusion and stenosis of multiple and bilateral precerebral arteries with cerebral infarction — (Use additional code to identify presence of hypertension)
435.2 Subclavian steal syndrome — (Use additional code to identify presence of hypertension)
440.8 Atherosclerosis of other specified arteries
442.81 Aneurysm of artery of neck
442.82 Aneurysm of subclavian artery
443.21 Dissection of carotid artery
443.29 Dissection of other artery
447.1 Stricture of artery
747.81 Congenital anomaly of cerebrovascular system
900.00 Injury to carotid artery, unspecified
901.1 Innominate and subclavian artery injury

ICD-9-CM Procedural
39.59 Other repair of vessel

35695
35695 Transposition and/or reimplantation; carotid to subclavian artery

ICD-9-CM Diagnostic
433.10 Occlusion and stenosis of carotid artery without mention of cerebral infarction — (Use additional code to identify presence of hypertension)
433.11 Occlusion and stenosis of carotid artery with cerebral infarction — (Use additional code to identify presence of hypertension)
433.30 Occlusion and stenosis of multiple and bilateral precerebral arteries without mention of cerebral infarction — (Use additional code to identify presence of hypertension)
433.31 Occlusion and stenosis of multiple and bilateral precerebral arteries with cerebral infarction — (Use additional code to identify presence of hypertension)
435.2 Subclavian steal syndrome — (Use additional code to identify presence of hypertension)
440.8 Atherosclerosis of other specified arteries
442.81 Aneurysm of artery of neck
442.82 Aneurysm of subclavian artery
443.21 Dissection of carotid artery
443.29 Dissection of other artery
447.1 Stricture of artery
747.81 Congenital anomaly of cerebrovascular system
900.00 Injury to carotid artery, unspecified
901.1 Innominate and subclavian artery injury

ICD-9-CM Procedural
39.59 Other repair of vessel

35697
35697 Reimplantation, visceral artery to infrarenal aortic prosthesis, each artery (List separately in addition to code for primary procedure)

ICD-9-CM Diagnostic
This is an add-on code. Refer to the corresponding primary procedure code for ICD-9 diagnosis code links.

ICD-9-CM Procedural
39.59 Other repair of vessel

35700
35700 Reoperation, femoral-popliteal or femoral (popliteal)-anterior tibial, posterior tibial, peroneal artery or other distal vessels, more than one month after original operation (List separately in addition to code for primary procedure)

ICD-9-CM Diagnostic
This is an add-on code. Refer to the corresponding primary procedure code for ICD-9 diagnosis code links.

ICD-9-CM Procedural
38.08 Incision of lower limb arteries

35701
35701 Exploration (not followed by surgical repair), with or without lysis of artery; carotid artery

ICD-9-CM Diagnostic
433.10 Occlusion and stenosis of carotid artery without mention of cerebral infarction — (Use additional code to identify presence of hypertension)
433.30 Occlusion and stenosis of multiple and bilateral precerebral arteries without mention of cerebral infarction — (Use additional code to identify presence of hypertension)
435.8 Other specified transient cerebral ischemias — (Use additional code to identify presence of hypertension)
437.0 Cerebral atherosclerosis — (Use additional code to identify presence of hypertension)
443.21 Dissection of carotid artery
447.1 Stricture of artery
780.02 Transient alteration of awareness
780.2 Syncope and collapse
780.31 Febrile convulsions
780.39 Other convulsions
780.4 Dizziness and giddiness
785.9 Other symptoms involving cardiovascular system
900.03 Internal carotid artery injury

ICD-9-CM Procedural
38.02 Incision of other vessels of head and neck
39.91 Freeing of vessel

35721
35721 Exploration (not followed by surgical repair), with or without lysis of artery; femoral artery

ICD-9-CM Diagnostic
250.70 Diabetes with peripheral circulatory disorders, type II or unspecified type, not stated as uncontrolled — (Use additional code to identify manifestation: 443.81, 785.4)
250.71 Diabetes with peripheral circulatory disorders, type I [juvenile type], not stated as uncontrolled — (Use additional code to identify manifestation: 443.81, 785.4)

250.72 Diabetes with peripheral circulatory disorders, type II or unspecified type, uncontrolled — (Use additional code to identify manifestation: 443.81, 785.4)
250.73 Diabetes with peripheral circulatory disorders, type I [juvenile type], uncontrolled — (Use additional code to identify manifestation: 443.81, 785.4)
440.20 Atherosclerosis of native arteries of the extremities, unspecified
440.21 Atherosclerosis of native arteries of the extremities with intermittent claudication
440.22 Atherosclerosis of native arteries of the extremities with rest pain
440.23 Atherosclerosis of native arteries of the extremities with ulceration — (Use additional code for any associated ulceration: 707.10-707.9)
440.29 Other atherosclerosis of native arteries of the extremities
442.3 Aneurysm of artery of lower extremity
443.29 Dissection of other artery
443.81 Peripheral angiopathy in diseases classified elsewhere — (Code first underlying disease, 250.7)
443.9 Unspecified peripheral vascular disease
444.22 Embolism and thrombosis of arteries of lower extremity
445.02 Atheroembolism of lower extremity
447.1 Stricture of artery
447.6 Unspecified arteritis
447.8 Other specified disorders of arteries and arterioles
707.10 Ulcer of lower limb, unspecified
707.11 Ulcer of thigh
707.12 Ulcer of calf
707.13 Ulcer of ankle
707.14 Ulcer of heel and midfoot
707.15 Ulcer of other part of foot
707.19 Ulcer of other part of lower limb
785.4 Gangrene — (Code first any associated underlying condition:250.7, 443.0)
894.1 Multiple and unspecified open wound of lower limb, complicated — (Use additional code to identify infection)
904.0 Common femoral artery injury
904.1 Superficial femoral artery injury
904.7 Injury to specified blood vessels of lower extremity, other
908.3 Late effect of injury to blood vessel of head, neck, and extremities
928.00 Crushing injury of thigh — (Use additional code to identify any associated injuries: 800-829, 850.0-854.1, 860.0-869.1)
998.9 Unspecified complication of procedure, not elsewhere classified

ICD-9-CM Procedural

38.08 Incision of lower limb arteries
39.91 Freeing of vessel

35741

35741 Exploration (not followed by surgical repair), with or without lysis of artery; popliteal artery

ICD-9-CM Diagnostic

250.70 Diabetes with peripheral circulatory disorders, type II or unspecified type, not stated as uncontrolled — (Use additional code to identify manifestation: 443.81, 785.4)
250.71 Diabetes with peripheral circulatory disorders, type I [juvenile type], not stated as uncontrolled — (Use additional code to identify manifestation: 443.81, 785.4)
250.72 Diabetes with peripheral circulatory disorders, type II or unspecified type, uncontrolled — (Use additional code to identify manifestation: 443.81, 785.4)
250.73 Diabetes with peripheral circulatory disorders, type I [juvenile type], uncontrolled — (Use additional code to identify manifestation: 443.81, 785.4)
440.20 Atherosclerosis of native arteries of the extremities, unspecified
440.21 Atherosclerosis of native arteries of the extremities with intermittent claudication
440.22 Atherosclerosis of native arteries of the extremities with rest pain
440.23 Atherosclerosis of native arteries of the extremities with ulceration — (Use additional code for any associated ulceration: 707.10-707.9)
440.24 Atherosclerosis of native arteries of the extremities with gangrene
440.29 Other atherosclerosis of native arteries of the extremities
443.81 Peripheral angiopathy in diseases classified elsewhere — (Code first underlying disease, 250.7)
443.9 Unspecified peripheral vascular disease
444.22 Embolism and thrombosis of arteries of lower extremity
444.9 Embolism and thrombosis of unspecified artery
445.02 Atheroembolism of lower extremity
447.1 Stricture of artery
447.6 Unspecified arteritis
447.8 Other specified disorders of arteries and arterioles
707.10 Ulcer of lower limb, unspecified
707.11 Ulcer of thigh
707.12 Ulcer of calf
707.13 Ulcer of ankle
707.14 Ulcer of heel and midfoot
707.15 Ulcer of other part of foot
707.19 Ulcer of other part of lower limb
785.4 Gangrene — (Code first any associated underlying condition:250.7, 443.0)
785.9 Other symptoms involving cardiovascular system
904.41 Popliteal artery injury
904.7 Injury to specified blood vessels of lower extremity, other
908.3 Late effect of injury to blood vessel of head, neck, and extremities
928.10 Crushing injury of lower leg — (Use additional code to identify any associated injuries: 800-829, 850.0-854.1, 860.0-869.1)

ICD-9-CM Procedural

38.08 Incision of lower limb arteries
39.91 Freeing of vessel

35761

35761 Exploration (not followed by surgical repair), with or without lysis of artery; other vessels

ICD-9-CM Diagnostic

440.21 Atherosclerosis of native arteries of the extremities with intermittent claudication
440.22 Atherosclerosis of native arteries of the extremities with rest pain
440.23 Atherosclerosis of native arteries of the extremities with ulceration — (Use additional code for any associated ulceration: 707.10-707.9)
440.24 Atherosclerosis of native arteries of the extremities with gangrene
440.29 Other atherosclerosis of native arteries of the extremities
442.0 Aneurysm of artery of upper extremity
442.1 Aneurysm of renal artery
442.83 Aneurysm of splenic artery
442.84 Aneurysm of other visceral artery
443.29 Dissection of other artery
444.21 Embolism and thrombosis of arteries of upper extremity
444.22 Embolism and thrombosis of arteries of lower extremity
444.89 Embolism and thrombosis of other specified artery
445.89 Atheroembolism of other site
447.6 Unspecified arteritis
448.1 Nevus, non-neoplastic
459.9 Unspecified circulatory system disorder
557.0 Acute vascular insufficiency of intestine
729.5 Pain in soft tissues of limb
785.4 Gangrene — (Code first any associated underlying condition:250.7, 443.0)
785.9 Other symptoms involving cardiovascular system
900.9 Injury to unspecified blood vessel of head and neck
902.9 Injury to blood vessel of abdomen and pelvis, unspecified
903.9 Injury to unspecified blood vessel of upper extremity
904.8 Injury to unspecified blood vessel of lower extremity

ICD-9-CM Procedural

38.00 Incision of vessel, unspecified site
39.91 Freeing of vessel

35800

35800 Exploration for postoperative hemorrhage, thrombosis or infection; neck

ICD-9-CM Diagnostic

433.10 Occlusion and stenosis of carotid artery without mention of cerebral infarction — (Use additional code to identify presence of hypertension)
433.11 Occlusion and stenosis of carotid artery with cerebral infarction — (Use additional code to identify presence of hypertension)
433.20 Occlusion and stenosis of vertebral artery without mention of cerebral infarction — (Use additional code to identify presence of hypertension)
433.21 Occlusion and stenosis of vertebral artery with cerebral infarction — (Use additional code to identify presence of hypertension)
433.30 Occlusion and stenosis of multiple and bilateral precerebral arteries without mention of cerebral infarction — (Use additional code to identify presence of hypertension)
433.31 Occlusion and stenosis of multiple and bilateral precerebral arteries with cerebral infarction — (Use additional code to identify presence of hypertension)
433.80 Occlusion and stenosis of other specified precerebral artery without mention of cerebral infarction — (Use additional code to identify presence of hypertension)
433.81 Occlusion and stenosis of other specified precerebral artery with cerebral infarction — (Use additional code to identify presence of hypertension)

Unspecified code
♀ Female diagnosis
Manifestation code
♂ Male diagnosis

958.2 Secondary and recurrent hemorrhage as an early complication of trauma
958.3 Posttraumatic wound infection not elsewhere classified
996.1 Mechanical complication of other vascular device, implant, and graft
996.60 Infection and inflammatory reaction due to unspecified device, implant, and graft — (Use additional code to identify specified infections) ▽
997.2 Peripheral vascular complications — (Use additional code to identify complications)
998.0 Postoperative shock, not elsewhere classified
998.11 Hemorrhage complicating a procedure
998.12 Hematoma complicating a procedure
998.13 Seroma complicating a procedure
998.31 Disruption of internal operation wound
998.51 Infected postoperative seroma — (Use additional code to identify organism)
998.59 Other postoperative infection — (Use additional code to identify infection)
998.83 Non-healing surgical wound

ICD-9-CM Procedural

38.02 Incision of other vessels of head and neck
39.41 Control of hemorrhage following vascular surgery
39.98 Control of hemorrhage, not otherwise specified

35820

35820 Exploration for postoperative hemorrhage, thrombosis or infection; chest

ICD-9-CM Diagnostic

415.11 Iatrogenic pulmonary embolism and infarction
440.0 Atherosclerosis of aorta
444.1 Embolism and thrombosis of thoracic aorta
445.89 Atheroembolism of other site
997.2 Peripheral vascular complications — (Use additional code to identify complications)
997.79 Vascular complications of other vessels — (Use additional code to identify complications)
998.11 Hemorrhage complicating a procedure
998.12 Hematoma complicating a procedure
998.13 Seroma complicating a procedure
998.31 Disruption of internal operation wound
998.51 Infected postoperative seroma — (Use additional code to identify organism)
998.59 Other postoperative infection — (Use additional code to identify infection)

ICD-9-CM Procedural

38.04 Incision of aorta
38.05 Incision of other thoracic vessels
39.41 Control of hemorrhage following vascular surgery
39.98 Control of hemorrhage, not otherwise specified

35840

35840 Exploration for postoperative hemorrhage, thrombosis or infection; abdomen

ICD-9-CM Diagnostic

444.81 Embolism and thrombosis of iliac artery
444.89 Embolism and thrombosis of other specified artery
445.89 Atheroembolism of other site
453.3 Embolism and thrombosis of renal vein
453.8 Embolism and thrombosis of other specified veins
557.0 Acute vascular insufficiency of intestine
593.81 Vascular disorders of kidney
997.2 Peripheral vascular complications — (Use additional code to identify complications)
997.4 Digestive system complication — (Use additional code to identify complications)
997.5 Urinary complications — (Use additional code to identify complications)
997.71 Vascular complications of mesenteric artery — (Use additional code to identify complications)
997.72 Vascular complications of renal artery — (Use additional code to identify complications)
997.79 Vascular complications of other vessels — (Use additional code to identify complications)
998.11 Hemorrhage complicating a procedure
998.12 Hematoma complicating a procedure
998.13 Seroma complicating a procedure
998.31 Disruption of internal operation wound
998.51 Infected postoperative seroma — (Use additional code to identify organism)
998.59 Other postoperative infection — (Use additional code to identify infection)

ICD-9-CM Procedural

38.00 Incision of vessel, unspecified site
38.06 Incision of abdominal arteries
39.41 Control of hemorrhage following vascular surgery
39.98 Control of hemorrhage, not otherwise specified
54.19 Other laparotomy

35860

35860 Exploration for postoperative hemorrhage, thrombosis or infection; extremity

ICD-9-CM Diagnostic

444.21 Embolism and thrombosis of arteries of upper extremity
444.22 Embolism and thrombosis of arteries of lower extremity
445.01 Atheroembolism of upper extremity
445.02 Atheroembolism of lower extremity
453.8 Embolism and thrombosis of other specified veins
997.2 Peripheral vascular complications — (Use additional code to identify complications)
998.11 Hemorrhage complicating a procedure
998.12 Hematoma complicating a procedure
998.13 Seroma complicating a procedure
998.31 Disruption of internal operation wound
998.51 Infected postoperative seroma — (Use additional code to identify organism)
998.59 Other postoperative infection — (Use additional code to identify infection)

ICD-9-CM Procedural

38.03 Incision of upper limb vessels
38.08 Incision of lower limb arteries
39.41 Control of hemorrhage following vascular surgery
39.98 Control of hemorrhage, not otherwise specified

35870

35870 Repair of graft-enteric fistula

ICD-9-CM Diagnostic

447.2 Rupture of artery
996.74 Other complications due to other vascular device, implant, and graft

ICD-9-CM Procedural

39.49 Other revision of vascular procedure
46.72 Closure of fistula of duodenum
46.74 Closure of fistula of small intestine, except duodenum
46.76 Closure of fistula of large intestine

35875–35876

35875 Thrombectomy of arterial or venous graft (other than hemodialysis graft or fistula);
35876 with revision of arterial or venous graft

ICD-9-CM Diagnostic

996.1 Mechanical complication of other vascular device, implant, and graft
996.74 Other complications due to other vascular device, implant, and graft

ICD-9-CM Procedural

38.00 Incision of vessel, unspecified site
38.01 Incision of intracranial vessels
38.02 Incision of other vessels of head and neck
38.03 Incision of upper limb vessels

35879–35881

35879 Revision, lower extremity arterial bypass, without thrombectomy, open; with vein patch angioplasty
35881 with segmental vein interposition

ICD-9-CM Diagnostic

440.30 Atheroslerosis of unspecified bypass graft of extremities ▽
440.31 Atheroslerosis of autologous vein bypass graft of extremities
440.32 Atheroslerosis of nonautologous biological bypass graft of extremities
996.1 Mechanical complication of other vascular device, implant, and graft
996.62 Infection and inflammatory reaction due to other vascular device, implant, and graft — (Use additional code to identify specified infections)
996.74 Other complications due to other vascular device, implant, and graft

ICD-9-CM Procedural

38.48 Resection of lower limb arteries with replacement

▽ Unspecified code ♀ Female diagnosis ☒ Manifestation code ♂ Male diagnosis

39.49 Other revision of vascular procedure
39.56 Repair of blood vessel with tissue patch graft

35901

35901 Excision of infected graft; neck

ICD-9-CM Diagnostic

996.52 Mechanical complication due to other tissue graft, not elsewhere classified
996.62 Infection and inflammatory reaction due to other vascular device, implant, and graft — (Use additional code to identify specified infections)
996.74 Other complications due to other vascular device, implant, and graft
997.2 Peripheral vascular complications — (Use additional code to identify complications)
998.59 Other postoperative infection — (Use additional code to identify infection)

ICD-9-CM Procedural

38.12 Endarterectomy of other vessels of head and neck
38.62 Other excision of other vessels of head and neck
39.49 Other revision of vascular procedure

35903

35903 Excision of infected graft; extremity

ICD-9-CM Diagnostic

996.52 Mechanical complication due to other tissue graft, not elsewhere classified
996.62 Infection and inflammatory reaction due to other vascular device, implant, and graft — (Use additional code to identify specified infections)
996.74 Other complications due to other vascular device, implant, and graft
997.2 Peripheral vascular complications — (Use additional code to identify complications)
998.59 Other postoperative infection — (Use additional code to identify infection)

ICD-9-CM Procedural

38.13 Endarterectomy of upper limb vessels
38.18 Endarterectomy of lower limb arteries
38.68 Other excision of lower limb arteries
39.49 Other revision of vascular procedure

35905

35905 Excision of infected graft; thorax

ICD-9-CM Diagnostic

996.52 Mechanical complication due to other tissue graft, not elsewhere classified
996.62 Infection and inflammatory reaction due to other vascular device, implant, and graft — (Use additional code to identify specified infections)
996.74 Other complications due to other vascular device, implant, and graft
997.2 Peripheral vascular complications — (Use additional code to identify complications)
998.59 Other postoperative infection — (Use additional code to identify infection)

ICD-9-CM Procedural

38.15 Endarterectomy of other thoracic vessels
38.65 Other excision of other thoracic vessel
39.49 Other revision of vascular procedure

35907

35907 Excision of infected graft; abdomen

ICD-9-CM Diagnostic

996.52 Mechanical complication due to other tissue graft, not elsewhere classified
996.62 Infection and inflammatory reaction due to other vascular device, implant, and graft — (Use additional code to identify specified infections)
996.74 Other complications due to other vascular device, implant, and graft
997.2 Peripheral vascular complications — (Use additional code to identify complications)
998.59 Other postoperative infection — (Use additional code to identify infection)

ICD-9-CM Procedural

38.16 Endarterectomy of abdominal arteries
38.36 Resection of abdominal arteries with anastomosis
38.66 Other excision of abdominal arteries
39.49 Other revision of vascular procedure

36000

36000 Introduction of needle or intracatheter, vein

ICD-9-CM Diagnostic

The application of this code is too broad to adequately present ICD-9-CM diagnostic code links here. Refer to your ICD-9-CM book.

ICD-9-CM Procedural

38.93 Venous catheterization, not elsewhere classified

36002

36002 Injection procedures (eg, thrombin) for percutaneous treatment of extremity pseudoaneurysm

ICD-9-CM Diagnostic

442.0 Aneurysm of artery of upper extremity
442.3 Aneurysm of artery of lower extremity
442.9 Other aneurysm of unspecified site ▽

ICD-9-CM Procedural

99.25 Injection or infusion of cancer chemotherapeutic substance

HCPCS Level II Supplies & Services

HCPCS Level II codes are used to report the supplies, durable medical equipment, and certain medical services provided on an outpatient basis. Because the procedure(s) represented on this page would be performed in an inpatient facility, no HCPCS Level II codes apply.

36005

36005 Injection procedure for extremity venography (including introduction of needle or intracatheter)

ICD-9-CM Diagnostic

451.0 Phlebitis and thrombophlebitis of superficial vessels of lower extremities — (Use additional E code to identify drug, if drug-induced)
451.11 Phlebitis and thrombophlebitis of femoral vein (deep) (superficial) — (Use additional E code to identify drug, if drug-induced)
451.19 Phlebitis and thrombophlebitis of other deep vessels of lower extremities — (Use additional E code to identify drug, if drug-induced)
451.2 Phlebitis and thrombophlebitis of lower extremities, unspecified — (Use additional E code to identify drug, if drug-induced) ▽
451.81 Phlebitis and thrombophlebitis of iliac vein — (Use additional E code to identify drug, if drug-induced)
451.82 Phlebitis and thrombophlebitis of superficial veins of upper extremities — (Use additional E code to identify drug, if drug-induced)
451.83 Phlebitis and thrombophlebitis of deep veins of upper extremities — (Use additional E code to identify drug, if drug-induced)
451.84 Phlebitis and thrombophlebitis of upper extremities, unspecified — (Use additional E code to identify drug, if drug-induced) ▽
453.40 Venous embolism and thrombosis of unspecified deep vessels of lower extremity
453.41 Venous embolism and thrombosis of deep vessels of proximal lower extremity
453.42 Venous embolism and thrombosis of deep vessels of distal lower extremity
453.8 Embolism and thrombosis of other specified veins
453.9 Embolism and thrombosis of unspecified site ▽
454.0 Varicose veins of lower extremities with ulcer
454.1 Varicose veins of lower extremities with inflammation
454.2 Varicose veins of lower extremities with ulcer and inflammation
454.8 Varicose veins of the lower extremities with other complications
454.9 Asymptomatic varicose veins
459.10 Postphlebitic syndrome without complications
459.11 Postphlebitic syndrome with ulcer
459.12 Postphlebitic syndrome with inflammation
459.13 Postphlebitic syndrome with ulcer and inflammation
459.19 Postphlebitic syndrome with other complication
459.2 Compression of vein
459.81 Unspecified venous (peripheral) insufficiency — (Use additional code for any associated ulceration: 707.10-707.9) ▽
996.74 Other complications due to other vascular device, implant, and graft

ICD-9-CM Procedural

38.93 Venous catheterization, not elsewhere classified

▽ Unspecified code ♀ Female diagnosis ☒ Manifestation code ♂ Male diagnosis

36010

36010 Introduction of catheter, superior or inferior vena cava

ICD-9-CM Diagnostic

The application of this code is too broad to adequately present ICD-9-CM diagnostic code links here. Refer to your ICD-9-CM book.

ICD-9-CM Procedural

38.93 Venous catheterization, not elsewhere classified

36011

36011 Selective catheter placement, venous system; first order branch (eg, renal vein, jugular vein)

ICD-9-CM Diagnostic

The application of this code is too broad to adequately present ICD-9-CM diagnostic code links here. Refer to your ICD-9-CM book.

ICD-9-CM Procedural

38.93 Venous catheterization, not elsewhere classified

36012

36012 Selective catheter placement, venous system; second order, or more selective, branch (eg, left adrenal vein, petrosal sinus)

ICD-9-CM Diagnostic

The application of this code is too broad to adequately present ICD-9-CM diagnostic code links here. Refer to your ICD-9-CM book.

ICD-9-CM Procedural

38.93 Venous catheterization, not elsewhere classified

36013

36013 Introduction of catheter, right heart or main pulmonary artery

ICD-9-CM Diagnostic

414.10 Aneurysm of heart — (Use additional code to identify presence of hypertension: 401.0-405.9)
416.0 Primary pulmonary hypertension
417.0 Arteriovenous fistula of pulmonary vessels
417.1 Aneurysm of pulmonary artery
417.8 Other specified disease of pulmonary circulation
424.2 Tricuspid valve disorders, specified as nonrheumatic
424.3 Pulmonary valve disorders
745.0 Bulbus cordis anomalies and anomalies of cardiac septal closure, common truncus
745.11 Transposition of great vessels, double outlet right ventricle
745.2 Tetralogy of Fallot
745.3 Bulbus cordis anomalies and anomalies of cardiac septal closure, common ventricle
745.4 Ventricular septal defect

ICD-9-CM Procedural

37.21 Right heart cardiac catheterization

36014–36015

36014 Selective catheter placement, left or right pulmonary artery
36015 Selective catheter placement, segmental or subsegmental pulmonary artery

ICD-9-CM Diagnostic

162.3 Malignant neoplasm of upper lobe, bronchus, or lung
162.4 Malignant neoplasm of middle lobe, bronchus, or lung
162.5 Malignant neoplasm of lower lobe, bronchus, or lung
162.8 Malignant neoplasm of other parts of bronchus or lung
162.9 Malignant neoplasm of bronchus and lung, unspecified site ▽
197.0 Secondary malignant neoplasm of lung
231.2 Carcinoma in situ of bronchus and lung
231.9 Carcinoma in situ of respiratory system, part unspecified ▽
415.0 Acute cor pulmonale
416.0 Primary pulmonary hypertension
416.8 Other chronic pulmonary heart diseases
416.9 Unspecified chronic pulmonary heart disease ▽
417.0 Arteriovenous fistula of pulmonary vessels
417.1 Aneurysm of pulmonary artery
417.8 Other specified disease of pulmonary circulation
417.9 Unspecified disease of pulmonary circulation ▽
424.3 Pulmonary valve disorders
425.4 Other primary cardiomyopathies
428.0 Congestive heart failure, unspecified ▽
428.1 Left heart failure
428.20 Unspecified systolic heart failure ▽
428.21 Acute systolic heart failure
428.22 Chronic systolic heart failure
428.23 Acute on chronic systolic heart failure
428.30 Unspecified diastolic heart failure ▽
428.31 Acute diastolic heart failure
428.32 Chronic diastolic heart failure
428.33 Acute on chronic diastolic heart failure
428.40 Unspecified combined systolic and diastolic heart failure ▽
428.41 Acute combined systolic and diastolic heart failure
428.42 Chronic combined systolic and diastolic heart failure
428.43 Acute on chronic combined systolic and diastolic heart failure
447.1 Stricture of artery
486 Pneumonia, organism unspecified ▽
496 Chronic airway obstruction, not elsewhere classified — (Note: This code is not to be used with any code from 491-493) ▽
511.9 Unspecified pleural effusion ▽
514 Pulmonary congestion and hypostasis
518.0 Pulmonary collapse
518.3 Pulmonary eosinophilia
518.89 Other diseases of lung, not elsewhere classified
519.8 Other diseases of respiratory system, not elsewhere classified
673.20 Obstetrical blood-clot embolism, unspecified as to episode of care ▽ ♀
673.21 Obstetrical blood-clot embolism, with delivery, with or without mention of antepartum condition ♀
673.22 Obstetrical blood-clot embolism, with mention of postpartum complication ♀
673.24 Obstetrical blood-clot embolism, postpartum ♀
745.0 Bulbus cordis anomalies and anomalies of cardiac septal closure, common truncus
745.10 Complete transposition of great vessels
745.11 Transposition of great vessels, double outlet right ventricle
745.2 Tetralogy of Fallot
745.3 Bulbus cordis anomalies and anomalies of cardiac septal closure, common ventricle
745.4 Ventricular septal defect
747.3 Congenital anomalies of pulmonary artery
786.09 Other dyspnea and respiratory abnormalities
786.3 Hemoptysis
786.59 Other chest pain
786.6 Swelling, mass, or lump in chest
786.9 Other symptoms involving respiratory system and chest
794.2 Nonspecific abnormal results of pulmonary system function study
794.30 Nonspecific abnormal unspecified cardiovascular function study ▽
V72.5 Radiological examination, not elsewhere classified — (Use additional code(s) to identify any special screening examination(s) performed: V73.0-V82.9)

ICD-9-CM Procedural

38.91 Arterial catheterization

36100

36100 Introduction of needle or intracatheter, carotid or vertebral artery

ICD-9-CM Diagnostic

430 Subarachnoid hemorrhage — (Use additional code to identify presence of hypertension)
433.10 Occlusion and stenosis of carotid artery without mention of cerebral infarction — (Use additional code to identify presence of hypertension)
433.11 Occlusion and stenosis of carotid artery with cerebral infarction — (Use additional code to identify presence of hypertension)
433.20 Occlusion and stenosis of vertebral artery without mention of cerebral infarction — (Use additional code to identify presence of hypertension)
433.21 Occlusion and stenosis of vertebral artery with cerebral infarction — (Use additional code to identify presence of hypertension)
433.30 Occlusion and stenosis of multiple and bilateral precerebral arteries without mention of cerebral infarction — (Use additional code to identify presence of hypertension)
433.31 Occlusion and stenosis of multiple and bilateral precerebral arteries with cerebral infarction — (Use additional code to identify presence of hypertension)
433.80 Occlusion and stenosis of other specified precerebral artery without mention of cerebral infarction — (Use additional code to identify presence of hypertension)

▽ Unspecified code
♀ Female diagnosis
☒ Manifestation code
♂ Male diagnosis

433.81 Occlusion and stenosis of other specified precerebral artery with cerebral infarction — (Use additional code to identify presence of hypertension)
433.90 Occlusion and stenosis of unspecified precerebral artery without mention of cerebral infarction — (Use additional code to identify presence of hypertension) ▽
433.91 Occlusion and stenosis of unspecified precerebral artery with cerebral infarction — (Use additional code to identify presence of hypertension) ▽
435.1 Vertebral artery syndrome — (Use additional code to identify presence of hypertension)
435.9 Unspecified transient cerebral ischemia — (Use additional code to identify presence of hypertension) ▽
436 Acute, but ill-defined, cerebrovascular disease — (Use additional code to identify presence of hypertension) ▽
437.1 Other generalized ischemic cerebrovascular disease — (Use additional code to identify presence of hypertension)
437.3 Cerebral aneurysm, nonruptured — (Use additional code to identify presence of hypertension)
437.9 Unspecified cerebrovascular disease — (Use additional code to identify presence of hypertension) ▽
442.81 Aneurysm of artery of neck
443.21 Dissection of carotid artery
443.24 Dissection of vertebral artery
682.1 Cellulitis and abscess of neck — (Use additional code to identify organism)
780.02 Transient alteration of awareness
780.09 Other alteration of consciousness
780.2 Syncope and collapse
780.4 Dizziness and giddiness
784.0 Headache
784.2 Swelling, mass, or lump in head and neck
853.00 Other and unspecified intracranial hemorrhage following injury, without mention of open intracranial wound, unspecified state of consciousness ▽
V71.7 Observation for suspected cardiovascular disease
V72.5 Radiological examination, not elsewhere classified — (Use additional code(s) to identify any special screening examination(s) performed: V73.0-V82.9)

ICD-9-CM Procedural

38.91 Arterial catheterization

36120

36120 Introduction of needle or intracatheter; retrograde brachial artery

ICD-9-CM Diagnostic

440.20 Atherosclerosis of native arteries of the extremities, unspecified ▽
440.21 Atherosclerosis of native arteries of the extremities with intermittent claudication
442.0 Aneurysm of artery of upper extremity
442.9 Other aneurysm of unspecified site ▽
443.29 Dissection of other artery
443.9 Unspecified peripheral vascular disease ▽
444.21 Embolism and thrombosis of arteries of upper extremity
444.9 Embolism and thrombosis of unspecified artery ▽
445.01 Atheroembolism of upper extremity
447.1 Stricture of artery
785.4 Gangrene — (Code first any associated underlying condition:250.7, 443.0)
785.9 Other symptoms involving cardiovascular system
927.02 Crushing injury of axillary region — (Use additional code to identify any associated injuries: 800-829, 850.0-854.1, 860.0-869.1)
927.03 Crushing injury of upper arm — (Use additional code to identify any associated injuries: 800-829, 850.0-854.1, 860.0-869.1)
V71.7 Observation for suspected cardiovascular disease
V72.5 Radiological examination, not elsewhere classified — (Use additional code(s) to identify any special screening examination(s) performed: V73.0-V82.9)

ICD-9-CM Procedural

38.91 Arterial catheterization

36140

36140 Introduction of needle or intracatheter; extremity artery

ICD-9-CM Diagnostic

195.4 Malignant neoplasm of upper limb
195.5 Malignant neoplasm of lower limb
228.00 Hemangioma of unspecified site ▽
250.70 Diabetes with peripheral circulatory disorders, type II or unspecified type, not stated as uncontrolled — (Use additional code to identify manifestation: 443.81, 785.4)
250.71 Diabetes with peripheral circulatory disorders, type I [juvenile type], not stated as uncontrolled — (Use additional code to identify manifestation: 443.81, 785.4)
250.72 Diabetes with peripheral circulatory disorders, type II or unspecified type, uncontrolled — (Use additional code to identify manifestation: 443.81, 785.4)
250.73 Diabetes with peripheral circulatory disorders, type I [juvenile type], uncontrolled — (Use additional code to identify manifestation: 443.81, 785.4)
354.0 Carpal tunnel syndrome
440.21 Atherosclerosis of native arteries of the extremities with intermittent claudication
440.22 Atherosclerosis of native arteries of the extremities with rest pain
440.23 Atherosclerosis of native arteries of the extremities with ulceration — (Use additional code for any associated ulceration: 707.10-707.9)
440.30 Atherosclerosis of unspecified bypass graft of extremities ▽
442.0 Aneurysm of artery of upper extremity
442.3 Aneurysm of artery of lower extremity
443.0 Raynaud's syndrome — (Use additional code to identify gangrene, 785.4)
443.1 Thromboangiitis obliterans (Buerger's disease)
443.29 Dissection of other artery
443.81 Peripheral angiopathy in diseases classified elsewhere — (Code first underlying disease, 250.7) ☒
443.89 Other peripheral vascular disease
444.21 Embolism and thrombosis of arteries of upper extremity
444.22 Embolism and thrombosis of arteries of lower extremity
445.01 Atheroembolism of upper extremity
445.02 Atheroembolism of lower extremity
747.60 Congenital anomaly of the peripheral vascular system, unspecified site ▽
785.4 Gangrene — (Code first any associated underlying condition:250.7, 443.0)

ICD-9-CM Procedural

38.91 Arterial catheterization

HCPCS Level II Supplies & Services

A4550 Surgical trays

36145

36145 Introduction of needle or intracatheter; arteriovenous shunt created for dialysis (cannula, fistula, or graft)

ICD-9-CM Diagnostic

250.40 Diabetes with renal manifestations, type II or unspecified type, not stated as uncontrolled — (Use additional code to identify manifestation: 581.81, 583.81)
250.41 Diabetes with renal manifestations, type I [juvenile type], not stated as uncontrolled — (Use additional code to identify manifestation: 581.81, 583.81)
250.42 Diabetes with renal manifestations, type II or unspecified type, uncontrolled — (Use additional code to identify manifestation: 581.81, 583.81)
250.43 Diabetes with renal manifestations, type I [juvenile type], uncontrolled — (Use additional code to identify manifestation: 581.81, 583.81)
250.70 Diabetes with peripheral circulatory disorders, type II or unspecified type, not stated as uncontrolled — (Use additional code to identify manifestation: 443.81, 785.4)
445.81 Atheroembolism of kidney — (Use additional code for any associated kidney failure: 584, 585)
584.5 Acute renal failure with lesion of tubular necrosis
584.6 Acute renal failure with lesion of renal cortical necrosis
584.7 Acute renal failure with lesion of renal medullary (papillary) necrosis
584.8 Acute renal failure with other specified pathological lesion in kidney
584.9 Unspecified acute renal failure ▽
585 Chronic renal failure — (Use additional code to identify manifestation: 357.4, 420.0)
586 Unspecified renal failure ▽
728.88 Rhabdomyolysis
996.1 Mechanical complication of other vascular device, implant, and graft
996.62 Infection and inflammatory reaction due to other vascular device, implant, and graft — (Use additional code to identify specified infections)
996.73 Other complications due to renal dialysis device, implant, and graft
V45.1 Renal dialysis status — (This code is intended for use when these conditions are recorded as diagnoses or problems)
V72.5 Radiological examination, not elsewhere classified — (Use additional code(s) to identify any special screening examination(s) performed: V73.0-V82.9)

ICD-9-CM Procedural

38.91 Arterial catheterization
38.93 Venous catheterization, not elsewhere classified

HCPCS Level II Supplies & Services

A4550 Surgical trays

G0365 Vessel mapping of vessels for hemodialysis access (services for preoperative vessel mapping prior to creation of hemodialysis access using an autogenous hemodialysis conduit, including arterial inflow and venous outflow)

36160

36160 Introduction of needle or intracatheter, aortic, translumbar

ICD-9-CM Diagnostic

440.0 Atherosclerosis of aorta
441.9 Aortic aneurysm of unspecified site without mention of rupture ▽
447.1 Stricture of artery
447.2 Rupture of artery

ICD-9-CM Procedural

38.91 Arterial catheterization

36200

36200 Introduction of catheter, aorta

ICD-9-CM Diagnostic

428.0 Congestive heart failure, unspecified ▽
428.1 Left heart failure
428.20 Unspecified systolic heart failure ▽
428.21 Acute systolic heart failure
428.22 Chronic systolic heart failure
428.23 Acute on chronic systolic heart failure
428.30 Unspecified diastolic heart failure ▽
428.31 Acute diastolic heart failure
428.32 Chronic diastolic heart failure
428.33 Acute on chronic diastolic heart failure
428.40 Unspecified combined systolic and diastolic heart failure ▽
428.41 Acute combined systolic and diastolic heart failure
428.42 Chronic combined systolic and diastolic heart failure
428.43 Acute on chronic combined systolic and diastolic heart failure
440.0 Atherosclerosis of aorta
441.9 Aortic aneurysm of unspecified site without mention of rupture ▽
444.0 Embolism and thrombosis of abdominal aorta
444.1 Embolism and thrombosis of thoracic aorta

ICD-9-CM Procedural

38.91 Arterial catheterization

36215–36218

36215 Selective catheter placement, arterial system; each first order thoracic or brachiocephalic branch, within a vascular family
36216 initial second order thoracic or brachiocephalic branch, within a vascular family
36217 initial third order or more selective thoracic or brachiocephalic branch, within a vascular family
36218 additional second order, third order, and beyond, thoracic or brachiocephalic branch, within a vascular family (List in addition to code for initial second or third order vessel as appropriate)

ICD-9-CM Diagnostic

162.3 Malignant neoplasm of upper lobe, bronchus, or lung
162.4 Malignant neoplasm of middle lobe, bronchus, or lung
162.5 Malignant neoplasm of lower lobe, bronchus, or lung
162.8 Malignant neoplasm of other parts of bronchus or lung
162.9 Malignant neoplasm of bronchus and lung, unspecified site ▽
191.0 Malignant neoplasm of cerebrum, except lobes and ventricles
191.1 Malignant neoplasm of frontal lobe of brain
191.2 Malignant neoplasm of temporal lobe of brain
191.3 Malignant neoplasm of parietal lobe of brain
191.4 Malignant neoplasm of occipital lobe of brain
191.5 Malignant neoplasm of ventricles of brain
191.6 Malignant neoplasm of cerebellum NOS
191.7 Malignant neoplasm of brain stem
191.8 Malignant neoplasm of other parts of brain
191.9 Malignant neoplasm of brain, unspecified site ▽
192.1 Malignant neoplasm of cerebral meninges
192.2 Malignant neoplasm of spinal cord
192.3 Malignant neoplasm of spinal meninges
192.8 Malignant neoplasm of other specified sites of nervous system
192.9 Malignant neoplasm of nervous system, part unspecified ▽
194.3 Malignant neoplasm of pituitary gland and craniopharyngeal duct — (Use additional code to identify any functional activity)
194.5 Malignant neoplasm of carotid body — (Use additional code to identify any functional activity)
197.0 Secondary malignant neoplasm of lung
198.3 Secondary malignant neoplasm of brain and spinal cord
199.1 Other malignant neoplasm of unspecified site
212.3 Benign neoplasm of bronchus and lung
225.0 Benign neoplasm of brain
225.2 Benign neoplasm of cerebral meninges
225.3 Benign neoplasm of spinal cord
225.4 Benign neoplasm of spinal meninges
225.8 Benign neoplasm of other specified sites of nervous system
225.9 Benign neoplasm of nervous system, part unspecified ▽
227.3 Benign neoplasm of pituitary gland and craniopharyngeal duct (pouch) — (Use additional code to identify any functional activity)
227.5 Benign neoplasm of carotid body — (Use additional code to identify any functional activity)
228.00 Hemangioma of unspecified site ▽
228.02 Hemangioma of intracranial structures
231.2 Carcinoma in situ of bronchus and lung
235.7 Neoplasm of uncertain behavior of trachea, bronchus, and lung
237.0 Neoplasm of uncertain behavior of pituitary gland and craniopharyngeal duct — (Use additional code to identify any functional activity)
237.3 Neoplasm of uncertain behavior of paraganglia
237.5 Neoplasm of uncertain behavior of brain and spinal cord
237.6 Neoplasm of uncertain behavior of meninges
238.9 Neoplasm of uncertain behavior, site unspecified ▽
239.1 Neoplasm of unspecified nature of respiratory system
239.6 Neoplasm of unspecified nature of brain
239.7 Neoplasm of unspecified nature of endocrine glands and other parts of nervous system
239.9 Neoplasm of unspecified nature, site unspecified ▽
331.4 Obstructive hydrocephalus
342.90 Unspecified hemiplegia affecting unspecified side ▽
342.91 Unspecified hemiplegia affecting dominant side ▽
342.92 Unspecified hemiplegia affecting nondominant side ▽
344.9 Unspecified paralysis ▽
346.90 Unspecified migraine without mention of intractable migraine ▽
348.0 Cerebral cysts
348.8 Other conditions of brain
348.9 Unspecified condition of brain ▽
411.1 Intermediate coronary syndrome — (Use additional code to identify presence of hypertension: 401.0-405.9)
414.00 Coronary atherosclerosis of unspecified type of vessel, native or graft — (Use additional code to identify presence of hypertension: 401.0-405.9) ▽
414.01 Coronary atherosclerosis of native coronary artery — (Use additional code to identify presence of hypertension: 401.0-405.9)
414.03 Coronary atherosclerosis of nonautologous biological bypass graft — (Use additional code to identify presence of hypertension: 401.0-405.9)
414.04 Coronary atherosclerosis of artery bypass graft — (Use additional code to identify presence of hypertension: 401.0-405.9)
414.05 Coronary atherosclerosis of unspecified type of bypass graft — (Use additional code to identify presence of hypertension: 401.0-405.9) ▽
414.06 Coronary atherosclerosis, of native coronary artery of transplanted heart — (Use additional code to identify presence of hypertension: 401.0-405.9)
414.07 Coronary atherosclerosis, of bypass graft (artery) (vein) of transplanted heart — (Use additional code to identify presence of hypertension: 401.0-405.9)
430 Subarachnoid hemorrhage — (Use additional code to identify presence of hypertension)
431 Intracerebral hemorrhage — (Use additional code to identify presence of hypertension)
432.0 Nontraumatic extradural hemorrhage — (Use additional code to identify presence of hypertension)
432.1 Subdural hemorrhage — (Use additional code to identify presence of hypertension)
432.9 Unspecified intracranial hemorrhage — (Use additional code to identify presence of hypertension) ▽
433.00 Occlusion and stenosis of basilar artery without mention of cerebral infarction — (Use additional code to identify presence of hypertension)
433.01 Occlusion and stenosis of basilar artery with cerebral infarction — (Use additional code to identify presence of hypertension)
433.10 Occlusion and stenosis of carotid artery without mention of cerebral infarction — (Use additional code to identify presence of hypertension)
433.11 Occlusion and stenosis of carotid artery with cerebral infarction — (Use additional code to identify presence of hypertension)

433.20 Occlusion and stenosis of vertebral artery without mention of cerebral infarction — (Use additional code to identify presence of hypertension)
433.21 Occlusion and stenosis of vertebral artery with cerebral infarction — (Use additional code to identify presence of hypertension)
433.30 Occlusion and stenosis of multiple and bilateral precerebral arteries without mention of cerebral infarction — (Use additional code to identify presence of hypertension)
433.31 Occlusion and stenosis of multiple and bilateral precerebral arteries with cerebral infarction — (Use additional code to identify presence of hypertension)
433.80 Occlusion and stenosis of other specified precerebral artery without mention of cerebral infarction — (Use additional code to identify presence of hypertension)
433.81 Occlusion and stenosis of other specified precerebral artery with cerebral infarction — (Use additional code to identify presence of hypertension)
433.90 Occlusion and stenosis of unspecified precerebral artery without mention of cerebral infarction — (Use additional code to identify presence of hypertension) ▽
433.91 Occlusion and stenosis of unspecified precerebral artery with cerebral infarction — (Use additional code to identify presence of hypertension) ▽
434.00 Cerebral thrombosis without mention of cerebral infarction — (Use additional code to identify presence of hypertension)
434.01 Cerebral thrombosis with cerebral infarction — (Use additional code to identify presence of hypertension)
434.10 Cerebral embolism without mention of cerebral infarction — (Use additional code to identify presence of hypertension)
434.11 Cerebral embolism with cerebral infarction — (Use additional code to identify presence of hypertension)
434.90 Unspecified cerebral artery occlusion without mention of cerebral infarction — (Use additional code to identify presence of hypertension) ▽
434.91 Unspecified cerebral artery occlusion with cerebral infarction — (Use additional code to identify presence of hypertension) ▽
435.0 Basilar artery syndrome — (Use additional code to identify presence of hypertension)
435.1 Vertebral artery syndrome — (Use additional code to identify presence of hypertension)
435.2 Subclavian steal syndrome — (Use additional code to identify presence of hypertension)
435.3 Vertebrobasilar artery syndrome — (Use additional code to identify presence of hypertension)
435.8 Other specified transient cerebral ischemias — (Use additional code to identify presence of hypertension)
435.9 Unspecified transient cerebral ischemia — (Use additional code to identify presence of hypertension) ▽
436 Acute, but ill-defined, cerebrovascular disease — (Use additional code to identify presence of hypertension) ▽
437.0 Cerebral atherosclerosis — (Use additional code to identify presence of hypertension)
437.1 Other generalized ischemic cerebrovascular disease — (Use additional code to identify presence of hypertension)
437.3 Cerebral aneurysm, nonruptured — (Use additional code to identify presence of hypertension)
437.8 Other ill-defined cerebrovascular disease — (Use additional code to identify presence of hypertension)
437.9 Unspecified cerebrovascular disease — (Use additional code to identify presence of hypertension) ▽
438.0 Cognitive deficits due to cerebrovascular disease — (Use additional code to identify presence of hypertension)
438.11 Aphasia due to cerebrovascular disease — (Use additional code to identify presence of hypertension)
438.19 Other speech and language deficits due to cerebrovascular disease — (Use additional code to identify presence of hypertension)
438.21 Hemiplegia affecting dominant side due to cerebrovascular disease — (Use additional code to identify presence of hypertension)
438.30 Monoplegia of upper limb affecting unspecified side due to cerebrovascular disease — (Use additional code to identify presence of hypertension) ▽
438.32 Monoplegia of upper limb affecting nondominant side due to cerebrovascular disease — (Use additional code to identify presence of hypertension)
438.41 Monoplegia of lower limb affecting dominant side due to cerebrovascular disease — (Use additional code to identify presence of hypertension)
438.50 Other paralytic syndrome affecting unspecified side due to cerebrovascular disease — (Use additional code to identify type of paralytic syndrome: 344.81, 344.00-344.09. Use additional code to identify presence of hypertension) ▽
438.52 Other paralytic syndrome affecting nondominant side due to cerebrovascular disease — (Use additional code to identify type of paralytic syndrome: 344.81, 344.00-344.09. Use additional code to identify presence of hypertension)
438.6 Alteration of sensations as late effect of cerebrovascular disease — (Use additional code to identify the altered sensation. Use additional code to identify presence of hypertension)
438.7 Disturbance of vision as late effect of cerebrovascular disease — (Use additional code to identify the visual disturbance. Use additional code to identify presence of hypertension)
438.82 Dysphagia due to cerebrovascular disease — (Use additional code to identify presence of hypertension)
438.83 Facial weakness as late effect of cerebrovascular disease — (Use additional code to identify presence of hypertension)
438.84 Ataxia as late effect of cerebrovascular disease — (Use additional code to identify presence of hypertension)
438.85 Vertigo as late effect of cerebrovascular disease — (Use additional code to identify presence of hypertension)
438.9 Unspecified late effects of cerebrovascular disease due to cerebrovascular disease — (Use additional code to identify presence of hypertension) ▽
440.0 Atherosclerosis of aorta
440.20 Atherosclerosis of native arteries of the extremities, unspecified ▽
440.22 Atherosclerosis of native arteries of the extremities with rest pain
440.8 Atherosclerosis of other specified arteries
440.9 Generalized and unspecified atherosclerosis ▽
442.81 Aneurysm of artery of neck
442.82 Aneurysm of subclavian artery
442.9 Other aneurysm of unspecified site ▽
443.21 Dissection of carotid artery
443.29 Dissection of other artery
443.89 Other peripheral vascular disease
443.9 Unspecified peripheral vascular disease ▽
444.21 Embolism and thrombosis of arteries of upper extremity
444.9 Embolism and thrombosis of unspecified artery ▽
445.01 Atheroembolism of upper extremity
445.89 Atheroembolism of other site
447.0 Arteriovenous fistula, acquired
447.1 Stricture of artery
447.2 Rupture of artery
447.6 Unspecified arteritis ▽
447.9 Unspecified disorders of arteries and arterioles ▽
459.9 Unspecified circulatory system disorder ▽
729.5 Pain in soft tissues of limb
729.81 Swelling of limb
742.4 Other specified congenital anomalies of brain
747.60 Congenital anomaly of the peripheral vascular system, unspecified site ▽
747.63 Congenital upper limb vessel anomaly
747.81 Congenital anomaly of cerebrovascular system
780.02 Transient alteration of awareness
780.03 Persistent vegetative state
780.09 Other alteration of consciousness
780.1 Hallucinations
780.2 Syncope and collapse
780.31 Febrile convulsions
780.39 Other convulsions
780.4 Dizziness and giddiness
780.6 Fever
780.79 Other malaise and fatigue
782.0 Disturbance of skin sensation
784.0 Headache
784.2 Swelling, mass, or lump in head and neck
784.3 Aphasia
785.9 Other symptoms involving cardiovascular system
786.50 Unspecified chest pain ▽
786.59 Other chest pain
786.6 Swelling, mass, or lump in chest
786.9 Other symptoms involving respiratory system and chest
793.0 Nonspecific abnormal findings on radiological and other examination of skull and head
793.2 Nonspecific abnormal findings on radiological and other examination of other intrathoracic organs
794.30 Nonspecific abnormal unspecified cardiovascular function study ▽
851.00 Cortex (cerebral) contusion without mention of open intracranial wound, state of consciousness unspecified ▽
851.01 Cortex (cerebral) contusion without mention of open intracranial wound, no loss of consciousness
851.02 Cortex (cerebral) contusion without mention of open intracranial wound, brief (less than 1 hour) loss of consciousness
851.03 Cortex (cerebral) contusion without mention of open intracranial wound, moderate (1-24 hours) loss of consciousness

▽ Unspecified code ♀ Female diagnosis ☒ Manifestation code ♂ Male diagnosis

851.04 Cortex (cerebral) contusion without mention of open intracranial wound, prolonged (more than 24 hours) loss of consciousness and return to pre-exisiting conscious level
851.05 Cortex (cerebral) contusion without mention of open intracranial wound, prolonged (more than 24 hours) loss of consciousness, without return to pre-existing conscious level
851.06 Cortex (cerebral) contusion without mention of open intracranial wound, loss of consciousness of unspecified duration
851.09 Cortex (cerebral) contusion without mention of open intracranial wound, unspecified concussion
851.10 Cortex (cerebral) contusion with open intracranial wound, unspecified state of consciousness
851.11 Cortex (cerebral) contusion with open intracranial wound, no loss of consciousness
851.12 Cortex (cerebral) contusion with open intracranial wound, brief (less than 1 hour) loss of consciousness
851.13 Cortex (cerebral) contusion with open intracranial wound, moderate (1-24 hours) loss of consciousness
851.14 Cortex (cerebral) contusion with open intracranial wound, prolonged (more than 24 hours) loss of consciousness and return to pre-existing conscious level
851.15 Cortex (cerebral) contusion with open intracranial wound, prolonged (more than 24 hours) loss of consciousness, without return to pre-existing conscious level
851.16 Cortex (cerebral) contusion with open intracranial wound, loss of consciousness of unspecified duration
851.19 Cortex (cerebral) contusion with open intracranial wound, unspecified concussion
851.20 Cortex (cerebral) laceration without mention of open intracranial wound, unspecified state of consciousness
851.21 Cortex (cerebral) laceration without mention of open intracranial wound, no loss of consciousness
851.22 Cortex (cerebral) laceration without mention of open intracranial wound, brief (less than 1 hour) loss of consciousness
851.23 Cortex (cerebral) laceration without mention of open intracranial wound, moderate (1-24 hours) loss of consciousness
851.24 Cortex (cerebral) laceration without mention of open intracranial wound, prolonged (more than 24 hours) loss of consciousness and return to pre-existing conscious level
851.25 Cortex (cerebral) laceration without mention of open intracranial wound, prolonged (more than 24 hours) loss of consciousness, without return to pre-existing conscious level
851.26 Cortex (cerebral) laceration without mention of open intracranial wound, loss of consciousness of unspecified duration
851.29 Cortex (cerebral) laceration without mention of open intracranial wound, unspecified concussion
851.30 Cortex (cerebral) laceration with open intracranial wound, unspecified state of consciousness
851.31 Cortex (cerebral) laceration with open intracranial wound, no loss of consciousness
851.32 Cortex (cerebral) laceration with open intracranial wound, brief (less than 1 hour) loss of consciousness
851.33 Cortex (cerebral) laceration with open intracranial wound, moderate (1-24 hours) loss of consciousness
851.34 Cortex (cerebral) laceration with open intracranial wound, prolonged (more than 24 hours) loss of consciousness and return to pre-existing conscious level
851.35 Cortex (cerebral) laceration with open intracranial wound, prolonged (more than 24 hours) loss of consciousness, without return to pre-existing conscious level
851.36 Cortex (cerebral) laceration with open intracranial wound, loss of consciousness of unspecified duration
851.39 Cortex (cerebral) laceration with open intracranial wound, unspecified concussion
851.40 Cerebellar or brain stem contusion without mention of open intracranial wound, unspecified state of consciousness
851.41 Cerebellar or brain stem contusion without mention of open intracranial wound, no loss of consciousness
851.42 Cerebellar or brain stem contusion without mention of open intracranial wound, brief (less than 1 hour) loss of consciousness
851.43 Cerebellar or brain stem contusion without mention of open intracranial wound, moderate (1-24 hours) loss of consciousness
851.44 Cerebellar or brain stem contusion without mention of open intracranial wound, prolonged (more than 24 hours) loss consciousness and return to pre-existing conscious level
851.45 Cerebellar or brain stem contusion without mention of open intracranial wound, prolonged (more than 24 hours) loss of consciousness, without return to pre-existing conscious level
851.46 Cerebellar or brain stem contusion without mention of open intracranial wound, loss of consciousness of unspecified duration
851.49 Cerebellar or brain stem contusion without mention of open intracranial wound, unspecified concussion
851.50 Cerebellar or brain stem contusion with open intracranial wound, unspecified state of consciousness
851.51 Cerebellar or brain stem contusion with open intracranial wound, no loss of consciousness
851.52 Cerebellar or brain stem contusion with open intracranial wound, brief (less than 1 hour) loss of consciousness
851.53 Cerebellar or brain stem contusion with open intracranial wound, moderate (1-24 hours) loss of consciousness
851.54 Cerebellar or brain stem contusion with open intracranial wound, prolonged (more than 24 hours) loss of consciousness and return to pre-existing conscious level
851.55 Cerebellar or brain stem contusion with open intracranial wound, prolonged (more than 24 hours) loss of consciousness, without return to pre-existing conscious level
851.56 Cerebellar or brain stem contusion with open intracranial wound, loss of consciousness of unspecified duration
851.59 Cerebellar or brain stem contusion with open intracranial wound, unspecified concussion
851.60 Cerebellar or brain stem laceration without mention of open intracranial wound, unspecified state of consciousness
851.61 Cerebellar or brain stem laceration without mention of open intracranial wound, no loss of consciousness
851.62 Cerebellar or brain stem laceration without mention of open intracranial wound, brief (less than 1 hour) loss of consciousness
851.63 Cerebellar or brain stem laceration without mention of open intracranial wound, moderate (1-24 hours) loss of consciousness
851.64 Cerebellar or brain stem laceration without mention of open intracranial wound, prolonged (more than 24 hours) loss of consciousness and return to pre-existing conscious leve
851.65 Cerebellar or brain stem laceration without mention of open intracranial wound, prolonged (more than 24 hours) loss of consciousness, without return to pre-existing conscious level
851.66 Cerebellar or brain stem laceration without mention of open intracranial wound, loss of consciousness of unspecified duration
851.69 Cerebellar or brain stem laceration without mention of open intracranial wound, unspecified concussion
851.70 Cerebellar or brain stem laceration with open intracranial wound, state of consciousness unspecified
851.71 Cerebellar or brain stem laceration with open intracranial wound, no loss of consciousness
851.72 Cerebellar or brain stem laceration with open intracranial wound, brief (less than one hour) loss of consciousness
851.73 Cerebellar or brain stem laceration with open intracranial wound, moderate (1-24 hours) loss of consciousness
851.74 Cerebellar or brain stem laceration with open intracranial wound, prolonged (more than 24 hours) loss of consciousness and return to pre-existing conscious level
851.75 Cerebellar or brain stem laceration with open intracranial wound, prolonged (more than 24 hours) loss of consciousness, without return to pre-existing conscious level
851.76 Cerebellar or brain stem laceration with open intracranial wound, loss of consciousness of unspecified duration
851.79 Cerebellar or brain stem laceration with open intracranial wound, unspecified concussion
851.80 Other and unspecified cerebral laceration and contusion, without mention of open intracranial wound, unspecified state of consciousness
851.81 Other and unspecified cerebral laceration and contusion, without mention of open intracranial wound, no loss of consciousness
851.82 Other and unspecified cerebral laceration and contusion, without mention of open intracranial wound, brief (less than 1 hour) loss of consciousness
851.83 Other and unspecified cerebral laceration and contusion, without mention of open intracranial wound, moderate (1-24 hours) loss of consciousness
851.84 Other and unspecified cerebral laceration and contusion, without mention of open intracranial wound, prolonged (more than 24 hours) loss of consciousness and return to preexisting conscious level
851.85 Other and unspecified cerebral laceration and contusion, without mention of open intracranial wound, prolonged (more than 24 hours) loss of consciousness, without return to pre-existing conscious level
851.86 Other and unspecified cerebral laceration and contusion, without mention of open intracranial wound, loss of consciousness of unspecified duration
851.89 Other and unspecified cerebral laceration and contusion, without mention of open intracranial wound, unspecified concussion

Unspecified code
♀ Female diagnosis
Manifestation code
♂ Male diagnosis

851.90 Other and unspecified cerebral laceration and contusion, with open intracranial wound, unspecified state of consciousness
851.91 Other and unspecified cerebral laceration and contusion, with open intracranial wound, no loss of consciousness
851.92 Other and unspecified cerebral laceration and contusion, with open intracranial wound, brief (less than 1 hour) loss of consciousness
851.93 Other and unspecified cerebral laceration and contusion, with open intracranial wound, moderate (1-24 hours) loss of consciousness
851.94 Other and unspecified cerebral laceration and contusion, with open intracranial wound, prolonged (more than 24 hours) loss of consciousness and return to pre-existing conscious level
851.95 Other and unspecified cerebral laceration and contusion, with open intracranial wound, prolonged (more than 24 hours) loss of consciousness, without return to pre-existing conscious level
851.96 Other and unspecified cerebral laceration and contusion, with open intracranial wound, loss of consciousness of unspecified duration
851.99 Other and unspecified cerebral laceration and contusion, with open intracranial wound, unspecified concussion
852.00 Subarachnoid hemorrhage following injury, without mention of open intracranial wound, unspecified state of consciousness
852.01 Subarachnoid hemorrhage following injury, without mention of open intracranial wound, no loss of consciousness
852.02 Subarachnoid hemorrhage following injury, without mention of open intracranial wound, brief (less than 1 hour) loss of consciousness
852.03 Subarachnoid hemorrhage following injury, without mention of open intracranial wound, moderate (1-24 hours) loss of consciousness
852.04 Subarachnoid hemorrhage following injury, without mention of open intracranial wound, prolonged (more than 24 hours) loss of consciousness and return to pre-existing conscious level
852.05 Subarachnoid hemorrhage following injury, without mention of open intracranial wound, prolonged (more than 24 hours) loss of consciousness, without return to pre-existing conscious level
852.06 Subarachnoid hemorrhage following injury, without mention of open intracranial wound, loss of consciousness of unspecified duration
852.09 Subarachnoid hemorrhage following injury, without mention of open intracranial wound, unspecified concussion
852.10 Subarachnoid hemorrhage following injury, with open intracranial wound, unspecified state of consciousness
852.11 Subarachnoid hemorrhage following injury, with open intracranial wound, no loss of consciousness
852.12 Subarachnoid hemorrhage following injury, with open intracranial wound, brief (less than 1 hour) loss of consciousness
852.13 Subarachnoid hemorrhage following injury, with open intracranial wound, moderate (1-24 hours) loss of consciousness
852.14 Subarachnoid hemorrhage following injury, with open intracranial wound, prolonged (more than 24 hours) loss of consciousness and return to pre-existing conscious level
852.15 Subarachnoid hemorrhage following injury, with open intracranial wound, prolonged (more than 24 hours) loss of consciousness, without return to pre-existing conscious level
852.16 Subarachnoid hemorrhage following injury, with open intracranial wound, loss of consciousness of unspecified duration
852.19 Subarachnoid hemorrhage following injury, with open intracranial wound, unspecified concussion
852.20 Subdural hemorrhage following injury, without mention of open intracranial wound, unspecified state of consciousness
852.21 Subdural hemorrhage following injury, without mention of open intracranial wound, no loss of consciousness
852.22 Subdural hemorrhage following injury, without mention of open intracranial wound, brief (less than one hour) loss of consciousness
852.23 Subdural hemorrhage following injury, without mention of open intracranial wound, moderate (1-24 hours) loss of consciousness
852.24 Subdural hemorrhage following injury, without mention of open intracranial wound, prolonged (more than 24 hours) loss of consciousness and return to pre-existing conscious level
852.25 Subdural hemorrhage following injury, without mention of open intracranial wound, prolonged (more than 24 hours) loss of consciousness, without return to pre-existing conscious level
852.26 Subdural hemorrhage following injury, without mention of open intracranial wound, loss of consciousness of unspecified duration
852.29 Subdural hemorrhage following injury, without mention of open intracranial wound, unspecified concussion
852.30 Subdural hemorrhage following injury, with open intracranial wound, state of consciousness unspecified
852.31 Subdural hemorrhage following injury, with open intracranial wound, no loss of consciousness
852.32 Subdural hemorrhage following injury, with open intracranial wound, brief (less than 1 hour) loss of consciousness
852.33 Subdural hemorrhage following injury, with open intracranial wound, moderate (1-24 hours) loss of consciousness
852.34 Subdural hemorrhage following injury, with open intracranial wound, prolonged (more than 24 hours) loss of consciousness and return to pre-existing conscious level
852.35 Subdural hemorrhage following injury, with open intracranial wound, prolonged (more than 24 hours) loss of consciousness, without return to pre-existing conscious level
852.36 Subdural hemorrhage following injury, with open intracranial wound, loss of consciousness of unspecified duration
852.39 Subdural hemorrhage following injury, with open intracranial wound, unspecified concussion
852.40 Extradural hemorrhage following injury, without mention of open intracranial wound, unspecified state of consciousness
852.41 Extradural hemorrhage following injury, without mention of open intracranial wound, no loss of consciousness
852.42 Extradural hemorrhage following injury, without mention of open intracranial wound, brief (less than 1 hour) loss of consciousness
852.43 Extradural hemorrhage following injury, without mention of open intracranial wound, moderate (1-24 hours) loss of consciousness
852.44 Extradural hemorrhage following injury, without mention of open intracranial wound, prolonged (more than 24 hours) loss of consciousness and return to pre-existing conscious level
852.45 Extradural hemorrhage following injury, without mention of open intracranial wound, prolonged (more than 24 hours) loss of consciousness, without return to pre-existing conscious level
852.46 Extradural hemorrhage following injury, without mention of open intracranial wound, loss of consciousness of unspecified duration
852.49 Extradural hemorrhage following injury, without mention of open intracranial wound, unspecified concussion
852.50 Extradural hemorrhage following injury, with open intracranial wound, state of consciousness unspecified
852.51 Extradural hemorrhage following injury, with open intracranial wound, no loss of consciousness
852.52 Extradural hemorrhage following injury, with open intracranial wound, brief (less than 1 hour) loss of consciousness
852.53 Extradural hemorrhage following injury, with open intracranial wound, moderate (1-24 hours) loss of consciousness
852.54 Extradural hemorrhage following injury, with open intracranial wound, prolonged (more than 24 hours) loss of consciousness and return to pre-existing conscious level
852.55 Extradural hemorrhage following injury, with open intracranial wound, prolonged (more than 24 hours) loss of consciousness, without return to pre-existing conscious level
852.56 Extradural hemorrhage following injury, with open intracranial wound, loss of consciousness of unspecified duration
852.59 Extradural hemorrhage following injury, with open intracranial wound, unspecifiedconcussion
853.00 Other and unspecified intracranial hemorrhage following injury, without mention of open intracranial wound, unspecified state of consciousness
853.01 Other and unspecified intracranial hemorrhage following injury, without mention of open intracranial wound, no loss of consciousness
853.02 Other and unspecified intracranial hemorrhage following injury, without mention of open intracranial wound, brief (less than 1 hour) loss of consciousness
853.03 Other and unspecified intracranial hemorrhage following injury, without mention of open intracranial wound, moderate (1-24 hours) loss of consciousness
853.04 Other and unspecified intracranial hemorrhage following injury, without mention of open intracranial wound, prolonged (more than 24 hours) loss of consciousness and return to preexisting conscious level
853.05 Other and unspecified intracranial hemorrhage following injury. Without mention of open intracranial wound, prolonged (more than 24 hours) loss of consciousness, without return to pre-existing conscious level
853.06 Other and unspecified intracranial hemorrhage following injury, without mention of open intracranial wound, loss of consciousness of unspecified duration
853.09 Other and unspecified intracranial hemorrhage following injury, without mention of open intracranial wound, unspecified concussion
853.10 Other and unspecified intracranial hemorrhage following injury, with open intracranial wound, unspecified state of consciousness
853.11 Other and unspecified intracranial hemorrhage following injury, with open intracranial wound, no loss of consciousness

Unspecified code
♀ Female diagnosis
Manifestation code
♂ Male diagnosis

853.12 Other and unspecified intracranial hemorrhage following injury, with open intracranial wound, brief (less than 1 hour) loss of consciousness
853.13 Other and unspecified intracranial hemorrhage following injury, with open intracranial wound, moderate (1-24 hours) loss of consciousness
853.14 Other and unspecified intracranial hemorrhage following injury, with open intracranial wound, prolonged (more than 24 hours) loss of consciousness and return to pre-existing conscious level
853.15 Other and unspecified intracranial hemorrhage following injury, with open intracranial wound, prolonged (more than 24 hours) loss of consciousness, without return to pre-existing conscious level
853.16 Other and unspecified intracranial hemorrhage following injury, with open intracranial wound, loss of consciousness of unspecified duration ▽
853.19 Other and unspecified intracranial hemorrhage following injury, with open intracranial wound, unspecified concussion ▽
854.00 Intracranial injury of other and unspecified nature, without mention of open intracranial wound, unspecified state of consciousness ▽
854.01 Intracranial injury of other and unspecified nature, without mention of open intracranial wound, no loss of consciousness
854.02 Intracranial injury of other and unspecified nature, without mention of open intracranial wound, brief (less than 1 hour) loss of consciousness
854.03 Intracranial injury of other and unspecified nature, without mention of open intracranial wound, moderate (1-24 hours) loss of consciousness
854.04 Intracranial injury of other and unspecified nature, without mention of open intracranial wound, prolonged (more than 24 hours) loss of consciousness and return to pre-existing conscious level
854.05 Intracranial injury of other and unspecified nature, without mention of open intracranial wound, prolonged (more than 24 hours) loss of consciousness, without return to pre-existing conscious level
854.06 Intracranial injury of other and unspecified nature, without mention of open intracranial wound, loss of consciousness of unspecified duration ▽
854.09 Intracranial injury of other and unspecified nature, without mention of open intracranial wound, unspecified concussion ▽
854.10 Intracranial injury of other and unspecified nature, with open intracranial wound, unspecified state of consciousness ▽
854.11 Intracranial injury of other and unspecified nature, with open intracranial wound, no loss of consciousness
854.12 Intracranial injury of other and unspecified nature, with open intracranial wound, brief (less than 1 hour) loss of consciousness
854.13 Intracranial injury of other and unspecified nature, with open intracranial wound, moderate (1-24 hours) loss of consciousness
854.14 Intracranial injury of other and unspecified nature, with open intracranial wound, prolonged (more than 24 hours) loss of consciousness and return to pre-existing conscious level
854.15 Intracranial injury of other and unspecified nature, with open intracranial wound, prolonged (more than 24 hours) loss of consciousness, without return to pre-existing conscious level
854.16 Intracranial injury of other and unspecified nature, with open intracranial wound, loss of consciousness of unspecified duration ▽
854.19 Intracranial injury of other and unspecified nature, with open intracranial wound, with unspecified concussion ▽
V72.5 Radiological examination, not elsewhere classified — (Use additional code(s) to identify any special screening examination(s) performed: V73.0-V82.9)

ICD-9-CM Procedural

38.91 Arterial catheterization

36245–36248

36245 Selective catheter placement, arterial system; each first order abdominal, pelvic, or lower extremity artery branch, within a vascular family
36246 initial second order abdominal, pelvic, or lower extremity artery branch, within a vascular family
36247 initial third order or more selective abdominal, pelvic, or lower extremity artery branch, within a vascular family
36248 additional second order, third order, and beyond, abdominal, pelvic, or lower extremity artery branch, within a vascular family (List in addition to code for initial second or third order vessel as appropriate)

ICD-9-CM Diagnostic

153.9 Malignant neoplasm of colon, unspecified site ▽
154.0 Malignant neoplasm of rectosigmoid junction
155.0 Malignant neoplasm of liver, primary
155.1 Malignant neoplasm of intrahepatic bile ducts
155.2 Malignant neoplasm of liver, not specified as primary or secondary ▽
157.9 Malignant neoplasm of pancreas, part unspecified ▽
195.2 Malignant neoplasm of abdomen
195.3 Malignant neoplasm of pelvis
195.5 Malignant neoplasm of lower limb
195.8 Malignant neoplasm of other specified sites
197.7 Secondary malignant neoplasm of liver
199.0 Disseminated malignant neoplasm
199.1 Other malignant neoplasm of unspecified site
211.7 Benign neoplasm of islets of Langerhans — (Use additional code to identify any functional activity)
228.04 Hemangioma of intra-abdominal structures
235.3 Neoplasm of uncertain behavior of liver and biliary passages
250.70 Diabetes with peripheral circulatory disorders, type II or unspecified type, not stated as uncontrolled — (Use additional code to identify manifestation: 443.81, 785.4)
250.71 Diabetes with peripheral circulatory disorders, type I [juvenile type], not stated as uncontrolled — (Use additional code to identify manifestation: 443.81, 785.4)
250.72 Diabetes with peripheral circulatory disorders, type II or unspecified type, uncontrolled — (Use additional code to identify manifestation: 443.81, 785.4)
250.73 Diabetes with peripheral circulatory disorders, type I [juvenile type], uncontrolled — (Use additional code to identify manifestation: 443.81, 785.4)
440.1 Atherosclerosis of renal artery
440.20 Atherosclerosis of native arteries of the extremities, unspecified ▽
440.21 Atherosclerosis of native arteries of the extremities with intermittent claudication
440.22 Atherosclerosis of native arteries of the extremities with rest pain
440.23 Atherosclerosis of native arteries of the extremities with ulceration — (Use additional code for any associated ulceration: 707.10-707.9)
440.24 Atherosclerosis of native arteries of the extremities with gangrene
440.29 Other atherosclerosis of native arteries of the extremities
440.30 Atheroslerosis of unspecified bypass graft of extremities ▽
440.31 Atheroslerosis of autologous vein bypass graft of extremities
440.32 Atheroslerosis of nonautologous biological bypass graft of extremities
440.8 Atherosclerosis of other specified arteries
440.9 Generalized and unspecified atherosclerosis ▽
441.4 Abdominal aneurysm without mention of rupture
442.0 Aneurysm of artery of upper extremity
442.1 Aneurysm of renal artery
442.2 Aneurysm of iliac artery
442.3 Aneurysm of artery of lower extremity
442.89 Aneurysm of other specified artery
442.9 Other aneurysm of unspecified site ▽
443.22 Dissection of iliac artery
443.23 Dissection of renal artery
443.29 Dissection of other artery
443.81 Peripheral angiopathy in diseases classified elsewhere — (Code first underlying disease, 250.7) ☒
443.9 Unspecified peripheral vascular disease ▽
444.22 Embolism and thrombosis of arteries of lower extremity
444.81 Embolism and thrombosis of iliac artery
444.89 Embolism and thrombosis of other specified artery
444.9 Embolism and thrombosis of unspecified artery ▽
445.02 Atheroembolism of lower extremity
445.81 Atheroembolism of kidney — (Use additional code for any associated kidney failure: 584, 585)
445.89 Atheroembolism of other site
447.0 Arteriovenous fistula, acquired
447.1 Stricture of artery
447.9 Unspecified disorders of arteries and arterioles ▽
459.9 Unspecified circulatory system disorder ▽
593.81 Vascular disorders of kidney
729.5 Pain in soft tissues of limb
747.60 Congenital anomaly of the peripheral vascular system, unspecified site ▽
747.64 Congenital lower limb vessel anomaly
747.89 Other specified congenital anomaly of circulatory system
780.71 Chronic fatigue syndrome
780.79 Other malaise and fatigue
782.0 Disturbance of skin sensation
782.4 Jaundice, unspecified, not of newborn ▽
785.4 Gangrene — (Code first any associated underlying condition:250.7, 443.0)
785.9 Other symptoms involving cardiovascular system
789.00 Abdominal pain, unspecified site ▽
789.01 Abdominal pain, right upper quadrant
789.02 Abdominal pain, left upper quadrant
789.03 Abdominal pain, right lower quadrant
789.04 Abdominal pain, left lower quadrant
789.05 Abdominal pain, periumbilic
789.06 Abdominal pain, epigastric

▽ Unspecified code ♀ Female diagnosis ☒ Manifestation code ♂ Male diagnosis

789.07 Abdominal pain, generalized
789.09 Abdominal pain, other specified site
789.30 Abdominal or pelvic swelling, mass or lump, unspecified site
789.31 Abdominal or pelvic swelling, mass, or lump, right upper quadrant
789.32 Abdominal or pelvic swelling, mass, or lump, left upper quadrant
789.33 Abdominal or pelvic swelling, mass, or lump, right lower quadrant
789.34 Abdominal or pelvic swelling, mass, or lump, left lower quadrant
789.35 Abdominal or pelvic swelling, mass or lump, periumbilic
789.36 Abdominal or pelvic swelling, mass, or lump, epigastric
789.37 Abdominal or pelvic swelling, mass, or lump, epigastric, generalized
789.39 Abdominal or pelvic swelling, mass, or lump, other specified site
794.30 Nonspecific abnormal unspecified cardiovascular function study
904.0 Common femoral artery injury
904.1 Superficial femoral artery injury
904.2 Femoral vein injury
904.3 Saphenous vein injury
904.41 Popliteal artery injury
904.42 Popliteal vein injury
904.51 Anterior tibial artery injury
904.52 Anterior tibial vein injury
904.53 Posterior tibial artery injury
904.54 Posterior tibial vein injury
904.6 Deep plantar blood vessels injury
904.7 Injury to specified blood vessels of lower extremity, other
904.8 Injury to unspecified blood vessel of lower extremity
904.9 Injury to blood vessels, unspecified site
906.4 Late effect of crushing
928.00 Crushing injury of thigh — (Use additional code to identify any associated injuries: 800-829, 850.0-854.1, 860.0-869.1)
928.01 Crushing injury of hip — (Use additional code to identify any associated injuries: 800-829, 850.0-854.1, 860.0-869.1)
928.10 Crushing injury of lower leg — (Use additional code to identify any associated injuries: 800-829, 850.0-854.1, 860.0-869.1)
928.11 Crushing injury of knee — (Use additional code to identify any associated injuries: 800-829, 850.0-854.1, 860.0-869.1)
928.20 Crushing injury of foot — (Use additional code to identify any associated injuries: 800-829, 850.0-854.1, 860.0-869.1)
928.21 Crushing injury of ankle — (Use additional code to identify any associated injuries: 800-829, 850.0-854.1, 860.0-869.1)
928.3 Crushing injury of toe(s) — (Use additional code to identify any associated injuries: 800-829, 850.0-854.1, 860.0-869.1)
928.8 Crushing injury of multiple sites of lower limb — (Use additional code to identify any associated injuries: 800-829, 850.0-854.1, 860.0-869.1)
928.9 Crushing injury of unspecified site of lower limb — (Use additional code to identify any associated injuries: 800-829, 850.0-854.1, 860.0-869.1)
929.0 Crushing injury of multiple sites, not elsewhere classified — (Use additional code to identify any associated injuries: 800-829, 850.0-854.1, 860.0-869.1)
929.9 Crushing injury of unspecified site — (Use additional code to identify any associated injuries: 800-829, 850.0-854.1, 860.0-869.1)
996.73 Other complications due to renal dialysis device, implant, and graft
996.95 Complications of reattached foot and toe(s)
996.96 Complications of reattached lower extremity, other and unspecified
996.99 Complications of other specified reattached body part
997.2 Peripheral vascular complications — (Use additional code to identify complications)
998.6 Persistent postoperative fistula, not elsewhere classified
999.2 Other vascular complications of medical care, not elsewhere classified
V72.5 Radiological examination, not elsewhere classified — (Use additional code(s) to identify any special screening examination(s) performed: V73.0-V82.9)
V82.89 Special screening for other specified conditions

ICD-9-CM Procedural

38.91 Arterial catheterization

36260–36262

36260 Insertion of implantable intra-arterial infusion pump (eg, for chemotherapy of liver)
36261 Revision of implanted intra-arterial infusion pump
36262 Removal of implanted intra-arterial infusion pump

ICD-9-CM Diagnostic

155.0 Malignant neoplasm of liver, primary
155.1 Malignant neoplasm of intrahepatic bile ducts
159.1 Malignant neoplasm of spleen, not elsewhere classified
159.8 Malignant neoplasm of other sites of digestive system and intra-abdominal organs
159.9 Malignant neoplasm of ill-defined sites of digestive organs and peritoneum
171.4 Malignant neoplasm of connective and other soft tissue of thorax
197.7 Secondary malignant neoplasm of liver
197.8 Secondary malignant neoplasm of other digestive organs and spleen
230.7 Carcinoma in situ of other and unspecified parts of intestine
230.8 Carcinoma in situ of liver and biliary system
230.9 Carcinoma in situ of other and unspecified digestive organs
235.3 Neoplasm of uncertain behavior of liver and biliary passages
235.5 Neoplasm of uncertain behavior of other and unspecified digestive organs
996.1 Mechanical complication of other vascular device, implant, and graft
996.62 Infection and inflammatory reaction due to other vascular device, implant, and graft — (Use additional code to identify specified infections)
996.74 Other complications due to other vascular device, implant, and graft
V58.81 Fitting and adjustment of vascular catheter

ICD-9-CM Procedural

38.91 Arterial catheterization
39.59 Other repair of vessel
86.06 Insertion of totally implantable infusion pump
86.09 Other incision of skin and subcutaneous tissue

36400–36405

36400 Venipuncture, under age 3 years, necessitating physicians skill, not to be used for routine venipuncture; femoral or jugular vein
36405 scalp vein

ICD-9-CM Diagnostic

The application of this code is too broad to adequately present ICD-9-CM diagnostic code links here. Refer to your ICD-9-CM book.

ICD-9-CM Procedural

38.99 Other puncture of vein

36406

36406 Venipuncture, under age 3 years, necessitating physician's skill, not to be used for routine venipuncture; other vein

ICD-9-CM Diagnostic

The application of this code is too broad to adequately present ICD-9-CM diagnostic code links here. Refer to your ICD-9-CM book.

ICD-9-CM Procedural

38.99 Other puncture of vein

36410

36410 Venipuncture, age 3 years or older, necessitating physician's skill (separate procedure), for diagnostic or therapeutic purposes (not to be used for routine venipuncture)

ICD-9-CM Diagnostic

The application of this code is too broad to adequately present ICD-9-CM diagnostic code links here. Refer to your ICD-9-CM book.

ICD-9-CM Procedural

38.99 Other puncture of vein

36415–36416

36415 Collection of venous blood by venipuncture
36416 Collection of capillary blood specimen (eg, finger, heel, ear stick)

ICD-9-CM Diagnostic

The application of this code is too broad to adequately present ICD-9-CM diagnostic code links here. Refer to your ICD-9-CM book.

ICD-9-CM Procedural

38.99 Other puncture of vein

36420–36425

36420 Venipuncture, cutdown; under age 1 year
36425 age 1 or over

ICD-9-CM Diagnostic

The application of this code is too broad to adequately present ICD-9-CM diagnostic code links here. Refer to your ICD-9-CM book.

ICD-9-CM Procedural

38.94 Venous cutdown

36430

36430 Transfusion, blood or blood components

ICD-9-CM Diagnostic

The application of this code is too broad to adequately present ICD-9-CM diagnostic code links here. Refer to your ICD-9-CM book.

ICD-9-CM Procedural

99.02 Transfusion of previously collected autologous blood
99.03 Other transfusion of whole blood
99.04 Transfusion of packed cells
99.05 Transfusion of platelets
99.07 Transfusion of other serum

HCPCS Level II Supplies & Services

A4750 Blood tubing, arterial or venous, for hemodialysis, each
P9010 Blood (whole), for transfusion, per unit
P9011 Blood (split unit), specify amount
P9012 Cryoprecipitate, each unit
P9016 Red blood cells, leukocytes reduced, each unit

36440

36440 Push transfusion, blood, 2 years or under

ICD-9-CM Diagnostic

The application of this code is too broad to adequately present ICD-9-CM diagnostic code links here. Refer to your ICD-9-CM book.

ICD-9-CM Procedural

99.03 Other transfusion of whole blood
99.04 Transfusion of packed cells
99.05 Transfusion of platelets
99.06 Transfusion of coagulation factors
99.07 Transfusion of other serum
99.08 Transfusion of blood expander

HCPCS Level II Supplies & Services

A4750 Blood tubing, arterial or venous, for hemodialysis, each
P9010 Blood (whole), for transfusion, per unit
P9011 Blood (split unit), specify amount

36450–36455

36450 Exchange transfusion, blood; newborn
36455 other than newborn

ICD-9-CM Diagnostic

The application of this code is too broad to adequately present ICD-9-CM diagnostic code links here. Refer to your ICD-9-CM book.

ICD-9-CM Procedural

99.01 Exchange transfusion

HCPCS Level II Supplies & Services

A4750 Blood tubing, arterial or venous, for hemodialysis, each
P9021 Red blood cells, each unit
P9022 Red blood cells, washed, each unit

36460

36460 Transfusion, intrauterine, fetal

ICD-9-CM Diagnostic

The application of this code is too broad to adequately present ICD-9-CM diagnostic code links here. Refer to your ICD-9-CM book.

ICD-9-CM Procedural

75.2 Intrauterine transfusion

36468

36468 Single or multiple injections of sclerosing solutions, spider veins (telangiectasia); limb or trunk

ICD-9-CM Diagnostic

448.0 Hereditary hemorrhagic telangiectasia
448.9 Other and unspecified capillary diseases ▽
V50.1 Other plastic surgery for unacceptable cosmetic appearance

ICD-9-CM Procedural

39.92 Injection of sclerosing agent into vein

HCPCS Level II Supplies & Services

A4550 Surgical trays
J7130 Hypertonic saline solution, 50 or 100 mEq, 20 cc vial

36469

36469 Single or multiple injections of sclerosing solutions, spider veins (telangiectasia); face

ICD-9-CM Diagnostic

448.0 Hereditary hemorrhagic telangiectasia
448.1 Nevus, non-neoplastic
448.9 Other and unspecified capillary diseases ▽
V50.1 Other plastic surgery for unacceptable cosmetic appearance

ICD-9-CM Procedural

39.92 Injection of sclerosing agent into vein

HCPCS Level II Supplies & Services

A4550 Surgical trays
J7130 Hypertonic saline solution, 50 or 100 mEq, 20 cc vial

36470–36471

36470 Injection of sclerosing solution; single vein
36471 multiple veins, same leg

ICD-9-CM Diagnostic

448.9 Other and unspecified capillary diseases ▽
454.0 Varicose veins of lower extremities with ulcer
454.1 Varicose veins of lower extremities with inflammation
454.2 Varicose veins of lower extremities with ulcer and inflammation
454.8 Varicose veins of the lower extremities with other complications
454.9 Asymptomatic varicose veins
459.10 Postphlebitic syndrome without complications
459.11 Postphlebitic syndrome with ulcer
459.12 Postphlebitic syndrome with inflammation
459.13 Postphlebitic syndrome with ulcer and inflammation
459.19 Postphlebitic syndrome with other complication
459.81 Unspecified venous (peripheral) insufficiency — (Use additional code for any associated ulceration: 707.10-707.9) ▽
459.9 Unspecified circulatory system disorder ▽
729.5 Pain in soft tissues of limb
729.81 Swelling of limb
782.3 Edema
V50.1 Other plastic surgery for unacceptable cosmetic appearance

ICD-9-CM Procedural

39.92 Injection of sclerosing agent into vein

HCPCS Level II Supplies & Services

A4550 Surgical trays
J7130 Hypertonic saline solution, 50 or 100 mEq, 20 cc vial

36475–36476

36475 Endovenous ablation therapy of incompetent vein, extremity, inclusive of all imaging guidance and monitoring, percutaneous, radiofrequency; first vein treated
36476 second and subsequent veins treated in a single extremity, each through separate access sites (List separately in addition to code for primary procedure)

ICD-9-CM Diagnostic

454.0 Varicose veins of lower extremities with ulcer
454.1 Varicose veins of lower extremities with inflammation
454.2 Varicose veins of lower extremities with ulcer and inflammation

▽ Unspecified code
♀ Female diagnosis
☒ Manifestation code
♂ Male diagnosis

454.8 Varicose veins of the lower extremities with other complications
454.9 Asymptomatic varicose veins

ICD-9-CM Procedural

38.83 Other surgical occlusion of upper limb vessels
38.89 Other surgical occlusion of lower limb veins

36478–36479

36478 Endovenous ablation therapy of incompetent vein, extremity, inclusive of all imaging guidance and monitoring, percutaneous, laser; first vein treated
36479 second and subsequent veins treated in a single extremity, each through separate access sites (List separately in addition to code for primary procedure)

ICD-9-CM Diagnostic

454.0 Varicose veins of lower extremities with ulcer
454.1 Varicose veins of lower extremities with inflammation
454.2 Varicose veins of lower extremities with ulcer and inflammation
454.8 Varicose veins of the lower extremities with other complications
454.9 Asymptomatic varicose veins

ICD-9-CM Procedural

38.83 Other surgical occlusion of upper limb vessels
38.89 Other surgical occlusion of lower limb veins

36481

36481 Percutaneous portal vein catheterization by any method

ICD-9-CM Diagnostic

The application of this code is too broad to adequately present ICD-9-CM diagnostic code links here. Refer to your ICD-9-CM book.

ICD-9-CM Procedural

38.93 Venous catheterization, not elsewhere classified

36500

36500 Venous catheterization for selective organ blood sampling

ICD-9-CM Diagnostic

The application of this code is too broad to adequately present ICD-9-CM diagnostic code links here. Refer to your ICD-9-CM book.

ICD-9-CM Procedural

38.93 Venous catheterization, not elsewhere classified
39.93 Insertion of vessel-to-vessel cannula

HCPCS Level II Supplies & Services

A4649 Surgical supply; miscellaneous

36510

36510 Catheterization of umbilical vein for diagnosis or therapy, newborn

ICD-9-CM Diagnostic

The application of this code is too broad to adequately present ICD-9-CM diagnostic code links here. Refer to your ICD-9-CM book.

ICD-9-CM Procedural

38.92 Umbilical vein catheterization

36511–36516

36511 Therapeutic apheresis; for white blood cells
36512 for red blood cells
36513 for platelets
36514 for plasma pheresis
36515 with extracorporeal immunoadsorption and plasma reinfusion
36516 with extracorporeal selective adsorption or selective filtration and plasma reinfusion

ICD-9-CM Diagnostic

170.0 Malignant neoplasm of bones of skull and face, except mandible
170.1 Malignant neoplasm of mandible
170.2 Malignant neoplasm of vertebral column, excluding sacrum and coccyx
170.3 Malignant neoplasm of ribs, sternum, and clavicle
170.4 Malignant neoplasm of scapula and long bones of upper limb
170.5 Malignant neoplasm of short bones of upper limb
170.6 Malignant neoplasm of pelvic bones, sacrum, and coccyx
170.7 Malignant neoplasm of long bones of lower limb
170.8 Malignant neoplasm of short bones of lower limb
170.9 Malignant neoplasm of bone and articular cartilage, site unspecified ▽
174.0 Malignant neoplasm of nipple and areola of female breast ♀
174.1 Malignant neoplasm of central portion of female breast ♀
174.2 Malignant neoplasm of upper-inner quadrant of female breast ♀
174.3 Malignant neoplasm of lower-inner quadrant of female breast ♀
174.4 Malignant neoplasm of upper-outer quadrant of female breast ♀
174.5 Malignant neoplasm of lower-outer quadrant of female breast ♀
174.6 Malignant neoplasm of axillary tail of female breast ♀
174.8 Malignant neoplasm of other specified sites of female breast ♀
174.9 Malignant neoplasm of breast (female), unspecified site ▽ ♀
183.0 Malignant neoplasm of ovary — (Use additional code to identify any functional activity) ♀
194.0 Malignant neoplasm of adrenal gland — (Use additional code to identify any functional activity)
194.4 Malignant neoplasm of pineal gland — (Use additional code to identify any functional activity)
200.10 Lymphosarcoma, unspecified site, extranodal and solid organ sites ▽
200.11 Lymphosarcoma of lymph nodes of head, face, and neck
200.12 Lymphosarcoma of intrathoracic lymph nodes
200.13 Lymphosarcoma of intra-abdominal lymph nodes
200.14 Lymphosarcoma of lymph nodes of axilla and upper limb
200.15 Lymphosarcoma of lymph nodes of inguinal region and lower limb
200.16 Lymphosarcoma of intrapelvic lymph nodes
200.17 Lymphosarcoma of spleen
200.18 Lymphosarcoma of lymph nodes of multiple sites
201.00 Hodgkin's paragranuloma, unspecified site, extranodal and solid organ sites ▽
201.01 Hodgkin's paragranuloma of lymph nodes of head, face, and neck
201.02 Hodgkin's paragranuloma of intrathoracic lymph nodes
201.03 Hodgkin's paragranuloma of intra-abdominal lymph nodes
201.04 Hodgkin's paragranuloma of lymph nodes of axilla and upper limb
201.05 Hodgkin's paragranuloma of lymph nodes of inguinal region and lower limb
201.06 Hodgkin's paragranuloma of intrapelvic lymph nodes
201.07 Hodgkin's paragranuloma of spleen
201.08 Hodgkin's paragranuloma of lymph nodes of multiple sites
201.10 Hodgkin's granuloma, unspecified site, extranodal and solid organ sites ▽
201.11 Hodgkin's granuloma of lymph nodes of head, face, and neck
201.12 Hodgkin's granuloma of intrathoracic lymph nodes
201.13 Hodgkin's granuloma of intra-abdominal lymph nodes
201.14 Hodgkin's granuloma of lymph nodes of axilla and upper limb
201.15 Hodgkin's granuloma of lymph nodes of inguinal region and lower limb
201.16 Hodgkin's granuloma of intrapelvic lymph nodes
201.17 Hodgkin's granuloma of spleen
201.18 Hodgkin's granuloma of lymph nodes of multiple sites
201.20 Hodgkin's sarcoma, unspecified site, extranodal and solid organ sites ▽
201.21 Hodgkin's sarcoma of lymph nodes of head, face, and neck
201.22 Hodgkin's sarcoma of intrathoracic lymph nodes
201.23 Hodgkin's sarcoma of intra-abdominal lymph nodes
201.24 Hodgkin's sarcoma of lymph nodes of axilla and upper limb
201.25 Hodgkin's sarcoma of lymph nodes of inguinal region and lower limb
201.26 Hodgkin's sarcoma of intrapelvic lymph nodes
201.27 Hodgkin's sarcoma of spleen
201.28 Hodgkin's sarcoma of lymph nodes of multiple sites
201.40 Hodgkin's disease, lymphocytic-histiocytic predominance, unspecified site, extranodal and solid organ sites ▽
201.41 Hodgkin's disease, lymphocytic-histiocytic predominance of lymph nodes of head, face, and neck
201.42 Hodgkin's disease, lymphocytic-histiocytic predominance of intrathoracic lymph nodes
201.43 Hodgkin's disease, lymphocytic-histiocytic predominance of intra-abdominal lymph nodes
201.44 Hodgkin's disease, lymphocytic-histiocytic predominance of lymph nodes of axilla and upper limb
201.45 Hodgkin's disease, lymphocytic-histiocytic predominance of lymph nodes of inguinal region and lower limb
201.46 Hodgkin's disease, lymphocytic-histiocytic predominance of intrapelvic lymph nodes
201.47 Hodgkin's disease, lymphocytic-histiocytic predominance of spleen
201.48 Hodgkin's disease, lymphocytic-histiocytic predominance of lymph nodes of multiple sites
201.50 Hodgkin's disease, nodular sclerosis, unspecified site, extranodal and solid organ sites ▽
201.51 Hodgkin's disease, nodular sclerosis, of lymph nodes of head, face, and neck
201.52 Hodgkin's disease, nodular sclerosis, of intrathoracic lymph nodes

201.53 Hodgkin's disease, nodular sclerosis, of intra-abdominal lymph nodes
201.54 Hodgkin's disease, nodular sclerosis, of lymph nodes of axilla and upper limb
201.55 Hodgkin's disease, nodular sclerosis, of lymph nodes of inguinal region and lower limb
201.56 Hodgkin's disease, nodular sclerosis, of intrapelvic lymph nodes
201.57 Hodgkin's disease, nodular sclerosis, of spleen
201.58 Hodgkin's disease, nodular sclerosis, of lymph nodes of multiple sites
201.60 Hodgkin's disease, mixed cellularity, unspecified site, extranodal and solid organ sites
201.61 Hodgkin's disease, mixed cellularity, involving lymph nodes of head, face, and neck
201.62 Hodgkin's disease, mixed cellularity, of intrathoracic lymph nodes
201.63 Hodgkin's disease, mixed cellularity, of intra-abdominal lymph nodes
201.64 Hodgkin's disease, mixed cellularity, of lymph nodes of axilla and upper limb
201.65 Hodgkin's disease, mixed cellularity, of lymph nodes of inguinal region and lower limb
201.66 Hodgkin's disease, mixed cellularity, of intrapelvic lymph nodes
201.67 Hodgkin's disease, mixed cellularity, of spleen
201.68 Hodgkin's disease, mixed cellularity, of lymph nodes of multiple sites
201.70 Hodgkin's disease, lymphocytic depletion, unspecified site, extranodal and solid organ sites
201.71 Hodgkin's disease, lymphocytic depletion, of lymph nodes of head, face, and neck
201.72 Hodgkin's disease, lymphocytic depletion, of intrathoracic lymph nodes
201.73 Hodgkin's disease, lymphocytic depletion, of intra-abdominal lymph nodes
201.74 Hodgkin's disease, lymphocytic depletion, of lymph nodes of axilla and upper limb
201.75 Hodgkin's disease, lymphocytic depletion, of lymph nodes of inguinal region and lower limb
201.76 Hodgkin's disease, lymphocytic depletion, of intrapelvic lymph nodes
201.77 Hodgkin's disease, lymphocytic depletion, of spleen
201.78 Hodgkin's disease, lymphocytic depletion, of lymph nodes of multiple sites
201.90 Hodgkin's disease, unspecified type, unspecified site, extranodal and solid organ sites
201.91 Hodgkin's disease, unspecified type, of lymph nodes of head, face, and neck
201.92 Hodgkin's disease, unspecified type, of intrathoracic lymph nodes
201.93 Hodgkin's disease, unspecified type, of intra-abdominal lymph nodes
201.94 Hodgkin's disease, unspecified type, of lymph nodes of axilla and upper limb
201.95 Hodgkin's disease, unspecified type, of lymph nodes of inguinal region and lower limb
201.96 Hodgkin's disease, unspecified type, of intrapelvic lymph nodes
201.97 Hodgkin's disease, unspecified type, of spleen
201.98 Hodgkin's disease, unspecified type, of lymph nodes of multiple sites
202.00 Nodular lymphoma, unspecified site, extranodal and solid organ sites
202.01 Nodular lymphoma of lymph nodes of head, face, and neck
202.02 Nodular lymphoma of intrathoracic lymph nodes
202.03 Nodular lymphoma of intra-abdominal lymph nodes
202.04 Nodular lymphoma of lymph nodes of axilla and upper limb
202.05 Nodular lymphoma of lymph nodes of inguinal region and lower limb
202.06 Nodular lymphoma of intrapelvic lymph nodes
202.07 Nodular lymphoma of spleen
202.08 Nodular lymphoma of lymph nodes of multiple sites
202.10 Mycosis fungoides, unspecified site, extranodal and solid organ sites
202.11 Mycosis fungoides of lymph nodes of head, face, and neck
202.12 Mycosis fungoides of intrathoracic lymph nodes
202.13 Mycosis fungoides of intra-abdominal lymph nodes
202.14 Mycosis fungoides of lymph nodes of axilla and upper limb
202.15 Mycosis fungoides of lymph nodes of inguinal region and lower limb
202.16 Mycosis fungoides of intrapelvic lymph nodes
202.17 Mycosis fungoides of spleen
202.18 Mycosis fungoides of lymph nodes of multiple sites
202.20 Sezary's disease, unspecified site, extranodal and solid organ sites
202.21 Sezary's disease of lymph nodes of head, face, and neck
202.22 Sezary's disease of intrathoracic lymph nodes
202.23 Sezary's disease of intra-abdominal lymph nodes
202.24 Sezary's disease of lymph nodes of axilla and upper limb
202.25 Sezary's disease of lymph nodes of inguinal region and lower limb
202.26 Sezary's disease of intrapelvic lymph nodes
202.27 Sezary's disease of spleen
202.28 Sezary's disease of lymph nodes of multiple sites
202.30 Malignant histiocytosis, unspecified site, extranodal and solid organ sites
202.31 Malignant histiocytosis of lymph nodes of head, face, and neck
202.32 Malignant histiocytosis of intrathoracic lymph nodes
202.33 Malignant histiocytosis of intra-abdominal lymph nodes
202.34 Malignant histiocytosis of lymph nodes of axilla and upper limb
202.35 Malignant histiocytosis of lymph nodes of inguinal region and lower limb
202.36 Malignant histiocytosis of intrapelvic lymph nodes
202.37 Malignant histiocytosis of spleen
202.38 Malignant histiocytosis of lymph nodes of multiple sites
202.40 Leukemic reticuloendotheliosis, unspecified site, extranodal and solid organ sites
202.41 Leukemic reticuloendotheliosis of lymph nodes of head, face, and neck
202.42 Leukemic reticuloendotheliosis of intrathoracic lymph nodes
202.43 Leukemic reticuloendotheliosis of intra-abdominal lymph nodes
202.44 Leukemic reticuloendotheliosis of lymph nodes of axilla and upper limb
202.45 Leukemic reticuloendotheliosis of lymph nodes of inguinal region and lower limb
202.46 Leukemic reticuloendotheliosis of intrapelvic lymph nodes
202.47 Leukemic reticuloendotheliosis of spleen
202.48 Leukemic reticuloendotheliosis of lymph nodes of multipes sites
202.50 Letterer-Siwe disease, unspecified site, extranodal and solid organ sites
202.51 Letterer-Siwe disease of lymph nodes of head, face, and neck
202.52 Letterer-Siwe disease of intrathoracic lymph nodes
202.53 Letterer-Siwe disease of intra-abdominal lymph nodes
202.54 Letterer-Siwe disease of lymph nodes of axilla and upper limb
202.55 Letterer-Siwe disease of lymph nodes of inguinal region and lower limb
202.56 Letterer-Siwe disease of intrapelvic lymph nodes
202.57 Letterer-Siwe disease of spleen
202.58 Letterer-Siwe disease of lymph nodes of multiple sites
202.60 Malignant mast cell tumors, unspecified site, extranodal and solid organ sites
202.61 Malignant mast cell tumors of lymph nodes of head, face, and neck
202.62 Malignant mast cell tumors of intrathoracic lymph nodes
202.63 Malignant mast cell tumors of intra-abdominal lymph nodes
202.64 Malignant mast cell tumors of lymph nodes of axilla and upper limb
202.65 Malignant mast cell tumors of lymph nodes of inguinal region and lower limb
202.66 Malignant mast cell tumors of intrapelvic lymph nodes
202.67 Malignant mast cell tumors of spleen
202.68 Malignant mast cell tumors of lymph nodes of multiple sites
202.80 Other malignant lymphomas, unspecified site, extranodal and solid organ sites
202.81 Other malignant lymphomas of lymph nodes of head, face, and neck
202.82 Other malignant lymphomas of intrathoracic lymph nodes
202.83 Other malignant lymphomas of intra-abdominal lymph nodes
202.84 Other malignant lymphomas of lymph nodes of axilla and upper limb
202.85 Other malignant lymphomas of lymph nodes of inguinal region and lower limb
202.86 Other malignant lymphomas of intrapelvic lymph nodes
202.87 Other malignant lymphomas of spleen
202.88 Other malignant lymphomas of lymph nodes of multiple sites
202.90 Other and unspecified malignant neoplasms of lymphoid and histiocytic tissue, unspecified site, extranodal and solid organ sites
202.91 Other and unspecified malignant neoplasms of lymphoid and histiocytic tissue of lymph nodes of head, face, and neck
202.92 Other and unspecified malignant neoplasms of lymphoid and histiocytic tissue of intrathoracic lymph nodes
202.93 Other and unspecified malignant neoplasms of lymphoid and histiocytic tissue of intra-abdominal lymph nodes
202.94 Other and unspecified malignant neoplasms of lymphoid and histiocytic tissue of lymph nodes of axilla and upper limb
202.95 Other and unspecified malignant neoplasms of lymphoid and histiocytic tissue of lymph nodes of inguinal region and lower limb
202.96 Other and unspecified malignant neoplasms of lymphoid and histiocytic tissue of intrapelvic lymph nodes
202.97 Other and unspecified malignant neoplasms of lymphoid and histiocytic tissue of spleen
202.98 Other and unspecified malignant neoplasms of lymphoid and histiocytic tissue of lymph nodes of multiple sites
203.00 Multiple myeloma without mention of remission
203.10 Plasma cell leukemia without mention of remission
203.80 Other immunoproliferative neoplasms without mention of remission
204.00 Acute lymphoid leukemia without mention of remission
205.00 Acute myeloid leukemia without mention of remission
208.00 Acute leukemia of unspecified cell type without mention of remission
239.3 Neoplasm of unspecified nature of breast
242.90 Thyrotoxicosis without mention of goiter or other cause, without mention of thyrotoxic crisis or storm
273.1 Monoclonal paraproteinemia — (Use additional code to identify any associated mental retardation)
273.2 Other paraproteinemias — (Use additional code to identify any associated mental retardation)

Unspecified code
Female diagnosis
Manifestation code
Male diagnosis

274.89 Gout with other specified manifestations — (Use additional code to identify any associated mental retardation. Use additional code to identify manifestations: 357.4, 364.11)
283.0 Autoimmune hemolytic anemias — (Use additional E code to identify cause, if drug-induced)
283.11 Hemolytic-uremic syndrome — (Use additional E code to identify cause)
287.1 Qualitative platelet defects
287.3 Primary thrombocytopenia
287.4 Secondary thrombocytopenia — (Use additional E code to identify cause)
287.5 Unspecified thrombocytopenia
340 Multiple sclerosis
341.9 Unspecified demyelinating disease of central nervous system
356.3 Refsum's disease
356.9 Unspecified hereditary and idiopathic peripheral neuropathy
357.1 Polyneuropathy in collagen vascular disease — (Code first underlying disease: 446.0, 710.0, 714.0)
357.3 Polyneuropathy in malignant disease — (Code first underlying disease: 140.0-208.9)
357.4 Polyneuropathy in other diseases classified elsewhere — (Code first underlying disease: 032.0-032.9, 135, 251.2, 265.0, 265.2, 266.0-266.9, 277.1, 277.3, 585)
357.81 Chronic inflammatory demyelinating polyneuritis
357.82 Critical illness polyneuropathy
357.89 Other inflammatory and toxic neuropathy
358.00 Myasthenia gravis without (acute) exacerbation
358.01 Myasthenia gravis with (acute) exacerbation
358.8 Other specified myoneural disorders
358.9 Unspecified myoneural disorders
446.21 Goodpasture's syndrome — (Use additional code to identify renal disease, 583.81)
446.6 Thrombotic microangiopathy
447.6 Unspecified arteritis
580.4 Acute glomerulonephritis with lesion of rapidly progressive glomerulonephritis
583.0 Nephritis and nephropathy, not specified as acute or chronic, with lesion of proliferative glomerulonephritis
583.4 Nephritis and nephropathy, not specified as acute or chronic, with lesion of rapidly progressive glomerulonephritis
584.7 Acute renal failure with lesion of renal medullary (papillary) necrosis
585 Chronic renal failure — (Use additional code to identify manifestation: 357.4, 420.0)
586 Unspecified renal failure
694.4 Pemphigus
710.0 Systemic lupus erythematosus — (Use additional code to identify manifestation: 424.91, 581.81, 582.81, 583.81)
710.1 Systemic sclerosis — (Use additional code to identify manifestation: 359.6, 517.2)
773.0 Hemolytic disease due to Rh isoimmunization of fetus or newborn
780.71 Chronic fatigue syndrome
780.79 Other malaise and fatigue
996.89 Complications of other transplanted organ — (Use additional code to identify nature of complication, 078.5)
997.99 Other complications affecting other specified body systems, NEC — (Use additional code to identify complications)
V42.81 Bone marrow replaced by transplant — (This code is intended for use when these conditions are recorded as diagnoses or problems)
V42.82 Peripheral stem cells replaced by transplant — (This code is intended for use when these conditions are recorded as diagnoses or problems)
V42.83 Pancreas replaced by transplant — (This code is intended for use when these conditions are recorded as diagnoses or problems)
V42.89 Other organ or tissue replaced by transplant — (This code is intended for use when these conditions are recorded as diagnoses or problems)

ICD-9-CM Procedural
99.71 Therapeutic plasmapheresis
99.72 Therapeutic leukopheresis
99.73 Therapeutic erythrocytapheresis
99.74 Therapeutic plateletpheresis
99.76 Extracorporeal immunoadsorption
99.78 Aquapheresis
99.79 Other therapeutic apheresis

HCPCS Level II Supplies & Services
HCPCS Level II codes are used to report the supplies, durable medical equipment, and certain medical services provided on an outpatient basis. Because the procedure(s) represented on this page would be performed in an inpatient facility, no HCPCS Level II codes apply.

36522
36522 Photopheresis, extracorporeal

ICD-9-CM Diagnostic
The application of this code is too broad to adequately present ICD-9-CM diagnostic code links here. Refer to your ICD-9-CM book.

ICD-9-CM Procedural
99.88 Therapeutic photopheresis

36540
36540 Collection of blood specimen from a completely implantable venous access device

ICD-9-CM Diagnostic
The application of this code is too broad to adequately present ICD-9-CM diagnostic code links here. Refer to your ICD-9-CM book.

ICD-9-CM Procedural
38.99 Other puncture of vein

HCPCS Level II Supplies & Services
A4550 Surgical trays

36550
36550 Declotting by thrombolytic agent of implanted vascular access device or catheter

ICD-9-CM Diagnostic
996.74 Other complications due to other vascular device, implant, and graft

ICD-9-CM Procedural
86.09 Other incision of skin and subcutaneous tissue

HCPCS Level II Supplies & Services
J2995 Injection, streptokinase, per 250,000 IU

36555–36556
36555 Insertion of non-tunneled centrally inserted central venous catheter; under 5 years of age
36556 age 5 years or older

ICD-9-CM Diagnostic
The application of this code is too broad to adequately present ICD-9-CM diagnostic code links here. Refer to your ICD-9-CM book.

ICD-9-CM Procedural
86.07 Insertion of totally implantable vascular access device (VAD)

36557–36558
36557 Insertion of tunneled centrally inserted central venous catheter, without subcutaneous port or pump; under 5 years of age
36558 age 5 years or older

ICD-9-CM Diagnostic
The application of this code is too broad to adequately present ICD-9-CM diagnostic code links here. Refer to your ICD-9-CM book.

ICD-9-CM Procedural
86.07 Insertion of totally implantable vascular access device (VAD)

36560–36561
36560 Insertion of tunneled centrally inserted central venous access device, with subcutaneous port; under 5 years of age
36561 age 5 years or older

ICD-9-CM Diagnostic
The application of this code is too broad to adequately present ICD-9-CM diagnostic code links here. Refer to your ICD-9-CM book.

ICD-9-CM Procedural
86.07 Insertion of totally implantable vascular access device (VAD)

36563–36566

36563 Insertion of tunneled centrally inserted central venous access device with subcutaneous pump
36565 Insertion of tunneled centrally inserted central venous access device, requiring two catheters via two separate venous access sites; without subcutaneous port or pump (eg, Tesio type catheter)
36566 with subcutaneous port(s)

ICD-9-CM Diagnostic
The application of this code is too broad to adequately present ICD-9-CM diagnostic code links here. Refer to your ICD-9-CM book.

ICD-9-CM Procedural
86.07 Insertion of totally implantable vascular access device (VAD)

36568–36569

36568 Insertion of peripherally inserted central venous catheter (PICC), without subcutaneous port or pump; under 5 years of age
36569 age 5 years or older

ICD-9-CM Diagnostic
The application of this code is too broad to adequately present ICD-9-CM diagnostic code links here. Refer to your ICD-9-CM book.

ICD-9-CM Procedural
86.07 Insertion of totally implantable vascular access device (VAD)

36570–36571

36570 Insertion of peripherally inserted central venous access device, with subcutaneous port; under 5 years of age
36571 age 5 years or older

ICD-9-CM Diagnostic
The application of this code is too broad to adequately present ICD-9-CM diagnostic code links here. Refer to your ICD-9-CM book.

ICD-9-CM Procedural
86.07 Insertion of totally implantable vascular access device (VAD)

36575–36576

36575 Repair of tunneled or non-tunneled central venous access catheter, without subcutaneous port or pump, central or peripheral insertion site
36576 Repair of central venous access device, with subcutaneous port or pump, central or peripheral insertion site

ICD-9-CM Diagnostic
996.1 Mechanical complication of other vascular device, implant, and graft

ICD-9-CM Procedural
86.09 Other incision of skin and subcutaneous tissue

36578

36578 Replacement, catheter only, of central venous access device, with subcutaneous port or pump, central or peripheral insertion site

ICD-9-CM Diagnostic
996.1 Mechanical complication of other vascular device, implant, and graft
996.62 Infection and inflammatory reaction due to other vascular device, implant, and graft — (Use additional code to identify specified infections)
996.74 Other complications due to other vascular device, implant, and graft
V53.90 Fitting and adjustment, Unspecified device ▽
V53.99 Fitting and adjustment, Other device

ICD-9-CM Procedural
86.09 Other incision of skin and subcutaneous tissue

36580–36581

36580 Replacement, complete, of a non-tunneled centrally inserted central venous catheter, without subcutaneous port or pump, through same venous access
36581 Replacement, complete, of a tunneled centrally inserted central venous catheter, without subcutaneous port or pump, through same venous access

ICD-9-CM Diagnostic
996.1 Mechanical complication of other vascular device, implant, and graft
996.62 Infection and inflammatory reaction due to other vascular device, implant, and graft — (Use additional code to identify specified infections)
996.74 Other complications due to other vascular device, implant, and graft
V53.90 Fitting and adjustment, Unspecified device ▽
V53.99 Fitting and adjustment, Other device

ICD-9-CM Procedural
86.07 Insertion of totally implantable vascular access device (VAD)

36582–36583

36582 Replacement, complete, of a tunneled centrally inserted central venous access device, with subcutaneous port, through same venous access
36583 Replacement, complete, of a tunneled centrally inserted central venous access device, with subcutaneous pump, through same venous access

ICD-9-CM Diagnostic
996.1 Mechanical complication of other vascular device, implant, and graft
996.62 Infection and inflammatory reaction due to other vascular device, implant, and graft — (Use additional code to identify specified infections)
996.74 Other complications due to other vascular device, implant, and graft
V53.90 Fitting and adjustment, Unspecified device ▽
V53.99 Fitting and adjustment, Other device

ICD-9-CM Procedural
86.07 Insertion of totally implantable vascular access device (VAD)

36584

36584 Replacement, complete, of a peripherally inserted central venous catheter (PICC), without subcutaneous port or pump, through same venous access

ICD-9-CM Diagnostic
996.1 Mechanical complication of other vascular device, implant, and graft
996.62 Infection and inflammatory reaction due to other vascular device, implant, and graft — (Use additional code to identify specified infections)
996.74 Other complications due to other vascular device, implant, and graft
V53.90 Fitting and adjustment, Unspecified device ▽
V53.99 Fitting and adjustment, Other device

ICD-9-CM Procedural
86.07 Insertion of totally implantable vascular access device (VAD)

36585

36585 Replacement, complete, of a peripherally inserted central venous access device, with subcutaneous port, through same venous access

ICD-9-CM Diagnostic
996.1 Mechanical complication of other vascular device, implant, and graft
996.62 Infection and inflammatory reaction due to other vascular device, implant, and graft — (Use additional code to identify specified infections)
996.74 Other complications due to other vascular device, implant, and graft
V53.90 Fitting and adjustment, Unspecified device ▽
V53.99 Fitting and adjustment, Other device

ICD-9-CM Procedural
86.07 Insertion of totally implantable vascular access device (VAD)

36589–36590

36589 Removal of tunneled central venous catheter, without subcutaneous port or pump
36590 Removal of tunneled central venous access device, with subcutaneous port or pump, central or peripheral insertion

ICD-9-CM Diagnostic
996.1 Mechanical complication of other vascular device, implant, and graft
996.62 Infection and inflammatory reaction due to other vascular device, implant, and graft — (Use additional code to identify specified infections)
996.74 Other complications due to other vascular device, implant, and graft

ICD-9-CM Procedural
86.09 Other incision of skin and subcutaneous tissue

36595–36596

36595 Mechanical removal of pericatheter obstructive material (eg, fibrin sheath) from central venous device via separate venous access
36596 Mechanical removal of intraluminal (intracatheter) obstructive material from central venous device through device lumen

ICD-9-CM Diagnostic

996.1 Mechanical complication of other vascular device, implant, and graft
996.62 Infection and inflammatory reaction due to other vascular device, implant, and graft — (Use additional code to identify specified infections)
996.74 Other complications due to other vascular device, implant, and graft

ICD-9-CM Procedural

86.09 Other incision of skin and subcutaneous tissue

36597

36597 Repositioning of previously placed central venous catheter under fluoroscopic guidance

ICD-9-CM Diagnostic

The application of this code is too broad to adequately present ICD-9-CM diagnostic code links here. Refer to your ICD-9-CM book.

ICD-9-CM Procedural

86.09 Other incision of skin and subcutaneous tissue
88.39 X-ray, other and unspecified

36600

36600 Arterial puncture, withdrawal of blood for diagnosis

ICD-9-CM Diagnostic

The application of this code is too broad to adequately present ICD-9-CM diagnostic code links here. Refer to your ICD-9-CM book.

ICD-9-CM Procedural

38.98 Other puncture of artery

HCPCS Level II Supplies & Services

A4649 Surgical supply; miscellaneous

36620–36625

36620 Arterial catheterization or cannulation for sampling, monitoring or transfusion (separate procedure); percutaneous
36625 cutdown

ICD-9-CM Diagnostic

The application of this code is too broad to adequately present ICD-9-CM diagnostic code links here. Refer to your ICD-9-CM book.

ICD-9-CM Procedural

38.91 Arterial catheterization

HCPCS Level II Supplies & Services

A4649 Surgical supply; miscellaneous

36640

36640 Arterial catheterization for prolonged infusion therapy (chemotherapy), cutdown

ICD-9-CM Diagnostic

The application of this code is too broad to adequately present ICD-9-CM diagnostic code links here. Refer to your ICD-9-CM book.

ICD-9-CM Procedural

38.91 Arterial catheterization

HCPCS Level II Supplies & Services

A4649 Surgical supply; miscellaneous

36660

36660 Catheterization, umbilical artery, newborn, for diagnosis or therapy

ICD-9-CM Diagnostic

The application of this code is too broad to adequately present ICD-9-CM diagnostic code links here. Refer to your ICD-9-CM book.

ICD-9-CM Procedural

38.91 Arterial catheterization

36680

36680 Placement of needle for intraosseous infusion

ICD-9-CM Diagnostic

276.0 Hyperosmolality and/or hypernatremia — (Use additional code to identify any associated mental retardation)
276.1 Hyposmolality and/or hyponatremia — (Use additional code to identify any associated mental retardation)
276.5 Volume depletion — (Use additional code to identify any associated mental retardation)

ICD-9-CM Procedural

41.92 Injection into bone marrow

36800

36800 Insertion of cannula for hemodialysis, other purpose (separate procedure); vein to vein

ICD-9-CM Diagnostic

250.40 Diabetes with renal manifestations, type II or unspecified type, not stated as uncontrolled — (Use additional code to identify manifestation: 581.81, 583.81)
250.41 Diabetes with renal manifestations, type I [juvenile type], not stated as uncontrolled — (Use additional code to identify manifestation: 581.81, 583.81)
250.42 Diabetes with renal manifestations, type II or unspecified type, uncontrolled — (Use additional code to identify manifestation: 581.81, 583.81)
250.43 Diabetes with renal manifestations, type I [juvenile type], uncontrolled — (Use additional code to identify manifestation: 581.81, 583.81)
403.91 Unspecified hypertensive renal disease with renal failure ▽
445.81 Atheroembolism of kidney — (Use additional code for any associated kidney failure: 584, 585)
580.4 Acute glomerulonephritis with lesion of rapidly progressive glomerulonephritis
580.9 Acute glomerulonephritis with unspecified pathological lesion in kidney ▽
581.1 Nephrotic syndrome with lesion of membranous glomerulonephritis
581.81 Nephrotic syndrome with other specified pathological lesion in kidney in diseases classified elsewhere — (Code first underlying disease: 084.9, 250.4, 277.3, 446.0, 710.0) ☒
582.0 Chronic glomerulonephritis with lesion of proliferative glomerulonephritis
582.1 Chronic glomerulonephritis with lesion of membranous glomerulonephritis
582.2 Chronic glomerulonephritis with lesion of membranoproliferative glomerulonephritis
582.4 Chronic glomerulonephritis with lesion of rapidly progressive glomerulonephritis
582.81 Chronic glomerulonephritis with other specified pathological lesion in kidney in diseases classified elsewhere — (Code first underlying disease: 277.3, 710.0) ☒
582.89 Other chronic glomerulonephritis with specified pathological lesion in kidney
582.9 Chronic glomerulonephritis with unspecified pathological lesion in kidney ▽
583.0 Nephritis and nephropathy, not specified as acute or chronic, with lesion of proliferative glomerulonephritis
583.1 Nephritis and nephropathy, not specified as acute or chronic, with lesion of membranous glomerulonephritis
583.2 Nephritis and nephropathy, not specified as acute or chronic, with lesion of membranoproliferative glomerulonephritis
583.4 Nephritis and nephropathy, not specified as acute or chronic, with lesion of rapidly progressive glomerulonephritis
583.6 Nephritis and nephropathy, not specified as acute or chronic, with lesion of renal cortical necrosis
583.7 Nephritis and nephropathy, not specified as acute or chronic, with lesion of renal medullary necrosis
583.81 Nephritis and nephropathy, not specified as acute or chronic, with other specified pathological lesion in kidney, in diseases classified elsewhere — (Code first underlying disease: 016.0, 098.19, 250.4, 277.3, 446.21, 710.0) ☒
583.89 Other nephritis and nephropathy, not specified as acute or chronic, with specified pathological lesion in kidney
583.9 Nephritis and nephropathy, not specified as acute or chronic, with unspecified pathological lesion in kidney ▽
584.5 Acute renal failure with lesion of tubular necrosis
584.6 Acute renal failure with lesion of renal cortical necrosis
584.7 Acute renal failure with lesion of renal medullary (papillary) necrosis
584.8 Acute renal failure with other specified pathological lesion in kidney
584.9 Unspecified acute renal failure ▽

585 Chronic renal failure — (Use additional code to identify manifestation: 357.4, 420.0)
586 Unspecified renal failure ▽
587 Unspecified renal sclerosis ▽
588.0 Renal osteodystrophy
588.81 Secondary hyperparathyroidism (of renal origin)
588.89 Other specified disorders resulting from impaired renal function
588.9 Unspecified disorder resulting from impaired renal function ▽
590.00 Chronic pyelonephritis without lesion of renal medullary necrosis — (Code, if applicable, any causal condition first. Use additional code to identify organism, such as E. coli, 041.4)
590.01 Chronic pyelonephritis with lesion of renal medullary necrosis — (Code, if applicable, any causal condition first. Use additional code to identify organism, such as E. coli, 041.4)
590.10 Acute pyelonephritis without lesion of renal medullary necrosis — (Use additional code to identify organism, such as E. coli, 041.4)
590.11 Acute pyelonephritis with lesion of renal medullary necrosis — (Use additional code to identify organism, such as E. coli, 041.4)
590.3 Pyeloureteritis cystica — (Use additional code to identify organism, such as E. coli, 041.4)
590.80 Unspecified pyelonephritis — (Use additional code to identify organism, such as E. coli, 041.4) ▽
590.81 Pyelitis or pyelonephritis in diseases classified elsewhere — (Code first underlying disease, 016.0. Use additional code to identify organism, such as E. coli, 041.4) ☒
590.9 Unspecified infection of kidney — (Use additional code to identify organism, such as E. coli, 041.4) ▽
593.81 Vascular disorders of kidney
728.88 Rhabdomyolysis
958.5 Traumatic anuria
996.81 Complications of transplanted kidney — (Use additional code to identify nature of complication, 078.5)

ICD-9-CM Procedural

39.27 Arteriovenostomy for renal dialysis
39.93 Insertion of vessel-to-vessel cannula

HCPCS Level II Supplies & Services

A4305 Disposable drug delivery system, flow rate of 50 ml or greater per hour
A4306 Disposable drug delivery system, flow rate of 5 ml or less per hour
A4550 Surgical trays
A4730 Fistula cannulation set for hemodialysis, each

36810

36810 Insertion of cannula for hemodialysis, other purpose (separate procedure); arteriovenous, external (Scribner type)

ICD-9-CM Diagnostic

250.40 Diabetes with renal manifestations, type II or unspecified type, not stated as uncontrolled — (Use additional code to identify manifestation: 581.81, 583.81)
250.41 Diabetes with renal manifestations, type I [juvenile type], not stated as uncontrolled — (Use additional code to identify manifestation: 581.81, 583.81)
250.42 Diabetes with renal manifestations, type II or unspecified type, uncontrolled — (Use additional code to identify manifestation: 581.81, 583.81)
250.43 Diabetes with renal manifestations, type I [juvenile type], uncontrolled — (Use additional code to identify manifestation: 581.81, 583.81)
403.91 Unspecified hypertensive renal disease with renal failure ▽
445.81 Atheroembolism of kidney — (Use additional code for any associated kidney failure: 584, 585)
580.4 Acute glomerulonephritis with lesion of rapidly progressive glomerulonephritis
580.9 Acute glomerulonephritis with unspecified pathological lesion in kidney ▽
581.1 Nephrotic syndrome with lesion of membranous glomerulonephritis
581.81 Nephrotic syndrome with other specified pathological lesion in kidney in diseases classified elsewhere — (Code first underlying disease: 084.9, 250.4, 277.3, 446.0, 710.0) ☒
582.0 Chronic glomerulonephritis with lesion of proliferative glomerulonephritis
582.1 Chronic glomerulonephritis with lesion of membranous glomerulonephritis
582.2 Chronic glomerulonephritis with lesion of membranoproliferative glomerulonephritis
582.4 Chronic glomerulonephritis with lesion of rapidly progressive glomerulonephritis
582.81 Chronic glomerulonephritis with other specified pathological lesion in kidney in diseases classified elsewhere — (Code first underlying disease: 277.3, 710.0) ☒
582.89 Other chronic glomerulonephritis with specified pathological lesion in kidney
582.9 Chronic glomerulonephritis with unspecified pathological lesion in kidney ▽
583.0 Nephritis and nephropathy, not specified as acute or chronic, with lesion of proliferative glomerulonephritis
583.1 Nephritis and nephropathy, not specified as acute or chronic, with lesion of membranous glomerulonephritis
583.2 Nephritis and nephropathy, not specified as acute or chronic, with lesion of membranoproliferative glomerulonephritis
583.4 Nephritis and nephropathy, not specified as acute or chronic, with lesion of rapidly progressive glomerulonephritis
583.6 Nephritis and nephropathy, not specified as acute or chronic, with lesion of renal cortical necrosis
583.7 Nephritis and nephropathy, not specified as acute or chronic, with lesion of renal medullary necrosis
583.81 Nephritis and nephropathy, not specified as acute or chronic, with other specified pathological lesion in kidney, in diseases classified elsewhere — (Code first underlying disease: 016.0, 098.19, 250.4, 277.3, 446.21, 710.0) ☒
583.89 Other nephritis and nephropathy, not specified as acute or chronic, with specified pathological lesion in kidney
583.9 Nephritis and nephropathy, not specified as acute or chronic, with unspecified pathological lesion in kidney ▽
584.5 Acute renal failure with lesion of tubular necrosis
584.6 Acute renal failure with lesion of renal cortical necrosis
584.7 Acute renal failure with lesion of renal medullary (papillary) necrosis
584.8 Acute renal failure with other specified pathological lesion in kidney
584.9 Unspecified acute renal failure ▽
585 Chronic renal failure — (Use additional code to identify manifestation: 357.4, 420.0)
586 Unspecified renal failure ▽
587 Unspecified renal sclerosis ▽
588.0 Renal osteodystrophy
588.81 Secondary hyperparathyroidism (of renal origin)
588.89 Other specified disorders resulting from impaired renal function
588.9 Unspecified disorder resulting from impaired renal function ▽
590.00 Chronic pyelonephritis without lesion of renal medullary necrosis — (Code, if applicable, any causal condition first. Use additional code to identify organism, such as E. coli, 041.4)
590.01 Chronic pyelonephritis with lesion of renal medullary necrosis — (Code, if applicable, any causal condition first. Use additional code to identify organism, such as E. coli, 041.4)
590.10 Acute pyelonephritis without lesion of renal medullary necrosis — (Use additional code to identify organism, such as E. coli, 041.4)
590.11 Acute pyelonephritis with lesion of renal medullary necrosis — (Use additional code to identify organism, such as E. coli, 041.4)
590.3 Pyeloureteritis cystica — (Use additional code to identify organism, such as E. coli, 041.4)
590.80 Unspecified pyelonephritis — (Use additional code to identify organism, such as E. coli, 041.4) ▽
590.81 Pyelitis or pyelonephritis in diseases classified elsewhere — (Code first underlying disease, 016.0. Use additional code to identify organism, such as E. coli, 041.4) ☒
590.9 Unspecified infection of kidney — (Use additional code to identify organism, such as E. coli, 041.4) ▽
593.81 Vascular disorders of kidney
728.88 Rhabdomyolysis
958.5 Traumatic anuria
996.81 Complications of transplanted kidney — (Use additional code to identify nature of complication, 078.5)

ICD-9-CM Procedural

39.27 Arteriovenostomy for renal dialysis
39.93 Insertion of vessel-to-vessel cannula

HCPCS Level II Supplies & Services

G0365 Vessel mapping of vessels for hemodialysis access (services for preoperative vessel mapping prior to creation of hemodialysis access using an autogenous hemodialysis conduit, including arterial inflow and venous outflow)

36815

36815 Insertion of cannula for hemodialysis, other purpose (separate procedure); arteriovenous, external revision, or closure

ICD-9-CM Diagnostic

250.40 Diabetes with renal manifestations, type II or unspecified type, not stated as uncontrolled — (Use additional code to identify manifestation: 581.81, 583.81)
250.41 Diabetes with renal manifestations, type I [juvenile type], not stated as uncontrolled — (Use additional code to identify manifestation: 581.81, 583.81)

▽ Unspecified code ☒ Manifestation code
♀ Female diagnosis ♂ Male diagnosis

250.42 Diabetes with renal manifestations, type II or unspecified type, uncontrolled — (Use additional code to identify manifestation: 581.81, 583.81)
250.43 Diabetes with renal manifestations, type I [juvenile type], uncontrolled — (Use additional code to identify manifestation: 581.81, 583.81)
403.91 Unspecified hypertensive renal disease with renal failure ▽
445.81 Atheroembolism of kidney — (Use additional code for any associated kidney failure: 584, 585)
580.4 Acute glomerulonephritis with lesion of rapidly progressive glomerulonephritis
580.9 Acute glomerulonephritis with unspecified pathological lesion in kidney ▽
581.1 Nephrotic syndrome with lesion of membranous glomerulonephritis
581.81 Nephrotic syndrome with other specified pathological lesion in kidney in diseases classified elsewhere — (Code first underlying disease: 084.9, 250.4, 277.3, 446.0, 710.0) ☒
582.0 Chronic glomerulonephritis with lesion of proliferative glomerulonephritis
582.1 Chronic glomerulonephritis with lesion of membranous glomerulonephritis
582.2 Chronic glomerulonephritis with lesion of membranoproliferative glomerulonephritis
582.4 Chronic glomerulonephritis with lesion of rapidly progressive glomerulonephritis
582.81 Chronic glomerulonephritis with other specified pathological lesion in kidney in diseases classified elsewhere — (Code first underlying disease: 277.3, 710.0) ☒
582.89 Other chronic glomerulonephritis with specified pathological lesion in kidney
582.9 Chronic glomerulonephritis with unspecified pathological lesion in kidney ▽
583.0 Nephritis and nephropathy, not specified as acute or chronic, with lesion of proliferative glomerulonephritis
583.1 Nephritis and nephropathy, not specified as acute or chronic, with lesion of membranous glomerulonephritis
583.2 Nephritis and nephropathy, not specified as acute or chronic, with lesion of membranoproliferative glomerulonephritis
583.4 Nephritis and nephropathy, not specified as acute or chronic, with lesion of rapidly progressive glomerulonephritis
583.6 Nephritis and nephropathy, not specified as acute or chronic, with lesion of renal cortical necrosis
583.7 Nephritis and nephropathy, not specified as acute or chronic, with lesion of renal medullary necrosis
583.81 Nephritis and nephropathy, not specified as acute or chronic, with other specified pathological lesion in kidney, in diseases classified elsewhere — (Code first underlying disease: 016.0, 098.19, 250.4, 277.3, 446.21, 710.0) ☒
583.89 Other nephritis and nephropathy, not specified as acute or chronic, with specified pathological lesion in kidney
583.9 Nephritis and nephropathy, not specified as acute or chronic, with unspecified pathological lesion in kidney ▽
584.5 Acute renal failure with lesion of tubular necrosis
584.6 Acute renal failure with lesion of renal cortical necrosis
584.7 Acute renal failure with lesion of renal medullary (papillary) necrosis
584.8 Acute renal failure with other specified pathological lesion in kidney
584.9 Unspecified acute renal failure ▽
585 Chronic renal failure — (Use additional code to identify manifestation: 357.4, 420.0)
586 Unspecified renal failure ▽
587 Unspecified renal sclerosis ▽
588.0 Renal osteodystrophy
588.81 Secondary hyperparathyroidism (of renal origin)
588.89 Other specified disorders resulting from impaired renal function
588.9 Unspecified disorder resulting from impaired renal function ▽
590.00 Chronic pyelonephritis without lesion of renal medullary necrosis — (Code, if applicable, any causal condition first. Use additional code to identify organism, such as E. coli, 041.4)
590.01 Chronic pyelonephritis with lesion of renal medullary necrosis — (Code, if applicable, any causal condition first. Use additional code to identify organism, such as E. coli, 041.4)
590.10 Acute pyelonephritis without lesion of renal medullary necrosis — (Use additional code to identify organism, such as E. coli, 041.4)
590.11 Acute pyelonephritis with lesion of renal medullary necrosis — (Use additional code to identify organism, such as E. coli, 041.4)
590.3 Pyeloureteritis cystica — (Use additional code to identify organism, such as E. coli, 041.4)
590.80 Unspecified pyelonephritis — (Use additional code to identify organism, such as E. coli, 041.4) ▽
590.81 Pyelitis or pyelonephritis in diseases classified elsewhere — (Code first underlying disease, 016.0. Use additional code to identify organism, such as E. coli, 041.4) ☒
590.9 Unspecified infection of kidney — (Use additional code to identify organism, such as E. coli, 041.4) ▽
593.81 Vascular disorders of kidney
728.88 Rhabdomyolysis
958.5 Traumatic anuria
996.81 Complications of transplanted kidney — (Use additional code to identify nature of complication, 078.5)

ICD-9-CM Procedural

39.27 Arteriovenostomy for renal dialysis
39.93 Insertion of vessel-to-vessel cannula

HCPCS Level II Supplies & Services

G0365 Vessel mapping of vessels for hemodialysis access (services for preoperative vessel mapping prior to creation of hemodialysis access using an autogenous hemodialysis conduit, including arterial inflow and venous outflow)

36818–36819

36818 Arteriovenous anastomosis, open; by upper arm cephalic vein transposition
36819 Arteriovenous anastomosis, open; by upper arm basilic vein transposition

ICD-9-CM Diagnostic

250.40 Diabetes with renal manifestations, type II or unspecified type, not stated as uncontrolled — (Use additional code to identify manifestation: 581.81, 583.81)
250.41 Diabetes with renal manifestations, type I [juvenile type], not stated as uncontrolled — (Use additional code to identify manifestation: 581.81, 583.81)
250.42 Diabetes with renal manifestations, type II or unspecified type, uncontrolled — (Use additional code to identify manifestation: 581.81, 583.81)
250.43 Diabetes with renal manifestations, type I [juvenile type], uncontrolled — (Use additional code to identify manifestation: 581.81, 583.81)
403.91 Unspecified hypertensive renal disease with renal failure ▽
445.81 Atheroembolism of kidney — (Use additional code for any associated kidney failure: 584, 585)
580.4 Acute glomerulonephritis with lesion of rapidly progressive glomerulonephritis
580.9 Acute glomerulonephritis with unspecified pathological lesion in kidney ▽
581.1 Nephrotic syndrome with lesion of membranous glomerulonephritis
581.81 Nephrotic syndrome with other specified pathological lesion in kidney in diseases classified elsewhere — (Code first underlying disease: 084.9, 250.4, 277.3, 446.0, 710.0) ☒
582.0 Chronic glomerulonephritis with lesion of proliferative glomerulonephritis
582.1 Chronic glomerulonephritis with lesion of membranous glomerulonephritis
582.2 Chronic glomerulonephritis with lesion of membranoproliferative glomerulonephritis
582.4 Chronic glomerulonephritis with lesion of rapidly progressive glomerulonephritis
582.81 Chronic glomerulonephritis with other specified pathological lesion in kidney in diseases classified elsewhere — (Code first underlying disease: 277.3, 710.0) ☒
582.89 Other chronic glomerulonephritis with specified pathological lesion in kidney
582.9 Chronic glomerulonephritis with unspecified pathological lesion in kidney ▽
583.0 Nephritis and nephropathy, not specified as acute or chronic, with lesion of proliferative glomerulonephritis
583.1 Nephritis and nephropathy, not specified as acute or chronic, with lesion of membranous glomerulonephritis
583.2 Nephritis and nephropathy, not specified as acute or chronic, with lesion of membranoproliferative glomerulonephritis
583.4 Nephritis and nephropathy, not specified as acute or chronic, with lesion of rapidly progressive glomerulonephritis
583.6 Nephritis and nephropathy, not specified as acute or chronic, with lesion of renal cortical necrosis
583.7 Nephritis and nephropathy, not specified as acute or chronic, with lesion of renal medullary necrosis
583.81 Nephritis and nephropathy, not specified as acute or chronic, with other specified pathological lesion in kidney, in diseases classified elsewhere — (Code first underlying disease: 016.0, 098.19, 250.4, 277.3, 446.21, 710.0) ☒
583.89 Other nephritis and nephropathy, not specified as acute or chronic, with specified pathological lesion in kidney
583.9 Nephritis and nephropathy, not specified as acute or chronic, with unspecified pathological lesion in kidney ▽
584.5 Acute renal failure with lesion of tubular necrosis
584.6 Acute renal failure with lesion of renal cortical necrosis
584.7 Acute renal failure with lesion of renal medullary (papillary) necrosis
584.8 Acute renal failure with other specified pathological lesion in kidney
584.9 Unspecified acute renal failure ▽
585 Chronic renal failure — (Use additional code to identify manifestation: 357.4, 420.0)
586 Unspecified renal failure ▽
587 Unspecified renal sclerosis ▽
588.0 Renal osteodystrophy

588.81 Secondary hyperparathyroidism (of renal origin)
588.89 Other specified disorders resulting from impaired renal function
588.9 Unspecified disorder resulting from impaired renal function ▽
590.00 Chronic pyelonephritis without lesion of renal medullary necrosis — (Code, if applicable, any causal condition first. Use additional code to identify organism, such as E. coli, 041.4)
590.01 Chronic pyelonephritis with lesion of renal medullary necrosis — (Code, if applicable, any causal condition first. Use additional code to identify organism, such as E. coli, 041.4)
590.10 Acute pyelonephritis without lesion of renal medullary necrosis — (Use additional code to identify organism, such as E. coli, 041.4)
590.11 Acute pyelonephritis with lesion of renal medullary necrosis — (Use additional code to identify organism, such as E. coli, 041.4)
590.3 Pyeloureteritis cystica — (Use additional code to identify organism, such as E. coli, 041.4)
590.80 Unspecified pyelonephritis — (Use additional code to identify organism, such as E. coli, 041.4) ▽
590.81 Pyelitis or pyelonephritis in diseases classified elsewhere — (Code first underlying disease, 016.0. Use additional code to identify organism, such as E. coli, 041.4) ☒
590.9 Unspecified infection of kidney — (Use additional code to identify organism, such as E. coli, 041.4) ▽
593.81 Vascular disorders of kidney
728.88 Rhabdomyolysis
958.5 Traumatic anuria
996.81 Complications of transplanted kidney — (Use additional code to identify nature of complication, 078.5)

ICD-9-CM Procedural
39.27 Arteriovenostomy for renal dialysis

36820
36820 Arteriovenous anastomosis, open; by forearm vein transposition

ICD-9-CM Diagnostic
250.40 Diabetes with renal manifestations, type II or unspecified type, not stated as uncontrolled — (Use additional code to identify manifestation: 581.81, 583.81)
250.41 Diabetes with renal manifestations, type I [juvenile type], not stated as uncontrolled — (Use additional code to identify manifestation: 581.81, 583.81)
250.42 Diabetes with renal manifestations, type II or unspecified type, uncontrolled — (Use additional code to identify manifestation: 581.81, 583.81)
250.43 Diabetes with renal manifestations, type I [juvenile type], uncontrolled — (Use additional code to identify manifestation: 581.81, 583.81)
403.91 Unspecified hypertensive renal disease with renal failure ▽
445.81 Atheroembolism of kidney — (Use additional code for any associated kidney failure: 584, 585)
580.4 Acute glomerulonephritis with lesion of rapidly progressive glomerulonephritis
580.9 Acute glomerulonephritis with unspecified pathological lesion in kidney ▽
581.1 Nephrotic syndrome with lesion of membranous glomerulonephritis
581.81 Nephrotic syndrome with other specified pathological lesion in kidney in diseases classified elsewhere — (Code first underlying disease: 084.9, 250.4, 277.3, 446.0, 710.0) ☒
582.0 Chronic glomerulonephritis with lesion of proliferative glomerulonephritis
582.1 Chronic glomerulonephritis with lesion of membranous glomerulonephritis
582.2 Chronic glomerulonephritis with lesion of membranoproliferative glomerulonephritis
582.4 Chronic glomerulonephritis with lesion of rapidly progressive glomerulonephritis
582.81 Chronic glomerulonephritis with other specified pathological lesion in kidney in diseases classified elsewhere — (Code first underlying disease: 277.3, 710.0) ☒
582.89 Other chronic glomerulonephritis with specified pathological lesion in kidney
582.9 Chronic glomerulonephritis with unspecified pathological lesion in kidney ▽
583.0 Nephritis and nephropathy, not specified as acute or chronic, with lesion of proliferative glomerulonephritis
583.1 Nephritis and nephropathy, not specified as acute or chronic, with lesion of membranous glomerulonephritis
583.2 Nephritis and nephropathy, not specified as acute or chronic, with lesion of membranoproliferative glomerulonephritis
583.4 Nephritis and nephropathy, not specified as acute or chronic, with lesion of rapidly progressive glomerulonephritis
583.6 Nephritis and nephropathy, not specified as acute or chronic, with lesion of renal cortical necrosis
583.7 Nephritis and nephropathy, not specified as acute or chronic, with lesion of renal medullary necrosis
583.81 Nephritis and nephropathy, not specified as acute or chronic, with other specified pathological lesion in kidney, in diseases classified elsewhere — (Code first underlying disease: 016.0, 098.19, 250.4, 277.3, 446.21, 710.0) ☒
583.89 Other nephritis and nephropathy, not specified as acute or chronic, with specified pathological lesion in kidney
583.9 Nephritis and nephropathy, not specified as acute or chronic, with unspecified pathological lesion in kidney ▽
584.5 Acute renal failure with lesion of tubular necrosis
584.6 Acute renal failure with lesion of renal cortical necrosis
584.7 Acute renal failure with lesion of renal medullary (papillary) necrosis
584.8 Acute renal failure with other specified pathological lesion in kidney
584.9 Unspecified acute renal failure ▽
585 Chronic renal failure — (Use additional code to identify manifestation: 357.4, 420.0)
586 Unspecified renal failure ▽
587 Unspecified renal sclerosis ▽
588.0 Renal osteodystrophy
588.81 Secondary hyperparathyroidism (of renal origin)
588.89 Other specified disorders resulting from impaired renal function
588.9 Unspecified disorder resulting from impaired renal function ▽
590.00 Chronic pyelonephritis without lesion of renal medullary necrosis — (Code, if applicable, any causal condition first. Use additional code to identify organism, such as E. coli, 041.4)
590.01 Chronic pyelonephritis with lesion of renal medullary necrosis — (Code, if applicable, any causal condition first. Use additional code to identify organism, such as E. coli, 041.4)
590.10 Acute pyelonephritis without lesion of renal medullary necrosis — (Use additional code to identify organism, such as E. coli, 041.4)
590.11 Acute pyelonephritis with lesion of renal medullary necrosis — (Use additional code to identify organism, such as E. coli, 041.4)
590.3 Pyeloureteritis cystica — (Use additional code to identify organism, such as E. coli, 041.4)
590.80 Unspecified pyelonephritis — (Use additional code to identify organism, such as E. coli, 041.4) ▽
590.81 Pyelitis or pyelonephritis in diseases classified elsewhere — (Code first underlying disease, 016.0. Use additional code to identify organism, such as E. coli, 041.4) ☒
590.9 Unspecified infection of kidney — (Use additional code to identify organism, such as E. coli, 041.4) ▽
593.81 Vascular disorders of kidney
728.88 Rhabdomyolysis
958.5 Traumatic anuria
996.81 Complications of transplanted kidney — (Use additional code to identify nature of complication, 078.5)

ICD-9-CM Procedural
39.27 Arteriovenostomy for renal dialysis

HCPCS Level II Supplies & Services
HCPCS Level II codes are used to report the supplies, durable medical equipment, and certain medical services provided on an outpatient basis. Because the procedure(s) represented on this page would be performed in an inpatient or outpatient facility, no HCPCS Level II codes apply.

36821
36821 Arteriovenous anastomosis, open; direct, any site (eg, Cimino type) (separate procedure)

ICD-9-CM Diagnostic
250.40 Diabetes with renal manifestations, type II or unspecified type, not stated as uncontrolled — (Use additional code to identify manifestation: 581.81, 583.81)
250.41 Diabetes with renal manifestations, type I [juvenile type], not stated as uncontrolled — (Use additional code to identify manifestation: 581.81, 583.81)
250.42 Diabetes with renal manifestations, type II or unspecified type, uncontrolled — (Use additional code to identify manifestation: 581.81, 583.81)
250.43 Diabetes with renal manifestations, type I [juvenile type], uncontrolled — (Use additional code to identify manifestation: 581.81, 583.81)
403.91 Unspecified hypertensive renal disease with renal failure ▽
445.81 Atheroembolism of kidney — (Use additional code for any associated kidney failure: 584, 585)
580.4 Acute glomerulonephritis with lesion of rapidly progressive glomerulonephritis
580.9 Acute glomerulonephritis with unspecified pathological lesion in kidney ▽
581.1 Nephrotic syndrome with lesion of membranous glomerulonephritis
581.81 Nephrotic syndrome with other specified pathological lesion in kidney in diseases classified elsewhere — (Code first underlying disease: 084.9, 250.4, 277.3, 446.0, 710.0) ☒

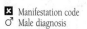

▽ Unspecified code
♀ Female diagnosis
☒ Manifestation code
♂ Male diagnosis

582.0 Chronic glomerulonephritis with lesion of proliferative glomerulonephritis
582.1 Chronic glomerulonephritis with lesion of membranous glomerulonephritis
582.2 Chronic glomerulonephritis with lesion of membranoproliferative glomerulonephritis
582.4 Chronic glomerulonephritis with lesion of rapidly progressive glomerulonephritis
582.81 Chronic glomerulonephritis with other specified pathological lesion in kidney in diseases classified elsewhere — (Code first underlying disease: 277.3, 710.0) ☒
582.89 Other chronic glomerulonephritis with specified pathological lesion in kidney
582.9 Chronic glomerulonephritis with unspecified pathological lesion in kidney ▽
583.0 Nephritis and nephropathy, not specified as acute or chronic, with lesion of proliferative glomerulonephritis
583.1 Nephritis and nephropathy, not specified as acute or chronic, with lesion of membranous glomerulonephritis
583.2 Nephritis and nephropathy, not specified as acute or chronic, with lesion of membranoproliferative glomerulonephritis
583.4 Nephritis and nephropathy, not specified as acute or chronic, with lesion of rapidly progressive glomerulonephritis
583.6 Nephritis and nephropathy, not specified as acute or chronic, with lesion of renal cortical necrosis
583.7 Nephritis and nephropathy, not specified as acute or chronic, with lesion of renal medullary necrosis
583.81 Nephritis and nephropathy, not specified as acute or chronic, with other specified pathological lesion in kidney, in diseases classified elsewhere — (Code first underlying disease: 016.0, 098.19, 250.4, 277.3, 446.21, 710.0) ☒
583.89 Other nephritis and nephropathy, not specified as acute or chronic, with specified pathological lesion in kidney
583.9 Nephritis and nephropathy, not specified as acute or chronic, with unspecified pathological lesion in kidney ▽
584.5 Acute renal failure with lesion of tubular necrosis
584.6 Acute renal failure with lesion of renal cortical necrosis
584.7 Acute renal failure with lesion of renal medullary (papillary) necrosis
584.8 Acute renal failure with other specified pathological lesion in kidney
584.9 Unspecified acute renal failure ▽
585 Chronic renal failure — (Use additional code to identify manifestation: 357.4, 420.0)
586 Unspecified renal failure ▽
587 Unspecified renal sclerosis ▽
588.0 Renal osteodystrophy
588.81 Secondary hyperparathyroidism (of renal origin)
588.89 Other specified disorders resulting from impaired renal function
588.9 Unspecified disorder resulting from impaired renal function ▽
590.00 Chronic pyelonephritis without lesion of renal medullary necrosis — (Code, if applicable, any causal condition first. Use additional code to identify organism, such as E. coli, 041.4)
590.01 Chronic pyelonephritis with lesion of renal medullary necrosis — (Code, if applicable, any causal condition first. Use additional code to identify organism, such as E. coli, 041.4)
590.10 Acute pyelonephritis without lesion of renal medullary necrosis — (Use additional code to identify organism, such as E. coli, 041.4)
590.11 Acute pyelonephritis with lesion of renal medullary necrosis — (Use additional code to identify organism, such as E. coli, 041.4)
590.3 Pyeloureteritis cystica — (Use additional code to identify organism, such as E. coli, 041.4)
590.80 Unspecified pyelonephritis — (Use additional code to identify organism, such as E. coli, 041.4) ▽
590.81 Pyelitis or pyelonephritis in diseases classified elsewhere — (Code first underlying disease, 016.0. Use additional code to identify organism, such as E. coli, 041.4) ☒
590.9 Unspecified infection of kidney — (Use additional code to identify organism, such as E. coli, 041.4) ▽
593.81 Vascular disorders of kidney
728.88 Rhabdomyolysis
958.5 Traumatic anuria
996.81 Complications of transplanted kidney — (Use additional code to identify nature of complication, 078.5)

ICD-9-CM Procedural

39.27 Arteriovenostomy for renal dialysis

36822

36822 Insertion of cannula(s) for prolonged extracorporeal circulation for cardiopulmonary insufficiency (ECMO) (separate procedure)

ICD-9-CM Diagnostic

428.0 Congestive heart failure, unspecified ▽
428.20 Unspecified systolic heart failure ▽
428.21 Acute systolic heart failure
428.22 Chronic systolic heart failure
428.23 Acute on chronic systolic heart failure
428.30 Unspecified diastolic heart failure ▽
428.31 Acute diastolic heart failure
428.32 Chronic diastolic heart failure
428.33 Acute on chronic diastolic heart failure
428.40 Unspecified combined systolic and diastolic heart failure ▽
428.41 Acute combined systolic and diastolic heart failure
428.42 Chronic combined systolic and diastolic heart failure
428.43 Acute on chronic combined systolic and diastolic heart failure
429.2 Unspecified cardiovascular disease — (Use additional code to identify presence of arteriosclerosis) ▽
429.4 Functional disturbances following cardiac surgery
518.5 Pulmonary insufficiency following trauma and surgery
518.81 Acute respiratory failure
518.82 Other pulmonary insufficiency, not elsewhere classified
746.09 Other congenital anomalies of pulmonary valve
746.89 Other specified congenital anomaly of heart
769 Respiratory distress syndrome in newborn
770.84 Respiratory failure of newborn
770.89 Other respiratory problems of newborn after birth
997.1 Cardiac complications — (Use additional code to identify complications)

ICD-9-CM Procedural

39.65 Extracorporeal membrane oxygenation (ECMO)

36823

36823 Insertion of arterial and venous cannula(s) for isolated extracorporeal circulation including regional chemotherapy perfusion to an extremity, with or without hyperthermia, with removal of cannula(s) and repair of arteriotomy and venotomy sites

ICD-9-CM Diagnostic

170.4 Malignant neoplasm of scapula and long bones of upper limb
170.5 Malignant neoplasm of short bones of upper limb
170.7 Malignant neoplasm of long bones of lower limb
170.8 Malignant neoplasm of short bones of lower limb
171.2 Malignant neoplasm of connective and other soft tissue of upper limb, including shoulder
171.3 Malignant neoplasm of connective and other soft tissue of lower limb, including hip
238.0 Neoplasm of uncertain behavior of bone and articular cartilage
238.1 Neoplasm of uncertain behavior of connective and other soft tissue ▽

ICD-9-CM Procedural

38.91 Arterial catheterization
38.93 Venous catheterization, not elsewhere classified
99.25 Injection or infusion of cancer chemotherapeutic substance

36825–36830

36825 Creation of arteriovenous fistula by other than direct arteriovenous anastomosis (separate procedure); autogenous graft
36830 nonautogenous graft (eg, biological collagen, thermoplastic graft)

ICD-9-CM Diagnostic

250.40 Diabetes with renal manifestations, type II or unspecified type, not stated as uncontrolled — (Use additional code to identify manifestation: 581.81, 583.81)
250.41 Diabetes with renal manifestations, type I [juvenile type], not stated as uncontrolled — (Use additional code to identify manifestation: 581.81, 583.81)
250.42 Diabetes with renal manifestations, type II or unspecified type, uncontrolled — (Use additional code to identify manifestation: 581.81, 583.81)
250.43 Diabetes with renal manifestations, type I [juvenile type], uncontrolled — (Use additional code to identify manifestation: 581.81, 583.81)
403.01 Malignant hypertensive renal disease with renal failure
403.91 Unspecified hypertensive renal disease with renal failure ▽
404.02 Malignant hypertensive heart and renal disease with renal failure
404.03 Malignant hypertensive heart and renal disease with heart failure and renal failure

▽ Unspecified code ♀ Female diagnosis ☒ Manifestation code ♂ Male diagnosis

405.01 Secondary renovascular hypertension, malignant

581.1 Nephrotic syndrome with lesion of membranous glomerulonephritis

581.81 Nephrotic syndrome with other specified pathological lesion in kidney in diseases classified elsewhere — (Code first underlying disease: 084.9, 250.4, 277.3, 446.0, 710.0) ☒

582.0 Chronic glomerulonephritis with lesion of proliferative glomerulonephritis

582.1 Chronic glomerulonephritis with lesion of membranous glomerulonephritis

582.2 Chronic glomerulonephritis with lesion of membranoproliferative glomerulonephritis

582.4 Chronic glomerulonephritis with lesion of rapidly progressive glomerulonephritis

582.81 Chronic glomerulonephritis with other specified pathological lesion in kidney in diseases classified elsewhere — (Code first underlying disease: 277.3, 710.0) ☒

582.89 Other chronic glomerulonephritis with specified pathological lesion in kidney

582.9 Chronic glomerulonephritis with unspecified pathological lesion in kidney ▽

583.0 Nephritis and nephropathy, not specified as acute or chronic, with lesion of proliferative glomerulonephritis

583.1 Nephritis and nephropathy, not specified as acute or chronic, with lesion of membranous glomerulonephritis

583.2 Nephritis and nephropathy, not specified as acute or chronic, with lesion of membranoproliferative glomerulonephritis

583.4 Nephritis and nephropathy, not specified as acute or chronic, with lesion of rapidly progressive glomerulonephritis

583.6 Nephritis and nephropathy, not specified as acute or chronic, with lesion of renal cortical necrosis

583.7 Nephritis and nephropathy, not specified as acute or chronic, with lesion of renal medullary necrosis

583.81 Nephritis and nephropathy, not specified as acute or chronic, with other specified pathological lesion in kidney, in diseases classified elsewhere — (Code first underlying disease: 016.0, 098.19, 250.4, 277.3, 446.21, 710.0) ☒

583.89 Other nephritis and nephropathy, not specified as acute or chronic, with specified pathological lesion in kidney

583.9 Nephritis and nephropathy, not specified as acute or chronic, with unspecified pathological lesion in kidney ▽

585 Chronic renal failure — (Use additional code to identify manifestation: 357.4, 420.0)

586 Unspecified renal failure ▽

587 Unspecified renal sclerosis ▽

588.0 Renal osteodystrophy

588.81 Secondary hyperparathyroidism (of renal origin)

588.89 Other specified disorders resulting from impaired renal function

588.9 Unspecified disorder resulting from impaired renal function ▽

590.00 Chronic pyelonephritis without lesion of renal medullary necrosis — (Code, if applicable, any causal condition first. Use additional code to identify organism, such as E. coli, 041.4)

590.01 Chronic pyelonephritis with lesion of renal medullary necrosis — (Code, if applicable, any causal condition first. Use additional code to identify organism, such as E. coli, 041.4)

590.3 Pyeloureteritis cystica — (Use additional code to identify organism, such as E. coli, 041.4)

590.80 Unspecified pyelonephritis — (Use additional code to identify organism, such as E. coli, 041.4) ▽

590.81 Pyelitis or pyelonephritis in diseases classified elsewhere — (Code first underlying disease, 016.0. Use additional code to identify organism, such as E. coli, 041.4) ☒

590.9 Unspecified infection of kidney — (Use additional code to identify organism, such as E. coli, 041.4) ▽

591 Hydronephrosis

593.81 Vascular disorders of kidney

958.5 Traumatic anuria

996.1 Mechanical complication of other vascular device, implant, and graft

996.73 Other complications due to renal dialysis device, implant, and graft

996.81 Complications of transplanted kidney — (Use additional code to identify nature of complication, 078.5)

V42.0 Kidney replaced by transplant — (This code is intended for use when these conditions are recorded as diagnoses or problems)

ICD-9-CM Procedural

39.27 Arteriovenostomy for renal dialysis

HCPCS Level II Supplies & Services

G0365 Vessel mapping of vessels for hemodialysis access (services for preoperative vessel mapping prior to creation of hemodialysis access using an autogenous hemodialysis conduit, including arterial inflow and venous outflow)

36831

36831 Thrombectomy, open, arteriovenous fistula without revision, autogenous or nonautogenous dialysis graft (separate procedure)

ICD-9-CM Diagnostic

403.91 Unspecified hypertensive renal disease with renal failure ▽

585 Chronic renal failure — (Use additional code to identify manifestation: 357.4, 420.0)

586 Unspecified renal failure ▽

996.73 Other complications due to renal dialysis device, implant, and graft

V45.1 Renal dialysis status — (This code is intended for use when these conditions are recorded as diagnoses or problems)

ICD-9-CM Procedural

38.03 Incision of upper limb vessels

HCPCS Level II Supplies & Services

G0365 Vessel mapping of vessels for hemodialysis access (services for preoperative vessel mapping prior to creation of hemodialysis access using an autogenous hemodialysis conduit, including arterial inflow and venous outflow)

36832–36833

36832 Revision, open, arteriovenous fistula; without thrombectomy, autogenous or nonautogenous dialysis graft (separate procedure)

36833 with thrombectomy, autogenous or nonautogenous dialysis graft (separate procedure)

ICD-9-CM Diagnostic

403.91 Unspecified hypertensive renal disease with renal failure ▽

585 Chronic renal failure — (Use additional code to identify manifestation: 357.4, 420.0)

586 Unspecified renal failure ▽

996.1 Mechanical complication of other vascular device, implant, and graft

996.62 Infection and inflammatory reaction due to other vascular device, implant, and graft — (Use additional code to identify specified infections)

996.73 Other complications due to renal dialysis device, implant, and graft

996.74 Other complications due to other vascular device, implant, and graft

996.81 Complications of transplanted kidney — (Use additional code to identify nature of complication, 078.5)

V42.0 Kidney replaced by transplant — (This code is intended for use when these conditions are recorded as diagnoses or problems)

V45.1 Renal dialysis status — (This code is intended for use when these conditions are recorded as diagnoses or problems)

V53.90 Fitting and adjustment, Unspecified device ▽

V53.99 Fitting and adjustment, Other device

ICD-9-CM Procedural

39.42 Revision of arteriovenous shunt for renal dialysis

39.49 Other revision of vascular procedure

39.94 Replacement of vessel-to-vessel cannula

HCPCS Level II Supplies & Services

G0365 Vessel mapping of vessels for hemodialysis access (services for preoperative vessel mapping prior to creation of hemodialysis access using an autogenous hemodialysis conduit, including arterial inflow and venous outflow)

36834

36834 Plastic repair of arteriovenous aneurysm (separate procedure)

ICD-9-CM Diagnostic

747.60 Congenital anomaly of the peripheral vascular system, unspecified site ▽

996.1 Mechanical complication of other vascular device, implant, and graft

V45.1 Renal dialysis status — (This code is intended for use when these conditions are recorded as diagnoses or problems)

ICD-9-CM Procedural

39.52 Other repair of aneurysm

36835

36835 Insertion of Thomas shunt (separate procedure)

ICD-9-CM Diagnostic

250.40 Diabetes with renal manifestations, type II or unspecified type, not stated as uncontrolled — (Use additional code to identify manifestation: 581.81, 583.81)

250.41 Diabetes with renal manifestations, type I [juvenile type], not stated as uncontrolled — (Use additional code to identify manifestation: 581.81, 583.81)

▽ Unspecified code
♀ Female diagnosis
☒ Manifestation code
♂ Male diagnosis

250.42 Diabetes with renal manifestations, type II or unspecified type, uncontrolled — (Use additional code to identify manifestation: 581.81, 583.81)
250.43 Diabetes with renal manifestations, type I [juvenile type], uncontrolled — (Use additional code to identify manifestation: 581.81, 583.81)
403.01 Malignant hypertensive renal disease with renal failure
403.91 Unspecified hypertensive renal disease with renal failure ▽
404.02 Malignant hypertensive heart and renal disease with renal failure
404.03 Malignant hypertensive heart and renal disease with heart failure and renal failure
405.01 Secondary renovascular hypertension, malignant
581.1 Nephrotic syndrome with lesion of membranous glomerulonephritis
581.81 Nephrotic syndrome with other specified pathological lesion in kidney in diseases classified elsewhere — (Code first underlying disease: 084.9, 250.4, 277.3, 446.0, 710.0) ☒
582.0 Chronic glomerulonephritis with lesion of proliferative glomerulonephritis
582.1 Chronic glomerulonephritis with lesion of membranous glomerulonephritis
582.2 Chronic glomerulonephritis with lesion of membranoproliferative glomerulonephritis
582.4 Chronic glomerulonephritis with lesion of rapidly progressive glomerulonephritis
582.81 Chronic glomerulonephritis with other specified pathological lesion in kidney in diseases classified elsewhere — (Code first underlying disease: 277.3, 710.0) ☒
582.89 Other chronic glomerulonephritis with specified pathological lesion in kidney
582.9 Chronic glomerulonephritis with unspecified pathological lesion in kidney ▽
583.0 Nephritis and nephropathy, not specified as acute or chronic, with lesion of proliferative glomerulonephritis
583.1 Nephritis and nephropathy, not specified as acute or chronic, with lesion of membranous glomerulonephritis
583.2 Nephritis and nephropathy, not specified as acute or chronic, with lesion of membranoproliferative glomerulonephritis
583.4 Nephritis and nephropathy, not specified as acute or chronic, with lesion of rapidly progressive glomerulonephritis
583.6 Nephritis and nephropathy, not specified as acute or chronic, with lesion of renal cortical necrosis
583.7 Nephritis and nephropathy, not specified as acute or chronic, with lesion of renal medullary necrosis
583.81 Nephritis and nephropathy, not specified as acute or chronic, with other specified pathological lesion in kidney, in diseases classified elsewhere — (Code first underlying disease: 016.0, 098.19, 250.4, 277.3, 446.21, 710.0) ☒
583.89 Other nephritis and nephropathy, not specified as acute or chronic, with specified pathological lesion in kidney
583.9 Nephritis and nephropathy, not specified as acute or chronic, with unspecified pathological lesion in kidney ▽
585 Chronic renal failure — (Use additional code to identify manifestation: 357.4, 420.0)
586 Unspecified renal failure ▽
587 Unspecified renal sclerosis ▽
588.0 Renal osteodystrophy
588.81 Secondary hyperparathyroidism (of renal origin)
588.89 Other specified disorders resulting from impaired renal function
588.9 Unspecified disorder resulting from impaired renal function ▽
590.00 Chronic pyelonephritis without lesion of renal medullary necrosis — (Code, if applicable, any causal condition first. Use additional code to identify organism, such as E. coli, 041.4)
590.01 Chronic pyelonephritis with lesion of renal medullary necrosis — (Code, if applicable, any causal condition first. Use additional code to identify organism, such as E. coli, 041.4)
590.3 Pyeloureteritis cystica — (Use additional code to identify organism, such as E. coli, 041.4)
590.80 Unspecified pyelonephritis — (Use additional code to identify organism, such as E. coli, 041.4) ▽
590.81 Pyelitis or pyelonephritis in diseases classified elsewhere — (Code first underlying disease, 016.0. Use additional code to identify organism, such as E. coli, 041.4) ☒
590.9 Unspecified infection of kidney — (Use additional code to identify organism, such as E. coli, 041.4) ▽
591 Hydronephrosis
593.81 Vascular disorders of kidney
958.5 Traumatic anuria
996.1 Mechanical complication of other vascular device, implant, and graft
996.73 Other complications due to renal dialysis device, implant, and graft
996.81 Complications of transplanted kidney — (Use additional code to identify nature of complication, 078.5)
V42.0 Kidney replaced by transplant — (This code is intended for use when these conditions are recorded as diagnoses or problems)

ICD-9-CM Procedural

39.27 Arteriovenostomy for renal dialysis

36838

36838 Distal revascularization and interval ligation (DRIL), upper extremity hemodialysis access (steal syndrome)

ICD-9-CM Diagnostic

435.2 Subclavian steal syndrome — (Use additional code to identify presence of hypertension)

ICD-9-CM Procedural

39.42 Revision of arteriovenous shunt for renal dialysis
39.53 Repair of arteriovenous fistula

36860–36861

36860 External cannula declotting (separate procedure); without balloon catheter
36861 with balloon catheter

ICD-9-CM Diagnostic

996.1 Mechanical complication of other vascular device, implant, and graft
996.73 Other complications due to renal dialysis device, implant, and graft
996.74 Other complications due to other vascular device, implant, and graft

ICD-9-CM Procedural

39.49 Other revision of vascular procedure

HCPCS Level II Supplies & Services

A4550 Surgical trays
J2995 Injection, streptokinase, per 250,000 IU

36870

36870 Thrombectomy, percutaneous, arteriovenous fistula, autogenous or nonautogenous graft (includes mechanical thrombus extraction and intra-graft thrombolysis)

ICD-9-CM Diagnostic

403.91 Unspecified hypertensive renal disease with renal failure ▽
585 Chronic renal failure — (Use additional code to identify manifestation: 357.4, 420.0)
586 Unspecified renal failure ▽
996.73 Other complications due to renal dialysis device, implant, and graft
V45.1 Renal dialysis status — (This code is intended for use when these conditions are recorded as diagnoses or problems)

ICD-9-CM Procedural

39.49 Other revision of vascular procedure

37140

37140 Venous anastomosis, open; portocaval

ICD-9-CM Diagnostic

452 Portal vein thrombosis
453.0 Budd-Chiari syndrome
456.20 Esophageal varices with bleeding in diseases classified elsewhere — (Code first underlying disease: 571.0-571.9, 572.3) ☒
459.2 Compression of vein
572.1 Portal pyemia
572.3 Portal hypertension

ICD-9-CM Procedural

39.1 Intra-abdominal venous shunt

37145

37145 Venous anastomosis, open; renoportal

ICD-9-CM Diagnostic

403.00 Malignant hypertensive renal disease without mention of renal failure
403.10 Benign hypertensive renal disease without mention of renal failure
452 Portal vein thrombosis
453.0 Budd-Chiari syndrome
453.3 Embolism and thrombosis of renal vein
578.9 Unspecified, hemorrhage of gastrointestinal tract ▽
586 Unspecified renal failure ▽

587 Unspecified renal sclerosis
593.81 Vascular disorders of kidney
747.62 Congenital renal vessel anomaly
747.69 Congenital anomaly of other specified site of peripheral vascular system
902.33 Portal vein injury

ICD-9-CM Procedural

39.1 Intra-abdominal venous shunt

37160

37160 Venous anastomosis, open; caval-mesenteric

ICD-9-CM Diagnostic

453.2 Embolism and thrombosis of vena cava
453.8 Embolism and thrombosis of other specified veins
557.0 Acute vascular insufficiency of intestine
557.1 Chronic vascular insufficiency of intestine
557.9 Unspecified vascular insufficiency of intestine

ICD-9-CM Procedural

39.1 Intra-abdominal venous shunt

37180

37180 Venous anastomosis, open; splenorenal, proximal

ICD-9-CM Diagnostic

453.3 Embolism and thrombosis of renal vein
453.8 Embolism and thrombosis of other specified veins
456.20 Esophageal varices with bleeding in diseases classified elsewhere — (Code first underlying disease: 571.0-571.9, 572.3)
459.2 Compression of vein
459.9 Unspecified circulatory system disorder
585 Chronic renal failure — (Use additional code to identify manifestation: 357.4, 420.0)
587 Unspecified renal sclerosis
865.01 Spleen hematoma, without rupture of capsule or mention of open wound into cavity

ICD-9-CM Procedural

39.1 Intra-abdominal venous shunt

37181

37181 Venous anastomosis, open; splenorenal, distal (selective decompression of esophagogastric varices, any technique)

ICD-9-CM Diagnostic

420.0 Acute pericarditis in diseases classified elsewhere — (Code first underlying disease: 017.9, 039.8, 066.8, 585)
453.3 Embolism and thrombosis of renal vein
453.8 Embolism and thrombosis of other specified veins
456.20 Esophageal varices with bleeding in diseases classified elsewhere — (Code first underlying disease: 571.0-571.9, 572.3)
459.2 Compression of vein
459.9 Unspecified circulatory system disorder
578.9 Unspecified, hemorrhage of gastrointestinal tract
585 Chronic renal failure — (Use additional code to identify manifestation: 357.4, 420.0)
587 Unspecified renal sclerosis
865.01 Spleen hematoma, without rupture of capsule or mention of open wound into cavity

ICD-9-CM Procedural

39.1 Intra-abdominal venous shunt

37182–37183

37182 Insertion of transvenous intrahepatic portosystemic shunt(s) (TIPS) (includes venous access, hepatic and portal vein catheterization, portography with hemodynamic evaluation, intrahepatic tract formation/dilatation, stent placement and all associated imaging guidance and documentation)
37183 Revision of transvenous intrahepatic portosystemic shunt(s) (TIPS) (includes venous access, hepatic and portal vein catheterization, portography with hemodynamic evaluation, intrahepatic tract recanulization/dilatation, stent placement and all associated imaging guidance and documentation)

ICD-9-CM Diagnostic

452 Portal vein thrombosis
453.0 Budd-Chiari syndrome
456.0 Esophageal varices with bleeding
456.1 Esophageal varices without mention of bleeding
456.20 Esophageal varices with bleeding in diseases classified elsewhere — (Code first underlying disease: 571.0-571.9, 572.3)
456.21 Esophageal varices without mention of bleeding in diseases classified elsewhere — (Code first underlying disease: 571.0-571.9, 572.3)
459.2 Compression of vein
572.1 Portal pyemia
572.3 Portal hypertension
789.5 Ascites
996.1 Mechanical complication of other vascular device, implant, and graft
996.62 Infection and inflammatory reaction due to other vascular device, implant, and graft — (Use additional code to identify specified infections)
996.74 Other complications due to other vascular device, implant, and graft
997.4 Digestive system complication — (Use additional code to identify complications)

ICD-9-CM Procedural

39.1 Intra-abdominal venous shunt

HCPCS Level II Supplies & Services

HCPCS Level II codes are used to report the supplies, durable medical equipment, and certain medical services provided on an outpatient basis. Because the procedure(s) represented on this page would be performed in an inpatient facility, no HCPCS Level II codes apply.

37195

37195 Thrombolysis, cerebral, by intravenous infusion

ICD-9-CM Diagnostic

434.00 Cerebral thrombosis without mention of cerebral infarction — (Use additional code to identify presence of hypertension)
434.01 Cerebral thrombosis with cerebral infarction — (Use additional code to identify presence of hypertension)
434.10 Cerebral embolism without mention of cerebral infarction — (Use additional code to identify presence of hypertension)
434.11 Cerebral embolism with cerebral infarction — (Use additional code to identify presence of hypertension)
434.90 Unspecified cerebral artery occlusion without mention of cerebral infarction — (Use additional code to identify presence of hypertension)
434.91 Unspecified cerebral artery occlusion with cerebral infarction — (Use additional code to identify presence of hypertension)
435.9 Unspecified transient cerebral ischemia — (Use additional code to identify presence of hypertension)
436 Acute, but ill-defined, cerebrovascular disease — (Use additional code to identify presence of hypertension)
997.02 Iatrogenic cerebrovascular infarction or hemorrhage — (Use additional code to identify complications)

ICD-9-CM Procedural

38.91 Arterial catheterization
88.41 Arteriography of cerebral arteries
99.10 Injection or infusion of thrombolytic agent
99.20 Injection or infusion of platelet inhibitor

37200

37200 Transcatheter biopsy

ICD-9-CM Diagnostic

The application of this code is too broad to adequately present ICD-9-CM diagnostic code links here. Refer to your ICD-9-CM book.

Unspecified code
Female diagnosis

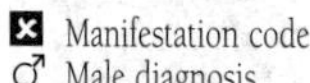

ICD-9-CM Procedural

38.21 Biopsy of blood vessel

37201–37202

37201 Transcatheter therapy, infusion for thrombolysis other than coronary
37202 Transcatheter therapy, infusion other than for thrombolysis, any type (eg, spasmolytic, vasoconstrictive)

ICD-9-CM Diagnostic

433.10 Occlusion and stenosis of carotid artery without mention of cerebral infarction — (Use additional code to identify presence of hypertension)
433.20 Occlusion and stenosis of vertebral artery without mention of cerebral infarction — (Use additional code to identify presence of hypertension)
433.30 Occlusion and stenosis of multiple and bilateral precerebral arteries without mention of cerebral infarction — (Use additional code to identify presence of hypertension)
433.80 Occlusion and stenosis of other specified precerebral artery without mention of cerebral infarction — (Use additional code to identify presence of hypertension)
434.00 Cerebral thrombosis without mention of cerebral infarction — (Use additional code to identify presence of hypertension)
435.0 Basilar artery syndrome — (Use additional code to identify presence of hypertension)
435.1 Vertebral artery syndrome — (Use additional code to identify presence of hypertension)
435.3 Vertebrobasilar artery syndrome — (Use additional code to identify presence of hypertension)
435.8 Other specified transient cerebral ischemias — (Use additional code to identify presence of hypertension)
435.9 Unspecified transient cerebral ischemia — (Use additional code to identify presence of hypertension) ▽
440.22 Atherosclerosis of native arteries of the extremities with rest pain
440.9 Generalized and unspecified atherosclerosis ▽
443.9 Unspecified peripheral vascular disease ▽
444.0 Embolism and thrombosis of abdominal aorta
444.21 Embolism and thrombosis of arteries of upper extremity
444.22 Embolism and thrombosis of arteries of lower extremity
444.81 Embolism and thrombosis of iliac artery
444.9 Embolism and thrombosis of unspecified artery ▽
445.01 Atheroembolism of upper extremity
445.02 Atheroembolism of lower extremity
445.81 Atheroembolism of kidney — (Use additional code for any associated kidney failure: 584, 585)
445.89 Atheroembolism of other site
447.1 Stricture of artery
447.9 Unspecified disorders of arteries and arterioles ▽
453.0 Budd-Chiari syndrome
453.2 Embolism and thrombosis of vena cava
453.3 Embolism and thrombosis of renal vein
453.40 Venous embolism and thrombosis of unspecified deep vessels of lower extremity
453.41 Venous embolism and thrombosis of deep vessels of proximal lower extremity
453.42 Venous embolism and thrombosis of deep vessels of distal lower extremity
453.8 Embolism and thrombosis of other specified veins
453.9 Embolism and thrombosis of unspecified site ▽
459.2 Compression of vein
729.5 Pain in soft tissues of limb
747.60 Congenital anomaly of the peripheral vascular system, unspecified site ▽
780.02 Transient alteration of awareness
780.2 Syncope and collapse
780.31 Febrile convulsions
780.39 Other convulsions
780.4 Dizziness and giddiness
996.1 Mechanical complication of other vascular device, implant, and graft
996.73 Other complications due to renal dialysis device, implant, and graft
996.74 Other complications due to other vascular device, implant, and graft
997.2 Peripheral vascular complications — (Use additional code to identify complications)
V72.5 Radiological examination, not elsewhere classified — (Use additional code(s) to identify any special screening examination(s) performed: V73.0-V82.9)

ICD-9-CM Procedural

00.17 Infusion of vasopressor agent
99.10 Injection or infusion of thrombolytic agent
99.20 Injection or infusion of platelet inhibitor
99.29 Injection or infusion of other therapeutic or prophylactic substance
99.77 Application or administration of adhesion barrier substance

HCPCS Level II Supplies & Services

C1884 Embolization protective system

37203

37203 Transcatheter retrieval, percutaneous, of intravascular foreign body (eg, fractured venous or arterial catheter)

ICD-9-CM Diagnostic

996.1 Mechanical complication of other vascular device, implant, and graft
996.73 Other complications due to renal dialysis device, implant, and graft
996.74 Other complications due to other vascular device, implant, and graft
998.4 Foreign body accidentally left during procedure, not elsewhere classified

ICD-9-CM Procedural

38.91 Arterial catheterization
38.93 Venous catheterization, not elsewhere classified
97.89 Removal of other therapeutic device

37204

37204 Transcatheter occlusion or embolization (eg, for tumor destruction, to achieve hemostasis, to occlude a vascular malformation), percutaneous, any method, non-central nervous system, non-head or neck

ICD-9-CM Diagnostic

151.0 Malignant neoplasm of cardia
151.1 Malignant neoplasm of pylorus
151.2 Malignant neoplasm of pyloric antrum
151.3 Malignant neoplasm of fundus of stomach
151.4 Malignant neoplasm of body of stomach
151.5 Malignant neoplasm of lesser curvature of stomach, unspecified ▽
151.6 Malignant neoplasm of greater curvature of stomach, unspecified ▽
151.8 Malignant neoplasm of other specified sites of stomach
151.9 Malignant neoplasm of stomach, unspecified site ▽
153.0 Malignant neoplasm of hepatic flexure
153.1 Malignant neoplasm of transverse colon
153.2 Malignant neoplasm of descending colon
153.3 Malignant neoplasm of sigmoid colon
153.4 Malignant neoplasm of cecum
153.5 Malignant neoplasm of appendix
153.6 Malignant neoplasm of ascending colon
153.7 Malignant neoplasm of splenic flexure
153.8 Malignant neoplasm of other specified sites of large intestine
153.9 Malignant neoplasm of colon, unspecified site ▽
154.0 Malignant neoplasm of rectosigmoid junction
154.1 Malignant neoplasm of rectum
154.2 Malignant neoplasm of anal canal
154.3 Malignant neoplasm of anus, unspecified site ▽
154.8 Malignant neoplasm of other sites of rectum, rectosigmoid junction, and anus
155.0 Malignant neoplasm of liver, primary
155.1 Malignant neoplasm of intrahepatic bile ducts
155.2 Malignant neoplasm of liver, not specified as primary or secondary ▽
156.0 Malignant neoplasm of gallbladder
156.1 Malignant neoplasm of extrahepatic bile ducts
156.2 Malignant neoplasm of ampulla of Vater
156.8 Malignant neoplasm of other specified sites of gallbladder and extrahepatic bile ducts
156.9 Malignant neoplasm of biliary tract, part unspecified site ▽
157.0 Malignant neoplasm of head of pancreas
157.1 Malignant neoplasm of body of pancreas
157.2 Malignant neoplasm of tail of pancreas
157.3 Malignant neoplasm of pancreatic duct
157.4 Malignant neoplasm of islets of Langerhans — (Use additional code to identify any functional activity)
157.8 Malignant neoplasm of other specified sites of pancreas
157.9 Malignant neoplasm of pancreas, part unspecified ▽
158.0 Malignant neoplasm of retroperitoneum
158.8 Malignant neoplasm of specified parts of peritoneum
158.9 Malignant neoplasm of peritoneum, unspecified ▽
159.0 Malignant neoplasm of intestinal tract, part unspecified ▽
159.1 Malignant neoplasm of spleen, not elsewhere classified
159.8 Malignant neoplasm of other sites of digestive system and intra-abdominal organs
159.9 Malignant neoplasm of ill-defined sites of digestive organs and peritoneum
162.3 Malignant neoplasm of upper lobe, bronchus, or lung
162.4 Malignant neoplasm of middle lobe, bronchus, or lung

162.5 Malignant neoplasm of lower lobe, bronchus, or lung
162.8 Malignant neoplasm of other parts of bronchus or lung
163.0 Malignant neoplasm of parietal pleura
163.1 Malignant neoplasm of visceral pleura
163.8 Malignant neoplasm of other specified sites of pleura
163.9 Malignant neoplasm of pleura, unspecified site ▽
164.0 Malignant neoplasm of thymus
164.1 Malignant neoplasm of heart
164.2 Malignant neoplasm of anterior mediastinum
164.3 Malignant neoplasm of posterior mediastinum
164.8 Malignant neoplasm of other parts of mediastinum
165.0 Malignant neoplasm of upper respiratory tract, part unspecified ▽
165.8 Malignant neoplasm of other sites within the respiratory system and intrathoracic organs
165.9 Malignant neoplasm of ill-defined sites within the respiratory system
171.2 Malignant neoplasm of connective and other soft tissue of upper limb, including shoulder
171.3 Malignant neoplasm of connective and other soft tissue of lower limb, including hip
171.4 Malignant neoplasm of connective and other soft tissue of thorax
171.5 Malignant neoplasm of connective and other soft tissue of abdomen
171.6 Malignant neoplasm of connective and other soft tissue of pelvis
171.7 Malignant neoplasm of connective and other soft tissue of trunk, unspecified site ▽
171.8 Malignant neoplasm of other specified sites of connective and other soft tissue
171.9 Malignant neoplasm of connective and other soft tissue, site unspecified ▽
189.0 Malignant neoplasm of kidney, except pelvis
189.1 Malignant neoplasm of renal pelvis
194.0 Malignant neoplasm of adrenal gland — (Use additional code to identify any functional activity)
195.1 Malignant neoplasm of thorax
195.2 Malignant neoplasm of abdomen
195.3 Malignant neoplasm of pelvis
195.4 Malignant neoplasm of upper limb
195.5 Malignant neoplasm of lower limb
195.8 Malignant neoplasm of other specified sites
197.0 Secondary malignant neoplasm of lung
197.1 Secondary malignant neoplasm of mediastinum
197.2 Secondary malignant neoplasm of pleura
197.4 Secondary malignant neoplasm of small intestine including duodenum
197.5 Secondary malignant neoplasm of large intestine and rectum
197.6 Secondary malignant neoplasm of retroperitoneum and peritoneum
197.7 Secondary malignant neoplasm of liver
197.8 Secondary malignant neoplasm of other digestive organs and spleen
198.0 Secondary malignant neoplasm of kidney
198.6 Secondary malignant neoplasm of ovary ♀
198.7 Secondary malignant neoplasm of adrenal gland
198.89 Secondary malignant neoplasm of other specified sites
199.0 Disseminated malignant neoplasm
211.0 Benign neoplasm of esophagus
211.1 Benign neoplasm of stomach
211.2 Benign neoplasm of duodenum, jejunum, and ileum
211.3 Benign neoplasm of colon
211.5 Benign neoplasm of liver and biliary passages
211.6 Benign neoplasm of pancreas, except islets of Langerhans
211.7 Benign neoplasm of islets of Langerhans — (Use additional code to identify any functional activity)
211.8 Benign neoplasm of retroperitoneum and peritoneum
211.9 Benign neoplasm of other and unspecified site of the digestive system ▽
212.3 Benign neoplasm of bronchus and lung
212.4 Benign neoplasm of pleura
212.5 Benign neoplasm of mediastinum
212.6 Benign neoplasm of thymus
212.7 Benign neoplasm of heart
212.8 Benign neoplasm of other specified sites of respiratory and intrathoracic organs
212.9 Benign neoplasm of respiratory and intrathoracic organs, site unspecified ▽
214.2 Lipoma of intrathoracic organs
214.3 Lipoma of intra-abdominal organs
215.2 Other benign neoplasm of connective and other soft tissue of upper limb, including shoulder
215.3 Other benign neoplasm of connective and other soft tissue of lower limb, including hip
215.4 Other benign neoplasm of connective and other soft tissue of thorax
215.5 Other benign neoplasm of connective and other soft tissue of abdomen
215.6 Other benign neoplasm of connective and other soft tissue of pelvis
215.7 Other benign neoplasm of connective and other soft tissue of trunk, unspecified ▽
215.8 Other benign neoplasm of connective and other soft tissue of other specified sites
215.9 Other benign neoplasm of connective and other soft tissue of unspecified site ▽
223.0 Benign neoplasm of kidney, except pelvis
223.1 Benign neoplasm of renal pelvis
223.9 Benign neoplasm of urinary organ, site unspecified ▽
227.0 Benign neoplasm of adrenal gland — (Use additional code to identify any functional activity)
227.6 Benign neoplasm of aortic body and other paraganglia — (Use additional code to identify any functional activity)
228.04 Hemangioma of intra-abdominal structures
230.2 Carcinoma in situ of stomach
230.7 Carcinoma in situ of other and unspecified parts of intestine ▽
230.8 Carcinoma in situ of liver and biliary system
230.9 Carcinoma in situ of other and unspecified digestive organs ▽
233.9 Carcinoma in situ of other and unspecified urinary organs ▽
442.0 Aneurysm of artery of upper extremity
442.1 Aneurysm of renal artery
442.2 Aneurysm of iliac artery
442.82 Aneurysm of subclavian artery
442.83 Aneurysm of splenic artery
442.84 Aneurysm of other visceral artery
442.89 Aneurysm of other specified artery
442.9 Other aneurysm of unspecified site ▽
447.0 Arteriovenous fistula, acquired
747.60 Congenital anomaly of the peripheral vascular system, unspecified site ▽
780.71 Chronic fatigue syndrome
780.79 Other malaise and fatigue
903.01 Axillary artery injury
903.3 Ulnar blood vessels injury
904.0 Common femoral artery injury
904.9 Injury to blood vessels, unspecified site ▽
958.2 Secondary and recurrent hemorrhage as an early complication of trauma
V72.5 Radiological examination, not elsewhere classified — (Use additional code(s) to identify any special screening examination(s) performed: V73.0-V82.9)

ICD-9-CM Procedural

38.80 Other surgical occlusion of vessels, unspecified site
38.84 Other surgical occlusion of abdominal aorta
38.86 Other surgical occlusion of abdominal arteries
39.53 Repair of arteriovenous fistula

37205–37206

37205 Transcatheter placement of an intravascular stent(s), (except coronary, carotid, and vertebral vessel), percutaneous; initial vessel
37206 each additional vessel (List separately in addition to code for primary procedure)

ICD-9-CM Diagnostic

440.20 Atherosclerosis of native arteries of the extremities, unspecified ▽
440.21 Atherosclerosis of native arteries of the extremities with intermittent claudication
440.22 Atherosclerosis of native arteries of the extremities with rest pain
440.23 Atherosclerosis of native arteries of the extremities with ulceration — (Use additional code for any associated ulceration: 707.10-707.9)
440.9 Generalized and unspecified atherosclerosis ▽

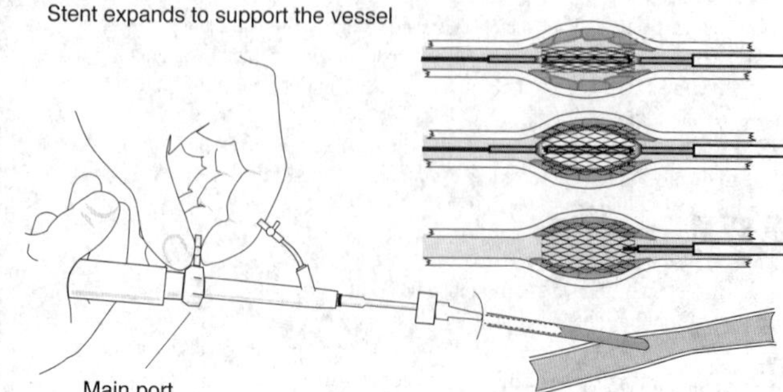
A catheter with a stent-transporting tip delivers a stent to the point where the vessel needs additional support
Stent Placement
Stent expands to support the vessel
Main port

▽ Unspecified code
♀ Female diagnosis
Manifestation code
♂ Male diagnosis

440.8 Atherosclerosis of other specified arteries
443.9 Unspecified peripheral vascular disease
444.21 Embolism and thrombosis of arteries of upper extremity
444.22 Embolism and thrombosis of arteries of lower extremity
444.81 Embolism and thrombosis of iliac artery
444.89 Embolism and thrombosis of other specified artery
444.9 Embolism and thrombosis of unspecified artery
445.01 Atheroembolism of upper extremity
445.02 Atheroembolism of lower extremity
445.89 Atheroembolism of other site
447.1 Stricture of artery
593.81 Vascular disorders of kidney
908.3 Late effect of injury to blood vessel of head, neck, and extremities
996.1 Mechanical complication of other vascular device, implant, and graft
996.73 Other complications due to renal dialysis device, implant, and graft
996.74 Other complications due to other vascular device, implant, and graft
V72.5 Radiological examination, not elsewhere classified — (Use additional code(s) to identify any special screening examination(s) performed: V73.0-V82.9)

ICD-9-CM Procedural

00.55 Insertion of drug-eluting peripheral vessel stent(s)
00.64 Percutaneous insertion of other precerebral (extracranial) artery stent(s)
00.65 Percutaneous insertion of intracranial vascular stent(s)
39.90 Insertion of non-drug-eluting peripheral vessel stents(s)

HCPCS Level II Supplies & Services

C1884 Embolization protective system

37207–37208

37207 Transcatheter placement of an intravascular stent(s), (non-coronary vessel), open; initial vessel
37208 each additional vessel (List separately in addition to code for primary procedure)

ICD-9-CM Diagnostic

433.10 Occlusion and stenosis of carotid artery without mention of cerebral infarction — (Use additional code to identify presence of hypertension)
433.20 Occlusion and stenosis of vertebral artery without mention of cerebral infarction — (Use additional code to identify presence of hypertension)
433.30 Occlusion and stenosis of multiple and bilateral precerebral arteries without mention of cerebral infarction — (Use additional code to identify presence of hypertension)
433.80 Occlusion and stenosis of other specified precerebral artery without mention of cerebral infarction — (Use additional code to identify presence of hypertension)
440.21 Atherosclerosis of native arteries of the extremities with intermittent claudication
440.22 Atherosclerosis of native arteries of the extremities with rest pain
440.8 Atherosclerosis of other specified arteries
440.9 Generalized and unspecified atherosclerosis
443.9 Unspecified peripheral vascular disease
444.21 Embolism and thrombosis of arteries of upper extremity
444.22 Embolism and thrombosis of arteries of lower extremity
444.89 Embolism and thrombosis of other specified artery
444.9 Embolism and thrombosis of unspecified artery
445.01 Atheroembolism of upper extremity
445.02 Atheroembolism of lower extremity
445.89 Atheroembolism of other site
447.1 Stricture of artery
908.3 Late effect of injury to blood vessel of head, neck, and extremities
996.1 Mechanical complication of other vascular device, implant, and graft
996.73 Other complications due to renal dialysis device, implant, and graft
996.74 Other complications due to other vascular device, implant, and graft

ICD-9-CM Procedural

00.55 Insertion of drug-eluting peripheral vessel stent(s)
39.90 Insertion of non-drug-eluting peripheral vessel stents(s)

HCPCS Level II Supplies & Services

C1884 Embolization protective system

37209

37209 Exchange of a previously placed arterial catheter during thrombolytic therapy

ICD-9-CM Diagnostic

433.10 Occlusion and stenosis of carotid artery without mention of cerebral infarction — (Use additional code to identify presence of hypertension)
433.20 Occlusion and stenosis of vertebral artery without mention of cerebral infarction — (Use additional code to identify presence of hypertension)
433.30 Occlusion and stenosis of multiple and bilateral precerebral arteries without mention of cerebral infarction — (Use additional code to identify presence of hypertension)
433.80 Occlusion and stenosis of other specified precerebral artery without mention of cerebral infarction — (Use additional code to identify presence of hypertension)
440.21 Atherosclerosis of native arteries of the extremities with intermittent claudication
440.22 Atherosclerosis of native arteries of the extremities with rest pain
440.8 Atherosclerosis of other specified arteries
447.1 Stricture of artery
908.3 Late effect of injury to blood vessel of head, neck, and extremities
996.1 Mechanical complication of other vascular device, implant, and graft
996.59 Mechanical complication due to other implant and internal device, not elsewhere classified
996.73 Other complications due to renal dialysis device, implant, and graft
996.74 Other complications due to other vascular device, implant, and graft

ICD-9-CM Procedural

38.91 Arterial catheterization

37215–37216

37215 Transcatheter placement of intravascular stent(s), cervical carotid artery, percutaneous; with distal embolic protection
37216 without distal embolic protection

ICD-9-CM Diagnostic

433.10 Occlusion and stenosis of carotid artery without mention of cerebral infarction — (Use additional code to identify presence of hypertension)
433.30 Occlusion and stenosis of multiple and bilateral precerebral arteries without mention of cerebral infarction — (Use additional code to identify presence of hypertension)
433.80 Occlusion and stenosis of other specified precerebral artery without mention of cerebral infarction — (Use additional code to identify presence of hypertension)
434.00 Cerebral thrombosis without mention of cerebral infarction — (Use additional code to identify presence of hypertension)
434.10 Cerebral embolism without mention of cerebral infarction — (Use additional code to identify presence of hypertension)
434.90 Unspecified cerebral artery occlusion without mention of cerebral infarction — (Use additional code to identify presence of hypertension)
435.8 Other specified transient cerebral ischemias — (Use additional code to identify presence of hypertension)
435.9 Unspecified transient cerebral ischemia — (Use additional code to identify presence of hypertension)
436 Acute, but ill-defined, cerebrovascular disease — (Use additional code to identify presence of hypertension)
437.0 Cerebral atherosclerosis — (Use additional code to identify presence of hypertension)
437.1 Other generalized ischemic cerebrovascular disease — (Use additional code to identify presence of hypertension)
437.3 Cerebral aneurysm, nonruptured — (Use additional code to identify presence of hypertension)
437.4 Cerebral arteritis — (Use additional code to identify presence of hypertension)
437.8 Other ill-defined cerebrovascular disease — (Use additional code to identify presence of hypertension)
438.0 Cognitive deficits due to cerebrovascular disease — (Use additional code to identify presence of hypertension)
438.10 Unspecified speech and language deficit due to cerebrovascular disease — (Use additional code to identify presence of hypertension)
438.11 Aphasia due to cerebrovascular disease — (Use additional code to identify presence of hypertension)
438.12 Dysphasia due to cerebrovascular disease — (Use additional code to identify presence of hypertension)
438.19 Other speech and language deficits due to cerebrovascular disease — (Use additional code to identify presence of hypertension)
438.20 Hemiplegia affecting unspecified side due to cerebrovascular disease — (Use additional code to identify presence of hypertension)
438.21 Hemiplegia affecting dominant side due to cerebrovascular disease — (Use additional code to identify presence of hypertension)
438.22 Hemiplegia affecting nondominant side due to cerebrovascular disease — (Use additional code to identify presence of hypertension)
438.30 Monoplegia of upper limb affecting unspecified side due to cerebrovascular disease — (Use additional code to identify presence of hypertension)
438.31 Monoplegia of upper limb affecting dominant side due to cerebrovascular disease — (Use additional code to identify presence of hypertension)

438.32 Monoplegia of upper limb affecting nondominant side due to cerebrovascular disease — (Use additional code to identify presence of hypertension)
438.40 Monoplegia of lower limb affecting unspecified side due to cerebrovascular disease — (Use additional code to identify presence of hypertension) ▽
438.41 Monoplegia of lower limb affecting dominant side due to cerebrovascular disease — (Use additional code to identify presence of hypertension)
438.42 Monoplegia of lower limb affecting nondominant side due to cerebrovascular disease — (Use additional code to identify presence of hypertension)
438.50 Other paralytic syndrome affecting unspecified side due to cerebrovascular disease — (Use additional code to identify type of paralytic syndrome: 344.81, 344.00-344.09. Use additional code to identify presence of hypertension) ▽
438.51 Other paralytic syndrome affecting dominant side due to cerebrovascular disease — (Use additional code to identify type of paralytic syndrome: 344.81, 344.00-344.09. Use additional code to identify presence of hypertension)
438.52 Other paralytic syndrome affecting nondominant side due to cerebrovascular disease — (Use additional code to identify type of paralytic syndrome: 344.81, 344.00-344.09. Use additional code to identify presence of hypertension)
438.53 Other paralytic syndrome, bilateral — (Use additional code to identify type of paralytic syndrome: 344.81, 344.00-344.09. Use additional code to identify presence of hypertension)
438.6 Alteration of sensations as late effect of cerebrovascular disease — (Use additional code to identify the altered sensation. Use additional code to identify presence of hypertension)
438.7 Disturbance of vision as late effect of cerebrovascular disease — (Use additional code to identify the visual disturbance. Use additional code to identify presence of hypertension)
438.81 Apraxia due to cerebrovascular disease — (Use additional code to identify presence of hypertension)
438.82 Dysphagia due to cerebrovascular disease — (Use additional code to identify presence of hypertension)
438.83 Facial weakness as late effect of cerebrovascular disease — (Use additional code to identify presence of hypertension)
438.84 Ataxia as late effect of cerebrovascular disease — (Use additional code to identify presence of hypertension)
438.85 Vertigo as late effect of cerebrovascular disease — (Use additional code to identify presence of hypertension)
438.89 Other late effects of cerebrovascular disease — (Use additional code to identify the late effect. Use additional code to identify presence of hypertension)
443.21 Dissection of carotid artery
447.1 Stricture of artery
908.3 Late effect of injury to blood vessel of head, neck, and extremities
996.1 Mechanical complication of other vascular device, implant, and graft
996.74 Other complications due to other vascular device, implant, and graft

ICD-9-CM Procedural

00.63 Percutaneous insertion of carotid artery stent(s)

HCPCS Level II Supplies & Services

C1884 Embolization protective system

37250–37251

37250 Intravascular ultrasound (non-coronary vessel) during diagnostic evaluation and/or therapeutic intervention; initial vessel (List separately in addition to code for primary procedure)
37251 each additional vessel (List separately in addition to code for primary procedure)

ICD-9-CM Diagnostic

This is an add-on code. Refer to the corresponding primary procedure code for ICD-9 diagnosis code links.

ICD-9-CM Procedural

00.01 Therapeutic ultrasound of vessels of head and neck
00.03 Therapeutic ultrasound of peripheral vascular vessels
00.09 Other therapeutic ultrasound
00.21 Intravascular imaging of extracranial cerebral vessels
00.22 Intravascular imaging of intrathoracic vessels
00.23 Intravascular imaging of peripheral vessels
00.25 Intravascular imaging of renal vessels
00.28 Intravascular imaging, other specified vessel(s)
00.29 Intravascular imaging, unspecified vessel(s)
88.77 Diagnostic ultrasound of peripheral vascular system

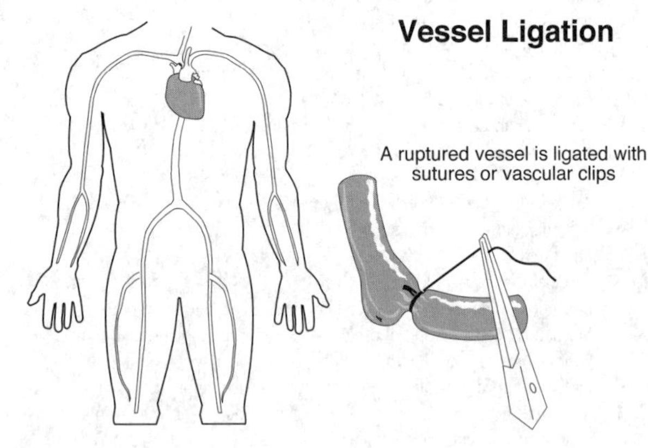

Vessel Ligation
A ruptured vessel is ligated with sutures or vascular clips

37500

37500 Vascular endoscopy, surgical, with ligation of perforator veins, subfascial (SEPS)

ICD-9-CM Diagnostic

454.0 Varicose veins of lower extremities with ulcer
454.1 Varicose veins of lower extremities with inflammation
454.2 Varicose veins of lower extremities with ulcer and inflammation
454.8 Varicose veins of the lower extremities with other complications
454.9 Asymptomatic varicose veins
459.10 Postphlebitic syndrome without complications
459.11 Postphlebitic syndrome with ulcer
459.12 Postphlebitic syndrome with inflammation
459.13 Postphlebitic syndrome with ulcer and inflammation
459.19 Postphlebitic syndrome with other complication
459.81 Unspecified venous (peripheral) insufficiency — (Use additional code for any associated ulceration: 707.10-707.9) ▽
707.10 Ulcer of lower limb, unspecified ▽
707.11 Ulcer of thigh
707.12 Ulcer of calf
707.13 Ulcer of ankle
707.14 Ulcer of heel and midfoot
707.15 Ulcer of other part of foot
707.19 Ulcer of other part of lower limb
729.5 Pain in soft tissues of limb

ICD-9-CM Procedural

38.59 Ligation and stripping of lower limb varicose veins
38.89 Other surgical occlusion of lower limb veins

HCPCS Level II Supplies & Services

HCPCS Level II codes are used to report the supplies, durable medical equipment, and certain medical services provided on an outpatient basis. Because the procedure(s) represented on this page would be performed in an inpatient or outpatient facility, no HCPCS Level II codes apply.

37565

37565 Ligation, internal jugular vein

ICD-9-CM Diagnostic

250.70 Diabetes with peripheral circulatory disorders, type II or unspecified type, not stated as uncontrolled — (Use additional code to identify manifestation: 443.81, 785.4)
250.71 Diabetes with peripheral circulatory disorders, type I [juvenile type], not stated as uncontrolled — (Use additional code to identify manifestation: 443.81, 785.4)
401.0 Essential hypertension, malignant
401.1 Essential hypertension, benign
401.9 Unspecified essential hypertension ▽
443.89 Other peripheral vascular disease
447.1 Stricture of artery
447.6 Unspecified arteritis ▽
447.8 Other specified disorders of arteries and arterioles
453.8 Embolism and thrombosis of other specified veins
459.0 Unspecified hemorrhage ▽
900.1 Internal jugular vein injury
998.11 Hemorrhage complicating a procedure
998.12 Hematoma complicating a procedure

▽ Unspecified code ♀ Female diagnosis ☒ Manifestation code ♂ Male diagnosis

998.13 Seroma complicating a procedure
998.2 Accidental puncture or laceration during procedure

ICD-9-CM Procedural

38.82 Other surgical occlusion of other vessels of head and neck

37600

37600 Ligation; external carotid artery

ICD-9-CM Diagnostic

250.70 Diabetes with peripheral circulatory disorders, type II or unspecified type, not stated as uncontrolled — (Use additional code to identify manifestation: 443.81, 785.4)
250.71 Diabetes with peripheral circulatory disorders, type I [juvenile type], not stated as uncontrolled — (Use additional code to identify manifestation: 443.81, 785.4)
401.0 Essential hypertension, malignant
401.1 Essential hypertension, benign
401.9 Unspecified essential hypertension
443.89 Other peripheral vascular disease
447.1 Stricture of artery
447.6 Unspecified arteritis
447.8 Other specified disorders of arteries and arterioles
459.0 Unspecified hemorrhage
478.29 Other disease of pharynx or nasopharynx
784.7 Epistaxis
900.02 External carotid artery injury
998.11 Hemorrhage complicating a procedure
998.12 Hematoma complicating a procedure
998.13 Seroma complicating a procedure
998.2 Accidental puncture or laceration during procedure

ICD-9-CM Procedural

21.06 Control of epistaxis by ligation of the external carotid artery
38.82 Other surgical occlusion of other vessels of head and neck

37605–37606

37605 Ligation; internal or common carotid artery
37606 internal or common carotid artery, with gradual occlusion, as with Selverstone or Crutchfield clamp

ICD-9-CM Diagnostic

250.70 Diabetes with peripheral circulatory disorders, type II or unspecified type, not stated as uncontrolled — (Use additional code to identify manifestation: 443.81, 785.4)
250.71 Diabetes with peripheral circulatory disorders, type I [juvenile type], not stated as uncontrolled — (Use additional code to identify manifestation: 443.81, 785.4)
401.0 Essential hypertension, malignant
401.9 Unspecified essential hypertension
435.9 Unspecified transient cerebral ischemia — (Use additional code to identify presence of hypertension)
442.81 Aneurysm of artery of neck
443.21 Dissection of carotid artery
443.89 Other peripheral vascular disease
447.1 Stricture of artery
447.6 Unspecified arteritis
447.8 Other specified disorders of arteries and arterioles
459.0 Unspecified hemorrhage
874.8 Open wound of other and unspecified parts of neck, without mention of complication — (Use additional code to identify infection)
900.01 Common carotid artery injury
900.03 Internal carotid artery injury
998.11 Hemorrhage complicating a procedure
998.12 Hematoma complicating a procedure
998.13 Seroma complicating a procedure
998.2 Accidental puncture or laceration during procedure

ICD-9-CM Procedural

38.82 Other surgical occlusion of other vessels of head and neck

37607

37607 Ligation or banding of angioaccess arteriovenous fistula

ICD-9-CM Diagnostic

996.73 Other complications due to renal dialysis device, implant, and graft
996.74 Other complications due to other vascular device, implant, and graft
V53.90 Fitting and adjustment, Unspecified device
V53.99 Fitting and adjustment, Other device
V58.81 Fitting and adjustment of vascular catheter

ICD-9-CM Procedural

38.82 Other surgical occlusion of other vessels of head and neck
39.49 Other revision of vascular procedure
39.53 Repair of arteriovenous fistula

37609

37609 Ligation or biopsy, temporal artery

ICD-9-CM Diagnostic

440.8 Atherosclerosis of other specified arteries
440.9 Generalized and unspecified atherosclerosis
446.5 Giant cell arteritis
447.6 Unspecified arteritis
459.9 Unspecified circulatory system disorder
747.81 Congenital anomaly of cerebrovascular system
780.2 Syncope and collapse
780.4 Dizziness and giddiness
780.6 Fever
784.0 Headache
784.2 Swelling, mass, or lump in head and neck
900.89 Injury to other specified blood vessels of head and neck
V71.89 Observation for other specified suspected conditions

ICD-9-CM Procedural

38.21 Biopsy of blood vessel
38.82 Other surgical occlusion of other vessels of head and neck

HCPCS Level II Supplies & Services

A4550 Surgical trays

37615

37615 Ligation, major artery (eg, post-traumatic, rupture); neck

ICD-9-CM Diagnostic

447.2 Rupture of artery
900.00 Injury to carotid artery, unspecified
900.01 Common carotid artery injury
900.02 External carotid artery injury
900.03 Internal carotid artery injury
900.82 Injury to multiple blood vessels of head and neck
900.89 Injury to other specified blood vessels of head and neck
998.11 Hemorrhage complicating a procedure
998.12 Hematoma complicating a procedure
998.13 Seroma complicating a procedure
998.2 Accidental puncture or laceration during procedure

ICD-9-CM Procedural

06.92 Ligation of thyroid vessels
38.82 Other surgical occlusion of other vessels of head and neck

37616

37616 Ligation, major artery (eg, post-traumatic, rupture); chest

ICD-9-CM Diagnostic

441.1 Thoracic aneurysm, ruptured
441.5 Aortic aneurysm of unspecified site, ruptured
447.2 Rupture of artery
901.0 Thoracic aorta injury
901.2 Superior vena cava injury
901.41 Pulmonary artery injury
908.4 Late effect of injury to blood vessel of thorax, abdomen, and pelvis
908.6 Late effect of certain complications of trauma
997.79 Vascular complications of other vessels — (Use additional code to identify complications)
998.11 Hemorrhage complicating a procedure

998.12 Hematoma complicating a procedure
998.13 Seroma complicating a procedure
998.2 Accidental puncture or laceration during procedure

ICD-9-CM Procedural

38.85 Other surgical occlusion of other thoracic vessel

37617

37617 Ligation, major artery (eg, post-traumatic, rupture); abdomen

ICD-9-CM Diagnostic

441.3 Abdominal aneurysm, ruptured
441.6 Thoracoabdominal aneurysm, ruptured
442.1 Aneurysm of renal artery
442.2 Aneurysm of iliac artery
442.84 Aneurysm of other visceral artery
902.0 Abdominal aorta injury
902.31 Injury to superior mesenteric vein and primary subdivisions
908.4 Late effect of injury to blood vessel of thorax, abdomen, and pelvis
908.6 Late effect of certain complications of trauma
997.71 Vascular complications of mesenteric artery — (Use additional code to identify complications)
997.72 Vascular complications of renal artery — (Use additional code to identify complications)
997.79 Vascular complications of other vessels — (Use additional code to identify complications)
998.11 Hemorrhage complicating a procedure
998.12 Hematoma complicating a procedure
998.13 Seroma complicating a procedure
998.2 Accidental puncture or laceration during procedure

ICD-9-CM Procedural

07.43 Ligation of adrenal vessels
38.86 Other surgical occlusion of abdominal arteries

37618

37618 Ligation, major artery (eg, post-traumatic, rupture); extremity

ICD-9-CM Diagnostic

881.10 Open wound of forearm, complicated — (Use additional code to identify infection)
903.01 Axillary artery injury
903.1 Brachial blood vessels injury
903.2 Radial blood vessels injury
903.3 Ulnar blood vessels injury
903.5 Digital blood vessels injury
903.8 Injury to specified blood vessels of upper extremity, other
904.0 Common femoral artery injury
904.1 Superficial femoral artery injury
904.41 Popliteal artery injury
904.51 Anterior tibial artery injury
904.53 Posterior tibial artery injury
904.6 Deep plantar blood vessels injury
996.1 Mechanical complication of other vascular device, implant, and graft
998.11 Hemorrhage complicating a procedure
998.12 Hematoma complicating a procedure
998.13 Seroma complicating a procedure
998.2 Accidental puncture or laceration during procedure

ICD-9-CM Procedural

38.83 Other surgical occlusion of upper limb vessels
38.88 Other surgical occlusion of lower limb arteries
38.89 Other surgical occlusion of lower limb veins

37620

37620 Interruption, partial or complete, of inferior vena cava by suture, ligation, plication, clip, extravascular, intravascular (umbrella device)

ICD-9-CM Diagnostic

414.9 Unspecified chronic ischemic heart disease — (Use additional code to identify presence of hypertension: 401.0-405.9) ▽
451.11 Phlebitis and thrombophlebitis of femoral vein (deep) (superficial) — (Use additional E code to identify drug, if drug-induced)
451.19 Phlebitis and thrombophlebitis of other deep vessels of lower extremities — (Use additional E code to identify drug, if drug-induced)
451.2 Phlebitis and thrombophlebitis of lower extremities, unspecified — (Use additional E code to identify drug, if drug-induced) ▽
451.81 Phlebitis and thrombophlebitis of iliac vein — (Use additional E code to identify drug, if drug-induced)
451.82 Phlebitis and thrombophlebitis of superficial veins of upper extremities — (Use additional E code to identify drug, if drug-induced)
451.83 Phlebitis and thrombophlebitis of deep veins of upper extremities — (Use additional E code to identify drug, if drug-induced)
451.84 Phlebitis and thrombophlebitis of upper extremities, unspecified — (Use additional E code to identify drug, if drug-induced) ▽
451.89 Phlebitis and thrombophlebitis of other site — (Use additional E code to identify drug, if drug-induced)
451.9 Phlebitis and thrombophlebitis of unspecified site — (Use additional E code to identify drug, if drug-induced) ▽
452 Portal vein thrombosis
453.0 Budd-Chiari syndrome
453.2 Embolism and thrombosis of vena cava
453.3 Embolism and thrombosis of renal vein
453.40 Venous embolism and thrombosis of unspecified deep vessels of lower extremity
453.41 Venous embolism and thrombosis of deep vessels of proximal lower extremity
453.42 Venous embolism and thrombosis of deep vessels of distal lower extremity
453.8 Embolism and thrombosis of other specified veins
453.9 Embolism and thrombosis of unspecified site ▽
459.9 Unspecified circulatory system disorder ▽
671.14 Varicose veins of vulva and perineum, postpartum ♀
902.10 Unspecified inferior vena cava injury ▽
998.2 Accidental puncture or laceration during procedure

ICD-9-CM Procedural

38.7 Interruption of the vena cava

37650

37650 Ligation of femoral vein

ICD-9-CM Diagnostic

451.11 Phlebitis and thrombophlebitis of femoral vein (deep) (superficial) — (Use additional E code to identify drug, if drug-induced)
451.2 Phlebitis and thrombophlebitis of lower extremities, unspecified — (Use additional E code to identify drug, if drug-induced) ▽
454.0 Varicose veins of lower extremities with ulcer
454.1 Varicose veins of lower extremities with inflammation
454.2 Varicose veins of lower extremities with ulcer and inflammation
454.8 Varicose veins of the lower extremities with other complications
454.9 Asymptomatic varicose veins
459.10 Postphlebitic syndrome without complications
459.11 Postphlebitic syndrome with ulcer
459.12 Postphlebitic syndrome with inflammation
459.13 Postphlebitic syndrome with ulcer and inflammation
459.19 Postphlebitic syndrome with other complication
459.81 Unspecified venous (peripheral) insufficiency — (Use additional code for any associated ulceration: 707.10-707.9) ▽
639.6 Embolism following abortion or ectopic and molar pregnancies ♀
904.2 Femoral vein injury
997.2 Peripheral vascular complications — (Use additional code to identify complications)
998.11 Hemorrhage complicating a procedure
998.12 Hematoma complicating a procedure
998.13 Seroma complicating a procedure
998.2 Accidental puncture or laceration during procedure

ICD-9-CM Procedural

38.89 Other surgical occlusion of lower limb veins

37660

37660 Ligation of common iliac vein

ICD-9-CM Diagnostic

442.2 Aneurysm of iliac artery
443.22 Dissection of iliac artery
451.81 Phlebitis and thrombophlebitis of iliac vein — (Use additional E code to identify drug, if drug-induced)
453.8 Embolism and thrombosis of other specified veins
902.54 Iliac vein injury
902.9 Injury to blood vessel of abdomen and pelvis, unspecified ▽

997.79 Vascular complications of other vessels — (Use additional code to identify complications)
998.11 Hemorrhage complicating a procedure
998.12 Hematoma complicating a procedure
998.13 Seroma complicating a procedure
998.2 Accidental puncture or laceration during procedure

ICD-9-CM Procedural

38.87 Other surgical occlusion of abdominal veins

37700

37700 Ligation and division of long saphenous vein at saphenofemoral junction, or distal interruptions

ICD-9-CM Diagnostic

454.0 Varicose veins of lower extremities with ulcer
454.1 Varicose veins of lower extremities with inflammation
454.2 Varicose veins of lower extremities with ulcer and inflammation
454.8 Varicose veins of the lower extremities with other complications
454.9 Asymptomatic varicose veins
459.10 Postphlebitic syndrome without complications
459.11 Postphlebitic syndrome with ulcer
459.12 Postphlebitic syndrome with inflammation
459.13 Postphlebitic syndrome with ulcer and inflammation
459.19 Postphlebitic syndrome with other complication
459.81 Unspecified venous (peripheral) insufficiency — (Use additional code for any associated ulceration: 707.10-707.9) ▽
707.10 Ulcer of lower limb, unspecified ▽
707.11 Ulcer of thigh
707.12 Ulcer of calf
707.13 Ulcer of ankle
707.14 Ulcer of heel and midfoot
707.15 Ulcer of other part of foot
707.19 Ulcer of other part of lower limb

ICD-9-CM Procedural

38.59 Ligation and stripping of lower limb varicose veins
38.89 Other surgical occlusion of lower limb veins

37720–37730

37720 Ligation and division and complete stripping of long or short saphenous veins
37730 Ligation and division and complete stripping of long and short saphenous veins

ICD-9-CM Diagnostic

454.0 Varicose veins of lower extremities with ulcer
454.1 Varicose veins of lower extremities with inflammation
454.2 Varicose veins of lower extremities with ulcer and inflammation
454.8 Varicose veins of the lower extremities with other complications
454.9 Asymptomatic varicose veins
459.10 Postphlebitic syndrome without complications
459.11 Postphlebitic syndrome with ulcer
459.12 Postphlebitic syndrome with inflammation
459.13 Postphlebitic syndrome with ulcer and inflammation
459.19 Postphlebitic syndrome with other complication
459.81 Unspecified venous (peripheral) insufficiency — (Use additional code for any associated ulceration: 707.10-707.9) ▽
707.10 Ulcer of lower limb, unspecified ▽
707.11 Ulcer of thigh
707.12 Ulcer of calf
707.13 Ulcer of ankle
707.14 Ulcer of heel and midfoot
707.15 Ulcer of other part of foot
707.19 Ulcer of other part of lower limb

ICD-9-CM Procedural

38.59 Ligation and stripping of lower limb varicose veins

37735

37735 Ligation and division and complete stripping of long or short saphenous veins with radical excision of ulcer and skin graft and/or interruption of communicating veins of lower leg, with excision of deep fascia

ICD-9-CM Diagnostic

454.0 Varicose veins of lower extremities with ulcer
454.1 Varicose veins of lower extremities with inflammation
454.2 Varicose veins of lower extremities with ulcer and inflammation
454.8 Varicose veins of the lower extremities with other complications
454.9 Asymptomatic varicose veins
459.10 Postphlebitic syndrome without complications
459.11 Postphlebitic syndrome with ulcer
459.12 Postphlebitic syndrome with inflammation
459.13 Postphlebitic syndrome with ulcer and inflammation
459.19 Postphlebitic syndrome with other complication
459.81 Unspecified venous (peripheral) insufficiency — (Use additional code for any associated ulceration: 707.10-707.9) ▽
707.10 Ulcer of lower limb, unspecified ▽
707.11 Ulcer of thigh
707.12 Ulcer of calf
707.13 Ulcer of ankle
707.14 Ulcer of heel and midfoot
707.15 Ulcer of other part of foot
707.19 Ulcer of other part of lower limb

ICD-9-CM Procedural

38.59 Ligation and stripping of lower limb varicose veins
86.4 Radical excision of skin lesion
86.60 Free skin graft, not otherwise specified
86.63 Full-thickness skin graft to other sites

37760

37760 Ligation of perforator veins, subfascial, radical (Linton type), with or without skin graft, open

ICD-9-CM Diagnostic

454.0 Varicose veins of lower extremities with ulcer
454.1 Varicose veins of lower extremities with inflammation
454.2 Varicose veins of lower extremities with ulcer and inflammation
454.8 Varicose veins of the lower extremities with other complications
454.9 Asymptomatic varicose veins
459.10 Postphlebitic syndrome without complications
459.11 Postphlebitic syndrome with ulcer
459.12 Postphlebitic syndrome with inflammation
459.13 Postphlebitic syndrome with ulcer and inflammation
459.19 Postphlebitic syndrome with other complication
459.81 Unspecified venous (peripheral) insufficiency — (Use additional code for any associated ulceration: 707.10-707.9) ▽
707.10 Ulcer of lower limb, unspecified ▽
707.11 Ulcer of thigh
707.12 Ulcer of calf
707.13 Ulcer of ankle
707.14 Ulcer of heel and midfoot
707.15 Ulcer of other part of foot
707.19 Ulcer of other part of lower limb
729.5 Pain in soft tissues of limb

ICD-9-CM Procedural

38.59 Ligation and stripping of lower limb varicose veins
38.89 Other surgical occlusion of lower limb veins
86.60 Free skin graft, not otherwise specified
86.63 Full-thickness skin graft to other sites

37765–37766

37765 Stab phlebectomy of varicose veins, one extremity; 10-20 stab incisions
37766 more than 20 incisions

ICD-9-CM Diagnostic

454.0 Varicose veins of lower extremities with ulcer
454.1 Varicose veins of lower extremities with inflammation
454.2 Varicose veins of lower extremities with ulcer and inflammation
454.8 Varicose veins of the lower extremities with other complications
454.9 Asymptomatic varicose veins

ICD-9-CM Procedural

38.59 Ligation and stripping of lower limb varicose veins

37780

37780 Ligation and division of short saphenous vein at saphenopopliteal junction (separate procedure)

ICD-9-CM Diagnostic

454.0 Varicose veins of lower extremities with ulcer
454.1 Varicose veins of lower extremities with inflammation
454.2 Varicose veins of lower extremities with ulcer and inflammation
454.8 Varicose veins of the lower extremities with other complications
454.9 Asymptomatic varicose veins
459.10 Postphlebitic syndrome without complications
459.11 Postphlebitic syndrome with ulcer
459.12 Postphlebitic syndrome with inflammation
459.13 Postphlebitic syndrome with ulcer and inflammation
459.19 Postphlebitic syndrome with other complication
459.81 Unspecified venous (peripheral) insufficiency — (Use additional code for any associated ulceration: 707.10-707.9) ▽
707.10 Ulcer of lower limb, unspecified ▽
707.11 Ulcer of thigh
707.12 Ulcer of calf
707.13 Ulcer of ankle
707.14 Ulcer of heel and midfoot
707.15 Ulcer of other part of foot
707.19 Ulcer of other part of lower limb
729.5 Pain in soft tissues of limb

ICD-9-CM Procedural

38.59 Ligation and stripping of lower limb varicose veins
38.89 Other surgical occlusion of lower limb veins

37785

37785 Ligation, division, and/or excision of varicose vein cluster(s), one leg

ICD-9-CM Diagnostic

454.0 Varicose veins of lower extremities with ulcer
454.1 Varicose veins of lower extremities with inflammation
454.2 Varicose veins of lower extremities with ulcer and inflammation
454.8 Varicose veins of the lower extremities with other complications
454.9 Asymptomatic varicose veins
459.10 Postphlebitic syndrome without complications
459.11 Postphlebitic syndrome with ulcer
459.12 Postphlebitic syndrome with inflammation
459.13 Postphlebitic syndrome with ulcer and inflammation
459.19 Postphlebitic syndrome with other complication
459.81 Unspecified venous (peripheral) insufficiency — (Use additional code for any associated ulceration: 707.10-707.9) ▽

ICD-9-CM Procedural

38.59 Ligation and stripping of lower limb varicose veins

37788

37788 Penile revascularization, artery, with or without vein graft

ICD-9-CM Diagnostic

250.70 Diabetes with peripheral circulatory disorders, type II or unspecified type, not stated as uncontrolled — (Use additional code to identify manifestation: 443.81, 785.4)
250.71 Diabetes with peripheral circulatory disorders, type I [juvenile type], not stated as uncontrolled — (Use additional code to identify manifestation: 443.81, 785.4)
250.72 Diabetes with peripheral circulatory disorders, type II or unspecified type, uncontrolled — (Use additional code to identify manifestation: 443.81, 785.4)
250.73 Diabetes with peripheral circulatory disorders, type I [juvenile type], uncontrolled — (Use additional code to identify manifestation: 443.81, 785.4)
250.80 Diabetes with other specified manifestations, type II or unspecified type, not stated as uncontrolled — (Use additional code to identify manifestation: 707.10-707.9, 731.8. Use additional E code to identify cause, if drug-induced)
250.81 Diabetes with other specified manifestations, type I [juvenile type], not stated as uncontrolled — (Use additional code to identify manifestation: 707.10-707.9, 731.8. Use additional E code to identify cause, if drug-induced)
250.82 Diabetes with other specified manifestations, type II or unspecified type, uncontrolled — (Use additional code to identify manifestation: 707.10-707.9, 731.8. Use additional E code to identify cause, if drug-induced)
250.83 Diabetes with other specified manifestations, type I [juvenile type], uncontrolled — (Use additional code to identify manifestation: 707.10-707.9, 731.8. Use additional E code to identify cause, if drug-induced)
443.81 Peripheral angiopathy in diseases classified elsewhere — (Code first underlying disease, 250.7) ☒
607.82 Vascular disorders of penis ♂
607.84 Impotence of organic origin ♂
902.87 Injury to multiple blood vessels of abdomen and pelvis
902.89 Injury to specified blood vessels of abdomen and pelvis, other
908.4 Late effect of injury to blood vessel of thorax, abdomen, and pelvis

ICD-9-CM Procedural

39.29 Other (peripheral) vascular shunt or bypass
39.31 Suture of artery
64.98 Other operations on penis

37790

37790 Penile venous occlusive procedure

ICD-9-CM Diagnostic

187.3 Malignant neoplasm of body of penis ♂
187.9 Malignant neoplasm of male genital organ, site unspecified ▽ ♂
250.70 Diabetes with peripheral circulatory disorders, type II or unspecified type, not stated as uncontrolled — (Use additional code to identify manifestation: 443.81, 785.4)
250.71 Diabetes with peripheral circulatory disorders, type I [juvenile type], not stated as uncontrolled — (Use additional code to identify manifestation: 443.81, 785.4)
250.72 Diabetes with peripheral circulatory disorders, type II or unspecified type, uncontrolled — (Use additional code to identify manifestation: 443.81, 785.4)
250.73 Diabetes with peripheral circulatory disorders, type I [juvenile type], uncontrolled — (Use additional code to identify manifestation: 443.81, 785.4)
250.80 Diabetes with other specified manifestations, type II or unspecified type, not stated as uncontrolled — (Use additional code to identify manifestation: 707.10-707.9, 731.8. Use additional E code to identify cause, if drug-induced)
250.81 Diabetes with other specified manifestations, type I [juvenile type], not stated as uncontrolled — (Use additional code to identify manifestation: 707.10-707.9, 731.8. Use additional E code to identify cause, if drug-induced)
250.82 Diabetes with other specified manifestations, type II or unspecified type, uncontrolled — (Use additional code to identify manifestation: 707.10-707.9, 731.8. Use additional E code to identify cause, if drug-induced)
250.83 Diabetes with other specified manifestations, type I [juvenile type], uncontrolled — (Use additional code to identify manifestation: 707.10-707.9, 731.8. Use additional E code to identify cause, if drug-induced)
443.81 Peripheral angiopathy in diseases classified elsewhere — (Code first underlying disease, 250.7) ☒
607.82 Vascular disorders of penis ♂
607.84 Impotence of organic origin ♂
608.83 Specified vascular disorder of male genital organs ♂
878.1 Open wound of penis, complicated — (Use additional code to identify infection) ♂
902.87 Injury to multiple blood vessels of abdomen and pelvis
902.89 Injury to specified blood vessels of abdomen and pelvis, other
908.4 Late effect of injury to blood vessel of thorax, abdomen, and pelvis

ICD-9-CM Procedural

39.29 Other (peripheral) vascular shunt or bypass
39.31 Suture of artery
64.98 Other operations on penis

▽ Unspecified code
♀ Female diagnosis
☒ Manifestation code
♂ Male diagnosis

Hemic and Lymphatic Systems

Spleen

38100–38102

- **38100** Splenectomy; total (separate procedure)
- **38101** partial (separate procedure)
- **38102** total, en bloc for extensive disease, in conjunction with other procedure (List in addition to code for primary procedure)

ICD-9-CM Diagnostic

- 159.1 Malignant neoplasm of spleen, not elsewhere classified
- 197.8 Secondary malignant neoplasm of other digestive organs and spleen
- 200.07 Reticulosarcoma of spleen
- 200.17 Lymphosarcoma of spleen
- 200.27 Burkitt's tumor or lymphoma of spleen
- 200.87 Other named variants of lymphosarcoma and reticulosarcoma of spleen
- 201.07 Hodgkin's paragranuloma of spleen
- 201.17 Hodgkin's granuloma of spleen
- 201.27 Hodgkin's sarcoma of spleen
- 201.47 Hodgkin's disease, lymphocytic-histiocytic predominance of spleen
- 201.57 Hodgkin's disease, nodular sclerosis, of spleen
- 201.67 Hodgkin's disease, mixed cellularity, of spleen
- 201.77 Hodgkin's disease, lymphocytic depletion, of spleen
- 201.90 Hodgkin's disease, unspecified type, unspecified site, extranodal and solid organ sites
- 201.97 Hodgkin's disease, unspecified type, of spleen
- 202.07 Nodular lymphoma of spleen
- 202.17 Mycosis fungoides of spleen
- 202.27 Sezary's disease of spleen
- 202.37 Malignant histiocytosis of spleen
- 202.47 Leukemic reticuloendotheliosis of spleen
- 202.57 Letterer-Siwe disease of spleen
- 202.67 Malignant mast cell tumors of spleen
- 202.80 Other malignant lymphomas, unspecified site, extranodal and solid organ sites
- 202.87 Other malignant lymphomas of spleen
- 202.97 Other and unspecified malignant neoplasms of lymphoid and histiocytic tissue of spleen
- 208.90 Unspecified leukemia without mention of remission
- 238.7 Neoplasm of uncertain behavior of other lymphatic and hematopoietic tissues
- 239.0 Neoplasm of unspecified nature of digestive system
- 282.0 Hereditary spherocytosis
- 283.0 Autoimmune hemolytic anemias — (Use additional E code to identify cause, if drug-induced)
- 287.3 Primary thrombocytopenia
- 287.5 Unspecified thrombocytopenia
- 289.4 Hypersplenism
- 289.50 Unspecified disease of spleen
- 289.51 Chronic congestive splenomegaly
- 289.52 Splenic sequestration — (Code first sickle-cell disease in crisis: 282.42, 282.62, 282.64, 282.69)
- 289.59 Other diseases of spleen
- 442.83 Aneurysm of splenic artery
- 443.29 Dissection of other artery
- 446.6 Thrombotic microangiopathy
- 789.00 Abdominal pain, unspecified site
- 789.02 Abdominal pain, left upper quadrant
- 789.07 Abdominal pain, generalized
- 789.09 Abdominal pain, other specified site
- 789.2 Splenomegaly
- 865.01 Spleen hematoma, without rupture of capsule or mention of open wound into cavity
- 865.02 Capsular tears to spleen, without major disruption of parenchyma or mention of open wound into cavity
- 865.03 Spleen laceration extending into parenchyma without mention of open wound into cavity
- 865.04 Massive parenchymal disruption of spleen without mention of open wound into cavity
- 865.09 Other spleen injury without mention of open wound into cavity
- 865.10 Unspecified spleen injury with open wound into cavity
- 865.11 Spleen hematoma, without rupture of capsule, with open wound into cavity
- 865.12 Capsular tears to spleen, without major disruption of parenchyma, with open wound into cavity
- 865.13 Spleen laceration extending into parenchyma, with open wound into cavity
- 865.14 Massive parenchyma disruption of spleen with open wound into cavity
- 865.19 Other spleen injury with open wound into cavity
- 998.2 Accidental puncture or laceration during procedure
- 998.89 Other specified complications
- 998.9 Unspecified complication of procedure, not elsewhere classified
- V64.41 Laparoscopic surgical procedure converted to open procedure

ICD-9-CM Procedural

- 41.42 Excision of lesion or tissue of spleen
- 41.43 Partial splenectomy
- 41.5 Total splenectomy

38115

- **38115** Repair of ruptured spleen (splenorrhaphy) with or without partial splenectomy

ICD-9-CM Diagnostic

- 289.59 Other diseases of spleen
- 767.8 Other specified birth trauma
- 865.01 Spleen hematoma, without rupture of capsule or mention of open wound into cavity
- 865.02 Capsular tears to spleen, without major disruption of parenchyma or mention of open wound into cavity
- 865.03 Spleen laceration extending into parenchyma without mention of open wound into cavity
- 865.04 Massive parenchymal disruption of spleen without mention of open wound into cavity
- 865.09 Other spleen injury without mention of open wound into cavity
- 865.11 Spleen hematoma, without rupture of capsule, with open wound into cavity
- 865.12 Capsular tears to spleen, without major disruption of parenchyma, with open wound into cavity
- 865.13 Spleen laceration extending into parenchyma, with open wound into cavity
- 865.14 Massive parenchyma disruption of spleen with open wound into cavity
- 865.19 Other spleen injury with open wound into cavity

ICD-9-CM Procedural

- 41.95 Repair and plastic operations on spleen

38120

- **38120** Laparoscopy, surgical, splenectomy

ICD-9-CM Diagnostic

- 159.1 Malignant neoplasm of spleen, not elsewhere classified
- 197.8 Secondary malignant neoplasm of other digestive organs and spleen
- 200.07 Reticulosarcoma of spleen
- 200.17 Lymphosarcoma of spleen
- 200.27 Burkitt's tumor or lymphoma of spleen
- 200.87 Other named variants of lymphosarcoma and reticulosarcoma of spleen
- 201.07 Hodgkin's paragranuloma of spleen
- 201.17 Hodgkin's granuloma of spleen
- 201.27 Hodgkin's sarcoma of spleen
- 201.47 Hodgkin's disease, lymphocytic-histiocytic predominance of spleen
- 201.57 Hodgkin's disease, nodular sclerosis, of spleen
- 201.67 Hodgkin's disease, mixed cellularity, of spleen
- 201.77 Hodgkin's disease, lymphocytic depletion, of spleen
- 201.90 Hodgkin's disease, unspecified type, unspecified site, extranodal and solid organ sites
- 201.97 Hodgkin's disease, unspecified type, of spleen
- 202.07 Nodular lymphoma of spleen
- 202.17 Mycosis fungoides of spleen

202.27 Sezary's disease of spleen
202.37 Malignant histiocytosis of spleen
202.47 Leukemic reticuloendotheliosis of spleen
202.57 Letterer-Siwe disease of spleen
202.67 Malignant mast cell tumors of spleen
202.80 Other malignant lymphomas, unspecified site, extranodal and solid organ sites
202.87 Other malignant lymphomas of spleen
202.97 Other and unspecified malignant neoplasms of lymphoid and histiocytic tissue of spleen
208.90 Unspecified leukemia without mention of remission
238.7 Neoplasm of uncertain behavior of other lymphatic and hematopoietic tissues
239.0 Neoplasm of unspecified nature of digestive system
282.0 Hereditary spherocytosis
283.0 Autoimmune hemolytic anemias — (Use additional E code to identify cause, if drug-induced)
287.3 Primary thrombocytopenia
287.5 Unspecified thrombocytopenia
289.4 Hypersplenism
289.50 Unspecified disease of spleen
289.51 Chronic congestive splenomegaly
289.52 Splenic sequestration — (Code first sickle-cell disease in crisis: 282.42, 282.62, 282.64, 282.69)
289.59 Other diseases of spleen
442.83 Aneurysm of splenic artery
446.6 Thrombotic microangiopathy
789.00 Abdominal pain, unspecified site
789.02 Abdominal pain, left upper quadrant
789.07 Abdominal pain, generalized
789.09 Abdominal pain, other specified site
789.2 Splenomegaly
865.01 Spleen hematoma, without rupture of capsule or mention of open wound into cavity
865.02 Capsular tears to spleen, without major disruption of parenchyma or mention of open wound into cavity
865.03 Spleen laceration extending into parenchyma without mention of open wound into cavity
865.04 Massive parenchymal disruption of spleen without mention of open wound into cavity
865.09 Other spleen injury without mention of open wound into cavity
865.10 Unspecified spleen injury with open wound into cavity
865.11 Spleen hematoma, without rupture of capsule, with open wound into cavity
865.12 Capsular tears to spleen, without major disruption of parenchyma, with open wound into cavity
865.13 Spleen laceration extending into parenchyma, with open wound into cavity
865.14 Massive parenchyma disruption of spleen with open wound into cavity
865.19 Other spleen injury with open wound into cavity
998.2 Accidental puncture or laceration during procedure
998.89 Other specified complications

ICD-9-CM Procedural

41.43 Partial splenectomy
41.5 Total splenectomy
41.93 Excision of accessory spleen

38200

38200 Injection procedure for splenoportography

ICD-9-CM Diagnostic

230.9 Carcinoma in situ of other and unspecified digestive organs
572.3 Portal hypertension
865.01 Spleen hematoma, without rupture of capsule or mention of open wound into cavity
865.09 Other spleen injury without mention of open wound into cavity

ICD-9-CM Procedural

41.39 Other diagnostic procedures on spleen
41.99 Other operations on spleen

38204

38204 Management of recipient hematopoietic progenitor cell donor search and cell acquisition

ICD-9-CM Diagnostic

The application of this code is too broad to adequately present ICD-9-CM diagnostic code links here. Refer to your ICD-9-CM book.

ICD-9-CM Procedural

41.98 Other operations on bone marrow

HCPCS Level II Supplies & Services

HCPCS Level II codes are used to report the supplies, durable medical equipment, and certain medical services provided on an outpatient basis. Because the procedure(s) represented on this page would be performed in an inpatient facility, no HCPCS Level II codes apply.

38205–38206

38205 Blood-derived hematopoietic progenitor cell harvesting for transplantation, per collection; allogenic
38206 autologous

ICD-9-CM Diagnostic

The application of this code is too broad to adequately present ICD-9-CM diagnostic code links here. Refer to your ICD-9-CM book.

ICD-9-CM Procedural

41.01 Autologous bone marrow transplant without purging
41.02 Allogeneic bone marrow transplant with purging
41.03 Allogeneic bone marrow transplant without purging
41.04 Autologous hematopoietic stem cell transplant without purging
41.05 Allogeneic hematopoietic stem cell transplant without purging
41.07 Autologous hematopoietic stem cell transplant with purging
41.08 Allogeneic hematopoietic stem cell transplant with purging
41.09 Autologous bone marrow transplant with purging

HCPCS Level II Supplies & Services

HCPCS Level II codes are used to report the supplies, durable medical equipment, and certain medical services provided on an outpatient basis. Because the procedure(s) represented on this page would be performed in an inpatient facility, no HCPCS Level II codes apply.

38207–38215

38207 Transplant preparation of hematopoietic progenitor cells; cryopreservation and storage
38208 thawing of previously frozen harvest, without washing
38209 thawing of previously frozen harvest, with washing
38210 specific cell depletion within harvest, T-cell depletion
38211 tumor cell depletion
38212 red blood cell removal
38213 platelet depletion
38214 plasma (volume) depletion
38215 cell concentration in plasma, mononuclear, or buffy coat layer

ICD-9-CM Diagnostic

The application of this code is too broad to adequately present ICD-9-CM diagnostic code links here. Refer to your ICD-9-CM book.

ICD-9-CM Procedural

41.00 Bone marrow transplant, not otherwise specified
41.02 Allogeneic bone marrow transplant with purging
41.07 Autologous hematopoietic stem cell transplant with purging
41.08 Allogeneic hematopoietic stem cell transplant with purging
41.09 Autologous bone marrow transplant with purging
41.98 Other operations on bone marrow

HCPCS Level II Supplies & Services

HCPCS Level II codes are used to report the supplies, durable medical equipment, and certain medical services provided on an outpatient basis. Because the procedure(s) represented on this page would be performed in an inpatient facility, no HCPCS Level II codes apply.

38220–38221

38220 Bone marrow; aspiration only
38221 biopsy, needle or trocar

ICD-9-CM Diagnostic

The application of this code is too broad to adequately present ICD-9-CM diagnostic code links here. Refer to your ICD-9-CM book.

ICD-9-CM Procedural

41.31 Biopsy of bone marrow
41.91 Aspiration of bone marrow from donor for transplant
99.79 Other therapeutic apheresis

HCPCS Level II Supplies & Services
HCPCS Level II codes are used to report the supplies, durable medical equipment, and certain medical services provided on an outpatient basis. Because the procedure(s) represented on this page would be performed in an inpatient or outpatient facility, no HCPCS Level II codes apply.

38230
38230 Bone marrow harvesting for transplantation

ICD-9-CM Diagnostic
V59.3 Bone marrow donor

ICD-9-CM Procedural
41.91 Aspiration of bone marrow from donor for transplant

38240–38242
38240 Bone marrow or blood-derived peripheral stem cell transplantation; allogenic
38241 autologous
38242 allogeneic donor lymphocyte infusions

ICD-9-CM Diagnostic
The application of this code is too broad to adequately present ICD-9-CM diagnostic code links here. Refer to your ICD-9-CM book.

ICD-9-CM Procedural
00.91 Transplant from live related donor
00.92 Transplant from live non-related donor
41.01 Autologous bone marrow transplant without purging
41.02 Allogeneic bone marrow transplant with purging
41.03 Allogeneic bone marrow transplant without purging
41.04 Autologous hematopoietic stem cell transplant without purging
41.05 Allogeneic hematopoietic stem cell transplant without purging
41.06 Cord blood stem cell transplant
41.07 Autologous hematopoietic stem cell transplant with purging
41.08 Allogeneic hematopoietic stem cell transplant with purging
41.09 Autologous bone marrow transplant with purging

HCPCS Level II Supplies & Services
HCPCS Level II codes are used to report the supplies, durable medical equipment, and certain medical services provided on an outpatient basis. Because the procedure(s) represented on this page would be performed in an inpatient facility, no HCPCS Level II codes apply.

Lymph Nodes and Lymphatic Channels

38300–38305
38300 Drainage of lymph node abscess or lymphadenitis; simple
38305 extensive

ICD-9-CM Diagnostic
289.1 Chronic lymphadenitis
289.2 Nonspecific mesenteric lymphadenitis
289.3 Lymphadenitis, unspecified, except mesenteric ▽
457.2 Lymphangitis
457.8 Other noninfectious disorders of lymphatic channels
683 Acute lymphadenitis — (Use additional code to identify organism)
784.2 Swelling, mass, or lump in head and neck

ICD-9-CM Procedural
40.0 Incision of lymphatic structures

38308
38308 Lymphangiotomy or other operations on lymphatic channels

ICD-9-CM Diagnostic
289.1 Chronic lymphadenitis
289.2 Nonspecific mesenteric lymphadenitis
289.3 Lymphadenitis, unspecified, except mesenteric ▽
457.2 Lymphangitis
457.8 Other noninfectious disorders of lymphatic channels
683 Acute lymphadenitis — (Use additional code to identify organism)
784.2 Swelling, mass, or lump in head and neck

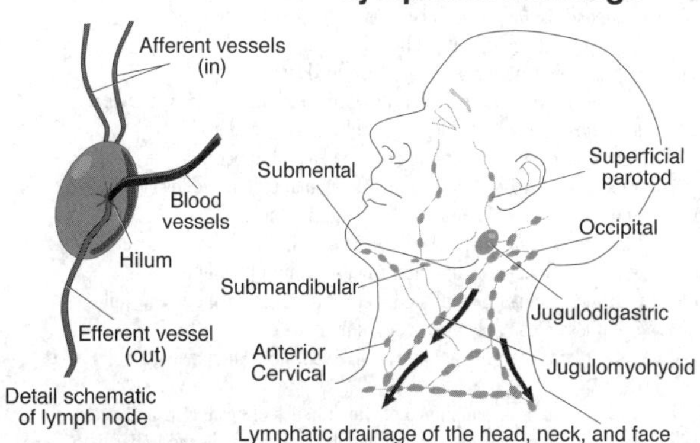

Lymphatic drainage of the head, neck, and face

ICD-9-CM Procedural
40.0 Incision of lymphatic structures
40.40 Radical neck dissection, not otherwise specified

38380
38380 Suture and/or ligation of thoracic duct; cervical approach

ICD-9-CM Diagnostic
289.1 Chronic lymphadenitis
289.3 Lymphadenitis, unspecified, except mesenteric ▽
457.2 Lymphangitis
457.8 Other noninfectious disorders of lymphatic channels

ICD-9-CM Procedural
40.63 Closure of fistula of thoracic duct
40.64 Ligation of thoracic duct

38381–38382
38381 Suture and/or ligation of thoracic duct; thoracic approach
38382 abdominal approach

ICD-9-CM Diagnostic
196.1 Secondary and unspecified malignant neoplasm of intrathoracic lymph nodes
202.82 Other malignant lymphomas of intrathoracic lymph nodes
289.1 Chronic lymphadenitis
289.3 Lymphadenitis, unspecified, except mesenteric ▽
457.2 Lymphangitis
457.8 Other noninfectious disorders of lymphatic channels

ICD-9-CM Procedural
40.63 Closure of fistula of thoracic duct
40.64 Ligation of thoracic duct

38500–38505
38500 Biopsy or excision of lymph node(s); open, superficial
38505 by needle, superficial (eg, cervical, inguinal, axillary)

ICD-9-CM Diagnostic
135 Sarcoidosis
172.5 Malignant melanoma of skin of trunk, except scrotum
172.6 Malignant melanoma of skin of upper limb, including shoulder
172.7 Malignant melanoma of skin of lower limb, including hip
172.8 Malignant melanoma of other specified sites of skin
180.9 Malignant neoplasm of cervix uteri, unspecified site ▽ ♀
182.0 Malignant neoplasm of corpus uteri, except isthmus ♀
185 Malignant neoplasm of prostate ♂
188.9 Malignant neoplasm of bladder, part unspecified ▽
196.0 Secondary and unspecified malignant neoplasm of lymph nodes of head, face, and neck
196.3 Secondary and unspecified malignant neoplasm of lymph nodes of axilla and upper limb
196.5 Secondary and unspecified malignant neoplasm of lymph nodes of inguinal region and lower limb
196.8 Secondary and unspecified malignant neoplasm of lymph nodes of multiple sites

196.9 Secondary and unspecified malignant neoplasm of lymph nodes, site unspecified ▽
198.89 Secondary malignant neoplasm of other specified sites
199.0 Disseminated malignant neoplasm
199.1 Other malignant neoplasm of unspecified site
200.00 Reticulosarcoma, unspecified site, extranodal and solid organ sites ▽
200.01 Reticulosarcoma of lymph nodes of head, face, and neck
200.04 Reticulosarcoma of lymph nodes of axilla and upper limb
200.05 Reticulosarcoma of lymph nodes of inguinal region and lower limb
200.08 Reticulosarcoma of lymph nodes of multiple sites
200.10 Lymphosarcoma, unspecified site, extranodal and solid organ sites ▽
200.14 Lymphosarcoma of lymph nodes of axilla and upper limb
200.15 Lymphosarcoma of lymph nodes of inguinal region and lower limb
200.18 Lymphosarcoma of lymph nodes of multiple sites
200.20 Burkitt's tumor or lymphoma, unspecified site, extranodal and solid organ sites ▽
200.21 Burkitt's tumor or lymphoma of lymph nodes of head, face, and neck
200.24 Burkitt's tumor or lymphoma of lymph nodes of axilla and upper limb
200.25 Burkitt's tumor or lymphoma of lymph nodes of inguinal region and lower limb
200.28 Burkitt's tumor or lymphoma of lymph nodes of multiple sites
201.00 Hodgkin's paragranuloma, unspecified site, extranodal and solid organ sites ▽
201.01 Hodgkin's paragranuloma of lymph nodes of head, face, and neck
201.04 Hodgkin's paragranuloma of lymph nodes of axilla and upper limb
201.05 Hodgkin's paragranuloma of lymph nodes of inguinal region and lower limb
201.08 Hodgkin's paragranuloma of lymph nodes of multiple sites
201.10 Hodgkin's granuloma, unspecified site, extranodal and solid organ sites ▽
201.11 Hodgkin's granuloma of lymph nodes of head, face, and neck
201.14 Hodgkin's granuloma of lymph nodes of axilla and upper limb
201.15 Hodgkin's granuloma of lymph nodes of inguinal region and lower limb
201.18 Hodgkin's granuloma of lymph nodes of multiple sites
201.20 Hodgkin's sarcoma, unspecified site, extranodal and solid organ sites ▽
201.24 Hodgkin's sarcoma of lymph nodes of axilla and upper limb
201.25 Hodgkin's sarcoma of lymph nodes of inguinal region and lower limb
201.28 Hodgkin's sarcoma of lymph nodes of multiple sites
201.40 Hodgkin's disease, lymphocytic-histiocytic predominance, unspecified site, extranodal and solid organ sites ▽
201.44 Hodgkin's disease, lymphocytic-histiocytic predominance of lymph nodes of axilla and upper limb
201.45 Hodgkin's disease, lymphocytic-histiocytic predominance of lymph nodes of inguinal region and lower limb
201.48 Hodgkin's disease, lymphocytic-histiocytic predominance of lymph nodes of multiple sites
201.51 Hodgkin's disease, nodular sclerosis, of lymph nodes of head, face, and neck
201.54 Hodgkin's disease, nodular sclerosis, of lymph nodes of axilla and upper limb
201.55 Hodgkin's disease, nodular sclerosis, of lymph nodes of inguinal region and lower limb
201.58 Hodgkin's disease, nodular sclerosis, of lymph nodes of multiple sites
201.60 Hodgkin's disease, mixed cellularity, unspecified site, extranodal and solid organ sites ▽
201.61 Hodgkin's disease, mixed cellularity, involving lymph nodes of head, face, and neck
201.65 Hodgkin's disease, mixed cellularity, of lymph nodes of inguinal region and lower limb
201.68 Hodgkin's disease, mixed cellularity, of lymph nodes of multiple sites
201.70 Hodgkin's disease, lymphocytic depletion, unspecified site, extranodal and solid organ sites ▽
201.71 Hodgkin's disease, lymphocytic depletion, of lymph nodes of head, face, and neck
201.74 Hodgkin's disease, lymphocytic depletion, of lymph nodes of axilla and upper limb
201.75 Hodgkin's disease, lymphocytic depletion, of lymph nodes of inguinal region and lower limb
201.78 Hodgkin's disease, lymphocytic depletion, of lymph nodes of multiple sites
201.90 Hodgkin's disease, unspecified type, unspecified site, extranodal and solid organ sites ▽
201.91 Hodgkin's disease, unspecified type, of lymph nodes of head, face, and neck ▽
201.94 Hodgkin's disease, unspecified type, of lymph nodes of axilla and upper limb ▽
201.95 Hodgkin's disease, unspecified type, of lymph nodes of inguinal region and lower limb ▽
201.98 Hodgkin's disease, unspecified type, of lymph nodes of multiple sites ▽
202.00 Nodular lymphoma, unspecified site, extranodal and solid organ sites ▽
202.01 Nodular lymphoma of lymph nodes of head, face, and neck
202.04 Nodular lymphoma of lymph nodes of axilla and upper limb
202.05 Nodular lymphoma of lymph nodes of inguinal region and lower limb
202.08 Nodular lymphoma of lymph nodes of multiple sites
202.10 Mycosis fungoides, unspecified site, extranodal and solid organ sites ▽
202.11 Mycosis fungoides of lymph nodes of head, face, and neck
202.14 Mycosis fungoides of lymph nodes of axilla and upper limb
202.15 Mycosis fungoides of lymph nodes of inguinal region and lower limb
202.18 Mycosis fungoides of lymph nodes of multiple sites
202.20 Sezary's disease, unspecified site, extranodal and solid organ sites ▽
202.21 Sezary's disease of lymph nodes of head, face, and neck
202.28 Sezary's disease of lymph nodes of multiple sites
202.30 Malignant histiocytosis, unspecified site, extranodal and solid organ sites ▽
202.31 Malignant histiocytosis of lymph nodes of head, face, and neck
202.34 Malignant histiocytosis of lymph nodes of axilla and upper limb
202.35 Malignant histiocytosis of lymph nodes of inguinal region and lower limb
202.38 Malignant histiocytosis of lymph nodes of multiple sites
202.40 Leukemic reticuloendotheliosis, unspecified site, extranodal and solid organ sites ▽
202.41 Leukemic reticuloendotheliosis of lymph nodes of head, face, and neck
202.44 Leukemic reticuloendotheliosis of lymph nodes of axilla and upper limb
202.45 Leukemic reticuloendotheliosis of lymph nodes of inguinal region and lower limb
202.48 Leukemic reticuloendotheliosis of lymph nodes of multipes sites
202.50 Letterer-Siwe disease, unspecified site, extranodal and solid organ sites ▽
202.51 Letterer-Siwe disease of lymph nodes of head, face, and neck
202.54 Letterer-Siwe disease of lymph nodes of axilla and upper limb
202.55 Letterer-Siwe disease of lymph nodes of inguinal region and lower limb
202.58 Letterer-Siwe disease of lymph nodes of multiple sites
202.60 Malignant mast cell tumors, unspecified site, extranodal and solid organ sites ▽
202.61 Malignant mast cell tumors of lymph nodes of head, face, and neck
202.64 Malignant mast cell tumors of lymph nodes of axilla and upper limb
202.65 Malignant mast cell tumors of lymph nodes of inguinal region and lower limb
202.68 Malignant mast cell tumors of lymph nodes of multiple sites
202.80 Other malignant lymphomas, unspecified site, extranodal and solid organ sites ▽
202.81 Other malignant lymphomas of lymph nodes of head, face, and neck
202.84 Other malignant lymphomas of lymph nodes of axilla and upper limb
202.85 Other malignant lymphomas of lymph nodes of inguinal region and lower limb
202.88 Other malignant lymphomas of lymph nodes of multiple sites
202.91 Other and unspecified malignant neoplasms of lymphoid and histiocytic tissue of lymph nodes of head, face, and neck ▽
202.94 Other and unspecified malignant neoplasms of lymphoid and histiocytic tissue of lymph nodes of axilla and upper limb ▽
202.95 Other and unspecified malignant neoplasms of lymphoid and histiocytic tissue of lymph nodes of inguinal region and lower limb ▽
202.98 Other and unspecified malignant neoplasms of lymphoid and histiocytic tissue of lymph nodes of multiple sites ▽
228.00 Hemangioma of unspecified site ▽
228.01 Hemangioma of skin and subcutaneous tissue
229.0 Benign neoplasm of lymph nodes
229.9 Benign neoplasm of unspecified site ▽
233.1 Carcinoma in situ of cervix uteri ♀
238.8 Neoplasm of uncertain behavior of other specified sites
239.8 Neoplasm of unspecified nature of other specified sites
239.9 Neoplasm of unspecified nature, site unspecified ▽
289.1 Chronic lymphadenitis
289.3 Lymphadenitis, unspecified, except mesenteric ▽
457.8 Other noninfectious disorders of lymphatic channels
683 Acute lymphadenitis — (Use additional code to identify organism)
782.2 Localized superficial swelling, mass, or lump
784.2 Swelling, mass, or lump in head and neck
785.6 Enlargement of lymph nodes

ICD-9-CM Procedural

40.11 Biopsy of lymphatic structure
40.23 Excision of axillary lymph node
40.24 Excision of inguinal lymph node
40.29 Simple excision of other lymphatic structure

HCPCS Level II Supplies & Services

A4550 Surgical trays

38510–38520

38510 Biopsy or excision of lymph node(s); open, deep cervical node(s)
38520 open, deep cervical node(s) with excision scalene fat pad

ICD-9-CM Diagnostic

142.9 Malignant neoplasm of salivary gland, unspecified ▽
144.9 Malignant neoplasm of floor of mouth, part unspecified ▽

▽ Unspecified code
♀ Female diagnosis
⊠ Manifestation code
♂ Male diagnosis

145.9	Malignant neoplasm of mouth, unspecified site ▽
146.9	Malignant neoplasm of oropharynx, unspecified site ▽
147.9	Malignant neoplasm of nasopharynx, unspecified site ▽
148.9	Malignant neoplasm of hypopharynx, unspecified site ▽
149.8	Malignant neoplasm of other sites within the lip and oral cavity
150.0	Malignant neoplasm of cervical esophagus
150.3	Malignant neoplasm of upper third of esophagus
150.9	Malignant neoplasm of esophagus, unspecified site ▽
161.9	Malignant neoplasm of larynx, unspecified site ▽
172.3	Malignant melanoma of skin of other and unspecified parts of face
172.4	Malignant melanoma of skin of scalp and neck
174.8	Malignant neoplasm of other specified sites of female breast ♀
174.9	Malignant neoplasm of breast (female), unspecified site ▽ ♀
176.5	Kaposi's sarcoma of lymph nodes
176.9	Kaposi's sarcoma of unspecified site ▽
196.0	Secondary and unspecified malignant neoplasm of lymph nodes of head, face, and neck
196.8	Secondary and unspecified malignant neoplasm of lymph nodes of multiple sites
196.9	Secondary and unspecified malignant neoplasm of lymph nodes, site unspecified ▽
198.89	Secondary malignant neoplasm of other specified sites
199.0	Disseminated malignant neoplasm
199.1	Other malignant neoplasm of unspecified site
200.00	Reticulosarcoma, unspecified site, extranodal and solid organ sites ▽
200.01	Reticulosarcoma of lymph nodes of head, face, and neck
200.10	Lymphosarcoma, unspecified site, extranodal and solid organ sites ▽
200.11	Lymphosarcoma of lymph nodes of head, face, and neck
200.20	Burkitt's tumor or lymphoma, unspecified site, extranodal and solid organ sites ▽
200.21	Burkitt's tumor or lymphoma of lymph nodes of head, face, and neck
200.80	Other named variants, unspecified site, extranodal and solid organ sites ▽
200.81	Other named variants of lymphosarcoma and reticulosarcoma of lymph nodes of head, face, and neck
201.00	Hodgkin's paragranuloma, unspecified site, extranodal and solid organ sites ▽
201.01	Hodgkin's paragranuloma of lymph nodes of head, face, and neck
201.10	Hodgkin's granuloma, unspecified site, extranodal and solid organ sites ▽
201.11	Hodgkin's granuloma of lymph nodes of head, face, and neck
201.20	Hodgkin's sarcoma, unspecified site, extranodal and solid organ sites ▽
201.21	Hodgkin's sarcoma of lymph nodes of head, face, and neck
201.40	Hodgkin's disease, lymphocytic-histiocytic predominance, unspecified site, extranodal and solid organ sites ▽
201.41	Hodgkin's disease, lymphocytic-histiocytic predominance of lymph nodes of head, face, and neck
201.50	Hodgkin's disease, nodular sclerosis, unspecified site, extranodal and solid organ sites ▽
201.51	Hodgkin's disease, nodular sclerosis, of lymph nodes of head, face, and neck
201.60	Hodgkin's disease, mixed cellularity, unspecified site, extranodal and solid organ sites ▽
201.61	Hodgkin's disease, mixed cellularity, involving lymph nodes of head, face, and neck
201.70	Hodgkin's disease, lymphocytic depletion, unspecified site, extranodal and solid organ sites ▽
201.71	Hodgkin's disease, lymphocytic depletion, of lymph nodes of head, face, and neck
201.90	Hodgkin's disease, unspecified type, unspecified site, extranodal and solid organ sites ▽
201.91	Hodgkin's disease, unspecified type, of lymph nodes of head, face, and neck ▽
202.00	Nodular lymphoma, unspecified site, extranodal and solid organ sites ▽
202.01	Nodular lymphoma of lymph nodes of head, face, and neck
202.10	Mycosis fungoides, unspecified site, extranodal and solid organ sites ▽
202.11	Mycosis fungoides of lymph nodes of head, face, and neck
202.20	Sezary's disease, unspecified site, extranodal and solid organ sites ▽
202.30	Malignant histiocytosis, unspecified site, extranodal and solid organ sites ▽
202.31	Malignant histiocytosis of lymph nodes of head, face, and neck
202.40	Leukemic reticuloendotheliosis, unspecified site, extranodal and solid organ sites ▽
202.41	Leukemic reticuloendotheliosis of lymph nodes of head, face, and neck
202.50	Letterer-Siwe disease, unspecified site, extranodal and solid organ sites ▽
202.51	Letterer-Siwe disease of lymph nodes of head, face, and neck
202.60	Malignant mast cell tumors, unspecified site, extranodal and solid organ sites ▽
202.61	Malignant mast cell tumors of lymph nodes of head, face, and neck
202.80	Other malignant lymphomas, unspecified site, extranodal and solid organ sites ▽
202.81	Other malignant lymphomas of lymph nodes of head, face, and neck
202.90	Other and unspecified malignant neoplasms of lymphoid and histiocytic tissue, unspecified site, extranodal and solid organ sites ▽
202.91	Other and unspecified malignant neoplasms of lymphoid and histiocytic tissue of lymph nodes of head, face, and neck ▽
229.0	Benign neoplasm of lymph nodes
229.8	Benign neoplasm of other specified sites
229.9	Benign neoplasm of unspecified site ▽
238.7	Neoplasm of uncertain behavior of other lymphatic and hematopoietic tissues
239.8	Neoplasm of unspecified nature of other specified sites
239.9	Neoplasm of unspecified nature, site unspecified ▽
289.1	Chronic lymphadenitis
457.8	Other noninfectious disorders of lymphatic channels
683	Acute lymphadenitis — (Use additional code to identify organism)
784.2	Swelling, mass, or lump in head and neck
785.6	Enlargement of lymph nodes
786.6	Swelling, mass, or lump in chest

ICD-9-CM Procedural

40.11	Biopsy of lymphatic structure
40.21	Excision of deep cervical lymph node

38525

38525 Biopsy or excision of lymph node(s); open, deep axillary node(s)

ICD-9-CM Diagnostic

172.5	Malignant melanoma of skin of trunk, except scrotum
172.6	Malignant melanoma of skin of upper limb, including shoulder
174.0	Malignant neoplasm of nipple and areola of female breast ♀
174.3	Malignant neoplasm of lower-inner quadrant of female breast ♀
174.4	Malignant neoplasm of upper-outer quadrant of female breast ♀
174.5	Malignant neoplasm of lower-outer quadrant of female breast ♀
174.6	Malignant neoplasm of axillary tail of female breast ♀
174.8	Malignant neoplasm of other specified sites of female breast ♀
175.9	Malignant neoplasm of other and unspecified sites of male breast ▽ ♂
195.1	Malignant neoplasm of thorax
196.3	Secondary and unspecified malignant neoplasm of lymph nodes of axilla and upper limb
198.89	Secondary malignant neoplasm of other specified sites
199.0	Disseminated malignant neoplasm
199.1	Other malignant neoplasm of unspecified site
200.00	Reticulosarcoma, unspecified site, extranodal and solid organ sites ▽
200.04	Reticulosarcoma of lymph nodes of axilla and upper limb
200.10	Lymphosarcoma, unspecified site, extranodal and solid organ sites ▽
200.14	Lymphosarcoma of lymph nodes of axilla and upper limb
200.20	Burkitt's tumor or lymphoma, unspecified site, extranodal and solid organ sites ▽
200.24	Burkitt's tumor or lymphoma of lymph nodes of axilla and upper limb
200.80	Other named variants, unspecified site, extranodal and solid organ sites ▽
200.84	Other named variants of lymphosarcoma and reticulosarcoma of lymph nodes of axilla and upper limb
201.00	Hodgkin's paragranuloma, unspecified site, extranodal and solid organ sites ▽
201.04	Hodgkin's paragranuloma of lymph nodes of axilla and upper limb
201.10	Hodgkin's granuloma, unspecified site, extranodal and solid organ sites ▽
201.14	Hodgkin's granuloma of lymph nodes of axilla and upper limb
201.20	Hodgkin's sarcoma, unspecified site, extranodal and solid organ sites ▽
201.24	Hodgkin's sarcoma of lymph nodes of axilla and upper limb
201.40	Hodgkin's disease, lymphocytic-histiocytic predominance, unspecified site, extranodal and solid organ sites ▽
201.44	Hodgkin's disease, lymphocytic-histiocytic predominance of lymph nodes of axilla and upper limb
201.50	Hodgkin's disease, nodular sclerosis, unspecified site, extranodal and solid organ sites ▽
201.54	Hodgkin's disease, nodular sclerosis, of lymph nodes of axilla and upper limb
201.60	Hodgkin's disease, mixed cellularity, unspecified site, extranodal and solid organ sites ▽
201.64	Hodgkin's disease, mixed cellularity, of lymph nodes of axilla and upper limb
201.70	Hodgkin's disease, lymphocytic depletion, unspecified site, extranodal and solid organ sites ▽
201.74	Hodgkin's disease, lymphocytic depletion, of lymph nodes of axilla and upper limb
201.90	Hodgkin's disease, unspecified type, unspecified site, extranodal and solid organ sites ▽
201.94	Hodgkin's disease, unspecified type, of lymph nodes of axilla and upper limb ▽
202.00	Nodular lymphoma, unspecified site, extranodal and solid organ sites ▽
202.04	Nodular lymphoma of lymph nodes of axilla and upper limb
202.10	Mycosis fungoides, unspecified site, extranodal and solid organ sites ▽

▽ Unspecified code ♀ Female diagnosis ☒ Manifestation code ♂ Male diagnosis

202.14 Mycosis fungoides of lymph nodes of axilla and upper limb
202.20 Sezary's disease, unspecified site, extranodal and solid organ sites ▽
202.24 Sezary's disease of lymph nodes of axilla and upper limb
202.30 Malignant histiocytosis, unspecified site, extranodal and solid organ sites ▽
202.34 Malignant histiocytosis of lymph nodes of axilla and upper limb
202.40 Leukemic reticuloendotheliosis, unspecified site, extranodal and solid organ sites ▽
202.44 Leukemic reticuloendotheliosis of lymph nodes of axilla and upper limb
202.50 Letterer-Siwe disease, unspecified site, extranodal and solid organ sites ▽
202.54 Letterer-Siwe disease of lymph nodes of axilla and upper limb
202.60 Malignant mast cell tumors, unspecified site, extranodal and solid organ sites ▽
202.64 Malignant mast cell tumors of lymph nodes of axilla and upper limb
202.80 Other malignant lymphomas, unspecified site, extranodal and solid organ sites ▽
202.84 Other malignant lymphomas of lymph nodes of axilla and upper limb
202.90 Other and unspecified malignant neoplasms of lymphoid and histiocytic tissue, unspecified site, extranodal and solid organ sites ▽
202.94 Other and unspecified malignant neoplasms of lymphoid and histiocytic tissue of lymph nodes of axilla and upper limb ▽
229.0 Benign neoplasm of lymph nodes
229.8 Benign neoplasm of other specified sites
229.9 Benign neoplasm of unspecified site ▽
238.7 Neoplasm of uncertain behavior of other lymphatic and hematopoietic tissues
239.8 Neoplasm of unspecified nature of other specified sites
239.9 Neoplasm of unspecified nature, site unspecified ▽
289.1 Chronic lymphadenitis
289.3 Lymphadenitis, unspecified, except mesenteric ▽
683 Acute lymphadenitis — (Use additional code to identify organism)
785.6 Enlargement of lymph nodes

ICD-9-CM Procedural

40.11 Biopsy of lymphatic structure
40.23 Excision of axillary lymph node

38530

38530 Biopsy or excision of lymph node(s); open, internal mammary node(s)

ICD-9-CM Diagnostic

170.3 Malignant neoplasm of ribs, sternum, and clavicle
171.4 Malignant neoplasm of connective and other soft tissue of thorax
174.0 Malignant neoplasm of nipple and areola of female breast ♀
174.1 Malignant neoplasm of central portion of female breast ♀
174.2 Malignant neoplasm of upper-inner quadrant of female breast ♀
174.3 Malignant neoplasm of lower-inner quadrant of female breast ♀
174.4 Malignant neoplasm of upper-outer quadrant of female breast ♀
174.5 Malignant neoplasm of lower-outer quadrant of female breast ♀
174.6 Malignant neoplasm of axillary tail of female breast ♀
174.8 Malignant neoplasm of other specified sites of female breast ♀
196.9 Secondary and unspecified malignant neoplasm of lymph nodes, site unspecified ▽
198.81 Secondary malignant neoplasm of breast
289.3 Lymphadenitis, unspecified, except mesenteric ▽

ICD-9-CM Procedural

40.22 Excision of internal mammary lymph node

38542

38542 Dissection, deep jugular node(s)

ICD-9-CM Diagnostic

142.1 Malignant neoplasm of submandibular gland
161.0 Malignant neoplasm of glottis
161.1 Malignant neoplasm of supraglottis
161.3 Malignant neoplasm of laryngeal cartilages
161.9 Malignant neoplasm of larynx, unspecified site ▽
193 Malignant neoplasm of thyroid gland — (Use additional code to identify any functional activity)
194.1 Malignant neoplasm of parathyroid gland — (Use additional code to identify any functional activity)
196.0 Secondary and unspecified malignant neoplasm of lymph nodes of head, face, and neck
200.01 Reticulosarcoma of lymph nodes of head, face, and neck
200.11 Lymphosarcoma of lymph nodes of head, face, and neck
201.01 Hodgkin's paragranuloma of lymph nodes of head, face, and neck
201.91 Hodgkin's disease, unspecified type, of lymph nodes of head, face, and neck ▽
228.1 Lymphangioma, any site
784.2 Swelling, mass, or lump in head and neck
785.6 Enlargement of lymph nodes

ICD-9-CM Procedural

30.4 Radical laryngectomy
40.3 Regional lymph node excision
40.40 Radical neck dissection, not otherwise specified
40.41 Radical neck dissection, unilateral
40.42 Radical neck dissection, bilateral

38550–38555

38550 Excision of cystic hygroma, axillary or cervical; without deep neurovascular dissection
38555 with deep neurovascular dissection

ICD-9-CM Diagnostic

228.1 Lymphangioma, any site

ICD-9-CM Procedural

40.29 Simple excision of other lymphatic structure
40.59 Radical excision of other lymph nodes

38562–38564

38562 Limited lymphadenectomy for staging (separate procedure); pelvic and para-aortic
38564 retroperitoneal (aortic and/or splenic)

ICD-9-CM Diagnostic

151.5 Malignant neoplasm of lesser curvature of stomach, unspecified ▽
151.8 Malignant neoplasm of other specified sites of stomach
152.0 Malignant neoplasm of duodenum
153.7 Malignant neoplasm of splenic flexure
154.0 Malignant neoplasm of rectosigmoid junction
154.1 Malignant neoplasm of rectum
156.1 Malignant neoplasm of extrahepatic bile ducts
157.8 Malignant neoplasm of other specified sites of pancreas
157.9 Malignant neoplasm of pancreas, part unspecified ▽
158.0 Malignant neoplasm of retroperitoneum
158.8 Malignant neoplasm of specified parts of peritoneum
159.1 Malignant neoplasm of spleen, not elsewhere classified
180.0 Malignant neoplasm of endocervix ♀
180.1 Malignant neoplasm of exocervix ♀
180.8 Malignant neoplasm of other specified sites of cervix ♀
180.9 Malignant neoplasm of cervix uteri, unspecified site ▽ ♀
181 Malignant neoplasm of placenta ♀
182.0 Malignant neoplasm of corpus uteri, except isthmus ♀
182.1 Malignant neoplasm of isthmus ♀
182.8 Malignant neoplasm of other specified sites of body of uterus ♀
183.0 Malignant neoplasm of ovary — (Use additional code to identify any functional activity) ♀
183.2 Malignant neoplasm of fallopian tube ♀
183.3 Malignant neoplasm of broad ligament of uterus ♀
183.4 Malignant neoplasm of parametrium of uterus ♀
183.5 Malignant neoplasm of round ligament of uterus ♀
183.8 Malignant neoplasm of other specified sites of uterine adnexa ♀
183.9 Malignant neoplasm of uterine adnexa, unspecified site ▽ ♀
185 Malignant neoplasm of prostate ♂
186.9 Malignant neoplasm of other and unspecified testis — (Use additional code to identify any functional activity) ▽ ♂
187.1 Malignant neoplasm of prepuce ♂
187.2 Malignant neoplasm of glans penis ♂
187.3 Malignant neoplasm of body of penis ♂
187.4 Malignant neoplasm of penis, part unspecified ▽ ♂
187.5 Malignant neoplasm of epididymis ♂
187.6 Malignant neoplasm of spermatic cord ♂
187.7 Malignant neoplasm of scrotum ♂
187.8 Malignant neoplasm of other specified sites of male genital organs ♂
187.9 Malignant neoplasm of male genital organ, site unspecified ▽ ♂
188.0 Malignant neoplasm of trigone of urinary bladder
188.1 Malignant neoplasm of dome of urinary bladder
188.2 Malignant neoplasm of lateral wall of urinary bladder
188.3 Malignant neoplasm of anterior wall of urinary bladder
188.4 Malignant neoplasm of posterior wall of urinary bladder
188.5 Malignant neoplasm of bladder neck
188.6 Malignant neoplasm of ureteric orifice

188.8	Malignant neoplasm of other specified sites of bladder
188.9	Malignant neoplasm of bladder, part unspecified ▽
189.0	Malignant neoplasm of kidney, except pelvis
189.1	Malignant neoplasm of renal pelvis
189.2	Malignant neoplasm of ureter
189.3	Malignant neoplasm of urethra
189.4	Malignant neoplasm of paraurethral glands
189.8	Malignant neoplasm of other specified sites of urinary organs
189.9	Malignant neoplasm of urinary organ, site unspecified ▽
195.3	Malignant neoplasm of pelvis
196.2	Secondary and unspecified malignant neoplasm of intra-abdominal lymph nodes
196.6	Secondary and unspecified malignant neoplasm of intrapelvic lymph nodes
197.5	Secondary malignant neoplasm of large intestine and rectum
197.6	Secondary malignant neoplasm of retroperitoneum and peritoneum
197.8	Secondary malignant neoplasm of other digestive organs and spleen
198.89	Secondary malignant neoplasm of other specified sites
201.90	Hodgkin's disease, unspecified type, unspecified site, extranodal and solid organ sites ▽
211.4	Benign neoplasm of rectum and anal canal
230.4	Carcinoma in situ of rectum
235.2	Neoplasm of uncertain behavior of stomach, intestines, and rectum
235.4	Neoplasm of uncertain behavior of retroperitoneum and peritoneum
235.5	Neoplasm of uncertain behavior of other and unspecified digestive organs ▽
238.8	Neoplasm of uncertain behavior of other specified sites
239.0	Neoplasm of unspecified nature of digestive system

ICD-9-CM Procedural

40.3	Regional lymph node excision
40.9	Other operations on lymphatic structures

38570–38572

38570	Laparoscopy, surgical; with retroperitoneal lymph node sampling (biopsy), single or multiple
38571	with bilateral total pelvic lymphadenectomy
38572	with bilateral total pelvic lymphadenectomy and peri-aortic lymph node sampling (biopsy), single or multiple

ICD-9-CM Diagnostic

153.9	Malignant neoplasm of colon, unspecified site ▽
154.0	Malignant neoplasm of rectosigmoid junction
154.1	Malignant neoplasm of rectum
180.9	Malignant neoplasm of cervix uteri, unspecified site ▽ ♀
182.0	Malignant neoplasm of corpus uteri, except isthmus ♀
183.0	Malignant neoplasm of ovary — (Use additional code to identify any functional activity) ♀
185	Malignant neoplasm of prostate ♂
196.2	Secondary and unspecified malignant neoplasm of intra-abdominal lymph nodes
196.6	Secondary and unspecified malignant neoplasm of intrapelvic lymph nodes
200.13	Lymphosarcoma of intra-abdominal lymph nodes
201.93	Hodgkin's disease, unspecified type, of intra-abdominal lymph nodes ▽
202.03	Nodular lymphoma of intra-abdominal lymph nodes
202.83	Other malignant lymphomas of intra-abdominal lymph nodes
238.8	Neoplasm of uncertain behavior of other specified sites
239.8	Neoplasm of unspecified nature of other specified sites
288.8	Other specified disease of white blood cells
289.1	Chronic lymphadenitis
289.3	Lymphadenitis, unspecified, except mesenteric ▽
457.8	Other noninfectious disorders of lymphatic channels
683	Acute lymphadenitis — (Use additional code to identify organism)
782.2	Localized superficial swelling, mass, or lump
785.6	Enlargement of lymph nodes

ICD-9-CM Procedural

40.11	Biopsy of lymphatic structure
40.3	Regional lymph node excision

38700

38700	Suprahyoid lymphadenectomy

ICD-9-CM Diagnostic

140.8	Malignant neoplasm of other sites of lip
141.9	Malignant neoplasm of tongue, unspecified site ▽
142.1	Malignant neoplasm of submandibular gland
142.2	Malignant neoplasm of sublingual gland
142.9	Malignant neoplasm of salivary gland, unspecified ▽
143.9	Malignant neoplasm of gum, unspecified site ▽
144.9	Malignant neoplasm of floor of mouth, part unspecified ▽
145.0	Malignant neoplasm of cheek mucosa
145.9	Malignant neoplasm of mouth, unspecified site ▽
146.9	Malignant neoplasm of oropharynx, unspecified site ▽
148.9	Malignant neoplasm of hypopharynx, unspecified site ▽
160.9	Malignant neoplasm of site of nasal cavities, middle ear, and accessory sinus, unspecified site ▽
161.0	Malignant neoplasm of glottis
161.1	Malignant neoplasm of supraglottis
161.3	Malignant neoplasm of laryngeal cartilages
161.8	Malignant neoplasm of other specified sites of larynx
161.9	Malignant neoplasm of larynx, unspecified site ▽
170.0	Malignant neoplasm of bones of skull and face, except mandible
170.1	Malignant neoplasm of mandible
172.9	Melanoma of skin, site unspecified ▽
196.0	Secondary and unspecified malignant neoplasm of lymph nodes of head, face, and neck
238.8	Neoplasm of uncertain behavior of other specified sites

ICD-9-CM Procedural

40.3	Regional lymph node excision

38720–38724

38720	Cervical lymphadenectomy (complete)
38724	Cervical lymphadenectomy (modified radical neck dissection)

ICD-9-CM Diagnostic

141.0	Malignant neoplasm of base of tongue
141.1	Malignant neoplasm of dorsal surface of tongue
141.2	Malignant neoplasm of tip and lateral border of tongue
141.3	Malignant neoplasm of ventral surface of tongue
141.4	Malignant neoplasm of anterior two-thirds of tongue, part unspecified ▽
141.5	Malignant neoplasm of junctional zone of tongue
141.6	Malignant neoplasm of lingual tonsil
141.9	Malignant neoplasm of tongue, unspecified site ▽
142.0	Malignant neoplasm of parotid gland
142.1	Malignant neoplasm of submandibular gland
142.2	Malignant neoplasm of sublingual gland
142.8	Malignant neoplasm of other major salivary glands
142.9	Malignant neoplasm of salivary gland, unspecified ▽
144.0	Malignant neoplasm of anterior portion of floor of mouth
144.1	Malignant neoplasm of lateral portion of floor of mouth
144.8	Malignant neoplasm of other sites of floor of mouth
144.9	Malignant neoplasm of floor of mouth, part unspecified ▽
145.0	Malignant neoplasm of cheek mucosa
145.1	Malignant neoplasm of vestibule of mouth
145.2	Malignant neoplasm of hard palate
145.3	Malignant neoplasm of soft palate
145.4	Malignant neoplasm of uvula
145.5	Malignant neoplasm of palate, unspecified ▽
145.6	Malignant neoplasm of retromolar area
145.8	Malignant neoplasm of other specified parts of mouth
145.9	Malignant neoplasm of mouth, unspecified site ▽
146.9	Malignant neoplasm of oropharynx, unspecified site ▽
148.0	Malignant neoplasm of postcricoid region of hypopharynx
148.1	Malignant neoplasm of pyriform sinus
148.2	Malignant neoplasm of aryepiglottic fold, hypopharyngeal aspect
148.3	Malignant neoplasm of posterior hypopharyngeal wall
148.8	Malignant neoplasm of other specified sites of hypopharynx
148.9	Malignant neoplasm of hypopharynx, unspecified site ▽
149.0	Malignant neoplasm of pharynx, unspecified ▽
149.1	Malignant neoplasm of Waldeyer's ring
149.8	Malignant neoplasm of other sites within the lip and oral cavity
149.9	Malignant neoplasm of ill-defined sites of lip and oral cavity
150.0	Malignant neoplasm of cervical esophagus
150.1	Malignant neoplasm of thoracic esophagus
150.3	Malignant neoplasm of upper third of esophagus
150.4	Malignant neoplasm of middle third of esophagus
150.8	Malignant neoplasm of other specified part of esophagus
150.9	Malignant neoplasm of esophagus, unspecified site ▽
161.0	Malignant neoplasm of glottis
161.1	Malignant neoplasm of supraglottis
161.2	Malignant neoplasm of subglottis
161.3	Malignant neoplasm of laryngeal cartilages

▽ Unspecified code ♀ Female diagnosis M Manifestation code ♂ Male diagnosis

161.8 Malignant neoplasm of other specified sites of larynx
161.9 Malignant neoplasm of larynx, unspecified site ▽
162.0 Malignant neoplasm of trachea
170.1 Malignant neoplasm of mandible
172.4 Malignant melanoma of skin of scalp and neck
173.4 Other malignant neoplasm of scalp and skin of neck
193 Malignant neoplasm of thyroid gland — (Use additional code to identify any functional activity)
194.1 Malignant neoplasm of parathyroid gland — (Use additional code to identify any functional activity)
194.5 Malignant neoplasm of carotid body — (Use additional code to identify any functional activity)
195.0 Malignant neoplasm of head, face, and neck
196.0 Secondary and unspecified malignant neoplasm of lymph nodes of head, face, and neck
198.89 Secondary malignant neoplasm of other specified sites
199.0 Disseminated malignant neoplasm
199.1 Other malignant neoplasm of unspecified site
238.8 Neoplasm of uncertain behavior of other specified sites
239.3 Neoplasm of unspecified nature of breast
239.8 Neoplasm of unspecified nature of other specified sites
784.2 Swelling, mass, or lump in head and neck
785.6 Enlargement of lymph nodes

ICD-9-CM Procedural

40.40 Radical neck dissection, not otherwise specified
40.41 Radical neck dissection, unilateral
40.42 Radical neck dissection, bilateral

38740–38745

38740 Axillary lymphadenectomy; superficial
38745 complete

ICD-9-CM Diagnostic

170.4 Malignant neoplasm of scapula and long bones of upper limb
170.5 Malignant neoplasm of short bones of upper limb
171.2 Malignant neoplasm of connective and other soft tissue of upper limb, including shoulder
172.6 Malignant melanoma of skin of upper limb, including shoulder
174.1 Malignant neoplasm of central portion of female breast ♀
174.2 Malignant neoplasm of upper-inner quadrant of female breast ♀
174.3 Malignant neoplasm of lower-inner quadrant of female breast ♀
174.4 Malignant neoplasm of upper-outer quadrant of female breast ♀
174.5 Malignant neoplasm of lower-outer quadrant of female breast ♀
174.6 Malignant neoplasm of axillary tail of female breast ♀
174.8 Malignant neoplasm of other specified sites of female breast ♀
174.9 Malignant neoplasm of breast (female), unspecified site ▽ ♀
175.9 Malignant neoplasm of other and unspecified sites of male breast ▽ ♂
176.5 Kaposi's sarcoma of lymph nodes
195.1 Malignant neoplasm of thorax
196.3 Secondary and unspecified malignant neoplasm of lymph nodes of axilla and upper limb
198.89 Secondary malignant neoplasm of other specified sites
199.1 Other malignant neoplasm of unspecified site
229.0 Benign neoplasm of lymph nodes
229.8 Benign neoplasm of other specified sites
233.0 Carcinoma in situ of breast
238.8 Neoplasm of uncertain behavior of other specified sites
239.3 Neoplasm of unspecified nature of breast
239.8 Neoplasm of unspecified nature of other specified sites
611.72 Lump or mass in breast
785.6 Enlargement of lymph nodes
793.80 Unspecified abnormal mammogram ▽
793.81 Mammographic microcalcification
793.89 Other abnormal findings on radiological examination of breast
V10.3 Personal history of malignant neoplasm of breast
V10.79 Personal history of other lymphatic and hematopoietic neoplasm
V10.82 Personal history of malignant melanoma of skin

ICD-9-CM Procedural

40.23 Excision of axillary lymph node
40.29 Simple excision of other lymphatic structure
40.51 Radical excision of axillary lymph nodes

38746

38746 Thoracic lymphadenectomy, regional, including mediastinal and peritracheal nodes (List separately in addition to code for primary procedure)

ICD-9-CM Diagnostic

This is an add-on code. Refer to the corresponding primary procedure code for ICD-9 diagnosis code links.

ICD-9-CM Procedural

40.3 Regional lymph node excision

38747

38747 Abdominal lymphadenectomy, regional, including celiac, gastric, portal, peripancreatic, with or without para-aortic and vena caval nodes (List separately in addition to code for primary procedure)

ICD-9-CM Diagnostic

This is an add-on code. Refer to the corresponding primary procedure code for ICD-9 diagnosis code links.

ICD-9-CM Procedural

40.3 Regional lymph node excision
40.53 Radical excision of iliac lymph nodes

38760–38765

38760 Inguinofemoral lymphadenectomy, superficial, including Cloquet's node (separate procedure)
38765 Inguinofemoral lymphadenectomy, superficial, in continuity with pelvic lymphadenectomy, including external iliac, hypogastric, and obturator nodes (separate procedure)

ICD-9-CM Diagnostic

154.0 Malignant neoplasm of rectosigmoid junction
154.1 Malignant neoplasm of rectum
172.5 Malignant melanoma of skin of trunk, except scrotum
172.7 Malignant melanoma of skin of lower limb, including hip
176.5 Kaposi's sarcoma of lymph nodes
180.0 Malignant neoplasm of endocervix ♀
180.1 Malignant neoplasm of exocervix ♀
180.8 Malignant neoplasm of other specified sites of cervix ♀
180.9 Malignant neoplasm of cervix uteri, unspecified site ▽ ♀
181 Malignant neoplasm of placenta ♀
182.0 Malignant neoplasm of corpus uteri, except isthmus ♀
182.1 Malignant neoplasm of isthmus ♀
182.8 Malignant neoplasm of other specified sites of body of uterus ♀
183.0 Malignant neoplasm of ovary — (Use additional code to identify any functional activity) ♀
183.2 Malignant neoplasm of fallopian tube ♀
183.3 Malignant neoplasm of broad ligament of uterus ♀
183.4 Malignant neoplasm of parametrium of uterus ♀
183.5 Malignant neoplasm of round ligament of uterus ♀
183.8 Malignant neoplasm of other specified sites of uterine adnexa ♀
183.9 Malignant neoplasm of uterine adnexa, unspecified site ▽ ♀
184.0 Malignant neoplasm of vagina ♀
184.1 Malignant neoplasm of labia majora ♀
184.2 Malignant neoplasm of labia minora ♀
184.3 Malignant neoplasm of clitoris ♀
184.4 Malignant neoplasm of vulva, unspecified site ▽ ♀
184.8 Malignant neoplasm of other specified sites of female genital organs ♀
184.9 Malignant neoplasm of female genital organ, site unspecified ▽ ♀
185 Malignant neoplasm of prostate ♂
186.9 Malignant neoplasm of other and unspecified testis — (Use additional code to identify any functional activity) ▽ ♂
187.1 Malignant neoplasm of prepuce ♂
187.2 Malignant neoplasm of glans penis ♂
187.3 Malignant neoplasm of body of penis ♂
187.4 Malignant neoplasm of penis, part unspecified ▽ ♂
187.5 Malignant neoplasm of epididymis ♂
187.6 Malignant neoplasm of spermatic cord ♂
187.7 Malignant neoplasm of scrotum ♂
187.8 Malignant neoplasm of other specified sites of male genital organs ♂
187.9 Malignant neoplasm of male genital organ, site unspecified ▽ ♂
188.0 Malignant neoplasm of trigone of urinary bladder
188.1 Malignant neoplasm of dome of urinary bladder
188.2 Malignant neoplasm of lateral wall of urinary bladder
188.3 Malignant neoplasm of anterior wall of urinary bladder

188.4 Malignant neoplasm of posterior wall of urinary bladder
188.5 Malignant neoplasm of bladder neck
188.6 Malignant neoplasm of ureteric orifice
188.8 Malignant neoplasm of other specified sites of bladder
188.9 Malignant neoplasm of bladder, part unspecified ▽
189.0 Malignant neoplasm of kidney, except pelvis
189.1 Malignant neoplasm of renal pelvis
189.2 Malignant neoplasm of ureter
189.3 Malignant neoplasm of urethra
189.4 Malignant neoplasm of paraurethral glands
189.8 Malignant neoplasm of other specified sites of urinary organs
189.9 Malignant neoplasm of urinary organ, site unspecified ▽
196.2 Secondary and unspecified malignant neoplasm of intra-abdominal lymph nodes
196.5 Secondary and unspecified malignant neoplasm of lymph nodes of inguinal region and lower limb
197.5 Secondary malignant neoplasm of large intestine and rectum
201.90 Hodgkin's disease, unspecified type, unspecified site, extranodal and solid organ sites ▽
202.85 Other malignant lymphomas of lymph nodes of inguinal region and lower limb
211.4 Benign neoplasm of rectum and anal canal
229.0 Benign neoplasm of lymph nodes
230.4 Carcinoma in situ of rectum
235.2 Neoplasm of uncertain behavior of stomach, intestines, and rectum
238.8 Neoplasm of uncertain behavior of other specified sites
239.0 Neoplasm of unspecified nature of digestive system
289.3 Lymphadenitis, unspecified, except mesenteric ▽
785.6 Enlargement of lymph nodes

ICD-9-CM Procedural

40.24 Excision of inguinal lymph node
40.3 Regional lymph node excision

38770

38770 Pelvic lymphadenectomy, including external iliac, hypogastric, and obturator nodes (separate procedure)

ICD-9-CM Diagnostic

154.0 Malignant neoplasm of rectosigmoid junction
154.1 Malignant neoplasm of rectum
172.5 Malignant melanoma of skin of trunk, except scrotum
172.7 Malignant melanoma of skin of lower limb, including hip
180.0 Malignant neoplasm of endocervix ♀
180.1 Malignant neoplasm of exocervix ♀
180.8 Malignant neoplasm of other specified sites of cervix ♀
180.9 Malignant neoplasm of cervix uteri, unspecified site ▽ ♀
182.0 Malignant neoplasm of corpus uteri, except isthmus ♀
182.1 Malignant neoplasm of isthmus ♀
182.8 Malignant neoplasm of other specified sites of body of uterus ♀
183.0 Malignant neoplasm of ovary — (Use additional code to identify any functional activity) ♀
183.2 Malignant neoplasm of fallopian tube ♀
183.3 Malignant neoplasm of broad ligament of uterus ♀
183.4 Malignant neoplasm of parametrium of uterus ♀
183.5 Malignant neoplasm of round ligament of uterus ♀
183.8 Malignant neoplasm of other specified sites of uterine adnexa ♀
183.9 Malignant neoplasm of uterine adnexa, unspecified site ▽ ♀
184.0 Malignant neoplasm of vagina ♀
184.1 Malignant neoplasm of labia majora ♀
184.2 Malignant neoplasm of labia minora ♀
184.3 Malignant neoplasm of clitoris ♀
184.4 Malignant neoplasm of vulva, unspecified site ▽ ♀
184.8 Malignant neoplasm of other specified sites of female genital organs ♀
184.9 Malignant neoplasm of female genital organ, site unspecified ▽ ♀
185 Malignant neoplasm of prostate ♂
186.9 Malignant neoplasm of other and unspecified testis — (Use additional code to identify any functional activity) ▽ ♂
187.1 Malignant neoplasm of prepuce ♂
187.2 Malignant neoplasm of glans penis ♂
187.3 Malignant neoplasm of body of penis ♂
187.4 Malignant neoplasm of penis, part unspecified ▽ ♂
187.5 Malignant neoplasm of epididymis ♂
187.6 Malignant neoplasm of spermatic cord ♂
187.7 Malignant neoplasm of scrotum ♂
187.8 Malignant neoplasm of other specified sites of male genital organs ♂
187.9 Malignant neoplasm of male genital organ, site unspecified ▽ ♂
188.0 Malignant neoplasm of trigone of urinary bladder
188.1 Malignant neoplasm of dome of urinary bladder
188.2 Malignant neoplasm of lateral wall of urinary bladder
188.3 Malignant neoplasm of anterior wall of urinary bladder
188.4 Malignant neoplasm of posterior wall of urinary bladder
188.5 Malignant neoplasm of bladder neck
188.6 Malignant neoplasm of ureteric orifice
188.7 Malignant neoplasm of urachus
188.8 Malignant neoplasm of other specified sites of bladder
188.9 Malignant neoplasm of bladder, part unspecified ▽
189.0 Malignant neoplasm of kidney, except pelvis
189.1 Malignant neoplasm of renal pelvis
189.2 Malignant neoplasm of ureter
189.3 Malignant neoplasm of urethra
189.4 Malignant neoplasm of paraurethral glands
189.9 Malignant neoplasm of urinary organ, site unspecified ▽
196.6 Secondary and unspecified malignant neoplasm of intrapelvic lymph nodes
198.89 Secondary malignant neoplasm of other specified sites
199.1 Other malignant neoplasm of unspecified site
238.8 Neoplasm of uncertain behavior of other specified sites
239.8 Neoplasm of unspecified nature of other specified sites

ICD-9-CM Procedural

40.53 Radical excision of iliac lymph nodes

38780

38780 Retroperitoneal transabdominal lymphadenectomy, extensive, including pelvic, aortic, and renal nodes (separate procedure)

ICD-9-CM Diagnostic

152.0 Malignant neoplasm of duodenum
153.7 Malignant neoplasm of splenic flexure
153.9 Malignant neoplasm of colon, unspecified site ▽
154.1 Malignant neoplasm of rectum
157.0 Malignant neoplasm of head of pancreas
157.1 Malignant neoplasm of body of pancreas
157.9 Malignant neoplasm of pancreas, part unspecified ▽
158.0 Malignant neoplasm of retroperitoneum
158.8 Malignant neoplasm of specified parts of peritoneum
180.0 Malignant neoplasm of endocervix ♀
180.1 Malignant neoplasm of exocervix ♀
180.8 Malignant neoplasm of other specified sites of cervix ♀
180.9 Malignant neoplasm of cervix uteri, unspecified site ▽ ♀
182.0 Malignant neoplasm of corpus uteri, except isthmus ♀
182.1 Malignant neoplasm of isthmus ♀
182.8 Malignant neoplasm of other specified sites of body of uterus ♀
183.0 Malignant neoplasm of ovary — (Use additional code to identify any functional activity) ♀
183.2 Malignant neoplasm of fallopian tube ♀
183.3 Malignant neoplasm of broad ligament of uterus ♀
183.4 Malignant neoplasm of parametrium of uterus ♀
183.5 Malignant neoplasm of round ligament of uterus ♀
183.8 Malignant neoplasm of other specified sites of uterine adnexa ♀
183.9 Malignant neoplasm of uterine adnexa, unspecified site ▽ ♀
185 Malignant neoplasm of prostate ♂
186.9 Malignant neoplasm of other and unspecified testis — (Use additional code to identify any functional activity) ▽ ♂
188.0 Malignant neoplasm of trigone of urinary bladder
188.1 Malignant neoplasm of dome of urinary bladder
188.2 Malignant neoplasm of lateral wall of urinary bladder
188.3 Malignant neoplasm of anterior wall of urinary bladder
188.4 Malignant neoplasm of posterior wall of urinary bladder
188.5 Malignant neoplasm of bladder neck
188.6 Malignant neoplasm of ureteric orifice
188.8 Malignant neoplasm of other specified sites of bladder
188.9 Malignant neoplasm of bladder, part unspecified ▽
189.0 Malignant neoplasm of kidney, except pelvis
189.1 Malignant neoplasm of renal pelvis
189.2 Malignant neoplasm of ureter
189.3 Malignant neoplasm of urethra
189.4 Malignant neoplasm of paraurethral glands
189.8 Malignant neoplasm of other specified sites of urinary organs
189.9 Malignant neoplasm of urinary organ, site unspecified ▽
194.0 Malignant neoplasm of adrenal gland — (Use additional code to identify any functional activity)

196.2 Secondary and unspecified malignant neoplasm of intra-abdominal lymph nodes
197.5 Secondary malignant neoplasm of large intestine and rectum
197.6 Secondary malignant neoplasm of retroperitoneum and peritoneum
197.8 Secondary malignant neoplasm of other digestive organs and spleen
235.4 Neoplasm of uncertain behavior of retroperitoneum and peritoneum
238.8 Neoplasm of uncertain behavior of other specified sites

ICD-9-CM Procedural

40.54 Radical groin dissection

38790

38790 Injection procedure; lymphangiography

ICD-9-CM Diagnostic

180.0 Malignant neoplasm of endocervix ♀
180.1 Malignant neoplasm of exocervix ♀
180.8 Malignant neoplasm of other specified sites of cervix ♀
180.9 Malignant neoplasm of cervix uteri, unspecified site ▽ ♀
186.0 Malignant neoplasm of undescended testis — (Use additional code to identify any functional activity) ♂
186.9 Malignant neoplasm of other and unspecified testis — (Use additional code to identify any functional activity) ▽ ♂
201.50 Hodgkin's disease, nodular sclerosis, unspecified site, extranodal and solid organ sites ▽
201.60 Hodgkin's disease, mixed cellularity, unspecified site, extranodal and solid organ sites ▽
201.70 Hodgkin's disease, lymphocytic depletion, unspecified site, extranodal and solid organ sites ▽
785.6 Enlargement of lymph nodes

ICD-9-CM Procedural

40.19 Other diagnostic procedures on lymphatic structures
87.34 Intrathoracic lymphangiogram

38792

38792 Injection procedure; for identification of sentinel node

ICD-9-CM Diagnostic

142.1 Malignant neoplasm of submandibular gland
161.0 Malignant neoplasm of glottis
161.1 Malignant neoplasm of supraglottis
161.3 Malignant neoplasm of laryngeal cartilages
161.9 Malignant neoplasm of larynx, unspecified site ▽
174.0 Malignant neoplasm of nipple and areola of female breast ♀
174.1 Malignant neoplasm of central portion of female breast ♀
174.2 Malignant neoplasm of upper-inner quadrant of female breast ♀
174.3 Malignant neoplasm of lower-inner quadrant of female breast ♀
174.4 Malignant neoplasm of upper-outer quadrant of female breast ♀
174.5 Malignant neoplasm of lower-outer quadrant of female breast ♀
174.6 Malignant neoplasm of axillary tail of female breast ♀
174.8 Malignant neoplasm of other specified sites of female breast ♀
174.9 Malignant neoplasm of breast (female), unspecified site ▽ ♀
193 Malignant neoplasm of thyroid gland — (Use additional code to identify any functional activity)
194.1 Malignant neoplasm of parathyroid gland — (Use additional code to identify any functional activity)
196.0 Secondary and unspecified malignant neoplasm of lymph nodes of head, face, and neck
196.1 Secondary and unspecified malignant neoplasm of intrathoracic lymph nodes
196.2 Secondary and unspecified malignant neoplasm of intra-abdominal lymph nodes
196.3 Secondary and unspecified malignant neoplasm of lymph nodes of axilla and upper limb
196.5 Secondary and unspecified malignant neoplasm of lymph nodes of inguinal region and lower limb
196.6 Secondary and unspecified malignant neoplasm of intrapelvic lymph nodes
196.8 Secondary and unspecified malignant neoplasm of lymph nodes of multiple sites
196.9 Secondary and unspecified malignant neoplasm of lymph nodes, site unspecified ▽
200.01 Reticulosarcoma of lymph nodes of head, face, and neck
200.11 Lymphosarcoma of lymph nodes of head, face, and neck
201.01 Hodgkin's paragranuloma of lymph nodes of head, face, and neck
201.91 Hodgkin's disease, unspecified type, of lymph nodes of head, face, and neck ▽
202.81 Other malignant lymphomas of lymph nodes of head, face, and neck
228.1 Lymphangioma, any site
784.2 Swelling, mass, or lump in head and neck
785.6 Enlargement of lymph nodes

ICD-9-CM Procedural

99.99 Other miscellaneous procedures

38794

38794 Cannulation, thoracic duct

ICD-9-CM Diagnostic

201.50 Hodgkin's disease, nodular sclerosis, unspecified site, extranodal and solid organ sites ▽
201.60 Hodgkin's disease, mixed cellularity, unspecified site, extranodal and solid organ sites ▽
201.70 Hodgkin's disease, lymphocytic depletion, unspecified site, extranodal and solid organ sites ▽
202.02 Nodular lymphoma of intrathoracic lymph nodes
202.22 Sezary's disease of intrathoracic lymph nodes
202.32 Malignant histiocytosis of intrathoracic lymph nodes
202.82 Other malignant lymphomas of intrathoracic lymph nodes
457.1 Other noninfectious lymphedema

ICD-9-CM Procedural

40.61 Cannulation of thoracic duct
40.9 Other operations on lymphatic structures

▽ Unspecified code
♀ Female diagnosis
☒ Manifestation code
♂ Male diagnosis

Mediastinum and Diaphragm

Mediastinum

39000

39000 Mediastinotomy with exploration, drainage, removal of foreign body, or biopsy; cervical approach

ICD-9-CM Diagnostic

164.0 Malignant neoplasm of thymus
164.2 Malignant neoplasm of anterior mediastinum
164.3 Malignant neoplasm of posterior mediastinum
212.5 Benign neoplasm of mediastinum
212.6 Benign neoplasm of thymus
235.8 Neoplasm of uncertain behavior of pleura, thymus, and mediastinum
513.1 Abscess of mediastinum
519.2 Mediastinitis
519.3 Other diseases of mediastinum, not elsewhere classified
860.2 Traumatic hemothorax without mention of open wound into thorax
860.3 Traumatic hemothorax with open wound into thorax
862.8 Injury to multiple and unspecified intrathoracic organs without mention of open wound into cavity
862.9 Injury to multiple and unspecified intrathoracic organs with open wound into cavity
901.9 Injury to unspecified blood vessel of thorax ▽
998.4 Foreign body accidentally left during procedure, not elsewhere classified

ICD-9-CM Procedural

34.1 Incision of mediastinum
34.26 Open biopsy of mediastinum

39010

39010 Mediastinotomy with exploration, drainage, removal of foreign body, or biopsy; transthoracic approach, including either transthoracic or median sternotomy

ICD-9-CM Diagnostic

164.2 Malignant neoplasm of anterior mediastinum
164.3 Malignant neoplasm of posterior mediastinum
164.9 Malignant neoplasm of mediastinum, part unspecified ▽
212.5 Benign neoplasm of mediastinum
513.1 Abscess of mediastinum
519.2 Mediastinitis
519.3 Other diseases of mediastinum, not elsewhere classified
793.1 Nonspecific abnormal findings on radiological and other examination of lung field
860.2 Traumatic hemothorax without mention of open wound into thorax
860.3 Traumatic hemothorax with open wound into thorax
862.8 Injury to multiple and unspecified intrathoracic organs without mention of open wound into cavity
862.9 Injury to multiple and unspecified intrathoracic organs with open wound into cavity
901.9 Injury to unspecified blood vessel of thorax ▽
998.11 Hemorrhage complicating a procedure

ICD-9-CM Procedural

34.1 Incision of mediastinum
34.26 Open biopsy of mediastinum
34.3 Excision or destruction of lesion or tissue of mediastinum

39200

39200 Excision of mediastinal cyst

ICD-9-CM Diagnostic

748.8 Other specified congenital anomaly of respiratory system
V64.42 Thoracoscopic surgical procedure converted to open procedure

ICD-9-CM Procedural

34.3 Excision or destruction of lesion or tissue of mediastinum

39220

39220 Excision of mediastinal tumor

ICD-9-CM Diagnostic

164.2 Malignant neoplasm of anterior mediastinum
164.3 Malignant neoplasm of posterior mediastinum
164.8 Malignant neoplasm of other parts of mediastinum
164.9 Malignant neoplasm of mediastinum, part unspecified ▽
212.5 Benign neoplasm of mediastinum
235.8 Neoplasm of uncertain behavior of pleura, thymus, and mediastinum

ICD-9-CM Procedural

34.3 Excision or destruction of lesion or tissue of mediastinum

39400

39400 Mediastinoscopy, with or without biopsy

ICD-9-CM Diagnostic

162.0 Malignant neoplasm of trachea
162.2 Malignant neoplasm of main bronchus
162.3 Malignant neoplasm of upper lobe, bronchus, or lung
162.4 Malignant neoplasm of middle lobe, bronchus, or lung
162.5 Malignant neoplasm of lower lobe, bronchus, or lung
162.8 Malignant neoplasm of other parts of bronchus or lung
162.9 Malignant neoplasm of bronchus and lung, unspecified site ▽
163.0 Malignant neoplasm of parietal pleura
163.1 Malignant neoplasm of visceral pleura
163.8 Malignant neoplasm of other specified sites of pleura
163.9 Malignant neoplasm of pleura, unspecified site ▽
164.0 Malignant neoplasm of thymus
164.2 Malignant neoplasm of anterior mediastinum
164.3 Malignant neoplasm of posterior mediastinum
164.8 Malignant neoplasm of other parts of mediastinum
164.9 Malignant neoplasm of mediastinum, part unspecified ▽
165.0 Malignant neoplasm of upper respiratory tract, part unspecified ▽
165.8 Malignant neoplasm of other sites within the respiratory system and intrathoracic organs
165.9 Malignant neoplasm of ill-defined sites within the respiratory system
195.1 Malignant neoplasm of thorax
196.1 Secondary and unspecified malignant neoplasm of intrathoracic lymph nodes
197.0 Secondary malignant neoplasm of lung
197.1 Secondary malignant neoplasm of mediastinum
197.2 Secondary malignant neoplasm of pleura
197.3 Secondary malignant neoplasm of other respiratory organs
198.89 Secondary malignant neoplasm of other specified sites
199.1 Other malignant neoplasm of unspecified site
200.00 Reticulosarcoma, unspecified site, extranodal and solid organ sites ▽
200.02 Reticulosarcoma of intrathoracic lymph nodes
200.08 Reticulosarcoma of lymph nodes of multiple sites
200.10 Lymphosarcoma, unspecified site, extranodal and solid organ sites ▽
200.12 Lymphosarcoma of intrathoracic lymph nodes
200.18 Lymphosarcoma of lymph nodes of multiple sites
200.20 Burkitt's tumor or lymphoma, unspecified site, extranodal and solid organ sites ▽
200.22 Burkitt's tumor or lymphoma of intrathoracic lymph nodes
200.28 Burkitt's tumor or lymphoma of lymph nodes of multiple sites
200.80 Other named variants, unspecified site, extranodal and solid organ sites ▽
200.82 Other named variants of lymphosarcoma and reticulosarcoma of intrathoracic lymph nodes
200.88 Other named variants of lymphosarcoma and reticulosarcoma of lymph nodes of multiple sites
201.00 Hodgkin's paragranuloma, unspecified site, extranodal and solid organ sites ▽
201.02 Hodgkin's paragranuloma of intrathoracic lymph nodes

201.08 Hodgkin's paragranuloma of lymph nodes of multiple sites
201.10 Hodgkin's granuloma, unspecified site, extranodal and solid organ sites ▽
201.12 Hodgkin's granuloma of intrathoracic lymph nodes
201.18 Hodgkin's granuloma of lymph nodes of multiple sites
201.20 Hodgkin's sarcoma, unspecified site, extranodal and solid organ sites ▽
201.22 Hodgkin's sarcoma of intrathoracic lymph nodes
201.28 Hodgkin's sarcoma of lymph nodes of multiple sites
201.40 Hodgkin's disease, lymphocytic-histiocytic predominance, unspecified site, extranodal and solid organ sites ▽
201.42 Hodgkin's disease, lymphocytic-histiocytic predominance of intrathoracic lymph nodes
201.48 Hodgkin's disease, lymphocytic-histiocytic predominance of lymph nodes of multiple sites
201.50 Hodgkin's disease, nodular sclerosis, unspecified site, extranodal and solid organ sites ▽
201.52 Hodgkin's disease, nodular sclerosis, of intrathoracic lymph nodes
201.58 Hodgkin's disease, nodular sclerosis, of lymph nodes of multiple sites
201.60 Hodgkin's disease, mixed cellularity, unspecified site, extranodal and solid organ sites ▽
201.62 Hodgkin's disease, mixed cellularity, of intrathoracic lymph nodes
201.68 Hodgkin's disease, mixed cellularity, of lymph nodes of multiple sites
201.70 Hodgkin's disease, lymphocytic depletion, unspecified site, extranodal and solid organ sites ▽
201.78 Hodgkin's disease, lymphocytic depletion, of lymph nodes of multiple sites
201.90 Hodgkin's disease, unspecified type, unspecified site, extranodal and solid organ sites ▽
201.92 Hodgkin's disease, unspecified type, of intrathoracic lymph nodes ▽
201.98 Hodgkin's disease, unspecified type, of lymph nodes of multiple sites ▽
202.00 Nodular lymphoma, unspecified site, extranodal and solid organ sites ▽
202.02 Nodular lymphoma of intrathoracic lymph nodes
202.08 Nodular lymphoma of lymph nodes of multiple sites
202.10 Mycosis fungoides, unspecified site, extranodal and solid organ sites ▽
202.12 Mycosis fungoides of intrathoracic lymph nodes
202.18 Mycosis fungoides of lymph nodes of multiple sites
202.20 Sezary's disease, unspecified site, extranodal and solid organ sites ▽
202.22 Sezary's disease of intrathoracic lymph nodes
202.28 Sezary's disease of lymph nodes of multiple sites
202.30 Malignant histiocytosis, unspecified site, extranodal and solid organ sites ▽
202.32 Malignant histiocytosis of intrathoracic lymph nodes
202.38 Malignant histiocytosis of lymph nodes of multiple sites
202.40 Leukemic reticuloendotheliosis, unspecified site, extranodal and solid organ sites ▽
202.42 Leukemic reticuloendotheliosis of intrathoracic lymph nodes
202.48 Leukemic reticuloendotheliosis of lymph nodes of multipes sites
202.50 Letterer-Siwe disease, unspecified site, extranodal and solid organ sites ▽
202.52 Letterer-Siwe disease of intrathoracic lymph nodes
202.58 Letterer-Siwe disease of lymph nodes of multiple sites
202.60 Malignant mast cell tumors, unspecified site, extranodal and solid organ sites ▽
202.62 Malignant mast cell tumors of intrathoracic lymph nodes
202.68 Malignant mast cell tumors of lymph nodes of multiple sites
202.80 Other malignant lymphomas, unspecified site, extranodal and solid organ sites ▽
202.82 Other malignant lymphomas of intrathoracic lymph nodes
202.88 Other malignant lymphomas of lymph nodes of multiple sites
202.90 Other and unspecified malignant neoplasms of lymphoid and histiocytic tissue, unspecified site, extranodal and solid organ sites ▽
202.92 Other and unspecified malignant neoplasms of lymphoid and histiocytic tissue of intrathoracic lymph nodes ▽
202.98 Other and unspecified malignant neoplasms of lymphoid and histiocytic tissue of lymph nodes of multiple sites ▽
212.2 Benign neoplasm of trachea
212.3 Benign neoplasm of bronchus and lung
212.4 Benign neoplasm of pleura
212.5 Benign neoplasm of mediastinum
212.6 Benign neoplasm of thymus
231.1 Carcinoma in situ of trachea
231.2 Carcinoma in situ of bronchus and lung
231.8 Carcinoma in situ of other specified parts of respiratory system
231.9 Carcinoma in situ of respiratory system, part unspecified ▽
235.7 Neoplasm of uncertain behavior of trachea, bronchus, and lung
235.8 Neoplasm of uncertain behavior of pleura, thymus, and mediastinum
235.9 Neoplasm of uncertain behavior of other and unspecified respiratory organs ▽
238.8 Neoplasm of uncertain behavior of other specified sites
239.1 Neoplasm of unspecified nature of respiratory system
239.8 Neoplasm of unspecified nature of other specified sites
254.8 Other specified diseases of thymus gland
496 Chronic airway obstruction, not elsewhere classified — (Note: This code is not to be used with any code from 491-493) ▽
519.2 Mediastinitis
519.3 Other diseases of mediastinum, not elsewhere classified
785.6 Enlargement of lymph nodes
786.50 Unspecified chest pain ▽
786.6 Swelling, mass, or lump in chest
793.2 Nonspecific abnormal findings on radiological and other examination of other intrathoracic organs

ICD-9-CM Procedural

34.22 Mediastinoscopy
34.25 Closed (percutaneous) (needle) biopsy of mediastinum
40.11 Biopsy of lymphatic structure

Diaphragm

39501

39501 Repair, laceration of diaphragm, any approach

ICD-9-CM Diagnostic

862.0 Diaphragm injury without mention of open wound into cavity
862.1 Diaphragm injury with open wound into cavity
998.2 Accidental puncture or laceration during procedure

ICD-9-CM Procedural

34.82 Suture of laceration of diaphragm
34.84 Other repair of diaphragm

39502

39502 Repair, paraesophageal hiatus hernia, transabdominal, with or without fundoplasty, vagotomy, and/or pyloroplasty, except neonatal

ICD-9-CM Diagnostic

551.3 Diaphragmatic hernia with gangrene
552.3 Diaphragmatic hernia with obstruction
553.3 Diaphragmatic hernia without mention of obstruction or gangrene
750.6 Congenital hiatus hernia

ICD-9-CM Procedural

44.00 Vagotomy, not otherwise specified
44.29 Other pyloroplasty
44.69 Other repair of stomach
53.7 Repair of diaphragmatic hernia, abdominal approach

39503

39503 Repair, neonatal diaphragmatic hernia, with or without chest tube insertion and with or without creation of ventral hernia

ICD-9-CM Diagnostic

756.6 Congenital anomaly of diaphragm

ICD-9-CM Procedural

53.80 Repair of diaphragmatic hernia with thoracic approach, not otherwise specified

39520–39531

39520 Repair, diaphragmatic hernia (esophageal hiatal); transthoracic
39530 combined, thoracoabdominal
39531 combined, thoracoabdominal, with dilation of stricture (with or without gastroplasty)

ICD-9-CM Diagnostic

551.3 Diaphragmatic hernia with gangrene
552.3 Diaphragmatic hernia with obstruction
553.3 Diaphragmatic hernia without mention of obstruction or gangrene

ICD-9-CM Procedural

44.69 Other repair of stomach
53.80 Repair of diaphragmatic hernia with thoracic approach, not otherwise specified

▽ Unspecified code ♀ Female diagnosis ☒ Manifestation code ♂ Male diagnosis

39540–39541

39540 Repair, diaphragmatic hernia (other than neonatal), traumatic; acute
39541 chronic

ICD-9-CM Diagnostic

551.3 Diaphragmatic hernia with gangrene
552.3 Diaphragmatic hernia with obstruction
553.3 Diaphragmatic hernia without mention of obstruction or gangrene
862.0 Diaphragm injury without mention of open wound into cavity

ICD-9-CM Procedural

53.7 Repair of diaphragmatic hernia, abdominal approach

39545

39545 Imbrication of diaphragm for eventration, transthoracic or transabdominal, paralytic or nonparalytic

ICD-9-CM Diagnostic

519.4 Disorders of diaphragm
551.3 Diaphragmatic hernia with gangrene
552.3 Diaphragmatic hernia with obstruction
553.3 Diaphragmatic hernia without mention of obstruction or gangrene
862.0 Diaphragm injury without mention of open wound into cavity

ICD-9-CM Procedural

34.84 Other repair of diaphragm
34.89 Other operations on diaphragm
53.9 Other hernia repair

39560–39561

39560 Resection, diaphragm; with simple repair (eg, primary suture)
39561 with complex repair (eg, prosthetic material, local muscle flap)

ICD-9-CM Diagnostic

171.4 Malignant neoplasm of connective and other soft tissue of thorax
198.89 Secondary malignant neoplasm of other specified sites
215.4 Other benign neoplasm of connective and other soft tissue of thorax
238.1 Neoplasm of uncertain behavior of connective and other soft tissue ▽
239.2 Neoplasms of unspecified nature of bone, soft tissue, and skin
519.4 Disorders of diaphragm
567.2 Other suppurative peritonitis
568.0 Peritoneal adhesions (postoperative) (postinfection)
568.89 Other specified disorder of peritoneum
756.6 Congenital anomaly of diaphragm
908.0 Late effect of internal injury to chest
998.31 Disruption of internal operation wound
998.4 Foreign body accidentally left during procedure, not elsewhere classified
998.51 Infected postoperative seroma — (Use additional code to identify organism)
998.59 Other postoperative infection — (Use additional code to identify infection)
998.6 Persistent postoperative fistula, not elsewhere classified
998.83 Non-healing surgical wound

ICD-9-CM Procedural

34.81 Excision of lesion or tissue of diaphragm
83.82 Graft of muscle or fascia

Digestive System

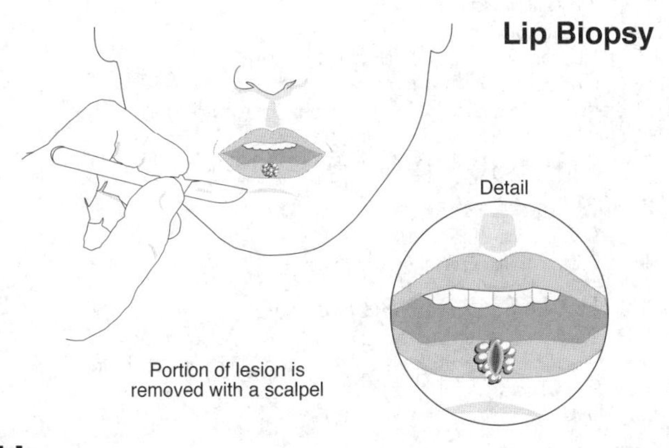

Lip Biopsy
Detail
Portion of lesion is removed with a scalpel

Lips

40490

40490	Biopsy of lip

ICD-9-CM Diagnostic

140.0	Malignant neoplasm of upper lip, vermilion border
140.1	Malignant neoplasm of lower lip, vermilion border
140.3	Malignant neoplasm of upper lip, inner aspect
140.4	Malignant neoplasm of lower lip, inner aspect
140.5	Malignant neoplasm of lip, inner aspect, unspecified as to upper or lower ▽
140.6	Malignant neoplasm of commissure of lip
140.8	Malignant neoplasm of other sites of lip
140.9	Malignant neoplasm of lip, vermilion border, unspecified as to upper or lower ▽
149.8	Malignant neoplasm of other sites within the lip and oral cavity
149.9	Malignant neoplasm of ill-defined sites of lip and oral cavity
172.0	Malignant melanoma of skin of lip
173.0	Other malignant neoplasm of skin of lip
195.0	Malignant neoplasm of head, face, and neck
198.2	Secondary malignant neoplasm of skin
198.89	Secondary malignant neoplasm of other specified sites
210.0	Benign neoplasm of lip
216.0	Benign neoplasm of skin of lip
230.0	Carcinoma in situ of lip, oral cavity, and pharynx
232.0	Carcinoma in situ of skin of lip
235.1	Neoplasm of uncertain behavior of lip, oral cavity, and pharynx
239.0	Neoplasm of unspecified nature of digestive system
239.2	Neoplasms of unspecified nature of bone, soft tissue, and skin
528.5	Diseases of lips
528.6	Leukoplakia of oral mucosa, including tongue
528.9	Other and unspecified diseases of the oral soft tissues ▽
692.79	Other dermatitis due to solar radiation
782.2	Localized superficial swelling, mass, or lump
784.2	Swelling, mass, or lump in head and neck
V10.02	Personal history of malignant neoplasm of other and unspecified parts of oral cavity and pharynx ▽
V84.09	Genetic susceptibility to other malignant neoplasm

ICD-9-CM Procedural

27.23	Biopsy of lip

HCPCS Level II Supplies & Services

A4305	Disposable drug delivery system, flow rate of 50 ml or greater per hour
A4306	Disposable drug delivery system, flow rate of 5 ml or less per hour
A4550	Surgical trays

40500

40500	Vermilionectomy (lip shave), with mucosal advancement

ICD-9-CM Diagnostic

140.0	Malignant neoplasm of upper lip, vermilion border
140.1	Malignant neoplasm of lower lip, vermilion border
140.3	Malignant neoplasm of upper lip, inner aspect
140.4	Malignant neoplasm of lower lip, inner aspect
140.5	Malignant neoplasm of lip, inner aspect, unspecified as to upper or lower ▽
140.6	Malignant neoplasm of commissure of lip
140.8	Malignant neoplasm of other sites of lip
140.9	Malignant neoplasm of lip, vermilion border, unspecified as to upper or lower ▽
172.0	Malignant melanoma of skin of lip
173.0	Other malignant neoplasm of skin of lip
210.0	Benign neoplasm of lip
216.0	Benign neoplasm of skin of lip
230.0	Carcinoma in situ of lip, oral cavity, and pharynx
528.5	Diseases of lips
528.6	Leukoplakia of oral mucosa, including tongue
528.9	Other and unspecified diseases of the oral soft tissues ▽
692.79	Other dermatitis due to solar radiation
709.2	Scar condition and fibrosis of skin
750.25	Congenital fistula of lip
750.9	Unspecified congenital anomaly of upper alimentary tract ▽
873.53	Open wound of lip, complicated — (Use additional code to identify infection)
906.0	Late effect of open wound of head, neck, and trunk
906.5	Late effect of burn of eye, face, head, and neck
908.9	Late effect of unspecified injury ▽
941.23	Blisters, with epidermal loss due to burn (second degree) of lip(s)
941.33	Full-thickness skin loss due to burn (third degree nos) of lip(s)
941.43	Deep necrosis of underlying tissues due to burn (deep third degree) of lip(s), without mention of loss of a body part
959.09	Injury of face and neck, other and unspecified
V50.1	Other plastic surgery for unacceptable cosmetic appearance
V51	Aftercare involving the use of plastic surgery
V84.09	Genetic susceptibility to other malignant neoplasm

ICD-9-CM Procedural

27.43	Other excision of lesion or tissue of lip

HCPCS Level II Supplies & Services

A4305	Disposable drug delivery system, flow rate of 50 ml or greater per hour
A4306	Disposable drug delivery system, flow rate of 5 ml or less per hour
A4550	Surgical trays

40510–40520

40510	Excision of lip; transverse wedge excision with primary closure
40520	V-excision with primary direct linear closure

ICD-9-CM Diagnostic

140.0	Malignant neoplasm of upper lip, vermilion border
140.1	Malignant neoplasm of lower lip, vermilion border
140.3	Malignant neoplasm of upper lip, inner aspect
140.4	Malignant neoplasm of lower lip, inner aspect
140.5	Malignant neoplasm of lip, inner aspect, unspecified as to upper or lower ▽
140.6	Malignant neoplasm of commissure of lip
140.8	Malignant neoplasm of other sites of lip
140.9	Malignant neoplasm of lip, vermilion border, unspecified as to upper or lower ▽
172.0	Malignant melanoma of skin of lip
173.0	Other malignant neoplasm of skin of lip
195.0	Malignant neoplasm of head, face, and neck
199.1	Other malignant neoplasm of unspecified site
210.0	Benign neoplasm of lip
214.0	Lipoma of skin and subcutaneous tissue of face

215.0 Other benign neoplasm of connective and other soft tissue of head, face, and neck
216.0 Benign neoplasm of skin of lip
228.00 Hemangioma of unspecified site ▽
230.0 Carcinoma in situ of lip, oral cavity, and pharynx
232.0 Carcinoma in situ of skin of lip
235.1 Neoplasm of uncertain behavior of lip, oral cavity, and pharynx
239.2 Neoplasms of unspecified nature of bone, soft tissue, and skin
528.5 Diseases of lips
692.79 Other dermatitis due to solar radiation
701.5 Other abnormal granulation tissue
709.2 Scar condition and fibrosis of skin
925.1 Crushing injury of face and scalp — (Use additional code to identify any associated injuries: 800-829, 850.0-854.1, 860.0-869.1)
V51 Aftercare involving the use of plastic surgery
V84.09 Genetic susceptibility to other malignant neoplasm

ICD-9-CM Procedural

27.42 Wide excision of lesion of lip
27.43 Other excision of lesion or tissue of lip

HCPCS Level II Supplies & Services

A4305 Disposable drug delivery system, flow rate of 50 ml or greater per hour
A4306 Disposable drug delivery system, flow rate of 5 ml or less per hour
A4550 Surgical trays

40525–40527

40525 Excision of lip; full thickness, reconstruction with local flap (eg, Estlander or fan)
40527 full thickness, reconstruction with cross lip flap (Abbe-Estlander)

ICD-9-CM Diagnostic

140.0 Malignant neoplasm of upper lip, vermilion border
140.1 Malignant neoplasm of lower lip, vermilion border
140.3 Malignant neoplasm of upper lip, inner aspect
140.4 Malignant neoplasm of lower lip, inner aspect
140.5 Malignant neoplasm of lip, inner aspect, unspecified as to upper or lower ▽
140.6 Malignant neoplasm of commissure of lip
140.8 Malignant neoplasm of other sites of lip
140.9 Malignant neoplasm of lip, vermilion border, unspecified as to upper or lower ▽
172.0 Malignant melanoma of skin of lip
173.0 Other malignant neoplasm of skin of lip
195.0 Malignant neoplasm of head, face, and neck
199.1 Other malignant neoplasm of unspecified site
210.0 Benign neoplasm of lip
216.0 Benign neoplasm of skin of lip
228.00 Hemangioma of unspecified site ▽
230.0 Carcinoma in situ of lip, oral cavity, and pharynx
232.0 Carcinoma in situ of skin of lip
235.1 Neoplasm of uncertain behavior of lip, oral cavity, and pharynx
528.5 Diseases of lips
925.1 Crushing injury of face and scalp — (Use additional code to identify any associated injuries: 800-829, 850.0-854.1, 860.0-869.1)
V84.09 Genetic susceptibility to other malignant neoplasm

ICD-9-CM Procedural

27.42 Wide excision of lesion of lip
27.43 Other excision of lesion or tissue of lip
27.55 Full-thickness skin graft to lip and mouth
27.57 Attachment of pedicle or flap graft to lip and mouth

HCPCS Level II Supplies & Services

A4305 Disposable drug delivery system, flow rate of 50 ml or greater per hour
A4306 Disposable drug delivery system, flow rate of 5 ml or less per hour
A4550 Surgical trays

40530

40530 Resection of lip, more than one-fourth, without reconstruction

ICD-9-CM Diagnostic

140.0 Malignant neoplasm of upper lip, vermilion border
140.1 Malignant neoplasm of lower lip, vermilion border
140.3 Malignant neoplasm of upper lip, inner aspect
140.4 Malignant neoplasm of lower lip, inner aspect
140.5 Malignant neoplasm of lip, inner aspect, unspecified as to upper or lower ▽
140.6 Malignant neoplasm of commissure of lip
140.8 Malignant neoplasm of other sites of lip
140.9 Malignant neoplasm of lip, vermilion border, unspecified as to upper or lower ▽
171.0 Malignant neoplasm of connective and other soft tissue of head, face, and neck
172.0 Malignant melanoma of skin of lip
173.0 Other malignant neoplasm of skin of lip
195.0 Malignant neoplasm of head, face, and neck
199.1 Other malignant neoplasm of unspecified site
210.0 Benign neoplasm of lip
216.0 Benign neoplasm of skin of lip
230.0 Carcinoma in situ of lip, oral cavity, and pharynx
232.0 Carcinoma in situ of skin of lip
235.1 Neoplasm of uncertain behavior of lip, oral cavity, and pharynx
528.5 Diseases of lips
V84.09 Genetic susceptibility to other malignant neoplasm

ICD-9-CM Procedural

27.42 Wide excision of lesion of lip
27.43 Other excision of lesion or tissue of lip

HCPCS Level II Supplies & Services

A4305 Disposable drug delivery system, flow rate of 50 ml or greater per hour
A4306 Disposable drug delivery system, flow rate of 5 ml or less per hour
A4550 Surgical trays

40650–40654

40650 Repair lip, full thickness; vermilion only
40652 up to half vertical height
40654 over one-half vertical height, or complex

ICD-9-CM Diagnostic

140.0 Malignant neoplasm of upper lip, vermilion border
140.1 Malignant neoplasm of lower lip, vermilion border
140.3 Malignant neoplasm of upper lip, inner aspect
140.4 Malignant neoplasm of lower lip, inner aspect
140.9 Malignant neoplasm of lip, vermilion border, unspecified as to upper or lower ▽
172.0 Malignant melanoma of skin of lip
173.0 Other malignant neoplasm of skin of lip
195.0 Malignant neoplasm of head, face, and neck
210.0 Benign neoplasm of lip
216.0 Benign neoplasm of skin of lip
228.00 Hemangioma of unspecified site ▽
232.0 Carcinoma in situ of skin of lip
528.5 Diseases of lips
709.2 Scar condition and fibrosis of skin
744.82 Microcheilia
873.40 Open wound of face, unspecified site, without mention of complication — (Use additional code to identify infection) ▽
873.43 Open wound of lip, without mention of complication — (Use additional code to identify infection)
873.50 Open wound of face, unspecified site, complicated — (Use additional code to identify infection) ▽
873.53 Open wound of lip, complicated — (Use additional code to identify infection)
873.59 Open wound of face, other and multiple sites, complicated — (Use additional code to identify infection)
906.0 Late effect of open wound of head, neck, and trunk
925.1 Crushing injury of face and scalp — (Use additional code to identify any associated injuries: 800-829, 850.0-854.1, 860.0-869.1)
941.23 Blisters, with epidermal loss due to burn (second degree) of lip(s)
959.09 Injury of face and neck, other and unspecified
998.32 Disruption of external operation wound
V51 Aftercare involving the use of plastic surgery
V84.09 Genetic susceptibility to other malignant neoplasm

ICD-9-CM Procedural

27.51 Suture of laceration of lip
27.59 Other plastic repair of mouth

HCPCS Level II Supplies & Services

A4305 Disposable drug delivery system, flow rate of 50 ml or greater per hour
A4306 Disposable drug delivery system, flow rate of 5 ml or less per hour
A4550 Surgical trays

▽ Unspecified code ♀ Female diagnosis ☒ Manifestation code ♂ Male diagnosis

40700

40700 Plastic repair of cleft lip/nasal deformity; primary, partial or complete, unilateral

ICD-9-CM Diagnostic

749.10 Unspecified cleft lip ▽
749.11 Unilateral cleft lip, complete
749.12 Unilateral cleft lip, incomplete
749.20 Unspecified cleft palate with cleft lip ▽
749.21 Unilateral cleft palate with cleft lip, complete
749.22 Unilateral cleft palate with cleft lip, incomplete
V13.69 Personal history of other congenital malformations

ICD-9-CM Procedural

27.54 Repair of cleft lip

40701–40702

40701 Plastic repair of cleft lip/nasal deformity; primary bilateral, one stage procedure
40702 primary bilateral, one of two stages

ICD-9-CM Diagnostic

749.13 Bilateral cleft lip, complete
749.14 Bilateral cleft lip, incomplete
749.23 Bilateral cleft palate with cleft lip, complete
749.24 Bilateral cleft palate with cleft lip, incomplete
749.25 Other combinations of cleft palate with cleft lip
V13.69 Personal history of other congenital malformations

ICD-9-CM Procedural

27.54 Repair of cleft lip

40720

40720 Plastic repair of cleft lip/nasal deformity; secondary, by recreation of defect and reclosure

ICD-9-CM Diagnostic

749.10 Unspecified cleft lip ▽
749.11 Unilateral cleft lip, complete
749.12 Unilateral cleft lip, incomplete
749.13 Bilateral cleft lip, complete
749.14 Bilateral cleft lip, incomplete
749.20 Unspecified cleft palate with cleft lip ▽
749.21 Unilateral cleft palate with cleft lip, complete
749.22 Unilateral cleft palate with cleft lip, incomplete
749.23 Bilateral cleft palate with cleft lip, complete
749.25 Other combinations of cleft palate with cleft lip
V13.69 Personal history of other congenital malformations

ICD-9-CM Procedural

27.54 Repair of cleft lip

40761

40761 Plastic repair of cleft lip/nasal deformity; with cross lip pedicle flap (Abbe-Estlander type), including sectioning and inserting of pedicle

ICD-9-CM Diagnostic

749.10 Unspecified cleft lip ▽
749.11 Unilateral cleft lip, complete
749.12 Unilateral cleft lip, incomplete
749.13 Bilateral cleft lip, complete
749.14 Bilateral cleft lip, incomplete
749.20 Unspecified cleft palate with cleft lip ▽
749.21 Unilateral cleft palate with cleft lip, complete
749.22 Unilateral cleft palate with cleft lip, incomplete
749.23 Bilateral cleft palate with cleft lip, complete
749.25 Other combinations of cleft palate with cleft lip
V13.69 Personal history of other congenital malformations

ICD-9-CM Procedural

27.54 Repair of cleft lip
27.57 Attachment of pedicle or flap graft to lip and mouth

Vestibule of Mouth

40800–40801

40800 Drainage of abscess, cyst, hematoma, vestibule of mouth; simple
40801 complicated

ICD-9-CM Diagnostic

478.24 Retropharyngeal abscess
520.6 Disturbances in tooth eruption
522.0 Pulpitis
522.5 Periapical abscess without sinus
523.3 Acute periodontitis
526.0 Developmental odontogenic cysts
526.1 Fissural cysts of jaw
528.3 Cellulitis and abscess of oral soft tissues
528.4 Cysts of oral soft tissues
567.2 Other suppurative peritonitis
682.0 Cellulitis and abscess of face — (Use additional code to identify organism)
780.6 Fever
782.2 Localized superficial swelling, mass, or lump
784.2 Swelling, mass, or lump in head and neck

ICD-9-CM Procedural

27.0 Drainage of face and floor of mouth

HCPCS Level II Supplies & Services

A4305 Disposable drug delivery system, flow rate of 50 ml or greater per hour
A4306 Disposable drug delivery system, flow rate of 5 ml or less per hour
A4550 Surgical trays

40804–40805

40804 Removal of embedded foreign body, vestibule of mouth; simple
40805 complicated

ICD-9-CM Diagnostic

709.4 Foreign body granuloma of skin and subcutaneous tissue
728.82 Foreign body granuloma of muscle
784.2 Swelling, mass, or lump in head and neck
873.70 Open wound of mouth, unspecified site, complicated — (Use additional code to identify infection) ▽
873.71 Open wound of buccal mucosa, complicated — (Use additional code to identify infection)
873.72 Open wound of gum (alveolar process), complicated — (Use additional code to identify infection)
873.74 Open wound of tongue and floor of mouth, complicated — (Use additional code to identify infection)
873.75 Open wound of palate, complicated — (Use additional code to identify infection)
873.79 Open wound of mouth, other and multiple sites, complicated — (Use additional code to identify infection)
935.0 Foreign body in mouth

ICD-9-CM Procedural

27.92 Incision of mouth, unspecified structure
98.01 Removal of intraluminal foreign body from mouth without incision

HCPCS Level II Supplies & Services

A4305 Disposable drug delivery system, flow rate of 50 ml or greater per hour
A4306 Disposable drug delivery system, flow rate of 5 ml or less per hour
A4550 Surgical trays

40806

40806 Incision of labial frenum (frenotomy)

ICD-9-CM Diagnostic

520.8 Other specified disorders of tooth development and eruption
523.20 Gingival recession, unspecified
523.21 Gingival recession, minimal
523.22 Gingival recession, moderate
523.23 Gingival recession, severe
523.24 Gingival recession, localized
523.25 Gingival recession, generalized
524.01 Maxillary hyperplasia
524.02 Mandibular hyperplasia

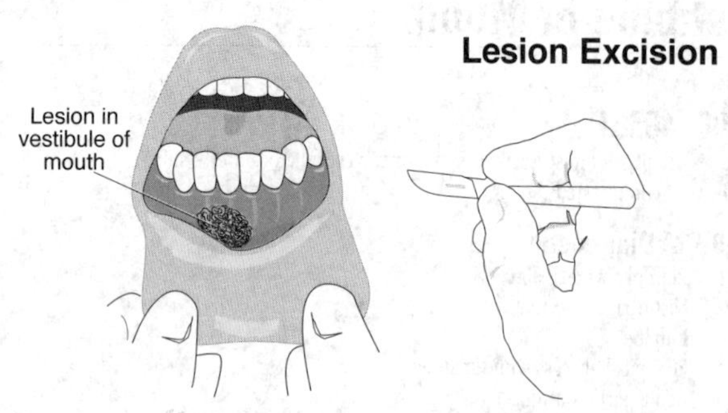

524.04 Mandibular hypoplasia
524.09 Other specified major anomaly of jaw size
524.12 Other jaw asymmetry
524.39 Other anomalies of tooth position
524.71 Alveolar maxillary hyperplasia
524.72 Alveolar mandibular hyperplasia
524.74 Alveolar mandibular hypoplasia
525.20 Unspecified atrophy of edentulous alveolar ridge
528.79 Other disturbances of oral epithelium, including tongue
744.9 Unspecified congenital anomaly of face and neck ▽
756.82 Accessory muscle

ICD-9-CM Procedural
27.91 Labial frenotomy

HCPCS Level II Supplies & Services
A4550 Surgical trays

40808
40808 Biopsy, vestibule of mouth

ICD-9-CM Diagnostic
140.3 Malignant neoplasm of upper lip, inner aspect
140.4 Malignant neoplasm of lower lip, inner aspect
140.5 Malignant neoplasm of lip, inner aspect, unspecified as to upper or lower ▽
140.6 Malignant neoplasm of commissure of lip
140.8 Malignant neoplasm of other sites of lip
140.9 Malignant neoplasm of lip, vermilion border, unspecified as to upper or lower ▽
144.8 Malignant neoplasm of other sites of floor of mouth
144.9 Malignant neoplasm of floor of mouth, part unspecified ▽
145.1 Malignant neoplasm of vestibule of mouth
145.8 Malignant neoplasm of other specified parts of mouth
145.9 Malignant neoplasm of mouth, unspecified site ▽
198.89 Secondary malignant neoplasm of other specified sites
210.4 Benign neoplasm of other and unspecified parts of mouth ▽
230.0 Carcinoma in situ of lip, oral cavity, and pharynx
235.1 Neoplasm of uncertain behavior of lip, oral cavity, and pharynx
239.0 Neoplasm of unspecified nature of digestive system
239.9 Neoplasm of unspecified nature, site unspecified ▽
522.8 Radicular cyst of dental pulp
528.0 Stomatitis
528.3 Cellulitis and abscess of oral soft tissues
528.6 Leukoplakia of oral mucosa, including tongue
528.79 Other disturbances of oral epithelium, including tongue
528.8 Oral submucosal fibrosis, including of tongue
528.9 Other and unspecified diseases of the oral soft tissues ▽
697.0 Lichen planus

ICD-9-CM Procedural
27.24 Biopsy of mouth, unspecified structure

HCPCS Level II Supplies & Services
A4550 Surgical trays

40810–40812
40810 Excision of lesion of mucosa and submucosa, vestibule of mouth; without repair
40812 with simple repair

ICD-9-CM Diagnostic
144.9 Malignant neoplasm of floor of mouth, part unspecified ▽
145.0 Malignant neoplasm of cheek mucosa
145.1 Malignant neoplasm of vestibule of mouth
145.8 Malignant neoplasm of other specified parts of mouth
145.9 Malignant neoplasm of mouth, unspecified site ▽
171.0 Malignant neoplasm of connective and other soft tissue of head, face, and neck
199.1 Other malignant neoplasm of unspecified site
210.0 Benign neoplasm of lip
214.8 Lipoma of other specified sites
214.9 Lipoma of unspecified site ▽
215.0 Other benign neoplasm of connective and other soft tissue of head, face, and neck
230.0 Carcinoma in situ of lip, oral cavity, and pharynx
235.1 Neoplasm of uncertain behavior of lip, oral cavity, and pharynx
239.0 Neoplasm of unspecified nature of digestive system
239.9 Neoplasm of unspecified nature, site unspecified ▽
527.6 Mucocele of salivary gland
528.4 Cysts of oral soft tissues
528.5 Diseases of lips
528.6 Leukoplakia of oral mucosa, including tongue
528.71 Minimal keratinized residual ridge mucosa
528.72 Excessive keratinized residual ridge mucosa
528.79 Other disturbances of oral epithelium, including tongue
528.8 Oral submucosal fibrosis, including of tongue
528.9 Other and unspecified diseases of the oral soft tissues ▽
682.0 Cellulitis and abscess of face — (Use additional code to identify organism)
697.0 Lichen planus
701.1 Acquired keratoderma
706.2 Sebaceous cyst
782.2 Localized superficial swelling, mass, or lump
784.2 Swelling, mass, or lump in head and neck

ICD-9-CM Procedural
27.49 Other excision of mouth

HCPCS Level II Supplies & Services
A4550 Surgical trays

40814–40816
40814 Excision of lesion of mucosa and submucosa, vestibule of mouth; with complex repair
40816 complex, with excision of underlying muscle

ICD-9-CM Diagnostic
140.4 Malignant neoplasm of lower lip, inner aspect
140.5 Malignant neoplasm of lip, inner aspect, unspecified as to upper or lower ▽
144.9 Malignant neoplasm of floor of mouth, part unspecified ▽
145.0 Malignant neoplasm of cheek mucosa
145.1 Malignant neoplasm of vestibule of mouth
145.8 Malignant neoplasm of other specified parts of mouth
145.9 Malignant neoplasm of mouth, unspecified site ▽
171.0 Malignant neoplasm of connective and other soft tissue of head, face, and neck
210.4 Benign neoplasm of other and unspecified parts of mouth ▽
214.8 Lipoma of other specified sites
215.0 Other benign neoplasm of connective and other soft tissue of head, face, and neck
230.0 Carcinoma in situ of lip, oral cavity, and pharynx
235.1 Neoplasm of uncertain behavior of lip, oral cavity, and pharynx
527.6 Mucocele of salivary gland
528.4 Cysts of oral soft tissues
528.6 Leukoplakia of oral mucosa, including tongue
528.71 Minimal keratinized residual ridge mucosa
528.72 Excessive keratinized residual ridge mucosa
528.79 Other disturbances of oral epithelium, including tongue
528.8 Oral submucosal fibrosis, including of tongue
528.9 Other and unspecified diseases of the oral soft tissues ▽
784.2 Swelling, mass, or lump in head and neck

ICD-9-CM Procedural
27.49 Other excision of mouth

▽ Unspecified code
♀ Female diagnosis
☒ Manifestation code
♂ Male diagnosis

83.32 Excision of lesion of muscle

HCPCS Level II Supplies & Services

A4305 Disposable drug delivery system, flow rate of 50 ml or greater per hour
A4306 Disposable drug delivery system, flow rate of 5 ml or less per hour
A4550 Surgical trays

40818

40818 Excision of mucosa of vestibule of mouth as donor graft

ICD-9-CM Diagnostic

140.8 Malignant neoplasm of other sites of lip
145.1 Malignant neoplasm of vestibule of mouth
210.3 Benign neoplasm of floor of mouth
230.0 Carcinoma in situ of lip, oral cavity, and pharynx
523.8 Other specified periodontal diseases
525.20 Unspecified atrophy of edentulous alveolar ridge
528.6 Leukoplakia of oral mucosa, including tongue
V10.02 Personal history of malignant neoplasm of other and unspecified parts of oral cavity and pharynx ▽
V51 Aftercare involving the use of plastic surgery

ICD-9-CM Procedural

86.69 Other skin graft to other sites

40819

40819 Excision of frenum, labial or buccal (frenumectomy, frenulectomy, frenectomy)

ICD-9-CM Diagnostic

140.3 Malignant neoplasm of upper lip, inner aspect
140.4 Malignant neoplasm of lower lip, inner aspect
140.5 Malignant neoplasm of lip, inner aspect, unspecified as to upper or lower ▽
140.8 Malignant neoplasm of other sites of lip
210.0 Benign neoplasm of lip
239.0 Neoplasm of unspecified nature of digestive system
520.8 Other specified disorders of tooth development and eruption
523.8 Other specified periodontal diseases
525.20 Unspecified atrophy of edentulous alveolar ridge
528.5 Diseases of lips
744.9 Unspecified congenital anomaly of face and neck ▽
750.26 Other specified congenital anomalies of mouth
750.8 Other specified congenital anomalies of upper alimentary tract
756.82 Accessory muscle

ICD-9-CM Procedural

27.41 Labial frenectomy

HCPCS Level II Supplies & Services

A4305 Disposable drug delivery system, flow rate of 50 ml or greater per hour
A4306 Disposable drug delivery system, flow rate of 5 ml or less per hour
A4550 Surgical trays

40820

40820 Destruction of lesion or scar of vestibule of mouth by physical methods (eg, laser, thermal, cryo, chemical)

ICD-9-CM Diagnostic

145.0 Malignant neoplasm of cheek mucosa
210.0 Benign neoplasm of lip
210.3 Benign neoplasm of floor of mouth
210.4 Benign neoplasm of other and unspecified parts of mouth ▽
228.09 Hemangioma of other sites
230.0 Carcinoma in situ of lip, oral cavity, and pharynx
235.1 Neoplasm of uncertain behavior of lip, oral cavity, and pharynx
239.0 Neoplasm of unspecified nature of digestive system
239.2 Neoplasms of unspecified nature of bone, soft tissue, and skin
528.2 Oral aphthae
528.4 Cysts of oral soft tissues
528.6 Leukoplakia of oral mucosa, including tongue
528.79 Other disturbances of oral epithelium, including tongue
528.8 Oral submucosal fibrosis, including of tongue
528.9 Other and unspecified diseases of the oral soft tissues ▽
709.2 Scar condition and fibrosis of skin
784.2 Swelling, mass, or lump in head and neck

ICD-9-CM Procedural

27.49 Other excision of mouth
27.99 Other operations on oral cavity

HCPCS Level II Supplies & Services

A4305 Disposable drug delivery system, flow rate of 50 ml or greater per hour
A4306 Disposable drug delivery system, flow rate of 5 ml or less per hour
A4550 Surgical trays

40830–40831

40830 Closure of laceration, vestibule of mouth; 2.5 cm or less
40831 over 2.5 cm or complex

ICD-9-CM Diagnostic

873.43 Open wound of lip, without mention of complication — (Use additional code to identify infection)
873.49 Open wound of face, other and multiple sites, without mention of complication — (Use additional code to identify infection)
873.53 Open wound of lip, complicated — (Use additional code to identify infection)
873.59 Open wound of face, other and multiple sites, complicated — (Use additional code to identify infection)
873.60 Open wound of mouth, unspecified site, without mention of complication — (Use additional code to identify infection) ▽
873.61 Open wound of buccal mucosa, without mention of complication — (Use additional code to identify infection)
873.62 Open wound of gum (alveolar process), without mention of complication — (Use additional code to identify infection)
873.64 Open wound of tongue and floor of mouth, without mention of complication — (Use additional code to identify infection)
873.65 Open wound of palate, without mention of complication — (Use additional code to identify infection)
873.69 Open wound of mouth, other and multiple sites, without mention of complication — (Use additional code to identify infection)
873.70 Open wound of mouth, unspecified site, complicated — (Use additional code to identify infection) ▽
873.71 Open wound of buccal mucosa, complicated — (Use additional code to identify infection)
873.72 Open wound of gum (alveolar process), complicated — (Use additional code to identify infection)
873.74 Open wound of tongue and floor of mouth, complicated — (Use additional code to identify infection)
873.75 Open wound of palate, complicated — (Use additional code to identify infection)
873.79 Open wound of mouth, other and multiple sites, complicated — (Use additional code to identify infection)
873.8 Other and unspecified open wound of head without mention of complication — (Use additional code to identify infection) ▽
873.9 Other and unspecified open wound of head, complicated — (Use additional code to identify infection) ▽
959.09 Injury of face and neck, other and unspecified

ICD-9-CM Procedural

27.52 Suture of laceration of other part of mouth

HCPCS Level II Supplies & Services

A4550 Surgical trays

40840–40844

40840 Vestibuloplasty; anterior
40842 posterior, unilateral
40843 posterior, bilateral
40844 entire arch

ICD-9-CM Diagnostic

386.12 Vestibular neuronitis
525.10 Unspecified acquired absence of teeth ▽
525.11 Loss of teeth due to trauma
525.12 Loss of teeth due to periodontal disease
525.13 Loss of teeth due to caries
525.19 Other loss of teeth
525.20 Unspecified atrophy of edentulous alveolar ridge
525.8 Other specified disorders of the teeth and supporting structures
528.9 Other and unspecified diseases of the oral soft tissues ▽
733.7 Algoneurodystrophy
750.26 Other specified congenital anomalies of mouth

873.59 Open wound of face, other and multiple sites, complicated — (Use additional code to identify infection)
905.0 Late effect of fracture of skull and face bones
906.0 Late effect of open wound of head, neck, and trunk
906.5 Late effect of burn of eye, face, head, and neck
908.9 Late effect of unspecified injury ▽
909.3 Late effect of complications of surgical and medical care
925.1 Crushing injury of face and scalp — (Use additional code to identify any associated injuries: 800-829, 850.0-854.1, 860.0-869.1)
947.0 Burn of mouth and pharynx
959.09 Injury of face and neck, other and unspecified
959.9 Injury, other and unspecified, unspecified site ▽
V41.6 Problems with swallowing and mastication — (This code is intended for use when these conditions are recorded as diagnoses or problems)

ICD-9-CM Procedural
24.91 Extension or deepening of buccolabial or lingual sulcus

HCPCS Level II Supplies & Services
A4305 Disposable drug delivery system, flow rate of 50 ml or greater per hour
A4306 Disposable drug delivery system, flow rate of 5 ml or less per hour
A4550 Surgical trays

40845
40845 Vestibuloplasty; complex (including ridge extension, muscle repositioning)

ICD-9-CM Diagnostic
230.0 Carcinoma in situ of lip, oral cavity, and pharynx
525.10 Unspecified acquired absence of teeth ▽
525.11 Loss of teeth due to trauma
525.12 Loss of teeth due to periodontal disease
525.13 Loss of teeth due to caries
525.19 Other loss of teeth
525.20 Unspecified atrophy of edentulous alveolar ridge
905.0 Late effect of fracture of skull and face bones
906.0 Late effect of open wound of head, neck, and trunk
906.8 Late effect of burns of other specified sites
947.0 Burn of mouth and pharynx
V10.02 Personal history of malignant neoplasm of other and unspecified parts of oral cavity and pharynx ▽
V41.6 Problems with swallowing and mastication — (This code is intended for use when these conditions are recorded as diagnoses or problems)
V50.1 Other plastic surgery for unacceptable cosmetic appearance
V51 Aftercare involving the use of plastic surgery

ICD-9-CM Procedural
24.91 Extension or deepening of buccolabial or lingual sulcus

Tongue and Floor of Mouth

41000
41000 Intraoral incision and drainage of abscess, cyst, or hematoma of tongue or floor of mouth; lingual

ICD-9-CM Diagnostic
528.3 Cellulitis and abscess of oral soft tissues
528.4 Cysts of oral soft tissues
529.0 Glossitis
529.6 Glossodynia
529.8 Other specified conditions of the tongue
750.19 Other congenital anomaly of tongue
780.6 Fever
784.2 Swelling, mass, or lump in head and neck
920 Contusion of face, scalp, and neck except eye(s)
958.3 Posttraumatic wound infection not elsewhere classified
998.12 Hematoma complicating a procedure
998.59 Other postoperative infection — (Use additional code to identify infection)

ICD-9-CM Procedural
25.94 Other glossotomy
27.0 Drainage of face and floor of mouth

HCPCS Level II Supplies & Services
A4305 Disposable drug delivery system, flow rate of 50 ml or greater per hour

Tongue and Oral Cavity

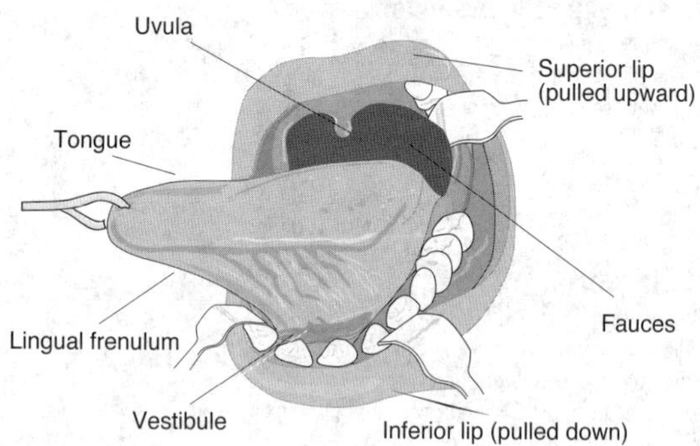

A4306 Disposable drug delivery system, flow rate of 5 ml or less per hour
A4550 Surgical trays

41005–41007
41005 Intraoral incision and drainage of abscess, cyst, or hematoma of tongue or floor of mouth; sublingual, superficial
41006 sublingual, deep, supramylohyoid
41007 submental space

ICD-9-CM Diagnostic
523.3 Acute periodontitis
526.0 Developmental odontogenic cysts
526.4 Inflammatory conditions of jaw
527.3 Abscess of salivary gland
527.6 Mucocele of salivary gland
528.3 Cellulitis and abscess of oral soft tissues
528.4 Cysts of oral soft tissues
529.0 Glossitis
529.6 Glossodynia
529.8 Other specified conditions of the tongue
750.19 Other congenital anomaly of tongue
750.26 Other specified congenital anomalies of mouth
780.6 Fever
784.2 Swelling, mass, or lump in head and neck
920 Contusion of face, scalp, and neck except eye(s)
958.3 Posttraumatic wound infection not elsewhere classified
998.12 Hematoma complicating a procedure
998.59 Other postoperative infection — (Use additional code to identify infection)

ICD-9-CM Procedural
25.94 Other glossotomy
27.0 Drainage of face and floor of mouth

HCPCS Level II Supplies & Services
A4305 Disposable drug delivery system, flow rate of 50 ml or greater per hour
A4306 Disposable drug delivery system, flow rate of 5 ml or less per hour
A4550 Surgical trays

41008
41008 Intraoral incision and drainage of abscess, cyst, or hematoma of tongue or floor of mouth; submandibular space

ICD-9-CM Diagnostic
526.4 Inflammatory conditions of jaw
528.3 Cellulitis and abscess of oral soft tissues
528.4 Cysts of oral soft tissues
528.9 Other and unspecified diseases of the oral soft tissues ▽
529.6 Glossodynia
529.8 Other specified conditions of the tongue
682.0 Cellulitis and abscess of face — (Use additional code to identify organism)
750.19 Other congenital anomaly of tongue
750.26 Other specified congenital anomalies of mouth
780.6 Fever
784.2 Swelling, mass, or lump in head and neck
920 Contusion of face, scalp, and neck except eye(s)
958.3 Posttraumatic wound infection not elsewhere classified
998.12 Hematoma complicating a procedure
998.59 Other postoperative infection — (Use additional code to identify infection)

▽ Unspecified code ♀ Female diagnosis ☒ Manifestation code ♂ Male diagnosis

ICD-9-CM Procedural
25.94 Other glossotomy
27.0 Drainage of face and floor of mouth

HCPCS Level II Supplies & Services
A4305 Disposable drug delivery system, flow rate of 50 ml or greater per hour
A4306 Disposable drug delivery system, flow rate of 5 ml or less per hour
A4550 Surgical trays

41009
41009 Intraoral incision and drainage of abscess, cyst, or hematoma of tongue or floor of mouth; masticator space

ICD-9-CM Diagnostic
522.5 Periapical abscess without sinus
522.7 Periapical abscess with sinus
523.3 Acute periodontitis
528.3 Cellulitis and abscess of oral soft tissues
528.4 Cysts of oral soft tissues
528.9 Other and unspecified diseases of the oral soft tissues ▽
529.6 Glossodynia
529.8 Other specified conditions of the tongue
682.0 Cellulitis and abscess of face — (Use additional code to identify organism)
750.26 Other specified congenital anomalies of mouth
784.2 Swelling, mass, or lump in head and neck
920 Contusion of face, scalp, and neck except eye(s)
958.3 Posttraumatic wound infection not elsewhere classified
998.12 Hematoma complicating a procedure
998.59 Other postoperative infection — (Use additional code to identify infection)

ICD-9-CM Procedural
25.94 Other glossotomy
27.0 Drainage of face and floor of mouth

HCPCS Level II Supplies & Services
A4305 Disposable drug delivery system, flow rate of 50 ml or greater per hour
A4306 Disposable drug delivery system, flow rate of 5 ml or less per hour
A4550 Surgical trays

41010
41010 Incision of lingual frenum (frenotomy)

ICD-9-CM Diagnostic
524.02 Mandibular hyperplasia
524.74 Alveolar mandibular hypoplasia
750.0 Tongue tie
750.12 Congenital adhesions of tongue

ICD-9-CM Procedural
25.91 Lingual frenotomy

HCPCS Level II Supplies & Services
A4550 Surgical trays

41015–41016
41015 Extraoral incision and drainage of abscess, cyst, or hematoma of floor of mouth; sublingual
41016 submental

ICD-9-CM Diagnostic
526.4 Inflammatory conditions of jaw
528.3 Cellulitis and abscess of oral soft tissues
528.4 Cysts of oral soft tissues
529.0 Glossitis
529.6 Glossodynia
529.8 Other specified conditions of the tongue
682.0 Cellulitis and abscess of face — (Use additional code to identify organism)
750.26 Other specified congenital anomalies of mouth
780.6 Fever
784.2 Swelling, mass, or lump in head and neck
920 Contusion of face, scalp, and neck except eye(s)
958.3 Posttraumatic wound infection not elsewhere classified
998.12 Hematoma complicating a procedure
998.59 Other postoperative infection — (Use additional code to identify infection)

ICD-9-CM Procedural
27.0 Drainage of face and floor of mouth

HCPCS Level II Supplies & Services
A4305 Disposable drug delivery system, flow rate of 50 ml or greater per hour
A4306 Disposable drug delivery system, flow rate of 5 ml or less per hour
A4550 Surgical trays

41017
41017 Extraoral incision and drainage of abscess, cyst, or hematoma of floor of mouth; submandibular

ICD-9-CM Diagnostic
526.4 Inflammatory conditions of jaw
528.3 Cellulitis and abscess of oral soft tissues
528.4 Cysts of oral soft tissues
528.9 Other and unspecified diseases of the oral soft tissues ▽
682.0 Cellulitis and abscess of face — (Use additional code to identify organism)
750.26 Other specified congenital anomalies of mouth
780.6 Fever
784.2 Swelling, mass, or lump in head and neck
920 Contusion of face, scalp, and neck except eye(s)
958.3 Posttraumatic wound infection not elsewhere classified
998.12 Hematoma complicating a procedure
998.59 Other postoperative infection — (Use additional code to identify infection)

ICD-9-CM Procedural
27.0 Drainage of face and floor of mouth

HCPCS Level II Supplies & Services
A4305 Disposable drug delivery system, flow rate of 50 ml or greater per hour
A4306 Disposable drug delivery system, flow rate of 5 ml or less per hour
A4550 Surgical trays

41018
41018 Extraoral incision and drainage of abscess, cyst, or hematoma of floor of mouth; masticator space

ICD-9-CM Diagnostic
522.5 Periapical abscess without sinus
522.7 Periapical abscess with sinus
523.3 Acute periodontitis
528.3 Cellulitis and abscess of oral soft tissues
528.4 Cysts of oral soft tissues
528.9 Other and unspecified diseases of the oral soft tissues ▽
682.0 Cellulitis and abscess of face — (Use additional code to identify organism)
750.26 Other specified congenital anomalies of mouth
780.6 Fever
784.2 Swelling, mass, or lump in head and neck
906.0 Late effect of open wound of head, neck, and trunk
920 Contusion of face, scalp, and neck except eye(s)
958.3 Posttraumatic wound infection not elsewhere classified
998.12 Hematoma complicating a procedure
998.59 Other postoperative infection — (Use additional code to identify infection)

ICD-9-CM Procedural
27.0 Drainage of face and floor of mouth
27.92 Incision of mouth, unspecified structure

HCPCS Level II Supplies & Services
A4305 Disposable drug delivery system, flow rate of 50 ml or greater per hour
A4306 Disposable drug delivery system, flow rate of 5 ml or less per hour
A4550 Surgical trays

41100–41105
41100 Biopsy of tongue; anterior two-thirds
41105 posterior one-third

ICD-9-CM Diagnostic
141.0 Malignant neoplasm of base of tongue
141.1 Malignant neoplasm of dorsal surface of tongue
141.2 Malignant neoplasm of tip and lateral border of tongue
141.3 Malignant neoplasm of ventral surface of tongue
141.4 Malignant neoplasm of anterior two-thirds of tongue, part unspecified ▽
141.5 Malignant neoplasm of junctional zone of tongue
141.8 Malignant neoplasm of other sites of tongue

- 141.9 Malignant neoplasm of tongue, unspecified site
- 198.89 Secondary malignant neoplasm of other specified sites
- 210.1 Benign neoplasm of tongue
- 228.00 Hemangioma of unspecified site
- 228.09 Hemangioma of other sites
- 230.0 Carcinoma in situ of lip, oral cavity, and pharynx
- 235.1 Neoplasm of uncertain behavior of lip, oral cavity, and pharynx
- 239.0 Neoplasm of unspecified nature of digestive system
- 239.2 Neoplasms of unspecified nature of bone, soft tissue, and skin
- 277.3 Amyloidosis — (Use additional code to identify any associated mental retardation)
- 528.6 Leukoplakia of oral mucosa, including tongue
- 528.79 Other disturbances of oral epithelium, including tongue
- 528.8 Oral submucosal fibrosis, including of tongue
- 528.9 Other and unspecified diseases of the oral soft tissues
- 529.0 Glossitis
- 529.6 Glossodynia
- 529.8 Other specified conditions of the tongue
- 697.0 Lichen planus
- 781.1 Disturbances of sensation of smell and taste
- 784.2 Swelling, mass, or lump in head and neck

ICD-9-CM Procedural
- 25.01 Closed (needle) biopsy of tongue
- 25.02 Open biopsy of tongue

HCPCS Level II Supplies & Services
- A4550 Surgical trays

41108
41108 Biopsy of floor of mouth

ICD-9-CM Diagnostic
- 144.0 Malignant neoplasm of anterior portion of floor of mouth
- 144.1 Malignant neoplasm of lateral portion of floor of mouth
- 144.8 Malignant neoplasm of other sites of floor of mouth
- 144.9 Malignant neoplasm of floor of mouth, part unspecified
- 145.9 Malignant neoplasm of mouth, unspecified site
- 198.89 Secondary malignant neoplasm of other specified sites
- 199.1 Other malignant neoplasm of unspecified site
- 210.3 Benign neoplasm of floor of mouth
- 210.4 Benign neoplasm of other and unspecified parts of mouth
- 228.00 Hemangioma of unspecified site
- 228.09 Hemangioma of other sites
- 230.0 Carcinoma in situ of lip, oral cavity, and pharynx
- 235.1 Neoplasm of uncertain behavior of lip, oral cavity, and pharynx
- 239.0 Neoplasm of unspecified nature of digestive system
- 528.6 Leukoplakia of oral mucosa, including tongue
- 528.79 Other disturbances of oral epithelium, including tongue
- 528.8 Oral submucosal fibrosis, including of tongue
- 528.9 Other and unspecified diseases of the oral soft tissues
- 697.0 Lichen planus

ICD-9-CM Procedural
- 27.24 Biopsy of mouth, unspecified structure

HCPCS Level II Supplies & Services
- A4550 Surgical trays

41110
41110 Excision of lesion of tongue without closure

ICD-9-CM Diagnostic
- 141.0 Malignant neoplasm of base of tongue
- 141.1 Malignant neoplasm of dorsal surface of tongue
- 141.2 Malignant neoplasm of tip and lateral border of tongue
- 141.3 Malignant neoplasm of ventral surface of tongue
- 141.4 Malignant neoplasm of anterior two-thirds of tongue, part unspecified
- 141.5 Malignant neoplasm of junctional zone of tongue
- 141.6 Malignant neoplasm of lingual tonsil
- 141.8 Malignant neoplasm of other sites of tongue
- 141.9 Malignant neoplasm of tongue, unspecified site
- 198.89 Secondary malignant neoplasm of other specified sites
- 210.1 Benign neoplasm of tongue
- 228.00 Hemangioma of unspecified site
- 228.09 Hemangioma of other sites
- 230.0 Carcinoma in situ of lip, oral cavity, and pharynx
- 235.1 Neoplasm of uncertain behavior of lip, oral cavity, and pharynx
- 239.0 Neoplasm of unspecified nature of digestive system
- 239.2 Neoplasms of unspecified nature of bone, soft tissue, and skin
- 528.6 Leukoplakia of oral mucosa, including tongue
- 528.79 Other disturbances of oral epithelium, including tongue
- 528.8 Oral submucosal fibrosis, including of tongue
- 528.9 Other and unspecified diseases of the oral soft tissues
- 529.0 Glossitis
- 529.8 Other specified conditions of the tongue
- 697.0 Lichen planus
- 784.2 Swelling, mass, or lump in head and neck

ICD-9-CM Procedural
- 25.1 Excision or destruction of lesion or tissue of tongue

HCPCS Level II Supplies & Services
- A4550 Surgical trays

41112–41114
41112 Excision of lesion of tongue with closure; anterior two-thirds
41113 posterior one-third
41114 with local tongue flap

ICD-9-CM Diagnostic
- 141.0 Malignant neoplasm of base of tongue
- 141.1 Malignant neoplasm of dorsal surface of tongue
- 141.2 Malignant neoplasm of tip and lateral border of tongue
- 141.3 Malignant neoplasm of ventral surface of tongue
- 141.4 Malignant neoplasm of anterior two-thirds of tongue, part unspecified
- 141.5 Malignant neoplasm of junctional zone of tongue
- 141.9 Malignant neoplasm of tongue, unspecified site
- 198.89 Secondary malignant neoplasm of other specified sites
- 210.1 Benign neoplasm of tongue
- 228.09 Hemangioma of other sites
- 230.0 Carcinoma in situ of lip, oral cavity, and pharynx
- 235.1 Neoplasm of uncertain behavior of lip, oral cavity, and pharynx
- 235.7 Neoplasm of uncertain behavior of trachea, bronchus, and lung
- 239.0 Neoplasm of unspecified nature of digestive system
- 528.6 Leukoplakia of oral mucosa, including tongue
- 528.79 Other disturbances of oral epithelium, including tongue
- 528.8 Oral submucosal fibrosis, including of tongue
- 528.9 Other and unspecified diseases of the oral soft tissues
- 529.0 Glossitis
- 529.8 Other specified conditions of the tongue
- 697.0 Lichen planus
- 784.2 Swelling, mass, or lump in head and neck

ICD-9-CM Procedural
- 25.1 Excision or destruction of lesion or tissue of tongue

HCPCS Level II Supplies & Services
- A4305 Disposable drug delivery system, flow rate of 50 ml or greater per hour
- A4306 Disposable drug delivery system, flow rate of 5 ml or less per hour
- A4550 Surgical trays

41115
41115 Excision of lingual frenum (frenectomy)

ICD-9-CM Diagnostic
- 141.3 Malignant neoplasm of ventral surface of tongue
- 145.1 Malignant neoplasm of vestibule of mouth
- 210.0 Benign neoplasm of lip
- 230.0 Carcinoma in situ of lip, oral cavity, and pharynx
- 235.1 Neoplasm of uncertain behavior of lip, oral cavity, and pharynx
- 528.9 Other and unspecified diseases of the oral soft tissues
- 529.6 Glossodynia
- 750.0 Tongue tie
- 750.12 Congenital adhesions of tongue

ICD-9-CM Procedural
- 25.92 Lingual frenectomy

HCPCS Level II Supplies & Services
- A4305 Disposable drug delivery system, flow rate of 50 ml or greater per hour
- A4306 Disposable drug delivery system, flow rate of 5 ml or less per hour
- A4550 Surgical trays

41116

41116 Excision, lesion of floor of mouth

ICD-9-CM Diagnostic

144.0 Malignant neoplasm of anterior portion of floor of mouth
144.1 Malignant neoplasm of lateral portion of floor of mouth
144.8 Malignant neoplasm of other sites of floor of mouth
144.9 Malignant neoplasm of floor of mouth, part unspecified ▽
145.9 Malignant neoplasm of mouth, unspecified site ▽
149.8 Malignant neoplasm of other sites within the lip and oral cavity
198.89 Secondary malignant neoplasm of other specified sites
210.3 Benign neoplasm of floor of mouth
210.4 Benign neoplasm of other and unspecified parts of mouth ▽
228.00 Hemangioma of unspecified site ▽
228.09 Hemangioma of other sites
230.0 Carcinoma in situ of lip, oral cavity, and pharynx
235.1 Neoplasm of uncertain behavior of lip, oral cavity, and pharynx
527.6 Mucocele of salivary gland
528.6 Leukoplakia of oral mucosa, including tongue
528.79 Other disturbances of oral epithelium, including tongue
528.9 Other and unspecified diseases of the oral soft tissues ▽
784.2 Swelling, mass, or lump in head and neck

ICD-9-CM Procedural

27.49 Other excision of mouth

HCPCS Level II Supplies & Services

A4305 Disposable drug delivery system, flow rate of 50 ml or greater per hour
A4306 Disposable drug delivery system, flow rate of 5 ml or less per hour
A4550 Surgical trays

41120–41130

41120 Glossectomy; less than one-half tongue
41130 hemiglossectomy

ICD-9-CM Diagnostic

141.0 Malignant neoplasm of base of tongue
141.1 Malignant neoplasm of dorsal surface of tongue
141.2 Malignant neoplasm of tip and lateral border of tongue
141.3 Malignant neoplasm of ventral surface of tongue
141.4 Malignant neoplasm of anterior two-thirds of tongue, part unspecified ▽
141.8 Malignant neoplasm of other sites of tongue
141.9 Malignant neoplasm of tongue, unspecified site ▽
144.9 Malignant neoplasm of floor of mouth, part unspecified ▽
149.0 Malignant neoplasm of pharynx, unspecified ▽
195.0 Malignant neoplasm of head, face, and neck
198.89 Secondary malignant neoplasm of other specified sites
210.1 Benign neoplasm of tongue
230.0 Carcinoma in situ of lip, oral cavity, and pharynx
235.1 Neoplasm of uncertain behavior of lip, oral cavity, and pharynx
750.15 Macroglossia

ICD-9-CM Procedural

25.2 Partial glossectomy

41135

41135 Glossectomy; partial, with unilateral radical neck dissection

ICD-9-CM Diagnostic

141.0 Malignant neoplasm of base of tongue
141.1 Malignant neoplasm of dorsal surface of tongue
141.2 Malignant neoplasm of tip and lateral border of tongue
141.3 Malignant neoplasm of ventral surface of tongue
141.4 Malignant neoplasm of anterior two-thirds of tongue, part unspecified ▽
141.5 Malignant neoplasm of junctional zone of tongue
141.6 Malignant neoplasm of lingual tonsil
141.8 Malignant neoplasm of other sites of tongue
141.9 Malignant neoplasm of tongue, unspecified site ▽
171.0 Malignant neoplasm of connective and other soft tissue of head, face, and neck
195.0 Malignant neoplasm of head, face, and neck
196.0 Secondary and unspecified malignant neoplasm of lymph nodes of head, face, and neck
198.89 Secondary malignant neoplasm of other specified sites
238.8 Neoplasm of uncertain behavior of other specified sites

ICD-9-CM Procedural

25.2 Partial glossectomy
40.41 Radical neck dissection, unilateral

41140–41145

41140 Glossectomy; complete or total, with or without tracheostomy, without radical neck dissection
41145 complete or total, with or without tracheostomy, with unilateral radical neck dissection

ICD-9-CM Diagnostic

141.0 Malignant neoplasm of base of tongue
141.1 Malignant neoplasm of dorsal surface of tongue
141.2 Malignant neoplasm of tip and lateral border of tongue
141.3 Malignant neoplasm of ventral surface of tongue
141.4 Malignant neoplasm of anterior two-thirds of tongue, part unspecified ▽
141.5 Malignant neoplasm of junctional zone of tongue
141.6 Malignant neoplasm of lingual tonsil
141.8 Malignant neoplasm of other sites of tongue
141.9 Malignant neoplasm of tongue, unspecified site ▽
171.0 Malignant neoplasm of connective and other soft tissue of head, face, and neck
195.0 Malignant neoplasm of head, face, and neck
196.0 Secondary and unspecified malignant neoplasm of lymph nodes of head, face, and neck
198.89 Secondary malignant neoplasm of other specified sites
238.8 Neoplasm of uncertain behavior of other specified sites
239.8 Neoplasm of unspecified nature of other specified sites

ICD-9-CM Procedural

25.3 Complete glossectomy
31.1 Temporary tracheostomy
31.21 Mediastinal tracheostomy
31.29 Other permanent tracheostomy
40.41 Radical neck dissection, unilateral

HCPCS Level II Supplies & Services

A7527 Tracheostomy/laryngectomy tube plug/stop, each

41150

41150 Glossectomy; composite procedure with resection floor of mouth and mandibular resection, without radical neck dissection

ICD-9-CM Diagnostic

141.0 Malignant neoplasm of base of tongue
141.1 Malignant neoplasm of dorsal surface of tongue
141.2 Malignant neoplasm of tip and lateral border of tongue
141.3 Malignant neoplasm of ventral surface of tongue
141.4 Malignant neoplasm of anterior two-thirds of tongue, part unspecified ▽
141.5 Malignant neoplasm of junctional zone of tongue
141.6 Malignant neoplasm of lingual tonsil
141.8 Malignant neoplasm of other sites of tongue
141.9 Malignant neoplasm of tongue, unspecified site ▽
144.0 Malignant neoplasm of anterior portion of floor of mouth
144.1 Malignant neoplasm of lateral portion of floor of mouth
144.8 Malignant neoplasm of other sites of floor of mouth
144.9 Malignant neoplasm of floor of mouth, part unspecified ▽
145.8 Malignant neoplasm of other specified parts of mouth
145.9 Malignant neoplasm of mouth, unspecified site ▽
170.1 Malignant neoplasm of mandible
195.0 Malignant neoplasm of head, face, and neck
196.0 Secondary and unspecified malignant neoplasm of lymph nodes of head, face, and neck
198.5 Secondary malignant neoplasm of bone and bone marrow
198.89 Secondary malignant neoplasm of other specified sites
235.1 Neoplasm of uncertain behavior of lip, oral cavity, and pharynx
238.0 Neoplasm of uncertain behavior of bone and articular cartilage
238.8 Neoplasm of uncertain behavior of other specified sites
239.0 Neoplasm of unspecified nature of digestive system

ICD-9-CM Procedural

25.2 Partial glossectomy
25.3 Complete glossectomy
27.49 Other excision of mouth
76.31 Partial mandibulectomy

41153

41153 Glossectomy; composite procedure with resection floor of mouth, with suprahyoid neck dissection

ICD-9-CM Diagnostic

141.0 Malignant neoplasm of base of tongue
141.1 Malignant neoplasm of dorsal surface of tongue
141.2 Malignant neoplasm of tip and lateral border of tongue
141.3 Malignant neoplasm of ventral surface of tongue
141.4 Malignant neoplasm of anterior two-thirds of tongue, part unspecified ▽
141.5 Malignant neoplasm of junctional zone of tongue
141.6 Malignant neoplasm of lingual tonsil
141.8 Malignant neoplasm of other sites of tongue
141.9 Malignant neoplasm of tongue, unspecified site ▽
142.2 Malignant neoplasm of sublingual gland
144.0 Malignant neoplasm of anterior portion of floor of mouth
144.1 Malignant neoplasm of lateral portion of floor of mouth
144.8 Malignant neoplasm of other sites of floor of mouth
144.9 Malignant neoplasm of floor of mouth, part unspecified ▽
145.8 Malignant neoplasm of other specified parts of mouth
170.1 Malignant neoplasm of mandible
195.0 Malignant neoplasm of head, face, and neck
196.0 Secondary and unspecified malignant neoplasm of lymph nodes of head, face, and neck
198.5 Secondary malignant neoplasm of bone and bone marrow
198.89 Secondary malignant neoplasm of other specified sites
235.0 Neoplasm of uncertain behavior of major salivary glands
235.1 Neoplasm of uncertain behavior of lip, oral cavity, and pharynx
238.0 Neoplasm of uncertain behavior of bone and articular cartilage
238.8 Neoplasm of uncertain behavior of other specified sites
239.0 Neoplasm of unspecified nature of digestive system

ICD-9-CM Procedural

25.2 Partial glossectomy
25.3 Complete glossectomy
27.49 Other excision of mouth
40.3 Regional lymph node excision

41155

41155 Glossectomy; composite procedure with resection floor of mouth, mandibular resection, and radical neck dissection (Commando type)

ICD-9-CM Diagnostic

141.0 Malignant neoplasm of base of tongue
141.1 Malignant neoplasm of dorsal surface of tongue
141.2 Malignant neoplasm of tip and lateral border of tongue
141.3 Malignant neoplasm of ventral surface of tongue
141.4 Malignant neoplasm of anterior two-thirds of tongue, part unspecified ▽
141.5 Malignant neoplasm of junctional zone of tongue
141.6 Malignant neoplasm of lingual tonsil
141.9 Malignant neoplasm of tongue, unspecified site ▽
143.1 Malignant neoplasm of lower gum
144.0 Malignant neoplasm of anterior portion of floor of mouth
144.1 Malignant neoplasm of lateral portion of floor of mouth
144.8 Malignant neoplasm of other sites of floor of mouth
144.9 Malignant neoplasm of floor of mouth, part unspecified ▽
145.8 Malignant neoplasm of other specified parts of mouth
146.9 Malignant neoplasm of oropharynx, unspecified site ▽
170.1 Malignant neoplasm of mandible
171.0 Malignant neoplasm of connective and other soft tissue of head, face, and neck
195.0 Malignant neoplasm of head, face, and neck
196.0 Secondary and unspecified malignant neoplasm of lymph nodes of head, face, and neck
198.5 Secondary malignant neoplasm of bone and bone marrow
198.89 Secondary malignant neoplasm of other specified sites
230.0 Carcinoma in situ of lip, oral cavity, and pharynx
235.1 Neoplasm of uncertain behavior of lip, oral cavity, and pharynx
238.0 Neoplasm of uncertain behavior of bone and articular cartilage
238.8 Neoplasm of uncertain behavior of other specified sites

ICD-9-CM Procedural

25.2 Partial glossectomy
25.3 Complete glossectomy
27.49 Other excision of mouth
40.42 Radical neck dissection, bilateral
76.31 Partial mandibulectomy

41250–41252

41250 Repair of laceration 2.5 cm or less; floor of mouth and/or anterior two-thirds of tongue
41251 posterior one-third of tongue
41252 Repair of laceration of tongue, floor of mouth, over 2.6 cm or complex

ICD-9-CM Diagnostic

873.64 Open wound of tongue and floor of mouth, without mention of complication — (Use additional code to identify infection)
873.69 Open wound of mouth, other and multiple sites, without mention of complication — (Use additional code to identify infection)
873.72 Open wound of gum (alveolar process), complicated — (Use additional code to identify infection)
873.74 Open wound of tongue and floor of mouth, complicated — (Use additional code to identify infection)
873.79 Open wound of mouth, other and multiple sites, complicated — (Use additional code to identify infection)
998.2 Accidental puncture or laceration during procedure
998.32 Disruption of external operation wound

ICD-9-CM Procedural

25.51 Suture of laceration of tongue
27.52 Suture of laceration of other part of mouth

HCPCS Level II Supplies & Services

A4305 Disposable drug delivery system, flow rate of 50 ml or greater per hour
A4306 Disposable drug delivery system, flow rate of 5 ml or less per hour
A4550 Surgical trays

41500

41500 Fixation of tongue, mechanical, other than suture (eg, K-wire)

ICD-9-CM Diagnostic

141.0 Malignant neoplasm of base of tongue
141.1 Malignant neoplasm of dorsal surface of tongue
141.2 Malignant neoplasm of tip and lateral border of tongue
141.3 Malignant neoplasm of ventral surface of tongue
141.4 Malignant neoplasm of anterior two-thirds of tongue, part unspecified ▽
141.5 Malignant neoplasm of junctional zone of tongue
141.9 Malignant neoplasm of tongue, unspecified site ▽
230.0 Carcinoma in situ of lip, oral cavity, and pharynx
235.1 Neoplasm of uncertain behavior of lip, oral cavity, and pharynx
529.8 Other specified conditions of the tongue
750.0 Tongue tie
750.15 Macroglossia
750.16 Microglossia
750.19 Other congenital anomaly of tongue
756.0 Congenital anomalies of skull and face bones

ICD-9-CM Procedural

25.59 Other repair and plastic operations on tongue

HCPCS Level II Supplies & Services

A4305 Disposable drug delivery system, flow rate of 50 ml or greater per hour
A4306 Disposable drug delivery system, flow rate of 5 ml or less per hour
A4550 Surgical trays

41510

41510 Suture of tongue to lip for micrognathia (Douglas type procedure)

ICD-9-CM Diagnostic

524.00 Unspecified major anomaly of jaw size ▽
524.03 Maxillary hypoplasia
524.04 Mandibular hypoplasia
524.06 Microgenia
524.10 Unspecified anomaly of relationship of jaw to cranial base ▽
524.73 Alveolar maxillary hypoplasia
524.74 Alveolar mandibular hypoplasia
750.15 Macroglossia

ICD-9-CM Procedural

25.59 Other repair and plastic operations on tongue

HCPCS Level II Supplies & Services

A4305 Disposable drug delivery system, flow rate of 50 ml or greater per hour
A4306 Disposable drug delivery system, flow rate of 5 ml or less per hour

▽ Unspecified code ♀ Female diagnosis ☒ Manifestation code ♂ Male diagnosis

A4550 Surgical trays

41520

41520 Frenoplasty (surgical revision of frenum, eg, with Z-plasty)

ICD-9-CM Diagnostic

524.02 Mandibular hyperplasia
524.04 Mandibular hypoplasia
529.8 Other specified conditions of the tongue
750.0 Tongue tie
750.10 Congenital anomaly of tongue, unspecified
750.12 Congenital adhesions of tongue
906.0 Late effect of open wound of head, neck, and trunk

ICD-9-CM Procedural

25.59 Other repair and plastic operations on tongue

HCPCS Level II Supplies & Services

A4305 Disposable drug delivery system, flow rate of 50 ml or greater per hour
A4306 Disposable drug delivery system, flow rate of 5 ml or less per hour
A4550 Surgical trays

Dentoalveolar Structures

41800

41800 Drainage of abscess, cyst, hematoma from dentoalveolar structures

ICD-9-CM Diagnostic

522.5 Periapical abscess without sinus
522.7 Periapical abscess with sinus
522.8 Radicular cyst of dental pulp
523.3 Acute periodontitis
526.0 Developmental odontogenic cysts
526.1 Fissural cysts of jaw
526.2 Other cysts of jaws
526.4 Inflammatory conditions of jaw
528.3 Cellulitis and abscess of oral soft tissues
528.4 Cysts of oral soft tissues
784.2 Swelling, mass, or lump in head and neck
925.1 Crushing injury of face and scalp — (Use additional code to identify any associated injuries: 800-829, 850.0-854.1, 860.0-869.1)
958.3 Posttraumatic wound infection not elsewhere classified
998.51 Infected postoperative seroma — (Use additional code to identify organism)
998.59 Other postoperative infection — (Use additional code to identify infection)

ICD-9-CM Procedural

24.0 Incision of gum or alveolar bone

HCPCS Level II Supplies & Services

A4550 Surgical trays

41805–41806

41805 Removal of embedded foreign body from dentoalveolar structures; soft tissues
41806 bone

ICD-9-CM Diagnostic

522.6 Chronic apical periodontitis
523.4 Chronic periodontitis
526.4 Inflammatory conditions of jaw
873.72 Open wound of gum (alveolar process), complicated — (Use additional code to identify infection)
873.73 Open wound of tooth (broken), complicated — (Use additional code to identify infection)
873.79 Open wound of mouth, other and multiple sites, complicated — (Use additional code to identify infection)
910.6 Face, neck, and scalp, except eye, superficial foreign body (splinter), without major open wound or mention of infection
910.7 Face, neck, and scalp except eye, superficial foreign body (splinter), without major open wound, infected
935.0 Foreign body in mouth
996.4 Mechanical complication of internal orthopedic device, implant, and graft
996.67 Infection and inflammatory reaction due to other internal orthopedic device, implant, and graft — (Use additional code to identify specified infections)
998.4 Foreign body accidentally left during procedure, not elsewhere classified
998.51 Infected postoperative seroma — (Use additional code to identify organism)
998.59 Other postoperative infection — (Use additional code to identify infection)

ICD-9-CM Procedural

24.0 Incision of gum or alveolar bone
98.22 Removal of other foreign body without incision from head and neck

HCPCS Level II Supplies & Services

A4305 Disposable drug delivery system, flow rate of 50 ml or greater per hour
A4306 Disposable drug delivery system, flow rate of 5 ml or less per hour
A4550 Surgical trays

41820

41820 Gingivectomy, excision gingiva, each quadrant

ICD-9-CM Diagnostic

143.0 Malignant neoplasm of upper gum
143.1 Malignant neoplasm of lower gum
143.8 Malignant neoplasm of other sites of gum
143.9 Malignant neoplasm of gum, unspecified site
198.89 Secondary malignant neoplasm of other specified sites
210.4 Benign neoplasm of other and unspecified parts of mouth
230.0 Carcinoma in situ of lip, oral cavity, and pharynx
235.1 Neoplasm of uncertain behavior of lip, oral cavity, and pharynx
239.0 Neoplasm of unspecified nature of digestive system
523.0 Acute gingivitis
523.1 Chronic gingivitis
523.3 Acute periodontitis
523.4 Chronic periodontitis
523.8 Other specified periodontal diseases
996.4 Mechanical complication of internal orthopedic device, implant, and graft
996.67 Infection and inflammatory reaction due to other internal orthopedic device, implant, and graft — (Use additional code to identify specified infections)

ICD-9-CM Procedural

24.31 Excision of lesion or tissue of gum

HCPCS Level II Supplies & Services

A4305 Disposable drug delivery system, flow rate of 50 ml or greater per hour
A4306 Disposable drug delivery system, flow rate of 5 ml or less per hour
A4550 Surgical trays

41821

41821 Operculectomy, excision pericoronal tissues

ICD-9-CM Diagnostic

520.6 Disturbances in tooth eruption
520.8 Other specified disorders of tooth development and eruption
521.6 Ankylosis of teeth
523.1 Chronic gingivitis
523.3 Acute periodontitis
523.4 Chronic periodontitis
528.6 Leukoplakia of oral mucosa, including tongue
528.9 Other and unspecified diseases of the oral soft tissues

ICD-9-CM Procedural

24.6 Exposure of tooth

Periodontal Disease

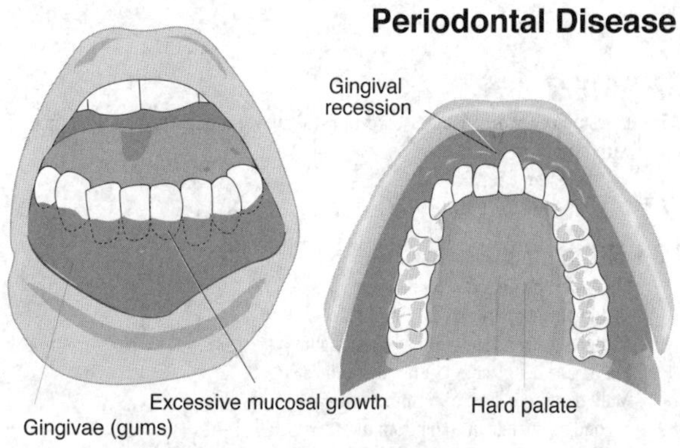

Gingivitis is an inflammatory response to bacteria on the teeth

HCPCS Level II Supplies & Services

A4305 Disposable drug delivery system, flow rate of 50 ml or greater per hour
A4306 Disposable drug delivery system, flow rate of 5 ml or less per hour
A4550 Surgical trays

41822

41822 Excision of fibrous tuberosities, dentoalveolar structures

ICD-9-CM Diagnostic

523.3 Acute periodontitis
523.4 Chronic periodontitis
523.8 Other specified periodontal diseases
524.70 Unspecified alveolar anomaly ▽
524.79 Other specified alveolar anomaly
524.89 Other specified dentofacial anomalies
524.9 Unspecified dentofacial anomalies ▽
525.8 Other specified disorders of the teeth and supporting structures
525.9 Unspecified disorder of the teeth and supporting structures ▽
526.89 Other specified disease of the jaws

ICD-9-CM Procedural

77.69 Local excision of lesion or tissue of other bone, except facial bones

HCPCS Level II Supplies & Services

A4305 Disposable drug delivery system, flow rate of 50 ml or greater per hour
A4306 Disposable drug delivery system, flow rate of 5 ml or less per hour
A4550 Surgical trays

41823

41823 Excision of osseous tuberosities, dentoalveolar structures

ICD-9-CM Diagnostic

210.4 Benign neoplasm of other and unspecified parts of mouth ▽
213.0 Benign neoplasm of bones of skull and face
520.6 Disturbances in tooth eruption
523.3 Acute periodontitis
523.4 Chronic periodontitis
523.8 Other specified periodontal diseases
523.9 Unspecified gingival and periodontal disease ▽
524.70 Unspecified alveolar anomaly ▽
524.79 Other specified alveolar anomaly
524.89 Other specified dentofacial anomalies
524.9 Unspecified dentofacial anomalies ▽
525.8 Other specified disorders of the teeth and supporting structures
525.9 Unspecified disorder of the teeth and supporting structures ▽
526.0 Developmental odontogenic cysts
526.81 Exostosis of jaw
526.89 Other specified disease of the jaws
528.9 Other and unspecified diseases of the oral soft tissues ▽
730.88 Other infections involving bone diseases classified elsewhere, other specified sites — (Code first underlying disease: 002.0, 015.0-015.9. Use additional code to identify organism) ☒

ICD-9-CM Procedural

77.69 Local excision of lesion or tissue of other bone, except facial bones

HCPCS Level II Supplies & Services

A4305 Disposable drug delivery system, flow rate of 50 ml or greater per hour
A4306 Disposable drug delivery system, flow rate of 5 ml or less per hour
A4550 Surgical trays

41825–41827

41825 Excision of lesion or tumor (except listed above), dentoalveolar structures; without repair
41826 with simple repair
41827 with complex repair

ICD-9-CM Diagnostic

143.0 Malignant neoplasm of upper gum
143.1 Malignant neoplasm of lower gum
143.8 Malignant neoplasm of other sites of gum
143.9 Malignant neoplasm of gum, unspecified site ▽
145.6 Malignant neoplasm of retromolar area
198.89 Secondary malignant neoplasm of other specified sites
210.4 Benign neoplasm of other and unspecified parts of mouth ▽
235.1 Neoplasm of uncertain behavior of lip, oral cavity, and pharynx
522.8 Radicular cyst of dental pulp
523.8 Other specified periodontal diseases
526.0 Developmental odontogenic cysts
526.1 Fissural cysts of jaw
526.2 Other cysts of jaws
526.3 Central giant cell (reparative) granuloma
528.4 Cysts of oral soft tissues
528.6 Leukoplakia of oral mucosa, including tongue
528.9 Other and unspecified diseases of the oral soft tissues ▽
784.2 Swelling, mass, or lump in head and neck

ICD-9-CM Procedural

24.31 Excision of lesion or tissue of gum
24.4 Excision of dental lesion of jaw

HCPCS Level II Supplies & Services

A4305 Disposable drug delivery system, flow rate of 50 ml or greater per hour
A4306 Disposable drug delivery system, flow rate of 5 ml or less per hour
A4550 Surgical trays

41828

41828 Excision of hyperplastic alveolar mucosa, each quadrant (specify)

ICD-9-CM Diagnostic

210.4 Benign neoplasm of other and unspecified parts of mouth ▽
523.8 Other specified periodontal diseases
528.9 Other and unspecified diseases of the oral soft tissues ▽
V54.89 Other orthopedic aftercare

ICD-9-CM Procedural

24.31 Excision of lesion or tissue of gum

41830

41830 Alveolectomy, including curettage of osteitis or sequestrectomy

ICD-9-CM Diagnostic

170.1 Malignant neoplasm of mandible
522.6 Chronic apical periodontitis
522.8 Radicular cyst of dental pulp
523.4 Chronic periodontitis
523.5 Periodontosis
525.8 Other specified disorders of the teeth and supporting structures
526.4 Inflammatory conditions of jaw
526.5 Alveolitis of jaw
784.2 Swelling, mass, or lump in head and neck
906.0 Late effect of open wound of head, neck, and trunk

ICD-9-CM Procedural

24.5 Alveoloplasty

41850

41850 Destruction of lesion (except excision), dentoalveolar structures

ICD-9-CM Diagnostic

143.0 Malignant neoplasm of upper gum
143.1 Malignant neoplasm of lower gum
170.1 Malignant neoplasm of mandible
210.4 Benign neoplasm of other and unspecified parts of mouth ▽
213.1 Benign neoplasm of lower jaw bone
228.00 Hemangioma of unspecified site ▽
230.0 Carcinoma in situ of lip, oral cavity, and pharynx
235.1 Neoplasm of uncertain behavior of lip, oral cavity, and pharynx
239.2 Neoplasms of unspecified nature of bone, soft tissue, and skin
520.6 Disturbances in tooth eruption
523.8 Other specified periodontal diseases
526.0 Developmental odontogenic cysts
526.89 Other specified disease of the jaws

ICD-9-CM Procedural

24.39 Other operations on gum

HCPCS Level II Supplies & Services

A4550 Surgical trays

▽ Unspecified code ☒ Manifestation code
♀ Female diagnosis ♂ Male diagnosis

41870

41870 Periodontal mucosal grafting

ICD-9-CM Diagnostic

143.0 Malignant neoplasm of upper gum
143.1 Malignant neoplasm of lower gum
210.4 Benign neoplasm of other and unspecified parts of mouth ▽
230.0 Carcinoma in situ of lip, oral cavity, and pharynx
520.6 Disturbances in tooth eruption
523.1 Chronic gingivitis
523.20 Gingival recession, unspecified
523.21 Gingival recession, minimal
523.22 Gingival recession, moderate
523.23 Gingival recession, severe
523.24 Gingival recession, localized
523.25 Gingival recession, generalized
523.4 Chronic periodontitis
523.5 Periodontosis
523.8 Other specified periodontal diseases
528.6 Leukoplakia of oral mucosa, including tongue
V10.02 Personal history of malignant neoplasm of other and unspecified parts of oral cavity and pharynx ▽
V51 Aftercare involving the use of plastic surgery

ICD-9-CM Procedural

24.39 Other operations on gum

41872

41872 Gingivoplasty, each quadrant (specify)

ICD-9-CM Diagnostic

520.6 Disturbances in tooth eruption
523.0 Acute gingivitis
523.1 Chronic gingivitis
523.20 Gingival recession, unspecified
523.21 Gingival recession, minimal
523.22 Gingival recession, moderate
523.23 Gingival recession, severe
523.24 Gingival recession, localized
523.25 Gingival recession, generalized
523.5 Periodontosis
523.8 Other specified periodontal diseases
873.62 Open wound of gum (alveolar process), without mention of complication — (Use additional code to identify infection)
873.72 Open wound of gum (alveolar process), complicated — (Use additional code to identify infection)
906.0 Late effect of open wound of head, neck, and trunk
996.60 Infection and inflammatory reaction due to unspecified device, implant, and graft — (Use additional code to identify specified infections) ▽

ICD-9-CM Procedural

24.2 Gingivoplasty

41874

41874 Alveoloplasty, each quadrant (specify)

ICD-9-CM Diagnostic

143.0 Malignant neoplasm of upper gum
143.1 Malignant neoplasm of lower gum
143.9 Malignant neoplasm of gum, unspecified site ▽
170.1 Malignant neoplasm of mandible
198.89 Secondary malignant neoplasm of other specified sites
210.4 Benign neoplasm of other and unspecified parts of mouth ▽
213.1 Benign neoplasm of lower jaw bone
230.0 Carcinoma in situ of lip, oral cavity, and pharynx
235.1 Neoplasm of uncertain behavior of lip, oral cavity, and pharynx
238.0 Neoplasm of uncertain behavior of bone and articular cartilage
522.4 Acute apical periodontitis of pulpal origin
523.20 Gingival recession, unspecified
523.21 Gingival recession, minimal
523.22 Gingival recession, moderate
523.23 Gingival recession, severe
523.24 Gingival recession, localized
523.25 Gingival recession, generalized
523.4 Chronic periodontitis
524.39 Other anomalies of tooth position
524.72 Alveolar mandibular hyperplasia
524.74 Alveolar mandibular hypoplasia
524.79 Other specified alveolar anomaly
525.0 Exfoliation of teeth due to systemic causes
525.10 Unspecified acquired absence of teeth ▽
525.11 Loss of teeth due to trauma
525.12 Loss of teeth due to periodontal disease
525.13 Loss of teeth due to caries
525.19 Other loss of teeth
526.4 Inflammatory conditions of jaw
784.2 Swelling, mass, or lump in head and neck
873.72 Open wound of gum (alveolar process), complicated — (Use additional code to identify infection)
996.67 Infection and inflammatory reaction due to other internal orthopedic device, implant, and graft — (Use additional code to identify specified infections)

ICD-9-CM Procedural

24.5 Alveoloplasty

Palate and Uvula

42000

42000 Drainage of abscess of palate, uvula

ICD-9-CM Diagnostic

526.4 Inflammatory conditions of jaw
528.3 Cellulitis and abscess of oral soft tissues
958.3 Posttraumatic wound infection not elsewhere classified

ICD-9-CM Procedural

27.1 Incision of palate
27.71 Incision of uvula

HCPCS Level II Supplies & Services

A4550 Surgical trays

42100

42100 Biopsy of palate, uvula

ICD-9-CM Diagnostic

145.2 Malignant neoplasm of hard palate
145.3 Malignant neoplasm of soft palate
145.4 Malignant neoplasm of uvula
145.5 Malignant neoplasm of palate, unspecified ▽
145.9 Malignant neoplasm of mouth, unspecified site ▽
147.3 Malignant neoplasm of anterior wall of nasopharynx
198.89 Secondary malignant neoplasm of other specified sites
210.4 Benign neoplasm of other and unspecified parts of mouth ▽
210.7 Benign neoplasm of nasopharynx
210.8 Benign neoplasm of hypopharynx
213.0 Benign neoplasm of bones of skull and face
229.9 Benign neoplasm of unspecified site ▽
230.0 Carcinoma in situ of lip, oral cavity, and pharynx
235.1 Neoplasm of uncertain behavior of lip, oral cavity, and pharynx
239.0 Neoplasm of unspecified nature of digestive system
528.0 Stomatitis
528.4 Cysts of oral soft tissues
528.6 Leukoplakia of oral mucosa, including tongue
528.79 Other disturbances of oral epithelium, including tongue
528.8 Oral submucosal fibrosis, including of tongue
528.9 Other and unspecified diseases of the oral soft tissues ▽
686.1 Pyogenic granuloma of skin and subcutaneous tissue
697.0 Lichen planus
784.2 Swelling, mass, or lump in head and neck
V10.89 Personal history of malignant neoplasm of other site

ICD-9-CM Procedural

27.21 Biopsy of bony palate
27.22 Biopsy of uvula and soft palate

HCPCS Level II Supplies & Services

A4550 Surgical trays

42104–42107

42104 Excision, lesion of palate, uvula; without closure
42106 with simple primary closure
42107 with local flap closure

ICD-9-CM Diagnostic

145.2 Malignant neoplasm of hard palate
145.3 Malignant neoplasm of soft palate
145.4 Malignant neoplasm of uvula
145.5 Malignant neoplasm of palate, unspecified
147.3 Malignant neoplasm of anterior wall of nasopharynx
198.89 Secondary malignant neoplasm of other specified sites
199.1 Other malignant neoplasm of unspecified site
210.4 Benign neoplasm of other and unspecified parts of mouth
210.7 Benign neoplasm of nasopharynx
215.0 Other benign neoplasm of connective and other soft tissue of head, face, and neck
228.1 Lymphangioma, any site
230.0 Carcinoma in situ of lip, oral cavity, and pharynx
235.1 Neoplasm of uncertain behavior of lip, oral cavity, and pharynx
239.0 Neoplasm of unspecified nature of digestive system
478.26 Cyst of pharynx or nasopharynx
526.1 Fissural cysts of jaw
528.3 Cellulitis and abscess of oral soft tissues
528.4 Cysts of oral soft tissues
528.6 Leukoplakia of oral mucosa, including tongue
528.79 Other disturbances of oral epithelium, including tongue
528.9 Other and unspecified diseases of the oral soft tissues
697.0 Lichen planus
750.26 Other specified congenital anomalies of mouth
784.2 Swelling, mass, or lump in head and neck

ICD-9-CM Procedural

27.31 Local excision or destruction of lesion or tissue of bony palate
27.69 Other plastic repair of palate
27.72 Excision of uvula
27.79 Other operations on uvula

HCPCS Level II Supplies & Services

A4305 Disposable drug delivery system, flow rate of 50 ml or greater per hour
A4306 Disposable drug delivery system, flow rate of 5 ml or less per hour
A4550 Surgical trays

42120

42120 Resection of palate or extensive resection of lesion

ICD-9-CM Diagnostic

145.2 Malignant neoplasm of hard palate
145.3 Malignant neoplasm of soft palate
145.5 Malignant neoplasm of palate, unspecified
145.9 Malignant neoplasm of mouth, unspecified site
147.3 Malignant neoplasm of anterior wall of nasopharynx
198.89 Secondary malignant neoplasm of other specified sites
210.3 Benign neoplasm of floor of mouth
210.4 Benign neoplasm of other and unspecified parts of mouth
210.7 Benign neoplasm of nasopharynx
214.9 Lipoma of unspecified site
215.0 Other benign neoplasm of connective and other soft tissue of head, face, and neck
228.1 Lymphangioma, any site
230.0 Carcinoma in situ of lip, oral cavity, and pharynx
235.1 Neoplasm of uncertain behavior of lip, oral cavity, and pharynx
239.0 Neoplasm of unspecified nature of digestive system
478.26 Cyst of pharynx or nasopharynx
526.1 Fissural cysts of jaw
528.3 Cellulitis and abscess of oral soft tissues
528.4 Cysts of oral soft tissues
528.6 Leukoplakia of oral mucosa, including tongue
528.9 Other and unspecified diseases of the oral soft tissues

ICD-9-CM Procedural

27.31 Local excision or destruction of lesion or tissue of bony palate
27.32 Wide excision or destruction of lesion or tissue of bony palate

42140

42140 Uvulectomy, excision of uvula

ICD-9-CM Diagnostic

145.4 Malignant neoplasm of uvula
198.89 Secondary malignant neoplasm of other specified sites
210.4 Benign neoplasm of other and unspecified parts of mouth
230.0 Carcinoma in situ of lip, oral cavity, and pharynx
235.1 Neoplasm of uncertain behavior of lip, oral cavity, and pharynx
239.0 Neoplasm of unspecified nature of digestive system
528.9 Other and unspecified diseases of the oral soft tissues
750.26 Other specified congenital anomalies of mouth
780.51 Insomnia with sleep apnea
780.53 Hypersomnia with sleep apnea
780.57 Other and unspecified sleep apnea
786.09 Other dyspnea and respiratory abnormalities

ICD-9-CM Procedural

27.72 Excision of uvula

HCPCS Level II Supplies & Services

A4305 Disposable drug delivery system, flow rate of 50 ml or greater per hour
A4306 Disposable drug delivery system, flow rate of 5 ml or less per hour
A4550 Surgical trays

42145

42145 Palatopharyngoplasty (eg, uvulopalatopharyngoplasty, uvulopharyngoplasty)

ICD-9-CM Diagnostic

145.2 Malignant neoplasm of hard palate
145.3 Malignant neoplasm of soft palate
145.4 Malignant neoplasm of uvula
145.5 Malignant neoplasm of palate, unspecified
146.2 Malignant neoplasm of tonsillar pillars (anterior) (posterior)
147.3 Malignant neoplasm of anterior wall of nasopharynx
149.0 Malignant neoplasm of pharynx, unspecified
198.89 Secondary malignant neoplasm of other specified sites
210.4 Benign neoplasm of other and unspecified parts of mouth
210.7 Benign neoplasm of nasopharynx
210.9 Benign neoplasm of pharynx, unspecified
230.0 Carcinoma in situ of lip, oral cavity, and pharynx
235.1 Neoplasm of uncertain behavior of lip, oral cavity, and pharynx
239.0 Neoplasm of unspecified nature of digestive system
496 Chronic airway obstruction, not elsewhere classified — (Note: This code is not to be used with any code from 491-493)
528.9 Other and unspecified diseases of the oral soft tissues
750.26 Other specified congenital anomalies of mouth
780.50 Unspecified sleep disturbance
780.53 Hypersomnia with sleep apnea
780.57 Other and unspecified sleep apnea
786.09 Other dyspnea and respiratory abnormalities
786.9 Other symptoms involving respiratory system and chest

ICD-9-CM Procedural

27.69 Other plastic repair of palate
27.73 Repair of uvula
29.4 Plastic operation on pharynx

42160

42160 Destruction of lesion, palate or uvula (thermal, cryo or chemical)

ICD-9-CM Diagnostic

145.2 Malignant neoplasm of hard palate
145.3 Malignant neoplasm of soft palate
145.4 Malignant neoplasm of uvula
145.5 Malignant neoplasm of palate, unspecified
147.3 Malignant neoplasm of anterior wall of nasopharynx
198.89 Secondary malignant neoplasm of other specified sites
210.4 Benign neoplasm of other and unspecified parts of mouth
210.7 Benign neoplasm of nasopharynx
230.0 Carcinoma in situ of lip, oral cavity, and pharynx
235.1 Neoplasm of uncertain behavior of lip, oral cavity, and pharynx
239.0 Neoplasm of unspecified nature of digestive system
528.9 Other and unspecified diseases of the oral soft tissues

Palatal Prosthesis

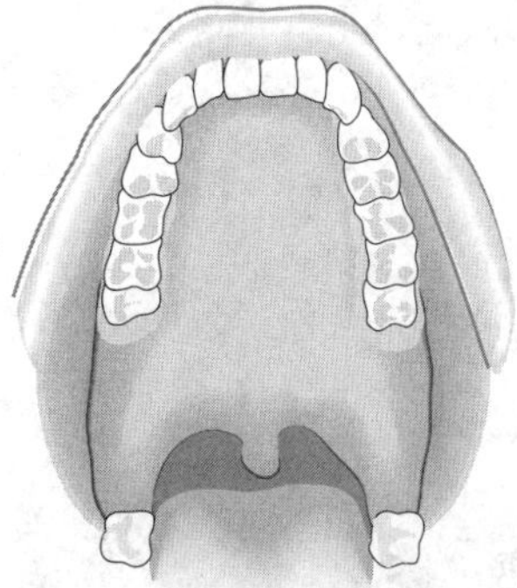
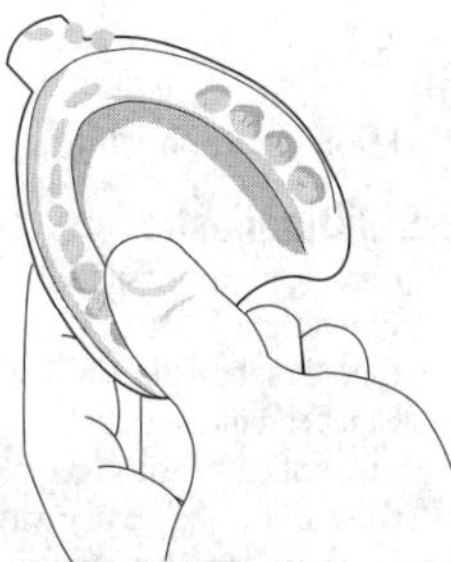

The doctor takes impressions of the upper jaw to customize a palatal prosthesis

ICD-9-CM Procedural
27.31 Local excision or destruction of lesion or tissue of bony palate
27.79 Other operations on uvula

HCPCS Level II Supplies & Services
A4305 Disposable drug delivery system, flow rate of 50 ml or greater per hour
A4306 Disposable drug delivery system, flow rate of 5 ml or less per hour
A4550 Surgical trays

42180–42182
42180 Repair, laceration of palate; up to 2 cm
42182 over 2 cm or complex

ICD-9-CM Diagnostic
873.65 Open wound of palate, without mention of complication — (Use additional code to identify infection)
873.69 Open wound of mouth, other and multiple sites, without mention of complication — (Use additional code to identify infection)
873.75 Open wound of palate, complicated — (Use additional code to identify infection)
879.8 Open wound(s) (multiple) of unspecified site(s), without mention of complication — (Use additional code to identify infection) ▽

ICD-9-CM Procedural
27.61 Suture of laceration of palate

HCPCS Level II Supplies & Services
A4305 Disposable drug delivery system, flow rate of 50 ml or greater per hour
A4306 Disposable drug delivery system, flow rate of 5 ml or less per hour
A4550 Surgical trays

42200
42200 Palatoplasty for cleft palate, soft and/or hard palate only

ICD-9-CM Diagnostic
749.00 Unspecified cleft palate ▽
749.01 Unilateral cleft palate, complete
749.02 Unilateral cleft palate, incomplete
749.03 Bilateral cleft palate, complete
749.04 Bilateral cleft palate, incomplete
749.13 Bilateral cleft lip, complete
749.14 Bilateral cleft lip, incomplete
749.20 Unspecified cleft palate with cleft lip ▽
749.21 Unilateral cleft palate with cleft lip, complete
749.22 Unilateral cleft palate with cleft lip, incomplete
749.23 Bilateral cleft palate with cleft lip, complete
749.24 Bilateral cleft palate with cleft lip, incomplete
749.25 Other combinations of cleft palate with cleft lip

ICD-9-CM Procedural
27.62 Correction of cleft palate

42205–42210
42205 Palatoplasty for cleft palate, with closure of alveolar ridge; soft tissue only
42210 with bone graft to alveolar ridge (includes obtaining graft)

ICD-9-CM Diagnostic
749.00 Unspecified cleft palate ▽
749.01 Unilateral cleft palate, complete
749.02 Unilateral cleft palate, incomplete
749.03 Bilateral cleft palate, complete
749.04 Bilateral cleft palate, incomplete
749.13 Bilateral cleft lip, complete
749.14 Bilateral cleft lip, incomplete
749.20 Unspecified cleft palate with cleft lip ▽
749.21 Unilateral cleft palate with cleft lip, complete
749.22 Unilateral cleft palate with cleft lip, incomplete
749.23 Bilateral cleft palate with cleft lip, complete
749.24 Bilateral cleft palate with cleft lip, incomplete
749.25 Other combinations of cleft palate with cleft lip

ICD-9-CM Procedural
27.62 Correction of cleft palate
76.91 Bone graft to facial bone
77.79 Excision of other bone for graft, except facial bones

42215
42215 Palatoplasty for cleft palate; major revision

ICD-9-CM Diagnostic
749.00 Unspecified cleft palate ▽
749.01 Unilateral cleft palate, complete
749.02 Unilateral cleft palate, incomplete
749.03 Bilateral cleft palate, complete
749.04 Bilateral cleft palate, incomplete
749.13 Bilateral cleft lip, complete
749.14 Bilateral cleft lip, incomplete
749.20 Unspecified cleft palate with cleft lip ▽
749.21 Unilateral cleft palate with cleft lip, complete
749.22 Unilateral cleft palate with cleft lip, incomplete
749.23 Bilateral cleft palate with cleft lip, complete
749.24 Bilateral cleft palate with cleft lip, incomplete
749.25 Other combinations of cleft palate with cleft lip
783.3 Feeding difficulties and mismanagement
784.49 Other voice disturbance

ICD-9-CM Procedural
27.63 Revision of cleft palate repair

42220
42220 Palatoplasty for cleft palate; secondary lengthening procedure

ICD-9-CM Diagnostic
749.00 Unspecified cleft palate ▽
749.01 Unilateral cleft palate, complete
749.02 Unilateral cleft palate, incomplete
749.03 Bilateral cleft palate, complete
749.04 Bilateral cleft palate, incomplete
749.13 Bilateral cleft lip, complete
749.14 Bilateral cleft lip, incomplete
749.20 Unspecified cleft palate with cleft lip ▽
749.21 Unilateral cleft palate with cleft lip, complete
749.22 Unilateral cleft palate with cleft lip, incomplete
749.23 Bilateral cleft palate with cleft lip, complete
749.24 Bilateral cleft palate with cleft lip, incomplete
749.25 Other combinations of cleft palate with cleft lip
783.3 Feeding difficulties and mismanagement
784.49 Other voice disturbance

ICD-9-CM Procedural
27.63 Revision of cleft palate repair

42225
42225 Palatoplasty for cleft palate; attachment pharyngeal flap

ICD-9-CM Diagnostic
749.00 Unspecified cleft palate ▽
749.01 Unilateral cleft palate, complete
749.02 Unilateral cleft palate, incomplete
749.03 Bilateral cleft palate, complete
749.04 Bilateral cleft palate, incomplete
749.13 Bilateral cleft lip, complete
749.14 Bilateral cleft lip, incomplete

749.20 Unspecified cleft palate with cleft lip ▽
749.21 Unilateral cleft palate with cleft lip, complete
749.22 Unilateral cleft palate with cleft lip, incomplete
749.23 Bilateral cleft palate with cleft lip, complete
749.24 Bilateral cleft palate with cleft lip, incomplete
749.25 Other combinations of cleft palate with cleft lip
783.3 Feeding difficulties and mismanagement
784.49 Other voice disturbance

ICD-9-CM Procedural

27.63 Revision of cleft palate repair

42226

42226 Lengthening of palate, and pharyngeal flap

ICD-9-CM Diagnostic

524.10 Unspecified anomaly of relationship of jaw to cranial base ▽
524.29 Other anomalies of dental arch relationship
524.50 Dentofacial functional abnormality, unspecified
524.59 Other dentofacial functional abnormalities
524.70 Unspecified alveolar anomaly ▽
524.73 Alveolar maxillary hypoplasia
524.79 Other specified alveolar anomaly
528.9 Other and unspecified diseases of the oral soft tissues ▽
749.23 Bilateral cleft palate with cleft lip, complete
750.29 Other specified congenital anomaly of pharynx
754.0 Congenital musculoskeletal deformities of skull, face, and jaw
783.3 Feeding difficulties and mismanagement

ICD-9-CM Procedural

27.63 Revision of cleft palate repair
27.69 Other plastic repair of palate

42227

42227 Lengthening of palate, with island flap

ICD-9-CM Diagnostic

524.10 Unspecified anomaly of relationship of jaw to cranial base ▽
524.29 Other anomalies of dental arch relationship
524.50 Dentofacial functional abnormality, unspecified
524.59 Other dentofacial functional abnormalities
524.70 Unspecified alveolar anomaly ▽
524.71 Alveolar maxillary hyperplasia
524.73 Alveolar maxillary hypoplasia
524.79 Other specified alveolar anomaly
528.9 Other and unspecified diseases of the oral soft tissues ▽
749.00 Unspecified cleft palate ▽
749.01 Unilateral cleft palate, complete
750.29 Other specified congenital anomaly of pharynx
754.0 Congenital musculoskeletal deformities of skull, face, and jaw
784.49 Other voice disturbance

ICD-9-CM Procedural

27.69 Other plastic repair of palate

42235

42235 Repair of anterior palate, including vomer flap

ICD-9-CM Diagnostic

145.2 Malignant neoplasm of hard palate
145.5 Malignant neoplasm of palate, unspecified ▽
147.3 Malignant neoplasm of anterior wall of nasopharynx
198.89 Secondary malignant neoplasm of other specified sites
230.0 Carcinoma in situ of lip, oral cavity, and pharynx
478.29 Other disease of pharynx or nasopharynx
526.89 Other specified disease of the jaws
749.00 Unspecified cleft palate ▽
749.22 Unilateral cleft palate with cleft lip, incomplete
749.23 Bilateral cleft palate with cleft lip, complete
783.3 Feeding difficulties and mismanagement
802.5 Malar and maxillary bones, open fracture
873.65 Open wound of palate, without mention of complication — (Use additional code to identify infection)
873.75 Open wound of palate, complicated — (Use additional code to identify infection)

ICD-9-CM Procedural

27.69 Other plastic repair of palate

42260

42260 Repair of nasolabial fistula

ICD-9-CM Diagnostic

473.0 Chronic maxillary sinusitis
473.2 Chronic ethmoidal sinusitis
473.3 Chronic sphenoidal sinusitis
473.8 Other chronic sinusitis
473.9 Unspecified sinusitis (chronic) ▽
478.1 Other diseases of nasal cavity and sinuses
519.8 Other diseases of respiratory system, not elsewhere classified
519.9 Unspecified disease of respiratory system ▽
528.3 Cellulitis and abscess of oral soft tissues
528.5 Diseases of lips
748.1 Other congenital anomaly of nose
750.25 Congenital fistula of lip
873.51 Open wound of cheek, complicated — (Use additional code to identify infection)
873.53 Open wound of lip, complicated — (Use additional code to identify infection)

ICD-9-CM Procedural

21.82 Closure of nasal fistula

42280–42281

42280 Maxillary impression for palatal prosthesis
42281 Insertion of pin-retained palatal prosthesis

ICD-9-CM Diagnostic

145.2 Malignant neoplasm of hard palate
145.5 Malignant neoplasm of palate, unspecified ▽
198.89 Secondary malignant neoplasm of other specified sites
230.0 Carcinoma in situ of lip, oral cavity, and pharynx
526.89 Other specified disease of the jaws
749.00 Unspecified cleft palate ▽
749.01 Unilateral cleft palate, complete
749.02 Unilateral cleft palate, incomplete
749.03 Bilateral cleft palate, complete
749.04 Bilateral cleft palate, incomplete
749.13 Bilateral cleft lip, complete
749.14 Bilateral cleft lip, incomplete
749.20 Unspecified cleft palate with cleft lip ▽
749.21 Unilateral cleft palate with cleft lip, complete
749.22 Unilateral cleft palate with cleft lip, incomplete
749.23 Bilateral cleft palate with cleft lip, complete
749.24 Bilateral cleft palate with cleft lip, incomplete
749.25 Other combinations of cleft palate with cleft lip
750.9 Unspecified congenital anomaly of upper alimentary tract ▽
873.65 Open wound of palate, without mention of complication — (Use additional code to identify infection)
873.75 Open wound of palate, complicated — (Use additional code to identify infection)
906.0 Late effect of open wound of head, neck, and trunk
V10.02 Personal history of malignant neoplasm of other and unspecified parts of oral cavity and pharynx ▽
V13.69 Personal history of other congenital malformations
V51 Aftercare involving the use of plastic surgery
V52.8 Fitting and adjustment of other specified prosthetic device

ICD-9-CM Procedural

27.64 Insertion of palatal implant
27.69 Other plastic repair of palate
99.99 Other miscellaneous procedures

Salivary Gland and Ducts

42300–42305

42300 Drainage of abscess; parotid, simple
42305 parotid, complicated

ICD-9-CM Diagnostic

527.2 Sialoadenitis
527.3 Abscess of salivary gland
528.3 Cellulitis and abscess of oral soft tissues
682.0 Cellulitis and abscess of face — (Use additional code to identify organism)
958.3 Posttraumatic wound infection not elsewhere classified

ICD-9-CM Procedural

26.0 Incision of salivary gland or duct

HCPCS Level II Supplies & Services

A4550 Surgical trays

42310–42320

42310 Drainage of abscess; submaxillary or sublingual, intraoral
42320 submaxillary, external

ICD-9-CM Diagnostic

527.2 Sialoadenitis
527.3 Abscess of salivary gland
527.4 Fistula of salivary gland
527.6 Mucocele of salivary gland
528.3 Cellulitis and abscess of oral soft tissues
682.0 Cellulitis and abscess of face — (Use additional code to identify organism)
958.3 Posttraumatic wound infection not elsewhere classified

ICD-9-CM Procedural

26.0 Incision of salivary gland or duct

HCPCS Level II Supplies & Services

A4305 Disposable drug delivery system, flow rate of 50 ml or greater per hour
A4306 Disposable drug delivery system, flow rate of 5 ml or less per hour
A4550 Surgical trays

42325–42326

42325 Fistulization of sublingual salivary cyst (ranula);
42326 with prosthesis

ICD-9-CM Diagnostic

527.6 Mucocele of salivary gland
750.26 Other specified congenital anomalies of mouth

ICD-9-CM Procedural

26.49 Other repair and plastic operations on salivary gland or duct

HCPCS Level II Supplies & Services

A4305 Disposable drug delivery system, flow rate of 50 ml or greater per hour
A4306 Disposable drug delivery system, flow rate of 5 ml or less per hour
A4550 Surgical trays

42330–42340

42330 Sialolithotomy; submandibular (submaxillary), sublingual or parotid, uncomplicated, intraoral
42335 submandibular (submaxillary), complicated, intraoral
42340 parotid, extraoral or complicated intraoral

ICD-9-CM Diagnostic

527.2 Sialoadenitis
527.5 Sialolithiasis
784.2 Swelling, mass, or lump in head and neck
793.4 Nonspecific abnormal findings on radiological and other examination of gastrointestinal tract

ICD-9-CM Procedural

26.0 Incision of salivary gland or duct

HCPCS Level II Supplies & Services

A4305 Disposable drug delivery system, flow rate of 50 ml or greater per hour
A4306 Disposable drug delivery system, flow rate of 5 ml or less per hour
A4550 Surgical trays

42400–42405

42400 Biopsy of salivary gland; needle
42405 incisional

ICD-9-CM Diagnostic

142.0 Malignant neoplasm of parotid gland
142.1 Malignant neoplasm of submandibular gland
142.2 Malignant neoplasm of sublingual gland
142.8 Malignant neoplasm of other major salivary glands
142.9 Malignant neoplasm of salivary gland, unspecified ▽
198.89 Secondary malignant neoplasm of other specified sites
210.2 Benign neoplasm of major salivary glands
230.0 Carcinoma in situ of lip, oral cavity, and pharynx
235.0 Neoplasm of uncertain behavior of major salivary glands
238.9 Neoplasm of uncertain behavior, site unspecified ▽
239.0 Neoplasm of unspecified nature of digestive system
239.8 Neoplasm of unspecified nature of other specified sites
359.6 Symptomatic inflammatory myopathy in diseases classified elsewhere — (Code first underlying disease: 135, 140.0-208.9, 277.3, 446.0, 710.0, 710.1, 710.2, 714.0) ☒
517.8 Lung involvement in other diseases classified elsewhere — (Code first underlying disease: 135, 277.3, 710.0, 710.2, 710.4) ☒
527.1 Hypertrophy of salivary gland
527.2 Sialoadenitis
527.3 Abscess of salivary gland
527.5 Sialolithiasis
527.8 Other specified diseases of the salivary glands
710.2 Sicca syndrome
784.2 Swelling, mass, or lump in head and neck
V41.5 Problems with smell and taste — (This code is intended for use when these conditions are recorded as diagnoses or problems)

ICD-9-CM Procedural

26.11 Closed (needle) biopsy of salivary gland or duct
26.12 Open biopsy of salivary gland or duct

HCPCS Level II Supplies & Services

A4305 Disposable drug delivery system, flow rate of 50 ml or greater per hour
A4306 Disposable drug delivery system, flow rate of 5 ml or less per hour
A4550 Surgical trays

42408

42408 Excision of sublingual salivary cyst (ranula)

ICD-9-CM Diagnostic

527.6 Mucocele of salivary gland
750.26 Other specified congenital anomalies of mouth

ICD-9-CM Procedural

26.29 Other excision of salivary gland lesion

HCPCS Level II Supplies & Services

A4305 Disposable drug delivery system, flow rate of 50 ml or greater per hour
A4306 Disposable drug delivery system, flow rate of 5 ml or less per hour
A4550 Surgical trays

42409

42409 Marsupialization of sublingual salivary cyst (ranula)

ICD-9-CM Diagnostic

527.6 Mucocele of salivary gland
750.26 Other specified congenital anomalies of mouth

ICD-9-CM Procedural

26.21 Marsupialization of salivary gland cyst

HCPCS Level II Supplies & Services

A4305 Disposable drug delivery system, flow rate of 50 ml or greater per hour
A4306 Disposable drug delivery system, flow rate of 5 ml or less per hour
A4550 Surgical trays

42410–42415

42410	Excision of parotid tumor or parotid gland; lateral lobe, without nerve dissection
42415	lateral lobe, with dissection and preservation of facial nerve

ICD-9-CM Diagnostic

142.0	Malignant neoplasm of parotid gland
142.9	Malignant neoplasm of salivary gland, unspecified ▽
198.89	Secondary malignant neoplasm of other specified sites
210.2	Benign neoplasm of major salivary glands
230.0	Carcinoma in situ of lip, oral cavity, and pharynx
235.0	Neoplasm of uncertain behavior of major salivary glands
239.0	Neoplasm of unspecified nature of digestive system
527.2	Sialoadenitis
527.6	Mucocele of salivary gland
784.2	Swelling, mass, or lump in head and neck
785.6	Enlargement of lymph nodes

ICD-9-CM Procedural

26.29	Other excision of salivary gland lesion
26.31	Partial sialoadenectomy

42420–42426

42420	Excision of parotid tumor or parotid gland; total, with dissection and preservation of facial nerve
42425	total, en bloc removal with sacrifice of facial nerve
42426	total, with unilateral radical neck dissection

ICD-9-CM Diagnostic

142.0	Malignant neoplasm of parotid gland
142.9	Malignant neoplasm of salivary gland, unspecified ▽
196.0	Secondary and unspecified malignant neoplasm of lymph nodes of head, face, and neck
198.89	Secondary malignant neoplasm of other specified sites
210.2	Benign neoplasm of major salivary glands
230.0	Carcinoma in situ of lip, oral cavity, and pharynx
235.0	Neoplasm of uncertain behavior of major salivary glands
239.0	Neoplasm of unspecified nature of digestive system
527.2	Sialoadenitis
527.6	Mucocele of salivary gland
784.2	Swelling, mass, or lump in head and neck
785.6	Enlargement of lymph nodes

ICD-9-CM Procedural

04.07	Other excision or avulsion of cranial and peripheral nerves
26.32	Complete sialoadenectomy
40.41	Radical neck dissection, unilateral

42440

42440	Excision of submandibular (submaxillary) gland

ICD-9-CM Diagnostic

142.1	Malignant neoplasm of submandibular gland
198.89	Secondary malignant neoplasm of other specified sites
210.2	Benign neoplasm of major salivary glands
230.0	Carcinoma in situ of lip, oral cavity, and pharynx
235.0	Neoplasm of uncertain behavior of major salivary glands
235.1	Neoplasm of uncertain behavior of lip, oral cavity, and pharynx
239.0	Neoplasm of unspecified nature of digestive system
527.1	Hypertrophy of salivary gland
527.2	Sialoadenitis
527.5	Sialolithiasis
527.6	Mucocele of salivary gland
527.8	Other specified diseases of the salivary glands
784.2	Swelling, mass, or lump in head and neck

ICD-9-CM Procedural

26.30	Sialoadenectomy, not otherwise specified
26.31	Partial sialoadenectomy
26.32	Complete sialoadenectomy

42450

42450	Excision of sublingual gland

ICD-9-CM Diagnostic

142.2	Malignant neoplasm of sublingual gland
144.9	Malignant neoplasm of floor of mouth, part unspecified ▽
198.89	Secondary malignant neoplasm of other specified sites
210.2	Benign neoplasm of major salivary glands
210.3	Benign neoplasm of floor of mouth
230.0	Carcinoma in situ of lip, oral cavity, and pharynx
235.0	Neoplasm of uncertain behavior of major salivary glands
235.1	Neoplasm of uncertain behavior of lip, oral cavity, and pharynx
239.0	Neoplasm of unspecified nature of digestive system
527.1	Hypertrophy of salivary gland
527.2	Sialoadenitis
527.5	Sialolithiasis
527.6	Mucocele of salivary gland
527.8	Other specified diseases of the salivary glands
784.2	Swelling, mass, or lump in head and neck
787.2	Dysphagia

ICD-9-CM Procedural

26.30	Sialoadenectomy, not otherwise specified
26.31	Partial sialoadenectomy
26.32	Complete sialoadenectomy

42500–42505

42500	Plastic repair of salivary duct, sialodochoplasty; primary or simple
42505	secondary or complicated

ICD-9-CM Diagnostic

527.2	Sialoadenitis
527.4	Fistula of salivary gland
527.5	Sialolithiasis
527.6	Mucocele of salivary gland
527.7	Disturbance of salivary secretion
527.8	Other specified diseases of the salivary glands
873.51	Open wound of cheek, complicated — (Use additional code to identify infection)
873.54	Open wound of jaw, complicated — (Use additional code to identify infection)
873.69	Open wound of mouth, other and multiple sites, without mention of complication — (Use additional code to identify infection)
873.79	Open wound of mouth, other and multiple sites, complicated — (Use additional code to identify infection)
906.0	Late effect of open wound of head, neck, and trunk
998.2	Accidental puncture or laceration during procedure

ICD-9-CM Procedural

26.49	Other repair and plastic operations on salivary gland or duct

HCPCS Level II Supplies & Services

A4305	Disposable drug delivery system, flow rate of 50 ml or greater per hour
A4306	Disposable drug delivery system, flow rate of 5 ml or less per hour
A4550	Surgical trays

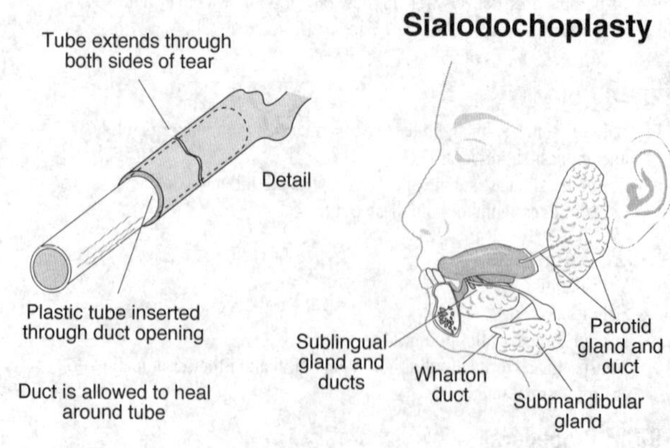

Sialodochoplasty
Tube extends through both sides of tear
Detail
Plastic tube inserted through duct opening
Duct is allowed to heal around tube
Sublingual gland and ducts
Wharton duct
Parotid gland and duct
Submandibular gland

▽ Unspecified code
♀ Female diagnosis
☒ Manifestation code
♂ Male diagnosis

42507–42510

42507 Parotid duct diversion, bilateral (Wilke type procedure);
42508 with excision of one submandibular gland
42509 with excision of both submandibular glands
42510 with ligation of both submandibular (Wharton's) ducts

ICD-9-CM Diagnostic

527.5 Sialolithiasis
527.7 Disturbance of salivary secretion
527.8 Other specified diseases of the salivary glands
873.51 Open wound of cheek, complicated — (Use additional code to identify infection)
873.59 Open wound of face, other and multiple sites, complicated — (Use additional code to identify infection)
873.61 Open wound of buccal mucosa, without mention of complication — (Use additional code to identify infection)
873.69 Open wound of mouth, other and multiple sites, without mention of complication — (Use additional code to identify infection)
873.71 Open wound of buccal mucosa, complicated — (Use additional code to identify infection)
873.79 Open wound of mouth, other and multiple sites, complicated — (Use additional code to identify infection)
906.0 Late effect of open wound of head, neck, and trunk

ICD-9-CM Procedural

26.31 Partial sialoadenectomy
26.32 Complete sialoadenectomy
26.49 Other repair and plastic operations on salivary gland or duct
26.99 Other operations on salivary gland or duct

42550

42550 Injection procedure for sialography

ICD-9-CM Diagnostic

142.0 Malignant neoplasm of parotid gland
142.1 Malignant neoplasm of submandibular gland
142.2 Malignant neoplasm of sublingual gland
142.8 Malignant neoplasm of other major salivary glands
142.9 Malignant neoplasm of salivary gland, unspecified ▽
144.9 Malignant neoplasm of floor of mouth, part unspecified ▽
210.2 Benign neoplasm of major salivary glands
210.3 Benign neoplasm of floor of mouth
210.4 Benign neoplasm of other and unspecified parts of mouth ▽
230.0 Carcinoma in situ of lip, oral cavity, and pharynx
235.0 Neoplasm of uncertain behavior of major salivary glands
235.1 Neoplasm of uncertain behavior of lip, oral cavity, and pharynx
239.0 Neoplasm of unspecified nature of digestive system
527.1 Hypertrophy of salivary gland
527.2 Sialoadenitis
527.5 Sialolithiasis
527.6 Mucocele of salivary gland
527.7 Disturbance of salivary secretion
527.8 Other specified diseases of the salivary glands
527.9 Unspecified disease of the salivary glands ▽
784.2 Swelling, mass, or lump in head and neck
787.2 Dysphagia
V72.5 Radiological examination, not elsewhere classified — (Use additional code(s) to identify any special screening examination(s) performed: V73.0-V82.9)

ICD-9-CM Procedural

26.19 Other diagnostic procedures on salivary glands and ducts
87.09 Other soft tissue x-ray of face, head, and neck

HCPCS Level II Supplies & Services

A4305 Disposable drug delivery system, flow rate of 50 ml or greater per hour
A4550 Surgical trays
A9525 Supply of low or iso-osmolar contrast material, 10 mg of iodine

42600

42600 Closure salivary fistula

ICD-9-CM Diagnostic

527.4 Fistula of salivary gland
750.24 Congenital fistula of salivary gland
998.6 Persistent postoperative fistula, not elsewhere classified

ICD-9-CM Procedural

26.42 Closure of salivary fistula

HCPCS Level II Supplies & Services

A4305 Disposable drug delivery system, flow rate of 50 ml or greater per hour
A4306 Disposable drug delivery system, flow rate of 5 ml or less per hour
A4550 Surgical trays

42650–42660

42650 Dilation salivary duct
42660 Dilation and catheterization of salivary duct, with or without injection

ICD-9-CM Diagnostic

210.2 Benign neoplasm of major salivary glands
235.0 Neoplasm of uncertain behavior of major salivary glands
527.2 Sialoadenitis
527.5 Sialolithiasis
527.7 Disturbance of salivary secretion
527.8 Other specified diseases of the salivary glands
784.2 Swelling, mass, or lump in head and neck

ICD-9-CM Procedural

26.91 Probing of salivary duct

HCPCS Level II Supplies & Services

A4305 Disposable drug delivery system, flow rate of 50 ml or greater per hour
A4306 Disposable drug delivery system, flow rate of 5 ml or less per hour
A4550 Surgical trays

42665

42665 Ligation salivary duct, intraoral

ICD-9-CM Diagnostic

527.2 Sialoadenitis
527.4 Fistula of salivary gland
527.5 Sialolithiasis
527.7 Disturbance of salivary secretion
527.8 Other specified diseases of the salivary glands

ICD-9-CM Procedural

26.99 Other operations on salivary gland or duct

HCPCS Level II Supplies & Services

A4305 Disposable drug delivery system, flow rate of 50 ml or greater per hour
A4306 Disposable drug delivery system, flow rate of 5 ml or less per hour
A4550 Surgical trays

Pharynx, Adenoids, and Tonsils

42700

42700 Incision and drainage abscess; peritonsillar

ICD-9-CM Diagnostic

462 Acute pharyngitis — (Use additional code to identify infectious organism)
463 Acute tonsillitis — (Use additional code to identify infectious organism)
474.00 Chronic tonsillitis
474.01 Chronic adenoiditis
474.02 Chronic tonsillitis and adenoiditis
474.10 Hypertrophy of tonsil with adenoids
474.11 Hypertrophy of tonsils alone
474.12 Hypertrophy of adenoids alone
474.8 Other chronic disease of tonsils and adenoids
475 Peritonsillar abscess — (Use additional code to identify infectious organism)
478.24 Retropharyngeal abscess
478.29 Other disease of pharynx or nasopharynx
784.2 Swelling, mass, or lump in head and neck

ICD-9-CM Procedural

28.0 Incision and drainage of tonsil and peritonsillar structures

HCPCS Level II Supplies & Services

A4305 Disposable drug delivery system, flow rate of 50 ml or greater per hour
A4306 Disposable drug delivery system, flow rate of 5 ml or less per hour
A4550 Surgical trays

▽ Unspecified code
♀ Female diagnosis
☒ Manifestation code
♂ Male diagnosis

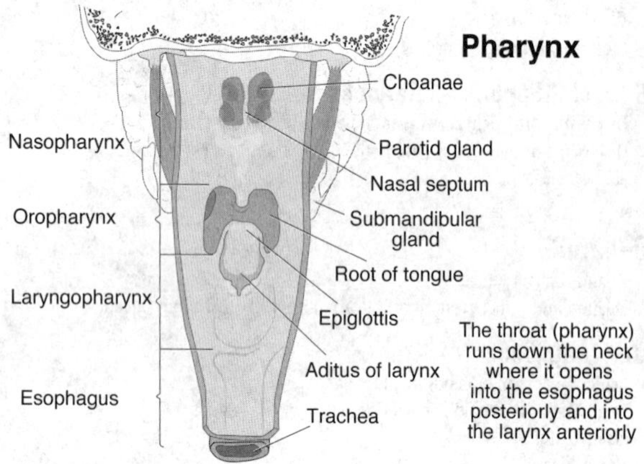

42720–42725

42720 Incision and drainage abscess; retropharyngeal or parapharyngeal, intraoral approach
42725 retropharyngeal or parapharyngeal, external approach

ICD-9-CM Diagnostic

475 Peritonsillar abscess — (Use additional code to identify infectious organism)
478.21 Cellulitis of pharynx or nasopharynx
478.22 Parapharyngeal abscess
478.24 Retropharyngeal abscess
478.29 Other disease of pharynx or nasopharynx

ICD-9-CM Procedural

28.0 Incision and drainage of tonsil and peritonsillar structures

HCPCS Level II Supplies & Services

A4305 Disposable drug delivery system, flow rate of 50 ml or greater per hour
A4306 Disposable drug delivery system, flow rate of 5 ml or less per hour
A4550 Surgical trays

42800–42802

42800 Biopsy; oropharynx
42802 hypopharynx

ICD-9-CM Diagnostic

146.0 Malignant neoplasm of tonsil
146.1 Malignant neoplasm of tonsillar fossa
146.2 Malignant neoplasm of tonsillar pillars (anterior) (posterior)
146.3 Malignant neoplasm of vallecula
146.4 Malignant neoplasm of anterior aspect of epiglottis
146.6 Malignant neoplasm of lateral wall of oropharynx
146.7 Malignant neoplasm of posterior wall of oropharynx
146.8 Malignant neoplasm of other specified sites of oropharynx
146.9 Malignant neoplasm of oropharynx, unspecified site ▽
148.0 Malignant neoplasm of postcricoid region of hypopharynx
148.1 Malignant neoplasm of pyriform sinus
148.2 Malignant neoplasm of aryepiglottic fold, hypopharyngeal aspect
148.3 Malignant neoplasm of posterior hypopharyngeal wall
148.8 Malignant neoplasm of other specified sites of hypopharynx
148.9 Malignant neoplasm of hypopharynx, unspecified site ▽
149.0 Malignant neoplasm of pharynx, unspecified ▽
149.8 Malignant neoplasm of other sites within the lip and oral cavity
149.9 Malignant neoplasm of ill-defined sites of lip and oral cavity
176.2 Kaposi's sarcoma of palate
176.8 Kaposi's sarcoma of other specified sites
196.0 Secondary and unspecified malignant neoplasm of lymph nodes of head, face, and neck
198.89 Secondary malignant neoplasm of other specified sites
202.81 Other malignant lymphomas of lymph nodes of head, face, and neck
210.5 Benign neoplasm of tonsil
210.6 Benign neoplasm of other parts of oropharynx
210.8 Benign neoplasm of hypopharynx
210.9 Benign neoplasm of pharynx, unspecified ▽
230.0 Carcinoma in situ of lip, oral cavity, and pharynx
235.1 Neoplasm of uncertain behavior of lip, oral cavity, and pharynx
239.0 Neoplasm of unspecified nature of digestive system
446.4 Wegener's granulomatosis
478.21 Cellulitis of pharynx or nasopharynx
478.22 Parapharyngeal abscess
478.24 Retropharyngeal abscess
478.26 Cyst of pharynx or nasopharynx
478.29 Other disease of pharynx or nasopharynx
528.2 Oral aphthae
528.6 Leukoplakia of oral mucosa, including tongue
528.9 Other and unspecified diseases of the oral soft tissues ▽

ICD-9-CM Procedural

29.12 Pharyngeal biopsy

HCPCS Level II Supplies & Services

A4305 Disposable drug delivery system, flow rate of 50 ml or greater per hour
A4306 Disposable drug delivery system, flow rate of 5 ml or less per hour
A4550 Surgical trays

42804–42806

42804 Biopsy; nasopharynx, visible lesion, simple
42806 nasopharynx, survey for unknown primary lesion

ICD-9-CM Diagnostic

147.0 Malignant neoplasm of superior wall of nasopharynx
147.1 Malignant neoplasm of posterior wall of nasopharynx
147.2 Malignant neoplasm of lateral wall of nasopharynx
147.3 Malignant neoplasm of anterior wall of nasopharynx
147.8 Malignant neoplasm of other specified sites of nasopharynx
147.9 Malignant neoplasm of nasopharynx, unspecified site ▽
149.0 Malignant neoplasm of pharynx, unspecified ▽
196.0 Secondary and unspecified malignant neoplasm of lymph nodes of head, face, and neck
198.89 Secondary malignant neoplasm of other specified sites
202.81 Other malignant lymphomas of lymph nodes of head, face, and neck
210.5 Benign neoplasm of tonsil
210.7 Benign neoplasm of nasopharynx
210.9 Benign neoplasm of pharynx, unspecified ▽
229.9 Benign neoplasm of unspecified site ▽
230.0 Carcinoma in situ of lip, oral cavity, and pharynx
235.1 Neoplasm of uncertain behavior of lip, oral cavity, and pharynx
239.0 Neoplasm of unspecified nature of digestive system
475 Peritonsillar abscess — (Use additional code to identify infectious organism)
478.0 Hypertrophy of nasal turbinates
478.21 Cellulitis of pharynx or nasopharynx
478.26 Cyst of pharynx or nasopharynx
478.29 Other disease of pharynx or nasopharynx

ICD-9-CM Procedural

29.12 Pharyngeal biopsy

HCPCS Level II Supplies & Services

A4305 Disposable drug delivery system, flow rate of 50 ml or greater per hour
A4306 Disposable drug delivery system, flow rate of 5 ml or less per hour
A4550 Surgical trays

42808

42808 Excision or destruction of lesion of pharynx, any method

ICD-9-CM Diagnostic

146.0 Malignant neoplasm of tonsil
147.0 Malignant neoplasm of superior wall of nasopharynx
147.1 Malignant neoplasm of posterior wall of nasopharynx
147.2 Malignant neoplasm of lateral wall of nasopharynx
147.3 Malignant neoplasm of anterior wall of nasopharynx
147.9 Malignant neoplasm of nasopharynx, unspecified site ▽
148.0 Malignant neoplasm of postcricoid region of hypopharynx
148.1 Malignant neoplasm of pyriform sinus
148.2 Malignant neoplasm of aryepiglottic fold, hypopharyngeal aspect
148.3 Malignant neoplasm of posterior hypopharyngeal wall
148.9 Malignant neoplasm of hypopharynx, unspecified site ▽
149.0 Malignant neoplasm of pharynx, unspecified ▽
198.89 Secondary malignant neoplasm of other specified sites
210.5 Benign neoplasm of tonsil
210.6 Benign neoplasm of other parts of oropharynx
210.7 Benign neoplasm of nasopharynx
210.8 Benign neoplasm of hypopharynx
210.9 Benign neoplasm of pharynx, unspecified ▽

▽ Unspecified code ♀ Female diagnosis ☒ Manifestation code ♂ Male diagnosis

230.0 Carcinoma in situ of lip, oral cavity, and pharynx
235.1 Neoplasm of uncertain behavior of lip, oral cavity, and pharynx
239.0 Neoplasm of unspecified nature of digestive system
478.26 Cyst of pharynx or nasopharynx
478.29 Other disease of pharynx or nasopharynx

ICD-9-CM Procedural
29.39 Other excision or destruction of lesion or tissue of pharynx

HCPCS Level II Supplies & Services
A4305 Disposable drug delivery system, flow rate of 50 ml or greater per hour
A4306 Disposable drug delivery system, flow rate of 5 ml or less per hour
A4550 Surgical trays

42809
42809 Removal of foreign body from pharynx

ICD-9-CM Diagnostic
784.1 Throat pain
873.70 Open wound of mouth, unspecified site, complicated — (Use additional code to identify infection) ▽
873.79 Open wound of mouth, other and multiple sites, complicated — (Use additional code to identify infection)
933.0 Foreign body in pharynx
998.4 Foreign body accidentally left during procedure, not elsewhere classified
998.7 Acute reaction to foreign substance accidentally left during procedure, not elsewhere classified

ICD-9-CM Procedural
29.0 Pharyngotomy
98.13 Removal of intraluminal foreign body from pharynx without incision

HCPCS Level II Supplies & Services
A4305 Disposable drug delivery system, flow rate of 50 ml or greater per hour
A4306 Disposable drug delivery system, flow rate of 5 ml or less per hour
A4550 Surgical trays

42810–42815
42810 Excision branchial cleft cyst or vestige, confined to skin and subcutaneous tissues
42815 Excision branchial cleft cyst, vestige, or fistula, extending beneath subcutaneous tissues and/or into pharynx

ICD-9-CM Diagnostic
744.41 Congenital branchial cleft sinus or fistula
744.42 Congenital branchial cleft cyst
744.43 Congenital cervical auricle
744.46 Congenital preauricular sinus or fistula
744.47 Congenital preauricular cyst
744.49 Other congenital branchial cleft cyst or fistula; preauricular sinus
744.89 Other specified congenital anomaly of face and neck

ICD-9-CM Procedural
29.2 Excision of branchial cleft cyst or vestige
29.52 Closure of branchial cleft fistula

HCPCS Level II Supplies & Services
A4305 Disposable drug delivery system, flow rate of 50 ml or greater per hour
A4306 Disposable drug delivery system, flow rate of 5 ml or less per hour
A4550 Surgical trays

42820–42821
42820 Tonsillectomy and adenoidectomy; under age 12
42821 age 12 or over

ICD-9-CM Diagnostic
034.0 Streptococcal sore throat
146.0 Malignant neoplasm of tonsil
210.5 Benign neoplasm of tonsil
463 Acute tonsillitis — (Use additional code to identify infectious organism)
472.0 Chronic rhinitis
472.1 Chronic pharyngitis
473.0 Chronic maxillary sinusitis
473.1 Chronic frontal sinusitis
473.2 Chronic ethmoidal sinusitis
473.8 Other chronic sinusitis
474.00 Chronic tonsillitis
474.01 Chronic adenoiditis
474.02 Chronic tonsillitis and adenoiditis
474.10 Hypertrophy of tonsil with adenoids
474.11 Hypertrophy of tonsils alone
474.12 Hypertrophy of adenoids alone
474.2 Adenoid vegetations
474.8 Other chronic disease of tonsils and adenoids
474.9 Unspecified chronic disease of tonsils and adenoids ▽
475 Peritonsillar abscess — (Use additional code to identify infectious organism)
478.1 Other diseases of nasal cavity and sinuses
519.8 Other diseases of respiratory system, not elsewhere classified
780.51 Insomnia with sleep apnea
780.53 Hypersomnia with sleep apnea
780.57 Other and unspecified sleep apnea ▽
780.59 Other sleep disturbances
786.09 Other dyspnea and respiratory abnormalities
V12.09 Personal history of other infectious and parasitic disease

ICD-9-CM Procedural
28.3 Tonsillectomy with adenoidectomy

42825–42826
42825 Tonsillectomy, primary or secondary; under age 12
42826 age 12 or over

ICD-9-CM Diagnostic
034.0 Streptococcal sore throat
146.0 Malignant neoplasm of tonsil
210.5 Benign neoplasm of tonsil
463 Acute tonsillitis — (Use additional code to identify infectious organism)
472.1 Chronic pharyngitis
473.0 Chronic maxillary sinusitis
473.1 Chronic frontal sinusitis
473.2 Chronic ethmoidal sinusitis
473.8 Other chronic sinusitis
473.9 Unspecified sinusitis (chronic) ▽
474.11 Hypertrophy of tonsils alone
474.8 Other chronic disease of tonsils and adenoids
475 Peritonsillar abscess — (Use additional code to identify infectious organism)
V12.09 Personal history of other infectious and parasitic disease

ICD-9-CM Procedural
28.2 Tonsillectomy without adenoidectomy

42830–42836
42830 Adenoidectomy, primary; under age 12
42831 age 12 or over
42835 Adenoidectomy, secondary; under age 12
42836 age 12 or over

ICD-9-CM Diagnostic
147.1 Malignant neoplasm of posterior wall of nasopharynx
198.89 Secondary malignant neoplasm of other specified sites
210.7 Benign neoplasm of nasopharynx
230.0 Carcinoma in situ of lip, oral cavity, and pharynx
235.1 Neoplasm of uncertain behavior of lip, oral cavity, and pharynx
239.0 Neoplasm of unspecified nature of digestive system
381.10 Simple or unspecified chronic serous otitis media
382.3 Unspecified chronic suppurative otitis media ▽
382.9 Unspecified otitis media ▽
472.2 Chronic nasopharyngitis
473.0 Chronic maxillary sinusitis
473.1 Chronic frontal sinusitis
473.2 Chronic ethmoidal sinusitis
473.8 Other chronic sinusitis
473.9 Unspecified sinusitis (chronic) ▽
474.01 Chronic adenoiditis
474.12 Hypertrophy of adenoids alone
474.2 Adenoid vegetations
474.8 Other chronic disease of tonsils and adenoids
474.9 Unspecified chronic disease of tonsils and adenoids ▽
478.1 Other diseases of nasal cavity and sinuses
478.29 Other disease of pharynx or nasopharynx
519.8 Other diseases of respiratory system, not elsewhere classified
786.09 Other dyspnea and respiratory abnormalities

ICD-9-CM Procedural
28.6 Adenoidectomy without tonsillectomy

42842–42845
42842 Radical resection of tonsil, tonsillar pillars, and/or retromolar trigone; without closure
42844 closure with local flap (eg, tongue, buccal)
42845 closure with other flap

ICD-9-CM Diagnostic
141.6 Malignant neoplasm of lingual tonsil
145.6 Malignant neoplasm of retromolar area
146.0 Malignant neoplasm of tonsil
146.1 Malignant neoplasm of tonsillar fossa
146.2 Malignant neoplasm of tonsillar pillars (anterior) (posterior)
146.3 Malignant neoplasm of vallecula
146.4 Malignant neoplasm of anterior aspect of epiglottis
146.5 Malignant neoplasm of junctional region of oropharynx
146.6 Malignant neoplasm of lateral wall of oropharynx
147.1 Malignant neoplasm of posterior wall of nasopharynx
198.89 Secondary malignant neoplasm of other specified sites
210.6 Benign neoplasm of other parts of oropharynx
210.7 Benign neoplasm of nasopharynx
230.0 Carcinoma in situ of lip, oral cavity, and pharynx
235.1 Neoplasm of uncertain behavior of lip, oral cavity, and pharynx
239.0 Neoplasm of unspecified nature of digestive system

ICD-9-CM Procedural
25.2 Partial glossectomy
25.4 Radical glossectomy
28.99 Other operations on tonsils and adenoids

42860
42860 Excision of tonsil tags

ICD-9-CM Diagnostic
474.8 Other chronic disease of tonsils and adenoids

ICD-9-CM Procedural
28.4 Excision of tonsil tag

42870
42870 Excision or destruction lingual tonsil, any method (separate procedure)

ICD-9-CM Diagnostic
141.6 Malignant neoplasm of lingual tonsil
198.89 Secondary malignant neoplasm of other specified sites
210.1 Benign neoplasm of tongue
230.0 Carcinoma in situ of lip, oral cavity, and pharynx
235.1 Neoplasm of uncertain behavior of lip, oral cavity, and pharynx
239.0 Neoplasm of unspecified nature of digestive system
463 Acute tonsillitis — (Use additional code to identify infectious organism)
474.00 Chronic tonsillitis
474.02 Chronic tonsillitis and adenoiditis
474.8 Other chronic disease of tonsils and adenoids
475 Peritonsillar abscess — (Use additional code to identify infectious organism)
744.89 Other specified congenital anomaly of face and neck

ICD-9-CM Procedural
28.5 Excision of lingual tonsil

42890
42890 Limited pharyngectomy

ICD-9-CM Diagnostic
146.0 Malignant neoplasm of tonsil
146.1 Malignant neoplasm of tonsillar fossa
146.2 Malignant neoplasm of tonsillar pillars (anterior) (posterior)
146.3 Malignant neoplasm of vallecula
146.4 Malignant neoplasm of anterior aspect of epiglottis
146.5 Malignant neoplasm of junctional region of oropharynx
146.6 Malignant neoplasm of lateral wall of oropharynx
146.7 Malignant neoplasm of posterior wall of oropharynx
146.8 Malignant neoplasm of other specified sites of oropharynx
147.1 Malignant neoplasm of posterior wall of nasopharynx
147.2 Malignant neoplasm of lateral wall of nasopharynx
147.3 Malignant neoplasm of anterior wall of nasopharynx
149.0 Malignant neoplasm of pharynx, unspecified ▽
198.89 Secondary malignant neoplasm of other specified sites
210.5 Benign neoplasm of tonsil
210.6 Benign neoplasm of other parts of oropharynx
210.7 Benign neoplasm of nasopharynx
210.8 Benign neoplasm of hypopharynx
230.0 Carcinoma in situ of lip, oral cavity, and pharynx
235.1 Neoplasm of uncertain behavior of lip, oral cavity, and pharynx
239.0 Neoplasm of unspecified nature of digestive system
472.1 Chronic pharyngitis
478.21 Cellulitis of pharynx or nasopharynx

ICD-9-CM Procedural
29.33 Pharyngectomy (partial)

42892–42894
42892 Resection of lateral pharyngeal wall or pyriform sinus, direct closure by advancement of lateral and posterior pharyngeal walls
42894 Resection of pharyngeal wall requiring closure with myocutaneous flap

ICD-9-CM Diagnostic
146.0 Malignant neoplasm of tonsil
146.1 Malignant neoplasm of tonsillar fossa
146.2 Malignant neoplasm of tonsillar pillars (anterior) (posterior)
146.3 Malignant neoplasm of vallecula
146.4 Malignant neoplasm of anterior aspect of epiglottis
146.5 Malignant neoplasm of junctional region of oropharynx
146.6 Malignant neoplasm of lateral wall of oropharynx
146.7 Malignant neoplasm of posterior wall of oropharynx
146.8 Malignant neoplasm of other specified sites of oropharynx
147.1 Malignant neoplasm of posterior wall of nasopharynx
147.2 Malignant neoplasm of lateral wall of nasopharynx
147.3 Malignant neoplasm of anterior wall of nasopharynx
148.1 Malignant neoplasm of pyriform sinus
149.0 Malignant neoplasm of pharynx, unspecified ▽
198.89 Secondary malignant neoplasm of other specified sites
210.4 Benign neoplasm of other and unspecified parts of mouth ▽
210.5 Benign neoplasm of tonsil
210.6 Benign neoplasm of other parts of oropharynx
210.7 Benign neoplasm of nasopharynx
210.8 Benign neoplasm of hypopharynx
230.0 Carcinoma in situ of lip, oral cavity, and pharynx
235.1 Neoplasm of uncertain behavior of lip, oral cavity, and pharynx
239.0 Neoplasm of unspecified nature of digestive system

ICD-9-CM Procedural
29.33 Pharyngectomy (partial)
29.4 Plastic operation on pharynx

42900
42900 Suture pharynx for wound or injury

ICD-9-CM Diagnostic
874.4 Open wound of pharynx, without mention of complication — (Use additional code to identify infection)
874.5 Open wound of pharynx, complicated — (Use additional code to identify infection)
959.01 Head injury, unspecified ▽
959.09 Injury of face and neck, other and unspecified
998.2 Accidental puncture or laceration during procedure

ICD-9-CM Procedural
29.51 Suture of laceration of pharynx

42950
42950 Pharyngoplasty (plastic or reconstructive operation on pharynx)

ICD-9-CM Diagnostic
146.0 Malignant neoplasm of tonsil
146.1 Malignant neoplasm of tonsillar fossa
146.2 Malignant neoplasm of tonsillar pillars (anterior) (posterior)
146.3 Malignant neoplasm of vallecula
146.4 Malignant neoplasm of anterior aspect of epiglottis

146.5 Malignant neoplasm of junctional region of oropharynx
146.6 Malignant neoplasm of lateral wall of oropharynx
146.7 Malignant neoplasm of posterior wall of oropharynx
146.8 Malignant neoplasm of other specified sites of oropharynx
147.0 Malignant neoplasm of superior wall of nasopharynx
147.1 Malignant neoplasm of posterior wall of nasopharynx
147.2 Malignant neoplasm of lateral wall of nasopharynx
147.3 Malignant neoplasm of anterior wall of nasopharynx
147.9 Malignant neoplasm of nasopharynx, unspecified site ▽
149.0 Malignant neoplasm of pharynx, unspecified ▽
198.89 Secondary malignant neoplasm of other specified sites
210.4 Benign neoplasm of other and unspecified parts of mouth ▽
210.5 Benign neoplasm of tonsil
210.6 Benign neoplasm of other parts of oropharynx
210.7 Benign neoplasm of nasopharynx
210.8 Benign neoplasm of hypopharynx
230.0 Carcinoma in situ of lip, oral cavity, and pharynx
235.1 Neoplasm of uncertain behavior of lip, oral cavity, and pharynx
239.0 Neoplasm of unspecified nature of digestive system
906.0 Late effect of open wound of head, neck, and trunk
906.5 Late effect of burn of eye, face, head, and neck
909.1 Late effect of toxic effects of nonmedical substances
909.2 Late effect of radiation
909.3 Late effect of complications of surgical and medical care
947.0 Burn of mouth and pharynx
V10.02 Personal history of malignant neoplasm of other and unspecified parts of oral cavity and pharynx ▽
V45.89 Other postsurgical status — (This code is intended for use when these conditions are recorded as diagnoses or problems)
V51 Aftercare involving the use of plastic surgery

ICD-9-CM Procedural
29.4 Plastic operation on pharynx

42953
42953 Pharyngoesophageal repair

ICD-9-CM Diagnostic
862.22 Esophagus injury without mention of open wound into cavity
862.32 Esophagus injury with open wound into cavity
874.4 Open wound of pharynx, without mention of complication — (Use additional code to identify infection)
874.5 Open wound of pharynx, complicated — (Use additional code to identify infection)
925.2 Crushing injury of neck — (Use additional code to identify any associated injuries: 800-829, 850.0-854.1, 860.0-869.1)
998.2 Accidental puncture or laceration during procedure
998.31 Disruption of internal operation wound
998.83 Non-healing surgical wound

ICD-9-CM Procedural
29.51 Suture of laceration of pharynx
42.82 Suture of laceration of esophagus

42955
42955 Pharyngostomy (fistulization of pharynx, external for feeding)

ICD-9-CM Diagnostic
146.0 Malignant neoplasm of tonsil
146.1 Malignant neoplasm of tonsillar fossa
146.2 Malignant neoplasm of tonsillar pillars (anterior) (posterior)
146.5 Malignant neoplasm of junctional region of oropharynx
146.6 Malignant neoplasm of lateral wall of oropharynx
146.7 Malignant neoplasm of posterior wall of oropharynx
146.9 Malignant neoplasm of oropharynx, unspecified site ▽
147.0 Malignant neoplasm of superior wall of nasopharynx
147.3 Malignant neoplasm of anterior wall of nasopharynx
147.9 Malignant neoplasm of nasopharynx, unspecified site ▽
148.0 Malignant neoplasm of postcricoid region of hypopharynx
148.1 Malignant neoplasm of pyriform sinus
148.3 Malignant neoplasm of posterior hypopharyngeal wall
148.8 Malignant neoplasm of other specified sites of hypopharynx
149.0 Malignant neoplasm of pharynx, unspecified ▽
150.0 Malignant neoplasm of cervical esophagus
150.3 Malignant neoplasm of upper third of esophagus
150.9 Malignant neoplasm of esophagus, unspecified site ▽
197.8 Secondary malignant neoplasm of other digestive organs and spleen
198.89 Secondary malignant neoplasm of other specified sites
210.6 Benign neoplasm of other parts of oropharynx
210.7 Benign neoplasm of nasopharynx
210.8 Benign neoplasm of hypopharynx
210.9 Benign neoplasm of pharynx, unspecified ▽
211.0 Benign neoplasm of esophagus
874.4 Open wound of pharynx, without mention of complication — (Use additional code to identify infection)
874.5 Open wound of pharynx, complicated — (Use additional code to identify infection)
947.0 Burn of mouth and pharynx
V10.02 Personal history of malignant neoplasm of other and unspecified parts of oral cavity and pharynx ▽
V45.89 Other postsurgical status — (This code is intended for use when these conditions are recorded as diagnoses or problems)

ICD-9-CM Procedural
29.99 Other operations on pharynx

42960–42962
42960 Control oropharyngeal hemorrhage, primary or secondary (eg, post-tonsillectomy); simple
42961 complicated, requiring hospitalization
42962 with secondary surgical intervention

ICD-9-CM Diagnostic
784.8 Hemorrhage from throat
998.11 Hemorrhage complicating a procedure
998.2 Accidental puncture or laceration during procedure

ICD-9-CM Procedural
28.7 Control of hemorrhage after tonsillectomy and adenoidectomy

HCPCS Level II Supplies & Services
A4305 Disposable drug delivery system, flow rate of 50 ml or greater per hour
A4306 Disposable drug delivery system, flow rate of 5 ml or less per hour
A4550 Surgical trays

42970–42972
42970 Control of nasopharyngeal hemorrhage, primary or secondary (eg, postadenoidectomy); simple, with posterior nasal packs, with or without anterior packs and/or cautery
42971 complicated, requiring hospitalization
42972 with secondary surgical intervention

ICD-9-CM Diagnostic
784.8 Hemorrhage from throat
998.11 Hemorrhage complicating a procedure
998.2 Accidental puncture or laceration during procedure

ICD-9-CM Procedural
28.7 Control of hemorrhage after tonsillectomy and adenoidectomy

HCPCS Level II Supplies & Services
A4305 Disposable drug delivery system, flow rate of 50 ml or greater per hour
A4306 Disposable drug delivery system, flow rate of 5 ml or less per hour
A4550 Surgical trays

Esophagus

43020
43020 Esophagotomy, cervical approach, with removal of foreign body

ICD-9-CM Diagnostic
530.3 Stricture and stenosis of esophagus
530.89 Other specified disorder of the esophagus
862.32 Esophagus injury with open wound into cavity
935.1 Foreign body in esophagus

ICD-9-CM Procedural
42.09 Other incision of esophagus

43030

43030 Cricopharyngeal myotomy

ICD-9-CM Diagnostic

147.1 Malignant neoplasm of posterior wall of nasopharynx
149.0 Malignant neoplasm of pharynx, unspecified
198.89 Secondary malignant neoplasm of other specified sites
210.7 Benign neoplasm of nasopharynx
210.9 Benign neoplasm of pharynx, unspecified
464.11 Acute tracheitis with obstruction
464.21 Acute laryngotracheitis with obstruction
478.29 Other disease of pharynx or nasopharynx
478.74 Stenosis of larynx

ICD-9-CM Procedural

29.31 Cricopharyngeal myotomy

43045

43045 Esophagotomy, thoracic approach, with removal of foreign body

ICD-9-CM Diagnostic

478.29 Other disease of pharynx or nasopharynx
530.3 Stricture and stenosis of esophagus
862.32 Esophagus injury with open wound into cavity
935.1 Foreign body in esophagus

ICD-9-CM Procedural

42.09 Other incision of esophagus

43100

43100 Excision of lesion, esophagus, with primary repair; cervical approach

ICD-9-CM Diagnostic

150.0 Malignant neoplasm of cervical esophagus
150.1 Malignant neoplasm of thoracic esophagus
150.3 Malignant neoplasm of upper third of esophagus
150.4 Malignant neoplasm of middle third of esophagus
150.8 Malignant neoplasm of other specified part of esophagus
150.9 Malignant neoplasm of esophagus, unspecified site
197.8 Secondary malignant neoplasm of other digestive organs and spleen
211.0 Benign neoplasm of esophagus
230.1 Carcinoma in situ of esophagus
235.5 Neoplasm of uncertain behavior of other and unspecified digestive organs
239.0 Neoplasm of unspecified nature of digestive system
530.89 Other specified disorder of the esophagus

ICD-9-CM Procedural

42.32 Local excision of other lesion or tissue of esophagus

43101

43101 Excision of lesion, esophagus, with primary repair; thoracic or abdominal approach

ICD-9-CM Diagnostic

150.0 Malignant neoplasm of cervical esophagus
150.1 Malignant neoplasm of thoracic esophagus
150.2 Malignant neoplasm of abdominal esophagus
150.3 Malignant neoplasm of upper third of esophagus
150.4 Malignant neoplasm of middle third of esophagus
150.5 Malignant neoplasm of lower third of esophagus
150.8 Malignant neoplasm of other specified part of esophagus
150.9 Malignant neoplasm of esophagus, unspecified site
197.8 Secondary malignant neoplasm of other digestive organs and spleen
211.0 Benign neoplasm of esophagus
230.1 Carcinoma in situ of esophagus
235.5 Neoplasm of uncertain behavior of other and unspecified digestive organs
239.0 Neoplasm of unspecified nature of digestive system
530.89 Other specified disorder of the esophagus

ICD-9-CM Procedural

42.32 Local excision of other lesion or tissue of esophagus

43107

43107 Total or near total esophagectomy, without thoracotomy; with pharyngogastrostomy or cervical esophagogastrostomy, with or without pyloroplasty (transhiatal)

ICD-9-CM Diagnostic

150.0 Malignant neoplasm of cervical esophagus
150.1 Malignant neoplasm of thoracic esophagus
150.2 Malignant neoplasm of abdominal esophagus
150.3 Malignant neoplasm of upper third of esophagus
150.4 Malignant neoplasm of middle third of esophagus
150.5 Malignant neoplasm of lower third of esophagus
150.8 Malignant neoplasm of other specified part of esophagus
150.9 Malignant neoplasm of esophagus, unspecified site
197.8 Secondary malignant neoplasm of other digestive organs and spleen
230.1 Carcinoma in situ of esophagus
235.5 Neoplasm of uncertain behavior of other and unspecified digestive organs
239.0 Neoplasm of unspecified nature of digestive system
456.0 Esophageal varices with bleeding
456.1 Esophageal varices without mention of bleeding
530.5 Dyskinesia of esophagus
530.84 Tracheoesophageal fistula
530.89 Other specified disorder of the esophagus
572.3 Portal hypertension
750.4 Other specified congenital anomaly of esophagus
750.9 Unspecified congenital anomaly of upper alimentary tract
862.22 Esophagus injury without mention of open wound into cavity
862.32 Esophagus injury with open wound into cavity
906.8 Late effect of burns of other specified sites
909.2 Late effect of radiation
947.2 Burn of esophagus
997.4 Digestive system complication — (Use additional code to identify complications)

ICD-9-CM Procedural

42.41 Partial esophagectomy
42.42 Total esophagectomy
42.62 Antesternal esophagogastrostomy
44.29 Other pyloroplasty

43108

43108 Total or near total esophagectomy, without thoracotomy; with colon interposition or small intestine reconstruction, including intestine mobilization, preparation and anastomosis(es)

ICD-9-CM Diagnostic

150.0 Malignant neoplasm of cervical esophagus
150.1 Malignant neoplasm of thoracic esophagus
150.2 Malignant neoplasm of abdominal esophagus
150.3 Malignant neoplasm of upper third of esophagus
150.4 Malignant neoplasm of middle third of esophagus
150.5 Malignant neoplasm of lower third of esophagus
150.8 Malignant neoplasm of other specified part of esophagus
150.9 Malignant neoplasm of esophagus, unspecified site
197.8 Secondary malignant neoplasm of other digestive organs and spleen
230.1 Carcinoma in situ of esophagus
235.5 Neoplasm of uncertain behavior of other and unspecified digestive organs
239.0 Neoplasm of unspecified nature of digestive system
456.0 Esophageal varices with bleeding
456.1 Esophageal varices without mention of bleeding
530.5 Dyskinesia of esophagus
530.84 Tracheoesophageal fistula
530.89 Other specified disorder of the esophagus
572.3 Portal hypertension
750.4 Other specified congenital anomaly of esophagus
750.9 Unspecified congenital anomaly of upper alimentary tract
862.22 Esophagus injury without mention of open wound into cavity
862.32 Esophagus injury with open wound into cavity
906.8 Late effect of burns of other specified sites
909.2 Late effect of radiation
947.2 Burn of esophagus
997.4 Digestive system complication — (Use additional code to identify complications)

ICD-9-CM Procedural

42.41 Partial esophagectomy

Unspecified code
♀ Female diagnosis
Manifestation code
♂ Male diagnosis

42.42 Total esophagectomy
42.63 Antesternal esophageal anastomosis with interposition of small bowel
42.65 Antesternal esophageal anastomosis with interposition of colon

43112

43112 Total or near total esophagectomy, with thoracotomy; with pharyngogastrostomy or cervical esophagogastrostomy, with or without pyloroplasty

ICD-9-CM Diagnostic

150.0 Malignant neoplasm of cervical esophagus
150.1 Malignant neoplasm of thoracic esophagus
150.2 Malignant neoplasm of abdominal esophagus
150.3 Malignant neoplasm of upper third of esophagus
150.4 Malignant neoplasm of middle third of esophagus
150.5 Malignant neoplasm of lower third of esophagus
150.8 Malignant neoplasm of other specified part of esophagus
150.9 Malignant neoplasm of esophagus, unspecified site ▽
197.8 Secondary malignant neoplasm of other digestive organs and spleen
230.1 Carcinoma in situ of esophagus
235.5 Neoplasm of uncertain behavior of other and unspecified digestive organs ▽
239.0 Neoplasm of unspecified nature of digestive system
456.0 Esophageal varices with bleeding
456.1 Esophageal varices without mention of bleeding
530.5 Dyskinesia of esophagus
530.84 Tracheoesophageal fistula
530.89 Other specified disorder of the esophagus
572.3 Portal hypertension
750.4 Other specified congenital anomaly of esophagus
750.9 Unspecified congenital anomaly of upper alimentary tract ▽
862.22 Esophagus injury without mention of open wound into cavity
862.32 Esophagus injury with open wound into cavity
906.8 Late effect of burns of other specified sites
909.1 Late effect of toxic effects of nonmedical substances
909.2 Late effect of radiation
947.2 Burn of esophagus
997.4 Digestive system complication — (Use additional code to identify complications)

ICD-9-CM Procedural

42.41 Partial esophagectomy
42.42 Total esophagectomy
42.52 Intrathoracic esophagogastrostomy
44.29 Other pyloroplasty

43113

43113 Total or near total esophagectomy, with thoracotomy; with colon interposition or small intestine reconstruction, including intestine mobilization, preparation, and anastomosis(es)

ICD-9-CM Diagnostic

150.0 Malignant neoplasm of cervical esophagus
150.1 Malignant neoplasm of thoracic esophagus
150.2 Malignant neoplasm of abdominal esophagus
150.3 Malignant neoplasm of upper third of esophagus
150.4 Malignant neoplasm of middle third of esophagus
150.5 Malignant neoplasm of lower third of esophagus
150.8 Malignant neoplasm of other specified part of esophagus
150.9 Malignant neoplasm of esophagus, unspecified site ▽
197.8 Secondary malignant neoplasm of other digestive organs and spleen
230.1 Carcinoma in situ of esophagus
235.5 Neoplasm of uncertain behavior of other and unspecified digestive organs ▽
239.0 Neoplasm of unspecified nature of digestive system
456.0 Esophageal varices with bleeding
456.1 Esophageal varices without mention of bleeding
530.5 Dyskinesia of esophagus
530.84 Tracheoesophageal fistula
530.89 Other specified disorder of the esophagus
572.3 Portal hypertension
750.4 Other specified congenital anomaly of esophagus
750.9 Unspecified congenital anomaly of upper alimentary tract ▽
862.22 Esophagus injury without mention of open wound into cavity
862.32 Esophagus injury with open wound into cavity
906.8 Late effect of burns of other specified sites
909.1 Late effect of toxic effects of nonmedical substances
909.2 Late effect of radiation
947.2 Burn of esophagus
997.4 Digestive system complication — (Use additional code to identify complications)

ICD-9-CM Procedural

42.41 Partial esophagectomy
42.42 Total esophagectomy
42.53 Intrathoracic esophageal anastomosis with interposition of small bowel
42.55 Intrathoracic esophageal anastomosis with interposition of colon

43116

43116 Partial esophagectomy, cervical, with free intestinal graft, including microvascular anastomosis, obtaining the graft and intestinal reconstruction

ICD-9-CM Diagnostic

150.0 Malignant neoplasm of cervical esophagus
150.1 Malignant neoplasm of thoracic esophagus
150.2 Malignant neoplasm of abdominal esophagus
150.3 Malignant neoplasm of upper third of esophagus
150.4 Malignant neoplasm of middle third of esophagus
150.5 Malignant neoplasm of lower third of esophagus
150.8 Malignant neoplasm of other specified part of esophagus
150.9 Malignant neoplasm of esophagus, unspecified site ▽
197.8 Secondary malignant neoplasm of other digestive organs and spleen
211.0 Benign neoplasm of esophagus
230.1 Carcinoma in situ of esophagus
235.5 Neoplasm of uncertain behavior of other and unspecified digestive organs ▽
239.0 Neoplasm of unspecified nature of digestive system
530.20 Ulcer of esophagus without bleeding — (Use additional E code to identify cause, if induced by chemical or drug)
530.21 Ulcer of esophagus with bleeding — (Use additional E code to identify cause, if induced by chemical or drug)
530.6 Diverticulum of esophagus, acquired
530.82 Esophageal hemorrhage
530.83 Esophageal leukoplakia
530.85 Barrett's esophagus
530.89 Other specified disorder of the esophagus

ICD-9-CM Procedural

42.41 Partial esophagectomy
42.63 Antesternal esophageal anastomosis with interposition of small bowel
42.65 Antesternal esophageal anastomosis with interposition of colon

43117

43117 Partial esophagectomy, distal two-thirds, with thoracotomy and separate abdominal incision, with or without proximal gastrectomy; with thoracic esophagogastrostomy, with or without pyloroplasty (Ivor Lewis)

ICD-9-CM Diagnostic

150.1 Malignant neoplasm of thoracic esophagus
150.2 Malignant neoplasm of abdominal esophagus
150.3 Malignant neoplasm of upper third of esophagus
150.4 Malignant neoplasm of middle third of esophagus
150.5 Malignant neoplasm of lower third of esophagus
150.8 Malignant neoplasm of other specified part of esophagus
151.0 Malignant neoplasm of cardia
151.9 Malignant neoplasm of stomach, unspecified site ▽
197.8 Secondary malignant neoplasm of other digestive organs and spleen
230.1 Carcinoma in situ of esophagus
235.5 Neoplasm of uncertain behavior of other and unspecified digestive organs ▽
239.0 Neoplasm of unspecified nature of digestive system
456.0 Esophageal varices with bleeding
456.1 Esophageal varices without mention of bleeding
530.20 Ulcer of esophagus without bleeding — (Use additional E code to identify cause, if induced by chemical or drug)
530.21 Ulcer of esophagus with bleeding — (Use additional E code to identify cause, if induced by chemical or drug)
530.6 Diverticulum of esophagus, acquired
530.82 Esophageal hemorrhage
530.85 Barrett's esophagus
530.89 Other specified disorder of the esophagus
531.20 Acute gastric ulcer with hemorrhage and perforation, without mention of obstruction — (Use additional E code to identify drug, if drug induced)

ICD-9-CM Procedural

42.41 Partial esophagectomy

42.52 Intrathoracic esophagogastrostomy
43.5 Partial gastrectomy with anastomosis to esophagus
44.29 Other pyloroplasty

43118

43118 Partial esophagectomy, distal two-thirds, with thoracotomy and separate abdominal incision, with or without proximal gastrectomy; with colon interposition or small intestine reconstruction, including intestine mobilization, preparation, and anastomosis(es)

ICD-9-CM Diagnostic

150.1 Malignant neoplasm of thoracic esophagus
150.2 Malignant neoplasm of abdominal esophagus
150.3 Malignant neoplasm of upper third of esophagus
150.4 Malignant neoplasm of middle third of esophagus
150.5 Malignant neoplasm of lower third of esophagus
150.8 Malignant neoplasm of other specified part of esophagus
151.0 Malignant neoplasm of cardia
151.9 Malignant neoplasm of stomach, unspecified site ▽
197.8 Secondary malignant neoplasm of other digestive organs and spleen
230.1 Carcinoma in situ of esophagus
235.5 Neoplasm of uncertain behavior of other and unspecified digestive organs ▽
239.0 Neoplasm of unspecified nature of digestive system
530.20 Ulcer of esophagus without bleeding — (Use additional E code to identify cause, if induced by chemical or drug)
530.21 Ulcer of esophagus with bleeding — (Use additional E code to identify cause, if induced by chemical or drug)
530.6 Diverticulum of esophagus, acquired
530.82 Esophageal hemorrhage
530.85 Barrett's esophagus
530.89 Other specified disorder of the esophagus
531.00 Acute gastric ulcer with hemorrhage, without mention of obstruction — (Use additional E code to identify drug, if drug induced)
531.20 Acute gastric ulcer with hemorrhage and perforation, without mention of obstruction — (Use additional E code to identify drug, if drug induced)
531.30 Acute gastric ulcer without mention of hemorrhage, perforation, or obstruction — (Use additional E code to identify drug, if drug induced)
531.40 Chronic or unspecified gastric ulcer with hemorrhage, without mention of obstruction — (Use additional E code to identify drug, if drug induced)
531.41 Chronic or unspecified gastric ulcer with hemorrhage and obstruction — (Use additional E code to identify drug, if drug induced)

ICD-9-CM Procedural

42.41 Partial esophagectomy
42.52 Intrathoracic esophagogastrostomy
42.53 Intrathoracic esophageal anastomosis with interposition of small bowel
42.55 Intrathoracic esophageal anastomosis with interposition of colon
43.5 Partial gastrectomy with anastomosis to esophagus

43121

43121 Partial esophagectomy, distal two-thirds, with thoracotomy only, with or without proximal gastrectomy, with thoracic esophagogastrostomy, with or without pyloroplasty

ICD-9-CM Diagnostic

150.1 Malignant neoplasm of thoracic esophagus
150.2 Malignant neoplasm of abdominal esophagus
150.3 Malignant neoplasm of upper third of esophagus
150.4 Malignant neoplasm of middle third of esophagus
150.5 Malignant neoplasm of lower third of esophagus
150.8 Malignant neoplasm of other specified part of esophagus
151.0 Malignant neoplasm of cardia
151.9 Malignant neoplasm of stomach, unspecified site ▽
197.8 Secondary malignant neoplasm of other digestive organs and spleen
230.1 Carcinoma in situ of esophagus
235.5 Neoplasm of uncertain behavior of other and unspecified digestive organs ▽
239.0 Neoplasm of unspecified nature of digestive system
456.0 Esophageal varices with bleeding
530.20 Ulcer of esophagus without bleeding — (Use additional E code to identify cause, if induced by chemical or drug)
530.21 Ulcer of esophagus with bleeding — (Use additional E code to identify cause, if induced by chemical or drug)
530.3 Stricture and stenosis of esophagus
530.4 Perforation of esophagus
530.5 Dyskinesia of esophagus
530.82 Esophageal hemorrhage
530.85 Barrett's esophagus
530.89 Other specified disorder of the esophagus
531.00 Acute gastric ulcer with hemorrhage, without mention of obstruction — (Use additional E code to identify drug, if drug induced)
531.20 Acute gastric ulcer with hemorrhage and perforation, without mention of obstruction — (Use additional E code to identify drug, if drug induced)
531.30 Acute gastric ulcer without mention of hemorrhage, perforation, or obstruction — (Use additional E code to identify drug, if drug induced)
531.40 Chronic or unspecified gastric ulcer with hemorrhage, without mention of obstruction — (Use additional E code to identify drug, if drug induced)
531.41 Chronic or unspecified gastric ulcer with hemorrhage and obstruction — (Use additional E code to identify drug, if drug induced)

ICD-9-CM Procedural

42.41 Partial esophagectomy
42.52 Intrathoracic esophagogastrostomy
43.5 Partial gastrectomy with anastomosis to esophagus
44.29 Other pyloroplasty

43122

43122 Partial esophagectomy, thoracoabdominal or abdominal approach, with or without proximal gastrectomy; with esophagogastrostomy, with or without pyloroplasty

ICD-9-CM Diagnostic

150.1 Malignant neoplasm of thoracic esophagus
150.2 Malignant neoplasm of abdominal esophagus
150.3 Malignant neoplasm of upper third of esophagus
150.4 Malignant neoplasm of middle third of esophagus
150.5 Malignant neoplasm of lower third of esophagus
150.8 Malignant neoplasm of other specified part of esophagus
151.0 Malignant neoplasm of cardia
151.9 Malignant neoplasm of stomach, unspecified site ▽
197.8 Secondary malignant neoplasm of other digestive organs and spleen
230.1 Carcinoma in situ of esophagus
235.5 Neoplasm of uncertain behavior of other and unspecified digestive organs ▽
239.0 Neoplasm of unspecified nature of digestive system
456.0 Esophageal varices with bleeding
530.20 Ulcer of esophagus without bleeding — (Use additional E code to identify cause, if induced by chemical or drug)
530.21 Ulcer of esophagus with bleeding — (Use additional E code to identify cause, if induced by chemical or drug)
530.3 Stricture and stenosis of esophagus
530.4 Perforation of esophagus
530.5 Dyskinesia of esophagus
530.81 Esophageal reflux
530.82 Esophageal hemorrhage
530.83 Esophageal leukoplakia
530.85 Barrett's esophagus
531.00 Acute gastric ulcer with hemorrhage, without mention of obstruction — (Use additional E code to identify drug, if drug induced)
531.20 Acute gastric ulcer with hemorrhage and perforation, without mention of obstruction — (Use additional E code to identify drug, if drug induced)
531.30 Acute gastric ulcer without mention of hemorrhage, perforation, or obstruction — (Use additional E code to identify drug, if drug induced)
531.40 Chronic or unspecified gastric ulcer with hemorrhage, without mention of obstruction — (Use additional E code to identify drug, if drug induced)
531.41 Chronic or unspecified gastric ulcer with hemorrhage and obstruction — (Use additional E code to identify drug, if drug induced)

ICD-9-CM Procedural

42.41 Partial esophagectomy
42.52 Intrathoracic esophagogastrostomy
43.5 Partial gastrectomy with anastomosis to esophagus
44.29 Other pyloroplasty

43123

43123 Partial esophagectomy, thoracoabdominal or abdominal approach, with or without proximal gastrectomy; with colon interposition or small intestine reconstruction, including intestine mobilization, preparation, and anastomosis(es)

ICD-9-CM Diagnostic

150.1 Malignant neoplasm of thoracic esophagus
150.2 Malignant neoplasm of abdominal esophagus
150.3 Malignant neoplasm of upper third of esophagus

▽ Unspecified code
♀ Female diagnosis
☒ Manifestation code
♂ Male diagnosis

150.4 Malignant neoplasm of middle third of esophagus
150.5 Malignant neoplasm of lower third of esophagus
150.8 Malignant neoplasm of other specified part of esophagus
150.9 Malignant neoplasm of esophagus, unspecified site
151.0 Malignant neoplasm of cardia
151.9 Malignant neoplasm of stomach, unspecified site
154.0 Malignant neoplasm of rectosigmoid junction
197.8 Secondary malignant neoplasm of other digestive organs and spleen
230.1 Carcinoma in situ of esophagus
235.5 Neoplasm of uncertain behavior of other and unspecified digestive organs
239.0 Neoplasm of unspecified nature of digestive system
530.20 Ulcer of esophagus without bleeding — (Use additional E code to identify cause, if induced by chemical or drug)
530.21 Ulcer of esophagus with bleeding — (Use additional E code to identify cause, if induced by chemical or drug)
530.4 Perforation of esophagus
530.82 Esophageal hemorrhage
530.83 Esophageal leukoplakia
530.85 Barrett's esophagus
530.89 Other specified disorder of the esophagus
531.00 Acute gastric ulcer with hemorrhage, without mention of obstruction — (Use additional E code to identify drug, if drug induced)
531.01 Acute gastric ulcer with hemorrhage and obstruction — (Use additional E code to identify drug, if drug induced)
531.10 Acute gastric ulcer with perforation, without mention of obstruction — (Use additional E code to identify drug, if drug induced)
531.11 Acute gastric ulcer with perforation and obstruction — (Use additional E code to identify drug, if drug induced)
531.20 Acute gastric ulcer with hemorrhage and perforation, without mention of obstruction — (Use additional E code to identify drug, if drug induced)
531.21 Acute gastric ulcer with hemorrhage, perforation, and obstruction — (Use additional E code to identify drug, if drug induced)
531.30 Acute gastric ulcer without mention of hemorrhage, perforation, or obstruction — (Use additional E code to identify drug, if drug induced)
531.31 Acute gastric ulcer without mention of hemorrhage or perforation, with obstruction — (Use additional E code to identify drug, if drug induced)
531.40 Chronic or unspecified gastric ulcer with hemorrhage, without mention of obstruction — (Use additional E code to identify drug, if drug induced)
531.41 Chronic or unspecified gastric ulcer with hemorrhage and obstruction — (Use additional E code to identify drug, if drug induced)

ICD-9-CM Procedural

42.41 Partial esophagectomy
42.52 Intrathoracic esophagogastrostomy
42.53 Intrathoracic esophageal anastomosis with interposition of small bowel
42.55 Intrathoracic esophageal anastomosis with interposition of colon

43124

43124 Total or partial esophagectomy, without reconstruction (any approach), with cervical esophagostomy

ICD-9-CM Diagnostic

150.0 Malignant neoplasm of cervical esophagus
150.1 Malignant neoplasm of thoracic esophagus
150.2 Malignant neoplasm of abdominal esophagus
150.3 Malignant neoplasm of upper third of esophagus
150.4 Malignant neoplasm of middle third of esophagus
150.5 Malignant neoplasm of lower third of esophagus
150.8 Malignant neoplasm of other specified part of esophagus
150.9 Malignant neoplasm of esophagus, unspecified site
197.8 Secondary malignant neoplasm of other digestive organs and spleen
230.1 Carcinoma in situ of esophagus
235.5 Neoplasm of uncertain behavior of other and unspecified digestive organs
239.0 Neoplasm of unspecified nature of digestive system
530.20 Ulcer of esophagus without bleeding — (Use additional E code to identify cause, if induced by chemical or drug)
530.21 Ulcer of esophagus with bleeding — (Use additional E code to identify cause, if induced by chemical or drug)
530.82 Esophageal hemorrhage
530.83 Esophageal leukoplakia
530.84 Tracheoesophageal fistula
530.85 Barrett's esophagus
530.89 Other specified disorder of the esophagus

ICD-9-CM Procedural

42.11 Cervical esophagostomy
42.41 Partial esophagectomy
42.42 Total esophagectomy
42.62 Antesternal esophagogastrostomy

43130

43130 Diverticulectomy of hypopharynx or esophagus, with or without myotomy; cervical approach

ICD-9-CM Diagnostic

530.6 Diverticulum of esophagus, acquired
750.27 Congenital diverticulum of pharynx
750.4 Other specified congenital anomaly of esophagus

ICD-9-CM Procedural

29.32 Pharyngeal diverticulectomy
42.31 Local excision of esophageal diverticulum

43135

43135 Diverticulectomy of hypopharynx or esophagus, with or without myotomy; thoracic approach

ICD-9-CM Diagnostic

530.6 Diverticulum of esophagus, acquired
750.27 Congenital diverticulum of pharynx
750.4 Other specified congenital anomaly of esophagus

ICD-9-CM Procedural

29.32 Pharyngeal diverticulectomy
42.31 Local excision of esophageal diverticulum

43200–43202

43200 Esophagoscopy, rigid or flexible; diagnostic, with or without collection of specimen(s) by brushing or washing (separate procedure)
43202 with biopsy, single or multiple
43201 with directed submucosal injection(s), any substance

ICD-9-CM Diagnostic

150.0 Malignant neoplasm of cervical esophagus
150.1 Malignant neoplasm of thoracic esophagus
150.2 Malignant neoplasm of abdominal esophagus
150.3 Malignant neoplasm of upper third of esophagus
150.4 Malignant neoplasm of middle third of esophagus
150.5 Malignant neoplasm of lower third of esophagus
150.8 Malignant neoplasm of other specified part of esophagus
150.9 Malignant neoplasm of esophagus, unspecified site
171.0 Malignant neoplasm of connective and other soft tissue of head, face, and neck
193 Malignant neoplasm of thyroid gland — (Use additional code to identify any functional activity)
195.0 Malignant neoplasm of head, face, and neck
196.0 Secondary and unspecified malignant neoplasm of lymph nodes of head, face, and neck
196.9 Secondary and unspecified malignant neoplasm of lymph nodes, site unspecified
197.8 Secondary malignant neoplasm of other digestive organs and spleen
198.89 Secondary malignant neoplasm of other specified sites
199.0 Disseminated malignant neoplasm
199.1 Other malignant neoplasm of unspecified site

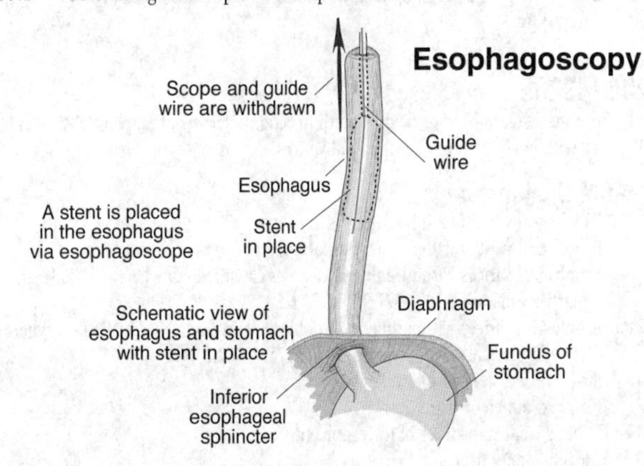
Esophagoscopy
Scope and guide wire are withdrawn
Guide wire
Esophagus
A stent is placed in the esophagus via esophagoscope
Stent in place
Schematic view of esophagus and stomach with stent in place
Diaphragm
Fundus of stomach
Inferior esophageal sphincter

202.81 Other malignant lymphomas of lymph nodes of head, face, and neck
211.0 Benign neoplasm of esophagus
211.9 Benign neoplasm of other and unspecified site of the digestive system ▽
230.1 Carcinoma in situ of esophagus
235.5 Neoplasm of uncertain behavior of other and unspecified digestive organs ▽
239.0 Neoplasm of unspecified nature of digestive system
263.0 Malnutrition of moderate degree
306.4 Gastrointestinal malfunction arising from mental factors
352.3 Disorders of pneumogastric (10th) nerve
448.0 Hereditary hemorrhagic telangiectasia
456.0 Esophageal varices with bleeding
456.1 Esophageal varices without mention of bleeding
530.0 Achalasia and cardiospasm
530.11 Reflux esophagitis — (Use additional E code to identify cause, if induced by chemical or drug)
530.12 Acute esophagitis — (Use additional E code to identify cause, if induced by chemical or drug)
530.19 Other esophagitis — (Use additional E code to identify cause, if induced by chemical or drug)
530.20 Ulcer of esophagus without bleeding — (Use additional E code to identify cause, if induced by chemical or drug)
530.21 Ulcer of esophagus with bleeding — (Use additional E code to identify cause, if induced by chemical or drug)
530.3 Stricture and stenosis of esophagus
530.4 Perforation of esophagus
530.5 Dyskinesia of esophagus
530.6 Diverticulum of esophagus, acquired
530.7 Gastroesophageal laceration-hemorrhage syndrome
530.81 Esophageal reflux
530.82 Esophageal hemorrhage
530.83 Esophageal leukoplakia
530.84 Tracheoesophageal fistula
530.85 Barrett's esophagus
530.89 Other specified disorder of the esophagus
530.9 Unspecified disorder of esophagus ▽
552.3 Diaphragmatic hernia with obstruction
553.3 Diaphragmatic hernia without mention of obstruction or gangrene
578.0 Hematemesis
578.1 Blood in stool
578.9 Unspecified, hemorrhage of gastrointestinal tract ▽
750.4 Other specified congenital anomaly of esophagus
750.9 Unspecified congenital anomaly of upper alimentary tract ▽
784.1 Throat pain
787.1 Heartburn
787.2 Dysphagia
793.4 Nonspecific abnormal findings on radiological and other examination of gastrointestinal tract
799.89 Other ill-defined conditions
862.22 Esophagus injury without mention of open wound into cavity

ICD-9-CM Procedural

42.23 Other esophagoscopy
42.24 Closed (endoscopic) biopsy of esophagus
42.33 Endoscopic excision or destruction of lesion or tissue of esophagus

HCPCS Level II Supplies & Services

A4270 Disposable endoscope sheath, each
A4305 Disposable drug delivery system, flow rate of 50 ml or greater per hour
A4306 Disposable drug delivery system, flow rate of 5 ml or less per hour
A4550 Surgical trays

43204–43205

43204 Esophagoscopy, rigid or flexible; with injection sclerosis of esophageal varices
43205 with band ligation of esophageal varices

ICD-9-CM Diagnostic

456.0 Esophageal varices with bleeding
456.1 Esophageal varices without mention of bleeding
456.20 Esophageal varices with bleeding in diseases classified elsewhere — (Code first underlying disease: 571.0-571.9, 572.3) ☒
456.21 Esophageal varices without mention of bleeding in diseases classified elsewhere — (Code first underlying disease: 571.0-571.9, 572.3) ☒
530.3 Stricture and stenosis of esophagus
530.82 Esophageal hemorrhage
530.89 Other specified disorder of the esophagus
571.0 Alcoholic fatty liver
571.1 Acute alcoholic hepatitis
571.2 Alcoholic cirrhosis of liver
571.3 Unspecified alcoholic liver damage ▽
571.40 Unspecified chronic hepatitis ▽
571.41 Chronic persistent hepatitis
571.49 Other chronic hepatitis
571.5 Cirrhosis of liver without mention of alcohol
571.6 Biliary cirrhosis
571.8 Other chronic nonalcoholic liver disease
571.9 Unspecified chronic liver disease without mention of alcohol ▽
572.3 Portal hypertension
578.0 Hematemesis

ICD-9-CM Procedural

42.33 Endoscopic excision or destruction of lesion or tissue of esophagus

43215

43215 Esophagoscopy, rigid or flexible; with removal of foreign body

ICD-9-CM Diagnostic

935.1 Foreign body in esophagus

ICD-9-CM Procedural

98.02 Removal of intraluminal foreign body from esophagus without incision

HCPCS Level II Supplies & Services

A4270 Disposable endoscope sheath, each
A4305 Disposable drug delivery system, flow rate of 50 ml or greater per hour
A4306 Disposable drug delivery system, flow rate of 5 ml or less per hour
A4550 Surgical trays

43216–43217

43216 Esophagoscopy, rigid or flexible; with removal of tumor(s), polyp(s), or other lesion(s) by hot biopsy forceps or bipolar cautery
43217 with removal of tumor(s), polyp(s), or other lesion(s) by snare technique

ICD-9-CM Diagnostic

150.0 Malignant neoplasm of cervical esophagus
150.1 Malignant neoplasm of thoracic esophagus
150.2 Malignant neoplasm of abdominal esophagus
150.3 Malignant neoplasm of upper third of esophagus
150.4 Malignant neoplasm of middle third of esophagus
150.5 Malignant neoplasm of lower third of esophagus
150.8 Malignant neoplasm of other specified part of esophagus
150.9 Malignant neoplasm of esophagus, unspecified site ▽
197.8 Secondary malignant neoplasm of other digestive organs and spleen
211.0 Benign neoplasm of esophagus
230.1 Carcinoma in situ of esophagus
235.5 Neoplasm of uncertain behavior of other and unspecified digestive organs ▽
239.0 Neoplasm of unspecified nature of digestive system
530.83 Esophageal leukoplakia
530.89 Other specified disorder of the esophagus

ICD-9-CM Procedural

42.33 Endoscopic excision or destruction of lesion or tissue of esophagus

HCPCS Level II Supplies & Services

A4270 Disposable endoscope sheath, each
A4305 Disposable drug delivery system, flow rate of 50 ml or greater per hour
A4306 Disposable drug delivery system, flow rate of 5 ml or less per hour
A4550 Surgical trays

43219

43219 Esophagoscopy, rigid or flexible; with insertion of plastic tube or stent

ICD-9-CM Diagnostic

150.0 Malignant neoplasm of cervical esophagus
150.1 Malignant neoplasm of thoracic esophagus
150.2 Malignant neoplasm of abdominal esophagus
150.3 Malignant neoplasm of upper third of esophagus
150.4 Malignant neoplasm of middle third of esophagus
150.5 Malignant neoplasm of lower third of esophagus
150.8 Malignant neoplasm of other specified part of esophagus
150.9 Malignant neoplasm of esophagus, unspecified site ▽
197.8 Secondary malignant neoplasm of other digestive organs and spleen
211.0 Benign neoplasm of esophagus

▽ Unspecified code ☒ Manifestation code
♀ Female diagnosis ♂ Male diagnosis

230.1 Carcinoma in situ of esophagus
235.5 Neoplasm of uncertain behavior of other and unspecified digestive organs ▽
239.0 Neoplasm of unspecified nature of digestive system
530.3 Stricture and stenosis of esophagus
530.89 Other specified disorder of the esophagus
750.3 Congenital tracheoesophageal fistula, esophageal atresia and stenosis

ICD-9-CM Procedural
42.81 Insertion of permanent tube into esophagus

43220–43226
43220 Esophagoscopy, rigid or flexible; with balloon dilation (less than 30 mm diameter)
43226 with insertion of guide wire followed by dilation over guide wire

ICD-9-CM Diagnostic
150.0 Malignant neoplasm of cervical esophagus
150.1 Malignant neoplasm of thoracic esophagus
150.2 Malignant neoplasm of abdominal esophagus
150.3 Malignant neoplasm of upper third of esophagus
150.4 Malignant neoplasm of middle third of esophagus
150.5 Malignant neoplasm of lower third of esophagus
150.8 Malignant neoplasm of other specified part of esophagus
151.0 Malignant neoplasm of cardia
197.8 Secondary malignant neoplasm of other digestive organs and spleen
199.1 Other malignant neoplasm of unspecified site
211.0 Benign neoplasm of esophagus
230.1 Carcinoma in situ of esophagus
235.5 Neoplasm of uncertain behavior of other and unspecified digestive organs ▽
239.0 Neoplasm of unspecified nature of digestive system
456.1 Esophageal varices without mention of bleeding
530.0 Achalasia and cardiospasm
530.11 Reflux esophagitis — (Use additional E code to identify cause, if induced by chemical or drug)
530.12 Acute esophagitis — (Use additional E code to identify cause, if induced by chemical or drug)
530.19 Other esophagitis — (Use additional E code to identify cause, if induced by chemical or drug)
530.3 Stricture and stenosis of esophagus
530.5 Dyskinesia of esophagus
530.81 Esophageal reflux
530.89 Other specified disorder of the esophagus
750.3 Congenital tracheoesophageal fistula, esophageal atresia and stenosis

ICD-9-CM Procedural
42.92 Dilation of esophagus

HCPCS Level II Supplies & Services
A4270 Disposable endoscope sheath, each
A4305 Disposable drug delivery system, flow rate of 50 ml or greater per hour
A4306 Disposable drug delivery system, flow rate of 5 ml or less per hour
A4550 Surgical trays

43227
43227 Esophagoscopy, rigid or flexible; with control of bleeding (eg, injection, bipolar cautery, unipolar cautery, laser, heater probe, stapler, plasma coagulator)

ICD-9-CM Diagnostic
150.0 Malignant neoplasm of cervical esophagus
150.1 Malignant neoplasm of thoracic esophagus
150.2 Malignant neoplasm of abdominal esophagus
150.3 Malignant neoplasm of upper third of esophagus
150.4 Malignant neoplasm of middle third of esophagus
150.5 Malignant neoplasm of lower third of esophagus
150.8 Malignant neoplasm of other specified part of esophagus
211.0 Benign neoplasm of esophagus
456.0 Esophageal varices with bleeding
456.20 Esophageal varices with bleeding in diseases classified elsewhere — (Code first underlying disease: 571.0-571.9, 572.3) ☒
530.21 Ulcer of esophagus with bleeding — (Use additional E code to identify cause, if induced by chemical or drug)
530.4 Perforation of esophagus
530.7 Gastroesophageal laceration-hemorrhage syndrome
530.81 Esophageal reflux
530.82 Esophageal hemorrhage
530.83 Esophageal leukoplakia
530.84 Tracheoesophageal fistula
530.85 Barrett's esophagus
530.89 Other specified disorder of the esophagus
571.0 Alcoholic fatty liver
571.1 Acute alcoholic hepatitis
571.2 Alcoholic cirrhosis of liver
571.3 Unspecified alcoholic liver damage ▽
571.40 Unspecified chronic hepatitis ▽
571.41 Chronic persistent hepatitis
571.9 Unspecified chronic liver disease without mention of alcohol ▽
572.3 Portal hypertension
998.11 Hemorrhage complicating a procedure
998.2 Accidental puncture or laceration during procedure

ICD-9-CM Procedural
42.33 Endoscopic excision or destruction of lesion or tissue of esophagus

43228
43228 Esophagoscopy, rigid or flexible; with ablation of tumor(s), polyp(s), or other lesion(s), not amenable to removal by hot biopsy forceps, bipolar cautery or snare technique

ICD-9-CM Diagnostic
150.0 Malignant neoplasm of cervical esophagus
150.1 Malignant neoplasm of thoracic esophagus
150.2 Malignant neoplasm of abdominal esophagus
150.3 Malignant neoplasm of upper third of esophagus
150.4 Malignant neoplasm of middle third of esophagus
150.5 Malignant neoplasm of lower third of esophagus
150.8 Malignant neoplasm of other specified part of esophagus
150.9 Malignant neoplasm of esophagus, unspecified site ▽
211.0 Benign neoplasm of esophagus
230.1 Carcinoma in situ of esophagus
235.5 Neoplasm of uncertain behavior of other and unspecified digestive organs ▽
239.0 Neoplasm of unspecified nature of digestive system
530.81 Esophageal reflux
530.83 Esophageal leukoplakia
530.84 Tracheoesophageal fistula
530.89 Other specified disorder of the esophagus

ICD-9-CM Procedural
42.33 Endoscopic excision or destruction of lesion or tissue of esophagus

43231
43231 Esophagoscopy, rigid or flexible; with endoscopic ultrasound examination

ICD-9-CM Diagnostic
150.0 Malignant neoplasm of cervical esophagus
150.1 Malignant neoplasm of thoracic esophagus
150.2 Malignant neoplasm of abdominal esophagus
150.3 Malignant neoplasm of upper third of esophagus
150.4 Malignant neoplasm of middle third of esophagus
150.5 Malignant neoplasm of lower third of esophagus
150.8 Malignant neoplasm of other specified part of esophagus
150.9 Malignant neoplasm of esophagus, unspecified site ▽
171.0 Malignant neoplasm of connective and other soft tissue of head, face, and neck
193 Malignant neoplasm of thyroid gland — (Use additional code to identify any functional activity)
195.0 Malignant neoplasm of head, face, and neck
196.0 Secondary and unspecified malignant neoplasm of lymph nodes of head, face, and neck
196.1 Secondary and unspecified malignant neoplasm of intrathoracic lymph nodes
196.9 Secondary and unspecified malignant neoplasm of lymph nodes, site unspecified ▽
197.8 Secondary malignant neoplasm of other digestive organs and spleen
198.89 Secondary malignant neoplasm of other specified sites
199.0 Disseminated malignant neoplasm
199.1 Other malignant neoplasm of unspecified site
202.81 Other malignant lymphomas of lymph nodes of head, face, and neck
211.0 Benign neoplasm of esophagus
211.9 Benign neoplasm of other and unspecified site of the digestive system ▽
230.1 Carcinoma in situ of esophagus
235.5 Neoplasm of uncertain behavior of other and unspecified digestive organs ▽
239.0 Neoplasm of unspecified nature of digestive system
263.0 Malnutrition of moderate degree
306.4 Gastrointestinal malfunction arising from mental factors

▽ Unspecified code ☒ Manifestation code
♀ Female diagnosis ♂ Male diagnosis

352.3 Disorders of pneumogastric (10th) nerve

448.0 Hereditary hemorrhagic telangiectasia

456.0 Esophageal varices with bleeding

456.1 Esophageal varices without mention of bleeding

530.0 Achalasia and cardiospasm

530.11 Reflux esophagitis — (Use additional E code to identify cause, if induced by chemical or drug)

530.12 Acute esophagitis — (Use additional E code to identify cause, if induced by chemical or drug)

530.19 Other esophagitis — (Use additional E code to identify cause, if induced by chemical or drug)

530.20 Ulcer of esophagus without bleeding — (Use additional E code to identify cause, if induced by chemical or drug)

530.21 Ulcer of esophagus with bleeding — (Use additional E code to identify cause, if induced by chemical or drug)

530.3 Stricture and stenosis of esophagus

530.4 Perforation of esophagus

530.5 Dyskinesia of esophagus

530.6 Diverticulum of esophagus, acquired

530.7 Gastroesophageal laceration-hemorrhage syndrome

530.81 Esophageal reflux

530.82 Esophageal hemorrhage

530.83 Esophageal leukoplakia

530.84 Tracheoesophageal fistula

530.85 Barrett's esophagus

530.89 Other specified disorder of the esophagus

530.9 Unspecified disorder of esophagus ▽

552.3 Diaphragmatic hernia with obstruction

553.3 Diaphragmatic hernia without mention of obstruction or gangrene

578.0 Hematemesis

578.9 Unspecified, hemorrhage of gastrointestinal tract ▽

750.4 Other specified congenital anomaly of esophagus

750.9 Unspecified congenital anomaly of upper alimentary tract ▽

784.1 Throat pain

787.1 Heartburn

787.2 Dysphagia

793.4 Nonspecific abnormal findings on radiological and other examination of gastrointestinal tract

799.89 Other ill-defined conditions

862.22 Esophagus injury without mention of open wound into cavity

ICD-9-CM Procedural

42.23 Other esophagoscopy

88.74 Diagnostic ultrasound of digestive system

43232

43232 Esophagoscopy, rigid or flexible; with transendoscopic ultrasound-guided intramural or transmural fine needle aspiration/biopsy(s)

ICD-9-CM Diagnostic

150.0 Malignant neoplasm of cervical esophagus

150.1 Malignant neoplasm of thoracic esophagus

150.2 Malignant neoplasm of abdominal esophagus

150.3 Malignant neoplasm of upper third of esophagus

150.4 Malignant neoplasm of middle third of esophagus

150.5 Malignant neoplasm of lower third of esophagus

150.8 Malignant neoplasm of other specified part of esophagus

150.9 Malignant neoplasm of esophagus, unspecified site ▽

171.0 Malignant neoplasm of connective and other soft tissue of head, face, and neck

193 Malignant neoplasm of thyroid gland — (Use additional code to identify any functional activity)

195.0 Malignant neoplasm of head, face, and neck

196.0 Secondary and unspecified malignant neoplasm of lymph nodes of head, face, and neck

196.1 Secondary and unspecified malignant neoplasm of intrathoracic lymph nodes

196.9 Secondary and unspecified malignant neoplasm of lymph nodes, site unspecified ▽

197.8 Secondary malignant neoplasm of other digestive organs and spleen

198.89 Secondary malignant neoplasm of other specified sites

199.0 Disseminated malignant neoplasm

199.1 Other malignant neoplasm of unspecified site

202.81 Other malignant lymphomas of lymph nodes of head, face, and neck

211.0 Benign neoplasm of esophagus

211.9 Benign neoplasm of other and unspecified site of the digestive system ▽

230.1 Carcinoma in situ of esophagus

235.5 Neoplasm of uncertain behavior of other and unspecified digestive organs ▽

239.0 Neoplasm of unspecified nature of digestive system

239.8 Neoplasm of unspecified nature of other specified sites

448.0 Hereditary hemorrhagic telangiectasia

530.0 Achalasia and cardiospasm

530.20 Ulcer of esophagus without bleeding — (Use additional E code to identify cause, if induced by chemical or drug)

530.21 Ulcer of esophagus with bleeding — (Use additional E code to identify cause, if induced by chemical or drug)

530.6 Diverticulum of esophagus, acquired

530.83 Esophageal leukoplakia

530.85 Barrett's esophagus

530.89 Other specified disorder of the esophagus

530.9 Unspecified disorder of esophagus ▽

578.0 Hematemesis

578.9 Unspecified, hemorrhage of gastrointestinal tract ▽

786.6 Swelling, mass, or lump in chest

787.2 Dysphagia

789.36 Abdominal or pelvic swelling, mass, or lump, epigastric

793.4 Nonspecific abnormal findings on radiological and other examination of gastrointestinal tract

799.89 Other ill-defined conditions

ICD-9-CM Procedural

42.24 Closed (endoscopic) biopsy of esophagus

88.74 Diagnostic ultrasound of digestive system

43234

43234 Upper gastrointestinal endoscopy, simple primary examination (eg, with small diameter flexible endoscope) (separate procedure)

ICD-9-CM Diagnostic

150.0 Malignant neoplasm of cervical esophagus

151.0 Malignant neoplasm of cardia

151.1 Malignant neoplasm of pylorus

151.2 Malignant neoplasm of pyloric antrum

151.3 Malignant neoplasm of fundus of stomach

151.4 Malignant neoplasm of body of stomach

151.5 Malignant neoplasm of lesser curvature of stomach, unspecified ▽

151.6 Malignant neoplasm of greater curvature of stomach, unspecified ▽

151.8 Malignant neoplasm of other specified sites of stomach

151.9 Malignant neoplasm of stomach, unspecified site ▽

211.1 Benign neoplasm of stomach

211.2 Benign neoplasm of duodenum, jejunum, and ileum

239.0 Neoplasm of unspecified nature of digestive system

456.1 Esophageal varices without mention of bleeding

530.11 Reflux esophagitis — (Use additional E code to identify cause, if induced by chemical or drug)

530.12 Acute esophagitis — (Use additional E code to identify cause, if induced by chemical or drug)

530.19 Other esophagitis — (Use additional E code to identify cause, if induced by chemical or drug)

530.20 Ulcer of esophagus without bleeding — (Use additional E code to identify cause, if induced by chemical or drug)

530.21 Ulcer of esophagus with bleeding — (Use additional E code to identify cause, if induced by chemical or drug)

530.3 Stricture and stenosis of esophagus

530.4 Perforation of esophagus

530.5 Dyskinesia of esophagus

530.6 Diverticulum of esophagus, acquired

530.81 Esophageal reflux

530.83 Esophageal leukoplakia

530.85 Barrett's esophagus

531.30 Acute gastric ulcer without mention of hemorrhage, perforation, or obstruction — (Use additional E code to identify drug, if drug induced)

531.31 Acute gastric ulcer without mention of hemorrhage or perforation, with obstruction — (Use additional E code to identify drug, if drug induced)

531.70 Chronic gastric ulcer without mention of hemorrhage, perforation, without mention of obstruction — (Use additional E code to identify drug, if drug induced)

531.71 Chronic gastric ulcer without mention of hemorrhage or perforation, with obstruction — (Use additional E code to identify drug, if drug induced)

531.90 Gastric ulcer, unspecified as acute or chronic, without mention of hemorrhage, perforation, or obstruction — (Use additional E code to identify drug, if drug induced) ▽

532.90 Duodenal ulcer, unspecified as acute or chronic, without hemorrhage, perforation, or obstruction — (Use additional E code to identify drug, if drug induced) ▽
533.70 Chronic peptic ulcer, unspecified site, without mention of hemorrhage, perforation, or obstruction — (Use additional E code to identify drug, if drug induced)
533.71 Chronic peptic ulcer of unspecified site without mention of hemorrhage or perforation, with obstruction — (Use additional E code to identify drug, if drug induced)
535.10 Atrophic gastritis without mention of hemorrhage
535.40 Other specified gastritis without mention of hemorrhage
535.60 Duodenitis without mention of hemorrhage
536.2 Persistent vomiting
537.4 Fistula of stomach or duodenum
537.84 Dieulafoy lesion (hemorrhagic) of stomach and duodenum
553.3 Diaphragmatic hernia without mention of obstruction or gangrene
578.0 Hematemesis
578.1 Blood in stool
750.6 Congenital hiatus hernia
751.5 Other congenital anomalies of intestine
783.0 Anorexia
783.3 Feeding difficulties and mismanagement
783.7 Adult failure to thrive
787.01 Nausea with vomiting
793.4 Nonspecific abnormal findings on radiological and other examination of gastrointestinal tract
V10.04 Personal history of malignant neoplasm of stomach

ICD-9-CM Procedural

44.13 Other gastroscopy

HCPCS Level II Supplies & Services

A4270 Disposable endoscope sheath, each
A4550 Surgical trays

43235–43236

43235 Upper gastrointestinal endoscopy including esophagus, stomach, and either the duodenum and/or jejunum as appropriate; diagnostic, with or without collection of specimen(s) by brushing or washing (separate procedure)
43236 with directed submucosal injection(s), any substance

ICD-9-CM Diagnostic

150.0 Malignant neoplasm of cervical esophagus
150.1 Malignant neoplasm of thoracic esophagus
150.2 Malignant neoplasm of abdominal esophagus
150.3 Malignant neoplasm of upper third of esophagus
150.4 Malignant neoplasm of middle third of esophagus
150.5 Malignant neoplasm of lower third of esophagus
150.8 Malignant neoplasm of other specified part of esophagus
150.9 Malignant neoplasm of esophagus, unspecified site ▽
151.0 Malignant neoplasm of cardia
151.1 Malignant neoplasm of pylorus
151.2 Malignant neoplasm of pyloric antrum
151.3 Malignant neoplasm of fundus of stomach
151.4 Malignant neoplasm of body of stomach
151.5 Malignant neoplasm of lesser curvature of stomach, unspecified ▽
151.6 Malignant neoplasm of greater curvature of stomach, unspecified ▽
151.8 Malignant neoplasm of other specified sites of stomach
151.9 Malignant neoplasm of stomach, unspecified site ▽
152.0 Malignant neoplasm of duodenum
152.1 Malignant neoplasm of jejunum
152.8 Malignant neoplasm of other specified sites of small intestine
152.9 Malignant neoplasm of small intestine, unspecified site ▽
159.9 Malignant neoplasm of ill-defined sites of digestive organs and peritoneum
197.4 Secondary malignant neoplasm of small intestine including duodenum
197.8 Secondary malignant neoplasm of other digestive organs and spleen
199.0 Disseminated malignant neoplasm
199.1 Other malignant neoplasm of unspecified site
211.0 Benign neoplasm of esophagus
211.1 Benign neoplasm of stomach
211.2 Benign neoplasm of duodenum, jejunum, and ileum
230.1 Carcinoma in situ of esophagus
230.2 Carcinoma in situ of stomach
235.2 Neoplasm of uncertain behavior of stomach, intestines, and rectum
239.0 Neoplasm of unspecified nature of digestive system
285.9 Unspecified anemia ▽
456.21 Esophageal varices without mention of bleeding in diseases classified elsewhere — (Code first underlying disease: 571.0-571.9, 572.3) ☒
530.0 Achalasia and cardiospasm
530.10 Unspecified esophagitis — (Use additional E code to identify cause, if induced by chemical or drug) ▽
530.11 Reflux esophagitis — (Use additional E code to identify cause, if induced by chemical or drug)
530.12 Acute esophagitis — (Use additional E code to identify cause, if induced by chemical or drug)
530.19 Other esophagitis — (Use additional E code to identify cause, if induced by chemical or drug)
530.20 Ulcer of esophagus without bleeding — (Use additional E code to identify cause, if induced by chemical or drug)
530.21 Ulcer of esophagus with bleeding — (Use additional E code to identify cause, if induced by chemical or drug)
530.3 Stricture and stenosis of esophagus
530.5 Dyskinesia of esophagus
530.6 Diverticulum of esophagus, acquired
530.7 Gastroesophageal laceration-hemorrhage syndrome
530.81 Esophageal reflux
530.82 Esophageal hemorrhage
530.83 Esophageal leukoplakia
530.84 Tracheoesophageal fistula
530.85 Barrett's esophagus
530.89 Other specified disorder of the esophagus
531.00 Acute gastric ulcer with hemorrhage, without mention of obstruction — (Use additional E code to identify drug, if drug induced)
531.01 Acute gastric ulcer with hemorrhage and obstruction — (Use additional E code to identify drug, if drug induced)
531.10 Acute gastric ulcer with perforation, without mention of obstruction — (Use additional E code to identify drug, if drug induced)
531.20 Acute gastric ulcer with hemorrhage and perforation, without mention of obstruction — (Use additional E code to identify drug, if drug induced)
531.30 Acute gastric ulcer without mention of hemorrhage, perforation, or obstruction — (Use additional E code to identify drug, if drug induced)
531.31 Acute gastric ulcer without mention of hemorrhage or perforation, with obstruction — (Use additional E code to identify drug, if drug induced)
531.40 Chronic or unspecified gastric ulcer with hemorrhage, without mention of obstruction — (Use additional E code to identify drug, if drug induced)
531.41 Chronic or unspecified gastric ulcer with hemorrhage and obstruction — (Use additional E code to identify drug, if drug induced)
531.50 Chronic or unspecified gastric ulcer with perforation, without mention of obstruction — (Use additional E code to identify drug, if drug induced)
531.51 Chronic or unspecified gastric ulcer with perforation and obstruction — (Use additional E code to identify drug, if drug induced)
531.60 Chronic or unspecified gastric ulcer with hemorrhage and perforation, without mention of obstruction — (Use additional E code to identify drug, if drug induced)
531.61 Chronic or unspecified gastric ulcer with hemorrhage, perforation, and obstruction — (Use additional E code to identify drug, if drug induced)
531.70 Chronic gastric ulcer without mention of hemorrhage, perforation, without mention of obstruction — (Use additional E code to identify drug, if drug induced)
531.71 Chronic gastric ulcer without mention of hemorrhage or perforation, with obstruction — (Use additional E code to identify drug, if drug induced)
531.90 Gastric ulcer, unspecified as acute or chronic, without mention of hemorrhage, perforation, or obstruction — (Use additional E code to identify drug, if drug induced) ▽
531.91 Gastric ulcer, unspecified as acute or chronic, without mention of hemorrhage or perforation, with obstruction — (Use additional E code to identify drug, if drug induced) ▽
532.00 Acute duodenal ulcer with hemorrhage, without mention of obstruction — (Use additional E code to identify drug, if drug induced)
532.01 Acute duodenal ulcer with hemorrhage and obstruction — (Use additional E code to identify drug, if drug induced)
532.10 Acute duodenal ulcer with perforation, without mention of obstruction — (Use additional E code to identify drug, if drug induced)
532.11 Acute duodenal ulcer with perforation and obstruction — (Use additional E code to identify drug, if drug induced)
532.20 Acute duodenal ulcer with hemorrhage and perforation, without mention of obstruction — (Use additional E code to identify drug, if drug induced)
532.21 Acute duodenal ulcer with hemorrhage, perforation, and obstruction — (Use additional E code to identify drug, if drug induced)
532.30 Acute duodenal ulcer without mention of hemorrhage, perforation, or obstruction — (Use additional E code to identify drug, if drug induced)

532.31 Acute duodenal ulcer without mention of hemorrhage or perforation, with obstruction — (Use additional E code to identify drug, if drug induced)
532.40 Chronic or unspecified duodenal ulcer with hemorrhage, without mention of obstruction — (Use additional E code to identify drug, if drug induced)
532.41 Chronic or unspecified duodenal ulcer with hemorrhage and obstruction — (Use additional E code to identify drug, if drug induced)
532.50 Chronic or unspecified duodenal ulcer with perforation, without mention of obstruction — (Use additional E code to identify drug, if drug induced)
532.51 Chronic or unspecified duodenal ulcer with perforation and obstruction — (Use additional E code to identify drug, if drug induced)
532.60 Chronic or unspecified duodenal ulcer with hemorrhage and perforation, without mention of obstruction — (Use additional E code to identify drug, if drug induced)
532.61 Chronic or unspecified duodenal ulcer with hemorrhage, perforation, and obstruction — (Use additional E code to identify drug, if drug induced)
532.70 Chronic duodenal ulcer without mention of hemorrhage, perforation, or obstruction — (Use additional E code to identify drug, if drug induced)
532.71 Chronic duodenal ulcer without mention of hemorrhage or perforation, with obstruction — (Use additional E code to identify drug, if drug induced)
532.90 Duodenal ulcer, unspecified as acute or chronic, without hemorrhage, perforation, or obstruction — (Use additional E code to identify drug, if drug induced)
532.91 Duodenal ulcer, unspecified as acute or chronic, without mention of hemorrhage or perforation, with obstruction — (Use additional E code to identify drug, if drug induced)
533.00 Acute peptic ulcer, unspecified site, with hemorrhage, without mention of obstruction — (Use additional E code to identify drug, if drug induced)
533.01 Acute peptic ulcer, unspecified site, with hemorrhage and obstruction — (Use additional E code to identify drug, if drug induced)
533.10 Acute peptic ulcer, unspecified site, with perforation, without mention of obstruction — (Use additional E code to identify drug, if drug induced)
533.11 Acute peptic ulcer, unspecified site, with perforation and obstruction — (Use additional E code to identify drug, if drug induced)
533.20 Acute peptic ulcer, unspecified site, with hemorrhage and perforation, without mention of obstruction — (Use additional E code to identify drug, if drug induced)
533.21 Acute peptic ulcer, unspecified site, with hemorrhage, perforation, and obstruction — (Use additional E code to identify drug, if drug induced)
533.30 Acute peptic ulcer, unspecified site, without mention of hemorrhage, perforation, or obstruction — (Use additional E code to identify drug, if drug induced)
533.31 Acute peptic ulcer, unspecified site, without mention of hemorrhage and perforation, with obstruction — (Use additional E code to identify drug, if drug induced)
533.40 Chronic or unspecified peptic ulcer, unspecified site, with hemorrhage, without mention of obstruction — (Use additional E code to identify drug, if drug induced)
533.41 Chronic or unspecified peptic ulcer, unspecified site, with hemorrhage and obstruction — (Use additional E code to identify drug, if drug induced)
533.50 Chronic or unspecified peptic ulcer, unspecified site, with perforation, without mention of obstruction — (Use additional E code to identify drug, if drug induced)
533.51 Chronic or unspecified peptic ulcer, unspecified site, with perforation and obstruction — (Use additional E code to identify drug, if drug induced)
533.60 Chronic or unspecified peptic ulcer, unspecified site, with hemorrhage and perforation, without mention of obstruction — (Use additional E code to identify drug, if drug induced)
533.61 Chronic or unspecified peptic ulcer, unspecified site, with hemorrhage, perforation, and obstruction — (Use additional E code to identify drug, if drug induced)
533.70 Chronic peptic ulcer, unspecified site, without mention of hemorrhage, perforation, or obstruction — (Use additional E code to identify drug, if drug induced)
533.71 Chronic peptic ulcer of unspecified site without mention of hemorrhage or perforation, with obstruction — (Use additional E code to identify drug, if drug induced)
533.90 Peptic ulcer, unspecified site, unspecified as acute or chronic, without mention of hemorrhage, perforation, or obstruction — (Use additional E code to identify drug, if drug induced)
533.91 Peptic ulcer, unspecified site, unspecified as acute or chronic, without mention of hemorrhage or perforation, with obstruction — (Use additional E code to identify drug, if drug induced)
534.00 Acute gastrojejunal ulcer with hemorrhage, without mention of obstruction
534.01 Acute gastrojejunal ulcer, with hemorrhage and obstruction
534.10 Acute gastrojejunal ulcer with perforation, without mention of obstruction
534.11 Acute gastrojejunal ulcer with perforation and obstruction
534.20 Acute gastrojejunal ulcer with hemorrhage and perforation, without mention of obstruction
534.21 Acute gastrojejunal ulcer with hemorrhage, perforation, and obstruction
534.30 Acute gastrojejunal ulcer without mention of hemorrhage, perforation, or obstruction
534.31 Acute gastrojejunal ulcer without mention of hemorrhage or perforation, with obstruction
534.40 Chronic or unspecified gastrojejunal ulcer with hemorrhage, without mention of obstruction
534.41 Chronic or unspecified gastrojejunal ulcer, with hemorrhage and obstruction
534.50 Chronic or unspecified gastrojejunal ulcer with perforation, without mention of obstruction
534.51 Chronic or unspecified gastrojejunal ulcer with perforation and obstruction
534.60 Chronic or unspecified gastrojejunal ulcer with hemorrhage and perforation, without mention of obstruction
534.61 Chronic or unspecified gastrojejunal ulcer with hemorrhage, perforation, and obstruction
534.70 Chronic gastrojejunal ulcer without mention of hemorrhage, perforation, or obstruction
534.71 Chronic gastrojejunal ulcer without mention of hemorrhage or perforation, with obstruction
534.90 Gastrojejunal ulcer, unspecified as acute or chronic, without mention of hemorrhage, perforation, or obstruction
534.91 Gastrojejunal ulcer, unspecified as acute or chronic, without mention of hemorrhage or perforation, with obstruction
535.00 Acute gastritis without mention of hemorrhage
535.01 Acute gastritis with hemorrhage
535.10 Atrophic gastritis without mention of hemorrhage
535.11 Atrophic gastritis with hemorrhage
535.20 Gastric mucosal hypertrophy without mention of hemorrhage
535.21 Gastric mucosal hypertrophy with hemorrhage
535.30 Alcoholic gastritis without mention of hemorrhage
535.31 Alcoholic gastritis with hemorrhage
535.40 Other specified gastritis without mention of hemorrhage
535.41 Other specified gastritis with hemorrhage
535.60 Duodenitis without mention of hemorrhage
535.61 Duodenitis with hemorrhage
536.0 Achlorhydria
536.1 Acute dilatation of stomach
536.2 Persistent vomiting
536.3 Gastroparesis
536.8 Dyspepsia and other specified disorders of function of stomach
536.9 Unspecified functional disorder of stomach
537.0 Acquired hypertrophic pyloric stenosis
537.1 Gastric diverticulum
537.2 Chronic duodenal ileus
537.3 Other obstruction of duodenum
537.4 Fistula of stomach or duodenum
537.5 Gastroptosis
537.6 Hourglass stricture or stenosis of stomach
537.81 Pylorospasm
537.82 Angiodysplasia of stomach and duodenum (without mention of hemorrhage)
537.83 Angiodysplasia of stomach and duodenum with hemorrhage
537.84 Dieulafoy lesion (hemorrhagic) of stomach and duodenum
537.89 Other specified disorder of stomach and duodenum
537.9 Unspecified disorder of stomach and duodenum
552.3 Diaphragmatic hernia with obstruction
553.3 Diaphragmatic hernia without mention of obstruction or gangrene
555.0 Regional enteritis of small intestine
558.1 Gastroenteritis and colitis due to radiation
558.2 Toxic gastroenteritis and colitis — (Use additional E code to identify cause)
558.3 Gastroenteritis and colitis, allergic — (Use additional code to identify type of food allergy: V15.01-V15.05)
558.9 Other and unspecified noninfectious gastroenteritis and colitis
569.5 Abscess of intestine
569.82 Ulceration of intestine
569.86 Dieulafoy lesion (hemorrhagic) of intestine
569.89 Other specified disorder of intestines
571.0 Alcoholic fatty liver
571.1 Acute alcoholic hepatitis
571.2 Alcoholic cirrhosis of liver
571.3 Unspecified alcoholic liver damage
571.40 Unspecified chronic hepatitis
571.41 Chronic persistent hepatitis
571.49 Other chronic hepatitis
571.5 Cirrhosis of liver without mention of alcohol

Unspecified code
♀ Female diagnosis
Manifestation code
♂ Male diagnosis

571.6 Biliary cirrhosis
571.8 Other chronic nonalcoholic liver disease
572.3 Portal hypertension
577.0 Acute pancreatitis
577.1 Chronic pancreatitis
578.0 Hematemesis
578.1 Blood in stool
579.0 Celiac disease
579.2 Blind loop syndrome
579.3 Other and unspecified postsurgical nonabsorption ▽
579.8 Other specified intestinal malabsorption
747.61 Congenital gastrointestinal vessel anomaly
750.3 Congenital tracheoesophageal fistula, esophageal atresia and stenosis
750.4 Other specified congenital anomaly of esophagus
750.5 Congenital hypertrophic pyloric stenosis
750.6 Congenital hiatus hernia
750.7 Other specified congenital anomalies of stomach
751.8 Other specified congenital anomalies of digestive system
783.0 Anorexia
783.21 Loss of weight
783.22 Underweight
783.7 Adult failure to thrive
784.1 Throat pain
787.1 Heartburn
787.2 Dysphagia
787.3 Flatulence, eructation, and gas pain
787.4 Visible peristalsis
787.5 Abnormal bowel sounds
787.99 Other symptoms involving digestive system
789.09 Abdominal pain, other specified site
792.1 Nonspecific abnormal finding in stool contents
793.4 Nonspecific abnormal findings on radiological and other examination of gastrointestinal tract
997.4 Digestive system complication — (Use additional code to identify complications)
V10.00 Personal history of malignant neoplasm of unspecified site in gastrointestinal tract ▽
V12.71 Personal history of peptic ulcer disease
V12.79 Personal history of other diseases of digestive disease
V16.0 Family history of malignant neoplasm of gastrointestinal tract
V18.5 Family history of digestive disorders
V67.00 Follow-up examination, following unspecified surgery ▽
V67.09 Follow-up examination, following other surgery
V67.59 Other follow-up examination
V67.9 Unspecified follow-up examination ▽
V71.1 Observation for suspected malignant neoplasm
V71.89 Observation for other specified suspected conditions

ICD-9-CM Procedural

42.23 Other esophagoscopy
42.33 Endoscopic excision or destruction of lesion or tissue of esophagus
43.41 Endoscopic excision or destruction of lesion or tissue of stomach
45.16 Esophagogastroduodenoscopy (EGD) with closed biopsy

HCPCS Level II Supplies & Services

A4270 Disposable endoscope sheath, each
A4550 Surgical trays

43237–43238

43237 Upper gastrointestinal endoscopy including esophagus, stomach, and either the duodenum and/or jejunum as appropriate; with endoscopic ultrasound examination limited to the esophagus

43238 with transendoscopic ultrasound-guided intramural or transmural fine needle aspiration/biopsy(s), esophagus (includes endoscopic ultrasound examination limited to the esophagus)

ICD-9-CM Diagnostic

150.0 Malignant neoplasm of cervical esophagus
150.1 Malignant neoplasm of thoracic esophagus
150.2 Malignant neoplasm of abdominal esophagus
150.3 Malignant neoplasm of upper third of esophagus
150.4 Malignant neoplasm of middle third of esophagus
150.5 Malignant neoplasm of lower third of esophagus
150.8 Malignant neoplasm of other specified part of esophagus
150.9 Malignant neoplasm of esophagus, unspecified site ▽
171.0 Malignant neoplasm of connective and other soft tissue of head, face, and neck
193 Malignant neoplasm of thyroid gland — (Use additional code to identify any functional activity)
195.0 Malignant neoplasm of head, face, and neck
196.0 Secondary and unspecified malignant neoplasm of lymph nodes of head, face, and neck
196.9 Secondary and unspecified malignant neoplasm of lymph nodes, site unspecified ▽
197.8 Secondary malignant neoplasm of other digestive organs and spleen
198.89 Secondary malignant neoplasm of other specified sites
199.0 Disseminated malignant neoplasm
199.1 Other malignant neoplasm of unspecified site
202.81 Other malignant lymphomas of lymph nodes of head, face, and neck
211.0 Benign neoplasm of esophagus
211.9 Benign neoplasm of other and unspecified site of the digestive system ▽
230.1 Carcinoma in situ of esophagus
235.5 Neoplasm of uncertain behavior of other and unspecified digestive organs ▽
239.0 Neoplasm of unspecified nature of digestive system
263.0 Malnutrition of moderate degree
306.4 Gastrointestinal malfunction arising from mental factors
352.3 Disorders of pneumogastric (10th) nerve
448.0 Hereditary hemorrhagic telangiectasia
456.0 Esophageal varices with bleeding
456.1 Esophageal varices without mention of bleeding
530.0 Achalasia and cardiospasm
530.11 Reflux esophagitis — (Use additional E code to identify cause, if induced by chemical or drug)
530.12 Acute esophagitis — (Use additional E code to identify cause, if induced by chemical or drug)
530.19 Other esophagitis — (Use additional E code to identify cause, if induced by chemical or drug)
530.20 Ulcer of esophagus without bleeding — (Use additional E code to identify cause, if induced by chemical or drug)
530.21 Ulcer of esophagus with bleeding — (Use additional E code to identify cause, if induced by chemical or drug)
530.3 Stricture and stenosis of esophagus
530.4 Perforation of esophagus
530.5 Dyskinesia of esophagus
530.6 Diverticulum of esophagus, acquired
530.7 Gastroesophageal laceration-hemorrhage syndrome
530.81 Esophageal reflux
530.82 Esophageal hemorrhage
530.83 Esophageal leukoplakia
530.84 Tracheoesophageal fistula
530.85 Barrett's esophagus
530.89 Other specified disorder of the esophagus
530.9 Unspecified disorder of esophagus ▽
552.3 Diaphragmatic hernia with obstruction
553.3 Diaphragmatic hernia without mention of obstruction or gangrene
578.0 Hematemesis
578.1 Blood in stool
578.9 Unspecified, hemorrhage of gastrointestinal tract ▽
750.4 Other specified congenital anomaly of esophagus
750.9 Unspecified congenital anomaly of upper alimentary tract ▽
784.1 Throat pain
787.1 Heartburn
787.2 Dysphagia
793.4 Nonspecific abnormal findings on radiological and other examination of gastrointestinal tract
799.89 Other ill-defined conditions
862.22 Esophagus injury without mention of open wound into cavity

ICD-9-CM Procedural

42.29 Other diagnostic procedures on esophagus
42.33 Endoscopic excision or destruction of lesion or tissue of esophagus
43.41 Endoscopic excision or destruction of lesion or tissue of stomach
45.16 Esophagogastroduodenoscopy (EGD) with closed biopsy

HCPCS Level II Supplies & Services

A4270 Disposable endoscope sheath, each
A4550 Surgical trays

43239

43239 Upper gastrointestinal endoscopy including esophagus, stomach, and either the duodenum and/or jejunum as appropriate; with biopsy, single or multiple

ICD-9-CM Diagnostic

150.0 Malignant neoplasm of cervical esophagus

150.1 Malignant neoplasm of thoracic esophagus

150.2 Malignant neoplasm of abdominal esophagus

150.3 Malignant neoplasm of upper third of esophagus

150.4 Malignant neoplasm of middle third of esophagus

150.5 Malignant neoplasm of lower third of esophagus

150.8 Malignant neoplasm of other specified part of esophagus

150.9 Malignant neoplasm of esophagus, unspecified site ▽

151.0 Malignant neoplasm of cardia

151.1 Malignant neoplasm of pylorus

151.2 Malignant neoplasm of pyloric antrum

151.3 Malignant neoplasm of fundus of stomach

151.4 Malignant neoplasm of body of stomach

151.5 Malignant neoplasm of lesser curvature of stomach, unspecified ▽

151.6 Malignant neoplasm of greater curvature of stomach, unspecified ▽

151.8 Malignant neoplasm of other specified sites of stomach

151.9 Malignant neoplasm of stomach, unspecified site ▽

152.0 Malignant neoplasm of duodenum

152.1 Malignant neoplasm of jejunum

152.8 Malignant neoplasm of other specified sites of small intestine

152.9 Malignant neoplasm of small intestine, unspecified site ▽

159.9 Malignant neoplasm of ill-defined sites of digestive organs and peritoneum

197.4 Secondary malignant neoplasm of small intestine including duodenum

197.8 Secondary malignant neoplasm of other digestive organs and spleen

199.0 Disseminated malignant neoplasm

199.1 Other malignant neoplasm of unspecified site

211.0 Benign neoplasm of esophagus

211.1 Benign neoplasm of stomach

211.2 Benign neoplasm of duodenum, jejunum, and ileum

230.1 Carcinoma in situ of esophagus

230.2 Carcinoma in situ of stomach

235.2 Neoplasm of uncertain behavior of stomach, intestines, and rectum

239.0 Neoplasm of unspecified nature of digestive system

285.9 Unspecified anemia ▽

456.21 Esophageal varices without mention of bleeding in diseases classified elsewhere — (Code first underlying disease: 571.0-571.9, 572.3) ☒

530.0 Achalasia and cardiospasm

530.10 Unspecified esophagitis — (Use additional E code to identify cause, if induced by chemical or drug) ▽

530.11 Reflux esophagitis — (Use additional E code to identify cause, if induced by chemical or drug)

530.12 Acute esophagitis — (Use additional E code to identify cause, if induced by chemical or drug)

530.19 Other esophagitis — (Use additional E code to identify cause, if induced by chemical or drug)

530.20 Ulcer of esophagus without bleeding — (Use additional E code to identify cause, if induced by chemical or drug)

530.21 Ulcer of esophagus with bleeding — (Use additional E code to identify cause, if induced by chemical or drug)

530.3 Stricture and stenosis of esophagus

530.5 Dyskinesia of esophagus

530.6 Diverticulum of esophagus, acquired

530.7 Gastroesophageal laceration-hemorrhage syndrome

530.81 Esophageal reflux

530.82 Esophageal hemorrhage

530.83 Esophageal leukoplakia

530.84 Tracheoesophageal fistula

530.85 Barrett's esophagus

530.89 Other specified disorder of the esophagus

531.00 Acute gastric ulcer with hemorrhage, without mention of obstruction — (Use additional E code to identify drug, if drug induced)

531.01 Acute gastric ulcer with hemorrhage and obstruction — (Use additional E code to identify drug, if drug induced)

531.10 Acute gastric ulcer with perforation, without mention of obstruction — (Use additional E code to identify drug, if drug induced)

531.20 Acute gastric ulcer with hemorrhage and perforation, without mention of obstruction — (Use additional E code to identify drug, if drug induced)

531.30 Acute gastric ulcer without mention of hemorrhage, perforation, or obstruction — (Use additional E code to identify drug, if drug induced)

531.31 Acute gastric ulcer without mention of hemorrhage or perforation, with obstruction — (Use additional E code to identify drug, if drug induced)

531.40 Chronic or unspecified gastric ulcer with hemorrhage, without mention of obstruction — (Use additional E code to identify drug, if drug induced)

531.41 Chronic or unspecified gastric ulcer with hemorrhage and obstruction — (Use additional E code to identify drug, if drug induced)

531.50 Chronic or unspecified gastric ulcer with perforation, without mention of obstruction — (Use additional E code to identify drug, if drug induced)

531.51 Chronic or unspecified gastric ulcer with perforation and obstruction — (Use additional E code to identify drug, if drug induced)

531.60 Chronic or unspecified gastric ulcer with hemorrhage and perforation, without mention of obstruction — (Use additional E code to identify drug, if drug induced)

531.61 Chronic or unspecified gastric ulcer with hemorrhage, perforation, and obstruction — (Use additional E code to identify drug, if drug induced)

531.70 Chronic gastric ulcer without mention of hemorrhage, perforation, without mention of obstruction — (Use additional E code to identify drug, if drug induced)

531.71 Chronic gastric ulcer without mention of hemorrhage or perforation, with obstruction — (Use additional E code to identify drug, if drug induced)

531.90 Gastric ulcer, unspecified as acute or chronic, without mention of hemorrhage, perforation, or obstruction — (Use additional E code to identify drug, if drug induced) ▽

531.91 Gastric ulcer, unspecified as acute or chronic, without mention of hemorrhage or perforation, with obstruction — (Use additional E code to identify drug, if drug induced) ▽

532.00 Acute duodenal ulcer with hemorrhage, without mention of obstruction — (Use additional E code to identify drug, if drug induced)

532.01 Acute duodenal ulcer with hemorrhage and obstruction — (Use additional E code to identify drug, if drug induced)

532.10 Acute duodenal ulcer with perforation, without mention of obstruction — (Use additional E code to identify drug, if drug induced)

532.11 Acute duodenal ulcer with perforation and obstruction — (Use additional E code to identify drug, if drug induced)

532.20 Acute duodenal ulcer with hemorrhage and perforation, without mention of obstruction — (Use additional E code to identify drug, if drug induced)

532.21 Acute duodenal ulcer with hemorrhage, perforation, and obstruction — (Use additional E code to identify drug, if drug induced)

532.30 Acute duodenal ulcer without mention of hemorrhage, perforation, or obstruction — (Use additional E code to identify drug, if drug induced)

532.31 Acute duodenal ulcer without mention of hemorrhage or perforation, with obstruction — (Use additional E code to identify drug, if drug induced)

532.40 Chronic or unspecified duodenal ulcer with hemorrhage, without mention of obstruction — (Use additional E code to identify drug, if drug induced)

532.41 Chronic or unspecified duodenal ulcer with hemorrhage and obstruction — (Use additional E code to identify drug, if drug induced)

532.50 Chronic or unspecified duodenal ulcer with perforation, without mention of obstruction — (Use additional E code to identify drug, if drug induced)

532.51 Chronic or unspecified duodenal ulcer with perforation and obstruction — (Use additional E code to identify drug, if drug induced)

532.60 Chronic or unspecified duodenal ulcer with hemorrhage and perforation, without mention of obstruction — (Use additional E code to identify drug, if drug induced)

532.61 Chronic or unspecified duodenal ulcer with hemorrhage, perforation, and obstruction — (Use additional E code to identify drug, if drug induced)

532.70 Chronic duodenal ulcer without mention of hemorrhage, perforation, or obstruction — (Use additional E code to identify drug, if drug induced)

532.71 Chronic duodenal ulcer without mention of hemorrhage or perforation, with obstruction — (Use additional E code to identify drug, if drug induced)

532.90 Duodenal ulcer, unspecified as acute or chronic, without hemorrhage, perforation, or obstruction — (Use additional E code to identify drug, if drug induced) ▽

532.91 Duodenal ulcer, unspecified as acute or chronic, without mention of hemorrhage or perforation, with obstruction — (Use additional E code to identify drug, if drug induced) ▽

533.00 Acute peptic ulcer, unspecified site, with hemorrhage, without mention of obstruction — (Use additional E code to identify drug, if drug induced)

533.01 Acute peptic ulcer, unspecified site, with hemorrhage and obstruction — (Use additional E code to identify drug, if drug induced)

533.10 Acute peptic ulcer, unspecified site, with perforation, without mention of obstruction — (Use additional E code to identify drug, if drug induced)

533.11 Acute peptic ulcer, unspecified site, with perforation and obstruction — (Use additional E code to identify drug, if drug induced)

533.20 Acute peptic ulcer, unspecified site, with hemorrhage and perforation, without mention of obstruction — (Use additional E code to identify drug, if drug induced)

533.21 Acute peptic ulcer, unspecified site, with hemorrhage, perforation, and obstruction — (Use additional E code to identify drug, if drug induced)

533.30 Acute peptic ulcer, unspecified site, without mention of hemorrhage, perforation, or obstruction — (Use additional E code to identify drug, if drug induced)
533.31 Acute peptic ulcer, unspecified site, without mention of hemorrhage and perforation, with obstruction — (Use additional E code to identify drug, if drug induced)
533.40 Chronic or unspecified peptic ulcer, unspecified site, with hemorrhage, without mention of obstruction — (Use additional E code to identify drug, if drug induced)
533.41 Chronic or unspecified peptic ulcer, unspecified site, with hemorrhage and obstruction — (Use additional E code to identify drug, if drug induced)
533.50 Chronic or unspecified peptic ulcer, unspecified site, with perforation, without mention of obstruction — (Use additional E code to identify drug, if drug induced)
533.51 Chronic or unspecified peptic ulcer, unspecified site, with perforation and obstruction — (Use additional E code to identify drug, if drug induced)
533.60 Chronic or unspecified peptic ulcer, unspecified site, with hemorrhage and perforation, without mention of obstruction — (Use additional E code to identify drug, if drug induced)
533.61 Chronic or unspecified peptic ulcer, unspecified site, with hemorrhage, perforation, and obstruction — (Use additional E code to identify drug, if drug induced)
533.70 Chronic peptic ulcer, unspecified site, without mention of hemorrhage, perforation, or obstruction — (Use additional E code to identify drug, if drug induced)
533.71 Chronic peptic ulcer of unspecified site without mention of hemorrhage or perforation, with obstruction — (Use additional E code to identify drug, if drug induced)
533.90 Peptic ulcer, unspecified site, unspecified as acute or chronic, without mention of hemorrhage, perforation, or obstruction — (Use additional E code to identify drug, if drug induced) ▽
533.91 Peptic ulcer, unspecified site, unspecified as acute or chronic, without mention of hemorrhage or perforation, with obstruction — (Use additional E code to identify drug, if drug induced) ▽
534.00 Acute gastrojejunal ulcer with hemorrhage, without mention of obstruction
534.01 Acute gastrojejunal ulcer, with hemorrhage and obstruction
534.10 Acute gastrojejunal ulcer with perforation, without mention of obstruction
534.11 Acute gastrojejunal ulcer with perforation and obstruction
534.20 Acute gastrojejunal ulcer with hemorrhage and perforation, without mention of obstruction
534.21 Acute gastrojejunal ulcer with hemorrhage, perforation, and obstruction
534.30 Acute gastrojejunal ulcer without mention of hemorrhage, perforation, or obstruction
534.31 Acute gastrojejunal ulcer without mention of hemorrhage or perforation, with obstruction
534.40 Chronic or unspecified gastrojejunal ulcer with hemorrhage, without mention of obstruction
534.41 Chronic or unspecified gastrojejunal ulcer, with hemorrhage and obstruction
534.50 Chronic or unspecified gastrojejunal ulcer with perforation, without mention of obstruction
534.51 Chronic or unspecified gastrojejunal ulcer with perforation and obstruction
534.60 Chronic or unspecified gastrojejunal ulcer with hemorrhage and perforation, without mention of obstruction
534.61 Chronic or unspecified gastrojejunal ulcer with hemorrhage, perforation, and obstruction
534.70 Chronic gastrojejunal ulcer without mention of hemorrhage, perforation, or obstruction
534.71 Chronic gastrojejunal ulcer without mention of hemorrhage or perforation, with obstruction
534.90 Gastrojejunal ulcer, unspecified as acute or chronic, without mention of hemorrhage, perforation, or obstruction ▽
534.91 Gastrojejunal ulcer, unspecified as acute or chronic, without mention of hemorrhage or perforation, with obstruction ▽
535.00 Acute gastritis without mention of hemorrhage
535.01 Acute gastritis with hemorrhage
535.10 Atrophic gastritis without mention of hemorrhage
535.11 Atrophic gastritis with hemorrhage
535.20 Gastric mucosal hypertrophy without mention of hemorrhage
535.21 Gastric mucosal hypertrophy with hemorrhage
535.30 Alcoholic gastritis without mention of hemorrhage
535.31 Alcoholic gastritis with hemorrhage
535.40 Other specified gastritis without mention of hemorrhage
535.41 Other specified gastritis with hemorrhage
535.60 Duodenitis without mention of hemorrhage
535.61 Duodenitis with hemorrhage
536.0 Achlorhydria
536.1 Acute dilatation of stomach
536.2 Persistent vomiting
536.3 Gastroparesis
536.8 Dyspepsia and other specified disorders of function of stomach
536.9 Unspecified functional disorder of stomach ▽
537.0 Acquired hypertrophic pyloric stenosis
537.1 Gastric diverticulum
537.2 Chronic duodenal ileus
537.3 Other obstruction of duodenum
537.4 Fistula of stomach or duodenum
537.5 Gastroptosis
537.6 Hourglass stricture or stenosis of stomach
537.81 Pylorospasm
537.82 Angiodysplasia of stomach and duodenum (without mention of hemorrhage)
537.83 Angiodysplasia of stomach and duodenum with hemorrhage
537.84 Dieulafoy lesion (hemorrhagic) of stomach and duodenum
537.89 Other specified disorder of stomach and duodenum
537.9 Unspecified disorder of stomach and duodenum ▽
552.3 Diaphragmatic hernia with obstruction
553.3 Diaphragmatic hernia without mention of obstruction or gangrene
555.0 Regional enteritis of small intestine
558.1 Gastroenteritis and colitis due to radiation
558.2 Toxic gastroenteritis and colitis — (Use additional E code to identify cause)
558.3 Gastroenteritis and colitis, allergic — (Use additional code to identify type of food allergy: V15.01-V15.05)
558.9 Other and unspecified noninfectious gastroenteritis and colitis ▽
569.5 Abscess of intestine
569.82 Ulceration of intestine
569.86 Dieulafoy lesion (hemorrhagic) of intestine
569.89 Other specified disorder of intestines
571.0 Alcoholic fatty liver
571.1 Acute alcoholic hepatitis
571.2 Alcoholic cirrhosis of liver
571.3 Unspecified alcoholic liver damage ▽
571.40 Unspecified chronic hepatitis ▽
571.41 Chronic persistent hepatitis
571.49 Other chronic hepatitis
571.5 Cirrhosis of liver without mention of alcohol
571.6 Biliary cirrhosis
571.8 Other chronic nonalcoholic liver disease
572.3 Portal hypertension
577.0 Acute pancreatitis
577.1 Chronic pancreatitis
578.0 Hematemesis
578.1 Blood in stool
579.0 Celiac disease
579.2 Blind loop syndrome
579.3 Other and unspecified postsurgical nonabsorption ▽
579.8 Other specified intestinal malabsorption
747.61 Congenital gastrointestinal vessel anomaly
750.3 Congenital tracheoesophageal fistula, esophageal atresia and stenosis
750.4 Other specified congenital anomaly of esophagus
750.5 Congenital hypertrophic pyloric stenosis
750.6 Congenital hiatus hernia
750.7 Other specified congenital anomalies of stomach
751.8 Other specified congenital anomalies of digestive system
783.0 Anorexia
783.21 Loss of weight
783.22 Underweight
783.7 Adult failure to thrive
784.1 Throat pain
787.1 Heartburn
787.2 Dysphagia
787.3 Flatulence, eructation, and gas pain
787.4 Visible peristalsis
787.5 Abnormal bowel sounds
787.99 Other symptoms involving digestive system
789.09 Abdominal pain, other specified site
792.1 Nonspecific abnormal finding in stool contents
793.4 Nonspecific abnormal findings on radiological and other examination of gastrointestinal tract
997.4 Digestive system complication — (Use additional code to identify complications)
V10.00 Personal history of malignant neoplasm of unspecified site in gastrointestinal tract ▽
V12.71 Personal history of peptic ulcer disease

V12.79 Personal history of other diseases of digestive disease
V16.0 Family history of malignant neoplasm of gastrointestinal tract
V18.5 Family history of digestive disorders
V67.00 Follow-up examination, following unspecified surgery ▽
V67.09 Follow-up examination, following other surgery
V67.59 Other follow-up examination
V67.9 Unspecified follow-up examination ▽
V71.1 Observation for suspected malignant neoplasm
V71.89 Observation for other specified suspected conditions

ICD-9-CM Procedural

42.23 Other esophagoscopy
42.33 Endoscopic excision or destruction of lesion or tissue of esophagus
43.41 Endoscopic excision or destruction of lesion or tissue of stomach
45.16 Esophagogastroduodenoscopy (EGD) with closed biopsy

HCPCS Level II Supplies & Services

A4270 Disposable endoscope sheath, each
A4550 Surgical trays

43240

43240 Upper gastrointestinal endoscopy including esophagus, stomach, and either the duodenum and/or jejunum as appropriate; with transmural drainage of pseudocyst

ICD-9-CM Diagnostic

577.2 Cyst and pseudocyst of pancreas

ICD-9-CM Procedural

45.13 Other endoscopy of small intestine
52.4 Internal drainage of pancreatic cyst

43241

43241 Upper gastrointestinal endoscopy including esophagus, stomach, and either the duodenum and/or jejunum as appropriate; with transendoscopic intraluminal tube or catheter placement

ICD-9-CM Diagnostic

150.1 Malignant neoplasm of thoracic esophagus
150.2 Malignant neoplasm of abdominal esophagus
150.3 Malignant neoplasm of upper third of esophagus
150.4 Malignant neoplasm of middle third of esophagus
150.5 Malignant neoplasm of lower third of esophagus
150.8 Malignant neoplasm of other specified part of esophagus
150.9 Malignant neoplasm of esophagus, unspecified site ▽
151.0 Malignant neoplasm of cardia
151.1 Malignant neoplasm of pylorus
151.2 Malignant neoplasm of pyloric antrum
151.3 Malignant neoplasm of fundus of stomach
151.4 Malignant neoplasm of body of stomach
151.5 Malignant neoplasm of lesser curvature of stomach, unspecified ▽
151.6 Malignant neoplasm of greater curvature of stomach, unspecified ▽
151.8 Malignant neoplasm of other specified sites of stomach
151.9 Malignant neoplasm of stomach, unspecified site ▽
152.0 Malignant neoplasm of duodenum
152.1 Malignant neoplasm of jejunum
152.2 Malignant neoplasm of ileum
152.8 Malignant neoplasm of other specified sites of small intestine
161.9 Malignant neoplasm of larynx, unspecified site ▽
197.4 Secondary malignant neoplasm of small intestine including duodenum
197.8 Secondary malignant neoplasm of other digestive organs and spleen
198.89 Secondary malignant neoplasm of other specified sites
211.1 Benign neoplasm of stomach
230.1 Carcinoma in situ of esophagus
230.2 Carcinoma in situ of stomach
239.8 Neoplasm of unspecified nature of other specified sites
261 Nutritional marasmus
262 Other severe protein-calorie malnutrition
263.0 Malnutrition of moderate degree
263.1 Malnutrition of mild degree
263.2 Arrested development following protein-calorie malnutrition
263.8 Other protein-calorie malnutrition
263.9 Unspecified protein-calorie malnutrition ▽
269.8 Other nutritional deficiency
269.9 Unspecified nutritional deficiency ▽
276.5 Volume depletion — (Use additional code to identify any associated mental retardation)
307.1 Anorexia nervosa
436 Acute, but ill-defined, cerebrovascular disease — (Use additional code to identify presence of hypertension) ▽
456.0 Esophageal varices with bleeding
519.00 Unspecified tracheostomy complication ▽
519.01 Infection of tracheostomy — (Use additional code to identify type of infection: 038.0-038.9, 682.1. Use additional code to identify organism: 041.00-041.9)
519.02 Mechanical complication of tracheostomy
519.09 Other tracheostomy complications
530.3 Stricture and stenosis of esophagus
530.4 Perforation of esophagus
530.5 Dyskinesia of esophagus
530.81 Esophageal reflux
531.00 Acute gastric ulcer with hemorrhage, without mention of obstruction — (Use additional E code to identify drug, if drug induced)
531.01 Acute gastric ulcer with hemorrhage and obstruction — (Use additional E code to identify drug, if drug induced)
531.10 Acute gastric ulcer with perforation, without mention of obstruction — (Use additional E code to identify drug, if drug induced)
531.11 Acute gastric ulcer with perforation and obstruction — (Use additional E code to identify drug, if drug induced)
531.20 Acute gastric ulcer with hemorrhage and perforation, without mention of obstruction — (Use additional E code to identify drug, if drug induced)
531.21 Acute gastric ulcer with hemorrhage, perforation, and obstruction — (Use additional E code to identify drug, if drug induced)
531.30 Acute gastric ulcer without mention of hemorrhage, perforation, or obstruction — (Use additional E code to identify drug, if drug induced)
531.31 Acute gastric ulcer without mention of hemorrhage or perforation, with obstruction — (Use additional E code to identify drug, if drug induced)
531.40 Chronic or unspecified gastric ulcer with hemorrhage, without mention of obstruction — (Use additional E code to identify drug, if drug induced)
531.41 Chronic or unspecified gastric ulcer with hemorrhage and obstruction — (Use additional E code to identify drug, if drug induced)
531.50 Chronic or unspecified gastric ulcer with perforation, without mention of obstruction — (Use additional E code to identify drug, if drug induced)
531.51 Chronic or unspecified gastric ulcer with perforation and obstruction — (Use additional E code to identify drug, if drug induced)
531.60 Chronic or unspecified gastric ulcer with hemorrhage and perforation, without mention of obstruction — (Use additional E code to identify drug, if drug induced)
531.61 Chronic or unspecified gastric ulcer with hemorrhage, perforation, and obstruction — (Use additional E code to identify drug, if drug induced)
531.70 Chronic gastric ulcer without mention of hemorrhage, perforation, without mention of obstruction — (Use additional E code to identify drug, if drug induced)
531.71 Chronic gastric ulcer without mention of hemorrhage or perforation, with obstruction — (Use additional E code to identify drug, if drug induced)
531.90 Gastric ulcer, unspecified as acute or chronic, without mention of hemorrhage, perforation, or obstruction — (Use additional E code to identify drug, if drug induced) ▽
531.91 Gastric ulcer, unspecified as acute or chronic, without mention of hemorrhage or perforation, with obstruction — (Use additional E code to identify drug, if drug induced) ▽
532.00 Acute duodenal ulcer with hemorrhage, without mention of obstruction — (Use additional E code to identify drug, if drug induced)
532.01 Acute duodenal ulcer with hemorrhage and obstruction — (Use additional E code to identify drug, if drug induced)
532.10 Acute duodenal ulcer with perforation, without mention of obstruction — (Use additional E code to identify drug, if drug induced)
532.11 Acute duodenal ulcer with perforation and obstruction — (Use additional E code to identify drug, if drug induced)
532.20 Acute duodenal ulcer with hemorrhage and perforation, without mention of obstruction — (Use additional E code to identify drug, if drug induced)
532.21 Acute duodenal ulcer with hemorrhage, perforation, and obstruction — (Use additional E code to identify drug, if drug induced)
532.30 Acute duodenal ulcer without mention of hemorrhage, perforation, or obstruction — (Use additional E code to identify drug, if drug induced)
532.31 Acute duodenal ulcer without mention of hemorrhage or perforation, with obstruction — (Use additional E code to identify drug, if drug induced)
532.40 Chronic or unspecified duodenal ulcer with hemorrhage, without mention of obstruction — (Use additional E code to identify drug, if drug induced)
532.41 Chronic or unspecified duodenal ulcer with hemorrhage and obstruction — (Use additional E code to identify drug, if drug induced)

▽ Unspecified code ♀ Female diagnosis ☒ Manifestation code ♂ Male diagnosis

532.50 Chronic or unspecified duodenal ulcer with perforation, without mention of obstruction — (Use additional E code to identify drug, if drug induced)
532.51 Chronic or unspecified duodenal ulcer with perforation and obstruction — (Use additional E code to identify drug, if drug induced)
532.60 Chronic or unspecified duodenal ulcer with hemorrhage and perforation, without mention of obstruction — (Use additional E code to identify drug, if drug induced)
532.61 Chronic or unspecified duodenal ulcer with hemorrhage, perforation, and obstruction — (Use additional E code to identify drug, if drug induced)
532.70 Chronic duodenal ulcer without mention of hemorrhage, perforation, or obstruction — (Use additional E code to identify drug, if drug induced)
532.71 Chronic duodenal ulcer without mention of hemorrhage or perforation, with obstruction — (Use additional E code to identify drug, if drug induced)
532.90 Duodenal ulcer, unspecified as acute or chronic, without hemorrhage, perforation, or obstruction — (Use additional E code to identify drug, if drug induced) ▽
532.91 Duodenal ulcer, unspecified as acute or chronic, without mention of hemorrhage or perforation, with obstruction — (Use additional E code to identify drug, if drug induced) ▽
533.00 Acute peptic ulcer, unspecified site, with hemorrhage, without mention of obstruction — (Use additional E code to identify drug, if drug induced)
533.01 Acute peptic ulcer, unspecified site, with hemorrhage and obstruction — (Use additional E code to identify drug, if drug induced)
533.10 Acute peptic ulcer, unspecified site, with perforation, without mention of obstruction — (Use additional E code to identify drug, if drug induced)
533.11 Acute peptic ulcer, unspecified site, with perforation and obstruction — (Use additional E code to identify drug, if drug induced)
533.20 Acute peptic ulcer, unspecified site, with hemorrhage and perforation, without mention of obstruction — (Use additional E code to identify drug, if drug induced)
533.21 Acute peptic ulcer, unspecified site, with hemorrhage, perforation, and obstruction — (Use additional E code to identify drug, if drug induced)
533.30 Acute peptic ulcer, unspecified site, without mention of hemorrhage, perforation, or obstruction — (Use additional E code to identify drug, if drug induced)
533.31 Acute peptic ulcer, unspecified site, without mention of hemorrhage and perforation, with obstruction — (Use additional E code to identify drug, if drug induced)
533.40 Chronic or unspecified peptic ulcer, unspecified site, with hemorrhage, without mention of obstruction — (Use additional E code to identify drug, if drug induced)
533.41 Chronic or unspecified peptic ulcer, unspecified site, with hemorrhage and obstruction — (Use additional E code to identify drug, if drug induced)
533.50 Chronic or unspecified peptic ulcer, unspecified site, with perforation, without mention of obstruction — (Use additional E code to identify drug, if drug induced)
533.51 Chronic or unspecified peptic ulcer, unspecified site, with perforation and obstruction — (Use additional E code to identify drug, if drug induced)
533.90 Peptic ulcer, unspecified site, unspecified as acute or chronic, without mention of hemorrhage, perforation, or obstruction — (Use additional E code to identify drug, if drug induced) ▽
535.50 Unspecified gastritis and gastroduodenitis without mention of hemorrhage ▽
535.60 Duodenitis without mention of hemorrhage
536.2 Persistent vomiting
536.8 Dyspepsia and other specified disorders of function of stomach
536.9 Unspecified functional disorder of stomach ▽
537.3 Other obstruction of duodenum
537.84 Dieulafoy lesion (hemorrhagic) of stomach and duodenum
537.89 Other specified disorder of stomach and duodenum
560.1 Paralytic ileus
560.2 Volvulus
560.89 Other specified intestinal obstruction
569.84 Angiodysplasia of intestine (without mention of hemorrhage)
569.86 Dieulafoy lesion (hemorrhagic) of intestine
578.9 Unspecified, hemorrhage of gastrointestinal tract ▽
707.9 Chronic ulcer of unspecified site ▽
750.5 Congenital hypertrophic pyloric stenosis
750.7 Other specified congenital anomalies of stomach
751.1 Congenital atresia and stenosis of small intestine
783.0 Anorexia
783.3 Feeding difficulties and mismanagement
783.40 Lack of normal physiological development, unspecified ▽
783.41 Failure to thrive
783.42 Delayed milestones
783.43 Short stature
783.7 Adult failure to thrive
787.01 Nausea with vomiting
787.2 Dysphagia
854.06 Intracranial injury of other and unspecified nature, without mention of open intracranial wound, loss of consciousness of unspecified duration ▽
947.2 Burn of esophagus
959.01 Head injury, unspecified ▽
994.2 Effects of hunger
997.4 Digestive system complication — (Use additional code to identify complications)

ICD-9-CM Procedural

42.81 Insertion of permanent tube into esophagus
45.13 Other endoscopy of small intestine
96.06 Insertion of Sengstaaken tube

HCPCS Level II Supplies & Services

A4270 Disposable endoscope sheath, each
A4305 Disposable drug delivery system, flow rate of 50 ml or greater per hour
A4306 Disposable drug delivery system, flow rate of 5 ml or less per hour
A4550 Surgical trays

43242

43242 Upper gastrointestinal endoscopy including esophagus, stomach, and either the duodenum and/or jejunum as appropriate; with transendoscopic ultrasound-guided intramural or transmural fine needle aspiration/biopsy(s) (includes endoscopic ultrasound examination of the esophagus, stomach, and either the duodenum and/or jejunum as appropriate)

ICD-9-CM Diagnostic

150.0 Malignant neoplasm of cervical esophagus
150.1 Malignant neoplasm of thoracic esophagus
150.2 Malignant neoplasm of abdominal esophagus
150.3 Malignant neoplasm of upper third of esophagus
150.4 Malignant neoplasm of middle third of esophagus
150.5 Malignant neoplasm of lower third of esophagus
150.8 Malignant neoplasm of other specified part of esophagus
150.9 Malignant neoplasm of esophagus, unspecified site ▽
151.0 Malignant neoplasm of cardia
151.1 Malignant neoplasm of pylorus
151.2 Malignant neoplasm of pyloric antrum
151.3 Malignant neoplasm of fundus of stomach
151.4 Malignant neoplasm of body of stomach
151.5 Malignant neoplasm of lesser curvature of stomach, unspecified ▽
151.6 Malignant neoplasm of greater curvature of stomach, unspecified ▽
151.8 Malignant neoplasm of other specified sites of stomach
151.9 Malignant neoplasm of stomach, unspecified site ▽
152.0 Malignant neoplasm of duodenum
152.1 Malignant neoplasm of jejunum
152.8 Malignant neoplasm of other specified sites of small intestine
152.9 Malignant neoplasm of small intestine, unspecified site ▽
155.0 Malignant neoplasm of liver, primary
155.1 Malignant neoplasm of intrahepatic bile ducts
156.0 Malignant neoplasm of gallbladder
156.1 Malignant neoplasm of extrahepatic bile ducts
156.2 Malignant neoplasm of ampulla of Vater
156.8 Malignant neoplasm of other specified sites of gallbladder and extrahepatic bile ducts
156.9 Malignant neoplasm of biliary tract, part unspecified site ▽
157.0 Malignant neoplasm of head of pancreas
157.1 Malignant neoplasm of body of pancreas
157.2 Malignant neoplasm of tail of pancreas
157.3 Malignant neoplasm of pancreatic duct
157.4 Malignant neoplasm of islets of Langerhans — (Use additional code to identify any functional activity)
157.8 Malignant neoplasm of other specified sites of pancreas
157.9 Malignant neoplasm of pancreas, part unspecified ▽
158.8 Malignant neoplasm of specified parts of peritoneum
159.8 Malignant neoplasm of other sites of digestive system and intra-abdominal organs
159.9 Malignant neoplasm of ill-defined sites of digestive organs and peritoneum
171.4 Malignant neoplasm of connective and other soft tissue of thorax
171.5 Malignant neoplasm of connective and other soft tissue of abdomen
195.1 Malignant neoplasm of thorax
195.2 Malignant neoplasm of abdomen
196.1 Secondary and unspecified malignant neoplasm of intrathoracic lymph nodes

196.2 Secondary and unspecified malignant neoplasm of intra-abdominal lymph nodes
197.4 Secondary malignant neoplasm of small intestine including duodenum
197.8 Secondary malignant neoplasm of other digestive organs and spleen
199.0 Disseminated malignant neoplasm
199.1 Other malignant neoplasm of unspecified site
211.0 Benign neoplasm of esophagus
211.1 Benign neoplasm of stomach
211.2 Benign neoplasm of duodenum, jejunum, and ileum
211.6 Benign neoplasm of pancreas, except islets of Langerhans
211.7 Benign neoplasm of islets of Langerhans — (Use additional code to identify any functional activity)
215.5 Other benign neoplasm of connective and other soft tissue of abdomen
230.1 Carcinoma in situ of esophagus
230.2 Carcinoma in situ of stomach
230.7 Carcinoma in situ of other and unspecified parts of intestine ▽
230.8 Carcinoma in situ of liver and biliary system
230.9 Carcinoma in situ of other and unspecified digestive organs ▽
235.2 Neoplasm of uncertain behavior of stomach, intestines, and rectum
235.3 Neoplasm of uncertain behavior of liver and biliary passages
235.4 Neoplasm of uncertain behavior of retroperitoneum and peritoneum
235.5 Neoplasm of uncertain behavior of other and unspecified digestive organs ▽
239.0 Neoplasm of unspecified nature of digestive system
239.8 Neoplasm of unspecified nature of other specified sites
786.6 Swelling, mass, or lump in chest
789.1 Hepatomegaly
789.30 Abdominal or pelvic swelling, mass or lump, unspecified site ▽
789.31 Abdominal or pelvic swelling, mass, or lump, right upper quadrant
789.32 Abdominal or pelvic swelling, mass, or lump, left upper quadrant
789.33 Abdominal or pelvic swelling, mass, or lump, right lower quadrant
789.34 Abdominal or pelvic swelling, mass, or lump, left lower quadrant
789.35 Abdominal or pelvic swelling, mass or lump, periumbilic
789.36 Abdominal or pelvic swelling, mass, or lump, epigastric
789.39 Abdominal or pelvic swelling, mass, or lump, other specified site

ICD-9-CM Procedural

42.29 Other diagnostic procedures on esophagus
45.16 Esophagogastroduodenoscopy (EGD) with closed biopsy

43243–43244

43243 Upper gastrointestinal endoscopy including esophagus, stomach, and either the duodenum and/or jejunum as appropriate; with injection sclerosis of esophageal and/or gastric varices
43244 Upper gastrointestinal endoscopy including esophagus, stomach, and either the duodenum and/or jejunum as appropriate; with band ligation of esophageal and/or gastric varices

ICD-9-CM Diagnostic

280.0 Iron deficiency anemia secondary to blood loss (chronic)
280.9 Unspecified iron deficiency anemia ▽
285.9 Unspecified anemia ▽
456.0 Esophageal varices with bleeding
456.1 Esophageal varices without mention of bleeding
456.20 Esophageal varices with bleeding in diseases classified elsewhere — (Code first underlying disease: 571.0-571.9, 572.3) ☒
456.21 Esophageal varices without mention of bleeding in diseases classified elsewhere — (Code first underlying disease: 571.0-571.9, 572.3) ☒
456.8 Varices of other sites
530.3 Stricture and stenosis of esophagus
530.7 Gastroesophageal laceration-hemorrhage syndrome
530.82 Esophageal hemorrhage
537.84 Dieulafoy lesion (hemorrhagic) of stomach and duodenum
569.86 Dieulafoy lesion (hemorrhagic) of intestine
571.0 Alcoholic fatty liver
571.1 Acute alcoholic hepatitis
571.2 Alcoholic cirrhosis of liver
571.3 Unspecified alcoholic liver damage ▽
571.40 Unspecified chronic hepatitis ▽
571.41 Chronic persistent hepatitis
571.5 Cirrhosis of liver without mention of alcohol
571.6 Biliary cirrhosis
571.8 Other chronic nonalcoholic liver disease
571.9 Unspecified chronic liver disease without mention of alcohol ▽
572.3 Portal hypertension
578.0 Hematemesis
578.1 Blood in stool
578.9 Unspecified, hemorrhage of gastrointestinal tract ▽
747.61 Congenital gastrointestinal vessel anomaly

ICD-9-CM Procedural

42.33 Endoscopic excision or destruction of lesion or tissue of esophagus
43.41 Endoscopic excision or destruction of lesion or tissue of stomach

HCPCS Level II Supplies & Services

A4270 Disposable endoscope sheath, each
A4305 Disposable drug delivery system, flow rate of 50 ml or greater per hour
A4306 Disposable drug delivery system, flow rate of 5 ml or less per hour
A4550 Surgical trays

43245

43245 Upper gastrointestinal endoscopy including esophagus, stomach, and either the duodenum and/or jejunum as appropriate; with dilation of gastric outlet for obstruction (eg, balloon, guide wire, bougie)

ICD-9-CM Diagnostic

151.4 Malignant neoplasm of body of stomach
151.9 Malignant neoplasm of stomach, unspecified site ▽
530.0 Achalasia and cardiospasm
530.10 Unspecified esophagitis — (Use additional E code to identify cause, if induced by chemical or drug) ▽
530.11 Reflux esophagitis — (Use additional E code to identify cause, if induced by chemical or drug)
530.12 Acute esophagitis — (Use additional E code to identify cause, if induced by chemical or drug)
530.19 Other esophagitis — (Use additional E code to identify cause, if induced by chemical or drug)
530.20 Ulcer of esophagus without bleeding — (Use additional E code to identify cause, if induced by chemical or drug)
530.81 Esophageal reflux
530.85 Barrett's esophagus
531.01 Acute gastric ulcer with hemorrhage and obstruction — (Use additional E code to identify drug, if drug induced)
531.11 Acute gastric ulcer with perforation and obstruction — (Use additional E code to identify drug, if drug induced)
531.21 Acute gastric ulcer with hemorrhage, perforation, and obstruction — (Use additional E code to identify drug, if drug induced)
531.31 Acute gastric ulcer without mention of hemorrhage or perforation, with obstruction — (Use additional E code to identify drug, if drug induced)
531.41 Chronic or unspecified gastric ulcer with hemorrhage and obstruction — (Use additional E code to identify drug, if drug induced)
531.51 Chronic or unspecified gastric ulcer with perforation and obstruction — (Use additional E code to identify drug, if drug induced)
531.61 Chronic or unspecified gastric ulcer with hemorrhage, perforation, and obstruction — (Use additional E code to identify drug, if drug induced)
531.71 Chronic gastric ulcer without mention of hemorrhage or perforation, with obstruction — (Use additional E code to identify drug, if drug induced)
531.91 Gastric ulcer, unspecified as acute or chronic, without mention of hemorrhage or perforation, with obstruction — (Use additional E code to identify drug, if drug induced) ▽
533.01 Acute peptic ulcer, unspecified site, with hemorrhage and obstruction — (Use additional E code to identify drug, if drug induced)
533.11 Acute peptic ulcer, unspecified site, with perforation and obstruction — (Use additional E code to identify drug, if drug induced)
533.21 Acute peptic ulcer, unspecified site, with hemorrhage, perforation, and obstruction — (Use additional E code to identify drug, if drug induced)
533.31 Acute peptic ulcer, unspecified site, without mention of hemorrhage and perforation, with obstruction — (Use additional E code to identify drug, if drug induced)
533.41 Chronic or unspecified peptic ulcer, unspecified site, with hemorrhage and obstruction — (Use additional E code to identify drug, if drug induced)
533.51 Chronic or unspecified peptic ulcer, unspecified site, with perforation and obstruction — (Use additional E code to identify drug, if drug induced)
533.61 Chronic or unspecified peptic ulcer, unspecified site, with hemorrhage, perforation, and obstruction — (Use additional E code to identify drug, if drug induced)
533.71 Chronic peptic ulcer of unspecified site without mention of hemorrhage or perforation, with obstruction — (Use additional E code to identify drug, if drug induced)
533.91 Peptic ulcer, unspecified site, unspecified as acute or chronic, without mention of hemorrhage or perforation, with obstruction — (Use additional E code to identify drug, if drug induced) ▽
535.00 Acute gastritis without mention of hemorrhage

535.40 Other specified gastritis without mention of hemorrhage
536.2 Persistent vomiting
537.0 Acquired hypertrophic pyloric stenosis
537.1 Gastric diverticulum
537.5 Gastroptosis
537.6 Hourglass stricture or stenosis of stomach
537.81 Pylorospasm
537.82 Angiodysplasia of stomach and duodenum (without mention of hemorrhage)
537.83 Angiodysplasia of stomach and duodenum with hemorrhage
537.89 Other specified disorder of stomach and duodenum
578.9 Unspecified, hemorrhage of gastrointestinal tract
750.5 Congenital hypertrophic pyloric stenosis
750.6 Congenital hiatus hernia
750.7 Other specified congenital anomalies of stomach
750.8 Other specified congenital anomalies of upper alimentary tract
750.9 Unspecified congenital anomaly of upper alimentary tract
751.8 Other specified congenital anomalies of digestive system
751.9 Unspecified congenital anomaly of digestive system
787.01 Nausea with vomiting
789.00 Abdominal pain, unspecified site
793.4 Nonspecific abnormal findings on radiological and other examination of gastrointestinal tract
997.4 Digestive system complication — (Use additional code to identify complications)

ICD-9-CM Procedural

44.22 Endoscopic dilation of pylorus

HCPCS Level II Supplies & Services

A4270 Disposable endoscope sheath, each
A4305 Disposable drug delivery system, flow rate of 50 ml or greater per hour
A4306 Disposable drug delivery system, flow rate of 5 ml or less per hour
A4550 Surgical trays

43246

43246 Upper gastrointestinal endoscopy including esophagus, stomach, and either the duodenum and/or jejunum as appropriate; with directed placement of percutaneous gastrostomy tube

ICD-9-CM Diagnostic

141.9 Malignant neoplasm of tongue, unspecified site
145.0 Malignant neoplasm of cheek mucosa
145.1 Malignant neoplasm of vestibule of mouth
145.2 Malignant neoplasm of hard palate
145.3 Malignant neoplasm of soft palate
145.4 Malignant neoplasm of uvula
145.5 Malignant neoplasm of palate, unspecified
145.6 Malignant neoplasm of retromolar area
145.8 Malignant neoplasm of other specified parts of mouth
145.9 Malignant neoplasm of mouth, unspecified site
146.0 Malignant neoplasm of tonsil
146.1 Malignant neoplasm of tonsillar fossa
146.2 Malignant neoplasm of tonsillar pillars (anterior) (posterior)
146.3 Malignant neoplasm of vallecula
146.4 Malignant neoplasm of anterior aspect of epiglottis
146.5 Malignant neoplasm of junctional region of oropharynx
146.6 Malignant neoplasm of lateral wall of oropharynx
146.7 Malignant neoplasm of posterior wall of oropharynx
146.8 Malignant neoplasm of other specified sites of oropharynx
146.9 Malignant neoplasm of oropharynx, unspecified site
150.3 Malignant neoplasm of upper third of esophagus
150.4 Malignant neoplasm of middle third of esophagus
150.5 Malignant neoplasm of lower third of esophagus
150.8 Malignant neoplasm of other specified part of esophagus
150.9 Malignant neoplasm of esophagus, unspecified site
151.9 Malignant neoplasm of stomach, unspecified site
152.8 Malignant neoplasm of other specified sites of small intestine
161.9 Malignant neoplasm of larynx, unspecified site
197.8 Secondary malignant neoplasm of other digestive organs and spleen
230.1 Carcinoma in situ of esophagus
230.2 Carcinoma in situ of stomach
261 Nutritional marasmus
262 Other severe protein-calorie malnutrition
263.0 Malnutrition of moderate degree
263.1 Malnutrition of mild degree
263.2 Arrested development following protein-calorie malnutrition
263.8 Other protein-calorie malnutrition
263.9 Unspecified protein-calorie malnutrition
269.9 Unspecified nutritional deficiency
276.5 Volume depletion — (Use additional code to identify any associated mental retardation)
307.1 Anorexia nervosa
335.20 Amyotrophic lateral sclerosis
348.1 Anoxic brain damage — (Use additional E code to identify cause)
436 Acute, but ill-defined, cerebrovascular disease — (Use additional code to identify presence of hypertension)
530.3 Stricture and stenosis of esophagus
531.60 Chronic or unspecified gastric ulcer with hemorrhage and perforation, without mention of obstruction — (Use additional E code to identify drug, if drug induced)
532.20 Acute duodenal ulcer with hemorrhage and perforation, without mention of obstruction — (Use additional E code to identify drug, if drug induced)
536.2 Persistent vomiting
537.2 Chronic duodenal ileus
537.3 Other obstruction of duodenum
578.9 Unspecified, hemorrhage of gastrointestinal tract
579.8 Other specified intestinal malabsorption
579.9 Unspecified intestinal malabsorption
780.2 Syncope and collapse
780.31 Febrile convulsions
780.39 Other convulsions
780.4 Dizziness and giddiness
780.52 Other insomnia
780.6 Fever
780.79 Other malaise and fatigue
780.8 Generalized hyperhidrosis
783.0 Anorexia
783.21 Loss of weight
783.22 Underweight
783.3 Feeding difficulties and mismanagement
783.7 Adult failure to thrive
783.9 Other symptoms concerning nutrition, metabolism, and development
787.01 Nausea with vomiting
787.2 Dysphagia
789.00 Abdominal pain, unspecified site
994.2 Effects of hunger
997.4 Digestive system complication — (Use additional code to identify complications)
V55.1 Attention to gastrostomy

ICD-9-CM Procedural

43.11 Percutaneous (endoscopic) gastrostomy (PEG)
44.32 Percutaneous [endoscopic] gastrojejunostomy

43247

43247 Upper gastrointestinal endoscopy including esophagus, stomach, and either the duodenum and/or jejunum as appropriate; with removal of foreign body

ICD-9-CM Diagnostic

935.1 Foreign body in esophagus
935.2 Foreign body in stomach
936 Foreign body in intestine and colon
938 Foreign body in digestive system, unspecified
996.79 Other complications due to other internal prosthetic device, implant, and graft
998.4 Foreign body accidentally left during procedure, not elsewhere classified

ICD-9-CM Procedural

42.23 Other esophagoscopy
44.13 Other gastroscopy
98.02 Removal of intraluminal foreign body from esophagus without incision
98.03 Removal of intraluminal foreign body from stomach and small intestine without incision

HCPCS Level II Supplies & Services

A4270 Disposable endoscope sheath, each
A4550 Surgical trays

43248–43249

43248 Upper gastrointestinal endoscopy including esophagus, stomach, and either the duodenum and/or jejunum as appropriate; with insertion of guide wire followed by dilation of esophagus over guide wire
43249 with balloon dilation of esophagus (less than 30 mm diameter)

ICD-9-CM Diagnostic

150.0 Malignant neoplasm of cervical esophagus
150.1 Malignant neoplasm of thoracic esophagus
150.3 Malignant neoplasm of upper third of esophagus
150.4 Malignant neoplasm of middle third of esophagus
150.5 Malignant neoplasm of lower third of esophagus
150.8 Malignant neoplasm of other specified part of esophagus
150.9 Malignant neoplasm of esophagus, unspecified site ▽
151.0 Malignant neoplasm of cardia
151.1 Malignant neoplasm of pylorus
151.2 Malignant neoplasm of pyloric antrum
151.3 Malignant neoplasm of fundus of stomach
151.4 Malignant neoplasm of body of stomach
151.5 Malignant neoplasm of lesser curvature of stomach, unspecified ▽
151.6 Malignant neoplasm of greater curvature of stomach, unspecified ▽
151.8 Malignant neoplasm of other specified sites of stomach
151.9 Malignant neoplasm of stomach, unspecified site ▽
197.8 Secondary malignant neoplasm of other digestive organs and spleen
211.0 Benign neoplasm of esophagus
211.1 Benign neoplasm of stomach
230.1 Carcinoma in situ of esophagus
235.5 Neoplasm of uncertain behavior of other and unspecified digestive organs ▽
239.0 Neoplasm of unspecified nature of digestive system
530.11 Reflux esophagitis — (Use additional E code to identify cause, if induced by chemical or drug)
530.12 Acute esophagitis — (Use additional E code to identify cause, if induced by chemical or drug)
530.19 Other esophagitis — (Use additional E code to identify cause, if induced by chemical or drug)
530.20 Ulcer of esophagus without bleeding — (Use additional E code to identify cause, if induced by chemical or drug)
530.3 Stricture and stenosis of esophagus
530.5 Dyskinesia of esophagus
530.81 Esophageal reflux
530.85 Barrett's esophagus
530.89 Other specified disorder of the esophagus
531.21 Acute gastric ulcer with hemorrhage, perforation, and obstruction — (Use additional E code to identify drug, if drug induced)
787.2 Dysphagia

ICD-9-CM Procedural

42.92 Dilation of esophagus

HCPCS Level II Supplies & Services

A4270 Disposable endoscope sheath, each
A4305 Disposable drug delivery system, flow rate of 50 ml or greater per hour
A4306 Disposable drug delivery system, flow rate of 5 ml or less per hour
A4550 Surgical trays

43250–43251

43250 Upper gastrointestinal endoscopy including esophagus, stomach, and either the duodenum and/or jejunum as appropriate; with removal of tumor(s), polyp(s), or other lesion(s) by hot biopsy forceps or bipolar cautery
43251 with removal of tumor(s), polyp(s), or other lesion(s) by snare technique

ICD-9-CM Diagnostic

150.0 Malignant neoplasm of cervical esophagus
150.1 Malignant neoplasm of thoracic esophagus
150.2 Malignant neoplasm of abdominal esophagus
150.3 Malignant neoplasm of upper third of esophagus
150.4 Malignant neoplasm of middle third of esophagus
150.5 Malignant neoplasm of lower third of esophagus
150.8 Malignant neoplasm of other specified part of esophagus
151.0 Malignant neoplasm of cardia
151.1 Malignant neoplasm of pylorus
151.2 Malignant neoplasm of pyloric antrum
151.3 Malignant neoplasm of fundus of stomach
151.4 Malignant neoplasm of body of stomach
151.5 Malignant neoplasm of lesser curvature of stomach, unspecified ▽
151.6 Malignant neoplasm of greater curvature of stomach, unspecified ▽
151.8 Malignant neoplasm of other specified sites of stomach
152.0 Malignant neoplasm of duodenum
152.1 Malignant neoplasm of jejunum
152.8 Malignant neoplasm of other specified sites of small intestine
197.4 Secondary malignant neoplasm of small intestine including duodenum
197.8 Secondary malignant neoplasm of other digestive organs and spleen
211.0 Benign neoplasm of esophagus
211.1 Benign neoplasm of stomach
211.2 Benign neoplasm of duodenum, jejunum, and ileum
211.9 Benign neoplasm of other and unspecified site of the digestive system ▽
230.2 Carcinoma in situ of stomach
230.7 Carcinoma in situ of other and unspecified parts of intestine ▽
235.2 Neoplasm of uncertain behavior of stomach, intestines, and rectum
235.5 Neoplasm of uncertain behavior of other and unspecified digestive organs ▽
530.9 Unspecified disorder of esophagus ▽
537.82 Angiodysplasia of stomach and duodenum (without mention of hemorrhage)
537.83 Angiodysplasia of stomach and duodenum with hemorrhage
537.89 Other specified disorder of stomach and duodenum

ICD-9-CM Procedural

42.33 Endoscopic excision or destruction of lesion or tissue of esophagus
43.41 Endoscopic excision or destruction of lesion or tissue of stomach
45.30 Endoscopic excision or destruction of lesion of duodenum
45.33 Local excision of lesion or tissue of small intestine, except duodenum

HCPCS Level II Supplies & Services

A4270 Disposable endoscope sheath, each
A4550 Surgical trays

43255

43255 Upper gastrointestinal endoscopy including esophagus, stomach, and either the duodenum and/or jejunum as appropriate; with control of bleeding, any method

ICD-9-CM Diagnostic

150.5 Malignant neoplasm of lower third of esophagus
150.8 Malignant neoplasm of other specified part of esophagus
150.9 Malignant neoplasm of esophagus, unspecified site ▽
151.0 Malignant neoplasm of cardia
151.1 Malignant neoplasm of pylorus
151.2 Malignant neoplasm of pyloric antrum
151.3 Malignant neoplasm of fundus of stomach
151.4 Malignant neoplasm of body of stomach
151.5 Malignant neoplasm of lesser curvature of stomach, unspecified ▽
151.6 Malignant neoplasm of greater curvature of stomach, unspecified ▽
151.8 Malignant neoplasm of other specified sites of stomach
151.9 Malignant neoplasm of stomach, unspecified site ▽
153.3 Malignant neoplasm of sigmoid colon
211.0 Benign neoplasm of esophagus
211.1 Benign neoplasm of stomach
211.2 Benign neoplasm of duodenum, jejunum, and ileum
211.3 Benign neoplasm of colon
280.0 Iron deficiency anemia secondary to blood loss (chronic)
285.1 Acute posthemorrhagic anemia
285.9 Unspecified anemia ▽
448.0 Hereditary hemorrhagic telangiectasia
448.9 Other and unspecified capillary diseases ▽
456.0 Esophageal varices with bleeding
456.20 Esophageal varices with bleeding in diseases classified elsewhere — (Code first underlying disease: 571.0-571.9, 572.3) ☒
530.21 Ulcer of esophagus with bleeding — (Use additional E code to identify cause, if induced by chemical or drug)
530.7 Gastroesophageal laceration-hemorrhage syndrome
530.81 Esophageal reflux
530.82 Esophageal hemorrhage
530.83 Esophageal leukoplakia
530.84 Tracheoesophageal fistula
530.85 Barrett's esophagus
530.89 Other specified disorder of the esophagus
530.9 Unspecified disorder of esophagus ▽
531.00 Acute gastric ulcer with hemorrhage, without mention of obstruction — (Use additional E code to identify drug, if drug induced)
531.01 Acute gastric ulcer with hemorrhage and obstruction — (Use additional E code to identify drug, if drug induced)
531.10 Acute gastric ulcer with perforation, without mention of obstruction — (Use additional E code to identify drug, if drug induced)

▽ Unspecified code ♀ Female diagnosis ☒ Manifestation code ♂ Male diagnosis

531.11 Acute gastric ulcer with perforation and obstruction — (Use additional E code to identify drug, if drug induced)
531.20 Acute gastric ulcer with hemorrhage and perforation, without mention of obstruction — (Use additional E code to identify drug, if drug induced)
531.21 Acute gastric ulcer with hemorrhage, perforation, and obstruction — (Use additional E code to identify drug, if drug induced)
531.30 Acute gastric ulcer without mention of hemorrhage, perforation, or obstruction — (Use additional E code to identify drug, if drug induced)
531.31 Acute gastric ulcer without mention of hemorrhage or perforation, with obstruction — (Use additional E code to identify drug, if drug induced)
531.40 Chronic or unspecified gastric ulcer with hemorrhage, without mention of obstruction — (Use additional E code to identify drug, if drug induced)
531.41 Chronic or unspecified gastric ulcer with hemorrhage and obstruction — (Use additional E code to identify drug, if drug induced)
531.50 Chronic or unspecified gastric ulcer with perforation, without mention of obstruction — (Use additional E code to identify drug, if drug induced)
531.51 Chronic or unspecified gastric ulcer with perforation and obstruction — (Use additional E code to identify drug, if drug induced)
531.60 Chronic or unspecified gastric ulcer with hemorrhage and perforation, without mention of obstruction — (Use additional E code to identify drug, if drug induced)
531.61 Chronic or unspecified gastric ulcer with hemorrhage, perforation, and obstruction — (Use additional E code to identify drug, if drug induced)
531.70 Chronic gastric ulcer without mention of hemorrhage, perforation, without mention of obstruction — (Use additional E code to identify drug, if drug induced)
531.71 Chronic gastric ulcer without mention of hemorrhage or perforation, with obstruction — (Use additional E code to identify drug, if drug induced)
531.90 Gastric ulcer, unspecified as acute or chronic, without mention of hemorrhage, perforation, or obstruction — (Use additional E code to identify drug, if drug induced) ▽
531.91 Gastric ulcer, unspecified as acute or chronic, without mention of hemorrhage or perforation, with obstruction — (Use additional E code to identify drug, if drug induced) ▽
533.00 Acute peptic ulcer, unspecified site, with hemorrhage, without mention of obstruction — (Use additional E code to identify drug, if drug induced)
533.10 Acute peptic ulcer, unspecified site, with perforation, without mention of obstruction — (Use additional E code to identify drug, if drug induced)
533.11 Acute peptic ulcer, unspecified site, with perforation and obstruction — (Use additional E code to identify drug, if drug induced)
533.20 Acute peptic ulcer, unspecified site, with hemorrhage and perforation, without mention of obstruction — (Use additional E code to identify drug, if drug induced)
533.21 Acute peptic ulcer, unspecified site, with hemorrhage, perforation, and obstruction — (Use additional E code to identify drug, if drug induced)
533.30 Acute peptic ulcer, unspecified site, without mention of hemorrhage, perforation, or obstruction — (Use additional E code to identify drug, if drug induced)
533.31 Acute peptic ulcer, unspecified site, without mention of hemorrhage and perforation, with obstruction — (Use additional E code to identify drug, if drug induced)
533.40 Chronic or unspecified peptic ulcer, unspecified site, with hemorrhage, without mention of obstruction — (Use additional E code to identify drug, if drug induced)
533.41 Chronic or unspecified peptic ulcer, unspecified site, with hemorrhage and obstruction — (Use additional E code to identify drug, if drug induced)
533.50 Chronic or unspecified peptic ulcer, unspecified site, with perforation, without mention of obstruction — (Use additional E code to identify drug, if drug induced)
533.51 Chronic or unspecified peptic ulcer, unspecified site, with perforation and obstruction — (Use additional E code to identify drug, if drug induced)
533.60 Chronic or unspecified peptic ulcer, unspecified site, with hemorrhage and perforation, without mention of obstruction — (Use additional E code to identify drug, if drug induced)
533.61 Chronic or unspecified peptic ulcer, unspecified site, with hemorrhage, perforation, and obstruction — (Use additional E code to identify drug, if drug induced)
533.70 Chronic peptic ulcer, unspecified site, without mention of hemorrhage, perforation, or obstruction — (Use additional E code to identify drug, if drug induced)
533.71 Chronic peptic ulcer of unspecified site without mention of hemorrhage or perforation, with obstruction — (Use additional E code to identify drug, if drug induced)
533.90 Peptic ulcer, unspecified site, unspecified as acute or chronic, without mention of hemorrhage, perforation, or obstruction — (Use additional E code to identify drug, if drug induced) ▽
533.91 Peptic ulcer, unspecified site, unspecified as acute or chronic, without mention of hemorrhage or perforation, with obstruction — (Use additional E code to identify drug, if drug induced) ▽
535.11 Atrophic gastritis with hemorrhage
535.51 Unspecified gastritis and gastroduodenitis with hemorrhage ▽
537.84 Dieulafoy lesion (hemorrhagic) of stomach and duodenum
569.85 Angiodysplasia of intestine with hemorrhage
569.86 Dieulafoy lesion (hemorrhagic) of intestine
571.0 Alcoholic fatty liver
571.1 Acute alcoholic hepatitis
571.2 Alcoholic cirrhosis of liver
571.3 Unspecified alcoholic liver damage ▽
571.40 Unspecified chronic hepatitis ▽
571.41 Chronic persistent hepatitis
571.49 Other chronic hepatitis
571.5 Cirrhosis of liver without mention of alcohol
571.6 Biliary cirrhosis
571.8 Other chronic nonalcoholic liver disease
571.9 Unspecified chronic liver disease without mention of alcohol ▽
572.3 Portal hypertension
578.0 Hematemesis
578.1 Blood in stool
578.9 Unspecified, hemorrhage of gastrointestinal tract ▽
747.60 Congenital anomaly of the peripheral vascular system, unspecified site ▽
787.01 Nausea with vomiting
789.00 Abdominal pain, unspecified site ▽
789.30 Abdominal or pelvic swelling, mass or lump, unspecified site ▽
792.1 Nonspecific abnormal finding in stool contents
V45.89 Other postsurgical status — (This code is intended for use when these conditions are recorded as diagnoses or problems)

ICD-9-CM Procedural

42.33 Endoscopic excision or destruction of lesion or tissue of esophagus
44.43 Endoscopic control of gastric or duodenal bleeding

43256

43256 Upper gastrointestinal endoscopy including esophagus, stomach, and either the duodenum and/or jejunum as appropriate; with transendoscopic stent placement (includes predilation)

ICD-9-CM Diagnostic

150.0 Malignant neoplasm of cervical esophagus
150.1 Malignant neoplasm of thoracic esophagus
150.3 Malignant neoplasm of upper third of esophagus
150.4 Malignant neoplasm of middle third of esophagus
150.5 Malignant neoplasm of lower third of esophagus
150.8 Malignant neoplasm of other specified part of esophagus
150.9 Malignant neoplasm of esophagus, unspecified site ▽
151.0 Malignant neoplasm of cardia
151.1 Malignant neoplasm of pylorus
151.2 Malignant neoplasm of pyloric antrum
151.3 Malignant neoplasm of fundus of stomach
151.4 Malignant neoplasm of body of stomach
151.5 Malignant neoplasm of lesser curvature of stomach, unspecified ▽
151.6 Malignant neoplasm of greater curvature of stomach, unspecified ▽
151.8 Malignant neoplasm of other specified sites of stomach
151.9 Malignant neoplasm of stomach, unspecified site ▽
152.0 Malignant neoplasm of duodenum
152.1 Malignant neoplasm of jejunum
196.1 Secondary and unspecified malignant neoplasm of intrathoracic lymph nodes
197.4 Secondary malignant neoplasm of small intestine including duodenum
197.8 Secondary malignant neoplasm of other digestive organs and spleen
211.0 Benign neoplasm of esophagus
211.1 Benign neoplasm of stomach
211.2 Benign neoplasm of duodenum, jejunum, and ileum
230.1 Carcinoma in situ of esophagus
230.7 Carcinoma in situ of other and unspecified parts of intestine ▽
235.5 Neoplasm of uncertain behavior of other and unspecified digestive organs ▽
239.0 Neoplasm of unspecified nature of digestive system
239.8 Neoplasm of unspecified nature of other specified sites
530.11 Reflux esophagitis — (Use additional E code to identify cause, if induced by chemical or drug)
530.12 Acute esophagitis — (Use additional E code to identify cause, if induced by chemical or drug)
530.19 Other esophagitis — (Use additional E code to identify cause, if induced by chemical or drug)

▽ Unspecified code ♀ Female diagnosis ☒ Manifestation code ♂ Male diagnosis

530.20 Ulcer of esophagus without bleeding — (Use additional E code to identify cause, if induced by chemical or drug)
530.21 Ulcer of esophagus with bleeding — (Use additional E code to identify cause, if induced by chemical or drug)
530.3 Stricture and stenosis of esophagus
530.5 Dyskinesia of esophagus
530.81 Esophageal reflux
530.85 Barrett's esophagus
530.89 Other specified disorder of the esophagus
537.0 Acquired hypertrophic pyloric stenosis
537.2 Chronic duodenal ileus
537.3 Other obstruction of duodenum
537.6 Hourglass stricture or stenosis of stomach
537.89 Other specified disorder of stomach and duodenum
557.1 Chronic vascular insufficiency of intestine
560.2 Volvulus
560.81 Intestinal or peritoneal adhesions with obstruction (postoperative) (postinfection)
560.89 Other specified intestinal obstruction
560.9 Unspecified intestinal obstruction ▽
568.0 Peritoneal adhesions (postoperative) (postinfection)
750.5 Congenital hypertrophic pyloric stenosis
750.7 Other specified congenital anomalies of stomach
751.1 Congenital atresia and stenosis of small intestine
787.2 Dysphagia
997.4 Digestive system complication — (Use additional code to identify complications)

ICD-9-CM Procedural

42.81 Insertion of permanent tube into esophagus

43257

43257 Upper gastrointestinal endoscopy including esophagus, stomach, and either the duodenum and/or jejunum as appropriate; with delivery of thermal energy to the muscle of lower esophageal sphincter and/or gastric cardia, for treatment of gastroesophageal reflux disease

ICD-9-CM Diagnostic

530.10 Unspecified esophagitis — (Use additional E code to identify cause, if induced by chemical or drug) ▽
530.11 Reflux esophagitis — (Use additional E code to identify cause, if induced by chemical or drug)
530.12 Acute esophagitis — (Use additional E code to identify cause, if induced by chemical or drug)
530.20 Ulcer of esophagus without bleeding — (Use additional E code to identify cause, if induced by chemical or drug)
530.21 Ulcer of esophagus with bleeding — (Use additional E code to identify cause, if induced by chemical or drug)
530.4 Perforation of esophagus
530.81 Esophageal reflux

ICD-9-CM Procedural

42.33 Endoscopic excision or destruction of lesion or tissue of esophagus
44.67 Laparoscopic procedures for creation of esophagogastric sphincteric competence
45.13 Other endoscopy of small intestine

43258

43258 Upper gastrointestinal endoscopy including esophagus, stomach, and either the duodenum and/or jejunum as appropriate; with ablation of tumor(s), polyp(s), or other lesion(s) not amenable to removal by hot biopsy forceps, bipolar cautery or snare technique

ICD-9-CM Diagnostic

150.0 Malignant neoplasm of cervical esophagus
150.1 Malignant neoplasm of thoracic esophagus
150.2 Malignant neoplasm of abdominal esophagus
150.3 Malignant neoplasm of upper third of esophagus
150.4 Malignant neoplasm of middle third of esophagus
150.5 Malignant neoplasm of lower third of esophagus
150.8 Malignant neoplasm of other specified part of esophagus
151.0 Malignant neoplasm of cardia
151.1 Malignant neoplasm of pylorus
151.2 Malignant neoplasm of pyloric antrum
151.3 Malignant neoplasm of fundus of stomach
151.4 Malignant neoplasm of body of stomach
151.5 Malignant neoplasm of lesser curvature of stomach, unspecified ▽
151.6 Malignant neoplasm of greater curvature of stomach, unspecified ▽
151.8 Malignant neoplasm of other specified sites of stomach
152.0 Malignant neoplasm of duodenum
152.1 Malignant neoplasm of jejunum
152.8 Malignant neoplasm of other specified sites of small intestine
197.4 Secondary malignant neoplasm of small intestine including duodenum
197.8 Secondary malignant neoplasm of other digestive organs and spleen
211.0 Benign neoplasm of esophagus
211.1 Benign neoplasm of stomach
211.2 Benign neoplasm of duodenum, jejunum, and ileum
211.9 Benign neoplasm of other and unspecified site of the digestive system ▽
230.2 Carcinoma in situ of stomach
230.7 Carcinoma in situ of other and unspecified parts of intestine ▽
235.2 Neoplasm of uncertain behavior of stomach, intestines, and rectum
235.5 Neoplasm of uncertain behavior of other and unspecified digestive organs ▽
530.9 Unspecified disorder of esophagus ▽
537.82 Angiodysplasia of stomach and duodenum (without mention of hemorrhage)
537.83 Angiodysplasia of stomach and duodenum with hemorrhage
537.89 Other specified disorder of stomach and duodenum

ICD-9-CM Procedural

42.33 Endoscopic excision or destruction of lesion or tissue of esophagus
43.41 Endoscopic excision or destruction of lesion or tissue of stomach
45.30 Endoscopic excision or destruction of lesion of duodenum
45.34 Other destruction of lesion of small intestine, except duodenum

HCPCS Level II Supplies & Services

A4270 Disposable endoscope sheath, each
A4305 Disposable drug delivery system, flow rate of 50 ml or greater per hour
A4306 Disposable drug delivery system, flow rate of 5 ml or less per hour
A4550 Surgical trays

43259

43259 Upper gastrointestinal endoscopy including esophagus, stomach, and either the duodenum and/or jejunum as appropriate; with endoscopic ultrasound examination, including the esophagus, stomach, and either the duodenum and/or jejunum as appropriate

ICD-9-CM Diagnostic

150.0 Malignant neoplasm of cervical esophagus
150.1 Malignant neoplasm of thoracic esophagus
150.2 Malignant neoplasm of abdominal esophagus
150.3 Malignant neoplasm of upper third of esophagus
150.4 Malignant neoplasm of middle third of esophagus
150.5 Malignant neoplasm of lower third of esophagus
150.8 Malignant neoplasm of other specified part of esophagus
151.0 Malignant neoplasm of cardia
151.1 Malignant neoplasm of pylorus
151.2 Malignant neoplasm of pyloric antrum
151.3 Malignant neoplasm of fundus of stomach
151.4 Malignant neoplasm of body of stomach
151.5 Malignant neoplasm of lesser curvature of stomach, unspecified ▽
151.6 Malignant neoplasm of greater curvature of stomach, unspecified ▽
151.8 Malignant neoplasm of other specified sites of stomach
152.0 Malignant neoplasm of duodenum
152.1 Malignant neoplasm of jejunum
197.8 Secondary malignant neoplasm of other digestive organs and spleen
211.1 Benign neoplasm of stomach
230.1 Carcinoma in situ of esophagus
230.2 Carcinoma in situ of stomach
230.9 Carcinoma in situ of other and unspecified digestive organs ▽
235.2 Neoplasm of uncertain behavior of stomach, intestines, and rectum
789.30 Abdominal or pelvic swelling, mass or lump, unspecified site ▽
789.31 Abdominal or pelvic swelling, mass, or lump, right upper quadrant
789.32 Abdominal or pelvic swelling, mass, or lump, left upper quadrant
789.33 Abdominal or pelvic swelling, mass, or lump, right lower quadrant
789.34 Abdominal or pelvic swelling, mass, or lump, left lower quadrant
789.35 Abdominal or pelvic swelling, mass or lump, periumbilic
789.36 Abdominal or pelvic swelling, mass, or lump, epigastric
789.37 Abdominal or pelvic swelling, mass, or lump, epigastric, generalized
789.39 Abdominal or pelvic swelling, mass, or lump, other specified site

ICD-9-CM Procedural

42.23 Other esophagoscopy
42.29 Other diagnostic procedures on esophagus
44.13 Other gastroscopy

▽ Unspecified code ♀ Female diagnosis ☒ Manifestation code ♂ Male diagnosis

45.13 Other endoscopy of small intestine

HCPCS Level II Supplies & Services

A4270 Disposable endoscope sheath, each
A4305 Disposable drug delivery system, flow rate of 50 ml or greater per hour
A4306 Disposable drug delivery system, flow rate of 5 ml or less per hour
A4550 Surgical trays

43260–43261

43260 Endoscopic retrograde cholangiopancreatography (ERCP); diagnostic, with or without collection of specimen(s) by brushing or washing (separate procedure)
43261 with biopsy, single or multiple

ICD-9-CM Diagnostic

155.1 Malignant neoplasm of intrahepatic bile ducts
156.0 Malignant neoplasm of gallbladder
156.1 Malignant neoplasm of extrahepatic bile ducts
156.2 Malignant neoplasm of ampulla of Vater
156.8 Malignant neoplasm of other specified sites of gallbladder and extrahepatic bile ducts
156.9 Malignant neoplasm of biliary tract, part unspecified site ▽
197.8 Secondary malignant neoplasm of other digestive organs and spleen
211.5 Benign neoplasm of liver and biliary passages
211.6 Benign neoplasm of pancreas, except islets of Langerhans
211.7 Benign neoplasm of islets of Langerhans — (Use additional code to identify any functional activity)
230.8 Carcinoma in situ of liver and biliary system
230.9 Carcinoma in situ of other and unspecified digestive organs ▽
235.3 Neoplasm of uncertain behavior of liver and biliary passages
235.5 Neoplasm of uncertain behavior of other and unspecified digestive organs ▽
239.0 Neoplasm of unspecified nature of digestive system
251.9 Unspecified disorder of pancreatic internal secretion ▽
277.4 Disorders of bilirubin excretion — (Use additional code to identify any associated mental retardation)
560.1 Paralytic ileus
560.31 Gallstone ileus
571.5 Cirrhosis of liver without mention of alcohol
571.6 Biliary cirrhosis
572.0 Abscess of liver
574.00 Calculus of gallbladder with acute cholecystitis, without mention of obstruction
574.01 Calculus of gallbladder with acute cholecystitis and obstruction
574.10 Calculus of gallbladder with other cholecystitis, without mention of obstruction
574.11 Calculus of gallbladder with other cholecystitis and obstruction
574.20 Calculus of gallbladder without mention of cholecystitis or obstruction
574.21 Calculus of gallbladder without mention of cholecystitis, with obstruction
574.30 Calculus of bile duct with acute cholecystitis without mention of obstruction
574.31 Calculus of bile duct with acute cholecystitis and obstruction
574.40 Calculus of bile duct with other cholecystitis, without mention of obstruction
574.41 Calculus of bile duct with other cholecystitis and obstruction
574.50 Calculus of bile duct without mention of cholecystitis or obstruction
574.51 Calculus of bile duct without mention of cholecystitis, with obstruction
575.0 Acute cholecystitis
575.2 Obstruction of gallbladder
575.3 Hydrops of gallbladder
575.4 Perforation of gallbladder
575.5 Fistula of gallbladder
575.6 Cholesterolosis of gallbladder
575.8 Other specified disorder of gallbladder
575.9 Unspecified disorder of gallbladder ▽
576.0 Postcholecystectomy syndrome
576.1 Cholangitis
576.2 Obstruction of bile duct
576.3 Perforation of bile duct
576.4 Fistula of bile duct
576.5 Spasm of sphincter of Oddi
576.8 Other specified disorders of biliary tract
577.0 Acute pancreatitis
577.1 Chronic pancreatitis
577.2 Cyst and pseudocyst of pancreas
577.8 Other specified disease of pancreas
578.9 Unspecified, hemorrhage of gastrointestinal tract ▽
751.60 Unspecified congenital anomaly of gallbladder, bile ducts, and liver ▽
751.61 Congenital biliary atresia
751.62 Congenital cystic disease of liver
751.69 Other congenital anomaly of gallbladder, bile ducts, and liver
751.7 Congenital anomalies of pancreas
780.6 Fever
782.4 Jaundice, unspecified, not of newborn ▽
783.0 Anorexia
783.21 Loss of weight
783.22 Underweight
783.7 Adult failure to thrive
790.5 Other nonspecific abnormal serum enzyme levels
793.4 Nonspecific abnormal findings on radiological and other examination of gastrointestinal tract
794.9 Nonspecific abnormal results of other specified function study
996.82 Complications of transplanted liver — (Use additional code to identify nature of complication, 078.5)
996.86 Complications of transplanted pancreas — (Use additional code to identify nature of complication, 078.5)
997.4 Digestive system complication — (Use additional code to identify complications)

ICD-9-CM Procedural

51.10 Endoscopic retrograde cholangiopancreatography (ERCP)
51.14 Other closed (endoscopic) biopsy of biliary duct or sphincter of Oddi
51.19 Other diagnostic procedures on biliary tract
51.88 Endoscopic removal of stone(s) from biliary tract
52.14 Closed (endoscopic) biopsy of pancreatic duct
52.19 Other diagnostic procedures on pancreas

43262–43263

43262 Endoscopic retrograde cholangiopancreatography (ERCP); with sphincterotomy/papillotomy
43263 with pressure measurement of sphincter of Oddi (pancreatic duct or common bile duct)

ICD-9-CM Diagnostic

155.1 Malignant neoplasm of intrahepatic bile ducts
156.0 Malignant neoplasm of gallbladder
156.1 Malignant neoplasm of extrahepatic bile ducts
156.2 Malignant neoplasm of ampulla of Vater
156.8 Malignant neoplasm of other specified sites of gallbladder and extrahepatic bile ducts
157.0 Malignant neoplasm of head of pancreas
157.1 Malignant neoplasm of body of pancreas
157.2 Malignant neoplasm of tail of pancreas
157.3 Malignant neoplasm of pancreatic duct
157.4 Malignant neoplasm of islets of Langerhans — (Use additional code to identify any functional activity)
157.8 Malignant neoplasm of other specified sites of pancreas
197.8 Secondary malignant neoplasm of other digestive organs and spleen
211.5 Benign neoplasm of liver and biliary passages
230.8 Carcinoma in situ of liver and biliary system
235.3 Neoplasm of uncertain behavior of liver and biliary passages
560.31 Gallstone ileus
571.5 Cirrhosis of liver without mention of alcohol
571.6 Biliary cirrhosis
574.00 Calculus of gallbladder with acute cholecystitis, without mention of obstruction
574.01 Calculus of gallbladder with acute cholecystitis and obstruction
574.11 Calculus of gallbladder with other cholecystitis and obstruction
574.20 Calculus of gallbladder without mention of cholecystitis or obstruction
574.21 Calculus of gallbladder without mention of cholecystitis, with obstruction
574.30 Calculus of bile duct with acute cholecystitis without mention of obstruction
574.31 Calculus of bile duct with acute cholecystitis and obstruction
574.40 Calculus of bile duct with other cholecystitis, without mention of obstruction
574.41 Calculus of bile duct with other cholecystitis and obstruction
574.50 Calculus of bile duct without mention of cholecystitis or obstruction
574.51 Calculus of bile duct without mention of cholecystitis, with obstruction
575.0 Acute cholecystitis
575.11 Chronic cholecystitis
575.12 Acute and chronic cholecystitis
575.2 Obstruction of gallbladder
575.3 Hydrops of gallbladder
575.4 Perforation of gallbladder
575.5 Fistula of gallbladder
575.6 Cholesterolosis of gallbladder
575.8 Other specified disorder of gallbladder
576.0 Postcholecystectomy syndrome
576.1 Cholangitis
576.2 Obstruction of bile duct
576.3 Perforation of bile duct

▽ Unspecified code
♀ Female diagnosis
☒ Manifestation code
♂ Male diagnosis

576.4 Fistula of bile duct
576.5 Spasm of sphincter of Oddi
576.8 Other specified disorders of biliary tract
577.0 Acute pancreatitis
577.1 Chronic pancreatitis
577.2 Cyst and pseudocyst of pancreas
577.8 Other specified disease of pancreas
751.69 Other congenital anomaly of gallbladder, bile ducts, and liver
751.7 Congenital anomalies of pancreas
782.4 Jaundice, unspecified, not of newborn
787.01 Nausea with vomiting
789.01 Abdominal pain, right upper quadrant
790.4 Nonspecific elevation of levels of transaminase or lactic acid dehydrogenase (LDH)
790.5 Other nonspecific abnormal serum enzyme levels
790.6 Other abnormal blood chemistry
793.4 Nonspecific abnormal findings on radiological and other examination of gastrointestinal tract
794.8 Nonspecific abnormal results of liver function study
996.82 Complications of transplanted liver — (Use additional code to identify nature of complication, 078.5)

ICD-9-CM Procedural

51.15 Pressure measurement of sphincter of Oddi
51.85 Endoscopic sphincterotomy and papillotomy

43264–43265

43264 Endoscopic retrograde cholangiopancreatography (ERCP); with endoscopic retrograde removal of calculus/calculi from biliary and/or pancreatic ducts
43265 with endoscopic retrograde destruction, lithotripsy of calculus/calculi, any method

ICD-9-CM Diagnostic

574.00 Calculus of gallbladder with acute cholecystitis, without mention of obstruction
574.01 Calculus of gallbladder with acute cholecystitis and obstruction
574.10 Calculus of gallbladder with other cholecystitis, without mention of obstruction
574.11 Calculus of gallbladder with other cholecystitis and obstruction
574.20 Calculus of gallbladder without mention of cholecystitis or obstruction
574.21 Calculus of gallbladder without mention of cholecystitis, with obstruction
574.30 Calculus of bile duct with acute cholecystitis without mention of obstruction
574.31 Calculus of bile duct with acute cholecystitis and obstruction
574.40 Calculus of bile duct with other cholecystitis, without mention of obstruction
574.41 Calculus of bile duct with other cholecystitis and obstruction
574.50 Calculus of bile duct without mention of cholecystitis or obstruction
574.51 Calculus of bile duct without mention of cholecystitis, with obstruction
576.2 Obstruction of bile duct
576.8 Other specified disorders of biliary tract
577.0 Acute pancreatitis
577.1 Chronic pancreatitis
577.2 Cyst and pseudocyst of pancreas
577.8 Other specified disease of pancreas
751.69 Other congenital anomaly of gallbladder, bile ducts, and liver
782.4 Jaundice, unspecified, not of newborn

ICD-9-CM Procedural

51.88 Endoscopic removal of stone(s) from biliary tract
52.94 Endoscopic removal of stone(s) from pancreatic duct
98.52 Extracorporeal shockwave lithotripsy (ESWL) of the gallbladder and/or bile duct
98.59 Extracorporeal shockwave lithotripsy (ESWL) of other sites

43267–43269

43264 Endoscopic retrograde cholangiopancreatography (ERCP); with endoscopic retrograde removal of calculus/calculi from biliary and/or pancreatic ducts
43268 with endoscopic retrograde insertion of tube or stent into bile or pancreatic duct
43269 with endoscopic retrograde removal of foreign body and/or change of tube or stent

ICD-9-CM Diagnostic

155.0 Malignant neoplasm of liver, primary
155.1 Malignant neoplasm of intrahepatic bile ducts
155.2 Malignant neoplasm of liver, not specified as primary or secondary
156.0 Malignant neoplasm of gallbladder
156.1 Malignant neoplasm of extrahepatic bile ducts
156.2 Malignant neoplasm of ampulla of Vater
156.8 Malignant neoplasm of other specified sites of gallbladder and extrahepatic bile ducts
156.9 Malignant neoplasm of biliary tract, part unspecified site
157.0 Malignant neoplasm of head of pancreas
157.1 Malignant neoplasm of body of pancreas
157.2 Malignant neoplasm of tail of pancreas
157.3 Malignant neoplasm of pancreatic duct
157.4 Malignant neoplasm of islets of Langerhans — (Use additional code to identify any functional activity)
157.8 Malignant neoplasm of other specified sites of pancreas
157.9 Malignant neoplasm of pancreas, part unspecified
197.8 Secondary malignant neoplasm of other digestive organs and spleen
211.5 Benign neoplasm of liver and biliary passages
230.8 Carcinoma in situ of liver and biliary system
235.3 Neoplasm of uncertain behavior of liver and biliary passages
239.0 Neoplasm of unspecified nature of digestive system
560.31 Gallstone ileus
570 Acute and subacute necrosis of liver
571.6 Biliary cirrhosis
574.00 Calculus of gallbladder with acute cholecystitis, without mention of obstruction
574.01 Calculus of gallbladder with acute cholecystitis and obstruction
574.10 Calculus of gallbladder with other cholecystitis, without mention of obstruction
574.11 Calculus of gallbladder with other cholecystitis and obstruction
574.20 Calculus of gallbladder without mention of cholecystitis or obstruction
574.21 Calculus of gallbladder without mention of cholecystitis, with obstruction
574.31 Calculus of bile duct with acute cholecystitis and obstruction
574.40 Calculus of bile duct with other cholecystitis, without mention of obstruction
574.41 Calculus of bile duct with other cholecystitis and obstruction
574.50 Calculus of bile duct without mention of cholecystitis or obstruction
574.51 Calculus of bile duct without mention of cholecystitis, with obstruction
575.0 Acute cholecystitis
575.11 Chronic cholecystitis
575.12 Acute and chronic cholecystitis
575.2 Obstruction of gallbladder
575.3 Hydrops of gallbladder
575.4 Perforation of gallbladder
575.5 Fistula of gallbladder
575.6 Cholesterolosis of gallbladder
575.8 Other specified disorder of gallbladder
576.0 Postcholecystectomy syndrome
576.1 Cholangitis
576.2 Obstruction of bile duct
576.3 Perforation of bile duct
576.4 Fistula of bile duct
576.5 Spasm of sphincter of Oddi
576.8 Other specified disorders of biliary tract
576.9 Unspecified disorder of biliary tract
577.0 Acute pancreatitis
577.1 Chronic pancreatitis
577.2 Cyst and pseudocyst of pancreas
577.8 Other specified disease of pancreas
751.69 Other congenital anomaly of gallbladder, bile ducts, and liver
751.7 Congenital anomalies of pancreas
782.4 Jaundice, unspecified, not of newborn
787.01 Nausea with vomiting
789.00 Abdominal pain, unspecified site
794.8 Nonspecific abnormal results of liver function study
996.59 Mechanical complication due to other implant and internal device, not elsewhere classified
996.69 Infection and inflammatory reaction due to other internal prosthetic device, implant, and graft — (Use additional code to identify specified infections)
996.79 Other complications due to other internal prosthetic device, implant, and graft
998.89 Other specified complications
V53.90 Fitting and adjustment, Unspecified device
V53.99 Fitting and adjustment, Other device

ICD-9-CM Procedural

51.86 Endoscopic insertion of nasobiliary drainage tube
51.87 Endoscopic insertion of stent (tube) into bile duct
51.95 Removal of prosthetic device from bile duct
52.93 Endoscopic insertion of stent (tube) into pancreatic duct
52.97 Endoscopic insertion of nasopancreatic drainage tube
97.05 Replacement of stent (tube) in biliary or pancreatic duct
97.55 Removal of T-tube, other bile duct tube, or liver tube

43271–43272

43271 Endoscopic retrograde cholangiopancreatography (ERCP); with endoscopic retrograde balloon dilation of ampulla, biliary and/or pancreatic duct(s)
43272 with ablation of tumor(s), polyp(s), or other lesion(s) not amenable to removal by hot biopsy forceps, bipolar cautery or snare technique

ICD-9-CM Diagnostic

155.1 Malignant neoplasm of intrahepatic bile ducts
155.2 Malignant neoplasm of liver, not specified as primary or secondary ▽
156.0 Malignant neoplasm of gallbladder
156.1 Malignant neoplasm of extrahepatic bile ducts
156.2 Malignant neoplasm of ampulla of Vater
156.8 Malignant neoplasm of other specified sites of gallbladder and extrahepatic bile ducts
156.9 Malignant neoplasm of biliary tract, part unspecified site ▽
157.9 Malignant neoplasm of pancreas, part unspecified ▽
197.8 Secondary malignant neoplasm of other digestive organs and spleen
211.5 Benign neoplasm of liver and biliary passages
211.6 Benign neoplasm of pancreas, except islets of Langerhans
230.8 Carcinoma in situ of liver and biliary system
230.9 Carcinoma in situ of other and unspecified digestive organs ▽
235.3 Neoplasm of uncertain behavior of liver and biliary passages
235.5 Neoplasm of uncertain behavior of other and unspecified digestive organs ▽
239.0 Neoplasm of unspecified nature of digestive system
574.00 Calculus of gallbladder with acute cholecystitis, without mention of obstruction
574.21 Calculus of gallbladder without mention of cholecystitis, with obstruction
574.50 Calculus of bile duct without mention of cholecystitis or obstruction
574.51 Calculus of bile duct without mention of cholecystitis, with obstruction
575.11 Chronic cholecystitis
575.12 Acute and chronic cholecystitis
575.2 Obstruction of gallbladder
575.3 Hydrops of gallbladder
575.4 Perforation of gallbladder
575.5 Fistula of gallbladder
575.6 Cholesterolosis of gallbladder
575.8 Other specified disorder of gallbladder
575.9 Unspecified disorder of gallbladder ▽
576.0 Postcholecystectomy syndrome
576.1 Cholangitis
576.2 Obstruction of bile duct
576.3 Perforation of bile duct
576.4 Fistula of bile duct
576.5 Spasm of sphincter of Oddi
576.8 Other specified disorders of biliary tract
577.0 Acute pancreatitis
577.1 Chronic pancreatitis
577.2 Cyst and pseudocyst of pancreas
577.8 Other specified disease of pancreas
751.7 Congenital anomalies of pancreas
782.4 Jaundice, unspecified, not of newborn ▽
794.8 Nonspecific abnormal results of liver function study
997.4 Digestive system complication — (Use additional code to identify complications)

ICD-9-CM Procedural

51.64 Endoscopic excision or destruction of lesion of biliary ducts or sphincter of Oddi
51.81 Dilation of sphincter of Oddi
51.84 Endoscopic dilation of ampulla and biliary duct
52.98 Endoscopic dilation of pancreatic duct

43280

43280 Laparoscopy, surgical, esophagogastric fundoplasty (eg, Nissen, Toupet procedures)

ICD-9-CM Diagnostic

150.4 Malignant neoplasm of middle third of esophagus
150.5 Malignant neoplasm of lower third of esophagus
150.8 Malignant neoplasm of other specified part of esophagus
150.9 Malignant neoplasm of esophagus, unspecified site ▽
151.0 Malignant neoplasm of cardia
197.8 Secondary malignant neoplasm of other digestive organs and spleen
230.1 Carcinoma in situ of esophagus
230.2 Carcinoma in situ of stomach
530.11 Reflux esophagitis — (Use additional E code to identify cause, if induced by chemical or drug)
530.12 Acute esophagitis — (Use additional E code to identify cause, if induced by chemical or drug)
530.20 Ulcer of esophagus without bleeding — (Use additional E code to identify cause, if induced by chemical or drug)
530.21 Ulcer of esophagus with bleeding — (Use additional E code to identify cause, if induced by chemical or drug)
530.3 Stricture and stenosis of esophagus
530.81 Esophageal reflux
530.85 Barrett's esophagus
552.3 Diaphragmatic hernia with obstruction
553.3 Diaphragmatic hernia without mention of obstruction or gangrene
750.3 Congenital tracheoesophageal fistula, esophageal atresia and stenosis
750.4 Other specified congenital anomaly of esophagus
756.6 Congenital anomaly of diaphragm
783.3 Feeding difficulties and mismanagement
787.2 Dysphagia
789.06 Abdominal pain, epigastric
789.07 Abdominal pain, generalized
789.09 Abdominal pain, other specified site
862.22 Esophagus injury without mention of open wound into cavity
908.1 Late effect of internal injury to intra-abdominal organs
908.6 Late effect of certain complications of trauma
909.3 Late effect of complications of surgical and medical care
925.2 Crushing injury of neck — (Use additional code to identify any associated injuries: 800-829, 850.0-854.1, 860.0-869.1)
997.4 Digestive system complication — (Use additional code to identify complications)
V47.3 Other digestive problems — (This code is intended for use when these conditions are recorded as diagnoses or problems)

ICD-9-CM Procedural

44.67 Laparoscopic procedures for creation of esophagogastric sphincteric competence

43300–43305

43300 Esophagoplasty (plastic repair or reconstruction), cervical approach; without repair of tracheoesophageal fistula
43305 with repair of tracheoesophageal fistula

ICD-9-CM Diagnostic

150.0 Malignant neoplasm of cervical esophagus
150.2 Malignant neoplasm of abdominal esophagus
150.3 Malignant neoplasm of upper third of esophagus
150.4 Malignant neoplasm of middle third of esophagus
150.5 Malignant neoplasm of lower third of esophagus
150.8 Malignant neoplasm of other specified part of esophagus
211.0 Benign neoplasm of esophagus
230.1 Carcinoma in situ of esophagus
235.5 Neoplasm of uncertain behavior of other and unspecified digestive organs ▽
239.0 Neoplasm of unspecified nature of digestive system
530.0 Achalasia and cardiospasm
530.11 Reflux esophagitis — (Use additional E code to identify cause, if induced by chemical or drug)
530.19 Other esophagitis — (Use additional E code to identify cause, if induced by chemical or drug)
530.20 Ulcer of esophagus without bleeding — (Use additional E code to identify cause, if induced by chemical or drug)
530.21 Ulcer of esophagus with bleeding — (Use additional E code to identify cause, if induced by chemical or drug)
530.3 Stricture and stenosis of esophagus
530.4 Perforation of esophagus
530.5 Dyskinesia of esophagus
530.6 Diverticulum of esophagus, acquired
530.7 Gastroesophageal laceration-hemorrhage syndrome
530.81 Esophageal reflux
530.82 Esophageal hemorrhage
530.83 Esophageal leukoplakia
530.84 Tracheoesophageal fistula
530.85 Barrett's esophagus
530.9 Unspecified disorder of esophagus ▽
750.3 Congenital tracheoesophageal fistula, esophageal atresia and stenosis
862.22 Esophagus injury without mention of open wound into cavity
862.32 Esophagus injury with open wound into cavity

ICD-9-CM Procedural

31.73 Closure of other fistula of trachea
42.89 Other repair of esophagus

43310–43312

43310 Esophagoplasty (plastic repair or reconstruction), thoracic approach; without repair of tracheoesophageal fistula
43312 with repair of tracheoesophageal fistula

ICD-9-CM Diagnostic

150.0 Malignant neoplasm of cervical esophagus
150.1 Malignant neoplasm of thoracic esophagus
150.2 Malignant neoplasm of abdominal esophagus
150.3 Malignant neoplasm of upper third of esophagus
150.4 Malignant neoplasm of middle third of esophagus
150.5 Malignant neoplasm of lower third of esophagus
150.8 Malignant neoplasm of other specified part of esophagus
211.0 Benign neoplasm of esophagus
230.1 Carcinoma in situ of esophagus
235.5 Neoplasm of uncertain behavior of other and unspecified digestive organs ▽
239.0 Neoplasm of unspecified nature of digestive system
530.0 Achalasia and cardiospasm
530.11 Reflux esophagitis — (Use additional E code to identify cause, if induced by chemical or drug)
530.19 Other esophagitis — (Use additional E code to identify cause, if induced by chemical or drug)
530.20 Ulcer of esophagus without bleeding — (Use additional E code to identify cause, if induced by chemical or drug)
530.21 Ulcer of esophagus with bleeding — (Use additional E code to identify cause, if induced by chemical or drug)
530.3 Stricture and stenosis of esophagus
530.4 Perforation of esophagus
530.5 Dyskinesia of esophagus
530.6 Diverticulum of esophagus, acquired
530.7 Gastroesophageal laceration-hemorrhage syndrome
530.81 Esophageal reflux
530.82 Esophageal hemorrhage
530.83 Esophageal leukoplakia
530.84 Tracheoesophageal fistula
530.85 Barrett's esophagus
530.9 Unspecified disorder of esophagus ▽
750.3 Congenital tracheoesophageal fistula, esophageal atresia and stenosis
862.22 Esophagus injury without mention of open wound into cavity
862.32 Esophagus injury with open wound into cavity

ICD-9-CM Procedural

31.73 Closure of other fistula of trachea
42.89 Other repair of esophagus

43313–43314

43313 Esophagoplasty for congenital defect (plastic repair or reconstruction), thoracic approach; without repair of congenital tracheoesophageal fistula
43314 with repair of congenital tracheoesophageal fistula

ICD-9-CM Diagnostic

750.3 Congenital tracheoesophageal fistula, esophageal atresia and stenosis
750.4 Other specified congenital anomaly of esophagus
750.6 Congenital hiatus hernia
750.7 Other specified congenital anomalies of stomach
750.8 Other specified congenital anomalies of upper alimentary tract
750.9 Unspecified congenital anomaly of upper alimentary tract ▽

ICD-9-CM Procedural

31.73 Closure of other fistula of trachea
42.89 Other repair of esophagus

43320

43320 Esophagogastrostomy (cardioplasty), with or without vagotomy and pyloroplasty, transabdominal or transthoracic approach

ICD-9-CM Diagnostic

150.0 Malignant neoplasm of cervical esophagus
150.2 Malignant neoplasm of abdominal esophagus
150.3 Malignant neoplasm of upper third of esophagus
150.4 Malignant neoplasm of middle third of esophagus
150.5 Malignant neoplasm of lower third of esophagus
150.9 Malignant neoplasm of esophagus, unspecified site ▽
151.0 Malignant neoplasm of cardia
197.8 Secondary malignant neoplasm of other digestive organs and spleen
230.1 Carcinoma in situ of esophagus
230.2 Carcinoma in situ of stomach
530.0 Achalasia and cardiospasm
530.11 Reflux esophagitis — (Use additional E code to identify cause, if induced by chemical or drug)
530.20 Ulcer of esophagus without bleeding — (Use additional E code to identify cause, if induced by chemical or drug)
530.21 Ulcer of esophagus with bleeding — (Use additional E code to identify cause, if induced by chemical or drug)
530.3 Stricture and stenosis of esophagus
530.4 Perforation of esophagus
530.85 Barrett's esophagus
750.3 Congenital tracheoesophageal fistula, esophageal atresia and stenosis
750.4 Other specified congenital anomaly of esophagus
862.32 Esophagus injury with open wound into cavity
925.2 Crushing injury of neck — (Use additional code to identify any associated injuries: 800-829, 850.0-854.1, 860.0-869.1)

ICD-9-CM Procedural

42.52 Intrathoracic esophagogastrostomy
44.02 Highly selective vagotomy
44.29 Other pyloroplasty

43324

43324 Esophagogastric fundoplasty (eg, Nissen, Belsey IV, Hill procedures)

ICD-9-CM Diagnostic

150.4 Malignant neoplasm of middle third of esophagus
150.5 Malignant neoplasm of lower third of esophagus
150.8 Malignant neoplasm of other specified part of esophagus
150.9 Malignant neoplasm of esophagus, unspecified site ▽
151.0 Malignant neoplasm of cardia
197.8 Secondary malignant neoplasm of other digestive organs and spleen
230.1 Carcinoma in situ of esophagus
230.2 Carcinoma in situ of stomach
530.11 Reflux esophagitis — (Use additional E code to identify cause, if induced by chemical or drug)
530.20 Ulcer of esophagus without bleeding — (Use additional E code to identify cause, if induced by chemical or drug)
530.21 Ulcer of esophagus with bleeding — (Use additional E code to identify cause, if induced by chemical or drug)
530.3 Stricture and stenosis of esophagus
530.81 Esophageal reflux
530.85 Barrett's esophagus
552.3 Diaphragmatic hernia with obstruction
553.3 Diaphragmatic hernia without mention of obstruction or gangrene
750.3 Congenital tracheoesophageal fistula, esophageal atresia and stenosis
750.4 Other specified congenital anomaly of esophagus
756.6 Congenital anomaly of diaphragm
783.3 Feeding difficulties and mismanagement
787.2 Dysphagia
789.06 Abdominal pain, epigastric
789.07 Abdominal pain, generalized
789.09 Abdominal pain, other specified site
862.22 Esophagus injury without mention of open wound into cavity
908.1 Late effect of internal injury to intra-abdominal organs
908.6 Late effect of certain complications of trauma
909.3 Late effect of complications of surgical and medical care
925.2 Crushing injury of neck — (Use additional code to identify any associated injuries: 800-829, 850.0-854.1, 860.0-869.1)
997.4 Digestive system complication — (Use additional code to identify complications)
V47.3 Other digestive problems — (This code is intended for use when these conditions are recorded as diagnoses or problems)
V64.41 Laparoscopic surgical procedure converted to open procedure

ICD-9-CM Procedural

44.65 Esophagogastroplasty
44.66 Other procedures for creation of esophagogastric sphincteric competence

43325

43325 Esophagogastric fundoplasty; with fundic patch (Thal-Nissen procedure)

ICD-9-CM Diagnostic

150.4 Malignant neoplasm of middle third of esophagus
150.5 Malignant neoplasm of lower third of esophagus
150.8 Malignant neoplasm of other specified part of esophagus

150.9 Malignant neoplasm of esophagus, unspecified site ▽
151.0 Malignant neoplasm of cardia
197.8 Secondary malignant neoplasm of other digestive organs and spleen
230.1 Carcinoma in situ of esophagus
230.2 Carcinoma in situ of stomach
530.11 Reflux esophagitis — (Use additional E code to identify cause, if induced by chemical or drug)
530.20 Ulcer of esophagus without bleeding — (Use additional E code to identify cause, if induced by chemical or drug)
530.21 Ulcer of esophagus with bleeding — (Use additional E code to identify cause, if induced by chemical or drug)
530.3 Stricture and stenosis of esophagus
530.81 Esophageal reflux
530.85 Barrett's esophagus
552.3 Diaphragmatic hernia with obstruction
553.3 Diaphragmatic hernia without mention of obstruction or gangrene
750.3 Congenital tracheoesophageal fistula, esophageal atresia and stenosis
750.4 Other specified congenital anomaly of esophagus
756.6 Congenital anomaly of diaphragm
783.3 Feeding difficulties and mismanagement
787.2 Dysphagia
789.06 Abdominal pain, epigastric
789.07 Abdominal pain, generalized
789.09 Abdominal pain, other specified site
862.22 Esophagus injury without mention of open wound into cavity
908.1 Late effect of internal injury to intra-abdominal organs
908.6 Late effect of certain complications of trauma
909.3 Late effect of complications of surgical and medical care
925.2 Crushing injury of neck — (Use additional code to identify any associated injuries: 800-829, 850.0-854.1, 860.0-869.1)
997.4 Digestive system complication — (Use additional code to identify complications)
V47.3 Other digestive problems — (This code is intended for use when these conditions are recorded as diagnoses or problems)
V64.41 Laparoscopic surgical procedure converted to open procedure

ICD-9-CM Procedural

44.66 Other procedures for creation of esophagogastric sphincteric competence
44.69 Other repair of stomach

43326

43326 Esophagogastric fundoplasty; with gastroplasty (eg, Collis)

ICD-9-CM Diagnostic

150.4 Malignant neoplasm of middle third of esophagus
150.5 Malignant neoplasm of lower third of esophagus
150.8 Malignant neoplasm of other specified part of esophagus
150.9 Malignant neoplasm of esophagus, unspecified site ▽
151.0 Malignant neoplasm of cardia
197.8 Secondary malignant neoplasm of other digestive organs and spleen
230.1 Carcinoma in situ of esophagus
230.2 Carcinoma in situ of stomach
530.11 Reflux esophagitis — (Use additional E code to identify cause, if induced by chemical or drug)
530.20 Ulcer of esophagus without bleeding — (Use additional E code to identify cause, if induced by chemical or drug)
530.21 Ulcer of esophagus with bleeding — (Use additional E code to identify cause, if induced by chemical or drug)
530.3 Stricture and stenosis of esophagus
530.81 Esophageal reflux
530.85 Barrett's esophagus
552.3 Diaphragmatic hernia with obstruction
553.3 Diaphragmatic hernia without mention of obstruction or gangrene
750.3 Congenital tracheoesophageal fistula, esophageal atresia and stenosis
750.4 Other specified congenital anomaly of esophagus
756.6 Congenital anomaly of diaphragm
783.3 Feeding difficulties and mismanagement
787.2 Dysphagia
789.06 Abdominal pain, epigastric
789.07 Abdominal pain, generalized
789.09 Abdominal pain, other specified site
862.22 Esophagus injury without mention of open wound into cavity
908.1 Late effect of internal injury to intra-abdominal organs
908.6 Late effect of certain complications of trauma
909.3 Late effect of complications of surgical and medical care
925.2 Crushing injury of neck — (Use additional code to identify any associated injuries: 800-829, 850.0-854.1, 860.0-869.1)
997.4 Digestive system complication — (Use additional code to identify complications)
V47.3 Other digestive problems — (This code is intended for use when these conditions are recorded as diagnoses or problems)
V64.41 Laparoscopic surgical procedure converted to open procedure

ICD-9-CM Procedural

44.66 Other procedures for creation of esophagogastric sphincteric competence
44.69 Other repair of stomach

43330–43331

43330 Esophagomyotomy (Heller type); abdominal approach
43331 thoracic approach

ICD-9-CM Diagnostic

150.0 Malignant neoplasm of cervical esophagus
150.1 Malignant neoplasm of thoracic esophagus
150.2 Malignant neoplasm of abdominal esophagus
150.3 Malignant neoplasm of upper third of esophagus
150.4 Malignant neoplasm of middle third of esophagus
150.5 Malignant neoplasm of lower third of esophagus
150.8 Malignant neoplasm of other specified part of esophagus
150.9 Malignant neoplasm of esophagus, unspecified site ▽
530.0 Achalasia and cardiospasm
530.11 Reflux esophagitis — (Use additional E code to identify cause, if induced by chemical or drug)
530.19 Other esophagitis — (Use additional E code to identify cause, if induced by chemical or drug)
530.20 Ulcer of esophagus without bleeding — (Use additional E code to identify cause, if induced by chemical or drug)
530.21 Ulcer of esophagus with bleeding — (Use additional E code to identify cause, if induced by chemical or drug)
530.3 Stricture and stenosis of esophagus
530.4 Perforation of esophagus
530.6 Diverticulum of esophagus, acquired
530.7 Gastroesophageal laceration-hemorrhage syndrome
530.81 Esophageal reflux
530.82 Esophageal hemorrhage
530.83 Esophageal leukoplakia
530.84 Tracheoesophageal fistula
530.85 Barrett's esophagus
530.89 Other specified disorder of the esophagus
552.3 Diaphragmatic hernia with obstruction
553.3 Diaphragmatic hernia without mention of obstruction or gangrene
750.4 Other specified congenital anomaly of esophagus
756.6 Congenital anomaly of diaphragm
V64.42 Thoracoscopic surgical procedure converted to open procedure

ICD-9-CM Procedural

42.7 Esophagomyotomy

43340–43341

43340 Esophagojejunostomy (without total gastrectomy); abdominal approach
43341 thoracic approach

ICD-9-CM Diagnostic

150.0 Malignant neoplasm of cervical esophagus
150.1 Malignant neoplasm of thoracic esophagus
150.2 Malignant neoplasm of abdominal esophagus
150.3 Malignant neoplasm of upper third of esophagus
150.4 Malignant neoplasm of middle third of esophagus
150.5 Malignant neoplasm of lower third of esophagus
150.8 Malignant neoplasm of other specified part of esophagus
150.9 Malignant neoplasm of esophagus, unspecified site ▽
151.0 Malignant neoplasm of cardia
151.3 Malignant neoplasm of fundus of stomach
151.4 Malignant neoplasm of body of stomach
235.5 Neoplasm of uncertain behavior of other and unspecified digestive organs ▽
239.0 Neoplasm of unspecified nature of digestive system
530.11 Reflux esophagitis — (Use additional E code to identify cause, if induced by chemical or drug)
530.20 Ulcer of esophagus without bleeding — (Use additional E code to identify cause, if induced by chemical or drug)

530.21 Ulcer of esophagus with bleeding — (Use additional E code to identify cause, if induced by chemical or drug)
530.3 Stricture and stenosis of esophagus
530.5 Dyskinesia of esophagus
530.6 Diverticulum of esophagus, acquired
530.85 Barrett's esophagus
531.40 Chronic or unspecified gastric ulcer with hemorrhage, without mention of obstruction — (Use additional E code to identify drug, if drug induced)
531.50 Chronic or unspecified gastric ulcer with perforation, without mention of obstruction — (Use additional E code to identify drug, if drug induced)
531.60 Chronic or unspecified gastric ulcer with hemorrhage and perforation, without mention of obstruction — (Use additional E code to identify drug, if drug induced)

ICD-9-CM Procedural

42.54 Other intrathoracic esophagoenterostomy

43350–43352

43350 Esophagostomy, fistulization of esophagus, external; abdominal approach
43351 thoracic approach
43352 cervical approach

ICD-9-CM Diagnostic

148.8 Malignant neoplasm of other specified sites of hypopharynx
148.9 Malignant neoplasm of hypopharynx, unspecified site ▽
149.0 Malignant neoplasm of pharynx, unspecified ▽
150.0 Malignant neoplasm of cervical esophagus
150.1 Malignant neoplasm of thoracic esophagus
150.2 Malignant neoplasm of abdominal esophagus
150.3 Malignant neoplasm of upper third of esophagus
150.8 Malignant neoplasm of other specified part of esophagus
150.9 Malignant neoplasm of esophagus, unspecified site ▽
197.8 Secondary malignant neoplasm of other digestive organs and spleen
230.1 Carcinoma in situ of esophagus
235.5 Neoplasm of uncertain behavior of other and unspecified digestive organs ▽
239.0 Neoplasm of unspecified nature of digestive system
530.0 Achalasia and cardiospasm
530.11 Reflux esophagitis — (Use additional E code to identify cause, if induced by chemical or drug)
530.12 Acute esophagitis — (Use additional E code to identify cause, if induced by chemical or drug)
530.19 Other esophagitis — (Use additional E code to identify cause, if induced by chemical or drug)
530.20 Ulcer of esophagus without bleeding — (Use additional E code to identify cause, if induced by chemical or drug)
530.21 Ulcer of esophagus with bleeding — (Use additional E code to identify cause, if induced by chemical or drug)
530.3 Stricture and stenosis of esophagus
530.4 Perforation of esophagus
530.5 Dyskinesia of esophagus
530.6 Diverticulum of esophagus, acquired
530.7 Gastroesophageal laceration-hemorrhage syndrome
530.81 Esophageal reflux
530.82 Esophageal hemorrhage
530.83 Esophageal leukoplakia
530.84 Tracheoesophageal fistula
530.85 Barrett's esophagus
530.9 Unspecified disorder of esophagus ▽
V10.03 Personal history of malignant neoplasm of esophagus

ICD-9-CM Procedural

42.10 Esophagostomy, not otherwise specified
42.11 Cervical esophagostomy
42.19 Other external fistulization of esophagus

43360

43360 Gastrointestinal reconstruction for previous esophagectomy, for obstructing esophageal lesion or fistula, or for previous esophageal exclusion; with stomach, with or without pyloroplasty

ICD-9-CM Diagnostic

150.0 Malignant neoplasm of cervical esophagus
150.1 Malignant neoplasm of thoracic esophagus
150.2 Malignant neoplasm of abdominal esophagus
150.3 Malignant neoplasm of upper third of esophagus
150.4 Malignant neoplasm of middle third of esophagus
150.5 Malignant neoplasm of lower third of esophagus
150.8 Malignant neoplasm of other specified part of esophagus
150.9 Malignant neoplasm of esophagus, unspecified site ▽
197.8 Secondary malignant neoplasm of other digestive organs and spleen
211.0 Benign neoplasm of esophagus
230.1 Carcinoma in situ of esophagus
235.5 Neoplasm of uncertain behavior of other and unspecified digestive organs ▽
239.0 Neoplasm of unspecified nature of digestive system
530.20 Ulcer of esophagus without bleeding — (Use additional E code to identify cause, if induced by chemical or drug)
530.21 Ulcer of esophagus with bleeding — (Use additional E code to identify cause, if induced by chemical or drug)
530.3 Stricture and stenosis of esophagus
530.6 Diverticulum of esophagus, acquired
530.84 Tracheoesophageal fistula
530.85 Barrett's esophagus
530.89 Other specified disorder of the esophagus

ICD-9-CM Procedural

42.19 Other external fistulization of esophagus
42.32 Local excision of other lesion or tissue of esophagus
42.58 Intrathoracic esophageal anastomosis with other interposition
42.84 Repair of esophageal fistula, not elsewhere classified
44.29 Other pyloroplasty

43361

43361 Gastrointestinal reconstruction for previous esophagectomy, for obstructing esophageal lesion or fistula, or for previous esophageal exclusion; with colon interposition or small intestine reconstruction, including intestine mobilization, preparation, and anastomosis(es)

ICD-9-CM Diagnostic

150.0 Malignant neoplasm of cervical esophagus
150.1 Malignant neoplasm of thoracic esophagus
150.2 Malignant neoplasm of abdominal esophagus
150.3 Malignant neoplasm of upper third of esophagus
150.4 Malignant neoplasm of middle third of esophagus
150.5 Malignant neoplasm of lower third of esophagus
150.8 Malignant neoplasm of other specified part of esophagus
150.9 Malignant neoplasm of esophagus, unspecified site ▽
197.8 Secondary malignant neoplasm of other digestive organs and spleen
211.0 Benign neoplasm of esophagus
230.1 Carcinoma in situ of esophagus
235.5 Neoplasm of uncertain behavior of other and unspecified digestive organs ▽
239.0 Neoplasm of unspecified nature of digestive system
530.20 Ulcer of esophagus without bleeding — (Use additional E code to identify cause, if induced by chemical or drug)
530.21 Ulcer of esophagus with bleeding — (Use additional E code to identify cause, if induced by chemical or drug)
530.3 Stricture and stenosis of esophagus
530.6 Diverticulum of esophagus, acquired
530.84 Tracheoesophageal fistula
530.85 Barrett's esophagus
530.89 Other specified disorder of the esophagus

ICD-9-CM Procedural

42.53 Intrathoracic esophageal anastomosis with interposition of small bowel
42.55 Intrathoracic esophageal anastomosis with interposition of colon
42.63 Antesternal esophageal anastomosis with interposition of small bowel
42.65 Antesternal esophageal anastomosis with interposition of colon

43400

43400 Ligation, direct, esophageal varices

ICD-9-CM Diagnostic

456.0 Esophageal varices with bleeding
456.1 Esophageal varices without mention of bleeding
456.20 Esophageal varices with bleeding in diseases classified elsewhere — (Code first underlying disease: 571.0-571.9, 572.3) ☒
456.21 Esophageal varices without mention of bleeding in diseases classified elsewhere — (Code first underlying disease: 571.0-571.9, 572.3) ☒
530.82 Esophageal hemorrhage
530.89 Other specified disorder of the esophagus
571.0 Alcoholic fatty liver
571.1 Acute alcoholic hepatitis
571.2 Alcoholic cirrhosis of liver

▽ Unspecified code ♀ Female diagnosis ☒ Manifestation code ♂ Male diagnosis

571.3 Unspecified alcoholic liver damage ▽
571.40 Unspecified chronic hepatitis ▽
571.41 Chronic persistent hepatitis
571.49 Other chronic hepatitis
571.5 Cirrhosis of liver without mention of alcohol
571.6 Biliary cirrhosis
571.8 Other chronic nonalcoholic liver disease
571.9 Unspecified chronic liver disease without mention of alcohol ▽
572.3 Portal hypertension

ICD-9-CM Procedural

42.91 Ligation of esophageal varices

43401

43401 Transection of esophagus with repair, for esophageal varices

ICD-9-CM Diagnostic

456.0 Esophageal varices with bleeding
456.1 Esophageal varices without mention of bleeding
456.20 Esophageal varices with bleeding in diseases classified elsewhere — (Code first underlying disease: 571.0-571.9, 572.3) ☒
456.21 Esophageal varices without mention of bleeding in diseases classified elsewhere — (Code first underlying disease: 571.0-571.9, 572.3) ☒
530.82 Esophageal hemorrhage
530.89 Other specified disorder of the esophagus
571.0 Alcoholic fatty liver
571.1 Acute alcoholic hepatitis
571.2 Alcoholic cirrhosis of liver
571.3 Unspecified alcoholic liver damage ▽
571.40 Unspecified chronic hepatitis ▽
571.41 Chronic persistent hepatitis
571.49 Other chronic hepatitis
571.5 Cirrhosis of liver without mention of alcohol
571.6 Biliary cirrhosis
571.8 Other chronic nonalcoholic liver disease
571.9 Unspecified chronic liver disease without mention of alcohol ▽
572.3 Portal hypertension

ICD-9-CM Procedural

42.99 Other operations on esophagus

43405

43405 Ligation or stapling at gastroesophageal junction for pre-existing esophageal perforation

ICD-9-CM Diagnostic

530.4 Perforation of esophagus
530.7 Gastroesophageal laceration-hemorrhage syndrome
862.22 Esophagus injury without mention of open wound into cavity
862.32 Esophagus injury with open wound into cavity
863.0 Stomach injury without mention of open wound into cavity
863.1 Stomach injury with open wound into cavity

ICD-9-CM Procedural

42.82 Suture of laceration of esophagus
42.89 Other repair of esophagus

43410

43410 Suture of esophageal wound or injury; cervical approach

ICD-9-CM Diagnostic

530.7 Gastroesophageal laceration-hemorrhage syndrome
862.22 Esophagus injury without mention of open wound into cavity
862.32 Esophagus injury with open wound into cavity
959.9 Injury, other and unspecified, unspecified site ▽
998.2 Accidental puncture or laceration during procedure

ICD-9-CM Procedural

42.82 Suture of laceration of esophagus

43415

43415 Suture of esophageal wound or injury; transthoracic or transabdominal approach

ICD-9-CM Diagnostic

530.7 Gastroesophageal laceration-hemorrhage syndrome
862.22 Esophagus injury without mention of open wound into cavity
862.32 Esophagus injury with open wound into cavity
959.9 Injury, other and unspecified, unspecified site ▽
998.2 Accidental puncture or laceration during procedure

ICD-9-CM Procedural

42.82 Suture of laceration of esophagus

43420

43420 Closure of esophagostomy or fistula; cervical approach

ICD-9-CM Diagnostic

530.0 Achalasia and cardiospasm
530.11 Reflux esophagitis — (Use additional E code to identify cause, if induced by chemical or drug)
530.20 Ulcer of esophagus without bleeding — (Use additional E code to identify cause, if induced by chemical or drug)
530.21 Ulcer of esophagus with bleeding — (Use additional E code to identify cause, if induced by chemical or drug)
530.4 Perforation of esophagus
530.5 Dyskinesia of esophagus
530.6 Diverticulum of esophagus, acquired
530.84 Tracheoesophageal fistula
530.85 Barrett's esophagus
530.89 Other specified disorder of the esophagus
750.3 Congenital tracheoesophageal fistula, esophageal atresia and stenosis
750.4 Other specified congenital anomaly of esophagus
862.32 Esophagus injury with open wound into cavity
959.9 Injury, other and unspecified, unspecified site ▽
V10.03 Personal history of malignant neoplasm of esophagus
V55.9 Attention to unspecified artificial opening ▽

ICD-9-CM Procedural

42.83 Closure of esophagostomy
42.84 Repair of esophageal fistula, not elsewhere classified

43425

43425 Closure of esophagostomy or fistula; transthoracic or transabdominal approach

ICD-9-CM Diagnostic

530.0 Achalasia and cardiospasm
530.11 Reflux esophagitis — (Use additional E code to identify cause, if induced by chemical or drug)
530.20 Ulcer of esophagus without bleeding — (Use additional E code to identify cause, if induced by chemical or drug)
530.21 Ulcer of esophagus with bleeding — (Use additional E code to identify cause, if induced by chemical or drug)
530.4 Perforation of esophagus
530.5 Dyskinesia of esophagus
530.6 Diverticulum of esophagus, acquired
530.84 Tracheoesophageal fistula
530.85 Barrett's esophagus
530.89 Other specified disorder of the esophagus
750.3 Congenital tracheoesophageal fistula, esophageal atresia and stenosis
750.4 Other specified congenital anomaly of esophagus
862.32 Esophagus injury with open wound into cavity
959.9 Injury, other and unspecified, unspecified site ▽
V10.03 Personal history of malignant neoplasm of esophagus
V55.9 Attention to unspecified artificial opening ▽

ICD-9-CM Procedural

42.83 Closure of esophagostomy
42.84 Repair of esophageal fistula, not elsewhere classified

43450–43453

43450 Dilation of esophagus, by unguided sound or bougie, single or multiple passes
43453 Dilation of esophagus, over guide wire

ICD-9-CM Diagnostic

150.0 Malignant neoplasm of cervical esophagus
150.1 Malignant neoplasm of thoracic esophagus
150.2 Malignant neoplasm of abdominal esophagus
150.3 Malignant neoplasm of upper third of esophagus
150.4 Malignant neoplasm of middle third of esophagus
150.5 Malignant neoplasm of lower third of esophagus
150.8 Malignant neoplasm of other specified part of esophagus
150.9 Malignant neoplasm of esophagus, unspecified site
211.0 Benign neoplasm of esophagus
235.5 Neoplasm of uncertain behavior of other and unspecified digestive organs
239.0 Neoplasm of unspecified nature of digestive system
530.0 Achalasia and cardiospasm
530.11 Reflux esophagitis — (Use additional E code to identify cause, if induced by chemical or drug)
530.12 Acute esophagitis — (Use additional E code to identify cause, if induced by chemical or drug)
530.19 Other esophagitis — (Use additional E code to identify cause, if induced by chemical or drug)
530.20 Ulcer of esophagus without bleeding — (Use additional E code to identify cause, if induced by chemical or drug)
530.21 Ulcer of esophagus with bleeding — (Use additional E code to identify cause, if induced by chemical or drug)
530.3 Stricture and stenosis of esophagus
530.4 Perforation of esophagus
530.5 Dyskinesia of esophagus
530.6 Diverticulum of esophagus, acquired
530.81 Esophageal reflux
530.82 Esophageal hemorrhage
530.83 Esophageal leukoplakia
530.84 Tracheoesophageal fistula
530.85 Barrett's esophagus
530.89 Other specified disorder of the esophagus
750.3 Congenital tracheoesophageal fistula, esophageal atresia and stenosis
750.4 Other specified congenital anomaly of esophagus
751.9 Unspecified congenital anomaly of digestive system
784.9 Other symptoms involving head and neck
787.2 Dysphagia
793.4 Nonspecific abnormal findings on radiological and other examination of gastrointestinal tract
935.1 Foreign body in esophagus
V10.03 Personal history of malignant neoplasm of esophagus

ICD-9-CM Procedural

42.92 Dilation of esophagus

HCPCS Level II Supplies & Services

A4270 Disposable endoscope sheath, each
A4305 Disposable drug delivery system, flow rate of 50 ml or greater per hour
A4306 Disposable drug delivery system, flow rate of 5 ml or less per hour
A4550 Surgical trays

43456

43456 Dilation of esophagus, by balloon or dilator, retrograde

ICD-9-CM Diagnostic

150.0 Malignant neoplasm of cervical esophagus
150.1 Malignant neoplasm of thoracic esophagus
150.2 Malignant neoplasm of abdominal esophagus
150.3 Malignant neoplasm of upper third of esophagus
150.4 Malignant neoplasm of middle third of esophagus
150.5 Malignant neoplasm of lower third of esophagus
150.8 Malignant neoplasm of other specified part of esophagus
150.9 Malignant neoplasm of esophagus, unspecified site
211.0 Benign neoplasm of esophagus
235.5 Neoplasm of uncertain behavior of other and unspecified digestive organs
239.0 Neoplasm of unspecified nature of digestive system
530.0 Achalasia and cardiospasm
530.11 Reflux esophagitis — (Use additional E code to identify cause, if induced by chemical or drug)
530.12 Acute esophagitis — (Use additional E code to identify cause, if induced by chemical or drug)
530.19 Other esophagitis — (Use additional E code to identify cause, if induced by chemical or drug)
530.20 Ulcer of esophagus without bleeding — (Use additional E code to identify cause, if induced by chemical or drug)
530.21 Ulcer of esophagus with bleeding — (Use additional E code to identify cause, if induced by chemical or drug)
530.3 Stricture and stenosis of esophagus
530.4 Perforation of esophagus
530.5 Dyskinesia of esophagus
530.6 Diverticulum of esophagus, acquired
530.81 Esophageal reflux
530.82 Esophageal hemorrhage
530.83 Esophageal leukoplakia
530.84 Tracheoesophageal fistula
530.85 Barrett's esophagus
530.89 Other specified disorder of the esophagus
750.3 Congenital tracheoesophageal fistula, esophageal atresia and stenosis
750.4 Other specified congenital anomaly of esophagus
751.9 Unspecified congenital anomaly of digestive system
784.9 Other symptoms involving head and neck
787.2 Dysphagia
793.4 Nonspecific abnormal findings on radiological and other examination of gastrointestinal tract
935.1 Foreign body in esophagus
V10.03 Personal history of malignant neoplasm of esophagus

ICD-9-CM Procedural

42.92 Dilation of esophagus

HCPCS Level II Supplies & Services

A4270 Disposable endoscope sheath, each
A4305 Disposable drug delivery system, flow rate of 50 ml or greater per hour
A4306 Disposable drug delivery system, flow rate of 5 ml or less per hour
A4550 Surgical trays

43458

43458 Dilation of esophagus with balloon (30 mm diameter or larger) for achalasia

ICD-9-CM Diagnostic

150.0 Malignant neoplasm of cervical esophagus
150.1 Malignant neoplasm of thoracic esophagus
150.2 Malignant neoplasm of abdominal esophagus
150.3 Malignant neoplasm of upper third of esophagus
150.4 Malignant neoplasm of middle third of esophagus
150.5 Malignant neoplasm of lower third of esophagus
150.8 Malignant neoplasm of other specified part of esophagus
150.9 Malignant neoplasm of esophagus, unspecified site
211.0 Benign neoplasm of esophagus
235.5 Neoplasm of uncertain behavior of other and unspecified digestive organs
239.0 Neoplasm of unspecified nature of digestive system
530.0 Achalasia and cardiospasm
530.11 Reflux esophagitis — (Use additional E code to identify cause, if induced by chemical or drug)
530.12 Acute esophagitis — (Use additional E code to identify cause, if induced by chemical or drug)
530.19 Other esophagitis — (Use additional E code to identify cause, if induced by chemical or drug)
530.20 Ulcer of esophagus without bleeding — (Use additional E code to identify cause, if induced by chemical or drug)
530.21 Ulcer of esophagus with bleeding — (Use additional E code to identify cause, if induced by chemical or drug)
530.3 Stricture and stenosis of esophagus
530.4 Perforation of esophagus
530.5 Dyskinesia of esophagus
530.6 Diverticulum of esophagus, acquired
530.81 Esophageal reflux
530.82 Esophageal hemorrhage
530.83 Esophageal leukoplakia
530.84 Tracheoesophageal fistula
530.85 Barrett's esophagus
530.89 Other specified disorder of the esophagus
750.3 Congenital tracheoesophageal fistula, esophageal atresia and stenosis
750.4 Other specified congenital anomaly of esophagus
751.9 Unspecified congenital anomaly of digestive system
784.9 Other symptoms involving head and neck
787.2 Dysphagia

Unspecified code
Female diagnosis
Manifestation code
Male diagnosis

793.4 Nonspecific abnormal findings on radiological and other examination of gastrointestinal tract
935.1 Foreign body in esophagus
V10.03 Personal history of malignant neoplasm of esophagus

ICD-9-CM Procedural

42.92 Dilation of esophagus

HCPCS Level II Supplies & Services

A4270 Disposable endoscope sheath, each
A4305 Disposable drug delivery system, flow rate of 50 ml or greater per hour
A4306 Disposable drug delivery system, flow rate of 5 ml or less per hour
A4550 Surgical trays

43460

43460 Esophagogastric tamponade, with balloon (Sengstaaken type)

ICD-9-CM Diagnostic

456.0 Esophageal varices with bleeding
456.1 Esophageal varices without mention of bleeding
456.20 Esophageal varices with bleeding in diseases classified elsewhere — (Code first underlying disease: 571.0-571.9, 572.3) ☒
456.21 Esophageal varices without mention of bleeding in diseases classified elsewhere — (Code first underlying disease: 571.0-571.9, 572.3) ☒
530.20 Ulcer of esophagus without bleeding — (Use additional E code to identify cause, if induced by chemical or drug)
530.21 Ulcer of esophagus with bleeding — (Use additional E code to identify cause, if induced by chemical or drug)
530.4 Perforation of esophagus
530.7 Gastroesophageal laceration-hemorrhage syndrome
530.82 Esophageal hemorrhage
530.85 Barrett's esophagus
571.0 Alcoholic fatty liver
571.1 Acute alcoholic hepatitis
571.2 Alcoholic cirrhosis of liver
571.3 Unspecified alcoholic liver damage ▽
571.40 Unspecified chronic hepatitis ▽
571.41 Chronic persistent hepatitis
571.5 Cirrhosis of liver without mention of alcohol
571.8 Other chronic nonalcoholic liver disease
572.3 Portal hypertension

ICD-9-CM Procedural

96.06 Insertion of Sengstaaken tube

HCPCS Level II Supplies & Services

A4305 Disposable drug delivery system, flow rate of 50 ml or greater per hour
A4306 Disposable drug delivery system, flow rate of 5 ml or less per hour
A4550 Surgical trays

43496

43496 Free jejunum transfer with microvascular anastomosis

ICD-9-CM Diagnostic

150.0 Malignant neoplasm of cervical esophagus
150.1 Malignant neoplasm of thoracic esophagus
150.2 Malignant neoplasm of abdominal esophagus
150.8 Malignant neoplasm of other specified part of esophagus
150.9 Malignant neoplasm of esophagus, unspecified site ▽
197.8 Secondary malignant neoplasm of other digestive organs and spleen
230.1 Carcinoma in situ of esophagus
235.5 Neoplasm of uncertain behavior of other and unspecified digestive organs ▽
239.0 Neoplasm of unspecified nature of digestive system

ICD-9-CM Procedural

45.62 Other partial resection of small intestine

Stomach

43500–43502

43500 Gastrotomy; with exploration or foreign body removal
43501 with suture repair of bleeding ulcer
43502 with suture repair of pre-existing esophagogastric laceration (eg, Mallory-Weiss)

ICD-9-CM Diagnostic

530.4 Perforation of esophagus
530.7 Gastroesophageal laceration-hemorrhage syndrome
530.89 Other specified disorder of the esophagus
531.00 Acute gastric ulcer with hemorrhage, without mention of obstruction — (Use additional E code to identify drug, if drug induced)
531.01 Acute gastric ulcer with hemorrhage and obstruction — (Use additional E code to identify drug, if drug induced)
531.20 Acute gastric ulcer with hemorrhage and perforation, without mention of obstruction — (Use additional E code to identify drug, if drug induced)
531.21 Acute gastric ulcer with hemorrhage, perforation, and obstruction — (Use additional E code to identify drug, if drug induced)
531.30 Acute gastric ulcer without mention of hemorrhage, perforation, or obstruction — (Use additional E code to identify drug, if drug induced)
531.31 Acute gastric ulcer without mention of hemorrhage or perforation, with obstruction — (Use additional E code to identify drug, if drug induced)
531.40 Chronic or unspecified gastric ulcer with hemorrhage, without mention of obstruction — (Use additional E code to identify drug, if drug induced)
531.41 Chronic or unspecified gastric ulcer with hemorrhage and obstruction — (Use additional E code to identify drug, if drug induced)
531.50 Chronic or unspecified gastric ulcer with perforation, without mention of obstruction — (Use additional E code to identify drug, if drug induced)
531.51 Chronic or unspecified gastric ulcer with perforation and obstruction — (Use additional E code to identify drug, if drug induced)
531.60 Chronic or unspecified gastric ulcer with hemorrhage and perforation, without mention of obstruction — (Use additional E code to identify drug, if drug induced)
531.61 Chronic or unspecified gastric ulcer with hemorrhage, perforation, and obstruction — (Use additional E code to identify drug, if drug induced)
531.70 Chronic gastric ulcer without mention of hemorrhage, perforation, without mention of obstruction — (Use additional E code to identify drug, if drug induced)
531.71 Chronic gastric ulcer without mention of hemorrhage or perforation, with obstruction — (Use additional E code to identify drug, if drug induced)
537.4 Fistula of stomach or duodenum
789.06 Abdominal pain, epigastric
789.07 Abdominal pain, generalized
789.36 Abdominal or pelvic swelling, mass, or lump, epigastric
793.4 Nonspecific abnormal findings on radiological and other examination of gastrointestinal tract
863.0 Stomach injury without mention of open wound into cavity
935.2 Foreign body in stomach
V12.71 Personal history of peptic ulcer disease

ICD-9-CM Procedural

42.82 Suture of laceration of esophagus
43.0 Gastrotomy
44.41 Suture of gastric ulcer site
44.49 Other control of hemorrhage of stomach or duodenum

43510

43510 Gastrotomy; with esophageal dilation and insertion of permanent intraluminal tube (eg, Celestin or Mousseaux-Barbin)

ICD-9-CM Diagnostic

150.0 Malignant neoplasm of cervical esophagus
150.1 Malignant neoplasm of thoracic esophagus
150.2 Malignant neoplasm of abdominal esophagus
150.3 Malignant neoplasm of upper third of esophagus
150.4 Malignant neoplasm of middle third of esophagus
150.5 Malignant neoplasm of lower third of esophagus
150.8 Malignant neoplasm of other specified part of esophagus
150.9 Malignant neoplasm of esophagus, unspecified site ▽
211.1 Benign neoplasm of stomach
230.1 Carcinoma in situ of esophagus
235.5 Neoplasm of uncertain behavior of other and unspecified digestive organs ▽

239.0 Neoplasm of unspecified nature of digestive system
530.0 Achalasia and cardiospasm
530.11 Reflux esophagitis — (Use additional E code to identify cause, if induced by chemical or drug)
530.12 Acute esophagitis — (Use additional E code to identify cause, if induced by chemical or drug)
530.19 Other esophagitis — (Use additional E code to identify cause, if induced by chemical or drug)
530.3 Stricture and stenosis of esophagus
530.5 Dyskinesia of esophagus
530.6 Diverticulum of esophagus, acquired
530.81 Esophageal reflux
530.89 Other specified disorder of the esophagus
750.3 Congenital tracheoesophageal fistula, esophageal atresia and stenosis
750.4 Other specified congenital anomaly of esophagus
751.9 Unspecified congenital anomaly of digestive system ▽
787.2 Dysphagia
V10.03 Personal history of malignant neoplasm of esophagus
V10.04 Personal history of malignant neoplasm of stomach

ICD-9-CM Procedural

42.81 Insertion of permanent tube into esophagus
42.92 Dilation of esophagus

43520

43520 Pyloromyotomy, cutting of pyloric muscle (Fredet-Ramstedt type operation)

ICD-9-CM Diagnostic

151.0 Malignant neoplasm of cardia
151.1 Malignant neoplasm of pylorus
151.2 Malignant neoplasm of pyloric antrum
151.3 Malignant neoplasm of fundus of stomach
537.0 Acquired hypertrophic pyloric stenosis
537.81 Pylorospasm
537.82 Angiodysplasia of stomach and duodenum (without mention of hemorrhage)
537.83 Angiodysplasia of stomach and duodenum with hemorrhage
537.89 Other specified disorder of stomach and duodenum
537.9 Unspecified disorder of stomach and duodenum ▽
750.5 Congenital hypertrophic pyloric stenosis

ICD-9-CM Procedural

43.3 Pyloromyotomy

43600–43605

43600 Biopsy of stomach; by capsule, tube, peroral (one or more specimens)
43605 by laparotomy

ICD-9-CM Diagnostic

151.0 Malignant neoplasm of cardia
151.1 Malignant neoplasm of pylorus
151.2 Malignant neoplasm of pyloric antrum
151.3 Malignant neoplasm of fundus of stomach
151.4 Malignant neoplasm of body of stomach
151.5 Malignant neoplasm of lesser curvature of stomach, unspecified ▽
151.6 Malignant neoplasm of greater curvature of stomach, unspecified ▽
151.8 Malignant neoplasm of other specified sites of stomach
211.1 Benign neoplasm of stomach
230.2 Carcinoma in situ of stomach
235.2 Neoplasm of uncertain behavior of stomach, intestines, and rectum
239.0 Neoplasm of unspecified nature of digestive system
531.70 Chronic gastric ulcer without mention of hemorrhage, perforation, without mention of obstruction — (Use additional E code to identify drug, if drug induced)
535.20 Gastric mucosal hypertrophy without mention of hemorrhage
535.50 Unspecified gastritis and gastroduodenitis without mention of hemorrhage ▽
536.1 Acute dilatation of stomach
536.2 Persistent vomiting
536.8 Dyspepsia and other specified disorders of function of stomach
537.1 Gastric diverticulum
537.81 Pylorospasm
537.82 Angiodysplasia of stomach and duodenum (without mention of hemorrhage)
537.83 Angiodysplasia of stomach and duodenum with hemorrhage
537.89 Other specified disorder of stomach and duodenum
750.5 Congenital hypertrophic pyloric stenosis
750.7 Other specified congenital anomalies of stomach
783.0 Anorexia
783.7 Adult failure to thrive
787.01 Nausea with vomiting
793.4 Nonspecific abnormal findings on radiological and other examination of gastrointestinal tract

ICD-9-CM Procedural

44.14 Closed [endoscopic] biopsy of stomach
44.15 Open biopsy of stomach

HCPCS Level II Supplies & Services

A4305 Disposable drug delivery system, flow rate of 50 ml or greater per hour
A4306 Disposable drug delivery system, flow rate of 5 ml or less per hour
A4550 Surgical trays

43610

43610 Excision, local; ulcer or benign tumor of stomach

ICD-9-CM Diagnostic

211.1 Benign neoplasm of stomach
531.00 Acute gastric ulcer with hemorrhage, without mention of obstruction — (Use additional E code to identify drug, if drug induced)
531.01 Acute gastric ulcer with hemorrhage and obstruction — (Use additional E code to identify drug, if drug induced)
531.10 Acute gastric ulcer with perforation, without mention of obstruction — (Use additional E code to identify drug, if drug induced)
531.11 Acute gastric ulcer with perforation and obstruction — (Use additional E code to identify drug, if drug induced)
531.20 Acute gastric ulcer with hemorrhage and perforation, without mention of obstruction — (Use additional E code to identify drug, if drug induced)
531.21 Acute gastric ulcer with hemorrhage, perforation, and obstruction — (Use additional E code to identify drug, if drug induced)
531.30 Acute gastric ulcer without mention of hemorrhage, perforation, or obstruction — (Use additional E code to identify drug, if drug induced)
531.31 Acute gastric ulcer without mention of hemorrhage or perforation, with obstruction — (Use additional E code to identify drug, if drug induced)
531.40 Chronic or unspecified gastric ulcer with hemorrhage, without mention of obstruction — (Use additional E code to identify drug, if drug induced)
531.41 Chronic or unspecified gastric ulcer with hemorrhage and obstruction — (Use additional E code to identify drug, if drug induced)
531.50 Chronic or unspecified gastric ulcer with perforation, without mention of obstruction — (Use additional E code to identify drug, if drug induced)
531.51 Chronic or unspecified gastric ulcer with perforation and obstruction — (Use additional E code to identify drug, if drug induced)
531.60 Chronic or unspecified gastric ulcer with hemorrhage and perforation, without mention of obstruction — (Use additional E code to identify drug, if drug induced)
531.61 Chronic or unspecified gastric ulcer with hemorrhage, perforation, and obstruction — (Use additional E code to identify drug, if drug induced)
531.70 Chronic gastric ulcer without mention of hemorrhage, perforation, without mention of obstruction — (Use additional E code to identify drug, if drug induced)
531.71 Chronic gastric ulcer without mention of hemorrhage or perforation, with obstruction — (Use additional E code to identify drug, if drug induced)
531.90 Gastric ulcer, unspecified as acute or chronic, without mention of hemorrhage, perforation, or obstruction — (Use additional E code to identify drug, if drug induced) ▽

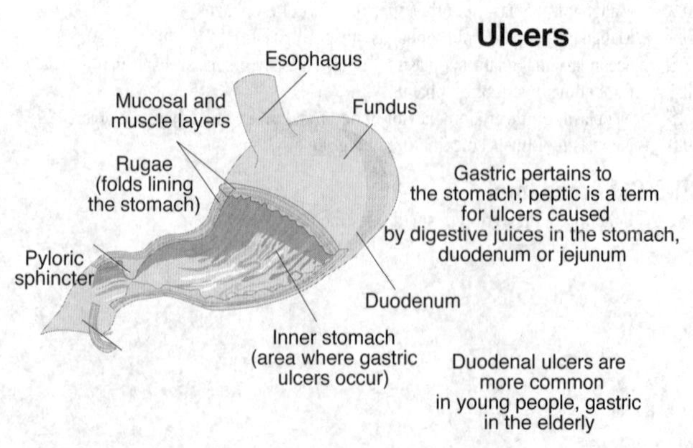
Ulcers
Esophagus
Mucosal and muscle layers
Fundus
Rugae (folds lining the stomach)
Gastric pertains to the stomach; peptic is a term for ulcers caused by digestive juices in the stomach, duodenum or jejunum
Pyloric sphincter
Duodenum
Inner stomach (area where gastric ulcers occur)
Duodenal ulcers are more common in young people, gastric in the elderly

▽ Unspecified code ♀ Female diagnosis ☒ Manifestation code ♂ Male diagnosis

531.91 Gastric ulcer, unspecified as acute or chronic, without mention of hemorrhage or perforation, with obstruction — (Use additional E code to identify drug, if drug induced)
533.00 Acute peptic ulcer, unspecified site, with hemorrhage, without mention of obstruction — (Use additional E code to identify drug, if drug induced)
533.01 Acute peptic ulcer, unspecified site, with hemorrhage and obstruction — (Use additional E code to identify drug, if drug induced)
533.10 Acute peptic ulcer, unspecified site, with perforation, without mention of obstruction — (Use additional E code to identify drug, if drug induced)
533.11 Acute peptic ulcer, unspecified site, with perforation and obstruction — (Use additional E code to identify drug, if drug induced)
533.20 Acute peptic ulcer, unspecified site, with hemorrhage and perforation, without mention of obstruction — (Use additional E code to identify drug, if drug induced)
533.21 Acute peptic ulcer, unspecified site, with hemorrhage, perforation, and obstruction — (Use additional E code to identify drug, if drug induced)
533.30 Acute peptic ulcer, unspecified site, without mention of hemorrhage, perforation, or obstruction — (Use additional E code to identify drug, if drug induced)
533.31 Acute peptic ulcer, unspecified site, without mention of hemorrhage and perforation, with obstruction — (Use additional E code to identify drug, if drug induced)
533.40 Chronic or unspecified peptic ulcer, unspecified site, with hemorrhage, without mention of obstruction — (Use additional E code to identify drug, if drug induced)
533.41 Chronic or unspecified peptic ulcer, unspecified site, with hemorrhage and obstruction — (Use additional E code to identify drug, if drug induced)
533.50 Chronic or unspecified peptic ulcer, unspecified site, with perforation, without mention of obstruction — (Use additional E code to identify drug, if drug induced)
533.51 Chronic or unspecified peptic ulcer, unspecified site, with perforation and obstruction — (Use additional E code to identify drug, if drug induced)
533.60 Chronic or unspecified peptic ulcer, unspecified site, with hemorrhage and perforation, without mention of obstruction — (Use additional E code to identify drug, if drug induced)
533.61 Chronic or unspecified peptic ulcer, unspecified site, with hemorrhage, perforation, and obstruction — (Use additional E code to identify drug, if drug induced)
533.70 Chronic peptic ulcer, unspecified site, without mention of hemorrhage, perforation, or obstruction — (Use additional E code to identify drug, if drug induced)
533.71 Chronic peptic ulcer of unspecified site without mention of hemorrhage or perforation, with obstruction — (Use additional E code to identify drug, if drug induced)
533.90 Peptic ulcer, unspecified site, unspecified as acute or chronic, without mention of hemorrhage, perforation, or obstruction — (Use additional E code to identify drug, if drug induced)
533.91 Peptic ulcer, unspecified site, unspecified as acute or chronic, without mention of hemorrhage or perforation, with obstruction — (Use additional E code to identify drug, if drug induced)

ICD-9-CM Procedural

43.42 Local excision of other lesion or tissue of stomach

43611

43611 Excision, local; malignant tumor of stomach

ICD-9-CM Diagnostic

151.0 Malignant neoplasm of cardia
151.1 Malignant neoplasm of pylorus
151.2 Malignant neoplasm of pyloric antrum
151.3 Malignant neoplasm of fundus of stomach
151.4 Malignant neoplasm of body of stomach
151.5 Malignant neoplasm of lesser curvature of stomach, unspecified
151.6 Malignant neoplasm of greater curvature of stomach, unspecified
151.8 Malignant neoplasm of other specified sites of stomach
151.9 Malignant neoplasm of stomach, unspecified site
197.8 Secondary malignant neoplasm of other digestive organs and spleen
230.2 Carcinoma in situ of stomach
235.2 Neoplasm of uncertain behavior of stomach, intestines, and rectum
239.0 Neoplasm of unspecified nature of digestive system

ICD-9-CM Procedural

43.42 Local excision of other lesion or tissue of stomach

43620

43620 Gastrectomy, total; with esophagoenterostomy

ICD-9-CM Diagnostic

151.0 Malignant neoplasm of cardia
151.1 Malignant neoplasm of pylorus
151.2 Malignant neoplasm of pyloric antrum
151.3 Malignant neoplasm of fundus of stomach
151.4 Malignant neoplasm of body of stomach
151.5 Malignant neoplasm of lesser curvature of stomach, unspecified
151.6 Malignant neoplasm of greater curvature of stomach, unspecified
151.8 Malignant neoplasm of other specified sites of stomach
151.9 Malignant neoplasm of stomach, unspecified site
197.8 Secondary malignant neoplasm of other digestive organs and spleen
211.1 Benign neoplasm of stomach
235.2 Neoplasm of uncertain behavior of stomach, intestines, and rectum
239.0 Neoplasm of unspecified nature of digestive system
531.00 Acute gastric ulcer with hemorrhage, without mention of obstruction — (Use additional E code to identify drug, if drug induced)
531.01 Acute gastric ulcer with hemorrhage and obstruction — (Use additional E code to identify drug, if drug induced)
531.10 Acute gastric ulcer with perforation, without mention of obstruction — (Use additional E code to identify drug, if drug induced)
531.11 Acute gastric ulcer with perforation and obstruction — (Use additional E code to identify drug, if drug induced)
531.20 Acute gastric ulcer with hemorrhage and perforation, without mention of obstruction — (Use additional E code to identify drug, if drug induced)
531.21 Acute gastric ulcer with hemorrhage, perforation, and obstruction — (Use additional E code to identify drug, if drug induced)
533.00 Acute peptic ulcer, unspecified site, with hemorrhage, without mention of obstruction — (Use additional E code to identify drug, if drug induced)
533.01 Acute peptic ulcer, unspecified site, with hemorrhage and obstruction — (Use additional E code to identify drug, if drug induced)
533.10 Acute peptic ulcer, unspecified site, with perforation, without mention of obstruction — (Use additional E code to identify drug, if drug induced)
533.11 Acute peptic ulcer, unspecified site, with perforation and obstruction — (Use additional E code to identify drug, if drug induced)
533.20 Acute peptic ulcer, unspecified site, with hemorrhage and perforation, without mention of obstruction — (Use additional E code to identify drug, if drug induced)
533.21 Acute peptic ulcer, unspecified site, with hemorrhage, perforation, and obstruction — (Use additional E code to identify drug, if drug induced)
533.30 Acute peptic ulcer, unspecified site, without mention of hemorrhage, perforation, or obstruction — (Use additional E code to identify drug, if drug induced)
533.31 Acute peptic ulcer, unspecified site, without mention of hemorrhage and perforation, with obstruction — (Use additional E code to identify drug, if drug induced)
533.40 Chronic or unspecified peptic ulcer, unspecified site, with hemorrhage, without mention of obstruction — (Use additional E code to identify drug, if drug induced)
533.41 Chronic or unspecified peptic ulcer, unspecified site, with hemorrhage and obstruction — (Use additional E code to identify drug, if drug induced)
533.50 Chronic or unspecified peptic ulcer, unspecified site, with perforation, without mention of obstruction — (Use additional E code to identify drug, if drug induced)
533.51 Chronic or unspecified peptic ulcer, unspecified site, with perforation and obstruction — (Use additional E code to identify drug, if drug induced)
533.60 Chronic or unspecified peptic ulcer, unspecified site, with hemorrhage and perforation, without mention of obstruction — (Use additional E code to identify drug, if drug induced)
533.61 Chronic or unspecified peptic ulcer, unspecified site, with hemorrhage, perforation, and obstruction — (Use additional E code to identify drug, if drug induced)
533.70 Chronic peptic ulcer, unspecified site, without mention of hemorrhage, perforation, or obstruction — (Use additional E code to identify drug, if drug induced)
533.71 Chronic peptic ulcer of unspecified site without mention of hemorrhage or perforation, with obstruction — (Use additional E code to identify drug, if drug induced)
533.90 Peptic ulcer, unspecified site, unspecified as acute or chronic, without mention of hemorrhage, perforation, or obstruction — (Use additional E code to identify drug, if drug induced)
533.91 Peptic ulcer, unspecified site, unspecified as acute or chronic, without mention of hemorrhage or perforation, with obstruction — (Use additional E code to identify drug, if drug induced)

863.0 Stomach injury without mention of open wound into cavity
863.1 Stomach injury with open wound into cavity

ICD-9-CM Procedural

43.91 Total gastrectomy with intestinal interposition
43.99 Other total gastrectomy

43621

43621 Gastrectomy, total; with Roux-en-Y reconstruction

ICD-9-CM Diagnostic

151.0 Malignant neoplasm of cardia
151.1 Malignant neoplasm of pylorus
151.2 Malignant neoplasm of pyloric antrum
151.3 Malignant neoplasm of fundus of stomach
151.4 Malignant neoplasm of body of stomach
151.5 Malignant neoplasm of lesser curvature of stomach, unspecified
151.6 Malignant neoplasm of greater curvature of stomach, unspecified
151.8 Malignant neoplasm of other specified sites of stomach
151.9 Malignant neoplasm of stomach, unspecified site
197.8 Secondary malignant neoplasm of other digestive organs and spleen
211.1 Benign neoplasm of stomach
235.2 Neoplasm of uncertain behavior of stomach, intestines, and rectum
239.0 Neoplasm of unspecified nature of digestive system
531.00 Acute gastric ulcer with hemorrhage, without mention of obstruction — (Use additional E code to identify drug, if drug induced)
531.01 Acute gastric ulcer with hemorrhage and obstruction — (Use additional E code to identify drug, if drug induced)
531.10 Acute gastric ulcer with perforation, without mention of obstruction — (Use additional E code to identify drug, if drug induced)
531.11 Acute gastric ulcer with perforation and obstruction — (Use additional E code to identify drug, if drug induced)
531.20 Acute gastric ulcer with hemorrhage and perforation, without mention of obstruction — (Use additional E code to identify drug, if drug induced)
531.21 Acute gastric ulcer with hemorrhage, perforation, and obstruction — (Use additional E code to identify drug, if drug induced)
533.00 Acute peptic ulcer, unspecified site, with hemorrhage, without mention of obstruction — (Use additional E code to identify drug, if drug induced)
533.01 Acute peptic ulcer, unspecified site, with hemorrhage and obstruction — (Use additional E code to identify drug, if drug induced)
533.10 Acute peptic ulcer, unspecified site, with perforation, without mention of obstruction — (Use additional E code to identify drug, if drug induced)
533.11 Acute peptic ulcer, unspecified site, with perforation and obstruction — (Use additional E code to identify drug, if drug induced)
533.20 Acute peptic ulcer, unspecified site, with hemorrhage and perforation, without mention of obstruction — (Use additional E code to identify drug, if drug induced)
533.21 Acute peptic ulcer, unspecified site, with hemorrhage, perforation, and obstruction — (Use additional E code to identify drug, if drug induced)
533.30 Acute peptic ulcer, unspecified site, without mention of hemorrhage, perforation, or obstruction — (Use additional E code to identify drug, if drug induced)
533.31 Acute peptic ulcer, unspecified site, without mention of hemorrhage and perforation, with obstruction — (Use additional E code to identify drug, if drug induced)
533.40 Chronic or unspecified peptic ulcer, unspecified site, with hemorrhage, without mention of obstruction — (Use additional E code to identify drug, if drug induced)
533.41 Chronic or unspecified peptic ulcer, unspecified site, with hemorrhage and obstruction — (Use additional E code to identify drug, if drug induced)
533.50 Chronic or unspecified peptic ulcer, unspecified site, with perforation, without mention of obstruction — (Use additional E code to identify drug, if drug induced)
533.51 Chronic or unspecified peptic ulcer, unspecified site, with perforation and obstruction — (Use additional E code to identify drug, if drug induced)
533.60 Chronic or unspecified peptic ulcer, unspecified site, with hemorrhage and perforation, without mention of obstruction — (Use additional E code to identify drug, if drug induced)
533.61 Chronic or unspecified peptic ulcer, unspecified site, with hemorrhage, perforation, and obstruction — (Use additional E code to identify drug, if drug induced)
533.70 Chronic peptic ulcer, unspecified site, without mention of hemorrhage, perforation, or obstruction — (Use additional E code to identify drug, if drug induced)
533.71 Chronic peptic ulcer of unspecified site without mention of hemorrhage or perforation, with obstruction — (Use additional E code to identify drug, if drug induced)
533.90 Peptic ulcer, unspecified site, unspecified as acute or chronic, without mention of hemorrhage, perforation, or obstruction — (Use additional E code to identify drug, if drug induced)
533.91 Peptic ulcer, unspecified site, unspecified as acute or chronic, without mention of hemorrhage or perforation, with obstruction — (Use additional E code to identify drug, if drug induced)
863.0 Stomach injury without mention of open wound into cavity
863.1 Stomach injury with open wound into cavity

ICD-9-CM Procedural

43.91 Total gastrectomy with intestinal interposition
43.99 Other total gastrectomy

43622

43622 Gastrectomy, total; with formation of intestinal pouch, any type

ICD-9-CM Diagnostic

151.0 Malignant neoplasm of cardia
151.1 Malignant neoplasm of pylorus
151.2 Malignant neoplasm of pyloric antrum
151.3 Malignant neoplasm of fundus of stomach
151.4 Malignant neoplasm of body of stomach
151.5 Malignant neoplasm of lesser curvature of stomach, unspecified
151.6 Malignant neoplasm of greater curvature of stomach, unspecified
151.8 Malignant neoplasm of other specified sites of stomach
151.9 Malignant neoplasm of stomach, unspecified site
197.8 Secondary malignant neoplasm of other digestive organs and spleen
211.1 Benign neoplasm of stomach
235.2 Neoplasm of uncertain behavior of stomach, intestines, and rectum
239.0 Neoplasm of unspecified nature of digestive system
531.00 Acute gastric ulcer with hemorrhage, without mention of obstruction — (Use additional E code to identify drug, if drug induced)
531.01 Acute gastric ulcer with hemorrhage and obstruction — (Use additional E code to identify drug, if drug induced)
531.10 Acute gastric ulcer with perforation, without mention of obstruction — (Use additional E code to identify drug, if drug induced)
531.11 Acute gastric ulcer with perforation and obstruction — (Use additional E code to identify drug, if drug induced)
531.20 Acute gastric ulcer with hemorrhage and perforation, without mention of obstruction — (Use additional E code to identify drug, if drug induced)
531.21 Acute gastric ulcer with hemorrhage, perforation, and obstruction — (Use additional E code to identify drug, if drug induced)
533.00 Acute peptic ulcer, unspecified site, with hemorrhage, without mention of obstruction — (Use additional E code to identify drug, if drug induced)
533.01 Acute peptic ulcer, unspecified site, with hemorrhage and obstruction — (Use additional E code to identify drug, if drug induced)
533.10 Acute peptic ulcer, unspecified site, with perforation, without mention of obstruction — (Use additional E code to identify drug, if drug induced)
533.11 Acute peptic ulcer, unspecified site, with perforation and obstruction — (Use additional E code to identify drug, if drug induced)
533.20 Acute peptic ulcer, unspecified site, with hemorrhage and perforation, without mention of obstruction — (Use additional E code to identify drug, if drug induced)
533.21 Acute peptic ulcer, unspecified site, with hemorrhage, perforation, and obstruction — (Use additional E code to identify drug, if drug induced)
533.30 Acute peptic ulcer, unspecified site, without mention of hemorrhage, perforation, or obstruction — (Use additional E code to identify drug, if drug induced)
533.31 Acute peptic ulcer, unspecified site, without mention of hemorrhage and perforation, with obstruction — (Use additional E code to identify drug, if drug induced)
533.40 Chronic or unspecified peptic ulcer, unspecified site, with hemorrhage, without mention of obstruction — (Use additional E code to identify drug, if drug induced)
533.41 Chronic or unspecified peptic ulcer, unspecified site, with hemorrhage and obstruction — (Use additional E code to identify drug, if drug induced)
533.50 Chronic or unspecified peptic ulcer, unspecified site, with perforation, without mention of obstruction — (Use additional E code to identify drug, if drug induced)
533.51 Chronic or unspecified peptic ulcer, unspecified site, with perforation and obstruction — (Use additional E code to identify drug, if drug induced)

533.60 Chronic or unspecified peptic ulcer, unspecified site, with hemorrhage and perforation, without mention of obstruction — (Use additional E code to identify drug, if drug induced)
533.61 Chronic or unspecified peptic ulcer, unspecified site, with hemorrhage, perforation, and obstruction — (Use additional E code to identify drug, if drug induced)
533.70 Chronic peptic ulcer, unspecified site, without mention of hemorrhage, perforation, or obstruction — (Use additional E code to identify drug, if drug induced)
533.71 Chronic peptic ulcer of unspecified site without mention of hemorrhage or perforation, with obstruction — (Use additional E code to identify drug, if drug induced)
533.90 Peptic ulcer, unspecified site, unspecified as acute or chronic, without mention of hemorrhage, perforation, or obstruction — (Use additional E code to identify drug, if drug induced) ▽
533.91 Peptic ulcer, unspecified site, unspecified as acute or chronic, without mention of hemorrhage or perforation, with obstruction — (Use additional E code to identify drug, if drug induced) ▽
863.0 Stomach injury without mention of open wound into cavity
863.1 Stomach injury with open wound into cavity

ICD-9-CM Procedural

43.91 Total gastrectomy with intestinal interposition
43.99 Other total gastrectomy

43631

43631 Gastrectomy, partial, distal; with gastroduodenostomy

ICD-9-CM Diagnostic

151.1 Malignant neoplasm of pylorus
151.2 Malignant neoplasm of pyloric antrum
151.4 Malignant neoplasm of body of stomach
151.8 Malignant neoplasm of other specified sites of stomach
151.9 Malignant neoplasm of stomach, unspecified site ▽
197.8 Secondary malignant neoplasm of other digestive organs and spleen
211.1 Benign neoplasm of stomach
235.2 Neoplasm of uncertain behavior of stomach, intestines, and rectum
239.0 Neoplasm of unspecified nature of digestive system
531.00 Acute gastric ulcer with hemorrhage, without mention of obstruction — (Use additional E code to identify drug, if drug induced)
531.01 Acute gastric ulcer with hemorrhage and obstruction — (Use additional E code to identify drug, if drug induced)
531.10 Acute gastric ulcer with perforation, without mention of obstruction — (Use additional E code to identify drug, if drug induced)
531.11 Acute gastric ulcer with perforation and obstruction — (Use additional E code to identify drug, if drug induced)
531.20 Acute gastric ulcer with hemorrhage and perforation, without mention of obstruction — (Use additional E code to identify drug, if drug induced)
531.21 Acute gastric ulcer with hemorrhage, perforation, and obstruction — (Use additional E code to identify drug, if drug induced)
531.40 Chronic or unspecified gastric ulcer with hemorrhage, without mention of obstruction — (Use additional E code to identify drug, if drug induced)
531.41 Chronic or unspecified gastric ulcer with hemorrhage and obstruction — (Use additional E code to identify drug, if drug induced)
531.50 Chronic or unspecified gastric ulcer with perforation, without mention of obstruction — (Use additional E code to identify drug, if drug induced)
531.51 Chronic or unspecified gastric ulcer with perforation and obstruction — (Use additional E code to identify drug, if drug induced)
531.60 Chronic or unspecified gastric ulcer with hemorrhage and perforation, without mention of obstruction — (Use additional E code to identify drug, if drug induced)
531.61 Chronic or unspecified gastric ulcer with hemorrhage, perforation, and obstruction — (Use additional E code to identify drug, if drug induced)
531.70 Chronic gastric ulcer without mention of hemorrhage, perforation, without mention of obstruction — (Use additional E code to identify drug, if drug induced)
531.71 Chronic gastric ulcer without mention of hemorrhage or perforation, with obstruction — (Use additional E code to identify drug, if drug induced)
531.90 Gastric ulcer, unspecified as acute or chronic, without mention of hemorrhage, perforation, or obstruction — (Use additional E code to identify drug, if drug induced) ▽
531.91 Gastric ulcer, unspecified as acute or chronic, without mention of hemorrhage or perforation, with obstruction — (Use additional E code to identify drug, if drug induced) ▽
533.00 Acute peptic ulcer, unspecified site, with hemorrhage, without mention of obstruction — (Use additional E code to identify drug, if drug induced)
533.01 Acute peptic ulcer, unspecified site, with hemorrhage and obstruction — (Use additional E code to identify drug, if drug induced)
533.10 Acute peptic ulcer, unspecified site, with perforation, without mention of obstruction — (Use additional E code to identify drug, if drug induced)
533.11 Acute peptic ulcer, unspecified site, with perforation and obstruction — (Use additional E code to identify drug, if drug induced)
533.20 Acute peptic ulcer, unspecified site, with hemorrhage and perforation, without mention of obstruction — (Use additional E code to identify drug, if drug induced)
533.21 Acute peptic ulcer, unspecified site, with hemorrhage, perforation, and obstruction — (Use additional E code to identify drug, if drug induced)
533.30 Acute peptic ulcer, unspecified site, without mention of hemorrhage, perforation, or obstruction — (Use additional E code to identify drug, if drug induced)
533.31 Acute peptic ulcer, unspecified site, without mention of hemorrhage and perforation, with obstruction — (Use additional E code to identify drug, if drug induced)
533.40 Chronic or unspecified peptic ulcer, unspecified site, with hemorrhage, without mention of obstruction — (Use additional E code to identify drug, if drug induced)
533.41 Chronic or unspecified peptic ulcer, unspecified site, with hemorrhage and obstruction — (Use additional E code to identify drug, if drug induced)
533.50 Chronic or unspecified peptic ulcer, unspecified site, with perforation, without mention of obstruction — (Use additional E code to identify drug, if drug induced)
533.51 Chronic or unspecified peptic ulcer, unspecified site, with perforation and obstruction — (Use additional E code to identify drug, if drug induced)
533.60 Chronic or unspecified peptic ulcer, unspecified site, with hemorrhage and perforation, without mention of obstruction — (Use additional E code to identify drug, if drug induced)
533.61 Chronic or unspecified peptic ulcer, unspecified site, with hemorrhage, perforation, and obstruction — (Use additional E code to identify drug, if drug induced)
533.70 Chronic peptic ulcer, unspecified site, without mention of hemorrhage, perforation, or obstruction — (Use additional E code to identify drug, if drug induced)
533.71 Chronic peptic ulcer of unspecified site without mention of hemorrhage or perforation, with obstruction — (Use additional E code to identify drug, if drug induced)
533.90 Peptic ulcer, unspecified site, unspecified as acute or chronic, without mention of hemorrhage, perforation, or obstruction — (Use additional E code to identify drug, if drug induced) ▽
533.91 Peptic ulcer, unspecified site, unspecified as acute or chronic, without mention of hemorrhage or perforation, with obstruction — (Use additional E code to identify drug, if drug induced) ▽
863.0 Stomach injury without mention of open wound into cavity
863.1 Stomach injury with open wound into cavity
997.4 Digestive system complication — (Use additional code to identify complications)

ICD-9-CM Procedural

43.6 Partial gastrectomy with anastomosis to duodenum

43632

43632 Gastrectomy, partial, distal; with gastrojejunostomy

ICD-9-CM Diagnostic

151.1 Malignant neoplasm of pylorus
151.2 Malignant neoplasm of pyloric antrum
151.4 Malignant neoplasm of body of stomach
151.8 Malignant neoplasm of other specified sites of stomach
151.9 Malignant neoplasm of stomach, unspecified site ▽
197.8 Secondary malignant neoplasm of other digestive organs and spleen
211.1 Benign neoplasm of stomach
235.2 Neoplasm of uncertain behavior of stomach, intestines, and rectum
239.0 Neoplasm of unspecified nature of digestive system
531.00 Acute gastric ulcer with hemorrhage, without mention of obstruction — (Use additional E code to identify drug, if drug induced)
531.01 Acute gastric ulcer with hemorrhage and obstruction — (Use additional E code to identify drug, if drug induced)
531.10 Acute gastric ulcer with perforation, without mention of obstruction — (Use additional E code to identify drug, if drug induced)
531.11 Acute gastric ulcer with perforation and obstruction — (Use additional E code to identify drug, if drug induced)
531.20 Acute gastric ulcer with hemorrhage and perforation, without mention of obstruction — (Use additional E code to identify drug, if drug induced)

531.21 Acute gastric ulcer with hemorrhage, perforation, and obstruction — (Use additional E code to identify drug, if drug induced)
531.40 Chronic or unspecified gastric ulcer with hemorrhage, without mention of obstruction — (Use additional E code to identify drug, if drug induced)
531.41 Chronic or unspecified gastric ulcer with hemorrhage and obstruction — (Use additional E code to identify drug, if drug induced)
531.50 Chronic or unspecified gastric ulcer with perforation, without mention of obstruction — (Use additional E code to identify drug, if drug induced)
531.51 Chronic or unspecified gastric ulcer with perforation and obstruction — (Use additional E code to identify drug, if drug induced)
531.60 Chronic or unspecified gastric ulcer with hemorrhage and perforation, without mention of obstruction — (Use additional E code to identify drug, if drug induced)
531.61 Chronic or unspecified gastric ulcer with hemorrhage, perforation, and obstruction — (Use additional E code to identify drug, if drug induced)
531.70 Chronic gastric ulcer without mention of hemorrhage, perforation, without mention of obstruction — (Use additional E code to identify drug, if drug induced)
531.71 Chronic gastric ulcer without mention of hemorrhage or perforation, with obstruction — (Use additional E code to identify drug, if drug induced)
531.90 Gastric ulcer, unspecified as acute or chronic, without mention of hemorrhage, perforation, or obstruction — (Use additional E code to identify drug, if drug induced) ▽
531.91 Gastric ulcer, unspecified as acute or chronic, without mention of hemorrhage or perforation, with obstruction — (Use additional E code to identify drug, if drug induced) ▽
533.00 Acute peptic ulcer, unspecified site, with hemorrhage, without mention of obstruction — (Use additional E code to identify drug, if drug induced)
533.01 Acute peptic ulcer, unspecified site, with hemorrhage and obstruction — (Use additional E code to identify drug, if drug induced)
533.10 Acute peptic ulcer, unspecified site, with perforation, without mention of obstruction — (Use additional E code to identify drug, if drug induced)
533.11 Acute peptic ulcer, unspecified site, with perforation and obstruction — (Use additional E code to identify drug, if drug induced)
533.20 Acute peptic ulcer, unspecified site, with hemorrhage and perforation, without mention of obstruction — (Use additional E code to identify drug, if drug induced)
533.21 Acute peptic ulcer, unspecified site, with hemorrhage, perforation, and obstruction — (Use additional E code to identify drug, if drug induced)
533.30 Acute peptic ulcer, unspecified site, without mention of hemorrhage, perforation, or obstruction — (Use additional E code to identify drug, if drug induced)
533.31 Acute peptic ulcer, unspecified site, without mention of hemorrhage and perforation, with obstruction — (Use additional E code to identify drug, if drug induced)
533.40 Chronic or unspecified peptic ulcer, unspecified site, with hemorrhage, without mention of obstruction — (Use additional E code to identify drug, if drug induced)
533.41 Chronic or unspecified peptic ulcer, unspecified site, with hemorrhage and obstruction — (Use additional E code to identify drug, if drug induced)
533.50 Chronic or unspecified peptic ulcer, unspecified site, with perforation, without mention of obstruction — (Use additional E code to identify drug, if drug induced)
533.51 Chronic or unspecified peptic ulcer, unspecified site, with perforation and obstruction — (Use additional E code to identify drug, if drug induced)
533.60 Chronic or unspecified peptic ulcer, unspecified site, with hemorrhage and perforation, without mention of obstruction — (Use additional E code to identify drug, if drug induced)
533.61 Chronic or unspecified peptic ulcer, unspecified site, with hemorrhage, perforation, and obstruction — (Use additional E code to identify drug, if drug induced)
533.70 Chronic peptic ulcer, unspecified site, without mention of hemorrhage, perforation, or obstruction — (Use additional E code to identify drug, if drug induced)
533.71 Chronic peptic ulcer of unspecified site without mention of hemorrhage or perforation, with obstruction — (Use additional E code to identify drug, if drug induced)
533.90 Peptic ulcer, unspecified site, unspecified as acute or chronic, without mention of hemorrhage, perforation, or obstruction — (Use additional E code to identify drug, if drug induced) ▽
533.91 Peptic ulcer, unspecified site, unspecified as acute or chronic, without mention of hemorrhage or perforation, with obstruction — (Use additional E code to identify drug, if drug induced) ▽
863.0 Stomach injury without mention of open wound into cavity
863.1 Stomach injury with open wound into cavity
997.4 Digestive system complication — (Use additional code to identify complications)

ICD-9-CM Procedural

43.7 Partial gastrectomy with anastomosis to jejunum

43633–43634

43633 Gastrectomy, partial, distal; with Roux-en-Y reconstruction
43634 with formation of intestinal pouch

ICD-9-CM Diagnostic

151.1 Malignant neoplasm of pylorus
151.2 Malignant neoplasm of pyloric antrum
151.4 Malignant neoplasm of body of stomach
151.8 Malignant neoplasm of other specified sites of stomach
151.9 Malignant neoplasm of stomach, unspecified site ▽
197.8 Secondary malignant neoplasm of other digestive organs and spleen
211.1 Benign neoplasm of stomach
235.2 Neoplasm of uncertain behavior of stomach, intestines, and rectum
239.0 Neoplasm of unspecified nature of digestive system
531.00 Acute gastric ulcer with hemorrhage, without mention of obstruction — (Use additional E code to identify drug, if drug induced)
531.01 Acute gastric ulcer with hemorrhage and obstruction — (Use additional E code to identify drug, if drug induced)
531.10 Acute gastric ulcer with perforation, without mention of obstruction — (Use additional E code to identify drug, if drug induced)
531.11 Acute gastric ulcer with perforation and obstruction — (Use additional E code to identify drug, if drug induced)
531.20 Acute gastric ulcer with hemorrhage and perforation, without mention of obstruction — (Use additional E code to identify drug, if drug induced)
531.21 Acute gastric ulcer with hemorrhage, perforation, and obstruction — (Use additional E code to identify drug, if drug induced)
531.40 Chronic or unspecified gastric ulcer with hemorrhage, without mention of obstruction — (Use additional E code to identify drug, if drug induced)
531.41 Chronic or unspecified gastric ulcer with hemorrhage and obstruction — (Use additional E code to identify drug, if drug induced)
531.50 Chronic or unspecified gastric ulcer with perforation, without mention of obstruction — (Use additional E code to identify drug, if drug induced)
531.51 Chronic or unspecified gastric ulcer with perforation and obstruction — (Use additional E code to identify drug, if drug induced)
531.60 Chronic or unspecified gastric ulcer with hemorrhage and perforation, without mention of obstruction — (Use additional E code to identify drug, if drug induced)
531.61 Chronic or unspecified gastric ulcer with hemorrhage, perforation, and obstruction — (Use additional E code to identify drug, if drug induced)
531.70 Chronic gastric ulcer without mention of hemorrhage, perforation, without mention of obstruction — (Use additional E code to identify drug, if drug induced)
531.71 Chronic gastric ulcer without mention of hemorrhage or perforation, with obstruction — (Use additional E code to identify drug, if drug induced)
531.90 Gastric ulcer, unspecified as acute or chronic, without mention of hemorrhage, perforation, or obstruction — (Use additional E code to identify drug, if drug induced) ▽
531.91 Gastric ulcer, unspecified as acute or chronic, without mention of hemorrhage or perforation, with obstruction — (Use additional E code to identify drug, if drug induced) ▽
533.00 Acute peptic ulcer, unspecified site, with hemorrhage, without mention of obstruction — (Use additional E code to identify drug, if drug induced)
533.01 Acute peptic ulcer, unspecified site, with hemorrhage and obstruction — (Use additional E code to identify drug, if drug induced)
533.10 Acute peptic ulcer, unspecified site, with perforation, without mention of obstruction — (Use additional E code to identify drug, if drug induced)
533.11 Acute peptic ulcer, unspecified site, with perforation and obstruction — (Use additional E code to identify drug, if drug induced)
533.20 Acute peptic ulcer, unspecified site, with hemorrhage and perforation, without mention of obstruction — (Use additional E code to identify drug, if drug induced)
533.21 Acute peptic ulcer, unspecified site, with hemorrhage, perforation, and obstruction — (Use additional E code to identify drug, if drug induced)
533.30 Acute peptic ulcer, unspecified site, without mention of hemorrhage, perforation, or obstruction — (Use additional E code to identify drug, if drug induced)
533.31 Acute peptic ulcer, unspecified site, without mention of hemorrhage and perforation, with obstruction — (Use additional E code to identify drug, if drug induced)

▽ Unspecified code ♀ Female diagnosis ☒ Manifestation code ♂ Male diagnosis

533.40 Chronic or unspecified peptic ulcer, unspecified site, with hemorrhage, without mention of obstruction — (Use additional E code to identify drug, if drug induced)
533.41 Chronic or unspecified peptic ulcer, unspecified site, with hemorrhage and obstruction — (Use additional E code to identify drug, if drug induced)
533.50 Chronic or unspecified peptic ulcer, unspecified site, with perforation, without mention of obstruction — (Use additional E code to identify drug, if drug induced)
533.51 Chronic or unspecified peptic ulcer, unspecified site, with perforation and obstruction — (Use additional E code to identify drug, if drug induced)
533.60 Chronic or unspecified peptic ulcer, unspecified site, with hemorrhage and perforation, without mention of obstruction — (Use additional E code to identify drug, if drug induced)
533.61 Chronic or unspecified peptic ulcer, unspecified site, with hemorrhage, perforation, and obstruction — (Use additional E code to identify drug, if drug induced)
533.70 Chronic peptic ulcer, unspecified site, without mention of hemorrhage, perforation, or obstruction — (Use additional E code to identify drug, if drug induced)
533.71 Chronic peptic ulcer of unspecified site without mention of hemorrhage or perforation, with obstruction — (Use additional E code to identify drug, if drug induced)
533.90 Peptic ulcer, unspecified site, unspecified as acute or chronic, without mention of hemorrhage, perforation, or obstruction — (Use additional E code to identify drug, if drug induced) ▽
533.91 Peptic ulcer, unspecified site, unspecified as acute or chronic, without mention of hemorrhage or perforation, with obstruction — (Use additional E code to identify drug, if drug induced) ▽
863.0 Stomach injury without mention of open wound into cavity
863.1 Stomach injury with open wound into cavity
997.4 Digestive system complication — (Use additional code to identify complications)

ICD-9-CM Procedural

43.7 Partial gastrectomy with anastomosis to jejunum

43635

43635 Vagotomy when performed with partial distal gastrectomy (List separately in addition to code(s) for primary procedure)

ICD-9-CM Diagnostic

This is an add-on code. Refer to the corresponding primary procedure code for ICD-9 diagnosis code links.

ICD-9-CM Procedural

44.01 Truncal vagotomy

43638–43639

43638 Gastrectomy, partial, proximal, thoracic or abdominal approach including esophagogastrostomy, with vagotomy;
43639 with pyloroplasty or pyloromyotomy

ICD-9-CM Diagnostic

151.0 Malignant neoplasm of cardia
151.2 Malignant neoplasm of pyloric antrum
151.4 Malignant neoplasm of body of stomach
151.8 Malignant neoplasm of other specified sites of stomach
151.9 Malignant neoplasm of stomach, unspecified site ▽
197.8 Secondary malignant neoplasm of other digestive organs and spleen
211.1 Benign neoplasm of stomach
230.2 Carcinoma in situ of stomach
235.2 Neoplasm of uncertain behavior of stomach, intestines, and rectum
239.0 Neoplasm of unspecified nature of digestive system
531.00 Acute gastric ulcer with hemorrhage, without mention of obstruction — (Use additional E code to identify drug, if drug induced)
531.01 Acute gastric ulcer with hemorrhage and obstruction — (Use additional E code to identify drug, if drug induced)
531.10 Acute gastric ulcer with perforation, without mention of obstruction — (Use additional E code to identify drug, if drug induced)
531.11 Acute gastric ulcer with perforation and obstruction — (Use additional E code to identify drug, if drug induced)
531.20 Acute gastric ulcer with hemorrhage and perforation, without mention of obstruction — (Use additional E code to identify drug, if drug induced)
531.21 Acute gastric ulcer with hemorrhage, perforation, and obstruction — (Use additional E code to identify drug, if drug induced)
531.30 Acute gastric ulcer without mention of hemorrhage, perforation, or obstruction — (Use additional E code to identify drug, if drug induced)
531.31 Acute gastric ulcer without mention of hemorrhage or perforation, with obstruction — (Use additional E code to identify drug, if drug induced)
531.40 Chronic or unspecified gastric ulcer with hemorrhage, without mention of obstruction — (Use additional E code to identify drug, if drug induced)
531.41 Chronic or unspecified gastric ulcer with hemorrhage and obstruction — (Use additional E code to identify drug, if drug induced)
531.50 Chronic or unspecified gastric ulcer with perforation, without mention of obstruction — (Use additional E code to identify drug, if drug induced)
531.51 Chronic or unspecified gastric ulcer with perforation and obstruction — (Use additional E code to identify drug, if drug induced)
531.60 Chronic or unspecified gastric ulcer with hemorrhage and perforation, without mention of obstruction — (Use additional E code to identify drug, if drug induced)
531.61 Chronic or unspecified gastric ulcer with hemorrhage, perforation, and obstruction — (Use additional E code to identify drug, if drug induced)
531.70 Chronic gastric ulcer without mention of hemorrhage, perforation, without mention of obstruction — (Use additional E code to identify drug, if drug induced)
531.71 Chronic gastric ulcer without mention of hemorrhage or perforation, with obstruction — (Use additional E code to identify drug, if drug induced)
531.90 Gastric ulcer, unspecified as acute or chronic, without mention of hemorrhage, perforation, or obstruction — (Use additional E code to identify drug, if drug induced) ▽
531.91 Gastric ulcer, unspecified as acute or chronic, without mention of hemorrhage or perforation, with obstruction — (Use additional E code to identify drug, if drug induced) ▽
533.00 Acute peptic ulcer, unspecified site, with hemorrhage, without mention of obstruction — (Use additional E code to identify drug, if drug induced)
533.01 Acute peptic ulcer, unspecified site, with hemorrhage and obstruction — (Use additional E code to identify drug, if drug induced)
533.10 Acute peptic ulcer, unspecified site, with perforation, without mention of obstruction — (Use additional E code to identify drug, if drug induced)
533.11 Acute peptic ulcer, unspecified site, with perforation and obstruction — (Use additional E code to identify drug, if drug induced)
533.20 Acute peptic ulcer, unspecified site, with hemorrhage and perforation, without mention of obstruction — (Use additional E code to identify drug, if drug induced)
533.21 Acute peptic ulcer, unspecified site, with hemorrhage, perforation, and obstruction — (Use additional E code to identify drug, if drug induced)
533.30 Acute peptic ulcer, unspecified site, without mention of hemorrhage, perforation, or obstruction — (Use additional E code to identify drug, if drug induced)
533.31 Acute peptic ulcer, unspecified site, without mention of hemorrhage and perforation, with obstruction — (Use additional E code to identify drug, if drug induced)
533.40 Chronic or unspecified peptic ulcer, unspecified site, with hemorrhage, without mention of obstruction — (Use additional E code to identify drug, if drug induced)
533.41 Chronic or unspecified peptic ulcer, unspecified site, with hemorrhage and obstruction — (Use additional E code to identify drug, if drug induced)
533.50 Chronic or unspecified peptic ulcer, unspecified site, with perforation, without mention of obstruction — (Use additional E code to identify drug, if drug induced)
533.51 Chronic or unspecified peptic ulcer, unspecified site, with perforation and obstruction — (Use additional E code to identify drug, if drug induced)
533.60 Chronic or unspecified peptic ulcer, unspecified site, with hemorrhage and perforation, without mention of obstruction — (Use additional E code to identify drug, if drug induced)
533.61 Chronic or unspecified peptic ulcer, unspecified site, with hemorrhage, perforation, and obstruction — (Use additional E code to identify drug, if drug induced)
533.70 Chronic peptic ulcer, unspecified site, without mention of hemorrhage, perforation, or obstruction — (Use additional E code to identify drug, if drug induced)
533.71 Chronic peptic ulcer of unspecified site without mention of hemorrhage or perforation, with obstruction — (Use additional E code to identify drug, if drug induced)
533.90 Peptic ulcer, unspecified site, unspecified as acute or chronic, without mention of hemorrhage, perforation, or obstruction — (Use additional E code to identify drug, if drug induced) ▽
533.91 Peptic ulcer, unspecified site, unspecified as acute or chronic, without mention of hemorrhage or perforation, with obstruction — (Use additional E code to identify drug, if drug induced) ▽
863.0 Stomach injury without mention of open wound into cavity

863.1 Stomach injury with open wound into cavity

ICD-9-CM Procedural

43.3 Pyloromyotomy
43.5 Partial gastrectomy with anastomosis to esophagus
44.00 Vagotomy, not otherwise specified
44.29 Other pyloroplasty

43640–43641

43640 Vagotomy including pyloroplasty, with or without gastrostomy; truncal or selective
43641 parietal cell (highly selective)

ICD-9-CM Diagnostic

151.1 Malignant neoplasm of pylorus
197.8 Secondary malignant neoplasm of other digestive organs and spleen
230.2 Carcinoma in situ of stomach
531.00 Acute gastric ulcer with hemorrhage, without mention of obstruction — (Use additional E code to identify drug, if drug induced)
531.01 Acute gastric ulcer with hemorrhage and obstruction — (Use additional E code to identify drug, if drug induced)
531.10 Acute gastric ulcer with perforation, without mention of obstruction — (Use additional E code to identify drug, if drug induced)
531.11 Acute gastric ulcer with perforation and obstruction — (Use additional E code to identify drug, if drug induced)
531.20 Acute gastric ulcer with hemorrhage and perforation, without mention of obstruction — (Use additional E code to identify drug, if drug induced)
531.40 Chronic or unspecified gastric ulcer with hemorrhage, without mention of obstruction — (Use additional E code to identify drug, if drug induced)
531.41 Chronic or unspecified gastric ulcer with hemorrhage and obstruction — (Use additional E code to identify drug, if drug induced)
531.50 Chronic or unspecified gastric ulcer with perforation, without mention of obstruction — (Use additional E code to identify drug, if drug induced)
531.51 Chronic or unspecified gastric ulcer with perforation and obstruction — (Use additional E code to identify drug, if drug induced)
531.60 Chronic or unspecified gastric ulcer with hemorrhage and perforation, without mention of obstruction — (Use additional E code to identify drug, if drug induced)
531.61 Chronic or unspecified gastric ulcer with hemorrhage, perforation, and obstruction — (Use additional E code to identify drug, if drug induced)
531.70 Chronic gastric ulcer without mention of hemorrhage, perforation, without mention of obstruction — (Use additional E code to identify drug, if drug induced)
531.71 Chronic gastric ulcer without mention of hemorrhage or perforation, with obstruction — (Use additional E code to identify drug, if drug induced)
531.90 Gastric ulcer, unspecified as acute or chronic, without mention of hemorrhage, perforation, or obstruction — (Use additional E code to identify drug, if drug induced) ▽
531.91 Gastric ulcer, unspecified as acute or chronic, without mention of hemorrhage or perforation, with obstruction — (Use additional E code to identify drug, if drug induced) ▽
532.00 Acute duodenal ulcer with hemorrhage, without mention of obstruction — (Use additional E code to identify drug, if drug induced)
532.01 Acute duodenal ulcer with hemorrhage and obstruction — (Use additional E code to identify drug, if drug induced)
532.10 Acute duodenal ulcer with perforation, without mention of obstruction — (Use additional E code to identify drug, if drug induced)
532.11 Acute duodenal ulcer with perforation and obstruction — (Use additional E code to identify drug, if drug induced)
532.20 Acute duodenal ulcer with hemorrhage and perforation, without mention of obstruction — (Use additional E code to identify drug, if drug induced)
532.21 Acute duodenal ulcer with hemorrhage, perforation, and obstruction — (Use additional E code to identify drug, if drug induced)
532.30 Acute duodenal ulcer without mention of hemorrhage, perforation, or obstruction — (Use additional E code to identify drug, if drug induced)
532.31 Acute duodenal ulcer without mention of hemorrhage or perforation, with obstruction — (Use additional E code to identify drug, if drug induced)
532.40 Chronic or unspecified duodenal ulcer with hemorrhage, without mention of obstruction — (Use additional E code to identify drug, if drug induced)
532.41 Chronic or unspecified duodenal ulcer with hemorrhage and obstruction — (Use additional E code to identify drug, if drug induced)
532.50 Chronic or unspecified duodenal ulcer with perforation, without mention of obstruction — (Use additional E code to identify drug, if drug induced)
532.51 Chronic or unspecified duodenal ulcer with perforation and obstruction — (Use additional E code to identify drug, if drug induced)
532.60 Chronic or unspecified duodenal ulcer with hemorrhage and perforation, without mention of obstruction — (Use additional E code to identify drug, if drug induced)
532.61 Chronic or unspecified duodenal ulcer with hemorrhage, perforation, and obstruction — (Use additional E code to identify drug, if drug induced)
532.71 Chronic duodenal ulcer without mention of hemorrhage or perforation, with obstruction — (Use additional E code to identify drug, if drug induced)
532.90 Duodenal ulcer, unspecified as acute or chronic, without hemorrhage, perforation, or obstruction — (Use additional E code to identify drug, if drug induced) ▽
532.91 Duodenal ulcer, unspecified as acute or chronic, without mention of hemorrhage or perforation, with obstruction — (Use additional E code to identify drug, if drug induced) ▽
533.00 Acute peptic ulcer, unspecified site, with hemorrhage, without mention of obstruction — (Use additional E code to identify drug, if drug induced)
533.01 Acute peptic ulcer, unspecified site, with hemorrhage and obstruction — (Use additional E code to identify drug, if drug induced)
533.10 Acute peptic ulcer, unspecified site, with perforation, without mention of obstruction — (Use additional E code to identify drug, if drug induced)
533.11 Acute peptic ulcer, unspecified site, with perforation and obstruction — (Use additional E code to identify drug, if drug induced)
533.20 Acute peptic ulcer, unspecified site, with hemorrhage and perforation, without mention of obstruction — (Use additional E code to identify drug, if drug induced)
533.21 Acute peptic ulcer, unspecified site, with hemorrhage, perforation, and obstruction — (Use additional E code to identify drug, if drug induced)
533.30 Acute peptic ulcer, unspecified site, without mention of hemorrhage, perforation, or obstruction — (Use additional E code to identify drug, if drug induced)
533.31 Acute peptic ulcer, unspecified site, without mention of hemorrhage and perforation, with obstruction — (Use additional E code to identify drug, if drug induced)
533.40 Chronic or unspecified peptic ulcer, unspecified site, with hemorrhage, without mention of obstruction — (Use additional E code to identify drug, if drug induced)
533.41 Chronic or unspecified peptic ulcer, unspecified site, with hemorrhage and obstruction — (Use additional E code to identify drug, if drug induced)
533.50 Chronic or unspecified peptic ulcer, unspecified site, with perforation, without mention of obstruction — (Use additional E code to identify drug, if drug induced)
533.51 Chronic or unspecified peptic ulcer, unspecified site, with perforation and obstruction — (Use additional E code to identify drug, if drug induced)
533.60 Chronic or unspecified peptic ulcer, unspecified site, with hemorrhage and perforation, without mention of obstruction — (Use additional E code to identify drug, if drug induced)
533.61 Chronic or unspecified peptic ulcer, unspecified site, with hemorrhage, perforation, and obstruction — (Use additional E code to identify drug, if drug induced)
533.70 Chronic peptic ulcer, unspecified site, without mention of hemorrhage, perforation, or obstruction — (Use additional E code to identify drug, if drug induced)
533.71 Chronic peptic ulcer of unspecified site without mention of hemorrhage or perforation, with obstruction — (Use additional E code to identify drug, if drug induced)
533.90 Peptic ulcer, unspecified site, unspecified as acute or chronic, without mention of hemorrhage, perforation, or obstruction — (Use additional E code to identify drug, if drug induced) ▽
533.91 Peptic ulcer, unspecified site, unspecified as acute or chronic, without mention of hemorrhage or perforation, with obstruction — (Use additional E code to identify drug, if drug induced) ▽
536.8 Dyspepsia and other specified disorders of function of stomach
536.9 Unspecified functional disorder of stomach ▽
537.0 Acquired hypertrophic pyloric stenosis
789.00 Abdominal pain, unspecified site ▽
789.06 Abdominal pain, epigastric
789.9 Other symptoms involving abdomen and pelvis

ICD-9-CM Procedural

43.19 Other gastrostomy
44.01 Truncal vagotomy
44.02 Highly selective vagotomy
44.03 Other selective vagotomy
44.29 Other pyloroplasty

▽ Unspecified code ☒ Manifestation code
♀ Female diagnosis ♂ Male diagnosis

43644–43645

43644 Laparoscopy, surgical, gastric restrictive procedure; with gastric bypass and Roux-en-Y gastroenterostomy (roux limb 150 cm or less)
43645 with gastric bypass and small intestine reconstruction to limit absorption

ICD-9-CM Diagnostic

244.9 Unspecified hypothyroidism ♥
253.8 Other disorders of the pituitary and other syndromes of diencephalohypophyseal origin
255.8 Other specified disorders of adrenal glands
259.9 Unspecified endocrine disorder ♥
278.00 Obesity, unspecified — (Use additional code to identify any associated mental retardation) ♥
278.01 Morbid obesity — (Use additional code to identify any associated mental retardation)

ICD-9-CM Procedural

44.38 Laparoscopic gastroenterostomy

43651–43652

43651 Laparoscopy, surgical; transection of vagus nerves, truncal
43652 transection of vagus nerves, selective or highly selective

ICD-9-CM Diagnostic

150.2 Malignant neoplasm of abdominal esophagus
151.1 Malignant neoplasm of pylorus
151.2 Malignant neoplasm of pyloric antrum
151.3 Malignant neoplasm of fundus of stomach
151.4 Malignant neoplasm of body of stomach
151.5 Malignant neoplasm of lesser curvature of stomach, unspecified ♥
151.6 Malignant neoplasm of greater curvature of stomach, unspecified ♥
151.8 Malignant neoplasm of other specified sites of stomach
151.9 Malignant neoplasm of stomach, unspecified site ♥
152.0 Malignant neoplasm of duodenum
152.1 Malignant neoplasm of jejunum
155.0 Malignant neoplasm of liver, primary
352.3 Disorders of pneumogastric (10th) nerve
531.70 Chronic gastric ulcer without mention of hemorrhage, perforation, without mention of obstruction — (Use additional E code to identify drug, if drug induced)
532.70 Chronic duodenal ulcer without mention of hemorrhage, perforation, or obstruction — (Use additional E code to identify drug, if drug induced)
533.70 Chronic peptic ulcer, unspecified site, without mention of hemorrhage, perforation, or obstruction — (Use additional E code to identify drug, if drug induced)
536.8 Dyspepsia and other specified disorders of function of stomach

ICD-9-CM Procedural

44.01 Truncal vagotomy
44.02 Highly selective vagotomy
44.03 Other selective vagotomy

43653

43653 Laparoscopy, surgical; gastrostomy, without construction of gastric tube (eg, Stamm procedure) (separate procedure)

ICD-9-CM Diagnostic

150.1 Malignant neoplasm of thoracic esophagus
150.2 Malignant neoplasm of abdominal esophagus
150.3 Malignant neoplasm of upper third of esophagus
150.4 Malignant neoplasm of middle third of esophagus
150.5 Malignant neoplasm of lower third of esophagus
150.8 Malignant neoplasm of other specified part of esophagus
150.9 Malignant neoplasm of esophagus, unspecified site ♥
151.0 Malignant neoplasm of cardia
151.1 Malignant neoplasm of pylorus
151.2 Malignant neoplasm of pyloric antrum
151.3 Malignant neoplasm of fundus of stomach
151.4 Malignant neoplasm of body of stomach
151.5 Malignant neoplasm of lesser curvature of stomach, unspecified ♥
151.6 Malignant neoplasm of greater curvature of stomach, unspecified ♥
151.8 Malignant neoplasm of other specified sites of stomach
151.9 Malignant neoplasm of stomach, unspecified site ♥
152.0 Malignant neoplasm of duodenum
152.1 Malignant neoplasm of jejunum
152.2 Malignant neoplasm of ileum
161.9 Malignant neoplasm of larynx, unspecified site ♥
197.4 Secondary malignant neoplasm of small intestine including duodenum
197.8 Secondary malignant neoplasm of other digestive organs and spleen
198.89 Secondary malignant neoplasm of other specified sites
211.1 Benign neoplasm of stomach
230.2 Carcinoma in situ of stomach
239.8 Neoplasm of unspecified nature of other specified sites
261 Nutritional marasmus
262 Other severe protein-calorie malnutrition
263.0 Malnutrition of moderate degree
263.1 Malnutrition of mild degree
263.2 Arrested development following protein-calorie malnutrition
263.8 Other protein-calorie malnutrition
276.5 Volume depletion — (Use additional code to identify any associated mental retardation)
307.1 Anorexia nervosa
436 Acute, but ill-defined, cerebrovascular disease — (Use additional code to identify presence of hypertension) ♥
519.00 Unspecified tracheostomy complication ♥
519.01 Infection of tracheostomy — (Use additional code to identify type of infection: 038.0-038.9, 682.1. Use additional code to identify organism: 041.00-041.9)
519.02 Mechanical complication of tracheostomy
519.09 Other tracheostomy complications
530.3 Stricture and stenosis of esophagus
530.4 Perforation of esophagus
530.5 Dyskinesia of esophagus
530.81 Esophageal reflux
531.00 Acute gastric ulcer with hemorrhage, without mention of obstruction — (Use additional E code to identify drug, if drug induced)
531.01 Acute gastric ulcer with hemorrhage and obstruction — (Use additional E code to identify drug, if drug induced)
531.10 Acute gastric ulcer with perforation, without mention of obstruction — (Use additional E code to identify drug, if drug induced)
531.11 Acute gastric ulcer with perforation and obstruction — (Use additional E code to identify drug, if drug induced)
531.20 Acute gastric ulcer with hemorrhage and perforation, without mention of obstruction — (Use additional E code to identify drug, if drug induced)
531.21 Acute gastric ulcer with hemorrhage, perforation, and obstruction — (Use additional E code to identify drug, if drug induced)
531.30 Acute gastric ulcer without mention of hemorrhage, perforation, or obstruction — (Use additional E code to identify drug, if drug induced)
531.31 Acute gastric ulcer without mention of hemorrhage or perforation, with obstruction — (Use additional E code to identify drug, if drug induced)
531.40 Chronic or unspecified gastric ulcer with hemorrhage, without mention of obstruction — (Use additional E code to identify drug, if drug induced)
531.41 Chronic or unspecified gastric ulcer with hemorrhage and obstruction — (Use additional E code to identify drug, if drug induced)
531.50 Chronic or unspecified gastric ulcer with perforation, without mention of obstruction — (Use additional E code to identify drug, if drug induced)
531.51 Chronic or unspecified gastric ulcer with perforation and obstruction — (Use additional E code to identify drug, if drug induced)
531.60 Chronic or unspecified gastric ulcer with hemorrhage and perforation, without mention of obstruction — (Use additional E code to identify drug, if drug induced)
531.61 Chronic or unspecified gastric ulcer with hemorrhage, perforation, and obstruction — (Use additional E code to identify drug, if drug induced)
531.70 Chronic gastric ulcer without mention of hemorrhage, perforation, without mention of obstruction — (Use additional E code to identify drug, if drug induced)
531.71 Chronic gastric ulcer without mention of hemorrhage or perforation, with obstruction — (Use additional E code to identify drug, if drug induced)
531.90 Gastric ulcer, unspecified as acute or chronic, without mention of hemorrhage, perforation, or obstruction — (Use additional E code to identify drug, if drug induced) ♥
531.91 Gastric ulcer, unspecified as acute or chronic, without mention of hemorrhage or perforation, with obstruction — (Use additional E code to identify drug, if drug induced) ♥
532.00 Acute duodenal ulcer with hemorrhage, without mention of obstruction — (Use additional E code to identify drug, if drug induced)
532.01 Acute duodenal ulcer with hemorrhage and obstruction — (Use additional E code to identify drug, if drug induced)
532.10 Acute duodenal ulcer with perforation, without mention of obstruction — (Use additional E code to identify drug, if drug induced)
532.11 Acute duodenal ulcer with perforation and obstruction — (Use additional E code to identify drug, if drug induced)

♥ Unspecified code ♀ Female diagnosis ☒ Manifestation code ♂ Male diagnosis

532.20 Acute duodenal ulcer with hemorrhage and perforation, without mention of obstruction — (Use additional E code to identify drug, if drug induced)
532.21 Acute duodenal ulcer with hemorrhage, perforation, and obstruction — (Use additional E code to identify drug, if drug induced)
532.30 Acute duodenal ulcer without mention of hemorrhage, perforation, or obstruction — (Use additional E code to identify drug, if drug induced)
532.31 Acute duodenal ulcer without mention of hemorrhage or perforation, with obstruction — (Use additional E code to identify drug, if drug induced)
532.40 Chronic or unspecified duodenal ulcer with hemorrhage, without mention of obstruction — (Use additional E code to identify drug, if drug induced)
532.41 Chronic or unspecified duodenal ulcer with hemorrhage and obstruction — (Use additional E code to identify drug, if drug induced)
532.50 Chronic or unspecified duodenal ulcer with perforation, without mention of obstruction — (Use additional E code to identify drug, if drug induced)
532.51 Chronic or unspecified duodenal ulcer with perforation and obstruction — (Use additional E code to identify drug, if drug induced)
532.60 Chronic or unspecified duodenal ulcer with hemorrhage and perforation, without mention of obstruction — (Use additional E code to identify drug, if drug induced)
532.61 Chronic or unspecified duodenal ulcer with hemorrhage, perforation, and obstruction — (Use additional E code to identify drug, if drug induced)
532.70 Chronic duodenal ulcer without mention of hemorrhage, perforation, or obstruction — (Use additional E code to identify drug, if drug induced)
532.71 Chronic duodenal ulcer without mention of hemorrhage or perforation, with obstruction — (Use additional E code to identify drug, if drug induced)
532.90 Duodenal ulcer, unspecified as acute or chronic, without hemorrhage, perforation, or obstruction — (Use additional E code to identify drug, if drug induced)
532.91 Duodenal ulcer, unspecified as acute or chronic, without mention of hemorrhage or perforation, with obstruction — (Use additional E code to identify drug, if drug induced)
533.00 Acute peptic ulcer, unspecified site, with hemorrhage, without mention of obstruction — (Use additional E code to identify drug, if drug induced)
533.01 Acute peptic ulcer, unspecified site, with hemorrhage and obstruction — (Use additional E code to identify drug, if drug induced)
533.10 Acute peptic ulcer, unspecified site, with perforation, without mention of obstruction — (Use additional E code to identify drug, if drug induced)
533.11 Acute peptic ulcer, unspecified site, with perforation and obstruction — (Use additional E code to identify drug, if drug induced)
533.20 Acute peptic ulcer, unspecified site, with hemorrhage and perforation, without mention of obstruction — (Use additional E code to identify drug, if drug induced)
533.21 Acute peptic ulcer, unspecified site, with hemorrhage, perforation, and obstruction — (Use additional E code to identify drug, if drug induced)
533.30 Acute peptic ulcer, unspecified site, without mention of hemorrhage, perforation, or obstruction — (Use additional E code to identify drug, if drug induced)
533.40 Chronic or unspecified peptic ulcer, unspecified site, with hemorrhage, without mention of obstruction — (Use additional E code to identify drug, if drug induced)
533.41 Chronic or unspecified peptic ulcer, unspecified site, with hemorrhage and obstruction — (Use additional E code to identify drug, if drug induced)
533.50 Chronic or unspecified peptic ulcer, unspecified site, with perforation, without mention of obstruction — (Use additional E code to identify drug, if drug induced)
533.51 Chronic or unspecified peptic ulcer, unspecified site, with perforation and obstruction — (Use additional E code to identify drug, if drug induced)
535.50 Unspecified gastritis and gastroduodenitis without mention of hemorrhage
536.9 Unspecified functional disorder of stomach
537.89 Other specified disorder of stomach and duodenum
578.9 Unspecified, hemorrhage of gastrointestinal tract
707.9 Chronic ulcer of unspecified site
750.5 Congenital hypertrophic pyloric stenosis
750.7 Other specified congenital anomalies of stomach
751.1 Congenital atresia and stenosis of small intestine
783.0 Anorexia
783.3 Feeding difficulties and mismanagement
783.7 Adult failure to thrive
787.01 Nausea with vomiting
787.2 Dysphagia
854.06 Intracranial injury of other and unspecified nature, without mention of open intracranial wound, loss of consciousness of unspecified duration
994.2 Effects of hunger
997.4 Digestive system complication — (Use additional code to identify complications)

ICD-9-CM Procedural

43.19 Other gastrostomy

43750

43750 Percutaneous placement of gastrostomy tube

ICD-9-CM Diagnostic

141.0 Malignant neoplasm of base of tongue
141.1 Malignant neoplasm of dorsal surface of tongue
141.2 Malignant neoplasm of tip and lateral border of tongue
141.3 Malignant neoplasm of ventral surface of tongue
141.4 Malignant neoplasm of anterior two-thirds of tongue, part unspecified
141.8 Malignant neoplasm of other sites of tongue
141.9 Malignant neoplasm of tongue, unspecified site
149.0 Malignant neoplasm of pharynx, unspecified
149.1 Malignant neoplasm of Waldeyer's ring
149.8 Malignant neoplasm of other sites within the lip and oral cavity
149.9 Malignant neoplasm of ill-defined sites of lip and oral cavity
150.0 Malignant neoplasm of cervical esophagus
150.1 Malignant neoplasm of thoracic esophagus
150.2 Malignant neoplasm of abdominal esophagus
150.3 Malignant neoplasm of upper third of esophagus
150.4 Malignant neoplasm of middle third of esophagus
150.5 Malignant neoplasm of lower third of esophagus
150.8 Malignant neoplasm of other specified part of esophagus
150.9 Malignant neoplasm of esophagus, unspecified site
151.0 Malignant neoplasm of cardia
151.1 Malignant neoplasm of pylorus
151.2 Malignant neoplasm of pyloric antrum
151.3 Malignant neoplasm of fundus of stomach
151.4 Malignant neoplasm of body of stomach
151.5 Malignant neoplasm of lesser curvature of stomach, unspecified
151.6 Malignant neoplasm of greater curvature of stomach, unspecified
151.8 Malignant neoplasm of other specified sites of stomach
151.9 Malignant neoplasm of stomach, unspecified site
161.9 Malignant neoplasm of larynx, unspecified site
197.8 Secondary malignant neoplasm of other digestive organs and spleen
199.1 Other malignant neoplasm of unspecified site
203.00 Multiple myeloma without mention of remission
210.9 Benign neoplasm of pharynx, unspecified
235.5 Neoplasm of uncertain behavior of other and unspecified digestive organs
250.30 Diabetes with other coma, type II or unspecified type, not stated as uncontrolled
250.31 Diabetes with other coma, type I [juvenile type], not stated as uncontrolled
250.32 Diabetes with other coma, type II or unspecified type, uncontrolled
250.33 Diabetes with other coma, type I [juvenile type], uncontrolled
260 Kwashiorkor
261 Nutritional marasmus
262 Other severe protein-calorie malnutrition
330.8 Other specified cerebral degenerations in childhood — (Use additional code to identify associated mental retardation)
330.9 Unspecified cerebral degeneration in childhood — (Use additional code to identify associated mental retardation)
335.20 Amyotrophic lateral sclerosis
348.1 Anoxic brain damage — (Use additional E code to identify cause)
436 Acute, but ill-defined, cerebrovascular disease — (Use additional code to identify presence of hypertension)
478.6 Edema of larynx
530.11 Reflux esophagitis — (Use additional E code to identify cause, if induced by chemical or drug)
530.12 Acute esophagitis — (Use additional E code to identify cause, if induced by chemical or drug)
530.19 Other esophagitis — (Use additional E code to identify cause, if induced by chemical or drug)
530.20 Ulcer of esophagus without bleeding — (Use additional E code to identify cause, if induced by chemical or drug)
530.21 Ulcer of esophagus with bleeding — (Use additional E code to identify cause, if induced by chemical or drug)
530.3 Stricture and stenosis of esophagus
530.4 Perforation of esophagus
530.5 Dyskinesia of esophagus
530.6 Diverticulum of esophagus, acquired
530.7 Gastroesophageal laceration-hemorrhage syndrome
530.81 Esophageal reflux
530.82 Esophageal hemorrhage
530.83 Esophageal leukoplakia

Unspecified code
♀ Female diagnosis
Manifestation code
♂ Male diagnosis

530.84 Tracheoesophageal fistula
530.85 Barrett's esophagus
530.89 Other specified disorder of the esophagus
536.8 Dyspepsia and other specified disorders of function of stomach
750.3 Congenital tracheoesophageal fistula, esophageal atresia and stenosis
780.01 Coma
783.0 Anorexia
783.21 Loss of weight
783.22 Underweight
783.3 Feeding difficulties and mismanagement
783.40 Lack of normal physiological development, unspecified ▽
783.7 Adult failure to thrive
787.01 Nausea with vomiting
787.02 Nausea alone
787.03 Vomiting alone
787.2 Dysphagia
789.00 Abdominal pain, unspecified site ▽
854.00 Intracranial injury of other and unspecified nature, without mention of open intracranial wound, unspecified state of consciousness ▽
854.05 Intracranial injury of other and unspecified nature, without mention of open intracranial wound, prolonged (more than 24 hours) loss of consciousness, without return to pre-existing conscious level
959.01 Head injury, unspecified ▽
998.59 Other postoperative infection — (Use additional code to identify infection)
V10.00 Personal history of malignant neoplasm of unspecified site in gastrointestinal tract ▽
V10.01 Personal history of malignant neoplasm of tongue
V10.02 Personal history of malignant neoplasm of other and unspecified parts of oral cavity and pharynx ▽
V10.03 Personal history of malignant neoplasm of esophagus
V10.21 Personal history of malignant neoplasm of larynx

ICD-9-CM Procedural

43.11 Percutaneous (endoscopic) gastrostomy (PEG)

HCPCS Level II Supplies & Services

A4305 Disposable drug delivery system, flow rate of 50 ml or greater per hour
A4550 Surgical trays
B4086 Gastrostomy/jejunostomy tube, any material, any type, (standard or low profile), each

43752

43752 Naso- or oro-gastric tube placement, requiring physician's skill and fluoroscopic guidance (includes fluoroscopy, image documentation and report)

ICD-9-CM Diagnostic

141.0 Malignant neoplasm of base of tongue
141.1 Malignant neoplasm of dorsal surface of tongue
141.2 Malignant neoplasm of tip and lateral border of tongue
141.3 Malignant neoplasm of ventral surface of tongue
141.4 Malignant neoplasm of anterior two-thirds of tongue, part unspecified ▽
141.8 Malignant neoplasm of other sites of tongue
141.9 Malignant neoplasm of tongue, unspecified site ▽
149.0 Malignant neoplasm of pharynx, unspecified ▽
149.1 Malignant neoplasm of Waldeyer's ring
149.8 Malignant neoplasm of other sites within the lip and oral cavity
149.9 Malignant neoplasm of ill-defined sites of lip and oral cavity
150.0 Malignant neoplasm of cervical esophagus
150.1 Malignant neoplasm of thoracic esophagus
150.2 Malignant neoplasm of abdominal esophagus
150.3 Malignant neoplasm of upper third of esophagus
150.4 Malignant neoplasm of middle third of esophagus
150.5 Malignant neoplasm of lower third of esophagus
150.8 Malignant neoplasm of other specified part of esophagus
150.9 Malignant neoplasm of esophagus, unspecified site ▽
151.0 Malignant neoplasm of cardia
151.1 Malignant neoplasm of pylorus
151.2 Malignant neoplasm of pyloric antrum
151.3 Malignant neoplasm of fundus of stomach
151.4 Malignant neoplasm of body of stomach
151.5 Malignant neoplasm of lesser curvature of stomach, unspecified ▽
151.6 Malignant neoplasm of greater curvature of stomach, unspecified ▽
151.8 Malignant neoplasm of other specified sites of stomach
151.9 Malignant neoplasm of stomach, unspecified site ▽
161.9 Malignant neoplasm of larynx, unspecified site ▽
197.8 Secondary malignant neoplasm of other digestive organs and spleen
199.1 Other malignant neoplasm of unspecified site
203.00 Multiple myeloma without mention of remission
210.9 Benign neoplasm of pharynx, unspecified ▽
235.5 Neoplasm of uncertain behavior of other and unspecified digestive organs ▽
250.30 Diabetes with other coma, type II or unspecified type, not stated as uncontrolled
250.31 Diabetes with other coma, type I [juvenile type], not stated as uncontrolled
250.32 Diabetes with other coma, type II or unspecified type, uncontrolled
250.33 Diabetes with other coma, type I [juvenile type], uncontrolled
260 Kwashiorkor
261 Nutritional marasmus
262 Other severe protein-calorie malnutrition
330.8 Other specified cerebral degenerations in childhood — (Use additional code to identify associated mental retardation)
330.9 Unspecified cerebral degeneration in childhood — (Use additional code to identify associated mental retardation) ▽
335.20 Amyotrophic lateral sclerosis
348.1 Anoxic brain damage — (Use additional E code to identify cause)
436 Acute, but ill-defined, cerebrovascular disease — (Use additional code to identify presence of hypertension) ▽
478.6 Edema of larynx
530.11 Reflux esophagitis — (Use additional E code to identify cause, if induced by chemical or drug)
530.12 Acute esophagitis — (Use additional E code to identify cause, if induced by chemical or drug)
530.19 Other esophagitis — (Use additional E code to identify cause, if induced by chemical or drug)
530.20 Ulcer of esophagus without bleeding — (Use additional E code to identify cause, if induced by chemical or drug)
530.21 Ulcer of esophagus with bleeding — (Use additional E code to identify cause, if induced by chemical or drug)
530.3 Stricture and stenosis of esophagus
530.4 Perforation of esophagus
530.5 Dyskinesia of esophagus
530.6 Diverticulum of esophagus, acquired
530.7 Gastroesophageal laceration-hemorrhage syndrome
530.81 Esophageal reflux
530.82 Esophageal hemorrhage
530.83 Esophageal leukoplakia
530.84 Tracheoesophageal fistula
530.85 Barrett's esophagus
530.89 Other specified disorder of the esophagus
536.8 Dyspepsia and other specified disorders of function of stomach
750.3 Congenital tracheoesophageal fistula, esophageal atresia and stenosis
780.01 Coma
783.0 Anorexia
783.21 Loss of weight
783.22 Underweight
783.3 Feeding difficulties and mismanagement
783.40 Lack of normal physiological development, unspecified ▽
783.7 Adult failure to thrive
787.01 Nausea with vomiting
787.02 Nausea alone
787.03 Vomiting alone
787.2 Dysphagia
789.00 Abdominal pain, unspecified site ▽
854.00 Intracranial injury of other and unspecified nature, without mention of open intracranial wound, unspecified state of consciousness ▽
854.05 Intracranial injury of other and unspecified nature, without mention of open intracranial wound, prolonged (more than 24 hours) loss of consciousness, without return to pre-existing conscious level
959.01 Head injury, unspecified ▽
998.59 Other postoperative infection — (Use additional code to identify infection)
V10.00 Personal history of malignant neoplasm of unspecified site in gastrointestinal tract ▽
V10.01 Personal history of malignant neoplasm of tongue
V10.02 Personal history of malignant neoplasm of other and unspecified parts of oral cavity and pharynx ▽
V10.03 Personal history of malignant neoplasm of esophagus
V10.21 Personal history of malignant neoplasm of larynx

ICD-9-CM Procedural

96.06 Insertion of Sengstaaken tube
96.07 Insertion of other (naso-)gastric tube
96.6 Enteral infusion of concentrated nutritional substances

HCPCS Level II Supplies & Services
A4305 Disposable drug delivery system, flow rate of 50 ml or greater per hour
A4550 Surgical trays
B4086 Gastrostomy/jejunostomy tube, any material, any type, (standard or low profile), each

43760
43760 Change of gastrostomy tube

ICD-9-CM Diagnostic
536.40 Unspecified gastrostomy complication ▽
536.41 Infection of gastrostomy — (Use additional code to specify type of infection: 038.0-038.9, 041.00-041.9. Use additional code to identify organism: 041.00-041.9)
536.42 Mechanical complication of gastrostomy
536.49 Other gastrostomy complications
682.2 Cellulitis and abscess of trunk — (Use additional code to identify organism)
V44.1 Gastrostomy status — (This code is intended for use when these conditions are recorded as diagnoses or problems)
V55.2 Attention to ileostomy

ICD-9-CM Procedural
97.02 Replacement of gastrostomy tube

HCPCS Level II Supplies & Services
A4550 Surgical trays

43761
43761 Repositioning of the gastric feeding tube, any method, through the duodenum for enteric nutrition

ICD-9-CM Diagnostic
V55.4 Attention to other artificial opening of digestive tract

ICD-9-CM Procedural
44.99 Other operations on stomach

HCPCS Level II Supplies & Services
B4034 Enteral feeding supply kit; syringe, per day
B4035 Enteral feeding supply kit; pump fed, per day
B4036 Enteral feeding supply kit; gravity fed, per day
B9000 Enteral nutrition infusion pump — without alarm
B9002 Enteral nutrition infusion pump — with alarm

43800
43800 Pyloroplasty

ICD-9-CM Diagnostic
537.0 Acquired hypertrophic pyloric stenosis
537.81 Pylorospasm
750.5 Congenital hypertrophic pyloric stenosis

ICD-9-CM Procedural
44.21 Dilation of pylorus by incision
44.22 Endoscopic dilation of pylorus
44.29 Other pyloroplasty

43810
43810 Gastroduodenostomy

ICD-9-CM Diagnostic
151.1 Malignant neoplasm of pylorus
151.5 Malignant neoplasm of lesser curvature of stomach, unspecified ▽
151.6 Malignant neoplasm of greater curvature of stomach, unspecified ▽
151.9 Malignant neoplasm of stomach, unspecified site ▽
152.0 Malignant neoplasm of duodenum
197.4 Secondary malignant neoplasm of small intestine including duodenum
230.7 Carcinoma in situ of other and unspecified parts of intestine ▽
235.2 Neoplasm of uncertain behavior of stomach, intestines, and rectum
531.00 Acute gastric ulcer with hemorrhage, without mention of obstruction — (Use additional E code to identify drug, if drug induced)
531.01 Acute gastric ulcer with hemorrhage and obstruction — (Use additional E code to identify drug, if drug induced)
531.10 Acute gastric ulcer with perforation, without mention of obstruction — (Use additional E code to identify drug, if drug induced)
531.11 Acute gastric ulcer with perforation and obstruction — (Use additional E code to identify drug, if drug induced)
531.20 Acute gastric ulcer with hemorrhage and perforation, without mention of obstruction — (Use additional E code to identify drug, if drug induced)
531.21 Acute gastric ulcer with hemorrhage, perforation, and obstruction — (Use additional E code to identify drug, if drug induced)
531.31 Acute gastric ulcer without mention of hemorrhage or perforation, with obstruction — (Use additional E code to identify drug, if drug induced)
531.40 Chronic or unspecified gastric ulcer with hemorrhage, without mention of obstruction — (Use additional E code to identify drug, if drug induced)
531.41 Chronic or unspecified gastric ulcer with hemorrhage and obstruction — (Use additional E code to identify drug, if drug induced)
531.50 Chronic or unspecified gastric ulcer with perforation, without mention of obstruction — (Use additional E code to identify drug, if drug induced)
531.51 Chronic or unspecified gastric ulcer with perforation and obstruction — (Use additional E code to identify drug, if drug induced)
531.60 Chronic or unspecified gastric ulcer with hemorrhage and perforation, without mention of obstruction — (Use additional E code to identify drug, if drug induced)
531.61 Chronic or unspecified gastric ulcer with hemorrhage, perforation, and obstruction — (Use additional E code to identify drug, if drug induced)
531.70 Chronic gastric ulcer without mention of hemorrhage, perforation, without mention of obstruction — (Use additional E code to identify drug, if drug induced)
531.71 Chronic gastric ulcer without mention of hemorrhage or perforation, with obstruction — (Use additional E code to identify drug, if drug induced)
531.90 Gastric ulcer, unspecified as acute or chronic, without mention of hemorrhage, perforation, or obstruction — (Use additional E code to identify drug, if drug induced) ▽
531.91 Gastric ulcer, unspecified as acute or chronic, without mention of hemorrhage or perforation, with obstruction — (Use additional E code to identify drug, if drug induced) ▽
532.00 Acute duodenal ulcer with hemorrhage, without mention of obstruction — (Use additional E code to identify drug, if drug induced)
532.01 Acute duodenal ulcer with hemorrhage and obstruction — (Use additional E code to identify drug, if drug induced)
532.10 Acute duodenal ulcer with perforation, without mention of obstruction — (Use additional E code to identify drug, if drug induced)
532.11 Acute duodenal ulcer with perforation and obstruction — (Use additional E code to identify drug, if drug induced)
532.20 Acute duodenal ulcer with hemorrhage and perforation, without mention of obstruction — (Use additional E code to identify drug, if drug induced)
532.21 Acute duodenal ulcer with hemorrhage, perforation, and obstruction — (Use additional E code to identify drug, if drug induced)
532.30 Acute duodenal ulcer without mention of hemorrhage, perforation, or obstruction — (Use additional E code to identify drug, if drug induced)
532.31 Acute duodenal ulcer without mention of hemorrhage or perforation, with obstruction — (Use additional E code to identify drug, if drug induced)
532.40 Chronic or unspecified duodenal ulcer with hemorrhage, without mention of obstruction — (Use additional E code to identify drug, if drug induced)
532.41 Chronic or unspecified duodenal ulcer with hemorrhage and obstruction — (Use additional E code to identify drug, if drug induced)
532.50 Chronic or unspecified duodenal ulcer with perforation, without mention of obstruction — (Use additional E code to identify drug, if drug induced)
532.51 Chronic or unspecified duodenal ulcer with perforation and obstruction — (Use additional E code to identify drug, if drug induced)
532.60 Chronic or unspecified duodenal ulcer with hemorrhage and perforation, without mention of obstruction — (Use additional E code to identify drug, if drug induced)
532.61 Chronic or unspecified duodenal ulcer with hemorrhage, perforation, and obstruction — (Use additional E code to identify drug, if drug induced)
532.70 Chronic duodenal ulcer without mention of hemorrhage, perforation, or obstruction — (Use additional E code to identify drug, if drug induced)
532.71 Chronic duodenal ulcer without mention of hemorrhage or perforation, with obstruction — (Use additional E code to identify drug, if drug induced)
532.90 Duodenal ulcer, unspecified as acute or chronic, without hemorrhage, perforation, or obstruction — (Use additional E code to identify drug, if drug induced) ▽
532.91 Duodenal ulcer, unspecified as acute or chronic, without mention of hemorrhage or perforation, with obstruction — (Use additional E code to identify drug, if drug induced) ▽
533.00 Acute peptic ulcer, unspecified site, with hemorrhage, without mention of obstruction — (Use additional E code to identify drug, if drug induced)
533.01 Acute peptic ulcer, unspecified site, with hemorrhage and obstruction — (Use additional E code to identify drug, if drug induced)

533.10 Acute peptic ulcer, unspecified site, with perforation, without mention of obstruction — (Use additional E code to identify drug, if drug induced)
533.11 Acute peptic ulcer, unspecified site, with perforation and obstruction — (Use additional E code to identify drug, if drug induced)
533.20 Acute peptic ulcer, unspecified site, with hemorrhage and perforation, without mention of obstruction — (Use additional E code to identify drug, if drug induced)
533.21 Acute peptic ulcer, unspecified site, with hemorrhage, perforation, and obstruction — (Use additional E code to identify drug, if drug induced)
533.30 Acute peptic ulcer, unspecified site, without mention of hemorrhage, perforation, or obstruction — (Use additional E code to identify drug, if drug induced)
533.31 Acute peptic ulcer, unspecified site, without mention of hemorrhage and perforation, with obstruction — (Use additional E code to identify drug, if drug induced)
533.40 Chronic or unspecified peptic ulcer, unspecified site, with hemorrhage, without mention of obstruction — (Use additional E code to identify drug, if drug induced)
533.41 Chronic or unspecified peptic ulcer, unspecified site, with hemorrhage and obstruction — (Use additional E code to identify drug, if drug induced)
533.50 Chronic or unspecified peptic ulcer, unspecified site, with perforation, without mention of obstruction — (Use additional E code to identify drug, if drug induced)
533.51 Chronic or unspecified peptic ulcer, unspecified site, with perforation and obstruction — (Use additional E code to identify drug, if drug induced)
533.60 Chronic or unspecified peptic ulcer, unspecified site, with hemorrhage and perforation, without mention of obstruction — (Use additional E code to identify drug, if drug induced)
533.61 Chronic or unspecified peptic ulcer, unspecified site, with hemorrhage, perforation, and obstruction — (Use additional E code to identify drug, if drug induced)
533.70 Chronic peptic ulcer, unspecified site, without mention of hemorrhage, perforation, or obstruction — (Use additional E code to identify drug, if drug induced)
533.71 Chronic peptic ulcer of unspecified site without mention of hemorrhage or perforation, with obstruction — (Use additional E code to identify drug, if drug induced)
533.90 Peptic ulcer, unspecified site, unspecified as acute or chronic, without mention of hemorrhage, perforation, or obstruction — (Use additional E code to identify drug, if drug induced) ▽
533.91 Peptic ulcer, unspecified site, unspecified as acute or chronic, without mention of hemorrhage or perforation, with obstruction — (Use additional E code to identify drug, if drug induced) ▽

ICD-9-CM Procedural

44.39 Other gastroenterostomy without gastrectomy

43820–43825

43820 Gastrojejunostomy; without vagotomy
43825 with vagotomy, any type

ICD-9-CM Diagnostic

151.8 Malignant neoplasm of other specified sites of stomach
151.9 Malignant neoplasm of stomach, unspecified site ▽
152.0 Malignant neoplasm of duodenum
152.1 Malignant neoplasm of jejunum
152.3 Malignant neoplasm of Meckel's diverticulum
152.8 Malignant neoplasm of other specified sites of small intestine
152.9 Malignant neoplasm of small intestine, unspecified site ▽
197.4 Secondary malignant neoplasm of small intestine including duodenum
197.8 Secondary malignant neoplasm of other digestive organs and spleen
199.0 Disseminated malignant neoplasm
230.7 Carcinoma in situ of other and unspecified parts of intestine ▽
235.2 Neoplasm of uncertain behavior of stomach, intestines, and rectum
531.00 Acute gastric ulcer with hemorrhage, without mention of obstruction — (Use additional E code to identify drug, if drug induced)
531.01 Acute gastric ulcer with hemorrhage and obstruction — (Use additional E code to identify drug, if drug induced)
531.10 Acute gastric ulcer with perforation, without mention of obstruction — (Use additional E code to identify drug, if drug induced)
531.11 Acute gastric ulcer with perforation and obstruction — (Use additional E code to identify drug, if drug induced)
531.20 Acute gastric ulcer with hemorrhage and perforation, without mention of obstruction — (Use additional E code to identify drug, if drug induced)
531.21 Acute gastric ulcer with hemorrhage, perforation, and obstruction — (Use additional E code to identify drug, if drug induced)
531.30 Acute gastric ulcer without mention of hemorrhage, perforation, or obstruction — (Use additional E code to identify drug, if drug induced)
531.31 Acute gastric ulcer without mention of hemorrhage or perforation, with obstruction — (Use additional E code to identify drug, if drug induced)
531.40 Chronic or unspecified gastric ulcer with hemorrhage, without mention of obstruction — (Use additional E code to identify drug, if drug induced)
531.41 Chronic or unspecified gastric ulcer with hemorrhage and obstruction — (Use additional E code to identify drug, if drug induced)
531.50 Chronic or unspecified gastric ulcer with perforation, without mention of obstruction — (Use additional E code to identify drug, if drug induced)
531.51 Chronic or unspecified gastric ulcer with perforation and obstruction — (Use additional E code to identify drug, if drug induced)
531.60 Chronic or unspecified gastric ulcer with hemorrhage and perforation, without mention of obstruction — (Use additional E code to identify drug, if drug induced)
531.61 Chronic or unspecified gastric ulcer with hemorrhage, perforation, and obstruction — (Use additional E code to identify drug, if drug induced)
531.70 Chronic gastric ulcer without mention of hemorrhage, perforation, without mention of obstruction — (Use additional E code to identify drug, if drug induced)
531.71 Chronic gastric ulcer without mention of hemorrhage or perforation, with obstruction — (Use additional E code to identify drug, if drug induced)
531.90 Gastric ulcer, unspecified as acute or chronic, without mention of hemorrhage, perforation, or obstruction — (Use additional E code to identify drug, if drug induced) ▽
531.91 Gastric ulcer, unspecified as acute or chronic, without mention of hemorrhage or perforation, with obstruction — (Use additional E code to identify drug, if drug induced) ▽
532.00 Acute duodenal ulcer with hemorrhage, without mention of obstruction — (Use additional E code to identify drug, if drug induced)
532.01 Acute duodenal ulcer with hemorrhage and obstruction — (Use additional E code to identify drug, if drug induced)
532.10 Acute duodenal ulcer with perforation, without mention of obstruction — (Use additional E code to identify drug, if drug induced)
532.11 Acute duodenal ulcer with perforation and obstruction — (Use additional E code to identify drug, if drug induced)
532.20 Acute duodenal ulcer with hemorrhage and perforation, without mention of obstruction — (Use additional E code to identify drug, if drug induced)
532.21 Acute duodenal ulcer with hemorrhage, perforation, and obstruction — (Use additional E code to identify drug, if drug induced)
532.30 Acute duodenal ulcer without mention of hemorrhage, perforation, or obstruction — (Use additional E code to identify drug, if drug induced)
532.31 Acute duodenal ulcer without mention of hemorrhage or perforation, with obstruction — (Use additional E code to identify drug, if drug induced)
532.40 Chronic or unspecified duodenal ulcer with hemorrhage, without mention of obstruction — (Use additional E code to identify drug, if drug induced)
532.41 Chronic or unspecified duodenal ulcer with hemorrhage and obstruction — (Use additional E code to identify drug, if drug induced)
532.50 Chronic or unspecified duodenal ulcer with perforation, without mention of obstruction — (Use additional E code to identify drug, if drug induced)
532.51 Chronic or unspecified duodenal ulcer with perforation and obstruction — (Use additional E code to identify drug, if drug induced)
532.60 Chronic or unspecified duodenal ulcer with hemorrhage and perforation, without mention of obstruction — (Use additional E code to identify drug, if drug induced)
532.61 Chronic or unspecified duodenal ulcer with hemorrhage, perforation, and obstruction — (Use additional E code to identify drug, if drug induced)
532.70 Chronic duodenal ulcer without mention of hemorrhage, perforation, or obstruction — (Use additional E code to identify drug, if drug induced)
532.71 Chronic duodenal ulcer without mention of hemorrhage or perforation, with obstruction — (Use additional E code to identify drug, if drug induced)
532.90 Duodenal ulcer, unspecified as acute or chronic, without hemorrhage, perforation, or obstruction — (Use additional E code to identify drug, if drug induced) ▽
532.91 Duodenal ulcer, unspecified as acute or chronic, without mention of hemorrhage or perforation, with obstruction — (Use additional E code to identify drug, if drug induced) ▽
533.00 Acute peptic ulcer, unspecified site, with hemorrhage, without mention of obstruction — (Use additional E code to identify drug, if drug induced)
533.01 Acute peptic ulcer, unspecified site, with hemorrhage and obstruction — (Use additional E code to identify drug, if drug induced)
533.10 Acute peptic ulcer, unspecified site, with perforation, without mention of obstruction — (Use additional E code to identify drug, if drug induced)
533.11 Acute peptic ulcer, unspecified site, with perforation and obstruction — (Use additional E code to identify drug, if drug induced)

533.20 Acute peptic ulcer, unspecified site, with hemorrhage and perforation, without mention of obstruction — (Use additional E code to identify drug, if drug induced)
533.21 Acute peptic ulcer, unspecified site, with hemorrhage, perforation, and obstruction — (Use additional E code to identify drug, if drug induced)
533.30 Acute peptic ulcer, unspecified site, without mention of hemorrhage, perforation, or obstruction — (Use additional E code to identify drug, if drug induced)
533.31 Acute peptic ulcer, unspecified site, without mention of hemorrhage and perforation, with obstruction — (Use additional E code to identify drug, if drug induced)
533.40 Chronic or unspecified peptic ulcer, unspecified site, with hemorrhage, without mention of obstruction — (Use additional E code to identify drug, if drug induced)
533.41 Chronic or unspecified peptic ulcer, unspecified site, with hemorrhage and obstruction — (Use additional E code to identify drug, if drug induced)
533.50 Chronic or unspecified peptic ulcer, unspecified site, with perforation, without mention of obstruction — (Use additional E code to identify drug, if drug induced)
533.51 Chronic or unspecified peptic ulcer, unspecified site, with perforation and obstruction — (Use additional E code to identify drug, if drug induced)
533.60 Chronic or unspecified peptic ulcer, unspecified site, with hemorrhage and perforation, without mention of obstruction — (Use additional E code to identify drug, if drug induced)
533.61 Chronic or unspecified peptic ulcer, unspecified site, with hemorrhage, perforation, and obstruction — (Use additional E code to identify drug, if drug induced)
533.70 Chronic peptic ulcer, unspecified site, without mention of hemorrhage, perforation, or obstruction — (Use additional E code to identify drug, if drug induced)
533.71 Chronic peptic ulcer of unspecified site without mention of hemorrhage or perforation, with obstruction — (Use additional E code to identify drug, if drug induced)
533.90 Peptic ulcer, unspecified site, unspecified as acute or chronic, without mention of hemorrhage, perforation, or obstruction — (Use additional E code to identify drug, if drug induced) ▽
533.91 Peptic ulcer, unspecified site, unspecified as acute or chronic, without mention of hemorrhage or perforation, with obstruction — (Use additional E code to identify drug, if drug induced) ▽
534.00 Acute gastrojejunal ulcer with hemorrhage, without mention of obstruction
534.01 Acute gastrojejunal ulcer, with hemorrhage and obstruction
534.10 Acute gastrojejunal ulcer with perforation, without mention of obstruction
534.11 Acute gastrojejunal ulcer with perforation and obstruction
534.20 Acute gastrojejunal ulcer with hemorrhage and perforation, without mention of obstruction
534.21 Acute gastrojejunal ulcer with hemorrhage, perforation, and obstruction
534.30 Acute gastrojejunal ulcer without mention of hemorrhage, perforation, or obstruction
534.31 Acute gastrojejunal ulcer without mention of hemorrhage or perforation, with obstruction
534.40 Chronic or unspecified gastrojejunal ulcer with hemorrhage, without mention of obstruction
534.41 Chronic or unspecified gastrojejunal ulcer, with hemorrhage and obstruction
537.0 Acquired hypertrophic pyloric stenosis

ICD-9-CM Procedural

44.01 Truncal vagotomy
44.02 Highly selective vagotomy
44.03 Other selective vagotomy
44.39 Other gastroenterostomy without gastrectomy

43830–43831

43830 Gastrostomy, open; without construction of gastric tube (eg, Stamm procedure) (separate procedure)
43831 neonatal, for feeding

ICD-9-CM Diagnostic

150.1 Malignant neoplasm of thoracic esophagus
150.2 Malignant neoplasm of abdominal esophagus
150.3 Malignant neoplasm of upper third of esophagus
150.4 Malignant neoplasm of middle third of esophagus
150.5 Malignant neoplasm of lower third of esophagus
150.8 Malignant neoplasm of other specified part of esophagus
150.9 Malignant neoplasm of esophagus, unspecified site ▽
151.0 Malignant neoplasm of cardia
151.1 Malignant neoplasm of pylorus
151.2 Malignant neoplasm of pyloric antrum
151.3 Malignant neoplasm of fundus of stomach
151.4 Malignant neoplasm of body of stomach
151.5 Malignant neoplasm of lesser curvature of stomach, unspecified ▽
151.6 Malignant neoplasm of greater curvature of stomach, unspecified ▽
151.8 Malignant neoplasm of other specified sites of stomach
151.9 Malignant neoplasm of stomach, unspecified site ▽
152.0 Malignant neoplasm of duodenum
152.1 Malignant neoplasm of jejunum
152.2 Malignant neoplasm of ileum
161.9 Malignant neoplasm of larynx, unspecified site ▽
197.4 Secondary malignant neoplasm of small intestine including duodenum
197.8 Secondary malignant neoplasm of other digestive organs and spleen
198.89 Secondary malignant neoplasm of other specified sites
211.1 Benign neoplasm of stomach
230.2 Carcinoma in situ of stomach
239.8 Neoplasm of unspecified nature of other specified sites
261 Nutritional marasmus
262 Other severe protein-calorie malnutrition
263.0 Malnutrition of moderate degree
263.1 Malnutrition of mild degree
263.2 Arrested development following protein-calorie malnutrition
263.8 Other protein-calorie malnutrition
276.5 Volume depletion — (Use additional code to identify any associated mental retardation)
307.1 Anorexia nervosa
436 Acute, but ill-defined, cerebrovascular disease — (Use additional code to identify presence of hypertension) ▽
519.00 Unspecified tracheostomy complication ▽
519.01 Infection of tracheostomy — (Use additional code to identify type of infection: 038.0-038.9, 682.1. Use additional code to identify organism: 041.00-041.9)
519.02 Mechanical complication of tracheostomy
519.09 Other tracheostomy complications
530.3 Stricture and stenosis of esophagus
530.4 Perforation of esophagus
530.5 Dyskinesia of esophagus
530.81 Esophageal reflux
531.00 Acute gastric ulcer with hemorrhage, without mention of obstruction — (Use additional E code to identify drug, if drug induced)
531.01 Acute gastric ulcer with hemorrhage and obstruction — (Use additional E code to identify drug, if drug induced)
531.10 Acute gastric ulcer with perforation, without mention of obstruction — (Use additional E code to identify drug, if drug induced)
531.11 Acute gastric ulcer with perforation and obstruction — (Use additional E code to identify drug, if drug induced)
531.20 Acute gastric ulcer with hemorrhage and perforation, without mention of obstruction — (Use additional E code to identify drug, if drug induced)
531.21 Acute gastric ulcer with hemorrhage, perforation, and obstruction — (Use additional E code to identify drug, if drug induced)
531.30 Acute gastric ulcer without mention of hemorrhage, perforation, or obstruction — (Use additional E code to identify drug, if drug induced)
531.31 Acute gastric ulcer without mention of hemorrhage or perforation, with obstruction — (Use additional E code to identify drug, if drug induced)
531.40 Chronic or unspecified gastric ulcer with hemorrhage, without mention of obstruction — (Use additional E code to identify drug, if drug induced)
531.41 Chronic or unspecified gastric ulcer with hemorrhage and obstruction — (Use additional E code to identify drug, if drug induced)
531.50 Chronic or unspecified gastric ulcer with perforation, without mention of obstruction — (Use additional E code to identify drug, if drug induced)
531.51 Chronic or unspecified gastric ulcer with perforation and obstruction — (Use additional E code to identify drug, if drug induced)
531.60 Chronic or unspecified gastric ulcer with hemorrhage and perforation, without mention of obstruction — (Use additional E code to identify drug, if drug induced)
531.61 Chronic or unspecified gastric ulcer with hemorrhage, perforation, and obstruction — (Use additional E code to identify drug, if drug induced)
531.70 Chronic gastric ulcer without mention of hemorrhage, perforation, without mention of obstruction — (Use additional E code to identify drug, if drug induced)
531.71 Chronic gastric ulcer without mention of hemorrhage or perforation, with obstruction — (Use additional E code to identify drug, if drug induced)
531.90 Gastric ulcer, unspecified as acute or chronic, without mention of hemorrhage, perforation, or obstruction — (Use additional E code to identify drug, if drug induced) ▽

531.91 Gastric ulcer, unspecified as acute or chronic, without mention of hemorrhage or perforation, with obstruction — (Use additional E code to identify drug, if drug induced) ▽
532.00 Acute duodenal ulcer with hemorrhage, without mention of obstruction — (Use additional E code to identify drug, if drug induced)
532.01 Acute duodenal ulcer with hemorrhage and obstruction — (Use additional E code to identify drug, if drug induced)
532.10 Acute duodenal ulcer with perforation, without mention of obstruction — (Use additional E code to identify drug, if drug induced)
532.11 Acute duodenal ulcer with perforation and obstruction — (Use additional E code to identify drug, if drug induced)
532.20 Acute duodenal ulcer with hemorrhage and perforation, without mention of obstruction — (Use additional E code to identify drug, if drug induced)
532.21 Acute duodenal ulcer with hemorrhage, perforation, and obstruction — (Use additional E code to identify drug, if drug induced)
532.30 Acute duodenal ulcer without mention of hemorrhage, perforation, or obstruction — (Use additional E code to identify drug, if drug induced)
532.31 Acute duodenal ulcer without mention of hemorrhage or perforation, with obstruction — (Use additional E code to identify drug, if drug induced)
532.40 Chronic or unspecified duodenal ulcer with hemorrhage, without mention of obstruction — (Use additional E code to identify drug, if drug induced)
532.41 Chronic or unspecified duodenal ulcer with hemorrhage and obstruction — (Use additional E code to identify drug, if drug induced)
532.50 Chronic or unspecified duodenal ulcer with perforation, without mention of obstruction — (Use additional E code to identify drug, if drug induced)
532.51 Chronic or unspecified duodenal ulcer with perforation and obstruction — (Use additional E code to identify drug, if drug induced)
532.60 Chronic or unspecified duodenal ulcer with hemorrhage and perforation, without mention of obstruction — (Use additional E code to identify drug, if drug induced)
532.61 Chronic or unspecified duodenal ulcer with hemorrhage, perforation, and obstruction — (Use additional E code to identify drug, if drug induced)
532.70 Chronic duodenal ulcer without mention of hemorrhage, perforation, or obstruction — (Use additional E code to identify drug, if drug induced)
532.71 Chronic duodenal ulcer without mention of hemorrhage or perforation, with obstruction — (Use additional E code to identify drug, if drug induced)
532.90 Duodenal ulcer, unspecified as acute or chronic, without hemorrhage, perforation, or obstruction — (Use additional E code to identify drug, if drug induced) ▽
532.91 Duodenal ulcer, unspecified as acute or chronic, without mention of hemorrhage or perforation, with obstruction — (Use additional E code to identify drug, if drug induced) ▽
533.00 Acute peptic ulcer, unspecified site, with hemorrhage, without mention of obstruction — (Use additional E code to identify drug, if drug induced)
533.01 Acute peptic ulcer, unspecified site, with hemorrhage and obstruction — (Use additional E code to identify drug, if drug induced)
533.10 Acute peptic ulcer, unspecified site, with perforation, without mention of obstruction — (Use additional E code to identify drug, if drug induced)
533.11 Acute peptic ulcer, unspecified site, with perforation and obstruction — (Use additional E code to identify drug, if drug induced)
533.20 Acute peptic ulcer, unspecified site, with hemorrhage and perforation, without mention of obstruction — (Use additional E code to identify drug, if drug induced)
533.21 Acute peptic ulcer, unspecified site, with hemorrhage, perforation, and obstruction — (Use additional E code to identify drug, if drug induced)
533.30 Acute peptic ulcer, unspecified site, without mention of hemorrhage, perforation, or obstruction — (Use additional E code to identify drug, if drug induced)
533.31 Acute peptic ulcer, unspecified site, without mention of hemorrhage and perforation, with obstruction — (Use additional E code to identify drug, if drug induced)
533.40 Chronic or unspecified peptic ulcer, unspecified site, with hemorrhage, without mention of obstruction — (Use additional E code to identify drug, if drug induced)
533.41 Chronic or unspecified peptic ulcer, unspecified site, with hemorrhage and obstruction — (Use additional E code to identify drug, if drug induced)
533.50 Chronic or unspecified peptic ulcer, unspecified site, with perforation, without mention of obstruction — (Use additional E code to identify drug, if drug induced)
533.51 Chronic or unspecified peptic ulcer, unspecified site, with perforation and obstruction — (Use additional E code to identify drug, if drug induced)
535.50 Unspecified gastritis and gastroduodenitis without mention of hemorrhage ▽
536.9 Unspecified functional disorder of stomach ▽
537.89 Other specified disorder of stomach and duodenum
578.9 Unspecified, hemorrhage of gastrointestinal tract ▽
707.9 Chronic ulcer of unspecified site ▽
750.5 Congenital hypertrophic pyloric stenosis
750.7 Other specified congenital anomalies of stomach
751.1 Congenital atresia and stenosis of small intestine
783.0 Anorexia
783.3 Feeding difficulties and mismanagement
783.40 Lack of normal physiological development, unspecified ▽
783.41 Failure to thrive
783.42 Delayed milestones
783.43 Short stature
783.7 Adult failure to thrive
787.01 Nausea with vomiting
787.2 Dysphagia
854.06 Intracranial injury of other and unspecified nature, without mention of open intracranial wound, loss of consciousness of unspecified duration ▽
959.01 Head injury, unspecified ▽
959.19 Other injury of other sites of trunk
994.2 Effects of hunger
997.4 Digestive system complication — (Use additional code to identify complications)
V64.41 Laparoscopic surgical procedure converted to open procedure

ICD-9-CM Procedural

43.19 Other gastrostomy

43832

43832 Gastrostomy, open; with construction of gastric tube (eg, Janeway procedure)

ICD-9-CM Diagnostic

146.2 Malignant neoplasm of tonsillar pillars (anterior) (posterior)
146.3 Malignant neoplasm of vallecula
146.5 Malignant neoplasm of junctional region of oropharynx
146.6 Malignant neoplasm of lateral wall of oropharynx
146.7 Malignant neoplasm of posterior wall of oropharynx
146.8 Malignant neoplasm of other specified sites of oropharynx
146.9 Malignant neoplasm of oropharynx, unspecified site ▽
148.0 Malignant neoplasm of postcricoid region of hypopharynx
148.1 Malignant neoplasm of pyriform sinus
148.3 Malignant neoplasm of posterior hypopharyngeal wall
148.8 Malignant neoplasm of other specified sites of hypopharynx
148.9 Malignant neoplasm of hypopharynx, unspecified site ▽
150.0 Malignant neoplasm of cervical esophagus
150.1 Malignant neoplasm of thoracic esophagus
150.2 Malignant neoplasm of abdominal esophagus
150.3 Malignant neoplasm of upper third of esophagus
150.4 Malignant neoplasm of middle third of esophagus
150.5 Malignant neoplasm of lower third of esophagus
150.8 Malignant neoplasm of other specified part of esophagus
150.9 Malignant neoplasm of esophagus, unspecified site ▽
151.0 Malignant neoplasm of cardia
151.1 Malignant neoplasm of pylorus
151.2 Malignant neoplasm of pyloric antrum
151.3 Malignant neoplasm of fundus of stomach
151.4 Malignant neoplasm of body of stomach
151.5 Malignant neoplasm of lesser curvature of stomach, unspecified ▽
151.8 Malignant neoplasm of other specified sites of stomach
151.9 Malignant neoplasm of stomach, unspecified site ▽
197.8 Secondary malignant neoplasm of other digestive organs and spleen
198.89 Secondary malignant neoplasm of other specified sites
211.1 Benign neoplasm of stomach
230.2 Carcinoma in situ of stomach
531.00 Acute gastric ulcer with hemorrhage, without mention of obstruction — (Use additional E code to identify drug, if drug induced)
531.01 Acute gastric ulcer with hemorrhage and obstruction — (Use additional E code to identify drug, if drug induced)
531.10 Acute gastric ulcer with perforation, without mention of obstruction — (Use additional E code to identify drug, if drug induced)
531.11 Acute gastric ulcer with perforation and obstruction — (Use additional E code to identify drug, if drug induced)
531.20 Acute gastric ulcer with hemorrhage and perforation, without mention of obstruction — (Use additional E code to identify drug, if drug induced)
531.21 Acute gastric ulcer with hemorrhage, perforation, and obstruction — (Use additional E code to identify drug, if drug induced)
531.30 Acute gastric ulcer without mention of hemorrhage, perforation, or obstruction — (Use additional E code to identify drug, if drug induced)
531.31 Acute gastric ulcer without mention of hemorrhage or perforation, with obstruction — (Use additional E code to identify drug, if drug induced)

531.40 Chronic or unspecified gastric ulcer with hemorrhage, without mention of obstruction — (Use additional E code to identify drug, if drug induced)
531.41 Chronic or unspecified gastric ulcer with hemorrhage and obstruction — (Use additional E code to identify drug, if drug induced)
531.50 Chronic or unspecified gastric ulcer with perforation, without mention of obstruction — (Use additional E code to identify drug, if drug induced)
531.51 Chronic or unspecified gastric ulcer with perforation and obstruction — (Use additional E code to identify drug, if drug induced)
531.60 Chronic or unspecified gastric ulcer with hemorrhage and perforation, without mention of obstruction — (Use additional E code to identify drug, if drug induced)
531.61 Chronic or unspecified gastric ulcer with hemorrhage, perforation, and obstruction — (Use additional E code to identify drug, if drug induced)
531.70 Chronic gastric ulcer without mention of hemorrhage, perforation, without mention of obstruction — (Use additional E code to identify drug, if drug induced)
531.71 Chronic gastric ulcer without mention of hemorrhage or perforation, with obstruction — (Use additional E code to identify drug, if drug induced)
531.90 Gastric ulcer, unspecified as acute or chronic, without mention of hemorrhage, perforation, or obstruction — (Use additional E code to identify drug, if drug induced) ▽
531.91 Gastric ulcer, unspecified as acute or chronic, without mention of hemorrhage or perforation, with obstruction — (Use additional E code to identify drug, if drug induced) ▽
533.00 Acute peptic ulcer, unspecified site, with hemorrhage, without mention of obstruction — (Use additional E code to identify drug, if drug induced)
533.01 Acute peptic ulcer, unspecified site, with hemorrhage and obstruction — (Use additional E code to identify drug, if drug induced)
533.10 Acute peptic ulcer, unspecified site, with perforation, without mention of obstruction — (Use additional E code to identify drug, if drug induced)
533.11 Acute peptic ulcer, unspecified site, with perforation and obstruction — (Use additional E code to identify drug, if drug induced)
533.20 Acute peptic ulcer, unspecified site, with hemorrhage and perforation, without mention of obstruction — (Use additional E code to identify drug, if drug induced)
533.21 Acute peptic ulcer, unspecified site, with hemorrhage, perforation, and obstruction — (Use additional E code to identify drug, if drug induced)
533.30 Acute peptic ulcer, unspecified site, without mention of hemorrhage, perforation, or obstruction — (Use additional E code to identify drug, if drug induced)
533.31 Acute peptic ulcer, unspecified site, without mention of hemorrhage and perforation, with obstruction — (Use additional E code to identify drug, if drug induced)
533.40 Chronic or unspecified peptic ulcer, unspecified site, with hemorrhage, without mention of obstruction — (Use additional E code to identify drug, if drug induced)
533.41 Chronic or unspecified peptic ulcer, unspecified site, with hemorrhage and obstruction — (Use additional E code to identify drug, if drug induced)
533.50 Chronic or unspecified peptic ulcer, unspecified site, with perforation, without mention of obstruction — (Use additional E code to identify drug, if drug induced)
533.51 Chronic or unspecified peptic ulcer, unspecified site, with perforation and obstruction — (Use additional E code to identify drug, if drug induced)
533.60 Chronic or unspecified peptic ulcer, unspecified site, with hemorrhage and perforation, without mention of obstruction — (Use additional E code to identify drug, if drug induced)
533.61 Chronic or unspecified peptic ulcer, unspecified site, with hemorrhage, perforation, and obstruction — (Use additional E code to identify drug, if drug induced)
533.70 Chronic peptic ulcer, unspecified site, without mention of hemorrhage, perforation, or obstruction — (Use additional E code to identify drug, if drug induced)
533.71 Chronic peptic ulcer of unspecified site without mention of hemorrhage or perforation, with obstruction — (Use additional E code to identify drug, if drug induced)
533.90 Peptic ulcer, unspecified site, unspecified as acute or chronic, without mention of hemorrhage, perforation, or obstruction — (Use additional E code to identify drug, if drug induced) ▽
533.91 Peptic ulcer, unspecified site, unspecified as acute or chronic, without mention of hemorrhage or perforation, with obstruction — (Use additional E code to identify drug, if drug induced) ▽
V64.41 Laparoscopic surgical procedure converted to open procedure

ICD-9-CM Procedural

43.19 Other gastrostomy

43840

43840 Gastrorrhaphy, suture of perforated duodenal or gastric ulcer, wound, or injury

ICD-9-CM Diagnostic

531.10 Acute gastric ulcer with perforation, without mention of obstruction — (Use additional E code to identify drug, if drug induced)
531.11 Acute gastric ulcer with perforation and obstruction — (Use additional E code to identify drug, if drug induced)
531.20 Acute gastric ulcer with hemorrhage and perforation, without mention of obstruction — (Use additional E code to identify drug, if drug induced)
531.21 Acute gastric ulcer with hemorrhage, perforation, and obstruction — (Use additional E code to identify drug, if drug induced)
531.50 Chronic or unspecified gastric ulcer with perforation, without mention of obstruction — (Use additional E code to identify drug, if drug induced)
531.51 Chronic or unspecified gastric ulcer with perforation and obstruction — (Use additional E code to identify drug, if drug induced)
531.60 Chronic or unspecified gastric ulcer with hemorrhage and perforation, without mention of obstruction — (Use additional E code to identify drug, if drug induced)
531.61 Chronic or unspecified gastric ulcer with hemorrhage, perforation, and obstruction — (Use additional E code to identify drug, if drug induced)
532.10 Acute duodenal ulcer with perforation, without mention of obstruction — (Use additional E code to identify drug, if drug induced)
532.11 Acute duodenal ulcer with perforation and obstruction — (Use additional E code to identify drug, if drug induced)
532.20 Acute duodenal ulcer with hemorrhage and perforation, without mention of obstruction — (Use additional E code to identify drug, if drug induced)
532.21 Acute duodenal ulcer with hemorrhage, perforation, and obstruction — (Use additional E code to identify drug, if drug induced)
532.50 Chronic or unspecified duodenal ulcer with perforation, without mention of obstruction — (Use additional E code to identify drug, if drug induced)
532.51 Chronic or unspecified duodenal ulcer with perforation and obstruction — (Use additional E code to identify drug, if drug induced)
532.60 Chronic or unspecified duodenal ulcer with hemorrhage and perforation, without mention of obstruction — (Use additional E code to identify drug, if drug induced)
532.61 Chronic or unspecified duodenal ulcer with hemorrhage, perforation, and obstruction — (Use additional E code to identify drug, if drug induced)
533.10 Acute peptic ulcer, unspecified site, with perforation, without mention of obstruction — (Use additional E code to identify drug, if drug induced)
533.20 Acute peptic ulcer, unspecified site, with hemorrhage and perforation, without mention of obstruction — (Use additional E code to identify drug, if drug induced)
533.21 Acute peptic ulcer, unspecified site, with hemorrhage, perforation, and obstruction — (Use additional E code to identify drug, if drug induced)
533.50 Chronic or unspecified peptic ulcer, unspecified site, with perforation, without mention of obstruction — (Use additional E code to identify drug, if drug induced)
533.51 Chronic or unspecified peptic ulcer, unspecified site, with perforation and obstruction — (Use additional E code to identify drug, if drug induced)
533.60 Chronic or unspecified peptic ulcer, unspecified site, with hemorrhage and perforation, without mention of obstruction — (Use additional E code to identify drug, if drug induced)
533.61 Chronic or unspecified peptic ulcer, unspecified site, with hemorrhage, perforation, and obstruction — (Use additional E code to identify drug, if drug induced)
534.10 Acute gastrojejunal ulcer with perforation, without mention of obstruction
534.11 Acute gastrojejunal ulcer with perforation and obstruction
534.20 Acute gastrojejunal ulcer with hemorrhage and perforation, without mention of obstruction
534.21 Acute gastrojejunal ulcer with hemorrhage, perforation, and obstruction
534.50 Chronic or unspecified gastrojejunal ulcer with perforation, without mention of obstruction
534.51 Chronic or unspecified gastrojejunal ulcer with perforation and obstruction
534.60 Chronic or unspecified gastrojejunal ulcer with hemorrhage and perforation, without mention of obstruction
534.61 Chronic or unspecified gastrojejunal ulcer with hemorrhage, perforation, and obstruction
535.00 Acute gastritis without mention of hemorrhage
535.01 Acute gastritis with hemorrhage
535.10 Atrophic gastritis without mention of hemorrhage
535.11 Atrophic gastritis with hemorrhage
535.20 Gastric mucosal hypertrophy without mention of hemorrhage
535.21 Gastric mucosal hypertrophy with hemorrhage
535.30 Alcoholic gastritis without mention of hemorrhage
535.31 Alcoholic gastritis with hemorrhage

535.40 Other specified gastritis without mention of hemorrhage
535.41 Other specified gastritis with hemorrhage
535.60 Duodenitis without mention of hemorrhage
535.61 Duodenitis with hemorrhage
536.0 Achlorhydria
536.1 Acute dilatation of stomach
536.2 Persistent vomiting
536.3 Gastroparesis
536.8 Dyspepsia and other specified disorders of function of stomach
537.4 Fistula of stomach or duodenum
537.84 Dieulafoy lesion (hemorrhagic) of stomach and duodenum
537.89 Other specified disorder of stomach and duodenum
569.83 Perforation of intestine
578.9 Unspecified, hemorrhage of gastrointestinal tract
863.1 Stomach injury with open wound into cavity

ICD-9-CM Procedural

44.41 Suture of gastric ulcer site
44.42 Suture of duodenal ulcer site
44.61 Suture of laceration of stomach

43842–43843

43842 Gastric restrictive procedure, without gastric bypass, for morbid obesity; vertical-banded gastroplasty
43843 other than vertical-banded gastroplasty

ICD-9-CM Diagnostic

244.9 Unspecified hypothyroidism
253.8 Other disorders of the pituitary and other syndromes of diencephalohypophyseal origin
255.8 Other specified disorders of adrenal glands
259.9 Unspecified endocrine disorder
278.00 Obesity, unspecified — (Use additional code to identify any associated mental retardation)
278.01 Morbid obesity — (Use additional code to identify any associated mental retardation)

ICD-9-CM Procedural

44.69 Other repair of stomach

43845

43845 Gastric restrictive procedure with partial gastrectomy, pylorus-preserving duodenoileostomy and ileoileostomy (50 to 100 cm common channel) to limit absorption (biliopancreatic diversion with duodenal switch)

ICD-9-CM Diagnostic

244.9 Unspecified hypothyroidism
253.8 Other disorders of the pituitary and other syndromes of diencephalohypophyseal origin
255.8 Other specified disorders of adrenal glands
259.9 Unspecified endocrine disorder
278.00 Obesity, unspecified — (Use additional code to identify any associated mental retardation)
278.01 Morbid obesity — (Use additional code to identify any associated mental retardation)

ICD-9-CM Procedural

43.89 Other partial gastrectomy
45.51 Isolation of segment of small intestine
45.91 Small-to-small intestinal anastomosis

43846–43847

43846 Gastric restrictive procedure, with gastric bypass for morbid obesity; with short limb (150 cm or less) Roux-en-Y gastroenterostomy
43847 with small intestine reconstruction to limit absorption

ICD-9-CM Diagnostic

244.9 Unspecified hypothyroidism
253.8 Other disorders of the pituitary and other syndromes of diencephalohypophyseal origin
255.8 Other specified disorders of adrenal glands
259.9 Unspecified endocrine disorder
278.00 Obesity, unspecified — (Use additional code to identify any associated mental retardation)
278.01 Morbid obesity — (Use additional code to identify any associated mental retardation)

ICD-9-CM Procedural

44.31 High gastric bypass

43848

43848 Revision of gastric restrictive procedure for morbid obesity (separate procedure)

ICD-9-CM Diagnostic

278.01 Morbid obesity — (Use additional code to identify any associated mental retardation)
564.2 Postgastric surgery syndromes
997.4 Digestive system complication — (Use additional code to identify complications)
998.59 Other postoperative infection — (Use additional code to identify infection)
998.89 Other specified complications
V45.3 Intestinal bypass or anastomosis status — (This code is intended for use when these conditions are recorded as diagnoses or problems)

ICD-9-CM Procedural

44.5 Revision of gastric anastomosis

43850–43855

43850 Revision of gastroduodenal anastomosis (gastroduodenostomy) with reconstruction; without vagotomy
43855 with vagotomy

ICD-9-CM Diagnostic

151.9 Malignant neoplasm of stomach, unspecified site
152.0 Malignant neoplasm of duodenum
152.1 Malignant neoplasm of jejunum
152.2 Malignant neoplasm of ileum
152.3 Malignant neoplasm of Meckel's diverticulum
152.8 Malignant neoplasm of other specified sites of small intestine
152.9 Malignant neoplasm of small intestine, unspecified site
197.8 Secondary malignant neoplasm of other digestive organs and spleen
211.1 Benign neoplasm of stomach
230.2 Carcinoma in situ of stomach
531.00 Acute gastric ulcer with hemorrhage, without mention of obstruction — (Use additional E code to identify drug, if drug induced)
531.10 Acute gastric ulcer with perforation, without mention of obstruction — (Use additional E code to identify drug, if drug induced)
531.11 Acute gastric ulcer with perforation and obstruction — (Use additional E code to identify drug, if drug induced)
531.20 Acute gastric ulcer with hemorrhage and perforation, without mention of obstruction — (Use additional E code to identify drug, if drug induced)
531.21 Acute gastric ulcer with hemorrhage, perforation, and obstruction — (Use additional E code to identify drug, if drug induced)
531.50 Chronic or unspecified gastric ulcer with perforation, without mention of obstruction — (Use additional E code to identify drug, if drug induced)
531.51 Chronic or unspecified gastric ulcer with perforation and obstruction — (Use additional E code to identify drug, if drug induced)
531.60 Chronic or unspecified gastric ulcer with hemorrhage and perforation, without mention of obstruction — (Use additional E code to identify drug, if drug induced)
531.61 Chronic or unspecified gastric ulcer with hemorrhage, perforation, and obstruction — (Use additional E code to identify drug, if drug induced)
532.00 Acute duodenal ulcer with hemorrhage, without mention of obstruction — (Use additional E code to identify drug, if drug induced)
532.10 Acute duodenal ulcer with perforation, without mention of obstruction — (Use additional E code to identify drug, if drug induced)
532.20 Acute duodenal ulcer with hemorrhage and perforation, without mention of obstruction — (Use additional E code to identify drug, if drug induced)
533.10 Acute peptic ulcer, unspecified site, with perforation, without mention of obstruction — (Use additional E code to identify drug, if drug induced)
533.11 Acute peptic ulcer, unspecified site, with perforation and obstruction — (Use additional E code to identify drug, if drug induced)
533.20 Acute peptic ulcer, unspecified site, with hemorrhage and perforation, without mention of obstruction — (Use additional E code to identify drug, if drug induced)
533.21 Acute peptic ulcer, unspecified site, with hemorrhage, perforation, and obstruction — (Use additional E code to identify drug, if drug induced)
533.50 Chronic or unspecified peptic ulcer, unspecified site, with perforation, without mention of obstruction — (Use additional E code to identify drug, if drug induced)

533.51 Chronic or unspecified peptic ulcer, unspecified site, with perforation and obstruction — (Use additional E code to identify drug, if drug induced)
533.60 Chronic or unspecified peptic ulcer, unspecified site, with hemorrhage and perforation, without mention of obstruction — (Use additional E code to identify drug, if drug induced)
533.61 Chronic or unspecified peptic ulcer, unspecified site, with hemorrhage, perforation, and obstruction — (Use additional E code to identify drug, if drug induced)
537.2 Chronic duodenal ileus
537.3 Other obstruction of duodenum
537.81 Pylorospasm
537.82 Angiodysplasia of stomach and duodenum (without mention of hemorrhage)
537.83 Angiodysplasia of stomach and duodenum with hemorrhage
537.89 Other specified disorder of stomach and duodenum
564.2 Postgastric surgery syndromes

ICD-9-CM Procedural

44.00 Vagotomy, not otherwise specified
44.01 Truncal vagotomy
44.02 Highly selective vagotomy
44.03 Other selective vagotomy
44.5 Revision of gastric anastomosis

43860–43865

43860 Revision of gastrojejunal anastomosis (gastrojejunostomy) with reconstruction, with or without partial gastrectomy or intestine resection; without vagotomy
43865 with vagotomy

ICD-9-CM Diagnostic

152.0 Malignant neoplasm of duodenum
197.4 Secondary malignant neoplasm of small intestine including duodenum
211.2 Benign neoplasm of duodenum, jejunum, and ileum
230.7 Carcinoma in situ of other and unspecified parts of intestine ▽
531.10 Acute gastric ulcer with perforation, without mention of obstruction — (Use additional E code to identify drug, if drug induced)
531.11 Acute gastric ulcer with perforation and obstruction — (Use additional E code to identify drug, if drug induced)
531.20 Acute gastric ulcer with hemorrhage and perforation, without mention of obstruction — (Use additional E code to identify drug, if drug induced)
531.21 Acute gastric ulcer with hemorrhage, perforation, and obstruction — (Use additional E code to identify drug, if drug induced)
531.50 Chronic or unspecified gastric ulcer with perforation, without mention of obstruction — (Use additional E code to identify drug, if drug induced)
531.51 Chronic or unspecified gastric ulcer with perforation and obstruction — (Use additional E code to identify drug, if drug induced)
531.61 Chronic or unspecified gastric ulcer with hemorrhage, perforation, and obstruction — (Use additional E code to identify drug, if drug induced)
533.10 Acute peptic ulcer, unspecified site, with perforation, without mention of obstruction — (Use additional E code to identify drug, if drug induced)
533.11 Acute peptic ulcer, unspecified site, with perforation and obstruction — (Use additional E code to identify drug, if drug induced)
533.20 Acute peptic ulcer, unspecified site, with hemorrhage and perforation, without mention of obstruction — (Use additional E code to identify drug, if drug induced)
533.21 Acute peptic ulcer, unspecified site, with hemorrhage, perforation, and obstruction — (Use additional E code to identify drug, if drug induced)
533.50 Chronic or unspecified peptic ulcer, unspecified site, with perforation, without mention of obstruction — (Use additional E code to identify drug, if drug induced)
533.51 Chronic or unspecified peptic ulcer, unspecified site, with perforation and obstruction — (Use additional E code to identify drug, if drug induced)
533.60 Chronic or unspecified peptic ulcer, unspecified site, with hemorrhage and perforation, without mention of obstruction — (Use additional E code to identify drug, if drug induced)
533.61 Chronic or unspecified peptic ulcer, unspecified site, with hemorrhage, perforation, and obstruction — (Use additional E code to identify drug, if drug induced)
534.00 Acute gastrojejunal ulcer with hemorrhage, without mention of obstruction
534.10 Acute gastrojejunal ulcer with perforation, without mention of obstruction
534.20 Acute gastrojejunal ulcer with hemorrhage and perforation, without mention of obstruction
534.30 Acute gastrojejunal ulcer without mention of hemorrhage, perforation, or obstruction
534.50 Chronic or unspecified gastrojejunal ulcer with perforation, without mention of obstruction
534.60 Chronic or unspecified gastrojejunal ulcer with hemorrhage and perforation, without mention of obstruction
534.70 Chronic gastrojejunal ulcer without mention of hemorrhage, perforation, or obstruction
560.81 Intestinal or peritoneal adhesions with obstruction (postoperative) (postinfection)
564.2 Postgastric surgery syndromes
997.4 Digestive system complication — (Use additional code to identify complications)

ICD-9-CM Procedural

43.7 Partial gastrectomy with anastomosis to jejunum
44.00 Vagotomy, not otherwise specified
44.01 Truncal vagotomy
44.02 Highly selective vagotomy
44.03 Other selective vagotomy
44.39 Other gastroenterostomy without gastrectomy

43870

43870 Closure of gastrostomy, surgical

ICD-9-CM Diagnostic

536.40 Unspecified gastrostomy complication ▽
536.41 Infection of gastrostomy — (Use additional code to specify type of infection: 038.0-038.9, 041.00-041.9. Use additional code to identify organism: 041.00-041.9)
536.42 Mechanical complication of gastrostomy
536.49 Other gastrostomy complications
V10.00 Personal history of malignant neoplasm of unspecified site in gastrointestinal tract ▽
V10.01 Personal history of malignant neoplasm of tongue
V10.02 Personal history of malignant neoplasm of other and unspecified parts of oral cavity and pharynx ▽
V10.04 Personal history of malignant neoplasm of stomach
V10.21 Personal history of malignant neoplasm of larynx
V55.1 Attention to gastrostomy

ICD-9-CM Procedural

44.62 Closure of gastrostomy

43880

43880 Closure of gastrocolic fistula

ICD-9-CM Diagnostic

537.4 Fistula of stomach or duodenum

ICD-9-CM Procedural

44.63 Closure of other gastric fistula

Intestines (Except Rectum)

44005

44005 Enterolysis (freeing of intestinal adhesion) (separate procedure)

ICD-9-CM Diagnostic

537.3 Other obstruction of duodenum
560.81 Intestinal or peritoneal adhesions with obstruction (postoperative) (postinfection)
560.9 Unspecified intestinal obstruction ▽
567.2 Other suppurative peritonitis
568.0 Peritoneal adhesions (postoperative) (postinfection)
568.81 Hemoperitoneum (nontraumatic)
569.81 Fistula of intestine, excluding rectum and anus
569.83 Perforation of intestine
569.9 Unspecified disorder of intestine ▽
614.6 Pelvic peritoneal adhesions, female (postoperative) (postinfection) — (Use additional code to identify any associated infertility, 628.2. Use additional code to identify organism: 041.0, 041.1) ♀
628.2 Female infertility of tubal origin — (Use additional code for any associated peritubal adhesions, 614.6) ♀
789.00 Abdominal pain, unspecified site ▽
789.01 Abdominal pain, right upper quadrant
789.02 Abdominal pain, left upper quadrant

▽ Unspecified code ♀ Female diagnosis ☒ Manifestation code ♂ Male diagnosis

Large Intestine

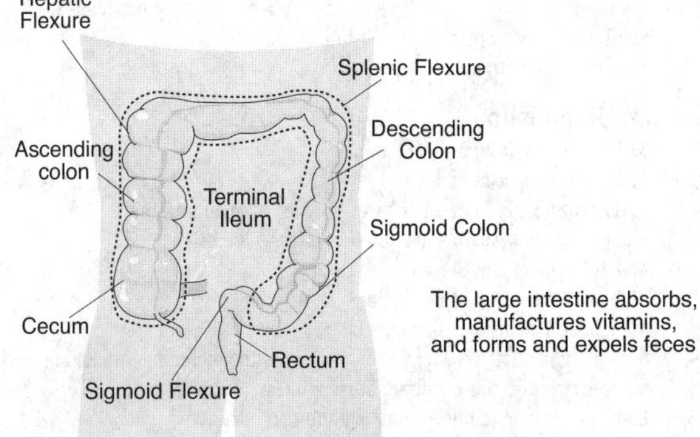

The large intestine absorbs, manufactures vitamins, and forms and expels feces

789.03 Abdominal pain, right lower quadrant
789.04 Abdominal pain, left lower quadrant
789.05 Abdominal pain, periumbilic
789.06 Abdominal pain, epigastric
789.07 Abdominal pain, generalized
789.09 Abdominal pain, other specified site
789.30 Abdominal or pelvic swelling, mass or lump, unspecified site ▽
789.31 Abdominal or pelvic swelling, mass, or lump, right upper quadrant
789.32 Abdominal or pelvic swelling, mass, or lump, left upper quadrant
789.33 Abdominal or pelvic swelling, mass, or lump, right lower quadrant
789.34 Abdominal or pelvic swelling, mass, or lump, left lower quadrant
789.35 Abdominal or pelvic swelling, mass or lump, periumbilic
789.36 Abdominal or pelvic swelling, mass, or lump, epigastric
789.37 Abdominal or pelvic swelling, mass, or lump, epigastric, generalized
789.39 Abdominal or pelvic swelling, mass, or lump, other specified site
997.4 Digestive system complication — (Use additional code to identify complications)
V45.72 Acquired absence of intestine (large) (small) — (This code is intended for use when these conditions are recorded as diagnoses or problems)
V64.41 Laparoscopic surgical procedure converted to open procedure

ICD-9-CM Procedural

54.59 Other lysis of peritoneal adhesions

44010

44010 Duodenotomy, for exploration, biopsy(s), or foreign body removal

ICD-9-CM Diagnostic

152.0 Malignant neoplasm of duodenum
197.4 Secondary malignant neoplasm of small intestine including duodenum
211.2 Benign neoplasm of duodenum, jejunum, and ileum
230.7 Carcinoma in situ of other and unspecified parts of intestine ▽
235.2 Neoplasm of uncertain behavior of stomach, intestines, and rectum
239.0 Neoplasm of unspecified nature of digestive system
936 Foreign body in intestine and colon

ICD-9-CM Procedural

45.01 Incision of duodenum
45.15 Open biopsy of small intestine

44015

44015 Tube or needle catheter jejunostomy for enteral alimentation, intraoperative, any method (List separately in addition to primary procedure)

ICD-9-CM Diagnostic

This is an add-on code. Refer to the corresponding primary procedure code for ICD-9 diagnosis code links.

ICD-9-CM Procedural

45.02 Other incision of small intestine
97.03 Replacement of tube or enterostomy device of small intestine

44020

44020 Enterotomy, small intestine, other than duodenum; for exploration, biopsy(s), or foreign body removal

ICD-9-CM Diagnostic

152.1 Malignant neoplasm of jejunum
152.2 Malignant neoplasm of ileum
197.4 Secondary malignant neoplasm of small intestine including duodenum
211.2 Benign neoplasm of duodenum, jejunum, and ileum
230.7 Carcinoma in situ of other and unspecified parts of intestine ▽
235.2 Neoplasm of uncertain behavior of stomach, intestines, and rectum
239.0 Neoplasm of unspecified nature of digestive system
560.31 Gallstone ileus
936 Foreign body in intestine and colon

ICD-9-CM Procedural

45.02 Other incision of small intestine
45.15 Open biopsy of small intestine

44021

44021 Enterotomy, small intestine, other than duodenum; for decompression (eg, Baker tube)

ICD-9-CM Diagnostic

152.1 Malignant neoplasm of jejunum
152.2 Malignant neoplasm of ileum
552.8 Hernia of other specified site, with obstruction
555.0 Regional enteritis of small intestine
560.1 Paralytic ileus
560.31 Gallstone ileus
560.81 Intestinal or peritoneal adhesions with obstruction (postoperative) (postinfection)
560.89 Other specified intestinal obstruction
560.9 Unspecified intestinal obstruction ▽
564.2 Postgastric surgery syndromes

ICD-9-CM Procedural

45.02 Other incision of small intestine

44025

44025 Colotomy, for exploration, biopsy(s), or foreign body removal

ICD-9-CM Diagnostic

153.0 Malignant neoplasm of hepatic flexure
153.1 Malignant neoplasm of transverse colon
153.2 Malignant neoplasm of descending colon
153.4 Malignant neoplasm of cecum
153.5 Malignant neoplasm of appendix
197.5 Secondary malignant neoplasm of large intestine and rectum
211.3 Benign neoplasm of colon
556.0 Ulcerative (chronic) enterocolitis
556.2 Ulcerative (chronic) proctitis
556.3 Ulcerative (chronic) proctosigmoiditis
556.4 Pseudopolyposis of colon
556.5 Left sided ulcerative (chronic) colitis
556.6 Universal ulcerative (chronic) colitis
556.8 Other ulcerative colitis
556.9 Unspecified ulcerative colitis ▽
560.81 Intestinal or peritoneal adhesions with obstruction (postoperative) (postinfection)
751.3 Hirschsprung's disease and other congenital functional disorders of colon
936 Foreign body in intestine and colon

ICD-9-CM Procedural

45.03 Incision of large intestine
45.26 Open biopsy of large intestine

44050–44055

44050 Reduction of volvulus, intussusception, internal hernia, by laparotomy
44055 Correction of malrotation by lysis of duodenal bands and/or reduction of midgut volvulus (eg, Ladd procedure)

ICD-9-CM Diagnostic

152.1 Malignant neoplasm of jejunum
152.2 Malignant neoplasm of ileum
152.3 Malignant neoplasm of Meckel's diverticulum
152.8 Malignant neoplasm of other specified sites of small intestine
152.9 Malignant neoplasm of small intestine, unspecified site ▽
153.0 Malignant neoplasm of hepatic flexure
153.1 Malignant neoplasm of transverse colon
153.2 Malignant neoplasm of descending colon

153.3 Malignant neoplasm of sigmoid colon
153.4 Malignant neoplasm of cecum
211.2 Benign neoplasm of duodenum, jejunum, and ileum
211.3 Benign neoplasm of colon
537.3 Other obstruction of duodenum
550.10 Inguinal hernia with obstruction, without mention of gangrene, unilateral or unspecified, (not specified as recurrent)
550.11 Inguinal hernia with obstruction, without mention of gangrene, recurrent unilateral or unspecified
550.12 Inguinal hernia with obstruction, without mention gangrene, bilateral, (not specified as recurrent)
550.90 Inguinal hernia without mention of obstruction or gangrene, unilateral or unspecified, (not specified as recurrent)
551.20 Unspecified ventral hernia with gangrene ▽
551.21 Incisional ventral hernia, with gangrene
552.00 Unilateral or unspecified femoral hernia with obstruction
552.8 Hernia of other specified site, with obstruction
552.9 Hernia of unspecified site, with obstruction ▽
553.1 Umbilical hernia without mention of obstruction or gangrene
553.8 Hernia of other specified sites of abdominal cavity without mention of obstruction or gangrene
553.9 Hernia of unspecified site of abdominal cavity without mention of obstruction or gangrene ▽
560.0 Intussusception
560.1 Paralytic ileus
560.2 Volvulus
560.81 Intestinal or peritoneal adhesions with obstruction (postoperative) (postinfection)
560.89 Other specified intestinal obstruction
560.9 Unspecified intestinal obstruction ▽
568.0 Peritoneal adhesions (postoperative) (postinfection)
751.1 Congenital atresia and stenosis of small intestine
751.4 Congenital anomalies of intestinal fixation

ICD-9-CM Procedural

46.81 Intra-abdominal manipulation of small intestine
46.82 Intra-abdominal manipulation of large intestine
54.95 Incision of peritoneum

44100

44100 Biopsy of intestine by capsule, tube, peroral (one or more specimens)

ICD-9-CM Diagnostic

152.0 Malignant neoplasm of duodenum
152.1 Malignant neoplasm of jejunum
152.2 Malignant neoplasm of ileum
152.8 Malignant neoplasm of other specified sites of small intestine
152.9 Malignant neoplasm of small intestine, unspecified site ▽
197.4 Secondary malignant neoplasm of small intestine including duodenum
211.2 Benign neoplasm of duodenum, jejunum, and ileum
230.7 Carcinoma in situ of other and unspecified parts of intestine ▽
235.2 Neoplasm of uncertain behavior of stomach, intestines, and rectum
239.0 Neoplasm of unspecified nature of digestive system
556.0 Ulcerative (chronic) enterocolitis
556.2 Ulcerative (chronic) proctitis
556.3 Ulcerative (chronic) proctosigmoiditis
556.4 Pseudopolyposis of colon
556.5 Left sided ulcerative (chronic) colitis
556.6 Universal ulcerative (chronic) colitis
556.8 Other ulcerative colitis
556.9 Unspecified ulcerative colitis ▽
578.1 Blood in stool
751.3 Hirschsprung's disease and other congenital functional disorders of colon
783.21 Loss of weight
783.22 Underweight
783.7 Adult failure to thrive
792.1 Nonspecific abnormal finding in stool contents
793.4 Nonspecific abnormal findings on radiological and other examination of gastrointestinal tract

ICD-9-CM Procedural

45.14 Closed [endoscopic] biopsy of small intestine

HCPCS Level II Supplies & Services

A4305 Disposable drug delivery system, flow rate of 50 ml or greater per hour
A4306 Disposable drug delivery system, flow rate of 5 ml or less per hour
A4550 Surgical trays

44110–44111

44110 Excision of one or more lesions of small or large intestine not requiring anastomosis, exteriorization, or fistulization; single enterotomy
44111 multiple enterotomies

ICD-9-CM Diagnostic

152.0 Malignant neoplasm of duodenum
152.2 Malignant neoplasm of ileum
152.8 Malignant neoplasm of other specified sites of small intestine
152.9 Malignant neoplasm of small intestine, unspecified site ▽
153.1 Malignant neoplasm of transverse colon
153.2 Malignant neoplasm of descending colon
153.3 Malignant neoplasm of sigmoid colon
197.4 Secondary malignant neoplasm of small intestine including duodenum
197.5 Secondary malignant neoplasm of large intestine and rectum
211.2 Benign neoplasm of duodenum, jejunum, and ileum
211.3 Benign neoplasm of colon
230.3 Carcinoma in situ of colon
230.4 Carcinoma in situ of rectum
230.7 Carcinoma in situ of other and unspecified parts of intestine ▽
235.2 Neoplasm of uncertain behavior of stomach, intestines, and rectum
560.81 Intestinal or peritoneal adhesions with obstruction (postoperative) (postinfection)
617.5 Endometriosis of intestine ♀
751.3 Hirschsprung's disease and other congenital functional disorders of colon

ICD-9-CM Procedural

45.31 Other local excision of lesion of duodenum
45.33 Local excision of lesion or tissue of small intestine, except duodenum
45.41 Excision of lesion or tissue of large intestine
45.61 Multiple segmental resection of small intestine

44120–44125

44120 Enterectomy, resection of small intestine; single resection and anastomosis
44121 each additional resection and anastomosis (List separately in addition to code for primary procedure)
44125 with enterostomy

ICD-9-CM Diagnostic

152.0 Malignant neoplasm of duodenum
152.1 Malignant neoplasm of jejunum
152.2 Malignant neoplasm of ileum
152.8 Malignant neoplasm of other specified sites of small intestine
152.9 Malignant neoplasm of small intestine, unspecified site ▽
197.4 Secondary malignant neoplasm of small intestine including duodenum
211.2 Benign neoplasm of duodenum, jejunum, and ileum
230.7 Carcinoma in situ of other and unspecified parts of intestine ▽
230.9 Carcinoma in situ of other and unspecified digestive organs ▽
235.2 Neoplasm of uncertain behavior of stomach, intestines, and rectum
239.0 Neoplasm of unspecified nature of digestive system
551.00 Femoral hernia with gangrene, unilateral or unspecified (not specified as recurrent)
551.21 Incisional ventral hernia, with gangrene
551.8 Hernia of other specified sites, with gangrene
551.9 Hernia of unspecified site, with gangrene ▽
552.00 Unilateral or unspecified femoral hernia with obstruction
552.21 Incisional hernia with obstruction
555.0 Regional enteritis of small intestine
555.9 Regional enteritis of unspecified site ▽
556.1 Ulcerative (chronic) ileocolitis
556.8 Other ulcerative colitis
556.9 Unspecified ulcerative colitis ▽
560.0 Intussusception
560.1 Paralytic ileus
560.2 Volvulus
560.81 Intestinal or peritoneal adhesions with obstruction (postoperative) (postinfection)
560.89 Other specified intestinal obstruction
560.9 Unspecified intestinal obstruction ▽
562.00 Diverticulosis of small intestine (without mention of hemorrhage) — (Use additional code to identify any associated peritonitis: 567.0-567.9)
562.01 Diverticulitis of small intestine (without mention of hemorrhage) — (Use additional code to identify any associated peritonitis: 567.0-567.9)
562.02 Diverticulosis of small intestine with hemorrhage — (Use additional code to identify any associated peritonitis: 567.0-567.9)

▽ Unspecified code
♀ Female diagnosis
☒ Manifestation code
♂ Male diagnosis

562.03 Divertulitis of small intestine with hemorrhage — (Use additional code to identify any associated peritonitis: 567.0-567.9)
567.0 Peritonitis in infectious diseases classified elsewhere — (Code first underlying disease) ☒
567.1 Pneumococcal peritonitis
567.2 Other suppurative peritonitis
567.8 Other specified peritonitis
567.9 Unspecified peritonitis ▽
569.5 Abscess of intestine
569.81 Fistula of intestine, excluding rectum and anus
569.82 Ulceration of intestine
569.83 Perforation of intestine
569.85 Angiodysplasia of intestine with hemorrhage
569.89 Other specified disorder of intestines
578.9 Unspecified, hemorrhage of gastrointestinal tract ▽
619.1 Digestive-genital tract fistula, female ♀
863.20 Small intestine injury, unspecified site, without mention of open wound into cavity ▽
863.21 Duodenum injury without mention of open wound into cavity
863.29 Other injury to small intestine without mention of open wound into cavity
863.30 Small intestine injury, unspecified site, with open wound into cavity ▽
863.31 Duodenum injury with open wound into cavity
863.39 Other injury to small intestine with open wound into cavity
863.80 Gastrointestinal tract injury, unspecified site, without mention of open wound into cavity ▽
863.89 Injury to other and unspecified gastrointestinal sites without mention of open wound into cavity
863.90 Gastrointestinal tract injury, unspecified site, with open wound into cavity ▽
863.99 Injury to other and unspecified gastrointestinal sites with open wound into cavity
997.4 Digestive system complication — (Use additional code to identify complications)
998.2 Accidental puncture or laceration during procedure
998.51 Infected postoperative seroma — (Use additional code to identify organism)
998.59 Other postoperative infection — (Use additional code to identify infection)
998.6 Persistent postoperative fistula, not elsewhere classified
V64.41 Laparoscopic surgical procedure converted to open procedure

ICD-9-CM Procedural

45.61 Multiple segmental resection of small intestine
45.62 Other partial resection of small intestine
46.01 Exteriorization of small intestine
46.03 Exteriorization of large intestine
46.20 Ileostomy, not otherwise specified
46.39 Other enterostomy

44126–44128

44126 Enterectomy, resection of small intestine for congenital atresia, single resection and anastomosis of proximal segment of intestine; without tapering
44127 with tapering
44128 each additional resection and anastomosis (List separately in addition to code for primary procedure)

ICD-9-CM Diagnostic

751.1 Congenital atresia and stenosis of small intestine
V64.41 Laparoscopic surgical procedure converted to open procedure

ICD-9-CM Procedural

45.62 Other partial resection of small intestine

44130

44130 Enteroenterostomy, anastomosis of intestine, with or without cutaneous enterostomy (separate procedure)

ICD-9-CM Diagnostic

152.0 Malignant neoplasm of duodenum
152.1 Malignant neoplasm of jejunum
152.2 Malignant neoplasm of ileum
152.3 Malignant neoplasm of Meckel's diverticulum
152.8 Malignant neoplasm of other specified sites of small intestine
152.9 Malignant neoplasm of small intestine, unspecified site ▽
197.4 Secondary malignant neoplasm of small intestine including duodenum
537.3 Other obstruction of duodenum
557.0 Acute vascular insufficiency of intestine
557.1 Chronic vascular insufficiency of intestine
560.0 Intussusception
560.1 Paralytic ileus
560.2 Volvulus
560.31 Gallstone ileus
560.39 Other impaction of intestine
560.81 Intestinal or peritoneal adhesions with obstruction (postoperative) (postinfection)
560.89 Other specified intestinal obstruction
560.9 Unspecified intestinal obstruction ▽
562.00 Diverticulosis of small intestine (without mention of hemorrhage) — (Use additional code to identify any associated peritonitis: 567.0-567.9)
562.01 Diverticulitis of small intestine (without mention of hemorrhage) — (Use additional code to identify any associated peritonitis: 567.0-567.9)
562.02 Diverticulosis of small intestine with hemorrhage — (Use additional code to identify any associated peritonitis: 567.0-567.9)
562.03 Divertulitis of small intestine with hemorrhage — (Use additional code to identify any associated peritonitis: 567.0-567.9)
564.3 Vomiting following gastrointestinal surgery
564.5 Functional diarrhea
564.81 Neurogenic bowel
564.89 Other functional disorders of intestine
567.0 Peritonitis in infectious diseases classified elsewhere — (Code first underlying disease) ☒
567.1 Pneumococcal peritonitis
567.2 Other suppurative peritonitis
567.8 Other specified peritonitis
567.9 Unspecified peritonitis ▽
568.0 Peritoneal adhesions (postoperative) (postinfection)
569.81 Fistula of intestine, excluding rectum and anus
569.82 Ulceration of intestine
569.83 Perforation of intestine
569.84 Angiodysplasia of intestine (without mention of hemorrhage)
569.85 Angiodysplasia of intestine with hemorrhage
569.89 Other specified disorder of intestines
569.9 Unspecified disorder of intestine ▽
578.1 Blood in stool
578.9 Unspecified, hemorrhage of gastrointestinal tract ▽
579.2 Blind loop syndrome
617.5 Endometriosis of intestine ♀
751.1 Congenital atresia and stenosis of small intestine
785.4 Gangrene — (Code first any associated underlying condition:250.7, 443.0)

ICD-9-CM Procedural

45.91 Small-to-small intestinal anastomosis
45.93 Other small-to-large intestinal anastomosis
45.94 Large-to-large intestinal anastomosis
46.01 Exteriorization of small intestine
46.03 Exteriorization of large intestine
46.10 Colostomy, not otherwise specified
46.20 Ileostomy, not otherwise specified
46.39 Other enterostomy

44132–44133

44132 Donor enterectomy (including cold preservation), open; from cadaver donor
44133 partial, from living donor

ICD-9-CM Diagnostic

V59.8 Donor of other specified organ or tissue

ICD-9-CM Procedural

45.62 Other partial resection of small intestine
45.63 Total removal of small intestine

44135–44136

44135 Intestinal allotransplantation; from cadaver donor
44136 from living donor

ICD-9-CM Diagnostic

152.0 Malignant neoplasm of duodenum
152.1 Malignant neoplasm of jejunum
152.2 Malignant neoplasm of ileum
152.8 Malignant neoplasm of other specified sites of small intestine
152.9 Malignant neoplasm of small intestine, unspecified site ▽
197.4 Secondary malignant neoplasm of small intestine including duodenum
551.00 Femoral hernia with gangrene, unilateral or unspecified (not specified as recurrent)
551.21 Incisional ventral hernia, with gangrene

551.8 Hernia of other specified sites, with gangrene
551.9 Hernia of unspecified site, with gangrene ▽
552.00 Unilateral or unspecified femoral hernia with obstruction
552.21 Incisional hernia with obstruction
555.0 Regional enteritis of small intestine
555.9 Regional enteritis of unspecified site ▽
556.1 Ulcerative (chronic) ileocolitis
556.8 Other ulcerative colitis
556.9 Unspecified ulcerative colitis ▽
560.0 Intussusception
560.1 Paralytic ileus
560.2 Volvulus
560.81 Intestinal or peritoneal adhesions with obstruction (postoperative) (postinfection)
560.89 Other specified intestinal obstruction
560.9 Unspecified intestinal obstruction ▽
562.00 Diverticulosis of small intestine (without mention of hemorrhage) — (Use additional code to identify any associated peritonitis: 567.0-567.9)
562.01 Diverticulitis of small intestine (without mention of hemorrhage) — (Use additional code to identify any associated peritonitis: 567.0-567.9)
562.02 Diverticulosis of small intestine with hemorrhage — (Use additional code to identify any associated peritonitis: 567.0-567.9)
562.03 Divertulitis of small intestine with hemorrhage — (Use additional code to identify any associated peritonitis: 567.0-567.9)
567.0 Peritonitis in infectious diseases classified elsewhere — (Code first underlying disease) ☒
567.1 Pneumococcal peritonitis
567.2 Other suppurative peritonitis
567.8 Other specified peritonitis
567.9 Unspecified peritonitis ▽
569.85 Angiodysplasia of intestine with hemorrhage
569.89 Other specified disorder of intestines
578.9 Unspecified, hemorrhage of gastrointestinal tract ▽
579.3 Other and unspecified postsurgical nonabsorption ▽
751.1 Congenital atresia and stenosis of small intestine
751.5 Other congenital anomalies of intestine
863.30 Small intestine injury, unspecified site, with open wound into cavity ▽
863.31 Duodenum injury with open wound into cavity
863.39 Other injury to small intestine with open wound into cavity
863.90 Gastrointestinal tract injury, unspecified site, with open wound into cavity ▽
863.99 Injury to other and unspecified gastrointestinal sites with open wound into cavity
997.4 Digestive system complication — (Use additional code to identify complications)
998.51 Infected postoperative seroma — (Use additional code to identify organism)
998.59 Other postoperative infection — (Use additional code to identify infection)

ICD-9-CM Procedural

46.97 Transplant of intestine

44137

44137 Removal of transplanted intestinal allograft, complete

ICD-9-CM Diagnostic

152.0 Malignant neoplasm of duodenum
152.1 Malignant neoplasm of jejunum
152.2 Malignant neoplasm of ileum
152.8 Malignant neoplasm of other specified sites of small intestine
152.9 Malignant neoplasm of small intestine, unspecified site ▽
197.4 Secondary malignant neoplasm of small intestine including duodenum
551.00 Femoral hernia with gangrene, unilateral or unspecified (not specified as recurrent)
551.21 Incisional ventral hernia, with gangrene
551.8 Hernia of other specified sites, with gangrene
551.9 Hernia of unspecified site, with gangrene ▽
552.00 Unilateral or unspecified femoral hernia with obstruction
552.21 Incisional hernia with obstruction
555.0 Regional enteritis of small intestine
555.9 Regional enteritis of unspecified site ▽
556.1 Ulcerative (chronic) ileocolitis
556.8 Other ulcerative colitis
556.9 Unspecified ulcerative colitis ▽
560.0 Intussusception
560.1 Paralytic ileus
560.2 Volvulus
560.81 Intestinal or peritoneal adhesions with obstruction (postoperative) (postinfection)
560.89 Other specified intestinal obstruction
560.9 Unspecified intestinal obstruction ▽
562.00 Diverticulosis of small intestine (without mention of hemorrhage) — (Use additional code to identify any associated peritonitis: 567.0-567.9)
562.01 Diverticulitis of small intestine (without mention of hemorrhage) — (Use additional code to identify any associated peritonitis: 567.0-567.9)
562.02 Diverticulosis of small intestine with hemorrhage — (Use additional code to identify any associated peritonitis: 567.0-567.9)
562.03 Divertulitis of small intestine with hemorrhage — (Use additional code to identify any associated peritonitis: 567.0-567.9)
567.0 Peritonitis in infectious diseases classified elsewhere — (Code first underlying disease) ☒
567.1 Pneumococcal peritonitis
567.2 Other suppurative peritonitis
567.8 Other specified peritonitis
567.9 Unspecified peritonitis ▽
569.85 Angiodysplasia of intestine with hemorrhage
569.89 Other specified disorder of intestines
578.9 Unspecified, hemorrhage of gastrointestinal tract ▽
579.3 Other and unspecified postsurgical nonabsorption ▽
751.1 Congenital atresia and stenosis of small intestine
751.5 Other congenital anomalies of intestine
863.30 Small intestine injury, unspecified site, with open wound into cavity ▽
863.31 Duodenum injury with open wound into cavity
863.39 Other injury to small intestine with open wound into cavity
863.90 Gastrointestinal tract injury, unspecified site, with open wound into cavity ▽
863.99 Injury to other and unspecified gastrointestinal sites with open wound into cavity
996.87 Complications of transplanted organ, intestine — (Use additional code to identify nature of complication, 078.5)
997.4 Digestive system complication — (Use additional code to identify complications)
998.51 Infected postoperative seroma — (Use additional code to identify organism)
998.59 Other postoperative infection — (Use additional code to identify infection)

ICD-9-CM Procedural

46.99 Other operations on intestines

44139

44139 Mobilization (take-down) of splenic flexure performed in conjunction with partial colectomy (List separately in addition to primary procedure)

ICD-9-CM Diagnostic

This is an add-on code. Refer to the corresponding primary procedure code for ICD-9 diagnosis code links.

ICD-9-CM Procedural

45.79 Other partial excision of large intestine
46.99 Other operations on intestines

44140

44140 Colectomy, partial; with anastomosis

ICD-9-CM Diagnostic

153.0 Malignant neoplasm of hepatic flexure
153.1 Malignant neoplasm of transverse colon
153.2 Malignant neoplasm of descending colon
153.3 Malignant neoplasm of sigmoid colon
153.4 Malignant neoplasm of cecum
153.6 Malignant neoplasm of ascending colon
153.7 Malignant neoplasm of splenic flexure
153.8 Malignant neoplasm of other specified sites of large intestine
153.9 Malignant neoplasm of colon, unspecified site ▽
154.0 Malignant neoplasm of rectosigmoid junction
154.1 Malignant neoplasm of rectum
154.8 Malignant neoplasm of other sites of rectum, rectosigmoid junction, and anus
159.0 Malignant neoplasm of intestinal tract, part unspecified ▽
197.4 Secondary malignant neoplasm of small intestine including duodenum
197.5 Secondary malignant neoplasm of large intestine and rectum
211.3 Benign neoplasm of colon
211.4 Benign neoplasm of rectum and anal canal
211.9 Benign neoplasm of other and unspecified site of the digestive system ▽
230.3 Carcinoma in situ of colon
230.4 Carcinoma in situ of rectum

▽ Unspecified code
♀ Female diagnosis
☒ Manifestation code
♂ Male diagnosis

235.2 Neoplasm of uncertain behavior of stomach, intestines, and rectum
239.0 Neoplasm of unspecified nature of digestive system
550.00 Inguinal hernia with gangrene, unilateral or unspecified, (not specified as recurrent)
551.1 Umbilical hernia with gangrene
552.8 Hernia of other specified site, with obstruction
555.1 Regional enteritis of large intestine
555.2 Regional enteritis of small intestine with large intestine
555.9 Regional enteritis of unspecified site ▽
556.0 Ulcerative (chronic) enterocolitis
556.1 Ulcerative (chronic) ileocolitis
556.2 Ulcerative (chronic) proctitis
556.3 Ulcerative (chronic) proctosigmoiditis
556.4 Pseudopolyposis of colon
556.5 Left sided ulcerative (chronic) colitis
556.6 Universal ulcerative (chronic) colitis
556.8 Other ulcerative colitis
556.9 Unspecified ulcerative colitis ▽
557.0 Acute vascular insufficiency of intestine
557.1 Chronic vascular insufficiency of intestine
557.9 Unspecified vascular insufficiency of intestine ▽
558.1 Gastroenteritis and colitis due to radiation
558.2 Toxic gastroenteritis and colitis — (Use additional E code to identify cause)
558.9 Other and unspecified noninfectious gastroenteritis and colitis ▽
560.0 Intussusception
560.1 Paralytic ileus
560.2 Volvulus
560.81 Intestinal or peritoneal adhesions with obstruction (postoperative) (postinfection)
560.89 Other specified intestinal obstruction
560.9 Unspecified intestinal obstruction ▽
562.10 Diverticulosis of colon (without mention of hemorrhage) — (Use additional code to identify any associated peritonitis: 567.0-567.9)
562.11 Diverticulitis of colon (without mention of hemorrhage) — (Use additional code to identify any associated peritonitis: 567.0-567.9)
562.12 Diverticulosis of colon with hemorrhage — (Use additional code to identify any associated peritonitis: 567.0-567.9)
562.13 Diverticulitis of colon with hemorrhage — (Use additional code to identify any associated peritonitis: 567.0-567.9)
564.7 Megacolon, other than Hirschsprung's
567.0 Peritonitis in infectious diseases classified elsewhere — (Code first underlying disease) ☒
567.1 Pneumococcal peritonitis
567.2 Other suppurative peritonitis
567.8 Other specified peritonitis
567.9 Unspecified peritonitis ▽
569.5 Abscess of intestine
569.81 Fistula of intestine, excluding rectum and anus
569.82 Ulceration of intestine
569.83 Perforation of intestine
569.84 Angiodysplasia of intestine (without mention of hemorrhage)
569.85 Angiodysplasia of intestine with hemorrhage
569.89 Other specified disorder of intestines
569.9 Unspecified disorder of intestine ▽
578.9 Unspecified, hemorrhage of gastrointestinal tract ▽
596.1 Intestinovesical fistula — (Use additional code to identify urinary incontinence: 625.6, 788.30-788.39)
619.1 Digestive-genital tract fistula, female ♀
751.5 Other congenital anomalies of intestine
751.8 Other specified congenital anomalies of digestive system
751.9 Unspecified congenital anomaly of digestive system ▽
787.99 Other symptoms involving digestive system
V64.41 Laparoscopic surgical procedure converted to open procedure

ICD-9-CM Procedural

45.79 Other partial excision of large intestine

44141

44141 Colectomy, partial; with skin level cecostomy or colostomy

ICD-9-CM Diagnostic

153.0 Malignant neoplasm of hepatic flexure
153.1 Malignant neoplasm of transverse colon
153.2 Malignant neoplasm of descending colon
153.3 Malignant neoplasm of sigmoid colon
153.4 Malignant neoplasm of cecum
153.5 Malignant neoplasm of appendix
153.6 Malignant neoplasm of ascending colon
153.7 Malignant neoplasm of splenic flexure
153.8 Malignant neoplasm of other specified sites of large intestine
153.9 Malignant neoplasm of colon, unspecified site ▽
154.0 Malignant neoplasm of rectosigmoid junction
154.1 Malignant neoplasm of rectum
211.3 Benign neoplasm of colon
211.4 Benign neoplasm of rectum and anal canal
235.2 Neoplasm of uncertain behavior of stomach, intestines, and rectum
239.0 Neoplasm of unspecified nature of digestive system
556.3 Ulcerative (chronic) proctosigmoiditis
556.4 Pseudopolyposis of colon
556.9 Unspecified ulcerative colitis ▽
557.0 Acute vascular insufficiency of intestine
557.1 Chronic vascular insufficiency of intestine
557.9 Unspecified vascular insufficiency of intestine ▽
560.0 Intussusception
560.1 Paralytic ileus
560.2 Volvulus
560.81 Intestinal or peritoneal adhesions with obstruction (postoperative) (postinfection)
560.89 Other specified intestinal obstruction
560.9 Unspecified intestinal obstruction ▽
562.10 Diverticulosis of colon (without mention of hemorrhage) — (Use additional code to identify any associated peritonitis: 567.0-567.9)
562.11 Diverticulitis of colon (without mention of hemorrhage) — (Use additional code to identify any associated peritonitis: 567.0-567.9)
562.12 Diverticulosis of colon with hemorrhage — (Use additional code to identify any associated peritonitis: 567.0-567.9)
562.13 Diverticulitis of colon with hemorrhage — (Use additional code to identify any associated peritonitis: 567.0-567.9)
564.7 Megacolon, other than Hirschsprung's
567.0 Peritonitis in infectious diseases classified elsewhere — (Code first underlying disease) ☒
567.1 Pneumococcal peritonitis
567.2 Other suppurative peritonitis
567.8 Other specified peritonitis
567.9 Unspecified peritonitis ▽
569.5 Abscess of intestine
569.81 Fistula of intestine, excluding rectum and anus
569.82 Ulceration of intestine
569.83 Perforation of intestine
569.84 Angiodysplasia of intestine (without mention of hemorrhage)
569.85 Angiodysplasia of intestine with hemorrhage
569.89 Other specified disorder of intestines
569.9 Unspecified disorder of intestine ▽
578.9 Unspecified, hemorrhage of gastrointestinal tract ▽
614.5 Acute or unspecified pelvic peritonitis, female — (Use additional code to identify organism: 041.0, 041.1) ♀
751.5 Other congenital anomalies of intestine
785.4 Gangrene — (Code first any associated underlying condition:250.7, 443.0)
863.29 Other injury to small intestine without mention of open wound into cavity
863.30 Small intestine injury, unspecified site, with open wound into cavity ▽
863.31 Duodenum injury with open wound into cavity
863.39 Other injury to small intestine with open wound into cavity
V64.41 Laparoscopic surgical procedure converted to open procedure

ICD-9-CM Procedural

45.73 Right hemicolectomy
45.74 Resection of transverse colon
45.75 Left hemicolectomy
45.76 Sigmoidectomy
46.03 Exteriorization of large intestine
46.04 Resection of exteriorized segment of large intestine
46.10 Colostomy, not otherwise specified
46.13 Permanent colostomy

44143

44143 Colectomy, partial; with end colostomy and closure of distal segment (Hartmann type procedure)

ICD-9-CM Diagnostic

153.0 Malignant neoplasm of hepatic flexure
153.1 Malignant neoplasm of transverse colon
153.2 Malignant neoplasm of descending colon

▽ Unspecified code ♀ Female diagnosis ☒ Manifestation code ♂ Male diagnosis

153.3 Malignant neoplasm of sigmoid colon
153.4 Malignant neoplasm of cecum
153.5 Malignant neoplasm of appendix
153.6 Malignant neoplasm of ascending colon
153.7 Malignant neoplasm of splenic flexure
153.8 Malignant neoplasm of other specified sites of large intestine
153.9 Malignant neoplasm of colon, unspecified site
154.0 Malignant neoplasm of rectosigmoid junction
154.1 Malignant neoplasm of rectum
154.8 Malignant neoplasm of other sites of rectum, rectosigmoid junction, and anus
159.0 Malignant neoplasm of intestinal tract, part unspecified
197.5 Secondary malignant neoplasm of large intestine and rectum
198.89 Secondary malignant neoplasm of other specified sites
199.1 Other malignant neoplasm of unspecified site
211.3 Benign neoplasm of colon
211.4 Benign neoplasm of rectum and anal canal
230.3 Carcinoma in situ of colon
230.4 Carcinoma in situ of rectum
235.2 Neoplasm of uncertain behavior of stomach, intestines, and rectum
239.0 Neoplasm of unspecified nature of digestive system
555.1 Regional enteritis of large intestine
555.2 Regional enteritis of small intestine with large intestine
555.9 Regional enteritis of unspecified site
556.0 Ulcerative (chronic) enterocolitis
556.1 Ulcerative (chronic) ileocolitis
556.2 Ulcerative (chronic) proctitis
556.3 Ulcerative (chronic) proctosigmoiditis
556.4 Pseudopolyposis of colon
556.5 Left sided ulcerative (chronic) colitis
556.6 Universal ulcerative (chronic) colitis
556.8 Other ulcerative colitis
556.9 Unspecified ulcerative colitis
557.0 Acute vascular insufficiency of intestine
557.1 Chronic vascular insufficiency of intestine
557.9 Unspecified vascular insufficiency of intestine
560.2 Volvulus
560.81 Intestinal or peritoneal adhesions with obstruction (postoperative) (postinfection)
560.89 Other specified intestinal obstruction
560.9 Unspecified intestinal obstruction
562.10 Diverticulosis of colon (without mention of hemorrhage) — (Use additional code to identify any associated peritonitis: 567.0-567.9)
562.11 Diverticulitis of colon (without mention of hemorrhage) — (Use additional code to identify any associated peritonitis: 567.0-567.9)
562.12 Diverticulosis of colon with hemorrhage — (Use additional code to identify any associated peritonitis: 567.0-567.9)
562.13 Diverticulitis of colon with hemorrhage — (Use additional code to identify any associated peritonitis: 567.0-567.9)
564.81 Neurogenic bowel
564.89 Other functional disorders of intestine
567.0 Peritonitis in infectious diseases classified elsewhere — (Code first underlying disease)
567.1 Pneumococcal peritonitis
567.2 Other suppurative peritonitis
567.8 Other specified peritonitis
567.9 Unspecified peritonitis
569.5 Abscess of intestine
569.81 Fistula of intestine, excluding rectum and anus
569.82 Ulceration of intestine
569.83 Perforation of intestine
569.84 Angiodysplasia of intestine (without mention of hemorrhage)
569.85 Angiodysplasia of intestine with hemorrhage
569.89 Other specified disorder of intestines
569.9 Unspecified disorder of intestine
578.1 Blood in stool
578.9 Unspecified, hemorrhage of gastrointestinal tract
596.1 Intestinovesical fistula — (Use additional code to identify urinary incontinence: 625.6, 788.30-788.39)
619.1 Digestive-genital tract fistula, female ♀
751.2 Congenital atresia and stenosis of large intestine, rectum, and anal canal
751.3 Hirschsprung's disease and other congenital functional disorders of colon
751.4 Congenital anomalies of intestinal fixation
751.5 Other congenital anomalies of intestine
751.8 Other specified congenital anomalies of digestive system
751.9 Unspecified congenital anomaly of digestive system
777.5 Necrotizing enterocolitis in fetus or newborn
777.6 Perinatal intestinal perforation
777.8 Other specified perinatal disorder of digestive system
777.9 Unspecified perinatal disorder of digestive system
789.00 Abdominal pain, unspecified site
789.01 Abdominal pain, right upper quadrant
789.02 Abdominal pain, left upper quadrant
789.03 Abdominal pain, right lower quadrant
789.04 Abdominal pain, left lower quadrant
789.05 Abdominal pain, periumbilic
789.06 Abdominal pain, epigastric
789.07 Abdominal pain, generalized
789.09 Abdominal pain, other specified site
789.30 Abdominal or pelvic swelling, mass or lump, unspecified site
789.31 Abdominal or pelvic swelling, mass, or lump, right upper quadrant
789.32 Abdominal or pelvic swelling, mass, or lump, left upper quadrant
789.33 Abdominal or pelvic swelling, mass, or lump, right lower quadrant
789.34 Abdominal or pelvic swelling, mass, or lump, left lower quadrant
789.35 Abdominal or pelvic swelling, mass or lump, periumbilic
789.36 Abdominal or pelvic swelling, mass, or lump, epigastric
789.37 Abdominal or pelvic swelling, mass, or lump, epigastric, generalized
789.39 Abdominal or pelvic swelling, mass, or lump, other specified site
789.9 Other symptoms involving abdomen and pelvis
793.4 Nonspecific abnormal findings on radiological and other examination of gastrointestinal tract
863.40 Colon injury unspecified site, without mention of open wound into cavity
863.41 Ascending (right) colon injury without mention of open wound into cavity
863.42 Transverse colon injury without mention of open wound into cavity
863.43 Descending (left) colon injury without mention of open wound into cavity
863.44 Sigmoid colon injury without mention of open wound into cavity
863.45 Rectum injury without mention of open wound into cavity
863.46 Injury to multiple sites in colon and rectum without mention of open wound into cavity
863.49 Other colon and rectum injury, without mention of open wound into cavity
863.50 Colon injury, unspecified site, with open wound into cavity
863.51 Ascending (right) colon injury with open wound into cavity
863.52 Transverse colon injury with open wound into cavity
863.53 Descending (left) colon injury with open wound into cavity
863.54 Sigmoid colon injury with open wound into cavity
863.55 Rectum injury with open wound into cavity
863.56 Injury to multiple sites in colon and rectum with open wound into cavity
863.59 Other injury to colon and rectum with open wound into cavity
863.80 Gastrointestinal tract injury, unspecified site, without mention of open wound into cavity
863.90 Gastrointestinal tract injury, unspecified site, with open wound into cavity
869.0 Internal injury to unspecified or ill-defined organs without mention of open wound into cavity
869.1 Internal injury to unspecified or ill-defined organs with open wound into cavity
936 Foreign body in intestine and colon
937 Foreign body in anus and rectum
938 Foreign body in digestive system, unspecified
997.4 Digestive system complication — (Use additional code to identify complications)
998.2 Accidental puncture or laceration during procedure
998.31 Disruption of internal operation wound
998.6 Persistent postoperative fistula, not elsewhere classified
998.9 Unspecified complication of procedure, not elsewhere classified
V64.41 Laparoscopic surgical procedure converted to open procedure

ICD-9-CM Procedural

45.72 Cecectomy
45.73 Right hemicolectomy
45.74 Resection of transverse colon
45.75 Left hemicolectomy

44144

44144 Colectomy, partial; with resection, with colostomy or ileostomy and creation of mucofistula

ICD-9-CM Diagnostic

153.0 Malignant neoplasm of hepatic flexure
153.1 Malignant neoplasm of transverse colon
153.2 Malignant neoplasm of descending colon
153.3 Malignant neoplasm of sigmoid colon
153.4 Malignant neoplasm of cecum
153.5 Malignant neoplasm of appendix
153.6 Malignant neoplasm of ascending colon

Unspecified code
♀ Female diagnosis
Manifestation code
♂ Male diagnosis

153.7 Malignant neoplasm of splenic flexure
153.8 Malignant neoplasm of other specified sites of large intestine
153.9 Malignant neoplasm of colon, unspecified site ▽
154.0 Malignant neoplasm of rectosigmoid junction
154.1 Malignant neoplasm of rectum
154.2 Malignant neoplasm of anal canal
159.0 Malignant neoplasm of intestinal tract, part unspecified ▽
197.5 Secondary malignant neoplasm of large intestine and rectum
198.89 Secondary malignant neoplasm of other specified sites
199.1 Other malignant neoplasm of unspecified site
211.3 Benign neoplasm of colon
211.4 Benign neoplasm of rectum and anal canal
230.3 Carcinoma in situ of colon
230.4 Carcinoma in situ of rectum
235.2 Neoplasm of uncertain behavior of stomach, intestines, and rectum
239.0 Neoplasm of unspecified nature of digestive system
550.00 Inguinal hernia with gangrene, unilateral or unspecified, (not specified as recurrent)
550.01 Inguinal hernia with gangrene, recurrent unilateral or unspecified inguinal hernia
550.02 Inguinal hernia with gangrene, bilateral
550.03 Inguinal hernia with gangrene, recurrent bilateral
550.10 Inguinal hernia with obstruction, without mention of gangrene, unilateral or unspecified, (not specified as recurrent)
550.11 Inguinal hernia with obstruction, without mention of gangrene, recurrent unilateral or unspecified
550.12 Inguinal hernia with obstruction, without mention gangrene, bilateral, (not specified as recurrent)
550.13 Inguinal hernia with obstruction, without mention of gangrene, recurrent bilateral
551.00 Femoral hernia with gangrene, unilateral or unspecified (not specified as recurrent)
551.01 Femoral hernia with gangrene, recurrent unilateral or unspecified
551.02 Femoral hernia with gangrene, bilateral, (not specified as recurrent)
551.03 Femoral hernia with gangrene, recurrent bilateral
551.1 Umbilical hernia with gangrene
551.21 Incisional ventral hernia, with gangrene
551.29 Other ventral hernia with gangrene
551.3 Diaphragmatic hernia with gangrene
551.8 Hernia of other specified sites, with gangrene
551.9 Hernia of unspecified site, with gangrene ▽
552.00 Unilateral or unspecified femoral hernia with obstruction
552.01 Recurrent unilateral or unspecified femoral hernia with obstruction
552.02 Bilateral femoral hernia with obstruction
552.03 Recurrent bilateral femoral hernia with obstruction
552.1 Umbilical hernia with obstruction
552.21 Incisional hernia with obstruction
552.29 Other ventral hernia with obstruction
552.3 Diaphragmatic hernia with obstruction
552.8 Hernia of other specified site, with obstruction
552.9 Hernia of unspecified site, with obstruction ▽
555.1 Regional enteritis of large intestine
555.9 Regional enteritis of unspecified site ▽
556.0 Ulcerative (chronic) enterocolitis
556.1 Ulcerative (chronic) ileocolitis
556.2 Ulcerative (chronic) proctitis
556.3 Ulcerative (chronic) proctosigmoiditis
556.4 Pseudopolyposis of colon
556.5 Left sided ulcerative (chronic) colitis
556.6 Universal ulcerative (chronic) colitis
556.8 Other ulcerative colitis
556.9 Unspecified ulcerative colitis ▽
557.0 Acute vascular insufficiency of intestine
557.1 Chronic vascular insufficiency of intestine
557.9 Unspecified vascular insufficiency of intestine ▽
560.2 Volvulus
560.81 Intestinal or peritoneal adhesions with obstruction (postoperative) (postinfection)
560.89 Other specified intestinal obstruction
560.9 Unspecified intestinal obstruction ▽
562.10 Diverticulosis of colon (without mention of hemorrhage) — (Use additional code to identify any associated peritonitis: 567.0-567.9)
562.11 Diverticulitis of colon (without mention of hemorrhage) — (Use additional code to identify any associated peritonitis: 567.0-567.9)
562.12 Diverticulosis of colon with hemorrhage — (Use additional code to identify any associated peritonitis: 567.0-567.9)
562.13 Diverticulitis of colon with hemorrhage — (Use additional code to identify any associated peritonitis: 567.0-567.9)
564.81 Neurogenic bowel
564.89 Other functional disorders of intestine
567.0 Peritonitis in infectious diseases classified elsewhere — (Code first underlying disease) ☒
567.1 Pneumococcal peritonitis
567.2 Other suppurative peritonitis
567.8 Other specified peritonitis
567.9 Unspecified peritonitis ▽
569.5 Abscess of intestine
569.81 Fistula of intestine, excluding rectum and anus
569.82 Ulceration of intestine
569.83 Perforation of intestine
569.84 Angiodysplasia of intestine (without mention of hemorrhage)
569.85 Angiodysplasia of intestine with hemorrhage
569.89 Other specified disorder of intestines
569.9 Unspecified disorder of intestine ▽
578.1 Blood in stool
578.9 Unspecified, hemorrhage of gastrointestinal tract ▽
596.1 Intestinovesical fistula — (Use additional code to identify urinary incontinence: 625.6, 788.30-788.39)
619.1 Digestive-genital tract fistula, female ♀
751.2 Congenital atresia and stenosis of large intestine, rectum, and anal canal
751.3 Hirschsprung's disease and other congenital functional disorders of colon
751.4 Congenital anomalies of intestinal fixation
751.5 Other congenital anomalies of intestine
777.5 Necrotizing enterocolitis in fetus or newborn
777.6 Perinatal intestinal perforation
777.8 Other specified perinatal disorder of digestive system
777.9 Unspecified perinatal disorder of digestive system ▽
789.01 Abdominal pain, right upper quadrant
789.02 Abdominal pain, left upper quadrant
789.03 Abdominal pain, right lower quadrant
789.04 Abdominal pain, left lower quadrant
789.05 Abdominal pain, periumbilic
789.06 Abdominal pain, epigastric
789.07 Abdominal pain, generalized
789.09 Abdominal pain, other specified site
789.31 Abdominal or pelvic swelling, mass, or lump, right upper quadrant
789.32 Abdominal or pelvic swelling, mass, or lump, left upper quadrant
789.33 Abdominal or pelvic swelling, mass, or lump, right lower quadrant
789.34 Abdominal or pelvic swelling, mass, or lump, left lower quadrant
789.35 Abdominal or pelvic swelling, mass or lump, periumbilic
789.36 Abdominal or pelvic swelling, mass, or lump, epigastric
789.37 Abdominal or pelvic swelling, mass, or lump, epigastric, generalized
789.39 Abdominal or pelvic swelling, mass, or lump, other specified site
789.9 Other symptoms involving abdomen and pelvis
793.4 Nonspecific abnormal findings on radiological and other examination of gastrointestinal tract
863.41 Ascending (right) colon injury without mention of open wound into cavity
863.42 Transverse colon injury without mention of open wound into cavity
863.43 Descending (left) colon injury without mention of open wound into cavity
863.44 Sigmoid colon injury without mention of open wound into cavity
863.45 Rectum injury without mention of open wound into cavity
863.46 Injury to multiple sites in colon and rectum without mention of open wound into cavity
863.49 Other colon and rectum injury, without mention of open wound into cavity
863.51 Ascending (right) colon injury with open wound into cavity
863.52 Transverse colon injury with open wound into cavity
863.53 Descending (left) colon injury with open wound into cavity
863.54 Sigmoid colon injury with open wound into cavity
863.55 Rectum injury with open wound into cavity
863.56 Injury to multiple sites in colon and rectum with open wound into cavity
863.59 Other injury to colon and rectum with open wound into cavity
869.0 Internal injury to unspecified or ill-defined organs without mention of open wound into cavity
869.1 Internal injury to unspecified or ill-defined organs with open wound into cavity
936 Foreign body in intestine and colon
937 Foreign body in anus and rectum
938 Foreign body in digestive system, unspecified ▽
997.4 Digestive system complication — (Use additional code to identify complications)
998.2 Accidental puncture or laceration during procedure
998.31 Disruption of internal operation wound
998.51 Infected postoperative seroma — (Use additional code to identify organism)

998.59 Other postoperative infection — (Use additional code to identify infection)
998.6 Persistent postoperative fistula, not elsewhere classified
V64.41 Laparoscopic surgical procedure converted to open procedure

ICD-9-CM Procedural

45.72 Cecectomy
45.73 Right hemicolectomy
45.74 Resection of transverse colon
45.75 Left hemicolectomy
45.76 Sigmoidectomy
45.79 Other partial excision of large intestine
46.01 Exteriorization of small intestine
46.03 Exteriorization of large intestine
46.10 Colostomy, not otherwise specified
46.11 Temporary colostomy
46.13 Permanent colostomy
46.21 Temporary ileostomy
46.22 Continent ileostomy
46.23 Other permanent ileostomy

44145–44146

44144 Colectomy, partial; with resection, with colostomy or ileostomy and creation of mucofistula
44146 with coloproctostomy (low pelvic anastomosis), with colostomy

ICD-9-CM Diagnostic

153.0 Malignant neoplasm of hepatic flexure
153.1 Malignant neoplasm of transverse colon
153.2 Malignant neoplasm of descending colon
153.3 Malignant neoplasm of sigmoid colon
153.4 Malignant neoplasm of cecum
153.5 Malignant neoplasm of appendix
153.6 Malignant neoplasm of ascending colon
153.7 Malignant neoplasm of splenic flexure
153.8 Malignant neoplasm of other specified sites of large intestine
153.9 Malignant neoplasm of colon, unspecified site ▽
154.0 Malignant neoplasm of rectosigmoid junction
154.1 Malignant neoplasm of rectum
154.2 Malignant neoplasm of anal canal
154.8 Malignant neoplasm of other sites of rectum, rectosigmoid junction, and anus
159.0 Malignant neoplasm of intestinal tract, part unspecified ▽
197.5 Secondary malignant neoplasm of large intestine and rectum
211.3 Benign neoplasm of colon
211.4 Benign neoplasm of rectum and anal canal
230.3 Carcinoma in situ of colon
230.4 Carcinoma in situ of rectum
230.9 Carcinoma in situ of other and unspecified digestive organs ▽
235.2 Neoplasm of uncertain behavior of stomach, intestines, and rectum
239.0 Neoplasm of unspecified nature of digestive system
555.1 Regional enteritis of large intestine
555.2 Regional enteritis of small intestine with large intestine
555.9 Regional enteritis of unspecified site ▽
556.0 Ulcerative (chronic) enterocolitis
556.1 Ulcerative (chronic) ileocolitis
556.2 Ulcerative (chronic) proctitis
556.3 Ulcerative (chronic) proctosigmoiditis
556.4 Pseudopolyposis of colon
556.5 Left sided ulcerative (chronic) colitis
556.6 Universal ulcerative (chronic) colitis
556.8 Other ulcerative colitis
556.9 Unspecified ulcerative colitis ▽
557.0 Acute vascular insufficiency of intestine
557.1 Chronic vascular insufficiency of intestine
557.9 Unspecified vascular insufficiency of intestine ▽
560.39 Other impaction of intestine
560.81 Intestinal or peritoneal adhesions with obstruction (postoperative) (postinfection)
560.89 Other specified intestinal obstruction
560.9 Unspecified intestinal obstruction ▽
562.10 Diverticulosis of colon (without mention of hemorrhage) — (Use additional code to identify any associated peritonitis: 567.0-567.9)
562.11 Diverticulitis of colon (without mention of hemorrhage) — (Use additional code to identify any associated peritonitis: 567.0-567.9)
562.12 Diverticulosis of colon with hemorrhage — (Use additional code to identify any associated peritonitis: 567.0-567.9)
562.13 Diverticulitis of colon with hemorrhage — (Use additional code to identify any associated peritonitis: 567.0-567.9)
564.7 Megacolon, other than Hirschsprung's
567.0 Peritonitis in infectious diseases classified elsewhere — (Code first underlying disease) ☒
567.1 Pneumococcal peritonitis
567.2 Other suppurative peritonitis
567.8 Other specified peritonitis
567.9 Unspecified peritonitis ▽
569.1 Rectal prolapse
569.81 Fistula of intestine, excluding rectum and anus
569.82 Ulceration of intestine
569.83 Perforation of intestine
569.84 Angiodysplasia of intestine (without mention of hemorrhage)
569.85 Angiodysplasia of intestine with hemorrhage
569.89 Other specified disorder of intestines
569.9 Unspecified disorder of intestine ▽
596.1 Intestinovesical fistula — (Use additional code to identify urinary incontinence: 625.6, 788.30-788.39)
619.1 Digestive-genital tract fistula, female ♀
751.8 Other specified congenital anomalies of digestive system
777.5 Necrotizing enterocolitis in fetus or newborn
777.6 Perinatal intestinal perforation
777.8 Other specified perinatal disorder of digestive system
787.99 Other symptoms involving digestive system
V64.41 Laparoscopic surgical procedure converted to open procedure

ICD-9-CM Procedural

45.75 Left hemicolectomy
45.76 Sigmoidectomy
45.94 Large-to-large intestinal anastomosis
46.03 Exteriorization of large intestine
46.10 Colostomy, not otherwise specified
46.11 Temporary colostomy
46.13 Permanent colostomy

44147

44147 Colectomy, partial; abdominal and transanal approach

ICD-9-CM Diagnostic

153.0 Malignant neoplasm of hepatic flexure
153.1 Malignant neoplasm of transverse colon
153.2 Malignant neoplasm of descending colon
153.3 Malignant neoplasm of sigmoid colon
153.4 Malignant neoplasm of cecum
153.5 Malignant neoplasm of appendix
153.6 Malignant neoplasm of ascending colon
153.7 Malignant neoplasm of splenic flexure
153.8 Malignant neoplasm of other specified sites of large intestine
153.9 Malignant neoplasm of colon, unspecified site ▽
154.0 Malignant neoplasm of rectosigmoid junction
154.1 Malignant neoplasm of rectum
154.2 Malignant neoplasm of anal canal
556.9 Unspecified ulcerative colitis ▽
560.81 Intestinal or peritoneal adhesions with obstruction (postoperative) (postinfection)
562.10 Diverticulosis of colon (without mention of hemorrhage) — (Use additional code to identify any associated peritonitis: 567.0-567.9)
562.11 Diverticulitis of colon (without mention of hemorrhage) — (Use additional code to identify any associated peritonitis: 567.0-567.9)
562.12 Diverticulosis of colon with hemorrhage — (Use additional code to identify any associated peritonitis: 567.0-567.9)
562.13 Diverticulitis of colon with hemorrhage — (Use additional code to identify any associated peritonitis: 567.0-567.9)
567.0 Peritonitis in infectious diseases classified elsewhere — (Code first underlying disease) ☒
567.1 Pneumococcal peritonitis
567.2 Other suppurative peritonitis
567.8 Other specified peritonitis
567.9 Unspecified peritonitis ▽
569.83 Perforation of intestine
569.84 Angiodysplasia of intestine (without mention of hemorrhage)
569.89 Other specified disorder of intestines
V64.41 Laparoscopic surgical procedure converted to open procedure

ICD-9-CM Procedural

45.75 Left hemicolectomy
45.76 Sigmoidectomy
45.79 Other partial excision of large intestine
45.94 Large-to-large intestinal anastomosis

44150

44150 Colectomy, total, abdominal, without proctectomy; with ileostomy or ileoproctostomy

ICD-9-CM Diagnostic

153.0 Malignant neoplasm of hepatic flexure
153.1 Malignant neoplasm of transverse colon
153.2 Malignant neoplasm of descending colon
153.3 Malignant neoplasm of sigmoid colon
153.4 Malignant neoplasm of cecum
153.5 Malignant neoplasm of appendix
153.6 Malignant neoplasm of ascending colon
153.7 Malignant neoplasm of splenic flexure
153.8 Malignant neoplasm of other specified sites of large intestine
153.9 Malignant neoplasm of colon, unspecified site ▽
154.0 Malignant neoplasm of rectosigmoid junction
154.1 Malignant neoplasm of rectum
197.5 Secondary malignant neoplasm of large intestine and rectum
211.3 Benign neoplasm of colon
211.4 Benign neoplasm of rectum and anal canal
230.3 Carcinoma in situ of colon
230.4 Carcinoma in situ of rectum
230.7 Carcinoma in situ of other and unspecified parts of intestine ▽
235.2 Neoplasm of uncertain behavior of stomach, intestines, and rectum
239.0 Neoplasm of unspecified nature of digestive system
556.0 Ulcerative (chronic) enterocolitis
556.1 Ulcerative (chronic) ileocolitis
556.2 Ulcerative (chronic) proctitis
556.3 Ulcerative (chronic) proctosigmoiditis
556.4 Pseudopolyposis of colon
556.5 Left sided ulcerative (chronic) colitis
556.6 Universal ulcerative (chronic) colitis
556.8 Other ulcerative colitis
556.9 Unspecified ulcerative colitis ▽
557.0 Acute vascular insufficiency of intestine
557.1 Chronic vascular insufficiency of intestine
557.9 Unspecified vascular insufficiency of intestine ▽
558.9 Other and unspecified noninfectious gastroenteritis and colitis ▽
560.9 Unspecified intestinal obstruction ▽
562.10 Diverticulosis of colon (without mention of hemorrhage) — (Use additional code to identify any associated peritonitis: 567.0-567.9)
562.11 Diverticulitis of colon (without mention of hemorrhage) — (Use additional code to identify any associated peritonitis: 567.0-567.9)
562.12 Diverticulosis of colon with hemorrhage — (Use additional code to identify any associated peritonitis: 567.0-567.9)
562.13 Diverticulitis of colon with hemorrhage — (Use additional code to identify any associated peritonitis: 567.0-567.9)
564.7 Megacolon, other than Hirschsprung's
564.81 Neurogenic bowel
564.89 Other functional disorders of intestine
567.0 Peritonitis in infectious diseases classified elsewhere — (Code first underlying disease) ☒
567.1 Pneumococcal peritonitis
567.2 Other suppurative peritonitis
567.8 Other specified peritonitis
567.9 Unspecified peritonitis ▽
569.82 Ulceration of intestine
569.83 Perforation of intestine
569.89 Other specified disorder of intestines
569.9 Unspecified disorder of intestine ▽
578.1 Blood in stool
578.9 Unspecified, hemorrhage of gastrointestinal tract ▽
751.3 Hirschsprung's disease and other congenital functional disorders of colon
777.1 Fetal and newborn meconium obstruction
777.5 Necrotizing enterocolitis in fetus or newborn
777.6 Perinatal intestinal perforation
777.8 Other specified perinatal disorder of digestive system
863.40 Colon injury unspecified site, without mention of open wound into cavity ▽
863.41 Ascending (right) colon injury without mention of open wound into cavity
863.42 Transverse colon injury without mention of open wound into cavity
863.43 Descending (left) colon injury without mention of open wound into cavity
863.44 Sigmoid colon injury without mention of open wound into cavity
863.45 Rectum injury without mention of open wound into cavity
863.46 Injury to multiple sites in colon and rectum without mention of open wound into cavity
863.49 Other colon and rectum injury, without mention of open wound into cavity
998.89 Other specified complications
V64.41 Laparoscopic surgical procedure converted to open procedure

ICD-9-CM Procedural

45.8 Total intra-abdominal colectomy
45.92 Anastomosis of small intestine to rectal stump
46.20 Ileostomy, not otherwise specified
46.23 Other permanent ileostomy

44151–44153

44151 Colectomy, total, abdominal, without proctectomy; with continent ileostomy
44152 with rectal mucosectomy, ileoanal anastomosis, with or without loop ileostomy
44153 with rectal mucosectomy, ileoanal anastomosis, creation of ileal reservoir (S or J), with or without loop ileostomy

ICD-9-CM Diagnostic

153.0 Malignant neoplasm of hepatic flexure
153.1 Malignant neoplasm of transverse colon
153.2 Malignant neoplasm of descending colon
153.3 Malignant neoplasm of sigmoid colon
153.4 Malignant neoplasm of cecum
153.5 Malignant neoplasm of appendix
153.6 Malignant neoplasm of ascending colon
153.7 Malignant neoplasm of splenic flexure
153.8 Malignant neoplasm of other specified sites of large intestine
153.9 Malignant neoplasm of colon, unspecified site ▽
154.0 Malignant neoplasm of rectosigmoid junction
154.1 Malignant neoplasm of rectum
197.5 Secondary malignant neoplasm of large intestine and rectum
211.3 Benign neoplasm of colon
211.4 Benign neoplasm of rectum and anal canal
230.3 Carcinoma in situ of colon
230.4 Carcinoma in situ of rectum
230.7 Carcinoma in situ of other and unspecified parts of intestine ▽
235.2 Neoplasm of uncertain behavior of stomach, intestines, and rectum
239.0 Neoplasm of unspecified nature of digestive system
556.0 Ulcerative (chronic) enterocolitis
556.1 Ulcerative (chronic) ileocolitis
556.2 Ulcerative (chronic) proctitis
556.3 Ulcerative (chronic) proctosigmoiditis
556.4 Pseudopolyposis of colon
556.5 Left sided ulcerative (chronic) colitis
556.6 Universal ulcerative (chronic) colitis
556.8 Other ulcerative colitis
556.9 Unspecified ulcerative colitis ▽
557.0 Acute vascular insufficiency of intestine
557.1 Chronic vascular insufficiency of intestine
557.9 Unspecified vascular insufficiency of intestine ▽
558.9 Other and unspecified noninfectious gastroenteritis and colitis ▽
560.9 Unspecified intestinal obstruction ▽
562.10 Diverticulosis of colon (without mention of hemorrhage) — (Use additional code to identify any associated peritonitis: 567.0-567.9)
562.11 Diverticulitis of colon (without mention of hemorrhage) — (Use additional code to identify any associated peritonitis: 567.0-567.9)
562.12 Diverticulosis of colon with hemorrhage — (Use additional code to identify any associated peritonitis: 567.0-567.9)
562.13 Diverticulitis of colon with hemorrhage — (Use additional code to identify any associated peritonitis: 567.0-567.9)
564.7 Megacolon, other than Hirschsprung's
564.81 Neurogenic bowel
564.89 Other functional disorders of intestine
567.0 Peritonitis in infectious diseases classified elsewhere — (Code first underlying disease) ☒
567.1 Pneumococcal peritonitis
567.2 Other suppurative peritonitis
567.8 Other specified peritonitis
567.9 Unspecified peritonitis ▽
569.82 Ulceration of intestine
569.83 Perforation of intestine

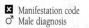

569.89 Other specified disorder of intestines
569.9 Unspecified disorder of intestine ▽
578.1 Blood in stool
578.9 Unspecified, hemorrhage of gastrointestinal tract ▽
751.3 Hirschsprung's disease and other congenital functional disorders of colon
777.1 Fetal and newborn meconium obstruction
777.5 Necrotizing enterocolitis in fetus or newborn
777.6 Perinatal intestinal perforation
777.8 Other specified perinatal disorder of digestive system
863.40 Colon injury unspecified site, without mention of open wound into cavity ▽
863.41 Ascending (right) colon injury without mention of open wound into cavity
863.42 Transverse colon injury without mention of open wound into cavity
863.43 Descending (left) colon injury without mention of open wound into cavity
863.44 Sigmoid colon injury without mention of open wound into cavity
863.45 Rectum injury without mention of open wound into cavity
863.46 Injury to multiple sites in colon and rectum without mention of open wound into cavity
863.49 Other colon and rectum injury, without mention of open wound into cavity
998.89 Other specified complications
V64.41 Laparoscopic surgical procedure converted to open procedure

ICD-9-CM Procedural

45.8 Total intra-abdominal colectomy
46.22 Continent ileostomy

44155–44156

44155 Colectomy, total, abdominal, with proctectomy; with ileostomy
44156 with continent ileostomy

ICD-9-CM Diagnostic

153.0 Malignant neoplasm of hepatic flexure
153.1 Malignant neoplasm of transverse colon
153.2 Malignant neoplasm of descending colon
153.3 Malignant neoplasm of sigmoid colon
153.4 Malignant neoplasm of cecum
153.5 Malignant neoplasm of appendix
153.6 Malignant neoplasm of ascending colon
153.7 Malignant neoplasm of splenic flexure
153.8 Malignant neoplasm of other specified sites of large intestine
153.9 Malignant neoplasm of colon, unspecified site ▽
154.0 Malignant neoplasm of rectosigmoid junction
154.1 Malignant neoplasm of rectum
197.5 Secondary malignant neoplasm of large intestine and rectum
211.3 Benign neoplasm of colon
211.4 Benign neoplasm of rectum and anal canal
230.3 Carcinoma in situ of colon
230.4 Carcinoma in situ of rectum
230.7 Carcinoma in situ of other and unspecified parts of intestine ▽
235.2 Neoplasm of uncertain behavior of stomach, intestines, and rectum
239.0 Neoplasm of unspecified nature of digestive system
555.1 Regional enteritis of large intestine
556.0 Ulcerative (chronic) enterocolitis
556.1 Ulcerative (chronic) ileocolitis
556.2 Ulcerative (chronic) proctitis
556.3 Ulcerative (chronic) proctosigmoiditis
556.4 Pseudopolyposis of colon
556.5 Left sided ulcerative (chronic) colitis
556.6 Universal ulcerative (chronic) colitis
556.8 Other ulcerative colitis
556.9 Unspecified ulcerative colitis ▽
557.0 Acute vascular insufficiency of intestine
557.1 Chronic vascular insufficiency of intestine
557.9 Unspecified vascular insufficiency of intestine ▽
560.9 Unspecified intestinal obstruction ▽
562.10 Diverticulosis of colon (without mention of hemorrhage) — (Use additional code to identify any associated peritonitis: 567.0-567.9)
562.11 Diverticulitis of colon (without mention of hemorrhage) — (Use additional code to identify any associated peritonitis: 567.0-567.9)
562.12 Diverticulosis of colon with hemorrhage — (Use additional code to identify any associated peritonitis: 567.0-567.9)
562.13 Diverticulitis of colon with hemorrhage — (Use additional code to identify any associated peritonitis: 567.0-567.9)
567.0 Peritonitis in infectious diseases classified elsewhere — (Code first underlying disease) ☒
567.1 Pneumococcal peritonitis
567.2 Other suppurative peritonitis
567.8 Other specified peritonitis
567.9 Unspecified peritonitis ▽
569.82 Ulceration of intestine
569.83 Perforation of intestine
569.89 Other specified disorder of intestines
578.1 Blood in stool
751.2 Congenital atresia and stenosis of large intestine, rectum, and anal canal
751.3 Hirschsprung's disease and other congenital functional disorders of colon
777.1 Fetal and newborn meconium obstruction
777.5 Necrotizing enterocolitis in fetus or newborn
777.6 Perinatal intestinal perforation
863.40 Colon injury unspecified site, without mention of open wound into cavity ▽
863.41 Ascending (right) colon injury without mention of open wound into cavity
863.42 Transverse colon injury without mention of open wound into cavity
863.43 Descending (left) colon injury without mention of open wound into cavity
863.44 Sigmoid colon injury without mention of open wound into cavity
863.45 Rectum injury without mention of open wound into cavity
863.46 Injury to multiple sites in colon and rectum without mention of open wound into cavity
863.49 Other colon and rectum injury, without mention of open wound into cavity
998.89 Other specified complications
V64.41 Laparoscopic surgical procedure converted to open procedure

ICD-9-CM Procedural

45.71 Multiple segmental resection of large intestine
45.73 Right hemicolectomy
45.8 Total intra-abdominal colectomy
46.20 Ileostomy, not otherwise specified
46.22 Continent ileostomy
48.5 Abdominoperineal resection of rectum

44160

44160 Colectomy, partial, with removal of terminal ileum with ileocolostomy

ICD-9-CM Diagnostic

152.2 Malignant neoplasm of ileum
152.3 Malignant neoplasm of Meckel's diverticulum
152.8 Malignant neoplasm of other specified sites of small intestine
152.9 Malignant neoplasm of small intestine, unspecified site ▽
153.0 Malignant neoplasm of hepatic flexure
153.1 Malignant neoplasm of transverse colon
153.2 Malignant neoplasm of descending colon
153.3 Malignant neoplasm of sigmoid colon
153.4 Malignant neoplasm of cecum
153.6 Malignant neoplasm of ascending colon
153.7 Malignant neoplasm of splenic flexure
153.8 Malignant neoplasm of other specified sites of large intestine
153.9 Malignant neoplasm of colon, unspecified site ▽
154.0 Malignant neoplasm of rectosigmoid junction
154.1 Malignant neoplasm of rectum
154.2 Malignant neoplasm of anal canal
154.3 Malignant neoplasm of anus, unspecified site ▽
154.8 Malignant neoplasm of other sites of rectum, rectosigmoid junction, and anus
197.4 Secondary malignant neoplasm of small intestine including duodenum
197.5 Secondary malignant neoplasm of large intestine and rectum
211.2 Benign neoplasm of duodenum, jejunum, and ileum
211.3 Benign neoplasm of colon
211.4 Benign neoplasm of rectum and anal canal
211.9 Benign neoplasm of other and unspecified site of the digestive system ▽
229.9 Benign neoplasm of unspecified site ▽
230.3 Carcinoma in situ of colon
235.2 Neoplasm of uncertain behavior of stomach, intestines, and rectum
239.0 Neoplasm of unspecified nature of digestive system
550.00 Inguinal hernia with gangrene, unilateral or unspecified, (not specified as recurrent)
551.1 Umbilical hernia with gangrene
552.8 Hernia of other specified site, with obstruction
555.1 Regional enteritis of large intestine
555.2 Regional enteritis of small intestine with large intestine
556.0 Ulcerative (chronic) enterocolitis
556.1 Ulcerative (chronic) ileocolitis
556.2 Ulcerative (chronic) proctitis
556.3 Ulcerative (chronic) proctosigmoiditis
556.8 Other ulcerative colitis
557.0 Acute vascular insufficiency of intestine
557.1 Chronic vascular insufficiency of intestine

557.9 Unspecified vascular insufficiency of intestine
558.1 Gastroenteritis and colitis due to radiation
558.2 Toxic gastroenteritis and colitis — (Use additional E code to identify cause)
558.9 Other and unspecified noninfectious gastroenteritis and colitis
560.0 Intussusception
560.1 Paralytic ileus
560.2 Volvulus
560.31 Gallstone ileus
560.39 Other impaction of intestine
560.81 Intestinal or peritoneal adhesions with obstruction (postoperative) (postinfection)
560.89 Other specified intestinal obstruction
560.9 Unspecified intestinal obstruction
562.10 Diverticulosis of colon (without mention of hemorrhage) — (Use additional code to identify any associated peritonitis: 567.0-567.9)
562.11 Diverticulitis of colon (without mention of hemorrhage) — (Use additional code to identify any associated peritonitis: 567.0-567.9)
562.12 Diverticulosis of colon with hemorrhage — (Use additional code to identify any associated peritonitis: 567.0-567.9)
562.13 Diverticulitis of colon with hemorrhage — (Use additional code to identify any associated peritonitis: 567.0-567.9)
564.7 Megacolon, other than Hirschsprung's
567.0 Peritonitis in infectious diseases classified elsewhere — (Code first underlying disease)
567.1 Pneumococcal peritonitis
567.2 Other suppurative peritonitis
567.8 Other specified peritonitis
567.9 Unspecified peritonitis
569.81 Fistula of intestine, excluding rectum and anus
569.82 Ulceration of intestine
569.83 Perforation of intestine
569.84 Angiodysplasia of intestine (without mention of hemorrhage)
569.85 Angiodysplasia of intestine with hemorrhage
569.89 Other specified disorder of intestines
569.9 Unspecified disorder of intestine
578.9 Unspecified, hemorrhage of gastrointestinal tract
596.1 Intestinovesical fistula — (Use additional code to identify urinary incontinence: 625.6, 788.30-788.39)
619.1 Digestive-genital tract fistula, female ♀
751.5 Other congenital anomalies of intestine
751.8 Other specified congenital anomalies of digestive system
751.9 Unspecified congenital anomaly of digestive system
V64.41 Laparoscopic surgical procedure converted to open procedure

ICD-9-CM Procedural

45.72 Cecectomy
45.73 Right hemicolectomy
45.74 Resection of transverse colon
45.75 Left hemicolectomy
45.93 Other small-to-large intestinal anastomosis

44200

44200 Laparoscopy, surgical; enterolysis (freeing of intestinal adhesion) (separate procedure)

ICD-9-CM Diagnostic

560.81 Intestinal or peritoneal adhesions with obstruction (postoperative) (postinfection)
568.0 Peritoneal adhesions (postoperative) (postinfection)
617.5 Endometriosis of intestine ♀
751.4 Congenital anomalies of intestinal fixation
789.00 Abdominal pain, unspecified site
789.01 Abdominal pain, right upper quadrant
789.02 Abdominal pain, left upper quadrant
789.03 Abdominal pain, right lower quadrant
789.04 Abdominal pain, left lower quadrant
789.05 Abdominal pain, periumbilic
789.06 Abdominal pain, epigastric
789.07 Abdominal pain, generalized
789.09 Abdominal pain, other specified site
789.30 Abdominal or pelvic swelling, mass or lump, unspecified site
789.31 Abdominal or pelvic swelling, mass, or lump, right upper quadrant
789.32 Abdominal or pelvic swelling, mass, or lump, left upper quadrant
789.33 Abdominal or pelvic swelling, mass, or lump, right lower quadrant
789.34 Abdominal or pelvic swelling, mass, or lump, left lower quadrant
789.35 Abdominal or pelvic swelling, mass or lump, periumbilic
789.36 Abdominal or pelvic swelling, mass, or lump, epigastric
789.37 Abdominal or pelvic swelling, mass, or lump, epigastric, generalized
789.39 Abdominal or pelvic swelling, mass, or lump, other specified site
908.1 Late effect of internal injury to intra-abdominal organs
908.2 Late effect of internal injury to other internal organs
908.6 Late effect of certain complications of trauma
909.3 Late effect of complications of surgical and medical care

ICD-9-CM Procedural

54.51 Laparoscopic lysis of peritoneal adhesions

44201

44201 Laparoscopy, surgical; jejunostomy (eg, for decompression or feeding)

ICD-9-CM Diagnostic

150.1 Malignant neoplasm of thoracic esophagus
150.2 Malignant neoplasm of abdominal esophagus
150.3 Malignant neoplasm of upper third of esophagus
150.4 Malignant neoplasm of middle third of esophagus
150.5 Malignant neoplasm of lower third of esophagus
150.8 Malignant neoplasm of other specified part of esophagus
150.9 Malignant neoplasm of esophagus, unspecified site
151.0 Malignant neoplasm of cardia
151.1 Malignant neoplasm of pylorus
151.2 Malignant neoplasm of pyloric antrum
151.3 Malignant neoplasm of fundus of stomach
151.4 Malignant neoplasm of body of stomach
151.5 Malignant neoplasm of lesser curvature of stomach, unspecified
151.6 Malignant neoplasm of greater curvature of stomach, unspecified
151.8 Malignant neoplasm of other specified sites of stomach
151.9 Malignant neoplasm of stomach, unspecified site
152.0 Malignant neoplasm of duodenum
152.1 Malignant neoplasm of jejunum
152.2 Malignant neoplasm of ileum
161.9 Malignant neoplasm of larynx, unspecified site
197.4 Secondary malignant neoplasm of small intestine including duodenum
197.8 Secondary malignant neoplasm of other digestive organs and spleen
198.89 Secondary malignant neoplasm of other specified sites
211.1 Benign neoplasm of stomach
230.2 Carcinoma in situ of stomach
239.8 Neoplasm of unspecified nature of other specified sites
261 Nutritional marasmus
262 Other severe protein-calorie malnutrition
263.0 Malnutrition of moderate degree
263.1 Malnutrition of mild degree
263.2 Arrested development following protein-calorie malnutrition
263.8 Other protein-calorie malnutrition
276.5 Volume depletion — (Use additional code to identify any associated mental retardation)
307.1 Anorexia nervosa
436 Acute, but ill-defined, cerebrovascular disease — (Use additional code to identify presence of hypertension)
519.00 Unspecified tracheostomy complication
519.01 Infection of tracheostomy — (Use additional code to identify type of infection: 038.0-038.9, 682.1. Use additional code to identify organism: 041.00-041.9)
519.02 Mechanical complication of tracheostomy
519.09 Other tracheostomy complications
530.3 Stricture and stenosis of esophagus
530.4 Perforation of esophagus
530.5 Dyskinesia of esophagus
530.81 Esophageal reflux
531.00 Acute gastric ulcer with hemorrhage, without mention of obstruction — (Use additional E code to identify drug, if drug induced)
531.01 Acute gastric ulcer with hemorrhage and obstruction — (Use additional E code to identify drug, if drug induced)
531.10 Acute gastric ulcer with perforation, without mention of obstruction — (Use additional E code to identify drug, if drug induced)
531.11 Acute gastric ulcer with perforation and obstruction — (Use additional E code to identify drug, if drug induced)
531.20 Acute gastric ulcer with hemorrhage and perforation, without mention of obstruction — (Use additional E code to identify drug, if drug induced)
531.21 Acute gastric ulcer with hemorrhage, perforation, and obstruction — (Use additional E code to identify drug, if drug induced)
531.30 Acute gastric ulcer without mention of hemorrhage, perforation, or obstruction — (Use additional E code to identify drug, if drug induced)

531.31 Acute gastric ulcer without mention of hemorrhage or perforation, with obstruction — (Use additional E code to identify drug, if drug induced)
531.40 Chronic or unspecified gastric ulcer with hemorrhage, without mention of obstruction — (Use additional E code to identify drug, if drug induced)
531.41 Chronic or unspecified gastric ulcer with hemorrhage and obstruction — (Use additional E code to identify drug, if drug induced)
531.50 Chronic or unspecified gastric ulcer with perforation, without mention of obstruction — (Use additional E code to identify drug, if drug induced)
531.51 Chronic or unspecified gastric ulcer with perforation and obstruction — (Use additional E code to identify drug, if drug induced)
531.60 Chronic or unspecified gastric ulcer with hemorrhage and perforation, without mention of obstruction — (Use additional E code to identify drug, if drug induced)
531.61 Chronic or unspecified gastric ulcer with hemorrhage, perforation, and obstruction — (Use additional E code to identify drug, if drug induced)
531.70 Chronic gastric ulcer without mention of hemorrhage, perforation, without mention of obstruction — (Use additional E code to identify drug, if drug induced)
531.71 Chronic gastric ulcer without mention of hemorrhage or perforation, with obstruction — (Use additional E code to identify drug, if drug induced)
531.90 Gastric ulcer, unspecified as acute or chronic, without mention of hemorrhage, perforation, or obstruction — (Use additional E code to identify drug, if drug induced) ▽
531.91 Gastric ulcer, unspecified as acute or chronic, without mention of hemorrhage or perforation, with obstruction — (Use additional E code to identify drug, if drug induced) ▽
532.00 Acute duodenal ulcer with hemorrhage, without mention of obstruction — (Use additional E code to identify drug, if drug induced)
532.01 Acute duodenal ulcer with hemorrhage and obstruction — (Use additional E code to identify drug, if drug induced)
532.10 Acute duodenal ulcer with perforation, without mention of obstruction — (Use additional E code to identify drug, if drug induced)
532.11 Acute duodenal ulcer with perforation and obstruction — (Use additional E code to identify drug, if drug induced)
532.20 Acute duodenal ulcer with hemorrhage and perforation, without mention of obstruction — (Use additional E code to identify drug, if drug induced)
532.21 Acute duodenal ulcer with hemorrhage, perforation, and obstruction — (Use additional E code to identify drug, if drug induced)
532.30 Acute duodenal ulcer without mention of hemorrhage, perforation, or obstruction — (Use additional E code to identify drug, if drug induced)
532.31 Acute duodenal ulcer without mention of hemorrhage or perforation, with obstruction — (Use additional E code to identify drug, if drug induced)
532.40 Chronic or unspecified duodenal ulcer with hemorrhage, without mention of obstruction — (Use additional E code to identify drug, if drug induced)
532.41 Chronic or unspecified duodenal ulcer with hemorrhage and obstruction — (Use additional E code to identify drug, if drug induced)
532.50 Chronic or unspecified duodenal ulcer with perforation, without mention of obstruction — (Use additional E code to identify drug, if drug induced)
532.51 Chronic or unspecified duodenal ulcer with perforation and obstruction — (Use additional E code to identify drug, if drug induced)
532.60 Chronic or unspecified duodenal ulcer with hemorrhage and perforation, without mention of obstruction — (Use additional E code to identify drug, if drug induced)
532.61 Chronic or unspecified duodenal ulcer with hemorrhage, perforation, and obstruction — (Use additional E code to identify drug, if drug induced)
532.70 Chronic duodenal ulcer without mention of hemorrhage, perforation, or obstruction — (Use additional E code to identify drug, if drug induced)
532.71 Chronic duodenal ulcer without mention of hemorrhage or perforation, with obstruction — (Use additional E code to identify drug, if drug induced)
532.90 Duodenal ulcer, unspecified as acute or chronic, without hemorrhage, perforation, or obstruction — (Use additional E code to identify drug, if drug induced) ▽
532.91 Duodenal ulcer, unspecified as acute or chronic, without mention of hemorrhage or perforation, with obstruction — (Use additional E code to identify drug, if drug induced) ▽
533.00 Acute peptic ulcer, unspecified site, with hemorrhage, without mention of obstruction — (Use additional E code to identify drug, if drug induced)
533.01 Acute peptic ulcer, unspecified site, with hemorrhage and obstruction — (Use additional E code to identify drug, if drug induced)
533.10 Acute peptic ulcer, unspecified site, with perforation, without mention of obstruction — (Use additional E code to identify drug, if drug induced)
533.11 Acute peptic ulcer, unspecified site, with perforation and obstruction — (Use additional E code to identify drug, if drug induced)
533.20 Acute peptic ulcer, unspecified site, with hemorrhage and perforation, without mention of obstruction — (Use additional E code to identify drug, if drug induced)
533.21 Acute peptic ulcer, unspecified site, with hemorrhage, perforation, and obstruction — (Use additional E code to identify drug, if drug induced)
533.30 Acute peptic ulcer, unspecified site, without mention of hemorrhage, perforation, or obstruction — (Use additional E code to identify drug, if drug induced)
533.40 Chronic or unspecified peptic ulcer, unspecified site, with hemorrhage, without mention of obstruction — (Use additional E code to identify drug, if drug induced)
533.41 Chronic or unspecified peptic ulcer, unspecified site, with hemorrhage and obstruction — (Use additional E code to identify drug, if drug induced)
533.50 Chronic or unspecified peptic ulcer, unspecified site, with perforation, without mention of obstruction — (Use additional E code to identify drug, if drug induced)
533.51 Chronic or unspecified peptic ulcer, unspecified site, with perforation and obstruction — (Use additional E code to identify drug, if drug induced)
535.50 Unspecified gastritis and gastroduodenitis without mention of hemorrhage ▽
536.9 Unspecified functional disorder of stomach ▽
537.89 Other specified disorder of stomach and duodenum
578.9 Unspecified, hemorrhage of gastrointestinal tract ▽
707.9 Chronic ulcer of unspecified site ▽
750.5 Congenital hypertrophic pyloric stenosis
750.7 Other specified congenital anomalies of stomach
751.1 Congenital atresia and stenosis of small intestine
783.0 Anorexia
783.3 Feeding difficulties and mismanagement
783.7 Adult failure to thrive
787.01 Nausea with vomiting
787.2 Dysphagia
854.06 Intracranial injury of other and unspecified nature, without mention of open intracranial wound, loss of consciousness of unspecified duration ▽
994.2 Effects of hunger
997.4 Digestive system complication — (Use additional code to identify complications)

ICD-9-CM Procedural

46.39 Other enterostomy

44202–44203

44202 Laparoscopy, surgical; enterectomy, resection of small intestine, single resection and anastomosis
44203 each additional small intestine resection and anastomosis (List separately in addition to code for primary procedure)

ICD-9-CM Diagnostic

152.0 Malignant neoplasm of duodenum
152.1 Malignant neoplasm of jejunum
152.2 Malignant neoplasm of ileum
152.8 Malignant neoplasm of other specified sites of small intestine
152.9 Malignant neoplasm of small intestine, unspecified site ▽
197.4 Secondary malignant neoplasm of small intestine including duodenum
211.2 Benign neoplasm of duodenum, jejunum, and ileum
230.7 Carcinoma in situ of other and unspecified parts of intestine ▽
230.9 Carcinoma in situ of other and unspecified digestive organs ▽
235.2 Neoplasm of uncertain behavior of stomach, intestines, and rectum
239.0 Neoplasm of unspecified nature of digestive system
551.00 Femoral hernia with gangrene, unilateral or unspecified (not specified as recurrent)
551.01 Femoral hernia with gangrene, recurrent unilateral or unspecified
551.02 Femoral hernia with gangrene, bilateral, (not specified as recurrent)
551.03 Femoral hernia with gangrene, recurrent bilateral
551.21 Incisional ventral hernia, with gangrene
551.8 Hernia of other specified sites, with gangrene
551.9 Hernia of unspecified site, with gangrene ▽
552.00 Unilateral or unspecified femoral hernia with obstruction
552.21 Incisional hernia with obstruction
555.0 Regional enteritis of small intestine
555.9 Regional enteritis of unspecified site ▽
556.1 Ulcerative (chronic) ileocolitis
560.0 Intussusception
560.1 Paralytic ileus
560.2 Volvulus
560.81 Intestinal or peritoneal adhesions with obstruction (postoperative) (postinfection)
560.89 Other specified intestinal obstruction
560.9 Unspecified intestinal obstruction ▽

▽ Unspecified code
♀ Female diagnosis
☒ Manifestation code
♂ Male diagnosis

562.00 Diverticulosis of small intestine (without mention of hemorrhage) — (Use additional code to identify any associated peritonitis: 567.0-567.9)
562.01 Diverticulitis of small intestine (without mention of hemorrhage) — (Use additional code to identify any associated peritonitis: 567.0-567.9)
562.02 Diverticulosis of small intestine with hemorrhage — (Use additional code to identify any associated peritonitis: 567.0-567.9)
562.03 Divertulitis of small intestine with hemorrhage — (Use additional code to identify any associated peritonitis: 567.0-567.9)
567.0 Peritonitis in infectious diseases classified elsewhere — (Code first underlying disease) ☒
567.1 Pneumococcal peritonitis
567.2 Other suppurative peritonitis
567.8 Other specified peritonitis
567.9 Unspecified peritonitis ▽
569.5 Abscess of intestine
569.81 Fistula of intestine, excluding rectum and anus
569.82 Ulceration of intestine
569.83 Perforation of intestine
569.85 Angiodysplasia of intestine with hemorrhage
569.89 Other specified disorder of intestines
578.9 Unspecified, hemorrhage of gastrointestinal tract ▽
619.1 Digestive-genital tract fistula, female ♀
863.20 Small intestine injury, unspecified site, without mention of open wound into cavity ▽
863.21 Duodenum injury without mention of open wound into cavity
863.29 Other injury to small intestine without mention of open wound into cavity
863.30 Small intestine injury, unspecified site, with open wound into cavity ▽
863.31 Duodenum injury with open wound into cavity
863.39 Other injury to small intestine with open wound into cavity
863.80 Gastrointestinal tract injury, unspecified site, without mention of open wound into cavity ▽
863.89 Injury to other and unspecified gastrointestinal sites without mention of open wound into cavity
863.90 Gastrointestinal tract injury, unspecified site, with open wound into cavity ▽
863.99 Injury to other and unspecified gastrointestinal sites with open wound into cavity
997.4 Digestive system complication — (Use additional code to identify complications)
998.2 Accidental puncture or laceration during procedure
998.51 Infected postoperative seroma — (Use additional code to identify organism)
998.59 Other postoperative infection — (Use additional code to identify infection)
998.6 Persistent postoperative fistula, not elsewhere classified

ICD-9-CM Procedural

45.62 Other partial resection of small intestine

44204–44205

44204 Laparoscopy, surgical; colectomy, partial, with anastomosis
44205 colectomy, partial, with removal of terminal ileum with ileocolostomy

ICD-9-CM Diagnostic

152.2 Malignant neoplasm of ileum
152.3 Malignant neoplasm of Meckel's diverticulum
152.8 Malignant neoplasm of other specified sites of small intestine
152.9 Malignant neoplasm of small intestine, unspecified site ▽
153.0 Malignant neoplasm of hepatic flexure
153.1 Malignant neoplasm of transverse colon
153.2 Malignant neoplasm of descending colon
153.3 Malignant neoplasm of sigmoid colon
153.4 Malignant neoplasm of cecum
153.6 Malignant neoplasm of ascending colon
153.7 Malignant neoplasm of splenic flexure
153.8 Malignant neoplasm of other specified sites of large intestine
153.9 Malignant neoplasm of colon, unspecified site ▽
154.0 Malignant neoplasm of rectosigmoid junction
154.1 Malignant neoplasm of rectum
154.2 Malignant neoplasm of anal canal
154.3 Malignant neoplasm of anus, unspecified site ▽
154.8 Malignant neoplasm of other sites of rectum, rectosigmoid junction, and anus
197.4 Secondary malignant neoplasm of small intestine including duodenum
197.5 Secondary malignant neoplasm of large intestine and rectum
211.2 Benign neoplasm of duodenum, jejunum, and ileum
211.3 Benign neoplasm of colon
211.4 Benign neoplasm of rectum and anal canal
211.9 Benign neoplasm of other and unspecified site of the digestive system ▽
229.9 Benign neoplasm of unspecified site ▽
230.3 Carcinoma in situ of colon
235.2 Neoplasm of uncertain behavior of stomach, intestines, and rectum
239.0 Neoplasm of unspecified nature of digestive system
550.00 Inguinal hernia with gangrene, unilateral or unspecified, (not specified as recurrent)
551.1 Umbilical hernia with gangrene
552.8 Hernia of other specified site, with obstruction
555.1 Regional enteritis of large intestine
555.2 Regional enteritis of small intestine with large intestine
556.0 Ulcerative (chronic) enterocolitis
556.1 Ulcerative (chronic) ileocolitis
556.2 Ulcerative (chronic) proctitis
556.3 Ulcerative (chronic) proctosigmoiditis
556.8 Other ulcerative colitis
557.0 Acute vascular insufficiency of intestine
557.1 Chronic vascular insufficiency of intestine
557.9 Unspecified vascular insufficiency of intestine ▽
558.1 Gastroenteritis and colitis due to radiation
558.2 Toxic gastroenteritis and colitis — (Use additional E code to identify cause)
558.9 Other and unspecified noninfectious gastroenteritis and colitis ▽
560.0 Intussusception
560.1 Paralytic ileus
560.2 Volvulus
560.31 Gallstone ileus
560.39 Other impaction of intestine
560.81 Intestinal or peritoneal adhesions with obstruction (postoperative) (postinfection)
560.89 Other specified intestinal obstruction
560.9 Unspecified intestinal obstruction ▽
562.10 Diverticulosis of colon (without mention of hemorrhage) — (Use additional code to identify any associated peritonitis: 567.0-567.9)
562.11 Diverticulitis of colon (without mention of hemorrhage) — (Use additional code to identify any associated peritonitis: 567.0-567.9)
562.12 Diverticulosis of colon with hemorrhage — (Use additional code to identify any associated peritonitis: 567.0-567.9)
562.13 Diverticulitis of colon with hemorrhage — (Use additional code to identify any associated peritonitis: 567.0-567.9)
564.7 Megacolon, other than Hirschsprung's
567.0 Peritonitis in infectious diseases classified elsewhere — (Code first underlying disease) ☒
567.1 Pneumococcal peritonitis
567.2 Other suppurative peritonitis
567.8 Other specified peritonitis
567.9 Unspecified peritonitis ▽
569.81 Fistula of intestine, excluding rectum and anus
569.82 Ulceration of intestine
569.83 Perforation of intestine
569.84 Angiodysplasia of intestine (without mention of hemorrhage)
569.85 Angiodysplasia of intestine with hemorrhage
569.89 Other specified disorder of intestines
569.9 Unspecified disorder of intestine ▽
578.9 Unspecified, hemorrhage of gastrointestinal tract ▽
596.1 Intestinovesical fistula — (Use additional code to identify urinary incontinence: 625.6, 788.30-788.39)
619.1 Digestive-genital tract fistula, female ♀
751.5 Other congenital anomalies of intestine
751.8 Other specified congenital anomalies of digestive system
751.9 Unspecified congenital anomaly of digestive system ▽

ICD-9-CM Procedural

45.72 Cecectomy
45.73 Right hemicolectomy
45.74 Resection of transverse colon
45.75 Left hemicolectomy
45.76 Sigmoidectomy
45.79 Other partial excision of large intestine

44206

44206 Laparoscopy, surgical; colectomy, partial, with end colostomy and closure of distal segment (Hartmann type procedure)

ICD-9-CM Diagnostic

153.0 Malignant neoplasm of hepatic flexure
153.1 Malignant neoplasm of transverse colon
153.2 Malignant neoplasm of descending colon
153.3 Malignant neoplasm of sigmoid colon

153.4	Malignant neoplasm of cecum
153.5	Malignant neoplasm of appendix
153.6	Malignant neoplasm of ascending colon
153.7	Malignant neoplasm of splenic flexure
153.8	Malignant neoplasm of other specified sites of large intestine
153.9	Malignant neoplasm of colon, unspecified site ▽
154.0	Malignant neoplasm of rectosigmoid junction
154.1	Malignant neoplasm of rectum
154.8	Malignant neoplasm of other sites of rectum, rectosigmoid junction, and anus
159.0	Malignant neoplasm of intestinal tract, part unspecified ▽
197.5	Secondary malignant neoplasm of large intestine and rectum
198.89	Secondary malignant neoplasm of other specified sites
199.1	Other malignant neoplasm of unspecified site
211.3	Benign neoplasm of colon
211.4	Benign neoplasm of rectum and anal canal
230.3	Carcinoma in situ of colon
230.4	Carcinoma in situ of rectum
235.2	Neoplasm of uncertain behavior of stomach, intestines, and rectum
239.0	Neoplasm of unspecified nature of digestive system
555.1	Regional enteritis of large intestine
555.2	Regional enteritis of small intestine with large intestine
555.9	Regional enteritis of unspecified site ▽
556.0	Ulcerative (chronic) enterocolitis
556.1	Ulcerative (chronic) ileocolitis
556.2	Ulcerative (chronic) proctitis
556.3	Ulcerative (chronic) proctosigmoiditis
556.4	Pseudopolyposis of colon
556.5	Left sided ulcerative (chronic) colitis
556.6	Universal ulcerative (chronic) colitis
556.8	Other ulcerative colitis
556.9	Unspecified ulcerative colitis ▽
557.0	Acute vascular insufficiency of intestine
557.1	Chronic vascular insufficiency of intestine
557.9	Unspecified vascular insufficiency of intestine ▽
560.2	Volvulus
560.81	Intestinal or peritoneal adhesions with obstruction (postoperative) (postinfection)
560.89	Other specified intestinal obstruction
560.9	Unspecified intestinal obstruction ▽
562.10	Diverticulosis of colon (without mention of hemorrhage) — (Use additional code to identify any associated peritonitis: 567.0-567.9)
562.11	Diverticulitis of colon (without mention of hemorrhage) — (Use additional code to identify any associated peritonitis: 567.0-567.9)
562.12	Diverticulosis of colon with hemorrhage — (Use additional code to identify any associated peritonitis: 567.0-567.9)
562.13	Diverticulitis of colon with hemorrhage — (Use additional code to identify any associated peritonitis: 567.0-567.9)
564.81	Neurogenic bowel
564.89	Other functional disorders of intestine
567.0	Peritonitis in infectious diseases classified elsewhere — (Code first underlying disease) ☒
567.1	Pneumococcal peritonitis
567.2	Other suppurative peritonitis
567.8	Other specified peritonitis
567.9	Unspecified peritonitis ▽
569.5	Abscess of intestine
569.81	Fistula of intestine, excluding rectum and anus
569.82	Ulceration of intestine
569.83	Perforation of intestine
569.84	Angiodysplasia of intestine (without mention of hemorrhage)
569.85	Angiodysplasia of intestine with hemorrhage
569.89	Other specified disorder of intestines
569.9	Unspecified disorder of intestine ▽
578.1	Blood in stool
578.9	Unspecified, hemorrhage of gastrointestinal tract ▽
596.1	Intestinovesical fistula — (Use additional code to identify urinary incontinence: 625.6, 788.30-788.39)
619.1	Digestive-genital tract fistula, female ♀
751.2	Congenital atresia and stenosis of large intestine, rectum, and anal canal
751.3	Hirschsprung's disease and other congenital functional disorders of colon
751.4	Congenital anomalies of intestinal fixation
751.5	Other congenital anomalies of intestine
751.8	Other specified congenital anomalies of digestive system
751.9	Unspecified congenital anomaly of digestive system ▽
777.5	Necrotizing enterocolitis in fetus or newborn
777.6	Perinatal intestinal perforation
777.8	Other specified perinatal disorder of digestive system
777.9	Unspecified perinatal disorder of digestive system ▽
789.00	Abdominal pain, unspecified site ▽
789.01	Abdominal pain, right upper quadrant
789.02	Abdominal pain, left upper quadrant
789.03	Abdominal pain, right lower quadrant
789.04	Abdominal pain, left lower quadrant
789.05	Abdominal pain, periumbilic
789.06	Abdominal pain, epigastric
789.07	Abdominal pain, generalized
789.09	Abdominal pain, other specified site
789.30	Abdominal or pelvic swelling, mass or lump, unspecified site ▽
789.31	Abdominal or pelvic swelling, mass, or lump, right upper quadrant
789.32	Abdominal or pelvic swelling, mass, or lump, left upper quadrant
789.33	Abdominal or pelvic swelling, mass, or lump, right lower quadrant
789.34	Abdominal or pelvic swelling, mass, or lump, left lower quadrant
789.35	Abdominal or pelvic swelling, mass or lump, periumbilic
789.36	Abdominal or pelvic swelling, mass, or lump, epigastric
789.37	Abdominal or pelvic swelling, mass, or lump, epigastric, generalized
789.39	Abdominal or pelvic swelling, mass, or lump, other specified site
789.9	Other symptoms involving abdomen and pelvis
793.4	Nonspecific abnormal findings on radiological and other examination of gastrointestinal tract
863.40	Colon injury unspecified site, without mention of open wound into cavity ▽
863.41	Ascending (right) colon injury without mention of open wound into cavity
863.42	Transverse colon injury without mention of open wound into cavity
863.43	Descending (left) colon injury without mention of open wound into cavity
863.44	Sigmoid colon injury without mention of open wound into cavity
863.45	Rectum injury without mention of open wound into cavity
863.46	Injury to multiple sites in colon and rectum without mention of open wound into cavity
863.49	Other colon and rectum injury, without mention of open wound into cavity
863.50	Colon injury, unspecified site, with open wound into cavity ▽
863.51	Ascending (right) colon injury with open wound into cavity
863.52	Transverse colon injury with open wound into cavity
863.53	Descending (left) colon injury with open wound into cavity
863.54	Sigmoid colon injury with open wound into cavity
863.55	Rectum injury with open wound into cavity
863.56	Injury to multiple sites in colon and rectum with open wound into cavity
863.59	Other injury to colon and rectum with open wound into cavity
863.80	Gastrointestinal tract injury, unspecified site, without mention of open wound into cavity ▽
863.90	Gastrointestinal tract injury, unspecified site, with open wound into cavity ▽
869.0	Internal injury to unspecified or ill-defined organs without mention of open wound into cavity
869.1	Internal injury to unspecified or ill-defined organs with open wound into cavity
936	Foreign body in intestine and colon
937	Foreign body in anus and rectum
938	Foreign body in digestive system, unspecified ▽
997.4	Digestive system complication — (Use additional code to identify complications)
998.2	Accidental puncture or laceration during procedure
998.31	Disruption of internal operation wound
998.6	Persistent postoperative fistula, not elsewhere classified
998.9	Unspecified complication of procedure, not elsewhere classified ▽

ICD-9-CM Procedural

45.72	Cecectomy
45.73	Right hemicolectomy
45.74	Resection of transverse colon
45.75	Left hemicolectomy

44207–44208

44207	Laparoscopy, surgical; colectomy, partial, with anastomosis, with coloproctostomy (low pelvic anastomosis)
44208	colectomy, partial, with anastomosis, with coloproctostomy (low pelvic anastomosis) with colostomy

ICD-9-CM Diagnostic

153.0	Malignant neoplasm of hepatic flexure
153.1	Malignant neoplasm of transverse colon
153.2	Malignant neoplasm of descending colon
153.3	Malignant neoplasm of sigmoid colon
153.4	Malignant neoplasm of cecum
153.5	Malignant neoplasm of appendix
153.6	Malignant neoplasm of ascending colon

▽ Unspecified code
♀ Female diagnosis
☒ Manifestation code
♂ Male diagnosis

153.7 Malignant neoplasm of splenic flexure
153.8 Malignant neoplasm of other specified sites of large intestine
153.9 Malignant neoplasm of colon, unspecified site
154.0 Malignant neoplasm of rectosigmoid junction
154.1 Malignant neoplasm of rectum
154.2 Malignant neoplasm of anal canal
154.8 Malignant neoplasm of other sites of rectum, rectosigmoid junction, and anus
159.0 Malignant neoplasm of intestinal tract, part unspecified
197.5 Secondary malignant neoplasm of large intestine and rectum
211.3 Benign neoplasm of colon
211.4 Benign neoplasm of rectum and anal canal
230.3 Carcinoma in situ of colon
230.4 Carcinoma in situ of rectum
230.9 Carcinoma in situ of other and unspecified digestive organs
235.2 Neoplasm of uncertain behavior of stomach, intestines, and rectum
239.0 Neoplasm of unspecified nature of digestive system
555.1 Regional enteritis of large intestine
555.2 Regional enteritis of small intestine with large intestine
555.9 Regional enteritis of unspecified site
556.0 Ulcerative (chronic) enterocolitis
556.1 Ulcerative (chronic) ileocolitis
556.2 Ulcerative (chronic) proctitis
556.3 Ulcerative (chronic) proctosigmoiditis
556.4 Pseudopolyposis of colon
556.5 Left sided ulcerative (chronic) colitis
556.6 Universal ulcerative (chronic) colitis
556.8 Other ulcerative colitis
556.9 Unspecified ulcerative colitis
557.0 Acute vascular insufficiency of intestine
557.1 Chronic vascular insufficiency of intestine
557.9 Unspecified vascular insufficiency of intestine
560.39 Other impaction of intestine
560.81 Intestinal or peritoneal adhesions with obstruction (postoperative) (postinfection)
560.89 Other specified intestinal obstruction
560.9 Unspecified intestinal obstruction
562.10 Diverticulosis of colon (without mention of hemorrhage) — (Use additional code to identify any associated peritonitis: 567.0-567.9)
562.11 Diverticulitis of colon (without mention of hemorrhage) — (Use additional code to identify any associated peritonitis: 567.0-567.9)
562.12 Diverticulosis of colon with hemorrhage — (Use additional code to identify any associated peritonitis: 567.0-567.9)
562.13 Diverticulitis of colon with hemorrhage — (Use additional code to identify any associated peritonitis: 567.0-567.9)
564.7 Megacolon, other than Hirschsprung's
567.0 Peritonitis in infectious diseases classified elsewhere — (Code first underlying disease)
567.1 Pneumococcal peritonitis
567.2 Other suppurative peritonitis
567.8 Other specified peritonitis
567.9 Unspecified peritonitis
569.1 Rectal prolapse
569.81 Fistula of intestine, excluding rectum and anus
569.82 Ulceration of intestine
569.83 Perforation of intestine
569.84 Angiodysplasia of intestine (without mention of hemorrhage)
569.85 Angiodysplasia of intestine with hemorrhage
569.89 Other specified disorder of intestines
569.9 Unspecified disorder of intestine
596.1 Intestinovesical fistula — (Use additional code to identify urinary incontinence: 625.6, 788.30-788.39)
619.1 Digestive-genital tract fistula, female ♀
751.8 Other specified congenital anomalies of digestive system
777.5 Necrotizing enterocolitis in fetus or newborn
777.6 Perinatal intestinal perforation
777.8 Other specified perinatal disorder of digestive system
787.99 Other symptoms involving digestive system

ICD-9-CM Procedural

45.75 Left hemicolectomy
45.76 Sigmoidectomy
45.94 Large-to-large intestinal anastomosis
46.03 Exteriorization of large intestine
46.11 Temporary colostomy
46.13 Permanent colostomy

HCPCS Level II Supplies & Services

HCPCS Level II codes are used to report the supplies, durable medical equipment, and certain medical services provided on an outpatient basis. Because the procedure(s) represented on this page would be performed in an inpatient facility, no HCPCS Level II codes apply.

44210

44210 Laparoscopy, surgical; colectomy, total, abdominal, without proctectomy, with ileostomy or ileoproctostomy

ICD-9-CM Diagnostic

153.0 Malignant neoplasm of hepatic flexure
153.1 Malignant neoplasm of transverse colon
153.2 Malignant neoplasm of descending colon
153.3 Malignant neoplasm of sigmoid colon
153.4 Malignant neoplasm of cecum
153.5 Malignant neoplasm of appendix
153.6 Malignant neoplasm of ascending colon
153.7 Malignant neoplasm of splenic flexure
153.8 Malignant neoplasm of other specified sites of large intestine
153.9 Malignant neoplasm of colon, unspecified site
154.0 Malignant neoplasm of rectosigmoid junction
154.1 Malignant neoplasm of rectum
197.5 Secondary malignant neoplasm of large intestine and rectum
211.3 Benign neoplasm of colon
211.4 Benign neoplasm of rectum and anal canal
230.3 Carcinoma in situ of colon
230.4 Carcinoma in situ of rectum
230.7 Carcinoma in situ of other and unspecified parts of intestine
235.2 Neoplasm of uncertain behavior of stomach, intestines, and rectum
239.0 Neoplasm of unspecified nature of digestive system
556.0 Ulcerative (chronic) enterocolitis
556.1 Ulcerative (chronic) ileocolitis
556.2 Ulcerative (chronic) proctitis
556.3 Ulcerative (chronic) proctosigmoiditis
556.4 Pseudopolyposis of colon
556.5 Left sided ulcerative (chronic) colitis
556.6 Universal ulcerative (chronic) colitis
556.8 Other ulcerative colitis
556.9 Unspecified ulcerative colitis
557.0 Acute vascular insufficiency of intestine
557.1 Chronic vascular insufficiency of intestine
557.9 Unspecified vascular insufficiency of intestine
558.9 Other and unspecified noninfectious gastroenteritis and colitis
560.9 Unspecified intestinal obstruction
562.10 Diverticulosis of colon (without mention of hemorrhage) — (Use additional code to identify any associated peritonitis: 567.0-567.9)
562.11 Diverticulitis of colon (without mention of hemorrhage) — (Use additional code to identify any associated peritonitis: 567.0-567.9)
562.12 Diverticulosis of colon with hemorrhage — (Use additional code to identify any associated peritonitis: 567.0-567.9)
562.13 Diverticulitis of colon with hemorrhage — (Use additional code to identify any associated peritonitis: 567.0-567.9)
564.7 Megacolon, other than Hirschsprung's
564.81 Neurogenic bowel
564.89 Other functional disorders of intestine
567.0 Peritonitis in infectious diseases classified elsewhere — (Code first underlying disease)
567.1 Pneumococcal peritonitis
567.2 Other suppurative peritonitis
567.8 Other specified peritonitis
567.9 Unspecified peritonitis
569.82 Ulceration of intestine
569.83 Perforation of intestine
569.89 Other specified disorder of intestines
569.9 Unspecified disorder of intestine
578.1 Blood in stool
578.9 Unspecified, hemorrhage of gastrointestinal tract
751.3 Hirschsprung's disease and other congenital functional disorders of colon
777.1 Fetal and newborn meconium obstruction
777.5 Necrotizing enterocolitis in fetus or newborn
777.6 Perinatal intestinal perforation
777.8 Other specified perinatal disorder of digestive system
863.40 Colon injury unspecified site, without mention of open wound into cavity
863.41 Ascending (right) colon injury without mention of open wound into cavity
863.42 Transverse colon injury without mention of open wound into cavity

863.43 Descending (left) colon injury without mention of open wound into cavity
863.44 Sigmoid colon injury without mention of open wound into cavity
863.45 Rectum injury without mention of open wound into cavity
863.46 Injury to multiple sites in colon and rectum without mention of open wound into cavity
863.49 Other colon and rectum injury, without mention of open wound into cavity
998.89 Other specified complications

ICD-9-CM Procedural

45.8 Total intra-abdominal colectomy
45.92 Anastomosis of small intestine to rectal stump
46.23 Other permanent ileostomy

HCPCS Level II Supplies & Services

HCPCS Level II codes are used to report the supplies, durable medical equipment, and certain medical services provided on an outpatient basis. Because the procedure(s) represented on this page would be performed in an inpatient facility, no HCPCS Level II codes apply.

44211

44211 Laparoscopy, surgical; colectomy, total, abdominal, with proctectomy, with ileoanal anastomosis, creation of ileal reservoir (S or J), with loop ileostomy, with or without rectal mucosectomy

ICD-9-CM Diagnostic

153.0 Malignant neoplasm of hepatic flexure
153.1 Malignant neoplasm of transverse colon
153.2 Malignant neoplasm of descending colon
153.3 Malignant neoplasm of sigmoid colon
153.4 Malignant neoplasm of cecum
153.5 Malignant neoplasm of appendix
153.6 Malignant neoplasm of ascending colon
153.7 Malignant neoplasm of splenic flexure
153.8 Malignant neoplasm of other specified sites of large intestine
153.9 Malignant neoplasm of colon, unspecified site ▽
154.0 Malignant neoplasm of rectosigmoid junction
154.1 Malignant neoplasm of rectum
197.5 Secondary malignant neoplasm of large intestine and rectum
211.3 Benign neoplasm of colon
211.4 Benign neoplasm of rectum and anal canal
230.3 Carcinoma in situ of colon
230.4 Carcinoma in situ of rectum
230.7 Carcinoma in situ of other and unspecified parts of intestine ▽
235.2 Neoplasm of uncertain behavior of stomach, intestines, and rectum
239.0 Neoplasm of unspecified nature of digestive system
556.0 Ulcerative (chronic) enterocolitis
556.1 Ulcerative (chronic) ileocolitis
556.2 Ulcerative (chronic) proctitis
556.3 Ulcerative (chronic) proctosigmoiditis
556.4 Pseudopolyposis of colon
556.5 Left sided ulcerative (chronic) colitis
556.6 Universal ulcerative (chronic) colitis
556.8 Other ulcerative colitis
556.9 Unspecified ulcerative colitis ▽
557.0 Acute vascular insufficiency of intestine
557.1 Chronic vascular insufficiency of intestine
557.9 Unspecified vascular insufficiency of intestine ▽
558.9 Other and unspecified noninfectious gastroenteritis and colitis ▽
560.9 Unspecified intestinal obstruction ▽
562.10 Diverticulosis of colon (without mention of hemorrhage) — (Use additional code to identify any associated peritonitis: 567.0-567.9)
562.11 Diverticulitis of colon (without mention of hemorrhage) — (Use additional code to identify any associated peritonitis: 567.0-567.9)
562.12 Diverticulosis of colon with hemorrhage — (Use additional code to identify any associated peritonitis: 567.0-567.9)
562.13 Diverticulitis of colon with hemorrhage — (Use additional code to identify any associated peritonitis: 567.0-567.9)
564.7 Megacolon, other than Hirschsprung's
564.81 Neurogenic bowel
564.89 Other functional disorders of intestine
567.0 Peritonitis in infectious diseases classified elsewhere — (Code first underlying disease) ☒
567.1 Pneumococcal peritonitis
567.2 Other suppurative peritonitis
567.8 Other specified peritonitis
567.9 Unspecified peritonitis ▽
569.82 Ulceration of intestine
569.83 Perforation of intestine
569.89 Other specified disorder of intestines
569.9 Unspecified disorder of intestine ▽
578.1 Blood in stool
578.9 Unspecified, hemorrhage of gastrointestinal tract ▽
751.3 Hirschsprung's disease and other congenital functional disorders of colon
777.1 Fetal and newborn meconium obstruction
777.5 Necrotizing enterocolitis in fetus or newborn
777.6 Perinatal intestinal perforation
777.8 Other specified perinatal disorder of digestive system
863.40 Colon injury unspecified site, without mention of open wound into cavity ▽
863.41 Ascending (right) colon injury without mention of open wound into cavity
863.42 Transverse colon injury without mention of open wound into cavity
863.43 Descending (left) colon injury without mention of open wound into cavity
863.44 Sigmoid colon injury without mention of open wound into cavity
863.45 Rectum injury without mention of open wound into cavity
863.46 Injury to multiple sites in colon and rectum without mention of open wound into cavity
863.49 Other colon and rectum injury, without mention of open wound into cavity
998.89 Other specified complications

ICD-9-CM Procedural

45.8 Total intra-abdominal colectomy
45.95 Anastomosis to anus
46.01 Exteriorization of small intestine
46.23 Other permanent ileostomy

44212

44212 Laparoscopy, surgical; colectomy, total, abdominal, with proctectomy, with ileostomy

ICD-9-CM Diagnostic

153.0 Malignant neoplasm of hepatic flexure
153.1 Malignant neoplasm of transverse colon
153.2 Malignant neoplasm of descending colon
153.3 Malignant neoplasm of sigmoid colon
153.4 Malignant neoplasm of cecum
153.5 Malignant neoplasm of appendix
153.6 Malignant neoplasm of ascending colon
153.7 Malignant neoplasm of splenic flexure
153.8 Malignant neoplasm of other specified sites of large intestine
153.9 Malignant neoplasm of colon, unspecified site ▽
154.0 Malignant neoplasm of rectosigmoid junction
154.1 Malignant neoplasm of rectum
197.5 Secondary malignant neoplasm of large intestine and rectum
211.3 Benign neoplasm of colon
211.4 Benign neoplasm of rectum and anal canal
230.3 Carcinoma in situ of colon
230.4 Carcinoma in situ of rectum
230.7 Carcinoma in situ of other and unspecified parts of intestine ▽
235.2 Neoplasm of uncertain behavior of stomach, intestines, and rectum
239.0 Neoplasm of unspecified nature of digestive system
555.1 Regional enteritis of large intestine
556.0 Ulcerative (chronic) enterocolitis
556.1 Ulcerative (chronic) ileocolitis
556.2 Ulcerative (chronic) proctitis
556.3 Ulcerative (chronic) proctosigmoiditis
556.4 Pseudopolyposis of colon
556.5 Left sided ulcerative (chronic) colitis
556.6 Universal ulcerative (chronic) colitis
556.8 Other ulcerative colitis
556.9 Unspecified ulcerative colitis ▽
557.0 Acute vascular insufficiency of intestine
557.1 Chronic vascular insufficiency of intestine
557.9 Unspecified vascular insufficiency of intestine ▽
560.9 Unspecified intestinal obstruction ▽
562.10 Diverticulosis of colon (without mention of hemorrhage) — (Use additional code to identify any associated peritonitis: 567.0-567.9)
562.11 Diverticulitis of colon (without mention of hemorrhage) — (Use additional code to identify any associated peritonitis: 567.0-567.9)
562.12 Diverticulosis of colon with hemorrhage — (Use additional code to identify any associated peritonitis: 567.0-567.9)
562.13 Diverticulitis of colon with hemorrhage — (Use additional code to identify any associated peritonitis: 567.0-567.9)

▽ Unspecified code ☒ Manifestation code
♀ Female diagnosis ♂ Male diagnosis

567.0 Peritonitis in infectious diseases classified elsewhere — (Code first underlying disease) ☒
567.1 Pneumococcal peritonitis
567.2 Other suppurative peritonitis
567.8 Other specified peritonitis
567.9 Unspecified peritonitis ▽
569.82 Ulceration of intestine
569.83 Perforation of intestine
569.89 Other specified disorder of intestines
578.1 Blood in stool
751.2 Congenital atresia and stenosis of large intestine, rectum, and anal canal
751.3 Hirschsprung's disease and other congenital functional disorders of colon
777.1 Fetal and newborn meconium obstruction
777.5 Necrotizing enterocolitis in fetus or newborn
777.6 Perinatal intestinal perforation
863.40 Colon injury unspecified site, without mention of open wound into cavity ▽
863.41 Ascending (right) colon injury without mention of open wound into cavity
863.42 Transverse colon injury without mention of open wound into cavity
863.43 Descending (left) colon injury without mention of open wound into cavity
863.44 Sigmoid colon injury without mention of open wound into cavity
863.45 Rectum injury without mention of open wound into cavity
863.46 Injury to multiple sites in colon and rectum without mention of open wound into cavity
863.49 Other colon and rectum injury, without mention of open wound into cavity
998.89 Other specified complications

ICD-9-CM Procedural

45.71 Multiple segmental resection of large intestine
45.73 Right hemicolectomy
45.8 Total intra-abdominal colectomy
46.23 Other permanent ileostomy
48.5 Abdominoperineal resection of rectum

44300

44300 Enterostomy or cecostomy, tube (eg, for decompression or feeding) (separate procedure)

ICD-9-CM Diagnostic

150.5 Malignant neoplasm of lower third of esophagus
150.8 Malignant neoplasm of other specified part of esophagus
150.9 Malignant neoplasm of esophagus, unspecified site ▽
151.0 Malignant neoplasm of cardia
151.1 Malignant neoplasm of pylorus
151.2 Malignant neoplasm of pyloric antrum
151.3 Malignant neoplasm of fundus of stomach
151.4 Malignant neoplasm of body of stomach
151.5 Malignant neoplasm of lesser curvature of stomach, unspecified ▽
151.6 Malignant neoplasm of greater curvature of stomach, unspecified ▽
151.8 Malignant neoplasm of other specified sites of stomach
151.9 Malignant neoplasm of stomach, unspecified site ▽
152.9 Malignant neoplasm of small intestine, unspecified site ▽
153.3 Malignant neoplasm of sigmoid colon
153.4 Malignant neoplasm of cecum
153.5 Malignant neoplasm of appendix
153.6 Malignant neoplasm of ascending colon
153.7 Malignant neoplasm of splenic flexure
153.8 Malignant neoplasm of other specified sites of large intestine
153.9 Malignant neoplasm of colon, unspecified site ▽
154.0 Malignant neoplasm of rectosigmoid junction
195.2 Malignant neoplasm of abdomen
197.4 Secondary malignant neoplasm of small intestine including duodenum
197.8 Secondary malignant neoplasm of other digestive organs and spleen
263.0 Malnutrition of moderate degree
263.1 Malnutrition of mild degree
263.2 Arrested development following protein-calorie malnutrition
263.8 Other protein-calorie malnutrition
263.9 Unspecified protein-calorie malnutrition ▽
330.8 Other specified cerebral degenerations in childhood — (Use additional code to identify associated mental retardation)
348.1 Anoxic brain damage — (Use additional E code to identify cause)
436 Acute, but ill-defined, cerebrovascular disease — (Use additional code to identify presence of hypertension) ▽
530.11 Reflux esophagitis — (Use additional E code to identify cause, if induced by chemical or drug)
530.12 Acute esophagitis — (Use additional E code to identify cause, if induced by chemical or drug)
530.19 Other esophagitis — (Use additional E code to identify cause, if induced by chemical or drug)
530.20 Ulcer of esophagus without bleeding — (Use additional E code to identify cause, if induced by chemical or drug)
530.21 Ulcer of esophagus with bleeding — (Use additional E code to identify cause, if induced by chemical or drug)
530.3 Stricture and stenosis of esophagus
530.4 Perforation of esophagus
530.5 Dyskinesia of esophagus
530.6 Diverticulum of esophagus, acquired
530.7 Gastroesophageal laceration-hemorrhage syndrome
530.81 Esophageal reflux
530.82 Esophageal hemorrhage
530.83 Esophageal leukoplakia
530.84 Tracheoesophageal fistula
530.85 Barrett's esophagus
530.89 Other specified disorder of the esophagus
531.00 Acute gastric ulcer with hemorrhage, without mention of obstruction — (Use additional E code to identify drug, if drug induced)
531.01 Acute gastric ulcer with hemorrhage and obstruction — (Use additional E code to identify drug, if drug induced)
531.10 Acute gastric ulcer with perforation, without mention of obstruction — (Use additional E code to identify drug, if drug induced)
531.11 Acute gastric ulcer with perforation and obstruction — (Use additional E code to identify drug, if drug induced)
531.20 Acute gastric ulcer with hemorrhage and perforation, without mention of obstruction — (Use additional E code to identify drug, if drug induced)
531.21 Acute gastric ulcer with hemorrhage, perforation, and obstruction — (Use additional E code to identify drug, if drug induced)
531.30 Acute gastric ulcer without mention of hemorrhage, perforation, or obstruction — (Use additional E code to identify drug, if drug induced)
531.31 Acute gastric ulcer without mention of hemorrhage or perforation, with obstruction — (Use additional E code to identify drug, if drug induced)
531.40 Chronic or unspecified gastric ulcer with hemorrhage, without mention of obstruction — (Use additional E code to identify drug, if drug induced)
531.41 Chronic or unspecified gastric ulcer with hemorrhage and obstruction — (Use additional E code to identify drug, if drug induced)
531.50 Chronic or unspecified gastric ulcer with perforation, without mention of obstruction — (Use additional E code to identify drug, if drug induced)
531.51 Chronic or unspecified gastric ulcer with perforation and obstruction — (Use additional E code to identify drug, if drug induced)
531.60 Chronic or unspecified gastric ulcer with hemorrhage and perforation, without mention of obstruction — (Use additional E code to identify drug, if drug induced)
531.61 Chronic or unspecified gastric ulcer with hemorrhage, perforation, and obstruction — (Use additional E code to identify drug, if drug induced)
531.70 Chronic gastric ulcer without mention of hemorrhage, perforation, without mention of obstruction — (Use additional E code to identify drug, if drug induced)
531.71 Chronic gastric ulcer without mention of hemorrhage or perforation, with obstruction — (Use additional E code to identify drug, if drug induced)
531.90 Gastric ulcer, unspecified as acute or chronic, without mention of hemorrhage, perforation, or obstruction — (Use additional E code to identify drug, if drug induced) ▽
531.91 Gastric ulcer, unspecified as acute or chronic, without mention of hemorrhage or perforation, with obstruction — (Use additional E code to identify drug, if drug induced) ▽
532.00 Acute duodenal ulcer with hemorrhage, without mention of obstruction — (Use additional E code to identify drug, if drug induced)
532.01 Acute duodenal ulcer with hemorrhage and obstruction — (Use additional E code to identify drug, if drug induced)
532.10 Acute duodenal ulcer with perforation, without mention of obstruction — (Use additional E code to identify drug, if drug induced)
532.11 Acute duodenal ulcer with perforation and obstruction — (Use additional E code to identify drug, if drug induced)
532.20 Acute duodenal ulcer with hemorrhage and perforation, without mention of obstruction — (Use additional E code to identify drug, if drug induced)
532.21 Acute duodenal ulcer with hemorrhage, perforation, and obstruction — (Use additional E code to identify drug, if drug induced)
532.30 Acute duodenal ulcer without mention of hemorrhage, perforation, or obstruction — (Use additional E code to identify drug, if drug induced)
532.31 Acute duodenal ulcer without mention of hemorrhage or perforation, with obstruction — (Use additional E code to identify drug, if drug induced)
532.40 Chronic or unspecified duodenal ulcer with hemorrhage, without mention of obstruction — (Use additional E code to identify drug, if drug induced)

532.41 Chronic or unspecified duodenal ulcer with hemorrhage and obstruction — (Use additional E code to identify drug, if drug induced)
532.50 Chronic or unspecified duodenal ulcer with perforation, without mention of obstruction — (Use additional E code to identify drug, if drug induced)
532.60 Chronic or unspecified duodenal ulcer with hemorrhage and perforation, without mention of obstruction — (Use additional E code to identify drug, if drug induced)
532.61 Chronic or unspecified duodenal ulcer with hemorrhage, perforation, and obstruction — (Use additional E code to identify drug, if drug induced)
532.70 Chronic duodenal ulcer without mention of hemorrhage, perforation, or obstruction — (Use additional E code to identify drug, if drug induced)
532.71 Chronic duodenal ulcer without mention of hemorrhage or perforation, with obstruction — (Use additional E code to identify drug, if drug induced)
532.90 Duodenal ulcer, unspecified as acute or chronic, without hemorrhage, perforation, or obstruction — (Use additional E code to identify drug, if drug induced) ▽
532.91 Duodenal ulcer, unspecified as acute or chronic, without mention of hemorrhage or perforation, with obstruction — (Use additional E code to identify drug, if drug induced) ▽
533.00 Acute peptic ulcer, unspecified site, with hemorrhage, without mention of obstruction — (Use additional E code to identify drug, if drug induced)
533.01 Acute peptic ulcer, unspecified site, with hemorrhage and obstruction — (Use additional E code to identify drug, if drug induced)
533.10 Acute peptic ulcer, unspecified site, with perforation, without mention of obstruction — (Use additional E code to identify drug, if drug induced)
533.11 Acute peptic ulcer, unspecified site, with perforation and obstruction — (Use additional E code to identify drug, if drug induced)
533.20 Acute peptic ulcer, unspecified site, with hemorrhage and perforation, without mention of obstruction — (Use additional E code to identify drug, if drug induced)
533.21 Acute peptic ulcer, unspecified site, with hemorrhage, perforation, and obstruction — (Use additional E code to identify drug, if drug induced)
533.30 Acute peptic ulcer, unspecified site, without mention of hemorrhage, perforation, or obstruction — (Use additional E code to identify drug, if drug induced)
533.31 Acute peptic ulcer, unspecified site, without mention of hemorrhage and perforation, with obstruction — (Use additional E code to identify drug, if drug induced)
533.40 Chronic or unspecified peptic ulcer, unspecified site, with hemorrhage, without mention of obstruction — (Use additional E code to identify drug, if drug induced)
533.41 Chronic or unspecified peptic ulcer, unspecified site, with hemorrhage and obstruction — (Use additional E code to identify drug, if drug induced)
533.50 Chronic or unspecified peptic ulcer, unspecified site, with perforation, without mention of obstruction — (Use additional E code to identify drug, if drug induced)
533.51 Chronic or unspecified peptic ulcer, unspecified site, with perforation and obstruction — (Use additional E code to identify drug, if drug induced)
533.60 Chronic or unspecified peptic ulcer, unspecified site, with hemorrhage and perforation, without mention of obstruction — (Use additional E code to identify drug, if drug induced)
533.61 Chronic or unspecified peptic ulcer, unspecified site, with hemorrhage, perforation, and obstruction — (Use additional E code to identify drug, if drug induced)
533.70 Chronic peptic ulcer, unspecified site, without mention of hemorrhage, perforation, or obstruction — (Use additional E code to identify drug, if drug induced)
533.71 Chronic peptic ulcer of unspecified site without mention of hemorrhage or perforation, with obstruction — (Use additional E code to identify drug, if drug induced)
533.90 Peptic ulcer, unspecified site, unspecified as acute or chronic, without mention of hemorrhage, perforation, or obstruction — (Use additional E code to identify drug, if drug induced) ▽
533.91 Peptic ulcer, unspecified site, unspecified as acute or chronic, without mention of hemorrhage or perforation, with obstruction — (Use additional E code to identify drug, if drug induced) ▽
537.4 Fistula of stomach or duodenum
557.0 Acute vascular insufficiency of intestine
560.1 Paralytic ileus
560.2 Volvulus
560.81 Intestinal or peritoneal adhesions with obstruction (postoperative) (postinfection)
560.9 Unspecified intestinal obstruction ▽
564.81 Neurogenic bowel
564.89 Other functional disorders of intestine
569.81 Fistula of intestine, excluding rectum and anus
569.82 Ulceration of intestine
569.83 Perforation of intestine
569.84 Angiodysplasia of intestine (without mention of hemorrhage)
569.85 Angiodysplasia of intestine with hemorrhage
569.89 Other specified disorder of intestines
783.21 Loss of weight
783.22 Underweight
783.3 Feeding difficulties and mismanagement
783.7 Adult failure to thrive
787.01 Nausea with vomiting
787.2 Dysphagia
793.4 Nonspecific abnormal findings on radiological and other examination of gastrointestinal tract
994.2 Effects of hunger

ICD-9-CM Procedural

46.10 Colostomy, not otherwise specified
46.39 Other enterostomy

44310

44310 Ileostomy or jejunostomy, non-tube (separate procedure)

ICD-9-CM Diagnostic

153.0 Malignant neoplasm of hepatic flexure
153.1 Malignant neoplasm of transverse colon
153.2 Malignant neoplasm of descending colon
153.3 Malignant neoplasm of sigmoid colon
153.4 Malignant neoplasm of cecum
153.5 Malignant neoplasm of appendix
153.6 Malignant neoplasm of ascending colon
153.7 Malignant neoplasm of splenic flexure
153.8 Malignant neoplasm of other specified sites of large intestine
153.9 Malignant neoplasm of colon, unspecified site ▽
154.0 Malignant neoplasm of rectosigmoid junction
211.2 Benign neoplasm of duodenum, jejunum, and ileum
211.3 Benign neoplasm of colon
211.4 Benign neoplasm of rectum and anal canal
230.4 Carcinoma in situ of rectum
230.7 Carcinoma in situ of other and unspecified parts of intestine ▽
235.2 Neoplasm of uncertain behavior of stomach, intestines, and rectum
239.0 Neoplasm of unspecified nature of digestive system
556.0 Ulcerative (chronic) enterocolitis
556.1 Ulcerative (chronic) ileocolitis
556.2 Ulcerative (chronic) proctitis
556.3 Ulcerative (chronic) proctosigmoiditis
556.4 Pseudopolyposis of colon
556.5 Left sided ulcerative (chronic) colitis
556.8 Other ulcerative colitis
556.9 Unspecified ulcerative colitis ▽
557.0 Acute vascular insufficiency of intestine
557.9 Unspecified vascular insufficiency of intestine ▽
560.2 Volvulus
562.10 Diverticulosis of colon (without mention of hemorrhage) — (Use additional code to identify any associated peritonitis: 567.0-567.9)
562.11 Diverticulitis of colon (without mention of hemorrhage) — (Use additional code to identify any associated peritonitis: 567.0-567.9)
562.12 Diverticulosis of colon with hemorrhage — (Use additional code to identify any associated peritonitis: 567.0-567.9)
562.13 Diverticulitis of colon with hemorrhage — (Use additional code to identify any associated peritonitis: 567.0-567.9)
564.7 Megacolon, other than Hirschsprung's
564.81 Neurogenic bowel
564.89 Other functional disorders of intestine
567.0 Peritonitis in infectious diseases classified elsewhere — (Code first underlying disease) ☒
567.1 Pneumococcal peritonitis
567.2 Other suppurative peritonitis
567.8 Other specified peritonitis
567.9 Unspecified peritonitis ▽
569.82 Ulceration of intestine
569.83 Perforation of intestine
569.89 Other specified disorder of intestines
777.1 Fetal and newborn meconium obstruction
777.5 Necrotizing enterocolitis in fetus or newborn
777.6 Perinatal intestinal perforation
863.40 Colon injury unspecified site, without mention of open wound into cavity ▽

▽ Unspecified code
♀ Female diagnosis
☒ Manifestation code
♂ Male diagnosis

863.41 Ascending (right) colon injury without mention of open wound into cavity
863.42 Transverse colon injury without mention of open wound into cavity
863.43 Descending (left) colon injury without mention of open wound into cavity
863.44 Sigmoid colon injury without mention of open wound into cavity
863.45 Rectum injury without mention of open wound into cavity
863.46 Injury to multiple sites in colon and rectum without mention of open wound into cavity
863.49 Other colon and rectum injury, without mention of open wound into cavity
998.89 Other specified complications
V64.41 Laparoscopic surgical procedure converted to open procedure

ICD-9-CM Procedural

46.20 Ileostomy, not otherwise specified
46.21 Temporary ileostomy

44312–44314

44312 Revision of ileostomy; simple (release of superficial scar) (separate procedure)
44314 complicated (reconstruction in-depth) (separate procedure)

ICD-9-CM Diagnostic

560.81 Intestinal or peritoneal adhesions with obstruction (postoperative) (postinfection)
569.60 Unspecified complication of colostomy or enterostomy ▽
569.61 Infection of colostomy or enterostomy — (Use additional code to identify organism: 041.00-041.9. Use additional code to specify type of infection: 038.0-038.9, 682.2)
569.62 Mechanical complication of colostomy and enterostomy
569.69 Other complication of colostomy or enterostomy
997.4 Digestive system complication — (Use additional code to identify complications)
V10.05 Personal history of malignant neoplasm of large intestine
V10.06 Personal history of malignant neoplasm of rectum, rectosigmoid junction, and anus
V44.2 Ileostomy status — (This code is intended for use when these conditions are recorded as diagnoses or problems)
V55.2 Attention to ileostomy

ICD-9-CM Procedural

46.40 Revision of intestinal stoma, not otherwise specified
46.41 Revision of stoma of small intestine

44316

44316 Continent ileostomy (Kock procedure) (separate procedure)

ICD-9-CM Diagnostic

153.0 Malignant neoplasm of hepatic flexure
153.1 Malignant neoplasm of transverse colon
153.2 Malignant neoplasm of descending colon
153.4 Malignant neoplasm of cecum
153.5 Malignant neoplasm of appendix
153.6 Malignant neoplasm of ascending colon
153.7 Malignant neoplasm of splenic flexure
153.8 Malignant neoplasm of other specified sites of large intestine
153.9 Malignant neoplasm of colon, unspecified site ▽
154.0 Malignant neoplasm of rectosigmoid junction
197.5 Secondary malignant neoplasm of large intestine and rectum
211.3 Benign neoplasm of colon
211.4 Benign neoplasm of rectum and anal canal
230.3 Carcinoma in situ of colon
230.4 Carcinoma in situ of rectum
230.7 Carcinoma in situ of other and unspecified parts of intestine ▽
235.2 Neoplasm of uncertain behavior of stomach, intestines, and rectum
239.0 Neoplasm of unspecified nature of digestive system
556.0 Ulcerative (chronic) enterocolitis
556.1 Ulcerative (chronic) ileocolitis
556.2 Ulcerative (chronic) proctitis
556.3 Ulcerative (chronic) proctosigmoiditis
556.4 Pseudopolyposis of colon
556.5 Left sided ulcerative (chronic) colitis
556.6 Universal ulcerative (chronic) colitis
556.8 Other ulcerative colitis
556.9 Unspecified ulcerative colitis ▽
557.0 Acute vascular insufficiency of intestine
557.1 Chronic vascular insufficiency of intestine
557.9 Unspecified vascular insufficiency of intestine ▽
562.10 Diverticulosis of colon (without mention of hemorrhage) — (Use additional code to identify any associated peritonitis: 567.0-567.9)
562.11 Diverticulitis of colon (without mention of hemorrhage) — (Use additional code to identify any associated peritonitis: 567.0-567.9)
562.12 Diverticulosis of colon with hemorrhage — (Use additional code to identify any associated peritonitis: 567.0-567.9)
562.13 Diverticulitis of colon with hemorrhage — (Use additional code to identify any associated peritonitis: 567.0-567.9)
564.7 Megacolon, other than Hirschsprung's
564.81 Neurogenic bowel
564.89 Other functional disorders of intestine
567.0 Peritonitis in infectious diseases classified elsewhere — (Code first underlying disease) ☒
567.1 Pneumococcal peritonitis
567.2 Other suppurative peritonitis
567.8 Other specified peritonitis
567.9 Unspecified peritonitis ▽
569.82 Ulceration of intestine
569.83 Perforation of intestine
569.89 Other specified disorder of intestines
777.1 Fetal and newborn meconium obstruction
777.5 Necrotizing enterocolitis in fetus or newborn
777.6 Perinatal intestinal perforation
863.40 Colon injury unspecified site, without mention of open wound into cavity ▽
863.41 Ascending (right) colon injury without mention of open wound into cavity
863.42 Transverse colon injury without mention of open wound into cavity
863.43 Descending (left) colon injury without mention of open wound into cavity
863.44 Sigmoid colon injury without mention of open wound into cavity
863.45 Rectum injury without mention of open wound into cavity
863.46 Injury to multiple sites in colon and rectum without mention of open wound into cavity
863.49 Other colon and rectum injury, without mention of open wound into cavity
998.89 Other specified complications

ICD-9-CM Procedural

46.22 Continent ileostomy

44320–44322

44320 Colostomy or skin level cecostomy; (separate procedure)
44322 with multiple biopsies (eg, for congenital megacolon) (separate procedure)

ICD-9-CM Diagnostic

151.9 Malignant neoplasm of stomach, unspecified site ▽
152.0 Malignant neoplasm of duodenum
152.1 Malignant neoplasm of jejunum
152.2 Malignant neoplasm of ileum
152.3 Malignant neoplasm of Meckel's diverticulum
152.8 Malignant neoplasm of other specified sites of small intestine
152.9 Malignant neoplasm of small intestine, unspecified site ▽
153.0 Malignant neoplasm of hepatic flexure
153.1 Malignant neoplasm of transverse colon
153.2 Malignant neoplasm of descending colon
153.3 Malignant neoplasm of sigmoid colon
153.4 Malignant neoplasm of cecum
153.9 Malignant neoplasm of colon, unspecified site ▽
154.0 Malignant neoplasm of rectosigmoid junction
154.1 Malignant neoplasm of rectum
154.2 Malignant neoplasm of anal canal
197.4 Secondary malignant neoplasm of small intestine including duodenum
197.5 Secondary malignant neoplasm of large intestine and rectum
199.1 Other malignant neoplasm of unspecified site
211.3 Benign neoplasm of colon
230.3 Carcinoma in situ of colon
230.4 Carcinoma in situ of rectum
230.9 Carcinoma in situ of other and unspecified digestive organs ▽
235.2 Neoplasm of uncertain behavior of stomach, intestines, and rectum
239.0 Neoplasm of unspecified nature of digestive system
532.10 Acute duodenal ulcer with perforation, without mention of obstruction — (Use additional E code to identify drug, if drug induced)
555.0 Regional enteritis of small intestine
555.1 Regional enteritis of large intestine
555.2 Regional enteritis of small intestine with large intestine
555.9 Regional enteritis of unspecified site ▽
556.0 Ulcerative (chronic) enterocolitis
556.1 Ulcerative (chronic) ileocolitis
556.2 Ulcerative (chronic) proctitis

▽ Unspecified code
♀ Female diagnosis
☒ Manifestation code
♂ Male diagnosis

556.3 Ulcerative (chronic) proctosigmoiditis
556.4 Pseudopolyposis of colon
556.5 Left sided ulcerative (chronic) colitis
556.6 Universal ulcerative (chronic) colitis
556.8 Other ulcerative colitis
556.9 Unspecified ulcerative colitis ▽
557.0 Acute vascular insufficiency of intestine
558.1 Gastroenteritis and colitis due to radiation
558.2 Toxic gastroenteritis and colitis — (Use additional E code to identify cause)
558.3 Gastroenteritis and colitis, allergic — (Use additional code to identify type of food allergy: V15.01-V15.05)
558.9 Other and unspecified noninfectious gastroenteritis and colitis ▽
560.1 Paralytic ileus
560.2 Volvulus
560.31 Gallstone ileus
560.39 Other impaction of intestine
560.81 Intestinal or peritoneal adhesions with obstruction (postoperative) (postinfection)
560.89 Other specified intestinal obstruction
560.9 Unspecified intestinal obstruction ▽
562.10 Diverticulosis of colon (without mention of hemorrhage) — (Use additional code to identify any associated peritonitis: 567.0-567.9)
562.11 Diverticulitis of colon (without mention of hemorrhage) — (Use additional code to identify any associated peritonitis: 567.0-567.9)
562.12 Diverticulosis of colon with hemorrhage — (Use additional code to identify any associated peritonitis: 567.0-567.9)
562.13 Diverticulitis of colon with hemorrhage — (Use additional code to identify any associated peritonitis: 567.0-567.9)
564.7 Megacolon, other than Hirschsprung's
564.81 Neurogenic bowel
564.89 Other functional disorders of intestine
565.1 Anal fistula
566 Abscess of anal and rectal regions
567.0 Peritonitis in infectious diseases classified elsewhere — (Code first underlying disease) ☒
567.1 Pneumococcal peritonitis
567.2 Other suppurative peritonitis
567.8 Other specified peritonitis
567.9 Unspecified peritonitis ▽
569.1 Rectal prolapse
569.2 Stenosis of rectum and anus
569.3 Hemorrhage of rectum and anus
569.41 Ulcer of anus and rectum
569.49 Other specified disorder of rectum and anus
569.5 Abscess of intestine
569.61 Infection of colostomy or enterostomy — (Use additional code to identify organism: 041.00-041.9. Use additional code to specify type of infection: 038.0-038.9, 682.2)
569.69 Other complication of colostomy or enterostomy
569.81 Fistula of intestine, excluding rectum and anus
569.82 Ulceration of intestine
569.83 Perforation of intestine
569.84 Angiodysplasia of intestine (without mention of hemorrhage)
569.85 Angiodysplasia of intestine with hemorrhage
569.89 Other specified disorder of intestines
578.9 Unspecified, hemorrhage of gastrointestinal tract ▽
596.1 Intestinovesical fistula — (Use additional code to identify urinary incontinence: 625.6, 788.30-788.39)
619.1 Digestive-genital tract fistula, female ♀
625.6 Female stress incontinence ♀
751.0 Meckel's diverticulum
751.1 Congenital atresia and stenosis of small intestine
751.2 Congenital atresia and stenosis of large intestine, rectum, and anal canal
751.3 Hirschsprung's disease and other congenital functional disorders of colon
751.4 Congenital anomalies of intestinal fixation
751.5 Other congenital anomalies of intestine
787.6 Incontinence of feces
863.55 Rectum injury with open wound into cavity

ICD-9-CM Procedural

46.03 Exteriorization of large intestine
46.10 Colostomy, not otherwise specified
46.11 Temporary colostomy
46.13 Permanent colostomy

44340–44345

44340 Revision of colostomy; simple (release of superficial scar) (separate procedure)
44345 complicated (reconstruction in-depth) (separate procedure)

ICD-9-CM Diagnostic

560.81 Intestinal or peritoneal adhesions with obstruction (postoperative) (postinfection)
569.60 Unspecified complication of colostomy or enterostomy ▽
569.61 Infection of colostomy or enterostomy — (Use additional code to identify organism: 041.00-041.9. Use additional code to specify type of infection: 038.0-038.9, 682.2)
569.62 Mechanical complication of colostomy and enterostomy
569.69 Other complication of colostomy or enterostomy
707.8 Chronic ulcer of other specified site
997.4 Digestive system complication — (Use additional code to identify complications)
998.2 Accidental puncture or laceration during procedure
998.31 Disruption of internal operation wound
998.32 Disruption of external operation wound
V10.05 Personal history of malignant neoplasm of large intestine
V10.06 Personal history of malignant neoplasm of rectum, rectosigmoid junction, and anus
V44.3 Colostomy status — (This code is intended for use when these conditions are recorded as diagnoses or problems)
V55.3 Attention to colostomy

ICD-9-CM Procedural

46.40 Revision of intestinal stoma, not otherwise specified
46.43 Other revision of stoma of large intestine

44346

44346 Revision of colostomy; with repair of paracolostomy hernia (separate procedure)

ICD-9-CM Diagnostic

560.81 Intestinal or peritoneal adhesions with obstruction (postoperative) (postinfection)
569.61 Infection of colostomy or enterostomy — (Use additional code to identify organism: 041.00-041.9. Use additional code to specify type of infection: 038.0-038.9, 682.2)
569.62 Mechanical complication of colostomy and enterostomy
569.69 Other complication of colostomy or enterostomy
707.8 Chronic ulcer of other specified site
997.4 Digestive system complication — (Use additional code to identify complications)
998.2 Accidental puncture or laceration during procedure
998.31 Disruption of internal operation wound
998.32 Disruption of external operation wound
V10.05 Personal history of malignant neoplasm of large intestine
V10.06 Personal history of malignant neoplasm of rectum, rectosigmoid junction, and anus
V44.3 Colostomy status — (This code is intended for use when these conditions are recorded as diagnoses or problems)
V55.3 Attention to colostomy

ICD-9-CM Procedural

46.40 Revision of intestinal stoma, not otherwise specified
46.42 Repair of pericolostomy hernia
46.43 Other revision of stoma of large intestine

44360–44361

44360 Small intestinal endoscopy, enteroscopy beyond second portion of duodenum, not including ileum; diagnostic, with or without collection of specimen(s) by brushing or washing (separate procedure)
44361 with biopsy, single or multiple

ICD-9-CM Diagnostic

152.0 Malignant neoplasm of duodenum
152.1 Malignant neoplasm of jejunum
152.9 Malignant neoplasm of small intestine, unspecified site ▽
197.4 Secondary malignant neoplasm of small intestine including duodenum
211.2 Benign neoplasm of duodenum, jejunum, and ileum
532.00 Acute duodenal ulcer with hemorrhage, without mention of obstruction — (Use additional E code to identify drug, if drug induced)
532.01 Acute duodenal ulcer with hemorrhage and obstruction — (Use additional E code to identify drug, if drug induced)

▽ Unspecified code
♀ Female diagnosis
☒ Manifestation code
♂ Male diagnosis

Pancreas and Small Intestine

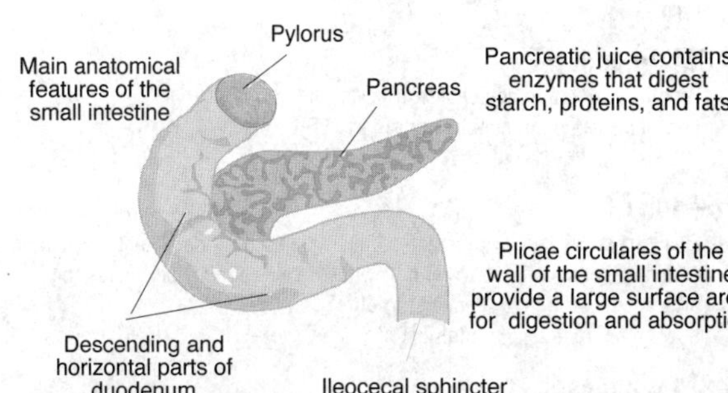
Main anatomical features of the small intestine
Pylorus
Pancreas
Pancreatic juice contains enzymes that digest starch, proteins, and fats
Plicae circulares of the wall of the small intestine provide a large surface area for digestion and absorption
Descending and horizontal parts of duodenum
Ileocecal sphincter origin of the large intestine

532.10 Acute duodenal ulcer with perforation, without mention of obstruction — (Use additional E code to identify drug, if drug induced)
532.11 Acute duodenal ulcer with perforation and obstruction — (Use additional E code to identify drug, if drug induced)
532.20 Acute duodenal ulcer with hemorrhage and perforation, without mention of obstruction — (Use additional E code to identify drug, if drug induced)
532.21 Acute duodenal ulcer with hemorrhage, perforation, and obstruction — (Use additional E code to identify drug, if drug induced)
532.30 Acute duodenal ulcer without mention of hemorrhage, perforation, or obstruction — (Use additional E code to identify drug, if drug induced)
532.31 Acute duodenal ulcer without mention of hemorrhage or perforation, with obstruction — (Use additional E code to identify drug, if drug induced)
532.90 Duodenal ulcer, unspecified as acute or chronic, without hemorrhage, perforation, or obstruction — (Use additional E code to identify drug, if drug induced) ▽
535.50 Unspecified gastritis and gastroduodenitis without mention of hemorrhage ▽
535.51 Unspecified gastritis and gastroduodenitis with hemorrhage ▽
535.60 Duodenitis without mention of hemorrhage
535.61 Duodenitis with hemorrhage
537.3 Other obstruction of duodenum
537.84 Dieulafoy lesion (hemorrhagic) of stomach and duodenum
555.2 Regional enteritis of small intestine with large intestine
569.86 Dieulafoy lesion (hemorrhagic) of intestine
578.0 Hematemesis
578.1 Blood in stool
578.9 Unspecified, hemorrhage of gastrointestinal tract ▽
579.9 Unspecified intestinal malabsorption ▽
751.0 Meckel's diverticulum
783.21 Loss of weight
783.22 Underweight
783.7 Adult failure to thrive
793.4 Nonspecific abnormal findings on radiological and other examination of gastrointestinal tract

ICD-9-CM Procedural
45.13 Other endoscopy of small intestine
45.14 Closed [endoscopic] biopsy of small intestine
45.16 Esophagogastroduodenoscopy (EGD) with closed biopsy

HCPCS Level II Supplies & Services
A4270 Disposable endoscope sheath, each
A4305 Disposable drug delivery system, flow rate of 50 ml or greater per hour
A4306 Disposable drug delivery system, flow rate of 5 ml or less per hour
A4550 Surgical trays

44363
44363 Small intestinal endoscopy, enteroscopy beyond second portion of duodenum, not including ileum; with removal of foreign body

ICD-9-CM Diagnostic
936 Foreign body in intestine and colon
998.4 Foreign body accidentally left during procedure, not elsewhere classified
998.7 Acute reaction to foreign substance accidentally left during procedure, not elsewhere classified

ICD-9-CM Procedural
98.03 Removal of intraluminal foreign body from stomach and small intestine without incision

HCPCS Level II Supplies & Services
A4270 Disposable endoscope sheath, each
A4305 Disposable drug delivery system, flow rate of 50 ml or greater per hour
A4306 Disposable drug delivery system, flow rate of 5 ml or less per hour
A4550 Surgical trays

44364–44365
44364 Small intestinal endoscopy, enteroscopy beyond second portion of duodenum, not including ileum; with removal of tumor(s), polyp(s), or other lesion(s) by snare technique
44365 with removal of tumor(s), polyp(s), or other lesion(s) by hot biopsy forceps or bipolar cautery

ICD-9-CM Diagnostic
152.0 Malignant neoplasm of duodenum
152.1 Malignant neoplasm of jejunum
197.4 Secondary malignant neoplasm of small intestine including duodenum
211.2 Benign neoplasm of duodenum, jejunum, and ileum
230.7 Carcinoma in situ of other and unspecified parts of intestine ▽
235.2 Neoplasm of uncertain behavior of stomach, intestines, and rectum
239.0 Neoplasm of unspecified nature of digestive system

ICD-9-CM Procedural
45.30 Endoscopic excision or destruction of lesion of duodenum

HCPCS Level II Supplies & Services
A4270 Disposable endoscope sheath, each
A4305 Disposable drug delivery system, flow rate of 50 ml or greater per hour
A4306 Disposable drug delivery system, flow rate of 5 ml or less per hour
A4550 Surgical trays

44366
44366 Small intestinal endoscopy, enteroscopy beyond second portion of duodenum, not including ileum; with control of bleeding (eg, injection, bipolar cautery, unipolar cautery, laser, heater probe, stapler, plasma coagulator)

ICD-9-CM Diagnostic
152.0 Malignant neoplasm of duodenum
152.1 Malignant neoplasm of jejunum
197.4 Secondary malignant neoplasm of small intestine including duodenum
211.2 Benign neoplasm of duodenum, jejunum, and ileum
532.00 Acute duodenal ulcer with hemorrhage, without mention of obstruction — (Use additional E code to identify drug, if drug induced)
532.01 Acute duodenal ulcer with hemorrhage and obstruction — (Use additional E code to identify drug, if drug induced)
532.21 Acute duodenal ulcer with hemorrhage, perforation, and obstruction — (Use additional E code to identify drug, if drug induced)
532.40 Chronic or unspecified duodenal ulcer with hemorrhage, without mention of obstruction — (Use additional E code to identify drug, if drug induced)
532.60 Chronic or unspecified duodenal ulcer with hemorrhage and perforation, without mention of obstruction — (Use additional E code to identify drug, if drug induced)
535.61 Duodenitis with hemorrhage
537.84 Dieulafoy lesion (hemorrhagic) of stomach and duodenum
537.89 Other specified disorder of stomach and duodenum
569.86 Dieulafoy lesion (hemorrhagic) of intestine

ICD-9-CM Procedural
44.43 Endoscopic control of gastric or duodenal bleeding

HCPCS Level II Supplies & Services
A4270 Disposable endoscope sheath, each
A4305 Disposable drug delivery system, flow rate of 50 ml or greater per hour
A4306 Disposable drug delivery system, flow rate of 5 ml or less per hour
A4550 Surgical trays

44369
44369 Small intestinal endoscopy, enteroscopy beyond second portion of duodenum, not including ileum; with ablation of tumor(s), polyp(s), or other lesion(s) not amenable to removal by hot biopsy forceps, bipolar cautery or snare technique

ICD-9-CM Diagnostic
152.0 Malignant neoplasm of duodenum
152.1 Malignant neoplasm of jejunum
197.4 Secondary malignant neoplasm of small intestine including duodenum

211.2 Benign neoplasm of duodenum, jejunum, and ileum
230.7 Carcinoma in situ of other and unspecified parts of intestine
235.2 Neoplasm of uncertain behavior of stomach, intestines, and rectum
239.0 Neoplasm of unspecified nature of digestive system

ICD-9-CM Procedural

45.30 Endoscopic excision or destruction of lesion of duodenum

HCPCS Level II Supplies & Services

A4270 Disposable endoscope sheath, each
A4305 Disposable drug delivery system, flow rate of 50 ml or greater per hour
A4306 Disposable drug delivery system, flow rate of 5 ml or less per hour
A4550 Surgical trays

44370

44370 Small intestinal endoscopy, enteroscopy beyond second portion of duodenum, not including ileum; with transendoscopic stent placement (includes predilation)

ICD-9-CM Diagnostic

152.0 Malignant neoplasm of duodenum
152.1 Malignant neoplasm of jejunum
152.8 Malignant neoplasm of other specified sites of small intestine
152.9 Malignant neoplasm of small intestine, unspecified site
196.2 Secondary and unspecified malignant neoplasm of intra-abdominal lymph nodes
197.4 Secondary malignant neoplasm of small intestine including duodenum
537.2 Chronic duodenal ileus
537.3 Other obstruction of duodenum
560.1 Paralytic ileus
560.2 Volvulus
560.81 Intestinal or peritoneal adhesions with obstruction (postoperative) (postinfection)
560.89 Other specified intestinal obstruction
560.9 Unspecified intestinal obstruction
751.1 Congenital atresia and stenosis of small intestine
997.4 Digestive system complication — (Use additional code to identify complications)

ICD-9-CM Procedural

45.13 Other endoscopy of small intestine
46.79 Other repair of intestine

44372–44373

44372 Small intestinal endoscopy, enteroscopy beyond second portion of duodenum, not including ileum; with placement of percutaneous jejunostomy tube
44373 with conversion of percutaneous gastrostomy tube to percutaneous jejunostomy tube

ICD-9-CM Diagnostic

146.9 Malignant neoplasm of oropharynx, unspecified site
148.9 Malignant neoplasm of hypopharynx, unspecified site
150.9 Malignant neoplasm of esophagus, unspecified site
151.9 Malignant neoplasm of stomach, unspecified site
152.0 Malignant neoplasm of duodenum
152.1 Malignant neoplasm of jejunum
261 Nutritional marasmus
262 Other severe protein-calorie malnutrition
348.1 Anoxic brain damage — (Use additional E code to identify cause)
530.0 Achalasia and cardiospasm
530.20 Ulcer of esophagus without bleeding — (Use additional E code to identify cause, if induced by chemical or drug)
530.21 Ulcer of esophagus with bleeding — (Use additional E code to identify cause, if induced by chemical or drug)
531.00 Acute gastric ulcer with hemorrhage, without mention of obstruction — (Use additional E code to identify drug, if drug induced)
531.01 Acute gastric ulcer with hemorrhage and obstruction — (Use additional E code to identify drug, if drug induced)
535.60 Duodenitis without mention of hemorrhage
535.61 Duodenitis with hemorrhage
537.0 Acquired hypertrophic pyloric stenosis
537.4 Fistula of stomach or duodenum
579.0 Celiac disease
579.1 Tropical sprue
579.2 Blind loop syndrome
579.8 Other specified intestinal malabsorption
751.2 Congenital atresia and stenosis of large intestine, rectum, and anal canal
751.3 Hirschsprung's disease and other congenital functional disorders of colon
V10.00 Personal history of malignant neoplasm of unspecified site in gastrointestinal tract

ICD-9-CM Procedural

44.32 Percutaneous [endoscopic] gastrojejunostomy
46.32 Percutaneous (endoscopic) jejunostomy (PEJ)

44376–44377

44376 Small intestinal endoscopy, enteroscopy beyond second portion of duodenum, including ileum; diagnostic, with or without collection of specimen(s) by brushing or washing (separate procedure)
44377 with biopsy, single or multiple

ICD-9-CM Diagnostic

152.0 Malignant neoplasm of duodenum
152.1 Malignant neoplasm of jejunum
152.2 Malignant neoplasm of ileum
197.4 Secondary malignant neoplasm of small intestine including duodenum
211.3 Benign neoplasm of colon
230.7 Carcinoma in situ of other and unspecified parts of intestine
235.2 Neoplasm of uncertain behavior of stomach, intestines, and rectum
239.0 Neoplasm of unspecified nature of digestive system
532.30 Acute duodenal ulcer without mention of hemorrhage, perforation, or obstruction — (Use additional E code to identify drug, if drug induced)
532.31 Acute duodenal ulcer without mention of hemorrhage or perforation, with obstruction — (Use additional E code to identify drug, if drug induced)
532.70 Chronic duodenal ulcer without mention of hemorrhage, perforation, or obstruction — (Use additional E code to identify drug, if drug induced)
532.71 Chronic duodenal ulcer without mention of hemorrhage or perforation, with obstruction — (Use additional E code to identify drug, if drug induced)
535.60 Duodenitis without mention of hemorrhage
535.61 Duodenitis with hemorrhage
537.84 Dieulafoy lesion (hemorrhagic) of stomach and duodenum
555.0 Regional enteritis of small intestine
555.2 Regional enteritis of small intestine with large intestine
560.2 Volvulus
560.81 Intestinal or peritoneal adhesions with obstruction (postoperative) (postinfection)
560.89 Other specified intestinal obstruction
564.5 Functional diarrhea
569.82 Ulceration of intestine
569.83 Perforation of intestine
569.86 Dieulafoy lesion (hemorrhagic) of intestine
578.1 Blood in stool
793.4 Nonspecific abnormal findings on radiological and other examination of gastrointestinal tract

ICD-9-CM Procedural

45.14 Closed [endoscopic] biopsy of small intestine
45.16 Esophagogastroduodenoscopy (EGD) with closed biopsy

HCPCS Level II Supplies & Services

A4270 Disposable endoscope sheath, each
A4305 Disposable drug delivery system, flow rate of 50 ml or greater per hour
A4306 Disposable drug delivery system, flow rate of 5 ml or less per hour
A4550 Surgical trays

44378

44378 Small intestinal endoscopy, enteroscopy beyond second portion of duodenum, including ileum; with control of bleeding (eg, injection, bipolar cautery, unipolar cautery, laser, heater probe, stapler, plasma coagulator)

ICD-9-CM Diagnostic

152.0 Malignant neoplasm of duodenum
152.1 Malignant neoplasm of jejunum
152.2 Malignant neoplasm of ileum
197.4 Secondary malignant neoplasm of small intestine including duodenum
211.2 Benign neoplasm of duodenum, jejunum, and ileum
230.7 Carcinoma in situ of other and unspecified parts of intestine
532.00 Acute duodenal ulcer with hemorrhage, without mention of obstruction — (Use additional E code to identify drug, if drug induced)
532.01 Acute duodenal ulcer with hemorrhage and obstruction — (Use additional E code to identify drug, if drug induced)

532.20 Acute duodenal ulcer with hemorrhage and perforation, without mention of obstruction — (Use additional E code to identify drug, if drug induced)
532.21 Acute duodenal ulcer with hemorrhage, perforation, and obstruction — (Use additional E code to identify drug, if drug induced)
532.40 Chronic or unspecified duodenal ulcer with hemorrhage, without mention of obstruction — (Use additional E code to identify drug, if drug induced)
532.41 Chronic or unspecified duodenal ulcer with hemorrhage and obstruction — (Use additional E code to identify drug, if drug induced)
532.60 Chronic or unspecified duodenal ulcer with hemorrhage and perforation, without mention of obstruction — (Use additional E code to identify drug, if drug induced)
532.61 Chronic or unspecified duodenal ulcer with hemorrhage, perforation, and obstruction — (Use additional E code to identify drug, if drug induced)
534.00 Acute gastrojejunal ulcer with hemorrhage, without mention of obstruction
534.40 Chronic or unspecified gastrojejunal ulcer with hemorrhage, without mention of obstruction
535.61 Duodenitis with hemorrhage
537.84 Dieulafoy lesion (hemorrhagic) of stomach and duodenum
537.89 Other specified disorder of stomach and duodenum
560.2 Volvulus
560.81 Intestinal or peritoneal adhesions with obstruction (postoperative) (postinfection)
564.5 Functional diarrhea
569.82 Ulceration of intestine
569.83 Perforation of intestine
569.86 Dieulafoy lesion (hemorrhagic) of intestine
578.1 Blood in stool

ICD-9-CM Procedural

44.43 Endoscopic control of gastric or duodenal bleeding
45.13 Other endoscopy of small intestine

HCPCS Level II Supplies & Services

A4270 Disposable endoscope sheath, each
A4305 Disposable drug delivery system, flow rate of 50 ml or greater per hour
A4306 Disposable drug delivery system, flow rate of 5 ml or less per hour
A4550 Surgical trays

44379

44379 Small intestinal endoscopy, enteroscopy beyond second portion of duodenum, including ileum; with transendoscopic stent placement (includes predilation)

ICD-9-CM Diagnostic

152.0 Malignant neoplasm of duodenum
152.1 Malignant neoplasm of jejunum
152.2 Malignant neoplasm of ileum
152.3 Malignant neoplasm of Meckel's diverticulum
152.8 Malignant neoplasm of other specified sites of small intestine
152.9 Malignant neoplasm of small intestine, unspecified site ▽
196.2 Secondary and unspecified malignant neoplasm of intra-abdominal lymph nodes
197.4 Secondary malignant neoplasm of small intestine including duodenum
537.2 Chronic duodenal ileus
537.3 Other obstruction of duodenum
560.1 Paralytic ileus
560.2 Volvulus
560.81 Intestinal or peritoneal adhesions with obstruction (postoperative) (postinfection)
560.89 Other specified intestinal obstruction
560.9 Unspecified intestinal obstruction ▽
751.1 Congenital atresia and stenosis of small intestine
997.4 Digestive system complication — (Use additional code to identify complications)

ICD-9-CM Procedural

45.13 Other endoscopy of small intestine
46.79 Other repair of intestine

44380–44382

44380 Ileoscopy, through stoma; diagnostic, with or without collection of specimen(s) by brushing or washing (separate procedure)
44382 with biopsy, single or multiple

ICD-9-CM Diagnostic

152.0 Malignant neoplasm of duodenum
152.1 Malignant neoplasm of jejunum
152.2 Malignant neoplasm of ileum
211.2 Benign neoplasm of duodenum, jejunum, and ileum
230.3 Carcinoma in situ of colon
555.0 Regional enteritis of small intestine
555.1 Regional enteritis of large intestine
555.2 Regional enteritis of small intestine with large intestine
555.9 Regional enteritis of unspecified site ▽
560.81 Intestinal or peritoneal adhesions with obstruction (postoperative) (postinfection)
564.1 Irritable bowel syndrome
569.61 Infection of colostomy or enterostomy — (Use additional code to identify organism: 041.00-041.9. Use additional code to specify type of infection: 038.0-038.9, 682.2)
569.69 Other complication of colostomy or enterostomy
578.1 Blood in stool
V10.00 Personal history of malignant neoplasm of unspecified site in gastrointestinal tract ▽

ICD-9-CM Procedural

45.12 Endoscopy of small intestine through artificial stoma
45.14 Closed [endoscopic] biopsy of small intestine

HCPCS Level II Supplies & Services

A4270 Disposable endoscope sheath, each
A4305 Disposable drug delivery system, flow rate of 50 ml or greater per hour
A4306 Disposable drug delivery system, flow rate of 5 ml or less per hour
A4550 Surgical trays

44383

44383 Ileoscopy, through stoma; with transendoscopic stent placement (includes predilation)

ICD-9-CM Diagnostic

152.0 Malignant neoplasm of duodenum
152.1 Malignant neoplasm of jejunum
152.2 Malignant neoplasm of ileum
196.2 Secondary and unspecified malignant neoplasm of intra-abdominal lymph nodes
197.4 Secondary malignant neoplasm of small intestine including duodenum
560.81 Intestinal or peritoneal adhesions with obstruction (postoperative) (postinfection)
560.89 Other specified intestinal obstruction
560.9 Unspecified intestinal obstruction ▽
751.1 Congenital atresia and stenosis of small intestine
997.4 Digestive system complication — (Use additional code to identify complications)

ICD-9-CM Procedural

45.12 Endoscopy of small intestine through artificial stoma
46.79 Other repair of intestine

44385–44386

44385 Endoscopic evaluation of small intestinal (abdominal or pelvic) pouch; diagnostic, with or without collection of specimen(s) by brushing or washing (separate procedure)
44386 with biopsy, single or multiple

ICD-9-CM Diagnostic

152.0 Malignant neoplasm of duodenum
152.1 Malignant neoplasm of jejunum
152.2 Malignant neoplasm of ileum
211.2 Benign neoplasm of duodenum, jejunum, and ileum
230.3 Carcinoma in situ of colon
555.0 Regional enteritis of small intestine
555.1 Regional enteritis of large intestine
555.2 Regional enteritis of small intestine with large intestine
555.9 Regional enteritis of unspecified site ▽
560.81 Intestinal or peritoneal adhesions with obstruction (postoperative) (postinfection)
560.89 Other specified intestinal obstruction
564.1 Irritable bowel syndrome
569.61 Infection of colostomy or enterostomy — (Use additional code to identify organism: 041.00-041.9. Use additional code to specify type of infection: 038.0-038.9, 682.2)
569.69 Other complication of colostomy or enterostomy
569.81 Fistula of intestine, excluding rectum and anus

569.82	Ulceration of intestine
569.83	Perforation of intestine
569.86	Dieulafoy lesion (hemorrhagic) of intestine
578.9	Unspecified, hemorrhage of gastrointestinal tract

ICD-9-CM Procedural

45.13	Other endoscopy of small intestine
45.14	Closed [endoscopic] biopsy of small intestine

HCPCS Level II Supplies & Services

A4270	Disposable endoscope sheath, each
A4305	Disposable drug delivery system, flow rate of 50 ml or greater per hour
A4306	Disposable drug delivery system, flow rate of 5 ml or less per hour
A4550	Surgical trays

44388–44389

44388	Colonoscopy through stoma; diagnostic, with or without collection of specimen(s) by brushing or washing (separate procedure)
44389	with biopsy, single or multiple

ICD-9-CM Diagnostic

153.0	Malignant neoplasm of hepatic flexure
153.1	Malignant neoplasm of transverse colon
153.2	Malignant neoplasm of descending colon
153.3	Malignant neoplasm of sigmoid colon
153.4	Malignant neoplasm of cecum
153.5	Malignant neoplasm of appendix
153.6	Malignant neoplasm of ascending colon
153.7	Malignant neoplasm of splenic flexure
153.8	Malignant neoplasm of other specified sites of large intestine
153.9	Malignant neoplasm of colon, unspecified site
154.0	Malignant neoplasm of rectosigmoid junction
154.1	Malignant neoplasm of rectum
154.2	Malignant neoplasm of anal canal
154.3	Malignant neoplasm of anus, unspecified site
154.8	Malignant neoplasm of other sites of rectum, rectosigmoid junction, and anus
197.5	Secondary malignant neoplasm of large intestine and rectum
211.3	Benign neoplasm of colon
211.4	Benign neoplasm of rectum and anal canal
230.3	Carcinoma in situ of colon
230.4	Carcinoma in situ of rectum
230.5	Carcinoma in situ of anal canal
230.6	Carcinoma in situ of anus, unspecified
230.7	Carcinoma in situ of other and unspecified parts of intestine
239.9	Neoplasm of unspecified nature, site unspecified
555.0	Regional enteritis of small intestine
555.2	Regional enteritis of small intestine with large intestine
555.9	Regional enteritis of unspecified site
556.0	Ulcerative (chronic) enterocolitis
556.1	Ulcerative (chronic) ileocolitis
556.2	Ulcerative (chronic) proctitis
556.3	Ulcerative (chronic) proctosigmoiditis
556.4	Pseudopolyposis of colon
556.5	Left sided ulcerative (chronic) colitis
556.6	Universal ulcerative (chronic) colitis
556.8	Other ulcerative colitis
556.9	Unspecified ulcerative colitis
557.0	Acute vascular insufficiency of intestine
557.1	Chronic vascular insufficiency of intestine
557.9	Unspecified vascular insufficiency of intestine
558.1	Gastroenteritis and colitis due to radiation
558.2	Toxic gastroenteritis and colitis — (Use additional E code to identify cause)
558.3	Gastroenteritis and colitis, allergic — (Use additional code to identify type of food allergy: V15.01-V15.05)
558.9	Other and unspecified noninfectious gastroenteritis and colitis
560.81	Intestinal or peritoneal adhesions with obstruction (postoperative) (postinfection)
560.89	Other specified intestinal obstruction
560.9	Unspecified intestinal obstruction
562.10	Diverticulosis of colon (without mention of hemorrhage) — (Use additional code to identify any associated peritonitis: 567.0-567.9)
562.11	Diverticulitis of colon (without mention of hemorrhage) — (Use additional code to identify any associated peritonitis: 567.0-567.9)
564.00	Unspecified constipation
564.01	Slow transit constipation
564.02	Outlet dysfunction constipation
564.09	Other constipation
564.7	Megacolon, other than Hirschsprung's
567.0	Peritonitis in infectious diseases classified elsewhere — (Code first underlying disease)
567.1	Pneumococcal peritonitis
567.2	Other suppurative peritonitis
567.8	Other specified peritonitis
567.9	Unspecified peritonitis
569.1	Rectal prolapse
569.2	Stenosis of rectum and anus
569.3	Hemorrhage of rectum and anus
569.41	Ulcer of anus and rectum
569.42	Anal or rectal pain
569.49	Other specified disorder of rectum and anus
569.5	Abscess of intestine
569.61	Infection of colostomy or enterostomy — (Use additional code to identify organism: 041.00-041.9. Use additional code to specify type of infection: 038.0-038.9, 682.2)
569.69	Other complication of colostomy or enterostomy
569.81	Fistula of intestine, excluding rectum and anus
569.82	Ulceration of intestine
569.83	Perforation of intestine
569.84	Angiodysplasia of intestine (without mention of hemorrhage)
569.85	Angiodysplasia of intestine with hemorrhage
569.86	Dieulafoy lesion (hemorrhagic) of intestine
569.89	Other specified disorder of intestines
569.9	Unspecified disorder of intestine
578.1	Blood in stool
578.9	Unspecified, hemorrhage of gastrointestinal tract
751.3	Hirschsprung's disease and other congenital functional disorders of colon
783.21	Loss of weight
783.22	Underweight
783.7	Adult failure to thrive
793.4	Nonspecific abnormal findings on radiological and other examination of gastrointestinal tract
V10.05	Personal history of malignant neoplasm of large intestine
V12.70	Personal history of unspecified digestive disease
V16.0	Family history of malignant neoplasm of gastrointestinal tract
V44.3	Colostomy status — (This code is intended for use when these conditions are recorded as diagnoses or problems)
V55.3	Attention to colostomy
V71.1	Observation for suspected malignant neoplasm

ICD-9-CM Procedural

45.22	Endoscopy of large intestine through artificial stoma
45.25	Closed [endoscopic] biopsy of large intestine

HCPCS Level II Supplies & Services

A4270	Disposable endoscope sheath, each
A4365	Adhesive remover wipes, any type, per 50
A4397	Irrigation supply; sleeve, each
A4398	Ostomy irrigation supply; bag, each
A4399	Ostomy irrigation supply; cone/catheter, including brush

44390

44390	Colonoscopy through stoma; with removal of foreign body

ICD-9-CM Diagnostic

936	Foreign body in intestine and colon
998.4	Foreign body accidentally left during procedure, not elsewhere classified
998.7	Acute reaction to foreign substance accidentally left during procedure, not elsewhere classified
V44.3	Colostomy status — (This code is intended for use when these conditions are recorded as diagnoses or problems)

ICD-9-CM Procedural

98.04	Removal of intraluminal foreign body from large intestine without incision

HCPCS Level II Supplies & Services

A4270	Disposable endoscope sheath, each
A4365	Adhesive remover wipes, any type, per 50
A4397	Irrigation supply; sleeve, each
A4398	Ostomy irrigation supply; bag, each
A4399	Ostomy irrigation supply; cone/catheter, including brush

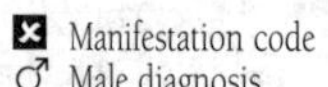

44391

44391 Colonoscopy through stoma; with control of bleeding (eg, injection, bipolar cautery, unipolar cautery, laser, heater probe, stapler, plasma coagulator)

ICD-9-CM Diagnostic

152.3 Malignant neoplasm of Meckel's diverticulum
152.8 Malignant neoplasm of other specified sites of small intestine
152.9 Malignant neoplasm of small intestine, unspecified site ▽
153.0 Malignant neoplasm of hepatic flexure
153.1 Malignant neoplasm of transverse colon
153.8 Malignant neoplasm of other specified sites of large intestine
153.9 Malignant neoplasm of colon, unspecified site ▽
154.0 Malignant neoplasm of rectosigmoid junction
154.1 Malignant neoplasm of rectum
197.5 Secondary malignant neoplasm of large intestine and rectum
230.3 Carcinoma in situ of colon
562.12 Diverticulosis of colon with hemorrhage — (Use additional code to identify any associated peritonitis: 567.0-567.9)
562.13 Diverticulitis of colon with hemorrhage — (Use additional code to identify any associated peritonitis: 567.0-567.9)
569.69 Other complication of colostomy or enterostomy
569.82 Ulceration of intestine
569.83 Perforation of intestine
569.85 Angiodysplasia of intestine with hemorrhage
569.86 Dieulafoy lesion (hemorrhagic) of intestine
578.1 Blood in stool
578.9 Unspecified, hemorrhage of gastrointestinal tract ▽
V44.3 Colostomy status — (This code is intended for use when these conditions are recorded as diagnoses or problems)

ICD-9-CM Procedural

45.43 Endoscopic destruction of other lesion or tissue of large intestine

HCPCS Level II Supplies & Services

A4270 Disposable endoscope sheath, each
A4365 Adhesive remover wipes, any type, per 50
A4397 Irrigation supply; sleeve, each
A4398 Ostomy irrigation supply; bag, each
A4399 Ostomy irrigation supply; cone/catheter, including brush

44392–44394

44392 Colonoscopy through stoma; with removal of tumor(s), polyp(s), or other lesion(s) by hot biopsy forceps or bipolar cautery
44393 with ablation of tumor(s), polyp(s), or other lesion(s) not amenable to removal by hot biopsy forceps, bipolar cautery or snare technique
44394 with removal of tumor(s), polyp(s), or other lesion(s) by snare technique

ICD-9-CM Diagnostic

152.0 Malignant neoplasm of duodenum
152.1 Malignant neoplasm of jejunum
152.2 Malignant neoplasm of ileum
152.3 Malignant neoplasm of Meckel's diverticulum
152.8 Malignant neoplasm of other specified sites of small intestine
152.9 Malignant neoplasm of small intestine, unspecified site ▽
153.0 Malignant neoplasm of hepatic flexure
153.1 Malignant neoplasm of transverse colon
153.2 Malignant neoplasm of descending colon
153.3 Malignant neoplasm of sigmoid colon
153.4 Malignant neoplasm of cecum
153.5 Malignant neoplasm of appendix
153.6 Malignant neoplasm of ascending colon
153.7 Malignant neoplasm of splenic flexure
153.8 Malignant neoplasm of other specified sites of large intestine
153.9 Malignant neoplasm of colon, unspecified site ▽
154.0 Malignant neoplasm of rectosigmoid junction
154.1 Malignant neoplasm of rectum
197.5 Secondary malignant neoplasm of large intestine and rectum
211.2 Benign neoplasm of duodenum, jejunum, and ileum
211.3 Benign neoplasm of colon
230.3 Carcinoma in situ of colon
230.7 Carcinoma in situ of other and unspecified parts of intestine ▽
235.2 Neoplasm of uncertain behavior of stomach, intestines, and rectum
560.81 Intestinal or peritoneal adhesions with obstruction (postoperative) (postinfection)
569.85 Angiodysplasia of intestine with hemorrhage
578.1 Blood in stool
V44.3 Colostomy status — (This code is intended for use when these conditions are recorded as diagnoses or problems)

ICD-9-CM Procedural

45.42 Endoscopic polypectomy of large intestine
45.43 Endoscopic destruction of other lesion or tissue of large intestine

HCPCS Level II Supplies & Services

A4270 Disposable endoscope sheath, each
A4365 Adhesive remover wipes, any type, per 50
A4397 Irrigation supply; sleeve, each
A4398 Ostomy irrigation supply; bag, each
A4399 Ostomy irrigation supply; cone/catheter, including brush

44397

44397 Colonoscopy through stoma; with transendoscopic stent placement (includes predilation)

ICD-9-CM Diagnostic

153.0 Malignant neoplasm of hepatic flexure
153.1 Malignant neoplasm of transverse colon
153.2 Malignant neoplasm of descending colon
153.3 Malignant neoplasm of sigmoid colon
153.4 Malignant neoplasm of cecum
153.5 Malignant neoplasm of appendix
153.6 Malignant neoplasm of ascending colon
153.7 Malignant neoplasm of splenic flexure
153.8 Malignant neoplasm of other specified sites of large intestine
153.9 Malignant neoplasm of colon, unspecified site ▽
154.0 Malignant neoplasm of rectosigmoid junction
154.1 Malignant neoplasm of rectum
197.5 Secondary malignant neoplasm of large intestine and rectum
560.81 Intestinal or peritoneal adhesions with obstruction (postoperative) (postinfection)
560.89 Other specified intestinal obstruction
560.9 Unspecified intestinal obstruction ▽
751.2 Congenital atresia and stenosis of large intestine, rectum, and anal canal
997.4 Digestive system complication — (Use additional code to identify complications)

ICD-9-CM Procedural

45.22 Endoscopy of large intestine through artificial stoma
46.79 Other repair of intestine

44500

44500 Introduction of long gastrointestinal tube (eg, Miller-Abbott) (separate procedure)

ICD-9-CM Diagnostic

The application of this code is too broad to adequately present ICD-9-CM diagnostic code links here. Refer to your ICD-9-CM book.

ICD-9-CM Procedural

96.08 Insertion of (naso-) intestinal tube

44602–44603

44602 Suture of small intestine (enterorrhaphy) for perforated ulcer, diverticulum, wound, injury or rupture; single perforation
44603 multiple perforations

ICD-9-CM Diagnostic

532.10 Acute duodenal ulcer with perforation, without mention of obstruction — (Use additional E code to identify drug, if drug induced)
532.11 Acute duodenal ulcer with perforation and obstruction — (Use additional E code to identify drug, if drug induced)
532.20 Acute duodenal ulcer with hemorrhage and perforation, without mention of obstruction — (Use additional E code to identify drug, if drug induced)
532.21 Acute duodenal ulcer with hemorrhage, perforation, and obstruction — (Use additional E code to identify drug, if drug induced)
532.50 Chronic or unspecified duodenal ulcer with perforation, without mention of obstruction — (Use additional E code to identify drug, if drug induced)
532.51 Chronic or unspecified duodenal ulcer with perforation and obstruction — (Use additional E code to identify drug, if drug induced)
532.60 Chronic or unspecified duodenal ulcer with hemorrhage and perforation, without mention of obstruction — (Use additional E code to identify drug, if drug induced)

532.61 Chronic or unspecified duodenal ulcer with hemorrhage, perforation, and obstruction — (Use additional E code to identify drug, if drug induced)
560.2 Volvulus
560.81 Intestinal or peritoneal adhesions with obstruction (postoperative) (postinfection)
560.89 Other specified intestinal obstruction
562.00 Diverticulosis of small intestine (without mention of hemorrhage) — (Use additional code to identify any associated peritonitis: 567.0-567.9)
562.01 Diverticulitis of small intestine (without mention of hemorrhage) — (Use additional code to identify any associated peritonitis: 567.0-567.9)
562.02 Diverticulosis of small intestine with hemorrhage — (Use additional code to identify any associated peritonitis: 567.0-567.9)
562.03 Divertulitis of small intestine with hemorrhage — (Use additional code to identify any associated peritonitis: 567.0-567.9)
567.0 Peritonitis in infectious diseases classified elsewhere — (Code first underlying disease) ☒
567.1 Pneumococcal peritonitis
567.2 Other suppurative peritonitis
567.8 Other specified peritonitis
567.9 Unspecified peritonitis ▽
569.81 Fistula of intestine, excluding rectum and anus
569.82 Ulceration of intestine
569.83 Perforation of intestine
569.84 Angiodysplasia of intestine (without mention of hemorrhage)
569.86 Dieulafoy lesion (hemorrhagic) of intestine
569.89 Other specified disorder of intestines
596.1 Intestinovesical fistula — (Use additional code to identify urinary incontinence: 625.6, 788.30-788.39)
863.20 Small intestine injury, unspecified site, without mention of open wound into cavity ▽
863.21 Duodenum injury without mention of open wound into cavity
863.30 Small intestine injury, unspecified site, with open wound into cavity ▽
863.31 Duodenum injury with open wound into cavity

ICD-9-CM Procedural

44.42 Suture of duodenal ulcer site
46.71 Suture of laceration of duodenum
46.73 Suture of laceration of small intestine, except duodenum
46.79 Other repair of intestine

44604–44605

44604 Suture of large intestine (colorrhaphy) for perforated ulcer, diverticulum, wound, injury or rupture (single or multiple perforations); without colostomy
44605 with colostomy

ICD-9-CM Diagnostic

540.0 Acute appendicitis with generalized peritonitis
540.1 Acute appendicitis with peritoneal abscess
556.0 Ulcerative (chronic) enterocolitis
556.1 Ulcerative (chronic) ileocolitis
556.2 Ulcerative (chronic) proctitis
556.3 Ulcerative (chronic) proctosigmoiditis
556.4 Pseudopolyposis of colon
556.5 Left sided ulcerative (chronic) colitis
556.6 Universal ulcerative (chronic) colitis
556.9 Unspecified ulcerative colitis ▽
560.2 Volvulus
562.10 Diverticulosis of colon (without mention of hemorrhage) — (Use additional code to identify any associated peritonitis: 567.0-567.9)
562.11 Diverticulitis of colon (without mention of hemorrhage) — (Use additional code to identify any associated peritonitis: 567.0-567.9)
562.12 Diverticulosis of colon with hemorrhage — (Use additional code to identify any associated peritonitis: 567.0-567.9)
562.13 Diverticulitis of colon with hemorrhage — (Use additional code to identify any associated peritonitis: 567.0-567.9)
567.0 Peritonitis in infectious diseases classified elsewhere — (Code first underlying disease) ☒
567.1 Pneumococcal peritonitis
567.2 Other suppurative peritonitis
567.8 Other specified peritonitis
567.9 Unspecified peritonitis ▽
569.81 Fistula of intestine, excluding rectum and anus
569.82 Ulceration of intestine
569.83 Perforation of intestine
569.84 Angiodysplasia of intestine (without mention of hemorrhage)
569.85 Angiodysplasia of intestine with hemorrhage
569.86 Dieulafoy lesion (hemorrhagic) of intestine
569.89 Other specified disorder of intestines
777.6 Perinatal intestinal perforation
863.40 Colon injury unspecified site, without mention of open wound into cavity ▽
863.41 Ascending (right) colon injury without mention of open wound into cavity
863.42 Transverse colon injury without mention of open wound into cavity
863.43 Descending (left) colon injury without mention of open wound into cavity
863.44 Sigmoid colon injury without mention of open wound into cavity
863.45 Rectum injury without mention of open wound into cavity
863.46 Injury to multiple sites in colon and rectum without mention of open wound into cavity
863.49 Other colon and rectum injury, without mention of open wound into cavity
863.50 Colon injury, unspecified site, with open wound into cavity ▽
863.52 Transverse colon injury with open wound into cavity
863.59 Other injury to colon and rectum with open wound into cavity

ICD-9-CM Procedural

46.03 Exteriorization of large intestine
46.11 Temporary colostomy
46.13 Permanent colostomy
46.75 Suture of laceration of large intestine
46.79 Other repair of intestine

44615

44615 Intestinal strictureplasty (enterotomy and enterorrhaphy) with or without dilation, for intestinal obstruction

ICD-9-CM Diagnostic

560.31 Gallstone ileus
560.81 Intestinal or peritoneal adhesions with obstruction (postoperative) (postinfection)
560.89 Other specified intestinal obstruction
560.9 Unspecified intestinal obstruction ▽
751.1 Congenital atresia and stenosis of small intestine
751.2 Congenital atresia and stenosis of large intestine, rectum, and anal canal
997.4 Digestive system complication — (Use additional code to identify complications)

ICD-9-CM Procedural

45.00 Incision of intestine, not otherwise specified
45.02 Other incision of small intestine
45.03 Incision of large intestine
46.73 Suture of laceration of small intestine, except duodenum
46.79 Other repair of intestine
46.85 Dilation of intestine

44620–44626

44620 Closure of enterostomy, large or small intestine;
44625 with resection and anastomosis other than colorectal
44626 with resection and colorectal anastomosis (eg, closure of Hartmann type procedure)

ICD-9-CM Diagnostic

560.81 Intestinal or peritoneal adhesions with obstruction (postoperative) (postinfection)
569.61 Infection of colostomy or enterostomy — (Use additional code to identify organism: 041.00-041.9. Use additional code to specify type of infection: 038.0-038.9, 682.2)
569.62 Mechanical complication of colostomy and enterostomy
569.69 Other complication of colostomy or enterostomy
V10.05 Personal history of malignant neoplasm of large intestine
V10.06 Personal history of malignant neoplasm of rectum, rectosigmoid junction, and anus
V10.09 Personal history of malignant neoplasm of other site in gastrointestinal tract
V55.2 Attention to ileostomy
V55.3 Attention to colostomy
V55.4 Attention to other artificial opening of digestive tract

ICD-9-CM Procedural

45.90 Intestinal anastomosis, not otherwise specified
45.94 Large-to-large intestinal anastomosis
46.50 Closure of intestinal stoma, not otherwise specified
46.51 Closure of stoma of small intestine
46.52 Closure of stoma of large intestine

▽ Unspecified code ♀ Female diagnosis ☒ Manifestation code ♂ Male diagnosis

44640

44640 Closure of intestinal cutaneous fistula

ICD-9-CM Diagnostic

537.4 Fistula of stomach or duodenum
569.81 Fistula of intestine, excluding rectum and anus
576.4 Fistula of bile duct
756.71 Prune belly syndrome
756.79 Other congenital anomalies of abdominal wall
998.6 Persistent postoperative fistula, not elsewhere classified

ICD-9-CM Procedural

46.72 Closure of fistula of duodenum
46.74 Closure of fistula of small intestine, except duodenum

44650

44650 Closure of enteroenteric or enterocolic fistula

ICD-9-CM Diagnostic

537.4 Fistula of stomach or duodenum
569.81 Fistula of intestine, excluding rectum and anus
576.4 Fistula of bile duct
751.5 Other congenital anomalies of intestine
998.6 Persistent postoperative fistula, not elsewhere classified

ICD-9-CM Procedural

46.72 Closure of fistula of duodenum
46.74 Closure of fistula of small intestine, except duodenum
46.76 Closure of fistula of large intestine
47.92 Closure of appendiceal fistula

44660–44661

44660 Closure of enterovesical fistula; without intestinal or bladder resection
44661 with intestine and/or bladder resection

ICD-9-CM Diagnostic

555.0 Regional enteritis of small intestine
555.1 Regional enteritis of large intestine
555.2 Regional enteritis of small intestine with large intestine
555.9 Regional enteritis of unspecified site ▽
562.11 Diverticulitis of colon (without mention of hemorrhage) — (Use additional code to identify any associated peritonitis: 567.0-567.9)
567.0 Peritonitis in infectious diseases classified elsewhere — (Code first underlying disease) ☒
567.1 Pneumococcal peritonitis
567.2 Other suppurative peritonitis
567.8 Other specified peritonitis
567.9 Unspecified peritonitis ▽
596.1 Intestinovesical fistula — (Use additional code to identify urinary incontinence: 625.6, 788.30-788.39)
998.6 Persistent postoperative fistula, not elsewhere classified

ICD-9-CM Procedural

45.62 Other partial resection of small intestine
45.79 Other partial excision of large intestine
57.6 Partial cystectomy
57.83 Repair of fistula involving bladder and intestine

44680

44680 Intestinal plication (separate procedure)

ICD-9-CM Diagnostic

560.81 Intestinal or peritoneal adhesions with obstruction (postoperative) (postinfection)
568.81 Hemoperitoneum (nontraumatic)
751.1 Congenital atresia and stenosis of small intestine
751.2 Congenital atresia and stenosis of large intestine, rectum, and anal canal
997.4 Digestive system complication — (Use additional code to identify complications)

ICD-9-CM Procedural

44.64 Gastropexy
46.60 Fixation of intestine, not otherwise specified
46.61 Fixation of small intestine to abdominal wall
46.62 Other fixation of small intestine
46.63 Fixation of large intestine to abdominal wall

44700

44700 Exclusion of small intestine from pelvis by mesh or other prosthesis, or native tissue (eg, bladder or omentum)

ICD-9-CM Diagnostic

151.0 Malignant neoplasm of cardia
151.1 Malignant neoplasm of pylorus
151.2 Malignant neoplasm of pyloric antrum
151.3 Malignant neoplasm of fundus of stomach
151.4 Malignant neoplasm of body of stomach
151.5 Malignant neoplasm of lesser curvature of stomach, unspecified ▽
151.6 Malignant neoplasm of greater curvature of stomach, unspecified ▽
151.8 Malignant neoplasm of other specified sites of stomach
151.9 Malignant neoplasm of stomach, unspecified site ▽
152.3 Malignant neoplasm of Meckel's diverticulum
153.0 Malignant neoplasm of hepatic flexure
153.1 Malignant neoplasm of transverse colon
153.2 Malignant neoplasm of descending colon
153.3 Malignant neoplasm of sigmoid colon
153.4 Malignant neoplasm of cecum
153.5 Malignant neoplasm of appendix
153.6 Malignant neoplasm of ascending colon
153.7 Malignant neoplasm of splenic flexure
153.8 Malignant neoplasm of other specified sites of large intestine
153.9 Malignant neoplasm of colon, unspecified site ▽
154.0 Malignant neoplasm of rectosigmoid junction
155.0 Malignant neoplasm of liver, primary
157.9 Malignant neoplasm of pancreas, part unspecified ▽
158.8 Malignant neoplasm of specified parts of peritoneum
158.9 Malignant neoplasm of peritoneum, unspecified ▽
179 Malignant neoplasm of uterus, part unspecified ▽ ♀
180.0 Malignant neoplasm of endocervix ♀
180.1 Malignant neoplasm of exocervix ♀
180.8 Malignant neoplasm of other specified sites of cervix ♀
182.0 Malignant neoplasm of corpus uteri, except isthmus ♀
182.1 Malignant neoplasm of isthmus ♀
182.8 Malignant neoplasm of other specified sites of body of uterus ♀
183.0 Malignant neoplasm of ovary — (Use additional code to identify any functional activity) ♀
185 Malignant neoplasm of prostate ♂
186.0 Malignant neoplasm of undescended testis — (Use additional code to identify any functional activity) ♂
186.9 Malignant neoplasm of other and unspecified testis — (Use additional code to identify any functional activity) ▽ ♂
188.0 Malignant neoplasm of trigone of urinary bladder
188.1 Malignant neoplasm of dome of urinary bladder
188.2 Malignant neoplasm of lateral wall of urinary bladder
188.3 Malignant neoplasm of anterior wall of urinary bladder
188.4 Malignant neoplasm of posterior wall of urinary bladder
188.5 Malignant neoplasm of bladder neck
188.6 Malignant neoplasm of ureteric orifice
188.7 Malignant neoplasm of urachus
188.8 Malignant neoplasm of other specified sites of bladder
188.9 Malignant neoplasm of bladder, part unspecified ▽
189.0 Malignant neoplasm of kidney, except pelvis
189.1 Malignant neoplasm of renal pelvis
189.2 Malignant neoplasm of ureter
196.2 Secondary and unspecified malignant neoplasm of intra-abdominal lymph nodes
196.6 Secondary and unspecified malignant neoplasm of intrapelvic lymph nodes
197.4 Secondary malignant neoplasm of small intestine including duodenum
197.5 Secondary malignant neoplasm of large intestine and rectum
197.6 Secondary malignant neoplasm of retroperitoneum and peritoneum
198.82 Secondary malignant neoplasm of genital organs
199.0 Disseminated malignant neoplasm
199.1 Other malignant neoplasm of unspecified site
201.46 Hodgkin's disease, lymphocytic-histiocytic predominance of intrapelvic lymph nodes
201.96 Hodgkin's disease, unspecified type, of intrapelvic lymph nodes ▽
202.53 Letterer-Siwe disease of intra-abdominal lymph nodes
202.56 Letterer-Siwe disease of intrapelvic lymph nodes
202.63 Malignant mast cell tumors of intra-abdominal lymph nodes
202.66 Malignant mast cell tumors of intrapelvic lymph nodes
202.83 Other malignant lymphomas of intra-abdominal lymph nodes

▽ Unspecified code ♀ Female diagnosis ☒ Manifestation code ♂ Male diagnosis

202.86 Other malignant lymphomas of intrapelvic lymph nodes

ICD-9-CM Procedural

46.62 Other fixation of small intestine
46.99 Other operations on intestines
54.74 Other repair of omentum

44701

44701 Intraoperative colonic lavage (List separately in addition to code for primary procedure)

ICD-9-CM Diagnostic

This is an add-on code. Refer to the corresponding primary procedure code for ICD-9 diagnosis code links.

ICD-9-CM Procedural

46.99 Other operations on intestines

HCPCS Level II Supplies & Services

The HCPCS Level II code(s) would be the same as the actual procedure performed because these are in-addition-to codes.

44715–44721

44715 Backbench standard preparation of cadaver or living donor intestine allograft prior to transplantation, including mobilization and fashioning of the superior mesenteric artery and vein
44720 Backbench reconstruction of cadaver or living donor intestine allograft prior to transplantation; venous anastomosis, each
44721 arterial anastomosis, each

ICD-9-CM Diagnostic

152.0 Malignant neoplasm of duodenum
152.1 Malignant neoplasm of jejunum
152.2 Malignant neoplasm of ileum
152.8 Malignant neoplasm of other specified sites of small intestine
152.9 Malignant neoplasm of small intestine, unspecified site ▽
197.4 Secondary malignant neoplasm of small intestine including duodenum
551.00 Femoral hernia with gangrene, unilateral or unspecified (not specified as recurrent)
551.21 Incisional ventral hernia, with gangrene
551.8 Hernia of other specified sites, with gangrene
551.9 Hernia of unspecified site, with gangrene ▽
552.00 Unilateral or unspecified femoral hernia with obstruction
552.21 Incisional hernia with obstruction
555.0 Regional enteritis of small intestine
555.9 Regional enteritis of unspecified site ▽
556.1 Ulcerative (chronic) ileocolitis
556.8 Other ulcerative colitis
556.9 Unspecified ulcerative colitis ▽
560.0 Intussusception
560.1 Paralytic ileus
560.2 Volvulus
560.81 Intestinal or peritoneal adhesions with obstruction (postoperative) (postinfection)
560.89 Other specified intestinal obstruction
560.9 Unspecified intestinal obstruction ▽
562.00 Diverticulosis of small intestine (without mention of hemorrhage) — (Use additional code to identify any associated peritonitis: 567.0-567.9)
562.01 Diverticulitis of small intestine (without mention of hemorrhage) — (Use additional code to identify any associated peritonitis: 567.0-567.9)
562.02 Diverticulosis of small intestine with hemorrhage — (Use additional code to identify any associated peritonitis: 567.0-567.9)
562.03 Divertulitis of small intestine with hemorrhage — (Use additional code to identify any associated peritonitis: 567.0-567.9)
567.0 Peritonitis in infectious diseases classified elsewhere — (Code first underlying disease) ☒
567.1 Pneumococcal peritonitis
567.2 Other suppurative peritonitis
567.8 Other specified peritonitis
567.9 Unspecified peritonitis ▽
569.85 Angiodysplasia of intestine with hemorrhage
569.89 Other specified disorder of intestines
578.9 Unspecified, hemorrhage of gastrointestinal tract ▽
579.3 Other and unspecified postsurgical nonabsorption ▽
751.1 Congenital atresia and stenosis of small intestine
751.5 Other congenital anomalies of intestine
863.30 Small intestine injury, unspecified site, with open wound into cavity ▽
863.31 Duodenum injury with open wound into cavity
863.39 Other injury to small intestine with open wound into cavity
863.90 Gastrointestinal tract injury, unspecified site, with open wound into cavity ▽
863.99 Injury to other and unspecified gastrointestinal sites with open wound into cavity
997.4 Digestive system complication — (Use additional code to identify complications)
998.51 Infected postoperative seroma — (Use additional code to identify organism)
998.59 Other postoperative infection — (Use additional code to identify infection)

ICD-9-CM Procedural

00.91 Transplant from live related donor
00.92 Transplant from live non-related donor
00.93 Transplant from cadaver
46.97 Transplant of intestine

Meckel's Diverticulum and the Messentery

44800

44800 Excision of Meckel's diverticulum (diverticulectomy) or omphalomesenteric duct

ICD-9-CM Diagnostic

152.3 Malignant neoplasm of Meckel's diverticulum
197.4 Secondary malignant neoplasm of small intestine including duodenum
567.0 Peritonitis in infectious diseases classified elsewhere — (Code first underlying disease) ☒
567.1 Pneumococcal peritonitis
567.2 Other suppurative peritonitis
567.8 Other specified peritonitis
567.9 Unspecified peritonitis ▽
751.0 Meckel's diverticulum

ICD-9-CM Procedural

45.33 Local excision of lesion or tissue of small intestine, except duodenum

44820

44820 Excision of lesion of mesentery (separate procedure)

ICD-9-CM Diagnostic

153.3 Malignant neoplasm of sigmoid colon
153.4 Malignant neoplasm of cecum
153.8 Malignant neoplasm of other specified sites of large intestine
158.8 Malignant neoplasm of specified parts of peritoneum
183.4 Malignant neoplasm of parametrium of uterus ♀
197.6 Secondary malignant neoplasm of retroperitoneum and peritoneum
211.8 Benign neoplasm of retroperitoneum and peritoneum
235.4 Neoplasm of uncertain behavior of retroperitoneum and peritoneum
239.0 Neoplasm of unspecified nature of digestive system
568.0 Peritoneal adhesions (postoperative) (postinfection)
568.81 Hemoperitoneum (nontraumatic)
568.82 Peritoneal effusion (chronic)
568.89 Other specified disorder of peritoneum
569.82 Ulceration of intestine

ICD-9-CM Procedural

54.4 Excision or destruction of peritoneal tissue

44850

44850 Suture of mesentery (separate procedure)

ICD-9-CM Diagnostic

152.9 Malignant neoplasm of small intestine, unspecified site ▽
153.9 Malignant neoplasm of colon, unspecified site ▽
158.8 Malignant neoplasm of specified parts of peritoneum
560.81 Intestinal or peritoneal adhesions with obstruction (postoperative) (postinfection)
863.20 Small intestine injury, unspecified site, without mention of open wound into cavity ▽

▽ Unspecified code
♀ Female diagnosis
☒ Manifestation code
♂ Male diagnosis

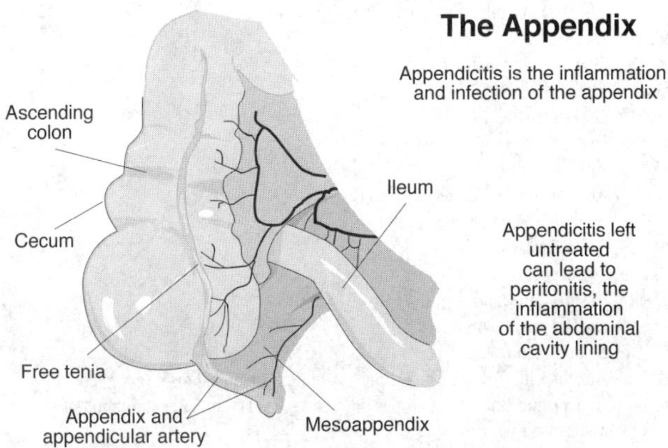
The Appendix
Appendicitis is the inflammation and infection of the appendix
Ascending colon
Ileum
Cecum
Appendicitis left untreated can lead to peritonitis, the inflammation of the abdominal cavity lining
Free tenia
Appendix and appendicular artery
Mesoappendix

863.30 Small intestine injury, unspecified site, with open wound into cavity ▽
863.40 Colon injury unspecified site, without mention of open wound into cavity ▽
863.50 Colon injury, unspecified site, with open wound into cavity ▽
863.89 Injury to other and unspecified gastrointestinal sites without mention of open wound into cavity
863.99 Injury to other and unspecified gastrointestinal sites with open wound into cavity

ICD-9-CM Procedural
54.75 Other repair of mesentery

Appendix

44900–44901
44900 Incision and drainage of appendiceal abscess; open
44901 percutaneous

ICD-9-CM Diagnostic
540.1 Acute appendicitis with peritoneal abscess
542 Other appendicitis

ICD-9-CM Procedural
47.2 Drainage of appendiceal abscess

44950–44955
44950 Appendectomy;
44955 when done for indicated purpose at time of other major procedure (not as separate procedure) (List separately in addition to code for primary procedure)

ICD-9-CM Diagnostic
153.5 Malignant neoplasm of appendix
540.9 Acute appendicitis without mention of peritonitis
541 Appendicitis, unqualified
542 Other appendicitis
543.0 Hyperplasia of appendix (lymphoid)
543.9 Other and unspecified diseases of appendix ▽
617.5 Endometriosis of intestine ♀
780.6 Fever
787.01 Nausea with vomiting
787.02 Nausea alone
787.03 Vomiting alone
787.99 Other symptoms involving digestive system
789.03 Abdominal pain, right lower quadrant
789.05 Abdominal pain, periumbilic
789.06 Abdominal pain, epigastric
789.07 Abdominal pain, generalized
789.09 Abdominal pain, other specified site
789.30 Abdominal or pelvic swelling, mass or lump, unspecified site ▽
789.33 Abdominal or pelvic swelling, mass, or lump, right lower quadrant
789.35 Abdominal or pelvic swelling, mass or lump, periumbilic
789.36 Abdominal or pelvic swelling, mass, or lump, epigastric
789.37 Abdominal or pelvic swelling, mass, or lump, epigastric, generalized
789.39 Abdominal or pelvic swelling, mass, or lump, other specified site
789.63 Abdominal tenderness, right lower quadrant
V50.49 Other prophylactic gland removal
V64.41 Laparoscopic surgical procedure converted to open procedure

ICD-9-CM Procedural
47.09 Other appendectomy
47.19 Other incidental appendectomy

44960
44960 Appendectomy; for ruptured appendix with abscess or generalized peritonitis

ICD-9-CM Diagnostic
540.0 Acute appendicitis with generalized peritonitis
540.1 Acute appendicitis with peritoneal abscess
780.6 Fever
789.00 Abdominal pain, unspecified site ▽
789.03 Abdominal pain, right lower quadrant
789.05 Abdominal pain, periumbilic
789.06 Abdominal pain, epigastric
789.07 Abdominal pain, generalized
789.09 Abdominal pain, other specified site
789.30 Abdominal or pelvic swelling, mass or lump, unspecified site ▽
789.33 Abdominal or pelvic swelling, mass, or lump, right lower quadrant
789.35 Abdominal or pelvic swelling, mass or lump, periumbilic
789.36 Abdominal or pelvic swelling, mass, or lump, epigastric
789.37 Abdominal or pelvic swelling, mass, or lump, epigastric, generalized
789.39 Abdominal or pelvic swelling, mass, or lump, other specified site
V64.41 Laparoscopic surgical procedure converted to open procedure

ICD-9-CM Procedural
47.09 Other appendectomy

44970
44970 Laparoscopy, surgical, appendectomy

ICD-9-CM Diagnostic
153.5 Malignant neoplasm of appendix
197.5 Secondary malignant neoplasm of large intestine and rectum
211.3 Benign neoplasm of colon
230.3 Carcinoma in situ of colon
235.2 Neoplasm of uncertain behavior of stomach, intestines, and rectum
239.0 Neoplasm of unspecified nature of digestive system
540.0 Acute appendicitis with generalized peritonitis
540.9 Acute appendicitis without mention of peritonitis
541 Appendicitis, unqualified
542 Other appendicitis
543.0 Hyperplasia of appendix (lymphoid)
543.9 Other and unspecified diseases of appendix ▽
789.03 Abdominal pain, right lower quadrant
789.05 Abdominal pain, periumbilic
789.07 Abdominal pain, generalized
789.09 Abdominal pain, other specified site
789.33 Abdominal or pelvic swelling, mass, or lump, right lower quadrant
789.35 Abdominal or pelvic swelling, mass or lump, periumbilic
789.37 Abdominal or pelvic swelling, mass, or lump, epigastric, generalized
789.39 Abdominal or pelvic swelling, mass, or lump, other specified site

ICD-9-CM Procedural
47.01 Laparoscopic appendectomy
47.11 Laparoscopic incidental appendectomy

Rectum

45000
45000 Transrectal drainage of pelvic abscess

ICD-9-CM Diagnostic
540.1 Acute appendicitis with peritoneal abscess
555.1 Regional enteritis of large intestine
560.81 Intestinal or peritoneal adhesions with obstruction (postoperative) (postinfection)
562.11 Diverticulitis of colon (without mention of hemorrhage) — (Use additional code to identify any associated peritonitis: 567.0-567.9)

567.0 Peritonitis in infectious diseases classified elsewhere — (Code first underlying disease) ☒
567.1 Pneumococcal peritonitis
567.2 Other suppurative peritonitis
567.8 Other specified peritonitis
567.9 Unspecified peritonitis ▽
569.5 Abscess of intestine
569.82 Ulceration of intestine
569.83 Perforation of intestine
614.3 Acute parametritis and pelvic cellulitis — (Use additional code to identify organism: 041.0, 041.1) ♀
614.4 Chronic or unspecified parametritis and pelvic cellulitis — (Use additional code to identify organism: 041.0, 041.1) ♀
614.5 Acute or unspecified pelvic peritonitis, female — (Use additional code to identify organism: 041.0, 041.1) ♀
614.8 Other specified inflammatory disease of female pelvic organs and tissues — (Use additional code to identify organism: 041.0, 041.1) ♀
639.0 Genital tract and pelvic infection following abortion or ectopic and molar pregnancies ♀

ICD-9-CM Procedural
48.0 Proctotomy

45005
45005 Incision and drainage of submucosal abscess, rectum

ICD-9-CM Diagnostic
566 Abscess of anal and rectal regions
998.51 Infected postoperative seroma — (Use additional code to identify organism)
998.59 Other postoperative infection — (Use additional code to identify infection)

ICD-9-CM Procedural
48.0 Proctotomy
48.81 Incision of perirectal tissue
49.91 Incision of anal septum

45020
45020 Incision and drainage of deep supralevator, pelvirectal, or retrorectal abscess

ICD-9-CM Diagnostic
555.1 Regional enteritis of large intestine
556.1 Ulcerative (chronic) ileocolitis
556.2 Ulcerative (chronic) proctitis
556.3 Ulcerative (chronic) proctosigmoiditis
556.4 Pseudopolyposis of colon
556.5 Left sided ulcerative (chronic) colitis
556.6 Universal ulcerative (chronic) colitis
556.8 Other ulcerative colitis
566 Abscess of anal and rectal regions
567.2 Other suppurative peritonitis
614.3 Acute parametritis and pelvic cellulitis — (Use additional code to identify organism: 041.0, 041.1) ♀
614.4 Chronic or unspecified parametritis and pelvic cellulitis — (Use additional code to identify organism: 041.0, 041.1) ♀
614.8 Other specified inflammatory disease of female pelvic organs and tissues — (Use additional code to identify organism: 041.0, 041.1) ♀
639.0 Genital tract and pelvic infection following abortion or ectopic and molar pregnancies ♀
998.51 Infected postoperative seroma — (Use additional code to identify organism)
998.59 Other postoperative infection — (Use additional code to identify infection)

ICD-9-CM Procedural
48.0 Proctotomy
48.81 Incision of perirectal tissue

45100
45100 Biopsy of anorectal wall, anal approach (eg, congenital megacolon)

ICD-9-CM Diagnostic
154.1 Malignant neoplasm of rectum
154.2 Malignant neoplasm of anal canal
154.3 Malignant neoplasm of anus, unspecified site ▽
197.5 Secondary malignant neoplasm of large intestine and rectum
211.4 Benign neoplasm of rectum and anal canal
230.4 Carcinoma in situ of rectum
239.0 Neoplasm of unspecified nature of digestive system
564.00 Unspecified constipation ▽
564.01 Slow transit constipation
564.02 Outlet dysfunction constipation
564.09 Other constipation
564.1 Irritable bowel syndrome
565.0 Anal fissure
566 Abscess of anal and rectal regions
569.0 Anal and rectal polyp
569.1 Rectal prolapse
569.2 Stenosis of rectum and anus
569.41 Ulcer of anus and rectum
569.42 Anal or rectal pain
578.1 Blood in stool
751.3 Hirschsprung's disease and other congenital functional disorders of colon
793.4 Nonspecific abnormal findings on radiological and other examination of gastrointestinal tract
V10.05 Personal history of malignant neoplasm of large intestine
V10.06 Personal history of malignant neoplasm of rectum, rectosigmoid junction, and anus

ICD-9-CM Procedural
48.24 Closed (endoscopic) biopsy of rectum
48.25 Open biopsy of rectum
49.23 Biopsy of anus

HCPCS Level II Supplies & Services
A4305 Disposable drug delivery system, flow rate of 50 ml or greater per hour
A4306 Disposable drug delivery system, flow rate of 5 ml or less per hour
A4550 Surgical trays

45108
45108 Anorectal myomectomy

ICD-9-CM Diagnostic
154.8 Malignant neoplasm of other sites of rectum, rectosigmoid junction, and anus
211.4 Benign neoplasm of rectum and anal canal
564.00 Unspecified constipation ▽
564.01 Slow transit constipation
564.02 Outlet dysfunction constipation
564.09 Other constipation
569.2 Stenosis of rectum and anus
569.49 Other specified disorder of rectum and anus
787.6 Incontinence of feces

ICD-9-CM Procedural
48.92 Anorectal myectomy

45110–45111
45110 Proctectomy; complete, combined abdominoperineal, with colostomy
45111 partial resection of rectum, transabdominal approach

ICD-9-CM Diagnostic
153.3 Malignant neoplasm of sigmoid colon
153.9 Malignant neoplasm of colon, unspecified site ▽
154.0 Malignant neoplasm of rectosigmoid junction
154.1 Malignant neoplasm of rectum
154.2 Malignant neoplasm of anal canal
154.8 Malignant neoplasm of other sites of rectum, rectosigmoid junction, and anus
197.5 Secondary malignant neoplasm of large intestine and rectum
211.3 Benign neoplasm of colon
230.3 Carcinoma in situ of colon
230.4 Carcinoma in situ of rectum
235.2 Neoplasm of uncertain behavior of stomach, intestines, and rectum
555.1 Regional enteritis of large intestine
556.0 Ulcerative (chronic) enterocolitis
556.1 Ulcerative (chronic) ileocolitis
556.2 Ulcerative (chronic) proctitis
556.3 Ulcerative (chronic) proctosigmoiditis
556.4 Pseudopolyposis of colon
556.5 Left sided ulcerative (chronic) colitis
556.6 Universal ulcerative (chronic) colitis
556.8 Other ulcerative colitis
556.9 Unspecified ulcerative colitis ▽
557.0 Acute vascular insufficiency of intestine
557.1 Chronic vascular insufficiency of intestine

557.9 Unspecified vascular insufficiency of intestine ▽
569.1 Rectal prolapse
751.3 Hirschsprung's disease and other congenital functional disorders of colon

ICD-9-CM Procedural
48.5 Abdominoperineal resection of rectum
48.69 Other resection of rectum

45112
45112 Proctectomy, combined abdominoperineal, pull-through procedure (eg, colo-anal anastomosis)

ICD-9-CM Diagnostic
153.3 Malignant neoplasm of sigmoid colon
153.9 Malignant neoplasm of colon, unspecified site ▽
154.0 Malignant neoplasm of rectosigmoid junction
154.1 Malignant neoplasm of rectum
230.3 Carcinoma in situ of colon
230.4 Carcinoma in situ of rectum
555.1 Regional enteritis of large intestine
555.9 Regional enteritis of unspecified site ▽
556.0 Ulcerative (chronic) enterocolitis
556.2 Ulcerative (chronic) proctitis
569.1 Rectal prolapse
751.3 Hirschsprung's disease and other congenital functional disorders of colon

ICD-9-CM Procedural
48.49 Other pull-through resection of rectum
48.5 Abdominoperineal resection of rectum
48.65 Duhamel resection of rectum

45113
45113 Proctectomy, partial, with rectal mucosectomy, ileoanal anastomosis, creation of ileal reservoir (S or J), with or without loop ileostomy

ICD-9-CM Diagnostic
153.9 Malignant neoplasm of colon, unspecified site ▽
154.0 Malignant neoplasm of rectosigmoid junction
154.1 Malignant neoplasm of rectum
154.2 Malignant neoplasm of anal canal
154.3 Malignant neoplasm of anus, unspecified site ▽
154.8 Malignant neoplasm of other sites of rectum, rectosigmoid junction, and anus
230.3 Carcinoma in situ of colon
230.4 Carcinoma in situ of rectum
235.2 Neoplasm of uncertain behavior of stomach, intestines, and rectum
555.1 Regional enteritis of large intestine
556.0 Ulcerative (chronic) enterocolitis
556.2 Ulcerative (chronic) proctitis
569.1 Rectal prolapse
751.3 Hirschsprung's disease and other congenital functional disorders of colon

ICD-9-CM Procedural
45.95 Anastomosis to anus
46.01 Exteriorization of small intestine

45114–45116
45114 Proctectomy, partial, with anastomosis; abdominal and transsacral approach
45116 transsacral approach only (Kraske type)

ICD-9-CM Diagnostic
153.9 Malignant neoplasm of colon, unspecified site ▽
154.0 Malignant neoplasm of rectosigmoid junction
154.1 Malignant neoplasm of rectum
154.2 Malignant neoplasm of anal canal
154.3 Malignant neoplasm of anus, unspecified site ▽
154.8 Malignant neoplasm of other sites of rectum, rectosigmoid junction, and anus
230.3 Carcinoma in situ of colon
230.4 Carcinoma in situ of rectum
555.1 Regional enteritis of large intestine
556.0 Ulcerative (chronic) enterocolitis
556.2 Ulcerative (chronic) proctitis
569.1 Rectal prolapse
751.3 Hirschsprung's disease and other congenital functional disorders of colon

ICD-9-CM Procedural
48.5 Abdominoperineal resection of rectum
48.69 Other resection of rectum

45119
45119 Proctectomy, combined abdominoperineal pull-through procedure (eg, colo-anal anastomosis), with creation of colonic reservoir (eg, J-pouch), with or without proximal diverting ostomy

ICD-9-CM Diagnostic
153.9 Malignant neoplasm of colon, unspecified site ▽
154.0 Malignant neoplasm of rectosigmoid junction
154.1 Malignant neoplasm of rectum
154.2 Malignant neoplasm of anal canal
154.3 Malignant neoplasm of anus, unspecified site ▽
154.8 Malignant neoplasm of other sites of rectum, rectosigmoid junction, and anus
230.3 Carcinoma in situ of colon
230.4 Carcinoma in situ of rectum
235.2 Neoplasm of uncertain behavior of stomach, intestines, and rectum
555.1 Regional enteritis of large intestine
556.0 Ulcerative (chronic) enterocolitis
556.2 Ulcerative (chronic) proctitis
569.1 Rectal prolapse
751.3 Hirschsprung's disease and other congenital functional disorders of colon

ICD-9-CM Procedural
48.49 Other pull-through resection of rectum
48.65 Duhamel resection of rectum

45120
45120 Proctectomy, complete (for congenital megacolon), abdominal and perineal approach; with pull-through procedure and anastomosis (eg, Swenson, Duhamel, or Soave type operation)

ICD-9-CM Diagnostic
751.3 Hirschsprung's disease and other congenital functional disorders of colon

ICD-9-CM Procedural
48.41 Soave submucosal resection of rectum
48.49 Other pull-through resection of rectum
48.65 Duhamel resection of rectum

45121
45121 Proctectomy, complete (for congenital megacolon), abdominal and perineal approach; with subtotal or total colectomy, with multiple biopsies

ICD-9-CM Diagnostic
751.3 Hirschsprung's disease and other congenital functional disorders of colon

ICD-9-CM Procedural
48.49 Other pull-through resection of rectum
48.5 Abdominoperineal resection of rectum

45123
45123 Proctectomy, partial, without anastomosis, perineal approach

ICD-9-CM Diagnostic
153.9 Malignant neoplasm of colon, unspecified site ▽
154.0 Malignant neoplasm of rectosigmoid junction
154.1 Malignant neoplasm of rectum
154.2 Malignant neoplasm of anal canal
154.3 Malignant neoplasm of anus, unspecified site ▽
154.8 Malignant neoplasm of other sites of rectum, rectosigmoid junction, and anus
230.3 Carcinoma in situ of colon
230.4 Carcinoma in situ of rectum
235.2 Neoplasm of uncertain behavior of stomach, intestines, and rectum
555.1 Regional enteritis of large intestine
556.0 Ulcerative (chronic) enterocolitis
556.2 Ulcerative (chronic) proctitis
569.1 Rectal prolapse
751.3 Hirschsprung's disease and other congenital functional disorders of colon

ICD-9-CM Procedural
48.69 Other resection of rectum

45126

45126 Pelvic exenteration for colorectal malignancy, with proctectomy (with or without colostomy), with removal of bladder and ureteral transplantations, and/or hysterectomy, or cervicectomy, with or without removal of tube(s), with or without removal of ovary(s), or any combination thereof

ICD-9-CM Diagnostic

153.0 Malignant neoplasm of hepatic flexure
153.1 Malignant neoplasm of transverse colon
153.2 Malignant neoplasm of descending colon
153.3 Malignant neoplasm of sigmoid colon
153.4 Malignant neoplasm of cecum
153.5 Malignant neoplasm of appendix
153.6 Malignant neoplasm of ascending colon
153.7 Malignant neoplasm of splenic flexure
153.8 Malignant neoplasm of other specified sites of large intestine
153.9 Malignant neoplasm of colon, unspecified site ▽
154.0 Malignant neoplasm of rectosigmoid junction
154.1 Malignant neoplasm of rectum
154.2 Malignant neoplasm of anal canal
154.3 Malignant neoplasm of anus, unspecified site ▽
154.8 Malignant neoplasm of other sites of rectum, rectosigmoid junction, and anus
197.5 Secondary malignant neoplasm of large intestine and rectum
198.1 Secondary malignant neoplasm of other urinary organs
198.6 Secondary malignant neoplasm of ovary ♀
198.82 Secondary malignant neoplasm of genital organs
198.89 Secondary malignant neoplasm of other specified sites
199.0 Disseminated malignant neoplasm
199.1 Other malignant neoplasm of unspecified site

ICD-9-CM Procedural

46.13 Permanent colostomy
68.8 Pelvic evisceration

45130–45135

45130 Excision of rectal procidentia, with anastomosis; perineal approach
45135 abdominal and perineal approach

ICD-9-CM Diagnostic

569.1 Rectal prolapse

ICD-9-CM Procedural

48.69 Other resection of rectum

45136

45136 Excision of ileoanal reservoir with ileostomy

ICD-9-CM Diagnostic

153.0 Malignant neoplasm of hepatic flexure
153.1 Malignant neoplasm of transverse colon
153.2 Malignant neoplasm of descending colon
153.3 Malignant neoplasm of sigmoid colon
153.4 Malignant neoplasm of cecum
153.5 Malignant neoplasm of appendix
153.6 Malignant neoplasm of ascending colon
153.7 Malignant neoplasm of splenic flexure
153.8 Malignant neoplasm of other specified sites of large intestine
153.9 Malignant neoplasm of colon, unspecified site ▽
154.0 Malignant neoplasm of rectosigmoid junction
154.1 Malignant neoplasm of rectum
197.5 Secondary malignant neoplasm of large intestine and rectum
211.3 Benign neoplasm of colon
211.4 Benign neoplasm of rectum and anal canal
230.3 Carcinoma in situ of colon
230.4 Carcinoma in situ of rectum
230.7 Carcinoma in situ of other and unspecified parts of intestine ▽
235.2 Neoplasm of uncertain behavior of stomach, intestines, and rectum
239.0 Neoplasm of unspecified nature of digestive system
556.0 Ulcerative (chronic) enterocolitis
556.1 Ulcerative (chronic) ileocolitis
556.2 Ulcerative (chronic) proctitis
556.3 Ulcerative (chronic) proctosigmoiditis
556.4 Pseudopolyposis of colon
556.5 Left sided ulcerative (chronic) colitis
556.6 Universal ulcerative (chronic) colitis
556.8 Other ulcerative colitis
556.9 Unspecified ulcerative colitis ▽
557.0 Acute vascular insufficiency of intestine
557.1 Chronic vascular insufficiency of intestine
557.9 Unspecified vascular insufficiency of intestine ▽
558.9 Other and unspecified noninfectious gastroenteritis and colitis ▽
560.9 Unspecified intestinal obstruction ▽
562.10 Diverticulosis of colon (without mention of hemorrhage) — (Use additional code to identify any associated peritonitis: 567.0-567.9)
562.11 Diverticulitis of colon (without mention of hemorrhage) — (Use additional code to identify any associated peritonitis: 567.0-567.9)
562.12 Diverticulosis of colon with hemorrhage — (Use additional code to identify any associated peritonitis: 567.0-567.9)
562.13 Diverticulitis of colon with hemorrhage — (Use additional code to identify any associated peritonitis: 567.0-567.9)
564.7 Megacolon, other than Hirschsprung's
564.81 Neurogenic bowel
564.89 Other functional disorders of intestine
567.0 Peritonitis in infectious diseases classified elsewhere — (Code first underlying disease) ☒
567.1 Pneumococcal peritonitis
567.2 Other suppurative peritonitis
567.8 Other specified peritonitis
567.9 Unspecified peritonitis ▽
569.82 Ulceration of intestine
569.83 Perforation of intestine
569.89 Other specified disorder of intestines
569.9 Unspecified disorder of intestine ▽
578.1 Blood in stool
578.9 Unspecified, hemorrhage of gastrointestinal tract ▽
751.3 Hirschsprung's disease and other congenital functional disorders of colon
777.1 Fetal and newborn meconium obstruction
777.5 Necrotizing enterocolitis in fetus or newborn
777.6 Perinatal intestinal perforation
777.8 Other specified perinatal disorder of digestive system
863.40 Colon injury unspecified site, without mention of open wound into cavity ▽
863.41 Ascending (right) colon injury without mention of open wound into cavity
863.42 Transverse colon injury without mention of open wound into cavity
863.43 Descending (left) colon injury without mention of open wound into cavity
863.44 Sigmoid colon injury without mention of open wound into cavity
863.45 Rectum injury without mention of open wound into cavity
863.46 Injury to multiple sites in colon and rectum without mention of open wound into cavity
863.49 Other colon and rectum injury, without mention of open wound into cavity
997.4 Digestive system complication — (Use additional code to identify complications)
998.59 Other postoperative infection — (Use additional code to identify infection)
998.89 Other specified complications

ICD-9-CM Procedural

46.23 Other permanent ileostomy
46.99 Other operations on intestines

45150

45150 Division of stricture of rectum

ICD-9-CM Diagnostic

569.2 Stenosis of rectum and anus
569.3 Hemorrhage of rectum and anus
569.42 Anal or rectal pain
569.49 Other specified disorder of rectum and anus
751.2 Congenital atresia and stenosis of large intestine, rectum, and anal canal
908.1 Late effect of internal injury to intra-abdominal organs
909.3 Late effect of complications of surgical and medical care
947.3 Burn of gastrointestinal tract
997.4 Digestive system complication — (Use additional code to identify complications)

ICD-9-CM Procedural

48.91 Incision of rectal stricture

▽ Unspecified code ♀ Female diagnosis ☒ Manifestation code ♂ Male diagnosis

45160–45170

45160 Excision of rectal tumor by proctotomy, transacral or transcoccygeal approach
45170 Excision of rectal tumor, transanal approach

ICD-9-CM Diagnostic

154.0 Malignant neoplasm of rectosigmoid junction
154.1 Malignant neoplasm of rectum
154.8 Malignant neoplasm of other sites of rectum, rectosigmoid junction, and anus
197.5 Secondary malignant neoplasm of large intestine and rectum
211.4 Benign neoplasm of rectum and anal canal
228.04 Hemangioma of intra-abdominal structures
230.4 Carcinoma in situ of rectum
235.2 Neoplasm of uncertain behavior of stomach, intestines, and rectum
239.0 Neoplasm of unspecified nature of digestive system
569.3 Hemorrhage of rectum and anus
569.49 Other specified disorder of rectum and anus
578.1 Blood in stool
751.5 Other congenital anomalies of intestine
787.99 Other symptoms involving digestive system

ICD-9-CM Procedural

48.0 Proctotomy
48.35 Local excision of rectal lesion or tissue
48.82 Excision of perirectal tissue

45190

45190 Destruction of rectal tumor (eg, electrodessication, electrosurgery, laser ablation, laser resection, cryosurgery) transanal approach

ICD-9-CM Diagnostic

154.0 Malignant neoplasm of rectosigmoid junction
154.1 Malignant neoplasm of rectum
154.8 Malignant neoplasm of other sites of rectum, rectosigmoid junction, and anus
197.5 Secondary malignant neoplasm of large intestine and rectum
211.4 Benign neoplasm of rectum and anal canal
228.04 Hemangioma of intra-abdominal structures
230.4 Carcinoma in situ of rectum
235.2 Neoplasm of uncertain behavior of stomach, intestines, and rectum
238.1 Neoplasm of uncertain behavior of connective and other soft tissue ▽
239.0 Neoplasm of unspecified nature of digestive system
569.3 Hemorrhage of rectum and anus
751.5 Other congenital anomalies of intestine
787.99 Other symptoms involving digestive system

ICD-9-CM Procedural

48.32 Other electrocoagulation of rectal lesion or tissue
48.33 Destruction of rectal lesion or tissue by laser
48.34 Destruction of rectal lesion or tissue by cryosurgery

45300–45305

45300 Proctosigmoidoscopy, rigid; diagnostic, with or without collection of specimen(s) by brushing or washing (separate procedure)
45303 with dilation (eg, balloon, guide wire, bougie)
45305 with biopsy, single or multiple

ICD-9-CM Diagnostic

153.3 Malignant neoplasm of sigmoid colon
153.8 Malignant neoplasm of other specified sites of large intestine

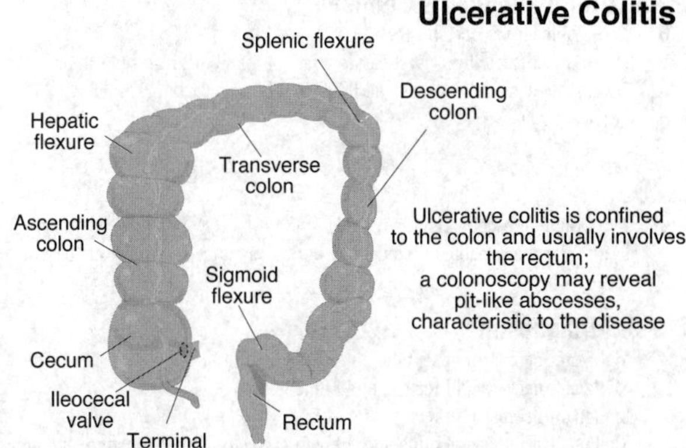

154.0 Malignant neoplasm of rectosigmoid junction
154.1 Malignant neoplasm of rectum
154.2 Malignant neoplasm of anal canal
154.3 Malignant neoplasm of anus, unspecified site ▽
154.8 Malignant neoplasm of other sites of rectum, rectosigmoid junction, and anus
197.5 Secondary malignant neoplasm of large intestine and rectum
211.3 Benign neoplasm of colon
211.4 Benign neoplasm of rectum and anal canal
230.3 Carcinoma in situ of colon
230.4 Carcinoma in situ of rectum
235.2 Neoplasm of uncertain behavior of stomach, intestines, and rectum
239.0 Neoplasm of unspecified nature of digestive system
455.0 Internal hemorrhoids without mention of complication
455.1 Internal thrombosed hemorrhoids
455.2 Internal hemorrhoids with other complication
455.3 External hemorrhoids without mention of complication
455.4 External thrombosed hemorrhoids
455.5 External hemorrhoids with other complication
455.6 Unspecified hemorrhoids without mention of complication ▽
455.7 Unspecified thrombosed hemorrhoids ▽
455.8 Unspecified hemorrhoids with other complication ▽
455.9 Residual hemorrhoidal skin tags
555.1 Regional enteritis of large intestine
555.9 Regional enteritis of unspecified site ▽
556.0 Ulcerative (chronic) enterocolitis
556.9 Unspecified ulcerative colitis ▽
557.1 Chronic vascular insufficiency of intestine
557.9 Unspecified vascular insufficiency of intestine ▽
558.1 Gastroenteritis and colitis due to radiation
558.2 Toxic gastroenteritis and colitis — (Use additional E code to identify cause)
558.3 Gastroenteritis and colitis, allergic — (Use additional code to identify type of food allergy: V15.01-V15.05)
558.9 Other and unspecified noninfectious gastroenteritis and colitis ▽
560.0 Intussusception
560.1 Paralytic ileus
560.2 Volvulus
560.30 Unspecified impaction of intestine ▽
560.31 Gallstone ileus
560.39 Other impaction of intestine
562.10 Diverticulosis of colon (without mention of hemorrhage) — (Use additional code to identify any associated peritonitis: 567.0-567.9)
562.13 Diverticulitis of colon with hemorrhage — (Use additional code to identify any associated peritonitis: 567.0-567.9)
564.00 Unspecified constipation ▽
564.01 Slow transit constipation
564.02 Outlet dysfunction constipation
564.09 Other constipation
564.1 Irritable bowel syndrome
564.5 Functional diarrhea
564.6 Anal spasm
564.81 Neurogenic bowel
564.89 Other functional disorders of intestine
565.0 Anal fissure
565.1 Anal fistula
566 Abscess of anal and rectal regions
567.0 Peritonitis in infectious diseases classified elsewhere — (Code first underlying disease) ☒
567.1 Pneumococcal peritonitis
567.2 Other suppurative peritonitis
567.8 Other specified peritonitis
567.9 Unspecified peritonitis ▽
569.0 Anal and rectal polyp
569.1 Rectal prolapse
569.2 Stenosis of rectum and anus
569.3 Hemorrhage of rectum and anus
569.41 Ulcer of anus and rectum
569.42 Anal or rectal pain
569.49 Other specified disorder of rectum and anus
569.81 Fistula of intestine, excluding rectum and anus
569.82 Ulceration of intestine
569.83 Perforation of intestine
569.84 Angiodysplasia of intestine (without mention of hemorrhage)
569.85 Angiodysplasia of intestine with hemorrhage
569.89 Other specified disorder of intestines
569.9 Unspecified disorder of intestine ▽
578.1 Blood in stool

698.0 Pruritus ani
780.99 Other general symptoms
783.21 Loss of weight
783.22 Underweight
783.7 Adult failure to thrive
787.3 Flatulence, eructation, and gas pain
787.6 Incontinence of feces
787.99 Other symptoms involving digestive system
789.00 Abdominal pain, unspecified site
789.01 Abdominal pain, right upper quadrant
789.02 Abdominal pain, left upper quadrant
789.03 Abdominal pain, right lower quadrant
789.04 Abdominal pain, left lower quadrant
789.05 Abdominal pain, periumbilic
789.06 Abdominal pain, epigastric
789.07 Abdominal pain, generalized
789.09 Abdominal pain, other specified site
789.30 Abdominal or pelvic swelling, mass or lump, unspecified site
789.31 Abdominal or pelvic swelling, mass, or lump, right upper quadrant
789.32 Abdominal or pelvic swelling, mass, or lump, left upper quadrant
789.33 Abdominal or pelvic swelling, mass, or lump, right lower quadrant
789.34 Abdominal or pelvic swelling, mass, or lump, left lower quadrant
789.35 Abdominal or pelvic swelling, mass or lump, periumbilic
789.36 Abdominal or pelvic swelling, mass, or lump, epigastric
789.37 Abdominal or pelvic swelling, mass, or lump, epigastric, generalized
789.39 Abdominal or pelvic swelling, mass, or lump, other specified site
792.1 Nonspecific abnormal finding in stool contents
793.4 Nonspecific abnormal findings on radiological and other examination of gastrointestinal tract
863.45 Rectum injury without mention of open wound into cavity
997.4 Digestive system complication — (Use additional code to identify complications)
V10.05 Personal history of malignant neoplasm of large intestine
V10.06 Personal history of malignant neoplasm of rectum, rectosigmoid junction, and anus
V12.70 Personal history of unspecified digestive disease
V12.72 Personal history of colonic polyps
V12.79 Personal history of other diseases of digestive disease
V76.41 Screening for malignant neoplasm of the rectum
V76.49 Special screening for malignant neoplasms, other sites

ICD-9-CM Procedural

48.23 Rigid proctosigmoidoscopy
48.24 Closed (endoscopic) biopsy of rectum
96.22 Dilation of rectum

HCPCS Level II Supplies & Services

A4270 Disposable endoscope sheath, each
A4305 Disposable drug delivery system, flow rate of 50 ml or greater per hour
A4306 Disposable drug delivery system, flow rate of 5 ml or less per hour
A4550 Surgical trays

45307

45307 Proctosigmoidoscopy, rigid; with removal of foreign body

ICD-9-CM Diagnostic

569.3 Hemorrhage of rectum and anus
569.42 Anal or rectal pain
569.49 Other specified disorder of rectum and anus
578.1 Blood in stool
793.4 Nonspecific abnormal findings on radiological and other examination of gastrointestinal tract
936 Foreign body in intestine and colon
937 Foreign body in anus and rectum

ICD-9-CM Procedural

98.04 Removal of intraluminal foreign body from large intestine without incision

HCPCS Level II Supplies & Services

A4270 Disposable endoscope sheath, each
A4305 Disposable drug delivery system, flow rate of 50 ml or greater per hour
A4306 Disposable drug delivery system, flow rate of 5 ml or less per hour
A4550 Surgical trays

45308–45315

45308 Proctosigmoidoscopy, rigid; with removal of single tumor, polyp, or other lesion by hot biopsy forceps or bipolar cautery
45309 with removal of single tumor, polyp, or other lesion by snare technique
45315 with removal of multiple tumors, polyps, or other lesions by hot biopsy forceps, bipolar cautery or snare technique

ICD-9-CM Diagnostic

153.3 Malignant neoplasm of sigmoid colon
153.8 Malignant neoplasm of other specified sites of large intestine
154.0 Malignant neoplasm of rectosigmoid junction
154.1 Malignant neoplasm of rectum
211.3 Benign neoplasm of colon
211.4 Benign neoplasm of rectum and anal canal
235.2 Neoplasm of uncertain behavior of stomach, intestines, and rectum
239.0 Neoplasm of unspecified nature of digestive system
556.0 Ulcerative (chronic) enterocolitis
569.0 Anal and rectal polyp
569.3 Hemorrhage of rectum and anus
569.42 Anal or rectal pain
569.49 Other specified disorder of rectum and anus
793.4 Nonspecific abnormal findings on radiological and other examination of gastrointestinal tract

ICD-9-CM Procedural

48.32 Other electrocoagulation of rectal lesion or tissue
48.36 [Endoscopic] polypectomy of rectum

HCPCS Level II Supplies & Services

A4270 Disposable endoscope sheath, each
A4305 Disposable drug delivery system, flow rate of 50 ml or greater per hour
A4306 Disposable drug delivery system, flow rate of 5 ml or less per hour
A4550 Surgical trays

45317

45317 Proctosigmoidoscopy, rigid; with control of bleeding (eg, injection, bipolar cautery, unipolar cautery, laser, heater probe, stapler, plasma coagulator)

ICD-9-CM Diagnostic

154.1 Malignant neoplasm of rectum
448.9 Other and unspecified capillary diseases
455.0 Internal hemorrhoids without mention of complication
455.2 Internal hemorrhoids with other complication
556.0 Ulcerative (chronic) enterocolitis
556.3 Ulcerative (chronic) proctosigmoiditis
557.0 Acute vascular insufficiency of intestine
562.12 Diverticulosis of colon with hemorrhage — (Use additional code to identify any associated peritonitis: 567.0-567.9)
562.13 Diverticulitis of colon with hemorrhage — (Use additional code to identify any associated peritonitis: 567.0-567.9)
569.3 Hemorrhage of rectum and anus
569.49 Other specified disorder of rectum and anus
569.85 Angiodysplasia of intestine with hemorrhage
578.1 Blood in stool
578.9 Unspecified, hemorrhage of gastrointestinal tract

ICD-9-CM Procedural

45.43 Endoscopic destruction of other lesion or tissue of large intestine
48.32 Other electrocoagulation of rectal lesion or tissue

HCPCS Level II Supplies & Services

A4270 Disposable endoscope sheath, each
A4305 Disposable drug delivery system, flow rate of 50 ml or greater per hour
A4306 Disposable drug delivery system, flow rate of 5 ml or less per hour
A4550 Surgical trays

45320

45320 Proctosigmoidoscopy, rigid; with ablation of tumor(s), polyp(s), or other lesion(s) not amenable to removal by hot biopsy forceps, bipolar cautery or snare technique (eg, laser)

ICD-9-CM Diagnostic

153.3 Malignant neoplasm of sigmoid colon
154.0 Malignant neoplasm of rectosigmoid junction
154.1 Malignant neoplasm of rectum
154.8 Malignant neoplasm of other sites of rectum, rectosigmoid junction, and anus

Unspecified code
♀ Female diagnosis
Manifestation code
♂ Male diagnosis

211.3 Benign neoplasm of colon
211.4 Benign neoplasm of rectum and anal canal
235.2 Neoplasm of uncertain behavior of stomach, intestines, and rectum
239.0 Neoplasm of unspecified nature of digestive system
569.3 Hemorrhage of rectum and anus
569.41 Ulcer of anus and rectum
569.49 Other specified disorder of rectum and anus

ICD-9-CM Procedural

45.42 Endoscopic polypectomy of large intestine
45.43 Endoscopic destruction of other lesion or tissue of large intestine
48.33 Destruction of rectal lesion or tissue by laser
48.36 [Endoscopic] polypectomy of rectum

45321

45321 Proctosigmoidoscopy, rigid; with decompression of volvulus

ICD-9-CM Diagnostic

211.3 Benign neoplasm of colon
560.2 Volvulus
787.3 Flatulence, eructation, and gas pain

ICD-9-CM Procedural

46.85 Dilation of intestine
48.0 Proctotomy

45327

45327 Proctosigmoidoscopy, rigid; with transendoscopic stent placement (includes predilation)

ICD-9-CM Diagnostic

153.3 Malignant neoplasm of sigmoid colon
153.8 Malignant neoplasm of other specified sites of large intestine
153.9 Malignant neoplasm of colon, unspecified site
154.0 Malignant neoplasm of rectosigmoid junction
154.1 Malignant neoplasm of rectum
197.5 Secondary malignant neoplasm of large intestine and rectum
560.81 Intestinal or peritoneal adhesions with obstruction (postoperative) (postinfection)
560.89 Other specified intestinal obstruction
560.9 Unspecified intestinal obstruction
751.2 Congenital atresia and stenosis of large intestine, rectum, and anal canal
997.4 Digestive system complication — (Use additional code to identify complications)

ICD-9-CM Procedural

46.79 Other repair of intestine
48.23 Rigid proctosigmoidoscopy

45330–45331

45330 Sigmoidoscopy, flexible; diagnostic, with or without collection of specimen(s) by brushing or washing (separate procedure)
45331 with biopsy, single or multiple

ICD-9-CM Diagnostic

153.2 Malignant neoplasm of descending colon
153.3 Malignant neoplasm of sigmoid colon
153.8 Malignant neoplasm of other specified sites of large intestine
153.9 Malignant neoplasm of colon, unspecified site
154.0 Malignant neoplasm of rectosigmoid junction
154.1 Malignant neoplasm of rectum
154.2 Malignant neoplasm of anal canal
154.3 Malignant neoplasm of anus, unspecified site
154.8 Malignant neoplasm of other sites of rectum, rectosigmoid junction, and anus
159.0 Malignant neoplasm of intestinal tract, part unspecified
159.9 Malignant neoplasm of ill-defined sites of digestive organs and peritoneum
197.5 Secondary malignant neoplasm of large intestine and rectum
199.0 Disseminated malignant neoplasm
199.1 Other malignant neoplasm of unspecified site
211.3 Benign neoplasm of colon
211.4 Benign neoplasm of rectum and anal canal
211.9 Benign neoplasm of other and unspecified site of the digestive system
230.3 Carcinoma in situ of colon
230.4 Carcinoma in situ of rectum
230.5 Carcinoma in situ of anal canal
230.6 Carcinoma in situ of anus, unspecified
230.7 Carcinoma in situ of other and unspecified parts of intestine
230.9 Carcinoma in situ of other and unspecified digestive organs
235.2 Neoplasm of uncertain behavior of stomach, intestines, and rectum
235.5 Neoplasm of uncertain behavior of other and unspecified digestive organs
239.0 Neoplasm of unspecified nature of digestive system
280.0 Iron deficiency anemia secondary to blood loss (chronic)
285.1 Acute posthemorrhagic anemia
285.8 Other specified anemias
306.4 Gastrointestinal malfunction arising from mental factors
455.0 Internal hemorrhoids without mention of complication
455.1 Internal thrombosed hemorrhoids
455.2 Internal hemorrhoids with other complication
455.3 External hemorrhoids without mention of complication
455.4 External thrombosed hemorrhoids
455.5 External hemorrhoids with other complication
455.6 Unspecified hemorrhoids without mention of complication
455.7 Unspecified thrombosed hemorrhoids
455.8 Unspecified hemorrhoids with other complication
455.9 Residual hemorrhoidal skin tags
555.1 Regional enteritis of large intestine
555.2 Regional enteritis of small intestine with large intestine
555.9 Regional enteritis of unspecified site
556.0 Ulcerative (chronic) enterocolitis
556.2 Ulcerative (chronic) proctitis
556.3 Ulcerative (chronic) proctosigmoiditis
556.4 Pseudopolyposis of colon
556.6 Universal ulcerative (chronic) colitis
556.8 Other ulcerative colitis
556.9 Unspecified ulcerative colitis
558.1 Gastroenteritis and colitis due to radiation
558.2 Toxic gastroenteritis and colitis — (Use additional E code to identify cause)
558.3 Gastroenteritis and colitis, allergic — (Use additional code to identify type of food allergy: V15.01-V15.05)
558.9 Other and unspecified noninfectious gastroenteritis and colitis
560.9 Unspecified intestinal obstruction
562.10 Diverticulosis of colon (without mention of hemorrhage) — (Use additional code to identify any associated peritonitis: 567.0-567.9)
562.11 Diverticulitis of colon (without mention of hemorrhage) — (Use additional code to identify any associated peritonitis: 567.0-567.9)
562.12 Diverticulosis of colon with hemorrhage — (Use additional code to identify any associated peritonitis: 567.0-567.9)
562.13 Diverticulitis of colon with hemorrhage — (Use additional code to identify any associated peritonitis: 567.0-567.9)
564.00 Unspecified constipation
564.01 Slow transit constipation
564.02 Outlet dysfunction constipation
564.09 Other constipation
564.1 Irritable bowel syndrome
564.4 Other postoperative functional disorders
564.5 Functional diarrhea
564.6 Anal spasm
564.7 Megacolon, other than Hirschsprung's
564.81 Neurogenic bowel
564.89 Other functional disorders of intestine
565.0 Anal fissure
565.1 Anal fistula
566 Abscess of anal and rectal regions
567.0 Peritonitis in infectious diseases classified elsewhere — (Code first underlying disease)
567.1 Pneumococcal peritonitis
567.2 Other suppurative peritonitis
567.8 Other specified peritonitis
567.9 Unspecified peritonitis
569.0 Anal and rectal polyp
569.1 Rectal prolapse
569.2 Stenosis of rectum and anus
569.3 Hemorrhage of rectum and anus
569.41 Ulcer of anus and rectum
569.42 Anal or rectal pain
569.49 Other specified disorder of rectum and anus
569.5 Abscess of intestine
569.60 Unspecified complication of colostomy or enterostomy
569.82 Ulceration of intestine
569.83 Perforation of intestine
569.84 Angiodysplasia of intestine (without mention of hemorrhage)

Unspecified code — Manifestation code
♀ Female diagnosis — ♂ Male diagnosis

569.85 Angiodysplasia of intestine with hemorrhage
569.89 Other specified disorder of intestines
578.1 Blood in stool
619.0 Urinary-genital tract fistula, female ♀
619.1 Digestive-genital tract fistula, female ♀
619.2 Genital tract-skin fistula, female ♀
619.8 Other specified fistula involving female genital tract ♀
619.9 Unspecified fistula involving female genital tract ▽ ♀
747.61 Congenital gastrointestinal vessel anomaly
751.2 Congenital atresia and stenosis of large intestine, rectum, and anal canal
751.3 Hirschsprung's disease and other congenital functional disorders of colon
751.4 Congenital anomalies of intestinal fixation
751.5 Other congenital anomalies of intestine
783.21 Loss of weight
783.22 Underweight
783.7 Adult failure to thrive
787.3 Flatulence, eructation, and gas pain
787.4 Visible peristalsis
787.5 Abnormal bowel sounds
787.6 Incontinence of feces
787.7 Abnormal feces
787.91 Diarrhea
787.99 Other symptoms involving digestive system
789.00 Abdominal pain, unspecified site ▽
789.03 Abdominal pain, right lower quadrant
789.04 Abdominal pain, left lower quadrant
789.07 Abdominal pain, generalized
789.09 Abdominal pain, other specified site
789.30 Abdominal or pelvic swelling, mass or lump, unspecified site ▽
789.33 Abdominal or pelvic swelling, mass, or lump, right lower quadrant
789.34 Abdominal or pelvic swelling, mass, or lump, left lower quadrant
789.37 Abdominal or pelvic swelling, mass, or lump, epigastric, generalized
789.39 Abdominal or pelvic swelling, mass, or lump, other specified site
789.5 Ascites
792.1 Nonspecific abnormal finding in stool contents
793.4 Nonspecific abnormal findings on radiological and other examination of gastrointestinal tract
996.87 Complications of transplanted organ, intestine — (Use additional code to identify nature of complication, 078.5)
997.4 Digestive system complication — (Use additional code to identify complications)
V10.00 Personal history of malignant neoplasm of unspecified site in gastrointestinal tract ▽
V10.06 Personal history of malignant neoplasm of rectum, rectosigmoid junction, and anus
V10.09 Personal history of malignant neoplasm of other site in gastrointestinal tract
V12.00 Personal history of unspecified infectious and parasitic disease ▽
V12.70 Personal history of unspecified digestive disease ▽
V12.72 Personal history of colonic polyps
V12.79 Personal history of other diseases of digestive disease
V16.0 Family history of malignant neoplasm of gastrointestinal tract
V18.5 Family history of digestive disorders
V44.2 Ileostomy status — (This code is intended for use when these conditions are recorded as diagnoses or problems)
V44.3 Colostomy status — (This code is intended for use when these conditions are recorded as diagnoses or problems)
V47.3 Other digestive problems — (This code is intended for use when these conditions are recorded as diagnoses or problems)
V55.3 Attention to colostomy
V67.00 Follow-up examination, following unspecified surgery ▽
V67.09 Follow-up examination, following other surgery
V72.85 Other specified examination — (Use additional code(s) to identify any special screening examination(s) performed: V73.0-V82.9)
V76.41 Screening for malignant neoplasm of the rectum
V76.49 Special screening for malignant neoplasms, other sites
V82.9 Screening for unspecified condition ▽

ICD-9-CM Procedural

45.24 Flexible sigmoidoscopy
45.25 Closed [endoscopic] biopsy of large intestine

HCPCS Level II Supplies & Services

A4270 Disposable endoscope sheath, each
A4305 Disposable drug delivery system, flow rate of 50 ml or greater per hour
A4306 Disposable drug delivery system, flow rate of 5 ml or less per hour
A4550 Surgical trays
G0104 Colorectal cancer screening; flexible sigmoidoscopy

45332

45332 Sigmoidoscopy, flexible; with removal of foreign body

ICD-9-CM Diagnostic

569.3 Hemorrhage of rectum and anus
569.42 Anal or rectal pain
578.1 Blood in stool
936 Foreign body in intestine and colon
937 Foreign body in anus and rectum

ICD-9-CM Procedural

45.24 Flexible sigmoidoscopy
98.05 Removal of intraluminal foreign body from rectum and anus without incision

HCPCS Level II Supplies & Services

A4270 Disposable endoscope sheath, each
A4305 Disposable drug delivery system, flow rate of 50 ml or greater per hour
A4306 Disposable drug delivery system, flow rate of 5 ml or less per hour
A4550 Surgical trays

45333

45333 Sigmoidoscopy, flexible; with removal of tumor(s), polyp(s), or other lesion(s) by hot biopsy forceps or bipolar cautery

ICD-9-CM Diagnostic

153.2 Malignant neoplasm of descending colon
153.3 Malignant neoplasm of sigmoid colon
153.4 Malignant neoplasm of cecum
153.5 Malignant neoplasm of appendix
153.6 Malignant neoplasm of ascending colon
153.7 Malignant neoplasm of splenic flexure
153.8 Malignant neoplasm of other specified sites of large intestine
154.0 Malignant neoplasm of rectosigmoid junction
154.1 Malignant neoplasm of rectum
211.3 Benign neoplasm of colon
211.4 Benign neoplasm of rectum and anal canal
211.9 Benign neoplasm of other and unspecified site of the digestive system ▽
230.3 Carcinoma in situ of colon
230.4 Carcinoma in situ of rectum
235.2 Neoplasm of uncertain behavior of stomach, intestines, and rectum
239.0 Neoplasm of unspecified nature of digestive system
455.0 Internal hemorrhoids without mention of complication
455.1 Internal thrombosed hemorrhoids
455.2 Internal hemorrhoids with other complication
455.3 External hemorrhoids without mention of complication
455.4 External thrombosed hemorrhoids
455.5 External hemorrhoids with other complication
455.6 Unspecified hemorrhoids without mention of complication ▽
455.7 Unspecified thrombosed hemorrhoids ▽
455.8 Unspecified hemorrhoids with other complication ▽
556.0 Ulcerative (chronic) enterocolitis
558.9 Other and unspecified noninfectious gastroenteritis and colitis ▽
562.10 Diverticulosis of colon (without mention of hemorrhage) — (Use additional code to identify any associated peritonitis: 567.0-567.9)
562.11 Diverticulitis of colon (without mention of hemorrhage) — (Use additional code to identify any associated peritonitis: 567.0-567.9)
562.12 Diverticulosis of colon with hemorrhage — (Use additional code to identify any associated peritonitis: 567.0-567.9)
562.13 Diverticulitis of colon with hemorrhage — (Use additional code to identify any associated peritonitis: 567.0-567.9)
564.00 Unspecified constipation ▽
564.01 Slow transit constipation
564.02 Outlet dysfunction constipation
564.09 Other constipation
564.1 Irritable bowel syndrome
564.7 Megacolon, other than Hirschsprung's
569.0 Anal and rectal polyp
569.1 Rectal prolapse
569.2 Stenosis of rectum and anus
569.3 Hemorrhage of rectum and anus
569.41 Ulcer of anus and rectum
578.1 Blood in stool
578.9 Unspecified, hemorrhage of gastrointestinal tract ▽
787.3 Flatulence, eructation, and gas pain
787.4 Visible peristalsis
787.5 Abnormal bowel sounds

▽ Unspecified code ♀ Female diagnosis ☒ Manifestation code ♂ Male diagnosis

787.6 Incontinence of feces
787.7 Abnormal feces
787.91 Diarrhea
787.99 Other symptoms involving digestive system
789.00 Abdominal pain, unspecified site ▽
793.4 Nonspecific abnormal findings on radiological and other examination of gastrointestinal tract
V10.05 Personal history of malignant neoplasm of large intestine
V10.06 Personal history of malignant neoplasm of rectum, rectosigmoid junction, and anus

ICD-9-CM Procedural

45.42 Endoscopic polypectomy of large intestine
45.43 Endoscopic destruction of other lesion or tissue of large intestine

HCPCS Level II Supplies & Services

A4270 Disposable endoscope sheath, each
A4305 Disposable drug delivery system, flow rate of 50 ml or greater per hour
A4306 Disposable drug delivery system, flow rate of 5 ml or less per hour
A4550 Surgical trays

45334

45334 Sigmoidoscopy, flexible; with control of bleeding (eg, injection, bipolar cautery, unipolar cautery, laser, heater probe, stapler, plasma coagulator)

ICD-9-CM Diagnostic

153.3 Malignant neoplasm of sigmoid colon
154.1 Malignant neoplasm of rectum
448.9 Other and unspecified capillary diseases ▽
455.1 Internal thrombosed hemorrhoids
455.2 Internal hemorrhoids with other complication
556.0 Ulcerative (chronic) enterocolitis
556.2 Ulcerative (chronic) proctitis
556.3 Ulcerative (chronic) proctosigmoiditis
557.0 Acute vascular insufficiency of intestine
562.12 Diverticulosis of colon with hemorrhage — (Use additional code to identify any associated peritonitis: 567.0-567.9)
562.13 Diverticulitis of colon with hemorrhage — (Use additional code to identify any associated peritonitis: 567.0-567.9)
569.3 Hemorrhage of rectum and anus
569.49 Other specified disorder of rectum and anus
578.1 Blood in stool
578.9 Unspecified, hemorrhage of gastrointestinal tract ▽
998.11 Hemorrhage complicating a procedure

ICD-9-CM Procedural

45.43 Endoscopic destruction of other lesion or tissue of large intestine

HCPCS Level II Supplies & Services

A4270 Disposable endoscope sheath, each
A4305 Disposable drug delivery system, flow rate of 50 ml or greater per hour
A4306 Disposable drug delivery system, flow rate of 5 ml or less per hour
A4550 Surgical trays

45335

45335 Sigmoidoscopy, flexible; with directed submucosal injection(s), any substance

ICD-9-CM Diagnostic

153.2 Malignant neoplasm of descending colon
153.3 Malignant neoplasm of sigmoid colon
153.8 Malignant neoplasm of other specified sites of large intestine
153.9 Malignant neoplasm of colon, unspecified site ▽
154.0 Malignant neoplasm of rectosigmoid junction
154.1 Malignant neoplasm of rectum
154.2 Malignant neoplasm of anal canal
154.3 Malignant neoplasm of anus, unspecified site ▽
154.8 Malignant neoplasm of other sites of rectum, rectosigmoid junction, and anus
159.0 Malignant neoplasm of intestinal tract, part unspecified ▽
159.9 Malignant neoplasm of ill-defined sites of digestive organs and peritoneum
197.5 Secondary malignant neoplasm of large intestine and rectum
199.0 Disseminated malignant neoplasm
199.1 Other malignant neoplasm of unspecified site
211.3 Benign neoplasm of colon
211.4 Benign neoplasm of rectum and anal canal
211.9 Benign neoplasm of other and unspecified site of the digestive system ▽
230.3 Carcinoma in situ of colon
230.4 Carcinoma in situ of rectum
230.5 Carcinoma in situ of anal canal
230.6 Carcinoma in situ of anus, unspecified ▽
230.7 Carcinoma in situ of other and unspecified parts of intestine ▽
235.2 Neoplasm of uncertain behavior of stomach, intestines, and rectum
235.5 Neoplasm of uncertain behavior of other and unspecified digestive organs ▽
239.0 Neoplasm of unspecified nature of digestive system
306.4 Gastrointestinal malfunction arising from mental factors
455.0 Internal hemorrhoids without mention of complication
455.1 Internal thrombosed hemorrhoids
455.2 Internal hemorrhoids with other complication
455.6 Unspecified hemorrhoids without mention of complication ▽
455.7 Unspecified thrombosed hemorrhoids ▽
455.8 Unspecified hemorrhoids with other complication ▽
455.9 Residual hemorrhoidal skin tags
555.1 Regional enteritis of large intestine
555.2 Regional enteritis of small intestine with large intestine
555.9 Regional enteritis of unspecified site ▽
556.0 Ulcerative (chronic) enterocolitis
556.2 Ulcerative (chronic) proctitis
556.3 Ulcerative (chronic) proctosigmoiditis
556.4 Pseudopolyposis of colon
556.6 Universal ulcerative (chronic) colitis
556.8 Other ulcerative colitis
556.9 Unspecified ulcerative colitis ▽
558.1 Gastroenteritis and colitis due to radiation
558.2 Toxic gastroenteritis and colitis — (Use additional E code to identify cause)
558.3 Gastroenteritis and colitis, allergic — (Use additional code to identify type of food allergy: V15.01-V15.05)
558.9 Other and unspecified noninfectious gastroenteritis and colitis ▽
562.10 Diverticulosis of colon (without mention of hemorrhage) — (Use additional code to identify any associated peritonitis: 567.0-567.9)
562.11 Diverticulitis of colon (without mention of hemorrhage) — (Use additional code to identify any associated peritonitis: 567.0-567.9)
562.12 Diverticulosis of colon with hemorrhage — (Use additional code to identify any associated peritonitis: 567.0-567.9)
562.13 Diverticulitis of colon with hemorrhage — (Use additional code to identify any associated peritonitis: 567.0-567.9)
564.00 Unspecified constipation ▽
564.01 Slow transit constipation
564.02 Outlet dysfunction constipation
564.09 Other constipation
564.1 Irritable bowel syndrome
564.4 Other postoperative functional disorders
564.5 Functional diarrhea
564.6 Anal spasm
564.7 Megacolon, other than Hirschsprung's
564.81 Neurogenic bowel
564.89 Other functional disorders of intestine
565.0 Anal fissure
565.1 Anal fistula
566 Abscess of anal and rectal regions
569.0 Anal and rectal polyp
569.2 Stenosis of rectum and anus
569.3 Hemorrhage of rectum and anus
569.41 Ulcer of anus and rectum
569.42 Anal or rectal pain
569.49 Other specified disorder of rectum and anus
569.5 Abscess of intestine
569.60 Unspecified complication of colostomy or enterostomy ▽
569.82 Ulceration of intestine
569.83 Perforation of intestine
569.84 Angiodysplasia of intestine (without mention of hemorrhage)
569.85 Angiodysplasia of intestine with hemorrhage
569.89 Other specified disorder of intestines
578.1 Blood in stool
619.1 Digestive-genital tract fistula, female ♀
747.61 Congenital gastrointestinal vessel anomaly
751.2 Congenital atresia and stenosis of large intestine, rectum, and anal canal
751.3 Hirschsprung's disease and other congenital functional disorders of colon
751.4 Congenital anomalies of intestinal fixation
751.5 Other congenital anomalies of intestine
787.3 Flatulence, eructation, and gas pain
787.4 Visible peristalsis
787.5 Abnormal bowel sounds
787.6 Incontinence of feces

787.7 Abnormal feces
787.91 Diarrhea
787.99 Other symptoms involving digestive system
789.00 Abdominal pain, unspecified site ▽
789.03 Abdominal pain, right lower quadrant
789.04 Abdominal pain, left lower quadrant
789.07 Abdominal pain, generalized
789.09 Abdominal pain, other specified site
789.5 Ascites
792.1 Nonspecific abnormal finding in stool contents
793.4 Nonspecific abnormal findings on radiological and other examination of gastrointestinal tract
996.87 Complications of transplanted organ, intestine — (Use additional code to identify nature of complication, 078.5)
997.4 Digestive system complication — (Use additional code to identify complications)
V47.3 Other digestive problems — (This code is intended for use when these conditions are recorded as diagnoses or problems)
V67.00 Follow-up examination, following unspecified surgery ▽
V67.09 Follow-up examination, following other surgery

ICD-9-CM Procedural

45.43 Endoscopic destruction of other lesion or tissue of large intestine

45337

45337 Sigmoidoscopy, flexible; with decompression of volvulus, any method

ICD-9-CM Diagnostic

560.2 Volvulus
787.3 Flatulence, eructation, and gas pain

ICD-9-CM Procedural

46.85 Dilation of intestine

45338–45339

45338 Sigmoidoscopy, flexible; with removal of tumor(s), polyp(s), or other lesion(s) by snare technique
45339 with ablation of tumor(s), polyp(s), or other lesion(s) not amenable to removal by hot biopsy forceps, bipolar cautery or snare technique

ICD-9-CM Diagnostic

153.2 Malignant neoplasm of descending colon
153.3 Malignant neoplasm of sigmoid colon
153.8 Malignant neoplasm of other specified sites of large intestine
154.0 Malignant neoplasm of rectosigmoid junction
154.1 Malignant neoplasm of rectum
154.8 Malignant neoplasm of other sites of rectum, rectosigmoid junction, and anus
211.3 Benign neoplasm of colon
211.4 Benign neoplasm of rectum and anal canal
230.3 Carcinoma in situ of colon
230.4 Carcinoma in situ of rectum
235.2 Neoplasm of uncertain behavior of stomach, intestines, and rectum
239.0 Neoplasm of unspecified nature of digestive system
556.0 Ulcerative (chronic) enterocolitis
569.0 Anal and rectal polyp
569.3 Hemorrhage of rectum and anus
569.41 Ulcer of anus and rectum
569.49 Other specified disorder of rectum and anus

ICD-9-CM Procedural

45.42 Endoscopic polypectomy of large intestine
45.43 Endoscopic destruction of other lesion or tissue of large intestine

HCPCS Level II Supplies & Services

A4270 Disposable endoscope sheath, each
A4305 Disposable drug delivery system, flow rate of 50 ml or greater per hour
A4306 Disposable drug delivery system, flow rate of 5 ml or less per hour
A4550 Surgical trays

45340

45340 Sigmoidoscopy, flexible; with dilation by balloon, 1 or more strictures

ICD-9-CM Diagnostic

560.81 Intestinal or peritoneal adhesions with obstruction (postoperative) (postinfection)
560.89 Other specified intestinal obstruction
560.9 Unspecified intestinal obstruction ▽
751.2 Congenital atresia and stenosis of large intestine, rectum, and anal canal
997.4 Digestive system complication — (Use additional code to identify complications)

ICD-9-CM Procedural

46.85 Dilation of intestine

HCPCS Level II Supplies & Services

HCPCS Level II codes are used to report the supplies, durable medical equipment, and certain medical services provided on an outpatient basis. Because the procedure(s) represented on this page would be performed in an inpatient or outpatient facility, no HCPCS Level II codes apply.

45341

45341 Sigmoidoscopy, flexible; with endoscopic ultrasound examination

ICD-9-CM Diagnostic

153.2 Malignant neoplasm of descending colon
153.3 Malignant neoplasm of sigmoid colon
153.8 Malignant neoplasm of other specified sites of large intestine
153.9 Malignant neoplasm of colon, unspecified site ▽
154.0 Malignant neoplasm of rectosigmoid junction
154.1 Malignant neoplasm of rectum
154.2 Malignant neoplasm of anal canal
154.3 Malignant neoplasm of anus, unspecified site ▽
154.8 Malignant neoplasm of other sites of rectum, rectosigmoid junction, and anus
159.0 Malignant neoplasm of intestinal tract, part unspecified ▽
159.9 Malignant neoplasm of ill-defined sites of digestive organs and peritoneum
196.2 Secondary and unspecified malignant neoplasm of intra-abdominal lymph nodes
197.5 Secondary malignant neoplasm of large intestine and rectum
199.0 Disseminated malignant neoplasm
199.1 Other malignant neoplasm of unspecified site
211.3 Benign neoplasm of colon
211.4 Benign neoplasm of rectum and anal canal
211.9 Benign neoplasm of other and unspecified site of the digestive system ▽
230.3 Carcinoma in situ of colon
230.4 Carcinoma in situ of rectum
230.5 Carcinoma in situ of anal canal
230.6 Carcinoma in situ of anus, unspecified ▽
230.7 Carcinoma in situ of other and unspecified parts of intestine ▽
230.9 Carcinoma in situ of other and unspecified digestive organs ▽
235.2 Neoplasm of uncertain behavior of stomach, intestines, and rectum
235.5 Neoplasm of uncertain behavior of other and unspecified digestive organs ▽
239.0 Neoplasm of unspecified nature of digestive system
280.0 Iron deficiency anemia secondary to blood loss (chronic)
285.1 Acute posthemorrhagic anemia
285.8 Other specified anemias
306.4 Gastrointestinal malfunction arising from mental factors
455.0 Internal hemorrhoids without mention of complication
455.1 Internal thrombosed hemorrhoids
455.2 Internal hemorrhoids with other complication
455.3 External hemorrhoids without mention of complication
455.4 External thrombosed hemorrhoids
455.5 External hemorrhoids with other complication
455.6 Unspecified hemorrhoids without mention of complication ▽
455.7 Unspecified thrombosed hemorrhoids ▽
455.8 Unspecified hemorrhoids with other complication ▽
455.9 Residual hemorrhoidal skin tags
555.1 Regional enteritis of large intestine
555.2 Regional enteritis of small intestine with large intestine
555.9 Regional enteritis of unspecified site ▽
556.0 Ulcerative (chronic) enterocolitis
556.2 Ulcerative (chronic) proctitis
556.3 Ulcerative (chronic) proctosigmoiditis
556.4 Pseudopolyposis of colon
556.6 Universal ulcerative (chronic) colitis
556.8 Other ulcerative colitis
556.9 Unspecified ulcerative colitis ▽
558.1 Gastroenteritis and colitis due to radiation
558.2 Toxic gastroenteritis and colitis — (Use additional E code to identify cause)
558.3 Gastroenteritis and colitis, allergic — (Use additional code to identify type of food allergy: V15.01-V15.05)
558.9 Other and unspecified noninfectious gastroenteritis and colitis ▽
560.9 Unspecified intestinal obstruction ▽

▽ Unspecified code ♀ Female diagnosis ☒ Manifestation code ♂ Male diagnosis

562.10 Diverticulosis of colon (without mention of hemorrhage) — (Use additional code to identify any associated peritonitis: 567.0-567.9)
562.11 Diverticulitis of colon (without mention of hemorrhage) — (Use additional code to identify any associated peritonitis: 567.0-567.9)
562.12 Diverticulosis of colon with hemorrhage — (Use additional code to identify any associated peritonitis: 567.0-567.9)
562.13 Diverticulitis of colon with hemorrhage — (Use additional code to identify any associated peritonitis: 567.0-567.9)
564.00 Unspecified constipation ▽
564.01 Slow transit constipation
564.02 Outlet dysfunction constipation
564.09 Other constipation
564.1 Irritable bowel syndrome
564.4 Other postoperative functional disorders
564.5 Functional diarrhea
564.6 Anal spasm
564.7 Megacolon, other than Hirschsprung's
564.81 Neurogenic bowel
564.89 Other functional disorders of intestine
565.0 Anal fissure
565.1 Anal fistula
566 Abscess of anal and rectal regions
567.0 Peritonitis in infectious diseases classified elsewhere — (Code first underlying disease) ☒
567.1 Pneumococcal peritonitis
567.2 Other suppurative peritonitis
567.8 Other specified peritonitis
567.9 Unspecified peritonitis ▽
569.0 Anal and rectal polyp
569.1 Rectal prolapse
569.2 Stenosis of rectum and anus
569.3 Hemorrhage of rectum and anus
569.41 Ulcer of anus and rectum
569.42 Anal or rectal pain
569.49 Other specified disorder of rectum and anus
569.5 Abscess of intestine
569.60 Unspecified complication of colostomy or enterostomy ▽
569.82 Ulceration of intestine
569.83 Perforation of intestine
569.84 Angiodysplasia of intestine (without mention of hemorrhage)
569.85 Angiodysplasia of intestine with hemorrhage
569.89 Other specified disorder of intestines
578.1 Blood in stool
619.0 Urinary-genital tract fistula, female ♀
619.1 Digestive-genital tract fistula, female ♀
619.2 Genital tract-skin fistula, female ♀
619.8 Other specified fistula involving female genital tract ♀
619.9 Unspecified fistula involving female genital tract ▽ ♀
747.61 Congenital gastrointestinal vessel anomaly
751.2 Congenital atresia and stenosis of large intestine, rectum, and anal canal
751.3 Hirschsprung's disease and other congenital functional disorders of colon
751.4 Congenital anomalies of intestinal fixation
751.5 Other congenital anomalies of intestine
783.21 Loss of weight
783.22 Underweight
783.7 Adult failure to thrive
787.3 Flatulence, eructation, and gas pain
787.4 Visible peristalsis
787.5 Abnormal bowel sounds
787.6 Incontinence of feces
787.7 Abnormal feces
787.91 Diarrhea
787.99 Other symptoms involving digestive system
789.00 Abdominal pain, unspecified site ▽
789.03 Abdominal pain, right lower quadrant
789.04 Abdominal pain, left lower quadrant
789.07 Abdominal pain, generalized
789.09 Abdominal pain, other specified site
789.30 Abdominal or pelvic swelling, mass or lump, unspecified site ▽
789.33 Abdominal or pelvic swelling, mass, or lump, right lower quadrant
789.34 Abdominal or pelvic swelling, mass, or lump, left lower quadrant
789.37 Abdominal or pelvic swelling, mass, or lump, epigastric, generalized
789.39 Abdominal or pelvic swelling, mass, or lump, other specified site
789.5 Ascites
792.1 Nonspecific abnormal finding in stool contents
793.4 Nonspecific abnormal findings on radiological and other examination of gastrointestinal tract
996.87 Complications of transplanted organ, intestine — (Use additional code to identify nature of complication, 078.5)
997.4 Digestive system complication — (Use additional code to identify complications)
V10.00 Personal history of malignant neoplasm of unspecified site in gastrointestinal tract ▽
V10.06 Personal history of malignant neoplasm of rectum, rectosigmoid junction, and anus
V10.09 Personal history of malignant neoplasm of other site in gastrointestinal tract
V12.00 Personal history of unspecified infectious and parasitic disease ▽
V12.70 Personal history of unspecified digestive disease ▽
V12.72 Personal history of colonic polyps
V12.79 Personal history of other diseases of digestive disease
V16.0 Family history of malignant neoplasm of gastrointestinal tract
V18.5 Family history of digestive disorders
V44.2 Ileostomy status — (This code is intended for use when these conditions are recorded as diagnoses or problems)
V44.3 Colostomy status — (This code is intended for use when these conditions are recorded as diagnoses or problems)
V47.3 Other digestive problems — (This code is intended for use when these conditions are recorded as diagnoses or problems)
V55.3 Attention to colostomy
V67.00 Follow-up examination, following unspecified surgery ▽
V67.09 Follow-up examination, following other surgery
V72.85 Other specified examination — (Use additional code(s) to identify any special screening examination(s) performed: V73.0-V82.9)
V76.41 Screening for malignant neoplasm of the rectum
V76.49 Special screening for malignant neoplasms, other sites
V82.9 Screening for unspecified condition ▽

ICD-9-CM Procedural

45.24 Flexible sigmoidoscopy
88.74 Diagnostic ultrasound of digestive system

45342

45342 Sigmoidoscopy, flexible; with transendoscopic ultrasound guided intramural or transmural fine needle aspiration/biopsy(s)

ICD-9-CM Diagnostic

153.2 Malignant neoplasm of descending colon
153.3 Malignant neoplasm of sigmoid colon
153.8 Malignant neoplasm of other specified sites of large intestine
153.9 Malignant neoplasm of colon, unspecified site ▽
154.0 Malignant neoplasm of rectosigmoid junction
154.1 Malignant neoplasm of rectum
154.2 Malignant neoplasm of anal canal
154.3 Malignant neoplasm of anus, unspecified site ▽
154.8 Malignant neoplasm of other sites of rectum, rectosigmoid junction, and anus
158.8 Malignant neoplasm of specified parts of peritoneum
158.9 Malignant neoplasm of peritoneum, unspecified ▽
159.0 Malignant neoplasm of intestinal tract, part unspecified ▽
159.9 Malignant neoplasm of ill-defined sites of digestive organs and peritoneum
195.2 Malignant neoplasm of abdomen
195.3 Malignant neoplasm of pelvis
196.2 Secondary and unspecified malignant neoplasm of intra-abdominal lymph nodes
196.5 Secondary and unspecified malignant neoplasm of lymph nodes of inguinal region and lower limb
196.6 Secondary and unspecified malignant neoplasm of intrapelvic lymph nodes
197.5 Secondary malignant neoplasm of large intestine and rectum
197.6 Secondary malignant neoplasm of retroperitoneum and peritoneum
199.0 Disseminated malignant neoplasm
199.1 Other malignant neoplasm of unspecified site
211.3 Benign neoplasm of colon
211.4 Benign neoplasm of rectum and anal canal
211.8 Benign neoplasm of retroperitoneum and peritoneum
211.9 Benign neoplasm of other and unspecified site of the digestive system ▽
230.3 Carcinoma in situ of colon
230.4 Carcinoma in situ of rectum
230.5 Carcinoma in situ of anal canal
230.6 Carcinoma in situ of anus, unspecified ▽
230.7 Carcinoma in situ of other and unspecified parts of intestine ▽
230.9 Carcinoma in situ of other and unspecified digestive organs ▽
235.2 Neoplasm of uncertain behavior of stomach, intestines, and rectum

▽ Unspecified code ☒ Manifestation code
♀ Female diagnosis ♂ Male diagnosis

235.4 Neoplasm of uncertain behavior of retroperitoneum and peritoneum
235.5 Neoplasm of uncertain behavior of other and unspecified digestive organs
239.0 Neoplasm of unspecified nature of digestive system
555.1 Regional enteritis of large intestine
555.2 Regional enteritis of small intestine with large intestine
555.9 Regional enteritis of unspecified site
556.0 Ulcerative (chronic) enterocolitis
556.2 Ulcerative (chronic) proctitis
556.3 Ulcerative (chronic) proctosigmoiditis
556.4 Pseudopolyposis of colon
556.6 Universal ulcerative (chronic) colitis
556.8 Other ulcerative colitis
556.9 Unspecified ulcerative colitis
562.10 Diverticulosis of colon (without mention of hemorrhage) — (Use additional code to identify any associated peritonitis: 567.0-567.9)
562.11 Diverticulitis of colon (without mention of hemorrhage) — (Use additional code to identify any associated peritonitis: 567.0-567.9)
562.12 Diverticulosis of colon with hemorrhage — (Use additional code to identify any associated peritonitis: 567.0-567.9)
562.13 Diverticulitis of colon with hemorrhage — (Use additional code to identify any associated peritonitis: 567.0-567.9)
569.0 Anal and rectal polyp
569.41 Ulcer of anus and rectum
569.49 Other specified disorder of rectum and anus
569.82 Ulceration of intestine
569.83 Perforation of intestine
569.89 Other specified disorder of intestines
578.1 Blood in stool
783.21 Loss of weight
789.30 Abdominal or pelvic swelling, mass or lump, unspecified site
789.33 Abdominal or pelvic swelling, mass, or lump, right lower quadrant
789.34 Abdominal or pelvic swelling, mass, or lump, left lower quadrant
789.39 Abdominal or pelvic swelling, mass, or lump, other specified site
793.4 Nonspecific abnormal findings on radiological and other examination of gastrointestinal tract
V10.00 Personal history of malignant neoplasm of unspecified site in gastrointestinal tract
V10.06 Personal history of malignant neoplasm of rectum, rectosigmoid junction, and anus
V10.09 Personal history of malignant neoplasm of other site in gastrointestinal tract
V12.00 Personal history of unspecified infectious and parasitic disease
V12.70 Personal history of unspecified digestive disease
V12.72 Personal history of colonic polyps
V12.79 Personal history of other diseases of digestive disease
V16.0 Family history of malignant neoplasm of gastrointestinal tract
V67.09 Follow-up examination, following other surgery
V76.41 Screening for malignant neoplasm of the rectum
V76.49 Special screening for malignant neoplasms, other sites
V82.9 Screening for unspecified condition

ICD-9-CM Procedural

45.25 Closed [endoscopic] biopsy of large intestine
88.74 Diagnostic ultrasound of digestive system

45345

45345 Sigmoidoscopy, flexible; with transendoscopic stent placement (includes predilation)

ICD-9-CM Diagnostic

153.2 Malignant neoplasm of descending colon
153.3 Malignant neoplasm of sigmoid colon
153.8 Malignant neoplasm of other specified sites of large intestine
153.9 Malignant neoplasm of colon, unspecified site
154.0 Malignant neoplasm of rectosigmoid junction
154.1 Malignant neoplasm of rectum
197.5 Secondary malignant neoplasm of large intestine and rectum
560.81 Intestinal or peritoneal adhesions with obstruction (postoperative) (postinfection)
560.89 Other specified intestinal obstruction
560.9 Unspecified intestinal obstruction
751.2 Congenital atresia and stenosis of large intestine, rectum, and anal canal
997.4 Digestive system complication — (Use additional code to identify complications)

ICD-9-CM Procedural

45.24 Flexible sigmoidoscopy
46.79 Other repair of intestine

45355

45355 Colonoscopy, rigid or flexible, transabdominal via colotomy, single or multiple

ICD-9-CM Diagnostic

153.0 Malignant neoplasm of hepatic flexure
153.1 Malignant neoplasm of transverse colon
153.2 Malignant neoplasm of descending colon
153.3 Malignant neoplasm of sigmoid colon
153.4 Malignant neoplasm of cecum
153.5 Malignant neoplasm of appendix
153.6 Malignant neoplasm of ascending colon
153.7 Malignant neoplasm of splenic flexure
153.8 Malignant neoplasm of other specified sites of large intestine
153.9 Malignant neoplasm of colon, unspecified site
154.0 Malignant neoplasm of rectosigmoid junction
154.1 Malignant neoplasm of rectum
154.2 Malignant neoplasm of anal canal
154.3 Malignant neoplasm of anus, unspecified site
197.5 Secondary malignant neoplasm of large intestine and rectum
199.0 Disseminated malignant neoplasm
199.1 Other malignant neoplasm of unspecified site
211.3 Benign neoplasm of colon
230.3 Carcinoma in situ of colon
230.4 Carcinoma in situ of rectum
230.5 Carcinoma in situ of anal canal
230.6 Carcinoma in situ of anus, unspecified
235.2 Neoplasm of uncertain behavior of stomach, intestines, and rectum
239.0 Neoplasm of unspecified nature of digestive system
280.0 Iron deficiency anemia secondary to blood loss (chronic)
280.9 Unspecified iron deficiency anemia
455.0 Internal hemorrhoids without mention of complication
455.2 Internal hemorrhoids with other complication
455.6 Unspecified hemorrhoids without mention of complication
455.8 Unspecified hemorrhoids with other complication
555.1 Regional enteritis of large intestine
555.2 Regional enteritis of small intestine with large intestine
555.9 Regional enteritis of unspecified site
556.0 Ulcerative (chronic) enterocolitis
556.1 Ulcerative (chronic) ileocolitis
556.2 Ulcerative (chronic) proctitis
556.3 Ulcerative (chronic) proctosigmoiditis
556.4 Pseudopolyposis of colon
556.5 Left sided ulcerative (chronic) colitis
556.6 Universal ulcerative (chronic) colitis
556.8 Other ulcerative colitis
557.0 Acute vascular insufficiency of intestine
557.1 Chronic vascular insufficiency of intestine
557.9 Unspecified vascular insufficiency of intestine
558.1 Gastroenteritis and colitis due to radiation
558.2 Toxic gastroenteritis and colitis — (Use additional E code to identify cause)
558.3 Gastroenteritis and colitis, allergic — (Use additional code to identify type of food allergy: V15.01-V15.05)
558.9 Other and unspecified noninfectious gastroenteritis and colitis
560.0 Intussusception
560.1 Paralytic ileus
560.2 Volvulus
560.39 Other impaction of intestine
560.89 Other specified intestinal obstruction
560.9 Unspecified intestinal obstruction
562.10 Diverticulosis of colon (without mention of hemorrhage) — (Use additional code to identify any associated peritonitis: 567.0-567.9)
562.11 Diverticulitis of colon (without mention of hemorrhage) — (Use additional code to identify any associated peritonitis: 567.0-567.9)
562.13 Diverticulitis of colon with hemorrhage — (Use additional code to identify any associated peritonitis: 567.0-567.9)
564.00 Unspecified constipation
564.01 Slow transit constipation
564.02 Outlet dysfunction constipation
564.09 Other constipation
564.1 Irritable bowel syndrome
564.4 Other postoperative functional disorders
564.5 Functional diarrhea
564.7 Megacolon, other than Hirschsprung's
564.81 Neurogenic bowel

Unspecified code
Female diagnosis
Manifestation code
Male diagnosis

564.89 Other functional disorders of intestine
565.0 Anal fissure
565.1 Anal fistula
566 Abscess of anal and rectal regions
567.0 Peritonitis in infectious diseases classified elsewhere — (Code first underlying disease) ☒
567.1 Pneumococcal peritonitis
567.2 Other suppurative peritonitis
567.8 Other specified peritonitis
567.9 Unspecified peritonitis ▽
569.0 Anal and rectal polyp
569.3 Hemorrhage of rectum and anus
569.42 Anal or rectal pain
569.49 Other specified disorder of rectum and anus
569.82 Ulceration of intestine
569.89 Other specified disorder of intestines
578.1 Blood in stool
578.9 Unspecified, hemorrhage of gastrointestinal tract ▽
579.0 Celiac disease
579.1 Tropical sprue
579.2 Blind loop syndrome
579.3 Other and unspecified postsurgical nonabsorption ▽
579.4 Pancreatic steatorrhea
579.8 Other specified intestinal malabsorption
747.61 Congenital gastrointestinal vessel anomaly
751.3 Hirschsprung's disease and other congenital functional disorders of colon
751.5 Other congenital anomalies of intestine
780.6 Fever
780.99 Other general symptoms
783.21 Loss of weight
783.22 Underweight
783.7 Adult failure to thrive
787.3 Flatulence, eructation, and gas pain
787.7 Abnormal feces
787.91 Diarrhea
787.99 Other symptoms involving digestive system
789.00 Abdominal pain, unspecified site ▽
789.01 Abdominal pain, right upper quadrant
789.02 Abdominal pain, left upper quadrant
789.03 Abdominal pain, right lower quadrant
789.04 Abdominal pain, left lower quadrant
789.05 Abdominal pain, periumbilic
789.06 Abdominal pain, epigastric
789.07 Abdominal pain, generalized
789.09 Abdominal pain, other specified site
789.30 Abdominal or pelvic swelling, mass or lump, unspecified site ▽
789.31 Abdominal or pelvic swelling, mass, or lump, right upper quadrant
789.32 Abdominal or pelvic swelling, mass, or lump, left upper quadrant
789.33 Abdominal or pelvic swelling, mass, or lump, right lower quadrant
789.34 Abdominal or pelvic swelling, mass, or lump, left lower quadrant
789.35 Abdominal or pelvic swelling, mass or lump, periumbilic
789.36 Abdominal or pelvic swelling, mass, or lump, epigastric
789.37 Abdominal or pelvic swelling, mass, or lump, epigastric, generalized
789.39 Abdominal or pelvic swelling, mass, or lump, other specified site
789.9 Other symptoms involving abdomen and pelvis
792.1 Nonspecific abnormal finding in stool contents
793.4 Nonspecific abnormal findings on radiological and other examination of gastrointestinal tract
997.4 Digestive system complication — (Use additional code to identify complications)
V10.05 Personal history of malignant neoplasm of large intestine
V10.06 Personal history of malignant neoplasm of rectum, rectosigmoid junction, and anus
V12.70 Personal history of unspecified digestive disease ▽
V12.72 Personal history of colonic polyps
V12.79 Personal history of other diseases of digestive disease
V16.0 Family history of malignant neoplasm of gastrointestinal tract
V18.5 Family history of digestive disorders
V45.89 Other postsurgical status — (This code is intended for use when these conditions are recorded as diagnoses or problems)
V47.3 Other digestive problems — (This code is intended for use when these conditions are recorded as diagnoses or problems)
V67.00 Follow-up examination, following unspecified surgery ▽
V67.09 Follow-up examination, following other surgery
V67.51 Follow-up examination following completed treatment with high-risk medications, not elsewhere classified
V71.1 Observation for suspected malignant neoplasm
V71.89 Observation for other specified suspected conditions
V71.9 Observation for unspecified suspected condition ▽

ICD-9-CM Procedural

45.21 Transabdominal endoscopy of large intestine
45.23 Colonoscopy

45378

45378 Colonoscopy, flexible, proximal to splenic flexure; diagnostic, with or without collection of specimen(s) by brushing or washing, with or without colon decompression (separate procedure)

ICD-9-CM Diagnostic

153.0 Malignant neoplasm of hepatic flexure
153.1 Malignant neoplasm of transverse colon
153.2 Malignant neoplasm of descending colon
153.3 Malignant neoplasm of sigmoid colon
153.4 Malignant neoplasm of cecum
153.5 Malignant neoplasm of appendix
153.6 Malignant neoplasm of ascending colon
153.7 Malignant neoplasm of splenic flexure
153.8 Malignant neoplasm of other specified sites of large intestine
153.9 Malignant neoplasm of colon, unspecified site ▽
154.0 Malignant neoplasm of rectosigmoid junction
154.1 Malignant neoplasm of rectum
154.2 Malignant neoplasm of anal canal
154.3 Malignant neoplasm of anus, unspecified site ▽
197.5 Secondary malignant neoplasm of large intestine and rectum
199.0 Disseminated malignant neoplasm
199.1 Other malignant neoplasm of unspecified site
211.3 Benign neoplasm of colon
230.3 Carcinoma in situ of colon
230.4 Carcinoma in situ of rectum
230.5 Carcinoma in situ of anal canal
230.6 Carcinoma in situ of anus, unspecified ▽
235.2 Neoplasm of uncertain behavior of stomach, intestines, and rectum
239.0 Neoplasm of unspecified nature of digestive system
280.0 Iron deficiency anemia secondary to blood loss (chronic)
280.9 Unspecified iron deficiency anemia ▽
455.0 Internal hemorrhoids without mention of complication
455.2 Internal hemorrhoids with other complication
455.6 Unspecified hemorrhoids without mention of complication ▽
455.8 Unspecified hemorrhoids with other complication ▽
555.1 Regional enteritis of large intestine
555.2 Regional enteritis of small intestine with large intestine
555.9 Regional enteritis of unspecified site ▽
556.0 Ulcerative (chronic) enterocolitis
556.1 Ulcerative (chronic) ileocolitis
556.2 Ulcerative (chronic) proctitis
556.3 Ulcerative (chronic) proctosigmoiditis
556.4 Pseudopolyposis of colon
556.5 Left sided ulcerative (chronic) colitis
556.6 Universal ulcerative (chronic) colitis
556.8 Other ulcerative colitis
557.0 Acute vascular insufficiency of intestine
557.1 Chronic vascular insufficiency of intestine
557.9 Unspecified vascular insufficiency of intestine ▽
558.1 Gastroenteritis and colitis due to radiation
558.2 Toxic gastroenteritis and colitis — (Use additional E code to identify cause)
558.3 Gastroenteritis and colitis, allergic — (Use additional code to identify type of food allergy: V15.01-V15.05)
558.9 Other and unspecified noninfectious gastroenteritis and colitis ▽
560.0 Intussusception
560.1 Paralytic ileus
560.2 Volvulus
560.39 Other impaction of intestine
560.89 Other specified intestinal obstruction
560.9 Unspecified intestinal obstruction ▽
562.10 Diverticulosis of colon (without mention of hemorrhage) — (Use additional code to identify any associated peritonitis: 567.0-567.9)
562.11 Diverticulitis of colon (without mention of hemorrhage) — (Use additional code to identify any associated peritonitis: 567.0-567.9)
562.13 Diverticulitis of colon with hemorrhage — (Use additional code to identify any associated peritonitis: 567.0-567.9)
564.00 Unspecified constipation ▽

564.01 Slow transit constipation
564.02 Outlet dysfunction constipation
564.09 Other constipation
564.1 Irritable bowel syndrome
564.4 Other postoperative functional disorders
564.5 Functional diarrhea
564.7 Megacolon, other than Hirschsprung's
564.81 Neurogenic bowel
564.89 Other functional disorders of intestine
565.0 Anal fissure
565.1 Anal fistula
566 Abscess of anal and rectal regions
567.0 Peritonitis in infectious diseases classified elsewhere — (Code first underlying disease) ☒
567.1 Pneumococcal peritonitis
567.2 Other suppurative peritonitis
567.8 Other specified peritonitis
567.9 Unspecified peritonitis ▽
569.0 Anal and rectal polyp
569.3 Hemorrhage of rectum and anus
569.42 Anal or rectal pain
569.49 Other specified disorder of rectum and anus
569.82 Ulceration of intestine
569.89 Other specified disorder of intestines
578.1 Blood in stool
578.9 Unspecified, hemorrhage of gastrointestinal tract ▽
579.0 Celiac disease
579.1 Tropical sprue
579.2 Blind loop syndrome
579.3 Other and unspecified postsurgical nonabsorption ▽
579.4 Pancreatic steatorrhea
579.8 Other specified intestinal malabsorption
747.61 Congenital gastrointestinal vessel anomaly
751.3 Hirschsprung's disease and other congenital functional disorders of colon
751.5 Other congenital anomalies of intestine
780.6 Fever
780.99 Other general symptoms
783.21 Loss of weight
783.22 Underweight
783.7 Adult failure to thrive
787.3 Flatulence, eructation, and gas pain
787.7 Abnormal feces
787.91 Diarrhea
787.99 Other symptoms involving digestive system
789.00 Abdominal pain, unspecified site ▽
789.01 Abdominal pain, right upper quadrant
789.02 Abdominal pain, left upper quadrant
789.03 Abdominal pain, right lower quadrant
789.04 Abdominal pain, left lower quadrant
789.05 Abdominal pain, periumbilic
789.06 Abdominal pain, epigastric
789.07 Abdominal pain, generalized
789.09 Abdominal pain, other specified site
789.30 Abdominal or pelvic swelling, mass or lump, unspecified site ▽
789.31 Abdominal or pelvic swelling, mass, or lump, right upper quadrant
789.32 Abdominal or pelvic swelling, mass, or lump, left upper quadrant
789.33 Abdominal or pelvic swelling, mass, or lump, right lower quadrant
789.34 Abdominal or pelvic swelling, mass, or lump, left lower quadrant
789.35 Abdominal or pelvic swelling, mass or lump, periumbilic
789.36 Abdominal or pelvic swelling, mass, or lump, epigastric
789.37 Abdominal or pelvic swelling, mass, or lump, epigastric, generalized
789.39 Abdominal or pelvic swelling, mass, or lump, other specified site
789.9 Other symptoms involving abdomen and pelvis
792.1 Nonspecific abnormal finding in stool contents
793.4 Nonspecific abnormal findings on radiological and other examination of gastrointestinal tract
997.4 Digestive system complication — (Use additional code to identify complications)
V10.05 Personal history of malignant neoplasm of large intestine
V10.06 Personal history of malignant neoplasm of rectum, rectosigmoid junction, and anus
V12.70 Personal history of unspecified digestive disease ▽
V12.72 Personal history of colonic polyps
V12.79 Personal history of other diseases of digestive disease
V16.0 Family history of malignant neoplasm of gastrointestinal tract
V18.5 Family history of digestive disorders
V45.89 Other postsurgical status — (This code is intended for use when these conditions are recorded as diagnoses or problems)
V47.3 Other digestive problems — (This code is intended for use when these conditions are recorded as diagnoses or problems)
V67.00 Follow-up examination, following unspecified surgery ▽
V67.09 Follow-up examination, following other surgery
V67.51 Follow-up examination following completed treatment with high-risk medications, not elsewhere classified
V71.1 Observation for suspected malignant neoplasm
V71.89 Observation for other specified suspected conditions
V71.9 Observation for unspecified suspected condition ▽

ICD-9-CM Procedural

45.23 Colonoscopy
45.25 Closed [endoscopic] biopsy of large intestine
46.85 Dilation of intestine

HCPCS Level II Supplies & Services

A4270 Disposable endoscope sheath, each
A4305 Disposable drug delivery system, flow rate of 50 ml or greater per hour
A4306 Disposable drug delivery system, flow rate of 5 ml or less per hour
G0105 Colorectal cancer screening; colonoscopy on individual at high risk
G0120 Colorectal cancer screening; alternative to G0105, screening colonoscopy, barium enema

45379

45379 Colonoscopy, flexible, proximal to splenic flexure; with removal of foreign body

ICD-9-CM Diagnostic

567.1 Pneumococcal peritonitis
567.2 Other suppurative peritonitis
567.8 Other specified peritonitis
567.9 Unspecified peritonitis ▽
569.3 Hemorrhage of rectum and anus
569.42 Anal or rectal pain
578.1 Blood in stool
793.4 Nonspecific abnormal findings on radiological and other examination of gastrointestinal tract
936 Foreign body in intestine and colon
938 Foreign body in digestive system, unspecified ▽

ICD-9-CM Procedural

45.23 Colonoscopy
98.04 Removal of intraluminal foreign body from large intestine without incision

HCPCS Level II Supplies & Services

A4270 Disposable endoscope sheath, each
A4305 Disposable drug delivery system, flow rate of 50 ml or greater per hour
A4306 Disposable drug delivery system, flow rate of 5 ml or less per hour
A4550 Surgical trays

45380

45380 Colonoscopy, flexible, proximal to splenic flexure; with biopsy, single or multiple

ICD-9-CM Diagnostic

153.1 Malignant neoplasm of transverse colon
153.2 Malignant neoplasm of descending colon
153.3 Malignant neoplasm of sigmoid colon
153.4 Malignant neoplasm of cecum
153.5 Malignant neoplasm of appendix
153.6 Malignant neoplasm of ascending colon
153.7 Malignant neoplasm of splenic flexure
153.8 Malignant neoplasm of other specified sites of large intestine
153.9 Malignant neoplasm of colon, unspecified site ▽
154.0 Malignant neoplasm of rectosigmoid junction
154.1 Malignant neoplasm of rectum
154.8 Malignant neoplasm of other sites of rectum, rectosigmoid junction, and anus
159.0 Malignant neoplasm of intestinal tract, part unspecified ▽
159.9 Malignant neoplasm of ill-defined sites of digestive organs and peritoneum
197.5 Secondary malignant neoplasm of large intestine and rectum
199.0 Disseminated malignant neoplasm
199.1 Other malignant neoplasm of unspecified site
211.3 Benign neoplasm of colon
211.4 Benign neoplasm of rectum and anal canal
228.1 Lymphangioma, any site

▽ Unspecified code ☒ Manifestation code
♀ Female diagnosis ♂ Male diagnosis

230.3 Carcinoma in situ of colon
230.4 Carcinoma in situ of rectum
230.5 Carcinoma in situ of anal canal
230.6 Carcinoma in situ of anus, unspecified ▽
235.2 Neoplasm of uncertain behavior of stomach, intestines, and rectum
235.5 Neoplasm of uncertain behavior of other and unspecified digestive organs ▽
239.0 Neoplasm of unspecified nature of digestive system
280.0 Iron deficiency anemia secondary to blood loss (chronic)
280.9 Unspecified iron deficiency anemia ▽
455.0 Internal hemorrhoids without mention of complication
555.1 Regional enteritis of large intestine
555.2 Regional enteritis of small intestine with large intestine
555.9 Regional enteritis of unspecified site ▽
556.0 Ulcerative (chronic) enterocolitis
556.1 Ulcerative (chronic) ileocolitis
556.2 Ulcerative (chronic) proctitis
556.3 Ulcerative (chronic) proctosigmoiditis
556.4 Pseudopolyposis of colon
556.5 Left sided ulcerative (chronic) colitis
556.6 Universal ulcerative (chronic) colitis
556.8 Other ulcerative colitis
558.1 Gastroenteritis and colitis due to radiation
558.2 Toxic gastroenteritis and colitis — (Use additional E code to identify cause)
558.3 Gastroenteritis and colitis, allergic — (Use additional code to identify type of food allergy: V15.01-V15.05)
558.9 Other and unspecified noninfectious gastroenteritis and colitis ▽
560.0 Intussusception
560.1 Paralytic ileus
560.2 Volvulus
560.31 Gallstone ileus
560.39 Other impaction of intestine
560.9 Unspecified intestinal obstruction ▽
562.10 Diverticulosis of colon (without mention of hemorrhage) — (Use additional code to identify any associated peritonitis: 567.0-567.9)
562.11 Diverticulitis of colon (without mention of hemorrhage) — (Use additional code to identify any associated peritonitis: 567.0-567.9)
564.00 Unspecified constipation ▽
564.01 Slow transit constipation
564.02 Outlet dysfunction constipation
564.09 Other constipation
564.1 Irritable bowel syndrome
564.4 Other postoperative functional disorders
564.5 Functional diarrhea
564.7 Megacolon, other than Hirschsprung's
567.0 Peritonitis in infectious diseases classified elsewhere — (Code first underlying disease) ☒
567.1 Pneumococcal peritonitis
567.2 Other suppurative peritonitis
567.8 Other specified peritonitis
567.9 Unspecified peritonitis ▽
569.0 Anal and rectal polyp
569.3 Hemorrhage of rectum and anus
569.49 Other specified disorder of rectum and anus
569.82 Ulceration of intestine
569.89 Other specified disorder of intestines
578.1 Blood in stool
578.9 Unspecified, hemorrhage of gastrointestinal tract ▽
780.99 Other general symptoms
783.21 Loss of weight
783.22 Underweight
783.7 Adult failure to thrive
787.3 Flatulence, eructation, and gas pain
787.7 Abnormal feces
787.91 Diarrhea
787.99 Other symptoms involving digestive system
789.00 Abdominal pain, unspecified site ▽
789.01 Abdominal pain, right upper quadrant
789.02 Abdominal pain, left upper quadrant
789.03 Abdominal pain, right lower quadrant
789.04 Abdominal pain, left lower quadrant
789.05 Abdominal pain, periumbilic
789.06 Abdominal pain, epigastric
789.07 Abdominal pain, generalized
789.09 Abdominal pain, other specified site
792.1 Nonspecific abnormal finding in stool contents
793.4 Nonspecific abnormal findings on radiological and other examination of gastrointestinal tract
V10.05 Personal history of malignant neoplasm of large intestine
V10.06 Personal history of malignant neoplasm of rectum, rectosigmoid junction, and anus
V12.70 Personal history of unspecified digestive disease ▽
V12.72 Personal history of colonic polyps
V12.79 Personal history of other diseases of digestive disease
V16.0 Family history of malignant neoplasm of gastrointestinal tract
V71.1 Observation for suspected malignant neoplasm
V71.9 Observation for unspecified suspected condition ▽

ICD-9-CM Procedural

45.25 Closed [endoscopic] biopsy of large intestine

HCPCS Level II Supplies & Services

A4270 Disposable endoscope sheath, each
A4305 Disposable drug delivery system, flow rate of 50 ml or greater per hour
A4306 Disposable drug delivery system, flow rate of 5 ml or less per hour
A4550 Surgical trays
G0105 Colorectal cancer screening; colonoscopy on individual at high risk

45381

45381 Colonoscopy, flexible, proximal to splenic flexure; with directed submucosal injection(s), any substance

ICD-9-CM Diagnostic

153.0 Malignant neoplasm of hepatic flexure
153.1 Malignant neoplasm of transverse colon
153.2 Malignant neoplasm of descending colon
153.3 Malignant neoplasm of sigmoid colon
153.4 Malignant neoplasm of cecum
153.5 Malignant neoplasm of appendix
153.6 Malignant neoplasm of ascending colon
153.7 Malignant neoplasm of splenic flexure
153.8 Malignant neoplasm of other specified sites of large intestine
153.9 Malignant neoplasm of colon, unspecified site ▽
154.0 Malignant neoplasm of rectosigmoid junction
154.1 Malignant neoplasm of rectum
154.2 Malignant neoplasm of anal canal
154.3 Malignant neoplasm of anus, unspecified site ▽
197.5 Secondary malignant neoplasm of large intestine and rectum
199.0 Disseminated malignant neoplasm
199.1 Other malignant neoplasm of unspecified site
211.3 Benign neoplasm of colon
230.3 Carcinoma in situ of colon
230.4 Carcinoma in situ of rectum
230.5 Carcinoma in situ of anal canal
230.6 Carcinoma in situ of anus, unspecified ▽
235.2 Neoplasm of uncertain behavior of stomach, intestines, and rectum
455.0 Internal hemorrhoids without mention of complication
455.1 Internal thrombosed hemorrhoids
455.2 Internal hemorrhoids with other complication
455.6 Unspecified hemorrhoids without mention of complication ▽
455.7 Unspecified thrombosed hemorrhoids ▽
455.8 Unspecified hemorrhoids with other complication ▽
555.1 Regional enteritis of large intestine
555.2 Regional enteritis of small intestine with large intestine
555.9 Regional enteritis of unspecified site ▽
556.0 Ulcerative (chronic) enterocolitis
556.1 Ulcerative (chronic) ileocolitis
556.2 Ulcerative (chronic) proctitis
556.3 Ulcerative (chronic) proctosigmoiditis
556.4 Pseudopolyposis of colon
556.5 Left sided ulcerative (chronic) colitis
556.6 Universal ulcerative (chronic) colitis
556.8 Other ulcerative colitis
558.1 Gastroenteritis and colitis due to radiation
558.2 Toxic gastroenteritis and colitis — (Use additional E code to identify cause)
558.3 Gastroenteritis and colitis, allergic — (Use additional code to identify type of food allergy: V15.01-V15.05)
558.9 Other and unspecified noninfectious gastroenteritis and colitis ▽
562.10 Diverticulosis of colon (without mention of hemorrhage) — (Use additional code to identify any associated peritonitis: 567.0-567.9)
562.11 Diverticulitis of colon (without mention of hemorrhage) — (Use additional code to identify any associated peritonitis: 567.0-567.9)

562.13 Diverticulitis of colon with hemorrhage — (Use additional code to identify any associated peritonitis: 567.0-567.9)
564.00 Unspecified constipation
564.01 Slow transit constipation
564.02 Outlet dysfunction constipation
564.09 Other constipation
564.1 Irritable bowel syndrome
564.4 Other postoperative functional disorders
564.5 Functional diarrhea
564.7 Megacolon, other than Hirschsprung's
564.81 Neurogenic bowel
564.89 Other functional disorders of intestine
565.0 Anal fissure
565.1 Anal fistula
566 Abscess of anal and rectal regions
569.0 Anal and rectal polyp
569.3 Hemorrhage of rectum and anus
569.42 Anal or rectal pain
569.49 Other specified disorder of rectum and anus
569.82 Ulceration of intestine
569.89 Other specified disorder of intestines
578.1 Blood in stool
578.9 Unspecified, hemorrhage of gastrointestinal tract
619.1 Digestive-genital tract fistula, female ♀
747.61 Congenital gastrointestinal vessel anomaly
751.2 Congenital atresia and stenosis of large intestine, rectum, and anal canal
751.3 Hirschsprung's disease and other congenital functional disorders of colon
751.5 Other congenital anomalies of intestine
787.3 Flatulence, eructation, and gas pain
787.7 Abnormal feces
787.91 Diarrhea
787.99 Other symptoms involving digestive system
789.00 Abdominal pain, unspecified site
789.01 Abdominal pain, right upper quadrant
789.02 Abdominal pain, left upper quadrant
789.03 Abdominal pain, right lower quadrant
789.04 Abdominal pain, left lower quadrant
789.05 Abdominal pain, periumbilic
789.06 Abdominal pain, epigastric
789.07 Abdominal pain, generalized
789.09 Abdominal pain, other specified site
792.1 Nonspecific abnormal finding in stool contents
793.4 Nonspecific abnormal findings on radiological and other examination of gastrointestinal tract
997.4 Digestive system complication — (Use additional code to identify complications)
V47.3 Other digestive problems — (This code is intended for use when these conditions are recorded as diagnoses or problems)
V67.00 Follow-up examination, following unspecified surgery
V67.09 Follow-up examination, following other surgery

ICD-9-CM Procedural

45.43 Endoscopic destruction of other lesion or tissue of large intestine

45382

45382 Colonoscopy, flexible, proximal to splenic flexure; with control of bleeding (eg, injection, bipolar cautery, unipolar cautery, laser, heater probe, stapler, plasma coagulator)

ICD-9-CM Diagnostic

153.7 Malignant neoplasm of splenic flexure
153.9 Malignant neoplasm of colon, unspecified site
211.3 Benign neoplasm of colon
448.9 Other and unspecified capillary diseases
455.2 Internal hemorrhoids with other complication
556.3 Ulcerative (chronic) proctosigmoiditis
556.9 Unspecified ulcerative colitis
557.0 Acute vascular insufficiency of intestine
557.1 Chronic vascular insufficiency of intestine
558.9 Other and unspecified noninfectious gastroenteritis and colitis
562.12 Diverticulosis of colon with hemorrhage — (Use additional code to identify any associated peritonitis: 567.0-567.9)
562.13 Diverticulitis of colon with hemorrhage — (Use additional code to identify any associated peritonitis: 567.0-567.9)
569.82 Ulceration of intestine
569.85 Angiodysplasia of intestine with hemorrhage
578.1 Blood in stool
578.9 Unspecified, hemorrhage of gastrointestinal tract
772.4 Fetal and neonatal gastrointestinal hemorrhage
789.00 Abdominal pain, unspecified site
789.01 Abdominal pain, right upper quadrant
789.02 Abdominal pain, left upper quadrant
789.03 Abdominal pain, right lower quadrant
789.04 Abdominal pain, left lower quadrant
789.05 Abdominal pain, periumbilic
789.06 Abdominal pain, epigastric
789.07 Abdominal pain, generalized
789.09 Abdominal pain, other specified site
789.30 Abdominal or pelvic swelling, mass or lump, unspecified site
793.4 Nonspecific abnormal findings on radiological and other examination of gastrointestinal tract

ICD-9-CM Procedural

45.43 Endoscopic destruction of other lesion or tissue of large intestine

HCPCS Level II Supplies & Services

A4270 Disposable endoscope sheath, each
A4305 Disposable drug delivery system, flow rate of 50 ml or greater per hour
A4306 Disposable drug delivery system, flow rate of 5 ml or less per hour
A4550 Surgical trays

45383–45385

45383 Colonoscopy, flexible, proximal to splenic flexure; with ablation of tumor(s), polyp(s), or other lesion(s) not amenable to removal by hot biopsy forceps, bipolar cautery or snare technique
45384 with removal of tumor(s), polyp(s), or other lesion(s) by hot biopsy forceps or bipolar cautery
45385 with removal of tumor(s), polyp(s), or other lesion(s) by snare technique

ICD-9-CM Diagnostic

153.0 Malignant neoplasm of hepatic flexure
153.1 Malignant neoplasm of transverse colon
153.2 Malignant neoplasm of descending colon
153.3 Malignant neoplasm of sigmoid colon
153.4 Malignant neoplasm of cecum
153.5 Malignant neoplasm of appendix
153.6 Malignant neoplasm of ascending colon
153.7 Malignant neoplasm of splenic flexure
153.8 Malignant neoplasm of other specified sites of large intestine
153.9 Malignant neoplasm of colon, unspecified site
154.0 Malignant neoplasm of rectosigmoid junction
154.1 Malignant neoplasm of rectum
154.2 Malignant neoplasm of anal canal
154.3 Malignant neoplasm of anus, unspecified site
199.1 Other malignant neoplasm of unspecified site
211.3 Benign neoplasm of colon
211.4 Benign neoplasm of rectum and anal canal
230.3 Carcinoma in situ of colon
230.4 Carcinoma in situ of rectum
230.5 Carcinoma in situ of anal canal
230.6 Carcinoma in situ of anus, unspecified
235.2 Neoplasm of uncertain behavior of stomach, intestines, and rectum
235.5 Neoplasm of uncertain behavior of other and unspecified digestive organs
239.0 Neoplasm of unspecified nature of digestive system
455.2 Internal hemorrhoids with other complication
556.0 Ulcerative (chronic) enterocolitis
556.1 Ulcerative (chronic) ileocolitis
556.2 Ulcerative (chronic) proctitis
556.3 Ulcerative (chronic) proctosigmoiditis
556.4 Pseudopolyposis of colon
556.5 Left sided ulcerative (chronic) colitis
556.6 Universal ulcerative (chronic) colitis
556.8 Other ulcerative colitis
556.9 Unspecified ulcerative colitis
558.9 Other and unspecified noninfectious gastroenteritis and colitis
562.10 Diverticulosis of colon (without mention of hemorrhage) — (Use additional code to identify any associated peritonitis: 567.0-567.9)
562.11 Diverticulitis of colon (without mention of hemorrhage) — (Use additional code to identify any associated peritonitis: 567.0-567.9)
564.00 Unspecified constipation
564.01 Slow transit constipation
564.02 Outlet dysfunction constipation

Unspecified code
♀ Female diagnosis
Manifestation code
♂ Male diagnosis

564.09 Other constipation
567.0 Peritonitis in infectious diseases classified elsewhere — (Code first underlying disease) ☒
567.1 Pneumococcal peritonitis
567.2 Other suppurative peritonitis
567.8 Other specified peritonitis
567.9 Unspecified peritonitis ▽
569.0 Anal and rectal polyp
569.3 Hemorrhage of rectum and anus
569.49 Other specified disorder of rectum and anus
569.84 Angiodysplasia of intestine (without mention of hemorrhage)
569.85 Angiodysplasia of intestine with hemorrhage
569.89 Other specified disorder of intestines
578.1 Blood in stool
783.21 Loss of weight
783.22 Underweight
787.7 Abnormal feces
787.91 Diarrhea
787.99 Other symptoms involving digestive system
789.00 Abdominal pain, unspecified site ▽
789.01 Abdominal pain, right upper quadrant
789.02 Abdominal pain, left upper quadrant
789.03 Abdominal pain, right lower quadrant
789.04 Abdominal pain, left lower quadrant
789.05 Abdominal pain, periumbilic
789.06 Abdominal pain, epigastric
789.07 Abdominal pain, generalized
789.09 Abdominal pain, other specified site
789.30 Abdominal or pelvic swelling, mass or lump, unspecified site ▽
789.31 Abdominal or pelvic swelling, mass, or lump, right upper quadrant
789.32 Abdominal or pelvic swelling, mass, or lump, left upper quadrant
789.33 Abdominal or pelvic swelling, mass, or lump, right lower quadrant
789.34 Abdominal or pelvic swelling, mass, or lump, left lower quadrant
789.35 Abdominal or pelvic swelling, mass or lump, periumbilic
789.36 Abdominal or pelvic swelling, mass, or lump, epigastric
789.37 Abdominal or pelvic swelling, mass, or lump, epigastric, generalized
789.39 Abdominal or pelvic swelling, mass, or lump, other specified site
792.1 Nonspecific abnormal finding in stool contents
793.4 Nonspecific abnormal findings on radiological and other examination of gastrointestinal tract
V10.05 Personal history of malignant neoplasm of large intestine
V10.06 Personal history of malignant neoplasm of rectum, rectosigmoid junction, and anus
V12.70 Personal history of unspecified digestive disease ▽
V12.72 Personal history of colonic polyps
V12.79 Personal history of other diseases of digestive disease
V71.89 Observation for other specified suspected conditions
V71.9 Observation for unspecified suspected condition ▽

ICD-9-CM Procedural

45.42 Endoscopic polypectomy of large intestine
45.43 Endoscopic destruction of other lesion or tissue of large intestine

HCPCS Level II Supplies & Services

A4270 Disposable endoscope sheath, each
A4305 Disposable drug delivery system, flow rate of 50 ml or greater per hour
A4306 Disposable drug delivery system, flow rate of 5 ml or less per hour
A4550 Surgical trays

45386

45386 Colonoscopy, flexible, proximal to splenic flexure; with dilation by balloon, 1 or more strictures

ICD-9-CM Diagnostic

560.81 Intestinal or peritoneal adhesions with obstruction (postoperative) (postinfection)
560.89 Other specified intestinal obstruction
560.9 Unspecified intestinal obstruction ▽
751.2 Congenital atresia and stenosis of large intestine, rectum, and anal canal
997.4 Digestive system complication — (Use additional code to identify complications)

ICD-9-CM Procedural

46.85 Dilation of intestine

45387

45387 Colonoscopy, flexible, proximal to splenic flexure; with transendoscopic stent placement (includes predilation)

ICD-9-CM Diagnostic

153.0 Malignant neoplasm of hepatic flexure
153.1 Malignant neoplasm of transverse colon
153.2 Malignant neoplasm of descending colon
153.3 Malignant neoplasm of sigmoid colon
153.4 Malignant neoplasm of cecum
153.5 Malignant neoplasm of appendix
153.6 Malignant neoplasm of ascending colon
153.7 Malignant neoplasm of splenic flexure
153.8 Malignant neoplasm of other specified sites of large intestine
153.9 Malignant neoplasm of colon, unspecified site ▽
154.0 Malignant neoplasm of rectosigmoid junction
154.1 Malignant neoplasm of rectum
197.5 Secondary malignant neoplasm of large intestine and rectum
560.81 Intestinal or peritoneal adhesions with obstruction (postoperative) (postinfection)
560.89 Other specified intestinal obstruction
560.9 Unspecified intestinal obstruction ▽
751.2 Congenital atresia and stenosis of large intestine, rectum, and anal canal
997.4 Digestive system complication — (Use additional code to identify complications)

ICD-9-CM Procedural

45.22 Endoscopy of large intestine through artificial stoma
46.79 Other repair of intestine

45391–45392

45391 Colonoscopy, flexible, proximal to splenic flexure; with endoscopic ultrasound examination
45392 with transendoscopic ultrasound guided intramural or transmural fine needle aspiration/biopsy(s)

ICD-9-CM Diagnostic

153.0 Malignant neoplasm of hepatic flexure
153.1 Malignant neoplasm of transverse colon
153.2 Malignant neoplasm of descending colon
153.3 Malignant neoplasm of sigmoid colon
153.4 Malignant neoplasm of cecum
153.5 Malignant neoplasm of appendix
153.6 Malignant neoplasm of ascending colon
153.7 Malignant neoplasm of splenic flexure
153.8 Malignant neoplasm of other specified sites of large intestine
153.9 Malignant neoplasm of colon, unspecified site ▽
154.0 Malignant neoplasm of rectosigmoid junction
154.1 Malignant neoplasm of rectum
154.2 Malignant neoplasm of anal canal
154.3 Malignant neoplasm of anus, unspecified site ▽
199.1 Other malignant neoplasm of unspecified site
211.3 Benign neoplasm of colon
211.4 Benign neoplasm of rectum and anal canal
230.3 Carcinoma in situ of colon
230.4 Carcinoma in situ of rectum
230.5 Carcinoma in situ of anal canal
230.6 Carcinoma in situ of anus, unspecified ▽
235.2 Neoplasm of uncertain behavior of stomach, intestines, and rectum
235.5 Neoplasm of uncertain behavior of other and unspecified digestive organs ▽
239.0 Neoplasm of unspecified nature of digestive system
277.3 Amyloidosis — (Use additional code to identify any associated mental retardation)
455.2 Internal hemorrhoids with other complication
555.9 Regional enteritis of unspecified site ▽
556.0 Ulcerative (chronic) enterocolitis
556.1 Ulcerative (chronic) ileocolitis
556.2 Ulcerative (chronic) proctitis
556.3 Ulcerative (chronic) proctosigmoiditis
556.4 Pseudopolyposis of colon
556.5 Left sided ulcerative (chronic) colitis
556.6 Universal ulcerative (chronic) colitis
556.8 Other ulcerative colitis
556.9 Unspecified ulcerative colitis ▽
558.9 Other and unspecified noninfectious gastroenteritis and colitis ▽

562.10 Diverticulosis of colon (without mention of hemorrhage) — (Use additional code to identify any associated peritonitis: 567.0-567.9)
562.11 Diverticulitis of colon (without mention of hemorrhage) — (Use additional code to identify any associated peritonitis: 567.0-567.9)
564.00 Unspecified constipation
564.01 Slow transit constipation
564.02 Outlet dysfunction constipation
564.09 Other constipation
564.7 Megacolon, other than Hirschsprung's
564.89 Other functional disorders of intestine
564.9 Unspecified functional disorder of intestine
567.0 Peritonitis in infectious diseases classified elsewhere — (Code first underlying disease) ☒
567.1 Pneumococcal peritonitis
567.2 Other suppurative peritonitis
567.8 Other specified peritonitis
567.9 Unspecified peritonitis
569.0 Anal and rectal polyp
569.3 Hemorrhage of rectum and anus
569.49 Other specified disorder of rectum and anus
569.5 Abscess of intestine
569.81 Fistula of intestine, excluding rectum and anus
569.82 Ulceration of intestine
569.83 Perforation of intestine
569.84 Angiodysplasia of intestine (without mention of hemorrhage)
569.85 Angiodysplasia of intestine with hemorrhage
569.89 Other specified disorder of intestines
569.9 Unspecified disorder of intestine
578.1 Blood in stool
751.3 Hirschsprung's disease and other congenital functional disorders of colon
783.21 Loss of weight
783.22 Underweight
787.7 Abnormal feces
787.91 Diarrhea
787.99 Other symptoms involving digestive system
789.00 Abdominal pain, unspecified site
789.01 Abdominal pain, right upper quadrant
789.02 Abdominal pain, left upper quadrant
789.03 Abdominal pain, right lower quadrant
789.04 Abdominal pain, left lower quadrant
789.05 Abdominal pain, periumbilic
789.06 Abdominal pain, epigastric
789.07 Abdominal pain, generalized
789.09 Abdominal pain, other specified site
789.30 Abdominal or pelvic swelling, mass or lump, unspecified site
789.31 Abdominal or pelvic swelling, mass, or lump, right upper quadrant
789.32 Abdominal or pelvic swelling, mass, or lump, left upper quadrant
789.33 Abdominal or pelvic swelling, mass, or lump, right lower quadrant
789.34 Abdominal or pelvic swelling, mass, or lump, left lower quadrant
789.35 Abdominal or pelvic swelling, mass or lump, periumbilic
789.36 Abdominal or pelvic swelling, mass, or lump, epigastric
789.37 Abdominal or pelvic swelling, mass, or lump, epigastric, generalized
789.39 Abdominal or pelvic swelling, mass, or lump, other specified site
792.1 Nonspecific abnormal finding in stool contents
793.4 Nonspecific abnormal findings on radiological and other examination of gastrointestinal tract
V10.05 Personal history of malignant neoplasm of large intestine
V10.06 Personal history of malignant neoplasm of rectum, rectosigmoid junction, and anus
V12.70 Personal history of unspecified digestive disease
V12.72 Personal history of colonic polyps
V12.79 Personal history of other diseases of digestive disease
V71.89 Observation for other specified suspected conditions
V71.9 Observation for unspecified suspected condition

ICD-9-CM Procedural

45.23 Colonoscopy
45.25 Closed [endoscopic] biopsy of large intestine
88.74 Diagnostic ultrasound of digestive system

HCPCS Level II Supplies & Services

A4270 Disposable endoscope sheath, each
A4305 Disposable drug delivery system, flow rate of 50 ml or greater per hour
A4306 Disposable drug delivery system, flow rate of 5 ml or less per hour
A4550 Surgical trays

45500

45500 Proctoplasty; for stenosis

ICD-9-CM Diagnostic

569.2 Stenosis of rectum and anus

ICD-9-CM Procedural

48.79 Other repair of rectum

45505

45505 Proctoplasty; for prolapse of mucous membrane

ICD-9-CM Diagnostic

569.1 Rectal prolapse

ICD-9-CM Procedural

48.79 Other repair of rectum

45520

45520 Perirectal injection of sclerosing solution for prolapse

ICD-9-CM Diagnostic

569.1 Rectal prolapse

ICD-9-CM Procedural

99.29 Injection or infusion of other therapeutic or prophylactic substance
99.77 Application or administration of adhesion barrier substance

HCPCS Level II Supplies & Services

A4305 Disposable drug delivery system, flow rate of 50 ml or greater per hour
A4306 Disposable drug delivery system, flow rate of 5 ml or less per hour
A4550 Surgical trays

45540

45540 Proctopexy for prolapse; abdominal approach

ICD-9-CM Diagnostic

569.1 Rectal prolapse

ICD-9-CM Procedural

48.75 Abdominal proctopexy

45541

45541 Proctopexy for prolapse; perineal approach

ICD-9-CM Diagnostic

569.1 Rectal prolapse

ICD-9-CM Procedural

48.76 Other proctopexy

45550

45550 Proctopexy combined with sigmoid resection, abdominal approach

ICD-9-CM Diagnostic

569.1 Rectal prolapse

ICD-9-CM Procedural

45.76 Sigmoidectomy
48.75 Abdominal proctopexy

45560

45560 Repair of rectocele (separate procedure)

ICD-9-CM Diagnostic

569.1 Rectal prolapse
569.49 Other specified disorder of rectum and anus
618.00 Prolapse of vaginal walls without mention of uterine prolapse, unspecified
618.04 Rectocele without mention of uterine prolapse
618.2 Uterovaginal prolapse, incomplete — (Use additional code to identify urinary incontinence: 625.6, 788.31, 788.33-788.39) ♀
618.3 Uterovaginal prolapse, complete — (Use additional code to identify urinary incontinence: 625.6, 788.31, 788.33-788.39) ♀

Unspecified code ☒ Manifestation code
♀ Female diagnosis ♂ Male diagnosis

618.4 Uterovaginal prolapse, unspecified — (Use additional code to identify urinary incontinence: 625.6, 788.31, 788.33-788.39) ▽ ♀
618.82 Incompetence or weakening of rectovaginal tissue

ICD-9-CM Procedural
70.52 Repair of rectocele

45562–45563
45562 Exploration, repair, and presacral drainage for rectal injury;
45563 with colostomy

ICD-9-CM Diagnostic
569.42 Anal or rectal pain
863.45 Rectum injury without mention of open wound into cavity
863.46 Injury to multiple sites in colon and rectum without mention of open wound into cavity
863.55 Rectum injury with open wound into cavity
863.56 Injury to multiple sites in colon and rectum with open wound into cavity

ICD-9-CM Procedural
46.11 Temporary colostomy
46.13 Permanent colostomy
48.69 Other resection of rectum
48.71 Suture of laceration of rectum
48.79 Other repair of rectum
75.62 Repair of current obstetric laceration of rectum and sphincter ani

45800–45805
45800 Closure of rectovesical fistula;
45805 with colostomy

ICD-9-CM Diagnostic
596.1 Intestinovesical fistula — (Use additional code to identify urinary incontinence: 625.6, 788.30-788.39)
625.6 Female stress incontinence ♀
753.8 Other specified congenital anomaly of bladder and urethra
788.30 Unspecified urinary incontinence ▽
788.31 Urge incontinence
788.32 Stress incontinence, male ♂
788.33 Mixed incontinence urge and stress (male)(female)
788.34 Incontinence without sensory awareness
788.35 Post-void dribbling
788.36 Nocturnal enuresis
788.37 Continuous leakage
788.39 Other urinary incontinence

ICD-9-CM Procedural
46.11 Temporary colostomy
46.13 Permanent colostomy
57.83 Repair of fistula involving bladder and intestine

45820–45825
45820 Closure of rectourethral fistula;
45825 with colostomy

ICD-9-CM Diagnostic
599.1 Urethral fistula
625.6 Female stress incontinence ♀
753.8 Other specified congenital anomaly of bladder and urethra
788.30 Unspecified urinary incontinence ▽
788.31 Urge incontinence
788.32 Stress incontinence, male ♂
788.33 Mixed incontinence urge and stress (male)(female)
788.34 Incontinence without sensory awareness
788.35 Post-void dribbling
788.36 Nocturnal enuresis
788.37 Continuous leakage
788.39 Other urinary incontinence

ICD-9-CM Procedural
46.03 Exteriorization of large intestine
46.10 Colostomy, not otherwise specified
46.11 Temporary colostomy
46.13 Permanent colostomy
58.43 Closure of other fistula of urethra

45900
45900 Reduction of procidentia (separate procedure) under anesthesia

ICD-9-CM Diagnostic
569.1 Rectal prolapse

ICD-9-CM Procedural
96.26 Manual reduction of rectal prolapse

HCPCS Level II Supplies & Services
A4305 Disposable drug delivery system, flow rate of 50 ml or greater per hour
A4306 Disposable drug delivery system, flow rate of 5 ml or less per hour
A4550 Surgical trays

45905
45905 Dilation of anal sphincter (separate procedure) under anesthesia other than local

ICD-9-CM Diagnostic
154.2 Malignant neoplasm of anal canal
211.4 Benign neoplasm of rectum and anal canal
455.2 Internal hemorrhoids with other complication
555.1 Regional enteritis of large intestine
564.6 Anal spasm
564.81 Neurogenic bowel
564.89 Other functional disorders of intestine
564.9 Unspecified functional disorder of intestine ▽
565.0 Anal fissure
565.1 Anal fistula
566 Abscess of anal and rectal regions
569.2 Stenosis of rectum and anus
569.41 Ulcer of anus and rectum
569.42 Anal or rectal pain
578.1 Blood in stool
751.2 Congenital atresia and stenosis of large intestine, rectum, and anal canal

ICD-9-CM Procedural
96.23 Dilation of anal sphincter

HCPCS Level II Supplies & Services
A4305 Disposable drug delivery system, flow rate of 50 ml or greater per hour
A4306 Disposable drug delivery system, flow rate of 5 ml or less per hour
A4550 Surgical trays

45910
45910 Dilation of rectal stricture (separate procedure) under anesthesia other than local

ICD-9-CM Diagnostic
154.2 Malignant neoplasm of anal canal
211.3 Benign neoplasm of colon
455.2 Internal hemorrhoids with other complication
564.00 Unspecified constipation ▽
564.02 Outlet dysfunction constipation
564.09 Other constipation
565.1 Anal fistula
569.2 Stenosis of rectum and anus
569.42 Anal or rectal pain
578.1 Blood in stool
751.2 Congenital atresia and stenosis of large intestine, rectum, and anal canal

ICD-9-CM Procedural
96.22 Dilation of rectum

HCPCS Level II Supplies & Services
A4305 Disposable drug delivery system, flow rate of 50 ml or greater per hour
A4306 Disposable drug delivery system, flow rate of 5 ml or less per hour
A4550 Surgical trays

45915
45915 Removal of fecal impaction or foreign body (separate procedure) under anesthesia

ICD-9-CM Diagnostic
560.1 Paralytic ileus
560.39 Other impaction of intestine

▽ Unspecified code
♀ Female diagnosis
☒ Manifestation code
♂ Male diagnosis

564.00 Unspecified constipation ▽
564.01 Slow transit constipation
564.02 Outlet dysfunction constipation
564.09 Other constipation
569.1 Rectal prolapse
569.2 Stenosis of rectum and anus
569.42 Anal or rectal pain
578.1 Blood in stool
787.5 Abnormal bowel sounds
937 Foreign body in anus and rectum

ICD-9-CM Procedural
96.38 Removal of impacted feces
98.05 Removal of intraluminal foreign body from rectum and anus without incision

HCPCS Level II Supplies & Services
A4305 Disposable drug delivery system, flow rate of 50 ml or greater per hour
A4306 Disposable drug delivery system, flow rate of 5 ml or less per hour
A4550 Surgical trays

Anus

46020
46020 Placement of seton

ICD-9-CM Diagnostic
565.1 Anal fistula
566 Abscess of anal and rectal regions
567.2 Other suppurative peritonitis
569.3 Hemorrhage of rectum and anus
569.42 Anal or rectal pain
569.5 Abscess of intestine
578.1 Blood in stool
751.5 Other congenital anomalies of intestine
958.3 Posttraumatic wound infection not elsewhere classified
998.51 Infected postoperative seroma — (Use additional code to identify organism)
998.59 Other postoperative infection — (Use additional code to identify infection)
998.6 Persistent postoperative fistula, not elsewhere classified

ICD-9-CM Procedural
49.99 Other operations on anus

HCPCS Level II Supplies & Services
A4550 Surgical trays

46030
46030 Removal of anal seton, other marker

ICD-9-CM Diagnostic
565.1 Anal fistula
566 Abscess of anal and rectal regions
619.1 Digestive-genital tract fistula, female ♀

ICD-9-CM Procedural
49.93 Other incision of anus

HCPCS Level II Supplies & Services
A4305 Disposable drug delivery system, flow rate of 50 ml or greater per hour
A4306 Disposable drug delivery system, flow rate of 5 ml or less per hour
A4550 Surgical trays

46040
46040 Incision and drainage of ischiorectal and/or perirectal abscess (separate procedure)

ICD-9-CM Diagnostic
455.5 External hemorrhoids with other complication
555.1 Regional enteritis of large intestine
555.2 Regional enteritis of small intestine with large intestine
555.9 Regional enteritis of unspecified site ▽
556.9 Unspecified ulcerative colitis ▽
562.11 Diverticulitis of colon (without mention of hemorrhage) — (Use additional code to identify any associated peritonitis: 567.0-567.9)
565.0 Anal fissure
565.1 Anal fistula
566 Abscess of anal and rectal regions
567.0 Peritonitis in infectious diseases classified elsewhere — (Code first underlying disease) ☒
567.1 Pneumococcal peritonitis
567.2 Other suppurative peritonitis
567.8 Other specified peritonitis
567.9 Unspecified peritonitis ▽
682.5 Cellulitis and abscess of buttock — (Use additional code to identify organism)
958.3 Posttraumatic wound infection not elsewhere classified
998.51 Infected postoperative seroma — (Use additional code to identify organism)
998.59 Other postoperative infection — (Use additional code to identify infection)

ICD-9-CM Procedural
48.81 Incision of perirectal tissue
49.01 Incision of perianal abscess

HCPCS Level II Supplies & Services
A4305 Disposable drug delivery system, flow rate of 50 ml or greater per hour
A4306 Disposable drug delivery system, flow rate of 5 ml or less per hour
A4550 Surgical trays

46045
46045 Incision and drainage of intramural, intramuscular, or submucosal abscess, transanal, under anesthesia

ICD-9-CM Diagnostic
555.1 Regional enteritis of large intestine
555.9 Regional enteritis of unspecified site ▽
562.11 Diverticulitis of colon (without mention of hemorrhage) — (Use additional code to identify any associated peritonitis: 567.0-567.9)
565.1 Anal fistula
566 Abscess of anal and rectal regions
567.0 Peritonitis in infectious diseases classified elsewhere — (Code first underlying disease) ☒
567.1 Pneumococcal peritonitis
567.2 Other suppurative peritonitis
567.8 Other specified peritonitis
567.9 Unspecified peritonitis ▽
680.5 Carbuncle and furuncle of buttock
682.2 Cellulitis and abscess of trunk — (Use additional code to identify organism)
682.5 Cellulitis and abscess of buttock — (Use additional code to identify organism)
958.3 Posttraumatic wound infection not elsewhere classified
998.51 Infected postoperative seroma — (Use additional code to identify organism)
998.59 Other postoperative infection — (Use additional code to identify infection)

ICD-9-CM Procedural
49.02 Other incision of perianal tissue
49.93 Other incision of anus

46050
46050 Incision and drainage, perianal abscess, superficial

ICD-9-CM Diagnostic
566 Abscess of anal and rectal regions
569.3 Hemorrhage of rectum and anus
680.5 Carbuncle and furuncle of buttock
958.3 Posttraumatic wound infection not elsewhere classified
998.51 Infected postoperative seroma — (Use additional code to identify organism)
998.59 Other postoperative infection — (Use additional code to identify infection)

ICD-9-CM Procedural
49.01 Incision of perianal abscess

HCPCS Level II Supplies & Services
A4305 Disposable drug delivery system, flow rate of 50 ml or greater per hour
A4306 Disposable drug delivery system, flow rate of 5 ml or less per hour
A4550 Surgical trays

▽ Unspecified code
♀ Female diagnosis
☒ Manifestation code
♂ Male diagnosis

46060

46060 Incision and drainage of ischiorectal or intramural abscess, with fistulectomy or fistulotomy, submuscular, with or without placement of seton

ICD-9-CM Diagnostic

562.11 Diverticulitis of colon (without mention of hemorrhage) — (Use additional code to identify any associated peritonitis: 567.0-567.9)
565.1 Anal fistula
566 Abscess of anal and rectal regions
567.0 Peritonitis in infectious diseases classified elsewhere — (Code first underlying disease) ☒
567.1 Pneumococcal peritonitis
567.2 Other suppurative peritonitis
567.8 Other specified peritonitis
567.9 Unspecified peritonitis ▽
569.42 Anal or rectal pain
569.49 Other specified disorder of rectum and anus
569.5 Abscess of intestine
682.2 Cellulitis and abscess of trunk — (Use additional code to identify organism)
682.5 Cellulitis and abscess of buttock — (Use additional code to identify organism)
958.3 Posttraumatic wound infection not elsewhere classified
998.51 Infected postoperative seroma — (Use additional code to identify organism)
998.59 Other postoperative infection — (Use additional code to identify infection)

ICD-9-CM Procedural

49.01 Incision of perianal abscess
49.02 Other incision of perianal tissue
49.11 Anal fistulotomy
49.12 Anal fistulectomy

HCPCS Level II Supplies & Services

A4305 Disposable drug delivery system, flow rate of 50 ml or greater per hour
A4306 Disposable drug delivery system, flow rate of 5 ml or less per hour
A4550 Surgical trays

46070

46070 Incision, anal septum (infant)

ICD-9-CM Diagnostic

751.5 Other congenital anomalies of intestine

ICD-9-CM Procedural

49.91 Incision of anal septum

HCPCS Level II Supplies & Services

A4305 Disposable drug delivery system, flow rate of 50 ml or greater per hour
A4306 Disposable drug delivery system, flow rate of 5 ml or less per hour
A4550 Surgical trays

46080

46080 Sphincterotomy, anal, division of sphincter (separate procedure)

ICD-9-CM Diagnostic

211.4 Benign neoplasm of rectum and anal canal
455.0 Internal hemorrhoids without mention of complication
455.1 Internal thrombosed hemorrhoids
455.2 Internal hemorrhoids with other complication
455.9 Residual hemorrhoidal skin tags
564.00 Unspecified constipation ▽
564.02 Outlet dysfunction constipation
564.09 Other constipation
565.0 Anal fissure
565.1 Anal fistula
569.0 Anal and rectal polyp
569.1 Rectal prolapse
569.2 Stenosis of rectum and anus
569.3 Hemorrhage of rectum and anus
569.41 Ulcer of anus and rectum
569.42 Anal or rectal pain
569.49 Other specified disorder of rectum and anus
578.1 Blood in stool

ICD-9-CM Procedural

49.51 Left lateral anal sphincterotomy
49.52 Posterior anal sphincterotomy
49.59 Other anal sphincterotomy

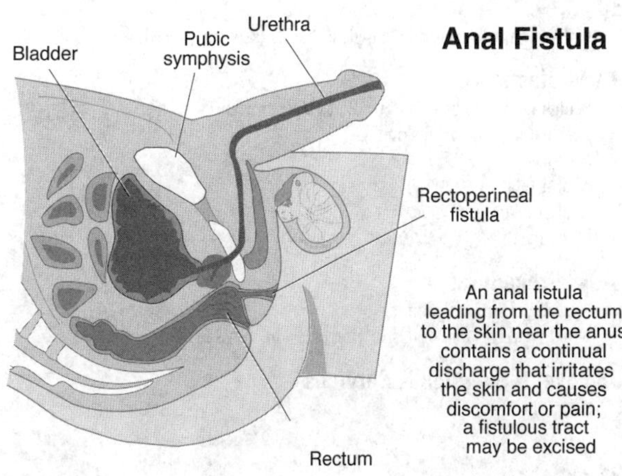

Anal Fistula

An anal fistula leading from the rectum to the skin near the anus contains a continual discharge that irritates the skin and causes discomfort or pain; a fistulous tract may be excised

46083

46083 Incision of thrombosed hemorrhoid, external

ICD-9-CM Diagnostic

455.4 External thrombosed hemorrhoids
569.42 Anal or rectal pain
578.1 Blood in stool

ICD-9-CM Procedural

49.47 Evacuation of thrombosed hemorrhoids

HCPCS Level II Supplies & Services

A4550 Surgical trays

46200

46200 Fissurectomy, with or without sphincterotomy

ICD-9-CM Diagnostic

555.1 Regional enteritis of large intestine
565.0 Anal fissure
565.1 Anal fistula
566 Abscess of anal and rectal regions
569.0 Anal and rectal polyp
569.1 Rectal prolapse
569.2 Stenosis of rectum and anus
569.3 Hemorrhage of rectum and anus
569.41 Ulcer of anus and rectum
569.42 Anal or rectal pain
569.49 Other specified disorder of rectum and anus
578.1 Blood in stool
751.2 Congenital atresia and stenosis of large intestine, rectum, and anal canal
751.5 Other congenital anomalies of intestine

ICD-9-CM Procedural

49.39 Other local excision or destruction of lesion or tissue of anus
49.51 Left lateral anal sphincterotomy
49.52 Posterior anal sphincterotomy

46210–46211

46210 Cryptectomy; single
46211 multiple (separate procedure)

ICD-9-CM Diagnostic

211.4 Benign neoplasm of rectum and anal canal
455.2 Internal hemorrhoids with other complication
565.1 Anal fistula
566 Abscess of anal and rectal regions
569.49 Other specified disorder of rectum and anus
578.1 Blood in stool

ICD-9-CM Procedural

49.39 Other local excision or destruction of lesion or tissue of anus

▽ Unspecified code ♀ Female diagnosis ☒ Manifestation code ♂ Male diagnosis

46220

46220 Papillectomy or excision of single tag, anus (separate procedure)

ICD-9-CM Diagnostic

216.5 Benign neoplasm of skin of trunk, except scrotum
455.9 Residual hemorrhoidal skin tags
565.0 Anal fissure
565.1 Anal fistula
569.42 Anal or rectal pain
578.1 Blood in stool

ICD-9-CM Procedural

49.03 Excision of perianal skin tags
49.39 Other local excision or destruction of lesion or tissue of anus

HCPCS Level II Supplies & Services

A4550 Surgical trays

46221

46221 Hemorrhoidectomy, by simple ligature (eg, rubber band)

ICD-9-CM Diagnostic

455.0 Internal hemorrhoids without mention of complication
455.1 Internal thrombosed hemorrhoids
455.2 Internal hemorrhoids with other complication
455.3 External hemorrhoids without mention of complication
455.4 External thrombosed hemorrhoids
455.5 External hemorrhoids with other complication
455.7 Unspecified thrombosed hemorrhoids ▽
455.9 Residual hemorrhoidal skin tags
569.1 Rectal prolapse
569.3 Hemorrhage of rectum and anus
569.41 Ulcer of anus and rectum
569.42 Anal or rectal pain
569.49 Other specified disorder of rectum and anus
578.1 Blood in stool

ICD-9-CM Procedural

49.45 Ligation of hemorrhoids

46230

46230 Excision of external hemorrhoid tags and/or multiple papillae

ICD-9-CM Diagnostic

455.3 External hemorrhoids without mention of complication
455.5 External hemorrhoids with other complication
455.9 Residual hemorrhoidal skin tags
565.0 Anal fissure
565.1 Anal fistula
569.0 Anal and rectal polyp
569.41 Ulcer of anus and rectum
569.49 Other specified disorder of rectum and anus
578.1 Blood in stool
787.99 Other symptoms involving digestive system

ICD-9-CM Procedural

49.03 Excision of perianal skin tags
49.46 Excision of hemorrhoids

HCPCS Level II Supplies & Services

A4550 Surgical trays

46250

46250 Hemorrhoidectomy, external, complete

ICD-9-CM Diagnostic

455.3 External hemorrhoids without mention of complication
455.4 External thrombosed hemorrhoids
455.5 External hemorrhoids with other complication
455.7 Unspecified thrombosed hemorrhoids ▽
455.9 Residual hemorrhoidal skin tags
569.3 Hemorrhage of rectum and anus
569.42 Anal or rectal pain
578.1 Blood in stool

ICD-9-CM Procedural

49.46 Excision of hemorrhoids

46255–46258

46255 Hemorrhoidectomy, internal and external, simple;
46257 with fissurectomy
46258 with fistulectomy, with or without fissurectomy

ICD-9-CM Diagnostic

211.4 Benign neoplasm of rectum and anal canal
455.0 Internal hemorrhoids without mention of complication
455.1 Internal thrombosed hemorrhoids
455.2 Internal hemorrhoids with other complication
455.3 External hemorrhoids without mention of complication
455.4 External thrombosed hemorrhoids
455.5 External hemorrhoids with other complication
455.7 Unspecified thrombosed hemorrhoids ▽
455.9 Residual hemorrhoidal skin tags
564.6 Anal spasm
565.0 Anal fissure
565.1 Anal fistula
566 Abscess of anal and rectal regions
569.3 Hemorrhage of rectum and anus
569.41 Ulcer of anus and rectum
569.42 Anal or rectal pain
578.1 Blood in stool
751.5 Other congenital anomalies of intestine

ICD-9-CM Procedural

49.12 Anal fistulectomy
49.39 Other local excision or destruction of lesion or tissue of anus
49.46 Excision of hemorrhoids

46260–46262

46260 Hemorrhoidectomy, internal and external, complex or extensive;
46261 with fissurectomy
46262 with fistulectomy, with or without fissurectomy

ICD-9-CM Diagnostic

455.0 Internal hemorrhoids without mention of complication
455.1 Internal thrombosed hemorrhoids
455.2 Internal hemorrhoids with other complication
455.3 External hemorrhoids without mention of complication
455.4 External thrombosed hemorrhoids
455.5 External hemorrhoids with other complication
455.7 Unspecified thrombosed hemorrhoids ▽
455.9 Residual hemorrhoidal skin tags
564.6 Anal spasm
565.0 Anal fissure
565.1 Anal fistula
566 Abscess of anal and rectal regions
569.3 Hemorrhage of rectum and anus
569.42 Anal or rectal pain
578.1 Blood in stool
751.5 Other congenital anomalies of intestine

ICD-9-CM Procedural

49.12 Anal fistulectomy
49.39 Other local excision or destruction of lesion or tissue of anus
49.46 Excision of hemorrhoids

46270–46285

46270 Surgical treatment of anal fistula (fistulectomy/fistulotomy); subcutaneous
46275 submuscular
46280 complex or multiple, with or without placement of seton
46285 second stage

ICD-9-CM Diagnostic

565.1 Anal fistula
566 Abscess of anal and rectal regions
569.3 Hemorrhage of rectum and anus
569.42 Anal or rectal pain
578.1 Blood in stool
751.5 Other congenital anomalies of intestine
998.6 Persistent postoperative fistula, not elsewhere classified

▽ Unspecified code ♀ Female diagnosis ☒ Manifestation code ♂ Male diagnosis

ICD-9-CM Procedural
49.11 Anal fistulotomy
49.12 Anal fistulectomy
49.73 Closure of anal fistula
49.93 Other incision of anus

46288
46288 Closure of anal fistula with rectal advancement flap

ICD-9-CM Diagnostic
555.9 Regional enteritis of unspecified site
565.1 Anal fistula
566 Abscess of anal and rectal regions
569.3 Hemorrhage of rectum and anus
569.42 Anal or rectal pain
569.49 Other specified disorder of rectum and anus
569.69 Other complication of colostomy or enterostomy
578.1 Blood in stool
751.5 Other congenital anomalies of intestine
998.6 Persistent postoperative fistula, not elsewhere classified

ICD-9-CM Procedural
49.73 Closure of anal fistula

46320
46320 Enucleation or excision of external thrombotic hemorrhoid

ICD-9-CM Diagnostic
455.4 External thrombosed hemorrhoids
569.3 Hemorrhage of rectum and anus
569.42 Anal or rectal pain
578.1 Blood in stool

ICD-9-CM Procedural
49.46 Excision of hemorrhoids
49.47 Evacuation of thrombosed hemorrhoids

HCPCS Level II Supplies & Services
A4305 Disposable drug delivery system, flow rate of 50 ml or greater per hour
A4306 Disposable drug delivery system, flow rate of 5 ml or less per hour
A4550 Surgical trays

46500
46500 Injection of sclerosing solution, hemorrhoids

ICD-9-CM Diagnostic
455.0 Internal hemorrhoids without mention of complication
455.1 Internal thrombosed hemorrhoids
455.2 Internal hemorrhoids with other complication
455.3 External hemorrhoids without mention of complication
455.4 External thrombosed hemorrhoids
455.5 External hemorrhoids with other complication
455.7 Unspecified thrombosed hemorrhoids
569.3 Hemorrhage of rectum and anus
569.42 Anal or rectal pain
578.1 Blood in stool

ICD-9-CM Procedural
49.42 Injection of hemorrhoids

HCPCS Level II Supplies & Services
A4550 Surgical trays

46600–46606
46600 Anoscopy; diagnostic, with or without collection of specimen(s) by brushing or washing (separate procedure)
46604 with dilation (eg, balloon, guide wire, bougie)
46606 with biopsy, single or multiple

ICD-9-CM Diagnostic
154.1 Malignant neoplasm of rectum
154.2 Malignant neoplasm of anal canal
154.3 Malignant neoplasm of anus, unspecified site
198.82 Secondary malignant neoplasm of genital organs
211.4 Benign neoplasm of rectum and anal canal
230.5 Carcinoma in situ of anal canal
235.5 Neoplasm of uncertain behavior of other and unspecified digestive organs
239.0 Neoplasm of unspecified nature of digestive system
455.0 Internal hemorrhoids without mention of complication
455.1 Internal thrombosed hemorrhoids
455.2 Internal hemorrhoids with other complication
455.3 External hemorrhoids without mention of complication
455.4 External thrombosed hemorrhoids
455.5 External hemorrhoids with other complication
455.7 Unspecified thrombosed hemorrhoids
455.9 Residual hemorrhoidal skin tags
555.1 Regional enteritis of large intestine
556.0 Ulcerative (chronic) enterocolitis
557.9 Unspecified vascular insufficiency of intestine
558.3 Gastroenteritis and colitis, allergic — (Use additional code to identify type of food allergy: V15.01-V15.05)
558.9 Other and unspecified noninfectious gastroenteritis and colitis
560.39 Other impaction of intestine
560.81 Intestinal or peritoneal adhesions with obstruction (postoperative) (postinfection)
560.89 Other specified intestinal obstruction
562.10 Diverticulosis of colon (without mention of hemorrhage) — (Use additional code to identify any associated peritonitis: 567.0-567.9)
562.11 Diverticulitis of colon (without mention of hemorrhage) — (Use additional code to identify any associated peritonitis: 567.0-567.9)
562.12 Diverticulosis of colon with hemorrhage — (Use additional code to identify any associated peritonitis: 567.0-567.9)
564.00 Unspecified constipation
564.01 Slow transit constipation
564.02 Outlet dysfunction constipation
564.09 Other constipation
564.1 Irritable bowel syndrome
564.6 Anal spasm
564.7 Megacolon, other than Hirschsprung's
564.81 Neurogenic bowel
564.89 Other functional disorders of intestine
565.0 Anal fissure
565.1 Anal fistula
566 Abscess of anal and rectal regions
567.0 Peritonitis in infectious diseases classified elsewhere — (Code first underlying disease)
567.1 Pneumococcal peritonitis
567.2 Other suppurative peritonitis
567.8 Other specified peritonitis
567.9 Unspecified peritonitis
569.1 Rectal prolapse
569.2 Stenosis of rectum and anus
569.3 Hemorrhage of rectum and anus
569.41 Ulcer of anus and rectum
569.42 Anal or rectal pain
569.49 Other specified disorder of rectum and anus
578.1 Blood in stool
698.0 Pruritus ani
751.2 Congenital atresia and stenosis of large intestine, rectum, and anal canal
787.3 Flatulence, eructation, and gas pain
787.6 Incontinence of feces
787.99 Other symptoms involving digestive system
V10.05 Personal history of malignant neoplasm of large intestine
V10.06 Personal history of malignant neoplasm of rectum, rectosigmoid junction, and anus
V70.0 Routine general medical examination at health care facility — (Use additional code(s) to identify any special screening examination(s) performed: V73.0-V82.9)

ICD-9-CM Procedural
49.21 Anoscopy
49.23 Biopsy of anus
96.23 Dilation of anal sphincter

HCPCS Level II Supplies & Services
A4270 Disposable endoscope sheath, each
A4305 Disposable drug delivery system, flow rate of 50 ml or greater per hour
A4306 Disposable drug delivery system, flow rate of 5 ml or less per hour
A4550 Surgical trays

46608

46608 Anoscopy; with removal of foreign body

ICD-9-CM Diagnostic

564.00 Unspecified constipation
564.01 Slow transit constipation
564.02 Outlet dysfunction constipation
564.09 Other constipation
564.6 Anal spasm
569.42 Anal or rectal pain
578.1 Blood in stool
937 Foreign body in anus and rectum

ICD-9-CM Procedural

49.21 Anoscopy
98.05 Removal of intraluminal foreign body from rectum and anus without incision

HCPCS Level II Supplies & Services

A4270 Disposable endoscope sheath, each
A4305 Disposable drug delivery system, flow rate of 50 ml or greater per hour
A4306 Disposable drug delivery system, flow rate of 5 ml or less per hour
A4550 Surgical trays

46610–46612

46610 Anoscopy; with removal of single tumor, polyp, or other lesion by hot biopsy forceps or bipolar cautery
46611 with removal of single tumor, polyp, or other lesion by snare technique
46612 with removal of multiple tumors, polyps, or other lesions by hot biopsy forceps, bipolar cautery or snare technique

ICD-9-CM Diagnostic

154.1 Malignant neoplasm of rectum
154.2 Malignant neoplasm of anal canal
154.8 Malignant neoplasm of other sites of rectum, rectosigmoid junction, and anus
211.4 Benign neoplasm of rectum and anal canal
230.8 Carcinoma in situ of liver and biliary system
235.5 Neoplasm of uncertain behavior of other and unspecified digestive organs
239.0 Neoplasm of unspecified nature of digestive system
569.0 Anal and rectal polyp
569.3 Hemorrhage of rectum and anus
569.41 Ulcer of anus and rectum
569.42 Anal or rectal pain
569.49 Other specified disorder of rectum and anus
578.1 Blood in stool
698.0 Pruritus ani
793.4 Nonspecific abnormal findings on radiological and other examination of gastrointestinal tract

ICD-9-CM Procedural

49.31 Endoscopic excision or destruction of lesion or tissue of anus

HCPCS Level II Supplies & Services

A4270 Disposable endoscope sheath, each
A4305 Disposable drug delivery system, flow rate of 50 ml or greater per hour
A4306 Disposable drug delivery system, flow rate of 5 ml or less per hour
A4550 Surgical trays

46614

46614 Anoscopy; with control of bleeding (eg, injection, bipolar cautery, unipolar cautery, laser, heater probe, stapler, plasma coagulator)

ICD-9-CM Diagnostic

154.1 Malignant neoplasm of rectum
154.2 Malignant neoplasm of anal canal
154.8 Malignant neoplasm of other sites of rectum, rectosigmoid junction, and anus
211.4 Benign neoplasm of rectum and anal canal
455.0 Internal hemorrhoids without mention of complication
455.1 Internal thrombosed hemorrhoids
455.2 Internal hemorrhoids with other complication
455.3 External hemorrhoids without mention of complication
455.4 External thrombosed hemorrhoids
455.5 External hemorrhoids with other complication
455.8 Unspecified hemorrhoids with other complication
558.9 Other and unspecified noninfectious gastroenteritis and colitis
569.3 Hemorrhage of rectum and anus
569.41 Ulcer of anus and rectum
998.11 Hemorrhage complicating a procedure

ICD-9-CM Procedural

49.95 Control of (postoperative) hemorrhage of anus

HCPCS Level II Supplies & Services

A4270 Disposable endoscope sheath, each
A4305 Disposable drug delivery system, flow rate of 50 ml or greater per hour
A4306 Disposable drug delivery system, flow rate of 5 ml or less per hour
A4550 Surgical trays

46615

46615 Anoscopy; with ablation of tumor(s), polyp(s), or other lesion(s) not amenable to removal by hot biopsy forceps, bipolar cautery or snare technique

ICD-9-CM Diagnostic

154.1 Malignant neoplasm of rectum
154.2 Malignant neoplasm of anal canal
154.8 Malignant neoplasm of other sites of rectum, rectosigmoid junction, and anus
211.4 Benign neoplasm of rectum and anal canal
230.5 Carcinoma in situ of anal canal
239.0 Neoplasm of unspecified nature of digestive system
558.9 Other and unspecified noninfectious gastroenteritis and colitis
569.0 Anal and rectal polyp
569.3 Hemorrhage of rectum and anus
569.41 Ulcer of anus and rectum
578.1 Blood in stool
787.99 Other symptoms involving digestive system

ICD-9-CM Procedural

49.31 Endoscopic excision or destruction of lesion or tissue of anus

HCPCS Level II Supplies & Services

A4270 Disposable endoscope sheath, each
A4305 Disposable drug delivery system, flow rate of 50 ml or greater per hour
A4306 Disposable drug delivery system, flow rate of 5 ml or less per hour
A4550 Surgical trays

46700–46705

46700 Anoplasty, plastic operation for stricture; adult
46705 infant

ICD-9-CM Diagnostic

564.00 Unspecified constipation
564.02 Outlet dysfunction constipation
564.09 Other constipation
569.2 Stenosis of rectum and anus
569.42 Anal or rectal pain
751.2 Congenital atresia and stenosis of large intestine, rectum, and anal canal
908.1 Late effect of internal injury to intra-abdominal organs
908.6 Late effect of certain complications of trauma

ICD-9-CM Procedural

49.79 Other repair of anal sphincter

46706

46706 Repair of anal fistula with fibrin glue

ICD-9-CM Diagnostic

565.1 Anal fistula
569.42 Anal or rectal pain
998.6 Persistent postoperative fistula, not elsewhere classified

ICD-9-CM Procedural

49.73 Closure of anal fistula

HCPCS Level II Supplies & Services

HCPCS Level II codes are used to report the supplies, durable medical equipment, and certain medical services provided on an outpatient basis. Because the procedure(s) represented on this page would be performed in an inpatient or outpatient facility, no HCPCS Level II codes apply.

46715

46715 Repair of low imperforate anus; with anoperineal fistula (cut-back procedure)

ICD-9-CM Diagnostic

751.2 Congenital atresia and stenosis of large intestine, rectum, and anal canal
751.8 Other specified congenital anomalies of digestive system

ICD-9-CM Procedural

49.11 Anal fistulotomy
49.79 Other repair of anal sphincter

46716

46716 Repair of low imperforate anus; with transposition of anoperineal or anovestibular fistula

ICD-9-CM Diagnostic

751.2 Congenital atresia and stenosis of large intestine, rectum, and anal canal
751.8 Other specified congenital anomalies of digestive system

ICD-9-CM Procedural

49.11 Anal fistulotomy
49.79 Other repair of anal sphincter

46730–46735

46730 Repair of high imperforate anus without fistula; perineal or sacroperineal approach
46735 combined transabdominal and sacroperineal approaches

ICD-9-CM Diagnostic

751.2 Congenital atresia and stenosis of large intestine, rectum, and anal canal
751.8 Other specified congenital anomalies of digestive system

ICD-9-CM Procedural

48.69 Other resection of rectum
49.79 Other repair of anal sphincter
49.99 Other operations on anus

46740–46742

46740 Repair of high imperforate anus with rectourethral or rectovaginal fistula; perineal or sacroperineal approach
46742 combined transabdominal and sacroperineal approaches

ICD-9-CM Diagnostic

751.2 Congenital atresia and stenosis of large intestine, rectum, and anal canal
753.8 Other specified congenital anomaly of bladder and urethra

ICD-9-CM Procedural

49.79 Other repair of anal sphincter
49.99 Other operations on anus
58.43 Closure of other fistula of urethra
70.73 Repair of rectovaginal fistula

46744–46748

46744 Repair of cloacal anomaly by anorectovaginoplasty and urethroplasty, sacroperineal approach
46746 Repair of cloacal anomaly by anorectovaginoplasty and urethroplasty, combined abdominal and sacroperineal approach;
46748 with vaginal lengthening by intestinal graft or pedicle flaps

ICD-9-CM Diagnostic

751.5 Other congenital anomalies of intestine
752.40 Unspecified congenital anomaly of cervix, vagina, and external female genitalia ▽ ♀
752.89 Other specified anomalies of genital organs
752.9 Unspecified congenital anomaly of genital organs ▽

ICD-9-CM Procedural

48.79 Other repair of rectum
49.79 Other repair of anal sphincter
56.89 Other repair of ureter
70.73 Repair of rectovaginal fistula
70.79 Other repair of vagina
71.9 Other operations on female genital organs

46750–46751

46750 Sphincteroplasty, anal, for incontinence or prolapse; adult
46751 child

ICD-9-CM Diagnostic

569.1 Rectal prolapse
578.1 Blood in stool
787.6 Incontinence of feces
863.45 Rectum injury without mention of open wound into cavity
863.55 Rectum injury with open wound into cavity

ICD-9-CM Procedural

49.79 Other repair of anal sphincter

HCPCS Level II Supplies & Services

A4520 Incontinence garment, any type, (e.g. brief, diaper), each

46753

46753 Graft (Thiersch operation) for rectal incontinence and/or prolapse

ICD-9-CM Diagnostic

569.1 Rectal prolapse
569.3 Hemorrhage of rectum and anus
578.1 Blood in stool
787.6 Incontinence of feces
863.45 Rectum injury without mention of open wound into cavity
863.55 Rectum injury with open wound into cavity

ICD-9-CM Procedural

49.79 Other repair of anal sphincter
49.94 Reduction of anal prolapse

HCPCS Level II Supplies & Services

A4520 Incontinence garment, any type, (e.g. brief, diaper), each

46754

46754 Removal of Thiersch wire or suture, anal canal

ICD-9-CM Diagnostic

569.1 Rectal prolapse
569.3 Hemorrhage of rectum and anus
578.1 Blood in stool
787.6 Incontinence of feces
863.45 Rectum injury without mention of open wound into cavity
863.55 Rectum injury with open wound into cavity
V45.89 Other postsurgical status — (This code is intended for use when these conditions are recorded as diagnoses or problems)
V58.3 Attention to surgical dressings and sutures
V58.49 Other specified aftercare following surgery — (This code should be used in conjunction with other aftercare codes to fully identify the reason for the aftercare encounter)

ICD-9-CM Procedural

49.99 Other operations on anus

HCPCS Level II Supplies & Services

A4305 Disposable drug delivery system, flow rate of 50 ml or greater per hour
A4306 Disposable drug delivery system, flow rate of 5 ml or less per hour
A4550 Surgical trays

46760

46760 Sphincteroplasty, anal, for incontinence, adult; muscle transplant

ICD-9-CM Diagnostic

569.1 Rectal prolapse
787.6 Incontinence of feces
863.45 Rectum injury without mention of open wound into cavity
863.55 Rectum injury with open wound into cavity

ICD-9-CM Procedural

49.74 Gracilis muscle transplant for anal incontinence

HCPCS Level II Supplies & Services

A4520 Incontinence garment, any type, (e.g. brief, diaper), each

▽ Unspecified code
♀ Female diagnosis
☒ Manifestation code
♂ Male diagnosis

46761–46762

46761 Sphincteroplasty, anal, for incontinence, adult; levator muscle imbrication (Park posterior anal repair)
46762 implantation artificial sphincter

ICD-9-CM Diagnostic

569.1 Rectal prolapse
787.6 Incontinence of feces
863.45 Rectum injury without mention of open wound into cavity
863.55 Rectum injury with open wound into cavity

ICD-9-CM Procedural

49.75 Implantation or revision of artificial anal sphincter
49.79 Other repair of anal sphincter

46900–46916

46900 Destruction of lesion(s), anus (eg, condyloma, papilloma, molluscum contagiosum, herpetic vesicle), simple; chemical
46910 electrodesiccation
46916 cryosurgery

ICD-9-CM Diagnostic

054.10 Unspecified genital herpes
078.0 Molluscum contagiosum
078.10 Unspecified viral warts
078.11 Condyloma acuminatum
078.19 Other specified viral warts
154.1 Malignant neoplasm of rectum
154.2 Malignant neoplasm of anal canal
154.3 Malignant neoplasm of anus, unspecified site
211.4 Benign neoplasm of rectum and anal canal
214.9 Lipoma of unspecified site
216.5 Benign neoplasm of skin of trunk, except scrotum
216.9 Benign neoplasm of skin, site unspecified
228.01 Hemangioma of skin and subcutaneous tissue
235.5 Neoplasm of uncertain behavior of other and unspecified digestive organs
238.2 Neoplasm of uncertain behavior of skin
239.0 Neoplasm of unspecified nature of digestive system
455.2 Internal hemorrhoids with other complication
569.3 Hemorrhage of rectum and anus
569.41 Ulcer of anus and rectum
569.42 Anal or rectal pain
578.1 Blood in stool

ICD-9-CM Procedural

49.39 Other local excision or destruction of lesion or tissue of anus

HCPCS Level II Supplies & Services

A4305 Disposable drug delivery system, flow rate of 50 ml or greater per hour
A4306 Disposable drug delivery system, flow rate of 5 ml or less per hour
A4550 Surgical trays

46917–46924

46917 Destruction of lesion(s), anus (eg, condyloma, papilloma, molluscum contagiosum, herpetic vesicle), simple; laser surgery
46922 surgical excision
46924 Destruction of lesion(s), anus (eg, condyloma, papilloma, molluscum contagiosum, herpetic vesicle), extensive (eg, laser surgery, electrosurgery, cryosurgery, chemosurgery)

ICD-9-CM Diagnostic

054.10 Unspecified genital herpes
078.0 Molluscum contagiosum
078.10 Unspecified viral warts
078.11 Condyloma acuminatum
078.19 Other specified viral warts
154.1 Malignant neoplasm of rectum
154.2 Malignant neoplasm of anal canal
154.3 Malignant neoplasm of anus, unspecified site
211.4 Benign neoplasm of rectum and anal canal
214.9 Lipoma of unspecified site
216.5 Benign neoplasm of skin of trunk, except scrotum
216.9 Benign neoplasm of skin, site unspecified
228.01 Hemangioma of skin and subcutaneous tissue
235.5 Neoplasm of uncertain behavior of other and unspecified digestive organs
238.2 Neoplasm of uncertain behavior of skin
239.0 Neoplasm of unspecified nature of digestive system
455.2 Internal hemorrhoids with other complication
569.3 Hemorrhage of rectum and anus
569.41 Ulcer of anus and rectum
569.42 Anal or rectal pain
578.1 Blood in stool

ICD-9-CM Procedural

49.39 Other local excision or destruction of lesion or tissue of anus

HCPCS Level II Supplies & Services

A4305 Disposable drug delivery system, flow rate of 50 ml or greater per hour
A4306 Disposable drug delivery system, flow rate of 5 ml or less per hour
A4550 Surgical trays

46934–46936

46934 Destruction of hemorrhoids, any method; internal
46935 external
46936 internal and external

ICD-9-CM Diagnostic

455.0 Internal hemorrhoids without mention of complication
455.1 Internal thrombosed hemorrhoids
455.2 Internal hemorrhoids with other complication
455.3 External hemorrhoids without mention of complication
455.4 External thrombosed hemorrhoids
455.5 External hemorrhoids with other complication
455.7 Unspecified thrombosed hemorrhoids
455.9 Residual hemorrhoidal skin tags
569.3 Hemorrhage of rectum and anus
569.42 Anal or rectal pain
578.1 Blood in stool

ICD-9-CM Procedural

49.43 Cauterization of hemorrhoids
49.44 Destruction of hemorrhoids by cryotherapy
49.49 Other procedures on hemorrhoids

HCPCS Level II Supplies & Services

A4305 Disposable drug delivery system, flow rate of 50 ml or greater per hour
A4306 Disposable drug delivery system, flow rate of 5 ml or less per hour
A4550 Surgical trays

46937–46938

46937 Cryosurgery of rectal tumor; benign
46938 malignant

ICD-9-CM Diagnostic

154.0 Malignant neoplasm of rectosigmoid junction
154.1 Malignant neoplasm of rectum
154.2 Malignant neoplasm of anal canal
154.8 Malignant neoplasm of other sites of rectum, rectosigmoid junction, and anus
211.4 Benign neoplasm of rectum and anal canal
569.3 Hemorrhage of rectum and anus
578.1 Blood in stool

ICD-9-CM Procedural

48.34 Destruction of rectal lesion or tissue by cryosurgery

HCPCS Level II Supplies & Services

A4305 Disposable drug delivery system, flow rate of 50 ml or greater per hour
A4306 Disposable drug delivery system, flow rate of 5 ml or less per hour
A4550 Surgical trays

46940–46942

46940 Curettage or cautery of anal fissure, including dilation of anal sphincter (separate procedure); initial
46942 subsequent

ICD-9-CM Diagnostic

564.00 Unspecified constipation
564.01 Slow transit constipation
564.02 Outlet dysfunction constipation
564.09 Other constipation
565.0 Anal fissure
569.3 Hemorrhage of rectum and anus

Unspecified code
Female diagnosis
Manifestation code
Male diagnosis

578.1 Blood in stool

ICD-9-CM Procedural

49.39 Other local excision or destruction of lesion or tissue of anus

HCPCS Level II Supplies & Services

A4305 Disposable drug delivery system, flow rate of 50 ml or greater per hour
A4306 Disposable drug delivery system, flow rate of 5 ml or less per hour
A4550 Surgical trays

46945–46946

46945 Ligation of internal hemorrhoids; single procedure
46946 multiple procedures

ICD-9-CM Diagnostic

455.0 Internal hemorrhoids without mention of complication
455.1 Internal thrombosed hemorrhoids
455.2 Internal hemorrhoids with other complication
569.3 Hemorrhage of rectum and anus
569.42 Anal or rectal pain
578.1 Blood in stool

ICD-9-CM Procedural

49.45 Ligation of hemorrhoids

HCPCS Level II Supplies & Services

A4305 Disposable drug delivery system, flow rate of 50 ml or greater per hour
A4306 Disposable drug delivery system, flow rate of 5 ml or less per hour
A4550 Surgical trays

46947

46947 Hemorrhoidopexy (eg, for prolapsing internal hemorrhoids) by stapling

ICD-9-CM Diagnostic

455.1 Internal thrombosed hemorrhoids
455.2 Internal hemorrhoids with other complication
569.3 Hemorrhage of rectum and anus
569.42 Anal or rectal pain
578.1 Blood in stool

ICD-9-CM Procedural

49.49 Other procedures on hemorrhoids

HCPCS Level II Supplies & Services

A4305 Disposable drug delivery system, flow rate of 50 ml or greater per hour
A4306 Disposable drug delivery system, flow rate of 5 ml or less per hour
A4550 Surgical trays

Liver

47000–47001

47000 Biopsy of liver, needle; percutaneous
47001 when done for indicated purpose at time of other major procedure (List separately in addition to code for primary procedure)

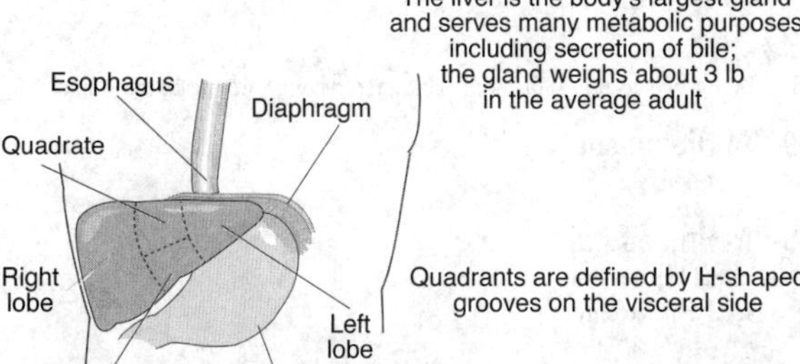
The Liver
The liver is the body's largest gland and serves many metabolic purposes including secretion of bile; the gland weighs about 3 lb in the average adult
Esophagus
Diaphragm
Quadrate
Right lobe
Left lobe
Caudate
Stomach
Quadrants are defined by H-shaped grooves on the visceral side

ICD-9-CM Diagnostic

155.0 Malignant neoplasm of liver, primary
155.1 Malignant neoplasm of intrahepatic bile ducts
155.2 Malignant neoplasm of liver, not specified as primary or secondary
195.2 Malignant neoplasm of abdomen
197.7 Secondary malignant neoplasm of liver
211.5 Benign neoplasm of liver and biliary passages
230.8 Carcinoma in situ of liver and biliary system
235.3 Neoplasm of uncertain behavior of liver and biliary passages
239.0 Neoplasm of unspecified nature of digestive system
277.3 Amyloidosis — (Use additional code to identify any associated mental retardation)
277.4 Disorders of bilirubin excretion — (Use additional code to identify any associated mental retardation)
570 Acute and subacute necrosis of liver
571.0 Alcoholic fatty liver
571.1 Acute alcoholic hepatitis
571.2 Alcoholic cirrhosis of liver
571.3 Unspecified alcoholic liver damage
571.41 Chronic persistent hepatitis
571.49 Other chronic hepatitis
571.5 Cirrhosis of liver without mention of alcohol
571.6 Biliary cirrhosis
571.8 Other chronic nonalcoholic liver disease
571.9 Unspecified chronic liver disease without mention of alcohol
572.0 Abscess of liver
572.1 Portal pyemia
572.2 Hepatic coma
572.4 Hepatorenal syndrome
572.8 Other sequelae of chronic liver disease
573.0 Chronic passive congestion of liver
573.1 Hepatitis in viral diseases classified elsewhere — (Code first underlying disease: 074.8, 075, 078.5)
573.2 Hepatitis in other infectious diseases classified elsewhere — (Code first underlying disease, 084.9)
573.3 Unspecified hepatitis — (Use additional E code to identify cause)
573.4 Hepatic infarction
573.8 Other specified disorders of liver
576.8 Other specified disorders of biliary tract
751.61 Congenital biliary atresia
751.62 Congenital cystic disease of liver
780.6 Fever
782.4 Jaundice, unspecified, not of newborn
789.00 Abdominal pain, unspecified site
789.01 Abdominal pain, right upper quadrant
789.02 Abdominal pain, left upper quadrant
789.03 Abdominal pain, right lower quadrant
789.04 Abdominal pain, left lower quadrant
789.05 Abdominal pain, periumbilic
789.06 Abdominal pain, epigastric
789.07 Abdominal pain, generalized
789.09 Abdominal pain, other specified site
789.1 Hepatomegaly
794.8 Nonspecific abnormal results of liver function study
864.01 Liver hematoma and contusion without mention of open wound into cavity
996.82 Complications of transplanted liver — (Use additional code to identify nature of complication, 078.5)
V42.7 Liver replaced by transplant — (This code is intended for use when these conditions are recorded as diagnoses or problems)

ICD-9-CM Procedural

50.11 Closed (percutaneous) (needle) biopsy of liver
50.12 Open biopsy of liver

47010–47011

47010 Hepatotomy; for open drainage of abscess or cyst, one or two stages
47011 for percutaneous drainage of abscess or cyst, one or two stages

ICD-9-CM Diagnostic

572.0 Abscess of liver
573.8 Other specified disorders of liver
751.62 Congenital cystic disease of liver

ICD-9-CM Procedural

50.0 Hepatotomy

Unspecified code | Manifestation code
Female diagnosis | Male diagnosis

47015

47015 Laparotomy, with aspiration and/or injection of hepatic parasitic (eg, amoebic or echinococcal) cyst(s) or abscess(es)

ICD-9-CM Diagnostic

006.3 Amebic liver abscess
122.0 Echinococcus granulosus infection of liver
122.5 Echinococcus multilocularis infection of liver
122.8 Unspecified echinococcus of liver ▽
572.0 Abscess of liver
573.8 Other specified disorders of liver

ICD-9-CM Procedural

50.94 Other injection of therapeutic substance into liver
54.19 Other laparotomy

47100

47100 Biopsy of liver, wedge

ICD-9-CM Diagnostic

155.0 Malignant neoplasm of liver, primary
155.1 Malignant neoplasm of intrahepatic bile ducts
155.2 Malignant neoplasm of liver, not specified as primary or secondary ▽
156.0 Malignant neoplasm of gallbladder
156.1 Malignant neoplasm of extrahepatic bile ducts
156.2 Malignant neoplasm of ampulla of Vater
156.8 Malignant neoplasm of other specified sites of gallbladder and extrahepatic bile ducts
156.9 Malignant neoplasm of biliary tract, part unspecified site ▽
157.0 Malignant neoplasm of head of pancreas
157.2 Malignant neoplasm of tail of pancreas
157.3 Malignant neoplasm of pancreatic duct
157.4 Malignant neoplasm of islets of Langerhans — (Use additional code to identify any functional activity)
157.8 Malignant neoplasm of other specified sites of pancreas
157.9 Malignant neoplasm of pancreas, part unspecified ▽
158.0 Malignant neoplasm of retroperitoneum
197.7 Secondary malignant neoplasm of liver
199.1 Other malignant neoplasm of unspecified site
211.5 Benign neoplasm of liver and biliary passages
211.6 Benign neoplasm of pancreas, except islets of Langerhans
230.8 Carcinoma in situ of liver and biliary system
235.3 Neoplasm of uncertain behavior of liver and biliary passages
277.3 Amyloidosis — (Use additional code to identify any associated mental retardation)
277.4 Disorders of bilirubin excretion — (Use additional code to identify any associated mental retardation)
287.3 Primary thrombocytopenia
570 Acute and subacute necrosis of liver
571.0 Alcoholic fatty liver
571.1 Acute alcoholic hepatitis
571.2 Alcoholic cirrhosis of liver
571.3 Unspecified alcoholic liver damage ▽
571.41 Chronic persistent hepatitis
571.49 Other chronic hepatitis
571.5 Cirrhosis of liver without mention of alcohol
571.6 Biliary cirrhosis
571.8 Other chronic nonalcoholic liver disease
571.9 Unspecified chronic liver disease without mention of alcohol ▽
572.0 Abscess of liver
572.1 Portal pyemia
572.3 Portal hypertension
572.4 Hepatorenal syndrome
573.0 Chronic passive congestion of liver
573.1 Hepatitis in viral diseases classified elsewhere — (Code first underlying disease: 074.8, 075, 078.5) ☒
573.2 Hepatitis in other infectious diseases classified elsewhere — (Code first underlying disease, 084.9) ☒
573.3 Unspecified hepatitis — (Use additional E code to identify cause) ▽
573.4 Hepatic infarction
573.8 Other specified disorders of liver
573.9 Unspecified disorder of liver ▽
576.8 Other specified disorders of biliary tract
751.60 Unspecified congenital anomaly of gallbladder, bile ducts, and liver ▽
751.61 Congenital biliary atresia
751.62 Congenital cystic disease of liver
751.69 Other congenital anomaly of gallbladder, bile ducts, and liver
782.4 Jaundice, unspecified, not of newborn ▽
789.00 Abdominal pain, unspecified site ▽
789.01 Abdominal pain, right upper quadrant
789.02 Abdominal pain, left upper quadrant
789.03 Abdominal pain, right lower quadrant
789.04 Abdominal pain, left lower quadrant
789.05 Abdominal pain, periumbilic
789.06 Abdominal pain, epigastric
789.07 Abdominal pain, generalized
789.09 Abdominal pain, other specified site
789.1 Hepatomegaly
789.2 Splenomegaly
789.30 Abdominal or pelvic swelling, mass or lump, unspecified site ▽
789.31 Abdominal or pelvic swelling, mass, or lump, right upper quadrant
789.36 Abdominal or pelvic swelling, mass, or lump, epigastric
789.39 Abdominal or pelvic swelling, mass, or lump, other specified site
794.8 Nonspecific abnormal results of liver function study
996.80 Complications of transplanted organ, unspecified site — (Use additional code to identify nature of complication, 078.5) ▽
996.82 Complications of transplanted liver — (Use additional code to identify nature of complication, 078.5)
V42.7 Liver replaced by transplant — (This code is intended for use when these conditions are recorded as diagnoses or problems)

ICD-9-CM Procedural

50.12 Open biopsy of liver

47120–47130

47120 Hepatectomy, resection of liver; partial lobectomy
47122 trisegmentectomy
47125 total left lobectomy
47130 total right lobectomy

ICD-9-CM Diagnostic

155.0 Malignant neoplasm of liver, primary
155.2 Malignant neoplasm of liver, not specified as primary or secondary ▽
197.7 Secondary malignant neoplasm of liver
211.5 Benign neoplasm of liver and biliary passages
230.8 Carcinoma in situ of liver and biliary system
235.3 Neoplasm of uncertain behavior of liver and biliary passages
239.0 Neoplasm of unspecified nature of digestive system
277.3 Amyloidosis — (Use additional code to identify any associated mental retardation)
277.4 Disorders of bilirubin excretion — (Use additional code to identify any associated mental retardation)
571.5 Cirrhosis of liver without mention of alcohol
571.6 Biliary cirrhosis
571.8 Other chronic nonalcoholic liver disease
572.0 Abscess of liver
573.8 Other specified disorders of liver
576.8 Other specified disorders of biliary tract
751.60 Unspecified congenital anomaly of gallbladder, bile ducts, and liver ▽
751.62 Congenital cystic disease of liver
751.69 Other congenital anomaly of gallbladder, bile ducts, and liver
782.4 Jaundice, unspecified, not of newborn ▽
789.1 Hepatomegaly

ICD-9-CM Procedural

50.22 Partial hepatectomy
50.3 Lobectomy of liver

47133

47133 Donor hepatectomy (including cold preservation), from cadaver donor

ICD-9-CM Diagnostic

V59.6 Liver donor

ICD-9-CM Procedural

50.22 Partial hepatectomy
50.4 Total hepatectomy

▽ Unspecified code ☒ Manifestation code
♀ Female diagnosis ♂ Male diagnosis

47135–47136

47135 Liver allotransplantation; orthotopic, partial or whole, from cadaver or living donor, any age
47136 heterotopic, partial or whole, from cadaver or living donor, any age

ICD-9-CM Diagnostic

155.0 Malignant neoplasm of liver, primary
197.7 Secondary malignant neoplasm of liver
273.4 Alpha-1-antitrypsin deficiency
570 Acute and subacute necrosis of liver
571.49 Other chronic hepatitis
571.5 Cirrhosis of liver without mention of alcohol
571.6 Biliary cirrhosis
571.8 Other chronic nonalcoholic liver disease
571.9 Unspecified chronic liver disease without mention of alcohol ▽
572.8 Other sequelae of chronic liver disease
573.8 Other specified disorders of liver
576.2 Obstruction of bile duct
576.8 Other specified disorders of biliary tract
751.61 Congenital biliary atresia
751.62 Congenital cystic disease of liver
751.69 Other congenital anomaly of gallbladder, bile ducts, and liver

ICD-9-CM Procedural

50.51 Auxiliary liver transplant
50.59 Other transplant of liver

47140–47142

47140 Donor hepatectomy (including cold preservation), from living donor; left lateral segment only (segments II and III)
47141 total left lobectomy (segments II, III and IV)
47142 total right lobectomy (segments V, VI, VII and VIII)

ICD-9-CM Diagnostic

V59.6 Liver donor

ICD-9-CM Procedural

50.22 Partial hepatectomy
50.3 Lobectomy of liver

47143–47145

47143 Backbench standard preparation of cadaver donor whole liver graft prior to allotransplantation, including cholecystectomy, if necessary, and dissection and removal of surrounding soft tissues to prepare the vena cava, portal vein, hepatic artery, and common bile duct for implantation; without trisegment or lobe split
47144 with trisegment split of whole liver graft into two partial liver grafts (ie, left lateral segment (segments II and III) and right trisegment (segments I and IV through VIII))
47145 with lobe split of whole liver graft into two partial liver grafts (ie, left lobe (segments II, III, and IV) and right lobe (segments I and V through VIII))

ICD-9-CM Diagnostic

155.0 Malignant neoplasm of liver, primary
197.7 Secondary malignant neoplasm of liver
273.4 Alpha-1-antitrypsin deficiency
570 Acute and subacute necrosis of liver
571.49 Other chronic hepatitis
571.5 Cirrhosis of liver without mention of alcohol
571.6 Biliary cirrhosis
571.8 Other chronic nonalcoholic liver disease
571.9 Unspecified chronic liver disease without mention of alcohol ▽
572.8 Other sequelae of chronic liver disease
573.8 Other specified disorders of liver
576.2 Obstruction of bile duct
576.8 Other specified disorders of biliary tract
751.61 Congenital biliary atresia
751.62 Congenital cystic disease of liver
751.69 Other congenital anomaly of gallbladder, bile ducts, and liver

ICD-9-CM Procedural

00.93 Transplant from cadaver
50.51 Auxiliary liver transplant
50.59 Other transplant of liver
50.99 Other operations on liver

47146–47147

47146 Backbench reconstruction of cadaver or living donor liver graft prior to allotransplantation; venous anastomosis, each
47147 arterial anastomosis, each

ICD-9-CM Diagnostic

155.0 Malignant neoplasm of liver, primary
197.7 Secondary malignant neoplasm of liver
273.4 Alpha-1-antitrypsin deficiency
570 Acute and subacute necrosis of liver
571.49 Other chronic hepatitis
571.5 Cirrhosis of liver without mention of alcohol
571.6 Biliary cirrhosis
571.8 Other chronic nonalcoholic liver disease
571.9 Unspecified chronic liver disease without mention of alcohol ▽
572.8 Other sequelae of chronic liver disease
573.8 Other specified disorders of liver
576.2 Obstruction of bile duct
576.8 Other specified disorders of biliary tract
751.61 Congenital biliary atresia
751.62 Congenital cystic disease of liver
751.69 Other congenital anomaly of gallbladder, bile ducts, and liver

ICD-9-CM Procedural

00.91 Transplant from live related donor
00.92 Transplant from live non-related donor
00.93 Transplant from cadaver
50.51 Auxiliary liver transplant
50.59 Other transplant of liver
50.99 Other operations on liver

47300

47300 Marsupialization of cyst or abscess of liver

ICD-9-CM Diagnostic

571.6 Biliary cirrhosis
572.0 Abscess of liver
573.8 Other specified disorders of liver
751.62 Congenital cystic disease of liver

ICD-9-CM Procedural

50.21 Marsupialization of lesion of liver

47350–47362

47350 Management of liver hemorrhage; simple suture of liver wound or injury
47360 complex suture of liver wound or injury, with or without hepatic artery ligation
47361 exploration of hepatic wound, extensive debridement, coagulation and/or suture, with or without packing of liver
47362 re-exploration of hepatic wound for removal of packing

ICD-9-CM Diagnostic

864.02 Liver laceration, minor, without mention of open wound into cavity
864.03 Liver laceration, moderate, without mention of open wound into cavity
864.04 Liver laceration, major, without mention of open wound into cavity
864.05 Liver injury without mention of open wound into cavity, unspecified laceration ▽
864.09 Other liver injury without mention of open wound into cavity
864.12 Liver laceration, minor, with open wound into cavity
864.13 Liver laceration, moderate, with open wound into cavity
864.14 Liver laceration, major, with open wound into cavity
864.19 Other liver injury with open wound into cavity
998.11 Hemorrhage complicating a procedure
998.2 Accidental puncture or laceration during procedure
998.31 Disruption of internal operation wound

ICD-9-CM Procedural

50.0 Hepatotomy
50.61 Closure of laceration of liver
50.69 Other repair of liver

▽ Unspecified code ♀ Female diagnosis ☒ Manifestation code ♂ Male diagnosis

47370–47371

47370 Laparoscopy, surgical, ablation of one or more liver tumor(s); radiofrequency
47371 cryosurgical

ICD-9-CM Diagnostic

155.0 Malignant neoplasm of liver, primary
155.2 Malignant neoplasm of liver, not specified as primary or secondary ▽
197.7 Secondary malignant neoplasm of liver
211.5 Benign neoplasm of liver and biliary passages
230.8 Carcinoma in situ of liver and biliary system
235.3 Neoplasm of uncertain behavior of liver and biliary passages
239.0 Neoplasm of unspecified nature of digestive system

ICD-9-CM Procedural

50.29 Other destruction of lesion of liver

47380–47382

47380 Ablation, open, of one or more liver tumor(s); radiofrequency
47381 cryosurgical
47382 Ablation, one or more liver tumor(s), percutaneous, radiofrequency

ICD-9-CM Diagnostic

155.0 Malignant neoplasm of liver, primary
155.2 Malignant neoplasm of liver, not specified as primary or secondary ▽
197.7 Secondary malignant neoplasm of liver
211.5 Benign neoplasm of liver and biliary passages
230.8 Carcinoma in situ of liver and biliary system
235.3 Neoplasm of uncertain behavior of liver and biliary passages
239.0 Neoplasm of unspecified nature of digestive system
V64.41 Laparoscopic surgical procedure converted to open procedure

ICD-9-CM Procedural

50.29 Other destruction of lesion of liver

Biliary Tract

47400

47400 Hepaticotomy or hepaticostomy with exploration, drainage, or removal of calculus

ICD-9-CM Diagnostic

574.50 Calculus of bile duct without mention of cholecystitis or obstruction
576.8 Other specified disorders of biliary tract

ICD-9-CM Procedural

51.59 Incision of other bile duct

47420–47425

47420 Choledochotomy or choledochostomy with exploration, drainage, or removal of calculus, with or without cholecystotomy; without transduodenal sphincterotomy or sphincteroplasty
47425 with transduodenal sphincterotomy or sphincteroplasty

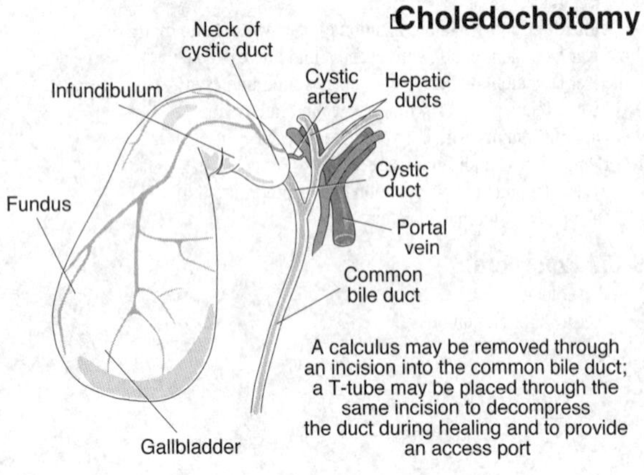

Choledochotomy
Neck of cystic duct
Infundibulum
Cystic artery
Hepatic ducts
Cystic duct
Fundus
Portal vein
Common bile duct
Gallbladder
A calculus may be removed through an incision into the common bile duct; a T-tube may be placed through the same incision to decompress the duct during healing and to provide an access port

ICD-9-CM Diagnostic

156.0 Malignant neoplasm of gallbladder
156.9 Malignant neoplasm of biliary tract, part unspecified site ▽
574.00 Calculus of gallbladder with acute cholecystitis, without mention of obstruction
574.01 Calculus of gallbladder with acute cholecystitis and obstruction
574.10 Calculus of gallbladder with other cholecystitis, without mention of obstruction
574.11 Calculus of gallbladder with other cholecystitis and obstruction
574.20 Calculus of gallbladder without mention of cholecystitis or obstruction
574.21 Calculus of gallbladder without mention of cholecystitis, with obstruction
574.30 Calculus of bile duct with acute cholecystitis without mention of obstruction
574.31 Calculus of bile duct with acute cholecystitis and obstruction
574.40 Calculus of bile duct with other cholecystitis, without mention of obstruction
574.41 Calculus of bile duct with other cholecystitis and obstruction
574.50 Calculus of bile duct without mention of cholecystitis or obstruction
574.51 Calculus of bile duct without mention of cholecystitis, with obstruction
574.60 Calculus of gallbladder and bile duct with acute cholecystitis, without mention of obstruction
574.61 Calculus of gallbladder and bile duct with acute cholecystitis, with obstruction
574.70 Calculus of gallbladder and bile duct with other cholecystitis, without mention of obstruction
574.71 Calculus of gallbladder and bile duct with other cholecystitis, with obstruction
574.80 Calculus of gallbladder and bile duct with acute and chronic cholecystitis, without mention of obstruction
574.81 Calculus of gallbladder and bile duct with acute and chronic cholecystitis, with obstruction
574.90 Calculus of gallbladder and bile duct without cholecystitis, without mention of obstruction
574.91 Calculus of gallbladder and bile duct without cholecystitis, with obstruction
576.5 Spasm of sphincter of Oddi
576.8 Other specified disorders of biliary tract
577.0 Acute pancreatitis
577.1 Chronic pancreatitis

ICD-9-CM Procedural

51.41 Common duct exploration for removal of calculus
51.51 Exploration of common bile duct
51.82 Pancreatic sphincterotomy
51.83 Pancreatic sphincteroplasty

47460

47460 Transduodenal sphincterotomy or sphincteroplasty, with or without transduodenal extraction of calculus (separate procedure)

ICD-9-CM Diagnostic

574.40 Calculus of bile duct with other cholecystitis, without mention of obstruction
574.41 Calculus of bile duct with other cholecystitis and obstruction
574.50 Calculus of bile duct without mention of cholecystitis or obstruction
574.51 Calculus of bile duct without mention of cholecystitis, with obstruction
576.2 Obstruction of bile duct
576.5 Spasm of sphincter of Oddi
576.8 Other specified disorders of biliary tract
577.1 Chronic pancreatitis
751.69 Other congenital anomaly of gallbladder, bile ducts, and liver
782.4 Jaundice, unspecified, not of newborn ▽
789.01 Abdominal pain, right upper quadrant
789.09 Abdominal pain, other specified site

ICD-9-CM Procedural

51.82 Pancreatic sphincterotomy
51.83 Pancreatic sphincteroplasty

47480

47480 Cholecystotomy or cholecystostomy with exploration, drainage, or removal of calculus (separate procedure)

ICD-9-CM Diagnostic

156.0 Malignant neoplasm of gallbladder
574.00 Calculus of gallbladder with acute cholecystitis, without mention of obstruction
574.01 Calculus of gallbladder with acute cholecystitis and obstruction
574.10 Calculus of gallbladder with other cholecystitis, without mention of obstruction
574.11 Calculus of gallbladder with other cholecystitis and obstruction
574.20 Calculus of gallbladder without mention of cholecystitis or obstruction
574.21 Calculus of gallbladder without mention of cholecystitis, with obstruction
575.0 Acute cholecystitis
575.10 Cholecystitis, unspecified ▽
575.11 Chronic cholecystitis

575.12 Acute and chronic cholecystitis
575.2 Obstruction of gallbladder
575.3 Hydrops of gallbladder
576.8 Other specified disorders of biliary tract

ICD-9-CM Procedural

51.03 Other cholecystostomy
51.04 Other cholecystotomy

47490

47490 Percutaneous cholecystostomy

ICD-9-CM Diagnostic

156.0 Malignant neoplasm of gallbladder
156.9 Malignant neoplasm of biliary tract, part unspecified site ▽
574.00 Calculus of gallbladder with acute cholecystitis, without mention of obstruction
574.20 Calculus of gallbladder without mention of cholecystitis or obstruction
575.0 Acute cholecystitis
575.11 Chronic cholecystitis
575.12 Acute and chronic cholecystitis
575.2 Obstruction of gallbladder
575.3 Hydrops of gallbladder
782.4 Jaundice, unspecified, not of newborn ▽

ICD-9-CM Procedural

51.01 Percutaneous aspiration of gallbladder

47500–47505

47500 Injection procedure for percutaneous transhepatic cholangiography
47505 Injection procedure for cholangiography through an existing catheter (eg, percutaneous transhepatic or T-tube)

ICD-9-CM Diagnostic

156.0 Malignant neoplasm of gallbladder
156.1 Malignant neoplasm of extrahepatic bile ducts
156.2 Malignant neoplasm of ampulla of Vater
156.8 Malignant neoplasm of other specified sites of gallbladder and extrahepatic bile ducts
156.9 Malignant neoplasm of biliary tract, part unspecified site ▽
157.9 Malignant neoplasm of pancreas, part unspecified ▽
195.2 Malignant neoplasm of abdomen
211.5 Benign neoplasm of liver and biliary passages
235.3 Neoplasm of uncertain behavior of liver and biliary passages
239.9 Neoplasm of unspecified nature, site unspecified ▽
573.4 Hepatic infarction
573.8 Other specified disorders of liver
574.10 Calculus of gallbladder with other cholecystitis, without mention of obstruction
574.11 Calculus of gallbladder with other cholecystitis and obstruction
574.20 Calculus of gallbladder without mention of cholecystitis or obstruction
574.21 Calculus of gallbladder without mention of cholecystitis, with obstruction
574.30 Calculus of bile duct with acute cholecystitis without mention of obstruction
574.31 Calculus of bile duct with acute cholecystitis and obstruction
574.40 Calculus of bile duct with other cholecystitis, without mention of obstruction
574.41 Calculus of bile duct with other cholecystitis and obstruction
574.50 Calculus of bile duct without mention of cholecystitis or obstruction
574.60 Calculus of gallbladder and bile duct with acute cholecystitis, without mention of obstruction
574.61 Calculus of gallbladder and bile duct with acute cholecystitis, with obstruction
574.70 Calculus of gallbladder and bile duct with other cholecystitis, without mention of obstruction
574.71 Calculus of gallbladder and bile duct with other cholecystitis, with obstruction
574.80 Calculus of gallbladder and bile duct with acute and chronic cholecystitis, without mention of obstruction
574.81 Calculus of gallbladder and bile duct with acute and chronic cholecystitis, with obstruction
574.90 Calculus of gallbladder and bile duct without cholecystitis, without mention of obstruction
574.91 Calculus of gallbladder and bile duct without cholecystitis, with obstruction
575.0 Acute cholecystitis
575.11 Chronic cholecystitis
575.12 Acute and chronic cholecystitis
575.2 Obstruction of gallbladder
575.3 Hydrops of gallbladder
575.4 Perforation of gallbladder
575.5 Fistula of gallbladder
575.6 Cholesterolosis of gallbladder
575.8 Other specified disorder of gallbladder
576.0 Postcholecystectomy syndrome
576.1 Cholangitis
576.2 Obstruction of bile duct
576.3 Perforation of bile duct
576.4 Fistula of bile duct
576.5 Spasm of sphincter of Oddi
576.8 Other specified disorders of biliary tract
751.69 Other congenital anomaly of gallbladder, bile ducts, and liver
782.4 Jaundice, unspecified, not of newborn ▽
V45.89 Other postsurgical status — (This code is intended for use when these conditions are recorded as diagnoses or problems)
V72.5 Radiological examination, not elsewhere classified — (Use additional code(s) to identify any special screening examination(s) performed: V73.0-V82.9)

ICD-9-CM Procedural

51.19 Other diagnostic procedures on biliary tract
87.51 Percutaneous hepatic cholangiogram
87.54 Other cholangiogram

47510–47511

47510 Introduction of percutaneous transhepatic catheter for biliary drainage
47511 Introduction of percutaneous transhepatic stent for internal and external biliary drainage

ICD-9-CM Diagnostic

155.0 Malignant neoplasm of liver, primary
155.1 Malignant neoplasm of intrahepatic bile ducts
155.2 Malignant neoplasm of liver, not specified as primary or secondary ▽
156.0 Malignant neoplasm of gallbladder
156.1 Malignant neoplasm of extrahepatic bile ducts
156.2 Malignant neoplasm of ampulla of Vater
156.8 Malignant neoplasm of other specified sites of gallbladder and extrahepatic bile ducts
156.9 Malignant neoplasm of biliary tract, part unspecified site ▽
211.5 Benign neoplasm of liver and biliary passages
572.0 Abscess of liver
572.1 Portal pyemia
572.2 Hepatic coma
572.3 Portal hypertension
572.4 Hepatorenal syndrome
573.1 Hepatitis in viral diseases classified elsewhere — (Code first underlying disease: 074.8, 075, 078.5) ☒
573.2 Hepatitis in other infectious diseases classified elsewhere — (Code first underlying disease, 084.9) ☒
573.4 Hepatic infarction
573.8 Other specified disorders of liver
574.00 Calculus of gallbladder with acute cholecystitis, without mention of obstruction
574.01 Calculus of gallbladder with acute cholecystitis and obstruction
574.10 Calculus of gallbladder with other cholecystitis, without mention of obstruction
574.11 Calculus of gallbladder with other cholecystitis and obstruction
574.20 Calculus of gallbladder without mention of cholecystitis or obstruction
574.21 Calculus of gallbladder without mention of cholecystitis, with obstruction
574.30 Calculus of bile duct with acute cholecystitis without mention of obstruction
574.31 Calculus of bile duct with acute cholecystitis and obstruction
574.40 Calculus of bile duct with other cholecystitis, without mention of obstruction
574.41 Calculus of bile duct with other cholecystitis and obstruction
574.50 Calculus of bile duct without mention of cholecystitis or obstruction
574.51 Calculus of bile duct without mention of cholecystitis, with obstruction
574.60 Calculus of gallbladder and bile duct with acute cholecystitis, without mention of obstruction
574.61 Calculus of gallbladder and bile duct with acute cholecystitis, with obstruction
574.70 Calculus of gallbladder and bile duct with other cholecystitis, without mention of obstruction
574.71 Calculus of gallbladder and bile duct with other cholecystitis, with obstruction
574.80 Calculus of gallbladder and bile duct with acute and chronic cholecystitis, without mention of obstruction
574.81 Calculus of gallbladder and bile duct with acute and chronic cholecystitis, with obstruction
574.90 Calculus of gallbladder and bile duct without cholecystitis, without mention of obstruction
574.91 Calculus of gallbladder and bile duct without cholecystitis, with obstruction
575.0 Acute cholecystitis
575.10 Cholecystitis, unspecified ▽
575.11 Chronic cholecystitis
575.12 Acute and chronic cholecystitis

575.2 Obstruction of gallbladder
575.3 Hydrops of gallbladder
575.4 Perforation of gallbladder
575.5 Fistula of gallbladder
575.6 Cholesterolosis of gallbladder
575.8 Other specified disorder of gallbladder
576.0 Postcholecystectomy syndrome
576.1 Cholangitis
576.2 Obstruction of bile duct
576.3 Perforation of bile duct
576.4 Fistula of bile duct
576.5 Spasm of sphincter of Oddi
576.8 Other specified disorders of biliary tract
782.4 Jaundice, unspecified, not of newborn ▽
868.02 Bile duct and gallbladder injury without mention of open wound into cavity
V58.82 Encounter for fitting and adjustment of non-vascular catheter NEC

ICD-9-CM Procedural

51.43 Insertion of choledochohepatic tube for decompression
51.98 Other percutaneous procedures on biliary tract
51.99 Other operations on biliary tract

47525–47530

47525 Change of percutaneous biliary drainage catheter
47530 Revision and/or reinsertion of transhepatic tube

ICD-9-CM Diagnostic

155.0 Malignant neoplasm of liver, primary
155.1 Malignant neoplasm of intrahepatic bile ducts
155.2 Malignant neoplasm of liver, not specified as primary or secondary ▽
156.0 Malignant neoplasm of gallbladder
156.1 Malignant neoplasm of extrahepatic bile ducts
156.2 Malignant neoplasm of ampulla of Vater
156.8 Malignant neoplasm of other specified sites of gallbladder and extrahepatic bile ducts
156.9 Malignant neoplasm of biliary tract, part unspecified site ▽
211.5 Benign neoplasm of liver and biliary passages
572.0 Abscess of liver
572.1 Portal pyemia
572.2 Hepatic coma
572.3 Portal hypertension
572.4 Hepatorenal syndrome
573.1 Hepatitis in viral diseases classified elsewhere — (Code first underlying disease: 074.8, 075, 078.5) ☒
573.2 Hepatitis in other infectious diseases classified elsewhere — (Code first underlying disease, 084.9) ☒
573.4 Hepatic infarction
573.8 Other specified disorders of liver
574.00 Calculus of gallbladder with acute cholecystitis, without mention of obstruction
574.01 Calculus of gallbladder with acute cholecystitis and obstruction
574.10 Calculus of gallbladder with other cholecystitis, without mention of obstruction
574.11 Calculus of gallbladder with other cholecystitis and obstruction
574.20 Calculus of gallbladder without mention of cholecystitis or obstruction
574.21 Calculus of gallbladder without mention of cholecystitis, with obstruction
574.30 Calculus of bile duct with acute cholecystitis without mention of obstruction
574.31 Calculus of bile duct with acute cholecystitis and obstruction
574.40 Calculus of bile duct with other cholecystitis, without mention of obstruction
574.41 Calculus of bile duct with other cholecystitis and obstruction
574.50 Calculus of bile duct without mention of cholecystitis or obstruction
574.51 Calculus of bile duct without mention of cholecystitis, with obstruction
574.60 Calculus of gallbladder and bile duct with acute cholecystitis, without mention of obstruction
574.61 Calculus of gallbladder and bile duct with acute cholecystitis, with obstruction
574.70 Calculus of gallbladder and bile duct with other cholecystitis, without mention of obstruction
574.71 Calculus of gallbladder and bile duct with other cholecystitis, with obstruction
574.80 Calculus of gallbladder and bile duct with acute and chronic cholecystitis, without mention of obstruction
574.81 Calculus of gallbladder and bile duct with acute and chronic cholecystitis, with obstruction
574.90 Calculus of gallbladder and bile duct without cholecystitis, without mention of obstruction
574.91 Calculus of gallbladder and bile duct without cholecystitis, with obstruction
575.0 Acute cholecystitis
575.10 Cholecystitis, unspecified ▽
575.11 Chronic cholecystitis
575.12 Acute and chronic cholecystitis
575.2 Obstruction of gallbladder
575.3 Hydrops of gallbladder
575.4 Perforation of gallbladder
575.5 Fistula of gallbladder
575.6 Cholesterolosis of gallbladder
575.8 Other specified disorder of gallbladder
576.0 Postcholecystectomy syndrome
576.1 Cholangitis
576.2 Obstruction of bile duct
576.3 Perforation of bile duct
576.4 Fistula of bile duct
576.5 Spasm of sphincter of Oddi
576.8 Other specified disorders of biliary tract
782.4 Jaundice, unspecified, not of newborn ▽
868.02 Bile duct and gallbladder injury without mention of open wound into cavity
V58.82 Encounter for fitting and adjustment of non-vascular catheter NEC

ICD-9-CM Procedural

97.05 Replacement of stent (tube) in biliary or pancreatic duct

47550

47550 Biliary endoscopy, intraoperative (choledochoscopy) (List separately in addition to code for primary procedure)

ICD-9-CM Diagnostic

This is an add-on code. Refer to the corresponding primary procedure code for ICD-9 diagnosis code links.

ICD-9-CM Procedural

51.11 Endoscopic retrograde cholangiography (ERC)

47552–47553

47552 Biliary endoscopy, percutaneous via T-tube or other tract; diagnostic, with or without collection of specimen(s) by brushing and/or washing (separate procedure)
47553 with biopsy, single or multiple

ICD-9-CM Diagnostic

156.0 Malignant neoplasm of gallbladder
156.1 Malignant neoplasm of extrahepatic bile ducts
156.8 Malignant neoplasm of other specified sites of gallbladder and extrahepatic bile ducts
156.9 Malignant neoplasm of biliary tract, part unspecified site ▽
197.8 Secondary malignant neoplasm of other digestive organs and spleen
211.8 Benign neoplasm of retroperitoneum and peritoneum
230.8 Carcinoma in situ of liver and biliary system
235.3 Neoplasm of uncertain behavior of liver and biliary passages
239.0 Neoplasm of unspecified nature of digestive system
575.0 Acute cholecystitis
576.8 Other specified disorders of biliary tract
782.4 Jaundice, unspecified, not of newborn ▽

ICD-9-CM Procedural

51.14 Other closed (endoscopic) biopsy of biliary duct or sphincter of Oddi
51.98 Other percutaneous procedures on biliary tract

47554

47554 Biliary endoscopy, percutaneous via T-tube or other tract; with removal of calculus/calculi

ICD-9-CM Diagnostic

574.00 Calculus of gallbladder with acute cholecystitis, without mention of obstruction
574.01 Calculus of gallbladder with acute cholecystitis and obstruction
574.10 Calculus of gallbladder with other cholecystitis, without mention of obstruction
574.11 Calculus of gallbladder with other cholecystitis and obstruction
574.20 Calculus of gallbladder without mention of cholecystitis or obstruction
574.21 Calculus of gallbladder without mention of cholecystitis, with obstruction
574.30 Calculus of bile duct with acute cholecystitis without mention of obstruction
574.31 Calculus of bile duct with acute cholecystitis and obstruction
574.40 Calculus of bile duct with other cholecystitis, without mention of obstruction
574.41 Calculus of bile duct with other cholecystitis and obstruction
574.50 Calculus of bile duct without mention of cholecystitis or obstruction
574.51 Calculus of bile duct without mention of cholecystitis, with obstruction

574.90 Calculus of gallbladder and bile duct without cholecystitis, without mention of obstruction
574.91 Calculus of gallbladder and bile duct without cholecystitis, with obstruction

ICD-9-CM Procedural
51.96 Percutaneous extraction of common duct stones

47555–47556
47555 Biliary endoscopy, percutaneous via T-tube or other tract; with dilation of biliary duct stricture(s) without stent
47556 with dilation of biliary duct stricture(s) with stent

ICD-9-CM Diagnostic
156.1 Malignant neoplasm of extrahepatic bile ducts
156.2 Malignant neoplasm of ampulla of Vater
156.8 Malignant neoplasm of other specified sites of gallbladder and extrahepatic bile ducts
156.9 Malignant neoplasm of biliary tract, part unspecified site ▽
211.5 Benign neoplasm of liver and biliary passages
230.8 Carcinoma in situ of liver and biliary system
235.3 Neoplasm of uncertain behavior of liver and biliary passages
239.0 Neoplasm of unspecified nature of digestive system
574.50 Calculus of bile duct without mention of cholecystitis or obstruction
576.2 Obstruction of bile duct

ICD-9-CM Procedural
51.87 Endoscopic insertion of stent (tube) into bile duct
51.98 Other percutaneous procedures on biliary tract

47560–47561
47560 Laparoscopy, surgical; with guided transhepatic cholangiography, without biopsy
47561 with guided transhepatic cholangiography with biopsy

ICD-9-CM Diagnostic
156.0 Malignant neoplasm of gallbladder
156.1 Malignant neoplasm of extrahepatic bile ducts
156.2 Malignant neoplasm of ampulla of Vater
156.8 Malignant neoplasm of other specified sites of gallbladder and extrahepatic bile ducts
156.9 Malignant neoplasm of biliary tract, part unspecified site ▽
157.9 Malignant neoplasm of pancreas, part unspecified ▽
195.2 Malignant neoplasm of abdomen
211.5 Benign neoplasm of liver and biliary passages
235.3 Neoplasm of uncertain behavior of liver and biliary passages
239.9 Neoplasm of unspecified nature, site unspecified ▽
573.4 Hepatic infarction
573.8 Other specified disorders of liver
574.10 Calculus of gallbladder with other cholecystitis, without mention of obstruction
574.11 Calculus of gallbladder with other cholecystitis and obstruction
574.20 Calculus of gallbladder without mention of cholecystitis or obstruction
574.21 Calculus of gallbladder without mention of cholecystitis, with obstruction
574.30 Calculus of bile duct with acute cholecystitis without mention of obstruction
574.31 Calculus of bile duct with acute cholecystitis and obstruction
574.40 Calculus of bile duct with other cholecystitis, without mention of obstruction
574.41 Calculus of bile duct with other cholecystitis and obstruction
574.50 Calculus of bile duct without mention of cholecystitis or obstruction
574.60 Calculus of gallbladder and bile duct with acute cholecystitis, without mention of obstruction
574.61 Calculus of gallbladder and bile duct with acute cholecystitis, with obstruction
574.70 Calculus of gallbladder and bile duct with other cholecystitis, without mention of obstruction
574.71 Calculus of gallbladder and bile duct with other cholecystitis, with obstruction
574.80 Calculus of gallbladder and bile duct with acute and chronic cholecystitis, without mention of obstruction
574.81 Calculus of gallbladder and bile duct with acute and chronic cholecystitis, with obstruction
574.90 Calculus of gallbladder and bile duct without cholecystitis, without mention of obstruction
574.91 Calculus of gallbladder and bile duct without cholecystitis, with obstruction
575.0 Acute cholecystitis
575.11 Chronic cholecystitis
575.12 Acute and chronic cholecystitis
575.2 Obstruction of gallbladder
575.3 Hydrops of gallbladder
575.4 Perforation of gallbladder
575.5 Fistula of gallbladder
575.6 Cholesterolosis of gallbladder
575.8 Other specified disorder of gallbladder
576.0 Postcholecystectomy syndrome
576.1 Cholangitis
576.2 Obstruction of bile duct
576.3 Perforation of bile duct
576.4 Fistula of bile duct
576.5 Spasm of sphincter of Oddi
576.8 Other specified disorders of biliary tract
751.69 Other congenital anomaly of gallbladder, bile ducts, and liver
782.4 Jaundice, unspecified, not of newborn ▽
V45.89 Other postsurgical status — (This code is intended for use when these conditions are recorded as diagnoses or problems)
V72.5 Radiological examination, not elsewhere classified — (Use additional code(s) to identify any special screening examination(s) performed: V73.0-V82.9)

ICD-9-CM Procedural
50.12 Open biopsy of liver
51.13 Open biopsy of gallbladder or bile ducts
87.53 Intraoperative cholangiogram

47562–47563
47562 Laparoscopy, surgical; cholecystectomy
47563 cholecystectomy with cholangiography

ICD-9-CM Diagnostic
156.0 Malignant neoplasm of gallbladder
156.8 Malignant neoplasm of other specified sites of gallbladder and extrahepatic bile ducts
197.8 Secondary malignant neoplasm of other digestive organs and spleen
211.5 Benign neoplasm of liver and biliary passages
230.8 Carcinoma in situ of liver and biliary system
235.3 Neoplasm of uncertain behavior of liver and biliary passages
239.0 Neoplasm of unspecified nature of digestive system
560.31 Gallstone ileus
571.5 Cirrhosis of liver without mention of alcohol
571.6 Biliary cirrhosis
574.00 Calculus of gallbladder with acute cholecystitis, without mention of obstruction
574.10 Calculus of gallbladder with other cholecystitis, without mention of obstruction
574.11 Calculus of gallbladder with other cholecystitis and obstruction
574.20 Calculus of gallbladder without mention of cholecystitis or obstruction
574.21 Calculus of gallbladder without mention of cholecystitis, with obstruction
574.30 Calculus of bile duct with acute cholecystitis without mention of obstruction
574.31 Calculus of bile duct with acute cholecystitis and obstruction
574.40 Calculus of bile duct with other cholecystitis, without mention of obstruction
574.41 Calculus of bile duct with other cholecystitis and obstruction
574.50 Calculus of bile duct without mention of cholecystitis or obstruction
574.51 Calculus of bile duct without mention of cholecystitis, with obstruction
574.60 Calculus of gallbladder and bile duct with acute cholecystitis, without mention of obstruction
574.61 Calculus of gallbladder and bile duct with acute cholecystitis, with obstruction
574.70 Calculus of gallbladder and bile duct with other cholecystitis, without mention of obstruction
574.71 Calculus of gallbladder and bile duct with other cholecystitis, with obstruction
574.80 Calculus of gallbladder and bile duct with acute and chronic cholecystitis, without mention of obstruction
574.81 Calculus of gallbladder and bile duct with acute and chronic cholecystitis, with obstruction
574.90 Calculus of gallbladder and bile duct without cholecystitis, without mention of obstruction
574.91 Calculus of gallbladder and bile duct without cholecystitis, with obstruction
575.0 Acute cholecystitis
575.11 Chronic cholecystitis
575.12 Acute and chronic cholecystitis
575.2 Obstruction of gallbladder
575.3 Hydrops of gallbladder
575.5 Fistula of gallbladder
575.6 Cholesterolosis of gallbladder
575.8 Other specified disorder of gallbladder
576.1 Cholangitis
576.8 Other specified disorders of biliary tract
782.4 Jaundice, unspecified, not of newborn ▽
789.01 Abdominal pain, right upper quadrant
789.06 Abdominal pain, epigastric
789.07 Abdominal pain, generalized

789.09 Abdominal pain, other specified site
789.30 Abdominal or pelvic swelling, mass or lump, unspecified site ▽
789.31 Abdominal or pelvic swelling, mass, or lump, right upper quadrant
789.36 Abdominal or pelvic swelling, mass, or lump, epigastric
789.37 Abdominal or pelvic swelling, mass, or lump, epigastric, generalized
789.39 Abdominal or pelvic swelling, mass, or lump, other specified site
793.3 Nonspecific abnormal findings on radiological and other examination of biliary tract
868.02 Bile duct and gallbladder injury without mention of open wound into cavity

ICD-9-CM Procedural
51.23 Laparoscopic cholecystectomy
51.24 Laparoscopic partial cholecystectomy
87.53 Intraoperative cholangiogram

47564
47564 Laparoscopy, surgical; cholecystectomy with exploration of common duct

ICD-9-CM Diagnostic
156.0 Malignant neoplasm of gallbladder
156.8 Malignant neoplasm of other specified sites of gallbladder and extrahepatic bile ducts
197.8 Secondary malignant neoplasm of other digestive organs and spleen
211.5 Benign neoplasm of liver and biliary passages
230.8 Carcinoma in situ of liver and biliary system
235.3 Neoplasm of uncertain behavior of liver and biliary passages
239.0 Neoplasm of unspecified nature of digestive system
560.31 Gallstone ileus
571.5 Cirrhosis of liver without mention of alcohol
571.6 Biliary cirrhosis
574.00 Calculus of gallbladder with acute cholecystitis, without mention of obstruction
574.10 Calculus of gallbladder with other cholecystitis, without mention of obstruction
574.11 Calculus of gallbladder with other cholecystitis and obstruction
574.20 Calculus of gallbladder without mention of cholecystitis or obstruction
574.50 Calculus of bile duct without mention of cholecystitis or obstruction
575.0 Acute cholecystitis
575.2 Obstruction of gallbladder
575.3 Hydrops of gallbladder
575.4 Perforation of gallbladder
575.5 Fistula of gallbladder
575.6 Cholesterolosis of gallbladder
575.8 Other specified disorder of gallbladder
576.1 Cholangitis
576.2 Obstruction of bile duct
576.8 Other specified disorders of biliary tract
782.4 Jaundice, unspecified, not of newborn ▽
789.01 Abdominal pain, right upper quadrant
789.06 Abdominal pain, epigastric
789.07 Abdominal pain, generalized
789.09 Abdominal pain, other specified site
789.30 Abdominal or pelvic swelling, mass or lump, unspecified site ▽
789.31 Abdominal or pelvic swelling, mass, or lump, right upper quadrant
789.36 Abdominal or pelvic swelling, mass, or lump, epigastric
789.37 Abdominal or pelvic swelling, mass, or lump, epigastric, generalized
789.39 Abdominal or pelvic swelling, mass, or lump, other specified site
793.3 Nonspecific abnormal findings on radiological and other examination of biliary tract
868.02 Bile duct and gallbladder injury without mention of open wound into cavity

ICD-9-CM Procedural
51.23 Laparoscopic cholecystectomy
51.41 Common duct exploration for removal of calculus
51.51 Exploration of common bile duct

47570
47570 Laparoscopy, surgical; cholecystoenterostomy

ICD-9-CM Diagnostic
155.0 Malignant neoplasm of liver, primary
155.1 Malignant neoplasm of intrahepatic bile ducts
156.0 Malignant neoplasm of gallbladder
156.9 Malignant neoplasm of biliary tract, part unspecified site ▽
157.0 Malignant neoplasm of head of pancreas
157.1 Malignant neoplasm of body of pancreas
211.5 Benign neoplasm of liver and biliary passages
571.5 Cirrhosis of liver without mention of alcohol
571.6 Biliary cirrhosis
574.00 Calculus of gallbladder with acute cholecystitis, without mention of obstruction
574.01 Calculus of gallbladder with acute cholecystitis and obstruction
574.10 Calculus of gallbladder with other cholecystitis, without mention of obstruction
574.11 Calculus of gallbladder with other cholecystitis and obstruction
574.20 Calculus of gallbladder without mention of cholecystitis or obstruction
574.21 Calculus of gallbladder without mention of cholecystitis, with obstruction
574.50 Calculus of bile duct without mention of cholecystitis or obstruction
575.2 Obstruction of gallbladder
575.8 Other specified disorder of gallbladder
576.1 Cholangitis
782.4 Jaundice, unspecified, not of newborn ▽

ICD-9-CM Procedural
51.32 Anastomosis of gallbladder to intestine

47600–47605
47600 Cholecystectomy;
47605 with cholangiography

ICD-9-CM Diagnostic
156.0 Malignant neoplasm of gallbladder
156.9 Malignant neoplasm of biliary tract, part unspecified site ▽
197.8 Secondary malignant neoplasm of other digestive organs and spleen
211.5 Benign neoplasm of liver and biliary passages
230.8 Carcinoma in situ of liver and biliary system
235.3 Neoplasm of uncertain behavior of liver and biliary passages
239.0 Neoplasm of unspecified nature of digestive system
560.31 Gallstone ileus
571.5 Cirrhosis of liver without mention of alcohol
571.6 Biliary cirrhosis
574.00 Calculus of gallbladder with acute cholecystitis, without mention of obstruction
574.01 Calculus of gallbladder with acute cholecystitis and obstruction
574.10 Calculus of gallbladder with other cholecystitis, without mention of obstruction
574.11 Calculus of gallbladder with other cholecystitis and obstruction
574.20 Calculus of gallbladder without mention of cholecystitis or obstruction
574.21 Calculus of gallbladder without mention of cholecystitis, with obstruction
574.30 Calculus of bile duct with acute cholecystitis without mention of obstruction
574.31 Calculus of bile duct with acute cholecystitis and obstruction
574.40 Calculus of bile duct with other cholecystitis, without mention of obstruction
574.41 Calculus of bile duct with other cholecystitis and obstruction
574.50 Calculus of bile duct without mention of cholecystitis or obstruction
574.51 Calculus of bile duct without mention of cholecystitis, with obstruction
574.60 Calculus of gallbladder and bile duct with acute cholecystitis, without mention of obstruction
574.61 Calculus of gallbladder and bile duct with acute cholecystitis, with obstruction
574.70 Calculus of gallbladder and bile duct with other cholecystitis, without mention of obstruction
574.71 Calculus of gallbladder and bile duct with other cholecystitis, with obstruction
574.80 Calculus of gallbladder and bile duct with acute and chronic cholecystitis, without mention of obstruction
574.81 Calculus of gallbladder and bile duct with acute and chronic cholecystitis, with obstruction
574.90 Calculus of gallbladder and bile duct without cholecystitis, without mention of obstruction
574.91 Calculus of gallbladder and bile duct without cholecystitis, with obstruction
575.0 Acute cholecystitis
575.11 Chronic cholecystitis
575.12 Acute and chronic cholecystitis
575.2 Obstruction of gallbladder
575.3 Hydrops of gallbladder
575.4 Perforation of gallbladder
575.5 Fistula of gallbladder
575.6 Cholesterolosis of gallbladder
575.8 Other specified disorder of gallbladder
576.1 Cholangitis
576.8 Other specified disorders of biliary tract
782.4 Jaundice, unspecified, not of newborn ▽
789.01 Abdominal pain, right upper quadrant
789.09 Abdominal pain, other specified site
789.31 Abdominal or pelvic swelling, mass, or lump, right upper quadrant
789.36 Abdominal or pelvic swelling, mass, or lump, epigastric
789.37 Abdominal or pelvic swelling, mass, or lump, epigastric, generalized
789.39 Abdominal or pelvic swelling, mass, or lump, other specified site
793.3 Nonspecific abnormal findings on radiological and other examination of biliary tract

868.02 Bile duct and gallbladder injury without mention of open wound into cavity
V64.41 Laparoscopic surgical procedure converted to open procedure

ICD-9-CM Procedural

51.21 Other partial cholecystectomy
51.22 Cholecystectomy
87.53 Intraoperative cholangiogram

47610–47620

47610 Cholecystectomy with exploration of common duct;
47612 with choledochoenterostomy
47620 with transduodenal sphincterotomy or sphincteroplasty, with or without cholangiography

ICD-9-CM Diagnostic

156.0 Malignant neoplasm of gallbladder
156.9 Malignant neoplasm of biliary tract, part unspecified site ▽
560.31 Gallstone ileus
574.00 Calculus of gallbladder with acute cholecystitis, without mention of obstruction
574.01 Calculus of gallbladder with acute cholecystitis and obstruction
574.10 Calculus of gallbladder with other cholecystitis, without mention of obstruction
574.11 Calculus of gallbladder with other cholecystitis and obstruction
574.20 Calculus of gallbladder without mention of cholecystitis or obstruction
574.21 Calculus of gallbladder without mention of cholecystitis, with obstruction
574.30 Calculus of bile duct with acute cholecystitis without mention of obstruction
574.31 Calculus of bile duct with acute cholecystitis and obstruction
574.40 Calculus of bile duct with other cholecystitis, without mention of obstruction
574.41 Calculus of bile duct with other cholecystitis and obstruction
574.50 Calculus of bile duct without mention of cholecystitis or obstruction
574.51 Calculus of bile duct without mention of cholecystitis, with obstruction
575.0 Acute cholecystitis
575.10 Cholecystitis, unspecified ▽
575.11 Chronic cholecystitis
575.12 Acute and chronic cholecystitis
575.2 Obstruction of gallbladder
575.9 Unspecified disorder of gallbladder ▽
576.8 Other specified disorders of biliary tract
782.4 Jaundice, unspecified, not of newborn ▽
789.00 Abdominal pain, unspecified site ▽
789.01 Abdominal pain, right upper quadrant
789.06 Abdominal pain, epigastric
789.07 Abdominal pain, generalized
793.3 Nonspecific abnormal findings on radiological and other examination of biliary tract
V64.41 Laparoscopic surgical procedure converted to open procedure

ICD-9-CM Procedural

51.22 Cholecystectomy
51.36 Choledochoenterostomy
51.41 Common duct exploration for removal of calculus
51.51 Exploration of common bile duct
51.82 Pancreatic sphincterotomy
51.83 Pancreatic sphincteroplasty
87.53 Intraoperative cholangiogram

47630

47630 Biliary duct stone extraction, percutaneous via T-tube tract, basket, or snare (eg, Burhenne technique)

ICD-9-CM Diagnostic

574.50 Calculus of bile duct without mention of cholecystitis or obstruction
574.51 Calculus of bile duct without mention of cholecystitis, with obstruction
574.90 Calculus of gallbladder and bile duct without cholecystitis, without mention of obstruction
574.91 Calculus of gallbladder and bile duct without cholecystitis, with obstruction
782.4 Jaundice, unspecified, not of newborn ▽

ICD-9-CM Procedural

51.98 Other percutaneous procedures on biliary tract

47700

47700 Exploration for congenital atresia of bile ducts, without repair, with or without liver biopsy, with or without cholangiography

ICD-9-CM Diagnostic

751.61 Congenital biliary atresia

ICD-9-CM Procedural

50.12 Open biopsy of liver
51.42 Common duct exploration for relief of other obstruction
87.53 Intraoperative cholangiogram

47701

47701 Portoenterostomy (eg, Kasai procedure)

ICD-9-CM Diagnostic

156.1 Malignant neoplasm of extrahepatic bile ducts
576.2 Obstruction of bile duct
751.61 Congenital biliary atresia

ICD-9-CM Procedural

51.37 Anastomosis of hepatic duct to gastrointestinal tract

47711–47712

47711 Excision of bile duct tumor, with or without primary repair of bile duct; extrahepatic
47712 intrahepatic

ICD-9-CM Diagnostic

155.1 Malignant neoplasm of intrahepatic bile ducts
156.1 Malignant neoplasm of extrahepatic bile ducts
156.9 Malignant neoplasm of biliary tract, part unspecified site ▽
197.8 Secondary malignant neoplasm of other digestive organs and spleen
211.5 Benign neoplasm of liver and biliary passages
230.8 Carcinoma in situ of liver and biliary system
235.3 Neoplasm of uncertain behavior of liver and biliary passages
239.0 Neoplasm of unspecified nature of digestive system

ICD-9-CM Procedural

51.69 Excision of other bile duct

47715

47715 Excision of choledochal cyst

ICD-9-CM Diagnostic

576.8 Other specified disorders of biliary tract
751.62 Congenital cystic disease of liver
751.69 Other congenital anomaly of gallbladder, bile ducts, and liver

ICD-9-CM Procedural

51.63 Other excision of common duct

47716

47716 Anastomosis, choledochal cyst, without excision

ICD-9-CM Diagnostic

576.8 Other specified disorders of biliary tract
751.62 Congenital cystic disease of liver
751.69 Other congenital anomaly of gallbladder, bile ducts, and liver

ICD-9-CM Procedural

51.39 Other bile duct anastomosis

47720–47741

47720 Cholecystoenterostomy; direct
47721 with gastroenterostomy
47740 Roux-en-Y
47741 Roux-en-Y with gastroenterostomy

ICD-9-CM Diagnostic

156.0 Malignant neoplasm of gallbladder
156.9 Malignant neoplasm of biliary tract, part unspecified site ▽
157.0 Malignant neoplasm of head of pancreas
157.1 Malignant neoplasm of body of pancreas

211.5 Benign neoplasm of liver and biliary passages
574.20 Calculus of gallbladder without mention of cholecystitis or obstruction
575.2 Obstruction of gallbladder
782.4 Jaundice, unspecified, not of newborn ▽
V64.41 Laparoscopic surgical procedure converted to open procedure

ICD-9-CM Procedural

44.39 Other gastroenterostomy without gastrectomy
51.32 Anastomosis of gallbladder to intestine
51.36 Choledochoenterostomy

47760–47765

47760 Anastomosis, of extrahepatic biliary ducts and gastrointestinal tract
47765 Anastomosis, of intrahepatic ducts and gastrointestinal tract

ICD-9-CM Diagnostic

156.9 Malignant neoplasm of biliary tract, part unspecified site ▽
211.5 Benign neoplasm of liver and biliary passages
576.2 Obstruction of bile duct
576.8 Other specified disorders of biliary tract

ICD-9-CM Procedural

51.37 Anastomosis of hepatic duct to gastrointestinal tract
51.39 Other bile duct anastomosis

47780–47785

47780 Anastomosis, Roux-en-Y, of extrahepatic biliary ducts and gastrointestinal tract
47785 Anastomosis, Roux-en-Y, of intrahepatic biliary ducts and gastrointestinal tract

ICD-9-CM Diagnostic

156.9 Malignant neoplasm of biliary tract, part unspecified site ▽
211.5 Benign neoplasm of liver and biliary passages
576.2 Obstruction of bile duct
576.8 Other specified disorders of biliary tract

ICD-9-CM Procedural

51.36 Choledochoenterostomy
51.37 Anastomosis of hepatic duct to gastrointestinal tract
51.39 Other bile duct anastomosis

47800

47800 Reconstruction, plastic, of extrahepatic biliary ducts with end-to-end anastomosis

ICD-9-CM Diagnostic

156.9 Malignant neoplasm of biliary tract, part unspecified site ▽
157.0 Malignant neoplasm of head of pancreas
157.1 Malignant neoplasm of body of pancreas
211.5 Benign neoplasm of liver and biliary passages
576.2 Obstruction of bile duct
576.8 Other specified disorders of biliary tract

ICD-9-CM Procedural

51.63 Other excision of common duct
51.69 Excision of other bile duct

47801

47801 Placement of choledochal stent

ICD-9-CM Diagnostic

156.9 Malignant neoplasm of biliary tract, part unspecified site ▽
211.5 Benign neoplasm of liver and biliary passages
576.2 Obstruction of bile duct
576.8 Other specified disorders of biliary tract
576.9 Unspecified disorder of biliary tract ▽

ICD-9-CM Procedural

51.87 Endoscopic insertion of stent (tube) into bile duct
97.05 Replacement of stent (tube) in biliary or pancreatic duct

47802

47802 U-tube hepaticoenterostomy

ICD-9-CM Diagnostic

155.0 Malignant neoplasm of liver, primary
197.7 Secondary malignant neoplasm of liver
571.5 Cirrhosis of liver without mention of alcohol
573.8 Other specified disorders of liver

ICD-9-CM Procedural

50.99 Other operations on liver
51.43 Insertion of choledochohepatic tube for decompression

47900

47900 Suture of extrahepatic biliary duct for pre-existing injury (separate procedure)

ICD-9-CM Diagnostic

868.02 Bile duct and gallbladder injury without mention of open wound into cavity
868.12 Bile duct and gallbladder injury, with open wound into cavity

ICD-9-CM Procedural

51.72 Choledochoplasty
51.79 Repair of other bile ducts

Pancreas

48000–48001

48000 Placement of drains, peripancreatic, for acute pancreatitis;
48001 with cholecystostomy, gastrostomy, and jejunostomy

ICD-9-CM Diagnostic

157.0 Malignant neoplasm of head of pancreas
157.1 Malignant neoplasm of body of pancreas
157.2 Malignant neoplasm of tail of pancreas
157.3 Malignant neoplasm of pancreatic duct
157.4 Malignant neoplasm of islets of Langerhans — (Use additional code to identify any functional activity)
157.8 Malignant neoplasm of other specified sites of pancreas
157.9 Malignant neoplasm of pancreas, part unspecified ▽
197.8 Secondary malignant neoplasm of other digestive organs and spleen
211.6 Benign neoplasm of pancreas, except islets of Langerhans
211.7 Benign neoplasm of islets of Langerhans — (Use additional code to identify any functional activity)
230.9 Carcinoma in situ of other and unspecified digestive organs ▽
235.5 Neoplasm of uncertain behavior of other and unspecified digestive organs ▽
239.0 Neoplasm of unspecified nature of digestive system
574.10 Calculus of gallbladder with other cholecystitis, without mention of obstruction
574.30 Calculus of bile duct with acute cholecystitis without mention of obstruction
574.40 Calculus of bile duct with other cholecystitis, without mention of obstruction
575.0 Acute cholecystitis
577.0 Acute pancreatitis
577.2 Cyst and pseudocyst of pancreas
577.8 Other specified disease of pancreas
863.81 Pancreas head injury without mention of open wound into cavity
863.82 Pancreas body injury without mention of open wound into cavity
863.84 Pancreas injury, multiple and unspecified sites, without mention of open wound into cavity
863.94 Pancreas injury, multiple and unspecified sites, with open wound into cavity
V64.41 Laparoscopic surgical procedure converted to open procedure

ICD-9-CM Procedural

43.19 Other gastrostomy
46.39 Other enterostomy
51.03 Other cholecystostomy
52.99 Other operations on pancreas

48005

48005 Resection or debridement of pancreas and peripancreatic tissue for acute necrotizing pancreatitis

ICD-9-CM Diagnostic

577.0 Acute pancreatitis
577.1 Chronic pancreatitis
577.2 Cyst and pseudocyst of pancreas
577.8 Other specified disease of pancreas
998.51 Infected postoperative seroma — (Use additional code to identify organism)
998.59 Other postoperative infection — (Use additional code to identify infection)

▽ Unspecified code
♀ Female diagnosis
☒ Manifestation code
♂ Male diagnosis

V42.83 Pancreas replaced by transplant — (This code is intended for use when these conditions are recorded as diagnoses or problems)

ICD-9-CM Procedural
52.22 Other excision or destruction of lesion or tissue of pancreas or pancreatic duct

48020
48020 Removal of pancreatic calculus

ICD-9-CM Diagnostic
577.8 Other specified disease of pancreas

ICD-9-CM Procedural
52.09 Other pancreatotomy

48100–48102
48100 Biopsy of pancreas, open (eg, fine needle aspiration, needle core biopsy, wedge biopsy)
48102 Biopsy of pancreas, percutaneous needle

ICD-9-CM Diagnostic
157.0 Malignant neoplasm of head of pancreas
157.1 Malignant neoplasm of body of pancreas
157.2 Malignant neoplasm of tail of pancreas
157.3 Malignant neoplasm of pancreatic duct
157.4 Malignant neoplasm of islets of Langerhans — (Use additional code to identify any functional activity)
157.8 Malignant neoplasm of other specified sites of pancreas
157.9 Malignant neoplasm of pancreas, part unspecified ▽
197.7 Secondary malignant neoplasm of liver
197.8 Secondary malignant neoplasm of other digestive organs and spleen
211.6 Benign neoplasm of pancreas, except islets of Langerhans
211.7 Benign neoplasm of islets of Langerhans — (Use additional code to identify any functional activity)
577.0 Acute pancreatitis
577.1 Chronic pancreatitis
577.2 Cyst and pseudocyst of pancreas
577.8 Other specified disease of pancreas
579.4 Pancreatic steatorrhea

ICD-9-CM Procedural
52.11 Closed (aspiration) (needle) (percutaneous) biopsy of pancreas
52.12 Open biopsy of pancreas

48120
48120 Excision of lesion of pancreas (eg, cyst, adenoma)

ICD-9-CM Diagnostic
157.0 Malignant neoplasm of head of pancreas
157.1 Malignant neoplasm of body of pancreas
157.2 Malignant neoplasm of tail of pancreas
157.3 Malignant neoplasm of pancreatic duct
157.4 Malignant neoplasm of islets of Langerhans — (Use additional code to identify any functional activity)
157.8 Malignant neoplasm of other specified sites of pancreas
157.9 Malignant neoplasm of pancreas, part unspecified ▽
197.8 Secondary malignant neoplasm of other digestive organs and spleen
211.6 Benign neoplasm of pancreas, except islets of Langerhans
211.7 Benign neoplasm of islets of Langerhans — (Use additional code to identify any functional activity)
230.9 Carcinoma in situ of other and unspecified digestive organs ▽
577.2 Cyst and pseudocyst of pancreas
V42.83 Pancreas replaced by transplant — (This code is intended for use when these conditions are recorded as diagnoses or problems)

ICD-9-CM Procedural
52.22 Other excision or destruction of lesion or tissue of pancreas or pancreatic duct

48140–48145
48140 Pancreatectomy, distal subtotal, with or without splenectomy; without pancreaticojejunostomy
48145 with pancreaticojejunostomy

ICD-9-CM Diagnostic
157.0 Malignant neoplasm of head of pancreas
157.1 Malignant neoplasm of body of pancreas
157.2 Malignant neoplasm of tail of pancreas
157.3 Malignant neoplasm of pancreatic duct
157.4 Malignant neoplasm of islets of Langerhans — (Use additional code to identify any functional activity)
157.8 Malignant neoplasm of other specified sites of pancreas
157.9 Malignant neoplasm of pancreas, part unspecified ▽
197.8 Secondary malignant neoplasm of other digestive organs and spleen
211.7 Benign neoplasm of islets of Langerhans — (Use additional code to identify any functional activity)
230.9 Carcinoma in situ of other and unspecified digestive organs ▽
577.0 Acute pancreatitis
577.1 Chronic pancreatitis
577.2 Cyst and pseudocyst of pancreas
577.8 Other specified disease of pancreas

ICD-9-CM Procedural
41.5 Total splenectomy
52.52 Distal pancreatectomy
52.96 Anastomosis of pancreas

48146
48146 Pancreatectomy, distal, near-total with preservation of duodenum (Child-type procedure)

ICD-9-CM Diagnostic
157.0 Malignant neoplasm of head of pancreas
157.1 Malignant neoplasm of body of pancreas
157.3 Malignant neoplasm of pancreatic duct
157.8 Malignant neoplasm of other specified sites of pancreas
577.1 Chronic pancreatitis
577.2 Cyst and pseudocyst of pancreas
577.8 Other specified disease of pancreas
863.81 Pancreas head injury without mention of open wound into cavity
863.82 Pancreas body injury without mention of open wound into cavity
863.84 Pancreas injury, multiple and unspecified sites, without mention of open wound into cavity
863.94 Pancreas injury, multiple and unspecified sites, with open wound into cavity
V42.83 Pancreas replaced by transplant — (This code is intended for use when these conditions are recorded as diagnoses or problems)

ICD-9-CM Procedural
52.52 Distal pancreatectomy

48148
48148 Excision of ampulla of Vater

ICD-9-CM Diagnostic
156.2 Malignant neoplasm of ampulla of Vater
197.8 Secondary malignant neoplasm of other digestive organs and spleen
211.5 Benign neoplasm of liver and biliary passages
230.8 Carcinoma in situ of liver and biliary system
235.3 Neoplasm of uncertain behavior of liver and biliary passages
V42.83 Pancreas replaced by transplant — (This code is intended for use when these conditions are recorded as diagnoses or problems)

ICD-9-CM Procedural
51.62 Excision of ampulla of Vater (with reimplantation of common duct)

48150–48152
48150 Pancreatectomy, proximal subtotal with total duodenectomy, partial gastrectomy, choledochoenterostomy and gastrojejunostomy (Whipple-type procedure); with pancreatojejunostomy
48152 without pancreatojejunostomy

ICD-9-CM Diagnostic
157.0 Malignant neoplasm of head of pancreas
157.1 Malignant neoplasm of body of pancreas
157.2 Malignant neoplasm of tail of pancreas
157.3 Malignant neoplasm of pancreatic duct
157.4 Malignant neoplasm of islets of Langerhans — (Use additional code to identify any functional activity)
157.8 Malignant neoplasm of other specified sites of pancreas
157.9 Malignant neoplasm of pancreas, part unspecified ▽
197.8 Secondary malignant neoplasm of other digestive organs and spleen

211.7 Benign neoplasm of islets of Langerhans — (Use additional code to identify any functional activity)
230.9 Carcinoma in situ of other and unspecified digestive organs ▽
577.1 Chronic pancreatitis
577.2 Cyst and pseudocyst of pancreas
577.8 Other specified disease of pancreas
863.81 Pancreas head injury without mention of open wound into cavity
863.82 Pancreas body injury without mention of open wound into cavity
863.84 Pancreas injury, multiple and unspecified sites, without mention of open wound into cavity
863.94 Pancreas injury, multiple and unspecified sites, with open wound into cavity

ICD-9-CM Procedural

52.7 Radical pancreaticoduodenectomy
52.96 Anastomosis of pancreas

48153–48154

48153 Pancreatectomy, proximal subtotal with near-total duodenectomy, choledochoenterostomy and duodenojejunostomy (pylorus-sparing, Whipple-type procedure); with pancreatojejunostomy
48154 without pancreatojejunostomy

ICD-9-CM Diagnostic

157.0 Malignant neoplasm of head of pancreas
157.1 Malignant neoplasm of body of pancreas
157.2 Malignant neoplasm of tail of pancreas
157.3 Malignant neoplasm of pancreatic duct
157.8 Malignant neoplasm of other specified sites of pancreas
577.0 Acute pancreatitis
577.1 Chronic pancreatitis
577.2 Cyst and pseudocyst of pancreas
577.8 Other specified disease of pancreas
863.81 Pancreas head injury without mention of open wound into cavity
863.82 Pancreas body injury without mention of open wound into cavity
863.84 Pancreas injury, multiple and unspecified sites, without mention of open wound into cavity
863.94 Pancreas injury, multiple and unspecified sites, with open wound into cavity

ICD-9-CM Procedural

52.7 Radical pancreaticoduodenectomy
52.96 Anastomosis of pancreas

48155–48160

48155 Pancreatectomy, total
48160 Pancreatectomy, total or subtotal, with autologous transplantation of pancreas or pancreatic islet cells

ICD-9-CM Diagnostic

157.0 Malignant neoplasm of head of pancreas
157.1 Malignant neoplasm of body of pancreas
157.2 Malignant neoplasm of tail of pancreas
157.3 Malignant neoplasm of pancreatic duct
157.4 Malignant neoplasm of islets of Langerhans — (Use additional code to identify any functional activity)
157.8 Malignant neoplasm of other specified sites of pancreas
157.9 Malignant neoplasm of pancreas, part unspecified ▽
197.8 Secondary malignant neoplasm of other digestive organs and spleen
230.9 Carcinoma in situ of other and unspecified digestive organs ▽
250.01 Diabetes mellitus without mention of complication, type I [juvenile type], not stated as uncontrolled
250.03 Diabetes mellitus without mention of complication, type I [juvenile type], uncontrolled
250.41 Diabetes with renal manifestations, type I [juvenile type], not stated as uncontrolled — (Use additional code to identify manifestation: 581.81, 583.81)
250.43 Diabetes with renal manifestations, type I [juvenile type], uncontrolled — (Use additional code to identify manifestation: 581.81, 583.81)
250.81 Diabetes with other specified manifestations, type I [juvenile type], not stated as uncontrolled — (Use additional code to identify manifestation: 707.10-707.9, 731.8. Use additional E code to identify cause, if drug-induced)
250.83 Diabetes with other specified manifestations, type I [juvenile type], uncontrolled — (Use additional code to identify manifestation: 707.10-707.9, 731.8. Use additional E code to identify cause, if drug-induced)
577.0 Acute pancreatitis
577.1 Chronic pancreatitis
577.2 Cyst and pseudocyst of pancreas
581.81 Nephrotic syndrome with other specified pathological lesion in kidney in diseases classified elsewhere — (Code first underlying disease: 084.9, 250.4, 277.3, 446.0, 710.0) ☒
583.81 Nephritis and nephropathy, not specified as acute or chronic, with other specified pathological lesion in kidney, in diseases classified elsewhere — (Code first underlying disease: 016.0, 098.19, 250.4, 277.3, 446.21, 710.0) ☒
V42.83 Pancreas replaced by transplant — (This code is intended for use when these conditions are recorded as diagnoses or problems)

ICD-9-CM Procedural

52.59 Other partial pancreatectomy
52.6 Total pancreatectomy
52.84 Autotransplantation of cells of islets of Langerhans

48180

48180 Pancreaticojejunostomy, side-to-side anastomosis (Puestow-type operation)

ICD-9-CM Diagnostic

577.1 Chronic pancreatitis
577.2 Cyst and pseudocyst of pancreas
577.8 Other specified disease of pancreas
V42.83 Pancreas replaced by transplant — (This code is intended for use when these conditions are recorded as diagnoses or problems)

ICD-9-CM Procedural

52.96 Anastomosis of pancreas

48400

48400 Injection procedure for intraoperative pancreatography (List separately in addition to code for primary procedure)

ICD-9-CM Diagnostic

This is an add-on code. Refer to the corresponding primary procedure code for ICD-9 diagnosis code links.

ICD-9-CM Procedural

52.19 Other diagnostic procedures on pancreas

HCPCS Level II Supplies & Services

The HCPCS Level II code(s) would be the same as the actual procedure performed because these are in-addition-to codes.

48500

48500 Marsupialization of pancreatic cyst

ICD-9-CM Diagnostic

577.2 Cyst and pseudocyst of pancreas
751.7 Congenital anomalies of pancreas
V42.83 Pancreas replaced by transplant — (This code is intended for use when these conditions are recorded as diagnoses or problems)

ICD-9-CM Procedural

52.3 Marsupialization of pancreatic cyst

48510–48511

48510 External drainage, pseudocyst of pancreas; open
48511 percutaneous

ICD-9-CM Diagnostic

577.2 Cyst and pseudocyst of pancreas
751.7 Congenital anomalies of pancreas

ICD-9-CM Procedural

52.01 Drainage of pancreatic cyst by catheter
52.09 Other pancreatotomy

48520

48520 Internal anastomosis of pancreatic cyst to gastrointestinal tract; direct

ICD-9-CM Diagnostic

577.1 Chronic pancreatitis
577.2 Cyst and pseudocyst of pancreas
577.8 Other specified disease of pancreas
751.7 Congenital anomalies of pancreas

▽ Unspecified code ☒ Manifestation code
♀ Female diagnosis ♂ Male diagnosis

ICD-9-CM Procedural
52.4 Internal drainage of pancreatic cyst

48540
48540 Internal anastomosis of pancreatic cyst to gastrointestinal tract; Roux-en-Y

ICD-9-CM Diagnostic
577.1 Chronic pancreatitis
577.2 Cyst and pseudocyst of pancreas
577.8 Other specified disease of pancreas
751.7 Congenital anomalies of pancreas

ICD-9-CM Procedural
52.4 Internal drainage of pancreatic cyst

48545–48547
48545 Pancreatorrhaphy for injury
48547 Duodenal exclusion with gastrojejunostomy for pancreatic injury

ICD-9-CM Diagnostic
863.80 Gastrointestinal tract injury, unspecified site, without mention of open wound into cavity ▽
863.81 Pancreas head injury without mention of open wound into cavity
863.82 Pancreas body injury without mention of open wound into cavity
863.83 Pancreas tail injury without mention of open wound into cavity
863.84 Pancreas injury, multiple and unspecified sites, without mention of open wound into cavity
863.90 Gastrointestinal tract injury, unspecified site, with open wound into cavity ▽
863.91 Pancreas head injury with open wound into cavity
863.92 Pancreas body injury with open wound into cavity
863.93 Pancreas tail injury with open wound into cavity
863.94 Pancreas injury, multiple and unspecified sites, with open wound into cavity

ICD-9-CM Procedural
44.39 Other gastroenterostomy without gastrectomy
52.95 Other repair of pancreas

48550
48550 Donor pancreatectomy (including cold preservation), with or without duodenal segment for transplantation

ICD-9-CM Diagnostic
V59.8 Donor of other specified organ or tissue

ICD-9-CM Procedural
52.6 Total pancreatectomy

48551–48552
48551 Backbench standard preparation of cadaver donor pancreas allograft prior to transplantation, including dissection of allograft from surrounding soft tissues, splenectomy, duodenotomy, ligation of bile duct, ligation of mesenteric vessels, and Y-graft arterial anastomoses from iliac artery to superior mesenteric artery and to splenic artery
48552 Backbench reconstruction of cadaver donor pancreas allograft prior to transplantation, venous anastomosis, each

ICD-9-CM Diagnostic
250.41 Diabetes with renal manifestations, type I [juvenile type], not stated as uncontrolled — (Use additional code to identify manifestation: 581.81, 583.81)
250.43 Diabetes with renal manifestations, type I [juvenile type], uncontrolled — (Use additional code to identify manifestation: 581.81, 583.81)
250.81 Diabetes with other specified manifestations, type I [juvenile type], not stated as uncontrolled — (Use additional code to identify manifestation: 707.10-707.9, 731.8. Use additional E code to identify cause, if drug-induced)
250.83 Diabetes with other specified manifestations, type I [juvenile type], uncontrolled — (Use additional code to identify manifestation: 707.10-707.9, 731.8. Use additional E code to identify cause, if drug-induced)
581.81 Nephrotic syndrome with other specified pathological lesion in kidney in diseases classified elsewhere — (Code first underlying disease: 084.9, 250.4, 277.3, 446.0, 710.0) ☒
583.81 Nephritis and nephropathy, not specified as acute or chronic, with other specified pathological lesion in kidney, in diseases classified elsewhere — (Code first underlying disease: 016.0, 098.19, 250.4, 277.3, 446.21, 710.0) ☒
586 Unspecified renal failure ▽
587 Unspecified renal sclerosis ▽
996.86 Complications of transplanted pancreas — (Use additional code to identify nature of complication, 078.5)

ICD-9-CM Procedural
00.93 Transplant from cadaver
52.83 Heterotransplant of pancreas
52.99 Other operations on pancreas

48554–48556
48554 Transplantation of pancreatic allograft
48556 Removal of transplanted pancreatic allograft

ICD-9-CM Diagnostic
250.41 Diabetes with renal manifestations, type I [juvenile type], not stated as uncontrolled — (Use additional code to identify manifestation: 581.81, 583.81)
250.43 Diabetes with renal manifestations, type I [juvenile type], uncontrolled — (Use additional code to identify manifestation: 581.81, 583.81)
250.81 Diabetes with other specified manifestations, type I [juvenile type], not stated as uncontrolled — (Use additional code to identify manifestation: 707.10-707.9, 731.8. Use additional E code to identify cause, if drug-induced)
250.83 Diabetes with other specified manifestations, type I [juvenile type], uncontrolled — (Use additional code to identify manifestation: 707.10-707.9, 731.8. Use additional E code to identify cause, if drug-induced)
581.81 Nephrotic syndrome with other specified pathological lesion in kidney in diseases classified elsewhere — (Code first underlying disease: 084.9, 250.4, 277.3, 446.0, 710.0) ☒
583.81 Nephritis and nephropathy, not specified as acute or chronic, with other specified pathological lesion in kidney, in diseases classified elsewhere — (Code first underlying disease: 016.0, 098.19, 250.4, 277.3, 446.21, 710.0) ☒
586 Unspecified renal failure ▽
587 Unspecified renal sclerosis ▽
996.86 Complications of transplanted pancreas — (Use additional code to identify nature of complication, 078.5)

ICD-9-CM Procedural
00.91 Transplant from live related donor
00.92 Transplant from live non-related donor
00.93 Transplant from cadaver
52.82 Homotransplant of pancreas
52.99 Other operations on pancreas

Abdomen, Peritoneum, and Omentum

49000
49000 Exploratory laparotomy, exploratory celiotomy with or without biopsy(s) (separate procedure)

ICD-9-CM Diagnostic
150.2 Malignant neoplasm of abdominal esophagus
150.5 Malignant neoplasm of lower third of esophagus
150.8 Malignant neoplasm of other specified part of esophagus
151.0 Malignant neoplasm of cardia
151.1 Malignant neoplasm of pylorus
151.2 Malignant neoplasm of pyloric antrum
151.3 Malignant neoplasm of fundus of stomach
151.4 Malignant neoplasm of body of stomach
151.5 Malignant neoplasm of lesser curvature of stomach, unspecified ▽
151.6 Malignant neoplasm of greater curvature of stomach, unspecified ▽
151.8 Malignant neoplasm of other specified sites of stomach
151.9 Malignant neoplasm of stomach, unspecified site ▽
152.0 Malignant neoplasm of duodenum
152.1 Malignant neoplasm of jejunum
152.2 Malignant neoplasm of ileum
152.3 Malignant neoplasm of Meckel's diverticulum
152.8 Malignant neoplasm of other specified sites of small intestine
152.9 Malignant neoplasm of small intestine, unspecified site ▽
153.0 Malignant neoplasm of hepatic flexure
153.1 Malignant neoplasm of transverse colon
153.2 Malignant neoplasm of descending colon
153.3 Malignant neoplasm of sigmoid colon
153.4 Malignant neoplasm of cecum
153.5 Malignant neoplasm of appendix
153.6 Malignant neoplasm of ascending colon

153.7 Malignant neoplasm of splenic flexure

153.8 Malignant neoplasm of other specified sites of large intestine

153.9 Malignant neoplasm of colon, unspecified site ▽

154.1 Malignant neoplasm of rectum

154.8 Malignant neoplasm of other sites of rectum, rectosigmoid junction, and anus

155.0 Malignant neoplasm of liver, primary

155.1 Malignant neoplasm of intrahepatic bile ducts

155.2 Malignant neoplasm of liver, not specified as primary or secondary ▽

156.0 Malignant neoplasm of gallbladder

156.1 Malignant neoplasm of extrahepatic bile ducts

156.2 Malignant neoplasm of ampulla of Vater

156.8 Malignant neoplasm of other specified sites of gallbladder and extrahepatic bile ducts

156.9 Malignant neoplasm of biliary tract, part unspecified site ▽

157.0 Malignant neoplasm of head of pancreas

157.1 Malignant neoplasm of body of pancreas

157.2 Malignant neoplasm of tail of pancreas

157.3 Malignant neoplasm of pancreatic duct

157.4 Malignant neoplasm of islets of Langerhans — (Use additional code to identify any functional activity)

157.8 Malignant neoplasm of other specified sites of pancreas

157.9 Malignant neoplasm of pancreas, part unspecified ▽

159.0 Malignant neoplasm of intestinal tract, part unspecified ▽

159.1 Malignant neoplasm of spleen, not elsewhere classified

159.8 Malignant neoplasm of other sites of digestive system and intra-abdominal organs

171.5 Malignant neoplasm of connective and other soft tissue of abdomen

171.6 Malignant neoplasm of connective and other soft tissue of pelvis

171.8 Malignant neoplasm of other specified sites of connective and other soft tissue

176.3 Kaposi's sarcoma of gastrointestinal sites

176.5 Kaposi's sarcoma of lymph nodes

179 Malignant neoplasm of uterus, part unspecified ▽ ♀

180.0 Malignant neoplasm of endocervix ♀

180.1 Malignant neoplasm of exocervix ♀

180.8 Malignant neoplasm of other specified sites of cervix ♀

180.9 Malignant neoplasm of cervix uteri, unspecified site ▽ ♀

182.0 Malignant neoplasm of corpus uteri, except isthmus ♀

182.1 Malignant neoplasm of isthmus ♀

182.8 Malignant neoplasm of other specified sites of body of uterus ♀

183.0 Malignant neoplasm of ovary — (Use additional code to identify any functional activity) ♀

183.2 Malignant neoplasm of fallopian tube ♀

183.3 Malignant neoplasm of broad ligament of uterus ♀

183.4 Malignant neoplasm of parametrium of uterus ♀

183.5 Malignant neoplasm of round ligament of uterus ♀

183.8 Malignant neoplasm of other specified sites of uterine adnexa ♀

183.9 Malignant neoplasm of uterine adnexa, unspecified site ▽ ♀

184.8 Malignant neoplasm of other specified sites of female genital organs ♀

184.9 Malignant neoplasm of female genital organ, site unspecified ▽ ♀

185 Malignant neoplasm of prostate ♂

187.3 Malignant neoplasm of body of penis ♂

187.5 Malignant neoplasm of epididymis ♂

187.6 Malignant neoplasm of spermatic cord ♂

187.8 Malignant neoplasm of other specified sites of male genital organs ♂

187.9 Malignant neoplasm of male genital organ, site unspecified ▽ ♂

188.0 Malignant neoplasm of trigone of urinary bladder

188.1 Malignant neoplasm of dome of urinary bladder

188.2 Malignant neoplasm of lateral wall of urinary bladder

188.3 Malignant neoplasm of anterior wall of urinary bladder

188.4 Malignant neoplasm of posterior wall of urinary bladder

188.5 Malignant neoplasm of bladder neck

188.6 Malignant neoplasm of ureteric orifice

188.8 Malignant neoplasm of other specified sites of bladder

188.9 Malignant neoplasm of bladder, part unspecified ▽

189.0 Malignant neoplasm of kidney, except pelvis

189.1 Malignant neoplasm of renal pelvis

189.2 Malignant neoplasm of ureter

189.3 Malignant neoplasm of urethra

189.4 Malignant neoplasm of paraurethral glands

189.8 Malignant neoplasm of other specified sites of urinary organs

189.9 Malignant neoplasm of urinary organ, site unspecified ▽

194.0 Malignant neoplasm of adrenal gland — (Use additional code to identify any functional activity)

195.2 Malignant neoplasm of abdomen

195.3 Malignant neoplasm of pelvis

196.2 Secondary and unspecified malignant neoplasm of intra-abdominal lymph nodes

196.6 Secondary and unspecified malignant neoplasm of intrapelvic lymph nodes

196.8 Secondary and unspecified malignant neoplasm of lymph nodes of multiple sites

196.9 Secondary and unspecified malignant neoplasm of lymph nodes, site unspecified ▽

197.4 Secondary malignant neoplasm of small intestine including duodenum

197.5 Secondary malignant neoplasm of large intestine and rectum

197.6 Secondary malignant neoplasm of retroperitoneum and peritoneum

197.7 Secondary malignant neoplasm of liver

197.8 Secondary malignant neoplasm of other digestive organs and spleen

198.0 Secondary malignant neoplasm of kidney

198.1 Secondary malignant neoplasm of other urinary organs

198.6 Secondary malignant neoplasm of ovary ♀

198.7 Secondary malignant neoplasm of adrenal gland

198.89 Secondary malignant neoplasm of other specified sites

199.0 Disseminated malignant neoplasm

200.00 Reticulosarcoma, unspecified site, extranodal and solid organ sites ▽

200.03 Reticulosarcoma of intra-abdominal lymph nodes

200.06 Reticulosarcoma of intrapelvic lymph nodes

200.07 Reticulosarcoma of spleen

200.08 Reticulosarcoma of lymph nodes of multiple sites

200.13 Lymphosarcoma of intra-abdominal lymph nodes

200.16 Lymphosarcoma of intrapelvic lymph nodes

200.17 Lymphosarcoma of spleen

200.18 Lymphosarcoma of lymph nodes of multiple sites

200.23 Burkitt's tumor or lymphoma of intra-abdominal lymph nodes

200.26 Burkitt's tumor or lymphoma of intrapelvic lymph nodes

200.27 Burkitt's tumor or lymphoma of spleen

200.28 Burkitt's tumor or lymphoma of lymph nodes of multiple sites

200.83 Other named variants of lymphosarcoma and reticulosarcoma of intra-abdominal lymph nodes

200.86 Other named variants of lymphosarcoma and reticulosarcoma of intrapelvic lymph nodes

200.87 Other named variants of lymphosarcoma and reticulosarcoma of spleen

200.88 Other named variants of lymphosarcoma and reticulosarcoma of lymph nodes of multiple sites

201.03 Hodgkin's paragranuloma of intra-abdominal lymph nodes

201.06 Hodgkin's paragranuloma of intrapelvic lymph nodes

201.07 Hodgkin's paragranuloma of spleen

201.08 Hodgkin's paragranuloma of lymph nodes of multiple sites

201.13 Hodgkin's granuloma of intra-abdominal lymph nodes

201.16 Hodgkin's granuloma of intrapelvic lymph nodes

201.17 Hodgkin's granuloma of spleen

201.18 Hodgkin's granuloma of lymph nodes of multiple sites

201.23 Hodgkin's sarcoma of intra-abdominal lymph nodes

201.26 Hodgkin's sarcoma of intrapelvic lymph nodes

201.27 Hodgkin's sarcoma of spleen

201.28 Hodgkin's sarcoma of lymph nodes of multiple sites

201.43 Hodgkin's disease, lymphocytic-histiocytic predominance of intra-abdominal lymph nodes

201.46 Hodgkin's disease, lymphocytic-histiocytic predominance of intrapelvic lymph nodes

201.47 Hodgkin's disease, lymphocytic-histiocytic predominance of spleen

201.48 Hodgkin's disease, lymphocytic-histiocytic predominance of lymph nodes of multiple sites

201.53 Hodgkin's disease, nodular sclerosis, of intra-abdominal lymph nodes

201.56 Hodgkin's disease, nodular sclerosis, of intrapelvic lymph nodes

201.57 Hodgkin's disease, nodular sclerosis, of spleen

201.58 Hodgkin's disease, nodular sclerosis, of lymph nodes of multiple sites

201.63 Hodgkin's disease, mixed cellularity, of intra-abdominal lymph nodes

201.66 Hodgkin's disease, mixed cellularity, of intrapelvic lymph nodes

201.67 Hodgkin's disease, mixed cellularity, of spleen

201.68 Hodgkin's disease, mixed cellularity, of lymph nodes of multiple sites

201.73 Hodgkin's disease, lymphocytic depletion, of intra-abdominal lymph nodes

201.76 Hodgkin's disease, lymphocytic depletion, of intrapelvic lymph nodes

201.77 Hodgkin's disease, lymphocytic depletion, of spleen

201.78 Hodgkin's disease, lymphocytic depletion, of lymph nodes of multiple sites

201.93 Hodgkin's disease, unspecified type, of intra-abdominal lymph nodes ▽

201.96 Hodgkin's disease, unspecified type, of intrapelvic lymph nodes ▽

201.97 Hodgkin's disease, unspecified type, of spleen ▽

201.98 Hodgkin's disease, unspecified type, of lymph nodes of multiple sites ▽

202.03 Nodular lymphoma of intra-abdominal lymph nodes

202.06 Nodular lymphoma of intrapelvic lymph nodes

202.07 Nodular lymphoma of spleen

▽ Unspecified code
♀ Female diagnosis
☒ Manifestation code
♂ Male diagnosis

202.08 Nodular lymphoma of lymph nodes of multiple sites
202.13 Mycosis fungoides of intra-abdominal lymph nodes
202.16 Mycosis fungoides of intrapelvic lymph nodes
202.17 Mycosis fungoides of spleen
202.18 Mycosis fungoides of lymph nodes of multiple sites
202.23 Sezary's disease of intra-abdominal lymph nodes
202.26 Sezary's disease of intrapelvic lymph nodes
202.27 Sezary's disease of spleen
202.28 Sezary's disease of lymph nodes of multiple sites
202.33 Malignant histiocytosis of intra-abdominal lymph nodes
202.36 Malignant histiocytosis of intrapelvic lymph nodes
202.37 Malignant histiocytosis of spleen
202.38 Malignant histiocytosis of lymph nodes of multiple sites
202.43 Leukemic reticuloendotheliosis of intra-abdominal lymph nodes
202.46 Leukemic reticuloendotheliosis of intrapelvic lymph nodes
202.47 Leukemic reticuloendotheliosis of spleen
202.48 Leukemic reticuloendotheliosis of lymph nodes of multipes sites
202.53 Letterer-Siwe disease of intra-abdominal lymph nodes
202.56 Letterer-Siwe disease of intrapelvic lymph nodes
202.57 Letterer-Siwe disease of spleen
202.58 Letterer-Siwe disease of lymph nodes of multiple sites
202.63 Malignant mast cell tumors of intra-abdominal lymph nodes
202.80 Other malignant lymphomas, unspecified site, extranodal and solid organ sites ▽
202.83 Other malignant lymphomas of intra-abdominal lymph nodes
202.86 Other malignant lymphomas of intrapelvic lymph nodes
202.87 Other malignant lymphomas of spleen
202.88 Other malignant lymphomas of lymph nodes of multiple sites
202.93 Other and unspecified malignant neoplasms of lymphoid and histiocytic tissue of intra-abdominal lymph nodes ▽
202.96 Other and unspecified malignant neoplasms of lymphoid and histiocytic tissue of intrapelvic lymph nodes ▽
202.97 Other and unspecified malignant neoplasms of lymphoid and histiocytic tissue of spleen ▽
202.98 Other and unspecified malignant neoplasms of lymphoid and histiocytic tissue of lymph nodes of multiple sites ▽
211.1 Benign neoplasm of stomach
211.2 Benign neoplasm of duodenum, jejunum, and ileum
211.3 Benign neoplasm of colon
211.8 Benign neoplasm of retroperitoneum and peritoneum
214.3 Lipoma of intra-abdominal organs
214.8 Lipoma of other specified sites
215.5 Other benign neoplasm of connective and other soft tissue of abdomen
215.6 Other benign neoplasm of connective and other soft tissue of pelvis
219.1 Benign neoplasm of corpus uteri ♀
219.8 Benign neoplasm of other specified parts of uterus ♀
220 Benign neoplasm of ovary — (Use additional code to identify any functional activity: 256.0-256.1) ♀
222.0 Benign neoplasm of testis — (Use additional code to identify any functional activity) ♂
222.2 Benign neoplasm of prostate ♂
222.3 Benign neoplasm of epididymis ♂
222.8 Benign neoplasm of other specified sites of male genital organs ♂
222.9 Benign neoplasm of male genital organ, site unspecified ▽ ♂
223.0 Benign neoplasm of kidney, except pelvis
223.1 Benign neoplasm of renal pelvis
223.2 Benign neoplasm of ureter
223.3 Benign neoplasm of bladder
223.81 Benign neoplasm of urethra
223.89 Benign neoplasm of other specified sites of urinary organs
223.9 Benign neoplasm of urinary organ, site unspecified ▽
227.0 Benign neoplasm of adrenal gland — (Use additional code to identify any functional activity)
227.6 Benign neoplasm of aortic body and other paraganglia — (Use additional code to identify any functional activity)
228.04 Hemangioma of intra-abdominal structures
228.1 Lymphangioma, any site
229.0 Benign neoplasm of lymph nodes
230.2 Carcinoma in situ of stomach
230.3 Carcinoma in situ of colon
230.4 Carcinoma in situ of rectum
230.7 Carcinoma in situ of other and unspecified parts of intestine ▽
230.8 Carcinoma in situ of liver and biliary system
230.9 Carcinoma in situ of other and unspecified digestive organs ▽
233.1 Carcinoma in situ of cervix uteri ♀
233.2 Carcinoma in situ of other and unspecified parts of uterus ▽ ♀
233.3 Carcinoma in situ of other and unspecified female genital organs ▽ ♀
233.4 Carcinoma in situ of prostate ♂
233.6 Carcinoma in situ of other and unspecified male genital organs ▽ ♂
233.7 Carcinoma in situ of bladder
233.9 Carcinoma in situ of other and unspecified urinary organs ▽
235.2 Neoplasm of uncertain behavior of stomach, intestines, and rectum
235.3 Neoplasm of uncertain behavior of liver and biliary passages
235.4 Neoplasm of uncertain behavior of retroperitoneum and peritoneum
235.5 Neoplasm of uncertain behavior of other and unspecified digestive organs ▽
236.0 Neoplasm of uncertain behavior of uterus ♀
236.1 Neoplasm of uncertain behavior of placenta ♀
236.2 Neoplasm of uncertain behavior of ovary — (Use additional code to identify any functional activity) ♀
236.3 Neoplasm of uncertain behavior of other and unspecified female genital organs ▽ ♀
236.5 Neoplasm of uncertain behavior of prostate ♂
236.7 Neoplasm of uncertain behavior of bladder
236.90 Neoplasm of uncertain behavior of urinary organ, unspecified ▽
236.91 Neoplasm of uncertain behavior of kidney and ureter
236.99 Neoplasm of uncertain behavior of other and unspecified urinary organs
237.2 Neoplasm of uncertain behavior of adrenal gland — (Use additional code to identify any functional activity)
237.3 Neoplasm of uncertain behavior of paraganglia
238.1 Neoplasm of uncertain behavior of connective and other soft tissue ▽
238.7 Neoplasm of uncertain behavior of other lymphatic and hematopoietic tissues
238.8 Neoplasm of uncertain behavior of other specified sites
238.9 Neoplasm of uncertain behavior, site unspecified ▽
239.0 Neoplasm of unspecified nature of digestive system
239.4 Neoplasm of unspecified nature of bladder
239.5 Neoplasm of unspecified nature of other genitourinary organs
239.8 Neoplasm of unspecified nature of other specified sites
239.9 Neoplasm of unspecified nature, site unspecified ▽
256.0 Hyperestrogenism ♀
256.1 Other ovarian hyperfunction ♀
256.4 Polycystic ovaries ♀
277.1 Disorders of porphyrin metabolism — (Use additional code to identify any associated mental retardation)
287.3 Primary thrombocytopenia
288.0 Agranulocytosis — (Use additional E code to identify drug or other cause)
289.1 Chronic lymphadenitis
289.2 Nonspecific mesenteric lymphadenitis
289.3 Lymphadenitis, unspecified, except mesenteric ▽
289.4 Hypersplenism
289.50 Unspecified disease of spleen ▽
289.51 Chronic congestive splenomegaly
289.52 Splenic sequestration — (Code first sickle-cell disease in crisis: 282.42, 282.62, 282.64, 282.69)
289.59 Other diseases of spleen
440.0 Atherosclerosis of aorta
440.1 Atherosclerosis of renal artery
440.8 Atherosclerosis of other specified arteries
440.9 Generalized and unspecified atherosclerosis ▽
441.02 Dissecting aortic aneurysm (any part), abdominal
441.03 Dissecting aortic aneurysm (any part), thoracoabdominal
441.9 Aortic aneurysm of unspecified site without mention of rupture ▽
442.1 Aneurysm of renal artery
442.83 Aneurysm of splenic artery
442.84 Aneurysm of other visceral artery
442.89 Aneurysm of other specified artery
442.9 Other aneurysm of unspecified site ▽
444.0 Embolism and thrombosis of abdominal aorta
444.89 Embolism and thrombosis of other specified artery
444.9 Embolism and thrombosis of unspecified artery ▽
447.0 Arteriovenous fistula, acquired
447.1 Stricture of artery
447.3 Hyperplasia of renal artery
447.5 Necrosis of artery
447.6 Unspecified arteritis ▽
447.8 Other specified disorders of arteries and arterioles
447.9 Unspecified disorders of arteries and arterioles ▽
452 Portal vein thrombosis
453.0 Budd-Chiari syndrome
453.1 Thrombophlebitis migrans
453.3 Embolism and thrombosis of renal vein
453.8 Embolism and thrombosis of other specified veins
456.5 Pelvic varices

457.8 Other noninfectious disorders of lymphatic channels
531.10 Acute gastric ulcer with perforation, without mention of obstruction — (Use additional E code to identify drug, if drug induced)
531.11 Acute gastric ulcer with perforation and obstruction — (Use additional E code to identify drug, if drug induced)
531.20 Acute gastric ulcer with hemorrhage and perforation, without mention of obstruction — (Use additional E code to identify drug, if drug induced)
531.31 Acute gastric ulcer without mention of hemorrhage or perforation, with obstruction — (Use additional E code to identify drug, if drug induced)
531.40 Chronic or unspecified gastric ulcer with hemorrhage, without mention of obstruction — (Use additional E code to identify drug, if drug induced)
531.41 Chronic or unspecified gastric ulcer with hemorrhage and obstruction — (Use additional E code to identify drug, if drug induced)
531.50 Chronic or unspecified gastric ulcer with perforation, without mention of obstruction — (Use additional E code to identify drug, if drug induced)
531.51 Chronic or unspecified gastric ulcer with perforation and obstruction — (Use additional E code to identify drug, if drug induced)
531.60 Chronic or unspecified gastric ulcer with hemorrhage and perforation, without mention of obstruction — (Use additional E code to identify drug, if drug induced)
531.61 Chronic or unspecified gastric ulcer with hemorrhage, perforation, and obstruction — (Use additional E code to identify drug, if drug induced)
531.90 Gastric ulcer, unspecified as acute or chronic, without mention of hemorrhage, perforation, or obstruction — (Use additional E code to identify drug, if drug induced) ▽
531.91 Gastric ulcer, unspecified as acute or chronic, without mention of hemorrhage or perforation, with obstruction — (Use additional E code to identify drug, if drug induced) ▽
532.00 Acute duodenal ulcer with hemorrhage, without mention of obstruction — (Use additional E code to identify drug, if drug induced)
532.01 Acute duodenal ulcer with hemorrhage and obstruction — (Use additional E code to identify drug, if drug induced)
532.10 Acute duodenal ulcer with perforation, without mention of obstruction — (Use additional E code to identify drug, if drug induced)
532.11 Acute duodenal ulcer with perforation and obstruction — (Use additional E code to identify drug, if drug induced)
532.20 Acute duodenal ulcer with hemorrhage and perforation, without mention of obstruction — (Use additional E code to identify drug, if drug induced)
532.21 Acute duodenal ulcer with hemorrhage, perforation, and obstruction — (Use additional E code to identify drug, if drug induced)
532.30 Acute duodenal ulcer without mention of hemorrhage, perforation, or obstruction — (Use additional E code to identify drug, if drug induced)
532.31 Acute duodenal ulcer without mention of hemorrhage or perforation, with obstruction — (Use additional E code to identify drug, if drug induced)
532.40 Chronic or unspecified duodenal ulcer with hemorrhage, without mention of obstruction — (Use additional E code to identify drug, if drug induced)
532.41 Chronic or unspecified duodenal ulcer with hemorrhage and obstruction — (Use additional E code to identify drug, if drug induced)
532.50 Chronic or unspecified duodenal ulcer with perforation, without mention of obstruction — (Use additional E code to identify drug, if drug induced)
532.51 Chronic or unspecified duodenal ulcer with perforation and obstruction — (Use additional E code to identify drug, if drug induced)
532.60 Chronic or unspecified duodenal ulcer with hemorrhage and perforation, without mention of obstruction — (Use additional E code to identify drug, if drug induced)
532.61 Chronic or unspecified duodenal ulcer with hemorrhage, perforation, and obstruction — (Use additional E code to identify drug, if drug induced)
532.90 Duodenal ulcer, unspecified as acute or chronic, without hemorrhage, perforation, or obstruction — (Use additional E code to identify drug, if drug induced) ▽
532.91 Duodenal ulcer, unspecified as acute or chronic, without mention of hemorrhage or perforation, with obstruction — (Use additional E code to identify drug, if drug induced) ▽
533.00 Acute peptic ulcer, unspecified site, with hemorrhage, without mention of obstruction — (Use additional E code to identify drug, if drug induced)
533.01 Acute peptic ulcer, unspecified site, with hemorrhage and obstruction — (Use additional E code to identify drug, if drug induced)
533.10 Acute peptic ulcer, unspecified site, with perforation, without mention of obstruction — (Use additional E code to identify drug, if drug induced)
533.11 Acute peptic ulcer, unspecified site, with perforation and obstruction — (Use additional E code to identify drug, if drug induced)
533.20 Acute peptic ulcer, unspecified site, with hemorrhage and perforation, without mention of obstruction — (Use additional E code to identify drug, if drug induced)
533.21 Acute peptic ulcer, unspecified site, with hemorrhage, perforation, and obstruction — (Use additional E code to identify drug, if drug induced)
533.30 Acute peptic ulcer, unspecified site, without mention of hemorrhage, perforation, or obstruction — (Use additional E code to identify drug, if drug induced)
533.31 Acute peptic ulcer, unspecified site, without mention of hemorrhage and perforation, with obstruction — (Use additional E code to identify drug, if drug induced)
533.40 Chronic or unspecified peptic ulcer, unspecified site, with hemorrhage, without mention of obstruction — (Use additional E code to identify drug, if drug induced)
533.41 Chronic or unspecified peptic ulcer, unspecified site, with hemorrhage and obstruction — (Use additional E code to identify drug, if drug induced)
533.60 Chronic or unspecified peptic ulcer, unspecified site, with hemorrhage and perforation, without mention of obstruction — (Use additional E code to identify drug, if drug induced)
533.61 Chronic or unspecified peptic ulcer, unspecified site, with hemorrhage, perforation, and obstruction — (Use additional E code to identify drug, if drug induced)
533.90 Peptic ulcer, unspecified site, unspecified as acute or chronic, without mention of hemorrhage, perforation, or obstruction — (Use additional E code to identify drug, if drug induced) ▽
533.91 Peptic ulcer, unspecified site, unspecified as acute or chronic, without mention of hemorrhage or perforation, with obstruction — (Use additional E code to identify drug, if drug induced) ▽
536.8 Dyspepsia and other specified disorders of function of stomach
537.0 Acquired hypertrophic pyloric stenosis
537.1 Gastric diverticulum
537.2 Chronic duodenal ileus
537.3 Other obstruction of duodenum
537.4 Fistula of stomach or duodenum
537.5 Gastroptosis
537.6 Hourglass stricture or stenosis of stomach
537.81 Pylorospasm
537.82 Angiodysplasia of stomach and duodenum (without mention of hemorrhage)
537.83 Angiodysplasia of stomach and duodenum with hemorrhage
537.84 Dieulafoy lesion (hemorrhagic) of stomach and duodenum
537.89 Other specified disorder of stomach and duodenum
537.9 Unspecified disorder of stomach and duodenum ▽
543.0 Hyperplasia of appendix (lymphoid)
543.9 Other and unspecified diseases of appendix ▽
553.8 Hernia of other specified sites of abdominal cavity without mention of obstruction or gangrene
557.9 Unspecified vascular insufficiency of intestine ▽
560.0 Intussusception
560.1 Paralytic ileus
560.2 Volvulus
560.30 Unspecified impaction of intestine ▽
560.31 Gallstone ileus
560.39 Other impaction of intestine
560.81 Intestinal or peritoneal adhesions with obstruction (postoperative) (postinfection)
560.89 Other specified intestinal obstruction
560.9 Unspecified intestinal obstruction ▽
562.00 Diverticulosis of small intestine (without mention of hemorrhage) — (Use additional code to identify any associated peritonitis: 567.0-567.9)
562.01 Diverticulitis of small intestine (without mention of hemorrhage) — (Use additional code to identify any associated peritonitis: 567.0-567.9)
567.0 Peritonitis in infectious diseases classified elsewhere — (Code first underlying disease) ☒
567.1 Pneumococcal peritonitis
567.2 Other suppurative peritonitis
567.8 Other specified peritonitis
567.9 Unspecified peritonitis ▽
568.0 Peritoneal adhesions (postoperative) (postinfection)
569.86 Dieulafoy lesion (hemorrhagic) of intestine
602.3 Dysplasia of prostate ♂
614.2 Salpingitis and oophoritis not specified as acute, subacute, or chronic — (Use additional code to identify organism: 041.0, 041.1) ♀
614.6 Pelvic peritoneal adhesions, female (postoperative) (postinfection) — (Use additional code to identify any associated infertility, 628.2. Use additional code to identify organism: 041.0, 041.1) ♀
617.3 Endometriosis of pelvic peritoneum ♀
620.2 Other and unspecified ovarian cyst ▽ ♀
625.8 Other specified symptom associated with female genital organs ♀
751.3 Hirschsprung's disease and other congenital functional disorders of colon
751.5 Other congenital anomalies of intestine
752.0 Congenital anomalies of ovaries ♀

▽ Unspecified code
♀ Female diagnosis
☒ Manifestation code
♂ Male diagnosis

752.10 Unspecified congenital anomaly of fallopian tubes and broad ligaments ▽ ♀
752.3 Other congenital anomaly of uterus ♀
753.8 Other specified congenital anomaly of bladder and urethra
789.00 Abdominal pain, unspecified site ▽
789.01 Abdominal pain, right upper quadrant
789.02 Abdominal pain, left upper quadrant
789.03 Abdominal pain, right lower quadrant
789.04 Abdominal pain, left lower quadrant
789.05 Abdominal pain, periumbilic
789.06 Abdominal pain, epigastric
789.07 Abdominal pain, generalized
789.09 Abdominal pain, other specified site
789.1 Hepatomegaly
789.2 Splenomegaly

ICD-9-CM Procedural

34.27 Biopsy of diaphragm
54.11 Exploratory laparotomy
54.23 Biopsy of peritoneum

49002

49002 Reopening of recent laparotomy

ICD-9-CM Diagnostic

553.21 Incisional hernia without mention of obstruction or gangrene
557.0 Acute vascular insufficiency of intestine
557.1 Chronic vascular insufficiency of intestine
560.81 Intestinal or peritoneal adhesions with obstruction (postoperative) (postinfection)
560.89 Other specified intestinal obstruction
567.2 Other suppurative peritonitis
567.8 Other specified peritonitis
568.81 Hemoperitoneum (nontraumatic)
568.9 Unspecified disorder of peritoneum ▽
614.6 Pelvic peritoneal adhesions, female (postoperative) (postinfection) — (Use additional code to identify any associated infertility, 628.2. Use additional code to identify organism: 041.0, 041.1) ♀
628.2 Female infertility of tubal origin — (Use additional code for any associated peritubal adhesions, 614.6) ♀
674.34 Other complication of obstetrical surgical wounds, postpartum condition or complication ♀
780.6 Fever
789.00 Abdominal pain, unspecified site ▽
789.01 Abdominal pain, right upper quadrant
789.02 Abdominal pain, left upper quadrant
789.03 Abdominal pain, right lower quadrant
789.04 Abdominal pain, left lower quadrant
789.05 Abdominal pain, periumbilic
789.06 Abdominal pain, epigastric
789.07 Abdominal pain, generalized
789.09 Abdominal pain, other specified site
789.1 Hepatomegaly
789.2 Splenomegaly
789.30 Abdominal or pelvic swelling, mass or lump, unspecified site ▽
789.31 Abdominal or pelvic swelling, mass, or lump, right upper quadrant
789.32 Abdominal or pelvic swelling, mass, or lump, left upper quadrant
789.33 Abdominal or pelvic swelling, mass, or lump, right lower quadrant
789.34 Abdominal or pelvic swelling, mass, or lump, left lower quadrant
789.35 Abdominal or pelvic swelling, mass or lump, periumbilic
789.36 Abdominal or pelvic swelling, mass, or lump, epigastric
789.37 Abdominal or pelvic swelling, mass, or lump, epigastric, generalized
789.39 Abdominal or pelvic swelling, mass, or lump, other specified site
996.80 Complications of transplanted organ, unspecified site — (Use additional code to identify nature of complication, 078.5) ▽
996.81 Complications of transplanted kidney — (Use additional code to identify nature of complication, 078.5)
996.82 Complications of transplanted liver — (Use additional code to identify nature of complication, 078.5)
996.86 Complications of transplanted pancreas — (Use additional code to identify nature of complication, 078.5)
996.87 Complications of transplanted organ, intestine — (Use additional code to identify nature of complication, 078.5)
996.89 Complications of other transplanted organ — (Use additional code to identify nature of complication, 078.5)
997.4 Digestive system complication — (Use additional code to identify complications)
997.5 Urinary complications — (Use additional code to identify complications)
998.11 Hemorrhage complicating a procedure
998.12 Hematoma complicating a procedure
998.13 Seroma complicating a procedure
998.31 Disruption of internal operation wound
998.32 Disruption of external operation wound
998.4 Foreign body accidentally left during procedure, not elsewhere classified
998.51 Infected postoperative seroma — (Use additional code to identify organism)
998.59 Other postoperative infection — (Use additional code to identify infection)
998.7 Acute reaction to foreign substance accidentally left during procedure, not elsewhere classified

ICD-9-CM Procedural

54.12 Reopening of recent laparotomy site

49010

49010 Exploration, retroperitoneal area with or without biopsy(s) (separate procedure)

ICD-9-CM Diagnostic

152.0 Malignant neoplasm of duodenum
157.0 Malignant neoplasm of head of pancreas
157.1 Malignant neoplasm of body of pancreas
157.2 Malignant neoplasm of tail of pancreas
157.3 Malignant neoplasm of pancreatic duct
157.4 Malignant neoplasm of islets of Langerhans — (Use additional code to identify any functional activity)
157.8 Malignant neoplasm of other specified sites of pancreas
157.9 Malignant neoplasm of pancreas, part unspecified ▽
158.0 Malignant neoplasm of retroperitoneum
158.8 Malignant neoplasm of specified parts of peritoneum
158.9 Malignant neoplasm of peritoneum, unspecified ▽
195.2 Malignant neoplasm of abdomen
197.4 Secondary malignant neoplasm of small intestine including duodenum
197.5 Secondary malignant neoplasm of large intestine and rectum
197.6 Secondary malignant neoplasm of retroperitoneum and peritoneum
197.7 Secondary malignant neoplasm of liver
198.89 Secondary malignant neoplasm of other specified sites
199.0 Disseminated malignant neoplasm
200.03 Reticulosarcoma of intra-abdominal lymph nodes
202.80 Other malignant lymphomas, unspecified site, extranodal and solid organ sites ▽
202.83 Other malignant lymphomas of intra-abdominal lymph nodes
211.8 Benign neoplasm of retroperitoneum and peritoneum
229.8 Benign neoplasm of other specified sites
235.4 Neoplasm of uncertain behavior of retroperitoneum and peritoneum
239.5 Neoplasm of unspecified nature of other genitourinary organs
569.5 Abscess of intestine
599.7 Hematuria
789.00 Abdominal pain, unspecified site ▽
789.01 Abdominal pain, right upper quadrant
789.02 Abdominal pain, left upper quadrant
789.03 Abdominal pain, right lower quadrant
789.04 Abdominal pain, left lower quadrant
789.05 Abdominal pain, periumbilic
789.06 Abdominal pain, epigastric
789.07 Abdominal pain, generalized
789.09 Abdominal pain, other specified site
789.30 Abdominal or pelvic swelling, mass or lump, unspecified site ▽
789.39 Abdominal or pelvic swelling, mass, or lump, other specified site
868.04 Retroperitoneum injury without mention of open wound into cavity
868.12 Bile duct and gallbladder injury, with open wound into cavity
868.13 Peritoneum injury with open wound into cavity
868.14 Retroperitoneum injury with open wound into cavity
879.3 Open wound of abdominal wall, anterior, complicated — (Use additional code to identify infection)
998.51 Infected postoperative seroma — (Use additional code to identify organism)
998.59 Other postoperative infection — (Use additional code to identify infection)
V45.89 Other postsurgical status — (This code is intended for use when these conditions are recorded as diagnoses or problems)

ICD-9-CM Procedural

54.0 Incision of abdominal wall
54.23 Biopsy of peritoneum

▽ Unspecified code
♀ Female diagnosis
☒ Manifestation code
♂ Male diagnosis

49020–49021

49020 Drainage of peritoneal abscess or localized peritonitis, exclusive of appendiceal abscess; open
49021 percutaneous

ICD-9-CM Diagnostic

151.9 Malignant neoplasm of stomach, unspecified site ▽
157.9 Malignant neoplasm of pancreas, part unspecified ▽
197.6 Secondary malignant neoplasm of retroperitoneum and peritoneum
198.89 Secondary malignant neoplasm of other specified sites
199.0 Disseminated malignant neoplasm
199.1 Other malignant neoplasm of unspecified site
537.4 Fistula of stomach or duodenum
537.82 Angiodysplasia of stomach and duodenum (without mention of hemorrhage)
537.83 Angiodysplasia of stomach and duodenum with hemorrhage
537.9 Unspecified disorder of stomach and duodenum ▽
555.9 Regional enteritis of unspecified site ▽
562.11 Diverticulitis of colon (without mention of hemorrhage) — (Use additional code to identify any associated peritonitis: 567.0-567.9)
562.13 Diverticulitis of colon with hemorrhage — (Use additional code to identify any associated peritonitis: 567.0-567.9)
567.0 Peritonitis in infectious diseases classified elsewhere — (Code first underlying disease) ☒
567.1 Pneumococcal peritonitis
567.2 Other suppurative peritonitis
567.8 Other specified peritonitis
567.9 Unspecified peritonitis ▽
568.81 Hemoperitoneum (nontraumatic)
568.82 Peritoneal effusion (chronic)
568.89 Other specified disorder of peritoneum
569.5 Abscess of intestine
569.83 Perforation of intestine
614.5 Acute or unspecified pelvic peritonitis, female — (Use additional code to identify organism: 041.0, 041.1) ♀
614.7 Other chronic pelvic peritonitis, female — (Use additional code to identify organism: 041.0, 041.1) ♀
670.00 Major puerperal infection, unspecified as to episode of care ▽ ♀
682.2 Cellulitis and abscess of trunk — (Use additional code to identify organism)
780.6 Fever
789.00 Abdominal pain, unspecified site ▽
789.30 Abdominal or pelvic swelling, mass or lump, unspecified site ▽
862.8 Injury to multiple and unspecified intrathoracic organs without mention of open wound into cavity
862.9 Injury to multiple and unspecified intrathoracic organs with open wound into cavity
863.95 Appendix injury with open wound into cavity
863.99 Injury to other and unspecified gastrointestinal sites with open wound into cavity
879.2 Open wound of abdominal wall, anterior, without mention of complication — (Use additional code to identify infection)
998.51 Infected postoperative seroma — (Use additional code to identify organism)
998.59 Other postoperative infection — (Use additional code to identify infection)
V45.89 Other postsurgical status — (This code is intended for use when these conditions are recorded as diagnoses or problems)

ICD-9-CM Procedural

54.19 Other laparotomy
54.91 Percutaneous abdominal drainage

49040–49041

49040 Drainage of subdiaphragmatic or subphrenic abscess; open
49041 percutaneous

ICD-9-CM Diagnostic

540.1 Acute appendicitis with peritoneal abscess
567.2 Other suppurative peritonitis
614.3 Acute parametritis and pelvic cellulitis — (Use additional code to identify organism: 041.0, 041.1) ♀
614.4 Chronic or unspecified parametritis and pelvic cellulitis — (Use additional code to identify organism: 041.0, 041.1) ♀
670.00 Major puerperal infection, unspecified as to episode of care ▽ ♀
670.02 Major puerperal infection, delivered, with mention of postpartum complication ♀
670.04 Major puerperal infection, postpartum ♀
998.59 Other postoperative infection — (Use additional code to identify infection)

ICD-9-CM Procedural

54.19 Other laparotomy
54.91 Percutaneous abdominal drainage

49060–49061

49060 Drainage of retroperitoneal abscess; open
49061 percutaneous

ICD-9-CM Diagnostic

540.1 Acute appendicitis with peritoneal abscess
555.9 Regional enteritis of unspecified site ▽
567.2 Other suppurative peritonitis
567.8 Other specified peritonitis
569.5 Abscess of intestine
577.0 Acute pancreatitis
590.2 Renal and perinephric abscess — (Use additional code to identify organism, such as E. coli, 041.4)
614.2 Salpingitis and oophoritis not specified as acute, subacute, or chronic — (Use additional code to identify organism: 041.0, 041.1) ♀
614.3 Acute parametritis and pelvic cellulitis — (Use additional code to identify organism: 041.0, 041.1) ♀
614.4 Chronic or unspecified parametritis and pelvic cellulitis — (Use additional code to identify organism: 041.0, 041.1) ♀
614.5 Acute or unspecified pelvic peritonitis, female — (Use additional code to identify organism: 041.0, 041.1) ♀
614.6 Pelvic peritoneal adhesions, female (postoperative) (postinfection) — (Use additional code to identify any associated infertility, 628.2. Use additional code to identify organism: 041.0, 041.1) ♀
614.7 Other chronic pelvic peritonitis, female — (Use additional code to identify organism: 041.0, 041.1) ♀
614.8 Other specified inflammatory disease of female pelvic organs and tissues — (Use additional code to identify organism: 041.0, 041.1) ♀
670.00 Major puerperal infection, unspecified as to episode of care ▽ ♀
670.02 Major puerperal infection, delivered, with mention of postpartum complication ♀
670.04 Major puerperal infection, postpartum ♀
998.59 Other postoperative infection — (Use additional code to identify infection)

ICD-9-CM Procedural

54.19 Other laparotomy
54.91 Percutaneous abdominal drainage

49062

49062 Drainage of extraperitoneal lymphocele to peritoneal cavity, open

ICD-9-CM Diagnostic

154.0 Malignant neoplasm of rectosigmoid junction
180.9 Malignant neoplasm of cervix uteri, unspecified site ▽ ♀
182.0 Malignant neoplasm of corpus uteri, except isthmus ♀
183.0 Malignant neoplasm of ovary — (Use additional code to identify any functional activity) ♀
185 Malignant neoplasm of prostate ♂
196.2 Secondary and unspecified malignant neoplasm of intra-abdominal lymph nodes
196.6 Secondary and unspecified malignant neoplasm of intrapelvic lymph nodes
200.13 Lymphosarcoma of intra-abdominal lymph nodes
201.93 Hodgkin's disease, unspecified type, of intra-abdominal lymph nodes ▽
202.03 Nodular lymphoma of intra-abdominal lymph nodes
202.83 Other malignant lymphomas of intra-abdominal lymph nodes
289.1 Chronic lymphadenitis
289.3 Lymphadenitis, unspecified, except mesenteric ▽
457.8 Other noninfectious disorders of lymphatic channels
683 Acute lymphadenitis — (Use additional code to identify organism)
782.2 Localized superficial swelling, mass, or lump
785.6 Enlargement of lymph nodes
996.81 Complications of transplanted kidney — (Use additional code to identify nature of complication, 078.5)
V42.0 Kidney replaced by transplant — (This code is intended for use when these conditions are recorded as diagnoses or problems)

ICD-9-CM Procedural

40.0 Incision of lymphatic structures

▽ Unspecified code ♀ Female diagnosis ☒ Manifestation code ♂ Male diagnosis

49080–49081

49080 Peritoneocentesis, abdominal paracentesis, or peritoneal lavage (diagnostic or therapeutic); initial
49081 subsequent

ICD-9-CM Diagnostic

151.8 Malignant neoplasm of other specified sites of stomach
151.9 Malignant neoplasm of stomach, unspecified site ▽
153.9 Malignant neoplasm of colon, unspecified site ▽
155.0 Malignant neoplasm of liver, primary
155.1 Malignant neoplasm of intrahepatic bile ducts
155.2 Malignant neoplasm of liver, not specified as primary or secondary ▽
156.0 Malignant neoplasm of gallbladder
156.1 Malignant neoplasm of extrahepatic bile ducts
156.2 Malignant neoplasm of ampulla of Vater
156.8 Malignant neoplasm of other specified sites of gallbladder and extrahepatic bile ducts
156.9 Malignant neoplasm of biliary tract, part unspecified site ▽
157.0 Malignant neoplasm of head of pancreas
157.1 Malignant neoplasm of body of pancreas
157.2 Malignant neoplasm of tail of pancreas
157.3 Malignant neoplasm of pancreatic duct
157.4 Malignant neoplasm of islets of Langerhans — (Use additional code to identify any functional activity)
157.8 Malignant neoplasm of other specified sites of pancreas
157.9 Malignant neoplasm of pancreas, part unspecified ▽
158.0 Malignant neoplasm of retroperitoneum
158.8 Malignant neoplasm of specified parts of peritoneum
158.9 Malignant neoplasm of peritoneum, unspecified ▽
183.0 Malignant neoplasm of ovary — (Use additional code to identify any functional activity) ♀
184.0 Malignant neoplasm of vagina ♀
195.2 Malignant neoplasm of abdomen
196.2 Secondary and unspecified malignant neoplasm of intra-abdominal lymph nodes
196.6 Secondary and unspecified malignant neoplasm of intrapelvic lymph nodes
197.6 Secondary malignant neoplasm of retroperitoneum and peritoneum
198.6 Secondary malignant neoplasm of ovary ♀
198.89 Secondary malignant neoplasm of other specified sites
199.0 Disseminated malignant neoplasm
199.1 Other malignant neoplasm of unspecified site
202.83 Other malignant lymphomas of intra-abdominal lymph nodes
233.3 Carcinoma in situ of other and unspecified female genital organs ▽ ♀
235.4 Neoplasm of uncertain behavior of retroperitoneum and peritoneum
236.3 Neoplasm of uncertain behavior of other and unspecified female genital organs ▽ ♀
239.8 Neoplasm of unspecified nature of other specified sites
239.9 Neoplasm of unspecified nature, site unspecified ▽
459.0 Unspecified hemorrhage ▽
540.0 Acute appendicitis with generalized peritonitis
540.1 Acute appendicitis with peritoneal abscess
540.9 Acute appendicitis without mention of peritonitis
541 Appendicitis, unqualified
542 Other appendicitis
543.0 Hyperplasia of appendix (lymphoid)
543.9 Other and unspecified diseases of appendix ▽
567.2 Other suppurative peritonitis
567.8 Other specified peritonitis
567.9 Unspecified peritonitis ▽
571.2 Alcoholic cirrhosis of liver
571.5 Cirrhosis of liver without mention of alcohol
571.6 Biliary cirrhosis
572.0 Abscess of liver
614.3 Acute parametritis and pelvic cellulitis — (Use additional code to identify organism: 041.0, 041.1) ♀
614.9 Unspecified inflammatory disease of female pelvic organs and tissues — (Use additional code to identify organism: 041.0, 041.1) ▽ ♀
780.6 Fever
787.01 Nausea with vomiting
789.00 Abdominal pain, unspecified site ▽
789.30 Abdominal or pelvic swelling, mass or lump, unspecified site ▽
789.5 Ascites
868.00 Injury to unspecified intra-abdominal organ without mention of open wound into cavity ▽
868.02 Bile duct and gallbladder injury without mention of open wound into cavity
868.03 Peritoneum injury without mention of open wound into cavity
868.13 Peritoneum injury with open wound into cavity
879.2 Open wound of abdominal wall, anterior, without mention of complication — (Use additional code to identify infection)
879.3 Open wound of abdominal wall, anterior, complicated — (Use additional code to identify infection)
879.4 Open wound of abdominal wall, lateral, without mention of complication — (Use additional code to identify infection)
879.5 Open wound of abdominal wall, lateral, complicated — (Use additional code to identify infection)
879.6 Open wound of other and unspecified parts of trunk, without mention of complication — (Use additional code to identify infection) ▽
879.7 Open wound of other and unspecified parts of trunk, complicated — (Use additional code to identify infection) ▽
879.8 Open wound(s) (multiple) of unspecified site(s), without mention of complication — (Use additional code to identify infection) ▽
879.9 Open wound(s) (multiple) of unspecified site(s), complicated — (Use additional code to identify infection) ▽
959.12 Other injury of abdomen
959.19 Other injury of other sites of trunk
998.51 Infected postoperative seroma — (Use additional code to identify organism)
998.59 Other postoperative infection — (Use additional code to identify infection)

ICD-9-CM Procedural

54.25 Peritoneal lavage
54.91 Percutaneous abdominal drainage

HCPCS Level II Supplies & Services

A4305 Disposable drug delivery system, flow rate of 50 ml or greater per hour
A4306 Disposable drug delivery system, flow rate of 5 ml or less per hour
A4550 Surgical trays

49085

49085 Removal of peritoneal foreign body from peritoneal cavity

ICD-9-CM Diagnostic

789.00 Abdominal pain, unspecified site ▽
868.10 Injury to unspecified intra-abdominal organ, with open wound into cavity ▽
868.13 Peritoneum injury with open wound into cavity
868.19 Injury to other and multiple intra-abdominal organs, with open wound into cavity
996.60 Infection and inflammatory reaction due to unspecified device, implant, and graft — (Use additional code to identify specified infections) ▽
996.62 Infection and inflammatory reaction due to other vascular device, implant, and graft — (Use additional code to identify specified infections)
996.70 Other complications due to unspecified device, implant, and graft ▽
998.4 Foreign body accidentally left during procedure, not elsewhere classified

ICD-9-CM Procedural

54.92 Removal of foreign body from peritoneal cavity

49180

49180 Biopsy, abdominal or retroperitoneal mass, percutaneous needle

ICD-9-CM Diagnostic

158.0 Malignant neoplasm of retroperitoneum
158.8 Malignant neoplasm of specified parts of peritoneum
158.9 Malignant neoplasm of peritoneum, unspecified ▽
159.8 Malignant neoplasm of other sites of digestive system and intra-abdominal organs
173.5 Other malignant neoplasm of skin of trunk, except scrotum
183.0 Malignant neoplasm of ovary — (Use additional code to identify any functional activity) ♀
183.8 Malignant neoplasm of other specified sites of uterine adnexa ♀
195.2 Malignant neoplasm of abdomen
196.2 Secondary and unspecified malignant neoplasm of intra-abdominal lymph nodes
196.6 Secondary and unspecified malignant neoplasm of intrapelvic lymph nodes
197.6 Secondary malignant neoplasm of retroperitoneum and peritoneum
198.89 Secondary malignant neoplasm of other specified sites
199.1 Other malignant neoplasm of unspecified site
202.80 Other malignant lymphomas, unspecified site, extranodal and solid organ sites ▽
211.8 Benign neoplasm of retroperitoneum and peritoneum
211.9 Benign neoplasm of other and unspecified site of the digestive system ▽
220 Benign neoplasm of ovary — (Use additional code to identify any functional activity: 256.0-256.1) ♀

▽ Unspecified code
♀ Female diagnosis
☒ Manifestation code
♂ Male diagnosis

227.6 Benign neoplasm of aortic body and other paraganglia — (Use additional code to identify any functional activity)
228.04 Hemangioma of intra-abdominal structures
235.4 Neoplasm of uncertain behavior of retroperitoneum and peritoneum
235.5 Neoplasm of uncertain behavior of other and unspecified digestive organs ▽
236.2 Neoplasm of uncertain behavior of ovary — (Use additional code to identify any functional activity) ♀
236.3 Neoplasm of uncertain behavior of other and unspecified female genital organs ▽ ♀
237.3 Neoplasm of uncertain behavior of paraganglia
238.8 Neoplasm of uncertain behavior of other specified sites
238.9 Neoplasm of uncertain behavior, site unspecified ▽
239.0 Neoplasm of unspecified nature of digestive system
239.7 Neoplasm of unspecified nature of endocrine glands and other parts of nervous system
239.9 Neoplasm of unspecified nature, site unspecified ▽
256.0 Hyperestrogenism ♀
256.1 Other ovarian hyperfunction ♀
614.6 Pelvic peritoneal adhesions, female (postoperative) (postinfection) — (Use additional code to identify any associated infertility, 628.2. Use additional code to identify organism: 041.0, 041.1) ♀
617.0 Endometriosis of uterus ♀
617.3 Endometriosis of pelvic peritoneum ♀
617.9 Endometriosis, site unspecified ▽ ♀
628.2 Female infertility of tubal origin — (Use additional code for any associated peritubal adhesions, 614.6) ♀
682.2 Cellulitis and abscess of trunk — (Use additional code to identify organism)
780.6 Fever
780.99 Other general symptoms
785.6 Enlargement of lymph nodes
787.99 Other symptoms involving digestive system
789.09 Abdominal pain, other specified site
789.30 Abdominal or pelvic swelling, mass or lump, unspecified site ▽
789.31 Abdominal or pelvic swelling, mass, or lump, right upper quadrant
789.32 Abdominal or pelvic swelling, mass, or lump, left upper quadrant
789.33 Abdominal or pelvic swelling, mass, or lump, right lower quadrant
789.34 Abdominal or pelvic swelling, mass, or lump, left lower quadrant
789.35 Abdominal or pelvic swelling, mass or lump, periumbilic
789.36 Abdominal or pelvic swelling, mass, or lump, epigastric
789.37 Abdominal or pelvic swelling, mass, or lump, epigastric, generalized
789.39 Abdominal or pelvic swelling, mass, or lump, other specified site
793.6 Nonspecific abnormal findings on radiological and other examination of abdominal area, including retroperitoneum
V72.5 Radiological examination, not elsewhere classified — (Use additional code(s) to identify any special screening examination(s) performed: V73.0-V82.9)

ICD-9-CM Procedural

54.24 Closed (percutaneous) (needle) biopsy of intra-abdominal mass

HCPCS Level II Supplies & Services

A4305 Disposable drug delivery system, flow rate of 50 ml or greater per hour
A4306 Disposable drug delivery system, flow rate of 5 ml or less per hour
A4550 Surgical trays

49200–49201

49200 Excision or destruction, open, intra-abdominal or retroperitoneal tumors or cysts or endometriomas;
49201 extensive

ICD-9-CM Diagnostic

154.0 Malignant neoplasm of rectosigmoid junction
158.0 Malignant neoplasm of retroperitoneum
158.8 Malignant neoplasm of specified parts of peritoneum
158.9 Malignant neoplasm of peritoneum, unspecified ▽
159.0 Malignant neoplasm of intestinal tract, part unspecified ▽
171.5 Malignant neoplasm of connective and other soft tissue of abdomen
171.6 Malignant neoplasm of connective and other soft tissue of pelvis
183.0 Malignant neoplasm of ovary — (Use additional code to identify any functional activity) ♀
183.3 Malignant neoplasm of broad ligament of uterus ♀
183.4 Malignant neoplasm of parametrium of uterus ♀
183.5 Malignant neoplasm of round ligament of uterus ♀
183.9 Malignant neoplasm of uterine adnexa, unspecified site ▽ ♀
194.0 Malignant neoplasm of adrenal gland — (Use additional code to identify any functional activity)
194.6 Malignant neoplasm of aortic body and other paraganglia — (Use additional code to identify any functional activity)
195.2 Malignant neoplasm of abdomen
195.3 Malignant neoplasm of pelvis
197.6 Secondary malignant neoplasm of retroperitoneum and peritoneum
198.89 Secondary malignant neoplasm of other specified sites
211.8 Benign neoplasm of retroperitoneum and peritoneum
211.9 Benign neoplasm of other and unspecified site of the digestive system ▽
214.3 Lipoma of intra-abdominal organs
214.8 Lipoma of other specified sites
228.04 Hemangioma of intra-abdominal structures
235.2 Neoplasm of uncertain behavior of stomach, intestines, and rectum
235.4 Neoplasm of uncertain behavior of retroperitoneum and peritoneum
237.3 Neoplasm of uncertain behavior of paraganglia
238.9 Neoplasm of uncertain behavior, site unspecified ▽
239.0 Neoplasm of unspecified nature of digestive system
239.9 Neoplasm of unspecified nature, site unspecified ▽
568.89 Other specified disorder of peritoneum
614.6 Pelvic peritoneal adhesions, female (postoperative) (postinfection) — (Use additional code to identify any associated infertility, 628.2. Use additional code to identify organism: 041.0, 041.1) ♀
617.0 Endometriosis of uterus ♀
617.1 Endometriosis of ovary ♀
617.2 Endometriosis of fallopian tube ♀
617.3 Endometriosis of pelvic peritoneum ♀
617.5 Endometriosis of intestine ♀
617.8 Endometriosis of other specified sites ♀
625.8 Other specified symptom associated with female genital organs ♀
789.00 Abdominal pain, unspecified site ▽
789.01 Abdominal pain, right upper quadrant
789.02 Abdominal pain, left upper quadrant
789.03 Abdominal pain, right lower quadrant
789.04 Abdominal pain, left lower quadrant
789.05 Abdominal pain, periumbilic
789.06 Abdominal pain, epigastric
789.07 Abdominal pain, generalized
789.09 Abdominal pain, other specified site
789.30 Abdominal or pelvic swelling, mass or lump, unspecified site ▽
789.31 Abdominal or pelvic swelling, mass, or lump, right upper quadrant
789.32 Abdominal or pelvic swelling, mass, or lump, left upper quadrant
789.33 Abdominal or pelvic swelling, mass, or lump, right lower quadrant
789.34 Abdominal or pelvic swelling, mass, or lump, left lower quadrant
789.35 Abdominal or pelvic swelling, mass or lump, periumbilic
789.36 Abdominal or pelvic swelling, mass, or lump, epigastric
789.37 Abdominal or pelvic swelling, mass, or lump, epigastric, generalized
789.39 Abdominal or pelvic swelling, mass, or lump, other specified site

ICD-9-CM Procedural

54.3 Excision or destruction of lesion or tissue of abdominal wall or umbilicus
54.4 Excision or destruction of peritoneal tissue

49215

49215 Excision of presacral or sacrococcygeal tumor

ICD-9-CM Diagnostic

170.6 Malignant neoplasm of pelvic bones, sacrum, and coccyx
171.6 Malignant neoplasm of connective and other soft tissue of pelvis
198.5 Secondary malignant neoplasm of bone and bone marrow
198.89 Secondary malignant neoplasm of other specified sites
213.6 Benign neoplasm of pelvic bones, sacrum, and coccyx
215.6 Other benign neoplasm of connective and other soft tissue of pelvis
238.0 Neoplasm of uncertain behavior of bone and articular cartilage
238.1 Neoplasm of uncertain behavior of connective and other soft tissue ▽
239.2 Neoplasms of unspecified nature of bone, soft tissue, and skin
782.2 Localized superficial swelling, mass, or lump

ICD-9-CM Procedural

54.4 Excision or destruction of peritoneal tissue
77.99 Total ostectomy of other bone, except facial bones

49220

49220 Staging laparotomy for Hodgkins disease or lymphoma (includes splenectomy, needle or open biopsies of both liver lobes, possibly also removal of abdominal nodes, abdominal node and/or bone marrow biopsies, ovarian repositioning)

ICD-9-CM Diagnostic

- 201.40 Hodgkin's disease, lymphocytic-histiocytic predominance, unspecified site, extranodal and solid organ sites ▽
- 201.41 Hodgkin's disease, lymphocytic-histiocytic predominance of lymph nodes of head, face, and neck
- 201.42 Hodgkin's disease, lymphocytic-histiocytic predominance of intrathoracic lymph nodes
- 201.43 Hodgkin's disease, lymphocytic-histiocytic predominance of intra-abdominal lymph nodes
- 201.44 Hodgkin's disease, lymphocytic-histiocytic predominance of lymph nodes of axilla and upper limb
- 201.45 Hodgkin's disease, lymphocytic-histiocytic predominance of lymph nodes of inguinal region and lower limb
- 201.46 Hodgkin's disease, lymphocytic-histiocytic predominance of intrapelvic lymph nodes
- 201.47 Hodgkin's disease, lymphocytic-histiocytic predominance of spleen
- 201.48 Hodgkin's disease, lymphocytic-histiocytic predominance of lymph nodes of multiple sites
- 201.50 Hodgkin's disease, nodular sclerosis, unspecified site, extranodal and solid organ sites ▽
- 201.51 Hodgkin's disease, nodular sclerosis, of lymph nodes of head, face, and neck
- 201.52 Hodgkin's disease, nodular sclerosis, of intrathoracic lymph nodes
- 201.70 Hodgkin's disease, lymphocytic depletion, unspecified site, extranodal and solid organ sites ▽
- 201.71 Hodgkin's disease, lymphocytic depletion, of lymph nodes of head, face, and neck
- 202.00 Nodular lymphoma, unspecified site, extranodal and solid organ sites ▽
- 202.08 Nodular lymphoma of lymph nodes of multiple sites
- 202.80 Other malignant lymphomas, unspecified site, extranodal and solid organ sites ▽
- 202.88 Other malignant lymphomas of lymph nodes of multiple sites

ICD-9-CM Procedural

- 40.3 Regional lymph node excision
- 41.31 Biopsy of bone marrow
- 45.19 Other diagnostic procedures on small intestine
- 50.11 Closed (percutaneous) (needle) biopsy of liver
- 50.12 Open biopsy of liver
- 54.11 Exploratory laparotomy

49250

49250 Umbilectomy, omphalectomy, excision of umbilicus (separate procedure)

ICD-9-CM Diagnostic

- 553.1 Umbilical hernia without mention of obstruction or gangrene
- 686.8 Other specified local infections of skin and subcutaneous tissue
- 728.84 Diastasis of muscle
- 771.4 Omphalitis of the newborn

ICD-9-CM Procedural

- 54.3 Excision or destruction of lesion or tissue of abdominal wall or umbilicus

49255

49255 Omentectomy, epiploectomy, resection of omentum (separate procedure)

ICD-9-CM Diagnostic

- 158.0 Malignant neoplasm of retroperitoneum
- 158.8 Malignant neoplasm of specified parts of peritoneum
- 159.0 Malignant neoplasm of intestinal tract, part unspecified ▽
- 159.9 Malignant neoplasm of ill-defined sites of digestive organs and peritoneum
- 171.5 Malignant neoplasm of connective and other soft tissue of abdomen
- 195.2 Malignant neoplasm of abdomen
- 195.8 Malignant neoplasm of other specified sites
- 196.2 Secondary and unspecified malignant neoplasm of intra-abdominal lymph nodes
- 197.4 Secondary malignant neoplasm of small intestine including duodenum
- 197.5 Secondary malignant neoplasm of large intestine and rectum
- 197.6 Secondary malignant neoplasm of retroperitoneum and peritoneum
- 197.7 Secondary malignant neoplasm of liver
- 197.8 Secondary malignant neoplasm of other digestive organs and spleen
- 198.82 Secondary malignant neoplasm of genital organs
- 198.89 Secondary malignant neoplasm of other specified sites
- 199.0 Disseminated malignant neoplasm
- 211.8 Benign neoplasm of retroperitoneum and peritoneum
- 211.9 Benign neoplasm of other and unspecified site of the digestive system ▽
- 235.4 Neoplasm of uncertain behavior of retroperitoneum and peritoneum
- 238.1 Neoplasm of uncertain behavior of connective and other soft tissue ▽
- 239.0 Neoplasm of unspecified nature of digestive system
- 239.8 Neoplasm of unspecified nature of other specified sites
- 567.2 Other suppurative peritonitis
- 568.0 Peritoneal adhesions (postoperative) (postinfection)
- 568.89 Other specified disorder of peritoneum
- 614.6 Pelvic peritoneal adhesions, female (postoperative) (postinfection) — (Use additional code to identify any associated infertility, 628.2. Use additional code to identify organism: 041.0, 041.1) ♀
- 628.2 Female infertility of tubal origin — (Use additional code for any associated peritubal adhesions, 614.6) ♀
- 789.00 Abdominal pain, unspecified site ▽
- 789.30 Abdominal or pelvic swelling, mass or lump, unspecified site ▽

ICD-9-CM Procedural

- 54.4 Excision or destruction of peritoneal tissue

49320

49320 Laparoscopy, abdomen, peritoneum, and omentum, diagnostic, with or without collection of specimen(s) by brushing or washing (separate procedure)

ICD-9-CM Diagnostic

- 151.1 Malignant neoplasm of pylorus
- 151.2 Malignant neoplasm of pyloric antrum
- 151.3 Malignant neoplasm of fundus of stomach
- 151.4 Malignant neoplasm of body of stomach
- 151.5 Malignant neoplasm of lesser curvature of stomach, unspecified ▽
- 151.6 Malignant neoplasm of greater curvature of stomach, unspecified ▽
- 151.8 Malignant neoplasm of other specified sites of stomach
- 151.9 Malignant neoplasm of stomach, unspecified site ▽
- 152.0 Malignant neoplasm of duodenum
- 152.1 Malignant neoplasm of jejunum
- 152.2 Malignant neoplasm of ileum
- 152.3 Malignant neoplasm of Meckel's diverticulum
- 152.8 Malignant neoplasm of other specified sites of small intestine
- 152.9 Malignant neoplasm of small intestine, unspecified site ▽
- 156.2 Malignant neoplasm of ampulla of Vater
- 156.8 Malignant neoplasm of other specified sites of gallbladder and extrahepatic bile ducts
- 156.9 Malignant neoplasm of biliary tract, part unspecified site ▽
- 157.0 Malignant neoplasm of head of pancreas
- 157.1 Malignant neoplasm of body of pancreas
- 157.2 Malignant neoplasm of tail of pancreas
- 157.4 Malignant neoplasm of islets of Langerhans — (Use additional code to identify any functional activity)
- 157.8 Malignant neoplasm of other specified sites of pancreas
- 157.9 Malignant neoplasm of pancreas, part unspecified ▽
- 158.0 Malignant neoplasm of retroperitoneum
- 158.8 Malignant neoplasm of specified parts of peritoneum
- 158.9 Malignant neoplasm of peritoneum, unspecified ▽
- 159.0 Malignant neoplasm of intestinal tract, part unspecified ▽
- 159.1 Malignant neoplasm of spleen, not elsewhere classified
- 159.8 Malignant neoplasm of other sites of digestive system and intra-abdominal organs
- 159.9 Malignant neoplasm of ill-defined sites of digestive organs and peritoneum
- 171.5 Malignant neoplasm of connective and other soft tissue of abdomen
- 171.6 Malignant neoplasm of connective and other soft tissue of pelvis
- 171.8 Malignant neoplasm of other specified sites of connective and other soft tissue
- 171.9 Malignant neoplasm of connective and other soft tissue, site unspecified ▽
- 180.0 Malignant neoplasm of endocervix ♀
- 180.1 Malignant neoplasm of exocervix ♀
- 180.8 Malignant neoplasm of other specified sites of cervix ♀
- 180.9 Malignant neoplasm of cervix uteri, unspecified site ▽ ♀
- 181 Malignant neoplasm of placenta ♀
- 182.0 Malignant neoplasm of corpus uteri, except isthmus ♀
- 182.1 Malignant neoplasm of isthmus ♀
- 182.8 Malignant neoplasm of other specified sites of body of uterus ♀
- 183.0 Malignant neoplasm of ovary — (Use additional code to identify any functional activity) ♀
- 183.2 Malignant neoplasm of fallopian tube ♀
- 183.3 Malignant neoplasm of broad ligament of uterus ♀

▽ Unspecified code ☒ Manifestation code
♀ Female diagnosis ♂ Male diagnosis

183.4 Malignant neoplasm of parametrium of uterus ♀
183.5 Malignant neoplasm of round ligament of uterus ♀
183.8 Malignant neoplasm of other specified sites of uterine adnexa ♀
183.9 Malignant neoplasm of uterine adnexa, unspecified site ▽ ♀
184.8 Malignant neoplasm of other specified sites of female genital organs ♀
184.9 Malignant neoplasm of female genital organ, site unspecified ▽ ♀
185 Malignant neoplasm of prostate ♂
187.8 Malignant neoplasm of other specified sites of male genital organs ♂
188.0 Malignant neoplasm of trigone of urinary bladder
188.1 Malignant neoplasm of dome of urinary bladder
188.2 Malignant neoplasm of lateral wall of urinary bladder
188.3 Malignant neoplasm of anterior wall of urinary bladder
188.4 Malignant neoplasm of posterior wall of urinary bladder
188.5 Malignant neoplasm of bladder neck
188.6 Malignant neoplasm of ureteric orifice
188.7 Malignant neoplasm of urachus
188.8 Malignant neoplasm of other specified sites of bladder
189.0 Malignant neoplasm of kidney, except pelvis
189.1 Malignant neoplasm of renal pelvis
189.2 Malignant neoplasm of ureter
189.8 Malignant neoplasm of other specified sites of urinary organs
194.0 Malignant neoplasm of adrenal gland — (Use additional code to identify any functional activity)
195.2 Malignant neoplasm of abdomen
195.3 Malignant neoplasm of pelvis
196.2 Secondary and unspecified malignant neoplasm of intra-abdominal lymph nodes
196.6 Secondary and unspecified malignant neoplasm of intrapelvic lymph nodes
197.4 Secondary malignant neoplasm of small intestine including duodenum
197.5 Secondary malignant neoplasm of large intestine and rectum
197.6 Secondary malignant neoplasm of retroperitoneum and peritoneum
197.7 Secondary malignant neoplasm of liver
197.8 Secondary malignant neoplasm of other digestive organs and spleen
198.0 Secondary malignant neoplasm of kidney
198.1 Secondary malignant neoplasm of other urinary organs
198.6 Secondary malignant neoplasm of ovary ♀
198.7 Secondary malignant neoplasm of adrenal gland
198.89 Secondary malignant neoplasm of other specified sites
199.0 Disseminated malignant neoplasm
200.03 Reticulosarcoma of intra-abdominal lymph nodes
200.06 Reticulosarcoma of intrapelvic lymph nodes
200.07 Reticulosarcoma of spleen
200.13 Lymphosarcoma of intra-abdominal lymph nodes
200.16 Lymphosarcoma of intrapelvic lymph nodes
200.17 Lymphosarcoma of spleen
200.23 Burkitt's tumor or lymphoma of intra-abdominal lymph nodes
200.26 Burkitt's tumor or lymphoma of intrapelvic lymph nodes
200.27 Burkitt's tumor or lymphoma of spleen
200.83 Other named variants of lymphosarcoma and reticulosarcoma of intra-abdominal lymph nodes
200.86 Other named variants of lymphosarcoma and reticulosarcoma of intrapelvic lymph nodes
201.03 Hodgkin's paragranuloma of intra-abdominal lymph nodes
201.06 Hodgkin's paragranuloma of intrapelvic lymph nodes
201.07 Hodgkin's paragranuloma of spleen
201.13 Hodgkin's granuloma of intra-abdominal lymph nodes
201.16 Hodgkin's granuloma of intrapelvic lymph nodes
201.17 Hodgkin's granuloma of spleen
201.18 Hodgkin's granuloma of lymph nodes of multiple sites
201.23 Hodgkin's sarcoma of intra-abdominal lymph nodes
201.26 Hodgkin's sarcoma of intrapelvic lymph nodes
201.27 Hodgkin's sarcoma of spleen
201.28 Hodgkin's sarcoma of lymph nodes of multiple sites
201.43 Hodgkin's disease, lymphocytic-histiocytic predominance of intra-abdominal lymph nodes
201.46 Hodgkin's disease, lymphocytic-histiocytic predominance of intrapelvic lymph nodes
201.47 Hodgkin's disease, lymphocytic-histiocytic predominance of spleen
201.53 Hodgkin's disease, nodular sclerosis, of intra-abdominal lymph nodes
201.56 Hodgkin's disease, nodular sclerosis, of intrapelvic lymph nodes
201.57 Hodgkin's disease, nodular sclerosis, of spleen
201.58 Hodgkin's disease, nodular sclerosis, of lymph nodes of multiple sites
201.63 Hodgkin's disease, mixed cellularity, of intra-abdominal lymph nodes
201.66 Hodgkin's disease, mixed cellularity, of intrapelvic lymph nodes
201.67 Hodgkin's disease, mixed cellularity, of spleen
201.68 Hodgkin's disease, mixed cellularity, of lymph nodes of multiple sites
201.73 Hodgkin's disease, lymphocytic depletion, of intra-abdominal lymph nodes
201.76 Hodgkin's disease, lymphocytic depletion, of intrapelvic lymph nodes
201.77 Hodgkin's disease, lymphocytic depletion, of spleen
201.78 Hodgkin's disease, lymphocytic depletion, of lymph nodes of multiple sites
201.93 Hodgkin's disease, unspecified type, of intra-abdominal lymph nodes ▽
201.96 Hodgkin's disease, unspecified type, of intrapelvic lymph nodes ▽
201.97 Hodgkin's disease, unspecified type, of spleen ▽
202.03 Nodular lymphoma of intra-abdominal lymph nodes
202.06 Nodular lymphoma of intrapelvic lymph nodes
202.07 Nodular lymphoma of spleen
202.08 Nodular lymphoma of lymph nodes of multiple sites
202.13 Mycosis fungoides of intra-abdominal lymph nodes
202.16 Mycosis fungoides of intrapelvic lymph nodes
202.17 Mycosis fungoides of spleen
202.23 Sezary's disease of intra-abdominal lymph nodes
202.26 Sezary's disease of intrapelvic lymph nodes
202.27 Sezary's disease of spleen
202.28 Sezary's disease of lymph nodes of multiple sites
202.30 Malignant histiocytosis, unspecified site, extranodal and solid organ sites ▽
202.33 Malignant histiocytosis of intra-abdominal lymph nodes
202.36 Malignant histiocytosis of intrapelvic lymph nodes
202.37 Malignant histiocytosis of spleen
202.40 Leukemic reticuloendotheliosis, unspecified site, extranodal and solid organ sites ▽
202.43 Leukemic reticuloendotheliosis of intra-abdominal lymph nodes
202.46 Leukemic reticuloendotheliosis of intrapelvic lymph nodes
202.47 Leukemic reticuloendotheliosis of spleen
202.53 Letterer-Siwe disease of intra-abdominal lymph nodes
202.56 Letterer-Siwe disease of intrapelvic lymph nodes
202.57 Letterer-Siwe disease of spleen
202.58 Letterer-Siwe disease of lymph nodes of multiple sites
202.63 Malignant mast cell tumors of intra-abdominal lymph nodes
202.66 Malignant mast cell tumors of intrapelvic lymph nodes
202.67 Malignant mast cell tumors of spleen
202.68 Malignant mast cell tumors of lymph nodes of multiple sites
202.83 Other malignant lymphomas of intra-abdominal lymph nodes
202.86 Other malignant lymphomas of intrapelvic lymph nodes
202.87 Other malignant lymphomas of spleen
202.88 Other malignant lymphomas of lymph nodes of multiple sites
202.93 Other and unspecified malignant neoplasms of lymphoid and histiocytic tissue of intra-abdominal lymph nodes ▽
202.96 Other and unspecified malignant neoplasms of lymphoid and histiocytic tissue of intrapelvic lymph nodes ▽
202.97 Other and unspecified malignant neoplasms of lymphoid and histiocytic tissue of spleen ▽
211.1 Benign neoplasm of stomach
211.2 Benign neoplasm of duodenum, jejunum, and ileum
211.3 Benign neoplasm of colon
211.4 Benign neoplasm of rectum and anal canal
211.5 Benign neoplasm of liver and biliary passages
211.6 Benign neoplasm of pancreas, except islets of Langerhans
211.7 Benign neoplasm of islets of Langerhans — (Use additional code to identify any functional activity)
211.8 Benign neoplasm of retroperitoneum and peritoneum
211.9 Benign neoplasm of other and unspecified site of the digestive system ▽
214.3 Lipoma of intra-abdominal organs
214.8 Lipoma of other specified sites
218.0 Submucous leiomyoma of uterus ♀
218.1 Intramural leiomyoma of uterus ♀
218.2 Subserous leiomyoma of uterus ♀
218.9 Leiomyoma of uterus, unspecified ▽ ♀
219.0 Benign neoplasm of cervix uteri ♀
219.1 Benign neoplasm of corpus uteri ♀
219.8 Benign neoplasm of other specified parts of uterus ♀
219.9 Benign neoplasm of uterus, part unspecified ▽ ♀
220 Benign neoplasm of ovary — (Use additional code to identify any functional activity: 256.0-256.1) ♀
221.0 Benign neoplasm of fallopian tube and uterine ligaments ♀
223.0 Benign neoplasm of kidney, except pelvis
223.1 Benign neoplasm of renal pelvis
223.2 Benign neoplasm of ureter
223.3 Benign neoplasm of bladder
227.0 Benign neoplasm of adrenal gland — (Use additional code to identify any functional activity)
227.6 Benign neoplasm of aortic body and other paraganglia — (Use additional code to identify any functional activity)

▽ Unspecified code
♀ Female diagnosis
☒ Manifestation code
♂ Male diagnosis

228.04 Hemangioma of intra-abdominal structures
228.1 Lymphangioma, any site
229.0 Benign neoplasm of lymph nodes
230.2 Carcinoma in situ of stomach
230.3 Carcinoma in situ of colon
230.4 Carcinoma in situ of rectum
230.7 Carcinoma in situ of other and unspecified parts of intestine ▽
230.8 Carcinoma in situ of liver and biliary system
230.9 Carcinoma in situ of other and unspecified digestive organs ▽
233.1 Carcinoma in situ of cervix uteri ♀
233.2 Carcinoma in situ of other and unspecified parts of uterus ▽ ♀
233.3 Carcinoma in situ of other and unspecified female genital organs ▽ ♀
233.4 Carcinoma in situ of prostate ♂
233.9 Carcinoma in situ of other and unspecified urinary organs ▽
235.2 Neoplasm of uncertain behavior of stomach, intestines, and rectum
235.3 Neoplasm of uncertain behavior of liver and biliary passages
236.0 Neoplasm of uncertain behavior of uterus ♀
236.2 Neoplasm of uncertain behavior of ovary — (Use additional code to identify any functional activity) ♀
236.3 Neoplasm of uncertain behavior of other and unspecified female genital organs ▽ ♀
236.7 Neoplasm of uncertain behavior of bladder
236.90 Neoplasm of uncertain behavior of urinary organ, unspecified ▽
236.91 Neoplasm of uncertain behavior of kidney and ureter
236.99 Neoplasm of uncertain behavior of other and unspecified urinary organs
237.2 Neoplasm of uncertain behavior of adrenal gland — (Use additional code to identify any functional activity)
237.3 Neoplasm of uncertain behavior of paraganglia
238.7 Neoplasm of uncertain behavior of other lymphatic and hematopoietic tissues
238.8 Neoplasm of uncertain behavior of other specified sites
238.9 Neoplasm of uncertain behavior, site unspecified ▽
239.0 Neoplasm of unspecified nature of digestive system
239.5 Neoplasm of unspecified nature of other genitourinary organs
239.7 Neoplasm of unspecified nature of endocrine glands and other parts of nervous system
239.8 Neoplasm of unspecified nature of other specified sites
239.9 Neoplasm of unspecified nature, site unspecified ▽
256.4 Polycystic ovaries ♀
256.8 Other ovarian dysfunction ♀
289.2 Nonspecific mesenteric lymphadenitis
289.3 Lymphadenitis, unspecified, except mesenteric ▽
289.4 Hypersplenism
289.51 Chronic congestive splenomegaly
289.52 Splenic sequestration — (Code first sickle-cell disease in crisis: 282.42, 282.62, 282.64, 282.69)
289.59 Other diseases of spleen
441.02 Dissecting aortic aneurysm (any part), abdominal
441.4 Abdominal aneurysm without mention of rupture
447.3 Hyperplasia of renal artery
447.4 Celiac artery compression syndrome
453.0 Budd-Chiari syndrome
453.1 Thrombophlebitis migrans
456.5 Pelvic varices
531.10 Acute gastric ulcer with perforation, without mention of obstruction — (Use additional E code to identify drug, if drug induced)
531.11 Acute gastric ulcer with perforation and obstruction — (Use additional E code to identify drug, if drug induced)
531.20 Acute gastric ulcer with hemorrhage and perforation, without mention of obstruction — (Use additional E code to identify drug, if drug induced)
531.21 Acute gastric ulcer with hemorrhage, perforation, and obstruction — (Use additional E code to identify drug, if drug induced)
531.50 Chronic or unspecified gastric ulcer with perforation, without mention of obstruction — (Use additional E code to identify drug, if drug induced)
531.51 Chronic or unspecified gastric ulcer with perforation and obstruction — (Use additional E code to identify drug, if drug induced)
531.60 Chronic or unspecified gastric ulcer with hemorrhage and perforation, without mention of obstruction — (Use additional E code to identify drug, if drug induced)
531.61 Chronic or unspecified gastric ulcer with hemorrhage, perforation, and obstruction — (Use additional E code to identify drug, if drug induced)
532.10 Acute duodenal ulcer with perforation, without mention of obstruction — (Use additional E code to identify drug, if drug induced)
532.11 Acute duodenal ulcer with perforation and obstruction — (Use additional E code to identify drug, if drug induced)
532.20 Acute duodenal ulcer with hemorrhage and perforation, without mention of obstruction — (Use additional E code to identify drug, if drug induced)
532.21 Acute duodenal ulcer with hemorrhage, perforation, and obstruction — (Use additional E code to identify drug, if drug induced)
532.50 Chronic or unspecified duodenal ulcer with perforation, without mention of obstruction — (Use additional E code to identify drug, if drug induced)
532.51 Chronic or unspecified duodenal ulcer with perforation and obstruction — (Use additional E code to identify drug, if drug induced)
532.60 Chronic or unspecified duodenal ulcer with hemorrhage and perforation, without mention of obstruction — (Use additional E code to identify drug, if drug induced)
532.61 Chronic or unspecified duodenal ulcer with hemorrhage, perforation, and obstruction — (Use additional E code to identify drug, if drug induced)
534.90 Gastrojejunal ulcer, unspecified as acute or chronic, without mention of hemorrhage, perforation, or obstruction ▽
534.91 Gastrojejunal ulcer, unspecified as acute or chronic, without mention of hemorrhage or perforation, with obstruction ▽
537.1 Gastric diverticulum
537.2 Chronic duodenal ileus
537.3 Other obstruction of duodenum
537.4 Fistula of stomach or duodenum
537.5 Gastroptosis
537.6 Hourglass stricture or stenosis of stomach
537.82 Angiodysplasia of stomach and duodenum (without mention of hemorrhage)
537.83 Angiodysplasia of stomach and duodenum with hemorrhage
537.89 Other specified disorder of stomach and duodenum
540.0 Acute appendicitis with generalized peritonitis
540.1 Acute appendicitis with peritoneal abscess
540.9 Acute appendicitis without mention of peritonitis
541 Appendicitis, unqualified
542 Other appendicitis
543.0 Hyperplasia of appendix (lymphoid)
543.9 Other and unspecified diseases of appendix ▽
550.00 Inguinal hernia with gangrene, unilateral or unspecified, (not specified as recurrent)
550.01 Inguinal hernia with gangrene, recurrent unilateral or unspecified inguinal hernia
550.02 Inguinal hernia with gangrene, bilateral
550.03 Inguinal hernia with gangrene, recurrent bilateral
550.10 Inguinal hernia with obstruction, without mention of gangrene, unilateral or unspecified, (not specified as recurrent)
550.11 Inguinal hernia with obstruction, without mention of gangrene, recurrent unilateral or unspecified
550.12 Inguinal hernia with obstruction, without mention gangrene, bilateral, (not specified as recurrent)
550.13 Inguinal hernia with obstruction, without mention of gangrene, recurrent bilateral
550.90 Inguinal hernia without mention of obstruction or gangrene, unilateral or unspecified, (not specified as recurrent)
550.91 Inguinal hernia without mention of obstruction or gangrene, recurrent unilateral or unspecified
550.92 Inguinal hernia without mention of obstruction or gangrene, bilateral, (not specified as recurrent)
550.93 Inguinal hernia without mention of obstruction or gangrene, recurrent bilateral
551.00 Femoral hernia with gangrene, unilateral or unspecified (not specified as recurrent)
551.01 Femoral hernia with gangrene, recurrent unilateral or unspecified
551.02 Femoral hernia with gangrene, bilateral, (not specified as recurrent)
551.1 Umbilical hernia with gangrene
551.21 Incisional ventral hernia, with gangrene
551.29 Other ventral hernia with gangrene
551.3 Diaphragmatic hernia with gangrene
551.8 Hernia of other specified sites, with gangrene
551.9 Hernia of unspecified site, with gangrene ▽
552.00 Unilateral or unspecified femoral hernia with obstruction
552.01 Recurrent unilateral or unspecified femoral hernia with obstruction
552.02 Bilateral femoral hernia with obstruction
552.03 Recurrent bilateral femoral hernia with obstruction
552.1 Umbilical hernia with obstruction
552.21 Incisional hernia with obstruction
552.29 Other ventral hernia with obstruction
552.3 Diaphragmatic hernia with obstruction
552.8 Hernia of other specified site, with obstruction
552.9 Hernia of unspecified site, with obstruction ▽
553.00 Unilateral or unspecified femoral hernia without mention of obstruction or gangrene, unilateral or unspecified
553.01 Femoral hernia without mention of obstruction or gangrene, recurrent unilateral or unspecified

553.02 Femoral hernia without mention of obstruction or gangrene, bilateral
553.03 Femoral hernia without mention of obstruction or gangrene, recurrent bilateral
553.1 Umbilical hernia without mention of obstruction or gangrene
553.21 Incisional hernia without mention of obstruction or gangrene
560.81 Intestinal or peritoneal adhesions with obstruction (postoperative) (postinfection)
560.89 Other specified intestinal obstruction
572.0 Abscess of liver
577.0 Acute pancreatitis
577.1 Chronic pancreatitis
577.2 Cyst and pseudocyst of pancreas
577.8 Other specified disease of pancreas
614.1 Chronic salpingitis and oophoritis — (Use additional code to identify organism: 041.0, 041.1) ♀
614.2 Salpingitis and oophoritis not specified as acute, subacute, or chronic — (Use additional code to identify organism: 041.0, 041.1) ♀
614.3 Acute parametritis and pelvic cellulitis — (Use additional code to identify organism: 041.0, 041.1) ♀
614.4 Chronic or unspecified parametritis and pelvic cellulitis — (Use additional code to identify organism: 041.0, 041.1) ♀
614.5 Acute or unspecified pelvic peritonitis, female — (Use additional code to identify organism: 041.0, 041.1) ♀
614.6 Pelvic peritoneal adhesions, female (postoperative) (postinfection) — (Use additional code to identify any associated infertility, 628.2. Use additional code to identify organism: 041.0, 041.1) ♀
614.7 Other chronic pelvic peritonitis, female — (Use additional code to identify organism: 041.0, 041.1) ♀
614.8 Other specified inflammatory disease of female pelvic organs and tissues — (Use additional code to identify organism: 041.0, 041.1) ♀
614.9 Unspecified inflammatory disease of female pelvic organs and tissues — (Use additional code to identify organism: 041.0, 041.1) ▽ ♀
617.1 Endometriosis of ovary ♀
617.2 Endometriosis of fallopian tube ♀
617.3 Endometriosis of pelvic peritoneum ♀
617.5 Endometriosis of intestine ♀
617.6 Endometriosis in scar of skin ♀
617.8 Endometriosis of other specified sites ♀
617.9 Endometriosis, site unspecified ▽ ♀
620.0 Follicular cyst of ovary ♀
620.1 Corpus luteum cyst or hematoma ♀
620.2 Other and unspecified ovarian cyst ▽ ♀
620.4 Prolapse or hernia of ovary and fallopian tube ♀
620.5 Torsion of ovary, ovarian pedicle, or fallopian tube ♀
620.6 Broad ligament laceration syndrome ♀
620.7 Hematoma of broad ligament ♀
620.8 Other noninflammatory disorder of ovary, fallopian tube, and broad ligament ♀
620.9 Unspecified noninflammatory disorder of ovary, fallopian tube, and broad ligament ▽ ♀
625.3 Dysmenorrhea ♀
625.5 Pelvic congestion syndrome ♀
625.8 Other specified symptom associated with female genital organs ♀
625.9 Unspecified symptom associated with female genital organs ▽ ♀
626.0 Absence of menstruation ♀
626.2 Excessive or frequent menstruation ♀
626.6 Metrorrhagia ♀
626.8 Other disorder of menstruation and other abnormal bleeding from female genital tract ♀
626.9 Unspecified disorder of menstruation and other abnormal bleeding from female genital tract ▽ ♀
627.1 Postmenopausal bleeding ♀
628.0 Female infertility associated with anovulation — (Use additional code for any associated Stein-Leventhal syndrome, 256.4) ♀
628.2 Female infertility of tubal origin — (Use additional code for any associated peritubal adhesions, 614.6) ♀
628.3 Female infertility of uterine origin — (Use additional code for any associated tuberculous endometriosis, 016.7) ♀
628.8 Female infertility of other specified origin ♀
628.9 Female infertility of unspecified origin ▽ ♀
629.0 Hematocele, female, not elsewhere classified ♀
629.9 Unspecified disorder of female genital organs ▽ ♀
632 Missed abortion — (Use additional code from category 639 to identify any associated complications) ♀
633.00 Abdominal pregnancy without intrauterine pregnancy — (Use additional code from category 639 to identify any associated complications) ♀
633.01 Abdominal pregnancy with intrauterine pregnancy — (Use additional code from category 639 to identify any associated complications) ♀
633.10 Tubal pregnancy without intrauterine pregnancy — (Use additional code from category 639 to identify any associated complications) ♀
633.11 Tubal pregnancy with intrauterine pregnancy — (Use additional code from category 639 to identify any associated complications) ♀
633.20 Ovarian pregnancy without intrauterine pregnancy — (Use additional code from category 639 to identify any associated complications) ♀
633.21 Ovarian pregnancy with intrauterine pregnancy — (Use additional code from category 639 to identify any associated complications) ♀
633.80 Other ectopic pregnancy without intrauterine pregnancy — (Use additional code from category 639 to identify any associated complications) ♀
633.81 Other ectopic pregnancy with intrauterine pregnancy — (Use additional code from category 639 to identify any associated complications) ♀
633.90 Unspecified ectopic pregnancy without intrauterine pregnancy — (Use additional code from category 639 to identify any associated complications) ▽ ♀
633.91 Unspecified ectopic pregnancy with intrauterine pregnancy — (Use additional code from category 639 to identify any associated complications) ▽ ♀
639.2 Damage to pelvic organs and tissues following abortion or ectopic and molar pregnancies ♀
752.0 Congenital anomalies of ovaries ♀
752.10 Unspecified congenital anomaly of fallopian tubes and broad ligaments ▽ ♀
752.11 Embryonic cyst of fallopian tubes and broad ligaments ♀
752.19 Other congenital anomaly of fallopian tubes and broad ligaments ♀
752.3 Other congenital anomaly of uterus ♀
780.6 Fever
789.00 Abdominal pain, unspecified site ▽
789.09 Abdominal pain, other specified site
789.30 Abdominal or pelvic swelling, mass or lump, unspecified site ▽
789.39 Abdominal or pelvic swelling, mass, or lump, other specified site
789.5 Ascites
793.6 Nonspecific abnormal findings on radiological and other examination of abdominal area, including retroperitoneum
795.00 Abnormal glandular Papanicolaou smear of cervix ▽ ♀
795.01 Papanicolaou smear of cervix with atypical squamous cells of undetermined significance (ASC-US) ♀
795.02 Papanicolaou smear of cervix with atypical squamous cells cannot exclude high grade squamous intraepithelial lesion (ASC-H) ♀
795.09 Other abnormal Papanicolaou smear of cervix and cervical HPV ♀
795.1 Nonspecific abnormal Papanicolaou smear of other site ▽

ICD-9-CM Procedural

54.21 Laparoscopy
54.23 Biopsy of peritoneum
54.24 Closed (percutaneous) (needle) biopsy of intra-abdominal mass
65.14 Other laparoscopic diagnostic procedures on ovaries

49321

49321 Laparoscopy, surgical; with biopsy (single or multiple)

ICD-9-CM Diagnostic

151.1 Malignant neoplasm of pylorus
151.2 Malignant neoplasm of pyloric antrum
151.3 Malignant neoplasm of fundus of stomach
151.4 Malignant neoplasm of body of stomach
151.5 Malignant neoplasm of lesser curvature of stomach, unspecified ▽
151.6 Malignant neoplasm of greater curvature of stomach, unspecified ▽
151.8 Malignant neoplasm of other specified sites of stomach
151.9 Malignant neoplasm of stomach, unspecified site ▽
152.0 Malignant neoplasm of duodenum
152.1 Malignant neoplasm of jejunum
152.2 Malignant neoplasm of ileum
152.3 Malignant neoplasm of Meckel's diverticulum
152.8 Malignant neoplasm of other specified sites of small intestine
152.9 Malignant neoplasm of small intestine, unspecified site ▽
156.2 Malignant neoplasm of ampulla of Vater
156.8 Malignant neoplasm of other specified sites of gallbladder and extrahepatic bile ducts
156.9 Malignant neoplasm of biliary tract, part unspecified site ▽
157.0 Malignant neoplasm of head of pancreas
157.1 Malignant neoplasm of body of pancreas
157.2 Malignant neoplasm of tail of pancreas
157.4 Malignant neoplasm of islets of Langerhans — (Use additional code to identify any functional activity)
157.8 Malignant neoplasm of other specified sites of pancreas

▽ Unspecified code
♀ Female diagnosis
☒ Manifestation code
♂ Male diagnosis

157.9 Malignant neoplasm of pancreas, part unspecified ▽
158.0 Malignant neoplasm of retroperitoneum
158.8 Malignant neoplasm of specified parts of peritoneum
158.9 Malignant neoplasm of peritoneum, unspecified ▽
159.0 Malignant neoplasm of intestinal tract, part unspecified ▽
159.1 Malignant neoplasm of spleen, not elsewhere classified
159.8 Malignant neoplasm of other sites of digestive system and intra-abdominal organs
159.9 Malignant neoplasm of ill-defined sites of digestive organs and peritoneum
171.5 Malignant neoplasm of connective and other soft tissue of abdomen
171.6 Malignant neoplasm of connective and other soft tissue of pelvis
171.8 Malignant neoplasm of other specified sites of connective and other soft tissue
171.9 Malignant neoplasm of connective and other soft tissue, site unspecified ▽
176.3 Kaposi's sarcoma of gastrointestinal sites
176.5 Kaposi's sarcoma of lymph nodes
179 Malignant neoplasm of uterus, part unspecified ▽ ♀
180.0 Malignant neoplasm of endocervix ♀
180.1 Malignant neoplasm of exocervix ♀
180.8 Malignant neoplasm of other specified sites of cervix ♀
180.9 Malignant neoplasm of cervix uteri, unspecified site ▽ ♀
181 Malignant neoplasm of placenta ♀
182.0 Malignant neoplasm of corpus uteri, except isthmus ♀
182.1 Malignant neoplasm of isthmus ♀
182.8 Malignant neoplasm of other specified sites of body of uterus ♀
183.0 Malignant neoplasm of ovary — (Use additional code to identify any functional activity) ♀
183.2 Malignant neoplasm of fallopian tube ♀
183.3 Malignant neoplasm of broad ligament of uterus ♀
183.4 Malignant neoplasm of parametrium of uterus ♀
183.5 Malignant neoplasm of round ligament of uterus ♀
183.8 Malignant neoplasm of other specified sites of uterine adnexa ♀
183.9 Malignant neoplasm of uterine adnexa, unspecified site ▽ ♀
184.8 Malignant neoplasm of other specified sites of female genital organs ♀
184.9 Malignant neoplasm of female genital organ, site unspecified ▽ ♀
185 Malignant neoplasm of prostate ♂
187.8 Malignant neoplasm of other specified sites of male genital organs ♂
187.9 Malignant neoplasm of male genital organ, site unspecified ▽ ♂
188.0 Malignant neoplasm of trigone of urinary bladder
188.1 Malignant neoplasm of dome of urinary bladder
188.2 Malignant neoplasm of lateral wall of urinary bladder
188.3 Malignant neoplasm of anterior wall of urinary bladder
188.4 Malignant neoplasm of posterior wall of urinary bladder
188.5 Malignant neoplasm of bladder neck
188.6 Malignant neoplasm of ureteric orifice
188.7 Malignant neoplasm of urachus
188.8 Malignant neoplasm of other specified sites of bladder
188.9 Malignant neoplasm of bladder, part unspecified ▽
189.0 Malignant neoplasm of kidney, except pelvis
189.1 Malignant neoplasm of renal pelvis
189.2 Malignant neoplasm of ureter
189.8 Malignant neoplasm of other specified sites of urinary organs
189.9 Malignant neoplasm of urinary organ, site unspecified ▽
194.0 Malignant neoplasm of adrenal gland — (Use additional code to identify any functional activity)
195.2 Malignant neoplasm of abdomen
195.3 Malignant neoplasm of pelvis
196.2 Secondary and unspecified malignant neoplasm of intra-abdominal lymph nodes
196.6 Secondary and unspecified malignant neoplasm of intrapelvic lymph nodes
196.8 Secondary and unspecified malignant neoplasm of lymph nodes of multiple sites
196.9 Secondary and unspecified malignant neoplasm of lymph nodes, site unspecified ▽
197.4 Secondary malignant neoplasm of small intestine including duodenum
197.5 Secondary malignant neoplasm of large intestine and rectum
197.6 Secondary malignant neoplasm of retroperitoneum and peritoneum
197.7 Secondary malignant neoplasm of liver
197.8 Secondary malignant neoplasm of other digestive organs and spleen
198.0 Secondary malignant neoplasm of kidney
198.1 Secondary malignant neoplasm of other urinary organs
198.6 Secondary malignant neoplasm of ovary ♀
198.7 Secondary malignant neoplasm of adrenal gland
198.89 Secondary malignant neoplasm of other specified sites
199.0 Disseminated malignant neoplasm
200.00 Reticulosarcoma, unspecified site, extranodal and solid organ sites ▽
200.03 Reticulosarcoma of intra-abdominal lymph nodes
200.06 Reticulosarcoma of intrapelvic lymph nodes
200.07 Reticulosarcoma of spleen
200.08 Reticulosarcoma of lymph nodes of multiple sites
200.10 Lymphosarcoma, unspecified site, extranodal and solid organ sites ▽
200.13 Lymphosarcoma of intra-abdominal lymph nodes
200.16 Lymphosarcoma of intrapelvic lymph nodes
200.17 Lymphosarcoma of spleen
200.18 Lymphosarcoma of lymph nodes of multiple sites
200.20 Burkitt's tumor or lymphoma, unspecified site, extranodal and solid organ sites ▽
200.23 Burkitt's tumor or lymphoma of intra-abdominal lymph nodes
200.26 Burkitt's tumor or lymphoma of intrapelvic lymph nodes
200.27 Burkitt's tumor or lymphoma of spleen
200.28 Burkitt's tumor or lymphoma of lymph nodes of multiple sites
200.80 Other named variants, unspecified site, extranodal and solid organ sites ▽
200.83 Other named variants of lymphosarcoma and reticulosarcoma of intra-abdominal lymph nodes
200.86 Other named variants of lymphosarcoma and reticulosarcoma of intrapelvic lymph nodes
201.03 Hodgkin's paragranuloma of intra-abdominal lymph nodes
201.06 Hodgkin's paragranuloma of intrapelvic lymph nodes
201.07 Hodgkin's paragranuloma of spleen
201.13 Hodgkin's granuloma of intra-abdominal lymph nodes
201.16 Hodgkin's granuloma of intrapelvic lymph nodes
201.17 Hodgkin's granuloma of spleen
201.18 Hodgkin's granuloma of lymph nodes of multiple sites
201.23 Hodgkin's sarcoma of intra-abdominal lymph nodes
201.26 Hodgkin's sarcoma of intrapelvic lymph nodes
201.27 Hodgkin's sarcoma of spleen
201.28 Hodgkin's sarcoma of lymph nodes of multiple sites
201.43 Hodgkin's disease, lymphocytic-histiocytic predominance of intra-abdominal lymph nodes
201.46 Hodgkin's disease, lymphocytic-histiocytic predominance of intrapelvic lymph nodes
201.47 Hodgkin's disease, lymphocytic-histiocytic predominance of spleen
201.53 Hodgkin's disease, nodular sclerosis, of intra-abdominal lymph nodes
201.56 Hodgkin's disease, nodular sclerosis, of intrapelvic lymph nodes
201.57 Hodgkin's disease, nodular sclerosis, of spleen
201.58 Hodgkin's disease, nodular sclerosis, of lymph nodes of multiple sites
201.63 Hodgkin's disease, mixed cellularity, of intra-abdominal lymph nodes
201.66 Hodgkin's disease, mixed cellularity, of intrapelvic lymph nodes
201.67 Hodgkin's disease, mixed cellularity, of spleen
201.68 Hodgkin's disease, mixed cellularity, of lymph nodes of multiple sites
201.73 Hodgkin's disease, lymphocytic depletion, of intra-abdominal lymph nodes
201.76 Hodgkin's disease, lymphocytic depletion, of intrapelvic lymph nodes
201.77 Hodgkin's disease, lymphocytic depletion, of spleen
201.78 Hodgkin's disease, lymphocytic depletion, of lymph nodes of multiple sites
201.93 Hodgkin's disease, unspecified type, of intra-abdominal lymph nodes ▽
201.96 Hodgkin's disease, unspecified type, of intrapelvic lymph nodes ▽
201.97 Hodgkin's disease, unspecified type, of spleen ▽
202.03 Nodular lymphoma of intra-abdominal lymph nodes
202.06 Nodular lymphoma of intrapelvic lymph nodes
202.07 Nodular lymphoma of spleen
202.08 Nodular lymphoma of lymph nodes of multiple sites
202.13 Mycosis fungoides of intra-abdominal lymph nodes
202.16 Mycosis fungoides of intrapelvic lymph nodes
202.17 Mycosis fungoides of spleen
202.23 Sezary's disease of intra-abdominal lymph nodes
202.26 Sezary's disease of intrapelvic lymph nodes
202.27 Sezary's disease of spleen
202.28 Sezary's disease of lymph nodes of multiple sites
202.30 Malignant histiocytosis, unspecified site, extranodal and solid organ sites ▽
202.33 Malignant histiocytosis of intra-abdominal lymph nodes
202.36 Malignant histiocytosis of intrapelvic lymph nodes
202.37 Malignant histiocytosis of spleen
202.40 Leukemic reticuloendotheliosis, unspecified site, extranodal and solid organ sites ▽
202.43 Leukemic reticuloendotheliosis of intra-abdominal lymph nodes
202.46 Leukemic reticuloendotheliosis of intrapelvic lymph nodes
202.47 Leukemic reticuloendotheliosis of spleen
202.53 Letterer-Siwe disease of intra-abdominal lymph nodes
202.56 Letterer-Siwe disease of intrapelvic lymph nodes
202.57 Letterer-Siwe disease of spleen
202.58 Letterer-Siwe disease of lymph nodes of multiple sites
202.63 Malignant mast cell tumors of intra-abdominal lymph nodes
202.66 Malignant mast cell tumors of intrapelvic lymph nodes

202.67 Malignant mast cell tumors of spleen

202.68 Malignant mast cell tumors of lymph nodes of multiple sites

202.83 Other malignant lymphomas of intra-abdominal lymph nodes

202.86 Other malignant lymphomas of intrapelvic lymph nodes

202.87 Other malignant lymphomas of spleen

202.88 Other malignant lymphomas of lymph nodes of multiple sites

202.93 Other and unspecified malignant neoplasms of lymphoid and histiocytic tissue of intra-abdominal lymph nodes ▽

202.96 Other and unspecified malignant neoplasms of lymphoid and histiocytic tissue of intrapelvic lymph nodes ▽

202.97 Other and unspecified malignant neoplasms of lymphoid and histiocytic tissue of spleen ▽

211.1 Benign neoplasm of stomach

211.2 Benign neoplasm of duodenum, jejunum, and ileum

211.3 Benign neoplasm of colon

211.4 Benign neoplasm of rectum and anal canal

211.5 Benign neoplasm of liver and biliary passages

211.6 Benign neoplasm of pancreas, except islets of Langerhans

211.7 Benign neoplasm of islets of Langerhans — (Use additional code to identify any functional activity)

211.8 Benign neoplasm of retroperitoneum and peritoneum

211.9 Benign neoplasm of other and unspecified site of the digestive system ▽

214.3 Lipoma of intra-abdominal organs

214.8 Lipoma of other specified sites

214.9 Lipoma of unspecified site ▽

218.0 Submucous leiomyoma of uterus ♀

218.1 Intramural leiomyoma of uterus ♀

218.2 Subserous leiomyoma of uterus ♀

218.9 Leiomyoma of uterus, unspecified ▽ ♀

219.0 Benign neoplasm of cervix uteri ♀

219.1 Benign neoplasm of corpus uteri ♀

219.8 Benign neoplasm of other specified parts of uterus ♀

219.9 Benign neoplasm of uterus, part unspecified ▽ ♀

220 Benign neoplasm of ovary — (Use additional code to identify any functional activity: 256.0-256.1) ♀

221.0 Benign neoplasm of fallopian tube and uterine ligaments ♀

221.8 Benign neoplasm of other specified sites of female genital organs ♀

222.2 Benign neoplasm of prostate ♂

223.0 Benign neoplasm of kidney, except pelvis

223.1 Benign neoplasm of renal pelvis

223.2 Benign neoplasm of ureter

223.3 Benign neoplasm of bladder

223.9 Benign neoplasm of urinary organ, site unspecified ▽

227.0 Benign neoplasm of adrenal gland — (Use additional code to identify any functional activity)

227.6 Benign neoplasm of aortic body and other paraganglia — (Use additional code to identify any functional activity)

228.04 Hemangioma of intra-abdominal structures

228.1 Lymphangioma, any site

229.0 Benign neoplasm of lymph nodes

229.8 Benign neoplasm of other specified sites

229.9 Benign neoplasm of unspecified site ▽

230.2 Carcinoma in situ of stomach

230.3 Carcinoma in situ of colon

230.4 Carcinoma in situ of rectum

230.7 Carcinoma in situ of other and unspecified parts of intestine ▽

230.8 Carcinoma in situ of liver and biliary system

230.9 Carcinoma in situ of other and unspecified digestive organs ▽

233.1 Carcinoma in situ of cervix uteri ♀

233.2 Carcinoma in situ of other and unspecified parts of uterus ▽ ♀

233.3 Carcinoma in situ of other and unspecified female genital organs ▽ ♀

233.4 Carcinoma in situ of prostate ♂

233.9 Carcinoma in situ of other and unspecified urinary organs ▽

235.2 Neoplasm of uncertain behavior of stomach, intestines, and rectum

235.3 Neoplasm of uncertain behavior of liver and biliary passages

236.0 Neoplasm of uncertain behavior of uterus ♀

236.2 Neoplasm of uncertain behavior of ovary — (Use additional code to identify any functional activity) ♀

236.3 Neoplasm of uncertain behavior of other and unspecified female genital organs ▽ ♀

236.7 Neoplasm of uncertain behavior of bladder

236.90 Neoplasm of uncertain behavior of urinary organ, unspecified ▽

236.91 Neoplasm of uncertain behavior of kidney and ureter

236.99 Neoplasm of uncertain behavior of other and unspecified urinary organs

237.2 Neoplasm of uncertain behavior of adrenal gland — (Use additional code to identify any functional activity)

237.3 Neoplasm of uncertain behavior of paraganglia

238.7 Neoplasm of uncertain behavior of other lymphatic and hematopoietic tissues

238.8 Neoplasm of uncertain behavior of other specified sites

238.9 Neoplasm of uncertain behavior, site unspecified ▽

239.0 Neoplasm of unspecified nature of digestive system

239.5 Neoplasm of unspecified nature of other genitourinary organs

239.7 Neoplasm of unspecified nature of endocrine glands and other parts of nervous system

239.8 Neoplasm of unspecified nature of other specified sites

239.9 Neoplasm of unspecified nature, site unspecified ▽

256.4 Polycystic ovaries ♀

289.2 Nonspecific mesenteric lymphadenitis

289.3 Lymphadenitis, unspecified, except mesenteric ▽

289.4 Hypersplenism

289.51 Chronic congestive splenomegaly

289.52 Splenic sequestration — (Code first sickle-cell disease in crisis: 282.42, 282.62, 282.64, 282.69)

289.59 Other diseases of spleen

577.0 Acute pancreatitis

577.1 Chronic pancreatitis

577.2 Cyst and pseudocyst of pancreas

577.8 Other specified disease of pancreas

614.1 Chronic salpingitis and oophoritis — (Use additional code to identify organism: 041.0, 041.1) ♀

614.2 Salpingitis and oophoritis not specified as acute, subacute, or chronic — (Use additional code to identify organism: 041.0, 041.1) ♀

614.3 Acute parametritis and pelvic cellulitis — (Use additional code to identify organism: 041.0, 041.1) ♀

614.4 Chronic or unspecified parametritis and pelvic cellulitis — (Use additional code to identify organism: 041.0, 041.1) ♀

614.5 Acute or unspecified pelvic peritonitis, female — (Use additional code to identify organism: 041.0, 041.1) ♀

614.7 Other chronic pelvic peritonitis, female — (Use additional code to identify organism: 041.0, 041.1) ♀

614.8 Other specified inflammatory disease of female pelvic organs and tissues — (Use additional code to identify organism: 041.0, 041.1) ♀

614.9 Unspecified inflammatory disease of female pelvic organs and tissues — (Use additional code to identify organism: 041.0, 041.1) ▽ ♀

617.1 Endometriosis of ovary ♀

617.2 Endometriosis of fallopian tube ♀

617.3 Endometriosis of pelvic peritoneum ♀

617.5 Endometriosis of intestine ♀

617.6 Endometriosis in scar of skin ♀

617.8 Endometriosis of other specified sites ♀

617.9 Endometriosis, site unspecified ▽ ♀

620.0 Follicular cyst of ovary ♀

620.1 Corpus luteum cyst or hematoma ♀

620.2 Other and unspecified ovarian cyst ▽ ♀

620.8 Other noninflammatory disorder of ovary, fallopian tube, and broad ligament ♀

620.9 Unspecified noninflammatory disorder of ovary, fallopian tube, and broad ligament ▽ ♀

625.8 Other specified symptom associated with female genital organs ♀

625.9 Unspecified symptom associated with female genital organs ▽ ♀

626.2 Excessive or frequent menstruation ♀

626.6 Metrorrhagia ♀

626.8 Other disorder of menstruation and other abnormal bleeding from female genital tract ♀

626.9 Unspecified disorder of menstruation and other abnormal bleeding from female genital tract ▽ ♀

627.1 Postmenopausal bleeding ♀

628.0 Female infertility associated with anovulation — (Use additional code for any associated Stein-Levanthal syndrome, 256.4) ♀

628.2 Female infertility of tubal origin — (Use additional code for any associated peritubal adhesions, 614.6) ♀

628.3 Female infertility of uterine origin — (Use additional code for any associated tuberculous endometriosis, 016.7) ♀

628.8 Female infertility of other specified origin ♀

628.9 Female infertility of unspecified origin ▽ ♀

629.0 Hematocele, female, not elsewhere classified ♀

629.9 Unspecified disorder of female genital organs ▽ ♀

752.11 Embryonic cyst of fallopian tubes and broad ligaments ♀

789.5 Ascites

793.6 Nonspecific abnormal findings on radiological and other examination of abdominal area, including retroperitoneum

795.00 Abnormal glandular Papanicolaou smear of cervix ▽ ♀

▽ Unspecified code
♀ Female diagnosis
☒ Manifestation code
♂ Male diagnosis

795.01 Papanicolaou smear of cervix with atypical squamous cells of undetermined significance (ASC-US) ♀
795.02 Papanicolaou smear of cervix with atypical squamous cells cannot exclude high grade squamous intraepithelial lesion (ASC-H) ♀
795.09 Other abnormal Papanicolaou smear of cervix and cervical HPV ♀
795.1 Nonspecific abnormal Papanicolaou smear of other site

ICD-9-CM Procedural

54.23 Biopsy of peritoneum
54.24 Closed (percutaneous) (needle) biopsy of intra-abdominal mass
65.14 Other laparoscopic diagnostic procedures on ovaries

49322

49322 Laparoscopy, surgical; with aspiration of cavity or cyst (eg, ovarian cyst) (single or multiple)

ICD-9-CM Diagnostic

179 Malignant neoplasm of uterus, part unspecified ♀
183.0 Malignant neoplasm of ovary — (Use additional code to identify any functional activity) ♀
183.2 Malignant neoplasm of fallopian tube ♀
183.4 Malignant neoplasm of parametrium of uterus ♀
183.9 Malignant neoplasm of uterine adnexa, unspecified site ♀
184.8 Malignant neoplasm of other specified sites of female genital organs ♀
199.0 Disseminated malignant neoplasm
199.1 Other malignant neoplasm of unspecified site
220 Benign neoplasm of ovary — (Use additional code to identify any functional activity: 256.0-256.1) ♀
256.0 Hyperestrogenism ♀
614.0 Acute salpingitis and oophoritis — (Use additional code to identify organism: 041.0, 041.1) ♀
614.1 Chronic salpingitis and oophoritis — (Use additional code to identify organism: 041.0, 041.1) ♀
614.2 Salpingitis and oophoritis not specified as acute, subacute, or chronic — (Use additional code to identify organism: 041.0, 041.1) ♀
614.3 Acute parametritis and pelvic cellulitis — (Use additional code to identify organism: 041.0, 041.1) ♀
614.4 Chronic or unspecified parametritis and pelvic cellulitis — (Use additional code to identify organism: 041.0, 041.1) ♀
614.6 Pelvic peritoneal adhesions, female (postoperative) (postinfection) — (Use additional code to identify any associated infertility, 628.2. Use additional code to identify organism: 041.0, 041.1) ♀
614.7 Other chronic pelvic peritonitis, female — (Use additional code to identify organism: 041.0, 041.1) ♀
614.8 Other specified inflammatory disease of female pelvic organs and tissues — (Use additional code to identify organism: 041.0, 041.1) ♀
617.0 Endometriosis of uterus ♀
617.1 Endometriosis of ovary ♀
617.2 Endometriosis of fallopian tube ♀
617.3 Endometriosis of pelvic peritoneum ♀
617.8 Endometriosis of other specified sites ♀
617.9 Endometriosis, site unspecified ♀
620.0 Follicular cyst of ovary ♀
620.1 Corpus luteum cyst or hematoma ♀
620.2 Other and unspecified ovarian cyst ♀
620.8 Other noninflammatory disorder of ovary, fallopian tube, and broad ligament ♀
621.0 Polyp of corpus uteri ♀
621.8 Other specified disorders of uterus, not elsewhere classified ♀
625.8 Other specified symptom associated with female genital organs ♀
625.9 Unspecified symptom associated with female genital organs ♀
627.0 Premenopausal menorrhagia ♀
628.2 Female infertility of tubal origin — (Use additional code for any associated peritubal adhesions, 614.6) ♀
780.6 Fever
789.00 Abdominal pain, unspecified site
789.01 Abdominal pain, right upper quadrant
789.02 Abdominal pain, left upper quadrant
789.03 Abdominal pain, right lower quadrant
789.04 Abdominal pain, left lower quadrant
789.30 Abdominal or pelvic swelling, mass or lump, unspecified site
789.31 Abdominal or pelvic swelling, mass, or lump, right upper quadrant
789.32 Abdominal or pelvic swelling, mass, or lump, left upper quadrant
789.33 Abdominal or pelvic swelling, mass, or lump, right lower quadrant
789.34 Abdominal or pelvic swelling, mass, or lump, left lower quadrant

ICD-9-CM Procedural

65.11 Aspiration biopsy of ovary
65.91 Aspiration of ovary
66.91 Aspiration of fallopian tube

49323

49323 Laparoscopy, surgical; with drainage of lymphocele to peritoneal cavity

ICD-9-CM Diagnostic

154.0 Malignant neoplasm of rectosigmoid junction
180.9 Malignant neoplasm of cervix uteri, unspecified site ♀
182.0 Malignant neoplasm of corpus uteri, except isthmus ♀
183.0 Malignant neoplasm of ovary — (Use additional code to identify any functional activity) ♀
185 Malignant neoplasm of prostate ♂
196.2 Secondary and unspecified malignant neoplasm of intra-abdominal lymph nodes
196.6 Secondary and unspecified malignant neoplasm of intrapelvic lymph nodes
200.13 Lymphosarcoma of intra-abdominal lymph nodes
201.93 Hodgkin's disease, unspecified type, of intra-abdominal lymph nodes
202.03 Nodular lymphoma of intra-abdominal lymph nodes
202.83 Other malignant lymphomas of intra-abdominal lymph nodes
289.1 Chronic lymphadenitis
289.3 Lymphadenitis, unspecified, except mesenteric
457.8 Other noninfectious disorders of lymphatic channels
683 Acute lymphadenitis — (Use additional code to identify organism)
782.2 Localized superficial swelling, mass, or lump
785.6 Enlargement of lymph nodes
996.81 Complications of transplanted kidney — (Use additional code to identify nature of complication, 078.5)
V42.0 Kidney replaced by transplant — (This code is intended for use when these conditions are recorded as diagnoses or problems)

ICD-9-CM Procedural

40.0 Incision of lymphatic structures

49329

49329 Unlisted laparoscopy procedure, abdomen, peritoneum and omentum

ICD-9-CM Diagnostic

The application of this code is too broad to adequately present ICD-9-CM diagnostic code links here. Refer to your ICD-9-CM book.

49400

49400 Injection of air or contrast into peritoneal cavity (separate procedure)

ICD-9-CM Diagnostic

The application of this code is too broad to adequately present ICD-9-CM diagnostic code links here. Refer to your ICD-9-CM book.

ICD-9-CM Procedural

33.33 Pneumoperitoneum for collapse of lung
54.29 Other diagnostic procedures on abdominal region
54.96 Injection of air into peritoneal cavity
88.11 Pelvic opaque dye contrast radiography
88.12 Pelvic gas contrast radiography
88.13 Other peritoneal pneumogram

HCPCS Level II Supplies & Services

A4305 Disposable drug delivery system, flow rate of 50 ml or greater per hour
A4550 Surgical trays
A9525 Supply of low or iso-osmolar contrast material, 10 mg of iodine

49419

49419 Insertion of intraperitoneal cannula or catheter, with subcutaneous reservoir, permanent (ie, totally implantable)

ICD-9-CM Diagnostic

151.0 Malignant neoplasm of cardia
151.1 Malignant neoplasm of pylorus
151.2 Malignant neoplasm of pyloric antrum
151.3 Malignant neoplasm of fundus of stomach
151.4 Malignant neoplasm of body of stomach
151.8 Malignant neoplasm of other specified sites of stomach
155.0 Malignant neoplasm of liver, primary

Unspecified code ♀ Female diagnosis ☒ Manifestation code ♂ Male diagnosis

158.0 Malignant neoplasm of retroperitoneum
158.8 Malignant neoplasm of specified parts of peritoneum
159.8 Malignant neoplasm of other sites of digestive system and intra-abdominal organs
159.9 Malignant neoplasm of ill-defined sites of digestive organs and peritoneum
182.0 Malignant neoplasm of corpus uteri, except isthmus ♀
182.1 Malignant neoplasm of isthmus ♀
182.8 Malignant neoplasm of other specified sites of body of uterus ♀
183.0 Malignant neoplasm of ovary — (Use additional code to identify any functional activity) ♀
183.2 Malignant neoplasm of fallopian tube ♀
183.5 Malignant neoplasm of round ligament of uterus ♀
183.8 Malignant neoplasm of other specified sites of uterine adnexa ♀
184.8 Malignant neoplasm of other specified sites of female genital organs ♀
197.6 Secondary malignant neoplasm of retroperitoneum and peritoneum
197.7 Secondary malignant neoplasm of liver
198.6 Secondary malignant neoplasm of ovary ♀
250.02 Diabetes mellitus without mention of complication, type II or unspecified type, uncontrolled
250.03 Diabetes mellitus without mention of complication, type I [juvenile type], uncontrolled
250.12 Diabetes with ketoacidosis, type II or unspecified type, uncontrolled
250.13 Diabetes with ketoacidosis, type I [juvenile type], uncontrolled
250.22 Diabetes with hyperosmolarity, type II or unspecified type, uncontrolled
250.23 Diabetes with hyperosmolarity, type I [juvenile type], uncontrolled
250.42 Diabetes with renal manifestations, type II or unspecified type, uncontrolled — (Use additional code to identify manifestation: 581.81, 583.81)
250.43 Diabetes with renal manifestations, type I [juvenile type], uncontrolled — (Use additional code to identify manifestation: 581.81, 583.81)
250.52 Diabetes with ophthalmic manifestations, type II or unspecified type, uncontrolled — (Use additional code to identify manifestation: 362.01, 362.02, 362.83, 365.44, 366.41, 369.0-369.9)
250.53 Diabetes with ophthalmic manifestations, type I [juvenile type], uncontrolled — (Use additional code to identify manifestation: 362.01, 362.02, 362.83, 365.44, 366.41, 369.0-369.9)
250.62 Diabetes with neurological manifestations, type II or unspecified type, uncontrolled — (Use additional code to identify manifestation: 337.1, 354.0-355.9, 357.2, 358.1, 713.5)
250.63 Diabetes with neurological manifestations, type I [juvenile type], uncontrolled — (Use additional code to identify manifestation: 337.1, 354.0-355.9, 357.2, 358.1, 713.5)
250.72 Diabetes with peripheral circulatory disorders, type II or unspecified type, uncontrolled — (Use additional code to identify manifestation: 443.81, 785.4)
250.73 Diabetes with peripheral circulatory disorders, type I [juvenile type], uncontrolled — (Use additional code to identify manifestation: 443.81, 785.4)
250.82 Diabetes with other specified manifestations, type II or unspecified type, uncontrolled — (Use additional code to identify manifestation: 707.10-707.9, 731.8. Use additional E code to identify cause, if drug-induced)
250.83 Diabetes with other specified manifestations, type I [juvenile type], uncontrolled — (Use additional code to identify manifestation: 707.10-707.9, 731.8. Use additional E code to identify cause, if drug-induced)
789.01 Abdominal pain, right upper quadrant
789.02 Abdominal pain, left upper quadrant
789.03 Abdominal pain, right lower quadrant
789.04 Abdominal pain, left lower quadrant
789.05 Abdominal pain, periumbilic
789.06 Abdominal pain, epigastric
789.07 Abdominal pain, generalized
789.09 Abdominal pain, other specified site

ICD-9-CM Procedural

54.99 Other operations of abdominal region

HCPCS Level II Supplies & Services

HCPCS Level II codes are used to report the supplies, durable medical equipment, and certain medical services provided on an outpatient basis. Because the procedure(s) represented on this page would be performed in an inpatient or outpatient facility, no HCPCS Level II codes apply.

49420–49421

49420 Insertion of intraperitoneal cannula or catheter for drainage or dialysis; temporary
49421 permanent

ICD-9-CM Diagnostic

250.40 Diabetes with renal manifestations, type II or unspecified type, not stated as uncontrolled — (Use additional code to identify manifestation: 581.81, 583.81)
250.41 Diabetes with renal manifestations, type I [juvenile type], not stated as uncontrolled — (Use additional code to identify manifestation: 581.81, 583.81)
250.42 Diabetes with renal manifestations, type II or unspecified type, uncontrolled — (Use additional code to identify manifestation: 581.81, 583.81)
250.43 Diabetes with renal manifestations, type I [juvenile type], uncontrolled — (Use additional code to identify manifestation: 581.81, 583.81)
445.81 Atheroembolism of kidney — (Use additional code for any associated kidney failure: 584, 585)
577.0 Acute pancreatitis
577.1 Chronic pancreatitis
577.2 Cyst and pseudocyst of pancreas
577.8 Other specified disease of pancreas
581.81 Nephrotic syndrome with other specified pathological lesion in kidney in diseases classified elsewhere — (Code first underlying disease: 084.9, 250.4, 277.3, 446.0, 710.0) ☒
581.9 Nephrotic syndrome with unspecified pathological lesion in kidney ▽
583.81 Nephritis and nephropathy, not specified as acute or chronic, with other specified pathological lesion in kidney, in diseases classified elsewhere — (Code first underlying disease: 016.0, 098.19, 250.4, 277.3, 446.21, 710.0) ☒
584.5 Acute renal failure with lesion of tubular necrosis
584.6 Acute renal failure with lesion of renal cortical necrosis
584.7 Acute renal failure with lesion of renal medullary (papillary) necrosis
584.8 Acute renal failure with other specified pathological lesion in kidney
584.9 Unspecified acute renal failure ▽
585 Chronic renal failure — (Use additional code to identify manifestation: 357.4, 420.0)
586 Unspecified renal failure ▽
728.88 Rhabdomyolysis
753.12 Congenital polycystic kidney, unspecified type ▽
789.00 Abdominal pain, unspecified site ▽
789.5 Ascites
998.51 Infected postoperative seroma — (Use additional code to identify organism)
998.59 Other postoperative infection — (Use additional code to identify infection)
V45.1 Renal dialysis status — (This code is intended for use when these conditions are recorded as diagnoses or problems)
V56.2 Fitting and adjustment of peritoneal dialysis catheter — (Use additional code for any concurrent peritoneal dialysis, V56.8. Use additional code to identify the associated condition)
V56.32 Encounter for adequacy testing for peritoneal dialysis — (Use additional code to identify the associated condition)
V56.8 Encounter other dialysis — (Use additional code to identify the associated condition)

ICD-9-CM Procedural

54.91 Percutaneous abdominal drainage

HCPCS Level II Supplies & Services

A4305 Disposable drug delivery system, flow rate of 50 ml or greater per hour
A4306 Disposable drug delivery system, flow rate of 5 ml or less per hour
A4550 Surgical trays

49422

49422 Removal of permanent intraperitoneal cannula or catheter

ICD-9-CM Diagnostic

577.0 Acute pancreatitis
577.1 Chronic pancreatitis
577.2 Cyst and pseudocyst of pancreas
577.8 Other specified disease of pancreas
996.56 Mechanical complications due to peritoneal dialysis catheter
996.68 Infection and inflammatory reaction due to peritoneal dialysis catheter — (Use additional code to identify specified infections)
996.73 Other complications due to renal dialysis device, implant, and graft
V56.2 Fitting and adjustment of peritoneal dialysis catheter — (Use additional code for any concurrent peritoneal dialysis, V56.8. Use additional code to identify the associated condition)
V56.32 Encounter for adequacy testing for peritoneal dialysis — (Use additional code to identify the associated condition)

▽ Unspecified code
♀ Female diagnosis

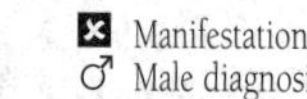

☒ Manifestation code
♂ Male diagnosis

ICD-9-CM Procedural
97.82 Removal of peritoneal drainage device

49423
49423 Exchange of previously placed abscess or cyst drainage catheter under radiological guidance (separate procedure)

ICD-9-CM Diagnostic
457.8 Other noninfectious disorders of lymphatic channels
540.1 Acute appendicitis with peritoneal abscess
567.2 Other suppurative peritonitis
567.8 Other specified peritonitis
568.89 Other specified disorder of peritoneum
569.5 Abscess of intestine
577.0 Acute pancreatitis
590.2 Renal and perinephric abscess — (Use additional code to identify organism, such as E. coli, 041.4)
614.2 Salpingitis and oophoritis not specified as acute, subacute, or chronic — (Use additional code to identify organism: 041.0, 041.1) ♀
614.3 Acute parametritis and pelvic cellulitis — (Use additional code to identify organism: 041.0, 041.1) ♀
614.4 Chronic or unspecified parametritis and pelvic cellulitis — (Use additional code to identify organism: 041.0, 041.1) ♀
614.5 Acute or unspecified pelvic peritonitis, female — (Use additional code to identify organism: 041.0, 041.1) ♀
751.8 Other specified congenital anomalies of digestive system
998.59 Other postoperative infection — (Use additional code to identify infection)

ICD-9-CM Procedural
97.15 Replacement of wound catheter

49424
49424 Contrast injection for assessment of abscess or cyst via previously placed drainage catheter or tube (separate procedure)

ICD-9-CM Diagnostic
457.8 Other noninfectious disorders of lymphatic channels
540.1 Acute appendicitis with peritoneal abscess
567.2 Other suppurative peritonitis
567.8 Other specified peritonitis
568.89 Other specified disorder of peritoneum
569.5 Abscess of intestine
577.0 Acute pancreatitis
590.2 Renal and perinephric abscess — (Use additional code to identify organism, such as E. coli, 041.4)
614.2 Salpingitis and oophoritis not specified as acute, subacute, or chronic — (Use additional code to identify organism: 041.0, 041.1) ♀
614.3 Acute parametritis and pelvic cellulitis — (Use additional code to identify organism: 041.0, 041.1) ♀
614.4 Chronic or unspecified parametritis and pelvic cellulitis — (Use additional code to identify organism: 041.0, 041.1) ♀
614.5 Acute or unspecified pelvic peritonitis, female — (Use additional code to identify organism: 041.0, 041.1) ♀
751.8 Other specified congenital anomalies of digestive system
998.59 Other postoperative infection — (Use additional code to identify infection)

ICD-9-CM Procedural
54.97 Injection of locally-acting therapeutic substance into peritoneal cavity

49425
49425 Insertion of peritoneal-venous shunt

ICD-9-CM Diagnostic
571.5 Cirrhosis of liver without mention of alcohol
577.0 Acute pancreatitis
577.1 Chronic pancreatitis
577.2 Cyst and pseudocyst of pancreas
577.8 Other specified disease of pancreas
789.5 Ascites

ICD-9-CM Procedural
54.94 Creation of peritoneovascular shunt

49426
49426 Revision of peritoneal-venous shunt

ICD-9-CM Diagnostic
789.5 Ascites
996.74 Other complications due to other vascular device, implant, and graft
998.59 Other postoperative infection — (Use additional code to identify infection)
V58.81 Fitting and adjustment of vascular catheter

ICD-9-CM Procedural
54.94 Creation of peritoneovascular shunt

49427
49427 Injection procedure (eg, contrast media) for evaluation of previously placed peritoneal-venous shunt

ICD-9-CM Diagnostic
789.5 Ascites
996.74 Other complications due to other vascular device, implant, and graft
998.59 Other postoperative infection — (Use additional code to identify infection)

ICD-9-CM Procedural
54.97 Injection of locally-acting therapeutic substance into peritoneal cavity

49428
49428 Ligation of peritoneal-venous shunt

ICD-9-CM Diagnostic
789.5 Ascites
996.74 Other complications due to other vascular device, implant, and graft
998.59 Other postoperative infection — (Use additional code to identify infection)
V58.81 Fitting and adjustment of vascular catheter

ICD-9-CM Procedural
54.99 Other operations of abdominal region

49429
49429 Removal of peritoneal-venous shunt

ICD-9-CM Diagnostic
789.5 Ascites
996.74 Other complications due to other vascular device, implant, and graft
998.51 Infected postoperative seroma — (Use additional code to identify organism)
998.59 Other postoperative infection — (Use additional code to identify infection)
V58.81 Fitting and adjustment of vascular catheter

ICD-9-CM Procedural
54.99 Other operations of abdominal region

49491–49492
49491 Repair, initial inguinal hernia, preterm infant (less than 37 weeks gestation at birth), performed from birth up to 50 weeks postconception age, with or without hydrocelectomy; reducible
49492 incarcerated or strangulated

ICD-9-CM Diagnostic
550.00 Inguinal hernia with gangrene, unilateral or unspecified, (not specified as recurrent)
550.02 Inguinal hernia with gangrene, bilateral
550.10 Inguinal hernia with obstruction, without mention of gangrene, unilateral or unspecified, (not specified as recurrent)
550.12 Inguinal hernia with obstruction, without mention gangrene, bilateral, (not specified as recurrent)
550.90 Inguinal hernia without mention of obstruction or gangrene, unilateral or unspecified, (not specified as recurrent)
550.92 Inguinal hernia without mention of obstruction or gangrene, bilateral, (not specified as recurrent)
603.0 Encysted hydrocele
603.1 Infected hydrocele — (Use additional code to identify organism)
603.8 Other specified type of hydrocele
603.9 Unspecified hydrocele ▽
778.6 Congenital hydrocele
V64.41 Laparoscopic surgical procedure converted to open procedure

Hernias

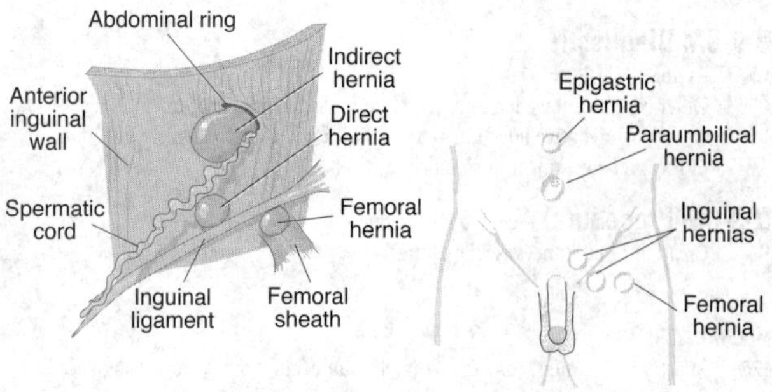

A hernia is a protrusion, usually through an abdominal wall containment; groin hernias are most common among both sexes and all age groups

ICD-9-CM Procedural

53.00 Unilateral repair of inguinal hernia, not otherwise specified
53.01 Unilateral repair of direct inguinal hernia
53.02 Unilateral repair of indirect inguinal hernia
53.03 Unilateral repair of direct inguinal hernia with graft or prosthesis
53.04 Unilateral repair of indirect inguinal hernia with graft or prosthesis
53.05 Unilateral repair of inguinal hernia with graft or prosthesis, not otherwise specified
53.11 Bilateral repair of direct inguinal hernia
53.12 Bilateral repair of indirect inguinal hernia
53.13 Bilateral repair of inguinal hernia, one direct and one indirect
53.14 Bilateral repair of direct inguinal hernia with graft or prosthesis
53.15 Bilateral repair of indirect inguinal hernia with graft or prosthesis
53.16 Bilateral repair of inguinal hernia, one direct and one indirect, with graft or prosthesis
53.17 Bilateral inguinal hernia repair with graft or prosthesis, not otherwise specified
63.1 Excision of varicocele and hydrocele of spermatic cord

49495–49496

49495 Repair, initial inguinal hernia, full term infant under age 6 months, or preterm infant over 50 weeks postconception age and under age 6 months at the time of surgery, with or without hydrocelectomy; reducible
49496 incarcerated or strangulated

ICD-9-CM Diagnostic

550.00 Inguinal hernia with gangrene, unilateral or unspecified, (not specified as recurrent)
550.02 Inguinal hernia with gangrene, bilateral
550.10 Inguinal hernia with obstruction, without mention of gangrene, unilateral or unspecified, (not specified as recurrent)
550.12 Inguinal hernia with obstruction, without mention gangrene, bilateral, (not specified as recurrent)
550.90 Inguinal hernia without mention of obstruction or gangrene, unilateral or unspecified, (not specified as recurrent)
550.92 Inguinal hernia without mention of obstruction or gangrene, bilateral, (not specified as recurrent)
603.0 Encysted hydrocele
603.1 Infected hydrocele — (Use additional code to identify organism)
603.8 Other specified type of hydrocele
603.9 Unspecified hydrocele
778.6 Congenital hydrocele
V64.41 Laparoscopic surgical procedure converted to open procedure

ICD-9-CM Procedural

53.00 Unilateral repair of inguinal hernia, not otherwise specified
53.01 Unilateral repair of direct inguinal hernia
53.02 Unilateral repair of indirect inguinal hernia
53.03 Unilateral repair of direct inguinal hernia with graft or prosthesis
53.04 Unilateral repair of indirect inguinal hernia with graft or prosthesis
53.05 Unilateral repair of inguinal hernia with graft or prosthesis, not otherwise specified
53.11 Bilateral repair of direct inguinal hernia
53.12 Bilateral repair of indirect inguinal hernia
53.13 Bilateral repair of inguinal hernia, one direct and one indirect
53.14 Bilateral repair of direct inguinal hernia with graft or prosthesis
53.15 Bilateral repair of indirect inguinal hernia with graft or prosthesis
53.16 Bilateral repair of inguinal hernia, one direct and one indirect, with graft or prosthesis
53.17 Bilateral inguinal hernia repair with graft or prosthesis, not otherwise specified
63.1 Excision of varicocele and hydrocele of spermatic cord

49500–49501

49500 Repair initial inguinal hernia, age 6 months to under 5 years, with or without hydrocelectomy; reducible
49501 incarcerated or strangulated

ICD-9-CM Diagnostic

550.00 Inguinal hernia with gangrene, unilateral or unspecified, (not specified as recurrent)
550.02 Inguinal hernia with gangrene, bilateral
550.10 Inguinal hernia with obstruction, without mention of gangrene, unilateral or unspecified, (not specified as recurrent)
550.12 Inguinal hernia with obstruction, without mention gangrene, bilateral, (not specified as recurrent)
550.90 Inguinal hernia without mention of obstruction or gangrene, unilateral or unspecified, (not specified as recurrent)
550.92 Inguinal hernia without mention of obstruction or gangrene, bilateral, (not specified as recurrent)
603.0 Encysted hydrocele
603.1 Infected hydrocele — (Use additional code to identify organism)
603.8 Other specified type of hydrocele
603.9 Unspecified hydrocele
778.6 Congenital hydrocele
V64.41 Laparoscopic surgical procedure converted to open procedure

ICD-9-CM Procedural

53.00 Unilateral repair of inguinal hernia, not otherwise specified
53.01 Unilateral repair of direct inguinal hernia
53.02 Unilateral repair of indirect inguinal hernia
53.03 Unilateral repair of direct inguinal hernia with graft or prosthesis
53.04 Unilateral repair of indirect inguinal hernia with graft or prosthesis
53.05 Unilateral repair of inguinal hernia with graft or prosthesis, not otherwise specified
53.11 Bilateral repair of direct inguinal hernia
53.12 Bilateral repair of indirect inguinal hernia
53.13 Bilateral repair of inguinal hernia, one direct and one indirect
53.14 Bilateral repair of direct inguinal hernia with graft or prosthesis
53.15 Bilateral repair of indirect inguinal hernia with graft or prosthesis
53.16 Bilateral repair of inguinal hernia, one direct and one indirect, with graft or prosthesis
53.17 Bilateral inguinal hernia repair with graft or prosthesis, not otherwise specified
53.9 Other hernia repair

49505–49507

49505 Repair initial inguinal hernia, age 5 years or over; reducible
49507 incarcerated or strangulated

ICD-9-CM Diagnostic

550.00 Inguinal hernia with gangrene, unilateral or unspecified, (not specified as recurrent)
550.02 Inguinal hernia with gangrene, bilateral
550.10 Inguinal hernia with obstruction, without mention of gangrene, unilateral or unspecified, (not specified as recurrent)
550.12 Inguinal hernia with obstruction, without mention gangrene, bilateral, (not specified as recurrent)
550.90 Inguinal hernia without mention of obstruction or gangrene, unilateral or unspecified, (not specified as recurrent)
550.92 Inguinal hernia without mention of obstruction or gangrene, bilateral, (not specified as recurrent)
V64.41 Laparoscopic surgical procedure converted to open procedure

ICD-9-CM Procedural

53.00 Unilateral repair of inguinal hernia, not otherwise specified
53.01 Unilateral repair of direct inguinal hernia
53.02 Unilateral repair of indirect inguinal hernia
53.03 Unilateral repair of direct inguinal hernia with graft or prosthesis
53.04 Unilateral repair of indirect inguinal hernia with graft or prosthesis
53.05 Unilateral repair of inguinal hernia with graft or prosthesis, not otherwise specified
53.11 Bilateral repair of direct inguinal hernia
53.12 Bilateral repair of indirect inguinal hernia
53.13 Bilateral repair of inguinal hernia, one direct and one indirect

Unspecified code
♀ Female diagnosis
Manifestation code
♂ Male diagnosis

53.14 Bilateral repair of direct inguinal hernia with graft or prosthesis
53.15 Bilateral repair of indirect inguinal hernia with graft or prosthesis
53.16 Bilateral repair of inguinal hernia, one direct and one indirect, with graft or prosthesis
53.17 Bilateral inguinal hernia repair with graft or prosthesis, not otherwise specified
53.9 Other hernia repair

49520–49521

49520 Repair recurrent inguinal hernia, any age; reducible
49521 incarcerated or strangulated

ICD-9-CM Diagnostic

550.01 Inguinal hernia with gangrene, recurrent unilateral or unspecified inguinal hernia
550.03 Inguinal hernia with gangrene, recurrent bilateral
550.11 Inguinal hernia with obstruction, without mention of gangrene, recurrent unilateral or unspecified
550.13 Inguinal hernia with obstruction, without mention of gangrene, recurrent bilateral
550.91 Inguinal hernia without mention of obstruction or gangrene, recurrent unilateral or unspecified
550.93 Inguinal hernia without mention of obstruction or gangrene, recurrent bilateral
V64.41 Laparoscopic surgical procedure converted to open procedure

ICD-9-CM Procedural

53.00 Unilateral repair of inguinal hernia, not otherwise specified
53.01 Unilateral repair of direct inguinal hernia
53.02 Unilateral repair of indirect inguinal hernia
53.03 Unilateral repair of direct inguinal hernia with graft or prosthesis
53.04 Unilateral repair of indirect inguinal hernia with graft or prosthesis
53.05 Unilateral repair of inguinal hernia with graft or prosthesis, not otherwise specified
53.11 Bilateral repair of direct inguinal hernia
53.12 Bilateral repair of indirect inguinal hernia
53.13 Bilateral repair of inguinal hernia, one direct and one indirect
53.14 Bilateral repair of direct inguinal hernia with graft or prosthesis
53.15 Bilateral repair of indirect inguinal hernia with graft or prosthesis
53.16 Bilateral repair of inguinal hernia, one direct and one indirect, with graft or prosthesis
53.17 Bilateral inguinal hernia repair with graft or prosthesis, not otherwise specified
53.9 Other hernia repair

49525

49525 Repair inguinal hernia, sliding, any age

ICD-9-CM Diagnostic

550.00 Inguinal hernia with gangrene, unilateral or unspecified, (not specified as recurrent)
550.01 Inguinal hernia with gangrene, recurrent unilateral or unspecified inguinal hernia
550.02 Inguinal hernia with gangrene, bilateral
550.03 Inguinal hernia with gangrene, recurrent bilateral
550.10 Inguinal hernia with obstruction, without mention of gangrene, unilateral or unspecified, (not specified as recurrent)
550.11 Inguinal hernia with obstruction, without mention of gangrene, recurrent unilateral or unspecified
550.12 Inguinal hernia with obstruction, without mention gangrene, bilateral, (not specified as recurrent)
550.13 Inguinal hernia with obstruction, without mention of gangrene, recurrent bilateral
550.90 Inguinal hernia without mention of obstruction or gangrene, unilateral or unspecified, (not specified as recurrent)
550.91 Inguinal hernia without mention of obstruction or gangrene, recurrent unilateral or unspecified
550.92 Inguinal hernia without mention of obstruction or gangrene, bilateral, (not specified as recurrent)
550.93 Inguinal hernia without mention of obstruction or gangrene, recurrent bilateral
V64.41 Laparoscopic surgical procedure converted to open procedure

ICD-9-CM Procedural

53.00 Unilateral repair of inguinal hernia, not otherwise specified
53.01 Unilateral repair of direct inguinal hernia
53.02 Unilateral repair of indirect inguinal hernia
53.03 Unilateral repair of direct inguinal hernia with graft or prosthesis
53.04 Unilateral repair of indirect inguinal hernia with graft or prosthesis
53.05 Unilateral repair of inguinal hernia with graft or prosthesis, not otherwise specified
53.11 Bilateral repair of direct inguinal hernia
53.12 Bilateral repair of indirect inguinal hernia
53.13 Bilateral repair of inguinal hernia, one direct and one indirect
53.14 Bilateral repair of direct inguinal hernia with graft or prosthesis
53.15 Bilateral repair of indirect inguinal hernia with graft or prosthesis
53.16 Bilateral repair of inguinal hernia, one direct and one indirect, with graft or prosthesis
53.17 Bilateral inguinal hernia repair with graft or prosthesis, not otherwise specified
53.9 Other hernia repair

49540

49540 Repair lumbar hernia

ICD-9-CM Diagnostic

551.8 Hernia of other specified sites, with gangrene
552.8 Hernia of other specified site, with obstruction
553.8 Hernia of other specified sites of abdominal cavity without mention of obstruction or gangrene

ICD-9-CM Procedural

53.9 Other hernia repair

49550–49553

49550 Repair initial femoral hernia, any age, reducible;
49553 incarcerated or strangulated

ICD-9-CM Diagnostic

551.00 Femoral hernia with gangrene, unilateral or unspecified (not specified as recurrent)
551.02 Femoral hernia with gangrene, bilateral, (not specified as recurrent)
552.00 Unilateral or unspecified femoral hernia with obstruction
552.02 Bilateral femoral hernia with obstruction
553.00 Unilateral or unspecified femoral hernia without mention of obstruction or gangrene, unilateral or unspecified
553.02 Femoral hernia without mention of obstruction or gangrene, bilateral

ICD-9-CM Procedural

53.21 Unilateral repair of femoral hernia with graft or prosthesis
53.29 Other unilateral femoral herniorrhaphy
53.31 Bilateral repair of femoral hernia with graft or prosthesis
53.39 Other bilateral femoral herniorrhaphy

49555–49557

49555 Repair recurrent femoral hernia; reducible
49557 incarcerated or strangulated

ICD-9-CM Diagnostic

551.01 Femoral hernia with gangrene, recurrent unilateral or unspecified
551.03 Femoral hernia with gangrene, recurrent bilateral
552.01 Recurrent unilateral or unspecified femoral hernia with obstruction
552.03 Recurrent bilateral femoral hernia with obstruction
553.01 Femoral hernia without mention of obstruction or gangrene, recurrent unilateral or unspecified
553.03 Femoral hernia without mention of obstruction or gangrene, recurrent bilateral

ICD-9-CM Procedural

53.21 Unilateral repair of femoral hernia with graft or prosthesis
53.29 Other unilateral femoral herniorrhaphy
53.31 Bilateral repair of femoral hernia with graft or prosthesis
53.39 Other bilateral femoral herniorrhaphy

49560–49566

49560 Repair initial incisional or ventral hernia; reducible
49561 incarcerated or strangulated
49565 Repair recurrent incisional or ventral hernia; reducible
49566 incarcerated or strangulated

ICD-9-CM Diagnostic

551.20 Unspecified ventral hernia with gangrene ▽
551.21 Incisional ventral hernia, with gangrene
552.20 Unspecified ventral hernia with obstruction ▽
552.21 Incisional hernia with obstruction
553.20 Unspecified ventral hernia without mention of obstruction or gangrene ▽

553.21 Incisional hernia without mention of obstruction or gangrene
789.00 Abdominal pain, unspecified site
789.01 Abdominal pain, right upper quadrant
789.02 Abdominal pain, left upper quadrant
789.03 Abdominal pain, right lower quadrant
789.04 Abdominal pain, left lower quadrant
789.05 Abdominal pain, periumbilic
789.06 Abdominal pain, epigastric
789.09 Abdominal pain, other specified site
789.30 Abdominal or pelvic swelling, mass or lump, unspecified site
789.31 Abdominal or pelvic swelling, mass, or lump, right upper quadrant
789.32 Abdominal or pelvic swelling, mass, or lump, left upper quadrant
789.33 Abdominal or pelvic swelling, mass, or lump, right lower quadrant
789.34 Abdominal or pelvic swelling, mass, or lump, left lower quadrant
789.35 Abdominal or pelvic swelling, mass or lump, periumbilic
789.36 Abdominal or pelvic swelling, mass, or lump, epigastric
789.39 Abdominal or pelvic swelling, mass, or lump, other specified site

ICD-9-CM Procedural

53.51 Incisional hernia repair
53.59 Repair of other hernia of anterior abdominal wall
53.61 Incisional hernia repair with prosthesis
53.69 Repair of other hernia of anterior abdominal wall with prosthesis

49568

49568 Implantation of mesh or other prosthesis for incisional or ventral hernia repair (List separately in addition to code for the incisional or ventral hernia repair)

ICD-9-CM Diagnostic

This is an add-on code. Refer to the corresponding primary procedure code for ICD-9 diagnosis code links.

ICD-9-CM Procedural

53.03 Unilateral repair of direct inguinal hernia with graft or prosthesis
53.04 Unilateral repair of indirect inguinal hernia with graft or prosthesis
53.05 Unilateral repair of inguinal hernia with graft or prosthesis, not otherwise specified
53.14 Bilateral repair of direct inguinal hernia with graft or prosthesis
53.15 Bilateral repair of indirect inguinal hernia with graft or prosthesis
53.16 Bilateral repair of inguinal hernia, one direct and one indirect, with graft or prosthesis
53.21 Unilateral repair of femoral hernia with graft or prosthesis
53.31 Bilateral repair of femoral hernia with graft or prosthesis
53.41 Repair of umbilical hernia with prosthesis
53.61 Incisional hernia repair with prosthesis
53.69 Repair of other hernia of anterior abdominal wall with prosthesis

49570–49572

49570 Repair epigastric hernia (eg, preperitoneal fat); reducible (separate procedure)
49572 incarcerated or strangulated

ICD-9-CM Diagnostic

551.29 Other ventral hernia with gangrene
552.29 Other ventral hernia with obstruction
553.29 Other ventral hernia without mention of obstruction or gangrene
789.06 Abdominal pain, epigastric

ICD-9-CM Procedural

53.59 Repair of other hernia of anterior abdominal wall
53.69 Repair of other hernia of anterior abdominal wall with prosthesis

49580–49587

49580 Repair umbilical hernia, under age 5 years; reducible
49582 incarcerated or strangulated
49585 Repair umbilical hernia, age 5 years or over; reducible
49587 incarcerated or strangulated

ICD-9-CM Diagnostic

551.1 Umbilical hernia with gangrene
552.1 Umbilical hernia with obstruction
553.1 Umbilical hernia without mention of obstruction or gangrene
756.79 Other congenital anomalies of abdominal wall
789.05 Abdominal pain, periumbilic
789.35 Abdominal or pelvic swelling, mass or lump, periumbilic

ICD-9-CM Procedural

53.41 Repair of umbilical hernia with prosthesis
53.49 Other umbilical herniorrhaphy

49590

49590 Repair spigelian hernia

ICD-9-CM Diagnostic

551.29 Other ventral hernia with gangrene
552.29 Other ventral hernia with obstruction
553.29 Other ventral hernia without mention of obstruction or gangrene
789.00 Abdominal pain, unspecified site

ICD-9-CM Procedural

53.59 Repair of other hernia of anterior abdominal wall

49600

49600 Repair of small omphalocele, with primary closure

ICD-9-CM Diagnostic

756.79 Other congenital anomalies of abdominal wall

ICD-9-CM Procedural

53.49 Other umbilical herniorrhaphy

49605–49606

49605 Repair of large omphalocele or gastroschisis; with or without prosthesis
49606 with removal of prosthesis, final reduction and closure, in operating room

ICD-9-CM Diagnostic

756.79 Other congenital anomalies of abdominal wall

ICD-9-CM Procedural

53.41 Repair of umbilical hernia with prosthesis
53.49 Other umbilical herniorrhaphy
54.71 Repair of gastroschisis

49610–49611

49610 Repair of omphalocele (Gross type operation); first stage
49611 second stage

ICD-9-CM Diagnostic

756.79 Other congenital anomalies of abdominal wall

ICD-9-CM Procedural

53.49 Other umbilical herniorrhaphy
54.71 Repair of gastroschisis

49650–49651

49650 Laparoscopy, surgical; repair initial inguinal hernia
49651 repair recurrent inguinal hernia

ICD-9-CM Diagnostic

550.90 Inguinal hernia without mention of obstruction or gangrene, unilateral or unspecified, (not specified as recurrent)
550.91 Inguinal hernia without mention of obstruction or gangrene, recurrent unilateral or unspecified
550.92 Inguinal hernia without mention of obstruction or gangrene, bilateral, (not specified as recurrent)
550.93 Inguinal hernia without mention of obstruction or gangrene, recurrent bilateral
789.03 Abdominal pain, right lower quadrant
789.04 Abdominal pain, left lower quadrant
789.07 Abdominal pain, generalized
789.09 Abdominal pain, other specified site
789.30 Abdominal or pelvic swelling, mass or lump, unspecified site

ICD-9-CM Procedural

53.00 Unilateral repair of inguinal hernia, not otherwise specified
53.01 Unilateral repair of direct inguinal hernia
53.02 Unilateral repair of indirect inguinal hernia
53.03 Unilateral repair of direct inguinal hernia with graft or prosthesis
53.04 Unilateral repair of indirect inguinal hernia with graft or prosthesis
53.05 Unilateral repair of inguinal hernia with graft or prosthesis, not otherwise specified

Unspecified code
♀ Female diagnosis
Manifestation code
♂ Male diagnosis

53.10 Bilateral repair of inguinal hernia, not otherwise specified
53.11 Bilateral repair of direct inguinal hernia
53.12 Bilateral repair of indirect inguinal hernia
53.13 Bilateral repair of inguinal hernia, one direct and one indirect
53.14 Bilateral repair of direct inguinal hernia with graft or prosthesis
53.15 Bilateral repair of indirect inguinal hernia with graft or prosthesis
53.16 Bilateral repair of inguinal hernia, one direct and one indirect, with graft or prosthesis
53.17 Bilateral inguinal hernia repair with graft or prosthesis, not otherwise specified

49900

49900 Suture, secondary, of abdominal wall for evisceration or dehiscence

ICD-9-CM Diagnostic

674.10 Disruption of cesarean wound, unspecified as to episode of care ♀
674.12 Disruption of cesarean wound, with delivery, with mention of postpartum complication ♀
674.14 Disruption of cesarean wound, postpartum ♀
674.30 Other complication of obstetrical surgical wounds, unspecified as to episode of care ♀
674.32 Other complication of obstetrical surgical wounds, with delivery, with mention of postpartum complication ♀
674.34 Other complication of obstetrical surgical wounds, postpartum condition or complication ♀
998.31 Disruption of internal operation wound
998.32 Disruption of external operation wound
998.83 Non-healing surgical wound

ICD-9-CM Procedural

54.61 Reclosure of postoperative disruption of abdominal wall
54.64 Suture of peritoneum

49904

49904 Omental flap, extra-abdominal (eg, for reconstruction of sternal and chest wall defects)

ICD-9-CM Diagnostic

162.9 Malignant neoplasm of bronchus and lung, unspecified site
171.4 Malignant neoplasm of connective and other soft tissue of thorax
172.5 Malignant melanoma of skin of trunk, except scrotum
174.0 Malignant neoplasm of nipple and areola of female breast ♀
174.1 Malignant neoplasm of central portion of female breast ♀
174.2 Malignant neoplasm of upper-inner quadrant of female breast ♀
174.3 Malignant neoplasm of lower-inner quadrant of female breast ♀
174.4 Malignant neoplasm of upper-outer quadrant of female breast ♀
174.5 Malignant neoplasm of lower-outer quadrant of female breast ♀
174.6 Malignant neoplasm of axillary tail of female breast ♀
174.8 Malignant neoplasm of other specified sites of female breast ♀
174.9 Malignant neoplasm of breast (female), unspecified site ♀
756.6 Congenital anomaly of diaphragm
756.70 Unspecified congenital anomaly of abdominal wall
875.0 Open wound of chest (wall), without mention of complication — (Use additional code to identify infection)
875.1 Open wound of chest (wall), complicated — (Use additional code to identify infection)
879.2 Open wound of abdominal wall, anterior, without mention of complication — (Use additional code to identify infection)
879.3 Open wound of abdominal wall, anterior, complicated — (Use additional code to identify infection)
879.4 Open wound of abdominal wall, lateral, without mention of complication — (Use additional code to identify infection)
879.5 Open wound of abdominal wall, lateral, complicated — (Use additional code to identify infection)
942.01 Burn of trunk, unspecified degree of breast
942.02 Burn of trunk, unspecified degree of chest wall, excluding breast and nipple
942.31 Full-thickness skin loss due to burn (third degree nos) of breast
942.32 Full-thickness skin loss due to burn (third degree nos) of chest wall, excluding breast and nipple
942.41 Deep necrosis of underlying tissues due to burn (deep third degree) of breast, without mention of loss of a body part
942.42 Deep necrosis of underlying tissues due to burn (deep third degree) of chest wall, excluding breast and nipple, without mention of loss of a body part
998.31 Disruption of internal operation wound
998.32 Disruption of external operation wound
998.83 Non-healing surgical wound

ICD-9-CM Procedural

34.79 Other repair of chest wall
53.9 Other hernia repair
54.74 Other repair of omentum

HCPCS Level II Supplies & Services

HCPCS Level II codes are used to report the supplies, durable medical equipment, and certain medical services provided on an outpatient basis. Because the procedure(s) represented on this page would be performed in an inpatient facility, no HCPCS Level II codes apply.

49905

49905 Omental flap, intra-abdominal (List separately in addition to code for primary procedure)

ICD-9-CM Diagnostic

This is an add-on code. Refer to the corresponding primary procedure code for ICD-9 diagnosis code links.

ICD-9-CM Procedural

34.79 Other repair of chest wall
53.9 Other hernia repair

HCPCS Level II Supplies & Services

The HCPCS Level II code(s) would be the same as the actual procedure performed because these are in-addition-to codes.

49906

49906 Free omental flap with microvascular anastomosis

ICD-9-CM Diagnostic

162.9 Malignant neoplasm of bronchus and lung, unspecified site
170.3 Malignant neoplasm of ribs, sternum, and clavicle
171.4 Malignant neoplasm of connective and other soft tissue of thorax
172.5 Malignant melanoma of skin of trunk, except scrotum
174.9 Malignant neoplasm of breast (female), unspecified site ♀
701.8 Other specified hypertrophic and atrophic condition of skin
701.9 Unspecified hypertrophic and atrophic condition of skin
756.3 Other congenital anomaly of ribs and sternum
756.6 Congenital anomaly of diaphragm
756.70 Unspecified congenital anomaly of abdominal wall
875.0 Open wound of chest (wall), without mention of complication — (Use additional code to identify infection)
875.1 Open wound of chest (wall), complicated — (Use additional code to identify infection)
879.2 Open wound of abdominal wall, anterior, without mention of complication — (Use additional code to identify infection)
879.3 Open wound of abdominal wall, anterior, complicated — (Use additional code to identify infection)
879.4 Open wound of abdominal wall, lateral, without mention of complication — (Use additional code to identify infection)
879.5 Open wound of abdominal wall, lateral, complicated — (Use additional code to identify infection)
942.02 Burn of trunk, unspecified degree of chest wall, excluding breast and nipple
942.32 Full-thickness skin loss due to burn (third degree nos) of chest wall, excluding breast and nipple
942.42 Deep necrosis of underlying tissues due to burn (deep third degree) of chest wall, excluding breast and nipple, without mention of loss of a body part
998.31 Disruption of internal operation wound
998.32 Disruption of external operation wound
998.83 Non-healing surgical wound

ICD-9-CM Procedural

36.39 Other heart revascularization
54.74 Other repair of omentum

Urinary System

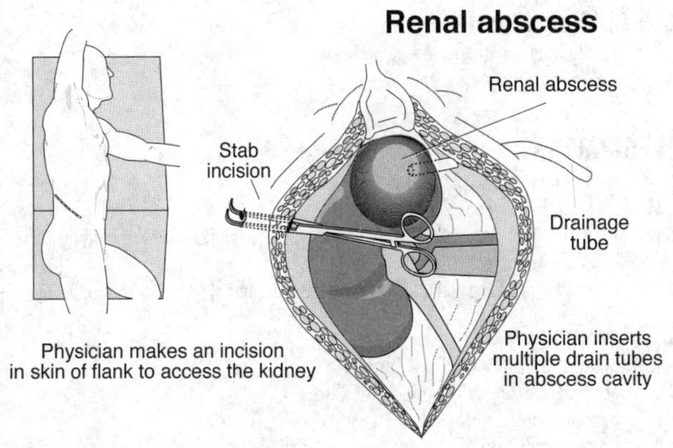
Renal abscess
Renal abscess
Stab incision
Drainage tube
Physician makes an incision in skin of flank to access the kidney
Physician inserts multiple drain tubes in abscess cavity

Kidney

50010

50010 Renal exploration, not necessitating other specific procedures

ICD-9-CM Diagnostic

189.0 Malignant neoplasm of kidney, except pelvis
189.1 Malignant neoplasm of renal pelvis
198.0 Secondary malignant neoplasm of kidney
223.1 Benign neoplasm of renal pelvis
233.9 Carcinoma in situ of other and unspecified urinary organs ▽
236.91 Neoplasm of uncertain behavior of kidney and ureter
239.5 Neoplasm of unspecified nature of other genitourinary organs
591 Hydronephrosis
593.0 Nephroptosis
593.1 Hypertrophy of kidney
593.2 Acquired cyst of kidney
593.81 Vascular disorders of kidney
593.9 Unspecified disorder of kidney and ureter ▽
866.00 Unspecified kidney injury without mention of open wound into cavity ▽
866.01 Kidney hematoma without rupture of capsule or mention of open wound into cavity
866.02 Kidney laceration without mention of open wound into cavity
866.03 Complete disruption of kidney parenchyma, without mention of open wound into cavity

ICD-9-CM Procedural

55.01 Nephrotomy
55.11 Pyelotomy

50020–50021

50020 Drainage of perirenal or renal abscess; open
50021 percutaneous

ICD-9-CM Diagnostic

590.2 Renal and perinephric abscess — (Use additional code to identify organism, such as E. coli, 041.4)
780.6 Fever
785.59 Other shock without mention of trauma
788.9 Other symptoms involving urinary system
996.80 Complications of transplanted organ, unspecified site — (Use additional code to identify nature of complication, 078.5) ▽
996.81 Complications of transplanted kidney — (Use additional code to identify nature of complication, 078.5)
998.51 Infected postoperative seroma — (Use additional code to identify organism)
998.59 Other postoperative infection — (Use additional code to identify infection)
V42.0 Kidney replaced by transplant — (This code is intended for use when these conditions are recorded as diagnoses or problems)

ICD-9-CM Procedural

55.01 Nephrotomy
55.92 Percutaneous aspiration of kidney (pelvis)
59.09 Other incision of perirenal or periureteral tissue

50040

50040 Nephrostomy, nephrotomy with drainage

ICD-9-CM Diagnostic

252.00 Hyperparathyroidism, unspecified
252.01 Primary hyperparathyroidism
252.02 Secondary hyperparathyroidism, non-renal
252.08 Other hyperparathyroidism
588.81 Secondary hyperparathyroidism (of renal origin)
588.89 Other specified disorders resulting from impaired renal function
590.10 Acute pyelonephritis without lesion of renal medullary necrosis — (Use additional code to identify organism, such as E. coli, 041.4)
590.11 Acute pyelonephritis with lesion of renal medullary necrosis — (Use additional code to identify organism, such as E. coli, 041.4)
590.2 Renal and perinephric abscess — (Use additional code to identify organism, such as E. coli, 041.4)
590.3 Pyeloureteritis cystica — (Use additional code to identify organism, such as E. coli, 041.4)
590.80 Unspecified pyelonephritis — (Use additional code to identify organism, such as E. coli, 041.4) ▽
592.0 Calculus of kidney
593.2 Acquired cyst of kidney
593.4 Other ureteric obstruction
593.70 Vesicoureteral reflux, unspecified or without reflex nephropathy
593.89 Other specified disorder of kidney and ureter
599.7 Hematuria
753.11 Congenital single renal cyst
753.13 Congenital polycystic kidney, autosomal dominant
753.14 Congenital polycystic kidney, autosomal recessive
753.15 Congenital renal dysplasia
753.16 Congenital medullary cystic kidney
753.17 Congenital medullary sponge kidney
753.19 Other specified congenital cystic kidney disease
753.20 Unspecified obstructive defect of renal pelvis and ureter ▽
753.21 Congenital obstruction of ureteropelvic junction
753.22 Congenital obstruction of ureterovesical junction
753.23 Congenital ureterocele
753.29 Other obstructive defect of renal pelvis and ureter
866.01 Kidney hematoma without rupture of capsule or mention of open wound into cavity
958.5 Traumatic anuria

ICD-9-CM Procedural

55.01 Nephrotomy
55.02 Nephrostomy

50045

50045 Nephrotomy, with exploration

ICD-9-CM Diagnostic

189.0 Malignant neoplasm of kidney, except pelvis
189.1 Malignant neoplasm of renal pelvis
198.0 Secondary malignant neoplasm of kidney
223.0 Benign neoplasm of kidney, except pelvis
223.1 Benign neoplasm of renal pelvis
233.9 Carcinoma in situ of other and unspecified urinary organs ▽
236.91 Neoplasm of uncertain behavior of kidney and ureter
239.5 Neoplasm of unspecified nature of other genitourinary organs
593.2 Acquired cyst of kidney
593.81 Vascular disorders of kidney
958.5 Traumatic anuria

ICD-9-CM Procedural

55.01 Nephrotomy

50060–50070

50060 Nephrolithotomy; removal of calculus
50065 secondary surgical operation for calculus
50070 complicated by congenital kidney abnormality

ICD-9-CM Diagnostic

252.00 Hyperparathyroidism, unspecified
252.01 Primary hyperparathyroidism
252.02 Secondary hyperparathyroidism, non-renal
252.08 Other hyperparathyroidism
588.81 Secondary hyperparathyroidism (of renal origin)
588.89 Other specified disorders resulting from impaired renal function
592.0 Calculus of kidney
592.9 Unspecified urinary calculus
599.7 Hematuria
753.21 Congenital obstruction of ureteropelvic junction
753.22 Congenital obstruction of ureterovesical junction
753.23 Congenital ureterocele
753.29 Other obstructive defect of renal pelvis and ureter
753.3 Other specified congenital anomalies of kidney
780.6 Fever
789.00 Abdominal pain, unspecified site
789.01 Abdominal pain, right upper quadrant
789.02 Abdominal pain, left upper quadrant
789.09 Abdominal pain, other specified site

ICD-9-CM Procedural

55.01 Nephrotomy

50075

50075 Nephrolithotomy; removal of large staghorn calculus filling renal pelvis and calyces (including anatrophic pyelolithotomy)

ICD-9-CM Diagnostic

252.00 Hyperparathyroidism, unspecified
252.01 Primary hyperparathyroidism
252.02 Secondary hyperparathyroidism, non-renal
252.08 Other hyperparathyroidism
588.81 Secondary hyperparathyroidism (of renal origin)
592.0 Calculus of kidney
592.9 Unspecified urinary calculus

ICD-9-CM Procedural

55.01 Nephrotomy
55.11 Pyelotomy

50080–50081

50080 Percutaneous nephrostolithotomy or pyelostolithotomy, with or without dilation, endoscopy, lithotripsy, stenting or basket extraction; up to 2 cm
50081 over 2 cm

ICD-9-CM Diagnostic

252.00 Hyperparathyroidism, unspecified
252.01 Primary hyperparathyroidism
252.02 Secondary hyperparathyroidism, non-renal
252.08 Other hyperparathyroidism
588.81 Secondary hyperparathyroidism (of renal origin)
588.89 Other specified disorders resulting from impaired renal function
592.0 Calculus of kidney
592.9 Unspecified urinary calculus
789.00 Abdominal pain, unspecified site
789.01 Abdominal pain, right upper quadrant
789.02 Abdominal pain, left upper quadrant
789.09 Abdominal pain, other specified site

ICD-9-CM Procedural

55.03 Percutaneous nephrostomy without fragmentation
55.04 Percutaneous nephrostomy with fragmentation

50100

50100 Transection or repositioning of aberrant renal vessels (separate procedure)

ICD-9-CM Diagnostic

593.3 Stricture or kinking of ureter
593.81 Vascular disorders of kidney
747.62 Congenital renal vessel anomaly
753.29 Other obstructive defect of renal pelvis and ureter
753.3 Other specified congenital anomalies of kidney

ICD-9-CM Procedural

39.55 Reimplantation of aberrant renal vessel
55.99 Other operations on kidney

50120–50135

50120 Pyelotomy; with exploration
50125 with drainage, pyelostomy
50130 with removal of calculus (pyelolithotomy, pelviolithotomy, including coagulum pyelolithotomy)
50135 complicated (eg, secondary operation, congenital kidney abnormality)

ICD-9-CM Diagnostic

189.1 Malignant neoplasm of renal pelvis
198.0 Secondary malignant neoplasm of kidney
223.1 Benign neoplasm of renal pelvis
233.9 Carcinoma in situ of other and unspecified urinary organs
236.91 Neoplasm of uncertain behavior of kidney and ureter
239.5 Neoplasm of unspecified nature of other genitourinary organs
252.00 Hyperparathyroidism, unspecified
252.01 Primary hyperparathyroidism
252.02 Secondary hyperparathyroidism, non-renal
252.08 Other hyperparathyroidism
588.81 Secondary hyperparathyroidism (of renal origin)
588.89 Other specified disorders resulting from impaired renal function
590.00 Chronic pyelonephritis without lesion of renal medullary necrosis — (Code, if applicable, any causal condition first. Use additional code to identify organism, such as E. coli, 041.4)
590.10 Acute pyelonephritis without lesion of renal medullary necrosis — (Use additional code to identify organism, such as E. coli, 041.4)
590.11 Acute pyelonephritis with lesion of renal medullary necrosis — (Use additional code to identify organism, such as E. coli, 041.4)
590.2 Renal and perinephric abscess — (Use additional code to identify organism, such as E. coli, 041.4)
590.3 Pyeloureteritis cystica — (Use additional code to identify organism, such as E. coli, 041.4)
592.0 Calculus of kidney
592.9 Unspecified urinary calculus
593.89 Other specified disorder of kidney and ureter
747.62 Congenital renal vessel anomaly
753.17 Congenital medullary sponge kidney
753.20 Unspecified obstructive defect of renal pelvis and ureter
753.21 Congenital obstruction of ureteropelvic junction
753.23 Congenital ureterocele
753.29 Other obstructive defect of renal pelvis and ureter
753.3 Other specified congenital anomalies of kidney

ICD-9-CM Procedural

55.11 Pyelotomy
55.12 Pyelostomy

50200–50205

50200 Renal biopsy; percutaneous, by trocar or needle
50205 by surgical exposure of kidney

ICD-9-CM Diagnostic

189.0 Malignant neoplasm of kidney, except pelvis
189.1 Malignant neoplasm of renal pelvis
198.0 Secondary malignant neoplasm of kidney
223.0 Benign neoplasm of kidney, except pelvis
223.1 Benign neoplasm of renal pelvis
228.09 Hemangioma of other sites
233.9 Carcinoma in situ of other and unspecified urinary organs
236.91 Neoplasm of uncertain behavior of kidney and ureter
239.5 Neoplasm of unspecified nature of other genitourinary organs
250.40 Diabetes with renal manifestations, type II or unspecified type, not stated as uncontrolled — (Use additional code to identify manifestation: 581.81, 583.81)

250.41 Diabetes with renal manifestations, type I [juvenile type], not stated as uncontrolled — (Use additional code to identify manifestation: 581.81, 583.81)
250.42 Diabetes with renal manifestations, type II or unspecified type, uncontrolled — (Use additional code to identify manifestation: 581.81, 583.81)
250.43 Diabetes with renal manifestations, type I [juvenile type], uncontrolled — (Use additional code to identify manifestation: 581.81, 583.81)
403.10 Benign hypertensive renal disease without mention of renal failure
403.11 Benign hypertensive renal disease with renal failure
445.81 Atheroembolism of kidney — (Use additional code for any associated kidney failure: 584, 585)
580.0 Acute glomerulonephritis with lesion of proliferative glomerulonephritis
580.89 Other acute glomerulonephritis with other specified pathological lesion in kidney
580.9 Acute glomerulonephritis with unspecified pathological lesion in kidney ▽
581.0 Nephrotic syndrome with lesion of proliferative glomerulonephritis
581.3 Nephrotic syndrome with lesion of minimal change glomerulonephritis
581.81 Nephrotic syndrome with other specified pathological lesion in kidney in diseases classified elsewhere — (Code first underlying disease: 084.9, 250.4, 277.3, 446.0, 710.0) ☒
581.9 Nephrotic syndrome with unspecified pathological lesion in kidney ▽
582.0 Chronic glomerulonephritis with lesion of proliferative glomerulonephritis
582.2 Chronic glomerulonephritis with lesion of membranoproliferative glomerulonephritis
582.4 Chronic glomerulonephritis with lesion of rapidly progressive glomerulonephritis
582.9 Chronic glomerulonephritis with unspecified pathological lesion in kidney ▽
583.0 Nephritis and nephropathy, not specified as acute or chronic, with lesion of proliferative glomerulonephritis
583.7 Nephritis and nephropathy, not specified as acute or chronic, with lesion of renal medullary necrosis
583.81 Nephritis and nephropathy, not specified as acute or chronic, with other specified pathological lesion in kidney, in diseases classified elsewhere — (Code first underlying disease: 016.0, 098.19, 250.4, 277.3, 446.21, 710.0) ☒
583.9 Nephritis and nephropathy, not specified as acute or chronic, with unspecified pathological lesion in kidney ▽
584.5 Acute renal failure with lesion of tubular necrosis
584.6 Acute renal failure with lesion of renal cortical necrosis
584.7 Acute renal failure with lesion of renal medullary (papillary) necrosis
584.8 Acute renal failure with other specified pathological lesion in kidney
584.9 Unspecified acute renal failure ▽
585 Chronic renal failure — (Use additional code to identify manifestation: 357.4, 420.0)
586 Unspecified renal failure ▽
588.0 Renal osteodystrophy
593.2 Acquired cyst of kidney
593.70 Vesicoureteral reflux, unspecified or without reflex nephropathy
593.9 Unspecified disorder of kidney and ureter ▽
599.7 Hematuria
728.88 Rhabdomyolysis
753.0 Congenital renal agenesis and dysgenesis
753.10 Unspecified congenital cystic kidney disease ▽
788.0 Renal colic
789.00 Abdominal pain, unspecified site ▽
789.09 Abdominal pain, other specified site
789.30 Abdominal or pelvic swelling, mass or lump, unspecified site ▽
789.39 Abdominal or pelvic swelling, mass, or lump, other specified site
791.0 Proteinuria
996.80 Complications of transplanted organ, unspecified site — (Use additional code to identify nature of complication, 078.5) ▽
996.81 Complications of transplanted kidney — (Use additional code to identify nature of complication, 078.5)
V42.0 Kidney replaced by transplant — (This code is intended for use when these conditions are recorded as diagnoses or problems)

ICD-9-CM Procedural

55.23 Closed (percutaneous) (needle) biopsy of kidney
55.24 Open biopsy of kidney

50220–50225

50220 Nephrectomy, including partial ureterectomy, any open approach including rib resection;
50225 complicated because of previous surgery on same kidney

ICD-9-CM Diagnostic

189.0 Malignant neoplasm of kidney, except pelvis
189.1 Malignant neoplasm of renal pelvis
189.2 Malignant neoplasm of ureter
189.8 Malignant neoplasm of other specified sites of urinary organs
198.0 Secondary malignant neoplasm of kidney
223.0 Benign neoplasm of kidney, except pelvis
223.1 Benign neoplasm of renal pelvis
223.2 Benign neoplasm of ureter
233.9 Carcinoma in situ of other and unspecified urinary organs ▽
236.91 Neoplasm of uncertain behavior of kidney and ureter
239.5 Neoplasm of unspecified nature of other genitourinary organs
403.01 Malignant hypertensive renal disease with renal failure
403.11 Benign hypertensive renal disease with renal failure
403.91 Unspecified hypertensive renal disease with renal failure ▽
404.02 Malignant hypertensive heart and renal disease with renal failure
404.12 Benign hypertensive heart and renal disease with renal failure
405.01 Secondary renovascular hypertension, malignant
405.91 Secondary renovascular hypertension, unspecified ▽
445.81 Atheroembolism of kidney — (Use additional code for any associated kidney failure: 584, 585)
580.0 Acute glomerulonephritis with lesion of proliferative glomerulonephritis
581.0 Nephrotic syndrome with lesion of proliferative glomerulonephritis
582.0 Chronic glomerulonephritis with lesion of proliferative glomerulonephritis
584.5 Acute renal failure with lesion of tubular necrosis
585 Chronic renal failure — (Use additional code to identify manifestation: 357.4, 420.0)
587 Unspecified renal sclerosis ▽
588.81 Secondary hyperparathyroidism (of renal origin)
588.89 Other specified disorders resulting from impaired renal function
590.00 Chronic pyelonephritis without lesion of renal medullary necrosis — (Code, if applicable, any causal condition first. Use additional code to identify organism, such as E. coli, 041.4)
590.01 Chronic pyelonephritis with lesion of renal medullary necrosis — (Code, if applicable, any causal condition first. Use additional code to identify organism, such as E. coli, 041.4)
591 Hydronephrosis
592.0 Calculus of kidney
593.4 Other ureteric obstruction
593.70 Vesicoureteral reflux, unspecified or without reflex nephropathy
593.71 Vesicoureteral reflux with reflux nephropathy, unilateral
593.72 Vesicoureteral reflux with reflux nephropathy, bilateral
593.73 Vesicoureteral reflux with reflux nephropathy, NOS
593.81 Vascular disorders of kidney
593.89 Other specified disorder of kidney and ureter
593.9 Unspecified disorder of kidney and ureter ▽
599.6 Unspecified urinary obstruction — (Use additional code to identify urinary incontinence: 625.6, 788.30-788.39) ▽
599.7 Hematuria
753.0 Congenital renal agenesis and dysgenesis
753.10 Unspecified congenital cystic kidney disease ▽
753.11 Congenital single renal cyst
753.12 Congenital polycystic kidney, unspecified type ▽
753.13 Congenital polycystic kidney, autosomal dominant
753.14 Congenital polycystic kidney, autosomal recessive
753.15 Congenital renal dysplasia
753.16 Congenital medullary cystic kidney
753.17 Congenital medullary sponge kidney
753.19 Other specified congenital cystic kidney disease
753.21 Congenital obstruction of ureteropelvic junction
753.23 Congenital ureterocele
753.29 Other obstructive defect of renal pelvis and ureter
866.02 Kidney laceration without mention of open wound into cavity
866.03 Complete disruption of kidney parenchyma, without mention of open wound into cavity
866.13 Complete disruption of kidney parenchyma, with open wound into cavity
879.3 Open wound of abdominal wall, anterior, complicated — (Use additional code to identify infection)
V64.41 Laparoscopic surgical procedure converted to open procedure

ICD-9-CM Procedural

55.51 Nephroureterectomy
55.52 Nephrectomy of remaining kidney
55.54 Bilateral nephrectomy

▽ Unspecified code ☒ Manifestation code
♀ Female diagnosis ♂ Male diagnosis

50230

50230 Nephrectomy, including partial ureterectomy, any open approach including rib resection; radical, with regional lymphadenectomy and/or vena caval thrombectomy

ICD-9-CM Diagnostic

189.0 Malignant neoplasm of kidney, except pelvis
189.1 Malignant neoplasm of renal pelvis
189.2 Malignant neoplasm of ureter
196.2 Secondary and unspecified malignant neoplasm of intra-abdominal lymph nodes
198.0 Secondary malignant neoplasm of kidney
198.1 Secondary malignant neoplasm of other urinary organs
199.1 Other malignant neoplasm of unspecified site
223.0 Benign neoplasm of kidney, except pelvis
223.1 Benign neoplasm of renal pelvis
223.2 Benign neoplasm of ureter
233.9 Carcinoma in situ of other and unspecified urinary organs ▽
236.91 Neoplasm of uncertain behavior of kidney and ureter
239.5 Neoplasm of unspecified nature of other genitourinary organs
403.01 Malignant hypertensive renal disease with renal failure
403.11 Benign hypertensive renal disease with renal failure
404.02 Malignant hypertensive heart and renal disease with renal failure
404.12 Benign hypertensive heart and renal disease with renal failure
445.81 Atheroembolism of kidney — (Use additional code for any associated kidney failure: 584, 585)
453.2 Embolism and thrombosis of vena cava
580.0 Acute glomerulonephritis with lesion of proliferative glomerulonephritis
581.0 Nephrotic syndrome with lesion of proliferative glomerulonephritis
582.0 Chronic glomerulonephritis with lesion of proliferative glomerulonephritis
584.5 Acute renal failure with lesion of tubular necrosis
585 Chronic renal failure — (Use additional code to identify manifestation: 357.4, 420.0)
587 Unspecified renal sclerosis ▽
588.81 Secondary hyperparathyroidism (of renal origin)
588.89 Other specified disorders resulting from impaired renal function
590.00 Chronic pyelonephritis without lesion of renal medullary necrosis — (Code, if applicable, any causal condition first. Use additional code to identify organism, such as E. coli, 041.4)
590.01 Chronic pyelonephritis with lesion of renal medullary necrosis — (Code, if applicable, any causal condition first. Use additional code to identify organism, such as E. coli, 041.4)
591 Hydronephrosis
592.0 Calculus of kidney
593.4 Other ureteric obstruction
593.70 Vesicoureteral reflux, unspecified or without reflex nephropathy
593.71 Vesicoureteral reflux with reflux nephropathy, unilateral
593.72 Vesicoureteral reflux with reflux nephropathy, bilateral
593.73 Vesicoureteral reflux with reflux nephropathy, NOS
593.81 Vascular disorders of kidney
593.89 Other specified disorder of kidney and ureter
593.9 Unspecified disorder of kidney and ureter ▽
599.6 Unspecified urinary obstruction — (Use additional code to identify urinary incontinence: 625.6, 788.30-788.39) ▽
599.7 Hematuria
753.0 Congenital renal agenesis and dysgenesis
753.10 Unspecified congenital cystic kidney disease ▽
753.11 Congenital single renal cyst
753.12 Congenital polycystic kidney, unspecified type ▽
753.13 Congenital polycystic kidney, autosomal dominant
753.14 Congenital polycystic kidney, autosomal recessive
753.15 Congenital renal dysplasia
753.16 Congenital medullary cystic kidney
753.17 Congenital medullary sponge kidney
753.19 Other specified congenital cystic kidney disease
753.21 Congenital obstruction of ureteropelvic junction
753.23 Congenital ureterocele
753.29 Other obstructive defect of renal pelvis and ureter
866.03 Complete disruption of kidney parenchyma, without mention of open wound into cavity
866.13 Complete disruption of kidney parenchyma, with open wound into cavity
V64.41 Laparoscopic surgical procedure converted to open procedure

ICD-9-CM Procedural

38.07 Incision of abdominal veins
40.3 Regional lymph node excision
55.51 Nephroureterectomy
55.52 Nephrectomy of remaining kidney
55.54 Bilateral nephrectomy

50234–50236

50234 Nephrectomy with total ureterectomy and bladder cuff; through same incision
50236 through separate incision

ICD-9-CM Diagnostic

188.6 Malignant neoplasm of ureteric orifice
189.0 Malignant neoplasm of kidney, except pelvis
189.1 Malignant neoplasm of renal pelvis
189.2 Malignant neoplasm of ureter
189.8 Malignant neoplasm of other specified sites of urinary organs
198.0 Secondary malignant neoplasm of kidney
198.1 Secondary malignant neoplasm of other urinary organs
223.0 Benign neoplasm of kidney, except pelvis
223.1 Benign neoplasm of renal pelvis
223.2 Benign neoplasm of ureter
233.9 Carcinoma in situ of other and unspecified urinary organs ▽
236.91 Neoplasm of uncertain behavior of kidney and ureter
239.5 Neoplasm of unspecified nature of other genitourinary organs
403.01 Malignant hypertensive renal disease with renal failure
403.11 Benign hypertensive renal disease with renal failure
403.91 Unspecified hypertensive renal disease with renal failure ▽
404.02 Malignant hypertensive heart and renal disease with renal failure
404.12 Benign hypertensive heart and renal disease with renal failure
405.01 Secondary renovascular hypertension, malignant
445.81 Atheroembolism of kidney — (Use additional code for any associated kidney failure: 584, 585)
580.0 Acute glomerulonephritis with lesion of proliferative glomerulonephritis
581.0 Nephrotic syndrome with lesion of proliferative glomerulonephritis
582.0 Chronic glomerulonephritis with lesion of proliferative glomerulonephritis
584.5 Acute renal failure with lesion of tubular necrosis
585 Chronic renal failure — (Use additional code to identify manifestation: 357.4, 420.0)
587 Unspecified renal sclerosis ▽
588.81 Secondary hyperparathyroidism (of renal origin)
588.89 Other specified disorders resulting from impaired renal function
590.00 Chronic pyelonephritis without lesion of renal medullary necrosis — (Code, if applicable, any causal condition first. Use additional code to identify organism, such as E. coli, 041.4)
590.01 Chronic pyelonephritis with lesion of renal medullary necrosis — (Code, if applicable, any causal condition first. Use additional code to identify organism, such as E. coli, 041.4)
591 Hydronephrosis
592.0 Calculus of kidney
593.4 Other ureteric obstruction
593.70 Vesicoureteral reflux, unspecified or without reflex nephropathy
593.71 Vesicoureteral reflux with reflux nephropathy, unilateral
593.72 Vesicoureteral reflux with reflux nephropathy, bilateral
593.73 Vesicoureteral reflux with reflux nephropathy, NOS
593.81 Vascular disorders of kidney
593.89 Other specified disorder of kidney and ureter
599.7 Hematuria
753.0 Congenital renal agenesis and dysgenesis
753.10 Unspecified congenital cystic kidney disease ▽
753.11 Congenital single renal cyst
753.12 Congenital polycystic kidney, unspecified type ▽
753.13 Congenital polycystic kidney, autosomal dominant
753.14 Congenital polycystic kidney, autosomal recessive
753.15 Congenital renal dysplasia
753.16 Congenital medullary cystic kidney
753.17 Congenital medullary sponge kidney
753.19 Other specified congenital cystic kidney disease
753.20 Unspecified obstructive defect of renal pelvis and ureter ▽
753.21 Congenital obstruction of ureteropelvic junction
753.22 Congenital obstruction of ureterovesical junction
753.23 Congenital ureterocele
753.29 Other obstructive defect of renal pelvis and ureter
866.02 Kidney laceration without mention of open wound into cavity
866.03 Complete disruption of kidney parenchyma, without mention of open wound into cavity
866.13 Complete disruption of kidney parenchyma, with open wound into cavity
V64.41 Laparoscopic surgical procedure converted to open procedure

ICD-9-CM Procedural
55.51 Nephroureterectomy
55.52 Nephrectomy of remaining kidney
55.54 Bilateral nephrectomy

50240
50240 Nephrectomy, partial

ICD-9-CM Diagnostic
189.0 Malignant neoplasm of kidney, except pelvis
189.1 Malignant neoplasm of renal pelvis
198.0 Secondary malignant neoplasm of kidney
223.0 Benign neoplasm of kidney, except pelvis
223.1 Benign neoplasm of renal pelvis
233.9 Carcinoma in situ of other and unspecified urinary organs ▽
236.91 Neoplasm of uncertain behavior of kidney and ureter
239.5 Neoplasm of unspecified nature of other genitourinary organs
587 Unspecified renal sclerosis ▽
591 Hydronephrosis
593.2 Acquired cyst of kidney
593.70 Vesicoureteral reflux, unspecified or without reflex nephropathy
593.71 Vesicoureteral reflux with reflux nephropathy, unilateral
593.72 Vesicoureteral reflux with reflux nephropathy, bilateral
593.73 Vesicoureteral reflux with reflux nephropathy, NOS
593.81 Vascular disorders of kidney
593.89 Other specified disorder of kidney and ureter
593.9 Unspecified disorder of kidney and ureter ▽
599.7 Hematuria
753.11 Congenital single renal cyst
753.12 Congenital polycystic kidney, unspecified type ▽
753.13 Congenital polycystic kidney, autosomal dominant
753.14 Congenital polycystic kidney, autosomal recessive
753.15 Congenital renal dysplasia
753.16 Congenital medullary cystic kidney
753.17 Congenital medullary sponge kidney
753.19 Other specified congenital cystic kidney disease
753.20 Unspecified obstructive defect of renal pelvis and ureter ▽
753.21 Congenital obstruction of ureteropelvic junction
753.22 Congenital obstruction of ureterovesical junction
753.23 Congenital ureterocele
753.29 Other obstructive defect of renal pelvis and ureter
866.00 Unspecified kidney injury without mention of open wound into cavity ▽
V64.41 Laparoscopic surgical procedure converted to open procedure

ICD-9-CM Procedural
55.4 Partial nephrectomy

50280–50290
50280 Excision or unroofing of cyst(s) of kidney
50290 Excision of perinephric cyst

ICD-9-CM Diagnostic
593.2 Acquired cyst of kidney
593.89 Other specified disorder of kidney and ureter
753.10 Unspecified congenital cystic kidney disease ▽
753.11 Congenital single renal cyst
753.12 Congenital polycystic kidney, unspecified type ▽
753.13 Congenital polycystic kidney, autosomal dominant
753.14 Congenital polycystic kidney, autosomal recessive
753.19 Other specified congenital cystic kidney disease

ICD-9-CM Procedural
55.39 Other local destruction or excision of renal lesion or tissue
59.91 Excision of perirenal or perivesical tissue

50300–50320
50300 Donor nephrectomy (including cold preservation); from cadaver donor, unilateral or bilateral
50320 open, from living donor

ICD-9-CM Diagnostic
V59.4 Kidney donor

ICD-9-CM Procedural
55.51 Nephroureterectomy
55.54 Bilateral nephrectomy

50323–50325
50323 Backbench standard preparation of cadaver donor renal allograft prior to transplantation, including dissection and removal of perinephric fat, diaphragmatic and retroperitoneal attachments, excision of adrenal gland, and preparation of ureter(s), renal vein(s), and renal artery(s), ligating branches, as necessary
50325 Backbench standard preparation of living donor renal allograft (open or laparoscopic) prior to transplantation, including dissection and removal of perinephric fat and preparation of ureter(s), renal vein(s), and renal artery(s), ligating branches, as necessary

ICD-9-CM Diagnostic
189.0 Malignant neoplasm of kidney, except pelvis
189.1 Malignant neoplasm of renal pelvis
198.0 Secondary malignant neoplasm of kidney
223.0 Benign neoplasm of kidney, except pelvis
236.91 Neoplasm of uncertain behavior of kidney and ureter
250.40 Diabetes with renal manifestations, type II or unspecified type, not stated as uncontrolled — (Use additional code to identify manifestation: 581.81, 583.81)
250.41 Diabetes with renal manifestations, type I [juvenile type], not stated as uncontrolled — (Use additional code to identify manifestation: 581.81, 583.81)
250.42 Diabetes with renal manifestations, type II or unspecified type, uncontrolled — (Use additional code to identify manifestation: 581.81, 583.81)
250.43 Diabetes with renal manifestations, type I [juvenile type], uncontrolled — (Use additional code to identify manifestation: 581.81, 583.81)
403.01 Malignant hypertensive renal disease with renal failure
403.11 Benign hypertensive renal disease with renal failure
403.91 Unspecified hypertensive renal disease with renal failure ▽
445.81 Atheroembolism of kidney — (Use additional code for any associated kidney failure: 584, 585)
580.0 Acute glomerulonephritis with lesion of proliferative glomerulonephritis
581.0 Nephrotic syndrome with lesion of proliferative glomerulonephritis
581.81 Nephrotic syndrome with other specified pathological lesion in kidney in diseases classified elsewhere — (Code first underlying disease: 084.9, 250.4, 277.3, 446.0, 710.0) ☒
582.0 Chronic glomerulonephritis with lesion of proliferative glomerulonephritis
583.81 Nephritis and nephropathy, not specified as acute or chronic, with other specified pathological lesion in kidney, in diseases classified elsewhere — (Code first underlying disease: 016.0, 098.19, 250.4, 277.3, 446.21, 710.0) ☒
584.5 Acute renal failure with lesion of tubular necrosis
585 Chronic renal failure — (Use additional code to identify manifestation: 357.4, 420.0)
586 Unspecified renal failure ▽
590.00 Chronic pyelonephritis without lesion of renal medullary necrosis — (Code, if applicable, any causal condition first. Use additional code to identify organism, such as E. coli, 041.4)
590.01 Chronic pyelonephritis with lesion of renal medullary necrosis — (Code, if applicable, any causal condition first. Use additional code to identify organism, such as E. coli, 041.4)
590.80 Unspecified pyelonephritis — (Use additional code to identify organism, such as E. coli, 041.4) ▽
593.70 Vesicoureteral reflux, unspecified or without reflex nephropathy
593.71 Vesicoureteral reflux with reflux nephropathy, unilateral
593.72 Vesicoureteral reflux with reflux nephropathy, bilateral
593.73 Vesicoureteral reflux with reflux nephropathy, NOS
593.81 Vascular disorders of kidney
753.12 Congenital polycystic kidney, unspecified type ▽
753.17 Congenital medullary sponge kidney
866.13 Complete disruption of kidney parenchyma, with open wound into cavity
996.81 Complications of transplanted kidney — (Use additional code to identify nature of complication, 078.5)

ICD-9-CM Procedural
00.91 Transplant from live related donor
00.92 Transplant from live non-related donor
00.93 Transplant from cadaver
55.69 Other kidney transplantation
55.99 Other operations on kidney

▽ Unspecified code ☒ Manifestation code
♀ Female diagnosis ♂ Male diagnosis

50327–50329

50327 Backbench reconstruction of cadaver or living donor renal allograft prior to transplantation; venous anastomosis, each
50328 arterial anastomosis, each
50329 ureteral anastomosis, each

ICD-9-CM Diagnostic

189.0 Malignant neoplasm of kidney, except pelvis
189.1 Malignant neoplasm of renal pelvis
198.0 Secondary malignant neoplasm of kidney
223.0 Benign neoplasm of kidney, except pelvis
236.91 Neoplasm of uncertain behavior of kidney and ureter
250.40 Diabetes with renal manifestations, type II or unspecified type, not stated as uncontrolled — (Use additional code to identify manifestation: 581.81, 583.81)
250.41 Diabetes with renal manifestations, type I [juvenile type], not stated as uncontrolled — (Use additional code to identify manifestation: 581.81, 583.81)
250.42 Diabetes with renal manifestations, type II or unspecified type, uncontrolled — (Use additional code to identify manifestation: 581.81, 583.81)
250.43 Diabetes with renal manifestations, type I [juvenile type], uncontrolled — (Use additional code to identify manifestation: 581.81, 583.81)
403.01 Malignant hypertensive renal disease with renal failure
403.11 Benign hypertensive renal disease with renal failure
403.91 Unspecified hypertensive renal disease with renal failure ▽
445.81 Atheroembolism of kidney — (Use additional code for any associated kidney failure: 584, 585)
580.0 Acute glomerulonephritis with lesion of proliferative glomerulonephritis
581.0 Nephrotic syndrome with lesion of proliferative glomerulonephritis
581.81 Nephrotic syndrome with other specified pathological lesion in kidney in diseases classified elsewhere — (Code first underlying disease: 084.9, 250.4, 277.3, 446.0, 710.0) ☒
582.0 Chronic glomerulonephritis with lesion of proliferative glomerulonephritis
583.81 Nephritis and nephropathy, not specified as acute or chronic, with other specified pathological lesion in kidney, in diseases classified elsewhere — (Code first underlying disease: 016.0, 098.19, 250.4, 277.3, 446.21, 710.0) ☒
584.5 Acute renal failure with lesion of tubular necrosis
585 Chronic renal failure — (Use additional code to identify manifestation: 357.4, 420.0)
586 Unspecified renal failure ▽
590.00 Chronic pyelonephritis without lesion of renal medullary necrosis — (Code, if applicable, any causal condition first. Use additional code to identify organism, such as E. coli, 041.4)
590.01 Chronic pyelonephritis with lesion of renal medullary necrosis — (Code, if applicable, any causal condition first. Use additional code to identify organism, such as E. coli, 041.4)
590.80 Unspecified pyelonephritis — (Use additional code to identify organism, such as E. coli, 041.4) ▽
593.70 Vesicoureteral reflux, unspecified or without reflex nephropathy
593.71 Vesicoureteral reflux with reflux nephropathy, unilateral
593.72 Vesicoureteral reflux with reflux nephropathy, bilateral
593.73 Vesicoureteral reflux with reflux nephropathy, NOS
593.81 Vascular disorders of kidney
753.12 Congenital polycystic kidney, unspecified type ▽
753.17 Congenital medullary sponge kidney
866.13 Complete disruption of kidney parenchyma, with open wound into cavity
996.81 Complications of transplanted kidney — (Use additional code to identify nature of complication, 078.5)

ICD-9-CM Procedural

00.91 Transplant from live related donor
00.92 Transplant from live non-related donor
00.93 Transplant from cadaver
55.69 Other kidney transplantation
55.99 Other operations on kidney

50340

50340 Recipient nephrectomy (separate procedure)

ICD-9-CM Diagnostic

189.0 Malignant neoplasm of kidney, except pelvis
189.1 Malignant neoplasm of renal pelvis
198.0 Secondary malignant neoplasm of kidney
223.0 Benign neoplasm of kidney, except pelvis
236.91 Neoplasm of uncertain behavior of kidney and ureter
250.40 Diabetes with renal manifestations, type II or unspecified type, not stated as uncontrolled — (Use additional code to identify manifestation: 581.81, 583.81)
250.41 Diabetes with renal manifestations, type I [juvenile type], not stated as uncontrolled — (Use additional code to identify manifestation: 581.81, 583.81)
250.42 Diabetes with renal manifestations, type II or unspecified type, uncontrolled — (Use additional code to identify manifestation: 581.81, 583.81)
250.43 Diabetes with renal manifestations, type I [juvenile type], uncontrolled — (Use additional code to identify manifestation: 581.81, 583.81)
403.01 Malignant hypertensive renal disease with renal failure
403.11 Benign hypertensive renal disease with renal failure
403.91 Unspecified hypertensive renal disease with renal failure ▽
445.81 Atheroembolism of kidney — (Use additional code for any associated kidney failure: 584, 585)
580.0 Acute glomerulonephritis with lesion of proliferative glomerulonephritis
581.0 Nephrotic syndrome with lesion of proliferative glomerulonephritis
581.81 Nephrotic syndrome with other specified pathological lesion in kidney in diseases classified elsewhere — (Code first underlying disease: 084.9, 250.4, 277.3, 446.0, 710.0) ☒
582.0 Chronic glomerulonephritis with lesion of proliferative glomerulonephritis
583.81 Nephritis and nephropathy, not specified as acute or chronic, with other specified pathological lesion in kidney, in diseases classified elsewhere — (Code first underlying disease: 016.0, 098.19, 250.4, 277.3, 446.21, 710.0) ☒
584.5 Acute renal failure with lesion of tubular necrosis
585 Chronic renal failure — (Use additional code to identify manifestation: 357.4, 420.0)
586 Unspecified renal failure ▽
590.00 Chronic pyelonephritis without lesion of renal medullary necrosis — (Code, if applicable, any causal condition first. Use additional code to identify organism, such as E. coli, 041.4)
590.01 Chronic pyelonephritis with lesion of renal medullary necrosis — (Code, if applicable, any causal condition first. Use additional code to identify organism, such as E. coli, 041.4)
590.80 Unspecified pyelonephritis — (Use additional code to identify organism, such as E. coli, 041.4) ▽
593.70 Vesicoureteral reflux, unspecified or without reflex nephropathy
593.71 Vesicoureteral reflux with reflux nephropathy, unilateral
593.72 Vesicoureteral reflux with reflux nephropathy, bilateral
593.73 Vesicoureteral reflux with reflux nephropathy, NOS
593.81 Vascular disorders of kidney
753.12 Congenital polycystic kidney, unspecified type ▽
753.17 Congenital medullary sponge kidney
866.13 Complete disruption of kidney parenchyma, with open wound into cavity
996.81 Complications of transplanted kidney — (Use additional code to identify nature of complication, 078.5)

ICD-9-CM Procedural

55.51 Nephroureterectomy
55.54 Bilateral nephrectomy

50360–50365

50360 Renal allotransplantation, implantation of graft; without recipient nephrectomy
50365 with recipient nephrectomy

ICD-9-CM Diagnostic

189.0 Malignant neoplasm of kidney, except pelvis
189.1 Malignant neoplasm of renal pelvis
198.0 Secondary malignant neoplasm of kidney
223.0 Benign neoplasm of kidney, except pelvis
236.91 Neoplasm of uncertain behavior of kidney and ureter
250.40 Diabetes with renal manifestations, type II or unspecified type, not stated as uncontrolled — (Use additional code to identify manifestation: 581.81, 583.81)
250.41 Diabetes with renal manifestations, type I [juvenile type], not stated as uncontrolled — (Use additional code to identify manifestation: 581.81, 583.81)
250.42 Diabetes with renal manifestations, type II or unspecified type, uncontrolled — (Use additional code to identify manifestation: 581.81, 583.81)
250.43 Diabetes with renal manifestations, type I [juvenile type], uncontrolled — (Use additional code to identify manifestation: 581.81, 583.81)
403.01 Malignant hypertensive renal disease with renal failure
403.11 Benign hypertensive renal disease with renal failure
403.91 Unspecified hypertensive renal disease with renal failure ▽
445.81 Atheroembolism of kidney — (Use additional code for any associated kidney failure: 584, 585)
580.0 Acute glomerulonephritis with lesion of proliferative glomerulonephritis
581.0 Nephrotic syndrome with lesion of proliferative glomerulonephritis
581.81 Nephrotic syndrome with other specified pathological lesion in kidney in diseases classified elsewhere — (Code first underlying disease: 084.9, 250.4, 277.3, 446.0, 710.0) ☒
582.0 Chronic glomerulonephritis with lesion of proliferative glomerulonephritis

▽ Unspecified code
♀ Female diagnosis
☒ Manifestation code
♂ Male diagnosis

583.81 Nephritis and nephropathy, not specified as acute or chronic, with other specified pathological lesion in kidney, in diseases classified elsewhere — (Code first underlying disease: 016.0, 098.19, 250.4, 277.3, 446.21, 710.0) ☒
584.5 Acute renal failure with lesion of tubular necrosis
585 Chronic renal failure — (Use additional code to identify manifestation: 357.4, 420.0)
586 Unspecified renal failure ▽
590.00 Chronic pyelonephritis without lesion of renal medullary necrosis — (Code, if applicable, any causal condition first. Use additional code to identify organism, such as E. coli, 041.4)
590.01 Chronic pyelonephritis with lesion of renal medullary necrosis — (Code, if applicable, any causal condition first. Use additional code to identify organism, such as E. coli, 041.4)
590.80 Unspecified pyelonephritis — (Use additional code to identify organism, such as E. coli, 041.4) ▽
593.70 Vesicoureteral reflux, unspecified or without reflex nephropathy
593.71 Vesicoureteral reflux with reflux nephropathy, unilateral
593.72 Vesicoureteral reflux with reflux nephropathy, bilateral
593.73 Vesicoureteral reflux with reflux nephropathy, NOS
593.81 Vascular disorders of kidney
753.12 Congenital polycystic kidney, unspecified type ▽
753.17 Congenital medullary sponge kidney
866.13 Complete disruption of kidney parenchyma, with open wound into cavity
996.81 Complications of transplanted kidney — (Use additional code to identify nature of complication, 078.5)

ICD-9-CM Procedural

55.51 Nephroureterectomy
55.54 Bilateral nephrectomy
55.69 Other kidney transplantation

50370

50370 Removal of transplanted renal allograft

ICD-9-CM Diagnostic

593.81 Vascular disorders of kidney
996.81 Complications of transplanted kidney — (Use additional code to identify nature of complication, 078.5)

ICD-9-CM Procedural

00.91 Transplant from live related donor
00.92 Transplant from live non-related donor
00.93 Transplant from cadaver
55.53 Removal of transplanted or rejected kidney

50380

50380 Renal autotransplantation, reimplantation of kidney

ICD-9-CM Diagnostic

405.01 Secondary renovascular hypertension, malignant
405.11 Secondary renovascular hypertension, benign
593.81 Vascular disorders of kidney
902.42 Renal vein injury
902.49 Renal blood vessel injury, other
996.81 Complications of transplanted kidney — (Use additional code to identify nature of complication, 078.5)
V10.52 Personal history of malignant neoplasm of kidney
V10.53 Personal history of malignant neoplasm, renal pelvis

ICD-9-CM Procedural

55.61 Renal autotransplantation

50390

50390 Aspiration and/or injection of renal cyst or pelvis by needle, percutaneous

ICD-9-CM Diagnostic

189.0 Malignant neoplasm of kidney, except pelvis
189.1 Malignant neoplasm of renal pelvis
586 Unspecified renal failure ▽
593.2 Acquired cyst of kidney
593.89 Other specified disorder of kidney and ureter
753.10 Unspecified congenital cystic kidney disease ▽
753.11 Congenital single renal cyst
753.20 Unspecified obstructive defect of renal pelvis and ureter ▽
753.21 Congenital obstruction of ureteropelvic junction
753.22 Congenital obstruction of ureterovesical junction
753.23 Congenital ureterocele
753.29 Other obstructive defect of renal pelvis and ureter
753.3 Other specified congenital anomalies of kidney

ICD-9-CM Procedural

55.92 Percutaneous aspiration of kidney (pelvis)
55.96 Other injection of therapeutic substance into kidney

HCPCS Level II Supplies & Services

A4550 Surgical trays

50391

50391 Instillation(s) of therapeutic agent into renal pelvis and/or ureter through established nephrostomy, pyelostomy or ureterostomy tube (eg, anticarcinogenic or antifungal agent)

ICD-9-CM Diagnostic

016.00 Tuberculosis of kidney, confirmation unspecified — (Use additional code to identify manifestation: 583.81, 590.81) ▽
118 Opportunistic mycoses — (Use additional code to identify manifestation: 321.0-321.1, 380.15, 711.6)
188.6 Malignant neoplasm of ureteric orifice
189.0 Malignant neoplasm of kidney, except pelvis
189.1 Malignant neoplasm of renal pelvis
189.2 Malignant neoplasm of ureter
198.0 Secondary malignant neoplasm of kidney
198.1 Secondary malignant neoplasm of other urinary organs
233.7 Carcinoma in situ of bladder
233.9 Carcinoma in situ of other and unspecified urinary organs ▽
236.7 Neoplasm of uncertain behavior of bladder
236.91 Neoplasm of uncertain behavior of kidney and ureter
239.5 Neoplasm of unspecified nature of other genitourinary organs
583.81 Nephritis and nephropathy, not specified as acute or chronic, with other specified pathological lesion in kidney, in diseases classified elsewhere — (Code first underlying disease: 016.0, 098.19, 250.4, 277.3, 446.21, 710.0) ☒
590.00 Chronic pyelonephritis without lesion of renal medullary necrosis — (Code, if applicable, any causal condition first. Use additional code to identify organism, such as E. coli, 041.4)
590.01 Chronic pyelonephritis with lesion of renal medullary necrosis — (Code, if applicable, any causal condition first. Use additional code to identify organism, such as E. coli, 041.4)
590.10 Acute pyelonephritis without lesion of renal medullary necrosis — (Use additional code to identify organism, such as E. coli, 041.4)
590.11 Acute pyelonephritis with lesion of renal medullary necrosis — (Use additional code to identify organism, such as E. coli, 041.4)
590.2 Renal and perinephric abscess — (Use additional code to identify organism, such as E. coli, 041.4)
590.3 Pyeloureteritis cystica — (Use additional code to identify organism, such as E. coli, 041.4)
590.80 Unspecified pyelonephritis — (Use additional code to identify organism, such as E. coli, 041.4) ▽
590.81 Pyelitis or pyelonephritis in diseases classified elsewhere — (Code first underlying disease, 016.0. Use additional code to identify organism, such as E. coli, 041.4) ☒
590.9 Unspecified infection of kidney — (Use additional code to identify organism, such as E. coli, 041.4) ▽

ICD-9-CM Procedural

55.96 Other injection of therapeutic substance into kidney
92.25 Teleradiotherapy using electrons
96.49 Other genitourinary instillation
99.22 Injection of other anti-infective

50392–50393

50392 Introduction of intracatheter or catheter into renal pelvis for drainage and/or injection, percutaneous
50393 Introduction of ureteral catheter or stent into ureter through renal pelvis for drainage and/or injection, percutaneous

ICD-9-CM Diagnostic

189.0 Malignant neoplasm of kidney, except pelvis
189.1 Malignant neoplasm of renal pelvis
198.0 Secondary malignant neoplasm of kidney
223.1 Benign neoplasm of renal pelvis
252.00 Hyperparathyroidism, unspecified

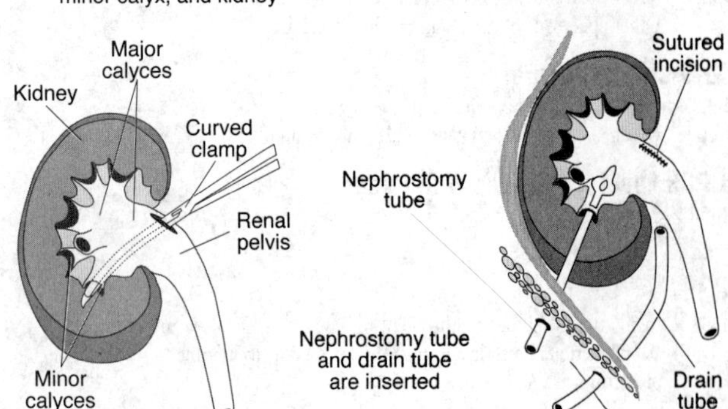

252.01 Primary hyperparathyroidism
252.02 Secondary hyperparathyroidism, non-renal
252.08 Other hyperparathyroidism
586 Unspecified renal failure ▽
588.81 Secondary hyperparathyroidism (of renal origin)
588.89 Other specified disorders resulting from impaired renal function
591 Hydronephrosis
592.0 Calculus of kidney
592.1 Calculus of ureter
592.9 Unspecified urinary calculus ▽
593.4 Other ureteric obstruction
593.89 Other specified disorder of kidney and ureter
753.20 Unspecified obstructive defect of renal pelvis and ureter ▽
753.21 Congenital obstruction of ureteropelvic junction
753.22 Congenital obstruction of ureterovesical junction
753.23 Congenital ureterocele
753.29 Other obstructive defect of renal pelvis and ureter
996.65 Infection and inflammatory reaction due to other genitourinary device, implant, and graft — (Use additional code to identify specified infections)
996.81 Complications of transplanted kidney — (Use additional code to identify nature of complication, 078.5)

ICD-9-CM Procedural

55.29 Other diagnostic procedures on kidney

HCPCS Level II Supplies & Services

A4550 Surgical trays

50394

50394 Injection procedure for pyelography (as nephrostogram, pyelostogram, antegrade pyeloureterograms) through nephrostomy or pyelostomy tube, or indwelling ureteral catheter

ICD-9-CM Diagnostic

189.0 Malignant neoplasm of kidney, except pelvis
189.1 Malignant neoplasm of renal pelvis
189.2 Malignant neoplasm of ureter
189.8 Malignant neoplasm of other specified sites of urinary organs
198.0 Secondary malignant neoplasm of kidney
198.1 Secondary malignant neoplasm of other urinary organs
199.0 Disseminated malignant neoplasm
199.1 Other malignant neoplasm of unspecified site
223.0 Benign neoplasm of kidney, except pelvis
223.1 Benign neoplasm of renal pelvis
223.2 Benign neoplasm of ureter
233.9 Carcinoma in situ of other and unspecified urinary organs ▽
236.91 Neoplasm of uncertain behavior of kidney and ureter
239.5 Neoplasm of unspecified nature of other genitourinary organs
252.00 Hyperparathyroidism, unspecified
252.01 Primary hyperparathyroidism
252.02 Secondary hyperparathyroidism, non-renal
252.08 Other hyperparathyroidism
357.4 Polyneuropathy in other diseases classified elsewhere — (Code first underlying disease: 032.0-032.9, 135, 251.2, 265.0, 265.2, 266.0-266.9, 277.1, 277.3, 585) ☒
585 Chronic renal failure — (Use additional code to identify manifestation: 357.4, 420.0)
586 Unspecified renal failure ▽
587 Unspecified renal sclerosis ▽
588.81 Secondary hyperparathyroidism (of renal origin)
588.89 Other specified disorders resulting from impaired renal function
590.00 Chronic pyelonephritis without lesion of renal medullary necrosis — (Code, if applicable, any causal condition first. Use additional code to identify organism, such as E. coli, 041.4)
590.01 Chronic pyelonephritis with lesion of renal medullary necrosis — (Code, if applicable, any causal condition first. Use additional code to identify organism, such as E. coli, 041.4)
590.3 Pyeloureteritis cystica — (Use additional code to identify organism, such as E. coli, 041.4)
591 Hydronephrosis
592.0 Calculus of kidney
592.9 Unspecified urinary calculus ▽
593.2 Acquired cyst of kidney
593.3 Stricture or kinking of ureter
593.4 Other ureteric obstruction
593.70 Vesicoureteral reflux, unspecified or without reflex nephropathy
593.71 Vesicoureteral reflux with reflux nephropathy, unilateral
593.72 Vesicoureteral reflux with reflux nephropathy, bilateral
593.73 Vesicoureteral reflux with reflux nephropathy, NOS
593.89 Other specified disorder of kidney and ureter
593.9 Unspecified disorder of kidney and ureter ▽
599.0 Urinary tract infection, site not specified — (Use additional code to identify organism, such as E. coli, 041.4) ▽
599.6 Unspecified urinary obstruction — (Use additional code to identify urinary incontinence: 625.6, 788.30-788.39) ▽
599.7 Hematuria
601.1 Chronic prostatitis — (Use additional code to identify organism: 041.0, 041.1) ♂
625.6 Female stress incontinence ♀
753.0 Congenital renal agenesis and dysgenesis
753.11 Congenital single renal cyst
753.12 Congenital polycystic kidney, unspecified type ▽
753.13 Congenital polycystic kidney, autosomal dominant
753.14 Congenital polycystic kidney, autosomal recessive
753.15 Congenital renal dysplasia
753.16 Congenital medullary cystic kidney
753.17 Congenital medullary sponge kidney
753.19 Other specified congenital cystic kidney disease
753.20 Unspecified obstructive defect of renal pelvis and ureter ▽
753.21 Congenital obstruction of ureteropelvic junction
753.22 Congenital obstruction of ureterovesical junction
753.23 Congenital ureterocele
753.29 Other obstructive defect of renal pelvis and ureter
753.9 Unspecified congenital anomaly of urinary system ▽
788.0 Renal colic
788.21 Incomplete bladder emptying
788.29 Other specified retention of urine
788.31 Urge incontinence
788.32 Stress incontinence, male ♂
788.33 Mixed incontinence urge and stress (male)(female)
788.34 Incontinence without sensory awareness
788.35 Post-void dribbling
788.36 Nocturnal enuresis
788.37 Continuous leakage
788.38 Overflow incontinence
788.39 Other urinary incontinence
788.41 Urinary frequency
788.42 Polyuria
788.43 Nocturia
788.9 Other symptoms involving urinary system
789.01 Abdominal pain, right upper quadrant
789.02 Abdominal pain, left upper quadrant
789.09 Abdominal pain, other specified site
789.31 Abdominal or pelvic swelling, mass, or lump, right upper quadrant
789.32 Abdominal or pelvic swelling, mass, or lump, left upper quadrant
789.39 Abdominal or pelvic swelling, mass, or lump, other specified site
791.9 Other nonspecific finding on examination of urine
793.5 Nonspecific abnormal findings on radiological and other examination of genitourinary organs
996.1 Mechanical complication of other vascular device, implant, and graft
996.59 Mechanical complication due to other implant and internal device, not elsewhere classified
996.76 Other complications due to genitourinary device, implant, and graft

996.81 Complications of transplanted kidney — (Use additional code to identify nature of complication, 078.5)
997.5 Urinary complications — (Use additional code to identify complications)

ICD-9-CM Procedural

55.96 Other injection of therapeutic substance into kidney
87.74 Retrograde pyelogram
87.75 Percutaneous pyelogram

HCPCS Level II Supplies & Services

A4550 Surgical trays

50395

50395 Introduction of guide into renal pelvis and/or ureter with dilation to establish nephrostomy tract, percutaneous

ICD-9-CM Diagnostic

189.1 Malignant neoplasm of renal pelvis
189.2 Malignant neoplasm of ureter
198.0 Secondary malignant neoplasm of kidney
198.1 Secondary malignant neoplasm of other urinary organs
223.1 Benign neoplasm of renal pelvis
223.2 Benign neoplasm of ureter
233.9 Carcinoma in situ of other and unspecified urinary organs ▽
236.91 Neoplasm of uncertain behavior of kidney and ureter
239.5 Neoplasm of unspecified nature of other genitourinary organs
252.00 Hyperparathyroidism, unspecified
252.01 Primary hyperparathyroidism
252.02 Secondary hyperparathyroidism, non-renal
252.08 Other hyperparathyroidism
588.81 Secondary hyperparathyroidism (of renal origin)
588.89 Other specified disorders resulting from impaired renal function
590.3 Pyeloureteritis cystica — (Use additional code to identify organism, such as E. coli, 041.4)
591 Hydronephrosis
592.0 Calculus of kidney
592.1 Calculus of ureter
592.9 Unspecified urinary calculus ▽
593.3 Stricture or kinking of ureter
593.4 Other ureteric obstruction
593.89 Other specified disorder of kidney and ureter
593.9 Unspecified disorder of kidney and ureter ▽
599.6 Unspecified urinary obstruction — (Use additional code to identify urinary incontinence: 625.6, 788.30-788.39) ▽
625.6 Female stress incontinence ♀
753.21 Congenital obstruction of ureteropelvic junction
753.22 Congenital obstruction of ureterovesical junction
753.23 Congenital ureterocele
753.29 Other obstructive defect of renal pelvis and ureter
788.30 Unspecified urinary incontinence ▽
788.31 Urge incontinence
788.32 Stress incontinence, male ♂
788.33 Mixed incontinence urge and stress (male)(female)
788.38 Overflow incontinence
996.81 Complications of transplanted kidney — (Use additional code to identify nature of complication, 078.5)

ICD-9-CM Procedural

55.03 Percutaneous nephrostomy without fragmentation

50396

50396 Manometric studies through nephrostomy or pyelostomy tube, or indwelling ureteral catheter

ICD-9-CM Diagnostic

591 Hydronephrosis
599.6 Unspecified urinary obstruction — (Use additional code to identify urinary incontinence: 625.6, 788.30-788.39) ▽
625.6 Female stress incontinence ♀
753.20 Unspecified obstructive defect of renal pelvis and ureter ▽
753.21 Congenital obstruction of ureteropelvic junction
753.22 Congenital obstruction of ureterovesical junction
753.23 Congenital ureterocele
753.29 Other obstructive defect of renal pelvis and ureter
788.21 Incomplete bladder emptying
788.29 Other specified retention of urine
788.30 Unspecified urinary incontinence ▽
788.31 Urge incontinence
788.32 Stress incontinence, male ♂
788.33 Mixed incontinence urge and stress (male)(female)
788.34 Incontinence without sensory awareness
788.35 Post-void dribbling
788.36 Nocturnal enuresis
788.37 Continuous leakage
788.38 Overflow incontinence
788.39 Other urinary incontinence

ICD-9-CM Procedural

89.21 Urinary manometry

HCPCS Level II Supplies & Services

A4550 Surgical trays

50398

50398 Change of nephrostomy or pyelostomy tube

ICD-9-CM Diagnostic

185 Malignant neoplasm of prostate ♂
188.0 Malignant neoplasm of trigone of urinary bladder
188.1 Malignant neoplasm of dome of urinary bladder
188.2 Malignant neoplasm of lateral wall of urinary bladder
188.3 Malignant neoplasm of anterior wall of urinary bladder
188.4 Malignant neoplasm of posterior wall of urinary bladder
188.5 Malignant neoplasm of bladder neck
188.8 Malignant neoplasm of other specified sites of bladder
188.9 Malignant neoplasm of bladder, part unspecified ▽
198.0 Secondary malignant neoplasm of kidney
198.1 Secondary malignant neoplasm of other urinary organs
198.82 Secondary malignant neoplasm of genital organs
223.0 Benign neoplasm of kidney, except pelvis
223.1 Benign neoplasm of renal pelvis
223.2 Benign neoplasm of ureter
223.3 Benign neoplasm of bladder
252.00 Hyperparathyroidism, unspecified
252.01 Primary hyperparathyroidism
252.02 Secondary hyperparathyroidism, non-renal
252.08 Other hyperparathyroidism
357.4 Polyneuropathy in other diseases classified elsewhere — (Code first underlying disease: 032.0-032.9, 135, 251.2, 265.0, 265.2, 266.0-266.9, 277.1, 277.3, 585) ☒
585 Chronic renal failure — (Use additional code to identify manifestation: 357.4, 420.0)
586 Unspecified renal failure ▽
588.81 Secondary hyperparathyroidism (of renal origin)
588.89 Other specified disorders resulting from impaired renal function
590.9 Unspecified infection of kidney — (Use additional code to identify organism, such as E. coli, 041.4) ▽
591 Hydronephrosis
592.0 Calculus of kidney
593.2 Acquired cyst of kidney
593.3 Stricture or kinking of ureter
593.4 Other ureteric obstruction
593.89 Other specified disorder of kidney and ureter
593.9 Unspecified disorder of kidney and ureter ▽
599.6 Unspecified urinary obstruction — (Use additional code to identify urinary incontinence: 625.6, 788.30-788.39) ▽
599.7 Hematuria
625.6 Female stress incontinence ♀
788.21 Incomplete bladder emptying
788.29 Other specified retention of urine
996.30 Mechanical complication of unspecified genitourinary device, implant, and graft ▽
996.64 Infection and inflammatory reaction due to indwelling urinary catheter — (Use additional code to identify specified infections: 038.0-038.9, 595.0-595.9)
996.65 Infection and inflammatory reaction due to other genitourinary device, implant, and graft — (Use additional code to identify specified infections)
996.79 Other complications due to other internal prosthetic device, implant, and graft
996.81 Complications of transplanted kidney — (Use additional code to identify nature of complication, 078.5)
997.5 Urinary complications — (Use additional code to identify complications)
V44.6 Status of other artificial opening of urinary tract — (This code is intended for use when these conditions are recorded as diagnoses or problems)

V55.6 Attention to other artificial opening of urinary tract

ICD-9-CM Procedural
55.93 Replacement of nephrostomy tube
55.94 Replacement of pyelostomy tube

HCPCS Level II Supplies & Services
A4550 Surgical trays

50400–50405
50400 Pyeloplasty (Foley Y-pyeloplasty), plastic operation on renal pelvis, with or without plastic operation on ureter, nephropexy, nephrostomy, pyelostomy, or ureteral splinting; simple
50405 complicated (congenital kidney abnormality, secondary pyeloplasty, solitary kidney, calycoplasty)

ICD-9-CM Diagnostic
588.81 Secondary hyperparathyroidism (of renal origin)
588.89 Other specified disorders resulting from impaired renal function
591 Hydronephrosis
592.0 Calculus of kidney
592.1 Calculus of ureter
593.3 Stricture or kinking of ureter
593.4 Other ureteric obstruction
593.5 Hydroureter
593.70 Vesicoureteral reflux, unspecified or without reflex nephropathy
593.71 Vesicoureteral reflux with reflux nephropathy, unilateral
593.72 Vesicoureteral reflux with reflux nephropathy, bilateral
593.73 Vesicoureteral reflux with reflux nephropathy, NOS
593.89 Other specified disorder of kidney and ureter
599.6 Unspecified urinary obstruction — (Use additional code to identify urinary incontinence: 625.6, 788.30-788.39) ▽
753.0 Congenital renal agenesis and dysgenesis
753.21 Congenital obstruction of ureteropelvic junction
753.22 Congenital obstruction of ureterovesical junction
753.23 Congenital ureterocele
753.29 Other obstructive defect of renal pelvis and ureter
V64.41 Laparoscopic surgical procedure converted to open procedure

ICD-9-CM Procedural
55.12 Pyelostomy
55.7 Nephropexy
55.87 Correction of ureteropelvic junction

50500
50500 Nephrorrhaphy, suture of kidney wound or injury

ICD-9-CM Diagnostic
866.02 Kidney laceration without mention of open wound into cavity
866.03 Complete disruption of kidney parenchyma, without mention of open wound into cavity
866.12 Kidney laceration with open wound into cavity
866.13 Complete disruption of kidney parenchyma, with open wound into cavity
998.2 Accidental puncture or laceration during procedure

ICD-9-CM Procedural
55.81 Suture of laceration of kidney

50520
50520 Closure of nephrocutaneous or pyelocutaneous fistula

ICD-9-CM Diagnostic
593.89 Other specified disorder of kidney and ureter
V55.6 Attention to other artificial opening of urinary tract

ICD-9-CM Procedural
55.83 Closure of other fistula of kidney

50525–50526
50525 Closure of nephrovisceral fistula (eg, renocolic), including visceral repair; abdominal approach
50526 thoracic approach

ICD-9-CM Diagnostic
593.89 Other specified disorder of kidney and ureter
619.0 Urinary-genital tract fistula, female ♀
753.7 Congenital anomalies of urachus

ICD-9-CM Procedural
55.83 Closure of other fistula of kidney

50540
50540 Symphysiotomy for horseshoe kidney with or without pyeloplasty and/or other plastic procedure, unilateral or bilateral (one operation)

ICD-9-CM Diagnostic
753.3 Other specified congenital anomalies of kidney

ICD-9-CM Procedural
55.85 Symphysiotomy for horseshoe kidney

50541–50542
50541 Laparoscopy, surgical; ablation of renal cysts
50542 ablation of renal mass lesion(s)

ICD-9-CM Diagnostic
189.0 Malignant neoplasm of kidney, except pelvis
189.1 Malignant neoplasm of renal pelvis
198.0 Secondary malignant neoplasm of kidney
223.0 Benign neoplasm of kidney, except pelvis
223.1 Benign neoplasm of renal pelvis
233.9 Carcinoma in situ of other and unspecified urinary organs ▽
236.91 Neoplasm of uncertain behavior of kidney and ureter
239.5 Neoplasm of unspecified nature of other genitourinary organs
587 Unspecified renal sclerosis ▽
591 Hydronephrosis
593.2 Acquired cyst of kidney
593.89 Other specified disorder of kidney and ureter
593.9 Unspecified disorder of kidney and ureter ▽
753.10 Unspecified congenital cystic kidney disease ▽
753.11 Congenital single renal cyst
753.12 Congenital polycystic kidney, unspecified type ▽
753.13 Congenital polycystic kidney, autosomal dominant
753.14 Congenital polycystic kidney, autosomal recessive
753.15 Congenital renal dysplasia
753.16 Congenital medullary cystic kidney
753.17 Congenital medullary sponge kidney
753.19 Other specified congenital cystic kidney disease

ICD-9-CM Procedural
55.39 Other local destruction or excision of renal lesion or tissue

HCPCS Level II Supplies & Services
HCPCS Level II codes are used to report the supplies, durable medical equipment, and certain medical services provided on an outpatient basis. Because the procedure(s) represented on this page would be performed in an inpatient facility, no HCPCS Level II codes apply.

50543
50543 Laparoscopy, surgical; partial nephrectomy

ICD-9-CM Diagnostic
189.0 Malignant neoplasm of kidney, except pelvis
189.1 Malignant neoplasm of renal pelvis
198.0 Secondary malignant neoplasm of kidney
223.0 Benign neoplasm of kidney, except pelvis
223.1 Benign neoplasm of renal pelvis
233.9 Carcinoma in situ of other and unspecified urinary organs ▽
236.91 Neoplasm of uncertain behavior of kidney and ureter
239.5 Neoplasm of unspecified nature of other genitourinary organs
587 Unspecified renal sclerosis ▽
591 Hydronephrosis
593.2 Acquired cyst of kidney
593.70 Vesicoureteral reflux, unspecified or without reflex nephropathy
593.71 Vesicoureteral reflux with reflux nephropathy, unilateral
593.72 Vesicoureteral reflux with reflux nephropathy, bilateral
593.73 Vesicoureteral reflux with reflux nephropathy, NOS
593.81 Vascular disorders of kidney
593.89 Other specified disorder of kidney and ureter
593.9 Unspecified disorder of kidney and ureter ▽

- 599.7 Hematuria
- 753.11 Congenital single renal cyst
- 753.12 Congenital polycystic kidney, unspecified type ▽
- 753.13 Congenital polycystic kidney, autosomal dominant
- 753.14 Congenital polycystic kidney, autosomal recessive
- 753.15 Congenital renal dysplasia
- 753.16 Congenital medullary cystic kidney
- 753.17 Congenital medullary sponge kidney
- 753.19 Other specified congenital cystic kidney disease
- 753.20 Unspecified obstructive defect of renal pelvis and ureter ▽
- 753.21 Congenital obstruction of ureteropelvic junction
- 753.22 Congenital obstruction of ureterovesical junction
- 753.23 Congenital ureterocele
- 753.29 Other obstructive defect of renal pelvis and ureter
- 866.00 Unspecified kidney injury without mention of open wound into cavity ▽

ICD-9-CM Procedural

- 55.4 Partial nephrectomy

HCPCS Level II Supplies & Services

HCPCS Level II codes are used to report the supplies, durable medical equipment, and certain medical services provided on an outpatient basis. Because the procedure(s) represented on this page would be performed in an inpatient facility, no HCPCS Level II codes apply.

50544

50544 Laparoscopy, surgical; pyeloplasty

ICD-9-CM Diagnostic

- 588.81 Secondary hyperparathyroidism (of renal origin)
- 588.89 Other specified disorders resulting from impaired renal function
- 591 Hydronephrosis
- 592.0 Calculus of kidney
- 592.1 Calculus of ureter
- 593.3 Stricture or kinking of ureter
- 593.4 Other ureteric obstruction
- 593.5 Hydroureter
- 593.70 Vesicoureteral reflux, unspecified or without reflex nephropathy
- 593.71 Vesicoureteral reflux with reflux nephropathy, unilateral
- 593.72 Vesicoureteral reflux with reflux nephropathy, bilateral
- 593.73 Vesicoureteral reflux with reflux nephropathy, NOS
- 593.89 Other specified disorder of kidney and ureter
- 599.6 Unspecified urinary obstruction — (Use additional code to identify urinary incontinence: 625.6, 788.30-788.39) ▽
- 753.0 Congenital renal agenesis and dysgenesis
- 753.21 Congenital obstruction of ureteropelvic junction
- 753.22 Congenital obstruction of ureterovesical junction
- 753.23 Congenital ureterocele
- 753.29 Other obstructive defect of renal pelvis and ureter

ICD-9-CM Procedural

- 55.87 Correction of ureteropelvic junction

50545

50545 Laparoscopy, surgical; radical nephrectomy (includes removal of Gerota's fascia and surrounding fatty tissue, removal of regional lymph nodes, and adrenalectomy)

ICD-9-CM Diagnostic

- 158.0 Malignant neoplasm of retroperitoneum
- 189.0 Malignant neoplasm of kidney, except pelvis
- 189.1 Malignant neoplasm of renal pelvis
- 194.0 Malignant neoplasm of adrenal gland — (Use additional code to identify any functional activity)
- 196.2 Secondary and unspecified malignant neoplasm of intra-abdominal lymph nodes
- 197.6 Secondary malignant neoplasm of retroperitoneum and peritoneum
- 198.0 Secondary malignant neoplasm of kidney
- 198.7 Secondary malignant neoplasm of adrenal gland
- 223.0 Benign neoplasm of kidney, except pelvis
- 223.1 Benign neoplasm of renal pelvis
- 233.9 Carcinoma in situ of other and unspecified urinary organs ▽
- 236.91 Neoplasm of uncertain behavior of kidney and ureter
- 239.5 Neoplasm of unspecified nature of other genitourinary organs
- 403.01 Malignant hypertensive renal disease with renal failure
- 403.11 Benign hypertensive renal disease with renal failure
- 403.91 Unspecified hypertensive renal disease with renal failure ▽
- 404.02 Malignant hypertensive heart and renal disease with renal failure
- 404.12 Benign hypertensive heart and renal disease with renal failure
- 405.01 Secondary renovascular hypertension, malignant
- 405.91 Secondary renovascular hypertension, unspecified ▽
- 445.81 Atheroembolism of kidney — (Use additional code for any associated kidney failure: 584, 585)
- 580.0 Acute glomerulonephritis with lesion of proliferative glomerulonephritis
- 580.4 Acute glomerulonephritis with lesion of rapidly progressive glomerulonephritis
- 581.0 Nephrotic syndrome with lesion of proliferative glomerulonephritis
- 581.1 Nephrotic syndrome with lesion of membranous glomerulonephritis
- 581.2 Nephrotic syndrome with lesion of membranoproliferative glomerulonephritis
- 582.0 Chronic glomerulonephritis with lesion of proliferative glomerulonephritis
- 582.1 Chronic glomerulonephritis with lesion of membranous glomerulonephritis
- 582.2 Chronic glomerulonephritis with lesion of membranoproliferative glomerulonephritis
- 582.4 Chronic glomerulonephritis with lesion of rapidly progressive glomerulonephritis
- 584.5 Acute renal failure with lesion of tubular necrosis
- 584.6 Acute renal failure with lesion of renal cortical necrosis
- 584.7 Acute renal failure with lesion of renal medullary (papillary) necrosis
- 585 Chronic renal failure — (Use additional code to identify manifestation: 357.4, 420.0)
- 587 Unspecified renal sclerosis ▽
- 588.81 Secondary hyperparathyroidism (of renal origin)
- 588.89 Other specified disorders resulting from impaired renal function
- 590.00 Chronic pyelonephritis without lesion of renal medullary necrosis — (Code, if applicable, any causal condition first. Use additional code to identify organism, such as E. coli, 041.4)
- 590.01 Chronic pyelonephritis with lesion of renal medullary necrosis — (Code, if applicable, any causal condition first. Use additional code to identify organism, such as E. coli, 041.4)
- 591 Hydronephrosis
- 592.0 Calculus of kidney
- 593.4 Other ureteric obstruction
- 593.70 Vesicoureteral reflux, unspecified or without reflex nephropathy
- 593.71 Vesicoureteral reflux with reflux nephropathy, unilateral
- 593.72 Vesicoureteral reflux with reflux nephropathy, bilateral
- 593.73 Vesicoureteral reflux with reflux nephropathy, NOS
- 593.81 Vascular disorders of kidney
- 593.89 Other specified disorder of kidney and ureter
- 593.9 Unspecified disorder of kidney and ureter ▽
- 599.6 Unspecified urinary obstruction — (Use additional code to identify urinary incontinence: 625.6, 788.30-788.39) ▽
- 599.7 Hematuria
- 728.88 Rhabdomyolysis
- 753.0 Congenital renal agenesis and dysgenesis
- 753.10 Unspecified congenital cystic kidney disease ▽
- 753.11 Congenital single renal cyst
- 753.12 Congenital polycystic kidney, unspecified type ▽
- 753.13 Congenital polycystic kidney, autosomal dominant
- 753.14 Congenital polycystic kidney, autosomal recessive
- 753.15 Congenital renal dysplasia
- 753.16 Congenital medullary cystic kidney
- 753.17 Congenital medullary sponge kidney
- 753.19 Other specified congenital cystic kidney disease
- 753.20 Unspecified obstructive defect of renal pelvis and ureter ▽
- 753.21 Congenital obstruction of ureteropelvic junction
- 753.23 Congenital ureterocele
- 753.29 Other obstructive defect of renal pelvis and ureter
- 866.02 Kidney laceration without mention of open wound into cavity
- 866.03 Complete disruption of kidney parenchyma, without mention of open wound into cavity
- 866.13 Complete disruption of kidney parenchyma, with open wound into cavity

ICD-9-CM Procedural

- 40.3 Regional lymph node excision
- 55.51 Nephroureterectomy

50546

50546 Laparoscopy, surgical; nephrectomy, including partial ureterectomy

ICD-9-CM Diagnostic

- 189.0 Malignant neoplasm of kidney, except pelvis
- 189.1 Malignant neoplasm of renal pelvis
- 198.0 Secondary malignant neoplasm of kidney

223.0 Benign neoplasm of kidney, except pelvis
223.1 Benign neoplasm of renal pelvis
233.9 Carcinoma in situ of other and unspecified urinary organs ▽
236.91 Neoplasm of uncertain behavior of kidney and ureter
239.5 Neoplasm of unspecified nature of other genitourinary organs
403.01 Malignant hypertensive renal disease with renal failure
403.11 Benign hypertensive renal disease with renal failure
403.91 Unspecified hypertensive renal disease with renal failure ▽
404.02 Malignant hypertensive heart and renal disease with renal failure
404.12 Benign hypertensive heart and renal disease with renal failure
405.01 Secondary renovascular hypertension, malignant
405.91 Secondary renovascular hypertension, unspecified ▽
445.81 Atheroembolism of kidney — (Use additional code for any associated kidney failure: 584, 585)
580.0 Acute glomerulonephritis with lesion of proliferative glomerulonephritis
580.4 Acute glomerulonephritis with lesion of rapidly progressive glomerulonephritis
581.0 Nephrotic syndrome with lesion of proliferative glomerulonephritis
581.1 Nephrotic syndrome with lesion of membranous glomerulonephritis
581.2 Nephrotic syndrome with lesion of membranoproliferative glomerulonephritis
582.0 Chronic glomerulonephritis with lesion of proliferative glomerulonephritis
582.1 Chronic glomerulonephritis with lesion of membranous glomerulonephritis
582.2 Chronic glomerulonephritis with lesion of membranoproliferative glomerulonephritis
582.4 Chronic glomerulonephritis with lesion of rapidly progressive glomerulonephritis
584.5 Acute renal failure with lesion of tubular necrosis
584.6 Acute renal failure with lesion of renal cortical necrosis
584.7 Acute renal failure with lesion of renal medullary (papillary) necrosis
585 Chronic renal failure — (Use additional code to identify manifestation: 357.4, 420.0)
587 Unspecified renal sclerosis ▽
588.81 Secondary hyperparathyroidism (of renal origin)
588.89 Other specified disorders resulting from impaired renal function
590.00 Chronic pyelonephritis without lesion of renal medullary necrosis — (Code, if applicable, any causal condition first. Use additional code to identify organism, such as E. coli, 041.4)
590.01 Chronic pyelonephritis with lesion of renal medullary necrosis — (Code, if applicable, any causal condition first. Use additional code to identify organism, such as E. coli, 041.4)
591 Hydronephrosis
592.0 Calculus of kidney
593.4 Other ureteric obstruction
593.70 Vesicoureteral reflux, unspecified or without reflex nephropathy
593.71 Vesicoureteral reflux with reflux nephropathy, unilateral
593.72 Vesicoureteral reflux with reflux nephropathy, bilateral
593.73 Vesicoureteral reflux with reflux nephropathy, NOS
593.81 Vascular disorders of kidney
593.89 Other specified disorder of kidney and ureter
593.9 Unspecified disorder of kidney and ureter ▽
599.6 Unspecified urinary obstruction — (Use additional code to identify urinary incontinence: 625.6, 788.30-788.39) ▽
599.7 Hematuria
728.88 Rhabdomyolysis
753.0 Congenital renal agenesis and dysgenesis
753.10 Unspecified congenital cystic kidney disease ▽
753.11 Congenital single renal cyst
753.12 Congenital polycystic kidney, unspecified type ▽
753.13 Congenital polycystic kidney, autosomal dominant
753.14 Congenital polycystic kidney, autosomal recessive
753.15 Congenital renal dysplasia
753.16 Congenital medullary cystic kidney
753.17 Congenital medullary sponge kidney
753.19 Other specified congenital cystic kidney disease
753.21 Congenital obstruction of ureteropelvic junction
753.23 Congenital ureterocele
753.29 Other obstructive defect of renal pelvis and ureter
866.02 Kidney laceration without mention of open wound into cavity
866.03 Complete disruption of kidney parenchyma, without mention of open wound into cavity
866.13 Complete disruption of kidney parenchyma, with open wound into cavity

ICD-9-CM Procedural

55.51 Nephroureterectomy

50547

50547 Laparoscopy, surgical; donor nephrectomy (including cold preservation), from living donor

ICD-9-CM Diagnostic

V59.4 Kidney donor

ICD-9-CM Procedural

55.51 Nephroureterectomy

50548

50548 Laparoscopy, surgical; nephrectomy with total ureterectomy

ICD-9-CM Diagnostic

188.6 Malignant neoplasm of ureteric orifice
189.0 Malignant neoplasm of kidney, except pelvis
189.1 Malignant neoplasm of renal pelvis
189.2 Malignant neoplasm of ureter
198.0 Secondary malignant neoplasm of kidney
198.1 Secondary malignant neoplasm of other urinary organs
223.0 Benign neoplasm of kidney, except pelvis
223.1 Benign neoplasm of renal pelvis
223.2 Benign neoplasm of ureter
233.9 Carcinoma in situ of other and unspecified urinary organs ▽
236.91 Neoplasm of uncertain behavior of kidney and ureter
239.5 Neoplasm of unspecified nature of other genitourinary organs
403.01 Malignant hypertensive renal disease with renal failure
403.11 Benign hypertensive renal disease with renal failure
403.91 Unspecified hypertensive renal disease with renal failure ▽
404.02 Malignant hypertensive heart and renal disease with renal failure
404.12 Benign hypertensive heart and renal disease with renal failure
405.01 Secondary renovascular hypertension, malignant
405.91 Secondary renovascular hypertension, unspecified ▽
445.81 Atheroembolism of kidney — (Use additional code for any associated kidney failure: 584, 585)
580.0 Acute glomerulonephritis with lesion of proliferative glomerulonephritis
580.4 Acute glomerulonephritis with lesion of rapidly progressive glomerulonephritis
581.0 Nephrotic syndrome with lesion of proliferative glomerulonephritis
581.1 Nephrotic syndrome with lesion of membranous glomerulonephritis
581.2 Nephrotic syndrome with lesion of membranoproliferative glomerulonephritis
582.0 Chronic glomerulonephritis with lesion of proliferative glomerulonephritis
582.1 Chronic glomerulonephritis with lesion of membranous glomerulonephritis
582.2 Chronic glomerulonephritis with lesion of membranoproliferative glomerulonephritis
582.4 Chronic glomerulonephritis with lesion of rapidly progressive glomerulonephritis
584.5 Acute renal failure with lesion of tubular necrosis
584.6 Acute renal failure with lesion of renal cortical necrosis
584.7 Acute renal failure with lesion of renal medullary (papillary) necrosis
585 Chronic renal failure — (Use additional code to identify manifestation: 357.4, 420.0)
587 Unspecified renal sclerosis ▽
588.81 Secondary hyperparathyroidism (of renal origin)
590.00 Chronic pyelonephritis without lesion of renal medullary necrosis — (Code, if applicable, any causal condition first. Use additional code to identify organism, such as E. coli, 041.4)
590.01 Chronic pyelonephritis with lesion of renal medullary necrosis — (Code, if applicable, any causal condition first. Use additional code to identify organism, such as E. coli, 041.4)
591 Hydronephrosis
592.0 Calculus of kidney
593.4 Other ureteric obstruction
593.70 Vesicoureteral reflux, unspecified or without reflex nephropathy
593.71 Vesicoureteral reflux with reflux nephropathy, unilateral
593.72 Vesicoureteral reflux with reflux nephropathy, bilateral
593.73 Vesicoureteral reflux with reflux nephropathy, NOS
593.81 Vascular disorders of kidney
593.89 Other specified disorder of kidney and ureter
593.9 Unspecified disorder of kidney and ureter ▽
599.6 Unspecified urinary obstruction — (Use additional code to identify urinary incontinence: 625.6, 788.30-788.39) ▽
599.7 Hematuria
728.88 Rhabdomyolysis
753.0 Congenital renal agenesis and dysgenesis
753.10 Unspecified congenital cystic kidney disease ▽
753.11 Congenital single renal cyst

▽ Unspecified code
♀ Female diagnosis
☒ Manifestation code
♂ Male diagnosis

753.12 Congenital polycystic kidney, unspecified type ▽
753.13 Congenital polycystic kidney, autosomal dominant
753.14 Congenital polycystic kidney, autosomal recessive
753.15 Congenital renal dysplasia
753.16 Congenital medullary cystic kidney
753.17 Congenital medullary sponge kidney
753.19 Other specified congenital cystic kidney disease
753.20 Unspecified obstructive defect of renal pelvis and ureter ▽
753.21 Congenital obstruction of ureteropelvic junction
753.23 Congenital ureterocele
753.29 Other obstructive defect of renal pelvis and ureter
866.02 Kidney laceration without mention of open wound into cavity
866.03 Complete disruption of kidney parenchyma, without mention of open wound into cavity
866.13 Complete disruption of kidney parenchyma, with open wound into cavity

ICD-9-CM Procedural

55.51 Nephroureterectomy

50551–50555

50551 Renal endoscopy through established nephrostomy or pyelostomy, with or without irrigation, instillation, or ureteropyelography, exclusive of radiologic service;
50553 with ureteral catheterization, with or without dilation of ureter
50555 with biopsy

ICD-9-CM Diagnostic

189.0 Malignant neoplasm of kidney, except pelvis
189.1 Malignant neoplasm of renal pelvis
198.0 Secondary malignant neoplasm of kidney
223.0 Benign neoplasm of kidney, except pelvis
223.1 Benign neoplasm of renal pelvis
233.9 Carcinoma in situ of other and unspecified urinary organs ▽
236.91 Neoplasm of uncertain behavior of kidney and ureter
239.5 Neoplasm of unspecified nature of other genitourinary organs
252.00 Hyperparathyroidism, unspecified
252.01 Primary hyperparathyroidism
252.02 Secondary hyperparathyroidism, non-renal
252.08 Other hyperparathyroidism
588.81 Secondary hyperparathyroidism (of renal origin)
592.0 Calculus of kidney
592.1 Calculus of ureter
593.3 Stricture or kinking of ureter
593.4 Other ureteric obstruction
593.81 Vascular disorders of kidney
593.89 Other specified disorder of kidney and ureter
599.6 Unspecified urinary obstruction — (Use additional code to identify urinary incontinence: 625.6, 788.30-788.39) ▽
753.20 Unspecified obstructive defect of renal pelvis and ureter ▽
753.21 Congenital obstruction of ureteropelvic junction
753.22 Congenital obstruction of ureterovesical junction
753.23 Congenital ureterocele
753.29 Other obstructive defect of renal pelvis and ureter
753.3 Other specified congenital anomalies of kidney
788.0 Renal colic
958.5 Traumatic anuria

ICD-9-CM Procedural

55.21 Nephroscopy
55.22 Pyeloscopy
55.23 Closed (percutaneous) (needle) biopsy of kidney
59.8 Ureteral catheterization

HCPCS Level II Supplies & Services

A4270 Disposable endoscope sheath, each
A9525 Supply of low or iso-osmolar contrast material, 10 mg of iodine

50557–50561

50557 Renal endoscopy through established nephrostomy or pyelostomy, with or without irrigation, instillation, or ureteropyelography, exclusive of radiologic service; with fulguration and/or incision, with or without biopsy
50561 with removal of foreign body or calculus

ICD-9-CM Diagnostic

189.0 Malignant neoplasm of kidney, except pelvis
189.1 Malignant neoplasm of renal pelvis
198.0 Secondary malignant neoplasm of kidney
223.0 Benign neoplasm of kidney, except pelvis
223.1 Benign neoplasm of renal pelvis
233.9 Carcinoma in situ of other and unspecified urinary organs ▽
236.91 Neoplasm of uncertain behavior of kidney and ureter
239.5 Neoplasm of unspecified nature of other genitourinary organs
252.00 Hyperparathyroidism, unspecified
252.01 Primary hyperparathyroidism
252.02 Secondary hyperparathyroidism, non-renal
252.08 Other hyperparathyroidism
588.81 Secondary hyperparathyroidism (of renal origin)
590.2 Renal and perinephric abscess — (Use additional code to identify organism, such as E. coli, 041.4)
592.0 Calculus of kidney
592.1 Calculus of ureter
592.9 Unspecified urinary calculus ▽
593.81 Vascular disorders of kidney
593.89 Other specified disorder of kidney and ureter
599.6 Unspecified urinary obstruction — (Use additional code to identify urinary incontinence: 625.6, 788.30-788.39) ▽
599.7 Hematuria
753.3 Other specified congenital anomalies of kidney
788.0 Renal colic
958.5 Traumatic anuria
996.30 Mechanical complication of unspecified genitourinary device, implant, and graft ▽
996.39 Mechanical complication of genitourinary device, implant, and graft, other
996.65 Infection and inflammatory reaction due to other genitourinary device, implant, and graft — (Use additional code to identify specified infections)
996.76 Other complications due to genitourinary device, implant, and graft
998.4 Foreign body accidentally left during procedure, not elsewhere classified

ICD-9-CM Procedural

55.03 Percutaneous nephrostomy without fragmentation
55.21 Nephroscopy
55.22 Pyeloscopy
55.23 Closed (percutaneous) (needle) biopsy of kidney
55.39 Other local destruction or excision of renal lesion or tissue

HCPCS Level II Supplies & Services

A4270 Disposable endoscope sheath, each
A9525 Supply of low or iso-osmolar contrast material, 10 mg of iodine

50562

50562 Renal endoscopy through established nephrostomy or pyelostomy, with or without irrigation, instillation, or ureteropyelography, exclusive of radiologic service; with resection of tumor

ICD-9-CM Diagnostic

189.0 Malignant neoplasm of kidney, except pelvis
189.1 Malignant neoplasm of renal pelvis
198.0 Secondary malignant neoplasm of kidney
223.0 Benign neoplasm of kidney, except pelvis
223.1 Benign neoplasm of renal pelvis
233.9 Carcinoma in situ of other and unspecified urinary organs ▽
236.91 Neoplasm of uncertain behavior of kidney and ureter
239.5 Neoplasm of unspecified nature of other genitourinary organs
593.2 Acquired cyst of kidney
593.89 Other specified disorder of kidney and ureter
599.7 Hematuria

ICD-9-CM Procedural

55.21 Nephroscopy
55.22 Pyeloscopy
55.39 Other local destruction or excision of renal lesion or tissue
55.4 Partial nephrectomy

HCPCS Level II Supplies & Services

HCPCS Level II codes are used to report the supplies, durable medical equipment, and certain medical services provided on an outpatient basis. Because the procedure(s) represented on this page would be performed in an inpatient facility, no HCPCS Level II codes apply.

50570–50574

50570 Renal endoscopy through nephrotomy or pyelotomy, with or without irrigation, instillation, or ureteropyelography, exclusive of radiologic service;
50572 with ureteral catheterization, with or without dilation of ureter
50574 with biopsy

ICD-9-CM Diagnostic

189.0 Malignant neoplasm of kidney, except pelvis
189.1 Malignant neoplasm of renal pelvis
198.0 Secondary malignant neoplasm of kidney
223.0 Benign neoplasm of kidney, except pelvis
223.1 Benign neoplasm of renal pelvis
233.9 Carcinoma in situ of other and unspecified urinary organs ▽
236.91 Neoplasm of uncertain behavior of kidney and ureter
239.5 Neoplasm of unspecified nature of other genitourinary organs
252.00 Hyperparathyroidism, unspecified
252.01 Primary hyperparathyroidism
252.02 Secondary hyperparathyroidism, non-renal
252.08 Other hyperparathyroidism
588.81 Secondary hyperparathyroidism (of renal origin)
592.0 Calculus of kidney
592.1 Calculus of ureter
593.3 Stricture or kinking of ureter
593.4 Other ureteric obstruction
593.81 Vascular disorders of kidney
593.89 Other specified disorder of kidney and ureter
599.6 Unspecified urinary obstruction — (Use additional code to identify urinary incontinence: 625.6, 788.30-788.39) ▽
753.20 Unspecified obstructive defect of renal pelvis and ureter ▽
753.21 Congenital obstruction of ureteropelvic junction
753.22 Congenital obstruction of ureterovesical junction
753.23 Congenital ureterocele
753.29 Other obstructive defect of renal pelvis and ureter
753.3 Other specified congenital anomalies of kidney
958.5 Traumatic anuria

ICD-9-CM Procedural

55.01 Nephrotomy
55.11 Pyelotomy
55.21 Nephroscopy
55.22 Pyeloscopy
55.23 Closed (percutaneous) (needle) biopsy of kidney
56.91 Dilation of ureteral meatus
59.8 Ureteral catheterization

50575

50575 Renal endoscopy through nephrotomy or pyelotomy, with or without irrigation, instillation, or ureteropyelography, exclusive of radiologic service; with endopyelotomy (includes cystoscopy, ureteroscopy, dilation of ureter and ureteral pelvic junction, incision of ureteral pelvic junction and insertion of endopyelotomy stent)

ICD-9-CM Diagnostic

189.0 Malignant neoplasm of kidney, except pelvis
189.1 Malignant neoplasm of renal pelvis
198.0 Secondary malignant neoplasm of kidney
223.1 Benign neoplasm of renal pelvis
593.4 Other ureteric obstruction
593.81 Vascular disorders of kidney
593.89 Other specified disorder of kidney and ureter
599.6 Unspecified urinary obstruction — (Use additional code to identify urinary incontinence: 625.6, 788.30-788.39) ▽
753.20 Unspecified obstructive defect of renal pelvis and ureter ▽
753.21 Congenital obstruction of ureteropelvic junction
753.22 Congenital obstruction of ureterovesical junction
753.23 Congenital ureterocele
753.29 Other obstructive defect of renal pelvis and ureter
753.3 Other specified congenital anomalies of kidney
958.5 Traumatic anuria

ICD-9-CM Procedural

55.01 Nephrotomy
55.11 Pyelotomy
55.21 Nephroscopy
55.22 Pyeloscopy
56.2 Ureterotomy
56.31 Ureteroscopy
56.91 Dilation of ureteral meatus
59.8 Ureteral catheterization

50576–50580

50576 Renal endoscopy through nephrotomy or pyelotomy, with or without irrigation, instillation, or ureteropyelography, exclusive of radiologic service; with fulguration and/or incision, with or without biopsy
50580 with removal of foreign body or calculus

ICD-9-CM Diagnostic

189.0 Malignant neoplasm of kidney, except pelvis
189.1 Malignant neoplasm of renal pelvis
198.0 Secondary malignant neoplasm of kidney
223.0 Benign neoplasm of kidney, except pelvis
223.1 Benign neoplasm of renal pelvis
233.9 Carcinoma in situ of other and unspecified urinary organs ▽
236.91 Neoplasm of uncertain behavior of kidney and ureter
239.5 Neoplasm of unspecified nature of other genitourinary organs
252.00 Hyperparathyroidism, unspecified
252.01 Primary hyperparathyroidism
252.02 Secondary hyperparathyroidism, non-renal
252.08 Other hyperparathyroidism
588.81 Secondary hyperparathyroidism (of renal origin)
590.2 Renal and perinephric abscess — (Use additional code to identify organism, such as E. coli, 041.4)
592.0 Calculus of kidney
592.1 Calculus of ureter
592.9 Unspecified urinary calculus ▽
593.4 Other ureteric obstruction
593.81 Vascular disorders of kidney
593.89 Other specified disorder of kidney and ureter
599.6 Unspecified urinary obstruction — (Use additional code to identify urinary incontinence: 625.6, 788.30-788.39) ▽
599.7 Hematuria
753.3 Other specified congenital anomalies of kidney
788.0 Renal colic
958.5 Traumatic anuria
996.30 Mechanical complication of unspecified genitourinary device, implant, and graft ▽
996.39 Mechanical complication of genitourinary device, implant, and graft, other
996.65 Infection and inflammatory reaction due to other genitourinary device, implant, and graft — (Use additional code to identify specified infections)
996.76 Other complications due to genitourinary device, implant, and graft
998.4 Foreign body accidentally left during procedure, not elsewhere classified

ICD-9-CM Procedural

55.01 Nephrotomy
55.03 Percutaneous nephrostomy without fragmentation
55.11 Pyelotomy
55.21 Nephroscopy
55.22 Pyeloscopy
55.23 Closed (percutaneous) (needle) biopsy of kidney
55.39 Other local destruction or excision of renal lesion or tissue

50590

50590 Lithotripsy, extracorporeal shock wave

ICD-9-CM Diagnostic

252.00 Hyperparathyroidism, unspecified
252.01 Primary hyperparathyroidism
252.02 Secondary hyperparathyroidism, non-renal
252.08 Other hyperparathyroidism
588.81 Secondary hyperparathyroidism (of renal origin)
592.0 Calculus of kidney
592.1 Calculus of ureter
592.9 Unspecified urinary calculus ▽
599.7 Hematuria
788.0 Renal colic

ICD-9-CM Procedural

98.51 Extracorporeal shockwave lithotripsy (ESWL) of the kidney, ureter and/or bladder

▽ Unspecified code
♀ Female diagnosis
☒ Manifestation code
♂ Male diagnosis

Ureter

50600

50600 Ureterotomy with exploration or drainage (separate procedure)

ICD-9-CM Diagnostic

189.2 Malignant neoplasm of ureter
198.1 Secondary malignant neoplasm of other urinary organs
223.2 Benign neoplasm of ureter
233.9 Carcinoma in situ of other and unspecified urinary organs ▽
236.91 Neoplasm of uncertain behavior of kidney and ureter
239.5 Neoplasm of unspecified nature of other genitourinary organs
591 Hydronephrosis
593.3 Stricture or kinking of ureter
593.4 Other ureteric obstruction
593.89 Other specified disorder of kidney and ureter
599.6 Unspecified urinary obstruction — (Use additional code to identify urinary incontinence: 625.6, 788.30-788.39) ▽
788.29 Other specified retention of urine
867.2 Ureter injury without mention of open wound into cavity
867.3 Ureter injury with open wound into cavity
998.2 Accidental puncture or laceration during procedure

ICD-9-CM Procedural

56.2 Ureterotomy

50605

50605 Ureterotomy for insertion of indwelling stent, all types

ICD-9-CM Diagnostic

189.2 Malignant neoplasm of ureter
198.1 Secondary malignant neoplasm of other urinary organs
223.2 Benign neoplasm of ureter
233.9 Carcinoma in situ of other and unspecified urinary organs ▽
236.91 Neoplasm of uncertain behavior of kidney and ureter
239.5 Neoplasm of unspecified nature of other genitourinary organs
591 Hydronephrosis
592.0 Calculus of kidney
592.1 Calculus of ureter
593.3 Stricture or kinking of ureter
593.4 Other ureteric obstruction
788.29 Other specified retention of urine

ICD-9-CM Procedural

56.2 Ureterotomy
59.8 Ureteral catheterization

50610–50630

50610 Ureterolithotomy; upper one-third of ureter
50620 middle one-third of ureter
50630 lower one-third of ureter

ICD-9-CM Diagnostic

592.1 Calculus of ureter
592.9 Unspecified urinary calculus ▽
593.4 Other ureteric obstruction
V64.41 Laparoscopic surgical procedure converted to open procedure

ICD-9-CM Procedural

56.2 Ureterotomy

50650

50650 Ureterectomy, with bladder cuff (separate procedure)

ICD-9-CM Diagnostic

180.9 Malignant neoplasm of cervix uteri, unspecified site ▽ ♀
182.0 Malignant neoplasm of corpus uteri, except isthmus ♀
182.1 Malignant neoplasm of isthmus ♀
188.0 Malignant neoplasm of trigone of urinary bladder
188.1 Malignant neoplasm of dome of urinary bladder
188.2 Malignant neoplasm of lateral wall of urinary bladder
188.3 Malignant neoplasm of anterior wall of urinary bladder
188.4 Malignant neoplasm of posterior wall of urinary bladder
188.5 Malignant neoplasm of bladder neck
188.6 Malignant neoplasm of ureteric orifice
188.7 Malignant neoplasm of urachus
189.2 Malignant neoplasm of ureter
198.1 Secondary malignant neoplasm of other urinary organs
223.2 Benign neoplasm of ureter
233.9 Carcinoma in situ of other and unspecified urinary organs ▽
236.91 Neoplasm of uncertain behavior of kidney and ureter
239.5 Neoplasm of unspecified nature of other genitourinary organs
593.89 Other specified disorder of kidney and ureter
867.2 Ureter injury without mention of open wound into cavity
867.3 Ureter injury with open wound into cavity

ICD-9-CM Procedural

56.40 Ureterectomy, not otherwise specified

50660

50660 Ureterectomy, total, ectopic ureter, combination abdominal, vaginal and/or perineal approach

ICD-9-CM Diagnostic

593.3 Stricture or kinking of ureter
753.22 Congenital obstruction of ureterovesical junction
753.29 Other obstructive defect of renal pelvis and ureter
753.4 Other specified congenital anomalies of ureter

ICD-9-CM Procedural

56.42 Total ureterectomy

50684

50684 Injection procedure for ureterography or ureteropyelography through ureterostomy or indwelling ureteral catheter

ICD-9-CM Diagnostic

189.1 Malignant neoplasm of renal pelvis
189.2 Malignant neoplasm of ureter
189.9 Malignant neoplasm of urinary organ, site unspecified ▽
198.0 Secondary malignant neoplasm of kidney
198.1 Secondary malignant neoplasm of other urinary organs
198.82 Secondary malignant neoplasm of genital organs
223.0 Benign neoplasm of kidney, except pelvis
223.1 Benign neoplasm of renal pelvis
223.2 Benign neoplasm of ureter
223.3 Benign neoplasm of bladder
223.9 Benign neoplasm of urinary organ, site unspecified ▽
233.9 Carcinoma in situ of other and unspecified urinary organs ▽
236.91 Neoplasm of uncertain behavior of kidney and ureter
239.5 Neoplasm of unspecified nature of other genitourinary organs
590.9 Unspecified infection of kidney — (Use additional code to identify organism, such as E. coli, 041.4) ▽
592.0 Calculus of kidney
592.1 Calculus of ureter
592.9 Unspecified urinary calculus ▽
593.4 Other ureteric obstruction
593.70 Vesicoureteral reflux, unspecified or without reflex nephropathy
593.71 Vesicoureteral reflux with reflux nephropathy, unilateral
593.72 Vesicoureteral reflux with reflux nephropathy, bilateral
593.73 Vesicoureteral reflux with reflux nephropathy, NOS
593.9 Unspecified disorder of kidney and ureter ▽
599.0 Urinary tract infection, site not specified — (Use additional code to identify organism, such as E. coli, 041.4) ▽
599.6 Unspecified urinary obstruction — (Use additional code to identify urinary incontinence: 625.6, 788.30-788.39) ▽
599.7 Hematuria
619.0 Urinary-genital tract fistula, female ♀
625.6 Female stress incontinence ♀
753.8 Other specified congenital anomaly of bladder and urethra
753.9 Unspecified congenital anomaly of urinary system ▽
788.0 Renal colic
788.8 Extravasation of urine
789.01 Abdominal pain, right upper quadrant
789.02 Abdominal pain, left upper quadrant
789.09 Abdominal pain, other specified site
789.31 Abdominal or pelvic swelling, mass, or lump, right upper quadrant
789.32 Abdominal or pelvic swelling, mass, or lump, left upper quadrant
789.39 Abdominal or pelvic swelling, mass, or lump, other specified site

ICD-9-CM Procedural

59.29 Other diagnostic procedures on perirenal tissue, perivesical tissue, and retroperitoneum
87.74 Retrograde pyelogram
87.76 Retrograde cystourethrogram

HCPCS Level II Supplies & Services

A4641 Supply of radiopharmaceutical diagnostic imaging agent, not otherwise classified
A4642 Supply of satumomab pendetide, radiopharmaceutical diagnostic imaging agent, per dose
A4647 Supply of paramagnetic contrast material (e.g., gadolinium)
A9525 Supply of low or iso-osmolar contrast material, 10 mg of iodine

50686

50686 Manometric studies through ureterostomy or indwelling ureteral catheter

ICD-9-CM Diagnostic

591 Hydronephrosis
593.3 Stricture or kinking of ureter
599.6 Unspecified urinary obstruction — (Use additional code to identify urinary incontinence: 625.6, 788.30-788.39) ▽
753.21 Congenital obstruction of ureteropelvic junction
753.22 Congenital obstruction of ureterovesical junction
753.23 Congenital ureterocele
753.29 Other obstructive defect of renal pelvis and ureter

ICD-9-CM Procedural

89.21 Urinary manometry

HCPCS Level II Supplies & Services

A4550 Surgical trays

50688

50688 Change of ureterostomy tube

ICD-9-CM Diagnostic

591 Hydronephrosis
996.59 Mechanical complication due to other implant and internal device, not elsewhere classified
V55.6 Attention to other artificial opening of urinary tract

ICD-9-CM Procedural

59.93 Replacement of ureterostomy tube

HCPCS Level II Supplies & Services

A4550 Surgical trays

50690

50690 Injection procedure for visualization of ileal conduit and/or ureteropyelography, exclusive of radiologic service

ICD-9-CM Diagnostic

189.0 Malignant neoplasm of kidney, except pelvis
189.1 Malignant neoplasm of renal pelvis
189.2 Malignant neoplasm of ureter
189.8 Malignant neoplasm of other specified sites of urinary organs
189.9 Malignant neoplasm of urinary organ, site unspecified ▽
198.0 Secondary malignant neoplasm of kidney
198.1 Secondary malignant neoplasm of other urinary organs
198.82 Secondary malignant neoplasm of genital organs
223.0 Benign neoplasm of kidney, except pelvis
223.1 Benign neoplasm of renal pelvis
223.2 Benign neoplasm of ureter
223.9 Benign neoplasm of urinary organ, site unspecified ▽
590.9 Unspecified infection of kidney — (Use additional code to identify organism, such as E. coli, 041.4) ▽
591 Hydronephrosis
592.0 Calculus of kidney
592.9 Unspecified urinary calculus ▽
593.4 Other ureteric obstruction
593.9 Unspecified disorder of kidney and ureter ▽
595.1 Chronic interstitial cystitis — (Use additional code to identify organism, such as E. coli, 041.4)
595.2 Other chronic cystitis — (Use additional code to identify organism, such as E. coli, 041.4)
599.0 Urinary tract infection, site not specified — (Use additional code to identify organism, such as E. coli, 041.4) ▽
599.6 Unspecified urinary obstruction — (Use additional code to identify urinary incontinence: 625.6, 788.30-788.39) ▽
599.7 Hematuria
753.8 Other specified congenital anomaly of bladder and urethra
753.9 Unspecified congenital anomaly of urinary system ▽
788.0 Renal colic
789.00 Abdominal pain, unspecified site ▽
789.01 Abdominal pain, right upper quadrant
789.02 Abdominal pain, left upper quadrant
789.09 Abdominal pain, other specified site
789.30 Abdominal or pelvic swelling, mass or lump, unspecified site ▽
789.32 Abdominal or pelvic swelling, mass, or lump, left upper quadrant
789.39 Abdominal or pelvic swelling, mass, or lump, other specified site
908.2 Late effect of internal injury to other internal organs
996.30 Mechanical complication of unspecified genitourinary device, implant, and graft ▽
996.76 Other complications due to genitourinary device, implant, and graft
997.5 Urinary complications — (Use additional code to identify complications)
V10.51 Personal history of malignant neoplasm of bladder
V10.52 Personal history of malignant neoplasm of kidney
V10.53 Personal history of malignant neoplasm, renal pelvis
V44.6 Status of other artificial opening of urinary tract — (This code is intended for use when these conditions are recorded as diagnoses or problems)

ICD-9-CM Procedural

59.29 Other diagnostic procedures on perirenal tissue, perivesical tissue, and retroperitoneum
87.73 Intravenous pyelogram
87.74 Retrograde pyelogram
87.75 Percutaneous pyelogram
87.78 Ileal conduitogram

HCPCS Level II Supplies & Services

A4641 Supply of radiopharmaceutical diagnostic imaging agent, not otherwise classified
A4642 Supply of satumomab pendetide, radiopharmaceutical diagnostic imaging agent, per dose
A4647 Supply of paramagnetic contrast material (e.g., gadolinium)
A9525 Supply of low or iso-osmolar contrast material, 10 mg of iodine

50700

50700 Ureteroplasty, plastic operation on ureter (eg, stricture)

ICD-9-CM Diagnostic

592.1 Calculus of ureter
593.3 Stricture or kinking of ureter
593.4 Other ureteric obstruction
593.89 Other specified disorder of kidney and ureter
599.6 Unspecified urinary obstruction — (Use additional code to identify urinary incontinence: 625.6, 788.30-788.39) ▽
614.9 Unspecified inflammatory disease of female pelvic organs and tissues — (Use additional code to identify organism: 041.0, 041.1) ▽ ♀
617.9 Endometriosis, site unspecified ▽ ♀
753.21 Congenital obstruction of ureteropelvic junction
753.22 Congenital obstruction of ureterovesical junction
753.23 Congenital ureterocele
753.29 Other obstructive defect of renal pelvis and ureter
997.5 Urinary complications — (Use additional code to identify complications)

ICD-9-CM Procedural

56.89 Other repair of ureter

50715

50715 Ureterolysis, with or without repositioning of ureter for retroperitoneal fibrosis

ICD-9-CM Diagnostic

593.4 Other ureteric obstruction
593.89 Other specified disorder of kidney and ureter

ICD-9-CM Procedural

59.02 Other lysis of perirenal or periureteral adhesions

▽ Unspecified code
♀ Female diagnosis
☒ Manifestation code
♂ Male diagnosis

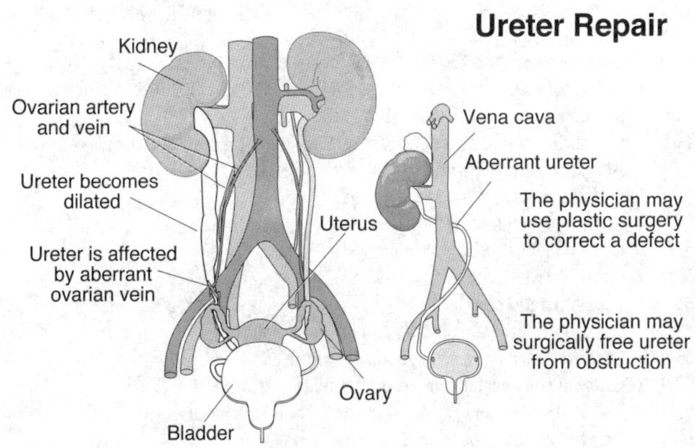
Ureter Repair
Kidney
Ovarian artery and vein
Ureter becomes dilated
Ureter is affected by aberrant ovarian vein
Uterus
Ovary
Bladder
Vena cava
Aberrant ureter
The physician may use plastic surgery to correct a defect
The physician may surgically free ureter from obstruction

50722

50722 Ureterolysis for ovarian vein syndrome

ICD-9-CM Diagnostic

593.4 Other ureteric obstruction
593.89 Other specified disorder of kidney and ureter

ICD-9-CM Procedural

59.02 Other lysis of perirenal or periureteral adhesions

50725

50725 Ureterolysis for retrocaval ureter, with reanastomosis of upper urinary tract or vena cava

ICD-9-CM Diagnostic

753.4 Other specified congenital anomalies of ureter

ICD-9-CM Procedural

56.79 Other anastomosis or bypass of ureter
59.02 Other lysis of perirenal or periureteral adhesions

HCPCS Level II Supplies & Services

A4349 Male external catheter, with or without adhesive, disposable, each

50727–50728

50727 Revision of urinary-cutaneous anastomosis (any type urostomy);
50728 with repair of fascial defect and hernia

ICD-9-CM Diagnostic

152.2 Malignant neoplasm of ileum
152.8 Malignant neoplasm of other specified sites of small intestine
153.4 Malignant neoplasm of cecum
188.0 Malignant neoplasm of trigone of urinary bladder
188.1 Malignant neoplasm of dome of urinary bladder
188.2 Malignant neoplasm of lateral wall of urinary bladder
188.3 Malignant neoplasm of anterior wall of urinary bladder
188.4 Malignant neoplasm of posterior wall of urinary bladder
188.5 Malignant neoplasm of bladder neck
188.6 Malignant neoplasm of ureteric orifice
188.8 Malignant neoplasm of other specified sites of bladder
188.9 Malignant neoplasm of bladder, part unspecified ▽
189.2 Malignant neoplasm of ureter
189.3 Malignant neoplasm of urethra
197.6 Secondary malignant neoplasm of retroperitoneum and peritoneum
560.81 Intestinal or peritoneal adhesions with obstruction (postoperative) (postinfection)
569.5 Abscess of intestine
569.60 Unspecified complication of colostomy or enterostomy ▽
569.61 Infection of colostomy or enterostomy — (Use additional code to identify organism: 041.00-041.9. Use additional code to specify type of infection: 038.0-038.9, 682.2)
569.62 Mechanical complication of colostomy and enterostomy
569.69 Other complication of colostomy or enterostomy
569.82 Ulceration of intestine
569.83 Perforation of intestine
569.89 Other specified disorder of intestines
569.9 Unspecified disorder of intestine ▽
593.3 Stricture or kinking of ureter
593.4 Other ureteric obstruction
593.89 Other specified disorder of kidney and ureter
599.6 Unspecified urinary obstruction — (Use additional code to identify urinary incontinence: 625.6, 788.30-788.39) ▽
614.6 Pelvic peritoneal adhesions, female (postoperative) (postinfection) — (Use additional code to identify any associated infertility, 628.2. Use additional code to identify organism: 041.0, 041.1) ♀
614.9 Unspecified inflammatory disease of female pelvic organs and tissues — (Use additional code to identify organism: 041.0, 041.1) ▽ ♀
682.2 Cellulitis and abscess of trunk — (Use additional code to identify organism)
707.8 Chronic ulcer of other specified site
997.5 Urinary complications — (Use additional code to identify complications)
V10.51 Personal history of malignant neoplasm of bladder
V55.6 Attention to other artificial opening of urinary tract

ICD-9-CM Procedural

56.52 Revision of cutaneous uretero-ileostomy
56.62 Revision of other cutaneous ureterostomy
56.72 Revision of ureterointestinal anastomosis
58.44 Reanastomosis of urethra

HCPCS Level II Supplies & Services

A4349 Male external catheter, with or without adhesive, disposable, each

50740

50740 Ureteropyelostomy, anastomosis of ureter and renal pelvis

ICD-9-CM Diagnostic

189.0 Malignant neoplasm of kidney, except pelvis
189.1 Malignant neoplasm of renal pelvis
198.0 Secondary malignant neoplasm of kidney
198.1 Secondary malignant neoplasm of other urinary organs
223.0 Benign neoplasm of kidney, except pelvis
223.1 Benign neoplasm of renal pelvis
593.3 Stricture or kinking of ureter
593.4 Other ureteric obstruction
593.89 Other specified disorder of kidney and ureter
599.6 Unspecified urinary obstruction — (Use additional code to identify urinary incontinence: 625.6, 788.30-788.39) ▽
753.10 Unspecified congenital cystic kidney disease ▽
753.19 Other specified congenital cystic kidney disease
753.20 Unspecified obstructive defect of renal pelvis and ureter ▽
753.21 Congenital obstruction of ureteropelvic junction
753.23 Congenital ureterocele
753.29 Other obstructive defect of renal pelvis and ureter

ICD-9-CM Procedural

55.86 Anastomosis of kidney

50750

50750 Ureterocalycostomy, anastomosis of ureter to renal calyx

ICD-9-CM Diagnostic

189.0 Malignant neoplasm of kidney, except pelvis
189.1 Malignant neoplasm of renal pelvis
198.0 Secondary malignant neoplasm of kidney
198.1 Secondary malignant neoplasm of other urinary organs
223.0 Benign neoplasm of kidney, except pelvis
223.1 Benign neoplasm of renal pelvis
593.3 Stricture or kinking of ureter
593.4 Other ureteric obstruction
593.89 Other specified disorder of kidney and ureter
599.6 Unspecified urinary obstruction — (Use additional code to identify urinary incontinence: 625.6, 788.30-788.39) ▽
753.10 Unspecified congenital cystic kidney disease ▽
753.19 Other specified congenital cystic kidney disease
753.20 Unspecified obstructive defect of renal pelvis and ureter ▽
753.21 Congenital obstruction of ureteropelvic junction
753.23 Congenital ureterocele
753.29 Other obstructive defect of renal pelvis and ureter

ICD-9-CM Procedural

55.86 Anastomosis of kidney

▽ Unspecified code
♀ Female diagnosis
☒ Manifestation code
♂ Male diagnosis

50760

50760 Ureteroureterostomy

ICD-9-CM Diagnostic

153.3 Malignant neoplasm of sigmoid colon
153.9 Malignant neoplasm of colon, unspecified site ▽
158.0 Malignant neoplasm of retroperitoneum
189.2 Malignant neoplasm of ureter
211.8 Benign neoplasm of retroperitoneum and peritoneum
593.3 Stricture or kinking of ureter
593.4 Other ureteric obstruction
753.21 Congenital obstruction of ureteropelvic junction
753.22 Congenital obstruction of ureterovesical junction
753.23 Congenital ureterocele
753.29 Other obstructive defect of renal pelvis and ureter
753.3 Other specified congenital anomalies of kidney
867.2 Ureter injury without mention of open wound into cavity
867.3 Ureter injury with open wound into cavity

ICD-9-CM Procedural

56.41 Partial ureterectomy
56.61 Formation of other cutaneous ureterostomy
56.75 Transureteroureterostomy

50770

50770 Transureteroureterostomy, anastomosis of ureter to contralateral ureter

ICD-9-CM Diagnostic

153.3 Malignant neoplasm of sigmoid colon
153.9 Malignant neoplasm of colon, unspecified site ▽
158.0 Malignant neoplasm of retroperitoneum
189.2 Malignant neoplasm of ureter
211.8 Benign neoplasm of retroperitoneum and peritoneum
593.3 Stricture or kinking of ureter
593.4 Other ureteric obstruction
753.21 Congenital obstruction of ureteropelvic junction
753.22 Congenital obstruction of ureterovesical junction
753.23 Congenital ureterocele
753.29 Other obstructive defect of renal pelvis and ureter
753.3 Other specified congenital anomalies of kidney
867.2 Ureter injury without mention of open wound into cavity
867.3 Ureter injury with open wound into cavity

ICD-9-CM Procedural

56.75 Transureteroureterostomy

50780–50785

50780 Ureteroneocystostomy; anastomosis of single ureter to bladder
50782 anastomosis of duplicated ureter to bladder
50783 with extensive ureteral tailoring
50785 with vesico-psoas hitch or bladder flap

ICD-9-CM Diagnostic

182.8 Malignant neoplasm of other specified sites of body of uterus ♀
185 Malignant neoplasm of prostate ♂
188.0 Malignant neoplasm of trigone of urinary bladder
188.9 Malignant neoplasm of bladder, part unspecified ▽
189.2 Malignant neoplasm of ureter
197.6 Secondary malignant neoplasm of retroperitoneum and peritoneum
198.1 Secondary malignant neoplasm of other urinary organs
223.2 Benign neoplasm of ureter
223.3 Benign neoplasm of bladder
236.90 Neoplasm of uncertain behavior of urinary organ, unspecified ▽
236.91 Neoplasm of uncertain behavior of kidney and ureter
236.99 Neoplasm of uncertain behavior of other and unspecified urinary organs
239.4 Neoplasm of unspecified nature of bladder
239.5 Neoplasm of unspecified nature of other genitourinary organs
344.61 Cauda equina syndrome with neurogenic bladder
591 Hydronephrosis
593.3 Stricture or kinking of ureter
593.4 Other ureteric obstruction
593.70 Vesicoureteral reflux, unspecified or without reflex nephropathy
593.71 Vesicoureteral reflux with reflux nephropathy, unilateral
593.72 Vesicoureteral reflux with reflux nephropathy, bilateral
593.73 Vesicoureteral reflux with reflux nephropathy, NOS
593.89 Other specified disorder of kidney and ureter
599.0 Urinary tract infection, site not specified — (Use additional code to identify organism, such as E. coli, 041.4) ▽
614.6 Pelvic peritoneal adhesions, female (postoperative) (postinfection) — (Use additional code to identify any associated infertility, 628.2. Use additional code to identify organism: 041.0, 041.1) ♀
614.9 Unspecified inflammatory disease of female pelvic organs and tissues — (Use additional code to identify organism: 041.0, 041.1) ▽ ♀
617.8 Endometriosis of other specified sites ♀
619.0 Urinary-genital tract fistula, female ♀
753.21 Congenital obstruction of ureteropelvic junction
753.22 Congenital obstruction of ureterovesical junction
753.23 Congenital ureterocele
753.29 Other obstructive defect of renal pelvis and ureter
753.4 Other specified congenital anomalies of ureter
753.9 Unspecified congenital anomaly of urinary system ▽
867.2 Ureter injury without mention of open wound into cavity
867.3 Ureter injury with open wound into cavity
867.7 Injury to other specified pelvic organs with open wound into cavity
867.8 Injury to unspecified pelvic organ without mention of open wound into cavity ▽
867.9 Injury to unspecified pelvic organ with open wound into cavity ▽
996.81 Complications of transplanted kidney — (Use additional code to identify nature of complication, 078.5)
998.2 Accidental puncture or laceration during procedure
V64.41 Laparoscopic surgical procedure converted to open procedure

ICD-9-CM Procedural

56.74 Ureteroneocystostomy

50800

50800 Ureteroenterostomy, direct anastomosis of ureter to intestine

ICD-9-CM Diagnostic

188.0 Malignant neoplasm of trigone of urinary bladder
188.1 Malignant neoplasm of dome of urinary bladder
188.2 Malignant neoplasm of lateral wall of urinary bladder
188.3 Malignant neoplasm of anterior wall of urinary bladder
188.4 Malignant neoplasm of posterior wall of urinary bladder
188.5 Malignant neoplasm of bladder neck
188.6 Malignant neoplasm of ureteric orifice
188.8 Malignant neoplasm of other specified sites of bladder
188.9 Malignant neoplasm of bladder, part unspecified ▽
189.2 Malignant neoplasm of ureter
198.1 Secondary malignant neoplasm of other urinary organs
589.0 Unilateral small kidney
592.1 Calculus of ureter
593.3 Stricture or kinking of ureter
593.4 Other ureteric obstruction
867.0 Bladder and urethra injury without mention of open wound into cavity
867.1 Bladder and urethra injury with open wound into cavity
867.2 Ureter injury without mention of open wound into cavity
867.3 Ureter injury with open wound into cavity
997.5 Urinary complications — (Use additional code to identify complications)

ICD-9-CM Procedural

56.71 Urinary diversion to intestine

50810

50810 Ureterosigmoidostomy, with creation of sigmoid bladder and establishment of abdominal or perineal colostomy, including intestine anastomosis

ICD-9-CM Diagnostic

188.0 Malignant neoplasm of trigone of urinary bladder
188.1 Malignant neoplasm of dome of urinary bladder
188.2 Malignant neoplasm of lateral wall of urinary bladder
188.3 Malignant neoplasm of anterior wall of urinary bladder
188.4 Malignant neoplasm of posterior wall of urinary bladder
188.5 Malignant neoplasm of bladder neck
188.6 Malignant neoplasm of ureteric orifice
188.7 Malignant neoplasm of urachus
188.8 Malignant neoplasm of other specified sites of bladder
188.9 Malignant neoplasm of bladder, part unspecified ▽
189.2 Malignant neoplasm of ureter
189.3 Malignant neoplasm of urethra
198.1 Secondary malignant neoplasm of other urinary organs
593.4 Other ureteric obstruction

▽ Unspecified code
♀ Female diagnosis
☒ Manifestation code
♂ Male diagnosis

595.82 Irradiation cystitis — (Use additional code to identify organism, such as E. coli, 041.4)
596.54 Neurogenic bladder, NOS — (Use additional code to identify urinary incontinence: 625.6, 788.30-788.39) ▽
596.8 Other specified disorder of bladder — (Use additional code to identify urinary incontinence: 625.6, 788.30-788.39)
753.5 Exstrophy of urinary bladder
753.8 Other specified congenital anomaly of bladder and urethra
867.0 Bladder and urethra injury without mention of open wound into cavity
867.1 Bladder and urethra injury with open wound into cavity
867.2 Ureter injury without mention of open wound into cavity
867.3 Ureter injury with open wound into cavity
997.5 Urinary complications — (Use additional code to identify complications)

ICD-9-CM Procedural

56.71 Urinary diversion to intestine

50815–50820

50815 Ureterocolon conduit, including intestine anastomosis
50820 Ureteroileal conduit (ileal bladder), including intestine anastomosis (Bricker operation)

ICD-9-CM Diagnostic

188.0 Malignant neoplasm of trigone of urinary bladder
188.1 Malignant neoplasm of dome of urinary bladder
188.2 Malignant neoplasm of lateral wall of urinary bladder
188.3 Malignant neoplasm of anterior wall of urinary bladder
188.4 Malignant neoplasm of posterior wall of urinary bladder
188.5 Malignant neoplasm of bladder neck
188.6 Malignant neoplasm of ureteric orifice
188.8 Malignant neoplasm of other specified sites of bladder
188.9 Malignant neoplasm of bladder, part unspecified ▽
189.2 Malignant neoplasm of ureter
189.3 Malignant neoplasm of urethra
198.1 Secondary malignant neoplasm of other urinary organs
591 Hydronephrosis
593.4 Other ureteric obstruction
595.82 Irradiation cystitis — (Use additional code to identify organism, such as E. coli, 041.4)
596.54 Neurogenic bladder, NOS — (Use additional code to identify urinary incontinence: 625.6, 788.30-788.39) ▽
596.8 Other specified disorder of bladder — (Use additional code to identify urinary incontinence: 625.6, 788.30-788.39)
753.5 Exstrophy of urinary bladder
753.8 Other specified congenital anomaly of bladder and urethra
867.0 Bladder and urethra injury without mention of open wound into cavity
867.1 Bladder and urethra injury with open wound into cavity

ICD-9-CM Procedural

56.51 Formation of cutaneous uretero-ileostomy
56.71 Urinary diversion to intestine

50825

50825 Continent diversion, including intestine anastomosis using any segment of small and/or large intestine (Kock pouch or Camey enterocystoplasty)

ICD-9-CM Diagnostic

188.0 Malignant neoplasm of trigone of urinary bladder
188.1 Malignant neoplasm of dome of urinary bladder
188.2 Malignant neoplasm of lateral wall of urinary bladder
188.3 Malignant neoplasm of anterior wall of urinary bladder
188.4 Malignant neoplasm of posterior wall of urinary bladder
188.5 Malignant neoplasm of bladder neck
188.6 Malignant neoplasm of ureteric orifice
188.8 Malignant neoplasm of other specified sites of bladder
188.9 Malignant neoplasm of bladder, part unspecified ▽
189.2 Malignant neoplasm of ureter
189.3 Malignant neoplasm of urethra
198.1 Secondary malignant neoplasm of other urinary organs
591 Hydronephrosis
593.4 Other ureteric obstruction
595.82 Irradiation cystitis — (Use additional code to identify organism, such as E. coli, 041.4)
596.54 Neurogenic bladder, NOS — (Use additional code to identify urinary incontinence: 625.6, 788.30-788.39) ▽
596.8 Other specified disorder of bladder — (Use additional code to identify urinary incontinence: 625.6, 788.30-788.39)
753.5 Exstrophy of urinary bladder
753.8 Other specified congenital anomaly of bladder and urethra
867.0 Bladder and urethra injury without mention of open wound into cavity
867.1 Bladder and urethra injury with open wound into cavity

ICD-9-CM Procedural

56.51 Formation of cutaneous uretero-ileostomy

50830

50830 Urinary undiversion (eg, taking down of ureteroileal conduit, ureterosigmoidostomy or ureteroenterostomy with ureteroureterostomy or ureteroneocystostomy)

ICD-9-CM Diagnostic

344.61 Cauda equina syndrome with neurogenic bladder
596.54 Neurogenic bladder, NOS — (Use additional code to identify urinary incontinence: 625.6, 788.30-788.39) ▽
753.21 Congenital obstruction of ureteropelvic junction
753.22 Congenital obstruction of ureterovesical junction
753.29 Other obstructive defect of renal pelvis and ureter
V10.50 Personal history of malignant neoplasm of unspecified urinary organ ▽
V10.51 Personal history of malignant neoplasm of bladder
V10.52 Personal history of malignant neoplasm of kidney
V10.53 Personal history of malignant neoplasm, renal pelvis
V10.59 Personal history of malignant neoplasm of other urinary organ
V13.00 Personal history of unspecified urinary disorder ▽
V13.09 Personal history of other disorder of urinary system
V15.3 Personal history of irradiation, presenting hazards to health
V15.5 Personal history of injury, presenting hazards to health
V55.5 Attention to cystostomy
V55.6 Attention to other artificial opening of urinary tract

ICD-9-CM Procedural

56.83 Closure of ureterostomy
57.99 Other operations on bladder

HCPCS Level II Supplies & Services

A4349 Male external catheter, with or without adhesive, disposable, each

50840

50840 Replacement of all or part of ureter by intestine segment, including intestine anastomosis

ICD-9-CM Diagnostic

189.2 Malignant neoplasm of ureter
344.61 Cauda equina syndrome with neurogenic bladder
592.1 Calculus of ureter
596.54 Neurogenic bladder, NOS — (Use additional code to identify urinary incontinence: 625.6, 788.30-788.39) ▽
596.8 Other specified disorder of bladder — (Use additional code to identify urinary incontinence: 625.6, 788.30-788.39)
617.8 Endometriosis of other specified sites ♀
867.2 Ureter injury without mention of open wound into cavity
867.3 Ureter injury with open wound into cavity
997.5 Urinary complications — (Use additional code to identify complications)

ICD-9-CM Procedural

56.89 Other repair of ureter

50845

50845 Cutaneous appendico-vesicostomy

ICD-9-CM Diagnostic

154.0 Malignant neoplasm of rectosigmoid junction
154.8 Malignant neoplasm of other sites of rectum, rectosigmoid junction, and anus
180.0 Malignant neoplasm of endocervix ♀
180.8 Malignant neoplasm of other specified sites of cervix ♀
185 Malignant neoplasm of prostate ♂
187.4 Malignant neoplasm of penis, part unspecified ▽ ♂
188.3 Malignant neoplasm of anterior wall of urinary bladder
188.5 Malignant neoplasm of bladder neck
189.3 Malignant neoplasm of urethra
189.8 Malignant neoplasm of other specified sites of urinary organs
198.1 Secondary malignant neoplasm of other urinary organs

▽ Unspecified code ♀ Female diagnosis ☒ Manifestation code ♂ Male diagnosis

223.3 Benign neoplasm of bladder
223.81 Benign neoplasm of urethra
233.1 Carcinoma in situ of cervix uteri ♀
233.7 Carcinoma in situ of bladder
233.9 Carcinoma in situ of other and unspecified urinary organs ▽
236.7 Neoplasm of uncertain behavior of bladder
236.99 Neoplasm of uncertain behavior of other and unspecified urinary organs
239.4 Neoplasm of unspecified nature of bladder
239.5 Neoplasm of unspecified nature of other genitourinary organs
344.61 Cauda equina syndrome with neurogenic bladder
592.0 Calculus of kidney
592.1 Calculus of ureter
593.4 Other ureteric obstruction
594.1 Other calculus in bladder
594.2 Calculus in urethra
595.89 Other specified types of cystitis — (Use additional code to identify organism, such as E. coli, 041.4)
596.0 Bladder neck obstruction — (Use additional code to identify urinary incontinence: 625.6, 788.30-788.39)
596.2 Vesical fistula, not elsewhere classified — (Use additional code to identify urinary incontinence: 625.6, 788.30-788.39)
596.3 Diverticulum of bladder — (Use additional code to identify urinary incontinence: 625.6, 788.30-788.39)
596.4 Atony of bladder — (Use additional code to identify urinary incontinence: 625.6, 788.30-788.39)
596.51 Hypertonicity of bladder — (Use additional code to identify urinary incontinence: 625.6, 788.30-788.39)
596.52 Low bladder compliance — (Use additional code to identify urinary incontinence: 625.6, 788.30-788.39)
596.53 Paralysis of bladder — (Use additional code to identify urinary incontinence: 625.6, 788.30-788.39)
596.54 Neurogenic bladder, NOS — (Use additional code to identify urinary incontinence: 625.6, 788.30-788.39) ▽
596.8 Other specified disorder of bladder — (Use additional code to identify urinary incontinence: 625.6, 788.30-788.39)
598.01 Urethral stricture due to infective diseases classified elsewhere — (Code first underlying disease: 095.8, 098.2, 120.0-120.9. Use additional code to identify urinary incontinence: 625.6, 788.30-788.39) ☒
599.1 Urethral fistula
599.2 Urethral diverticulum
599.6 Unspecified urinary obstruction — (Use additional code to identify urinary incontinence: 625.6, 788.30-788.39) ▽
599.7 Hematuria
599.84 Other specified disorders of urethra — (Use additional code to identify urinary incontinence: 625.6, 788.30-788.39)
600.01 Hypertrophy (benign) of prostate with urinary obstruction — (Use additional code to identify urinary incontinence: 788.30-788.39) ♂
600.11 Nodular prostate with urinary obstruction — (Use additional code to identify urinary incontinence: 788.30-788.39) ♂
600.21 Benign localized hyperplasia of prostate with urinary obstruction — (Use additional code to identify urinary incontinence: 788.30-788.39) ♂
600.91 Hyperplasia of prostate, unspecified, with urinary obstruction — (Use additional code to identify urinary incontinence: 788.30-788.39) ▽ ♂
602.1 Congestion or hemorrhage of prostate ♂
607.2 Other inflammatory disorders of penis — (Use additional code to identify organism) ♂
618.1 Uterine prolapse without mention of vaginal wall prolapse — (Use additional code to identify urinary incontinence: 625.6, 788.31, 788.33-788.39) ♀
618.2 Uterovaginal prolapse, incomplete — (Use additional code to identify urinary incontinence: 625.6, 788.31, 788.33-788.39) ♀
618.3 Uterovaginal prolapse, complete — (Use additional code to identify urinary incontinence: 625.6, 788.31, 788.33-788.39) ♀
618.4 Uterovaginal prolapse, unspecified — (Use additional code to identify urinary incontinence: 625.6, 788.31, 788.33-788.39) ▽ ♀
618.5 Prolapse of vaginal vault after hysterectomy — (Use additional code to identify urinary incontinence: 625.6, 788.31, 788.33-788.39) ♀
618.6 Vaginal enterocele, congenital or acquired — (Use additional code to identify urinary incontinence: 625.6, 788.31, 788.33-788.39) ♀
618.7 Genital prolapse, old laceration of muscles of pelvic floor — (Use additional code to identify urinary incontinence: 625.6, 788.31, 788.33-788.39) ♀
618.9 Unspecified genital prolapse — (Use additional code to identify urinary incontinence: 625.6, 788.31, 788.33-788.39) ▽ ♀
619.0 Urinary-genital tract fistula, female ♀
625.6 Female stress incontinence ♀
625.9 Unspecified symptom associated with female genital organs ▽ ♀
788.0 Renal colic
788.20 Unspecified retention of urine ▽
788.29 Other specified retention of urine
788.30 Unspecified urinary incontinence ▽
788.31 Urge incontinence
788.32 Stress incontinence, male ♂
788.33 Mixed incontinence urge and stress (male)(female)
788.38 Overflow incontinence
788.39 Other urinary incontinence
788.8 Extravasation of urine
789.30 Abdominal or pelvic swelling, mass or lump, unspecified site ▽
808.8 Unspecified closed fracture of pelvis ▽
867.0 Bladder and urethra injury without mention of open wound into cavity
867.1 Bladder and urethra injury with open wound into cavity
867.2 Ureter injury without mention of open wound into cavity
867.3 Ureter injury with open wound into cavity
867.8 Injury to unspecified pelvic organ without mention of open wound into cavity ▽
867.9 Injury to unspecified pelvic organ with open wound into cavity ▽
878.0 Open wound of penis, without mention of complication — (Use additional code to identify infection) ♂
878.1 Open wound of penis, complicated — (Use additional code to identify infection) ♂
879.8 Open wound(s) (multiple) of unspecified site(s), without mention of complication — (Use additional code to identify infection) ▽
879.9 Open wound(s) (multiple) of unspecified site(s), complicated — (Use additional code to identify infection) ▽
942.05 Burn of trunk, unspecified degree of genitalia ▽
996.30 Mechanical complication of unspecified genitourinary device, implant, and graft ▽
996.31 Mechanical complication due to urethral (indwelling) catheter
996.39 Mechanical complication of genitourinary device, implant, and graft, other
996.64 Infection and inflammatory reaction due to indwelling urinary catheter — (Use additional code to identify specified infections: 038.0-038.9, 595.0-595.9)
996.65 Infection and inflammatory reaction due to other genitourinary device, implant, and graft — (Use additional code to identify specified infections)
996.76 Other complications due to genitourinary device, implant, and graft
997.5 Urinary complications — (Use additional code to identify complications)
998.2 Accidental puncture or laceration during procedure
998.51 Infected postoperative seroma — (Use additional code to identify organism)
998.59 Other postoperative infection — (Use additional code to identify infection)
V55.5 Attention to cystostomy

ICD-9-CM Procedural

47.91 Appendicostomy
57.21 Vesicostomy

50860

50860 Ureterostomy, transplantation of ureter to skin

ICD-9-CM Diagnostic

188.0 Malignant neoplasm of trigone of urinary bladder
188.1 Malignant neoplasm of dome of urinary bladder
188.2 Malignant neoplasm of lateral wall of urinary bladder
188.3 Malignant neoplasm of anterior wall of urinary bladder
188.4 Malignant neoplasm of posterior wall of urinary bladder
188.5 Malignant neoplasm of bladder neck
188.6 Malignant neoplasm of ureteric orifice
188.8 Malignant neoplasm of other specified sites of bladder
344.61 Cauda equina syndrome with neurogenic bladder
592.1 Calculus of ureter
593.4 Other ureteric obstruction
596.0 Bladder neck obstruction — (Use additional code to identify urinary incontinence: 625.6, 788.30-788.39)
596.51 Hypertonicity of bladder — (Use additional code to identify urinary incontinence: 625.6, 788.30-788.39)
596.52 Low bladder compliance — (Use additional code to identify urinary incontinence: 625.6, 788.30-788.39)
596.53 Paralysis of bladder — (Use additional code to identify urinary incontinence: 625.6, 788.30-788.39)
596.54 Neurogenic bladder, NOS — (Use additional code to identify urinary incontinence: 625.6, 788.30-788.39) ▽
753.21 Congenital obstruction of ureteropelvic junction
753.22 Congenital obstruction of ureterovesical junction
753.29 Other obstructive defect of renal pelvis and ureter
753.6 Congenital atresia and stenosis of urethra and bladder neck

▽ Unspecified code
♀ Female diagnosis
☒ Manifestation code
♂ Male diagnosis

ICD-9-CM Procedural
56.61 Formation of other cutaneous ureterostomy

50900
50900 Ureterorrhaphy, suture of ureter (separate procedure)

ICD-9-CM Diagnostic
867.2 Ureter injury without mention of open wound into cavity
867.3 Ureter injury with open wound into cavity
E870.0 Accidental cut, puncture, perforation, or hemorrhage during surgical operation

ICD-9-CM Procedural
56.82 Suture of laceration of ureter

50920
50920 Closure of ureterocutaneous fistula

ICD-9-CM Diagnostic
593.82 Ureteral fistula
593.9 Unspecified disorder of kidney and ureter ▽
753.4 Other specified congenital anomalies of ureter

ICD-9-CM Procedural
56.84 Closure of other fistula of ureter

50930
50930 Closure of ureterovisceral fistula (including visceral repair)

ICD-9-CM Diagnostic
593.82 Ureteral fistula
593.9 Unspecified disorder of kidney and ureter ▽
596.2 Vesical fistula, not elsewhere classified — (Use additional code to identify urinary incontinence: 625.6, 788.30-788.39)
619.0 Urinary-genital tract fistula, female ♀
753.4 Other specified congenital anomalies of ureter

ICD-9-CM Procedural
56.84 Closure of other fistula of ureter

50940
50940 Deligation of ureter

ICD-9-CM Diagnostic
591 Hydronephrosis
593.4 Other ureteric obstruction
593.89 Other specified disorder of kidney and ureter
753.3 Other specified congenital anomalies of kidney
753.4 Other specified congenital anomalies of ureter
867.2 Ureter injury without mention of open wound into cavity
867.3 Ureter injury with open wound into cavity
996.81 Complications of transplanted kidney — (Use additional code to identify nature of complication, 078.5)
V58.3 Attention to surgical dressings and sutures
V58.49 Other specified aftercare following surgery — (This code should be used in conjunction with other aftercare codes to fully identify the reason for the aftercare encounter)

ICD-9-CM Procedural
56.86 Removal of ligature from ureter

50945
50945 Laparoscopy, surgical; ureterolithotomy

ICD-9-CM Diagnostic
592.1 Calculus of ureter
592.9 Unspecified urinary calculus ▽
593.4 Other ureteric obstruction

ICD-9-CM Procedural
56.2 Ureterotomy

50947–50948
50947 Laparoscopy, surgical; ureteroneocystostomy with cystoscopy and ureteral stent placement
50948 ureteroneocystostomy without cystoscopy and ureteral stent placement

ICD-9-CM Diagnostic
344.61 Cauda equina syndrome with neurogenic bladder
591 Hydronephrosis
593.3 Stricture or kinking of ureter
593.4 Other ureteric obstruction
593.5 Hydroureter
593.70 Vesicoureteral reflux, unspecified or without reflex nephropathy
593.71 Vesicoureteral reflux with reflux nephropathy, unilateral
593.72 Vesicoureteral reflux with reflux nephropathy, bilateral
593.73 Vesicoureteral reflux with reflux nephropathy, NOS
593.89 Other specified disorder of kidney and ureter
593.9 Unspecified disorder of kidney and ureter ▽
599.0 Urinary tract infection, site not specified — (Use additional code to identify organism, such as E. coli, 041.4) ▽
753.21 Congenital obstruction of ureteropelvic junction
753.22 Congenital obstruction of ureterovesical junction
753.23 Congenital ureterocele
753.29 Other obstructive defect of renal pelvis and ureter
753.4 Other specified congenital anomalies of ureter
753.9 Unspecified congenital anomaly of urinary system ▽

ICD-9-CM Procedural
56.74 Ureteroneocystostomy
59.8 Ureteral catheterization

50951–50955
50951 Ureteral endoscopy through established ureterostomy, with or without irrigation, instillation, or ureteropyelography, exclusive of radiologic service;
50953 with ureteral catheterization, with or without dilation of ureter
50955 with biopsy

ICD-9-CM Diagnostic
188.6 Malignant neoplasm of ureteric orifice
189.2 Malignant neoplasm of ureter
198.0 Secondary malignant neoplasm of kidney
198.1 Secondary malignant neoplasm of other urinary organs
223.1 Benign neoplasm of renal pelvis
223.2 Benign neoplasm of ureter
233.3 Carcinoma in situ of other and unspecified female genital organs ▽ ♀
233.7 Carcinoma in situ of bladder
233.9 Carcinoma in situ of other and unspecified urinary organs ▽
236.7 Neoplasm of uncertain behavior of bladder
236.91 Neoplasm of uncertain behavior of kidney and ureter
592.1 Calculus of ureter
593.3 Stricture or kinking of ureter
593.4 Other ureteric obstruction
593.5 Hydroureter
593.82 Ureteral fistula
593.89 Other specified disorder of kidney and ureter
599.7 Hematuria
753.21 Congenital obstruction of ureteropelvic junction
753.22 Congenital obstruction of ureterovesical junction
753.23 Congenital ureterocele
753.29 Other obstructive defect of renal pelvis and ureter

ICD-9-CM Procedural
56.31 Ureteroscopy
56.33 Closed endoscopic biopsy of ureter
56.91 Dilation of ureteral meatus
59.8 Ureteral catheterization

HCPCS Level II Supplies & Services
A4270 Disposable endoscope sheath, each
A9525 Supply of low or iso-osmolar contrast material, 10 mg of iodine

50957–50961

50957 Ureteral endoscopy through established ureterostomy, with or without irrigation, instillation, or ureteropyelography, exclusive of radiologic service; with fulguration and/or incision, with or without biopsy
50961 with removal of foreign body or calculus

ICD-9-CM Diagnostic

188.6 Malignant neoplasm of ureteric orifice
189.2 Malignant neoplasm of ureter
198.0 Secondary malignant neoplasm of kidney
198.1 Secondary malignant neoplasm of other urinary organs
223.1 Benign neoplasm of renal pelvis
223.2 Benign neoplasm of ureter
233.3 Carcinoma in situ of other and unspecified female genital organs ▽ ♀
233.7 Carcinoma in situ of bladder
233.9 Carcinoma in situ of other and unspecified urinary organs ▽
236.7 Neoplasm of uncertain behavior of bladder
236.91 Neoplasm of uncertain behavior of kidney and ureter
252.00 Hyperparathyroidism, unspecified
252.01 Primary hyperparathyroidism
252.02 Secondary hyperparathyroidism, non-renal
252.08 Other hyperparathyroidism
588.81 Secondary hyperparathyroidism (of renal origin)
592.0 Calculus of kidney
592.1 Calculus of ureter
592.9 Unspecified urinary calculus ▽
593.3 Stricture or kinking of ureter
593.4 Other ureteric obstruction
593.5 Hydroureter
593.82 Ureteral fistula
593.89 Other specified disorder of kidney and ureter
753.21 Congenital obstruction of ureteropelvic junction
753.22 Congenital obstruction of ureterovesical junction
753.23 Congenital ureterocele
753.29 Other obstructive defect of renal pelvis and ureter
996.30 Mechanical complication of unspecified genitourinary device, implant, and graft ▽
996.39 Mechanical complication of genitourinary device, implant, and graft, other
996.65 Infection and inflammatory reaction due to other genitourinary device, implant, and graft — (Use additional code to identify specified infections)
996.76 Other complications due to genitourinary device, implant, and graft
998.4 Foreign body accidentally left during procedure, not elsewhere classified

ICD-9-CM Procedural

56.2 Ureterotomy
56.31 Ureteroscopy
56.33 Closed endoscopic biopsy of ureter
56.99 Other operations on ureter

HCPCS Level II Supplies & Services

A4270 Disposable endoscope sheath, each
A9525 Supply of low or iso-osmolar contrast material, 10 mg of iodine

50970–50974

50970 Ureteral endoscopy through ureterotomy, with or without irrigation, instillation, or ureteropyelography, exclusive of radiologic service;
50972 with ureteral catheterization, with or without dilation of ureter
50974 with biopsy

ICD-9-CM Diagnostic

188.6 Malignant neoplasm of ureteric orifice
189.1 Malignant neoplasm of renal pelvis
189.2 Malignant neoplasm of ureter
198.0 Secondary malignant neoplasm of kidney
198.1 Secondary malignant neoplasm of other urinary organs
223.1 Benign neoplasm of renal pelvis
223.2 Benign neoplasm of ureter
223.3 Benign neoplasm of bladder
233.7 Carcinoma in situ of bladder
233.9 Carcinoma in situ of other and unspecified urinary organs ▽
236.7 Neoplasm of uncertain behavior of bladder
236.91 Neoplasm of uncertain behavior of kidney and ureter
239.4 Neoplasm of unspecified nature of bladder
239.5 Neoplasm of unspecified nature of other genitourinary organs
592.0 Calculus of kidney
592.1 Calculus of ureter
593.3 Stricture or kinking of ureter
593.4 Other ureteric obstruction
593.5 Hydroureter
593.82 Ureteral fistula
593.89 Other specified disorder of kidney and ureter
599.7 Hematuria
753.21 Congenital obstruction of ureteropelvic junction
753.22 Congenital obstruction of ureterovesical junction
753.23 Congenital ureterocele
753.29 Other obstructive defect of renal pelvis and ureter
788.0 Renal colic
789.01 Abdominal pain, right upper quadrant
789.02 Abdominal pain, left upper quadrant

ICD-9-CM Procedural

56.2 Ureterotomy
56.31 Ureteroscopy
56.33 Closed endoscopic biopsy of ureter
56.91 Dilation of ureteral meatus
59.8 Ureteral catheterization

50976–50980

50976 Ureteral endoscopy through ureterotomy, with or without irrigation, instillation, or ureteropyelography, exclusive of radiologic service; with fulguration and/or incision, with or without biopsy
50980 with removal of foreign body or calculus

ICD-9-CM Diagnostic

188.6 Malignant neoplasm of ureteric orifice
189.1 Malignant neoplasm of renal pelvis
189.2 Malignant neoplasm of ureter
198.0 Secondary malignant neoplasm of kidney
198.1 Secondary malignant neoplasm of other urinary organs
223.1 Benign neoplasm of renal pelvis
223.2 Benign neoplasm of ureter
223.3 Benign neoplasm of bladder
233.7 Carcinoma in situ of bladder
233.9 Carcinoma in situ of other and unspecified urinary organs ▽
236.7 Neoplasm of uncertain behavior of bladder
236.91 Neoplasm of uncertain behavior of kidney and ureter
239.4 Neoplasm of unspecified nature of bladder
239.5 Neoplasm of unspecified nature of other genitourinary organs
252.00 Hyperparathyroidism, unspecified
252.01 Primary hyperparathyroidism
252.02 Secondary hyperparathyroidism, non-renal
252.08 Other hyperparathyroidism
588.81 Secondary hyperparathyroidism (of renal origin)
592.0 Calculus of kidney
592.1 Calculus of ureter
592.9 Unspecified urinary calculus ▽
593.3 Stricture or kinking of ureter
593.4 Other ureteric obstruction
593.5 Hydroureter
593.82 Ureteral fistula
593.89 Other specified disorder of kidney and ureter
753.21 Congenital obstruction of ureteropelvic junction
753.22 Congenital obstruction of ureterovesical junction
753.23 Congenital ureterocele
753.29 Other obstructive defect of renal pelvis and ureter
996.39 Mechanical complication of genitourinary device, implant, and graft, other
996.65 Infection and inflammatory reaction due to other genitourinary device, implant, and graft — (Use additional code to identify specified infections)
996.76 Other complications due to genitourinary device, implant, and graft
998.4 Foreign body accidentally left during procedure, not elsewhere classified

ICD-9-CM Procedural

56.2 Ureterotomy
56.31 Ureteroscopy
56.33 Closed endoscopic biopsy of ureter
56.99 Other operations on ureter

Bladder

51000–51010

51000 Aspiration of bladder by needle
51005 Aspiration of bladder; by trocar or intracatheter
51010 with insertion of suprapubic catheter

ICD-9-CM Diagnostic

185 Malignant neoplasm of prostate ♂
188.0 Malignant neoplasm of trigone of urinary bladder
188.2 Malignant neoplasm of lateral wall of urinary bladder
188.3 Malignant neoplasm of anterior wall of urinary bladder
188.4 Malignant neoplasm of posterior wall of urinary bladder
188.5 Malignant neoplasm of bladder neck
188.6 Malignant neoplasm of ureteric orifice
344.61 Cauda equina syndrome with neurogenic bladder
590.00 Chronic pyelonephritis without lesion of renal medullary necrosis — (Code, if applicable, any causal condition first. Use additional code to identify organism, such as E. coli, 041.4)
590.3 Pyeloureteritis cystica — (Use additional code to identify organism, such as E. coli, 041.4)
590.81 Pyelitis or pyelonephritis in diseases classified elsewhere — (Code first underlying disease, 016.0. Use additional code to identify organism, such as E. coli, 041.4) ☒
593.70 Vesicoureteral reflux, unspecified or without reflex nephropathy
595.0 Acute cystitis — (Use additional code to identify organism, such as E. coli, 041.4)
595.1 Chronic interstitial cystitis — (Use additional code to identify organism, such as E. coli, 041.4)
595.3 Trigonitis — (Use additional code to identify organism, such as E. coli, 041.4)
595.4 Cystitis in diseases classified elsewhere — (Code first underlying disease: 006.8, 039.8, 120.0-120.9, 122.3, 122.6. Use additional code to identify organism, such as E. coli, 041.4) ☒
599.0 Urinary tract infection, site not specified — (Use additional code to identify organism, such as E. coli, 041.4) ▽
599.7 Hematuria
618.9 Unspecified genital prolapse — (Use additional code to identify urinary incontinence: 625.6, 788.31, 788.33-788.39) ▽ ♀
625.6 Female stress incontinence ♀
752.61 Hypospadias ♂
752.62 Epispadias ♂
752.63 Congenital chordee ♂
752.64 Micropenis ♂
752.65 Hidden penis ♂
752.69 Other penile anomalies ♂
753.6 Congenital atresia and stenosis of urethra and bladder neck
771.82 Urinary tract infection of newborn — (Use additional code to identify organism)
771.89 Other infections specific to the perinatal period — (Use additional code to identify organism)
783.5 Polydipsia
788.1 Dysuria
788.20 Unspecified retention of urine ▽
788.21 Incomplete bladder emptying
788.29 Other specified retention of urine
788.41 Urinary frequency
788.42 Polyuria
788.43 Nocturia
788.63 Urgency of urination
867.0 Bladder and urethra injury without mention of open wound into cavity

ICD-9-CM Procedural

57.11 Percutaneous aspiration of bladder
57.18 Other suprapubic cystostomy

HCPCS Level II Supplies & Services

A4550 Surgical trays

51020–51030

51020 Cystotomy or cystostomy; with fulguration and/or insertion of radioactive material
51030 with cryosurgical destruction of intravesical lesion

ICD-9-CM Diagnostic

188.0 Malignant neoplasm of trigone of urinary bladder
188.1 Malignant neoplasm of dome of urinary bladder
188.2 Malignant neoplasm of lateral wall of urinary bladder
188.3 Malignant neoplasm of anterior wall of urinary bladder
188.4 Malignant neoplasm of posterior wall of urinary bladder
188.5 Malignant neoplasm of bladder neck
188.6 Malignant neoplasm of ureteric orifice
188.7 Malignant neoplasm of urachus
188.8 Malignant neoplasm of other specified sites of bladder
198.1 Secondary malignant neoplasm of other urinary organs
223.3 Benign neoplasm of bladder
233.7 Carcinoma in situ of bladder
236.7 Neoplasm of uncertain behavior of bladder
239.4 Neoplasm of unspecified nature of bladder
596.9 Unspecified disorder of bladder — (Use additional code to identify urinary incontinence: 625.6, 788.30-788.39) ▽

ICD-9-CM Procedural

57.18 Other suprapubic cystostomy
92.27 Implantation or insertion of radioactive elements

51040

51040 Cystostomy, cystotomy with drainage

ICD-9-CM Diagnostic

185 Malignant neoplasm of prostate ♂
187.4 Malignant neoplasm of penis, part unspecified ▽ ♂
188.0 Malignant neoplasm of trigone of urinary bladder
188.2 Malignant neoplasm of lateral wall of urinary bladder
188.3 Malignant neoplasm of anterior wall of urinary bladder
188.4 Malignant neoplasm of posterior wall of urinary bladder
188.5 Malignant neoplasm of bladder neck
188.6 Malignant neoplasm of ureteric orifice
344.61 Cauda equina syndrome with neurogenic bladder
590.00 Chronic pyelonephritis without lesion of renal medullary necrosis — (Code, if applicable, any causal condition first. Use additional code to identify organism, such as E. coli, 041.4)
590.3 Pyeloureteritis cystica — (Use additional code to identify organism, such as E. coli, 041.4)
590.81 Pyelitis or pyelonephritis in diseases classified elsewhere — (Code first underlying disease, 016.0. Use additional code to identify organism, such as E. coli, 041.4) ☒
593.70 Vesicoureteral reflux, unspecified or without reflex nephropathy
595.0 Acute cystitis — (Use additional code to identify organism, such as E. coli, 041.4)
595.1 Chronic interstitial cystitis — (Use additional code to identify organism, such as E. coli, 041.4)
595.3 Trigonitis — (Use additional code to identify organism, such as E. coli, 041.4)
595.4 Cystitis in diseases classified elsewhere — (Code first underlying disease: 006.8, 039.8, 120.0-120.9, 122.3, 122.6. Use additional code to identify organism, such as E. coli, 041.4) ☒
598.01 Urethral stricture due to infective diseases classified elsewhere — (Code first underlying disease: 095.8, 098.2, 120.0-120.9. Use additional code to identify urinary incontinence: 625.6, 788.30-788.39) ☒
599.0 Urinary tract infection, site not specified — (Use additional code to identify organism, such as E. coli, 041.4) ▽
599.1 Urethral fistula
599.6 Unspecified urinary obstruction — (Use additional code to identify urinary incontinence: 625.6, 788.30-788.39) ▽
599.7 Hematuria
600.01 Hypertrophy (benign) of prostate with urinary obstruction — (Use additional code to identify urinary incontinence: 788.30-788.39) ♂
600.11 Nodular prostate with urinary obstruction — (Use additional code to identify urinary incontinence: 788.30-788.39) ♂
600.21 Benign localized hyperplasia of prostate with urinary obstruction — (Use additional code to identify urinary incontinence: 788.30-788.39) ♂
600.91 Hyperplasia of prostate, unspecified, with urinary obstruction — (Use additional code to identify urinary incontinence: 788.30-788.39) ▽ ♂
618.01 Cystocele without mention of uterine prolapse, midline
618.02 Cystocele without mention of uterine prolapse, lateral

▽ Unspecified code
♀ Female diagnosis
☒ Manifestation code
♂ Male diagnosis

618.9 Unspecified genital prolapse — (Use additional code to identify urinary incontinence: 625.6, 788.31, 788.33-788.39) ▽ ♀
625.6 Female stress incontinence ♀
752.61 Hypospadias ♂
752.62 Epispadias ♂
752.63 Congenital chordee ♂
752.64 Micropenis ♂
752.65 Hidden penis ♂
752.69 Other penile anomalies ♂
753.6 Congenital atresia and stenosis of urethra and bladder neck
771.82 Urinary tract infection of newborn — (Use additional code to identify organism)
771.89 Other infections specific to the perinatal period — (Use additional code to identify organism)
788.1 Dysuria
788.20 Unspecified retention of urine ▽
788.21 Incomplete bladder emptying
788.29 Other specified retention of urine
788.41 Urinary frequency
788.42 Polyuria
788.43 Nocturia
867.0 Bladder and urethra injury without mention of open wound into cavity

ICD-9-CM Procedural
57.18 Other suprapubic cystostomy
57.19 Other cystotomy

51045
51045 Cystotomy, with insertion of ureteral catheter or stent (separate procedure)

ICD-9-CM Diagnostic
592.1 Calculus of ureter
593.3 Stricture or kinking of ureter
593.4 Other ureteric obstruction
593.5 Hydroureter
593.82 Ureteral fistula
599.6 Unspecified urinary obstruction — (Use additional code to identify urinary incontinence: 625.6, 788.30-788.39) ▽
599.7 Hematuria
867.2 Ureter injury without mention of open wound into cavity
867.3 Ureter injury with open wound into cavity

ICD-9-CM Procedural
57.19 Other cystotomy

51050
51050 Cystolithotomy, cystotomy with removal of calculus, without vesical neck resection

ICD-9-CM Diagnostic
594.1 Other calculus in bladder
594.2 Calculus in urethra
594.8 Other lower urinary tract calculus
594.9 Unspecified calculus of lower urinary tract ▽

ICD-9-CM Procedural
57.19 Other cystotomy

51060–51065
51060 Transvesical ureterolithotomy
51065 Cystotomy, with calculus basket extraction and/or ultrasonic or electrohydraulic fragmentation of ureteral calculus

ICD-9-CM Diagnostic
592.1 Calculus of ureter
592.9 Unspecified urinary calculus ▽
594.1 Other calculus in bladder
V64.41 Laparoscopic surgical procedure converted to open procedure

ICD-9-CM Procedural
56.2 Ureterotomy
57.19 Other cystotomy

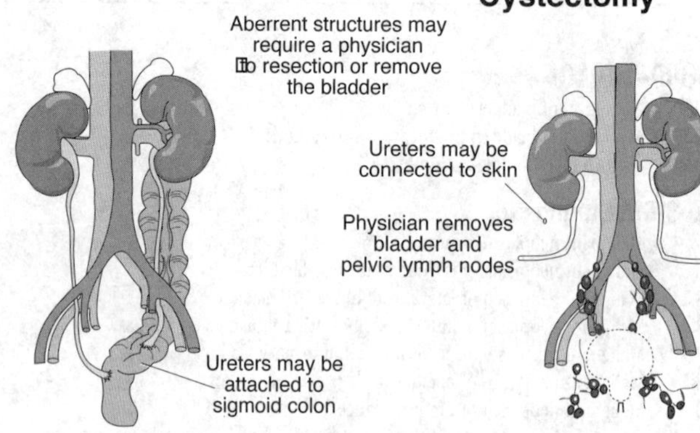
Cystectomy
Aberrent structures may require a physician to resection or remove the bladder
Ureters may be connected to skin
Physician removes bladder and pelvic lymph nodes
Ureters may be attached to sigmoid colon

51080
51080 Drainage of perivesical or prevesical space abscess

ICD-9-CM Diagnostic
595.89 Other specified types of cystitis — (Use additional code to identify organism, such as E. coli, 041.4)
614.3 Acute parametritis and pelvic cellulitis — (Use additional code to identify organism: 041.0, 041.1) ♀
614.4 Chronic or unspecified parametritis and pelvic cellulitis — (Use additional code to identify organism: 041.0, 041.1) ♀
997.5 Urinary complications — (Use additional code to identify complications)
998.51 Infected postoperative seroma — (Use additional code to identify organism)
998.59 Other postoperative infection — (Use additional code to identify infection)

ICD-9-CM Procedural
59.19 Other incision of perivesical tissue
59.92 Other operations on perirenal or perivesical tissue

51500
51500 Excision of urachal cyst or sinus, with or without umbilical hernia repair

ICD-9-CM Diagnostic
551.1 Umbilical hernia with gangrene
552.1 Umbilical hernia with obstruction
553.1 Umbilical hernia without mention of obstruction or gangrene
753.7 Congenital anomalies of urachus

ICD-9-CM Procedural
57.51 Excision of urachus

51520
51520 Cystotomy; for simple excision of vesical neck (separate procedure)

ICD-9-CM Diagnostic
188.5 Malignant neoplasm of bladder neck
198.1 Secondary malignant neoplasm of other urinary organs
223.3 Benign neoplasm of bladder
233.7 Carcinoma in situ of bladder
236.7 Neoplasm of uncertain behavior of bladder
239.4 Neoplasm of unspecified nature of bladder
595.1 Chronic interstitial cystitis — (Use additional code to identify organism, such as E. coli, 041.4)
598.01 Urethral stricture due to infective diseases classified elsewhere — (Code first underlying disease: 095.8, 098.2, 120.0-120.9. Use additional code to identify urinary incontinence: 625.6, 788.30-788.39) ☒
598.1 Traumatic urethral stricture — (Use additional code to identify urinary incontinence: 625.6, 788.30-788.39)
598.2 Postoperative urethral stricture — (Use additional code to identify urinary incontinence: 625.6, 788.30-788.39)
598.9 Unspecified urethral stricture — (Use additional code to identify urinary incontinence: 625.6, 788.30-788.39) ▽
625.6 Female stress incontinence ♀
788.30 Unspecified urinary incontinence ▽
788.31 Urge incontinence
788.32 Stress incontinence, male ♂
788.33 Mixed incontinence urge and stress (male)(female)

▽ Unspecified code
♀ Female diagnosis
☒ Manifestation code
♂ Male diagnosis

788.34 Incontinence without sensory awareness
788.35 Post-void dribbling
788.36 Nocturnal enuresis
788.37 Continuous leakage
788.38 Overflow incontinence

ICD-9-CM Procedural
57.59 Open excision or destruction of other lesion or tissue of bladder

51525
51525 Cystotomy; for excision of bladder diverticulum, single or multiple (separate procedure)

ICD-9-CM Diagnostic
596.3 Diverticulum of bladder — (Use additional code to identify urinary incontinence: 625.6, 788.30-788.39)
625.6 Female stress incontinence ♀
788.30 Unspecified urinary incontinence ▽
788.31 Urge incontinence
788.32 Stress incontinence, male ♂
788.33 Mixed incontinence urge and stress (male)(female)
788.34 Incontinence without sensory awareness
788.35 Post-void dribbling
788.36 Nocturnal enuresis
788.37 Continuous leakage
788.38 Overflow incontinence
788.39 Other urinary incontinence

ICD-9-CM Procedural
57.59 Open excision or destruction of other lesion or tissue of bladder

51530
51530 Cystotomy; for excision of bladder tumor

ICD-9-CM Diagnostic
188.0 Malignant neoplasm of trigone of urinary bladder
188.1 Malignant neoplasm of dome of urinary bladder
188.2 Malignant neoplasm of lateral wall of urinary bladder
188.3 Malignant neoplasm of anterior wall of urinary bladder
188.4 Malignant neoplasm of posterior wall of urinary bladder
188.5 Malignant neoplasm of bladder neck
188.6 Malignant neoplasm of ureteric orifice
188.7 Malignant neoplasm of urachus
188.9 Malignant neoplasm of bladder, part unspecified ▽
198.1 Secondary malignant neoplasm of other urinary organs
223.3 Benign neoplasm of bladder
233.7 Carcinoma in situ of bladder
236.7 Neoplasm of uncertain behavior of bladder
239.4 Neoplasm of unspecified nature of bladder

ICD-9-CM Procedural
57.59 Open excision or destruction of other lesion or tissue of bladder

51535
51535 Cystotomy for excision, incision, or repair of ureterocele

ICD-9-CM Diagnostic
593.70 Vesicoureteral reflux, unspecified or without reflex nephropathy
593.71 Vesicoureteral reflux with reflux nephropathy, unilateral
593.72 Vesicoureteral reflux with reflux nephropathy, bilateral
593.73 Vesicoureteral reflux with reflux nephropathy, NOS
593.89 Other specified disorder of kidney and ureter
753.23 Congenital ureterocele

ICD-9-CM Procedural
56.2 Ureterotomy
56.41 Partial ureterectomy
56.89 Other repair of ureter

51550–51555
51550 Cystectomy, partial; simple
51555 complicated (eg, postradiation, previous surgery, difficult location)

ICD-9-CM Diagnostic
152.2 Malignant neoplasm of ileum
153.9 Malignant neoplasm of colon, unspecified site ▽
188.0 Malignant neoplasm of trigone of urinary bladder
188.1 Malignant neoplasm of dome of urinary bladder
188.2 Malignant neoplasm of lateral wall of urinary bladder
188.3 Malignant neoplasm of anterior wall of urinary bladder
188.4 Malignant neoplasm of posterior wall of urinary bladder
188.5 Malignant neoplasm of bladder neck
188.6 Malignant neoplasm of ureteric orifice
188.8 Malignant neoplasm of other specified sites of bladder
188.9 Malignant neoplasm of bladder, part unspecified ▽
198.1 Secondary malignant neoplasm of other urinary organs
223.3 Benign neoplasm of bladder
233.7 Carcinoma in situ of bladder
238.8 Neoplasm of uncertain behavior of other specified sites
344.61 Cauda equina syndrome with neurogenic bladder
595.2 Other chronic cystitis — (Use additional code to identify organism, such as E. coli, 041.4)
596.1 Intestinovesical fistula — (Use additional code to identify urinary incontinence: 625.6, 788.30-788.39)
596.3 Diverticulum of bladder — (Use additional code to identify urinary incontinence: 625.6, 788.30-788.39)
625.6 Female stress incontinence ♀
789.30 Abdominal or pelvic swelling, mass or lump, unspecified site ▽
909.2 Late effect of radiation
V45.89 Other postsurgical status — (This code is intended for use when these conditions are recorded as diagnoses or problems)

ICD-9-CM Procedural
57.6 Partial cystectomy

51565
51565 Cystectomy, partial, with reimplantation of ureter(s) into bladder (ureteroneocystostomy)

ICD-9-CM Diagnostic
152.2 Malignant neoplasm of ileum
153.9 Malignant neoplasm of colon, unspecified site ▽
188.0 Malignant neoplasm of trigone of urinary bladder
188.1 Malignant neoplasm of dome of urinary bladder
188.2 Malignant neoplasm of lateral wall of urinary bladder
188.3 Malignant neoplasm of anterior wall of urinary bladder
188.4 Malignant neoplasm of posterior wall of urinary bladder
188.5 Malignant neoplasm of bladder neck
188.6 Malignant neoplasm of ureteric orifice
188.7 Malignant neoplasm of urachus
188.8 Malignant neoplasm of other specified sites of bladder
188.9 Malignant neoplasm of bladder, part unspecified ▽
198.1 Secondary malignant neoplasm of other urinary organs
223.3 Benign neoplasm of bladder
233.7 Carcinoma in situ of bladder
238.8 Neoplasm of uncertain behavior of other specified sites
344.61 Cauda equina syndrome with neurogenic bladder
595.2 Other chronic cystitis — (Use additional code to identify organism, such as E. coli, 041.4)
596.1 Intestinovesical fistula — (Use additional code to identify urinary incontinence: 625.6, 788.30-788.39)
596.3 Diverticulum of bladder — (Use additional code to identify urinary incontinence: 625.6, 788.30-788.39)
625.6 Female stress incontinence ♀
789.30 Abdominal or pelvic swelling, mass or lump, unspecified site ▽
909.2 Late effect of radiation
V45.89 Other postsurgical status — (This code is intended for use when these conditions are recorded as diagnoses or problems)

ICD-9-CM Procedural
56.74 Ureteroneocystostomy
57.6 Partial cystectomy

51570–51575
51570 Cystectomy, complete; (separate procedure)
51575 with bilateral pelvic lymphadenectomy, including external iliac, hypogastric, and obturator nodes

ICD-9-CM Diagnostic
153.9 Malignant neoplasm of colon, unspecified site ▽

185 Malignant neoplasm of prostate ♂
188.0 Malignant neoplasm of trigone of urinary bladder
188.1 Malignant neoplasm of dome of urinary bladder
188.2 Malignant neoplasm of lateral wall of urinary bladder
188.3 Malignant neoplasm of anterior wall of urinary bladder
188.4 Malignant neoplasm of posterior wall of urinary bladder
188.8 Malignant neoplasm of other specified sites of bladder
188.9 Malignant neoplasm of bladder, part unspecified ▽
196.6 Secondary and unspecified malignant neoplasm of intrapelvic lymph nodes
198.1 Secondary malignant neoplasm of other urinary organs
236.7 Neoplasm of uncertain behavior of bladder
236.99 Neoplasm of uncertain behavior of other and unspecified urinary organs
239.5 Neoplasm of unspecified nature of other genitourinary organs
595.1 Chronic interstitial cystitis — (Use additional code to identify organism, such as E. coli, 041.4)

ICD-9-CM Procedural

40.3 Regional lymph node excision
40.50 Radical excision of lymph nodes, not otherwise specified
57.71 Radical cystectomy
57.79 Other total cystectomy

51580–51585

51580 Cystectomy, complete, with ureterosigmoidostomy or ureterocutaneous transplantations;
51585 with bilateral pelvic lymphadenectomy, including external iliac, hypogastric, and obturator nodes

ICD-9-CM Diagnostic

185 Malignant neoplasm of prostate ♂
188.0 Malignant neoplasm of trigone of urinary bladder
188.1 Malignant neoplasm of dome of urinary bladder
188.2 Malignant neoplasm of lateral wall of urinary bladder
188.3 Malignant neoplasm of anterior wall of urinary bladder
188.4 Malignant neoplasm of posterior wall of urinary bladder
188.8 Malignant neoplasm of other specified sites of bladder
188.9 Malignant neoplasm of bladder, part unspecified ▽
196.6 Secondary and unspecified malignant neoplasm of intrapelvic lymph nodes
198.1 Secondary malignant neoplasm of other urinary organs
236.7 Neoplasm of uncertain behavior of bladder
239.4 Neoplasm of unspecified nature of bladder
595.1 Chronic interstitial cystitis — (Use additional code to identify organism, such as E. coli, 041.4)

ICD-9-CM Procedural

40.3 Regional lymph node excision
40.50 Radical excision of lymph nodes, not otherwise specified
56.51 Formation of cutaneous uretero-ileostomy
56.61 Formation of other cutaneous ureterostomy
56.71 Urinary diversion to intestine
57.71 Radical cystectomy

51590–51595

51590 Cystectomy, complete, with ureteroileal conduit or sigmoid bladder, including intestine anastomosis;
51595 with bilateral pelvic lymphadenectomy, including external iliac, hypogastric, and obturator nodes

ICD-9-CM Diagnostic

185 Malignant neoplasm of prostate ♂
188.0 Malignant neoplasm of trigone of urinary bladder
188.1 Malignant neoplasm of dome of urinary bladder
188.2 Malignant neoplasm of lateral wall of urinary bladder
188.3 Malignant neoplasm of anterior wall of urinary bladder
188.4 Malignant neoplasm of posterior wall of urinary bladder
188.8 Malignant neoplasm of other specified sites of bladder
188.9 Malignant neoplasm of bladder, part unspecified ▽
196.6 Secondary and unspecified malignant neoplasm of intrapelvic lymph nodes
198.1 Secondary malignant neoplasm of other urinary organs
236.7 Neoplasm of uncertain behavior of bladder
239.4 Neoplasm of unspecified nature of bladder

ICD-9-CM Procedural

40.3 Regional lymph node excision
40.50 Radical excision of lymph nodes, not otherwise specified
56.51 Formation of cutaneous uretero-ileostomy
56.71 Urinary diversion to intestine
57.71 Radical cystectomy

51596

51596 Cystectomy, complete, with continent diversion, any open technique, using any segment of small and/or large intestine to construct neobladder

ICD-9-CM Diagnostic

185 Malignant neoplasm of prostate ♂
187.8 Malignant neoplasm of other specified sites of male genital organs ♂
187.9 Malignant neoplasm of male genital organ, site unspecified ▽ ♂
188.0 Malignant neoplasm of trigone of urinary bladder
188.1 Malignant neoplasm of dome of urinary bladder
188.2 Malignant neoplasm of lateral wall of urinary bladder
188.3 Malignant neoplasm of anterior wall of urinary bladder
188.4 Malignant neoplasm of posterior wall of urinary bladder
188.8 Malignant neoplasm of other specified sites of bladder
188.9 Malignant neoplasm of bladder, part unspecified ▽
198.1 Secondary malignant neoplasm of other urinary organs
236.7 Neoplasm of uncertain behavior of bladder
239.4 Neoplasm of unspecified nature of bladder
595.1 Chronic interstitial cystitis — (Use additional code to identify organism, such as E. coli, 041.4)

ICD-9-CM Procedural

56.51 Formation of cutaneous uretero-ileostomy
57.71 Radical cystectomy

51597

51597 Pelvic exenteration, complete, for vesical, prostatic or urethral malignancy, with removal of bladder and ureteral transplantations, with or without hysterectomy and/or abdominoperineal resection of rectum and colon and colostomy, or any combination thereof

ICD-9-CM Diagnostic

185 Malignant neoplasm of prostate ♂
188.0 Malignant neoplasm of trigone of urinary bladder
188.1 Malignant neoplasm of dome of urinary bladder
188.2 Malignant neoplasm of lateral wall of urinary bladder
188.3 Malignant neoplasm of anterior wall of urinary bladder
188.4 Malignant neoplasm of posterior wall of urinary bladder
188.5 Malignant neoplasm of bladder neck
188.6 Malignant neoplasm of ureteric orifice
188.8 Malignant neoplasm of other specified sites of bladder
188.9 Malignant neoplasm of bladder, part unspecified ▽
189.3 Malignant neoplasm of urethra
197.5 Secondary malignant neoplasm of large intestine and rectum
198.1 Secondary malignant neoplasm of other urinary organs
198.6 Secondary malignant neoplasm of ovary ♀
198.82 Secondary malignant neoplasm of genital organs

ICD-9-CM Procedural

40.3 Regional lymph node excision
40.54 Radical groin dissection
46.13 Permanent colostomy
48.5 Abdominoperineal resection of rectum
56.61 Formation of other cutaneous ureterostomy
56.71 Urinary diversion to intestine
57.71 Radical cystectomy
68.8 Pelvic evisceration

51600–51610

51600 Injection procedure for cystography or voiding urethrocystography
51605 Injection procedure and placement of chain for contrast and/or chain urethrocystography
51610 Injection procedure for retrograde urethrocystography

ICD-9-CM Diagnostic

098.0 Gonococcal infection (acute) of lower genitourinary tract
185 Malignant neoplasm of prostate ♂
188.0 Malignant neoplasm of trigone of urinary bladder
188.1 Malignant neoplasm of dome of urinary bladder
188.2 Malignant neoplasm of lateral wall of urinary bladder
188.3 Malignant neoplasm of anterior wall of urinary bladder
188.4 Malignant neoplasm of posterior wall of urinary bladder

188.5 Malignant neoplasm of bladder neck
188.6 Malignant neoplasm of ureteric orifice
188.7 Malignant neoplasm of urachus
188.8 Malignant neoplasm of other specified sites of bladder
188.9 Malignant neoplasm of bladder, part unspecified ▽
199.0 Disseminated malignant neoplasm
199.1 Other malignant neoplasm of unspecified site
223.3 Benign neoplasm of bladder
223.81 Benign neoplasm of urethra
223.89 Benign neoplasm of other specified sites of urinary organs
239.4 Neoplasm of unspecified nature of bladder
344.61 Cauda equina syndrome with neurogenic bladder
357.4 Polyneuropathy in other diseases classified elsewhere — (Code first underlying disease: 032.0-032.9, 135, 251.2, 265.0, 265.2, 266.0-266.9, 277.1, 277.3, 585) ☒
585 Chronic renal failure — (Use additional code to identify manifestation: 357.4, 420.0)
586 Unspecified renal failure ▽
590.10 Acute pyelonephritis without lesion of renal medullary necrosis — (Use additional code to identify organism, such as E. coli, 041.4)
590.9 Unspecified infection of kidney — (Use additional code to identify organism, such as E. coli, 041.4) ▽
591 Hydronephrosis
592.0 Calculus of kidney
592.1 Calculus of ureter
592.9 Unspecified urinary calculus ▽
593.4 Other ureteric obstruction
593.70 Vesicoureteral reflux, unspecified or without reflex nephropathy
593.71 Vesicoureteral reflux with reflux nephropathy, unilateral
593.72 Vesicoureteral reflux with reflux nephropathy, bilateral
593.73 Vesicoureteral reflux with reflux nephropathy, NOS
593.9 Unspecified disorder of kidney and ureter ▽
594.0 Calculus in diverticulum of bladder
594.1 Other calculus in bladder
594.2 Calculus in urethra
594.8 Other lower urinary tract calculus
594.9 Unspecified calculus of lower urinary tract ▽
595.0 Acute cystitis — (Use additional code to identify organism, such as E. coli, 041.4)
595.2 Other chronic cystitis — (Use additional code to identify organism, such as E. coli, 041.4)
595.3 Trigonitis — (Use additional code to identify organism, such as E. coli, 041.4)
595.4 Cystitis in diseases classified elsewhere — (Code first underlying disease: 006.8, 039.8, 120.0-120.9, 122.3, 122.6. Use additional code to identify organism, such as E. coli, 041.4) ☒
595.81 Cystitis cystica — (Use additional code to identify organism, such as E. coli, 041.4)
595.82 Irradiation cystitis — (Use additional code to identify organism, such as E. coli, 041.4)
595.89 Other specified types of cystitis — (Use additional code to identify organism, such as E. coli, 041.4)
595.9 Unspecified cystitis — (Use additional code to identify organism, such as E. coli, 041.4) ▽
596.1 Intestinovesical fistula — (Use additional code to identify urinary incontinence: 625.6, 788.30-788.39)
596.2 Vesical fistula, not elsewhere classified — (Use additional code to identify urinary incontinence: 625.6, 788.30-788.39)
596.3 Diverticulum of bladder — (Use additional code to identify urinary incontinence: 625.6, 788.30-788.39)
596.4 Atony of bladder — (Use additional code to identify urinary incontinence: 625.6, 788.30-788.39)
596.51 Hypertonicity of bladder — (Use additional code to identify urinary incontinence: 625.6, 788.30-788.39)
596.52 Low bladder compliance — (Use additional code to identify urinary incontinence: 625.6, 788.30-788.39)
596.53 Paralysis of bladder — (Use additional code to identify urinary incontinence: 625.6, 788.30-788.39)
596.54 Neurogenic bladder, NOS — (Use additional code to identify urinary incontinence: 625.6, 788.30-788.39) ▽
596.55 Detrusor sphincter dyssynergia — (Use additional code to identify urinary incontinence: 625.6, 788.30-788.39)
596.59 Other functional disorder of bladder — (Use additional code to identify urinary incontinence: 625.6, 788.30-788.39)
597.81 Urethral syndrome NOS
597.89 Other urethritis
598.00 Urethral stricture due to unspecified infection — (Use additional code to identify urinary incontinence: 625.6, 788.30-788.39) ▽
598.01 Urethral stricture due to infective diseases classified elsewhere — (Code first underlying disease: 095.8, 098.2, 120.0-120.9. Use additional code to identify urinary incontinence: 625.6, 788.30-788.39) ☒
598.1 Traumatic urethral stricture — (Use additional code to identify urinary incontinence: 625.6, 788.30-788.39)
598.2 Postoperative urethral stricture — (Use additional code to identify urinary incontinence: 625.6, 788.30-788.39)
598.8 Other specified causes of urethral stricture — (Use additional code to identify urinary incontinence: 625.6, 788.30-788.39)
598.9 Unspecified urethral stricture — (Use additional code to identify urinary incontinence: 625.6, 788.30-788.39) ▽
599.0 Urinary tract infection, site not specified — (Use additional code to identify organism, such as E. coli, 041.4) ▽
599.1 Urethral fistula
599.6 Unspecified urinary obstruction — (Use additional code to identify urinary incontinence: 625.6, 788.30-788.39) ▽
599.7 Hematuria
599.81 Urethral hypermobility — (Use additional code to identify urinary incontinence: 625.6, 788.30-788.39)
599.82 Intrinsic (urethral) sphincter deficiency (ISD) — (Use additional code to identify urinary incontinence: 625.6, 788.30-788.39)
599.83 Urethral instability — (Use additional code to identify urinary incontinence: 625.6, 788.30-788.39)
599.84 Other specified disorders of urethra — (Use additional code to identify urinary incontinence: 625.6, 788.30-788.39)
599.89 Other specified disorders of urinary tract — (Use additional code to identify urinary incontinence: 625.6, 788.30-788.39)
600.00 Hypertrophy (benign) of prostate without urinary obstruction — (Use additional code to identify urinary incontinence: 788.30-788.39) ♂
600.01 Hypertrophy (benign) of prostate with urinary obstruction — (Use additional code to identify urinary incontinence: 788.30-788.39) ♂
600.10 Nodular prostate without urinary obstruction — (Use additional code to identify urinary incontinence: 788.30-788.39) ♂
600.11 Nodular prostate with urinary obstruction — (Use additional code to identify urinary incontinence: 788.30-788.39) ♂
600.20 Benign localized hyperplasia of prostate without urinary obstruction — (Use additional code to identify urinary incontinence: 788.30-788.39) ♂
600.21 Benign localized hyperplasia of prostate with urinary obstruction — (Use additional code to identify urinary incontinence: 788.30-788.39) ♂
600.3 Cyst of prostate — (Use additional code to identify urinary incontinence: 788.30-788.39) ♂
600.90 Hyperplasia of prostate, unspecified, without urinary obstruction — (Use additional code to identify urinary incontinence: 788.30-788.39) ▽ ♂
600.91 Hyperplasia of prostate, unspecified, with urinary obstruction — (Use additional code to identify urinary incontinence: 788.30-788.39) ▽ ♂
601.1 Chronic prostatitis — (Use additional code to identify organism: 041.0, 041.1) ♂
601.9 Unspecified prostatitis — (Use additional code to identify organism: 041.0, 041.1) ▽ ♂
618.01 Cystocele without mention of uterine prolapse, midline
618.02 Cystocele without mention of uterine prolapse, lateral
618.03 Urethrocele without mention of uterine prolapse
619.0 Urinary-genital tract fistula, female ♀
625.6 Female stress incontinence ♀
753.5 Exstrophy of urinary bladder
753.6 Congenital atresia and stenosis of urethra and bladder neck
753.8 Other specified congenital anomaly of bladder and urethra
753.9 Unspecified congenital anomaly of urinary system ▽
788.0 Renal colic
788.1 Dysuria
788.21 Incomplete bladder emptying
788.29 Other specified retention of urine
788.31 Urge incontinence
788.32 Stress incontinence, male ♂
788.33 Mixed incontinence urge and stress (male)(female)
788.34 Incontinence without sensory awareness
788.35 Post-void dribbling
788.36 Nocturnal enuresis
788.37 Continuous leakage
788.38 Overflow incontinence
788.39 Other urinary incontinence
788.41 Urinary frequency
788.42 Polyuria
788.43 Nocturia

▽ Unspecified code
♀ Female diagnosis
☒ Manifestation code
♂ Male diagnosis

788.5 Oliguria and anuria
788.61 Splitting of urinary stream
788.62 Slowing of urinary stream
788.63 Urgency of urination
788.69 Other abnormality of urination
788.7 Urethral discharge
788.8 Extravasation of urine
788.9 Other symptoms involving urinary system
789.03 Abdominal pain, right lower quadrant
789.04 Abdominal pain, left lower quadrant
789.05 Abdominal pain, periumbilic
789.07 Abdominal pain, generalized
789.09 Abdominal pain, other specified site
789.30 Abdominal or pelvic swelling, mass or lump, unspecified site ▽
789.33 Abdominal or pelvic swelling, mass, or lump, right lower quadrant
789.34 Abdominal or pelvic swelling, mass, or lump, left lower quadrant
789.35 Abdominal or pelvic swelling, mass or lump, periumbilic
789.37 Abdominal or pelvic swelling, mass, or lump, epigastric, generalized
789.39 Abdominal or pelvic swelling, mass, or lump, other specified site
793.5 Nonspecific abnormal findings on radiological and other examination of genitourinary organs
867.0 Bladder and urethra injury without mention of open wound into cavity
867.1 Bladder and urethra injury with open wound into cavity
959.12 Other injury of abdomen
959.19 Other injury of other sites of trunk
997.5 Urinary complications — (Use additional code to identify complications)
V10.51 Personal history of malignant neoplasm of bladder
V42.0 Kidney replaced by transplant — (This code is intended for use when these conditions are recorded as diagnoses or problems)
V45.89 Other postsurgical status — (This code is intended for use when these conditions are recorded as diagnoses or problems)
V55.5 Attention to cystostomy
V55.6 Attention to other artificial opening of urinary tract
V67.00 Follow-up examination, following unspecified surgery ▽
V67.09 Follow-up examination, following other surgery
V67.1 Radiotherapy follow-up examination

ICD-9-CM Procedural

87.76 Retrograde cystourethrogram
87.77 Other cystogram

HCPCS Level II Supplies & Services

A4641 Supply of radiopharmaceutical diagnostic imaging agent, not otherwise classified
A4642 Supply of satumomab pendetide, radiopharmaceutical diagnostic imaging agent, per dose
A9525 Supply of low or iso-osmolar contrast material, 10 mg of iodine

51700

51700 Bladder irrigation, simple, lavage and/or instillation

ICD-9-CM Diagnostic

185 Malignant neoplasm of prostate ♂
188.0 Malignant neoplasm of trigone of urinary bladder
188.1 Malignant neoplasm of dome of urinary bladder
188.2 Malignant neoplasm of lateral wall of urinary bladder
188.3 Malignant neoplasm of anterior wall of urinary bladder
188.4 Malignant neoplasm of posterior wall of urinary bladder
188.5 Malignant neoplasm of bladder neck
188.6 Malignant neoplasm of ureteric orifice
188.7 Malignant neoplasm of urachus
188.8 Malignant neoplasm of other specified sites of bladder
188.9 Malignant neoplasm of bladder, part unspecified ▽
233.7 Carcinoma in situ of bladder
344.61 Cauda equina syndrome with neurogenic bladder
593.3 Stricture or kinking of ureter
595.0 Acute cystitis — (Use additional code to identify organism, such as E. coli, 041.4)
595.1 Chronic interstitial cystitis — (Use additional code to identify organism, such as E. coli, 041.4)
595.2 Other chronic cystitis — (Use additional code to identify organism, such as E. coli, 041.4)
595.3 Trigonitis — (Use additional code to identify organism, such as E. coli, 041.4)
595.4 Cystitis in diseases classified elsewhere — (Code first underlying disease: 006.8, 039.8, 120.0-120.9, 122.3, 122.6. Use additional code to identify organism, such as E. coli, 041.4) ☒
595.81 Cystitis cystica — (Use additional code to identify organism, such as E. coli, 041.4)
595.82 Irradiation cystitis — (Use additional code to identify organism, such as E. coli, 041.4)
595.89 Other specified types of cystitis — (Use additional code to identify organism, such as E. coli, 041.4)
595.9 Unspecified cystitis — (Use additional code to identify organism, such as E. coli, 041.4) ▽
596.0 Bladder neck obstruction — (Use additional code to identify urinary incontinence: 625.6, 788.30-788.39)
596.4 Atony of bladder — (Use additional code to identify urinary incontinence: 625.6, 788.30-788.39)
596.7 Hemorrhage into bladder wall — (Use additional code to identify urinary incontinence: 625.6, 788.30-788.39)
596.8 Other specified disorder of bladder — (Use additional code to identify urinary incontinence: 625.6, 788.30-788.39)
597.80 Unspecified urethritis ▽
597.81 Urethral syndrome NOS
598.00 Urethral stricture due to unspecified infection — (Use additional code to identify urinary incontinence: 625.6, 788.30-788.39) ▽
598.01 Urethral stricture due to infective diseases classified elsewhere — (Code first underlying disease: 095.8, 098.2, 120.0-120.9. Use additional code to identify urinary incontinence: 625.6, 788.30-788.39) ☒
598.1 Traumatic urethral stricture — (Use additional code to identify urinary incontinence: 625.6, 788.30-788.39)
598.2 Postoperative urethral stricture — (Use additional code to identify urinary incontinence: 625.6, 788.30-788.39)
598.8 Other specified causes of urethral stricture — (Use additional code to identify urinary incontinence: 625.6, 788.30-788.39)
598.9 Unspecified urethral stricture — (Use additional code to identify urinary incontinence: 625.6, 788.30-788.39) ▽
599.0 Urinary tract infection, site not specified — (Use additional code to identify organism, such as E. coli, 041.4) ▽
599.7 Hematuria
600.01 Hypertrophy (benign) of prostate with urinary obstruction — (Use additional code to identify urinary incontinence: 788.30-788.39) ♂
600.11 Nodular prostate with urinary obstruction — (Use additional code to identify urinary incontinence: 788.30-788.39) ♂
600.21 Benign localized hyperplasia of prostate with urinary obstruction — (Use additional code to identify urinary incontinence: 788.30-788.39) ♂
600.3 Cyst of prostate — (Use additional code to identify urinary incontinence: 788.30-788.39) ♂
600.91 Hyperplasia of prostate, unspecified, with urinary obstruction — (Use additional code to identify urinary incontinence: 788.30-788.39) ▽ ♂
601.1 Chronic prostatitis — (Use additional code to identify organism: 041.0, 041.1) ♂
618.01 Cystocele without mention of uterine prolapse, midline
618.02 Cystocele without mention of uterine prolapse, lateral
618.03 Urethrocele without mention of uterine prolapse
625.6 Female stress incontinence ♀
788.21 Incomplete bladder emptying
788.29 Other specified retention of urine
788.41 Urinary frequency
788.42 Polyuria
V55.5 Attention to cystostomy

ICD-9-CM Procedural

96.47 Irrigation of cystostomy
96.49 Other genitourinary instillation

HCPCS Level II Supplies & Services

A4313 Insertion tray without drainage bag with indwelling catheter, Foley type, three-way, for continuous irrigation
A4316 Insertion tray with drainage bag with indwelling catheter, Foley type, three-way, for continuous irrigation
A4320 Irrigation tray with bulb or piston syringe, any purpose
A4321 Therapeutic agent for urinary catheter irrigation
A4322 Irrigation syringe, bulb or piston, each

▽ Unspecified code
♀ Female diagnosis
☒ Manifestation code
♂ Male diagnosis

51701–51703

51701 Insertion of non-indwelling bladder catheter (eg, straight catheterization for residual urine)
51702 Insertion of temporary indwelling bladder catheter; simple (eg, Foley)
51703 complicated (eg, altered anatomy, fractured catheter/balloon)

ICD-9-CM Diagnostic

185 Malignant neoplasm of prostate ♂
188.0 Malignant neoplasm of trigone of urinary bladder
188.1 Malignant neoplasm of dome of urinary bladder
188.2 Malignant neoplasm of lateral wall of urinary bladder
188.3 Malignant neoplasm of anterior wall of urinary bladder
188.4 Malignant neoplasm of posterior wall of urinary bladder
188.5 Malignant neoplasm of bladder neck
188.6 Malignant neoplasm of ureteric orifice
188.7 Malignant neoplasm of urachus
188.8 Malignant neoplasm of other specified sites of bladder
188.9 Malignant neoplasm of bladder, part unspecified ▽
189.0 Malignant neoplasm of kidney, except pelvis
189.1 Malignant neoplasm of renal pelvis
189.2 Malignant neoplasm of ureter
189.3 Malignant neoplasm of urethra
189.4 Malignant neoplasm of paraurethral glands
189.8 Malignant neoplasm of other specified sites of urinary organs
233.7 Carcinoma in situ of bladder
344.61 Cauda equina syndrome with neurogenic bladder
589.9 Unspecified small kidney ▽
593.3 Stricture or kinking of ureter
594.0 Calculus in diverticulum of bladder
594.1 Other calculus in bladder
594.2 Calculus in urethra
594.8 Other lower urinary tract calculus
595.0 Acute cystitis — (Use additional code to identify organism, such as E. coli, 041.4)
595.1 Chronic interstitial cystitis — (Use additional code to identify organism, such as E. coli, 041.4)
595.2 Other chronic cystitis — (Use additional code to identify organism, such as E. coli, 041.4)
595.3 Trigonitis — (Use additional code to identify organism, such as E. coli, 041.4)
595.4 Cystitis in diseases classified elsewhere — (Code first underlying disease: 006.8, 039.8, 120.0-120.9, 122.3, 122.6. Use additional code to identify organism, such as E. coli, 041.4) ☒
595.81 Cystitis cystica — (Use additional code to identify organism, such as E. coli, 041.4)
595.89 Other specified types of cystitis — (Use additional code to identify organism, such as E. coli, 041.4)
596.4 Atony of bladder — (Use additional code to identify urinary incontinence: 625.6, 788.30-788.39)
596.51 Hypertonicity of bladder — (Use additional code to identify urinary incontinence: 625.6, 788.30-788.39)
596.52 Low bladder compliance — (Use additional code to identify urinary incontinence: 625.6, 788.30-788.39)
596.53 Paralysis of bladder — (Use additional code to identify urinary incontinence: 625.6, 788.30-788.39)
596.8 Other specified disorder of bladder — (Use additional code to identify urinary incontinence: 625.6, 788.30-788.39)
597.80 Unspecified urethritis ▽
597.81 Urethral syndrome NOS
598.00 Urethral stricture due to unspecified infection — (Use additional code to identify urinary incontinence: 625.6, 788.30-788.39) ▽
598.01 Urethral stricture due to infective diseases classified elsewhere — (Code first underlying disease: 095.8, 098.2, 120.0-120.9. Use additional code to identify urinary incontinence: 625.6, 788.30-788.39) ☒
598.1 Traumatic urethral stricture — (Use additional code to identify urinary incontinence: 625.6, 788.30-788.39)
598.2 Postoperative urethral stricture — (Use additional code to identify urinary incontinence: 625.6, 788.30-788.39)
598.8 Other specified causes of urethral stricture — (Use additional code to identify urinary incontinence: 625.6, 788.30-788.39)
598.9 Unspecified urethral stricture — (Use additional code to identify urinary incontinence: 625.6, 788.30-788.39) ▽
599.1 Urethral fistula
599.2 Urethral diverticulum
599.3 Urethral caruncle
599.4 Urethral false passage
599.5 Prolapsed urethral mucosa
599.7 Hematuria
600.00 Hypertrophy (benign) of prostate without urinary obstruction — (Use additional code to identify urinary incontinence: 788.30-788.39) ♂
600.01 Hypertrophy (benign) of prostate with urinary obstruction — (Use additional code to identify urinary incontinence: 788.30-788.39) ♂
600.10 Nodular prostate without urinary obstruction — (Use additional code to identify urinary incontinence: 788.30-788.39) ♂
600.11 Nodular prostate with urinary obstruction — (Use additional code to identify urinary incontinence: 788.30-788.39) ♂
600.20 Benign localized hyperplasia of prostate without urinary obstruction — (Use additional code to identify urinary incontinence: 788.30-788.39) ♂
600.21 Benign localized hyperplasia of prostate with urinary obstruction — (Use additional code to identify urinary incontinence: 788.30-788.39) ♂
600.3 Cyst of prostate — (Use additional code to identify urinary incontinence: 788.30-788.39) ♂
600.90 Hyperplasia of prostate, unspecified, without urinary obstruction — (Use additional code to identify urinary incontinence: 788.30-788.39) ▽ ♂
600.91 Hyperplasia of prostate, unspecified, with urinary obstruction — (Use additional code to identify urinary incontinence: 788.30-788.39) ▽ ♂
601.1 Chronic prostatitis — (Use additional code to identify organism: 041.0, 041.1) ♂
618.00 Prolapse of vaginal walls without mention of uterine prolapse, unspecified
618.01 Cystocele without mention of uterine prolapse, midline
618.02 Cystocele without mention of uterine prolapse, lateral
618.03 Urethrocele without mention of uterine prolapse
618.04 Rectocele without mention of uterine prolapse
618.05 Perineocele without mention of uterine prolapse
618.09 Other prolapse of vaginal walls without mention of uterine prolapse
618.81 Incompetence or weakening of pubocervical tissue
618.82 Incompetence or weakening of rectovaginal tissue
618.83 Pelvic muscle wasting
618.89 Other specified genital prolapse
625.6 Female stress incontinence ♀
788.1 Dysuria
788.21 Incomplete bladder emptying
788.29 Other specified retention of urine
788.30 Unspecified urinary incontinence ▽
788.37 Continuous leakage
788.38 Overflow incontinence
788.41 Urinary frequency
788.42 Polyuria
867.0 Bladder and urethra injury without mention of open wound into cavity
867.1 Bladder and urethra injury with open wound into cavity
952.4 Cauda equina spinal cord injury without spinal bone injury
997.5 Urinary complications — (Use additional code to identify complications)

ICD-9-CM Procedural

57.94 Insertion of indwelling urinary catheter
57.95 Replacement of indwelling urinary catheter
57.99 Other operations on bladder

HCPCS Level II Supplies & Services

A4310 Insertion tray without drainage bag and without catheter (accessories only)
A4311 Insertion tray without drainage bag with indwelling catheter, Foley type, two-way latex with coating (Teflon, silicone, silicone elastomer or hydrophilic, etc.)
A4312 Insertion tray without drainage bag with indwelling catheter, Foley type, two-way, all silicone
A4313 Insertion tray without drainage bag with indwelling catheter, Foley type, three-way, for continuous irrigation
A4314 Insertion tray with drainage bag with indwelling catheter, Foley type, two-way latex with coating (Teflon, silicone, silicone elastomer or hydrophilic, etc.)

51705–51710

51705 Change of cystostomy tube; simple
51710 complicated

ICD-9-CM Diagnostic

185 Malignant neoplasm of prostate ♂
188.0 Malignant neoplasm of trigone of urinary bladder
188.1 Malignant neoplasm of dome of urinary bladder
188.2 Malignant neoplasm of lateral wall of urinary bladder
188.3 Malignant neoplasm of anterior wall of urinary bladder
188.4 Malignant neoplasm of posterior wall of urinary bladder
188.5 Malignant neoplasm of bladder neck
188.6 Malignant neoplasm of ureteric orifice
188.7 Malignant neoplasm of urachus

▽ Unspecified code
♀ Female diagnosis
☒ Manifestation code
♂ Male diagnosis

188.8 Malignant neoplasm of other specified sites of bladder
188.9 Malignant neoplasm of bladder, part unspecified ▽
344.1 Paraplegia
344.61 Cauda equina syndrome with neurogenic bladder
555.0 Regional enteritis of small intestine
596.0 Bladder neck obstruction — (Use additional code to identify urinary incontinence: 625.6, 788.30-788.39)
596.1 Intestinovesical fistula — (Use additional code to identify urinary incontinence: 625.6, 788.30-788.39)
596.2 Vesical fistula, not elsewhere classified — (Use additional code to identify urinary incontinence: 625.6, 788.30-788.39)
596.3 Diverticulum of bladder — (Use additional code to identify urinary incontinence: 625.6, 788.30-788.39)
596.4 Atony of bladder — (Use additional code to identify urinary incontinence: 625.6, 788.30-788.39)
596.51 Hypertonicity of bladder — (Use additional code to identify urinary incontinence: 625.6, 788.30-788.39)
596.52 Low bladder compliance — (Use additional code to identify urinary incontinence: 625.6, 788.30-788.39)
596.53 Paralysis of bladder — (Use additional code to identify urinary incontinence: 625.6, 788.30-788.39)
596.54 Neurogenic bladder, NOS — (Use additional code to identify urinary incontinence: 625.6, 788.30-788.39) ▽
596.55 Detrusor sphincter dyssynergia — (Use additional code to identify urinary incontinence: 625.6, 788.30-788.39)
596.59 Other functional disorder of bladder — (Use additional code to identify urinary incontinence: 625.6, 788.30-788.39)
596.7 Hemorrhage into bladder wall — (Use additional code to identify urinary incontinence: 625.6, 788.30-788.39)
596.8 Other specified disorder of bladder — (Use additional code to identify urinary incontinence: 625.6, 788.30-788.39)
598.1 Traumatic urethral stricture — (Use additional code to identify urinary incontinence: 625.6, 788.30-788.39)
599.0 Urinary tract infection, site not specified — (Use additional code to identify organism, such as E. coli, 041.4) ▽
599.1 Urethral fistula
599.2 Urethral diverticulum
599.7 Hematuria
600.01 Hypertrophy (benign) of prostate with urinary obstruction — (Use additional code to identify urinary incontinence: 788.30-788.39) ♂
600.11 Nodular prostate with urinary obstruction — (Use additional code to identify urinary incontinence: 788.30-788.39) ♂
600.21 Benign localized hyperplasia of prostate with urinary obstruction — (Use additional code to identify urinary incontinence: 788.30-788.39) ♂
600.3 Cyst of prostate — (Use additional code to identify urinary incontinence: 788.30-788.39) ♂
600.91 Hyperplasia of prostate, unspecified, with urinary obstruction — (Use additional code to identify urinary incontinence: 788.30-788.39) ▽ ♂
625.6 Female stress incontinence ♀
788.20 Unspecified retention of urine ▽
788.21 Incomplete bladder emptying
788.29 Other specified retention of urine
788.30 Unspecified urinary incontinence ▽
788.31 Urge incontinence
788.32 Stress incontinence, male ♂
788.33 Mixed incontinence urge and stress (male)(female)
788.38 Overflow incontinence
788.39 Other urinary incontinence
996.39 Mechanical complication of genitourinary device, implant, and graft, other
996.65 Infection and inflammatory reaction due to other genitourinary device, implant, and graft — (Use additional code to identify specified infections)
996.76 Other complications due to genitourinary device, implant, and graft
V10.51 Personal history of malignant neoplasm of bladder
V55.5 Attention to cystostomy

ICD-9-CM Procedural

59.94 Replacement of cystostomy tube

HCPCS Level II Supplies & Services

A4550 Surgical trays

51715

51715 Endoscopic injection of implant material into the submucosal tissues of the urethra and/or bladder neck

ICD-9-CM Diagnostic

185 Malignant neoplasm of prostate ♂
188.9 Malignant neoplasm of bladder, part unspecified ▽
344.1 Paraplegia
596.0 Bladder neck obstruction — (Use additional code to identify urinary incontinence: 625.6, 788.30-788.39)
596.4 Atony of bladder — (Use additional code to identify urinary incontinence: 625.6, 788.30-788.39)
596.51 Hypertonicity of bladder — (Use additional code to identify urinary incontinence: 625.6, 788.30-788.39)
596.52 Low bladder compliance — (Use additional code to identify urinary incontinence: 625.6, 788.30-788.39)
596.53 Paralysis of bladder — (Use additional code to identify urinary incontinence: 625.6, 788.30-788.39)
596.54 Neurogenic bladder, NOS — (Use additional code to identify urinary incontinence: 625.6, 788.30-788.39) ▽
596.55 Detrusor sphincter dyssynergia — (Use additional code to identify urinary incontinence: 625.6, 788.30-788.39)
599.1 Urethral fistula
625.6 Female stress incontinence ♀
788.29 Other specified retention of urine
788.32 Stress incontinence, male ♂
996.39 Mechanical complication of genitourinary device, implant, and graft, other
V10.46 Personal history of malignant neoplasm of prostate ♂

ICD-9-CM Procedural

59.72 Injection of implant into urethra and/or bladder neck

51720

51720 Bladder instillation of anticarcinogenic agent (including detention time)

ICD-9-CM Diagnostic

188.0 Malignant neoplasm of trigone of urinary bladder
188.1 Malignant neoplasm of dome of urinary bladder
188.2 Malignant neoplasm of lateral wall of urinary bladder
188.3 Malignant neoplasm of anterior wall of urinary bladder
188.4 Malignant neoplasm of posterior wall of urinary bladder
188.5 Malignant neoplasm of bladder neck
188.6 Malignant neoplasm of ureteric orifice
188.7 Malignant neoplasm of urachus
188.8 Malignant neoplasm of other specified sites of bladder
188.9 Malignant neoplasm of bladder, part unspecified ▽
198.1 Secondary malignant neoplasm of other urinary organs
233.7 Carcinoma in situ of bladder
233.9 Carcinoma in situ of other and unspecified urinary organs ▽
V58.1 Chemotherapy

ICD-9-CM Procedural

96.49 Other genitourinary instillation
99.25 Injection or infusion of cancer chemotherapeutic substance

HCPCS Level II Supplies & Services

J9031 BCG live (intravesical), per instillation
J9340 Thiotepa, 15 mg

51725–51726

51725 Simple cystometrogram (CMG) (eg, spinal manometer)
51726 Complex cystometrogram (eg, calibrated electronic equipment)

ICD-9-CM Diagnostic

185 Malignant neoplasm of prostate ♂
344.61 Cauda equina syndrome with neurogenic bladder
595.1 Chronic interstitial cystitis — (Use additional code to identify organism, such as E. coli, 041.4)
595.2 Other chronic cystitis — (Use additional code to identify organism, such as E. coli, 041.4)
595.3 Trigonitis — (Use additional code to identify organism, such as E. coli, 041.4)
595.4 Cystitis in diseases classified elsewhere — (Code first underlying disease: 006.8, 039.8, 120.0-120.9, 122.3, 122.6. Use additional code to identify organism, such as E. coli, 041.4) ☒
595.81 Cystitis cystica — (Use additional code to identify organism, such as E. coli, 041.4)

595.82 Irradiation cystitis — (Use additional code to identify organism, such as E. coli, 041.4)
595.89 Other specified types of cystitis — (Use additional code to identify organism, such as E. coli, 041.4)
596.0 Bladder neck obstruction — (Use additional code to identify urinary incontinence: 625.6, 788.30-788.39)
596.1 Intestinovesical fistula — (Use additional code to identify urinary incontinence: 625.6, 788.30-788.39)
596.2 Vesical fistula, not elsewhere classified — (Use additional code to identify urinary incontinence: 625.6, 788.30-788.39)
596.3 Diverticulum of bladder — (Use additional code to identify urinary incontinence: 625.6, 788.30-788.39)
596.4 Atony of bladder — (Use additional code to identify urinary incontinence: 625.6, 788.30-788.39)
596.51 Hypertonicity of bladder — (Use additional code to identify urinary incontinence: 625.6, 788.30-788.39)
596.52 Low bladder compliance — (Use additional code to identify urinary incontinence: 625.6, 788.30-788.39)
596.53 Paralysis of bladder — (Use additional code to identify urinary incontinence: 625.6, 788.30-788.39)
596.54 Neurogenic bladder, NOS — (Use additional code to identify urinary incontinence: 625.6, 788.30-788.39) ▽
596.55 Detrusor sphincter dyssynergia — (Use additional code to identify urinary incontinence: 625.6, 788.30-788.39)
596.59 Other functional disorder of bladder — (Use additional code to identify urinary incontinence: 625.6, 788.30-788.39)
598.00 Urethral stricture due to unspecified infection — (Use additional code to identify urinary incontinence: 625.6, 788.30-788.39) ▽
598.1 Traumatic urethral stricture — (Use additional code to identify urinary incontinence: 625.6, 788.30-788.39)
598.2 Postoperative urethral stricture — (Use additional code to identify urinary incontinence: 625.6, 788.30-788.39)
598.8 Other specified causes of urethral stricture — (Use additional code to identify urinary incontinence: 625.6, 788.30-788.39)
598.9 Unspecified urethral stricture — (Use additional code to identify urinary incontinence: 625.6, 788.30-788.39) ▽
599.0 Urinary tract infection, site not specified — (Use additional code to identify organism, such as E. coli, 041.4) ▽
599.6 Unspecified urinary obstruction — (Use additional code to identify urinary incontinence: 625.6, 788.30-788.39) ▽
599.7 Hematuria
600.00 Hypertrophy (benign) of prostate without urinary obstruction — (Use additional code to identify urinary incontinence: 788.30-788.39) ♂
600.01 Hypertrophy (benign) of prostate with urinary obstruction — (Use additional code to identify urinary incontinence: 788.30-788.39) ♂
600.10 Nodular prostate without urinary obstruction — (Use additional code to identify urinary incontinence: 788.30-788.39) ♂
600.11 Nodular prostate with urinary obstruction — (Use additional code to identify urinary incontinence: 788.30-788.39) ♂
600.20 Benign localized hyperplasia of prostate without urinary obstruction — (Use additional code to identify urinary incontinence: 788.30-788.39) ♂
600.21 Benign localized hyperplasia of prostate with urinary obstruction — (Use additional code to identify urinary incontinence: 788.30-788.39) ♂
600.3 Cyst of prostate — (Use additional code to identify urinary incontinence: 788.30-788.39) ♂
600.90 Hyperplasia of prostate, unspecified, without urinary obstruction — (Use additional code to identify urinary incontinence: 788.30-788.39) ▽ ♂
600.91 Hyperplasia of prostate, unspecified, with urinary obstruction — (Use additional code to identify urinary incontinence: 788.30-788.39) ▽ ♂
601.1 Chronic prostatitis — (Use additional code to identify organism: 041.0, 041.1) ♂
618.00 Prolapse of vaginal walls without mention of uterine prolapse, unspecified
618.01 Cystocele without mention of uterine prolapse, midline
618.02 Cystocele without mention of uterine prolapse, lateral
618.03 Urethrocele without mention of uterine prolapse
618.09 Other prolapse of vaginal walls without mention of uterine prolapse
618.1 Uterine prolapse without mention of vaginal wall prolapse — (Use additional code to identify urinary incontinence: 625.6, 788.31, 788.33-788.39) ♀
618.2 Uterovaginal prolapse, incomplete — (Use additional code to identify urinary incontinence: 625.6, 788.31, 788.33-788.39) ♀
618.3 Uterovaginal prolapse, complete — (Use additional code to identify urinary incontinence: 625.6, 788.31, 788.33-788.39) ♀
618.4 Uterovaginal prolapse, unspecified — (Use additional code to identify urinary incontinence: 625.6, 788.31, 788.33-788.39) ▽ ♀
618.5 Prolapse of vaginal vault after hysterectomy — (Use additional code to identify urinary incontinence: 625.6, 788.31, 788.33-788.39) ♀
618.6 Vaginal enterocele, congenital or acquired — (Use additional code to identify urinary incontinence: 625.6, 788.31, 788.33-788.39) ♀
618.7 Genital prolapse, old laceration of muscles of pelvic floor — (Use additional code to identify urinary incontinence: 625.6, 788.31, 788.33-788.39) ♀
618.81 Incompetence or weakening of pubocervical tissue
618.82 Incompetence or weakening of rectovaginal tissue
618.83 Pelvic muscle wasting
618.89 Other specified genital prolapse
618.9 Unspecified genital prolapse — (Use additional code to identify urinary incontinence: 625.6, 788.31, 788.33-788.39) ▽ ♀
619.0 Urinary-genital tract fistula, female ♀
625.6 Female stress incontinence ♀
741.90 Spina bifida without mention of hydrocephalus, unspecified region ▽
753.5 Exstrophy of urinary bladder
753.6 Congenital atresia and stenosis of urethra and bladder neck
753.8 Other specified congenital anomaly of bladder and urethra
788.1 Dysuria
788.20 Unspecified retention of urine ▽
788.21 Incomplete bladder emptying
788.29 Other specified retention of urine
788.30 Unspecified urinary incontinence ▽
788.31 Urge incontinence
788.32 Stress incontinence, male ♂
788.33 Mixed incontinence urge and stress (male)(female)
788.34 Incontinence without sensory awareness
788.35 Post-void dribbling
788.36 Nocturnal enuresis
788.37 Continuous leakage
788.38 Overflow incontinence
788.39 Other urinary incontinence
788.41 Urinary frequency
788.42 Polyuria
788.43 Nocturia
788.61 Splitting of urinary stream
788.62 Slowing of urinary stream
788.63 Urgency of urination
788.69 Other abnormality of urination
788.9 Other symptoms involving urinary system
V67.00 Follow-up examination, following unspecified surgery ▽
V67.09 Follow-up examination, following other surgery

ICD-9-CM Procedural

89.22 Cystometrogram

HCPCS Level II Supplies & Services

A4550 Surgical trays

51736–51741

51736 Simple uroflowmetry (UFR) (eg, stop-watch flow rate, mechanical uroflowmeter)
51741 Complex uroflowmetry (eg, calibrated electronic equipment)

ICD-9-CM Diagnostic

185 Malignant neoplasm of prostate ♂
344.61 Cauda equina syndrome with neurogenic bladder
595.1 Chronic interstitial cystitis — (Use additional code to identify organism, such as E. coli, 041.4)
595.2 Other chronic cystitis — (Use additional code to identify organism, such as E. coli, 041.4)
595.3 Trigonitis — (Use additional code to identify organism, such as E. coli, 041.4)
595.4 Cystitis in diseases classified elsewhere — (Code first underlying disease: 006.8, 039.8, 120.0-120.9, 122.3, 122.6. Use additional code to identify organism, such as E. coli, 041.4) ☒
595.81 Cystitis cystica — (Use additional code to identify organism, such as E. coli, 041.4)
595.82 Irradiation cystitis — (Use additional code to identify organism, such as E. coli, 041.4)
595.89 Other specified types of cystitis — (Use additional code to identify organism, such as E. coli, 041.4)
595.9 Unspecified cystitis — (Use additional code to identify organism, such as E. coli, 041.4) ▽
596.0 Bladder neck obstruction — (Use additional code to identify urinary incontinence: 625.6, 788.30-788.39)
596.1 Intestinovesical fistula — (Use additional code to identify urinary incontinence: 625.6, 788.30-788.39)

▽ Unspecified code
♀ Female diagnosis
☒ Manifestation code
♂ Male diagnosis

596.2 Vesical fistula, not elsewhere classified — (Use additional code to identify urinary incontinence: 625.6, 788.30-788.39)
596.3 Diverticulum of bladder — (Use additional code to identify urinary incontinence: 625.6, 788.30-788.39)
596.4 Atony of bladder — (Use additional code to identify urinary incontinence: 625.6, 788.30-788.39)
596.51 Hypertonicity of bladder — (Use additional code to identify urinary incontinence: 625.6, 788.30-788.39)
596.52 Low bladder compliance — (Use additional code to identify urinary incontinence: 625.6, 788.30-788.39)
596.53 Paralysis of bladder — (Use additional code to identify urinary incontinence: 625.6, 788.30-788.39)
596.54 Neurogenic bladder, NOS — (Use additional code to identify urinary incontinence: 625.6, 788.30-788.39) ▽
596.55 Detrusor sphincter dyssynergia — (Use additional code to identify urinary incontinence: 625.6, 788.30-788.39)
596.59 Other functional disorder of bladder — (Use additional code to identify urinary incontinence: 625.6, 788.30-788.39)
596.8 Other specified disorder of bladder — (Use additional code to identify urinary incontinence: 625.6, 788.30-788.39)
598.00 Urethral stricture due to unspecified infection — (Use additional code to identify urinary incontinence: 625.6, 788.30-788.39) ▽
598.1 Traumatic urethral stricture — (Use additional code to identify urinary incontinence: 625.6, 788.30-788.39)
598.2 Postoperative urethral stricture — (Use additional code to identify urinary incontinence: 625.6, 788.30-788.39)
598.8 Other specified causes of urethral stricture — (Use additional code to identify urinary incontinence: 625.6, 788.30-788.39)
599.0 Urinary tract infection, site not specified — (Use additional code to identify organism, such as E. coli, 041.4) ▽
599.7 Hematuria
600.00 Hypertrophy (benign) of prostate without urinary obstruction — (Use additional code to identify urinary incontinence: 788.30-788.39) ♂
600.01 Hypertrophy (benign) of prostate with urinary obstruction — (Use additional code to identify urinary incontinence: 788.30-788.39) ♂
600.10 Nodular prostate without urinary obstruction — (Use additional code to identify urinary incontinence: 788.30-788.39) ♂
600.11 Nodular prostate with urinary obstruction — (Use additional code to identify urinary incontinence: 788.30-788.39) ♂
600.20 Benign localized hyperplasia of prostate without urinary obstruction — (Use additional code to identify urinary incontinence: 788.30-788.39) ♂
600.21 Benign localized hyperplasia of prostate with urinary obstruction — (Use additional code to identify urinary incontinence: 788.30-788.39) ♂
600.3 Cyst of prostate — (Use additional code to identify urinary incontinence: 788.30-788.39) ♂
600.90 Hyperplasia of prostate, unspecified, without urinary obstruction — (Use additional code to identify urinary incontinence: 788.30-788.39) ▽ ♂
600.91 Hyperplasia of prostate, unspecified, with urinary obstruction — (Use additional code to identify urinary incontinence: 788.30-788.39) ▽ ♂
601.1 Chronic prostatitis — (Use additional code to identify organism: 041.0, 041.1) ♂
618.00 Prolapse of vaginal walls without mention of uterine prolapse, unspecified
618.01 Cystocele without mention of uterine prolapse, midline
618.02 Cystocele without mention of uterine prolapse, lateral
618.03 Urethrocele without mention of uterine prolapse
618.09 Other prolapse of vaginal walls without mention of uterine prolapse
618.1 Uterine prolapse without mention of vaginal wall prolapse — (Use additional code to identify urinary incontinence: 625.6, 788.31, 788.33-788.39) ♀
618.2 Uterovaginal prolapse, incomplete — (Use additional code to identify urinary incontinence: 625.6, 788.31, 788.33-788.39) ♀
618.3 Uterovaginal prolapse, complete — (Use additional code to identify urinary incontinence: 625.6, 788.31, 788.33-788.39) ♀
618.4 Uterovaginal prolapse, unspecified — (Use additional code to identify urinary incontinence: 625.6, 788.31, 788.33-788.39) ▽ ♀
618.5 Prolapse of vaginal vault after hysterectomy — (Use additional code to identify urinary incontinence: 625.6, 788.31, 788.33-788.39) ♀
618.6 Vaginal enterocele, congenital or acquired — (Use additional code to identify urinary incontinence: 625.6, 788.31, 788.33-788.39) ♀
618.7 Genital prolapse, old laceration of muscles of pelvic floor — (Use additional code to identify urinary incontinence: 625.6, 788.31, 788.33-788.39) ♀
618.81 Incompetence or weakening of pubocervical tissue
618.82 Incompetence or weakening of rectovaginal tissue
618.83 Pelvic muscle wasting
618.89 Other specified genital prolapse
618.9 Unspecified genital prolapse — (Use additional code to identify urinary incontinence: 625.6, 788.31, 788.33-788.39) ▽ ♀
619.0 Urinary-genital tract fistula, female ♀
625.6 Female stress incontinence ♀
741.90 Spina bifida without mention of hydrocephalus, unspecified region ▽
753.5 Exstrophy of urinary bladder
753.6 Congenital atresia and stenosis of urethra and bladder neck
753.8 Other specified congenital anomaly of bladder and urethra
788.1 Dysuria
788.21 Incomplete bladder emptying
788.29 Other specified retention of urine
788.31 Urge incontinence
788.32 Stress incontinence, male ♂
788.33 Mixed incontinence urge and stress (male)(female)
788.34 Incontinence without sensory awareness
788.35 Post-void dribbling
788.36 Nocturnal enuresis
788.37 Continuous leakage
788.38 Overflow incontinence
788.39 Other urinary incontinence
788.41 Urinary frequency
788.42 Polyuria
788.43 Nocturia
788.61 Splitting of urinary stream
788.62 Slowing of urinary stream
788.63 Urgency of urination
788.69 Other abnormality of urination
788.9 Other symptoms involving urinary system
V67.00 Follow-up examination, following unspecified surgery ▽
V67.09 Follow-up examination, following other surgery

ICD-9-CM Procedural

89.24 Uroflowmetry (UFR)

HCPCS Level II Supplies & Services

A4550 Surgical trays

51772

51772 Urethral pressure profile studies (UPP) (urethral closure pressure profile), any technique

ICD-9-CM Diagnostic

185 Malignant neoplasm of prostate ♂
344.61 Cauda equina syndrome with neurogenic bladder
595.2 Other chronic cystitis — (Use additional code to identify organism, such as E. coli, 041.4)
595.3 Trigonitis — (Use additional code to identify organism, such as E. coli, 041.4)
595.4 Cystitis in diseases classified elsewhere — (Code first underlying disease: 006.8, 039.8, 120.0-120.9, 122.3, 122.6. Use additional code to identify organism, such as E. coli, 041.4) ☒
595.81 Cystitis cystica — (Use additional code to identify organism, such as E. coli, 041.4)
595.82 Irradiation cystitis — (Use additional code to identify organism, such as E. coli, 041.4)
595.89 Other specified types of cystitis — (Use additional code to identify organism, such as E. coli, 041.4)
596.0 Bladder neck obstruction — (Use additional code to identify urinary incontinence: 625.6, 788.30-788.39)
596.1 Intestinovesical fistula — (Use additional code to identify urinary incontinence: 625.6, 788.30-788.39)
596.2 Vesical fistula, not elsewhere classified — (Use additional code to identify urinary incontinence: 625.6, 788.30-788.39)
596.3 Diverticulum of bladder — (Use additional code to identify urinary incontinence: 625.6, 788.30-788.39)
596.4 Atony of bladder — (Use additional code to identify urinary incontinence: 625.6, 788.30-788.39)
596.51 Hypertonicity of bladder — (Use additional code to identify urinary incontinence: 625.6, 788.30-788.39)
596.52 Low bladder compliance — (Use additional code to identify urinary incontinence: 625.6, 788.30-788.39)
596.53 Paralysis of bladder — (Use additional code to identify urinary incontinence: 625.6, 788.30-788.39)
596.54 Neurogenic bladder, NOS — (Use additional code to identify urinary incontinence: 625.6, 788.30-788.39) ▽
596.55 Detrusor sphincter dyssynergia — (Use additional code to identify urinary incontinence: 625.6, 788.30-788.39)
596.59 Other functional disorder of bladder — (Use additional code to identify urinary incontinence: 625.6, 788.30-788.39)

▽ Unspecified code ☒ Manifestation code
♀ Female diagnosis ♂ Male diagnosis

598.00 Urethral stricture due to unspecified infection — (Use additional code to identify urinary incontinence: 625.6, 788.30-788.39) ▽
598.1 Traumatic urethral stricture — (Use additional code to identify urinary incontinence: 625.6, 788.30-788.39)
598.2 Postoperative urethral stricture — (Use additional code to identify urinary incontinence: 625.6, 788.30-788.39)
598.8 Other specified causes of urethral stricture — (Use additional code to identify urinary incontinence: 625.6, 788.30-788.39)
599.0 Urinary tract infection, site not specified — (Use additional code to identify organism, such as E. coli, 041.4) ▽
599.7 Hematuria
600.00 Hypertrophy (benign) of prostate without urinary obstruction — (Use additional code to identify urinary incontinence: 788.30-788.39) ♂
600.01 Hypertrophy (benign) of prostate with urinary obstruction — (Use additional code to identify urinary incontinence: 788.30-788.39) ♂
600.10 Nodular prostate without urinary obstruction — (Use additional code to identify urinary incontinence: 788.30-788.39) ♂
600.11 Nodular prostate with urinary obstruction — (Use additional code to identify urinary incontinence: 788.30-788.39) ♂
600.20 Benign localized hyperplasia of prostate without urinary obstruction — (Use additional code to identify urinary incontinence: 788.30-788.39) ♂
600.21 Benign localized hyperplasia of prostate with urinary obstruction — (Use additional code to identify urinary incontinence: 788.30-788.39) ♂
600.3 Cyst of prostate — (Use additional code to identify urinary incontinence: 788.30-788.39) ♂
600.90 Hyperplasia of prostate, unspecified, without urinary obstruction — (Use additional code to identify urinary incontinence: 788.30-788.39) ▽ ♂
600.91 Hyperplasia of prostate, unspecified, with urinary obstruction — (Use additional code to identify urinary incontinence: 788.30-788.39) ▽ ♂
618.00 Prolapse of vaginal walls without mention of uterine prolapse, unspecified
618.01 Cystocele without mention of uterine prolapse, midline
618.02 Cystocele without mention of uterine prolapse, lateral
618.03 Urethrocele without mention of uterine prolapse
618.05 Perineocele without mention of uterine prolapse
618.1 Uterine prolapse without mention of vaginal wall prolapse — (Use additional code to identify urinary incontinence: 625.6, 788.31, 788.33-788.39) ♀
618.2 Uterovaginal prolapse, incomplete — (Use additional code to identify urinary incontinence: 625.6, 788.31, 788.33-788.39) ♀
618.3 Uterovaginal prolapse, complete — (Use additional code to identify urinary incontinence: 625.6, 788.31, 788.33-788.39) ♀
618.4 Uterovaginal prolapse, unspecified — (Use additional code to identify urinary incontinence: 625.6, 788.31, 788.33-788.39) ▽ ♀
618.5 Prolapse of vaginal vault after hysterectomy — (Use additional code to identify urinary incontinence: 625.6, 788.31, 788.33-788.39) ♀
618.6 Vaginal enterocele, congenital or acquired — (Use additional code to identify urinary incontinence: 625.6, 788.31, 788.33-788.39) ♀
618.7 Genital prolapse, old laceration of muscles of pelvic floor — (Use additional code to identify urinary incontinence: 625.6, 788.31, 788.33-788.39) ♀
618.81 Incompetence or weakening of pubocervical tissue
618.82 Incompetence or weakening of rectovaginal tissue
618.83 Pelvic muscle wasting
618.89 Other specified genital prolapse
618.9 Unspecified genital prolapse — (Use additional code to identify urinary incontinence: 625.6, 788.31, 788.33-788.39) ▽ ♀
625.6 Female stress incontinence ♀
741.90 Spina bifida without mention of hydrocephalus, unspecified region ▽
753.5 Exstrophy of urinary bladder
753.6 Congenital atresia and stenosis of urethra and bladder neck
753.8 Other specified congenital anomaly of bladder and urethra
753.9 Unspecified congenital anomaly of urinary system ▽
788.1 Dysuria
788.21 Incomplete bladder emptying
788.29 Other specified retention of urine
788.31 Urge incontinence
788.32 Stress incontinence, male ♂
788.33 Mixed incontinence urge and stress (male)(female)
788.34 Incontinence without sensory awareness
788.35 Post-void dribbling
788.36 Nocturnal enuresis
788.37 Continuous leakage
788.38 Overflow incontinence
788.39 Other urinary incontinence
788.41 Urinary frequency
788.42 Polyuria
788.43 Nocturia
788.61 Splitting of urinary stream
788.62 Slowing of urinary stream
788.63 Urgency of urination
788.69 Other abnormality of urination
788.9 Other symptoms involving urinary system
V67.00 Follow-up examination, following unspecified surgery ▽
V67.09 Follow-up examination, following other surgery

ICD-9-CM Procedural

89.25 Urethral pressure profile (UPP)

HCPCS Level II Supplies & Services

A4550 Surgical trays

51784–51785

51784 Electromyography studies (EMG) of anal or urethral sphincter, other than needle, any technique
51785 Needle electromyography studies (EMG) of anal or urethral sphincter, any technique

ICD-9-CM Diagnostic

185 Malignant neoplasm of prostate ♂
344.61 Cauda equina syndrome with neurogenic bladder
564.6 Anal spasm
595.1 Chronic interstitial cystitis — (Use additional code to identify organism, such as E. coli, 041.4)
595.2 Other chronic cystitis — (Use additional code to identify organism, such as E. coli, 041.4)
595.3 Trigonitis — (Use additional code to identify organism, such as E. coli, 041.4)
595.4 Cystitis in diseases classified elsewhere — (Code first underlying disease: 006.8, 039.8, 120.0-120.9, 122.3, 122.6. Use additional code to identify organism, such as E. coli, 041.4) ☒
595.81 Cystitis cystica — (Use additional code to identify organism, such as E. coli, 041.4)
595.82 Irradiation cystitis — (Use additional code to identify organism, such as E. coli, 041.4)
595.89 Other specified types of cystitis — (Use additional code to identify organism, such as E. coli, 041.4)
596.0 Bladder neck obstruction — (Use additional code to identify urinary incontinence: 625.6, 788.30-788.39)
596.1 Intestinovesical fistula — (Use additional code to identify urinary incontinence: 625.6, 788.30-788.39)
596.2 Vesical fistula, not elsewhere classified — (Use additional code to identify urinary incontinence: 625.6, 788.30-788.39)
596.3 Diverticulum of bladder — (Use additional code to identify urinary incontinence: 625.6, 788.30-788.39)
596.4 Atony of bladder — (Use additional code to identify urinary incontinence: 625.6, 788.30-788.39)
596.51 Hypertonicity of bladder — (Use additional code to identify urinary incontinence: 625.6, 788.30-788.39)
596.52 Low bladder compliance — (Use additional code to identify urinary incontinence: 625.6, 788.30-788.39)
596.53 Paralysis of bladder — (Use additional code to identify urinary incontinence: 625.6, 788.30-788.39)
596.54 Neurogenic bladder, NOS — (Use additional code to identify urinary incontinence: 625.6, 788.30-788.39) ▽
596.55 Detrusor sphincter dyssynergia — (Use additional code to identify urinary incontinence: 625.6, 788.30-788.39)
596.59 Other functional disorder of bladder — (Use additional code to identify urinary incontinence: 625.6, 788.30-788.39)
596.8 Other specified disorder of bladder — (Use additional code to identify urinary incontinence: 625.6, 788.30-788.39)
598.1 Traumatic urethral stricture — (Use additional code to identify urinary incontinence: 625.6, 788.30-788.39)
598.2 Postoperative urethral stricture — (Use additional code to identify urinary incontinence: 625.6, 788.30-788.39)
598.8 Other specified causes of urethral stricture — (Use additional code to identify urinary incontinence: 625.6, 788.30-788.39)
599.0 Urinary tract infection, site not specified — (Use additional code to identify organism, such as E. coli, 041.4) ▽
599.7 Hematuria
600.00 Hypertrophy (benign) of prostate without urinary obstruction — (Use additional code to identify urinary incontinence: 788.30-788.39) ♂
600.01 Hypertrophy (benign) of prostate with urinary obstruction — (Use additional code to identify urinary incontinence: 788.30-788.39) ♂
600.10 Nodular prostate without urinary obstruction — (Use additional code to identify urinary incontinence: 788.30-788.39) ♂

▽ Unspecified code
♀ Female diagnosis
☒ Manifestation code
♂ Male diagnosis

600.11 Nodular prostate with urinary obstruction — (Use additional code to identify urinary incontinence: 788.30-788.39) ♂
600.20 Benign localized hyperplasia of prostate without urinary obstruction — (Use additional code to identify urinary incontinence: 788.30-788.39) ♂
600.21 Benign localized hyperplasia of prostate with urinary obstruction — (Use additional code to identify urinary incontinence: 788.30-788.39) ♂
600.3 Cyst of prostate — (Use additional code to identify urinary incontinence: 788.30-788.39) ♂
600.90 Hyperplasia of prostate, unspecified, without urinary obstruction — (Use additional code to identify urinary incontinence: 788.30-788.39) ▽ ♂
600.91 Hyperplasia of prostate, unspecified, with urinary obstruction — (Use additional code to identify urinary incontinence: 788.30-788.39) ▽ ♂
601.1 Chronic prostatitis — (Use additional code to identify organism: 041.0, 041.1) ♂
618.00 Prolapse of vaginal walls without mention of uterine prolapse, unspecified
618.01 Cystocele without mention of uterine prolapse, midline
618.02 Cystocele without mention of uterine prolapse, lateral
618.03 Urethrocele without mention of uterine prolapse
618.04 Rectocele without mention of uterine prolapse
618.05 Perineocele without mention of uterine prolapse
618.09 Other prolapse of vaginal walls without mention of uterine prolapse
618.1 Uterine prolapse without mention of vaginal wall prolapse — (Use additional code to identify urinary incontinence: 625.6, 788.31, 788.33-788.39) ♀
618.2 Uterovaginal prolapse, incomplete — (Use additional code to identify urinary incontinence: 625.6, 788.31, 788.33-788.39) ♀
618.3 Uterovaginal prolapse, complete — (Use additional code to identify urinary incontinence: 625.6, 788.31, 788.33-788.39) ♀
618.4 Uterovaginal prolapse, unspecified — (Use additional code to identify urinary incontinence: 625.6, 788.31, 788.33-788.39) ▽ ♀
618.5 Prolapse of vaginal vault after hysterectomy — (Use additional code to identify urinary incontinence: 625.6, 788.31, 788.33-788.39) ♀
618.6 Vaginal enterocele, congenital or acquired — (Use additional code to identify urinary incontinence: 625.6, 788.31, 788.33-788.39) ♀
618.7 Genital prolapse, old laceration of muscles of pelvic floor — (Use additional code to identify urinary incontinence: 625.6, 788.31, 788.33-788.39) ♀
618.81 Incompetence or weakening of pubocervical tissue
618.82 Incompetence or weakening of rectovaginal tissue
618.83 Pelvic muscle wasting
618.89 Other specified genital prolapse
618.9 Unspecified genital prolapse — (Use additional code to identify urinary incontinence: 625.6, 788.31, 788.33-788.39) ▽ ♀
625.6 Female stress incontinence ♀
728.2 Muscular wasting and disuse atrophy, not elsewhere classified
741.90 Spina bifida without mention of hydrocephalus, unspecified region ▽
753.5 Exstrophy of urinary bladder
753.6 Congenital atresia and stenosis of urethra and bladder neck
753.8 Other specified congenital anomaly of bladder and urethra
787.6 Incontinence of feces
787.91 Diarrhea
787.99 Other symptoms involving digestive system
788.1 Dysuria
788.21 Incomplete bladder emptying
788.29 Other specified retention of urine
788.31 Urge incontinence
788.32 Stress incontinence, male ♂
788.33 Mixed incontinence urge and stress (male)(female)
788.34 Incontinence without sensory awareness
788.35 Post-void dribbling
788.36 Nocturnal enuresis
788.37 Continuous leakage
788.38 Overflow incontinence
788.39 Other urinary incontinence
788.41 Urinary frequency
788.42 Polyuria
788.43 Nocturia
788.61 Splitting of urinary stream
788.62 Slowing of urinary stream
788.63 Urgency of urination
788.69 Other abnormality of urination
788.9 Other symptoms involving urinary system
V47.4 Other urinary problems — (This code is intended for use when these conditions are recorded as diagnoses or problems)
V67.00 Follow-up examination, following unspecified surgery ▽
V67.09 Follow-up examination, following other surgery
V71.1 Observation for suspected malignant neoplasm
V71.89 Observation for other specified suspected conditions
V71.9 Observation for unspecified suspected condition ▽

ICD-9-CM Procedural

89.23 Urethral sphincter electromyogram

HCPCS Level II Supplies & Services

A4550 Surgical trays

51792

51792 Stimulus evoked response (eg, measurement of bulbocavernosus reflex latency time)

ICD-9-CM Diagnostic

344.61 Cauda equina syndrome with neurogenic bladder
440.9 Generalized and unspecified atherosclerosis ▽
596.51 Hypertonicity of bladder — (Use additional code to identify urinary incontinence: 625.6, 788.30-788.39)
600.00 Hypertrophy (benign) of prostate without urinary obstruction — (Use additional code to identify urinary incontinence: 788.30-788.39) ♂
600.01 Hypertrophy (benign) of prostate with urinary obstruction — (Use additional code to identify urinary incontinence: 788.30-788.39) ♂
600.10 Nodular prostate without urinary obstruction — (Use additional code to identify urinary incontinence: 788.30-788.39) ♂
600.11 Nodular prostate with urinary obstruction — (Use additional code to identify urinary incontinence: 788.30-788.39) ♂
600.20 Benign localized hyperplasia of prostate without urinary obstruction — (Use additional code to identify urinary incontinence: 788.30-788.39) ♂
600.21 Benign localized hyperplasia of prostate with urinary obstruction — (Use additional code to identify urinary incontinence: 788.30-788.39) ♂
600.3 Cyst of prostate — (Use additional code to identify urinary incontinence: 788.30-788.39) ♂
600.90 Hyperplasia of prostate, unspecified, without urinary obstruction — (Use additional code to identify urinary incontinence: 788.30-788.39) ▽ ♂
600.91 Hyperplasia of prostate, unspecified, with urinary obstruction — (Use additional code to identify urinary incontinence: 788.30-788.39) ▽ ♂
607.84 Impotence of organic origin ♂
608.83 Specified vascular disorder of male genital organs ♂
782.0 Disturbance of skin sensation
788.32 Stress incontinence, male ♂
788.39 Other urinary incontinence
788.41 Urinary frequency

ICD-9-CM Procedural

89.29 Other nonoperative genitourinary system measurements

HCPCS Level II Supplies & Services

A4550 Surgical trays

51795–51797

51795 Voiding pressure studies (VP); bladder voiding pressure, any technique
51797 intra-abdominal voiding pressure (AP) (rectal, gastric, intraperitoneal)

ICD-9-CM Diagnostic

185 Malignant neoplasm of prostate ♂
280.9 Unspecified iron deficiency anemia ▽
344.61 Cauda equina syndrome with neurogenic bladder
595.1 Chronic interstitial cystitis — (Use additional code to identify organism, such as E. coli, 041.4)
595.2 Other chronic cystitis — (Use additional code to identify organism, such as E. coli, 041.4)
595.3 Trigonitis — (Use additional code to identify organism, such as E. coli, 041.4)
595.4 Cystitis in diseases classified elsewhere — (Code first underlying disease: 006.8, 039.8, 120.0-120.9, 122.3, 122.6. Use additional code to identify organism, such as E. coli, 041.4) ☒
595.81 Cystitis cystica — (Use additional code to identify organism, such as E. coli, 041.4)
595.82 Irradiation cystitis — (Use additional code to identify organism, such as E. coli, 041.4)
595.89 Other specified types of cystitis — (Use additional code to identify organism, such as E. coli, 041.4)
596.0 Bladder neck obstruction — (Use additional code to identify urinary incontinence: 625.6, 788.30-788.39)
596.1 Intestinovesical fistula — (Use additional code to identify urinary incontinence: 625.6, 788.30-788.39)
596.2 Vesical fistula, not elsewhere classified — (Use additional code to identify urinary incontinence: 625.6, 788.30-788.39)

▽ Unspecified code ☒ Manifestation code
♀ Female diagnosis ♂ Male diagnosis

596.3 Diverticulum of bladder — (Use additional code to identify urinary incontinence: 625.6, 788.30-788.39)
596.4 Atony of bladder — (Use additional code to identify urinary incontinence: 625.6, 788.30-788.39)
596.51 Hypertonicity of bladder — (Use additional code to identify urinary incontinence: 625.6, 788.30-788.39)
596.52 Low bladder compliance — (Use additional code to identify urinary incontinence: 625.6, 788.30-788.39)
596.53 Paralysis of bladder — (Use additional code to identify urinary incontinence: 625.6, 788.30-788.39)
596.54 Neurogenic bladder, NOS — (Use additional code to identify urinary incontinence: 625.6, 788.30-788.39) ▽
596.55 Detrusor sphincter dyssynergia — (Use additional code to identify urinary incontinence: 625.6, 788.30-788.39)
596.59 Other functional disorder of bladder — (Use additional code to identify urinary incontinence: 625.6, 788.30-788.39)
596.8 Other specified disorder of bladder — (Use additional code to identify urinary incontinence: 625.6, 788.30-788.39)
597.81 Urethral syndrome NOS
598.00 Urethral stricture due to unspecified infection — (Use additional code to identify urinary incontinence: 625.6, 788.30-788.39) ▽
598.1 Traumatic urethral stricture — (Use additional code to identify urinary incontinence: 625.6, 788.30-788.39)
598.2 Postoperative urethral stricture — (Use additional code to identify urinary incontinence: 625.6, 788.30-788.39)
598.8 Other specified causes of urethral stricture — (Use additional code to identify urinary incontinence: 625.6, 788.30-788.39)
599.0 Urinary tract infection, site not specified — (Use additional code to identify organism, such as E. coli, 041.4) ▽
599.6 Unspecified urinary obstruction — (Use additional code to identify urinary incontinence: 625.6, 788.30-788.39) ▽
599.7 Hematuria
600.00 Hypertrophy (benign) of prostate without urinary obstruction — (Use additional code to identify urinary incontinence: 788.30-788.39) ♂
600.01 Hypertrophy (benign) of prostate with urinary obstruction — (Use additional code to identify urinary incontinence: 788.30-788.39) ♂
600.10 Nodular prostate without urinary obstruction — (Use additional code to identify urinary incontinence: 788.30-788.39) ♂
600.11 Nodular prostate with urinary obstruction — (Use additional code to identify urinary incontinence: 788.30-788.39) ♂
600.20 Benign localized hyperplasia of prostate without urinary obstruction — (Use additional code to identify urinary incontinence: 788.30-788.39) ♂
600.21 Benign localized hyperplasia of prostate with urinary obstruction — (Use additional code to identify urinary incontinence: 788.30-788.39) ♂
600.3 Cyst of prostate — (Use additional code to identify urinary incontinence: 788.30-788.39) ♂
600.90 Hyperplasia of prostate, unspecified, without urinary obstruction — (Use additional code to identify urinary incontinence: 788.30-788.39) ▽ ♂
600.91 Hyperplasia of prostate, unspecified, with urinary obstruction — (Use additional code to identify urinary incontinence: 788.30-788.39) ▽ ♂
601.1 Chronic prostatitis — (Use additional code to identify organism: 041.0, 041.1) ♂
602.9 Unspecified disorder of prostate ▽ ♂
618.00 Prolapse of vaginal walls without mention of uterine prolapse, unspecified
618.01 Cystocele without mention of uterine prolapse, midline
618.02 Cystocele without mention of uterine prolapse, lateral
618.03 Urethrocele without mention of uterine prolapse
618.05 Perineocele without mention of uterine prolapse
618.1 Uterine prolapse without mention of vaginal wall prolapse — (Use additional code to identify urinary incontinence: 625.6, 788.31, 788.33-788.39) ♀
618.2 Uterovaginal prolapse, incomplete — (Use additional code to identify urinary incontinence: 625.6, 788.31, 788.33-788.39) ♀
618.3 Uterovaginal prolapse, complete — (Use additional code to identify urinary incontinence: 625.6, 788.31, 788.33-788.39) ♀
618.4 Uterovaginal prolapse, unspecified — (Use additional code to identify urinary incontinence: 625.6, 788.31, 788.33-788.39) ▽ ♀
618.5 Prolapse of vaginal vault after hysterectomy — (Use additional code to identify urinary incontinence: 625.6, 788.31, 788.33-788.39) ♀
618.6 Vaginal enterocele, congenital or acquired — (Use additional code to identify urinary incontinence: 625.6, 788.31, 788.33-788.39) ♀
618.7 Genital prolapse, old laceration of muscles of pelvic floor — (Use additional code to identify urinary incontinence: 625.6, 788.31, 788.33-788.39) ♀
618.81 Incompetence or weakening of pubocervical tissue
618.82 Incompetence or weakening of rectovaginal tissue
625.5 Pelvic congestion syndrome ♀
625.6 Female stress incontinence ♀
741.90 Spina bifida without mention of hydrocephalus, unspecified region ▽
753.5 Exstrophy of urinary bladder
753.6 Congenital atresia and stenosis of urethra and bladder neck
753.8 Other specified congenital anomaly of bladder and urethra
788.1 Dysuria
788.21 Incomplete bladder emptying
788.29 Other specified retention of urine
788.31 Urge incontinence
788.32 Stress incontinence, male ♂
788.33 Mixed incontinence urge and stress (male)(female)
788.34 Incontinence without sensory awareness
788.35 Post-void dribbling
788.36 Nocturnal enuresis
788.37 Continuous leakage
788.38 Overflow incontinence
788.39 Other urinary incontinence
788.41 Urinary frequency
788.42 Polyuria
788.43 Nocturia
788.61 Splitting of urinary stream
788.62 Slowing of urinary stream
788.63 Urgency of urination
788.69 Other abnormality of urination
788.9 Other symptoms involving urinary system
V67.00 Follow-up examination, following unspecified surgery ▽
V67.09 Follow-up examination, following other surgery

ICD-9-CM Procedural

89.29 Other nonoperative genitourinary system measurements

HCPCS Level II Supplies & Services

A4550 Surgical trays

51798

51798 Measurement of post-voiding residual urine and/or bladder capacity by ultrasound, non-imaging

ICD-9-CM Diagnostic

596.4 Atony of bladder — (Use additional code to identify urinary incontinence: 625.6, 788.30-788.39)
596.54 Neurogenic bladder, NOS — (Use additional code to identify urinary incontinence: 625.6, 788.30-788.39) ▽
625.6 Female stress incontinence ♀
788.0 Renal colic
788.1 Dysuria
788.20 Unspecified retention of urine ▽
788.21 Incomplete bladder emptying
788.29 Other specified retention of urine
788.30 Unspecified urinary incontinence ▽
788.31 Urge incontinence
788.32 Stress incontinence, male ♂
788.33 Mixed incontinence urge and stress (male)(female)
788.34 Incontinence without sensory awareness
788.35 Post-void dribbling
788.36 Nocturnal enuresis
788.37 Continuous leakage
788.38 Overflow incontinence
788.39 Other urinary incontinence
788.41 Urinary frequency
788.42 Polyuria
788.43 Nocturia
788.5 Oliguria and anuria
788.62 Slowing of urinary stream
788.63 Urgency of urination
788.69 Other abnormality of urination
788.7 Urethral discharge
788.8 Extravasation of urine
788.9 Other symptoms involving urinary system

ICD-9-CM Procedural

89.29 Other nonoperative genitourinary system measurements

51800

51800 Cystoplasty or cystourethroplasty, plastic operation on bladder and/or vesical neck (anterior Y-plasty, vesical fundus resection), any procedure, with or without wedge resection of posterior vesical neck

ICD-9-CM Diagnostic

185 Malignant neoplasm of prostate ♂
593.70 Vesicoureteral reflux, unspecified or without reflex nephropathy
593.71 Vesicoureteral reflux with reflux nephropathy, unilateral
593.72 Vesicoureteral reflux with reflux nephropathy, bilateral
593.73 Vesicoureteral reflux with reflux nephropathy, NOS
596.2 Vesical fistula, not elsewhere classified — (Use additional code to identify urinary incontinence: 625.6, 788.30-788.39)
598.00 Urethral stricture due to unspecified infection — (Use additional code to identify urinary incontinence: 625.6, 788.30-788.39) ▽
598.01 Urethral stricture due to infective diseases classified elsewhere — (Code first underlying disease: 095.8, 098.2, 120.0-120.9. Use additional code to identify urinary incontinence: 625.6, 788.30-788.39) ☒
598.1 Traumatic urethral stricture — (Use additional code to identify urinary incontinence: 625.6, 788.30-788.39)
598.2 Postoperative urethral stricture — (Use additional code to identify urinary incontinence: 625.6, 788.30-788.39)
598.9 Unspecified urethral stricture — (Use additional code to identify urinary incontinence: 625.6, 788.30-788.39) ▽
625.6 Female stress incontinence ♀
788.30 Unspecified urinary incontinence ▽
788.31 Urge incontinence
788.32 Stress incontinence, male ♂
788.33 Mixed incontinence urge and stress (male)(female)
788.34 Incontinence without sensory awareness

ICD-9-CM Procedural

56.74 Ureteroneocystostomy
57.85 Cystourethroplasty and plastic repair of bladder neck

51820

51820 Cystourethroplasty with unilateral or bilateral ureteroneocystostomy

ICD-9-CM Diagnostic

185 Malignant neoplasm of prostate ♂
595.1 Chronic interstitial cystitis — (Use additional code to identify organism, such as E. coli, 041.4)
595.81 Cystitis cystica — (Use additional code to identify organism, such as E. coli, 041.4)
595.89 Other specified types of cystitis — (Use additional code to identify organism, such as E. coli, 041.4)
596.2 Vesical fistula, not elsewhere classified — (Use additional code to identify urinary incontinence: 625.6, 788.30-788.39)
598.00 Urethral stricture due to unspecified infection — (Use additional code to identify urinary incontinence: 625.6, 788.30-788.39) ▽
598.01 Urethral stricture due to infective diseases classified elsewhere — (Code first underlying disease: 095.8, 098.2, 120.0-120.9. Use additional code to identify urinary incontinence: 625.6, 788.30-788.39) ☒
598.1 Traumatic urethral stricture — (Use additional code to identify urinary incontinence: 625.6, 788.30-788.39)
598.2 Postoperative urethral stricture — (Use additional code to identify urinary incontinence: 625.6, 788.30-788.39)
598.9 Unspecified urethral stricture — (Use additional code to identify urinary incontinence: 625.6, 788.30-788.39) ▽
625.6 Female stress incontinence ♀
753.5 Exstrophy of urinary bladder
788.30 Unspecified urinary incontinence ▽
788.31 Urge incontinence
788.32 Stress incontinence, male ♂
788.33 Mixed incontinence urge and stress (male)(female)
788.34 Incontinence without sensory awareness

ICD-9-CM Procedural

56.74 Ureteroneocystostomy
57.85 Cystourethroplasty and plastic repair of bladder neck

51840–51841

51840 Anterior vesicourethropexy, or urethropexy (eg, Marshall-Marchetti-Krantz, Burch); simple
51841 complicated (eg, secondary repair)

ICD-9-CM Diagnostic

599.5 Prolapsed urethral mucosa
618.00 Prolapse of vaginal walls without mention of uterine prolapse, unspecified
618.01 Cystocele without mention of uterine prolapse, midline
618.02 Cystocele without mention of uterine prolapse, lateral
618.03 Urethrocele without mention of uterine prolapse
618.1 Uterine prolapse without mention of vaginal wall prolapse — (Use additional code to identify urinary incontinence: 625.6, 788.31, 788.33-788.39) ♀
618.2 Uterovaginal prolapse, incomplete — (Use additional code to identify urinary incontinence: 625.6, 788.31, 788.33-788.39) ♀
618.3 Uterovaginal prolapse, complete — (Use additional code to identify urinary incontinence: 625.6, 788.31, 788.33-788.39) ♀
618.4 Uterovaginal prolapse, unspecified — (Use additional code to identify urinary incontinence: 625.6, 788.31, 788.33-788.39) ▽ ♀
618.5 Prolapse of vaginal vault after hysterectomy — (Use additional code to identify urinary incontinence: 625.6, 788.31, 788.33-788.39) ♀
618.6 Vaginal enterocele, congenital or acquired — (Use additional code to identify urinary incontinence: 625.6, 788.31, 788.33-788.39) ♀
618.81 Incompetence or weakening of pubocervical tissue
625.5 Pelvic congestion syndrome ♀
625.6 Female stress incontinence ♀
625.8 Other specified symptom associated with female genital organs ♀
788.30 Unspecified urinary incontinence ▽
788.31 Urge incontinence
788.33 Mixed incontinence urge and stress (male)(female)
788.34 Incontinence without sensory awareness
788.35 Post-void dribbling
788.36 Nocturnal enuresis
788.37 Continuous leakage
788.38 Overflow incontinence
788.39 Other urinary incontinence

ICD-9-CM Procedural

59.5 Retropubic urethral suspension
59.79 Other repair of urinary stress incontinence

51845

51845 Abdomino-vaginal vesical neck suspension, with or without endoscopic control (eg, Stamey, Raz, modified Pereyra)

ICD-9-CM Diagnostic

599.5 Prolapsed urethral mucosa
618.00 Prolapse of vaginal walls without mention of uterine prolapse, unspecified
618.01 Cystocele without mention of uterine prolapse, midline
618.02 Cystocele without mention of uterine prolapse, lateral
618.03 Urethrocele without mention of uterine prolapse
618.1 Uterine prolapse without mention of vaginal wall prolapse — (Use additional code to identify urinary incontinence: 625.6, 788.31, 788.33-788.39) ♀
618.2 Uterovaginal prolapse, incomplete — (Use additional code to identify urinary incontinence: 625.6, 788.31, 788.33-788.39) ♀
618.3 Uterovaginal prolapse, complete — (Use additional code to identify urinary incontinence: 625.6, 788.31, 788.33-788.39) ♀
618.4 Uterovaginal prolapse, unspecified — (Use additional code to identify urinary incontinence: 625.6, 788.31, 788.33-788.39) ▽ ♀
618.5 Prolapse of vaginal vault after hysterectomy — (Use additional code to identify urinary incontinence: 625.6, 788.31, 788.33-788.39) ♀
618.6 Vaginal enterocele, congenital or acquired — (Use additional code to identify urinary incontinence: 625.6, 788.31, 788.33-788.39) ♀
618.7 Genital prolapse, old laceration of muscles of pelvic floor — (Use additional code to identify urinary incontinence: 625.6, 788.31, 788.33-788.39) ♀
618.81 Incompetence or weakening of pubocervical tissue
618.9 Unspecified genital prolapse — (Use additional code to identify urinary incontinence: 625.6, 788.31, 788.33-788.39) ▽ ♀
625.5 Pelvic congestion syndrome ♀
625.6 Female stress incontinence ♀
753.8 Other specified congenital anomaly of bladder and urethra
788.30 Unspecified urinary incontinence ▽
788.32 Stress incontinence, male ♂
788.33 Mixed incontinence urge and stress (male)(female)
788.34 Incontinence without sensory awareness
788.35 Post-void dribbling

▽ Unspecified code
♀ Female diagnosis
☒ Manifestation code
♂ Male diagnosis

788.36 Nocturnal enuresis
788.37 Continuous leakage
788.38 Overflow incontinence

ICD-9-CM Procedural

59.6 Paraurethral suspension

51860–51865

51860 Cystorrhaphy, suture of bladder wound, injury or rupture; simple
51865 complicated

ICD-9-CM Diagnostic

596.6 Nontraumatic rupture of bladder — (Use additional code to identify urinary incontinence: 625.6, 788.30-788.39)
634.21 Incomplete spontaneous abortion complicated by damage to pelvic organs or tissues ♀
634.22 Complete spontaneous abortion complicated by damage to pelvic organs or tissues ♀
635.21 Legally induced abortion complicated by damage to pelvic organs or tissues, incomplete ♀
635.22 Complete legally induced abortion complicated by damage to pelvic organs or tissues ♀
636.21 Incomplete illegally induced abortion complicated by damage to pelvic organs or tissues ♀
636.22 Complete illegally induced abortion complicated by damage to pelvic organs or tissues ♀
637.21 Legally unspecified abortion, incomplete, complicated by damage to pelvic organs or tissues ♀
637.22 Legally unspecified abortion, complete, complicated by damage to pelvic organs or tissues ♀
638.2 Failed attempted abortion complicated by damage to pelvic organs or tissues ♀
867.0 Bladder and urethra injury without mention of open wound into cavity
867.1 Bladder and urethra injury with open wound into cavity
998.2 Accidental puncture or laceration during procedure

ICD-9-CM Procedural

57.81 Suture of laceration of bladder
75.61 Repair of current obstetric laceration of bladder and urethra

51880

51880 Closure of cystostomy (separate procedure)

ICD-9-CM Diagnostic

V10.51 Personal history of malignant neoplasm of bladder
V55.5 Attention to cystostomy

ICD-9-CM Procedural

57.82 Closure of cystostomy

HCPCS Level II Supplies & Services

A4305 Disposable drug delivery system, flow rate of 50 ml or greater per hour
A4306 Disposable drug delivery system, flow rate of 5 ml or less per hour
A4550 Surgical trays

51900

51900 Closure of vesicovaginal fistula, abdominal approach

ICD-9-CM Diagnostic

619.0 Urinary-genital tract fistula, female ♀

ICD-9-CM Procedural

57.84 Repair of other fistula of bladder

51920–51925

51920 Closure of vesicouterine fistula;
51925 with hysterectomy

ICD-9-CM Diagnostic

182.8 Malignant neoplasm of other specified sites of body of uterus ♀
183.9 Malignant neoplasm of uterine adnexa, unspecified site ▽ ♀
615.9 Unspecified inflammatory disease of uterus — (Use additional code to identify organism: 041.0, 041.1) ▽ ♀
617.0 Endometriosis of uterus ♀
619.0 Urinary-genital tract fistula, female ♀
621.30 Endometrial hyperplasia, unspecified
621.31 Simple endometrial hyperplasia without atypia
621.32 Complex endometrial hyperplasia without atypia
621.33 Endometrial hyperplasia with atypia

ICD-9-CM Procedural

57.84 Repair of other fistula of bladder
68.59 Other vaginal hysterectomy

51940

51940 Closure, exstrophy of bladder

ICD-9-CM Diagnostic

753.5 Exstrophy of urinary bladder

ICD-9-CM Procedural

57.86 Repair of bladder exstrophy

51960

51960 Enterocystoplasty, including intestinal anastomosis

ICD-9-CM Diagnostic

344.61 Cauda equina syndrome with neurogenic bladder
596.51 Hypertonicity of bladder — (Use additional code to identify urinary incontinence: 625.6, 788.30-788.39)
596.52 Low bladder compliance — (Use additional code to identify urinary incontinence: 625.6, 788.30-788.39)
596.54 Neurogenic bladder, NOS — (Use additional code to identify urinary incontinence: 625.6, 788.30-788.39) ▽
596.8 Other specified disorder of bladder — (Use additional code to identify urinary incontinence: 625.6, 788.30-788.39)
753.5 Exstrophy of urinary bladder

ICD-9-CM Procedural

45.52 Isolation of segment of large intestine
57.87 Reconstruction of urinary bladder

51980

51980 Cutaneous vesicostomy

ICD-9-CM Diagnostic

233.4 Carcinoma in situ of prostate ♂
344.61 Cauda equina syndrome with neurogenic bladder
596.0 Bladder neck obstruction — (Use additional code to identify urinary incontinence: 625.6, 788.30-788.39)
596.51 Hypertonicity of bladder — (Use additional code to identify urinary incontinence: 625.6, 788.30-788.39)
596.9 Unspecified disorder of bladder — (Use additional code to identify urinary incontinence: 625.6, 788.30-788.39) ▽
598.8 Other specified causes of urethral stricture — (Use additional code to identify urinary incontinence: 625.6, 788.30-788.39)
598.9 Unspecified urethral stricture — (Use additional code to identify urinary incontinence: 625.6, 788.30-788.39) ▽
625.6 Female stress incontinence ♀
752.61 Hypospadias ♂
752.62 Epispadias ♂
752.63 Congenital chordee ♂
752.64 Micropenis ♂
752.65 Hidden penis ♂
752.69 Other penile anomalies ♂
753.6 Congenital atresia and stenosis of urethra and bladder neck

ICD-9-CM Procedural

57.21 Vesicostomy
57.22 Revision or closure of vesicostomy

HCPCS Level II Supplies & Services

A4550 Surgical trays

51990–51992

51990 Laparoscopy, surgical; urethral suspension for stress incontinence
51992 sling operation for stress incontinence (eg, fascia or synthetic)

ICD-9-CM Diagnostic

599.5 Prolapsed urethral mucosa
618.00 Prolapse of vaginal walls without mention of uterine prolapse, unspecified

618.01 Cystocele without mention of uterine prolapse, midline
618.02 Cystocele without mention of uterine prolapse, lateral
618.03 Urethrocele without mention of uterine prolapse
618.1 Uterine prolapse without mention of vaginal wall prolapse — (Use additional code to identify urinary incontinence: 625.6, 788.31, 788.33-788.39) ♀
618.2 Uterovaginal prolapse, incomplete — (Use additional code to identify urinary incontinence: 625.6, 788.31, 788.33-788.39) ♀
618.3 Uterovaginal prolapse, complete — (Use additional code to identify urinary incontinence: 625.6, 788.31, 788.33-788.39) ♀
618.4 Uterovaginal prolapse, unspecified — (Use additional code to identify urinary incontinence: 625.6, 788.31, 788.33-788.39) ▽ ♀
618.5 Prolapse of vaginal vault after hysterectomy — (Use additional code to identify urinary incontinence: 625.6, 788.31, 788.33-788.39) ♀
618.6 Vaginal enterocele, congenital or acquired — (Use additional code to identify urinary incontinence: 625.6, 788.31, 788.33-788.39) ♀
618.81 Incompetence or weakening of pubocervical tissue
625.5 Pelvic congestion syndrome ♀
625.6 Female stress incontinence ♀
625.8 Other specified symptom associated with female genital organs ♀
788.30 Unspecified urinary incontinence ▽
788.31 Urge incontinence
788.33 Mixed incontinence urge and stress (male)(female)
788.34 Incontinence without sensory awareness
788.35 Post-void dribbling
788.36 Nocturnal enuresis
788.37 Continuous leakage
788.38 Overflow incontinence
788.39 Other urinary incontinence

ICD-9-CM Procedural

59.5 Retropubic urethral suspension

52000

52000 Cystourethroscopy (separate procedure)

ICD-9-CM Diagnostic

185 Malignant neoplasm of prostate ♂
188.0 Malignant neoplasm of trigone of urinary bladder
188.1 Malignant neoplasm of dome of urinary bladder
188.2 Malignant neoplasm of lateral wall of urinary bladder
188.3 Malignant neoplasm of anterior wall of urinary bladder
188.4 Malignant neoplasm of posterior wall of urinary bladder
188.5 Malignant neoplasm of bladder neck
188.6 Malignant neoplasm of ureteric orifice
188.8 Malignant neoplasm of other specified sites of bladder
188.9 Malignant neoplasm of bladder, part unspecified ▽
189.3 Malignant neoplasm of urethra
199.0 Disseminated malignant neoplasm
199.1 Other malignant neoplasm of unspecified site
233.4 Carcinoma in situ of prostate ♂
233.7 Carcinoma in situ of bladder
233.9 Carcinoma in situ of other and unspecified urinary organs ▽
236.5 Neoplasm of uncertain behavior of prostate ♂
236.6 Neoplasm of uncertain behavior of other and unspecified male genital organs ▽ ♂
236.7 Neoplasm of uncertain behavior of bladder
239.4 Neoplasm of unspecified nature of bladder

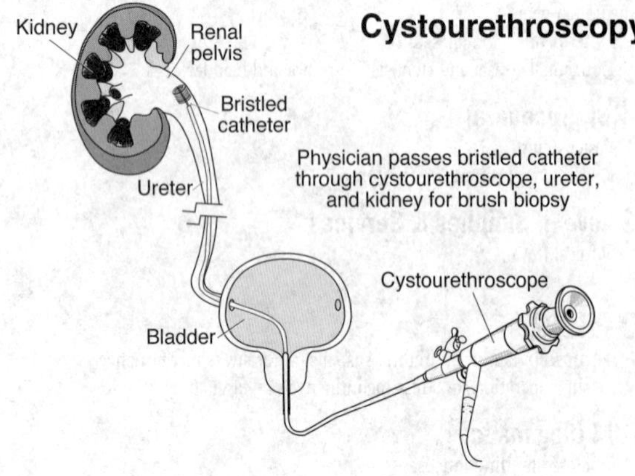
Cystourethroscopy
Kidney
Renal pelvis
Bristled catheter
Physician passes bristled catheter through cystourethroscope, ureter, and kidney for brush biopsy
Ureter
Cystourethroscope
Bladder

239.5 Neoplasm of unspecified nature of other genitourinary organs
344.61 Cauda equina syndrome with neurogenic bladder
590.00 Chronic pyelonephritis without lesion of renal medullary necrosis — (Code, if applicable, any causal condition first. Use additional code to identify organism, such as E. coli, 041.4)
591 Hydronephrosis
592.9 Unspecified urinary calculus ▽
594.1 Other calculus in bladder
595.0 Acute cystitis — (Use additional code to identify organism, such as E. coli, 041.4)
595.1 Chronic interstitial cystitis — (Use additional code to identify organism, such as E. coli, 041.4)
595.2 Other chronic cystitis — (Use additional code to identify organism, such as E. coli, 041.4)
595.3 Trigonitis — (Use additional code to identify organism, such as E. coli, 041.4)
595.81 Cystitis cystica — (Use additional code to identify organism, such as E. coli, 041.4)
595.82 Irradiation cystitis — (Use additional code to identify organism, such as E. coli, 041.4)
595.89 Other specified types of cystitis — (Use additional code to identify organism, such as E. coli, 041.4)
596.0 Bladder neck obstruction — (Use additional code to identify urinary incontinence: 625.6, 788.30-788.39)
596.1 Intestinovesical fistula — (Use additional code to identify urinary incontinence: 625.6, 788.30-788.39)
596.2 Vesical fistula, not elsewhere classified — (Use additional code to identify urinary incontinence: 625.6, 788.30-788.39)
596.3 Diverticulum of bladder — (Use additional code to identify urinary incontinence: 625.6, 788.30-788.39)
596.51 Hypertonicity of bladder — (Use additional code to identify urinary incontinence: 625.6, 788.30-788.39)
596.52 Low bladder compliance — (Use additional code to identify urinary incontinence: 625.6, 788.30-788.39)
596.53 Paralysis of bladder — (Use additional code to identify urinary incontinence: 625.6, 788.30-788.39)
596.54 Neurogenic bladder, NOS — (Use additional code to identify urinary incontinence: 625.6, 788.30-788.39) ▽
596.55 Detrusor sphincter dyssynergia — (Use additional code to identify urinary incontinence: 625.6, 788.30-788.39)
596.59 Other functional disorder of bladder — (Use additional code to identify urinary incontinence: 625.6, 788.30-788.39)
596.6 Nontraumatic rupture of bladder — (Use additional code to identify urinary incontinence: 625.6, 788.30-788.39)
596.7 Hemorrhage into bladder wall — (Use additional code to identify urinary incontinence: 625.6, 788.30-788.39)
596.8 Other specified disorder of bladder — (Use additional code to identify urinary incontinence: 625.6, 788.30-788.39)
597.0 Urethral abscess
597.80 Unspecified urethritis ▽
597.81 Urethral syndrome NOS
597.89 Other urethritis
598.00 Urethral stricture due to unspecified infection — (Use additional code to identify urinary incontinence: 625.6, 788.30-788.39) ▽
598.01 Urethral stricture due to infective diseases classified elsewhere — (Code first underlying disease: 095.8, 098.2, 120.0-120.9. Use additional code to identify urinary incontinence: 625.6, 788.30-788.39) ⊠
598.1 Traumatic urethral stricture — (Use additional code to identify urinary incontinence: 625.6, 788.30-788.39)
598.2 Postoperative urethral stricture — (Use additional code to identify urinary incontinence: 625.6, 788.30-788.39)
598.8 Other specified causes of urethral stricture — (Use additional code to identify urinary incontinence: 625.6, 788.30-788.39)
599.0 Urinary tract infection, site not specified — (Use additional code to identify organism, such as E. coli, 041.4) ▽
599.1 Urethral fistula
599.2 Urethral diverticulum
599.3 Urethral caruncle
599.4 Urethral false passage
599.5 Prolapsed urethral mucosa
599.7 Hematuria
599.81 Urethral hypermobility — (Use additional code to identify urinary incontinence: 625.6, 788.30-788.39)
599.82 Intrinsic (urethral) sphincter deficiency (ISD) — (Use additional code to identify urinary incontinence: 625.6, 788.30-788.39)
599.83 Urethral instability — (Use additional code to identify urinary incontinence: 625.6, 788.30-788.39)

▽ Unspecified code
♀ Female diagnosis
⊠ Manifestation code
♂ Male diagnosis

599.84 Other specified disorders of urethra — (Use additional code to identify urinary incontinence: 625.6, 788.30-788.39)
599.89 Other specified disorders of urinary tract — (Use additional code to identify urinary incontinence: 625.6, 788.30-788.39)
600.00 Hypertrophy (benign) of prostate without urinary obstruction — (Use additional code to identify urinary incontinence: 788.30-788.39) ♂
600.01 Hypertrophy (benign) of prostate with urinary obstruction — (Use additional code to identify urinary incontinence: 788.30-788.39) ♂
600.10 Nodular prostate without urinary obstruction — (Use additional code to identify urinary incontinence: 788.30-788.39) ♂
600.11 Nodular prostate with urinary obstruction — (Use additional code to identify urinary incontinence: 788.30-788.39) ♂
600.20 Benign localized hyperplasia of prostate without urinary obstruction — (Use additional code to identify urinary incontinence: 788.30-788.39) ♂
600.21 Benign localized hyperplasia of prostate with urinary obstruction — (Use additional code to identify urinary incontinence: 788.30-788.39) ♂
600.3 Cyst of prostate — (Use additional code to identify urinary incontinence: 788.30-788.39) ♂
600.90 Hyperplasia of prostate, unspecified, without urinary obstruction — (Use additional code to identify urinary incontinence: 788.30-788.39) ▽ ♂
600.91 Hyperplasia of prostate, unspecified, with urinary obstruction — (Use additional code to identify urinary incontinence: 788.30-788.39) ▽ ♂
601.0 Acute prostatitis — (Use additional code to identify organism: 041.0, 041.1) ♂
601.1 Chronic prostatitis — (Use additional code to identify organism: 041.0, 041.1) ♂
601.8 Other specified inflammatory disease of prostate — (Use additional code to identify organism: 041.0, 041.1) ♂
602.0 Calculus of prostate ♂
602.1 Congestion or hemorrhage of prostate ♂
602.3 Dysplasia of prostate ♂
602.8 Other specified disorder of prostate ♂
607.84 Impotence of organic origin ♂
619.0 Urinary-genital tract fistula, female ♀
625.6 Female stress incontinence ♀
753.5 Exstrophy of urinary bladder
753.6 Congenital atresia and stenosis of urethra and bladder neck
753.8 Other specified congenital anomaly of bladder and urethra
788.0 Renal colic
788.1 Dysuria
788.21 Incomplete bladder emptying
788.29 Other specified retention of urine
788.30 Unspecified urinary incontinence ▽
788.31 Urge incontinence
788.32 Stress incontinence, male ♂
788.33 Mixed incontinence urge and stress (male)(female)
788.34 Incontinence without sensory awareness
788.35 Post-void dribbling
788.36 Nocturnal enuresis
788.37 Continuous leakage
788.38 Overflow incontinence
788.39 Other urinary incontinence
788.41 Urinary frequency
788.42 Polyuria
788.43 Nocturia
788.5 Oliguria and anuria
788.63 Urgency of urination
788.69 Other abnormality of urination
788.7 Urethral discharge
788.8 Extravasation of urine
789.00 Abdominal pain, unspecified site ▽
789.01 Abdominal pain, right upper quadrant
789.02 Abdominal pain, left upper quadrant
789.07 Abdominal pain, generalized
789.09 Abdominal pain, other specified site
789.30 Abdominal or pelvic swelling, mass or lump, unspecified site ▽
789.31 Abdominal or pelvic swelling, mass, or lump, right upper quadrant
789.32 Abdominal or pelvic swelling, mass, or lump, left upper quadrant
789.37 Abdominal or pelvic swelling, mass, or lump, epigastric, generalized
789.39 Abdominal or pelvic swelling, mass, or lump, other specified site
793.5 Nonspecific abnormal findings on radiological and other examination of genitourinary organs
867.1 Bladder and urethra injury with open wound into cavity
939.0 Foreign body in bladder and urethra
V10.46 Personal history of malignant neoplasm of prostate ♂
V10.51 Personal history of malignant neoplasm of bladder
V71.1 Observation for suspected malignant neoplasm
V76.3 Screening for malignant neoplasm of the bladder

ICD-9-CM Procedural

57.32 Other cystoscopy

HCPCS Level II Supplies & Services

A4270 Disposable endoscope sheath, each
A4550 Surgical trays

52001

52001 Cystourethroscopy with irrigation and evacuation of multiple obstructing clots

ICD-9-CM Diagnostic

185 Malignant neoplasm of prostate ♂
188.0 Malignant neoplasm of trigone of urinary bladder
188.1 Malignant neoplasm of dome of urinary bladder
188.2 Malignant neoplasm of lateral wall of urinary bladder
188.3 Malignant neoplasm of anterior wall of urinary bladder
188.4 Malignant neoplasm of posterior wall of urinary bladder
188.5 Malignant neoplasm of bladder neck
188.6 Malignant neoplasm of ureteric orifice
188.8 Malignant neoplasm of other specified sites of bladder
188.9 Malignant neoplasm of bladder, part unspecified ▽
189.3 Malignant neoplasm of urethra
199.0 Disseminated malignant neoplasm
199.1 Other malignant neoplasm of unspecified site
233.4 Carcinoma in situ of prostate ♂
233.7 Carcinoma in situ of bladder
233.9 Carcinoma in situ of other and unspecified urinary organs ▽
236.5 Neoplasm of uncertain behavior of prostate ♂
236.6 Neoplasm of uncertain behavior of other and unspecified male genital organs ▽ ♂
236.7 Neoplasm of uncertain behavior of bladder
239.4 Neoplasm of unspecified nature of bladder
239.5 Neoplasm of unspecified nature of other genitourinary organs
344.61 Cauda equina syndrome with neurogenic bladder
590.00 Chronic pyelonephritis without lesion of renal medullary necrosis — (Code, if applicable, any causal condition first. Use additional code to identify organism, such as E. coli, 041.4)
591 Hydronephrosis
592.9 Unspecified urinary calculus ▽
594.1 Other calculus in bladder
595.0 Acute cystitis — (Use additional code to identify organism, such as E. coli, 041.4)
595.1 Chronic interstitial cystitis — (Use additional code to identify organism, such as E. coli, 041.4)
595.2 Other chronic cystitis — (Use additional code to identify organism, such as E. coli, 041.4)
595.3 Trigonitis — (Use additional code to identify organism, such as E. coli, 041.4)
595.81 Cystitis cystica — (Use additional code to identify organism, such as E. coli, 041.4)
595.82 Irradiation cystitis — (Use additional code to identify organism, such as E. coli, 041.4)
595.89 Other specified types of cystitis — (Use additional code to identify organism, such as E. coli, 041.4)
596.0 Bladder neck obstruction — (Use additional code to identify urinary incontinence: 625.6, 788.30-788.39)
596.1 Intestinovesical fistula — (Use additional code to identify urinary incontinence: 625.6, 788.30-788.39)
596.2 Vesical fistula, not elsewhere classified — (Use additional code to identify urinary incontinence: 625.6, 788.30-788.39)
596.3 Diverticulum of bladder — (Use additional code to identify urinary incontinence: 625.6, 788.30-788.39)
596.51 Hypertonicity of bladder — (Use additional code to identify urinary incontinence: 625.6, 788.30-788.39)
596.52 Low bladder compliance — (Use additional code to identify urinary incontinence: 625.6, 788.30-788.39)
596.53 Paralysis of bladder — (Use additional code to identify urinary incontinence: 625.6, 788.30-788.39)
596.54 Neurogenic bladder, NOS — (Use additional code to identify urinary incontinence: 625.6, 788.30-788.39) ▽
596.55 Detrusor sphincter dyssynergia — (Use additional code to identify urinary incontinence: 625.6, 788.30-788.39)
596.59 Other functional disorder of bladder — (Use additional code to identify urinary incontinence: 625.6, 788.30-788.39)

596.6 Nontraumatic rupture of bladder — (Use additional code to identify urinary incontinence: 625.6, 788.30-788.39)
596.7 Hemorrhage into bladder wall — (Use additional code to identify urinary incontinence: 625.6, 788.30-788.39)
596.8 Other specified disorder of bladder — (Use additional code to identify urinary incontinence: 625.6, 788.30-788.39)
597.0 Urethral abscess
597.80 Unspecified urethritis ▽
597.81 Urethral syndrome NOS
597.89 Other urethritis
598.00 Urethral stricture due to unspecified infection — (Use additional code to identify urinary incontinence: 625.6, 788.30-788.39) ▽
598.01 Urethral stricture due to infective diseases classified elsewhere — (Code first underlying disease: 095.8, 098.2, 120.0-120.9. Use additional code to identify urinary incontinence: 625.6, 788.30-788.39) ☒
598.1 Traumatic urethral stricture — (Use additional code to identify urinary incontinence: 625.6, 788.30-788.39)
598.2 Postoperative urethral stricture — (Use additional code to identify urinary incontinence: 625.6, 788.30-788.39)
598.8 Other specified causes of urethral stricture — (Use additional code to identify urinary incontinence: 625.6, 788.30-788.39)
599.0 Urinary tract infection, site not specified — (Use additional code to identify organism, such as E. coli, 041.4) ▽
599.1 Urethral fistula
599.2 Urethral diverticulum
599.3 Urethral caruncle
599.4 Urethral false passage
599.5 Prolapsed urethral mucosa
599.7 Hematuria
599.81 Urethral hypermobility — (Use additional code to identify urinary incontinence: 625.6, 788.30-788.39)
599.82 Intrinsic (urethral) sphincter deficiency (ISD) — (Use additional code to identify urinary incontinence: 625.6, 788.30-788.39)
599.83 Urethral instability — (Use additional code to identify urinary incontinence: 625.6, 788.30-788.39)
599.84 Other specified disorders of urethra — (Use additional code to identify urinary incontinence: 625.6, 788.30-788.39)
599.89 Other specified disorders of urinary tract — (Use additional code to identify urinary incontinence: 625.6, 788.30-788.39)
600.00 Hypertrophy (benign) of prostate without urinary obstruction — (Use additional code to identify urinary incontinence: 788.30-788.39) ♂
600.01 Hypertrophy (benign) of prostate with urinary obstruction — (Use additional code to identify urinary incontinence: 788.30-788.39) ♂
600.10 Nodular prostate without urinary obstruction — (Use additional code to identify urinary incontinence: 788.30-788.39) ♂
600.11 Nodular prostate with urinary obstruction — (Use additional code to identify urinary incontinence: 788.30-788.39) ♂
600.20 Benign localized hyperplasia of prostate without urinary obstruction — (Use additional code to identify urinary incontinence: 788.30-788.39) ♂
600.21 Benign localized hyperplasia of prostate with urinary obstruction — (Use additional code to identify urinary incontinence: 788.30-788.39) ♂
600.3 Cyst of prostate — (Use additional code to identify urinary incontinence: 788.30-788.39) ♂
600.90 Hyperplasia of prostate, unspecified, without urinary obstruction — (Use additional code to identify urinary incontinence: 788.30-788.39) ▽ ♂
600.91 Hyperplasia of prostate, unspecified, with urinary obstruction — (Use additional code to identify urinary incontinence: 788.30-788.39) ▽ ♂
601.0 Acute prostatitis — (Use additional code to identify organism: 041.0, 041.1) ♂
601.1 Chronic prostatitis — (Use additional code to identify organism: 041.0, 041.1) ♂
601.8 Other specified inflammatory disease of prostate — (Use additional code to identify organism: 041.0, 041.1) ♂
602.0 Calculus of prostate ♂
602.1 Congestion or hemorrhage of prostate ♂
602.3 Dysplasia of prostate ♂
602.8 Other specified disorder of prostate ♂
607.84 Impotence of organic origin ♂
619.0 Urinary-genital tract fistula, female ♀
625.6 Female stress incontinence ♀
753.5 Exstrophy of urinary bladder
753.6 Congenital atresia and stenosis of urethra and bladder neck
753.8 Other specified congenital anomaly of bladder and urethra
788.0 Renal colic
788.1 Dysuria
788.21 Incomplete bladder emptying
788.29 Other specified retention of urine
788.30 Unspecified urinary incontinence ▽
788.31 Urge incontinence
788.32 Stress incontinence, male ♂
788.33 Mixed incontinence urge and stress (male)(female)
788.34 Incontinence without sensory awareness
788.35 Post-void dribbling
788.36 Nocturnal enuresis
788.37 Continuous leakage
788.38 Overflow incontinence
788.39 Other urinary incontinence
788.41 Urinary frequency
788.42 Polyuria
788.43 Nocturia
788.5 Oliguria and anuria
788.63 Urgency of urination
788.69 Other abnormality of urination
788.7 Urethral discharge
788.8 Extravasation of urine
789.00 Abdominal pain, unspecified site ▽
789.01 Abdominal pain, right upper quadrant
789.02 Abdominal pain, left upper quadrant
789.07 Abdominal pain, generalized
789.09 Abdominal pain, other specified site
789.30 Abdominal or pelvic swelling, mass or lump, unspecified site ▽
789.31 Abdominal or pelvic swelling, mass, or lump, right upper quadrant
789.32 Abdominal or pelvic swelling, mass, or lump, left upper quadrant
789.37 Abdominal or pelvic swelling, mass, or lump, epigastric, generalized
789.39 Abdominal or pelvic swelling, mass, or lump, other specified site
793.5 Nonspecific abnormal findings on radiological and other examination of genitourinary organs
867.1 Bladder and urethra injury with open wound into cavity
939.0 Foreign body in bladder and urethra
V10.46 Personal history of malignant neoplasm of prostate ♂
V10.51 Personal history of malignant neoplasm of bladder
V71.1 Observation for suspected malignant neoplasm
V76.3 Screening for malignant neoplasm of the bladder

ICD-9-CM Procedural

57.99 Other operations on bladder

52005–52007

52005 Cystourethroscopy, with ureteral catheterization, with or without irrigation, instillation, or ureteropyelography, exclusive of radiologic service;
52007 with brush biopsy of ureter and/or renal pelvis

ICD-9-CM Diagnostic

185 Malignant neoplasm of prostate ♂
188.0 Malignant neoplasm of trigone of urinary bladder
188.1 Malignant neoplasm of dome of urinary bladder
188.2 Malignant neoplasm of lateral wall of urinary bladder
188.3 Malignant neoplasm of anterior wall of urinary bladder
188.4 Malignant neoplasm of posterior wall of urinary bladder
188.5 Malignant neoplasm of bladder neck
188.6 Malignant neoplasm of ureteric orifice
188.8 Malignant neoplasm of other specified sites of bladder
188.9 Malignant neoplasm of bladder, part unspecified ▽
189.1 Malignant neoplasm of renal pelvis
189.2 Malignant neoplasm of ureter
189.3 Malignant neoplasm of urethra
198.0 Secondary malignant neoplasm of kidney
198.1 Secondary malignant neoplasm of other urinary organs
199.1 Other malignant neoplasm of unspecified site
222.2 Benign neoplasm of prostate ♂
223.0 Benign neoplasm of kidney, except pelvis
223.1 Benign neoplasm of renal pelvis
223.3 Benign neoplasm of bladder
223.81 Benign neoplasm of urethra
223.89 Benign neoplasm of other specified sites of urinary organs
223.9 Benign neoplasm of urinary organ, site unspecified ▽
233.7 Carcinoma in situ of bladder
233.9 Carcinoma in situ of other and unspecified urinary organs ▽
236.5 Neoplasm of uncertain behavior of prostate ♂
236.7 Neoplasm of uncertain behavior of bladder
239.4 Neoplasm of unspecified nature of bladder
239.5 Neoplasm of unspecified nature of other genitourinary organs
344.61 Cauda equina syndrome with neurogenic bladder

▽ Unspecified code
♀ Female diagnosis
☒ Manifestation code
♂ Male diagnosis

591 Hydronephrosis
592.0 Calculus of kidney
592.1 Calculus of ureter
593.0 Nephroptosis
593.1 Hypertrophy of kidney
593.2 Acquired cyst of kidney
593.3 Stricture or kinking of ureter
593.4 Other ureteric obstruction
593.5 Hydroureter
593.70 Vesicoureteral reflux, unspecified or without reflex nephropathy
593.71 Vesicoureteral reflux with reflux nephropathy, unilateral
593.72 Vesicoureteral reflux with reflux nephropathy, bilateral
593.73 Vesicoureteral reflux with reflux nephropathy, NOS
593.81 Vascular disorders of kidney
593.82 Ureteral fistula
593.89 Other specified disorder of kidney and ureter
594.0 Calculus in diverticulum of bladder
594.1 Other calculus in bladder
594.2 Calculus in urethra
594.8 Other lower urinary tract calculus
595.0 Acute cystitis — (Use additional code to identify organism, such as E. coli, 041.4)
595.1 Chronic interstitial cystitis — (Use additional code to identify organism, such as E. coli, 041.4)
595.2 Other chronic cystitis — (Use additional code to identify organism, such as E. coli, 041.4)
595.3 Trigonitis — (Use additional code to identify organism, such as E. coli, 041.4)
595.81 Cystitis cystica — (Use additional code to identify organism, such as E. coli, 041.4)
595.82 Irradiation cystitis — (Use additional code to identify organism, such as E. coli, 041.4)
595.89 Other specified types of cystitis — (Use additional code to identify organism, such as E. coli, 041.4)
596.0 Bladder neck obstruction — (Use additional code to identify urinary incontinence: 625.6, 788.30-788.39)
596.1 Intestinovesical fistula — (Use additional code to identify urinary incontinence: 625.6, 788.30-788.39)
596.2 Vesical fistula, not elsewhere classified — (Use additional code to identify urinary incontinence: 625.6, 788.30-788.39)
596.3 Diverticulum of bladder — (Use additional code to identify urinary incontinence: 625.6, 788.30-788.39)
596.51 Hypertonicity of bladder — (Use additional code to identify urinary incontinence: 625.6, 788.30-788.39)
596.6 Nontraumatic rupture of bladder — (Use additional code to identify urinary incontinence: 625.6, 788.30-788.39)
596.7 Hemorrhage into bladder wall — (Use additional code to identify urinary incontinence: 625.6, 788.30-788.39)
596.8 Other specified disorder of bladder — (Use additional code to identify urinary incontinence: 625.6, 788.30-788.39)
598.00 Urethral stricture due to unspecified infection — (Use additional code to identify urinary incontinence: 625.6, 788.30-788.39) ▽
598.01 Urethral stricture due to infective diseases classified elsewhere — (Code first underlying disease: 095.8, 098.2, 120.0-120.9. Use additional code to identify urinary incontinence: 625.6, 788.30-788.39) ☒
598.1 Traumatic urethral stricture — (Use additional code to identify urinary incontinence: 625.6, 788.30-788.39)
598.2 Postoperative urethral stricture — (Use additional code to identify urinary incontinence: 625.6, 788.30-788.39)
598.8 Other specified causes of urethral stricture — (Use additional code to identify urinary incontinence: 625.6, 788.30-788.39)
599.0 Urinary tract infection, site not specified — (Use additional code to identify organism, such as E. coli, 041.4) ▽
599.7 Hematuria
600.00 Hypertrophy (benign) of prostate without urinary obstruction — (Use additional code to identify urinary incontinence: 788.30-788.39) ♂
600.01 Hypertrophy (benign) of prostate with urinary obstruction — (Use additional code to identify urinary incontinence: 788.30-788.39) ♂
600.10 Nodular prostate without urinary obstruction — (Use additional code to identify urinary incontinence: 788.30-788.39) ♂
600.11 Nodular prostate with urinary obstruction — (Use additional code to identify urinary incontinence: 788.30-788.39) ♂
600.20 Benign localized hyperplasia of prostate without urinary obstruction — (Use additional code to identify urinary incontinence: 788.30-788.39) ♂
600.21 Benign localized hyperplasia of prostate with urinary obstruction — (Use additional code to identify urinary incontinence: 788.30-788.39) ♂
600.3 Cyst of prostate — (Use additional code to identify urinary incontinence: 788.30-788.39) ♂
600.90 Hyperplasia of prostate, unspecified, without urinary obstruction — (Use additional code to identify urinary incontinence: 788.30-788.39) ▽ ♂
600.91 Hyperplasia of prostate, unspecified, with urinary obstruction — (Use additional code to identify urinary incontinence: 788.30-788.39) ▽ ♂
601.0 Acute prostatitis — (Use additional code to identify organism: 041.0, 041.1) ♂
601.1 Chronic prostatitis — (Use additional code to identify organism: 041.0, 041.1) ♂
601.8 Other specified inflammatory disease of prostate — (Use additional code to identify organism: 041.0, 041.1) ♂
625.6 Female stress incontinence ♀
625.9 Unspecified symptom associated with female genital organs ▽ ♀
753.0 Congenital renal agenesis and dysgenesis
753.11 Congenital single renal cyst
753.12 Congenital polycystic kidney, unspecified type ▽
753.13 Congenital polycystic kidney, autosomal dominant
753.14 Congenital polycystic kidney, autosomal recessive
753.15 Congenital renal dysplasia
753.16 Congenital medullary cystic kidney
753.17 Congenital medullary sponge kidney
753.19 Other specified congenital cystic kidney disease
753.21 Congenital obstruction of ureteropelvic junction
753.22 Congenital obstruction of ureterovesical junction
753.23 Congenital ureterocele
753.29 Other obstructive defect of renal pelvis and ureter
753.3 Other specified congenital anomalies of kidney
753.4 Other specified congenital anomalies of ureter
753.5 Exstrophy of urinary bladder
753.6 Congenital atresia and stenosis of urethra and bladder neck
753.8 Other specified congenital anomaly of bladder and urethra
788.0 Renal colic
788.1 Dysuria
788.21 Incomplete bladder emptying
788.29 Other specified retention of urine
788.31 Urge incontinence
788.32 Stress incontinence, male ♂
788.33 Mixed incontinence urge and stress (male)(female)
788.34 Incontinence without sensory awareness
788.35 Post-void dribbling
788.36 Nocturnal enuresis
788.37 Continuous leakage
788.38 Overflow incontinence
788.39 Other urinary incontinence
788.41 Urinary frequency
788.42 Polyuria
788.43 Nocturia
788.5 Oliguria and anuria
788.61 Splitting of urinary stream
788.62 Slowing of urinary stream
788.63 Urgency of urination
788.69 Other abnormality of urination
788.7 Urethral discharge
788.8 Extravasation of urine
788.9 Other symptoms involving urinary system
789.00 Abdominal pain, unspecified site ▽
789.01 Abdominal pain, right upper quadrant
789.02 Abdominal pain, left upper quadrant
789.07 Abdominal pain, generalized
789.09 Abdominal pain, other specified site
789.30 Abdominal or pelvic swelling, mass or lump, unspecified site ▽
789.31 Abdominal or pelvic swelling, mass, or lump, right upper quadrant
789.32 Abdominal or pelvic swelling, mass, or lump, left upper quadrant
789.37 Abdominal or pelvic swelling, mass, or lump, epigastric, generalized
789.39 Abdominal or pelvic swelling, mass, or lump, other specified site
793.5 Nonspecific abnormal findings on radiological and other examination of genitourinary organs
939.0 Foreign body in bladder and urethra

ICD-9-CM Procedural

56.33 Closed endoscopic biopsy of ureter
56.39 Other diagnostic procedures on ureter
57.32 Other cystoscopy
59.8 Ureteral catheterization
87.74 Retrograde pyelogram

▽ Unspecified code
♀ Female diagnosis
☒ Manifestation code
♂ Male diagnosis

HCPCS Level II Supplies & Services

A4270 Disposable endoscope sheath, each
A4550 Surgical trays

52010

52010 Cystourethroscopy, with ejaculatory duct catheterization, with or without irrigation, instillation, or duct radiography, exclusive of radiologic service

ICD-9-CM Diagnostic

600.00 Hypertrophy (benign) of prostate without urinary obstruction — (Use additional code to identify urinary incontinence: 788.30-788.39) ♂
600.01 Hypertrophy (benign) of prostate with urinary obstruction — (Use additional code to identify urinary incontinence: 788.30-788.39) ♂
600.10 Nodular prostate without urinary obstruction — (Use additional code to identify urinary incontinence: 788.30-788.39) ♂
600.11 Nodular prostate with urinary obstruction — (Use additional code to identify urinary incontinence: 788.30-788.39) ♂
600.20 Benign localized hyperplasia of prostate without urinary obstruction — (Use additional code to identify urinary incontinence: 788.30-788.39) ♂
600.21 Benign localized hyperplasia of prostate with urinary obstruction — (Use additional code to identify urinary incontinence: 788.30-788.39) ♂
600.3 Cyst of prostate — (Use additional code to identify urinary incontinence: 788.30-788.39) ♂
600.90 Hyperplasia of prostate, unspecified, without urinary obstruction — (Use additional code to identify urinary incontinence: 788.30-788.39) ▽ ♂
600.91 Hyperplasia of prostate, unspecified, with urinary obstruction — (Use additional code to identify urinary incontinence: 788.30-788.39) ▽ ♂
606.8 Infertility due to extratesticular causes ♂
607.84 Impotence of organic origin ♂
608.82 Hematospermia ♂
608.83 Specified vascular disorder of male genital organs ♂
753.9 Unspecified congenital anomaly of urinary system ▽

ICD-9-CM Procedural

57.32 Other cystoscopy
87.99 Other x-ray of male genital organs

HCPCS Level II Supplies & Services

A4270 Disposable endoscope sheath, each
A4550 Surgical trays

52204

52204 Cystourethroscopy, with biopsy

ICD-9-CM Diagnostic

185 Malignant neoplasm of prostate ♂
188.0 Malignant neoplasm of trigone of urinary bladder
188.1 Malignant neoplasm of dome of urinary bladder
188.2 Malignant neoplasm of lateral wall of urinary bladder
188.3 Malignant neoplasm of anterior wall of urinary bladder
188.4 Malignant neoplasm of posterior wall of urinary bladder
188.5 Malignant neoplasm of bladder neck
188.6 Malignant neoplasm of ureteric orifice
188.8 Malignant neoplasm of other specified sites of bladder
188.9 Malignant neoplasm of bladder, part unspecified ▽
189.0 Malignant neoplasm of kidney, except pelvis
189.1 Malignant neoplasm of renal pelvis
189.2 Malignant neoplasm of ureter
189.3 Malignant neoplasm of urethra
199.0 Disseminated malignant neoplasm
199.1 Other malignant neoplasm of unspecified site
223.3 Benign neoplasm of bladder
223.81 Benign neoplasm of urethra
233.4 Carcinoma in situ of prostate ♂
233.7 Carcinoma in situ of bladder
233.9 Carcinoma in situ of other and unspecified urinary organs ▽
236.5 Neoplasm of uncertain behavior of prostate ♂
236.6 Neoplasm of uncertain behavior of other and unspecified male genital organs ▽ ♂
236.7 Neoplasm of uncertain behavior of bladder
239.4 Neoplasm of unspecified nature of bladder
239.5 Neoplasm of unspecified nature of other genitourinary organs
593.89 Other specified disorder of kidney and ureter
594.1 Other calculus in bladder
595.0 Acute cystitis — (Use additional code to identify organism, such as E. coli, 041.4)
595.1 Chronic interstitial cystitis — (Use additional code to identify organism, such as E. coli, 041.4)
595.2 Other chronic cystitis — (Use additional code to identify organism, such as E. coli, 041.4)
595.3 Trigonitis — (Use additional code to identify organism, such as E. coli, 041.4)
595.4 Cystitis in diseases classified elsewhere — (Code first underlying disease: 006.8, 039.8, 120.0-120.9, 122.3, 122.6. Use additional code to identify organism, such as E. coli, 041.4) ☒
595.81 Cystitis cystica — (Use additional code to identify organism, such as E. coli, 041.4)
595.82 Irradiation cystitis — (Use additional code to identify organism, such as E. coli, 041.4)
595.89 Other specified types of cystitis — (Use additional code to identify organism, such as E. coli, 041.4)
595.9 Unspecified cystitis — (Use additional code to identify organism, such as E. coli, 041.4) ▽
596.0 Bladder neck obstruction — (Use additional code to identify urinary incontinence: 625.6, 788.30-788.39)
596.3 Diverticulum of bladder — (Use additional code to identify urinary incontinence: 625.6, 788.30-788.39)
596.9 Unspecified disorder of bladder — (Use additional code to identify urinary incontinence: 625.6, 788.30-788.39) ▽
597.0 Urethral abscess
597.81 Urethral syndrome NOS
597.89 Other urethritis
598.00 Urethral stricture due to unspecified infection — (Use additional code to identify urinary incontinence: 625.6, 788.30-788.39) ▽
598.01 Urethral stricture due to infective diseases classified elsewhere — (Code first underlying disease: 095.8, 098.2, 120.0-120.9. Use additional code to identify urinary incontinence: 625.6, 788.30-788.39) ☒
598.1 Traumatic urethral stricture — (Use additional code to identify urinary incontinence: 625.6, 788.30-788.39)
598.2 Postoperative urethral stricture — (Use additional code to identify urinary incontinence: 625.6, 788.30-788.39)
598.8 Other specified causes of urethral stricture — (Use additional code to identify urinary incontinence: 625.6, 788.30-788.39)
599.0 Urinary tract infection, site not specified — (Use additional code to identify organism, such as E. coli, 041.4) ▽
599.1 Urethral fistula
599.2 Urethral diverticulum
599.3 Urethral caruncle
599.4 Urethral false passage
599.5 Prolapsed urethral mucosa
599.7 Hematuria
599.81 Urethral hypermobility — (Use additional code to identify urinary incontinence: 625.6, 788.30-788.39)
599.82 Intrinsic (urethral) sphincter deficiency (ISD) — (Use additional code to identify urinary incontinence: 625.6, 788.30-788.39)
599.83 Urethral instability — (Use additional code to identify urinary incontinence: 625.6, 788.30-788.39)
599.84 Other specified disorders of urethra — (Use additional code to identify urinary incontinence: 625.6, 788.30-788.39)
599.89 Other specified disorders of urinary tract — (Use additional code to identify urinary incontinence: 625.6, 788.30-788.39)
600.00 Hypertrophy (benign) of prostate without urinary obstruction — (Use additional code to identify urinary incontinence: 788.30-788.39) ♂
600.01 Hypertrophy (benign) of prostate with urinary obstruction — (Use additional code to identify urinary incontinence: 788.30-788.39) ♂
600.10 Nodular prostate without urinary obstruction — (Use additional code to identify urinary incontinence: 788.30-788.39) ♂
600.11 Nodular prostate with urinary obstruction — (Use additional code to identify urinary incontinence: 788.30-788.39) ♂
600.20 Benign localized hyperplasia of prostate without urinary obstruction — (Use additional code to identify urinary incontinence: 788.30-788.39) ♂
600.21 Benign localized hyperplasia of prostate with urinary obstruction — (Use additional code to identify urinary incontinence: 788.30-788.39) ♂
600.3 Cyst of prostate — (Use additional code to identify urinary incontinence: 788.30-788.39) ♂
600.90 Hyperplasia of prostate, unspecified, without urinary obstruction — (Use additional code to identify urinary incontinence: 788.30-788.39) ▽ ♂
600.91 Hyperplasia of prostate, unspecified, with urinary obstruction — (Use additional code to identify urinary incontinence: 788.30-788.39) ▽ ♂
601.0 Acute prostatitis — (Use additional code to identify organism: 041.0, 041.1) ♂
601.1 Chronic prostatitis — (Use additional code to identify organism: 041.0, 041.1) ♂

▽ Unspecified code ☒ Manifestation code
♀ Female diagnosis ♂ Male diagnosis

601.8 Other specified inflammatory disease of prostate — (Use additional code to identify organism: 041.0, 041.1) ♂
601.9 Unspecified prostatitis — (Use additional code to identify organism: 041.0, 041.1) ▽ ♂
602.0 Calculus of prostate ♂
602.1 Congestion or hemorrhage of prostate ♂
602.3 Dysplasia of prostate ♂
602.8 Other specified disorder of prostate ♂
602.9 Unspecified disorder of prostate ▽ ♂
607.84 Impotence of organic origin ♂
619.0 Urinary-genital tract fistula, female ♀
753.6 Congenital atresia and stenosis of urethra and bladder neck
753.8 Other specified congenital anomaly of bladder and urethra
788.1 Dysuria
788.20 Unspecified retention of urine ▽
788.21 Incomplete bladder emptying
788.29 Other specified retention of urine
788.30 Unspecified urinary incontinence ▽
788.31 Urge incontinence
788.32 Stress incontinence, male ♂
788.33 Mixed incontinence urge and stress (male)(female)
788.34 Incontinence without sensory awareness
788.35 Post-void dribbling
788.36 Nocturnal enuresis
788.37 Continuous leakage
788.39 Other urinary incontinence
788.41 Urinary frequency
788.42 Polyuria
788.43 Nocturia
788.5 Oliguria and anuria
788.61 Splitting of urinary stream
788.62 Slowing of urinary stream
788.63 Urgency of urination
788.69 Other abnormality of urination
788.7 Urethral discharge
788.8 Extravasation of urine
788.9 Other symptoms involving urinary system
793.5 Nonspecific abnormal findings on radiological and other examination of genitourinary organs
939.0 Foreign body in bladder and urethra
V10.46 Personal history of malignant neoplasm of prostate ♂
V10.51 Personal history of malignant neoplasm of bladder
V47.4 Other urinary problems — (This code is intended for use when these conditions are recorded as diagnoses or problems)
V67.59 Other follow-up examination
V71.1 Observation for suspected malignant neoplasm
V71.89 Observation for other specified suspected conditions
V76.3 Screening for malignant neoplasm of the bladder

ICD-9-CM Procedural

57.33 Closed (transurethral) biopsy of bladder

HCPCS Level II Supplies & Services

A4270 Disposable endoscope sheath, each
A4305 Disposable drug delivery system, flow rate of 50 ml or greater per hour
A4306 Disposable drug delivery system, flow rate of 5 ml or less per hour
A4550 Surgical trays

52214

52214 Cystourethroscopy, with fulguration (including cryosurgery or laser surgery) of trigone, bladder neck, prostatic fossa, urethra, or periurethral glands

ICD-9-CM Diagnostic

185 Malignant neoplasm of prostate ♂
188.0 Malignant neoplasm of trigone of urinary bladder
188.1 Malignant neoplasm of dome of urinary bladder
188.5 Malignant neoplasm of bladder neck
188.9 Malignant neoplasm of bladder, part unspecified ▽
189.3 Malignant neoplasm of urethra
195.3 Malignant neoplasm of pelvis
198.1 Secondary malignant neoplasm of other urinary organs
198.89 Secondary malignant neoplasm of other specified sites
223.3 Benign neoplasm of bladder
223.81 Benign neoplasm of urethra
223.9 Benign neoplasm of urinary organ, site unspecified ▽
229.8 Benign neoplasm of other specified sites
233.7 Carcinoma in situ of bladder
233.9 Carcinoma in situ of other and unspecified urinary organs ▽
236.7 Neoplasm of uncertain behavior of bladder
236.99 Neoplasm of uncertain behavior of other and unspecified urinary organs
238.8 Neoplasm of uncertain behavior of other specified sites
239.4 Neoplasm of unspecified nature of bladder
239.5 Neoplasm of unspecified nature of other genitourinary organs
239.8 Neoplasm of unspecified nature of other specified sites
595.1 Chronic interstitial cystitis — (Use additional code to identify organism, such as E. coli, 041.4)
595.82 Irradiation cystitis — (Use additional code to identify organism, such as E. coli, 041.4)
596.2 Vesical fistula, not elsewhere classified — (Use additional code to identify urinary incontinence: 625.6, 788.30-788.39)
596.7 Hemorrhage into bladder wall — (Use additional code to identify urinary incontinence: 625.6, 788.30-788.39)
596.8 Other specified disorder of bladder — (Use additional code to identify urinary incontinence: 625.6, 788.30-788.39)
597.81 Urethral syndrome NOS
598.9 Unspecified urethral stricture — (Use additional code to identify urinary incontinence: 625.6, 788.30-788.39) ▽
599.2 Urethral diverticulum
599.3 Urethral caruncle
599.7 Hematuria
625.6 Female stress incontinence ♀
788.1 Dysuria
788.29 Other specified retention of urine
788.41 Urinary frequency
788.42 Polyuria
788.43 Nocturia
788.9 Other symptoms involving urinary system

ICD-9-CM Procedural

57.49 Other transurethral excision or destruction of lesion or tissue of bladder
58.31 Endoscopic excision or destruction of lesion or tissue of urethra

HCPCS Level II Supplies & Services

A4270 Disposable endoscope sheath, each
A4305 Disposable drug delivery system, flow rate of 50 ml or greater per hour
A4306 Disposable drug delivery system, flow rate of 5 ml or less per hour
A4550 Surgical trays

52224

52224 Cystourethroscopy, with fulguration (including cryosurgery or laser surgery) or treatment of MINOR (less than 0.5 cm) lesion(s) with or without biopsy

ICD-9-CM Diagnostic

185 Malignant neoplasm of prostate ♂
188.0 Malignant neoplasm of trigone of urinary bladder
188.1 Malignant neoplasm of dome of urinary bladder
188.2 Malignant neoplasm of lateral wall of urinary bladder
188.3 Malignant neoplasm of anterior wall of urinary bladder
188.4 Malignant neoplasm of posterior wall of urinary bladder
188.5 Malignant neoplasm of bladder neck
188.6 Malignant neoplasm of ureteric orifice
188.7 Malignant neoplasm of urachus
188.8 Malignant neoplasm of other specified sites of bladder
188.9 Malignant neoplasm of bladder, part unspecified ▽
189.3 Malignant neoplasm of urethra
189.9 Malignant neoplasm of urinary organ, site unspecified ▽
198.1 Secondary malignant neoplasm of other urinary organs
223.3 Benign neoplasm of bladder
223.81 Benign neoplasm of urethra
223.89 Benign neoplasm of other specified sites of urinary organs
223.9 Benign neoplasm of urinary organ, site unspecified ▽
233.7 Carcinoma in situ of bladder
236.7 Neoplasm of uncertain behavior of bladder
236.99 Neoplasm of uncertain behavior of other and unspecified urinary organs
239.4 Neoplasm of unspecified nature of bladder
595.0 Acute cystitis — (Use additional code to identify organism, such as E. coli, 041.4)
595.1 Chronic interstitial cystitis — (Use additional code to identify organism, such as E. coli, 041.4)
595.3 Trigonitis — (Use additional code to identify organism, such as E. coli, 041.4)

595.4 Cystitis in diseases classified elsewhere — (Code first underlying disease: 006.8, 039.8, 120.0-120.9, 122.3, 122.6. Use additional code to identify organism, such as E. coli, 041.4) ☒
595.81 Cystitis cystica — (Use additional code to identify organism, such as E. coli, 041.4)
595.82 Irradiation cystitis — (Use additional code to identify organism, such as E. coli, 041.4)
596.3 Diverticulum of bladder — (Use additional code to identify urinary incontinence: 625.6, 788.30-788.39)
596.8 Other specified disorder of bladder — (Use additional code to identify urinary incontinence: 625.6, 788.30-788.39)
599.3 Urethral caruncle
599.7 Hematuria
601.1 Chronic prostatitis — (Use additional code to identify organism: 041.0, 041.1) ♂
788.29 Other specified retention of urine
788.43 Nocturia
V10.51 Personal history of malignant neoplasm of bladder

ICD-9-CM Procedural
57.49 Other transurethral excision or destruction of lesion or tissue of bladder

HCPCS Level II Supplies & Services
A4270 Disposable endoscope sheath, each
A4305 Disposable drug delivery system, flow rate of 50 ml or greater per hour
A4306 Disposable drug delivery system, flow rate of 5 ml or less per hour
A4550 Surgical trays

52234–52240
52234 Cystourethroscopy, with fulguration (including cryosurgery or laser surgery) and/or resection of; SMALL bladder tumor(s) (0.5 up to 2.0 cm)
52235 MEDIUM bladder tumor(s) (2.0 to 5.0 cm)
52240 LARGE bladder tumor(s)

ICD-9-CM Diagnostic
188.0 Malignant neoplasm of trigone of urinary bladder
188.1 Malignant neoplasm of dome of urinary bladder
188.2 Malignant neoplasm of lateral wall of urinary bladder
188.3 Malignant neoplasm of anterior wall of urinary bladder
188.4 Malignant neoplasm of posterior wall of urinary bladder
188.5 Malignant neoplasm of bladder neck
188.6 Malignant neoplasm of ureteric orifice
188.7 Malignant neoplasm of urachus
188.8 Malignant neoplasm of other specified sites of bladder
188.9 Malignant neoplasm of bladder, part unspecified ▽
189.8 Malignant neoplasm of other specified sites of urinary organs
198.1 Secondary malignant neoplasm of other urinary organs
223.3 Benign neoplasm of bladder
233.7 Carcinoma in situ of bladder
236.7 Neoplasm of uncertain behavior of bladder
239.4 Neoplasm of unspecified nature of bladder
595.0 Acute cystitis — (Use additional code to identify organism, such as E. coli, 041.4)
595.1 Chronic interstitial cystitis — (Use additional code to identify organism, such as E. coli, 041.4)
595.3 Trigonitis — (Use additional code to identify organism, such as E. coli, 041.4)
595.4 Cystitis in diseases classified elsewhere — (Code first underlying disease: 006.8, 039.8, 120.0-120.9, 122.3, 122.6. Use additional code to identify organism, such as E. coli, 041.4) ☒
595.81 Cystitis cystica — (Use additional code to identify organism, such as E. coli, 041.4)
595.82 Irradiation cystitis — (Use additional code to identify organism, such as E. coli, 041.4)
599.7 Hematuria
V10.51 Personal history of malignant neoplasm of bladder

ICD-9-CM Procedural
57.49 Other transurethral excision or destruction of lesion or tissue of bladder

HCPCS Level II Supplies & Services
A4270 Disposable endoscope sheath, each
A4305 Disposable drug delivery system, flow rate of 50 ml or greater per hour
A4306 Disposable drug delivery system, flow rate of 5 ml or less per hour
A4550 Surgical trays

52250
52250 Cystourethroscopy with insertion of radioactive substance, with or without biopsy or fulguration

ICD-9-CM Diagnostic
188.0 Malignant neoplasm of trigone of urinary bladder
188.1 Malignant neoplasm of dome of urinary bladder
188.2 Malignant neoplasm of lateral wall of urinary bladder
188.3 Malignant neoplasm of anterior wall of urinary bladder
188.4 Malignant neoplasm of posterior wall of urinary bladder
188.5 Malignant neoplasm of bladder neck
188.6 Malignant neoplasm of ureteric orifice
188.7 Malignant neoplasm of urachus
188.9 Malignant neoplasm of bladder, part unspecified ▽
189.3 Malignant neoplasm of urethra

ICD-9-CM Procedural
57.32 Other cystoscopy
57.33 Closed (transurethral) biopsy of bladder
57.49 Other transurethral excision or destruction of lesion or tissue of bladder
92.27 Implantation or insertion of radioactive elements

HCPCS Level II Supplies & Services
A4550 Surgical trays

52260–52265
52260 Cystourethroscopy, with dilation of bladder for interstitial cystitis; general or conduction (spinal) anesthesia
52265 local anesthesia

ICD-9-CM Diagnostic
595.1 Chronic interstitial cystitis — (Use additional code to identify organism, such as E. coli, 041.4)
599.7 Hematuria
788.1 Dysuria
788.41 Urinary frequency

ICD-9-CM Procedural
57.92 Dilation of bladder neck

HCPCS Level II Supplies & Services
A4270 Disposable endoscope sheath, each
A4305 Disposable drug delivery system, flow rate of 50 ml or greater per hour
A4306 Disposable drug delivery system, flow rate of 5 ml or less per hour
A4550 Surgical trays

52270–52276
52270 Cystourethroscopy, with internal urethrotomy; female
52275 male
52276 Cystourethroscopy with direct vision internal urethrotomy

ICD-9-CM Diagnostic
185 Malignant neoplasm of prostate ♂
344.61 Cauda equina syndrome with neurogenic bladder
590.80 Unspecified pyelonephritis — (Use additional code to identify organism, such as E. coli, 041.4) ▽
595.0 Acute cystitis — (Use additional code to identify organism, such as E. coli, 041.4)
595.1 Chronic interstitial cystitis — (Use additional code to identify organism, such as E. coli, 041.4)
595.2 Other chronic cystitis — (Use additional code to identify organism, such as E. coli, 041.4)
595.3 Trigonitis — (Use additional code to identify organism, such as E. coli, 041.4)
595.4 Cystitis in diseases classified elsewhere — (Code first underlying disease: 006.8, 039.8, 120.0-120.9, 122.3, 122.6. Use additional code to identify organism, such as E. coli, 041.4) ☒
595.81 Cystitis cystica — (Use additional code to identify organism, such as E. coli, 041.4)
595.82 Irradiation cystitis — (Use additional code to identify organism, such as E. coli, 041.4)
595.89 Other specified types of cystitis — (Use additional code to identify organism, such as E. coli, 041.4)
595.9 Unspecified cystitis — (Use additional code to identify organism, such as E. coli, 041.4) ▽
596.8 Other specified disorder of bladder — (Use additional code to identify urinary incontinence: 625.6, 788.30-788.39)

597.0 Urethral abscess
598.00 Urethral stricture due to unspecified infection — (Use additional code to identify urinary incontinence: 625.6, 788.30-788.39) ▽
598.01 Urethral stricture due to infective diseases classified elsewhere — (Code first underlying disease: 095.8, 098.2, 120.0-120.9. Use additional code to identify urinary incontinence: 625.6, 788.30-788.39) ☒
598.1 Traumatic urethral stricture — (Use additional code to identify urinary incontinence: 625.6, 788.30-788.39)
598.2 Postoperative urethral stricture — (Use additional code to identify urinary incontinence: 625.6, 788.30-788.39)
598.8 Other specified causes of urethral stricture — (Use additional code to identify urinary incontinence: 625.6, 788.30-788.39)
598.9 Unspecified urethral stricture — (Use additional code to identify urinary incontinence: 625.6, 788.30-788.39) ▽
599.1 Urethral fistula
599.2 Urethral diverticulum
599.3 Urethral caruncle
599.6 Unspecified urinary obstruction — (Use additional code to identify urinary incontinence: 625.6, 788.30-788.39) ▽
599.7 Hematuria
600.00 Hypertrophy (benign) of prostate without urinary obstruction — (Use additional code to identify urinary incontinence: 788.30-788.39) ♂
600.01 Hypertrophy (benign) of prostate with urinary obstruction — (Use additional code to identify urinary incontinence: 788.30-788.39) ♂
600.10 Nodular prostate without urinary obstruction — (Use additional code to identify urinary incontinence: 788.30-788.39) ♂
600.11 Nodular prostate with urinary obstruction — (Use additional code to identify urinary incontinence: 788.30-788.39) ♂
600.20 Benign localized hyperplasia of prostate without urinary obstruction — (Use additional code to identify urinary incontinence: 788.30-788.39) ♂
600.21 Benign localized hyperplasia of prostate with urinary obstruction — (Use additional code to identify urinary incontinence: 788.30-788.39) ♂
600.3 Cyst of prostate — (Use additional code to identify urinary incontinence: 788.30-788.39) ♂
600.90 Hyperplasia of prostate, unspecified, without urinary obstruction — (Use additional code to identify urinary incontinence: 788.30-788.39) ▽ ♂
600.91 Hyperplasia of prostate, unspecified, with urinary obstruction — (Use additional code to identify urinary incontinence: 788.30-788.39) ▽ ♂
605 Redundant prepuce and phimosis ♂
625.6 Female stress incontinence ♀
753.6 Congenital atresia and stenosis of urethra and bladder neck
788.9 Other symptoms involving urinary system
867.0 Bladder and urethra injury without mention of open wound into cavity
996.76 Other complications due to genitourinary device, implant, and graft

ICD-9-CM Procedural

57.32 Other cystoscopy
58.5 Release of urethral stricture

HCPCS Level II Supplies & Services

A4270 Disposable endoscope sheath, each
A4305 Disposable drug delivery system, flow rate of 50 ml or greater per hour
A4306 Disposable drug delivery system, flow rate of 5 ml or less per hour
A4550 Surgical trays

52277

52277 Cystourethroscopy, with resection of external sphincter (sphincterotomy)

ICD-9-CM Diagnostic

344.61 Cauda equina syndrome with neurogenic bladder
596.51 Hypertonicity of bladder — (Use additional code to identify urinary incontinence: 625.6, 788.30-788.39)
596.54 Neurogenic bladder, NOS — (Use additional code to identify urinary incontinence: 625.6, 788.30-788.39) ▽
625.6 Female stress incontinence ♀

ICD-9-CM Procedural

57.32 Other cystoscopy
57.91 Sphincterotomy of bladder

HCPCS Level II Supplies & Services

A4270 Disposable endoscope sheath, each
A4305 Disposable drug delivery system, flow rate of 50 ml or greater per hour
A4306 Disposable drug delivery system, flow rate of 5 ml or less per hour
A4550 Surgical trays

52281–52282

52281 Cystourethroscopy, with calibration and/or dilation of urethral stricture or stenosis, with or without meatotomy, with or without injection procedure for cystography, male or female
52282 Cystourethroscopy, with insertion of urethral stent

ICD-9-CM Diagnostic

185 Malignant neoplasm of prostate ♂
222.2 Benign neoplasm of prostate ♂
233.4 Carcinoma in situ of prostate ♂
236.5 Neoplasm of uncertain behavior of prostate ♂
596.0 Bladder neck obstruction — (Use additional code to identify urinary incontinence: 625.6, 788.30-788.39)
597.89 Other urethritis
598.00 Urethral stricture due to unspecified infection — (Use additional code to identify urinary incontinence: 625.6, 788.30-788.39) ▽
598.01 Urethral stricture due to infective diseases classified elsewhere — (Code first underlying disease: 095.8, 098.2, 120.0-120.9. Use additional code to identify urinary incontinence: 625.6, 788.30-788.39) ☒
598.1 Traumatic urethral stricture — (Use additional code to identify urinary incontinence: 625.6, 788.30-788.39)
598.2 Postoperative urethral stricture — (Use additional code to identify urinary incontinence: 625.6, 788.30-788.39)
598.8 Other specified causes of urethral stricture — (Use additional code to identify urinary incontinence: 625.6, 788.30-788.39)
598.9 Unspecified urethral stricture — (Use additional code to identify urinary incontinence: 625.6, 788.30-788.39) ▽
599.1 Urethral fistula
599.2 Urethral diverticulum
599.3 Urethral caruncle
599.4 Urethral false passage
599.5 Prolapsed urethral mucosa
599.6 Unspecified urinary obstruction — (Use additional code to identify urinary incontinence: 625.6, 788.30-788.39) ▽
600.00 Hypertrophy (benign) of prostate without urinary obstruction — (Use additional code to identify urinary incontinence: 788.30-788.39) ♂
600.01 Hypertrophy (benign) of prostate with urinary obstruction — (Use additional code to identify urinary incontinence: 788.30-788.39) ♂
600.10 Nodular prostate without urinary obstruction — (Use additional code to identify urinary incontinence: 788.30-788.39) ♂
600.11 Nodular prostate with urinary obstruction — (Use additional code to identify urinary incontinence: 788.30-788.39) ♂
600.20 Benign localized hyperplasia of prostate without urinary obstruction — (Use additional code to identify urinary incontinence: 788.30-788.39) ♂
600.21 Benign localized hyperplasia of prostate with urinary obstruction — (Use additional code to identify urinary incontinence: 788.30-788.39) ♂
600.3 Cyst of prostate — (Use additional code to identify urinary incontinence: 788.30-788.39) ♂
600.90 Hyperplasia of prostate, unspecified, without urinary obstruction — (Use additional code to identify urinary incontinence: 788.30-788.39) ▽ ♂
600.91 Hyperplasia of prostate, unspecified, with urinary obstruction — (Use additional code to identify urinary incontinence: 788.30-788.39) ▽ ♂
601.1 Chronic prostatitis — (Use additional code to identify organism: 041.0, 041.1) ♂
601.9 Unspecified prostatitis — (Use additional code to identify organism: 041.0, 041.1) ▽ ♂
602.3 Dysplasia of prostate ♂
753.6 Congenital atresia and stenosis of urethra and bladder neck
788.29 Other specified retention of urine

ICD-9-CM Procedural

57.32 Other cystoscopy
58.5 Release of urethral stricture
58.99 Other operations on urethra and periurethral tissue
87.77 Other cystogram

HCPCS Level II Supplies & Services

A4270 Disposable endoscope sheath, each
A4305 Disposable drug delivery system, flow rate of 50 ml or greater per hour
A4306 Disposable drug delivery system, flow rate of 5 ml or less per hour
A4550 Surgical trays

▽ Unspecified code ☒ Manifestation code
♀ Female diagnosis ♂ Male diagnosis

52283

52283 Cystourethroscopy, with steroid injection into stricture

ICD-9-CM Diagnostic

596.0 Bladder neck obstruction — (Use additional code to identify urinary incontinence: 625.6, 788.30-788.39)
598.00 Urethral stricture due to unspecified infection — (Use additional code to identify urinary incontinence: 625.6, 788.30-788.39) ▽
598.01 Urethral stricture due to infective diseases classified elsewhere — (Code first underlying disease: 095.8, 098.2, 120.0-120.9. Use additional code to identify urinary incontinence: 625.6, 788.30-788.39) ☒
598.1 Traumatic urethral stricture — (Use additional code to identify urinary incontinence: 625.6, 788.30-788.39)
598.2 Postoperative urethral stricture — (Use additional code to identify urinary incontinence: 625.6, 788.30-788.39)
598.8 Other specified causes of urethral stricture — (Use additional code to identify urinary incontinence: 625.6, 788.30-788.39)
598.9 Unspecified urethral stricture — (Use additional code to identify urinary incontinence: 625.6, 788.30-788.39) ▽
599.6 Unspecified urinary obstruction — (Use additional code to identify urinary incontinence: 625.6, 788.30-788.39) ▽

ICD-9-CM Procedural

57.32 Other cystoscopy
99.23 Injection of steroid

HCPCS Level II Supplies & Services

A4270 Disposable endoscope sheath, each
A4305 Disposable drug delivery system, flow rate of 50 ml or greater per hour
A4306 Disposable drug delivery system, flow rate of 5 ml or less per hour
A4550 Surgical trays

52285

52285 Cystourethroscopy for treatment of the female urethral syndrome with any or all of the following: urethral meatotomy, urethral dilation, internal urethrotomy, lysis of urethrovaginal septal fibrosis, lateral incisions of the bladder neck, and fulguration of polyp(s) of urethra, bladder neck, and/or trigone

ICD-9-CM Diagnostic

595.0 Acute cystitis — (Use additional code to identify organism, such as E. coli, 041.4)
595.1 Chronic interstitial cystitis — (Use additional code to identify organism, such as E. coli, 041.4)
595.2 Other chronic cystitis — (Use additional code to identify organism, such as E. coli, 041.4)
595.3 Trigonitis — (Use additional code to identify organism, such as E. coli, 041.4)
595.4 Cystitis in diseases classified elsewhere — (Code first underlying disease: 006.8, 039.8, 120.0-120.9, 122.3, 122.6. Use additional code to identify organism, such as E. coli, 041.4) ☒
595.89 Other specified types of cystitis — (Use additional code to identify organism, such as E. coli, 041.4)
595.9 Unspecified cystitis — (Use additional code to identify organism, such as E. coli, 041.4) ▽
596.0 Bladder neck obstruction — (Use additional code to identify urinary incontinence: 625.6, 788.30-788.39)
597.0 Urethral abscess
597.80 Unspecified urethritis ▽
597.81 Urethral syndrome NOS
597.89 Other urethritis
598.1 Traumatic urethral stricture — (Use additional code to identify urinary incontinence: 625.6, 788.30-788.39)
598.2 Postoperative urethral stricture — (Use additional code to identify urinary incontinence: 625.6, 788.30-788.39)
599.0 Urinary tract infection, site not specified — (Use additional code to identify organism, such as E. coli, 041.4) ▽
599.1 Urethral fistula
599.3 Urethral caruncle
599.7 Hematuria
599.89 Other specified disorders of urinary tract — (Use additional code to identify urinary incontinence: 625.6, 788.30-788.39)
625.6 Female stress incontinence ♀
780.99 Other general symptoms
788.29 Other specified retention of urine

ICD-9-CM Procedural

57.32 Other cystoscopy
58.31 Endoscopic excision or destruction of lesion or tissue of urethra
58.5 Release of urethral stricture
58.6 Dilation of urethra

52290

52290 Cystourethroscopy; with ureteral meatotomy, unilateral or bilateral

ICD-9-CM Diagnostic

593.3 Stricture or kinking of ureter
593.4 Other ureteric obstruction
753.22 Congenital obstruction of ureterovesical junction
753.23 Congenital ureterocele
753.29 Other obstructive defect of renal pelvis and ureter

ICD-9-CM Procedural

56.1 Ureteral meatotomy
56.39 Other diagnostic procedures on ureter
57.32 Other cystoscopy

HCPCS Level II Supplies & Services

A4550 Surgical trays

52300–52301

52300 Cystourethroscopy; with resection or fulguration of orthotopic ureterocele(s), unilateral or bilateral
52301 with resection or fulguration of ectopic ureterocele(s), unilateral or bilateral

ICD-9-CM Diagnostic

593.89 Other specified disorder of kidney and ureter
753.23 Congenital ureterocele

ICD-9-CM Procedural

56.41 Partial ureterectomy
57.49 Other transurethral excision or destruction of lesion or tissue of bladder

HCPCS Level II Supplies & Services

A4550 Surgical trays

52305

52305 Cystourethroscopy; with incision or resection of orifice of bladder diverticulum, single or multiple

ICD-9-CM Diagnostic

596.3 Diverticulum of bladder — (Use additional code to identify urinary incontinence: 625.6, 788.30-788.39)

ICD-9-CM Procedural

57.32 Other cystoscopy
57.49 Other transurethral excision or destruction of lesion or tissue of bladder

HCPCS Level II Supplies & Services

A4550 Surgical trays

52310–52315

52310 Cystourethroscopy, with removal of foreign body, calculus, or ureteral stent from urethra or bladder (separate procedure); simple
52315 complicated

ICD-9-CM Diagnostic

594.1 Other calculus in bladder
594.2 Calculus in urethra
594.9 Unspecified calculus of lower urinary tract ▽
939.0 Foreign body in bladder and urethra
939.9 Foreign body in unspecified site in genitourinary tract ▽
996.39 Mechanical complication of genitourinary device, implant, and graft, other
996.65 Infection and inflammatory reaction due to other genitourinary device, implant, and graft — (Use additional code to identify specified infections)
996.76 Other complications due to genitourinary device, implant, and graft

ICD-9-CM Procedural

57.0 Transurethral clearance of bladder
57.32 Other cystoscopy
57.99 Other operations on bladder
97.62 Removal of ureterostomy tube and ureteral catheter
98.19 Removal of intraluminal foreign body from urethra without incision

▽ Unspecified code ☒ Manifestation code
♀ Female diagnosis ♂ Male diagnosis

HCPCS Level II Supplies & Services

A4270 Disposable endoscope sheath, each
A4305 Disposable drug delivery system, flow rate of 50 ml or greater per hour
A4306 Disposable drug delivery system, flow rate of 5 ml or less per hour
A4550 Surgical trays

52317–52318

52317 Litholapaxy: crushing or fragmentation of calculus by any means in bladder and removal of fragments; simple or small (less than 2.5 cm)
52318 complicated or large (over 2.5 cm)

ICD-9-CM Diagnostic

594.0 Calculus in diverticulum of bladder
594.1 Other calculus in bladder

ICD-9-CM Procedural

57.0 Transurethral clearance of bladder
57.19 Other cystotomy
57.99 Other operations on bladder
59.95 Ultrasonic fragmentation of urinary stones
98.19 Removal of intraluminal foreign body from urethra without incision

52320–52330

52320 Cystourethroscopy (including ureteral catheterization); with removal of ureteral calculus
52325 with fragmentation of ureteral calculus (eg, ultrasonic or electro-hydraulic technique)
52327 with subureteric injection of implant material
52330 with manipulation, without removal of ureteral calculus

ICD-9-CM Diagnostic

591 Hydronephrosis
592.1 Calculus of ureter
593.3 Stricture or kinking of ureter
593.4 Other ureteric obstruction
593.5 Hydroureter
593.89 Other specified disorder of kidney and ureter
599.7 Hematuria
788.0 Renal colic

ICD-9-CM Procedural

56.0 Transurethral removal of obstruction from ureter and renal pelvis
57.32 Other cystoscopy
59.95 Ultrasonic fragmentation of urinary stones

52332

52332 Cystourethroscopy, with insertion of indwelling ureteral stent (eg, Gibbons or double-J type)

ICD-9-CM Diagnostic

188.0 Malignant neoplasm of trigone of urinary bladder
188.1 Malignant neoplasm of dome of urinary bladder
188.2 Malignant neoplasm of lateral wall of urinary bladder
188.3 Malignant neoplasm of anterior wall of urinary bladder
189.2 Malignant neoplasm of ureter
198.1 Secondary malignant neoplasm of other urinary organs
223.2 Benign neoplasm of ureter
223.3 Benign neoplasm of bladder
223.9 Benign neoplasm of urinary organ, site unspecified ▽
236.7 Neoplasm of uncertain behavior of bladder
236.91 Neoplasm of uncertain behavior of kidney and ureter
239.4 Neoplasm of unspecified nature of bladder
239.5 Neoplasm of unspecified nature of other genitourinary organs
591 Hydronephrosis
592.0 Calculus of kidney
592.1 Calculus of ureter
593.3 Stricture or kinking of ureter
593.4 Other ureteric obstruction
593.89 Other specified disorder of kidney and ureter
599.6 Unspecified urinary obstruction — (Use additional code to identify urinary incontinence: 625.6, 788.30-788.39) ▽
599.7 Hematuria
599.89 Other specified disorders of urinary tract — (Use additional code to identify urinary incontinence: 625.6, 788.30-788.39)
619.0 Urinary-genital tract fistula, female ♀
753.4 Other specified congenital anomalies of ureter
788.0 Renal colic
867.2 Ureter injury without mention of open wound into cavity
867.3 Ureter injury with open wound into cavity
996.59 Mechanical complication due to other implant and internal device, not elsewhere classified

ICD-9-CM Procedural

57.32 Other cystoscopy
59.8 Ureteral catheterization

HCPCS Level II Supplies & Services

A4270 Disposable endoscope sheath, each
A4305 Disposable drug delivery system, flow rate of 50 ml or greater per hour
A4306 Disposable drug delivery system, flow rate of 5 ml or less per hour
A4550 Surgical trays

52334

52334 Cystourethroscopy with insertion of ureteral guide wire through kidney to establish a percutaneous nephrostomy, retrograde

ICD-9-CM Diagnostic

188.0 Malignant neoplasm of trigone of urinary bladder
188.1 Malignant neoplasm of dome of urinary bladder
188.2 Malignant neoplasm of lateral wall of urinary bladder
188.3 Malignant neoplasm of anterior wall of urinary bladder
188.4 Malignant neoplasm of posterior wall of urinary bladder
188.5 Malignant neoplasm of bladder neck
188.6 Malignant neoplasm of ureteric orifice
188.8 Malignant neoplasm of other specified sites of bladder
188.9 Malignant neoplasm of bladder, part unspecified ▽
189.0 Malignant neoplasm of kidney, except pelvis
189.1 Malignant neoplasm of renal pelvis
189.2 Malignant neoplasm of ureter
236.7 Neoplasm of uncertain behavior of bladder
590.2 Renal and perinephric abscess — (Use additional code to identify organism, such as E. coli, 041.4)
590.3 Pyeloureteritis cystica — (Use additional code to identify organism, such as E. coli, 041.4)
591 Hydronephrosis
592.0 Calculus of kidney
592.1 Calculus of ureter
593.3 Stricture or kinking of ureter
593.4 Other ureteric obstruction
593.89 Other specified disorder of kidney and ureter
596.8 Other specified disorder of bladder — (Use additional code to identify urinary incontinence: 625.6, 788.30-788.39)
599.6 Unspecified urinary obstruction — (Use additional code to identify urinary incontinence: 625.6, 788.30-788.39) ▽
599.7 Hematuria
753.21 Congenital obstruction of ureteropelvic junction
753.22 Congenital obstruction of ureterovesical junction
753.29 Other obstructive defect of renal pelvis and ureter
788.0 Renal colic

ICD-9-CM Procedural

55.03 Percutaneous nephrostomy without fragmentation
57.32 Other cystoscopy

52341–52343

52341 Cystourethroscopy; with treatment of ureteral stricture (eg, balloon dilation, laser, electrocautery, and incision)
52342 with treatment of ureteropelvic junction stricture (eg, balloon dilation, laser, electrocautery, and incision)
52343 with treatment of intra-renal stricture (eg, balloon dilation, laser, electrocautery, and incision)

ICD-9-CM Diagnostic

591 Hydronephrosis
593.3 Stricture or kinking of ureter
593.5 Hydroureter
593.89 Other specified disorder of kidney and ureter
753.20 Unspecified obstructive defect of renal pelvis and ureter ▽
753.21 Congenital obstruction of ureteropelvic junction
753.22 Congenital obstruction of ureterovesical junction
753.29 Other obstructive defect of renal pelvis and ureter

753.3 Other specified congenital anomalies of kidney

ICD-9-CM Procedural

56.2 Ureterotomy
57.32 Other cystoscopy
59.8 Ureteral catheterization

52344–52346

52344 Cystourethroscopy with ureteroscopy; with treatment of ureteral stricture (eg, balloon dilation, laser, electrocautery, and incision)
52345 with treatment of ureteropelvic junction stricture (eg, balloon dilation, laser, electrocautery, and incision)
52346 with treatment of intra-renal stricture (eg, balloon dilation, laser, electrocautery, and incision)

ICD-9-CM Diagnostic

591 Hydronephrosis
593.3 Stricture or kinking of ureter
593.5 Hydroureter
593.89 Other specified disorder of kidney and ureter
753.20 Unspecified obstructive defect of renal pelvis and ureter ▽
753.21 Congenital obstruction of ureteropelvic junction
753.22 Congenital obstruction of ureterovesical junction
753.29 Other obstructive defect of renal pelvis and ureter
753.3 Other specified congenital anomalies of kidney

ICD-9-CM Procedural

56.2 Ureterotomy
56.31 Ureteroscopy
57.32 Other cystoscopy
59.8 Ureteral catheterization

52351

52351 Cystourethroscopy, with ureteroscopy and/or pyeloscopy; diagnostic

ICD-9-CM Diagnostic

188.0 Malignant neoplasm of trigone of urinary bladder
188.1 Malignant neoplasm of dome of urinary bladder
188.2 Malignant neoplasm of lateral wall of urinary bladder
188.3 Malignant neoplasm of anterior wall of urinary bladder
188.4 Malignant neoplasm of posterior wall of urinary bladder
188.5 Malignant neoplasm of bladder neck
188.6 Malignant neoplasm of ureteric orifice
188.7 Malignant neoplasm of urachus
188.8 Malignant neoplasm of other specified sites of bladder
188.9 Malignant neoplasm of bladder, part unspecified ▽
189.0 Malignant neoplasm of kidney, except pelvis
189.1 Malignant neoplasm of renal pelvis
189.2 Malignant neoplasm of ureter
198.0 Secondary malignant neoplasm of kidney
198.1 Secondary malignant neoplasm of other urinary organs
223.0 Benign neoplasm of kidney, except pelvis
233.7 Carcinoma in situ of bladder
233.9 Carcinoma in situ of other and unspecified urinary organs ▽
236.7 Neoplasm of uncertain behavior of bladder
236.90 Neoplasm of uncertain behavior of urinary organ, unspecified ▽
236.91 Neoplasm of uncertain behavior of kidney and ureter
236.99 Neoplasm of uncertain behavior of other and unspecified urinary organs
239.5 Neoplasm of unspecified nature of other genitourinary organs
591 Hydronephrosis
592.0 Calculus of kidney
592.1 Calculus of ureter
593.3 Stricture or kinking of ureter
593.4 Other ureteric obstruction
593.5 Hydroureter
593.89 Other specified disorder of kidney and ureter
599.6 Unspecified urinary obstruction — (Use additional code to identify urinary incontinence: 625.6, 788.30-788.39) ▽
599.7 Hematuria
753.20 Unspecified obstructive defect of renal pelvis and ureter ▽
753.21 Congenital obstruction of ureteropelvic junction
753.22 Congenital obstruction of ureterovesical junction
753.23 Congenital ureterocele
753.29 Other obstructive defect of renal pelvis and ureter
788.0 Renal colic
788.1 Dysuria
789.00 Abdominal pain, unspecified site ▽
789.01 Abdominal pain, right upper quadrant
789.02 Abdominal pain, left upper quadrant
793.5 Nonspecific abnormal findings on radiological and other examination of genitourinary organs

ICD-9-CM Procedural

55.22 Pyeloscopy
56.31 Ureteroscopy
57.32 Other cystoscopy

52352–52353

52352 Cystourethroscopy, with ureteroscopy and/or pyeloscopy; with removal or manipulation of calculus (ureteral catheterization is included)
52353 with lithotripsy (ureteral catheterization is included)

ICD-9-CM Diagnostic

591 Hydronephrosis
592.0 Calculus of kidney
592.1 Calculus of ureter
593.5 Hydroureter
594.1 Other calculus in bladder
599.7 Hematuria
788.0 Renal colic
789.01 Abdominal pain, right upper quadrant
789.02 Abdominal pain, left upper quadrant

ICD-9-CM Procedural

55.22 Pyeloscopy
56.0 Transurethral removal of obstruction from ureter and renal pelvis
56.31 Ureteroscopy

52354–52355

52354 Cystourethroscopy, with ureteroscopy and/or pyeloscopy; with biopsy and/or fulguration of ureteral or renal pelvic lesion
52355 with resection of ureteral or renal pelvic tumor

ICD-9-CM Diagnostic

188.6 Malignant neoplasm of ureteric orifice
189.1 Malignant neoplasm of renal pelvis
189.2 Malignant neoplasm of ureter
198.0 Secondary malignant neoplasm of kidney
198.1 Secondary malignant neoplasm of other urinary organs
223.1 Benign neoplasm of renal pelvis
223.2 Benign neoplasm of ureter
233.9 Carcinoma in situ of other and unspecified urinary organs ▽
236.7 Neoplasm of uncertain behavior of bladder
236.91 Neoplasm of uncertain behavior of kidney and ureter
239.4 Neoplasm of unspecified nature of bladder
239.5 Neoplasm of unspecified nature of other genitourinary organs
590.3 Pyeloureteritis cystica — (Use additional code to identify organism, such as E. coli, 041.4)
593.4 Other ureteric obstruction
593.89 Other specified disorder of kidney and ureter
599.7 Hematuria
788.1 Dysuria
793.5 Nonspecific abnormal findings on radiological and other examination of genitourinary organs

ICD-9-CM Procedural

55.22 Pyeloscopy
55.23 Closed (percutaneous) (needle) biopsy of kidney
55.39 Other local destruction or excision of renal lesion or tissue
55.4 Partial nephrectomy
56.31 Ureteroscopy
56.33 Closed endoscopic biopsy of ureter
56.99 Other operations on ureter
57.32 Other cystoscopy
57.33 Closed (transurethral) biopsy of bladder
57.49 Other transurethral excision or destruction of lesion or tissue of bladder
58.23 Biopsy of urethra
58.31 Endoscopic excision or destruction of lesion or tissue of urethra
58.39 Other local excision or destruction of lesion or tissue of urethra

▽ Unspecified code ♀ Female diagnosis ☒ Manifestation code ♂ Male diagnosis

52400

52400 Cystourethroscopy with incision, fulguration, or resection of congenital posterior urethral valves, or congenital obstructive hypertrophic mucosal folds

ICD-9-CM Diagnostic

596.4 Atony of bladder — (Use additional code to identify urinary incontinence: 625.6, 788.30-788.39)
596.8 Other specified disorder of bladder — (Use additional code to identify urinary incontinence: 625.6, 788.30-788.39)
599.7 Hematuria
753.6 Congenital atresia and stenosis of urethra and bladder neck
753.8 Other specified congenital anomaly of bladder and urethra
753.9 Unspecified congenital anomaly of urinary system ▽
788.20 Unspecified retention of urine ▽

ICD-9-CM Procedural

57.19 Other cystotomy
57.32 Other cystoscopy
57.49 Other transurethral excision or destruction of lesion or tissue of bladder
58.0 Urethrotomy
58.31 Endoscopic excision or destruction of lesion or tissue of urethra

HCPCS Level II Supplies & Services

A4550 Surgical trays

52402

52402 Cystourethroscopy with transurethral resection or incision of ejaculatory ducts

ICD-9-CM Diagnostic

187.8 Malignant neoplasm of other specified sites of male genital organs ♂
198.82 Secondary malignant neoplasm of genital organs
222.8 Benign neoplasm of other specified sites of male genital organs ♂
233.6 Carcinoma in situ of other and unspecified male genital organs ▽ ♂
236.6 Neoplasm of uncertain behavior of other and unspecified male genital organs ▽ ♂
239.5 Neoplasm of unspecified nature of other genitourinary organs
600.00 Hypertrophy (benign) of prostate without urinary obstruction — (Use additional code to identify urinary incontinence: 788.30-788.39) ♂
600.01 Hypertrophy (benign) of prostate with urinary obstruction — (Use additional code to identify urinary incontinence: 788.30-788.39) ♂
600.10 Nodular prostate without urinary obstruction — (Use additional code to identify urinary incontinence: 788.30-788.39) ♂
600.11 Nodular prostate with urinary obstruction — (Use additional code to identify urinary incontinence: 788.30-788.39) ♂
600.20 Benign localized hyperplasia of prostate without urinary obstruction — (Use additional code to identify urinary incontinence: 788.30-788.39) ♂
600.21 Benign localized hyperplasia of prostate with urinary obstruction — (Use additional code to identify urinary incontinence: 788.30-788.39) ♂
600.90 Hyperplasia of prostate, unspecified, without urinary obstruction — (Use additional code to identify urinary incontinence: 788.30-788.39) ▽ ♂
600.91 Hyperplasia of prostate, unspecified, with urinary obstruction — (Use additional code to identify urinary incontinence: 788.30-788.39) ▽ ♂
606.0 Azoospermia ♂
606.1 Oligospermia ♂
606.8 Infertility due to extratesticular causes ♂
607.84 Impotence of organic origin ♂
608.4 Other inflammatory disorder of male genital organs — (Use additional code to identify organism) ♂
608.81 Specified disorder of male genital organs in diseases classified elsewhere — (Code first underlying disease: 016.5, 125.0-125.9) ☒ ♂
608.82 Hematospermia ♂
608.83 Specified vascular disorder of male genital organs ♂
608.85 Stricture of male genital organs ♂
608.89 Other specified disorder of male genital organs ♂
752.9 Unspecified congenital anomaly of genital organs ▽
V26.21 Fertility testing
V26.29 Other investigation and testing

ICD-9-CM Procedural

57.32 Other cystoscopy
60.72 Incision of seminal vesicle
60.73 Excision of seminal vesicle
60.79 Other operations on seminal vesicles

52450

52450 Transurethral incision of prostate

ICD-9-CM Diagnostic

185 Malignant neoplasm of prostate ♂
596.0 Bladder neck obstruction — (Use additional code to identify urinary incontinence: 625.6, 788.30-788.39)
600.00 Hypertrophy (benign) of prostate without urinary obstruction — (Use additional code to identify urinary incontinence: 788.30-788.39) ♂
600.01 Hypertrophy (benign) of prostate with urinary obstruction — (Use additional code to identify urinary incontinence: 788.30-788.39) ♂
600.10 Nodular prostate without urinary obstruction — (Use additional code to identify urinary incontinence: 788.30-788.39) ♂
600.11 Nodular prostate with urinary obstruction — (Use additional code to identify urinary incontinence: 788.30-788.39) ♂
600.20 Benign localized hyperplasia of prostate without urinary obstruction — (Use additional code to identify urinary incontinence: 788.30-788.39) ♂
600.21 Benign localized hyperplasia of prostate with urinary obstruction — (Use additional code to identify urinary incontinence: 788.30-788.39) ♂
600.3 Cyst of prostate — (Use additional code to identify urinary incontinence: 788.30-788.39) ♂
600.90 Hyperplasia of prostate, unspecified, without urinary obstruction — (Use additional code to identify urinary incontinence: 788.30-788.39) ▽ ♂
600.91 Hyperplasia of prostate, unspecified, with urinary obstruction — (Use additional code to identify urinary incontinence: 788.30-788.39) ▽ ♂
601.1 Chronic prostatitis — (Use additional code to identify organism: 041.0, 041.1) ♂
601.9 Unspecified prostatitis — (Use additional code to identify organism: 041.0, 041.1) ▽ ♂
788.20 Unspecified retention of urine ▽
788.21 Incomplete bladder emptying
788.29 Other specified retention of urine
788.30 Unspecified urinary incontinence ▽
788.31 Urge incontinence
788.32 Stress incontinence, male ♂
788.33 Mixed incontinence urge and stress (male)(female)
788.34 Incontinence without sensory awareness
788.35 Post-void dribbling
788.36 Nocturnal enuresis
788.37 Continuous leakage
788.39 Other urinary incontinence

ICD-9-CM Procedural

60.0 Incision of prostate

52500

52500 Transurethral resection of bladder neck (separate procedure)

ICD-9-CM Diagnostic

185 Malignant neoplasm of prostate ♂
223.3 Benign neoplasm of bladder
236.7 Neoplasm of uncertain behavior of bladder
596.0 Bladder neck obstruction — (Use additional code to identify urinary incontinence: 625.6, 788.30-788.39)
596.4 Atony of bladder — (Use additional code to identify urinary incontinence: 625.6, 788.30-788.39)
596.8 Other specified disorder of bladder — (Use additional code to identify urinary incontinence: 625.6, 788.30-788.39)
599.1 Urethral fistula
599.2 Urethral diverticulum
599.3 Urethral caruncle
599.4 Urethral false passage
599.7 Hematuria
599.81 Urethral hypermobility — (Use additional code to identify urinary incontinence: 625.6, 788.30-788.39)
600.00 Hypertrophy (benign) of prostate without urinary obstruction — (Use additional code to identify urinary incontinence: 788.30-788.39) ♂
600.01 Hypertrophy (benign) of prostate with urinary obstruction — (Use additional code to identify urinary incontinence: 788.30-788.39) ♂
600.10 Nodular prostate without urinary obstruction — (Use additional code to identify urinary incontinence: 788.30-788.39) ♂
600.11 Nodular prostate with urinary obstruction — (Use additional code to identify urinary incontinence: 788.30-788.39) ♂
600.20 Benign localized hyperplasia of prostate without urinary obstruction — (Use additional code to identify urinary incontinence: 788.30-788.39) ♂

▽ Unspecified code
♀ Female diagnosis
☒ Manifestation code
♂ Male diagnosis

600.21 Benign localized hyperplasia of prostate with urinary obstruction — (Use additional code to identify urinary incontinence: 788.30-788.39) ♂
600.3 Cyst of prostate — (Use additional code to identify urinary incontinence: 788.30-788.39) ♂
600.90 Hyperplasia of prostate, unspecified, without urinary obstruction — (Use additional code to identify urinary incontinence: 788.30-788.39) ▽ ♂
600.91 Hyperplasia of prostate, unspecified, with urinary obstruction — (Use additional code to identify urinary incontinence: 788.30-788.39) ▽ ♂
753.6 Congenital atresia and stenosis of urethra and bladder neck
753.9 Unspecified congenital anomaly of urinary system ▽
788.1 Dysuria
788.21 Incomplete bladder emptying
788.29 Other specified retention of urine

ICD-9-CM Procedural

57.49 Other transurethral excision or destruction of lesion or tissue of bladder

52510

52510 Transurethral balloon dilation of the prostatic urethra

ICD-9-CM Diagnostic

598.00 Urethral stricture due to unspecified infection — (Use additional code to identify urinary incontinence: 625.6, 788.30-788.39) ▽
598.01 Urethral stricture due to infective diseases classified elsewhere — (Code first underlying disease: 095.8, 098.2, 120.0-120.9. Use additional code to identify urinary incontinence: 625.6, 788.30-788.39) ☒
598.1 Traumatic urethral stricture — (Use additional code to identify urinary incontinence: 625.6, 788.30-788.39)
598.2 Postoperative urethral stricture — (Use additional code to identify urinary incontinence: 625.6, 788.30-788.39)
598.9 Unspecified urethral stricture — (Use additional code to identify urinary incontinence: 625.6, 788.30-788.39) ▽
599.1 Urethral fistula
599.2 Urethral diverticulum
599.3 Urethral caruncle
599.4 Urethral false passage
599.5 Prolapsed urethral mucosa
599.6 Unspecified urinary obstruction — (Use additional code to identify urinary incontinence: 625.6, 788.30-788.39) ▽
599.7 Hematuria
600.00 Hypertrophy (benign) of prostate without urinary obstruction — (Use additional code to identify urinary incontinence: 788.30-788.39) ♂
600.01 Hypertrophy (benign) of prostate with urinary obstruction — (Use additional code to identify urinary incontinence: 788.30-788.39) ♂
600.10 Nodular prostate without urinary obstruction — (Use additional code to identify urinary incontinence: 788.30-788.39) ♂
600.11 Nodular prostate with urinary obstruction — (Use additional code to identify urinary incontinence: 788.30-788.39) ♂
600.20 Benign localized hyperplasia of prostate without urinary obstruction — (Use additional code to identify urinary incontinence: 788.30-788.39) ♂
600.21 Benign localized hyperplasia of prostate with urinary obstruction — (Use additional code to identify urinary incontinence: 788.30-788.39) ♂
600.3 Cyst of prostate — (Use additional code to identify urinary incontinence: 788.30-788.39) ♂
600.90 Hyperplasia of prostate, unspecified, without urinary obstruction — (Use additional code to identify urinary incontinence: 788.30-788.39) ▽ ♂
600.91 Hyperplasia of prostate, unspecified, with urinary obstruction — (Use additional code to identify urinary incontinence: 788.30-788.39) ▽ ♂
602.8 Other specified disorder of prostate ♂

ICD-9-CM Procedural

60.95 Transurethral balloon dilation of the prostatic urethra

52601

52601 Transurethral electrosurgical resection of prostate, including control of postoperative bleeding, complete (vasectomy, meatotomy, cystourethroscopy, urethral calibration and/or dilation, and internal urethrotomy are included)

ICD-9-CM Diagnostic

185 Malignant neoplasm of prostate ♂
222.2 Benign neoplasm of prostate ♂
233.4 Carcinoma in situ of prostate ♂
236.5 Neoplasm of uncertain behavior of prostate ♂
591 Hydronephrosis
596.0 Bladder neck obstruction — (Use additional code to identify urinary incontinence: 625.6, 788.30-788.39)
598.9 Unspecified urethral stricture — (Use additional code to identify urinary incontinence: 625.6, 788.30-788.39) ▽
599.6 Unspecified urinary obstruction — (Use additional code to identify urinary incontinence: 625.6, 788.30-788.39) ▽
599.7 Hematuria
600.00 Hypertrophy (benign) of prostate without urinary obstruction — (Use additional code to identify urinary incontinence: 788.30-788.39) ♂
600.01 Hypertrophy (benign) of prostate with urinary obstruction — (Use additional code to identify urinary incontinence: 788.30-788.39) ♂
600.10 Nodular prostate without urinary obstruction — (Use additional code to identify urinary incontinence: 788.30-788.39) ♂
600.11 Nodular prostate with urinary obstruction — (Use additional code to identify urinary incontinence: 788.30-788.39) ♂
600.20 Benign localized hyperplasia of prostate without urinary obstruction — (Use additional code to identify urinary incontinence: 788.30-788.39) ♂
600.21 Benign localized hyperplasia of prostate with urinary obstruction — (Use additional code to identify urinary incontinence: 788.30-788.39) ♂
600.3 Cyst of prostate — (Use additional code to identify urinary incontinence: 788.30-788.39) ♂
600.90 Hyperplasia of prostate, unspecified, without urinary obstruction — (Use additional code to identify urinary incontinence: 788.30-788.39) ▽ ♂
600.91 Hyperplasia of prostate, unspecified, with urinary obstruction — (Use additional code to identify urinary incontinence: 788.30-788.39) ▽ ♂
601.0 Acute prostatitis — (Use additional code to identify organism: 041.0, 041.1) ♂
601.1 Chronic prostatitis — (Use additional code to identify organism: 041.0, 041.1) ♂
601.9 Unspecified prostatitis — (Use additional code to identify organism: 041.0, 041.1) ▽ ♂
602.3 Dysplasia of prostate ♂
602.9 Unspecified disorder of prostate ▽ ♂
788.20 Unspecified retention of urine ▽
788.21 Incomplete bladder emptying
788.29 Other specified retention of urine
788.39 Other urinary incontinence
V84.03 Genetic susceptibility to malignant neoplasm of prostate
V84.09 Genetic susceptibility to other malignant neoplasm

ICD-9-CM Procedural

60.21 Transurethral (ultrasound) guided laser induced prostatectomy (TULIP)
60.29 Other transurethral prostatectomy

52606

52606 Transurethral fulguration for postoperative bleeding occurring after the usual follow-up time

ICD-9-CM Diagnostic

596.7 Hemorrhage into bladder wall — (Use additional code to identify urinary incontinence: 625.6, 788.30-788.39)
599.7 Hematuria
997.5 Urinary complications — (Use additional code to identify complications)
998.11 Hemorrhage complicating a procedure

ICD-9-CM Procedural

60.94 Control of (postoperative) hemorrhage of prostate

52612–52614

52612 Transurethral resection of prostate; first stage of two-stage resection (partial resection)
52614 second stage of two-stage resection (resection completed)

ICD-9-CM Diagnostic

185 Malignant neoplasm of prostate ♂
198.82 Secondary malignant neoplasm of genital organs
222.2 Benign neoplasm of prostate ♂
233.4 Carcinoma in situ of prostate ♂
236.5 Neoplasm of uncertain behavior of prostate ♂
239.5 Neoplasm of unspecified nature of other genitourinary organs
600.00 Hypertrophy (benign) of prostate without urinary obstruction — (Use additional code to identify urinary incontinence: 788.30-788.39) ♂
600.01 Hypertrophy (benign) of prostate with urinary obstruction — (Use additional code to identify urinary incontinence: 788.30-788.39) ♂
600.10 Nodular prostate without urinary obstruction — (Use additional code to identify urinary incontinence: 788.30-788.39) ♂
600.11 Nodular prostate with urinary obstruction — (Use additional code to identify urinary incontinence: 788.30-788.39) ♂

▽ Unspecified code ♀ Female diagnosis ☒ Manifestation code ♂ Male diagnosis

600.20 Benign localized hyperplasia of prostate without urinary obstruction — (Use additional code to identify urinary incontinence: 788.30-788.39) ♂
600.21 Benign localized hyperplasia of prostate with urinary obstruction — (Use additional code to identify urinary incontinence: 788.30-788.39) ♂
600.3 Cyst of prostate — (Use additional code to identify urinary incontinence: 788.30-788.39) ♂
600.90 Hyperplasia of prostate, unspecified, without urinary obstruction — (Use additional code to identify urinary incontinence: 788.30-788.39) ▽ ♂
600.91 Hyperplasia of prostate, unspecified, with urinary obstruction — (Use additional code to identify urinary incontinence: 788.30-788.39) ▽ ♂
601.0 Acute prostatitis — (Use additional code to identify organism: 041.0, 041.1) ♂
601.1 Chronic prostatitis — (Use additional code to identify organism: 041.0, 041.1) ♂
601.2 Abscess of prostate — (Use additional code to identify organism: 041.0, 041.1) ♂
601.3 Prostatocystitis — (Use additional code to identify organism: 041.0, 041.1) ♂
601.4 Prostatitis in diseases classified elsewhere — (Code first underlying disease: 016.5, 039.8, 095.8, 116.0. Use additional code to identify organism: 041.0, 041.1) ☒ ♂
601.9 Unspecified prostatitis — (Use additional code to identify organism: 041.0, 041.1) ▽ ♂
602.3 Dysplasia of prostate ♂
788.20 Unspecified retention of urine ▽
788.21 Incomplete bladder emptying
788.29 Other specified retention of urine
788.39 Other urinary incontinence
V84.03 Genetic susceptibility to malignant neoplasm of prostate
V84.09 Genetic susceptibility to other malignant neoplasm

ICD-9-CM Procedural

60.29 Other transurethral prostatectomy

52620–52630

52620 Transurethral resection; of residual obstructive tissue after 90 days postoperative
52630 of regrowth of obstructive tissue longer than one year postoperative

ICD-9-CM Diagnostic

185 Malignant neoplasm of prostate ♂
188.9 Malignant neoplasm of bladder, part unspecified ▽
222.2 Benign neoplasm of prostate ♂
233.4 Carcinoma in situ of prostate ♂
236.5 Neoplasm of uncertain behavior of prostate ♂
591 Hydronephrosis
596.0 Bladder neck obstruction — (Use additional code to identify urinary incontinence: 625.6, 788.30-788.39)
598.9 Unspecified urethral stricture — (Use additional code to identify urinary incontinence: 625.6, 788.30-788.39) ▽
599.6 Unspecified urinary obstruction — (Use additional code to identify urinary incontinence: 625.6, 788.30-788.39) ▽
600.00 Hypertrophy (benign) of prostate without urinary obstruction — (Use additional code to identify urinary incontinence: 788.30-788.39) ♂
600.01 Hypertrophy (benign) of prostate with urinary obstruction — (Use additional code to identify urinary incontinence: 788.30-788.39) ♂
600.10 Nodular prostate without urinary obstruction — (Use additional code to identify urinary incontinence: 788.30-788.39) ♂
600.11 Nodular prostate with urinary obstruction — (Use additional code to identify urinary incontinence: 788.30-788.39) ♂
600.20 Benign localized hyperplasia of prostate without urinary obstruction — (Use additional code to identify urinary incontinence: 788.30-788.39) ♂
600.21 Benign localized hyperplasia of prostate with urinary obstruction — (Use additional code to identify urinary incontinence: 788.30-788.39) ♂
600.3 Cyst of prostate — (Use additional code to identify urinary incontinence: 788.30-788.39) ♂
600.90 Hyperplasia of prostate, unspecified, without urinary obstruction — (Use additional code to identify urinary incontinence: 788.30-788.39) ▽ ♂
600.91 Hyperplasia of prostate, unspecified, with urinary obstruction — (Use additional code to identify urinary incontinence: 788.30-788.39) ▽ ♂
601.0 Acute prostatitis — (Use additional code to identify organism: 041.0, 041.1) ♂
601.1 Chronic prostatitis — (Use additional code to identify organism: 041.0, 041.1) ♂
601.9 Unspecified prostatitis — (Use additional code to identify organism: 041.0, 041.1) ▽ ♂
602.3 Dysplasia of prostate ♂
602.9 Unspecified disorder of prostate ▽ ♂
788.20 Unspecified retention of urine ▽
788.21 Incomplete bladder emptying
788.29 Other specified retention of urine
788.39 Other urinary incontinence

ICD-9-CM Procedural

60.29 Other transurethral prostatectomy

52640

52640 Transurethral resection; of postoperative bladder neck contracture

ICD-9-CM Diagnostic

596.0 Bladder neck obstruction — (Use additional code to identify urinary incontinence: 625.6, 788.30-788.39)
598.2 Postoperative urethral stricture — (Use additional code to identify urinary incontinence: 625.6, 788.30-788.39)
599.6 Unspecified urinary obstruction — (Use additional code to identify urinary incontinence: 625.6, 788.30-788.39) ▽
788.20 Unspecified retention of urine ▽
788.21 Incomplete bladder emptying
788.29 Other specified retention of urine
788.30 Unspecified urinary incontinence ▽
788.31 Urge incontinence
788.32 Stress incontinence, male ♂
788.33 Mixed incontinence urge and stress (male)(female)
788.34 Incontinence without sensory awareness
788.35 Post-void dribbling
788.36 Nocturnal enuresis
788.37 Continuous leakage
788.38 Overflow incontinence
788.39 Other urinary incontinence

ICD-9-CM Procedural

57.49 Other transurethral excision or destruction of lesion or tissue of bladder

52647–52648

52647 Non-contact laser coagulation of prostate, including control of postoperative bleeding, complete (vasectomy, meatotomy, cystourethroscopy, urethral calibration and/or dilation, and internal urethrotomy are included)
52648 Contact laser vaporization with or without transurethral resection of prostate, including control of postoperative bleeding, complete (vasectomy, meatotomy, cystourethroscopy, urethral calibration and/or dilation, and internal urethrotomy are included)

ICD-9-CM Diagnostic

185 Malignant neoplasm of prostate ♂
188.9 Malignant neoplasm of bladder, part unspecified ▽
198.82 Secondary malignant neoplasm of genital organs
222.2 Benign neoplasm of prostate ♂
233.4 Carcinoma in situ of prostate ♂
236.5 Neoplasm of uncertain behavior of prostate ♂
239.5 Neoplasm of unspecified nature of other genitourinary organs
591 Hydronephrosis
596.0 Bladder neck obstruction — (Use additional code to identify urinary incontinence: 625.6, 788.30-788.39)
600.00 Hypertrophy (benign) of prostate without urinary obstruction — (Use additional code to identify urinary incontinence: 788.30-788.39) ♂
600.01 Hypertrophy (benign) of prostate with urinary obstruction — (Use additional code to identify urinary incontinence: 788.30-788.39) ♂
600.10 Nodular prostate without urinary obstruction — (Use additional code to identify urinary incontinence: 788.30-788.39) ♂
600.11 Nodular prostate with urinary obstruction — (Use additional code to identify urinary incontinence: 788.30-788.39) ♂
600.20 Benign localized hyperplasia of prostate without urinary obstruction — (Use additional code to identify urinary incontinence: 788.30-788.39) ♂
600.21 Benign localized hyperplasia of prostate with urinary obstruction — (Use additional code to identify urinary incontinence: 788.30-788.39) ♂
600.3 Cyst of prostate — (Use additional code to identify urinary incontinence: 788.30-788.39) ♂
600.90 Hyperplasia of prostate, unspecified, without urinary obstruction — (Use additional code to identify urinary incontinence: 788.30-788.39) ▽ ♂
600.91 Hyperplasia of prostate, unspecified, with urinary obstruction — (Use additional code to identify urinary incontinence: 788.30-788.39) ▽ ♂
601.0 Acute prostatitis — (Use additional code to identify organism: 041.0, 041.1) ♂
601.1 Chronic prostatitis — (Use additional code to identify organism: 041.0, 041.1) ♂
601.2 Abscess of prostate — (Use additional code to identify organism: 041.0, 041.1) ♂

601.3 Prostatocystitis — (Use additional code to identify organism: 041.0, 041.1) ♂
601.4 Prostatitis in diseases classified elsewhere — (Code first underlying disease: 016.5, 039.8, 095.8, 116.0. Use additional code to identify organism: 041.0, 041.1) ☒ ♂
601.8 Other specified inflammatory disease of prostate — (Use additional code to identify organism: 041.0, 041.1) ♂
602.3 Dysplasia of prostate ♂
788.20 Unspecified retention of urine ▽

ICD-9-CM Procedural
60.21 Transurethral (ultrasound) guided laser induced prostatectomy (TULIP)
60.61 Local excision of lesion of prostate
60.93 Repair of prostate
60.94 Control of (postoperative) hemorrhage of prostate

52700
52700 Transurethral drainage of prostatic abscess

ICD-9-CM Diagnostic
601.0 Acute prostatitis — (Use additional code to identify organism: 041.0, 041.1) ♂
601.1 Chronic prostatitis — (Use additional code to identify organism: 041.0, 041.1) ♂
601.2 Abscess of prostate — (Use additional code to identify organism: 041.0, 041.1) ♂
601.3 Prostatocystitis — (Use additional code to identify organism: 041.0, 041.1) ♂
601.4 Prostatitis in diseases classified elsewhere — (Code first underlying disease: 016.5, 039.8, 095.8, 116.0. Use additional code to identify organism: 041.0, 041.1) ☒ ♂
601.8 Other specified inflammatory disease of prostate — (Use additional code to identify organism: 041.0, 041.1) ♂
601.9 Unspecified prostatitis — (Use additional code to identify organism: 041.0, 041.1) ▽ ♂

ICD-9-CM Procedural
60.0 Incision of prostate

Urethra

53000–53010
53000 Urethrotomy or urethrostomy, external (separate procedure); pendulous urethra
53010 perineal urethra, external

ICD-9-CM Diagnostic
597.81 Urethral syndrome NOS
598.00 Urethral stricture due to unspecified infection — (Use additional code to identify urinary incontinence: 625.6, 788.30-788.39) ▽
598.01 Urethral stricture due to infective diseases classified elsewhere — (Code first underlying disease: 095.8, 098.2, 120.0-120.9. Use additional code to identify urinary incontinence: 625.6, 788.30-788.39) ☒
598.1 Traumatic urethral stricture — (Use additional code to identify urinary incontinence: 625.6, 788.30-788.39)
598.2 Postoperative urethral stricture — (Use additional code to identify urinary incontinence: 625.6, 788.30-788.39)
598.8 Other specified causes of urethral stricture — (Use additional code to identify urinary incontinence: 625.6, 788.30-788.39)
598.9 Unspecified urethral stricture — (Use additional code to identify urinary incontinence: 625.6, 788.30-788.39) ▽
599.84 Other specified disorders of urethra — (Use additional code to identify urinary incontinence: 625.6, 788.30-788.39)
600.00 Hypertrophy (benign) of prostate without urinary obstruction — (Use additional code to identify urinary incontinence: 788.30-788.39) ♂
600.01 Hypertrophy (benign) of prostate with urinary obstruction — (Use additional code to identify urinary incontinence: 788.30-788.39) ♂
600.10 Nodular prostate without urinary obstruction — (Use additional code to identify urinary incontinence: 788.30-788.39) ♂
600.11 Nodular prostate with urinary obstruction — (Use additional code to identify urinary incontinence: 788.30-788.39) ♂
600.20 Benign localized hyperplasia of prostate without urinary obstruction — (Use additional code to identify urinary incontinence: 788.30-788.39) ♂
600.21 Benign localized hyperplasia of prostate with urinary obstruction — (Use additional code to identify urinary incontinence: 788.30-788.39) ♂
600.3 Cyst of prostate — (Use additional code to identify urinary incontinence: 788.30-788.39) ♂
600.90 Hyperplasia of prostate, unspecified, without urinary obstruction — (Use additional code to identify urinary incontinence: 788.30-788.39) ▽ ♂
600.91 Hyperplasia of prostate, unspecified, with urinary obstruction — (Use additional code to identify urinary incontinence: 788.30-788.39) ▽ ♂

ICD-9-CM Procedural
58.0 Urethrotomy

53020–53025
53020 Meatotomy, cutting of meatus (separate procedure); except infant
53025 infant

ICD-9-CM Diagnostic
598.00 Urethral stricture due to unspecified infection — (Use additional code to identify urinary incontinence: 625.6, 788.30-788.39) ▽
598.01 Urethral stricture due to infective diseases classified elsewhere — (Code first underlying disease: 095.8, 098.2, 120.0-120.9. Use additional code to identify urinary incontinence: 625.6, 788.30-788.39) ☒
598.1 Traumatic urethral stricture — (Use additional code to identify urinary incontinence: 625.6, 788.30-788.39)
598.2 Postoperative urethral stricture — (Use additional code to identify urinary incontinence: 625.6, 788.30-788.39)
598.8 Other specified causes of urethral stricture — (Use additional code to identify urinary incontinence: 625.6, 788.30-788.39)
607.1 Balanoposthitis — (Use additional code to identify organism) ♂
608.89 Other specified disorder of male genital organs ♂
752.61 Hypospadias ♂
752.62 Epispadias ♂
752.63 Congenital chordee ♂
752.64 Micropenis ♂
752.69 Other penile anomalies ♂
752.81 Scrotal transposition
753.6 Congenital atresia and stenosis of urethra and bladder neck
788.29 Other specified retention of urine

ICD-9-CM Procedural
58.1 Urethral meatotomy

HCPCS Level II Supplies & Services
A4305 Disposable drug delivery system, flow rate of 50 ml or greater per hour
A4306 Disposable drug delivery system, flow rate of 5 ml or less per hour
A4550 Surgical trays

53040–53060
53040 Drainage of deep periurethral abscess
53060 Drainage of Skene's gland abscess or cyst

ICD-9-CM Diagnostic
597.0 Urethral abscess
599.89 Other specified disorders of urinary tract — (Use additional code to identify urinary incontinence: 625.6, 788.30-788.39)

ICD-9-CM Procedural
58.91 Incision of periurethral tissue
71.09 Other incision of vulva and perineum

HCPCS Level II Supplies & Services
A4305 Disposable drug delivery system, flow rate of 50 ml or greater per hour
A4306 Disposable drug delivery system, flow rate of 5 ml or less per hour
A4550 Surgical trays

53080–53085
53080 Drainage of perineal urinary extravasation; uncomplicated (separate procedure)
53085 complicated

ICD-9-CM Diagnostic
788.8 Extravasation of urine

ICD-9-CM Procedural
59.92 Other operations on perirenal or perivesical tissue

HCPCS Level II Supplies & Services
A4305 Disposable drug delivery system, flow rate of 50 ml or greater per hour
A4306 Disposable drug delivery system, flow rate of 5 ml or less per hour
A4349 Male external catheter, with or without adhesive, disposable, each
A4550 Surgical trays

53200

53200 Biopsy of urethra

ICD-9-CM Diagnostic

188.5 Malignant neoplasm of bladder neck
188.9 Malignant neoplasm of bladder, part unspecified ▽
189.3 Malignant neoplasm of urethra
198.1 Secondary malignant neoplasm of other urinary organs
233.9 Carcinoma in situ of other and unspecified urinary organs ▽
239.5 Neoplasm of unspecified nature of other genitourinary organs
597.0 Urethral abscess
597.81 Urethral syndrome NOS
598.01 Urethral stricture due to infective diseases classified elsewhere — (Code first underlying disease: 095.8, 098.2, 120.0-120.9. Use additional code to identify urinary incontinence: 625.6, 788.30-788.39) ☒
598.2 Postoperative urethral stricture — (Use additional code to identify urinary incontinence: 625.6, 788.30-788.39)
598.8 Other specified causes of urethral stricture — (Use additional code to identify urinary incontinence: 625.6, 788.30-788.39)
598.9 Unspecified urethral stricture — (Use additional code to identify urinary incontinence: 625.6, 788.30-788.39) ▽
599.7 Hematuria
625.6 Female stress incontinence ♀

ICD-9-CM Procedural

58.23 Biopsy of urethra

HCPCS Level II Supplies & Services

A4550 Surgical trays

53210–53220

53210 Urethrectomy, total, including cystostomy; female
53215 male
53220 Excision or fulguration of carcinoma of urethra

ICD-9-CM Diagnostic

185 Malignant neoplasm of prostate ♂
188.5 Malignant neoplasm of bladder neck
189.3 Malignant neoplasm of urethra
198.1 Secondary malignant neoplasm of other urinary organs
233.7 Carcinoma in situ of bladder
233.9 Carcinoma in situ of other and unspecified urinary organs ▽
236.7 Neoplasm of uncertain behavior of bladder
236.99 Neoplasm of uncertain behavior of other and unspecified urinary organs
239.4 Neoplasm of unspecified nature of bladder
239.5 Neoplasm of unspecified nature of other genitourinary organs

ICD-9-CM Procedural

58.39 Other local excision or destruction of lesion or tissue of urethra

53230–53240

53230 Excision of urethral diverticulum (separate procedure); female
53235 male
53240 Marsupialization of urethral diverticulum, male or female

ICD-9-CM Diagnostic

599.2 Urethral diverticulum

ICD-9-CM Procedural

58.39 Other local excision or destruction of lesion or tissue of urethra

53250

53250 Excision of bulbourethral gland (Cowper's gland)

ICD-9-CM Diagnostic

597.0 Urethral abscess
597.89 Other urethritis

ICD-9-CM Procedural

58.92 Excision of periurethral tissue

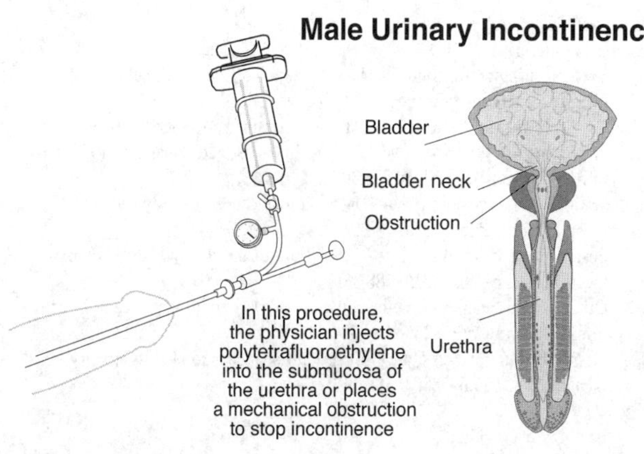
Male Urinary Incontinence
Bladder
Bladder neck
Obstruction
Urethra
In this procedure, the physician injects polytetrafluoroethylene into the submucosa of the urethra or places a mechanical obstruction to stop incontinence

53260–53275

53260 Excision or fulguration; urethral polyp(s), distal urethra
53265 urethral caruncle
53270 Skene's glands
53275 urethral prolapse

ICD-9-CM Diagnostic

597.89 Other urethritis
599.3 Urethral caruncle
599.5 Prolapsed urethral mucosa
599.81 Urethral hypermobility — (Use additional code to identify urinary incontinence: 625.6, 788.30-788.39)
599.89 Other specified disorders of urinary tract — (Use additional code to identify urinary incontinence: 625.6, 788.30-788.39)
599.9 Unspecified disorder of urethra and urinary tract ▽
753.8 Other specified congenital anomaly of bladder and urethra

ICD-9-CM Procedural

58.39 Other local excision or destruction of lesion or tissue of urethra
71.3 Other local excision or destruction of vulva and perineum

53400–53405

53400 Urethroplasty; first stage, for fistula, diverticulum, or stricture (eg, Johannsen type)
53405 second stage (formation of urethra), including urinary diversion

ICD-9-CM Diagnostic

597.81 Urethral syndrome NOS
598.00 Urethral stricture due to unspecified infection — (Use additional code to identify urinary incontinence: 625.6, 788.30-788.39) ▽
598.01 Urethral stricture due to infective diseases classified elsewhere — (Code first underlying disease: 095.8, 098.2, 120.0-120.9. Use additional code to identify urinary incontinence: 625.6, 788.30-788.39) ☒
598.1 Traumatic urethral stricture — (Use additional code to identify urinary incontinence: 625.6, 788.30-788.39)
598.2 Postoperative urethral stricture — (Use additional code to identify urinary incontinence: 625.6, 788.30-788.39)
598.8 Other specified causes of urethral stricture — (Use additional code to identify urinary incontinence: 625.6, 788.30-788.39)
598.9 Unspecified urethral stricture — (Use additional code to identify urinary incontinence: 625.6, 788.30-788.39) ▽
599.1 Urethral fistula
599.2 Urethral diverticulum

ICD-9-CM Procedural

58.46 Other reconstruction of urethra

HCPCS Level II Supplies & Services

A4349 Male external catheter, with or without adhesive, disposable, each

53410

53410 Urethroplasty, one-stage reconstruction of male anterior urethra

ICD-9-CM Diagnostic

188.5 Malignant neoplasm of bladder neck
189.3 Malignant neoplasm of urethra
597.0 Urethral abscess

597.81 Urethral syndrome NOS
597.89 Other urethritis
598.00 Urethral stricture due to unspecified infection — (Use additional code to identify urinary incontinence: 625.6, 788.30-788.39) ▽
598.01 Urethral stricture due to infective diseases classified elsewhere — (Code first underlying disease: 095.8, 098.2, 120.0-120.9. Use additional code to identify urinary incontinence: 625.6, 788.30-788.39) ☒
598.1 Traumatic urethral stricture — (Use additional code to identify urinary incontinence: 625.6, 788.30-788.39)
598.2 Postoperative urethral stricture — (Use additional code to identify urinary incontinence: 625.6, 788.30-788.39)
598.8 Other specified causes of urethral stricture — (Use additional code to identify urinary incontinence: 625.6, 788.30-788.39)
598.9 Unspecified urethral stricture — (Use additional code to identify urinary incontinence: 625.6, 788.30-788.39) ▽
599.1 Urethral fistula
599.2 Urethral diverticulum
752.61 Hypospadias ♂
752.62 Epispadias ♂
752.63 Congenital chordee ♂
752.64 Micropenis ♂
752.65 Hidden penis ♂
752.69 Other penile anomalies ♂
752.81 Scrotal transposition

ICD-9-CM Procedural

58.46 Other reconstruction of urethra

53415

53415 Urethroplasty, transpubic or perineal, one stage, for reconstruction or repair of prostatic or membranous urethra

ICD-9-CM Diagnostic

185 Malignant neoplasm of prostate ♂
188.5 Malignant neoplasm of bladder neck
189.3 Malignant neoplasm of urethra
598.00 Urethral stricture due to unspecified infection — (Use additional code to identify urinary incontinence: 625.6, 788.30-788.39) ▽
598.01 Urethral stricture due to infective diseases classified elsewhere — (Code first underlying disease: 095.8, 098.2, 120.0-120.9. Use additional code to identify urinary incontinence: 625.6, 788.30-788.39) ☒
598.1 Traumatic urethral stricture — (Use additional code to identify urinary incontinence: 625.6, 788.30-788.39)
598.2 Postoperative urethral stricture — (Use additional code to identify urinary incontinence: 625.6, 788.30-788.39)
598.8 Other specified causes of urethral stricture — (Use additional code to identify urinary incontinence: 625.6, 788.30-788.39)
598.9 Unspecified urethral stricture — (Use additional code to identify urinary incontinence: 625.6, 788.30-788.39) ▽
599.1 Urethral fistula
599.2 Urethral diverticulum
599.84 Other specified disorders of urethra — (Use additional code to identify urinary incontinence: 625.6, 788.30-788.39)
600.00 Hypertrophy (benign) of prostate without urinary obstruction — (Use additional code to identify urinary incontinence: 788.30-788.39) ♂
600.01 Hypertrophy (benign) of prostate with urinary obstruction — (Use additional code to identify urinary incontinence: 788.30-788.39) ♂
600.10 Nodular prostate without urinary obstruction — (Use additional code to identify urinary incontinence: 788.30-788.39) ♂
600.11 Nodular prostate with urinary obstruction — (Use additional code to identify urinary incontinence: 788.30-788.39) ♂
600.20 Benign localized hyperplasia of prostate without urinary obstruction — (Use additional code to identify urinary incontinence: 788.30-788.39) ♂
600.21 Benign localized hyperplasia of prostate with urinary obstruction — (Use additional code to identify urinary incontinence: 788.30-788.39) ♂
600.3 Cyst of prostate — (Use additional code to identify urinary incontinence: 788.30-788.39) ♂
600.90 Hyperplasia of prostate, unspecified, without urinary obstruction — (Use additional code to identify urinary incontinence: 788.30-788.39) ▽ ♂
600.91 Hyperplasia of prostate, unspecified, with urinary obstruction — (Use additional code to identify urinary incontinence: 788.30-788.39) ▽ ♂
752.61 Hypospadias ♂
752.62 Epispadias ♂
752.63 Congenital chordee ♂
752.64 Micropenis ♂
752.65 Hidden penis ♂
752.69 Other penile anomalies ♂
752.81 Scrotal transposition

ICD-9-CM Procedural

58.46 Other reconstruction of urethra

53420–53425

53420 Urethroplasty, two-stage reconstruction or repair of prostatic or membranous urethra; first stage
53425 second stage

ICD-9-CM Diagnostic

185 Malignant neoplasm of prostate ♂
188.5 Malignant neoplasm of bladder neck
189.3 Malignant neoplasm of urethra
598.00 Urethral stricture due to unspecified infection — (Use additional code to identify urinary incontinence: 625.6, 788.30-788.39) ▽
598.01 Urethral stricture due to infective diseases classified elsewhere — (Code first underlying disease: 095.8, 098.2, 120.0-120.9. Use additional code to identify urinary incontinence: 625.6, 788.30-788.39) ☒
598.1 Traumatic urethral stricture — (Use additional code to identify urinary incontinence: 625.6, 788.30-788.39)
598.2 Postoperative urethral stricture — (Use additional code to identify urinary incontinence: 625.6, 788.30-788.39)
598.8 Other specified causes of urethral stricture — (Use additional code to identify urinary incontinence: 625.6, 788.30-788.39)
598.9 Unspecified urethral stricture — (Use additional code to identify urinary incontinence: 625.6, 788.30-788.39) ▽
599.1 Urethral fistula
599.2 Urethral diverticulum
599.5 Prolapsed urethral mucosa
599.84 Other specified disorders of urethra — (Use additional code to identify urinary incontinence: 625.6, 788.30-788.39)
600.00 Hypertrophy (benign) of prostate without urinary obstruction — (Use additional code to identify urinary incontinence: 788.30-788.39) ♂
600.01 Hypertrophy (benign) of prostate with urinary obstruction — (Use additional code to identify urinary incontinence: 788.30-788.39) ♂
600.10 Nodular prostate without urinary obstruction — (Use additional code to identify urinary incontinence: 788.30-788.39) ♂
600.11 Nodular prostate with urinary obstruction — (Use additional code to identify urinary incontinence: 788.30-788.39) ♂
600.20 Benign localized hyperplasia of prostate without urinary obstruction — (Use additional code to identify urinary incontinence: 788.30-788.39) ♂
600.21 Benign localized hyperplasia of prostate with urinary obstruction — (Use additional code to identify urinary incontinence: 788.30-788.39) ♂
600.3 Cyst of prostate — (Use additional code to identify urinary incontinence: 788.30-788.39) ♂
600.90 Hyperplasia of prostate, unspecified, without urinary obstruction — (Use additional code to identify urinary incontinence: 788.30-788.39) ▽ ♂
600.91 Hyperplasia of prostate, unspecified, with urinary obstruction — (Use additional code to identify urinary incontinence: 788.30-788.39) ▽ ♂
752.61 Hypospadias ♂
752.62 Epispadias ♂
752.63 Congenital chordee ♂
752.64 Micropenis ♂
752.65 Hidden penis ♂
752.69 Other penile anomalies ♂
752.81 Scrotal transposition

ICD-9-CM Procedural

58.46 Other reconstruction of urethra

53430

53430 Urethroplasty, reconstruction of female urethra

ICD-9-CM Diagnostic

188.5 Malignant neoplasm of bladder neck
189.3 Malignant neoplasm of urethra
598.01 Urethral stricture due to infective diseases classified elsewhere — (Code first underlying disease: 095.8, 098.2, 120.0-120.9. Use additional code to identify urinary incontinence: 625.6, 788.30-788.39) ☒
598.1 Traumatic urethral stricture — (Use additional code to identify urinary incontinence: 625.6, 788.30-788.39)
598.2 Postoperative urethral stricture — (Use additional code to identify urinary incontinence: 625.6, 788.30-788.39)

▽ Unspecified code
♀ Female diagnosis
☒ Manifestation code
♂ Male diagnosis

598.8 Other specified causes of urethral stricture — (Use additional code to identify urinary incontinence: 625.6, 788.30-788.39)
598.9 Unspecified urethral stricture — (Use additional code to identify urinary incontinence: 625.6, 788.30-788.39) ▽
599.89 Other specified disorders of urinary tract — (Use additional code to identify urinary incontinence: 625.6, 788.30-788.39)
625.6 Female stress incontinence ♀

ICD-9-CM Procedural
58.46 Other reconstruction of urethra

53431
53431 Urethroplasty with tubularization of posterior urethra and/or lower bladder for incontinence (eg, Tenago, Leadbetter procedure)

ICD-9-CM Diagnostic
598.8 Other specified causes of urethral stricture — (Use additional code to identify urinary incontinence: 625.6, 788.30-788.39)
625.6 Female stress incontinence ♀
788.30 Unspecified urinary incontinence ▽
788.31 Urge incontinence
788.32 Stress incontinence, male ♂
788.33 Mixed incontinence urge and stress (male)(female)
788.34 Incontinence without sensory awareness
788.35 Post-void dribbling
788.36 Nocturnal enuresis
788.37 Continuous leakage
788.38 Overflow incontinence
788.39 Other urinary incontinence

ICD-9-CM Procedural
58.49 Other repair of urethra

53440
53440 Sling operation for correction of male urinary incontinence (eg, fascia or synthetic)

ICD-9-CM Diagnostic
598.8 Other specified causes of urethral stricture — (Use additional code to identify urinary incontinence: 625.6, 788.30-788.39)
788.30 Unspecified urinary incontinence ▽
788.31 Urge incontinence
788.32 Stress incontinence, male ♂
788.33 Mixed incontinence urge and stress (male)(female)
788.34 Incontinence without sensory awareness
788.35 Post-void dribbling
788.36 Nocturnal enuresis
788.37 Continuous leakage
788.38 Overflow incontinence
788.39 Other urinary incontinence

ICD-9-CM Procedural
57.99 Other operations on bladder

HCPCS Level II Supplies & Services
A4349 Male external catheter, with or without adhesive, disposable, each

53442
53442 Removal or revision of sling for male urinary incontinence (eg, fascia or synthetic)

ICD-9-CM Diagnostic
598.8 Other specified causes of urethral stricture — (Use additional code to identify urinary incontinence: 625.6, 788.30-788.39)
788.31 Urge incontinence
788.32 Stress incontinence, male ♂
788.33 Mixed incontinence urge and stress (male)(female)
788.34 Incontinence without sensory awareness
788.35 Post-void dribbling
788.36 Nocturnal enuresis
788.37 Continuous leakage
788.38 Overflow incontinence
788.39 Other urinary incontinence
996.39 Mechanical complication of genitourinary device, implant, and graft, other
996.76 Other complications due to genitourinary device, implant, and graft

ICD-9-CM Procedural
58.99 Other operations on urethra and periurethral tissue

HCPCS Level II Supplies & Services
A4349 Male external catheter, with or without adhesive, disposable, each

53444
53444 Insertion of tandem cuff (dual cuff)

ICD-9-CM Diagnostic
598.8 Other specified causes of urethral stricture — (Use additional code to identify urinary incontinence: 625.6, 788.30-788.39)
625.6 Female stress incontinence ♀
753.6 Congenital atresia and stenosis of urethra and bladder neck
788.30 Unspecified urinary incontinence ▽
788.31 Urge incontinence
788.32 Stress incontinence, male ♂
788.33 Mixed incontinence urge and stress (male)(female)
788.34 Incontinence without sensory awareness
788.35 Post-void dribbling
788.36 Nocturnal enuresis
788.37 Continuous leakage
788.38 Overflow incontinence
788.39 Other urinary incontinence

ICD-9-CM Procedural
58.93 Implantation of artificial urinary sphincter (AUS)

53445
53445 Insertion of inflatable urethral/bladder neck sphincter, including placement of pump, reservoir, and cuff

ICD-9-CM Diagnostic
598.8 Other specified causes of urethral stricture — (Use additional code to identify urinary incontinence: 625.6, 788.30-788.39)
625.6 Female stress incontinence ♀
753.5 Exstrophy of urinary bladder
753.6 Congenital atresia and stenosis of urethra and bladder neck
788.30 Unspecified urinary incontinence ▽
788.31 Urge incontinence
788.32 Stress incontinence, male ♂
788.33 Mixed incontinence urge and stress (male)(female)
788.34 Incontinence without sensory awareness
788.35 Post-void dribbling
788.36 Nocturnal enuresis
788.37 Continuous leakage
788.38 Overflow incontinence
788.39 Other urinary incontinence
V10.46 Personal history of malignant neoplasm of prostate ♂

ICD-9-CM Procedural
58.93 Implantation of artificial urinary sphincter (AUS)

53446
53446 Removal of inflatable urethral/bladder neck sphincter, including pump, reservoir, and cuff

ICD-9-CM Diagnostic
996.39 Mechanical complication of genitourinary device, implant, and graft, other
996.65 Infection and inflammatory reaction due to other genitourinary device, implant, and graft — (Use additional code to identify specified infections)
996.76 Other complications due to genitourinary device, implant, and graft
997.5 Urinary complications — (Use additional code to identify complications)

ICD-9-CM Procedural
58.99 Other operations on urethra and periurethral tissue

53447
53447 Removal and replacement of inflatable urethral/bladder neck sphincter including pump, reservoir, and cuff at the same operative session

ICD-9-CM Diagnostic
625.6 Female stress incontinence ♀
788.30 Unspecified urinary incontinence ▽
788.31 Urge incontinence

788.32 Stress incontinence, male ♂
788.33 Mixed incontinence urge and stress (male)(female)
788.34 Incontinence without sensory awareness
788.35 Post-void dribbling
788.36 Nocturnal enuresis
788.37 Continuous leakage
788.38 Overflow incontinence
788.39 Other urinary incontinence
996.39 Mechanical complication of genitourinary device, implant, and graft, other
996.65 Infection and inflammatory reaction due to other genitourinary device, implant, and graft — (Use additional code to identify specified infections)
996.76 Other complications due to genitourinary device, implant, and graft
997.5 Urinary complications — (Use additional code to identify complications)
V53.6 Fitting and adjustment of urinary device

ICD-9-CM Procedural

58.99 Other operations on urethra and periurethral tissue

53448

53448 Removal and replacement of inflatable urethral/bladder neck sphincter including pump, reservoir, and cuff through an infected field at the same operative session including irrigation and debridement of infected tissue

ICD-9-CM Diagnostic

595.89 Other specified types of cystitis — (Use additional code to identify organism, such as E. coli, 041.4)
596.8 Other specified disorder of bladder — (Use additional code to identify urinary incontinence: 625.6, 788.30-788.39)
597.0 Urethral abscess
597.80 Unspecified urethritis ▽
597.89 Other urethritis
625.6 Female stress incontinence ♀
788.30 Unspecified urinary incontinence ▽
788.31 Urge incontinence
788.32 Stress incontinence, male ♂
788.33 Mixed incontinence urge and stress (male)(female)
788.34 Incontinence without sensory awareness
788.35 Post-void dribbling
788.36 Nocturnal enuresis
788.37 Continuous leakage
788.38 Overflow incontinence
788.39 Other urinary incontinence
996.65 Infection and inflammatory reaction due to other genitourinary device, implant, and graft — (Use additional code to identify specified infections)
996.76 Other complications due to genitourinary device, implant, and graft
997.5 Urinary complications — (Use additional code to identify complications)
998.59 Other postoperative infection — (Use additional code to identify infection)

ICD-9-CM Procedural

58.93 Implantation of artificial urinary sphincter (AUS)

53449

53449 Repair of inflatable urethral/bladder neck sphincter, including pump, reservoir, and cuff

ICD-9-CM Diagnostic

996.39 Mechanical complication of genitourinary device, implant, and graft, other

ICD-9-CM Procedural

58.99 Other operations on urethra and periurethral tissue

53450–53460

53450 Urethromeatoplasty, with mucosal advancement
53460 Urethromeatoplasty, with partial excision of distal urethral segment (Richardson type procedure)

ICD-9-CM Diagnostic

598.00 Urethral stricture due to unspecified infection — (Use additional code to identify urinary incontinence: 625.6, 788.30-788.39) ▽
598.01 Urethral stricture due to infective diseases classified elsewhere — (Code first underlying disease: 095.8, 098.2, 120.0-120.9. Use additional code to identify urinary incontinence: 625.6, 788.30-788.39) ☒
598.1 Traumatic urethral stricture — (Use additional code to identify urinary incontinence: 625.6, 788.30-788.39)
598.2 Postoperative urethral stricture — (Use additional code to identify urinary incontinence: 625.6, 788.30-788.39)
598.8 Other specified causes of urethral stricture — (Use additional code to identify urinary incontinence: 625.6, 788.30-788.39)
598.9 Unspecified urethral stricture — (Use additional code to identify urinary incontinence: 625.6, 788.30-788.39) ▽
599.1 Urethral fistula
599.2 Urethral diverticulum
599.3 Urethral caruncle
599.4 Urethral false passage
599.5 Prolapsed urethral mucosa
599.9 Unspecified disorder of urethra and urinary tract ▽
607.1 Balanoposthitis — (Use additional code to identify organism) ♂
607.81 Balanitis xerotica obliterans ♂
752.61 Hypospadias ♂
752.62 Epispadias ♂
752.81 Scrotal transposition
753.6 Congenital atresia and stenosis of urethra and bladder neck

ICD-9-CM Procedural

58.39 Other local excision or destruction of lesion or tissue of urethra
58.47 Urethral meatoplasty
58.49 Other repair of urethra

53500

53500 Urethrolysis, transvaginal, secondary, open, including cystourethroscopy (eg, postsurgical obstruction, scarring)

ICD-9-CM Diagnostic

597.81 Urethral syndrome NOS
598.00 Urethral stricture due to unspecified infection — (Use additional code to identify urinary incontinence: 625.6, 788.30-788.39) ▽
598.01 Urethral stricture due to infective diseases classified elsewhere — (Code first underlying disease: 095.8, 098.2, 120.0-120.9. Use additional code to identify urinary incontinence: 625.6, 788.30-788.39) ☒
598.1 Traumatic urethral stricture — (Use additional code to identify urinary incontinence: 625.6, 788.30-788.39)
598.2 Postoperative urethral stricture — (Use additional code to identify urinary incontinence: 625.6, 788.30-788.39)
598.8 Other specified causes of urethral stricture — (Use additional code to identify urinary incontinence: 625.6, 788.30-788.39)
598.9 Unspecified urethral stricture — (Use additional code to identify urinary incontinence: 625.6, 788.30-788.39) ▽

ICD-9-CM Procedural

58.5 Release of urethral stricture

53502–53515

53502 Urethrorrhaphy, suture of urethral wound or injury, female
53505 Urethrorrhaphy, suture of urethral wound or injury; penile
53510 perineal
53515 prostatomembranous

ICD-9-CM Diagnostic

599.84 Other specified disorders of urethra — (Use additional code to identify urinary incontinence: 625.6, 788.30-788.39)
634.22 Complete spontaneous abortion complicated by damage to pelvic organs or tissues ♀
635.21 Legally induced abortion complicated by damage to pelvic organs or tissues, incomplete ♀
635.22 Complete legally induced abortion complicated by damage to pelvic organs or tissues ♀
636.21 Incomplete illegally induced abortion complicated by damage to pelvic organs or tissues ♀
636.22 Complete illegally induced abortion complicated by damage to pelvic organs or tissues ♀
637.21 Legally unspecified abortion, incomplete, complicated by damage to pelvic organs or tissues ♀
637.22 Legally unspecified abortion, complete, complicated by damage to pelvic organs or tissues ♀
638.2 Failed attempted abortion complicated by damage to pelvic organs or tissues ♀
639.2 Damage to pelvic organs and tissues following abortion or ectopic and molar pregnancies ♀
665.51 Other injury to pelvic organs, with delivery ♀
665.54 Other injury to pelvic organs, postpartum ♀
867.0 Bladder and urethra injury without mention of open wound into cavity

▽ Unspecified code ♀ Female diagnosis ☒ Manifestation code ♂ Male diagnosis

867.1 Bladder and urethra injury with open wound into cavity
878.0 Open wound of penis, without mention of complication — (Use additional code to identify infection) ♂
878.1 Open wound of penis, complicated — (Use additional code to identify infection) ♂
998.2 Accidental puncture or laceration during procedure

ICD-9-CM Procedural

58.41 Suture of laceration of urethra
75.61 Repair of current obstetric laceration of bladder and urethra

HCPCS Level II Supplies & Services

A4305 Disposable drug delivery system, flow rate of 50 ml or greater per hour
A4306 Disposable drug delivery system, flow rate of 5 ml or less per hour
A4550 Surgical trays

53520

53520 Closure of urethrostomy or urethrocutaneous fistula, male (separate procedure)

ICD-9-CM Diagnostic

599.1 Urethral fistula
V10.51 Personal history of malignant neoplasm of bladder
V10.59 Personal history of malignant neoplasm of other urinary organ
V13.09 Personal history of other disorder of urinary system
V15.3 Personal history of irradiation, presenting hazards to health
V15.5 Personal history of injury, presenting hazards to health
V55.5 Attention to cystostomy
V55.6 Attention to other artificial opening of urinary tract

ICD-9-CM Procedural

58.42 Closure of urethrostomy

53600–53605

53600 Dilation of urethral stricture by passage of sound or urethral dilator, male; initial
53601 subsequent
53605 Dilation of urethral stricture or vesical neck by passage of sound or urethral dilator, male, general or conduction (spinal) anesthesia

ICD-9-CM Diagnostic

185 Malignant neoplasm of prostate ♂
596.0 Bladder neck obstruction — (Use additional code to identify urinary incontinence: 625.6, 788.30-788.39)
597.81 Urethral syndrome NOS
598.00 Urethral stricture due to unspecified infection — (Use additional code to identify urinary incontinence: 625.6, 788.30-788.39) ▽
598.01 Urethral stricture due to infective diseases classified elsewhere — (Code first underlying disease: 095.8, 098.2, 120.0-120.9. Use additional code to identify urinary incontinence: 625.6, 788.30-788.39) ☒
598.1 Traumatic urethral stricture — (Use additional code to identify urinary incontinence: 625.6, 788.30-788.39)
598.2 Postoperative urethral stricture — (Use additional code to identify urinary incontinence: 625.6, 788.30-788.39)
598.8 Other specified causes of urethral stricture — (Use additional code to identify urinary incontinence: 625.6, 788.30-788.39)
598.9 Unspecified urethral stricture — (Use additional code to identify urinary incontinence: 625.6, 788.30-788.39) ▽
600.00 Hypertrophy (benign) of prostate without urinary obstruction — (Use additional code to identify urinary incontinence: 788.30-788.39) ♂
600.01 Hypertrophy (benign) of prostate with urinary obstruction — (Use additional code to identify urinary incontinence: 788.30-788.39) ♂
600.10 Nodular prostate without urinary obstruction — (Use additional code to identify urinary incontinence: 788.30-788.39) ♂
600.11 Nodular prostate with urinary obstruction — (Use additional code to identify urinary incontinence: 788.30-788.39) ♂
600.20 Benign localized hyperplasia of prostate without urinary obstruction — (Use additional code to identify urinary incontinence: 788.30-788.39) ♂
600.21 Benign localized hyperplasia of prostate with urinary obstruction — (Use additional code to identify urinary incontinence: 788.30-788.39) ♂
600.3 Cyst of prostate — (Use additional code to identify urinary incontinence: 788.30-788.39) ♂
600.90 Hyperplasia of prostate, unspecified, without urinary obstruction — (Use additional code to identify urinary incontinence: 788.30-788.39) ▽ ♂
600.91 Hyperplasia of prostate, unspecified, with urinary obstruction — (Use additional code to identify urinary incontinence: 788.30-788.39) ▽ ♂
601.1 Chronic prostatitis — (Use additional code to identify organism: 041.0, 041.1) ♂
601.9 Unspecified prostatitis — (Use additional code to identify organism: 041.0, 041.1) ▽ ♂
753.6 Congenital atresia and stenosis of urethra and bladder neck
788.29 Other specified retention of urine

ICD-9-CM Procedural

57.92 Dilation of bladder neck
58.6 Dilation of urethra

HCPCS Level II Supplies & Services

A4550 Surgical trays

53620–53621

53620 Dilation of urethral stricture by passage of filiform and follower, male; initial
53621 subsequent

ICD-9-CM Diagnostic

185 Malignant neoplasm of prostate ♂
596.0 Bladder neck obstruction — (Use additional code to identify urinary incontinence: 625.6, 788.30-788.39)
596.8 Other specified disorder of bladder — (Use additional code to identify urinary incontinence: 625.6, 788.30-788.39)
597.81 Urethral syndrome NOS
598.00 Urethral stricture due to unspecified infection — (Use additional code to identify urinary incontinence: 625.6, 788.30-788.39) ▽
598.01 Urethral stricture due to infective diseases classified elsewhere — (Code first underlying disease: 095.8, 098.2, 120.0-120.9. Use additional code to identify urinary incontinence: 625.6, 788.30-788.39) ☒
598.1 Traumatic urethral stricture — (Use additional code to identify urinary incontinence: 625.6, 788.30-788.39)
598.2 Postoperative urethral stricture — (Use additional code to identify urinary incontinence: 625.6, 788.30-788.39)
598.8 Other specified causes of urethral stricture — (Use additional code to identify urinary incontinence: 625.6, 788.30-788.39)
598.9 Unspecified urethral stricture — (Use additional code to identify urinary incontinence: 625.6, 788.30-788.39) ▽
599.6 Unspecified urinary obstruction — (Use additional code to identify urinary incontinence: 625.6, 788.30-788.39) ▽
599.7 Hematuria
600.00 Hypertrophy (benign) of prostate without urinary obstruction — (Use additional code to identify urinary incontinence: 788.30-788.39) ♂
600.01 Hypertrophy (benign) of prostate with urinary obstruction — (Use additional code to identify urinary incontinence: 788.30-788.39) ♂
600.10 Nodular prostate without urinary obstruction — (Use additional code to identify urinary incontinence: 788.30-788.39) ♂
600.11 Nodular prostate with urinary obstruction — (Use additional code to identify urinary incontinence: 788.30-788.39) ♂
600.20 Benign localized hyperplasia of prostate without urinary obstruction — (Use additional code to identify urinary incontinence: 788.30-788.39) ♂
600.21 Benign localized hyperplasia of prostate with urinary obstruction — (Use additional code to identify urinary incontinence: 788.30-788.39) ♂
600.3 Cyst of prostate — (Use additional code to identify urinary incontinence: 788.30-788.39) ♂
600.90 Hyperplasia of prostate, unspecified, without urinary obstruction — (Use additional code to identify urinary incontinence: 788.30-788.39) ▽ ♂
600.91 Hyperplasia of prostate, unspecified, with urinary obstruction — (Use additional code to identify urinary incontinence: 788.30-788.39) ▽ ♂
601.0 Acute prostatitis — (Use additional code to identify organism: 041.0, 041.1) ♂
601.1 Chronic prostatitis — (Use additional code to identify organism: 041.0, 041.1) ♂
601.9 Unspecified prostatitis — (Use additional code to identify organism: 041.0, 041.1) ▽ ♂
753.6 Congenital atresia and stenosis of urethra and bladder neck
788.20 Unspecified retention of urine ▽
788.29 Other specified retention of urine

ICD-9-CM Procedural

58.6 Dilation of urethra

HCPCS Level II Supplies & Services

A4550 Surgical trays

▽ Unspecified code ♀ Female diagnosis ☒ Manifestation code ♂ Male diagnosis

53660–53665

53660 Dilation of female urethra including suppository and/or instillation; initial
53661 subsequent
53665 Dilation of female urethra, general or conduction (spinal) anesthesia

ICD-9-CM Diagnostic

595.1 Chronic interstitial cystitis — (Use additional code to identify organism, such as E. coli, 041.4)
595.2 Other chronic cystitis — (Use additional code to identify organism, such as E. coli, 041.4)
595.3 Trigonitis — (Use additional code to identify organism, such as E. coli, 041.4)
597.80 Unspecified urethritis ▽
597.81 Urethral syndrome NOS
597.89 Other urethritis
598.00 Urethral stricture due to unspecified infection — (Use additional code to identify urinary incontinence: 625.6, 788.30-788.39) ▽
598.01 Urethral stricture due to infective diseases classified elsewhere — (Code first underlying disease: 095.8, 098.2, 120.0-120.9. Use additional code to identify urinary incontinence: 625.6, 788.30-788.39) ☒
598.1 Traumatic urethral stricture — (Use additional code to identify urinary incontinence: 625.6, 788.30-788.39)
598.2 Postoperative urethral stricture — (Use additional code to identify urinary incontinence: 625.6, 788.30-788.39)
598.8 Other specified causes of urethral stricture — (Use additional code to identify urinary incontinence: 625.6, 788.30-788.39)
599.82 Intrinsic (urethral) sphincter deficiency (ISD) — (Use additional code to identify urinary incontinence: 625.6, 788.30-788.39)
599.83 Urethral instability — (Use additional code to identify urinary incontinence: 625.6, 788.30-788.39)
599.89 Other specified disorders of urinary tract — (Use additional code to identify urinary incontinence: 625.6, 788.30-788.39)
599.9 Unspecified disorder of urethra and urinary tract ▽
625.6 Female stress incontinence ♀
753.6 Congenital atresia and stenosis of urethra and bladder neck
788.1 Dysuria
788.20 Unspecified retention of urine ▽
788.21 Incomplete bladder emptying
788.29 Other specified retention of urine

ICD-9-CM Procedural

58.6 Dilation of urethra
96.49 Other genitourinary instillation

HCPCS Level II Supplies & Services

A4550 Surgical trays

53850–53853

53850 Transurethral destruction of prostate tissue; by microwave thermotherapy
53852 by radiofrequency thermotherapy
53853 by water-induced thermotherapy

ICD-9-CM Diagnostic

185 Malignant neoplasm of prostate ♂
198.82 Secondary malignant neoplasm of genital organs
222.2 Benign neoplasm of prostate ♂
233.4 Carcinoma in situ of prostate ♂
236.5 Neoplasm of uncertain behavior of prostate ♂
239.5 Neoplasm of unspecified nature of other genitourinary organs
600.00 Hypertrophy (benign) of prostate without urinary obstruction — (Use additional code to identify urinary incontinence: 788.30-788.39) ♂
600.01 Hypertrophy (benign) of prostate with urinary obstruction — (Use additional code to identify urinary incontinence: 788.30-788.39) ♂
600.10 Nodular prostate without urinary obstruction — (Use additional code to identify urinary incontinence: 788.30-788.39) ♂
600.11 Nodular prostate with urinary obstruction — (Use additional code to identify urinary incontinence: 788.30-788.39) ♂
600.20 Benign localized hyperplasia of prostate without urinary obstruction — (Use additional code to identify urinary incontinence: 788.30-788.39) ♂
600.21 Benign localized hyperplasia of prostate with urinary obstruction — (Use additional code to identify urinary incontinence: 788.30-788.39) ♂
600.3 Cyst of prostate — (Use additional code to identify urinary incontinence: 788.30-788.39) ♂
600.90 Hyperplasia of prostate, unspecified, without urinary obstruction — (Use additional code to identify urinary incontinence: 788.30-788.39) ▽ ♂
600.91 Hyperplasia of prostate, unspecified, with urinary obstruction — (Use additional code to identify urinary incontinence: 788.30-788.39) ▽ ♂
602.3 Dysplasia of prostate ♂

ICD-9-CM Procedural

60.29 Other transurethral prostatectomy
60.97 Other transurethral destruction of prostate tissue by other thermotherapy

HCPCS Level II Supplies & Services

A4305 Disposable drug delivery system, flow rate of 50 ml or greater per hour
A4306 Disposable drug delivery system, flow rate of 5 ml or less per hour
A4550 Surgical trays

53899

53899 Unlisted procedure, urinary system

ICD-9-CM Diagnostic

The application of this code is too broad to adequately present ICD-9-CM diagnostic code links here. Refer to your ICD-9-CM book.

▽ Unspecified code
♀ Female diagnosis
☒ Manifestation code
♂ Male diagnosis

Male Genital System

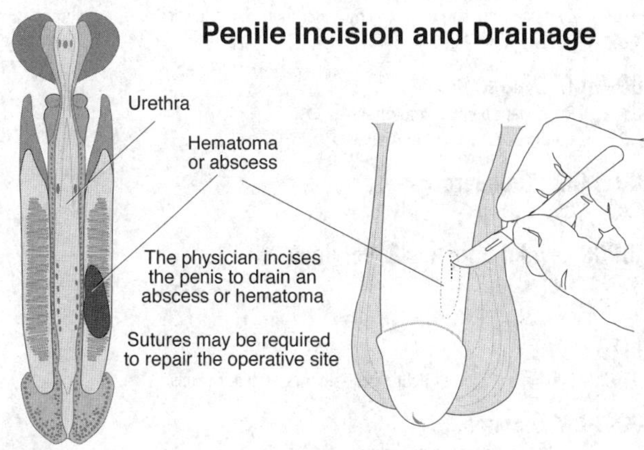

Penile Incision and Drainage
Urethra
Hematoma or abscess
The physician incises the penis to drain an abscess or hematoma
Sutures may be required to repair the operative site

Penis

54000–54001

54000 Slitting of prepuce, dorsal or lateral (separate procedure); newborn
54001 except newborn

ICD-9-CM Diagnostic

605 Redundant prepuce and phimosis ♂

ICD-9-CM Procedural

64.91 Dorsal or lateral slit of prepuce

HCPCS Level II Supplies & Services

A4550 Surgical trays

54015

54015 Incision and drainage of penis, deep

ICD-9-CM Diagnostic

098.0 Gonococcal infection (acute) of lower genitourinary tract
098.2 Gonococcal infections, chronic, of lower genitourinary tract
607.2 Other inflammatory disorders of penis — (Use additional code to identify organism) ♂
607.82 Vascular disorders of penis ♂
607.85 Peyronie's disease ♂
607.89 Other specified disorder of penis ♂

ICD-9-CM Procedural

64.92 Incision of penis

HCPCS Level II Supplies & Services

A4550 Surgical trays

54050–54056

54050 Destruction of lesion(s), penis (eg, condyloma, papilloma, molluscum contagiosum, herpetic vesicle), simple; chemical
54055 electrodesiccation
54056 cryosurgery

ICD-9-CM Diagnostic

054.13 Herpetic infection of penis ♂
078.0 Molluscum contagiosum
078.11 Condyloma acuminatum
078.19 Other specified viral warts
187.8 Malignant neoplasm of other specified sites of male genital organs ♂
198.82 Secondary malignant neoplasm of genital organs
222.1 Benign neoplasm of penis ♂
233.6 Carcinoma in situ of other and unspecified male genital organs ▽ ♂
239.5 Neoplasm of unspecified nature of other genitourinary organs
709.8 Other specified disorder of skin
709.9 Unspecified disorder of skin and subcutaneous tissue ▽

ICD-9-CM Procedural

64.2 Local excision or destruction of lesion of penis

HCPCS Level II Supplies & Services

A4550 Surgical trays

54057–54065

54057 Destruction of lesion(s), penis (eg, condyloma, papilloma, molluscum contagiosum, herpetic vesicle), simple; laser surgery
54060 surgical excision
54065 Destruction of lesion(s), penis (eg, condyloma, papilloma, molluscum contagiosum, herpetic vesicle), extensive (eg, laser surgery, electrosurgery, cryosurgery, chemosurgery)

ICD-9-CM Diagnostic

054.13 Herpetic infection of penis ♂
078.0 Molluscum contagiosum
078.11 Condyloma acuminatum
078.19 Other specified viral warts
187.8 Malignant neoplasm of other specified sites of male genital organs ♂
198.82 Secondary malignant neoplasm of genital organs
222.1 Benign neoplasm of penis ♂
233.6 Carcinoma in situ of other and unspecified male genital organs ▽ ♂
239.5 Neoplasm of unspecified nature of other genitourinary organs
709.8 Other specified disorder of skin
709.9 Unspecified disorder of skin and subcutaneous tissue ▽

ICD-9-CM Procedural

64.2 Local excision or destruction of lesion of penis

HCPCS Level II Supplies & Services

A4550 Surgical trays

54100–54105

54100 Biopsy of penis; (separate procedure)
54105 deep structures

ICD-9-CM Diagnostic

187.1 Malignant neoplasm of prepuce ♂
187.2 Malignant neoplasm of glans penis ♂
187.3 Malignant neoplasm of body of penis ♂
187.4 Malignant neoplasm of penis, part unspecified ▽ ♂
187.9 Malignant neoplasm of male genital organ, site unspecified ▽ ♂
198.82 Secondary malignant neoplasm of genital organs
222.1 Benign neoplasm of penis ♂
233.5 Carcinoma in situ of penis ♂
236.6 Neoplasm of uncertain behavior of other and unspecified male genital organs ▽ ♂
239.5 Neoplasm of unspecified nature of other genitourinary organs
607.0 Leukoplakia of penis ♂
607.85 Peyronie's disease ♂
607.89 Other specified disorder of penis ♂
686.1 Pyogenic granuloma of skin and subcutaneous tissue

ICD-9-CM Procedural

64.11 Biopsy of penis

HCPCS Level II Supplies & Services

A4550 Surgical trays

54110–54112

54110 Excision of penile plaque (Peyronie disease);
54111 with graft to 5 cm in length
54112 with graft greater than 5 cm in length

ICD-9-CM Diagnostic

607.85 Peyronie's disease ♂

ICD-9-CM Procedural

64.2 Local excision or destruction of lesion of penis
64.49 Other repair of penis

54115

54115 Removal foreign body from deep penile tissue (eg, plastic implant)

ICD-9-CM Diagnostic

939.3 Foreign body in penis ♂
996.39 Mechanical complication of genitourinary device, implant, and graft, other
996.65 Infection and inflammatory reaction due to other genitourinary device, implant, and graft — (Use additional code to identify specified infections)

ICD-9-CM Procedural

64.92 Incision of penis
64.96 Removal of internal prosthesis of penis

54120–54125

54120 Amputation of penis; partial
54125 complete

ICD-9-CM Diagnostic

187.1 Malignant neoplasm of prepuce ♂
187.2 Malignant neoplasm of glans penis ♂
187.3 Malignant neoplasm of body of penis ♂
187.4 Malignant neoplasm of penis, part unspecified ▽ ♂
187.9 Malignant neoplasm of male genital organ, site unspecified ▽ ♂
198.89 Secondary malignant neoplasm of other specified sites
222.1 Benign neoplasm of penis ♂
233.5 Carcinoma in situ of penis ♂
878.0 Open wound of penis, without mention of complication — (Use additional code to identify infection) ♂
878.1 Open wound of penis, complicated — (Use additional code to identify infection) ♂
942.35 Full-thickness skin loss due to burn (third degree nos) of genitalia
942.45 Deep necrosis of underlying tissues due to burn (deep third degree) of genitalia, without mention of loss of a body part
948.00 Burn (any degree) involving less than 10% of body surface with third degree burn of less than 10% or unspecified amount

ICD-9-CM Procedural

64.3 Amputation of penis

54130–54135

54130 Amputation of penis, radical; with bilateral inguinofemoral lymphadenectomy
54135 in continuity with bilateral pelvic lymphadenectomy, including external iliac, hypogastric and obturator nodes

ICD-9-CM Diagnostic

187.1 Malignant neoplasm of prepuce ♂
187.2 Malignant neoplasm of glans penis ♂
187.3 Malignant neoplasm of body of penis ♂
187.4 Malignant neoplasm of penis, part unspecified ▽ ♂
187.9 Malignant neoplasm of male genital organ, site unspecified ▽ ♂
196.2 Secondary and unspecified malignant neoplasm of intra-abdominal lymph nodes
196.5 Secondary and unspecified malignant neoplasm of lymph nodes of inguinal region and lower limb
196.6 Secondary and unspecified malignant neoplasm of intrapelvic lymph nodes
198.82 Secondary malignant neoplasm of genital organs
233.5 Carcinoma in situ of penis ♂
236.6 Neoplasm of uncertain behavior of other and unspecified male genital organs ▽ ♂
238.8 Neoplasm of uncertain behavior of other specified sites
239.5 Neoplasm of unspecified nature of other genitourinary organs
239.8 Neoplasm of unspecified nature of other specified sites

ICD-9-CM Procedural

40.50 Radical excision of lymph nodes, not otherwise specified
40.53 Radical excision of iliac lymph nodes
64.3 Amputation of penis

54150–54161

54150 Circumcision, using clamp or other device; newborn
54152 except newborn
54160 Circumcision, surgical excision other than clamp, device or dorsal slit; newborn
54161 except newborn

ICD-9-CM Diagnostic

605 Redundant prepuce and phimosis ♂
V50.2 Routine or ritual circumcision ♂

ICD-9-CM Procedural

64.0 Circumcision

HCPCS Level II Supplies & Services

A4550 Surgical trays

54162

54162 Lysis or excision of penile post-circumcision adhesions

ICD-9-CM Diagnostic

605 Redundant prepuce and phimosis ♂
709.2 Scar condition and fibrosis of skin
998.9 Unspecified complication of procedure, not elsewhere classified ▽

ICD-9-CM Procedural

64.93 Division of penile adhesions

HCPCS Level II Supplies & Services

A4550 Surgical trays

54163

54163 Repair incomplete circumcision

ICD-9-CM Diagnostic

605 Redundant prepuce and phimosis ♂
V50.1 Other plastic surgery for unacceptable cosmetic appearance
V50.2 Routine or ritual circumcision ♂

ICD-9-CM Procedural

64.0 Circumcision

HCPCS Level II Supplies & Services

A4550 Surgical trays

54164

54164 Frenulotomy of penis

ICD-9-CM Diagnostic

607.85 Peyronie's disease ♂
607.89 Other specified disorder of penis ♂
752.63 Congenital chordee ♂
752.69 Other penile anomalies ♂

ICD-9-CM Procedural

64.98 Other operations on penis

HCPCS Level II Supplies & Services

A4550 Surgical trays

54200–54205

54200 Injection procedure for Peyronie disease;
54205 with surgical exposure of plaque

ICD-9-CM Diagnostic

607.85 Peyronie's disease ♂

ICD-9-CM Procedural

64.92 Incision of penis
64.98 Other operations on penis
99.29 Injection or infusion of other therapeutic or prophylactic substance

▽ Unspecified code
♀ Female diagnosis
☒ Manifestation code
♂ Male diagnosis

99.77 Application or administration of adhesion barrier substance

HCPCS Level II Supplies & Services
A4550 Surgical trays

54220
54220 Irrigation of corpora cavernosa for priapism

ICD-9-CM Diagnostic
607.3 Priapism ♂

ICD-9-CM Procedural
64.98 Other operations on penis

HCPCS Level II Supplies & Services
A4550 Surgical trays

54230–54235
54230 Injection procedure for corpora cavernosography
54231 Dynamic cavernosometry, including intracavernosal injection of vasoactive drugs (eg, papaverine, phentolamine)
54235 Injection of corpora cavernosa with pharmacologic agent(s) (eg, papaverine, phentolamine)

ICD-9-CM Diagnostic
257.2 Other testicular hypofunction ♂
302.72 Psychosexual dysfunction with inhibited sexual excitement
607.3 Priapism ♂
607.82 Vascular disorders of penis ♂
607.84 Impotence of organic origin ♂
607.85 Peyronie's disease ♂
607.89 Other specified disorder of penis ♂
V41.7 Problems with sexual function — (This code is intended for use when these conditions are recorded as diagnoses or problems)

ICD-9-CM Procedural
64.19 Other diagnostic procedures on penis
87.99 Other x-ray of male genital organs
99.29 Injection or infusion of other therapeutic or prophylactic substance
99.77 Application or administration of adhesion barrier substance

HCPCS Level II Supplies & Services
A4550 Surgical trays
A9525 Supply of low or iso-osmolar contrast material, 10 mg of iodine
J2440 Injection, papaverine HCl, up to 60 mg
J2760 Injection, phentolamine mesylate, up to 5 mg

54240–54250
54240 Penile plethysmography
54250 Nocturnal penile tumescence and/or rigidity test

ICD-9-CM Diagnostic
257.2 Other testicular hypofunction ♂
302.72 Psychosexual dysfunction with inhibited sexual excitement
607.2 Other inflammatory disorders of penis — (Use additional code to identify organism) ♂
607.3 Priapism ♂
607.81 Balanitis xerotica obliterans ♂
607.82 Vascular disorders of penis ♂
607.83 Edema of penis ♂
607.84 Impotence of organic origin ♂
607.85 Peyronie's disease ♂
607.89 Other specified disorder of penis ♂
V41.7 Problems with sexual function — (This code is intended for use when these conditions are recorded as diagnoses or problems)

ICD-9-CM Procedural
89.29 Other nonoperative genitourinary system measurements
89.58 Plethysmogram

HCPCS Level II Supplies & Services
A4550 Surgical trays

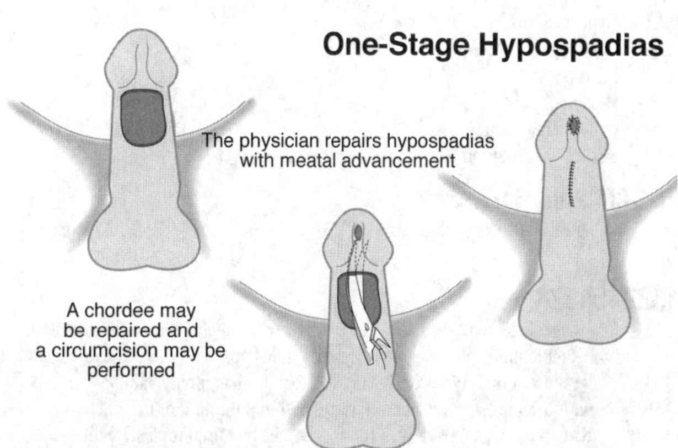
One-Stage Hypospadias
The physician repairs hypospadias with meatal advancement
A chordee may be repaired and a circumcision may be performed

54300–54304
54300 Plastic operation of penis for straightening of chordee (eg, hypospadias), with or without mobilization of urethra
54304 Plastic operation on penis for correction of chordee or for first stage hypospadias repair with or without transplantation of prepuce and/or skin flaps

ICD-9-CM Diagnostic
607.89 Other specified disorder of penis ♂
752.61 Hypospadias ♂
752.63 Congenital chordee ♂
752.69 Other penile anomalies ♂
752.81 Scrotal transposition

ICD-9-CM Procedural
58.45 Repair of hypospadias or epispadias
64.42 Release of chordee
64.49 Other repair of penis

54308–54312
54308 Urethroplasty for second stage hypospadias repair (including urinary diversion); less than 3 cm
54312 greater than 3 cm

ICD-9-CM Diagnostic
607.89 Other specified disorder of penis ♂
752.61 Hypospadias ♂
752.63 Congenital chordee ♂
752.69 Other penile anomalies ♂
752.81 Scrotal transposition

ICD-9-CM Procedural
58.45 Repair of hypospadias or epispadias

HCPCS Level II Supplies & Services
A4349 Male external catheter, with or without adhesive, disposable, each

54316
54316 Urethroplasty for second stage hypospadias repair (including urinary diversion) with free skin graft obtained from site other than genitalia

ICD-9-CM Diagnostic
607.89 Other specified disorder of penis ♂
752.61 Hypospadias ♂
752.63 Congenital chordee ♂
752.69 Other penile anomalies ♂
752.81 Scrotal transposition

ICD-9-CM Procedural
58.45 Repair of hypospadias or epispadias

HCPCS Level II Supplies & Services
A4349 Male external catheter, with or without adhesive, disposable, each

54318
54318 Urethroplasty for third stage hypospadias repair to release penis from scrotum (eg, third stage Cecil repair)

ICD-9-CM Diagnostic
607.89 Other specified disorder of penis ♂

752.61 Hypospadias ♂
752.63 Congenital chordee ♂
752.64 Micropenis ♂
752.65 Hidden penis ♂
752.69 Other penile anomalies ♂
752.81 Scrotal transposition

ICD-9-CM Procedural

58.46 Other reconstruction of urethra

54322–54328

54322 One stage distal hypospadias repair (with or without chordee or circumcision); with simple meatal advancement (eg, Magpi, V-flap)
54324 with urethroplasty by local skin flaps (eg, flip-flap, prepucial flap)
54326 with urethroplasty by local skin flaps and mobilization of urethra
54328 with extensive dissection to correct chordee and urethroplasty with local skin flaps, skin graft patch, and/or island flap

ICD-9-CM Diagnostic

607.89 Other specified disorder of penis ♂
752.61 Hypospadias ♂
752.63 Congenital chordee ♂
752.69 Other penile anomalies ♂
752.81 Scrotal transposition

ICD-9-CM Procedural

58.45 Repair of hypospadias or epispadias
64.42 Release of chordee

54332–54336

54332 One stage proximal penile or penoscrotal hypospadias repair requiring extensive dissection to correct chordee and urethroplasty by use of skin graft tube and/or island flap
54336 One stage perineal hypospadias repair requiring extensive dissection to correct chordee and urethroplasty by use of skin graft tube and/or island flap

ICD-9-CM Diagnostic

607.89 Other specified disorder of penis ♂
752.61 Hypospadias ♂
752.63 Congenital chordee ♂
752.69 Other penile anomalies ♂
752.81 Scrotal transposition

ICD-9-CM Procedural

58.45 Repair of hypospadias or epispadias
64.42 Release of chordee

54340–54348

54340 Repair of hypospadias complications (ie, fistula, stricture, diverticula); by closure, incision, or excision, simple
54344 requiring mobilization of skin flaps and urethroplasty with flap or patch graft
54348 requiring extensive dissection and urethroplasty with flap, patch or tubed graft (includes urinary diversion)

ICD-9-CM Diagnostic

598.2 Postoperative urethral stricture — (Use additional code to identify urinary incontinence: 625.6, 788.30-788.39)
599.1 Urethral fistula
599.2 Urethral diverticulum
605 Redundant prepuce and phimosis ♂
607.89 Other specified disorder of penis ♂
752.61 Hypospadias ♂
752.63 Congenital chordee ♂
752.81 Scrotal transposition
753.8 Other specified congenital anomaly of bladder and urethra
788.29 Other specified retention of urine
996.39 Mechanical complication of genitourinary device, implant, and graft, other
996.65 Infection and inflammatory reaction due to other genitourinary device, implant, and graft — (Use additional code to identify specified infections)
997.5 Urinary complications — (Use additional code to identify complications)
997.99 Other complications affecting other specified body systems, NEC — (Use additional code to identify complications)
998.59 Other postoperative infection — (Use additional code to identify infection)
998.6 Persistent postoperative fistula, not elsewhere classified
998.83 Non-healing surgical wound
998.89 Other specified complications
V13.61 Personal history of hypospadias ♂

ICD-9-CM Procedural

58.0 Urethrotomy
58.39 Other local excision or destruction of lesion or tissue of urethra
58.43 Closure of other fistula of urethra
58.6 Dilation of urethra

HCPCS Level II Supplies & Services

A4305 Disposable drug delivery system, flow rate of 50 ml or greater per hour
A4306 Disposable drug delivery system, flow rate of 5 ml or less per hour
A4349 Male external catheter, with or without adhesive, disposable, each
A4550 Surgical trays

54352

54352 Repair of hypospadias cripple requiring extensive dissection and excision of previously constructed structures including re-release of chordee and reconstruction of urethra and penis by use of local skin as grafts and island flaps and skin brought in as flaps or grafts

ICD-9-CM Diagnostic

598.2 Postoperative urethral stricture — (Use additional code to identify urinary incontinence: 625.6, 788.30-788.39)
599.1 Urethral fistula
599.2 Urethral diverticulum
605 Redundant prepuce and phimosis ♂
752.61 Hypospadias ♂
752.63 Congenital chordee ♂
752.81 Scrotal transposition
753.8 Other specified congenital anomaly of bladder and urethra
788.29 Other specified retention of urine
996.39 Mechanical complication of genitourinary device, implant, and graft, other
996.65 Infection and inflammatory reaction due to other genitourinary device, implant, and graft — (Use additional code to identify specified infections)
997.5 Urinary complications — (Use additional code to identify complications)
998.59 Other postoperative infection — (Use additional code to identify infection)
998.6 Persistent postoperative fistula, not elsewhere classified
998.83 Non-healing surgical wound
998.89 Other specified complications
V13.61 Personal history of hypospadias ♂
V13.69 Personal history of other congenital malformations

ICD-9-CM Procedural

58.0 Urethrotomy
58.39 Other local excision or destruction of lesion or tissue of urethra
58.43 Closure of other fistula of urethra
58.45 Repair of hypospadias or epispadias
58.49 Other repair of urethra
58.6 Dilation of urethra
64.42 Release of chordee

54360

54360 Plastic operation on penis to correct angulation

ICD-9-CM Diagnostic

098.2 Gonococcal infections, chronic, of lower genitourinary tract
607.85 Peyronie's disease ♂
607.89 Other specified disorder of penis ♂
752.62 Epispadias ♂
752.63 Congenital chordee ♂
752.69 Other penile anomalies ♂
996.39 Mechanical complication of genitourinary device, implant, and graft, other
996.65 Infection and inflammatory reaction due to other genitourinary device, implant, and graft — (Use additional code to identify specified infections)
V13.61 Personal history of hypospadias ♂
V13.69 Personal history of other congenital malformations

ICD-9-CM Procedural

64.49 Other repair of penis

Unspecified code
♀ Female diagnosis
Manifestation code
♂ Male diagnosis

54380–54390

54380 Plastic operation on penis for epispadias distal to external sphincter;
54385 with incontinence
54390 with exstrophy of bladder

ICD-9-CM Diagnostic

752.62 Epispadias ♂
753.5 Exstrophy of urinary bladder
788.37 Continuous leakage
788.39 Other urinary incontinence

ICD-9-CM Procedural

57.86 Repair of bladder exstrophy
58.45 Repair of hypospadias or epispadias
64.49 Other repair of penis

54400–54401

54400 Insertion of penile prosthesis; non-inflatable (semi-rigid)
54401 inflatable (self-contained)

ICD-9-CM Diagnostic

227.3 Benign neoplasm of pituitary gland and craniopharyngeal duct (pouch) — (Use additional code to identify any functional activity)
250.60 Diabetes with neurological manifestations, type II or unspecified type, not stated as uncontrolled — (Use additional code to identify manifestation: 337.1, 354.0-355.9, 357.2, 358.1, 713.5)
250.61 Diabetes with neurological manifestations, type I [juvenile type], not stated as uncontrolled — (Use additional code to identify manifestation: 337.1, 354.0-355.9, 357.2, 358.1, 713.5)
250.70 Diabetes with peripheral circulatory disorders, type II or unspecified type, not stated as uncontrolled — (Use additional code to identify manifestation: 443.81, 785.4)
250.71 Diabetes with peripheral circulatory disorders, type I [juvenile type], not stated as uncontrolled — (Use additional code to identify manifestation: 443.81, 785.4)
253.1 Other and unspecified anterior pituitary hyperfunction ▽
257.2 Other testicular hypofunction ♂
302.72 Psychosexual dysfunction with inhibited sexual excitement
337.1 Peripheral autonomic neuropathy in disorders classified elsewhere — (Code first underlying disease: 250.6, 277.3) ☒
443.81 Peripheral angiopathy in diseases classified elsewhere — (Code first underlying disease, 250.7) ☒
600.00 Hypertrophy (benign) of prostate without urinary obstruction — (Use additional code to identify urinary incontinence: 788.30-788.39) ♂
600.10 Nodular prostate without urinary obstruction — (Use additional code to identify urinary incontinence: 788.30-788.39) ♂
600.20 Benign localized hyperplasia of prostate without urinary obstruction — (Use additional code to identify urinary incontinence: 788.30-788.39) ♂
600.3 Cyst of prostate — (Use additional code to identify urinary incontinence: 788.30-788.39) ♂
600.90 Hyperplasia of prostate, unspecified, without urinary obstruction — (Use additional code to identify urinary incontinence: 788.30-788.39) ▽ ♂
607.81 Balanitis xerotica obliterans ♂
607.82 Vascular disorders of penis ♂
607.84 Impotence of organic origin ♂
607.89 Other specified disorder of penis ♂
608.83 Specified vascular disorder of male genital organs ♂
608.89 Other specified disorder of male genital organs ♂
752.89 Other specified anomalies of genital organs
907.2 Late effect of spinal cord injury
V10.46 Personal history of malignant neoplasm of prostate ♂
V52.8 Fitting and adjustment of other specified prosthetic device

ICD-9-CM Procedural

64.95 Insertion or replacement of non-inflatable penile prosthesis
64.97 Insertion or replacement of inflatable penile prosthesis

54405

54405 Insertion of multi-component, inflatable penile prosthesis, including placement of pump, cylinders, and reservoir

ICD-9-CM Diagnostic

227.3 Benign neoplasm of pituitary gland and craniopharyngeal duct (pouch) — (Use additional code to identify any functional activity)
250.60 Diabetes with neurological manifestations, type II or unspecified type, not stated as uncontrolled — (Use additional code to identify manifestation: 337.1, 354.0-355.9, 357.2, 358.1, 713.5)
250.61 Diabetes with neurological manifestations, type I [juvenile type], not stated as uncontrolled — (Use additional code to identify manifestation: 337.1, 354.0-355.9, 357.2, 358.1, 713.5)
250.70 Diabetes with peripheral circulatory disorders, type II or unspecified type, not stated as uncontrolled — (Use additional code to identify manifestation: 443.81, 785.4)
250.71 Diabetes with peripheral circulatory disorders, type I [juvenile type], not stated as uncontrolled — (Use additional code to identify manifestation: 443.81, 785.4)
253.1 Other and unspecified anterior pituitary hyperfunction ▽
257.2 Other testicular hypofunction ♂
302.72 Psychosexual dysfunction with inhibited sexual excitement
337.1 Peripheral autonomic neuropathy in disorders classified elsewhere — (Code first underlying disease: 250.6, 277.3) ☒
443.81 Peripheral angiopathy in diseases classified elsewhere — (Code first underlying disease, 250.7) ☒
600.00 Hypertrophy (benign) of prostate without urinary obstruction — (Use additional code to identify urinary incontinence: 788.30-788.39) ♂
600.10 Nodular prostate without urinary obstruction — (Use additional code to identify urinary incontinence: 788.30-788.39) ♂
600.20 Benign localized hyperplasia of prostate without urinary obstruction — (Use additional code to identify urinary incontinence: 788.30-788.39) ♂
600.3 Cyst of prostate — (Use additional code to identify urinary incontinence: 788.30-788.39) ♂
600.90 Hyperplasia of prostate, unspecified, without urinary obstruction — (Use additional code to identify urinary incontinence: 788.30-788.39) ▽ ♂
607.81 Balanitis xerotica obliterans ♂
607.82 Vascular disorders of penis ♂
607.84 Impotence of organic origin ♂
607.89 Other specified disorder of penis ♂
608.83 Specified vascular disorder of male genital organs ♂
608.89 Other specified disorder of male genital organs ♂
752.89 Other specified anomalies of genital organs
907.2 Late effect of spinal cord injury
V10.46 Personal history of malignant neoplasm of prostate ♂
V52.8 Fitting and adjustment of other specified prosthetic device

ICD-9-CM Procedural

64.97 Insertion or replacement of inflatable penile prosthesis

54406

54406 Removal of all components of a multi-component, inflatable penile prosthesis without replacement of prosthesis

ICD-9-CM Diagnostic

187.5 Malignant neoplasm of epididymis ♂
187.6 Malignant neoplasm of spermatic cord ♂
187.8 Malignant neoplasm of other specified sites of male genital organs ♂
233.6 Carcinoma in situ of other and unspecified male genital organs ▽ ♂
597.0 Urethral abscess
597.80 Unspecified urethritis ▽
597.89 Other urethritis
603.1 Infected hydrocele — (Use additional code to identify organism)
604.0 Orchitis, epididymitis, and epididymo-orchitis, with abscess — (Use additional code to identify organism: 041.0, 041.1, 041.4) ♂
604.90 Unspecified orchitis and epididymitis — (Use additional code to identify organism: 041.0, 041.1, 041.4) ▽ ♂
604.91 Orchitis and epididymitis in disease classified elsewhere — (Code first underlying disease: 032.89, 095.8, 125.0-125.9. Use additional code to identify organism: 041.0, 041.1, 041.4) ☒ ♂
607.1 Balanoposthitis — (Use additional code to identify organism) ♂
607.2 Other inflammatory disorders of penis — (Use additional code to identify organism) ♂
607.81 Balanitis xerotica obliterans ♂
607.83 Edema of penis ♂
608.0 Seminal vesiculitis — (Use additional code to identify organism) ♂
608.1 Spermatocele ♂
608.4 Other inflammatory disorder of male genital organs — (Use additional code to identify organism) ♂
608.81 Specified disorder of male genital organs in diseases classified elsewhere — (Code first underlying disease: 016.5, 125.0-125.9) ☒ ♂
608.86 Edema of male genital organs ♂
867.1 Bladder and urethra injury with open wound into cavity

867.7 Injury to other specified pelvic organs with open wound into cavity
878.1 Open wound of penis, complicated — (Use additional code to identify infection) ♂
878.3 Open wound of scrotum and testes, complicated — (Use additional code to identify infection) ♂
996.39 Mechanical complication of genitourinary device, implant, and graft, other
996.65 Infection and inflammatory reaction due to other genitourinary device, implant, and graft — (Use additional code to identify specified infections)
996.76 Other complications due to genitourinary device, implant, and graft
998.59 Other postoperative infection — (Use additional code to identify infection)
V52.8 Fitting and adjustment of other specified prosthetic device

ICD-9-CM Procedural

64.96 Removal of internal prosthesis of penis

HCPCS Level II Supplies & Services

HCPCS Level II codes are used to report the supplies, durable medical equipment, and certain medical services provided on an outpatient basis. Because the procedure(s) represented on this page would be performed in an inpatient or outpatient facility, no HCPCS Level II codes apply.

54408

54408 Repair of component(s) of a multi-component, inflatable penile prosthesis

ICD-9-CM Diagnostic

996.39 Mechanical complication of genitourinary device, implant, and graft, other

ICD-9-CM Procedural

64.99 Other operations on male genital organs

HCPCS Level II Supplies & Services

HCPCS Level II codes are used to report the supplies, durable medical equipment, and certain medical services provided on an outpatient basis. Because the procedure(s) represented on this page would be performed in an inpatient or outpatient facility, no HCPCS Level II codes apply.

54410

54410 Removal and replacement of all component(s) of a multi-component, inflatable penile prosthesis at the same operative session

ICD-9-CM Diagnostic

227.3 Benign neoplasm of pituitary gland and craniopharyngeal duct (pouch) — (Use additional code to identify any functional activity)
250.60 Diabetes with neurological manifestations, type II or unspecified type, not stated as uncontrolled — (Use additional code to identify manifestation: 337.1, 354.0-355.9, 357.2, 358.1, 713.5)
250.61 Diabetes with neurological manifestations, type I [juvenile type], not stated as uncontrolled — (Use additional code to identify manifestation: 337.1, 354.0-355.9, 357.2, 358.1, 713.5)
250.70 Diabetes with peripheral circulatory disorders, type II or unspecified type, not stated as uncontrolled — (Use additional code to identify manifestation: 443.81, 785.4)
250.71 Diabetes with peripheral circulatory disorders, type I [juvenile type], not stated as uncontrolled — (Use additional code to identify manifestation: 443.81, 785.4)
253.1 Other and unspecified anterior pituitary hyperfunction ▽
257.2 Other testicular hypofunction ♂
302.72 Psychosexual dysfunction with inhibited sexual excitement
337.1 Peripheral autonomic neuropathy in disorders classified elsewhere — (Code first underlying disease: 250.6, 277.3) ☒
443.81 Peripheral angiopathy in diseases classified elsewhere — (Code first underlying disease, 250.7) ☒
607.82 Vascular disorders of penis ♂
607.84 Impotence of organic origin ♂
607.89 Other specified disorder of penis ♂
608.83 Specified vascular disorder of male genital organs ♂
608.89 Other specified disorder of male genital organs ♂
752.89 Other specified anomalies of genital organs
907.2 Late effect of spinal cord injury
996.39 Mechanical complication of genitourinary device, implant, and graft, other
996.65 Infection and inflammatory reaction due to other genitourinary device, implant, and graft — (Use additional code to identify specified infections)
996.76 Other complications due to genitourinary device, implant, and graft
V10.46 Personal history of malignant neoplasm of prostate ♂
V45.77 Acquired absence of organ, genital organs — (This code is intended for use when these conditions are recorded as diagnoses or problems)
V52.8 Fitting and adjustment of other specified prosthetic device

ICD-9-CM Procedural

64.97 Insertion or replacement of inflatable penile prosthesis

54411

54411 Removal and replacement of all components of a multi-component inflatable penile prosthesis through an infected field at the same operative session, including irrigation and debridement of infected tissue

ICD-9-CM Diagnostic

227.3 Benign neoplasm of pituitary gland and craniopharyngeal duct (pouch) — (Use additional code to identify any functional activity)
250.60 Diabetes with neurological manifestations, type II or unspecified type, not stated as uncontrolled — (Use additional code to identify manifestation: 337.1, 354.0-355.9, 357.2, 358.1, 713.5)
250.61 Diabetes with neurological manifestations, type I [juvenile type], not stated as uncontrolled — (Use additional code to identify manifestation: 337.1, 354.0-355.9, 357.2, 358.1, 713.5)
250.70 Diabetes with peripheral circulatory disorders, type II or unspecified type, not stated as uncontrolled — (Use additional code to identify manifestation: 443.81, 785.4)
250.71 Diabetes with peripheral circulatory disorders, type I [juvenile type], not stated as uncontrolled — (Use additional code to identify manifestation: 443.81, 785.4)
253.1 Other and unspecified anterior pituitary hyperfunction ▽
257.2 Other testicular hypofunction ♂
302.72 Psychosexual dysfunction with inhibited sexual excitement
337.1 Peripheral autonomic neuropathy in disorders classified elsewhere — (Code first underlying disease: 250.6, 277.3) ☒
443.81 Peripheral angiopathy in diseases classified elsewhere — (Code first underlying disease, 250.7) ☒
597.0 Urethral abscess
597.80 Unspecified urethritis ▽
597.89 Other urethritis
603.1 Infected hydrocele — (Use additional code to identify organism)
604.0 Orchitis, epididymitis, and epididymo-orchitis, with abscess — (Use additional code to identify organism: 041.0, 041.1, 041.4) ♂
604.90 Unspecified orchitis and epididymitis — (Use additional code to identify organism: 041.0, 041.1, 041.4) ▽ ♂
604.91 Orchitis and epididymitis in disease classified elsewhere — (Code first underlying disease: 032.89, 095.8, 125.0-125.9. Use additional code to identify organism: 041.0, 041.1, 041.4) ☒ ♂
607.1 Balanoposthitis — (Use additional code to identify organism) ♂
607.2 Other inflammatory disorders of penis — (Use additional code to identify organism) ♂
607.81 Balanitis xerotica obliterans ♂
607.82 Vascular disorders of penis ♂
607.84 Impotence of organic origin ♂
607.89 Other specified disorder of penis ♂
608.0 Seminal vesiculitis — (Use additional code to identify organism) ♂
608.4 Other inflammatory disorder of male genital organs — (Use additional code to identify organism) ♂
608.81 Specified disorder of male genital organs in diseases classified elsewhere — (Code first underlying disease: 016.5, 125.0-125.9) ☒ ♂
608.83 Specified vascular disorder of male genital organs ♂
608.89 Other specified disorder of male genital organs ♂
752.89 Other specified anomalies of genital organs
907.2 Late effect of spinal cord injury
996.65 Infection and inflammatory reaction due to other genitourinary device, implant, and graft — (Use additional code to identify specified infections)
996.76 Other complications due to genitourinary device, implant, and graft
998.59 Other postoperative infection — (Use additional code to identify infection)
V10.46 Personal history of malignant neoplasm of prostate ♂
V52.8 Fitting and adjustment of other specified prosthetic device

ICD-9-CM Procedural

64.97 Insertion or replacement of inflatable penile prosthesis
86.22 Excisional debridement of wound, infection, or burn

HCPCS Level II Supplies & Services

HCPCS Level II codes are used to report the supplies, durable medical equipment, and certain medical services provided on an outpatient basis. Because the procedure(s) represented on this page would be performed in an inpatient or outpatient facility, no HCPCS Level II codes apply.

▽ Unspecified code ☒ Manifestation code
♀ Female diagnosis ♂ Male diagnosis

54415

54415 Removal of non-inflatable (semi-rigid) or inflatable (self-contained) penile prosthesis, without replacement of prosthesis

ICD-9-CM Diagnostic

187.5 Malignant neoplasm of epididymis ♂
187.6 Malignant neoplasm of spermatic cord ♂
187.8 Malignant neoplasm of other specified sites of male genital organs ♂
233.6 Carcinoma in situ of other and unspecified male genital organs ▽ ♂
597.0 Urethral abscess
597.80 Unspecified urethritis ▽
597.89 Other urethritis
603.1 Infected hydrocele — (Use additional code to identify organism)
604.0 Orchitis, epididymitis, and epididymo-orchitis, with abscess — (Use additional code to identify organism: 041.0, 041.1, 041.4) ♂
604.90 Unspecified orchitis and epididymitis — (Use additional code to identify organism: 041.0, 041.1, 041.4) ▽ ♂
604.91 Orchitis and epididymitis in disease classified elsewhere — (Code first underlying disease: 032.89, 095.8, 125.0-125.9. Use additional code to identify organism: 041.0, 041.1, 041.4) ☒ ♂
607.1 Balanoposthitis — (Use additional code to identify organism) ♂
607.2 Other inflammatory disorders of penis — (Use additional code to identify organism) ♂
607.81 Balanitis xerotica obliterans ♂
607.83 Edema of penis ♂
608.0 Seminal vesiculitis — (Use additional code to identify organism) ♂
608.1 Spermatocele ♂
608.4 Other inflammatory disorder of male genital organs — (Use additional code to identify organism) ♂
608.81 Specified disorder of male genital organs in diseases classified elsewhere — (Code first underlying disease: 016.5, 125.0-125.9) ☒ ♂
608.86 Edema of male genital organs ♂
867.1 Bladder and urethra injury with open wound into cavity
867.7 Injury to other specified pelvic organs with open wound into cavity
878.1 Open wound of penis, complicated — (Use additional code to identify infection) ♂
878.3 Open wound of scrotum and testes, complicated — (Use additional code to identify infection) ♂
996.39 Mechanical complication of genitourinary device, implant, and graft, other
996.65 Infection and inflammatory reaction due to other genitourinary device, implant, and graft — (Use additional code to identify specified infections)
996.76 Other complications due to genitourinary device, implant, and graft
998.59 Other postoperative infection — (Use additional code to identify infection)
V52.8 Fitting and adjustment of other specified prosthetic device

ICD-9-CM Procedural

64.96 Removal of internal prosthesis of penis

HCPCS Level II Supplies & Services

HCPCS Level II codes are used to report the supplies, durable medical equipment, and certain medical services provided on an outpatient basis. Because the procedure(s) represented on this page would be performed in an inpatient or outpatient facility, no HCPCS Level II codes apply.

54416

54416 Removal and replacement of non-inflatable (semi-rigid) or inflatable (self-contained) penile prosthesis at the same operative session

ICD-9-CM Diagnostic

227.3 Benign neoplasm of pituitary gland and craniopharyngeal duct (pouch) — (Use additional code to identify any functional activity)
250.60 Diabetes with neurological manifestations, type II or unspecified type, not stated as uncontrolled — (Use additional code to identify manifestation: 337.1, 354.0-355.9, 357.2, 358.1, 713.5)
250.61 Diabetes with neurological manifestations, type I [juvenile type], not stated as uncontrolled — (Use additional code to identify manifestation: 337.1, 354.0-355.9, 357.2, 358.1, 713.5)
250.70 Diabetes with peripheral circulatory disorders, type II or unspecified type, not stated as uncontrolled — (Use additional code to identify manifestation: 443.81, 785.4)
250.71 Diabetes with peripheral circulatory disorders, type I [juvenile type], not stated as uncontrolled — (Use additional code to identify manifestation: 443.81, 785.4)
253.1 Other and unspecified anterior pituitary hyperfunction ▽
257.2 Other testicular hypofunction ♂
302.72 Psychosexual dysfunction with inhibited sexual excitement
337.1 Peripheral autonomic neuropathy in disorders classified elsewhere — (Code first underlying disease: 250.6, 277.3) ☒
443.81 Peripheral angiopathy in diseases classified elsewhere — (Code first underlying disease, 250.7) ☒
607.82 Vascular disorders of penis ♂
607.84 Impotence of organic origin ♂
607.89 Other specified disorder of penis ♂
608.83 Specified vascular disorder of male genital organs ♂
608.89 Other specified disorder of male genital organs ♂
752.89 Other specified anomalies of genital organs
907.2 Late effect of spinal cord injury
996.39 Mechanical complication of genitourinary device, implant, and graft, other
996.65 Infection and inflammatory reaction due to other genitourinary device, implant, and graft — (Use additional code to identify specified infections)
996.76 Other complications due to genitourinary device, implant, and graft
V10.46 Personal history of malignant neoplasm of prostate ♂
V52.8 Fitting and adjustment of other specified prosthetic device

ICD-9-CM Procedural

64.95 Insertion or replacement of non-inflatable penile prosthesis
64.97 Insertion or replacement of inflatable penile prosthesis

HCPCS Level II Supplies & Services

HCPCS Level II codes are used to report the supplies, durable medical equipment, and certain medical services provided on an outpatient basis. Because the procedure(s) represented on this page would be performed in an inpatient or outpatient facility, no HCPCS Level II codes apply.

54417

54417 Removal and replacement of non-inflatable (semi-rigid) or inflatable (self-contained) penile prosthesis through an infected field at the same operative session, including irrigation and debridement of infected tissue

ICD-9-CM Diagnostic

227.3 Benign neoplasm of pituitary gland and craniopharyngeal duct (pouch) — (Use additional code to identify any functional activity)
250.60 Diabetes with neurological manifestations, type II or unspecified type, not stated as uncontrolled — (Use additional code to identify manifestation: 337.1, 354.0-355.9, 357.2, 358.1, 713.5)
250.61 Diabetes with neurological manifestations, type I [juvenile type], not stated as uncontrolled — (Use additional code to identify manifestation: 337.1, 354.0-355.9, 357.2, 358.1, 713.5)
250.70 Diabetes with peripheral circulatory disorders, type II or unspecified type, not stated as uncontrolled — (Use additional code to identify manifestation: 443.81, 785.4)
250.71 Diabetes with peripheral circulatory disorders, type I [juvenile type], not stated as uncontrolled — (Use additional code to identify manifestation: 443.81, 785.4)
253.1 Other and unspecified anterior pituitary hyperfunction ▽
257.2 Other testicular hypofunction ♂
302.72 Psychosexual dysfunction with inhibited sexual excitement
337.1 Peripheral autonomic neuropathy in disorders classified elsewhere — (Code first underlying disease: 250.6, 277.3) ☒
443.81 Peripheral angiopathy in diseases classified elsewhere — (Code first underlying disease, 250.7) ☒
597.0 Urethral abscess
597.80 Unspecified urethritis ▽
597.89 Other urethritis
603.1 Infected hydrocele — (Use additional code to identify organism)
604.0 Orchitis, epididymitis, and epididymo-orchitis, with abscess — (Use additional code to identify organism: 041.0, 041.1, 041.4) ♂
604.90 Unspecified orchitis and epididymitis — (Use additional code to identify organism: 041.0, 041.1, 041.4) ▽ ♂
604.91 Orchitis and epididymitis in disease classified elsewhere — (Code first underlying disease: 032.89, 095.8, 125.0-125.9. Use additional code to identify organism: 041.0, 041.1, 041.4) ☒ ♂
607.1 Balanoposthitis — (Use additional code to identify organism) ♂
607.2 Other inflammatory disorders of penis — (Use additional code to identify organism) ♂
607.81 Balanitis xerotica obliterans ♂
607.82 Vascular disorders of penis ♂
607.84 Impotence of organic origin ♂
607.89 Other specified disorder of penis ♂
608.0 Seminal vesiculitis — (Use additional code to identify organism) ♂
608.4 Other inflammatory disorder of male genital organs — (Use additional code to identify organism) ♂

▽ Unspecified code ☒ Manifestation code
♀ Female diagnosis ♂ Male diagnosis

608.81 Specified disorder of male genital organs in diseases classified elsewhere — (Code first underlying disease: 016.5, 125.0-125.9) ☒ ♂
608.83 Specified vascular disorder of male genital organs ♂
608.89 Other specified disorder of male genital organs ♂
752.89 Other specified anomalies of genital organs
907.2 Late effect of spinal cord injury
996.65 Infection and inflammatory reaction due to other genitourinary device, implant, and graft — (Use additional code to identify specified infections)
996.76 Other complications due to genitourinary device, implant, and graft
998.59 Other postoperative infection — (Use additional code to identify infection)
V10.46 Personal history of malignant neoplasm of prostate ♂
V45.77 Acquired absence of organ, genital organs — (This code is intended for use when these conditions are recorded as diagnoses or problems)
V52.8 Fitting and adjustment of other specified prosthetic device

ICD-9-CM Procedural

64.95 Insertion or replacement of non-inflatable penile prosthesis
64.97 Insertion or replacement of inflatable penile prosthesis
86.22 Excisional debridement of wound, infection, or burn

54420–54435

54420 Corpora cavernosa-saphenous vein shunt (priapism operation), unilateral or bilateral
54430 Corpora cavernosa-corpus spongiosum shunt (priapism operation), unilateral or bilateral
54435 Corpora cavernosa-glans penis fistulization (eg, biopsy needle, Winter procedure, rongeur, or punch) for priapism

ICD-9-CM Diagnostic

607.3 Priapism ♂

ICD-9-CM Procedural

64.98 Other operations on penis

HCPCS Level II Supplies & Services

A4305 Disposable drug delivery system, flow rate of 50 ml or greater per hour
A4306 Disposable drug delivery system, flow rate of 5 ml or less per hour
A4550 Surgical trays

54440

54440 Plastic operation of penis for injury

ICD-9-CM Diagnostic

878.0 Open wound of penis, without mention of complication — (Use additional code to identify infection) ♂
878.1 Open wound of penis, complicated — (Use additional code to identify infection) ♂
959.13 Other injury, Fracture of corpus cavernosum penis
959.14 Other injury of external genitals

ICD-9-CM Procedural

64.41 Suture of laceration of penis
64.43 Construction of penis
64.44 Reconstruction of penis
64.49 Other repair of penis

54450

54450 Foreskin manipulation including lysis of preputial adhesions and stretching

ICD-9-CM Diagnostic

605 Redundant prepuce and phimosis ♂
752.89 Other specified anomalies of genital organs

ICD-9-CM Procedural

64.93 Division of penile adhesions
64.98 Other operations on penis
99.95 Stretching of foreskin

HCPCS Level II Supplies & Services

A4550 Surgical trays

Testis

54500–54505

54500 Biopsy of testis, needle (separate procedure)
54505 Biopsy of testis, incisional (separate procedure)

ICD-9-CM Diagnostic

186.0 Malignant neoplasm of undescended testis — (Use additional code to identify any functional activity) ♂
186.9 Malignant neoplasm of other and unspecified testis — (Use additional code to identify any functional activity) ▽ ♂
198.82 Secondary malignant neoplasm of genital organs
222.0 Benign neoplasm of testis — (Use additional code to identify any functional activity) ♂
233.6 Carcinoma in situ of other and unspecified male genital organs ▽ ♂
236.4 Neoplasm of uncertain behavior of testis — (Use additional code to identify any functional activity) ♂
239.5 Neoplasm of unspecified nature of other genitourinary organs
257.2 Other testicular hypofunction ♂
606.0 Azoospermia ♂
606.1 Oligospermia ♂
608.2 Torsion of testis ♂
608.3 Atrophy of testis ♂
608.81 Specified disorder of male genital organs in diseases classified elsewhere — (Code first underlying disease: 016.5, 125.0-125.9) ☒ ♂
608.82 Hematospermia ♂
608.89 Other specified disorder of male genital organs ♂

ICD-9-CM Procedural

62.11 Closed (percutaneous) (needle) biopsy of testis
62.12 Open biopsy of testis

HCPCS Level II Supplies & Services

A4550 Surgical trays

54512

54512 Excision of extraparenchymal lesion of testis

ICD-9-CM Diagnostic

186.0 Malignant neoplasm of undescended testis — (Use additional code to identify any functional activity) ♂
186.9 Malignant neoplasm of other and unspecified testis — (Use additional code to identify any functional activity) ▽ ♂
198.82 Secondary malignant neoplasm of genital organs
222.0 Benign neoplasm of testis — (Use additional code to identify any functional activity) ♂
233.6 Carcinoma in situ of other and unspecified male genital organs ▽ ♂
236.4 Neoplasm of uncertain behavior of testis — (Use additional code to identify any functional activity) ♂
239.5 Neoplasm of unspecified nature of other genitourinary organs
608.4 Other inflammatory disorder of male genital organs — (Use additional code to identify organism) ♂
608.89 Other specified disorder of male genital organs ♂
608.9 Unspecified disorder of male genital organs ▽ ♂

ICD-9-CM Procedural

62.2 Excision or destruction of testicular lesion

HCPCS Level II Supplies & Services

A4550 Surgical trays

54520

54520 Orchiectomy, simple (including subcapsular), with or without testicular prosthesis, scrotal or inguinal approach

ICD-9-CM Diagnostic

185 Malignant neoplasm of prostate ♂
186.0 Malignant neoplasm of undescended testis — (Use additional code to identify any functional activity) ♂
186.9 Malignant neoplasm of other and unspecified testis — (Use additional code to identify any functional activity) ▽ ♂
198.82 Secondary malignant neoplasm of genital organs
222.0 Benign neoplasm of testis — (Use additional code to identify any functional activity) ♂

▽ Unspecified code
♀ Female diagnosis
☒ Manifestation code
♂ Male diagnosis

233.6 Carcinoma in situ of other and unspecified male genital organs ▽ ♂
239.5 Neoplasm of unspecified nature of other genitourinary organs
604.0 Orchitis, epididymitis, and epididymo-orchitis, with abscess — (Use additional code to identify organism: 041.0, 041.1, 041.4) ♂
604.91 Orchitis and epididymitis in disease classified elsewhere — (Code first underlying disease: 032.89, 095.8, 125.0-125.9. Use additional code to identify organism: 041.0, 041.1, 041.4) ☒ ♂
604.99 Other orchitis, epididymitis, and epididymo-orchitis, without mention of abscess — (Use additional code to identify organism: 041.0, 041.1, 041.4) ♂
608.2 Torsion of testis ♂
608.3 Atrophy of testis ♂
608.4 Other inflammatory disorder of male genital organs — (Use additional code to identify organism) ♂
608.81 Specified disorder of male genital organs in diseases classified elsewhere — (Code first underlying disease: 016.5, 125.0-125.9) ☒ ♂
608.83 Specified vascular disorder of male genital organs ♂
608.89 Other specified disorder of male genital organs ♂
752.51 Undescended testis ♂
752.52 Retractile testis ♂
752.81 Scrotal transposition
878.2 Open wound of scrotum and testes, without mention of complication — (Use additional code to identify infection) ♂
878.3 Open wound of scrotum and testes, complicated — (Use additional code to identify infection) ♂
926.0 Crushing injury of external genitalia — (Use additional code to identify any associated injuries: 800-829, 850.0-854.1, 860.0-869.1)
V50.49 Other prophylactic gland removal
V64.41 Laparoscopic surgical procedure converted to open procedure

ICD-9-CM Procedural

62.3 Unilateral orchiectomy
62.41 Removal of both testes at same operative episode
62.42 Removal of remaining testis
62.7 Insertion of testicular prosthesis

54522

54522 Orchiectomy, partial

ICD-9-CM Diagnostic

186.0 Malignant neoplasm of undescended testis — (Use additional code to identify any functional activity) ♂
186.9 Malignant neoplasm of other and unspecified testis — (Use additional code to identify any functional activity) ▽ ♂
198.82 Secondary malignant neoplasm of genital organs
222.0 Benign neoplasm of testis — (Use additional code to identify any functional activity) ♂
233.6 Carcinoma in situ of other and unspecified male genital organs ▽ ♂
239.5 Neoplasm of unspecified nature of other genitourinary organs
604.0 Orchitis, epididymitis, and epididymo-orchitis, with abscess — (Use additional code to identify organism: 041.0, 041.1, 041.4) ♂
604.91 Orchitis and epididymitis in disease classified elsewhere — (Code first underlying disease: 032.89, 095.8, 125.0-125.9. Use additional code to identify organism: 041.0, 041.1, 041.4) ☒ ♂
604.99 Other orchitis, epididymitis, and epididymo-orchitis, without mention of abscess — (Use additional code to identify organism: 041.0, 041.1, 041.4) ♂
608.2 Torsion of testis ♂
608.4 Other inflammatory disorder of male genital organs — (Use additional code to identify organism) ♂
608.81 Specified disorder of male genital organs in diseases classified elsewhere — (Code first underlying disease: 016.5, 125.0-125.9) ☒ ♂
608.83 Specified vascular disorder of male genital organs ♂
608.89 Other specified disorder of male genital organs ♂
878.2 Open wound of scrotum and testes, without mention of complication — (Use additional code to identify infection) ♂
878.3 Open wound of scrotum and testes, complicated — (Use additional code to identify infection) ♂
926.0 Crushing injury of external genitalia — (Use additional code to identify any associated injuries: 800-829, 850.0-854.1, 860.0-869.1)
V64.41 Laparoscopic surgical procedure converted to open procedure

ICD-9-CM Procedural

62.3 Unilateral orchiectomy

54530–54535

54530 Orchiectomy, radical, for tumor; inguinal approach
54535 with abdominal exploration

ICD-9-CM Diagnostic

186.0 Malignant neoplasm of undescended testis — (Use additional code to identify any functional activity) ♂
186.9 Malignant neoplasm of other and unspecified testis — (Use additional code to identify any functional activity) ▽ ♂
187.5 Malignant neoplasm of epididymis ♂
187.8 Malignant neoplasm of other specified sites of male genital organs ♂
198.82 Secondary malignant neoplasm of genital organs
233.6 Carcinoma in situ of other and unspecified male genital organs ▽ ♂
236.4 Neoplasm of uncertain behavior of testis — (Use additional code to identify any functional activity) ♂
239.5 Neoplasm of unspecified nature of other genitourinary organs
V64.41 Laparoscopic surgical procedure converted to open procedure

ICD-9-CM Procedural

62.3 Unilateral orchiectomy
62.41 Removal of both testes at same operative episode
62.42 Removal of remaining testis

54550–54560

54550 Exploration for undescended testis (inguinal or scrotal area)
54560 Exploration for undescended testis with abdominal exploration

ICD-9-CM Diagnostic

752.51 Undescended testis ♂
752.52 Retractile testis ♂
752.81 Scrotal transposition

ICD-9-CM Procedural

62.0 Incision of testis

54600

54600 Reduction of torsion of testis, surgical, with or without fixation of contralateral testis

ICD-9-CM Diagnostic

608.2 Torsion of testis ♂

ICD-9-CM Procedural

63.52 Reduction of torsion of testis or spermatic cord

54620

54620 Fixation of contralateral testis (separate procedure)

ICD-9-CM Diagnostic

608.81 Specified disorder of male genital organs in diseases classified elsewhere — (Code first underlying disease: 016.5, 125.0-125.9) ☒ ♂
608.89 Other specified disorder of male genital organs ♂

ICD-9-CM Procedural

62.5 Orchiopexy

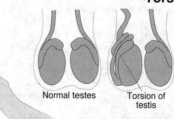

Torsion of Testis

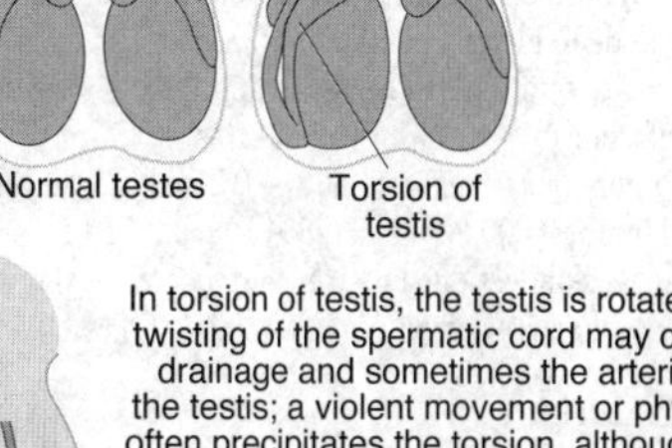

In torsion of testis, the testis is rotated upon itself; twisting of the spermatic cord may cut off venous drainage and sometimes the arterial supply to the testis; a violent movement or physical trauma often precipitates the torsion, although incomplete descent and other abnormalities may be predisposing factors

▽ Unspecified code
♀ Female diagnosis
☒ Manifestation code
♂ Male diagnosis

54640–54650

54640 Orchiopexy, inguinal approach, with or without hernia repair
54650 Orchiopexy, abdominal approach, for intra-abdominal testis (eg, Fowler-Stephens)

ICD-9-CM Diagnostic

550.90 Inguinal hernia without mention of obstruction or gangrene, unilateral or unspecified, (not specified as recurrent)
608.2 Torsion of testis ♂
608.89 Other specified disorder of male genital organs ♂
752.51 Undescended testis ♂
752.52 Retractile testis ♂
752.81 Scrotal transposition
752.89 Other specified anomalies of genital organs
V64.41 Laparoscopic surgical procedure converted to open procedure

ICD-9-CM Procedural

62.5 Orchiopexy

54660

54660 Insertion of testicular prosthesis (separate procedure)

ICD-9-CM Diagnostic

608.89 Other specified disorder of male genital organs ♂
752.51 Undescended testis ♂
752.52 Retractile testis ♂
752.9 Unspecified congenital anomaly of genital organs ▽
V10.47 Personal history of malignant neoplasm of testis ♂
V45.89 Other postsurgical status — (This code is intended for use when these conditions are recorded as diagnoses or problems)
V52.8 Fitting and adjustment of other specified prosthetic device

ICD-9-CM Procedural

62.7 Insertion of testicular prosthesis

54670

54670 Suture or repair of testicular injury

ICD-9-CM Diagnostic

878.2 Open wound of scrotum and testes, without mention of complication — (Use additional code to identify infection) ♂
878.3 Open wound of scrotum and testes, complicated — (Use additional code to identify infection) ♂
926.0 Crushing injury of external genitalia — (Use additional code to identify any associated injuries: 800-829, 850.0-854.1, 860.0-869.1)

ICD-9-CM Procedural

62.61 Suture of laceration of testis

HCPCS Level II Supplies & Services

A4550 Surgical trays

54680

54680 Transplantation of testis(es) to thigh (because of scrotal destruction)

ICD-9-CM Diagnostic

187.7 Malignant neoplasm of scrotum ♂
198.82 Secondary malignant neoplasm of genital organs
222.4 Benign neoplasm of scrotum ♂
233.6 Carcinoma in situ of other and unspecified male genital organs ▽ ♂
878.2 Open wound of scrotum and testes, without mention of complication — (Use additional code to identify infection) ♂
878.3 Open wound of scrotum and testes, complicated — (Use additional code to identify infection) ♂
926.0 Crushing injury of external genitalia — (Use additional code to identify any associated injuries: 800-829, 850.0-854.1, 860.0-869.1)
942.35 Full-thickness skin loss due to burn (third degree nos) of genitalia
959.14 Other injury of external genitals

ICD-9-CM Procedural

62.99 Other operations on testes

54690

54690 Laparoscopy, surgical; orchiectomy

ICD-9-CM Diagnostic

186.0 Malignant neoplasm of undescended testis — (Use additional code to identify any functional activity) ♂
186.9 Malignant neoplasm of other and unspecified testis — (Use additional code to identify any functional activity) ▽ ♂
198.82 Secondary malignant neoplasm of genital organs
222.0 Benign neoplasm of testis — (Use additional code to identify any functional activity) ♂
233.6 Carcinoma in situ of other and unspecified male genital organs ▽ ♂
236.4 Neoplasm of uncertain behavior of testis — (Use additional code to identify any functional activity) ♂
239.5 Neoplasm of unspecified nature of other genitourinary organs
608.2 Torsion of testis ♂
608.3 Atrophy of testis ♂
608.83 Specified vascular disorder of male genital organs ♂
608.89 Other specified disorder of male genital organs ♂
V50.49 Other prophylactic gland removal

ICD-9-CM Procedural

62.3 Unilateral orchiectomy
62.41 Removal of both testes at same operative episode
62.42 Removal of remaining testis

54692

54692 Laparoscopy, surgical; orchiopexy for intra-abdominal testis

ICD-9-CM Diagnostic

752.51 Undescended testis ♂
752.52 Retractile testis ♂
752.81 Scrotal transposition

ICD-9-CM Procedural

62.5 Orchiopexy

Epididymis

54700

54700 Incision and drainage of epididymis, testis and/or scrotal space (eg, abscess or hematoma)

ICD-9-CM Diagnostic

604.0 Orchitis, epididymitis, and epididymo-orchitis, with abscess — (Use additional code to identify organism: 041.0, 041.1, 041.4) ♂
608.82 Hematospermia ♂
608.83 Specified vascular disorder of male genital organs ♂
922.4 Contusion of genital organs
998.12 Hematoma complicating a procedure

ICD-9-CM Procedural

61.0 Incision and drainage of scrotum and tunica vaginalis
62.0 Incision of testis

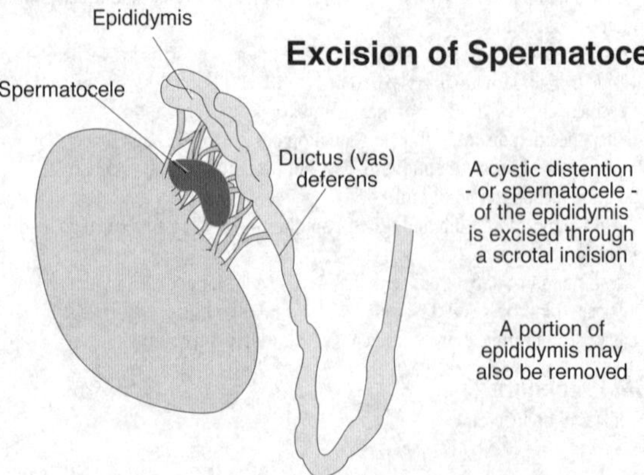
Excision of Spermatocele
Epididymis
Spermatocele
Ductus (vas) deferens
A cystic distention - or spermatocele - of the epididymis is excised through a scrotal incision
A portion of epididymis may also be removed

▽ Unspecified code
♀ Female diagnosis
☒ Manifestation code
♂ Male diagnosis

HCPCS Level II Supplies & Services

A4550 Surgical trays

54800–54820

54800 Biopsy of epididymis, needle
54820 Exploration of epididymis, with or without biopsy

ICD-9-CM Diagnostic

187.5 Malignant neoplasm of epididymis ♂
198.82 Secondary malignant neoplasm of genital organs
222.3 Benign neoplasm of epididymis ♂
233.6 Carcinoma in situ of other and unspecified male genital organs ▽ ♂
236.6 Neoplasm of uncertain behavior of other and unspecified male genital organs ▽ ♂
239.5 Neoplasm of unspecified nature of other genitourinary organs
604.90 Unspecified orchitis and epididymitis — (Use additional code to identify organism: 041.0, 041.1, 041.4) ▽ ♂
604.91 Orchitis and epididymitis in disease classified elsewhere — (Code first underlying disease: 032.89, 095.8, 125.0-125.9. Use additional code to identify organism: 041.0, 041.1, 041.4) ☒ ♂

ICD-9-CM Procedural

63.01 Biopsy of spermatic cord, epididymis, or vas deferens
63.92 Epididymotomy

HCPCS Level II Supplies & Services

A4550 Surgical trays

54830

54830 Excision of local lesion of epididymis

ICD-9-CM Diagnostic

187.5 Malignant neoplasm of epididymis ♂
198.82 Secondary malignant neoplasm of genital organs
222.3 Benign neoplasm of epididymis ♂
233.6 Carcinoma in situ of other and unspecified male genital organs ▽ ♂
236.6 Neoplasm of uncertain behavior of other and unspecified male genital organs ▽ ♂
239.5 Neoplasm of unspecified nature of other genitourinary organs
608.89 Other specified disorder of male genital organs ♂

ICD-9-CM Procedural

63.2 Excision of cyst of epididymis
63.3 Excision of other lesion or tissue of spermatic cord and epididymis

HCPCS Level II Supplies & Services

A4550 Surgical trays

54840

54840 Excision of spermatocele, with or without epididymectomy

ICD-9-CM Diagnostic

608.1 Spermatocele ♂

ICD-9-CM Procedural

63.3 Excision of other lesion or tissue of spermatic cord and epididymis
63.4 Epididymectomy

54860–54861

54860 Epididymectomy; unilateral
54861 bilateral

ICD-9-CM Diagnostic

187.5 Malignant neoplasm of epididymis ♂
198.82 Secondary malignant neoplasm of genital organs
214.8 Lipoma of other specified sites
222.3 Benign neoplasm of epididymis ♂
233.6 Carcinoma in situ of other and unspecified male genital organs ▽ ♂
236.6 Neoplasm of uncertain behavior of other and unspecified male genital organs ▽ ♂
239.5 Neoplasm of unspecified nature of other genitourinary organs
604.90 Unspecified orchitis and epididymitis — (Use additional code to identify organism: 041.0, 041.1, 041.4) ▽ ♂
604.91 Orchitis and epididymitis in disease classified elsewhere — (Code first underlying disease: 032.89, 095.8, 125.0-125.9. Use additional code to identify organism: 041.0, 041.1, 041.4) ☒ ♂
604.99 Other orchitis, epididymitis, and epididymo-orchitis, without mention of abscess — (Use additional code to identify organism: 041.0, 041.1, 041.4) ♂
608.81 Specified disorder of male genital organs in diseases classified elsewhere — (Code first underlying disease: 016.5, 125.0-125.9) ☒ ♂
608.89 Other specified disorder of male genital organs ♂

ICD-9-CM Procedural

63.4 Epididymectomy

54900–54901

54900 Epididymovasostomy, anastomosis of epididymis to vas deferens; unilateral
54901 bilateral

ICD-9-CM Diagnostic

606.0 Azoospermia ♂
606.1 Oligospermia ♂
606.8 Infertility due to extratesticular causes ♂
752.9 Unspecified congenital anomaly of genital organs ▽

ICD-9-CM Procedural

63.83 Epididymovasostomy

Tunica Vaginalis

55000

55000 Puncture aspiration of hydrocele, tunica vaginalis, with or without injection of medication

ICD-9-CM Diagnostic

603.0 Encysted hydrocele
603.1 Infected hydrocele — (Use additional code to identify organism)
603.8 Other specified type of hydrocele
603.9 Unspecified hydrocele ▽
608.84 Chylocele of tunica vaginalis ♂
778.6 Congenital hydrocele

ICD-9-CM Procedural

61.91 Percutaneous aspiration of tunica vaginalis

HCPCS Level II Supplies & Services

A4550 Surgical trays

55040–55041

55040 Excision of hydrocele; unilateral
55041 bilateral

ICD-9-CM Diagnostic

603.0 Encysted hydrocele
603.1 Infected hydrocele — (Use additional code to identify organism)
603.8 Other specified type of hydrocele
603.9 Unspecified hydrocele ▽
778.6 Congenital hydrocele

ICD-9-CM Procedural

61.2 Excision of hydrocele (of tunica vaginalis)

55060

55060 Repair of tunica vaginalis hydrocele (Bottle type)

ICD-9-CM Diagnostic

603.0 Encysted hydrocele
603.1 Infected hydrocele — (Use additional code to identify organism)
603.8 Other specified type of hydrocele
603.9 Unspecified hydrocele ▽
608.84 Chylocele of tunica vaginalis ♂
778.6 Congenital hydrocele

ICD-9-CM Procedural

61.2 Excision of hydrocele (of tunica vaginalis)

Scrotum

55100

55100 Drainage of scrotal wall abscess

ICD-9-CM Diagnostic

608.4 Other inflammatory disorder of male genital organs — (Use additional code to identify organism) ♂

ICD-9-CM Procedural

61.0 Incision and drainage of scrotum and tunica vaginalis

HCPCS Level II Supplies & Services

A4550 Surgical trays

55110

55110 Scrotal exploration

ICD-9-CM Diagnostic

187.7 Malignant neoplasm of scrotum ♂
198.82 Secondary malignant neoplasm of genital organs
222.4 Benign neoplasm of scrotum ♂
233.6 Carcinoma in situ of other and unspecified male genital organs ▽ ♂
236.6 Neoplasm of uncertain behavior of other and unspecified male genital organs ▽ ♂
239.5 Neoplasm of unspecified nature of other genitourinary organs
257.2 Other testicular hypofunction ♂
456.4 Scrotal varices ♂
604.0 Orchitis, epididymitis, and epididymo-orchitis, with abscess — (Use additional code to identify organism: 041.0, 041.1, 041.4) ♂
604.91 Orchitis and epididymitis in disease classified elsewhere — (Code first underlying disease: 032.89, 095.8, 125.0-125.9. Use additional code to identify organism: 041.0, 041.1, 041.4) ☒ ♂
604.99 Other orchitis, epididymitis, and epididymo-orchitis, without mention of abscess — (Use additional code to identify organism: 041.0, 041.1, 041.4) ♂
608.2 Torsion of testis ♂
608.4 Other inflammatory disorder of male genital organs — (Use additional code to identify organism) ♂
608.81 Specified disorder of male genital organs in diseases classified elsewhere — (Code first underlying disease: 016.5, 125.0-125.9) ☒ ♂
608.82 Hematospermia ♂
608.83 Specified vascular disorder of male genital organs ♂
608.84 Chylocele of tunica vaginalis ♂
608.85 Stricture of male genital organs ♂
608.89 Other specified disorder of male genital organs ♂
752.81 Scrotal transposition
752.89 Other specified anomalies of genital organs
996.39 Mechanical complication of genitourinary device, implant, and graft, other
996.65 Infection and inflammatory reaction due to other genitourinary device, implant, and graft — (Use additional code to identify specified infections)
996.76 Other complications due to genitourinary device, implant, and graft
998.2 Accidental puncture or laceration during procedure
998.51 Infected postoperative seroma — (Use additional code to identify organism)
998.59 Other postoperative infection — (Use additional code to identify infection)
998.89 Other specified complications

ICD-9-CM Procedural

61.0 Incision and drainage of scrotum and tunica vaginalis

HCPCS Level II Supplies & Services

A4550 Surgical trays

55120

55120 Removal of foreign body in scrotum

ICD-9-CM Diagnostic

709.4 Foreign body granuloma of skin and subcutaneous tissue
729.6 Residual foreign body in soft tissue
878.2 Open wound of scrotum and testes, without mention of complication — (Use additional code to identify infection) ♂
878.3 Open wound of scrotum and testes, complicated — (Use additional code to identify infection) ♂
911.6 Trunk, superficial foreign body (splinter), without major open wound and without mention of infection
911.7 Trunk, superficial foreign body (splinter), without major open wound, infected
998.4 Foreign body accidentally left during procedure, not elsewhere classified

ICD-9-CM Procedural

61.0 Incision and drainage of scrotum and tunica vaginalis
98.24 Removal of foreign body from scrotum or penis without incision

HCPCS Level II Supplies & Services

A4550 Surgical trays

55150

55150 Resection of scrotum

ICD-9-CM Diagnostic

187.7 Malignant neoplasm of scrotum ♂
198.82 Secondary malignant neoplasm of genital organs
222.4 Benign neoplasm of scrotum ♂
233.6 Carcinoma in situ of other and unspecified male genital organs ▽ ♂
236.6 Neoplasm of uncertain behavior of other and unspecified male genital organs ▽ ♂
239.5 Neoplasm of unspecified nature of other genitourinary organs
608.89 Other specified disorder of male genital organs ♂
878.2 Open wound of scrotum and testes, without mention of complication — (Use additional code to identify infection) ♂
878.3 Open wound of scrotum and testes, complicated — (Use additional code to identify infection) ♂

ICD-9-CM Procedural

61.3 Excision or destruction of lesion or tissue of scrotum

55175–55180

55175 Scrotoplasty; simple
55180 complicated

ICD-9-CM Diagnostic

187.7 Malignant neoplasm of scrotum ♂
198.82 Secondary malignant neoplasm of genital organs
222.4 Benign neoplasm of scrotum ♂
233.6 Carcinoma in situ of other and unspecified male genital organs ▽ ♂
236.6 Neoplasm of uncertain behavior of other and unspecified male genital organs ▽ ♂
239.5 Neoplasm of unspecified nature of other genitourinary organs
608.89 Other specified disorder of male genital organs ♂
878.2 Open wound of scrotum and testes, without mention of complication — (Use additional code to identify infection) ♂
878.3 Open wound of scrotum and testes, complicated — (Use additional code to identify infection) ♂

ICD-9-CM Procedural

61.49 Other repair of scrotum and tunica vaginalis

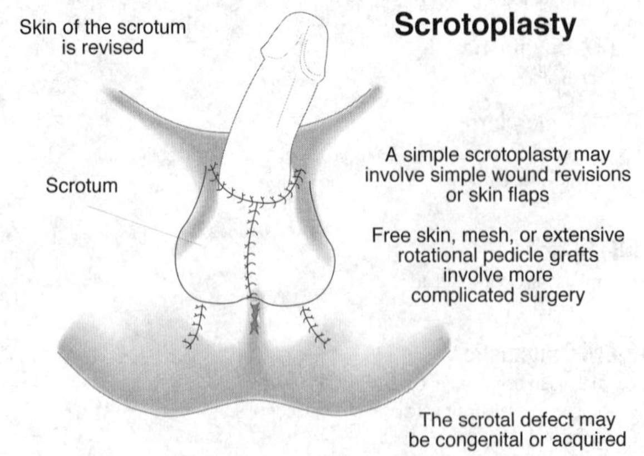
Skin of the scrotum is revised
Scrotoplasty
A simple scrotoplasty may involve simple wound revisions or skin flaps
Scrotum
Free skin, mesh, or extensive rotational pedicle grafts involve more complicated surgery
The scrotal defect may be congenital or acquired

▽ Unspecified code ♀ Female diagnosis ☒ Manifestation code ♂ Male diagnosis

Vas Deferens

55200

55200 Vasotomy, cannulization with or without incision of vas, unilateral or bilateral (separate procedure)

ICD-9-CM Diagnostic

302.72 Psychosexual dysfunction with inhibited sexual excitement
606.0 Azoospermia ♂
606.1 Oligospermia ♂
606.8 Infertility due to extratesticular causes ♂
607.84 Impotence of organic origin ♂
608.4 Other inflammatory disorder of male genital organs — (Use additional code to identify organism) ♂
608.81 Specified disorder of male genital organs in diseases classified elsewhere — (Code first underlying disease: 016.5, 125.0-125.9) ☒ ♂
608.82 Hematospermia ♂
608.83 Specified vascular disorder of male genital organs ♂
608.85 Stricture of male genital organs ♂
608.89 Other specified disorder of male genital organs ♂
V26.21 Fertility testing
V26.22 Aftercare following sterilization reversal
V26.29 Other investigation and testing

ICD-9-CM Procedural

63.6 Vasotomy

HCPCS Level II Supplies & Services

A4550 Surgical trays

55250

55250 Vasectomy, unilateral or bilateral (separate procedure), including postoperative semen examination(s)

ICD-9-CM Diagnostic

V25.2 Sterilization

ICD-9-CM Procedural

63.73 Vasectomy

HCPCS Level II Supplies & Services

A4550 Surgical trays

55300

55300 Vasotomy for vasograms, seminal vesiculograms, or epididymograms, unilateral or bilateral

ICD-9-CM Diagnostic

187.6 Malignant neoplasm of spermatic cord ♂
198.82 Secondary malignant neoplasm of genital organs
222.8 Benign neoplasm of other specified sites of male genital organs ♂
233.6 Carcinoma in situ of other and unspecified male genital organs ▽ ♂
302.72 Psychosexual dysfunction with inhibited sexual excitement
606.0 Azoospermia ♂
606.1 Oligospermia ♂
606.8 Infertility due to extratesticular causes ♂
607.84 Impotence of organic origin ♂
608.4 Other inflammatory disorder of male genital organs — (Use additional code to identify organism) ♂
608.81 Specified disorder of male genital organs in diseases classified elsewhere — (Code first underlying disease: 016.5, 125.0-125.9) ☒ ♂
608.82 Hematospermia ♂
608.83 Specified vascular disorder of male genital organs ♂
608.85 Stricture of male genital organs ♂
608.89 Other specified disorder of male genital organs ♂
V26.21 Fertility testing
V26.22 Aftercare following sterilization reversal
V26.29 Other investigation and testing

ICD-9-CM Procedural

63.6 Vasotomy
87.91 Contrast seminal vesiculogram
87.92 Other x-ray of prostate and seminal vesicles
87.93 Contrast epididymogram

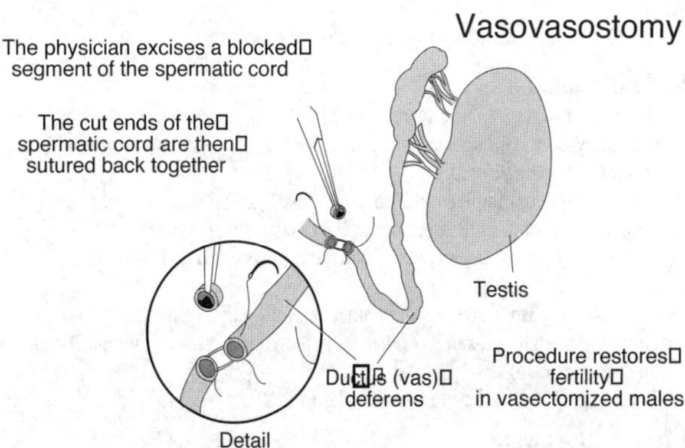
Vasovasostomy
The physician excises a blocked segment of the spermatic cord
The cut ends of the spermatic cord are then sutured back together
Testis
Ductus (vas) deferens
Procedure restores fertility in vasectomized males
Detail

87.94 Contrast vasogram
87.95 Other x-ray of epididymis and vas deferens

HCPCS Level II Supplies & Services

A4550 Surgical trays
A9525 Supply of low or iso-osmolar contrast material, 10 mg of iodine

55400

55400 Vasovasostomy, vasovasorrhaphy

ICD-9-CM Diagnostic

V26.0 Tuboplasty or vasoplasty after previous sterilization
V26.52 Vasectomy sterilization status ♂

ICD-9-CM Procedural

63.81 Suture of laceration of vas deferens and epididymis
63.82 Reconstruction of surgically divided vas deferens
63.89 Other repair of vas deferens and epididymis

55450

55450 Ligation (percutaneous) of vas deferens, unilateral or bilateral (separate procedure)

ICD-9-CM Diagnostic

V25.2 Sterilization

ICD-9-CM Procedural

63.71 Ligation of vas deferens

HCPCS Level II Supplies & Services

A4550 Surgical trays

Spermatic Cord

55500

55500 Excision of hydrocele of spermatic cord, unilateral (separate procedure)

ICD-9-CM Diagnostic

603.0 Encysted hydrocele
603.1 Infected hydrocele — (Use additional code to identify organism)
603.8 Other specified type of hydrocele
603.9 Unspecified hydrocele ▽
778.6 Congenital hydrocele

ICD-9-CM Procedural

63.1 Excision of varicocele and hydrocele of spermatic cord

HCPCS Level II Supplies & Services

A4305 Disposable drug delivery system, flow rate of 50 ml or greater per hour
A4306 Disposable drug delivery system, flow rate of 5 ml or less per hour
A4550 Surgical trays

55520

55520 Excision of lesion of spermatic cord (separate procedure)

ICD-9-CM Diagnostic

187.6 Malignant neoplasm of spermatic cord ♂
198.82 Secondary malignant neoplasm of genital organs
214.4 Lipoma of spermatic cord ♂
222.8 Benign neoplasm of other specified sites of male genital organs ♂
233.6 Carcinoma in situ of other and unspecified male genital organs ▽ ♂
236.6 Neoplasm of uncertain behavior of other and unspecified male genital organs ▽ ♂
239.5 Neoplasm of unspecified nature of other genitourinary organs
608.4 Other inflammatory disorder of male genital organs — (Use additional code to identify organism) ♂
608.89 Other specified disorder of male genital organs ♂

ICD-9-CM Procedural

63.3 Excision of other lesion or tissue of spermatic cord and epididymis

HCPCS Level II Supplies & Services

A4305 Disposable drug delivery system, flow rate of 50 ml or greater per hour
A4306 Disposable drug delivery system, flow rate of 5 ml or less per hour
A4550 Surgical trays

55530–55535

55530 Excision of varicocele or ligation of spermatic veins for varicocele; (separate procedure)
55535 abdominal approach

ICD-9-CM Diagnostic

456.4 Scrotal varices ♂
V64.41 Laparoscopic surgical procedure converted to open procedure

ICD-9-CM Procedural

63.1 Excision of varicocele and hydrocele of spermatic cord
63.72 Ligation of spermatic cord

55540

55540 Excision of varicocele or ligation of spermatic veins for varicocele; with hernia repair

ICD-9-CM Diagnostic

456.4 Scrotal varices ♂
V64.41 Laparoscopic surgical procedure converted to open procedure

ICD-9-CM Procedural

53.01 Unilateral repair of direct inguinal hernia
53.02 Unilateral repair of indirect inguinal hernia
53.03 Unilateral repair of direct inguinal hernia with graft or prosthesis
63.1 Excision of varicocele and hydrocele of spermatic cord
63.72 Ligation of spermatic cord

55550

55550 Laparoscopy, surgical, with ligation of spermatic veins for varicocele

ICD-9-CM Diagnostic

456.4 Scrotal varices ♂
606.8 Infertility due to extratesticular causes ♂

ICD-9-CM Procedural

63.1 Excision of varicocele and hydrocele of spermatic cord

Seminal Vesicles

55600–55605

55600 Vesiculotomy;
55605 complicated

ICD-9-CM Diagnostic

187.8 Malignant neoplasm of other specified sites of male genital organs ♂
198.82 Secondary malignant neoplasm of genital organs
222.8 Benign neoplasm of other specified sites of male genital organs ♂
233.6 Carcinoma in situ of other and unspecified male genital organs ▽ ♂
236.6 Neoplasm of uncertain behavior of other and unspecified male genital organs ▽ ♂
239.5 Neoplasm of unspecified nature of other genitourinary organs
608.0 Seminal vesiculitis — (Use additional code to identify organism) ♂
608.82 Hematospermia ♂
608.83 Specified vascular disorder of male genital organs ♂
608.85 Stricture of male genital organs ♂
608.89 Other specified disorder of male genital organs ♂

ICD-9-CM Procedural

60.72 Incision of seminal vesicle

55650

55650 Vesiculectomy, any approach

ICD-9-CM Diagnostic

187.8 Malignant neoplasm of other specified sites of male genital organs ♂
198.82 Secondary malignant neoplasm of genital organs
222.8 Benign neoplasm of other specified sites of male genital organs ♂
233.6 Carcinoma in situ of other and unspecified male genital organs ▽ ♂
236.6 Neoplasm of uncertain behavior of other and unspecified male genital organs ▽ ♂
239.5 Neoplasm of unspecified nature of other genitourinary organs
608.0 Seminal vesiculitis — (Use additional code to identify organism) ♂
608.83 Specified vascular disorder of male genital organs ♂
608.85 Stricture of male genital organs ♂
608.89 Other specified disorder of male genital organs ♂

ICD-9-CM Procedural

60.73 Excision of seminal vesicle

55680

55680 Excision of Mullerian duct cyst

ICD-9-CM Diagnostic

752.89 Other specified anomalies of genital organs

ICD-9-CM Procedural

60.73 Excision of seminal vesicle

Prostate

55700–55705

55700 Biopsy, prostate; needle or punch, single or multiple, any approach
55705 incisional, any approach

ICD-9-CM Diagnostic

185 Malignant neoplasm of prostate ♂
198.82 Secondary malignant neoplasm of genital organs
222.2 Benign neoplasm of prostate ♂
233.4 Carcinoma in situ of prostate ♂
236.5 Neoplasm of uncertain behavior of prostate ♂
239.5 Neoplasm of unspecified nature of other genitourinary organs
600.00 Hypertrophy (benign) of prostate without urinary obstruction — (Use additional code to identify urinary incontinence: 788.30-788.39) ♂
600.01 Hypertrophy (benign) of prostate with urinary obstruction — (Use additional code to identify urinary incontinence: 788.30-788.39) ♂
600.10 Nodular prostate without urinary obstruction — (Use additional code to identify urinary incontinence: 788.30-788.39) ♂
600.11 Nodular prostate with urinary obstruction — (Use additional code to identify urinary incontinence: 788.30-788.39) ♂
600.20 Benign localized hyperplasia of prostate without urinary obstruction — (Use additional code to identify urinary incontinence: 788.30-788.39) ♂
600.21 Benign localized hyperplasia of prostate with urinary obstruction — (Use additional code to identify urinary incontinence: 788.30-788.39) ♂
600.3 Cyst of prostate — (Use additional code to identify urinary incontinence: 788.30-788.39) ♂
600.90 Hyperplasia of prostate, unspecified, without urinary obstruction — (Use additional code to identify urinary incontinence: 788.30-788.39) ▽ ♂
600.91 Hyperplasia of prostate, unspecified, with urinary obstruction — (Use additional code to identify urinary incontinence: 788.30-788.39) ▽ ♂

601.0 Acute prostatitis — (Use additional code to identify organism: 041.0, 041.1) ♂
601.1 Chronic prostatitis — (Use additional code to identify organism: 041.0, 041.1) ♂
601.2 Abscess of prostate — (Use additional code to identify organism: 041.0, 041.1) ♂
601.3 Prostatocystitis — (Use additional code to identify organism: 041.0, 041.1) ♂
601.4 Prostatitis in diseases classified elsewhere — (Code first underlying disease: 016.5, 039.8, 095.8, 116.0. Use additional code to identify organism: 041.0, 041.1) ⊠ ♂
601.8 Other specified inflammatory disease of prostate — (Use additional code to identify organism: 041.0, 041.1) ♂
602.0 Calculus of prostate ♂
602.1 Congestion or hemorrhage of prostate ♂
602.2 Atrophy of prostate ♂
602.3 Dysplasia of prostate ♂
602.8 Other specified disorder of prostate ♂
788.29 Other specified retention of urine
788.41 Urinary frequency
788.42 Polyuria
788.43 Nocturia
790.93 Elevated prostate specific antigen (PSA) ♂
793.5 Nonspecific abnormal findings on radiological and other examination of genitourinary organs
V10.46 Personal history of malignant neoplasm of prostate ♂
V71.1 Observation for suspected malignant neoplasm

ICD-9-CM Procedural

60.11 Closed (percutaneous) (needle) biopsy of prostate
60.12 Open biopsy of prostate
60.91 Percutaneous aspiration of prostate

HCPCS Level II Supplies & Services

A4550 Surgical trays

55720–55725

55720 Prostatotomy, external drainage of prostatic abscess, any approach; simple
55725 complicated

ICD-9-CM Diagnostic

098.12 Gonococcal prostatitis (acute) ♂
098.32 Gonococcal prostatitis, chronic ♂
601.2 Abscess of prostate — (Use additional code to identify organism: 041.0, 041.1) ♂

ICD-9-CM Procedural

60.0 Incision of prostate
60.81 Incision of periprostatic tissue

HCPCS Level II Supplies & Services

A4305 Disposable drug delivery system, flow rate of 50 ml or greater per hour
A4306 Disposable drug delivery system, flow rate of 5 ml or less per hour
A4550 Surgical trays

55801

55801 Prostatectomy, perineal, subtotal (including control of postoperative bleeding, vasectomy, meatotomy, urethral calibration and/or dilation, and internal urethrotomy)

Perineal Prostatectomy

Internal and external iliac nodes
Common iliac nodes
Superficial inguinal nodes
Obturator node
Prostate

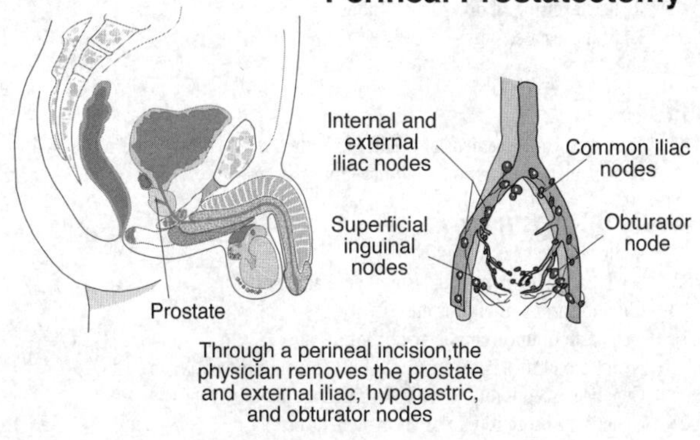

Through a perineal incision, the physician removes the prostate and external iliac, hypogastric, and obturator nodes

ICD-9-CM Diagnostic

185 Malignant neoplasm of prostate ♂
198.82 Secondary malignant neoplasm of genital organs
222.2 Benign neoplasm of prostate ♂
233.4 Carcinoma in situ of prostate ♂
236.5 Neoplasm of uncertain behavior of prostate ♂
239.5 Neoplasm of unspecified nature of other genitourinary organs
600.00 Hypertrophy (benign) of prostate without urinary obstruction — (Use additional code to identify urinary incontinence: 788.30-788.39) ♂
600.01 Hypertrophy (benign) of prostate with urinary obstruction — (Use additional code to identify urinary incontinence: 788.30-788.39) ♂
600.10 Nodular prostate without urinary obstruction — (Use additional code to identify urinary incontinence: 788.30-788.39) ♂
600.11 Nodular prostate with urinary obstruction — (Use additional code to identify urinary incontinence: 788.30-788.39) ♂
600.20 Benign localized hyperplasia of prostate without urinary obstruction — (Use additional code to identify urinary incontinence: 788.30-788.39) ♂
600.21 Benign localized hyperplasia of prostate with urinary obstruction — (Use additional code to identify urinary incontinence: 788.30-788.39) ♂
600.3 Cyst of prostate — (Use additional code to identify urinary incontinence: 788.30-788.39) ♂
600.90 Hyperplasia of prostate, unspecified, without urinary obstruction — (Use additional code to identify urinary incontinence: 788.30-788.39) ▽ ♂
600.91 Hyperplasia of prostate, unspecified, with urinary obstruction — (Use additional code to identify urinary incontinence: 788.30-788.39) ▽ ♂
601.0 Acute prostatitis — (Use additional code to identify organism: 041.0, 041.1) ♂
601.1 Chronic prostatitis — (Use additional code to identify organism: 041.0, 041.1) ♂
601.2 Abscess of prostate — (Use additional code to identify organism: 041.0, 041.1) ♂
601.3 Prostatocystitis — (Use additional code to identify organism: 041.0, 041.1) ♂
601.4 Prostatitis in diseases classified elsewhere — (Code first underlying disease: 016.5, 039.8, 095.8, 116.0. Use additional code to identify organism: 041.0, 041.1) ⊠ ♂
601.8 Other specified inflammatory disease of prostate — (Use additional code to identify organism: 041.0, 041.1) ♂
602.0 Calculus of prostate ♂
602.2 Atrophy of prostate ♂
602.3 Dysplasia of prostate ♂
602.8 Other specified disorder of prostate ♂
V84.03 Genetic susceptibility to malignant neoplasm of prostate
v84.09 Genetic susceptibility to other malignant neoplasm

ICD-9-CM Procedural

60.62 Perineal prostatectomy
60.82 Excision of periprostatic tissue

55810–55812

55810 Prostatectomy, perineal radical;
55812 with lymph node biopsy(s) (limited pelvic lymphadenectomy)

ICD-9-CM Diagnostic

185 Malignant neoplasm of prostate ♂
196.6 Secondary and unspecified malignant neoplasm of intrapelvic lymph nodes
198.82 Secondary malignant neoplasm of genital organs
233.4 Carcinoma in situ of prostate ♂
236.5 Neoplasm of uncertain behavior of prostate ♂
239.5 Neoplasm of unspecified nature of other genitourinary organs
601.0 Acute prostatitis — (Use additional code to identify organism: 041.0, 041.1) ♂
601.1 Chronic prostatitis — (Use additional code to identify organism: 041.0, 041.1) ♂
601.2 Abscess of prostate — (Use additional code to identify organism: 041.0, 041.1) ♂
601.3 Prostatocystitis — (Use additional code to identify organism: 041.0, 041.1) ♂
601.4 Prostatitis in diseases classified elsewhere — (Code first underlying disease: 016.5, 039.8, 095.8, 116.0. Use additional code to identify organism: 041.0, 041.1) ⊠ ♂
601.8 Other specified inflammatory disease of prostate — (Use additional code to identify organism: 041.0, 041.1) ♂
602.0 Calculus of prostate ♂
602.2 Atrophy of prostate ♂
602.3 Dysplasia of prostate ♂
602.8 Other specified disorder of prostate ♂
V84.03 Genetic susceptibility to malignant neoplasm of prostate
V84.09 Genetic susceptibility to other malignant neoplasm

ICD-9-CM Procedural

40.11 Biopsy of lymphatic structure
40.3 Regional lymph node excision
60.5 Radical prostatectomy

55815

55815 Prostatectomy, perineal radical; with bilateral pelvic lymphadenectomy, including external iliac, hypogastric and obturator nodes

ICD-9-CM Diagnostic

185 Malignant neoplasm of prostate ♂
196.6 Secondary and unspecified malignant neoplasm of intrapelvic lymph nodes
198.82 Secondary malignant neoplasm of genital organs
233.4 Carcinoma in situ of prostate ♂
236.5 Neoplasm of uncertain behavior of prostate ♂
239.5 Neoplasm of unspecified nature of other genitourinary organs
601.0 Acute prostatitis — (Use additional code to identify organism: 041.0, 041.1) ♂
601.1 Chronic prostatitis — (Use additional code to identify organism: 041.0, 041.1) ♂
601.2 Abscess of prostate — (Use additional code to identify organism: 041.0, 041.1) ♂
601.3 Prostatocystitis — (Use additional code to identify organism: 041.0, 041.1) ♂
601.4 Prostatitis in diseases classified elsewhere — (Code first underlying disease: 016.5, 039.8, 095.8, 116.0. Use additional code to identify organism: 041.0, 041.1) ☒ ♂
601.8 Other specified inflammatory disease of prostate — (Use additional code to identify organism: 041.0, 041.1) ♂
602.0 Calculus of prostate ♂
602.2 Atrophy of prostate ♂
602.3 Dysplasia of prostate ♂
602.8 Other specified disorder of prostate ♂
V84.03 Genetic susceptibility to malignant neoplasm of prostate
V84.09 Genetic susceptibility to other malignant neoplasm

ICD-9-CM Procedural

40.53 Radical excision of iliac lymph nodes
40.59 Radical excision of other lymph nodes
60.5 Radical prostatectomy

55821–55831

55821 Prostatectomy (including control of postoperative bleeding, vasectomy, meatotomy, urethral calibration and/or dilation, and internal urethrotomy); suprapubic, subtotal, one or two stages
55831 retropubic, subtotal

ICD-9-CM Diagnostic

185 Malignant neoplasm of prostate ♂
198.82 Secondary malignant neoplasm of genital organs
222.2 Benign neoplasm of prostate ♂
233.4 Carcinoma in situ of prostate ♂
236.5 Neoplasm of uncertain behavior of prostate ♂
239.5 Neoplasm of unspecified nature of other genitourinary organs
600.00 Hypertrophy (benign) of prostate without urinary obstruction — (Use additional code to identify urinary incontinence: 788.30-788.39) ♂
600.01 Hypertrophy (benign) of prostate with urinary obstruction — (Use additional code to identify urinary incontinence: 788.30-788.39) ♂
600.10 Nodular prostate without urinary obstruction — (Use additional code to identify urinary incontinence: 788.30-788.39) ♂
600.11 Nodular prostate with urinary obstruction — (Use additional code to identify urinary incontinence: 788.30-788.39) ♂
600.20 Benign localized hyperplasia of prostate without urinary obstruction — (Use additional code to identify urinary incontinence: 788.30-788.39) ♂
600.21 Benign localized hyperplasia of prostate with urinary obstruction — (Use additional code to identify urinary incontinence: 788.30-788.39) ♂
600.3 Cyst of prostate — (Use additional code to identify urinary incontinence: 788.30-788.39) ♂
600.90 Hyperplasia of prostate, unspecified, without urinary obstruction — (Use additional code to identify urinary incontinence: 788.30-788.39) ▽ ♂
600.91 Hyperplasia of prostate, unspecified, with urinary obstruction — (Use additional code to identify urinary incontinence: 788.30-788.39) ▽ ♂
601.0 Acute prostatitis — (Use additional code to identify organism: 041.0, 041.1) ♂
601.1 Chronic prostatitis — (Use additional code to identify organism: 041.0, 041.1) ♂
601.2 Abscess of prostate — (Use additional code to identify organism: 041.0, 041.1) ♂
601.3 Prostatocystitis — (Use additional code to identify organism: 041.0, 041.1) ♂
601.4 Prostatitis in diseases classified elsewhere — (Code first underlying disease: 016.5, 039.8, 095.8, 116.0. Use additional code to identify organism: 041.0, 041.1) ☒ ♂
601.8 Other specified inflammatory disease of prostate — (Use additional code to identify organism: 041.0, 041.1) ♂
602.0 Calculus of prostate ♂
602.2 Atrophy of prostate ♂
602.3 Dysplasia of prostate ♂
602.8 Other specified disorder of prostate ♂
788.20 Unspecified retention of urine ▽
788.21 Incomplete bladder emptying
788.29 Other specified retention of urine
V84.03 Genetic susceptibility to malignant neoplasm of prostate
V84.09 Genetic susceptibility to other malignant neoplasm

ICD-9-CM Procedural

60.3 Suprapubic prostatectomy
60.4 Retropubic prostatectomy

55840–55842

55840 Prostatectomy, retropubic radical, with or without nerve sparing;
55842 with lymph node biopsy(s) (limited pelvic lymphadenectomy)

ICD-9-CM Diagnostic

185 Malignant neoplasm of prostate ♂
196.6 Secondary and unspecified malignant neoplasm of intrapelvic lymph nodes
198.82 Secondary malignant neoplasm of genital organs
233.4 Carcinoma in situ of prostate ♂
236.5 Neoplasm of uncertain behavior of prostate ♂
239.5 Neoplasm of unspecified nature of other genitourinary organs
V64.41 Laparoscopic surgical procedure converted to open procedure
V84.03 Genetic susceptibility to malignant neoplasm of prostate
V84.09 Genetic susceptibility to other malignant neoplasm

ICD-9-CM Procedural

40.11 Biopsy of lymphatic structure
40.3 Regional lymph node excision
60.5 Radical prostatectomy

55845

55845 Prostatectomy, retropubic radical, with or without nerve sparing; with bilateral pelvic lymphadenectomy, including external iliac, hypogastric, and obturator nodes

ICD-9-CM Diagnostic

185 Malignant neoplasm of prostate ♂
196.6 Secondary and unspecified malignant neoplasm of intrapelvic lymph nodes
198.82 Secondary malignant neoplasm of genital organs
233.4 Carcinoma in situ of prostate ♂
236.5 Neoplasm of uncertain behavior of prostate ♂
239.5 Neoplasm of unspecified nature of other genitourinary organs
V64.41 Laparoscopic surgical procedure converted to open procedure
V84.03 Genetic susceptibility to malignant neoplasm of prostate
V84.09 Genetic susceptibility to other malignant neoplasm

ICD-9-CM Procedural

40.3 Regional lymph node excision
40.53 Radical excision of iliac lymph nodes
40.59 Radical excision of other lymph nodes
60.5 Radical prostatectomy

55859

55859 Transperineal placement of needles or catheters into prostate for interstitial radioelement application, with or without cystoscopy

ICD-9-CM Diagnostic

185 Malignant neoplasm of prostate ♂
198.82 Secondary malignant neoplasm of genital organs
233.4 Carcinoma in situ of prostate ♂
236.5 Neoplasm of uncertain behavior of prostate ♂
239.5 Neoplasm of unspecified nature of other genitourinary organs
V84.03 Genetic susceptibility to malignant neoplasm of prostate
V84.09 Genetic susceptibility to other malignant neoplasm

▽ Unspecified code
♀ Female diagnosis
☒ Manifestation code
♂ Male diagnosis

ICD-9-CM Procedural

60.99 Other operations on prostate
92.27 Implantation or insertion of radioactive elements

55860–55865

55860 Exposure of prostate, any approach, for insertion of radioactive substance;
55862 with lymph node biopsy(s) (limited pelvic lymphadenectomy)
55865 with bilateral pelvic lymphadenectomy, including external iliac, hypogastric and obturator nodes

ICD-9-CM Diagnostic

185 Malignant neoplasm of prostate ♂
196.6 Secondary and unspecified malignant neoplasm of intrapelvic lymph nodes
198.82 Secondary malignant neoplasm of genital organs
233.4 Carcinoma in situ of prostate ♂
236.5 Neoplasm of uncertain behavior of prostate ♂
239.5 Neoplasm of unspecified nature of other genitourinary organs
V84.03 Genetic susceptibility to malignant neoplasm of prostate
V84.09 Genetic susceptibility to other malignant neoplasm

ICD-9-CM Procedural

40.11 Biopsy of lymphatic structure
40.3 Regional lymph node excision
40.53 Radical excision of iliac lymph nodes
60.0 Incision of prostate

55866

55866 Laparoscopy, surgical prostatectomy, retropubic radical, including nerve sparing

ICD-9-CM Diagnostic

185 Malignant neoplasm of prostate ♂
196.6 Secondary and unspecified malignant neoplasm of intrapelvic lymph nodes
198.82 Secondary malignant neoplasm of genital organs
233.4 Carcinoma in situ of prostate ♂
236.5 Neoplasm of uncertain behavior of prostate ♂
239.5 Neoplasm of unspecified nature of other genitourinary organs
V84.03 Genetic susceptibility to malignant neoplasm of prostate
V84.09 Genetic susceptibility to other malignant neoplasm

ICD-9-CM Procedural

60.5 Radical prostatectomy

HCPCS Level II Supplies & Services

HCPCS Level II codes are used to report the supplies, durable medical equipment, and certain medical services provided on an outpatient basis. Because the procedure(s) represented on this page would be performed in an inpatient facility, no HCPCS Level II codes apply.

55870

55870 Electroejaculation

ICD-9-CM Diagnostic

302.72 Psychosexual dysfunction with inhibited sexual excitement
344.00 Unspecified quadriplegia ▽
344.01 Quadriplegia and quadriparesis, C1-C4, complete
344.02 Quadriplegia and quadriparesis, C1-C4, incomplete
344.03 Quadriplegia and quadriparesis, C5-C7, complete
344.04 C5-C7, incomplete
344.09 Other quadriplegia and quadriparesis
344.1 Paraplegia
607.84 Impotence of organic origin ♂
608.87 Retrograde ejaculation ♂

ICD-9-CM Procedural

99.96 Collection of sperm for artificial insemination

HCPCS Level II Supplies & Services

A4550 Surgical trays

55873

55873 Cryosurgical ablation of the prostate (includes ultrasonic guidance for interstitial cryosurgical probe placement)

ICD-9-CM Diagnostic

185 Malignant neoplasm of prostate ♂
198.82 Secondary malignant neoplasm of genital organs
222.2 Benign neoplasm of prostate ♂
233.4 Carcinoma in situ of prostate ♂
236.5 Neoplasm of uncertain behavior of prostate ♂
239.5 Neoplasm of unspecified nature of other genitourinary organs
600.00 Hypertrophy (benign) of prostate without urinary obstruction — (Use additional code to identify urinary incontinence: 788.30-788.39) ♂
600.01 Hypertrophy (benign) of prostate with urinary obstruction — (Use additional code to identify urinary incontinence: 788.30-788.39) ♂
600.10 Nodular prostate without urinary obstruction — (Use additional code to identify urinary incontinence: 788.30-788.39) ♂
600.11 Nodular prostate with urinary obstruction — (Use additional code to identify urinary incontinence: 788.30-788.39) ♂
600.20 Benign localized hyperplasia of prostate without urinary obstruction — (Use additional code to identify urinary incontinence: 788.30-788.39) ♂
600.21 Benign localized hyperplasia of prostate with urinary obstruction — (Use additional code to identify urinary incontinence: 788.30-788.39) ♂
600.3 Cyst of prostate — (Use additional code to identify urinary incontinence: 788.30-788.39) ♂
600.90 Hyperplasia of prostate, unspecified, without urinary obstruction — (Use additional code to identify urinary incontinence: 788.30-788.39) ▽ ♂
600.91 Hyperplasia of prostate, unspecified, with urinary obstruction — (Use additional code to identify urinary incontinence: 788.30-788.39) ▽ ♂
601.0 Acute prostatitis — (Use additional code to identify organism: 041.0, 041.1) ♂
601.1 Chronic prostatitis — (Use additional code to identify organism: 041.0, 041.1) ♂
601.2 Abscess of prostate — (Use additional code to identify organism: 041.0, 041.1) ♂
601.3 Prostatocystitis — (Use additional code to identify organism: 041.0, 041.1) ♂
601.4 Prostatitis in diseases classified elsewhere — (Code first underlying disease: 016.5, 039.8, 095.8, 116.0. Use additional code to identify organism: 041.0, 041.1) ☒ ♂
601.8 Other specified inflammatory disease of prostate — (Use additional code to identify organism: 041.0, 041.1) ♂
602.0 Calculus of prostate ♂
602.2 Atrophy of prostate ♂
602.3 Dysplasia of prostate ♂
602.8 Other specified disorder of prostate ♂
V84.03 Genetic susceptibility to malignant neoplasm of prostate
V84.09 Genetic susceptibility to other malignant neoplasm

ICD-9-CM Procedural

60.62 Perineal prostatectomy

▽ Unspecified code
♀ Female diagnosis
☒ Manifestation code
♂ Male diagnosis

Intersex Surgery

55970

55970 Intersex surgery; male to female

ICD-9-CM Diagnostic

302.50 Trans-sexualism with unspecified sexual history ▽
302.51 Trans-sexualism with asexual history
302.52 Trans-sexualism with homosexual history
302.53 Trans-sexualism with heterosexual history
302.6 Gender identity disorder in children
302.85 Gender identity disorder in adolescents or adults
752.7 Indeterminate sex and pseudohermaphroditism
752.89 Other specified anomalies of genital organs
758.81 Other conditions due to sex chromosome anomalies

ICD-9-CM Procedural

62.41 Removal of both testes at same operative episode
64.3 Amputation of penis
64.5 Operations for sex transformation, not elsewhere classified
64.99 Other operations on male genital organs

55980

55980 Intersex surgery; female to male

ICD-9-CM Diagnostic

302.50 Trans-sexualism with unspecified sexual history ▽
302.51 Trans-sexualism with asexual history
302.52 Trans-sexualism with homosexual history
302.53 Trans-sexualism with heterosexual history
302.6 Gender identity disorder in children
302.85 Gender identity disorder in adolescents or adults
752.7 Indeterminate sex and pseudohermaphroditism
752.89 Other specified anomalies of genital organs
758.81 Other conditions due to sex chromosome anomalies

ICD-9-CM Procedural

62.7 Insertion of testicular prosthesis
64.43 Construction of penis
64.5 Operations for sex transformation, not elsewhere classified
64.97 Insertion or replacement of inflatable penile prosthesis

Female Genital System

Vulva, Perineum and Introitus

56405

56405 Incision and drainage of vulva or perineal abscess

ICD-9-CM Diagnostic

597.0 Urethral abscess
614.4 Chronic or unspecified parametritis and pelvic cellulitis — (Use additional code to identify organism: 041.0, 041.1) ♀
616.4 Other abscess of vulva — (Use additional code to identify organism: 041.0, 041.1) ♀
616.9 Unspecified inflammatory disease of cervix, vagina, and vulva — (Use additional code to identify organism: 041.0, 041.1) ▽ ♀
682.2 Cellulitis and abscess of trunk — (Use additional code to identify organism)
752.49 Other congenital anomaly of cervix, vagina, and external female genitalia ♀

ICD-9-CM Procedural

71.09 Other incision of vulva and perineum

HCPCS Level II Supplies & Services

A4550 Surgical trays

56420

56420 Incision and drainage of Bartholin's gland abscess

ICD-9-CM Diagnostic

616.3 Abscess of Bartholin's gland — (Use additional code to identify organism: 041.0, 041.1) ♀

ICD-9-CM Procedural

71.22 Incision of Bartholin's gland (cyst)

HCPCS Level II Supplies & Services

A4550 Surgical trays

56440

56440 Marsupialization of Bartholin's gland cyst

ICD-9-CM Diagnostic

616.2 Cyst of Bartholin's gland — (Use additional code to identify organism: 041.0, 041.1) ♀
616.3 Abscess of Bartholin's gland — (Use additional code to identify organism: 041.0, 041.1) ♀

ICD-9-CM Procedural

71.23 Marsupialization of Bartholin's gland (cyst)

HCPCS Level II Supplies & Services

A4550 Surgical trays

56441

56441 Lysis of labial adhesions

ICD-9-CM Diagnostic

624.4 Old laceration or scarring of vulva ♀
752.49 Other congenital anomaly of cervix, vagina, and external female genitalia ♀

ICD-9-CM Procedural

71.01 Lysis of vulvar adhesions

HCPCS Level II Supplies & Services

A4550 Surgical trays

56501–56515

56501 Destruction of lesion(s), vulva; simple (eg, laser surgery, electrosurgery, cryosurgery, chemosurgery)
56515 extensive (eg, laser surgery, electrosurgery, cryosurgery, chemosurgery)

ICD-9-CM Diagnostic

054.11 Herpetic vulvovaginitis ♀
054.12 Herpetic ulceration of vulva ♀
078.11 Condyloma acuminatum
078.19 Other specified viral warts
184.4 Malignant neoplasm of vulva, unspecified site ▽ ♀
198.82 Secondary malignant neoplasm of genital organs
221.2 Benign neoplasm of vulva ♀
228.01 Hemangioma of skin and subcutaneous tissue
233.3 Carcinoma in situ of other and unspecified female genital organs ▽ ♀
236.3 Neoplasm of uncertain behavior of other and unspecified female genital organs ▽ ♀
239.5 Neoplasm of unspecified nature of other genitourinary organs
456.6 Vulval varices ♀
616.8 Other specified inflammatory disease of cervix, vagina, and vulva — (Use additional code to identify organism: 041.0, 041.1) ♀
624.0 Dystrophy of vulva ♀
624.6 Polyp of labia and vulva ♀
624.8 Other specified noninflammatory disorder of vulva and perineum ♀
625.8 Other specified symptom associated with female genital organs ♀
698.1 Pruritus of genital organs
701.0 Circumscribed scleroderma
701.5 Other abnormal granulation tissue
709.9 Unspecified disorder of skin and subcutaneous tissue ▽
752.49 Other congenital anomaly of cervix, vagina, and external female genitalia ♀

ICD-9-CM Procedural

71.3 Other local excision or destruction of vulva and perineum

HCPCS Level II Supplies & Services

A4305 Disposable drug delivery system, flow rate of 50 ml or greater per hour
A4306 Disposable drug delivery system, flow rate of 5 ml or less per hour
A4550 Surgical trays

56605–56606

56605 Biopsy of vulva or perineum (separate procedure); one lesion
56606 each separate additional lesion (List separately in addition to code for primary procedure)

ICD-9-CM Diagnostic

054.11 Herpetic vulvovaginitis ♀
054.12 Herpetic ulceration of vulva ♀
078.11 Condyloma acuminatum
078.19 Other specified viral warts
172.5 Malignant melanoma of skin of trunk, except scrotum
173.5 Other malignant neoplasm of skin of trunk, except scrotum
184.4 Malignant neoplasm of vulva, unspecified site ▽ ♀
195.3 Malignant neoplasm of pelvis
198.2 Secondary malignant neoplasm of skin
198.82 Secondary malignant neoplasm of genital organs
198.89 Secondary malignant neoplasm of other specified sites
214.9 Lipoma of unspecified site ▽
216.5 Benign neoplasm of skin of trunk, except scrotum
221.2 Benign neoplasm of vulva ♀
232.5 Carcinoma in situ of skin of trunk, except scrotum
233.3 Carcinoma in situ of other and unspecified female genital organs ▽ ♀
234.8 Carcinoma in situ of other specified sites
236.3 Neoplasm of uncertain behavior of other and unspecified female genital organs ▽ ♀
238.2 Neoplasm of uncertain behavior of skin
239.2 Neoplasms of unspecified nature of bone, soft tissue, and skin
239.5 Neoplasm of unspecified nature of other genitourinary organs

▽ Unspecified code
♀ Female diagnosis
☒ Manifestation code
♂ Male diagnosis

567.9 Unspecified peritonitis ▽
616.10 Unspecified vaginitis and vulvovaginitis — (Use additional code to identify organism: 041.0, 041.1, 041.4) ▽ ♀
624.0 Dystrophy of vulva ♀
624.8 Other specified noninflammatory disorder of vulva and perineum ♀
625.8 Other specified symptom associated with female genital organs ♀
629.8 Other specified disorder of female genital organs ♀
709.9 Unspecified disorder of skin and subcutaneous tissue ▽
752.49 Other congenital anomaly of cervix, vagina, and external female genitalia ♀

ICD-9-CM Procedural

71.11 Biopsy of vulva

HCPCS Level II Supplies & Services

A4550 Surgical trays

56620–56625

56620 Vulvectomy simple; partial
56625 complete

ICD-9-CM Diagnostic

171.6 Malignant neoplasm of connective and other soft tissue of pelvis
172.5 Malignant melanoma of skin of trunk, except scrotum
173.5 Other malignant neoplasm of skin of trunk, except scrotum
184.4 Malignant neoplasm of vulva, unspecified site ▽ ♀
198.82 Secondary malignant neoplasm of genital organs
199.1 Other malignant neoplasm of unspecified site
221.2 Benign neoplasm of vulva ♀
233.3 Carcinoma in situ of other and unspecified female genital organs ▽ ♀
236.3 Neoplasm of uncertain behavior of other and unspecified female genital organs ▽ ♀
239.5 Neoplasm of unspecified nature of other genitourinary organs
616.4 Other abscess of vulva — (Use additional code to identify organism: 041.0, 041.1) ♀
623.0 Dysplasia of vagina ♀
624.3 Hypertrophy of labia ♀
624.8 Other specified noninflammatory disorder of vulva and perineum ♀
698.1 Pruritus of genital organs
701.0 Circumscribed scleroderma
752.40 Unspecified congenital anomaly of cervix, vagina, and external female genitalia ▽ ♀
752.41 Embryonic cyst of cervix, vagina, and external female genitalia ♀
752.49 Other congenital anomaly of cervix, vagina, and external female genitalia ♀
752.89 Other specified anomalies of genital organs
752.9 Unspecified congenital anomaly of genital organs ▽
V84.09 Genetic susceptibility to other malignant neoplasm

ICD-9-CM Procedural

71.61 Unilateral vulvectomy
71.62 Bilateral vulvectomy

HCPCS Level II Supplies & Services

A4305 Disposable drug delivery system, flow rate of 50 ml or greater per hour
A4306 Disposable drug delivery system, flow rate of 5 ml or less per hour
A4550 Surgical trays

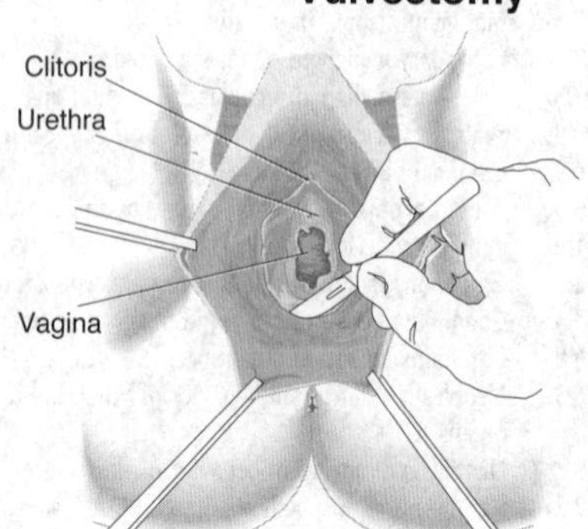
Vulvectomy
The distal portions of the urethra and vagina may be excised with the labia
The physician may also remove skin, subcutaneous fatty tissue, and deeper tissues
Clitoris
Urethra
Vagina

56630–56632

56630 Vulvectomy, radical, partial;
56631 with unilateral inguinofemoral lymphadenectomy
56632 with bilateral inguinofemoral lymphadenectomy

ICD-9-CM Diagnostic

171.6 Malignant neoplasm of connective and other soft tissue of pelvis
172.5 Malignant melanoma of skin of trunk, except scrotum
173.5 Other malignant neoplasm of skin of trunk, except scrotum
184.4 Malignant neoplasm of vulva, unspecified site ▽ ♀
196.5 Secondary and unspecified malignant neoplasm of lymph nodes of inguinal region and lower limb
198.82 Secondary malignant neoplasm of genital organs
233.3 Carcinoma in situ of other and unspecified female genital organs ▽ ♀
236.3 Neoplasm of uncertain behavior of other and unspecified female genital organs ▽ ♀
239.5 Neoplasm of unspecified nature of other genitourinary organs
239.8 Neoplasm of unspecified nature of other specified sites
752.40 Unspecified congenital anomaly of cervix, vagina, and external female genitalia ▽ ♀
752.41 Embryonic cyst of cervix, vagina, and external female genitalia ♀
752.49 Other congenital anomaly of cervix, vagina, and external female genitalia ♀
752.89 Other specified anomalies of genital organs
752.9 Unspecified congenital anomaly of genital organs ▽
V84.09 Genetic susceptibility to other malignant neoplasm

ICD-9-CM Procedural

40.3 Regional lymph node excision
71.5 Radical vulvectomy

56633–56637

56633 Vulvectomy, radical, complete;
56634 with unilateral inguinofemoral lymphadenectomy
56637 with bilateral inguinofemoral lymphadenectomy

ICD-9-CM Diagnostic

171.6 Malignant neoplasm of connective and other soft tissue of pelvis
172.5 Malignant melanoma of skin of trunk, except scrotum
173.5 Other malignant neoplasm of skin of trunk, except scrotum
184.4 Malignant neoplasm of vulva, unspecified site ▽ ♀
196.5 Secondary and unspecified malignant neoplasm of lymph nodes of inguinal region and lower limb
198.82 Secondary malignant neoplasm of genital organs
233.3 Carcinoma in situ of other and unspecified female genital organs ▽ ♀
236.3 Neoplasm of uncertain behavior of other and unspecified female genital organs ▽ ♀
239.5 Neoplasm of unspecified nature of other genitourinary organs
239.8 Neoplasm of unspecified nature of other specified sites
752.40 Unspecified congenital anomaly of cervix, vagina, and external female genitalia ▽ ♀
752.41 Embryonic cyst of cervix, vagina, and external female genitalia ♀
752.49 Other congenital anomaly of cervix, vagina, and external female genitalia ♀
752.89 Other specified anomalies of genital organs
V84.09 Genetic susceptibility to other malignant neoplasm

ICD-9-CM Procedural

40.3 Regional lymph node excision
71.5 Radical vulvectomy

56640

56640 Vulvectomy, radical, complete, with inguinofemoral, iliac, and pelvic lymphadenectomy

ICD-9-CM Diagnostic

171.6 Malignant neoplasm of connective and other soft tissue of pelvis
172.5 Malignant melanoma of skin of trunk, except scrotum
173.5 Other malignant neoplasm of skin of trunk, except scrotum
184.4 Malignant neoplasm of vulva, unspecified site ▽ ♀
196.5 Secondary and unspecified malignant neoplasm of lymph nodes of inguinal region and lower limb
196.6 Secondary and unspecified malignant neoplasm of intrapelvic lymph nodes
198.82 Secondary malignant neoplasm of genital organs
233.3 Carcinoma in situ of other and unspecified female genital organs ▽ ♀
236.3 Neoplasm of uncertain behavior of other and unspecified female genital organs ▽ ♀
239.5 Neoplasm of unspecified nature of other genitourinary organs

▽ Unspecified code
♀ Female diagnosis
☒ Manifestation code
♂ Male diagnosis

239.8 Neoplasm of unspecified nature of other specified sites
V84.09 Genetic susceptibility to other malignant neoplasm

ICD-9-CM Procedural
40.59 Radical excision of other lymph nodes
71.5 Radical vulvectomy

56700
56700 Partial hymenectomy or revision of hymenal ring

ICD-9-CM Diagnostic
184.0 Malignant neoplasm of vagina ♀
198.82 Secondary malignant neoplasm of genital organs
221.1 Benign neoplasm of vagina ♀
233.3 Carcinoma in situ of other and unspecified female genital organs ▽ ♀
236.3 Neoplasm of uncertain behavior of other and unspecified female genital organs ▽ ♀
614.9 Unspecified inflammatory disease of female pelvic organs and tissues — (Use additional code to identify organism: 041.0, 041.1) ▽ ♀
623.3 Tight hymenal ring ♀
625.0 Dyspareunia ♀
629.8 Other specified disorder of female genital organs ♀
752.40 Unspecified congenital anomaly of cervix, vagina, and external female genitalia ▽ ♀
752.41 Embryonic cyst of cervix, vagina, and external female genitalia ♀
752.42 Imperforate hymen ♀
752.49 Other congenital anomaly of cervix, vagina, and external female genitalia ♀
752.89 Other specified anomalies of genital organs
752.9 Unspecified congenital anomaly of genital organs ▽

ICD-9-CM Procedural
70.31 Hymenectomy
70.76 Hymenorrhaphy

HCPCS Level II Supplies & Services
A4550 Surgical trays

56720
56720 Hymenotomy, simple incision

ICD-9-CM Diagnostic
623.3 Tight hymenal ring ♀
752.42 Imperforate hymen ♀
752.49 Other congenital anomaly of cervix, vagina, and external female genitalia ♀

ICD-9-CM Procedural
70.11 Hymenotomy

HCPCS Level II Supplies & Services
A4550 Surgical trays

56740
56740 Excision of Bartholin's gland or cyst

ICD-9-CM Diagnostic
616.2 Cyst of Bartholin's gland — (Use additional code to identify organism: 041.0, 041.1) ♀
616.3 Abscess of Bartholin's gland — (Use additional code to identify organism: 041.0, 041.1) ♀

ICD-9-CM Procedural
71.24 Excision or other destruction of Bartholin's gland (cyst)

HCPCS Level II Supplies & Services
A4550 Surgical trays

56800
56800 Plastic repair of introitus

ICD-9-CM Diagnostic
623.2 Stricture or atresia of vagina — (Use additional E code to identify any external cause) ♀
624.4 Old laceration or scarring of vulva ♀
629.20 Female genital mutilation status, unspecified
629.21 Female genital mutilation, Type I status
629.22 Female genital mutilation, Type II status
629.23 Female genital mutilation, Type III status
752.40 Unspecified congenital anomaly of cervix, vagina, and external female genitalia ▽ ♀
752.49 Other congenital anomaly of cervix, vagina, and external female genitalia ♀
759.9 Unspecified congenital anomaly ▽

ICD-9-CM Procedural
71.79 Other repair of vulva and perineum

56805
56805 Clitoroplasty for intersex state

ICD-9-CM Diagnostic
255.2 Adrenogenital disorders

ICD-9-CM Procedural
71.4 Operations on clitoris

56810
56810 Perineoplasty, repair of perineum, nonobstetrical (separate procedure)

ICD-9-CM Diagnostic
184.8 Malignant neoplasm of other specified sites of female genital organs ♀
195.3 Malignant neoplasm of pelvis
198.89 Secondary malignant neoplasm of other specified sites
229.8 Benign neoplasm of other specified sites
234.8 Carcinoma in situ of other specified sites
238.8 Neoplasm of uncertain behavior of other specified sites
239.8 Neoplasm of unspecified nature of other specified sites
618.05 Perineocele without mention of uterine prolapse
618.7 Genital prolapse, old laceration of muscles of pelvic floor — (Use additional code to identify urinary incontinence: 625.6, 788.31, 788.33-788.39) ♀
618.9 Unspecified genital prolapse — (Use additional code to identify urinary incontinence: 625.6, 788.31, 788.33-788.39) ▽ ♀
625.0 Dyspareunia ♀
625.6 Female stress incontinence ♀
629.20 Female genital mutilation status, unspecified
629.21 Female genital mutilation, Type I status
629.22 Female genital mutilation, Type II status
629.23 Female genital mutilation, Type III status
701.0 Circumscribed scleroderma
752.40 Unspecified congenital anomaly of cervix, vagina, and external female genitalia ▽ ♀
752.41 Embryonic cyst of cervix, vagina, and external female genitalia ♀
752.49 Other congenital anomaly of cervix, vagina, and external female genitalia ♀
879.6 Open wound of other and unspecified parts of trunk, without mention of complication — (Use additional code to identify infection) ▽
879.7 Open wound of other and unspecified parts of trunk, complicated — (Use additional code to identify infection) ▽
959.14 Other injury of external genitals
959.19 Other injury of other sites of trunk

ICD-9-CM Procedural
71.79 Other repair of vulva and perineum

56820–56821
56820 Colposcopy of the vulva;
56821 with biopsy(s)

ICD-9-CM Diagnostic
054.11 Herpetic vulvovaginitis ♀
054.12 Herpetic ulceration of vulva ♀
078.11 Condyloma acuminatum
078.19 Other specified viral warts
184.1 Malignant neoplasm of labia majora ♀
184.2 Malignant neoplasm of labia minora ♀
184.3 Malignant neoplasm of clitoris ♀
184.4 Malignant neoplasm of vulva, unspecified site ▽ ♀
198.82 Secondary malignant neoplasm of genital organs
221.2 Benign neoplasm of vulva ♀
228.01 Hemangioma of skin and subcutaneous tissue
233.3 Carcinoma in situ of other and unspecified female genital organs ▽ ♀
236.3 Neoplasm of uncertain behavior of other and unspecified female genital organs ▽ ♀
239.5 Neoplasm of unspecified nature of other genitourinary organs

▽ Unspecified code
♀ Female diagnosis
☒ Manifestation code
♂ Male diagnosis

456.6 Vulval varices ♀
616.10 Unspecified vaginitis and vulvovaginitis — (Use additional code to identify organism: 041.0, 041.1, 041.4) ♀
616.11 Vaginitis and vulvovaginitis in diseases classified elsewhere — (Code first underlying disease, 127.4.) ♀
616.2 Cyst of Bartholin's gland — (Use additional code to identify organism: 041.0, 041.1) ♀
616.3 Abscess of Bartholin's gland — (Use additional code to identify organism: 041.0, 041.1) ♀
616.4 Other abscess of vulva — (Use additional code to identify organism: 041.0, 041.1) ♀
616.50 Unspecified ulceration of vulva — (Use additional code to identify organism: 041.0, 041.1) ♀
616.51 Ulceration of vulva in disease classified elsewhere — (Code first underlying disease: 016.7, 136.1.) ♀
616.8 Other specified inflammatory disease of cervix, vagina, and vulva — (Use additional code to identify organism: 041.0, 041.1) ♀
616.9 Unspecified inflammatory disease of cervix, vagina, and vulva — (Use additional code to identify organism: 041.0, 041.1) ♀
617.8 Endometriosis of other specified sites ♀
624.0 Dystrophy of vulva ♀
624.1 Atrophy of vulva ♀
624.2 Hypertrophy of clitoris ♀
624.3 Hypertrophy of labia ♀
624.4 Old laceration or scarring of vulva ♀
624.5 Hematoma of vulva ♀
624.6 Polyp of labia and vulva ♀
624.8 Other specified noninflammatory disorder of vulva and perineum ♀
624.9 Unspecified noninflammatory disorder of vulva and perineum ♀
625.8 Other specified symptom associated with female genital organs ♀
625.9 Unspecified symptom associated with female genital organs ♀
654.80 Congenital or acquired abnormality of vulva, unspecified as to episode of care in pregnancy — (Code first any associated obstructed labor, 660.2) ♀
654.81 Congenital or acquired abnormality of vulva, with delivery — (Code first any associated obstructed labor, 660.2) ♀
654.82 Congenital or acquired abnormality of vulva, delivered, with mention of postpartum complication — (Code first any associated obstructed labor, 660.2) ♀
654.83 Congenital or acquired abnormality of vulva, antepartum condition or complication — (Code first any associated obstructed labor, 660.2) ♀
654.84 Congenital or acquired abnormality of vulva, postpartum condition or complication — (Code first any associated obstructed labor, 660.2) ♀
698.1 Pruritus of genital organs
701.0 Circumscribed scleroderma
701.5 Other abnormal granulation tissue
709.9 Unspecified disorder of skin and subcutaneous tissue
752.40 Unspecified congenital anomaly of cervix, vagina, and external female genitalia ♀
752.41 Embryonic cyst of cervix, vagina, and external female genitalia ♀
752.42 Imperforate hymen ♀
752.49 Other congenital anomaly of cervix, vagina, and external female genitalia ♀
V13.29 Personal history of other genital system and obstetric disorders
V67.00 Follow-up examination, following unspecified surgery
V67.09 Follow-up examination, following other surgery
V71.5 Observation following alleged rape or seduction
V71.6 Observation following other inflicted injury

ICD-9-CM Procedural

71.11 Biopsy of vulva
71.19 Other diagnostic procedures on vulva

HCPCS Level II Supplies & Services

A4550 Surgical trays

Vagina

57000

57000 Colpotomy; with exploration

ICD-9-CM Diagnostic

184.0 Malignant neoplasm of vagina ♀
198.82 Secondary malignant neoplasm of genital organs
221.1 Benign neoplasm of vagina ♀
236.3 Neoplasm of uncertain behavior of other and unspecified female genital organs ♀
239.5 Neoplasm of unspecified nature of other genitourinary organs
616.10 Unspecified vaginitis and vulvovaginitis — (Use additional code to identify organism: 041.0, 041.1, 041.4) ♀
623.8 Other specified noninflammatory disorder of vagina ♀
623.9 Unspecified noninflammatory disorder of vagina ♀
625.3 Dysmenorrhea ♀

ICD-9-CM Procedural

70.12 Culdotomy

HCPCS Level II Supplies & Services

A4550 Surgical trays

57010

57010 Colpotomy; with drainage of pelvic abscess

ICD-9-CM Diagnostic

614.3 Acute parametritis and pelvic cellulitis — (Use additional code to identify organism: 041.0, 041.1) ♀
614.4 Chronic or unspecified parametritis and pelvic cellulitis — (Use additional code to identify organism: 041.0, 041.1) ♀
616.10 Unspecified vaginitis and vulvovaginitis — (Use additional code to identify organism: 041.0, 041.1, 041.4) ♀
998.51 Infected postoperative seroma — (Use additional code to identify organism)
998.59 Other postoperative infection — (Use additional code to identify infection)

ICD-9-CM Procedural

70.14 Other vaginotomy

HCPCS Level II Supplies & Services

A4305 Disposable drug delivery system, flow rate of 50 ml or greater per hour
A4306 Disposable drug delivery system, flow rate of 5 ml or less per hour
A4550 Surgical trays

57020

57020 Colpocentesis (separate procedure)

ICD-9-CM Diagnostic

184.0 Malignant neoplasm of vagina ♀
198.82 Secondary malignant neoplasm of genital organs
221.1 Benign neoplasm of vagina ♀
233.3 Carcinoma in situ of other and unspecified female genital organs ♀
236.3 Neoplasm of uncertain behavior of other and unspecified female genital organs ♀
239.5 Neoplasm of unspecified nature of other genitourinary organs
614.9 Unspecified inflammatory disease of female pelvic organs and tissues — (Use additional code to identify organism: 041.0, 041.1) ♀
752.40 Unspecified congenital anomaly of cervix, vagina, and external female genitalia ♀
752.41 Embryonic cyst of cervix, vagina, and external female genitalia ♀
752.49 Other congenital anomaly of cervix, vagina, and external female genitalia ♀
878.6 Open wound of vagina, without mention of complication — (Use additional code to identify infection) ♀
878.7 Open wound of vagina, complicated — (Use additional code to identify infection) ♀

ICD-9-CM Procedural

70.0 Culdocentesis

HCPCS Level II Supplies & Services

A4305 Disposable drug delivery system, flow rate of 50 ml or greater per hour
A4306 Disposable drug delivery system, flow rate of 5 ml or less per hour
A4550 Surgical trays

57022–57023

57022 Incision and drainage of vaginal hematoma; obstetrical/postpartum
57023 non-obstetrical (eg, post-trauma, spontaneous bleeding)

ICD-9-CM Diagnostic

623.6 Vaginal hematoma ♀
665.70 Pelvic hematoma, unspecified as to episode of care ♀
665.71 Pelvic hematoma, with delivery ♀
665.72 Pelvic hematoma, delivered with postpartum complication ♀
665.74 Pelvic hematoma, postpartum ♀

Unspecified code
♀ Female diagnosis
Manifestation code
♂ Male diagnosis

922.4 Contusion of genital organs

ICD-9-CM Procedural

70.14 Other vaginotomy
75.91 Evacuation of obstetrical incisional hematoma of perineum
75.92 Evacuation of other hematoma of vulva or vagina

HCPCS Level II Supplies & Services

A4550 Surgical trays

57061–57065

57061 Destruction of vaginal lesion(s); simple (eg, laser surgery, electrosurgery, cryosurgery, chemosurgery)
57065 extensive (eg, laser surgery, electrosurgery, cryosurgery, chemosurgery)

ICD-9-CM Diagnostic

078.11 Condyloma acuminatum
078.19 Other specified viral warts
184.0 Malignant neoplasm of vagina ♀
198.82 Secondary malignant neoplasm of genital organs
221.1 Benign neoplasm of vagina ♀
236.3 Neoplasm of uncertain behavior of other and unspecified female genital organs ▽ ♀
239.5 Neoplasm of unspecified nature of other genitourinary organs
616.8 Other specified inflammatory disease of cervix, vagina, and vulva — (Use additional code to identify organism: 041.0, 041.1) ♀
616.9 Unspecified inflammatory disease of cervix, vagina, and vulva — (Use additional code to identify organism: 041.0, 041.1) ▽ ♀
623.0 Dysplasia of vagina ♀
623.1 Leukoplakia of vagina ♀
623.5 Leukorrhea, not specified as infective ♀
623.7 Polyp of vagina ♀
623.8 Other specified noninflammatory disorder of vagina ♀
624.0 Dystrophy of vulva ♀
624.8 Other specified noninflammatory disorder of vulva and perineum ♀
701.5 Other abnormal granulation tissue

ICD-9-CM Procedural

70.13 Lysis of intraluminal adhesions of vagina
70.32 Excision or destruction of lesion of cul-de-sac
70.33 Excision or destruction of lesion of vagina

HCPCS Level II Supplies & Services

A4305 Disposable drug delivery system, flow rate of 50 ml or greater per hour
A4306 Disposable drug delivery system, flow rate of 5 ml or less per hour
A4550 Surgical trays

57100–57105

57100 Biopsy of vaginal mucosa; simple (separate procedure)
57105 extensive, requiring suture (including cysts)

ICD-9-CM Diagnostic

054.11 Herpetic vulvovaginitis ♀
078.11 Condyloma acuminatum
078.19 Other specified viral warts
098.0 Gonococcal infection (acute) of lower genitourinary tract
184.0 Malignant neoplasm of vagina ♀
198.82 Secondary malignant neoplasm of genital organs
221.1 Benign neoplasm of vagina ♀
236.3 Neoplasm of uncertain behavior of other and unspecified female genital organs ▽ ♀
239.5 Neoplasm of unspecified nature of other genitourinary organs
616.10 Unspecified vaginitis and vulvovaginitis — (Use additional code to identify organism: 041.0, 041.1, 041.4) ▽ ♀
616.8 Other specified inflammatory disease of cervix, vagina, and vulva — (Use additional code to identify organism: 041.0, 041.1) ♀
623.0 Dysplasia of vagina ♀
623.1 Leukoplakia of vagina ♀
623.5 Leukorrhea, not specified as infective ♀
623.7 Polyp of vagina ♀
623.8 Other specified noninflammatory disorder of vagina ♀
625.8 Other specified symptom associated with female genital organs ♀
627.3 Postmenopausal atrophic vaginitis ♀
698.1 Pruritus of genital organs
701.5 Other abnormal granulation tissue
752.41 Embryonic cyst of cervix, vagina, and external female genitalia ♀
752.49 Other congenital anomaly of cervix, vagina, and external female genitalia ♀
795.1 Nonspecific abnormal Papanicolaou smear of other site ▽
V67.1 Radiotherapy follow-up examination

ICD-9-CM Procedural

70.23 Biopsy of cul-de-sac
70.24 Vaginal biopsy

HCPCS Level II Supplies & Services

A4550 Surgical trays

57106–57109

57106 Vaginectomy, partial removal of vaginal wall;
57107 with removal of paravaginal tissue (radical vaginectomy)
57109 with removal of paravaginal tissue (radical vaginectomy) with bilateral total pelvic lymphadenectomy and para-aortic lymph node sampling (biopsy)

ICD-9-CM Diagnostic

184.0 Malignant neoplasm of vagina ♀
184.1 Malignant neoplasm of labia majora ♀
184.2 Malignant neoplasm of labia minora ♀
184.4 Malignant neoplasm of vulva, unspecified site ▽ ♀
184.8 Malignant neoplasm of other specified sites of female genital organs ♀
184.9 Malignant neoplasm of female genital organ, site unspecified ▽ ♀
196.2 Secondary and unspecified malignant neoplasm of intra-abdominal lymph nodes
198.82 Secondary malignant neoplasm of genital organs
221.1 Benign neoplasm of vagina ♀
233.3 Carcinoma in situ of other and unspecified female genital organs ▽ ♀
236.3 Neoplasm of uncertain behavior of other and unspecified female genital organs ▽ ♀
239.5 Neoplasm of unspecified nature of other genitourinary organs
616.10 Unspecified vaginitis and vulvovaginitis — (Use additional code to identify organism: 041.0, 041.1, 041.4) ▽ ♀
616.11 Vaginitis and vulvovaginitis in diseases classified elsewhere — (Code first underlying disease, 127.4.) ☒ ♀
616.9 Unspecified inflammatory disease of cervix, vagina, and vulva — (Use additional code to identify organism: 041.0, 041.1) ▽ ♀
618.00 Prolapse of vaginal walls without mention of uterine prolapse, unspecified
618.4 Uterovaginal prolapse, unspecified — (Use additional code to identify urinary incontinence: 625.6, 788.31, 788.33-788.39) ▽ ♀
618.89 Other specified genital prolapse
623.2 Stricture or atresia of vagina — (Use additional E code to identify any external cause) ♀
752.49 Other congenital anomaly of cervix, vagina, and external female genitalia ♀
V84.02 Genetic susceptibility to malignant neoplasm of ovary
V84.04 Genetic susceptibility to malignant neoplasm of endometrium
V84.09 Genetic susceptibility to other malignant neoplasm

ICD-9-CM Procedural

40.3 Regional lymph node excision
70.4 Obliteration and total excision of vagina

57110–57112

57110 Vaginectomy, complete removal of vaginal wall;
57111 with removal of paravaginal tissue (radical vaginectomy)
57112 with removal of paravaginal tissue (radical vaginectomy) with bilateral total pelvic lymphadenectomy and para-aortic lymph node sampling (biopsy)

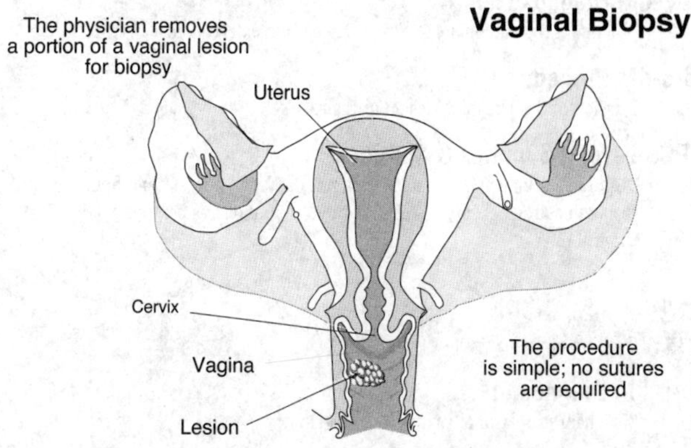
Vaginal Biopsy
The physician removes a portion of a vaginal lesion for biopsy
Uterus
Cervix
Vagina
Lesion
The procedure is simple; no sutures are required

ICD-9-CM Diagnostic

184.0 Malignant neoplasm of vagina ♀
184.1 Malignant neoplasm of labia majora ♀
184.2 Malignant neoplasm of labia minora ♀
184.4 Malignant neoplasm of vulva, unspecified site ▽ ♀
184.8 Malignant neoplasm of other specified sites of female genital organs ♀
184.9 Malignant neoplasm of female genital organ, site unspecified ▽ ♀
196.2 Secondary and unspecified malignant neoplasm of intra-abdominal lymph nodes
198.82 Secondary malignant neoplasm of genital organs
221.1 Benign neoplasm of vagina ♀
233.3 Carcinoma in situ of other and unspecified female genital organs ▽ ♀
236.3 Neoplasm of uncertain behavior of other and unspecified female genital organs ▽ ♀
239.5 Neoplasm of unspecified nature of other genitourinary organs
616.10 Unspecified vaginitis and vulvovaginitis — (Use additional code to identify organism: 041.0, 041.1, 041.4) ▽ ♀
616.11 Vaginitis and vulvovaginitis in diseases classified elsewhere — (Code first underlying disease, 127.4.) ☒ ♀
616.8 Other specified inflammatory disease of cervix, vagina, and vulva — (Use additional code to identify organism: 041.0, 041.1) ♀
616.9 Unspecified inflammatory disease of cervix, vagina, and vulva — (Use additional code to identify organism: 041.0, 041.1) ▽ ♀
618.00 Prolapse of vaginal walls without mention of uterine prolapse, unspecified
618.4 Uterovaginal prolapse, unspecified — (Use additional code to identify urinary incontinence: 625.6, 788.31, 788.33-788.39) ▽ ♀
623.2 Stricture or atresia of vagina — (Use additional E code to identify any external cause) ♀
752.49 Other congenital anomaly of cervix, vagina, and external female genitalia ♀
V84.01 Genetic susceptibility to malignant neoplasm of breast
V84.02 Genetic susceptibility to malignant neoplasm of ovary
V84.04 Genetic susceptibility to malignant neoplasm of endometrium
V84.09 Genetic susceptibility to other malignant neoplasm

ICD-9-CM Procedural

40.3 Regional lymph node excision
70.4 Obliteration and total excision of vagina

57120

57120 Colpocleisis (Le Fort type)

ICD-9-CM Diagnostic

184.0 Malignant neoplasm of vagina ♀
198.82 Secondary malignant neoplasm of genital organs
221.1 Benign neoplasm of vagina ♀
233.3 Carcinoma in situ of other and unspecified female genital organs ▽ ♀
236.3 Neoplasm of uncertain behavior of other and unspecified female genital organs ▽ ♀
239.5 Neoplasm of unspecified nature of other genitourinary organs
618.4 Uterovaginal prolapse, unspecified — (Use additional code to identify urinary incontinence: 625.6, 788.31, 788.33-788.39) ▽ ♀
752.49 Other congenital anomaly of cervix, vagina, and external female genitalia ♀

ICD-9-CM Procedural

70.8 Obliteration of vaginal vault

57130

57130 Excision of vaginal septum

ICD-9-CM Diagnostic

752.49 Other congenital anomaly of cervix, vagina, and external female genitalia ♀

ICD-9-CM Procedural

70.33 Excision or destruction of lesion of vagina

HCPCS Level II Supplies & Services

A4305 Disposable drug delivery system, flow rate of 50 ml or greater per hour
A4306 Disposable drug delivery system, flow rate of 5 ml or less per hour
A4550 Surgical trays

57135

57135 Excision of vaginal cyst or tumor

ICD-9-CM Diagnostic

184.0 Malignant neoplasm of vagina ♀
198.82 Secondary malignant neoplasm of genital organs
221.1 Benign neoplasm of vagina ♀
233.3 Carcinoma in situ of other and unspecified female genital organs ▽ ♀
236.3 Neoplasm of uncertain behavior of other and unspecified female genital organs ▽ ♀
239.5 Neoplasm of unspecified nature of other genitourinary organs
623.7 Polyp of vagina ♀
623.8 Other specified noninflammatory disorder of vagina ♀
752.41 Embryonic cyst of cervix, vagina, and external female genitalia ♀

ICD-9-CM Procedural

70.33 Excision or destruction of lesion of vagina

HCPCS Level II Supplies & Services

A4305 Disposable drug delivery system, flow rate of 50 ml or greater per hour
A4306 Disposable drug delivery system, flow rate of 5 ml or less per hour
A4550 Surgical trays

57150

57150 Irrigation of vagina and/or application of medicament for treatment of bacterial, parasitic, or fungoid disease

ICD-9-CM Diagnostic

054.11 Herpetic vulvovaginitis ♀
112.1 Candidiasis of vulva and vagina — (Use additional code to identify manifestation: 321.0-321.1, 380.15, 711.6) ♀
127.4 Enterobiasis
131.01 Trichomonal vulvovaginitis ♀
616.0 Cervicitis and endocervicitis — (Use additional code to identify organism: 041.0, 041.1) ♀
616.10 Unspecified vaginitis and vulvovaginitis — (Use additional code to identify organism: 041.0, 041.1, 041.4) ▽ ♀
616.11 Vaginitis and vulvovaginitis in diseases classified elsewhere — (Code first underlying disease, 127.4.) ☒ ♀
623.5 Leukorrhea, not specified as infective ♀

ICD-9-CM Procedural

96.44 Vaginal douche
96.49 Other genitourinary instillation

HCPCS Level II Supplies & Services

A4550 Surgical trays

57155

57155 Insertion of uterine tandems and/or vaginal ovoids for clinical brachytherapy

ICD-9-CM Diagnostic

179 Malignant neoplasm of uterus, part unspecified ▽ ♀
180.0 Malignant neoplasm of endocervix ♀
180.1 Malignant neoplasm of exocervix ♀
180.8 Malignant neoplasm of other specified sites of cervix ♀
180.9 Malignant neoplasm of cervix uteri, unspecified site ▽ ♀
182.0 Malignant neoplasm of corpus uteri, except isthmus ♀
182.1 Malignant neoplasm of isthmus ♀
182.8 Malignant neoplasm of other specified sites of body of uterus ♀
184.0 Malignant neoplasm of vagina ♀
184.8 Malignant neoplasm of other specified sites of female genital organs ♀
184.9 Malignant neoplasm of female genital organ, site unspecified ▽ ♀
198.82 Secondary malignant neoplasm of genital organs
233.1 Carcinoma in situ of cervix uteri ♀
233.2 Carcinoma in situ of other and unspecified parts of uterus ▽ ♀
233.3 Carcinoma in situ of other and unspecified female genital organs ▽ ♀
236.0 Neoplasm of uncertain behavior of uterus ♀
236.3 Neoplasm of uncertain behavior of other and unspecified female genital organs ▽ ♀

ICD-9-CM Procedural

92.27 Implantation or insertion of radioactive elements

HCPCS Level II Supplies & Services

HCPCS Level II codes are used to report the supplies, durable medical equipment, and certain medical services provided on an outpatient basis. Because the procedure(s) represented on this page would be performed in an inpatient or outpatient facility, no HCPCS Level II codes apply.

▽ Unspecified code
♀ Female diagnosis
☒ Manifestation code
♂ Male diagnosis

57160

57160 Fitting and insertion of pessary or other intravaginal support device

ICD-9-CM Diagnostic

618.00 Prolapse of vaginal walls without mention of uterine prolapse, unspecified
618.09 Other prolapse of vaginal walls without mention of uterine prolapse
618.1 Uterine prolapse without mention of vaginal wall prolapse — (Use additional code to identify urinary incontinence: 625.6, 788.31, 788.33-788.39) ♀
618.2 Uterovaginal prolapse, incomplete — (Use additional code to identify urinary incontinence: 625.6, 788.31, 788.33-788.39) ♀
618.3 Uterovaginal prolapse, complete — (Use additional code to identify urinary incontinence: 625.6, 788.31, 788.33-788.39) ♀
618.4 Uterovaginal prolapse, unspecified — (Use additional code to identify urinary incontinence: 625.6, 788.31, 788.33-788.39) ▽ ♀
618.5 Prolapse of vaginal vault after hysterectomy — (Use additional code to identify urinary incontinence: 625.6, 788.31, 788.33-788.39) ♀
618.6 Vaginal enterocele, congenital or acquired — (Use additional code to identify urinary incontinence: 625.6, 788.31, 788.33-788.39) ♀
618.89 Other specified genital prolapse
618.9 Unspecified genital prolapse — (Use additional code to identify urinary incontinence: 625.6, 788.31, 788.33-788.39) ▽ ♀
625.6 Female stress incontinence ♀
878.6 Open wound of vagina, without mention of complication — (Use additional code to identify infection) ♀
878.7 Open wound of vagina, complicated — (Use additional code to identify infection) ♀

ICD-9-CM Procedural

96.18 Insertion of other vaginal pessary
97.25 Replacement of other vaginal pessary

HCPCS Level II Supplies & Services

A4561 Pessary, rubber, any type
A4562 Pessary, non rubber, any type

57170

57170 Diaphragm or cervical cap fitting with instructions

ICD-9-CM Diagnostic

V24.2 Routine postpartum follow-up ♀
V25.02 General counseling for initiation of other contraceptive measures
V25.09 Other general counseling and advice for contraceptive management
V25.49 Surveillance of other previously prescribed contraceptive method

ICD-9-CM Procedural

96.17 Insertion of vaginal diaphragm
97.24 Replacement and refitting of vaginal diaphragm

HCPCS Level II Supplies & Services

A4261 Cervical cap for contraceptive use

57180

57180 Introduction of any hemostatic agent or pack for spontaneous or traumatic nonobstetrical vaginal hemorrhage (separate procedure)

ICD-9-CM Diagnostic

623.8 Other specified noninflammatory disorder of vagina ♀
626.9 Unspecified disorder of menstruation and other abnormal bleeding from female genital tract ▽ ♀
867.4 Uterus injury without mention of open wound into cavity ♀
878.6 Open wound of vagina, without mention of complication — (Use additional code to identify infection) ♀
878.7 Open wound of vagina, complicated — (Use additional code to identify infection) ♀
996.32 Mechanical complication due to intrauterine contraceptive device ♀
996.76 Other complications due to genitourinary device, implant, and graft
998.11 Hemorrhage complicating a procedure

ICD-9-CM Procedural

96.14 Vaginal packing
97.26 Replacement of vaginal or vulvar packing or drain

HCPCS Level II Supplies & Services

A4550 Surgical trays

57200–57210

57200 Colporrhaphy, suture of injury of vagina (nonobstetrical)
57210 Colpoperineorrhaphy, suture of injury of vagina and/or perineum (nonobstetrical)

ICD-9-CM Diagnostic

629.20 Female genital mutilation status, unspecified
629.21 Female genital mutilation, Type I status
629.22 Female genital mutilation, Type II status
629.23 Female genital mutilation, Type III status
878.4 Open wound of vulva, without mention of complication — (Use additional code to identify infection) ♀
878.5 Open wound of vulva, complicated — (Use additional code to identify infection) ♀
878.6 Open wound of vagina, without mention of complication — (Use additional code to identify infection) ♀
878.7 Open wound of vagina, complicated — (Use additional code to identify infection) ♀
878.8 Open wound of other and unspecified parts of genital organs, without mention of complication — (Use additional code to identify infection) ▽
878.9 Open wound of other and unspecified parts of genital organs, complicated — (Use additional code to identify infection) ▽
911.6 Trunk, superficial foreign body (splinter), without major open wound and without mention of infection
911.7 Trunk, superficial foreign body (splinter), without major open wound, infected
926.0 Crushing injury of external genitalia — (Use additional code to identify any associated injuries: 800-829, 850.0-854.1, 860.0-869.1)
939.2 Foreign body in vulva and vagina ♀
939.9 Foreign body in unspecified site in genitourinary tract ▽
959.14 Other injury of external genitals
995.53 Child sexual abuse
995.83 Adult sexual abuse — (Use additional code to identify any associated injury and perpetrator)

ICD-9-CM Procedural

70.71 Suture of laceration of vagina

HCPCS Level II Supplies & Services

A4305 Disposable drug delivery system, flow rate of 50 ml or greater per hour
A4306 Disposable drug delivery system, flow rate of 5 ml or less per hour
A4550 Surgical trays

57220

57220 Plastic operation on urethral sphincter, vaginal approach (eg, Kelly urethral plication)

ICD-9-CM Diagnostic

599.81 Urethral hypermobility — (Use additional code to identify urinary incontinence: 625.6, 788.30-788.39)
599.82 Intrinsic (urethral) sphincter deficiency (ISD) — (Use additional code to identify urinary incontinence: 625.6, 788.30-788.39)
599.83 Urethral instability — (Use additional code to identify urinary incontinence: 625.6, 788.30-788.39)
599.84 Other specified disorders of urethra — (Use additional code to identify urinary incontinence: 625.6, 788.30-788.39)
599.89 Other specified disorders of urinary tract — (Use additional code to identify urinary incontinence: 625.6, 788.30-788.39)
625.6 Female stress incontinence ♀

ICD-9-CM Procedural

59.3 Plication of urethrovesical junction

57230

57230 Plastic repair of urethrocele

ICD-9-CM Diagnostic

618.00 Prolapse of vaginal walls without mention of uterine prolapse, unspecified
618.01 Cystocele without mention of uterine prolapse, midline
618.02 Cystocele without mention of uterine prolapse, lateral
618.03 Urethrocele without mention of uterine prolapse
618.2 Uterovaginal prolapse, incomplete — (Use additional code to identify urinary incontinence: 625.6, 788.31, 788.33-788.39) ♀
618.3 Uterovaginal prolapse, complete — (Use additional code to identify urinary incontinence: 625.6, 788.31, 788.33-788.39) ♀
618.4 Uterovaginal prolapse, unspecified — (Use additional code to identify urinary incontinence: 625.6, 788.31, 788.33-788.39) ▽ ♀

▽ Unspecified code
♀ Female diagnosis
☒ Manifestation code
♂ Male diagnosis

ICD-9-CM Procedural
70.51 Repair of cystocele

57240
57240 Anterior colporrhaphy, repair of cystocele with or without repair of urethrocele

ICD-9-CM Diagnostic
618.00 Prolapse of vaginal walls without mention of uterine prolapse, unspecified
618.01 Cystocele without mention of uterine prolapse, midline
618.02 Cystocele without mention of uterine prolapse, lateral
618.03 Urethrocele without mention of uterine prolapse
618.2 Uterovaginal prolapse, incomplete — (Use additional code to identify urinary incontinence: 625.6, 788.31, 788.33-788.39) ♀
618.3 Uterovaginal prolapse, complete — (Use additional code to identify urinary incontinence: 625.6, 788.31, 788.33-788.39) ♀
618.4 Uterovaginal prolapse, unspecified — (Use additional code to identify urinary incontinence: 625.6, 788.31, 788.33-788.39) ♀
618.89 Other specified genital prolapse
625.6 Female stress incontinence ♀

ICD-9-CM Procedural
70.51 Repair of cystocele

57250
57250 Posterior colporrhaphy, repair of rectocele with or without perineorrhaphy

ICD-9-CM Diagnostic
618.00 Prolapse of vaginal walls without mention of uterine prolapse, unspecified
618.04 Rectocele without mention of uterine prolapse
618.05 Perineocele without mention of uterine prolapse
618.2 Uterovaginal prolapse, incomplete — (Use additional code to identify urinary incontinence: 625.6, 788.31, 788.33-788.39) ♀
618.3 Uterovaginal prolapse, complete — (Use additional code to identify urinary incontinence: 625.6, 788.31, 788.33-788.39) ♀
618.4 Uterovaginal prolapse, unspecified — (Use additional code to identify urinary incontinence: 625.6, 788.31, 788.33-788.39) ♀
618.5 Prolapse of vaginal vault after hysterectomy — (Use additional code to identify urinary incontinence: 625.6, 788.31, 788.33-788.39) ♀
618.6 Vaginal enterocele, congenital or acquired — (Use additional code to identify urinary incontinence: 625.6, 788.31, 788.33-788.39) ♀
618.7 Genital prolapse, old laceration of muscles of pelvic floor — (Use additional code to identify urinary incontinence: 625.6, 788.31, 788.33-788.39) ♀
618.82 Incompetence or weakening of rectovaginal tissue
625.6 Female stress incontinence ♀
788.33 Mixed incontinence urge and stress (male)(female)

ICD-9-CM Procedural
70.52 Repair of rectocele

57260–57265
57260 Combined anteroposterior colporrhaphy;
57265 with enterocele repair

ICD-9-CM Diagnostic
618.00 Prolapse of vaginal walls without mention of uterine prolapse, unspecified
618.04 Rectocele without mention of uterine prolapse
618.05 Perineocele without mention of uterine prolapse
618.09 Other prolapse of vaginal walls without mention of uterine prolapse
618.2 Uterovaginal prolapse, incomplete — (Use additional code to identify urinary incontinence: 625.6, 788.31, 788.33-788.39) ♀
618.3 Uterovaginal prolapse, complete — (Use additional code to identify urinary incontinence: 625.6, 788.31, 788.33-788.39) ♀
618.4 Uterovaginal prolapse, unspecified — (Use additional code to identify urinary incontinence: 625.6, 788.31, 788.33-788.39) ♀
618.5 Prolapse of vaginal vault after hysterectomy — (Use additional code to identify urinary incontinence: 625.6, 788.31, 788.33-788.39) ♀
618.6 Vaginal enterocele, congenital or acquired — (Use additional code to identify urinary incontinence: 625.6, 788.31, 788.33-788.39) ♀
618.7 Genital prolapse, old laceration of muscles of pelvic floor — (Use additional code to identify urinary incontinence: 625.6, 788.31, 788.33-788.39) ♀
618.81 Incompetence or weakening of pubocervical tissue
618.82 Incompetence or weakening of rectovaginal tissue
618.89 Other specified genital prolapse
625.6 Female stress incontinence ♀
788.33 Mixed incontinence urge and stress (male)(female)

ICD-9-CM Procedural
70.50 Repair of cystocele and rectocele
70.92 Other operations on cul-de-sac

57267
57267 Insertion of mesh or other prosthesis for repair of pelvic floor defect, each site (anterior, posterior compartment), vaginal approach (List separately in addition to code for primary procedure)

ICD-9-CM Diagnostic
This is an add-on code. Refer to the corresponding primary procedure code for ICD-9 diagnosis code links.

ICD-9-CM Procedural
70.79 Other repair of vagina

57268–57270
57268 Repair of enterocele, vaginal approach (separate procedure)
57270 Repair of enterocele, abdominal approach (separate procedure)

ICD-9-CM Diagnostic
618.6 Vaginal enterocele, congenital or acquired — (Use additional code to identify urinary incontinence: 625.6, 788.31, 788.33-788.39) ♀
625.6 Female stress incontinence ♀

ICD-9-CM Procedural
70.92 Other operations on cul-de-sac

57280
57280 Colpopexy, abdominal approach

ICD-9-CM Diagnostic
618.00 Prolapse of vaginal walls without mention of uterine prolapse, unspecified
618.03 Urethrocele without mention of uterine prolapse
618.04 Rectocele without mention of uterine prolapse
618.05 Perineocele without mention of uterine prolapse
618.09 Other prolapse of vaginal walls without mention of uterine prolapse
618.1 Uterine prolapse without mention of vaginal wall prolapse — (Use additional code to identify urinary incontinence: 625.6, 788.31, 788.33-788.39) ♀
618.2 Uterovaginal prolapse, incomplete — (Use additional code to identify urinary incontinence: 625.6, 788.31, 788.33-788.39) ♀
618.3 Uterovaginal prolapse, complete — (Use additional code to identify urinary incontinence: 625.6, 788.31, 788.33-788.39) ♀
618.4 Uterovaginal prolapse, unspecified — (Use additional code to identify urinary incontinence: 625.6, 788.31, 788.33-788.39) ♀
618.5 Prolapse of vaginal vault after hysterectomy — (Use additional code to identify urinary incontinence: 625.6, 788.31, 788.33-788.39) ♀
618.81 Incompetence or weakening of pubocervical tissue
618.82 Incompetence or weakening of rectovaginal tissue
618.89 Other specified genital prolapse
625.6 Female stress incontinence ♀

ICD-9-CM Procedural
70.77 Vaginal suspension and fixation

57282–57283
57282 Colpopexy, vaginal; extra-peritoneal approach (sacrospinous, iliococcygeus)
57283 intra-peritoneal approach (uterosacral, levator myorrhaphy)

ICD-9-CM Diagnostic
618.00 Prolapse of vaginal walls without mention of uterine prolapse, unspecified
618.01 Cystocele without mention of uterine prolapse, midline
618.02 Cystocele without mention of uterine prolapse, lateral
618.03 Urethrocele without mention of uterine prolapse
618.04 Rectocele without mention of uterine prolapse
618.05 Perineocele without mention of uterine prolapse
618.09 Other prolapse of vaginal walls without mention of uterine prolapse
618.1 Uterine prolapse without mention of vaginal wall prolapse — (Use additional code to identify urinary incontinence: 625.6, 788.31, 788.33-788.39) ♀
618.2 Uterovaginal prolapse, incomplete — (Use additional code to identify urinary incontinence: 625.6, 788.31, 788.33-788.39) ♀
618.3 Uterovaginal prolapse, complete — (Use additional code to identify urinary incontinence: 625.6, 788.31, 788.33-788.39) ♀
618.4 Uterovaginal prolapse, unspecified — (Use additional code to identify urinary incontinence: 625.6, 788.31, 788.33-788.39) ♀

Unspecified code
♀ Female diagnosis
Manifestation code
♂ Male diagnosis

618.5 Prolapse of vaginal vault after hysterectomy — (Use additional code to identify urinary incontinence: 625.6, 788.31, 788.33-788.39) ♀
618.7 Genital prolapse, old laceration of muscles of pelvic floor — (Use additional code to identify urinary incontinence: 625.6, 788.31, 788.33-788.39) ♀
618.81 Incompetence or weakening of pubocervical tissue
618.82 Incompetence or weakening of rectovaginal tissue
618.83 Pelvic muscle wasting
618.89 Other specified genital prolapse
625.6 Female stress incontinence ♀
788.30 Unspecified urinary incontinence ▽
788.33 Mixed incontinence urge and stress (male)(female)
788.38 Overflow incontinence

ICD-9-CM Procedural
70.77 Vaginal suspension and fixation

57284
57284 Paravaginal defect repair (including repair of cystocele, stress urinary incontinence, and/or incomplete vaginal prolapse)

ICD-9-CM Diagnostic
618.00 Prolapse of vaginal walls without mention of uterine prolapse, unspecified
618.01 Cystocele without mention of uterine prolapse, midline
618.02 Cystocele without mention of uterine prolapse, lateral
618.09 Other prolapse of vaginal walls without mention of uterine prolapse
618.1 Uterine prolapse without mention of vaginal wall prolapse — (Use additional code to identify urinary incontinence: 625.6, 788.31, 788.33-788.39) ♀
618.2 Uterovaginal prolapse, incomplete — (Use additional code to identify urinary incontinence: 625.6, 788.31, 788.33-788.39) ♀
618.3 Uterovaginal prolapse, complete — (Use additional code to identify urinary incontinence: 625.6, 788.31, 788.33-788.39) ♀
618.4 Uterovaginal prolapse, unspecified — (Use additional code to identify urinary incontinence: 625.6, 788.31, 788.33-788.39) ▽ ♀
618.5 Prolapse of vaginal vault after hysterectomy — (Use additional code to identify urinary incontinence: 625.6, 788.31, 788.33-788.39) ♀
618.82 Incompetence or weakening of rectovaginal tissue
618.89 Other specified genital prolapse
625.6 Female stress incontinence ♀

ICD-9-CM Procedural
70.51 Repair of cystocele
70.77 Vaginal suspension and fixation

57287
57287 Removal or revision of sling for stress incontinence (eg, fascia or synthetic)

ICD-9-CM Diagnostic
625.6 Female stress incontinence ♀
996.39 Mechanical complication of genitourinary device, implant, and graft, other
996.65 Infection and inflammatory reaction due to other genitourinary device, implant, and graft — (Use additional code to identify specified infections)
996.76 Other complications due to genitourinary device, implant, and graft
V53.6 Fitting and adjustment of urinary device

ICD-9-CM Procedural
59.79 Other repair of urinary stress incontinence

57288
57288 Sling operation for stress incontinence (eg, fascia or synthetic)

ICD-9-CM Diagnostic
625.6 Female stress incontinence ♀
V64.41 Laparoscopic surgical procedure converted to open procedure

ICD-9-CM Procedural
59.4 Suprapubic sling operation
59.71 Levator muscle operation for urethrovesical suspension
70.77 Vaginal suspension and fixation

57289
57289 Pereyra procedure, including anterior colporrhaphy

ICD-9-CM Diagnostic
618.00 Prolapse of vaginal walls without mention of uterine prolapse, unspecified
618.01 Cystocele without mention of uterine prolapse, midline
618.02 Cystocele without mention of uterine prolapse, lateral
618.03 Urethrocele without mention of uterine prolapse
618.05 Perineocele without mention of uterine prolapse
618.09 Other prolapse of vaginal walls without mention of uterine prolapse
618.1 Uterine prolapse without mention of vaginal wall prolapse — (Use additional code to identify urinary incontinence: 625.6, 788.31, 788.33-788.39) ♀
618.2 Uterovaginal prolapse, incomplete — (Use additional code to identify urinary incontinence: 625.6, 788.31, 788.33-788.39) ♀
618.3 Uterovaginal prolapse, complete — (Use additional code to identify urinary incontinence: 625.6, 788.31, 788.33-788.39) ♀
618.4 Uterovaginal prolapse, unspecified — (Use additional code to identify urinary incontinence: 625.6, 788.31, 788.33-788.39) ▽ ♀
625.6 Female stress incontinence ♀

ICD-9-CM Procedural
59.6 Paraurethral suspension
70.51 Repair of cystocele

57291–57292
57291 Construction of artificial vagina; without graft
57292 with graft

ICD-9-CM Diagnostic
184.0 Malignant neoplasm of vagina ♀
198.82 Secondary malignant neoplasm of genital organs
221.1 Benign neoplasm of vagina ♀
233.3 Carcinoma in situ of other and unspecified female genital organs ▽ ♀
236.3 Neoplasm of uncertain behavior of other and unspecified female genital organs ▽ ♀
239.5 Neoplasm of unspecified nature of other genitourinary organs
752.49 Other congenital anomaly of cervix, vagina, and external female genitalia ♀
959.12 Other injury of abdomen
959.19 Other injury of other sites of trunk
V51 Aftercare involving the use of plastic surgery

ICD-9-CM Procedural
70.61 Vaginal construction
86.63 Full-thickness skin graft to other sites
86.69 Other skin graft to other sites

57300
57300 Closure of rectovaginal fistula; vaginal or transanal approach

ICD-9-CM Diagnostic
619.1 Digestive-genital tract fistula, female ♀
677 Late effect of complication of pregnancy, childbirth, and the puerperium — (Code first any sequelae) ♀

ICD-9-CM Procedural
70.73 Repair of rectovaginal fistula

57305–57307
57305 Closure of rectovaginal fistula; abdominal approach
57307 abdominal approach, with concomitant colostomy

ICD-9-CM Diagnostic
619.1 Digestive-genital tract fistula, female ♀
677 Late effect of complication of pregnancy, childbirth, and the puerperium — (Code first any sequelae) ♀

ICD-9-CM Procedural
46.10 Colostomy, not otherwise specified
70.73 Repair of rectovaginal fistula

57308
57308 Closure of rectovaginal fistula; transperineal approach, with perineal body reconstruction, with or without levator plication

ICD-9-CM Diagnostic
619.1 Digestive-genital tract fistula, female ♀
677 Late effect of complication of pregnancy, childbirth, and the puerperium — (Code first any sequelae) ♀

ICD-9-CM Procedural
70.73 Repair of rectovaginal fistula

57310–57311

57310 Closure of urethrovaginal fistula;
57311 with bulbocavernosus transplant

ICD-9-CM Diagnostic

619.0 Urinary-genital tract fistula, female ♀
677 Late effect of complication of pregnancy, childbirth, and the puerperium — (Code first any sequelae) ♀

ICD-9-CM Procedural

58.43 Closure of other fistula of urethra

57320–57330

57320 Closure of vesicovaginal fistula; vaginal approach
57330 transvesical and vaginal approach

ICD-9-CM Diagnostic

619.0 Urinary-genital tract fistula, female ♀
677 Late effect of complication of pregnancy, childbirth, and the puerperium — (Code first any sequelae) ♀

ICD-9-CM Procedural

57.84 Repair of other fistula of bladder

57335

57335 Vaginoplasty for intersex state

ICD-9-CM Diagnostic

255.2 Adrenogenital disorders
752.40 Unspecified congenital anomaly of cervix, vagina, and external female genitalia ▽ ♀

ICD-9-CM Procedural

70.79 Other repair of vagina

57400

57400 Dilation of vagina under anesthesia

ICD-9-CM Diagnostic

616.8 Other specified inflammatory disease of cervix, vagina, and vulva — (Use additional code to identify organism: 041.0, 041.1) ♀
623.2 Stricture or atresia of vagina — (Use additional E code to identify any external cause) ♀
752.49 Other congenital anomaly of cervix, vagina, and external female genitalia ♀

ICD-9-CM Procedural

96.16 Other vaginal dilation

HCPCS Level II Supplies & Services

A4305 Disposable drug delivery system, flow rate of 50 ml or greater per hour
A4306 Disposable drug delivery system, flow rate of 5 ml or less per hour
A4550 Surgical trays

57410

57410 Pelvic examination under anesthesia

ICD-9-CM Diagnostic

179 Malignant neoplasm of uterus, part unspecified ▽ ♀
180.0 Malignant neoplasm of endocervix ♀
180.1 Malignant neoplasm of exocervix ♀
180.8 Malignant neoplasm of other specified sites of cervix ♀
182.0 Malignant neoplasm of corpus uteri, except isthmus ♀
182.1 Malignant neoplasm of isthmus ♀
182.8 Malignant neoplasm of other specified sites of body of uterus ♀
183.0 Malignant neoplasm of ovary — (Use additional code to identify any functional activity) ♀
183.8 Malignant neoplasm of other specified sites of uterine adnexa ♀
198.82 Secondary malignant neoplasm of genital organs
218.0 Submucous leiomyoma of uterus ♀
218.1 Intramural leiomyoma of uterus ♀
218.2 Subserous leiomyoma of uterus ♀
219.0 Benign neoplasm of cervix uteri ♀
219.1 Benign neoplasm of corpus uteri ♀
219.8 Benign neoplasm of other specified parts of uterus ♀
219.9 Benign neoplasm of uterus, part unspecified ▽ ♀
220 Benign neoplasm of ovary — (Use additional code to identify any functional activity: 256.0-256.1) ♀
233.1 Carcinoma in situ of cervix uteri ♀
233.2 Carcinoma in situ of other and unspecified parts of uterus ▽ ♀
236.0 Neoplasm of uncertain behavior of uterus ♀
236.2 Neoplasm of uncertain behavior of ovary — (Use additional code to identify any functional activity) ♀
239.5 Neoplasm of unspecified nature of other genitourinary organs
256.0 Hyperestrogenism ♀
614.1 Chronic salpingitis and oophoritis — (Use additional code to identify organism: 041.0, 041.1) ♀
614.6 Pelvic peritoneal adhesions, female (postoperative) (postinfection) — (Use additional code to identify any associated infertility, 628.2. Use additional code to identify organism: 041.0, 041.1) ♀
614.9 Unspecified inflammatory disease of female pelvic organs and tissues — (Use additional code to identify organism: 041.0, 041.1) ▽ ♀
616.0 Cervicitis and endocervicitis — (Use additional code to identify organism: 041.0, 041.1) ♀
616.10 Unspecified vaginitis and vulvovaginitis — (Use additional code to identify organism: 041.0, 041.1, 041.4) ▽ ♀
617.0 Endometriosis of uterus ♀
617.1 Endometriosis of ovary ♀
617.3 Endometriosis of pelvic peritoneum ♀
617.4 Endometriosis of rectovaginal septum and vagina ♀
617.5 Endometriosis of intestine ♀
618.00 Prolapse of vaginal walls without mention of uterine prolapse, unspecified
618.09 Other prolapse of vaginal walls without mention of uterine prolapse
618.1 Uterine prolapse without mention of vaginal wall prolapse — (Use additional code to identify urinary incontinence: 625.6, 788.31, 788.33-788.39) ♀
618.81 Incompetence or weakening of pubocervical tissue
618.83 Pelvic muscle wasting
618.89 Other specified genital prolapse
620.0 Follicular cyst of ovary ♀
620.1 Corpus luteum cyst or hematoma ♀
620.2 Other and unspecified ovarian cyst ▽ ♀
620.4 Prolapse or hernia of ovary and fallopian tube ♀
620.5 Torsion of ovary, ovarian pedicle, or fallopian tube ♀
620.8 Other noninflammatory disorder of ovary, fallopian tube, and broad ligament ♀
621.0 Polyp of corpus uteri ♀
621.1 Chronic subinvolution of uterus ♀
621.2 Hypertrophy of uterus ♀
621.30 Endometrial hyperplasia, unspecified
621.31 Simple endometrial hyperplasia without atypia
621.32 Complex endometrial hyperplasia without atypia
621.33 Endometrial hyperplasia with atypia
621.5 Intrauterine synechiae ♀
621.6 Malposition of uterus ♀
621.7 Chronic inversion of uterus ♀
621.8 Other specified disorders of uterus, not elsewhere classified ♀
622.10 Dysplasia of cervix, unspecified
622.11 Mild dysplasia of cervix
622.12 Moderate dysplasia of cervix
622.4 Stricture and stenosis of cervix ♀
622.7 Mucous polyp of cervix ♀
623.5 Leukorrhea, not specified as infective ♀
623.7 Polyp of vagina ♀
623.8 Other specified noninflammatory disorder of vagina ♀
625.0 Dyspareunia ♀
625.1 Vaginismus ♀
625.3 Dysmenorrhea ♀
625.5 Pelvic congestion syndrome ♀
625.6 Female stress incontinence ♀
625.8 Other specified symptom associated with female genital organs ♀
626.0 Absence of menstruation ♀
626.1 Scanty or infrequent menstruation ♀
626.2 Excessive or frequent menstruation ♀
626.4 Irregular menstrual cycle ♀
626.6 Metrorrhagia ♀
626.8 Other disorder of menstruation and other abnormal bleeding from female genital tract ♀
627.1 Postmenopausal bleeding ♀
627.9 Unspecified menopausal and postmenopausal disorder ▽ ♀
628.2 Female infertility of tubal origin — (Use additional code for any associated peritubal adhesions, 614.6) ♀

▽ Unspecified code
♀ Female diagnosis
☒ Manifestation code
♂ Male diagnosis

631 Other abnormal product of conception — (Use additional code from category 639 to identify any associated complications) ♀
632 Missed abortion — (Use additional code from category 639 to identify any associated complications) ♀
633.10 Tubal pregnancy without intrauterine pregnancy — (Use additional code from category 639 to identify any associated complications) ♀
633.11 Tubal pregnancy with intrauterine pregnancy — (Use additional code from category 639 to identify any associated complications) ♀
752.11 Embryonic cyst of fallopian tubes and broad ligaments ♀
789.03 Abdominal pain, right lower quadrant
789.04 Abdominal pain, left lower quadrant
789.05 Abdominal pain, periumbilic
789.07 Abdominal pain, generalized
789.09 Abdominal pain, other specified site
789.30 Abdominal or pelvic swelling, mass or lump, unspecified site ▽
789.31 Abdominal or pelvic swelling, mass, or lump, right upper quadrant
789.32 Abdominal or pelvic swelling, mass, or lump, left upper quadrant
789.33 Abdominal or pelvic swelling, mass, or lump, right lower quadrant
789.34 Abdominal or pelvic swelling, mass, or lump, left lower quadrant
795.00 Abnormal glandular Papanicolaou smear of cervix ▽ ♀
795.01 Papanicolaou smear of cervix with atypical squamous cells of undetermined significance (ASC-US) ♀
795.02 Papanicolaou smear of cervix with atypical squamous cells cannot exclude high grade squamous intraepithelial lesion (ASC-H) ♀
795.03 Papanicolaou smear of cervix with low grade squamous intraepithelial lesion (LGSIL)
795.04 Papanicolaou smear of cervix with high grade squamous intraepithelial lesion (HGSIL)
795.05 Cervical high risk human papillomavirus (HPV) DNA test positive
795.08 Nonspecific abnormal papanicolaou smear of cervix, unsatisfactory smear
795.09 Other abnormal Papanicolaou smear of cervix and cervical HPV ♀
795.1 Nonspecific abnormal Papanicolaou smear of other site ▽
V25.2 Sterilization
V71.5 Observation following alleged rape or seduction
V72.31 Routine gynecological examination

ICD-9-CM Procedural

70.29 Other diagnostic procedures on vagina and cul-de-sac
89.26 Gynecological examination

HCPCS Level II Supplies & Services

A4305 Disposable drug delivery system, flow rate of 50 ml or greater per hour
A4306 Disposable drug delivery system, flow rate of 5 ml or less per hour
A4550 Surgical trays

57415

57415 Removal of impacted vaginal foreign body (separate procedure) under anesthesia

ICD-9-CM Diagnostic

939.2 Foreign body in vulva and vagina ♀

ICD-9-CM Procedural

98.17 Removal of intraluminal foreign body from vagina without incision

HCPCS Level II Supplies & Services

A4305 Disposable drug delivery system, flow rate of 50 ml or greater per hour
A4306 Disposable drug delivery system, flow rate of 5 ml or less per hour
A4550 Surgical trays

57420–57421

57420 Colposcopy of the entire vagina, with cervix if present;
57421 with biopsy(s)

ICD-9-CM Diagnostic

054.11 Herpetic vulvovaginitis ♀
180.0 Malignant neoplasm of endocervix ♀
180.1 Malignant neoplasm of exocervix ♀
180.8 Malignant neoplasm of other specified sites of cervix ♀
180.9 Malignant neoplasm of cervix uteri, unspecified site ▽ ♀
184.0 Malignant neoplasm of vagina ♀
184.8 Malignant neoplasm of other specified sites of female genital organs ♀
184.9 Malignant neoplasm of female genital organ, site unspecified ▽ ♀
198.82 Secondary malignant neoplasm of genital organs
199.1 Other malignant neoplasm of unspecified site
221.1 Benign neoplasm of vagina ♀
221.8 Benign neoplasm of other specified sites of female genital organs ♀
221.9 Benign neoplasm of female genital organ, site unspecified ▽ ♀
233.3 Carcinoma in situ of other and unspecified female genital organs ▽ ♀
236.0 Neoplasm of uncertain behavior of uterus ♀
236.3 Neoplasm of uncertain behavior of other and unspecified female genital organs ▽ ♀
238.9 Neoplasm of uncertain behavior, site unspecified ▽
239.5 Neoplasm of unspecified nature of other genitourinary organs
616.0 Cervicitis and endocervicitis — (Use additional code to identify organism: 041.0, 041.1) ♀
616.10 Unspecified vaginitis and vulvovaginitis — (Use additional code to identify organism: 041.0, 041.1, 041.4) ▽ ♀
616.11 Vaginitis and vulvovaginitis in diseases classified elsewhere — (Code first underlying disease, 127.4.) ☒ ♀
616.2 Cyst of Bartholin's gland — (Use additional code to identify organism: 041.0, 041.1) ♀
616.3 Abscess of Bartholin's gland — (Use additional code to identify organism: 041.0, 041.1) ♀
616.8 Other specified inflammatory disease of cervix, vagina, and vulva — (Use additional code to identify organism: 041.0, 041.1) ♀
617.4 Endometriosis of rectovaginal septum and vagina ♀
617.9 Endometriosis, site unspecified ▽ ♀
623.0 Dysplasia of vagina ♀
623.1 Leukoplakia of vagina ♀
623.2 Stricture or atresia of vagina — (Use additional E code to identify any external cause) ♀
623.4 Old vaginal laceration ♀
623.5 Leukorrhea, not specified as infective ♀
623.6 Vaginal hematoma ♀
623.7 Polyp of vagina ♀
623.8 Other specified noninflammatory disorder of vagina ♀
623.9 Unspecified noninflammatory disorder of vagina ▽ ♀
625.0 Dyspareunia ♀
625.1 Vaginismus ♀
625.3 Dysmenorrhea ♀
625.8 Other specified symptom associated with female genital organs ♀
625.9 Unspecified symptom associated with female genital organs ▽ ♀
626.0 Absence of menstruation ♀
626.1 Scanty or infrequent menstruation ♀
626.2 Excessive or frequent menstruation ♀
626.3 Puberty bleeding ♀
626.4 Irregular menstrual cycle ♀
626.5 Ovulation bleeding ♀
626.6 Metrorrhagia ♀
626.7 Postcoital bleeding ♀
626.8 Other disorder of menstruation and other abnormal bleeding from female genital tract ♀
626.9 Unspecified disorder of menstruation and other abnormal bleeding from female genital tract ▽ ♀
627.0 Premenopausal menorrhagia ♀
627.1 Postmenopausal bleeding ♀
627.2 Symptomatic menopausal or female climacteric states ♀
627.3 Postmenopausal atrophic vaginitis ♀
627.4 Symptomatic states associated with artificial menopause ♀
654.70 Congenital or acquired abnormality of vagina, unspecified as to episode of care in pregnancy — (Code first any associated obstructed labor, 660.2) ▽ ♀
654.71 Congenital or acquired abnormality of vagina, with delivery — (Code first any associated obstructed labor, 660.2) ♀
654.72 Congenital or acquired abnormality of vagina, delivered, with mention of postpartum complication — (Code first any associated obstructed labor, 660.2) ♀
654.73 Congenital or acquired abnormality of vagina, antepartum condition or complication — (Code first any associated obstructed labor, 660.2) ♀
654.74 Congenital or acquired abnormality of vagina, postpartum condition or complication — (Code first any associated obstructed labor, 660.2) ♀
752.40 Unspecified congenital anomaly of cervix, vagina, and external female genitalia ▽ ♀
752.41 Embryonic cyst of cervix, vagina, and external female genitalia ♀
752.49 Other congenital anomaly of cervix, vagina, and external female genitalia ♀
789.00 Abdominal pain, unspecified site ▽
789.01 Abdominal pain, right upper quadrant
789.02 Abdominal pain, left upper quadrant
789.03 Abdominal pain, right lower quadrant
789.04 Abdominal pain, left lower quadrant
789.30 Abdominal or pelvic swelling, mass or lump, unspecified site ▽
789.31 Abdominal or pelvic swelling, mass, or lump, right upper quadrant

▽ Unspecified code
♀ Female diagnosis
☒ Manifestation code
♂ Male diagnosis

789.32 Abdominal or pelvic swelling, mass, or lump, left upper quadrant
789.33 Abdominal or pelvic swelling, mass, or lump, right lower quadrant
789.34 Abdominal or pelvic swelling, mass, or lump, left lower quadrant
795.1 Nonspecific abnormal Papanicolaou smear of other site ▽
795.39 Other nonspecific positive culture findings
796.0 Nonspecific abnormal toxicological findings
V10.40 Personal history of malignant neoplasm of unspecified female genital organ ▽ ♀
V10.41 Personal history of malignant neoplasm of cervix uteri ♀
V10.42 Personal history of malignant neoplasm of other parts of uterus ♀
V10.44 Personal history of malignant neoplasm of other female genital organs ♀
V13.29 Personal history of other genital system and obstetric disorders
V67.00 Follow-up examination, following unspecified surgery ▽
V67.01 Following surgery follow-up vaginal pap smear — (Use additional code to identify condition: V10.40-V10.44, V45.77) ♀
V67.09 Follow-up examination, following other surgery
V71.5 Observation following alleged rape or seduction
V71.6 Observation following other inflicted injury
V76.47 Special screening for malignant neoplasms, vagina — (Use additional code to identify acquired absence of uterus, V45.77) ♀
V84.02 Genetic susceptibility to malignant neoplasm of ovary
V84.04 Genetic susceptibility to malignant neoplasm of endometrium
V84.09 Genetic susceptibility to other malignant neoplasm

ICD-9-CM Procedural

70.21 Vaginoscopy
70.23 Biopsy of cul-de-sac
70.24 Vaginal biopsy

HCPCS Level II Supplies & Services

A4550 Surgical trays

57425

57425 Laparoscopy, surgical, colpopexy (suspension of vaginal apex)

ICD-9-CM Diagnostic

618.00 Prolapse of vaginal walls without mention of uterine prolapse, unspecified
618.09 Other prolapse of vaginal walls without mention of uterine prolapse
618.1 Uterine prolapse without mention of vaginal wall prolapse — (Use additional code to identify urinary incontinence: 625.6, 788.31, 788.33-788.39) ♀
618.2 Uterovaginal prolapse, incomplete — (Use additional code to identify urinary incontinence: 625.6, 788.31, 788.33-788.39) ♀
618.3 Uterovaginal prolapse, complete — (Use additional code to identify urinary incontinence: 625.6, 788.31, 788.33-788.39) ♀
618.4 Uterovaginal prolapse, unspecified — (Use additional code to identify urinary incontinence: 625.6, 788.31, 788.33-788.39) ▽ ♀
618.5 Prolapse of vaginal vault after hysterectomy — (Use additional code to identify urinary incontinence: 625.6, 788.31, 788.33-788.39) ♀
618.82 Incompetence or weakening of rectovaginal tissue
618.89 Other specified genital prolapse
625.6 Female stress incontinence ♀

ICD-9-CM Procedural

70.77 Vaginal suspension and fixation

57452–57461

57452 Colposcopy of the cervix including upper/adjacent vagina;
57454 with biopsy(s) of the cervix and endocervical curettage
57455 with biopsy(s) of the cervix
57456 with endocervical curettage
57460 with loop electrode biopsy(s) of the cervix
57461 with loop electrode conization of the cervix

ICD-9-CM Diagnostic

180.0 Malignant neoplasm of endocervix ♀
180.1 Malignant neoplasm of exocervix ♀
180.8 Malignant neoplasm of other specified sites of cervix ♀
180.9 Malignant neoplasm of cervix uteri, unspecified site ▽ ♀
182.0 Malignant neoplasm of corpus uteri, except isthmus ♀
182.1 Malignant neoplasm of isthmus ♀
182.8 Malignant neoplasm of other specified sites of body of uterus ♀
184.0 Malignant neoplasm of vagina ♀
198.82 Secondary malignant neoplasm of genital organs
199.1 Other malignant neoplasm of unspecified site
219.0 Benign neoplasm of cervix uteri ♀
221.2 Benign neoplasm of vulva ♀
221.8 Benign neoplasm of other specified sites of female genital organs ♀
233.1 Carcinoma in situ of cervix uteri ♀
233.3 Carcinoma in situ of other and unspecified female genital organs ▽ ♀
236.0 Neoplasm of uncertain behavior of uterus ♀
236.3 Neoplasm of uncertain behavior of other and unspecified female genital organs ▽ ♀
239.5 Neoplasm of unspecified nature of other genitourinary organs
616.0 Cervicitis and endocervicitis — (Use additional code to identify organism: 041.0, 041.1) ♀
616.10 Unspecified vaginitis and vulvovaginitis — (Use additional code to identify organism: 041.0, 041.1, 041.4) ▽ ♀
616.11 Vaginitis and vulvovaginitis in diseases classified elsewhere — (Code first underlying disease, 127.4.) ☒ ♀
616.8 Other specified inflammatory disease of cervix, vagina, and vulva — (Use additional code to identify organism: 041.0, 041.1) ♀
616.9 Unspecified inflammatory disease of cervix, vagina, and vulva — (Use additional code to identify organism: 041.0, 041.1) ▽ ♀
617.4 Endometriosis of rectovaginal septum and vagina ♀
617.9 Endometriosis, site unspecified ▽ ♀
622.0 Erosion and ectropion of cervix ♀
622.10 Dysplasia of cervix, unspecified
622.11 Mild dysplasia of cervix
622.12 Moderate dysplasia of cervix
622.2 Leukoplakia of cervix (uteri) ♀
622.3 Old laceration of cervix ♀
622.4 Stricture and stenosis of cervix ♀
622.5 Incompetence of cervix ♀
622.6 Hypertrophic elongation of cervix ♀
622.7 Mucous polyp of cervix ♀
622.8 Other specified noninflammatory disorder of cervix ♀
622.9 Unspecified noninflammatory disorder of cervix ▽ ♀
625.0 Dyspareunia ♀
625.3 Dysmenorrhea ♀
625.8 Other specified symptom associated with female genital organs ♀
625.9 Unspecified symptom associated with female genital organs ▽ ♀
626.0 Absence of menstruation ♀
626.1 Scanty or infrequent menstruation ♀
626.2 Excessive or frequent menstruation ♀
626.3 Puberty bleeding ♀
626.4 Irregular menstrual cycle ♀
626.5 Ovulation bleeding ♀
626.6 Metrorrhagia ♀
626.7 Postcoital bleeding ♀
626.8 Other disorder of menstruation and other abnormal bleeding from female genital tract ♀
626.9 Unspecified disorder of menstruation and other abnormal bleeding from female genital tract ▽ ♀
627.0 Premenopausal menorrhagia ♀
627.1 Postmenopausal bleeding ♀
627.4 Symptomatic states associated with artificial menopause ♀
654.60 Other congenital or acquired abnormality of cervix, unspecified as to episode of care in pregnancy — (Code first any associated obstructed labor, 660.2) ▽ ♀
654.61 Other congenital or acquired abnormality of cervix, with delivery — (Code first any associated obstructed labor, 660.2) ♀
654.62 Other congenital or acquired abnormality of cervix, delivered, with mention of postpartum complication — (Code first any associated obstructed labor, 660.2) ♀
654.63 Other congenital or acquired abnormality of cervix, antepartum condition or complication — (Code first any associated obstructed labor, 660.2) ♀
654.64 Other congenital or acquired abnormality of cervix, postpartum condition or complication — (Code first any associated obstructed labor, 660.2) ♀
752.40 Unspecified congenital anomaly of cervix, vagina, and external female genitalia ▽ ♀
752.41 Embryonic cyst of cervix, vagina, and external female genitalia ♀
752.49 Other congenital anomaly of cervix, vagina, and external female genitalia ♀
789.00 Abdominal pain, unspecified site ▽
789.01 Abdominal pain, right upper quadrant
789.02 Abdominal pain, left upper quadrant
789.03 Abdominal pain, right lower quadrant
789.04 Abdominal pain, left lower quadrant
789.30 Abdominal or pelvic swelling, mass or lump, unspecified site ▽
789.31 Abdominal or pelvic swelling, mass, or lump, right upper quadrant
789.32 Abdominal or pelvic swelling, mass, or lump, left upper quadrant
789.33 Abdominal or pelvic swelling, mass, or lump, right lower quadrant
789.34 Abdominal or pelvic swelling, mass, or lump, left lower quadrant
795.00 Abnormal glandular Papanicolaou smear of cervix ▽ ♀

▽ Unspecified code
♀ Female diagnosis
☒ Manifestation code
♂ Male diagnosis

795.01 Papanicolaou smear of cervix with atypical squamous cells of undetermined significance (ASC-US) ♀
795.02 Papanicolaou smear of cervix with atypical squamous cells cannot exclude high grade squamous intraepithelial lesion (ASC-H) ♀
795.03 Papanicolaou smear of cervix with low grade squamous intraepithelial lesion (LGSIL)
795.04 Papanicolaou smear of cervix with high grade squamous intraepithelial lesion (HGSIL)
795.05 Cervical high risk human papillomavirus (HPV) DNA test positive
795.08 Nonspecific abnormal papanicolaou smear of cervix, unsatisfactory smear
795.09 Other abnormal Papanicolaou smear of cervix and cervical HPV ♀
795.1 Nonspecific abnormal Papanicolaou smear of other site
795.39 Other nonspecific positive culture findings
796.0 Nonspecific abnormal toxicological findings
V10.40 Personal history of malignant neoplasm of unspecified female genital organ ♀
V10.41 Personal history of malignant neoplasm of cervix uteri ♀
V10.42 Personal history of malignant neoplasm of other parts of uterus ♀
V13.29 Personal history of other genital system and obstetric disorders
V67.00 Follow-up examination, following unspecified surgery
V67.09 Follow-up examination, following other surgery
V71.5 Observation following alleged rape or seduction
V71.6 Observation following other inflicted injury
V76.2 Screening for malignant neoplasm of the cervix ♀
V84.02 Genetic susceptibility to malignant neoplasm of ovary
V84.04 Genetic susceptibility to malignant neoplasm of endometrium
V84.09 Genetic susceptibility to other malignant neoplasm

ICD-9-CM Procedural
67.11 Endocervical biopsy
67.12 Other cervical biopsy
67.32 Destruction of lesion of cervix by cauterization
70.21 Vaginoscopy

HCPCS Level II Supplies & Services
A4305 Disposable drug delivery system, flow rate of 50 ml or greater per hour
A4306 Disposable drug delivery system, flow rate of 5 ml or less per hour
A4480 VABRA aspirator
A4550 Surgical trays

57500
57500 Biopsy, single or multiple, or local excision of lesion, with or without fulguration (separate procedure)

ICD-9-CM Diagnostic
180.0 Malignant neoplasm of endocervix ♀
180.1 Malignant neoplasm of exocervix ♀
180.8 Malignant neoplasm of other specified sites of cervix ♀
180.9 Malignant neoplasm of cervix uteri, unspecified site ♀
182.0 Malignant neoplasm of corpus uteri, except isthmus ♀
198.82 Secondary malignant neoplasm of genital organs
218.2 Subserous leiomyoma of uterus ♀
218.9 Leiomyoma of uterus, unspecified ♀
219.0 Benign neoplasm of cervix uteri ♀
221.8 Benign neoplasm of other specified sites of female genital organs ♀
221.9 Benign neoplasm of female genital organ, site unspecified ♀
228.00 Hemangioma of unspecified site
228.01 Hemangioma of skin and subcutaneous tissue
229.8 Benign neoplasm of other specified sites
233.1 Carcinoma in situ of cervix uteri ♀
236.0 Neoplasm of uncertain behavior of uterus ♀
239.5 Neoplasm of unspecified nature of other genitourinary organs
616.0 Cervicitis and endocervicitis — (Use additional code to identify organism: 041.0, 041.1) ♀
617.0 Endometriosis of uterus ♀
622.0 Erosion and ectropion of cervix ♀
622.10 Dysplasia of cervix, unspecified
622.11 Mild dysplasia of cervix
622.12 Moderate dysplasia of cervix
622.2 Leukoplakia of cervix (uteri) ♀
622.7 Mucous polyp of cervix ♀
622.8 Other specified noninflammatory disorder of cervix ♀
623.5 Leukorrhea, not specified as infective ♀
623.7 Polyp of vagina ♀
623.8 Other specified noninflammatory disorder of vagina ♀
625.3 Dysmenorrhea ♀

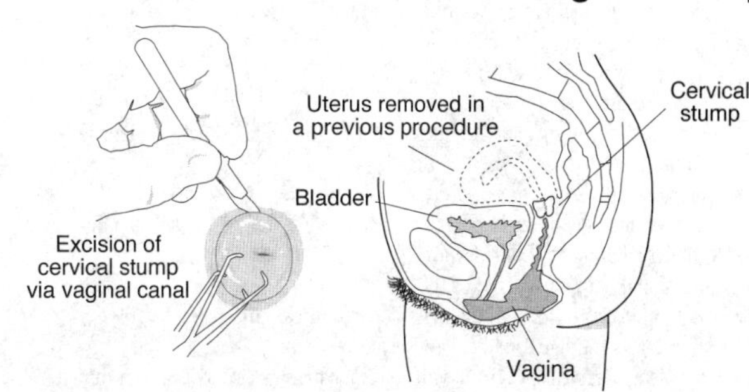

625.8 Other specified symptom associated with female genital organs ♀
626.2 Excessive or frequent menstruation ♀
626.4 Irregular menstrual cycle ♀
626.6 Metrorrhagia ♀
626.8 Other disorder of menstruation and other abnormal bleeding from female genital tract ♀
795.00 Abnormal glandular Papanicolaou smear of cervix ♀
795.01 Papanicolaou smear of cervix with atypical squamous cells of undetermined significance (ASC-US) ♀
795.02 Papanicolaou smear of cervix with atypical squamous cells cannot exclude high grade squamous intraepithelial lesion (ASC-H) ♀
795.03 Papanicolaou smear of cervix with low grade squamous intraepithelial lesion (LGSIL)
795.04 Papanicolaou smear of cervix with high grade squamous intraepithelial lesion (HGSIL)
795.05 Cervical high risk human papillomavirus (HPV) DNA test positive
795.08 Nonspecific abnormal papanicolaou smear of cervix, unsatisfactory smear
795.09 Other abnormal Papanicolaou smear of cervix and cervical HPV ♀
V76.2 Screening for malignant neoplasm of the cervix ♀
V84.02 Genetic susceptibility to malignant neoplasm of ovary
V84.04 Genetic susceptibility to malignant neoplasm of endometrium
V84.09 Genetic susceptibility to other malignant neoplasm

ICD-9-CM Procedural
67.11 Endocervical biopsy
67.12 Other cervical biopsy
67.31 Marsupialization of cervical cyst
67.39 Other excision or destruction of lesion or tissue of cervix

HCPCS Level II Supplies & Services
A4550 Surgical trays

57505
57505 Endocervical curettage (not done as part of a dilation and curettage)

ICD-9-CM Diagnostic
180.0 Malignant neoplasm of endocervix ♀
180.8 Malignant neoplasm of other specified sites of cervix ♀
218.0 Submucous leiomyoma of uterus ♀
218.2 Subserous leiomyoma of uterus ♀
218.9 Leiomyoma of uterus, unspecified ♀
219.0 Benign neoplasm of cervix uteri ♀
233.1 Carcinoma in situ of cervix uteri ♀
236.0 Neoplasm of uncertain behavior of uterus ♀
616.0 Cervicitis and endocervicitis — (Use additional code to identify organism: 041.0, 041.1) ♀
616.8 Other specified inflammatory disease of cervix, vagina, and vulva — (Use additional code to identify organism: 041.0, 041.1) ♀
617.0 Endometriosis of uterus ♀
622.0 Erosion and ectropion of cervix ♀
622.10 Dysplasia of cervix, unspecified
622.11 Mild dysplasia of cervix
622.12 Moderate dysplasia of cervix
622.2 Leukoplakia of cervix (uteri) ♀
622.7 Mucous polyp of cervix ♀
622.8 Other specified noninflammatory disorder of cervix ♀
623.0 Dysplasia of vagina ♀
623.1 Leukoplakia of vagina ♀
623.5 Leukorrhea, not specified as infective ♀

Unspecified code
♀ Female diagnosis
Manifestation code
♂ Male diagnosis

623.8 Other specified noninflammatory disorder of vagina ♀
625.3 Dysmenorrhea ♀
626.0 Absence of menstruation ♀
626.2 Excessive or frequent menstruation ♀
626.4 Irregular menstrual cycle ♀
626.6 Metrorrhagia ♀
626.8 Other disorder of menstruation and other abnormal bleeding from female genital tract ♀
627.1 Postmenopausal bleeding ♀
752.49 Other congenital anomaly of cervix, vagina, and external female genitalia ♀
759.0 Congenital anomalies of spleen
789.00 Abdominal pain, unspecified site
789.30 Abdominal or pelvic swelling, mass or lump, unspecified site
795.00 Abnormal glandular Papanicolaou smear of cervix ♀
795.01 Papanicolaou smear of cervix with atypical squamous cells of undetermined significance (ASC-US) ♀
795.02 Papanicolaou smear of cervix with atypical squamous cells cannot exclude high grade squamous intraepithelial lesion (ASC-H) ♀
795.03 Papanicolaou smear of cervix with low grade squamous intraepithelial lesion (LGSIL)
795.04 Papanicolaou smear of cervix with high grade squamous intraepithelial lesion (HGSIL)
795.05 Cervical high risk human papillomavirus (HPV) DNA test positive
795.08 Nonspecific abnormal papanicolaou smear of cervix, unsatisfactory smear
795.09 Other abnormal Papanicolaou smear of cervix and cervical HPV ♀
795.1 Nonspecific abnormal Papanicolaou smear of other site
795.39 Other nonspecific positive culture findings
V84.02 Genetic susceptibility to malignant neoplasm of ovary
V84.04 Genetic susceptibility to malignant neoplasm of endometrium
V84.09 Genetic susceptibility to other malignant neoplasm

ICD-9-CM Procedural

69.09 Other dilation and curettage of uterus

HCPCS Level II Supplies & Services

A4305 Disposable drug delivery system, flow rate of 50 ml or greater per hour
A4306 Disposable drug delivery system, flow rate of 5 ml or less per hour
A4550 Surgical trays

57510–57513

57510 Cautery of cervix; electro or thermal
57511 cryocautery, initial or repeat
57513 laser ablation

ICD-9-CM Diagnostic

180.1 Malignant neoplasm of exocervix ♀
180.8 Malignant neoplasm of other specified sites of cervix ♀
219.0 Benign neoplasm of cervix uteri ♀
233.1 Carcinoma in situ of cervix uteri ♀
236.0 Neoplasm of uncertain behavior of uterus ♀
239.5 Neoplasm of unspecified nature of other genitourinary organs
616.0 Cervicitis and endocervicitis — (Use additional code to identify organism: 041.0, 041.1) ♀
616.8 Other specified inflammatory disease of cervix, vagina, and vulva — (Use additional code to identify organism: 041.0, 041.1) ♀
617.0 Endometriosis of uterus ♀
622.0 Erosion and ectropion of cervix ♀
622.10 Dysplasia of cervix, unspecified
622.11 Mild dysplasia of cervix
622.12 Moderate dysplasia of cervix
622.2 Leukoplakia of cervix (uteri) ♀
622.6 Hypertrophic elongation of cervix ♀
622.7 Mucous polyp of cervix ♀
622.8 Other specified noninflammatory disorder of cervix ♀
625.0 Dyspareunia ♀
625.3 Dysmenorrhea ♀
626.2 Excessive or frequent menstruation ♀
626.6 Metrorrhagia ♀
626.7 Postcoital bleeding ♀
626.8 Other disorder of menstruation and other abnormal bleeding from female genital tract ♀
627.1 Postmenopausal bleeding ♀
752.40 Unspecified congenital anomaly of cervix, vagina, and external female genitalia ♀
752.49 Other congenital anomaly of cervix, vagina, and external female genitalia ♀
795.00 Abnormal glandular Papanicolaou smear of cervix ♀
795.01 Papanicolaou smear of cervix with atypical squamous cells of undetermined significance (ASC-US) ♀
795.02 Papanicolaou smear of cervix with atypical squamous cells cannot exclude high grade squamous intraepithelial lesion (ASC-H) ♀
795.03 Papanicolaou smear of cervix with low grade squamous intraepithelial lesion (LGSIL)
795.04 Papanicolaou smear of cervix with high grade squamous intraepithelial lesion (HGSIL)
795.05 Cervical high risk human papillomavirus (HPV) DNA test positive
795.08 Nonspecific abnormal papanicolaou smear of cervix, unsatisfactory smear
795.09 Other abnormal Papanicolaou smear of cervix and cervical HPV ♀
V84.02 Genetic susceptibility to malignant neoplasm of ovary
V84.04 Genetic susceptibility to malignant neoplasm of endometrium
V84.09 Genetic susceptibility to other malignant neoplasm

ICD-9-CM Procedural

67.32 Destruction of lesion of cervix by cauterization
67.33 Destruction of lesion of cervix by cryosurgery
67.39 Other excision or destruction of lesion or tissue of cervix

HCPCS Level II Supplies & Services

A4305 Disposable drug delivery system, flow rate of 50 ml or greater per hour
A4306 Disposable drug delivery system, flow rate of 5 ml or less per hour
A4550 Surgical trays

57520–57522

57520 Conization of cervix, with or without fulguration, with or without dilation and curettage, with or without repair; cold knife or laser
57522 loop electrode excision

ICD-9-CM Diagnostic

180.0 Malignant neoplasm of endocervix ♀
180.1 Malignant neoplasm of exocervix ♀
180.8 Malignant neoplasm of other specified sites of cervix ♀
180.9 Malignant neoplasm of cervix uteri, unspecified site ♀
198.82 Secondary malignant neoplasm of genital organs
199.1 Other malignant neoplasm of unspecified site
219.0 Benign neoplasm of cervix uteri ♀
233.1 Carcinoma in situ of cervix uteri ♀
233.3 Carcinoma in situ of other and unspecified female genital organs ♀
236.0 Neoplasm of uncertain behavior of uterus ♀
239.5 Neoplasm of unspecified nature of other genitourinary organs
616.0 Cervicitis and endocervicitis — (Use additional code to identify organism: 041.0, 041.1) ♀
622.0 Erosion and ectropion of cervix ♀
622.10 Dysplasia of cervix, unspecified
622.11 Mild dysplasia of cervix
622.12 Moderate dysplasia of cervix
622.6 Hypertrophic elongation of cervix ♀
622.7 Mucous polyp of cervix ♀
622.8 Other specified noninflammatory disorder of cervix ♀
623.0 Dysplasia of vagina ♀
625.3 Dysmenorrhea ♀
625.9 Unspecified symptom associated with female genital organs ♀
626.2 Excessive or frequent menstruation ♀
626.4 Irregular menstrual cycle ♀
626.6 Metrorrhagia ♀
626.8 Other disorder of menstruation and other abnormal bleeding from female genital tract ♀
627.1 Postmenopausal bleeding ♀
795.00 Abnormal glandular Papanicolaou smear of cervix ♀
795.01 Papanicolaou smear of cervix with atypical squamous cells of undetermined significance (ASC-US) ♀
795.02 Papanicolaou smear of cervix with atypical squamous cells cannot exclude high grade squamous intraepithelial lesion (ASC-H) ♀
795.03 Papanicolaou smear of cervix with low grade squamous intraepithelial lesion (LGSIL)
795.04 Papanicolaou smear of cervix with high grade squamous intraepithelial lesion (HGSIL)
795.05 Cervical high risk human papillomavirus (HPV) DNA test positive
795.08 Nonspecific abnormal papanicolaou smear of cervix, unsatisfactory smear
795.09 Other abnormal Papanicolaou smear of cervix and cervical HPV ♀
V84.02 Genetic susceptibility to malignant neoplasm of ovary
V84.04 Genetic susceptibility to malignant neoplasm of endometrium
V84.09 Genetic susceptibility to other malignant neoplasm

ICD-9-CM Procedural
67.2 Conization of cervix
67.32 Destruction of lesion of cervix by cauterization
69.09 Other dilation and curettage of uterus

HCPCS Level II Supplies & Services
A4305 Disposable drug delivery system, flow rate of 50 ml or greater per hour
A4306 Disposable drug delivery system, flow rate of 5 ml or less per hour
A4550 Surgical trays

57530–57531
57530 Trachelectomy (cervicectomy), amputation of cervix (separate procedure)
57531 Radical trachelectomy, with bilateral total pelvic lymphadenectomy and para-aortic lymph node sampling biopsy, with or without removal of tube(s), with or without removal of ovary(s)

ICD-9-CM Diagnostic
180.0 Malignant neoplasm of endocervix ♀
180.1 Malignant neoplasm of exocervix ♀
180.8 Malignant neoplasm of other specified sites of cervix ♀
196.2 Secondary and unspecified malignant neoplasm of intra-abdominal lymph nodes
196.6 Secondary and unspecified malignant neoplasm of intrapelvic lymph nodes
219.0 Benign neoplasm of cervix uteri ♀
233.1 Carcinoma in situ of cervix uteri ♀
236.0 Neoplasm of uncertain behavior of uterus ♀
239.5 Neoplasm of unspecified nature of other genitourinary organs
622.10 Dysplasia of cervix, unspecified
622.11 Mild dysplasia of cervix
622.12 Moderate dysplasia of cervix
795.00 Abnormal glandular Papanicolaou smear of cervix ▽ ♀
795.01 Papanicolaou smear of cervix with atypical squamous cells of undetermined significance (ASC-US) ♀
795.02 Papanicolaou smear of cervix with atypical squamous cells cannot exclude high grade squamous intraepithelial lesion (ASC-H) ♀
795.03 Papanicolaou smear of cervix with low grade squamous intraepithelial lesion (LGSIL)
795.09 Other abnormal Papanicolaou smear of cervix and cervical HPV ♀
V10.42 Personal history of malignant neoplasm of other parts of uterus ♀
V84.01 Genetic susceptibility to malignant neoplasm of breast
V84.02 Genetic susceptibility to malignant neoplasm of ovary
V84.04 Genetic susceptibility to malignant neoplasm of endometrium
V84.09 Genetic susceptibility to other malignant neoplasm

ICD-9-CM Procedural
40.53 Radical excision of iliac lymph nodes
40.59 Radical excision of other lymph nodes
65.39 Other unilateral oophorectomy
65.49 Other unilateral salpingo-oophorectomy
65.51 Other removal of both ovaries at same operative episode
65.61 Other removal of both ovaries and tubes at same operative episode
65.62 Other removal of remaining ovary and tube
66.4 Total unilateral salpingectomy
66.51 Removal of both fallopian tubes at same operative episode
66.52 Removal of remaining fallopian tube
67.4 Amputation of cervix

57540–57545
57540 Excision of cervical stump, abdominal approach;
57545 with pelvic floor repair

ICD-9-CM Diagnostic
180.0 Malignant neoplasm of endocervix ♀
180.1 Malignant neoplasm of exocervix ♀
180.8 Malignant neoplasm of other specified sites of cervix ♀
219.0 Benign neoplasm of cervix uteri ♀
233.1 Carcinoma in situ of cervix uteri ♀
236.0 Neoplasm of uncertain behavior of uterus ♀
239.5 Neoplasm of unspecified nature of other genitourinary organs
618.7 Genital prolapse, old laceration of muscles of pelvic floor — (Use additional code to identify urinary incontinence: 625.6, 788.31, 788.33-788.39) ♀
622.0 Erosion and ectropion of cervix ♀
622.10 Dysplasia of cervix, unspecified
622.11 Mild dysplasia of cervix
622.12 Moderate dysplasia of cervix
625.6 Female stress incontinence ♀
795.00 Abnormal glandular Papanicolaou smear of cervix ▽ ♀
795.01 Papanicolaou smear of cervix with atypical squamous cells of undetermined significance (ASC-US) ♀
795.02 Papanicolaou smear of cervix with atypical squamous cells cannot exclude high grade squamous intraepithelial lesion (ASC-H) ♀
795.04 Papanicolaou smear of cervix with high grade squamous intraepithelial lesion (HGSIL)
795.05 Cervical high risk human papillomavirus (HPV) DNA test positive
795.08 Nonspecific abnormal papanicolaou smear of cervix, unsatisfactory smear
795.09 Other abnormal Papanicolaou smear of cervix and cervical HPV ♀
V84.02 Genetic susceptibility to malignant neoplasm of ovary
V84.04 Genetic susceptibility to malignant neoplasm of endometrium
V84.09 Genetic susceptibility to other malignant neoplasm

ICD-9-CM Procedural
67.4 Amputation of cervix
70.79 Other repair of vagina

57550
57550 Excision of cervical stump, vaginal approach;

ICD-9-CM Diagnostic
180.0 Malignant neoplasm of endocervix ♀
180.1 Malignant neoplasm of exocervix ♀
180.8 Malignant neoplasm of other specified sites of cervix ♀
219.0 Benign neoplasm of cervix uteri ♀
233.1 Carcinoma in situ of cervix uteri ♀
236.0 Neoplasm of uncertain behavior of uterus ♀
239.5 Neoplasm of unspecified nature of other genitourinary organs
622.0 Erosion and ectropion of cervix ♀
622.10 Dysplasia of cervix, unspecified
622.11 Mild dysplasia of cervix
622.12 Moderate dysplasia of cervix
795.00 Abnormal glandular Papanicolaou smear of cervix ▽ ♀
795.01 Papanicolaou smear of cervix with atypical squamous cells of undetermined significance (ASC-US) ♀
795.02 Papanicolaou smear of cervix with atypical squamous cells cannot exclude high grade squamous intraepithelial lesion (ASC-H) ♀
795.03 Papanicolaou smear of cervix with low grade squamous intraepithelial lesion (LGSIL)
795.04 Papanicolaou smear of cervix with high grade squamous intraepithelial lesion (HGSIL)
795.05 Cervical high risk human papillomavirus (HPV) DNA test positive
795.08 Nonspecific abnormal papanicolaou smear of cervix, unsatisfactory smear
795.09 Other abnormal Papanicolaou smear of cervix and cervical HPV ♀
V84.02 Genetic susceptibility to malignant neoplasm of ovary
V84.04 Genetic susceptibility to malignant neoplasm of endometrium
V84.09 Genetic susceptibility to other malignant neoplasm

ICD-9-CM Procedural
67.4 Amputation of cervix

57555–57556
57555 Excision of cervical stump, vaginal approach; with anterior and/or posterior repair
57556 with repair of enterocele

ICD-9-CM Diagnostic
180.0 Malignant neoplasm of endocervix ♀
180.1 Malignant neoplasm of exocervix ♀
180.8 Malignant neoplasm of other specified sites of cervix ♀
219.0 Benign neoplasm of cervix uteri ♀
233.1 Carcinoma in situ of cervix uteri ♀
236.0 Neoplasm of uncertain behavior of uterus ♀
239.5 Neoplasm of unspecified nature of other genitourinary organs
617.0 Endometriosis of uterus ♀
618.00 Prolapse of vaginal walls without mention of uterine prolapse, unspecified
618.03 Urethrocele without mention of uterine prolapse
618.04 Rectocele without mention of uterine prolapse
618.05 Perineocele without mention of uterine prolapse
618.1 Uterine prolapse without mention of vaginal wall prolapse — (Use additional code to identify urinary incontinence: 625.6, 788.31, 788.33-788.39) ♀
618.2 Uterovaginal prolapse, incomplete — (Use additional code to identify urinary incontinence: 625.6, 788.31, 788.33-788.39) ♀

▽ Unspecified code ♀ Female diagnosis ☒ Manifestation code ♂ Male diagnosis

618.5 Prolapse of vaginal vault after hysterectomy — (Use additional code to identify urinary incontinence: 625.6, 788.31, 788.33-788.39) ♀
618.6 Vaginal enterocele, congenital or acquired — (Use additional code to identify urinary incontinence: 625.6, 788.31, 788.33-788.39) ♀
618.81 Incompetence or weakening of pubocervical tissue
618.82 Incompetence or weakening of rectovaginal tissue
622.0 Erosion and ectropion of cervix ♀
622.10 Dysplasia of cervix, unspecified
622.11 Mild dysplasia of cervix
622.12 Moderate dysplasia of cervix
622.2 Leukoplakia of cervix (uteri) ♀
622.8 Other specified noninflammatory disorder of cervix ♀
625.6 Female stress incontinence ♀
795.00 Abnormal glandular Papanicolaou smear of cervix ▽ ♀
795.01 Papanicolaou smear of cervix with atypical squamous cells of undetermined significance (ASC-US) ♀
795.02 Papanicolaou smear of cervix with atypical squamous cells cannot exclude high grade squamous intraepithelial lesion (ASC-H) ♀
795.03 Papanicolaou smear of cervix with low grade squamous intraepithelial lesion (LGSIL)
795.04 Papanicolaou smear of cervix with high grade squamous intraepithelial lesion (HGSIL)
795.05 Cervical high risk human papillomavirus (HPV) DNA test positive
795.08 Nonspecific abnormal papanicolaou smear of cervix, unsatisfactory smear
795.09 Other abnormal Papanicolaou smear of cervix and cervical HPV ♀
V84.02 Genetic susceptibility to malignant neoplasm of ovary
V84.04 Genetic susceptibility to malignant neoplasm of endometrium
V84.09 Genetic susceptibility to other malignant neoplasm

ICD-9-CM Procedural

67.4 Amputation of cervix
70.50 Repair of cystocele and rectocele
70.92 Other operations on cul-de-sac

57700

57700 Cerclage of uterine cervix, nonobstetrical

ICD-9-CM Diagnostic

622.5 Incompetence of cervix ♀
654.54 Cervical incompetence, postpartum condition or complication — (Code first any associated obstructed labor, 660.2) ♀
867.4 Uterus injury without mention of open wound into cavity ♀

ICD-9-CM Procedural

67.59 Other repair of cervical os

HCPCS Level II Supplies & Services

A4550 Surgical trays

57720

57720 Trachelorrhaphy, plastic repair of uterine cervix, vaginal approach

ICD-9-CM Diagnostic

622.3 Old laceration of cervix ♀
622.5 Incompetence of cervix ♀
665.31 Laceration of cervix, with delivery ♀
665.34 Laceration of cervix, postpartum ♀
867.4 Uterus injury without mention of open wound into cavity ♀

ICD-9-CM Procedural

67.69 Other repair of cervix

57800

57800 Dilation of cervical canal, instrumental (separate procedure)

ICD-9-CM Diagnostic

622.4 Stricture and stenosis of cervix ♀
622.8 Other specified noninflammatory disorder of cervix ♀
626.8 Other disorder of menstruation and other abnormal bleeding from female genital tract ♀
628.4 Female infertility of cervical or vaginal origin ♀
789.00 Abdominal pain, unspecified site ▽

ICD-9-CM Procedural

67.0 Dilation of cervical canal

HCPCS Level II Supplies & Services

A4550 Surgical trays

57820

57820 Dilation and curettage of cervical stump

ICD-9-CM Diagnostic

180.0 Malignant neoplasm of endocervix ♀
180.8 Malignant neoplasm of other specified sites of cervix ♀
233.1 Carcinoma in situ of cervix uteri ♀
236.0 Neoplasm of uncertain behavior of uterus ♀
239.5 Neoplasm of unspecified nature of other genitourinary organs
616.0 Cervicitis and endocervicitis — (Use additional code to identify organism: 041.0, 041.1) ♀
617.0 Endometriosis of uterus ♀
622.0 Erosion and ectropion of cervix ♀
622.10 Dysplasia of cervix, unspecified
622.11 Mild dysplasia of cervix
622.12 Moderate dysplasia of cervix
622.2 Leukoplakia of cervix (uteri) ♀
622.4 Stricture and stenosis of cervix ♀
622.7 Mucous polyp of cervix ♀
622.8 Other specified noninflammatory disorder of cervix ♀
627.1 Postmenopausal bleeding ♀

ICD-9-CM Procedural

69.09 Other dilation and curettage of uterus

HCPCS Level II Supplies & Services

A4550 Surgical trays

Corpus Uteri

58100

58100 Endometrial sampling (biopsy) with or without endocervical sampling (biopsy), without cervical dilation, any method (separate procedure)

ICD-9-CM Diagnostic

179 Malignant neoplasm of uterus, part unspecified ▽ ♀
180.0 Malignant neoplasm of endocervix ♀
180.1 Malignant neoplasm of exocervix ♀
180.8 Malignant neoplasm of other specified sites of cervix ♀
180.9 Malignant neoplasm of cervix uteri, unspecified site ▽ ♀
182.0 Malignant neoplasm of corpus uteri, except isthmus ♀
182.8 Malignant neoplasm of other specified sites of body of uterus ♀
184.9 Malignant neoplasm of female genital organ, site unspecified ▽ ♀
198.89 Secondary malignant neoplasm of other specified sites
199.1 Other malignant neoplasm of unspecified site
218.0 Submucous leiomyoma of uterus ♀
218.1 Intramural leiomyoma of uterus ♀
219.8 Benign neoplasm of other specified parts of uterus ♀
219.9 Benign neoplasm of uterus, part unspecified ▽ ♀
221.9 Benign neoplasm of female genital organ, site unspecified ▽ ♀
233.1 Carcinoma in situ of cervix uteri ♀
233.3 Carcinoma in situ of other and unspecified female genital organs ▽ ♀
239.5 Neoplasm of unspecified nature of other genitourinary organs
239.9 Neoplasm of unspecified nature, site unspecified ▽
256.31 Premature menopause ♀
256.39 Other ovarian failure ♀
256.4 Polycystic ovaries ♀
615.0 Acute inflammatory disease of uterus, except cervix — (Use additional code to identify organism: 041.0, 041.1) ♀
615.1 Chronic inflammatory disease of uterus, except cervix — (Use additional code to identify organism: 041.0, 041.1) ♀
616.0 Cervicitis and endocervicitis — (Use additional code to identify organism: 041.0, 041.1) ♀
617.0 Endometriosis of uterus ♀
617.8 Endometriosis of other specified sites ♀
617.9 Endometriosis, site unspecified ▽ ♀
621.0 Polyp of corpus uteri ♀
621.2 Hypertrophy of uterus ♀
621.30 Endometrial hyperplasia, unspecified
621.31 Simple endometrial hyperplasia without atypia

621.32 Complex endometrial hyperplasia without atypia
621.33 Endometrial hyperplasia with atypia
621.4 Hematometra ♀
621.5 Intrauterine synechiae ♀
621.8 Other specified disorders of uterus, not elsewhere classified ♀
622.10 Dysplasia of cervix, unspecified
622.11 Mild dysplasia of cervix
622.12 Moderate dysplasia of cervix
622.4 Stricture and stenosis of cervix ♀
622.7 Mucous polyp of cervix ♀
623.5 Leukorrhea, not specified as infective ♀
623.7 Polyp of vagina ♀
623.8 Other specified noninflammatory disorder of vagina ♀
625.1 Vaginismus ♀
625.3 Dysmenorrhea ♀
625.8 Other specified symptom associated with female genital organs ♀
626.0 Absence of menstruation ♀
626.1 Scanty or infrequent menstruation ♀
626.2 Excessive or frequent menstruation ♀
626.3 Puberty bleeding ♀
626.4 Irregular menstrual cycle ♀
626.5 Ovulation bleeding ♀
626.6 Metrorrhagia ♀
626.8 Other disorder of menstruation and other abnormal bleeding from female genital tract ♀
627.1 Postmenopausal bleeding ♀
627.2 Symptomatic menopausal or female climacteric states ♀
627.3 Postmenopausal atrophic vaginitis ♀
627.8 Other specified menopausal and postmenopausal disorder ♀
628.0 Female infertility associated with anovulation — (Use additional code for any associated Stein-Levanthal syndrome, 256.4) ♀
628.3 Female infertility of uterine origin — (Use additional code for any associated tuberculous endometriosis, 016.7) ♀
628.4 Female infertility of cervical or vaginal origin ♀
628.8 Female infertility of other specified origin ♀
629.0 Hematocele, female, not elsewhere classified ♀
646.30 Pregnancy complication, habitual aborter unspecified as to episode of care ▽ ♀
677 Late effect of complication of pregnancy, childbirth, and the puerperium — (Code first any sequelae) ♀
789.30 Abdominal or pelvic swelling, mass or lump, unspecified site ▽
795.00 Abnormal glandular Papanicolaou smear of cervix ▽ ♀
795.01 Papanicolaou smear of cervix with atypical squamous cells of undetermined significance (ASC-US) ♀
795.02 Papanicolaou smear of cervix with atypical squamous cells cannot exclude high grade squamous intraepithelial lesion (ASC-H) ♀
795.03 Papanicolaou smear of cervix with low grade squamous intraepithelial lesion (LGSIL)
795.04 Papanicolaou smear of cervix with high grade squamous intraepithelial lesion (HGSIL)
795.05 Cervical high risk human papillomavirus (HPV) DNA test positive
795.08 Nonspecific abnormal papanicolaou smear of cervix, unsatisfactory smear
795.09 Other abnormal Papanicolaou smear of cervix and cervical HPV ♀
795.1 Nonspecific abnormal Papanicolaou smear of other site ▽

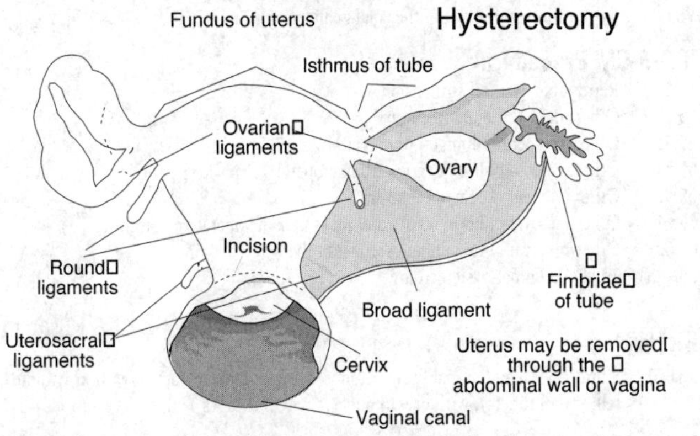

795.39 Other nonspecific positive culture findings
795.4 Other nonspecific abnormal histological findings
V84.02 Genetic susceptibility to malignant neoplasm of ovary
V84.04 Genetic susceptibility to malignant neoplasm of endometrium
V84.09 Genetic susceptibility to other malignant neoplasm

ICD-9-CM Procedural

67.11 Endocervical biopsy
67.12 Other cervical biopsy
68.13 Open biopsy of uterus
68.16 Closed biopsy of uterus

HCPCS Level II Supplies & Services

A4550 Surgical trays

58120

58120 Dilation and curettage, diagnostic and/or therapeutic (nonobstetrical)

ICD-9-CM Diagnostic

179 Malignant neoplasm of uterus, part unspecified ▽ ♀
180.0 Malignant neoplasm of endocervix ♀
180.1 Malignant neoplasm of exocervix ♀
180.8 Malignant neoplasm of other specified sites of cervix ♀
180.9 Malignant neoplasm of cervix uteri, unspecified site ▽ ♀
182.0 Malignant neoplasm of corpus uteri, except isthmus ♀
182.1 Malignant neoplasm of isthmus ♀
182.8 Malignant neoplasm of other specified sites of body of uterus ♀
184.0 Malignant neoplasm of vagina ♀
198.82 Secondary malignant neoplasm of genital organs
218.0 Submucous leiomyoma of uterus ♀
218.1 Intramural leiomyoma of uterus ♀
218.9 Leiomyoma of uterus, unspecified ▽ ♀
233.1 Carcinoma in situ of cervix uteri ♀
233.2 Carcinoma in situ of other and unspecified parts of uterus ▽ ♀
233.3 Carcinoma in situ of other and unspecified female genital organs ▽ ♀
236.0 Neoplasm of uncertain behavior of uterus ♀
239.5 Neoplasm of unspecified nature of other genitourinary organs
615.1 Chronic inflammatory disease of uterus, except cervix — (Use additional code to identify organism: 041.0, 041.1) ♀
616.0 Cervicitis and endocervicitis — (Use additional code to identify organism: 041.0, 041.1) ♀
616.10 Unspecified vaginitis and vulvovaginitis — (Use additional code to identify organism: 041.0, 041.1, 041.4) ▽ ♀
617.0 Endometriosis of uterus ♀
617.9 Endometriosis, site unspecified ▽ ♀
621.0 Polyp of corpus uteri ♀
621.2 Hypertrophy of uterus ♀
621.30 Endometrial hyperplasia, unspecified
621.31 Simple endometrial hyperplasia without atypia
621.32 Complex endometrial hyperplasia without atypia
621.33 Endometrial hyperplasia with atypia
621.8 Other specified disorders of uterus, not elsewhere classified ♀
622.10 Dysplasia of cervix, unspecified
622.11 Mild dysplasia of cervix
622.12 Moderate dysplasia of cervix
622.4 Stricture and stenosis of cervix ♀
622.7 Mucous polyp of cervix ♀
623.8 Other specified noninflammatory disorder of vagina ♀
625.0 Dyspareunia ♀
625.3 Dysmenorrhea ♀
625.8 Other specified symptom associated with female genital organs ♀
626.0 Absence of menstruation ♀
626.1 Scanty or infrequent menstruation ♀
626.2 Excessive or frequent menstruation ♀
626.3 Puberty bleeding ♀
626.4 Irregular menstrual cycle ♀
626.6 Metrorrhagia ♀
626.8 Other disorder of menstruation and other abnormal bleeding from female genital tract ♀
627.0 Premenopausal menorrhagia ♀
627.1 Postmenopausal bleeding ♀
628.9 Female infertility of unspecified origin ▽ ♀
677 Late effect of complication of pregnancy, childbirth, and the puerperium — (Code first any sequelae) ♀
V84.02 Genetic susceptibility to malignant neoplasm of ovary
V84.04 Genetic susceptibility to malignant neoplasm of endometrium
V84.09 Genetic susceptibility to other malignant neoplasm

ICD-9-CM Procedural

69.09 Other dilation and curettage of uterus

HCPCS Level II Supplies & Services

A4305 Disposable drug delivery system, flow rate of 50 ml or greater per hour
A4306 Disposable drug delivery system, flow rate of 5 ml or less per hour
A4550 Surgical trays

58140–58146

58140 Myomectomy, excision of fibroid tumor(s) of uterus, 1 to 4 intramural myoma(s) with total weight of 250 grams or less and/or removal of surface myomas; abdominal approach
58145 Myomectomy, excision of fibroid tumor(s) of uterus, 1 to 4 intramural myoma(s) with total weight of 250 grams or less and/or removal of surface myomas; vaginal approach
58146 Myomectomy, excision of fibroid tumor(s) of uterus, 5 or more intramural myomas and/or intramural myomas with total weight greater than 250 grams, abdominal approach

ICD-9-CM Diagnostic

218.0 Submucous leiomyoma of uterus ♀
218.1 Intramural leiomyoma of uterus ♀
218.2 Subserous leiomyoma of uterus ♀
218.9 Leiomyoma of uterus, unspecified ▽ ♀
V64.41 Laparoscopic surgical procedure converted to open procedure

ICD-9-CM Procedural

68.29 Other excision or destruction of lesion of uterus

HCPCS Level II Supplies & Services

HCPCS Level II codes are used to report the supplies, durable medical equipment, and certain medical services provided on an outpatient basis. Because the procedure(s) represented on this page would be performed in an inpatient facility, no HCPCS Level II codes apply.

58150–58152

58150 Total abdominal hysterectomy (corpus and cervix), with or without removal of tube(s), with or without removal of ovary(s);
58152 with colpo-urethrocystopexy (eg, Marshall-Marchetti-Krantz, Burch)

ICD-9-CM Diagnostic

179 Malignant neoplasm of uterus, part unspecified ▽ ♀
180.0 Malignant neoplasm of endocervix ♀
180.9 Malignant neoplasm of cervix uteri, unspecified site ▽ ♀
182.0 Malignant neoplasm of corpus uteri, except isthmus ♀
182.1 Malignant neoplasm of isthmus ♀
182.8 Malignant neoplasm of other specified sites of body of uterus ♀
183.0 Malignant neoplasm of ovary — (Use additional code to identify any functional activity) ♀
183.2 Malignant neoplasm of fallopian tube ♀
183.8 Malignant neoplasm of other specified sites of uterine adnexa ♀
183.9 Malignant neoplasm of uterine adnexa, unspecified site ▽ ♀
184.9 Malignant neoplasm of female genital organ, site unspecified ▽ ♀
198.6 Secondary malignant neoplasm of ovary ♀
198.82 Secondary malignant neoplasm of genital organs
199.1 Other malignant neoplasm of unspecified site
218.0 Submucous leiomyoma of uterus ♀
218.1 Intramural leiomyoma of uterus ♀
218.2 Subserous leiomyoma of uterus ♀
233.1 Carcinoma in situ of cervix uteri ♀
233.2 Carcinoma in situ of other and unspecified parts of uterus ▽ ♀
233.3 Carcinoma in situ of other and unspecified female genital organs ▽ ♀
236.0 Neoplasm of uncertain behavior of uterus ♀
236.1 Neoplasm of uncertain behavior of placenta ♀
236.2 Neoplasm of uncertain behavior of ovary — (Use additional code to identify any functional activity) ♀
236.3 Neoplasm of uncertain behavior of other and unspecified female genital organs ▽ ♀
239.5 Neoplasm of unspecified nature of other genitourinary organs
256.0 Hyperestrogenism ♀
614.1 Chronic salpingitis and oophoritis — (Use additional code to identify organism: 041.0, 041.1) ♀
614.2 Salpingitis and oophoritis not specified as acute, subacute, or chronic — (Use additional code to identify organism: 041.0, 041.1) ♀
614.3 Acute parametritis and pelvic cellulitis — (Use additional code to identify organism: 041.0, 041.1) ♀
614.4 Chronic or unspecified parametritis and pelvic cellulitis — (Use additional code to identify organism: 041.0, 041.1) ♀
614.5 Acute or unspecified pelvic peritonitis, female — (Use additional code to identify organism: 041.0, 041.1) ♀
614.6 Pelvic peritoneal adhesions, female (postoperative) (postinfection) — (Use additional code to identify any associated infertility, 628.2. Use additional code to identify organism: 041.0, 041.1) ♀
617.0 Endometriosis of uterus ♀
617.1 Endometriosis of ovary ♀
617.2 Endometriosis of fallopian tube ♀
617.3 Endometriosis of pelvic peritoneum ♀
617.9 Endometriosis, site unspecified ▽ ♀
618.01 Cystocele without mention of uterine prolapse, midline
618.02 Cystocele without mention of uterine prolapse, lateral
618.03 Urethrocele without mention of uterine prolapse
618.09 Other prolapse of vaginal walls without mention of uterine prolapse
618.1 Uterine prolapse without mention of vaginal wall prolapse — (Use additional code to identify urinary incontinence: 625.6, 788.31, 788.33-788.39) ♀
618.2 Uterovaginal prolapse, incomplete — (Use additional code to identify urinary incontinence: 625.6, 788.31, 788.33-788.39) ♀
618.3 Uterovaginal prolapse, complete — (Use additional code to identify urinary incontinence: 625.6, 788.31, 788.33-788.39) ♀
618.4 Uterovaginal prolapse, unspecified — (Use additional code to identify urinary incontinence: 625.6, 788.31, 788.33-788.39) ▽ ♀
620.0 Follicular cyst of ovary ♀
620.1 Corpus luteum cyst or hematoma ♀
620.2 Other and unspecified ovarian cyst ▽ ♀
620.8 Other noninflammatory disorder of ovary, fallopian tube, and broad ligament ♀
621.0 Polyp of corpus uteri ♀
621.2 Hypertrophy of uterus ♀
621.30 Endometrial hyperplasia, unspecified
621.31 Simple endometrial hyperplasia without atypia
621.32 Complex endometrial hyperplasia without atypia
621.33 Endometrial hyperplasia with atypia
621.8 Other specified disorders of uterus, not elsewhere classified ♀
622.10 Dysplasia of cervix, unspecified
622.11 Mild dysplasia of cervix
622.12 Moderate dysplasia of cervix
625.3 Dysmenorrhea ♀
625.5 Pelvic congestion syndrome ♀
625.6 Female stress incontinence ♀
625.8 Other specified symptom associated with female genital organs ♀
626.2 Excessive or frequent menstruation ♀
626.6 Metrorrhagia ♀
626.8 Other disorder of menstruation and other abnormal bleeding from female genital tract ♀
627.1 Postmenopausal bleeding ♀
627.2 Symptomatic menopausal or female climacteric states ♀
677 Late effect of complication of pregnancy, childbirth, and the puerperium — (Code first any sequelae) ♀
752.2 Congenital doubling of uterus ♀
752.3 Other congenital anomaly of uterus ♀
789.00 Abdominal pain, unspecified site ▽
789.30 Abdominal or pelvic swelling, mass or lump, unspecified site ▽
V84.02 Genetic susceptibility to malignant neoplasm of ovary
V84.04 Genetic susceptibility to malignant neoplasm of endometrium
V84.09 Genetic susceptibility to other malignant neoplasm

ICD-9-CM Procedural

59.5 Retropubic urethral suspension
65.39 Other unilateral oophorectomy
65.49 Other unilateral salpingo-oophorectomy
65.51 Other removal of both ovaries at same operative episode
65.52 Other removal of remaining ovary
65.61 Other removal of both ovaries and tubes at same operative episode
65.62 Other removal of remaining ovary and tube
68.4 Total abdominal hysterectomy

58180

58180 Supracervical abdominal hysterectomy (subtotal hysterectomy), with or without removal of tube(s), with or without removal of ovary(s)

ICD-9-CM Diagnostic

182.0 Malignant neoplasm of corpus uteri, except isthmus ♀
182.1 Malignant neoplasm of isthmus ♀
182.8 Malignant neoplasm of other specified sites of body of uterus ♀
183.8 Malignant neoplasm of other specified sites of uterine adnexa ♀

▽ Unspecified code
♀ Female diagnosis
☒ Manifestation code
♂ Male diagnosis

183.9 Malignant neoplasm of uterine adnexa, unspecified site ▽ ♀
184.8 Malignant neoplasm of other specified sites of female genital organs ♀
218.0 Submucous leiomyoma of uterus ♀
218.1 Intramural leiomyoma of uterus ♀
218.2 Subserous leiomyoma of uterus ♀
236.0 Neoplasm of uncertain behavior of uterus ♀
236.3 Neoplasm of uncertain behavior of other and unspecified female genital organs ▽ ♀
239.5 Neoplasm of unspecified nature of other genitourinary organs
617.0 Endometriosis of uterus ♀
617.1 Endometriosis of ovary ♀
617.2 Endometriosis of fallopian tube ♀
618.1 Uterine prolapse without mention of vaginal wall prolapse — (Use additional code to identify urinary incontinence: 625.6, 788.31, 788.33-788.39) ♀
625.3 Dysmenorrhea ♀
626.8 Other disorder of menstruation and other abnormal bleeding from female genital tract ♀
677 Late effect of complication of pregnancy, childbirth, and the puerperium — (Code first any sequelae) ♀
V84.02 Genetic susceptibility to malignant neoplasm of ovary
V84.04 Genetic susceptibility to malignant neoplasm of endometrium
V84.09 Genetic susceptibility to other malignant neoplasm

ICD-9-CM Procedural

65.39 Other unilateral oophorectomy
65.49 Other unilateral salpingo-oophorectomy
65.51 Other removal of both ovaries at same operative episode
65.52 Other removal of remaining ovary
65.61 Other removal of both ovaries and tubes at same operative episode
65.62 Other removal of remaining ovary and tube
68.39 Other subtotal abdominal hysterectomy, NOS

58200

58200 Total abdominal hysterectomy, including partial vaginectomy, with para-aortic and pelvic lymph node sampling, with or without removal of tube(s), with or without removal of ovary(s)

ICD-9-CM Diagnostic

179 Malignant neoplasm of uterus, part unspecified ▽ ♀
180.0 Malignant neoplasm of endocervix ♀
180.1 Malignant neoplasm of exocervix ♀
180.8 Malignant neoplasm of other specified sites of cervix ♀
182.0 Malignant neoplasm of corpus uteri, except isthmus ♀
182.1 Malignant neoplasm of isthmus ♀
182.8 Malignant neoplasm of other specified sites of body of uterus ♀
183.0 Malignant neoplasm of ovary — (Use additional code to identify any functional activity) ♀
183.2 Malignant neoplasm of fallopian tube ♀
183.3 Malignant neoplasm of broad ligament of uterus ♀
183.4 Malignant neoplasm of parametrium of uterus ♀
183.5 Malignant neoplasm of round ligament of uterus ♀
183.8 Malignant neoplasm of other specified sites of uterine adnexa ♀
183.9 Malignant neoplasm of uterine adnexa, unspecified site ▽ ♀
184.0 Malignant neoplasm of vagina ♀
184.8 Malignant neoplasm of other specified sites of female genital organs ♀
196.2 Secondary and unspecified malignant neoplasm of intra-abdominal lymph nodes
196.6 Secondary and unspecified malignant neoplasm of intrapelvic lymph nodes
196.8 Secondary and unspecified malignant neoplasm of lymph nodes of multiple sites
198.82 Secondary malignant neoplasm of genital organs
233.1 Carcinoma in situ of cervix uteri ♀
236.0 Neoplasm of uncertain behavior of uterus ♀
236.2 Neoplasm of uncertain behavior of ovary — (Use additional code to identify any functional activity) ♀
238.8 Neoplasm of uncertain behavior of other specified sites
239.5 Neoplasm of unspecified nature of other genitourinary organs
239.8 Neoplasm of unspecified nature of other specified sites
V84.02 Genetic susceptibility to malignant neoplasm of ovary
V84.04 Genetic susceptibility to malignant neoplasm of endometrium
V84.09 Genetic susceptibility to other malignant neoplasm

ICD-9-CM Procedural

40.11 Biopsy of lymphatic structure
65.39 Other unilateral oophorectomy
65.49 Other unilateral salpingo-oophorectomy
65.51 Other removal of both ovaries at same operative episode
65.52 Other removal of remaining ovary
65.61 Other removal of both ovaries and tubes at same operative episode
65.62 Other removal of remaining ovary and tube
68.4 Total abdominal hysterectomy
70.8 Obliteration of vaginal vault

58210

58210 Radical abdominal hysterectomy, with bilateral total pelvic lymphadenectomy and para-aortic lymph node sampling (biopsy), with or without removal of tube(s), with or without removal of ovary(s)

ICD-9-CM Diagnostic

179 Malignant neoplasm of uterus, part unspecified ▽ ♀
180.0 Malignant neoplasm of endocervix ♀
180.1 Malignant neoplasm of exocervix ♀
180.8 Malignant neoplasm of other specified sites of cervix ♀
182.0 Malignant neoplasm of corpus uteri, except isthmus ♀
182.1 Malignant neoplasm of isthmus ♀
182.8 Malignant neoplasm of other specified sites of body of uterus ♀
183.0 Malignant neoplasm of ovary — (Use additional code to identify any functional activity) ♀
183.2 Malignant neoplasm of fallopian tube ♀
183.3 Malignant neoplasm of broad ligament of uterus ♀
183.4 Malignant neoplasm of parametrium of uterus ♀
183.5 Malignant neoplasm of round ligament of uterus ♀
183.8 Malignant neoplasm of other specified sites of uterine adnexa ♀
183.9 Malignant neoplasm of uterine adnexa, unspecified site ▽ ♀
184.0 Malignant neoplasm of vagina ♀
184.8 Malignant neoplasm of other specified sites of female genital organs ♀
196.2 Secondary and unspecified malignant neoplasm of intra-abdominal lymph nodes
196.6 Secondary and unspecified malignant neoplasm of intrapelvic lymph nodes
196.8 Secondary and unspecified malignant neoplasm of lymph nodes of multiple sites
198.82 Secondary malignant neoplasm of genital organs
233.1 Carcinoma in situ of cervix uteri ♀
236.0 Neoplasm of uncertain behavior of uterus ♀
236.2 Neoplasm of uncertain behavior of ovary — (Use additional code to identify any functional activity) ♀
238.8 Neoplasm of uncertain behavior of other specified sites
239.5 Neoplasm of unspecified nature of other genitourinary organs
239.8 Neoplasm of unspecified nature of other specified sites
V84.02 Genetic susceptibility to malignant neoplasm of ovary
V84.04 Genetic susceptibility to malignant neoplasm of endometrium
V84.09 Genetic susceptibility to other malignant neoplasm

ICD-9-CM Procedural

40.11 Biopsy of lymphatic structure
40.3 Regional lymph node excision
40.59 Radical excision of other lymph nodes
65.39 Other unilateral oophorectomy
65.49 Other unilateral salpingo-oophorectomy
65.51 Other removal of both ovaries at same operative episode
65.52 Other removal of remaining ovary
65.61 Other removal of both ovaries and tubes at same operative episode
65.62 Other removal of remaining ovary and tube
68.6 Radical abdominal hysterectomy

58240

58240 Pelvic exenteration for gynecologic malignancy, with total abdominal hysterectomy or cervicectomy, with or without removal of tube(s), with or without removal of ovary(s), with removal of bladder and ureteral transplantations, and/or abdominoperineal resection of rectum and colon and colostomy, or any combination thereof

ICD-9-CM Diagnostic

179 Malignant neoplasm of uterus, part unspecified ▽ ♀
180.0 Malignant neoplasm of endocervix ♀
180.1 Malignant neoplasm of exocervix ♀
180.8 Malignant neoplasm of other specified sites of cervix ♀
182.0 Malignant neoplasm of corpus uteri, except isthmus ♀
182.1 Malignant neoplasm of isthmus ♀
182.8 Malignant neoplasm of other specified sites of body of uterus ♀
183.0 Malignant neoplasm of ovary — (Use additional code to identify any functional activity) ♀

▽ Unspecified code ♀ Female diagnosis ☒ Manifestation code ♂ Male diagnosis

183.2 Malignant neoplasm of fallopian tube ♀
183.3 Malignant neoplasm of broad ligament of uterus ♀
183.4 Malignant neoplasm of parametrium of uterus ♀
183.5 Malignant neoplasm of round ligament of uterus ♀
183.8 Malignant neoplasm of other specified sites of uterine adnexa ♀
183.9 Malignant neoplasm of uterine adnexa, unspecified site ▽ ♀
184.0 Malignant neoplasm of vagina ♀
184.8 Malignant neoplasm of other specified sites of female genital organs ♀
184.9 Malignant neoplasm of female genital organ, site unspecified ▽ ♀
197.5 Secondary malignant neoplasm of large intestine and rectum
198.1 Secondary malignant neoplasm of other urinary organs
198.6 Secondary malignant neoplasm of ovary ♀
198.82 Secondary malignant neoplasm of genital organs
199.0 Disseminated malignant neoplasm
199.1 Other malignant neoplasm of unspecified site
V84.02 Genetic susceptibility to malignant neoplasm of ovary
V84.04 Genetic susceptibility to malignant neoplasm of endometrium
V84.09 Genetic susceptibility to other malignant neoplasm

ICD-9-CM Procedural

40.3 Regional lymph node excision
40.59 Radical excision of other lymph nodes
46.13 Permanent colostomy
56.61 Formation of other cutaneous ureterostomy
68.8 Pelvic evisceration

58260–58263

58260 Vaginal hysterectomy, for uterus 250 grams or less;
58262 with removal of tube(s), and/or ovary(s)
58263 with removal of tube(s), and/or ovary(s), with repair of enterocele

ICD-9-CM Diagnostic

180.0 Malignant neoplasm of endocervix ♀
180.1 Malignant neoplasm of exocervix ♀
180.8 Malignant neoplasm of other specified sites of cervix ♀
180.9 Malignant neoplasm of cervix uteri, unspecified site ▽ ♀
181 Malignant neoplasm of placenta ♀
182.0 Malignant neoplasm of corpus uteri, except isthmus ♀
182.1 Malignant neoplasm of isthmus ♀
182.8 Malignant neoplasm of other specified sites of body of uterus ♀
183.0 Malignant neoplasm of ovary — (Use additional code to identify any functional activity) ♀
183.8 Malignant neoplasm of other specified sites of uterine adnexa ♀
183.9 Malignant neoplasm of uterine adnexa, unspecified site ▽ ♀
198.6 Secondary malignant neoplasm of ovary ♀
199.1 Other malignant neoplasm of unspecified site
218.0 Submucous leiomyoma of uterus ♀
218.1 Intramural leiomyoma of uterus ♀
218.2 Subserous leiomyoma of uterus ♀
218.9 Leiomyoma of uterus, unspecified ▽ ♀
233.1 Carcinoma in situ of cervix uteri ♀
233.2 Carcinoma in situ of other and unspecified parts of uterus ▽ ♀
233.3 Carcinoma in situ of other and unspecified female genital organs ▽ ♀
236.0 Neoplasm of uncertain behavior of uterus ♀
236.2 Neoplasm of uncertain behavior of ovary — (Use additional code to identify any functional activity) ♀
236.3 Neoplasm of uncertain behavior of other and unspecified female genital organs ▽ ♀
239.5 Neoplasm of unspecified nature of other genitourinary organs
553.9 Hernia of unspecified site of abdominal cavity without mention of obstruction or gangrene ▽
614.4 Chronic or unspecified parametritis and pelvic cellulitis — (Use additional code to identify organism: 041.0, 041.1) ♀
614.9 Unspecified inflammatory disease of female pelvic organs and tissues — (Use additional code to identify organism: 041.0, 041.1) ▽ ♀
617.0 Endometriosis of uterus ♀
617.9 Endometriosis, site unspecified ▽ ♀
618.1 Uterine prolapse without mention of vaginal wall prolapse — (Use additional code to identify urinary incontinence: 625.6, 788.31, 788.33-788.39) ♀
618.2 Uterovaginal prolapse, incomplete — (Use additional code to identify urinary incontinence: 625.6, 788.31, 788.33-788.39) ♀
618.3 Uterovaginal prolapse, complete — (Use additional code to identify urinary incontinence: 625.6, 788.31, 788.33-788.39) ♀
618.4 Uterovaginal prolapse, unspecified — (Use additional code to identify urinary incontinence: 625.6, 788.31, 788.33-788.39) ▽ ♀
618.6 Vaginal enterocele, congenital or acquired — (Use additional code to identify urinary incontinence: 625.6, 788.31, 788.33-788.39) ♀
618.9 Unspecified genital prolapse — (Use additional code to identify urinary incontinence: 625.6, 788.31, 788.33-788.39) ▽ ♀
621.0 Polyp of corpus uteri ♀
621.2 Hypertrophy of uterus ♀
621.30 Endometrial hyperplasia, unspecified
621.31 Simple endometrial hyperplasia without atypia
621.32 Complex endometrial hyperplasia without atypia
621.33 Endometrial hyperplasia with atypia
621.6 Malposition of uterus ♀
621.8 Other specified disorders of uterus, not elsewhere classified ♀
621.9 Unspecified disorder of uterus ▽ ♀
622.10 Dysplasia of cervix, unspecified
622.11 Mild dysplasia of cervix
622.12 Moderate dysplasia of cervix
625.3 Dysmenorrhea ♀
625.6 Female stress incontinence ♀
625.8 Other specified symptom associated with female genital organs ♀
626.2 Excessive or frequent menstruation ♀
626.6 Metrorrhagia ♀
626.8 Other disorder of menstruation and other abnormal bleeding from female genital tract ♀
626.9 Unspecified disorder of menstruation and other abnormal bleeding from female genital tract ▽ ♀
627.1 Postmenopausal bleeding ♀
677 Late effect of complication of pregnancy, childbirth, and the puerperium — (Code first any sequelae) ♀
788.33 Mixed incontinence urge and stress (male)(female)
789.30 Abdominal or pelvic swelling, mass or lump, unspecified site ▽
V50.49 Other prophylactic gland removal
V84.02 Genetic susceptibility to malignant neoplasm of ovary
V84.04 Genetic susceptibility to malignant neoplasm of endometrium
V84.09 Genetic susceptibility to other malignant neoplasm

ICD-9-CM Procedural

65.39 Other unilateral oophorectomy
65.49 Other unilateral salpingo-oophorectomy
65.51 Other removal of both ovaries at same operative episode
65.52 Other removal of remaining ovary
65.61 Other removal of both ovaries and tubes at same operative episode
65.62 Other removal of remaining ovary and tube
68.59 Other vaginal hysterectomy
70.92 Other operations on cul-de-sac

58267

58267 Vaginal hysterectomy, for uterus 250 grams or less; with colpo-urethrocystopexy (Marshall-Marchetti-Krantz type, Pereyra type) with or without endoscopic control

ICD-9-CM Diagnostic

180.0 Malignant neoplasm of endocervix ♀
180.1 Malignant neoplasm of exocervix ♀
180.8 Malignant neoplasm of other specified sites of cervix ♀
182.0 Malignant neoplasm of corpus uteri, except isthmus ♀
182.1 Malignant neoplasm of isthmus ♀
182.8 Malignant neoplasm of other specified sites of body of uterus ♀
218.0 Submucous leiomyoma of uterus ♀
218.1 Intramural leiomyoma of uterus ♀
218.2 Subserous leiomyoma of uterus ♀
218.9 Leiomyoma of uterus, unspecified ▽ ♀
614.4 Chronic or unspecified parametritis and pelvic cellulitis — (Use additional code to identify organism: 041.0, 041.1) ♀
614.9 Unspecified inflammatory disease of female pelvic organs and tissues — (Use additional code to identify organism: 041.0, 041.1) ▽ ♀
617.0 Endometriosis of uterus ♀
618.00 Prolapse of vaginal walls without mention of uterine prolapse, unspecified
618.01 Cystocele without mention of uterine prolapse, midline
618.02 Cystocele without mention of uterine prolapse, lateral
618.03 Urethrocele without mention of uterine prolapse
618.09 Other prolapse of vaginal walls without mention of uterine prolapse
618.1 Uterine prolapse without mention of vaginal wall prolapse — (Use additional code to identify urinary incontinence: 625.6, 788.31, 788.33-788.39) ♀
618.2 Uterovaginal prolapse, incomplete — (Use additional code to identify urinary incontinence: 625.6, 788.31, 788.33-788.39) ♀

618.3 Uterovaginal prolapse, complete — (Use additional code to identify urinary incontinence: 625.6, 788.31, 788.33-788.39) ♀
618.4 Uterovaginal prolapse, unspecified — (Use additional code to identify urinary incontinence: 625.6, 788.31, 788.33-788.39) ▽ ♀
625.3 Dysmenorrhea ♀
625.6 Female stress incontinence ♀
626.2 Excessive or frequent menstruation ♀
626.8 Other disorder of menstruation and other abnormal bleeding from female genital tract ♀
788.33 Mixed incontinence urge and stress (male)(female)
V84.02 Genetic susceptibility to malignant neoplasm of ovary
V84.04 Genetic susceptibility to malignant neoplasm of endometrium
V84.09 Genetic susceptibility to other malignant neoplasm

ICD-9-CM Procedural

59.5 Retropubic urethral suspension
68.59 Other vaginal hysterectomy

58270

58270 Vaginal hysterectomy, for uterus 250 grams or less; with repair of enterocele

ICD-9-CM Diagnostic

180.0 Malignant neoplasm of endocervix ♀
180.1 Malignant neoplasm of exocervix ♀
182.0 Malignant neoplasm of corpus uteri, except isthmus ♀
182.1 Malignant neoplasm of isthmus ♀
182.8 Malignant neoplasm of other specified sites of body of uterus ♀
218.0 Submucous leiomyoma of uterus ♀
218.1 Intramural leiomyoma of uterus ♀
218.2 Subserous leiomyoma of uterus ♀
218.9 Leiomyoma of uterus, unspecified ▽ ♀
233.1 Carcinoma in situ of cervix uteri ♀
618.04 Rectocele without mention of uterine prolapse
618.1 Uterine prolapse without mention of vaginal wall prolapse — (Use additional code to identify urinary incontinence: 625.6, 788.31, 788.33-788.39) ♀
618.2 Uterovaginal prolapse, incomplete — (Use additional code to identify urinary incontinence: 625.6, 788.31, 788.33-788.39) ♀
618.3 Uterovaginal prolapse, complete — (Use additional code to identify urinary incontinence: 625.6, 788.31, 788.33-788.39) ♀
618.4 Uterovaginal prolapse, unspecified — (Use additional code to identify urinary incontinence: 625.6, 788.31, 788.33-788.39) ▽ ♀
618.6 Vaginal enterocele, congenital or acquired — (Use additional code to identify urinary incontinence: 625.6, 788.31, 788.33-788.39) ♀
618.83 Pelvic muscle wasting
618.9 Unspecified genital prolapse — (Use additional code to identify urinary incontinence: 625.6, 788.31, 788.33-788.39) ▽ ♀
621.30 Endometrial hyperplasia, unspecified
621.31 Simple endometrial hyperplasia without atypia
621.32 Complex endometrial hyperplasia without atypia
621.33 Endometrial hyperplasia with atypia
622.10 Dysplasia of cervix, unspecified
622.11 Mild dysplasia of cervix
622.12 Moderate dysplasia of cervix
625.3 Dysmenorrhea ♀
625.6 Female stress incontinence ♀
626.2 Excessive or frequent menstruation ♀
626.6 Metrorrhagia ♀
626.8 Other disorder of menstruation and other abnormal bleeding from female genital tract ♀
627.1 Postmenopausal bleeding ♀
788.33 Mixed incontinence urge and stress (male)(female)
V84.02 Genetic susceptibility to malignant neoplasm of ovary
V84.04 Genetic susceptibility to malignant neoplasm of endometrium
V84.09 Genetic susceptibility to other malignant neoplasm

ICD-9-CM Procedural

68.59 Other vaginal hysterectomy
70.92 Other operations on cul-de-sac

58275–58280

58275 Vaginal hysterectomy, with total or partial vaginectomy;
58280 with repair of enterocele

ICD-9-CM Diagnostic

180.0 Malignant neoplasm of endocervix ♀
180.1 Malignant neoplasm of exocervix ♀
180.8 Malignant neoplasm of other specified sites of cervix ♀
182.0 Malignant neoplasm of corpus uteri, except isthmus ♀
182.1 Malignant neoplasm of isthmus ♀
182.8 Malignant neoplasm of other specified sites of body of uterus ♀
184.0 Malignant neoplasm of vagina ♀
218.0 Submucous leiomyoma of uterus ♀
218.1 Intramural leiomyoma of uterus ♀
218.2 Subserous leiomyoma of uterus ♀
618.00 Prolapse of vaginal walls without mention of uterine prolapse, unspecified
618.09 Other prolapse of vaginal walls without mention of uterine prolapse
618.1 Uterine prolapse without mention of vaginal wall prolapse — (Use additional code to identify urinary incontinence: 625.6, 788.31, 788.33-788.39) ♀
618.2 Uterovaginal prolapse, incomplete — (Use additional code to identify urinary incontinence: 625.6, 788.31, 788.33-788.39) ♀
618.3 Uterovaginal prolapse, complete — (Use additional code to identify urinary incontinence: 625.6, 788.31, 788.33-788.39) ♀
618.6 Vaginal enterocele, congenital or acquired — (Use additional code to identify urinary incontinence: 625.6, 788.31, 788.33-788.39) ♀
618.82 Incompetence or weakening of rectovaginal tissue
621.2 Hypertrophy of uterus ♀
625.3 Dysmenorrhea ♀
625.6 Female stress incontinence ♀
626.2 Excessive or frequent menstruation ♀
626.6 Metrorrhagia ♀
626.8 Other disorder of menstruation and other abnormal bleeding from female genital tract ♀
788.33 Mixed incontinence urge and stress (male)(female)
V84.02 Genetic susceptibility to malignant neoplasm of ovary
V84.04 Genetic susceptibility to malignant neoplasm of endometrium
V84.09 Genetic susceptibility to other malignant neoplasm

ICD-9-CM Procedural

68.59 Other vaginal hysterectomy
70.4 Obliteration and total excision of vagina
70.8 Obliteration of vaginal vault
70.92 Other operations on cul-de-sac

58285

58285 Vaginal hysterectomy, radical (Schauta type operation)

ICD-9-CM Diagnostic

180.0 Malignant neoplasm of endocervix ♀
180.1 Malignant neoplasm of exocervix ♀
180.8 Malignant neoplasm of other specified sites of cervix ♀
182.0 Malignant neoplasm of corpus uteri, except isthmus ♀
182.1 Malignant neoplasm of isthmus ♀
182.8 Malignant neoplasm of other specified sites of body of uterus ♀
183.2 Malignant neoplasm of fallopian tube ♀
183.3 Malignant neoplasm of broad ligament of uterus ♀
183.4 Malignant neoplasm of parametrium of uterus ♀
183.5 Malignant neoplasm of round ligament of uterus ♀
183.8 Malignant neoplasm of other specified sites of uterine adnexa ♀
198.82 Secondary malignant neoplasm of genital organs
236.0 Neoplasm of uncertain behavior of uterus ♀
239.5 Neoplasm of unspecified nature of other genitourinary organs
618.1 Uterine prolapse without mention of vaginal wall prolapse — (Use additional code to identify urinary incontinence: 625.6, 788.31, 788.33-788.39) ♀
618.2 Uterovaginal prolapse, incomplete — (Use additional code to identify urinary incontinence: 625.6, 788.31, 788.33-788.39) ♀
618.3 Uterovaginal prolapse, complete — (Use additional code to identify urinary incontinence: 625.6, 788.31, 788.33-788.39) ♀
618.4 Uterovaginal prolapse, unspecified — (Use additional code to identify urinary incontinence: 625.6, 788.31, 788.33-788.39) ▽ ♀
618.83 Pelvic muscle wasting
618.89 Other specified genital prolapse
625.6 Female stress incontinence ♀
V84.02 Genetic susceptibility to malignant neoplasm of ovary
V84.04 Genetic susceptibility to malignant neoplasm of endometrium
V84.09 Genetic susceptibility to other malignant neoplasm

ICD-9-CM Procedural

68.7 Radical vaginal hysterectomy

▽ Unspecified code
♀ Female diagnosis
☒ Manifestation code
♂ Male diagnosis

58290–58292

58290 Vaginal hysterectomy, for uterus greater than 250 grams;
58291 with removal of tube(s) and/or ovary(s)
58292 with removal of tube(s) and/or ovary(s), with repair of enterocele

ICD-9-CM Diagnostic

180.0 Malignant neoplasm of endocervix ♀
180.1 Malignant neoplasm of exocervix ♀
180.8 Malignant neoplasm of other specified sites of cervix ♀
180.9 Malignant neoplasm of cervix uteri, unspecified site ▽ ♀
181 Malignant neoplasm of placenta ♀
182.0 Malignant neoplasm of corpus uteri, except isthmus ♀
182.1 Malignant neoplasm of isthmus ♀
182.8 Malignant neoplasm of other specified sites of body of uterus ♀
183.0 Malignant neoplasm of ovary — (Use additional code to identify any functional activity) ♀
183.8 Malignant neoplasm of other specified sites of uterine adnexa ♀
183.9 Malignant neoplasm of uterine adnexa, unspecified site ▽ ♀
198.6 Secondary malignant neoplasm of ovary ♀
199.1 Other malignant neoplasm of unspecified site
218.0 Submucous leiomyoma of uterus ♀
218.1 Intramural leiomyoma of uterus ♀
218.2 Subserous leiomyoma of uterus ♀
218.9 Leiomyoma of uterus, unspecified ▽ ♀
233.1 Carcinoma in situ of cervix uteri ♀
233.2 Carcinoma in situ of other and unspecified parts of uterus ▽ ♀
233.3 Carcinoma in situ of other and unspecified female genital organs ▽ ♀
236.0 Neoplasm of uncertain behavior of uterus ♀
236.2 Neoplasm of uncertain behavior of ovary — (Use additional code to identify any functional activity) ♀
236.3 Neoplasm of uncertain behavior of other and unspecified female genital organs ▽ ♀
239.5 Neoplasm of unspecified nature of other genitourinary organs
553.9 Hernia of unspecified site of abdominal cavity without mention of obstruction or gangrene ▽
614.4 Chronic or unspecified parametritis and pelvic cellulitis — (Use additional code to identify organism: 041.0, 041.1) ♀
614.9 Unspecified inflammatory disease of female pelvic organs and tissues — (Use additional code to identify organism: 041.0, 041.1) ▽ ♀
617.0 Endometriosis of uterus ♀
617.9 Endometriosis, site unspecified ▽ ♀
618.1 Uterine prolapse without mention of vaginal wall prolapse — (Use additional code to identify urinary incontinence: 625.6, 788.31, 788.33-788.39) ♀
618.2 Uterovaginal prolapse, incomplete — (Use additional code to identify urinary incontinence: 625.6, 788.31, 788.33-788.39) ♀
618.3 Uterovaginal prolapse, complete — (Use additional code to identify urinary incontinence: 625.6, 788.31, 788.33-788.39) ♀
618.4 Uterovaginal prolapse, unspecified — (Use additional code to identify urinary incontinence: 625.6, 788.31, 788.33-788.39) ▽ ♀
618.6 Vaginal enterocele, congenital or acquired — (Use additional code to identify urinary incontinence: 625.6, 788.31, 788.33-788.39) ♀
618.82 Incompetence or weakening of rectovaginal tissue
618.9 Unspecified genital prolapse — (Use additional code to identify urinary incontinence: 625.6, 788.31, 788.33-788.39) ▽ ♀
621.0 Polyp of corpus uteri ♀
621.2 Hypertrophy of uterus ♀
621.30 Endometrial hyperplasia, unspecified
621.31 Simple endometrial hyperplasia without atypia
621.32 Complex endometrial hyperplasia without atypia
621.33 Endometrial hyperplasia with atypia
621.6 Malposition of uterus ♀
621.8 Other specified disorders of uterus, not elsewhere classified ♀
621.9 Unspecified disorder of uterus ▽ ♀
622.10 Dysplasia of cervix, unspecified
622.11 Mild dysplasia of cervix
622.12 Moderate dysplasia of cervix
625.3 Dysmenorrhea ♀
625.6 Female stress incontinence ♀
625.8 Other specified symptom associated with female genital organs ♀
625.9 Unspecified symptom associated with female genital organs ▽ ♀
626.2 Excessive or frequent menstruation ♀
626.6 Metrorrhagia ♀
626.8 Other disorder of menstruation and other abnormal bleeding from female genital tract ♀
626.9 Unspecified disorder of menstruation and other abnormal bleeding from female genital tract ▽ ♀
627.1 Postmenopausal bleeding ♀
677 Late effect of complication of pregnancy, childbirth, and the puerperium — (Code first any sequelae) ♀
788.33 Mixed incontinence urge and stress (male)(female)
789.30 Abdominal or pelvic swelling, mass or lump, unspecified site ▽
V50.49 Other prophylactic gland removal
V84.02 Genetic susceptibility to malignant neoplasm of ovary
V84.04 Genetic susceptibility to malignant neoplasm of endometrium
V84.09 Genetic susceptibility to other malignant neoplasm

ICD-9-CM Procedural

65.39 Other unilateral oophorectomy
65.49 Other unilateral salpingo-oophorectomy
65.51 Other removal of both ovaries at same operative episode
65.52 Other removal of remaining ovary
65.61 Other removal of both ovaries and tubes at same operative episode
65.62 Other removal of remaining ovary and tube
68.59 Other vaginal hysterectomy
70.92 Other operations on cul-de-sac

HCPCS Level II Supplies & Services

HCPCS Level II codes are used to report the supplies, durable medical equipment, and certain medical services provided on an outpatient basis. Because the procedure(s) represented on this page would be performed in an inpatient facility, no HCPCS Level II codes apply.

58293

58293 Vaginal hysterectomy, for uterus greater than 250 grams; with colpo-urethrocystopexy (Marshall-Marchetti-Krantz type, Pereyra type) with or without endoscopic control

ICD-9-CM Diagnostic

180.0 Malignant neoplasm of endocervix ♀
180.1 Malignant neoplasm of exocervix ♀
180.8 Malignant neoplasm of other specified sites of cervix ♀
182.0 Malignant neoplasm of corpus uteri, except isthmus ♀
182.1 Malignant neoplasm of isthmus ♀
182.8 Malignant neoplasm of other specified sites of body of uterus ♀
218.0 Submucous leiomyoma of uterus ♀
218.1 Intramural leiomyoma of uterus ♀
218.2 Subserous leiomyoma of uterus ♀
218.9 Leiomyoma of uterus, unspecified ▽ ♀
614.4 Chronic or unspecified parametritis and pelvic cellulitis — (Use additional code to identify organism: 041.0, 041.1) ♀
614.9 Unspecified inflammatory disease of female pelvic organs and tissues — (Use additional code to identify organism: 041.0, 041.1) ▽ ♀
617.0 Endometriosis of uterus ♀
618.00 Prolapse of vaginal walls without mention of uterine prolapse, unspecified
618.01 Cystocele without mention of uterine prolapse, midline
618.02 Cystocele without mention of uterine prolapse, lateral
618.03 Urethrocele without mention of uterine prolapse
618.09 Other prolapse of vaginal walls without mention of uterine prolapse
618.1 Uterine prolapse without mention of vaginal wall prolapse — (Use additional code to identify urinary incontinence: 625.6, 788.31, 788.33-788.39) ♀
618.2 Uterovaginal prolapse, incomplete — (Use additional code to identify urinary incontinence: 625.6, 788.31, 788.33-788.39) ♀
618.3 Uterovaginal prolapse, complete — (Use additional code to identify urinary incontinence: 625.6, 788.31, 788.33-788.39) ♀
618.4 Uterovaginal prolapse, unspecified — (Use additional code to identify urinary incontinence: 625.6, 788.31, 788.33-788.39) ▽ ♀
625.3 Dysmenorrhea ♀
625.6 Female stress incontinence ♀
626.2 Excessive or frequent menstruation ♀
626.8 Other disorder of menstruation and other abnormal bleeding from female genital tract ♀
788.33 Mixed incontinence urge and stress (male)(female)
V84.02 Genetic susceptibility to malignant neoplasm of ovary
V84.04 Genetic susceptibility to malignant neoplasm of endometrium
V84.09 Genetic susceptibility to other malignant neoplasm

ICD-9-CM Procedural

59.5 Retropubic urethral suspension
68.59 Other vaginal hysterectomy

HCPCS Level II Supplies & Services

HCPCS Level II codes are used to report the supplies, durable medical equipment, and certain medical services provided on an outpatient basis. Because the procedure(s) represented on this page would be performed in an inpatient facility, no HCPCS Level II codes apply.

58294

58294 Vaginal hysterectomy, for uterus greater than 250 grams; with repair of enterocele

ICD-9-CM Diagnostic

180.0 Malignant neoplasm of endocervix ♀
180.1 Malignant neoplasm of exocervix ♀
182.0 Malignant neoplasm of corpus uteri, except isthmus ♀
182.1 Malignant neoplasm of isthmus ♀
182.8 Malignant neoplasm of other specified sites of body of uterus ♀
218.0 Submucous leiomyoma of uterus ♀
218.1 Intramural leiomyoma of uterus ♀
218.2 Subserous leiomyoma of uterus ♀
218.9 Leiomyoma of uterus, unspecified ♀
233.1 Carcinoma in situ of cervix uteri ♀
618.00 Prolapse of vaginal walls without mention of uterine prolapse, unspecified
618.1 Uterine prolapse without mention of vaginal wall prolapse — (Use additional code to identify urinary incontinence: 625.6, 788.31, 788.33-788.39) ♀
618.2 Uterovaginal prolapse, incomplete — (Use additional code to identify urinary incontinence: 625.6, 788.31, 788.33-788.39) ♀
618.3 Uterovaginal prolapse, complete — (Use additional code to identify urinary incontinence: 625.6, 788.31, 788.33-788.39) ♀
618.4 Uterovaginal prolapse, unspecified — (Use additional code to identify urinary incontinence: 625.6, 788.31, 788.33-788.39) ♀
618.6 Vaginal enterocele, congenital or acquired — (Use additional code to identify urinary incontinence: 625.6, 788.31, 788.33-788.39) ♀
618.82 Incompetence or weakening of rectovaginal tissue
618.9 Unspecified genital prolapse — (Use additional code to identify urinary incontinence: 625.6, 788.31, 788.33-788.39) ♀
621.30 Endometrial hyperplasia, unspecified
621.31 Simple endometrial hyperplasia without atypia
621.32 Complex endometrial hyperplasia without atypia
621.33 Endometrial hyperplasia with atypia
622.10 Dysplasia of cervix, unspecified
622.11 Mild dysplasia of cervix
622.12 Moderate dysplasia of cervix
625.3 Dysmenorrhea ♀
625.6 Female stress incontinence ♀
626.2 Excessive or frequent menstruation ♀
626.6 Metrorrhagia ♀
626.8 Other disorder of menstruation and other abnormal bleeding from female genital tract ♀
627.1 Postmenopausal bleeding ♀
788.33 Mixed incontinence urge and stress (male)(female)
V84.02 Genetic susceptibility to malignant neoplasm of ovary
V84.04 Genetic susceptibility to malignant neoplasm of endometrium
V84.09 Genetic susceptibility to other malignant neoplasm

ICD-9-CM Procedural

68.59 Other vaginal hysterectomy
70.92 Other operations on cul-de-sac

58300–58301

58300 Insertion of intrauterine device (IUD)
58301 Removal of intrauterine device (IUD)

ICD-9-CM Diagnostic

996.32 Mechanical complication due to intrauterine contraceptive device ♀
996.65 Infection and inflammatory reaction due to other genitourinary device, implant, and graft — (Use additional code to identify specified infections)
996.76 Other complications due to genitourinary device, implant, and graft
V25.1 Insertion of intrauterine contraceptive device ♀
V25.42 Surveillance of previously prescribed intrauterine contraceptive device ♀

ICD-9-CM Procedural

69.7 Insertion of intrauterine contraceptive device
97.71 Removal of intrauterine contraceptive device

HCPCS Level II Supplies & Services

A4550 Surgical trays
J7300 Intrauterine copper contraceptive
J7302 Levonorgestrel-releasing intrauterine contraceptive system, 52 mg

58321–58322

58321 Artificial insemination; intra-cervical
58322 intra-uterine

ICD-9-CM Diagnostic

606.0 Azoospermia ♂
606.1 Oligospermia ♂
606.8 Infertility due to extratesticular causes ♂
606.9 Unspecified male infertility ♂
622.4 Stricture and stenosis of cervix ♀
628.0 Female infertility associated with anovulation — (Use additional code for any associated Stein-Leventhal syndrome, 256.4) ♀
628.1 Female infertility of pituitary-hypothalamic origin — (Code first underlying disease: 253.0-253.4, 253.8) ♀
628.4 Female infertility of cervical or vaginal origin ♀
628.8 Female infertility of other specified origin ♀
628.9 Female infertility of unspecified origin ♀
V26.1 Artificial insemination ♀

ICD-9-CM Procedural

69.92 Artificial insemination

HCPCS Level II Supplies & Services

A4550 Surgical trays

58323

58323 Sperm washing for artificial insemination

ICD-9-CM Diagnostic

606.0 Azoospermia ♂
606.1 Oligospermia ♂
606.8 Infertility due to extratesticular causes ♂
606.9 Unspecified male infertility ♂
622.4 Stricture and stenosis of cervix ♀
628.0 Female infertility associated with anovulation — (Use additional code for any associated Stein-Leventhal syndrome, 256.4) ♀
628.1 Female infertility of pituitary-hypothalamic origin — (Code first underlying disease: 253.0-253.4, 253.8) ♀
628.4 Female infertility of cervical or vaginal origin ♀
628.8 Female infertility of other specified origin ♀
628.9 Female infertility of unspecified origin ♀
V26.1 Artificial insemination ♀

ICD-9-CM Procedural

99.99 Other miscellaneous procedures

HCPCS Level II Supplies & Services

A4649 Surgical supply; miscellaneous

58340

58340 Catheterization and introduction of saline or contrast material for saline infusion sonohysterography (SIS) or hysterosalpingography

ICD-9-CM Diagnostic

218.0 Submucous leiomyoma of uterus ♀
218.1 Intramural leiomyoma of uterus ♀
218.2 Subserous leiomyoma of uterus ♀
218.9 Leiomyoma of uterus, unspecified ♀
256.31 Premature menopause ♀
256.39 Other ovarian failure ♀
256.4 Polycystic ovaries ♀
256.8 Other ovarian dysfunction ♀
259.9 Unspecified endocrine disorder
614.1 Chronic salpingitis and oophoritis — (Use additional code to identify organism: 041.0, 041.1) ♀
614.2 Salpingitis and oophoritis not specified as acute, subacute, or chronic — (Use additional code to identify organism: 041.0, 041.1) ♀
614.6 Pelvic peritoneal adhesions, female (postoperative) (postinfection) — (Use additional code to identify any associated infertility, 628.2. Use additional code to identify organism: 041.0, 041.1) ♀
614.9 Unspecified inflammatory disease of female pelvic organs and tissues — (Use additional code to identify organism: 041.0, 041.1) ♀
617.0 Endometriosis of uterus ♀

617.1 Endometriosis of ovary ♀
617.2 Endometriosis of fallopian tube ♀
617.3 Endometriosis of pelvic peritoneum ♀
617.9 Endometriosis, site unspecified ▽ ♀
620.5 Torsion of ovary, ovarian pedicle, or fallopian tube ♀
620.8 Other noninflammatory disorder of ovary, fallopian tube, and broad ligament ♀
621.1 Chronic subinvolution of uterus ♀
621.2 Hypertrophy of uterus ♀
625.3 Dysmenorrhea ♀
625.5 Pelvic congestion syndrome ♀
626.0 Absence of menstruation ♀
626.1 Scanty or infrequent menstruation ♀
626.2 Excessive or frequent menstruation ♀
626.4 Irregular menstrual cycle ♀
626.6 Metrorrhagia ♀
628.0 Female infertility associated with anovulation — (Use additional code for any associated Stein-Levanthal syndrome, 256.4) ♀
628.2 Female infertility of tubal origin — (Use additional code for any associated peritubal adhesions, 614.6) ♀
628.3 Female infertility of uterine origin — (Use additional code for any associated tuberculous endometriosis, 016.7) ♀
628.8 Female infertility of other specified origin ♀
628.9 Female infertility of unspecified origin ▽ ♀
629.0 Hematocele, female, not elsewhere classified ♀
752.2 Congenital doubling of uterus ♀
752.3 Other congenital anomaly of uterus ♀
789.00 Abdominal pain, unspecified site ▽
789.30 Abdominal or pelvic swelling, mass or lump, unspecified site ▽
793.5 Nonspecific abnormal findings on radiological and other examination of genitourinary organs
998.2 Accidental puncture or laceration during procedure
V13.29 Personal history of other genital system and obstetric disorders
V26.0 Tuboplasty or vasoplasty after previous sterilization
V26.21 Fertility testing
V26.22 Aftercare following sterilization reversal
V26.29 Other investigation and testing
V71.89 Observation for other specified suspected conditions
V72.5 Radiological examination, not elsewhere classified — (Use additional code(s) to identify any special screening examination(s) performed: V73.0-V82.9)

ICD-9-CM Procedural

68.19 Other diagnostic procedures on uterus and supporting structures
87.82 Gas contrast hysterosalpingogram
87.83 Opaque dye contrast hysterosalpingogram
87.84 Percutaneous hysterogram

58345

58345 Transcervical introduction of fallopian tube catheter for diagnosis and/or re-establishing patency (any method), with or without hysterosalpingography

ICD-9-CM Diagnostic

256.4 Polycystic ovaries ♀
256.8 Other ovarian dysfunction ♀
614.1 Chronic salpingitis and oophoritis — (Use additional code to identify organism: 041.0, 041.1) ♀
614.2 Salpingitis and oophoritis not specified as acute, subacute, or chronic — (Use additional code to identify organism: 041.0, 041.1) ♀
614.6 Pelvic peritoneal adhesions, female (postoperative) (postinfection) — (Use additional code to identify any associated infertility, 628.2. Use additional code to identify organism: 041.0, 041.1) ♀
617.2 Endometriosis of fallopian tube ♀
620.8 Other noninflammatory disorder of ovary, fallopian tube, and broad ligament ♀
621.1 Chronic subinvolution of uterus ♀
621.2 Hypertrophy of uterus ♀
621.30 Endometrial hyperplasia, unspecified
621.31 Simple endometrial hyperplasia without atypia
621.32 Complex endometrial hyperplasia without atypia
621.33 Endometrial hyperplasia with atypia
621.7 Chronic inversion of uterus ♀
622.4 Stricture and stenosis of cervix ♀
622.8 Other specified noninflammatory disorder of cervix ♀
628.2 Female infertility of tubal origin — (Use additional code for any associated peritubal adhesions, 614.6) ♀
628.8 Female infertility of other specified origin ♀
628.9 Female infertility of unspecified origin ▽ ♀
752.19 Other congenital anomaly of fallopian tubes and broad ligaments ♀
V26.21 Fertility testing
V26.22 Aftercare following sterilization reversal
V26.29 Other investigation and testing

ICD-9-CM Procedural

66.79 Other repair of fallopian tube
66.8 Insufflation of fallopian tube
66.95 Insufflation of therapeutic agent into fallopian tubes
66.96 Dilation of fallopian tube
87.85 Other x-ray of fallopian tubes and uterus

58346

58346 Insertion of Heyman capsules for clinical brachytherapy

ICD-9-CM Diagnostic

179 Malignant neoplasm of uterus, part unspecified ▽ ♀
180.0 Malignant neoplasm of endocervix ♀
180.1 Malignant neoplasm of exocervix ♀
180.8 Malignant neoplasm of other specified sites of cervix ♀
180.9 Malignant neoplasm of cervix uteri, unspecified site ▽ ♀
182.0 Malignant neoplasm of corpus uteri, except isthmus ♀
182.1 Malignant neoplasm of isthmus ♀
182.8 Malignant neoplasm of other specified sites of body of uterus ♀
198.82 Secondary malignant neoplasm of genital organs
233.1 Carcinoma in situ of cervix uteri ♀
233.2 Carcinoma in situ of other and unspecified parts of uterus ▽ ♀
233.3 Carcinoma in situ of other and unspecified female genital organs ▽ ♀
236.0 Neoplasm of uncertain behavior of uterus ♀
236.3 Neoplasm of uncertain behavior of other and unspecified female genital organs ▽ ♀

ICD-9-CM Procedural

92.27 Implantation or insertion of radioactive elements

HCPCS Level II Supplies & Services

HCPCS Level II codes are used to report the supplies, durable medical equipment, and certain medical services provided on an outpatient basis. Because the procedure(s) represented on this page would be performed in an inpatient or outpatient facility, no HCPCS Level II codes apply.

58350

58350 Chromotubation of oviduct, including materials

ICD-9-CM Diagnostic

614.1 Chronic salpingitis and oophoritis — (Use additional code to identify organism: 041.0, 041.1) ♀
614.2 Salpingitis and oophoritis not specified as acute, subacute, or chronic — (Use additional code to identify organism: 041.0, 041.1) ♀
614.3 Acute parametritis and pelvic cellulitis — (Use additional code to identify organism: 041.0, 041.1) ♀
614.4 Chronic or unspecified parametritis and pelvic cellulitis — (Use additional code to identify organism: 041.0, 041.1) ♀
614.5 Acute or unspecified pelvic peritonitis, female — (Use additional code to identify organism: 041.0, 041.1) ♀
614.6 Pelvic peritoneal adhesions, female (postoperative) (postinfection) — (Use additional code to identify any associated infertility, 628.2. Use additional code to identify organism: 041.0, 041.1) ♀
617.0 Endometriosis of uterus ♀
617.2 Endometriosis of fallopian tube ♀
617.3 Endometriosis of pelvic peritoneum ♀
617.8 Endometriosis of other specified sites ♀
620.0 Follicular cyst of ovary ♀
620.2 Other and unspecified ovarian cyst ▽ ♀
620.3 Acquired atrophy of ovary and fallopian tube ♀
620.8 Other noninflammatory disorder of ovary, fallopian tube, and broad ligament ♀
625.3 Dysmenorrhea ♀
628.2 Female infertility of tubal origin — (Use additional code for any associated peritubal adhesions, 614.6) ♀
628.8 Female infertility of other specified origin ♀
628.9 Female infertility of unspecified origin ▽ ♀
752.19 Other congenital anomaly of fallopian tubes and broad ligaments ♀
V26.21 Fertility testing

V26.22 Aftercare following sterilization reversal
V26.29 Other investigation and testing

ICD-9-CM Procedural

66.8 Insufflation of fallopian tube
66.95 Insufflation of therapeutic agent into fallopian tubes

58353–58356

58353 Endometrial ablation, thermal, without hysteroscopic guidance
58356 Endometrial cryoablation with ultrasonic guidance, including endometrial curettage, when performed

ICD-9-CM Diagnostic

617.0 Endometriosis of uterus ♀
617.9 Endometriosis, site unspecified ▽ ♀
626.2 Excessive or frequent menstruation ♀
626.6 Metrorrhagia ♀
626.8 Other disorder of menstruation and other abnormal bleeding from female genital tract ♀
627.1 Postmenopausal bleeding ♀

ICD-9-CM Procedural

68.23 Endometrial ablation
69.09 Other dilation and curettage of uterus
69.59 Other aspiration curettage of uterus
88.79 Other diagnostic ultrasound

HCPCS Level II Supplies & Services

A4550 Surgical trays

58400–58410

58400 Uterine suspension, with or without shortening of round ligaments, with or without shortening of sacrouterine ligaments; (separate procedure)
58410 with presacral sympathectomy

ICD-9-CM Diagnostic

618.00 Prolapse of vaginal walls without mention of uterine prolapse, unspecified
618.1 Uterine prolapse without mention of vaginal wall prolapse — (Use additional code to identify urinary incontinence: 625.6, 788.31, 788.33-788.39) ♀
618.2 Uterovaginal prolapse, incomplete — (Use additional code to identify urinary incontinence: 625.6, 788.31, 788.33-788.39) ♀
618.3 Uterovaginal prolapse, complete — (Use additional code to identify urinary incontinence: 625.6, 788.31, 788.33-788.39) ♀
618.81 Incompetence or weakening of pubocervical tissue
618.89 Other specified genital prolapse
621.6 Malposition of uterus ♀
621.7 Chronic inversion of uterus ♀
625.0 Dyspareunia ♀
625.3 Dysmenorrhea ♀
625.6 Female stress incontinence ♀
625.8 Other specified symptom associated with female genital organs ♀
625.9 Unspecified symptom associated with female genital organs ▽ ♀

ICD-9-CM Procedural

05.24 Presacral sympathectomy
69.21 Interposition operation of uterine supporting structures
69.22 Other uterine suspension
69.29 Other repair of uterus and supporting structures
69.98 Other operations on supporting structures of uterus

58520

58520 Hysterorrhaphy, repair of ruptured uterus (nonobstetrical)

ICD-9-CM Diagnostic

621.8 Other specified disorders of uterus, not elsewhere classified ♀
867.4 Uterus injury without mention of open wound into cavity ♀
867.5 Uterus injury with open wound into cavity ♀

ICD-9-CM Procedural

69.29 Other repair of uterus and supporting structures
69.49 Other repair of uterus

58540

58540 Hysteroplasty, repair of uterine anomaly (Strassman type)

ICD-9-CM Diagnostic

621.5 Intrauterine synechiae ♀
621.8 Other specified disorders of uterus, not elsewhere classified ♀
752.2 Congenital doubling of uterus ♀
752.3 Other congenital anomaly of uterus ♀

ICD-9-CM Procedural

68.22 Incision or excision of congenital septum of uterus
69.23 Vaginal repair of chronic inversion of uterus
69.49 Other repair of uterus

58545–58546

58545 Laparoscopy, surgical, myomectomy, excision; 1 to 4 intramural myomas with total weight of 250 grams or less and/or removal of surface myomas
58546 5 or more intramural myomas and/or intramural myomas with total weight greater than 250 grams

ICD-9-CM Diagnostic

218.0 Submucous leiomyoma of uterus ♀
218.1 Intramural leiomyoma of uterus ♀
218.2 Subserous leiomyoma of uterus ♀
218.9 Leiomyoma of uterus, unspecified ▽ ♀

ICD-9-CM Procedural

68.29 Other excision or destruction of lesion of uterus

HCPCS Level II Supplies & Services

HCPCS Level II codes are used to report the supplies, durable medical equipment, and certain medical services provided on an outpatient basis. Because the procedure(s) represented on this page would be performed in an inpatient facility, no HCPCS Level II codes apply.

58550–58554

58550 Laparoscopy surgical, with vaginal hysterectomy, for uterus 250 grams or less;
58552 with removal of tube(s) and/or ovary(s)
58553 Laparoscopy, surgical, with vaginal hysterectomy, for uterus greater than 250 grams;
58554 with removal of tube(s) and/or ovary(s)

ICD-9-CM Diagnostic

180.0 Malignant neoplasm of endocervix ♀
180.1 Malignant neoplasm of exocervix ♀
180.8 Malignant neoplasm of other specified sites of cervix ♀
180.9 Malignant neoplasm of cervix uteri, unspecified site ▽ ♀
181 Malignant neoplasm of placenta ♀
182.0 Malignant neoplasm of corpus uteri, except isthmus ♀
182.1 Malignant neoplasm of isthmus ♀
182.8 Malignant neoplasm of other specified sites of body of uterus ♀
183.0 Malignant neoplasm of ovary — (Use additional code to identify any functional activity) ♀
183.8 Malignant neoplasm of other specified sites of uterine adnexa ♀
183.9 Malignant neoplasm of uterine adnexa, unspecified site ▽ ♀
198.6 Secondary malignant neoplasm of ovary ♀
199.1 Other malignant neoplasm of unspecified site
218.0 Submucous leiomyoma of uterus ♀
218.1 Intramural leiomyoma of uterus ♀
218.2 Subserous leiomyoma of uterus ♀
218.9 Leiomyoma of uterus, unspecified ▽ ♀
233.1 Carcinoma in situ of cervix uteri ♀
233.2 Carcinoma in situ of other and unspecified parts of uterus ▽ ♀
233.3 Carcinoma in situ of other and unspecified female genital organs ▽ ♀
236.0 Neoplasm of uncertain behavior of uterus ♀
236.2 Neoplasm of uncertain behavior of ovary — (Use additional code to identify any functional activity) ♀
236.3 Neoplasm of uncertain behavior of other and unspecified female genital organs ▽ ♀
239.5 Neoplasm of unspecified nature of other genitourinary organs
553.9 Hernia of unspecified site of abdominal cavity without mention of obstruction or gangrene ▽
614.4 Chronic or unspecified parametritis and pelvic cellulitis — (Use additional code to identify organism: 041.0, 041.1) ♀
614.9 Unspecified inflammatory disease of female pelvic organs and tissues — (Use additional code to identify organism: 041.0, 041.1) ▽ ♀

617.0 Endometriosis of uterus ♀
617.9 Endometriosis, site unspecified ▽ ♀
618.00 Prolapse of vaginal walls without mention of uterine prolapse, unspecified
618.1 Uterine prolapse without mention of vaginal wall prolapse — (Use additional code to identify urinary incontinence: 625.6, 788.31, 788.33-788.39) ♀
618.2 Uterovaginal prolapse, incomplete — (Use additional code to identify urinary incontinence: 625.6, 788.31, 788.33-788.39) ♀
618.3 Uterovaginal prolapse, complete — (Use additional code to identify urinary incontinence: 625.6, 788.31, 788.33-788.39) ♀
618.4 Uterovaginal prolapse, unspecified — (Use additional code to identify urinary incontinence: 625.6, 788.31, 788.33-788.39) ▽ ♀
618.89 Other specified genital prolapse
618.9 Unspecified genital prolapse — (Use additional code to identify urinary incontinence: 625.6, 788.31, 788.33-788.39) ▽ ♀
621.0 Polyp of corpus uteri ♀
621.2 Hypertrophy of uterus ♀
621.30 Endometrial hyperplasia, unspecified
621.31 Simple endometrial hyperplasia without atypia
621.32 Complex endometrial hyperplasia without atypia
621.33 Endometrial hyperplasia with atypia
621.6 Malposition of uterus ♀
621.8 Other specified disorders of uterus, not elsewhere classified ♀
621.9 Unspecified disorder of uterus ▽ ♀
622.10 Dysplasia of cervix, unspecified
622.11 Mild dysplasia of cervix
622.12 Moderate dysplasia of cervix
625.3 Dysmenorrhea ♀
625.6 Female stress incontinence ♀
625.8 Other specified symptom associated with female genital organs ♀
625.9 Unspecified symptom associated with female genital organs ▽ ♀
626.2 Excessive or frequent menstruation ♀
626.6 Metrorrhagia ♀
626.8 Other disorder of menstruation and other abnormal bleeding from female genital tract ♀
626.9 Unspecified disorder of menstruation and other abnormal bleeding from female genital tract ▽ ♀
627.1 Postmenopausal bleeding ♀
677 Late effect of complication of pregnancy, childbirth, and the puerperium — (Code first any sequelae) ♀
788.33 Mixed incontinence urge and stress (male)(female)
789.30 Abdominal or pelvic swelling, mass or lump, unspecified site ▽
V50.49 Other prophylactic gland removal
V84.02 Genetic susceptibility to malignant neoplasm of ovary
V84.04 Genetic susceptibility to malignant neoplasm of endometrium
V84.09 Genetic susceptibility to other malignant neoplasm

ICD-9-CM Procedural

65.31 Laparoscopic unilateral oophorectomy
65.41 Laparoscopic unilateral salpingo-oophorectomy
65.53 Laparoscopic removal of both ovaries at same operative episode
65.54 Laparoscopic removal of remaining ovary
65.63 Laparoscopic removal of both ovaries and tubes at same operative episode
65.64 Laparoscopic removal of remaining ovary and tube
68.31 Laparoscopic supracervical hysterectomy [LSH]
68.51 Laparoscopically assisted vaginal hysterectomy (LAVH)

HCPCS Level II Supplies & Services

HCPCS Level II codes are used to report the supplies, durable medical equipment, and certain medical services provided on an outpatient basis. Because the procedure(s) represented on this page would be performed in an inpatient facility, no HCPCS Level II codes apply.

58555

58555 Hysteroscopy, diagnostic (separate procedure)

ICD-9-CM Diagnostic

179 Malignant neoplasm of uterus, part unspecified ▽ ♀
180.0 Malignant neoplasm of endocervix ♀
180.1 Malignant neoplasm of exocervix ♀
180.8 Malignant neoplasm of other specified sites of cervix ♀
180.9 Malignant neoplasm of cervix uteri, unspecified site ▽ ♀
182.0 Malignant neoplasm of corpus uteri, except isthmus ♀
182.1 Malignant neoplasm of isthmus ♀
183.2 Malignant neoplasm of fallopian tube ♀
183.3 Malignant neoplasm of broad ligament of uterus ♀
183.4 Malignant neoplasm of parametrium of uterus ♀
183.5 Malignant neoplasm of round ligament of uterus ♀
183.8 Malignant neoplasm of other specified sites of uterine adnexa ♀
183.9 Malignant neoplasm of uterine adnexa, unspecified site ▽ ♀
198.82 Secondary malignant neoplasm of genital organs
218.0 Submucous leiomyoma of uterus ♀
218.1 Intramural leiomyoma of uterus ♀
218.2 Subserous leiomyoma of uterus ♀
218.9 Leiomyoma of uterus, unspecified ▽ ♀
219.0 Benign neoplasm of cervix uteri ♀
219.1 Benign neoplasm of corpus uteri ♀
219.8 Benign neoplasm of other specified parts of uterus ♀
219.9 Benign neoplasm of uterus, part unspecified ▽ ♀
221.0 Benign neoplasm of fallopian tube and uterine ligaments ♀
221.8 Benign neoplasm of other specified sites of female genital organs ♀
233.1 Carcinoma in situ of cervix uteri ♀
233.2 Carcinoma in situ of other and unspecified parts of uterus ▽ ♀
233.3 Carcinoma in situ of other and unspecified female genital organs ▽ ♀
236.0 Neoplasm of uncertain behavior of uterus ♀
236.3 Neoplasm of uncertain behavior of other and unspecified female genital organs ▽ ♀
239.5 Neoplasm of unspecified nature of other genitourinary organs
614.4 Chronic or unspecified parametritis and pelvic cellulitis — (Use additional code to identify organism: 041.0, 041.1) ♀
615.0 Acute inflammatory disease of uterus, except cervix — (Use additional code to identify organism: 041.0, 041.1) ♀
615.1 Chronic inflammatory disease of uterus, except cervix — (Use additional code to identify organism: 041.0, 041.1) ♀
616.0 Cervicitis and endocervicitis — (Use additional code to identify organism: 041.0, 041.1) ♀
617.0 Endometriosis of uterus ♀
618.1 Uterine prolapse without mention of vaginal wall prolapse — (Use additional code to identify urinary incontinence: 625.6, 788.31, 788.33-788.39) ♀
621.0 Polyp of corpus uteri ♀
621.2 Hypertrophy of uterus ♀
621.30 Endometrial hyperplasia, unspecified
621.31 Simple endometrial hyperplasia without atypia
621.32 Complex endometrial hyperplasia without atypia
621.33 Endometrial hyperplasia with atypia
621.4 Hematometra ♀
621.5 Intrauterine synechiae ♀
621.8 Other specified disorders of uterus, not elsewhere classified ♀
622.10 Dysplasia of cervix, unspecified
622.11 Mild dysplasia of cervix
622.12 Moderate dysplasia of cervix
623.8 Other specified noninflammatory disorder of vagina ♀
625.3 Dysmenorrhea ♀
626.0 Absence of menstruation ♀
626.2 Excessive or frequent menstruation ♀
626.4 Irregular menstrual cycle ♀
626.6 Metrorrhagia ♀
626.8 Other disorder of menstruation and other abnormal bleeding from female genital tract ♀
627.0 Premenopausal menorrhagia ♀
627.1 Postmenopausal bleeding ♀
628.3 Female infertility of uterine origin — (Use additional code for any associated tuberculous endometriosis, 016.7) ♀
628.9 Female infertility of unspecified origin ▽ ♀
629.0 Hematocele, female, not elsewhere classified ♀
629.1 Hydrocele, canal of Nuck ♀
629.8 Other specified disorder of female genital organs ♀
789.00 Abdominal pain, unspecified site ▽
789.01 Abdominal pain, right upper quadrant
789.02 Abdominal pain, left upper quadrant
789.03 Abdominal pain, right lower quadrant
789.04 Abdominal pain, left lower quadrant
789.30 Abdominal or pelvic swelling, mass or lump, unspecified site ▽
789.31 Abdominal or pelvic swelling, mass, or lump, right upper quadrant
789.32 Abdominal or pelvic swelling, mass, or lump, left upper quadrant
789.33 Abdominal or pelvic swelling, mass, or lump, right lower quadrant
789.34 Abdominal or pelvic swelling, mass, or lump, left lower quadrant
V26.21 Fertility testing
V26.29 Other investigation and testing
V84.02 Genetic susceptibility to malignant neoplasm of ovary
V84.04 Genetic susceptibility to malignant neoplasm of endometrium
V84.09 Genetic susceptibility to other malignant neoplasm

▽ Unspecified code
♀ Female diagnosis
☒ Manifestation code
♂ Male diagnosis

ICD-9-CM Procedural

68.12 Hysteroscopy

HCPCS Level II Supplies & Services

A4550 Surgical trays

58558

58558 Hysteroscopy, surgical; with sampling (biopsy) of endometrium and/or polypectomy, with or without D & C

ICD-9-CM Diagnostic

179 Malignant neoplasm of uterus, part unspecified ▽ ♀
180.0 Malignant neoplasm of endocervix ♀
180.1 Malignant neoplasm of exocervix ♀
180.8 Malignant neoplasm of other specified sites of cervix ♀
180.9 Malignant neoplasm of cervix uteri, unspecified site ▽ ♀
182.0 Malignant neoplasm of corpus uteri, except isthmus ♀
182.1 Malignant neoplasm of isthmus ♀
182.8 Malignant neoplasm of other specified sites of body of uterus ♀
199.1 Other malignant neoplasm of unspecified site
218.0 Submucous leiomyoma of uterus ♀
218.1 Intramural leiomyoma of uterus ♀
218.2 Subserous leiomyoma of uterus ♀
219.0 Benign neoplasm of cervix uteri ♀
219.1 Benign neoplasm of corpus uteri ♀
219.8 Benign neoplasm of other specified parts of uterus ♀
219.9 Benign neoplasm of uterus, part unspecified ▽ ♀
233.1 Carcinoma in situ of cervix uteri ♀
233.2 Carcinoma in situ of other and unspecified parts of uterus ▽ ♀
233.3 Carcinoma in situ of other and unspecified female genital organs ▽ ♀
236.0 Neoplasm of uncertain behavior of uterus ♀
236.3 Neoplasm of uncertain behavior of other and unspecified female genital organs ▽ ♀
239.5 Neoplasm of unspecified nature of other genitourinary organs
256.9 Unspecified ovarian dysfunction ▽ ♀
614.6 Pelvic peritoneal adhesions, female (postoperative) (postinfection) — (Use additional code to identify any associated infertility, 628.2. Use additional code to identify organism: 041.0, 041.1) ♀
617.0 Endometriosis of uterus ♀
617.1 Endometriosis of ovary ♀
617.3 Endometriosis of pelvic peritoneum ♀
617.9 Endometriosis, site unspecified ▽ ♀
618.1 Uterine prolapse without mention of vaginal wall prolapse — (Use additional code to identify urinary incontinence: 625.6, 788.31, 788.33-788.39) ♀
621.0 Polyp of corpus uteri ♀
621.2 Hypertrophy of uterus ♀
621.30 Endometrial hyperplasia, unspecified
621.31 Simple endometrial hyperplasia without atypia
621.32 Complex endometrial hyperplasia without atypia
621.33 Endometrial hyperplasia with atypia
622.10 Dysplasia of cervix, unspecified
622.11 Mild dysplasia of cervix
622.12 Moderate dysplasia of cervix
622.4 Stricture and stenosis of cervix ♀
622.7 Mucous polyp of cervix ♀
625.3 Dysmenorrhea ♀
625.6 Female stress incontinence ♀
625.8 Other specified symptom associated with female genital organs ♀
626.0 Absence of menstruation ♀
626.2 Excessive or frequent menstruation ♀
626.4 Irregular menstrual cycle ♀
626.6 Metrorrhagia ♀
626.8 Other disorder of menstruation and other abnormal bleeding from female genital tract ♀
627.0 Premenopausal menorrhagia ♀
627.1 Postmenopausal bleeding ♀
628.2 Female infertility of tubal origin — (Use additional code for any associated peritubal adhesions, 614.6) ♀
628.3 Female infertility of uterine origin — (Use additional code for any associated tuberculous endometriosis, 016.7) ♀
628.4 Female infertility of cervical or vaginal origin ♀
628.8 Female infertility of other specified origin ♀
628.9 Female infertility of unspecified origin ▽ ♀
789.30 Abdominal or pelvic swelling, mass or lump, unspecified site ▽
789.31 Abdominal or pelvic swelling, mass, or lump, right upper quadrant
789.32 Abdominal or pelvic swelling, mass, or lump, left upper quadrant
789.33 Abdominal or pelvic swelling, mass, or lump, right lower quadrant
789.34 Abdominal or pelvic swelling, mass, or lump, left lower quadrant
795.00 Abnormal glandular Papanicolaou smear of cervix ▽ ♀
795.01 Papanicolaou smear of cervix with atypical squamous cells of undetermined significance (ASC-US) ♀
795.02 Papanicolaou smear of cervix with atypical squamous cells cannot exclude high grade squamous intraepithelial lesion (ASC-H) ♀
795.03 Papanicolaou smear of cervix with low grade squamous intraepithelial lesion (LGSIL)
795.04 Papanicolaou smear of cervix with high grade squamous intraepithelial lesion (HGSIL)
795.05 Cervical high risk human papillomavirus (HPV) DNA test positive
795.08 Nonspecific abnormal papanicolaou smear of cervix, unsatisfactory smear
795.09 Other abnormal Papanicolaou smear of cervix and cervical HPV ♀
795.1 Nonspecific abnormal Papanicolaou smear of other site ▽
795.39 Other nonspecific positive culture findings
V26.21 Fertility testing
V84.02 Genetic susceptibility to malignant neoplasm of ovary
V84.04 Genetic susceptibility to malignant neoplasm of endometrium
V84.09 Genetic susceptibility to other malignant neoplasm

ICD-9-CM Procedural

68.16 Closed biopsy of uterus
68.29 Other excision or destruction of lesion of uterus
69.09 Other dilation and curettage of uterus

58559–58560

58559 Hysteroscopy, surgical; with lysis of intrauterine adhesions (any method)
58560 with division or resection of intrauterine septum (any method)

ICD-9-CM Diagnostic

621.5 Intrauterine synechiae ♀
626.2 Excessive or frequent menstruation ♀
752.2 Congenital doubling of uterus ♀
752.3 Other congenital anomaly of uterus ♀
908.1 Late effect of internal injury to intra-abdominal organs
908.2 Late effect of internal injury to other internal organs
908.6 Late effect of certain complications of trauma
909.3 Late effect of complications of surgical and medical care

ICD-9-CM Procedural

68.21 Division of endometrial synechiae
68.22 Incision or excision of congenital septum of uterus

58561

58561 Hysteroscopy, surgical; with removal of leiomyomata

ICD-9-CM Diagnostic

218.0 Submucous leiomyoma of uterus ♀
218.1 Intramural leiomyoma of uterus ♀
218.2 Subserous leiomyoma of uterus ♀
218.9 Leiomyoma of uterus, unspecified ▽ ♀
626.2 Excessive or frequent menstruation ♀
626.6 Metrorrhagia ♀

ICD-9-CM Procedural

68.29 Other excision or destruction of lesion of uterus

58562

58562 Hysteroscopy, surgical; with removal of impacted foreign body

ICD-9-CM Diagnostic

939.1 Foreign body in uterus, any part ♀
996.32 Mechanical complication due to intrauterine contraceptive device ♀
996.65 Infection and inflammatory reaction due to other genitourinary device, implant, and graft — (Use additional code to identify specified infections)

ICD-9-CM Procedural

97.71 Removal of intrauterine contraceptive device
98.16 Removal of intraluminal foreign body from uterus without incision

58563

58563 Hysteroscopy, surgical; with endometrial ablation (eg, endometrial resection, electrosurgical ablation, thermoablation)

ICD-9-CM Diagnostic

617.0 Endometriosis of uterus ♀
617.9 Endometriosis, site unspecified ▽ ♀
626.2 Excessive or frequent menstruation ♀
626.6 Metrorrhagia ♀
626.8 Other disorder of menstruation and other abnormal bleeding from female genital tract ♀
627.1 Postmenopausal bleeding ♀

ICD-9-CM Procedural

68.23 Endometrial ablation

58565

58565 Hysteroscopy, surgical; with bilateral fallopian tube cannulation to induce occlusion by placement of permanent implants

ICD-9-CM Diagnostic

659.41 Grand multiparity, delivered, with or without mention of antepartum condition ♀
V25.2 Sterilization
V61.5 Multiparity

ICD-9-CM Procedural

66.29 Other bilateral endoscopic destruction or occlusion of fallopian tubes

Oviduct/Ovary

58600–58605

58600 Ligation or transection of fallopian tube(s), abdominal or vaginal approach, unilateral or bilateral
58605 Ligation or transection of fallopian tube(s), abdominal or vaginal approach, postpartum, unilateral or bilateral, during same hospitalization (separate procedure)

ICD-9-CM Diagnostic

659.41 Grand multiparity, delivered, with or without mention of antepartum condition ♀
V25.2 Sterilization
V61.5 Multiparity

ICD-9-CM Procedural

66.32 Other bilateral ligation and division of fallopian tubes

58611

58611 Ligation or transection of fallopian tube(s) when done at the time of cesarean delivery or intra-abdominal surgery (not a separate procedure) (List separately in addition to code for primary procedure)

ICD-9-CM Diagnostic

V25.2 Sterilization
V61.5 Multiparity

ICD-9-CM Procedural

66.32 Other bilateral ligation and division of fallopian tubes

58615

58615 Occlusion of fallopian tube(s) by device (eg, band, clip, Falope ring) vaginal or suprapubic approach

ICD-9-CM Diagnostic

V25.2 Sterilization
V61.5 Multiparity

ICD-9-CM Procedural

66.31 Other bilateral ligation and crushing of fallopian tubes
66.39 Other bilateral destruction or occlusion of fallopian tubes
66.92 Unilateral destruction or occlusion of fallopian tube

58660

58660 Laparoscopy, surgical; with lysis of adhesions (salpingolysis, ovariolysis) (separate procedure)

ICD-9-CM Diagnostic

568.0 Peritoneal adhesions (postoperative) (postinfection)
568.89 Other specified disorder of peritoneum
614.1 Chronic salpingitis and oophoritis — (Use additional code to identify organism: 041.0, 041.1) ♀
614.2 Salpingitis and oophoritis not specified as acute, subacute, or chronic — (Use additional code to identify organism: 041.0, 041.1) ♀
614.5 Acute or unspecified pelvic peritonitis, female — (Use additional code to identify organism: 041.0, 041.1) ♀
614.6 Pelvic peritoneal adhesions, female (postoperative) (postinfection) — (Use additional code to identify any associated infertility, 628.2. Use additional code to identify organism: 041.0, 041.1) ♀
614.9 Unspecified inflammatory disease of female pelvic organs and tissues — (Use additional code to identify organism: 041.0, 041.1) ▽ ♀
617.0 Endometriosis of uterus ♀
617.1 Endometriosis of ovary ♀
617.2 Endometriosis of fallopian tube ♀
617.3 Endometriosis of pelvic peritoneum ♀
617.8 Endometriosis of other specified sites ♀
625.3 Dysmenorrhea ♀
625.8 Other specified symptom associated with female genital organs ♀
628.2 Female infertility of tubal origin — (Use additional code for any associated peritubal adhesions, 614.6) ♀
628.3 Female infertility of uterine origin — (Use additional code for any associated tuberculous endometriosis, 016.7) ♀
628.8 Female infertility of other specified origin ♀
628.9 Female infertility of unspecified origin ▽ ♀
789.00 Abdominal pain, unspecified site ▽
789.01 Abdominal pain, right upper quadrant
789.02 Abdominal pain, left upper quadrant
789.03 Abdominal pain, right lower quadrant
789.04 Abdominal pain, left lower quadrant
789.05 Abdominal pain, periumbilic
789.30 Abdominal or pelvic swelling, mass or lump, unspecified site ▽
789.31 Abdominal or pelvic swelling, mass, or lump, right upper quadrant
789.32 Abdominal or pelvic swelling, mass, or lump, left upper quadrant
789.33 Abdominal or pelvic swelling, mass, or lump, right lower quadrant
789.34 Abdominal or pelvic swelling, mass, or lump, left lower quadrant

ICD-9-CM Procedural

65.81 Laparoscpic lysis of adhesions of ovary and fallopian tube

58661

58661 Laparoscopy, surgical; with removal of adnexal structures (partial or total oophorectomy and/or salpingectomy)

ICD-9-CM Diagnostic

183.0 Malignant neoplasm of ovary — (Use additional code to identify any functional activity) ♀
183.2 Malignant neoplasm of fallopian tube ♀
183.8 Malignant neoplasm of other specified sites of uterine adnexa ♀
198.6 Secondary malignant neoplasm of ovary ♀
220 Benign neoplasm of ovary — (Use additional code to identify any functional activity: 256.0-256.1) ♀
221.0 Benign neoplasm of fallopian tube and uterine ligaments ♀
221.8 Benign neoplasm of other specified sites of female genital organs ♀
233.3 Carcinoma in situ of other and unspecified female genital organs ▽ ♀
236.2 Neoplasm of uncertain behavior of ovary — (Use additional code to identify any functional activity) ♀
236.3 Neoplasm of uncertain behavior of other and unspecified female genital organs ▽ ♀
239.5 Neoplasm of unspecified nature of other genitourinary organs
256.0 Hyperestrogenism ♀
614.1 Chronic salpingitis and oophoritis — (Use additional code to identify organism: 041.0, 041.1) ♀
614.2 Salpingitis and oophoritis not specified as acute, subacute, or chronic — (Use additional code to identify organism: 041.0, 041.1) ♀
614.6 Pelvic peritoneal adhesions, female (postoperative) (postinfection) — (Use additional code to identify any associated infertility, 628.2. Use additional code to identify organism: 041.0, 041.1) ♀
617.1 Endometriosis of ovary ♀
617.2 Endometriosis of fallopian tube ♀

▽ Unspecified code ☒ Manifestation code
♀ Female diagnosis ♂ Male diagnosis

617.3 Endometriosis of pelvic peritoneum ♀
617.9 Endometriosis, site unspecified ♀
620.0 Follicular cyst of ovary ♀
620.1 Corpus luteum cyst or hematoma ♀
620.2 Other and unspecified ovarian cyst ♀
620.5 Torsion of ovary, ovarian pedicle, or fallopian tube ♀
628.2 Female infertility of tubal origin — (Use additional code for any associated peritubal adhesions, 614.6) ♀
789.00 Abdominal pain, unspecified site
789.01 Abdominal pain, right upper quadrant
789.02 Abdominal pain, left upper quadrant
789.03 Abdominal pain, right lower quadrant
789.04 Abdominal pain, left lower quadrant
789.30 Abdominal or pelvic swelling, mass or lump, unspecified site
789.31 Abdominal or pelvic swelling, mass, or lump, right upper quadrant
789.32 Abdominal or pelvic swelling, mass, or lump, left upper quadrant
789.33 Abdominal or pelvic swelling, mass, or lump, right lower quadrant
789.34 Abdominal or pelvic swelling, mass, or lump, left lower quadrant
V84.02 Genetic susceptibility to malignant neoplasm of ovary
V84.04 Genetic susceptibility to malignant neoplasm of endometrium
V84.09 Genetic susceptibility to other malignant neoplasm

ICD-9-CM Procedural

65.24 Laparoscopic wedge resection of ovary
65.31 Laparoscopic unilateral oophorectomy
65.41 Laparoscopic unilateral salpingo-oophorectomy
65.53 Laparoscopic removal of both ovaries at same operative episode
65.54 Laparoscopic removal of remaining ovary
65.63 Laparoscopic removal of both ovaries and tubes at same operative episode
65.64 Laparoscopic removal of remaining ovary and tube
66.4 Total unilateral salpingectomy
66.51 Removal of both fallopian tubes at same operative episode
66.52 Removal of remaining fallopian tube
66.62 Salpingectomy with removal of tubal pregnancy
66.63 Bilateral partial salpingectomy, not otherwise specified
66.69 Other partial salpingectomy

58662

58662 Laparoscopy, surgical; with fulguration or excision of lesions of the ovary, pelvic viscera, or peritoneal surface by any method

ICD-9-CM Diagnostic

158.8 Malignant neoplasm of specified parts of peritoneum
158.9 Malignant neoplasm of peritoneum, unspecified
159.8 Malignant neoplasm of other sites of digestive system and intra-abdominal organs
197.6 Secondary malignant neoplasm of retroperitoneum and peritoneum
211.8 Benign neoplasm of retroperitoneum and peritoneum
219.1 Benign neoplasm of corpus uteri ♀
220 Benign neoplasm of ovary — (Use additional code to identify any functional activity: 256.0-256.1) ♀
221.0 Benign neoplasm of fallopian tube and uterine ligaments ♀
235.4 Neoplasm of uncertain behavior of retroperitoneum and peritoneum
256.4 Polycystic ovaries ♀
568.89 Other specified disorder of peritoneum
614.6 Pelvic peritoneal adhesions, female (postoperative) (postinfection) — (Use additional code to identify any associated infertility, 628.2. Use additional code to identify organism: 041.0, 041.1) ♀
617.0 Endometriosis of uterus ♀
617.1 Endometriosis of ovary ♀
617.2 Endometriosis of fallopian tube ♀
617.3 Endometriosis of pelvic peritoneum ♀
617.8 Endometriosis of other specified sites ♀
617.9 Endometriosis, site unspecified ♀
620.0 Follicular cyst of ovary ♀
620.1 Corpus luteum cyst or hematoma ♀
620.2 Other and unspecified ovarian cyst ♀
620.8 Other noninflammatory disorder of ovary, fallopian tube, and broad ligament ♀
621.0 Polyp of corpus uteri ♀
621.30 Endometrial hyperplasia, unspecified
621.31 Simple endometrial hyperplasia without atypia
621.32 Complex endometrial hyperplasia without atypia
621.33 Endometrial hyperplasia with atypia
625.3 Dysmenorrhea ♀
625.8 Other specified symptom associated with female genital organs ♀
628.0 Female infertility associated with anovulation — (Use additional code for any associated Stein-Levanthal syndrome, 256.4) ♀
628.2 Female infertility of tubal origin — (Use additional code for any associated peritubal adhesions, 614.6) ♀
628.3 Female infertility of uterine origin — (Use additional code for any associated tuberculous endometriosis, 016.7) ♀
628.8 Female infertility of other specified origin ♀
752.11 Embryonic cyst of fallopian tubes and broad ligaments ♀
789.00 Abdominal pain, unspecified site
789.01 Abdominal pain, right upper quadrant
789.02 Abdominal pain, left upper quadrant
789.03 Abdominal pain, right lower quadrant
789.04 Abdominal pain, left lower quadrant
789.30 Abdominal or pelvic swelling, mass or lump, unspecified site
789.31 Abdominal or pelvic swelling, mass, or lump, right upper quadrant
789.32 Abdominal or pelvic swelling, mass, or lump, left upper quadrant
789.33 Abdominal or pelvic swelling, mass, or lump, right lower quadrant
789.34 Abdominal or pelvic swelling, mass, or lump, left lower quadrant
V84.02 Genetic susceptibility to malignant neoplasm of ovary
V84.04 Genetic susceptibility to malignant neoplasm of endometrium
V84.09 Genetic susceptibility to other malignant neoplasm

ICD-9-CM Procedural

54.4 Excision or destruction of peritoneal tissue
65.25 Other laparoscopic local excision or destruction of ovary
69.19 Other excision or destruction of uterus and supporting structures

58670–58671

58670 Laparoscopy, surgical; with fulguration of oviducts (with or without transection)
58671 with occlusion of oviducts by device (eg, band, clip, or Falope ring)

ICD-9-CM Diagnostic

V25.2 Sterilization
V61.5 Multiparity

ICD-9-CM Procedural

66.21 Bilateral endoscopic ligation and crushing of fallopian tubes
66.22 Bilateral endoscopic ligation and division of fallopian tubes
66.29 Other bilateral endoscopic destruction or occlusion of fallopian tubes

58672

58672 Laparoscopy, surgical; with fimbrioplasty

ICD-9-CM Diagnostic

614.1 Chronic salpingitis and oophoritis — (Use additional code to identify organism: 041.0, 041.1) ♀
614.2 Salpingitis and oophoritis not specified as acute, subacute, or chronic — (Use additional code to identify organism: 041.0, 041.1) ♀
614.4 Chronic or unspecified parametritis and pelvic cellulitis — (Use additional code to identify organism: 041.0, 041.1) ♀
614.6 Pelvic peritoneal adhesions, female (postoperative) (postinfection) — (Use additional code to identify any associated infertility, 628.2. Use additional code to identify organism: 041.0, 041.1) ♀
614.8 Other specified inflammatory disease of female pelvic organs and tissues — (Use additional code to identify organism: 041.0, 041.1) ♀
617.2 Endometriosis of fallopian tube ♀
628.2 Female infertility of tubal origin — (Use additional code for any associated peritubal adhesions, 614.6) ♀
752.19 Other congenital anomaly of fallopian tubes and broad ligaments ♀

ICD-9-CM Procedural

66.79 Other repair of fallopian tube

58673

58673 Laparoscopy, surgical; with salpingostomy (salpingoneostomy)

ICD-9-CM Diagnostic

139.8 Late effects of other and unspecified infectious and parasitic diseases
614.1 Chronic salpingitis and oophoritis — (Use additional code to identify organism: 041.0, 041.1) ♀
614.2 Salpingitis and oophoritis not specified as acute, subacute, or chronic — (Use additional code to identify organism: 041.0, 041.1) ♀
614.4 Chronic or unspecified parametritis and pelvic cellulitis — (Use additional code to identify organism: 041.0, 041.1) ♀

614.6 Pelvic peritoneal adhesions, female (postoperative) (postinfection) — (Use additional code to identify any associated infertility, 628.2. Use additional code to identify organism: 041.0, 041.1) ♀
614.8 Other specified inflammatory disease of female pelvic organs and tissues — (Use additional code to identify organism: 041.0, 041.1) ♀
617.2 Endometriosis of fallopian tube ♀
628.2 Female infertility of tubal origin — (Use additional code for any associated peritubal adhesions, 614.6) ♀
908.2 Late effect of internal injury to other internal organs
V51 Aftercare involving the use of plastic surgery

ICD-9-CM Procedural

66.02 Salpingostomy

58700

58700 Salpingectomy, complete or partial, unilateral or bilateral (separate procedure)

ICD-9-CM Diagnostic

183.2 Malignant neoplasm of fallopian tube ♀
198.82 Secondary malignant neoplasm of genital organs
221.0 Benign neoplasm of fallopian tube and uterine ligaments ♀
233.3 Carcinoma in situ of other and unspecified female genital organs ▽ ♀
236.3 Neoplasm of uncertain behavior of other and unspecified female genital organs ▽ ♀
239.5 Neoplasm of unspecified nature of other genitourinary organs
614.1 Chronic salpingitis and oophoritis — (Use additional code to identify organism: 041.0, 041.1) ♀
614.2 Salpingitis and oophoritis not specified as acute, subacute, or chronic — (Use additional code to identify organism: 041.0, 041.1) ♀
617.2 Endometriosis of fallopian tube ♀
620.4 Prolapse or hernia of ovary and fallopian tube ♀
620.5 Torsion of ovary, ovarian pedicle, or fallopian tube ♀
789.00 Abdominal pain, unspecified site ▽
V50.49 Other prophylactic gland removal
V84.02 Genetic susceptibility to malignant neoplasm of ovary
V84.04 Genetic susceptibility to malignant neoplasm of endometrium
V84.09 Genetic susceptibility to other malignant neoplasm

ICD-9-CM Procedural

66.4 Total unilateral salpingectomy
66.51 Removal of both fallopian tubes at same operative episode
66.52 Removal of remaining fallopian tube
66.63 Bilateral partial salpingectomy, not otherwise specified
66.69 Other partial salpingectomy

58720

58720 Salpingo-oophorectomy, complete or partial, unilateral or bilateral (separate procedure)

ICD-9-CM Diagnostic

183.0 Malignant neoplasm of ovary — (Use additional code to identify any functional activity) ♀
183.2 Malignant neoplasm of fallopian tube ♀
198.6 Secondary malignant neoplasm of ovary ♀
198.89 Secondary malignant neoplasm of other specified sites
199.1 Other malignant neoplasm of unspecified site
220 Benign neoplasm of ovary — (Use additional code to identify any functional activity: 256.0-256.1) ♀
221.0 Benign neoplasm of fallopian tube and uterine ligaments ♀
233.3 Carcinoma in situ of other and unspecified female genital organs ▽ ♀
236.2 Neoplasm of uncertain behavior of ovary — (Use additional code to identify any functional activity) ♀
236.3 Neoplasm of uncertain behavior of other and unspecified female genital organs ▽ ♀
239.5 Neoplasm of unspecified nature of other genitourinary organs
256.0 Hyperestrogenism ♀
256.4 Polycystic ovaries ♀
614.0 Acute salpingitis and oophoritis — (Use additional code to identify organism: 041.0, 041.1) ♀
614.1 Chronic salpingitis and oophoritis — (Use additional code to identify organism: 041.0, 041.1) ♀
614.2 Salpingitis and oophoritis not specified as acute, subacute, or chronic — (Use additional code to identify organism: 041.0, 041.1) ♀
614.6 Pelvic peritoneal adhesions, female (postoperative) (postinfection) — (Use additional code to identify any associated infertility, 628.2. Use additional code to identify organism: 041.0, 041.1) ♀
617.1 Endometriosis of ovary ♀
617.2 Endometriosis of fallopian tube ♀
620.0 Follicular cyst of ovary ♀
620.1 Corpus luteum cyst or hematoma ♀
620.2 Other and unspecified ovarian cyst ▽ ♀
620.4 Prolapse or hernia of ovary and fallopian tube ♀
620.5 Torsion of ovary, ovarian pedicle, or fallopian tube ♀
620.8 Other noninflammatory disorder of ovary, fallopian tube, and broad ligament ♀
625.3 Dysmenorrhea ♀
625.8 Other specified symptom associated with female genital organs ♀
626.2 Excessive or frequent menstruation ♀
626.8 Other disorder of menstruation and other abnormal bleeding from female genital tract ♀
628.2 Female infertility of tubal origin — (Use additional code for any associated peritubal adhesions, 614.6) ♀
752.0 Congenital anomalies of ovaries ♀
752.10 Unspecified congenital anomaly of fallopian tubes and broad ligaments ▽ ♀
752.11 Embryonic cyst of fallopian tubes and broad ligaments ♀
V84.02 Genetic susceptibility to malignant neoplasm of ovary
V84.04 Genetic susceptibility to malignant neoplasm of endometrium
V84.09 Genetic susceptibility to other malignant neoplasm

ICD-9-CM Procedural

65.49 Other unilateral salpingo-oophorectomy
65.61 Other removal of both ovaries and tubes at same operative episode
65.62 Other removal of remaining ovary and tube

58740

58740 Lysis of adhesions (salpingolysis, ovariolysis)

ICD-9-CM Diagnostic

614.1 Chronic salpingitis and oophoritis — (Use additional code to identify organism: 041.0, 041.1) ♀
614.2 Salpingitis and oophoritis not specified as acute, subacute, or chronic — (Use additional code to identify organism: 041.0, 041.1) ♀
614.5 Acute or unspecified pelvic peritonitis, female — (Use additional code to identify organism: 041.0, 041.1) ♀
614.6 Pelvic peritoneal adhesions, female (postoperative) (postinfection) — (Use additional code to identify any associated infertility, 628.2. Use additional code to identify organism: 041.0, 041.1) ♀
617.0 Endometriosis of uterus ♀
617.1 Endometriosis of ovary ♀
617.2 Endometriosis of fallopian tube ♀
617.3 Endometriosis of pelvic peritoneum ♀
625.3 Dysmenorrhea ♀
625.8 Other specified symptom associated with female genital organs ♀
626.2 Excessive or frequent menstruation ♀
628.2 Female infertility of tubal origin — (Use additional code for any associated peritubal adhesions, 614.6) ♀
628.8 Female infertility of other specified origin ♀
752.19 Other congenital anomaly of fallopian tubes and broad ligaments ♀
789.01 Abdominal pain, right upper quadrant
789.02 Abdominal pain, left upper quadrant
789.03 Abdominal pain, right lower quadrant
789.04 Abdominal pain, left lower quadrant
789.31 Abdominal or pelvic swelling, mass, or lump, right upper quadrant
789.32 Abdominal or pelvic swelling, mass, or lump, left upper quadrant
789.33 Abdominal or pelvic swelling, mass, or lump, right lower quadrant
789.34 Abdominal or pelvic swelling, mass, or lump, left lower quadrant
V64.41 Laparoscopic surgical procedure converted to open procedure

ICD-9-CM Procedural

65.89 Other lysis of adhesions of ovary and fallopian tube

58750

58750 Tubotubal anastomosis

ICD-9-CM Diagnostic

221.0 Benign neoplasm of fallopian tube and uterine ligaments ♀
614.1 Chronic salpingitis and oophoritis — (Use additional code to identify organism: 041.0, 041.1) ♀
614.2 Salpingitis and oophoritis not specified as acute, subacute, or chronic — (Use additional code to identify organism: 041.0, 041.1) ♀

614.6 Pelvic peritoneal adhesions, female (postoperative) (postinfection) — (Use additional code to identify any associated infertility, 628.2. Use additional code to identify organism: 041.0, 041.1) ♀
614.7 Other chronic pelvic peritonitis, female — (Use additional code to identify organism: 041.0, 041.1) ♀
614.8 Other specified inflammatory disease of female pelvic organs and tissues — (Use additional code to identify organism: 041.0, 041.1) ♀
628.2 Female infertility of tubal origin — (Use additional code for any associated peritubal adhesions, 614.6) ♀
628.8 Female infertility of other specified origin ♀
628.9 Female infertility of unspecified origin ▽ ♀
752.19 Other congenital anomaly of fallopian tubes and broad ligaments ♀
V26.0 Tuboplasty or vasoplasty after previous sterilization

ICD-9-CM Procedural

66.73 Salpingo-salpingostomy

58752

58752 Tubouterine implantation

ICD-9-CM Diagnostic

221.0 Benign neoplasm of fallopian tube and uterine ligaments ♀
614.1 Chronic salpingitis and oophoritis — (Use additional code to identify organism: 041.0, 041.1) ♀
614.2 Salpingitis and oophoritis not specified as acute, subacute, or chronic — (Use additional code to identify organism: 041.0, 041.1) ♀
614.6 Pelvic peritoneal adhesions, female (postoperative) (postinfection) — (Use additional code to identify any associated infertility, 628.2. Use additional code to identify organism: 041.0, 041.1) ♀
614.7 Other chronic pelvic peritonitis, female — (Use additional code to identify organism: 041.0, 041.1) ♀
614.8 Other specified inflammatory disease of female pelvic organs and tissues — (Use additional code to identify organism: 041.0, 041.1) ♀
628.2 Female infertility of tubal origin — (Use additional code for any associated peritubal adhesions, 614.6) ♀
752.19 Other congenital anomaly of fallopian tubes and broad ligaments ♀
V26.0 Tuboplasty or vasoplasty after previous sterilization

ICD-9-CM Procedural

66.74 Salpingo-uterostomy

58760

58760 Fimbrioplasty

ICD-9-CM Diagnostic

614.1 Chronic salpingitis and oophoritis — (Use additional code to identify organism: 041.0, 041.1) ♀
614.2 Salpingitis and oophoritis not specified as acute, subacute, or chronic — (Use additional code to identify organism: 041.0, 041.1) ♀
614.3 Acute parametritis and pelvic cellulitis — (Use additional code to identify organism: 041.0, 041.1) ♀
614.4 Chronic or unspecified parametritis and pelvic cellulitis — (Use additional code to identify organism: 041.0, 041.1) ♀
614.5 Acute or unspecified pelvic peritonitis, female — (Use additional code to identify organism: 041.0, 041.1) ♀
614.6 Pelvic peritoneal adhesions, female (postoperative) (postinfection) — (Use additional code to identify any associated infertility, 628.2. Use additional code to identify organism: 041.0, 041.1) ♀
614.8 Other specified inflammatory disease of female pelvic organs and tissues — (Use additional code to identify organism: 041.0, 041.1) ♀
617.2 Endometriosis of fallopian tube ♀
628.2 Female infertility of tubal origin — (Use additional code for any associated peritubal adhesions, 614.6) ♀
752.19 Other congenital anomaly of fallopian tubes and broad ligaments ♀
909.3 Late effect of complications of surgical and medical care
V64.41 Laparoscopic surgical procedure converted to open procedure

ICD-9-CM Procedural

66.79 Other repair of fallopian tube

58770

58770 Salpingostomy (salpingoneostomy)

ICD-9-CM Diagnostic

221.0 Benign neoplasm of fallopian tube and uterine ligaments ♀
256.9 Unspecified ovarian dysfunction ▽ ♀
614.1 Chronic salpingitis and oophoritis — (Use additional code to identify organism: 041.0, 041.1) ♀
614.2 Salpingitis and oophoritis not specified as acute, subacute, or chronic — (Use additional code to identify organism: 041.0, 041.1) ♀
614.3 Acute parametritis and pelvic cellulitis — (Use additional code to identify organism: 041.0, 041.1) ♀
614.4 Chronic or unspecified parametritis and pelvic cellulitis — (Use additional code to identify organism: 041.0, 041.1) ♀
614.5 Acute or unspecified pelvic peritonitis, female — (Use additional code to identify organism: 041.0, 041.1) ♀
614.6 Pelvic peritoneal adhesions, female (postoperative) (postinfection) — (Use additional code to identify any associated infertility, 628.2. Use additional code to identify organism: 041.0, 041.1) ♀
614.8 Other specified inflammatory disease of female pelvic organs and tissues — (Use additional code to identify organism: 041.0, 041.1) ♀
617.2 Endometriosis of fallopian tube ♀
620.9 Unspecified noninflammatory disorder of ovary, fallopian tube, and broad ligament ▽ ♀
625.9 Unspecified symptom associated with female genital organs ▽ ♀
628.2 Female infertility of tubal origin — (Use additional code for any associated peritubal adhesions, 614.6) ♀
908.2 Late effect of internal injury to other internal organs
909.3 Late effect of complications of surgical and medical care
V64.41 Laparoscopic surgical procedure converted to open procedure

ICD-9-CM Procedural

66.02 Salpingostomy
66.72 Salpingo-oophorostomy

Ovary

58800–58805

58800 Drainage of ovarian cyst(s), unilateral or bilateral, (separate procedure); vaginal approach
58805 abdominal approach

ICD-9-CM Diagnostic

220 Benign neoplasm of ovary — (Use additional code to identify any functional activity: 256.0-256.1) ♀
256.4 Polycystic ovaries ♀
620.0 Follicular cyst of ovary ♀
620.1 Corpus luteum cyst or hematoma ♀
620.2 Other and unspecified ovarian cyst ▽ ♀
789.31 Abdominal or pelvic swelling, mass, or lump, right upper quadrant
789.32 Abdominal or pelvic swelling, mass, or lump, left upper quadrant
789.33 Abdominal or pelvic swelling, mass, or lump, right lower quadrant
789.34 Abdominal or pelvic swelling, mass, or lump, left lower quadrant
V84.02 Genetic susceptibility to malignant neoplasm of ovary
V84.04 Genetic susceptibility to malignant neoplasm of endometrium
V84.09 Genetic susceptibility to other malignant neoplasm

ICD-9-CM Procedural

65.09 Other oophorectomy
65.91 Aspiration of ovary
65.93 Manual rupture of ovarian cyst

58820–58822

58820 Drainage of ovarian abscess; vaginal approach, open
58822 abdominal approach

ICD-9-CM Diagnostic

614.0 Acute salpingitis and oophoritis — (Use additional code to identify organism: 041.0, 041.1) ♀
614.1 Chronic salpingitis and oophoritis — (Use additional code to identify organism: 041.0, 041.1) ♀
614.2 Salpingitis and oophoritis not specified as acute, subacute, or chronic — (Use additional code to identify organism: 041.0, 041.1) ♀
614.3 Acute parametritis and pelvic cellulitis — (Use additional code to identify organism: 041.0, 041.1) ♀
614.4 Chronic or unspecified parametritis and pelvic cellulitis — (Use additional code to identify organism: 041.0, 041.1) ♀
780.6 Fever

789.01 Abdominal pain, right upper quadrant
789.02 Abdominal pain, left upper quadrant
789.03 Abdominal pain, right lower quadrant
789.04 Abdominal pain, left lower quadrant
789.31 Abdominal or pelvic swelling, mass, or lump, right upper quadrant
789.32 Abdominal or pelvic swelling, mass, or lump, left upper quadrant
789.33 Abdominal or pelvic swelling, mass, or lump, right lower quadrant
789.34 Abdominal or pelvic swelling, mass, or lump, left lower quadrant
998.51 Infected postoperative seroma — (Use additional code to identify organism)
998.59 Other postoperative infection — (Use additional code to identify infection)

ICD-9-CM Procedural
65.09 Other oophorectomy
65.11 Aspiration biopsy of ovary
65.91 Aspiration of ovary

58823
58823 Drainage of pelvic abscess, transvaginal or transrectal approach, percutaneous (eg, ovarian, pericolic)

ICD-9-CM Diagnostic
614.0 Acute salpingitis and oophoritis — (Use additional code to identify organism: 041.0, 041.1) ♀
614.1 Chronic salpingitis and oophoritis — (Use additional code to identify organism: 041.0, 041.1) ♀
614.2 Salpingitis and oophoritis not specified as acute, subacute, or chronic — (Use additional code to identify organism: 041.0, 041.1) ♀
614.3 Acute parametritis and pelvic cellulitis — (Use additional code to identify organism: 041.0, 041.1) ♀
614.4 Chronic or unspecified parametritis and pelvic cellulitis — (Use additional code to identify organism: 041.0, 041.1) ♀
780.6 Fever
789.01 Abdominal pain, right upper quadrant
789.02 Abdominal pain, left upper quadrant
789.03 Abdominal pain, right lower quadrant
789.04 Abdominal pain, left lower quadrant
789.33 Abdominal or pelvic swelling, mass, or lump, right lower quadrant
789.34 Abdominal or pelvic swelling, mass, or lump, left lower quadrant
998.51 Infected postoperative seroma — (Use additional code to identify organism)
998.59 Other postoperative infection — (Use additional code to identify infection)

ICD-9-CM Procedural
54.91 Percutaneous abdominal drainage
65.91 Aspiration of ovary

58825
58825 Transposition, ovary(s)

ICD-9-CM Diagnostic
153.3 Malignant neoplasm of sigmoid colon
153.8 Malignant neoplasm of other specified sites of large intestine
154.0 Malignant neoplasm of rectosigmoid junction
154.1 Malignant neoplasm of rectum
154.8 Malignant neoplasm of other sites of rectum, rectosigmoid junction, and anus
158.0 Malignant neoplasm of retroperitoneum
158.8 Malignant neoplasm of specified parts of peritoneum
188.0 Malignant neoplasm of trigone of urinary bladder
188.1 Malignant neoplasm of dome of urinary bladder
188.2 Malignant neoplasm of lateral wall of urinary bladder
188.3 Malignant neoplasm of anterior wall of urinary bladder

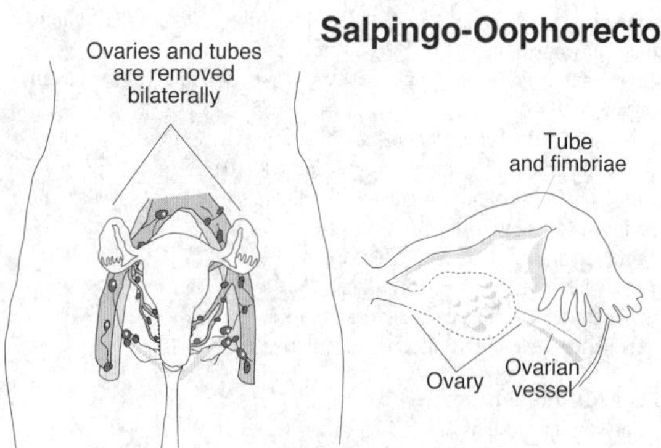

188.4 Malignant neoplasm of posterior wall of urinary bladder
188.5 Malignant neoplasm of bladder neck
189.2 Malignant neoplasm of ureter
189.3 Malignant neoplasm of urethra
752.0 Congenital anomalies of ovaries ♀

ICD-9-CM Procedural
65.99 Other operations on ovary

58900
58900 Biopsy of ovary, unilateral or bilateral (separate procedure)

ICD-9-CM Diagnostic
183.0 Malignant neoplasm of ovary — (Use additional code to identify any functional activity) ♀
183.8 Malignant neoplasm of other specified sites of uterine adnexa ♀
198.82 Secondary malignant neoplasm of genital organs
220 Benign neoplasm of ovary — (Use additional code to identify any functional activity: 256.0-256.1) ♀
236.2 Neoplasm of uncertain behavior of ovary — (Use additional code to identify any functional activity) ♀
239.5 Neoplasm of unspecified nature of other genitourinary organs
256.0 Hyperestrogenism ♀
617.1 Endometriosis of ovary ♀
620.0 Follicular cyst of ovary ♀
620.1 Corpus luteum cyst or hematoma ♀
620.2 Other and unspecified ovarian cyst ▽ ♀
620.8 Other noninflammatory disorder of ovary, fallopian tube, and broad ligament ♀
789.01 Abdominal pain, right upper quadrant
789.02 Abdominal pain, left upper quadrant
789.03 Abdominal pain, right lower quadrant
789.04 Abdominal pain, left lower quadrant
789.30 Abdominal or pelvic swelling, mass or lump, unspecified site ▽
789.31 Abdominal or pelvic swelling, mass, or lump, right upper quadrant
789.32 Abdominal or pelvic swelling, mass, or lump, left upper quadrant
789.33 Abdominal or pelvic swelling, mass, or lump, right lower quadrant
789.34 Abdominal or pelvic swelling, mass, or lump, left lower quadrant
V84.02 Genetic susceptibility to malignant neoplasm of ovary
V84.04 Genetic susceptibility to malignant neoplasm of endometrium
V84.09 Genetic susceptibility to other malignant neoplasm

ICD-9-CM Procedural
65.11 Aspiration biopsy of ovary
65.12 Other biopsy of ovary

58920
58920 Wedge resection or bisection of ovary, unilateral or bilateral

ICD-9-CM Diagnostic
220 Benign neoplasm of ovary — (Use additional code to identify any functional activity: 256.0-256.1) ♀
256.0 Hyperestrogenism ♀
256.1 Other ovarian hyperfunction ♀
256.4 Polycystic ovaries ♀
256.8 Other ovarian dysfunction ♀
620.0 Follicular cyst of ovary ♀
620.1 Corpus luteum cyst or hematoma ♀

▽ Unspecified code
♀ Female diagnosis
☒ Manifestation code
♂ Male diagnosis

620.2 Other and unspecified ovarian cyst ▽ ♀
789.31 Abdominal or pelvic swelling, mass, or lump, right upper quadrant
789.32 Abdominal or pelvic swelling, mass, or lump, left upper quadrant
789.33 Abdominal or pelvic swelling, mass, or lump, right lower quadrant
789.34 Abdominal or pelvic swelling, mass, or lump, left lower quadrant

ICD-9-CM Procedural
65.22 Wedge resection of ovary
65.29 Other local excision or destruction of ovary

58925
58925 Ovarian cystectomy, unilateral or bilateral

ICD-9-CM Diagnostic
220 Benign neoplasm of ovary — (Use additional code to identify any functional activity: 256.0-256.1) ♀
236.2 Neoplasm of uncertain behavior of ovary — (Use additional code to identify any functional activity) ♀
256.0 Hyperestrogenism ♀
256.4 Polycystic ovaries ♀
620.0 Follicular cyst of ovary ♀
620.1 Corpus luteum cyst or hematoma ♀
620.2 Other and unspecified ovarian cyst ▽ ♀
625.8 Other specified symptom associated with female genital organs ♀
625.9 Unspecified symptom associated with female genital organs ▽ ♀
752.11 Embryonic cyst of fallopian tubes and broad ligaments ♀
789.01 Abdominal pain, right upper quadrant
789.02 Abdominal pain, left upper quadrant
789.03 Abdominal pain, right lower quadrant
789.04 Abdominal pain, left lower quadrant
789.31 Abdominal or pelvic swelling, mass, or lump, right upper quadrant
789.32 Abdominal or pelvic swelling, mass, or lump, left upper quadrant
789.33 Abdominal or pelvic swelling, mass, or lump, right lower quadrant
789.34 Abdominal or pelvic swelling, mass, or lump, left lower quadrant

ICD-9-CM Procedural
65.21 Marsupialization of ovarian cyst
65.29 Other local excision or destruction of ovary

58940
58940 Oophorectomy, partial or total, unilateral or bilateral;

ICD-9-CM Diagnostic
183.0 Malignant neoplasm of ovary — (Use additional code to identify any functional activity) ♀
198.6 Secondary malignant neoplasm of ovary ♀
220 Benign neoplasm of ovary — (Use additional code to identify any functional activity: 256.0-256.1) ♀
233.3 Carcinoma in situ of other and unspecified female genital organs ▽ ♀
236.2 Neoplasm of uncertain behavior of ovary — (Use additional code to identify any functional activity) ♀
239.5 Neoplasm of unspecified nature of other genitourinary organs
256.0 Hyperestrogenism ♀
617.1 Endometriosis of ovary ♀
620.0 Follicular cyst of ovary ♀
620.1 Corpus luteum cyst or hematoma ♀
620.2 Other and unspecified ovarian cyst ▽ ♀
620.5 Torsion of ovary, ovarian pedicle, or fallopian tube ♀
620.8 Other noninflammatory disorder of ovary, fallopian tube, and broad ligament ♀
625.8 Other specified symptom associated with female genital organs ♀
625.9 Unspecified symptom associated with female genital organs ▽ ♀
752.11 Embryonic cyst of fallopian tubes and broad ligaments ♀
789.01 Abdominal pain, right upper quadrant
789.02 Abdominal pain, left upper quadrant
789.03 Abdominal pain, right lower quadrant
789.04 Abdominal pain, left lower quadrant
789.31 Abdominal or pelvic swelling, mass, or lump, right upper quadrant
789.32 Abdominal or pelvic swelling, mass, or lump, left upper quadrant
789.33 Abdominal or pelvic swelling, mass, or lump, right lower quadrant
789.34 Abdominal or pelvic swelling, mass, or lump, left lower quadrant
V50.42 Prophylactic ovary removal ♀
V64.41 Laparoscopic surgical procedure converted to open procedure
V84.02 Genetic susceptibility to malignant neoplasm of ovary
V84.04 Genetic susceptibility to malignant neoplasm of endometrium
V84.09 Genetic susceptibility to other malignant neoplasm

ICD-9-CM Procedural
65.21 Marsupialization of ovarian cyst
65.29 Other local excision or destruction of ovary
65.39 Other unilateral oophorectomy
65.51 Other removal of both ovaries at same operative episode
65.52 Other removal of remaining ovary

58943
58943 Oophorectomy, partial or total, unilateral or bilateral; for ovarian, tubal or primary peritoneal malignancy, with para-aortic and pelvic lymph node biopsies, peritoneal washings, peritoneal biopsies, diaphragmatic assessments, with or without salpingectomy(s), with or without omentectomy

ICD-9-CM Diagnostic
183.0 Malignant neoplasm of ovary — (Use additional code to identify any functional activity) ♀
183.8 Malignant neoplasm of other specified sites of uterine adnexa ♀
196.6 Secondary and unspecified malignant neoplasm of intrapelvic lymph nodes
197.6 Secondary malignant neoplasm of retroperitoneum and peritoneum
198.6 Secondary malignant neoplasm of ovary ♀
236.2 Neoplasm of uncertain behavior of ovary — (Use additional code to identify any functional activity) ♀
V84.02 Genetic susceptibility to malignant neoplasm of ovary
V84.04 Genetic susceptibility to malignant neoplasm of endometrium
V84.09 Genetic susceptibility to other malignant neoplasm

ICD-9-CM Procedural
40.11 Biopsy of lymphatic structure
54.23 Biopsy of peritoneum
54.4 Excision or destruction of peritoneal tissue
65.29 Other local excision or destruction of ovary
65.39 Other unilateral oophorectomy
65.49 Other unilateral salpingo-oophorectomy
65.51 Other removal of both ovaries at same operative episode
65.52 Other removal of remaining ovary
65.61 Other removal of both ovaries and tubes at same operative episode
65.62 Other removal of remaining ovary and tube

58950
58950 Resection of ovarian, tubal or primary peritoneal malignancy with bilateral salpingo-oophorectomy and omentectomy;

ICD-9-CM Diagnostic
158.8 Malignant neoplasm of specified parts of peritoneum
158.9 Malignant neoplasm of peritoneum, unspecified ▽
183.0 Malignant neoplasm of ovary — (Use additional code to identify any functional activity) ♀
183.2 Malignant neoplasm of fallopian tube ♀
183.8 Malignant neoplasm of other specified sites of uterine adnexa ♀
198.6 Secondary malignant neoplasm of ovary ♀
198.82 Secondary malignant neoplasm of genital organs
235.4 Neoplasm of uncertain behavior of retroperitoneum and peritoneum
236.2 Neoplasm of uncertain behavior of ovary — (Use additional code to identify any functional activity) ♀
236.3 Neoplasm of uncertain behavior of other and unspecified female genital organs ▽ ♀
V84.02 Genetic susceptibility to malignant neoplasm of ovary
V84.04 Genetic susceptibility to malignant neoplasm of endometrium
V84.09 Genetic susceptibility to other malignant neoplasm

ICD-9-CM Procedural
54.4 Excision or destruction of peritoneal tissue
65.61 Other removal of both ovaries and tubes at same operative episode

58951
58951 Resection of ovarian, tubal or primary peritoneal malignancy with bilateral salpingo-oophorectomy and omentectomy; with total abdominal hysterectomy, pelvic and limited para-aortic lymphadenectomy

ICD-9-CM Diagnostic
158.8 Malignant neoplasm of specified parts of peritoneum
158.9 Malignant neoplasm of peritoneum, unspecified ▽

183.0 Malignant neoplasm of ovary — (Use additional code to identify any functional activity) ♀
183.2 Malignant neoplasm of fallopian tube ♀
183.8 Malignant neoplasm of other specified sites of uterine adnexa ♀
196.2 Secondary and unspecified malignant neoplasm of intra-abdominal lymph nodes
196.6 Secondary and unspecified malignant neoplasm of intrapelvic lymph nodes
198.6 Secondary malignant neoplasm of ovary ♀
198.82 Secondary malignant neoplasm of genital organs
235.4 Neoplasm of uncertain behavior of retroperitoneum and peritoneum
236.2 Neoplasm of uncertain behavior of ovary — (Use additional code to identify any functional activity) ♀
236.3 Neoplasm of uncertain behavior of other and unspecified female genital organs ▽ ♀
V84.02 Genetic susceptibility to malignant neoplasm of ovary
V84.04 Genetic susceptibility to malignant neoplasm of endometrium
V84.09 Genetic susceptibility to other malignant neoplasm

ICD-9-CM Procedural

40.3 Regional lymph node excision
54.4 Excision or destruction of peritoneal tissue
65.61 Other removal of both ovaries and tubes at same operative episode
68.4 Total abdominal hysterectomy

58952

58952 Resection of ovarian, tubal or primary peritoneal malignancy with bilateral salpingo-oophorectomy and omentectomy; with radical dissection for debulking (ie, radical excision or destruction, intra-abdominal or retroperitoneal tumors)

ICD-9-CM Diagnostic

158.8 Malignant neoplasm of specified parts of peritoneum
158.9 Malignant neoplasm of peritoneum, unspecified ▽
183.0 Malignant neoplasm of ovary — (Use additional code to identify any functional activity) ♀
183.2 Malignant neoplasm of fallopian tube ♀
183.8 Malignant neoplasm of other specified sites of uterine adnexa ♀
197.6 Secondary malignant neoplasm of retroperitoneum and peritoneum
198.6 Secondary malignant neoplasm of ovary ♀
198.82 Secondary malignant neoplasm of genital organs
198.89 Secondary malignant neoplasm of other specified sites
199.0 Disseminated malignant neoplasm
199.1 Other malignant neoplasm of unspecified site
235.4 Neoplasm of uncertain behavior of retroperitoneum and peritoneum
236.2 Neoplasm of uncertain behavior of ovary — (Use additional code to identify any functional activity) ♀
236.3 Neoplasm of uncertain behavior of other and unspecified female genital organs ▽ ♀
V84.02 Genetic susceptibility to malignant neoplasm of ovary
V84.04 Genetic susceptibility to malignant neoplasm of endometrium
V84.09 Genetic susceptibility to other malignant neoplasm

ICD-9-CM Procedural

54.4 Excision or destruction of peritoneal tissue
65.61 Other removal of both ovaries and tubes at same operative episode

58953

58953 Bilateral salpingo-oophorectomy with omentectomy, total abdominal hysterectomy and radical dissection for debulking;

ICD-9-CM Diagnostic

158.8 Malignant neoplasm of specified parts of peritoneum
158.9 Malignant neoplasm of peritoneum, unspecified ▽
183.0 Malignant neoplasm of ovary — (Use additional code to identify any functional activity) ♀
183.2 Malignant neoplasm of fallopian tube ♀
183.8 Malignant neoplasm of other specified sites of uterine adnexa ♀
197.6 Secondary malignant neoplasm of retroperitoneum and peritoneum
198.6 Secondary malignant neoplasm of ovary ♀
198.82 Secondary malignant neoplasm of genital organs
198.89 Secondary malignant neoplasm of other specified sites
235.4 Neoplasm of uncertain behavior of retroperitoneum and peritoneum
236.2 Neoplasm of uncertain behavior of ovary — (Use additional code to identify any functional activity) ♀
236.3 Neoplasm of uncertain behavior of other and unspecified female genital organs ▽ ♀
V84.02 Genetic susceptibility to malignant neoplasm of ovary
V84.04 Genetic susceptibility to malignant neoplasm of endometrium
V84.09 Genetic susceptibility to other malignant neoplasm

ICD-9-CM Procedural

54.4 Excision or destruction of peritoneal tissue
68.6 Radical abdominal hysterectomy

HCPCS Level II Supplies & Services

HCPCS Level II codes are used to report the supplies, durable medical equipment, and certain medical services provided on an outpatient basis. Because the procedure(s) represented on this page would be performed in an inpatient facility, no HCPCS Level II codes apply.

58954

58954 Bilateral salpingo-oophorectomy with omentectomy, total abdominal hysterectomy and radical dissection for debulking; with pelvic lymphadenectomy and limited para-aortic lymphadenectomy

ICD-9-CM Diagnostic

158.8 Malignant neoplasm of specified parts of peritoneum
158.9 Malignant neoplasm of peritoneum, unspecified ▽
183.0 Malignant neoplasm of ovary — (Use additional code to identify any functional activity) ♀
183.2 Malignant neoplasm of fallopian tube ♀
183.8 Malignant neoplasm of other specified sites of uterine adnexa ♀
196.2 Secondary and unspecified malignant neoplasm of intra-abdominal lymph nodes
196.6 Secondary and unspecified malignant neoplasm of intrapelvic lymph nodes
197.6 Secondary malignant neoplasm of retroperitoneum and peritoneum
198.6 Secondary malignant neoplasm of ovary ♀
198.82 Secondary malignant neoplasm of genital organs
198.89 Secondary malignant neoplasm of other specified sites
235.4 Neoplasm of uncertain behavior of retroperitoneum and peritoneum
236.2 Neoplasm of uncertain behavior of ovary — (Use additional code to identify any functional activity) ♀
236.3 Neoplasm of uncertain behavior of other and unspecified female genital organs ▽ ♀
V84.02 Genetic susceptibility to malignant neoplasm of ovary
V84.04 Genetic susceptibility to malignant neoplasm of endometrium
V84.09 Genetic susceptibility to other malignant neoplasm

ICD-9-CM Procedural

40.3 Regional lymph node excision
54.4 Excision or destruction of peritoneal tissue
65.61 Other removal of both ovaries and tubes at same operative episode
68.6 Radical abdominal hysterectomy

HCPCS Level II Supplies & Services

HCPCS Level II codes are used to report the supplies, durable medical equipment, and certain medical services provided on an outpatient basis. Because the procedure(s) represented on this page would be performed in an inpatient facility, no HCPCS Level II codes apply.

58956

58956 Bilateral salpingo-oophorectomy with total omentectomy, total abdominal hysterectomy for malignancy

ICD-9-CM Diagnostic

158.8 Malignant neoplasm of specified parts of peritoneum
179 Malignant neoplasm of uterus, part unspecified ▽ ♀
180.0 Malignant neoplasm of endocervix ♀
180.1 Malignant neoplasm of exocervix ♀
180.8 Malignant neoplasm of other specified sites of cervix ♀
180.9 Malignant neoplasm of cervix uteri, unspecified site ▽ ♀
182.0 Malignant neoplasm of corpus uteri, except isthmus ♀
182.1 Malignant neoplasm of isthmus ♀
182.8 Malignant neoplasm of other specified sites of body of uterus ♀
183.0 Malignant neoplasm of ovary — (Use additional code to identify any functional activity) ♀
183.2 Malignant neoplasm of fallopian tube ♀
183.3 Malignant neoplasm of broad ligament of uterus ♀
183.4 Malignant neoplasm of parametrium of uterus ♀
183.5 Malignant neoplasm of round ligament of uterus ♀
183.8 Malignant neoplasm of other specified sites of uterine adnexa ♀
183.9 Malignant neoplasm of uterine adnexa, unspecified site ▽ ♀
184.0 Malignant neoplasm of vagina ♀

▽ Unspecified code
♀ Female diagnosis
☒ Manifestation code
♂ Male diagnosis

184.8 Malignant neoplasm of other specified sites of female genital organs ♀
184.9 Malignant neoplasm of female genital organ, site unspecified ▽ ♀
197.5 Secondary malignant neoplasm of large intestine and rectum
197.6 Secondary malignant neoplasm of retroperitoneum and peritoneum
198.1 Secondary malignant neoplasm of other urinary organs
198.6 Secondary malignant neoplasm of ovary ♀
198.82 Secondary malignant neoplasm of genital organs
199.0 Disseminated malignant neoplasm
199.1 Other malignant neoplasm of unspecified site
V84.02 Genetic susceptibility to malignant neoplasm of ovary
V84.04 Genetic susceptibility to malignant neoplasm of endometrium
V84.09 Genetic susceptibility to other malignant neoplasm

ICD-9-CM Procedural

54.4 Excision or destruction of peritoneal tissue
65.61 Other removal of both ovaries and tubes at same operative episode
68.4 Total abdominal hysterectomy

58960

58960 Laparotomy, for staging or restaging of ovarian, tubal or primary peritoneal malignancy (second look), with or without omentectomy, peritoneal washing, biopsy of abdominal and pelvic peritoneum, diaphragmatic assessment with pelvic and limited para-aortic lymphadenectomy

ICD-9-CM Diagnostic

183.0 Malignant neoplasm of ovary — (Use additional code to identify any functional activity) ♀
183.8 Malignant neoplasm of other specified sites of uterine adnexa ♀
196.6 Secondary and unspecified malignant neoplasm of intrapelvic lymph nodes
197.6 Secondary malignant neoplasm of retroperitoneum and peritoneum
198.6 Secondary malignant neoplasm of ovary ♀
198.89 Secondary malignant neoplasm of other specified sites
236.2 Neoplasm of uncertain behavior of ovary — (Use additional code to identify any functional activity) ♀
V10.43 Personal history of malignant neoplasm of ovary ♀
V84.02 Genetic susceptibility to malignant neoplasm of ovary
V84.04 Genetic susceptibility to malignant neoplasm of endometrium
V84.09 Genetic susceptibility to other malignant neoplasm

ICD-9-CM Procedural

40.3 Regional lymph node excision
54.11 Exploratory laparotomy
54.12 Reopening of recent laparotomy site
54.23 Biopsy of peritoneum

In Vitro Fertilization

58970

58970 Follicle puncture for oocyte retrieval, any method

ICD-9-CM Diagnostic

256.4 Polycystic ovaries ♀
614.5 Acute or unspecified pelvic peritonitis, female — (Use additional code to identify organism: 041.0, 041.1) ♀
614.6 Pelvic peritoneal adhesions, female (postoperative) (postinfection) — (Use additional code to identify any associated infertility, 628.2. Use additional code to identify organism: 041.0, 041.1) ♀
617.0 Endometriosis of uterus ♀
617.3 Endometriosis of pelvic peritoneum ♀
628.0 Female infertility associated with anovulation — (Use additional code for any associated Stein-Levanthal syndrome, 256.4) ♀
628.1 Female infertility of pituitary-hypothalamic origin — (Code first underlying disease: 253.0-253.4, 253.8) ☒ ♀
628.2 Female infertility of tubal origin — (Use additional code for any associated peritubal adhesions, 614.6) ♀
628.3 Female infertility of uterine origin — (Use additional code for any associated tuberculous endometriosis, 016.7) ♀
628.4 Female infertility of cervical or vaginal origin ♀
628.8 Female infertility of other specified origin ♀
628.9 Female infertility of unspecified origin ▽ ♀
V26.8 Other specified procreative management

ICD-9-CM Procedural

65.99 Other operations on ovary

HCPCS Level II Supplies & Services

A4305 Disposable drug delivery system, flow rate of 50 ml or greater per hour
A4306 Disposable drug delivery system, flow rate of 5 ml or less per hour
A4550 Surgical trays

58974

58974 Embryo transfer, intrauterine

ICD-9-CM Diagnostic

256.39 Other ovarian failure ♀
256.4 Polycystic ovaries ♀
256.8 Other ovarian dysfunction ♀
614.6 Pelvic peritoneal adhesions, female (postoperative) (postinfection) — (Use additional code to identify any associated infertility, 628.2. Use additional code to identify organism: 041.0, 041.1) ♀
628.0 Female infertility associated with anovulation — (Use additional code for any associated Stein-Levanthal syndrome, 256.4) ♀
628.1 Female infertility of pituitary-hypothalamic origin — (Code first underlying disease: 253.0-253.4, 253.8) ☒ ♀
628.2 Female infertility of tubal origin — (Use additional code for any associated peritubal adhesions, 614.6) ♀
628.3 Female infertility of uterine origin — (Use additional code for any associated tuberculous endometriosis, 016.7) ♀
628.4 Female infertility of cervical or vaginal origin ♀
628.8 Female infertility of other specified origin ♀
628.9 Female infertility of unspecified origin ▽ ♀
V26.8 Other specified procreative management

ICD-9-CM Procedural

71.9 Other operations on female genital organs

HCPCS Level II Supplies & Services

A4305 Disposable drug delivery system, flow rate of 50 ml or greater per hour
A4306 Disposable drug delivery system, flow rate of 5 ml or less per hour
A4550 Surgical trays

58976

58976 Gamete, zygote, or embryo intrafallopian transfer, any method

ICD-9-CM Diagnostic

256.39 Other ovarian failure ♀
256.4 Polycystic ovaries ♀
617.1 Endometriosis of ovary ♀
628.0 Female infertility associated with anovulation — (Use additional code for any associated Stein-Levanthal syndrome, 256.4) ♀
628.1 Female infertility of pituitary-hypothalamic origin — (Code first underlying disease: 253.0-253.4, 253.8) ☒ ♀
628.2 Female infertility of tubal origin — (Use additional code for any associated peritubal adhesions, 614.6) ♀
628.8 Female infertility of other specified origin ♀
628.9 Female infertility of unspecified origin ▽ ♀
V26.8 Other specified procreative management

ICD-9-CM Procedural

71.9 Other operations on female genital organs

HCPCS Level II Supplies & Services

A4305 Disposable drug delivery system, flow rate of 50 ml or greater per hour
A4306 Disposable drug delivery system, flow rate of 5 ml or less per hour
A4550 Surgical trays

Maternity Care and Delivery

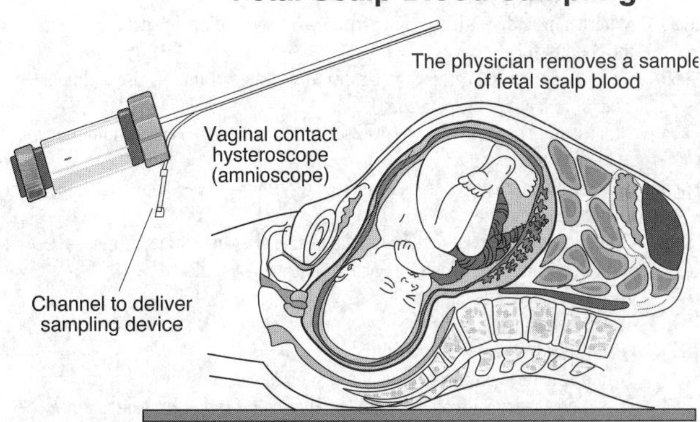

59000

59000 Amniocentesis; diagnostic

ICD-9-CM Diagnostic

642.03 Benign essential hypertension antepartum ♀
644.03 Threatened premature labor, antepartum ♀
645.13 Post term pregnancy, antepartum condition or complication ♀
645.23 Prolonged pregnancy, delivered, antepartum condition or complication ♀
646.03 Papyraceous fetus, antepartum ♀
646.13 Edema or excessive weight gain, antepartum ♀
646.83 Other specifed complication, antepartum ♀
648.03 Maternal diabetes mellitus, antepartum — (Use additional code(s) to identify the condition) ♀
648.93 Other current maternal conditions classifiable elsewhere, antepartum — (Use additional code(s) to identify the condition) ♀
651.03 Twin pregnancy, antepartum ♀
651.13 Triplet pregnancy, antepartum ♀
651.23 Quadruplet pregnancy, antepartum ♀
651.33 Twin pregnancy with fetal loss and retention of one fetus, antepartum ♀
651.43 Triplet pregnancy with fetal loss and retention of one or more, antepartum ♀
651.53 Quadruplet pregnancy with fetal loss and retention of one or more, antepartum ♀
651.63 Other multiple pregnancy with fetal loss and retention of one or more fetus(es), antepartum ♀
651.83 Other specified multiple gestation, antepartum ♀
655.03 Central nervous system malformation in fetus, antepartum ♀
655.13 Chromosomal abnormality in fetus, affecting management of mother, antepartum ♀
655.23 Hereditary disease in family possibly affecting fetus, affecting management of mother, antepartum condition or complication ♀
655.33 Suspected damage to fetus from viral disease in mother, affecting management of mother, antepartum condition or complication ♀
655.43 Suspected damage to fetus from other disease in mother, affecting management of mother, antepartum condition or complication ♀
655.53 Suspected damage to fetus from drugs, affecting management of mother, antepartum ♀
655.63 Suspected damage to fetus from radiation, affecting management of mother, antepartum condition or complication ♀
655.73 Decreased fetal movements, affecting management of mother, antepartum condition or complication ♀
655.83 Other known or suspected fetal abnormality, not elsewhere classified, affecting management of mother, antepartum condition or complication ♀
655.93 Unspecified fetal abnormality affecting management of mother, antepartum condition or complication ▽ ♀
656.03 Fetal-maternal hemorrhage, antepartum condition or complication ♀
656.13 Rhesus isoimmunization affecting management of mother, antepartum condition ♀
656.23 Isoimmunization from other and unspecified blood-group incompatibility, affecting management of mother, antepartum ♀
656.53 Poor fetal growth, affecting management of mother, antepartum condition or complication ♀
656.83 Other specified fetal and placental problems affecting management of mother, antepartum ♀
657.03 Polyhydramnios, antepartum complication ♀
658.03 Oligohydramnios, antepartum ♀
658.43 Infection of amniotic cavity, antepartum ♀
658.83 Other problem associated with amniotic cavity and membranes, antepartum ♀
659.53 Elderly primigravida, antepartum ♀
659.63 Elderly multigravida, with antepartum condition or complication ♀
741.90 Spina bifida without mention of hydrocephalus, unspecified region ▽
758.0 Down's syndrome
758.1 Patau's syndrome
758.2 Edwards' syndrome
758.31 Cri-du-chat syndrome
758.32 Velo-cardio-facial syndrome
758.33 Autosomal deletion syndromes, other microdeletions
758.39 Autosomal deletion syndromes, other autosomal deletions
758.4 Balanced autosomal translocation in normal individual
758.5 Other conditions due to autosomal anomalies
758.6 Gonadal dysgenesis
758.7 Klinefelter's syndrome ♂
758.9 Conditions due to anomaly of unspecified chromosome ▽
762.7 Fetus or newborn affected by chorioamnionitis
762.8 Fetus or newborn affected by other specified abnormalities of chorion and amnion
792.3 Nonspecific abnormal finding in amniotic fluid ♀
795.2 Nonspecific abnormal findings on chromosomal analysis
V13.29 Personal history of other genital system and obstetric disorders
V18.4 Family history of mental retardation
V19.5 Family history of congenital anomalies
V19.7 Family history of consanguinity
V23.41 Supervision of pregnancy with history of pre-term labor ♀
V23.49 Supervision of pregnancy with other poor obstetric history ♀
V23.81 Supervision of high-risk pregnancy of elderly primigravida ♀
V23.82 Supervision of high-risk pregnancy of elderly multigravida ♀
V23.89 Supervision of other high-risk pregnancy ♀
V28.0 Antenatal screening for chromosomal anomalies by amniocentesis ♀
V28.1 Antenatal screening for raised alpha-fetoprotein levels in amniotic fluid ♀
V28.2 Other antenatal screening based on amniocentesis ♀
V28.5 Antenatal screening for isoimmunization
V28.8 Other specified antenatal screening

ICD-9-CM Procedural

75.1 Diagnostic amniocentesis

HCPCS Level II Supplies & Services

A4305 Disposable drug delivery system, flow rate of 50 ml or greater per hour
A4306 Disposable drug delivery system, flow rate of 5 ml or less per hour
A4550 Surgical trays

59001

59001 Amniocentesis; therapeutic amniotic fluid reduction (includes ultrasound guidance)

ICD-9-CM Diagnostic

657.00 Polyhydramnios, unspecified as to episode of care ▽ ♀
657.01 Polyhydramnios, with delivery ♀
657.03 Polyhydramnios, antepartum complication ♀

ICD-9-CM Procedural

75.99 Other obstetric operations

HCPCS Level II Supplies & Services

HCPCS Level II codes are used to report the supplies, durable medical equipment, and certain medical services provided on an outpatient basis. Because the procedure(s) represented on this page would be performed in an inpatient or outpatient facility, no HCPCS Level II codes apply.

59012

59012 Cordocentesis (intrauterine), any method

ICD-9-CM Diagnostic

646.13 Edema or excessive weight gain, antepartum ♀
646.83 Other specifed complication, antepartum ☒ ♀
655.13 Chromosomal abnormality in fetus, affecting management of mother, antepartum ♀
655.23 Hereditary disease in family possibly affecting fetus, affecting management of mother, antepartum condition or complication ♀
655.33 Suspected damage to fetus from viral disease in mother, affecting management of mother, antepartum condition or complication ♀
655.43 Suspected damage to fetus from other disease in mother, affecting management of mother, antepartum condition or complication ♀
656.03 Fetal-maternal hemorrhage, antepartum condition or complication ♀
658.43 Infection of amniotic cavity, antepartum ♀
659.53 Elderly primigravida, antepartum ♀
759.83 Fragile X syndrome
762.7 Fetus or newborn affected by chorioamnionitis
762.8 Fetus or newborn affected by other specified abnormalities of chorion and amnion
772.0 Fetal blood loss
V23.81 Supervision of high-risk pregnancy of elderly primigravida ♀
V23.82 Supervision of high-risk pregnancy of elderly multigravida ♀

ICD-9-CM Procedural

75.35 Other diagnostic procedures on fetus and amnion

59015

59015 Chorionic villus sampling, any method

ICD-9-CM Diagnostic

646.03 Papyraceous fetus, antepartum ♀
655.13 Chromosomal abnormality in fetus, affecting management of mother, antepartum ♀
655.23 Hereditary disease in family possibly affecting fetus, affecting management of mother, antepartum condition or complication ♀
655.33 Suspected damage to fetus from viral disease in mother, affecting management of mother, antepartum condition or complication ♀
655.43 Suspected damage to fetus from other disease in mother, affecting management of mother, antepartum condition or complication ♀
655.83 Other known or suspected fetal abnormality, not elsewhere classified, affecting management of mother, antepartum condition or complication ♀
655.93 Unspecified fetal abnormality affecting management of mother, antepartum condition or complication ▽ ♀
659.53 Elderly primigravida, antepartum ♀
659.63 Elderly multigravida, with antepartum condition or complication ♀
V13.69 Personal history of other congenital malformations
V19.5 Family history of congenital anomalies
V23.81 Supervision of high-risk pregnancy of elderly primigravida ♀
V23.89 Supervision of other high-risk pregnancy ♀
V28.8 Other specified antenatal screening

ICD-9-CM Procedural

75.35 Other diagnostic procedures on fetus and amnion

59020

59020 Fetal contraction stress test

ICD-9-CM Diagnostic

642.03 Benign essential hypertension antepartum ♀
642.13 Hypertension secondary to renal disease, antepartum ♀
642.23 Other pre-existing hypertension, antepartum ♀
642.33 Transient hypertension of pregnancy, antepartum ♀
642.43 Mild or unspecified pre-eclampsia, antepartum ♀
642.53 Severe pre-eclampsia, antepartum ♀
642.73 Pre-eclampsia or eclampsia superimposed on pre-existing hypertension, antepartum ♀
642.93 Unspecified hypertension antepartum ▽ ♀
643.13 Hyperemesis gravidarum with metabolic disturbance, antepartum ♀
643.23 Late vomiting of pregnancy, antepartum ♀
643.83 Other vomiting complicating pregnancy, antepartum — (Use additional code to specify cause) ♀
643.93 Unspecified vomiting of pregnancy, antepartum ▽ ♀
645.13 Post term pregnancy, antepartum condition or complication ♀
645.23 Prolonged pregnancy, delivered, antepartum condition or complication ♀
646.13 Edema or excessive weight gain, antepartum ♀
646.23 Unspecified antepartum renal disease ▽ ♀
646.83 Other specifed complication, antepartum ♀
646.93 Unspecified complication of pregnancy, antepartum ▽ ♀
648.03 Maternal diabetes mellitus, antepartum — (Use additional code(s) to identify the condition) ♀
648.33 Maternal drug dependence, antepartum — (Use additional code(s) to identify the condition) ♀
648.53 Maternal congenital cardiovascular disorders, antepartum — (Use additional code(s) to identify the condition) ♀
648.63 Other maternal cardiovascular diseases, antepartum — (Use additional code(s) to identify the condition) ♀
648.83 Abnormal maternal glucose tolerance, antepartum — (Use additional code(s) to identify the condition) ♀
648.93 Other current maternal conditions classifiable elsewhere, antepartum — (Use additional code(s) to identify the condition) ♀
651.03 Twin pregnancy, antepartum ♀
651.13 Triplet pregnancy, antepartum ♀
651.23 Quadruplet pregnancy, antepartum ♀
651.33 Twin pregnancy with fetal loss and retention of one fetus, antepartum ♀
651.43 Triplet pregnancy with fetal loss and retention of one or more, antepartum ♀
651.53 Quadruplet pregnancy with fetal loss and retention of one or more, antepartum ♀
651.63 Other multiple pregnancy with fetal loss and retention of one or more fetus(es), antepartum ♀
651.83 Other specified multiple gestation, antepartum ♀
651.93 Unspecified multiple gestation, antepartum ▽ ♀
654.23 Previous cesarean delivery, antepartum condition or complication — (Code first any associated obstructed labor, 660.2) ♀
655.03 Central nervous system malformation in fetus, antepartum ♀
655.13 Chromosomal abnormality in fetus, affecting management of mother, antepartum ♀
655.23 Hereditary disease in family possibly affecting fetus, affecting management of mother, antepartum condition or complication ♀
655.33 Suspected damage to fetus from viral disease in mother, affecting management of mother, antepartum condition or complication ♀
655.43 Suspected damage to fetus from other disease in mother, affecting management of mother, antepartum condition or complication ♀
655.53 Suspected damage to fetus from drugs, affecting management of mother, antepartum ♀
655.63 Suspected damage to fetus from radiation, affecting management of mother, antepartum condition or complication ♀
655.83 Other known or suspected fetal abnormality, not elsewhere classified, affecting management of mother, antepartum condition or complication ♀
655.93 Unspecified fetal abnormality affecting management of mother, antepartum condition or complication ▽ ♀
656.03 Fetal-maternal hemorrhage, antepartum condition or complication ♀
656.13 Rhesus isoimmunization affecting management of mother, antepartum condition ♀
656.23 Isoimmunization from other and unspecified blood-group incompatibility, affecting management of mother, antepartum ♀
656.33 Fetal distress affecting management of mother, antepartum ♀
656.53 Poor fetal growth, affecting management of mother, antepartum condition or complication ♀
656.63 Excessive fetal growth affecting management of mother, antepartum ♀
656.83 Other specified fetal and placental problems affecting management of mother, antepartum ♀
656.93 Unspecified fetal and placental problem affecting management of mother, antepartum ▽ ♀
657.03 Polyhydramnios, antepartum complication ♀
658.03 Oligohydramnios, antepartum ♀
659.53 Elderly primigravida, antepartum ♀
659.63 Elderly multigravida, with antepartum condition or complication ♀
659.73 Abnormality in fetal heart rate or rhythm, antepartum condition or complication ♀
V22.0 Supervision of normal first pregnancy ♀
V22.1 Supervision of other normal pregnancy ♀
V23.0 Pregnancy with history of infertility ♀
V23.1 Pregnancy with history of trophoblastic disease ♀
V23.2 Pregnancy with history of abortion ♀
V23.3 Pregnancy with grand multiparity ♀

V23.41 Supervision of pregnancy with history of pre-term labor ♀
V23.49 Supervision of pregnancy with other poor obstetric history ♀
V23.5 Pregnancy with other poor reproductive history ♀
V23.7 Insufficient prenatal care ♀
V23.81 Supervision of high-risk pregnancy of elderly primigravida ♀
V23.82 Supervision of high-risk pregnancy of elderly multigravida ♀
V23.83 Supervision of high-risk pregnancy of young primigravida ♀
V23.84 Supervision of high-risk pregnancy of young multigravida ♀
V23.89 Supervision of other high-risk pregnancy ♀
V71.89 Observation for other specified suspected conditions

ICD-9-CM Procedural

75.34 Other fetal monitoring

HCPCS Level II Supplies & Services

A4649 Surgical supply; miscellaneous

59025

59025 Fetal non-stress test

ICD-9-CM Diagnostic

641.03 Placenta previa without hemorrhage, antepartum ♀
641.83 Other antepartum hemorrhage, antepartum ♀
642.03 Benign essential hypertension antepartum ♀
642.13 Hypertension secondary to renal disease, antepartum ♀
642.23 Other pre-existing hypertension, antepartum ♀
642.33 Transient hypertension of pregnancy, antepartum ♀
642.43 Mild or unspecified pre-eclampsia, antepartum ♀
642.53 Severe pre-eclampsia, antepartum ♀
642.63 Eclampsia, antepartum ♀
642.73 Pre-eclampsia or eclampsia superimposed on pre-existing hypertension, antepartum ♀
642.93 Unspecified hypertension antepartum ▽ ♀
643.13 Hyperemesis gravidarum with metabolic disturbance, antepartum ♀
643.23 Late vomiting of pregnancy, antepartum ♀
643.83 Other vomiting complicating pregnancy, antepartum — (Use additional code to specify cause) ♀
643.93 Unspecified vomiting of pregnancy, antepartum ▽ ♀
644.03 Threatened premature labor, antepartum ♀
644.13 Other threatened labor, antepartum ♀
645.13 Post term pregnancy, antepartum condition or complication ♀
645.23 Prolonged pregnancy, delivered, antepartum condition or complication ♀
646.13 Edema or excessive weight gain, antepartum ♀
646.23 Unspecified antepartum renal disease ▽ ♀
646.73 Liver disorders antepartum ♀
646.83 Other specifed complication, antepartum ♀
646.93 Unspecified complication of pregnancy, antepartum ▽ ♀
647.23 Other antepartum maternal venereal disease, previous postpartum condition — (Use additional code(s) to further specify complication) ♀
647.53 Maternal rubella, antepartum — (Use additional code(s) to further specify complication) ♀
647.63 Other maternal viral disease, antepartum — (Use additional code(s) to further specify complication) ♀
647.83 Other specified maternal infectious and parasitic disease, antepartum — (Use additional code(s) to further specify complication) ♀
647.93 Unspecified maternal infection or infestation, antepartum — (Use additional code(s) to further specify complication) ▽ ♀
648.03 Maternal diabetes mellitus, antepartum — (Use additional code(s) to identify the condition) ♀
648.13 Maternal thyroid dysfunction, antepartum condition or complication — (Use additional code(s) to identify the condition) ♀
648.23 Maternal anemia, antepartum — (Use additional code(s) to identify the condition) ♀
648.33 Maternal drug dependence, antepartum — (Use additional code(s) to identify the condition) ♀
648.43 Maternal mental disorders, antepartum — (Use additional code(s) to identify the condition) ♀
648.53 Maternal congenital cardiovascular disorders, antepartum — (Use additional code(s) to identify the condition) ♀
648.63 Other maternal cardiovascular diseases, antepartum — (Use additional code(s) to identify the condition) ♀
648.83 Abnormal maternal glucose tolerance, antepartum — (Use additional code(s) to identify the condition) ♀
648.93 Other current maternal conditions classifiable elsewhere, antepartum — (Use additional code(s) to identify the condition) ♀
651.03 Twin pregnancy, antepartum ♀
651.13 Triplet pregnancy, antepartum ♀
651.23 Quadruplet pregnancy, antepartum ♀
651.33 Twin pregnancy with fetal loss and retention of one fetus, antepartum ♀
651.43 Triplet pregnancy with fetal loss and retention of one or more, antepartum ♀
651.53 Quadruplet pregnancy with fetal loss and retention of one or more, antepartum ♀
651.63 Other multiple pregnancy with fetal loss and retention of one or more fetus(es), antepartum ♀
651.83 Other specified multiple gestation, antepartum ♀
651.93 Unspecified multiple gestation, antepartum ▽ ♀
655.03 Central nervous system malformation in fetus, antepartum ♀
655.13 Chromosomal abnormality in fetus, affecting management of mother, antepartum ♀
655.23 Hereditary disease in family possibly affecting fetus, affecting management of mother, antepartum condition or complication ♀
655.33 Suspected damage to fetus from viral disease in mother, affecting management of mother, antepartum condition or complication ♀
655.43 Suspected damage to fetus from other disease in mother, affecting management of mother, antepartum condition or complication ♀
655.53 Suspected damage to fetus from drugs, affecting management of mother, antepartum ♀
655.63 Suspected damage to fetus from radiation, affecting management of mother, antepartum condition or complication ♀
655.83 Other known or suspected fetal abnormality, not elsewhere classified, affecting management of mother, antepartum condition or complication ♀
655.93 Unspecified fetal abnormality affecting management of mother, antepartum condition or complication ▽ ♀
656.23 Isoimmunization from other and unspecified blood-group incompatibility, affecting management of mother, antepartum ♀
656.33 Fetal distress affecting management of mother, antepartum ♀
656.53 Poor fetal growth, affecting management of mother, antepartum condition or complication ♀
656.63 Excessive fetal growth affecting management of mother, antepartum ♀
656.73 Other placental conditions affecting management of mother, antepartum ♀
656.83 Other specified fetal and placental problems affecting management of mother, antepartum ♀
656.93 Unspecified fetal and placental problem affecting management of mother, antepartum ▽ ♀
657.03 Polyhydramnios, antepartum complication ♀
658.03 Oligohydramnios, antepartum ♀
658.13 Premature rupture of membranes in pregnancy, antepartum ♀
658.23 Delayed delivery after spontaneous or unspecified rupture of membranes, antepartum ♀
658.33 Delayed delivery after artificial rupture of membranes, antepartum ♀
658.43 Infection of amniotic cavity, antepartum ♀
659.03 Failed mechanical induction of labor, antepartum ♀
659.13 Failed medical or unspecified induction of labor, antepartum ♀
659.23 Unspecified maternal pyrexia, antepartum ♀
659.43 Grand multiparity with current pregnancy, antepartum ♀
659.53 Elderly primigravida, antepartum ♀
659.63 Elderly multigravida, with antepartum condition or complication ♀
659.73 Abnormality in fetal heart rate or rhythm, antepartum condition or complication ♀
V22.0 Supervision of normal first pregnancy ♀
V22.1 Supervision of other normal pregnancy ♀
V23.0 Pregnancy with history of infertility ♀
V23.1 Pregnancy with history of trophoblastic disease ♀
V23.2 Pregnancy with history of abortion ♀
V23.3 Pregnancy with grand multiparity ♀
V23.41 Supervision of pregnancy with history of pre-term labor ♀
V23.49 Supervision of pregnancy with other poor obstetric history ♀
V23.5 Pregnancy with other poor reproductive history ♀
V23.7 Insufficient prenatal care ♀
V23.81 Supervision of high-risk pregnancy of elderly primigravida ♀
V23.82 Supervision of high-risk pregnancy of elderly multigravida ♀
V23.83 Supervision of high-risk pregnancy of young primigravida ♀
V23.84 Supervision of high-risk pregnancy of young multigravida ♀
V23.89 Supervision of other high-risk pregnancy ♀
V23.9 Unspecified high-risk pregnancy ▽ ♀

ICD-9-CM Procedural

75.34 Other fetal monitoring

HCPCS Level II Supplies & Services

A4649 Surgical supply; miscellaneous

59030

59030 Fetal scalp blood sampling

ICD-9-CM Diagnostic

642.41 Mild or unspecified pre-eclampsia, with delivery ♀
642.43 Mild or unspecified pre-eclampsia, antepartum ♀
642.51 Severe pre-eclampsia, with delivery ♀
642.53 Severe pre-eclampsia, antepartum ♀
642.61 Eclampsia, with delivery ♀
642.63 Eclampsia, antepartum ♀
642.71 Pre-eclampsia or eclampsia superimposed on pre-existing hypertension, with delivery ♀
642.73 Pre-eclampsia or eclampsia superimposed on pre-existing hypertension, antepartum ♀
648.01 Maternal diabetes mellitus with delivery — (Use additional code(s) to identify the condition) ♀
648.03 Maternal diabetes mellitus, antepartum — (Use additional code(s) to identify the condition) ♀
656.11 Rhesus isoimmunization affecting management of mother, delivered ♀
656.13 Rhesus isoimmunization affecting management of mother, antepartum condition ♀
656.31 Fetal distress affecting management of mother, delivered ♀
656.33 Fetal distress affecting management of mother, antepartum ♀
656.71 Other placental conditions affecting management of mother, delivered ♀
656.73 Other placental conditions affecting management of mother, antepartum ♀
658.31 Delayed delivery after artificial rupture of membranes, delivered ♀
658.33 Delayed delivery after artificial rupture of membranes, antepartum ♀
659.71 Abnormality in fetal heart rate or rhythm, delivered, with or without mention of antepartum condition ♀
659.73 Abnormality in fetal heart rate or rhythm, antepartum condition or complication ♀
661.01 Primary uterine inertia, with delivery ♀
661.03 Primary uterine inertia, antepartum ♀
661.11 Secondary uterine inertia, with delivery ♀
661.13 Secondary uterine inertia, antepartum ♀
661.21 Other and unspecified uterine inertia, with delivery ▽ ♀
661.23 Other and unspecified uterine inertia, antepartum ▽ ♀
661.41 Hypertonic, incoordinate, or prolonged uterine contractions, with delivery ♀
661.43 Hypertonic, incoordinate, or prolonged uterine contractions, antepartum ♀
662.01 Prolonged first stage of labor, delivered ♀
662.03 Prolonged first stage of labor, antepartum ♀
662.11 Unspecified prolonged labor, delivered ▽ ♀
662.13 Unspecified prolonged labor, antepartum ▽ ♀
662.21 Prolonged second stage of labor, delivered ♀
662.23 Prolonged second stage of labor, antepartum ♀

ICD-9-CM Procedural

75.33 Fetal blood sampling and biopsy

HCPCS Level II Supplies & Services

A4649 Surgical supply; miscellaneous

59050–59051

59050 Fetal monitoring during labor by consulting physician (ie, non-attending physician) with written report; supervision and interpretation
59051 interpretation only

ICD-9-CM Diagnostic

641.01 Placenta previa without hemorrhage, with delivery ♀
641.03 Placenta previa without hemorrhage, antepartum ♀
641.11 Hemorrhage from placenta previa, with delivery ♀
641.13 Hemorrhage from placenta previa, antepartum ♀
641.21 Premature separation of placenta, with delivery ♀
641.23 Premature separation of placenta, antepartum ♀
641.31 Antepartum hemorrhage associated with coagulation defects, with delivery ♀
641.33 Antepartum hemorrhage associated with coagulation defect, antepartumm ♀
641.81 Other antepartum hemorrhage, with delivery ♀
641.83 Other antepartum hemorrhage, antepartum ♀
642.01 Benign essential hypertension with delivery ♀
642.03 Benign essential hypertension antepartum ♀
642.11 Hypertension secondary to renal disease, with delivery ♀
642.13 Hypertension secondary to renal disease, antepartum ♀
642.21 Other pre-existing hypertension, with delivery ♀
642.23 Other pre-existing hypertension, antepartum ♀
642.31 Transient hypertension of pregnancy, with delivery ♀
642.33 Transient hypertension of pregnancy, antepartum ♀
642.41 Mild or unspecified pre-eclampsia, with delivery ♀
642.43 Mild or unspecified pre-eclampsia, antepartum ♀
642.51 Severe pre-eclampsia, with delivery ♀
642.53 Severe pre-eclampsia, antepartum ♀
642.61 Eclampsia, with delivery ♀
642.63 Eclampsia, antepartum ♀
642.71 Pre-eclampsia or eclampsia superimposed on pre-existing hypertension, with delivery ♀
642.73 Pre-eclampsia or eclampsia superimposed on pre-existing hypertension, antepartum ♀
642.91 Unspecified hypertension, with delivery ▽ ♀
642.93 Unspecified hypertension antepartum ▽ ♀
643.11 Hyperemesis gravidarum with metabolic disturbance, delivered ♀
643.13 Hyperemesis gravidarum with metabolic disturbance, antepartum ♀
643.21 Late vomiting of pregnancy, delivered ♀
643.23 Late vomiting of pregnancy, antepartum ♀
643.81 Other vomiting complicating pregnancy, delivered — (Use additional code to specify cause) ♀
643.83 Other vomiting complicating pregnancy, antepartum — (Use additional code to specify cause) ♀
643.91 Unspecified vomiting of pregnancy, delivered ▽ ♀
643.93 Unspecified vomiting of pregnancy, antepartum ▽ ♀
645.11 Post term pregnancy, delivered, with or without mention of antepartum condition ♀
645.13 Post term pregnancy, antepartum condition or complication ♀
645.21 Prolonged pregnancy, delivered, with or without mention of antepartum condition ♀
645.23 Prolonged pregnancy, delivered, antepartum condition or complication ♀
646.11 Edema or excessive weight gain in pregnancy, with delivery, with or without mention of antepartum complication ♀
646.13 Edema or excessive weight gain, antepartum ♀
646.21 Unspecified renal disease in pregnancy, with delivery ▽ ♀
646.23 Unspecified antepartum renal disease ▽ ♀
646.31 Pregnancy complication, habitual aborter with or without mention of antepartum condition ♀
646.33 Habitual aborter, antepartum condition or complication ♀
646.71 Liver disorders in pregnancy, with delivery ♀
646.73 Liver disorders antepartum ♀
646.81 Other specified complication of pregnancy, with delivery ♀
646.83 Other specifed complication, antepartum ♀
646.91 Unspecified complication of pregnancy, with delivery ▽ ♀
646.93 Unspecified complication of pregnancy, antepartum ▽ ♀
647.01 Maternal syphilis, complicating pregnancy, with delivery — (Use additional code(s) to further specify complication) ♀
647.03 Maternal syphilis, antepartum — (Use additional code(s) to further specify complication) ♀
647.11 Maternal gonorrhea with delivery — (Use additional code(s) to further specify complication) ♀
647.13 Maternal gonorrhea, antepartum — (Use additional code(s) to further specify complication) ♀
647.21 Other maternal venereal diseases with delivery — (Use additional code(s) to further specify complication) ♀
647.23 Other antepartum maternal venereal disease, previous postpartum condition — (Use additional code(s) to further specify complication) ♀
647.31 Maternal tuberculosis with delivery — (Use additional code(s) to further specify complication) ♀
647.33 Maternal tuberculosis, antepartum — (Use additional code(s) to further specify complication) ♀
647.51 Maternal rubella with delivery — (Use additional code(s) to further specify complication) ♀
647.53 Maternal rubella, antepartum — (Use additional code(s) to further specify complication) ♀
647.61 Other maternal viral disease with delivery — (Use additional code(s) to further specify complication) ♀
647.63 Other maternal viral disease, antepartum — (Use additional code(s) to further specify complication) ♀
647.81 Other specified maternal infectious and parasitic disease with delivery — (Use additional code(s) to further specify complication) ♀
647.83 Other specified maternal infectious and parasitic disease, antepartum — (Use additional code(s) to further specify complication) ♀
647.91 Unspecified maternal infection or infestation with delivery — (Use additional code(s) to further specify complication) ▽ ♀
647.93 Unspecified maternal infection or infestation, antepartum — (Use additional code(s) to further specify complication) ▽ ♀
648.01 Maternal diabetes mellitus with delivery — (Use additional code(s) to identify the condition) ♀

▽ Unspecified code
♀ Female diagnosis
☒ Manifestation code
♂ Male diagnosis

648.03 Maternal diabetes mellitus, antepartum — (Use additional code(s) to identify the condition) ♀
648.11 Maternal thyroid dysfunction with delivery, with or without mention of antepartum condition — (Use additional code(s) to identify the condition) ♀
648.13 Maternal thyroid dysfunction, antepartum condition or complication — (Use additional code(s) to identify the condition) ♀
648.21 Maternal anemia, with delivery — (Use additional code(s) to identify the condition) ♀
648.23 Maternal anemia, antepartum — (Use additional code(s) to identify the condition) ♀
648.31 Maternal drug dependence, with delivery — (Use additional code(s) to identify the condition) ♀
648.33 Maternal drug dependence, antepartum — (Use additional code(s) to identify the condition) ♀
648.51 Maternal congenital cardiovascular disorders, with delivery — (Use additional code(s) to identify the condition) ♀
648.53 Maternal congenital cardiovascular disorders, antepartum — (Use additional code(s) to identify the condition) ♀
648.61 Other maternal cardiovascular diseases, with delivery — (Use additional code(s) to identify the condition) ♀
648.63 Other maternal cardiovascular diseases, antepartum — (Use additional code(s) to identify the condition) ♀
648.81 Abnormal maternal glucose tolerance, with delivery — (Use additional code(s) to identify the condition) ♀
648.83 Abnormal maternal glucose tolerance, antepartum — (Use additional code(s) to identify the condition) ♀
648.91 Other current maternal conditions classifiable elsewhere, with delivery — (Use additional code(s) to identify the condition) ♀
648.93 Other current maternal conditions classifiable elsewhere, antepartum — (Use additional code(s) to identify the condition) ♀
651.01 Twin pregnancy, delivered ♀
651.03 Twin pregnancy, antepartum ♀
651.11 Triplet pregnancy, delivered ♀
651.13 Triplet pregnancy, antepartum ♀
651.21 Quadruplet pregnancy, delivered ♀
651.23 Quadruplet pregnancy, antepartum ♀
651.31 Twin pregnancy with fetal loss and retention of one fetus, delivered ♀
651.33 Twin pregnancy with fetal loss and retention of one fetus, antepartum ♀
651.41 Triplet pregnancy with fetal loss and retention of one or more, delivered ♀
651.43 Triplet pregnancy with fetal loss and retention of one or more, antepartum ♀
651.51 Quadruplet pregnancy with fetal loss and retention of one or more, delivered ♀
651.53 Quadruplet pregnancy with fetal loss and retention of one or more, antepartum ♀
651.61 Other multiple pregnancy with fetal loss and retention of one or more fetus(es), delivered ♀
651.63 Other multiple pregnancy with fetal loss and retention of one or more fetus(es), antepartum ♀
651.81 Other specified multiple gestation, delivered ♀
651.83 Other specified multiple gestation, antepartum ♀
651.91 Unspecified multiple gestation, delivered ▽ ♀
651.93 Unspecified multiple gestation, antepartum ▽ ♀
654.41 Other abnormalities in shape or position of gravid uterus and of neighboring structures, delivered — (Code first any associated obstructed labor, 660.2) ♀
655.01 Central nervous system malformation in fetus, with delivery ♀
655.03 Central nervous system malformation in fetus, antepartum ♀
655.11 Chromosomal abnormality in fetus, affecting management of mother, with delivery ♀
655.13 Chromosomal abnormality in fetus, affecting management of mother, antepartum ♀
655.21 Hereditary disease in family possibly affecting fetus, affecting management of mother, with delivery ♀
655.23 Hereditary disease in family possibly affecting fetus, affecting management of mother, antepartum condition or complication ♀
655.31 Suspected damage to fetus from viral disease in mother, affecting management of mother, with delivery ♀
655.33 Suspected damage to fetus from viral disease in mother, affecting management of mother, antepartum condition or complication ♀
655.41 Suspected damage to fetus from other disease in mother, affecting management of mother, with delivery ♀
655.43 Suspected damage to fetus from other disease in mother, affecting management of mother, antepartum condition or complication ♀
655.51 Suspected damage to fetus from drugs, affecting management of mother, delivered ♀
655.53 Suspected damage to fetus from drugs, affecting management of mother, antepartum ♀
655.61 Suspected damage to fetus from radiation, affecting management of mother, delivered ♀
655.63 Suspected damage to fetus from radiation, affecting management of mother, antepartum condition or complication ♀
655.81 Other known or suspected fetal abnormality, not elsewhere classified, affecting management of mother, delivery ♀
655.83 Other known or suspected fetal abnormality, not elsewhere classified, affecting management of mother, antepartum condition or complication ♀
655.91 Unspecified fetal abnormality affecting management of mother, delivery ▽ ♀
655.93 Unspecified fetal abnormality affecting management of mother, antepartum condition or complication ▽ ♀
656.01 Fetal-maternal hemorrhage, with delivery ♀
656.11 Rhesus isoimmunization affecting management of mother, delivered ♀
656.13 Rhesus isoimmunization affecting management of mother, antepartum condition ♀
656.21 Isoimmunization from other and unspecified blood-group incompatibility, affecting management of mother, delivered ♀
656.23 Isoimmunization from other and unspecified blood-group incompatibility, affecting management of mother, antepartum ♀
656.31 Fetal distress affecting management of mother, delivered ♀
656.33 Fetal distress affecting management of mother, antepartum ♀
656.51 Poor fetal growth, affecting management of mother, delivered ♀
656.53 Poor fetal growth, affecting management of mother, antepartum condition or complication ♀
656.61 Excessive fetal growth affecting management of mother, delivered ♀
656.63 Excessive fetal growth affecting management of mother, antepartum ♀
656.71 Other placental conditions affecting management of mother, delivered ♀
656.73 Other placental conditions affecting management of mother, antepartum ♀
656.81 Other specified fetal and placental problems affecting management of mother, delivered ♀
656.83 Other specified fetal and placental problems affecting management of mother, antepartum ♀
656.91 Unspecified fetal and placental problem affecting management of mother, delivered ▽ ♀
656.93 Unspecified fetal and placental problem affecting management of mother, antepartum ▽ ♀
657.01 Polyhydramnios, with delivery ♀
657.03 Polyhydramnios, antepartum complication ♀
658.01 Oligohydramnios, delivered ♀
658.03 Oligohydramnios, antepartum ♀
658.11 Premature rupture of membranes in pregnancy, delivered ♀
658.13 Premature rupture of membranes in pregnancy, antepartum ♀
658.21 Delayed delivery after spontaneous or unspecified rupture of membranes, delivered ♀
658.23 Delayed delivery after spontaneous or unspecified rupture of membranes, antepartum ♀
658.31 Delayed delivery after artificial rupture of membranes, delivered ♀
658.33 Delayed delivery after artificial rupture of membranes, antepartum ♀
658.41 Infection of amniotic cavity, delivered ♀
658.43 Infection of amniotic cavity, antepartum ♀
659.01 Failed mechanical induction of labor, delivered ♀
659.03 Failed mechanical induction of labor, antepartum ♀
659.11 Failed medical or unspecified induction of labor, delivered ♀
659.13 Failed medical or unspecified induction of labor, antepartum ♀
659.21 Unspecified maternal pyrexia during labor, delivered ♀
659.23 Unspecified maternal pyrexia, antepartum ♀
659.31 Generalized infection during labor, delivered ♀
659.33 Generalized infection during labor, antepartum ♀
659.41 Grand multiparity, delivered, with or without mention of antepartum condition ♀
659.43 Grand multiparity with current pregnancy, antepartum ♀
659.51 Elderly primigravida, delivered ♀
659.53 Elderly primigravida, antepartum ♀
659.61 Elderly multigravida, delivered, with mention of antepartum condition ♀
659.63 Elderly multigravida, with antepartum condition or complication ♀
659.71 Abnormality in fetal heart rate or rhythm, delivered, with or without mention of antepartum condition ♀
659.73 Abnormality in fetal heart rate or rhythm, antepartum condition or complication ♀
660.61 Unspecified failed trial of labor, delivered ▽ ♀
660.63 Unspecified failed trial of labor, antepartum ▽ ♀
661.11 Secondary uterine inertia, with delivery ♀
661.13 Secondary uterine inertia, antepartum ♀
661.21 Other and unspecified uterine inertia, with delivery ▽ ♀
661.23 Other and unspecified uterine inertia, antepartum ▽ ♀
661.41 Hypertonic, incoordinate, or prolonged uterine contractions, with delivery ♀

661.43 Hypertonic, incoordinate, or prolonged uterine contractions, antepartum ♀
662.01 Prolonged first stage of labor, delivered ♀
662.03 Prolonged first stage of labor, antepartum ♀
662.11 Unspecified prolonged labor, delivered ▽ ♀
662.13 Unspecified prolonged labor, antepartum ▽ ♀
662.21 Prolonged second stage of labor, delivered ♀
662.23 Prolonged second stage of labor, antepartum ♀
V23.3 Pregnancy with grand multiparity ♀
V23.41 Supervision of pregnancy with history of pre-term labor ♀
V23.49 Supervision of pregnancy with other poor obstetric history ♀
V23.5 Pregnancy with other poor reproductive history ♀
V23.7 Insufficient prenatal care ♀
V23.81 Supervision of high-risk pregnancy of elderly primigravida ♀
V23.82 Supervision of high-risk pregnancy of elderly multigravida ♀
V23.83 Supervision of high-risk pregnancy of young primigravida ♀
V23.84 Supervision of high-risk pregnancy of young multigravida ♀
V23.89 Supervision of other high-risk pregnancy ♀
V23.9 Unspecified high-risk pregnancy ▽ ♀

ICD-9-CM Procedural

75.34 Other fetal monitoring

HCPCS Level II Supplies & Services

A4649 Surgical supply; miscellaneous

59070

59070 Transabdominal amnioinfusion, including ultrasound guidance

ICD-9-CM Diagnostic

656.83 Other specified fetal and placental problems affecting management of mother, antepartum ♀
658.03 Oligohydramnios, antepartum ♀
658.43 Infection of amniotic cavity, antepartum ♀
659.73 Abnormality in fetal heart rate or rhythm, antepartum condition or complication ♀
663.13 Cord around neck, with compression, complicating labor and delivery, antepartum ♀
663.23 Other and unspecified cord entanglement, with compression, complicating labor and delivery, antepartum ▽ ♀

ICD-9-CM Procedural

75.37 Amnioinfusion

59072

59072 Fetal umbilical cord occlusion, including ultrasound guidance

ICD-9-CM Diagnostic

651.03 Twin pregnancy, antepartum ♀
651.13 Triplet pregnancy, antepartum ♀
651.23 Quadruplet pregnancy, antepartum ♀
651.83 Other specified multiple gestation, antepartum ♀
653.73 Other fetal abnormality causing disproportion, antepartum — (Code first any associated obstructed labor, 660.1) ♀
657.03 Polyhydramnios, antepartum complication ♀
658.03 Oligohydramnios, antepartum ♀
658.83 Other problem associated with amniotic cavity and membranes, antepartum ♀

ICD-9-CM Procedural

75.35 Other diagnostic procedures on fetus and amnion

59074–59076

59074 Fetal fluid drainage (eg, vesicocentesis, thoracocentesis, paracentesis), including ultrasound guidance
59076 Fetal shunt placement, including ultrasound guidance

ICD-9-CM Diagnostic

078.5 Cytomegaloviral disease — (Use additional code to identify manifestation: 484.1, 573.1)
647.63 Other maternal viral disease, antepartum — (Use additional code(s) to further specify complication) ♀
653.73 Other fetal abnormality causing disproportion, antepartum — (Code first any associated obstructed labor, 660.1) ♀
655.33 Suspected damage to fetus from viral disease in mother, affecting management of mother, antepartum condition or complication ♀
655.83 Other known or suspected fetal abnormality, not elsewhere classified, affecting management of mother, antepartum condition or complication ♀
656.83 Other specified fetal and placental problems affecting management of mother, antepartum ♀
657.03 Polyhydramnios, antepartum complication ♀

ICD-9-CM Procedural

75.35 Other diagnostic procedures on fetus and amnion

59100

59100 Hysterotomy, abdominal (eg, for hydatidiform mole, abortion)

ICD-9-CM Diagnostic

630 Hydatidiform mole — (Use additional code from category 639 to identify any associated complications) ♀
631 Other abnormal product of conception — (Use additional code from category 639 to identify any associated complications) ♀
632 Missed abortion — (Use additional code from category 639 to identify any associated complications) ♀
655.01 Central nervous system malformation in fetus, with delivery ♀
655.03 Central nervous system malformation in fetus, antepartum ♀
655.11 Chromosomal abnormality in fetus, affecting management of mother, with delivery ♀
655.13 Chromosomal abnormality in fetus, affecting management of mother, antepartum ♀
655.21 Hereditary disease in family possibly affecting fetus, affecting management of mother, with delivery ♀
655.23 Hereditary disease in family possibly affecting fetus, affecting management of mother, antepartum condition or complication ♀
655.31 Suspected damage to fetus from viral disease in mother, affecting management of mother, with delivery ♀
655.33 Suspected damage to fetus from viral disease in mother, affecting management of mother, antepartum condition or complication ♀
655.41 Suspected damage to fetus from other disease in mother, affecting management of mother, with delivery ♀
655.43 Suspected damage to fetus from other disease in mother, affecting management of mother, antepartum condition or complication ♀
655.51 Suspected damage to fetus from drugs, affecting management of mother, delivered ♀
655.53 Suspected damage to fetus from drugs, affecting management of mother, antepartum ♀
655.61 Suspected damage to fetus from radiation, affecting management of mother, delivered ♀
655.63 Suspected damage to fetus from radiation, affecting management of mother, antepartum condition or complication ♀
655.71 Decreased fetal movements, affecting management of mother, delivered ♀
655.73 Decreased fetal movements, affecting management of mother, antepartum condition or complication ♀
655.81 Other known or suspected fetal abnormality, not elsewhere classified, affecting management of mother, delivery ♀
655.83 Other known or suspected fetal abnormality, not elsewhere classified, affecting management of mother, antepartum condition or complication ♀
655.91 Unspecified fetal abnormality affecting management of mother, delivery ▽ ♀
655.93 Unspecified fetal abnormality affecting management of mother, antepartum condition or complication ▽ ♀
656.41 Intrauterine death affecting management of mother, delivered ♀
656.43 Intrauterine death affecting management of mother, antepartum ♀
659.51 Elderly primigravida, delivered ♀
659.53 Elderly primigravida, antepartum ♀
659.61 Elderly multigravida, delivered, with mention of antepartum condition ♀
659.63 Elderly multigravida, with antepartum condition or complication ♀
V13.1 Personal history of trophoblastic disease ♀
V19.5 Family history of congenital anomalies
V23.1 Pregnancy with history of trophoblastic disease ♀
V61.7 Other unwanted pregnancy ♀

ICD-9-CM Procedural

68.0 Hysterotomy
74.91 Hysterotomy to terminate pregnancy
75.33 Fetal blood sampling and biopsy

▽ Unspecified code
♀ Female diagnosis
☒ Manifestation code
♂ Male diagnosis

59120–59121

59120 Surgical treatment of ectopic pregnancy; tubal or ovarian, requiring salpingectomy and/or oophorectomy, abdominal or vaginal approach
59121 tubal or ovarian, without salpingectomy and/or oophorectomy

ICD-9-CM Diagnostic

633.10 Tubal pregnancy without intrauterine pregnancy — (Use additional code from category 639 to identify any associated complications) ♀
633.11 Tubal pregnancy with intrauterine pregnancy — (Use additional code from category 639 to identify any associated complications) ♀
633.20 Ovarian pregnancy without intrauterine pregnancy — (Use additional code from category 639 to identify any associated complications) ♀
633.21 Ovarian pregnancy with intrauterine pregnancy — (Use additional code from category 639 to identify any associated complications) ♀
633.80 Other ectopic pregnancy without intrauterine pregnancy — (Use additional code from category 639 to identify any associated complications) ♀
633.81 Other ectopic pregnancy with intrauterine pregnancy — (Use additional code from category 639 to identify any associated complications) ♀
633.90 Unspecified ectopic pregnancy without intrauterine pregnancy — (Use additional code from category 639 to identify any associated complications) ▽ ♀
633.91 Unspecified ectopic pregnancy with intrauterine pregnancy — (Use additional code from category 639 to identify any associated complications) ▽ ♀
639.0 Genital tract and pelvic infection following abortion or ectopic and molar pregnancies ♀
639.1 Delayed or excessive hemorrhage following abortion or ectopic and molar pregnancies ♀
639.2 Damage to pelvic organs and tissues following abortion or ectopic and molar pregnancies ♀
639.3 Renal failure following abortion or ectopic and molar pregnancies ♀
639.8 Other specified complication following abortion or ectopic and molar pregnancies ♀
639.9 Unspecified complication following abortion or ectopic and molar pregnancies ▽ ♀
789.00 Abdominal pain, unspecified site ▽
789.03 Abdominal pain, right lower quadrant
789.04 Abdominal pain, left lower quadrant
V64.41 Laparoscopic surgical procedure converted to open procedure

ICD-9-CM Procedural

65.22 Wedge resection of ovary
65.39 Other unilateral oophorectomy
65.49 Other unilateral salpingo-oophorectomy
66.62 Salpingectomy with removal of tubal pregnancy

59130

59130 Surgical treatment of ectopic pregnancy; abdominal pregnancy

ICD-9-CM Diagnostic

633.00 Abdominal pregnancy without intrauterine pregnancy — (Use additional code from category 639 to identify any associated complications) ♀
633.01 Abdominal pregnancy with intrauterine pregnancy — (Use additional code from category 639 to identify any associated complications) ♀
633.80 Other ectopic pregnancy without intrauterine pregnancy — (Use additional code from category 639 to identify any associated complications) ♀
633.81 Other ectopic pregnancy with intrauterine pregnancy — (Use additional code from category 639 to identify any associated complications) ♀
639.0 Genital tract and pelvic infection following abortion or ectopic and molar pregnancies ♀
639.1 Delayed or excessive hemorrhage following abortion or ectopic and molar pregnancies ♀
639.2 Damage to pelvic organs and tissues following abortion or ectopic and molar pregnancies ♀
639.3 Renal failure following abortion or ectopic and molar pregnancies ♀
639.8 Other specified complication following abortion or ectopic and molar pregnancies ♀
639.9 Unspecified complication following abortion or ectopic and molar pregnancies ▽ ♀

ICD-9-CM Procedural

74.3 Removal of extratubal ectopic pregnancy
75.99 Other obstetric operations

59135–59140

59135 Surgical treatment of ectopic pregnancy; interstitial, uterine pregnancy requiring total hysterectomy
59136 interstitial, uterine pregnancy with partial resection of uterus
59140 cervical, with evacuation

ICD-9-CM Diagnostic

633.80 Other ectopic pregnancy without intrauterine pregnancy — (Use additional code from category 639 to identify any associated complications) ♀
633.81 Other ectopic pregnancy with intrauterine pregnancy — (Use additional code from category 639 to identify any associated complications) ♀
633.90 Unspecified ectopic pregnancy without intrauterine pregnancy — (Use additional code from category 639 to identify any associated complications) ▽ ♀
633.91 Unspecified ectopic pregnancy with intrauterine pregnancy — (Use additional code from category 639 to identify any associated complications) ▽ ♀
639.0 Genital tract and pelvic infection following abortion or ectopic and molar pregnancies ♀
639.1 Delayed or excessive hemorrhage following abortion or ectopic and molar pregnancies ♀
639.2 Damage to pelvic organs and tissues following abortion or ectopic and molar pregnancies ♀
639.3 Renal failure following abortion or ectopic and molar pregnancies ♀
639.8 Other specified complication following abortion or ectopic and molar pregnancies ♀
639.9 Unspecified complication following abortion or ectopic and molar pregnancies ▽ ♀

ICD-9-CM Procedural

68.39 Other subtotal abdominal hysterectomy, NOS
68.4 Total abdominal hysterectomy
74.3 Removal of extratubal ectopic pregnancy

59150–59151

59150 Laparoscopic treatment of ectopic pregnancy; without salpingectomy and/or oophorectomy
59151 with salpingectomy and/or oophorectomy

ICD-9-CM Diagnostic

633.00 Abdominal pregnancy without intrauterine pregnancy — (Use additional code from category 639 to identify any associated complications) ♀
633.01 Abdominal pregnancy with intrauterine pregnancy — (Use additional code from category 639 to identify any associated complications) ♀
633.10 Tubal pregnancy without intrauterine pregnancy — (Use additional code from category 639 to identify any associated complications) ♀
633.11 Tubal pregnancy with intrauterine pregnancy — (Use additional code from category 639 to identify any associated complications) ♀
633.20 Ovarian pregnancy without intrauterine pregnancy — (Use additional code from category 639 to identify any associated complications) ♀
633.21 Ovarian pregnancy with intrauterine pregnancy — (Use additional code from category 639 to identify any associated complications) ♀
633.80 Other ectopic pregnancy without intrauterine pregnancy — (Use additional code from category 639 to identify any associated complications) ♀
633.81 Other ectopic pregnancy with intrauterine pregnancy — (Use additional code from category 639 to identify any associated complications) ♀
633.90 Unspecified ectopic pregnancy without intrauterine pregnancy — (Use additional code from category 639 to identify any associated complications) ▽ ♀
633.91 Unspecified ectopic pregnancy with intrauterine pregnancy — (Use additional code from category 639 to identify any associated complications) ▽ ♀
639.0 Genital tract and pelvic infection following abortion or ectopic and molar pregnancies ♀
639.1 Delayed or excessive hemorrhage following abortion or ectopic and molar pregnancies ♀
639.2 Damage to pelvic organs and tissues following abortion or ectopic and molar pregnancies ♀
639.3 Renal failure following abortion or ectopic and molar pregnancies ♀
639.8 Other specified complication following abortion or ectopic and molar pregnancies ♀
639.9 Unspecified complication following abortion or ectopic and molar pregnancies ▽ ♀
789.00 Abdominal pain, unspecified site ▽
789.03 Abdominal pain, right lower quadrant
789.04 Abdominal pain, left lower quadrant

ICD-9-CM Procedural

65.01 Laparoscopic oophorotomy
65.31 Laparoscopic unilateral oophorectomy
65.54 Laparoscopic removal of remaining ovary
66.01 Salpingotomy
66.4 Total unilateral salpingectomy
66.62 Salpingectomy with removal of tubal pregnancy

59160

59160 Curettage, postpartum

ICD-9-CM Diagnostic

666.00 Third-stage postpartum hemorrhage, unspecified as to episode of care ♀
666.02 Third-stage postpartum hemorrhage, with delivery ♀
666.04 Third-stage postpartum hemorrhage, postpartum ♀
666.10 Other immediate postpartum hemorrhage, unspecified as to episode of care ▽ ♀
666.12 Other immediate postpartum hemorrhage, with delivery ♀
666.14 Other immediate postpartum hemorrhage, postpartum ♀
666.20 Delayed and secondary postpartum hemorrhage, unspecified as to episode of care ♀
666.22 Delayed and secondary postpartum hemorrhage, with delivery ♀
666.24 Delayed and secondary postpartum hemorrhage, postpartum ♀
666.30 Postpartum coagulation defects, unspecified as to episode of care ♀
666.32 Postpartum coagulation defects, with delivery ♀
666.34 Postpartum coagulation defects, postpartum ♀
667.00 Retained placenta without hemorrhage, unspecified as to episode of care ♀
667.02 Retained placenta without hemorrhage, with delivery, with mention of postpartum complication ♀
667.04 Retained placenta without hemorrhage, postpartum condition or complication ♀
667.10 Retained portions of placenta or membranes, without hemorrhage, unspecified as to episode of care ♀
667.12 Retained portions of placenta or membranes, without hemorrhage, delivered, with mention of postpartum complication ♀
667.14 Retained portions of placenta or membranes, without hemorrhage, postpartum condition or complication ♀

ICD-9-CM Procedural

69.02 Dilation and curettage following delivery or abortion
69.52 Aspiration curettage following delivery or abortion

HCPCS Level II Supplies & Services

A4305 Disposable drug delivery system, flow rate of 50 ml or greater per hour
A4306 Disposable drug delivery system, flow rate of 5 ml or less per hour
A4550 Surgical trays

59200

59200 Insertion of cervical dilator (eg, laminaria, prostaglandin) (separate procedure)

ICD-9-CM Diagnostic

645.11 Post term pregnancy, delivered, with or without mention of antepartum condition ♀
645.13 Post term pregnancy, antepartum condition or complication ♀
645.21 Prolonged pregnancy, delivered, with or without mention of antepartum condition ♀
645.23 Prolonged pregnancy, delivered, antepartum condition or complication ♀
658.10 Premature rupture of membranes in pregnancy, unspecified as to episode of care ▽ ♀
658.11 Premature rupture of membranes in pregnancy, delivered ♀
658.13 Premature rupture of membranes in pregnancy, antepartum ♀
658.20 Delayed delivery after spontaneous or unspecified rupture of membranes, unspecified as to episode of care ▽ ♀
658.21 Delayed delivery after spontaneous or unspecified rupture of membranes, delivered ♀
658.23 Delayed delivery after spontaneous or unspecified rupture of membranes, antepartum ♀
658.30 Delayed delivery after artificial rupture of membranes, unspecified as to episode of care ▽ ♀
658.31 Delayed delivery after artificial rupture of membranes, delivered ♀
658.33 Delayed delivery after artificial rupture of membranes, antepartum ♀
658.90 Unspecified problem associated with amniotic cavity and membranes, unspecified as to episode of care ▽ ♀
658.91 Unspecified problem associated with amniotic cavity and membranes, delivered ▽ ♀
658.93 Unspecified problem associated with amniotic cavity and membranes, antepartum ▽ ♀
659.10 Failed medical or unspecified induction of labor, unspecified as to episode of care ▽ ♀
659.11 Failed medical or unspecified induction of labor, delivered ♀
659.13 Failed medical or unspecified induction of labor, antepartum ♀
661.00 Primary uterine inertia, unspecified as to episode of care ▽ ♀
661.01 Primary uterine inertia, with delivery ♀
661.03 Primary uterine inertia, antepartum ♀
661.10 Secondary uterine inertia, unspecified as to episode of care ▽ ♀
661.13 Secondary uterine inertia, antepartum ♀
661.20 Other and unspecified uterine inertia, unspecified as to episode of care ▽ ♀
661.23 Other and unspecified uterine inertia, antepartum ▽ ♀
661.40 Hypertonic, incoordinate, or prolonged uterine contractions, unspecified as to episode of care ▽ ♀
661.41 Hypertonic, incoordinate, or prolonged uterine contractions, with delivery ♀
661.43 Hypertonic, incoordinate, or prolonged uterine contractions, antepartum ♀
661.90 Unspecified abnormality of labor, unspecified as to episode of care ▽ ♀
661.91 Unspecified abnormality of labor, with delivery ▽ ♀
661.93 Unspecified abnormality of labor, antepartum ▽ ♀
662.00 Prolonged first stage of labor, unspecified as to episode of care ▽ ♀
662.03 Prolonged first stage of labor, antepartum ♀

ICD-9-CM Procedural

69.93 Insertion of laminaria
73.1 Other surgical induction of labor

HCPCS Level II Supplies & Services

A4649 Surgical supply; miscellaneous

59300

59300 Episiotomy or vaginal repair, by other than attending physician

ICD-9-CM Diagnostic

664.01 First-degree perineal laceration, with delivery ♀
664.04 First-degree perineal laceration, postpartum ♀
664.11 Second-degree perineal laceration, with delivery ♀
664.14 Second-degree perineal laceration, postpartum ♀
664.21 Third-degree perineal laceration, with delivery ♀
664.24 Third-degree perineal laceration, postpartum ♀
664.31 Fourth-degree perineal laceration, with delivery ♀
664.34 Fourth-degree perineal laceration, postpartum ♀
664.41 Unspecified perineal laceration, with delivery ▽ ♀
664.44 Unspecified perineal laceration, postpartum ▽ ♀
665.41 High vaginal laceration, with delivery ♀
665.44 High vaginal laceration, postpartum ♀

ICD-9-CM Procedural

73.6 Episiotomy
75.69 Repair of other current obstetric laceration

HCPCS Level II Supplies & Services

A4550 Surgical trays

59320–59325

59320 Cerclage of cervix, during pregnancy; vaginal
59325 abdominal

ICD-9-CM Diagnostic

622.3 Old laceration of cervix ♀
654.50 Cervical incompetence, unspecified as to episode of care in pregnancy — (Code first any associated obstructed labor, 660.2) ▽ ♀
654.53 Cervical incompetence, antepartum condition or complication — (Code first any associated obstructed labor, 660.2) ♀
654.60 Other congenital or acquired abnormality of cervix, unspecified as to episode of care in pregnancy — (Code first any associated obstructed labor, 660.2) ▽ ♀
654.63 Other congenital or acquired abnormality of cervix, antepartum condition or complication — (Code first any associated obstructed labor, 660.2) ♀
654.90 Other and unspecified abnormality of organs and soft tissues of pelvis, unspecified as to episode of care in pregnancy — (Code first any associated obstructed labor, 660.2) ▽ ♀
654.93 Other and unspecified abnormality of organs and soft tissues of pelvis, antepartum condition or complication — (Code first any associated obstructed labor, 660.2) ▽ ♀
V23.2 Pregnancy with history of abortion ♀
V23.81 Supervision of high-risk pregnancy of elderly primigravida ♀

▽ Unspecified code
♀ Female diagnosis
☒ Manifestation code
♂ Male diagnosis

V23.82 Supervision of high-risk pregnancy of elderly multigravida ♀
V23.83 Supervision of high-risk pregnancy of young primigravida ♀
V23.84 Supervision of high-risk pregnancy of young multigravida ♀
V23.89 Supervision of other high-risk pregnancy ♀

ICD-9-CM Procedural

67.51 Transabdominal cerclage of cervix
67.59 Other repair of cervical os

HCPCS Level II Supplies & Services

A4305 Disposable drug delivery system, flow rate of 50 ml or greater per hour
A4306 Disposable drug delivery system, flow rate of 5 ml or less per hour
A4550 Surgical trays

59350

59350 Hysterorrhaphy of ruptured uterus

ICD-9-CM Diagnostic

654.20 Previous cesarean delivery, unspecified as to episode of care or not applicable — (Code first any associated obstructed labor, 660.2) ▽ ♀
654.21 Previous cesarean delivery, delivered, with or without mention of antepartum condition — (Code first any associated obstructed labor, 660.2) ♀
654.23 Previous cesarean delivery, antepartum condition or complication — (Code first any associated obstructed labor, 660.2) ♀
665.00 Rupture of uterus before onset of labor, unspecified as to episode of care ▽ ♀
665.01 Rupture of uterus before onset of labor, with delivery ♀
665.03 Rupture of uterus before onset of labor, antepartum ♀
665.10 Rupture of uterus during labor, unspecified as to episode ▽ ♀
665.11 Rupture of uterus during labor, with delivery ♀

ICD-9-CM Procedural

69.41 Suture of laceration of uterus
75.50 Repair of current obstetric laceration of uterus, not otherwise specified
75.52 Repair of current obstetric laceration of corpus uteri

59400–59410

59400 Routine obstetric care including antepartum care, vaginal delivery (with or without episiotomy, and/or forceps) and postpartum care
59409 Vaginal delivery only (with or without episiotomy and/or forceps);
59410 including postpartum care

ICD-9-CM Diagnostic

640.01 Threatened abortion, delivered ♀
641.01 Placenta previa without hemorrhage, with delivery ♀
641.11 Hemorrhage from placenta previa, with delivery ♀
641.21 Premature separation of placenta, with delivery ♀
641.31 Antepartum hemorrhage associated with coagulation defects, with delivery ♀
641.81 Other antepartum hemorrhage, with delivery ♀
641.91 Unspecified antepartum hemorrhage, with delivery ▽ ♀
642.01 Benign essential hypertension with delivery ♀
642.11 Hypertension secondary to renal disease, with delivery ♀
642.21 Other pre-existing hypertension, with delivery ♀
642.31 Transient hypertension of pregnancy, with delivery ♀
642.41 Mild or unspecified pre-eclampsia, with delivery ♀
642.51 Severe pre-eclampsia, with delivery ♀
642.61 Eclampsia, with delivery ♀
642.71 Pre-eclampsia or eclampsia superimposed on pre-existing hypertension, with delivery ♀
642.91 Unspecified hypertension, with delivery ▽ ♀
643.01 Mild hyperemesis gravidarum, delivered ♀
643.11 Hyperemesis gravidarum with metabolic disturbance, delivered ♀
643.21 Late vomiting of pregnancy, delivered ♀
643.81 Other vomiting complicating pregnancy, delivered — (Use additional code to specify cause) ♀
644.21 Early onset of delivery, delivered, with or without mention of antepartum condition ♀
645.11 Post term pregnancy, delivered, with or without mention of antepartum condition ♀
645.21 Prolonged pregnancy, delivered, with or without mention of antepartum condition ♀
646.01 Papyraceous fetus, delivered, with or without mention of antepartum condition ♀
646.11 Edema or excessive weight gain in pregnancy, with delivery, with or without mention of antepartum complication ♀
646.21 Unspecified renal disease in pregnancy, with delivery ▽ ♀
646.31 Pregnancy complication, habitual aborter with or without mention of antepartum condition ♀
646.41 Peripheral neuritis in pregnancy, with delivery ♀
646.51 Asymptomatic bacteriuria in pregnancy, with delivery ♀
646.61 Infections of genitourinary tract in pregnancy, with delivery ♀
646.71 Liver disorders in pregnancy, with delivery ♀
646.81 Other specified complication of pregnancy, with delivery ♀
646.91 Unspecified complication of pregnancy, with delivery ▽ ♀
647.01 Maternal syphilis, complicating pregnancy, with delivery — (Use additional code(s) to further specify complication) ♀
647.11 Maternal gonorrhea with delivery — (Use additional code(s) to further specify complication) ♀
647.21 Other maternal venereal diseases with delivery — (Use additional code(s) to further specify complication) ♀
647.31 Maternal tuberculosis with delivery — (Use additional code(s) to further specify complication) ♀
647.41 Maternal malaria with delivery — (Use additional code(s) to further specify complication) ♀
647.51 Maternal rubella with delivery — (Use additional code(s) to further specify complication) ♀
647.61 Other maternal viral disease with delivery — (Use additional code(s) to further specify complication) ♀
647.81 Other specified maternal infectious and parasitic disease with delivery — (Use additional code(s) to further specify complication) ♀
647.91 Unspecified maternal infection or infestation with delivery — (Use additional code(s) to further specify complication) ▽ ♀
648.01 Maternal diabetes mellitus with delivery — (Use additional code(s) to identify the condition) ♀
648.11 Maternal thyroid dysfunction with delivery, with or without mention of antepartum condition — (Use additional code(s) to identify the condition) ♀
648.21 Maternal anemia, with delivery — (Use additional code(s) to identify the condition) ♀
648.31 Maternal drug dependence, with delivery — (Use additional code(s) to identify the condition) ♀
648.41 Maternal mental disorders, with delivery — (Use additional code(s) to identify the condition) ♀
648.51 Maternal congenital cardiovascular disorders, with delivery — (Use additional code(s) to identify the condition) ♀
648.61 Other maternal cardiovascular diseases, with delivery — (Use additional code(s) to identify the condition) ♀
648.71 Bone and joint disorders of maternal back, pelvis, and lower limbs, with delivery — (Use additional code(s) to identify the condition) ♀
648.81 Abnormal maternal glucose tolerance, with delivery — (Use additional code(s) to identify the condition) ♀
648.91 Other current maternal conditions classifiable elsewhere, with delivery — (Use additional code(s) to identify the condition) ♀
650 Normal delivery — (This code is for use as a single diagnosis code and is not to be used with any other code in the range 630-676. Use additional code to indicate outcome of delivery, V27.0.) ♀
651.01 Twin pregnancy, delivered ♀
651.11 Triplet pregnancy, delivered ♀
651.21 Quadruplet pregnancy, delivered ♀
651.31 Twin pregnancy with fetal loss and retention of one fetus, delivered ♀
651.41 Triplet pregnancy with fetal loss and retention of one or more, delivered ♀
651.51 Quadruplet pregnancy with fetal loss and retention of one or more, delivered ♀
651.61 Other multiple pregnancy with fetal loss and retention of one or more fetus(es), delivered ♀
651.81 Other specified multiple gestation, delivered ♀
651.91 Unspecified multiple gestation, delivered ▽ ♀
652.11 Breech or other malpresentation successfully converted to cephalic presentation, delivered — (Code first any associated obstructed labor, 660.0) ♀
652.21 Breech presentation without mention of version, delivered — (Code first any associated obstructed labor, 660.0) ♀
652.41 Fetal face or brow presentation, delivered — (Code first any associated obstructed labor, 660.0) ♀
652.71 Prolapsed arm of fetus, delivered — (Code first any associated obstructed labor, 660.0) ♀
652.81 Other specified malposition or malpresentation of fetus, delivered — (Code first any associated obstructed labor, 660.0) ♀
652.91 Unspecified malposition or malpresentation of fetus, delivered — (Code first any associated obstructed labor, 660.0) ▽ ♀
654.01 Congenital abnormalities of pregnant uterus, delivered — (Code first any associated obstructed labor, 660.2) ♀
654.11 Tumors of body of uterus, delivered — (Code first any associated obstructed labor, 660.2) ♀

▽ Unspecified code
♀ Female diagnosis
☒ Manifestation code
♂ Male diagnosis

654.31 Retroverted and incarcerated gravid uterus, delivered — (Code first any associated obstructed labor, 660.2) ♀
654.41 Other abnormalities in shape or position of gravid uterus and of neighboring structures, delivered — (Code first any associated obstructed labor, 660.2) ♀
654.51 Cervical incompetence, delivered — (Code first any associated obstructed labor, 660.2) ♀
654.61 Other congenital or acquired abnormality of cervix, with delivery — (Code first any associated obstructed labor, 660.2) ♀
654.71 Congenital or acquired abnormality of vagina, with delivery — (Code first any associated obstructed labor, 660.2) ♀
654.81 Congenital or acquired abnormality of vulva, with delivery — (Code first any associated obstructed labor, 660.2) ♀
654.91 Other and unspecified abnormality of organs and soft tissues of pelvis, with delivery — (Code first any associated obstructed labor, 660.2) ▽ ♀
655.01 Central nervous system malformation in fetus, with delivery ♀
655.11 Chromosomal abnormality in fetus, affecting management of mother, with delivery ♀
655.21 Hereditary disease in family possibly affecting fetus, affecting management of mother, with delivery ♀
655.31 Suspected damage to fetus from viral disease in mother, affecting management of mother, with delivery ♀
655.41 Suspected damage to fetus from other disease in mother, affecting management of mother, with delivery ♀
655.81 Other known or suspected fetal abnormality, not elsewhere classified, affecting management of mother, delivery ♀
655.91 Unspecified fetal abnormality affecting management of mother, delivery ▽ ♀
656.01 Fetal-maternal hemorrhage, with delivery ♀
656.11 Rhesus isoimmunization affecting management of mother, delivered ♀
656.21 Isoimmunization from other and unspecified blood-group incompatibility, affecting management of mother, delivered ♀
656.31 Fetal distress affecting management of mother, delivered ♀
656.41 Intrauterine death affecting management of mother, delivered ♀
656.51 Poor fetal growth, affecting management of mother, delivered ♀
656.61 Excessive fetal growth affecting management of mother, delivered ♀
656.71 Other placental conditions affecting management of mother, delivered ♀
656.81 Other specified fetal and placental problems affecting management of mother, delivered ♀
656.91 Unspecified fetal and placental problem affecting management of mother, delivered ▽ ♀
657.01 Polyhydramnios, with delivery ♀
658.01 Oligohydramnios, delivered ♀
658.11 Premature rupture of membranes in pregnancy, delivered ♀
658.21 Delayed delivery after spontaneous or unspecified rupture of membranes, delivered ♀
658.31 Delayed delivery after artificial rupture of membranes, delivered ♀
658.41 Infection of amniotic cavity, delivered ♀
658.81 Other problem associated with amniotic cavity and membranes, delivered ♀
658.91 Unspecified problem associated with amniotic cavity and membranes, delivered ▽ ♀
659.21 Unspecified maternal pyrexia during labor, delivered ♀
659.31 Generalized infection during labor, delivered ♀
659.41 Grand multiparity, delivered, with or without mention of antepartum condition ♀
659.51 Elderly primigravida, delivered ♀
659.61 Elderly multigravida, delivered, with mention of antepartum condition ♀
659.81 Other specified indication for care or intervention related to labor and delivery, delivered ♀
659.91 Unspecified indication for care or intervention related to labor and delivery, delivered ▽ ♀
660.81 Other causes of obstructed labor, delivered ♀
661.31 Precipitate labor, with delivery ♀
662.01 Prolonged first stage of labor, delivered ♀
662.21 Prolonged second stage of labor, delivered ♀
662.31 Delayed delivery of second twin, triplet, etc., delivered ♀
663.11 Cord around neck, with compression, complicating labor and delivery, delivered ♀
663.31 Other and unspecified cord entanglement, without mention of compression, complicating labor and delivery, delivered ▽ ♀
663.41 Short cord complicating labor and delivery, delivered ♀
663.61 Vascular lesions of cord complicating labor and delivery, delivered ♀
663.81 Other umbilical cord complications during labor and delivery, delivered ♀
663.91 Unspecified umbilical cord complication during labor and delivery, delivered ▽ ♀
664.01 First-degree perineal laceration, with delivery ♀
664.11 Second-degree perineal laceration, with delivery ♀
664.21 Third-degree perineal laceration, with delivery ♀
664.31 Fourth-degree perineal laceration, with delivery ♀
664.41 Unspecified perineal laceration, with delivery ▽ ♀
664.51 Vulvar and perineal hematoma, with delivery ♀
664.80 Other specified trauma to perineum and vulva, unspecified as to episode of care in pregnancy ▽ ♀
664.81 Other specified trauma to perineum and vulva, with delivery ♀
664.91 Unspecified trauma to perineum and vulva, with delivery ▽ ♀
665.31 Laceration of cervix, with delivery ♀
665.41 High vaginal laceration, with delivery ♀
665.51 Other injury to pelvic organs, with delivery ♀
665.61 Damage to pelvic joints and ligaments, with delivery ♀
665.71 Pelvic hematoma, with delivery ♀
665.81 Other specified obstetrical trauma, with delivery ♀
665.91 Unspecified obstetrical trauma, with delivery ▽ ♀
666.02 Third-stage postpartum hemorrhage, with delivery ♀
666.12 Other immediate postpartum hemorrhage, with delivery ♀
666.22 Delayed and secondary postpartum hemorrhage, with delivery ♀
667.02 Retained placenta without hemorrhage, with delivery, with mention of postpartum complication ♀
668.01 Pulmonary complications of the administration of anesthesia or other sedation in labor and delivery, delivered — (Use additional code(s) to further specify complication) ♀
668.11 Cardiac complications of the administration of anesthesia or other sedation in labor and delivery, delivered — (Use additional code(s) to further specify complication) ♀
668.21 Central nervous system complications of the administration of anesthesia or other sedation in labor and delivery, delivered — (Use additional code(s) to further specify complication) ♀
668.81 Other complications of the administration of anesthesia or other sedation in labor and delivery, delivered — (Use additional code(s) to further specify complication) ♀
668.91 Unspecified complication of the administration of anesthesia or other sedation in labor and delivery, delivered — (Use additional code(s) to further specify complication) ▽ ♀
669.01 Maternal distress, with delivery, with or without mention of antepartum condition ♀
669.11 Shock during or following labor and delivery, with delivery, with or without mention of antepartum condition ♀
669.21 Maternal hypotension syndrome, with delivery, with or without mention of antepartum condition ♀
669.51 Forceps or vacuum extractor delivery without mention of indication, delivered, with or without mention of antepartum condition ♀
669.81 Other complication of labor and delivery, delivered, with or without mention of antepartum condition ♀
671.01 Varicose veins of legs, with delivery, with or without mention of antepartum condition ♀
671.81 Other venous complication, with delivery, with or without mention of antepartum condition ♀
671.82 Other venous complication, with delivery, with mention of postpartum complication ♀
676.01 Retracted nipple, delivered, with or without mention of antepartum condition ♀
676.02 Retracted nipple, delivered, with mention of postpartum complication ♀
676.21 Engorgement of breasts, delivered, with or without mention of antepartum condition ♀
676.22 Engorgement of breasts, delivered, with mention of postpartum complication ♀
676.31 Other and unspecified disorder of breast associated with childbirth, delivered, with or without mention of antepartum condition ▽ ♀
676.32 Other and unspecified disorder of breast associated with childbirth, delivered, with mention of postpartum complication ▽ ♀
676.41 Failure of lactation, with delivery, with or without mention of antepartum condition ♀
676.42 Failure of lactation, with delivery, with mention of postpartum complication ♀
676.51 Suppressed lactation, with delivery, with or without mention of antepartum condition ♀
676.52 Suppressed lactation, with delivery, with mention of postpartum complication ♀
676.91 Unspecified disorder of lactation, with delivery, with or without mention of antepartum condition ▽ ♀
676.92 Unspecified disorder of lactation, with delivery, with mention of postpartum complication ▽ ♀
V22.0 Supervision of normal first pregnancy ♀
V22.1 Supervision of other normal pregnancy ♀
V23.0 Pregnancy with history of infertility ♀
V23.2 Pregnancy with history of abortion ♀

▽ Unspecified code ♀ Female diagnosis ☒ Manifestation code ♂ Male diagnosis

V23.81 Supervision of high-risk pregnancy of elderly primigravida ♀
V23.82 Supervision of high-risk pregnancy of elderly multigravida ♀
V23.83 Supervision of high-risk pregnancy of young primigravida ♀
V23.84 Supervision of high-risk pregnancy of young multigravida ♀
V23.89 Supervision of other high-risk pregnancy ♀
V24.0 Postpartum care and examination immediately after delivery ♀
V24.1 Postpartum care and examination of lactating mother ♀
V24.2 Routine postpartum follow-up ♀
V27.0 Outcome of delivery, single liveborn — (This code is intended for the coding of the outcome of delivery on the mother's record) ♀
V27.1 Outcome of delivery, single stillborn — (This code is intended for the coding of the outcome of delivery on the mother's record) ♀
V27.2 Outcome of delivery, twins, both liveborn — (This code is intended for the coding of the outcome of delivery on the mother's record) ♀
V27.3 Outcome of delivery, twins, one liveborn and one stillborn — (This code is intended for the coding of the outcome of delivery on the mother's record) ♀
V27.4 Outcome of delivery, twins, both stillborn — (This code is intended for the coding of the outcome of delivery on the mother's record) ♀
V27.5 Outcome of delivery, other multiple birth, all liveborn — (This code is intended for the coding of the outcome of delivery on the mother's record) ♀
V27.6 Outcome of delivery, other multiple birth, some liveborn — (This code is intended for the coding of the outcome of delivery on the mother's record) ♀
V27.7 Outcome of delivery, other multiple birth, all stillborn — (This code is intended for the coding of the outcome of delivery on the mother's record) ♀
V27.9 Outcome of delivery, unspecified — (This code is intended for the coding of the outcome of delivery on the mother's record) ▽ ♀

ICD-9-CM Procedural

72.0 Low forceps operation
72.1 Low forceps operation with episiotomy
72.21 Mid forceps operation with episiotomy
72.29 Other mid forceps operation
72.31 High forceps operation with episiotomy
72.39 Other high forceps operation
72.4 Forceps rotation of fetal head
72.51 Partial breech extraction with forceps to aftercoming head
72.52 Other partial breech extraction
72.53 Total breech extraction with forceps to aftercoming head
72.54 Other total breech extraction
72.6 Forceps application to aftercoming head
72.71 Vacuum extraction with episiotomy
72.79 Other vacuum extraction
72.8 Other specified instrumental delivery
72.9 Unspecified instrumental delivery
73.01 Induction of labor by artificial rupture of membranes
73.09 Other artificial rupture of membranes
73.4 Medical induction of labor
73.59 Other manually assisted delivery

59412

59412 External cephalic version, with or without tocolysis

ICD-9-CM Diagnostic

652.10 Breech or other malpresentation successfully converted to cephalic presentation, unspecified as to episode of care — (Code first any associated obstructed labor, 660.0) ▽ ♀
652.11 Breech or other malpresentation successfully converted to cephalic presentation, delivered — (Code first any associated obstructed labor, 660.0) ♀
652.13 Breech or other malpresentation successfully converted to cephalic presentation, antepartum — (Code first any associated obstructed labor, 660.0) ♀
652.21 Breech presentation without mention of version, delivered — (Code first any associated obstructed labor, 660.0) ♀
652.23 Breech presentation without mention of version, antepartum — (Code first any associated obstructed labor, 660.0) ♀

ICD-9-CM Procedural

72.51 Partial breech extraction with forceps to aftercoming head
73.21 Internal and combined version without extraction
73.22 Internal and combined version with extraction
73.51 Manual rotation of fetal head
73.59 Other manually assisted delivery
73.6 Episiotomy
73.91 External version to assist delivery

59414

59414 Delivery of placenta (separate procedure)

ICD-9-CM Diagnostic

666.02 Third-stage postpartum hemorrhage, with delivery ♀
666.04 Third-stage postpartum hemorrhage, postpartum ♀
666.22 Delayed and secondary postpartum hemorrhage, with delivery ♀
666.24 Delayed and secondary postpartum hemorrhage, postpartum ♀
667.02 Retained placenta without hemorrhage, with delivery, with mention of postpartum complication ♀
667.04 Retained placenta without hemorrhage, postpartum condition or complication ♀
667.12 Retained portions of placenta or membranes, without hemorrhage, delivered, with mention of postpartum complication ♀
667.14 Retained portions of placenta or membranes, without hemorrhage, postpartum condition or complication ♀
V27.0 Outcome of delivery, single liveborn — (This code is intended for the coding of the outcome of delivery on the mother's record) ♀
V27.1 Outcome of delivery, single stillborn — (This code is intended for the coding of the outcome of delivery on the mother's record) ♀
V27.2 Outcome of delivery, twins, both liveborn — (This code is intended for the coding of the outcome of delivery on the mother's record) ♀
V27.3 Outcome of delivery, twins, one liveborn and one stillborn — (This code is intended for the coding of the outcome of delivery on the mother's record) ♀
V27.4 Outcome of delivery, twins, both stillborn — (This code is intended for the coding of the outcome of delivery on the mother's record) ♀

ICD-9-CM Procedural

73.59 Other manually assisted delivery
75.4 Manual removal of retained placenta

59425–59426

59425 Antepartum care only; 4-6 visits
59426 7 or more visits

ICD-9-CM Diagnostic

632 Missed abortion — (Use additional code from category 639 to identify any associated complications) ♀
634.00 Unspecified spontaneous abortion complicated by genital tract and pelvic infection ▽ ♀
634.01 Incomplete spontaneous abortion complicated by genital tract and pelvic infection ♀
634.02 Complete spontaneous abortion complicated by genital tract and pelvic infection ♀
634.10 Unspecified spontaneous abortion complicated by delayed or excessive hemorrhage ▽ ♀
634.11 Incomplete spontaneous abortion complicated by delayed or excessive hemorrhage ♀
634.12 Complete spontaneous abortion complicated by delayed or excessive hemorrhage ♀
634.20 Unspecified spontaneous abortion complicated by damage to pelvic organs or tissues ▽ ♀
634.21 Incomplete spontaneous abortion complicated by damage to pelvic organs or tissues ♀
634.22 Complete spontaneous abortion complicated by damage to pelvic organs or tissues ♀
634.30 Unspecified spontaneous abortion complicated by renal failure ▽ ♀
634.31 Incomplete spontaneous abortion complicated by renal failure ♀
634.32 Complete spontaneous abortion complicated by renal failure ♀
634.40 Unspecified spontaneous abortion complicated by metabolic disorder ▽ ♀
634.41 Incomplete spontaneous abortion complicated by metabolic disorder ♀
634.42 Complete spontaneous abortion complicated by metabolic disorder ♀
634.50 Unspecified spontaneous abortion complicated by shock ▽ ♀
634.51 Incomplete spontaneous abortion complicated by shock ♀
634.52 Complete spontaneous abortion complicated by shock ♀
634.60 Unspecified spontaneous abortion complicated by embolism ▽ ♀
634.61 Incomplete spontaneous abortion complicated by embolism ♀
634.62 Complete spontaneous abortion complicated by embolism ♀
634.70 Unspecified spontaneous abortion with other specified complications ▽ ♀
634.71 Incomplete spontaneous abortion with other specified complications ♀
634.72 Complete spontaneous abortion with other specified complications ♀
634.80 Unspecified spontaneous abortion with unspecified complication ▽ ♀
634.81 Incomplete spontaneous abortion with unspecified complication ▽ ♀
634.82 Complete spontaneous abortion with unspecified complication ▽ ♀
634.90 Unspecified spontaneous abortion without mention of complication ▽ ♀
634.91 Incomplete spontaneous abortion without mention of complication ♀

634.92 Complete spontaneous abortion without mention of complication ♀
635.00 Unspecified legally induced abortion complicated by genital tract and pelvic infection ♀
635.01 Incomplete legally induced abortion complicated by genital tract and pelvic infection ♀
635.02 Complete legally induced abortion complicated by genital tract and pelvic infection ♀
635.10 Unspecified legally induced abortion complicated by delayed or excessive hemorrhage ♀
635.11 Incomplete legally induced abortion complicated by delayed or excessive hemorrhage ♀
635.12 Complete legally induced abortion complicated by delayed or excessive hemorrhage ♀
635.20 Unspecified legally induced abortion complicated by damage to pelvic organs or tissues ♀
635.21 Legally induced abortion complicated by damage to pelvic organs or tissues, incomplete ♀
635.22 Complete legally induced abortion complicated by damage to pelvic organs or tissues ♀
635.30 Unspecified legally induced abortion complicated by renal failure ♀
635.31 Incomplete legally induced abortion complicated by renal failure ♀
635.32 Complete legally induced abortion complicated by renal failure ♀
635.40 Unspecified legally induced abortion complicated by metabolic disorder ♀
635.41 Incomplete legally induced abortion complicated by metabolic disorder ♀
635.42 Complete legally induced abortion complicated by metabolic disorder ♀
635.50 Unspecified legally induced abortion complicated by shock ♀
635.51 Legally induced abortion, complicated by shock, incomplete ♀
635.52 Complete legally induced abortion complicated by shock ♀
635.60 Unspecified legally induced abortion complicated by embolism ♀
635.61 Incomplete legally induced abortion complicated by embolism ♀
635.62 Complete legally induced abortion complicated by embolism ♀
635.70 Unspecified legally induced abortion with other specified complications ♀
635.71 Incomplete legally induced abortion with other specified complications ♀
635.72 Complete legally induced abortion with other specified complications ♀
635.80 Unspecified legally induced abortion with unspecified complication ♀
635.81 Incomplete legally induced abortion with unspecified complication ♀
635.82 Complete legally induced abortion with unspecified complication ♀
635.90 Unspecified legally induced abortion without mention of complication ♀
635.91 Incomplete legally induced abortion without mention of complication ♀
635.92 Complete legally induced abortion without mention of complication ♀
642.03 Benign essential hypertension antepartum ♀
642.13 Hypertension secondary to renal disease, antepartum ♀
642.23 Other pre-existing hypertension, antepartum ♀
642.33 Transient hypertension of pregnancy, antepartum ♀
642.43 Mild or unspecified pre-eclampsia, antepartum ♀
642.53 Severe pre-eclampsia, antepartum ♀
642.63 Eclampsia, antepartum ♀
642.73 Pre-eclampsia or eclampsia superimposed on pre-existing hypertension, antepartum ♀
642.93 Unspecified hypertension antepartum ♀
643.03 Mild hyperemesis gravidarum, antepartum ♀
643.13 Hyperemesis gravidarum with metabolic disturbance, antepartum ♀
643.23 Late vomiting of pregnancy, antepartum ♀
643.83 Other vomiting complicating pregnancy, antepartum — (Use additional code to specify cause) ♀
643.93 Unspecified vomiting of pregnancy, antepartum ♀
646.53 Asymptomatic bacteriuria antepartum ♀
648.13 Maternal thyroid dysfunction, antepartum condition or complication — (Use additional code(s) to identify the condition) ♀
648.83 Abnormal maternal glucose tolerance, antepartum — (Use additional code(s) to identify the condition) ♀
652.23 Breech presentation without mention of version, antepartum — (Code first any associated obstructed labor, 660.0) ♀
654.13 Tumors of body of uterus, antepartum condition or complication — (Code first any associated obstructed labor, 660.2) ♀
654.43 Other abnormalities in shape or position of gravid uterus and of neighboring structures, antepartum — (Code first any associated obstructed labor, 660.2) ♀
654.53 Cervical incompetence, antepartum condition or complication — (Code first any associated obstructed labor, 660.2) ♀
654.73 Congenital or acquired abnormality of vagina, antepartum condition or complication — (Code first any associated obstructed labor, 660.2) ♀
654.83 Congenital or acquired abnormality of vulva, antepartum condition or complication — (Code first any associated obstructed labor, 660.2) ♀
654.93 Other and unspecified abnormality of organs and soft tissues of pelvis, antepartum condition or complication — (Code first any associated obstructed labor, 660.2) ♀
655.13 Chromosomal abnormality in fetus, affecting management of mother, antepartum ♀
655.23 Hereditary disease in family possibly affecting fetus, affecting management of mother, antepartum condition or complication ♀
655.33 Suspected damage to fetus from viral disease in mother, affecting management of mother, antepartum condition or complication ♀
655.43 Suspected damage to fetus from other disease in mother, affecting management of mother, antepartum condition or complication ♀
655.63 Suspected damage to fetus from radiation, affecting management of mother, antepartum condition or complication ♀
655.83 Other known or suspected fetal abnormality, not elsewhere classified, affecting management of mother, antepartum condition or complication ♀
655.93 Unspecified fetal abnormality affecting management of mother, antepartum condition or complication ♀
656.43 Intrauterine death affecting management of mother, antepartum ♀
656.53 Poor fetal growth, affecting management of mother, antepartum condition or complication ♀
656.63 Excessive fetal growth affecting management of mother, antepartum ♀
657.03 Polyhydramnios, antepartum complication ♀
658.03 Oligohydramnios, antepartum ♀
658.13 Premature rupture of membranes in pregnancy, antepartum ♀
659.43 Grand multiparity with current pregnancy, antepartum ♀
659.53 Elderly primigravida, antepartum ♀
659.63 Elderly multigravida, with antepartum condition or complication ♀
669.23 Maternal hypotension syndrome, antepartum ♀
671.03 Varicose veins of legs, antepartum ♀
671.83 Other venous complication, antepartum ♀
676.03 Retracted nipple, antepartum condition or complication ♀
676.23 Engorgement of breast, antepartum ♀
676.33 Other and unspecified disorder of breast associated with childbirth, antepartum condition or complication ♀
V22.0 Supervision of normal first pregnancy ♀
V22.1 Supervision of other normal pregnancy ♀
V23.81 Supervision of high-risk pregnancy of elderly primigravida ♀
V23.82 Supervision of high-risk pregnancy of elderly multigravida ♀
V23.83 Supervision of high-risk pregnancy of young primigravida ♀
V23.84 Supervision of high-risk pregnancy of young multigravida ♀
V23.89 Supervision of other high-risk pregnancy ♀

ICD-9-CM Procedural

89.04 Other interview and evaluation
89.26 Gynecological examination

HCPCS Level II Supplies & Services

A4649 Surgical supply; miscellaneous

59430

59430 Postpartum care only (separate procedure)

ICD-9-CM Diagnostic

V24.0 Postpartum care and examination immediately after delivery ♀
V24.1 Postpartum care and examination of lactating mother ♀
V24.2 Routine postpartum follow-up ♀
V72.31 Routine gynecological examination

ICD-9-CM Procedural

89.04 Other interview and evaluation
89.26 Gynecological examination

HCPCS Level II Supplies & Services

A4649 Surgical supply; miscellaneous

59510–59515

59510 Routine obstetric care including antepartum care, cesarean delivery, and postpartum care
59514 Cesarean delivery only;
59515 including postpartum care

ICD-9-CM Diagnostic

640.01 Threatened abortion, delivered ♀
640.91 Unspecified hemorrhage in early pregnancy, delivered ♀
641.01 Placenta previa without hemorrhage, with delivery ♀
641.11 Hemorrhage from placenta previa, with delivery ♀

Unspecified code ♀ Female diagnosis ☒ Manifestation code ♂ Male diagnosis

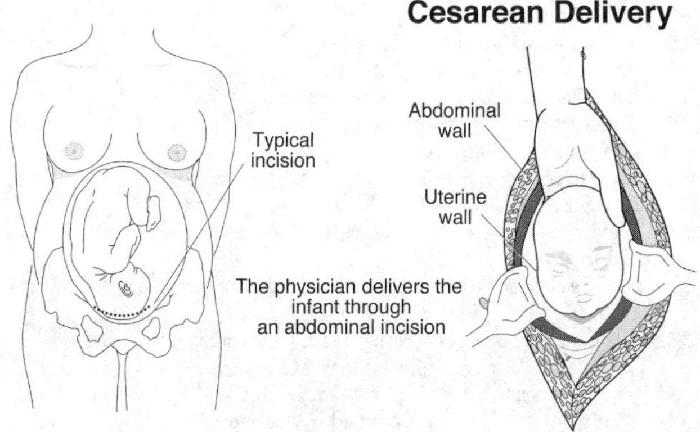
Cesarean Delivery
Typical incision
Abdominal wall
Uterine wall
The physician delivers the infant through an abdominal incision

641.21 Premature separation of placenta, with delivery ♀
641.31 Antepartum hemorrhage associated with coagulation defects, with delivery ♀
641.81 Other antepartum hemorrhage, with delivery ♀
641.91 Unspecified antepartum hemorrhage, with delivery ▽ ♀
642.01 Benign essential hypertension with delivery ♀
642.11 Hypertension secondary to renal disease, with delivery ♀
642.21 Other pre-existing hypertension, with delivery ♀
642.31 Transient hypertension of pregnancy, with delivery ♀
642.41 Mild or unspecified pre-eclampsia, with delivery ♀
642.51 Severe pre-eclampsia, with delivery ♀
642.61 Eclampsia, with delivery ♀
642.71 Pre-eclampsia or eclampsia superimposed on pre-existing hypertension, with delivery ♀
642.91 Unspecified hypertension, with delivery ▽ ♀
643.01 Mild hyperemesis gravidarum, delivered ♀
643.11 Hyperemesis gravidarum with metabolic disturbance, delivered ♀
643.21 Late vomiting of pregnancy, delivered ♀
643.81 Other vomiting complicating pregnancy, delivered — (Use additional code to specify cause) ♀
643.91 Unspecified vomiting of pregnancy, delivered ▽ ♀
644.21 Early onset of delivery, delivered, with or without mention of antepartum condition ♀
645.11 Post term pregnancy, delivered, with or without mention of antepartum condition ♀
645.21 Prolonged pregnancy, delivered, with or without mention of antepartum condition ♀
646.01 Papyraceous fetus, delivered, with or without mention of antepartum condition ♀
646.11 Edema or excessive weight gain in pregnancy, with delivery, with or without mention of antepartum complication ♀
646.21 Unspecified renal disease in pregnancy, with delivery ▽ ♀
646.23 Unspecified antepartum renal disease ▽ ♀
646.41 Peripheral neuritis in pregnancy, with delivery ♀
646.51 Asymptomatic bacteriuria in pregnancy, with delivery ♀
646.61 Infections of genitourinary tract in pregnancy, with delivery ♀
646.71 Liver disorders in pregnancy, with delivery ♀
646.81 Other specified complication of pregnancy, with delivery ♀
646.91 Unspecified complication of pregnancy, with delivery ▽ ♀
647.01 Maternal syphilis, complicating pregnancy, with delivery — (Use additional code(s) to further specify complication) ♀
647.11 Maternal gonorrhea with delivery — (Use additional code(s) to further specify complication) ♀
647.21 Other maternal venereal diseases with delivery — (Use additional code(s) to further specify complication) ♀
647.31 Maternal tuberculosis with delivery — (Use additional code(s) to further specify complication) ♀
647.41 Maternal malaria with delivery — (Use additional code(s) to further specify complication) ♀
647.51 Maternal rubella with delivery — (Use additional code(s) to further specify complication) ♀
647.61 Other maternal viral disease with delivery — (Use additional code(s) to further specify complication) ♀
647.81 Other specified maternal infectious and parasitic disease with delivery — (Use additional code(s) to further specify complication) ♀
647.91 Unspecified maternal infection or infestation with delivery — (Use additional code(s) to further specify complication) ▽ ♀
648.01 Maternal diabetes mellitus with delivery — (Use additional code(s) to identify the condition) ♀
648.11 Maternal thyroid dysfunction with delivery, with or without mention of antepartum condition — (Use additional code(s) to identify the condition) ♀
648.21 Maternal anemia, with delivery — (Use additional code(s) to identify the condition) ♀
648.31 Maternal drug dependence, with delivery — (Use additional code(s) to identify the condition) ♀
648.41 Maternal mental disorders, with delivery — (Use additional code(s) to identify the condition) ♀
648.51 Maternal congenital cardiovascular disorders, with delivery — (Use additional code(s) to identify the condition) ♀
648.61 Other maternal cardiovascular diseases, with delivery — (Use additional code(s) to identify the condition) ♀
648.71 Bone and joint disorders of maternal back, pelvis, and lower limbs, with delivery — (Use additional code(s) to identify the condition) ♀
648.81 Abnormal maternal glucose tolerance, with delivery — (Use additional code(s) to identify the condition) ♀
648.91 Other current maternal conditions classifiable elsewhere, with delivery — (Use additional code(s) to identify the condition) ♀
651.01 Twin pregnancy, delivered ♀
651.11 Triplet pregnancy, delivered ♀
651.21 Quadruplet pregnancy, delivered ♀
651.31 Twin pregnancy with fetal loss and retention of one fetus, delivered ♀
651.41 Triplet pregnancy with fetal loss and retention of one or more, delivered ♀
651.51 Quadruplet pregnancy with fetal loss and retention of one or more, delivered ♀
651.61 Other multiple pregnancy with fetal loss and retention of one or more fetus(es), delivered ♀
651.81 Other specified multiple gestation, delivered ♀
651.91 Unspecified multiple gestation, delivered ▽ ♀
652.01 Unstable lie of fetus, delivered — (Code first any associated obstructed labor, 660.0) ♀
652.11 Breech or other malpresentation successfully converted to cephalic presentation, delivered — (Code first any associated obstructed labor, 660.0) ♀
652.21 Breech presentation without mention of version, delivered — (Code first any associated obstructed labor, 660.0) ♀
652.31 Transverse or oblique fetal presentation, delivered — (Code first any associated obstructed labor, 660.0) ♀
652.41 Fetal face or brow presentation, delivered — (Code first any associated obstructed labor, 660.0) ♀
652.51 High fetal head at term, delivered — (Code first any associated obstructed labor, 660.0) ♀
652.61 Multiple gestation with malpresentation of one fetus or more, delivered — (Code first any associated obstructed labor, 660.0) ♀
652.71 Prolapsed arm of fetus, delivered — (Code first any associated obstructed labor, 660.0) ♀
652.81 Other specified malposition or malpresentation of fetus, delivered — (Code first any associated obstructed labor, 660.0) ♀
652.91 Unspecified malposition or malpresentation of fetus, delivered — (Code first any associated obstructed labor, 660.0) ▽ ♀
653.01 Major abnormality of bony pelvis, not further specified, delivered — (Code first any associated obstructed labor, 660.1) ♀
653.11 Generally contracted pelvis in pregnancy, delivered — (Code first any associated obstructed labor, 660.1) ♀
653.21 Inlet contraction of pelvis in pregnancy, delivered — (Code first any associated obstructed labor, 660.1) ♀
653.31 Outlet contraction of pelvis in pregnancy, delivered — (Code first any associated obstructed labor, 660.1) ♀
653.41 Fetopelvic disproportion, delivered — (Code first any associated obstructed labor, 660.1) ♀
653.51 Unusually large fetus causing disproportion, delivered — (Code first any associated obstructed labor, 660.1) ♀
653.61 Hydrocephalic fetus causing disproportion, delivered — (Code first any associated obstructed labor, 660.1) ♀
653.71 Other fetal abnormality causing disproportion, delivered — (Code first any associated obstructed labor, 660.1) ♀
654.01 Congenital abnormalities of pregnant uterus, delivered — (Code first any associated obstructed labor, 660.2) ♀
654.11 Tumors of body of uterus, delivered — (Code first any associated obstructed labor, 660.2) ♀
654.21 Previous cesarean delivery, delivered, with or without mention of antepartum condition — (Code first any associated obstructed labor, 660.2) ♀
654.31 Retroverted and incarcerated gravid uterus, delivered — (Code first any associated obstructed labor, 660.2) ♀
654.41 Other abnormalities in shape or position of gravid uterus and of neighboring structures, delivered — (Code first any associated obstructed labor, 660.2) ♀

▽ Unspecified code ♀ Female diagnosis ☒ Manifestation code ♂ Male diagnosis

654.51 Cervical incompetence, delivered — (Code first any associated obstructed labor, 660.2) ♀
654.61 Other congenital or acquired abnormality of cervix, with delivery — (Code first any associated obstructed labor, 660.2) ♀
654.71 Congenital or acquired abnormality of vagina, with delivery — (Code first any associated obstructed labor, 660.2) ♀
654.81 Congenital or acquired abnormality of vulva, with delivery — (Code first any associated obstructed labor, 660.2) ♀
654.84 Congenital or acquired abnormality of vulva, postpartum condition or complication — (Code first any associated obstructed labor, 660.2) ♀
654.91 Other and unspecified abnormality of organs and soft tissues of pelvis, with delivery — (Code first any associated obstructed labor, 660.2) ▽ ♀
655.01 Central nervous system malformation in fetus, with delivery ♀
655.11 Chromosomal abnormality in fetus, affecting management of mother, with delivery ♀
655.21 Hereditary disease in family possibly affecting fetus, affecting management of mother, with delivery ♀
655.31 Suspected damage to fetus from viral disease in mother, affecting management of mother, with delivery ♀
655.41 Suspected damage to fetus from other disease in mother, affecting management of mother, with delivery ♀
655.51 Suspected damage to fetus from drugs, affecting management of mother, delivered ♀
655.61 Suspected damage to fetus from radiation, affecting management of mother, delivered ♀
655.81 Other known or suspected fetal abnormality, not elsewhere classified, affecting management of mother, delivery ♀
655.91 Unspecified fetal abnormality affecting management of mother, delivery ▽ ♀
656.01 Fetal-maternal hemorrhage, with delivery ♀
656.11 Rhesus isoimmunization affecting management of mother, delivered ♀
656.21 Isoimmunization from other and unspecified blood-group incompatibility, affecting management of mother, delivered ♀
656.31 Fetal distress affecting management of mother, delivered ♀
656.41 Intrauterine death affecting management of mother, delivered ♀
656.51 Poor fetal growth, affecting management of mother, delivered ♀
656.61 Excessive fetal growth affecting management of mother, delivered ♀
656.71 Other placental conditions affecting management of mother, delivered ♀
656.81 Other specified fetal and placental problems affecting management of mother, delivered ♀
656.91 Unspecified fetal and placental problem affecting management of mother, delivered ▽ ♀
657.01 Polyhydramnios, with delivery ♀
658.01 Oligohydramnios, delivered ♀
658.11 Premature rupture of membranes in pregnancy, delivered ♀
658.21 Delayed delivery after spontaneous or unspecified rupture of membranes, delivered ♀
658.31 Delayed delivery after artificial rupture of membranes, delivered ♀
658.41 Infection of amniotic cavity, delivered ♀
658.81 Other problem associated with amniotic cavity and membranes, delivered ♀
658.91 Unspecified problem associated with amniotic cavity and membranes, delivered ▽ ♀
659.01 Failed mechanical induction of labor, delivered ♀
659.11 Failed medical or unspecified induction of labor, delivered ♀
659.21 Unspecified maternal pyrexia during labor, delivered ♀
659.31 Generalized infection during labor, delivered ♀
659.41 Grand multiparity, delivered, with or without mention of antepartum condition ♀
659.51 Elderly primigravida, delivered ♀
659.61 Elderly multigravida, delivered, with mention of antepartum condition ♀
659.81 Other specified indication for care or intervention related to labor and delivery, delivered ♀
659.91 Unspecified indication for care or intervention related to labor and delivery, delivered ▽ ♀
660.01 Obstruction caused by malposition of fetus at onset of labor, delivered — (Use additional code from 652.0-652.9 to identify condition) ♀
660.11 Obstruction by bony pelvis during labor and delivery, delivered — (Use additional code from 653.0-653.9 to identify condition) ♀
660.21 Obstruction by abnormal pelvic soft tissues during laborand delivery, delivered — (Use additional code from 654.0-654.9 to identify condition) ♀
660.31 Deep transverse arrest and persistent occipitoposterior position during labor and deliver, delivered ♀
660.41 Shoulder (girdle) dystocia during labor and deliver, delivered ♀
660.51 Locked twins, delivered ♀
660.61 Unspecified failed trial of labor, delivered ▽ ♀
660.71 Unspecified failed forceps or vacuum extractor, delivered ▽ ♀
660.81 Other causes of obstructed labor, delivered ♀
660.91 Unspecified obstructed labor, with delivery ▽ ♀
661.01 Primary uterine inertia, with delivery ♀
661.11 Secondary uterine inertia, with delivery ♀
661.21 Other and unspecified uterine inertia, with delivery ▽ ♀
662.01 Prolonged first stage of labor, delivered ♀
662.21 Prolonged second stage of labor, delivered ♀
662.31 Delayed delivery of second twin, triplet, etc., delivered ♀
663.01 Prolapse of cord, complicating labor and delivery, delivered ♀
663.11 Cord around neck, with compression, complicating labor and delivery, delivered ♀
663.21 Other and unspecified cord entanglement, with compression, complicating labor and delivery, delivered ▽ ♀
663.31 Other and unspecified cord entanglement, without mention of compression, complicating labor and delivery, delivered ▽ ♀
663.41 Short cord complicating labor and delivery, delivered ♀
663.51 Vasa previa complicating labor and delivery, delivered ♀
663.61 Vascular lesions of cord complicating labor and delivery, delivered ♀
663.81 Other umbilical cord complications during labor and delivery, delivered ♀
663.91 Unspecified umbilical cord complication during labor and delivery, delivered ▽ ♀
665.01 Rupture of uterus before onset of labor, with delivery ♀
665.11 Rupture of uterus during labor, with delivery ♀
665.22 Inversion of uterus, delivered with postpartum complication ♀
665.81 Other specified obstetrical trauma, with delivery ♀
665.82 Other specified obstetrical trauma, delivered, with postpartum ♀
665.91 Unspecified obstetrical trauma, with delivery ▽ ♀
665.92 Unspecified obstetrical trauma, delivered, with postpartum complication ▽ ♀
666.02 Third-stage postpartum hemorrhage, with delivery ♀
666.12 Other immediate postpartum hemorrhage, with delivery ♀
667.02 Retained placenta without hemorrhage, with delivery, with mention of postpartum complication ♀
667.12 Retained portions of placenta or membranes, without hemorrhage, delivered, with mention of postpartum complication ♀
668.01 Pulmonary complications of the administration of anesthesia or other sedation in labor and delivery, delivered — (Use additional code(s) to further specify complication) ♀
668.11 Cardiac complications of the administration of anesthesia or other sedation in labor and delivery, delivered — (Use additional code(s) to further specify complication) ♀
668.21 Central nervous system complications of the administration of anesthesia or other sedation in labor and delivery, delivered — (Use additional code(s) to further specify complication) ♀
668.81 Other complications of the administration of anesthesia or other sedation in labor and delivery, delivered — (Use additional code(s) to further specify complication) ♀
668.91 Unspecified complication of the administration of anesthesia or other sedation in labor and delivery, delivered — (Use additional code(s) to further specify complication) ▽ ♀
669.01 Maternal distress, with delivery, with or without mention of antepartum condition ♀
669.02 Maternal distress, with delivery, with mention of postpartum complication ♀
669.11 Shock during or following labor and delivery, with delivery, with or without mention of antepartum condition ♀
669.12 Shock during or following labor and delivery, with delivery, with mention of postpartum complication ♀
669.21 Maternal hypotension syndrome, with delivery, with or without mention of antepartum condition ♀
669.32 Acute renal failure with delivery, with mention of postpartum complication ♀
669.41 Other complications of obstetrical surgery and procedures, with delivery, with or without mention of antepartum condition ♀
669.42 Other complications of obstetrical surgery and procedures, with delivery, with mention of postpartum complication ♀
669.51 Forceps or vacuum extractor delivery without mention of indication, delivered, with or without mention of antepartum condition ♀
669.61 Breech extraction, without mention of indication, delivered, with or without mention of antepartum condition ♀
669.71 Cesarean delivery, without mention of indication, delivered, with or without mention of antepartum condition ♀
669.81 Other complication of labor and delivery, delivered, with or without mention of antepartum condition ♀
669.91 Unspecified complication of labor and delivery, with delivery, with or without mention of antepartum condition ▽ ♀
671.01 Varicose veins of legs, with delivery, with or without mention of antepartum condition ♀
671.81 Other venous complication, with delivery, with or without mention of antepartum condition ♀

▽ Unspecified code ♀ Female diagnosis ☒ Manifestation code ♂ Male diagnosis

671.82 Other venous complication, with delivery, with mention of postpartum complication ♀
676.01 Retracted nipple, delivered, with or without mention of antepartum condition ♀
676.02 Retracted nipple, delivered, with mention of postpartum complication ♀
676.21 Engorgement of breasts, delivered, with or without mention of antepartum condition ♀
676.22 Engorgement of breasts, delivered, with mention of postpartum complication ♀
676.31 Other and unspecified disorder of breast associated with childbirth, delivered, with or without mention of antepartum condition ▽ ♀
676.32 Other and unspecified disorder of breast associated with childbirth, delivered, with mention of postpartum complication ▽ ♀
676.41 Failure of lactation, with delivery, with or without mention of antepartum condition ♀
676.42 Failure of lactation, with delivery, with mention of postpartum complication ♀
676.51 Suppressed lactation, with delivery, with or without mention of antepartum condition ♀
676.52 Suppressed lactation, with delivery, with mention of postpartum complication ♀
676.91 Unspecified disorder of lactation, with delivery, with or without mention of antepartum condition ▽ ♀
676.92 Unspecified disorder of lactation, with delivery, with mention of postpartum complication ▽ ♀
V23.0 Pregnancy with history of infertility ♀
V23.1 Pregnancy with history of trophoblastic disease ♀
V23.2 Pregnancy with history of abortion ♀
V23.3 Pregnancy with grand multiparity ♀
V23.41 Supervision of pregnancy with history of pre-term labor ♀
V23.49 Supervision of pregnancy with other poor obstetric history ♀
V23.5 Pregnancy with other poor reproductive history ♀
V23.7 Insufficient prenatal care ♀
V23.81 Supervision of high-risk pregnancy of elderly primigravida ♀
V23.82 Supervision of high-risk pregnancy of elderly multigravida ♀
V23.83 Supervision of high-risk pregnancy of young primigravida ♀
V23.84 Supervision of high-risk pregnancy of young multigravida ♀
V23.89 Supervision of other high-risk pregnancy ♀
V23.9 Unspecified high-risk pregnancy ▽ ♀
V24.0 Postpartum care and examination immediately after delivery ♀
V24.1 Postpartum care and examination of lactating mother ♀
V24.2 Routine postpartum follow-up ♀
V27.0 Outcome of delivery, single liveborn — (This code is intended for the coding of the outcome of delivery on the mother's record) ♀
V27.1 Outcome of delivery, single stillborn — (This code is intended for the coding of the outcome of delivery on the mother's record) ♀
V27.2 Outcome of delivery, twins, both liveborn — (This code is intended for the coding of the outcome of delivery on the mother's record) ♀
V27.3 Outcome of delivery, twins, one liveborn and one stillborn — (This code is intended for the coding of the outcome of delivery on the mother's record) ♀
V27.4 Outcome of delivery, twins, both stillborn — (This code is intended for the coding of the outcome of delivery on the mother's record) ♀
V27.5 Outcome of delivery, other multiple birth, all liveborn — (This code is intended for the coding of the outcome of delivery on the mother's record) ♀
V27.6 Outcome of delivery, other multiple birth, some liveborn — (This code is intended for the coding of the outcome of delivery on the mother's record) ♀
V27.7 Outcome of delivery, other multiple birth, all stillborn — (This code is intended for the coding of the outcome of delivery on the mother's record) ♀
V27.9 Outcome of delivery, unspecified — (This code is intended for the coding of the outcome of delivery on the mother's record) ▽ ♀

ICD-9-CM Procedural

73.3 Failed forceps
74.0 Classical cesarean section
74.1 Low cervical cesarean section
74.2 Extraperitoneal cesarean section
74.4 Cesarean section of other specified type

59525

59525 Subtotal or total hysterectomy after cesarean delivery (List separately in addition to code for primary procedure)

ICD-9-CM Diagnostic

180.0 Malignant neoplasm of endocervix ♀
180.1 Malignant neoplasm of exocervix ♀
182.0 Malignant neoplasm of corpus uteri, except isthmus ♀
182.8 Malignant neoplasm of other specified sites of body of uterus ♀
183.2 Malignant neoplasm of fallopian tube ♀
183.3 Malignant neoplasm of broad ligament of uterus ♀
183.4 Malignant neoplasm of parametrium of uterus ♀
614.7 Other chronic pelvic peritonitis, female — (Use additional code to identify organism: 041.0, 041.1) ♀
614.8 Other specified inflammatory disease of female pelvic organs and tissues — (Use additional code to identify organism: 041.0, 041.1) ♀
615.0 Acute inflammatory disease of uterus, except cervix — (Use additional code to identify organism: 041.0, 041.1) ♀
615.1 Chronic inflammatory disease of uterus, except cervix — (Use additional code to identify organism: 041.0, 041.1) ♀
615.9 Unspecified inflammatory disease of uterus — (Use additional code to identify organism: 041.0, 041.1) ▽ ♀
617.0 Endometriosis of uterus ♀
626.8 Other disorder of menstruation and other abnormal bleeding from female genital tract ♀
654.11 Tumors of body of uterus, delivered — (Code first any associated obstructed labor, 660.2) ♀
654.31 Retroverted and incarcerated gravid uterus, delivered — (Code first any associated obstructed labor, 660.2) ♀
665.01 Rupture of uterus before onset of labor, with delivery ♀
665.11 Rupture of uterus during labor, with delivery ♀
666.12 Other immediate postpartum hemorrhage, with delivery ♀

ICD-9-CM Procedural

68.39 Other subtotal abdominal hysterectomy, NOS
68.4 Total abdominal hysterectomy
68.9 Other and unspecified hysterectomy

59610–59614

59610 Routine obstetric care including antepartum care, vaginal delivery (with or without episiotomy, and/or forceps) and postpartum care, after previous cesarean delivery
59612 Vaginal delivery only, after previous cesarean delivery (with or without episiotomy and/or forceps);
59614 including postpartum care

ICD-9-CM Diagnostic

640.01 Threatened abortion, delivered ♀
640.91 Unspecified hemorrhage in early pregnancy, delivered ▽ ♀
641.01 Placenta previa without hemorrhage, with delivery ♀
641.11 Hemorrhage from placenta previa, with delivery ♀
641.21 Premature separation of placenta, with delivery ♀
641.31 Antepartum hemorrhage associated with coagulation defects, with delivery ♀
641.81 Other antepartum hemorrhage, with delivery ♀
641.91 Unspecified antepartum hemorrhage, with delivery ▽ ♀
642.01 Benign essential hypertension with delivery ♀
642.11 Hypertension secondary to renal disease, with delivery ♀
642.21 Other pre-existing hypertension, with delivery ♀
642.31 Transient hypertension of pregnancy, with delivery ♀
642.41 Mild or unspecified pre-eclampsia, with delivery ♀
642.51 Severe pre-eclampsia, with delivery ♀
642.61 Eclampsia, with delivery ♀
642.71 Pre-eclampsia or eclampsia superimposed on pre-existing hypertension, with delivery ♀
642.91 Unspecified hypertension, with delivery ▽ ♀
643.01 Mild hyperemesis gravidarum, delivered ♀
643.11 Hyperemesis gravidarum with metabolic disturbance, delivered ♀
643.21 Late vomiting of pregnancy, delivered ♀
643.81 Other vomiting complicating pregnancy, delivered — (Use additional code to specify cause) ♀
643.91 Unspecified vomiting of pregnancy, delivered ▽ ♀
644.21 Early onset of delivery, delivered, with or without mention of antepartum condition ♀
645.11 Post term pregnancy, delivered, with or without mention of antepartum condition ♀
645.21 Prolonged pregnancy, delivered, with or without mention of antepartum condition ♀
646.01 Papyraceous fetus, delivered, with or without mention of antepartum condition ♀
646.11 Edema or excessive weight gain in pregnancy, with delivery, with or without mention of antepartum complication ♀
646.21 Unspecified renal disease in pregnancy, with delivery ▽ ♀
646.31 Pregnancy complication, habitual aborter with or without mention of antepartum condition ♀
646.41 Peripheral neuritis in pregnancy, with delivery ♀

646.51 Asymptomatic bacteriuria in pregnancy, with delivery ♀
646.61 Infections of genitourinary tract in pregnancy, with delivery ♀
646.71 Liver disorders in pregnancy, with delivery ♀
646.81 Other specified complication of pregnancy, with delivery ♀
646.91 Unspecified complication of pregnancy, with delivery ▽ ♀
647.01 Maternal syphilis, complicating pregnancy, with delivery — (Use additional code(s) to further specify complication) ♀
647.11 Maternal gonorrhea with delivery — (Use additional code(s) to further specify complication) ♀
647.21 Other maternal venereal diseases with delivery — (Use additional code(s) to further specify complication) ♀
647.31 Maternal tuberculosis with delivery — (Use additional code(s) to further specify complication) ♀
647.41 Maternal malaria with delivery — (Use additional code(s) to further specify complication) ♀
647.51 Maternal rubella with delivery — (Use additional code(s) to further specify complication) ♀
647.61 Other maternal viral disease with delivery — (Use additional code(s) to further specify complication) ♀
647.81 Other specified maternal infectious and parasitic disease with delivery — (Use additional code(s) to further specify complication) ♀
647.91 Unspecified maternal infection or infestation with delivery — (Use additional code(s) to further specify complication) ▽ ♀
648.01 Maternal diabetes mellitus with delivery — (Use additional code(s) to identify the condition) ♀
648.11 Maternal thyroid dysfunction with delivery, with or without mention of antepartum condition — (Use additional code(s) to identify the condition) ♀
648.21 Maternal anemia, with delivery — (Use additional code(s) to identify the condition) ♀
648.31 Maternal drug dependence, with delivery — (Use additional code(s) to identify the condition) ♀
648.41 Maternal mental disorders, with delivery — (Use additional code(s) to identify the condition) ♀
648.51 Maternal congenital cardiovascular disorders, with delivery — (Use additional code(s) to identify the condition) ♀
648.61 Other maternal cardiovascular diseases, with delivery — (Use additional code(s) to identify the condition) ♀
648.71 Bone and joint disorders of maternal back, pelvis, and lower limbs, with delivery — (Use additional code(s) to identify the condition) ♀
648.81 Abnormal maternal glucose tolerance, with delivery — (Use additional code(s) to identify the condition) ♀
648.91 Other current maternal conditions classifiable elsewhere, with delivery — (Use additional code(s) to identify the condition) ♀
651.01 Twin pregnancy, delivered ♀
651.21 Quadruplet pregnancy, delivered ♀
651.31 Twin pregnancy with fetal loss and retention of one fetus, delivered ♀
651.41 Triplet pregnancy with fetal loss and retention of one or more, delivered ♀
651.51 Quadruplet pregnancy with fetal loss and retention of one or more, delivered ♀
651.61 Other multiple pregnancy with fetal loss and retention of one or more fetus(es), delivered ♀
651.81 Other specified multiple gestation, delivered ♀
651.91 Unspecified multiple gestation, delivered ▽ ♀
652.11 Breech or other malpresentation successfully converted to cephalic presentation, delivered — (Code first any associated obstructed labor, 660.0) ♀
652.21 Breech presentation without mention of version, delivered — (Code first any associated obstructed labor, 660.0) ♀
652.41 Fetal face or brow presentation, delivered — (Code first any associated obstructed labor, 660.0) ♀
652.71 Prolapsed arm of fetus, delivered — (Code first any associated obstructed labor, 660.0) ♀
652.81 Other specified malposition or malpresentation of fetus, delivered — (Code first any associated obstructed labor, 660.0) ♀
652.91 Unspecified malposition or malpresentation of fetus, delivered — (Code first any associated obstructed labor, 660.0) ▽ ♀
654.01 Congenital abnormalities of pregnant uterus, delivered — (Code first any associated obstructed labor, 660.2) ♀
654.11 Tumors of body of uterus, delivered — (Code first any associated obstructed labor, 660.2) ♀
654.21 Previous cesarean delivery, delivered, with or without mention of antepartum condition — (Code first any associated obstructed labor, 660.2) ♀
654.31 Retroverted and incarcerated gravid uterus, delivered — (Code first any associated obstructed labor, 660.2) ♀
654.41 Other abnormalities in shape or position of gravid uterus and of neighboring structures, delivered — (Code first any associated obstructed labor, 660.2) ♀
654.51 Cervical incompetence, delivered — (Code first any associated obstructed labor, 660.2) ♀
654.61 Other congenital or acquired abnormality of cervix, with delivery — (Code first any associated obstructed labor, 660.2) ♀
654.71 Congenital or acquired abnormality of vagina, with delivery — (Code first any associated obstructed labor, 660.2) ♀
654.81 Congenital or acquired abnormality of vulva, with delivery — (Code first any associated obstructed labor, 660.2) ♀
654.91 Other and unspecified abnormality of organs and soft tissues of pelvis, with delivery — (Code first any associated obstructed labor, 660.2) ▽ ♀
655.01 Central nervous system malformation in fetus, with delivery ♀
655.11 Chromosomal abnormality in fetus, affecting management of mother, with delivery ♀
655.21 Hereditary disease in family possibly affecting fetus, affecting management of mother, with delivery ♀
655.31 Suspected damage to fetus from viral disease in mother, affecting management of mother, with delivery ♀
655.41 Suspected damage to fetus from other disease in mother, affecting management of mother, with delivery ♀
655.81 Other known or suspected fetal abnormality, not elsewhere classified, affecting management of mother, delivery ♀
655.91 Unspecified fetal abnormality affecting management of mother, delivery ▽ ♀
656.01 Fetal-maternal hemorrhage, with delivery ♀
656.11 Rhesus isoimmunization affecting management of mother, delivered ♀
656.21 Isoimmunization from other and unspecified blood-group incompatibility, affecting management of mother, delivered ♀
656.31 Fetal distress affecting management of mother, delivered ♀
656.41 Intrauterine death affecting management of mother, delivered ♀
656.51 Poor fetal growth, affecting management of mother, delivered ♀
656.61 Excessive fetal growth affecting management of mother, delivered ♀
656.71 Other placental conditions affecting management of mother, delivered ♀
656.81 Other specified fetal and placental problems affecting management of mother, delivered ♀
656.91 Unspecified fetal and placental problem affecting management of mother, delivered ▽ ♀
657.01 Polyhydramnios, with delivery ♀
658.01 Oligohydramnios, delivered ♀
658.11 Premature rupture of membranes in pregnancy, delivered ♀
658.21 Delayed delivery after spontaneous or unspecified rupture of membranes, delivered ♀
658.31 Delayed delivery after artificial rupture of membranes, delivered ♀
658.41 Infection of amniotic cavity, delivered ♀
658.81 Other problem associated with amniotic cavity and membranes, delivered ♀
658.91 Unspecified problem associated with amniotic cavity and membranes, delivered ▽ ♀
659.21 Unspecified maternal pyrexia during labor, delivered ♀
659.31 Generalized infection during labor, delivered ♀
659.41 Grand multiparity, delivered, with or without mention of antepartum condition ♀
659.51 Elderly primigravida, delivered ♀
659.61 Elderly multigravida, delivered, with mention of antepartum condition ♀
659.81 Other specified indication for care or intervention related to labor and delivery, delivered ♀
659.91 Unspecified indication for care or intervention related to labor and delivery, delivered ▽ ♀
660.81 Other causes of obstructed labor, delivered ♀
661.31 Precipitate labor, with delivery ♀
662.01 Prolonged first stage of labor, delivered ♀
662.21 Prolonged second stage of labor, delivered ♀
662.31 Delayed delivery of second twin, triplet, etc., delivered ♀
663.11 Cord around neck, with compression, complicating labor and delivery, delivered ♀
663.31 Other and unspecified cord entanglement, without mention of compression, complicating labor and delivery, delivered ▽ ♀
663.41 Short cord complicating labor and delivery, delivered ♀
663.61 Vascular lesions of cord complicating labor and delivery, delivered ♀
663.81 Other umbilical cord complications during labor and delivery, delivered ♀
663.91 Unspecified umbilical cord complication during labor and delivery, delivered ▽ ♀
664.01 First-degree perineal laceration, with delivery ♀
664.11 Second-degree perineal laceration, with delivery ♀
664.21 Third-degree perineal laceration, with delivery ♀
664.31 Fourth-degree perineal laceration, with delivery ♀
664.41 Unspecified perineal laceration, with delivery ▽ ♀
664.51 Vulvar and perineal hematoma, with delivery ♀
664.81 Other specified trauma to perineum and vulva, with delivery ♀

664.91 Unspecified trauma to perineum and vulva, with delivery ▽ ♀
665.31 Laceration of cervix, with delivery ♀
665.41 High vaginal laceration, with delivery ♀
665.51 Other injury to pelvic organs, with delivery ♀
665.61 Damage to pelvic joints and ligaments, with delivery ♀
665.71 Pelvic hematoma, with delivery ♀
665.81 Other specified obstetrical trauma, with delivery ♀
665.91 Unspecified obstetrical trauma, with delivery ▽ ♀
666.02 Third-stage postpartum hemorrhage, with delivery ♀
666.12 Other immediate postpartum hemorrhage, with delivery ♀
666.22 Delayed and secondary postpartum hemorrhage, with delivery ♀
667.02 Retained placenta without hemorrhage, with delivery, with mention of postpartum complication ♀
668.01 Pulmonary complications of the administration of anesthesia or other sedation in labor and delivery, delivered — (Use additional code(s) to further specify complication) ♀
668.11 Cardiac complications of the administration of anesthesia or other sedation in labor and delivery, delivered — (Use additional code(s) to further specify complication) ♀
668.21 Central nervous system complications of the administration of anesthesia or other sedation in labor and delivery, delivered — (Use additional code(s) to further specify complication) ♀
668.81 Other complications of the administration of anesthesia or other sedation in labor and delivery, delivered — (Use additional code(s) to further specify complication) ♀
668.91 Unspecified complication of the administration of anesthesia or other sedation in labor and delivery, delivered — (Use additional code(s) to further specify complication) ▽ ♀
669.01 Maternal distress, with delivery, with or without mention of antepartum condition ♀
669.11 Shock during or following labor and delivery, with delivery, with or without mention of antepartum condition ♀
669.21 Maternal hypotension syndrome, with delivery, with or without mention of antepartum condition ♀
669.41 Other complications of obstetrical surgery and procedures, with delivery, with or without mention of antepartum condition ♀
669.51 Forceps or vacuum extractor delivery without mention of indication, delivered, with or without mention of antepartum condition ♀
669.61 Breech extraction, without mention of indication, delivered, with or without mention of antepartum condition ♀
669.81 Other complication of labor and delivery, delivered, with or without mention of antepartum condition ♀
669.91 Unspecified complication of labor and delivery, with delivery, with or without mention of antepartum condition ▽ ♀
671.01 Varicose veins of legs, with delivery, with or without mention of antepartum condition ♀
671.81 Other venous complication, with delivery, with or without mention of antepartum condition ♀
671.82 Other venous complication, with delivery, with mention of postpartum complication ♀
676.01 Retracted nipple, delivered, with or without mention of antepartum condition ♀
676.02 Retracted nipple, delivered, with mention of postpartum complication ♀
676.04 Retracted nipple, postpartum condition or complication ♀
676.21 Engorgement of breasts, delivered, with or without mention of antepartum condition ♀
676.22 Engorgement of breasts, delivered, with mention of postpartum complication ♀
676.31 Other and unspecified disorder of breast associated with childbirth, delivered, with or without mention of antepartum condition ▽ ♀
676.32 Other and unspecified disorder of breast associated with childbirth, delivered, with mention of postpartum complication ▽ ♀
676.41 Failure of lactation, with delivery, with or without mention of antepartum condition ♀
676.42 Failure of lactation, with delivery, with mention of postpartum complication ♀
676.51 Suppressed lactation, with delivery, with or without mention of antepartum condition ♀
676.52 Suppressed lactation, with delivery, with mention of postpartum complication ♀
676.91 Unspecified disorder of lactation, with delivery, with or without mention of antepartum condition ▽ ♀
676.92 Unspecified disorder of lactation, with delivery, with mention of postpartum complication ▽ ♀
V22.1 Supervision of other normal pregnancy ♀
V23.0 Pregnancy with history of infertility ♀
V23.2 Pregnancy with history of abortion ♀
V23.41 Supervision of pregnancy with history of pre-term labor ♀
V23.49 Supervision of pregnancy with other poor obstetric history ♀
V23.82 Supervision of high-risk pregnancy of elderly multigravida ♀
V23.84 Supervision of high-risk pregnancy of young multigravida ♀
V23.89 Supervision of other high-risk pregnancy ♀
V24.0 Postpartum care and examination immediately after delivery ♀
V24.1 Postpartum care and examination of lactating mother ♀
V24.2 Routine postpartum follow-up ♀
V27.0 Outcome of delivery, single liveborn — (This code is intended for the coding of the outcome of delivery on the mother's record) ♀
V27.1 Outcome of delivery, single stillborn — (This code is intended for the coding of the outcome of delivery on the mother's record) ♀
V27.2 Outcome of delivery, twins, both liveborn — (This code is intended for the coding of the outcome of delivery on the mother's record) ♀
V27.3 Outcome of delivery, twins, one liveborn and one stillborn — (This code is intended for the coding of the outcome of delivery on the mother's record) ♀
V27.4 Outcome of delivery, twins, both stillborn — (This code is intended for the coding of the outcome of delivery on the mother's record) ♀
V27.5 Outcome of delivery, other multiple birth, all liveborn — (This code is intended for the coding of the outcome of delivery on the mother's record) ♀
V27.6 Outcome of delivery, other multiple birth, some liveborn — (This code is intended for the coding of the outcome of delivery on the mother's record) ♀
V27.7 Outcome of delivery, other multiple birth, all stillborn — (This code is intended for the coding of the outcome of delivery on the mother's record) ♀

ICD-9-CM Procedural

72.0 Low forceps operation
72.1 Low forceps operation with episiotomy
72.21 Mid forceps operation with episiotomy
72.29 Other mid forceps operation
72.31 High forceps operation with episiotomy
72.39 Other high forceps operation
72.4 Forceps rotation of fetal head
72.51 Partial breech extraction with forceps to aftercoming head
72.52 Other partial breech extraction
72.53 Total breech extraction with forceps to aftercoming head
72.54 Other total breech extraction
72.6 Forceps application to aftercoming head
72.71 Vacuum extraction with episiotomy
72.79 Other vacuum extraction
72.8 Other specified instrumental delivery
72.9 Unspecified instrumental delivery
73.01 Induction of labor by artificial rupture of membranes
73.09 Other artificial rupture of membranes
73.4 Medical induction of labor
73.59 Other manually assisted delivery

59618–59622

59618 Routine obstetric care including antepartum care, cesarean delivery, and postpartum care, following attempted vaginal delivery after previous cesarean delivery
59620 Cesarean delivery only, following attempted vaginal delivery after previous cesarean delivery;
59622 including postpartum care

ICD-9-CM Diagnostic

640.01 Threatened abortion, delivered ♀
640.91 Unspecified hemorrhage in early pregnancy, delivered ▽ ♀
641.01 Placenta previa without hemorrhage, with delivery ♀
641.11 Hemorrhage from placenta previa, with delivery ♀
641.21 Premature separation of placenta, with delivery ♀
641.31 Antepartum hemorrhage associated with coagulation defects, with delivery ♀
641.81 Other antepartum hemorrhage, with delivery ♀
641.91 Unspecified antepartum hemorrhage, with delivery ▽ ♀
642.01 Benign essential hypertension with delivery ♀
642.11 Hypertension secondary to renal disease, with delivery ♀
642.21 Other pre-existing hypertension, with delivery ♀
642.31 Transient hypertension of pregnancy, with delivery ♀
642.41 Mild or unspecified pre-eclampsia, with delivery ♀
642.51 Severe pre-eclampsia, with delivery ♀
642.61 Eclampsia, with delivery ♀
642.71 Pre-eclampsia or eclampsia superimposed on pre-existing hypertension, with delivery ♀
642.91 Unspecified hypertension, with delivery ▽ ♀
643.01 Mild hyperemesis gravidarum, delivered ♀
643.11 Hyperemesis gravidarum with metabolic disturbance, delivered ♀

643.21 Late vomiting of pregnancy, delivered ♀
643.81 Other vomiting complicating pregnancy, delivered — (Use additional code to specify cause) ♀
643.91 Unspecified vomiting of pregnancy, delivered ▽ ♀
644.21 Early onset of delivery, delivered, with or without mention of antepartum condition ♀
645.11 Post term pregnancy, delivered, with or without mention of antepartum condition ♀
645.21 Prolonged pregnancy, delivered, with or without mention of antepartum condition ♀
646.01 Papyraceous fetus, delivered, with or without mention of antepartum condition ♀
646.11 Edema or excessive weight gain in pregnancy, with delivery, with or without mention of antepartum complication ♀
646.21 Unspecified renal disease in pregnancy, with delivery ▽ ♀
646.31 Pregnancy complication, habitual aborter with or without mention of antepartum condition ♀
646.41 Peripheral neuritis in pregnancy, with delivery ♀
646.51 Asymptomatic bacteriuria in pregnancy, with delivery ♀
646.61 Infections of genitourinary tract in pregnancy, with delivery ♀
646.71 Liver disorders in pregnancy, with delivery ♀
646.81 Other specified complication of pregnancy, with delivery ♀
646.91 Unspecified complication of pregnancy, with delivery ▽ ♀
647.01 Maternal syphilis, complicating pregnancy, with delivery — (Use additional code(s) to further specify complication) ♀
647.11 Maternal gonorrhea with delivery — (Use additional code(s) to further specify complication) ♀
647.21 Other maternal venereal diseases with delivery — (Use additional code(s) to further specify complication) ♀
647.31 Maternal tuberculosis with delivery — (Use additional code(s) to further specify complication) ♀
647.41 Maternal malaria with delivery — (Use additional code(s) to further specify complication) ♀
647.51 Maternal rubella with delivery — (Use additional code(s) to further specify complication) ♀
647.61 Other maternal viral disease with delivery — (Use additional code(s) to further specify complication) ♀
647.81 Other specified maternal infectious and parasitic disease with delivery — (Use additional code(s) to further specify complication) ♀
647.91 Unspecified maternal infection or infestation with delivery — (Use additional code(s) to further specify complication) ▽ ♀
648.01 Maternal diabetes mellitus with delivery — (Use additional code(s) to identify the condition) ♀
648.11 Maternal thyroid dysfunction with delivery, with or without mention of antepartum condition — (Use additional code(s) to identify the condition) ♀
648.21 Maternal anemia, with delivery — (Use additional code(s) to identify the condition) ♀
648.31 Maternal drug dependence, with delivery — (Use additional code(s) to identify the condition) ♀
648.41 Maternal mental disorders, with delivery — (Use additional code(s) to identify the condition) ♀
648.51 Maternal congenital cardiovascular disorders, with delivery — (Use additional code(s) to identify the condition) ♀
648.61 Other maternal cardiovascular diseases, with delivery — (Use additional code(s) to identify the condition) ♀
648.71 Bone and joint disorders of maternal back, pelvis, and lower limbs, with delivery — (Use additional code(s) to identify the condition) ♀
648.81 Abnormal maternal glucose tolerance, with delivery — (Use additional code(s) to identify the condition) ♀
648.91 Other current maternal conditions classifiable elsewhere, with delivery — (Use additional code(s) to identify the condition) ♀
651.01 Twin pregnancy, delivered ♀
651.11 Triplet pregnancy, delivered ♀
651.21 Quadruplet pregnancy, delivered ♀
651.31 Twin pregnancy with fetal loss and retention of one fetus, delivered ♀
651.41 Triplet pregnancy with fetal loss and retention of one or more, delivered ♀
651.51 Quadruplet pregnancy with fetal loss and retention of one or more, delivered ♀
651.61 Other multiple pregnancy with fetal loss and retention of one or more fetus(es), delivered ♀
651.81 Other specified multiple gestation, delivered ♀
651.91 Unspecified multiple gestation, delivered ▽ ♀
652.01 Unstable lie of fetus, delivered — (Code first any associated obstructed labor, 660.0) ♀
652.11 Breech or other malpresentation successfully converted to cephalic presentation, delivered — (Code first any associated obstructed labor, 660.0) ♀
652.21 Breech presentation without mention of version, delivered — (Code first any associated obstructed labor, 660.0) ♀
652.31 Transverse or oblique fetal presentation, delivered — (Code first any associated obstructed labor, 660.0) ♀
652.41 Fetal face or brow presentation, delivered — (Code first any associated obstructed labor, 660.0) ♀
652.51 High fetal head at term, delivered — (Code first any associated obstructed labor, 660.0) ♀
652.61 Multiple gestation with malpresentation of one fetus or more, delivered — (Code first any associated obstructed labor, 660.0) ♀
652.71 Prolapsed arm of fetus, delivered — (Code first any associated obstructed labor, 660.0) ♀
652.81 Other specified malposition or malpresentation of fetus, delivered — (Code first any associated obstructed labor, 660.0) ♀
652.91 Unspecified malposition or malpresentation of fetus, delivered — (Code first any associated obstructed labor, 660.0) ▽ ♀
653.01 Major abnormality of bony pelvis, not further specified, delivered — (Code first any associated obstructed labor, 660.1) ♀
653.11 Generally contracted pelvis in pregnancy, delivered — (Code first any associated obstructed labor, 660.1) ♀
653.21 Inlet contraction of pelvis in pregnancy, delivered — (Code first any associated obstructed labor, 660.1) ♀
653.31 Outlet contraction of pelvis in pregnancy, delivered — (Code first any associated obstructed labor, 660.1) ♀
653.41 Fetopelvic disproportion, delivered — (Code first any associated obstructed labor, 660.1) ♀
653.51 Unusually large fetus causing disproportion, delivered — (Code first any associated obstructed labor, 660.1) ♀
653.61 Hydrocephalic fetus causing disproportion, delivered — (Code first any associated obstructed labor, 660.1) ♀
653.71 Other fetal abnormality causing disproportion, delivered — (Code first any associated obstructed labor, 660.1) ♀
654.01 Congenital abnormalities of pregnant uterus, delivered — (Code first any associated obstructed labor, 660.2) ♀
654.11 Tumors of body of uterus, delivered — (Code first any associated obstructed labor, 660.2) ♀
654.21 Previous cesarean delivery, delivered, with or without mention of antepartum condition — (Code first any associated obstructed labor, 660.2) ♀
654.31 Retroverted and incarcerated gravid uterus, delivered — (Code first any associated obstructed labor, 660.2) ♀
654.41 Other abnormalities in shape or position of gravid uterus and of neighboring structures, delivered — (Code first any associated obstructed labor, 660.2) ♀
654.51 Cervical incompetence, delivered — (Code first any associated obstructed labor, 660.2) ♀
654.61 Other congenital or acquired abnormality of cervix, with delivery — (Code first any associated obstructed labor, 660.2) ♀
654.71 Congenital or acquired abnormality of vagina, with delivery — (Code first any associated obstructed labor, 660.2) ♀
654.81 Congenital or acquired abnormality of vulva, with delivery — (Code first any associated obstructed labor, 660.2) ♀
654.91 Other and unspecified abnormality of organs and soft tissues of pelvis, with delivery — (Code first any associated obstructed labor, 660.2) ▽ ♀
655.01 Central nervous system malformation in fetus, with delivery ♀
655.11 Chromosomal abnormality in fetus, affecting management of mother, with delivery ♀
655.21 Hereditary disease in family possibly affecting fetus, affecting management of mother, with delivery ♀
655.31 Suspected damage to fetus from viral disease in mother, affecting management of mother, with delivery ♀
655.41 Suspected damage to fetus from other disease in mother, affecting management of mother, with delivery ♀
655.51 Suspected damage to fetus from drugs, affecting management of mother, delivered ♀
655.61 Suspected damage to fetus from radiation, affecting management of mother, delivered ♀
655.81 Other known or suspected fetal abnormality, not elsewhere classified, affecting management of mother, delivery ♀
655.91 Unspecified fetal abnormality affecting management of mother, delivery ▽ ♀
656.01 Fetal-maternal hemorrhage, with delivery ♀
656.11 Rhesus isoimmunization affecting management of mother, delivered ♀
656.21 Isoimmunization from other and unspecified blood-group incompatibility, affecting management of mother, delivered ♀
656.31 Fetal distress affecting management of mother, delivered ♀
656.41 Intrauterine death affecting management of mother, delivered ♀
656.51 Poor fetal growth, affecting management of mother, delivered ♀
656.61 Excessive fetal growth affecting management of mother, delivered ♀

▽ Unspecified code
♀ Female diagnosis
☒ Manifestation code
♂ Male diagnosis

656.71 Other placental conditions affecting management of mother, delivered ♀
656.81 Other specified fetal and placental problems affecting management of mother, delivered ♀
656.91 Unspecified fetal and placental problem affecting management of mother, delivered ▽ ♀
657.01 Polyhydramnios, with delivery ♀
658.01 Oligohydramnios, delivered ♀
658.11 Premature rupture of membranes in pregnancy, delivered ♀
658.21 Delayed delivery after spontaneous or unspecified rupture of membranes, delivered ♀
658.31 Delayed delivery after artificial rupture of membranes, delivered ♀
658.41 Infection of amniotic cavity, delivered ♀
658.81 Other problem associated with amniotic cavity and membranes, delivered ♀
658.91 Unspecified problem associated with amniotic cavity and membranes, delivered ▽ ♀
659.01 Failed mechanical induction of labor, delivered ♀
659.11 Failed medical or unspecified induction of labor, delivered ♀
659.21 Unspecified maternal pyrexia during labor, delivered ♀
659.31 Generalized infection during labor, delivered ♀
659.41 Grand multiparity, delivered, with or without mention of antepartum condition ♀
659.51 Elderly primigravida, delivered ♀
659.61 Elderly multigravida, delivered, with mention of antepartum condition ♀
659.81 Other specified indication for care or intervention related to labor and delivery, delivered ♀
659.91 Unspecified indication for care or intervention related to labor and delivery, delivered ▽ ♀
660.01 Obstruction caused by malposition of fetus at onset of labor, delivered — (Use additional code from 652.0-652.9 to identify condition) ♀
660.11 Obstruction by bony pelvis during labor and delivery, delivered — (Use additional code from 653.0-653.9 to identify condition) ♀
660.21 Obstruction by abnormal pelvic soft tissues during laborand delivery, delivered — (Use additional code from 654.0-654.9 to identify condition) ♀
660.31 Deep transverse arrest and persistent occipitoposterior position during labor and deliver, delivered ♀
660.41 Shoulder (girdle) dystocia during labor and deliver, delivered ♀
660.51 Locked twins, delivered ♀
660.61 Unspecified failed trial of labor, delivered ▽ ♀
660.71 Unspecified failed forceps or vacuum extractor, delivered ▽ ♀
660.81 Other causes of obstructed labor, delivered ♀
660.91 Unspecified obstructed labor, with delivery ▽ ♀
661.01 Primary uterine inertia, with delivery ♀
661.11 Secondary uterine inertia, with delivery ♀
661.21 Other and unspecified uterine inertia, with delivery ▽ ♀
662.01 Prolonged first stage of labor, delivered ♀
662.21 Prolonged second stage of labor, delivered ♀
662.31 Delayed delivery of second twin, triplet, etc., delivered ♀
663.01 Prolapse of cord, complicating labor and delivery, delivered ♀
663.11 Cord around neck, with compression, complicating labor and delivery, delivered ♀
663.21 Other and unspecified cord entanglement, with compression, complicating labor and delivery, delivered ▽ ♀
663.31 Other and unspecified cord entanglement, without mention of compression, complicating labor and delivery, delivered ▽ ♀
663.41 Short cord complicating labor and delivery, delivered ♀
663.51 Vasa previa complicating labor and delivery, delivered ♀
663.61 Vascular lesions of cord complicating labor and delivery, delivered ♀
663.81 Other umbilical cord complications during labor and delivery, delivered ♀
663.91 Unspecified umbilical cord complication during labor and delivery, delivered ▽ ♀
665.01 Rupture of uterus before onset of labor, with delivery ♀
665.11 Rupture of uterus during labor, with delivery ♀
665.22 Inversion of uterus, delivered with postpartum complication ♀
665.81 Other specified obstetrical trauma, with delivery ♀
665.82 Other specified obstetrical trauma, delivered, with postpartum ♀
665.91 Unspecified obstetrical trauma, with delivery ▽ ♀
665.92 Unspecified obstetrical trauma, delivered, with postpartum complication ▽ ♀
666.02 Third-stage postpartum hemorrhage, with delivery ♀
666.12 Other immediate postpartum hemorrhage, with delivery ♀
667.02 Retained placenta without hemorrhage, with delivery, with mention of postpartum complication ♀
667.12 Retained portions of placenta or membranes, without hemorrhage, delivered, with mention of postpartum complication ♀
668.01 Pulmonary complications of the administration of anesthesia or other sedation in labor and delivery, delivered — (Use additional code(s) to further specify complication) ♀
668.11 Cardiac complications of the administration of anesthesia or other sedation in labor and delivery, delivered — (Use additional code(s) to further specify complication) ♀
668.21 Central nervous system complications of the administration of anesthesia or other sedation in labor and delivery, delivered — (Use additional code(s) to further specify complication) ♀
668.81 Other complications of the administration of anesthesia or other sedation in labor and delivery, delivered — (Use additional code(s) to further specify complication) ♀
668.91 Unspecified complication of the administration of anesthesia or other sedation in labor and delivery, delivered — (Use additional code(s) to further specify complication) ▽ ♀
669.01 Maternal distress, with delivery, with or without mention of antepartum condition ♀
669.02 Maternal distress, with delivery, with mention of postpartum complication ♀
669.11 Shock during or following labor and delivery, with delivery, with or without mention of antepartum condition ♀
669.12 Shock during or following labor and delivery, with delivery, with mention of postpartum complication ♀
669.21 Maternal hypotension syndrome, with delivery, with or without mention of antepartum condition ♀
669.32 Acute renal failure with delivery, with mention of postpartum complication ♀
669.41 Other complications of obstetrical surgery and procedures, with delivery, with or without mention of antepartum condition ♀
669.42 Other complications of obstetrical surgery and procedures, with delivery, with mention of postpartum complication ♀
669.51 Forceps or vacuum extractor delivery without mention of indication, delivered, with or without mention of antepartum condition ♀
669.61 Breech extraction, without mention of indication, delivered, with or without mention of antepartum condition ♀
669.71 Cesarean delivery, without mention of indication, delivered, with or without mention of antepartum condition ♀
669.81 Other complication of labor and delivery, delivered, with or without mention of antepartum condition ♀
669.91 Unspecified complication of labor and delivery, with delivery, with or without mention of antepartum condition ▽ ♀
671.01 Varicose veins of legs, with delivery, with or without mention of antepartum condition ♀
671.81 Other venous complication, with delivery, with or without mention of antepartum condition ♀
671.82 Other venous complication, with delivery, with mention of postpartum complication ♀
676.01 Retracted nipple, delivered, with or without mention of antepartum condition ♀
676.02 Retracted nipple, delivered, with mention of postpartum complication ♀
676.21 Engorgement of breasts, delivered, with or without mention of antepartum condition ♀
676.22 Engorgement of breasts, delivered, with mention of postpartum complication ♀
676.31 Other and unspecified disorder of breast associated with childbirth, delivered, with or without mention of antepartum condition ▽ ♀
676.32 Other and unspecified disorder of breast associated with childbirth, delivered, with mention of postpartum complication ▽ ♀
676.41 Failure of lactation, with delivery, with or without mention of antepartum condition ♀
676.42 Failure of lactation, with delivery, with mention of postpartum complication ♀
676.51 Suppressed lactation, with delivery, with or without mention of antepartum condition ♀
676.52 Suppressed lactation, with delivery, with mention of postpartum complication ♀
676.91 Unspecified disorder of lactation, with delivery, with or without mention of antepartum condition ▽ ♀
676.92 Unspecified disorder of lactation, with delivery, with mention of postpartum complication ▽ ♀
V23.0 Pregnancy with history of infertility ♀
V23.1 Pregnancy with history of trophoblastic disease ♀
V23.2 Pregnancy with history of abortion ♀
V23.3 Pregnancy with grand multiparity ♀
V23.41 Supervision of pregnancy with history of pre-term labor ♀
V23.49 Supervision of pregnancy with other poor obstetric history ♀
V23.5 Pregnancy with other poor reproductive history ♀
V23.7 Insufficient prenatal care ♀
V23.82 Supervision of high-risk pregnancy of elderly multigravida ♀
V23.84 Supervision of high-risk pregnancy of young multigravida ♀
V23.89 Supervision of other high-risk pregnancy ♀
V23.9 Unspecified high-risk pregnancy ▽ ♀

V24.0 Postpartum care and examination immediately after delivery ♀
V24.1 Postpartum care and examination of lactating mother ♀
V24.2 Routine postpartum follow-up ♀
V27.0 Outcome of delivery, single liveborn — (This code is intended for the coding of the outcome of delivery on the mother's record) ♀
V27.1 Outcome of delivery, single stillborn — (This code is intended for the coding of the outcome of delivery on the mother's record) ♀
V27.2 Outcome of delivery, twins, both liveborn — (This code is intended for the coding of the outcome of delivery on the mother's record) ♀
V27.3 Outcome of delivery, twins, one liveborn and one stillborn — (This code is intended for the coding of the outcome of delivery on the mother's record) ♀
V27.4 Outcome of delivery, twins, both stillborn — (This code is intended for the coding of the outcome of delivery on the mother's record) ♀

ICD-9-CM Procedural

73.3 Failed forceps
74.0 Classical cesarean section
74.1 Low cervical cesarean section
74.4 Cesarean section of other specified type

59812

59812 Treatment of incomplete abortion, any trimester, completed surgically

ICD-9-CM Diagnostic

634.01 Incomplete spontaneous abortion complicated by genital tract and pelvic infection ♀
634.11 Incomplete spontaneous abortion complicated by delayed or excessive hemorrhage ♀
634.21 Incomplete spontaneous abortion complicated by damage to pelvic organs or tissues ♀
634.31 Incomplete spontaneous abortion complicated by renal failure ♀
634.41 Incomplete spontaneous abortion complicated by metabolic disorder ♀
634.51 Incomplete spontaneous abortion complicated by shock ♀
634.61 Incomplete spontaneous abortion complicated by embolism ♀
634.71 Incomplete spontaneous abortion with other specified complications ♀
634.81 Incomplete spontaneous abortion with unspecified complication ▽ ♀
634.91 Incomplete spontaneous abortion without mention of complication ♀
635.01 Incomplete legally induced abortion complicated by genital tract and pelvic infection ♀
635.11 Incomplete legally induced abortion complicated by delayed or excessive hemorrhage ♀
635.21 Legally induced abortion complicated by damage to pelvic organs or tissues, incomplete ♀
635.31 Incomplete legally induced abortion complicated by renal failure ♀
635.41 Incomplete legally induced abortion complicated by metabolic disorder ♀
635.51 Legally induced abortion, complicated by shock, incomplete ♀
635.61 Incomplete legally induced abortion complicated by embolism ♀
635.71 Incomplete legally induced abortion with other specified complications ♀
635.81 Incomplete legally induced abortion with unspecified complication ▽ ♀
635.91 Incomplete legally induced abortion without mention of complication ♀
636.01 Incomplete illegally induced abortion complicated by genital tractm and pelvic infection ♀
636.11 Incomplete illegally induced abortion complicated by delayed or excessive hemorrhage ♀
636.21 Incomplete illegally induced abortion complicated by damage to pelvic organs or tissues ♀
636.31 Incomplete illegally induced abortion complicated by renal failure ♀
636.41 Incomplete illegally induced abortion complicated by metabolic disorder ♀
636.51 Incomplete illegally induced abortion complicated by shock ♀
636.61 Incomplete illegally induced abortion complicated by embolism ♀
636.71 Incomplete illegally induced abortion with other specified complications ♀
636.81 Incomplete illegally induced abortion with unspecified complication ▽ ♀
636.91 Incomplete illegally induced abortion without mention of complication ♀
637.01 Legally unspecified abortion, incomplete, complicated by genital tract and pelvic infection ♀
637.11 Legally unspecified abortion, incomplete, complicated by delayed or excessive hemorrhage ♀
637.21 Legally unspecified abortion, incomplete, complicated by damage to pelvic organs or tissues ♀
637.31 Legally unspecified abortion, incomplete, complicated by renal failure ♀
637.41 Legally unspecified abortion, incomplete, complicated by metabolic disorder ♀
637.51 Legally unspecified abortion, incomplete, complicated by shock ♀
637.61 Legally unspecified abortion, incomplete, complicated by embolism ♀
637.71 Legally unspecified abortion, incomplete, with other specified complications ♀
637.81 Legally unspecified abortion, incomplete, with unspecified complication ▽ ♀
637.91 Legally unspecified abortion, incomplete, without mention of complication ♀

ICD-9-CM Procedural

69.02 Dilation and curettage following delivery or abortion

HCPCS Level II Supplies & Services

A4305 Disposable drug delivery system, flow rate of 50 ml or greater per hour
A4306 Disposable drug delivery system, flow rate of 5 ml or less per hour
A4550 Surgical trays

59820–59821

59820 Treatment of missed abortion, completed surgically; first trimester
59821 second trimester

ICD-9-CM Diagnostic

632 Missed abortion — (Use additional code from category 639 to identify any associated complications) ♀
656.41 Intrauterine death affecting management of mother, delivered ♀
656.43 Intrauterine death affecting management of mother, antepartum ♀

ICD-9-CM Procedural

69.02 Dilation and curettage following delivery or abortion

HCPCS Level II Supplies & Services

A4305 Disposable drug delivery system, flow rate of 50 ml or greater per hour
A4306 Disposable drug delivery system, flow rate of 5 ml or less per hour
A4550 Surgical trays

59830

59830 Treatment of septic abortion, completed surgically

ICD-9-CM Diagnostic

634.01 Incomplete spontaneous abortion complicated by genital tract and pelvic infection ♀
634.71 Incomplete spontaneous abortion with other specified complications ♀
634.81 Incomplete spontaneous abortion with unspecified complication ▽ ♀
634.91 Incomplete spontaneous abortion without mention of complication ♀
635.01 Incomplete legally induced abortion complicated by genital tract and pelvic infection ♀
635.81 Incomplete legally induced abortion with unspecified complication ▽ ♀
635.91 Incomplete legally induced abortion without mention of complication ♀
636.01 Incomplete illegally induced abortion complicated by genital tractm and pelvic infection ♀
636.71 Incomplete illegally induced abortion with other specified complications ♀
636.81 Incomplete illegally induced abortion with unspecified complication ▽ ♀
636.91 Incomplete illegally induced abortion without mention of complication ♀
637.01 Legally unspecified abortion, incomplete, complicated by genital tract and pelvic infection ♀
637.71 Legally unspecified abortion, incomplete, with other specified complications ♀
637.81 Legally unspecified abortion, incomplete, with unspecified complication ▽ ♀
638.0 Failed attempted abortion complicated by genital tract and pelvic infection ♀
638.7 Failed attempted abortion with other specified complication ♀
656.41 Intrauterine death affecting management of mother, delivered ♀
656.43 Intrauterine death affecting management of mother, antepartum ♀

ICD-9-CM Procedural

69.02 Dilation and curettage following delivery or abortion

59840–59841

59840 Induced abortion, by dilation and curettage
59841 Induced abortion, by dilation and evacuation

ICD-9-CM Diagnostic

635.00 Unspecified legally induced abortion complicated by genital tract and pelvic infection ▽ ♀
635.01 Incomplete legally induced abortion complicated by genital tract and pelvic infection ♀
635.02 Complete legally induced abortion complicated by genital tract and pelvic infection ♀
635.10 Unspecified legally induced abortion complicated by delayed or excessive hemorrhage ▽ ♀
635.11 Incomplete legally induced abortion complicated by delayed or excessive hemorrhage ♀
635.12 Complete legally induced abortion complicated by delayed or excessive hemorrhage ♀
635.20 Unspecified legally induced abortion complicated by damage to pelvic organs or tissues ▽ ♀

635.21 Legally induced abortion complicated by damage to pelvic organs or tissues, incomplete ♀
635.22 Complete legally induced abortion complicated by damage to pelvic organs or tissues ♀
635.30 Unspecified legally induced abortion complicated by renal failure ▽ ♀
635.31 Incomplete legally induced abortion complicated by renal failure ♀
635.32 Complete legally induced abortion complicated by renal failure ♀
635.40 Unspecified legally induced abortion complicated by metabolic disorder ▽ ♀
635.41 Incomplete legally induced abortion complicated by metabolic disorder ♀
635.42 Complete legally induced abortion complicated by metabolic disorder ♀
635.50 Unspecified legally induced abortion complicated by shock ▽ ♀
635.51 Legally induced abortion, complicated by shock, incomplete ♀
635.52 Complete legally induced abortion complicated by shock ♀
635.60 Unspecified legally induced abortion complicated by embolism ▽ ♀
635.61 Incomplete legally induced abortion complicated by embolism ♀
635.62 Complete legally induced abortion complicated by embolism ♀
635.70 Unspecified legally induced abortion with other specified complications ▽ ♀
635.71 Incomplete legally induced abortion with other specified complications ♀
635.72 Complete legally induced abortion with other specified complications ♀
635.80 Unspecified legally induced abortion with unspecified complication ▽ ♀
635.81 Incomplete legally induced abortion with unspecified complication ▽ ♀
635.82 Complete legally induced abortion with unspecified complication ▽ ♀
635.90 Unspecified legally induced abortion without mention of complication ♀
635.91 Incomplete legally induced abortion without mention of complication ♀
635.92 Complete legally induced abortion without mention of complication ♀
646.03 Papyraceous fetus, antepartum ♀
646.23 Unspecified antepartum renal disease ▽ ♀
655.00 Central nervous system malformation in fetus, unspecified as to episode of care in pregnancy ▽ ♀
655.03 Central nervous system malformation in fetus, antepartum ♀
655.10 Chromosomal abnormality in fetus, affecting management of mother, unspecified as to episode of care in pregnancy ▽ ♀
655.13 Chromosomal abnormality in fetus, affecting management of mother, antepartum ♀
655.20 Hereditary disease in family possibly affecting fetus, affecting management of mother, unspecified as to episode of care in pregnancy ▽ ♀
655.30 Suspected damage to fetus from viral disease in mother, affecting management of mother, unspecified as to episode of care in pregnancy ▽ ♀
655.33 Suspected damage to fetus from viral disease in mother, affecting management of mother, antepartum condition or complication ♀
655.40 Suspected damage to fetus from other disease in mother, affecting management of mother, unspecified as to episode of care in pregnancy ▽ ♀
655.43 Suspected damage to fetus from other disease in mother, affecting management of mother, antepartum condition or complication ♀
655.50 Suspected damage to fetus from drugs, affecting management of mother, unspecified as to episode of care ▽ ♀
655.53 Suspected damage to fetus from drugs, affecting management of mother, antepartum ♀
655.60 Suspected damage to fetus from radiation, affecting management of mother, unspecified as to episode of care ▽ ♀
655.63 Suspected damage to fetus from radiation, affecting management of mother, antepartum condition or complication ♀
655.80 Other known or suspected fetal abnormality, not elsewhere classified, affecting management of mother, unspecified as to episode of care ▽ ♀
655.83 Other known or suspected fetal abnormality, not elsewhere classified, affecting management of mother, antepartum condition or complication ♀
655.90 Unspecified fetal abnormality affecting management of mother, unspecified as to episode of care ▽ ♀
655.93 Unspecified fetal abnormality affecting management of mother, antepartum condition or complication ▽ ♀
656.23 Isoimmunization from other and unspecified blood-group incompatibility, affecting management of mother, antepartum ♀
656.43 Intrauterine death affecting management of mother, antepartum ♀
659.63 Elderly multigravida, with antepartum condition or complication ♀
V61.7 Other unwanted pregnancy ♀

ICD-9-CM Procedural

69.01 Dilation and curettage for termination of pregnancy
69.51 Aspiration curettage of uterus for termination of pregnancy
69.99 Other operations on cervix and uterus

HCPCS Level II Supplies & Services

A4305 Disposable drug delivery system, flow rate of 50 ml or greater per hour
A4306 Disposable drug delivery system, flow rate of 5 ml or less per hour
A4550 Surgical trays

59850–59852

59850 Induced abortion, by one or more intra-amniotic injections (amniocentesis-injections), including hospital admission and visits, delivery of fetus and secundines;
59851 with dilation and curettage and/or evacuation
59852 with hysterotomy (failed intra-amniotic injection)

ICD-9-CM Diagnostic

635.00 Unspecified legally induced abortion complicated by genital tract and pelvic infection ▽ ♀
635.01 Incomplete legally induced abortion complicated by genital tract and pelvic infection ♀
635.02 Complete legally induced abortion complicated by genital tract and pelvic infection ♀
635.10 Unspecified legally induced abortion complicated by delayed or excessive hemorrhage ▽ ♀
635.11 Incomplete legally induced abortion complicated by delayed or excessive hemorrhage ♀
635.12 Complete legally induced abortion complicated by delayed or excessive hemorrhage ♀
635.20 Unspecified legally induced abortion complicated by damage to pelvic organs or tissues ▽ ♀
635.21 Legally induced abortion complicated by damage to pelvic organs or tissues, incomplete ♀
635.22 Complete legally induced abortion complicated by damage to pelvic organs or tissues ♀
635.30 Unspecified legally induced abortion complicated by renal failure ▽ ♀
635.31 Incomplete legally induced abortion complicated by renal failure ♀
635.32 Complete legally induced abortion complicated by renal failure ♀
635.40 Unspecified legally induced abortion complicated by metabolic disorder ▽ ♀
635.41 Incomplete legally induced abortion complicated by metabolic disorder ♀
635.42 Complete legally induced abortion complicated by metabolic disorder ♀
635.50 Unspecified legally induced abortion complicated by shock ▽ ♀
635.51 Legally induced abortion, complicated by shock, incomplete ♀
635.52 Complete legally induced abortion complicated by shock ♀
635.60 Unspecified legally induced abortion complicated by embolism ▽ ♀
635.61 Incomplete legally induced abortion complicated by embolism ♀
635.62 Complete legally induced abortion complicated by embolism ♀
635.70 Unspecified legally induced abortion with other specified complications ▽ ♀
635.71 Incomplete legally induced abortion with other specified complications ♀
635.72 Complete legally induced abortion with other specified complications ♀
635.80 Unspecified legally induced abortion with unspecified complication ▽ ♀
635.81 Incomplete legally induced abortion with unspecified complication ▽ ♀
635.82 Complete legally induced abortion with unspecified complication ▽ ♀
635.90 Unspecified legally induced abortion without mention of complication ♀
635.91 Incomplete legally induced abortion without mention of complication ♀
635.92 Complete legally induced abortion without mention of complication ♀
638.0 Failed attempted abortion complicated by genital tract and pelvic infection ♀
638.1 Failed attempted abortion complicated by delayed or excessive hemorrhage ♀
638.2 Failed attempted abortion complicated by damage to pelvic organs or tissues ♀
638.3 Failed attempted abortion complicated by renal failure ♀
638.4 Failed attempted abortion complicated by metabolic disorder ♀
638.5 Failed attempted abortion complicated by shock ♀
638.6 Failed attempted abortion complicated by embolism ♀
638.7 Failed attempted abortion with other specified complication ♀
638.8 Failed attempted abortion with unspecified complication ▽ ♀
638.9 Failed attempted abortion without mention of complication ♀
646.03 Papyraceous fetus, antepartum ♀
646.23 Unspecified antepartum renal disease ▽ ♀
648.40 Maternal mental disorders, complicating pregnancy, childbirth, or the puerperium, unspecified as to episode of care — (Use additional code(s) to identify the condition) ▽ ♀
648.41 Maternal mental disorders, with delivery — (Use additional code(s) to identify the condition) ♀
648.43 Maternal mental disorders, antepartum — (Use additional code(s) to identify the condition) ♀
655.00 Central nervous system malformation in fetus, unspecified as to episode of care in pregnancy ▽ ♀
655.01 Central nervous system malformation in fetus, with delivery ♀
655.03 Central nervous system malformation in fetus, antepartum ♀
655.10 Chromosomal abnormality in fetus, affecting management of mother, unspecified as to episode of care in pregnancy ▽ ♀
655.13 Chromosomal abnormality in fetus, affecting management of mother, antepartum ♀
655.20 Hereditary disease in family possibly affecting fetus, affecting management of mother, unspecified as to episode of care in pregnancy ▽ ♀

655.21 Hereditary disease in family possibly affecting fetus, affecting management of mother, with delivery ♀

655.23 Hereditary disease in family possibly affecting fetus, affecting management of mother, antepartum condition or complication ♀

655.80 Other known or suspected fetal abnormality, not elsewhere classified, affecting management of mother, unspecified as to episode of care ▽ ♀

655.81 Other known or suspected fetal abnormality, not elsewhere classified, affecting management of mother, delivery ♀

655.83 Other known or suspected fetal abnormality, not elsewhere classified, affecting management of mother, antepartum condition or complication ♀

655.90 Unspecified fetal abnormality affecting management of mother, unspecified as to episode of care ▽ ♀

655.91 Unspecified fetal abnormality affecting management of mother, delivery ▽ ♀

655.93 Unspecified fetal abnormality affecting management of mother, antepartum condition or complication ▽ ♀

656.40 Intrauterine death affecting management of mother, unspecified as to episode of care ▽ ♀

656.41 Intrauterine death affecting management of mother, delivered ♀

656.43 Intrauterine death affecting management of mother, antepartum ♀

659.63 Elderly multigravida, with antepartum condition or complication ♀

V19.5 Family history of congenital anomalies

V61.7 Other unwanted pregnancy ♀

ICD-9-CM Procedural

69.01 Dilation and curettage for termination of pregnancy

69.51 Aspiration curettage of uterus for termination of pregnancy

74.91 Hysterotomy to terminate pregnancy

75.0 Intra-amniotic injection for abortion

59855–59857

59855 Induced abortion, by one or more vaginal suppositories (eg, prostaglandin) with or without cervical dilation (eg, laminaria), including hospital admission and visits, delivery of fetus and secundines;

59856 with dilation and curettage and/or evacuation

59857 with hysterotomy (failed medical evacuation)

ICD-9-CM Diagnostic

635.00 Unspecified legally induced abortion complicated by genital tract and pelvic infection ▽ ♀

635.01 Incomplete legally induced abortion complicated by genital tract and pelvic infection ♀

635.02 Complete legally induced abortion complicated by genital tract and pelvic infection ♀

635.10 Unspecified legally induced abortion complicated by delayed or excessive hemorrhage ▽ ♀

635.11 Incomplete legally induced abortion complicated by delayed or excessive hemorrhage ♀

635.12 Complete legally induced abortion complicated by delayed or excessive hemorrhage ♀

635.20 Unspecified legally induced abortion complicated by damage to pelvic organs or tissues ▽ ♀

635.21 Legally induced abortion complicated by damage to pelvic organs or tissues, incomplete ♀

635.22 Complete legally induced abortion complicated by damage to pelvic organs or tissues ♀

635.30 Unspecified legally induced abortion complicated by renal failure ▽ ♀

635.31 Incomplete legally induced abortion complicated by renal failure ♀

635.32 Complete legally induced abortion complicated by renal failure ♀

635.40 Unspecified legally induced abortion complicated by metabolic disorder ▽ ♀

635.41 Incomplete legally induced abortion complicated by metabolic disorder ♀

635.42 Complete legally induced abortion complicated by metabolic disorder ♀

635.50 Unspecified legally induced abortion complicated by shock ▽ ♀

635.51 Legally induced abortion, complicated by shock, incomplete ♀

635.52 Complete legally induced abortion complicated by shock ♀

635.60 Unspecified legally induced abortion complicated by embolism ▽ ♀

635.61 Incomplete legally induced abortion complicated by embolism ♀

635.62 Complete legally induced abortion complicated by embolism ♀

635.70 Unspecified legally induced abortion with other specified complications ▽ ♀

635.71 Incomplete legally induced abortion with other specified complications ♀

635.72 Complete legally induced abortion with other specified complications ♀

635.80 Unspecified legally induced abortion with unspecified complication ▽ ♀

635.81 Incomplete legally induced abortion with unspecified complication ▽ ♀

635.82 Complete legally induced abortion with unspecified complication ▽ ♀

635.90 Unspecified legally induced abortion without mention of complication ♀

635.91 Incomplete legally induced abortion without mention of complication ♀

635.92 Complete legally induced abortion without mention of complication ♀

638.0 Failed attempted abortion complicated by genital tract and pelvic infection ♀

638.1 Failed attempted abortion complicated by delayed or excessive hemorrhage ♀

638.2 Failed attempted abortion complicated by damage to pelvic organs or tissues ♀

638.3 Failed attempted abortion complicated by renal failure ♀

638.4 Failed attempted abortion complicated by metabolic disorder ♀

638.5 Failed attempted abortion complicated by shock ♀

638.6 Failed attempted abortion complicated by embolism ♀

638.7 Failed attempted abortion with other specified complication ♀

638.8 Failed attempted abortion with unspecified complication ▽ ♀

638.9 Failed attempted abortion without mention of complication ♀

646.03 Papyraceous fetus, antepartum ♀

646.23 Unspecified antepartum renal disease ▽ ♀

648.40 Maternal mental disorders, complicating pregnancy, childbirth, or the puerperium, unspecified as to episode of care — (Use additional code(s) to identify the condition) ▽ ♀

648.41 Maternal mental disorders, with delivery — (Use additional code(s) to identify the condition) ♀

648.43 Maternal mental disorders, antepartum — (Use additional code(s) to identify the condition) ♀

655.00 Central nervous system malformation in fetus, unspecified as to episode of care in pregnancy ▽ ♀

655.01 Central nervous system malformation in fetus, with delivery ♀

655.03 Central nervous system malformation in fetus, antepartum ♀

655.10 Chromosomal abnormality in fetus, affecting management of mother, unspecified as to episode of care in pregnancy ▽ ♀

655.13 Chromosomal abnormality in fetus, affecting management of mother, antepartum ♀

655.20 Hereditary disease in family possibly affecting fetus, affecting management of mother, unspecified as to episode of care in pregnancy ▽ ♀

655.21 Hereditary disease in family possibly affecting fetus, affecting management of mother, with delivery ♀

655.23 Hereditary disease in family possibly affecting fetus, affecting management of mother, antepartum condition or complication ♀

655.80 Other known or suspected fetal abnormality, not elsewhere classified, affecting management of mother, unspecified as to episode of care ▽ ♀

655.81 Other known or suspected fetal abnormality, not elsewhere classified, affecting management of mother, delivery ♀

655.83 Other known or suspected fetal abnormality, not elsewhere classified, affecting management of mother, antepartum condition or complication ♀

655.90 Unspecified fetal abnormality affecting management of mother, unspecified as to episode of care ▽ ♀

655.91 Unspecified fetal abnormality affecting management of mother, delivery ▽ ♀

655.93 Unspecified fetal abnormality affecting management of mother, antepartum condition or complication ▽ ♀

656.40 Intrauterine death affecting management of mother, unspecified as to episode of care ▽ ♀

656.41 Intrauterine death affecting management of mother, delivered ♀

656.43 Intrauterine death affecting management of mother, antepartum ♀

659.63 Elderly multigravida, with antepartum condition or complication ♀

V19.5 Family history of congenital anomalies

V61.7 Other unwanted pregnancy ♀

ICD-9-CM Procedural

69.01 Dilation and curettage for termination of pregnancy

69.51 Aspiration curettage of uterus for termination of pregnancy

69.93 Insertion of laminaria

74.91 Hysterotomy to terminate pregnancy

96.49 Other genitourinary instillation

59866

59866 Multifetal pregnancy reduction(s) (MPR)

ICD-9-CM Diagnostic

651.13 Triplet pregnancy, antepartum ♀

651.23 Quadruplet pregnancy, antepartum ♀

651.83 Other specified multiple gestation, antepartum ♀

651.93 Unspecified multiple gestation, antepartum ▽ ♀

V23.0 Pregnancy with history of infertility ♀

V23.41 Supervision of pregnancy with history of pre-term labor ♀

V23.49 Supervision of pregnancy with other poor obstetric history ♀

V23.5 Pregnancy with other poor reproductive history ♀

V23.81 Supervision of high-risk pregnancy of elderly primigravida ♀

V23.82 Supervision of high-risk pregnancy of elderly multigravida ♀

V23.83 Supervision of high-risk pregnancy of young primigravida ♀

V23.84 Supervision of high-risk pregnancy of young multigravida ♀

V23.89 Supervision of other high-risk pregnancy ♀

ICD-9-CM Procedural

75.0 Intra-amniotic injection for abortion
75.99 Other obstetric operations

59870

59870 Uterine evacuation and curettage for hydatidiform mole

ICD-9-CM Diagnostic

630 Hydatidiform mole — (Use additional code from category 639 to identify any associated complications) ♀

ICD-9-CM Procedural

69.01 Dilation and curettage for termination of pregnancy
69.02 Dilation and curettage following delivery or abortion
69.59 Other aspiration curettage of uterus

HCPCS Level II Supplies & Services

A4305 Disposable drug delivery system, flow rate of 50 ml or greater per hour
A4306 Disposable drug delivery system, flow rate of 5 ml or less per hour
A4550 Surgical trays

59871

59871 Removal of cerclage suture under anesthesia (other than local)

ICD-9-CM Diagnostic

622.3 Old laceration of cervix ♀
654.53 Cervical incompetence, antepartum condition or complication — (Code first any associated obstructed labor, 660.2) ♀
654.63 Other congenital or acquired abnormality of cervix, antepartum condition or complication — (Code first any associated obstructed labor, 660.2) ♀
654.93 Other and unspecified abnormality of organs and soft tissues of pelvis, antepartum condition or complication — (Code first any associated obstructed labor, 660.2) ▽ ♀
V23.2 Pregnancy with history of abortion ♀
V23.81 Supervision of high-risk pregnancy of elderly primigravida ♀
V23.82 Supervision of high-risk pregnancy of elderly multigravida ♀
V23.83 Supervision of high-risk pregnancy of young primigravida ♀
V23.84 Supervision of high-risk pregnancy of young multigravida ♀
V23.89 Supervision of other high-risk pregnancy ♀

ICD-9-CM Procedural

69.96 Removal of cerclage material from cervix

▽ Unspecified code
♀ Female diagnosis
☒ Manifestation code
♂ Male diagnosis

Endocrine System

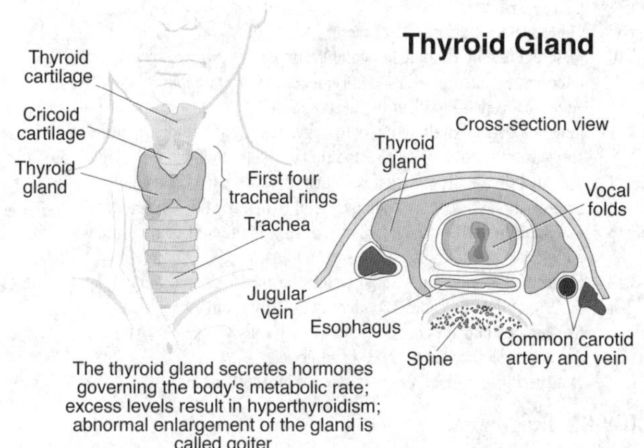

The thyroid gland secretes hormones governing the body's metabolic rate; excess levels result in hyperthyroidism; abnormal enlargement of the gland is called goiter

Thyroid Gland

60000

60000 Incision and drainage of thyroglossal duct cyst, infected

ICD-9-CM Diagnostic

759.2 Congenital anomalies of other endocrine glands
780.6 Fever
784.2 Swelling, mass, or lump in head and neck

ICD-9-CM Procedural

06.09 Other incision of thyroid field

HCPCS Level II Supplies & Services

A4305 Disposable drug delivery system, flow rate of 50 ml or greater per hour
A4306 Disposable drug delivery system, flow rate of 5 ml or less per hour
A4550 Surgical trays

60001

60001 Aspiration and/or injection, thyroid cyst

ICD-9-CM Diagnostic

246.2 Cyst of thyroid
648.11 Maternal thyroid dysfunction with delivery, with or without mention of antepartum condition — (Use additional code(s) to identify the condition) ♀
648.12 Maternal thyroid dysfunction with delivery, with current postpartum complication — (Use additional code(s) to identify the condition) ♀
648.13 Maternal thyroid dysfunction, antepartum condition or complication — (Use additional code(s) to identify the condition) ♀
648.14 Maternal thyroid dysfunction, previous postpartum condition or complication — (Use additional code(s) to identify the condition) ♀
V10.29 Personal history of malignant neoplasm of other respiratory and intrathoracic organs
V18.1 Family history of other endocrine and metabolic diseases

ICD-9-CM Procedural

06.01 Aspiration of thyroid field
06.98 Other operations on thyroid glands

HCPCS Level II Supplies & Services

A4305 Disposable drug delivery system, flow rate of 50 ml or greater per hour
A4306 Disposable drug delivery system, flow rate of 5 ml or less per hour
A4550 Surgical trays

60100

60100 Biopsy thyroid, percutaneous core needle

ICD-9-CM Diagnostic

193 Malignant neoplasm of thyroid gland — (Use additional code to identify any functional activity)
198.89 Secondary malignant neoplasm of other specified sites
226 Benign neoplasm of thyroid glands — (Use additional code to identify any functional activity)
234.8 Carcinoma in situ of other specified sites
237.4 Neoplasm of uncertain behavior of other and unspecified endocrine glands ▽
239.7 Neoplasm of unspecified nature of endocrine glands and other parts of nervous system
240.0 Goiter, specified as simple
240.9 Goiter, unspecified ▽
241.0 Nontoxic uninodular goiter
241.1 Nontoxic multinodular goiter
241.9 Unspecified nontoxic nodular goiter ▽
242.10 Toxic uninodular goiter without mention of thyrotoxic crisis or storm
242.11 Toxic uninodular goiter with mention of thyrotoxic crisis or storm
242.20 Toxic multinodular goiter without mention of thyrotoxic crisis or storm
242.21 Toxic multinodular goiter with mention of thyrotoxic crisis or storm
242.30 Toxic nodular goiter, unspecified type, without mention of thyrotoxic crisis or storm ▽
242.31 Toxic nodular goiter, unspecified type, with mention of thyrotoxic crisis or storm ▽
242.40 Thyrotoxicosis from ectopic thyroid nodule without mention of thyrotoxic crisis or storm
242.41 Thyrotoxicosis from ectopic thyroid nodule with mention of thyrotoxic crisis or storm
245.0 Acute thyroiditis — (Use additional code to identify organism)
245.1 Subacute thyroiditis
245.2 Chronic lymphocytic thyroiditis
245.3 Chronic fibrous thyroiditis
245.4 Iatrogenic thyroiditis — (Use additional code to identify cause)
245.8 Other and unspecified chronic thyroiditis ▽
245.9 Unspecified thyroiditis ▽
246.2 Cyst of thyroid
246.8 Other specified disorders of thyroid
648.10 Maternal thyroid dysfunction complicating pregnancy, childbirth, or the puerperium, unspecified as to episode of care or not applicable — (Use additional code(s) to identify the condition) ▽ ♀
648.11 Maternal thyroid dysfunction with delivery, with or without mention of antepartum condition — (Use additional code(s) to identify the condition) ♀
648.12 Maternal thyroid dysfunction with delivery, with current postpartum complication — (Use additional code(s) to identify the condition) ♀
648.13 Maternal thyroid dysfunction, antepartum condition or complication — (Use additional code(s) to identify the condition) ♀
648.14 Maternal thyroid dysfunction, previous postpartum condition or complication — (Use additional code(s) to identify the condition) ♀
759.2 Congenital anomalies of other endocrine glands
784.2 Swelling, mass, or lump in head and neck
794.5 Nonspecific abnormal results of thyroid function study
794.6 Nonspecific abnormal results of other endocrine function study
V10.29 Personal history of malignant neoplasm of other respiratory and intrathoracic organs

ICD-9-CM Procedural

06.11 Closed (percutaneous) (needle) biopsy of thyroid gland

HCPCS Level II Supplies & Services

A4305 Disposable drug delivery system, flow rate of 50 ml or greater per hour
A4306 Disposable drug delivery system, flow rate of 5 ml or less per hour
A4550 Surgical trays

▽ Unspecified code
♀ Female diagnosis
☒ Manifestation code
♂ Male diagnosis

60200

60200 Excision of cyst or adenoma of thyroid, or transection of isthmus

ICD-9-CM Diagnostic

226 Benign neoplasm of thyroid glands — (Use additional code to identify any functional activity)
237.4 Neoplasm of uncertain behavior of other and unspecified endocrine glands ▽
240.9 Goiter, unspecified ▽
241.0 Nontoxic uninodular goiter
241.1 Nontoxic multinodular goiter
241.9 Unspecified nontoxic nodular goiter ▽
242.00 Toxic diffuse goiter without mention of thyrotoxic crisis or storm
242.01 Toxic diffuse goiter with mention of thyrotoxic crisis or storm
242.10 Toxic uninodular goiter without mention of thyrotoxic crisis or storm
242.11 Toxic uninodular goiter with mention of thyrotoxic crisis or storm
242.20 Toxic multinodular goiter without mention of thyrotoxic crisis or storm
242.21 Toxic multinodular goiter with mention of thyrotoxic crisis or storm
242.30 Toxic nodular goiter, unspecified type, without mention of thyrotoxic crisis or storm ▽
242.31 Toxic nodular goiter, unspecified type, with mention of thyrotoxic crisis or storm ▽
242.40 Thyrotoxicosis from ectopic thyroid nodule without mention of thyrotoxic crisis or storm
242.41 Thyrotoxicosis from ectopic thyroid nodule with mention of thyrotoxic crisis or storm
242.80 Thyrotoxicosis of other specified origin without mention of thyrotoxic crisis or storm — (Use additional E code to identify cause, if drug-induced)
242.81 Thyrotoxicosis of other specified origin with mention of thyrotoxic crisis or storm — (Use additional E code to identify cause, if drug-induced)
242.90 Thyrotoxicosis without mention of goiter or other cause, without mention of thyrotoxic crisis or storm
242.91 Thyrotoxicosis without mention of goiter or other cause, with mention of thyrotoxic crisis or storm
245.8 Other and unspecified chronic thyroiditis ▽
246.2 Cyst of thyroid
784.2 Swelling, mass, or lump in head and neck

ICD-9-CM Procedural

06.31 Excision of lesion of thyroid
06.39 Other partial thyroidectomy
06.91 Division of thyroid isthmus

HCPCS Level II Supplies & Services

A4305 Disposable drug delivery system, flow rate of 50 ml or greater per hour
A4306 Disposable drug delivery system, flow rate of 5 ml or less per hour
A4550 Surgical trays

60210–60212

60210 Partial thyroid lobectomy, unilateral; with or without isthmusectomy
60212 with contralateral subtotal lobectomy, including isthmusectomy

ICD-9-CM Diagnostic

193 Malignant neoplasm of thyroid gland — (Use additional code to identify any functional activity)
198.89 Secondary malignant neoplasm of other specified sites
226 Benign neoplasm of thyroid glands — (Use additional code to identify any functional activity)
234.8 Carcinoma in situ of other specified sites
237.4 Neoplasm of uncertain behavior of other and unspecified endocrine glands ▽
239.7 Neoplasm of unspecified nature of endocrine glands and other parts of nervous system
240.0 Goiter, specified as simple
240.9 Goiter, unspecified ▽
241.0 Nontoxic uninodular goiter
241.1 Nontoxic multinodular goiter
241.9 Unspecified nontoxic nodular goiter ▽
242.10 Toxic uninodular goiter without mention of thyrotoxic crisis or storm
242.11 Toxic uninodular goiter with mention of thyrotoxic crisis or storm
242.20 Toxic multinodular goiter without mention of thyrotoxic crisis or storm
242.21 Toxic multinodular goiter with mention of thyrotoxic crisis or storm
242.30 Toxic nodular goiter, unspecified type, without mention of thyrotoxic crisis or storm ▽
242.31 Toxic nodular goiter, unspecified type, with mention of thyrotoxic crisis or storm ▽
242.40 Thyrotoxicosis from ectopic thyroid nodule without mention of thyrotoxic crisis or storm
242.41 Thyrotoxicosis from ectopic thyroid nodule with mention of thyrotoxic crisis or storm
245.0 Acute thyroiditis — (Use additional code to identify organism)
245.1 Subacute thyroiditis
245.2 Chronic lymphocytic thyroiditis
245.3 Chronic fibrous thyroiditis
245.4 Iatrogenic thyroiditis — (Use additional code to identify cause)
245.8 Other and unspecified chronic thyroiditis ▽
245.9 Unspecified thyroiditis ▽
246.2 Cyst of thyroid
246.8 Other specified disorders of thyroid
648.10 Maternal thyroid dysfunction complicating pregnancy, childbirth, or the puerperium, unspecified as to episode of care or not applicable — (Use additional code(s) to identify the condition) ▽ ♀
648.11 Maternal thyroid dysfunction with delivery, with or without mention of antepartum condition — (Use additional code(s) to identify the condition) ♀
648.12 Maternal thyroid dysfunction with delivery, with current postpartum complication — (Use additional code(s) to identify the condition) ♀
648.13 Maternal thyroid dysfunction, antepartum condition or complication — (Use additional code(s) to identify the condition) ♀
648.14 Maternal thyroid dysfunction, previous postpartum condition or complication — (Use additional code(s) to identify the condition) ♀
759.2 Congenital anomalies of other endocrine glands
784.2 Swelling, mass, or lump in head and neck
794.5 Nonspecific abnormal results of thyroid function study

ICD-9-CM Procedural

06.2 Unilateral thyroid lobectomy
06.39 Other partial thyroidectomy

60220–60225

60220 Total thyroid lobectomy, unilateral; with or without isthmusectomy
60225 with contralateral subtotal lobectomy, including isthmusectomy

ICD-9-CM Diagnostic

193 Malignant neoplasm of thyroid gland — (Use additional code to identify any functional activity)
195.0 Malignant neoplasm of head, face, and neck
198.89 Secondary malignant neoplasm of other specified sites
226 Benign neoplasm of thyroid glands — (Use additional code to identify any functional activity)
234.8 Carcinoma in situ of other specified sites
237.4 Neoplasm of uncertain behavior of other and unspecified endocrine glands ▽
239.7 Neoplasm of unspecified nature of endocrine glands and other parts of nervous system
240.0 Goiter, specified as simple
240.9 Goiter, unspecified ▽
241.0 Nontoxic uninodular goiter
241.1 Nontoxic multinodular goiter
241.9 Unspecified nontoxic nodular goiter ▽
242.10 Toxic uninodular goiter without mention of thyrotoxic crisis or storm
242.20 Toxic multinodular goiter without mention of thyrotoxic crisis or storm
245.2 Chronic lymphocytic thyroiditis
245.3 Chronic fibrous thyroiditis
245.4 Iatrogenic thyroiditis — (Use additional code to identify cause)
245.8 Other and unspecified chronic thyroiditis ▽
245.9 Unspecified thyroiditis ▽
648.10 Maternal thyroid dysfunction complicating pregnancy, childbirth, or the puerperium, unspecified as to episode of care or not applicable — (Use additional code(s) to identify the condition) ▽ ♀
648.11 Maternal thyroid dysfunction with delivery, with or without mention of antepartum condition — (Use additional code(s) to identify the condition) ♀
648.12 Maternal thyroid dysfunction with delivery, with current postpartum complication — (Use additional code(s) to identify the condition) ♀
648.13 Maternal thyroid dysfunction, antepartum condition or complication — (Use additional code(s) to identify the condition) ♀
648.14 Maternal thyroid dysfunction, previous postpartum condition or complication — (Use additional code(s) to identify the condition) ♀
784.2 Swelling, mass, or lump in head and neck

ICD-9-CM Procedural

06.2 Unilateral thyroid lobectomy
06.39 Other partial thyroidectomy

60240

60240 Thyroidectomy, total or complete

ICD-9-CM Diagnostic

193 Malignant neoplasm of thyroid gland — (Use additional code to identify any functional activity)
198.89 Secondary malignant neoplasm of other specified sites
226 Benign neoplasm of thyroid glands — (Use additional code to identify any functional activity)
234.8 Carcinoma in situ of other specified sites
237.4 Neoplasm of uncertain behavior of other and unspecified endocrine glands ▽
239.1 Neoplasm of unspecified nature of respiratory system
239.7 Neoplasm of unspecified nature of endocrine glands and other parts of nervous system
240.9 Goiter, unspecified ▽
241.0 Nontoxic uninodular goiter
241.1 Nontoxic multinodular goiter
241.9 Unspecified nontoxic nodular goiter ▽
242.00 Toxic diffuse goiter without mention of thyrotoxic crisis or storm
242.01 Toxic diffuse goiter with mention of thyrotoxic crisis or storm
242.10 Toxic uninodular goiter without mention of thyrotoxic crisis or storm
242.20 Toxic multinodular goiter without mention of thyrotoxic crisis or storm
242.21 Toxic multinodular goiter with mention of thyrotoxic crisis or storm
242.90 Thyrotoxicosis without mention of goiter or other cause, without mention of thyrotoxic crisis or storm
242.91 Thyrotoxicosis without mention of goiter or other cause, with mention of thyrotoxic crisis or storm
245.2 Chronic lymphocytic thyroiditis
245.8 Other and unspecified chronic thyroiditis ▽
245.9 Unspecified thyroiditis ▽
784.2 Swelling, mass, or lump in head and neck

ICD-9-CM Procedural

06.4 Complete thyroidectomy

60252–60254

60252 Thyroidectomy, total or subtotal for malignancy; with limited neck dissection
60254 with radical neck dissection

ICD-9-CM Diagnostic

161.0 Malignant neoplasm of glottis
161.1 Malignant neoplasm of supraglottis
161.2 Malignant neoplasm of subglottis
161.3 Malignant neoplasm of laryngeal cartilages
161.8 Malignant neoplasm of other specified sites of larynx
193 Malignant neoplasm of thyroid gland — (Use additional code to identify any functional activity)
196.0 Secondary and unspecified malignant neoplasm of lymph nodes of head, face, and neck
198.89 Secondary malignant neoplasm of other specified sites
200.01 Reticulosarcoma of lymph nodes of head, face, and neck
234.8 Carcinoma in situ of other specified sites
237.4 Neoplasm of uncertain behavior of other and unspecified endocrine glands ▽
238.8 Neoplasm of uncertain behavior of other specified sites
239.7 Neoplasm of unspecified nature of endocrine glands and other parts of nervous system
239.8 Neoplasm of unspecified nature of other specified sites

ICD-9-CM Procedural

06.39 Other partial thyroidectomy
06.4 Complete thyroidectomy
40.3 Regional lymph node excision
40.41 Radical neck dissection, unilateral

60260

60260 Thyroidectomy, removal of all remaining thyroid tissue following previous removal of a portion of thyroid

ICD-9-CM Diagnostic

161.3 Malignant neoplasm of laryngeal cartilages
193 Malignant neoplasm of thyroid gland — (Use additional code to identify any functional activity)
197.3 Secondary malignant neoplasm of other respiratory organs
198.89 Secondary malignant neoplasm of other specified sites
231.0 Carcinoma in situ of larynx
234.8 Carcinoma in situ of other specified sites
237.4 Neoplasm of uncertain behavior of other and unspecified endocrine glands ▽
239.7 Neoplasm of unspecified nature of endocrine glands and other parts of nervous system

ICD-9-CM Procedural

06.4 Complete thyroidectomy

60270–60271

60270 Thyroidectomy, including substernal thyroid; sternal split or transthoracic approach
60271 cervical approach

ICD-9-CM Diagnostic

193 Malignant neoplasm of thyroid gland — (Use additional code to identify any functional activity)
202.00 Nodular lymphoma, unspecified site, extranodal and solid organ sites ▽
226 Benign neoplasm of thyroid glands — (Use additional code to identify any functional activity)
237.4 Neoplasm of uncertain behavior of other and unspecified endocrine glands ▽
239.7 Neoplasm of unspecified nature of endocrine glands and other parts of nervous system
240.0 Goiter, specified as simple
240.9 Goiter, unspecified ▽
241.9 Unspecified nontoxic nodular goiter ▽
242.00 Toxic diffuse goiter without mention of thyrotoxic crisis or storm
242.01 Toxic diffuse goiter with mention of thyrotoxic crisis or storm
242.10 Toxic uninodular goiter without mention of thyrotoxic crisis or storm
242.11 Toxic uninodular goiter with mention of thyrotoxic crisis or storm
242.20 Toxic multinodular goiter without mention of thyrotoxic crisis or storm
242.40 Thyrotoxicosis from ectopic thyroid nodule without mention of thyrotoxic crisis or storm

ICD-9-CM Procedural

06.50 Substernal thyroidectomy, not otherwise specified
06.51 Partial substernal thyroidectomy
06.52 Complete substernal thyroidectomy

60280–60281

60280 Excision of thyroglossal duct cyst or sinus;
60281 recurrent

ICD-9-CM Diagnostic

759.2 Congenital anomalies of other endocrine glands

ICD-9-CM Procedural

06.7 Excision of thyroglossal duct or tract

Parathyroid, Thymus, Adrenal Gland, Pancreas, and Carotid Body

60500–60505

60500 Parathyroidectomy or exploration of parathyroid(s);
60502 re-exploration
60505 with mediastinal exploration, sternal split or transthoracic approach

ICD-9-CM Diagnostic

194.1 Malignant neoplasm of parathyroid gland — (Use additional code to identify any functional activity)
196.1 Secondary and unspecified malignant neoplasm of intrathoracic lymph nodes
198.89 Secondary malignant neoplasm of other specified sites
227.1 Benign neoplasm of parathyroid gland — (Use additional code to identify any functional activity)
234.8 Carcinoma in situ of other specified sites
237.4 Neoplasm of uncertain behavior of other and unspecified endocrine glands ▽
238.8 Neoplasm of uncertain behavior of other specified sites
239.7 Neoplasm of unspecified nature of endocrine glands and other parts of nervous system
239.8 Neoplasm of unspecified nature of other specified sites
252.00 Hyperparathyroidism, unspecified
252.01 Primary hyperparathyroidism
252.02 Secondary hyperparathyroidism, non-renal

252.08 Other hyperparathyroidism
252.1 Hypoparathyroidism
275.40 Unspecified disorder of calcium metabolism — (Use additional code to identify any associated mental retardation) ▽
275.41 Hypocalcemia — (Use additional code to identify any associated mental retardation)
275.42 Hypercalcemia — (Use additional code to identify any associated mental retardation)
275.49 Other disorders of calcium metabolism — (Use additional code to identify any associated mental retardation)

ICD-9-CM Procedural
06.02 Reopening of wound of thyroid field
06.81 Complete parathyroidectomy
06.89 Other parathyroidectomy

60512
60512 Parathyroid autotransplantation (List separately in addition to code for primary procedure)

ICD-9-CM Diagnostic
This is an add-on code. Refer to the corresponding primary procedure code for ICD-9 diagnosis code links.

ICD-9-CM Procedural
06.95 Parathyroid tissue reimplantation

60520
60520 Thymectomy, partial or total; transcervical approach (separate procedure)

ICD-9-CM Diagnostic
164.0 Malignant neoplasm of thymus
196.1 Secondary and unspecified malignant neoplasm of intrathoracic lymph nodes
198.89 Secondary malignant neoplasm of other specified sites
212.6 Benign neoplasm of thymus
235.8 Neoplasm of uncertain behavior of pleura, thymus, and mediastinum
238.8 Neoplasm of uncertain behavior of other specified sites
239.8 Neoplasm of unspecified nature of other specified sites
279.2 Combined immunity deficiency — (Use additional code to identify any associated mental retardation)
358.00 Myasthenia gravis without (acute) exacerbation
358.01 Myasthenia gravis with (acute) exacerbation
759.2 Congenital anomalies of other endocrine glands
786.6 Swelling, mass, or lump in chest

ICD-9-CM Procedural
07.80 Thymectomy, not otherwise specified
07.81 Partial excision of thymus
07.82 Total excision of thymus

60521–60522
60521 Thymectomy, partial or total; sternal split or transthoracic approach, without radical mediastinal dissection (separate procedure)
60522 sternal split or transthoracic approach, with radical mediastinal dissection (separate procedure)

ICD-9-CM Diagnostic
164.0 Malignant neoplasm of thymus
196.1 Secondary and unspecified malignant neoplasm of intrathoracic lymph nodes
198.89 Secondary malignant neoplasm of other specified sites
212.6 Benign neoplasm of thymus
235.8 Neoplasm of uncertain behavior of pleura, thymus, and mediastinum
238.8 Neoplasm of uncertain behavior of other specified sites
239.8 Neoplasm of unspecified nature of other specified sites
279.2 Combined immunity deficiency — (Use additional code to identify any associated mental retardation)
358.00 Myasthenia gravis without (acute) exacerbation
358.01 Myasthenia gravis with (acute) exacerbation
759.2 Congenital anomalies of other endocrine glands
786.6 Swelling, mass, or lump in chest

ICD-9-CM Procedural
07.80 Thymectomy, not otherwise specified
07.81 Partial excision of thymus
07.82 Total excision of thymus

60540–60545
60540 Adrenalectomy, partial or complete, or exploration of adrenal gland with or without biopsy, transabdominal, lumbar or dorsal (separate procedure);
60545 with excision of adjacent retroperitoneal tumor

ICD-9-CM Diagnostic
189.0 Malignant neoplasm of kidney, except pelvis
189.1 Malignant neoplasm of renal pelvis
194.0 Malignant neoplasm of adrenal gland — (Use additional code to identify any functional activity)
197.6 Secondary malignant neoplasm of retroperitoneum and peritoneum
197.7 Secondary malignant neoplasm of liver
198.7 Secondary malignant neoplasm of adrenal gland
211.8 Benign neoplasm of retroperitoneum and peritoneum
227.0 Benign neoplasm of adrenal gland — (Use additional code to identify any functional activity)
234.8 Carcinoma in situ of other specified sites
235.4 Neoplasm of uncertain behavior of retroperitoneum and peritoneum
237.2 Neoplasm of uncertain behavior of adrenal gland — (Use additional code to identify any functional activity)
239.0 Neoplasm of unspecified nature of digestive system
239.7 Neoplasm of unspecified nature of endocrine glands and other parts of nervous system
255.0 Cushing's syndrome — (Use additional E code to identify cause, if drug-induced)
255.10 Primary aldosteronism
255.11 Glucocorticoid-remediable aldosteronism
255.12 Conn's syndrome
255.13 Bartter's syndrome
255.14 Other secondary aldosteronism
255.2 Adrenogenital disorders
255.3 Other corticoadrenal overactivity
255.4 Corticoadrenal insufficiency
255.5 Other adrenal hypofunction
255.6 Medulloadrenal hyperfunction
V64.41 Laparoscopic surgical procedure converted to open procedure

ICD-9-CM Procedural
07.00 Exploration of adrenal field, not otherwise specified
07.01 Unilateral exploration of adrenal field
07.02 Bilateral exploration of adrenal field
07.12 Open biopsy of adrenal gland
07.22 Unilateral adrenalectomy
07.29 Other partial adrenalectomy
07.3 Bilateral adrenalectomy
54.4 Excision or destruction of peritoneal tissue

60600–60605
60600 Excision of carotid body tumor; without excision of carotid artery
60605 with excision of carotid artery

ICD-9-CM Diagnostic
194.5 Malignant neoplasm of carotid body — (Use additional code to identify any functional activity)
198.89 Secondary malignant neoplasm of other specified sites
227.5 Benign neoplasm of carotid body — (Use additional code to identify any functional activity)
239.7 Neoplasm of unspecified nature of endocrine glands and other parts of nervous system

ICD-9-CM Procedural
39.8 Operations on carotid body and other vascular bodies

60650
60650 Laparoscopy, surgical, with adrenalectomy, partial or complete, or exploration of adrenal gland with or without biopsy, transabdominal, lumbar or dorsal

ICD-9-CM Diagnostic
189.0 Malignant neoplasm of kidney, except pelvis
189.1 Malignant neoplasm of renal pelvis
194.0 Malignant neoplasm of adrenal gland — (Use additional code to identify any functional activity)
197.7 Secondary malignant neoplasm of liver
198.7 Secondary malignant neoplasm of adrenal gland
227.0 Benign neoplasm of adrenal gland — (Use additional code to identify any functional activity)

▽ Unspecified code ♀ Female diagnosis ☒ Manifestation code ♂ Male diagnosis

234.8 Carcinoma in situ of other specified sites
237.2 Neoplasm of uncertain behavior of adrenal gland — (Use additional code to identify any functional activity)
239.7 Neoplasm of unspecified nature of endocrine glands and other parts of nervous system
255.0 Cushing's syndrome — (Use additional E code to identify cause, if drug-induced)
255.10 Primary aldosteronism
255.11 Glucocorticoid-remediable aldosteronism
255.12 Conn's syndrome
255.13 Bartter's syndrome
255.14 Other secondary aldosteronism
255.2 Adrenogenital disorders
255.3 Other corticoadrenal overactivity
255.4 Corticoadrenal insufficiency
255.5 Other adrenal hypofunction
255.6 Medulloadrenal hyperfunction

ICD-9-CM Procedural

07.00 Exploration of adrenal field, not otherwise specified
07.01 Unilateral exploration of adrenal field
07.02 Bilateral exploration of adrenal field
07.11 Closed (percutaneous) (needle) biopsy of adrenal gland
07.22 Unilateral adrenalectomy
07.29 Other partial adrenalectomy
07.3 Bilateral adrenalectomy

Nervous System

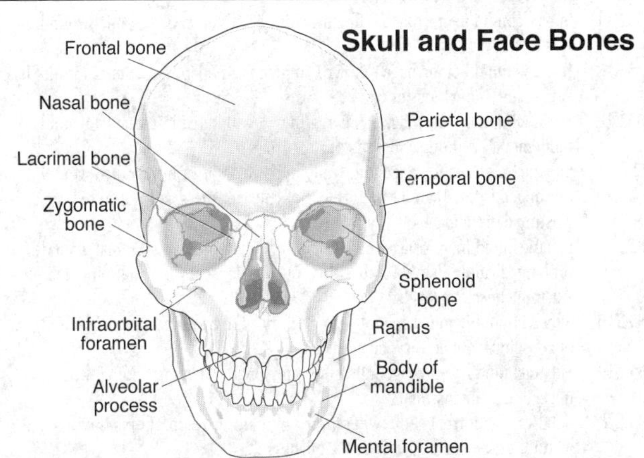

Skull, Meninges, and Brain

61000–61001

61000 Subdural tap through fontanelle, or suture, infant, unilateral or bilateral; initial
61001 subsequent taps

ICD-9-CM Diagnostic

324.0 Intracranial abscess
331.3 Communicating hydrocephalus
331.4 Obstructive hydrocephalus
741.01 Spina bifida with hydrocephalus, cervical region
742.3 Congenital hydrocephalus
742.4 Other specified congenital anomalies of brain
771.2 Other congenital infection specific to the perinatal period
780.6 Fever
854.00 Intracranial injury of other and unspecified nature, without mention of open intracranial wound, unspecified state of consciousness ▽
907.0 Late effect of intracranial injury without mention of skull fracture

ICD-9-CM Procedural

01.09 Other cranial puncture

HCPCS Level II Supplies & Services

A4550 Surgical trays

61020–61026

61020 Ventricular puncture through previous burr hole, fontanelle, suture, or implanted ventricular catheter/reservoir; without injection
61026 with injection of medication or other substance for diagnosis or treatment

ICD-9-CM Diagnostic

324.0 Intracranial abscess
331.3 Communicating hydrocephalus
331.4 Obstructive hydrocephalus
854.00 Intracranial injury of other and unspecified nature, without mention of open intracranial wound, unspecified state of consciousness ▽
907.0 Late effect of intracranial injury without mention of skull fracture

ICD-9-CM Procedural

01.02 Ventriculopuncture through previously implanted catheter
01.09 Other cranial puncture

61050–61055

61050 Cisternal or lateral cervical (C1-C2) puncture; without injection (separate procedure)
61055 with injection of medication or other substance for diagnosis or treatment (eg, C1-C2)

ICD-9-CM Diagnostic

321.1 Meningitis in other fungal diseases — (Code first underlying disease: 110.0-118) ☒
321.2 Meningitis due to viruses not elsewhere classified — (Code first underlying disease: 060.0-066.9) ☒
321.3 Meningitis due to trypanosomiasis — (Code first underlying disease: 086.0-086.9) ☒
321.4 Meningitis in sarcoidosis — (Code first underlying disease, 135) ☒
321.8 Meningitis due to other nonbacterial organisms classified elsewhere — (Code first underlying disease) ☒
324.1 Intraspinal abscess
324.9 Intracranial and intraspinal abscess of unspecified site ▽
331.3 Communicating hydrocephalus
331.4 Obstructive hydrocephalus
349.81 Cerebrospinal fluid rhinorrhea
368.2 Diplopia
722.71 Intervertebral cervical disc disorder with myelopathy, cervical region
723.0 Spinal stenosis in cervical region
723.1 Cervicalgia
723.3 Cervicobrachial syndrome (diffuse)
723.8 Other syndromes affecting cervical region
780.2 Syncope and collapse
780.4 Dizziness and giddiness
780.6 Fever
784.0 Headache
996.2 Mechanical complication of nervous system device, implant, and graft
996.63 Infection and inflammatory reaction due to nervous system device, implant, and graft — (Use additional code to identify specified infections)
996.75 Other complications due to nervous system device, implant, and graft
997.01 Central nervous system complication — (Use additional code to identify complications)
998.2 Accidental puncture or laceration during procedure
V45.2 Presence of cerebrospinal fluid drainage device — (This code is intended for use when these conditions are recorded as diagnoses or problems)
V67.00 Follow-up examination, following unspecified surgery ▽
V67.09 Follow-up examination, following other surgery
V67.1 Radiotherapy follow-up examination
V67.2 Chemotherapy follow-up examination
V67.51 Follow-up examination following completed treatment with high-risk medications, not elsewhere classified
V67.59 Other follow-up examination
V67.6 Combined treatment follow-up examination

ICD-9-CM Procedural

01.01 Cisternal puncture

61070

61070 Puncture of shunt tubing or reservoir for aspiration or injection procedure

ICD-9-CM Diagnostic

191.5 Malignant neoplasm of ventricles of brain
191.8 Malignant neoplasm of other parts of brain
198.3 Secondary malignant neoplasm of brain and spinal cord
322.0 Nonpyogenic meningitis
324.9 Intracranial and intraspinal abscess of unspecified site ▽
331.3 Communicating hydrocephalus
331.4 Obstructive hydrocephalus
996.2 Mechanical complication of nervous system device, implant, and graft
996.63 Infection and inflammatory reaction due to nervous system device, implant, and graft — (Use additional code to identify specified infections)
996.75 Other complications due to nervous system device, implant, and graft

V45.89 Other postsurgical status — (This code is intended for use when these conditions are recorded as diagnoses or problems)
V67.00 Follow-up examination, following unspecified surgery ▽
V67.09 Follow-up examination, following other surgery
V67.1 Radiotherapy follow-up examination
V67.2 Chemotherapy follow-up examination
V67.51 Follow-up examination following completed treatment with high-risk medications, not elsewhere classified
V67.59 Other follow-up examination

ICD-9-CM Procedural

01.02 Ventriculopuncture through previously implanted catheter
02.41 Irrigation and exploration of ventricular shunt
03.92 Injection of other agent into spinal canal

HCPCS Level II Supplies & Services

A9525 Supply of low or iso-osmolar contrast material, 10 mg of iodine

61105–61108

61105 Twist drill hole for subdural or ventricular puncture;
61107 for implanting ventricular catheter or pressure recording device
61108 for evacuation and/or drainage of subdural hematoma

ICD-9-CM Diagnostic

191.1 Malignant neoplasm of frontal lobe of brain
191.2 Malignant neoplasm of temporal lobe of brain
191.3 Malignant neoplasm of parietal lobe of brain
191.4 Malignant neoplasm of occipital lobe of brain
191.5 Malignant neoplasm of ventricles of brain
191.6 Malignant neoplasm of cerebellum NOS
191.7 Malignant neoplasm of brain stem
191.8 Malignant neoplasm of other parts of brain
191.9 Malignant neoplasm of brain, unspecified site ▽
192.1 Malignant neoplasm of cerebral meninges
198.3 Secondary malignant neoplasm of brain and spinal cord
225.0 Benign neoplasm of brain
225.2 Benign neoplasm of cerebral meninges
237.5 Neoplasm of uncertain behavior of brain and spinal cord
239.6 Neoplasm of unspecified nature of brain
324.0 Intracranial abscess
331.3 Communicating hydrocephalus
331.4 Obstructive hydrocephalus
348.5 Cerebral edema
430 Subarachnoid hemorrhage — (Use additional code to identify presence of hypertension)
431 Intracerebral hemorrhage — (Use additional code to identify presence of hypertension)
432.1 Subdural hemorrhage — (Use additional code to identify presence of hypertension)
432.9 Unspecified intracranial hemorrhage — (Use additional code to identify presence of hypertension) ▽
437.3 Cerebral aneurysm, nonruptured — (Use additional code to identify presence of hypertension)
742.3 Congenital hydrocephalus
747.81 Congenital anomaly of cerebrovascular system
767.0 Subdural and cerebral hemorrhage, birth trauma — (Use additional code to identify cause)
800.24 Closed fracture of vault of skull with subarachnoid, subdural, and extradural hemorrhage, prolonged (more than 24 hours) loss of consciousness and return to pre-existing conscious level
851.05 Cortex (cerebral) contusion without mention of open intracranial wound, prolonged (more than 24 hours) loss of consciousness, without return to pre-existing conscious level
852.00 Subarachnoid hemorrhage following injury, without mention of open intracranial wound, unspecified state of consciousness ▽
852.01 Subarachnoid hemorrhage following injury, without mention of open intracranial wound, no loss of consciousness
852.02 Subarachnoid hemorrhage following injury, without mention of open intracranial wound, brief (less than 1 hour) loss of consciousness
852.03 Subarachnoid hemorrhage following injury, without mention of open intracranial wound, moderate (1-24 hours) loss of consciousness
852.04 Subarachnoid hemorrhage following injury, without mention of open intracranial wound, prolonged (more than 24 hours) loss of consciousness and return to pre-existing conscious level
852.05 Subarachnoid hemorrhage following injury, without mention of open intracranial wound, prolonged (more than 24 hours) loss of consciousness, without return to pre-existing conscious level
852.06 Subarachnoid hemorrhage following injury, without mention of open intracranial wound, loss of consciousness of unspecified duration ▽
852.09 Subarachnoid hemorrhage following injury, without mention of open intracranial wound, unspecified concussion ▽
852.10 Subarachnoid hemorrhage following injury, with open intracranial wound, unspecified state of consciousness ▽
852.11 Subarachnoid hemorrhage following injury, with open intracranial wound, no loss of consciousness
852.12 Subarachnoid hemorrhage following injury, with open intracranial wound, brief (less than 1 hour) loss of consciousness
852.13 Subarachnoid hemorrhage following injury, with open intracranial wound, moderate (1-24 hours) loss of consciousness
852.14 Subarachnoid hemorrhage following injury, with open intracranial wound, prolonged (more than 24 hours) loss of consciousness and return to pre-existing conscious level
852.15 Subarachnoid hemorrhage following injury, with open intracranial wound, prolonged (more than 24 hours) loss of consciousness, without return to pre-existing conscious level
852.16 Subarachnoid hemorrhage following injury, with open intracranial wound, loss of consciousness of unspecified duration ▽
852.19 Subarachnoid hemorrhage following injury, with open intracranial wound, unspecified concussion ▽
852.20 Subdural hemorrhage following injury, without mention of open intracranial wound, unspecified state of consciousness ▽
852.21 Subdural hemorrhage following injury, without mention of open intracranial wound, no loss of consciousness
852.22 Subdural hemorrhage following injury, without mention of open intracranial wound, brief (less than one hour) loss of consciousness
852.23 Subdural hemorrhage following injury, without mention of open intracranial wound, moderate (1-24 hours) loss of consciousness
852.24 Subdural hemorrhage following injury, without mention of open intracranial wound, prolonged (more than 24 hours) loss of consciousness and return to pre-existing conscious level
852.25 Subdural hemorrhage following injury, without mention of open intracranial wound, prolonged (more than 24 hours) loss of consciousness, without return to pre-existing conscious level
852.26 Subdural hemorrhage following injury, without mention of open intracranial wound, loss of consciousness of unspecified duration ▽
852.29 Subdural hemorrhage following injury, without mention of open intracranial wound, unspecified concussion ▽
852.30 Subdural hemorrhage following injury, with open intracranial wound, state of consciousness unspecified ▽
852.31 Subdural hemorrhage following injury, with open intracranial wound, no loss of consciousness
852.32 Subdural hemorrhage following injury, with open intracranial wound, brief (less than 1 hour) loss of consciousness
852.33 Subdural hemorrhage following injury, with open intracranial wound, moderate (1-24 hours) loss of consciousness
852.34 Subdural hemorrhage following injury, with open intracranial wound, prolonged (more than 24 hours) loss of consciousness and return to pre-existing conscious level
852.35 Subdural hemorrhage following injury, with open intracranial wound, prolonged (more than 24 hours) loss of consciousness, without return to pre-existing conscious level
852.36 Subdural hemorrhage following injury, with open intracranial wound, loss of consciousness of unspecified duration ▽
852.39 Subdural hemorrhage following injury, with open intracranial wound, unspecified concussion ▽
852.40 Extradural hemorrhage following injury, without mention of open intracranial wound, unspecified state of consciousness ▽
852.41 Extradural hemorrhage following injury, without mention of open intracranial wound, no loss of consciousness
852.42 Extradural hemorrhage following injury, without mention of open intracranial wound, brief (less than 1 hour) loss of consciousness
852.43 Extradural hemorrhage following injury, without mention of open intracranial wound, moderate (1-24 hours) loss of consciousness
852.44 Extradural hemorrhage following injury, without mention of open intracranial wound, prolonged (more than 24 hours) loss of consciousness and return to pre-existing conscious level
852.45 Extradural hemorrhage following injury, without mention of open intracranial wound, prolonged (more than 24 hours) loss of consciousness, without return to pre-existing conscious level

▽ Unspecified code
♀ Female diagnosis
☒ Manifestation code
♂ Male diagnosis

852.46 Extradural hemorrhage following injury, without mention of open intracranial wound, loss of consciousness of unspecified duration ▽
852.49 Extradural hemorrhage following injury, without mention of open intracranial wound, unspecified concussion ▽
852.50 Extradural hemorrhage following injury, with open intracranial wound, state of consciousness unspecified ▽
852.51 Extradural hemorrhage following injury, with open intracranial wound, no loss of consciousness
852.52 Extradural hemorrhage following injury, with open intracranial wound, brief (less than 1 hour) loss of consciousness
852.53 Extradural hemorrhage following injury, with open intracranial wound, moderate (1-24 hours) loss of consciousness
852.54 Extradural hemorrhage following injury, with open intracranial wound, prolonged (more than 24 hours) loss of consciousness and return to pre-existing conscious level
852.55 Extradural hemorrhage following injury, with open intracranial wound, prolonged (more than 24 hours) loss of consciousness, without return to pre-existing conscious level
852.56 Extradural hemorrhage following injury, with open intracranial wound, loss of consciousness of unspecified duration ▽
852.59 Extradural hemorrhage following injury, with open intracranial wound, unspecifiedconcussion ▽
853.00 Other and unspecified intracranial hemorrhage following injury, without mention of open intracranial wound, unspecified state of consciousness ▽
853.01 Other and unspecified intracranial hemorrhage following injury, without mention of open intracranial wound, no loss of consciousness
853.02 Other and unspecified intracranial hemorrhage following injury, without mention of open intracranial wound, brief (less than 1 hour) loss of consciousness
853.03 Other and unspecified intracranial hemorrhage following injury, without mention of open intracranial wound, moderate (1-24 hours) loss of consciousness
853.04 Other and unspecified intracranial hemorrhage following injury, without mention of open intracranial wound, prolonged (more than 24 hours) loss of consciousness and return to preexisting conscious level
853.05 Other and unspecified intracranial hemorrhage following injury. Without mention of open intracranial wound, prolonged (more than 24 hours) loss of consciousness, without return to pre-existing conscious level
853.06 Other and unspecified intracranial hemorrhage following injury, without mention of open intracranial wound, loss of consciousness of unspecified duration ▽
853.09 Other and unspecified intracranial hemorrhage following injury, without mention of open intracranial wound, unspecified concussion ▽
853.10 Other and unspecified intracranial hemorrhage following injury, with open intracranial wound, unspecified state of consciousness ▽
853.11 Other and unspecified intracranial hemorrhage following injury, with open intracranial wound, no loss of consciousness
853.12 Other and unspecified intracranial hemorrhage following injury, with open intracranial wound, brief (less than 1 hour) loss of consciousness
853.13 Other and unspecified intracranial hemorrhage following injury, with open intracranial wound, moderate (1-24 hours) loss of consciousness
853.14 Other and unspecified intracranial hemorrhage following injury, with open intracranial wound, prolonged (more than 24 hours) loss of consciousness and return to pre-existing conscious level
853.15 Other and unspecified intracranial hemorrhage following injury, with open intracranial wound, prolonged (more than 24 hours) loss of consciousness, without return to pre-existing conscious level
853.16 Other and unspecified intracranial hemorrhage following injury, with open intracranial wound, loss of consciousness of unspecified duration ▽
853.19 Other and unspecified intracranial hemorrhage following injury, with open intracranial wound, unspecified concussion ▽
854.00 Intracranial injury of other and unspecified nature, without mention of open intracranial wound, unspecified state of consciousness ▽
854.01 Intracranial injury of other and unspecified nature, without mention of open intracranial wound, no loss of consciousness
854.02 Intracranial injury of other and unspecified nature, without mention of open intracranial wound, brief (less than 1 hour) loss of consciousness
854.03 Intracranial injury of other and unspecified nature, without mention of open intracranial wound, moderate (1-24 hours) loss of consciousness
854.04 Intracranial injury of other and unspecified nature, without mention of open intracranial wound, prolonged (more than 24 hours) loss of consciousness and return to pre-existing conscious level
854.05 Intracranial injury of other and unspecified nature, without mention of open intracranial wound, prolonged (more than 24 hours) loss of consciousness, without return to pre-existing conscious level
854.06 Intracranial injury of other and unspecified nature, without mention of open intracranial wound, loss of consciousness of unspecified duration ▽
854.09 Intracranial injury of other and unspecified nature, without mention of open intracranial wound, unspecified concussion ▽
854.10 Intracranial injury of other and unspecified nature, with open intracranial wound, unspecified state of consciousness ▽
854.11 Intracranial injury of other and unspecified nature, with open intracranial wound, no loss of consciousness
854.12 Intracranial injury of other and unspecified nature, with open intracranial wound, brief (less than 1 hour) loss of consciousness
854.13 Intracranial injury of other and unspecified nature, with open intracranial wound, moderate (1-24 hours) loss of consciousness
854.14 Intracranial injury of other and unspecified nature, with open intracranial wound, prolonged (more than 24 hours) loss of consciousness and return to pre-existing conscious level
854.15 Intracranial injury of other and unspecified nature, with open intracranial wound, prolonged (more than 24 hours) loss of consciousness, without return to pre-existing conscious level
854.16 Intracranial injury of other and unspecified nature, with open intracranial wound, loss of consciousness of unspecified duration ▽
854.19 Intracranial injury of other and unspecified nature, with open intracranial wound, with unspecified concussion ▽
958.2 Secondary and recurrent hemorrhage as an early complication of trauma
996.63 Infection and inflammatory reaction due to nervous system device, implant, and graft — (Use additional code to identify specified infections)

ICD-9-CM Procedural

01.09 Other cranial puncture
01.18 Other diagnostic procedures on brain and cerebral meninges
01.31 Incision of cerebral meninges
02.31 Ventricular shunt to structure in head and neck
02.39 Other operations to establish drainage of ventricle

61120

61120 Burr hole(s) for ventricular puncture (including injection of gas, contrast media, dye, or radioactive material)

ICD-9-CM Diagnostic

191.9 Malignant neoplasm of brain, unspecified site ▽
225.0 Benign neoplasm of brain
239.6 Neoplasm of unspecified nature of brain
331.3 Communicating hydrocephalus
331.4 Obstructive hydrocephalus
349.89 Other specified disorder of nervous system
349.9 Unspecified disorders of nervous system ▽
388.61 Cerebrospinal fluid otorrhea
430 Subarachnoid hemorrhage — (Use additional code to identify presence of hypertension)
431 Intracerebral hemorrhage — (Use additional code to identify presence of hypertension)
803.10 Other closed skull fracture with cerebral laceration and contusion, unspecified state of consciousness ▽
803.20 Other closed skull fracture with subarachnoid, subdural, and extradural hemorrhage, unspecified state of consciousness ▽
803.60 Other open skull fracture with cerebral laceration and contusion, unspecified state of consciousness ▽

ICD-9-CM Procedural

01.18 Other diagnostic procedures on brain and cerebral meninges
01.24 Other craniotomy

61140

61140 Burr hole(s) or trephine; with biopsy of brain or intracranial lesion

ICD-9-CM Diagnostic

191.0 Malignant neoplasm of cerebrum, except lobes and ventricles
191.1 Malignant neoplasm of frontal lobe of brain
191.2 Malignant neoplasm of temporal lobe of brain
191.3 Malignant neoplasm of parietal lobe of brain
191.4 Malignant neoplasm of occipital lobe of brain
191.5 Malignant neoplasm of ventricles of brain
191.6 Malignant neoplasm of cerebellum NOS
191.7 Malignant neoplasm of brain stem
191.8 Malignant neoplasm of other parts of brain
191.9 Malignant neoplasm of brain, unspecified site ▽
192.1 Malignant neoplasm of cerebral meninges

198.3 Secondary malignant neoplasm of brain and spinal cord
198.4 Secondary malignant neoplasm of other parts of nervous system
199.1 Other malignant neoplasm of unspecified site
225.0 Benign neoplasm of brain
237.5 Neoplasm of uncertain behavior of brain and spinal cord
239.6 Neoplasm of unspecified nature of brain
239.7 Neoplasm of unspecified nature of endocrine glands and other parts of nervous system
324.0 Intracranial abscess
348.0 Cerebral cysts

ICD-9-CM Procedural

01.11 Closed (percutaneous) (needle) biopsy of cerebral meninges
01.12 Open biopsy of cerebral meninges
01.13 Closed (percutaneous) (needle) biopsy of brain
01.14 Open biopsy of brain

61150–61151

61150 Burr hole(s) or trephine; with drainage of brain abscess or cyst
61151 with subsequent tapping (aspiration) of intracranial abscess or cyst

ICD-9-CM Diagnostic

324.0 Intracranial abscess
324.9 Intracranial and intraspinal abscess of unspecified site ▽
348.0 Cerebral cysts
349.1 Nervous system complications from surgically implanted device
742.4 Other specified congenital anomalies of brain

ICD-9-CM Procedural

01.09 Other cranial puncture
01.21 Incision and drainage of cranial sinus
01.24 Other craniotomy
01.31 Incision of cerebral meninges
01.39 Other incision of brain

61154

61154 Burr hole(s) with evacuation and/or drainage of hematoma, extradural or subdural

ICD-9-CM Diagnostic

432.0 Nontraumatic extradural hemorrhage — (Use additional code to identify presence of hypertension)
432.1 Subdural hemorrhage — (Use additional code to identify presence of hypertension)
852.04 Subarachnoid hemorrhage following injury, without mention of open intracranial wound, prolonged (more than 24 hours) loss of consciousness and return to pre-existing conscious level
852.20 Subdural hemorrhage following injury, without mention of open intracranial wound, unspecified state of consciousness ▽
852.21 Subdural hemorrhage following injury, without mention of open intracranial wound, no loss of consciousness
852.22 Subdural hemorrhage following injury, without mention of open intracranial wound, brief (less than one hour) loss of consciousness
852.23 Subdural hemorrhage following injury, without mention of open intracranial wound, moderate (1-24 hours) loss of consciousness
852.24 Subdural hemorrhage following injury, without mention of open intracranial wound, prolonged (more than 24 hours) loss of consciousness and return to pre-existing conscious level
852.25 Subdural hemorrhage following injury, without mention of open intracranial wound, prolonged (more than 24 hours) loss of consciousness, without return to pre-existing conscious level
852.26 Subdural hemorrhage following injury, without mention of open intracranial wound, loss of consciousness of unspecified duration ▽
852.29 Subdural hemorrhage following injury, without mention of open intracranial wound, unspecified concussion ▽
852.30 Subdural hemorrhage following injury, with open intracranial wound, state of consciousness unspecified ▽
852.31 Subdural hemorrhage following injury, with open intracranial wound, no loss of consciousness
852.32 Subdural hemorrhage following injury, with open intracranial wound, brief (less than 1 hour) loss of consciousness
852.33 Subdural hemorrhage following injury, with open intracranial wound, moderate (1-24 hours) loss of consciousness
852.34 Subdural hemorrhage following injury, with open intracranial wound, prolonged (more than 24 hours) loss of consciousness and return to pre-existing conscious level
852.35 Subdural hemorrhage following injury, with open intracranial wound, prolonged (more than 24 hours) loss of consciousness, without return to pre-existing conscious level
852.36 Subdural hemorrhage following injury, with open intracranial wound, loss of consciousness of unspecified duration ▽
852.39 Subdural hemorrhage following injury, with open intracranial wound, unspecified concussion ▽
852.40 Extradural hemorrhage following injury, without mention of open intracranial wound, unspecified state of consciousness ▽
852.41 Extradural hemorrhage following injury, without mention of open intracranial wound, no loss of consciousness
852.42 Extradural hemorrhage following injury, without mention of open intracranial wound, brief (less than 1 hour) loss of consciousness
852.43 Extradural hemorrhage following injury, without mention of open intracranial wound, moderate (1-24 hours) loss of consciousness
852.44 Extradural hemorrhage following injury, without mention of open intracranial wound, prolonged (more than 24 hours) loss of consciousness and return to pre-existing conscious level
852.45 Extradural hemorrhage following injury, without mention of open intracranial wound, prolonged (more than 24 hours) loss of consciousness, without return to pre-existing conscious level
852.46 Extradural hemorrhage following injury, without mention of open intracranial wound, loss of consciousness of unspecified duration ▽
852.49 Extradural hemorrhage following injury, without mention of open intracranial wound, unspecified concussion ▽
852.50 Extradural hemorrhage following injury, with open intracranial wound, state of consciousness unspecified ▽
852.51 Extradural hemorrhage following injury, with open intracranial wound, no loss of consciousness
852.52 Extradural hemorrhage following injury, with open intracranial wound, brief (less than 1 hour) loss of consciousness
852.53 Extradural hemorrhage following injury, with open intracranial wound, moderate (1-24 hours) loss of consciousness
852.54 Extradural hemorrhage following injury, with open intracranial wound, prolonged (more than 24 hours) loss of consciousness and return to pre-existing conscious level
852.55 Extradural hemorrhage following injury, with open intracranial wound, prolonged (more than 24 hours) loss of consciousness, without return to pre-existing conscious level
852.56 Extradural hemorrhage following injury, with open intracranial wound, loss of consciousness of unspecified duration ▽
852.59 Extradural hemorrhage following injury, with open intracranial wound, unspecifiedconcussion ▽
854.00 Intracranial injury of other and unspecified nature, without mention of open intracranial wound, unspecified state of consciousness ▽
854.01 Intracranial injury of other and unspecified nature, without mention of open intracranial wound, no loss of consciousness
854.02 Intracranial injury of other and unspecified nature, without mention of open intracranial wound, brief (less than 1 hour) loss of consciousness
854.03 Intracranial injury of other and unspecified nature, without mention of open intracranial wound, moderate (1-24 hours) loss of consciousness
854.04 Intracranial injury of other and unspecified nature, without mention of open intracranial wound, prolonged (more than 24 hours) loss of consciousness and return to pre-existing conscious level
854.05 Intracranial injury of other and unspecified nature, without mention of open intracranial wound, prolonged (more than 24 hours) loss of consciousness, without return to pre-existing conscious level
854.06 Intracranial injury of other and unspecified nature, without mention of open intracranial wound, loss of consciousness of unspecified duration ▽
854.09 Intracranial injury of other and unspecified nature, without mention of open intracranial wound, unspecified concussion ▽
854.10 Intracranial injury of other and unspecified nature, with open intracranial wound, unspecified state of consciousness ▽
854.11 Intracranial injury of other and unspecified nature, with open intracranial wound, no loss of consciousness
854.12 Intracranial injury of other and unspecified nature, with open intracranial wound, brief (less than 1 hour) loss of consciousness
854.13 Intracranial injury of other and unspecified nature, with open intracranial wound, moderate (1-24 hours) loss of consciousness
854.14 Intracranial injury of other and unspecified nature, with open intracranial wound, prolonged (more than 24 hours) loss of consciousness and return to pre-existing conscious level
854.15 Intracranial injury of other and unspecified nature, with open intracranial wound, prolonged (more than 24 hours) loss of consciousness, without return to pre-existing conscious level

854.16 Intracranial injury of other and unspecified nature, with open intracranial wound, loss of consciousness of unspecified duration
854.19 Intracranial injury of other and unspecified nature, with open intracranial wound, with unspecified concussion
997.02 Iatrogenic cerebrovascular infarction or hemorrhage — (Use additional code to identify complications)

ICD-9-CM Procedural

01.24 Other craniotomy
01.31 Incision of cerebral meninges

61156–61210

61156 Burr hole(s); with aspiration of hematoma or cyst, intracerebral
61210 for implanting ventricular catheter, reservoir, EEG electrode(s) or pressure recording device (separate procedure)

ICD-9-CM Diagnostic

191.1 Malignant neoplasm of frontal lobe of brain
191.2 Malignant neoplasm of temporal lobe of brain
191.3 Malignant neoplasm of parietal lobe of brain
191.4 Malignant neoplasm of occipital lobe of brain
191.5 Malignant neoplasm of ventricles of brain
191.6 Malignant neoplasm of cerebellum NOS
191.7 Malignant neoplasm of brain stem
191.8 Malignant neoplasm of other parts of brain
191.9 Malignant neoplasm of brain, unspecified site
192.1 Malignant neoplasm of cerebral meninges
198.3 Secondary malignant neoplasm of brain and spinal cord
225.0 Benign neoplasm of brain
225.2 Benign neoplasm of cerebral meninges
239.6 Neoplasm of unspecified nature of brain
324.0 Intracranial abscess
331.3 Communicating hydrocephalus
331.4 Obstructive hydrocephalus
345.01 Generalized nonconvulsive epilepsy with intractable epilepsy
345.10 Generalized convulsive epilepsy without mention of intractable epilepsy
345.11 Generalized convulsive epilepsy with intractable epilepsy
345.2 Epileptic petit mal status
345.40 Partial epilepsy with impairment of consciousness, without mention of intractable epilepsy
345.41 Partial epilepsy with impairment of consciousness, with intractable epilepsy
345.50 Partial epilepsy without mention of impairment of consciousness, without mention of intractable epilepsy
345.51 Partial epilepsy without mention of impairment of consciousness, with intractable epilepsy
345.60 Infantile spasms without mention of intractable epilepsy
345.61 Infantile spasms with intractable epilepsy
345.70 Epilepsia partialis continua without mention of intractable epilepsy
345.71 Epilepsia partialis continua with intractable epilepsy
345.80 Other forms of epilepsy without mention of intractable epilepsy
345.81 Other forms of epilepsy with intractable epilepsy
345.90 Unspecified epilepsy without mention of intractable epilepsy
345.91 Unspecified epilepsy with intractable epilepsy
348.0 Cerebral cysts
348.5 Cerebral edema
430 Subarachnoid hemorrhage — (Use additional code to identify presence of hypertension)
431 Intracerebral hemorrhage — (Use additional code to identify presence of hypertension)
432.1 Subdural hemorrhage — (Use additional code to identify presence of hypertension)
432.9 Unspecified intracranial hemorrhage — (Use additional code to identify presence of hypertension)
742.4 Other specified congenital anomalies of brain
747.81 Congenital anomaly of cerebrovascular system
767.0 Subdural and cerebral hemorrhage, birth trauma — (Use additional code to identify cause)
780.01 Coma
780.39 Other convulsions
800.24 Closed fracture of vault of skull with subarachnoid, subdural, and extradural hemorrhage, prolonged (more than 24 hours) loss of consciousness and return to pre-existing conscious level
800.70 Open fracture of vault of skull with subarachnoid, subdural, and extradural hemorrhage, unspecified state of consciousness
800.71 Open fracture of vault of skull with subarachnoid, subdural, and extradural hemorrhage, no loss of consciousness
800.72 Open fracture of vault of skull with subarachnoid, subdural, and extradural hemorrhage, brief (less than one hour) loss of consciousness
800.73 Open fracture of vault of skull with subarachnoid, subdural, and extradural hemorrhage, moderate (1-24 hours) loss of consciousness
800.74 Open fracture of vault of skull with subarachnoid, subdural, and extradural hemorrhage, prolonged (more than 24 hours) loss of consciousness and return to pre-existing conscious level
800.75 Open fracture of vault of skull with subarachnoid, subdural, and extradural hemorrhage, prolonged (more than 24 hours) loss of consciousness, without return to pre-existing conscious level
800.76 Open fracture of vault of skull with subarachnoid, subdural, and extradural hemorrhage, loss of consciousness of unspecified duration
800.79 Open fracture of vault of skull with subarachnoid, subdural, and extradural hemorrhage, unspecified concussion
803.30 Other closed skull fracture with other and unspecified intracranial hemorrhage, unspecified state of unconsciousness
803.31 Other closed skull fracture with other and unspecified intracranial hemorrhage, no loss of consciousness
803.32 Other closed skull fracture with other and unspecified intracranial hemorrhage, brief (less than one hour) loss of consciousness
803.33 Other closed skull fracture with other and unspecified intracranial hemorrhage, moderate (1-24 hours) loss of consciousness
803.34 Other closed skull fracture with other and unspecified intracranial hemorrhage, prolonged (more than 24 hours) loss of consciousness and return to pre-existing conscious level
803.35 Other closed skull fracture with other and unspecified intracranial hemorrhage, prolonged (more than 24 hours) loss of consciousness, without return to pre-existing conscious level
803.36 Other closed skull fracture with other and unspecified intracranial hemorrhage, loss of consciousness of unspecified duration
803.39 Other closed skull fracture with other and unspecified intracranial hemorrhage, unspecified concussion
852.00 Subarachnoid hemorrhage following injury, without mention of open intracranial wound, unspecified state of consciousness
852.01 Subarachnoid hemorrhage following injury, without mention of open intracranial wound, no loss of consciousness
852.02 Subarachnoid hemorrhage following injury, without mention of open intracranial wound, brief (less than 1 hour) loss of consciousness
852.03 Subarachnoid hemorrhage following injury, without mention of open intracranial wound, moderate (1-24 hours) loss of consciousness
852.04 Subarachnoid hemorrhage following injury, without mention of open intracranial wound, prolonged (more than 24 hours) loss of consciousness and return to pre-existing conscious level
852.05 Subarachnoid hemorrhage following injury, without mention of open intracranial wound, prolonged (more than 24 hours) loss of consciousness, without return to pre-existing conscious level
852.06 Subarachnoid hemorrhage following injury, without mention of open intracranial wound, loss of consciousness of unspecified duration
852.09 Subarachnoid hemorrhage following injury, without mention of open intracranial wound, unspecified concussion
852.10 Subarachnoid hemorrhage following injury, with open intracranial wound, unspecified state of consciousness
852.11 Subarachnoid hemorrhage following injury, with open intracranial wound, no loss of consciousness
852.12 Subarachnoid hemorrhage following injury, with open intracranial wound, brief (less than 1 hour) loss of consciousness
852.13 Subarachnoid hemorrhage following injury, with open intracranial wound, moderate (1-24 hours) loss of consciousness
852.14 Subarachnoid hemorrhage following injury, with open intracranial wound, prolonged (more than 24 hours) loss of consciousness and return to pre-existing conscious level
852.15 Subarachnoid hemorrhage following injury, with open intracranial wound, prolonged (more than 24 hours) loss of consciousness, without return to pre-existing conscious level
852.16 Subarachnoid hemorrhage following injury, with open intracranial wound, loss of consciousness of unspecified duration
852.19 Subarachnoid hemorrhage following injury, with open intracranial wound, unspecified concussion
852.20 Subdural hemorrhage following injury, without mention of open intracranial wound, unspecified state of consciousness
852.21 Subdural hemorrhage following injury, without mention of open intracranial wound, no loss of consciousness
852.22 Subdural hemorrhage following injury, without mention of open intracranial wound, brief (less than one hour) loss of consciousness
852.23 Subdural hemorrhage following injury, without mention of open intracranial wound, moderate (1-24 hours) loss of consciousness

852.24 Subdural hemorrhage following injury, without mention of open intracranial wound, prolonged (more than 24 hours) loss of consciousness and return to pre-existing conscious level
852.25 Subdural hemorrhage following injury, without mention of open intracranial wound, prolonged (more than 24 hours) loss of consciousness, without return to pre-existing conscious level
852.26 Subdural hemorrhage following injury, without mention of open intracranial wound, loss of consciousness of unspecified duration ▽
852.29 Subdural hemorrhage following injury, without mention of open intracranial wound, unspecified concussion ▽
852.30 Subdural hemorrhage following injury, with open intracranial wound, state of consciousness unspecified ▽
852.31 Subdural hemorrhage following injury, with open intracranial wound, no loss of consciousness
852.32 Subdural hemorrhage following injury, with open intracranial wound, brief (less than 1 hour) loss of consciousness
852.33 Subdural hemorrhage following injury, with open intracranial wound, moderate (1-24 hours) loss of consciousness
852.34 Subdural hemorrhage following injury, with open intracranial wound, prolonged (more than 24 hours) loss of consciousness and return to pre-existing conscious level
852.35 Subdural hemorrhage following injury, with open intracranial wound, prolonged (more than 24 hours) loss of consciousness, without return to pre-existing conscious level
852.36 Subdural hemorrhage following injury, with open intracranial wound, loss of consciousness of unspecified duration ▽
852.39 Subdural hemorrhage following injury, with open intracranial wound, unspecified concussion ▽
852.40 Extradural hemorrhage following injury, without mention of open intracranial wound, unspecified state of consciousness ▽
852.41 Extradural hemorrhage following injury, without mention of open intracranial wound, no loss of consciousness
852.42 Extradural hemorrhage following injury, without mention of open intracranial wound, brief (less than 1 hour) loss of consciousness
852.43 Extradural hemorrhage following injury, without mention of open intracranial wound, moderate (1-24 hours) loss of consciousness
852.44 Extradural hemorrhage following injury, without mention of open intracranial wound, prolonged (more than 24 hours) loss of consciousness and return to pre-existing conscious level
852.45 Extradural hemorrhage following injury, without mention of open intracranial wound, prolonged (more than 24 hours) loss of consciousness, without return to pre-existing conscious level
852.46 Extradural hemorrhage following injury, without mention of open intracranial wound, loss of consciousness of unspecified duration ▽
852.49 Extradural hemorrhage following injury, without mention of open intracranial wound, unspecified concussion ▽
852.50 Extradural hemorrhage following injury, with open intracranial wound, state of consciousness unspecified ▽
852.51 Extradural hemorrhage following injury, with open intracranial wound, no loss of consciousness
852.52 Extradural hemorrhage following injury, with open intracranial wound, brief (less than 1 hour) loss of consciousness
852.53 Extradural hemorrhage following injury, with open intracranial wound, moderate (1-24 hours) loss of consciousness
852.54 Extradural hemorrhage following injury, with open intracranial wound, prolonged (more than 24 hours) loss of consciousness and return to pre-existing conscious level
852.55 Extradural hemorrhage following injury, with open intracranial wound, prolonged (more than 24 hours) loss of consciousness, without return to pre-existing conscious level
852.56 Extradural hemorrhage following injury, with open intracranial wound, loss of consciousness of unspecified duration ▽
852.59 Extradural hemorrhage following injury, with open intracranial wound, unspecifiedconcussion ▽
996.2 Mechanical complication of nervous system device, implant, and graft
996.63 Infection and inflammatory reaction due to nervous system device, implant, and graft — (Use additional code to identify specified infections)
997.09 Other nervous system complications — (Use additional code to identify complications)

ICD-9-CM Procedural

01.18 Other diagnostic procedures on brain and cerebral meninges
01.24 Other craniotomy
02.2 Ventriculostomy
02.93 Implantation or replacement of intracranial neurostimulator lead(s)

61215

61215 Insertion of subcutaneous reservoir, pump or continuous infusion system for connection to ventricular catheter

ICD-9-CM Diagnostic

191.3 Malignant neoplasm of parietal lobe of brain
191.9 Malignant neoplasm of brain, unspecified site ▽
198.3 Secondary malignant neoplasm of brain and spinal cord
198.4 Secondary malignant neoplasm of other parts of nervous system
199.1 Other malignant neoplasm of unspecified site
202.81 Other malignant lymphomas of lymph nodes of head, face, and neck
237.5 Neoplasm of uncertain behavior of brain and spinal cord

ICD-9-CM Procedural

86.06 Insertion of totally implantable infusion pump

61250–61253

61250 Burr hole(s) or trephine, supratentorial, exploratory, not followed by other surgery
61253 Burr hole(s) or trephine, infratentorial, unilateral or bilateral

ICD-9-CM Diagnostic

326 Late effects of intracranial abscess or pyogenic infection — (Use additional code to identify condition: 331.4, 342.00-342.92, 344.00-344.9)
348.4 Compression of brain
430 Subarachnoid hemorrhage — (Use additional code to identify presence of hypertension)
432.1 Subdural hemorrhage — (Use additional code to identify presence of hypertension)
742.9 Unspecified congenital anomaly of brain, spinal cord, and nervous system ▽
747.81 Congenital anomaly of cerebrovascular system
767.0 Subdural and cerebral hemorrhage, birth trauma — (Use additional code to identify cause)
803.30 Other closed skull fracture with other and unspecified intracranial hemorrhage, unspecified state of unconsciousness ▽
803.31 Other closed skull fracture with other and unspecified intracranial hemorrhage, no loss of consciousness ▽
803.32 Other closed skull fracture with other and unspecified intracranial hemorrhage, brief (less than one hour) loss of consciousness ▽
803.33 Other closed skull fracture with other and unspecified intracranial hemorrhage, moderate (1-24 hours) loss of consciousness ▽
803.34 Other closed skull fracture with other and unspecified intracranial hemorrhage, prolonged (more than 24 hours) loss of consciousness and return to pre-existing conscious level ▽
803.35 Other closed skull fracture with other and unspecified intracranial hemorrhage, prolonged (more than 24 hours) loss of consciousness, without return to pre-existing conscious level ▽
803.36 Other closed skull fracture with other and unspecified intracranial hemorrhage, loss of consciousness of unspecified duration ▽
803.39 Other closed skull fracture with other and unspecified intracranial hemorrhage, unspecified concussion ▽
852.20 Subdural hemorrhage following injury, without mention of open intracranial wound, unspecified state of consciousness ▽
853.10 Other and unspecified intracranial hemorrhage following injury, with open intracranial wound, unspecified state of consciousness ▽

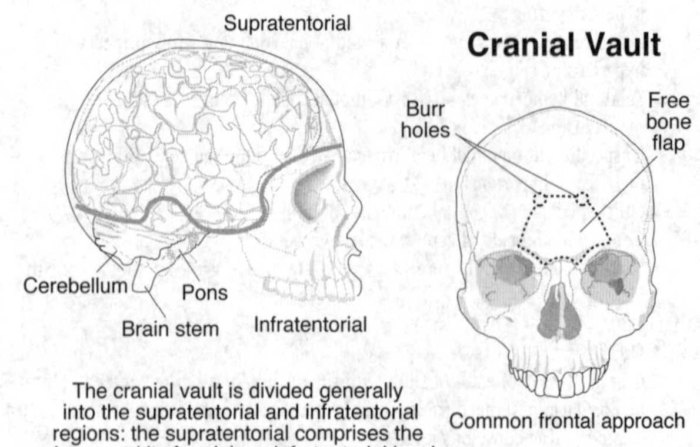

The cranial vault is divided generally into the supratentorial and infratentorial regions: the supratentorial comprises the cerebrum and its four lobes; infratentorial involves the cerebellum and the brain stem

Common frontal approach

▽ Unspecified code ☒ Manifestation code
♀ Female diagnosis ♂ Male diagnosis

ICD-9-CM Procedural

01.24 Other craniotomy
07.51 Exploration of pineal field
07.52 Incision of pineal gland
07.71 Exploration of pituitary fossa
07.72 Incision of pituitary gland

61304–61305

61304 Craniectomy or craniotomy, exploratory; supratentorial
61305 infratentorial (posterior fossa)

ICD-9-CM Diagnostic

191.0 Malignant neoplasm of cerebrum, except lobes and ventricles
191.1 Malignant neoplasm of frontal lobe of brain
191.2 Malignant neoplasm of temporal lobe of brain
191.3 Malignant neoplasm of parietal lobe of brain
191.4 Malignant neoplasm of occipital lobe of brain
191.5 Malignant neoplasm of ventricles of brain
191.6 Malignant neoplasm of cerebellum NOS
191.7 Malignant neoplasm of brain stem
191.8 Malignant neoplasm of other parts of brain
198.3 Secondary malignant neoplasm of brain and spinal cord
225.0 Benign neoplasm of brain
225.1 Benign neoplasm of cranial nerves
225.2 Benign neoplasm of cerebral meninges
239.6 Neoplasm of unspecified nature of brain
239.7 Neoplasm of unspecified nature of endocrine glands and other parts of nervous system
324.0 Intracranial abscess
348.4 Compression of brain
349.81 Cerebrospinal fluid rhinorrhea
388.61 Cerebrospinal fluid otorrhea
430 Subarachnoid hemorrhage — (Use additional code to identify presence of hypertension)
431 Intracerebral hemorrhage — (Use additional code to identify presence of hypertension)
432.0 Nontraumatic extradural hemorrhage — (Use additional code to identify presence of hypertension)
432.1 Subdural hemorrhage — (Use additional code to identify presence of hypertension)
432.9 Unspecified intracranial hemorrhage — (Use additional code to identify presence of hypertension) ▽
437.3 Cerebral aneurysm, nonruptured — (Use additional code to identify presence of hypertension)
767.0 Subdural and cerebral hemorrhage, birth trauma — (Use additional code to identify cause)
784.0 Headache
800.00 Closed fracture of vault of skull without mention of intracranial injury, unspecified state of consciousness ▽
800.01 Closed fracture of vault of skull without mention of intracranial injury, no loss of consciousness
800.02 Closed fracture of vault of skull without mention of intracranial injury, brief (less than one hour) loss of consciousness
800.03 Closed fracture of vault of skull without mention of intracranial injury, moderate (1-24 hours) loss of consciousness
800.04 Closed fracture of vault of skull without mention of intracranial injury, prolonged (more than 24 hours) loss of consciousness and return to pre-existing conscious level
800.05 Closed fracture of vault of skull without mention of intracranial injury, prolonged (more than 24 hours) loss of consciousness, without return to pre-existing conscious level
800.06 Closed fracture of vault of skull without mention of intracranial injury, loss of consciousness of unspecified duration ▽
800.09 Closed fracture of vault of skull without mention of intracranial injury, unspecified concussion ▽
800.10 Closed fracture of vault of skull with cerebral laceration and contusion, unspecified state of consciousness ▽
800.11 Closed fracture of vault of skull with cerebral laceration and contusion, no loss of consciousness
800.12 Closed fracture of vault of skull with cerebral laceration and contusion, brief (less than one hour) loss of consciousness
800.13 Closed fracture of vault of skull with cerebral laceration and contusion, moderate (1-24 hours) loss of consciousness
800.14 Closed fracture of vault of skull with cerebral laceration and contusion, prolonged (more than 24 hours) loss of consciousness and return to pre-existing conscious level
800.15 Closed fracture of vault of skull with cerebral laceration and contusion, prolonged (more than 24 hours) loss of consciousness, without return to pre-existing conscious level
800.16 Closed fracture of vault of skull with cerebral laceration and contusion, loss of consciousness of unspecified duration ▽
800.19 Closed fracture of vault of skull with cerebral laceration and contusion, unspecified concussion ▽
800.20 Closed fracture of vault of skull with subarachnoid, subdural, and extradural hemorrhage, unspecified state of consciousness ▽
800.21 Closed fracture of vault of skull with subarachnoid, subdural, and extradural hemorrhage, no loss of consciousness
800.22 Closed fracture of vault of skull with subarachnoid, subdural, and extradural hemorrhage, brief (less than one hour) loss of consciousness
800.23 Closed fracture of vault of skull with subarachnoid, subdural, and extradural hemorrhage, moderate (1-24 hours) loss of consciousness
800.24 Closed fracture of vault of skull with subarachnoid, subdural, and extradural hemorrhage, prolonged (more than 24 hours) loss of consciousness and return to pre-existing conscious level
800.25 Closed fracture of vault of skull with subarachnoid, subdural, and extradural hemorrhage, prolonged (more than 24 hours) loss of consciousness, without return to pre-existing conscious level
800.26 Closed fracture of vault of skull with subarachnoid, subdural, and extradural hemorrhage, loss of consciousness of unspecified duration ▽
800.29 Closed fracture of vault of skull with subarachnoid, subdural, and extradural hemorrhage, unspecified concussion ▽
800.30 Closed fracture of vault of skull with other and unspecified intracranial hemorrhage, unspecified state of consciousness ▽
800.31 Closed fracture of vault of skull with other and unspecified intracranial hemorrhage, no loss of consciousness ▽
800.32 Closed fracture of vault of skull with other and unspecified intracranial hemorrhage, brief (less than one hour) loss of consciousness ▽
800.33 Closed fracture of vault of skull with other and unspecified intracranial hemorrhage, moderate (1-24 hours) loss of consciousness ▽
800.34 Closed fracture of vault of skull with other and unspecified intracranial hemorrhage, prolonged (more than 24 hours) loss of consciousness and return to pre-existing conscious level ▽
800.35 Closed fracture of vault of skull with other and unspecified intracranial hemorrhage, prolonged (more than 24 hours) loss of consciousness, without return to pre-existing conscious level ▽
800.36 Closed fracture of vault of skull with other and unspecified intracranial hemorrhage, loss of consciousness of unspecified duration ▽
800.40 Closed fracture of vault of skull with intracranial injury of other and unspecified nature, unspecified state of consciousness ▽
800.41 Closed fracture of vault of skull with intracranial injury of other and unspecified nature, no loss of consciousness ▽
800.42 Closed fracture of vault of skull with intracranial injury of other and unspecified nature, brief (less than one hour) loss of consciousness ▽
800.43 Closed fracture of vault of skull with intracranial injury of other and unspecified nature, moderate (1-24 hours) loss of consciousness ▽
800.44 Closed fracture of vault of skull with intracranial injury of other and unspecified nature, prolonged (more than 24 hours) loss of consciousness and return to pre-existing conscious level ▽
800.45 Closed fracture of vault of skull with intracranial injury of other and unspecified nature, prolonged (more than 24 hours) loss of consciousness, without return to pre-existing conscious level ▽
800.46 Closed fracture of vault of skull with intracranial injury of other and unspecified nature, loss of consciousness of unspecified duration ▽
800.49 Closed fracture of vault of skull with intracranial injury of other and unspecified nature, unspecified concussion ▽
800.50 Open fracture of vault of skull without mention of intracranial injury, unspecified state of consciousness ▽
800.51 Open fracture of vault of skull without mention of intracranial injury, no loss of consciousness
800.52 Open fracture of vault of skull without mention of intracranial injury, brief (less than one hour) loss of consciousness
800.53 Open fracture of vault of skull without mention of intracranial injury, moderate (1-24 hours) loss of consciousness
800.54 Open fracture of vault of skull without mention of intracranial injury, prolonged (more than 24 hours) loss of consciousness and return to pre-existing conscious level
800.55 Open fracture of vault of skull without mention of intracranial injury, prolonged (more than 24 hours) loss of consciousness, without return to pre-existing conscious level
800.56 Open fracture of vault of skull without mention of intracranial injury, loss of consciousness of unspecified duration ▽

800.59 Open fracture of vault of skull without mention of intracranial injury, unspecified concussion ▽
800.60 Open fracture of vault of skull with cerebral laceration and contusion, unspecified state of consciousness ▽
800.61 Open fracture of vault of skull with cerebral laceration and contusion, no loss of consciousness
800.62 Open fracture of vault of skull with cerebral laceration and contusion, brief (less than one hour) loss of consciousness
800.63 Open fracture of vault of skull with cerebral laceration and contusion, moderate (1-24 hours) loss of consciousness
800.64 Open fracture of vault of skull with cerebral laceration and contusion, prolonged (more than 24 hours) loss of consciousness and return to pre-existing conscious level
800.65 Open fracture of vault of skull with cerebral laceration and contusion, prolonged (more than 24 hours) loss of consciousness, without return to pre-existing conscious level
800.66 Open fracture of vault of skull with cerebral laceration and contusion, loss of consciousness of unspecified duration ▽
800.69 Open fracture of vault of skull with cerebral laceration and contusion, unspecified concussion ▽
800.70 Open fracture of vault of skull with subarachnoid, subdural, and extradural hemorrhage, unspecified state of consciousness ▽
800.71 Open fracture of vault of skull with subarachnoid, subdural, and extradural hemorrhage, no loss of consciousness
800.72 Open fracture of vault of skull with subarachnoid, subdural, and extradural hemorrhage, brief (less than one hour) loss of consciousness
800.73 Open fracture of vault of skull with subarachnoid, subdural, and extradural hemorrhage, moderate (1-24 hours) loss of consciousness
800.74 Open fracture of vault of skull with subarachnoid, subdural, and extradural hemorrhage, prolonged (more than 24 hours) loss of consciousness and return to pre-existing conscious level
800.75 Open fracture of vault of skull with subarachnoid, subdural, and extradural hemorrhage, prolonged (more than 24 hours) loss of consciousness, without return to pre-existing conscious level
800.76 Open fracture of vault of skull with subarachnoid, subdural, and extradural hemorrhage, loss of consciousness of unspecified duration ▽
800.79 Open fracture of vault of skull with subarachnoid, subdural, and extradural hemorrhage, unspecified concussion ▽
800.80 Open fracture of vault of skull with other and unspecified intracranial hemorrhage, unspecified state of consciousness ▽
800.81 Open fracture of vault of skull with other and unspecified intracranial hemorrhage, no loss of consciousness ▽
800.82 Open fracture of vault of skull with other and unspecified intracranial hemorrhage, brief (less than one hour) loss of consciousness ▽
800.83 Open fracture of vault of skull with other and unspecified intracranial hemorrhage, moderate (1-24 hours) loss of consciousness ▽
800.84 Open fracture of vault of skull with other and unspecified intracranial hemorrhage, prolonged (more than 24 hours) loss of consciousness and return to pre-existing conscious level ▽
800.85 Open fracture of vault of skull with other and unspecified intracranial hemorrhage, prolonged (more than 24 hours) loss of consciousness, without return to pre-existing conscious level ▽
800.86 Open fracture of vault of skull with other and unspecified intracranial hemorrhage, loss of consciousness of unspecified duration ▽
800.89 Open fracture of vault of skull with other and unspecified intracranial hemorrhage, unspecified concussion ▽
800.90 Open fracture of vault of skull with intracranial injury of other and unspecified nature, unspecified state of consciousness ▽
800.91 Open fracture of vault of skull with intracranial injury of other and unspecified nature, no loss of consciousness ▽
800.92 Open fracture of vault of skull with intracranial injury of other and unspecified nature, brief (less than one hour) loss of consciousness ▽
800.93 Open fracture of vault of skull with intracranial injury of other and unspecified nature, moderate (1-24 hours) loss of consciousness ▽
800.94 Open fracture of vault of skull with intracranial injury of other and unspecified nature, prolonged (more than 24 hours) loss of consciousness and return to pre-existing conscious level ▽
800.95 Open fracture of vault of skull with intracranial injury of other and unspecified nature, prolonged (more than 24 hours) loss of consciousness, without return to pre-existing conscious level ▽
800.96 Open fracture of vault of skull with intracranial injury of other and unspecified nature, loss of consciousness of unspecified duration ▽
800.99 Open fracture of vault of skull with intracranial injury of other and unspecified nature, unspecified concussion ▽
801.00 Closed fracture of base of skull without mention of intracranial injury, unspecified state of consciousness ▽
801.01 Closed fracture of base of skull without mention of intracranial injury, no loss of consciousness
801.02 Closed fracture of base of skull without mention of intracranial injury, brief (less than one hour) loss of consciousness
801.03 Closed fracture of base of skull without mention of intracranial injury, moderate (1-24 hours) loss of consciousness
801.04 Closed fracture of base of skull without mention of intracranial injury, prolonged (more than 24 hours) loss of consciousness and return to pre-existing conscious level
801.05 Closed fracture of base of skull without mention of intracranial injury, prolonged (more than 24 hours) loss of consciousness, without return to pre-existing conscious level
801.06 Closed fracture of base of skull without mention of intracranial injury, loss of consciousness of unspecified duration ▽
801.09 Closed fracture of base of skull without mention of intracranial injury, unspecified concussion ▽
801.10 Closed fracture of base of skull with cerebral laceration and contusion, unspecified state of consciousness ▽
801.11 Closed fracture of base of skull with cerebral laceration and contusion, no loss of consciousness
801.12 Closed fracture of base of skull with cerebral laceration and contusion, brief (less than one hour) loss of consciousness
801.13 Closed fracture of base of skull with cerebral laceration and contusion, moderate (1-24 hours) loss of consciousness
801.14 Closed fracture of base of skull with cerebral laceration and contusion, prolonged (more than 24 hours) loss of consciousness and return to pre-existing conscious level
801.15 Closed fracture of base of skull with cerebral laceration and contusion, prolonged (more than 24 hours) loss of consciousness, without return to pre-existing conscious level
801.16 Closed fracture of base of skull with cerebral laceration and contusion, loss of consciousness of unspecified duration ▽
801.19 Closed fracture of base of skull with cerebral laceration and contusion, unspecified concussion ▽
801.20 Closed fracture of base of skull with subarachnoid, subdural, and extradural hemorrhage, unspecified state of consciousness ▽
801.21 Closed fracture of base of skull with subarachnoid, subdural, and extradural hemorrhage, no loss of consciousness
801.22 Closed fracture of base of skull with subarachnoid, subdural, and extradural hemorrhage, brief (less than one hour) loss of consciousness
801.23 Closed fracture of base of skull with subarachnoid, subdural, and extradural hemorrhage, moderate (1-24 hours) loss of consciousness
801.24 Closed fracture of base of skull with subarachnoid, subdural, and extradural hemorrhage, prolonged (more than 24 hours) loss of consciousness and return to pre-existing conscious level
801.25 Closed fracture of base of skull with subarachnoid, subdural, and extradural hemorrhage, prolonged (more than 24 hours) loss of consciousness, without return to pre-existing conscious level
801.26 Closed fracture of base of skull with subarachnoid, subdural, and extradural hemorrhage, loss of consciousness of unspecified duration ▽
801.29 Closed fracture of base of skull with subarachnoid, subdural, and extradural hemorrhage, unspecified concussion ▽
801.30 Closed fracture of base of skull with other and unspecified intracranial hemorrhage, unspecified state of consciousness ▽
801.31 Closed fracture of base of skull with other and unspecified intracranial hemorrhage, no loss of consciousness ▽
801.32 Closed fracture of base of skull with other and unspecified intracranial hemorrhage, brief (less than one hour) loss of consciousness ▽
801.33 Closed fracture of base of skull with other and unspecified intracranial hemorrhage, moderate (1-24 hours) loss of consciousness ▽
801.34 Closed fracture of base of skull with other and unspecified intracranial hemorrhage, prolonged (more than 24 hours) loss of consciousness and return to pre-existing conscious level ▽
801.35 Closed fracture of base of skull with other and unspecified intracranial hemorrhage, prolonged (more than 24 hours) loss of consciousness, without return to pre-existing conscious level ▽
801.36 Closed fracture of base of skull with other and unspecified intracranial hemorrhage, loss of consciousness of unspecified duration ▽
801.39 Closed fracture of base of skull with other and unspecified intracranial hemorrhage, unspecified concussion ▽
801.40 Closed fracture of base of skull with intracranial injury of other and unspecified nature, unspecified state of consciousness ▽
801.41 Closed fracture of base of skull with intracranial injury of other and unspecified nature, no loss of consciousness ▽
801.42 Closed fracture of base of skull with intracranial injury of other and unspecified nature, brief (less than one hour) loss of consciousness ▽

801.43 Closed fracture of base of skull with intracranial injury of other and unspecified nature, moderate (1-24 hours) loss of consciousness
801.44 Closed fracture of base of skull with intracranial injury of other and unspecified nature, prolonged (more than 24 hours) loss of consciousness and return to pre-existing conscious level
801.45 Closed fracture of base of skull with intracranial injury of other and unspecified nature, prolonged (more than 24 hours) loss of consciousness, without return to pre-existing conscious level
801.46 Closed fracture of base of skull with intracranial injury of other and unspecified nature, loss of consciousness of unspecified duration
801.49 Closed fracture of base of skull with intracranial injury of other and unspecified nature, unspecified concussion
801.50 Open fracture of base of skull without mention of intracranial injury, unspecified state of consciousness
801.51 Open fracture of base of skull without mention of intracranial injury, no loss of consciousness
801.52 Open fracture of base of skull without mention of intracranial injury, brief (less than one hour) loss of consciousness
801.53 Open fracture of base of skull without mention of intracranial injury, moderate (1-24 hours) loss of consciousness
801.54 Open fracture of base of skull without mention of intracranial injury, prolonged (more than 24 hours) loss of consciousness and return to pre-existing conscious level
801.55 Open fracture of base of skull without mention of intracranial injury, prolonged (more than 24 hours) loss of consciousness, without return to pre-existing conscious level
801.56 Open fracture of base of skull without mention of intracranial injury, loss of consciousness of unspecified duration
801.59 Open fracture of base of skull without mention of intracranial injury, unspecified concussion
801.60 Open fracture of base of skull with cerebral laceration and contusion, unspecified state of consciousness
801.61 Open fracture of base of skull with cerebral laceration and contusion, no loss of consciousness
801.62 Open fracture of base of skull with cerebral laceration and contusion, brief (less than one hour) loss of consciousness
801.63 Open fracture of base of skull with cerebral laceration and contusion, moderate (1-24 hours) loss of consciousness
801.64 Open fracture of base of skull with cerebral laceration and contusion, prolonged (more than 24 hours) loss of consciousness and return to pre-existing conscious level
801.65 Open fracture of base of skull with cerebral laceration and contusion, prolonged (more than 24 hours) loss of consciousness, without return to pre-existing conscious level
801.66 Open fracture of base of skull with cerebral laceration and contusion, loss of consciousness of unspecified duration
801.69 Open fracture of base of skull with cerebral laceration and contusion, unspecified concussion
801.70 Open fracture of base of skull with subarachnoid, subdural, and extradural hemorrhage, unspecified state of consciousness
801.71 Open fracture of base of skull with subarachnoid, subdural, and extradural hemorrhage, no loss of consciousness
801.72 Open fracture of base of skull with subarachnoid, subdural, and extradural hemorrhage, brief (less than one hour) loss of consciousness
801.73 Open fracture of base of skull with subarachnoid, subdural, and extradural hemorrhage, moderate (1-24 hours) loss of consciousness
801.74 Open fracture of base of skull with subarachnoid, subdural, and extradural hemorrhage, prolonged (more than 24 hours) loss of consciousness and return to pre-existing conscious level
801.75 Open fracture of base of skull with subarachnoid, subdural, and extradural hemorrhage, prolonged (more than 24 hours) loss of consciousness, without return to pre-existing conscious level
801.76 Open fracture of base of skull with subarachnoid, subdural, and extradural hemorrhage, loss of consciousness of unspecified duration
801.79 Open fracture of base of skull with subarachnoid, subdural, and extradural hemorrhage, unspecified concussion
801.80 Open fracture of base of skull with other and unspecified intracranial hemorrhage, unspecified state of consciousness
801.81 Open fracture of base of skull with other and unspecified intracranial hemorrhage, no loss of consciousness
801.82 Open fracture of base of skull with other and unspecified intracranial hemorrhage, brief (less than one hour) loss of consciousness
801.83 Open fracture of base of skull with other and unspecified intracranial hemorrhage, moderate (1-24 hours) loss of consciousness
801.84 Open fracture of base of skull with other and unspecified intracranial hemorrhage, prolonged (more than 24 hours) loss of consciousness and return to pre-existing conscious level
801.85 Open fracture of base of skull with other and unspecified intracranial hemorrhage, prolonged (more than 24 hours) loss of consciousness, without return to pre-existing conscious level
801.86 Open fracture of base of skull with other and unspecified intracranial hemorrhage, loss of consciousness of unspecified duration
801.89 Open fracture of base of skull with other and unspecified intracranial hemorrhage, unspecified concussion
801.90 Open fracture of base of skull with intracranial injury of other and unspecified nature, unspecified state of consciousness
801.91 Open fracture of base of skull with intracranial injury of other and unspecified nature, no loss of consciousness
801.92 Open fracture of base of skull with intracranial injury of other and unspecified nature, brief (less than one hour) loss of consciousness
801.93 Open fracture of base of skull with intracranial injury of other and unspecified nature, moderate (1-24 hours) loss of consciousness
801.94 Open fracture of base of skull with intracranial injury of other and unspecified nature, prolonged (more than 24 hours) loss of consciousness and return to pre-existing conscious level
801.95 Open fracture of base of skull with intracranial injury of other and unspecified nature, prolonged (more than 24 hours) loss of consciousness, without return to pre-existing conscious level
801.96 Open fracture of base of skull with intracranial injury of other and unspecified nature, loss of consciousness of unspecified duration
801.99 Open fracture of base of skull with intracranial injury of other and unspecified nature, unspecified concussion
803.00 Other closed skull fracture without mention of intracranial injury, unspecified state of consciousness
803.01 Other closed skull fracture without mention of intracranial injury, no loss of consciousness
803.02 Other closed skull fracture without mention of intracranial injury, brief (less than one hour) loss of consciousness
803.03 Other closed skull fracture without mention of intracranial injury, moderate (1-24 hours) loss of consciousness
803.04 Other closed skull fracture without mention of intracranial injury, prolonged (more than 24 hours) loss of consciousness and return to pre-existing conscious level
803.05 Other closed skull fracture without mention of intracranial injury, prolonged (more than 24 hours) loss of consciousness, without return to pre-existing conscious level
803.06 Other closed skull fracture without mention of intracranial injury, loss of consciousness of unspecified duration
803.09 Other closed skull fracture without mention of intracranial injury, unspecified concussion
803.10 Other closed skull fracture with cerebral laceration and contusion, unspecified state of consciousness
803.11 Other closed skull fracture with cerebral laceration and contusion, no loss of consciousness
803.12 Other closed skull fracture with cerebral laceration and contusion, brief (less than one hour) loss of consciousness
803.13 Other closed skull fracture with cerebral laceration and contusion, moderate (1-24 hours) loss of consciousness
803.14 Other closed skull fracture with cerebral laceration and contusion, prolonged (more than 24 hours) loss of consciousness and return to pre-existing conscious level
803.15 Other closed skull fracture with cerebral laceration and contusion, prolonged (more than 24 hours) loss of consciousness, without return to pre-existing conscious level
803.16 Other closed skull fracture with cerebral laceration and contusion, loss of consciousness of unspecified duration
803.19 Other closed skull fracture with cerebral laceration and contusion, unspecified concussion
803.20 Other closed skull fracture with subarachnoid, subdural, and extradural hemorrhage, unspecified state of consciousness
803.21 Other closed skull fracture with subarachnoid, subdural, and extradural hemorrhage, no loss of consciousness
803.22 Other closed skull fracture with subarachnoid, subdural, and extradural hemorrhage, brief (less than one hour) loss of consciousness
803.23 Other closed skull fracture with subarachnoid, subdural, and extradural hemorrhage, moderate (1-24 hours) loss of consciousness
803.24 Other closed skull fracture with subarachnoid, subdural, and extradural hemorrhage, prolonged (more than 24 hours) loss of consciousness and return to pre-existing conscious level

803.25 Other closed skull fracture with subarachnoid, subdural, and extradural hemorrhage, prolonged (more than 24 hours) loss of consciousness, without return to pre-existing conscious level
803.26 Other closed skull fracture with subarachnoid, subdural, and extradural hemorrhage, loss of consciousness of unspecified duration ▽
803.29 Other closed skull fracture with subarachnoid, subdural, and extradural hemorrhage, unspecified concussion ▽
803.30 Other closed skull fracture with other and unspecified intracranial hemorrhage, unspecified state of unconsciousness ▽
803.31 Other closed skull fracture with other and unspecified intracranial hemorrhage, no loss of consciousness ▽
803.32 Other closed skull fracture with other and unspecified intracranial hemorrhage, brief (less than one hour) loss of consciousness ▽
803.33 Other closed skull fracture with other and unspecified intracranial hemorrhage, moderate (1-24 hours) loss of consciousness ▽
803.34 Other closed skull fracture with other and unspecified intracranial hemorrhage, prolonged (more than 24 hours) loss of consciousness and return to pre-existing conscious level ▽
803.35 Other closed skull fracture with other and unspecified intracranial hemorrhage, prolonged (more than 24 hours) loss of consciousness, without return to pre-existing conscious level ▽
803.36 Other closed skull fracture with other and unspecified intracranial hemorrhage, loss of consciousness of unspecified duration ▽
803.39 Other closed skull fracture with other and unspecified intracranial hemorrhage, unspecified concussion ▽
803.40 Other closed skull fracture with intracranial injury of other and unspecified nature, unspecified state of consciousness ▽
803.41 Other closed skull fracture with intracranial injury of other and unspecified nature, no loss of consciousness ▽
803.42 Other closed skull fracture with intracranial injury of other and unspecified nature, brief (less than one hour) loss of consciousness ▽
803.43 Other closed skull fracture with intracranial injury of other and unspecified nature, moderate (1-24 hours) loss of consciousness ▽
803.44 Other closed skull fracture with intracranial injury of other and unspecified nature, prolonged (more than 24 hours) loss of consciousness and return to pre-existing conscious level ▽
803.45 Other closed skull fracture with intracranial injury of other and unspecified nature, prolonged (more than 24 hours) loss of consciousness, without return to pre-existing conscious level ▽
803.46 Other closed skull fracture with intracranial injury of other and unspecified nature, loss of consciousness of unspecified duration ▽
803.49 Other closed skull fracture with intracranial injury of other and unspecified nature, unspecified concussion ▽
803.50 Other open skull fracture without mention of injury, state of consciousness unspecified ▽
803.51 Other open skull fracture without mention of intracranial injury, no loss of consciousness
803.52 Other open skull fracture without mention of intracranial injury, brief (less than one hour) loss of consciousness
803.53 Other open skull fracture without mention of intracranial injury, moderate (1-24 hours) loss of consciousness
803.54 Other open skull fracture without mention of intracranial injury, prolonged (more than 24 hours) loss of consciousness and return to pre-existing conscious level
803.55 Other open skull fracture without mention of intracranial injury, prolonged (more than 24 hours) loss of consciousness, without return to pre-existing conscious level
803.56 Other open skull fracture without mention of intracranial injury, loss of consciousness of unspecified duration ▽
803.59 Other open skull fracture without mention of intracranial injury, unspecified concussion ▽
803.60 Other open skull fracture with cerebral laceration and contusion, unspecified state of consciousness ▽
803.61 Other open skull fracture with cerebral laceration and contusion, no loss of consciousness
803.62 Other open skull fracture with cerebral laceration and contusion, brief (less than one hour) loss of consciousness
803.63 Other open skull fracture with cerebral laceration and contusion, moderate (1-24 hours) loss of consciousness
803.64 Other open skull fracture with cerebral laceration and contusion, prolonged (more than 24 hours) loss of consciousness and return to pre-existing conscious level
803.65 Other open skull fracture with cerebral laceration and contusion, prolonged (more than 24 hours) loss of consciousness, without return to pre-existing conscious level
803.66 Other open skull fracture with cerebral laceration and contusion, loss of consciousness of unspecified duration ▽
803.69 Other open skull fracture with cerebral laceration and contusion, unspecified concussion ▽
803.70 Other open skull fracture with subarachnoid, subdural, and extradural hemorrhage, unspecified state of consciousness ▽
803.71 Other open skull fracture with subarachnoid, subdural, and extradural hemorrhage, no loss of consciousness
803.72 Other open skull fracture with subarachnoid, subdural, and extradural hemorrhage, brief (less than one hour) loss of consciousness
803.73 Other open skull fracture with subarachnoid, subdural, and extradural hemorrhage, moderate (1-24 hours) loss of consciousness
803.74 Other open skull fracture with subarachnoid, subdural, and extradural hemorrhage, prolonged (more than 24 hours) loss of consciousness and return to pre-existing conscious level
803.75 Other open skull fracture with subarachnoid, subdural, and extradural hemorrhage, prolonged (more than 24 hours) loss of consciousness, without return to pre-existing conscious level
803.76 Other open skull fracture with subarachnoid, subdural, and extradural hemorrhage, loss of consciousness of unspecified duration ▽
803.79 Other open skull fracture with subarachnoid, subdural, and extradural hemorrhage, unspecified concussion ▽
803.80 Other open skull fracture with other and unspecified intracranial hemorrhage, unspecified state of consciousness ▽
803.81 Other open skull fracture with other and unspecified intracranial hemorrhage, no loss of consciousness ▽
803.82 Other open skull fracture with other and unspecified intracranial hemorrhage, brief (less than one hour) loss of consciousness ▽
803.83 Other open skull fracture with other and unspecified intracranial hemorrhage, moderate (1-24 hours) loss of consciousness ▽
803.84 Other open skull fracture with other and unspecified intracranial hemorrhage, prolonged (more than 24 hours) loss of consciousness and return to pre-existing conscious level ▽
803.85 Other open skull fracture with other and unspecified intracranial hemorrhage, prolonged (more than 24 hours) loss of consciousness, without return to pre-existing conscious level ▽
803.86 Other open skull fracture with other and unspecified intracranial hemorrhage, loss of consciousness of unspecified duration ▽
803.89 Other open skull fracture with other and unspecified intracranial hemorrhage, unspecified concussion ▽
803.90 Other open skull fracture with intracranial injury of other and unspecified nature, unspecified state of consciousness ▽
803.91 Other open skull fracture with intracranial injury of other and unspecified nature, no loss of consciousness ▽
803.92 Other open skull fracture with intracranial injury of other and unspecified nature, brief (less than one hour) loss of consciousness ▽
803.93 Other open skull fracture with intracranial injury of other and unspecified nature, moderate (1-24 hours) loss of consciousness ▽
803.94 Other open skull fracture with intracranial injury of other and unspecified nature, prolonged (more than 24 hours) loss of consciousness and return to pre-existing conscious level ▽
803.95 Other open skull fracture with intracranial injury of other and unspecified nature, prolonged (more than 24 hours) loss of consciousness, without return to pre-existing conscious level ▽
803.96 Other open skull fracture with intracranial injury of other and unspecified nature, loss of consciousness of unspecified duration ▽
803.99 Other open skull fracture with intracranial injury of other and unspecified nature, unspecified concussion ▽
804.00 Closed fractures involving skull or face with other bones, without mention of intracranial injury, unspecified state of consciousness ▽
804.01 Closed fractures involving skull or face with other bones, without mention of intracranial injury, no loss of consciousness
804.02 Closed fractures involving skull or face with other bones, without mention of intracranial injury, brief (less than one hour) loss of consciousness
804.03 Closed fractures involving skull or face with other bones, without mention of intracranial injury, moderate (1-24 hours) loss of consciousness
804.04 Closed fractures involving skull or face with other bones, without mention or intracranial injury, prolonged (more than 24 hours) loss of consciousness and return to pre-existing conscious level
804.05 Closed fractures involving skull of face with other bones, without mention of intracranial injury, prolonged (more than 24 hours) loss of consciousness, without return to pre-existing conscious level
804.06 Closed fractures involving skull of face with other bones, without mention of intracranial injury, loss of consciousness of unspecified duration ▽
804.09 Closed fractures involving skull of face with other bones, without mention of intracranial injury, unspecified concussion ▽

804.10 Closed fractures involving skull or face with other bones, with cerebral laceration and contusion, unspecified state of consciousness

804.11 Closed fractures involving skull or face with other bones, with cerebral laceration and contusion, no loss of consciousness

804.12 Closed fractures involving skull or face with other bones, with cerebral laceration and contusion, brief (less than one hour) loss of consciousness

804.13 Closed fractures involving skull or face with other bones, with cerebral laceration and contusion, moderate (1-24 hours) loss of consciousness

804.14 Closed fractures involving skull or face with other bones, with cerebral laceration and contusion, prolonged (more than 24 hours) loss of consciousness and return to pre-existing conscious level

804.15 Closed fractures involving skull or face with other bones, with cerebral laceration and contusion, prolonged (more than 24 hours) loss of consciousness, without return to pre-existing conscious level

804.16 Closed fractures involving skull or face with other bones, with cerebral laceration and contusion, loss of consciousness of unspecified duration

804.19 Closed fractures involving skull or face with other bones, with cerebral laceration and contusion, unspecified concussion

804.20 Closed fractures involving skull or face with other bones with subarachnoid, subdural, and extradural hemorrhage, unspecified state of consciousness

804.21 Closed fractures involving skull or face with other bones with subarachnoid, subdural, and extradural hemorrhage, no loss of consciousness

804.22 Closed fractures involving skull or face with other bones with subarachnoid, subdural, and extradural hemorrhage, brief (less than one hour) loss of consciousness

804.23 Closed fractures involving skull or face with other bones with subarachnoid, subdural, and extradural hemorrhage, moderate (1-24 hours) loss of consciousness

804.24 Closed fractures involving skull or face with other bones with subarachnoid, subdural, and extradural hemorrhage, prolonged (more than 24 hours) loss of consciousness and return to pre-existing conscious level

804.25 Closed fractures involving skull or face with other bones with subarachnoid, subdural, and extradural hemorrhage, prolonged (more than 24 hours) loss of consciousness, without return to pre-existing conscious level

804.26 Closed fractures involving skull or face with other bones with subarachnoid, subdural, and extradural hemorrhage, loss of consciousness of unspecified duration

804.29 Closed fractures involving skull or face with other bones with subarachnoid, subdural, and extradural hemorrhage, unspecified concussion

804.30 Closed fractures involving skull or face with other bones, with other and unspecified intracranial hemorrhage, unspecified state of consciousness

804.31 Closed fractures involving skull or face with other bones, with other and unspecified intracranial hemorrhage, no loss of consciousness

804.32 Closed fractures involving skull or face with other bones, with other and unspecified intracranial hemorrhage, brief (less than one hour) loss of consciousness

804.33 Closed fractures involving skull or face with other bones, with other and unspecified intracranial hemorrrhage, moderate (1-24 hours) loss of consciousness

804.34 Closed fractures involving skull or face with other bones, with other and unspecified intracranial hemorrhage, prolonged (more than 24 hours) loss of consciousness and return to preexisting conscious level

804.35 Closed fractures involving skull or face with other bones, with other and unspecified intracranial hemorrhage, prolonged (more than 24 hours) loss of consciousness, without return to pre-existing conscious level

804.36 Closed fractures involving skull or face with other bones, with other and unspecified intracranial hemorrhage, loss of consciousness of unspecified duration

804.39 Closed fractures involving skull or face with other bones, with other and unspecified intracranial hemorrhage, unspecified concussion

804.40 Closed fractures involving skull or face with other bones, with intracranial injury of other and unspecified nature, unspecified state of consciousness

804.41 Closed fractures involving skull or face with other bones, with intracranial injury of other and unspecified nature, no loss of consciousness

804.42 Closed fractures involving skull or face with other bones, with intracranial injury of other and unspecified nature, brief (less than one hour) loss of consciousness

804.43 Closed fractures involving skull or face with other bones, with intracranial injury of other and unspecified nature, moderate (1-24 hours) loss of consciousness

804.44 Closed fractures involving skull or face with other bones, with intracranial injury of other and unspecified nature, prolonged (more than 24 hours) loss of consciousness and return to pre-existing conscious level

804.45 Closed fractures involving skull or face with other bones, with intracranial injury of other and unspecified nature, prolonged (more than 24 hours) loss of consciousness, without return to pre-existing conscious level

804.46 Closed fractures involving skull or face with other bones, with intracranial injury of other and unspecified nature, loss of consciousness of unspecified duration

804.49 Closed fractures involving skull or face with other bones, with intracranial injury of other and unspecified nature, unspecified concussion

804.50 Open fractures involving skull or face with other bones, without mention of intracranial injury, unspecified state of consciousness

804.51 Open fractures involving skull or face with other bones, without mention of intracranial injury, no loss of consciousness

804.52 Open fractures involving skull or face with other bones, without mention of intracranial injury, brief (less than one hour) loss of consciousness

804.54 Open fractures involving skull or face with other bones, without mention of intracranial injury, prolonged (more than 24 hours) loss of consciousness and return to pre-existing conscious level

804.55 Open fractures involving skull or face with other bones, without mention of intracranial injury, prolonged (more than 24 hours) loss of consciousness, without return to pre-existing conscious level

804.56 Open fractures involving skull or face with other bones, without mention of intracranial injury, loss of consciousness of unspecified duration

804.59 Open fractures involving skull or face with other bones, without mention of intracranial injury, unspecified concussion

804.60 Open fractures involving skull or face with other bones, with cerebral laceration and contusion, unspecified state of consciousness

804.61 Open fractures involving skull or face with other bones, with cerebral laceration and contusion, no loss of consciousness

804.62 Open fractures involving skull or face with other bones, with cerebral laceration and contusion, brief (less than one hour) loss of consciousness

804.63 Open fractures involving skull or face with other bones, with cerebral laceration and contusion, moderate (1-24 hours) loss of consciousness

804.64 Open fractures involving skull or face with other bones, with cerebral laceration and contusion, prolonged (more than 24 hours) loss of consciousness and return to pre-existing conscious level

804.65 Open fractures involving skull or face with other bones, with cerebral laceration and contusion, prolonged (more than 24 hours) loss of consciousness, without return to pre-existing conscious level

804.66 Open fractures involving skull or face with other bones, with cerebral laceration and contusion, loss of consciousness of unspecified duration

804.69 Open fractures involving skull or face with other bones, with cerebral laceration and contusion, unspecified concussion

804.70 Open fractures involving skull or face with other bones with subarachnoid, subdural, and extradural hemorrhage, unspecified state of consciousness

804.71 Open fractures involving skull or face with other bones with subarachnoid, subdural, and extradural hemorrhage, no loss of consciousness

804.72 Open fractures involving skull or face with other bones with subarachnoid, subdural, and extradural hemorrhage, brief (less than one hour) loss of consciousness

804.73 Open fractures involving skull or face with other bones with subarachnoid, subdural, and extradural hemorrhage, moderate (1-24 hours) loss of consciousness

804.74 Open fractures involving skull or face with other bones with subarachnoid, subdural, and extradural hemorrhage, prolonged (more than 24 hours) loss of consciousness and return to pre-existing conscious level

804.75 Open fractures involving skull or face with other bones with subarachnoid, subdural, and extradural hemorrhage, prolonged (more than 24 hours) loss of consciousness, without return to pre-existing conscious level

804.76 Open fractures involving skull or face with other bones with subarachnoid, subdural, and extradural hemorrhage, loss of consciousness of unspecified duration

804.79 Open fractures involving skull or face with other bones with subarachnoid, subdural, and extradural hemorrhage, unspecified concussion

804.80 Open fractures involving skull or face with other bones, with other and unspecified intracranial hemorrhage, unspecified state of consciousness

804.81 Open fractures involving skull or face with other bones, with other and unspecified intracranial hemorrhage, no loss of consciousness

804.82 Open fractures involving skull or face with other bones, with other and unspecified intracranial hemorrhage, brief (less than one hour) loss of consciousness

804.83 Open fractures involving skull or face with other bones, with other and unspecified intracranial hemorrhage, moderate (1-24 hours) loss of consciousness

804.84 Open fractures involving skull or face with other bones, with other and unspecified intracranial hemorrhage, prolonged (more than 24 hours) loss of consciousness and return to pre-existing conscious level

804.85 Open fractures involving skull or face with other bones, with other and unspecified intracranial hemorrhage, prolonged (more than 24 hours) loss of consciousness, without return to pre-existing conscious level

804.86 Open fractures involving skull or face with other bones, with other and unspecified intracranial hemorrhage, loss of consciousness of unspecified duration
804.89 Open fractures involving skull or face with other bones, with other and unspecified intracranial hemorrhage, unspecified concussion
804.90 Open fractures involving skull or face with other bones, with intracranial injury of other and unspecified nature, unspecified state of consciousness
804.91 Open fractures involving skull or face with other bones, with intracranial injury of other and unspecified nature, no loss of consciousness
804.92 Open fractures involving skull or face with other bones, with intracranial injury of other and unspecified nature, brief (less than one hour) loss of consciousness
804.93 Open fractures involving skull or face with other bones, with intracranial injury of other and unspecified nature, moderate (1-24 hours) loss of consciousness
804.94 Open fractures involving skull or face with other bones, with intracranial injury of other and unspecified nature, prolonged (more than 24 hours) loss of consciousness and return to pre-existing conscious level
804.95 Open fractures involving skull or face with other bones, with intracranial injury of other and unspecified nature, prolonged (more than 24 hours) loss of consciousness, without return to pre-existing level
804.96 Open fractures involving skull or face with other bones, with intracranial injury of other and unspecified nature, loss of consciousness of unspecified duration
804.99 Open fractures involving skull or face with other bones, with intracranial injury of other and unspecified nature, unspecified concussion
854.05 Intracranial injury of other and unspecified nature, without mention of open intracranial wound, prolonged (more than 24 hours) loss of consciousness, without return to pre-existing conscious level
854.06 Intracranial injury of other and unspecified nature, without mention of open intracranial wound, loss of consciousness of unspecified duration
854.09 Intracranial injury of other and unspecified nature, without mention of open intracranial wound, unspecified concussion
854.10 Intracranial injury of other and unspecified nature, with open intracranial wound, unspecified state of consciousness
854.11 Intracranial injury of other and unspecified nature, with open intracranial wound, no loss of consciousness
854.12 Intracranial injury of other and unspecified nature, with open intracranial wound, brief (less than 1 hour) loss of consciousness
854.13 Intracranial injury of other and unspecified nature, with open intracranial wound, moderate (1-24 hours) loss of consciousness
854.14 Intracranial injury of other and unspecified nature, with open intracranial wound, prolonged (more than 24 hours) loss of consciousness and return to pre-existing conscious level
854.15 Intracranial injury of other and unspecified nature, with open intracranial wound, prolonged (more than 24 hours) loss of consciousness, without return to pre-existing conscious level
854.16 Intracranial injury of other and unspecified nature, with open intracranial wound, loss of consciousness of unspecified duration
854.19 Intracranial injury of other and unspecified nature, with open intracranial wound, with unspecified concussion

ICD-9-CM Procedural

01.24 Other craniotomy
01.25 Other craniectomy
07.51 Exploration of pineal field
07.52 Incision of pineal gland
07.71 Exploration of pituitary fossa
07.72 Incision of pituitary gland

61312–61313

61312 Craniectomy or craniotomy for evacuation of hematoma, supratentorial; extradural or subdural
61313 intracerebral

ICD-9-CM Diagnostic

348.4 Compression of brain
431 Intracerebral hemorrhage — (Use additional code to identify presence of hypertension)
432.0 Nontraumatic extradural hemorrhage — (Use additional code to identify presence of hypertension)
432.1 Subdural hemorrhage — (Use additional code to identify presence of hypertension)
432.9 Unspecified intracranial hemorrhage — (Use additional code to identify presence of hypertension)
747.81 Congenital anomaly of cerebrovascular system
800.20 Closed fracture of vault of skull with subarachnoid, subdural, and extradural hemorrhage, unspecified state of consciousness
800.21 Closed fracture of vault of skull with subarachnoid, subdural, and extradural hemorrhage, no loss of consciousness
800.22 Closed fracture of vault of skull with subarachnoid, subdural, and extradural hemorrhage, brief (less than one hour) loss of consciousness
800.23 Closed fracture of vault of skull with subarachnoid, subdural, and extradural hemorrhage, moderate (1-24 hours) loss of consciousness
800.24 Closed fracture of vault of skull with subarachnoid, subdural, and extradural hemorrhage, prolonged (more than 24 hours) loss of consciousness and return to pre-existing conscious level
800.25 Closed fracture of vault of skull with subarachnoid, subdural, and extradural hemorrhage, prolonged (more than 24 hours) loss of consciousness, without return to pre-existing conscious level
800.26 Closed fracture of vault of skull with subarachnoid, subdural, and extradural hemorrhage, loss of consciousness of unspecified duration
800.29 Closed fracture of vault of skull with subarachnoid, subdural, and extradural hemorrhage, unspecified concussion
800.30 Closed fracture of vault of skull with other and unspecified intracranial hemorrhage, unspecified state of consciousness
800.70 Open fracture of vault of skull with subarachnoid, subdural, and extradural hemorrhage, unspecified state of consciousness
800.71 Open fracture of vault of skull with subarachnoid, subdural, and extradural hemorrhage, no loss of consciousness
800.72 Open fracture of vault of skull with subarachnoid, subdural, and extradural hemorrhage, brief (less than one hour) loss of consciousness
800.73 Open fracture of vault of skull with subarachnoid, subdural, and extradural hemorrhage, moderate (1-24 hours) loss of consciousness
800.74 Open fracture of vault of skull with subarachnoid, subdural, and extradural hemorrhage, prolonged (more than 24 hours) loss of consciousness and return to pre-existing conscious level
800.75 Open fracture of vault of skull with subarachnoid, subdural, and extradural hemorrhage, prolonged (more than 24 hours) loss of consciousness, without return to pre-existing conscious level
800.76 Open fracture of vault of skull with subarachnoid, subdural, and extradural hemorrhage, loss of consciousness of unspecified duration
800.79 Open fracture of vault of skull with subarachnoid, subdural, and extradural hemorrhage, unspecified concussion
851.00 Cortex (cerebral) contusion without mention of open intracranial wound, state of consciousness unspecified
851.02 Cortex (cerebral) contusion without mention of open intracranial wound, brief (less than 1 hour) loss of consciousness
851.03 Cortex (cerebral) contusion without mention of open intracranial wound, moderate (1-24 hours) loss of consciousness
851.04 Cortex (cerebral) contusion without mention of open intracranial wound, prolonged (more than 24 hours) loss of consciousness and return to pre-exisiting conscious level
851.05 Cortex (cerebral) contusion without mention of open intracranial wound, prolonged (more than 24 hours) loss of consciousness, without return to pre-existing conscious level
851.06 Cortex (cerebral) contusion without mention of open intracranial wound, loss of consciousness of unspecified duration
851.09 Cortex (cerebral) contusion without mention of open intracranial wound, unspecified concussion
851.80 Other and unspecified cerebral laceration and contusion, without mention of open intracranial wound, unspecified state of consciousness
851.81 Other and unspecified cerebral laceration and contusion, without mention of open intracranial wound, no loss of consciousness
851.82 Other and unspecified cerebral laceration and contusion, without mention of open intracranial wound, brief (less than 1 hour) loss of consciousness
851.83 Other and unspecified cerebral laceration and contusion, without mention of open intracranial wound, moderate (1-24 hours) loss of consciousness
851.84 Other and unspecified cerebral laceration and contusion, without mention of open intracranial wound, prolonged (more than 24 hours) loss of consciousness and return to preexisting conscious level
851.85 Other and unspecified cerebral laceration and contusion, without mention of open intracranial wound, prolonged (more than 24 hours) loss of consciousness, without return to pre-existing conscious level
851.86 Other and unspecified cerebral laceration and contusion, without mention of open intracranial wound, loss of consciousness of unspecified duration
851.89 Other and unspecified cerebral laceration and contusion, without mention of open intracranial wound, unspecified concussion
852.20 Subdural hemorrhage following injury, without mention of open intracranial wound, unspecified state of consciousness
852.21 Subdural hemorrhage following injury, without mention of open intracranial wound, no loss of consciousness

Unspecified code
Female diagnosis
Manifestation code
Male diagnosis

852.22 Subdural hemorrhage following injury, without mention of open intracranial wound, brief (less than one hour) loss of consciousness
852.23 Subdural hemorrhage following injury, without mention of open intracranial wound, moderate (1-24 hours) loss of consciousness
852.24 Subdural hemorrhage following injury, without mention of open intracranial wound, prolonged (more than 24 hours) loss of consciousness and return to pre-existing conscious level
852.25 Subdural hemorrhage following injury, without mention of open intracranial wound, prolonged (more than 24 hours) loss of consciousness, without return to pre-existing conscious level
852.26 Subdural hemorrhage following injury, without mention of open intracranial wound, loss of consciousness of unspecified duration
852.29 Subdural hemorrhage following injury, without mention of open intracranial wound, unspecified concussion
852.40 Extradural hemorrhage following injury, without mention of open intracranial wound, unspecified state of consciousness
852.41 Extradural hemorrhage following injury, without mention of open intracranial wound, no loss of consciousness
852.42 Extradural hemorrhage following injury, without mention of open intracranial wound, brief (less than 1 hour) loss of consciousness
852.43 Extradural hemorrhage following injury, without mention of open intracranial wound, moderate (1-24 hours) loss of consciousness
852.44 Extradural hemorrhage following injury, without mention of open intracranial wound, prolonged (more than 24 hours) loss of consciousness and return to pre-existing conscious level
852.45 Extradural hemorrhage following injury, without mention of open intracranial wound, prolonged (more than 24 hours) loss of consciousness, without return to pre-existing conscious level
852.46 Extradural hemorrhage following injury, without mention of open intracranial wound, loss of consciousness of unspecified duration
852.49 Extradural hemorrhage following injury, without mention of open intracranial wound, unspecified concussion
853.00 Other and unspecified intracranial hemorrhage following injury, without mention of open intracranial wound, unspecified state of consciousness
853.01 Other and unspecified intracranial hemorrhage following injury, without mention of open intracranial wound, no loss of consciousness
853.02 Other and unspecified intracranial hemorrhage following injury, without mention of open intracranial wound, brief (less than 1 hour) loss of consciousness
853.03 Other and unspecified intracranial hemorrhage following injury, without mention of open intracranial wound, moderate (1-24 hours) loss of consciousness
853.04 Other and unspecified intracranial hemorrhage following injury, without mention of open intracranial wound, prolonged (more than 24 hours) loss of consciousness and return to preexisting conscious level
853.05 Other and unspecified intracranial hemorrhage following injury. Without mention of open intracranial wound, prolonged (more than 24 hours) loss of consciousness, without return to pre-existing conscious level
853.06 Other and unspecified intracranial hemorrhage following injury, without mention of open intracranial wound, loss of consciousness of unspecified duration
853.09 Other and unspecified intracranial hemorrhage following injury, without mention of open intracranial wound, unspecified concussion
853.10 Other and unspecified intracranial hemorrhage following injury, with open intracranial wound, unspecified state of consciousness
853.11 Other and unspecified intracranial hemorrhage following injury, with open intracranial wound, no loss of consciousness
853.12 Other and unspecified intracranial hemorrhage following injury, with open intracranial wound, brief (less than 1 hour) loss of consciousness
853.13 Other and unspecified intracranial hemorrhage following injury, with open intracranial wound, moderate (1-24 hours) loss of consciousness
853.14 Other and unspecified intracranial hemorrhage following injury, with open intracranial wound, prolonged (more than 24 hours) loss of consciousness and return to pre-existing conscious level
853.15 Other and unspecified intracranial hemorrhage following injury, with open intracranial wound, prolonged (more than 24 hours) loss of consciousness, without return to pre-existing conscious level
853.16 Other and unspecified intracranial hemorrhage following injury, with open intracranial wound, loss of consciousness of unspecified duration
853.19 Other and unspecified intracranial hemorrhage following injury, with open intracranial wound, unspecified concussion

ICD-9-CM Procedural

01.24 Other craniotomy
01.31 Incision of cerebral meninges
01.39 Other incision of brain

61314–61315

61314 Craniectomy or craniotomy for evacuation of hematoma, infratentorial; extradural or subdural
61315 intracerebellar

ICD-9-CM Diagnostic

348.4 Compression of brain
431 Intracerebral hemorrhage — (Use additional code to identify presence of hypertension)
432.0 Nontraumatic extradural hemorrhage — (Use additional code to identify presence of hypertension)
432.1 Subdural hemorrhage — (Use additional code to identify presence of hypertension)
432.9 Unspecified intracranial hemorrhage — (Use additional code to identify presence of hypertension)
747.81 Congenital anomaly of cerebrovascular system
801.20 Closed fracture of base of skull with subarachnoid, subdural, and extradural hemorrhage, unspecified state of consciousness
801.21 Closed fracture of base of skull with subarachnoid, subdural, and extradural hemorrhage, no loss of consciousness
801.22 Closed fracture of base of skull with subarachnoid, subdural, and extradural hemorrhage, brief (less than one hour) loss of consciousness
801.23 Closed fracture of base of skull with subarachnoid, subdural, and extradural hemorrhage, moderate (1-24 hours) loss of consciousness
801.24 Closed fracture of base of skull with subarachnoid, subdural, and extradural hemorrhage, prolonged (more than 24 hours) loss of consciousness and return to pre-existing conscious level
801.25 Closed fracture of base of skull with subarachnoid, subdural, and extradural hemorrhage, prolonged (more than 24 hours) loss of consciousness, without return to pre-existing conscious level
801.26 Closed fracture of base of skull with subarachnoid, subdural, and extradural hemorrhage, loss of consciousness of unspecified duration
801.29 Closed fracture of base of skull with subarachnoid, subdural, and extradural hemorrhage, unspecified concussion
801.70 Open fracture of base of skull with subarachnoid, subdural, and extradural hemorrhage, unspecified state of consciousness
801.72 Open fracture of base of skull with subarachnoid, subdural, and extradural hemorrhage, brief (less than one hour) loss of consciousness
801.73 Open fracture of base of skull with subarachnoid, subdural, and extradural hemorrhage, moderate (1-24 hours) loss of consciousness
801.74 Open fracture of base of skull with subarachnoid, subdural, and extradural hemorrhage, prolonged (more than 24 hours) loss of consciousness and return to pre-existing conscious level
801.75 Open fracture of base of skull with subarachnoid, subdural, and extradural hemorrhage, prolonged (more than 24 hours) loss of consciousness, without return to pre-existing conscious level
801.76 Open fracture of base of skull with subarachnoid, subdural, and extradural hemorrhage, loss of consciousness of unspecified duration
801.79 Open fracture of base of skull with subarachnoid, subdural, and extradural hemorrhage, unspecified concussion
851.03 Cortex (cerebral) contusion without mention of open intracranial wound, moderate (1-24 hours) loss of consciousness
851.40 Cerebellar or brain stem contusion without mention of open intracranial wound, unspecified state of consciousness
851.41 Cerebellar or brain stem contusion without mention of open intracranial wound, no loss of consciousness
851.42 Cerebellar or brain stem contusion without mention of open intracranial wound, brief (less than 1 hour) loss of consciousness
851.43 Cerebellar or brain stem contusion without mention of open intracranial wound, moderate (1-24 hours) loss of consciousness
851.44 Cerebellar or brain stem contusion without mention of open intracranial wound, prolonged (more than 24 hours) loss consciousness and return to pre-existing conscious level
851.45 Cerebellar or brain stem contusion without mention of open intracranial wound, prolonged (more than 24 hours) loss of consciousness, without return to pre-existing conscious level
851.46 Cerebellar or brain stem contusion without mention of open intracranial wound, loss of consciousness of unspecified duration
851.49 Cerebellar or brain stem contusion without mention of open intracranial wound, unspecified concussion
851.50 Cerebellar or brain stem contusion with open intracranial wound, unspecified state of consciousness
851.51 Cerebellar or brain stem contusion with open intracranial wound, no loss of consciousness
851.52 Cerebellar or brain stem contusion with open intracranial wound, brief (less than 1 hour) loss of consciousness

851.53 Cerebellar or brain stem contusion with open intracranial wound, moderate (1-24 hours) loss of consciousness
851.54 Cerebellar or brain stem contusion with open intracranial wound, prolonged (more than 24 hours) loss of consciousness and return to pre-existing conscious level
851.55 Cerebellar or brain stem contusion with open intracranial wound, prolonged (more than 24 hours) loss of consciousness, without return to pre-existing conscious level
851.56 Cerebellar or brain stem contusion with open intracranial wound, loss of consciousness of unspecified duration
851.59 Cerebellar or brain stem contusion with open intracranial wound, unspecified concussion
852.20 Subdural hemorrhage following injury, without mention of open intracranial wound, unspecified state of consciousness
852.21 Subdural hemorrhage following injury, without mention of open intracranial wound, no loss of consciousness
852.22 Subdural hemorrhage following injury, without mention of open intracranial wound, brief (less than one hour) loss of consciousness
852.23 Subdural hemorrhage following injury, without mention of open intracranial wound, moderate (1-24 hours) loss of consciousness
852.24 Subdural hemorrhage following injury, without mention of open intracranial wound, prolonged (more than 24 hours) loss of consciousness and return to pre-existing conscious level
852.25 Subdural hemorrhage following injury, without mention of open intracranial wound, prolonged (more than 24 hours) loss of consciousness, without return to pre-existing conscious level
852.26 Subdural hemorrhage following injury, without mention of open intracranial wound, loss of consciousness of unspecified duration
852.29 Subdural hemorrhage following injury, without mention of open intracranial wound, unspecified concussion
852.30 Subdural hemorrhage following injury, with open intracranial wound, state of consciousness unspecified
852.31 Subdural hemorrhage following injury, with open intracranial wound, no loss of consciousness
852.32 Subdural hemorrhage following injury, with open intracranial wound, brief (less than 1 hour) loss of consciousness
852.33 Subdural hemorrhage following injury, with open intracranial wound, moderate (1-24 hours) loss of consciousness
852.34 Subdural hemorrhage following injury, with open intracranial wound, prolonged (more than 24 hours) loss of consciousness and return to pre-existing conscious level
852.35 Subdural hemorrhage following injury, with open intracranial wound, prolonged (more than 24 hours) loss of consciousness, without return to pre-existing conscious level
852.36 Subdural hemorrhage following injury, with open intracranial wound, loss of consciousness of unspecified duration
852.39 Subdural hemorrhage following injury, with open intracranial wound, unspecified concussion
852.40 Extradural hemorrhage following injury, without mention of open intracranial wound, unspecified state of consciousness
852.41 Extradural hemorrhage following injury, without mention of open intracranial wound, no loss of consciousness
852.42 Extradural hemorrhage following injury, without mention of open intracranial wound, brief (less than 1 hour) loss of consciousness
852.43 Extradural hemorrhage following injury, without mention of open intracranial wound, moderate (1-24 hours) loss of consciousness
852.44 Extradural hemorrhage following injury, without mention of open intracranial wound, prolonged (more than 24 hours) loss of consciousness and return to pre-existing conscious level
852.45 Extradural hemorrhage following injury, without mention of open intracranial wound, prolonged (more than 24 hours) loss of consciousness, without return to pre-existing conscious level
852.46 Extradural hemorrhage following injury, without mention of open intracranial wound, loss of consciousness of unspecified duration
852.49 Extradural hemorrhage following injury, without mention of open intracranial wound, unspecified concussion
852.50 Extradural hemorrhage following injury, with open intracranial wound, state of consciousness unspecified
852.51 Extradural hemorrhage following injury, with open intracranial wound, no loss of consciousness
852.52 Extradural hemorrhage following injury, with open intracranial wound, brief (less than 1 hour) loss of consciousness
852.53 Extradural hemorrhage following injury, with open intracranial wound, moderate (1-24 hours) loss of consciousness
852.54 Extradural hemorrhage following injury, with open intracranial wound, prolonged (more than 24 hours) loss of consciousness and return to pre-existing conscious level
852.55 Extradural hemorrhage following injury, with open intracranial wound, prolonged (more than 24 hours) loss of consciousness, without return to pre-existing conscious level
852.56 Extradural hemorrhage following injury, with open intracranial wound, loss of consciousness of unspecified duration
852.59 Extradural hemorrhage following injury, with open intracranial wound, unspecifiedconcussion
853.00 Other and unspecified intracranial hemorrhage following injury, without mention of open intracranial wound, unspecified state of consciousness
853.10 Other and unspecified intracranial hemorrhage following injury, with open intracranial wound, unspecified state of consciousness

ICD-9-CM Procedural

01.24 Other craniotomy
01.31 Incision of cerebral meninges
01.39 Other incision of brain

61316

61316 Incision and subcutaneous placement of cranial bone graft (List separately in addition to code for primary procedure)

ICD-9-CM Diagnostic

This is an add-on code. Refer to the corresponding primary procedure code for ICD-9 diagnosis code links.

ICD-9-CM Procedural

02.03 Formation of cranial bone flap

HCPCS Level II Supplies & Services

The HCPCS Level II code(s) would be the same as the actual procedure performed because these are in-addition-to codes.

61320–61321

61320 Craniectomy or craniotomy, drainage of intracranial abscess; supratentorial
61321 infratentorial

ICD-9-CM Diagnostic

324.0 Intracranial abscess
324.9 Intracranial and intraspinal abscess of unspecified site
998.59 Other postoperative infection — (Use additional code to identify infection)

ICD-9-CM Procedural

01.24 Other craniotomy
01.31 Incision of cerebral meninges
01.39 Other incision of brain

61322–61323

61322 Craniectomy or craniotomy, decompressive, with or without duraplasty, for treatment of intracranial hypertension, without evacuation of associated intraparenchymal hematoma; without lobectomy
61323 with lobectomy

ICD-9-CM Diagnostic

191.0 Malignant neoplasm of cerebrum, except lobes and ventricles
191.1 Malignant neoplasm of frontal lobe of brain
191.2 Malignant neoplasm of temporal lobe of brain
191.3 Malignant neoplasm of parietal lobe of brain
191.4 Malignant neoplasm of occipital lobe of brain
191.5 Malignant neoplasm of ventricles of brain
191.9 Malignant neoplasm of brain, unspecified site
225.0 Benign neoplasm of brain
227.3 Benign neoplasm of pituitary gland and craniopharyngeal duct (pouch) — (Use additional code to identify any functional activity)
237.5 Neoplasm of uncertain behavior of brain and spinal cord
239.6 Neoplasm of unspecified nature of brain
323.0 Encephalitis in viral diseases classified elsewhere — (Code first underlying disease: 073.7, 075, 078.3)
324.0 Intracranial abscess
331.3 Communicating hydrocephalus
331.4 Obstructive hydrocephalus
348.2 Benign intracranial hypertension
348.30 Encephalopathy, unspecified
348.4 Compression of brain

Unspecified code
Female diagnosis
Manifestation code
Male diagnosis

348.5 Cerebral edema
348.9 Unspecified condition of brain ▽
430 Subarachnoid hemorrhage — (Use additional code to identify presence of hypertension)
431 Intracerebral hemorrhage — (Use additional code to identify presence of hypertension)
432.0 Nontraumatic extradural hemorrhage — (Use additional code to identify presence of hypertension)
432.1 Subdural hemorrhage — (Use additional code to identify presence of hypertension)
432.9 Unspecified intracranial hemorrhage — (Use additional code to identify presence of hypertension) ▽
741.00 Spina bifida with hydrocephalus, unspecified region ▽
742.3 Congenital hydrocephalus
800.10 Closed fracture of vault of skull with cerebral laceration and contusion, unspecified state of consciousness ▽
800.11 Closed fracture of vault of skull with cerebral laceration and contusion, no loss of consciousness
800.12 Closed fracture of vault of skull with cerebral laceration and contusion, brief (less than one hour) loss of consciousness
800.13 Closed fracture of vault of skull with cerebral laceration and contusion, moderate (1-24 hours) loss of consciousness
800.14 Closed fracture of vault of skull with cerebral laceration and contusion, prolonged (more than 24 hours) loss of consciousness and return to pre-existing conscious level
800.15 Closed fracture of vault of skull with cerebral laceration and contusion, prolonged (more than 24 hours) loss of consciousness, without return to pre-existing conscious level
800.16 Closed fracture of vault of skull with cerebral laceration and contusion, loss of consciousness of unspecified duration ▽
800.19 Closed fracture of vault of skull with cerebral laceration and contusion, unspecified concussion ▽
800.20 Closed fracture of vault of skull with subarachnoid, subdural, and extradural hemorrhage, unspecified state of consciousness ▽
800.21 Closed fracture of vault of skull with subarachnoid, subdural, and extradural hemorrhage, no loss of consciousness
800.22 Closed fracture of vault of skull with subarachnoid, subdural, and extradural hemorrhage, brief (less than one hour) loss of consciousness
800.23 Closed fracture of vault of skull with subarachnoid, subdural, and extradural hemorrhage, moderate (1-24 hours) loss of consciousness
800.24 Closed fracture of vault of skull with subarachnoid, subdural, and extradural hemorrhage, prolonged (more than 24 hours) loss of consciousness and return to pre-existing conscious level
800.25 Closed fracture of vault of skull with subarachnoid, subdural, and extradural hemorrhage, prolonged (more than 24 hours) loss of consciousness, without return to pre-existing conscious level
800.26 Closed fracture of vault of skull with subarachnoid, subdural, and extradural hemorrhage, loss of consciousness of unspecified duration ▽
800.29 Closed fracture of vault of skull with subarachnoid, subdural, and extradural hemorrhage, unspecified concussion ▽
800.30 Closed fracture of vault of skull with other and unspecified intracranial hemorrhage, unspecified state of consciousness ▽
800.31 Closed fracture of vault of skull with other and unspecified intracranial hemorrhage, no loss of consciousness ▽
800.32 Closed fracture of vault of skull with other and unspecified intracranial hemorrhage, brief (less than one hour) loss of consciousness ▽
800.33 Closed fracture of vault of skull with other and unspecified intracranial hemorrhage, moderate (1-24 hours) loss of consciousness ▽
800.34 Closed fracture of vault of skull with other and unspecified intracranial hemorrhage, prolonged (more than 24 hours) loss of consciousness and return to pre-existing conscious level ▽
800.35 Closed fracture of vault of skull with other and unspecified intracranial hemorrhage, prolonged (more than 24 hours) loss of consciousness, without return to pre-existing conscious level ▽
800.36 Closed fracture of vault of skull with other and unspecified intracranial hemorrhage, loss of consciousness of unspecified duration ▽
800.39 Closed fracture of vault of skull with other and unspecified intracranial hemorrhage, unspecified concussion ▽
801.10 Closed fracture of base of skull with cerebral laceration and contusion, unspecified state of consciousness ▽
801.11 Closed fracture of base of skull with cerebral laceration and contusion, no loss of consciousness
801.12 Closed fracture of base of skull with cerebral laceration and contusion, brief (less than one hour) loss of consciousness
801.13 Closed fracture of base of skull with cerebral laceration and contusion, moderate (1-24 hours) loss of consciousness
801.14 Closed fracture of base of skull with cerebral laceration and contusion, prolonged (more than 24 hours) loss of consciousness and return to pre-existing conscious level
801.15 Closed fracture of base of skull with cerebral laceration and contusion, prolonged (more than 24 hours) loss of consciousness, without return to pre-existing conscious level
801.16 Closed fracture of base of skull with cerebral laceration and contusion, loss of consciousness of unspecified duration ▽
801.19 Closed fracture of base of skull with cerebral laceration and contusion, unspecified concussion ▽
801.20 Closed fracture of base of skull with subarachnoid, subdural, and extradural hemorrhage, unspecified state of consciousness ▽
801.21 Closed fracture of base of skull with subarachnoid, subdural, and extradural hemorrhage, no loss of consciousness
801.22 Closed fracture of base of skull with subarachnoid, subdural, and extradural hemorrhage, brief (less than one hour) loss of consciousness
801.23 Closed fracture of base of skull with subarachnoid, subdural, and extradural hemorrhage, moderate (1-24 hours) loss of consciousness
801.24 Closed fracture of base of skull with subarachnoid, subdural, and extradural hemorrhage, prolonged (more than 24 hours) loss of consciousness and return to pre-existing conscious level
801.25 Closed fracture of base of skull with subarachnoid, subdural, and extradural hemorrhage, prolonged (more than 24 hours) loss of consciousness, without return to pre-existing conscious level
801.26 Closed fracture of base of skull with subarachnoid, subdural, and extradural hemorrhage, loss of consciousness of unspecified duration ▽
801.29 Closed fracture of base of skull with subarachnoid, subdural, and extradural hemorrhage, unspecified concussion ▽
801.30 Closed fracture of base of skull with other and unspecified intracranial hemorrhage, unspecified state of consciousness ▽
801.31 Closed fracture of base of skull with other and unspecified intracranial hemorrhage, no loss of consciousness ▽
801.32 Closed fracture of base of skull with other and unspecified intracranial hemorrhage, brief (less than one hour) loss of consciousness ▽
801.33 Closed fracture of base of skull with other and unspecified intracranial hemorrhage, moderate (1-24 hours) loss of consciousness ▽
801.34 Closed fracture of base of skull with other and unspecified intracranial hemorrhage, prolonged (more than 24 hours) loss of consciousness and return to pre-existing conscious level ▽
801.35 Closed fracture of base of skull with other and unspecified intracranial hemorrhage, prolonged (more than 24 hours) loss of consciousness, without return to pre-existing conscious level ▽
801.36 Closed fracture of base of skull with other and unspecified intracranial hemorrhage, loss of consciousness of unspecified duration ▽
801.39 Closed fracture of base of skull with other and unspecified intracranial hemorrhage, unspecified concussion ▽
851.00 Cortex (cerebral) contusion without mention of open intracranial wound, state of consciousness unspecified ▽
851.01 Cortex (cerebral) contusion without mention of open intracranial wound, no loss of consciousness
851.02 Cortex (cerebral) contusion without mention of open intracranial wound, brief (less than 1 hour) loss of consciousness
851.03 Cortex (cerebral) contusion without mention of open intracranial wound, moderate (1-24 hours) loss of consciousness
851.04 Cortex (cerebral) contusion without mention of open intracranial wound, prolonged (more than 24 hours) loss of consciousness and return to pre-exisiting conscious level
851.05 Cortex (cerebral) contusion without mention of open intracranial wound, prolonged (more than 24 hours) loss of consciousness, without return to pre-existing conscious level
851.06 Cortex (cerebral) contusion without mention of open intracranial wound, loss of consciousness of unspecified duration ▽
851.09 Cortex (cerebral) contusion without mention of open intracranial wound, unspecified concussion ▽
851.40 Cerebellar or brain stem contusion without mention of open intracranial wound, unspecified state of consciousness ▽
851.41 Cerebellar or brain stem contusion without mention of open intracranial wound, no loss of consciousness
851.42 Cerebellar or brain stem contusion without mention of open intracranial wound, brief (less than 1 hour) loss of consciousness
851.43 Cerebellar or brain stem contusion without mention of open intracranial wound, moderate (1-24 hours) loss of consciousness
851.44 Cerebellar or brain stem contusion without mention of open intracranial wound, prolonged (more than 24 hours) loss consciousness and return to pre-existing conscious level

851.45 Cerebellar or brain stem contusion without mention of open intracranial wound, prolonged (more than 24 hours) loss of consciousness, without return to pre-existing conscious level
851.46 Cerebellar or brain stem contusion without mention of open intracranial wound, loss of consciousness of unspecified duration
851.49 Cerebellar or brain stem contusion without mention of open intracranial wound, unspecified concussion
852.00 Subarachnoid hemorrhage following injury, without mention of open intracranial wound, unspecified state of consciousness
852.01 Subarachnoid hemorrhage following injury, without mention of open intracranial wound, no loss of consciousness
852.02 Subarachnoid hemorrhage following injury, without mention of open intracranial wound, brief (less than 1 hour) loss of consciousness
852.03 Subarachnoid hemorrhage following injury, without mention of open intracranial wound, moderate (1-24 hours) loss of consciousness
852.04 Subarachnoid hemorrhage following injury, without mention of open intracranial wound, prolonged (more than 24 hours) loss of consciousness and return to pre-existing conscious level
852.05 Subarachnoid hemorrhage following injury, without mention of open intracranial wound, prolonged (more than 24 hours) loss of consciousness, without return to pre-existing conscious level
852.06 Subarachnoid hemorrhage following injury, without mention of open intracranial wound, loss of consciousness of unspecified duration
852.09 Subarachnoid hemorrhage following injury, without mention of open intracranial wound, unspecified concussion
852.20 Subdural hemorrhage following injury, without mention of open intracranial wound, unspecified state of consciousness
852.21 Subdural hemorrhage following injury, without mention of open intracranial wound, no loss of consciousness
852.22 Subdural hemorrhage following injury, without mention of open intracranial wound, brief (less than one hour) loss of consciousness
852.23 Subdural hemorrhage following injury, without mention of open intracranial wound, moderate (1-24 hours) loss of consciousness
852.24 Subdural hemorrhage following injury, without mention of open intracranial wound, prolonged (more than 24 hours) loss of consciousness and return to pre-existing conscious level
852.25 Subdural hemorrhage following injury, without mention of open intracranial wound, prolonged (more than 24 hours) loss of consciousness, without return to pre-existing conscious level
852.26 Subdural hemorrhage following injury, without mention of open intracranial wound, loss of consciousness of unspecified duration
852.29 Subdural hemorrhage following injury, without mention of open intracranial wound, unspecified concussion
852.40 Extradural hemorrhage following injury, without mention of open intracranial wound, unspecified state of consciousness
852.41 Extradural hemorrhage following injury, without mention of open intracranial wound, no loss of consciousness
852.42 Extradural hemorrhage following injury, without mention of open intracranial wound, brief (less than 1 hour) loss of consciousness
852.43 Extradural hemorrhage following injury, without mention of open intracranial wound, moderate (1-24 hours) loss of consciousness
852.44 Extradural hemorrhage following injury, without mention of open intracranial wound, prolonged (more than 24 hours) loss of consciousness and return to pre-existing conscious level
852.45 Extradural hemorrhage following injury, without mention of open intracranial wound, prolonged (more than 24 hours) loss of consciousness, without return to pre-existing conscious level
852.46 Extradural hemorrhage following injury, without mention of open intracranial wound, loss of consciousness of unspecified duration
852.49 Extradural hemorrhage following injury, without mention of open intracranial wound, unspecified concussion

ICD-9-CM Procedural

01.24 Other craniotomy
01.25 Other craniectomy
01.53 Lobectomy of brain
01.59 Other excision or destruction of lesion or tissue of brain

HCPCS Level II Supplies & Services

HCPCS Level II codes are used to report the supplies, durable medical equipment, and certain medical services provided on an outpatient basis. Because the procedure(s) represented on this page would be performed in an inpatient facility, no HCPCS Level II codes apply.

61330

61330 Decompression of orbit only, transcranial approach

ICD-9-CM Diagnostic

191.9 Malignant neoplasm of brain, unspecified site
202.81 Other malignant lymphomas of lymph nodes of head, face, and neck
213.0 Benign neoplasm of bones of skull and face
224.0 Benign neoplasm of eyeball, except conjunctiva, cornea, retina, and choroid
239.6 Neoplasm of unspecified nature of brain
348.2 Benign intracranial hypertension
348.5 Cerebral edema
377.39 Other optic neuritis
747.81 Congenital anomaly of cerebrovascular system
756.0 Congenital anomalies of skull and face bones
854.05 Intracranial injury of other and unspecified nature, without mention of open intracranial wound, prolonged (more than 24 hours) loss of consciousness, without return to pre-existing conscious level

ICD-9-CM Procedural

01.24 Other craniotomy
16.09 Other orbitotomy

61332–61333

61332 Exploration of orbit (transcranial approach); with biopsy
61333 with removal of lesion

ICD-9-CM Diagnostic

170.0 Malignant neoplasm of bones of skull and face, except mandible
190.1 Malignant neoplasm of orbit
190.9 Malignant neoplasm of eye, part unspecified
198.4 Secondary malignant neoplasm of other parts of nervous system
198.5 Secondary malignant neoplasm of bone and bone marrow
213.0 Benign neoplasm of bones of skull and face
224.1 Benign neoplasm of orbit
228.02 Hemangioma of intracranial structures
234.0 Carcinoma in situ of eye
238.0 Neoplasm of uncertain behavior of bone and articular cartilage
238.8 Neoplasm of uncertain behavior of other specified sites
239.2 Neoplasms of unspecified nature of bone, soft tissue, and skin
239.8 Neoplasm of unspecified nature of other specified sites
341.0 Neuromyelitis optica
367.52 Total or complete internal ophthalmoplegia
378.72 Progressive external ophthalmoplegia
743.66 Specified congenital anomaly of orbit

ICD-9-CM Procedural

01.24 Other craniotomy
16.09 Other orbitotomy
16.23 Biopsy of eyeball and orbit
16.92 Excision of lesion of orbit

61334

61334 Exploration of orbit (transcranial approach); with removal of foreign body

ICD-9-CM Diagnostic

870.4 Penetrating wound of orbit with foreign body — (Use additional code to identify infection)
871.5 Penetration of eyeball with magnetic foreign body — (Use additional code to identify infection)

ICD-9-CM Procedural

16.09 Other orbitotomy
16.1 Removal of penetrating foreign body from eye, not otherwise specified

61340

61340 Subtemporal cranial decompression (pseudotumor cerebri, slit ventricle syndrome)

ICD-9-CM Diagnostic

331.3 Communicating hydrocephalus
331.4 Obstructive hydrocephalus
348.2 Benign intracranial hypertension
741.00 Spina bifida with hydrocephalus, unspecified region
741.01 Spina bifida with hydrocephalus, cervical region
741.02 Spina bifida with hydrocephalus, dorsal (thoracic) region

741.03 Spina bifida with hydrocephalus, lumbar region
742.3 Congenital hydrocephalus
996.75 Other complications due to nervous system device, implant, and graft

ICD-9-CM Procedural
01.24 Other craniotomy

61343
61343 Craniectomy, suboccipital with cervical laminectomy for decompression of medulla and spinal cord, with or without dural graft (eg, Arnold-Chiari malformation)

ICD-9-CM Diagnostic
336.0 Syringomyelia and syringobulbia
336.9 Unspecified disease of spinal cord ▽
348.4 Compression of brain
741.01 Spina bifida with hydrocephalus, cervical region
742.0 Encephalocele
742.2 Congenital reduction deformities of brain
742.59 Other specified congenital anomaly of spinal cord
742.9 Unspecified congenital anomaly of brain, spinal cord, and nervous system ▽
756.10 Congenital anomaly of spine, unspecified ▽
756.4 Chondrodystrophy
784.0 Headache

ICD-9-CM Procedural
03.09 Other exploration and decompression of spinal canal

61345
61345 Other cranial decompression, posterior fossa

ICD-9-CM Diagnostic
191.9 Malignant neoplasm of brain, unspecified site ▽
202.81 Other malignant lymphomas of lymph nodes of head, face, and neck
237.5 Neoplasm of uncertain behavior of brain and spinal cord
323.0 Encephalitis in viral diseases classified elsewhere — (Code first underlying disease: 073.7, 075, 078.3) ☒
437.0 Cerebral atherosclerosis — (Use additional code to identify presence of hypertension)
437.3 Cerebral aneurysm, nonruptured — (Use additional code to identify presence of hypertension)
741.00 Spina bifida with hydrocephalus, unspecified region ▽
742.53 Hydromyelia
850.4 Concussion with prolonged (more than 24 hours) loss of consciousness, without return to pre-existing conscious level

ICD-9-CM Procedural
01.24 Other craniotomy

61440
61440 Craniotomy for section of tentorium cerebelli (separate procedure)

ICD-9-CM Diagnostic
148.3 Malignant neoplasm of posterior hypopharyngeal wall
191.6 Malignant neoplasm of cerebellum NOS
191.9 Malignant neoplasm of brain, unspecified site ▽
192.1 Malignant neoplasm of cerebral meninges
198.3 Secondary malignant neoplasm of brain and spinal cord
225.0 Benign neoplasm of brain
225.1 Benign neoplasm of cranial nerves
225.2 Benign neoplasm of cerebral meninges
237.5 Neoplasm of uncertain behavior of brain and spinal cord
239.6 Neoplasm of unspecified nature of brain
322.2 Chronic meningitis
324.0 Intracranial abscess
326 Late effects of intracranial abscess or pyogenic infection — (Use additional code to identify condition: 331.4, 342.00-342.92, 344.00-344.9)
331.4 Obstructive hydrocephalus
346.00 Classical migraine without mention of intractable migraine
348.0 Cerebral cysts
747.81 Congenital anomaly of cerebrovascular system

ICD-9-CM Procedural
01.32 Lobotomy and tractotomy

61450
61450 Craniectomy, subtemporal, for section, compression, or decompression of sensory root of gasserian ganglion

ICD-9-CM Diagnostic
192.0 Malignant neoplasm of cranial nerves
195.0 Malignant neoplasm of head, face, and neck
350.1 Trigeminal neuralgia
350.2 Atypical face pain
738.19 Other specified acquired deformity of head
756.0 Congenital anomalies of skull and face bones

ICD-9-CM Procedural
04.05 Gasserian ganglionectomy
04.42 Other cranial nerve decompression

61458
61458 Craniectomy, suboccipital; for exploration or decompression of cranial nerves

ICD-9-CM Diagnostic
225.1 Benign neoplasm of cranial nerves
350.1 Trigeminal neuralgia
350.8 Other specified trigeminal nerve disorders
351.8 Other facial nerve disorders
352.1 Glossopharyngeal neuralgia
386.01 Active Meniere's disease, cochleovestibular

ICD-9-CM Procedural
04.42 Other cranial nerve decompression

61460
61460 Craniectomy, suboccipital; for section of one or more cranial nerves

ICD-9-CM Diagnostic
350.1 Trigeminal neuralgia
351.8 Other facial nerve disorders
352.1 Glossopharyngeal neuralgia
355.9 Mononeuritis of unspecified site ▽
386.01 Active Meniere's disease, cochleovestibular
386.19 Other and unspecified peripheral vertigo
386.2 Vertigo of central origin

ICD-9-CM Procedural
04.02 Division of trigeminal nerve
04.03 Division or crushing of other cranial and peripheral nerves

61470
61470 Craniectomy, suboccipital; for medullary tractotomy

ICD-9-CM Diagnostic
346.80 Other forms of migraine without mention of intractable migraine
350.1 Trigeminal neuralgia
352.1 Glossopharyngeal neuralgia
352.6 Multiple cranial nerve palsies
386.03 Active Meniere's disease, vestibular
723.1 Cervicalgia

ICD-9-CM Procedural
01.32 Lobotomy and tractotomy

61480
61480 Craniectomy, suboccipital; for mesencephalic tractotomy or pedunculotomy

ICD-9-CM Diagnostic
346.80 Other forms of migraine without mention of intractable migraine
350.1 Trigeminal neuralgia
350.2 Atypical face pain
352.1 Glossopharyngeal neuralgia
352.6 Multiple cranial nerve palsies
386.03 Active Meniere's disease, vestibular
723.1 Cervicalgia

ICD-9-CM Procedural
01.32 Lobotomy and tractotomy

▽ Unspecified code
♀ Female diagnosis
☒ Manifestation code
♂ Male diagnosis

61490

61490 Craniotomy for lobotomy, including cingulotomy

ICD-9-CM Diagnostic

191.1 Malignant neoplasm of frontal lobe of brain
191.2 Malignant neoplasm of temporal lobe of brain
191.3 Malignant neoplasm of parietal lobe of brain
191.4 Malignant neoplasm of occipital lobe of brain
198.3 Secondary malignant neoplasm of brain and spinal cord
225.0 Benign neoplasm of brain
237.5 Neoplasm of uncertain behavior of brain and spinal cord
239.6 Neoplasm of unspecified nature of brain
296.33 Major depressive disorder, recurrent episode, severe, without mention of psychotic behavior — (Use additional code to identify any associated physical disease, injury, or condition affecting the brain)
300.09 Other anxiety states
300.3 Obsessive-compulsive disorders
723.1 Cervicalgia

ICD-9-CM Procedural

01.32 Lobotomy and tractotomy

61500–61501

61500 Craniectomy; with excision of tumor or other bone lesion of skull
61501 for osteomyelitis

ICD-9-CM Diagnostic

170.0 Malignant neoplasm of bones of skull and face, except mandible
198.5 Secondary malignant neoplasm of bone and bone marrow
213.0 Benign neoplasm of bones of skull and face
238.0 Neoplasm of uncertain behavior of bone and articular cartilage
239.2 Neoplasms of unspecified nature of bone, soft tissue, and skin
730.18 Chronic osteomyelitis, other specified sites — (Use additional code to identify organism, 041.1)
730.28 Unspecified osteomyelitis, other specified sites — (Use additional code to identify organism, 041.1) ▽
733.21 Solitary bone cyst
733.22 Aneurysmal bone cyst
733.29 Other cyst of bone
733.3 Hyperostosis of skull

ICD-9-CM Procedural

01.6 Excision of lesion of skull
77.09 Sequestrectomy of other bone, except facial bones

61510

61510 Craniectomy, trephination, bone flap craniotomy; for excision of brain tumor, supratentorial, except meningioma

ICD-9-CM Diagnostic

191.0 Malignant neoplasm of cerebrum, except lobes and ventricles
191.1 Malignant neoplasm of frontal lobe of brain
191.2 Malignant neoplasm of temporal lobe of brain
191.3 Malignant neoplasm of parietal lobe of brain
191.4 Malignant neoplasm of occipital lobe of brain
191.5 Malignant neoplasm of ventricles of brain
191.8 Malignant neoplasm of other parts of brain
198.3 Secondary malignant neoplasm of brain and spinal cord
198.4 Secondary malignant neoplasm of other parts of nervous system
225.0 Benign neoplasm of brain
225.1 Benign neoplasm of cranial nerves
228.02 Hemangioma of intracranial structures
237.5 Neoplasm of uncertain behavior of brain and spinal cord
238.1 Neoplasm of uncertain behavior of connective and other soft tissue ▽
239.6 Neoplasm of unspecified nature of brain

ICD-9-CM Procedural

01.59 Other excision or destruction of lesion or tissue of brain
07.59 Other operations on pineal gland

61512

61512 Craniectomy, trephination, bone flap craniotomy; for excision of meningioma, supratentorial

ICD-9-CM Diagnostic

192.1 Malignant neoplasm of cerebral meninges
225.2 Benign neoplasm of cerebral meninges
237.6 Neoplasm of uncertain behavior of meninges

ICD-9-CM Procedural

01.51 Excision of lesion or tissue of cerebral meninges

61514

61514 Craniectomy, trephination, bone flap craniotomy; for excision of brain abscess, supratentorial

ICD-9-CM Diagnostic

324.0 Intracranial abscess

ICD-9-CM Procedural

01.59 Other excision or destruction of lesion or tissue of brain

61516

61516 Craniectomy, trephination, bone flap craniotomy; for excision or fenestration of cyst, supratentorial

ICD-9-CM Diagnostic

331.4 Obstructive hydrocephalus
348.0 Cerebral cysts
742.4 Other specified congenital anomalies of brain

ICD-9-CM Procedural

01.59 Other excision or destruction of lesion or tissue of brain

61517

61517 Implantation of brain intracavitary chemotherapy agent (List separately in addition to code for primary procedure)

ICD-9-CM Diagnostic

This is an add-on code. Refer to the corresponding primary procedure code for ICD-9 diagnosis code links.

ICD-9-CM Procedural

00.10 Implantation of chemotherapeutic agent

HCPCS Level II Supplies & Services

The HCPCS Level II code(s) would be the same as the actual procedure performed because these are in-addition-to codes.

61518

61518 Craniectomy for excision of brain tumor, infratentorial or posterior fossa; except meningioma, cerebellopontine angle tumor, or midline tumor at base of skull

ICD-9-CM Diagnostic

191.6 Malignant neoplasm of cerebellum NOS
191.7 Malignant neoplasm of brain stem
191.9 Malignant neoplasm of brain, unspecified site ▽
192.8 Malignant neoplasm of other specified sites of nervous system
198.3 Secondary malignant neoplasm of brain and spinal cord
225.0 Benign neoplasm of brain
225.1 Benign neoplasm of cranial nerves
237.5 Neoplasm of uncertain behavior of brain and spinal cord
239.6 Neoplasm of unspecified nature of brain

ICD-9-CM Procedural

01.59 Other excision or destruction of lesion or tissue of brain

61519

61519 Craniectomy for excision of brain tumor, infratentorial or posterior fossa; meningioma

ICD-9-CM Diagnostic

192.1 Malignant neoplasm of cerebral meninges
225.2 Benign neoplasm of cerebral meninges

237.6 Neoplasm of uncertain behavior of meninges

ICD-9-CM Procedural

01.51 Excision of lesion or tissue of cerebral meninges

61520

61520 Craniectomy for excision of brain tumor, infratentorial or posterior fossa; cerebellopontine angle tumor

ICD-9-CM Diagnostic

191.6 Malignant neoplasm of cerebellum NOS
198.3 Secondary malignant neoplasm of brain and spinal cord
225.0 Benign neoplasm of brain
225.1 Benign neoplasm of cranial nerves
228.02 Hemangioma of intracranial structures
237.3 Neoplasm of uncertain behavior of paraganglia
237.5 Neoplasm of uncertain behavior of brain and spinal cord
237.72 Neurofibromatosis, Type 2 (acoustic neurofibromatosis)
239.6 Neoplasm of unspecified nature of brain

ICD-9-CM Procedural

01.59 Other excision or destruction of lesion or tissue of brain
04.01 Excision of acoustic neuroma

61521

61521 Craniectomy for excision of brain tumor, infratentorial or posterior fossa; midline tumor at base of skull

ICD-9-CM Diagnostic

191.7 Malignant neoplasm of brain stem
191.8 Malignant neoplasm of other parts of brain
198.3 Secondary malignant neoplasm of brain and spinal cord
225.0 Benign neoplasm of brain
225.1 Benign neoplasm of cranial nerves
225.2 Benign neoplasm of cerebral meninges
225.8 Benign neoplasm of other specified sites of nervous system
225.9 Benign neoplasm of nervous system, part unspecified ▽
237.5 Neoplasm of uncertain behavior of brain and spinal cord
239.6 Neoplasm of unspecified nature of brain

ICD-9-CM Procedural

01.59 Other excision or destruction of lesion or tissue of brain

61522

61522 Craniectomy, infratentorial or posterior fossa; for excision of brain abscess

ICD-9-CM Diagnostic

324.0 Intracranial abscess

ICD-9-CM Procedural

01.59 Other excision or destruction of lesion or tissue of brain

61524

61524 Craniectomy, infratentorial or posterior fossa; for excision or fenestration of cyst

ICD-9-CM Diagnostic

348.0 Cerebral cysts
742.4 Other specified congenital anomalies of brain

ICD-9-CM Procedural

01.59 Other excision or destruction of lesion or tissue of brain

61526–61530

61526 Craniectomy, bone flap craniotomy, transtemporal (mastoid) for excision of cerebellopontine angle tumor;
61530 combined with middle/posterior fossa craniotomy/craniectomy

ICD-9-CM Diagnostic

191.6 Malignant neoplasm of cerebellum NOS
198.3 Secondary malignant neoplasm of brain and spinal cord
225.0 Benign neoplasm of brain
225.1 Benign neoplasm of cranial nerves
228.02 Hemangioma of intracranial structures
237.3 Neoplasm of uncertain behavior of paraganglia
237.5 Neoplasm of uncertain behavior of brain and spinal cord
237.72 Neurofibromatosis, Type 2 (acoustic neurofibromatosis)
239.6 Neoplasm of unspecified nature of brain

ICD-9-CM Procedural

01.59 Other excision or destruction of lesion or tissue of brain
04.01 Excision of acoustic neuroma

61531

61531 Subdural implantation of strip electrodes through one or more burr or trephine hole(s) for long term seizure monitoring

ICD-9-CM Diagnostic

345.00 Generalized nonconvulsive epilepsy without mention of intractable epilepsy
345.01 Generalized nonconvulsive epilepsy with intractable epilepsy
345.10 Generalized convulsive epilepsy without mention of intractable epilepsy
345.11 Generalized convulsive epilepsy with intractable epilepsy
345.2 Epileptic petit mal status
345.3 Epileptic grand mal status
345.40 Partial epilepsy with impairment of consciousness, without mention of intractable epilepsy
345.41 Partial epilepsy with impairment of consciousness, with intractable epilepsy
345.50 Partial epilepsy without mention of impairment of consciousness, without mention of intractable epilepsy
345.51 Partial epilepsy without mention of impairment of consciousness, with intractable epilepsy
345.70 Epilepsia partialis continua without mention of intractable epilepsy
345.71 Epilepsia partialis continua with intractable epilepsy
345.80 Other forms of epilepsy without mention of intractable epilepsy
345.81 Other forms of epilepsy with intractable epilepsy
345.90 Unspecified epilepsy without mention of intractable epilepsy ▽
345.91 Unspecified epilepsy with intractable epilepsy ▽

ICD-9-CM Procedural

02.93 Implantation or replacement of intracranial neurostimulator lead(s)

61533

61533 Craniotomy with elevation of bone flap; for subdural implantation of an electrode array, for long term seizure monitoring

ICD-9-CM Diagnostic

345.00 Generalized nonconvulsive epilepsy without mention of intractable epilepsy
345.01 Generalized nonconvulsive epilepsy with intractable epilepsy
345.10 Generalized convulsive epilepsy without mention of intractable epilepsy
345.11 Generalized convulsive epilepsy with intractable epilepsy
345.2 Epileptic petit mal status
345.3 Epileptic grand mal status
345.40 Partial epilepsy with impairment of consciousness, without mention of intractable epilepsy
345.41 Partial epilepsy with impairment of consciousness, with intractable epilepsy
345.50 Partial epilepsy without mention of impairment of consciousness, without mention of intractable epilepsy
345.51 Partial epilepsy without mention of impairment of consciousness, with intractable epilepsy
345.70 Epilepsia partialis continua without mention of intractable epilepsy
345.71 Epilepsia partialis continua with intractable epilepsy
345.80 Other forms of epilepsy without mention of intractable epilepsy
345.81 Other forms of epilepsy with intractable epilepsy
345.90 Unspecified epilepsy without mention of intractable epilepsy ▽
345.91 Unspecified epilepsy with intractable epilepsy ▽

ICD-9-CM Procedural

02.93 Implantation or replacement of intracranial neurostimulator lead(s)

61534

61534 Craniotomy with elevation of bone flap; for excision of epileptogenic focus without electrocorticography during surgery

ICD-9-CM Diagnostic

345.00 Generalized nonconvulsive epilepsy without mention of intractable epilepsy
345.01 Generalized nonconvulsive epilepsy with intractable epilepsy
345.10 Generalized convulsive epilepsy without mention of intractable epilepsy
345.11 Generalized convulsive epilepsy with intractable epilepsy
345.2 Epileptic petit mal status
345.3 Epileptic grand mal status

▽ Unspecified code ♀ Female diagnosis ☒ Manifestation code ♂ Male diagnosis

345.40 Partial epilepsy with impairment of consciousness, without mention of intractable epilepsy
345.41 Partial epilepsy with impairment of consciousness, with intractable epilepsy
345.50 Partial epilepsy without mention of impairment of consciousness, without mention of intractable epilepsy
345.51 Partial epilepsy without mention of impairment of consciousness, with intractable epilepsy
345.70 Epilepsia partialis continua without mention of intractable epilepsy
345.71 Epilepsia partialis continua with intractable epilepsy
345.80 Other forms of epilepsy without mention of intractable epilepsy
345.81 Other forms of epilepsy with intractable epilepsy
345.90 Unspecified epilepsy without mention of intractable epilepsy ▽
345.91 Unspecified epilepsy with intractable epilepsy ▽

ICD-9-CM Procedural

01.59 Other excision or destruction of lesion or tissue of brain

61535

61535 Craniotomy with elevation of bone flap; for removal of epidural or subdural electrode array, without excision of cerebral tissue (separate procedure)

ICD-9-CM Diagnostic

345.00 Generalized nonconvulsive epilepsy without mention of intractable epilepsy
345.01 Generalized nonconvulsive epilepsy with intractable epilepsy
345.10 Generalized convulsive epilepsy without mention of intractable epilepsy
345.11 Generalized convulsive epilepsy with intractable epilepsy
345.2 Epileptic petit mal status
345.3 Epileptic grand mal status
345.40 Partial epilepsy with impairment of consciousness, without mention of intractable epilepsy
345.41 Partial epilepsy with impairment of consciousness, with intractable epilepsy
345.50 Partial epilepsy without mention of impairment of consciousness, without mention of intractable epilepsy
345.51 Partial epilepsy without mention of impairment of consciousness, with intractable epilepsy
345.70 Epilepsia partialis continua without mention of intractable epilepsy
345.71 Epilepsia partialis continua with intractable epilepsy
345.80 Other forms of epilepsy without mention of intractable epilepsy
345.81 Other forms of epilepsy with intractable epilepsy
345.90 Unspecified epilepsy without mention of intractable epilepsy ▽
345.91 Unspecified epilepsy with intractable epilepsy ▽
996.2 Mechanical complication of nervous system device, implant, and graft
996.63 Infection and inflammatory reaction due to nervous system device, implant, and graft — (Use additional code to identify specified infections)
996.75 Other complications due to nervous system device, implant, and graft
V53.02 Neuropacemaker (brain) (peripheral nerve) (spinal cord)

ICD-9-CM Procedural

01.22 Removal of intracranial neurostimulator lead(s)

61536

61536 Craniotomy with elevation of bone flap; for excision of cerebral epileptogenic focus, with electrocorticography during surgery (includes removal of electrode array)

ICD-9-CM Diagnostic

345.00 Generalized nonconvulsive epilepsy without mention of intractable epilepsy
345.01 Generalized nonconvulsive epilepsy with intractable epilepsy
345.10 Generalized convulsive epilepsy without mention of intractable epilepsy
345.11 Generalized convulsive epilepsy with intractable epilepsy
345.2 Epileptic petit mal status
345.3 Epileptic grand mal status
345.40 Partial epilepsy with impairment of consciousness, without mention of intractable epilepsy
345.41 Partial epilepsy with impairment of consciousness, with intractable epilepsy
345.50 Partial epilepsy without mention of impairment of consciousness, without mention of intractable epilepsy
345.51 Partial epilepsy without mention of impairment of consciousness, with intractable epilepsy
345.70 Epilepsia partialis continua without mention of intractable epilepsy
345.71 Epilepsia partialis continua with intractable epilepsy
345.80 Other forms of epilepsy without mention of intractable epilepsy
345.81 Other forms of epilepsy with intractable epilepsy
345.90 Unspecified epilepsy without mention of intractable epilepsy ▽
345.91 Unspecified epilepsy with intractable epilepsy ▽

ICD-9-CM Procedural

01.24 Other craniotomy
01.59 Other excision or destruction of lesion or tissue of brain

61537–61540

61537 Craniotomy with elevation of bone flap; for lobectomy, temporal lobe, without electrocorticography during surgery
61538 for lobectomy, temporal lobe, with electrocorticography during surgery
61539 for lobectomy, other than temporal lobe, partial or total, with electrocorticography during surgery
61540 for lobectomy, other than temporal lobe, partial or total, without electrocorticography during surgery

ICD-9-CM Diagnostic

191.1 Malignant neoplasm of frontal lobe of brain
191.2 Malignant neoplasm of temporal lobe of brain
191.3 Malignant neoplasm of parietal lobe of brain
191.4 Malignant neoplasm of occipital lobe of brain
191.9 Malignant neoplasm of brain, unspecified site ▽
198.3 Secondary malignant neoplasm of brain and spinal cord
225.0 Benign neoplasm of brain
228.02 Hemangioma of intracranial structures
237.5 Neoplasm of uncertain behavior of brain and spinal cord
239.6 Neoplasm of unspecified nature of brain
345.00 Generalized nonconvulsive epilepsy without mention of intractable epilepsy
345.01 Generalized nonconvulsive epilepsy with intractable epilepsy
345.10 Generalized convulsive epilepsy without mention of intractable epilepsy
345.11 Generalized convulsive epilepsy with intractable epilepsy
345.2 Epileptic petit mal status
345.3 Epileptic grand mal status
345.40 Partial epilepsy with impairment of consciousness, without mention of intractable epilepsy
345.41 Partial epilepsy with impairment of consciousness, with intractable epilepsy
345.50 Partial epilepsy without mention of impairment of consciousness, without mention of intractable epilepsy
345.51 Partial epilepsy without mention of impairment of consciousness, with intractable epilepsy
345.70 Epilepsia partialis continua without mention of intractable epilepsy
345.71 Epilepsia partialis continua with intractable epilepsy
345.80 Other forms of epilepsy without mention of intractable epilepsy
345.81 Other forms of epilepsy with intractable epilepsy
345.90 Unspecified epilepsy without mention of intractable epilepsy ▽
345.91 Unspecified epilepsy with intractable epilepsy ▽

ICD-9-CM Procedural

01.53 Lobectomy of brain
01.59 Other excision or destruction of lesion or tissue of brain

61541

61541 Craniotomy with elevation of bone flap; for transection of corpus callosum

ICD-9-CM Diagnostic

198.3 Secondary malignant neoplasm of brain and spinal cord
225.0 Benign neoplasm of brain
237.5 Neoplasm of uncertain behavior of brain and spinal cord
239.6 Neoplasm of unspecified nature of brain
345.00 Generalized nonconvulsive epilepsy without mention of intractable epilepsy
345.01 Generalized nonconvulsive epilepsy with intractable epilepsy
345.10 Generalized convulsive epilepsy without mention of intractable epilepsy
345.11 Generalized convulsive epilepsy with intractable epilepsy
345.2 Epileptic petit mal status
345.3 Epileptic grand mal status
345.40 Partial epilepsy with impairment of consciousness, without mention of intractable epilepsy
345.41 Partial epilepsy with impairment of consciousness, with intractable epilepsy
345.50 Partial epilepsy without mention of impairment of consciousness, without mention of intractable epilepsy
345.51 Partial epilepsy without mention of impairment of consciousness, with intractable epilepsy
345.70 Epilepsia partialis continua without mention of intractable epilepsy
345.71 Epilepsia partialis continua with intractable epilepsy
345.80 Other forms of epilepsy without mention of intractable epilepsy
345.81 Other forms of epilepsy with intractable epilepsy
345.90 Unspecified epilepsy without mention of intractable epilepsy ▽
345.91 Unspecified epilepsy with intractable epilepsy ▽

▽ Unspecified code ♀ Female diagnosis ☒ Manifestation code ♂ Male diagnosis

348.0 Cerebral cysts
742.4 Other specified congenital anomalies of brain

ICD-9-CM Procedural

01.32 Lobotomy and tractotomy

61542–61543

61542 Craniotomy with elevation of bone flap; for total hemispherectomy
61543 for partial or subtotal (functional) hemispherectomy

ICD-9-CM Diagnostic

191.2 Malignant neoplasm of temporal lobe of brain
198.3 Secondary malignant neoplasm of brain and spinal cord
225.0 Benign neoplasm of brain
237.5 Neoplasm of uncertain behavior of brain and spinal cord
239.6 Neoplasm of unspecified nature of brain
345.00 Generalized nonconvulsive epilepsy without mention of intractable epilepsy
345.01 Generalized nonconvulsive epilepsy with intractable epilepsy
345.10 Generalized convulsive epilepsy without mention of intractable epilepsy
345.11 Generalized convulsive epilepsy with intractable epilepsy
345.2 Epileptic petit mal status
345.3 Epileptic grand mal status
345.40 Partial epilepsy with impairment of consciousness, without mention of intractable epilepsy
345.41 Partial epilepsy with impairment of consciousness, with intractable epilepsy
345.50 Partial epilepsy without mention of impairment of consciousness, without mention of intractable epilepsy
345.51 Partial epilepsy without mention of impairment of consciousness, with intractable epilepsy
345.70 Epilepsia partialis continua without mention of intractable epilepsy
345.71 Epilepsia partialis continua with intractable epilepsy
345.80 Other forms of epilepsy without mention of intractable epilepsy
345.81 Other forms of epilepsy with intractable epilepsy
345.90 Unspecified epilepsy without mention of intractable epilepsy ▽
345.91 Unspecified epilepsy with intractable epilepsy ▽

ICD-9-CM Procedural

01.52 Hemispherectomy

61544

61544 Craniotomy with elevation of bone flap; for excision or coagulation of choroid plexus

ICD-9-CM Diagnostic

191.5 Malignant neoplasm of ventricles of brain
198.3 Secondary malignant neoplasm of brain and spinal cord
225.0 Benign neoplasm of brain
237.5 Neoplasm of uncertain behavior of brain and spinal cord
239.6 Neoplasm of unspecified nature of brain
331.3 Communicating hydrocephalus
741.00 Spina bifida with hydrocephalus, unspecified region ▽
742.3 Congenital hydrocephalus

ICD-9-CM Procedural

02.14 Choroid plexectomy

61545

61545 Craniotomy with elevation of bone flap; for excision of craniopharyngioma

ICD-9-CM Diagnostic

237.0 Neoplasm of uncertain behavior of pituitary gland and craniopharyngeal duct — (Use additional code to identify any functional activity)

ICD-9-CM Procedural

01.59 Other excision or destruction of lesion or tissue of brain

61546–61548

61546 Craniotomy for hypophysectomy or excision of pituitary tumor, intracranial approach
61548 Hypophysectomy or excision of pituitary tumor, transnasal or transseptal approach, nonstereotactic

ICD-9-CM Diagnostic

194.3 Malignant neoplasm of pituitary gland and craniopharyngeal duct — (Use additional code to identify any functional activity)
227.3 Benign neoplasm of pituitary gland and craniopharyngeal duct (pouch) — (Use additional code to identify any functional activity)
237.0 Neoplasm of uncertain behavior of pituitary gland and craniopharyngeal duct — (Use additional code to identify any functional activity)
239.7 Neoplasm of unspecified nature of endocrine glands and other parts of nervous system
253.0 Acromegaly and gigantism
253.1 Other and unspecified anterior pituitary hyperfunction ▽
253.2 Panhypopituitarism
253.3 Pituitary dwarfism
253.4 Other anterior pituitary disorders
253.5 Diabetes insipidus
253.6 Other disorders of neurohypophysis
253.7 Iatrogenic pituitary disorders — (Use additional E code to identify cause)
253.8 Other disorders of the pituitary and other syndromes of diencephalohypophyseal origin
253.9 Unspecified disorder of the pituitary gland and its hypothalamic control ▽

ICD-9-CM Procedural

07.61 Partial excision of pituitary gland, transfrontal approach
07.62 Partial excision of pituitary gland, transsphenoidal approach
07.63 Partial excision of pituitary gland, unspecified approach
07.64 Total excision of pituitary gland, transfrontal approach
07.65 Total excision of pituitary gland, transsphenoidal approach
07.68 Total excision of pituitary gland, other specified approach
07.69 Total excision of pituitary gland, unspecified approach

61550–61552

61550 Craniectomy for craniosynostosis; single cranial suture
61552 multiple cranial sutures

ICD-9-CM Diagnostic

756.0 Congenital anomalies of skull and face bones

ICD-9-CM Procedural

02.01 Opening of cranial suture

61556–61557

61556 Craniotomy for craniosynostosis; frontal or parietal bone flap
61557 bifrontal bone flap

ICD-9-CM Diagnostic

756.0 Congenital anomalies of skull and face bones

ICD-9-CM Procedural

01.24 Other craniotomy

61558–61559

61558 Extensive craniectomy for multiple cranial suture craniosynostosis (eg, cloverleaf skull); not requiring bone grafts
61559 recontouring with multiple osteotomies and bone autografts (eg, barrel-stave procedure) (includes obtaining grafts)

ICD-9-CM Diagnostic

756.0 Congenital anomalies of skull and face bones
756.59 Other congenital osteodystrophy

ICD-9-CM Procedural

02.01 Opening of cranial suture
02.04 Bone graft to skull

61563–61564

61563 Excision, intra and extracranial, benign tumor of cranial bone (eg, fibrous dysplasia); without optic nerve decompression
61564 with optic nerve decompression

ICD-9-CM Diagnostic

213.0 Benign neoplasm of bones of skull and face

ICD-9-CM Procedural

01.6 Excision of lesion of skull
04.42 Other cranial nerve decompression

▽ Unspecified code ♀ Female diagnosis ☒ Manifestation code ♂ Male diagnosis

61566–61567

61566 Craniotomy with elevation of bone flap; for selective amygdalohippocampectomy
61567 for multiple subpial transections, with electrocorticography during surgery

ICD-9-CM Diagnostic

345.41 Partial epilepsy with impairment of consciousness, with intractable epilepsy

61570–61571

61570 Craniectomy or craniotomy; with excision of foreign body from brain
61571 with treatment of penetrating wound of brain

ICD-9-CM Diagnostic

800.61 Open fracture of vault of skull with cerebral laceration and contusion, no loss of consciousness
800.62 Open fracture of vault of skull with cerebral laceration and contusion, brief (less than one hour) loss of consciousness
800.63 Open fracture of vault of skull with cerebral laceration and contusion, moderate (1-24 hours) loss of consciousness
800.64 Open fracture of vault of skull with cerebral laceration and contusion, prolonged (more than 24 hours) loss of consciousness and return to pre-existing conscious level
800.65 Open fracture of vault of skull with cerebral laceration and contusion, prolonged (more than 24 hours) loss of consciousness, without return to pre-existing conscious level
800.66 Open fracture of vault of skull with cerebral laceration and contusion, loss of consciousness of unspecified duration ▽
800.69 Open fracture of vault of skull with cerebral laceration and contusion, unspecified concussion ▽
800.71 Open fracture of vault of skull with subarachnoid, subdural, and extradural hemorrhage, no loss of consciousness
800.74 Open fracture of vault of skull with subarachnoid, subdural, and extradural hemorrhage, prolonged (more than 24 hours) loss of consciousness and return to pre-existing conscious level
801.61 Open fracture of base of skull with cerebral laceration and contusion, no loss of consciousness
801.62 Open fracture of base of skull with cerebral laceration and contusion, brief (less than one hour) loss of consciousness
801.63 Open fracture of base of skull with cerebral laceration and contusion, moderate (1-24 hours) loss of consciousness
801.64 Open fracture of base of skull with cerebral laceration and contusion, prolonged (more than 24 hours) loss of consciousness and return to pre-existing conscious level
801.65 Open fracture of base of skull with cerebral laceration and contusion, prolonged (more than 24 hours) loss of consciousness, without return to pre-existing conscious level
801.66 Open fracture of base of skull with cerebral laceration and contusion, loss of consciousness of unspecified duration ▽
801.69 Open fracture of base of skull with cerebral laceration and contusion, unspecified concussion ▽
851.12 Cortex (cerebral) contusion with open intracranial wound, brief (less than 1 hour) loss of consciousness
851.16 Cortex (cerebral) contusion with open intracranial wound, loss of consciousness of unspecified duration ▽
851.31 Cortex (cerebral) laceration with open intracranial wound, no loss of consciousness
851.32 Cortex (cerebral) laceration with open intracranial wound, brief (less than 1 hour) loss of consciousness
851.33 Cortex (cerebral) laceration with open intracranial wound, moderate (1-24 hours) loss of consciousness
851.36 Cortex (cerebral) laceration with open intracranial wound, loss of consciousness of unspecified duration ▽
851.90 Other and unspecified cerebral laceration and contusion, with open intracranial wound, unspecified state of consciousness ▽
852.34 Subdural hemorrhage following injury, with open intracranial wound, prolonged (more than 24 hours) loss of consciousness and return to pre-existing conscious level
852.51 Extradural hemorrhage following injury, with open intracranial wound, no loss of consciousness
852.52 Extradural hemorrhage following injury, with open intracranial wound, brief (less than 1 hour) loss of consciousness
852.56 Extradural hemorrhage following injury, with open intracranial wound, loss of consciousness of unspecified duration ▽
853.11 Other and unspecified intracranial hemorrhage following injury, with open intracranial wound, no loss of consciousness
853.12 Other and unspecified intracranial hemorrhage following injury, with open intracranial wound, brief (less than 1 hour) loss of consciousness
854.10 Intracranial injury of other and unspecified nature, with open intracranial wound, unspecified state of consciousness ▽
854.11 Intracranial injury of other and unspecified nature, with open intracranial wound, no loss of consciousness
854.12 Intracranial injury of other and unspecified nature, with open intracranial wound, brief (less than 1 hour) loss of consciousness
854.13 Intracranial injury of other and unspecified nature, with open intracranial wound, moderate (1-24 hours) loss of consciousness
854.14 Intracranial injury of other and unspecified nature, with open intracranial wound, prolonged (more than 24 hours) loss of consciousness and return to pre-existing conscious level
854.15 Intracranial injury of other and unspecified nature, with open intracranial wound, prolonged (more than 24 hours) loss of consciousness, without return to pre-existing conscious level
854.16 Intracranial injury of other and unspecified nature, with open intracranial wound, loss of consciousness of unspecified duration ▽
854.19 Intracranial injury of other and unspecified nature, with open intracranial wound, with unspecified concussion ▽

ICD-9-CM Procedural

01.39 Other incision of brain
02.92 Repair of brain

61575–61576

61575 Transoral approach to skull base, brain stem or upper spinal cord for biopsy, decompression or excision of lesion;
61576 requiring splitting of tongue and/or mandible (including tracheostomy)

ICD-9-CM Diagnostic

170.0 Malignant neoplasm of bones of skull and face, except mandible
191.7 Malignant neoplasm of brain stem
192.2 Malignant neoplasm of spinal cord
198.3 Secondary malignant neoplasm of brain and spinal cord
198.5 Secondary malignant neoplasm of bone and bone marrow
213.0 Benign neoplasm of bones of skull and face
225.0 Benign neoplasm of brain
225.2 Benign neoplasm of cerebral meninges
237.5 Neoplasm of uncertain behavior of brain and spinal cord
238.0 Neoplasm of uncertain behavior of bone and articular cartilage
239.6 Neoplasm of unspecified nature of brain
721.0 Cervical spondylosis without myelopathy
721.1 Cervical spondylosis with myelopathy
756.12 Congenital spondylolisthesis
756.15 Congenital fusion of spine (vertebra)

ICD-9-CM Procedural

01.14 Open biopsy of brain
01.59 Other excision or destruction of lesion or tissue of brain
03.32 Biopsy of spinal cord or spinal meninges

HCPCS Level II Supplies & Services

A7527 Tracheostomy/laryngectomy tube plug/stop, each

61580

61580 Craniofacial approach to anterior cranial fossa; extradural, including lateral rhinotomy, ethmoidectomy, sphenoidectomy, without maxillectomy or orbital exenteration

ICD-9-CM Diagnostic

160.0 Malignant neoplasm of nasal cavities
160.3 Malignant neoplasm of ethmoidal sinus
160.5 Malignant neoplasm of sphenoidal sinus
160.8 Malignant neoplasm of other sites of nasal cavities, middle ear, and accessory sinuses
170.0 Malignant neoplasm of bones of skull and face, except mandible
190.0 Malignant neoplasm of eyeball, except conjunctiva, cornea, retina, and choroid
191.0 Malignant neoplasm of cerebrum, except lobes and ventricles
192.0 Malignant neoplasm of cranial nerves
192.1 Malignant neoplasm of cerebral meninges
196.0 Secondary and unspecified malignant neoplasm of lymph nodes of head, face, and neck
197.3 Secondary malignant neoplasm of other respiratory organs
198.4 Secondary malignant neoplasm of other parts of nervous system
225.1 Benign neoplasm of cranial nerves

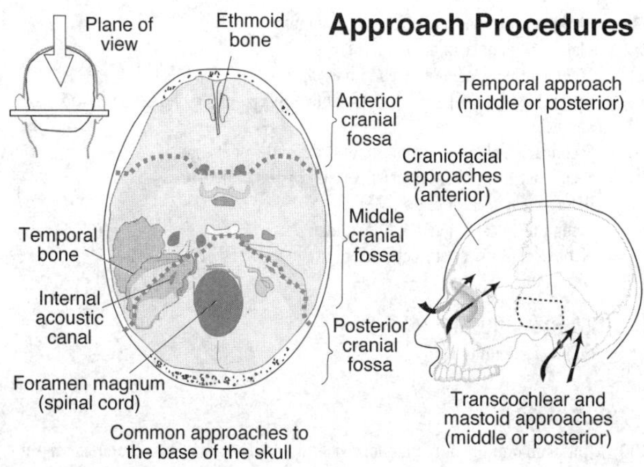

225.2 Benign neoplasm of cerebral meninges
237.6 Neoplasm of uncertain behavior of meninges
239.7 Neoplasm of unspecified nature of endocrine glands and other parts of nervous system
324.0 Intracranial abscess
349.81 Cerebrospinal fluid rhinorrhea
430 Subarachnoid hemorrhage — (Use additional code to identify presence of hypertension)
437.3 Cerebral aneurysm, nonruptured — (Use additional code to identify presence of hypertension)
747.81 Congenital anomaly of cerebrovascular system

ICD-9-CM Procedural

01.24 Other craniotomy
21.1 Incision of nose
22.63 Ethmoidectomy
22.64 Sphenoidectomy

61581

61581 Craniofacial approach to anterior cranial fossa; extradural, including lateral rhinotomy, orbital exenteration, ethmoidectomy, sphenoidectomy and/or maxillectomy

ICD-9-CM Diagnostic

160.0 Malignant neoplasm of nasal cavities
160.3 Malignant neoplasm of ethmoidal sinus
160.5 Malignant neoplasm of sphenoidal sinus
160.8 Malignant neoplasm of other sites of nasal cavities, middle ear, and accessory sinuses
170.0 Malignant neoplasm of bones of skull and face, except mandible
190.0 Malignant neoplasm of eyeball, except conjunctiva, cornea, retina, and choroid
191.0 Malignant neoplasm of cerebrum, except lobes and ventricles
192.0 Malignant neoplasm of cranial nerves
192.1 Malignant neoplasm of cerebral meninges
196.0 Secondary and unspecified malignant neoplasm of lymph nodes of head, face, and neck
197.3 Secondary malignant neoplasm of other respiratory organs
198.4 Secondary malignant neoplasm of other parts of nervous system
225.1 Benign neoplasm of cranial nerves
225.2 Benign neoplasm of cerebral meninges
237.6 Neoplasm of uncertain behavior of meninges
239.7 Neoplasm of unspecified nature of endocrine glands and other parts of nervous system
324.0 Intracranial abscess
349.81 Cerebrospinal fluid rhinorrhea
430 Subarachnoid hemorrhage — (Use additional code to identify presence of hypertension)
437.3 Cerebral aneurysm, nonruptured — (Use additional code to identify presence of hypertension)
747.81 Congenital anomaly of cerebrovascular system

ICD-9-CM Procedural

01.24 Other craniotomy
16.59 Other exenteration of orbit
21.1 Incision of nose
22.62 Excision of lesion of maxillary sinus with other approach
22.63 Ethmoidectomy
22.64 Sphenoidectomy

61582

61582 Craniofacial approach to anterior cranial fossa; extradural, including unilateral or bifrontal craniotomy, elevation of frontal lobe(s), osteotomy of base of anterior cranial fossa

ICD-9-CM Diagnostic

170.0 Malignant neoplasm of bones of skull and face, except mandible
191.0 Malignant neoplasm of cerebrum, except lobes and ventricles
191.1 Malignant neoplasm of frontal lobe of brain
191.8 Malignant neoplasm of other parts of brain
192.0 Malignant neoplasm of cranial nerves
192.1 Malignant neoplasm of cerebral meninges
198.3 Secondary malignant neoplasm of brain and spinal cord
198.4 Secondary malignant neoplasm of other parts of nervous system
225.0 Benign neoplasm of brain
225.1 Benign neoplasm of cranial nerves
225.2 Benign neoplasm of cerebral meninges
237.0 Neoplasm of uncertain behavior of pituitary gland and craniopharyngeal duct — (Use additional code to identify any functional activity)
237.5 Neoplasm of uncertain behavior of brain and spinal cord
237.6 Neoplasm of uncertain behavior of meninges
239.6 Neoplasm of unspecified nature of brain
239.7 Neoplasm of unspecified nature of endocrine glands and other parts of nervous system
324.0 Intracranial abscess
349.81 Cerebrospinal fluid rhinorrhea
430 Subarachnoid hemorrhage — (Use additional code to identify presence of hypertension)
437.3 Cerebral aneurysm, nonruptured — (Use additional code to identify presence of hypertension)
747.81 Congenital anomaly of cerebrovascular system

ICD-9-CM Procedural

01.24 Other craniotomy

61583

61583 Craniofacial approach to anterior cranial fossa; intradural, including unilateral or bifrontal craniotomy, elevation or resection of frontal lobe, osteotomy of base of anterior cranial fossa

ICD-9-CM Diagnostic

170.0 Malignant neoplasm of bones of skull and face, except mandible
191.0 Malignant neoplasm of cerebrum, except lobes and ventricles
191.1 Malignant neoplasm of frontal lobe of brain
191.8 Malignant neoplasm of other parts of brain
192.0 Malignant neoplasm of cranial nerves
192.1 Malignant neoplasm of cerebral meninges
198.3 Secondary malignant neoplasm of brain and spinal cord
198.4 Secondary malignant neoplasm of other parts of nervous system
225.0 Benign neoplasm of brain
225.2 Benign neoplasm of cerebral meninges
237.0 Neoplasm of uncertain behavior of pituitary gland and craniopharyngeal duct — (Use additional code to identify any functional activity)
237.5 Neoplasm of uncertain behavior of brain and spinal cord
239.6 Neoplasm of unspecified nature of brain
324.0 Intracranial abscess
349.81 Cerebrospinal fluid rhinorrhea
430 Subarachnoid hemorrhage — (Use additional code to identify presence of hypertension)
437.3 Cerebral aneurysm, nonruptured — (Use additional code to identify presence of hypertension)
747.81 Congenital anomaly of cerebrovascular system

ICD-9-CM Procedural

01.24 Other craniotomy

61584

61584 Orbitocranial approach to anterior cranial fossa, extradural, including supraorbital ridge osteotomy and elevation of frontal and/or temporal lobe(s); without orbital exenteration

ICD-9-CM Diagnostic

160.8 Malignant neoplasm of other sites of nasal cavities, middle ear, and accessory sinuses
170.0 Malignant neoplasm of bones of skull and face, except mandible
190.0 Malignant neoplasm of eyeball, except conjunctiva, cornea, retina, and choroid

190.1 Malignant neoplasm of orbit
190.8 Malignant neoplasm of other specified sites of eye
191.0 Malignant neoplasm of cerebrum, except lobes and ventricles
191.1 Malignant neoplasm of frontal lobe of brain
191.2 Malignant neoplasm of temporal lobe of brain
191.8 Malignant neoplasm of other parts of brain
192.0 Malignant neoplasm of cranial nerves
192.1 Malignant neoplasm of cerebral meninges
192.3 Malignant neoplasm of spinal meninges
198.3 Secondary malignant neoplasm of brain and spinal cord
198.4 Secondary malignant neoplasm of other parts of nervous system
213.0 Benign neoplasm of bones of skull and face
225.0 Benign neoplasm of brain
225.2 Benign neoplasm of cerebral meninges
237.5 Neoplasm of uncertain behavior of brain and spinal cord
324.0 Intracranial abscess
430 Subarachnoid hemorrhage — (Use additional code to identify presence of hypertension)
437.3 Cerebral aneurysm, nonruptured — (Use additional code to identify presence of hypertension)
747.81 Congenital anomaly of cerebrovascular system

ICD-9-CM Procedural

01.24 Other craniotomy
77.30 Other division of bone, unspecified site

61585

61585 Orbitocranial approach to anterior cranial fossa, extradural, including supraorbital ridge osteotomy and elevation of frontal and/or temporal lobe(s); with orbital exenteration

ICD-9-CM Diagnostic

160.8 Malignant neoplasm of other sites of nasal cavities, middle ear, and accessory sinuses
170.0 Malignant neoplasm of bones of skull and face, except mandible
190.0 Malignant neoplasm of eyeball, except conjunctiva, cornea, retina, and choroid
190.1 Malignant neoplasm of orbit
190.8 Malignant neoplasm of other specified sites of eye
191.0 Malignant neoplasm of cerebrum, except lobes and ventricles
191.1 Malignant neoplasm of frontal lobe of brain
191.2 Malignant neoplasm of temporal lobe of brain
191.8 Malignant neoplasm of other parts of brain
191.9 Malignant neoplasm of brain, unspecified site ▽
192.0 Malignant neoplasm of cranial nerves
192.1 Malignant neoplasm of cerebral meninges
196.0 Secondary and unspecified malignant neoplasm of lymph nodes of head, face, and neck
198.3 Secondary malignant neoplasm of brain and spinal cord
198.4 Secondary malignant neoplasm of other parts of nervous system
225.0 Benign neoplasm of brain
225.2 Benign neoplasm of cerebral meninges
237.5 Neoplasm of uncertain behavior of brain and spinal cord
324.0 Intracranial abscess
430 Subarachnoid hemorrhage — (Use additional code to identify presence of hypertension)
437.3 Cerebral aneurysm, nonruptured — (Use additional code to identify presence of hypertension)
747.81 Congenital anomaly of cerebrovascular system

ICD-9-CM Procedural

01.24 Other craniotomy

61586

61586 Bicoronal, transzygomatic and/or LeFort I osteotomy approach to anterior cranial fossa with or without internal fixation, without bone graft

ICD-9-CM Diagnostic

160.8 Malignant neoplasm of other sites of nasal cavities, middle ear, and accessory sinuses
170.0 Malignant neoplasm of bones of skull and face, except mandible
190.0 Malignant neoplasm of eyeball, except conjunctiva, cornea, retina, and choroid
190.1 Malignant neoplasm of orbit
190.8 Malignant neoplasm of other specified sites of eye
191.0 Malignant neoplasm of cerebrum, except lobes and ventricles
191.1 Malignant neoplasm of frontal lobe of brain
191.2 Malignant neoplasm of temporal lobe of brain
191.8 Malignant neoplasm of other parts of brain
192.0 Malignant neoplasm of cranial nerves
192.1 Malignant neoplasm of cerebral meninges
196.0 Secondary and unspecified malignant neoplasm of lymph nodes of head, face, and neck
198.3 Secondary malignant neoplasm of brain and spinal cord
198.4 Secondary malignant neoplasm of other parts of nervous system
225.0 Benign neoplasm of brain
225.2 Benign neoplasm of cerebral meninges
237.5 Neoplasm of uncertain behavior of brain and spinal cord
324.0 Intracranial abscess

ICD-9-CM Procedural

01.24 Other craniotomy

61590–61591

61590 Infratemporal pre-auricular approach to middle cranial fossa (parapharyngeal space, infratemporal and midline skull base, nasopharynx), with or without disarticulation of the mandible, including parotidectomy, craniotomy, decompression and/or mobilization of the facial nerve and/or petrous carotid artery

61591 Infratemporal post-auricular approach to middle cranial fossa (internal auditory meatus, petrous apex, tentorium, cavernous sinus, parasellar area, infratemporal fossa) including mastoidectomy, resection of sigmoid sinus, with or without decompression and/or mobilization of contents of auditory canal or petrous carotid artery

ICD-9-CM Diagnostic

160.1 Malignant neoplasm of auditory tube, middle ear, and mastoid air cells
170.0 Malignant neoplasm of bones of skull and face, except mandible
191.2 Malignant neoplasm of temporal lobe of brain
191.3 Malignant neoplasm of parietal lobe of brain
191.9 Malignant neoplasm of brain, unspecified site ▽
194.3 Malignant neoplasm of pituitary gland and craniopharyngeal duct — (Use additional code to identify any functional activity)
196.0 Secondary and unspecified malignant neoplasm of lymph nodes of head, face, and neck
198.3 Secondary malignant neoplasm of brain and spinal cord
198.4 Secondary malignant neoplasm of other parts of nervous system
198.5 Secondary malignant neoplasm of bone and bone marrow
198.89 Secondary malignant neoplasm of other specified sites
212.0 Benign neoplasm of nasal cavities, middle ear, and accessory sinuses
213.0 Benign neoplasm of bones of skull and face
225.0 Benign neoplasm of brain
225.1 Benign neoplasm of cranial nerves
225.2 Benign neoplasm of cerebral meninges
237.0 Neoplasm of uncertain behavior of pituitary gland and craniopharyngeal duct — (Use additional code to identify any functional activity)
237.3 Neoplasm of uncertain behavior of paraganglia
237.5 Neoplasm of uncertain behavior of brain and spinal cord
239.6 Neoplasm of unspecified nature of brain
324.0 Intracranial abscess
430 Subarachnoid hemorrhage — (Use additional code to identify presence of hypertension)
437.3 Cerebral aneurysm, nonruptured — (Use additional code to identify presence of hypertension)
747.81 Congenital anomaly of cerebrovascular system

ICD-9-CM Procedural

01.24 Other craniotomy
04.42 Other cranial nerve decompression
20.49 Other mastoidectomy
26.30 Sialoadenectomy, not otherwise specified

61592

61592 Orbitocranial zygomatic approach to middle cranial fossa (cavernous sinus and carotid artery, clivus, basilar artery or petrous apex) including osteotomy of zygoma, craniotomy, extra- or intradural elevation of temporal lobe

ICD-9-CM Diagnostic

147.0 Malignant neoplasm of superior wall of nasopharynx
147.8 Malignant neoplasm of other specified sites of nasopharynx
170.0 Malignant neoplasm of bones of skull and face, except mandible
191.2 Malignant neoplasm of temporal lobe of brain
191.3 Malignant neoplasm of parietal lobe of brain
191.7 Malignant neoplasm of brain stem

▽ Unspecified code ♀ Female diagnosis
☒ Manifestation code ♂ Male diagnosis

191.8 Malignant neoplasm of other parts of brain
191.9 Malignant neoplasm of brain, unspecified site
198.3 Secondary malignant neoplasm of brain and spinal cord
198.4 Secondary malignant neoplasm of other parts of nervous system
210.7 Benign neoplasm of nasopharynx
225.0 Benign neoplasm of brain
225.2 Benign neoplasm of cerebral meninges
237.5 Neoplasm of uncertain behavior of brain and spinal cord
239.6 Neoplasm of unspecified nature of brain
324.0 Intracranial abscess
430 Subarachnoid hemorrhage — (Use additional code to identify presence of hypertension)
437.3 Cerebral aneurysm, nonruptured — (Use additional code to identify presence of hypertension)
747.81 Congenital anomaly of cerebrovascular system

ICD-9-CM Procedural

01.24 Other craniotomy
77.30 Other division of bone, unspecified site

61595

61595 Transtemporal approach to posterior cranial fossa, jugular foramen or midline skull base, including mastoidectomy, decompression of sigmoid sinus and/or facial nerve, with or without mobilization

ICD-9-CM Diagnostic

191.7 Malignant neoplasm of brain stem
191.8 Malignant neoplasm of other parts of brain
192.0 Malignant neoplasm of cranial nerves
198.3 Secondary malignant neoplasm of brain and spinal cord
198.5 Secondary malignant neoplasm of bone and bone marrow
213.0 Benign neoplasm of bones of skull and face
225.0 Benign neoplasm of brain
225.1 Benign neoplasm of cranial nerves
225.2 Benign neoplasm of cerebral meninges
237.5 Neoplasm of uncertain behavior of brain and spinal cord
238.0 Neoplasm of uncertain behavior of bone and articular cartilage
239.6 Neoplasm of unspecified nature of brain
239.7 Neoplasm of unspecified nature of endocrine glands and other parts of nervous system
324.0 Intracranial abscess
430 Subarachnoid hemorrhage — (Use additional code to identify presence of hypertension)
437.3 Cerebral aneurysm, nonruptured — (Use additional code to identify presence of hypertension)
747.81 Congenital anomaly of cerebrovascular system

ICD-9-CM Procedural

01.59 Other excision or destruction of lesion or tissue of brain
04.42 Other cranial nerve decompression
20.49 Other mastoidectomy

61596

61596 Transcochlear approach to posterior cranial fossa, jugular foramen or midline skull base, including labyrinthectomy, decompression, with or without mobilization of facial nerve and/or petrous carotid artery

ICD-9-CM Diagnostic

170.0 Malignant neoplasm of bones of skull and face, except mandible
191.7 Malignant neoplasm of brain stem
191.8 Malignant neoplasm of other parts of brain
191.9 Malignant neoplasm of brain, unspecified site
192.0 Malignant neoplasm of cranial nerves
198.3 Secondary malignant neoplasm of brain and spinal cord
198.4 Secondary malignant neoplasm of other parts of nervous system
198.5 Secondary malignant neoplasm of bone and bone marrow
213.0 Benign neoplasm of bones of skull and face
225.0 Benign neoplasm of brain
225.1 Benign neoplasm of cranial nerves
225.2 Benign neoplasm of cerebral meninges
237.3 Neoplasm of uncertain behavior of paraganglia
237.5 Neoplasm of uncertain behavior of brain and spinal cord
238.0 Neoplasm of uncertain behavior of bone and articular cartilage
239.6 Neoplasm of unspecified nature of brain
239.7 Neoplasm of unspecified nature of endocrine glands and other parts of nervous system
324.0 Intracranial abscess
430 Subarachnoid hemorrhage — (Use additional code to identify presence of hypertension)
437.3 Cerebral aneurysm, nonruptured — (Use additional code to identify presence of hypertension)
747.81 Congenital anomaly of cerebrovascular system

ICD-9-CM Procedural

04.42 Other cranial nerve decompression
20.79 Other incision, excision, and destruction of inner ear

61597

61597 Transcondylar (far lateral) approach to posterior cranial fossa, jugular foramen or midline skull base, including occipital condylectomy, mastoidectomy, resection of C1-C3 vertebral body(s), decompression of vertebral artery, with or without mobilization

ICD-9-CM Diagnostic

170.2 Malignant neoplasm of vertebral column, excluding sacrum and coccyx
191.6 Malignant neoplasm of cerebellum NOS
191.7 Malignant neoplasm of brain stem
192.0 Malignant neoplasm of cranial nerves
198.3 Secondary malignant neoplasm of brain and spinal cord
198.4 Secondary malignant neoplasm of other parts of nervous system
198.5 Secondary malignant neoplasm of bone and bone marrow
213.0 Benign neoplasm of bones of skull and face
225.0 Benign neoplasm of brain
225.1 Benign neoplasm of cranial nerves
225.2 Benign neoplasm of cerebral meninges
228.02 Hemangioma of intracranial structures
237.5 Neoplasm of uncertain behavior of brain and spinal cord
238.0 Neoplasm of uncertain behavior of bone and articular cartilage
239.2 Neoplasms of unspecified nature of bone, soft tissue, and skin
239.6 Neoplasm of unspecified nature of brain
324.0 Intracranial abscess
430 Subarachnoid hemorrhage — (Use additional code to identify presence of hypertension)
437.3 Cerebral aneurysm, nonruptured — (Use additional code to identify presence of hypertension)
747.81 Congenital anomaly of cerebrovascular system

ICD-9-CM Procedural

20.49 Other mastoidectomy
77.89 Other partial ostectomy of other bone, except facial bones

61598

61598 Transpetrosal approach to posterior cranial fossa, clivus or foramen magnum, including ligation of superior petrosal sinus and/or sigmoid sinus

ICD-9-CM Diagnostic

170.0 Malignant neoplasm of bones of skull and face, except mandible
170.2 Malignant neoplasm of vertebral column, excluding sacrum and coccyx
191.7 Malignant neoplasm of brain stem
192.0 Malignant neoplasm of cranial nerves
198.3 Secondary malignant neoplasm of brain and spinal cord
198.4 Secondary malignant neoplasm of other parts of nervous system
198.5 Secondary malignant neoplasm of bone and bone marrow
213.0 Benign neoplasm of bones of skull and face
225.0 Benign neoplasm of brain
225.1 Benign neoplasm of cranial nerves
225.2 Benign neoplasm of cerebral meninges
228.02 Hemangioma of intracranial structures
237.3 Neoplasm of uncertain behavior of paraganglia
237.5 Neoplasm of uncertain behavior of brain and spinal cord
238.0 Neoplasm of uncertain behavior of bone and articular cartilage
239.6 Neoplasm of unspecified nature of brain
430 Subarachnoid hemorrhage — (Use additional code to identify presence of hypertension)
437.3 Cerebral aneurysm, nonruptured — (Use additional code to identify presence of hypertension)
747.81 Congenital anomaly of cerebrovascular system

ICD-9-CM Procedural

01.59 Other excision or destruction of lesion or tissue of brain

61600–61601

61600 Resection or excision of neoplastic, vascular or infectious lesion of base of anterior cranial fossa; extradural
61601 intradural, including dural repair, with or without graft

ICD-9-CM Diagnostic

170.0 Malignant neoplasm of bones of skull and face, except mandible
191.0 Malignant neoplasm of cerebrum, except lobes and ventricles
191.1 Malignant neoplasm of frontal lobe of brain
191.8 Malignant neoplasm of other parts of brain
192.0 Malignant neoplasm of cranial nerves
192.1 Malignant neoplasm of cerebral meninges
198.3 Secondary malignant neoplasm of brain and spinal cord
198.4 Secondary malignant neoplasm of other parts of nervous system
198.5 Secondary malignant neoplasm of bone and bone marrow
225.0 Benign neoplasm of brain
225.1 Benign neoplasm of cranial nerves
225.2 Benign neoplasm of cerebral meninges
237.0 Neoplasm of uncertain behavior of pituitary gland and craniopharyngeal duct — (Use additional code to identify any functional activity)
237.5 Neoplasm of uncertain behavior of brain and spinal cord
237.6 Neoplasm of uncertain behavior of meninges
239.6 Neoplasm of unspecified nature of brain
239.7 Neoplasm of unspecified nature of endocrine glands and other parts of nervous system
324.0 Intracranial abscess
349.81 Cerebrospinal fluid rhinorrhea
430 Subarachnoid hemorrhage — (Use additional code to identify presence of hypertension)
437.3 Cerebral aneurysm, nonruptured — (Use additional code to identify presence of hypertension)
437.8 Other ill-defined cerebrovascular disease — (Use additional code to identify presence of hypertension)
437.9 Unspecified cerebrovascular disease — (Use additional code to identify presence of hypertension) ▽
747.81 Congenital anomaly of cerebrovascular system

ICD-9-CM Procedural

01.24 Other craniotomy
01.51 Excision of lesion or tissue of cerebral meninges

61605–61606

61605 Resection or excision of neoplastic, vascular or infectious lesion of infratemporal fossa, parapharyngeal space, petrous apex; extradural
61606 intradural, including dural repair, with or without graft

ICD-9-CM Diagnostic

170.0 Malignant neoplasm of bones of skull and face, except mandible
191.2 Malignant neoplasm of temporal lobe of brain
191.3 Malignant neoplasm of parietal lobe of brain
191.9 Malignant neoplasm of brain, unspecified site ▽
192.0 Malignant neoplasm of cranial nerves
194.3 Malignant neoplasm of pituitary gland and craniopharyngeal duct — (Use additional code to identify any functional activity)
198.3 Secondary malignant neoplasm of brain and spinal cord
198.4 Secondary malignant neoplasm of other parts of nervous system
225.0 Benign neoplasm of brain
225.1 Benign neoplasm of cranial nerves
225.2 Benign neoplasm of cerebral meninges
237.5 Neoplasm of uncertain behavior of brain and spinal cord
239.6 Neoplasm of unspecified nature of brain
324.0 Intracranial abscess
430 Subarachnoid hemorrhage — (Use additional code to identify presence of hypertension)
437.3 Cerebral aneurysm, nonruptured — (Use additional code to identify presence of hypertension)
437.8 Other ill-defined cerebrovascular disease — (Use additional code to identify presence of hypertension)
747.81 Congenital anomaly of cerebrovascular system

ICD-9-CM Procedural

01.24 Other craniotomy
01.51 Excision of lesion or tissue of cerebral meninges

61607–61608

61607 Resection or excision of neoplastic, vascular or infectious lesion of parasellar area, cavernous sinus, clivus or midline skull base; extradural
61608 intradural, including dural repair, with or without graft

ICD-9-CM Diagnostic

170.0 Malignant neoplasm of bones of skull and face, except mandible
191.7 Malignant neoplasm of brain stem
191.8 Malignant neoplasm of other parts of brain
192.0 Malignant neoplasm of cranial nerves
194.3 Malignant neoplasm of pituitary gland and craniopharyngeal duct — (Use additional code to identify any functional activity)
198.3 Secondary malignant neoplasm of brain and spinal cord
198.5 Secondary malignant neoplasm of bone and bone marrow
225.0 Benign neoplasm of brain
225.1 Benign neoplasm of cranial nerves
225.2 Benign neoplasm of cerebral meninges
237.0 Neoplasm of uncertain behavior of pituitary gland and craniopharyngeal duct — (Use additional code to identify any functional activity)
237.5 Neoplasm of uncertain behavior of brain and spinal cord
239.7 Neoplasm of unspecified nature of endocrine glands and other parts of nervous system
324.0 Intracranial abscess
325 Phlebitis and thrombophlebitis of intracranial venous sinuses
430 Subarachnoid hemorrhage — (Use additional code to identify presence of hypertension)
437.3 Cerebral aneurysm, nonruptured — (Use additional code to identify presence of hypertension)
437.8 Other ill-defined cerebrovascular disease — (Use additional code to identify presence of hypertension)
478.1 Other diseases of nasal cavity and sinuses
747.81 Congenital anomaly of cerebrovascular system

ICD-9-CM Procedural

01.51 Excision of lesion or tissue of cerebral meninges
01.6 Excision of lesion of skull

61609–61612

61609 Transection or ligation, carotid artery in cavernous sinus; without repair (List separately in addition to code for primary procedure)
61610 with repair by anastomosis or graft (List separately in addition to code for primary procedure)
61611 Transection or ligation, carotid artery in petrous canal; without repair (List separately in addition to code for primary procedure)
61612 with repair by anastomosis or graft (List separately in addition to code for primary procedure)

ICD-9-CM Diagnostic

This is an add-on code. Refer to the corresponding primary procedure code for ICD-9 diagnosis code links.

ICD-9-CM Procedural

38.82 Other surgical occlusion of other vessels of head and neck

61613

61613 Obliteration of carotid aneurysm, arteriovenous malformation, or carotid-cavernous fistula by dissection within cavernous sinus

ICD-9-CM Diagnostic

430 Subarachnoid hemorrhage — (Use additional code to identify presence of hypertension)
437.3 Cerebral aneurysm, nonruptured — (Use additional code to identify presence of hypertension)
747.81 Congenital anomaly of cerebrovascular system
853.00 Other and unspecified intracranial hemorrhage following injury, without mention of open intracranial wound, unspecified state of consciousness ▽
900.82 Injury to multiple blood vessels of head and neck

ICD-9-CM Procedural

38.60 Other excision of vessels, unspecified site
38.82 Other surgical occlusion of other vessels of head and neck
39.52 Other repair of aneurysm
39.53 Repair of arteriovenous fistula

61615–61616

61615 Resection or excision of neoplastic, vascular or infectious lesion of base of posterior cranial fossa, jugular foramen, foramen magnum, or C1-C3 vertebral bodies; extradural

61616 intradural, including dural repair, with or without graft

ICD-9-CM Diagnostic

170.0 Malignant neoplasm of bones of skull and face, except mandible
170.2 Malignant neoplasm of vertebral column, excluding sacrum and coccyx
191.7 Malignant neoplasm of brain stem
191.8 Malignant neoplasm of other parts of brain
191.9 Malignant neoplasm of brain, unspecified site ▽
192.0 Malignant neoplasm of cranial nerves
198.3 Secondary malignant neoplasm of brain and spinal cord
198.5 Secondary malignant neoplasm of bone and bone marrow
213.2 Benign neoplasm of vertebral column, excluding sacrum and coccyx
225.0 Benign neoplasm of brain
225.1 Benign neoplasm of cranial nerves
225.2 Benign neoplasm of cerebral meninges
228.02 Hemangioma of intracranial structures
237.3 Neoplasm of uncertain behavior of paraganglia
237.5 Neoplasm of uncertain behavior of brain and spinal cord
238.0 Neoplasm of uncertain behavior of bone and articular cartilage
239.2 Neoplasms of unspecified nature of bone, soft tissue, and skin
239.6 Neoplasm of unspecified nature of brain
239.7 Neoplasm of unspecified nature of endocrine glands and other parts of nervous system
324.0 Intracranial abscess
348.0 Cerebral cysts
437.1 Other generalized ischemic cerebrovascular disease — (Use additional code to identify presence of hypertension)
437.8 Other ill-defined cerebrovascular disease — (Use additional code to identify presence of hypertension)
437.9 Unspecified cerebrovascular disease — (Use additional code to identify presence of hypertension) ▽
747.81 Congenital anomaly of cerebrovascular system

ICD-9-CM Procedural

01.24 Other craniotomy
01.51 Excision of lesion or tissue of cerebral meninges
01.6 Excision of lesion of skull
77.69 Local excision of lesion or tissue of other bone, except facial bones

61618–61619

61618 Secondary repair of dura for cerebrospinal fluid leak, anterior, middle or posterior cranial fossa following surgery of the skull base; by free tissue graft (eg, pericranium, fascia, tensor fascia lata, adipose tissue, homologous or synthetic grafts)

61619 by local or regionalized vascularized pedicle flap or myocutaneous flap (including galea, temporalis, frontalis or occipitalis muscle)

ICD-9-CM Diagnostic

349.81 Cerebrospinal fluid rhinorrhea
388.61 Cerebrospinal fluid otorrhea
997.00 Unspecified nervous system complication — (Use additional code to identify complications) ▽
998.2 Accidental puncture or laceration during procedure

ICD-9-CM Procedural

02.12 Other repair of cerebral meninges

61623

61623 Endovascular temporary balloon arterial occlusion, head or neck (extracranial/intracranial) including selective catheterization of vessel to be occluded, positioning and inflation of occlusion balloon, concomitant neurological monitoring, and radiologic supervision and interpretation of all angiography required for balloon occlusion and to exclude vascular injury post occlusion

ICD-9-CM Diagnostic

171.0 Malignant neoplasm of connective and other soft tissue of head, face, and neck
198.89 Secondary malignant neoplasm of other specified sites
215.0 Other benign neoplasm of connective and other soft tissue of head, face, and neck
228.00 Hemangioma of unspecified site ▽
228.09 Hemangioma of other sites
238.1 Neoplasm of uncertain behavior of connective and other soft tissue ▽
239.2 Neoplasms of unspecified nature of bone, soft tissue, and skin
442.81 Aneurysm of artery of neck
447.0 Arteriovenous fistula, acquired
747.60 Congenital anomaly of the peripheral vascular system, unspecified site ▽
747.69 Congenital anomaly of other specified site of peripheral vascular system
900.02 External carotid artery injury

ICD-9-CM Procedural

38.82 Other surgical occlusion of other vessels of head and neck

61624

61624 Transcatheter permanent occlusion or embolization (eg, for tumor destruction, to achieve hemostasis, to occlude a vascular malformation), percutaneous, any method; central nervous system (intracranial, spinal cord)

ICD-9-CM Diagnostic

191.0 Malignant neoplasm of cerebrum, except lobes and ventricles
191.1 Malignant neoplasm of frontal lobe of brain
191.2 Malignant neoplasm of temporal lobe of brain
191.3 Malignant neoplasm of parietal lobe of brain
191.4 Malignant neoplasm of occipital lobe of brain
191.5 Malignant neoplasm of ventricles of brain
191.6 Malignant neoplasm of cerebellum NOS
191.8 Malignant neoplasm of other parts of brain
191.9 Malignant neoplasm of brain, unspecified site ▽
192.1 Malignant neoplasm of cerebral meninges
192.2 Malignant neoplasm of spinal cord
198.3 Secondary malignant neoplasm of brain and spinal cord
198.4 Secondary malignant neoplasm of other parts of nervous system
225.0 Benign neoplasm of brain
225.2 Benign neoplasm of cerebral meninges
225.3 Benign neoplasm of spinal cord
225.4 Benign neoplasm of spinal meninges
225.8 Benign neoplasm of other specified sites of nervous system
228.02 Hemangioma of intracranial structures
237.5 Neoplasm of uncertain behavior of brain and spinal cord
237.6 Neoplasm of uncertain behavior of meninges
239.6 Neoplasm of unspecified nature of brain
239.7 Neoplasm of unspecified nature of endocrine glands and other parts of nervous system
430 Subarachnoid hemorrhage — (Use additional code to identify presence of hypertension)
431 Intracerebral hemorrhage — (Use additional code to identify presence of hypertension)
437.3 Cerebral aneurysm, nonruptured — (Use additional code to identify presence of hypertension)
747.81 Congenital anomaly of cerebrovascular system
747.82 Congenital spinal vessel anomaly

ICD-9-CM Procedural

38.81 Other surgical occlusion of intracranial vessels
38.82 Other surgical occlusion of other vessels of head and neck

61626

61626 Transcatheter permanent occlusion or embolization (eg, for tumor destruction, to achieve hemostasis, to occlude a vascular malformation), percutaneous, any method; non-central nervous system, head or neck (extracranial, brachiocephalic branch)

ICD-9-CM Diagnostic

171.0 Malignant neoplasm of connective and other soft tissue of head, face, and neck
198.89 Secondary malignant neoplasm of other specified sites
215.0 Other benign neoplasm of connective and other soft tissue of head, face, and neck
228.00 Hemangioma of unspecified site ▽
228.09 Hemangioma of other sites
238.1 Neoplasm of uncertain behavior of connective and other soft tissue ▽
239.2 Neoplasms of unspecified nature of bone, soft tissue, and skin
442.81 Aneurysm of artery of neck
447.0 Arteriovenous fistula, acquired
747.60 Congenital anomaly of the peripheral vascular system, unspecified site ▽
747.69 Congenital anomaly of other specified site of peripheral vascular system
900.02 External carotid artery injury

ICD-9-CM Procedural
38.82 Other surgical occlusion of other vessels of head and neck

61680–61682
61680 Surgery of intracranial arteriovenous malformation; supratentorial, simple
61682 supratentorial, complex

ICD-9-CM Diagnostic
228.02 Hemangioma of intracranial structures
437.3 Cerebral aneurysm, nonruptured — (Use additional code to identify presence of hypertension)
437.8 Other ill-defined cerebrovascular disease — (Use additional code to identify presence of hypertension)
747.81 Congenital anomaly of cerebrovascular system

ICD-9-CM Procedural
38.31 Resection of intracranial vessels with anastomosis
38.41 Resection of intracranial vessels with replacement

61684–61686
61684 Surgery of intracranial arteriovenous malformation; infratentorial, simple
61686 infratentorial, complex

ICD-9-CM Diagnostic
228.02 Hemangioma of intracranial structures
437.3 Cerebral aneurysm, nonruptured — (Use additional code to identify presence of hypertension)
437.8 Other ill-defined cerebrovascular disease — (Use additional code to identify presence of hypertension)
747.81 Congenital anomaly of cerebrovascular system

ICD-9-CM Procedural
38.31 Resection of intracranial vessels with anastomosis
38.41 Resection of intracranial vessels with replacement
38.42 Resection of other vessels of head and neck with replacement

61690–61692
61690 Surgery of intracranial arteriovenous malformation; dural, simple
61692 dural, complex

ICD-9-CM Diagnostic
228.02 Hemangioma of intracranial structures
437.8 Other ill-defined cerebrovascular disease — (Use additional code to identify presence of hypertension)
747.81 Congenital anomaly of cerebrovascular system
900.9 Injury to unspecified blood vessel of head and neck ▽

ICD-9-CM Procedural
02.13 Ligation of meningeal vessel
38.31 Resection of intracranial vessels with anastomosis
38.41 Resection of intracranial vessels with replacement
38.42 Resection of other vessels of head and neck with replacement

61697–61698
61697 Surgery of complex intracranial aneurysm, intracranial approach; carotid circulation
61698 vertebrobasilar circulation

ICD-9-CM Diagnostic
430 Subarachnoid hemorrhage — (Use additional code to identify presence of hypertension)
437.3 Cerebral aneurysm, nonruptured — (Use additional code to identify presence of hypertension)
747.81 Congenital anomaly of cerebrovascular system
900.01 Common carotid artery injury
900.82 Injury to multiple blood vessels of head and neck
900.89 Injury to other specified blood vessels of head and neck

ICD-9-CM Procedural
38.31 Resection of intracranial vessels with anastomosis
38.41 Resection of intracranial vessels with replacement

61700
61700 Surgery of simple intracranial aneurysm, intracranial approach; carotid circulation

ICD-9-CM Diagnostic
430 Subarachnoid hemorrhage — (Use additional code to identify presence of hypertension)
437.3 Cerebral aneurysm, nonruptured — (Use additional code to identify presence of hypertension)
747.81 Congenital anomaly of cerebrovascular system
900.01 Common carotid artery injury
900.82 Injury to multiple blood vessels of head and neck

ICD-9-CM Procedural
38.31 Resection of intracranial vessels with anastomosis
38.41 Resection of intracranial vessels with replacement

61702
61702 Surgery of simple intracranial aneurysm, intracranial approach; vertebrobasilar circulation

ICD-9-CM Diagnostic
430 Subarachnoid hemorrhage — (Use additional code to identify presence of hypertension)
437.3 Cerebral aneurysm, nonruptured — (Use additional code to identify presence of hypertension)
747.81 Congenital anomaly of cerebrovascular system
900.89 Injury to other specified blood vessels of head and neck

ICD-9-CM Procedural
38.31 Resection of intracranial vessels with anastomosis
38.41 Resection of intracranial vessels with replacement

61703
61703 Surgery of intracranial aneurysm, cervical approach by application of occluding clamp to cervical carotid artery (Selverstone-Crutchfield type)

ICD-9-CM Diagnostic
430 Subarachnoid hemorrhage — (Use additional code to identify presence of hypertension)
437.3 Cerebral aneurysm, nonruptured — (Use additional code to identify presence of hypertension)
747.81 Congenital anomaly of cerebrovascular system

ICD-9-CM Procedural
38.31 Resection of intracranial vessels with anastomosis
38.32 Resection of other vessels of head and neck with anastomosis
38.81 Other surgical occlusion of intracranial vessels

61705–61710
61705 Surgery of aneurysm, vascular malformation or carotid-cavernous fistula; by intracranial and cervical occlusion of carotid artery
61708 by intracranial electrothrombosis
61710 by intra-arterial embolization, injection procedure, or balloon catheter

ICD-9-CM Diagnostic
430 Subarachnoid hemorrhage — (Use additional code to identify presence of hypertension)
437.3 Cerebral aneurysm, nonruptured — (Use additional code to identify presence of hypertension)
442.81 Aneurysm of artery of neck
443.21 Dissection of carotid artery
747.69 Congenital anomaly of other specified site of peripheral vascular system
747.81 Congenital anomaly of cerebrovascular system
853.00 Other and unspecified intracranial hemorrhage following injury, without mention of open intracranial wound, unspecified state of consciousness ▽
900.82 Injury to multiple blood vessels of head and neck

ICD-9-CM Procedural
38.31 Resection of intracranial vessels with anastomosis
38.32 Resection of other vessels of head and neck with anastomosis
38.81 Other surgical occlusion of intracranial vessels

▽ Unspecified code ♀ Female diagnosis ☒ Manifestation code ♂ Male diagnosis

61711

61711 Anastomosis, arterial, extracranial-intracranial (eg, middle cerebral/cortical) arteries

ICD-9-CM Diagnostic

433.10 Occlusion and stenosis of carotid artery without mention of cerebral infarction — (Use additional code to identify presence of hypertension)
437.0 Cerebral atherosclerosis — (Use additional code to identify presence of hypertension)
437.3 Cerebral aneurysm, nonruptured — (Use additional code to identify presence of hypertension)
442.9 Other aneurysm of unspecified site ▽
747.81 Congenital anomaly of cerebrovascular system

ICD-9-CM Procedural

38.31 Resection of intracranial vessels with anastomosis
38.32 Resection of other vessels of head and neck with anastomosis

61720–61735

61720 Creation of lesion by stereotactic method, including burr hole(s) and localizing and recording techniques, single or multiple stages; globus pallidus or thalamus
61735 subcortical structure(s) other than globus pallidus or thalamus

ICD-9-CM Diagnostic

239.6 Neoplasm of unspecified nature of brain
300.3 Obsessive-compulsive disorders
332.0 Paralysis agitans
333.0 Other degenerative diseases of the basal ganglia
333.5 Other choreas — (Use additional E code to identify drug, if drug-induced)
340 Multiple sclerosis
343.1 Hemiplegic infantile cerebral palsy
729.2 Unspecified neuralgia, neuritis, and radiculitis ▽
782.0 Disturbance of skin sensation
854.00 Intracranial injury of other and unspecified nature, without mention of open intracranial wound, unspecified state of consciousness ▽
854.19 Intracranial injury of other and unspecified nature, with open intracranial wound, with unspecified concussion ▽

ICD-9-CM Procedural

01.39 Other incision of brain
01.41 Operations on thalamus
01.42 Operations on globus pallidus
07.61 Partial excision of pituitary gland, transfrontal approach

61750–61751

61750 Stereotactic biopsy, aspiration, or excision, including burr hole(s), for intracranial lesion;
61751 with computed tomography and/or magnetic resonance guidance

ICD-9-CM Diagnostic

191.1 Malignant neoplasm of frontal lobe of brain
191.2 Malignant neoplasm of temporal lobe of brain
191.3 Malignant neoplasm of parietal lobe of brain
191.4 Malignant neoplasm of occipital lobe of brain
191.7 Malignant neoplasm of brain stem
191.9 Malignant neoplasm of brain, unspecified site ▽
198.3 Secondary malignant neoplasm of brain and spinal cord
225.0 Benign neoplasm of brain
237.5 Neoplasm of uncertain behavior of brain and spinal cord
239.6 Neoplasm of unspecified nature of brain
324.0 Intracranial abscess
330.0 Leukodystrophy — (Use additional code to identify associated mental retardation)
340 Multiple sclerosis
431 Intracerebral hemorrhage — (Use additional code to identify presence of hypertension)

ICD-9-CM Procedural

01.09 Other cranial puncture
01.13 Closed (percutaneous) (needle) biopsy of brain
87.03 Computerized axial tomography of head
88.91 Magnetic resonance imaging of brain and brain stem
88.96 Other intraoperative magnetic resonance imaging
92.30 Stereotactic radiosurgery, not otherwise specified

61760

61760 Stereotactic implantation of depth electrodes into the cerebrum for long term seizure monitoring

ICD-9-CM Diagnostic

345.10 Generalized convulsive epilepsy without mention of intractable epilepsy
345.11 Generalized convulsive epilepsy with intractable epilepsy
345.3 Epileptic grand mal status
345.40 Partial epilepsy with impairment of consciousness, without mention of intractable epilepsy
345.41 Partial epilepsy with impairment of consciousness, with intractable epilepsy
345.80 Other forms of epilepsy without mention of intractable epilepsy
345.81 Other forms of epilepsy with intractable epilepsy

ICD-9-CM Procedural

02.93 Implantation or replacement of intracranial neurostimulator lead(s)

61770

61770 Stereotactic localization, including burr hole(s), with insertion of catheter(s) or probe(s) for placement of radiation source

ICD-9-CM Diagnostic

191.0 Malignant neoplasm of cerebrum, except lobes and ventricles
191.1 Malignant neoplasm of frontal lobe of brain
191.2 Malignant neoplasm of temporal lobe of brain
191.3 Malignant neoplasm of parietal lobe of brain
191.4 Malignant neoplasm of occipital lobe of brain
191.5 Malignant neoplasm of ventricles of brain
191.6 Malignant neoplasm of cerebellum NOS
191.7 Malignant neoplasm of brain stem
191.8 Malignant neoplasm of other parts of brain
194.3 Malignant neoplasm of pituitary gland and craniopharyngeal duct — (Use additional code to identify any functional activity)
198.3 Secondary malignant neoplasm of brain and spinal cord
198.89 Secondary malignant neoplasm of other specified sites
234.8 Carcinoma in situ of other specified sites
237.0 Neoplasm of uncertain behavior of pituitary gland and craniopharyngeal duct — (Use additional code to identify any functional activity)

ICD-9-CM Procedural

01.24 Other craniotomy
87.03 Computerized axial tomography of head
93.59 Other immobilization, pressure, and attention to wound

61790–61791

61790 Creation of lesion by stereotactic method, percutaneous, by neurolytic agent (eg, alcohol, thermal, electrical, radiofrequency); gasserian ganglion
61791 trigeminal medullary tract

ICD-9-CM Diagnostic

192.0 Malignant neoplasm of cranial nerves
195.0 Malignant neoplasm of head, face, and neck
198.4 Secondary malignant neoplasm of other parts of nervous system
350.1 Trigeminal neuralgia
350.2 Atypical face pain
350.8 Other specified trigeminal nerve disorders

ICD-9-CM Procedural

04.05 Gasserian ganglionectomy
04.2 Destruction of cranial and peripheral nerves

61793

61793 Stereotactic radiosurgery (particle beam, gamma ray or linear accelerator), one or more sessions

ICD-9-CM Diagnostic

191.0 Malignant neoplasm of cerebrum, except lobes and ventricles
191.1 Malignant neoplasm of frontal lobe of brain
191.2 Malignant neoplasm of temporal lobe of brain
191.3 Malignant neoplasm of parietal lobe of brain
191.4 Malignant neoplasm of occipital lobe of brain
191.5 Malignant neoplasm of ventricles of brain
191.6 Malignant neoplasm of cerebellum NOS
191.7 Malignant neoplasm of brain stem
192.1 Malignant neoplasm of cerebral meninges

194.3 Malignant neoplasm of pituitary gland and craniopharyngeal duct — (Use additional code to identify any functional activity)
198.3 Secondary malignant neoplasm of brain and spinal cord
225.0 Benign neoplasm of brain
225.1 Benign neoplasm of cranial nerves
225.2 Benign neoplasm of cerebral meninges
227.3 Benign neoplasm of pituitary gland and craniopharyngeal duct (pouch) — (Use additional code to identify any functional activity)
237.0 Neoplasm of uncertain behavior of pituitary gland and craniopharyngeal duct — (Use additional code to identify any functional activity)
237.5 Neoplasm of uncertain behavior of brain and spinal cord
239.6 Neoplasm of unspecified nature of brain

ICD-9-CM Procedural

92.31 Single source photon radiosurgery
92.32 Multi-source photon radiosurgery
92.33 Particulate radiosurgery
93.59 Other immobilization, pressure, and attention to wound

61795

61795 Stereotactic computer assisted volumetric (navigational) procedure, intracranial, extracranial, or spinal (List separately in addition to code for primary procedure)

ICD-9-CM Diagnostic

This is an add-on code. Refer to the corresponding primary procedure code for ICD-9 diagnosis code links.

ICD-9-CM Procedural

00.31 Computer assisted surgery with CT/CTA
00.32 Computer assisted surgery with MR/MRA
00.33 Computer assisted surgery with fluoroscopy
00.34 Imageless computer assisted surgery
00.35 Computer assisted surgery with multiple datasets
00.39 Other computer assisted surgery

61850

61850 Twist drill or burr hole(s) for implantation of neurostimulator electrodes, cortical

ICD-9-CM Diagnostic

296.33 Major depressive disorder, recurrent episode, severe, without mention of psychotic behavior — (Use additional code to identify any associated physical disease, injury, or condition affecting the brain)
300.3 Obsessive-compulsive disorders
345.11 Generalized convulsive epilepsy with intractable epilepsy
350.2 Atypical face pain
723.1 Cervicalgia
729.2 Unspecified neuralgia, neuritis, and radiculitis ▽
782.0 Disturbance of skin sensation
784.0 Headache

ICD-9-CM Procedural

02.93 Implantation or replacement of intracranial neurostimulator lead(s)

61860

61860 Craniectomy or craniotomy for implantation of neurostimulator electrodes, cerebral, cortical

ICD-9-CM Diagnostic

296.33 Major depressive disorder, recurrent episode, severe, without mention of psychotic behavior — (Use additional code to identify any associated physical disease, injury, or condition affecting the brain)
300.3 Obsessive-compulsive disorders
307.48 Repetitive intrusions of sleep
343.3 Monoplegic infantile cerebral palsy
344.40 Monoplegia of upper limb affecting unspecified side ▽
344.41 Monoplegia of upper limb affecting dominant side
344.42 Monoplegia of upper limb affecting nondominant side
345.11 Generalized convulsive epilepsy with intractable epilepsy
345.40 Partial epilepsy with impairment of consciousness, without mention of intractable epilepsy
346.01 Classical migraine with intractable migraine, so stated
346.11 Common migraine with intractable migraine, so stated
346.20 Variants of migraine without mention of intractable migraine
348.1 Anoxic brain damage — (Use additional E code to identify cause)
350.1 Trigeminal neuralgia
350.2 Atypical face pain
433.21 Occlusion and stenosis of vertebral artery with cerebral infarction — (Use additional code to identify presence of hypertension)
723.1 Cervicalgia
729.2 Unspecified neuralgia, neuritis, and radiculitis ▽
782.4 Jaundice, unspecified, not of newborn ▽
784.0 Headache

ICD-9-CM Procedural

02.93 Implantation or replacement of intracranial neurostimulator lead(s)

61863–61864

61863 Twist drill, burr hole, craniotomy, or craniectomy with stereotactic implantation of neurostimulator electrode array in subcortical site (eg, thalamus, globus pallidus, subthalamic nucleus, periventricular, periaqueductal gray), without use of intraoperative microelectrode recording; first array
61864 each additional array (List separately in addition to primary procedure)

ICD-9-CM Diagnostic

296.33 Major depressive disorder, recurrent episode, severe, without mention of psychotic behavior — (Use additional code to identify any associated physical disease, injury, or condition affecting the brain)
300.3 Obsessive-compulsive disorders
307.48 Repetitive intrusions of sleep
332.0 Paralysis agitans
333.1 Essential and other specified forms of tremor — (Use additional E code to identify drug, if drug-induced)
343.3 Monoplegic infantile cerebral palsy
344.41 Monoplegia of upper limb affecting dominant side
344.42 Monoplegia of upper limb affecting nondominant side
345.11 Generalized convulsive epilepsy with intractable epilepsy
346.01 Classical migraine with intractable migraine, so stated
346.11 Common migraine with intractable migraine, so stated
348.1 Anoxic brain damage — (Use additional E code to identify cause)
350.1 Trigeminal neuralgia

ICD-9-CM Procedural

02.93 Implantation or replacement of intracranial neurostimulator lead(s)

61867–61868

61867 Twist drill, burr hole, craniotomy, or craniectomy with stereotactic implantation of neurostimulator electrode array in subcortical site (eg, thalamus, globus pallidus, subthalamic nucleus, periventricular, periaqueductal gray), with use of intraoperative microelectrode recording; first array
61868 each additional array (List separately in addition to primary procedure)

ICD-9-CM Diagnostic

296.33 Major depressive disorder, recurrent episode, severe, without mention of psychotic behavior — (Use additional code to identify any associated physical disease, injury, or condition affecting the brain)
300.3 Obsessive-compulsive disorders
307.48 Repetitive intrusions of sleep
332.0 Paralysis agitans
333.1 Essential and other specified forms of tremor — (Use additional E code to identify drug, if drug-induced)
343.3 Monoplegic infantile cerebral palsy
344.41 Monoplegia of upper limb affecting dominant side
344.42 Monoplegia of upper limb affecting nondominant side
345.11 Generalized convulsive epilepsy with intractable epilepsy
346.01 Classical migraine with intractable migraine, so stated
346.11 Common migraine with intractable migraine, so stated
348.1 Anoxic brain damage — (Use additional E code to identify cause)
350.1 Trigeminal neuralgia

ICD-9-CM Procedural

02.93 Implantation or replacement of intracranial neurostimulator lead(s)

61870–61875

61870 Craniectomy for implantation of neurostimulator electrodes, cerebellar; cortical
61875 subcortical

ICD-9-CM Diagnostic

307.48 Repetitive intrusions of sleep

332.0 Paralysis agitans
333.1 Essential and other specified forms of tremor — (Use additional E code to identify drug, if drug-induced)
343.3 Monoplegic infantile cerebral palsy
344.41 Monoplegia of upper limb affecting dominant side
344.42 Monoplegia of upper limb affecting nondominant side
345.11 Generalized convulsive epilepsy with intractable epilepsy
346.01 Classical migraine with intractable migraine, so stated
346.11 Common migraine with intractable migraine, so stated
346.20 Variants of migraine without mention of intractable migraine
348.1 Anoxic brain damage — (Use additional E code to identify cause)
350.1 Trigeminal neuralgia
350.2 Atypical face pain
433.21 Occlusion and stenosis of vertebral artery with cerebral infarction — (Use additional code to identify presence of hypertension)

ICD-9-CM Procedural

02.93 Implantation or replacement of intracranial neurostimulator lead(s)

61880

61880 Revision or removal of intracranial neurostimulator electrodes

ICD-9-CM Diagnostic

307.81 Tension headache
307.89 Other pain disorder related to psychological factors
332.0 Paralysis agitans
345.10 Generalized convulsive epilepsy without mention of intractable epilepsy
345.2 Epileptic petit mal status
345.3 Epileptic grand mal status
345.40 Partial epilepsy with impairment of consciousness, without mention of intractable epilepsy
350.1 Trigeminal neuralgia
996.2 Mechanical complication of nervous system device, implant, and graft
996.63 Infection and inflammatory reaction due to nervous system device, implant, and graft — (Use additional code to identify specified infections)
996.75 Other complications due to nervous system device, implant, and graft
998.51 Infected postoperative seroma — (Use additional code to identify organism)
998.59 Other postoperative infection — (Use additional code to identify infection)
V53.02 Neuropacemaker (brain) (peripheral nerve) (spinal cord)

ICD-9-CM Procedural

01.22 Removal of intracranial neurostimulator lead(s)
02.99 Other operations on skull, brain, and cerebral meninges

61885–61886

61885 Insertion or replacement of cranial neurostimulator pulse generator or receiver, direct or inductive coupling; with connection to a single electrode array
61886 with connection to two or more electrode arrays

ICD-9-CM Diagnostic

296.33 Major depressive disorder, recurrent episode, severe, without mention of psychotic behavior — (Use additional code to identify any associated physical disease, injury, or condition affecting the brain)
300.3 Obsessive-compulsive disorders
332.0 Paralysis agitans
333.1 Essential and other specified forms of tremor — (Use additional E code to identify drug, if drug-induced)
345.01 Generalized nonconvulsive epilepsy with intractable epilepsy
345.11 Generalized convulsive epilepsy with intractable epilepsy
345.41 Partial epilepsy with impairment of consciousness, with intractable epilepsy
345.51 Partial epilepsy without mention of impairment of consciousness, with intractable epilepsy
345.91 Unspecified epilepsy with intractable epilepsy ▽
350.2 Atypical face pain
723.1 Cervicalgia
729.2 Unspecified neuralgia, neuritis, and radiculitis ▽
780.39 Other convulsions
996.2 Mechanical complication of nervous system device, implant, and graft
996.63 Infection and inflammatory reaction due to nervous system device, implant, and graft — (Use additional code to identify specified infections)
996.75 Other complications due to nervous system device, implant, and graft
997.00 Unspecified nervous system complication — (Use additional code to identify complications) ▽

ICD-9-CM Procedural

86.94 Insertion or replacement of single array neurostimulator pulse generator
86.95 Insertion or replacement of dual array neurostimulator pulse generator

61888

61888 Revision or removal of cranial neurostimulator pulse generator or receiver

ICD-9-CM Diagnostic

307.81 Tension headache
307.89 Other pain disorder related to psychological factors
332.0 Paralysis agitans
345.10 Generalized convulsive epilepsy without mention of intractable epilepsy
345.2 Epileptic petit mal status
345.3 Epileptic grand mal status
350.1 Trigeminal neuralgia
996.2 Mechanical complication of nervous system device, implant, and graft
996.63 Infection and inflammatory reaction due to nervous system device, implant, and graft — (Use additional code to identify specified infections)
996.75 Other complications due to nervous system device, implant, and graft
998.51 Infected postoperative seroma — (Use additional code to identify organism)
998.59 Other postoperative infection — (Use additional code to identify infection)
V53.02 Neuropacemaker (brain) (peripheral nerve) (spinal cord)

ICD-9-CM Procedural

02.99 Other operations on skull, brain, and cerebral meninges
86.05 Incision with removal of foreign body or device from skin and subcutaneous tissue

62000–62010

62000 Elevation of depressed skull fracture; simple, extradural
62005 compound or comminuted, extradural
62010 with repair of dura and/or debridement of brain

ICD-9-CM Diagnostic

800.02 Closed fracture of vault of skull without mention of intracranial injury, brief (less than one hour) loss of consciousness
800.10 Closed fracture of vault of skull with cerebral laceration and contusion, unspecified state of consciousness ▽
800.13 Closed fracture of vault of skull with cerebral laceration and contusion, moderate (1-24 hours) loss of consciousness
800.16 Closed fracture of vault of skull with cerebral laceration and contusion, loss of consciousness of unspecified duration ▽
800.21 Closed fracture of vault of skull with subarachnoid, subdural, and extradural hemorrhage, no loss of consciousness
800.26 Closed fracture of vault of skull with subarachnoid, subdural, and extradural hemorrhage, loss of consciousness of unspecified duration ▽
800.41 Closed fracture of vault of skull with intracranial injury of other and unspecified nature, no loss of consciousness ▽
800.46 Closed fracture of vault of skull with intracranial injury of other and unspecified nature, loss of consciousness of unspecified duration ▽
800.50 Open fracture of vault of skull without mention of intracranial injury, unspecified state of consciousness ▽
800.56 Open fracture of vault of skull without mention of intracranial injury, loss of consciousness of unspecified duration ▽
800.60 Open fracture of vault of skull with cerebral laceration and contusion, unspecified state of consciousness ▽
800.63 Open fracture of vault of skull with cerebral laceration and contusion, moderate (1-24 hours) loss of consciousness
800.65 Open fracture of vault of skull with cerebral laceration and contusion, prolonged (more than 24 hours) loss of consciousness, without return to pre-existing conscious level
800.66 Open fracture of vault of skull with cerebral laceration and contusion, loss of consciousness of unspecified duration ▽
800.76 Open fracture of vault of skull with subarachnoid, subdural, and extradural hemorrhage, loss of consciousness of unspecified duration ▽
801.01 Closed fracture of base of skull without mention of intracranial injury, no loss of consciousness
801.23 Closed fracture of base of skull with subarachnoid, subdural, and extradural hemorrhage, moderate (1-24 hours) loss of consciousness
801.46 Closed fracture of base of skull with intracranial injury of other and unspecified nature, loss of consciousness of unspecified duration ▽
801.50 Open fracture of base of skull without mention of intracranial injury, unspecified state of consciousness ▽
801.51 Open fracture of base of skull without mention of intracranial injury, no loss of consciousness
801.56 Open fracture of base of skull without mention of intracranial injury, loss of consciousness of unspecified duration ▽

801.66 Open fracture of base of skull with cerebral laceration and contusion, loss of consciousness of unspecified duration
801.76 Open fracture of base of skull with subarachnoid, subdural, and extradural hemorrhage, loss of consciousness of unspecified duration
803.11 Other closed skull fracture with cerebral laceration and contusion, no loss of consciousness
803.21 Other closed skull fracture with subarachnoid, subdural, and extradural hemorrhage, no loss of consciousness
803.26 Other closed skull fracture with subarachnoid, subdural, and extradural hemorrhage, loss of consciousness of unspecified duration
803.50 Other open skull fracture without mention of injury, state of consciousness unspecified
803.51 Other open skull fracture without mention of intracranial injury, no loss of consciousness
803.56 Other open skull fracture without mention of intracranial injury, loss of consciousness of unspecified duration
803.61 Other open skull fracture with cerebral laceration and contusion, no loss of consciousness
803.66 Other open skull fracture with cerebral laceration and contusion, loss of consciousness of unspecified duration
804.12 Closed fractures involving skull or face with other bones, with cerebral laceration and contusion, brief (less than one hour) loss of consciousness
804.56 Open fractures involving skull or face with other bones, without mention of intracranial injury, loss of consciousness of unspecified duration
804.66 Open fractures involving skull or face with other bones, with cerebral laceration and contusion, loss of consciousness of unspecified duration

ICD-9-CM Procedural
01.59 Other excision or destruction of lesion or tissue of brain
02.02 Elevation of skull fracture fragments

62100
62100 Craniotomy for repair of dural/cerebrospinal fluid leak, including surgery for rhinorrhea/otorrhea

ICD-9-CM Diagnostic
349.81 Cerebrospinal fluid rhinorrhea
388.61 Cerebrospinal fluid otorrhea
800.43 Closed fracture of vault of skull with intracranial injury of other and unspecified nature, moderate (1-24 hours) loss of consciousness
800.56 Open fracture of vault of skull without mention of intracranial injury, loss of consciousness of unspecified duration
800.66 Open fracture of vault of skull with cerebral laceration and contusion, loss of consciousness of unspecified duration
801.22 Closed fracture of base of skull with subarachnoid, subdural, and extradural hemorrhage, brief (less than one hour) loss of consciousness
801.41 Closed fracture of base of skull with intracranial injury of other and unspecified nature, no loss of consciousness
801.46 Closed fracture of base of skull with intracranial injury of other and unspecified nature, loss of consciousness of unspecified duration
997.01 Central nervous system complication — (Use additional code to identify complications)
998.2 Accidental puncture or laceration during procedure

ICD-9-CM Procedural
02.11 Simple suture of dura mater of brain
02.12 Other repair of cerebral meninges

62115–62117
62115 Reduction of craniomegalic skull (eg, treated hydrocephalus); not requiring bone grafts or cranioplasty
62116 with simple cranioplasty
62117 requiring craniotomy and reconstruction with or without bone graft (includes obtaining grafts)

ICD-9-CM Diagnostic
331.3 Communicating hydrocephalus
331.4 Obstructive hydrocephalus
733.3 Hyperostosis of skull
738.12 Zygomatic hypoplasia
738.19 Other specified acquired deformity of head
741.00 Spina bifida with hydrocephalus, unspecified region
742.3 Congenital hydrocephalus

ICD-9-CM Procedural
02.01 Opening of cranial suture
02.04 Bone graft to skull
02.06 Other cranial osteoplasty

62120–62121
62120 Repair of encephalocele, skull vault, including cranioplasty
62121 Craniotomy for repair of encephalocele, skull base

ICD-9-CM Diagnostic
742.0 Encephalocele
742.3 Congenital hydrocephalus
905.0 Late effect of fracture of skull and face bones

ICD-9-CM Procedural
02.12 Other repair of cerebral meninges

62140–62141
62140 Cranioplasty for skull defect; up to 5 cm diameter
62141 larger than 5 cm diameter

ICD-9-CM Diagnostic
738.11 Zygomatic hyperplasia
740.0 Anencephalus
741.00 Spina bifida with hydrocephalus, unspecified region
742.1 Microcephalus
742.3 Congenital hydrocephalus
754.0 Congenital musculoskeletal deformities of skull, face, and jaw
756.0 Congenital anomalies of skull and face bones
800.65 Open fracture of vault of skull with cerebral laceration and contusion, prolonged (more than 24 hours) loss of consciousness, without return to pre-existing conscious level
800.75 Open fracture of vault of skull with subarachnoid, subdural, and extradural hemorrhage, prolonged (more than 24 hours) loss of consciousness, without return to pre-existing conscious level
905.0 Late effect of fracture of skull and face bones

ICD-9-CM Procedural
02.06 Other cranial osteoplasty

62142
62142 Removal of bone flap or prosthetic plate of skull

ICD-9-CM Diagnostic
170.0 Malignant neoplasm of bones of skull and face, except mandible
738.19 Other specified acquired deformity of head
996.60 Infection and inflammatory reaction due to unspecified device, implant, and graft — (Use additional code to identify specified infections)
996.63 Infection and inflammatory reaction due to nervous system device, implant, and graft — (Use additional code to identify specified infections)

ICD-9-CM Procedural
02.06 Other cranial osteoplasty
02.07 Removal of skull plate

62143
62143 Replacement of bone flap or prosthetic plate of skull

ICD-9-CM Diagnostic
170.0 Malignant neoplasm of bones of skull and face, except mandible
738.19 Other specified acquired deformity of head
800.65 Open fracture of vault of skull with cerebral laceration and contusion, prolonged (more than 24 hours) loss of consciousness, without return to pre-existing conscious level
800.75 Open fracture of vault of skull with subarachnoid, subdural, and extradural hemorrhage, prolonged (more than 24 hours) loss of consciousness, without return to pre-existing conscious level
905.0 Late effect of fracture of skull and face bones
907.0 Late effect of intracranial injury without mention of skull fracture
996.60 Infection and inflammatory reaction due to unspecified device, implant, and graft — (Use additional code to identify specified infections)
996.63 Infection and inflammatory reaction due to nervous system device, implant, and graft — (Use additional code to identify specified infections)

ICD-9-CM Procedural
02.05 Insertion of skull plate
02.06 Other cranial osteoplasty

Unspecified code
Female diagnosis
Manifestation code
Male diagnosis

62145

62145 Cranioplasty for skull defect with reparative brain surgery

ICD-9-CM Diagnostic

170.0 Malignant neoplasm of bones of skull and face, except mandible
738.19 Other specified acquired deformity of head
742.4 Other specified congenital anomalies of brain
756.0 Congenital anomalies of skull and face bones
800.66 Open fracture of vault of skull with cerebral laceration and contusion, loss of consciousness of unspecified duration ▽
801.06 Closed fracture of base of skull without mention of intracranial injury, loss of consciousness of unspecified duration ▽
801.66 Open fracture of base of skull with cerebral laceration and contusion, loss of consciousness of unspecified duration ▽
803.66 Other open skull fracture with cerebral laceration and contusion, loss of consciousness of unspecified duration ▽

ICD-9-CM Procedural

02.06 Other cranial osteoplasty

62146–62147

62146 Cranioplasty with autograft (includes obtaining bone grafts); up to 5 cm diameter
62147 larger than 5 cm diameter

ICD-9-CM Diagnostic

170.0 Malignant neoplasm of bones of skull and face, except mandible
738.19 Other specified acquired deformity of head
742.4 Other specified congenital anomalies of brain
756.0 Congenital anomalies of skull and face bones
800.66 Open fracture of vault of skull with cerebral laceration and contusion, loss of consciousness of unspecified duration ▽
801.06 Closed fracture of base of skull without mention of intracranial injury, loss of consciousness of unspecified duration ▽
801.66 Open fracture of base of skull with cerebral laceration and contusion, loss of consciousness of unspecified duration ▽
803.61 Other open skull fracture with cerebral laceration and contusion, no loss of consciousness
854.06 Intracranial injury of other and unspecified nature, without mention of open intracranial wound, loss of consciousness of unspecified duration ▽

ICD-9-CM Procedural

02.04 Bone graft to skull
02.06 Other cranial osteoplasty

62148

62148 Incision and retrieval of subcutaneous cranial bone graft for cranioplasty (List separately in addition to code for primary procedure)

ICD-9-CM Diagnostic

This is an add-on code. Refer to the corresponding primary procedure code for ICD-9 diagnosis code links.

ICD-9-CM Procedural

02.03 Formation of cranial bone flap
02.06 Other cranial osteoplasty

HCPCS Level II Supplies & Services

The HCPCS Level II code(s) would be the same as the actual procedure performed because these are in-addition-to codes.

62160

62160 Neuroendoscopy, intracranial, for placement or replacement of ventricular catheter and attachment to shunt system or external drainage (List separately in addition to code for primary procedure)

ICD-9-CM Diagnostic

This is an add-on code. Refer to the corresponding primary procedure code for ICD-9 diagnosis code links.

ICD-9-CM Procedural

02.31 Ventricular shunt to structure in head and neck
02.32 Ventricular shunt to circulatory system
02.33 Ventricular shunt to thoracic cavity
02.34 Ventricular shunt to abdominal cavity and organs
02.35 Ventricular shunt to urinary system
02.39 Other operations to establish drainage of ventricle
02.42 Replacement of ventricular shunt

HCPCS Level II Supplies & Services

The HCPCS Level II code(s) would be the same as the actual procedure performed because these are in-addition-to codes.

62161–62162

62161 Neuroendoscopy, intracranial; with dissection of adhesions, fenestration of septum pellucidum or intraventricular cysts (including placement, replacement, or removal of ventricular catheter)
62162 with fenestration or excision of colloid cyst, including placement of external ventricular catheter for drainage

ICD-9-CM Diagnostic

348.0 Cerebral cysts
349.2 Disorders of meninges, not elsewhere classified ▽
742.4 Other specified congenital anomalies of brain

ICD-9-CM Procedural

01.59 Other excision or destruction of lesion or tissue of brain

HCPCS Level II Supplies & Services

HCPCS Level II codes are used to report the supplies, durable medical equipment, and certain medical services provided on an outpatient basis. Because the procedure(s) represented on this page would be performed in an inpatient facility, no HCPCS Level II codes apply.

62163

62163 Neuroendoscopy, intracranial; with retrieval of foreign body

ICD-9-CM Diagnostic

851.10 Cortex (cerebral) contusion with open intracranial wound, unspecified state of consciousness ▽
851.11 Cortex (cerebral) contusion with open intracranial wound, no loss of consciousness
851.12 Cortex (cerebral) contusion with open intracranial wound, brief (less than 1 hour) loss of consciousness
851.13 Cortex (cerebral) contusion with open intracranial wound, moderate (1-24 hours) loss of consciousness
851.14 Cortex (cerebral) contusion with open intracranial wound, prolonged (more than 24 hours) loss of consciousness and return to pre-existing conscious level
851.15 Cortex (cerebral) contusion with open intracranial wound, prolonged (more than 24 hours) loss of consciousness, without return to pre-existing conscious level
851.16 Cortex (cerebral) contusion with open intracranial wound, loss of consciousness of unspecified duration ▽
851.19 Cortex (cerebral) contusion with open intracranial wound, unspecified concussion ▽
851.30 Cortex (cerebral) laceration with open intracranial wound, unspecified state of consciousness ▽
851.31 Cortex (cerebral) laceration with open intracranial wound, no loss of consciousness
851.32 Cortex (cerebral) laceration with open intracranial wound, brief (less than 1 hour) loss of consciousness
851.33 Cortex (cerebral) laceration with open intracranial wound, moderate (1-24 hours) loss of consciousness
851.34 Cortex (cerebral) laceration with open intracranial wound, prolonged (more than 24 hours) loss of consciousness and return to pre-existing conscious level
851.35 Cortex (cerebral) laceration with open intracranial wound, prolonged (more than 24 hours) loss of consciousness, without return to pre-existing conscious level
851.36 Cortex (cerebral) laceration with open intracranial wound, loss of consciousness of unspecified duration ▽
851.39 Cortex (cerebral) laceration with open intracranial wound, unspecified concussion ▽
851.50 Cerebellar or brain stem contusion with open intracranial wound, unspecified state of consciousness ▽
851.51 Cerebellar or brain stem contusion with open intracranial wound, no loss of consciousness
851.52 Cerebellar or brain stem contusion with open intracranial wound, brief (less than 1 hour) loss of consciousness
851.53 Cerebellar or brain stem contusion with open intracranial wound, moderate (1-24 hours) loss of consciousness

▽ Unspecified code ♀ Female diagnosis ☒ Manifestation code ♂ Male diagnosis

851.54 Cerebellar or brain stem contusion with open intracranial wound, prolonged (more than 24 hours) loss of consciousness and return to pre-existing conscious level
851.55 Cerebellar or brain stem contusion with open intracranial wound, prolonged (more than 24 hours) loss of consciousness, without return to pre-existing conscious level
851.56 Cerebellar or brain stem contusion with open intracranial wound, loss of consciousness of unspecified duration
851.59 Cerebellar or brain stem contusion with open intracranial wound, unspecified concussion
851.70 Cerebellar or brain stem laceration with open intracranial wound, state of consciousness unspecified
851.71 Cerebellar or brain stem laceration with open intracranial wound, no loss of consciousness
851.72 Cerebellar or brain stem laceration with open intracranial wound, brief (less than one hour) loss of consciousness
851.73 Cerebellar or brain stem laceration with open intracranial wound, moderate (1-24 hours) loss of consciousness
851.74 Cerebellar or brain stem laceration with open intracranial wound, prolonged (more than 24 hours) loss of consciousness and return to pre-existing conscious level
851.75 Cerebellar or brain stem laceration with open intracranial wound, prolonged (more than 24 hours) loss of consciousness, without return to pre-existing conscious level
851.76 Cerebellar or brain stem laceration with open intracranial wound, loss of consciousness of unspecified duration
851.79 Cerebellar or brain stem laceration with open intracranial wound, unspecified concussion
851.90 Other and unspecified cerebral laceration and contusion, with open intracranial wound, unspecified state of consciousness
851.91 Other and unspecified cerebral laceration and contusion, with open intracranial wound, no loss of consciousness
851.92 Other and unspecified cerebral laceration and contusion, with open intracranial wound, brief (less than 1 hour) loss of consciousness
851.93 Other and unspecified cerebral laceration and contusion, with open intracranial wound, moderate (1-24 hours) loss of consciousness
851.94 Other and unspecified cerebral laceration and contusion, with open intracranial wound, prolonged (more than 24 hours) loss of consciousness and return to pre-existing conscious level
851.95 Other and unspecified cerebral laceration and contusion, with open intracranial wound, prolonged (more than 24 hours) loss of consciousness, without return to pre-existing conscious level
851.96 Other and unspecified cerebral laceration and contusion, with open intracranial wound, loss of consciousness of unspecified duration
851.99 Other and unspecified cerebral laceration and contusion, with open intracranial wound, unspecified concussion
852.10 Subarachnoid hemorrhage following injury, with open intracranial wound, unspecified state of consciousness
852.11 Subarachnoid hemorrhage following injury, with open intracranial wound, no loss of consciousness
852.12 Subarachnoid hemorrhage following injury, with open intracranial wound, brief (less than 1 hour) loss of consciousness
852.13 Subarachnoid hemorrhage following injury, with open intracranial wound, moderate (1-24 hours) loss of consciousness
852.14 Subarachnoid hemorrhage following injury, with open intracranial wound, prolonged (more than 24 hours) loss of consciousness and return to pre-existing conscious level
852.15 Subarachnoid hemorrhage following injury, with open intracranial wound, prolonged (more than 24 hours) loss of consciousness, without return to pre-existing conscious level
852.16 Subarachnoid hemorrhage following injury, with open intracranial wound, loss of consciousness of unspecified duration
852.19 Subarachnoid hemorrhage following injury, with open intracranial wound, unspecified concussion
852.30 Subdural hemorrhage following injury, with open intracranial wound, state of consciousness unspecified
852.31 Subdural hemorrhage following injury, with open intracranial wound, no loss of consciousness
852.32 Subdural hemorrhage following injury, with open intracranial wound, brief (less than 1 hour) loss of consciousness
852.33 Subdural hemorrhage following injury, with open intracranial wound, moderate (1-24 hours) loss of consciousness
852.34 Subdural hemorrhage following injury, with open intracranial wound, prolonged (more than 24 hours) loss of consciousness and return to pre-existing conscious level
852.35 Subdural hemorrhage following injury, with open intracranial wound, prolonged (more than 24 hours) loss of consciousness, without return to pre-existing conscious level
852.36 Subdural hemorrhage following injury, with open intracranial wound, loss of consciousness of unspecified duration
852.39 Subdural hemorrhage following injury, with open intracranial wound, unspecified concussion
852.50 Extradural hemorrhage following injury, with open intracranial wound, state of consciousness unspecified
852.51 Extradural hemorrhage following injury, with open intracranial wound, no loss of consciousness
852.52 Extradural hemorrhage following injury, with open intracranial wound, brief (less than 1 hour) loss of consciousness
852.53 Extradural hemorrhage following injury, with open intracranial wound, moderate (1-24 hours) loss of consciousness
852.54 Extradural hemorrhage following injury, with open intracranial wound, prolonged (more than 24 hours) loss of consciousness and return to pre-existing conscious level
852.55 Extradural hemorrhage following injury, with open intracranial wound, prolonged (more than 24 hours) loss of consciousness, without return to pre-existing conscious level
852.56 Extradural hemorrhage following injury, with open intracranial wound, loss of consciousness of unspecified duration
852.59 Extradural hemorrhage following injury, with open intracranial wound, unspecifiedconcussion
853.10 Other and unspecified intracranial hemorrhage following injury, with open intracranial wound, unspecified state of consciousness
853.11 Other and unspecified intracranial hemorrhage following injury, with open intracranial wound, no loss of consciousness
853.12 Other and unspecified intracranial hemorrhage following injury, with open intracranial wound, brief (less than 1 hour) loss of consciousness
853.13 Other and unspecified intracranial hemorrhage following injury, with open intracranial wound, moderate (1-24 hours) loss of consciousness
853.14 Other and unspecified intracranial hemorrhage following injury, with open intracranial wound, prolonged (more than 24 hours) loss of consciousness and return to pre-existing conscious level
853.15 Other and unspecified intracranial hemorrhage following injury, with open intracranial wound, prolonged (more than 24 hours) loss of consciousness, without return to pre-existing conscious level
853.16 Other and unspecified intracranial hemorrhage following injury, with open intracranial wound, loss of consciousness of unspecified duration
853.19 Other and unspecified intracranial hemorrhage following injury, with open intracranial wound, unspecified concussion
854.10 Intracranial injury of other and unspecified nature, with open intracranial wound, unspecified state of consciousness
854.11 Intracranial injury of other and unspecified nature, with open intracranial wound, no loss of consciousness
854.12 Intracranial injury of other and unspecified nature, with open intracranial wound, brief (less than 1 hour) loss of consciousness
854.13 Intracranial injury of other and unspecified nature, with open intracranial wound, moderate (1-24 hours) loss of consciousness
854.14 Intracranial injury of other and unspecified nature, with open intracranial wound, prolonged (more than 24 hours) loss of consciousness and return to pre-existing conscious level
854.15 Intracranial injury of other and unspecified nature, with open intracranial wound, prolonged (more than 24 hours) loss of consciousness, without return to pre-existing conscious level
854.16 Intracranial injury of other and unspecified nature, with open intracranial wound, loss of consciousness of unspecified duration
854.19 Intracranial injury of other and unspecified nature, with open intracranial wound, with unspecified concussion

ICD-9-CM Procedural

01.24 Other craniotomy
01.39 Other incision of brain

HCPCS Level II Supplies & Services

HCPCS Level II codes are used to report the supplies, durable medical equipment, and certain medical services provided on an outpatient basis. Because the procedure(s) represented on this page would be performed in an inpatient facility, no HCPCS Level II codes apply.

Unspecified code
Female diagnosis
Manifestation code
Male diagnosis

62164

62164 Neuroendoscopy, intracranial; with excision of brain tumor, including placement of external ventricular catheter for drainage

ICD-9-CM Diagnostic

191.0 Malignant neoplasm of cerebrum, except lobes and ventricles
191.1 Malignant neoplasm of frontal lobe of brain
191.2 Malignant neoplasm of temporal lobe of brain
191.3 Malignant neoplasm of parietal lobe of brain
191.4 Malignant neoplasm of occipital lobe of brain
191.5 Malignant neoplasm of ventricles of brain
191.6 Malignant neoplasm of cerebellum NOS
191.7 Malignant neoplasm of brain stem
191.8 Malignant neoplasm of other parts of brain
191.9 Malignant neoplasm of brain, unspecified site ▽
192.0 Malignant neoplasm of cranial nerves
192.1 Malignant neoplasm of cerebral meninges
192.8 Malignant neoplasm of other specified sites of nervous system
198.3 Secondary malignant neoplasm of brain and spinal cord
225.0 Benign neoplasm of brain
225.1 Benign neoplasm of cranial nerves
237.5 Neoplasm of uncertain behavior of brain and spinal cord
239.6 Neoplasm of unspecified nature of brain

ICD-9-CM Procedural

01.59 Other excision or destruction of lesion or tissue of brain

HCPCS Level II Supplies & Services

HCPCS Level II codes are used to report the supplies, durable medical equipment, and certain medical services provided on an outpatient basis. Because the procedure(s) represented on this page would be performed in an inpatient facility, no HCPCS Level II codes apply.

62165

62165 Neuroendoscopy, intracranial; with excision of pituitary tumor, transnasal or trans-sphenoidal approach

ICD-9-CM Diagnostic

194.3 Malignant neoplasm of pituitary gland and craniopharyngeal duct — (Use additional code to identify any functional activity)
227.3 Benign neoplasm of pituitary gland and craniopharyngeal duct (pouch) — (Use additional code to identify any functional activity)
237.0 Neoplasm of uncertain behavior of pituitary gland and craniopharyngeal duct — (Use additional code to identify any functional activity)
239.7 Neoplasm of unspecified nature of endocrine glands and other parts of nervous system
253.0 Acromegaly and gigantism
253.1 Other and unspecified anterior pituitary hyperfunction ▽
253.2 Panhypopituitarism
253.3 Pituitary dwarfism
253.4 Other anterior pituitary disorders
253.5 Diabetes insipidus
253.6 Other disorders of neurohypophysis
253.7 Iatrogenic pituitary disorders — (Use additional E code to identify cause)
253.8 Other disorders of the pituitary and other syndromes of diencephalohypophyseal origin
253.9 Unspecified disorder of the pituitary gland and its hypothalamic control ▽

ICD-9-CM Procedural

07.62 Partial excision of pituitary gland, transsphenoidal approach
07.63 Partial excision of pituitary gland, unspecified approach

HCPCS Level II Supplies & Services

HCPCS Level II codes are used to report the supplies, durable medical equipment, and certain medical services provided on an outpatient basis. Because the procedure(s) represented on this page would be performed in an inpatient facility, no HCPCS Level II codes apply.

62180

62180 Ventriculocisternostomy (Torkildsen type operation)

ICD-9-CM Diagnostic

191.5 Malignant neoplasm of ventricles of brain
237.5 Neoplasm of uncertain behavior of brain and spinal cord
331.3 Communicating hydrocephalus
331.4 Obstructive hydrocephalus
348.2 Benign intracranial hypertension
741.01 Spina bifida with hydrocephalus, cervical region
742.3 Congenital hydrocephalus

ICD-9-CM Procedural

02.2 Ventriculostomy
02.31 Ventricular shunt to structure in head and neck

62190

62190 Creation of shunt; subarachnoid/subdural-atrial, -jugular, -auricular

ICD-9-CM Diagnostic

331.3 Communicating hydrocephalus
331.4 Obstructive hydrocephalus
741.01 Spina bifida with hydrocephalus, cervical region
742.3 Congenital hydrocephalus
905.0 Late effect of fracture of skull and face bones

ICD-9-CM Procedural

02.32 Ventricular shunt to circulatory system

62192

62192 Creation of shunt; subarachnoid/subdural-peritoneal, -pleural, other terminus

ICD-9-CM Diagnostic

331.3 Communicating hydrocephalus
331.4 Obstructive hydrocephalus
741.03 Spina bifida with hydrocephalus, lumbar region
742.3 Congenital hydrocephalus
905.0 Late effect of fracture of skull and face bones

ICD-9-CM Procedural

02.31 Ventricular shunt to structure in head and neck
02.33 Ventricular shunt to thoracic cavity
02.34 Ventricular shunt to abdominal cavity and organs
02.35 Ventricular shunt to urinary system
02.39 Other operations to establish drainage of ventricle

62194

62194 Replacement or irrigation, subarachnoid/subdural catheter

ICD-9-CM Diagnostic

331.3 Communicating hydrocephalus
331.4 Obstructive hydrocephalus
741.03 Spina bifida with hydrocephalus, lumbar region
742.3 Congenital hydrocephalus
905.0 Late effect of fracture of skull and face bones
996.2 Mechanical complication of nervous system device, implant, and graft
996.63 Infection and inflammatory reaction due to nervous system device, implant, and graft — (Use additional code to identify specified infections)
V53.01 Fitting and adjustment of cerebral ventricular (communicating) shunt

ICD-9-CM Procedural

02.41 Irrigation and exploration of ventricular shunt
02.42 Replacement of ventricular shunt

HCPCS Level II Supplies & Services

A4550 Surgical trays

62200–62201

62200 Ventriculocisternostomy, third ventricle;
62201 stereotactic, neuroendoscopic method

ICD-9-CM Diagnostic

331.3 Communicating hydrocephalus
331.4 Obstructive hydrocephalus
741.01 Spina bifida with hydrocephalus, cervical region
741.03 Spina bifida with hydrocephalus, lumbar region
742.3 Congenital hydrocephalus
772.10 Intraventricular hemorrhage, unspecified grade ▽
772.11 Intraventricular hemorrhage, Grade I
772.12 Intraventricular hemorrhage, Grade II
772.13 Intraventricular hemorrhage, Grade III
772.14 Intraventricular hemorrhage, Grade IV
996.2 Mechanical complication of nervous system device, implant, and graft

▽ Unspecified code ♀ Female diagnosis ☒ Manifestation code ♂ Male diagnosis

996.63 Infection and inflammatory reaction due to nervous system device, implant, and graft — (Use additional code to identify specified infections)

ICD-9-CM Procedural

02.2 Ventriculostomy

62220

62220 Creation of shunt; ventriculo-atrial, -jugular, -auricular

ICD-9-CM Diagnostic

225.2 Benign neoplasm of cerebral meninges
331.3 Communicating hydrocephalus
331.4 Obstructive hydrocephalus
741.03 Spina bifida with hydrocephalus, lumbar region
742.3 Congenital hydrocephalus
907.0 Late effect of intracranial injury without mention of skull fracture
996.2 Mechanical complication of nervous system device, implant, and graft
996.63 Infection and inflammatory reaction due to nervous system device, implant, and graft — (Use additional code to identify specified infections)

ICD-9-CM Procedural

02.31 Ventricular shunt to structure in head and neck
02.32 Ventricular shunt to circulatory system

62223

62223 Creation of shunt; ventriculo-peritoneal, -pleural, other terminus

ICD-9-CM Diagnostic

191.5 Malignant neoplasm of ventricles of brain
191.6 Malignant neoplasm of cerebellum NOS
198.3 Secondary malignant neoplasm of brain and spinal cord
225.0 Benign neoplasm of brain
225.2 Benign neoplasm of cerebral meninges
225.8 Benign neoplasm of other specified sites of nervous system
225.9 Benign neoplasm of nervous system, part unspecified ▽
239.6 Neoplasm of unspecified nature of brain
331.3 Communicating hydrocephalus
331.4 Obstructive hydrocephalus
348.0 Cerebral cysts
348.2 Benign intracranial hypertension
741.01 Spina bifida with hydrocephalus, cervical region
741.03 Spina bifida with hydrocephalus, lumbar region
742.3 Congenital hydrocephalus
772.10 Intraventricular hemorrhage, unspecified grade ▽
772.11 Intraventricular hemorrhage, Grade I
772.12 Intraventricular hemorrhage, Grade II
772.13 Intraventricular hemorrhage, Grade III
772.14 Intraventricular hemorrhage, Grade IV
907.0 Late effect of intracranial injury without mention of skull fracture
996.2 Mechanical complication of nervous system device, implant, and graft

ICD-9-CM Procedural

02.33 Ventricular shunt to thoracic cavity
02.34 Ventricular shunt to abdominal cavity and organs
02.35 Ventricular shunt to urinary system
02.39 Other operations to establish drainage of ventricle

62225–62230

62225 Replacement or irrigation, ventricular catheter
62230 Replacement or revision of cerebrospinal fluid shunt, obstructed valve, or distal catheter in shunt system

ICD-9-CM Diagnostic

331.3 Communicating hydrocephalus
331.4 Obstructive hydrocephalus
741.03 Spina bifida with hydrocephalus, lumbar region
742.3 Congenital hydrocephalus
772.10 Intraventricular hemorrhage, unspecified grade ▽
772.11 Intraventricular hemorrhage, Grade I
772.12 Intraventricular hemorrhage, Grade II
772.13 Intraventricular hemorrhage, Grade III
772.14 Intraventricular hemorrhage, Grade IV
907.0 Late effect of intracranial injury without mention of skull fracture
996.2 Mechanical complication of nervous system device, implant, and graft
996.63 Infection and inflammatory reaction due to nervous system device, implant, and graft — (Use additional code to identify specified infections)
996.75 Other complications due to nervous system device, implant, and graft
V53.01 Fitting and adjustment of cerebral ventricular (communicating) shunt

ICD-9-CM Procedural

02.41 Irrigation and exploration of ventricular shunt
02.42 Replacement of ventricular shunt

HCPCS Level II Supplies & Services

A4550 Surgical trays

62252

62252 Reprogramming of programmable cerebrospinal shunt

ICD-9-CM Diagnostic

331.3 Communicating hydrocephalus
331.4 Obstructive hydrocephalus
741.03 Spina bifida with hydrocephalus, lumbar region
742.3 Congenital hydrocephalus
772.10 Intraventricular hemorrhage, unspecified grade ▽
772.11 Intraventricular hemorrhage, Grade I
772.12 Intraventricular hemorrhage, Grade II
772.13 Intraventricular hemorrhage, Grade III
772.14 Intraventricular hemorrhage, Grade IV
907.0 Late effect of intracranial injury without mention of skull fracture
V53.01 Fitting and adjustment of cerebral ventricular (communicating) shunt

ICD-9-CM Procedural

89.05 Diagnostic interview and evaluation, not otherwise specified

HCPCS Level II Supplies & Services

A4550 Surgical trays

62256–62258

62256 Removal of complete cerebrospinal fluid shunt system; without replacement
62258 with replacement by similar or other shunt at same operation

ICD-9-CM Diagnostic

331.3 Communicating hydrocephalus
331.4 Obstructive hydrocephalus
348.2 Benign intracranial hypertension
741.01 Spina bifida with hydrocephalus, cervical region
741.03 Spina bifida with hydrocephalus, lumbar region
742.3 Congenital hydrocephalus
772.10 Intraventricular hemorrhage, unspecified grade ▽
772.11 Intraventricular hemorrhage, Grade I
772.12 Intraventricular hemorrhage, Grade II
772.13 Intraventricular hemorrhage, Grade III
772.14 Intraventricular hemorrhage, Grade IV
996.2 Mechanical complication of nervous system device, implant, and graft
996.63 Infection and inflammatory reaction due to nervous system device, implant, and graft — (Use additional code to identify specified infections)
V53.01 Fitting and adjustment of cerebral ventricular (communicating) shunt

ICD-9-CM Procedural

02.42 Replacement of ventricular shunt
02.43 Removal of ventricular shunt

Spine and Spinal Cord

62263–62264

62263 Percutaneous lysis of epidural adhesions using solution injection (eg, hypertonic saline, enzyme) or mechanical means (eg, catheter) including radiologic localization (includes contrast when administered), multiple adhesiolysis sessions; 2 or more days
62264 1 day

ICD-9-CM Diagnostic

349.2 Disorders of meninges, not elsewhere classified ▽
742.59 Other specified congenital anomaly of spinal cord

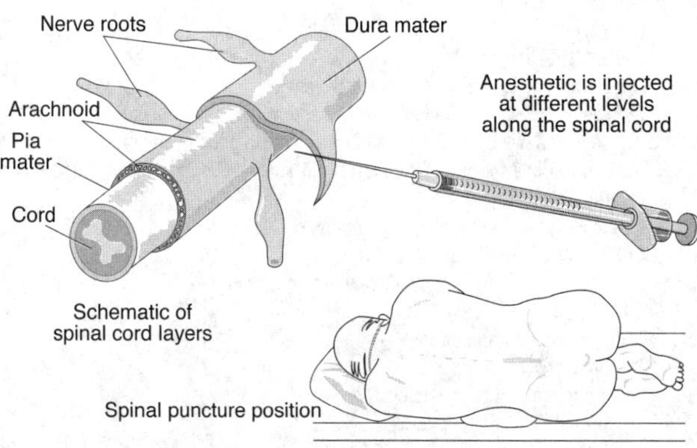

ICD-9-CM Procedural

03.90 Insertion of catheter into spinal canal for infusion of therapeutic or palliative substances
03.91 Injection of anesthetic into spinal canal for analgesia
03.92 Injection of other agent into spinal canal
03.96 Percutaneous denervation of facet
86.09 Other incision of skin and subcutaneous tissue

62268

62268 Percutaneous aspiration, spinal cord cyst or syrinx

ICD-9-CM Diagnostic

324.1 Intraspinal abscess
336.0 Syringomyelia and syringobulbia
349.2 Disorders of meninges, not elsewhere classified ▽

ICD-9-CM Procedural

03.99 Other operations on spinal cord and spinal canal structures

62269

62269 Biopsy of spinal cord, percutaneous needle

ICD-9-CM Diagnostic

192.2 Malignant neoplasm of spinal cord
198.3 Secondary malignant neoplasm of brain and spinal cord
225.3 Benign neoplasm of spinal cord
237.5 Neoplasm of uncertain behavior of brain and spinal cord
324.1 Intraspinal abscess
336.0 Syringomyelia and syringobulbia
340 Multiple sclerosis
349.2 Disorders of meninges, not elsewhere classified ▽

ICD-9-CM Procedural

03.32 Biopsy of spinal cord or spinal meninges

62270

62270 Spinal puncture, lumbar, diagnostic

ICD-9-CM Diagnostic

170.2 Malignant neoplasm of vertebral column, excluding sacrum and coccyx
191.5 Malignant neoplasm of ventricles of brain
191.8 Malignant neoplasm of other parts of brain
191.9 Malignant neoplasm of brain, unspecified site ▽
192.2 Malignant neoplasm of spinal cord
192.3 Malignant neoplasm of spinal meninges
192.8 Malignant neoplasm of other specified sites of nervous system
192.9 Malignant neoplasm of nervous system, part unspecified ▽
198.3 Secondary malignant neoplasm of brain and spinal cord
198.4 Secondary malignant neoplasm of other parts of nervous system
198.5 Secondary malignant neoplasm of bone and bone marrow
199.0 Disseminated malignant neoplasm
199.1 Other malignant neoplasm of unspecified site
225.0 Benign neoplasm of brain
225.2 Benign neoplasm of cerebral meninges
225.3 Benign neoplasm of spinal cord
225.4 Benign neoplasm of spinal meninges
225.8 Benign neoplasm of other specified sites of nervous system
225.9 Benign neoplasm of nervous system, part unspecified ▽
237.5 Neoplasm of uncertain behavior of brain and spinal cord
237.6 Neoplasm of uncertain behavior of meninges
238.7 Neoplasm of uncertain behavior of other lymphatic and hematopoietic tissues
239.6 Neoplasm of unspecified nature of brain
239.7 Neoplasm of unspecified nature of endocrine glands and other parts of nervous system
293.0 Delirium due to conditions classified elsewhere — (Code first the associated physical or neurological condition)
293.1 Subacute delirium — (Code first the associated physical or neurological condition)
303.00 Acute alcoholic intoxication, unspecified drunkenness — (Use additional code to identify any associated condition: 291.0-291.9, 304.00-304.93, 331.7, 345.00-345.91, 535.3, 571.1, 571.2, 571.3) ▽
303.01 Acute alcoholic intoxication, continuous drunkenness — (Use additional code to identify any associated condition: 291.0-291.9, 304.00-304.93, 331.7, 345.00-345.91, 535.3, 571.1, 571.2, 571.3)
303.02 Acute alcoholic intoxication, episodic drunkenness — (Use additional code to identify any associated condition: 291.0-291.9, 304.00-304.93, 331.7, 345.00-345.91, 535.3, 571.1, 571.2, 571.3)
303.03 Acute alcoholic intoxication, in remission — (Use additional code to identify any associated condition: 291.0-291.9, 304.00-304.93, 331.7, 345.00-345.91, 535.3, 571.1, 571.2, 571.3)
303.90 Other and unspecified alcohol dependence, unspecified drunkenness — (Use additional code to identify any associated condition: 291.0-291.9, 304.00-304.93, 331.7, 345.00-345.91, 535.3, 571.1, 571.2, 571.3) ▽
303.91 Other and unspecified alcohol dependence, continuous drunkenness — (Use additional code to identify any associated condition: 291.0-291.9, 304.00-304.93, 331.7, 345.00-345.91, 535.3, 571.1, 571.2, 571.3) ▽
303.92 Other and unspecified alcohol dependence, episodic drunkenness — (Use additional code to identify any associated condition: 291.0-291.9, 304.00-304.93, 331.7, 345.00-345.91, 535.3, 571.1, 571.2, 571.3) ▽
303.93 Other and unspecified alcohol dependence, in remission — (Use additional code to identify any associated condition: 291.0-291.9, 304.00-304.93, 331.7, 345.00-345.91, 535.3, 571.1, 571.2, 571.3) ▽
320.0 Hemophilus meningitis
320.1 Pneumococcal meningitis
320.2 Streptococcal meningitis
320.3 Staphylococcal meningitis
320.7 Meningitis in other bacterial diseases classified elsewhere — (Code first underlying disease: 002.0, 027.0, 033.0-033.9, 039.8) ☒
320.81 Anaerobic meningitis
320.82 Meningitis due to gram-negative bacteria, not elsewhere classified
320.89 Meningitis due to other specified bacteria
320.9 Meningitis due to unspecified bacterium ▽
321.0 Cryptococcal meningitis — (Code first underlying disease, 117.5) ☒
321.1 Meningitis in other fungal diseases — (Code first underlying disease: 110.0-118) ☒
321.2 Meningitis due to viruses not elsewhere classified — (Code first underlying disease: 060.0-066.9) ☒
321.3 Meningitis due to trypanosomiasis — (Code first underlying disease: 086.0-086.9) ☒
321.4 Meningitis in sarcoidosis — (Code first underlying disease, 135) ☒
321.8 Meningitis due to other nonbacterial organisms classified elsewhere — (Code first underlying disease) ☒
322.0 Nonpyogenic meningitis
322.1 Eosinophilic meningitis
322.2 Chronic meningitis
322.9 Unspecified meningitis ▽
323.0 Encephalitis in viral diseases classified elsewhere — (Code first underlying disease: 073.7, 075, 078.3) ☒
323.1 Encephalitis in rickettsial diseases classified elsewhere — (Code first underlying disease: 080-083.9) ☒
323.2 Encephalitis in protozoal diseases classified elsewhere — (Code first underlying disease: 084.0-084.9, 086.0-086.9) ☒
323.4 Other encephalitis due to infection classified elsewhere — (Code first underlying disease) ☒
323.5 Encephalitis following immunization procedures — (Use additional E code to identify vaccine)
323.6 Postinfectious encephalitis — (Code first underlying disease) ☒
323.7 Toxic encephalitis — (Code first underlying cause: 961.3, 982.1, 984.0-984.9, 985.0, 985.8) ☒
323.8 Other causes of encephalitis
323.9 Unspecified cause of encephalitis ▽
324.0 Intracranial abscess
324.1 Intraspinal abscess

▽ Unspecified code ☒ Manifestation code
♀ Female diagnosis ♂ Male diagnosis

324.9 Intracranial and intraspinal abscess of unspecified site ▽
331.3 Communicating hydrocephalus
331.4 Obstructive hydrocephalus
332.0 Paralysis agitans
333.6 Idiopathic torsion dystonia
334.0 Friedreich's ataxia
334.1 Hereditary spastic paraplegia
334.2 Primary cerebellar degeneration
334.3 Other cerebellar ataxia — (Use additional E code to identify drug, if drug-induced)
334.4 Cerebellar ataxia in diseases classified elsewhere — (Code first underlying disease: 140.0-239.9, 244.0-244.9, 303.00-303.93) ☒
334.8 Other spinocerebellar diseases
334.9 Unspecified spinocerebellar disease ▽
335.0 Werdnig-Hoffmann disease
335.10 Unspecified spinal muscular atrophy ▽
335.11 Kugelberg-Welander disease
335.19 Other spinal muscular atrophy
335.20 Amyotrophic lateral sclerosis
335.21 Progressive muscular atrophy
335.22 Progressive bulbar palsy
335.23 Pseudobulbar palsy
335.24 Primary lateral sclerosis
335.29 Other motor neuron diseases
335.8 Other anterior horn cell diseases
335.9 Unspecified anterior horn cell disease ▽
336.0 Syringomyelia and syringobulbia
336.2 Subacute combined degeneration of spinal cord in diseases classified elsewhere — (Code first underlying disease: 266.2, 281.0, 281.1) ☒
336.3 Myelopathy in other diseases classified elsewhere — (Code first underlying disease: 140.0-239.9) ☒
336.8 Other myelopathy — (Use additional E code to identify cause)
336.9 Unspecified disease of spinal cord ▽
340 Multiple sclerosis
341.8 Other demyelinating diseases of central nervous system
341.9 Unspecified demyelinating disease of central nervous system ▽
342.90 Unspecified hemiplegia affecting unspecified side ▽
342.91 Unspecified hemiplegia affecting dominant side ▽
342.92 Unspecified hemiplegia affecting nondominant side ▽
344.00 Unspecified quadriplegia ▽
344.30 Monoplegia of lower limb affecting unspecified side ▽
344.31 Monoplegia of lower limb affecting dominant side
344.32 Monoplegia of lower limb affecting nondominant side
344.9 Unspecified paralysis ▽
348.2 Benign intracranial hypertension
348.30 Encephalopathy, unspecified ▽
348.9 Unspecified condition of brain ▽
349.82 Toxic encephalopathy — (Use additional E code to identify cause)
349.89 Other specified disorder of nervous system
357.0 Acute infective polyneuritis
430 Subarachnoid hemorrhage — (Use additional code to identify presence of hypertension)
432.1 Subdural hemorrhage — (Use additional code to identify presence of hypertension)
432.9 Unspecified intracranial hemorrhage — (Use additional code to identify presence of hypertension) ▽
434.91 Unspecified cerebral artery occlusion with cerebral infarction — (Use additional code to identify presence of hypertension) ▽
435.9 Unspecified transient cerebral ischemia — (Use additional code to identify presence of hypertension) ▽
436 Acute, but ill-defined, cerebrovascular disease — (Use additional code to identify presence of hypertension) ▽
437.2 Hypertensive encephalopathy — (Use additional code to identify presence of hypertension)
437.3 Cerebral aneurysm, nonruptured — (Use additional code to identify presence of hypertension)
437.4 Cerebral arteritis — (Use additional code to identify presence of hypertension)
437.5 Moyamoya disease — (Use additional code to identify presence of hypertension)
437.6 Nonpyogenic thrombosis of intracranial venous sinus — (Use additional code to identify presence of hypertension)
437.7 Transient global amnesia — (Use additional code to identify presence of hypertension)
437.8 Other ill-defined cerebrovascular disease — (Use additional code to identify presence of hypertension)
437.9 Unspecified cerebrovascular disease — (Use additional code to identify presence of hypertension) ▽
724.2 Lumbago
724.5 Unspecified backache ▽
747.81 Congenital anomaly of cerebrovascular system
771.81 Septicemia (sepsis) of newborn — (Use additional code to identify organism)
771.83 Bacteremia of newborn — (Use additional code to identify organism)
771.89 Other infections specific to the perinatal period — (Use additional code to identify organism)
777.2 Neonatal intestinal obstruction due to inspissated milk
779.0 Convulsions in newborn
779.1 Other and unspecified cerebral irritability in newborn ▽
780.01 Coma
780.02 Transient alteration of awareness
780.03 Persistent vegetative state
780.09 Other alteration of consciousness
780.2 Syncope and collapse
780.31 Febrile convulsions
780.39 Other convulsions
780.4 Dizziness and giddiness
780.6 Fever
781.3 Lack of coordination
781.6 Meningismus
782.0 Disturbance of skin sensation
784.0 Headache
785.52 Septic shock — (Code first systemic inflammatory response syndrome due to infectious process with organ dysfunction, 995.92)
790.7 Bacteremia — (Use additional code to identify organism)
792.0 Nonspecific abnormal finding in cerebrospinal fluid
901.89 Injury to specified blood vessels of thorax, other
961.3 Poisoning by quinoline and hydroxyquinoline derivatives — (Use additional code to specify the effects of the poisoning)
982.1 Toxic effect of carbon tetrachloride — (Use additional code to specify the nature of the toxic effect)
984.0 Toxic effect of inorganic lead compounds — (Use additional code to specify the nature of the toxic effect)
984.1 Toxic effect of organic lead compounds — (Use additional code to specify the nature of the toxic effect)
984.8 Toxic effect of other lead compounds — (Use additional code to specify the nature of the toxic effect)
984.9 Toxic effect of unspecified lead compound — (Use additional code to specify the nature of the toxic effect) ▽
985.0 Toxic effect of mercury and its compounds — (Use additional code to specify the nature of the toxic effect)
985.8 Toxic effect of other specified metals — (Use additional code to specify the nature of the toxic effect)
997.01 Central nervous system complication — (Use additional code to identify complications)
997.02 Iatrogenic cerebrovascular infarction or hemorrhage — (Use additional code to identify complications)
997.09 Other nervous system complications — (Use additional code to identify complications)
V71.89 Observation for other specified suspected conditions
V71.9 Observation for unspecified suspected condition ▽

ICD-9-CM Procedural

03.31 Spinal tap

HCPCS Level II Supplies & Services

A4550 Surgical trays

62272

62272 Spinal puncture, therapeutic, for drainage of cerebrospinal fluid (by needle or catheter)

ICD-9-CM Diagnostic

191.0 Malignant neoplasm of cerebrum, except lobes and ventricles
225.2 Benign neoplasm of cerebral meninges
225.3 Benign neoplasm of spinal cord
322.9 Unspecified meningitis ▽
324.0 Intracranial abscess
324.1 Intraspinal abscess
325 Phlebitis and thrombophlebitis of intracranial venous sinuses
340 Multiple sclerosis
348.4 Compression of brain
742.0 Encephalocele

▽ Unspecified code ☒ Manifestation code
♀ Female diagnosis ♂ Male diagnosis

781.6 Meningismus
997.09 Other nervous system complications — (Use additional code to identify complications)

ICD-9-CM Procedural
03.31 Spinal tap

HCPCS Level II Supplies & Services
A4550 Surgical trays

62273
62273 Injection, epidural, of blood or clot patch

ICD-9-CM Diagnostic
349.0 Reaction to spinal or lumbar puncture
784.0 Headache
997.09 Other nervous system complications — (Use additional code to identify complications)

ICD-9-CM Procedural
03.95 Spinal blood patch

HCPCS Level II Supplies & Services
A4550 Surgical trays

62280–62282
62280 Injection/infusion of neurolytic substance (eg, alcohol, phenol, iced saline solutions), with or without other therapeutic substance; subarachnoid
62281 epidural, cervical or thoracic
62282 epidural, lumbar, sacral (caudal)

ICD-9-CM Diagnostic
333.83 Spasmodic torticollis — (Use additional E code to identify drug, if drug-induced)
337.0 Idiopathic peripheral autonomic neuropathy
337.22 Reflex sympathetic dystrophy of the lower limb
337.9 Unspecified disorder of autonomic nervous system ▽
340 Multiple sclerosis
353.1 Lumbosacral plexus lesions
353.4 Lumbosacral root lesions, not elsewhere classified
354.4 Causalgia of upper limb
354.5 Mononeuritis multiplex
355.71 Causalgia of lower limb
715.98 Osteoarthrosis, unspecified whether generalized or localized, other specified sites ▽
722.52 Degeneration of lumbar or lumbosacral intervertebral disc
722.83 Postlaminectomy syndrome, lumbar region
724.02 Spinal stenosis of lumbar region
724.2 Lumbago
724.3 Sciatica
724.4 Thoracic or lumbosacral neuritis or radiculitis, unspecified ▽
724.6 Disorders of sacrum
729.2 Unspecified neuralgia, neuritis, and radiculitis ▽

ICD-9-CM Procedural
03.8 Injection of destructive agent into spinal canal
03.92 Injection of other agent into spinal canal

62284
62284 Injection procedure for myelography and/or computed tomography, spinal (other than C1-C2 and posterior fossa)

ICD-9-CM Diagnostic
170.2 Malignant neoplasm of vertebral column, excluding sacrum and coccyx
191.5 Malignant neoplasm of ventricles of brain
191.8 Malignant neoplasm of other parts of brain
192.2 Malignant neoplasm of spinal cord
192.3 Malignant neoplasm of spinal meninges
192.8 Malignant neoplasm of other specified sites of nervous system
198.3 Secondary malignant neoplasm of brain and spinal cord
198.4 Secondary malignant neoplasm of other parts of nervous system
198.5 Secondary malignant neoplasm of bone and bone marrow
199.0 Disseminated malignant neoplasm
213.2 Benign neoplasm of vertebral column, excluding sacrum and coccyx
225.3 Benign neoplasm of spinal cord
225.4 Benign neoplasm of spinal meninges
225.8 Benign neoplasm of other specified sites of nervous system
237.5 Neoplasm of uncertain behavior of brain and spinal cord
237.6 Neoplasm of uncertain behavior of meninges
237.70 Neurofibromatosis, unspecified ▽
237.71 Neurofibromatosis, Type 1 (von Recklinghausen's disease)
237.72 Neurofibromatosis, Type 2 (acoustic neurofibromatosis)
238.0 Neoplasm of uncertain behavior of bone and articular cartilage
239.2 Neoplasms of unspecified nature of bone, soft tissue, and skin
239.8 Neoplasm of unspecified nature of other specified sites
324.1 Intraspinal abscess
336.0 Syringomyelia and syringobulbia
344.01 Quadriplegia and quadriparesis, C1-C4, complete
344.02 Quadriplegia and quadriparesis, C1-C4, incomplete
344.03 Quadriplegia and quadriparesis, C5-C7, complete
344.04 C5-C7, incomplete
344.09 Other quadriplegia and quadriparesis
344.1 Paraplegia
344.60 Cauda equina syndrome without mention of neurogenic bladder
349.1 Nervous system complications from surgically implanted device
349.2 Disorders of meninges, not elsewhere classified ▽
349.89 Other specified disorder of nervous system
353.1 Lumbosacral plexus lesions
359.1 Hereditary progressive muscular dystrophy
721.0 Cervical spondylosis without myelopathy
721.1 Cervical spondylosis with myelopathy
721.2 Thoracic spondylosis without myelopathy
721.3 Lumbosacral spondylosis without myelopathy
721.41 Spondylosis with myelopathy, thoracic region
721.42 Spondylosis with myelopathy, lumbar region
721.5 Kissing spine
721.6 Ankylosing vertebral hyperostosis
721.7 Traumatic spondylopathy
721.8 Other allied disorders of spine
722.0 Displacement of cervical intervertebral disc without myelopathy
722.10 Displacement of lumbar intervertebral disc without myelopathy
722.11 Displacement of thoracic intervertebral disc without myelopathy
722.4 Degeneration of cervical intervertebral disc
722.51 Degeneration of thoracic or thoracolumbar intervertebral disc
722.52 Degeneration of lumbar or lumbosacral intervertebral disc
722.6 Degeneration of intervertebral disc, site unspecified ▽
722.71 Intervertebral cervical disc disorder with myelopathy, cervical region
722.72 Intervertebral thoracic disc disorder with myelopathy, thoracic region
722.73 Intervertebral lumbar disc disorder with myelopathy, lumbar region
722.81 Postlaminectomy syndrome, cervical region
722.82 Postlaminectomy syndrome, thoracic region
722.83 Postlaminectomy syndrome, lumbar region
722.91 Other and unspecified disc disorder of cervical region
722.92 Other and unspecified disc disorder of thoracic region
722.93 Other and unspecified disc disorder of lumbar region
723.0 Spinal stenosis in cervical region
723.1 Cervicalgia
723.4 Brachial neuritis or radiculitis nos
723.5 Torticollis, unspecified ▽
723.6 Panniculitis specified as affecting neck
723.7 Ossification of posterior longitudinal ligament in cervical region
723.9 Unspecified musculoskeletal disorders and symptoms referable to neck ▽
724.02 Spinal stenosis of lumbar region
724.09 Spinal stenosis, other region other than cervical
724.1 Pain in thoracic spine
724.2 Lumbago
724.3 Sciatica
724.4 Thoracic or lumbosacral neuritis or radiculitis, unspecified ▽
724.5 Unspecified backache ▽
724.6 Disorders of sacrum
724.70 Unspecified disorder of coccyx ▽
724.71 Hypermobility of coccyx
724.79 Other disorder of coccyx
724.8 Other symptoms referable to back
724.9 Other unspecified back disorder
729.2 Unspecified neuralgia, neuritis, and radiculitis ▽
729.5 Pain in soft tissues of limb
733.13 Pathologic fracture of vertebrae
733.90 Disorder of bone and cartilage, unspecified ▽
733.95 Stress fracture of other bone
738.4 Acquired spondylolisthesis
738.5 Other acquired deformity of back or spine

▽ Unspecified code ♀ Female diagnosis ☒ Manifestation code ♂ Male diagnosis

739.1 Nonallopathic lesion of cervical region, not elsewhere classified

739.2 Nonallopathic lesion of thoracic region, not elsewhere classified

739.3 Nonallopathic lesion of lumbar region, not elsewhere classified

741.01 Spina bifida with hydrocephalus, cervical region

741.02 Spina bifida with hydrocephalus, dorsal (thoracic) region

741.03 Spina bifida with hydrocephalus, lumbar region

741.92 Spina bifida without mention of hydrocephalus, dorsal (thoracic) region

741.93 Spina bifida without mention of hydrocephalus, lumbar region

756.10 Congenital anomaly of spine, unspecified ▽

756.11 Congenital spondylolysis, lumbosacral region

756.12 Congenital spondylolisthesis

756.13 Congenital absence of vertebra

756.14 Hemivertebra

756.15 Congenital fusion of spine (vertebra)

756.16 Klippel-Feil syndrome

756.17 Spina bifida occulta

756.19 Other congenital anomaly of spine

784.9 Other symptoms involving head and neck

793.7 Nonspecific abnormal findings on radiological and other examination of musculoskeletal system

805.10 Open fracture of cervical vertebra, unspecified level without mention of spinal cord injury ▽

805.11 Open fracture of first cervical vertebra without mention of spinal cord injury

805.12 Open fracture of second cervical vertebra without mention of spinal cord injury

805.13 Open fracture of third cervical vertebra without mention of spinal cord injury

805.14 Open fracture of fourth cervical vertebra without mention of spinal cord injury

805.15 Open fracture of fifth cervical vertebra without mention of spinal cord injury

805.16 Open fracture of sixth cervical vertebra without mention of spinal cord injury

805.17 Open fracture of seventh cervical vertebra without mention of spinal cord injury

805.18 Open fracture of multiple cervical vertebrae without mention of spinal cord injury

805.2 Closed fracture of dorsal (thoracic) vertebra without mention of spinal cord injury

805.3 Open fracture of dorsal (thoracic) vertebra without mention of spinal cord injury

805.4 Closed fracture of lumbar vertebra without mention of spinal cord injury

805.5 Open fracture of lumbar vertebra without mention of spinal cord injury

805.6 Closed fracture of sacrum and coccyx without mention of spinal cord injury

805.7 Open fracture of sacrum and coccyx without mention of spinal cord injury

806.00 Closed fracture of C1-C4 level with unspecified spinal cord injury ▽

806.01 Closed fracture of C1-C4 level with complete lesion of cord

806.02 Closed fracture of C1-C4 level with anterior cord syndrome

806.03 Closed fracture of C1-C4 level with central cord syndrome

806.04 Closed fracture of C1-C4 level with other specified spinal cord injury

806.05 Closed fracture of C5-C7 level with unspecified spinal cord injury ▽

806.06 Closed fracture of C5-C7 level with complete lesion of cord

806.07 Closed fracture of C5-C7 level with anterior cord syndrome

806.08 Closed fracture of C5-C7 level with central cord syndrome

806.09 Closed fracture of C5-C7 level with other specified spinal cord injury

806.10 Open fracture of C1-C4 level with unspecified spinal cord injury ▽

806.11 Open fracture of C1-C4 level with complete lesion of cord

806.12 Open fracture of C1-C4 level with anterior cord syndrome

806.13 Open fracture of C1-C4 level with central cord syndrome

806.14 Open fracture of C1-C4 level with other specified spinal cord injury

806.15 Open fracture of C5-C7 level with unspecified spinal cord injury ▽

806.16 Open fracture of C5-C7 level with complete lesion of cord

806.17 Open fracture of C5-C7 level with anterior cord syndrome

806.18 Open fracture of C5-C7 level with central cord syndrome

806.19 Open fracture of C5-C7 level with other specified spinal cord injury

806.20 Closed fracture of T1-T6 level with unspecified spinal cord injury ▽

806.21 Closed fracture of T1-T6 level with complete lesion of cord

806.22 Closed fracture of T1-T6 level with anterior cord syndrome

806.23 Closed fracture of T1-T6 level with central cord syndrome

806.24 Closed fracture of T1-T6 level with other specified spinal cord injury

806.25 Closed fracture of T7-T12 level with unspecified spinal cord injury ▽

806.26 Closed fracture of T7-T12 level with complete lesion of cord

806.27 Closed fracture of T7-T12 level with anterior cord syndrome

806.28 Closed fracture of T7-T12 level with central cord syndrome

806.29 Closed fracture of T7-T12 level with other specified spinal cord injury

806.30 Open fracture of T1-T6 level with unspecified spinal cord injury ▽

806.31 Open fracture of T1-T6 level with complete lesion of cord

806.32 Open fracture of T1-T6 level with anterior cord syndrome

806.33 Open fracture of T1-T6 level with central cord syndrome

806.34 Open fracture of T1-T6 level with other specified spinal cord injury

806.35 Open fracture of T7-T12 level with unspecified spinal cord injury ▽

806.36 Open fracture of T7-T12 level with complete lesion of cord

806.37 Open fracture of T7-T12 level with anterior cord syndrome

806.38 Open fracture of T7-T12 level with central cord syndrome

806.39 Open fracture of T7-T12 level with other specified spinal cord injury

806.4 Closed fracture of lumbar spine with spinal cord injury

806.5 Open fracture of lumbar spine with spinal cord injury

839.01 Closed dislocation, first cervical vertebra

839.02 Closed dislocation, second cervical vertebra

839.03 Closed dislocation, third cervical vertebra

839.04 Closed dislocation, fourth cervical vertebra

839.05 Closed dislocation, fifth cervical vertebra

839.06 Closed dislocation, sixth cervical vertebra

839.07 Closed dislocation, seventh cervical vertebra

839.08 Closed dislocation, multiple cervical vertebrae

839.11 Open dislocation, first cervical vertebra

839.12 Open dislocation, second cervical vertebra

839.13 Open dislocation, third cervical vertebra

839.14 Open dislocation, fourth cervical vertebra

839.15 Open dislocation, fifth cervical vertebra

839.16 Open dislocation, sixth cervical vertebra

839.17 Open dislocation, seventh cervical vertebra

839.18 Open dislocation, multiple cervical vertebrae

839.20 Closed dislocation, lumbar vertebra

839.21 Closed dislocation, thoracic vertebra

839.30 Open dislocation, lumbar vertebra

839.31 Open dislocation, thoracic vertebra

846.0 Sprain and strain of lumbosacral (joint) (ligament)

846.9 Unspecified site of sacroiliac region sprain and strain ▽

847.0 Neck sprain and strain

847.1 Thoracic sprain and strain

847.2 Lumbar sprain and strain

847.9 Sprain and strain of unspecified site of back ▽

905.1 Late effect of fracture of spine and trunk without mention of spinal cord lesion

907.2 Late effect of spinal cord injury

952.00 C1-C4 level spinal cord injury, unspecified ▽

952.01 C1-C4 level with complete lesion of spinal cord

952.02 C1-C4 level with anterior cord syndrome

952.03 C1-C4 level with central cord syndrome

952.04 C1-C4 level with other specified spinal cord injury

952.05 C5-C7 level spinal cord injury, unspecified ▽

952.06 C5-C7 level with complete lesion of spinal cord

952.07 C5-C7 level with anterior cord syndrome

952.08 C5-C7 level with central cord syndrome

952.09 C5-C7 level with other specified spinal cord injury

952.10 T1-T6 level spinal cord injury, unspecified ▽

952.11 T1-T6 level with complete lesion of spinal cord

952.12 T1-T6 level with anterior cord syndrome

952.13 T1-T6 level with central cord syndrome

952.14 T1-T6 level with other specified spinal cord injury

952.15 T7-T12 level spinal cord injury, unspecified ▽

952.16 T7-T12 level with complete lesion of spinal cord

952.17 T7-T12 level with anterior cord syndrome

952.18 T7-T12 level with central cord syndrome

952.19 T7-T12 level with other specified spinal cord injury

952.2 Lumbar spinal cord injury without spinal bone injury

952.3 Sacral spinal cord injury without spinal bone injury

952.4 Cauda equina spinal cord injury without spinal bone injury

952.8 Multiple sites of spinal cord injury without spinal bone injury

953.0 Injury to cervical nerve root

953.1 Injury to dorsal nerve root

953.2 Injury to lumbar nerve root

953.3 Injury to sacral nerve root

953.4 Injury to brachial plexus

953.5 Injury to lumbosacral plexus

953.8 Injury to multiple sites of nerve roots and spinal plexus

959.09 Injury of face and neck, other and unspecified

959.19 Other injury of other sites of trunk

996.4 Mechanical complication of internal orthopedic device, implant, and graft

996.63 Infection and inflammatory reaction due to nervous system device, implant, and graft — (Use additional code to identify specified infections)

996.67 Infection and inflammatory reaction due to other internal orthopedic device, implant, and graft — (Use additional code to identify specified infections)

996.75 Other complications due to nervous system device, implant, and graft

996.78 Other complications due to other internal orthopedic device, implant, and graft

ICD-9-CM Procedural

03.92 Injection of other agent into spinal canal

87.21 Contrast myelogram
88.38 Other computerized axial tomography

HCPCS Level II Supplies & Services

A4550 Surgical trays
A9525 Supply of low or iso-osmolar contrast material, 10 mg of iodine
J2175 Injection, meperidine HCl, per 100 mg
J2400 Injection, chloroprocaine HCl, per 30 ml

62287

62287 Aspiration or decompression procedure, percutaneous, of nucleus pulposus of intervertebral disk, any method, single or multiple levels, lumbar (eg, manual or automated percutaneous diskectomy, percutaneous laser diskectomy)

ICD-9-CM Diagnostic

722.10 Displacement of lumbar intervertebral disc without myelopathy
722.73 Intervertebral lumbar disc disorder with myelopathy, lumbar region
722.93 Other and unspecified disc disorder of lumbar region
724.2 Lumbago
724.4 Thoracic or lumbosacral neuritis or radiculitis, unspecified ▽
724.5 Unspecified backache ▽

ICD-9-CM Procedural

80.59 Other destruction of intervertebral disc

62290–62291

62290 Injection procedure for diskography, each level; lumbar
62291 cervical or thoracic

ICD-9-CM Diagnostic

719.48 Pain in joint, other specified sites
721.0 Cervical spondylosis without myelopathy
721.1 Cervical spondylosis with myelopathy
721.2 Thoracic spondylosis without myelopathy
721.3 Lumbosacral spondylosis without myelopathy
721.41 Spondylosis with myelopathy, thoracic region
721.42 Spondylosis with myelopathy, lumbar region
722.0 Displacement of cervical intervertebral disc without myelopathy
722.10 Displacement of lumbar intervertebral disc without myelopathy
722.11 Displacement of thoracic intervertebral disc without myelopathy
722.31 Schmorl's nodes, thoracic region
722.32 Schmorl's nodes, lumbar region
722.4 Degeneration of cervical intervertebral disc
722.51 Degeneration of thoracic or thoracolumbar intervertebral disc
722.52 Degeneration of lumbar or lumbosacral intervertebral disc
722.71 Intervertebral cervical disc disorder with myelopathy, cervical region
722.72 Intervertebral thoracic disc disorder with myelopathy, thoracic region
722.73 Intervertebral lumbar disc disorder with myelopathy, lumbar region
722.82 Postlaminectomy syndrome, thoracic region
722.83 Postlaminectomy syndrome, lumbar region
722.91 Other and unspecified disc disorder of cervical region
722.92 Other and unspecified disc disorder of thoracic region
722.93 Other and unspecified disc disorder of lumbar region
723.1 Cervicalgia
723.4 Brachial neuritis or radiculitis nos
724.01 Spinal stenosis of thoracic region
724.02 Spinal stenosis of lumbar region
724.1 Pain in thoracic spine
724.2 Lumbago
724.4 Thoracic or lumbosacral neuritis or radiculitis, unspecified ▽
724.5 Unspecified backache ▽
724.9 Other unspecified back disorder
729.5 Pain in soft tissues of limb
756.10 Congenital anomaly of spine, unspecified ▽
756.19 Other congenital anomaly of spine

ICD-9-CM Procedural

03.92 Injection of other agent into spinal canal
87.22 Other x-ray of cervical spine
87.24 Other x-ray of lumbosacral spine

HCPCS Level II Supplies & Services

A4550 Surgical trays
A9525 Supply of low or iso-osmolar contrast material, 10 mg of iodine

62292

62292 Injection procedure for chemonucleolysis, including diskography, intervertebral disk, single or multiple levels, lumbar

ICD-9-CM Diagnostic

722.10 Displacement of lumbar intervertebral disc without myelopathy
722.51 Degeneration of thoracic or thoracolumbar intervertebral disc
722.73 Intervertebral lumbar disc disorder with myelopathy, lumbar region
722.93 Other and unspecified disc disorder of lumbar region
724.2 Lumbago
724.4 Thoracic or lumbosacral neuritis or radiculitis, unspecified ▽
724.5 Unspecified backache ▽

ICD-9-CM Procedural

03.6 Lysis of adhesions of spinal cord and nerve roots
80.52 Intervertebral chemonucleolysis
80.59 Other destruction of intervertebral disc
87.29 Other x-ray of spine

62294

62294 Injection procedure, arterial, for occlusion of arteriovenous malformation, spinal

ICD-9-CM Diagnostic

442.89 Aneurysm of other specified artery
747.82 Congenital spinal vessel anomaly

ICD-9-CM Procedural

03.99 Other operations on spinal cord and spinal canal structures

62310

62310 Injection, single (not via indwelling catheter), not including neurolytic substances, with or without contrast (for either localization or epidurography), of diagnostic or therapeutic substance(s) (including anesthetic, antispasmodic, opioid, steroid, other solution), epidural or subarachnoid; cervical or thoracic

ICD-9-CM Diagnostic

340 Multiple sclerosis
721.0 Cervical spondylosis without myelopathy
721.1 Cervical spondylosis with myelopathy
721.2 Thoracic spondylosis without myelopathy
721.41 Spondylosis with myelopathy, thoracic region
722.0 Displacement of cervical intervertebral disc without myelopathy
722.11 Displacement of thoracic intervertebral disc without myelopathy
722.31 Schmorl's nodes, thoracic region
722.4 Degeneration of cervical intervertebral disc
722.51 Degeneration of thoracic or thoracolumbar intervertebral disc
722.71 Intervertebral cervical disc disorder with myelopathy, cervical region
722.72 Intervertebral thoracic disc disorder with myelopathy, thoracic region
722.81 Postlaminectomy syndrome, cervical region
722.82 Postlaminectomy syndrome, thoracic region
722.91 Other and unspecified disc disorder of cervical region
722.92 Other and unspecified disc disorder of thoracic region
723.0 Spinal stenosis in cervical region
723.1 Cervicalgia
723.2 Cervicocranial syndrome
723.3 Cervicobrachial syndrome (diffuse)
723.4 Brachial neuritis or radiculitis nos
723.8 Other syndromes affecting cervical region
724.01 Spinal stenosis of thoracic region
724.4 Thoracic or lumbosacral neuritis or radiculitis, unspecified ▽
733.20 Unspecified cyst of bone (localized) ▽
847.0 Neck sprain and strain
847.1 Thoracic sprain and strain

ICD-9-CM Procedural

03.91 Injection of anesthetic into spinal canal for analgesia
03.92 Injection of other agent into spinal canal

62311

62311 Injection, single (not via indwelling catheter), not including neurolytic substances, with or without contrast (for either localization or epidurography), of diagnostic or therapeutic substance(s) (including anesthetic, antispasmodic, opioid, steroid, other solution), epidural or subarachnoid; lumbar, sacral (caudal)

ICD-9-CM Diagnostic

340 Multiple sclerosis
721.3 Lumbosacral spondylosis without myelopathy
721.42 Spondylosis with myelopathy, lumbar region
722.10 Displacement of lumbar intervertebral disc without myelopathy
722.32 Schmorl's nodes, lumbar region
722.51 Degeneration of thoracic or thoracolumbar intervertebral disc
722.52 Degeneration of lumbar or lumbosacral intervertebral disc
722.73 Intervertebral lumbar disc disorder with myelopathy, lumbar region
722.83 Postlaminectomy syndrome, lumbar region
722.93 Other and unspecified disc disorder of lumbar region
724.02 Spinal stenosis of lumbar region
724.2 Lumbago
724.3 Sciatica
724.4 Thoracic or lumbosacral neuritis or radiculitis, unspecified
724.5 Unspecified backache
724.6 Disorders of sacrum
733.20 Unspecified cyst of bone (localized)
733.21 Solitary bone cyst
846.0 Sprain and strain of lumbosacral (joint) (ligament)
847.2 Lumbar sprain and strain
847.3 Sprain and strain of sacrum

ICD-9-CM Procedural

03.91 Injection of anesthetic into spinal canal for analgesia
03.92 Injection of other agent into spinal canal

62318

62318 Injection, including catheter placement, continuous infusion or intermittent bolus, not including neurolytic substances, with or without contrast (for either localization or epidurography), of diagnostic or therapeutic substance(s) (including anesthetic, antispasmodic, opioid, steroid, other solution), epidural or subarachnoid; cervical or thoracic

ICD-9-CM Diagnostic

340 Multiple sclerosis
721.0 Cervical spondylosis without myelopathy
721.1 Cervical spondylosis with myelopathy
721.2 Thoracic spondylosis without myelopathy
721.41 Spondylosis with myelopathy, thoracic region
722.0 Displacement of cervical intervertebral disc without myelopathy
722.11 Displacement of thoracic intervertebral disc without myelopathy
722.31 Schmorl's nodes, thoracic region
722.4 Degeneration of cervical intervertebral disc
722.51 Degeneration of thoracic or thoracolumbar intervertebral disc
722.71 Intervertebral cervical disc disorder with myelopathy, cervical region
722.72 Intervertebral thoracic disc disorder with myelopathy, thoracic region
722.81 Postlaminectomy syndrome, cervical region
722.82 Postlaminectomy syndrome, thoracic region
722.91 Other and unspecified disc disorder of cervical region
722.92 Other and unspecified disc disorder of thoracic region
723.0 Spinal stenosis in cervical region
723.1 Cervicalgia
723.2 Cervicocranial syndrome
723.3 Cervicobrachial syndrome (diffuse)
723.4 Brachial neuritis or radiculitis nos
723.8 Other syndromes affecting cervical region
724.01 Spinal stenosis of thoracic region
724.4 Thoracic or lumbosacral neuritis or radiculitis, unspecified
733.20 Unspecified cyst of bone (localized)
733.21 Solitary bone cyst
847.0 Neck sprain and strain
847.1 Thoracic sprain and strain

ICD-9-CM Procedural

03.90 Insertion of catheter into spinal canal for infusion of therapeutic or palliative substances
03.91 Injection of anesthetic into spinal canal for analgesia
03.92 Injection of other agent into spinal canal

62319

62319 Injection, including catheter placement, continuous infusion or intermittent bolus, not including neurolytic substances, with or without contrast (for either localization or epidurography), of diagnostic or therapeutic substance(s) (including anesthetic, antispasmodic, opioid, steroid, other solution), epidural or subarachnoid; lumbar, sacral (caudal)

ICD-9-CM Diagnostic

340 Multiple sclerosis
721.3 Lumbosacral spondylosis without myelopathy
721.42 Spondylosis with myelopathy, lumbar region
722.10 Displacement of lumbar intervertebral disc without myelopathy
722.32 Schmorl's nodes, lumbar region
722.51 Degeneration of thoracic or thoracolumbar intervertebral disc
722.52 Degeneration of lumbar or lumbosacral intervertebral disc
722.73 Intervertebral lumbar disc disorder with myelopathy, lumbar region
722.83 Postlaminectomy syndrome, lumbar region
722.93 Other and unspecified disc disorder of lumbar region
724.02 Spinal stenosis of lumbar region
724.2 Lumbago
724.3 Sciatica
724.4 Thoracic or lumbosacral neuritis or radiculitis, unspecified
724.5 Unspecified backache
724.6 Disorders of sacrum
733.20 Unspecified cyst of bone (localized)
733.21 Solitary bone cyst
846.0 Sprain and strain of lumbosacral (joint) (ligament)
847.2 Lumbar sprain and strain
847.3 Sprain and strain of sacrum

ICD-9-CM Procedural

03.90 Insertion of catheter into spinal canal for infusion of therapeutic or palliative substances
03.91 Injection of anesthetic into spinal canal for analgesia
03.92 Injection of other agent into spinal canal

62350–62355

62350 Implantation, revision or repositioning of tunneled intrathecal or epidural catheter, for long-term medication administration via an external pump or implantable reservoir/infusion pump; without laminectomy
62351 with laminectomy
62355 Removal of previously implanted intrathecal or epidural catheter

ICD-9-CM Diagnostic

191.7 Malignant neoplasm of brain stem
192.2 Malignant neoplasm of spinal cord
192.3 Malignant neoplasm of spinal meninges
198.3 Secondary malignant neoplasm of brain and spinal cord
199.0 Disseminated malignant neoplasm
199.1 Other malignant neoplasm of unspecified site
202.80 Other malignant lymphomas, unspecified site, extranodal and solid organ sites
202.90 Other and unspecified malignant neoplasms of lymphoid and histiocytic tissue, unspecified site, extranodal and solid organ sites
722.81 Postlaminectomy syndrome, cervical region
722.82 Postlaminectomy syndrome, thoracic region
722.83 Postlaminectomy syndrome, lumbar region
723.1 Cervicalgia
724.1 Pain in thoracic spine
724.2 Lumbago
996.2 Mechanical complication of nervous system device, implant, and graft
996.63 Infection and inflammatory reaction due to nervous system device, implant, and graft — (Use additional code to identify specified infections)
996.75 Other complications due to nervous system device, implant, and graft
V53.09 Fitting and adjustment of other devices related to nervous system and special senses

ICD-9-CM Procedural

03.02 Reopening of laminectomy site
03.09 Other exploration and decompression of spinal canal
03.90 Insertion of catheter into spinal canal for infusion of therapeutic or palliative substances
03.99 Other operations on spinal cord and spinal canal structures

Unspecified code
Female diagnosis
Manifestation code
Male diagnosis

62360–62365

62360 Implantation or replacement of device for intrathecal or epidural drug infusion; subcutaneous reservoir
62361 non-programmable pump
62362 programmable pump, including preparation of pump, with or without programming
62365 Removal of subcutaneous reservoir or pump, previously implanted for intrathecal or epidural infusion

ICD-9-CM Diagnostic

191.7 Malignant neoplasm of brain stem
192.2 Malignant neoplasm of spinal cord
192.3 Malignant neoplasm of spinal meninges
198.3 Secondary malignant neoplasm of brain and spinal cord
202.80 Other malignant lymphomas, unspecified site, extranodal and solid organ sites ▽
202.90 Other and unspecified malignant neoplasms of lymphoid and histiocytic tissue, unspecified site, extranodal and solid organ sites ▽
722.81 Postlaminectomy syndrome, cervical region
722.82 Postlaminectomy syndrome, thoracic region
722.83 Postlaminectomy syndrome, lumbar region
723.1 Cervicalgia
724.1 Pain in thoracic spine
724.2 Lumbago
996.2 Mechanical complication of nervous system device, implant, and graft
996.63 Infection and inflammatory reaction due to nervous system device, implant, and graft — (Use additional code to identify specified infections)
996.75 Other complications due to nervous system device, implant, and graft
V53.09 Fitting and adjustment of other devices related to nervous system and special senses

ICD-9-CM Procedural

86.06 Insertion of totally implantable infusion pump
86.09 Other incision of skin and subcutaneous tissue

62367–62368

62367 Electronic analysis of programmable, implanted pump for intrathecal or epidural drug infusion (includes evaluation of reservoir status, alarm status, drug prescription status); without reprogramming
62368 with reprogramming

ICD-9-CM Diagnostic

191.7 Malignant neoplasm of brain stem
192.2 Malignant neoplasm of spinal cord
192.3 Malignant neoplasm of spinal meninges
198.3 Secondary malignant neoplasm of brain and spinal cord
202.80 Other malignant lymphomas, unspecified site, extranodal and solid organ sites ▽
202.90 Other and unspecified malignant neoplasms of lymphoid and histiocytic tissue, unspecified site, extranodal and solid organ sites ▽
722.81 Postlaminectomy syndrome, cervical region
722.82 Postlaminectomy syndrome, thoracic region
722.83 Postlaminectomy syndrome, lumbar region
723.1 Cervicalgia
724.1 Pain in thoracic spine
724.2 Lumbago 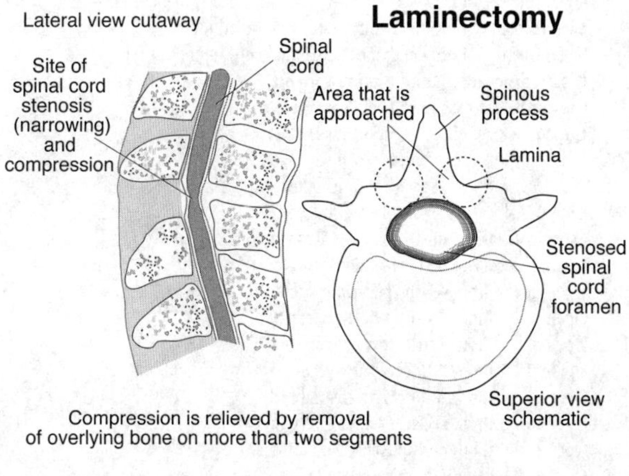
996.2 Mechanical complication of nervous system device, implant, and graft
996.63 Infection and inflammatory reaction due to nervous system device, implant, and graft — (Use additional code to identify specified infections)
996.75 Other complications due to nervous system device, implant, and graft
V53.09 Fitting and adjustment of other devices related to nervous system and special senses

ICD-9-CM Procedural

86.06 Insertion of totally implantable infusion pump

Laminectomy

Lateral view cutaway
Site of spinal cord stenosis (narrowing) and compression
Spinal cord
Area that is approached
Spinous process
Lamina
Stenosed spinal cord foramen
Superior view schematic

Compression is relieved by removal of overlying bone on more than two segments

63001–63011

63001 Laminectomy with exploration and/or decompression of spinal cord and/or cauda equina, without facetectomy, foraminotomy or diskectomy, (eg, spinal stenosis), one or two vertebral segments; cervical
63003 thoracic
63005 lumbar, except for spondylolisthesis
63011 sacral

ICD-9-CM Diagnostic

344.60 Cauda equina syndrome without mention of neurogenic bladder
353.1 Lumbosacral plexus lesions
355.0 Lesion of sciatic nerve
715.98 Osteoarthrosis, unspecified whether generalized or localized, other specified sites ▽
719.48 Pain in joint, other specified sites
720.0 Ankylosing spondylitis
720.2 Sacroiliitis, not elsewhere classified
721.0 Cervical spondylosis without myelopathy
721.1 Cervical spondylosis with myelopathy
721.2 Thoracic spondylosis without myelopathy
721.3 Lumbosacral spondylosis without myelopathy
721.41 Spondylosis with myelopathy, thoracic region
721.42 Spondylosis with myelopathy, lumbar region
722.0 Displacement of cervical intervertebral disc without myelopathy
722.10 Displacement of lumbar intervertebral disc without myelopathy
722.52 Degeneration of lumbar or lumbosacral intervertebral disc
722.71 Intervertebral cervical disc disorder with myelopathy, cervical region
722.73 Intervertebral lumbar disc disorder with myelopathy, lumbar region
722.83 Postlaminectomy syndrome, lumbar region
722.91 Other and unspecified disc disorder of cervical region
722.93 Other and unspecified disc disorder of lumbar region
723.0 Spinal stenosis in cervical region
723.1 Cervicalgia
723.4 Brachial neuritis or radiculitis nos
724.01 Spinal stenosis of thoracic region
724.02 Spinal stenosis of lumbar region
724.09 Spinal stenosis, other region other than cervical
724.1 Pain in thoracic spine
724.2 Lumbago
724.3 Sciatica
724.4 Thoracic or lumbosacral neuritis or radiculitis, unspecified ▽
724.6 Disorders of sacrum
728.5 Hypermobility syndrome
729.2 Unspecified neuralgia, neuritis, and radiculitis ▽
729.4 Unspecified fasciitis ▽
738.2 Acquired deformity of neck
738.4 Acquired spondylolisthesis
756.10 Congenital anomaly of spine, unspecified ▽
756.11 Congenital spondylolysis, lumbosacral region
805.10 Open fracture of cervical vertebra, unspecified level without mention of spinal cord injury ▽
805.2 Closed fracture of dorsal (thoracic) vertebra without mention of spinal cord injury
805.3 Open fracture of dorsal (thoracic) vertebra without mention of spinal cord injury
805.4 Closed fracture of lumbar vertebra without mention of spinal cord injury
805.5 Open fracture of lumbar vertebra without mention of spinal cord injury
805.6 Closed fracture of sacrum and coccyx without mention of spinal cord injury
805.7 Open fracture of sacrum and coccyx without mention of spinal cord injury
806.00 Closed fracture of C1-C4 level with unspecified spinal cord injury ▽
806.20 Closed fracture of T1-T6 level with unspecified spinal cord injury ▽
806.4 Closed fracture of lumbar spine with spinal cord injury
806.5 Open fracture of lumbar spine with spinal cord injury
806.60 Closed fracture of sacrum and coccyx with unspecified spinal cord injury ▽
806.69 Closed fracture of sacrum and coccyx with other spinal cord injury
806.70 Open fracture of sacrum and coccyx with unspecified spinal cord injury ▽

806.79 Open fracture of sacrum and coccyx with other spinal cord injury
839.00 Closed dislocation, unspecified cervical vertebra ▽
839.10 Open dislocation, unspecified cervical vertebra ▽
905.1 Late effect of fracture of spine and trunk without mention of spinal cord lesion
907.2 Late effect of spinal cord injury
952.2 Lumbar spinal cord injury without spinal bone injury
952.3 Sacral spinal cord injury without spinal bone injury
953.3 Injury to sacral nerve root
953.5 Injury to lumbosacral plexus

ICD-9-CM Procedural

03.09 Other exploration and decompression of spinal canal

63012

63012 Laminectomy with removal of abnormal facets and/or pars inter-articularis with decompression of cauda equina and nerve roots for spondylolisthesis, lumbar (Gill type procedure)

ICD-9-CM Diagnostic

721.3 Lumbosacral spondylosis without myelopathy
721.42 Spondylosis with myelopathy, lumbar region
724.2 Lumbago
724.4 Thoracic or lumbosacral neuritis or radiculitis, unspecified ▽
724.5 Unspecified backache ▽
738.4 Acquired spondylolisthesis
756.11 Congenital spondylolysis, lumbosacral region
756.12 Congenital spondylolisthesis

ICD-9-CM Procedural

03.09 Other exploration and decompression of spinal canal

63015–63017

63015 Laminectomy with exploration and/or decompression of spinal cord and/or cauda equina, without facetectomy, foraminotomy or diskectomy, (eg, spinal stenosis), more than 2 vertebral segments; cervical
63016 thoracic
63017 lumbar

ICD-9-CM Diagnostic

720.0 Ankylosing spondylitis
721.0 Cervical spondylosis without myelopathy
721.1 Cervical spondylosis with myelopathy
721.2 Thoracic spondylosis without myelopathy
721.3 Lumbosacral spondylosis without myelopathy
721.41 Spondylosis with myelopathy, thoracic region
721.42 Spondylosis with myelopathy, lumbar region
722.10 Displacement of lumbar intervertebral disc without myelopathy
722.83 Postlaminectomy syndrome, lumbar region
722.93 Other and unspecified disc disorder of lumbar region
723.0 Spinal stenosis in cervical region
723.4 Brachial neuritis or radiculitis nos
723.7 Ossification of posterior longitudinal ligament in cervical region
724.01 Spinal stenosis of thoracic region
724.02 Spinal stenosis of lumbar region
724.1 Pain in thoracic spine
724.2 Lumbago
724.3 Sciatica
724.4 Thoracic or lumbosacral neuritis or radiculitis, unspecified ▽
724.5 Unspecified backache ▽
724.9 Other unspecified back disorder
729.2 Unspecified neuralgia, neuritis, and radiculitis ▽
738.4 Acquired spondylolisthesis
756.11 Congenital spondylolysis, lumbosacral region
756.12 Congenital spondylolisthesis
756.19 Other congenital anomaly of spine
805.00 Closed fracture of cervical vertebra, unspecified level without mention of spinal cord injury ▽
805.10 Open fracture of cervical vertebra, unspecified level without mention of spinal cord injury ▽
805.2 Closed fracture of dorsal (thoracic) vertebra without mention of spinal cord injury
805.3 Open fracture of dorsal (thoracic) vertebra without mention of spinal cord injury
805.4 Closed fracture of lumbar vertebra without mention of spinal cord injury
805.5 Open fracture of lumbar vertebra without mention of spinal cord injury
806.00 Closed fracture of C1-C4 level with unspecified spinal cord injury ▽
806.19 Open fracture of C5-C7 level with other specified spinal cord injury
806.20 Closed fracture of T1-T6 level with unspecified spinal cord injury ▽
806.30 Open fracture of T1-T6 level with unspecified spinal cord injury ▽
806.4 Closed fracture of lumbar spine with spinal cord injury
806.5 Open fracture of lumbar spine with spinal cord injury
846.0 Sprain and strain of lumbosacral (joint) (ligament)
905.1 Late effect of fracture of spine and trunk without mention of spinal cord lesion
905.6 Late effect of dislocation
907.2 Late effect of spinal cord injury
907.3 Late effect of injury to nerve root(s), spinal plexus(es), and other nerves of trunk
952.2 Lumbar spinal cord injury without spinal bone injury
953.0 Injury to cervical nerve root
953.1 Injury to dorsal nerve root
953.2 Injury to lumbar nerve root
953.5 Injury to lumbosacral plexus

ICD-9-CM Procedural

03.09 Other exploration and decompression of spinal canal

63020–63035

63020 Laminotomy (hemilaminectomy), with decompression of nerve root(s), including partial facetectomy, foraminotomy and/or excision of herniated intervertebral disk; one interspace, cervical
63030 one interspace, lumbar (including open or endoscopically-assisted approach)
63035 each additional interspace, cervical or lumbar (List separately in addition to code for primary procedure)

ICD-9-CM Diagnostic

721.0 Cervical spondylosis without myelopathy
721.1 Cervical spondylosis with myelopathy
721.3 Lumbosacral spondylosis without myelopathy
721.42 Spondylosis with myelopathy, lumbar region
722.0 Displacement of cervical intervertebral disc without myelopathy
722.10 Displacement of lumbar intervertebral disc without myelopathy
722.51 Degeneration of thoracic or thoracolumbar intervertebral disc
722.52 Degeneration of lumbar or lumbosacral intervertebral disc
722.71 Intervertebral cervical disc disorder with myelopathy, cervical region
722.73 Intervertebral lumbar disc disorder with myelopathy, lumbar region
723.0 Spinal stenosis in cervical region
723.1 Cervicalgia
723.4 Brachial neuritis or radiculitis nos
723.7 Ossification of posterior longitudinal ligament in cervical region
724.02 Spinal stenosis of lumbar region
724.2 Lumbago
724.3 Sciatica
724.4 Thoracic or lumbosacral neuritis or radiculitis, unspecified ▽
724.9 Other unspecified back disorder
738.4 Acquired spondylolisthesis
756.10 Congenital anomaly of spine, unspecified ▽
756.11 Congenital spondylolysis, lumbosacral region
756.12 Congenital spondylolisthesis
756.19 Other congenital anomaly of spine
805.4 Closed fracture of lumbar vertebra without mention of spinal cord injury
805.5 Open fracture of lumbar vertebra without mention of spinal cord injury
806.00 Closed fracture of C1-C4 level with unspecified spinal cord injury ▽
806.10 Open fracture of C1-C4 level with unspecified spinal cord injury ▽
806.19 Open fracture of C5-C7 level with other specified spinal cord injury
806.4 Closed fracture of lumbar spine with spinal cord injury
806.5 Open fracture of lumbar spine with spinal cord injury
839.03 Closed dislocation, third cervical vertebra
839.04 Closed dislocation, fourth cervical vertebra
839.05 Closed dislocation, fifth cervical vertebra
839.06 Closed dislocation, sixth cervical vertebra
839.07 Closed dislocation, seventh cervical vertebra
839.08 Closed dislocation, multiple cervical vertebrae
839.10 Open dislocation, unspecified cervical vertebra ▽
839.11 Open dislocation, first cervical vertebra
839.12 Open dislocation, second cervical vertebra
839.13 Open dislocation, third cervical vertebra
839.14 Open dislocation, fourth cervical vertebra
839.15 Open dislocation, fifth cervical vertebra
839.16 Open dislocation, sixth cervical vertebra
839.17 Open dislocation, seventh cervical vertebra
839.18 Open dislocation, multiple cervical vertebrae
839.20 Closed dislocation, lumbar vertebra

▽ Unspecified code
♀ Female diagnosis
☒ Manifestation code
♂ Male diagnosis

905.1 Late effect of fracture of spine and trunk without mention of spinal cord lesion
907.2 Late effect of spinal cord injury
952.00 C1-C4 level spinal cord injury, unspecified ▽
952.2 Lumbar spinal cord injury without spinal bone injury
953.2 Injury to lumbar nerve root

ICD-9-CM Procedural

80.51 Excision of intervertebral disc

63040–63044

63040 Laminotomy (hemilaminectomy), with decompression of nerve root(s), including partial facetectomy, foraminotomy and/or excision of herniated intervertebral disk, reexploration, single interspace; cervical
63042 lumbar
63043 each additional cervical interspace (List separately in addition to code for primary procedure)
63044 each additional lumbar interspace (List separately in addition to code for primary procedure)

ICD-9-CM Diagnostic

721.0 Cervical spondylosis without myelopathy
721.1 Cervical spondylosis with myelopathy
721.3 Lumbosacral spondylosis without myelopathy
721.42 Spondylosis with myelopathy, lumbar region
722.0 Displacement of cervical intervertebral disc without myelopathy
722.10 Displacement of lumbar intervertebral disc without myelopathy
722.4 Degeneration of cervical intervertebral disc
722.52 Degeneration of lumbar or lumbosacral intervertebral disc
722.71 Intervertebral cervical disc disorder with myelopathy, cervical region
722.73 Intervertebral lumbar disc disorder with myelopathy, lumbar region
722.81 Postlaminectomy syndrome, cervical region
722.83 Postlaminectomy syndrome, lumbar region
722.93 Other and unspecified disc disorder of lumbar region
723.0 Spinal stenosis in cervical region
723.1 Cervicalgia
723.4 Brachial neuritis or radiculitis nos
724.02 Spinal stenosis of lumbar region
724.4 Thoracic or lumbosacral neuritis or radiculitis, unspecified ▽
756.11 Congenital spondylolysis, lumbosacral region
756.12 Congenital spondylolisthesis
805.00 Closed fracture of cervical vertebra, unspecified level without mention of spinal cord injury ▽
805.10 Open fracture of cervical vertebra, unspecified level without mention of spinal cord injury ▽
806.00 Closed fracture of C1-C4 level with unspecified spinal cord injury ▽
806.10 Open fracture of C1-C4 level with unspecified spinal cord injury ▽
806.4 Closed fracture of lumbar spine with spinal cord injury
806.5 Open fracture of lumbar spine with spinal cord injury
839.00 Closed dislocation, unspecified cervical vertebra ▽
839.10 Open dislocation, unspecified cervical vertebra ▽
907.3 Late effect of injury to nerve root(s), spinal plexus(es), and other nerves of trunk
909.3 Late effect of complications of surgical and medical care
952.2 Lumbar spinal cord injury without spinal bone injury
953.2 Injury to lumbar nerve root
953.5 Injury to lumbosacral plexus
V45.4 Arthrodesis status — (This code is intended for use when these conditions are recorded as diagnoses or problems)

ICD-9-CM Procedural

03.02 Reopening of laminectomy site
80.51 Excision of intervertebral disc

63045–63048

63045 Laminectomy, facetectomy and foraminotomy (unilateral or bilateral with decompression of spinal cord, cauda equina and/or nerve root(s), (eg, spinal or lateral recess stenosis), single vertebral segment; cervical
63046 thoracic
63047 lumbar
63048 each additional segment, cervical, thoracic, or lumbar (List separately in addition to code for primary procedure)

ICD-9-CM Diagnostic

721.0 Cervical spondylosis without myelopathy
721.1 Cervical spondylosis with myelopathy
721.2 Thoracic spondylosis without myelopathy
721.3 Lumbosacral spondylosis without myelopathy
721.41 Spondylosis with myelopathy, thoracic region
721.42 Spondylosis with myelopathy, lumbar region
722.10 Displacement of lumbar intervertebral disc without myelopathy
722.51 Degeneration of thoracic or thoracolumbar intervertebral disc
722.52 Degeneration of lumbar or lumbosacral intervertebral disc
722.71 Intervertebral cervical disc disorder with myelopathy, cervical region
722.72 Intervertebral thoracic disc disorder with myelopathy, thoracic region
722.73 Intervertebral lumbar disc disorder with myelopathy, lumbar region
722.83 Postlaminectomy syndrome, lumbar region
722.93 Other and unspecified disc disorder of lumbar region
723.0 Spinal stenosis in cervical region
723.1 Cervicalgia
723.4 Brachial neuritis or radiculitis nos
723.7 Ossification of posterior longitudinal ligament in cervical region
724.01 Spinal stenosis of thoracic region
724.02 Spinal stenosis of lumbar region
724.1 Pain in thoracic spine
724.4 Thoracic or lumbosacral neuritis or radiculitis, unspecified ▽
724.9 Other unspecified back disorder
729.2 Unspecified neuralgia, neuritis, and radiculitis ▽
738.4 Acquired spondylolisthesis
756.11 Congenital spondylolysis, lumbosacral region
756.12 Congenital spondylolisthesis
805.2 Closed fracture of dorsal (thoracic) vertebra without mention of spinal cord injury
805.3 Open fracture of dorsal (thoracic) vertebra without mention of spinal cord injury
805.4 Closed fracture of lumbar vertebra without mention of spinal cord injury
805.5 Open fracture of lumbar vertebra without mention of spinal cord injury
806.00 Closed fracture of C1-C4 level with unspecified spinal cord injury ▽
806.10 Open fracture of C1-C4 level with unspecified spinal cord injury ▽
806.20 Closed fracture of T1-T6 level with unspecified spinal cord injury ▽
806.30 Open fracture of T1-T6 level with unspecified spinal cord injury ▽
806.4 Closed fracture of lumbar spine with spinal cord injury
806.5 Open fracture of lumbar spine with spinal cord injury
839.00 Closed dislocation, unspecified cervical vertebra ▽
839.10 Open dislocation, unspecified cervical vertebra ▽
839.21 Closed dislocation, thoracic vertebra
839.31 Open dislocation, thoracic vertebra
952.00 C1-C4 level spinal cord injury, unspecified ▽
952.10 T1-T6 level spinal cord injury, unspecified ▽
952.2 Lumbar spinal cord injury without spinal bone injury
953.1 Injury to dorsal nerve root
953.2 Injury to lumbar nerve root

ICD-9-CM Procedural

03.09 Other exploration and decompression of spinal canal

63050–63051

63050 Laminoplasty, cervical, with decompression of the spinal cord, two or more vertebral segments;
63051 with reconstruction of the posterior bony elements (including the application of bridging bone graft and non-segmental fixation devices (eg, wire, suture, mini-plates), when performed)

ICD-9-CM Diagnostic

720.0 Ankylosing spondylitis
721.1 Cervical spondylosis with myelopathy
722.71 Intervertebral cervical disc disorder with myelopathy, cervical region
723.0 Spinal stenosis in cervical region
723.1 Cervicalgia
723.4 Brachial neuritis or radiculitis nos
756.10 Congenital anomaly of spine, unspecified ▽
756.19 Other congenital anomaly of spine
905.1 Late effect of fracture of spine and trunk without mention of spinal cord lesion

ICD-9-CM Procedural

03.09 Other exploration and decompression of spinal canal
03.59 Other repair and plastic operations on spinal cord structures

63055–63057

63055 Transpedicular approach with decompression of spinal cord, equina and/or nerve root(s) (eg, herniated intervertebral disk), single segment; thoracic
63056 lumbar (including transfacet, or lateral extraforaminal approach) (eg, far lateral herniated intervertebral disk)
63057 each additional segment, thoracic or lumbar (List separately in addition to code for primary procedure)

ICD-9-CM Diagnostic

722.10 Displacement of lumbar intervertebral disc without myelopathy
722.11 Displacement of thoracic intervertebral disc without myelopathy
722.51 Degeneration of thoracic or thoracolumbar intervertebral disc
722.52 Degeneration of lumbar or lumbosacral intervertebral disc
722.72 Intervertebral thoracic disc disorder with myelopathy, thoracic region
722.73 Intervertebral lumbar disc disorder with myelopathy, lumbar region
724.01 Spinal stenosis of thoracic region
724.02 Spinal stenosis of lumbar region
724.3 Sciatica
724.4 Thoracic or lumbosacral neuritis or radiculitis, unspecified ▽
729.2 Unspecified neuralgia, neuritis, and radiculitis ▽
729.5 Pain in soft tissues of limb
733.13 Pathologic fracture of vertebrae
733.95 Stress fracture of other bone
805.2 Closed fracture of dorsal (thoracic) vertebra without mention of spinal cord injury
805.3 Open fracture of dorsal (thoracic) vertebra without mention of spinal cord injury
805.4 Closed fracture of lumbar vertebra without mention of spinal cord injury
805.5 Open fracture of lumbar vertebra without mention of spinal cord injury
806.20 Closed fracture of T1-T6 level with unspecified spinal cord injury ▽
806.30 Open fracture of T1-T6 level with unspecified spinal cord injury ▽
806.4 Closed fracture of lumbar spine with spinal cord injury
806.5 Open fracture of lumbar spine with spinal cord injury

ICD-9-CM Procedural

03.09 Other exploration and decompression of spinal canal

63064–63066

63064 Costovertebral approach with decompression of spinal cord or nerve root(s), (eg, herniated intervertebral disk), thoracic; single segment
63066 each additional segment (List separately in addition to code for primary procedure)

ICD-9-CM Diagnostic

722.11 Displacement of thoracic intervertebral disc without myelopathy
722.51 Degeneration of thoracic or thoracolumbar intervertebral disc
722.72 Intervertebral thoracic disc disorder with myelopathy, thoracic region
722.92 Other and unspecified disc disorder of thoracic region
724.01 Spinal stenosis of thoracic region
738.4 Acquired spondylolisthesis
756.12 Congenital spondylolisthesis
805.2 Closed fracture of dorsal (thoracic) vertebra without mention of spinal cord injury
805.3 Open fracture of dorsal (thoracic) vertebra without mention of spinal cord injury
806.20 Closed fracture of T1-T6 level with unspecified spinal cord injury ▽
806.21 Closed fracture of T1-T6 level with complete lesion of cord
806.30 Open fracture of T1-T6 level with unspecified spinal cord injury ▽
952.19 T7-T12 level with other specified spinal cord injury

ICD-9-CM Procedural

03.09 Other exploration and decompression of spinal canal

63075–63076

63075 Diskectomy, anterior, with decompression of spinal cord and/or nerve root(s), including osteophytectomy; cervical, single interspace
63076 cervical, each additional interspace (List separately in addition to code for primary procedure)

ICD-9-CM Diagnostic

721.0 Cervical spondylosis without myelopathy
721.1 Cervical spondylosis with myelopathy
721.8 Other allied disorders of spine
722.0 Displacement of cervical intervertebral disc without myelopathy
722.4 Degeneration of cervical intervertebral disc
722.71 Intervertebral cervical disc disorder with myelopathy, cervical region

Vertebral Corpectomy

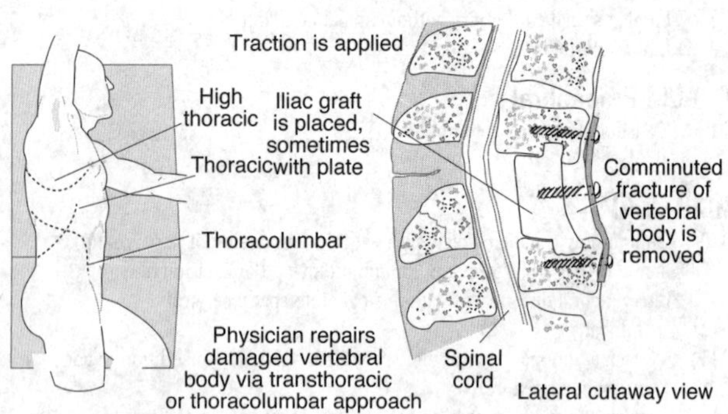

722.91 Other and unspecified disc disorder of cervical region
723.0 Spinal stenosis in cervical region
723.1 Cervicalgia
723.2 Cervicocranial syndrome
723.3 Cervicobrachial syndrome (diffuse)
723.4 Brachial neuritis or radiculitis nos
723.7 Ossification of posterior longitudinal ligament in cervical region
729.5 Pain in soft tissues of limb
738.4 Acquired spondylolisthesis
738.5 Other acquired deformity of back or spine
756.10 Congenital anomaly of spine, unspecified ▽
756.19 Other congenital anomaly of spine
839.03 Closed dislocation, third cervical vertebra
839.04 Closed dislocation, fourth cervical vertebra
839.05 Closed dislocation, fifth cervical vertebra
839.06 Closed dislocation, sixth cervical vertebra
839.07 Closed dislocation, seventh cervical vertebra
839.08 Closed dislocation, multiple cervical vertebrae
839.11 Open dislocation, first cervical vertebra
839.12 Open dislocation, second cervical vertebra
839.13 Open dislocation, third cervical vertebra
839.14 Open dislocation, fourth cervical vertebra
839.15 Open dislocation, fifth cervical vertebra
839.16 Open dislocation, sixth cervical vertebra
839.17 Open dislocation, seventh cervical vertebra
839.18 Open dislocation, multiple cervical vertebrae
905.1 Late effect of fracture of spine and trunk without mention of spinal cord lesion
907.2 Late effect of spinal cord injury
952.00 C1-C4 level spinal cord injury, unspecified ▽
952.09 C5-C7 level with other specified spinal cord injury

ICD-9-CM Procedural

80.51 Excision of intervertebral disc

63077–63078

63077 Diskectomy, anterior, with decompression of spinal cord and/or nerve root(s), including osteophytectomy; thoracic, single interspace
63078 thoracic, each additional interspace (List separately in addition to code for primary procedure)

ICD-9-CM Diagnostic

721.2 Thoracic spondylosis without myelopathy
721.41 Spondylosis with myelopathy, thoracic region
721.8 Other allied disorders of spine
722.11 Displacement of thoracic intervertebral disc without myelopathy
722.51 Degeneration of thoracic or thoracolumbar intervertebral disc
722.72 Intervertebral thoracic disc disorder with myelopathy, thoracic region
722.92 Other and unspecified disc disorder of thoracic region
724.01 Spinal stenosis of thoracic region
724.1 Pain in thoracic spine
729.2 Unspecified neuralgia, neuritis, and radiculitis ▽
754.2 Congenital musculoskeletal deformity of spine
952.10 T1-T6 level spinal cord injury, unspecified ▽

ICD-9-CM Procedural

80.51 Excision of intervertebral disc

▽ Unspecified code
♀ Female diagnosis
☒ Manifestation code
♂ Male diagnosis

63081–63082

63081 Vertebral corpectomy (vertebral body resection), partial or complete, anterior approach with decompression of spinal cord and/or nerve root(s); cervical, single segment

63082 cervical, each additional segment (List separately in addition to code for primary procedure)

ICD-9-CM Diagnostic

170.2 Malignant neoplasm of vertebral column, excluding sacrum and coccyx
721.0 Cervical spondylosis without myelopathy
721.1 Cervical spondylosis with myelopathy
722.0 Displacement of cervical intervertebral disc without myelopathy
722.4 Degeneration of cervical intervertebral disc
722.71 Intervertebral cervical disc disorder with myelopathy, cervical region
722.91 Other and unspecified disc disorder of cervical region
723.0 Spinal stenosis in cervical region
723.1 Cervicalgia
723.4 Brachial neuritis or radiculitis nos
730.28 Unspecified osteomyelitis, other specified sites — (Use additional code to identify organism, 041.1) ▽
756.10 Congenital anomaly of spine, unspecified ▽
756.12 Congenital spondylolisthesis
806.00 Closed fracture of C1-C4 level with unspecified spinal cord injury ▽
806.10 Open fracture of C1-C4 level with unspecified spinal cord injury ▽

ICD-9-CM Procedural

03.09 Other exploration and decompression of spinal canal
03.59 Other repair and plastic operations on spinal cord structures

63085–63086

63085 Vertebral corpectomy (vertebral body resection), partial or complete, transthoracic approach with decompression of spinal cord and/or nerve root(s); thoracic, single segment

63086 thoracic, each additional segment (List separately in addition to code for primary procedure)

ICD-9-CM Diagnostic

170.2 Malignant neoplasm of vertebral column, excluding sacrum and coccyx
721.2 Thoracic spondylosis without myelopathy
721.41 Spondylosis with myelopathy, thoracic region
722.11 Displacement of thoracic intervertebral disc without myelopathy
722.51 Degeneration of thoracic or thoracolumbar intervertebral disc
722.72 Intervertebral thoracic disc disorder with myelopathy, thoracic region
724.1 Pain in thoracic spine
724.4 Thoracic or lumbosacral neuritis or radiculitis, unspecified ▽
729.2 Unspecified neuralgia, neuritis, and radiculitis ▽
730.28 Unspecified osteomyelitis, other specified sites — (Use additional code to identify organism, 041.1) ▽
805.2 Closed fracture of dorsal (thoracic) vertebra without mention of spinal cord injury
805.3 Open fracture of dorsal (thoracic) vertebra without mention of spinal cord injury
806.20 Closed fracture of T1-T6 level with unspecified spinal cord injury ▽
806.30 Open fracture of T1-T6 level with unspecified spinal cord injury ▽

ICD-9-CM Procedural

03.09 Other exploration and decompression of spinal canal
03.59 Other repair and plastic operations on spinal cord structures

63087–63088

63087 Vertebral corpectomy (vertebral body resection), partial or complete, combined thoracolumbar approach with decompression of spinal cord, cauda equina or nerve root(s), lower thoracic or lumbar; single segment

63088 each additional segment (List separately in addition to code for primary procedure)

ICD-9-CM Diagnostic

170.2 Malignant neoplasm of vertebral column, excluding sacrum and coccyx
721.2 Thoracic spondylosis without myelopathy
721.41 Spondylosis with myelopathy, thoracic region
722.10 Displacement of lumbar intervertebral disc without myelopathy
722.11 Displacement of thoracic intervertebral disc without myelopathy
722.51 Degeneration of thoracic or thoracolumbar intervertebral disc
722.52 Degeneration of lumbar or lumbosacral intervertebral disc
722.72 Intervertebral thoracic disc disorder with myelopathy, thoracic region
722.73 Intervertebral lumbar disc disorder with myelopathy, lumbar region
722.93 Other and unspecified disc disorder of lumbar region
724.02 Spinal stenosis of lumbar region
724.4 Thoracic or lumbosacral neuritis or radiculitis, unspecified ▽
730.28 Unspecified osteomyelitis, other specified sites — (Use additional code to identify organism, 041.1) ▽
805.2 Closed fracture of dorsal (thoracic) vertebra without mention of spinal cord injury
805.3 Open fracture of dorsal (thoracic) vertebra without mention of spinal cord injury
805.4 Closed fracture of lumbar vertebra without mention of spinal cord injury
805.5 Open fracture of lumbar vertebra without mention of spinal cord injury
806.25 Closed fracture of T7-T12 level with unspecified spinal cord injury ▽
806.35 Open fracture of T7-T12 level with unspecified spinal cord injury ▽
806.4 Closed fracture of lumbar spine with spinal cord injury
806.5 Open fracture of lumbar spine with spinal cord injury

ICD-9-CM Procedural

03.09 Other exploration and decompression of spinal canal
03.59 Other repair and plastic operations on spinal cord structures

63090–63091

63090 Vertebral corpectomy (vertebral body resection), partial or complete, transperitoneal or retroperitoneal approach with decompression of spinal cord, cauda equina or nerve root(s), lower thoracic, lumbar, or sacral; single segment

63091 each additional segment (List separately in addition to code for primary procedure)

ICD-9-CM Diagnostic

170.2 Malignant neoplasm of vertebral column, excluding sacrum and coccyx
170.6 Malignant neoplasm of pelvic bones, sacrum, and coccyx
721.2 Thoracic spondylosis without myelopathy
721.3 Lumbosacral spondylosis without myelopathy
721.41 Spondylosis with myelopathy, thoracic region
722.10 Displacement of lumbar intervertebral disc without myelopathy
722.11 Displacement of thoracic intervertebral disc without myelopathy
722.51 Degeneration of thoracic or thoracolumbar intervertebral disc
722.52 Degeneration of lumbar or lumbosacral intervertebral disc
722.72 Intervertebral thoracic disc disorder with myelopathy, thoracic region
722.73 Intervertebral lumbar disc disorder with myelopathy, lumbar region
722.93 Other and unspecified disc disorder of lumbar region
724.02 Spinal stenosis of lumbar region
724.4 Thoracic or lumbosacral neuritis or radiculitis, unspecified ▽
724.6 Disorders of sacrum
730.28 Unspecified osteomyelitis, other specified sites — (Use additional code to identify organism, 041.1) ▽
738.4 Acquired spondylolisthesis
805.2 Closed fracture of dorsal (thoracic) vertebra without mention of spinal cord injury
805.3 Open fracture of dorsal (thoracic) vertebra without mention of spinal cord injury
805.4 Closed fracture of lumbar vertebra without mention of spinal cord injury
805.5 Open fracture of lumbar vertebra without mention of spinal cord injury
806.25 Closed fracture of T7-T12 level with unspecified spinal cord injury ▽
806.35 Open fracture of T7-T12 level with unspecified spinal cord injury ▽
806.4 Closed fracture of lumbar spine with spinal cord injury
806.5 Open fracture of lumbar spine with spinal cord injury

ICD-9-CM Procedural

03.09 Other exploration and decompression of spinal canal
03.59 Other repair and plastic operations on spinal cord structures

63101–63103

63101 Vertebral corpectomy (vertebral body resection), partial or complete, lateral extracavitary approach with decompression of spinal cord and/or nerve root(s) (eg, for tumor or retropulsed bone fragments); thoracic, single segment

63102 lumbar, single segment

63103 thoracic or lumbar, each additional segment (List separately in addition to code for primary procedure)

ICD-9-CM Diagnostic

170.2 Malignant neoplasm of vertebral column, excluding sacrum and coccyx
721.2 Thoracic spondylosis without myelopathy
721.41 Spondylosis with myelopathy, thoracic region
722.10 Displacement of lumbar intervertebral disc without myelopathy
722.11 Displacement of thoracic intervertebral disc without myelopathy
722.51 Degeneration of thoracic or thoracolumbar intervertebral disc

722.52 Degeneration of lumbar or lumbosacral intervertebral disc
722.72 Intervertebral thoracic disc disorder with myelopathy, thoracic region
722.73 Intervertebral lumbar disc disorder with myelopathy, lumbar region
722.93 Other and unspecified disc disorder of lumbar region
724.02 Spinal stenosis of lumbar region
724.1 Pain in thoracic spine
724.4 Thoracic or lumbosacral neuritis or radiculitis, unspecified ▽
730.28 Unspecified osteomyelitis, other specified sites — (Use additional code to identify organism, 041.1) ▽
805.2 Closed fracture of dorsal (thoracic) vertebra without mention of spinal cord injury
805.3 Open fracture of dorsal (thoracic) vertebra without mention of spinal cord injury
805.4 Closed fracture of lumbar vertebra without mention of spinal cord injury
805.5 Open fracture of lumbar vertebra without mention of spinal cord injury
806.20 Closed fracture of T1-T6 level with unspecified spinal cord injury ▽
806.25 Closed fracture of T7-T12 level with unspecified spinal cord injury ▽
806.30 Open fracture of T1-T6 level with unspecified spinal cord injury ▽
806.35 Open fracture of T7-T12 level with unspecified spinal cord injury ▽
806.4 Closed fracture of lumbar spine with spinal cord injury
806.5 Open fracture of lumbar spine with spinal cord injury

ICD-9-CM Procedural

03.09 Other exploration and decompression of spinal canal
03.59 Other repair and plastic operations on spinal cord structures

63170

63170 Laminectomy with myelotomy (eg, Bischof or DREZ type), cervical, thoracic, or thoracolumbar

ICD-9-CM Diagnostic

336.0 Syringomyelia and syringobulbia
353.6 Phantom limb (syndrome)
724.1 Pain in thoracic spine
724.2 Lumbago
724.4 Thoracic or lumbosacral neuritis or radiculitis, unspecified ▽
724.5 Unspecified backache ▽
741.01 Spina bifida with hydrocephalus, cervical region
741.02 Spina bifida with hydrocephalus, dorsal (thoracic) region
741.03 Spina bifida with hydrocephalus, lumbar region
741.91 Spina bifida without mention of hydrocephalus, cervical region
741.92 Spina bifida without mention of hydrocephalus, dorsal (thoracic) region
741.93 Spina bifida without mention of hydrocephalus, lumbar region

ICD-9-CM Procedural

03.09 Other exploration and decompression of spinal canal
03.29 Other chordotomy

63172–63173

63172 Laminectomy with drainage of intramedullary cyst/syrinx; to subarachnoid space
63173 to peritoneal or pleural space

ICD-9-CM Diagnostic

336.0 Syringomyelia and syringobulbia
349.2 Disorders of meninges, not elsewhere classified ▽

ICD-9-CM Procedural

03.09 Other exploration and decompression of spinal canal
03.79 Other shunt of spinal theca

63180–63182

63180 Laminectomy and section of dentate ligaments, with or without dural graft, cervical; one or two segments
63182 more than two segments

ICD-9-CM Diagnostic

353.2 Cervical root lesions, not elsewhere classified
354.5 Mononeuritis multiplex
723.1 Cervicalgia
723.4 Brachial neuritis or radiculitis nos

ICD-9-CM Procedural

03.09 Other exploration and decompression of spinal canal

63185–63190

63185 Laminectomy with rhizotomy; one or two segments
63190 more than two segments

ICD-9-CM Diagnostic

343.9 Unspecified infantile cerebral palsy ▽
720.2 Sacroiliitis, not elsewhere classified
723.1 Cervicalgia
723.4 Brachial neuritis or radiculitis nos
724.1 Pain in thoracic spine
724.2 Lumbago
724.3 Sciatica
724.4 Thoracic or lumbosacral neuritis or radiculitis, unspecified ▽
724.6 Disorders of sacrum
729.1 Unspecified myalgia and myositis ▽
729.2 Unspecified neuralgia, neuritis, and radiculitis ▽
729.5 Pain in soft tissues of limb
786.52 Painful respiration

ICD-9-CM Procedural

03.09 Other exploration and decompression of spinal canal
03.1 Division of intraspinal nerve root

63191

63191 Laminectomy with section of spinal accessory nerve

ICD-9-CM Diagnostic

333.83 Spasmodic torticollis — (Use additional E code to identify drug, if drug-induced)
334.1 Hereditary spastic paraplegia
343.0 Diplegic infantile cerebral palsy
343.8 Other specified infantile cerebral palsy
343.9 Unspecified infantile cerebral palsy ▽
724.1 Pain in thoracic spine
724.3 Sciatica
724.4 Thoracic or lumbosacral neuritis or radiculitis, unspecified ▽
724.6 Disorders of sacrum
729.1 Unspecified myalgia and myositis ▽
729.2 Unspecified neuralgia, neuritis, and radiculitis ▽
739.4 Nonallopathic lesion of sacral region, not elsewhere classified
781.0 Abnormal involuntary movements
786.52 Painful respiration

ICD-9-CM Procedural

03.09 Other exploration and decompression of spinal canal
03.59 Other repair and plastic operations on spinal cord structures
04.04 Other incision of cranial and peripheral nerves

63194–63195

63194 Laminectomy with cordotomy, with section of one spinothalamic tract, one stage; cervical
63195 thoracic

ICD-9-CM Diagnostic

333.83 Spasmodic torticollis — (Use additional E code to identify drug, if drug-induced)
334.1 Hereditary spastic paraplegia
343.0 Diplegic infantile cerebral palsy
343.8 Other specified infantile cerebral palsy
343.9 Unspecified infantile cerebral palsy ▽
724.1 Pain in thoracic spine
724.4 Thoracic or lumbosacral neuritis or radiculitis, unspecified ▽
729.1 Unspecified myalgia and myositis ▽
729.2 Unspecified neuralgia, neuritis, and radiculitis ▽
781.0 Abnormal involuntary movements
781.7 Tetany

ICD-9-CM Procedural

03.09 Other exploration and decompression of spinal canal
03.29 Other chordotomy

63196–63199

63196 Laminectomy with cordotomy, with section of both spinothalamic tracts, one stage; cervical
63197 thoracic
63198 Laminectomy with cordotomy with section of both spinothalamic tracts, two stages within 14 days; cervical
63199 thoracic

ICD-9-CM Diagnostic

333.83 Spasmodic torticollis — (Use additional E code to identify drug, if drug-induced)
334.1 Hereditary spastic paraplegia
343.0 Diplegic infantile cerebral palsy
343.8 Other specified infantile cerebral palsy
343.9 Unspecified infantile cerebral palsy
724.1 Pain in thoracic spine
724.4 Thoracic or lumbosacral neuritis or radiculitis, unspecified
729.1 Unspecified myalgia and myositis
729.2 Unspecified neuralgia, neuritis, and radiculitis
781.0 Abnormal involuntary movements
781.7 Tetany

ICD-9-CM Procedural

03.09 Other exploration and decompression of spinal canal
03.29 Other chordotomy

63200

63200 Laminectomy, with release of tethered spinal cord, lumbar

ICD-9-CM Diagnostic

741.01 Spina bifida with hydrocephalus, cervical region
741.02 Spina bifida with hydrocephalus, dorsal (thoracic) region
741.03 Spina bifida with hydrocephalus, lumbar region
741.91 Spina bifida without mention of hydrocephalus, cervical region
741.92 Spina bifida without mention of hydrocephalus, dorsal (thoracic) region
741.93 Spina bifida without mention of hydrocephalus, lumbar region
742.53 Hydromyelia
742.59 Other specified congenital anomaly of spinal cord
756.10 Congenital anomaly of spine, unspecified
756.11 Congenital spondylolysis, lumbosacral region
756.12 Congenital spondylolisthesis
756.13 Congenital absence of vertebra
756.15 Congenital fusion of spine (vertebra)

ICD-9-CM Procedural

03.09 Other exploration and decompression of spinal canal
03.29 Other chordotomy

63250–63252

63250 Laminectomy for excision or occlusion of arteriovenous malformation of spinal cord; cervical
63251 thoracic
63252 thoracolumbar

ICD-9-CM Diagnostic

747.82 Congenital spinal vessel anomaly

ICD-9-CM Procedural

03.09 Other exploration and decompression of spinal canal
03.39 Other diagnostic procedures on spinal cord and spinal canal structures
03.59 Other repair and plastic operations on spinal cord structures

63265–63268

63265 Laminectomy for excision or evacuation of intraspinal lesion other than neoplasm, extradural; cervical
63266 thoracic
63267 lumbar
63268 sacral

ICD-9-CM Diagnostic

324.1 Intraspinal abscess
336.1 Vascular myelopathies

ICD-9-CM Procedural

03.4 Excision or destruction of lesion of spinal cord or spinal meninges

63270–63273

63270 Laminectomy for excision of intraspinal lesion other than neoplasm, intradural; cervical
63271 thoracic
63272 lumbar
63273 sacral

ICD-9-CM Diagnostic

324.1 Intraspinal abscess
349.2 Disorders of meninges, not elsewhere classified

ICD-9-CM Procedural

03.4 Excision or destruction of lesion of spinal cord or spinal meninges

63275–63278

63275 Laminectomy for biopsy/excision of intraspinal neoplasm; extradural, cervical
63276 extradural, thoracic
63277 extradural, lumbar
63278 extradural, sacral

ICD-9-CM Diagnostic

192.2 Malignant neoplasm of spinal cord
192.3 Malignant neoplasm of spinal meninges
198.3 Secondary malignant neoplasm of brain and spinal cord
199.0 Disseminated malignant neoplasm
225.3 Benign neoplasm of spinal cord
237.5 Neoplasm of uncertain behavior of brain and spinal cord
237.6 Neoplasm of uncertain behavior of meninges
239.7 Neoplasm of unspecified nature of endocrine glands and other parts of nervous system

ICD-9-CM Procedural

03.32 Biopsy of spinal cord or spinal meninges
03.4 Excision or destruction of lesion of spinal cord or spinal meninges

63280–63283

63280 Laminectomy for biopsy/excision of intraspinal neoplasm; intradural, extramedullary, cervical
63281 intradural, extramedullary, thoracic
63282 intradural, extramedullary, lumbar
63283 intradural, sacral

ICD-9-CM Diagnostic

192.2 Malignant neoplasm of spinal cord
192.3 Malignant neoplasm of spinal meninges
198.3 Secondary malignant neoplasm of brain and spinal cord
199.0 Disseminated malignant neoplasm
225.3 Benign neoplasm of spinal cord
225.4 Benign neoplasm of spinal meninges
237.5 Neoplasm of uncertain behavior of brain and spinal cord
237.6 Neoplasm of uncertain behavior of meninges
239.7 Neoplasm of unspecified nature of endocrine glands and other parts of nervous system

ICD-9-CM Procedural

03.32 Biopsy of spinal cord or spinal meninges
03.4 Excision or destruction of lesion of spinal cord or spinal meninges

63285–63290

63285 Laminectomy for biopsy/excision of intraspinal neoplasm; intradural, intramedullary, cervical
63286 intradural, intramedullary, thoracic
63287 intradural, intramedullary, thoracolumbar
63290 combined extradural-intradural lesion, any level

ICD-9-CM Diagnostic

192.2 Malignant neoplasm of spinal cord
192.3 Malignant neoplasm of spinal meninges
198.3 Secondary malignant neoplasm of brain and spinal cord
199.0 Disseminated malignant neoplasm
225.3 Benign neoplasm of spinal cord
225.4 Benign neoplasm of spinal meninges
237.5 Neoplasm of uncertain behavior of brain and spinal cord
237.6 Neoplasm of uncertain behavior of meninges

239.7 Neoplasm of unspecified nature of endocrine glands and other parts of nervous system

ICD-9-CM Procedural

03.32 Biopsy of spinal cord or spinal meninges
03.4 Excision or destruction of lesion of spinal cord or spinal meninges

63295

63295 Osteoplastic reconstruction of dorsal spinal elements, following primary intraspinal procedure (List separately in addition to code for primary procedure)

ICD-9-CM Diagnostic

This is an add-on code. Refer to the corresponding primary procedure code for ICD-9 diagnosis code links.

ICD-9-CM Procedural

03.59 Other repair and plastic operations on spinal cord structures

63300–63303

63300 Vertebral corpectomy (vertebral body resection), partial or complete, for excision of intraspinal lesion, single segment; extradural, cervical
63301 extradural, thoracic by transthoracic approach
63302 extradural, thoracic by thoracolumbar approach
63303 extradural, lumbar or sacral by transperitoneal or retroperitoneal approach

ICD-9-CM Diagnostic

192.2 Malignant neoplasm of spinal cord
192.3 Malignant neoplasm of spinal meninges
198.3 Secondary malignant neoplasm of brain and spinal cord
199.0 Disseminated malignant neoplasm
225.3 Benign neoplasm of spinal cord
225.4 Benign neoplasm of spinal meninges
237.5 Neoplasm of uncertain behavior of brain and spinal cord
237.6 Neoplasm of uncertain behavior of meninges
239.7 Neoplasm of unspecified nature of endocrine glands and other parts of nervous system
324.1 Intraspinal abscess
336.1 Vascular myelopathies

ICD-9-CM Procedural

03.39 Other diagnostic procedures on spinal cord and spinal canal structures
03.4 Excision or destruction of lesion of spinal cord or spinal meninges
03.6 Lysis of adhesions of spinal cord and nerve roots

63304–63307

63304 Vertebral corpectomy (vertebral body resection), partial or complete, for excision of intraspinal lesion, single segment; intradural, cervical
63305 intradural, thoracic by transthoracic approach
63306 intradural, thoracic by thoracolumbar approach
63307 intradural, lumbar or sacral by transperitoneal or retroperitoneal approach

ICD-9-CM Diagnostic

192.2 Malignant neoplasm of spinal cord
192.3 Malignant neoplasm of spinal meninges
198.3 Secondary malignant neoplasm of brain and spinal cord
199.0 Disseminated malignant neoplasm
225.3 Benign neoplasm of spinal cord
225.4 Benign neoplasm of spinal meninges
237.5 Neoplasm of uncertain behavior of brain and spinal cord
237.6 Neoplasm of uncertain behavior of meninges
239.7 Neoplasm of unspecified nature of endocrine glands and other parts of nervous system
324.1 Intraspinal abscess
336.1 Vascular myelopathies

ICD-9-CM Procedural

03.39 Other diagnostic procedures on spinal cord and spinal canal structures
03.4 Excision or destruction of lesion of spinal cord or spinal meninges
03.6 Lysis of adhesions of spinal cord and nerve roots

63308

63308 Vertebral corpectomy (vertebral body resection), partial or complete, for excision of intraspinal lesion, single segment; each additional segment (List separately in addition to codes for single segment)

ICD-9-CM Diagnostic

This is an add-on code. Refer to the corresponding primary procedure code for ICD-9 diagnosis code links.

ICD-9-CM Procedural

03.39 Other diagnostic procedures on spinal cord and spinal canal structures
03.4 Excision or destruction of lesion of spinal cord or spinal meninges
03.6 Lysis of adhesions of spinal cord and nerve roots

63600–63615

63600 Creation of lesion of spinal cord by stereotactic method, percutaneous, any modality (including stimulation and/or recording)
63610 Stereotactic stimulation of spinal cord, percutaneous, separate procedure not followed by other surgery
63615 Stereotactic biopsy, aspiration, or excision of lesion, spinal cord

ICD-9-CM Diagnostic

192.2 Malignant neoplasm of spinal cord
192.3 Malignant neoplasm of spinal meninges
198.3 Secondary malignant neoplasm of brain and spinal cord
225.3 Benign neoplasm of spinal cord
237.5 Neoplasm of uncertain behavior of brain and spinal cord
239.7 Neoplasm of unspecified nature of endocrine glands and other parts of nervous system
332.0 Paralysis agitans
332.1 Secondary Parkinsonism — (Use additional E code to identify drug, if drug-induced)
336.1 Vascular myelopathies
722.2 Displacement of intervertebral disc, site unspecified, without myelopathy 🔻
722.52 Degeneration of lumbar or lumbosacral intervertebral disc
722.73 Intervertebral lumbar disc disorder with myelopathy, lumbar region
722.82 Postlaminectomy syndrome, thoracic region
724.02 Spinal stenosis of lumbar region
724.4 Thoracic or lumbosacral neuritis or radiculitis, unspecified 🔻
729.5 Pain in soft tissues of limb
781.2 Abnormality of gait
781.3 Lack of coordination
953.2 Injury to lumbar nerve root

ICD-9-CM Procedural

03.21 Percutaneous chordotomy
03.32 Biopsy of spinal cord or spinal meninges
03.39 Other diagnostic procedures on spinal cord and spinal canal structures
03.4 Excision or destruction of lesion of spinal cord or spinal meninges
03.92 Injection of other agent into spinal canal

63650

63650 Percutaneous implantation of neurostimulator electrode array, epidural

ICD-9-CM Diagnostic

150.0 Malignant neoplasm of cervical esophagus
171.3 Malignant neoplasm of connective and other soft tissue of lower limb, including hip
171.5 Malignant neoplasm of connective and other soft tissue of abdomen
171.6 Malignant neoplasm of connective and other soft tissue of pelvis
171.8 Malignant neoplasm of other specified sites of connective and other soft tissue
176.3 Kaposi's sarcoma of gastrointestinal sites
180.0 Malignant neoplasm of endocervix ♀
180.1 Malignant neoplasm of exocervix ♀
180.8 Malignant neoplasm of other specified sites of cervix ♀
182.0 Malignant neoplasm of corpus uteri, except isthmus ♀
182.1 Malignant neoplasm of isthmus ♀
182.8 Malignant neoplasm of other specified sites of body of uterus ♀
183.0 Malignant neoplasm of ovary — (Use additional code to identify any functional activity) ♀
183.2 Malignant neoplasm of fallopian tube ♀
183.3 Malignant neoplasm of broad ligament of uterus ♀
183.4 Malignant neoplasm of parametrium of uterus ♀
183.5 Malignant neoplasm of round ligament of uterus ♀
183.8 Malignant neoplasm of other specified sites of uterine adnexa ♀
184.0 Malignant neoplasm of vagina ♀

🔻 Unspecified code ♀ Female diagnosis ☒ Manifestation code ♂ Male diagnosis

184.8 Malignant neoplasm of other specified sites of female genital organs ♀
186.0 Malignant neoplasm of undescended testis — (Use additional code to identify any functional activity) ♂
188.0 Malignant neoplasm of trigone of urinary bladder
188.1 Malignant neoplasm of dome of urinary bladder
188.2 Malignant neoplasm of lateral wall of urinary bladder
188.3 Malignant neoplasm of anterior wall of urinary bladder
188.4 Malignant neoplasm of posterior wall of urinary bladder
188.5 Malignant neoplasm of bladder neck
188.6 Malignant neoplasm of ureteric orifice
188.7 Malignant neoplasm of urachus
188.8 Malignant neoplasm of other specified sites of bladder
189.0 Malignant neoplasm of kidney, except pelvis
189.1 Malignant neoplasm of renal pelvis
189.2 Malignant neoplasm of ureter
189.3 Malignant neoplasm of urethra
189.4 Malignant neoplasm of paraurethral glands
189.8 Malignant neoplasm of other specified sites of urinary organs
192.2 Malignant neoplasm of spinal cord
192.3 Malignant neoplasm of spinal meninges
192.8 Malignant neoplasm of other specified sites of nervous system
195.2 Malignant neoplasm of abdomen
195.3 Malignant neoplasm of pelvis
195.5 Malignant neoplasm of lower limb
195.8 Malignant neoplasm of other specified sites
196.2 Secondary and unspecified malignant neoplasm of intra-abdominal lymph nodes
196.3 Secondary and unspecified malignant neoplasm of lymph nodes of axilla and upper limb
196.5 Secondary and unspecified malignant neoplasm of lymph nodes of inguinal region and lower limb
196.6 Secondary and unspecified malignant neoplasm of intrapelvic lymph nodes
196.8 Secondary and unspecified malignant neoplasm of lymph nodes of multiple sites
197.4 Secondary malignant neoplasm of small intestine including duodenum
197.5 Secondary malignant neoplasm of large intestine and rectum
197.6 Secondary malignant neoplasm of retroperitoneum and peritoneum
197.7 Secondary malignant neoplasm of liver
197.8 Secondary malignant neoplasm of other digestive organs and spleen
198.1 Secondary malignant neoplasm of other urinary organs
198.3 Secondary malignant neoplasm of brain and spinal cord
198.5 Secondary malignant neoplasm of bone and bone marrow
198.6 Secondary malignant neoplasm of ovary ♀
198.82 Secondary malignant neoplasm of genital organs
198.89 Secondary malignant neoplasm of other specified sites
199.0 Disseminated malignant neoplasm
337.0 Idiopathic peripheral autonomic neuropathy
337.20 Unspecified reflex sympathetic dystrophy ▽
337.21 Reflex sympathetic dystrophy of the upper limb
337.22 Reflex sympathetic dystrophy of the lower limb
337.29 Reflex sympathetic dystrophy of other specified site
337.9 Unspecified disorder of autonomic nervous system ▽
344.1 Paraplegia
353.0 Brachial plexus lesions
353.1 Lumbosacral plexus lesions
353.2 Cervical root lesions, not elsewhere classified
353.3 Thoracic root lesions, not elsewhere classified
353.4 Lumbosacral root lesions, not elsewhere classified
353.5 Neuralgic amyotrophy
353.6 Phantom limb (syndrome)
353.8 Other nerve root and plexus disorders
354.4 Causalgia of upper limb
354.5 Mononeuritis multiplex
354.8 Other mononeuritis of upper limb
354.9 Unspecified mononeuritis of upper limb ▽
355.0 Lesion of sciatic nerve
355.1 Meralgia paresthetica
355.2 Other lesion of femoral nerve
355.3 Lesion of lateral popliteal nerve
355.4 Lesion of medial popliteal nerve
355.6 Lesion of plantar nerve
355.71 Causalgia of lower limb
355.8 Unspecified mononeuritis of lower limb ▽
577.0 Acute pancreatitis
577.1 Chronic pancreatitis
577.9 Unspecified disease of pancreas ▽
721.3 Lumbosacral spondylosis without myelopathy
722.52 Degeneration of lumbar or lumbosacral intervertebral disc
722.73 Intervertebral lumbar disc disorder with myelopathy, lumbar region
722.81 Postlaminectomy syndrome, cervical region
722.82 Postlaminectomy syndrome, thoracic region
722.83 Postlaminectomy syndrome, lumbar region
723.1 Cervicalgia
723.4 Brachial neuritis or radiculitis nos
723.9 Unspecified musculoskeletal disorders and symptoms referable to neck ▽
724.02 Spinal stenosis of lumbar region
724.1 Pain in thoracic spine
724.2 Lumbago
724.3 Sciatica
724.4 Thoracic or lumbosacral neuritis or radiculitis, unspecified ▽
724.79 Other disorder of coccyx
729.2 Unspecified neuralgia, neuritis, and radiculitis ▽
729.5 Pain in soft tissues of limb
731.0 Osteitis deformans without mention of bone tumor
905.1 Late effect of fracture of spine and trunk without mention of spinal cord lesion
905.2 Late effect of fracture of upper extremities
905.3 Late effect of fracture of neck of femur
905.4 Late effect of fracture of lower extremities
905.5 Late effect of fracture of multiple and unspecified bones
907.2 Late effect of spinal cord injury
907.3 Late effect of injury to nerve root(s), spinal plexus(es), and other nerves of trunk
907.4 Late effect of injury to peripheral nerve of shoulder girdle and upper limb
907.5 Late effect of injury to peripheral nerve of pelvic girdle and lower limb
907.9 Late effect of injury to other and unspecified nerve ▽
908.6 Late effect of certain complications of trauma
908.9 Late effect of unspecified injury ▽
953.2 Injury to lumbar nerve root

ICD-9-CM Procedural

03.93 Implantation or replacement of spinal neurostimulator lead(s)

63655

63655 Laminectomy for implantation of neurostimulator electrodes, plate/paddle, epidural

ICD-9-CM Diagnostic

150.0 Malignant neoplasm of cervical esophagus
171.3 Malignant neoplasm of connective and other soft tissue of lower limb, including hip
171.5 Malignant neoplasm of connective and other soft tissue of abdomen
171.6 Malignant neoplasm of connective and other soft tissue of pelvis
171.8 Malignant neoplasm of other specified sites of connective and other soft tissue
176.3 Kaposi's sarcoma of gastrointestinal sites
180.0 Malignant neoplasm of endocervix ♀
180.1 Malignant neoplasm of exocervix ♀
180.8 Malignant neoplasm of other specified sites of cervix ♀
182.0 Malignant neoplasm of corpus uteri, except isthmus ♀
182.1 Malignant neoplasm of isthmus ♀
182.8 Malignant neoplasm of other specified sites of body of uterus ♀
183.0 Malignant neoplasm of ovary — (Use additional code to identify any functional activity) ♀
183.2 Malignant neoplasm of fallopian tube ♀
183.3 Malignant neoplasm of broad ligament of uterus ♀
183.4 Malignant neoplasm of parametrium of uterus ♀
183.5 Malignant neoplasm of round ligament of uterus ♀
183.8 Malignant neoplasm of other specified sites of uterine adnexa ♀
184.0 Malignant neoplasm of vagina ♀
184.8 Malignant neoplasm of other specified sites of female genital organs ♀
186.0 Malignant neoplasm of undescended testis — (Use additional code to identify any functional activity) ♂
188.0 Malignant neoplasm of trigone of urinary bladder
188.1 Malignant neoplasm of dome of urinary bladder
188.2 Malignant neoplasm of lateral wall of urinary bladder
188.3 Malignant neoplasm of anterior wall of urinary bladder
188.4 Malignant neoplasm of posterior wall of urinary bladder
188.5 Malignant neoplasm of bladder neck
188.6 Malignant neoplasm of ureteric orifice
188.7 Malignant neoplasm of urachus
188.8 Malignant neoplasm of other specified sites of bladder
189.0 Malignant neoplasm of kidney, except pelvis
189.1 Malignant neoplasm of renal pelvis

▽ Unspecified code ♀ Female diagnosis ☒ Manifestation code ♂ Male diagnosis

189.2	Malignant neoplasm of ureter
189.3	Malignant neoplasm of urethra
189.4	Malignant neoplasm of paraurethral glands
189.8	Malignant neoplasm of other specified sites of urinary organs
192.2	Malignant neoplasm of spinal cord
192.3	Malignant neoplasm of spinal meninges
192.8	Malignant neoplasm of other specified sites of nervous system
195.2	Malignant neoplasm of abdomen
195.3	Malignant neoplasm of pelvis
195.5	Malignant neoplasm of lower limb
195.8	Malignant neoplasm of other specified sites
196.2	Secondary and unspecified malignant neoplasm of intra-abdominal lymph nodes
196.3	Secondary and unspecified malignant neoplasm of lymph nodes of axilla and upper limb
196.5	Secondary and unspecified malignant neoplasm of lymph nodes of inguinal region and lower limb
196.6	Secondary and unspecified malignant neoplasm of intrapelvic lymph nodes
196.8	Secondary and unspecified malignant neoplasm of lymph nodes of multiple sites
197.4	Secondary malignant neoplasm of small intestine including duodenum
197.5	Secondary malignant neoplasm of large intestine and rectum
197.6	Secondary malignant neoplasm of retroperitoneum and peritoneum
197.7	Secondary malignant neoplasm of liver
197.8	Secondary malignant neoplasm of other digestive organs and spleen
198.1	Secondary malignant neoplasm of other urinary organs
198.3	Secondary malignant neoplasm of brain and spinal cord
198.5	Secondary malignant neoplasm of bone and bone marrow
198.6	Secondary malignant neoplasm of ovary ♀
198.82	Secondary malignant neoplasm of genital organs
198.89	Secondary malignant neoplasm of other specified sites
199.0	Disseminated malignant neoplasm
337.0	Idiopathic peripheral autonomic neuropathy
337.20	Unspecified reflex sympathetic dystrophy ▽
337.21	Reflex sympathetic dystrophy of the upper limb
337.22	Reflex sympathetic dystrophy of the lower limb
337.29	Reflex sympathetic dystrophy of other specified site
337.9	Unspecified disorder of autonomic nervous system ▽
344.1	Paraplegia
353.0	Brachial plexus lesions
353.1	Lumbosacral plexus lesions
353.2	Cervical root lesions, not elsewhere classified
353.3	Thoracic root lesions, not elsewhere classified
353.4	Lumbosacral root lesions, not elsewhere classified
353.5	Neuralgic amyotrophy
353.6	Phantom limb (syndrome)
353.8	Other nerve root and plexus disorders
354.4	Causalgia of upper limb
354.5	Mononeuritis multiplex
354.8	Other mononeuritis of upper limb
354.9	Unspecified mononeuritis of upper limb ▽
355.0	Lesion of sciatic nerve
355.1	Meralgia paresthetica
355.2	Other lesion of femoral nerve
355.3	Lesion of lateral popliteal nerve
355.4	Lesion of medial popliteal nerve
355.6	Lesion of plantar nerve
355.71	Causalgia of lower limb
355.8	Unspecified mononeuritis of lower limb ▽
577.0	Acute pancreatitis
577.1	Chronic pancreatitis
577.9	Unspecified disease of pancreas ▽
721.3	Lumbosacral spondylosis without myelopathy
722.52	Degeneration of lumbar or lumbosacral intervertebral disc
722.73	Intervertebral lumbar disc disorder with myelopathy, lumbar region
722.81	Postlaminectomy syndrome, cervical region
722.82	Postlaminectomy syndrome, thoracic region
722.83	Postlaminectomy syndrome, lumbar region
723.1	Cervicalgia
723.4	Brachial neuritis or radiculitis nos
723.9	Unspecified musculoskeletal disorders and symptoms referable to neck ▽
724.02	Spinal stenosis of lumbar region
724.1	Pain in thoracic spine
724.2	Lumbago
724.3	Sciatica
724.4	Thoracic or lumbosacral neuritis or radiculitis, unspecified ▽
724.79	Other disorder of coccyx
729.2	Unspecified neuralgia, neuritis, and radiculitis ▽
729.5	Pain in soft tissues of limb
731.0	Osteitis deformans without mention of bone tumor
905.1	Late effect of fracture of spine and trunk without mention of spinal cord lesion
905.2	Late effect of fracture of upper extremities
905.3	Late effect of fracture of neck of femur
905.4	Late effect of fracture of lower extremities
905.5	Late effect of fracture of multiple and unspecified bones
907.2	Late effect of spinal cord injury
907.3	Late effect of injury to nerve root(s), spinal plexus(es), and other nerves of trunk
907.4	Late effect of injury to peripheral nerve of shoulder girdle and upper limb
907.5	Late effect of injury to peripheral nerve of pelvic girdle and lower limb
907.9	Late effect of injury to other and unspecified nerve ▽
908.6	Late effect of certain complications of trauma
908.9	Late effect of unspecified injury ▽
953.2	Injury to lumbar nerve root

ICD-9-CM Procedural

03.09	Other exploration and decompression of spinal canal
03.93	Implantation or replacement of spinal neurostimulator lead(s)

63660

63660 Revision or removal of spinal neurostimulator electrode percutaneous array(s) or plate/paddle(s)

ICD-9-CM Diagnostic

349.1	Nervous system complications from surgically implanted device
353.8	Other nerve root and plexus disorders
443.9	Unspecified peripheral vascular disease ▽
722.2	Displacement of intervertebral disc, site unspecified, without myelopathy ▽
722.83	Postlaminectomy syndrome, lumbar region
724.2	Lumbago
724.4	Thoracic or lumbosacral neuritis or radiculitis, unspecified ▽
729.5	Pain in soft tissues of limb
953.2	Injury to lumbar nerve root
996.2	Mechanical complication of nervous system device, implant, and graft
996.63	Infection and inflammatory reaction due to nervous system device, implant, and graft — (Use additional code to identify specified infections)
996.75	Other complications due to nervous system device, implant, and graft
V53.02	Neuropacemaker (brain) (peripheral nerve) (spinal cord)

ICD-9-CM Procedural

03.94	Removal of spinal neurostimulator lead(s)

63685

63685 Insertion or replacement of spinal neurostimulator pulse generator or receiver, direct or inductive coupling

ICD-9-CM Diagnostic

053.19	Other herpes zoster with nervous system complications
322.9	Unspecified meningitis ▽
337.21	Reflex sympathetic dystrophy of the upper limb
337.22	Reflex sympathetic dystrophy of the lower limb
337.29	Reflex sympathetic dystrophy of other specified site
353.3	Thoracic root lesions, not elsewhere classified
353.4	Lumbosacral root lesions, not elsewhere classified
353.6	Phantom limb (syndrome)
353.8	Other nerve root and plexus disorders
354.4	Causalgia of upper limb
355.71	Causalgia of lower limb
440.22	Atherosclerosis of native arteries of the extremities with rest pain
721.2	Thoracic spondylosis without myelopathy
721.3	Lumbosacral spondylosis without myelopathy
722.10	Displacement of lumbar intervertebral disc without myelopathy
722.11	Displacement of thoracic intervertebral disc without myelopathy
722.2	Displacement of intervertebral disc, site unspecified, without myelopathy ▽
722.51	Degeneration of thoracic or thoracolumbar intervertebral disc
722.52	Degeneration of lumbar or lumbosacral intervertebral disc
722.81	Postlaminectomy syndrome, cervical region
722.82	Postlaminectomy syndrome, thoracic region
722.83	Postlaminectomy syndrome, lumbar region
723.4	Brachial neuritis or radiculitis nos
724.2	Lumbago
724.4	Thoracic or lumbosacral neuritis or radiculitis, unspecified ▽

▽ Unspecified code
♀ Female diagnosis
☒ Manifestation code
♂ Male diagnosis

729.2 Unspecified neuralgia, neuritis, and radiculitis ▽
952.4 Cauda equina spinal cord injury without spinal bone injury
953.2 Injury to lumbar nerve root
996.2 Mechanical complication of nervous system device, implant, and graft
996.63 Infection and inflammatory reaction due to nervous system device, implant, and graft — (Use additional code to identify specified infections)
996.75 Other complications due to nervous system device, implant, and graft

ICD-9-CM Procedural

86.94 Insertion or replacement of single array neurostimulator pulse generator
86.95 Insertion or replacement of dual array neurostimulator pulse generator
86.96 Insertion or replacement of other neurostimulator pulse generator

63688

63688 Revision or removal of implanted spinal neurostimulator pulse generator or receiver

ICD-9-CM Diagnostic

349.1 Nervous system complications from surgically implanted device
353.8 Other nerve root and plexus disorders
721.3 Lumbosacral spondylosis without myelopathy
722.2 Displacement of intervertebral disc, site unspecified, without myelopathy ▽
722.83 Postlaminectomy syndrome, lumbar region
724.2 Lumbago
724.4 Thoracic or lumbosacral neuritis or radiculitis, unspecified ▽
729.5 Pain in soft tissues of limb
953.2 Injury to lumbar nerve root
996.2 Mechanical complication of nervous system device, implant, and graft
996.63 Infection and inflammatory reaction due to nervous system device, implant, and graft — (Use additional code to identify specified infections)

ICD-9-CM Procedural

86.05 Incision with removal of foreign body or device from skin and subcutaneous tissue

63700–63702

63700 Repair of meningocele; less than 5 cm diameter
63702 larger than 5 cm diameter

ICD-9-CM Diagnostic

331.4 Obstructive hydrocephalus
741.01 Spina bifida with hydrocephalus, cervical region
741.02 Spina bifida with hydrocephalus, dorsal (thoracic) region
741.03 Spina bifida with hydrocephalus, lumbar region
741.91 Spina bifida without mention of hydrocephalus, cervical region
741.92 Spina bifida without mention of hydrocephalus, dorsal (thoracic) region
741.93 Spina bifida without mention of hydrocephalus, lumbar region

ICD-9-CM Procedural

03.51 Repair of spinal meningocele

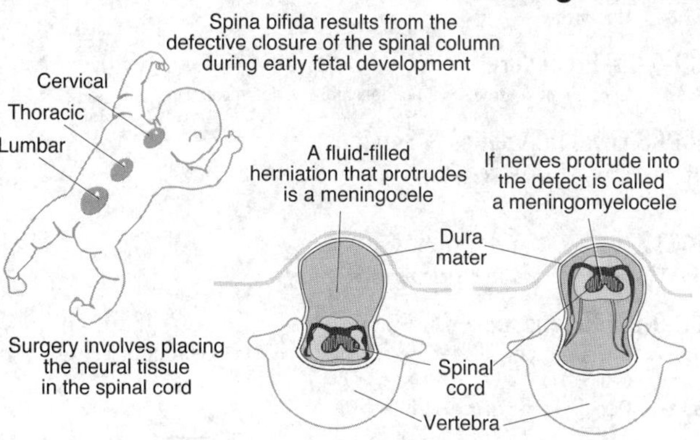
Meningocele
Spina bifida results from the defective closure of the spinal column during early fetal development
Cervical
Thoracic
Lumbar
A fluid-filled herniation that protrudes is a meningocele
If nerves protrude into the defect is called a meningomyelocele
Dura mater
Surgery involves placing the neural tissue in the spinal cord
Spinal cord
Vertebra

63704–63706

63704 Repair of myelomeningocele; less than 5 cm diameter
63706 larger than 5 cm diameter

ICD-9-CM Diagnostic

741.01 Spina bifida with hydrocephalus, cervical region
741.02 Spina bifida with hydrocephalus, dorsal (thoracic) region
741.03 Spina bifida with hydrocephalus, lumbar region
741.91 Spina bifida without mention of hydrocephalus, cervical region
741.92 Spina bifida without mention of hydrocephalus, dorsal (thoracic) region
741.93 Spina bifida without mention of hydrocephalus, lumbar region

ICD-9-CM Procedural

03.52 Repair of spinal myelomeningocele
03.59 Other repair and plastic operations on spinal cord structures

63707–63709

63707 Repair of dural/cerebrospinal fluid leak, not requiring laminectomy
63709 Repair of dural/cerebrospinal fluid leak or pseudomeningocele, with laminectomy

ICD-9-CM Diagnostic

996.75 Other complications due to nervous system device, implant, and graft
997.09 Other nervous system complications — (Use additional code to identify complications)
998.2 Accidental puncture or laceration during procedure
998.31 Disruption of internal operation wound
998.6 Persistent postoperative fistula, not elsewhere classified

ICD-9-CM Procedural

02.12 Other repair of cerebral meninges
03.09 Other exploration and decompression of spinal canal
03.59 Other repair and plastic operations on spinal cord structures

63710

63710 Dural graft, spinal

ICD-9-CM Diagnostic

225.2 Benign neoplasm of cerebral meninges
237.5 Neoplasm of uncertain behavior of brain and spinal cord
996.75 Other complications due to nervous system device, implant, and graft
998.31 Disruption of internal operation wound

ICD-9-CM Procedural

02.12 Other repair of cerebral meninges

63740–63741

63740 Creation of shunt, lumbar, subarachnoid-peritoneal, -pleural, or other; including laminectomy
63741 percutaneous, not requiring laminectomy

ICD-9-CM Diagnostic

331.3 Communicating hydrocephalus
331.4 Obstructive hydrocephalus
348.2 Benign intracranial hypertension
742.3 Congenital hydrocephalus

ICD-9-CM Procedural

03.09 Other exploration and decompression of spinal canal
03.71 Spinal subarachnoid-peritoneal shunt
03.72 Spinal subarachnoid-ureteral shunt
03.79 Other shunt of spinal theca

63744

63744 Replacement, irrigation or revision of lumbosubarachnoid shunt

ICD-9-CM Diagnostic

348.2 Benign intracranial hypertension
996.1 Mechanical complication of other vascular device, implant, and graft
996.2 Mechanical complication of nervous system device, implant, and graft
996.63 Infection and inflammatory reaction due to nervous system device, implant, and graft — (Use additional code to identify specified infections)
996.75 Other complications due to nervous system device, implant, and graft

ICD-9-CM Procedural

03.97 Revision of spinal thecal shunt
03.99 Other operations on spinal cord and spinal canal structures

HCPCS Level II Supplies & Services

A4305 Disposable drug delivery system, flow rate of 50 ml or greater per hour
A4306 Disposable drug delivery system, flow rate of 5 ml or less per hour
A4550 Surgical trays

63746

63746 Removal of entire lumbosubarachnoid shunt system without replacement

ICD-9-CM Diagnostic

348.2 Benign intracranial hypertension
996.1 Mechanical complication of other vascular device, implant, and graft
996.2 Mechanical complication of nervous system device, implant, and graft
996.63 Infection and inflammatory reaction due to nervous system device, implant, and graft — (Use additional code to identify specified infections)
996.75 Other complications due to nervous system device, implant, and graft

ICD-9-CM Procedural

03.98 Removal of spinal thecal shunt
03.99 Other operations on spinal cord and spinal canal structures

Extracranial Nerves, Peripheral Nerves, and Autonomic Nervous System

64400

64400 Injection, anesthetic agent; trigeminal nerve, any division or branch

ICD-9-CM Diagnostic

350.1 Trigeminal neuralgia
350.2 Atypical face pain
729.1 Unspecified myalgia and myositis

ICD-9-CM Procedural

04.81 Injection of anesthetic into peripheral nerve for analgesia

HCPCS Level II Supplies & Services

J2400 Injection, chloroprocaine HCl, per 30 ml

64402

64402 Injection, anesthetic agent; facial nerve

ICD-9-CM Diagnostic

333.81 Blepharospasm — (Use additional E code to identify drug, if drug-induced)
350.2 Atypical face pain
351.0 Bell's palsy
351.1 Geniculate ganglionitis
351.8 Other facial nerve disorders

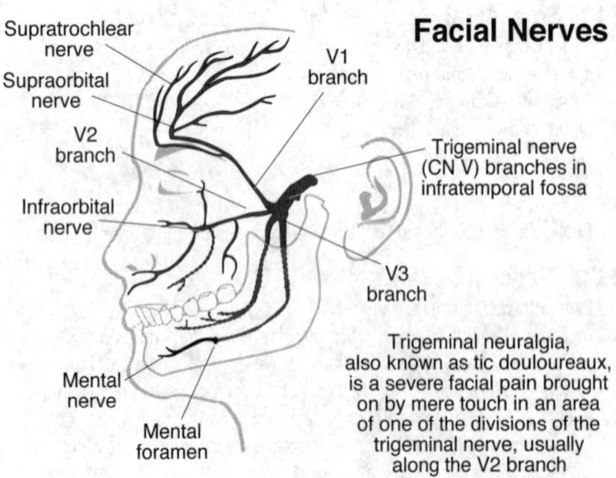
Facial Nerves
Supratrochlear nerve
Supraorbital nerve
V1 branch
V2 branch
Trigeminal nerve (CN V) branches in infratemporal fossa
Infraorbital nerve
V3 branch
Mental nerve
Mental foramen
Trigeminal neuralgia, also known as tic douloureux, is a severe facial pain brought on by mere touch in an area of one of the divisions of the trigeminal nerve, usually along the V2 branch

352.9 Unspecified disorder of cranial nerves
525.3 Retained dental root
526.4 Inflammatory conditions of jaw
691.8 Other atopic dermatitis and related conditions
784.0 Headache
873.41 Open wound of cheek, without mention of complication — (Use additional code to identify infection)
873.42 Open wound of forehead, without mention of complication — (Use additional code to identify infection)
873.43 Open wound of lip, without mention of complication — (Use additional code to identify infection)
873.44 Open wound of jaw, without mention of complication — (Use additional code to identify infection)

ICD-9-CM Procedural

04.81 Injection of anesthetic into peripheral nerve for analgesia

HCPCS Level II Supplies & Services

J2400 Injection, chloroprocaine HCl, per 30 ml

64405

64405 Injection, anesthetic agent; greater occipital nerve

ICD-9-CM Diagnostic

353.2 Cervical root lesions, not elsewhere classified
353.8 Other nerve root and plexus disorders
729.2 Unspecified neuralgia, neuritis, and radiculitis

ICD-9-CM Procedural

04.81 Injection of anesthetic into peripheral nerve for analgesia

HCPCS Level II Supplies & Services

J2400 Injection, chloroprocaine HCl, per 30 ml

64408

64408 Injection, anesthetic agent; vagus nerve

ICD-9-CM Diagnostic

352.3 Disorders of pneumogastric (10th) nerve
536.1 Acute dilatation of stomach

ICD-9-CM Procedural

04.81 Injection of anesthetic into peripheral nerve for analgesia

HCPCS Level II Supplies & Services

J2400 Injection, chloroprocaine HCl, per 30 ml

64410

64410 Injection, anesthetic agent; phrenic nerve

ICD-9-CM Diagnostic

353.2 Cervical root lesions, not elsewhere classified
519.4 Disorders of diaphragm
786.8 Hiccough

ICD-9-CM Procedural

04.81 Injection of anesthetic into peripheral nerve for analgesia

HCPCS Level II Supplies & Services

J2400 Injection, chloroprocaine HCl, per 30 ml

64412

64412 Injection, anesthetic agent; spinal accessory nerve

ICD-9-CM Diagnostic

333.83 Spasmodic torticollis — (Use additional E code to identify drug, if drug-induced)
352.4 Disorders of accessory (11th) nerve

ICD-9-CM Procedural

03.91 Injection of anesthetic into spinal canal for analgesia
04.81 Injection of anesthetic into peripheral nerve for analgesia

HCPCS Level II Supplies & Services

J2400 Injection, chloroprocaine HCl, per 30 ml

Unspecified code
♀ Female diagnosis
Manifestation code
♂ Male diagnosis

64413

64413 Injection, anesthetic agent; cervical plexus

ICD-9-CM Diagnostic

346.00 Classical migraine without mention of intractable migraine
346.01 Classical migraine with intractable migraine, so stated
346.10 Common migraine without mention of intractable migraine
721.0 Cervical spondylosis without myelopathy
721.1 Cervical spondylosis with myelopathy
722.0 Displacement of cervical intervertebral disc without myelopathy
722.4 Degeneration of cervical intervertebral disc
723.1 Cervicalgia
723.2 Cervicocranial syndrome
723.3 Cervicobrachial syndrome (diffuse)
723.4 Brachial neuritis or radiculitis nos
847.0 Neck sprain and strain
847.1 Thoracic sprain and strain

ICD-9-CM Procedural

04.81 Injection of anesthetic into peripheral nerve for analgesia

HCPCS Level II Supplies & Services

J2400 Injection, chloroprocaine HCl, per 30 ml

64415–64417

64415 Injection, anesthetic agent; brachial plexus, single
64417 axillary nerve
64416 brachial plexus, continuous infusion by catheter (including catheter placement) including daily management for anesthetic agent administration

ICD-9-CM Diagnostic

337.21 Reflex sympathetic dystrophy of the upper limb
353.0 Brachial plexus lesions
354.4 Causalgia of upper limb
357.81 Chronic inflammatory demyelinating polyneuritis
357.89 Other inflammatory and toxic neuropathy
716.11 Traumatic arthropathy, shoulder region
719.41 Pain in joint, shoulder region
719.42 Pain in joint, upper arm
723.4 Brachial neuritis or radiculitis nos
729.1 Unspecified myalgia and myositis ▽
729.5 Pain in soft tissues of limb
840.4 Rotator cuff (capsule) sprain and strain
953.4 Injury to brachial plexus

ICD-9-CM Procedural

04.81 Injection of anesthetic into peripheral nerve for analgesia

HCPCS Level II Supplies & Services

J2400 Injection, chloroprocaine HCl, per 30 ml

64418

64418 Injection, anesthetic agent; suprascapular nerve

ICD-9-CM Diagnostic

357.81 Chronic inflammatory demyelinating polyneuritis
357.89 Other inflammatory and toxic neuropathy
718.31 Recurrent dislocation of shoulder joint
719.41 Pain in joint, shoulder region
723.1 Cervicalgia
723.4 Brachial neuritis or radiculitis nos
726.11 Calcifying tendinitis of shoulder
728.85 Spasm of muscle
729.1 Unspecified myalgia and myositis ▽
729.2 Unspecified neuralgia, neuritis, and radiculitis ▽
729.5 Pain in soft tissues of limb

ICD-9-CM Procedural

04.81 Injection of anesthetic into peripheral nerve for analgesia

HCPCS Level II Supplies & Services

J2400 Injection, chloroprocaine HCl, per 30 ml

64420–64421

64420 Injection, anesthetic agent; intercostal nerve, single
64421 intercostal nerves, multiple, regional block

ICD-9-CM Diagnostic

162.4 Malignant neoplasm of middle lobe, bronchus, or lung
162.9 Malignant neoplasm of bronchus and lung, unspecified site ▽
174.0 Malignant neoplasm of nipple and areola of female breast ♀
174.1 Malignant neoplasm of central portion of female breast ♀
174.2 Malignant neoplasm of upper-inner quadrant of female breast ♀
174.3 Malignant neoplasm of lower-inner quadrant of female breast ♀
174.4 Malignant neoplasm of upper-outer quadrant of female breast ♀
174.5 Malignant neoplasm of lower-outer quadrant of female breast ♀
174.6 Malignant neoplasm of axillary tail of female breast ♀
174.8 Malignant neoplasm of other specified sites of female breast ♀
174.9 Malignant neoplasm of breast (female), unspecified site ▽ ♀
175.0 Malignant neoplasm of nipple and areola of male breast ♂
197.0 Secondary malignant neoplasm of lung
197.1 Secondary malignant neoplasm of mediastinum
197.2 Secondary malignant neoplasm of pleura
198.5 Secondary malignant neoplasm of bone and bone marrow
353.8 Other nerve root and plexus disorders
354.8 Other mononeuritis of upper limb
357.81 Chronic inflammatory demyelinating polyneuritis
357.89 Other inflammatory and toxic neuropathy
357.9 Unspecified inflammatory and toxic neuropathy ▽
724.1 Pain in thoracic spine
729.1 Unspecified myalgia and myositis ▽
729.2 Unspecified neuralgia, neuritis, and radiculitis ▽
733.99 Other disorders of bone and cartilage
786.52 Painful respiration
807.00 Closed fracture of rib(s), unspecified ▽
807.01 Closed fracture of one rib
807.02 Closed fracture of two ribs
807.03 Closed fracture of three ribs
807.04 Closed fracture of four ribs
807.05 Closed fracture of five ribs
807.06 Closed fracture of six ribs
807.07 Closed fracture of seven ribs
807.08 Closed fracture of eight or more ribs
807.09 Closed fracture of multiple ribs, unspecified ▽
807.10 Open fracture of rib(s), unspecified ▽
807.11 Open fracture of one rib
807.12 Open fracture of two ribs
807.13 Open fracture of three ribs
807.14 Open fracture of four ribs
807.15 Open fracture of five ribs
807.16 Open fracture of six ribs
807.17 Open fracture of seven ribs
807.18 Open fracture of eight or more ribs
807.19 Open fracture of multiple ribs, unspecified ▽
807.2 Closed fracture of sternum
807.3 Open fracture of sternum
922.1 Contusion of chest wall
957.9 Injury to nerves, unspecified site ▽

ICD-9-CM Procedural

04.81 Injection of anesthetic into peripheral nerve for analgesia

HCPCS Level II Supplies & Services

J2400 Injection, chloroprocaine HCl, per 30 ml

64425

64425 Injection, anesthetic agent; ilioinguinal, iliohypogastric nerves

ICD-9-CM Diagnostic

185 Malignant neoplasm of prostate ♂
195.2 Malignant neoplasm of abdomen
337.9 Unspecified disorder of autonomic nervous system ▽
355.1 Meralgia paresthetica
355.2 Other lesion of femoral nerve
355.3 Lesion of lateral popliteal nerve
355.4 Lesion of medial popliteal nerve
355.5 Tarsal tunnel syndrome
355.6 Lesion of plantar nerve
355.79 Other mononeuritis of lower limb

▽ Unspecified code ♀ Female diagnosis ☒ Manifestation code ♂ Male diagnosis

355.8 Unspecified mononeuritis of lower limb ▽
355.9 Mononeuritis of unspecified site ▽
550.90 Inguinal hernia without mention of obstruction or gangrene, unilateral or unspecified, (not specified as recurrent)
603.8 Other specified type of hydrocele
607.1 Balanoposthitis — (Use additional code to identify organism) ♂
608.1 Spermatocele ♂
721.42 Spondylosis with myelopathy, lumbar region
724.2 Lumbago
729.2 Unspecified neuralgia, neuritis, and radiculitis ▽
729.5 Pain in soft tissues of limb

ICD-9-CM Procedural

04.81 Injection of anesthetic into peripheral nerve for analgesia

HCPCS Level II Supplies & Services

J2400 Injection, chloroprocaine HCl, per 30 ml

64430–64435

64430 Injection, anesthetic agent; pudendal nerve
64435 paracervical (uterine) nerve

ICD-9-CM Diagnostic

218.0 Submucous leiomyoma of uterus ♀
218.1 Intramural leiomyoma of uterus ♀
218.2 Subserous leiomyoma of uterus ♀
218.9 Leiomyoma of uterus, unspecified ▽ ♀
219.0 Benign neoplasm of cervix uteri ♀
219.1 Benign neoplasm of corpus uteri ♀
219.8 Benign neoplasm of other specified parts of uterus ♀
219.9 Benign neoplasm of uterus, part unspecified ▽ ♀
221.0 Benign neoplasm of fallopian tube and uterine ligaments ♀
239.5 Neoplasm of unspecified nature of other genitourinary organs
616.0 Cervicitis and endocervicitis — (Use additional code to identify organism: 041.0, 041.1) ♀
616.2 Cyst of Bartholin's gland — (Use additional code to identify organism: 041.0, 041.1) ♀
622.10 Dysplasia of cervix, unspecified
622.11 Mild dysplasia of cervix
622.12 Moderate dysplasia of cervix
622.7 Mucous polyp of cervix ♀
625.3 Dysmenorrhea ♀
626.2 Excessive or frequent menstruation ♀
626.4 Irregular menstrual cycle ♀
626.6 Metrorrhagia ♀
626.8 Other disorder of menstruation and other abnormal bleeding from female genital tract ♀
626.9 Unspecified disorder of menstruation and other abnormal bleeding from female genital tract ▽ ♀
627.0 Premenopausal menorrhagia ♀
627.1 Postmenopausal bleeding ♀
628.3 Female infertility of uterine origin — (Use additional code for any associated tuberculous endometriosis, 016.7) ♀
632 Missed abortion — (Use additional code from category 639 to identify any associated complications) ♀
635.00 Unspecified legally induced abortion complicated by genital tract and pelvic infection ▽ ♀
635.01 Incomplete legally induced abortion complicated by genital tract and pelvic infection ♀
635.02 Complete legally induced abortion complicated by genital tract and pelvic infection ♀
635.10 Unspecified legally induced abortion complicated by delayed or excessive hemorrhage ▽ ♀
635.11 Incomplete legally induced abortion complicated by delayed or excessive hemorrhage ♀
635.12 Complete legally induced abortion complicated by delayed or excessive hemorrhage ♀
635.20 Unspecified legally induced abortion complicated by damage to pelvic organs or tissues ▽ ♀
635.21 Legally induced abortion complicated by damage to pelvic organs or tissues, incomplete ♀
635.22 Complete legally induced abortion complicated by damage to pelvic organs or tissues ♀
635.30 Unspecified legally induced abortion complicated by renal failure ▽ ♀
635.31 Incomplete legally induced abortion complicated by renal failure ♀
635.32 Complete legally induced abortion complicated by renal failure ♀
635.40 Unspecified legally induced abortion complicated by metabolic disorder ▽ ♀
635.41 Incomplete legally induced abortion complicated by metabolic disorder ♀
635.42 Complete legally induced abortion complicated by metabolic disorder ♀
635.50 Unspecified legally induced abortion complicated by shock ▽ ♀
635.51 Legally induced abortion, complicated by shock, incomplete ♀
635.52 Complete legally induced abortion complicated by shock ♀
635.60 Unspecified legally induced abortion complicated by embolism ▽ ♀
635.61 Incomplete legally induced abortion complicated by embolism ♀
635.62 Complete legally induced abortion complicated by embolism ♀
635.70 Unspecified legally induced abortion with other specified complications ▽ ♀
635.71 Incomplete legally induced abortion with other specified complications ♀
635.72 Complete legally induced abortion with other specified complications ♀
635.80 Unspecified legally induced abortion with unspecified complication ▽ ♀
635.81 Incomplete legally induced abortion with unspecified complication ▽ ♀
635.82 Complete legally induced abortion with unspecified complication ▽ ♀
635.90 Unspecified legally induced abortion without mention of complication ♀
635.91 Incomplete legally induced abortion without mention of complication ♀
635.92 Complete legally induced abortion without mention of complication ♀
637.00 Abortion, unspecified as to completion or legality, complicated by genital tract and pelvic infection ▽ ♀
637.01 Legally unspecified abortion, incomplete, complicated by genital tract and pelvic infection ♀
637.02 Legally unspecified abortion, complete, complicated by genital tract and pelvic infection ♀
637.10 Abortion, unspecified as to completion or legality, complicated by delayed or excessive hemorrhage ▽ ♀
637.11 Legally unspecified abortion, incomplete, complicated by delayed or excessive hemorrhage ♀
637.12 Legally unspecified abortion, complete, complicated by delayed or excessive hemorrhage ♀
637.20 Abortion, unspecified as to completion or legality, complicated by damage to pelvic organs or tissues ▽ ♀
637.21 Legally unspecified abortion, incomplete, complicated by damage to pelvic organs or tissues ♀
637.22 Legally unspecified abortion, complete, complicated by damage to pelvic organs or tissues ♀
637.30 Abortion, unspecified as to completion or legality, complicated by renal failure ▽ ♀
637.31 Legally unspecified abortion, incomplete, complicated by renal failure ♀
637.32 Legally unspecified abortion, complete, complicated by renal failure ♀
637.40 Abortion, unspecified as to completeness or legality, complicated by metabolic disorder ▽ ♀
637.41 Legally unspecified abortion, incomplete, complicated by metabolic disorder ♀
637.42 Legally unspecified abortion, complete, complicated by metabolic disorder ♀
637.50 Abortion, unspecified as to completion or legality, complicated by shock ▽ ♀
637.51 Legally unspecified abortion, incomplete, complicated by shock ♀
637.52 Legally unspecified abortion, complete, complicated by shock ♀
637.60 Abortion, unspecified as to completion or legality, complicated by embolism ▽ ♀
637.61 Legally unspecified abortion, incomplete, complicated by embolism ♀
637.62 Legally unspecified abortion, complete, complicated by embolism ♀
637.70 Abortion, unspecified as to completion or legality, with other specified complications ▽ ♀
637.71 Legally unspecified abortion, incomplete, with other specified complications ♀
637.72 Legally unspecified abortion, complete, with other specified complications ♀
637.80 Abortion, unspecified as to completion or legality, with unspecified complication ▽ ♀
637.81 Legally unspecified abortion, incomplete, with unspecified complication ▽ ♀
637.82 Legally unspecified abortion, complete, with unspecified complication ▽ ♀
637.90 Unspecified type of abortion, unspecified as to completion or legality, without mention of complication ♀
637.91 Legally unspecified abortion, incomplete, without mention of complication ♀
637.92 Legally unspecified abortion, complete, without mention of complication ♀
638.0 Failed attempted abortion complicated by genital tract and pelvic infection ♀
638.1 Failed attempted abortion complicated by delayed or excessive hemorrhage ♀
638.2 Failed attempted abortion complicated by damage to pelvic organs or tissues ♀
638.3 Failed attempted abortion complicated by renal failure ♀
638.4 Failed attempted abortion complicated by metabolic disorder ♀
638.5 Failed attempted abortion complicated by shock ♀
638.6 Failed attempted abortion complicated by embolism ♀
638.7 Failed attempted abortion with other specified complication ♀
638.8 Failed attempted abortion with unspecified complication ▽ ♀
638.9 Failed attempted abortion without mention of complication ♀
646.31 Pregnancy complication, habitual aborter with or without mention of antepartum condition ♀

▽ Unspecified code
♀ Female diagnosis
☒ Manifestation code
♂ Male diagnosis

650 Normal delivery — (This code is for use as a single diagnosis code and is not to be used with any other code in the range 630-676. Use additional code to indicate outcome of delivery, V27.0.) ♀
652.11 Breech or other malpresentation successfully converted to cephalic presentation, delivered — (Code first any associated obstructed labor, 660.0) ♀
652.13 Breech or other malpresentation successfully converted to cephalic presentation, antepartum — (Code first any associated obstructed labor, 660.0) ♀
656.31 Fetal distress affecting management of mother, delivered ♀
658.11 Premature rupture of membranes in pregnancy, delivered ♀
658.31 Delayed delivery after artificial rupture of membranes, delivered ♀
660.01 Obstruction caused by malposition of fetus at onset of labor, delivered — (Use additional code from 652.0-652.9 to identify condition) ♀
660.03 Obstruction caused by malposition of fetus at onset of labor, antepartum — (Use additional code from 652.0-652.9 to identify condition) ♀
664.01 First-degree perineal laceration, with delivery ♀

ICD-9-CM Procedural
04.81 Injection of anesthetic into peripheral nerve for analgesia

HCPCS Level II Supplies & Services
A4550 Surgical trays
J2400 Injection, chloroprocaine HCl, per 30 ml

64445–64446
64445 Injection, anesthetic agent; sciatic nerve, single
64446 sciatic nerve, continuous infusion by catheter, (including catheter placement) including daily management for anesthetic agent administration

ICD-9-CM Diagnostic
355.0 Lesion of sciatic nerve
355.79 Other mononeuritis of lower limb
357.81 Chronic inflammatory demyelinating polyneuritis
357.89 Other inflammatory and toxic neuropathy
719.45 Pain in joint, pelvic region and thigh
720.2 Sacroiliitis, not elsewhere classified
721.42 Spondylosis with myelopathy, lumbar region
722.10 Displacement of lumbar intervertebral disc without myelopathy
722.52 Degeneration of lumbar or lumbosacral intervertebral disc
722.83 Postlaminectomy syndrome, lumbar region
724.02 Spinal stenosis of lumbar region
724.2 Lumbago
724.3 Sciatica
724.4 Thoracic or lumbosacral neuritis or radiculitis, unspecified ▽
729.1 Unspecified myalgia and myositis ▽
729.2 Unspecified neuralgia, neuritis, and radiculitis ▽
729.5 Pain in soft tissues of limb

ICD-9-CM Procedural
04.81 Injection of anesthetic into peripheral nerve for analgesia

HCPCS Level II Supplies & Services
J2400 Injection, chloroprocaine HCl, per 30 ml

64447–64448
64447 Injection, anesthetic agent; femoral nerve, single
64448 Injection, anesthetic agent; femoral nerve, continuous infusion by catheter (including catheter placement) including daily management for anesthetic agent administration

ICD-9-CM Diagnostic
355.1 Meralgia paresthetica
355.2 Other lesion of femoral nerve
355.71 Causalgia of lower limb
355.79 Other mononeuritis of lower limb
719.45 Pain in joint, pelvic region and thigh
726.5 Enthesopathy of hip region
726.61 Pes anserinus tendinitis or bursitis
726.62 Tibial collateral ligament bursitis
726.63 Fibular collateral ligament bursitis
726.65 Prepatellar bursitis
726.69 Other enthesopathy of knee
729.1 Unspecified myalgia and myositis ▽
729.2 Unspecified neuralgia, neuritis, and radiculitis ▽
729.5 Pain in soft tissues of limb

ICD-9-CM Procedural
04.81 Injection of anesthetic into peripheral nerve for analgesia

64449
64449 Injection, anesthetic agent; lumbar plexus, posterior approach, continuous infusion by catheter (including catheter placement) including daily management for anesthetic agent administration

ICD-9-CM Diagnostic
353.1 Lumbosacral plexus lesions
353.4 Lumbosacral root lesions, not elsewhere classified
353.6 Phantom limb (syndrome)
353.8 Other nerve root and plexus disorders
355.0 Lesion of sciatic nerve
355.79 Other mononeuritis of lower limb
719.45 Pain in joint, pelvic region and thigh
719.48 Pain in joint, other specified sites
720.0 Ankylosing spondylitis
720.1 Spinal enthesopathy
721.3 Lumbosacral spondylosis without myelopathy
721.42 Spondylosis with myelopathy, lumbar region
721.6 Ankylosing vertebral hyperostosis
721.7 Traumatic spondylopathy
722.10 Displacement of lumbar intervertebral disc without myelopathy
722.32 Schmorl's nodes, lumbar region
722.52 Degeneration of lumbar or lumbosacral intervertebral disc
722.73 Intervertebral lumbar disc disorder with myelopathy, lumbar region
722.83 Postlaminectomy syndrome, lumbar region
722.93 Other and unspecified disc disorder of lumbar region
724.02 Spinal stenosis of lumbar region
724.2 Lumbago
724.3 Sciatica
724.4 Thoracic or lumbosacral neuritis or radiculitis, unspecified ▽
724.5 Unspecified backache ▽
724.6 Disorders of sacrum
724.8 Other symptoms referable to back
724.9 Other unspecified back disorder
729.2 Unspecified neuralgia, neuritis, and radiculitis ▽
739.3 Nonallopathic lesion of lumbar region, not elsewhere classified
739.4 Nonallopathic lesion of sacral region, not elsewhere classified
756.12 Congenital spondylolisthesis
847.2 Lumbar sprain and strain
847.3 Sprain and strain of sacrum

ICD-9-CM Procedural
04.81 Injection of anesthetic into peripheral nerve for analgesia

64450
64450 Injection, anesthetic agent; other peripheral nerve or branch

ICD-9-CM Diagnostic
The application of this code is too broad to adequately present ICD-9-CM diagnostic code links here. Refer to your ICD-9-CM book.

ICD-9-CM Procedural
04.81 Injection of anesthetic into peripheral nerve for analgesia

HCPCS Level II Supplies & Services
J2400 Injection, chloroprocaine HCl, per 30 ml

64470–64472
64470 Injection, anesthetic agent and/or steroid, paravertebral facet joint or facet joint nerve; cervical or thoracic, single level
64472 cervical or thoracic, each additional level (List separately in addition to code for primary procedure)

ICD-9-CM Diagnostic
353.2 Cervical root lesions, not elsewhere classified
353.3 Thoracic root lesions, not elsewhere classified
353.5 Neuralgic amyotrophy
353.6 Phantom limb (syndrome)
353.8 Other nerve root and plexus disorders
720.0 Ankylosing spondylitis
720.1 Spinal enthesopathy
721.0 Cervical spondylosis without myelopathy

▽ Unspecified code ♀ Female diagnosis ☒ Manifestation code ♂ Male diagnosis

721.1 Cervical spondylosis with myelopathy
721.2 Thoracic spondylosis without myelopathy
721.41 Spondylosis with myelopathy, thoracic region
721.6 Ankylosing vertebral hyperostosis
721.7 Traumatic spondylopathy
722.0 Displacement of cervical intervertebral disc without myelopathy
722.11 Displacement of thoracic intervertebral disc without myelopathy
722.31 Schmorl's nodes, thoracic region
722.4 Degeneration of cervical intervertebral disc
722.51 Degeneration of thoracic or thoracolumbar intervertebral disc
722.71 Intervertebral cervical disc disorder with myelopathy, cervical region
722.72 Intervertebral thoracic disc disorder with myelopathy, thoracic region
722.81 Postlaminectomy syndrome, cervical region
722.82 Postlaminectomy syndrome, thoracic region
722.91 Other and unspecified disc disorder of cervical region
722.92 Other and unspecified disc disorder of thoracic region
723.0 Spinal stenosis in cervical region
723.1 Cervicalgia
723.2 Cervicocranial syndrome
723.3 Cervicobrachial syndrome (diffuse)
723.4 Brachial neuritis or radiculitis nos
723.6 Panniculitis specified as affecting neck
723.8 Other syndromes affecting cervical region
723.9 Unspecified musculoskeletal disorders and symptoms referable to neck ▽
724.01 Spinal stenosis of thoracic region
724.1 Pain in thoracic spine
724.4 Thoracic or lumbosacral neuritis or radiculitis, unspecified ▽
729.2 Unspecified neuralgia, neuritis, and radiculitis ▽
739.0 Nonallopathic lesion of head region, not elsewhere classified
847.0 Neck sprain and strain
847.1 Thoracic sprain and strain

ICD-9-CM Procedural
03.92 Injection of other agent into spinal canal
04.81 Injection of anesthetic into peripheral nerve for analgesia

HCPCS Level II Supplies & Services
J2400 Injection, chloroprocaine HCl, per 30 ml

64475–64476
64475 Injection, anesthetic agent and/or steroid, paravertebral facet joint or facet joint nerve; lumbar or sacral, single level
64476 lumbar or sacral, each additional level (List separately in addition to code for primary procedure)

ICD-9-CM Diagnostic
353.1 Lumbosacral plexus lesions
353.4 Lumbosacral root lesions, not elsewhere classified
353.6 Phantom limb (syndrome)
353.8 Other nerve root and plexus disorders
355.0 Lesion of sciatic nerve
355.79 Other mononeuritis of lower limb
719.45 Pain in joint, pelvic region and thigh
719.48 Pain in joint, other specified sites
720.0 Ankylosing spondylitis
720.1 Spinal enthesopathy
721.3 Lumbosacral spondylosis without myelopathy
721.42 Spondylosis with myelopathy, lumbar region
721.6 Ankylosing vertebral hyperostosis
721.7 Traumatic spondylopathy
722.10 Displacement of lumbar intervertebral disc without myelopathy
722.32 Schmorl's nodes, lumbar region
722.52 Degeneration of lumbar or lumbosacral intervertebral disc
722.73 Intervertebral lumbar disc disorder with myelopathy, lumbar region
722.83 Postlaminectomy syndrome, lumbar region
722.93 Other and unspecified disc disorder of lumbar region
724.02 Spinal stenosis of lumbar region
724.2 Lumbago
724.3 Sciatica
724.4 Thoracic or lumbosacral neuritis or radiculitis, unspecified ▽
724.5 Unspecified backache ▽
724.6 Disorders of sacrum
724.8 Other symptoms referable to back
724.9 Other unspecified back disorder
729.2 Unspecified neuralgia, neuritis, and radiculitis ▽
739.3 Nonallopathic lesion of lumbar region, not elsewhere classified
739.4 Nonallopathic lesion of sacral region, not elsewhere classified
756.12 Congenital spondylolisthesis
847.2 Lumbar sprain and strain
847.3 Sprain and strain of sacrum

ICD-9-CM Procedural
03.92 Injection of other agent into spinal canal
04.81 Injection of anesthetic into peripheral nerve for analgesia

HCPCS Level II Supplies & Services
J2400 Injection, chloroprocaine HCl, per 30 ml

64479–64480
64479 Injection, anesthetic agent and/or steroid, transforaminal epidural; cervical or thoracic, single level
64480 cervical or thoracic, each additional level (List separately in addition to code for primary procedure)

ICD-9-CM Diagnostic
353.2 Cervical root lesions, not elsewhere classified
353.3 Thoracic root lesions, not elsewhere classified
353.5 Neuralgic amyotrophy
353.6 Phantom limb (syndrome)
353.8 Other nerve root and plexus disorders
720.0 Ankylosing spondylitis
720.1 Spinal enthesopathy
721.0 Cervical spondylosis without myelopathy
721.1 Cervical spondylosis with myelopathy
721.2 Thoracic spondylosis without myelopathy
721.41 Spondylosis with myelopathy, thoracic region
721.6 Ankylosing vertebral hyperostosis
721.7 Traumatic spondylopathy
722.0 Displacement of cervical intervertebral disc without myelopathy
722.11 Displacement of thoracic intervertebral disc without myelopathy
722.31 Schmorl's nodes, thoracic region
722.4 Degeneration of cervical intervertebral disc
722.51 Degeneration of thoracic or thoracolumbar intervertebral disc
722.71 Intervertebral cervical disc disorder with myelopathy, cervical region
722.72 Intervertebral thoracic disc disorder with myelopathy, thoracic region
722.81 Postlaminectomy syndrome, cervical region
722.82 Postlaminectomy syndrome, thoracic region
722.91 Other and unspecified disc disorder of cervical region
722.92 Other and unspecified disc disorder of thoracic region
723.0 Spinal stenosis in cervical region
723.1 Cervicalgia
723.2 Cervicocranial syndrome
723.3 Cervicobrachial syndrome (diffuse)
723.4 Brachial neuritis or radiculitis nos
723.6 Panniculitis specified as affecting neck
723.8 Other syndromes affecting cervical region
723.9 Unspecified musculoskeletal disorders and symptoms referable to neck ▽
724.01 Spinal stenosis of thoracic region
724.1 Pain in thoracic spine
724.4 Thoracic or lumbosacral neuritis or radiculitis, unspecified ▽
729.2 Unspecified neuralgia, neuritis, and radiculitis ▽
739.0 Nonallopathic lesion of head region, not elsewhere classified
847.0 Neck sprain and strain
847.1 Thoracic sprain and strain

ICD-9-CM Procedural
03.91 Injection of anesthetic into spinal canal for analgesia
03.92 Injection of other agent into spinal canal

HCPCS Level II Supplies & Services
J2400 Injection, chloroprocaine HCl, per 30 ml

64483–64484
64483 Injection, anesthetic agent and/or steroid, transforaminal epidural; lumbar or sacral, single level
64484 lumbar or sacral, each additional level (List separately in addition to code for primary procedure)

ICD-9-CM Diagnostic
353.1 Lumbosacral plexus lesions
353.4 Lumbosacral root lesions, not elsewhere classified
353.6 Phantom limb (syndrome)

▽ Unspecified code ♀ Female diagnosis ☒ Manifestation code ♂ Male diagnosis

353.8 Other nerve root and plexus disorders
355.0 Lesion of sciatic nerve
355.79 Other mononeuritis of lower limb
719.45 Pain in joint, pelvic region and thigh
719.48 Pain in joint, other specified sites
720.0 Ankylosing spondylitis
720.1 Spinal enthesopathy
721.3 Lumbosacral spondylosis without myelopathy
721.42 Spondylosis with myelopathy, lumbar region
721.6 Ankylosing vertebral hyperostosis
721.7 Traumatic spondylopathy
722.10 Displacement of lumbar intervertebral disc without myelopathy
722.32 Schmorl's nodes, lumbar region
722.52 Degeneration of lumbar or lumbosacral intervertebral disc
722.73 Intervertebral lumbar disc disorder with myelopathy, lumbar region
722.83 Postlaminectomy syndrome, lumbar region
722.93 Other and unspecified disc disorder of lumbar region
724.02 Spinal stenosis of lumbar region
724.2 Lumbago
724.3 Sciatica
724.4 Thoracic or lumbosacral neuritis or radiculitis, unspecified ▽
724.5 Unspecified backache ▽
724.6 Disorders of sacrum
724.8 Other symptoms referable to back
724.9 Other unspecified back disorder
729.2 Unspecified neuralgia, neuritis, and radiculitis ▽
739.3 Nonallopathic lesion of lumbar region, not elsewhere classified
739.4 Nonallopathic lesion of sacral region, not elsewhere classified
756.12 Congenital spondylolisthesis
847.2 Lumbar sprain and strain
847.3 Sprain and strain of sacrum

ICD-9-CM Procedural
03.91 Injection of anesthetic into spinal canal for analgesia
03.92 Injection of other agent into spinal canal

HCPCS Level II Supplies & Services
J2400 Injection, chloroprocaine HCl, per 30 ml

64505
64505 Injection, anesthetic agent; sphenopalatine ganglion

ICD-9-CM Diagnostic
350.2 Atypical face pain
524.62 Arthralgia of temporomandibular joint
784.0 Headache
830.1 Open dislocation of jaw
848.1 Sprain and strain of jaw

ICD-9-CM Procedural
05.31 Injection of anesthetic into sympathetic nerve for analgesia

HCPCS Level II Supplies & Services
J2400 Injection, chloroprocaine HCl, per 30 ml

64508
64508 Injection, anesthetic agent; carotid sinus (separate procedure)

ICD-9-CM Diagnostic
333.0 Other degenerative diseases of the basal ganglia
337.0 Idiopathic peripheral autonomic neuropathy

ICD-9-CM Procedural
05.31 Injection of anesthetic into sympathetic nerve for analgesia

HCPCS Level II Supplies & Services
J2400 Injection, chloroprocaine HCl, per 30 ml

64510–64520
64510 Injection, anesthetic agent; stellate ganglion (cervical sympathetic)
64520 lumbar or thoracic (paravertebral sympathetic)

ICD-9-CM Diagnostic
307.81 Tension headache
337.0 Idiopathic peripheral autonomic neuropathy
337.21 Reflex sympathetic dystrophy of the upper limb
337.22 Reflex sympathetic dystrophy of the lower limb
337.29 Reflex sympathetic dystrophy of other specified site
346.01 Classical migraine with intractable migraine, so stated
354.4 Causalgia of upper limb
354.5 Mononeuritis multiplex
354.9 Unspecified mononeuritis of upper limb ▽
355.8 Unspecified mononeuritis of lower limb ▽
355.9 Mononeuritis of unspecified site ▽
719.41 Pain in joint, shoulder region
719.42 Pain in joint, upper arm
719.44 Pain in joint, hand
719.45 Pain in joint, pelvic region and thigh
719.46 Pain in joint, lower leg
723.1 Cervicalgia
723.2 Cervicocranial syndrome
723.3 Cervicobrachial syndrome (diffuse)
723.4 Brachial neuritis or radiculitis nos
724.2 Lumbago
724.5 Unspecified backache ▽
729.2 Unspecified neuralgia, neuritis, and radiculitis ▽
729.5 Pain in soft tissues of limb

ICD-9-CM Procedural
05.31 Injection of anesthetic into sympathetic nerve for analgesia

HCPCS Level II Supplies & Services
J2400 Injection, chloroprocaine HCl, per 30 ml

64517
64517 Injection, anesthetic agent; superior hypogastric plexus

ICD-9-CM Diagnostic
617.0 Endometriosis of uterus ♀
617.1 Endometriosis of ovary ♀
617.2 Endometriosis of fallopian tube ♀
617.3 Endometriosis of pelvic peritoneum ♀
617.4 Endometriosis of rectovaginal septum and vagina ♀
617.5 Endometriosis of intestine ♀
617.8 Endometriosis of other specified sites ♀
617.9 Endometriosis, site unspecified ▽ ♀
625.0 Dyspareunia ♀
625.2 Mittelschmerz ♀
625.3 Dysmenorrhea ♀
625.9 Unspecified symptom associated with female genital organs ▽ ♀

ICD-9-CM Procedural
05.31 Injection of anesthetic into sympathetic nerve for analgesia

64530
64530 Injection, anesthetic agent; celiac plexus, with or without radiologic monitoring

ICD-9-CM Diagnostic
157.0 Malignant neoplasm of head of pancreas
157.1 Malignant neoplasm of body of pancreas
157.2 Malignant neoplasm of tail of pancreas
157.3 Malignant neoplasm of pancreatic duct
157.4 Malignant neoplasm of islets of Langerhans — (Use additional code to identify any functional activity)
157.8 Malignant neoplasm of other specified sites of pancreas
157.9 Malignant neoplasm of pancreas, part unspecified ▽
577.0 Acute pancreatitis
577.1 Chronic pancreatitis
786.51 Precordial pain
789.00 Abdominal pain, unspecified site ▽
789.01 Abdominal pain, right upper quadrant
789.02 Abdominal pain, left upper quadrant
789.06 Abdominal pain, epigastric
789.07 Abdominal pain, generalized
789.09 Abdominal pain, other specified site

ICD-9-CM Procedural
05.31 Injection of anesthetic into sympathetic nerve for analgesia

64550

64550 Application of surface (transcutaneous) neurostimulator

ICD-9-CM Diagnostic

354.4 Causalgia of upper limb
719.46 Pain in joint, lower leg
722.11 Displacement of thoracic intervertebral disc without myelopathy
723.1 Cervicalgia
723.4 Brachial neuritis or radiculitis nos
724.2 Lumbago
724.3 Sciatica
729.1 Unspecified myalgia and myositis ▽
729.2 Unspecified neuralgia, neuritis, and radiculitis ▽
846.0 Sprain and strain of lumbosacral (joint) (ligament)

ICD-9-CM Procedural

04.19 Other diagnostic procedures on cranial and peripheral nerves and ganglia

HCPCS Level II Supplies & Services

E0720 TENS, two lead, localized stimulation
E0730 Transcutaneous electrical nerve stimulation device, four or more leads, for multiple nerve stimulation
E0731 Form-fitting conductive garment for delivery of TENS or NMES (with conductive fibers separated from the patient's skin by layers of fabric)
E0744 Neuromuscular stimulator for scoliosis
E0745 Neuromuscular stimulator, electronic shock unit

64553–64565

64553 Percutaneous implantation of neurostimulator electrodes; cranial nerve
64555 peripheral nerve (excludes sacral nerve)
64560 autonomic nerve
64565 neuromuscular

ICD-9-CM Diagnostic

The application of this code is too broad to adequately present ICD-9-CM diagnostic code links here. Refer to your ICD-9-CM book.

ICD-9-CM Procedural

02.93 Implantation or replacement of intracranial neurostimulator lead(s)
04.92 Implantation or replacement of peripheral neurostimulator lead(s)
04.99 Other operations on cranial and peripheral nerves

HCPCS Level II Supplies & Services

E0752 Implantable neurostimulator electrode, each

64573–64581

64573 Incision for implantation of neurostimulator electrodes; cranial nerve
64575 peripheral nerve (excludes sacral nerve)
64577 autonomic nerve
64580 neuromuscular
64581 sacral nerve (transforaminal placement)

ICD-9-CM Diagnostic

The application of this code is too broad to adequately present ICD-9-CM diagnostic code links here. Refer to your ICD-9-CM book.

ICD-9-CM Procedural

02.93 Implantation or replacement of intracranial neurostimulator lead(s)
04.92 Implantation or replacement of peripheral neurostimulator lead(s)
04.99 Other operations on cranial and peripheral nerves

HCPCS Level II Supplies & Services

E0752 Implantable neurostimulator electrode, each

64585

64585 Revision or removal of peripheral neurostimulator electrodes

ICD-9-CM Diagnostic

996.2 Mechanical complication of nervous system device, implant, and graft
996.63 Infection and inflammatory reaction due to nervous system device, implant, and graft — (Use additional code to identify specified infections)
996.75 Other complications due to nervous system device, implant, and graft

ICD-9-CM Procedural

04.93 Removal of peripheral neurostimulator lead(s)

64590–64595

64590 Insertion or replacement of peripheral neurostimulator pulse generator or receiver, direct or inductive coupling
64595 Revision or removal of peripheral neurostimulator pulse generator or receiver

ICD-9-CM Diagnostic

250.60 Diabetes with neurological manifestations, type II or unspecified type, not stated as uncontrolled — (Use additional code to identify manifestation: 337.1, 354.0-355.9, 357.2, 358.1, 713.5)
250.61 Diabetes with neurological manifestations, type I [juvenile type], not stated as uncontrolled — (Use additional code to identify manifestation: 337.1, 354.0-355.9, 357.2, 358.1, 713.5)
250.62 Diabetes with neurological manifestations, type II or unspecified type, uncontrolled — (Use additional code to identify manifestation: 337.1, 354.0-355.9, 357.2, 358.1, 713.5)
250.63 Diabetes with neurological manifestations, type I [juvenile type], uncontrolled — (Use additional code to identify manifestation: 337.1, 354.0-355.9, 357.2, 358.1, 713.5)
337.1 Peripheral autonomic neuropathy in disorders classified elsewhere — (Code first underlying disease: 250.6, 277.3) ☒
337.20 Unspecified reflex sympathetic dystrophy ▽
337.22 Reflex sympathetic dystrophy of the lower limb
337.29 Reflex sympathetic dystrophy of other specified site
354.5 Mononeuritis multiplex
355.1 Meralgia paresthetica
355.2 Other lesion of femoral nerve
355.3 Lesion of lateral popliteal nerve
355.4 Lesion of medial popliteal nerve
355.71 Causalgia of lower limb
355.79 Other mononeuritis of lower limb
355.8 Unspecified mononeuritis of lower limb ▽
356.0 Hereditary peripheral neuropathy
356.3 Refsum's disease
356.4 Idiopathic progressive polyneuropathy
356.8 Other specified idiopathic peripheral neuropathy
357.2 Polyneuropathy in diabetes — (Code first underlying disease: 250.6) ☒
357.3 Polyneuropathy in malignant disease — (Code first underlying disease: 140.0-208.9) ☒
595.1 Chronic interstitial cystitis — (Use additional code to identify organism, such as E. coli, 041.4)
596.55 Detrusor sphincter dyssynergia — (Use additional code to identify urinary incontinence: 625.6, 788.30-788.39)
596.59 Other functional disorder of bladder — (Use additional code to identify urinary incontinence: 625.6, 788.30-788.39)
788.20 Unspecified retention of urine ▽
788.21 Incomplete bladder emptying
788.31 Urge incontinence
788.33 Mixed incontinence urge and stress (male)(female)
788.34 Incontinence without sensory awareness
788.41 Urinary frequency
996.2 Mechanical complication of nervous system device, implant, and graft
996.63 Infection and inflammatory reaction due to nervous system device, implant, and graft — (Use additional code to identify specified infections)
996.75 Other complications due to nervous system device, implant, and graft

ICD-9-CM Procedural

86.05 Incision with removal of foreign body or device from skin and subcutaneous tissue
86.94 Insertion or replacement of single array neurostimulator pulse generator
86.95 Insertion or replacement of dual array neurostimulator pulse generator
86.96 Insertion or replacement of other neurostimulator pulse generator

HCPCS Level II Supplies & Services

E0752 Implantable neurostimulator electrode, each

64600

64600 Destruction by neurolytic agent, trigeminal nerve; supraorbital, infraorbital, mental, or inferior alveolar branch

ICD-9-CM Diagnostic

171.0 Malignant neoplasm of connective and other soft tissue of head, face, and neck
225.1 Benign neoplasm of cranial nerves
238.1 Neoplasm of uncertain behavior of connective and other soft tissue ▽
239.2 Neoplasms of unspecified nature of bone, soft tissue, and skin
350.1 Trigeminal neuralgia
350.2 Atypical face pain

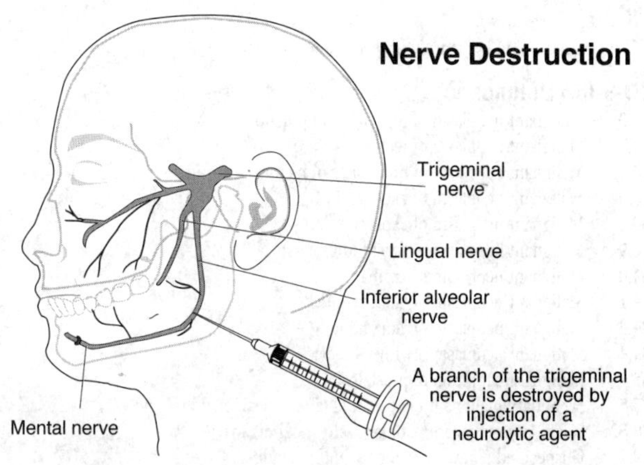
Nerve Destruction
Trigeminal nerve
Lingual nerve
Inferior alveolar nerve
A branch of the trigeminal nerve is destroyed by injection of a neurolytic agent
Mental nerve

350.8 Other specified trigeminal nerve disorders
907.1 Late effect of injury to cranial nerve
951.2 Injury to trigeminal nerve

ICD-9-CM Procedural
04.2 Destruction of cranial and peripheral nerves

HCPCS Level II Supplies & Services
A4550 Surgical trays

64605–64610
64605 Destruction by neurolytic agent, trigeminal nerve; second and third division branches at foramen ovale
64610 second and third division branches at foramen ovale under radiologic monitoring

ICD-9-CM Diagnostic
171.0 Malignant neoplasm of connective and other soft tissue of head, face, and neck
225.1 Benign neoplasm of cranial nerves
238.1 Neoplasm of uncertain behavior of connective and other soft tissue ▽
239.2 Neoplasms of unspecified nature of bone, soft tissue, and skin
350.1 Trigeminal neuralgia
350.2 Atypical face pain
350.8 Other specified trigeminal nerve disorders
907.1 Late effect of injury to cranial nerve
951.2 Injury to trigeminal nerve

ICD-9-CM Procedural
04.2 Destruction of cranial and peripheral nerves

64612–64613
64612 Chemodenervation of muscle(s); muscle(s) innervated by facial nerve (eg, for blepharospasm, hemifacial spasm)
64613 cervical spinal muscle(s) (eg, for spasmodic torticollis)

ICD-9-CM Diagnostic
333.3 Tics of organic origin — (Use additional E code to identify drug, if drug-induced)
333.6 Idiopathic torsion dystonia
333.81 Blepharospasm — (Use additional E code to identify drug, if drug-induced)
333.82 Orofacial dyskinesia — (Use additional E code to identify drug, if drug-induced)
333.83 Spasmodic torticollis — (Use additional E code to identify drug, if drug-induced)
333.89 Other fragments of torsion dystonia — (Use additional E code to identify drug, if drug-induced)
340 Multiple sclerosis
350.2 Atypical face pain
351.8 Other facial nerve disorders
781.0 Abnormal involuntary movements

ICD-9-CM Procedural
04.2 Destruction of cranial and peripheral nerves

HCPCS Level II Supplies & Services
A4550 Surgical trays
J0585 Botulinum toxin type A, per unit
J0587 Botulinum toxin type B, per 100 units

64614
64614 Chemodenervation of muscle(s); extremity(s) and/or trunk muscle(s) (eg, for dystonia, cerebral palsy, multiple sclerosis)

ICD-9-CM Diagnostic
333.0 Other degenerative diseases of the basal ganglia
333.1 Essential and other specified forms of tremor — (Use additional E code to identify drug, if drug-induced)
333.2 Myoclonus — (Use additional E code to identify drug, if drug-induced)
333.3 Tics of organic origin — (Use additional E code to identify drug, if drug-induced)
333.4 Huntington's chorea
333.5 Other choreas — (Use additional E code to identify drug, if drug-induced)
333.6 Idiopathic torsion dystonia
333.7 Symptomatic torsion dystonia — (Use additional E code to identify drug, if drug-induced)
333.84 Organic writers' cramp — (Use additional E code to identify drug, if drug-induced)
333.89 Other fragments of torsion dystonia — (Use additional E code to identify drug, if drug-induced)
333.90 Unspecified extrapyramidal disease and abnormal movement disorder ▽
333.91 Stiff-man syndrome
333.92 Neuroleptic malignant syndrome — (Use additional E code to identify drug)
333.93 Benign shuddering attacks
333.99 Other extrapyramidal disease and abnormal movement disorder
340 Multiple sclerosis
341.1 Schilder's disease
341.8 Other demyelinating diseases of central nervous system
341.9 Unspecified demyelinating disease of central nervous system ▽
342.10 Spastic hemiplegia affecting unspecified side ▽
342.11 Spastic hemiplegia affecting dominant side
342.12 Spastic hemiplegia affecting nondominant side
343.0 Diplegic infantile cerebral palsy
343.1 Hemiplegic infantile cerebral palsy
343.2 Quadriplegic infantile cerebral palsy
343.3 Monoplegic infantile cerebral palsy
343.4 Infantile hemiplegia
343.8 Other specified infantile cerebral palsy
343.9 Unspecified infantile cerebral palsy ▽
344.89 Other specified paralytic syndrome
781.0 Abnormal involuntary movements

ICD-9-CM Procedural
04.2 Destruction of cranial and peripheral nerves

HCPCS Level II Supplies & Services
A4550 Surgical trays
J0585 Botulinum toxin type A, per unit

64620
64620 Destruction by neurolytic agent, intercostal nerve

ICD-9-CM Diagnostic
355.9 Mononeuritis of unspecified site ▽
729.2 Unspecified neuralgia, neuritis, and radiculitis ▽
786.52 Painful respiration

ICD-9-CM Procedural
04.2 Destruction of cranial and peripheral nerves

HCPCS Level II Supplies & Services
A4550 Surgical trays

64622–64623
64622 Destruction by neurolytic agent, paravertebral facet joint nerve; lumbar or sacral, single level
64623 lumbar or sacral, each additional level (List separately in addition to code for primary procedure)

ICD-9-CM Diagnostic
353.1 Lumbosacral plexus lesions
353.4 Lumbosacral root lesions, not elsewhere classified
353.6 Phantom limb (syndrome)
353.8 Other nerve root and plexus disorders
355.0 Lesion of sciatic nerve
355.79 Other mononeuritis of lower limb

719.45 Pain in joint, pelvic region and thigh
719.48 Pain in joint, other specified sites
720.0 Ankylosing spondylitis
720.1 Spinal enthesopathy
721.3 Lumbosacral spondylosis without myelopathy
721.42 Spondylosis with myelopathy, lumbar region
721.6 Ankylosing vertebral hyperostosis
721.7 Traumatic spondylopathy
722.10 Displacement of lumbar intervertebral disc without myelopathy
722.32 Schmorl's nodes, lumbar region
722.52 Degeneration of lumbar or lumbosacral intervertebral disc
722.73 Intervertebral lumbar disc disorder with myelopathy, lumbar region
722.83 Postlaminectomy syndrome, lumbar region
722.93 Other and unspecified disc disorder of lumbar region
724.02 Spinal stenosis of lumbar region
724.2 Lumbago
724.3 Sciatica
724.4 Thoracic or lumbosacral neuritis or radiculitis, unspecified ▽
724.5 Unspecified backache ▽
724.8 Other symptoms referable to back
724.9 Other unspecified back disorder
729.2 Unspecified neuralgia, neuritis, and radiculitis ▽
739.3 Nonallopathic lesion of lumbar region, not elsewhere classified
739.4 Nonallopathic lesion of sacral region, not elsewhere classified
756.12 Congenital spondylolisthesis

ICD-9-CM Procedural

04.2 Destruction of cranial and peripheral nerves

64626–64627

64626 Destruction by neurolytic agent, paravertebral facet joint nerve; cervical or thoracic, single level
64627 cervical or thoracic, each additional level (List separately in addition to code for primary procedure)

ICD-9-CM Diagnostic

353.2 Cervical root lesions, not elsewhere classified
353.3 Thoracic root lesions, not elsewhere classified
353.5 Neuralgic amyotrophy
353.6 Phantom limb (syndrome)
353.8 Other nerve root and plexus disorders
720.0 Ankylosing spondylitis
720.1 Spinal enthesopathy
721.0 Cervical spondylosis without myelopathy
721.1 Cervical spondylosis with myelopathy
721.2 Thoracic spondylosis without myelopathy
721.41 Spondylosis with myelopathy, thoracic region
721.6 Ankylosing vertebral hyperostosis
721.7 Traumatic spondylopathy
722.0 Displacement of cervical intervertebral disc without myelopathy
722.11 Displacement of thoracic intervertebral disc without myelopathy
722.31 Schmorl's nodes, thoracic region
722.4 Degeneration of cervical intervertebral disc
722.51 Degeneration of thoracic or thoracolumbar intervertebral disc
722.71 Intervertebral cervical disc disorder with myelopathy, cervical region
722.72 Intervertebral thoracic disc disorder with myelopathy, thoracic region
722.81 Postlaminectomy syndrome, cervical region
722.82 Postlaminectomy syndrome, thoracic region
722.91 Other and unspecified disc disorder of cervical region
722.92 Other and unspecified disc disorder of thoracic region
723.0 Spinal stenosis in cervical region
723.1 Cervicalgia
723.2 Cervicocranial syndrome
723.3 Cervicobrachial syndrome (diffuse)
723.4 Brachial neuritis or radiculitis nos
723.6 Panniculitis specified as affecting neck
723.8 Other syndromes affecting cervical region
723.9 Unspecified musculoskeletal disorders and symptoms referable to neck ▽
724.01 Spinal stenosis of thoracic region
724.1 Pain in thoracic spine
724.4 Thoracic or lumbosacral neuritis or radiculitis, unspecified ▽
729.2 Unspecified neuralgia, neuritis, and radiculitis ▽
739.0 Nonallopathic lesion of head region, not elsewhere classified

ICD-9-CM Procedural

04.2 Destruction of cranial and peripheral nerves

64630

64630 Destruction by neurolytic agent; pudendal nerve

ICD-9-CM Diagnostic

154.0 Malignant neoplasm of rectosigmoid junction
154.1 Malignant neoplasm of rectum
154.8 Malignant neoplasm of other sites of rectum, rectosigmoid junction, and anus
180.0 Malignant neoplasm of endocervix ♀
180.1 Malignant neoplasm of exocervix ♀
180.9 Malignant neoplasm of cervix uteri, unspecified site ▽ ♀
184.0 Malignant neoplasm of vagina ♀
184.1 Malignant neoplasm of labia majora ♀
184.2 Malignant neoplasm of labia minora ♀
184.4 Malignant neoplasm of vulva, unspecified site ▽ ♀
185 Malignant neoplasm of prostate ♂
197.5 Secondary malignant neoplasm of large intestine and rectum
198.82 Secondary malignant neoplasm of genital organs
729.2 Unspecified neuralgia, neuritis, and radiculitis ▽

ICD-9-CM Procedural

04.2 Destruction of cranial and peripheral nerves

64640

64640 Destruction by neurolytic agent; other peripheral nerve or branch

ICD-9-CM Diagnostic

The application of this code is too broad to adequately present ICD-9-CM diagnostic code links here. Refer to your ICD-9-CM book.

ICD-9-CM Procedural

04.2 Destruction of cranial and peripheral nerves

64680

64680 Destruction by neurolytic agent, with or without radiologic monitoring; celiac plexus

ICD-9-CM Diagnostic

157.0 Malignant neoplasm of head of pancreas
157.1 Malignant neoplasm of body of pancreas
157.2 Malignant neoplasm of tail of pancreas
157.3 Malignant neoplasm of pancreatic duct
157.4 Malignant neoplasm of islets of Langerhans — (Use additional code to identify any functional activity)
577.1 Chronic pancreatitis
577.8 Other specified disease of pancreas

ICD-9-CM Procedural

05.32 Injection of neurolytic agent into sympathetic nerve

64681

64681 Destruction by neurolytic agent, with or without radiologic monitoring; superior hypogastric plexus

ICD-9-CM Diagnostic

617.0 Endometriosis of uterus ♀
617.1 Endometriosis of ovary ♀
617.2 Endometriosis of fallopian tube ♀
617.3 Endometriosis of pelvic peritoneum ♀
617.4 Endometriosis of rectovaginal septum and vagina ♀
617.5 Endometriosis of intestine ♀
617.8 Endometriosis of other specified sites ♀
617.9 Endometriosis, site unspecified ▽ ♀
625.0 Dyspareunia ♀
625.2 Mittelschmerz ♀
625.3 Dysmenorrhea ♀
625.9 Unspecified symptom associated with female genital organs ▽ ♀

ICD-9-CM Procedural

05.32 Injection of neurolytic agent into sympathetic nerve

▽ Unspecified code ♀ Female diagnosis ☒ Manifestation code ♂ Male diagnosis

64702–64704

64702 Neuroplasty; digital, one or both, same digit
64704 nerve of hand or foot

ICD-9-CM Diagnostic

354.2 Lesion of ulnar nerve
354.3 Lesion of radial nerve
354.4 Causalgia of upper limb
355.4 Lesion of medial popliteal nerve
355.5 Tarsal tunnel syndrome
355.6 Lesion of plantar nerve
355.71 Causalgia of lower limb
355.79 Other mononeuritis of lower limb
355.8 Unspecified mononeuritis of lower limb ▽
709.2 Scar condition and fibrosis of skin
711.44 Arthropathy, associated with other bacterial diseases, hand — (Code first underlying disease, such as: diseases classifiable to 010-040 (except 036.82), 090-099 (except 098.50)) ☒
718.54 Ankylosis of hand joint
719.44 Pain in joint, hand
719.47 Pain in joint, ankle and foot
719.64 Other symptoms referable to hand joint
727.03 Trigger finger (acquired)
727.05 Other tenosynovitis of hand and wrist
727.42 Ganglion of tendon sheath
727.81 Contracture of tendon (sheath)
728.6 Contracture of palmar fascia
728.71 Plantar fascial fibromatosis
729.2 Unspecified neuralgia, neuritis, and radiculitis ▽
729.5 Pain in soft tissues of limb
736.21 Boutonniere deformity
736.22 Swan-neck deformity
755.12 Syndactyly of fingers with fusion of bone
755.13 Syndactyly of toes without fusion of bone
755.14 Syndactyly of toes with fusion of bone
782.0 Disturbance of skin sensation
906.1 Late effect of open wound of extremities without mention of tendon injury
907.4 Late effect of injury to peripheral nerve of shoulder girdle and upper limb
907.5 Late effect of injury to peripheral nerve of pelvic girdle and lower limb
907.9 Late effect of injury to other and unspecified nerve ▽
908.6 Late effect of certain complications of trauma
908.9 Late effect of unspecified injury ▽
909.3 Late effect of complications of surgical and medical care
955.6 Injury to digital nerve, upper limb
955.7 Injury to other specified nerve(s) of shoulder girdle and upper limb
955.8 Injury to multiple nerves of shoulder girdle and upper limb
955.9 Injury to unspecified nerve of shoulder girdle and upper limb ▽
957.8 Injury to multiple nerves in several parts

ICD-9-CM Procedural

04.49 Other peripheral nerve or ganglion decompression or lysis of adhesions
04.79 Other neuroplasty

HCPCS Level II Supplies & Services

A4550 Surgical trays

64708–64712

64708 Neuroplasty, major peripheral nerve, arm or leg; other than specified
64712 sciatic nerve

ICD-9-CM Diagnostic

353.9 Unspecified nerve root and plexus disorder ▽
354.3 Lesion of radial nerve
354.4 Causalgia of upper limb
354.9 Unspecified mononeuritis of upper limb ▽
355.0 Lesion of sciatic nerve
355.71 Causalgia of lower limb
355.79 Other mononeuritis of lower limb
355.8 Unspecified mononeuritis of lower limb ▽
729.5 Pain in soft tissues of limb
782.0 Disturbance of skin sensation
906.1 Late effect of open wound of extremities without mention of tendon injury
907.4 Late effect of injury to peripheral nerve of shoulder girdle and upper limb
907.5 Late effect of injury to peripheral nerve of pelvic girdle and lower limb
907.9 Late effect of injury to other and unspecified nerve ▽
908.6 Late effect of certain complications of trauma
908.9 Late effect of unspecified injury ▽
909.3 Late effect of complications of surgical and medical care
955.0 Injury to axillary nerve
955.1 Injury to median nerve
955.2 Injury to ulnar nerve
955.3 Injury to radial nerve
955.4 Injury to musculocutaneous nerve
955.7 Injury to other specified nerve(s) of shoulder girdle and upper limb
955.8 Injury to multiple nerves of shoulder girdle and upper limb
955.9 Injury to unspecified nerve of shoulder girdle and upper limb ▽
956.0 Injury to sciatic nerve
956.1 Injury to femoral nerve
956.2 Injury to posterior tibial nerve
956.3 Injury to peroneal nerve
956.4 Injury to cutaneous sensory nerve, lower limb
956.5 Injury to other specified nerve(s) of pelvic girdle and lower limb
956.8 Injury to multiple nerves of pelvic girdle and lower limb
956.9 Injury to unspecified nerve of pelvic girdle and lower limb ▽
957.8 Injury to multiple nerves in several parts
996.75 Other complications due to nervous system device, implant, and graft
998.2 Accidental puncture or laceration during procedure

ICD-9-CM Procedural

04.49 Other peripheral nerve or ganglion decompression or lysis of adhesions
04.79 Other neuroplasty

64713

64713 Neuroplasty, major peripheral nerve, arm or leg; brachial plexus

ICD-9-CM Diagnostic

353.0 Brachial plexus lesions
723.4 Brachial neuritis or radiculitis nos
953.4 Injury to brachial plexus
996.75 Other complications due to nervous system device, implant, and graft

ICD-9-CM Procedural

04.79 Other neuroplasty

64714

64714 Neuroplasty, major peripheral nerve, arm or leg; lumbar plexus

ICD-9-CM Diagnostic

353.1 Lumbosacral plexus lesions
724.2 Lumbago
724.4 Thoracic or lumbosacral neuritis or radiculitis, unspecified ▽
729.5 Pain in soft tissues of limb
953.5 Injury to lumbosacral plexus
996.75 Other complications due to nervous system device, implant, and graft

ICD-9-CM Procedural

04.79 Other neuroplasty

64716

64716 Neuroplasty and/or transposition; cranial nerve (specify)

ICD-9-CM Diagnostic

171.0 Malignant neoplasm of connective and other soft tissue of head, face, and neck
225.1 Benign neoplasm of cranial nerves
350.1 Trigeminal neuralgia
350.2 Atypical face pain
350.8 Other specified trigeminal nerve disorders
350.9 Unspecified trigeminal nerve disorder ▽
351.0 Bell's palsy
352.1 Glossopharyngeal neuralgia
352.6 Multiple cranial nerve palsies
907.1 Late effect of injury to cranial nerve
951.2 Injury to trigeminal nerve
951.4 Injury to facial nerve
998.2 Accidental puncture or laceration during procedure

ICD-9-CM Procedural

04.41 Decompression of trigeminal nerve root
04.6 Transposition of cranial and peripheral nerves
04.79 Other neuroplasty

64718

64718 Neuroplasty and/or transposition; ulnar nerve at elbow

ICD-9-CM Diagnostic

354.2 Lesion of ulnar nerve
354.5 Mononeuritis multiplex
356.8 Other specified idiopathic peripheral neuropathy
718.42 Contracture of upper arm joint
719.42 Pain in joint, upper arm
723.4 Brachial neuritis or radiculitis nos
727.41 Ganglion of joint
729.5 Pain in soft tissues of limb
782.0 Disturbance of skin sensation
906.1 Late effect of open wound of extremities without mention of tendon injury
907.4 Late effect of injury to peripheral nerve of shoulder girdle and upper limb
908.9 Late effect of unspecified injury ▽
909.3 Late effect of complications of surgical and medical care
955.2 Injury to ulnar nerve
955.9 Injury to unspecified nerve of shoulder girdle and upper limb ▽
996.75 Other complications due to nervous system device, implant, and graft

ICD-9-CM Procedural

04.49 Other peripheral nerve or ganglion decompression or lysis of adhesions
04.6 Transposition of cranial and peripheral nerves
04.79 Other neuroplasty

64719–64721

64719 Neuroplasty and/or transposition; ulnar nerve at wrist
64721 median nerve at carpal tunnel

ICD-9-CM Diagnostic

354.0 Carpal tunnel syndrome
354.2 Lesion of ulnar nerve
354.5 Mononeuritis multiplex
357.1 Polyneuropathy in collagen vascular disease — (Code first underlying disease: 446.0, 710.0, 714.0) ☒
359.6 Symptomatic inflammatory myopathy in diseases classified elsewhere — (Code first underlying disease: 135, 140.0-208.9, 277.3, 446.0, 710.0, 710.1, 710.2, 714.0) ☒
714.0 Rheumatoid arthritis — (Use additional code to identify manifestation: 357.1, 359.6)
715.94 Osteoarthrosis, unspecified whether generalized or localized, hand ▽
716.14 Traumatic arthropathy, hand
719.44 Pain in joint, hand
723.4 Brachial neuritis or radiculitis nos
726.4 Enthesopathy of wrist and carpus
727.04 Radial styloid tenosynovitis
727.41 Ganglion of joint
728.6 Contracture of palmar fascia
729.5 Pain in soft tissues of limb
782.0 Disturbance of skin sensation
794.17 Nonspecific abnormal electromyogram (EMG)
906.1 Late effect of open wound of extremities without mention of tendon injury
907.4 Late effect of injury to peripheral nerve of shoulder girdle and upper limb
908.9 Late effect of unspecified injury ▽
909.3 Late effect of complications of surgical and medical care
955.1 Injury to median nerve
955.2 Injury to ulnar nerve

ICD-9-CM Procedural

04.43 Release of carpal tunnel
04.49 Other peripheral nerve or ganglion decompression or lysis of adhesions
04.6 Transposition of cranial and peripheral nerves
04.79 Other neuroplasty

64722

64722 Decompression; unspecified nerve(s) (specify)

ICD-9-CM Diagnostic

The application of this code is too broad to adequately present ICD-9-CM diagnostic code links here. Refer to your ICD-9-CM book.

ICD-9-CM Procedural

04.42 Other cranial nerve decompression
04.49 Other peripheral nerve or ganglion decompression or lysis of adhesions

64726

64726 Decompression; plantar digital nerve

ICD-9-CM Diagnostic

355.5 Tarsal tunnel syndrome
355.6 Lesion of plantar nerve
355.71 Causalgia of lower limb

ICD-9-CM Procedural

04.49 Other peripheral nerve or ganglion decompression or lysis of adhesions

HCPCS Level II Supplies & Services

A4550 Surgical trays

64727

64727 Internal neurolysis, requiring use of operating microscope (List separately in addition to code for neuroplasty) (Neuroplasty includes external neurolysis)

ICD-9-CM Diagnostic

This is an add-on code. Refer to the corresponding primary procedure code for ICD-9 diagnosis code links.

ICD-9-CM Procedural

04.41 Decompression of trigeminal nerve root
04.42 Other cranial nerve decompression
04.43 Release of carpal tunnel
04.49 Other peripheral nerve or ganglion decompression or lysis of adhesions
04.6 Transposition of cranial and peripheral nerves
04.79 Other neuroplasty

64732

64732 Transection or avulsion of; supraorbital nerve

ICD-9-CM Diagnostic

190.1 Malignant neoplasm of orbit
238.8 Neoplasm of uncertain behavior of other specified sites
802.6 Orbital floor (blow-out), closed fracture
870.3 Penetrating wound of orbit, without mention of foreign body — (Use additional code to identify infection)
871.1 Ocular laceration with prolapse or exposure of intraocular tissue — (Use additional code to identify infection)
873.52 Open wound of forehead, complicated — (Use additional code to identify infection)
925.1 Crushing injury of face and scalp — (Use additional code to identify any associated injuries: 800-829, 850.0-854.1, 860.0-869.1)
959.01 Head injury, unspecified ▽
959.09 Injury of face and neck, other and unspecified

ICD-9-CM Procedural

04.07 Other excision or avulsion of cranial and peripheral nerves

64734

64734 Transection or avulsion of; infraorbital nerve

ICD-9-CM Diagnostic

171.0 Malignant neoplasm of connective and other soft tissue of head, face, and neck
225.1 Benign neoplasm of cranial nerves
238.1 Neoplasm of uncertain behavior of connective and other soft tissue ▽
239.2 Neoplasms of unspecified nature of bone, soft tissue, and skin
350.1 Trigeminal neuralgia
350.2 Atypical face pain
350.8 Other specified trigeminal nerve disorders
729.6 Residual foreign body in soft tissue
784.2 Swelling, mass, or lump in head and neck
907.1 Late effect of injury to cranial nerve
925.1 Crushing injury of face and scalp — (Use additional code to identify any associated injuries: 800-829, 850.0-854.1, 860.0-869.1)
951.2 Injury to trigeminal nerve

ICD-9-CM Procedural

04.07 Other excision or avulsion of cranial and peripheral nerves

▽ Unspecified code ♀ Female diagnosis ☒ Manifestation code ♂ Male diagnosis

64736

64736 Transection or avulsion of; mental nerve

ICD-9-CM Diagnostic

171.0 Malignant neoplasm of connective and other soft tissue of head, face, and neck
225.1 Benign neoplasm of cranial nerves
238.1 Neoplasm of uncertain behavior of connective and other soft tissue ▽
239.2 Neoplasms of unspecified nature of bone, soft tissue, and skin
350.1 Trigeminal neuralgia
350.2 Atypical face pain
350.8 Other specified trigeminal nerve disorders
784.0 Headache
907.1 Late effect of injury to cranial nerve
951.2 Injury to trigeminal nerve

ICD-9-CM Procedural

04.07 Other excision or avulsion of cranial and peripheral nerves

64738

64738 Transection or avulsion of; inferior alveolar nerve by osteotomy

ICD-9-CM Diagnostic

171.0 Malignant neoplasm of connective and other soft tissue of head, face, and neck
225.1 Benign neoplasm of cranial nerves
238.1 Neoplasm of uncertain behavior of connective and other soft tissue ▽
239.2 Neoplasms of unspecified nature of bone, soft tissue, and skin
350.1 Trigeminal neuralgia
350.2 Atypical face pain
907.1 Late effect of injury to cranial nerve
951.2 Injury to trigeminal nerve

ICD-9-CM Procedural

04.07 Other excision or avulsion of cranial and peripheral nerves

64740

64740 Transection or avulsion of; lingual nerve

ICD-9-CM Diagnostic

171.0 Malignant neoplasm of connective and other soft tissue of head, face, and neck
225.1 Benign neoplasm of cranial nerves
238.1 Neoplasm of uncertain behavior of connective and other soft tissue ▽
239.2 Neoplasms of unspecified nature of bone, soft tissue, and skin
350.1 Trigeminal neuralgia
350.8 Other specified trigeminal nerve disorders
729.6 Residual foreign body in soft tissue
907.1 Late effect of injury to cranial nerve
951.2 Injury to trigeminal nerve

ICD-9-CM Procedural

04.07 Other excision or avulsion of cranial and peripheral nerves

64742

64742 Transection or avulsion of; facial nerve, differential or complete

ICD-9-CM Diagnostic

192.0 Malignant neoplasm of cranial nerves
237.9 Neoplasm of uncertain behavior of other and unspecified parts of nervous system ▽
350.2 Atypical face pain
351.1 Geniculate ganglionitis
729.2 Unspecified neuralgia, neuritis, and radiculitis ▽
784.2 Swelling, mass, or lump in head and neck
802.8 Other facial bones, closed fracture
873.51 Open wound of cheek, complicated — (Use additional code to identify infection)
925.1 Crushing injury of face and scalp — (Use additional code to identify any associated injuries: 800-829, 850.0-854.1, 860.0-869.1)
959.01 Head injury, unspecified ▽
959.09 Injury of face and neck, other and unspecified

ICD-9-CM Procedural

04.07 Other excision or avulsion of cranial and peripheral nerves

64744

64744 Transection or avulsion of; greater occipital nerve

ICD-9-CM Diagnostic

237.5 Neoplasm of uncertain behavior of brain and spinal cord
346.21 Variants of migraine with intractable migraine, so stated
353.2 Cervical root lesions, not elsewhere classified
729.2 Unspecified neuralgia, neuritis, and radiculitis ▽
805.01 Closed fracture of first cervical vertebra without mention of spinal cord injury
847.0 Neck sprain and strain
925.2 Crushing injury of neck — (Use additional code to identify any associated injuries: 800-829, 850.0-854.1, 860.0-869.1)
959.01 Head injury, unspecified ▽
959.09 Injury of face and neck, other and unspecified

ICD-9-CM Procedural

04.07 Other excision or avulsion of cranial and peripheral nerves

64746

64746 Transection or avulsion of; phrenic nerve

ICD-9-CM Diagnostic

519.4 Disorders of diaphragm
786.8 Hiccough

ICD-9-CM Procedural

04.07 Other excision or avulsion of cranial and peripheral nerves
33.31 Destruction of phrenic nerve for collapse of lung

64752–64760

64752 Transection or avulsion of; vagus nerve (vagotomy), transthoracic
64755 vagus nerves limited to proximal stomach (selective proximal vagotomy, proximal gastric vagotomy, parietal cell vagotomy, supra- or highly selective vagotomy)
64760 vagus nerve (vagotomy), abdominal

ICD-9-CM Diagnostic

150.2 Malignant neoplasm of abdominal esophagus
155.0 Malignant neoplasm of liver, primary
159.1 Malignant neoplasm of spleen, not elsewhere classified
192.0 Malignant neoplasm of cranial nerves
235.2 Neoplasm of uncertain behavior of stomach, intestines, and rectum
237.71 Neurofibromatosis, Type 1 (von Recklinghausen's disease)
237.9 Neoplasm of uncertain behavior of other and unspecified parts of nervous system ▽
352.3 Disorders of pneumogastric (10th) nerve
531.70 Chronic gastric ulcer without mention of hemorrhage, perforation, without mention of obstruction — (Use additional E code to identify drug, if drug induced)
533.40 Chronic or unspecified peptic ulcer, unspecified site, with hemorrhage, without mention of obstruction — (Use additional E code to identify drug, if drug induced)
750.3 Congenital tracheoesophageal fistula, esophageal atresia and stenosis
951.8 Injury to other specified cranial nerves
V64.41 Laparoscopic surgical procedure converted to open procedure

ICD-9-CM Procedural

04.07 Other excision or avulsion of cranial and peripheral nerves
44.00 Vagotomy, not otherwise specified
44.01 Truncal vagotomy
44.02 Highly selective vagotomy
44.03 Other selective vagotomy

64761

64761 Transection or avulsion of; pudendal nerve

ICD-9-CM Diagnostic

198.82 Secondary malignant neoplasm of genital organs
236.3 Neoplasm of uncertain behavior of other and unspecified female genital organs ▽ ♀
623.2 Stricture or atresia of vagina — (Use additional E code to identify any external cause) ♀
625.0 Dyspareunia ♀
669.81 Other complication of labor and delivery, delivered, with or without mention of antepartum condition ♀

▽ Unspecified code
♀ Female diagnosis
☒ Manifestation code
♂ Male diagnosis

956.5 Injury to other specified nerve(s) of pelvic girdle and lower limb

ICD-9-CM Procedural

04.07 Other excision or avulsion of cranial and peripheral nerves

64763–64766

64763 Transection or avulsion of obturator nerve, extrapelvic, with or without adductor tenotomy

64766 Transection or avulsion of obturator nerve, intrapelvic, with or without adductor tenotomy

ICD-9-CM Diagnostic

171.3 Malignant neoplasm of connective and other soft tissue of lower limb, including hip
198.89 Secondary malignant neoplasm of other specified sites
215.3 Other benign neoplasm of connective and other soft tissue of lower limb, including hip
225.8 Benign neoplasm of other specified sites of nervous system
237.71 Neurofibromatosis, Type 1 (von Recklinghausen's disease)
238.1 Neoplasm of uncertain behavior of connective and other soft tissue
239.2 Neoplasms of unspecified nature of bone, soft tissue, and skin
351.1 Geniculate ganglionitis
353.6 Phantom limb (syndrome)
355.71 Causalgia of lower limb
355.9 Mononeuritis of unspecified site
729.2 Unspecified neuralgia, neuritis, and radiculitis
907.5 Late effect of injury to peripheral nerve of pelvic girdle and lower limb
956.5 Injury to other specified nerve(s) of pelvic girdle and lower limb

ICD-9-CM Procedural

04.07 Other excision or avulsion of cranial and peripheral nerves
83.12 Adductor tenotomy of hip

64771

64771 Transection or avulsion of other cranial nerve, extradural

ICD-9-CM Diagnostic

171.0 Malignant neoplasm of connective and other soft tissue of head, face, and neck
192.0 Malignant neoplasm of cranial nerves
350.2 Atypical face pain
351.1 Geniculate ganglionitis
352.0 Disorders of olfactory (1st) nerve
729.2 Unspecified neuralgia, neuritis, and radiculitis
784.2 Swelling, mass, or lump in head and neck
803.09 Other closed skull fracture without mention of intracranial injury, unspecified concussion
925.1 Crushing injury of face and scalp — (Use additional code to identify any associated injuries: 800-829, 850.0-854.1, 860.0-869.1)
951.2 Injury to trigeminal nerve
959.01 Head injury, unspecified
959.09 Injury of face and neck, other and unspecified

ICD-9-CM Procedural

04.07 Other excision or avulsion of cranial and peripheral nerves

64772

64772 Transection or avulsion of other spinal nerve, extradural

ICD-9-CM Diagnostic

237.71 Neurofibromatosis, Type 1 (von Recklinghausen's disease)
353.6 Phantom limb (syndrome)
354.4 Causalgia of upper limb
355.1 Meralgia paresthetica
716.15 Traumatic arthropathy, pelvic region and thigh
729.2 Unspecified neuralgia, neuritis, and radiculitis
879.4 Open wound of abdominal wall, lateral, without mention of complication — (Use additional code to identify infection)
926.11 Crushing injury of back — (Use additional code to identify any associated injuries: 800-829, 850.0-854.1, 860.0-869.1)
953.4 Injury to brachial plexus
954.1 Injury to other sympathetic nerve, excluding shoulder and pelvic girdles
955.3 Injury to radial nerve

ICD-9-CM Procedural

03.1 Division of intraspinal nerve root
04.07 Other excision or avulsion of cranial and peripheral nerves
07.42 Division of nerves to adrenal glands

64774

64774 Excision of neuroma; cutaneous nerve, surgically identifiable

ICD-9-CM Diagnostic

The application of this code is too broad to adequately present ICD-9-CM diagnostic code links here. Refer to your ICD-9-CM book.

ICD-9-CM Procedural

04.07 Other excision or avulsion of cranial and peripheral nerves

64776–64778

64776 Excision of neuroma; digital nerve, one or both, same digit

64778 digital nerve, each additional digit (List separately in addition to code for primary procedure)

ICD-9-CM Diagnostic

237.70 Neurofibromatosis, unspecified
354.9 Unspecified mononeuritis of upper limb
355.6 Lesion of plantar nerve
356.4 Idiopathic progressive polyneuropathy
782.2 Localized superficial swelling, mass, or lump

ICD-9-CM Procedural

04.07 Other excision or avulsion of cranial and peripheral nerves

HCPCS Level II Supplies & Services

A4550 Surgical trays

64782–64783

64782 Excision of neuroma; hand or foot, except digital nerve

64783 hand or foot, each additional nerve, except same digit (List separately in addition to code for primary procedure)

ICD-9-CM Diagnostic

215.2 Other benign neoplasm of connective and other soft tissue of upper limb, including shoulder
215.3 Other benign neoplasm of connective and other soft tissue of lower limb, including hip
354.8 Other mononeuritis of upper limb
355.8 Unspecified mononeuritis of lower limb
729.2 Unspecified neuralgia, neuritis, and radiculitis
729.5 Pain in soft tissues of limb
782.0 Disturbance of skin sensation
782.2 Localized superficial swelling, mass, or lump
955.7 Injury to other specified nerve(s) of shoulder girdle and upper limb
955.8 Injury to multiple nerves of shoulder girdle and upper limb
955.9 Injury to unspecified nerve of shoulder girdle and upper limb
956.5 Injury to other specified nerve(s) of pelvic girdle and lower limb
956.8 Injury to multiple nerves of pelvic girdle and lower limb
956.9 Injury to unspecified nerve of pelvic girdle and lower limb

ICD-9-CM Procedural

04.07 Other excision or avulsion of cranial and peripheral nerves

HCPCS Level II Supplies & Services

A4550 Surgical trays

64784

64784 Excision of neuroma; major peripheral nerve, except sciatic

ICD-9-CM Diagnostic

215.2 Other benign neoplasm of connective and other soft tissue of upper limb, including shoulder
215.3 Other benign neoplasm of connective and other soft tissue of lower limb, including hip
353.6 Phantom limb (syndrome)
729.5 Pain in soft tissues of limb

ICD-9-CM Procedural

04.06 Other cranial or peripheral ganglionectomy
04.07 Other excision or avulsion of cranial and peripheral nerves

64786

64786 Excision of neuroma; sciatic nerve

ICD-9-CM Diagnostic

215.3 Other benign neoplasm of connective and other soft tissue of lower limb, including hip
237.70 Neurofibromatosis, unspecified ▽
355.0 Lesion of sciatic nerve
355.71 Causalgia of lower limb
724.3 Sciatica
729.5 Pain in soft tissues of limb

ICD-9-CM Procedural

04.06 Other cranial or peripheral ganglionectomy
04.07 Other excision or avulsion of cranial and peripheral nerves

64787

64787 Implantation of nerve end into bone or muscle (List separately in addition to neuroma excision)

ICD-9-CM Diagnostic

This is an add-on code. Refer to the corresponding primary procedure code for ICD-9 diagnosis code links.

ICD-9-CM Procedural

04.07 Other excision or avulsion of cranial and peripheral nerves

64788–64792

64788 Excision of neurofibroma or neurolemmoma; cutaneous nerve
64790 major peripheral nerve
64792 extensive (including malignant type)

ICD-9-CM Diagnostic

171.0 Malignant neoplasm of connective and other soft tissue of head, face, and neck
171.2 Malignant neoplasm of connective and other soft tissue of upper limb, including shoulder
171.3 Malignant neoplasm of connective and other soft tissue of lower limb, including hip
171.4 Malignant neoplasm of connective and other soft tissue of thorax
171.5 Malignant neoplasm of connective and other soft tissue of abdomen
171.6 Malignant neoplasm of connective and other soft tissue of pelvis
171.7 Malignant neoplasm of connective and other soft tissue of trunk, unspecified site ▽
171.9 Malignant neoplasm of connective and other soft tissue, site unspecified ▽
215.0 Other benign neoplasm of connective and other soft tissue of head, face, and neck
215.2 Other benign neoplasm of connective and other soft tissue of upper limb, including shoulder
215.3 Other benign neoplasm of connective and other soft tissue of lower limb, including hip
215.4 Other benign neoplasm of connective and other soft tissue of thorax
215.5 Other benign neoplasm of connective and other soft tissue of abdomen
215.6 Other benign neoplasm of connective and other soft tissue of pelvis
215.7 Other benign neoplasm of connective and other soft tissue of trunk, unspecified ▽
215.9 Other benign neoplasm of connective and other soft tissue of unspecified site ▽
237.70 Neurofibromatosis, unspecified ▽
237.71 Neurofibromatosis, Type 1 (von Recklinghausen's disease)
237.72 Neurofibromatosis, Type 2 (acoustic neurofibromatosis)
238.1 Neoplasm of uncertain behavior of connective and other soft tissue ▽
353.9 Unspecified nerve root and plexus disorder ▽
354.3 Lesion of radial nerve
354.8 Other mononeuritis of upper limb
354.9 Unspecified mononeuritis of upper limb ▽
355.6 Lesion of plantar nerve
355.71 Causalgia of lower limb
355.9 Mononeuritis of unspecified site ▽
729.5 Pain in soft tissues of limb

ICD-9-CM Procedural

04.07 Other excision or avulsion of cranial and peripheral nerves

64795

64795 Biopsy of nerve

ICD-9-CM Diagnostic

171.0 Malignant neoplasm of connective and other soft tissue of head, face, and neck
195.0 Malignant neoplasm of head, face, and neck
198.4 Secondary malignant neoplasm of other parts of nervous system
215.0 Other benign neoplasm of connective and other soft tissue of head, face, and neck
234.8 Carcinoma in situ of other specified sites
237.70 Neurofibromatosis, unspecified ▽
238.1 Neoplasm of uncertain behavior of connective and other soft tissue ▽
239.2 Neoplasms of unspecified nature of bone, soft tissue, and skin
350.8 Other specified trigeminal nerve disorders

ICD-9-CM Procedural

04.12 Open biopsy of cranial or peripheral nerve or ganglion
04.19 Other diagnostic procedures on cranial and peripheral nerves and ganglia
05.11 Biopsy of sympathetic nerve or ganglion

HCPCS Level II Supplies & Services

A4305 Disposable drug delivery system, flow rate of 50 ml or greater per hour
A4306 Disposable drug delivery system, flow rate of 5 ml or less per hour
A4550 Surgical trays

64802–64804

64802 Sympathectomy, cervical
64804 Sympathectomy, cervicothoracic

ICD-9-CM Diagnostic

198.89 Secondary malignant neoplasm of other specified sites
238.1 Neoplasm of uncertain behavior of connective and other soft tissue ▽
239.2 Neoplasms of unspecified nature of bone, soft tissue, and skin
277.3 Amyloidosis — (Use additional code to identify any associated mental retardation)
337.1 Peripheral autonomic neuropathy in disorders classified elsewhere — (Code first underlying disease: 250.6, 277.3) ☒
353.2 Cervical root lesions, not elsewhere classified
353.3 Thoracic root lesions, not elsewhere classified
354.4 Causalgia of upper limb
354.5 Mononeuritis multiplex
780.8 Generalized hyperhidrosis

ICD-9-CM Procedural

05.22 Cervical sympathectomy

64809

64809 Sympathectomy, thoracolumbar

ICD-9-CM Diagnostic

198.89 Secondary malignant neoplasm of other specified sites
238.1 Neoplasm of uncertain behavior of connective and other soft tissue ▽
239.2 Neoplasms of unspecified nature of bone, soft tissue, and skin
353.1 Lumbosacral plexus lesions
353.3 Thoracic root lesions, not elsewhere classified
355.71 Causalgia of lower limb
724.4 Thoracic or lumbosacral neuritis or radiculitis, unspecified ▽

ICD-9-CM Procedural

05.23 Lumbar sympathectomy

64818

64818 Sympathectomy, lumbar

ICD-9-CM Diagnostic

238.1 Neoplasm of uncertain behavior of connective and other soft tissue ▽
239.2 Neoplasms of unspecified nature of bone, soft tissue, and skin
337.9 Unspecified disorder of autonomic nervous system ▽
353.1 Lumbosacral plexus lesions
353.4 Lumbosacral root lesions, not elsewhere classified
354.4 Causalgia of upper limb
724.4 Thoracic or lumbosacral neuritis or radiculitis, unspecified ▽
729.5 Pain in soft tissues of limb
736.71 Acquired equinovarus deformity

▽ Unspecified code ☒ Manifestation code
♀ Female diagnosis ♂ Male diagnosis

ICD-9-CM Procedural

05.23 Lumbar sympathectomy

64820–64823

64820 Sympathectomy; digital arteries, each digit
64821 radial artery
64822 ulnar artery
64823 superficial palmar arch

ICD-9-CM Diagnostic

277.3 Amyloidosis — (Use additional code to identify any associated mental retardation)
337.1 Peripheral autonomic neuropathy in disorders classified elsewhere — (Code first underlying disease: 250.6, 277.3) ☒
354.2 Lesion of ulnar nerve
354.3 Lesion of radial nerve
354.4 Causalgia of upper limb
354.5 Mononeuritis multiplex
354.8 Other mononeuritis of upper limb
354.9 Unspecified mononeuritis of upper limb ▽
729.5 Pain in soft tissues of limb

ICD-9-CM Procedural

05.25 Periarterial sympathectomy
05.29 Other sympathectomy and ganglionectomy

64831–64832

64831 Suture of digital nerve, hand or foot; one nerve
64832 each additional digital nerve (List separately in addition to code for primary procedure)

ICD-9-CM Diagnostic

816.11 Open fracture of middle or proximal phalanx or phalanges of hand
882.2 Open wound of hand except finger(s) alone, with tendon involvement — (Use additional code to identify infection)
883.0 Open wound of finger(s), without mention of complication — (Use additional code to identify infection)
883.2 Open wound of finger(s), with tendon involvement — (Use additional code to identify infection)
892.1 Open wound of foot except toe(s) alone, complicated — (Use additional code to identify infection)
893.0 Open wound of toe(s), without mention of complication — (Use additional code to identify infection)
893.2 Open wound of toe(s), with tendon involvement — (Use additional code to identify infection)
927.20 Crushing injury of hand(s) — (Use additional code to identify any associated injuries: 800-829, 850.0-854.1, 860.0-869.1)
927.3 Crushing injury of finger(s) — (Use additional code to identify any associated injuries: 800-829, 850.0-854.1, 860.0-869.1)
928.3 Crushing injury of toe(s) — (Use additional code to identify any associated injuries: 800-829, 850.0-854.1, 860.0-869.1)
955.6 Injury to digital nerve, upper limb
956.5 Injury to other specified nerve(s) of pelvic girdle and lower limb
959.5 Injury, other and unspecified, finger

ICD-9-CM Procedural

04.3 Suture of cranial and peripheral nerves

HCPCS Level II Supplies & Services

A4550 Surgical trays

64834–64837

64834 Suture of one nerve, hand or foot; common sensory nerve
64835 median motor thenar
64836 ulnar motor
64837 Suture of each additional nerve, hand or foot (List separately in addition to code for primary procedure)

ICD-9-CM Diagnostic

881.02 Open wound of wrist, without mention of complication — (Use additional code to identify infection)
881.22 Open wound of wrist, with tendon involvement — (Use additional code to identify infection)
882.0 Open wound of hand except finger(s) alone, without mention of complication — (Use additional code to identify infection)
883.0 Open wound of finger(s), without mention of complication — (Use additional code to identify infection)
892.0 Open wound of foot except toe(s) alone, without mention of complication — (Use additional code to identify infection)
893.0 Open wound of toe(s), without mention of complication — (Use additional code to identify infection)
927.21 Crushing injury of wrist — (Use additional code to identify any associated injuries: 800-829, 850.0-854.1, 860.0-869.1)
928.20 Crushing injury of foot — (Use additional code to identify any associated injuries: 800-829, 850.0-854.1, 860.0-869.1)
955.1 Injury to median nerve
955.2 Injury to ulnar nerve
955.5 Injury to cutaneous sensory nerve, upper limb
956.4 Injury to cutaneous sensory nerve, lower limb
956.5 Injury to other specified nerve(s) of pelvic girdle and lower limb
959.4 Injury, other and unspecified, hand, except finger

ICD-9-CM Procedural

04.3 Suture of cranial and peripheral nerves

HCPCS Level II Supplies & Services

A4550 Surgical trays

64840

64840 Suture of posterior tibial nerve

ICD-9-CM Diagnostic

891.0 Open wound of knee, leg (except thigh), and ankle, without mention of complication — (Use additional code to identify infection)
928.10 Crushing injury of lower leg — (Use additional code to identify any associated injuries: 800-829, 850.0-854.1, 860.0-869.1)
928.11 Crushing injury of knee — (Use additional code to identify any associated injuries: 800-829, 850.0-854.1, 860.0-869.1)
956.2 Injury to posterior tibial nerve

ICD-9-CM Procedural

04.3 Suture of cranial and peripheral nerves

HCPCS Level II Supplies & Services

A4550 Surgical trays

64856–64859

64856 Suture of major peripheral nerve, arm or leg, except sciatic; including transposition
64857 without transposition
64858 Suture of sciatic nerve
64859 Suture of each additional major peripheral nerve (List separately in addition to code for primary procedure)

ICD-9-CM Diagnostic

880.03 Open wound of upper arm, without mention of complication — (Use additional code to identify infection)
880.23 Open wound of upper arm, with tendon involvement — (Use additional code to identify infection)
881.02 Open wound of wrist, without mention of complication — (Use additional code to identify infection)
881.22 Open wound of wrist, with tendon involvement — (Use additional code to identify infection)
884.0 Multiple and unspecified open wound of upper limb, without mention of complication — (Use additional code to identify infection)
890.0 Open wound of hip and thigh, without mention of complication — (Use additional code to identify infection)
890.2 Open wound of hip and thigh, with tendon involvement — (Use additional code to identify infection)
891.0 Open wound of knee, leg (except thigh), and ankle, without mention of complication — (Use additional code to identify infection)
891.2 Open wound of knee, leg (except thigh), and ankle, with tendon involvement — (Use additional code to identify infection)
927.8 Crushing injury of multiple sites of upper limb — (Use additional code to identify any associated injuries: 800-829, 850.0-854.1, 860.0-869.1)
928.00 Crushing injury of thigh — (Use additional code to identify any associated injuries: 800-829, 850.0-854.1, 860.0-869.1)
928.10 Crushing injury of lower leg — (Use additional code to identify any associated injuries: 800-829, 850.0-854.1, 860.0-869.1)
955.0 Injury to axillary nerve
955.1 Injury to median nerve

955.2 Injury to ulnar nerve
955.3 Injury to radial nerve
955.7 Injury to other specified nerve(s) of shoulder girdle and upper limb
956.0 Injury to sciatic nerve
956.1 Injury to femoral nerve
956.3 Injury to peroneal nerve
956.5 Injury to other specified nerve(s) of pelvic girdle and lower limb

ICD-9-CM Procedural

04.3 Suture of cranial and peripheral nerves
04.6 Transposition of cranial and peripheral nerves

64861

64861 Suture of; brachial plexus

ICD-9-CM Diagnostic

880.03 Open wound of upper arm, without mention of complication — (Use additional code to identify infection)
927.00 Crushing injury of shoulder region — (Use additional code to identify any associated injuries: 800-829, 850.0-854.1, 860.0-869.1)
953.4 Injury to brachial plexus

ICD-9-CM Procedural

04.3 Suture of cranial and peripheral nerves

64862

64862 Suture of; lumbar plexus

ICD-9-CM Diagnostic

876.0 Open wound of back, without mention of complication — (Use additional code to identify infection)
876.1 Open wound of back, complicated — (Use additional code to identify infection)
877.0 Open wound of buttock, without mention of complication — (Use additional code to identify infection)
877.1 Open wound of buttock, complicated — (Use additional code to identify infection)
926.11 Crushing injury of back — (Use additional code to identify any associated injuries: 800-829, 850.0-854.1, 860.0-869.1)
953.5 Injury to lumbosacral plexus

ICD-9-CM Procedural

04.3 Suture of cranial and peripheral nerves

64864–64865

64864 Suture of facial nerve; extracranial
64865 infratemporal, with or without grafting

ICD-9-CM Diagnostic

872.8 Open wound of ear, part unspecified, without mention of complication — (Use additional code to identify infection) ▽
873.40 Open wound of face, unspecified site, without mention of complication — (Use additional code to identify infection) ▽
873.42 Open wound of forehead, without mention of complication — (Use additional code to identify infection)
873.50 Open wound of face, unspecified site, complicated — (Use additional code to identify infection) ▽
925.1 Crushing injury of face and scalp — (Use additional code to identify any associated injuries: 800-829, 850.0-854.1, 860.0-869.1)
951.4 Injury to facial nerve

ICD-9-CM Procedural

04.3 Suture of cranial and peripheral nerves
04.5 Cranial or peripheral nerve graft

64866–64870

64866 Anastomosis; facial-spinal accessory
64868 facial-hypoglossal
64870 facial-phrenic

ICD-9-CM Diagnostic

277.3 Amyloidosis — (Use additional code to identify any associated mental retardation)
307.0 Stuttering
351.0 Bell's palsy
352.4 Disorders of accessory (11th) nerve
352.5 Disorders of hypoglossal (12th) nerve
352.6 Multiple cranial nerve palsies
355.9 Mononeuritis of unspecified site ▽
357.4 Polyneuropathy in other diseases classified elsewhere — (Code first underlying disease: 032.0-032.9, 135, 251.2, 265.0, 265.2, 266.0-266.9, 277.1, 277.3, 585) ☒
527.8 Other specified diseases of the salivary glands
529.8 Other specified conditions of the tongue
782.62 Flushing
784.5 Other speech disturbance
803.90 Other open skull fracture with intracranial injury of other and unspecified nature, unspecified state of consciousness ▽
951.4 Injury to facial nerve
951.6 Injury to accessory nerve
951.7 Injury to hypoglossal nerve

ICD-9-CM Procedural

04.71 Hypoglossal-facial anastomosis
04.72 Accessory-facial anastomosis
04.74 Other anastomosis of cranial or peripheral nerve

64872–64876

64872 Suture of nerve; requiring secondary or delayed suture (list separately in addition to code for primary neurorrhaphy)
64874 requiring extensive mobilization, or transposition of nerve (list separately in addition to code for nerve suture)
64876 requiring shortening of bone of extremity (list separately in addition to code for nerve suture)

ICD-9-CM Diagnostic

This is an add-on code. Refer to the corresponding primary procedure code for ICD-9 diagnosis code links.

ICD-9-CM Procedural

04.3 Suture of cranial and peripheral nerves
04.6 Transposition of cranial and peripheral nerves
04.76 Repair of old traumatic injury of cranial and peripheral nerves
05.81 Repair of sympathetic nerve or ganglion
78.29 Limb shortening procedures, other

HCPCS Level II Supplies & Services

The HCPCS Level II code(s) would be the same as the actual procedure performed because these are in-addition-to codes.

64885–64886

64885 Nerve graft (includes obtaining graft), head or neck; up to 4 cm in length
64886 more than 4 cm in length

ICD-9-CM Diagnostic

171.0 Malignant neoplasm of connective and other soft tissue of head, face, and neck
225.1 Benign neoplasm of cranial nerves
873.54 Open wound of jaw, complicated — (Use additional code to identify infection)
905.0 Late effect of fracture of skull and face bones
906.0 Late effect of open wound of head, neck, and trunk
907.1 Late effect of injury to cranial nerve
951.2 Injury to trigeminal nerve
951.4 Injury to facial nerve
951.7 Injury to hypoglossal nerve
951.8 Injury to other specified cranial nerves

ICD-9-CM Procedural

04.5 Cranial or peripheral nerve graft

64890–64891

64890 Nerve graft (includes obtaining graft), single strand, hand or foot; up to 4 cm length
64891 more than 4 cm length

ICD-9-CM Diagnostic

171.2 Malignant neoplasm of connective and other soft tissue of upper limb, including shoulder
171.3 Malignant neoplasm of connective and other soft tissue of lower limb, including hip
215.2 Other benign neoplasm of connective and other soft tissue of upper limb, including shoulder

▽ Unspecified code ☒ Manifestation code
♀ Female diagnosis ♂ Male diagnosis

215.3 Other benign neoplasm of connective and other soft tissue of lower limb, including hip
238.1 Neoplasm of uncertain behavior of connective and other soft tissue ▽
239.2 Neoplasms of unspecified nature of bone, soft tissue, and skin
277.3 Amyloidosis — (Use additional code to identify any associated mental retardation)
354.0 Carpal tunnel syndrome
354.5 Mononeuritis multiplex
355.6 Lesion of plantar nerve
356.0 Hereditary peripheral neuropathy
356.4 Idiopathic progressive polyneuropathy
357.81 Chronic inflammatory demyelinating polyneuritis
357.82 Critical illness polyneuropathy
357.89 Other inflammatory and toxic neuropathy
359.6 Symptomatic inflammatory myopathy in diseases classified elsewhere — (Code first underlying disease: 135, 140.0-208.9, 277.3, 446.0, 710.0, 710.1, 710.2, 714.0) ☒
446.0 Polyarteritis nodosa
710.0 Systemic lupus erythematosus — (Use additional code to identify manifestation: 424.91, 581.81, 582.81, 583.81)
710.1 Systemic sclerosis — (Use additional code to identify manifestation: 359.6, 517.2)
710.2 Sicca syndrome
714.0 Rheumatoid arthritis — (Use additional code to identify manifestation: 357.1, 359.6)
882.1 Open wound of hand except finger(s) alone, complicated — (Use additional code to identify infection)
883.1 Open wound of finger(s), complicated — (Use additional code to identify infection)
892.1 Open wound of foot except toe(s) alone, complicated — (Use additional code to identify infection)
893.1 Open wound of toe(s), complicated — (Use additional code to identify infection)
927.20 Crushing injury of hand(s) — (Use additional code to identify any associated injuries: 800-829, 850.0-854.1, 860.0-869.1)
927.3 Crushing injury of finger(s) — (Use additional code to identify any associated injuries: 800-829, 850.0-854.1, 860.0-869.1)
928.20 Crushing injury of foot — (Use additional code to identify any associated injuries: 800-829, 850.0-854.1, 860.0-869.1)
928.3 Crushing injury of toe(s) — (Use additional code to identify any associated injuries: 800-829, 850.0-854.1, 860.0-869.1)

ICD-9-CM Procedural

04.5 Cranial or peripheral nerve graft

64892–64893

64892 Nerve graft (includes obtaining graft), single strand, arm or leg; up to 4 cm length
64893 more than 4 cm length

ICD-9-CM Diagnostic

171.2 Malignant neoplasm of connective and other soft tissue of upper limb, including shoulder
171.3 Malignant neoplasm of connective and other soft tissue of lower limb, including hip
215.2 Other benign neoplasm of connective and other soft tissue of upper limb, including shoulder
215.3 Other benign neoplasm of connective and other soft tissue of lower limb, including hip
238.1 Neoplasm of uncertain behavior of connective and other soft tissue ▽
239.2 Neoplasms of unspecified nature of bone, soft tissue, and skin
354.3 Lesion of radial nerve
355.0 Lesion of sciatic nerve
880.13 Open wound of upper arm, complicated — (Use additional code to identify infection)
881.10 Open wound of forearm, complicated — (Use additional code to identify infection)
890.1 Open wound of hip and thigh, complicated — (Use additional code to identify infection)
891.1 Open wound of knee, leg (except thigh), and ankle, complicated — (Use additional code to identify infection)
927.03 Crushing injury of upper arm — (Use additional code to identify any associated injuries: 800-829, 850.0-854.1, 860.0-869.1)
927.10 Crushing injury of forearm — (Use additional code to identify any associated injuries: 800-829, 850.0-854.1, 860.0-869.1)
928.00 Crushing injury of thigh — (Use additional code to identify any associated injuries: 800-829, 850.0-854.1, 860.0-869.1)
928.10 Crushing injury of lower leg — (Use additional code to identify any associated injuries: 800-829, 850.0-854.1, 860.0-869.1)
956.0 Injury to sciatic nerve

ICD-9-CM Procedural

04.5 Cranial or peripheral nerve graft

64895–64896

64895 Nerve graft (includes obtaining graft), multiple strands (cable), hand or foot; up to 4 cm length
64896 more than 4 cm length

ICD-9-CM Diagnostic

171.2 Malignant neoplasm of connective and other soft tissue of upper limb, including shoulder
171.3 Malignant neoplasm of connective and other soft tissue of lower limb, including hip
215.2 Other benign neoplasm of connective and other soft tissue of upper limb, including shoulder
215.3 Other benign neoplasm of connective and other soft tissue of lower limb, including hip
238.1 Neoplasm of uncertain behavior of connective and other soft tissue ▽
239.2 Neoplasms of unspecified nature of bone, soft tissue, and skin
277.3 Amyloidosis — (Use additional code to identify any associated mental retardation)
354.5 Mononeuritis multiplex
356.0 Hereditary peripheral neuropathy
356.4 Idiopathic progressive polyneuropathy
357.81 Chronic inflammatory demyelinating polyneuritis
357.82 Critical illness polyneuropathy
357.89 Other inflammatory and toxic neuropathy
359.6 Symptomatic inflammatory myopathy in diseases classified elsewhere — (Code first underlying disease: 135, 140.0-208.9, 277.3, 446.0, 710.0, 710.1, 710.2, 714.0) ☒
446.0 Polyarteritis nodosa
710.0 Systemic lupus erythematosus — (Use additional code to identify manifestation: 424.91, 581.81, 582.81, 583.81)
710.1 Systemic sclerosis — (Use additional code to identify manifestation: 359.6, 517.2)
710.2 Sicca syndrome
714.0 Rheumatoid arthritis — (Use additional code to identify manifestation: 357.1, 359.6)
882.1 Open wound of hand except finger(s) alone, complicated — (Use additional code to identify infection)
883.1 Open wound of finger(s), complicated — (Use additional code to identify infection)
892.1 Open wound of foot except toe(s) alone, complicated — (Use additional code to identify infection)
893.1 Open wound of toe(s), complicated — (Use additional code to identify infection)
927.20 Crushing injury of hand(s) — (Use additional code to identify any associated injuries: 800-829, 850.0-854.1, 860.0-869.1)
927.3 Crushing injury of finger(s) — (Use additional code to identify any associated injuries: 800-829, 850.0-854.1, 860.0-869.1)
928.20 Crushing injury of foot — (Use additional code to identify any associated injuries: 800-829, 850.0-854.1, 860.0-869.1)
928.3 Crushing injury of toe(s) — (Use additional code to identify any associated injuries: 800-829, 850.0-854.1, 860.0-869.1)
955.8 Injury to multiple nerves of shoulder girdle and upper limb
956.8 Injury to multiple nerves of pelvic girdle and lower limb

ICD-9-CM Procedural

04.5 Cranial or peripheral nerve graft

64897–64898

64897 Nerve graft (includes obtaining graft), multiple strands (cable), arm or leg; up to 4 cm length
64898 more than 4 cm length

ICD-9-CM Diagnostic

171.2 Malignant neoplasm of connective and other soft tissue of upper limb, including shoulder
171.3 Malignant neoplasm of connective and other soft tissue of lower limb, including hip

▽ Unspecified code ♀ Female diagnosis ☒ Manifestation code ♂ Male diagnosis

215.2 Other benign neoplasm of connective and other soft tissue of upper limb, including shoulder
215.3 Other benign neoplasm of connective and other soft tissue of lower limb, including hip
238.1 Neoplasm of uncertain behavior of connective and other soft tissue ▽
239.2 Neoplasms of unspecified nature of bone, soft tissue, and skin
277.3 Amyloidosis — (Use additional code to identify any associated mental retardation)
354.5 Mononeuritis multiplex
356.0 Hereditary peripheral neuropathy
356.4 Idiopathic progressive polyneuropathy
357.81 Chronic inflammatory demyelinating polyneuritis
357.82 Critical illness polyneuropathy
357.89 Other inflammatory and toxic neuropathy
359.6 Symptomatic inflammatory myopathy in diseases classified elsewhere — (Code first underlying disease: 135, 140.0-208.9, 277.3, 446.0, 710.0, 710.1, 710.2, 714.0) ☒
446.0 Polyarteritis nodosa
710.0 Systemic lupus erythematosus — (Use additional code to identify manifestation: 424.91, 581.81, 582.81, 583.81)
710.1 Systemic sclerosis — (Use additional code to identify manifestation: 359.6, 517.2)
710.2 Sicca syndrome
714.0 Rheumatoid arthritis — (Use additional code to identify manifestation: 357.1, 359.6)
881.10 Open wound of forearm, complicated — (Use additional code to identify infection)
891.0 Open wound of knee, leg (except thigh), and ankle, without mention of complication — (Use additional code to identify infection)
927.03 Crushing injury of upper arm — (Use additional code to identify any associated injuries: 800-829, 850.0-854.1, 860.0-869.1)
928.10 Crushing injury of lower leg — (Use additional code to identify any associated injuries: 800-829, 850.0-854.1, 860.0-869.1)
955.7 Injury to other specified nerve(s) of shoulder girdle and upper limb
956.5 Injury to other specified nerve(s) of pelvic girdle and lower limb

ICD-9-CM Procedural

04.5 Cranial or peripheral nerve graft

64901–64902

64901 Nerve graft, each additional nerve; single strand (List separately in addition to code for primary procedure)
64902 multiple strands (cable) (List separately in addition to code for primary procedure)

ICD-9-CM Diagnostic

This is an add-on code. Refer to the corresponding primary procedure code for ICD-9 diagnosis code links.

ICD-9-CM Procedural

04.5 Cranial or peripheral nerve graft

64905–64907

64905 Nerve pedicle transfer; first stage
64907 second stage

ICD-9-CM Diagnostic

The application of this code is too broad to adequately present ICD-9-CM diagnostic code links here. Refer to your ICD-9-CM book.

ICD-9-CM Procedural

04.5 Cranial or peripheral nerve graft

Eye and Ocular Adnexa

Eyeball

65091–65093

65091 Evisceration of ocular contents; without implant
65093 with implant

ICD-9-CM Diagnostic

360.00 Unspecified purulent endophthalmitis ▽
360.01 Acute endophthalmitis
360.02 Panophthalmitis
360.13 Parasitic endophthalmitis NOS
360.41 Blind hypotensive eye
360.42 Blind hypertensive eye
871.1 Ocular laceration with prolapse or exposure of intraocular tissue — (Use additional code to identify infection)
871.2 Rupture of eye with partial loss of intraocular tissue — (Use additional code to identify infection)
871.5 Penetration of eyeball with magnetic foreign body — (Use additional code to identify infection)
871.6 Penetration of eyeball with (nonmagnetic) foreign body — (Use additional code to identify infection)
V43.0 Eye globe replaced by other means — (This code is intended for use when these conditions are recorded as diagnoses or problems)
V52.2 Fitting and adjustment of artificial eye

ICD-9-CM Procedural

16.31 Removal of ocular contents with synchronous implant into scleral shell
16.39 Other evisceration of eyeball

HCPCS Level II Supplies & Services

V2623 Prosthetic eye, plastic, custom

65101–65105

65101 Enucleation of eye; without implant
65103 with implant, muscles not attached to implant
65105 with implant, muscles attached to implant

ICD-9-CM Diagnostic

190.0 Malignant neoplasm of eyeball, except conjunctiva, cornea, retina, and choroid
190.3 Malignant neoplasm of conjunctiva
190.4 Malignant neoplasm of cornea
190.5 Malignant neoplasm of retina
190.6 Malignant neoplasm of choroid
190.8 Malignant neoplasm of other specified sites of eye
234.0 Carcinoma in situ of eye
360.41 Blind hypotensive eye
360.42 Blind hypertensive eye
376.51 Enophthalmos due to atrophy of orbital tissue
376.52 Enophthalmos due to trauma or surgery
871.2 Rupture of eye with partial loss of intraocular tissue — (Use additional code to identify infection)
871.3 Avulsion of eye — (Use additional code to identify infection)
871.5 Penetration of eyeball with magnetic foreign body — (Use additional code to identify infection)
871.6 Penetration of eyeball with (nonmagnetic) foreign body — (Use additional code to identify infection)
V43.0 Eye globe replaced by other means — (This code is intended for use when these conditions are recorded as diagnoses or problems)
V52.2 Fitting and adjustment of artificial eye

ICD-9-CM Procedural

16.41 Enucleation of eyeball with synchronous implant into Tenon's capsule with attachment of muscles
16.42 Enucleation of eyeball with other synchronous implant
16.49 Other enucleation of eyeball

65110–65114

65110 Exenteration of orbit (does not include skin graft), removal of orbital contents; only
65112 with therapeutic removal of bone
65114 with muscle or myocutaneous flap

ICD-9-CM Diagnostic

170.0 Malignant neoplasm of bones of skull and face, except mandible
172.1 Malignant melanoma of skin of eyelid, including canthus
190.0 Malignant neoplasm of eyeball, except conjunctiva, cornea, retina, and choroid
190.2 Malignant neoplasm of lacrimal gland
190.3 Malignant neoplasm of conjunctiva
190.4 Malignant neoplasm of cornea
190.5 Malignant neoplasm of retina
190.6 Malignant neoplasm of choroid
190.8 Malignant neoplasm of other specified sites of eye

ICD-9-CM Procedural

16.51 Exenteration of orbit with removal of adjacent structures
16.52 Exenteration of orbit with therapeutic removal of orbital bone
16.59 Other exenteration of orbit
83.82 Graft of muscle or fascia

65125

65125 Modification of ocular implant with placement or replacement of pegs (eg, drilling receptacle for prosthesis appendage) (separate procedure)

ICD-9-CM Diagnostic

360.89 Other disorders of globe
996.59 Mechanical complication due to other implant and internal device, not elsewhere classified
V10.84 Personal history of malignant neoplasm of eye
V52.2 Fitting and adjustment of artificial eye

ICD-9-CM Procedural

16.69 Other secondary procedures after removal of eyeball
95.34 Ocular prosthetics

HCPCS Level II Supplies & Services

V2623 Prosthetic eye, plastic, custom

65130–65140

65130 Insertion of ocular implant secondary; after evisceration, in scleral shell
65135 after enucleation, muscles not attached to implant
65140 after enucleation, muscles attached to implant

ICD-9-CM Diagnostic

360.89 Other disorders of globe
V10.84 Personal history of malignant neoplasm of eye
V43.0 Eye globe replaced by other means — (This code is intended for use when these conditions are recorded as diagnoses or problems)
V52.2 Fitting and adjustment of artificial eye

ICD-9-CM Procedural

16.61 Secondary insertion of ocular implant

HCPCS Level II Supplies & Services

V2623 Prosthetic eye, plastic, custom

65150–65155

65150 Reinsertion of ocular implant; with or without conjunctival graft
65155 with use of foreign material for reinforcement and/or attachment of muscles to implant

ICD-9-CM Diagnostic

360.89 Other disorders of globe

996.59 Mechanical complication due to other implant and internal device, not elsewhere classified
998.51 Infected postoperative seroma — (Use additional code to identify organism)
998.59 Other postoperative infection — (Use additional code to identify infection)
V10.84 Personal history of malignant neoplasm of eye
V52.2 Fitting and adjustment of artificial eye

ICD-9-CM Procedural
10.42 Reconstruction of conjunctival cul-de-sac with free graft
10.43 Other reconstruction of conjunctival cul-de-sac
10.44 Other free graft to conjunctiva
16.62 Revision and reinsertion of ocular implant

HCPCS Level II Supplies & Services
V2623 Prosthetic eye, plastic, custom

65175
65175 Removal of ocular implant

ICD-9-CM Diagnostic
376.00 Unspecified acute inflammation of orbit
376.10 Unspecified chronic inflammation of orbit
379.91 Pain in or around eye
996.59 Mechanical complication due to other implant and internal device, not elsewhere classified
996.69 Infection and inflammatory reaction due to other internal prosthetic device, implant, and graft — (Use additional code to identify specified infections)
998.31 Disruption of internal operation wound
998.51 Infected postoperative seroma — (Use additional code to identify organism)
998.59 Other postoperative infection — (Use additional code to identify infection)

ICD-9-CM Procedural
16.71 Removal of ocular implant
97.31 Removal of eye prosthesis

HCPCS Level II Supplies & Services
V2623 Prosthetic eye, plastic, custom

65205–65210
65205 Removal of foreign body, external eye; conjunctival superficial
65210 conjunctival embedded (includes concretions), subconjunctival, or scleral nonperforating

ICD-9-CM Diagnostic
918.2 Superficial injury of conjunctiva
918.9 Other and unspecified superficial injuries of eye
930.1 Foreign body in conjunctival sac
930.8 Foreign body in other and combined sites on external eye

ICD-9-CM Procedural
10.0 Removal of embedded foreign body from conjunctiva by incision
98.21 Removal of superficial foreign body from eye without incision
98.22 Removal of other foreign body without incision from head and neck

HCPCS Level II Supplies & Services
A4550 Surgical trays
A6410 Eye pad, sterile, each
A6411 Eye pad, non-sterile, each
A6412 Eye patch, occlusive, each

65220–65222
65220 Removal of foreign body, external eye; corneal, without slit lamp
65222 corneal, with slit lamp

ICD-9-CM Diagnostic
918.1 Superficial injury of cornea
918.9 Other and unspecified superficial injuries of eye
930.0 Foreign body in cornea
930.8 Foreign body in other and combined sites on external eye

ICD-9-CM Procedural
11.1 Incision of cornea
98.21 Removal of superficial foreign body from eye without incision

HCPCS Level II Supplies & Services
A4550 Surgical trays
A6410 Eye pad, sterile, each
A6411 Eye pad, non-sterile, each
A6412 Eye patch, occlusive, each

65235
65235 Removal of foreign body, intraocular; from anterior chamber of eye or lens

ICD-9-CM Diagnostic
360.51 Foreign body, magnetic, in anterior chamber of eye
360.52 Foreign body, magnetic, in iris or ciliary body
360.53 Foreign body, magnetic, in lens
360.59 Intraocular foreign body, magnetic, in other or multiple sites
360.60 Foreign body, intraocular, unspecified
360.61 Foreign body in anterior chamber
360.62 Foreign body in iris or ciliary body
360.63 Foreign body in lens
360.69 Foreign body in other or multiple sites of eye
871.5 Penetration of eyeball with magnetic foreign body — (Use additional code to identify infection)
871.6 Penetration of eyeball with (nonmagnetic) foreign body — (Use additional code to identify infection)

ICD-9-CM Procedural
12.00 Removal of intraocular foreign body from anterior segment of eye, not otherwise specified
12.01 Removal of intraocular foreign body from anterior segment of eye with use of magnet
12.02 Removal of intraocular foreign body from anterior segment of eye without use of magnet
13.01 Removal of foreign body from lens with use of magnet

HCPCS Level II Supplies & Services
A4550 Surgical trays
A6410 Eye pad, sterile, each
A6411 Eye pad, non-sterile, each
A6412 Eye patch, occlusive, each

65260
65260 Removal of foreign body, intraocular; from posterior segment, magnetic extraction, anterior or posterior route

ICD-9-CM Diagnostic
360.50 Foreign body, magnetic, intraocular, unspecified
360.54 Foreign body, magnetic, in vitreous
360.55 Foreign body, magnetic, in posterior wall
360.59 Intraocular foreign body, magnetic, in other or multiple sites
871.5 Penetration of eyeball with magnetic foreign body — (Use additional code to identify infection)

ICD-9-CM Procedural
14.01 Removal of foreign body from posterior segment of eye with use of magnet

HCPCS Level II Supplies & Services
A4550 Surgical trays
A6410 Eye pad, sterile, each
A6411 Eye pad, non-sterile, each
A6412 Eye patch, occlusive, each

65265
65265 Removal of foreign body, intraocular; from posterior segment, nonmagnetic extraction

ICD-9-CM Diagnostic
360.60 Foreign body, intraocular, unspecified
360.64 Foreign body in vitreous
360.65 Foreign body in posterior wall of eye
360.69 Foreign body in other or multiple sites of eye
870.4 Penetrating wound of orbit with foreign body — (Use additional code to identify infection)
871.6 Penetration of eyeball with (nonmagnetic) foreign body — (Use additional code to identify infection)

ICD-9-CM Procedural
14.02 Removal of foreign body from posterior segment of eye without use of magnet

HCPCS Level II Supplies & Services

A4550 Surgical trays
A6410 Eye pad, sterile, each
A6411 Eye pad, non-sterile, each
A6412 Eye patch, occlusive, each

65270–65273

65270 Repair of laceration; conjunctiva, with or without nonperforating laceration sclera, direct closure
65272 conjunctiva, by mobilization and rearrangement, without hospitalization
65273 conjunctiva, by mobilization and rearrangement, with hospitalization

ICD-9-CM Diagnostic

871.0 Ocular laceration without prolapse of intraocular tissue — (Use additional code to identify infection)
871.4 Unspecified laceration of eye — (Use additional code to identify infection) ▽
871.9 Unspecified open wound of eyeball — (Use additional code to identify infection) ▽
918.2 Superficial injury of conjunctiva

ICD-9-CM Procedural

10.6 Repair of laceration of conjunctiva
12.81 Suture of laceration of sclera

HCPCS Level II Supplies & Services

A4550 Surgical trays
A6410 Eye pad, sterile, each
A6411 Eye pad, non-sterile, each
A6412 Eye patch, occlusive, each

65275–65285

65275 Repair of laceration; cornea, nonperforating, with or without removal foreign body
65280 cornea and/or sclera, perforating, not involving uveal tissue
65285 cornea and/or sclera, perforating, with reposition or resection of uveal tissue

ICD-9-CM Diagnostic

871.0 Ocular laceration without prolapse of intraocular tissue — (Use additional code to identify infection)
871.1 Ocular laceration with prolapse or exposure of intraocular tissue — (Use additional code to identify infection)
871.4 Unspecified laceration of eye — (Use additional code to identify infection) ▽
871.7 Unspecified ocular penetration — (Use additional code to identify infection) ▽
871.9 Unspecified open wound of eyeball — (Use additional code to identify infection) ▽
918.1 Superficial injury of cornea
930.0 Foreign body in cornea
930.1 Foreign body in conjunctival sac
930.8 Foreign body in other and combined sites on external eye

ICD-9-CM Procedural

11.51 Suture of corneal laceration
12.81 Suture of laceration of sclera
12.97 Other operations on iris
12.98 Other operations on ciliary body

HCPCS Level II Supplies & Services

A4305 Disposable drug delivery system, flow rate of 50 ml or greater per hour
A4306 Disposable drug delivery system, flow rate of 5 ml or less per hour
A4550 Surgical trays
A6410 Eye pad, sterile, each
A6411 Eye pad, non-sterile, each

65286

65286 Repair of laceration; application of tissue glue, wounds of cornea and/or sclera

ICD-9-CM Diagnostic

871.0 Ocular laceration without prolapse of intraocular tissue — (Use additional code to identify infection)
871.1 Ocular laceration with prolapse or exposure of intraocular tissue — (Use additional code to identify infection)
871.4 Unspecified laceration of eye — (Use additional code to identify infection) ▽
871.7 Unspecified ocular penetration — (Use additional code to identify infection) ▽
871.9 Unspecified open wound of eyeball — (Use additional code to identify infection) ▽
918.1 Superficial injury of cornea

ICD-9-CM Procedural

11.59 Other repair of cornea
12.89 Other operations on sclera
16.82 Repair of rupture of eyeball

HCPCS Level II Supplies & Services

A4305 Disposable drug delivery system, flow rate of 50 ml or greater per hour
A4306 Disposable drug delivery system, flow rate of 5 ml or less per hour
A4550 Surgical trays
A6410 Eye pad, sterile, each
A6411 Eye pad, non-sterile, each

65290

65290 Repair of wound, extraocular muscle, tendon and/or Tenon's capsule

ICD-9-CM Diagnostic

870.4 Penetrating wound of orbit with foreign body — (Use additional code to identify infection)
870.8 Other specified open wound of ocular adnexa — (Use additional code to identify infection)
871.6 Penetration of eyeball with (nonmagnetic) foreign body — (Use additional code to identify infection)

ICD-9-CM Procedural

16.81 Repair of wound of orbit
16.89 Other repair of injury of eyeball or orbit

Anterior Segment

65400–65410

65400 Excision of lesion, cornea (keratectomy, lamellar, partial), except pterygium
65410 Biopsy of cornea

ICD-9-CM Diagnostic

190.4 Malignant neoplasm of cornea
198.4 Secondary malignant neoplasm of other parts of nervous system
224.4 Benign neoplasm of cornea
234.0 Carcinoma in situ of eye
238.8 Neoplasm of uncertain behavior of other specified sites
239.8 Neoplasm of unspecified nature of other specified sites
370.01 Marginal corneal ulcer
370.03 Central corneal ulcer
370.55 Corneal abscess
371.00 Unspecified corneal opacity ▽
371.10 Unspecified corneal deposit ▽
371.11 Anterior pigmentations of cornea
371.12 Stromal pigmentations of cornea
371.13 Posterior pigmentations of cornea
371.14 Kayser-Fleischer ring
371.15 Other deposits of cornea associated with metabolic disorders
371.16 Argentous deposits of cornea
371.70 Unspecified corneal deformity ▽
371.89 Other corneal disorder

ICD-9-CM Procedural

11.22 Biopsy of cornea
11.49 Other removal or destruction of corneal lesion

HCPCS Level II Supplies & Services

A4550 Surgical trays
A6410 Eye pad, sterile, each
A6411 Eye pad, non-sterile, each
A6412 Eye patch, occlusive, each

65420–65426

65420 Excision or transposition of pterygium; without graft
65426 with graft

ICD-9-CM Diagnostic

372.40 Unspecified pterygium ▽
372.41 Peripheral ptergium, stationary

372.42 Peripheral pterygium, progressive
372.43 Central pterygium
372.44 Double pterygium
372.45 Recurrent pterygium
372.52 Pseudopterygium

ICD-9-CM Procedural

11.31 Transposition of pterygium
11.32 Excision of pterygium with corneal graft
11.39 Other excision of pterygium

HCPCS Level II Supplies & Services

A4305 Disposable drug delivery system, flow rate of 50 ml or greater per hour
A4306 Disposable drug delivery system, flow rate of 5 ml or less per hour
A4550 Surgical trays
A6410 Eye pad, sterile, each
A6411 Eye pad, non-sterile, each

65430

65430 Scraping of cornea, diagnostic, for smear and/or culture

ICD-9-CM Diagnostic

017.30 Tuberculosis of eye, confirmation unspecified — (Use additional code to identify manifestation: 363.13, 364.11, 370.31, 370.59, 379.09) ▽
017.32 Tuberculosis of eye, bacteriological or histological examination unknown (at present) — (Use additional code to identify manifestation: 363.13, 364.11, 370.31, 370.59, 379.09)
017.33 Tuberculosis of eye, tubercle bacilli found (in sputum) by microscopy — (Use additional code to identify manifestation: 363.13, 364.11, 370.31, 370.59, 379.09)
017.34 Tuberculosis of eye, tubercle bacilli not found (in sputum) by microscopy, but found by bacterial culture — (Use additional code to identify manifestation: 363.13, 364.11, 370.31, 370.59, 379.09)
017.35 Tuberculosis of eye, tubercle bacilli not found by bacteriological examination, but tuberculosis confirmed histologically — (Use additional code to identify manifestation: 363.13, 364.11, 370.31, 370.59, 379.09)
017.36 Tuberculosis of eye, tubercle bacilli not found by bacteriological or histological examination, but tuberculosis confirmed by other methods [inoculation of animals] — (Use additional code to identify manifestation: 363.13, 364.11, 370.31, 370.59, 379.09)
053.21 Herpes zoster keratoconjunctivitis
054.42 Dendritic keratitis
054.43 Herpes simplex disciform keratitis
077.1 Epidemic keratoconjunctivitis
090.3 Syphilitic interstitial keratitis
098.43 Gonococcal keratitis
370.00 Unspecified corneal ulcer ▽
370.01 Marginal corneal ulcer
370.03 Central corneal ulcer
370.21 Punctate keratitis
370.22 Macular keratitis
370.23 Filamentary keratitis
370.31 Phlyctenular keratoconjunctivitis — (Use additional code for any associated tuberculosis, 017.3)
370.40 Unspecified keratoconjunctivitis ▽
370.44 Keratitis or keratoconjunctivitis in exanthema — (Code first underlying condition: 050.0-052.9) ☒
370.49 Other unspecified keratoconjunctivitis
370.52 Diffuse interstitial keratitis
370.54 Sclerosing keratitis
370.55 Corneal abscess
370.8 Other forms of keratitis
371.00 Unspecified corneal opacity ▽
371.10 Unspecified corneal deposit ▽
371.70 Unspecified corneal deformity ▽
371.89 Other corneal disorder

ICD-9-CM Procedural

11.21 Scraping of cornea for smear or culture

HCPCS Level II Supplies & Services

A4305 Disposable drug delivery system, flow rate of 50 ml or greater per hour
A4306 Disposable drug delivery system, flow rate of 5 ml or less per hour
A4550 Surgical trays
A6410 Eye pad, sterile, each
A6411 Eye pad, non-sterile, each

65435–65436

65435 Removal of corneal epithelium; with or without chemocauterization (abrasion, curettage)
65436 with application of chelating agent (eg, EDTA)

ICD-9-CM Diagnostic

053.29 Other ophthalmic herpes zoster complications
054.43 Herpes simplex disciform keratitis
364.10 Unspecified chronic iridocyclitis ▽
371.40 Unspecified corneal degeneration ▽
371.41 Senile corneal changes
371.42 Recurrent erosion of cornea
371.43 Band-shaped keratopathy
371.44 Other calcerous degenerations of cornea
371.45 Keratomalacia NOS
371.46 Nodular degeneration of cornea
371.48 Peripheral degenerations of cornea
371.49 Other corneal degenerations
940.2 Alkaline chemical burn of cornea and conjunctival sac
940.3 Acid chemical burn of cornea and conjunctival sac
940.4 Other burn of cornea and conjunctival sac

ICD-9-CM Procedural

11.31 Transposition of pterygium
11.41 Mechanical removal of corneal epithelium
11.49 Other removal or destruction of corneal lesion

HCPCS Level II Supplies & Services

A4305 Disposable drug delivery system, flow rate of 50 ml or greater per hour
A4306 Disposable drug delivery system, flow rate of 5 ml or less per hour
A4550 Surgical trays
A4612 Battery cables; replacement for patient-owned ventilator
A6410 Eye pad, sterile, each

65450

65450 Destruction of lesion of cornea by cryotherapy, photocoagulation or thermocauterization

ICD-9-CM Diagnostic

054.43 Herpes simplex disciform keratitis
090.3 Syphilitic interstitial keratitis
190.4 Malignant neoplasm of cornea
224.4 Benign neoplasm of cornea
234.0 Carcinoma in situ of eye
238.8 Neoplasm of uncertain behavior of other specified sites
238.9 Neoplasm of uncertain behavior, site unspecified ▽
370.00 Unspecified corneal ulcer ▽
370.55 Corneal abscess
371.70 Unspecified corneal deformity ▽
371.89 Other corneal disorder

ICD-9-CM Procedural

11.42 Thermocauterization of corneal lesion
11.43 Cryotherapy of corneal lesion
11.49 Other removal or destruction of corneal lesion

HCPCS Level II Supplies & Services

A4305 Disposable drug delivery system, flow rate of 50 ml or greater per hour
A4306 Disposable drug delivery system, flow rate of 5 ml or less per hour
A4550 Surgical trays
A6410 Eye pad, sterile, each
A6411 Eye pad, non-sterile, each

65600

65600 Multiple punctures of anterior cornea (eg, for corneal erosion, tattoo)

ICD-9-CM Diagnostic

054.43 Herpes simplex disciform keratitis
090.3 Syphilitic interstitial keratitis
370.00 Unspecified corneal ulcer ▽
370.50 Unspecified interstitial keratitis ▽
370.55 Corneal abscess
371.40 Unspecified corneal degeneration ▽
371.41 Senile corneal changes
371.42 Recurrent erosion of cornea
371.43 Band-shaped keratopathy

▽ Unspecified code ♀ Female diagnosis ☒ Manifestation code ♂ Male diagnosis

Corneal Disease

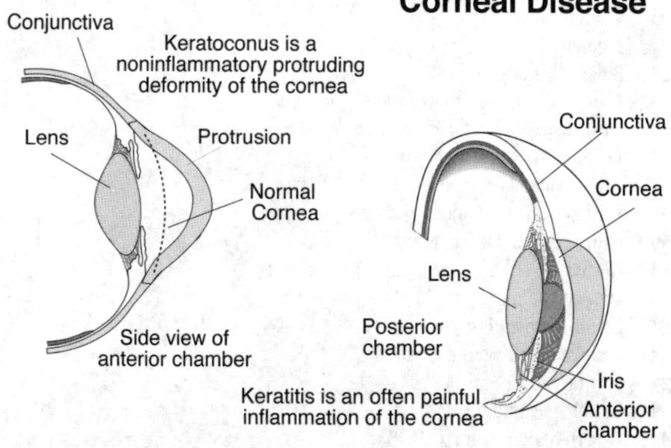

371.44 Other calcerous degenerations of cornea
371.45 Keratomalacia NOS
371.46 Nodular degeneration of cornea
371.48 Peripheral degenerations of cornea
371.49 Other corneal degenerations
371.70 Unspecified corneal deformity ▽
371.89 Other corneal disorder

ICD-9-CM Procedural
11.91 Tattooing of cornea

HCPCS Level II Supplies & Services
A4550 Surgical trays
A6410 Eye pad, sterile, each
A6411 Eye pad, non-sterile, each
A6412 Eye patch, occlusive, each

65710
65710 Keratoplasty (corneal transplant); lamellar

ICD-9-CM Diagnostic
371.01 Minor opacity of cornea
371.02 Peripheral opacity of cornea
371.03 Central opacity of cornea
371.11 Anterior pigmentations of cornea
371.12 Stromal pigmentations of cornea
371.13 Posterior pigmentations of cornea
371.30 Unspecified corneal membrane change ▽
371.41 Senile corneal changes
371.60 Unspecified keratoconus ▽
371.61 Keratoconus, stable condition
371.62 Keratoconus, acute hydrops
743.41 Congenital anomaly of corneal size and shape

ICD-9-CM Procedural
11.61 Lamellar keratoplasty with autograft
11.62 Other lamellar keratoplasty

HCPCS Level II Supplies & Services
C1818 Integrated keratoprosthesis

65730–65755
65730 Keratoplasty (corneal transplant); penetrating (except in aphakia)
65750 penetrating (in aphakia)
65755 penetrating (in pseudophakia)

ICD-9-CM Diagnostic
264.6 Vitamin A deficiency with xerophthalmic scars of cornea
370.06 Perforated corneal ulcer
370.63 Deep vascularization of cornea
370.8 Other forms of keratitis
371.02 Peripheral opacity of cornea
371.03 Central opacity of cornea
371.04 Adherent leucoma
371.11 Anterior pigmentations of cornea
371.16 Argentous deposits of cornea
371.20 Unspecified corneal edema ▽
371.23 Bullous keratopathy
371.31 Folds and rupture of Bowman's membrane
371.46 Nodular degeneration of cornea
371.53 Granular corneal dystrophy
371.60 Unspecified keratoconus ▽
371.62 Keratoconus, acute hydrops
379.31 Aphakia
743.35 Congenital aphakia
743.41 Congenital anomaly of corneal size and shape
743.42 Congenital corneal opacity, interfering with vision
871.0 Ocular laceration without prolapse of intraocular tissue — (Use additional code to identify infection)
871.1 Ocular laceration with prolapse or exposure of intraocular tissue — (Use additional code to identify infection)
871.5 Penetration of eyeball with magnetic foreign body — (Use additional code to identify infection)
871.6 Penetration of eyeball with (nonmagnetic) foreign body — (Use additional code to identify infection)
871.9 Unspecified open wound of eyeball — (Use additional code to identify infection) ▽
940.2 Alkaline chemical burn of cornea and conjunctival sac
996.51 Mechanical complication due to corneal graft
V43.1 Lens replaced by other means — (This code is intended for use when these conditions are recorded as diagnoses or problems)

ICD-9-CM Procedural
11.63 Penetrating keratoplasty with autograft
11.64 Other penetrating keratoplasty

HCPCS Level II Supplies & Services
C1818 Integrated keratoprosthesis

65760
65760 Keratomileusis

ICD-9-CM Diagnostic
367.89 Other disorders of refraction and accommodation
367.9 Unspecified disorder of refraction and accommodation ▽
371.61 Keratoconus, stable condition
371.62 Keratoconus, acute hydrops
371.70 Unspecified corneal deformity ▽

ICD-9-CM Procedural
11.71 Keratomileusis

HCPCS Level II Supplies & Services
C1818 Integrated keratoprosthesis
V2785 Processing, preserving and transporting corneal tissue

65765
65765 Keratophakia

ICD-9-CM Diagnostic
367.1 Myopia
367.89 Other disorders of refraction and accommodation
367.9 Unspecified disorder of refraction and accommodation ▽

ICD-9-CM Procedural
11.72 Keratophakia

65767
65767 Epikeratoplasty

ICD-9-CM Diagnostic
367.1 Myopia
367.89 Other disorders of refraction and accommodation
367.9 Unspecified disorder of refraction and accommodation ▽
371.61 Keratoconus, stable condition
379.31 Aphakia
743.35 Congenital aphakia
996.53 Mechanical complication due to ocular lens prosthesis

ICD-9-CM Procedural
11.76 Epikeratophakia

65770

65770 Keratoprosthesis

ICD-9-CM Diagnostic

076.1 Active stage trachoma
694.61 Benign mucous membrane pemphigoid with ocular involvement
695.1 Erythema multiforme
871.0 Ocular laceration without prolapse of intraocular tissue — (Use additional code to identify infection)
871.2 Rupture of eye with partial loss of intraocular tissue — (Use additional code to identify infection)
906.5 Late effect of burn of eye, face, head, and neck
940.2 Alkaline chemical burn of cornea and conjunctival sac
940.3 Acid chemical burn of cornea and conjunctival sac
940.4 Other burn of cornea and conjunctival sac
996.51 Mechanical complication due to corneal graft

ICD-9-CM Procedural

11.73 Keratoprosthesis

65771

65771 Radial keratotomy

ICD-9-CM Diagnostic

367.1 Myopia
367.20 Unspecified astigmatism ▽
367.22 Irregular astigmatism

ICD-9-CM Procedural

11.75 Radial keratotomy

HCPCS Level II Supplies & Services

A4305 Disposable drug delivery system, flow rate of 50 ml or greater per hour
A4306 Disposable drug delivery system, flow rate of 5 ml or less per hour
A4550 Surgical trays
A6410 Eye pad, sterile, each
A6411 Eye pad, non-sterile, each
C1818 Integrated keratoprosthesis

65772–65775

65772 Corneal relaxing incision for correction of surgically induced astigmatism
65775 Corneal wedge resection for correction of surgically induced astigmatism

ICD-9-CM Diagnostic

367.21 Regular astigmatism
367.22 Irregular astigmatism
996.51 Mechanical complication due to corneal graft
V42.5 Cornea replaced by transplant — (This code is intended for use when these conditions are recorded as diagnoses or problems)
V45.69 Other states following surgery of eye and adnexa — (This code is intended for use when these conditions are recorded as diagnoses or problems)

ICD-9-CM Procedural

11.79 Other reconstructive surgery on cornea

HCPCS Level II Supplies & Services

A4305 Disposable drug delivery system, flow rate of 50 ml or greater per hour
A4306 Disposable drug delivery system, flow rate of 5 ml or less per hour
A4550 Surgical trays
A6410 Eye pad, sterile, each
A6411 Eye pad, non-sterile, each

65780–65782

65780 Ocular surface reconstruction; amniotic membrane transplantation
65781 limbal stem cell allograft (eg, cadaveric or living donor)
65782 limbal conjunctival autograft (includes obtaining graft)

ICD-9-CM Diagnostic

190.3 Malignant neoplasm of conjunctiva
198.4 Secondary malignant neoplasm of other parts of nervous system
224.3 Benign neoplasm of conjunctiva
234.0 Carcinoma in situ of eye
238.8 Neoplasm of uncertain behavior of other specified sites
239.8 Neoplasm of unspecified nature of other specified sites
370.00 Unspecified corneal ulcer ▽
370.01 Marginal corneal ulcer
370.02 Ring corneal ulcer
370.03 Central corneal ulcer
370.07 Mooren's ulcer
371.23 Bullous keratopathy
371.24 Corneal edema due to wearing of contact lenses
371.40 Unspecified corneal degeneration ▽
371.42 Recurrent erosion of cornea
371.43 Band-shaped keratopathy
371.48 Peripheral degenerations of cornea
371.49 Other corneal degenerations
371.82 Corneal disorder due to contact lens
372.40 Unspecified pterygium ▽
372.41 Peripheral ptergium, stationary
372.42 Peripheral pterygium, progressive
372.43 Central pterygium
372.44 Double pterygium
372.45 Recurrent pterygium
372.50 Unspecified conjunctival degeneration ▽
372.52 Pseudopterygium
372.53 Conjunctival xerosis
372.54 Conjunctival concretions
372.63 Symblepharon
374.44 Sensory disorders of eyelid
695.1 Erythema multiforme
743.45 Aniridia
940.0 Chemical burn of eyelids and periocular area
940.1 Other burns of eyelids and periocular area
940.2 Alkaline chemical burn of cornea and conjunctival sac
940.3 Acid chemical burn of cornea and conjunctival sac
940.4 Other burn of cornea and conjunctival sac
940.9 Unspecified burn of eye and adnexa ▽
941.03 Burn of unspecified degree of lip(s) ▽
941.12 Erythema due to burn (first degree) of eye (with other parts face, head, and neck)
941.22 Blisters, with epidermal loss due to burn (second degree) of eye (with other parts of face, head, and neck)
941.32 Full-thickness skin loss due to burn (third degree nos) of eye (with other parts of face, head, and neck)

ICD-9-CM Procedural

11.79 Other reconstructive surgery on cornea

65800–65805

65800 Paracentesis of anterior chamber of eye (separate procedure); with diagnostic aspiration of aqueous
65805 with therapeutic release of aqueous

ICD-9-CM Diagnostic

054.44 Herpes simplex iridocyclitis
091.50 Early syphilis, syphilitic uveitis, unspecified ▽
091.52 Early syphilis, syphilitic iridocyclitis (secondary)
098.41 Gonococcal iridocyclitis
364.00 Unspecified acute and subacute iridocyclitis ▽
364.01 Primary iridocyclitis
364.02 Recurrent iridocyclitis
364.03 Secondary iridocyclitis, infectious
364.04 Secondary iridocyclitis, noninfectious
364.05 Hypopyon
365.22 Acute angle-closure glaucoma
365.59 Glaucoma associated with other lens disorders — (Use additional code for associated disorder: 379.33, 379.34, 743.36)
365.62 Glaucoma associated with ocular inflammations — (Use additional code for associated disorder: 364.00-364.3, 364.22)
365.64 Glaucoma associated with tumors or cysts — (Use additional code for associated disorder: 190.0-190.9, 224.0-224.9, 364.61)
365.65 Glaucoma associated with ocular trauma — (Use additional code for associated condition: 364.77, 921.3)
365.83 Aqueous misdirection

ICD-9-CM Procedural

12.21 Diagnostic aspiration of anterior chamber of eye
12.91 Therapeutic evacuation of anterior chamber

HCPCS Level II Supplies & Services

A4305 Disposable drug delivery system, flow rate of 50 ml or greater per hour
A4306 Disposable drug delivery system, flow rate of 5 ml or less per hour
A4550 Surgical trays

A6410 Eye pad, sterile, each
A6411 Eye pad, non-sterile, each

65810

65810 Paracentesis of anterior chamber of eye (separate procedure); with removal of vitreous and/or discission of anterior hyaloid membrane, with or without air injection

ICD-9-CM Diagnostic

364.74 Adhesions and disruptions of pupillary membranes
365.61 Glaucoma associated with pupillary block — (Use additional code for associated disorder, 364.74)
365.83 Aqueous misdirection
379.26 Vitreous prolapse

ICD-9-CM Procedural

12.91 Therapeutic evacuation of anterior chamber

65815

65815 Paracentesis of anterior chamber of eye (separate procedure); with removal of blood, with or without irrigation and/or air injection

ICD-9-CM Diagnostic

364.41 Hyphema
364.61 Implantation cysts of iris, ciliary body, and anterior chamber
365.64 Glaucoma associated with tumors or cysts — (Use additional code for associated disorder: 190.0-190.9, 224.0-224.9, 364.61)
365.83 Aqueous misdirection
921.3 Contusion of eyeball

ICD-9-CM Procedural

12.91 Therapeutic evacuation of anterior chamber

HCPCS Level II Supplies & Services

A4305 Disposable drug delivery system, flow rate of 50 ml or greater per hour
A4306 Disposable drug delivery system, flow rate of 5 ml or less per hour
A4550 Surgical trays
A6410 Eye pad, sterile, each
A6411 Eye pad, non-sterile, each

65820

65820 Goniotomy

ICD-9-CM Diagnostic

237.70 Neurofibromatosis, unspecified ▽
237.71 Neurofibromatosis, Type 1 (von Recklinghausen's disease)
365.11 Primary open-angle glaucoma
365.12 Low tension open-angle glaucoma
365.13 Pigmentary open-angle glaucoma
365.14 Open-angle glaucoma of childhood
365.15 Residual stage of open angle glaucoma
365.41 Glaucoma associated with chamber angle anomalies — (Code first associated disorder, 743.44) ☒
365.44 Glaucoma associated with systemic syndromes — (Code first associated disease: 237.7, 759.6) ☒
365.83 Aqueous misdirection
743.20 Unspecified buphthalmos ▽
743.21 Simple buphthalmos
743.22 Buphthalmos associated with other ocular anomaly
743.44 Specified congenital anomaly of anterior chamber, chamber angle, and related structures
759.6 Other congenital hamartoses, not elsewhere classified

ICD-9-CM Procedural

12.52 Goniotomy without goniopuncture
12.53 Goniotomy with goniopuncture

HCPCS Level II Supplies & Services

A4305 Disposable drug delivery system, flow rate of 50 ml or greater per hour
A4306 Disposable drug delivery system, flow rate of 5 ml or less per hour
A4550 Surgical trays
A6410 Eye pad, sterile, each
A6411 Eye pad, non-sterile, each

65850

65850 Trabeculotomy ab externo

ICD-9-CM Diagnostic

237.70 Neurofibromatosis, unspecified ▽
237.71 Neurofibromatosis, Type 1 (von Recklinghausen's disease)
365.10 Unspecified open-angle glaucoma ▽
365.11 Primary open-angle glaucoma
365.12 Low tension open-angle glaucoma
365.13 Pigmentary open-angle glaucoma
365.14 Open-angle glaucoma of childhood
365.15 Residual stage of open angle glaucoma
365.41 Glaucoma associated with chamber angle anomalies — (Code first associated disorder, 743.44) ☒
365.44 Glaucoma associated with systemic syndromes — (Code first associated disease: 237.7, 759.6) ☒
365.60 Glaucoma associated with unspecified ocular disorder ▽
365.83 Aqueous misdirection
371.11 Anterior pigmentations of cornea
371.12 Stromal pigmentations of cornea
743.44 Specified congenital anomaly of anterior chamber, chamber angle, and related structures
759.6 Other congenital hamartoses, not elsewhere classified

ICD-9-CM Procedural

12.54 Trabeculotomy ab externo

HCPCS Level II Supplies & Services

A4305 Disposable drug delivery system, flow rate of 50 ml or greater per hour
A4306 Disposable drug delivery system, flow rate of 5 ml or less per hour
A4550 Surgical trays
A6410 Eye pad, sterile, each
A6411 Eye pad, non-sterile, each

65855

65855 Trabeculoplasty by laser surgery, one or more sessions (defined treatment series)

ICD-9-CM Diagnostic

365.01 Borderline glaucoma, open angle with borderline findings
365.10 Unspecified open-angle glaucoma ▽
365.11 Primary open-angle glaucoma
365.13 Pigmentary open-angle glaucoma
365.15 Residual stage of open angle glaucoma
365.52 Pseudoexfoliation glaucoma — (Use additional code for associated pseudoexfoliation of capsule, 366.11)
365.60 Glaucoma associated with unspecified ocular disorder ▽
365.83 Aqueous misdirection
365.9 Unspecified glaucoma ▽
366.11 Pseudoexfoliation of lens capsule

ICD-9-CM Procedural

12.59 Other facilitation of intraocular circulation

HCPCS Level II Supplies & Services

A4305 Disposable drug delivery system, flow rate of 50 ml or greater per hour
A4306 Disposable drug delivery system, flow rate of 5 ml or less per hour
A4550 Surgical trays
A6410 Eye pad, sterile, each
A6411 Eye pad, non-sterile, each

65860

65860 Severing adhesions of anterior segment, laser technique (separate procedure)

ICD-9-CM Diagnostic

364.70 Unspecified adhesions of iris ▽
364.72 Anterior synechiae
364.73 Goniosynechiae

ICD-9-CM Procedural

12.39 Other iridoplasty

HCPCS Level II Supplies & Services

A4305 Disposable drug delivery system, flow rate of 50 ml or greater per hour
A4306 Disposable drug delivery system, flow rate of 5 ml or less per hour
A4550 Surgical trays
A6410 Eye pad, sterile, each

A6411 Eye pad, non-sterile, each

65865

65865 Severing adhesions of anterior segment of eye, incisional technique (with or without injection of air or liquid) (separate procedure); goniosynechiae

ICD-9-CM Diagnostic

364.01 Primary iridocyclitis
364.02 Recurrent iridocyclitis
364.10 Unspecified chronic iridocyclitis ▽
364.70 Unspecified adhesions of iris ▽
364.73 Goniosynechiae
365.23 Chronic angle-closure glaucoma
365.83 Aqueous misdirection

ICD-9-CM Procedural

12.31 Lysis of goniosynechiae

HCPCS Level II Supplies & Services

A4305 Disposable drug delivery system, flow rate of 50 ml or greater per hour
A4306 Disposable drug delivery system, flow rate of 5 ml or less per hour
A4550 Surgical trays
A6410 Eye pad, sterile, each
A6411 Eye pad, non-sterile, each

65870–65875

65870 Severing adhesions of anterior segment of eye, incisional technique (with or without injection of air or liquid) (separate procedure); anterior synechiae, except goniosynechiae
65875 posterior synechiae

ICD-9-CM Diagnostic

364.70 Unspecified adhesions of iris ▽
364.71 Posterior synechiae
364.72 Anterior synechiae

ICD-9-CM Procedural

12.32 Lysis of other anterior synechiae
12.33 Lysis of posterior synechiae

HCPCS Level II Supplies & Services

A4305 Disposable drug delivery system, flow rate of 50 ml or greater per hour
A4306 Disposable drug delivery system, flow rate of 5 ml or less per hour
A4550 Surgical trays
A6410 Eye pad, sterile, each
A6411 Eye pad, non-sterile, each

65880

65880 Severing adhesions of anterior segment of eye, incisional technique (with or without injection of air or liquid) (separate procedure); corneovitreal adhesions

ICD-9-CM Diagnostic

362.53 Cystoid macular degeneration of retina
364.70 Unspecified adhesions of iris ▽
371.00 Unspecified corneal opacity ▽
371.01 Minor opacity of cornea
371.02 Peripheral opacity of cornea
371.03 Central opacity of cornea
371.04 Adherent leucoma
379.29 Other disorders of vitreous
379.31 Aphakia

ICD-9-CM Procedural

12.34 Lysis of corneovitreal adhesions

HCPCS Level II Supplies & Services

A4305 Disposable drug delivery system, flow rate of 50 ml or greater per hour
A4306 Disposable drug delivery system, flow rate of 5 ml or less per hour
A4550 Surgical trays
A6410 Eye pad, sterile, each
A6411 Eye pad, non-sterile, each

65900

65900 Removal of epithelial downgrowth, anterior chamber of eye

ICD-9-CM Diagnostic

364.61 Implantation cysts of iris, ciliary body, and anterior chamber
906.0 Late effect of open wound of head, neck, and trunk
996.51 Mechanical complication due to corneal graft
996.53 Mechanical complication due to ocular lens prosthesis
996.69 Infection and inflammatory reaction due to other internal prosthetic device, implant, and graft — (Use additional code to identify specified infections)
996.79 Other complications due to other internal prosthetic device, implant, and graft
998.89 Other specified complications

ICD-9-CM Procedural

12.93 Removal or destruction of epithelial downgrowth from anterior chamber

HCPCS Level II Supplies & Services

A4305 Disposable drug delivery system, flow rate of 50 ml or greater per hour
A4306 Disposable drug delivery system, flow rate of 5 ml or less per hour
A4550 Surgical trays
A6410 Eye pad, sterile, each
A6411 Eye pad, non-sterile, each

65920

65920 Removal of implanted material, anterior segment of eye

ICD-9-CM Diagnostic

364.04 Secondary iridocyclitis, noninfectious
364.23 Lens-induced iridocyclitis
364.41 Hyphema
365.9 Unspecified glaucoma ▽
996.53 Mechanical complication due to ocular lens prosthesis
996.69 Infection and inflammatory reaction due to other internal prosthetic device, implant, and graft — (Use additional code to identify specified infections)
996.79 Other complications due to other internal prosthetic device, implant, and graft

ICD-9-CM Procedural

13.8 Removal of implanted lens

HCPCS Level II Supplies & Services

A4305 Disposable drug delivery system, flow rate of 50 ml or greater per hour
A4306 Disposable drug delivery system, flow rate of 5 ml or less per hour
A4550 Surgical trays
A6410 Eye pad, sterile, each
A6411 Eye pad, non-sterile, each

65930

65930 Removal of blood clot, anterior segment of eye

ICD-9-CM Diagnostic

364.41 Hyphema
364.42 Rubeosis iridis
364.77 Recession of chamber angle of eye
365.65 Glaucoma associated with ocular trauma — (Use additional code for associated condition: 364.77, 921.3)
372.72 Conjunctival hemorrhage
871.4 Unspecified laceration of eye — (Use additional code to identify infection) ▽
871.5 Penetration of eyeball with magnetic foreign body — (Use additional code to identify infection)
871.6 Penetration of eyeball with (nonmagnetic) foreign body — (Use additional code to identify infection)
871.7 Unspecified ocular penetration — (Use additional code to identify infection) ▽
871.9 Unspecified open wound of eyeball — (Use additional code to identify infection) ▽
921.3 Contusion of eyeball
996.79 Other complications due to other internal prosthetic device, implant, and graft
998.11 Hemorrhage complicating a procedure
998.12 Hematoma complicating a procedure

ICD-9-CM Procedural

12.91 Therapeutic evacuation of anterior chamber

HCPCS Level II Supplies & Services

A4305 Disposable drug delivery system, flow rate of 50 ml or greater per hour
A4306 Disposable drug delivery system, flow rate of 5 ml or less per hour
A4550 Surgical trays

▽ Unspecified code
♀ Female diagnosis
☒ Manifestation code
♂ Male diagnosis

A6410 Eye pad, sterile, each
A6411 Eye pad, non-sterile, each

66020–66030

66020 Injection, anterior chamber of eye (separate procedure); air or liquid
66030 medication

ICD-9-CM Diagnostic

360.00 Unspecified purulent endophthalmitis ▽
360.01 Acute endophthalmitis
360.34 Flat anterior chamber of eye
364.01 Primary iridocyclitis
364.3 Unspecified iridocyclitis ▽
364.73 Goniosynechiae
365.22 Acute angle-closure glaucoma
365.83 Aqueous misdirection

ICD-9-CM Procedural

12.92 Injection into anterior chamber

HCPCS Level II Supplies & Services

J7051 Sterile saline or water, up to 5 cc

66130

66130 Excision of lesion, sclera

ICD-9-CM Diagnostic

190.0 Malignant neoplasm of eyeball, except conjunctiva, cornea, retina, and choroid
198.4 Secondary malignant neoplasm of other parts of nervous system
224.0 Benign neoplasm of eyeball, except conjunctiva, cornea, retina, and choroid
234.0 Carcinoma in situ of eye
238.8 Neoplasm of uncertain behavior of other specified sites
239.8 Neoplasm of unspecified nature of other specified sites
379.19 Other scleral disorder

ICD-9-CM Procedural

12.84 Excision or destruction of lesion of sclera

HCPCS Level II Supplies & Services

A4305 Disposable drug delivery system, flow rate of 50 ml or greater per hour
A4306 Disposable drug delivery system, flow rate of 5 ml or less per hour
A4550 Surgical trays

66150–66155

66150 Fistulization of sclera for glaucoma; trephination with iridectomy
66155 thermocauterization with iridectomy

ICD-9-CM Diagnostic

364.51 Essential or progressive iris atrophy
365.20 Unspecified primary angle-closure glaucoma ▽
365.21 Intermittent angle-closure glaucoma
365.22 Acute angle-closure glaucoma
365.23 Chronic angle-closure glaucoma
365.24 Residual stage of angle-closure glaucoma
365.42 Glaucoma associated with anomalies of iris — (Code first associated disorder: 364.51, 743.45) ☒
365.51 Phacolytic glaucoma — (Use additional code for associated hypermature cataract, 366.18)
365.52 Pseudoexfoliation glaucoma — (Use additional code for associated pseudoexfoliation of capsule, 366.11)
365.83 Aqueous misdirection
366.11 Pseudoexfoliation of lens capsule
366.18 Hypermature senile cataract
743.45 Aniridia

ICD-9-CM Procedural

12.61 Trephination of sclera with iridectomy
12.62 Thermocauterization of sclera with iridectomy

66160

66160 Fistulization of sclera for glaucoma; sclerectomy with punch or scissors, with iridectomy

ICD-9-CM Diagnostic

364.51 Essential or progressive iris atrophy
365.11 Primary open-angle glaucoma
365.20 Unspecified primary angle-closure glaucoma ▽
365.21 Intermittent angle-closure glaucoma
365.22 Acute angle-closure glaucoma
365.23 Chronic angle-closure glaucoma
365.24 Residual stage of angle-closure glaucoma
365.42 Glaucoma associated with anomalies of iris — (Code first associated disorder: 364.51, 743.45) ☒
365.51 Phacolytic glaucoma — (Use additional code for associated hypermature cataract, 366.18)
365.52 Pseudoexfoliation glaucoma — (Use additional code for associated pseudoexfoliation of capsule, 366.11)
365.83 Aqueous misdirection
366.11 Pseudoexfoliation of lens capsule
366.18 Hypermature senile cataract
743.45 Aniridia

ICD-9-CM Procedural

12.65 Other scleral fistulization with iridectomy

66165

66165 Fistulization of sclera for glaucoma; iridencleisis or iridotasis

ICD-9-CM Diagnostic

364.51 Essential or progressive iris atrophy
365.11 Primary open-angle glaucoma
365.20 Unspecified primary angle-closure glaucoma ▽
365.21 Intermittent angle-closure glaucoma
365.22 Acute angle-closure glaucoma
365.23 Chronic angle-closure glaucoma
365.24 Residual stage of angle-closure glaucoma
365.42 Glaucoma associated with anomalies of iris — (Code first associated disorder: 364.51, 743.45) ☒
365.51 Phacolytic glaucoma — (Use additional code for associated hypermature cataract, 366.18)
365.52 Pseudoexfoliation glaucoma — (Use additional code for associated pseudoexfoliation of capsule, 366.11)
365.83 Aqueous misdirection
366.11 Pseudoexfoliation of lens capsule
366.18 Hypermature senile cataract
743.45 Aniridia

ICD-9-CM Procedural

12.63 Iridencleisis and iridotasis
12.79 Other glaucoma procedures

66170–66172

66170 Fistulization of sclera for glaucoma; trabeculectomy ab externo in absence of previous surgery
66172 trabeculectomy ab externo with scarring from previous ocular surgery or trauma (includes injection of antifibrotic agents)

ICD-9-CM Diagnostic

364.51 Essential or progressive iris atrophy
365.10 Unspecified open-angle glaucoma ▽
365.11 Primary open-angle glaucoma
365.12 Low tension open-angle glaucoma
365.13 Pigmentary open-angle glaucoma
365.14 Open-angle glaucoma of childhood
365.15 Residual stage of open angle glaucoma
365.20 Unspecified primary angle-closure glaucoma ▽
365.21 Intermittent angle-closure glaucoma
365.23 Chronic angle-closure glaucoma
365.24 Residual stage of angle-closure glaucoma
365.42 Glaucoma associated with anomalies of iris — (Code first associated disorder: 364.51, 743.45) ☒
365.52 Pseudoexfoliation glaucoma — (Use additional code for associated pseudoexfoliation of capsule, 366.11)
365.60 Glaucoma associated with unspecified ocular disorder ▽
365.83 Aqueous misdirection
365.9 Unspecified glaucoma ▽
366.11 Pseudoexfoliation of lens capsule
743.45 Aniridia

ICD-9-CM Procedural

12.64 Trabeculectomy ab externo

66180–66185

66180 Aqueous shunt to extraocular reservoir (eg, Molteno, Schocket, Denver-Krupin)
66185 Revision of aqueous shunt to extraocular reservoir

ICD-9-CM Diagnostic

362.35 Central vein occlusion of retina
364.41 Hyphema
364.51 Essential or progressive iris atrophy
365.11 Primary open-angle glaucoma
365.20 Unspecified primary angle-closure glaucoma ▽
365.21 Intermittent angle-closure glaucoma
365.23 Chronic angle-closure glaucoma
365.24 Residual stage of angle-closure glaucoma
365.42 Glaucoma associated with anomalies of iris — (Code first associated disorder: 364.51, 743.45) ☒
365.63 Glaucoma associated with vascular disorders of eye — (Use additional code for associated disorder: 362.35, 364.41)
365.83 Aqueous misdirection
743.45 Aniridia
996.59 Mechanical complication due to other implant and internal device, not elsewhere classified

ICD-9-CM Procedural

12.66 Postoperative revision of scleral fistulization procedure
12.69 Other scleral fistulizing procedure

66220–66225

66220 Repair of scleral staphyloma; without graft
66225 with graft

ICD-9-CM Diagnostic

379.11 Scleral ectasia
379.12 Staphyloma posticum
379.13 Equatorial staphyloma
379.14 Anterior staphyloma, localized
379.15 Ring staphyloma

ICD-9-CM Procedural

12.85 Repair of scleral staphyloma with graft
12.86 Other repair of scleral staphyloma

HCPCS Level II Supplies & Services

A4305 Disposable drug delivery system, flow rate of 50 ml or greater per hour
A4306 Disposable drug delivery system, flow rate of 5 ml or less per hour
A4550 Surgical trays

66250

66250 Revision or repair of operative wound of anterior segment, any type, early or late, major or minor procedure

ICD-9-CM Diagnostic

996.59 Mechanical complication due to other implant and internal device, not elsewhere classified
996.69 Infection and inflammatory reaction due to other internal prosthetic device, implant, and graft — (Use additional code to identify specified infections)
996.79 Other complications due to other internal prosthetic device, implant, and graft
998.31 Disruption of internal operation wound
998.59 Other postoperative infection — (Use additional code to identify infection)

ICD-9-CM Procedural

11.52 Repair of postoperative wound dehiscence of cornea
12.82 Repair of scleral fistula
12.83 Revision of operative wound of anterior segment, not elsewhere classified
12.99 Other operations on anterior chamber

HCPCS Level II Supplies & Services

A4550 Surgical trays

66500–66505

66500 Iridotomy by stab incision (separate procedure); except transfixion
66505 with transfixion as for iris bombe

ICD-9-CM Diagnostic

364.51 Essential or progressive iris atrophy
364.74 Adhesions and disruptions of pupillary membranes
365.20 Unspecified primary angle-closure glaucoma ▽
365.21 Intermittent angle-closure glaucoma
365.22 Acute angle-closure glaucoma
365.23 Chronic angle-closure glaucoma
365.24 Residual stage of angle-closure glaucoma
365.42 Glaucoma associated with anomalies of iris — (Code first associated disorder: 364.51, 743.45) ☒
365.61 Glaucoma associated with pupillary block — (Use additional code for associated disorder, 364.74)
365.83 Aqueous misdirection
743.45 Aniridia

ICD-9-CM Procedural

12.11 Iridotomy with transfixion
12.12 Other iridotomy

HCPCS Level II Supplies & Services

A4305 Disposable drug delivery system, flow rate of 50 ml or greater per hour
A4306 Disposable drug delivery system, flow rate of 5 ml or less per hour
A4550 Surgical trays

66600–66605

66600 Iridectomy, with corneoscleral or corneal section; for removal of lesion
66605 with cyclectomy

ICD-9-CM Diagnostic

190.0 Malignant neoplasm of eyeball, except conjunctiva, cornea, retina, and choroid
198.4 Secondary malignant neoplasm of other parts of nervous system
224.0 Benign neoplasm of eyeball, except conjunctiva, cornea, retina, and choroid
224.4 Benign neoplasm of cornea
234.0 Carcinoma in situ of eye
238.8 Neoplasm of uncertain behavior of other specified sites
239.8 Neoplasm of unspecified nature of other specified sites
364.60 Idiopathic cysts of iris, ciliary body, and anterior chamber
364.62 Exudative cysts of iris or anterior chamber

ICD-9-CM Procedural

12.14 Other iridectomy
12.40 Removal of lesion of anterior segment of eye, not otherwise specified
12.42 Excision of lesion of iris
12.44 Excision of lesion of ciliary body

66625

66625 Iridectomy, with corneoscleral or corneal section; peripheral for glaucoma (separate procedure)

ICD-9-CM Diagnostic

364.51 Essential or progressive iris atrophy
364.74 Adhesions and disruptions of pupillary membranes
365.02 Borderline glaucoma with anatomical narrow angle
365.20 Unspecified primary angle-closure glaucoma ▽
365.21 Intermittent angle-closure glaucoma
365.22 Acute angle-closure glaucoma
365.23 Chronic angle-closure glaucoma
365.24 Residual stage of angle-closure glaucoma
365.42 Glaucoma associated with anomalies of iris — (Code first associated disorder: 364.51, 743.45) ☒
365.61 Glaucoma associated with pupillary block — (Use additional code for associated disorder, 364.74)
365.83 Aqueous misdirection
743.45 Aniridia

ICD-9-CM Procedural

12.14 Other iridectomy

66630

66630 Iridectomy, with corneoscleral or corneal section; sector for glaucoma (separate procedure)

ICD-9-CM Diagnostic

364.51 Essential or progressive iris atrophy
364.74 Adhesions and disruptions of pupillary membranes
365.20 Unspecified primary angle-closure glaucoma ▽
365.21 Intermittent angle-closure glaucoma
365.22 Acute angle-closure glaucoma
365.23 Chronic angle-closure glaucoma
365.24 Residual stage of angle-closure glaucoma

365.42 Glaucoma associated with anomalies of iris — (Code first associated disorder: 364.51, 743.45) ☒
365.61 Glaucoma associated with pupillary block — (Use additional code for associated disorder, 364.74)
365.83 Aqueous misdirection
365.9 Unspecified glaucoma ▽
743.45 Aniridia

ICD-9-CM Procedural

12.14 Other iridectomy
12.39 Other iridoplasty

66635

66635 Iridectomy, with corneoscleral or corneal section; optical (separate procedure)

ICD-9-CM Diagnostic

364.75 Pupillary abnormalities
379.40 Unspecified abnormal pupillary function ▽
379.42 Miosis (persistent), not due to miotics
379.45 Argyll Robertson pupil, atypical

ICD-9-CM Procedural

12.14 Other iridectomy
12.39 Other iridoplasty

66680

66680 Repair of iris, ciliary body (as for iridodialysis)

ICD-9-CM Diagnostic

364.51 Essential or progressive iris atrophy
364.52 Iridoschisis
364.53 Pigmentary iris degeneration
364.54 Degeneration of pupillary margin
364.55 Miotic cysts of pupillary margin
364.56 Degenerative changes of chamber angle
364.57 Degenerative changes of ciliary body
364.75 Pupillary abnormalities
364.76 Iridodialysis
364.8 Other disorders of iris and ciliary body
871.1 Ocular laceration with prolapse or exposure of intraocular tissue — (Use additional code to identify infection)

ICD-9-CM Procedural

12.39 Other iridoplasty

66682

66682 Suture of iris, ciliary body (separate procedure) with retrieval of suture through small incision (eg, McCannel suture)

ICD-9-CM Diagnostic

364.51 Essential or progressive iris atrophy
364.52 Iridoschisis
364.53 Pigmentary iris degeneration
364.54 Degeneration of pupillary margin
364.55 Miotic cysts of pupillary margin
364.56 Degenerative changes of chamber angle
364.57 Degenerative changes of ciliary body
364.75 Pupillary abnormalities
364.76 Iridodialysis
364.8 Other disorders of iris and ciliary body
871.1 Ocular laceration with prolapse or exposure of intraocular tissue — (Use additional code to identify infection)

ICD-9-CM Procedural

12.39 Other iridoplasty

HCPCS Level II Supplies & Services

A4305 Disposable drug delivery system, flow rate of 50 ml or greater per hour
A4306 Disposable drug delivery system, flow rate of 5 ml or less per hour
A4550 Surgical trays

66700–66711

66700 Ciliary body destruction; diathermy
66710 cyclophotocoagulation, transscleral
66711 cyclophotocoagulation, endoscopic

ICD-9-CM Diagnostic

362.35 Central vein occlusion of retina
364.41 Hyphema
365.11 Primary open-angle glaucoma
365.23 Chronic angle-closure glaucoma
365.41 Glaucoma associated with chamber angle anomalies — (Code first associated disorder, 743.44) ☒
365.60 Glaucoma associated with unspecified ocular disorder ▽
365.63 Glaucoma associated with vascular disorders of eye — (Use additional code for associated disorder: 362.35, 364.41)
365.83 Aqueous misdirection
365.9 Unspecified glaucoma ▽
743.44 Specified congenital anomaly of anterior chamber, chamber angle, and related structures

ICD-9-CM Procedural

12.71 Cyclodiathermy
12.73 Cyclophotocoagulation

HCPCS Level II Supplies & Services

A4305 Disposable drug delivery system, flow rate of 50 ml or greater per hour
A4306 Disposable drug delivery system, flow rate of 5 ml or less per hour
A4550 Surgical trays

66720

66720 Ciliary body destruction; cryotherapy

ICD-9-CM Diagnostic

360.42 Blind hypertensive eye
365.02 Borderline glaucoma with anatomical narrow angle
365.04 Borderline glaucoma with ocular hypertension
365.10 Unspecified open-angle glaucoma ▽
365.11 Primary open-angle glaucoma
365.12 Low tension open-angle glaucoma
365.13 Pigmentary open-angle glaucoma
365.14 Open-angle glaucoma of childhood
365.15 Residual stage of open angle glaucoma
365.20 Unspecified primary angle-closure glaucoma ▽
365.21 Intermittent angle-closure glaucoma
365.22 Acute angle-closure glaucoma
365.23 Chronic angle-closure glaucoma
365.24 Residual stage of angle-closure glaucoma
365.63 Glaucoma associated with vascular disorders of eye — (Use additional code for associated disorder: 362.35, 364.41)
365.83 Aqueous misdirection

ICD-9-CM Procedural

12.72 Cyclocryotherapy

HCPCS Level II Supplies & Services

A4305 Disposable drug delivery system, flow rate of 50 ml or greater per hour
A4306 Disposable drug delivery system, flow rate of 5 ml or less per hour
A4550 Surgical trays

66740

66740 Ciliary body destruction; cyclodialysis

ICD-9-CM Diagnostic

364.51 Essential or progressive iris atrophy
365.02 Borderline glaucoma with anatomical narrow angle
365.04 Borderline glaucoma with ocular hypertension
365.10 Unspecified open-angle glaucoma ▽
365.11 Primary open-angle glaucoma
365.12 Low tension open-angle glaucoma
365.13 Pigmentary open-angle glaucoma
365.14 Open-angle glaucoma of childhood
365.15 Residual stage of open angle glaucoma
365.20 Unspecified primary angle-closure glaucoma ▽
365.21 Intermittent angle-closure glaucoma
365.22 Acute angle-closure glaucoma
365.23 Chronic angle-closure glaucoma

▽ Unspecified code ♀ Female diagnosis ☒ Manifestation code ♂ Male diagnosis

365.24 Residual stage of angle-closure glaucoma
365.42 Glaucoma associated with anomalies of iris — (Code first associated disorder: 364.51, 743.45) ☒
365.43 Glaucoma associated with other anterior segment anomalies — (Code first associated disorder, 743.41) ☒
365.44 Glaucoma associated with systemic syndromes — (Code first associated disease: 237.7, 759.6) ☒
365.83 Aqueous misdirection
743.41 Congenital anomaly of corneal size and shape
743.45 Aniridia

ICD-9-CM Procedural
12.55 Cyclodialysis

HCPCS Level II Supplies & Services
A4305 Disposable drug delivery system, flow rate of 50 ml or greater per hour
A4306 Disposable drug delivery system, flow rate of 5 ml or less per hour
A4550 Surgical trays

66761
66761 Iridotomy/iridectomy by laser surgery (eg, for glaucoma) (one or more sessions)

ICD-9-CM Diagnostic
364.51 Essential or progressive iris atrophy
365.20 Unspecified primary angle-closure glaucoma ▽
365.21 Intermittent angle-closure glaucoma
365.22 Acute angle-closure glaucoma
365.23 Chronic angle-closure glaucoma
365.24 Residual stage of angle-closure glaucoma
365.42 Glaucoma associated with anomalies of iris — (Code first associated disorder: 364.51, 743.45) ☒
365.43 Glaucoma associated with other anterior segment anomalies — (Code first associated disorder, 743.41) ☒
365.83 Aqueous misdirection
743.41 Congenital anomaly of corneal size and shape
743.45 Aniridia

ICD-9-CM Procedural
12.12 Other iridotomy
12.59 Other facilitation of intraocular circulation

HCPCS Level II Supplies & Services
A4305 Disposable drug delivery system, flow rate of 50 ml or greater per hour
A4306 Disposable drug delivery system, flow rate of 5 ml or less per hour
A4550 Surgical trays

66762
66762 Iridoplasty by photocoagulation (one or more sessions) (eg, for improvement of vision, for widening of anterior chamber angle)

ICD-9-CM Diagnostic
364.75 Pupillary abnormalities
364.76 Iridodialysis
364.77 Recession of chamber angle of eye
365.11 Primary open-angle glaucoma
365.83 Aqueous misdirection
379.42 Miosis (persistent), not due to miotics
871.1 Ocular laceration with prolapse or exposure of intraocular tissue — (Use additional code to identify infection)

ICD-9-CM Procedural
12.35 Coreoplasty
12.39 Other iridoplasty

HCPCS Level II Supplies & Services
A4305 Disposable drug delivery system, flow rate of 50 ml or greater per hour
A4306 Disposable drug delivery system, flow rate of 5 ml or less per hour
A4550 Surgical trays

66770
66770 Destruction of cyst or lesion iris or ciliary body (nonexcisional procedure)

ICD-9-CM Diagnostic
190.0 Malignant neoplasm of eyeball, except conjunctiva, cornea, retina, and choroid
198.4 Secondary malignant neoplasm of other parts of nervous system
224.0 Benign neoplasm of eyeball, except conjunctiva, cornea, retina, and choroid
234.0 Carcinoma in situ of eye
238.8 Neoplasm of uncertain behavior of other specified sites
239.8 Neoplasm of unspecified nature of other specified sites
364.55 Miotic cysts of pupillary margin
364.60 Idiopathic cysts of iris, ciliary body, and anterior chamber
364.61 Implantation cysts of iris, ciliary body, and anterior chamber
364.62 Exudative cysts of iris or anterior chamber
364.64 Exudative cyst of pars plana

ICD-9-CM Procedural
12.41 Destruction of lesion of iris, nonexcisional
12.43 Destruction of lesion of ciliary body, nonexcisional

HCPCS Level II Supplies & Services
A4305 Disposable drug delivery system, flow rate of 50 ml or greater per hour
A4306 Disposable drug delivery system, flow rate of 5 ml or less per hour
A4550 Surgical trays

66820
66820 Discission of secondary membranous cataract (opacified posterior lens capsule and/or anterior hyaloid); stab incision technique (Ziegler or Wheeler knife)

ICD-9-CM Diagnostic
366.50 Unspecified after-cataract ▽
366.51 Soemmering's ring
366.52 Other after-cataract, not obscuring vision
366.53 After-cataract, obscuring vision
996.53 Mechanical complication due to ocular lens prosthesis

ICD-9-CM Procedural
13.64 Discission of secondary membrane (after cataract)
13.66 Mechanical fragmentation of secondary membrane (after cataract)

HCPCS Level II Supplies & Services
A4305 Disposable drug delivery system, flow rate of 50 ml or greater per hour
A4306 Disposable drug delivery system, flow rate of 5 ml or less per hour
A4550 Surgical trays

66821
66821 Discission of secondary membranous cataract (opacified posterior lens capsule and/or anterior hyaloid); laser surgery (eg, YAG laser) (one or more stages)

ICD-9-CM Diagnostic
366.50 Unspecified after-cataract ▽
366.51 Soemmering's ring
366.52 Other after-cataract, not obscuring vision
366.53 After-cataract, obscuring vision
996.53 Mechanical complication due to ocular lens prosthesis

ICD-9-CM Procedural
13.64 Discission of secondary membrane (after cataract)

HCPCS Level II Supplies & Services
A4305 Disposable drug delivery system, flow rate of 50 ml or greater per hour
A4306 Disposable drug delivery system, flow rate of 5 ml or less per hour
A4550 Surgical trays

66825
66825 Repositioning of intraocular lens prosthesis, requiring an incision (separate procedure)

ICD-9-CM Diagnostic
996.53 Mechanical complication due to ocular lens prosthesis
V43.1 Lens replaced by other means — (This code is intended for use when these conditions are recorded as diagnoses or problems)
V45.61 Cataract extraction status — (Use additional code for associated artificial lens staus, V43.1)
V45.69 Other states following surgery of eye and adnexa — (This code is intended for use when these conditions are recorded as diagnoses or problems)

ICD-9-CM Procedural
13.9 Other operations on lens

▽ Unspecified code ♀ Female diagnosis ☒ Manifestation code ♂ Male diagnosis

Congenital Anomalies of Eye

A congenital keyhole pupil is also called a coloboma of the iris

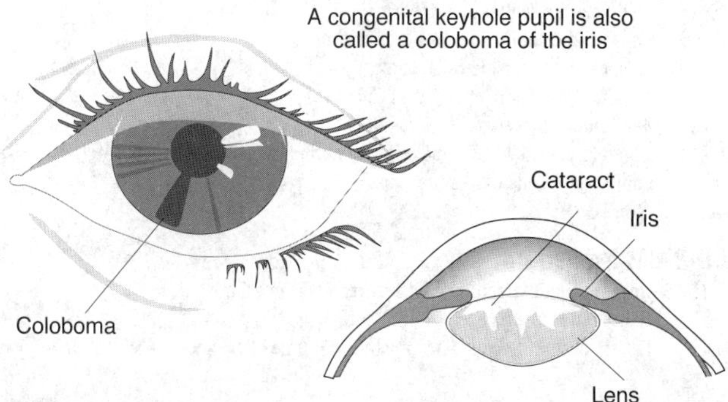

66830

66830 Removal of secondary membranous cataract (opacified posterior lens capsule and/or anterior hyaloid) with corneo-scleral section, with or without iridectomy (iridocapsulotomy, iridocapsulectomy)

ICD-9-CM Diagnostic

366.50 Unspecified after-cataract
366.51 Soemmering's ring
366.52 Other after-cataract, not obscuring vision
366.53 After-cataract, obscuring vision

ICD-9-CM Procedural

13.65 Excision of secondary membrane (after cataract)

HCPCS Level II Supplies & Services

A4305 Disposable drug delivery system, flow rate of 50 ml or greater per hour
A4306 Disposable drug delivery system, flow rate of 5 ml or less per hour
A4550 Surgical trays

66840

66840 Removal of lens material; aspiration technique, one or more stages

ICD-9-CM Diagnostic

366.00 Unspecified nonsenile cataract
366.20 Unspecified traumatic cataract
366.46 Cataract associated with radiation and other physical influences — (Use additional E code to identify cause)

ICD-9-CM Procedural

13.3 Extracapsular extraction of lens by simple aspiration (and irrigation) technique
13.41 Phacoemulsification and aspiration of cataract

HCPCS Level II Supplies & Services

A4305 Disposable drug delivery system, flow rate of 50 ml or greater per hour
A4306 Disposable drug delivery system, flow rate of 5 ml or less per hour
A4550 Surgical trays

66850

66850 Removal of lens material; phacofragmentation technique (mechanical or ultrasonic) (eg, phacoemulsification), with aspiration

ICD-9-CM Diagnostic

366.00 Unspecified nonsenile cataract
366.04 Nuclear cataract, nonsenile
366.10 Unspecified senile cataract
366.12 Incipient cataract
366.13 Anterior subcapsular polar senile cataract
366.19 Other and combined forms of senile cataract
366.21 Localized traumatic opacities of cataract
366.22 Total traumatic cataract
366.46 Cataract associated with radiation and other physical influences — (Use additional E code to identify cause)
366.8 Other cataract

ICD-9-CM Procedural

13.41 Phacoemulsification and aspiration of cataract
13.43 Mechanical phacofragmentation and other aspiration of cataract

HCPCS Level II Supplies & Services

A4305 Disposable drug delivery system, flow rate of 50 ml or greater per hour
A4306 Disposable drug delivery system, flow rate of 5 ml or less per hour
A4550 Surgical trays

66852

66852 Removal of lens material; pars plana approach, with or without vitrectomy

ICD-9-CM Diagnostic

366.00 Unspecified nonsenile cataract
366.04 Nuclear cataract, nonsenile
366.10 Unspecified senile cataract
366.12 Incipient cataract
366.13 Anterior subcapsular polar senile cataract
366.14 Posterior subcapsular polar senile cataract
366.15 Cortical senile cataract
366.16 Nuclear sclerosis
366.17 Total or mature senile cataract
366.18 Hypermature senile cataract
366.19 Other and combined forms of senile cataract
366.20 Unspecified traumatic cataract
366.21 Localized traumatic opacities of cataract
366.22 Total traumatic cataract
366.46 Cataract associated with radiation and other physical influences — (Use additional E code to identify cause)
366.8 Other cataract

ICD-9-CM Procedural

13.42 Mechanical phacofragmentation and aspiration of cataract by posterior route
14.74 Other mechanical vitrectomy

66920

66920 Removal of lens material; intracapsular

ICD-9-CM Diagnostic

366.00 Unspecified nonsenile cataract
366.04 Nuclear cataract, nonsenile
366.10 Unspecified senile cataract
366.11 Pseudoexfoliation of lens capsule
366.12 Incipient cataract
366.13 Anterior subcapsular polar senile cataract
366.14 Posterior subcapsular polar senile cataract
366.15 Cortical senile cataract
366.16 Nuclear sclerosis
366.17 Total or mature senile cataract
366.18 Hypermature senile cataract
366.19 Other and combined forms of senile cataract
366.20 Unspecified traumatic cataract
366.21 Localized traumatic opacities of cataract
366.22 Total traumatic cataract
366.46 Cataract associated with radiation and other physical influences — (Use additional E code to identify cause)
366.8 Other cataract
379.32 Subluxation of lens
379.33 Anterior dislocation of lens
379.34 Posterior dislocation of lens
379.39 Other disorders of lens

ICD-9-CM Procedural

13.11 Intracapsular extraction of lens by temporal inferior route
13.19 Other intracapsular extraction of lens

66930

66930 Removal of lens material; intracapsular, for dislocated lens

ICD-9-CM Diagnostic

379.32 Subluxation of lens

ICD-9-CM Procedural

13.11 Intracapsular extraction of lens by temporal inferior route
13.19 Other intracapsular extraction of lens

66940

66940 Removal of lens material; extracapsular (other than 66840, 66850, 66852)

ICD-9-CM Diagnostic

366.00 Unspecified nonsenile cataract ▽
366.04 Nuclear cataract, nonsenile
366.10 Unspecified senile cataract ▽
366.12 Incipient cataract
366.13 Anterior subcapsular polar senile cataract
366.14 Posterior subcapsular polar senile cataract
366.15 Cortical senile cataract
366.16 Nuclear sclerosis
366.17 Total or mature senile cataract
366.18 Hypermature senile cataract
366.19 Other and combined forms of senile cataract
366.20 Unspecified traumatic cataract ▽
366.21 Localized traumatic opacities of cataract
366.22 Total traumatic cataract
366.46 Cataract associated with radiation and other physical influences — (Use additional E code to identify cause)
366.8 Other cataract

ICD-9-CM Procedural

13.2 Extracapsular extraction of lens by linear extraction technique
13.51 Extracapsular extraction of lens by temporal inferior route
13.59 Other extracapsular extraction of lens

66982

66982 Extracapsular cataract removal with insertion of intraocular lens prosthesis (one stage procedure), manual or mechanical technique (eg, irrigation and aspiration or phacoemulsification), complex, requiring devices or techniques not generally used in routine cataract surgery (eg, iris expansion device, suture support for intraocular lens, or primary posterior capsulorrhexis) or performed on patients in the amblyogenic developmental stage

ICD-9-CM Diagnostic

366.00 Unspecified nonsenile cataract ▽
366.04 Nuclear cataract, nonsenile
366.10 Unspecified senile cataract ▽
366.12 Incipient cataract
366.13 Anterior subcapsular polar senile cataract
366.14 Posterior subcapsular polar senile cataract
366.15 Cortical senile cataract
366.16 Nuclear sclerosis
366.17 Total or mature senile cataract
366.18 Hypermature senile cataract
366.19 Other and combined forms of senile cataract
366.20 Unspecified traumatic cataract ▽
366.21 Localized traumatic opacities of cataract
366.22 Total traumatic cataract
366.46 Cataract associated with radiation and other physical influences — (Use additional E code to identify cause)
366.8 Other cataract
743.30 Unspecified congenital cataract ▽
743.31 Congenital capsular and subcapsular cataract
743.32 Congenital cortical and zonular cataract
743.33 Congenital nuclear cataract

ICD-9-CM Procedural

13.3 Extracapsular extraction of lens by simple aspiration (and irrigation) technique
13.41 Phacoemulsification and aspiration of cataract
13.43 Mechanical phacofragmentation and other aspiration of cataract
13.71 Insertion of intraocular lens prosthesis at time of cataract extraction, one-stage

66983

66983 Intracapsular cataract extraction with insertion of intraocular lens prosthesis (one stage procedure)

ICD-9-CM Diagnostic

366.00 Unspecified nonsenile cataract ▽
366.04 Nuclear cataract, nonsenile
366.10 Unspecified senile cataract ▽
366.12 Incipient cataract
366.13 Anterior subcapsular polar senile cataract
366.14 Posterior subcapsular polar senile cataract
366.15 Cortical senile cataract
366.16 Nuclear sclerosis
366.17 Total or mature senile cataract
366.18 Hypermature senile cataract
366.19 Other and combined forms of senile cataract
366.20 Unspecified traumatic cataract ▽
366.21 Localized traumatic opacities of cataract
366.22 Total traumatic cataract
366.46 Cataract associated with radiation and other physical influences — (Use additional E code to identify cause)
366.8 Other cataract

ICD-9-CM Procedural

13.11 Intracapsular extraction of lens by temporal inferior route
13.19 Other intracapsular extraction of lens
13.71 Insertion of intraocular lens prosthesis at time of cataract extraction, one-stage

66984

66984 Extracapsular cataract removal with insertion of intraocular lens prosthesis (one stage procedure), manual or mechanical technique (eg, irrigation and aspiration or phacoemulsification)

ICD-9-CM Diagnostic

366.00 Unspecified nonsenile cataract ▽
366.04 Nuclear cataract, nonsenile
366.10 Unspecified senile cataract ▽
366.12 Incipient cataract
366.13 Anterior subcapsular polar senile cataract
366.14 Posterior subcapsular polar senile cataract
366.15 Cortical senile cataract
366.16 Nuclear sclerosis
366.17 Total or mature senile cataract
366.18 Hypermature senile cataract
366.19 Other and combined forms of senile cataract
366.20 Unspecified traumatic cataract ▽
366.21 Localized traumatic opacities of cataract
366.22 Total traumatic cataract
366.46 Cataract associated with radiation and other physical influences — (Use additional E code to identify cause)
366.8 Other cataract
743.30 Unspecified congenital cataract ▽
743.31 Congenital capsular and subcapsular cataract
743.32 Congenital cortical and zonular cataract
743.33 Congenital nuclear cataract

ICD-9-CM Procedural

13.3 Extracapsular extraction of lens by simple aspiration (and irrigation) technique
13.41 Phacoemulsification and aspiration of cataract
13.43 Mechanical phacofragmentation and other aspiration of cataract
13.71 Insertion of intraocular lens prosthesis at time of cataract extraction, one-stage

66985

66985 Insertion of intraocular lens prosthesis (secondary implant), not associated with concurrent cataract removal

ICD-9-CM Diagnostic

379.31 Aphakia
743.35 Congenital aphakia
V43.1 Lens replaced by other means — (This code is intended for use when these conditions are recorded as diagnoses or problems)
V45.61 Cataract extraction status — (Use additional code for associated artificial lens staus, V43.1)
V45.69 Other states following surgery of eye and adnexa — (This code is intended for use when these conditions are recorded as diagnoses or problems)

ICD-9-CM Procedural

13.70 Insertion of pseudophakos, not otherwise specified
13.72 Secondary insertion of intraocular lens prosthesis

66986

66986 Exchange of intraocular lens

ICD-9-CM Diagnostic

364.10 Unspecified chronic iridocyclitis ▽
996.53 Mechanical complication due to ocular lens prosthesis

V43.1 Lens replaced by other means — (This code is intended for use when these conditions are recorded as diagnoses or problems)
V45.61 Cataract extraction status — (Use additional code for associated artificial lens staus, V43.1)
V45.69 Other states following surgery of eye and adnexa — (This code is intended for use when these conditions are recorded as diagnoses or problems)

ICD-9-CM Procedural

13.70 Insertion of pseudophakos, not otherwise specified
13.8 Removal of implanted lens

66990

66990 Use of ophthalmic endoscope (List separately in addition to code for primary procedure)

ICD-9-CM Diagnostic

This is an add-on code. Refer to the corresponding primary procedure code for ICD-9 diagnosis code links.

HCPCS Level II Supplies & Services

The HCPCS Level II code(s) would be the same as the actual procedure performed because these are in-addition-to codes.

Posterior Segment

67005–67010

67005 Removal of vitreous, anterior approach (open sky technique or limbal incision); partial removal
67010 subtotal removal with mechanical vitrectomy

ICD-9-CM Diagnostic

360.19 Other endophthalmitis
379.21 Vitreous degeneration
379.22 Crystalline deposits in vitreous
379.23 Vitreous hemorrhage
379.25 Vitreous membranes and strands
379.26 Vitreous prolapse
379.29 Other disorders of vitreous
871.1 Ocular laceration with prolapse or exposure of intraocular tissue — (Use additional code to identify infection)
997.99 Other complications affecting other specified body systems, NEC — (Use additional code to identify complications)
998.31 Disruption of internal operation wound
998.9 Unspecified complication of procedure, not elsewhere classified ▽

ICD-9-CM Procedural

14.71 Removal of vitreous, anterior approach
14.73 Mechanical vitrectomy by anterior approach

HCPCS Level II Supplies & Services

A4305 Disposable drug delivery system, flow rate of 50 ml or greater per hour
A4306 Disposable drug delivery system, flow rate of 5 ml or less per hour
A4550 Surgical trays

67015

67015 Aspiration or release of vitreous, subretinal or choroidal fluid, pars plana approach (posterior sclerotomy)

ICD-9-CM Diagnostic

362.40 Unspecified retinal layer separation ▽
363.61 Unspecified choroidal hemorrhage ▽
363.62 Expulsive choroidal hemorrhage
363.63 Choroidal rupture
363.70 Unspecified choroidal detachment ▽
363.71 Serous choroidal detachment
363.72 Hemorrhagic choroidal detachment

ICD-9-CM Procedural

14.11 Diagnostic aspiration of vitreous
14.71 Removal of vitreous, anterior approach

HCPCS Level II Supplies & Services

A4305 Disposable drug delivery system, flow rate of 50 ml or greater per hour
A4306 Disposable drug delivery system, flow rate of 5 ml or less per hour
A4550 Surgical trays

67025–67028

67025 Injection of vitreous substitute, pars plana or limbal approach, (fluid-gas exchange), with or without aspiration (separate procedure)
67027 Implantation of intravitreal drug delivery system (eg, ganciclovir implant), includes concomitant removal of vitreous
67028 Intravitreal injection of a pharmacologic agent (separate procedure)

ICD-9-CM Diagnostic

042 Human immunodeficiency virus [HIV] — (Use additional code(s) to identify all manifestations of HIV. Use additional code to identify HIV-2 infection, 079.53.)
078.5 Cytomegaloviral disease — (Use additional code to identify manifestation: 484.1, 573.1)
360.00 Unspecified purulent endophthalmitis ▽
360.01 Acute endophthalmitis
360.02 Panophthalmitis
360.03 Chronic endophthalmitis
360.04 Vitreous abscess
361.00 Retinal detachment with retinal defect, unspecified ▽
361.01 Recent retinal detachment, partial, with single defect
361.02 Recent retinal detachment, partial, with multiple defects
361.03 Recent retinal detachment, partial, with giant tear
361.04 Recent retinal detachment, partial, with retinal dialysis
361.05 Recent retinal detachment, total or subtotal
361.06 Old retinal detachment, partial
361.07 Old retinal detachment, total or subtotal
361.81 Traction detachment of retina
363.00 Unspecified focal chorioretinitis ▽
363.01 Focal choroiditis and chorioretinitis, juxtapapillary
363.03 Focal choroiditis and chorioretinitis of other posterior pole
363.04 Focal choroiditis and chorioretinitis, peripheral
363.05 Focal retinitis and retinochoroiditis, juxtapapillary
363.06 Focal retinitis and retinochoroiditis, macular or paramacular
363.07 Focal retinitis and retinochoroiditis of other posterior pole
363.08 Focal retinitis and retinochoroiditis, peripheral
363.10 Unspecified disseminated chorioretinitis ▽
363.11 Disseminated choroiditis and chorioretinitis, posterior pole
363.12 Disseminated choroiditis and chorioretinitis, peripheral
363.13 Disseminated choroiditis and chorioretinitis, generalized — (Code first any underlying disease, 017.3) ☒
363.14 Disseminated retinitis and retinochoroiditis, metastatic
363.20 Unspecified chorioretinitis ▽

ICD-9-CM Procedural

14.75 Injection of vitreous substitute
14.79 Other operations on vitreous
14.9 Other operations on retina, choroid, and posterior chamber

HCPCS Level II Supplies & Services

A4305 Disposable drug delivery system, flow rate of 50 ml or greater per hour
A4306 Disposable drug delivery system, flow rate of 5 ml or less per hour
A4550 Surgical trays

67030–67031

67030 Discission of vitreous strands (without removal), pars plana approach
67031 Severing of vitreous strands, vitreous face adhesions, sheets, membranes or opacities, laser surgery (one or more stages)

ICD-9-CM Diagnostic

379.24 Other vitreous opacities
379.25 Vitreous membranes and strands
379.29 Other disorders of vitreous

ICD-9-CM Procedural

14.79 Other operations on vitreous

HCPCS Level II Supplies & Services

A4305 Disposable drug delivery system, flow rate of 50 ml or greater per hour
A4306 Disposable drug delivery system, flow rate of 5 ml or less per hour
A4550 Surgical trays

67036–67038

67036 Vitrectomy, mechanical, pars plana approach;
67038 with epiretinal membrane stripping

ICD-9-CM Diagnostic

250.50 Diabetes with ophthalmic manifestations, type II or unspecified type, not stated as uncontrolled — (Use additional code to identify manifestation: 362.01, 362.02, 362.83, 365.44, 366.41, 369.0-369.9)
250.51 Diabetes with ophthalmic manifestations, type I [juvenile type], not stated as uncontrolled — (Use additional code to identify manifestation: 362.01, 362.02, 362.83, 365.44, 366.41, 369.0-369.9)
250.52 Diabetes with ophthalmic manifestations, type II or unspecified type, uncontrolled — (Use additional code to identify manifestation: 362.01, 362.02, 362.83, 365.44, 366.41, 369.0-369.9)
250.53 Diabetes with ophthalmic manifestations, type I [juvenile type], uncontrolled — (Use additional code to identify manifestation: 362.01, 362.02, 362.83, 365.44, 366.41, 369.0-369.9)
360.00 Unspecified purulent endophthalmitis ▽
360.01 Acute endophthalmitis
360.02 Panophthalmitis
360.03 Chronic endophthalmitis
360.04 Vitreous abscess
360.13 Parasitic endophthalmitis NOS
360.19 Other endophthalmitis
361.30 Unspecified retinal defect ▽
361.33 Multiple defects of retina without detachment
362.01 Background diabetic retinopathy — (Code first diabetes, 250.5x) ⊠
362.02 Proliferative diabetic retinopathy — (Code first diabetes, 250.5x) ⊠
362.54 Macular cyst, hole, or pseudohole of retina
362.56 Macular puckering of retina
362.83 Retinal edema
363.32 Other macular scars of chorioretina
365.44 Glaucoma associated with systemic syndromes — (Code first associated disease: 237.7, 759.6) ⊠
365.83 Aqueous misdirection
366.41 Diabetic cataract — (Code first diabetes, 250.5X) ⊠
369.00 Blindness of both eyes, impairment level not further specified ▽
369.01 Better eye: total vision impairment; lesser eye: total vision impairment
369.02 Better eye: near-total vision impairment; lesser eye: not further specified ▽
369.03 Better eye: near-total vision impairment; lesser eye: total vision impairment
369.04 Better eye: near-total vision impairment; lesser eye: near-total vision impairment
369.05 Better eye: profound vision impairment; lesser eye: not further specified ▽
369.06 Better eye: profound vision impairment; lesser eye: total vision impairment
369.07 Better eye: profound vision impairment; lesser eye: near-total vision impairment
369.08 Better eye: profound vision impairment; lesser eye: profound vision impairment
369.10 Profound, moderate or severe vision impairment, not further specified ▽
369.11 Better eye: severe vision impairment; lesser eye: blind, not further specified ▽
369.12 Better eye: severe vision impairment; lesser eye: total vision impairment
369.13 Better eye: severe vision impairment; lesser eye: near-total vision impairment
369.14 Better eye: severe vision impairment; lesser eye: profound vision impairment
369.15 Better eye: moderate vision impairment; lesser eye: blind, not further specified ▽
369.16 Better eye: moderate vision impairment; lesser eye: total vision impairment
369.17 Better eye: moderate vision impairment; lesser eye: near-total vision impairment
369.18 Better eye: moderate vision impairment; lesser eye: profound vision impairment
369.20 Vision impairment, both eyes, impairment level not further specified ▽
369.21 Better eye: severe vision impairment; lesser eye; impairment not further specified ▽
369.22 Better eye: severe vision impairment; lesser eye: severe vision impairment
369.23 Better eye: moderate vision impairment; lesser eye: impairment not further specified ▽
369.24 Better eye: moderate vision impairment; lesser eye: severe vision impairment
369.25 Better eye: moderate vision impairment; lesser eye: moderate vision impairment
369.3 Unqualified visual loss, both eyes
369.4 Legal blindness, as defined in USA
369.60 Impairment level not further specified ▽
369.61 One eye: total vision impairment; other eye: not specified ▽
369.62 One eye: total vision impairment; other eye: near-normal vision
369.64 One eye: near-total vision impairment; other eye: vision not specified ▽
369.65 One eye: near-total vision impairment; other eye: near-normal vision
369.66 One eye: near-total vision impairment; other eye: normal vision
369.67 One eye: profound vision impairment; other eye: vision not specified ▽
369.68 One eye: profound vision impairment; other eye: near-normal vision
369.69 One eye: profound vision impairment; other eye: normal vision
369.70 Low vision, one eye, not otherwise specified ▽
369.71 One eye: severe vision impairment; other eye: vision not specified ▽
369.72 One eye: severe vision impairment; other eye: near-normal vision
369.73 One eye: severe vision impairment; other eye: normal vision
369.74 One eye: moderate vision impairment; other eye: vision not specified ▽
369.75 One eye: moderate vision impairment; other eye: near-normal vision
369.76 One eye: moderate vision impairment; other eye: normal vision
369.8 Unqualified visual loss, one eye
369.9 Unspecified visual loss ▽
379.22 Crystalline deposits in vitreous
379.23 Vitreous hemorrhage
379.24 Other vitreous opacities
379.25 Vitreous membranes and strands
379.26 Vitreous prolapse
743.51 Vitreous anomaly, congenital
997.99 Other complications affecting other specified body systems, NEC — (Use additional code to identify complications)

ICD-9-CM Procedural

14.74 Other mechanical vitrectomy
14.9 Other operations on retina, choroid, and posterior chamber

HCPCS Level II Supplies & Services

A4305 Disposable drug delivery system, flow rate of 50 ml or greater per hour
A4306 Disposable drug delivery system, flow rate of 5 ml or less per hour
A4550 Surgical trays

67039–67040

67039 Vitrectomy, mechanical, pars plana approach; with focal endolaser photocoagulation
67040 with endolaser panretinal photocoagulation

ICD-9-CM Diagnostic

250.50 Diabetes with ophthalmic manifestations, type II or unspecified type, not stated as uncontrolled — (Use additional code to identify manifestation: 362.01, 362.02, 362.83, 365.44, 366.41, 369.0-369.9)
250.51 Diabetes with ophthalmic manifestations, type I [juvenile type], not stated as uncontrolled — (Use additional code to identify manifestation: 362.01, 362.02, 362.83, 365.44, 366.41, 369.0-369.9)
250.52 Diabetes with ophthalmic manifestations, type II or unspecified type, uncontrolled — (Use additional code to identify manifestation: 362.01, 362.02, 362.83, 365.44, 366.41, 369.0-369.9)
250.53 Diabetes with ophthalmic manifestations, type I [juvenile type], uncontrolled — (Use additional code to identify manifestation: 362.01, 362.02, 362.83, 365.44, 366.41, 369.0-369.9)
361.30 Unspecified retinal defect ▽
361.33 Multiple defects of retina without detachment
361.81 Traction detachment of retina
362.01 Background diabetic retinopathy — (Code first diabetes, 250.5x) ⊠
362.02 Proliferative diabetic retinopathy — (Code first diabetes, 250.5x) ⊠
362.14 Retinal microaneurysms NOS
362.54 Macular cyst, hole, or pseudohole of retina
362.56 Macular puckering of retina
362.83 Retinal edema
363.32 Other macular scars of chorioretina
365.44 Glaucoma associated with systemic syndromes — (Code first associated disease: 237.7, 759.6) ⊠
365.83 Aqueous misdirection
366.41 Diabetic cataract — (Code first diabetes, 250.5X) ⊠
369.00 Blindness of both eyes, impairment level not further specified ▽
369.01 Better eye: total vision impairment; lesser eye: total vision impairment
369.02 Better eye: near-total vision impairment; lesser eye: not further specified ▽
369.03 Better eye: near-total vision impairment; lesser eye: total vision impairment
369.04 Better eye: near-total vision impairment; lesser eye: near-total vision impairment
369.05 Better eye: profound vision impairment; lesser eye: not further specified ▽
369.06 Better eye: profound vision impairment; lesser eye: total vision impairment
369.07 Better eye: profound vision impairment; lesser eye: near-total vision impairment
369.08 Better eye: profound vision impairment; lesser eye: profound vision impairment
369.10 Profound, moderate or severe vision impairment, not further specified ▽
369.11 Better eye: severe vision impairment; lesser eye: blind, not further specified ▽
369.12 Better eye: severe vision impairment; lesser eye: total vision impairment
369.13 Better eye: severe vision impairment; lesser eye: near-total vision impairment
369.14 Better eye: severe vision impairment; lesser eye: profound vision impairment
369.15 Better eye: moderate vision impairment; lesser eye: blind, not further specified ▽
369.16 Better eye: moderate vision impairment; lesser eye: total vision impairment
369.17 Better eye: moderate vision impairment; lesser eye: near-total vision impairment
369.18 Better eye: moderate vision impairment; lesser eye: profound vision impairment

▽ Unspecified code
♀ Female diagnosis
⊠ Manifestation code
♂ Male diagnosis

369.20	Vision impairment, both eyes, impairment level not further specified ▽
369.21	Better eye: severe vision impairment; lesser eye; impairment not further specified ▽
369.22	Better eye: severe vision impairment; lesser eye: severe vision impairment
369.23	Better eye: moderate vision impairment; lesser eye: impairment not further specified ▽
369.24	Better eye: moderate vision impairment; lesser eye: severe vision impairment
369.25	Better eye: moderate vision impairment; lesser eye: moderate vision impairment
369.3	Unqualified visual loss, both eyes
369.4	Legal blindness, as defined in USA
369.60	Impairment level not further specified ▽
369.61	One eye: total vision impairment; other eye: not specified ▽
369.62	One eye: total vision impairment; other eye: near-normal vision
369.64	One eye: near-total vision impairment; other eye: vision not specified ▽
369.65	One eye: near-total vision impairment; other eye: near-normal vision
369.66	One eye: near-total vision impairment; other eye: normal vision
369.67	One eye: profound vision impairment; other eye: vision not specified ▽
369.68	One eye: profound vision impairment; other eye: near-normal vision
369.69	One eye: profound vision impairment; other eye: normal vision
369.70	Low vision, one eye, not otherwise specified ▽
369.71	One eye: severe vision impairment; other eye: vision not specified ▽
369.72	One eye: severe vision impairment; other eye: near-normal vision
369.73	One eye: severe vision impairment; other eye: normal vision
369.74	One eye: moderate vision impairment; other eye: vision not specified ▽
369.75	One eye: moderate vision impairment; other eye: near-normal vision
369.76	One eye: moderate vision impairment; other eye: normal vision
369.8	Unqualified visual loss, one eye
379.24	Other vitreous opacities

ICD-9-CM Procedural

14.33	Repair of retinal tear by xenon arc photocoagulation
14.34	Repair of retinal tear by laser photocoagulation
14.53	Repair of retinal detachment with xenon arc photocoagulation
14.54	Repair of retinal detachment with laser photocoagulation

HCPCS Level II Supplies & Services

A4305	Disposable drug delivery system, flow rate of 50 ml or greater per hour
A4306	Disposable drug delivery system, flow rate of 5 ml or less per hour
A4550	Surgical trays

67101

67101 Repair of retinal detachment, one or more sessions; cryotherapy or diathermy, with or without drainage of subretinal fluid

ICD-9-CM Diagnostic

361.00	Retinal detachment with retinal defect, unspecified ▽
361.02	Recent retinal detachment, partial, with multiple defects
361.03	Recent retinal detachment, partial, with giant tear
361.04	Recent retinal detachment, partial, with retinal dialysis
361.05	Recent retinal detachment, total or subtotal
361.06	Old retinal detachment, partial
361.07	Old retinal detachment, total or subtotal
361.2	Serous retinal detachment
361.30	Unspecified retinal defect ▽
361.81	Traction detachment of retina
361.89	Other forms of retinal detachment
361.9	Unspecified retinal detachment ▽

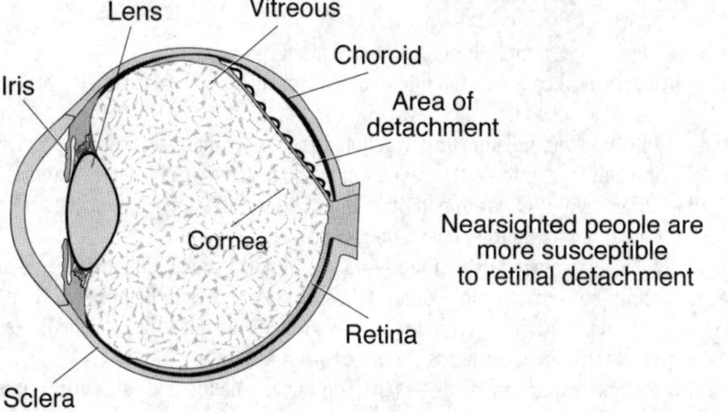

ICD-9-CM Procedural

14.51	Repair of retinal detachment with diathermy
14.52	Repair of retinal detachment with cryotherapy

HCPCS Level II Supplies & Services

A4305	Disposable drug delivery system, flow rate of 50 ml or greater per hour
A4306	Disposable drug delivery system, flow rate of 5 ml or less per hour
A4550	Surgical trays
C1814	Retinal tamponade device, silicone oil

67105

67105 Repair of retinal detachment, one or more sessions; photocoagulation, with or without drainage of subretinal fluid

ICD-9-CM Diagnostic

361.00	Retinal detachment with retinal defect, unspecified ▽
361.01	Recent retinal detachment, partial, with single defect
361.02	Recent retinal detachment, partial, with multiple defects
361.03	Recent retinal detachment, partial, with giant tear
361.04	Recent retinal detachment, partial, with retinal dialysis
361.05	Recent retinal detachment, total or subtotal
361.06	Old retinal detachment, partial
361.07	Old retinal detachment, total or subtotal
361.2	Serous retinal detachment
361.81	Traction detachment of retina
361.89	Other forms of retinal detachment
361.9	Unspecified retinal detachment ▽
362.42	Serous detachment of retinal pigment epithelium
362.43	Hemorrhagic detachment of retinal pigment epithelium

ICD-9-CM Procedural

14.35	Repair of retinal tear by photocoagulation of unspecified type
14.53	Repair of retinal detachment with xenon arc photocoagulation
14.54	Repair of retinal detachment with laser photocoagulation

HCPCS Level II Supplies & Services

A4305	Disposable drug delivery system, flow rate of 50 ml or greater per hour
A4306	Disposable drug delivery system, flow rate of 5 ml or less per hour
A4550	Surgical trays
C1814	Retinal tamponade device, silicone oil

67107

67107 Repair of retinal detachment; scleral buckling (such as lamellar scleral dissection, imbrication or encircling procedure), with or without implant, with or without cryotherapy, photocoagulation, and drainage of subretinal fluid

ICD-9-CM Diagnostic

361.00	Retinal detachment with retinal defect, unspecified ▽
361.01	Recent retinal detachment, partial, with single defect
361.02	Recent retinal detachment, partial, with multiple defects
361.03	Recent retinal detachment, partial, with giant tear
361.04	Recent retinal detachment, partial, with retinal dialysis
361.05	Recent retinal detachment, total or subtotal
361.06	Old retinal detachment, partial
361.07	Old retinal detachment, total or subtotal
361.2	Serous retinal detachment
361.81	Traction detachment of retina
361.89	Other forms of retinal detachment
361.9	Unspecified retinal detachment ▽
362.42	Serous detachment of retinal pigment epithelium
362.43	Hemorrhagic detachment of retinal pigment epithelium

ICD-9-CM Procedural

14.41	Scleral buckling with implant
14.49	Other scleral buckling

HCPCS Level II Supplies & Services

A4305	Disposable drug delivery system, flow rate of 50 ml or greater per hour
A4306	Disposable drug delivery system, flow rate of 5 ml or less per hour
A4550	Surgical trays
C1814	Retinal tamponade device, silicone oil

▽ Unspecified code ⊠ Manifestation code
♀ Female diagnosis ♂ Male diagnosis

67108

67108 Repair of retinal detachment; with vitrectomy, any method, with or without air or gas tamponade, focal endolaser photocoagulation, cryotherapy, drainage of subretinal fluid, scleral buckling, and/or removal of lens by same technique

ICD-9-CM Diagnostic

361.00 Retinal detachment with retinal defect, unspecified ▽
361.01 Recent retinal detachment, partial, with single defect
361.02 Recent retinal detachment, partial, with multiple defects
361.03 Recent retinal detachment, partial, with giant tear
361.04 Recent retinal detachment, partial, with retinal dialysis
361.05 Recent retinal detachment, total or subtotal
361.06 Old retinal detachment, partial
361.07 Old retinal detachment, total or subtotal
361.2 Serous retinal detachment
361.81 Traction detachment of retina
361.89 Other forms of retinal detachment
361.9 Unspecified retinal detachment ▽
362.42 Serous detachment of retinal pigment epithelium
362.43 Hemorrhagic detachment of retinal pigment epithelium
379.23 Vitreous hemorrhage

ICD-9-CM Procedural

13.9 Other operations on lens
14.49 Other scleral buckling
14.51 Repair of retinal detachment with diathermy
14.52 Repair of retinal detachment with cryotherapy
14.53 Repair of retinal detachment with xenon arc photocoagulation
14.54 Repair of retinal detachment with laser photocoagulation
14.71 Removal of vitreous, anterior approach
14.72 Other removal of vitreous
14.73 Mechanical vitrectomy by anterior approach
14.74 Other mechanical vitrectomy

HCPCS Level II Supplies & Services

A4305 Disposable drug delivery system, flow rate of 50 ml or greater per hour
A4306 Disposable drug delivery system, flow rate of 5 ml or less per hour
A4550 Surgical trays
C1814 Retinal tamponade device, silicone oil

67110–67112

67110 Repair of retinal detachment; by injection of air or other gas (eg, pneumatic retinopexy)
67112 by scleral buckling or vitrectomy, on patient having previous ipsilateral retinal detachment repair(s) using scleral buckling or vitrectomy techniques

ICD-9-CM Diagnostic

361.00 Retinal detachment with retinal defect, unspecified ▽
361.01 Recent retinal detachment, partial, with single defect
361.02 Recent retinal detachment, partial, with multiple defects
361.03 Recent retinal detachment, partial, with giant tear
361.04 Recent retinal detachment, partial, with retinal dialysis
361.05 Recent retinal detachment, total or subtotal
361.06 Old retinal detachment, partial
361.07 Old retinal detachment, total or subtotal
361.2 Serous retinal detachment
361.81 Traction detachment of retina
361.89 Other forms of retinal detachment
361.9 Unspecified retinal detachment ▽
362.42 Serous detachment of retinal pigment epithelium
362.43 Hemorrhagic detachment of retinal pigment epithelium
362.56 Macular puckering of retina

ICD-9-CM Procedural

14.59 Other repair of retinal detachment
14.9 Other operations on retina, choroid, and posterior chamber

HCPCS Level II Supplies & Services

A4305 Disposable drug delivery system, flow rate of 50 ml or greater per hour
A4306 Disposable drug delivery system, flow rate of 5 ml or less per hour
A4550 Surgical trays
C1814 Retinal tamponade device, silicone oil

67115

67115 Release of encircling material (posterior segment)

ICD-9-CM Diagnostic

996.59 Mechanical complication due to other implant and internal device, not elsewhere classified
996.69 Infection and inflammatory reaction due to other internal prosthetic device, implant, and graft — (Use additional code to identify specified infections)
996.79 Other complications due to other internal prosthetic device, implant, and graft
V45.69 Other states following surgery of eye and adnexa — (This code is intended for use when these conditions are recorded as diagnoses or problems)

ICD-9-CM Procedural

14.6 Removal of surgically implanted material from posterior segment of eye

HCPCS Level II Supplies & Services

A4305 Disposable drug delivery system, flow rate of 50 ml or greater per hour
A4306 Disposable drug delivery system, flow rate of 5 ml or less per hour
A4550 Surgical trays

67120

67120 Removal of implanted material, posterior segment; extraocular

ICD-9-CM Diagnostic

361.00 Retinal detachment with retinal defect, unspecified ▽
361.01 Recent retinal detachment, partial, with single defect
361.02 Recent retinal detachment, partial, with multiple defects
361.03 Recent retinal detachment, partial, with giant tear
361.04 Recent retinal detachment, partial, with retinal dialysis
361.05 Recent retinal detachment, total or subtotal
361.06 Old retinal detachment, partial
361.07 Old retinal detachment, total or subtotal
361.89 Other forms of retinal detachment
368.2 Diplopia
378.60 Unspecified mechanical strabismus ▽
996.59 Mechanical complication due to other implant and internal device, not elsewhere classified
996.69 Infection and inflammatory reaction due to other internal prosthetic device, implant, and graft — (Use additional code to identify specified infections)
998.31 Disruption of internal operation wound
998.51 Infected postoperative seroma — (Use additional code to identify organism)
998.59 Other postoperative infection — (Use additional code to identify infection)
V43.1 Lens replaced by other means — (This code is intended for use when these conditions are recorded as diagnoses or problems)
V45.61 Cataract extraction status — (Use additional code for associated artificial lens staus, V43.1)
V45.69 Other states following surgery of eye and adnexa — (This code is intended for use when these conditions are recorded as diagnoses or problems)

ICD-9-CM Procedural

14.6 Removal of surgically implanted material from posterior segment of eye

HCPCS Level II Supplies & Services

A4305 Disposable drug delivery system, flow rate of 50 ml or greater per hour
A4306 Disposable drug delivery system, flow rate of 5 ml or less per hour
A4550 Surgical trays

67121

67121 Removal of implanted material, posterior segment; intraocular

ICD-9-CM Diagnostic

379.31 Aphakia
996.53 Mechanical complication due to ocular lens prosthesis
996.59 Mechanical complication due to other implant and internal device, not elsewhere classified
996.69 Infection and inflammatory reaction due to other internal prosthetic device, implant, and graft — (Use additional code to identify specified infections)
996.79 Other complications due to other internal prosthetic device, implant, and graft
998.31 Disruption of internal operation wound
998.51 Infected postoperative seroma — (Use additional code to identify organism)
998.59 Other postoperative infection — (Use additional code to identify infection)
V43.1 Lens replaced by other means — (This code is intended for use when these conditions are recorded as diagnoses or problems)
V45.61 Cataract extraction status — (Use additional code for associated artificial lens staus, V43.1)

V45.69 Other states following surgery of eye and adnexa — (This code is intended for use when these conditions are recorded as diagnoses or problems)

ICD-9-CM Procedural

14.6 Removal of surgically implanted material from posterior segment of eye

HCPCS Level II Supplies & Services

A4305 Disposable drug delivery system, flow rate of 50 ml or greater per hour
A4306 Disposable drug delivery system, flow rate of 5 ml or less per hour
A4550 Surgical trays

67141

67141 Prophylaxis of retinal detachment (eg, retinal break, lattice degeneration) without drainage, one or more sessions; cryotherapy, diathermy

ICD-9-CM Diagnostic

361.06 Old retinal detachment, partial
361.07 Old retinal detachment, total or subtotal
361.30 Unspecified retinal defect ▽
361.31 Round hole of retina without detachment
361.32 Horseshoe tear of retina without detachment
361.33 Multiple defects of retina without detachment
362.60 Unspecified peripheral retinal degeneration ▽
362.61 Paving stone degeneration of peripheral retina
362.62 Microcystoid degeneration of peripheral retina
362.63 Lattice degeneration of peripheral retina
362.64 Senile reticular degeneration of peripheral retina

ICD-9-CM Procedural

14.31 Repair of retinal tear by diathermy
14.32 Repair of retinal tear by cryotherapy
14.51 Repair of retinal detachment with diathermy
14.52 Repair of retinal detachment with cryotherapy

HCPCS Level II Supplies & Services

A4305 Disposable drug delivery system, flow rate of 50 ml or greater per hour
A4306 Disposable drug delivery system, flow rate of 5 ml or less per hour
A4550 Surgical trays
C1814 Retinal tamponade device, silicone oil

67145

67145 Prophylaxis of retinal detachment (eg, retinal break, lattice degeneration) without drainage, one or more sessions; photocoagulation (laser or xenon arc)

ICD-9-CM Diagnostic

361.00 Retinal detachment with retinal defect, unspecified ▽
361.01 Recent retinal detachment, partial, with single defect
361.06 Old retinal detachment, partial
361.07 Old retinal detachment, total or subtotal
361.30 Unspecified retinal defect ▽
361.31 Round hole of retina without detachment
361.32 Horseshoe tear of retina without detachment
361.33 Multiple defects of retina without detachment
362.60 Unspecified peripheral retinal degeneration ▽
362.61 Paving stone degeneration of peripheral retina
362.62 Microcystoid degeneration of peripheral retina
362.63 Lattice degeneration of peripheral retina
362.64 Senile reticular degeneration of peripheral retina

ICD-9-CM Procedural

14.33 Repair of retinal tear by xenon arc photocoagulation
14.34 Repair of retinal tear by laser photocoagulation
14.53 Repair of retinal detachment with xenon arc photocoagulation
14.54 Repair of retinal detachment with laser photocoagulation

HCPCS Level II Supplies & Services

A4305 Disposable drug delivery system, flow rate of 50 ml or greater per hour
A4306 Disposable drug delivery system, flow rate of 5 ml or less per hour
A4550 Surgical trays
C1814 Retinal tamponade device, silicone oil

67208

67208 Destruction of localized lesion of retina (eg, macular edema, tumors), one or more sessions; cryotherapy, diathermy

ICD-9-CM Diagnostic

190.5 Malignant neoplasm of retina
190.6 Malignant neoplasm of choroid
198.4 Secondary malignant neoplasm of other parts of nervous system
224.5 Benign neoplasm of retina
224.6 Benign neoplasm of choroid
228.03 Hemangioma of retina
234.0 Carcinoma in situ of eye
238.8 Neoplasm of uncertain behavior of other specified sites
239.8 Neoplasm of unspecified nature of other specified sites
362.12 Exudative retinopathy
362.31 Central artery occlusion of retina
362.35 Central vein occlusion of retina
362.41 Central serous retinopathy
362.42 Serous detachment of retinal pigment epithelium
362.43 Hemorrhagic detachment of retinal pigment epithelium
362.50 Macular degeneration (senile) of retina, unspecified ▽
362.51 Nonexudative senile macular degeneration of retina
362.52 Exudative senile macular degeneration of retina
362.54 Macular cyst, hole, or pseudohole of retina

ICD-9-CM Procedural

14.21 Destruction of chorioretinal lesion by diathermy
14.22 Destruction of chorioretinal lesion by cryotherapy

HCPCS Level II Supplies & Services

A4305 Disposable drug delivery system, flow rate of 50 ml or greater per hour
A4306 Disposable drug delivery system, flow rate of 5 ml or less per hour
A4550 Surgical trays
C1814 Retinal tamponade device, silicone oil

67210

67210 Destruction of localized lesion of retina (eg, macular edema, tumors), one or more sessions; photocoagulation

ICD-9-CM Diagnostic

190.5 Malignant neoplasm of retina
190.6 Malignant neoplasm of choroid
190.9 Malignant neoplasm of eye, part unspecified ▽
224.5 Benign neoplasm of retina
224.6 Benign neoplasm of choroid
228.03 Hemangioma of retina
238.8 Neoplasm of uncertain behavior of other specified sites
239.8 Neoplasm of unspecified nature of other specified sites
362.01 Background diabetic retinopathy — (Code first diabetes, 250.5x) ☒
362.02 Proliferative diabetic retinopathy — (Code first diabetes, 250.5x) ☒
362.12 Exudative retinopathy
362.31 Central artery occlusion of retina
362.35 Central vein occlusion of retina
362.36 Venous tributary (branch) occlusion of retina
362.37 Venous engorgement of retina
362.41 Central serous retinopathy
362.42 Serous detachment of retinal pigment epithelium
362.43 Hemorrhagic detachment of retinal pigment epithelium
362.50 Macular degeneration (senile) of retina, unspecified ▽
362.51 Nonexudative senile macular degeneration of retina
362.52 Exudative senile macular degeneration of retina
362.54 Macular cyst, hole, or pseudohole of retina
362.82 Retinal exudates and deposits
362.83 Retinal edema
363.40 Unspecified choroidal degeneration ▽

ICD-9-CM Procedural

14.23 Destruction of chorioretinal lesion by xenon arc photocoagulation
14.24 Destruction of chorioretinal lesion by laser photocoagulation

HCPCS Level II Supplies & Services

A4305 Disposable drug delivery system, flow rate of 50 ml or greater per hour
A4306 Disposable drug delivery system, flow rate of 5 ml or less per hour
A4550 Surgical trays

▽ Unspecified code ☒ Manifestation code
♀ Female diagnosis ♂ Male diagnosis

67218

67218 Destruction of localized lesion of retina (eg, macular edema, tumors), one or more sessions; radiation by implantation of source (includes removal of source)

ICD-9-CM Diagnostic

190.5 Malignant neoplasm of retina
190.6 Malignant neoplasm of choroid
190.9 Malignant neoplasm of eye, part unspecified
198.4 Secondary malignant neoplasm of other parts of nervous system
224.5 Benign neoplasm of retina
224.6 Benign neoplasm of choroid
228.03 Hemangioma of retina
234.0 Carcinoma in situ of eye
238.8 Neoplasm of uncertain behavior of other specified sites
239.8 Neoplasm of unspecified nature of other specified sites
362.50 Macular degeneration (senile) of retina, unspecified
362.51 Nonexudative senile macular degeneration of retina
362.52 Exudative senile macular degeneration of retina
362.53 Cystoid macular degeneration of retina
362.54 Macular cyst, hole, or pseudohole of retina

ICD-9-CM Procedural

14.26 Destruction of chorioretinal lesion by radiation therapy
14.27 Destruction of chorioretinal lesion by implantation of radiation source

HCPCS Level II Supplies & Services

A4305 Disposable drug delivery system, flow rate of 50 ml or greater per hour
A4306 Disposable drug delivery system, flow rate of 5 ml or less per hour
A4550 Surgical trays
C1814 Retinal tamponade device, silicone oil

67220

67220 Destruction of localized lesion of choroid (eg, choroidal neovascularization); photocoagulation (eg, laser), one or more sessions

ICD-9-CM Diagnostic

190.6 Malignant neoplasm of choroid
198.4 Secondary malignant neoplasm of other parts of nervous system
224.6 Benign neoplasm of choroid
228.09 Hemangioma of other sites
234.0 Carcinoma in situ of eye
238.8 Neoplasm of uncertain behavior of other specified sites
239.8 Neoplasm of unspecified nature of other specified sites
362.16 Retinal neovascularization NOS
362.52 Exudative senile macular degeneration of retina
363.30 Unspecified chorioretinal scar
363.31 Solar retinopathy
363.32 Other macular scars of chorioretina
363.33 Other scars of posterior pole of chorioretina
363.34 Peripheral scars of the chorioretina
363.35 Disseminated scars of the chorioretina
363.40 Unspecified choroidal degeneration

ICD-9-CM Procedural

14.23 Destruction of chorioretinal lesion by xenon arc photocoagulation
14.24 Destruction of chorioretinal lesion by laser photocoagulation

HCPCS Level II Supplies & Services

A4305 Disposable drug delivery system, flow rate of 50 ml or greater per hour
A4306 Disposable drug delivery system, flow rate of 5 ml or less per hour
A4550 Surgical trays
G0186 Destruction of localized lesion of choroid (for example, choroidal neovascularization); photocoagulation, feeder vessel technique (one or more sessions)
J3490 Unclassified drugs

67221–67225

67221 Destruction of localized lesion of choroid (eg, choroidal neovascularization); photodynamic therapy (includes intravenous infusion)
67225 photodynamic therapy, second eye, at single session (List separately in addition to code for primary eye treatment)

ICD-9-CM Diagnostic

190.6 Malignant neoplasm of choroid
198.4 Secondary malignant neoplasm of other parts of nervous system
224.6 Benign neoplasm of choroid
228.09 Hemangioma of other sites
234.0 Carcinoma in situ of eye
238.8 Neoplasm of uncertain behavior of other specified sites
239.8 Neoplasm of unspecified nature of other specified sites
362.16 Retinal neovascularization NOS
362.52 Exudative senile macular degeneration of retina
363.30 Unspecified chorioretinal scar
363.31 Solar retinopathy
363.32 Other macular scars of chorioretina
363.33 Other scars of posterior pole of chorioretina
363.34 Peripheral scars of the chorioretina
363.35 Disseminated scars of the chorioretina
363.40 Unspecified choroidal degeneration

ICD-9-CM Procedural

14.29 Other destruction of chorioretinal lesion

HCPCS Level II Supplies & Services

A4305 Disposable drug delivery system, flow rate of 50 ml or greater per hour
A4306 Disposable drug delivery system, flow rate of 5 ml or less per hour
A4550 Surgical trays
G0186 Destruction of localized lesion of choroid (for example, choroidal neovascularization); photocoagulation, feeder vessel technique (one or more sessions)
J3395 Injection, verteporfin, 15 mg

67227–67228

67227 Destruction of extensive or progressive retinopathy (eg, diabetic retinopathy), one or more sessions; cryotherapy, diathermy
67228 photocoagulation (laser or xenon arc)

ICD-9-CM Diagnostic

250.50 Diabetes with ophthalmic manifestations, type II or unspecified type, not stated as uncontrolled — (Use additional code to identify manifestation: 362.01, 362.02, 362.83, 365.44, 366.41, 369.0-369.9)
250.51 Diabetes with ophthalmic manifestations, type I [juvenile type], not stated as uncontrolled — (Use additional code to identify manifestation: 362.01, 362.02, 362.83, 365.44, 366.41, 369.0-369.9)
250.52 Diabetes with ophthalmic manifestations, type II or unspecified type, uncontrolled — (Use additional code to identify manifestation: 362.01, 362.02, 362.83, 365.44, 366.41, 369.0-369.9)
250.53 Diabetes with ophthalmic manifestations, type I [juvenile type], uncontrolled — (Use additional code to identify manifestation: 362.01, 362.02, 362.83, 365.44, 366.41, 369.0-369.9)
362.01 Background diabetic retinopathy — (Code first diabetes, 250.5x)
362.02 Proliferative diabetic retinopathy — (Code first diabetes, 250.5x)
362.21 Retrolental fibroplasia
362.29 Other nondiabetic proliferative retinopathy
362.83 Retinal edema
365.44 Glaucoma associated with systemic syndromes — (Code first associated disease: 237.7, 759.6)
365.83 Aqueous misdirection
366.41 Diabetic cataract — (Code first diabetes, 250.5X)
369.00 Blindness of both eyes, impairment level not further specified
369.01 Better eye: total vision impairment; lesser eye: total vision impairment
369.02 Better eye: near-total vision impairment; lesser eye: not further specified
369.03 Better eye: near-total vision impairment; lesser eye: total vision impairment
369.04 Better eye: near-total vision impairment; lesser eye: near-total vision impairment
369.05 Better eye: profound vision impairment; lesser eye: not further specified
369.06 Better eye: profound vision impairment; lesser eye: total vision impairment
369.07 Better eye: profound vision impairment; lesser eye: near-total vision impairment
369.08 Better eye: profound vision impairment; lesser eye: profound vision impairment
369.10 Profound, moderate or severe vision impairment, not further specified
369.11 Better eye: severe vision impairment; lesser eye: blind, not further specified
369.12 Better eye: severe vision impairment; lesser eye: total vision impairment
369.13 Better eye: severe vision impairment; lesser eye: near-total vision impairment
369.14 Better eye: severe vision impairment; lesser eye: profound vision impairment
369.15 Better eye: moderate vision impairment; lesser eye: blind, not further specified
369.16 Better eye: moderate vision impairment; lesser eye: total vision impairment
369.17 Better eye: moderate vision impairment; lesser eye: near-total vision impairment
369.18 Better eye: moderate vision impairment; lesser eye: profound vision impairment
369.20 Vision impairment, both eyes, impairment level not further specified
369.21 Better eye: severe vision impairment; lesser eye; impairment not further specified
369.22 Better eye: severe vision impairment; lesser eye: severe vision impairment

Unspecified code
♀ Female diagnosis
Manifestation code
♂ Male diagnosis

369.23 Better eye: moderate vision impairment; lesser eye: impairment not further specified
369.24 Better eye: moderate vision impairment; lesser eye: severe vision impairment
369.25 Better eye: moderate vision impairment; lesser eye: moderate vision impairment
369.3 Unqualified visual loss, both eyes
369.4 Legal blindness, as defined in USA
369.60 Impairment level not further specified
369.61 One eye: total vision impairment; other eye: not specified
369.62 One eye: total vision impairment; other eye: near-normal vision
369.64 One eye: near-total vision impairment; other eye: vision not specified
369.65 One eye: near-total vision impairment; other eye: near-normal vision
369.66 One eye: near-total vision impairment; other eye: normal vision
369.67 One eye: profound vision impairment; other eye: vision not specified
369.68 One eye: profound vision impairment; other eye: near-normal vision
369.69 One eye: profound vision impairment; other eye: normal vision
369.70 Low vision, one eye, not otherwise specified
369.71 One eye: severe vision impairment; other eye: vision not specified
369.72 One eye: severe vision impairment; other eye: near-normal vision
369.73 One eye: severe vision impairment; other eye: normal vision
369.74 One eye: moderate vision impairment; other eye: vision not specified
369.75 One eye: moderate vision impairment; other eye: near-normal vision
369.76 One eye: moderate vision impairment; other eye: normal vision
369.8 Unqualified visual loss, one eye

ICD-9-CM Procedural

14.21 Destruction of chorioretinal lesion by diathermy
14.22 Destruction of chorioretinal lesion by cryotherapy
14.23 Destruction of chorioretinal lesion by xenon arc photocoagulation
14.24 Destruction of chorioretinal lesion by laser photocoagulation
14.25 Destruction of chorioretinal lesion by photocoagulation of unspecified type

HCPCS Level II Supplies & Services

A4305 Disposable drug delivery system, flow rate of 50 ml or greater per hour
A4306 Disposable drug delivery system, flow rate of 5 ml or less per hour
A4550 Surgical trays

67250–67255

67250 Scleral reinforcement (separate procedure); without graft
67255 with graft

ICD-9-CM Diagnostic

871.0 Ocular laceration without prolapse of intraocular tissue — (Use additional code to identify infection)
871.1 Ocular laceration with prolapse or exposure of intraocular tissue — (Use additional code to identify infection)
918.9 Other and unspecified superficial injuries of eye
921.3 Contusion of eyeball

ICD-9-CM Procedural

12.87 Scleral reinforcement with graft
12.88 Other scleral reinforcement

HCPCS Level II Supplies & Services

A4305 Disposable drug delivery system, flow rate of 50 ml or greater per hour
A4306 Disposable drug delivery system, flow rate of 5 ml or less per hour
A4550 Surgical trays

Ocular Adnexa

67311–67312

67311 Strabismus surgery, recession or resection procedure; one horizontal muscle
67312 two horizontal muscles

ICD-9-CM Diagnostic

368.2 Diplopia
378.00 Unspecified esotropia
378.01 Monocular esotropia
378.02 Monocular esotropia with A pattern
378.03 Monocular esotropia with V pattern
378.05 Alternating esotropia
378.11 Monocular exotropia
378.12 Monocular exotropia with A pattern
378.13 Monocular exotropia with V pattern
378.14 Monocular exotropia with other noncomitancies
378.15 Alternating exotropia
378.16 Alternating exotropia with A pattern
378.17 Alternating exotropia with V pattern
378.18 Alternating exotropia with other noncomitancies
378.21 Intermittent esotropia, monocular
378.22 Intermittent esotropia, alternating
378.23 Intermittent exotropia, monocular
378.24 Intermittent exotropia, alternating
378.35 Accommodative component in esotropia
378.51 Paralytic strabismus, third or oculomotor nerve palsy, partial
378.54 Paralytic strabismus, sixth or abducens nerve palsy
378.73 Strabismus in other neuromuscular disorders
781.93 Ocular torticollis

ICD-9-CM Procedural

15.11 Recession of one extraocular muscle
15.12 Advancement of one extraocular muscle
15.13 Resection of one extraocular muscle
15.3 Operations on two or more extraocular muscles involving temporary detachment from globe, one or both eyes

HCPCS Level II Supplies & Services

A4305 Disposable drug delivery system, flow rate of 50 ml or greater per hour
A4306 Disposable drug delivery system, flow rate of 5 ml or less per hour
A4550 Surgical trays

67314–67316

67314 Strabismus surgery, recession or resection procedure; one vertical muscle (excluding superior oblique)
67316 two or more vertical muscles (excluding superior oblique)

ICD-9-CM Diagnostic

368.2 Diplopia
378.11 Monocular exotropia
378.12 Monocular exotropia with A pattern
378.13 Monocular exotropia with V pattern
378.14 Monocular exotropia with other noncomitancies
378.15 Alternating exotropia
378.16 Alternating exotropia with A pattern
378.17 Alternating exotropia with V pattern
378.18 Alternating exotropia with other noncomitancies
378.21 Intermittent esotropia, monocular
378.22 Intermittent esotropia, alternating
378.23 Intermittent exotropia, monocular
378.24 Intermittent exotropia, alternating
378.31 Hypertropia
378.32 Hypotropia
378.45 Alternating hyperphoria
378.51 Paralytic strabismus, third or oculomotor nerve palsy, partial
378.55 Paralytic strabismus, external ophthalmoplegia
378.61 Mechanical strabismus from Brown's (tendon) sheath syndrome
378.87 Other dissociated deviation of eye movements
378.9 Unspecified disorder of eye movements
781.93 Ocular torticollis
802.6 Orbital floor (blow-out), closed fracture
802.7 Orbital floor (blow-out), open fracture

ICD-9-CM Procedural

15.11 Recession of one extraocular muscle
15.13 Resection of one extraocular muscle
15.3 Operations on two or more extraocular muscles involving temporary detachment from globe, one or both eyes

HCPCS Level II Supplies & Services

A4305 Disposable drug delivery system, flow rate of 50 ml or greater per hour
A4306 Disposable drug delivery system, flow rate of 5 ml or less per hour
A4550 Surgical trays

67318

67318 Strabismus surgery, any procedure, superior oblique muscle

ICD-9-CM Diagnostic

368.2 Diplopia
378.31 Hypertropia
378.33 Cyclotropia
378.51 Paralytic strabismus, third or oculomotor nerve palsy, partial

378.52 Paralytic strabismus, third or oculomotor nerve palsy, total
378.53 Paralytic strabismus, fourth or trochlear nerve palsy
378.55 Paralytic strabismus, external ophthalmoplegia
378.61 Mechanical strabismus from Brown's (tendon) sheath syndrome
378.71 Duane's syndrome
378.81 Palsy of conjugate gaze
378.9 Unspecified disorder of eye movements
781.93 Ocular torticollis

ICD-9-CM Procedural

15.11 Recession of one extraocular muscle
15.13 Resection of one extraocular muscle

HCPCS Level II Supplies & Services

A4305 Disposable drug delivery system, flow rate of 50 ml or greater per hour
A4306 Disposable drug delivery system, flow rate of 5 ml or less per hour
A4550 Surgical trays

67320

67320 Transposition procedure (eg, for paretic extraocular muscle), any extraocular muscle (specify) (List separately in addition to code for primary procedure)

ICD-9-CM Diagnostic

This is an add-on code. Refer to the corresponding primary procedure code for ICD-9 diagnosis code links.

ICD-9-CM Procedural

15.5 Transposition of extraocular muscles

HCPCS Level II Supplies & Services

The HCPCS Level II code(s) would be the same as the actual procedure performed because these are in-addition-to codes.

67331

67331 Strabismus surgery on patient with previous eye surgery or injury that did not involve the extraocular muscles (List separately in addition to code for primary procedure)

ICD-9-CM Diagnostic

The ICD•9 Diagnostic code(s) would be the same as the actual procedure performed because these are in-addition-to codes.

ICD-9-CM Procedural

15.19 Other operations on one extraocular muscle involving temporary detachment from globe
15.29 Other operations on one extraocular muscle
15.3 Operations on two or more extraocular muscles involving temporary detachment from globe, one or both eyes
15.5 Transposition of extraocular muscles
15.6 Revision of extraocular muscle surgery

HCPCS Level II Supplies & Services

The HCPCS Level II code(s) would be the same as the actual procedure performed because these are in-addition-to codes.

67332

67332 Strabismus surgery on patient with scarring of extraocular muscles (eg, prior ocular injury, strabismus or retinal detachment surgery) or restrictive myopathy (eg, dysthyroid ophthalmopathy) (List separately in addition to code for primary procedure)

ICD-9-CM Diagnostic

The ICD•9 Diagnostic code(s) would be the same as the actual procedure performed because these are in-addition-to codes.

ICD-9-CM Procedural

15.6 Revision of extraocular muscle surgery
15.9 Other operations on extraocular muscles and tendons

HCPCS Level II Supplies & Services

The HCPCS Level II code(s) would be the same as the actual procedure performed because these are in-addition-to codes.

67334

67334 Strabismus surgery by posterior fixation suture technique, with or without muscle recession (List separately in addition to code for primary procedure)

ICD-9-CM Diagnostic

This is an add-on code. Refer to the corresponding primary procedure code for ICD-9 diagnosis code links.

ICD-9-CM Procedural

15.11 Recession of one extraocular muscle
15.13 Resection of one extraocular muscle
15.9 Other operations on extraocular muscles and tendons

HCPCS Level II Supplies & Services

The HCPCS Level II code(s) would be the same as the actual procedure performed because these are in-addition-to codes.

67335

67335 Placement of adjustable suture(s) during strabismus surgery, including postoperative adjustment(s) of suture(s) (List separately in addition to code for specific strabismus surgery)

ICD-9-CM Diagnostic

This is an add-on code. Refer to the corresponding primary procedure code for ICD-9 diagnosis code links.

ICD-9-CM Procedural

15.4 Other operations on two or more extraocular muscles, one or both eyes
15.9 Other operations on extraocular muscles and tendons

HCPCS Level II Supplies & Services

The HCPCS Level II code(s) would be the same as the actual procedure performed because these are in-addition-to codes.

67340

67340 Strabismus surgery involving exploration and/or repair of detached extraocular muscle(s) (List separately in addition to code for primary procedure)

ICD-9-CM Diagnostic

This is an add-on code. Refer to the corresponding primary procedure code for ICD-9 diagnosis code links.

ICD-9-CM Procedural

15.6 Revision of extraocular muscle surgery
15.7 Repair of injury of extraocular muscle

HCPCS Level II Supplies & Services

The HCPCS Level II code(s) would be the same as the actual procedure performed because these are in-addition-to codes.

67343

67343 Release of extensive scar tissue without detaching extraocular muscle (separate procedure)

ICD-9-CM Diagnostic

373.8 Other inflammations of eyelids
378.01 Monocular esotropia
378.10 Unspecified exotropia
378.21 Intermittent esotropia, monocular
378.60 Unspecified mechanical strabismus
379.91 Pain in or around eye
379.92 Swelling or mass of eye
728.89 Other disorder of muscle, ligament, and fascia — (Use additional E code to identify drug, if drug-induced)
921.2 Contusion of orbital tissues

ICD-9-CM Procedural

15.29 Other operations on one extraocular muscle

HCPCS Level II Supplies & Services

A4305 Disposable drug delivery system, flow rate of 50 ml or greater per hour
A4306 Disposable drug delivery system, flow rate of 5 ml or less per hour
A4550 Surgical trays

67345

67345 Chemodenervation of extraocular muscle

ICD-9-CM Diagnostic

378.00 Unspecified esotropia ▽
378.01 Monocular esotropia
378.02 Monocular esotropia with A pattern
378.03 Monocular esotropia with V pattern
378.04 Monocular esotropia with other noncomitancies
378.05 Alternating esotropia
378.06 Alternating esotropia with A pattern
378.07 Alternating esotropia with V pattern
378.08 Alternating esotropia with other noncomitancies
378.10 Unspecified exotropia ▽
378.11 Monocular exotropia
378.12 Monocular exotropia with A pattern
378.13 Monocular exotropia with V pattern
378.14 Monocular exotropia with other noncomitancies
378.15 Alternating exotropia
378.16 Alternating exotropia with A pattern
378.17 Alternating exotropia with V pattern
378.18 Alternating exotropia with other noncomitancies
378.54 Paralytic strabismus, sixth or abducens nerve palsy

ICD-9-CM Procedural

15.29 Other operations on one extraocular muscle

HCPCS Level II Supplies & Services

A4305 Disposable drug delivery system, flow rate of 50 ml or greater per hour
A4306 Disposable drug delivery system, flow rate of 5 ml or less per hour
A4550 Surgical trays

67350

67350 Biopsy of extraocular muscle

ICD-9-CM Diagnostic

190.1 Malignant neoplasm of orbit
198.4 Secondary malignant neoplasm of other parts of nervous system
224.1 Benign neoplasm of orbit
234.0 Carcinoma in situ of eye
238.8 Neoplasm of uncertain behavior of other specified sites
239.8 Neoplasm of unspecified nature of other specified sites

ICD-9-CM Procedural

15.01 Biopsy of extraocular muscle or tendon

HCPCS Level II Supplies & Services

A4305 Disposable drug delivery system, flow rate of 50 ml or greater per hour
A4306 Disposable drug delivery system, flow rate of 5 ml or less per hour
A4550 Surgical trays

67400–67405

67400 Orbitotomy without bone flap (frontal or transconjunctival approach); for exploration, with or without biopsy
67405 with drainage only

ICD-9-CM Diagnostic

190.1 Malignant neoplasm of orbit
198.4 Secondary malignant neoplasm of other parts of nervous system
200.11 Lymphosarcoma of lymph nodes of head, face, and neck
224.0 Benign neoplasm of eyeball, except conjunctiva, cornea, retina, and choroid
239.8 Neoplasm of unspecified nature of other specified sites
362.35 Central vein occlusion of retina
368.11 Sudden visual loss
368.8 Other specified visual disturbances
373.9 Unspecified inflammation of eyelid ▽
375.03 Chronic enlargement of lacrimal gland
376.01 Orbital cellulitis
376.32 Orbital hemorrhage
377.39 Other optic neuritis
377.41 Ischemic optic neuropathy
379.91 Pain in or around eye
379.92 Swelling or mass of eye
379.93 Redness or discharge of eye

ICD-9-CM Procedural

16.09 Other orbitotomy
16.23 Biopsy of eyeball and orbit
77.49 Biopsy of other bone, except facial bones

67412–67413

67412 Orbitotomy without bone flap (frontal or transconjunctival approach); with removal of lesion
67413 with removal of foreign body

ICD-9-CM Diagnostic

190.1 Malignant neoplasm of orbit
213.0 Benign neoplasm of bones of skull and face
216.3 Benign neoplasm of skin of other and unspecified parts of face ▽
224.1 Benign neoplasm of orbit
228.01 Hemangioma of skin and subcutaneous tissue
228.09 Hemangioma of other sites
237.70 Neurofibromatosis, unspecified ▽
238.8 Neoplasm of uncertain behavior of other specified sites
239.2 Neoplasms of unspecified nature of bone, soft tissue, and skin
239.8 Neoplasm of unspecified nature of other specified sites
375.12 Other lacrimal cysts and cystic degeneration
376.01 Orbital cellulitis
376.6 Retained (old) foreign body following penetrating wound of orbit
376.81 Orbital cysts
379.92 Swelling or mass of eye
802.8 Other facial bones, closed fracture
870.4 Penetrating wound of orbit with foreign body — (Use additional code to identify infection)
930.8 Foreign body in other and combined sites on external eye
930.9 Foreign body in unspecified site on external eye ▽

ICD-9-CM Procedural

16.09 Other orbitotomy
16.1 Removal of penetrating foreign body from eye, not otherwise specified

67414

67414 Orbitotomy without bone flap (frontal or transconjunctival approach); with removal of bone for decompression

ICD-9-CM Diagnostic

224.1 Benign neoplasm of orbit
242.00 Toxic diffuse goiter without mention of thyrotoxic crisis or storm
246.9 Unspecified disorder of thyroid ▽
368.8 Other specified visual disturbances
374.41 Eyelid retraction or lag
376.21 Thyrotoxic exophthalmos ☒
378.9 Unspecified disorder of eye movements ▽
473.8 Other chronic sinusitis

ICD-9-CM Procedural

16.09 Other orbitotomy

67415

67415 Fine needle aspiration of orbital contents

ICD-9-CM Diagnostic

041.01 Streptococcus infection in conditions classified elsewhere and of unspecified site, group A — (Note: This code is to be used as an additional code to identify the bacterial agent in diseases classified elsewhere and bacterial infections of unspecified nature or site)
041.10 Unspecified staphylococcus infection in conditions classified elsewhere and of unspecified site — (Note: This code is to be used as an additional code to identify the bacterial agent in diseases classified elsewhere and bacterial infections of unspecified nature or site) ▽
041.11 Staphylococcus aureus infection in conditions classified elsewhere and of unspecified site — (Note: This code is to be used as an additional code to identify the bacterial agent in diseases classified elsewhere and bacterial infections of unspecified nature or site)
190.1 Malignant neoplasm of orbit
198.4 Secondary malignant neoplasm of other parts of nervous system
224.1 Benign neoplasm of orbit
234.0 Carcinoma in situ of eye
238.8 Neoplasm of uncertain behavior of other specified sites
368.8 Other specified visual disturbances

▽ Unspecified code
♀ Female diagnosis
☒ Manifestation code
♂ Male diagnosis

376.01 Orbital cellulitis
376.30 Unspecified exophthalmos ▽
376.33 Orbital edema or congestion
378.9 Unspecified disorder of eye movements ▽

ICD-9-CM Procedural
16.22 Diagnostic aspiration of orbit

HCPCS Level II Supplies & Services
A4550 Surgical trays

67420–67430
67420 Orbitotomy with bone flap or window, lateral approach (eg, Kroenlein); with removal of lesion
67430 with removal of foreign body

ICD-9-CM Diagnostic
190.1 Malignant neoplasm of orbit
213.0 Benign neoplasm of bones of skull and face
216.3 Benign neoplasm of skin of other and unspecified parts of face ▽
224.1 Benign neoplasm of orbit
228.01 Hemangioma of skin and subcutaneous tissue
228.09 Hemangioma of other sites
237.70 Neurofibromatosis, unspecified ▽
238.8 Neoplasm of uncertain behavior of other specified sites
239.2 Neoplasms of unspecified nature of bone, soft tissue, and skin
239.8 Neoplasm of unspecified nature of other specified sites
376.41 Hypertelorism of orbit
376.6 Retained (old) foreign body following penetrating wound of orbit
870.4 Penetrating wound of orbit with foreign body — (Use additional code to identify infection)
930.8 Foreign body in other and combined sites on external eye
930.9 Foreign body in unspecified site on external eye ▽

ICD-9-CM Procedural
16.01 Orbitotomy with bone flap
16.1 Removal of penetrating foreign body from eye, not otherwise specified

67440
67440 Orbitotomy with bone flap or window, lateral approach (eg, Kroenlein); with drainage

ICD-9-CM Diagnostic
224.1 Benign neoplasm of orbit
242.00 Toxic diffuse goiter without mention of thyrotoxic crisis or storm
368.8 Other specified visual disturbances
369.9 Unspecified visual loss ▽
376.01 Orbital cellulitis
376.21 Thyrotoxic exophthalmos ☒
376.31 Constant exophthalmos
376.41 Hypertelorism of orbit
376.52 Enophthalmos due to trauma or surgery
377.39 Other optic neuritis
377.41 Ischemic optic neuropathy
377.49 Other disorder of optic nerve
473.2 Chronic ethmoidal sinusitis

ICD-9-CM Procedural
16.01 Orbitotomy with bone flap

67445
67445 Orbitotomy with bone flap or window, lateral approach (eg, Kroenlein); with removal of bone for decompression

ICD-9-CM Diagnostic
242.01 Toxic diffuse goiter with mention of thyrotoxic crisis or storm
368.11 Sudden visual loss
369.00 Blindness of both eyes, impairment level not further specified ▽
376.21 Thyrotoxic exophthalmos ☒
802.6 Orbital floor (blow-out), closed fracture

ICD-9-CM Procedural
16.01 Orbitotomy with bone flap

67450
67450 Orbitotomy with bone flap or window, lateral approach (eg, Kroenlein); for exploration, with or without biopsy

ICD-9-CM Diagnostic
190.1 Malignant neoplasm of orbit
198.4 Secondary malignant neoplasm of other parts of nervous system
224.1 Benign neoplasm of orbit
234.0 Carcinoma in situ of eye
238.8 Neoplasm of uncertain behavior of other specified sites
239.8 Neoplasm of unspecified nature of other specified sites
379.91 Pain in or around eye
379.92 Swelling or mass of eye
379.93 Redness or discharge of eye

ICD-9-CM Procedural
16.01 Orbitotomy with bone flap
16.23 Biopsy of eyeball and orbit

67500–67505
67500 Retrobulbar injection; medication (separate procedure, does not include supply of medication)
67505 alcohol

ICD-9-CM Diagnostic
115.92 Unspecified Histoplasmosis retinitis — (Use additional code to identify manifestation: 321.0-321.1, 380.15, 711.6) ▽
135 Sarcoidosis
250.50 Diabetes with ophthalmic manifestations, type II or unspecified type, not stated as uncontrolled — (Use additional code to identify manifestation: 362.01, 362.02, 362.83, 365.44, 366.41, 369.0-369.9)
250.51 Diabetes with ophthalmic manifestations, type I [juvenile type], not stated as uncontrolled — (Use additional code to identify manifestation: 362.01, 362.02, 362.83, 365.44, 366.41, 369.0-369.9)
250.52 Diabetes with ophthalmic manifestations, type II or unspecified type, uncontrolled — (Use additional code to identify manifestation: 362.01, 362.02, 362.83, 365.44, 366.41, 369.0-369.9)
250.53 Diabetes with ophthalmic manifestations, type I [juvenile type], uncontrolled — (Use additional code to identify manifestation: 362.01, 362.02, 362.83, 365.44, 366.41, 369.0-369.9)
360.41 Blind hypotensive eye
360.42 Blind hypertensive eye
361.9 Unspecified retinal detachment ▽
362.01 Background diabetic retinopathy — (Code first diabetes, 250.5x) ☒
362.16 Retinal neovascularization NOS
362.53 Cystoid macular degeneration of retina
362.57 Drusen (degenerative) of retina
362.83 Retinal edema
363.21 Pars planitis
364.11 Chronic iridocyclitis in diseases classified elsewhere — (Code first underlying disease: 017.3, 135) ☒
364.3 Unspecified iridocyclitis ▽
364.42 Rubeosis iridis
365.11 Primary open-angle glaucoma
365.83 Aqueous misdirection
366.10 Unspecified senile cataract ▽
371.23 Bullous keratopathy
996.80 Complications of transplanted organ, unspecified site — (Use additional code to identify nature of complication, 078.5) ▽

ICD-9-CM Procedural
16.91 Retrobulbar injection of therapeutic agent

HCPCS Level II Supplies & Services
A4550 Surgical trays

67515
67515 Injection of medication or other substance into Tenon's capsule

ICD-9-CM Diagnostic
115.02 Histoplasma capsulatum retinitis — (Use additional code to identify manifestation: 321.0-321.1, 380.15, 711.6)
115.92 Unspecified Histoplasmosis retinitis — (Use additional code to identify manifestation: 321.0-321.1, 380.15, 711.6) ▽
361.89 Other forms of retinal detachment
362.36 Venous tributary (branch) occlusion of retina

362.52 Exudative senile macular degeneration of retina
362.53 Cystoid macular degeneration of retina
362.83 Retinal edema
363.21 Pars planitis
364.01 Primary iridocyclitis
364.02 Recurrent iridocyclitis
364.10 Unspecified chronic iridocyclitis ▽
364.3 Unspecified iridocyclitis ▽
366.16 Nuclear sclerosis
373.12 Hordeolum internum
379.91 Pain in or around eye

ICD-9-CM Procedural

16.99 Other operations on eyeball

HCPCS Level II Supplies & Services

A4550 Surgical trays

67550–67560

67550 Orbital implant (implant outside muscle cone); insertion
67560 removal or revision

ICD-9-CM Diagnostic

996.59 Mechanical complication due to other implant and internal device, not elsewhere classified
996.69 Infection and inflammatory reaction due to other internal prosthetic device, implant, and graft — (Use additional code to identify specified infections)
996.79 Other complications due to other internal prosthetic device, implant, and graft
V10.84 Personal history of malignant neoplasm of eye
V43.0 Eye globe replaced by other means — (This code is intended for use when these conditions are recorded as diagnoses or problems)
V52.2 Fitting and adjustment of artificial eye

ICD-9-CM Procedural

16.02 Orbitotomy with insertion of orbital implant
16.69 Other secondary procedures after removal of eyeball
16.72 Removal of orbital implant
97.31 Removal of eye prosthesis

HCPCS Level II Supplies & Services

A4550 Surgical trays

67570

67570 Optic nerve decompression (eg, incision or fenestration of optic nerve sheath)

ICD-9-CM Diagnostic

348.2 Benign intracranial hypertension
362.35 Central vein occlusion of retina
365.83 Aqueous misdirection
365.9 Unspecified glaucoma ▽
377.01 Papilledema associated with increased intracranial pressure
377.39 Other optic neuritis
377.41 Ischemic optic neuropathy

ICD-9-CM Procedural

04.42 Other cranial nerve decompression

67700

67700 Blepharotomy, drainage of abscess, eyelid

ICD-9-CM Diagnostic

373.11 Hordeolum externum
373.12 Hordeolum internum
373.13 Abscess of eyelid
373.9 Unspecified inflammation of eyelid ▽
374.84 Cysts of eyelids
374.9 Unspecified disorder of eyelid ▽
376.01 Orbital cellulitis

ICD-9-CM Procedural

08.01 Incision of lid margin
08.09 Other incision of eyelid

HCPCS Level II Supplies & Services

A4550 Surgical trays

67710

67710 Severing of tarsorrhaphy

ICD-9-CM Diagnostic

351.9 Unspecified facial nerve disorder ▽
370.21 Punctate keratitis
370.22 Macular keratitis
370.35 Neurotrophic keratoconjunctivitis
371.70 Unspecified corneal deformity ▽
907.1 Late effect of injury to cranial nerve
951.4 Injury to facial nerve
V58.3 Attention to surgical dressings and sutures
V58.49 Other specified aftercare following surgery — (This code should be used in conjunction with other aftercare codes to fully identify the reason for the aftercare encounter)

ICD-9-CM Procedural

08.02 Severing of blepharorrhaphy

HCPCS Level II Supplies & Services

A4305 Disposable drug delivery system, flow rate of 50 ml or greater per hour
A4306 Disposable drug delivery system, flow rate of 5 ml or less per hour
A4550 Surgical trays

67715

67715 Canthotomy (separate procedure)

ICD-9-CM Diagnostic

374.46 Blepharophimosis

ICD-9-CM Procedural

08.51 Canthotomy

HCPCS Level II Supplies & Services

A4305 Disposable drug delivery system, flow rate of 50 ml or greater per hour
A4306 Disposable drug delivery system, flow rate of 5 ml or less per hour
A4550 Surgical trays

67800–67808

67800 Excision of chalazion; single
67801 multiple, same lid
67805 multiple, different lids
67808 under general anesthesia and/or requiring hospitalization, single or multiple

ICD-9-CM Diagnostic

373.2 Chalazion

ICD-9-CM Procedural

08.21 Excision of chalazion

HCPCS Level II Supplies & Services

A4305 Disposable drug delivery system, flow rate of 50 ml or greater per hour
A4306 Disposable drug delivery system, flow rate of 5 ml or less per hour
A4550 Surgical trays

67810

67810 Biopsy of eyelid

ICD-9-CM Diagnostic

171.0 Malignant neoplasm of connective and other soft tissue of head, face, and neck
172.1 Malignant melanoma of skin of eyelid, including canthus
173.1 Other malignant neoplasm of skin of eyelid, including canthus
198.2 Secondary malignant neoplasm of skin
198.89 Secondary malignant neoplasm of other specified sites
215.0 Other benign neoplasm of connective and other soft tissue of head, face, and neck
216.1 Benign neoplasm of eyelid, including canthus
228.00 Hemangioma of unspecified site ▽
228.01 Hemangioma of skin and subcutaneous tissue
232.1 Carcinoma in situ of eyelid, including canthus
238.1 Neoplasm of uncertain behavior of connective and other soft tissue ▽
238.2 Neoplasm of uncertain behavior of skin
239.2 Neoplasms of unspecified nature of bone, soft tissue, and skin
239.9 Neoplasm of unspecified nature, site unspecified ▽
272.0 Pure hypercholesterolemia — (Use additional code to identify any associated mental retardation)

272.1 Pure hyperglyceridemia — (Use additional code to identify any associated mental retardation)
272.2 Mixed hyperlipidemia — (Use additional code to identify any associated mental retardation)
272.3 Hyperchylomicronemia — (Use additional code to identify any associated mental retardation)
272.4 Other and unspecified hyperlipidemia — (Use additional code to identify any associated mental retardation) ▽
272.5 Lipoprotein deficiencies — (Use additional code to identify any associated mental retardation)
272.6 Lipodystrophy — (Use additional code to identify any associated mental retardation. Use additional E code to identify cause, if iatrogenic)
272.7 Lipidoses — (Use additional code to identify any associated mental retardation)
272.9 Unspecified disorder of lipoid metabolism — (Use additional code to identify any associated mental retardation) ▽
373.2 Chalazion
373.9 Unspecified inflammation of eyelid ▽
374.51 Xanthelasma of eyelid — (Code first underlying condition: 272.0-272.9) ☒
374.84 Cysts of eyelids
379.92 Swelling or mass of eye
696.1 Other psoriasis and similar disorders
701.9 Unspecified hypertrophic and atrophic condition of skin ▽

ICD-9-CM Procedural
08.11 Biopsy of eyelid

HCPCS Level II Supplies & Services
A4550 Surgical trays

67820–67825
67820 Correction of trichiasis; epilation, by forceps only
67825 epilation by other than forceps (eg, by electrosurgery, cryotherapy, laser surgery)

ICD-9-CM Diagnostic
374.01 Senile entropion
374.04 Cicatricial entropion
374.05 Trichiasis of eyelid without entropion
374.54 Hypertrichosis of eyelid
374.89 Other disorders of eyelid
379.91 Pain in or around eye
743.63 Other specified congenital anomaly of eyelid
918.1 Superficial injury of cornea

ICD-9-CM Procedural
08.59 Other adjustment of lid position
08.91 Electrosurgical epilation of eyelid
08.92 Cryosurgical epilation of eyelid
08.93 Other epilation of eyelid

HCPCS Level II Supplies & Services
A4305 Disposable drug delivery system, flow rate of 50 ml or greater per hour
A4306 Disposable drug delivery system, flow rate of 5 ml or less per hour
A4550 Surgical trays

67830–67835
67830 Correction of trichiasis; incision of lid margin
67835 incision of lid margin, with free mucous membrane graft

ICD-9-CM Diagnostic
374.01 Senile entropion
374.04 Cicatricial entropion
374.05 Trichiasis of eyelid without entropion
374.54 Hypertrichosis of eyelid
374.89 Other disorders of eyelid
379.91 Pain in or around eye
743.63 Other specified congenital anomaly of eyelid
918.1 Superficial injury of cornea

ICD-9-CM Procedural
08.59 Other adjustment of lid position
08.93 Other epilation of eyelid

HCPCS Level II Supplies & Services
A4305 Disposable drug delivery system, flow rate of 50 ml or greater per hour
A4306 Disposable drug delivery system, flow rate of 5 ml or less per hour
A4550 Surgical trays

67840
67840 Excision of lesion of eyelid (except chalazion) without closure or with simple direct closure

ICD-9-CM Diagnostic
172.1 Malignant melanoma of skin of eyelid, including canthus
173.1 Other malignant neoplasm of skin of eyelid, including canthus
214.0 Lipoma of skin and subcutaneous tissue of face
215.0 Other benign neoplasm of connective and other soft tissue of head, face, and neck
216.1 Benign neoplasm of eyelid, including canthus
228.01 Hemangioma of skin and subcutaneous tissue
232.1 Carcinoma in situ of eyelid, including canthus
238.1 Neoplasm of uncertain behavior of connective and other soft tissue ▽
238.2 Neoplasm of uncertain behavior of skin
239.2 Neoplasms of unspecified nature of bone, soft tissue, and skin
372.51 Pinguecula
372.52 Pseudopterygium
372.54 Conjunctival concretions
372.56 Conjunctival deposits
372.61 Granuloma of conjunctiva
372.62 Localized adhesions and strands of conjunctiva
373.11 Hordeolum externum
373.12 Hordeolum internum
373.9 Unspecified inflammation of eyelid ▽
374.51 Xanthelasma of eyelid — (Code first underlying condition: 272.0-272.9) ☒
374.84 Cysts of eyelids
374.89 Other disorders of eyelid
702.0 Actinic keratosis
702.11 Inflamed seborrheic keratosis
702.19 Other seborrheic keratosis
706.2 Sebaceous cyst

ICD-9-CM Procedural
08.20 Removal of lesion of eyelid, not otherwise specified

HCPCS Level II Supplies & Services
A4305 Disposable drug delivery system, flow rate of 50 ml or greater per hour
A4306 Disposable drug delivery system, flow rate of 5 ml or less per hour
A4550 Surgical trays

67850
67850 Destruction of lesion of lid margin (up to 1 cm)

ICD-9-CM Diagnostic
173.1 Other malignant neoplasm of skin of eyelid, including canthus
216.1 Benign neoplasm of eyelid, including canthus
232.1 Carcinoma in situ of eyelid, including canthus
238.2 Neoplasm of uncertain behavior of skin
239.2 Neoplasms of unspecified nature of bone, soft tissue, and skin
373.2 Chalazion
373.9 Unspecified inflammation of eyelid ▽
374.05 Trichiasis of eyelid without entropion
374.84 Cysts of eyelids
379.92 Swelling or mass of eye
701.1 Acquired keratoderma
701.9 Unspecified hypertrophic and atrophic condition of skin ▽
706.2 Sebaceous cyst

ICD-9-CM Procedural
08.22 Excision of other minor lesion of eyelid

HCPCS Level II Supplies & Services
A4305 Disposable drug delivery system, flow rate of 50 ml or greater per hour
A4306 Disposable drug delivery system, flow rate of 5 ml or less per hour
A4550 Surgical trays

67875
67875 Temporary closure of eyelids by suture (eg, Frost suture)

ICD-9-CM Diagnostic
173.1 Other malignant neoplasm of skin of eyelid, including canthus
370.04 Hypopyon ulcer
370.06 Perforated corneal ulcer
370.20 Unspecified superficial keratitis ▽
370.34 Exposure keratoconjunctivitis

370.9 Unspecified keratitis
371.40 Unspecified corneal degeneration
372.73 Conjunctival edema
374.05 Trichiasis of eyelid without entropion
374.10 Unspecified ectropion
374.14 Cicatricial ectropion
374.23 Cicatricial lagophthalmos
374.41 Eyelid retraction or lag
378.55 Paralytic strabismus, external ophthalmoplegia

ICD-9-CM Procedural
08.99 Other operations on eyelids

HCPCS Level II Supplies & Services
A4550 Surgical trays

67880–67882
67880 Construction of intermarginal adhesions, median tarsorrhaphy, or canthorrhaphy;
67882 with transposition of tarsal plate

ICD-9-CM Diagnostic
351.0 Bell's palsy
351.9 Unspecified facial nerve disorder
370.01 Marginal corneal ulcer
370.06 Perforated corneal ulcer
370.20 Unspecified superficial keratitis
370.33 Keratoconjunctivitis sicca, not specified as Sjögren's
370.34 Exposure keratoconjunctivitis
370.35 Neurotrophic keratoconjunctivitis
370.40 Unspecified keratoconjunctivitis
371.03 Central opacity of cornea
371.40 Unspecified corneal degeneration
371.42 Recurrent erosion of cornea
374.11 Senile ectropion
374.14 Cicatricial ectropion
374.21 Paralytic lagophthalmos
374.22 Mechanical lagophthalmos
374.34 Blepharochalasis
374.41 Eyelid retraction or lag
378.55 Paralytic strabismus, external ophthalmoplegia
906.5 Late effect of burn of eye, face, head, and neck
918.1 Superficial injury of cornea

ICD-9-CM Procedural
08.52 Blepharorrhaphy
08.69 Other reconstruction of eyelid with flaps or grafts

67900
67900 Repair of brow ptosis (supraciliary, mid-forehead or coronal approach)

ICD-9-CM Diagnostic
351.9 Unspecified facial nerve disorder
374.21 Paralytic lagophthalmos
374.30 Unspecified ptosis of eyelid
374.31 Paralytic ptosis
374.32 Myogenic ptosis
374.33 Mechanical ptosis
374.34 Blepharochalasis
374.50 Unspecified degenerative disorder of eyelid
376.30 Unspecified exophthalmos
709.2 Scar condition and fibrosis of skin
709.3 Degenerative skin disorder
743.62 Congenital deformity of eyelid
998.9 Unspecified complication of procedure, not elsewhere classified

ICD-9-CM Procedural
08.36 Repair of blepharoptosis by other techniques
08.59 Other adjustment of lid position

HCPCS Level II Supplies & Services
A4305 Disposable drug delivery system, flow rate of 50 ml or greater per hour
A4306 Disposable drug delivery system, flow rate of 5 ml or less per hour
A4550 Surgical trays

Repair of Brow Ptosis

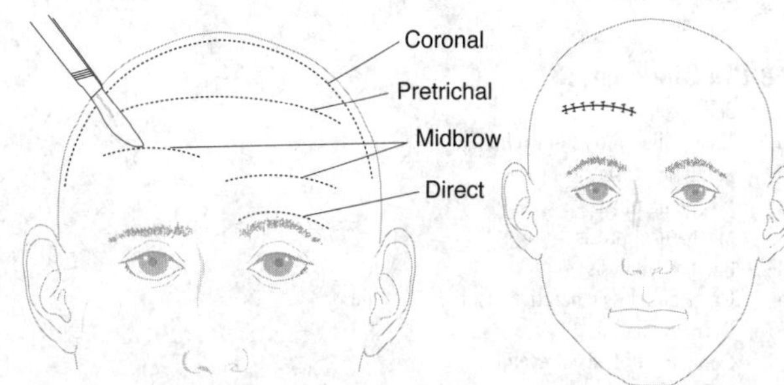

The incision may be made in any of several locations; the incision is repaired by suture

Droopy brow is fixed above the supraorbital rim

67901
67901 Repair of blepharoptosis; frontalis muscle technique with suture or other material

ICD-9-CM Diagnostic
374.30 Unspecified ptosis of eyelid
374.31 Paralytic ptosis
374.32 Myogenic ptosis
374.33 Mechanical ptosis
374.34 Blepharochalasis
378.72 Progressive external ophthalmoplegia
701.8 Other specified hypertrophic and atrophic condition of skin
743.61 Congenital ptosis of eyelid

ICD-9-CM Procedural
08.31 Repair of blepharoptosis by frontalis muscle technique with suture

HCPCS Level II Supplies & Services
A4305 Disposable drug delivery system, flow rate of 50 ml or greater per hour
A4306 Disposable drug delivery system, flow rate of 5 ml or less per hour
A4550 Surgical trays

67902
67902 Repair of blepharoptosis; frontalis muscle technique with fascial sling (includes obtaining fascia)

ICD-9-CM Diagnostic
374.30 Unspecified ptosis of eyelid
374.31 Paralytic ptosis
374.32 Myogenic ptosis
374.33 Mechanical ptosis
374.34 Blepharochalasis
378.55 Paralytic strabismus, external ophthalmoplegia
743.61 Congenital ptosis of eyelid

ICD-9-CM Procedural
08.32 Repair of blepharoptosis by frontalis muscle technique with fascial sling

67903
67903 Repair of blepharoptosis; (tarso) levator resection or advancement, internal approach

ICD-9-CM Diagnostic
374.30 Unspecified ptosis of eyelid
374.31 Paralytic ptosis
374.32 Myogenic ptosis
374.33 Mechanical ptosis
374.34 Blepharochalasis
743.61 Congenital ptosis of eyelid
951.0 Injury to oculomotor nerve

ICD-9-CM Procedural
08.33 Repair of blepharoptosis by resection or advancement of levator muscle or aponeurosis
08.34 Repair of blepharoptosis by other levator muscle techniques
08.35 Repair of blepharoptosis by tarsal technique

67904

67904 Repair of blepharoptosis; (tarso) levator resection or advancement, external approach

ICD-9-CM Diagnostic

351.0 Bell's palsy
374.30 Unspecified ptosis of eyelid
374.31 Paralytic ptosis
374.32 Myogenic ptosis
374.33 Mechanical ptosis
374.34 Blepharochalasis
374.50 Unspecified degenerative disorder of eyelid
374.87 Dermatochalasis
743.61 Congenital ptosis of eyelid

ICD-9-CM Procedural

08.33 Repair of blepharoptosis by resection or advancement of levator muscle or aponeurosis
08.34 Repair of blepharoptosis by other levator muscle techniques
08.35 Repair of blepharoptosis by tarsal technique

67906

67906 Repair of blepharoptosis; superior rectus technique with fascial sling (includes obtaining fascia)

ICD-9-CM Diagnostic

374.30 Unspecified ptosis of eyelid
374.31 Paralytic ptosis
374.32 Myogenic ptosis
374.33 Mechanical ptosis
374.34 Blepharochalasis
701.8 Other specified hypertrophic and atrophic condition of skin
743.61 Congenital ptosis of eyelid

ICD-9-CM Procedural

08.36 Repair of blepharoptosis by other techniques

67908

67908 Repair of blepharoptosis; conjunctivo-tarso-Muller's muscle-levator resection (eg, Fasanella-Servat type)

ICD-9-CM Diagnostic

374.30 Unspecified ptosis of eyelid
374.31 Paralytic ptosis
374.32 Myogenic ptosis
374.33 Mechanical ptosis
374.34 Blepharochalasis
743.61 Congenital ptosis of eyelid
743.62 Congenital deformity of eyelid

ICD-9-CM Procedural

08.33 Repair of blepharoptosis by resection or advancement of levator muscle or aponeurosis

67909

67909 Reduction of overcorrection of ptosis

ICD-9-CM Diagnostic

374.30 Unspecified ptosis of eyelid
374.31 Paralytic ptosis
374.32 Myogenic ptosis
374.33 Mechanical ptosis
374.34 Blepharochalasis
374.41 Eyelid retraction or lag
743.61 Congenital ptosis of eyelid

ICD-9-CM Procedural

08.37 Reduction of overcorrection of ptosis

HCPCS Level II Supplies & Services

A4305 Disposable drug delivery system, flow rate of 50 ml or greater per hour
A4306 Disposable drug delivery system, flow rate of 5 ml or less per hour
A4550 Surgical trays

67911

67911 Correction of lid retraction

ICD-9-CM Diagnostic

333.81 Blepharospasm — (Use additional E code to identify drug, if drug-induced)
351.0 Bell's palsy
370.34 Exposure keratoconjunctivitis
374.20 Unspecified lagophthalmos
374.21 Paralytic lagophthalmos
374.22 Mechanical lagophthalmos
374.23 Cicatricial lagophthalmos
374.41 Eyelid retraction or lag
374.89 Other disorders of eyelid
376.21 Thyrotoxic exophthalmos
743.62 Congenital deformity of eyelid
906.5 Late effect of burn of eye, face, head, and neck

ICD-9-CM Procedural

08.38 Correction of lid retraction
08.59 Other adjustment of lid position

67912

67912 Correction of lagophthalmos, with implantation of upper eyelid lid load (eg, gold weight)

ICD-9-CM Diagnostic

374.20 Unspecified lagophthalmos
374.21 Paralytic lagophthalmos
374.22 Mechanical lagophthalmos
374.23 Cicatricial lagophthalmos

ICD-9-CM Procedural

08.59 Other adjustment of lid position

67914

67914 Repair of ectropion; suture

ICD-9-CM Diagnostic

374.10 Unspecified ectropion
374.11 Senile ectropion
374.12 Mechanical ectropion
374.13 Spastic ectropion
374.14 Cicatricial ectropion
375.51 Eversion of lacrimal punctum

ICD-9-CM Procedural

08.42 Repair of entropion or ectropion by suture technique

HCPCS Level II Supplies & Services

A4305 Disposable drug delivery system, flow rate of 50 ml or greater per hour
A4306 Disposable drug delivery system, flow rate of 5 ml or less per hour
A4550 Surgical trays

67915

67915 Repair of ectropion; thermocauterization

ICD-9-CM Diagnostic

374.10 Unspecified ectropion
374.11 Senile ectropion
374.12 Mechanical ectropion
374.13 Spastic ectropion
374.14 Cicatricial ectropion
375.51 Eversion of lacrimal punctum

ICD-9-CM Procedural

08.41 Repair of entropion or ectropion by thermocauterization

HCPCS Level II Supplies & Services

A4305 Disposable drug delivery system, flow rate of 50 ml or greater per hour
A4306 Disposable drug delivery system, flow rate of 5 ml or less per hour
A4550 Surgical trays

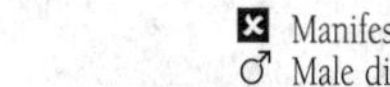

Manifestation code
Male diagnosis

67916

67916 Repair of ectropion; excision tarsal wedge

ICD-9-CM Diagnostic

374.10 Unspecified ectropion ▽
374.11 Senile ectropion
374.12 Mechanical ectropion
374.13 Spastic ectropion
374.14 Cicatricial ectropion
374.30 Unspecified ptosis of eyelid ▽
374.34 Blepharochalasis
375.51 Eversion of lacrimal punctum
728.4 Laxity of ligament

ICD-9-CM Procedural

08.43 Repair of entropion or ectropion with wedge resection

HCPCS Level II Supplies & Services

A4305 Disposable drug delivery system, flow rate of 50 ml or greater per hour
A4306 Disposable drug delivery system, flow rate of 5 ml or less per hour
A4550 Surgical trays

67917

67917 Repair of ectropion; extensive (eg, tarsal strip operations)

ICD-9-CM Diagnostic

333.81 Blepharospasm — (Use additional E code to identify drug, if drug-induced)
370.34 Exposure keratoconjunctivitis
374.11 Senile ectropion
374.12 Mechanical ectropion
374.13 Spastic ectropion
374.14 Cicatricial ectropion
374.32 Myogenic ptosis
374.34 Blepharochalasis
374.41 Eyelid retraction or lag
374.50 Unspecified degenerative disorder of eyelid ▽
374.9 Unspecified disorder of eyelid ▽
375.52 Stenosis of lacrimal punctum
376.41 Hypertelorism of orbit
743.62 Congenital deformity of eyelid

ICD-9-CM Procedural

08.44 Repair of entropion or ectropion with lid reconstruction
08.49 Other repair of entropion or ectropion

67921–67924

67921 Repair of entropion; suture
67922 thermocauterization
67923 excision tarsal wedge
67924 extensive (eg, tarsal strip or capsulopalpebral fascia repairs operation)

ICD-9-CM Diagnostic

374.01 Senile entropion
374.02 Mechanical entropion
374.03 Spastic entropion
374.04 Cicatricial entropion
374.34 Blepharochalasis
374.89 Other disorders of eyelid

ICD-9-CM Procedural

08.42 Repair of entropion or ectropion by suture technique
08.44 Repair of entropion or ectropion with lid reconstruction
08.49 Other repair of entropion or ectropion

HCPCS Level II Supplies & Services

A4305 Disposable drug delivery system, flow rate of 50 ml or greater per hour
A4306 Disposable drug delivery system, flow rate of 5 ml or less per hour
A4550 Surgical trays

67930–67935

67930 Suture of recent wound, eyelid, involving lid margin, tarsus, and/or palpebral conjunctiva direct closure; partial thickness
67935 full thickness

ICD-9-CM Diagnostic

870.0 Laceration of skin of eyelid and periocular area — (Use additional code to identify infection)
870.1 Laceration of eyelid, full-thickness, not involving lacrimal passages — (Use additional code to identify infection)
870.2 Laceration of eyelid involving lacrimal passages — (Use additional code to identify infection)
870.8 Other specified open wound of ocular adnexa — (Use additional code to identify infection)

ICD-9-CM Procedural

08.71 Reconstruction of eyelid involving lid margin, partial-thickness
08.82 Repair of laceration involving lid margin, partial-thickness
08.84 Repair of laceration of eyelid involving lid margin, full-thickness
08.99 Other operations on eyelids

HCPCS Level II Supplies & Services

A4305 Disposable drug delivery system, flow rate of 50 ml or greater per hour
A4306 Disposable drug delivery system, flow rate of 5 ml or less per hour
A4550 Surgical trays

67938

67938 Removal of embedded foreign body, eyelid

ICD-9-CM Diagnostic

374.86 Retained foreign body of eyelid
379.91 Pain in or around eye
870.0 Laceration of skin of eyelid and periocular area — (Use additional code to identify infection)
870.1 Laceration of eyelid, full-thickness, not involving lacrimal passages — (Use additional code to identify infection)
918.1 Superficial injury of cornea
930.1 Foreign body in conjunctival sac
930.2 Foreign body in lacrimal punctum
930.8 Foreign body in other and combined sites on external eye
930.9 Foreign body in unspecified site on external eye ▽
998.4 Foreign body accidentally left during procedure, not elsewhere classified

ICD-9-CM Procedural

08.99 Other operations on eyelids

HCPCS Level II Supplies & Services

A4305 Disposable drug delivery system, flow rate of 50 ml or greater per hour
A4306 Disposable drug delivery system, flow rate of 5 ml or less per hour
A4550 Surgical trays

67950

67950 Canthoplasty (reconstruction of canthus)

ICD-9-CM Diagnostic

173.1 Other malignant neoplasm of skin of eyelid, including canthus
216.1 Benign neoplasm of eyelid, including canthus
232.1 Carcinoma in situ of eyelid, including canthus
238.2 Neoplasm of uncertain behavior of skin
239.2 Neoplasms of unspecified nature of bone, soft tissue, and skin
333.81 Blepharospasm — (Use additional E code to identify drug, if drug-induced)
374.10 Unspecified ectropion ▽
374.11 Senile ectropion
374.14 Cicatricial ectropion
374.20 Unspecified lagophthalmos ▽
374.22 Mechanical lagophthalmos
374.41 Eyelid retraction or lag
374.46 Blepharophimosis
376.36 Lateral displacement of globe of eye
376.41 Hypertelorism of orbit
376.50 Enophthalmos, unspecified as to cause ▽
376.51 Enophthalmos due to atrophy of orbital tissue
376.52 Enophthalmos due to trauma or surgery
743.62 Congenital deformity of eyelid
802.6 Orbital floor (blow-out), closed fracture

▽ Unspecified code
♀ Female diagnosis
☒ Manifestation code
♂ Male diagnosis

870.0 Laceration of skin of eyelid and periocular area — (Use additional code to identify infection)
870.1 Laceration of eyelid, full-thickness, not involving lacrimal passages — (Use additional code to identify infection)
870.2 Laceration of eyelid involving lacrimal passages — (Use additional code to identify infection)
870.8 Other specified open wound of ocular adnexa — (Use additional code to identify infection)
906.0 Late effect of open wound of head, neck, and trunk
906.5 Late effect of burn of eye, face, head, and neck
940.0 Chemical burn of eyelids and periocular area
940.1 Other burns of eyelids and periocular area
V10.82 Personal history of malignant melanoma of skin
V10.83 Personal history of other malignant neoplasm of skin
V10.84 Personal history of malignant neoplasm of eye

ICD-9-CM Procedural

08.59 Other adjustment of lid position

HCPCS Level II Supplies & Services

A4305 Disposable drug delivery system, flow rate of 50 ml or greater per hour
A4306 Disposable drug delivery system, flow rate of 5 ml or less per hour
A4550 Surgical trays

67961–67966

67961 Excision and repair of eyelid, involving lid margin, tarsus, conjunctiva, canthus, or full thickness, may include preparation for skin graft or pedicle flap with adjacent tissue transfer or rearrangement; up to one-fourth of lid margin
67966 over one-fourth of lid margin

ICD-9-CM Diagnostic

171.0 Malignant neoplasm of connective and other soft tissue of head, face, and neck
172.1 Malignant melanoma of skin of eyelid, including canthus
173.1 Other malignant neoplasm of skin of eyelid, including canthus
198.2 Secondary malignant neoplasm of skin
198.89 Secondary malignant neoplasm of other specified sites
214.0 Lipoma of skin and subcutaneous tissue of face
215.0 Other benign neoplasm of connective and other soft tissue of head, face, and neck
216.1 Benign neoplasm of eyelid, including canthus
232.1 Carcinoma in situ of eyelid, including canthus
238.1 Neoplasm of uncertain behavior of connective and other soft tissue ▽
238.2 Neoplasm of uncertain behavior of skin
239.2 Neoplasms of unspecified nature of bone, soft tissue, and skin
372.64 Scarring of conjunctiva
373.9 Unspecified inflammation of eyelid ▽
374.05 Trichiasis of eyelid without entropion
374.11 Senile ectropion
374.12 Mechanical ectropion
374.13 Spastic ectropion
374.14 Cicatricial ectropion
374.21 Paralytic lagophthalmos
709.2 Scar condition and fibrosis of skin
728.4 Laxity of ligament
743.62 Congenital deformity of eyelid
940.0 Chemical burn of eyelids and periocular area
940.1 Other burns of eyelids and periocular area

ICD-9-CM Procedural

08.61 Reconstruction of eyelid with skin flap or graft
08.73 Reconstruction of eyelid involving lid margin, full-thickness
08.74 Other reconstruction of eyelid, full-thickness

HCPCS Level II Supplies & Services

A4305 Disposable drug delivery system, flow rate of 50 ml or greater per hour
A4306 Disposable drug delivery system, flow rate of 5 ml or less per hour
A4550 Surgical trays

67971–67974

67971 Reconstruction of eyelid, full thickness by transfer of tarsoconjunctival flap from opposing eyelid; up to two-thirds of eyelid, one stage or first stage
67973 total eyelid, lower, one stage or first stage
67974 total eyelid, upper, one stage or first stage

ICD-9-CM Diagnostic

171.0 Malignant neoplasm of connective and other soft tissue of head, face, and neck
172.1 Malignant melanoma of skin of eyelid, including canthus
173.1 Other malignant neoplasm of skin of eyelid, including canthus
198.2 Secondary malignant neoplasm of skin
198.89 Secondary malignant neoplasm of other specified sites
214.0 Lipoma of skin and subcutaneous tissue of face
215.0 Other benign neoplasm of connective and other soft tissue of head, face, and neck
216.1 Benign neoplasm of eyelid, including canthus
232.1 Carcinoma in situ of eyelid, including canthus
238.1 Neoplasm of uncertain behavior of connective and other soft tissue ▽
238.2 Neoplasm of uncertain behavior of skin
239.2 Neoplasms of unspecified nature of bone, soft tissue, and skin
372.64 Scarring of conjunctiva
373.9 Unspecified inflammation of eyelid ▽
374.05 Trichiasis of eyelid without entropion
374.10 Unspecified ectropion ▽
374.11 Senile ectropion
374.12 Mechanical ectropion
374.13 Spastic ectropion
374.14 Cicatricial ectropion
374.21 Paralytic lagophthalmos
374.9 Unspecified disorder of eyelid ▽
709.2 Scar condition and fibrosis of skin
728.4 Laxity of ligament
743.62 Congenital deformity of eyelid
940.0 Chemical burn of eyelids and periocular area
940.1 Other burns of eyelids and periocular area
V10.82 Personal history of malignant melanoma of skin
V10.83 Personal history of other malignant neoplasm of skin
V10.84 Personal history of malignant neoplasm of eye

ICD-9-CM Procedural

08.64 Reconstruction of eyelid with tarsoconjunctival flap
08.74 Other reconstruction of eyelid, full-thickness

67975

67975 Reconstruction of eyelid, full thickness by transfer of tarsoconjunctival flap from opposing eyelid; second stage

ICD-9-CM Diagnostic

171.0 Malignant neoplasm of connective and other soft tissue of head, face, and neck
172.1 Malignant melanoma of skin of eyelid, including canthus
173.1 Other malignant neoplasm of skin of eyelid, including canthus
198.2 Secondary malignant neoplasm of skin
198.89 Secondary malignant neoplasm of other specified sites
214.0 Lipoma of skin and subcutaneous tissue of face
215.0 Other benign neoplasm of connective and other soft tissue of head, face, and neck
216.1 Benign neoplasm of eyelid, including canthus
232.1 Carcinoma in situ of eyelid, including canthus
238.1 Neoplasm of uncertain behavior of connective and other soft tissue ▽
238.2 Neoplasm of uncertain behavior of skin
239.2 Neoplasms of unspecified nature of bone, soft tissue, and skin
372.64 Scarring of conjunctiva
373.9 Unspecified inflammation of eyelid ▽
374.05 Trichiasis of eyelid without entropion
374.10 Unspecified ectropion ▽
374.11 Senile ectropion
374.12 Mechanical ectropion
374.13 Spastic ectropion
374.14 Cicatricial ectropion
374.21 Paralytic lagophthalmos
374.9 Unspecified disorder of eyelid ▽
709.2 Scar condition and fibrosis of skin
728.4 Laxity of ligament
743.62 Congenital deformity of eyelid
940.0 Chemical burn of eyelids and periocular area
940.1 Other burns of eyelids and periocular area
V10.82 Personal history of malignant melanoma of skin
V10.83 Personal history of other malignant neoplasm of skin
V10.84 Personal history of malignant neoplasm of eye

ICD-9-CM Procedural

08.64 Reconstruction of eyelid with tarsoconjunctival flap
08.74 Other reconstruction of eyelid, full-thickness

▽ Unspecified code ♀ Female diagnosis ☒ Manifestation code ♂ Male diagnosis

Conjunctiva

68020

68020 Incision of conjunctiva, drainage of cyst

ICD-9-CM Diagnostic

372.54 Conjunctival concretions
372.75 Conjunctival cysts
373.11 Hordeolum externum
373.13 Abscess of eyelid
373.2 Chalazion
374.84 Cysts of eyelids
706.2 Sebaceous cyst
871.0 Ocular laceration without prolapse of intraocular tissue — (Use additional code to identify infection)

ICD-9-CM Procedural

10.1 Other incision of conjunctiva

HCPCS Level II Supplies & Services

A4550 Surgical trays

68040

68040 Expression of conjunctival follicles (eg, for trachoma)

ICD-9-CM Diagnostic

076.0 Initial stage trachoma
076.1 Active stage trachoma
076.9 Unspecified trachoma ▽
139.1 Late effects of trachoma
372.55 Conjunctival pigmentations
372.61 Granuloma of conjunctiva
372.64 Scarring of conjunctiva
373.6 Parasitic infestation of eyelid — (Code first underlying disease: 085.0-085.9, 125.2, 125.3, 132.0) ☒

ICD-9-CM Procedural

10.1 Other incision of conjunctiva

HCPCS Level II Supplies & Services

A4550 Surgical trays

68100

68100 Biopsy of conjunctiva

ICD-9-CM Diagnostic

173.1 Other malignant neoplasm of skin of eyelid, including canthus
190.3 Malignant neoplasm of conjunctiva
198.4 Secondary malignant neoplasm of other parts of nervous system
216.1 Benign neoplasm of eyelid, including canthus
224.3 Benign neoplasm of conjunctiva
234.0 Carcinoma in situ of eye
238.8 Neoplasm of uncertain behavior of other specified sites
239.8 Neoplasm of unspecified nature of other specified sites
370.33 Keratoconjunctivitis sicca, not specified as Sjögren's
372.51 Pinguecula
372.75 Conjunctival cysts
372.9 Unspecified disorder of conjunctiva ▽
694.61 Benign mucous membrane pemphigoid with ocular involvement

ICD-9-CM Procedural

10.21 Biopsy of conjunctiva

HCPCS Level II Supplies & Services

A4550 Surgical trays

68110–68115

68110 Excision of lesion, conjunctiva; up to 1 cm
68115 over 1 cm

ICD-9-CM Diagnostic

190.3 Malignant neoplasm of conjunctiva
198.4 Secondary malignant neoplasm of other parts of nervous system
224.3 Benign neoplasm of conjunctiva
234.0 Carcinoma in situ of eye
238.8 Neoplasm of uncertain behavior of other specified sites
239.8 Neoplasm of unspecified nature of other specified sites
372.03 Other mucopurulent conjunctivitis
372.15 Parasitic conjunctivitis — (Code first underlying disease: 085.5, 125.0-125.9) ☒
372.40 Unspecified pterygium ▽
372.45 Recurrent pterygium
372.51 Pinguecula
372.61 Granuloma of conjunctiva
372.71 Hyperemia of conjunctiva
372.74 Vascular abnormalities of conjunctiva
372.75 Conjunctival cysts
372.81 Conjunctivochalasis
372.89 Other disorders of conjunctiva
372.9 Unspecified disorder of conjunctiva ▽
694.61 Benign mucous membrane pemphigoid with ocular involvement

ICD-9-CM Procedural

10.31 Excision of lesion or tissue of conjunctiva

HCPCS Level II Supplies & Services

A4550 Surgical trays

68130

68130 Excision of lesion, conjunctiva; with adjacent sclera

ICD-9-CM Diagnostic

190.0 Malignant neoplasm of eyeball, except conjunctiva, cornea, retina, and choroid
190.3 Malignant neoplasm of conjunctiva
198.4 Secondary malignant neoplasm of other parts of nervous system
224.0 Benign neoplasm of eyeball, except conjunctiva, cornea, retina, and choroid
224.3 Benign neoplasm of conjunctiva
234.0 Carcinoma in situ of eye
238.8 Neoplasm of uncertain behavior of other specified sites
239.8 Neoplasm of unspecified nature of other specified sites
369.9 Unspecified visual loss ▽
370.32 Limbar and corneal involvement in vernal conjunctivitis — (Use additional code for vernal conjunctivitis, 372.13)
372.45 Recurrent pterygium
372.51 Pinguecula
372.61 Granuloma of conjunctiva
372.71 Hyperemia of conjunctiva
372.74 Vascular abnormalities of conjunctiva
372.75 Conjunctival cysts
372.9 Unspecified disorder of conjunctiva ▽
694.61 Benign mucous membrane pemphigoid with ocular involvement

ICD-9-CM Procedural

10.31 Excision of lesion or tissue of conjunctiva
12.84 Excision or destruction of lesion of sclera

HCPCS Level II Supplies & Services

A4550 Surgical trays

68135

68135 Destruction of lesion, conjunctiva

ICD-9-CM Diagnostic

190.3 Malignant neoplasm of conjunctiva
198.4 Secondary malignant neoplasm of other parts of nervous system
224.3 Benign neoplasm of conjunctiva
234.0 Carcinoma in situ of eye
238.8 Neoplasm of uncertain behavior of other specified sites
239.8 Neoplasm of unspecified nature of other specified sites
372.61 Granuloma of conjunctiva
372.62 Localized adhesions and strands of conjunctiva
372.64 Scarring of conjunctiva
372.71 Hyperemia of conjunctiva
372.74 Vascular abnormalities of conjunctiva
372.75 Conjunctival cysts
694.61 Benign mucous membrane pemphigoid with ocular involvement

ICD-9-CM Procedural

10.32 Destruction of lesion of conjunctiva

▽ Unspecified code
♀ Female diagnosis
☒ Manifestation code
♂ Male diagnosis

HCPCS Level II Supplies & Services

A4550 Surgical trays

68200

68200 Subconjunctival injection

ICD-9-CM Diagnostic

190.3 Malignant neoplasm of conjunctiva
224.3 Benign neoplasm of conjunctiva
234.0 Carcinoma in situ of eye
238.8 Neoplasm of uncertain behavior of other specified sites
239.8 Neoplasm of unspecified nature of other specified sites
370.34 Exposure keratoconjunctivitis
372.10 Unspecified chronic conjunctivitis ▽
372.61 Granuloma of conjunctiva
372.71 Hyperemia of conjunctiva
372.74 Vascular abnormalities of conjunctiva
372.75 Conjunctival cysts
372.81 Conjunctivochalasis
372.89 Other disorders of conjunctiva
379.00 Unspecified scleritis ▽
694.61 Benign mucous membrane pemphigoid with ocular involvement

ICD-9-CM Procedural

10.91 Subconjunctival injection

HCPCS Level II Supplies & Services

A4550 Surgical trays

68320–68325

68320 Conjunctivoplasty; with conjunctival graft or extensive rearrangement
68325 with buccal mucous membrane graft (includes obtaining graft)

ICD-9-CM Diagnostic

190.3 Malignant neoplasm of conjunctiva
198.4 Secondary malignant neoplasm of other parts of nervous system
224.3 Benign neoplasm of conjunctiva
234.0 Carcinoma in situ of eye
238.8 Neoplasm of uncertain behavior of other specified sites
239.8 Neoplasm of unspecified nature of other specified sites
360.32 Ocular fistula causing hypotony
360.89 Other disorders of globe
372.40 Unspecified pterygium ▽
372.61 Granuloma of conjunctiva
372.64 Scarring of conjunctiva
372.75 Conjunctival cysts
374.04 Cicatricial entropion
374.05 Trichiasis of eyelid without entropion
374.11 Senile ectropion
374.14 Cicatricial ectropion
376.9 Unspecified disorder of orbit ▽
379.11 Scleral ectasia
743.62 Congenital deformity of eyelid
743.69 Other congenital anomalies of eyelids, lacrimal system, and orbit
870.1 Laceration of eyelid, full-thickness, not involving lacrimal passages — (Use additional code to identify infection)
871.0 Ocular laceration without prolapse of intraocular tissue — (Use additional code to identify infection)
871.1 Ocular laceration with prolapse or exposure of intraocular tissue — (Use additional code to identify infection)
871.4 Unspecified laceration of eye — (Use additional code to identify infection) ▽
940.2 Alkaline chemical burn of cornea and conjunctival sac
940.3 Acid chemical burn of cornea and conjunctival sac
940.4 Other burn of cornea and conjunctival sac
996.59 Mechanical complication due to other implant and internal device, not elsewhere classified
V10.84 Personal history of malignant neoplasm of eye

ICD-9-CM Procedural

10.42 Reconstruction of conjunctival cul-de-sac with free graft
10.44 Other free graft to conjunctiva
10.49 Other conjunctivoplasty

68326–68328

68326 Conjunctivoplasty, reconstruction cul-de-sac; with conjunctival graft or extensive rearrangement
68328 with buccal mucous membrane graft (includes obtaining graft)

ICD-9-CM Diagnostic

190.3 Malignant neoplasm of conjunctiva
198.4 Secondary malignant neoplasm of other parts of nervous system
224.3 Benign neoplasm of conjunctiva
234.0 Carcinoma in situ of eye
238.8 Neoplasm of uncertain behavior of other specified sites
239.8 Neoplasm of unspecified nature of other specified sites
360.32 Ocular fistula causing hypotony
360.89 Other disorders of globe
372.61 Granuloma of conjunctiva
372.64 Scarring of conjunctiva
372.75 Conjunctival cysts
374.04 Cicatricial entropion
374.05 Trichiasis of eyelid without entropion
374.11 Senile ectropion
374.14 Cicatricial ectropion
376.9 Unspecified disorder of orbit ▽
743.62 Congenital deformity of eyelid
743.69 Other congenital anomalies of eyelids, lacrimal system, and orbit
870.1 Laceration of eyelid, full-thickness, not involving lacrimal passages — (Use additional code to identify infection)
871.0 Ocular laceration without prolapse of intraocular tissue — (Use additional code to identify infection)
871.1 Ocular laceration with prolapse or exposure of intraocular tissue — (Use additional code to identify infection)
871.4 Unspecified laceration of eye — (Use additional code to identify infection) ▽
940.2 Alkaline chemical burn of cornea and conjunctival sac
940.3 Acid chemical burn of cornea and conjunctival sac
940.4 Other burn of cornea and conjunctival sac
996.59 Mechanical complication due to other implant and internal device, not elsewhere classified
V10.84 Personal history of malignant neoplasm of eye

ICD-9-CM Procedural

10.42 Reconstruction of conjunctival cul-de-sac with free graft
10.43 Other reconstruction of conjunctival cul-de-sac

68330–68340

68330 Repair of symblepharon; conjunctivoplasty, without graft
68335 with free graft conjunctiva or buccal mucous membrane (includes obtaining graft)
68340 division of symblepharon, with or without insertion of conformer or contact lens

ICD-9-CM Diagnostic

372.63 Symblepharon

ICD-9-CM Procedural

10.41 Repair of symblepharon with free graft
10.49 Other conjunctivoplasty
10.5 Lysis of adhesions of conjunctiva and eyelid

68360

68360 Conjunctival flap; bridge or partial (separate procedure)

ICD-9-CM Diagnostic

190.3 Malignant neoplasm of conjunctiva
198.4 Secondary malignant neoplasm of other parts of nervous system
224.3 Benign neoplasm of conjunctiva
234.0 Carcinoma in situ of eye
238.8 Neoplasm of uncertain behavior of other specified sites
239.8 Neoplasm of unspecified nature of other specified sites
351.0 Bell's palsy
360.32 Ocular fistula causing hypotony
370.06 Perforated corneal ulcer
371.23 Bullous keratopathy
372.40 Unspecified pterygium ▽
372.45 Recurrent pterygium
372.61 Granuloma of conjunctiva
372.64 Scarring of conjunctiva
372.75 Conjunctival cysts

▽ Unspecified code ♀ Female diagnosis
☒ Manifestation code ♂ Male diagnosis

374.20 Unspecified lagophthalmos
743.69 Other congenital anomalies of eyelids, lacrimal system, and orbit
870.1 Laceration of eyelid, full-thickness, not involving lacrimal passages — (Use additional code to identify infection)
871.0 Ocular laceration without prolapse of intraocular tissue — (Use additional code to identify infection)
871.4 Unspecified laceration of eye — (Use additional code to identify infection)
998.32 Disruption of external operation wound
V10.84 Personal history of malignant neoplasm of eye

ICD-9-CM Procedural
10.49 Other conjunctivoplasty
11.53 Repair of corneal laceration or wound with conjunctival flap

68362
68362 Conjunctival flap; total (such as Gunderson thin flap or purse string flap)

ICD-9-CM Diagnostic
190.3 Malignant neoplasm of conjunctiva
198.4 Secondary malignant neoplasm of other parts of nervous system
224.3 Benign neoplasm of conjunctiva
234.0 Carcinoma in situ of eye
238.8 Neoplasm of uncertain behavior of other specified sites
239.8 Neoplasm of unspecified nature of other specified sites
351.0 Bell's palsy
360.32 Ocular fistula causing hypotony
370.06 Perforated corneal ulcer
371.23 Bullous keratopathy
371.82 Corneal disorder due to contact lens
372.45 Recurrent pterygium
372.61 Granuloma of conjunctiva
372.64 Scarring of conjunctiva
372.75 Conjunctival cysts
374.20 Unspecified lagophthalmos
743.69 Other congenital anomalies of eyelids, lacrimal system, and orbit
870.1 Laceration of eyelid, full-thickness, not involving lacrimal passages — (Use additional code to identify infection)
871.0 Ocular laceration without prolapse of intraocular tissue — (Use additional code to identify infection)
871.4 Unspecified laceration of eye — (Use additional code to identify infection)
996.67 Infection and inflammatory reaction due to other internal orthopedic device, implant, and graft — (Use additional code to identify specified infections)
998.32 Disruption of external operation wound
V10.84 Personal history of malignant neoplasm of eye

ICD-9-CM Procedural
10.49 Other conjunctivoplasty
11.53 Repair of corneal laceration or wound with conjunctival flap

68371
68371 Harvesting conjunctival allograft, living donor

ICD-9-CM Diagnostic
V59.8 Donor of other specified organ or tissue

ICD-9-CM Procedural
10.99 Other operations on conjunctiva

68400
68400 Incision, drainage of lacrimal gland

ICD-9-CM Diagnostic
375.00 Unspecified dacryoadenitis
375.01 Acute dacryoadenitis
375.02 Chronic dacryoadenitis
375.03 Chronic enlargement of lacrimal gland
375.31 Acute canaliculitis, lacrimal
375.32 Acute dacryocystitis
375.33 Phlegmonous dacryocystitis
375.55 Obstruction of nasolacrimal duct, neonatal
743.64 Specified congenital anomaly of lacrimal gland
743.65 Specified congenital anomaly of lacrimal passages

ICD-9-CM Procedural
09.0 Incision of lacrimal gland

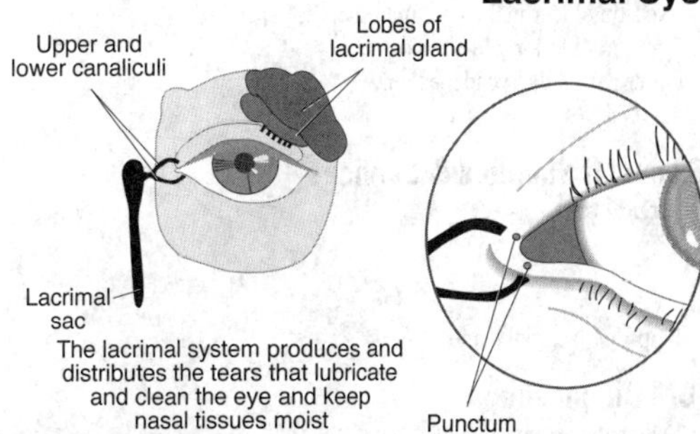
Lacrimal System
Upper and lower canaliculi
Lobes of lacrimal gland
Lacrimal sac
The lacrimal system produces and distributes the tears that lubricate and clean the eye and keep nasal tissues moist
Punctum
Tears are released into the eye through the lacrimal punctum
Deposits can form stones in the lacrimal canals; these stones are called dacryoliths

HCPCS Level II Supplies & Services
A4550 Surgical trays

68420
68420 Incision, drainage of lacrimal sac (dacryocystotomy or dacryocystostomy)

ICD-9-CM Diagnostic
216.1 Benign neoplasm of eyelid, including canthus
375.01 Acute dacryoadenitis
375.02 Chronic dacryoadenitis
375.03 Chronic enlargement of lacrimal gland
375.30 Unspecified dacryocystitis
375.31 Acute canaliculitis, lacrimal
375.32 Acute dacryocystitis
375.33 Phlegmonous dacryocystitis
375.54 Stenosis of lacrimal sac
375.55 Obstruction of nasolacrimal duct, neonatal
375.56 Stenosis of nasolacrimal duct, acquired
375.57 Dacryolith
376.01 Orbital cellulitis
743.64 Specified congenital anomaly of lacrimal gland
743.65 Specified congenital anomaly of lacrimal passages

ICD-9-CM Procedural
09.53 Incision of lacrimal sac

HCPCS Level II Supplies & Services
A4550 Surgical trays

68440
68440 Snip incision of lacrimal punctum

ICD-9-CM Diagnostic
375.15 Unspecified tear film insufficiency
375.20 Epiphora, unspecified as to cause
375.31 Acute canaliculitis, lacrimal
375.41 Chronic canaliculitis
375.42 Chronic dacryocystitis
375.52 Stenosis of lacrimal punctum
375.56 Stenosis of nasolacrimal duct, acquired
375.9 Unspecified disorder of lacrimal system

ICD-9-CM Procedural
09.51 Incision of lacrimal punctum

HCPCS Level II Supplies & Services
A4550 Surgical trays

68500–68505
68500 Excision of lacrimal gland (dacryoadenectomy), except for tumor; total
68505 partial

ICD-9-CM Diagnostic
375.03 Chronic enlargement of lacrimal gland
375.12 Other lacrimal cysts and cystic degeneration
375.13 Primary lacrimal atrophy
375.14 Secondary lacrimal atrophy
375.21 Epiphora due to excess lacrimation

Unspecified code
♀ Female diagnosis
Manifestation code
♂ Male diagnosis

ICD-9-CM Procedural
09.20 Excision of lacrimal gland, not otherwise specified
09.21 Excision of lesion of lacrimal gland
09.22 Other partial dacryoadenectomy
09.23 Total dacryoadenectomy

HCPCS Level II Supplies & Services
A4550 Surgical trays

68510
68510 Biopsy of lacrimal gland

ICD-9-CM Diagnostic
190.2 Malignant neoplasm of lacrimal gland
224.2 Benign neoplasm of lacrimal gland
234.0 Carcinoma in situ of eye
238.8 Neoplasm of uncertain behavior of other specified sites
239.8 Neoplasm of unspecified nature of other specified sites

ICD-9-CM Procedural
09.11 Biopsy of lacrimal gland

HCPCS Level II Supplies & Services
A4550 Surgical trays

68520
68520 Excision of lacrimal sac (dacryocystectomy)

ICD-9-CM Diagnostic
190.7 Malignant neoplasm of lacrimal duct
224.7 Benign neoplasm of lacrimal duct
234.0 Carcinoma in situ of eye
238.8 Neoplasm of uncertain behavior of other specified sites
239.8 Neoplasm of unspecified nature of other specified sites
375.30 Unspecified dacryocystitis
375.53 Stenosis of lacrimal canaliculi
375.54 Stenosis of lacrimal sac

ICD-9-CM Procedural
09.6 Excision of lacrimal sac and passage

68525
68525 Biopsy of lacrimal sac

ICD-9-CM Diagnostic
190.7 Malignant neoplasm of lacrimal duct
224.7 Benign neoplasm of lacrimal duct
234.0 Carcinoma in situ of eye
238.8 Neoplasm of uncertain behavior of other specified sites
239.8 Neoplasm of unspecified nature of other specified sites

ICD-9-CM Procedural
09.12 Biopsy of lacrimal sac

HCPCS Level II Supplies & Services
A4550 Surgical trays

68530
68530 Removal of foreign body or dacryolith, lacrimal passages

ICD-9-CM Diagnostic
375.57 Dacryolith
930.2 Foreign body in lacrimal punctum
930.8 Foreign body in other and combined sites on external eye

ICD-9-CM Procedural
09.99 Other operations on lacrimal system

HCPCS Level II Supplies & Services
A4305 Disposable drug delivery system, flow rate of 50 ml or greater per hour
A4306 Disposable drug delivery system, flow rate of 5 ml or less per hour
A4550 Surgical trays

68540–68550
68540 Excision of lacrimal gland tumor; frontal approach
68550 involving osteotomy

ICD-9-CM Diagnostic
190.2 Malignant neoplasm of lacrimal gland
224.2 Benign neoplasm of lacrimal gland
234.0 Carcinoma in situ of eye
238.8 Neoplasm of uncertain behavior of other specified sites
239.8 Neoplasm of unspecified nature of other specified sites

ICD-9-CM Procedural
09.21 Excision of lesion of lacrimal gland
09.23 Total dacryoadenectomy
76.69 Other facial bone repair

HCPCS Level II Supplies & Services
A4305 Disposable drug delivery system, flow rate of 50 ml or greater per hour
A4306 Disposable drug delivery system, flow rate of 5 ml or less per hour
A4550 Surgical trays

68700
68700 Plastic repair of canaliculi

ICD-9-CM Diagnostic
173.1 Other malignant neoplasm of skin of eyelid, including canthus
190.7 Malignant neoplasm of lacrimal duct
224.7 Benign neoplasm of lacrimal duct
234.0 Carcinoma in situ of eye
238.8 Neoplasm of uncertain behavior of other specified sites
239.8 Neoplasm of unspecified nature of other specified sites
370.33 Keratoconjunctivitis sicca, not specified as Sjögren's
374.10 Unspecified ectropion
374.11 Senile ectropion
375.15 Unspecified tear film insufficiency
375.20 Epiphora, unspecified as to cause
375.21 Epiphora due to excess lacrimation
375.22 Epiphora due to insufficient drainage
375.30 Unspecified dacryocystitis
375.31 Acute canaliculitis, lacrimal
375.32 Acute dacryocystitis
375.33 Phlegmonous dacryocystitis
375.42 Chronic dacryocystitis
375.52 Stenosis of lacrimal punctum
375.53 Stenosis of lacrimal canaliculi
375.54 Stenosis of lacrimal sac
375.55 Obstruction of nasolacrimal duct, neonatal
375.56 Stenosis of nasolacrimal duct, acquired
743.65 Specified congenital anomaly of lacrimal passages
870.1 Laceration of eyelid, full-thickness, not involving lacrimal passages — (Use additional code to identify infection)
870.2 Laceration of eyelid involving lacrimal passages — (Use additional code to identify infection)
870.8 Other specified open wound of ocular adnexa — (Use additional code to identify infection)

ICD-9-CM Procedural
09.73 Repair of canaliculus

HCPCS Level II Supplies & Services
A4305 Disposable drug delivery system, flow rate of 50 ml or greater per hour
A4306 Disposable drug delivery system, flow rate of 5 ml or less per hour
A4550 Surgical trays

68705
68705 Correction of everted punctum, cautery

ICD-9-CM Diagnostic
375.51 Eversion of lacrimal punctum

ICD-9-CM Procedural
09.71 Correction of everted punctum

HCPCS Level II Supplies & Services
A4550 Surgical trays

Unspecified code
♀ Female diagnosis
Manifestation code
♂ Male diagnosis

68720

68720 Dacryocystorhinostomy (fistulization of lacrimal sac to nasal cavity)

ICD-9-CM Diagnostic

375.20 Epiphora, unspecified as to cause ▽
375.22 Epiphora due to insufficient drainage
375.31 Acute canaliculitis, lacrimal
375.32 Acute dacryocystitis
375.33 Phlegmonous dacryocystitis
375.42 Chronic dacryocystitis
375.43 Lacrimal mucocele
375.53 Stenosis of lacrimal canaliculi
375.54 Stenosis of lacrimal sac
375.55 Obstruction of nasolacrimal duct, neonatal
375.56 Stenosis of nasolacrimal duct, acquired
743.65 Specified congenital anomaly of lacrimal passages

ICD-9-CM Procedural

09.81 Dacryocystorhinostomy (DCR)

68745–68750

68745 Conjunctivorhinostomy (fistulization of conjunctiva to nasal cavity); without tube
68750 with insertion of tube or stent

ICD-9-CM Diagnostic

375.20 Epiphora, unspecified as to cause ▽
375.22 Epiphora due to insufficient drainage
375.31 Acute canaliculitis, lacrimal
375.32 Acute dacryocystitis
375.33 Phlegmonous dacryocystitis
375.42 Chronic dacryocystitis
375.43 Lacrimal mucocele
375.53 Stenosis of lacrimal canaliculi
375.54 Stenosis of lacrimal sac
375.55 Obstruction of nasolacrimal duct, neonatal
375.56 Stenosis of nasolacrimal duct, acquired
743.65 Specified congenital anomaly of lacrimal passages

ICD-9-CM Procedural

09.82 Conjunctivocystorhinostomy
09.83 Conjunctivorhinostomy with insertion of tube or stent

68760

68760 Closure of the lacrimal punctum; by thermocauterization, ligation, or laser surgery

ICD-9-CM Diagnostic

370.20 Unspecified superficial keratitis ▽
370.21 Punctate keratitis
370.23 Filamentary keratitis
370.33 Keratoconjunctivitis sicca, not specified as Sjögren's
370.34 Exposure keratoconjunctivitis
370.8 Other forms of keratitis
371.42 Recurrent erosion of cornea
371.51 Juvenile epithelial corneal dystrophy
371.52 Other anterior corneal dystrophies
371.53 Granular corneal dystrophy
371.54 Lattice corneal dystrophy
371.55 Macular corneal dystrophy
371.56 Other stromal corneal dystrophies
371.57 Endothelial corneal dystrophy
371.58 Other posterior corneal dystrophies
374.41 Eyelid retraction or lag
375.00 Unspecified dacryoadenitis ▽
375.15 Unspecified tear film insufficiency ▽
710.2 Sicca syndrome

ICD-9-CM Procedural

09.72 Other repair of punctum
09.91 Obliteration of lacrimal punctum

HCPCS Level II Supplies & Services

A4550 Surgical trays

68761

68761 Closure of the lacrimal punctum; by plug, each

ICD-9-CM Diagnostic

370.21 Punctate keratitis
370.23 Filamentary keratitis
370.33 Keratoconjunctivitis sicca, not specified as Sjögren's
370.34 Exposure keratoconjunctivitis
370.8 Other forms of keratitis
370.9 Unspecified keratitis ▽
371.42 Recurrent erosion of cornea
373.31 Eczematous dermatitis of eyelid
374.41 Eyelid retraction or lag
375.15 Unspecified tear film insufficiency ▽
710.2 Sicca syndrome

ICD-9-CM Procedural

09.91 Obliteration of lacrimal punctum

HCPCS Level II Supplies & Services

A4262 Temporary, absorbable lacrimal duct implant, each
A4263 Permanent, long-term, nondissolvable lacrimal duct implant, each

68770

68770 Closure of lacrimal fistula (separate procedure)

ICD-9-CM Diagnostic

375.61 Lacrimal fistula

ICD-9-CM Procedural

09.99 Other operations on lacrimal system

HCPCS Level II Supplies & Services

A4305 Disposable drug delivery system, flow rate of 50 ml or greater per hour
A4306 Disposable drug delivery system, flow rate of 5 ml or less per hour
A4550 Surgical trays

68801

68801 Dilation of lacrimal punctum, with or without irrigation

ICD-9-CM Diagnostic

375.20 Epiphora, unspecified as to cause ▽
375.22 Epiphora due to insufficient drainage
375.31 Acute canaliculitis, lacrimal
375.32 Acute dacryocystitis
375.33 Phlegmonous dacryocystitis
375.42 Chronic dacryocystitis
375.43 Lacrimal mucocele
375.52 Stenosis of lacrimal punctum
375.53 Stenosis of lacrimal canaliculi
375.54 Stenosis of lacrimal sac
375.55 Obstruction of nasolacrimal duct, neonatal
375.56 Stenosis of nasolacrimal duct, acquired
375.57 Dacryolith
375.61 Lacrimal fistula
375.69 Other change of lacrimal passages
375.81 Granuloma of lacrimal passages
375.89 Other disorder of lacrimal system
743.65 Specified congenital anomaly of lacrimal passages

ICD-9-CM Procedural

09.41 Probing of lacrimal punctum

HCPCS Level II Supplies & Services

A4305 Disposable drug delivery system, flow rate of 50 ml or greater per hour
A4306 Disposable drug delivery system, flow rate of 5 ml or less per hour
A4550 Surgical trays

68810–68815

68810 Probing of nasolacrimal duct, with or without irrigation;
68811 requiring general anesthesia
68815 with insertion of tube or stent

ICD-9-CM Diagnostic

370.33 Keratoconjunctivitis sicca, not specified as Sjögren's
375.31 Acute canaliculitis, lacrimal

375.32 Acute dacryocystitis
375.33 Phlegmonous dacryocystitis
375.42 Chronic dacryocystitis
375.43 Lacrimal mucocele
375.52 Stenosis of lacrimal punctum
375.54 Stenosis of lacrimal sac
375.55 Obstruction of nasolacrimal duct, neonatal
375.56 Stenosis of nasolacrimal duct, acquired
375.57 Dacryolith
375.61 Lacrimal fistula
375.69 Other change of lacrimal passages
375.81 Granuloma of lacrimal passages
375.89 Other disorder of lacrimal system
743.65 Specified congenital anomaly of lacrimal passages

ICD-9-CM Procedural
09.43 Probing of nasolacrimal duct
09.44 Intubation of nasolacrimal duct

HCPCS Level II Supplies & Services
A4262 Temporary, absorbable lacrimal duct implant, each
A4263 Permanent, long-term, nondissolvable lacrimal duct implant, each
A4305 Disposable drug delivery system, flow rate of 50 ml or greater per hour
A4306 Disposable drug delivery system, flow rate of 5 ml or less per hour
A4550 Surgical trays

68840
68840 Probing of lacrimal canaliculi, with or without irrigation

ICD-9-CM Diagnostic
375.21 Epiphora due to excess lacrimation
375.22 Epiphora due to insufficient drainage
375.30 Unspecified dacryocystitis ▽
375.32 Acute dacryocystitis
375.42 Chronic dacryocystitis
375.51 Eversion of lacrimal punctum
375.52 Stenosis of lacrimal punctum
375.53 Stenosis of lacrimal canaliculi
375.55 Obstruction of nasolacrimal duct, neonatal
375.56 Stenosis of nasolacrimal duct, acquired

ICD-9-CM Procedural
09.42 Probing of lacrimal canaliculi

HCPCS Level II Supplies & Services
A4305 Disposable drug delivery system, flow rate of 50 ml or greater per hour
A4306 Disposable drug delivery system, flow rate of 5 ml or less per hour
A4550 Surgical trays

68850
68850 Injection of contrast medium for dacryocystography

ICD-9-CM Diagnostic
375.54 Stenosis of lacrimal sac
375.56 Stenosis of nasolacrimal duct, acquired
375.57 Dacryolith
375.9 Unspecified disorder of lacrimal system ▽
743.65 Specified congenital anomaly of lacrimal passages
930.2 Foreign body in lacrimal punctum

ICD-9-CM Procedural
09.19 Other diagnostic procedures on lacrimal system
87.05 Contrast dacryocystogram

HCPCS Level II Supplies & Services
A9525 Supply of low or iso-osmolar contrast material, 10 mg of iodine

Auditory System

External Ear

69000–69005

69000 Drainage external ear, abscess or hematoma; simple
69005 complicated

ICD-9-CM Diagnostic

380.10 Unspecified infective otitis externa ▽
380.11 Acute infection of pinna
380.31 Hematoma of auricle or pinna
680.0 Carbuncle and furuncle of face
706.2 Sebaceous cyst
738.7 Cauliflower ear
872.11 Open wound of auricle, complicated — (Use additional code to identify infection)
920 Contusion of face, scalp, and neck except eye(s)
998.51 Infected postoperative seroma — (Use additional code to identify organism)
998.59 Other postoperative infection — (Use additional code to identify infection)

ICD-9-CM Procedural

18.09 Other incision of external ear

HCPCS Level II Supplies & Services

A4305 Disposable drug delivery system, flow rate of 50 ml or greater per hour
A4306 Disposable drug delivery system, flow rate of 5 ml or less per hour
A4550 Surgical trays

69020

69020 Drainage external auditory canal, abscess

ICD-9-CM Diagnostic

380.10 Unspecified infective otitis externa ▽
380.16 Other chronic infective otitis externa
380.21 Cholesteatoma of external ear
380.22 Other acute otitis externa
380.23 Other chronic otitis externa
680.0 Carbuncle and furuncle of face
872.12 Open wound of auditory canal, complicated — (Use additional code to identify infection)

ICD-9-CM Procedural

18.02 Incision of external auditory canal

HCPCS Level II Supplies & Services

A4305 Disposable drug delivery system, flow rate of 50 ml or greater per hour
A4306 Disposable drug delivery system, flow rate of 5 ml or less per hour
A4550 Surgical trays

69090

69090 Ear piercing

ICD-9-CM Diagnostic

V50.3 Ear piercing

ICD-9-CM Procedural

18.01 Piercing of ear lobe

HCPCS Level II Supplies & Services

A4550 Surgical trays

69100

69100 Biopsy external ear

ICD-9-CM Diagnostic

171.0 Malignant neoplasm of connective and other soft tissue of head, face, and neck
172.2 Malignant melanoma of skin of ear and external auditory canal
173.2 Other malignant neoplasm of skin of ear and external auditory canal
198.2 Secondary malignant neoplasm of skin
198.89 Secondary malignant neoplasm of other specified sites
215.0 Other benign neoplasm of connective and other soft tissue of head, face, and neck
216.2 Benign neoplasm of ear and external auditory canal
232.2 Carcinoma in situ of skin of ear and external auditory canal
238.1 Neoplasm of uncertain behavior of connective and other soft tissue ▽
238.2 Neoplasm of uncertain behavior of skin
239.2 Neoplasms of unspecified nature of bone, soft tissue, and skin
380.01 Acute perichondritis of pinna
701.5 Other abnormal granulation tissue
702.0 Actinic keratosis

ICD-9-CM Procedural

18.12 Biopsy of external ear

HCPCS Level II Supplies & Services

A4305 Disposable drug delivery system, flow rate of 50 ml or greater per hour
A4306 Disposable drug delivery system, flow rate of 5 ml or less per hour
A4550 Surgical trays

69105

69105 Biopsy external auditory canal

ICD-9-CM Diagnostic

171.0 Malignant neoplasm of connective and other soft tissue of head, face, and neck
172.2 Malignant melanoma of skin of ear and external auditory canal
173.2 Other malignant neoplasm of skin of ear and external auditory canal
198.2 Secondary malignant neoplasm of skin
198.89 Secondary malignant neoplasm of other specified sites
215.0 Other benign neoplasm of connective and other soft tissue of head, face, and neck
216.2 Benign neoplasm of ear and external auditory canal
232.2 Carcinoma in situ of skin of ear and external auditory canal
238.1 Neoplasm of uncertain behavior of connective and other soft tissue ▽
238.2 Neoplasm of uncertain behavior of skin
239.2 Neoplasms of unspecified nature of bone, soft tissue, and skin
380.21 Cholesteatoma of external ear
380.23 Other chronic otitis externa
701.5 Other abnormal granulation tissue
709.4 Foreign body granuloma of skin and subcutaneous tissue

ICD-9-CM Procedural

18.12 Biopsy of external ear

HCPCS Level II Supplies & Services

A4305 Disposable drug delivery system, flow rate of 50 ml or greater per hour
A4306 Disposable drug delivery system, flow rate of 5 ml or less per hour
A4550 Surgical trays

69110–69120

69110 Excision external ear; partial, simple repair
69120 complete amputation

ICD-9-CM Diagnostic

171.0 Malignant neoplasm of connective and other soft tissue of head, face, and neck
172.2 Malignant melanoma of skin of ear and external auditory canal
173.2 Other malignant neoplasm of skin of ear and external auditory canal
198.2 Secondary malignant neoplasm of skin
198.89 Secondary malignant neoplasm of other specified sites
215.0 Other benign neoplasm of connective and other soft tissue of head, face, and neck
216.2 Benign neoplasm of ear and external auditory canal
232.2 Carcinoma in situ of skin of ear and external auditory canal
238.1 Neoplasm of uncertain behavior of connective and other soft tissue ▽

238.2 Neoplasm of uncertain behavior of skin
239.2 Neoplasms of unspecified nature of bone, soft tissue, and skin
380.21 Cholesteatoma of external ear
709.4 Foreign body granuloma of skin and subcutaneous tissue
738.7 Cauliflower ear
872.01 Open wound of auricle, without mention of complication — (Use additional code to identify infection)
925.1 Crushing injury of face and scalp — (Use additional code to identify any associated injuries: 800-829, 850.0-854.1, 860.0-869.1)
959.01 Head injury, unspecified
959.09 Injury of face and neck, other and unspecified

ICD-9-CM Procedural

18.29 Excision or destruction of other lesion of external ear
18.39 Other excision of external ear

HCPCS Level II Supplies & Services

A4305 Disposable drug delivery system, flow rate of 50 ml or greater per hour
A4306 Disposable drug delivery system, flow rate of 5 ml or less per hour
A4550 Surgical trays

69140

69140 Excision exostosis(es), external auditory canal

ICD-9-CM Diagnostic

380.81 Exostosis of external ear canal

ICD-9-CM Procedural

18.29 Excision or destruction of other lesion of external ear

HCPCS Level II Supplies & Services

A4305 Disposable drug delivery system, flow rate of 50 ml or greater per hour
A4306 Disposable drug delivery system, flow rate of 5 ml or less per hour
A4550 Surgical trays

69145

69145 Excision soft tissue lesion, external auditory canal

ICD-9-CM Diagnostic

171.0 Malignant neoplasm of connective and other soft tissue of head, face, and neck
172.2 Malignant melanoma of skin of ear and external auditory canal
173.2 Other malignant neoplasm of skin of ear and external auditory canal
198.2 Secondary malignant neoplasm of skin
198.89 Secondary malignant neoplasm of other specified sites
214.9 Lipoma of unspecified site
215.0 Other benign neoplasm of connective and other soft tissue of head, face, and neck
216.2 Benign neoplasm of ear and external auditory canal
232.2 Carcinoma in situ of skin of ear and external auditory canal
238.1 Neoplasm of uncertain behavior of connective and other soft tissue
238.2 Neoplasm of uncertain behavior of skin
239.2 Neoplasms of unspecified nature of bone, soft tissue, and skin
380.21 Cholesteatoma of external ear
380.23 Other chronic otitis externa
680.0 Carbuncle and furuncle of face
701.5 Other abnormal granulation tissue
706.2 Sebaceous cyst

ICD-9-CM Procedural

18.29 Excision or destruction of other lesion of external ear

HCPCS Level II Supplies & Services

A4305 Disposable drug delivery system, flow rate of 50 ml or greater per hour
A4306 Disposable drug delivery system, flow rate of 5 ml or less per hour
A4550 Surgical trays

69150–69155

69150 Radical excision external auditory canal lesion; without neck dissection
69155 with neck dissection

ICD-9-CM Diagnostic

171.0 Malignant neoplasm of connective and other soft tissue of head, face, and neck
172.2 Malignant melanoma of skin of ear and external auditory canal
173.2 Other malignant neoplasm of skin of ear and external auditory canal
198.2 Secondary malignant neoplasm of skin
198.89 Secondary malignant neoplasm of other specified sites
216.2 Benign neoplasm of ear and external auditory canal
232.2 Carcinoma in situ of skin of ear and external auditory canal
238.2 Neoplasm of uncertain behavior of skin
239.2 Neoplasms of unspecified nature of bone, soft tissue, and skin
380.14 Malignant otitis externa

ICD-9-CM Procedural

18.31 Radical excision of lesion of external ear
40.40 Radical neck dissection, not otherwise specified

69200–69205

69200 Removal foreign body from external auditory canal; without general anesthesia
69205 with general anesthesia

ICD-9-CM Diagnostic

931 Foreign body in ear

ICD-9-CM Procedural

18.9 Other operations on external ear
98.11 Removal of intraluminal foreign body from ear without incision

HCPCS Level II Supplies & Services

A4305 Disposable drug delivery system, flow rate of 50 ml or greater per hour
A4306 Disposable drug delivery system, flow rate of 5 ml or less per hour
A4550 Surgical trays

69210

69210 Removal impacted cerumen (separate procedure), one or both ears

ICD-9-CM Diagnostic

380.4 Impacted cerumen

ICD-9-CM Procedural

96.52 Irrigation of ear

HCPCS Level II Supplies & Services

A4550 Surgical trays

69220–69222

69220 Debridement, mastoidectomy cavity, simple (eg, routine cleaning)
69222 Debridement, mastoidectomy cavity, complex (eg, with anesthesia or more than routine cleaning)

ICD-9-CM Diagnostic

382.9 Unspecified otitis media
383.00 Acute mastoiditis without complications
383.1 Chronic mastoiditis
383.30 Unspecified postmastoidectomy complication
383.32 Recurrent cholesteatoma of postmastoidectomy cavity
383.33 Granulations of postmastoidectomy cavity
383.89 Other disorder of mastoid
385.30 Unspecified cholesteatoma
385.31 Cholesteatoma of attic
385.33 Cholesteatoma of middle ear and mastoid
388.60 Unspecified otorrhea

ICD-9-CM Procedural

86.28 Nonexcisional debridement of wound, infection, or burn

HCPCS Level II Supplies & Services

A4305 Disposable drug delivery system, flow rate of 50 ml or greater per hour
A4306 Disposable drug delivery system, flow rate of 5 ml or less per hour
A4550 Surgical trays

69300

69300 Otoplasty, protruding ear, with or without size reduction

ICD-9-CM Diagnostic

380.32 Acquired deformities of auricle or pinna
744.22 Macrotia
744.29 Other congenital anomaly of ear
V50.1 Other plastic surgery for unacceptable cosmetic appearance

ICD-9-CM Procedural

18.5 Surgical correction of prominent ear

Unspecified code
♀ Female diagnosis
Manifestation code
♂ Male diagnosis

HCPCS Level II Supplies & Services

A4305 Disposable drug delivery system, flow rate of 50 ml or greater per hour
A4306 Disposable drug delivery system, flow rate of 5 ml or less per hour
A4550 Surgical trays

69310

69310 Reconstruction of external auditory canal (meatoplasty) (eg, for stenosis due to injury, infection) (separate procedure)

ICD-9-CM Diagnostic

380.23 Other chronic otitis externa
380.50 Acquired stenosis of external ear canal unspecified as to cause ▽
380.51 Acquired stenosis of external ear canal secondary to trauma
380.52 Acquired stenosis of external ear canal secondary to surgery
380.53 Acquired stenosis of external ear canal secondary to inflammation

ICD-9-CM Procedural

18.6 Reconstruction of external auditory canal

69320

69320 Reconstruction external auditory canal for congenital atresia, single stage

ICD-9-CM Diagnostic

744.02 Other congenital anomaly of external ear causing impairment of hearing

ICD-9-CM Procedural

18.6 Reconstruction of external auditory canal

Middle Ear

69400–69401

69400 Eustachian tube inflation, transnasal; with catheterization
69401 without catheterization

ICD-9-CM Diagnostic

381.10 Simple or unspecified chronic serous otitis media
381.20 Simple or unspecified chronic mucoid otitis media
381.29 Other chronic mucoid otitis media
381.3 Other and unspecified chronic nonsuppurative otitis media ▽
381.50 Unspecified Eustachian salpingitis ▽
381.51 Acute Eustachian salpingitis
381.52 Chronic Eustachian salpingitis
381.60 Unspecified obstruction of Eustachian tube ▽
381.61 Osseous obstruction of Eustachian tube
381.62 Intrinsic cartilagenous obstruction of Eustachian tube
381.63 Extrinsic cartilagenous obstruction of Eustachian tube
381.81 Dysfunction of Eustachian tube

ICD-9-CM Procedural

20.8 Operations on Eustachian tube

HCPCS Level II Supplies & Services

A4305 Disposable drug delivery system, flow rate of 50 ml or greater per hour
A4306 Disposable drug delivery system, flow rate of 5 ml or less per hour
A4550 Surgical trays

69405

69405 Eustachian tube catheterization, transtympanic

ICD-9-CM Diagnostic

381.10 Simple or unspecified chronic serous otitis media
381.20 Simple or unspecified chronic mucoid otitis media
381.29 Other chronic mucoid otitis media
381.3 Other and unspecified chronic nonsuppurative otitis media ▽
381.50 Unspecified Eustachian salpingitis ▽
381.51 Acute Eustachian salpingitis
381.52 Chronic Eustachian salpingitis
381.60 Unspecified obstruction of Eustachian tube ▽
381.61 Osseous obstruction of Eustachian tube
381.62 Intrinsic cartilagenous obstruction of Eustachian tube
381.63 Extrinsic cartilagenous obstruction of Eustachian tube
381.81 Dysfunction of Eustachian tube

ICD-9-CM Procedural

20.8 Operations on Eustachian tube

HCPCS Level II Supplies & Services

A4305 Disposable drug delivery system, flow rate of 50 ml or greater per hour
A4306 Disposable drug delivery system, flow rate of 5 ml or less per hour
A4550 Surgical trays

69410

69410 Focal application of phase control substance, middle ear (baffle technique)

ICD-9-CM Diagnostic

380.21 Cholesteatoma of external ear
380.4 Impacted cerumen
381.61 Osseous obstruction of Eustachian tube
381.62 Intrinsic cartilagenous obstruction of Eustachian tube
381.63 Extrinsic cartilagenous obstruction of Eustachian tube
381.81 Dysfunction of Eustachian tube

ICD-9-CM Procedural

20.99 Other operations on middle and inner ear

69420–69421

69420 Myringotomy including aspiration and/or eustachian tube inflation
69421 Myringotomy including aspiration and/or eustachian tube inflation requiring general anesthesia

ICD-9-CM Diagnostic

381.01 Acute serous otitis media
381.02 Acute mucoid otitis media
381.03 Acute sanguinous otitis media
381.04 Acute allergic serous otitis media
381.05 Acute allergic mucoid otitis media
381.06 Acute allergic sanguinous otitis media
381.10 Simple or unspecified chronic serous otitis media
381.19 Other chronic serous otitis media
381.20 Simple or unspecified chronic mucoid otitis media
381.29 Other chronic mucoid otitis media
381.3 Other and unspecified chronic nonsuppurative otitis media ▽
381.4 Nonsuppurative otitis media, not specified as acute or chronic ▽
381.81 Dysfunction of Eustachian tube
381.89 Other disorders of Eustachian tube
382.00 Acute suppurative otitis media without spontaneous rupture of eardrum
382.3 Unspecified chronic suppurative otitis media ▽
383.00 Acute mastoiditis without complications
383.01 Subperiosteal abscess of mastoid
383.02 Acute mastoiditis with other complications
385.89 Other disorders of middle ear and mastoid
389.03 Conductive hearing loss, middle ear

ICD-9-CM Procedural

20.09 Other myringotomy
20.8 Operations on Eustachian tube

HCPCS Level II Supplies & Services

A4305 Disposable drug delivery system, flow rate of 50 ml or greater per hour
A4306 Disposable drug delivery system, flow rate of 5 ml or less per hour
A4550 Surgical trays

69424

69424 Ventilating tube removal requiring general anesthesia

ICD-9-CM Diagnostic

381.10 Simple or unspecified chronic serous otitis media
381.20 Simple or unspecified chronic mucoid otitis media
381.29 Other chronic mucoid otitis media
381.3 Other and unspecified chronic nonsuppurative otitis media ▽
381.4 Nonsuppurative otitis media, not specified as acute or chronic ▽
381.81 Dysfunction of Eustachian tube
382.00 Acute suppurative otitis media without spontaneous rupture of eardrum
382.1 Chronic tubotympanic suppurative otitis media
382.2 Chronic atticoantral suppurative otitis media
385.83 Retained foreign body of middle ear
388.60 Unspecified otorrhea ▽
388.71 Otogenic pain

996.69 Infection and inflammatory reaction due to other internal prosthetic device, implant, and graft — (Use additional code to identify specified infections)
996.79 Other complications due to other internal prosthetic device, implant, and graft
V53.09 Fitting and adjustment of other devices related to nervous system and special senses
V58.49 Other specified aftercare following surgery — (This code should be used in conjunction with other aftercare codes to fully identify the reason for the aftercare encounter)

ICD-9-CM Procedural
20.1 Removal of tympanostomy tube

HCPCS Level II Supplies & Services
A4305 Disposable drug delivery system, flow rate of 50 ml or greater per hour
A4306 Disposable drug delivery system, flow rate of 5 ml or less per hour
A4550 Surgical trays

69433–69436
69433 Tympanostomy (requiring insertion of ventilating tube), local or topical anesthesia
69436 Tympanostomy (requiring insertion of ventilating tube), general anesthesia

ICD-9-CM Diagnostic
381.00 Unspecified acute nonsuppurative otitis media ▽
381.01 Acute serous otitis media
381.10 Simple or unspecified chronic serous otitis media
381.19 Other chronic serous otitis media
381.20 Simple or unspecified chronic mucoid otitis media
381.29 Other chronic mucoid otitis media
381.3 Other and unspecified chronic nonsuppurative otitis media ▽
381.4 Nonsuppurative otitis media, not specified as acute or chronic ▽
381.7 Patulous Eustachian tube
381.81 Dysfunction of Eustachian tube
382.00 Acute suppurative otitis media without spontaneous rupture of eardrum
382.1 Chronic tubotympanic suppurative otitis media
382.3 Unspecified chronic suppurative otitis media ▽
384.81 Atrophic flaccid tympanic membrane
389.02 Conductive hearing loss, tympanic membrane
996.59 Mechanical complication due to other implant and internal device, not elsewhere classified
996.69 Infection and inflammatory reaction due to other internal prosthetic device, implant, and graft — (Use additional code to identify specified infections)
996.79 Other complications due to other internal prosthetic device, implant, and graft

ICD-9-CM Procedural
20.01 Myringotomy with insertion of tube

HCPCS Level II Supplies & Services
A4305 Disposable drug delivery system, flow rate of 50 ml or greater per hour
A4306 Disposable drug delivery system, flow rate of 5 ml or less per hour
A4550 Surgical trays

69440
69440 Middle ear exploration through postauricular or ear canal incision

ICD-9-CM Diagnostic
384.21 Central perforation of tympanic membrane
384.22 Attic perforation of tympanic membrane
384.23 Other marginal perforation of tympanic membrane
384.24 Multiple perforations of tympanic membrane
384.25 Total perforation of tympanic membrane
384.81 Atrophic flaccid tympanic membrane
384.82 Atrophic nonflaccid tympanic membrane
385.01 Tympanosclerosis involving tympanic membrane only
385.02 Tympanosclerosis involving tympanic membrane and ear ossicles
385.03 Tympanosclerosis involving tympanic membrane, ear ossicles, and middle ear
385.09 Tympanosclerosis involving other combination of structures
385.10 Adhesive middle ear disease, unspecified as to involvement ▽
385.19 Other middle ear adhesions and combinations
385.23 Discontinuity or dislocation of ear ossicles
385.32 Cholesteatoma of middle ear
385.83 Retained foreign body of middle ear
385.89 Other disorders of middle ear and mastoid
386.41 Round window fistula
386.42 Oval window fistula
386.48 Labyrinthine fistula of combined sites
389.03 Conductive hearing loss, middle ear
389.2 Mixed conductive and sensorineural hearing loss
872.61 Open wound of ear drum, without mention of complication — (Use additional code to identify infection)
872.62 Open wound of ossicles, without mention of complication — (Use additional code to identify infection)
872.71 Open wound of ear drum, complicated — (Use additional code to identify infection)

ICD-9-CM Procedural
20.09 Other myringotomy
20.39 Other diagnostic procedures on middle and inner ear

69450
69450 Tympanolysis, transcanal

ICD-9-CM Diagnostic
385.10 Adhesive middle ear disease, unspecified as to involvement ▽
385.11 Adhesions of drum head to incus
385.12 Adhesions of drum head to stapes
385.13 Adhesions of drum head to promontorium
385.19 Other middle ear adhesions and combinations
389.03 Conductive hearing loss, middle ear
389.08 Conductive hearing loss of combined types
389.2 Mixed conductive and sensorineural hearing loss

ICD-9-CM Procedural
20.23 Incision of middle ear

HCPCS Level II Supplies & Services
A4305 Disposable drug delivery system, flow rate of 50 ml or greater per hour
A4306 Disposable drug delivery system, flow rate of 5 ml or less per hour
A4550 Surgical trays

69501
69501 Transmastoid antrotomy (simple mastoidectomy)

ICD-9-CM Diagnostic
383.00 Acute mastoiditis without complications
383.01 Subperiosteal abscess of mastoid
383.02 Acute mastoiditis with other complications
383.1 Chronic mastoiditis
383.9 Unspecified mastoiditis ▽
385.30 Unspecified cholesteatoma ▽

ICD-9-CM Procedural
20.41 Simple mastoidectomy

69502
69502 Mastoidectomy; complete

ICD-9-CM Diagnostic
383.00 Acute mastoiditis without complications
383.01 Subperiosteal abscess of mastoid
383.02 Acute mastoiditis with other complications
383.1 Chronic mastoiditis
383.21 Acute petrositis

Mastoid Process

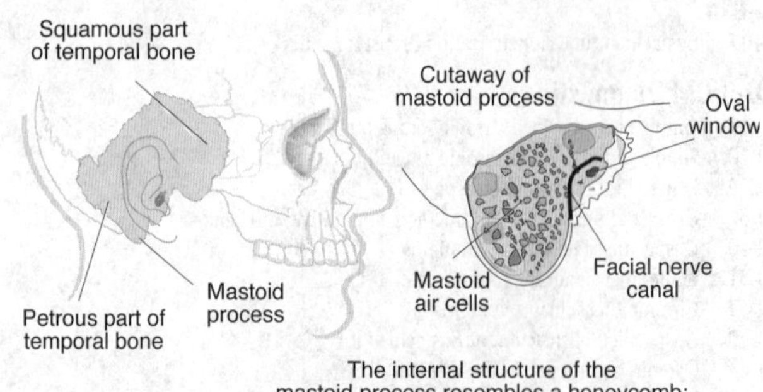

The internal structure of the mastoid process resembles a honeycomb; infections of the middle ear sometimes spread to the mastoid cells

383.22 Chronic petrositis
383.9 Unspecified mastoiditis
385.30 Unspecified cholesteatoma
385.33 Cholesteatoma of middle ear and mastoid
385.35 Diffuse cholesteatosis of middle ear and mastoid

ICD-9-CM Procedural
20.49 Other mastoidectomy

69505
69505 Mastoidectomy; modified radical

ICD-9-CM Diagnostic
383.1 Chronic mastoiditis
383.20 Unspecified petrositis
383.21 Acute petrositis
383.22 Chronic petrositis
383.89 Other disorder of mastoid
385.30 Unspecified cholesteatoma
385.31 Cholesteatoma of attic
385.33 Cholesteatoma of middle ear and mastoid
385.35 Diffuse cholesteatosis of middle ear and mastoid

ICD-9-CM Procedural
20.49 Other mastoidectomy

69511
69511 Mastoidectomy; radical

ICD-9-CM Diagnostic
160.1 Malignant neoplasm of auditory tube, middle ear, and mastoid air cells
197.3 Secondary malignant neoplasm of other respiratory organs
231.8 Carcinoma in situ of other specified parts of respiratory system
235.9 Neoplasm of uncertain behavior of other and unspecified respiratory organs
237.3 Neoplasm of uncertain behavior of paraganglia
239.1 Neoplasm of unspecified nature of respiratory system
383.1 Chronic mastoiditis
383.20 Unspecified petrositis
383.21 Acute petrositis
383.22 Chronic petrositis
383.89 Other disorder of mastoid
385.30 Unspecified cholesteatoma
385.31 Cholesteatoma of attic
385.33 Cholesteatoma of middle ear and mastoid
385.35 Diffuse cholesteatosis of middle ear and mastoid

ICD-9-CM Procedural
20.42 Radical mastoidectomy

69530
69530 Petrous apicectomy including radical mastoidectomy

ICD-9-CM Diagnostic
383.20 Unspecified petrositis
383.21 Acute petrositis
383.22 Chronic petrositis
385.21 Impaired mobility of malleus
385.30 Unspecified cholesteatoma
385.33 Cholesteatoma of middle ear and mastoid
385.35 Diffuse cholesteatosis of middle ear and mastoid
744.29 Other congenital anomaly of ear

ICD-9-CM Procedural
20.22 Incision of petrous pyramid air cells
20.42 Radical mastoidectomy
20.59 Other excision of middle ear

69535
69535 Resection temporal bone, external approach

ICD-9-CM Diagnostic
160.1 Malignant neoplasm of auditory tube, middle ear, and mastoid air cells
170.0 Malignant neoplasm of bones of skull and face, except mandible
171.0 Malignant neoplasm of connective and other soft tissue of head, face, and neck
172.2 Malignant melanoma of skin of ear and external auditory canal
197.3 Secondary malignant neoplasm of other respiratory organs
198.5 Secondary malignant neoplasm of bone and bone marrow
235.9 Neoplasm of uncertain behavior of other and unspecified respiratory organs

ICD-9-CM Procedural
20.59 Other excision of middle ear

69540
69540 Excision aural polyp

ICD-9-CM Diagnostic
385.30 Unspecified cholesteatoma
385.31 Cholesteatoma of attic
385.32 Cholesteatoma of middle ear
385.33 Cholesteatoma of middle ear and mastoid

ICD-9-CM Procedural
20.51 Excision of lesion of middle ear

HCPCS Level II Supplies & Services
A4305 Disposable drug delivery system, flow rate of 50 ml or greater per hour
A4306 Disposable drug delivery system, flow rate of 5 ml or less per hour
A4550 Surgical trays

69550
69550 Excision aural glomus tumor; transcanal

ICD-9-CM Diagnostic
194.6 Malignant neoplasm of aortic body and other paraganglia — (Use additional code to identify any functional activity)
212.0 Benign neoplasm of nasal cavities, middle ear, and accessory sinuses
216.2 Benign neoplasm of ear and external auditory canal
237.3 Neoplasm of uncertain behavior of paraganglia

ICD-9-CM Procedural
20.51 Excision of lesion of middle ear

HCPCS Level II Supplies & Services
A4305 Disposable drug delivery system, flow rate of 50 ml or greater per hour
A4306 Disposable drug delivery system, flow rate of 5 ml or less per hour
A4550 Surgical trays

69552
69552 Excision aural glomus tumor; transmastoid

ICD-9-CM Diagnostic
194.6 Malignant neoplasm of aortic body and other paraganglia — (Use additional code to identify any functional activity)
212.0 Benign neoplasm of nasal cavities, middle ear, and accessory sinuses
216.2 Benign neoplasm of ear and external auditory canal
237.3 Neoplasm of uncertain behavior of paraganglia

ICD-9-CM Procedural
20.51 Excision of lesion of middle ear

69554
69554 Excision aural glomus tumor; extended (extratemporal)

ICD-9-CM Diagnostic
194.6 Malignant neoplasm of aortic body and other paraganglia — (Use additional code to identify any functional activity)
212.0 Benign neoplasm of nasal cavities, middle ear, and accessory sinuses
216.2 Benign neoplasm of ear and external auditory canal
237.3 Neoplasm of uncertain behavior of paraganglia

ICD-9-CM Procedural
20.51 Excision of lesion of middle ear

69601
69601 Revision mastoidectomy; resulting in complete mastoidectomy

ICD-9-CM Diagnostic
383.01 Subperiosteal abscess of mastoid
383.02 Acute mastoiditis with other complications

383.1 Chronic mastoiditis
383.21 Acute petrositis
383.22 Chronic petrositis
383.30 Unspecified postmastoidectomy complication ▽
383.31 Mucosal cyst of postmastoidectomy cavity
383.32 Recurrent cholesteatoma of postmastoidectomy cavity
383.33 Granulations of postmastoidectomy cavity
383.81 Postauricular fistula
383.9 Unspecified mastoiditis ▽
385.30 Unspecified cholesteatoma ▽
385.33 Cholesteatoma of middle ear and mastoid

ICD-9-CM Procedural
20.49 Other mastoidectomy
20.92 Revision of mastoidectomy

69602
69602 Revision mastoidectomy; resulting in modified radical mastoidectomy

ICD-9-CM Diagnostic
383.01 Subperiosteal abscess of mastoid
383.02 Acute mastoiditis with other complications
383.1 Chronic mastoiditis
383.21 Acute petrositis
383.22 Chronic petrositis
383.30 Unspecified postmastoidectomy complication ▽
383.32 Recurrent cholesteatoma of postmastoidectomy cavity
383.33 Granulations of postmastoidectomy cavity
385.24 Partial loss or necrosis of ear ossicles
385.30 Unspecified cholesteatoma ▽
385.31 Cholesteatoma of attic
385.33 Cholesteatoma of middle ear and mastoid
385.35 Diffuse cholesteatosis of middle ear and mastoid

ICD-9-CM Procedural
20.49 Other mastoidectomy
20.92 Revision of mastoidectomy

69603
69603 Revision mastoidectomy; resulting in radical mastoidectomy

ICD-9-CM Diagnostic
381.3 Other and unspecified chronic nonsuppurative otitis media ▽
383.01 Subperiosteal abscess of mastoid
383.02 Acute mastoiditis with other complications
383.1 Chronic mastoiditis
383.20 Unspecified petrositis ▽
383.21 Acute petrositis
383.22 Chronic petrositis
383.30 Unspecified postmastoidectomy complication ▽
383.32 Recurrent cholesteatoma of postmastoidectomy cavity
383.81 Postauricular fistula
385.30 Unspecified cholesteatoma ▽
385.31 Cholesteatoma of attic
385.33 Cholesteatoma of middle ear and mastoid
385.35 Diffuse cholesteatosis of middle ear and mastoid

ICD-9-CM Procedural
20.42 Radical mastoidectomy
20.92 Revision of mastoidectomy

69604
69604 Revision mastoidectomy; resulting in tympanoplasty

ICD-9-CM Diagnostic
381.10 Simple or unspecified chronic serous otitis media
381.3 Other and unspecified chronic nonsuppurative otitis media ▽
382.1 Chronic tubotympanic suppurative otitis media
382.2 Chronic atticoantral suppurative otitis media
382.3 Unspecified chronic suppurative otitis media ▽
383.02 Acute mastoiditis with other complications
383.1 Chronic mastoiditis
383.30 Unspecified postmastoidectomy complication ▽
383.32 Recurrent cholesteatoma of postmastoidectomy cavity
383.33 Granulations of postmastoidectomy cavity
384.21 Central perforation of tympanic membrane
384.24 Multiple perforations of tympanic membrane
385.31 Cholesteatoma of attic

ICD-9-CM Procedural
19.4 Myringoplasty
19.6 Revision of tympanoplasty
20.49 Other mastoidectomy
20.92 Revision of mastoidectomy

69605
69605 Revision mastoidectomy; with apicectomy

ICD-9-CM Diagnostic
383.1 Chronic mastoiditis
383.21 Acute petrositis
383.22 Chronic petrositis
383.32 Recurrent cholesteatoma of postmastoidectomy cavity
385.30 Unspecified cholesteatoma ▽
385.33 Cholesteatoma of middle ear and mastoid
385.35 Diffuse cholesteatosis of middle ear and mastoid

ICD-9-CM Procedural
20.49 Other mastoidectomy
20.59 Other excision of middle ear
20.92 Revision of mastoidectomy

69610–69620
69610 Tympanic membrane repair, with or without site preparation of perforation for closure, with or without patch
69620 Myringoplasty (surgery confined to drumhead and donor area)

ICD-9-CM Diagnostic
381.02 Acute mucoid otitis media
382.1 Chronic tubotympanic suppurative otitis media
382.2 Chronic atticoantral suppurative otitis media
382.3 Unspecified chronic suppurative otitis media ▽
384.20 Unspecified perforation of tympanic membrane ▽
384.21 Central perforation of tympanic membrane
384.22 Attic perforation of tympanic membrane
384.23 Other marginal perforation of tympanic membrane
384.24 Multiple perforations of tympanic membrane
384.25 Total perforation of tympanic membrane
389.02 Conductive hearing loss, tympanic membrane
872.61 Open wound of ear drum, without mention of complication — (Use additional code to identify infection)
872.71 Open wound of ear drum, complicated — (Use additional code to identify infection)
996.59 Mechanical complication due to other implant and internal device, not elsewhere classified
996.79 Other complications due to other internal prosthetic device, implant, and graft

ICD-9-CM Procedural
19.4 Myringoplasty
19.52 Type II tympanoplasty

HCPCS Level II Supplies & Services
A4305 Disposable drug delivery system, flow rate of 50 ml or greater per hour
A4306 Disposable drug delivery system, flow rate of 5 ml or less per hour
A4550 Surgical trays

69631
69631 Tympanoplasty without mastoidectomy (including canalplasty, atticotomy and/or middle ear surgery), initial or revision; without ossicular chain reconstruction

ICD-9-CM Diagnostic
381.03 Acute sanguinous otitis media
381.10 Simple or unspecified chronic serous otitis media
381.3 Other and unspecified chronic nonsuppurative otitis media ▽
381.4 Nonsuppurative otitis media, not specified as acute or chronic ▽
382.00 Acute suppurative otitis media without spontaneous rupture of eardrum
382.1 Chronic tubotympanic suppurative otitis media
382.2 Chronic atticoantral suppurative otitis media
382.3 Unspecified chronic suppurative otitis media ▽
384.20 Unspecified perforation of tympanic membrane ▽

384.21 Central perforation of tympanic membrane
384.22 Attic perforation of tympanic membrane
384.23 Other marginal perforation of tympanic membrane
384.24 Multiple perforations of tympanic membrane
384.25 Total perforation of tympanic membrane
384.81 Atrophic flaccid tympanic membrane
385.32 Cholesteatoma of middle ear
389.02 Conductive hearing loss, tympanic membrane

ICD-9-CM Procedural

19.52 Type II tympanoplasty

69632

69632 Tympanoplasty without mastoidectomy (including canalplasty, atticotomy and/or middle ear surgery), initial or revision; with ossicular chain reconstruction (eg, postfenestration)

ICD-9-CM Diagnostic

382.00 Acute suppurative otitis media without spontaneous rupture of eardrum
382.01 Acute suppurative otitis media with spontaneous rupture of eardrum
382.3 Unspecified chronic suppurative otitis media ▽
384.20 Unspecified perforation of tympanic membrane ▽
384.25 Total perforation of tympanic membrane
384.81 Atrophic flaccid tympanic membrane
385.02 Tympanosclerosis involving tympanic membrane and ear ossicles
385.21 Impaired mobility of malleus
385.22 Impaired mobility of other ear ossicles
385.23 Discontinuity or dislocation of ear ossicles
385.24 Partial loss or necrosis of ear ossicles
385.31 Cholesteatoma of attic
385.32 Cholesteatoma of middle ear
385.33 Cholesteatoma of middle ear and mastoid
389.02 Conductive hearing loss, tympanic membrane
389.03 Conductive hearing loss, middle ear
744.02 Other congenital anomaly of external ear causing impairment of hearing
801.00 Closed fracture of base of skull without mention of intracranial injury, unspecified state of consciousness ▽

ICD-9-CM Procedural

18.6 Reconstruction of external auditory canal
19.3 Other operations on ossicular chain
19.53 Type III tympanoplasty
19.54 Type IV tympanoplasty

69633

69633 Tympanoplasty without mastoidectomy (including canalplasty, atticotomy and/or middle ear surgery), initial or revision; with ossicular chain reconstruction and synthetic prosthesis (eg, partial ossicular replacement prosthesis (PORP), total ossicular replacement prosthesis (TORP))

ICD-9-CM Diagnostic

382.00 Acute suppurative otitis media without spontaneous rupture of eardrum
382.01 Acute suppurative otitis media with spontaneous rupture of eardrum
382.3 Unspecified chronic suppurative otitis media ▽
384.20 Unspecified perforation of tympanic membrane ▽
384.25 Total perforation of tympanic membrane
384.81 Atrophic flaccid tympanic membrane
385.02 Tympanosclerosis involving tympanic membrane and ear ossicles
385.03 Tympanosclerosis involving tympanic membrane, ear ossicles, and middle ear
385.09 Tympanosclerosis involving other combination of structures
385.21 Impaired mobility of malleus
385.22 Impaired mobility of other ear ossicles
385.23 Discontinuity or dislocation of ear ossicles
385.24 Partial loss or necrosis of ear ossicles
385.31 Cholesteatoma of attic
385.32 Cholesteatoma of middle ear
385.33 Cholesteatoma of middle ear and mastoid
389.00 Unspecified conductive hearing loss ▽
389.02 Conductive hearing loss, tympanic membrane
389.03 Conductive hearing loss, middle ear
744.02 Other congenital anomaly of external ear causing impairment of hearing
744.04 Congenital anomalies of ear ossicles
801.00 Closed fracture of base of skull without mention of intracranial injury, unspecified state of consciousness ▽

ICD-9-CM Procedural

19.3 Other operations on ossicular chain
19.53 Type III tympanoplasty
19.54 Type IV tympanoplasty

69635

69635 Tympanoplasty with antrotomy or mastoidotomy (including canalplasty, atticotomy, middle ear surgery, and/or tympanic membrane repair); without ossicular chain reconstruction

ICD-9-CM Diagnostic

382.01 Acute suppurative otitis media with spontaneous rupture of eardrum
382.1 Chronic tubotympanic suppurative otitis media
382.2 Chronic atticoantral suppurative otitis media
382.3 Unspecified chronic suppurative otitis media ▽
383.1 Chronic mastoiditis
384.20 Unspecified perforation of tympanic membrane ▽
384.21 Central perforation of tympanic membrane
384.22 Attic perforation of tympanic membrane
384.23 Other marginal perforation of tympanic membrane
384.24 Multiple perforations of tympanic membrane
384.25 Total perforation of tympanic membrane
384.81 Atrophic flaccid tympanic membrane
385.32 Cholesteatoma of middle ear
385.33 Cholesteatoma of middle ear and mastoid
389.02 Conductive hearing loss, tympanic membrane
389.03 Conductive hearing loss, middle ear
744.02 Other congenital anomaly of external ear causing impairment of hearing
801.00 Closed fracture of base of skull without mention of intracranial injury, unspecified state of consciousness ▽

ICD-9-CM Procedural

19.52 Type II tympanoplasty

69636

69636 Tympanoplasty with antrotomy or mastoidotomy (including canalplasty, atticotomy, middle ear surgery, and/or tympanic membrane repair); with ossicular chain reconstruction

ICD-9-CM Diagnostic

382.01 Acute suppurative otitis media with spontaneous rupture of eardrum
382.1 Chronic tubotympanic suppurative otitis media
382.2 Chronic atticoantral suppurative otitis media
382.3 Unspecified chronic suppurative otitis media ▽
384.20 Unspecified perforation of tympanic membrane ▽
384.21 Central perforation of tympanic membrane
384.22 Attic perforation of tympanic membrane
384.23 Other marginal perforation of tympanic membrane
384.24 Multiple perforations of tympanic membrane
384.25 Total perforation of tympanic membrane
384.81 Atrophic flaccid tympanic membrane
385.02 Tympanosclerosis involving tympanic membrane and ear ossicles
385.21 Impaired mobility of malleus
385.22 Impaired mobility of other ear ossicles
385.23 Discontinuity or dislocation of ear ossicles
385.24 Partial loss or necrosis of ear ossicles
389.02 Conductive hearing loss, tympanic membrane
389.03 Conductive hearing loss, middle ear
389.08 Conductive hearing loss of combined types
389.2 Mixed conductive and sensorineural hearing loss
744.02 Other congenital anomaly of external ear causing impairment of hearing
801.00 Closed fracture of base of skull without mention of intracranial injury, unspecified state of consciousness ▽

ICD-9-CM Procedural

19.3 Other operations on ossicular chain
19.52 Type II tympanoplasty
19.53 Type III tympanoplasty
19.54 Type IV tympanoplasty

69637

69637 Tympanoplasty with antrotomy or mastoidotomy (including canalplasty, atticotomy, middle ear surgery, and/or tympanic membrane repair); with ossicular chain reconstruction and synthetic prosthesis (eg, partial ossicular replacement prosthesis (PORP), total ossicular replacement prosthesis (TORP))

ICD-9-CM Diagnostic

382.01 Acute suppurative otitis media with spontaneous rupture of eardrum
382.1 Chronic tubotympanic suppurative otitis media
382.2 Chronic atticoantral suppurative otitis media
384.20 Unspecified perforation of tympanic membrane ▽
384.21 Central perforation of tympanic membrane
384.22 Attic perforation of tympanic membrane
384.23 Other marginal perforation of tympanic membrane
384.24 Multiple perforations of tympanic membrane
384.25 Total perforation of tympanic membrane
384.81 Atrophic flaccid tympanic membrane
385.02 Tympanosclerosis involving tympanic membrane and ear ossicles
385.21 Impaired mobility of malleus
385.22 Impaired mobility of other ear ossicles
385.23 Discontinuity or dislocation of ear ossicles
385.24 Partial loss or necrosis of ear ossicles
389.02 Conductive hearing loss, tympanic membrane
389.03 Conductive hearing loss, middle ear
389.08 Conductive hearing loss of combined types
389.2 Mixed conductive and sensorineural hearing loss
744.02 Other congenital anomaly of external ear causing impairment of hearing
801.00 Closed fracture of base of skull without mention of intracranial injury, unspecified state of consciousness ▽

ICD-9-CM Procedural

19.52 Type II tympanoplasty
19.53 Type III tympanoplasty
19.54 Type IV tympanoplasty

69641

69641 Tympanoplasty with mastoidectomy (including canalplasty, middle ear surgery, tympanic membrane repair); without ossicular chain reconstruction

ICD-9-CM Diagnostic

382.1 Chronic tubotympanic suppurative otitis media
382.2 Chronic atticoantral suppurative otitis media
382.3 Unspecified chronic suppurative otitis media ▽
383.1 Chronic mastoiditis
384.21 Central perforation of tympanic membrane
384.22 Attic perforation of tympanic membrane
384.23 Other marginal perforation of tympanic membrane
385.32 Cholesteatoma of middle ear
385.33 Cholesteatoma of middle ear and mastoid
387.0 Otosclerosis involving oval window, nonobliterative
387.1 Otosclerosis involving oval window, obliterative
387.2 Cochlear otosclerosis
387.8 Other otosclerosis
389.02 Conductive hearing loss, tympanic membrane
389.03 Conductive hearing loss, middle ear

ICD-9-CM Procedural

19.52 Type II tympanoplasty

69642

69642 Tympanoplasty with mastoidectomy (including canalplasty, middle ear surgery, tympanic membrane repair); with ossicular chain reconstruction

ICD-9-CM Diagnostic

381.19 Other chronic serous otitis media
381.29 Other chronic mucoid otitis media
382.01 Acute suppurative otitis media with spontaneous rupture of eardrum
382.3 Unspecified chronic suppurative otitis media ▽
384.20 Unspecified perforation of tympanic membrane ▽
384.25 Total perforation of tympanic membrane
384.81 Atrophic flaccid tympanic membrane
385.02 Tympanosclerosis involving tympanic membrane and ear ossicles
385.21 Impaired mobility of malleus
385.22 Impaired mobility of other ear ossicles
385.23 Discontinuity or dislocation of ear ossicles
385.24 Partial loss or necrosis of ear ossicles
385.32 Cholesteatoma of middle ear
389.02 Conductive hearing loss, tympanic membrane
389.03 Conductive hearing loss, middle ear
389.08 Conductive hearing loss of combined types
389.2 Mixed conductive and sensorineural hearing loss

ICD-9-CM Procedural

19.3 Other operations on ossicular chain
19.53 Type III tympanoplasty
19.54 Type IV tympanoplasty

69643

69643 Tympanoplasty with mastoidectomy (including canalplasty, middle ear surgery, tympanic membrane repair); with intact or reconstructed wall, without ossicular chain reconstruction

ICD-9-CM Diagnostic

382.1 Chronic tubotympanic suppurative otitis media
382.2 Chronic atticoantral suppurative otitis media
382.3 Unspecified chronic suppurative otitis media ▽
383.1 Chronic mastoiditis
384.21 Central perforation of tympanic membrane
384.22 Attic perforation of tympanic membrane
384.23 Other marginal perforation of tympanic membrane
384.25 Total perforation of tympanic membrane
385.32 Cholesteatoma of middle ear
385.33 Cholesteatoma of middle ear and mastoid
387.0 Otosclerosis involving oval window, nonobliterative
387.1 Otosclerosis involving oval window, obliterative
387.2 Cochlear otosclerosis
387.8 Other otosclerosis
389.02 Conductive hearing loss, tympanic membrane
389.03 Conductive hearing loss, middle ear

ICD-9-CM Procedural

18.6 Reconstruction of external auditory canal
19.52 Type II tympanoplasty
20.41 Simple mastoidectomy
20.49 Other mastoidectomy

69644

69644 Tympanoplasty with mastoidectomy (including canalplasty, middle ear surgery, tympanic membrane repair); with intact or reconstructed canal wall, with ossicular chain reconstruction

ICD-9-CM Diagnostic

382.01 Acute suppurative otitis media with spontaneous rupture of eardrum
382.1 Chronic tubotympanic suppurative otitis media
382.2 Chronic atticoantral suppurative otitis media
383.1 Chronic mastoiditis
384.22 Attic perforation of tympanic membrane
384.25 Total perforation of tympanic membrane
384.81 Atrophic flaccid tympanic membrane
385.02 Tympanosclerosis involving tympanic membrane and ear ossicles
385.03 Tympanosclerosis involving tympanic membrane, ear ossicles, and middle ear
385.21 Impaired mobility of malleus
385.22 Impaired mobility of other ear ossicles
385.23 Discontinuity or dislocation of ear ossicles
385.24 Partial loss or necrosis of ear ossicles
385.32 Cholesteatoma of middle ear
385.33 Cholesteatoma of middle ear and mastoid
389.02 Conductive hearing loss, tympanic membrane
389.03 Conductive hearing loss, middle ear

ICD-9-CM Procedural

19.3 Other operations on ossicular chain
19.53 Type III tympanoplasty
19.54 Type IV tympanoplasty

69645

69645 Tympanoplasty with mastoidectomy (including canalplasty, middle ear surgery, tympanic membrane repair); radical or complete, without ossicular chain reconstruction

ICD-9-CM Diagnostic

382.1 Chronic tubotympanic suppurative otitis media
382.2 Chronic atticoantral suppurative otitis media
382.3 Unspecified chronic suppurative otitis media ▽
383.1 Chronic mastoiditis
384.22 Attic perforation of tympanic membrane
385.32 Cholesteatoma of middle ear
385.33 Cholesteatoma of middle ear and mastoid

ICD-9-CM Procedural

19.52 Type II tympanoplasty

69646

69646 Tympanoplasty with mastoidectomy (including canalplasty, middle ear surgery, tympanic membrane repair); radical or complete, with ossicular chain reconstruction

ICD-9-CM Diagnostic

382.01 Acute suppurative otitis media with spontaneous rupture of eardrum
382.1 Chronic tubotympanic suppurative otitis media
382.2 Chronic atticoantral suppurative otitis media
384.22 Attic perforation of tympanic membrane
384.25 Total perforation of tympanic membrane
384.81 Atrophic flaccid tympanic membrane
385.02 Tympanosclerosis involving tympanic membrane and ear ossicles
385.21 Impaired mobility of malleus
385.22 Impaired mobility of other ear ossicles
385.23 Discontinuity or dislocation of ear ossicles
385.24 Partial loss or necrosis of ear ossicles
385.32 Cholesteatoma of middle ear
389.02 Conductive hearing loss, tympanic membrane
389.03 Conductive hearing loss, middle ear
389.08 Conductive hearing loss of combined types
389.2 Mixed conductive and sensorineural hearing loss

ICD-9-CM Procedural

19.3 Other operations on ossicular chain
19.53 Type III tympanoplasty
19.54 Type IV tympanoplasty

69650

69650 Stapes mobilization

ICD-9-CM Diagnostic

387.0 Otosclerosis involving oval window, nonobliterative
387.8 Other otosclerosis
387.9 Unspecified otosclerosis ▽
389.00 Unspecified conductive hearing loss ▽
389.08 Conductive hearing loss of combined types

ICD-9-CM Procedural

19.0 Stapes mobilization

69660–69661

69660 Stapedectomy or stapedotomy with reestablishment of ossicular continuity, with or without use of foreign material;
69661 with footplate drill out

ICD-9-CM Diagnostic

385.03 Tympanosclerosis involving tympanic membrane, ear ossicles, and middle ear
385.09 Tympanosclerosis involving other combination of structures
385.10 Adhesive middle ear disease, unspecified as to involvement ▽
385.12 Adhesions of drum head to stapes
385.19 Other middle ear adhesions and combinations
385.22 Impaired mobility of other ear ossicles
385.23 Discontinuity or dislocation of ear ossicles
385.24 Partial loss or necrosis of ear ossicles
387.0 Otosclerosis involving oval window, nonobliterative
387.1 Otosclerosis involving oval window, obliterative
387.8 Other otosclerosis
387.9 Unspecified otosclerosis ▽
389.00 Unspecified conductive hearing loss ▽
389.02 Conductive hearing loss, tympanic membrane
389.03 Conductive hearing loss, middle ear
389.08 Conductive hearing loss of combined types
389.10 Unspecified sensorineural hearing loss ▽
389.18 Sensorineural hearing loss of combined types
389.9 Unspecified hearing loss ▽
744.04 Congenital anomalies of ear ossicles
744.09 Other congenital anomalies of ear causing impairment of hearing

ICD-9-CM Procedural

19.11 Stapedectomy with incus replacement
19.19 Other stapedectomy

69662

69662 Revision of stapedectomy or stapedotomy

ICD-9-CM Diagnostic

385.03 Tympanosclerosis involving tympanic membrane, ear ossicles, and middle ear
385.09 Tympanosclerosis involving other combination of structures
385.10 Adhesive middle ear disease, unspecified as to involvement ▽
385.12 Adhesions of drum head to stapes
385.19 Other middle ear adhesions and combinations
385.22 Impaired mobility of other ear ossicles
385.23 Discontinuity or dislocation of ear ossicles
385.24 Partial loss or necrosis of ear ossicles
387.0 Otosclerosis involving oval window, nonobliterative
387.8 Other otosclerosis
389.08 Conductive hearing loss of combined types
389.18 Sensorineural hearing loss of combined types
744.04 Congenital anomalies of ear ossicles
744.09 Other congenital anomalies of ear causing impairment of hearing
996.70 Other complications due to unspecified device, implant, and graft ▽
996.79 Other complications due to other internal prosthetic device, implant, and graft

ICD-9-CM Procedural

19.19 Other stapedectomy
19.21 Revision of stapedectomy with incus replacement
19.29 Other revision of stapedectomy

69666

69666 Repair oval window fistula

ICD-9-CM Diagnostic

385.30 Unspecified cholesteatoma ▽
386.10 Unspecified peripheral vertigo ▽
386.42 Oval window fistula
386.48 Labyrinthine fistula of combined sites
388.61 Cerebrospinal fluid otorrhea
389.18 Sensorineural hearing loss of combined types

ICD-9-CM Procedural

20.93 Repair of oval and round windows

69667

69667 Repair round window fistula

ICD-9-CM Diagnostic

386.10 Unspecified peripheral vertigo ▽
386.41 Round window fistula
386.48 Labyrinthine fistula of combined sites
388.61 Cerebrospinal fluid otorrhea
389.18 Sensorineural hearing loss of combined types

ICD-9-CM Procedural

20.93 Repair of oval and round windows

69670

69670 Mastoid obliteration (separate procedure)

ICD-9-CM Diagnostic

382.9 Unspecified otitis media ▽
383.1 Chronic mastoiditis

▽ Unspecified code
♀ Female diagnosis
☒ Manifestation code
♂ Male diagnosis

383.30 Unspecified postmastoidectomy complication ▽
383.31 Mucosal cyst of postmastoidectomy cavity
383.32 Recurrent cholesteatoma of postmastoidectomy cavity
385.30 Unspecified cholesteatoma ▽
385.33 Cholesteatoma of middle ear and mastoid
388.61 Cerebrospinal fluid otorrhea

ICD-9-CM Procedural

19.9 Other repair of middle ear

69676

69676 Tympanic neurectomy

ICD-9-CM Diagnostic

352.1 Glossopharyngeal neuralgia
388.5 Disorders of acoustic nerve
388.71 Otogenic pain
527.7 Disturbance of salivary secretion

ICD-9-CM Procedural

20.91 Tympanosympathectomy

69700

69700 Closure postauricular fistula, mastoid (separate procedure)

ICD-9-CM Diagnostic

383.81 Postauricular fistula

ICD-9-CM Procedural

19.9 Other repair of middle ear

69710

69710 Implantation or replacement of electromagnetic bone conduction hearing device in temporal bone

ICD-9-CM Diagnostic

388.12 Noise-induced hearing loss
389.00 Unspecified conductive hearing loss ▽
389.01 Conductive hearing loss, external ear
389.02 Conductive hearing loss, tympanic membrane
389.03 Conductive hearing loss, middle ear
389.04 Conductive hearing loss, inner ear
389.08 Conductive hearing loss of combined types
744.02 Other congenital anomaly of external ear causing impairment of hearing
996.60 Infection and inflammatory reaction due to unspecified device, implant, and graft — (Use additional code to identify specified infections) ▽
996.79 Other complications due to other internal prosthetic device, implant, and graft

ICD-9-CM Procedural

20.95 Implantation of electromagnetic hearing device

69711

69711 Removal or repair of electromagnetic bone conduction hearing device in temporal bone

ICD-9-CM Diagnostic

388.12 Noise-induced hearing loss
389.00 Unspecified conductive hearing loss ▽
389.01 Conductive hearing loss, external ear
389.02 Conductive hearing loss, tympanic membrane
389.03 Conductive hearing loss, middle ear
389.04 Conductive hearing loss, inner ear
389.08 Conductive hearing loss of combined types
389.8 Other specified forms of hearing loss
744.02 Other congenital anomaly of external ear causing impairment of hearing
996.69 Infection and inflammatory reaction due to other internal prosthetic device, implant, and graft — (Use additional code to identify specified infections)
996.79 Other complications due to other internal prosthetic device, implant, and graft
V53.09 Fitting and adjustment of other devices related to nervous system and special senses

ICD-9-CM Procedural

20.99 Other operations on middle and inner ear

69714–69715

69714 Implantation, osseointegrated implant, temporal bone, with percutaneous attachment to external speech processor/cochlear stimulator; without mastoidectomy
69715 with mastoidectomy

ICD-9-CM Diagnostic

389.10 Unspecified sensorineural hearing loss ▽
389.11 Sensory hearing loss
389.12 Neural hearing loss
389.2 Mixed conductive and sensorineural hearing loss
389.7 Deaf mutism, not elsewhere classifiable
389.8 Other specified forms of hearing loss
389.9 Unspecified hearing loss ▽

ICD-9-CM Procedural

20.98 Implantation or replacement of cochlear prosthetic device, multiple channel

69717–69718

69717 Replacement (including removal of existing device), osseointegrated implant, temporal bone, with percutaneous attachment to external speech processor/cochlear stimulator; without mastoidectomy
69718 with mastoidectomy

ICD-9-CM Diagnostic

389.10 Unspecified sensorineural hearing loss ▽
389.11 Sensory hearing loss
389.12 Neural hearing loss
389.2 Mixed conductive and sensorineural hearing loss
389.7 Deaf mutism, not elsewhere classifiable
389.8 Other specified forms of hearing loss
389.9 Unspecified hearing loss ▽
996.59 Mechanical complication due to other implant and internal device, not elsewhere classified
996.69 Infection and inflammatory reaction due to other internal prosthetic device, implant, and graft — (Use additional code to identify specified infections)
996.79 Other complications due to other internal prosthetic device, implant, and graft
V53.09 Fitting and adjustment of other devices related to nervous system and special senses

ICD-9-CM Procedural

20.98 Implantation or replacement of cochlear prosthetic device, multiple channel

69720–69725

69720 Decompression facial nerve, intratemporal; lateral to geniculate ganglion
69725 including medial to geniculate ganglion

ICD-9-CM Diagnostic

351.0 Bell's palsy
351.8 Other facial nerve disorders
351.9 Unspecified facial nerve disorder ▽
383.1 Chronic mastoiditis
385.33 Cholesteatoma of middle ear and mastoid
386.33 Suppurative labyrinthitis
801.00 Closed fracture of base of skull without mention of intracranial injury, unspecified state of consciousness ▽
801.01 Closed fracture of base of skull without mention of intracranial injury, no loss of consciousness
801.02 Closed fracture of base of skull without mention of intracranial injury, brief (less than one hour) loss of consciousness
801.03 Closed fracture of base of skull without mention of intracranial injury, moderate (1-24 hours) loss of consciousness
801.04 Closed fracture of base of skull without mention of intracranial injury, prolonged (more than 24 hours) loss of consciousness and return to pre-existing conscious level
801.05 Closed fracture of base of skull without mention of intracranial injury, prolonged (more than 24 hours) loss of consciousness, without return to pre-existing conscious level
801.06 Closed fracture of base of skull without mention of intracranial injury, loss of consciousness of unspecified duration ▽
801.09 Closed fracture of base of skull without mention of intracranial injury, unspecified concussion ▽
801.50 Open fracture of base of skull without mention of intracranial injury, unspecified state of consciousness ▽
854.00 Intracranial injury of other and unspecified nature, without mention of open intracranial wound, unspecified state of consciousness ▽

▽ Unspecified code ♀ Female diagnosis ☒ Manifestation code ♂ Male diagnosis

854.10 Intracranial injury of other and unspecified nature, with open intracranial wound, unspecified state of consciousness
951.4 Injury to facial nerve

ICD-9-CM Procedural

04.42 Other cranial nerve decompression

69740–69745

69740 Suture facial nerve, intratemporal, with or without graft or decompression; lateral to geniculate ganglion
69745 including medial to geniculate ganglion

ICD-9-CM Diagnostic

225.1 Benign neoplasm of cranial nerves
351.0 Bell's palsy
351.8 Other facial nerve disorders
351.9 Unspecified facial nerve disorder
383.30 Unspecified postmastoidectomy complication
386.33 Suppurative labyrinthitis
801.00 Closed fracture of base of skull without mention of intracranial injury, unspecified state of consciousness
801.01 Closed fracture of base of skull without mention of intracranial injury, no loss of consciousness
801.02 Closed fracture of base of skull without mention of intracranial injury, brief (less than one hour) loss of consciousness
801.03 Closed fracture of base of skull without mention of intracranial injury, moderate (1-24 hours) loss of consciousness
801.04 Closed fracture of base of skull without mention of intracranial injury, prolonged (more than 24 hours) loss of consciousness and return to pre-existing conscious level
801.05 Closed fracture of base of skull without mention of intracranial injury, prolonged (more than 24 hours) loss of consciousness, without return to pre-existing conscious level
801.06 Closed fracture of base of skull without mention of intracranial injury, loss of consciousness of unspecified duration
801.09 Closed fracture of base of skull without mention of intracranial injury, unspecified concussion
801.50 Open fracture of base of skull without mention of intracranial injury, unspecified state of consciousness
854.00 Intracranial injury of other and unspecified nature, without mention of open intracranial wound, unspecified state of consciousness
854.10 Intracranial injury of other and unspecified nature, with open intracranial wound, unspecified state of consciousness
951.4 Injury to facial nerve
998.2 Accidental puncture or laceration during procedure

ICD-9-CM Procedural

04.3 Suture of cranial and peripheral nerves

Inner Ear

69801–69802

69801 Labyrinthotomy, with or without cryosurgery including other nonexcisional destructive procedures or perfusion of vestibuloactive drugs (single or multiple perfusions); transcanal
69802 with mastoidectomy

ICD-9-CM Diagnostic

322.9 Unspecified meningitis
386.01 Active Meniere's disease, cochleovestibular
386.03 Active Meniere's disease, vestibular
386.10 Unspecified peripheral vertigo
386.19 Other and unspecified peripheral vertigo
386.50 Unspecified labyrinthine dysfunction
386.8 Other disorders of labyrinth
386.9 Unspecified vertiginous syndromes and labyrinthine disorders

ICD-9-CM Procedural

20.41 Simple mastoidectomy
20.72 Injection into inner ear
20.79 Other incision, excision, and destruction of inner ear

69805–69806

69805 Endolymphatic sac operation; without shunt
69806 with shunt

ICD-9-CM Diagnostic

322.9 Unspecified meningitis
386.01 Active Meniere's disease, cochleovestibular
386.03 Active Meniere's disease, vestibular
386.10 Unspecified peripheral vertigo
386.19 Other and unspecified peripheral vertigo
386.50 Unspecified labyrinthine dysfunction
386.58 Other forms and combinations of labyrinthine dysfunction
386.8 Other disorders of labyrinth
386.9 Unspecified vertiginous syndromes and labyrinthine disorders

ICD-9-CM Procedural

20.71 Endolymphatic shunt
20.79 Other incision, excision, and destruction of inner ear

69820

69820 Fenestration semicircular canal

ICD-9-CM Diagnostic

387.0 Otosclerosis involving oval window, nonobliterative
387.1 Otosclerosis involving oval window, obliterative
387.8 Other otosclerosis
387.9 Unspecified otosclerosis
389.00 Unspecified conductive hearing loss
389.08 Conductive hearing loss of combined types
389.12 Neural hearing loss
389.2 Mixed conductive and sensorineural hearing loss
744.02 Other congenital anomaly of external ear causing impairment of hearing

ICD-9-CM Procedural

20.61 Fenestration of inner ear (initial)

69840

69840 Revision fenestration operation

ICD-9-CM Diagnostic

387.0 Otosclerosis involving oval window, nonobliterative
387.1 Otosclerosis involving oval window, obliterative
387.2 Cochlear otosclerosis
387.8 Other otosclerosis
389.08 Conductive hearing loss of combined types
389.11 Sensory hearing loss
389.12 Neural hearing loss
389.2 Mixed conductive and sensorineural hearing loss
389.8 Other specified forms of hearing loss

ICD-9-CM Procedural

20.62 Revision of fenestration of inner ear

69905

69905 Labyrinthectomy; transcanal

ICD-9-CM Diagnostic

322.9 Unspecified meningitis
386.01 Active Meniere's disease, cochleovestibular
386.03 Active Meniere's disease, vestibular
386.10 Unspecified peripheral vertigo
386.19 Other and unspecified peripheral vertigo
386.50 Unspecified labyrinthine dysfunction
386.51 Hyperactive labyrinth, unilateral
386.58 Other forms and combinations of labyrinthine dysfunction
386.8 Other disorders of labyrinth
386.9 Unspecified vertiginous syndromes and labyrinthine disorders

ICD-9-CM Procedural

20.79 Other incision, excision, and destruction of inner ear

69910

69910 Labyrinthectomy; with mastoidectomy

ICD-9-CM Diagnostic

383.02 Acute mastoiditis with other complications
383.32 Recurrent cholesteatoma of postmastoidectomy cavity
385.35 Diffuse cholesteatosis of middle ear and mastoid
386.01 Active Meniere's disease, cochleovestibular
386.02 Active Meniere's disease, cochlear
386.03 Active Meniere's disease, vestibular
386.10 Unspecified peripheral vertigo ▽
386.12 Vestibular neuronitis
386.19 Other and unspecified peripheral vertigo
386.2 Vertigo of central origin
386.33 Suppurative labyrinthitis
386.48 Labyrinthine fistula of combined sites
386.50 Unspecified labyrinthine dysfunction ▽
386.9 Unspecified vertiginous syndromes and labyrinthine disorders ▽

ICD-9-CM Procedural

20.41 Simple mastoidectomy
20.79 Other incision, excision, and destruction of inner ear

69915

69915 Vestibular nerve section, translabyrinthine approach

ICD-9-CM Diagnostic

383.02 Acute mastoiditis with other complications
383.32 Recurrent cholesteatoma of postmastoidectomy cavity
385.35 Diffuse cholesteatosis of middle ear and mastoid
386.01 Active Meniere's disease, cochleovestibular
386.02 Active Meniere's disease, cochlear
386.03 Active Meniere's disease, vestibular
386.10 Unspecified peripheral vertigo ▽
386.12 Vestibular neuronitis
386.19 Other and unspecified peripheral vertigo
386.2 Vertigo of central origin
386.48 Labyrinthine fistula of combined sites
386.50 Unspecified labyrinthine dysfunction ▽
386.8 Other disorders of labyrinth
386.9 Unspecified vertiginous syndromes and labyrinthine disorders ▽

ICD-9-CM Procedural

20.41 Simple mastoidectomy
20.79 Other incision, excision, and destruction of inner ear

69930

69930 Cochlear device implantation, with or without mastoidectomy

ICD-9-CM Diagnostic

385.9 Unspecified disorder of middle ear and mastoid ▽
386.02 Active Meniere's disease, cochlear
389.08 Conductive hearing loss of combined types
389.10 Unspecified sensorineural hearing loss ▽
389.11 Sensory hearing loss
389.18 Sensorineural hearing loss of combined types
389.2 Mixed conductive and sensorineural hearing loss
389.7 Deaf mutism, not elsewhere classifiable
389.9 Unspecified hearing loss ▽

ICD-9-CM Procedural

20.96 Implantation or replacement of cochlear prosthetic device, not otherwise specified
20.97 Implantation or replacement of cochlear prosthetic device, single channel
20.98 Implantation or replacement of cochlear prosthetic device, multiple channel

HCPCS Level II Supplies & Services

L8614 Cochlear device/system
L8615 Headset/headpiece for use with cochlear implant device, replacement
L8616 Microphone for use with cochlear implant device, replacement
L8617 Transmitting coil for use with cochlear implant device, replacement
L8618 Transmitter cable for use with cochlear implant device, replacement
L8619 Cochlear implant external speech processor, replacement
L8620 Lithium ion battery for use with cochlear implant device, replacement, each
L8621 Zinc air battery for use with cochlear implant device, replacement, each
L8622 Alkaline battery for use with cochlear implant device, any size, replacement, each

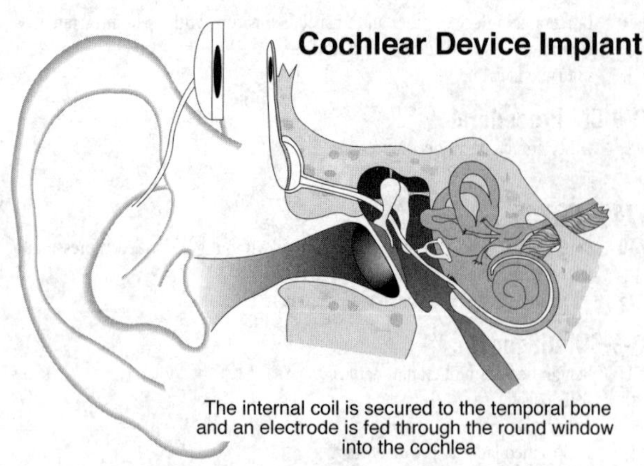

The internal coil is secured to the temporal bone and an electrode is fed through the round window into the cochlea

Temporal Bone, Middle Fossa Approach

69950

69950 Vestibular nerve section, transcranial approach

ICD-9-CM Diagnostic

322.9 Unspecified meningitis ▽
386.01 Active Meniere's disease, cochleovestibular
386.03 Active Meniere's disease, vestibular
386.10 Unspecified peripheral vertigo ▽
386.12 Vestibular neuronitis
386.19 Other and unspecified peripheral vertigo
386.50 Unspecified labyrinthine dysfunction ▽
386.8 Other disorders of labyrinth
386.9 Unspecified vertiginous syndromes and labyrinthine disorders ▽

ICD-9-CM Procedural

20.79 Other incision, excision, and destruction of inner ear

69955

69955 Total facial nerve decompression and/or repair (may include graft)

ICD-9-CM Diagnostic

237.3 Neoplasm of uncertain behavior of paraganglia
351.0 Bell's palsy
351.1 Geniculate ganglionitis
351.8 Other facial nerve disorders
351.9 Unspecified facial nerve disorder ▽
385.33 Cholesteatoma of middle ear and mastoid
801.00 Closed fracture of base of skull without mention of intracranial injury, unspecified state of consciousness ▽
801.50 Open fracture of base of skull without mention of intracranial injury, unspecified state of consciousness ▽
951.4 Injury to facial nerve

ICD-9-CM Procedural

04.42 Other cranial nerve decompression

69960

69960 Decompression internal auditory canal

ICD-9-CM Diagnostic

225.1 Benign neoplasm of cranial nerves
225.2 Benign neoplasm of cerebral meninges
381.52 Chronic Eustachian salpingitis
381.61 Osseous obstruction of Eustachian tube
381.62 Intrinsic cartilagenous obstruction of Eustachian tube
381.63 Extrinsic cartilagenous obstruction of Eustachian tube
385.03 Tympanosclerosis involving tympanic membrane, ear ossicles, and middle ear
385.32 Cholesteatoma of middle ear
385.82 Cholesterin granuloma of middle ear
385.83 Retained foreign body of middle ear

▽ Unspecified code ♀ Female diagnosis ☒ Manifestation code ♂ Male diagnosis

801.00 Closed fracture of base of skull without mention of intracranial injury, unspecified state of consciousness ▽

ICD-9-CM Procedural

04.42 Other cranial nerve decompression

69970

69970 Removal of tumor, temporal bone

ICD-9-CM Diagnostic

170.0 Malignant neoplasm of bones of skull and face, except mandible
213.0 Benign neoplasm of bones of skull and face
238.0 Neoplasm of uncertain behavior of bone and articular cartilage
239.2 Neoplasms of unspecified nature of bone, soft tissue, and skin

ICD-9-CM Procedural

01.6 Excision of lesion of skull

Operating Microscope

69990

69990 Microsurgical techniques, requiring use of operating microscope (List separately in addition to code for primary procedure)

ICD-9-CM Diagnostic

This is an add-on code. Refer to the corresponding primary procedure code for ICD-9 diagnosis code links.

HCPCS Level II Supplies & Services

The HCPCS Level II code(s) would be the same as the actual procedure performed because these are in-addition-to codes.

Appendix A

Add-On Codes

0036T Placement of proximal or distal extension prosthesis for endovascular repair of descending thoracic aortic aneurysm, pseudoaneurysm or dissection; each additional extension (List separately in addition to code for primary procedure)

0049T Prolonged extracorporeal percutaneous transseptal ventricular assist device, greater than 24 hours, each subsequent 24 hour period (List separately in addition to code for primary procedure)

0054T Computer-assisted musculoskeletal surgical navigational orthopedic procedure, with image-guidance based on fluoroscopic images (List separately in addition to code for primary procedure)

0055T Computer-assisted musculoskeletal surgical navigational orthopedic procedure, with image-guidance based on CT/MRI images (List separately in addition to code for primary procedure)

0056T Computer assisted musculoskeletal surgical navigational orthopedic procedure, image-less (List separately in addition to code for primary procedure)

0063T Percutaneous intradiscal annuloplasty, any method, unilateral or bilateral including fluoroscopic guidance; one or more additional levels (List separately in addition to 0062T for primary procedure)

0068T Acoustic heart sound recording and computer analysis; with interpretation and report (List separately in addition to codes for electrocardiography)

0069T Acoustic heart sound recording and computer analysis; acoustic heart sound recording and computer analysis only (List separately in addition to codes for electrocardiography)

0070T Acoustic heart sound recording and computer analysis; interpretation and report only (List separately in addition to codes for electrocardiography)

0076T Transcatheter placement of extracranial vertebral or intrathoracic carotid artery stent(s), including radiologic supervision and interpretation, percutaneous; each additional vessel (List separately in addition to code for primary procedure)

0079T Placement of visceral extension prosthesis for endovascular repair of abdominal aortic aneurysm involving visceral vessels, each visceral branch (List separately in addition to code for primary procedure)

0081T Placement of visceral extension prosthesis for endovascular repair of abdominal aortic aneurysm involving visceral vessels, each visceral branch, radiological supervision and interpretation (List separately in addition to code for primary procedure)

01953 Anesthesia for second and third degree burn excision or debridement with or without skin grafting, any site, for total body surface area (TBSA) treated during anesthesia and surgery; each additional nine percent total body surface area or part thereof (List separately in addition to code for primary procedure)

01968 Anesthesia for cesarean delivery following neuraxial labor analgesia/anesthesia (List separately in addition to code for primary procedure performed)

01969 Anesthesia for cesarean hysterectomy following neuraxial labor analgesia/anesthesia (List separately in addition to code for primary procedure performed)

11001 Debridement of extensive eczematous or infected skin; each additional 10% of the body surface (List separately in addition to code for primary procedure)

11008 Removal of prosthetic material or mesh, abdominal wall for necrotizing soft tissue infection (List separately in addition to code for primary procedure)

11101 Biopsy of skin, subcutaneous tissue and/or mucous membrane (including simple closure), unless otherwise listed; each separate/additional lesion (List separately in addition to code for primary procedure)

11201 Removal of skin tags, multiple fibrocutaneous tags, any area; each additional ten lesions (List separately in addition to code for primary procedure)

11732 Avulsion of nail plate, partial or complete, simple; each additional nail plate (List separately in addition to code for primary procedure)

11922 Tattooing, intradermal introduction of insoluble opaque pigments to correct color defects of skin, including micropigmentation; each additional 20.0 sq. cm (List separately in addition to code for primary procedure)

13102 Repair, complex, trunk; each additional 5 cm or less (List separately in addition to code for primary procedure)

13122 Repair, complex, scalp, arms, and/or legs; each additional 5 cm or less (List separately in addition to code for primary procedure)

13133 Repair, complex, forehead, cheeks, chin, mouth, neck, axillae, genitalia, hands and/or feet; each additional 5 cm or less (List separately in addition to code for primary procedure)

13153 Repair, complex, eyelids, nose, ears and/or lips; each additional 5 cm or less (List separately in addition to code for primary procedure)

15001 Surgical preparation or creation of recipient site by excision of open wounds, burn eschar, or scar (including subcutaneous tissues); each additional 100 sq. cm or each additional one percent of body area of infants and children (List separately in addition to code for primary procedure)

15101 Split graft, trunk, arms, legs; each additional 100 sq. cm, or each additional one percent of body area of infants and children, or part thereof (List separately in addition to code for primary procedure)

15121 Split graft, face, scalp, eyelids, mouth, neck, ears, orbits, genitalia, hands, feet and/or multiple digits; each additional 100 sq. cm, or each additional one percent of body area of infants and children, or part thereof (List separately in addition to code for primary procedure)

15201 Full thickness graft, free, including direct closure of donor site, trunk; each additional 20 sq. cm (List separately in addition to code for primary procedure)

15221 Full thickness graft, free, including direct closure of donor site, scalp, arms, and/or legs; each additional 20 sq. cm (List separately in addition to code for primary procedure)

15241 Full thickness graft, free, including direct closure of donor site, forehead, cheeks, chin, mouth, neck, axillae, genitalia, hands, and/or feet; each additional 20 sq. cm (List separately in addition to code for primary procedure)

15261 Full thickness graft, free, including direct closure of donor site, nose, ears, eyelids, and/or lips; each additional 20 sq. cm (List separately in addition to code for primary procedure)

15343 Application of bilaminate skin substitute/neodermis; each additional 25 sq. cm (List separately in addition to code for primary procedure)

15351 Application of allograft, skin; each additional 100 sq. cm (List separately in addition to code for primary procedure)

15401 Application of xenograft, skin; each additional 100 sq. cm (List separately in addition to code for primary procedure)

15787 Abrasion; each additional four lesions or less (List separately in addition to code for primary procedure)

16036 Escharotomy; each additional incision (List separately in addition to code for primary procedure)

17003 Destruction (eg, laser surgery, electrosurgery, cryosurgery, chemosurgery, surgical curettement), all benign or premalignant lesions (eg, actinic keratoses) other than skin tags or cutaneous vascular proliferative lesions; second through 14 lesions, each (List separately in addition to code for first lesion)

17310 Chemosurgery (Mohs micrographic technique), including removal of all gross tumor, surgical excision of tissue specimens, mapping, color coding of specimens, microscopic examination of specimens by the surgeon, and complete histopathologic preparation including the first routine stain (eg, hematoxylin and eosin, toluidine blue); each additional specimen, after the first 5 specimens, fixed or fresh tissue, any stage (List separately in addition to code for primary procedure)

19001 Puncture aspiration of cyst of breast; each additional cyst (List separately in addition to code for primary procedure)

19126 Excision of breast lesion identified by preoperative placement of radiological marker, open; each additional lesion separately identified by a preoperative radiological marker (List separately in addition to code for primary procedure)

19291 Preoperative placement of needle localization wire, breast; each additional lesion (List separately in addition to code for primary procedure)

19295 Image guided placement, metallic localization clip, percutaneous, during breast biopsy (List separately in addition to code for primary procedure)

19297 Placement of radiotherapy afterloading balloon catheter into the breast for interstitial radioelement application following partial mastectomy, includes imaging guidance; concurrent with partial mastectomy (List separately in addition to code for primary procedure)

22103 Partial excision of posterior vertebral component (eg, spinous process, lamina or facet) for intrinsic bony lesion, single vertebral segment; each additional segment (List separately in addition to code for primary procedure)

22116 Partial excision of vertebral body, for intrinsic bony lesion, without decompression of spinal cord or nerve root(s), single vertebral segment; each additional vertebral segment (List separately in addition to code for primary procedure)

22216 Osteotomy of spine, posterior or posterolateral approach, one vertebral segment; each additional vertebral segment (List separately in addition to primary procedure)

22226 Osteotomy of spine, including diskectomy, anterior approach, single vertebral segment; each additional vertebral segment (List separately in addition to code for primary procedure)

22328 Open treatment and/or reduction of vertebral fracture(s) and/or dislocation(s), posterior approach, one fractured vertebrae or dislocated segment; each additional fractured vertebrae or dislocated segment (List separately in addition to code for primary procedure)

22522 Percutaneous vertebroplasty, one vertebral body, unilateral or bilateral injection; each additional thoracic or lumbar vertebral body (List separately in addition to code for primary procedure)

22534 Arthrodesis, lateral extracavitary technique, including minimal diskectomy to prepare interspace (other than for decompression); thoracic or lumbar, each additional vertebral segment (List separately in addition to code for primary procedure)

22585 Arthrodesis, anterior interbody technique, including minimal diskectomy to prepare interspace (other than for decompression); each additional interspace (List separately in addition to code for primary procedure)

22614 Arthrodesis, posterior or posterolateral technique, single level; each additional vertebral segment (List separately in addition to code for primary procedure)

22632 Arthrodesis, posterior interbody technique, including laminectomy and/or diskectomy to prepare interspace (other than for decompression), single interspace; each additional interspace (List separately in addition to code for primary procedure)

26125 Fasciectomy, partial palmar with release of single digit including proximal interphalangeal joint, with or without Z-plasty, other local tissue rearrangement, or skin grafting (includes obtaining graft); each additional digit (List separately in addition to code for primary procedure)

26861 Arthrodesis, interphalangeal joint, with or without internal fixation; each additional interphalangeal joint (List separately in addition to code for primary procedure)

26863 Arthrodesis, interphalangeal joint, with or without internal fixation; with autograft (includes obtaining graft), each additional joint (List separately in addition to code for primary procedure)

27358 Excision or curettage of bone cyst or benign tumor of femur; with internal fixation (List in addition to code for primary procedure)

27692 Transfer or transplant of single tendon (with muscle redirection or rerouting); each additional tendon (List separately in addition to code for primary procedure)

31620 Endobronchial ultrasound (EBUS) during bronchoscopic diagnostic or therapeutic intervention(s) (List separately in addition to code for primary procedure(s))

31632 Bronchoscopy, rigid or flexible, with or without fluoroscopic guidance; with transbronchial lung biopsy(s), each additional lobe (List separately in addition to code for primary procedure)

31633 Bronchoscopy, rigid or flexible, with or without fluoroscopic guidance; with transbronchial needle aspiration biopsy(s), each additional lobe (List separately in addition to code for primary procedure)

31637 Bronchoscopy, rigid or flexible, with or without fluoroscopic guidance; each additional major bronchus stented (List separately in addition to code for primary procedure)

32501 Resection and repair of portion of bronchus (bronchoplasty) when performed at time of lobectomy or segmentectomy (List separately in addition to code for primary procedure)

33141 Transmyocardial laser revascularization, by thoracotomy; performed at the time of other open cardiac procedure(s) (List separately in addition to code for primary procedure)

33225 Insertion of pacing electrode, cardiac venous system, for left ventricular pacing, at time of insertion of pacing cardioverter-defibrillator or pacemaker pulse generator (including upgrade to dual chamber system) (List separately in addition to code for primary procedure)

33508 Endoscopy, surgical, including video-assisted harvest of vein(s) for coronary artery bypass procedure (List separately in addition to code for primary procedure)

33530 Reoperation, coronary artery bypass procedure or valve procedure, more than one month after original operation (List separately in addition to code for primary procedure)

33572 Coronary endarterectomy, open, any method, of left anterior descending, circumflex, or right coronary artery performed in conjunction with coronary artery bypass graft procedure, each vessel (List separately in addition to primary procedure)

33924 Ligation and takedown of a systemic-to-pulmonary artery shunt, performed in conjunction with a congenital heart procedure (List separately in addition to code for primary procedure)

33961 Prolonged extracorporeal circulation for cardiopulmonary insufficiency; each additional 24 hours (List separately in addition to code for primary procedure)

34808 Endovascular placement of iliac artery occlusion device (List separately in addition to code for primary procedure)

34813 Placement of femoral-femoral prosthetic graft during endovascular aortic aneurysm repair (List separately in addition to code for primary procedure)

34826 Placement of proximal or distal extension prosthesis for endovascular repair of infrarenal abdominal aortic or iliac aneurysm, false aneurysm, or dissection; each additional vessel (List separately in addition to code for primary procedure)

35390 Reoperation, carotid, thromboendarterectomy, more than one month after original operation (List separately in addition to code for primary procedure)

35400 Angioscopy (non-coronary vessels or grafts) during therapeutic intervention (List separately in addition to code for primary procedure)

35500 Harvest of upper extremity vein, one segment, for lower extremity or coronary artery bypass procedure (List separately in addition to code for primary procedure)

35572 Harvest of femoropopliteal vein, one segment, for vascular reconstruction procedure (eg, aortic, vena caval, coronary, peripheral artery) (List separately in addition to code for primary procedure)

35681 Bypass graft; composite, prosthetic and vein (List separately in addition to code for primary procedure)

35682 Bypass graft; autogenous composite, two segments of veins from two locations (List separately in addition to code for primary procedure)

35683 Bypass graft; autogenous composite, three or more segments of vein from two or more locations (List separately in addition to code for primary procedure)

35685 Placement of vein patch or cuff at distal anastomosis of bypass graft, synthetic conduit (List separately in addition to code for primary procedure)

35686 Creation of distal arteriovenous fistula during lower extremity bypass surgery (non-hemodialysis) (List separately in addition to code for primary procedure)

35697 Reimplantation, visceral artery to infrarenal aortic prosthesis, each artery (List separately in addition to code for primary procedure)

35700 Reoperation, femoral-popliteal or femoral (popliteal)-anterior tibial, posterior tibial, peroneal artery or other distal vessels, more than one month after original operation (List separately in addition to code for primary procedure)

36218 Selective catheter placement, arterial system; additional second order, third order, and beyond, thoracic or brachiocephalic branch, within a vascular family (List in addition to code for initial second or third order vessel as appropriate)

36248 Selective catheter placement, arterial system; additional second order, third order, and beyond, abdominal, pelvic, or lower extremity artery branch, within a vascular family (List in addition to code for initial second or third order vessel as appropriate)

36476 Endovenous ablation therapy of incompetent vein, extremity, inclusive of all imaging guidance and monitoring, percutaneous, radiofrequency; second and subsequent veins treated in a single extremity, each through separate access sites (List separately in addition to code for primary procedure)

36479 Endovenous ablation therapy of incompetent vein, extremity, inclusive of all imaging guidance and monitoring, percutaneous, laser; second and subsequent veins treated in a single extremity, each through separate access sites (List separately in addition to code for primary procedure)

37206 Transcatheter placement of an intravascular stent(s), (except coronary, carotid, and vertebral vessel), percutaneous; each additional vessel (List separately in addition to code for primary procedure)

37208 Transcatheter placement of an intravascular stent(s), (non-coronary vessel), open; each additional vessel (List separately in addition to code for primary procedure)

37250 Intravascular ultrasound (non-coronary vessel) during diagnostic evaluation and/or therapeutic intervention; initial vessel (List separately in addition to code for primary procedure)

37251 Intravascular ultrasound (non-coronary vessel) during diagnostic evaluation and/or therapeutic intervention; each additional vessel (List separately in addition to code for primary procedure)

38102 Splenectomy; total, en bloc for extensive disease, in conjunction with other procedure (List in addition to code for primary procedure)

38746 Thoracic lymphadenectomy, regional, including mediastinal and peritracheal nodes (List separately in addition to code for primary procedure)

38747 Abdominal lymphadenectomy, regional, including celiac, gastric, portal, peripancreatic, with or without para-aortic and vena caval nodes (List separately in addition to code for primary procedure)

43635 Vagotomy when performed with partial distal gastrectomy (List separately in addition to code(s) for primary procedure)

44015 Tube or needle catheter jejunostomy for enteral alimentation, intraoperative, any method (List separately in addition to primary procedure)

44121 Enterectomy, resection of small intestine; each additional resection and anastomosis (List separately in addition to code for primary procedure)

44128 Enterectomy, resection of small intestine for congenital atresia, single resection and anastomosis of proximal segment of intestine; each additional resection and anastomosis (List separately in addition to code for primary procedure)

44139 Mobilization (take-down) of splenic flexure performed in conjunction with partial colectomy (List separately in addition to primary procedure)

44203 Laparoscopy, surgical; each additional small intestine resection and anastomosis (List separately in addition to code for primary procedure)

44701 Intraoperative colonic lavage (List separately in addition to code for primary procedure)

44955 Appendectomy; when done for indicated purpose at time of other major procedure (not as separate procedure) (List separately in addition to code for primary procedure)

47001 Biopsy of liver, needle; when done for indicated purpose at time of other major procedure (List separately in addition to code for primary procedure)

47550 Biliary endoscopy, intraoperative (choledochoscopy) (List separately in addition to code for primary procedure)

48400 Injection procedure for intraoperative pancreatography (List separately in addition to code for primary procedure)

49568 Implantation of mesh or other prosthesis for incisional or ventral hernia repair (List separately in addition to code for the incisional or ventral hernia repair)

49905 Omental flap, intra-abdominal (List separately in addition to code for primary procedure)

56606 Biopsy of vulva or perineum (separate procedure); each separate additional lesion (List separately in addition to code for primary procedure)

57267 Insertion of mesh or other prosthesis for repair of pelvic floor defect, each site (anterior, posterior compartment), vaginal approach (List separately in addition to code for primary procedure)

58611 Ligation or transection of fallopian tube(s) when done at the time of cesarean delivery or intra-abdominal surgery (not a separate procedure) (List separately in addition to code for primary procedure)

59525 Subtotal or total hysterectomy after cesarean delivery (List separately in addition to code for primary procedure)

60512 Parathyroid autotransplantation (List separately in addition to code for primary procedure)

61316 Incision and subcutaneous placement of cranial bone graft (List separately in addition to code for primary procedure)

61517 Implantation of brain intracavitary chemotherapy agent (List separately in addition to code for primary procedure)

61609 Transection or ligation, carotid artery in cavernous sinus; without repair (List separately in addition to code for primary procedure)

61610 Transection or ligation, carotid artery in cavernous sinus; with repair by anastomosis or graft (List separately in addition to code for primary procedure)

61611 Transection or ligation, carotid artery in petrous canal; without repair (List separately in addition to code for primary procedure)

61612 Transection or ligation, carotid artery in petrous canal; with repair by anastomosis or graft (List separately in addition to code for primary procedure)

61795 Stereotactic computer assisted volumetric (navigational) procedure, intracranial, extracranial, or spinal (List separately in addition to code for primary procedure)

61864 Twist drill, burr hole, craniotomy, or craniectomy with stereotactic implantation of neurostimulator electrode array in subcortical site (eg, thalamus, globus pallidus, subthalamic nucleus, periventricular, periaqueductal gray), without use of intraoperative microelectrode recording; each additional array (List separately in addition to primary procedure)

61868 Twist drill, burr hole, craniotomy, or craniectomy with stereotactic implantation of neurostimulator electrode array in subcortical site (eg, thalamus, globus pallidus, subthalamic nucleus, periventricular, periaqueductal gray), with use of intraoperative microelectrode recording; each additional array (List separately in addition to primary procedure)

62148 Incision and retrieval of subcutaneous cranial bone graft for cranioplasty (List separately in addition to code for primary procedure)

62160 Neuroendoscopy, intracranial, for placement or replacement of ventricular catheter and attachment to shunt system or external drainage (List separately in addition to code for primary procedure)

63035 Laminotomy (hemilaminectomy), with decompression of nerve root(s), including partial facetectomy, foraminotomy and/or excision of herniated intervertebral disk; each additional interspace, cervical or lumbar (List separately in addition to code for primary procedure)

63043 Laminotomy (hemilaminectomy), with decompression of nerve root(s), including partial facetectomy, foraminotomy and/or excision of herniated intervertebral disk, reexploration, single interspace; each additional cervical interspace (List separately in addition to code for primary procedure)

63044 Laminotomy (hemilaminectomy), with decompression of nerve root(s), including partial facetectomy, foraminotomy and/or excision of herniated intervertebral disk, reexploration, single interspace; each additional lumbar interspace (List separately in addition to code for primary procedure)

63048 Laminectomy, facetectomy and foraminotomy (unilateral or bilateral with decompression of spinal cord, cauda equina and/or nerve root(s), (eg, spinal or lateral recess stenosis)), single vertebral segment; each additional segment, cervical, thoracic, or lumbar (List separately in addition to code for primary procedure)

63057 Transpedicular approach with decompression of spinal cord, equina and/or nerve root(s) (eg, herniated intervertebral disk), single segment; each additional segment, thoracic or lumbar (List separately in addition to code for primary procedure)

63066 Costovertebral approach with decompression of spinal cord or nerve root(s), (eg, herniated intervertebral disk), thoracic; each additional segment (List separately in addition to code for primary procedure)

63076 Diskectomy, anterior, with decompression of spinal cord and/or nerve root(s), including osteophytectomy; cervical, each additional interspace (List separately in addition to code for primary procedure)

63078 Diskectomy, anterior, with decompression of spinal cord and/or nerve root(s), including osteophytectomy; thoracic, each additional interspace (List separately in addition to code for primary procedure)

63082 Vertebral corpectomy (vertebral body resection), partial or complete, anterior approach with decompression of spinal cord and/or nerve root(s); cervical, each additional segment (List separately in addition to code for primary procedure)

63086 Vertebral corpectomy (vertebral body resection), partial or complete, transthoracic approach with decompression of spinal cord and/or nerve root(s); thoracic, each additional segment (List separately in addition to code for primary procedure)

63088 Vertebral corpectomy (vertebral body resection), partial or complete, combined thoracolumbar approach with decompression of spinal cord, cauda equina or nerve root(s), lower thoracic or lumbar; each additional segment (List separately in addition to code for primary procedure)

63091 Vertebral corpectomy (vertebral body resection), partial or complete, transperitoneal or retroperitoneal approach with decompression of spinal cord, cauda equina or nerve root(s), lower thoracic, lumbar, or sacral; each additional segment (List separately in addition to code for primary procedure)

63103 Vertebral corpectomy (vertebral body resection), partial or complete, lateral extracavitary approach with decompression of spinal cord and/or nerve root(s) (eg, for tumor or retropulsed bone fragments); thoracic or lumbar, each additional segment (List separately in addition to code for primary procedure)

63295 Osteoplastic reconstruction of dorsal spinal elements, following primary intraspinal procedure (List separately in addition to code for primary procedure)

63308 Vertebral corpectomy (vertebral body resection), partial or complete, for excision of intraspinal lesion, single segment; each additional segment (List separately in addition to codes for single segment)

64472 Injection, anesthetic agent and/or steroid, paravertebral facet joint or facet joint nerve; cervical or thoracic, each additional level (List separately in addition to code for primary procedure)

64476 Injection, anesthetic agent and/or steroid, paravertebral facet joint or facet joint nerve; lumbar or sacral, each additional level (List separately in addition to code for primary procedure)

64480 Injection, anesthetic agent and/or steroid, transforaminal epidural; cervical or thoracic, each additional level (List separately in addition to code for primary procedure)

64484 Injection, anesthetic agent and/or steroid, transforaminal epidural; lumbar or sacral, each additional level (List separately in addition to code for primary procedure)

64623 Destruction by neurolytic agent, paravertebral facet joint nerve; lumbar or sacral, each additional level (List separately in addition to code for primary procedure)

64627 Destruction by neurolytic agent, paravertebral facet joint nerve; cervical or thoracic, each additional level (List separately in addition to code for primary procedure)

64727 Internal neurolysis, requiring use of operating microscope (List separately in addition to code for neuroplasty) (Neuroplasty includes external neurolysis)

64778 Excision of neuroma; digital nerve, each additional digit (List separately in addition to code for primary procedure)

64783 Excision of neuroma; hand or foot, each additional nerve, except same digit (List separately in addition to code for primary procedure)

64787 Implantation of nerve end into bone or muscle (List separately in addition to neuroma excision)

64832 Suture of digital nerve, hand or foot; each additional digital nerve (List separately in addition to code for primary procedure)

64837 Suture of each additional nerve, hand or foot (List separately in addition to code for primary procedure)

64859 Suture of each additional major peripheral nerve (List separately in addition to code for primary procedure)

64872 Suture of nerve; requiring secondary or delayed suture (List separately in addition to code for primary neurorrhaphy)

64874 Suture of nerve; requiring extensive mobilization, or transposition of nerve (List separately in addition to code for nerve suture)

64876 Suture of nerve; requiring shortening of bone of extremity (List separately in addition to code for nerve suture)

64901 Nerve graft, each additional nerve; single strand (List separately in addition to code for primary procedure)

64902 Nerve graft, each additional nerve; multiple strands (cable) (List separately in addition to code for primary procedure)

66990 Use of ophthalmic endoscope (List separately in addition to code for primary procedure)

67225 Destruction of localized lesion of choroid (eg, choroidal neovascularization); photodynamic therapy, second eye, at single session (List separately in addition to code for primary eye treatment)

67320 Transposition procedure (eg, for paretic extraocular muscle), any extraocular muscle (specify) (List separately in addition to code for primary procedure)

67331 Strabismus surgery on patient with previous eye surgery or injury that did not involve the extraocular muscles (List separately in addition to code for primary procedure)

67332 Strabismus surgery on patient with scarring of extraocular muscles (eg, prior ocular injury, strabismus or retinal detachment surgery) or restrictive myopathy (eg, dysthyroid ophthalmopathy) (List separately in addition to code for primary procedure)

67334 Strabismus surgery by posterior fixation suture technique, with or without muscle recession (List separately in addition to code for primary procedure)

67335 Placement of adjustable suture(s) during strabismus surgery, including postoperative adjustment(s) of suture(s) (List separately in addition to code for specific strabismus surgery)

67340 Strabismus surgery involving exploration and/or repair of detached extraocular muscle(s) (List separately in addition to code for primary procedure)

69990 Microsurgical techniques, requiring use of operating microscope (List separately in addition to code for primary procedure)

74301 Cholangiography and/or pancreatography; additional set intraoperative, radiological supervision and interpretation (List separately in addition to code for primary procedure)

75774 Angiography, selective, each additional vessel studied after basic examination, radiological supervision and interpretation (List separately in addition to code for primary procedure)

75946 Intravascular ultrasound (non-coronary vessel), radiological supervision and interpretation; each additional non-coronary vessel (List separately in addition to code for primary procedure)

75964 Transluminal balloon angioplasty, each additional peripheral artery, radiological supervision and interpretation (List separately in addition to code for primary procedure)

75968 Transluminal balloon angioplasty, each additional visceral artery, radiological supervision and interpretation (List separately in addition to code for primary procedure)

75993 Transluminal atherectomy, each additional peripheral artery, radiological supervision and interpretation (List separately in addition to code for primary procedure)

75996 Transluminal atherectomy, each additional visceral artery, radiological supervision and interpretation (List separately in addition to code for primary procedure)

75998 Fluoroscopic guidance for central venous access device placement, replacement (catheter only or complete), or removal (includes fluoroscopic guidance for vascular access and catheter manipulation, any necessary contrast injections through access site or catheter with related venography radiologic supervision and interpretation, and radiographic documentation of final catheter position) (List separately in addition to code for primary procedure)

76082 Computer aided detection (computer algorithm analysis of digital image data for lesion detection) with further physician review for interpretation, with or without digitization of film radiographic images; diagnostic mammography (List separately in addition to code for primary procedure)

76083 Computer aided detection (computer algorithm analysis of digital image data for lesion detection) with further physician review for interpretation, with or without digitization of film radiographic images; screening mammography (List separately in addition to code for primary procedure)

76125 Cineradiography/videoradiography to complement routine examination (List separately in addition to code for primary procedure)

76802 Ultrasound, pregnant uterus, real time with image documentation, fetal and maternal evaluation, first trimester (<14 weeks 0 days), transabdominal approach; each additional gestation (List separately in addition to code for primary procedure)

76810 Ultrasound, pregnant uterus, real time with image documentation, fetal and maternal evaluation, after first trimester (> or = 14 weeks 0 days), transabdominal approach; each additional gestation (List separately in addition to code for primary procedure)

76812 Ultrasound, pregnant uterus, real time with image documentation, fetal and maternal evaluation plus detailed fetal anatomic examination, transabdominal approach; each additional gestation (List separately in addition to code for primary procedure)

76937 Ultrasound guidance for vascular access requiring ultrasound evaluation of potential access sites, documentation of selected vessel patency, concurrent realtime ultrasound visualization of vascular needle entry, with permanent recording and reporting (List separately in addition to code for primary procedure)

78020 Thyroid carcinoma metastases uptake (List separately in addition to code for primary procedure)

78478 Myocardial perfusion study with wall motion, qualitative or quantitative study (List separately in addition to code for primary procedure)

78480 Myocardial perfusion study with ejection fraction (List separately in addition to code for primary procedure)

78496 Cardiac blood pool imaging, gated equilibrium, single study, at rest, with right ventricular ejection fraction by first pass technique (List separately in addition to code for primary procedure)

87187 Susceptibility studies, antimicrobial agent; microdilution or agar dilution, minimum lethal concentration (MLC), each plate (List separately in addition to code for primary procedure)

87904 Infectious agent phenotype analysis by nucleic acid (DNA or RNA) with drug resistance tissue culture analysis, HIV 1; each additional 1 through 5 drugs tested (List separately in addition to code for primary procedure)

88141 Cytopathology, cervical or vaginal (any reporting system), requiring interpretation by physician (List separately in addition to code for technical service)

88155 Cytopathology, slides, cervical or vaginal, definitive hormonal evaluation (eg, maturation index, karyopyknotic index, estrogenic index) (List separately in addition to code(s) for other technical and interpretation services)

88185 Flow cytometry, cell surface, cytoplasmic, or nuclear marker, technical component only; each additional marker (List separately in addition to code for first marker)

88311 Decalcification procedure (List separately in addition to code for surgical pathology examination)

88312 Special stains (List separately in addition to code for primary service); Group I for microorganisms (eg, Gridley, acid fast, methenamine silver), each

88313 Special stains (List separately in addition to code for primary service); Group II, all other, (eg, iron, trichrome), except immunocytochemistry and immunoperoxidase stains, each

88314 Special stains (List separately in addition to code for primary service); histochemical staining with frozen section(s)

90466 Immunization administration under 8 years of age (includes percutaneous, intradermal, subcutaneous, or intramuscular injections) when the physician counsels the patient/family; each additional injection (single or combination vaccine/toxoid), per day (List separately in addition to code for primary procedure)

90468 Immunization administration under age 8 years (includes intranasal or oral routes of administration) when the physician counsels the patient/family; each additional administration (single or combination vaccine/toxoid), per day (List separately in addition to code for primary procedure)

90472 Immunization administration (includes percutaneous, intradermal, subcutaneous, or intramuscular injections); each additional vaccine (single or combination vaccine/toxoid) (List separately in addition to code for primary procedure)

90474 Immunization administration by intranasal or oral route; each additional vaccine (single or combination vaccine/toxoid) (List separately in addition to code for primary procedure)

90781 Intravenous infusion for therapy/diagnosis, administered by physician or under direct supervision of physician; each additional hour, up to eight (8) hours (List separately in addition to code for primary procedure)

92547 Use of vertical electrodes (List separately in addition to code for primary procedure)

92608 Evaluation for prescription for speech-generating augmentative and alternative communication device, face-to-face with the patient; each additional 30 minutes (List separately in addition to code for primary procedure)

92973 Percutaneous transluminal coronary thrombectomy (List separately in addition to code for primary procedure)

92974 Transcatheter placement of radiation delivery device for subsequent coronary intravascular brachytherapy (List separately in addition to code for primary procedure)

92978 Intravascular ultrasound (coronary vessel or graft) during diagnostic evaluation and/or therapeutic intervention including imaging supervision, interpretation and report; initial vessel (List separately in addition to code for primary procedure)

92979 Intravascular ultrasound (coronary vessel or graft) during diagnostic evaluation and/or therapeutic intervention including imaging supervision, interpretation and report; each additional vessel (List separately in addition to code for primary procedure)

92981 Transcatheter placement of an intracoronary stent(s), percutaneous, with or without other therapeutic intervention, any method; each additional vessel (List separately in addition to code for primary procedure)

92984 Percutaneous transluminal coronary balloon angioplasty; each additional vessel (List separately in addition to code for primary procedure)

92996 Percutaneous transluminal coronary atherectomy, by mechanical or other method, with or without balloon angioplasty; each additional vessel (List separately in addition to code for primary procedure)

92998 Percutaneous transluminal pulmonary artery balloon angioplasty; each additional vessel (List separately in addition to code for primary procedure)

93320 Doppler echocardiography, pulsed wave and/or continuous wave with spectral display (List separately in addition to codes for echocardiographic imaging); complete

93321 Doppler echocardiography, pulsed wave and/or continuous wave with spectral display (List separately in addition to codes for echocardiographic imaging); follow-up or limited study (List separately in addition to codes for echocardiographic imaging)

93325 Doppler echocardiography color flow velocity mapping (List separately in addition to codes for echocardiography)

93571 Intravascular Doppler velocity and/or pressure derived coronary flow reserve measurement (coronary vessel or graft) during coronary angiography including pharmacologically induced stress; initial vessel (List separately in addition to code for primary procedure)

93572 Intravascular Doppler velocity and/or pressure derived coronary flow reserve measurement (coronary vessel or graft) during coronary angiography including pharmacologically induced stress; each additional vessel (List separately in addition to code for primary procedure)

93609 Intraventricular and/or intra-atrial mapping of tachycardia site(s) with catheter manipulation to record from multiple sites to identify origin of tachycardia (List separately in addition to code for primary procedure)

93613 Intracardiac electrophysiologic 3-dimensional mapping (List separately in addition to code for primary procedure)

93621 Comprehensive electrophysiologic evaluation including insertion and repositioning of multiple electrode catheters with induction or attempted induction of arrhythmia; with left atrial pacing and recording from coronary sinus or left atrium (List separately in addition to code for primary procedure)

93622 Comprehensive electrophysiologic evaluation including insertion and repositioning of multiple electrode catheters with induction or attempted induction of arrhythmia; with left ventricular pacing and recording (List separately in addition to code for primary procedure)

93623 Programmed stimulation and pacing after intravenous drug infusion (List separately in addition to code for primary procedure)

93662 Intracardiac echocardiography during therapeutic/diagnostic intervention, including imaging supervision and interpretation (List separately in addition to code for primary procedure)

95920 Intraoperative neurophysiology testing, per hour (List separately in addition to code for primary procedure)

95962 Functional cortical and subcortical mapping by stimulation and/or recording of electrodes on brain surface, or of depth electrodes, to provoke seizures or identify vital brain structures; each additional hour of physician attendance (List separately in addition to code for primary procedure)

95967 Magnetoencephalography (MEG), recording and analysis; for evoked magnetic fields, each additional modality (eg, sensory, motor, language, or visual cortex localization) (List separately in addition to code for primary procedure)

95973 Electronic analysis of implanted neurostimulator pulse generator system (eg, rate, pulse amplitude and duration, configuration of wave form, battery status, electrode selectability, output modulation, cycling, impedance and patient compliance measurements); complex spinal cord, or peripheral (except cranial nerve) neurostimulator pulse generator/transmitter, with intraoperative or subsequent programming, each additional 30 minutes after first hour (List separately in addition to code for primary procedure)

95975 Electronic analysis of implanted neurostimulator pulse generator system (eg, rate, pulse amplitude and duration, configuration of wave form, battery status, electrode selectability, output modulation, cycling, impedance and patient compliance measurements); complex cranial nerve neurostimulator pulse generator/transmitter, with intraoperative or subsequent programming, each additional 30 minutes after first hour (List separately in addition to code for primary procedure)

95979 Electronic analysis of implanted neurostimulator pulse generator system (eg, rate, pulse amplitude and duration, battery status, electrode selectability and polarity, impedance and patient compliance measurements), complex deep brain neurostimulator pulse generator/transmitter, with initial or subsequent programming; each additional 30 minutes after first hour (List separately in addition to code for primary procedure)

96412 Chemotherapy administration, intravenous; infusion technique, one to 8 hours, each additional hour (List separately in addition to code for primary procedure)

96423 Chemotherapy administration, intra-arterial; infusion technique, one to 8 hours, each additional hour (List separately in addition to code for primary procedure)

96570 Photodynamic therapy by endoscopic application of light to ablate abnormal tissue via activation of photosensitive drug(s); first 30 minutes (List separately in addition to code for endoscopy or bronchoscopy procedures of lung and esophagus)

96571 Photodynamic therapy by endoscopic application of light to ablate abnormal tissue via activation of photosensitive drug(s); each additional 15 minutes (List separately in addition to code for endoscopy or bronchoscopy procedures of lung and esophagus)

97546 Work hardening/conditioning; each additional hour (List separately in addition to code for primary procedure)

97811 Acupuncture, one or more needles, without electrical stimulation; each additional 15 minutes of personal one-on-one contact with the patient, with re-insertion of needle(s) (List separately in addition to code for primary procedure)

97814 Acupuncture, one or more needles, with electrical stimulation; each additional 15 minutes of personal one-on-one contact with the patient (List separately in addition to code for primary procedure)

99100 Anesthesia for patient of extreme age, under 1 year and over 70 (List separately in addition to code for primary anesthesia procedure)

99116 Anesthesia complicated by utilization of total body hypothermia (List separately in addition to code for primary anesthesia procedure)

99135 Anesthesia complicated by utilization of controlled hypotension (List separately in addition to code for primary anesthesia procedure)

99140 Anesthesia complicated by emergency conditions (specify) (List separately in addition to code for primary anesthesia procedure)

99290 Critical care services delivered by a physician, face-to-face, during an interfacility transport of critically ill or critically injured pediatric patient, 24 months of age or less; each additional 30 minutes (List separately in addition to code for primary service)

99292 Critical care, evaluation and management of the critically ill or critically injured patient; each additional 30 minutes (List separately in addition to code for primary service)

99354 Prolonged physician service in the office or other outpatient setting requiring direct (face-to-face) patient contact beyond the usual service (eg, prolonged care and treatment of an acute asthmatic patient in an outpatient setting); first hour (List separately in addition to code for office or other outpatient Evaluation and Management service)

99355 Prolonged physician service in the office or other outpatient setting requiring direct (face-to-face) patient contact beyond the usual service (eg, prolonged care and treatment of an acute asthmatic patient in an outpatient setting); each additional 30 minutes (List separately in addition to code for prolonged physician service)

99356 Prolonged physician service in the inpatient setting, requiring direct (face-to-face) patient contact beyond the usual service (eg, maternal fetal monitoring for high risk delivery or other physiological monitoring, prolonged care of an acutely ill inpatient); first hour (List separately in addition to code for inpatient Evaluation and Management service)

99357 Prolonged physician service in the inpatient setting, requiring direct (face-to-face) patient contact beyond the usual service (eg, maternal fetal monitoring for high risk delivery or other physiological monitoring, prolonged care of an acutely ill inpatient); each additional 30 minutes (List separately in addition to code for prolonged physician service)

99358 Prolonged evaluation and management service before and/or after direct (face-to-face) patient care (eg, review of extensive records and tests, communication with other professionals and/or the patient/family); first hour (List separately in addition to code(s) for other physician service(s) and/or inpatient or outpatient Evaluation and Management service)

99359 Prolonged evaluation and management service before and/or after direct (face-to-face) patient care (eg, review of extensive records and tests, communication with other professionals and/or the patient/family); each additional 30 minutes (List separately in addition to code for prolonged physician service)

99602 Home infusion/specialty drug administration, per visit (up to 2 hours); each additional hour (List separately in addition to primary procedure)

Modifier 51 Exempt

17004 Destruction (eg, laser surgery, electrosurgery, cryosurgery, chemosurgery, surgical curettement), all benign or premalignant lesions (eg, actinic keratoses) other than skin tags or cutaneous vascular proliferative lesions, 15 or more lesions

17304 Chemosurgery (Mohs micrographic technique), including removal of all gross tumor, surgical excision of tissue specimens, mapping, color coding of specimens, microscopic examination of specimens by the surgeon, and complete histopathologic preparation including the first routine stain (eg, hematoxylin and eosin, toluidine blue); first stage, fresh tissue technique, up to 5 specimens

17305 Chemosurgery (Mohs micrographic technique), including removal of all gross tumor, surgical excision of tissue specimens, mapping, color coding of specimens, microscopic examination of specimens by the surgeon, and complete histopathologic preparation including the first routine stain (eg, hematoxylin and eosin, toluidine blue); second stage, fixed or fresh tissue, up to 5 specimens

17306 Chemosurgery (Mohs micrographic technique), including removal of all gross tumor, surgical excision of tissue specimens, mapping, color coding of specimens, microscopic examination of specimens by the surgeon, and complete histopathologic preparation including the first routine stain (eg, hematoxylin and eosin, toluidine blue); third stage, fixed or fresh tissue, up to 5 specimens

17307 Chemosurgery (Mohs micrographic technique), including removal of all gross tumor, surgical excision of tissue specimens, mapping, color coding of specimens, microscopic examination of specimens by the surgeon, and complete histopathologic preparation including the first routine stain (eg, hematoxylin and eosin, toluidine blue); additional stage(s), up to 5 specimens, each stage

20660 Application of cranial tongs, caliper, or stereotactic frame, including removal (separate procedure)

20690 Application of a uniplane (pins or wires in one plane), unilateral, external fixation system

20692 Application of a multiplane (pins or wires in more than one plane), unilateral, external fixation system (eg, Ilizarov, Monticelli type)

20900 Bone graft, any donor area; minor or small (eg, dowel or button)

20902 Bone graft, any donor area; major or large

20910 Cartilage graft; costochondral

20912 Cartilage graft; nasal septum

20920 Fascia lata graft; by stripper

20922 Fascia lata graft; by incision and area exposure, complex or sheet

20924 Tendon graft, from a distance (eg, palmaris, toe extensor, plantaris)

20926 Tissue grafts, other (eg, paratenon, fat, dermis)

20930 Allograft for spine surgery only; morselized

20931 Allograft for spine surgery only; structural

20936 Autograft for spine surgery only (includes harvesting the graft); local (eg, ribs, spinous process, or laminar fragments) obtained from same incision

20937 Autograft for spine surgery only (includes harvesting the graft); morselized (through separate skin or fascial incision)

20938 Autograft for spine surgery only (includes harvesting the graft); structural, bicortical or tricortical (through separate skin or fascial incision)

20974 Electrical stimulation to aid bone healing; noninvasive (nonoperative)

20975 Electrical stimulation to aid bone healing; invasive (operative)

22840 Posterior non-segmental instrumentation (eg, Harrington rod technique, pedicle fixation across one interspace, atlantoaxial transarticular screw fixation, sublaminar wiring at C1, facet screw fixation)

22841 Internal spinal fixation by wiring of spinous processes

22842 Posterior segmental instrumentation (eg, pedicle fixation, dual rods with multiple hooks and sublaminar wires); 3 to 6 vertebral segments

22843 Posterior segmental instrumentation (eg, pedicle fixation, dual rods with multiple hooks and sublaminar wires); 7 to 12 vertebral segments

22844 Posterior segmental instrumentation (eg, pedicle fixation, dual rods with multiple hooks and sublaminar wires); 13 or more vertebral segments

22845 Anterior instrumentation; 2 to 3 vertebral segments

22846 Anterior instrumentation; 4 to 7 vertebral segments

22847 Anterior instrumentation; 8 or more vertebral segments

22848 Pelvic fixation (attachment of caudal end of instrumentation to pelvic bony structures) other than sacrum

22851 Application of intervertebral biomechanical device(s) (eg, synthetic cage(s), threaded bone dowel(s), methylmethacrylate) to vertebral defect or interspace

31500 Intubation, endotracheal, emergency procedure

32000 Thoracentesis, puncture of pleural cavity for aspiration, initial or subsequent

32002 Thoracentesis with insertion of tube with or without water seal (eg, for pneumothorax) (separate procedure)

32020 Tube thoracostomy with or without water seal (eg, for abscess, hemothorax, empyema) (separate procedure)

33517 Coronary artery bypass, using venous graft(s) and arterial graft(s); single vein graft (List separately in addition to code for arterial graft)

33518 Coronary artery bypass, using venous graft(s) and arterial graft(s); two venous grafts (List separately in addition to code for arterial graft)

33519 Coronary artery bypass, using venous graft(s) and arterial graft(s); three venous grafts (List separately in addition to code for arterial graft)

33521 Coronary artery bypass, using venous graft(s) and arterial graft(s); four venous grafts (List separately in addition to code for arterial graft)

33522 Coronary artery bypass, using venous graft(s) and arterial graft(s); five venous grafts (List separately in addition to code for arterial graft)

33523 Coronary artery bypass, using venous graft(s) and arterial graft(s); six or more venous grafts (List separately in addition to code for arterial graft)

35600 Harvest of upper extremity artery, one segment, for coronary artery bypass procedure

36620 Arterial catheterization or cannulation for sampling, monitoring or transfusion (separate procedure); percutaneous

36660 Catheterization, umbilical artery, newborn, for diagnosis or therapy

38792 Injection procedure; for identification of sentinel node

44500 Introduction of long gastrointestinal tube (eg, Miller-Abbott) (separate procedure)

44720 Backbench reconstruction of cadaver or living donor intestine allograft prior to transplantation; venous anastomosis, each

44721 Backbench reconstruction of cadaver or living donor intestine allograft prior to transplantation; arterial anastomosis, each

47146 Backbench reconstruction of cadaver or living donor liver graft prior to allotransplantation; venous anastomosis, each

47147 Backbench reconstruction of cadaver or living donor liver graft prior to allotransplantation; arterial anastomosis, each

48552 Backbench reconstruction of cadaver donor pancreas allograft prior to transplantation, venous anastomosis, each

50327 Backbench reconstruction of cadaver or living donor renal allograft prior to transplantation; venous anastomosis, each

50328 Backbench reconstruction of cadaver or living donor renal allograft prior to transplantation; arterial anastomosis, each

50329 Backbench reconstruction of cadaver or living donor renal allograft prior to transplantation; ureteral anastomosis, each

61107 Twist drill hole for subdural or ventricular puncture; for implanting ventricular catheter or pressure recording device

61210 Burr hole(s); for implanting ventricular catheter, reservoir, EEG electrode(s) or pressure recording device (separate procedure)

62284 Injection procedure for myelography and/or computed tomography, spinal (other than C1-C2 and posterior fossa)

90281 Immune globulin (Ig), human, for intramuscular use

90283 Immune globulin (IgIV), human, for intravenous use

90287 Botulinum antitoxin, equine, any route

90288 Botulism immune globulin, human, for intravenous use

90291 Cytomegalovirus immune globulin (CMV-IgIV), human, for intravenous use

90296 Diphtheria antitoxin, equine, any route

90371 Hepatitis B immune globulin (HBIg), human, for intramuscular use

90375 Rabies immune globulin (RIg), human, for intramuscular and/or subcutaneous use

90376 Rabies immune globulin, heat-treated (RIg-HT), human, for intramuscular and/or subcutaneous use

90378 Respiratory syncytial virus immune globulin (RSV-IgIM), for intramuscular use, 50 mg, each

90379 Respiratory syncytial virus immune globulin (RSV-IgIV), human, for intravenous use

90384 Rho(D) immune globulin (RhIg), human, full-dose, for intramuscular use

90385 Rho(D) immune globulin (RhIg), human, mini-dose, for intramuscular use

90386 Rho(D) immune globulin (RhIgIV), human, for intravenous use

90389 Tetanus immune globulin (TIg), human, for intramuscular use

90393 Vaccinia immune globulin, human, for intramuscular use

90396 Varicella-zoster immune globulin, human, for intramuscular use

90399 Unlisted immune globulin

90476 Adenovirus vaccine, type 4, live, for oral use

90477 Adenovirus vaccine, type 7, live, for oral use

90581 Anthrax vaccine, for subcutaneous use

90585 Bacillus Calmette-Guerin vaccine (BCG) for tuberculosis, live, for percutaneous use

90586 Bacillus Calmette-Guerin vaccine (BCG) for bladder cancer, live, for intravesical use

90632 Hepatitis A vaccine, adult dosage, for intramuscular use

90633 Hepatitis A vaccine, pediatric/adolescent dosage-2 dose schedule, for intramuscular use

90634 Hepatitis A vaccine, pediatric/adolescent dosage-3 dose schedule, for intramuscular use
90636 Hepatitis A and hepatitis B vaccine (HepA-HepB), adult dosage, for intramuscular use
90645 Hemophilus influenza b vaccine (Hib), HbOC conjugate (4 dose schedule), for intramuscular use
90646 Hemophilus influenza b vaccine (Hib), PRP-D conjugate, for booster use only, intramuscular use
90647 Hemophilus influenza b vaccine (Hib), PRP-OMP conjugate (3 dose schedule), for intramuscular use
90648 Hemophilus influenza b vaccine (Hib), PRP-T conjugate (4 dose schedule), for intramuscular use
90655 Influenza virus vaccine, split virus, preservative free, for children 6-35 months of age, for intramuscular use
90656 Influenza virus vaccine, split virus, preservative free, for use in individuals 3 years and above, for intramuscular use
90657 Influenza virus vaccine, split virus, for children 6-35 months of age, for intramuscular use
90658 Influenza virus vaccine, split virus, for use in individuals 3 years of age and above, for intramuscular use
90660 Influenza virus vaccine, live, for intranasal use
90665 Lyme disease vaccine, adult dosage, for intramuscular use
90669 Pneumococcal conjugate vaccine, polyvalent, for children under 5 years, for intramuscular use
90675 Rabies vaccine, for intramuscular use
90676 Rabies vaccine, for intradermal use
90680 Rotavirus vaccine, tetravalent, live, for oral use
90690 Typhoid vaccine, live, oral
90691 Typhoid vaccine, Vi capsular polysaccharide (ViCPs), for intramuscular use
90692 Typhoid vaccine, heat- and phenol-inactivated (H-P), for subcutaneous or intradermal use
90693 Typhoid vaccine, acetone-killed, dried (AKD), for subcutaneous use (U.S. military)
90698 Diphtheria, tetanus toxoids, acellular pertussis vaccine, haemophilus influenza Type B, and poliovirus vaccine, inactivated (DTaP - Hib - IPV), for intramuscular use
90700 Diphtheria, tetanus toxoids, and acellular pertussis vaccine (DTaP), for use in individuals younger than 7 years, for intramuscular use
90701 Diphtheria, tetanus toxoids, and whole cell pertussis vaccine (DTP), for intramuscular use
90702 Diphtheria and tetanus toxoids (DT) adsorbed for use in individuals younger than 7 years, for intramuscular use
90703 Tetanus toxoid adsorbed, for intramuscular use
90704 Mumps virus vaccine, live, for subcutaneous use
90705 Measles virus vaccine, live, for subcutaneous use
90706 Rubella virus vaccine, live, for subcutaneous use
90707 Measles, mumps and rubella virus vaccine (MMR), live, for subcutaneous use
90708 Measles and rubella virus vaccine, live, for subcutaneous use
90710 Measles, mumps, rubella, and varicella vaccine (MMRV), live, for subcutaneous use
90712 Poliovirus vaccine, (any type(s)) (OPV), live, for oral use
90713 Poliovirus vaccine, inactivated, (IPV), for subcutaneous use
90715 Tetanus, diphtheria toxoids and acellular pertussis vaccine (TdaP), for use in individuals 7 years or older, for intramuscular use
90716 Varicella virus vaccine, live, for subcutaneous use
90717 Yellow fever vaccine, live, for subcutaneous use
90718 Tetanus and diphtheria toxoids (Td) adsorbed for use in individuals 7 years or older, for intramuscular use
90719 Diphtheria toxoid, for intramuscular use
90720 Diphtheria, tetanus toxoids, and whole cell pertussis vaccine and Hemophilus influenza B vaccine (DTP-Hib), for intramuscular use
90721 Diphtheria, tetanus toxoids, and acellular pertussis vaccine and Hemophilus influenza B vaccine (DtaP-Hib), for intramuscular use
90723 Diphtheria, tetanus toxoids, acellular pertussis vaccine, Hepatitis B, and poliovirus vaccine, inactivated (DtaP-HepB-IPV), for intramuscular use
90725 Cholera vaccine for injectable use
90727 Plague vaccine, for intramuscular use
90732 Pneumococcal polysaccharide vaccine, 23-valent, adult or immunosuppressed patient dosage, for use in individuals 2 years or older, for subcutaneous or intramuscular use
90733 Meningococcal polysaccharide vaccine (any group(s)), for subcutaneous use
90734 Meningococcal conjugate vaccine, serogroups A, C, Y and W-135 (tetravalent), for intramuscular use
90735 Japanese encephalitis virus vaccine, for subcutaneous use
90740 Hepatitis B vaccine, dialysis or immunosuppressed patient dosage (3 dose schedule), for intramuscular use
90743 Hepatitis B vaccine, adolescent (2 dose schedule), for intramuscular use
90744 Hepatitis B vaccine, pediatric/adolescent dosage (3 dose schedule), for intramuscular use
90746 Hepatitis B vaccine, adult dosage, for intramuscular use
90747 Hepatitis B vaccine, dialysis or immunosuppressed patient dosage (4 dose schedule), for intramuscular use
90748 Hepatitis B and Hemophilus influenza b vaccine (HepB-Hib), for intramuscular use
90749 Unlisted vaccine/toxoid
93501 Right heart catheterization
93503 Insertion and placement of flow directed catheter (eg, Swan-Ganz) for monitoring purposes
93505 Endomyocardial biopsy
93508 Catheter placement in coronary artery(s), arterial coronary conduit(s), and/or venous coronary bypass graft(s) for coronary angiography without concomitant left heart catheterization
93510 Left heart catheterization, retrograde, from the brachial artery, axillary artery or femoral artery; percutaneous
93511 Left heart catheterization, retrograde, from the brachial artery, axillary artery or femoral artery; by cutdown
93514 Left heart catheterization by left ventricular puncture
93524 Combined transseptal and retrograde left heart catheterization
93526 Combined right heart catheterization and retrograde left heart catheterization
93527 Combined right heart catheterization and transseptal left heart catheterization through intact septum (with or without retrograde left heart catheterization)
93528 Combined right heart catheterization with left ventricular puncture (with or without retrograde left heart catheterization)
93529 Combined right heart catheterization and left heart catheterization through existing septal opening (with or without retrograde left heart catheterization)
93530 Right heart catheterization, for congenital cardiac anomalies
93531 Combined right heart catheterization and retrograde left heart catheterization, for congenital cardiac anomalies
93532 Combined right heart catheterization and transseptal left heart catheterization through intact septum with or without retrograde left heart catheterization, for congenital cardiac anomalies
93533 Combined right heart catheterization and transseptal left heart catheterization through existing septal opening, with or without retrograde left heart catheterization, for congenital cardiac anomalies
93539 Injection procedure during cardiac catheterization; for selective opacification of arterial conduits (eg, internal mammary), whether native or used for bypass
93540 Injection procedure during cardiac catheterization; for selective opacification of aortocoronary venous bypass grafts, one or more coronary arteries
93541 Injection procedure during cardiac catheterization; for pulmonary angiography
93542 Injection procedure during cardiac catheterization; for selective right ventricular or right atrial angiography
93543 Injection procedure during cardiac catheterization; for selective left ventricular or left atrial angiography
93544 Injection procedure during cardiac catheterization; for aortography
93545 Injection procedure during cardiac catheterization; for selective coronary angiography (injection of radiopaque material may be by hand)
93555 Imaging supervision, interpretation and report for injection procedure(s) during cardiac catheterization; ventricular and/or atrial angiography
93556 Imaging supervision, interpretation and report for injection procedure(s) during cardiac catheterization; pulmonary angiography, aortography, and/or selective coronary angiography including venous bypass grafts and arterial conduits (whether native or used in bypass)
93600 Bundle of His recording
93602 Intra-atrial recording
93603 Right ventricular recording
93610 Intra-atrial pacing
93612 Intraventricular pacing
93615 Esophageal recording of atrial electrogram with or without ventricular electrogram(s);
93616 Esophageal recording of atrial electrogram with or without ventricular electrogram(s); with pacing
93618 Induction of arrhythmia by electrical pacing
93619 Comprehensive electrophysiologic evaluation with right atrial pacing and recording, right ventricular pacing and recording, His bundle recording, including insertion and repositioning of multiple electrode catheters, without induction or attempted induction of arrhythmia
93620 Comprehensive electrophysiologic evaluation including insertion and repositioning of multiple electrode catheters with induction or attempted induction of arrhythmia; with right atrial pacing and recording, right ventricular pacing and recording, His bundle recording

93624 Electrophysiologic follow-up study with pacing and recording to test effectiveness of therapy, including induction or attempted induction of arrhythmia
93631 Intra-operative epicardial and endocardial pacing and mapping to localize the site of tachycardia or zone of slow conduction for surgical correction
93640 Electrophysiologic evaluation of single or dual chamber pacing cardioverter-defibrillator leads including defibrillation threshold evaluation (induction of arrhythmia, evaluation of sensing and pacing for arrhythmia termination) at time of initial implantation or replacement;
93641 Electrophysiologic evaluation of single or dual chamber pacing cardioverter-defibrillator leads including defibrillation threshold evaluation (induction of arrhythmia, evaluation of sensing and pacing for arrhythmia termination) at time of initial implantation or replacement; with testing of single or dual chamber pacing cardioverter-defibrillator pulse generator
93642 Electrophysiologic evaluation of single or dual chamber pacing cardioverter-defibrillator (includes defibrillation threshold evaluation, induction of arrhythmia, evaluation of sensing and pacing for arrhythmia termination, and programming or reprogramming of sensing or therapeutic parameters)
93650 Intracardiac catheter ablation of atrioventricular node function, atrioventricular conduction for creation of complete heart block, with or without temporary pacemaker placement
93651 Intracardiac catheter ablation of arrhythmogenic focus; for treatment of supraventricular tachycardia by ablation of fast or slow atrioventricular pathways, accessory atrioventricular connections or other atrial foci, singly or in combination
93652 Intracardiac catheter ablation of arrhythmogenic focus; for treatment of ventricular tachycardia
93660 Evaluation of cardiovascular function with tilt table evaluation, with continuous ECG monitoring and intermittent blood pressure monitoring, with or without pharmacological intervention
95900 Nerve conduction, amplitude and latency/velocity study, each nerve; motor, without F-wave study
95903 Nerve conduction, amplitude and latency/velocity study, each nerve; motor, with F-wave study
95904 Nerve conduction, amplitude and latency/velocity study, each nerve; sensory
99141 Sedation with or without analgesia (conscious sedation); intravenous, intramuscular or inhalation
99142 Sedation with or without analgesia (conscious sedation); oral, rectal and/or intranasal

Modifier 63 Exempt

30545 Repair choanal atresia; transpalatine
31520 Laryngoscopy direct, with or without tracheoscopy; diagnostic, newborn
33401 Valvuloplasty, aortic valve; open, with inflow occlusion
33403 Valvuloplasty, aortic valve; using transventricular dilation, with cardiopulmonary bypass
33472 Valvotomy, pulmonary valve, open heart; with inflow occlusion
33502 Repair of anomalous coronary artery; by ligation
33503 Repair of anomalous coronary artery; by graft, without cardiopulmonary bypass
33505 Repair of anomalous coronary artery; with construction of intrapulmonary artery tunnel (Takeuchi procedure)
33506 Repair of anomalous coronary artery; by translocation from pulmonary artery to aorta
33610 Repair of complex cardiac anomalies (eg, single ventricle with subaortic obstruction) by surgical enlargement of ventricular septal defect
33611 Repair of double outlet right ventricle with intraventricular tunnel repair;
33619 Repair of single ventricle with aortic outflow obstruction and aortic arch hypoplasia (hypoplastic left heart syndrome) (eg, Norwood procedure)
33647 Repair of atrial septal defect and ventricular septal defect, with direct or patch closure
33670 Repair of complete atrioventricular canal, with or without prosthetic valve
33690 Banding of pulmonary artery
33694 Complete repair tetralogy of Fallot without pulmonary atresia; with transannular patch
33730 Complete repair of anomalous venous return (supracardiac, intracardiac, or infracardiac types)
33732 Repair of cor triatriatum or supravalvular mitral ring by resection of left atrial membrane
33735 Atrial septectomy or septostomy; closed heart (Blalock-Hanlon type operation)
33736 Atrial septectomy or septostomy; open heart with cardiopulmonary bypass
33750 Shunt; subclavian to pulmonary artery (Blalock-Taussig type operation)
33755 Shunt; ascending aorta to pulmonary artery (Waterston type operation)
33762 Shunt; descending aorta to pulmonary artery (Potts-Smith type operation)
33778 Repair of transposition of the great arteries, aortic pulmonary artery reconstruction (eg, Jatene type);
33786 Total repair, truncus arteriosus (Rastelli type operation)
33918 Repair of pulmonary atresia with ventricular septal defect, by unifocalization of pulmonary arteries; without cardiopulmonary bypass
33919 Repair of pulmonary atresia with ventricular septal defect, by unifocalization of pulmonary arteries; with cardiopulmonary bypass
33922 Transection of pulmonary artery with cardiopulmonary bypass
33960 Prolonged extracorporeal circulation for cardiopulmonary insufficiency; initial 24 hours
33961 Prolonged extracorporeal circulation for cardiopulmonary insufficiency; each additional 24 hours (List separately in addition to code for primary procedure)
36415 Collection of venous blood by venipuncture
36420 Venipuncture, cutdown; under age 1 year
36450 Exchange transfusion, blood; newborn
36460 Transfusion, intrauterine, fetal
36510 Catheterization of umbilical vein for diagnosis or therapy, newborn
36660 Catheterization, umbilical artery, newborn, for diagnosis or therapy
39503 Repair, neonatal diaphragmatic hernia, with or without chest tube insertion and with or without creation of ventral hernia
43313 Esophagoplasty for congenital defect (plastic repair or reconstruction), thoracic approach; without repair of congenital tracheoesophageal fistula
43314 Esophagoplasty for congenital defect (plastic repair or reconstruction), thoracic approach; with repair of congenital tracheoesophageal fistula
43520 Pyloromyotomy, cutting of pyloric muscle (Fredet-Ramstedt type operation)
43831 Gastrostomy, open; neonatal, for feeding
44055 Correction of malrotation by lysis of duodenal bands and/or reduction of midgut volvulus (eg, Ladd procedure)
44126 Enterectomy, resection of small intestine for congenital atresia, single resection and anastomosis of proximal segment of intestine; without tapering
44127 Enterectomy, resection of small intestine for congenital atresia, single resection and anastomosis of proximal segment of intestine; with tapering
44128 Enterectomy, resection of small intestine for congenital atresia, single resection and anastomosis of proximal segment of intestine; each additional resection and anastomosis (List separately in addition to code for primary procedure)
46070 Incision, anal septum (infant)
46705 Anoplasty, plastic operation for stricture; infant
46715 Repair of low imperforate anus; with anoperineal fistula (cut-back procedure)
46716 Repair of low imperforate anus; with transposition of anoperineal or anovestibular fistula
46730 Repair of high imperforate anus without fistula; perineal or sacroperineal approach
46735 Repair of high imperforate anus without fistula; combined transabdominal and sacroperineal approaches
46740 Repair of high imperforate anus with rectourethral or rectovaginal fistula; perineal or sacroperineal approach
46742 Repair of high imperforate anus with rectourethral or rectovaginal fistula; combined transabdominal and sacroperineal approaches
46744 Repair of cloacal anomaly by anorectovaginoplasty and urethroplasty, sacroperineal approach
47700 Exploration for congenital atresia of bile ducts, without repair, with or without liver biopsy, with or without cholangiography
47701 Portoenterostomy (eg, Kasai procedure)
49215 Excision of presacral or sacrococcygeal tumor
49491 Repair, initial inguinal hernia, preterm infant (less than 37 weeks gestation at birth), performed from birth up to 50 weeks postconception age, with or without hydrocelectomy; reducible
49492 Repair, initial inguinal hernia, preterm infant (less than 37 weeks gestation at birth), performed from birth up to 50 weeks postconception age, with or without hydrocelectomy; incarcerated or strangulated
49495 Repair, initial inguinal hernia, full term infant under age 6 months, or preterm infant over 50 weeks postconception age and under age 6 months at the time of surgery, with or without hydrocelectomy; reducible
49496 Repair, initial inguinal hernia, full term infant under age 6 months, or preterm infant over 50 weeks postconception age and under age 6 months at the time of surgery, with or without hydrocelectomy; incarcerated or strangulated
49600 Repair of small omphalocele, with primary closure
49605 Repair of large omphalocele or gastroschisis; with or without prosthesis
49606 Repair of large omphalocele or gastroschisis; with removal of prosthesis, final reduction and closure, in operating room
49610 Repair of omphalocele (Gross type operation); first stage
49611 Repair of omphalocele (Gross type operation); second stage
53025 Meatotomy, cutting of meatus (separate procedure); infant
54000 Slitting of prepuce, dorsal or lateral (separate procedure); newborn
54150 Circumcision, using clamp or other device; newborn
54160 Circumcision, surgical excision other than clamp, device or dorsal slit; newborn
63700 Repair of meningocele; less than 5 cm diameter
63702 Repair of meningocele; larger than 5 cm diameter

63704 Repair of myelomeningocele; less than 5 cm diameter
63706 Repair of myelomeningocele; larger than 5 cm diameter
65820 Goniotomy

Conscious Sedation

19298 Placement of radiotherapy afterloading brachytherapy catheters (multiple tube and button type) into the breast for interstitial radioelement application following (at the time of or subsequent to) partial mastectomy, includes imaging guidance
20982 Ablation, bone tumor(s) (eg, osteoid osteoma, metastasis) radiofrequency, percutaneous, including computed tomographic guidance
31615 Tracheobronchoscopy through established tracheostomy incision
31620 Endobronchial ultrasound (EBUS) during bronchoscopic diagnostic or therapeutic intervention(s) (List separately in addition to code for primary procedure(s))
31622 Bronchoscopy, rigid or flexible, with or without fluoroscopic guidance; diagnostic, with or without cell washing (separate procedure)
31623 Bronchoscopy, rigid or flexible, with or without fluoroscopic guidance; with brushing or protected brushings
31624 Bronchoscopy, rigid or flexible, with or without fluoroscopic guidance; with bronchial alveolar lavage
31625 Bronchoscopy, rigid or flexible, with or without fluoroscopic guidance; with bronchial or endobronchial biopsy(s), single or multiple sites
31628 Bronchoscopy, rigid or flexible, with or without fluoroscopic guidance; with transbronchial lung biopsy(s), single lobe
31629 Bronchoscopy, rigid or flexible, with or without fluoroscopic guidance; with transbronchial needle aspiration biopsy(s), trachea, main stem and/or lobar bronchus(i)
31635 Bronchoscopy, rigid or flexible, with or without fluoroscopic guidance; with removal of foreign body
31645 Bronchoscopy, (rigid or flexible); with therapeutic aspiration of tracheobronchial tree, initial (eg, drainage of lung abscess)
31646 Bronchoscopy, (rigid or flexible); with therapeutic aspiration of tracheobronchial tree, subsequent
31656 Bronchoscopy, (rigid or flexible); with injection of contrast material for segmental bronchography (fiberscope only)
31725 Catheter aspiration (separate procedure); tracheobronchial with fiberscope, bedside
32019 Insertion of indwelling tunneled pleural catheter with cuff
32020 Tube thoracostomy with or without water seal (eg, for abscess, hemothorax, empyema) (separate procedure)
32201 Pneumonostomy; with percutaneous drainage of abscess or cyst
33010 Pericardiocentesis; initial
33011 Pericardiocentesis; subsequent
33206 Insertion or replacement of permanent pacemaker with transvenous electrode(s); atrial
33207 Insertion or replacement of permanent pacemaker with transvenous electrode(s); ventricular
33208 Insertion or replacement of permanent pacemaker with transvenous electrode(s); atrial and ventricular
33210 Insertion or replacement of temporary transvenous single chamber cardiac electrode or pacemaker catheter (separate procedure)
33211 Insertion or replacement of temporary transvenous dual chamber pacing electrodes (separate procedure)
33212 Insertion or replacement of pacemaker pulse generator only; single chamber, atrial or ventricular
33213 Insertion or replacement of pacemaker pulse generator only; dual chamber
33214 Upgrade of implanted pacemaker system, conversion of single chamber system to dual chamber system (includes removal of previously placed pulse generator, testing of existing lead, insertion of new lead, insertion of new pulse generator)
33216 Insertion of a transvenous electrode; single chamber (one electrode) permanent pacemaker or single chamber pacing cardioverter-defibrillator
33217 Insertion of a transvenous electrode; dual chamber (two electrodes) permanent pacemaker or dual chamber pacing cardioverter-defibrillator
33218 Repair of single transvenous electrode for a single chamber, permanent pacemaker or single chamber pacing cardioverter-defibrillator
33220 Repair of two transvenous electrodes for a dual chamber permanent pacemaker or dual chamber pacing cardioverter-defibrillator
33222 Revision or relocation of skin pocket for pacemaker
33223 Revision of skin pocket for single or dual chamber pacing cardioverter-defibrillator
33233 Removal of permanent pacemaker pulse generator
33234 Removal of transvenous pacemaker electrode(s); single lead system, atrial or ventricular
33235 Removal of transvenous pacemaker electrode(s); dual lead system
33240 Insertion of single or dual chamber pacing cardioverter-defibrillator pulse generator
33241 Subcutaneous removal of single or dual chamber pacing cardioverter-defibrillator pulse generator
33244 Removal of single or dual chamber pacing cardioverter-defibrillator electrode(s); by transvenous extraction
33249 Insertion or repositioning of electrode lead(s) for single or dual chamber pacing cardioverter-defibrillator and insertion of pulse generator
35470 Transluminal balloon angioplasty, percutaneous; tibioperoneal trunk or branches, each vessel
35471 Transluminal balloon angioplasty, percutaneous; renal or visceral artery
35472 Transluminal balloon angioplasty, percutaneous; aortic
35473 Transluminal balloon angioplasty, percutaneous; iliac
35474 Transluminal balloon angioplasty, percutaneous; femoral-popliteal
35475 Transluminal balloon angioplasty, percutaneous; brachiocephalic trunk or branches, each vessel
35476 Transluminal balloon angioplasty, percutaneous; venous
36555 Insertion of non-tunneled centrally inserted central venous catheter; under 5 years of age
36557 Insertion of tunneled centrally inserted central venous catheter, without subcutaneous port or pump; under 5 years of age
36558 Insertion of tunneled centrally inserted central venous catheter, without subcutaneous port or pump; age 5 years or older
36560 Insertion of tunneled centrally inserted central venous access device, with subcutaneous port; under 5 years of age
36561 Insertion of tunneled centrally inserted central venous access device, with subcutaneous port; age 5 years or older
36563 Insertion of tunneled centrally inserted central venous access device with subcutaneous pump
36565 Insertion of tunneled centrally inserted central venous access device, requiring two catheters via two separate venous access sites; without subcutaneous port or pump (eg, Tesio type catheter)
36566 Insertion of tunneled centrally inserted central venous access device, requiring two catheters via two separate venous access sites; with subcutaneous port(s)
36568 Insertion of peripherally inserted central venous catheter (PICC), without subcutaneous port or pump; under 5 years of age
36570 Insertion of peripherally inserted central venous access device, with subcutaneous port; under 5 years of age
36571 Insertion of peripherally inserted central venous access device, with subcutaneous port; age 5 years or older
36576 Repair of central venous access device, with subcutaneous port or pump, central or peripheral insertion site
36578 Replacement, catheter only, of central venous access device, with subcutaneous port or pump, central or peripheral insertion site
36581 Replacement, complete, of a tunneled centrally inserted central venous catheter, without subcutaneous port or pump, through same venous access
36582 Replacement, complete, of a tunneled centrally inserted central venous access device, with subcutaneous port, through same venous access
36583 Replacement, complete, of a tunneled centrally inserted central venous access device, with subcutaneous pump, through same venous access
36585 Replacement, complete, of a peripherally inserted central venous access device, with subcutaneous port, through same venous access
36590 Removal of tunneled central venous access device, with subcutaneous port or pump, central or peripheral insertion
36870 Thrombectomy, percutaneous, arteriovenous fistula, autogenous or nonautogenous graft (includes mechanical thrombus extraction and intra-graft thrombolysis)
37203 Transcatheter retrieval, percutaneous, of intravascular foreign body (eg, fractured venous or arterial catheter)
37215 Transcatheter placement of intravascular stent(s), cervical carotid artery, percutaneous; with distal embolic protection
37216 Transcatheter placement of intravascular stent(s), cervical carotid artery, percutaneous; without distal embolic protection
43200 Esophagoscopy, rigid or flexible; diagnostic, with or without collection of specimen(s) by brushing or washing (separate procedure)
43201 Esophagoscopy, rigid or flexible; with directed submucosal injection(s), any substance
43202 Esophagoscopy, rigid or flexible; with biopsy, single or multiple
43204 Esophagoscopy, rigid or flexible; with injection sclerosis of esophageal varices
43205 Esophagoscopy, rigid or flexible; with band ligation of esophageal varices
43215 Esophagoscopy, rigid or flexible; with removal of foreign body
43216 Esophagoscopy, rigid or flexible; with removal of tumor(s), polyp(s), or other lesion(s) by hot biopsy forceps or bipolar cautery
43217 Esophagoscopy, rigid or flexible; with removal of tumor(s), polyp(s), or other lesion(s) by snare technique
43219 Esophagoscopy, rigid or flexible; with insertion of plastic tube or stent

43220 Esophagoscopy, rigid or flexible; with balloon dilation (less than 30 mm diameter)
43226 Esophagoscopy, rigid or flexible; with insertion of guide wire followed by dilation over guide wire
43227 Esophagoscopy, rigid or flexible; with control of bleeding (eg, injection, bipolar cautery, unipolar cautery, laser, heater probe, stapler, plasma coagulator)
43228 Esophagoscopy, rigid or flexible; with ablation of tumor(s), polyp(s), or other lesion(s), not amenable to removal by hot biopsy forceps, bipolar cautery or snare technique
43231 Esophagoscopy, rigid or flexible; with endoscopic ultrasound examination
43232 Esophagoscopy, rigid or flexible; with transendoscopic ultrasound-guided intramural or transmural fine needle aspiration/biopsy(s)
43234 Upper gastrointestinal endoscopy, simple primary examination (eg, with small diameter flexible endoscope) (separate procedure)
43235 Upper gastrointestinal endoscopy including esophagus, stomach, and either the duodenum and/or jejunum as appropriate; diagnostic, with or without collection of specimen(s) by brushing or washing (separate procedure)
43236 Upper gastrointestinal endoscopy including esophagus, stomach, and either the duodenum and/or jejunum as appropriate; with directed submucosal injection(s), any substance
43239 Upper gastrointestinal endoscopy including esophagus, stomach, and either the duodenum and/or jejunum as appropriate; with biopsy, single or multiple
43240 Upper gastrointestinal endoscopy including esophagus, stomach, and either the duodenum and/or jejunum as appropriate; with transmural drainage of pseudocyst
43241 Upper gastrointestinal endoscopy including esophagus, stomach, and either the duodenum and/or jejunum as appropriate; with transendoscopic intraluminal tube or catheter placement
43242 Upper gastrointestinal endoscopy including esophagus, stomach, and either the duodenum and/or jejunum as appropriate; with transendoscopic ultrasound-guided intramural or transmural fine needle aspiration/biopsy(s) (includes endoscopic ultrasound examination of the esophagus, stomach, and either the duodenum and/or jejunum as appropriate)
43243 Upper gastrointestinal endoscopy including esophagus, stomach, and either the duodenum and/or jejunum as appropriate; with injection sclerosis of esophageal and/or gastric varices
43244 Upper gastrointestinal endoscopy including esophagus, stomach, and either the duodenum and/or jejunum as appropriate; with band ligation of esophageal and/or gastric varices
43245 Upper gastrointestinal endoscopy including esophagus, stomach, and either the duodenum and/or jejunum as appropriate; with dilation of gastric outlet for obstruction (eg, balloon, guide wire, bougie)
43246 Upper gastrointestinal endoscopy including esophagus, stomach, and either the duodenum and/or jejunum as appropriate; with directed placement of percutaneous gastrostomy tube
43247 Upper gastrointestinal endoscopy including esophagus, stomach, and either the duodenum and/or jejunum as appropriate; with removal of foreign body
43248 Upper gastrointestinal endoscopy including esophagus, stomach, and either the duodenum and/or jejunum as appropriate; with insertion of guide wire followed by dilation of esophagus over guide wire
43249 Upper gastrointestinal endoscopy including esophagus, stomach, and either the duodenum and/or jejunum as appropriate; with balloon dilation of esophagus (less than 30 mm diameter)
43250 Upper gastrointestinal endoscopy including esophagus, stomach, and either the duodenum and/or jejunum as appropriate; with removal of tumor(s), polyp(s), or other lesion(s) by hot biopsy forceps or bipolar cautery
43251 Upper gastrointestinal endoscopy including esophagus, stomach, and either the duodenum and/or jejunum as appropriate; with removal of tumor(s), polyp(s), or other lesion(s) by snare technique
43255 Upper gastrointestinal endoscopy including esophagus, stomach, and either the duodenum and/or jejunum as appropriate; with control of bleeding, any method
43256 Upper gastrointestinal endoscopy including esophagus, stomach, and either the duodenum and/or jejunum as appropriate; with transendoscopic stent placement (includes predilation)
43257 Upper gastrointestinal endoscopy including esophagus, stomach, and either the duodenum and/or jejunum as appropriate; with delivery of thermal energy to the muscle of lower esophageal sphincter and/or gastric cardia, for treatment of gastroesophageal reflux disease
43258 Upper gastrointestinal endoscopy including esophagus, stomach, and either the duodenum and/or jejunum as appropriate; with ablation of tumor(s), polyp(s), or other lesion(s) not amenable to removal by hot biopsy forceps, bipolar cautery or snare technique
43259 Upper gastrointestinal endoscopy including esophagus, stomach, and either the duodenum and/or jejunum as appropriate; with endoscopic ultrasound examination, including the esophagus, stomach, and either the duodenum and/or jejunum as appropriate
43260 Endoscopic retrograde cholangiopancreatography (ERCP); diagnostic, with or without collection of specimen(s) by brushing or washing (separate procedure)
43261 Endoscopic retrograde cholangiopancreatography (ERCP); with biopsy, single or multiple
43262 Endoscopic retrograde cholangiopancreatography (ERCP); with sphincterotomy/papillotomy
43263 Endoscopic retrograde cholangiopancreatography (ERCP); with pressure measurement of sphincter of Oddi (pancreatic duct or common bile duct)
43264 Endoscopic retrograde cholangiopancreatography (ERCP); with endoscopic retrograde removal of calculus/calculi from biliary and/or pancreatic ducts
43265 Endoscopic retrograde cholangiopancreatography (ERCP); with endoscopic retrograde destruction, lithotripsy of calculus/calculi, any method
43267 Endoscopic retrograde cholangiopancreatography (ERCP); with endoscopic retrograde insertion of nasobiliary or nasopancreatic drainage tube
43268 Endoscopic retrograde cholangiopancreatography (ERCP); with endoscopic retrograde insertion of tube or stent into bile or pancreatic duct
43269 Endoscopic retrograde cholangiopancreatography (ERCP); with endoscopic retrograde removal of foreign body and/or change of tube or stent
43271 Endoscopic retrograde cholangiopancreatography (ERCP); with endoscopic retrograde balloon dilation of ampulla, biliary and/or pancreatic duct(s)
43272 Endoscopic retrograde cholangiopancreatography (ERCP); with ablation of tumor(s), polyp(s), or other lesion(s) not amenable to removal by hot biopsy forceps, bipolar cautery or snare technique
43453 Dilation of esophagus, over guide wire
43456 Dilation of esophagus, by balloon or dilator, retrograde
43458 Dilation of esophagus with balloon (30 mm diameter or larger) for achalasia
44360 Small intestinal endoscopy, enteroscopy beyond second portion of duodenum, not including ileum; diagnostic, with or without collection of specimen(s) by brushing or washing (separate procedure)
44361 Small intestinal endoscopy, enteroscopy beyond second portion of duodenum, not including ileum; with biopsy, single or multiple
44363 Small intestinal endoscopy, enteroscopy beyond second portion of duodenum, not including ileum; with removal of foreign body
44364 Small intestinal endoscopy, enteroscopy beyond second portion of duodenum, not including ileum; with removal of tumor(s), polyp(s), or other lesion(s) by snare technique
44365 Small intestinal endoscopy, enteroscopy beyond second portion of duodenum, not including ileum; with removal of tumor(s), polyp(s), or other lesion(s) by hot biopsy forceps or bipolar cautery
44366 Small intestinal endoscopy, enteroscopy beyond second portion of duodenum, not including ileum; with control of bleeding (eg, injection, bipolar cautery, unipolar cautery, laser, heater probe, stapler, plasma coagulator)
44369 Small intestinal endoscopy, enteroscopy beyond second portion of duodenum, not including ileum; with ablation of tumor(s), polyp(s), or other lesion(s) not amenable to removal by hot biopsy forceps, bipolar cautery or snare technique
44370 Small intestinal endoscopy, enteroscopy beyond second portion of duodenum, not including ileum; with transendoscopic stent placement (includes predilation)
44372 Small intestinal endoscopy, enteroscopy beyond second portion of duodenum, not including ileum; with placement of percutaneous jejunostomy tube
44373 Small intestinal endoscopy, enteroscopy beyond second portion of duodenum, not including ileum; with conversion of percutaneous gastrostomy tube to percutaneous jejunostomy tube
44376 Small intestinal endoscopy, enteroscopy beyond second portion of duodenum, including ileum; diagnostic, with or without collection of specimen(s) by brushing or washing (separate procedure)
44377 Small intestinal endoscopy, enteroscopy beyond second portion of duodenum, including ileum; with biopsy, single or multiple
44378 Small intestinal endoscopy, enteroscopy beyond second portion of duodenum, including ileum; with control of bleeding (eg, injection, bipolar cautery, unipolar cautery, laser, heater probe, stapler, plasma coagulator)
44379 Small intestinal endoscopy, enteroscopy beyond second portion of duodenum, including ileum; with transendoscopic stent placement (includes predilation)
44380 Ileoscopy, through stoma; diagnostic, with or without collection of specimen(s) by brushing or washing (separate procedure)
44382 Ileoscopy, through stoma; with biopsy, single or multiple
44383 Ileoscopy, through stoma; with transendoscopic stent placement (includes predilation)
44385 Endoscopic evaluation of small intestinal (abdominal or pelvic) pouch; diagnostic, with or without collection of specimen(s) by brushing or washing (separate procedure)

44386 Endoscopic evaluation of small intestinal (abdominal or pelvic) pouch; with biopsy, single or multiple
44388 Colonoscopy through stoma; diagnostic, with or without collection of specimen(s) by brushing or washing (separate procedure)
44389 Colonoscopy through stoma; with biopsy, single or multiple
44390 Colonoscopy through stoma; with removal of foreign body
44391 Colonoscopy through stoma; with control of bleeding (eg, injection, bipolar cautery, unipolar cautery, laser, heater probe, stapler, plasma coagulator)
44392 Colonoscopy through stoma; with removal of tumor(s), polyp(s), or other lesion(s) by hot biopsy forceps or bipolar cautery
44393 Colonoscopy through stoma; with ablation of tumor(s), polyp(s), or other lesion(s) not amenable to removal by hot biopsy forceps, bipolar cautery or snare technique
44394 Colonoscopy through stoma; with removal of tumor(s), polyp(s), or other lesion(s) by snare technique
44397 Colonoscopy through stoma; with transendoscopic stent placement (includes predilation)
44500 Introduction of long gastrointestinal tube (eg, Miller-Abbott) (separate procedure)
44901 Incision and drainage of appendiceal abscess; percutaneous
45303 Proctosigmoidoscopy, rigid; with dilation (eg, balloon, guide wire, bougie)
45305 Proctosigmoidoscopy, rigid; with biopsy, single or multiple
45307 Proctosigmoidoscopy, rigid; with removal of foreign body
45308 Proctosigmoidoscopy, rigid; with removal of single tumor, polyp, or other lesion by hot biopsy forceps or bipolar cautery
45309 Proctosigmoidoscopy, rigid; with removal of single tumor, polyp, or other lesion by snare technique
45315 Proctosigmoidoscopy, rigid; with removal of multiple tumors, polyps, or other lesions by hot biopsy forceps, bipolar cautery or snare technique
45317 Proctosigmoidoscopy, rigid; with control of bleeding (eg, injection, bipolar cautery, unipolar cautery, laser, heater probe, stapler, plasma coagulator)
45320 Proctosigmoidoscopy, rigid; with ablation of tumor(s), polyp(s), or other lesion(s) not amenable to removal by hot biopsy forceps, bipolar cautery or snare technique (eg, laser)
45327 Proctosigmoidoscopy, rigid; with transendoscopic stent placement (includes predilation)
45332 Sigmoidoscopy, flexible; with removal of foreign body
45333 Sigmoidoscopy, flexible; with removal of tumor(s), polyp(s), or other lesion(s) by hot biopsy forceps or bipolar cautery
45334 Sigmoidoscopy, flexible; with control of bleeding (eg, injection, bipolar cautery, unipolar cautery, laser, heater probe, stapler, plasma coagulator)
45337 Sigmoidoscopy, flexible; with decompression of volvulus, any method
45338 Sigmoidoscopy, flexible; with removal of tumor(s), polyp(s), or other lesion(s) by snare technique
45339 Sigmoidoscopy, flexible; with ablation of tumor(s), polyp(s), or other lesion(s) not amenable to removal by hot biopsy forceps, bipolar cautery or snare technique
45340 Sigmoidoscopy, flexible; with dilation by balloon, 1 or more strictures
45341 Sigmoidoscopy, flexible; with endoscopic ultrasound examination
45342 Sigmoidoscopy, flexible; with transendoscopic ultrasound guided intramural or transmural fine needle aspiration/biopsy(s)
45345 Sigmoidoscopy, flexible; with transendoscopic stent placement (includes predilation)
45355 Colonoscopy, rigid or flexible, transabdominal via colotomy, single or multiple
45378 Colonoscopy, flexible, proximal to splenic flexure; diagnostic, with or without collection of specimen(s) by brushing or washing, with or without colon decompression (separate procedure)
45379 Colonoscopy, flexible, proximal to splenic flexure; with removal of foreign body
45380 Colonoscopy, flexible, proximal to splenic flexure; with biopsy, single or multiple
45381 Colonoscopy, flexible, proximal to splenic flexure; with directed submucosal injection(s), any substance
45382 Colonoscopy, flexible, proximal to splenic flexure; with control of bleeding (eg, injection, bipolar cautery, unipolar cautery, laser, heater probe, stapler, plasma coagulator)
45383 Colonoscopy, flexible, proximal to splenic flexure; with ablation of tumor(s), polyp(s), or other lesion(s) not amenable to removal by hot biopsy forceps, bipolar cautery or snare technique
45384 Colonoscopy, flexible, proximal to splenic flexure; with removal of tumor(s), polyp(s), or other lesion(s) by hot biopsy forceps or bipolar cautery
45385 Colonoscopy, flexible, proximal to splenic flexure; with removal of tumor(s), polyp(s), or other lesion(s) by snare technique
45386 Colonoscopy, flexible, proximal to splenic flexure; with dilation by balloon, 1 or more strictures
45387 Colonoscopy, flexible, proximal to splenic flexure; with transendoscopic stent placement (includes predilation)
45391 Colonoscopy, flexible, proximal to splenic flexure; with endoscopic ultrasound examination
45392 Colonoscopy, flexible, proximal to splenic flexure; with transendoscopic ultrasound guided intramural or transmural fine needle aspiration/biopsy(s)
47011 Hepatotomy; for percutaneous drainage of abscess or cyst, one or two stages
48511 External drainage, pseudocyst of pancreas; percutaneous
49021 Drainage of peritoneal abscess or localized peritonitis, exclusive of appendiceal abscess; percutaneous
49041 Drainage of subdiaphragmatic or subphrenic abscess; percutaneous
49061 Drainage of retroperitoneal abscess; percutaneous
50021 Drainage of perirenal or renal abscess; percutaneous
58823 Drainage of pelvic abscess, transvaginal or transrectal approach, percutaneous (eg, ovarian, pericolic)
66720 Ciliary body destruction; cryotherapy
77600 Hyperthermia, externally generated; superficial (ie, heating to a depth of 4 cm or less)
77605 Hyperthermia, externally generated; deep (ie, heating to depths greater than 4 cm)
77610 Hyperthermia generated by interstitial probe(s); 5 or fewer interstitial applicators
77615 Hyperthermia generated by interstitial probe(s); more than 5 interstitial applicators
92953 Temporary transcutaneous pacing
92960 Cardioversion, elective, electrical conversion of arrhythmia; external
92961 Cardioversion, elective, electrical conversion of arrhythmia; internal (separate procedure)
92973 Percutaneous transluminal coronary thrombectomy (List separately in addition to code for primary procedure)
92974 Transcatheter placement of radiation delivery device for subsequent coronary intravascular brachytherapy (List separately in addition to code for primary procedure)
92975 Thrombolysis, coronary; by intracoronary infusion, including selective coronary angiography
92978 Intravascular ultrasound (coronary vessel or graft) during diagnostic evaluation and/or therapeutic intervention including imaging supervision, interpretation and report; initial vessel (List separately in addition to code for primary procedure)
92979 Intravascular ultrasound (coronary vessel or graft) during diagnostic evaluation and/or therapeutic intervention including imaging supervision, interpretation and report; each additional vessel (List separately in addition to code for primary procedure)
92980 Transcatheter placement of an intracoronary stent(s), percutaneous, with or without other therapeutic intervention, any method; single vessel
92981 Transcatheter placement of an intracoronary stent(s), percutaneous, with or without other therapeutic intervention, any method; each additional vessel (List separately in addition to code for primary procedure)
92982 Percutaneous transluminal coronary balloon angioplasty; single vessel
92984 Percutaneous transluminal coronary balloon angioplasty; each additional vessel (List separately in addition to code for primary procedure)
92986 Percutaneous balloon valvuloplasty; aortic valve
92987 Percutaneous balloon valvuloplasty; mitral valve
92995 Percutaneous transluminal coronary atherectomy, by mechanical or other method, with or without balloon angioplasty; single vessel
92996 Percutaneous transluminal coronary atherectomy, by mechanical or other method, with or without balloon angioplasty; each additional vessel (List separately in addition to code for primary procedure)
93312 Echocardiography, transesophageal, real time with image documentation (2D) (with or without M-mode recording); including probe placement, image acquisition, interpretation and report
93313 Echocardiography, transesophageal, real time with image documentation (2D) (with or without M-mode recording); placement of transesophageal probe only
93314 Echocardiography, transesophageal, real time with image documentation (2D) (with or without M-mode recording); image acquisition, interpretation and report only
93315 Transesophageal echocardiography for congenital cardiac anomalies; including probe placement, image acquisition, interpretation and report
93316 Transesophageal echocardiography for congenital cardiac anomalies; placement of transesophageal probe only
93317 Transesophageal echocardiography for congenital cardiac anomalies; image acquisition, interpretation and report only
93318 Echocardiography, transesophageal (TEE) for monitoring purposes, including probe placement, real time 2-dimensional image acquisition and interpretation leading to ongoing (continuous) assessment of (dynamically changing) cardiac pumping function and to therapeutic measures on an immediate time basis
93501 Right heart catheterization
93505 Endomyocardial biopsy

93508 Catheter placement in coronary artery(s), arterial coronary conduit(s), and/or venous coronary bypass graft(s) for coronary angiography without concomitant left heart catheterization
93510 Left heart catheterization, retrograde, from the brachial artery, axillary artery or femoral artery; percutaneous
93511 Left heart catheterization, retrograde, from the brachial artery, axillary artery or femoral artery; by cutdown
93514 Left heart catheterization by left ventricular puncture
93524 Combined transseptal and retrograde left heart catheterization
93526 Combined right heart catheterization and retrograde left heart catheterization
93527 Combined right heart catheterization and transseptal left heart catheterization through intact septum (with or without retrograde left heart catheterization)
93528 Combined right heart catheterization with left ventricular puncture (with or without retrograde left heart catheterization)
93529 Combined right heart catheterization and left heart catheterization through existing septal opening (with or without retrograde left heart catheterization)
93530 Right heart catheterization, for congenital cardiac anomalies
93539 Injection procedure during cardiac catheterization; for selective opacification of arterial conduits (eg, internal mammary), whether native or used for bypass
93540 Injection procedure during cardiac catheterization; for selective opacification of aortocoronary venous bypass grafts, one or more coronary arteries
93541 Injection procedure during cardiac catheterization; for pulmonary angiography
93542 Injection procedure during cardiac catheterization; for selective right ventricular or right atrial angiography
93543 Injection procedure during cardiac catheterization; for selective left ventricular or left atrial angiography
93544 Injection procedure during cardiac catheterization; for aortography
93545 Injection procedure during cardiac catheterization; for selective coronary angiography (injection of radiopaque material may be by hand)
93555 Imaging supervision, interpretation and report for injection procedure(s) during cardiac catheterization; ventricular and/or atrial angiography
93556 Imaging supervision, interpretation and report for injection procedure(s) during cardiac catheterization; pulmonary angiography, aortography, and/or selective coronary angiography including venous bypass grafts and arterial conduits (whether native or used in bypass)
93561 Indicator dilution studies such as dye or thermal dilution, including arterial and/or venous catheterization; with cardiac output measurement (separate procedure)
93562 Indicator dilution studies such as dye or thermal dilution, including arterial and/or venous catheterization; subsequent measurement of cardiac output
93571 Intravascular Doppler velocity and/or pressure derived coronary flow reserve measurement (coronary vessel or graft) during coronary angiography including pharmacologically induced stress; initial vessel (List separately in addition to code for primary procedure)
93572 Intravascular Doppler velocity and/or pressure derived coronary flow reserve measurement (coronary vessel or graft) during coronary angiography including pharmacologically induced stress; each additional vessel (List separately in addition to code for primary procedure)
93609 Intraventricular and/or intra-atrial mapping of tachycardia site(s) with catheter manipulation to record from multiple sites to identify origin of tachycardia (List separately in addition to code for primary procedure)
93613 Intracardiac electrophysiologic 3-dimensional mapping (List separately in addition to code for primary procedure)
93615 Esophageal recording of atrial electrogram with or without ventricular electrogram(s);
93616 Esophageal recording of atrial electrogram with or without ventricular electrogram(s); with pacing
93618 Induction of arrhythmia by electrical pacing
93619 Comprehensive electrophysiologic evaluation with right atrial pacing and recording, right ventricular pacing and recording, His bundle recording, including insertion and repositioning of multiple electrode catheters, without induction or attempted induction of arrhythmia
93620 Comprehensive electrophysiologic evaluation including insertion and repositioning of multiple electrode catheters with induction or attempted induction of arrhythmia; with right atrial pacing and recording, right ventricular pacing and recording, His bundle recording
93621 Comprehensive electrophysiologic evaluation including insertion and repositioning of multiple electrode catheters with induction or attempted induction of arrhythmia; with left atrial pacing and recording from coronary sinus or left atrium (List separately in addition to code for primary procedure)
93622 Comprehensive electrophysiologic evaluation including insertion and repositioning of multiple electrode catheters with induction or attempted induction of arrhythmia; with left ventricular pacing and recording (List separately in addition to code for primary procedure)
93624 Electrophysiologic follow-up study with pacing and recording to test effectiveness of therapy, including induction or attempted induction of arrhythmia
93640 Electrophysiologic evaluation of single or dual chamber pacing cardioverter-defibrillator leads including defibrillation threshold evaluation (induction of arrhythmia, evaluation of sensing and pacing for arrhythmia termination) at time of initial implantation or replacement;
93641 Electrophysiologic evaluation of single or dual chamber pacing cardioverter-defibrillator leads including defibrillation threshold evaluation (induction of arrhythmia, evaluation of sensing and pacing for arrhythmia termination) at time of initial implantation or replacement; with testing of single or dual chamber pacing cardioverter-defibrillator pulse generator
93642 Electrophysiologic evaluation of single or dual chamber pacing cardioverter-defibrillator (includes defibrillation threshold evaluation, induction of arrhythmia, evaluation of sensing and pacing for arrhythmia termination, and programming or reprogramming of sensing or therapeutic parameters)
93650 Intracardiac catheter ablation of atrioventricular node function, atrioventricular conduction for creation of complete heart block, with or without temporary pacemaker placement
93651 Intracardiac catheter ablation of arrhythmogenic focus; for treatment of supraventricular tachycardia by ablation of fast or slow atrioventricular pathways, accessory atrioventricular connections or other atrial foci, singly or in combination
93652 Intracardiac catheter ablation of arrhythmogenic focus; for treatment of ventricular tachycardia

Appendix B

Unlisted Codes

01999 Unlisted anesthesia procedure(s)
15999 Unlisted procedure, excision pressure ulcer
17999 Unlisted procedure, skin, mucous membrane and subcutaneous tissue
19499 Unlisted procedure, breast
20999 Unlisted procedure, musculoskeletal system, general
21089 Unlisted maxillofacial prosthetic procedure
21299 Unlisted craniofacial and maxillofacial procedure
21499 Unlisted musculoskeletal procedure, head
21899 Unlisted procedure, neck or thorax
22899 Unlisted procedure, spine
22999 Unlisted procedure, abdomen, musculoskeletal system
23929 Unlisted procedure, shoulder
24999 Unlisted procedure, humerus or elbow
25999 Unlisted procedure, forearm or wrist
26989 Unlisted procedure, hands or fingers
27299 Unlisted procedure, pelvis or hip joint
27599 Unlisted procedure, femur or knee
27899 Unlisted procedure, leg or ankle
28899 Unlisted procedure, foot or toes
29799 Unlisted procedure, casting or strapping
29999 Unlisted procedure, arthroscopy
30999 Unlisted procedure, nose
31299 Unlisted procedure, accessory sinuses
31599 Unlisted procedure, larynx
31899 Unlisted procedure, trachea, bronchi
32999 Unlisted procedure, lungs and pleura
33999 Unlisted procedure, cardiac surgery
36299 Unlisted procedure, vascular injection
37501 Unlisted vascular endoscopy procedure
37799 Unlisted procedure, vascular surgery
38129 Unlisted laparoscopy procedure, spleen
38589 Unlisted laparoscopy procedure, lymphatic system
38999 Unlisted procedure, hemic or lymphatic system
39499 Unlisted procedure, mediastinum
39599 Unlisted procedure, diaphragm
40799 Unlisted procedure, lips
40899 Unlisted procedure, vestibule of mouth
41599 Unlisted procedure, tongue, floor of mouth
41899 Unlisted procedure, dentoalveolar structures
42299 Unlisted procedure, palate, uvula
42699 Unlisted procedure, salivary glands or ducts
42999 Unlisted procedure, pharynx, adenoids, or tonsils
43289 Unlisted laparoscopy procedure, esophagus
43499 Unlisted procedure, esophagus
43659 Unlisted laparoscopy procedure, stomach
43999 Unlisted procedure, stomach
44238 Unlisted laparoscopy procedure, intestine (except rectum)
44239 Unlisted laparoscopy procedure, rectum
44799 Unlisted procedure, intestine
44899 Unlisted procedure, Meckel's diverticulum and the mesentery
44979 Unlisted laparoscopy procedure, appendix
45999 Unlisted procedure, rectum
46999 Unlisted procedure, anus
47379 Unlisted laparoscopic procedure, liver
47399 Unlisted procedure, liver
47579 Unlisted laparoscopy procedure, biliary tract
47999 Unlisted procedure, biliary tract
48999 Unlisted procedure, pancreas
49329 Unlisted laparoscopy procedure, abdomen, peritoneum and omentum
49659 Unlisted laparoscopy procedure, hernioplasty, herniorrhaphy, herniotomy
49999 Unlisted procedure, abdomen, peritoneum and omentum
50549 Unlisted laparoscopy procedure, renal
50949 Unlisted laparoscopy procedure, ureter
53899 Unlisted procedure, urinary system
54699 Unlisted laparoscopy procedure, testis
55559 Unlisted laparoscopy procedure, spermatic cord
55899 Unlisted procedure, male genital system
58578 Unlisted laparoscopy procedure, uterus
58579 Unlisted hysteroscopy procedure, uterus
58679 Unlisted laparoscopy procedure, oviduct, ovary
58999 Unlisted procedure, female genital system (nonobstetrical)
59897 Unlisted fetal invasive procedure, including ultrasound guidance
59898 Unlisted laparoscopy procedure, maternity care and delivery
59899 Unlisted procedure, maternity care and delivery
60659 Unlisted laparoscopy procedure, endocrine system
60699 Unlisted procedure, endocrine system
64999 Unlisted procedure, nervous system
66999 Unlisted procedure, anterior segment of eye
67299 Unlisted procedure, posterior segment
67399 Unlisted procedure, ocular muscle
67599 Unlisted procedure, orbit
67999 Unlisted procedure, eyelids
68399 Unlisted procedure, conjunctiva
68899 Unlisted procedure, lacrimal system
69399 Unlisted procedure, external ear
69799 Unlisted procedure, middle ear
69949 Unlisted procedure, inner ear
69979 Unlisted procedure, temporal bone, middle fossa approach
76496 Unlisted fluoroscopic procedure (eg, diagnostic, interventional)
76497 Unlisted computed tomography procedure (eg, diagnostic, interventional)
76498 Unlisted magnetic resonance procedure (eg, diagnostic, interventional)
76499 Unlisted diagnostic radiographic procedure
76999 Unlisted ultrasound procedure (eg, diagnostic, interventional)
77299 Unlisted procedure, therapeutic radiology clinical treatment planning
77399 Unlisted procedure, medical radiation physics, dosimetry and treatment devices, and special services
77499 Unlisted procedure, therapeutic radiology treatment management
77799 Unlisted procedure, clinical brachytherapy
78099 Unlisted endocrine procedure, diagnostic nuclear medicine
78199 Unlisted hematopoietic, reticuloendothelial and lymphatic procedure, diagnostic nuclear medicine
78299 Unlisted gastrointestinal procedure, diagnostic nuclear medicine
78399 Unlisted musculoskeletal procedure, diagnostic nuclear medicine
78499 Unlisted cardiovascular procedure, diagnostic nuclear medicine
78599 Unlisted respiratory procedure, diagnostic nuclear medicine
78699 Unlisted nervous system procedure, diagnostic nuclear medicine
78799 Unlisted genitourinary procedure, diagnostic nuclear medicine
78999 Unlisted miscellaneous procedure, diagnostic nuclear medicine
79999 Radiopharmaceutical therapy, unlisted procedure
81099 Unlisted urinalysis procedure
84999 Unlisted chemistry procedure
85999 Unlisted hematology and coagulation procedure
86586 Unlisted antigen, each
86849 Unlisted immunology procedure
86999 Unlisted transfusion medicine procedure
87999 Unlisted microbiology procedure
88099 Unlisted necropsy (autopsy) procedure
88199 Unlisted cytopathology procedure
88299 Unlisted cytogenetic study
88399 Unlisted surgical pathology procedure
89240 Unlisted miscellaneous pathology test
90399 Unlisted immune globulin
90749 Unlisted vaccine/toxoid
90799 Unlisted therapeutic, prophylactic or diagnostic injection
90899 Unlisted psychiatric service or procedure
90999 Unlisted dialysis procedure, inpatient or outpatient
91299 Unlisted diagnostic gastroenterology procedure
92499 Unlisted ophthalmological service or procedure
92700 Unlisted otorhinolaryngological service or procedure
93799 Unlisted cardiovascular service or procedure
94799 Unlisted pulmonary service or procedure
95199 Unlisted allergy/clinical immunologic service or procedure

95999	Unlisted neurological or neuromuscular diagnostic procedure
96549	Unlisted chemotherapy procedure
96999	Unlisted special dermatological service or procedure
97039	Unlisted modality (specify type and time if constant attendance)
97139	Unlisted therapeutic procedure (specify)
97799	Unlisted physical medicine/rehabilitation service or procedure
99199	Unlisted special service, procedure or report
99429	Unlisted preventive medicine service
99499	Unlisted evaluation and management service
99600	Unlisted home visit service or procedure

Appendix C

CPT Modifiers

This list includes all of the modifiers applicable to CPT codes.

21 **Prolonged Evaluation and Management Services:** When the face-to-face or floor/unit service(s) provided is prolonged or otherwise greater than that usually required for the highest level of evaluation and management service within a given category, it may be identified by adding modifier 21 to the evaluation and management code number. A report may also be appropriate.

22 **Unusual Procedural Services:** When the service(s) provided is greater than that usually required for the listed procedure, it may be identified by adding modifier 22 to the usual procedure number. A report may also be appropriate.

23 **Unusual Anesthesia:** Occasionally, a procedure, which usually requires either no anesthesia or local anesthesia, because of unusual circumstances must be done under general anesthesia. This circumstance may be reported by adding modifier 23 to the procedure code of the basic service.

24 **Unrelated Evaluation and Management Service by the Same Physician During a Postoperative Period:** The physician may need to indicate that an evaluation and management service was performed during a postoperative period for a reason(s) unrelated to the original procedure. This circumstance may be reported by adding modifier 24 to the appropriate level of E/M service.

25 **Significant, Separately Identifiable Evaluation and Management Service by the Same Physician on the Same Day of the Procedure or Other Service:** The physician may need to indicate that on the day a procedure or service identified by a CPT code was performed, the patients condition required a significant, separately identifiable E/M service above and beyond the other service provided or beyond the usual preoperative and postoperative care associated with the procedure that was performed. The E/M service may be prompted by the symptom or condition for which the procedure and/or service was provided. As such, different diagnoses are not required for reporting of the E/M services on the same date. This circumstance may be reported by adding modifier 25 to the appropriate level of E/M service. Note: This modifier is not used to report an E/M service that resulted in a decision to perform surgery. See modifier 57.

26 **Professional Component:** Certain procedures are a combination of a physician component and a technical component. When the physician component is reported separately, the service may be identified by adding modifier 26 to the usual procedure number.

32 **Mandated Services:** Services related to mandated consultation and/or related services (eg, PRO, third party payer, governmental, legislative, or regulatory requirement) may be identified by adding modifier 32 to the basic procedure.

47 **Anesthesia by Surgeon:** Regional or general anesthesia provided by the surgeon may be reported by adding modifier 47 to the basic service. (This does not include local anesthesia.) Note: Modifier 47 would not be used as a modifier for the anesthesia procedures 00100-01999.

50 **Bilateral Procedure:** Unless otherwise identified in the listings, bilateral procedures that are performed at the same operative session should be identified by adding modifier 50 to the appropriate five digit code.

51 **Multiple Procedures:** When multiple procedures, other than Evaluation and Management Services, are performed at the same session by the same provider, the primary procedure or service may be reported as listed. The additional procedure(s) or service(s) may be identified by appending modifier 51 to the additional procedure or service code(s). Note: This modifier should not be appended to designated "add-on" codes.

52 **Reduced Services:** Under certain circumstances a service or procedure is partially reduced or eliminated at the physicians discretion. Under these circumstances the service provided can be identified by its usual procedure number and the addition of modifier 52, signifying that the service is reduced. This provides a means of reporting reduced services without disturbing the identification of the basic service. Note: For hospital outpatient reporting of a previously scheduled procedure/service that is partially reduced or cancelled as a result of extenuating circumstances or those that threaten the well-being of the patient prior to or after administration of anesthesia, see modifiers 73 and 74 (see modifiers approved for ASC hospital outpatient use).

53 **Discontinued Procedure:** Under certain circumstances, the physician may elect to terminate a surgical or

diagnostic procedure. Due to extenuating circumstances or those that threaten the well being of the patient, it may be necessary to indicate that a surgical or diagnostic procedure was started but discontinued. This circumstance may be reported by adding modifier 53 to the code reported by the physician for the discontinued procedure. Note: This modifier is not used to report the elective cancellation of a procedure prior to the patients anesthesia induction and/or surgical preparation in the operating suite. For outpatient hospital/ambulatory surgery center (ASC) reporting of a previously scheduled procedure/service that is partially reduced or cancelled as a result of extenuating circumstances or those that threaten the well being of the patient prior to or after administration of anesthesia, see modifiers 73 and 74 (see modifiers approved for ASC hospital outpatient use).

54 **Surgical Care Only:** When one physician performs a surgical procedure and another provides preoperative and/or postoperative management, surgical services may be identified by adding modifier 54 to the usual procedure number.

55 **Postoperative Management Only:** When one physician performs the postoperative management and another physician has performed the surgical procedure, the postoperative component may be identified by adding modifier 55 to the usual procedure number.

56 **Preoperative Management Only:** When one physician performs the preoperative care and evaluation and another physician performs the surgical procedure, the preoperative component may be identified by adding modifier 56 to the usual procedure number.

57 **Decision for Surgery:** An evaluation and management service that resulted in the initial decision to perform the surgery may be identified by adding modifier 57 to the appropriate level of E/M service.

58 **Staged or Related Procedure or Service by the Same Physician During the Postoperative Period:** The physician may need to indicate that the performance of a procedure or service during the postoperative period was: a) planned prospectively at the time of the original procedure (staged); b) more extensive than the original procedure; or c) for therapy following a diagnostic surgical procedure. This circumstance may be reported by adding modifier 58 to the staged or related procedure. Note: This modifier is not used to report the treatment of a problem that requires a return to the operating room. See modifier 78.

59 **Distinct Procedural Service:** Under certain circumstances, the physician may need to indicate that a procedure or service was distinct or independent from other services performed on the same day. Modifier 59 is used to identify procedures/services that are not normally reported together, but are appropriate under the circumstances. This may represent a different session or patient encounter, different procedure or surgery, different site or organ system, separate incision/excision, separate lesion, or separate injury (or area of injury in extensive injuries) not ordinarily encountered or performed on the same day by the same physician. However, when another already established modifier is appropriate it should be used rather than modifier 59. Only if no more descriptive modifier is available, and the use of modifier 59 best explains the circumstances, should modifier 59 be used.

62 **Two Surgeons:** When two surgeons work together as primary surgeons performing distinct part(s) of a procedure, each surgeon should report his/her distinct operative work by adding modifier 62 to the procedure code and any associated add-on code(s) for that procedure as long as both surgeons continue to work together as primary surgeons. Each surgeon should report the co-surgery once using the same procedure code. If an additional procedure(s) (including an add-on procedure(s)) is performed during the same surgical session, a separate code(s) may be reported with the modifier 62 added. Note: If a co-surgeon acts as an assistant in the performance of an additional procedure(s) during the same surgical session, the service(s) may be reported using a separate procedure code(s) with modifier 80 or modifier 82 added, as appropriate.

63 **Procedure Performed on Infants less than 4 kg:** Procedures performed on neonates and infants up to a present body weight of 4 kg may involve significantly increased complexity and physician work commonly associated with these patients. This circumstance may be reported by adding the modifier 63 to the procedure number. Note: Unless otherwise designated, this modifier may only be appended to procedures/services listed in the 20000-69999 code series. Modifier 63 should not be appended to any CPT codes in the E/M, Anesthesia, Radiology, Pathology/Laboratory or Medicine sections.

66 **Surgical Team:** Under some circumstances, highly complex procedures (requiring the concomitant services of several physicians, often of different specialties, plus other highly skilled, specially trained personnel, various types of complex equipment) are carried out under the "surgical team" concept. Such circumstances may be identified by each participating physician with the addition of modifier 66 to the basic procedure number used for reporting services.

76 **Repeat Procedure by Same Physician:** The physician may need to indicate that a procedure or service was repeated subsequent to the original procedure or service. This circumstance may be reported by adding

modifier 76 to the repeated procedure/service.

77 **Repeat Procedure by Another Physician:** The physician may need to indicate that a basic procedure or service performed by another physician had to be repeated. This situation may be reported by adding modifier 77 to the repeated procedure/service.

78 **Return to the Operating Room for a Related Procedure During the Postoperative Period:** The physician may need to indicate that another procedure was performed during the postoperative period of the initial procedure. When this subsequent procedure is related to the first, and requires the use of the operating room, it may be reported by adding modifier 78 to the related procedure. (For repeat procedures on the same day, see modifier 76.)

79 **Unrelated Procedure or Service by the Same Physician During the Postoperative Period:** The physician may need to indicate that the performance of a procedure or service during the postoperative period was unrelated to the original procedure. This circumstance may be reported by using modifier 79. (For repeat procedures on the same day, see modifier 76.)

80 **Assistant Surgeon:** Surgical assistant services may be identified by adding modifier 80 to the usual procedure number(s).

81 **Minimum Assistant Surgeon:** Minimum surgical assistant services are identified by adding modifier 81 to the usual procedure number.

82 **Assistant Surgeon (when qualified resident surgeon not available):** The unavailability of a qualified resident surgeon is a prerequisite for use of modifier 82 appended to the usual procedure code number(s).

90 **Reference (Outside) Laboratory:** When laboratory procedures are performed by a party other than the treating or reporting physician, the procedure may be identified by adding modifier 90 to the usual procedure number.

91 **Repeat Clinical Diagnostic Laboratory Test:** In the course of treatment of the patient, it may be necessary to repeat the same laboratory test on the same day to obtain subsequent (multiple) test results. Under these circumstances, the laboratory test performed can be identified by its usual procedure number and the addition of modifier 91. Note: This modifier may not be used when tests are rerun to confirm initial results; due to testing problems with specimens or equipment; or for any other reason when a normal, one-time, reportable result is all that is required. This modifier may not be used when another code(s) describes a series of test results (eg, glucose tolerance tests, evocative/suppression testing). This modifier may only be used for a laboratory test(s) performed more than once on the same day on the same patient.

99 **Multiple Modifiers:** Under certain circumstances two or more modifiers may be necessary to completely delineate a service. In such situations, modifier 99 should be added to the basic procedure and other applicable modifiers may be listed as part of the description of the service.

Level II (HCPCS/National) Modifiers

Anatomical Modifiers

E1 Upper left, eyelid

E2 Lower left, eyelid

E3 Upper right, eyelid

E4 Lower right, eyelid

F1 Left hand, second digit

F2 Left hand, third digit

F3 Left hand, fourth digit

F4 Left hand, fifth digit

F5 Right hand, thumb

F6 Right hand, second digit

F7 Right hand, third digit

F8 Right hand, fourth digit

F9 Right hand, fifth digit

FA Left hand, thumb

LT Left side (used to identify procedures performed on the left side of the body)

RT Right side (used to identify procedures performed on the right side of the body)

T1 Left foot, second digit

T2 Left foot, third digit

T3 Left foot, fourth digit

T4 Left foot, fifth digit

T5 Right foot, great toe

T6 Right foot, second digit

T7 Right foot, third digit

T8 Right foot, fourth digit

T9 Right foot, fifth digit

TA Left foot, great toe

Ambulance Modifiers

GM Multiple patients on one ambulance trip

QM Ambulance service provided under arrangement by a provider of services

QN Ambulance service furnished directly by a provider of services

QL Patient pronounced dead after ambulance called

Anesthesia Modifiers

AA Anesthesia services performed personally by anesthesiologist

AD Medical supervision by a physician: more than four concurrent anesthesia procedures

G8 Monitored anesthesia care (MAC) for deep complex, complicated, or markedly invasive surgical procedure

G9 Monitored anesthesia care for patient who has history of severe cardio-pulmonary condition

QK Medical direction of two, three, or four concurrent anesthesia procedures involving qualified individuals

QS Monitored anesthesia care service

QY Medical direction of one certified registered nurse anesthetist (CRNA) by an anesthesiologist

QZ CRNA service: without medical direction by a physician

Coronary Artery Modifiers

LC Left circumflex coronary artery (Hospitals use with codes 92980-92984, 92995, 92996)

LD Left anterior descending coronary artery (Hospitals use with codes 92980-92984, 92995, 92996)

RC Right coronary artery (Hospitals use with codes 92980-92984, 92995, 92996)

Ophthalmology Modifiers

AP Determination of refractive state was not performed in the course of diagnostic ophthalmological examination

LS FDA-monitored intraocular lens implant

PL Progressive addition lenses

VP Aphakic patient

Professional Services

AH Clinical psychologist

AJ Clinical social worker

AM Physician, team member service

AS Physician assistant, nurse practitioner, or clinical nurse specialist services for assistant at surgery

AT Acute treatment (this modifier should be used when reporting service 98940, 98941, 98942)

CA Procedure payable only in the inpatient setting when performed emergently on an outpatient who expires prior to admission

CB Service ordered by a renal dialysis facility (RDF) physician as part of the esrd beneficiarys dialysis benefit, is not part of the composite rate, and is separately reimbursable

CC Procedure code change (use CC when the procedure code submitted was changed either for administrative reasons or because an incorrect code was filed)

EP Service provided as part of medicaid early periodic screening diagnosis and treatment (EPSDT) program

ET Emergency services

G7 Pregnancy resulted from rape or incest or pregnancy certified by physician as life threatening

GA Waiver of liability statement on file

GB Claim being resubmitted for payment because it is no longer covered under a global payment demonstration

GC This service has been performed in part by a resident under the direction of a teaching physician

GE This service has been performed by a resident without the presence of a teaching physician under the primary care exception

GF Non-physician (e.g. nurse practitioner (NP), certified registered nurse anaesthetist (CRNA), certified registered nurse (CRN), clinical nurse specialist (CNS), physician assistant (PA)) services in a critical access hospital

GG Performance and payment of a screening mammogram and diagnostic mammogram on the same patient, same day

GH Diagnostic mammogram converted from screening mammogram on same day

GJ "OPT OUT" physician or practitioner emergency or urgent service

GK Actual item/service ordered byphysician, item associated with GA or GZ modifier

GL Medically unnecessary upgrade provided instead of standard item, no charge, no advance beneficiary notice (ABN)

GN Service delivered personally by a speech-language pathologist or under an outpatient speech-language pathology plan of care

GO Service delivered personally by an occupational therapist or under an outpatient occupational therapy plan of care

GP Service delivered personally by a physical therapist or under an outpatient physical therapy plan of care

GQ Via asynchronous telecommunications system

GT Via interactive audio and video telecommunication systems

GV Attending physician not employed or paid under arrangement by the patients hospice provider

GW Service not related to the hospice patients terminal condition

GY Item or service statutorily excluded or does not meet the definition of any medicare benefit

GZ Item or service expected to be denied as not reasonable and necessary

H9 Court-ordered

HA Child/adolescent program

HB Adult program, non geriatric

HC Adult program, geriatric

HD Pregnant/parenting womens program

HE Mental health program

HF Substance abuse program

HG Opioid addiction treatment program

HH Integrated mental health/substance abuse program

HI Integrated mental health and mental retardation/developmental disabilities program

HJ Employee assistance program

HK Specialized mental health programs for high-risk populations

HL Intern

HM Less than bachelor degree level

HN Bachelors degree level

HO Masters degree level

HP Doctoral level

HQ Group setting

HR Family/couple with client present

HS Family/couple without client present

HT Multi-disciplinary team

HU Funded by child welfare agency

HV Funded state addictions agency

HW Funded by state mental health agency

HX Funded by county/local agency

HY Funded by juvenile justice agency

HZ Funded by criminal justice agency

KB Beneficiary requested upgrade for ABN, more than four modifiers identified on claim

KX Specific required documentation on file

KZ New coverage not implemented by managed care

Q4 Service for ordering/referring physician qualifies as a service exemption

Q5 Service furnished by a substitute physician under a reciprocal billing arrangement

Q6 Service furnished by a locum tenens physician

QB Physician providing service in a rural HPSA

QJ Services/items provided to a prisoner or patient in state or local custody, however the state or local government, as applicable, meets the requirements in 42 cfr 411.4 (b)

QP Documentation is on file showing that the laboratory test(s) was ordered individually or ordered as a CPT-recognized panel other than automated profile codes 80002-80019, G0058, G0059, and G0060

QQ Claim submitted with a written statement of intent

QR Repeat laboratory test performed on the same day

QS Monitored anesthesia care service

QV Item or service provided as routine care in a Medicare qualifying clinical trial

QW CLIA waived test

QX CRNA service: with medical direction by a physician

QY Medical direction of one certified registered nurse anesthetist (CRNA) by an anesthesiologist

QZ CRNA service: without medical direction by a physician

SA Nurse practitioner rendering service in collaboration with a physician

SB Nurse Midwife

SC Medically necessary service or supply

SD Services provided by registered nurse with specialized, highly technical home infusion training

SE State and/or federally funded programs/services

SG Ambulatory surgical center (ASC) facility service

SH Second concurrently administered infusion therapy

SJ Third or more concurrently administered infusion therapy

SK Member of high risk population (use only with codes for immunization)

SL State supplied vaccine

SM Second surgical opinion

SN Third surgical opinion

SQ Item ordered by home health

ST Related to trauma or injury

SU Procedure performed in physicians office (to denote use of facility and equipment)

TC Technical component. Under certain circumstances, a charge may be made for the technical component alone. Under those circumstances the technical component charge is identified by adding modifier TC to the usual procedure number. Technical component charges are institutional charges and not billed separately by physicians. However, portable x-ray suppliers only bill for technical component and should utilize modifier TC. The charge data from portable x-ray suppliers will then be used to build customary and prevailing profiles.

TD RN

TE LPN/LVN

TF Intermediate level of care

TG Complex/high level of care

TH Obstetrical treatment/services, prenatal or postpartum

TJ Program group, child and/or adolescent

TL Early intervention/individualized family service plan (IFSP)

TM Individualized education program (IEP)

TN Rural/outside providers customary service area

TP Medical transport, unloaded vehicle

TQ Basic life support transport by a volunteer ambulance provider

TS Follow-up service

TT Individualized service provided to more than one patient in same setting

TU Special payment rate, overtime

TV Special payment rates, holidays/weekends

U1 Medicaid level of care 1, as defined by each state

U2 Medicaid level of care 2, as defined by each state

U3 Medicaid level of care 3, as defined by each state

U4 Medicaid level of care 4, as defined by each state

U5 Medicaid level of care 5, as defined by each state

U6 Medicaid level of care 6, as defined by each state

U7 Medicaid level of care 7, as defined by each state

U8 Medicaid level of care 8, as defined by each state

U9 Medicaid level of care 9, as defined by each state

UA Medicaid level of care 10, as defined by each state

UB Medicaid level of care 11, as defined by each state

UC Medicaid level of care 12, as defined by each state

UD Medicaid level of care 13, as defined by each state

UF Services provided in the morning

UG Services provided in the afternoon

UH Services provided in the evening

UJ Services provided at night

UK Services provided on behalf of the client to someone other than the client (collateral relationship)

UN Two patients served

UP Three patients served

UQ Four patients served

UR Five patients served

US Six or more patients served

ESRD Modifiers

EJ Subsequent claims for a defined course of therapy, e.g., EPO, sodium hyaluronate, infliximab

EM Emergency reserve supply (for ESRD benefit only)

G1 Most recent urea reduction ratio (URR) reading of less than 60

G2 Most recent urea reduction ration (URR) reading of 60 to 64.9

G3 Most recent urea reduction ratio (URR) reading of 65 to 69.9

G4 Most recent urea reduction ratio (URR) reading of 70 to 74.9

G5 Most recent urea reduction ratio (URR) reading of 75 or greater

G6 ESRD patient for whom less than six dialysis sessions have been provided in a month

Q3 Live kidney donor: services associated with postoperative medical complications directly related to the donation

Dental Modifiers

ET Emergency services (dental procedures performed in emergency situations should show the modifier ET)